P9-CRS-026

ROSAI AND ACKERMAN'S

SURGICAL PATHOLOGY

TENTH EDITION

Commissioning Editor: *Michael Houston*
Development Editor: *Joanne Scott*
Editorial Assistant: *Kirsten Lowson*
Project Manager: *Joannah Duncan*
Design: *Charles Gray*
Illustration Manager: *Bruce Hogarth*
Illustrator: *Lynda Payne*
Marketing Manager(s) (USA/UK): *Tracie Pasker/Gaynor Jones*

Cover illustrations: Volume 1: Figures 4.79b, 8.23, 9.63, 13.17, 17.135, 9.38, 17.137a, 12.23c
Volume 2: Figures 19.251, 19.299a, 20.36, 20.113, 21.42, 21.100, 28.68, 28.93

ROSAI AND ACKERMAN'S

SURGICAL PATHOLOGY

TENTH EDITION

VOLUME 2

JUAN ROSAI MD

Director, International Center for Oncologic
Pathology Consultations
Centro Diagnostico Italiano (CDI)
Milan, Italy

Senior Pathology Consultant
Laboratory Corporation of America® Holdings
Burlington, NC, USA

Adjunct Professor, Department of Pathology
Weill Cornell Medical College
New York, NY, USA

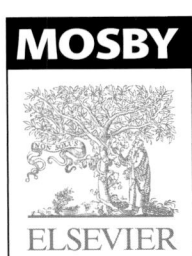

Edinburgh London New York Oxford Philadelphia St Louis Sydney Toronto

MOSBY
ELSEVIER
Mosby is an imprint of Elsevier Inc.

First edition 1953
Second edition 1959
Third edition 1964
Fourth edition 1968
Fifth edition 1974
Sixth edition 1981
Seventh edition 1989
Eighth edition 1996
Ninth edition 2004

British Library Cataloguing in Publication Data
Rosai, Juan, 1940–
Rosai and Ackerman's surgical pathology – 10th ed.
1. Pathology, Surgical.
I. Title II. Surgical pathology III. Ackerman, Lauren
Vedder, 1905–1993
617'.07–dc22

ISBN-13: 9780323069694

British Library Cataloguing in Publication Data
A catalogue record for this book is available from the British Library

Library of Congress Cataloging in Publication Data
A catalog record for this book is available from the Library of Congress

Printed in China
Last digit is the print number: 9 8 7 6 5 4 3 2 1

Contents

John KC Chan contributed the molecular genetic sections for Chapters 1–8, 10–22, 24–27, 30, 31.

Preface
to the tenth edition

The seven years that have elapsed between the current and the previous editions of this book have seen momentous changes taking place in the practice of surgical pathology. Immunohistochemistry has continued its notable expansion and has become an indispensable adjunct for the practice of the specialty. It has truly transformed the practice of surgical pathology in a fashion that no other technique has done before or after. Newcomers to the specialty take it for granted when ordering their panels, without pausing to think that only forty years ago none of this was available to the brave pathologists who based all of their diagnoses and other considerations on patterns of growth and cellular features seen in hematoxylin-stained slides, with the occasional modest help provided by one or another 'special stain'.

We are now in the midst of another transformation, resulting from the application to surgical pathology specimens of the enormous amount of new knowledge derived from the molecular genetic revolution. The potential and – in some instances – the already tangible benefits of this technology are too obvious to be emphasized. It may instead be instructive to reflect on the effect that this barrage of new information is having on the approach to surgical pathology by the new generation of practitioners, and the danger that the tradition of meticulous gross and microscopic examination upon which surgical pathology has been built may be gradually eroding. Some of this may be inevitable and is perhaps not altogether undesirable, yet the amount of information that this time-honored examination can still provide is so rich and dependable that one recoils at the thought of it being belittled or altogether ignored. With that caveat in mind, this edition dutifully incorporates the many promising results reached with the new technologies (emphasizing those in which a clinical validation has occurred), but always matching them against the results and conclusions derived from the morphology-based approach that has served pathologists so well for so long.

This difficult integration task has been carried out in most chapters by Dr John KC Chan, a brilliant representative of that emerging and still sparse cadre of surgical pathologists who combine a superb knowledge of conventional pathology with an understanding of the principles, possible applications and potential pitfalls of molecular genetic techniques.

Another important change that has taken place during this period concerns the increasing demands for standardization, compliance with regulatory controls and legal accountability, which have prompted various pathology organizations to produce sets of guidelines to help us navigate through an increasingly complicated terrain.

Yet another significant development concerns the pervasive influence acquired by electronic information systems in practically all activities that take place in the surgical pathology laboratory, rendering some degree of computer literacy indispensable to those wishing to practice the specialty.

It has not been easy to accommodate this rapidly changing and continuously expanding universe within the confines of the covers of this book. The amount of information that had to be reviewed, even if often of a merely confirmatory or plainly repetitive nature, was daunting, and the trend for the establishment of subspecialties in surgical pathology – each with its own rites and lingo – has accelerated. The sum of these factors has made the production of this book a heavy burden, to the point of making one wonder on more than one occasion whether it had grown beyond the capabilities of an individual. Yet, as you can see, despite it all, another edition has been completed, once again for the most part written by one author, in the continuing hope that whatever expertise is inevitably missing as a result may be compensated by what somebody in a related context referred to as 'the ultimate simplicity of one voice speaking'. Along those lines, a constant attempt has been made to preserve as much as possible the pragmatic flavor initially given to this work by its peerless begetter, Dr Lauren V Ackerman (1905-1993).

This goal of coherence notwithstanding, it became increasingly obvious that there were highly specialized areas (mainly but not exclusively in the non-neoplastic field) that could not have been covered adequately without the contribution of experts. I was fortunate in being able to secure once again the collaboration of outstanding individuals (listed on the contributors' page) for this purpose, and I am extremely grateful to them for their willingness in lending their considerable expertise to this effort.

A book that has gone through so many editions is bound to contain strata of text and illustrative material that have been contributed by somebody at some point, to subsequently being covered by other strata from somebody else, but whose original source will still be identifiable to the initiated. Among the several past contributors, I would like to mention Dr Morton E Smith (Chapter 30), Dr

Robert E Vickers (Chapter 6), and Dr John Morrow (sections on information systems on surgical pathology and model for an automated anatomic pathology system, Chapter 1).

Thanks are also due to the many colleagues and associates who generously contributed illustrative material from their own files or who pointed out inaccuracies, omissions, duplications, and typographical errors. Among them, I would like to single out for the magnitude of their contributions the following: Dr Fabio Facchetti, Brescia, Italy; Dr Robert Erlandson, South Berlington, Vermont, Dr Robin A Cooke, Brisbane, Australia; Dr Juan José Segura, San José, Costa Rica; Dr Pedro J Grases Galofré, Barcelona, Spain; Dr Michele Bisceglia, San Giovanni Rotondo, Italy; and Ms Loredana Alasio, Former Chief Cytotechnologist at the National Cancer Institute of Milan. I would also like to thank Dr Francesca Bono, Monza, Italy, for her help in producing the long list of immunohistochemical markers listed in Chapter 3.

Each of the editions of this book in which I have been involved has been written at a different place: the fifth at Washington University (St Louis), the sixth at the University of Minnesota (Minneapolis), the seventh at Yale University (New Haven), the eighth at Memorial Sloan-Kettering Cancer Center (New York), the ninth at the National Cancer Institute (Milan), and the current one at the Centro Diagnostico Italiano (Milan). In each place I have learned a great deal from my colleagues and have incorporated many of their comments and suggestions. I am most grateful to the countless staff pathologists, pathology residents, and pathology fellows from each of these places who have unwittingly contributed to the book in this fashion. I suspect that some of them will recognize themselves in some of the statements. These dear colleagues are too numerous to be named individually. I hope it will suffice if in their stead I were to name Drs Tshering Dorji and Giovanni Fellegara, my two latest associates, in representation of the entire group.

Once again, the contribution made by my wife, Dr Maria Luisa Carcangiu, has been colossal. It has encompassed every aspect of the book production, including innumerable conceptual and practical suggestions, tedious proof-readings of the text and double-checking of references, not to speak of the psychological support in the many moments of near collapse.

Finally, my thanks also go to Mrs Armanda Locatelli, the Assistant who collaborated in this effort from the beginning to the end, with accuracy, speed, and utmost dedication.

So, here it is for you, my fellow surgical pathologist, hoping that it will provide you with some assistance in carrying out our demanding, stressful, wonderful job.

Juan Rosai MD
Milan, Italy, 2011

Preface
to the first edition

This book can be only an introduction to the vast field of surgical pathology: the pathology of the living. It does not pretend to replace in any way the textbooks to general pathology, its purpose being merely to supplement them, assuming that the reader has a background in or access to those texts. The contents are not as complete as they might be because emphasis has been placed on the common rather than the rare lesions and are, to a great extent, based on the author's personal experiences.

This book has been written for the medical student as well as for those physicians who are daily intimately concerned with surgical pathology. This must of necessity include not only the surgeon and the pathologist, but also those physicians in other fields who are affected by its decisions, such as the radiologist and the internist. Gross pathology has been stressed throughout with an attempt to correlate the gross findings with the clinical observations. The many illustrations have been selected as typical of the various surgical conditions, although in a few instances the author has been unable to resist showing some of the more interesting rare lesions he has encountered. Concluding each chapter there is a bibliography listing those references which are not only relatively recent and readily available, but also those which will lead the reader to a more detailed knowledge of the subject.

Dr Zola K Cooper, Assistant Professor of Pathology and Surgical Pathology, has written one of the sections on Skin, and Dr David E Smith, Assistant Professor of Pathology and Surgical Pathology, has written the chapter on Central Nervous System. Both of these members of the Department are particularly well qualified for their respective roles because of their background and present responsibilities in these fields. Their efforts on my behalf are most gratefully acknowledged.

Many members of the Surgical Staff at Barnes Hospital have given much help both knowingly and unwittingly. I am particularly grateful to Dr Charles L Eckert, Associate Professor of Surgery, for letting me bother him rather constantly with my questions and for giving freely of his experience. Dr Richard Johnson, who succeeded me as Pathologist at the Ellis Fischel State Cancer Hospital, agreeably made available all the material there, and Dr Franz Leidler, Pathologist at the Veterans Hospital, has been most cooperative.

Thanks must be given to Dr HR McCarroll, Assistant Professor of Orthopedics, for constructively criticizing the chapter on Bone and Joint, and to Dr CA Waldron for helping me with the chapters related to the Oral Cavity. Among other faculty friends and colleagues who were especially helpful, I would like to mention Dr Carl E Lischer, Dr Eugene M Bricker, Dr Heinz Haffner, Dr Thomas H Burford, Dr Carl A Moyer, Dr Evarts A Graham, Dr Robert Elman, Dr Edward H Reinhard, Dr J Albert Key, Dr Glover H Copher, Dr Margaret G Smith, and Dr Robert A Moore.

Mr Cramer K Lewis, of our Department of Illustration, has been very patient with my demands, and his efforts and skill have been invaluable. Miss Marion Murphy, in charge of our Medical Library, and her associates gave untiringly of their time.

Because of recent advances in anesthesia, antibiotics, and pre- and postoperative care, modern surgery permits the radical excision of portions or all of various organs. There is a need today for contemplative surgeons, men with a rich background in the fundamental sciences, whether chemistry, physiology, or pathology. The modern surgeon should not ask himself, "Can I get away with this operation?" but rather, "What does the future hold for this patient?" It is hoped that this book may contribute in some small fashion toward the acquisition of this attitude.

Lauren V Ackerman MD
St. Louis, Missouri, USA
1953

List of Contributors

JOHN KC CHAN MD
Consultant Pathologist
Department of Pathology
Queen Elizabeth Hospital
Kowloon, Hong Kong, SAR China

DANIEL A ARBER MD
Professor and Associate Chair (Clinical Services) of Pathology
Department of Pathology
Stanford University
Stanford, CA, USA

RICHARD D BRUNNING MD
Professor Emeritus
Department of Laboratory Medicine and Pathology
University of Minnesota
Minneapolis, MN, USA

VALEER J DESMET MD PHD
Emeritus Professor of Histology and Pathology
Department of Pathology
University Hospital St Rafael
Leuven, Belgium

BK KLEINSCHMIDT-DEMASTERS MD
Professor of Pathology, Neurology and Neurosurgery
Department of Pathology
University of Colorado Health Sciences Center
Denver, CO, USA

NELSON G ORDÓÑEZ MD
Professor of Pathology
Department of Pathology
The University of Texas MD Anderson Cancer Center
Houston, TX, USA

MARC K ROSENBLUM MD
Chief, Neuropathology and Autopsy Service
Founder's Chair
Department of Pathology
Memorial Sloan-Kettering Cancer Center
Professor of Pathology and Laboratory Medicine
Weill Medical College, Cornell University
New York, NY, USA

GIOVANNI TALLINI MD
Professor of Pathology
Bologna University School of Medicine
Anatomic Pathology-Bellaria Hospital
Bologna, Italy

Dedication

This book is dedicated to four gentlemen of pathology:

Ellis S Benson
Allan J Murray
Stanton L Eversole, Jr
Julio H Happa

With deep gratitude for their support and friendship

Juan Rosai

Female reproductive system

Vulva, Vagina, Uterus–cervix, Uterus–corpus, Fallopian tube (including broad and round ligaments), Ovary, Placenta

19

Vulva

CHAPTER CONTENTS

Normal anatomy

The vulva is composed of the following anatomic structures: mons pubis, clitoris, labia minora, labia majora, vulvar vestibule and vestibulovaginal bulbs, urethral meatus, hymen, Bartholin and Skene glands and ducts, and vaginal introitus.[1,4]

The *labia majora* are lined by keratinized skin containing all the cutaneous adnexa: hair follicles, sebaceous glands, apocrine glands, and sweat (eccrine) glands.[3] The *labia minora* are covered by nonkeratinized stratified squamous epithelium on their vestibular surfaces but have a thin keratinized layer on their lateral side. Skin adnexa are usually absent in them, but on occasions one encounters both sweat and sebaceous glands.

Bartholin gland is the major vestibular gland and has a tubuloalveolar structure. It is made up of acini composed of mucus-secreting columnar cells and a duct lined by transitional epithelium.[2] *Minor vestibular glands* are of simple tubular type and are lined with a mucus-secreting columnar epithelium that merges with the stratified squamous epithelium of the vestibule.

Skene or *periurethral glands* are analogous to the male prostate gland; they are lined by a pseudostratified mucus-secreting columnar epithelium that merges with the transitional-type epithelium of the ducts, which in turn joins with the stratified squamous epithelium of the vestibule.

The *hymen* is lined by nonkeratinized stratified squamous epithelium on both surfaces.

The *clitoris* contains erectile tissue similar to that present in the corpora cavernosa of the penis.

Most of the vulvar lymph vessels drain to the superficial inguinal nodes, but those in the clitoris empty directly into the deep chain.

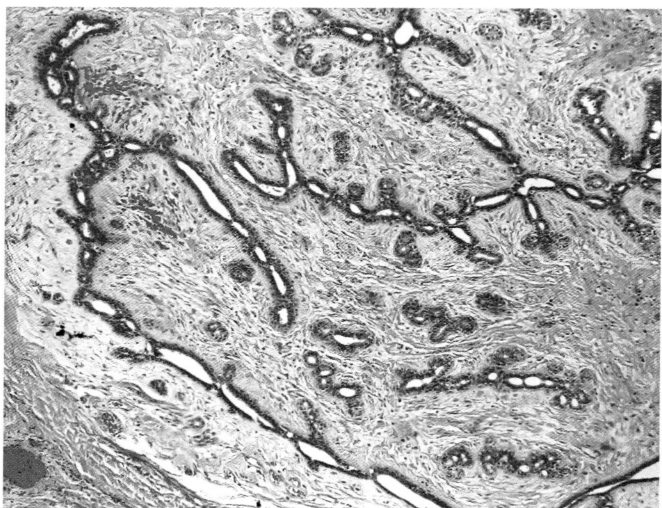

Fig. 19.1 Fibroadenoma of vulva arising from ectopic breast tissue.

Ectopic breast and related lesions

Ectopic mammary tissue can occur in the vulvar region, along the primitive milk line that extends in the embryo from the axilla to the groin. This tissue is subject to many of the physiologic and pathologic changes that occur in the normally situated breast and some that seem peculiar to this location. These include swelling and secretion of milk during pregnancy, cysts,[18] peculiar hyperplastic changes,[11] so-called pseudoangiomatous stromal hyperplasia (PASH; see Chapter 20),[13] fibroadenoma (including the juvenile type),[6,13,16] (Fig. 19.1) phylloides tumor,[7,17] and carcinoma.[9,14,15,18] Most of the latter have been of ductal type, including some of its variants (such as mucinous and tubulolobular carcinoma).[5,8,12] Mammary-type vulvar carcinoma has been reported in association with bilateral breast carcinoma.[10]

In addition, it is likely that ectopic mammary tissue is the source of the common benign vulvar tumor known as papillary hidradenoma (see p. 1409).

Inflammatory diseases

Syphilis in women often manifests itself initially in the vulvar region. The fully developed syphilitic chancre is composed microscopically of plasma cells, lymphocytes, and histiocytes, and is covered by a zone of ulceration infiltrated by neutrophils and necrotic debris. The microscopic appearance is not entirely specific, but the combination of numerous plasma cells and endarteritis should alert to the diagnosis. Sometimes, the possibility of syphilis is first suggested on the basis of the microscopic examination of an enlarged inguinal lymph node if this node shows a combination of capsular and pericapsular fibrosis, follicular hyperplasia, plasma cell infiltration, and endarteritis. The latter feature, which represents the most useful clue to the diagnosis, is particularly well seen in or outside the nodal capsule (see Chapter 21).

Granuloma inguinale (donovanosis) is a chronic infection caused by *Calymmatobacterium granulomatis*, a gram-negative, nonmotile, encapsulated bacillus.[22,31,38] It begins as a soft elevated granulomatous area that enlarges very slowly by peripheral extension and ulcerates. Microscopically, there is a dense dermal inflammatory infiltrate composed of histiocytes and plasma cells, with a scattering of small abscesses.[35] The diagnosis rests on the demonstration of Donovan bodies, which appear as small round encapsulated bodies inside the cytoplasm of the histiocytes. They can be seen in hematoxylin–eosin sections but are best demonstrated with Giemsa or Warthin–Starry stains. Pronounced pseudoepitheliomatous hyperplasia, which may accompany chronic lesions, should be distinguished from the very rare squamous cell carcinoma that may arise in such areas.[19] The infection can spread to the retroperitoneum and simulate a soft tissue neoplasm.[21]

Lymphogranuloma venereum is a venereal disease produced by *Chlamydia* organisms corresponding to serotypes L1, L2, and L3.[30,32,40] It mainly affects lymph vessels and lymphoid tissue. The initial small ulcer at a site of venereal contact often goes unnoticed. The first clinical manifestation is swelling of inguinal lymph nodes caused by stellate abscesses surrounded by pale epithelioid cells.[27] There is extensive scarring as the disease progresses, often leading to fistulas and strictures of the urethra, vagina, and rectum. The diagnosis can be confirmed by intradermal skin test (Frei test), complement fixation test, or immunofluorescence.[24] Serum immunoglobulin levels are usually markedly elevated. Rainey[34] reported 11 cases of squamous cell carcinoma or adenocarcinoma engrafted on lymphogranulomatous strictures. Most of the tumors were located in the anorectal area.

Crohn disease can involve the vulvar region.[20,28,29,39] In some cases, the vulvar lesions are associated with perineal disease and fistula formation, whereas in others they are separated from the anal lesions by normal tissue. Grossly, erythematous areas appear that later ulcerate. Microscopically, noncaseating granulomas may be found. The process reported as *vulvitis granulomatosa* is probably related to Crohn disease, in that some of the patients have subsequently developed either intestinal Crohn disease or cheilitis granulomatosa.[25]

Behçet disease can, rarely, involve the vulvar region, where it presents as a microscopically nonspecific ulceration.[26,37]

Necrotizing fasciitis of the vulva may be seen in diabetic women. It is associated with a high mortality rate; wide excision of the diseased tissue is the treatment of choice.[36]

Vulvar vestibulitis is a disorder characterized microscopically by a chronic inflammatory infiltrate predominantly involving the mucosal lamina propria and the periglandular/periductal connective tissue of the vestibular region.[33] There is no evidence of human papilloma virus (HPV) involvement.[23]

So-called 'chronic vulvar dystrophies'

There exists a group of vulvar diseases that are pathogenetically unrelated but that have several features in common at the clinical level. They usually present as irregular patchy areas of thickened skin, often accompanied by severe pruritus. The color is usually white, in which case the clinically descriptive term *leukoplakia* has traditionally been used. In other instances, the lesions are red or a mixture of both colors. They are easily traumatized and excoriated. In some of these lesions the vulvar soft tissues are atrophied and shrunken, in which case the term *kraurosis* has been employed.

In the presence of a lesion with some of these clinical features, it is essential to reach a specific diagnosis, and this often necessitates the performance of a biopsy.[48] Multiple biopsies are necessary if the lesion is large or varies in appearance from place to place. The differential diagnosis includes the following categories:

1 Specific dermatoses such as psoriasis, lichen planus, and lichen simplex chronicus (see Chapter 4).[41]
2 Squamous intraepithelial lesions (see p. 1403).

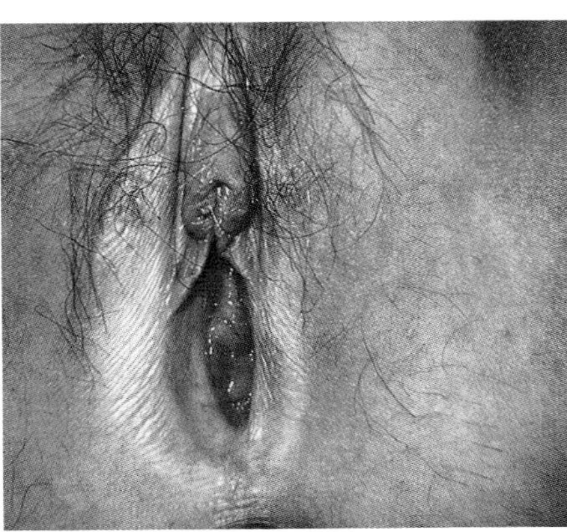

Fig. 19.2 Clinical appearance of vulvar lichen sclerosus.

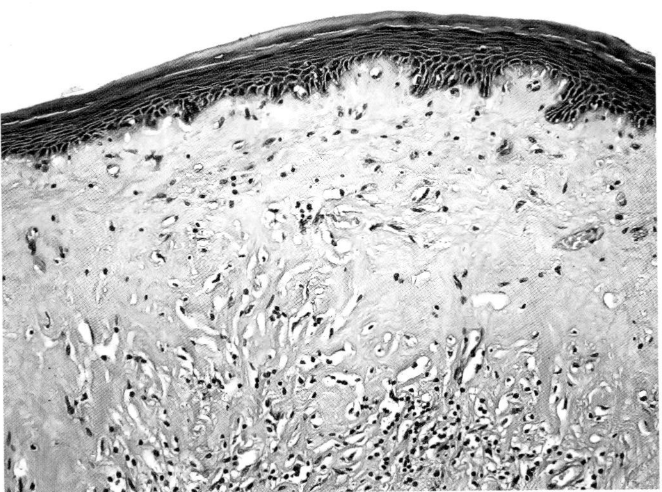

Fig. 19.3 Lichen sclerosus et atrophicus of vulva. A thick hypocellular edematous layer is bounded by atrophic epidermis on one side and inflamed stroma on the other.

3 So-called 'chronic vulvar dystrophy'. In turn, this highly questionable term[41,50] encompasses two diseases, which, although sometimes coexisting, should be regarded as separate: lichen sclerosus and keratosis.

Lichen sclerosus (et atrophicus) of the vulva may occur in any age group, including children[46] (Fig. 19.2). In the latter group, the vulvar region represents the most common location, and there is a high incidence of spontaneous involution at the time of puberty.[49] The microscopic features are similar but not identical to those seen in this disorder when it occurs elsewhere in the skin (see Chapter 4) (Fig. 19.3). It has been stated that the minimal histologic criteria for the microscopic diagnosis of lichen sclerosus are the presence of a vacuolar interface reaction pattern in conjunction with dermal sclerosis (homogenized and hyalinized eosinophilic collagen bundles) of any thickness in between the inflammatory infiltrate and the epithelium and/or vessel walls.[43] In the early stages, lichen sclerosus may be difficult to diagnose. The alterations may be very subtle and often more prominent in adnexal structures than in the interfollicular skin.[53] These changes may be difficult to distinguish from those of lichen planus.[44] The overlying epidermis is characteristically atrophic, but on occasions it may show foci of

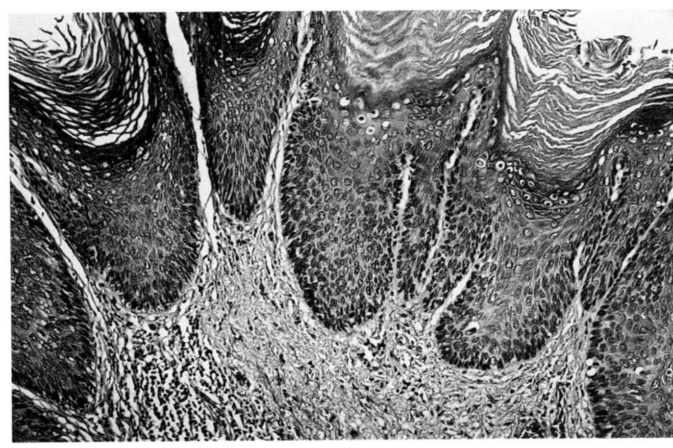

Fig. 19.4 Marked squamous cell hyperplasia (keratosis) of vulva associated with papillomatosis and chronic inflammation of the underlying stroma. There is no significant atypia.

pseudoepitheliomatous hyperplasia.[51] The curious fact that the dermal lymphocytic infiltrate shows a monoclonal gamma-T-cell receptor rearrangement has been documented.[54]

A highly controversial issue is the possible precancerous nature of lichen sclerosus. In one series, squamous cell carcinoma developed in only one of 92 patients,[45] and in another it was found in 12 (4%) of 290 patients followed for a mean period of 12.5 years.[57] The consensus is that if an increased risk exists, it must be of a very low magnitude.[42] The cases of lichen sclerosus associated with carcinoma show thickening of the epidermis and some degree of basal atypia (especially in the areas adjacent to the carcinoma), suggesting that there is a superimposed vulvar intraepithelial neoplasia (VIN).[56] This is supported by the fact that cases of carcinoma-associated lichen sclerosus tend to show an overexpression of P53.[42]

Keratosis (squamous hyperplasia) is characterized microscopically by acanthosis, prominent stratum granulosum, and hyperkeratosis, often associated with mild dermal chronic inflammatory infiltrate (Fig. 19.4). An important criterion for the use of this term without a qualifier is the *absence of atypia*. If this criterion is followed, keratosis does not represent a precancerous condition, a belief supported by the fact that such lesions are not clonal and are devoid of *TP53* mutations.[47] The situation may be slightly different for the condition that has been named *vulvar acanthosis with altered differentiation*, which is characterized by marked acanthosis, a variable verruciform architecture, loss of the granular layer, cytoplasmic pallor at the surface, and multilayered parakeratosis. It has been suggested that this keratosis variant (which is consistently negative for HPV) may be a precursor or a risk factor for verrucous carcinoma.[52]

Occasionally, the features of lichen sclerosus and squamous hyperplasia are seen to coexist, in which case the term *mixed vulvar dystrophy* has been used.[55] Furthermore, the changes of VIN are sometimes superimposed on any of these conditions. Failure to appreciate the existence of these various combinations is probably responsible for the widely different figures given regarding the precancerous connotations of these various entities.[55]

Human papilloma virus and vulvar pathology

The role of human papilloma virus (HPV) in vulvar pathology is analogous to the one it plays in the vagina and cervix, and is discussed in detail in connection with the latter (see p. 1442). In the vulva, this includes condyloma (acuminatum and flat), VIN, invasive squamous cell carcinoma and several of its microscopic subtypes[58] (including those arising in the urethra), and verrucous carcinoma.[60] Immunostaining for p16^{INK4a} is an effective way to identify HPV-positive lesions.[58,59]

From a practical standpoint, it is important to classify these conditions separately in view of their widely different natural history and treatment.

Condyloma and seborrheic keratosis

Vulvar **condyloma** is a venereal disease caused by HPV, usually type 6. The better known form is **condyloma acuminatum,** which is characterized grossly by one or several soft elevated masses of variable size (Fig. 19.5). Microscopically there is a complicated papillary arrangement of well-differentiated undulating squamous epithelium supported by delicate, well-vascularized connective tissue stalks containing mononuclear inflammatory cells (mainly CD4+ and CD8+ cells)[66] (Figs 19.6 and 19.7).

The other form of condyloma, which is actually much more common, is the **flat condyloma** (not to be confused with the *condyloma latum* of syphilis). The cytologic features are similar in both forms. Koilocytosis of the malpighian epithelium (see p. 1443) and lymphocytic infiltration of the stroma are regular features (Fig. 19.8). Koilocytosis refers to the combination of perinuclear cytoplasmic clearing and wrinkling of the nuclear membrane (nuclear 'raisins'). As a rule, this change is not as florid in vulvar condylomas as it tends to be in condylomas of the cervix. A typical condyloma shows minimal basal or parabasal cell atypia, orderly maturation, and a smooth transition to koilocytotic intermediate and superficial cells; mitoses may be numerous but are all typical.[61,68] In contrast, the lesions of VIN exhibit abnormal mitoses and nuclear pleomorphism, enlargement, and hyperchromasia in the basal and parabasal cell layers (see later section). The increased proliferative activity of condyloma (in contrast to fibroepithelial polyp and squamous papilloma) can be easily appreciated with the Ki-67/MIB-1 stain.[69] The DNA content of condylomas is diploid and polyploid (including tetraploidy and octaploidy), in contrast to the aneuploid pattern seen in most cases of VIN.[71]

Sometimes one sees verrucopapillary vulvar lesions in children or adults that lack the cytologic markers of condyloma; these are

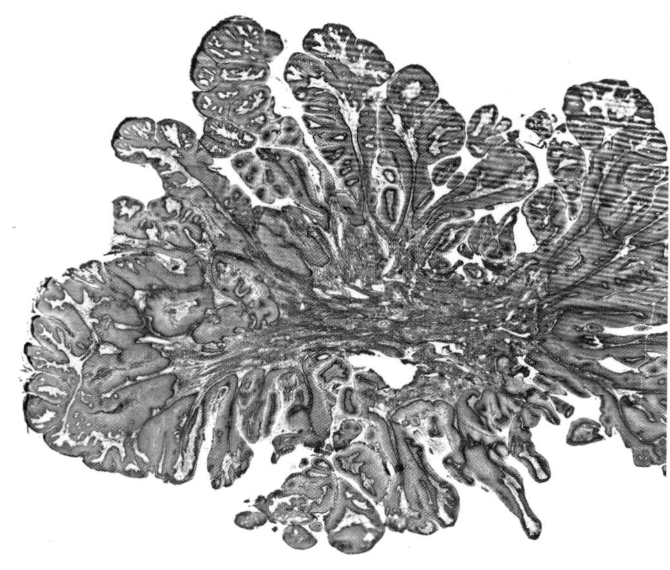

Fig. 19.6 Whole mount of condyloma acuminatum of vulva.

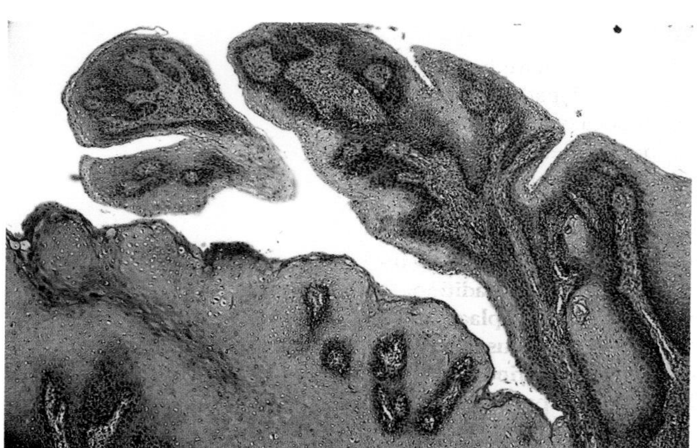

Fig. 19.7 Papillomatous shape of vulvar condyloma.

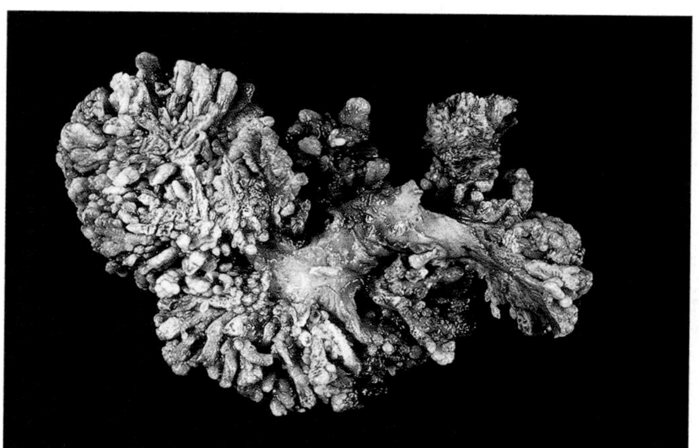

Fig. 19.5 Large condyloma of vulva.

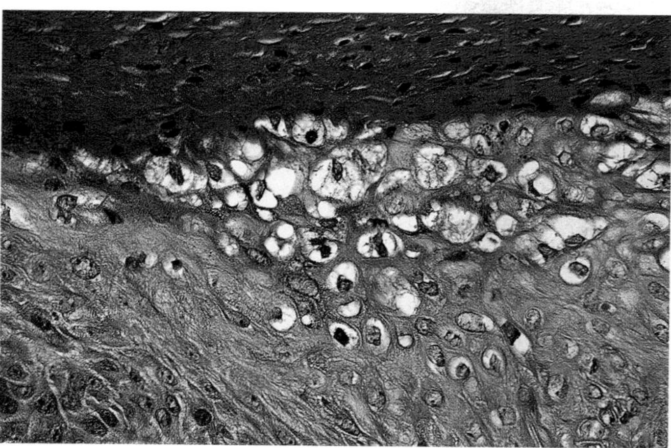

Fig. 19.8 Prominent koilocytotic changes in vulvar epithelium.

often referred to as *squamous papillomas* and usually contain genital HPV types by polymerase chain reaction (PCR).[64] Conversely, there may be multinucleated atypia of the epithelial squamous cells associated with reactive conditions in the absence of HPV infection.[65] Another vulvar lesion which needs to be discussed here is the process morphologically indistinguishable from cutaneous seborrheic keratosis, which in this particular location is frequently associated with HPV infection.[63] The differential diagnosis of condyloma also includes a lesion characterized by *epidermolytic hyperkeratosis*, which could be related to Darier disease or represent a form of Hailey–Hailey disease.[70] The acantholysis is usually suprabasal, but we have also seen it at the level of the granular layer.

The traditional therapy for condyloma consisted of podophyllin application. Microscopically, this results in epidermal pallor, necrosis of keratinocytes, and marked increase in mitosis; these changes wane after 72 hours and are essentially gone by 1 week.[72] Occasionally, similar microscopic changes are seen in the absence of podophyllin therapy.[67] The treatment of choice of these lesions at present is with carbon dioxide laser.[62]

Squamous intraepithelial lesions

The spectrum of abnormalities seen in atypical proliferative squamous lesions of the vulvar skin and generically designated as **vulvar intraepithelial neoplasia (VIN)** is wider than that exhibited by equivalent lesions in the vagina (VaIN) or cervix (CIN).[81,86] Traditionally, they have been segregated into subtypes on the basis of clinical and pathologic features.[78,94] However, both the International Society for the Study of Vulvovaginal Disease and the International Society of Gynecological Pathologists recommend the use of the term VIN, its division into three grades (VIN I, VIN II, VIN III), and the avoidance of terms such as carcinoma in situ, dysplasia, or eponyms (which still need to be mentioned to retain a link with the many classic studies on the subject).

The type of VIN traditionally known as *Bowen disease* presents as a slightly elevated, plaque-like lesion with a red velvety appearance (Fig. 19.9).[73] It is usually centered in the labia majora, and it may extend to the perineum and anus. Microscopically, there is hyperkeratosis and parakeratosis, acanthosis, and a variable number of multinucleated dyskeratotic cells and abnormal mitoses involving the entire thickness of the epidermis, therefore corresponding to a CIN III-type lesion (Fig. 19.10). The acrotrichium (intraepidermal portion of the hair follicle) is often involved, whereas the acrosyringium (intraepidermal portion of the sweat gland) is usually spared.[92,97] On occasion, the tumor cells are arranged in a nested pattern and/or have a clear cytoplasm, thus simulating Paget disease.[74,95]

The type of VIN designated as *bowenoid papulosis* presents as multiple, often pigmented, papules in or near the vulva of young patients. Clinically, they resemble verrucae, small condylomas, or nevi, but microscopically they show a degree of cytologic atypia approaching that of Bowen disease.[89] The distinction is largely made on clinical grounds, but some microscopic differences have been described, the most important being that in bowenoid papulosis the dysplastic cells are present in a background of relatively orderly epithelial maturation and that the acrotrichium is usually spared.[92,102] Spontaneous regression has been observed, and response to conservative therapy is the rule, even if recurrences are common.[75]

The similarities in morphologic appearance, ploidy pattern, and P53 expression between Bowen disease and bowenoid papulosis, their occasional coexistence,[76] and the fact that both are statistically associated with HPV[107] (see below) suggest an etiologic and pathogenetic link between the two. This has led to the proposal to group them under the term *bowenoid dysplasia*[102] and to incorporate them into the VIN concept, while still acknowledging the important differences they exhibit in age of appearance and risk of development of invasive carcinoma.[82] According to this proposal, such lesions could be diagnosed as *VIN, Bowen disease type* and *VIN, bowenoid papulosis type*, respectively. Another proposed morphologic approach is to divide VIN into two types: *warty* or *bowenoid* (which includes both Bowen disease and bowenoid papulosis) and *basaloid* or *undifferentiated*. The latter type, which resembles CIN III, shows a lesser degree of association with HPV than the warty type.[91] Yet another scheme, *which is the one currently favored* despite the proposals of yet additional schemes,[98] is to divide VIN into:

1 *Classic type.* It includes Bowen disease, bowenoid papulosis, warty VIN, carcinoma in situ, and basaloid VIN. It is consistently associated with HPV infection (p16 positive), has a predilection for young women, is frequently associated with other HPV-positive tumors of the lower genital tract, and is typically associated with invasive squamous cell carcinomas of basaloid or warty type.[96]

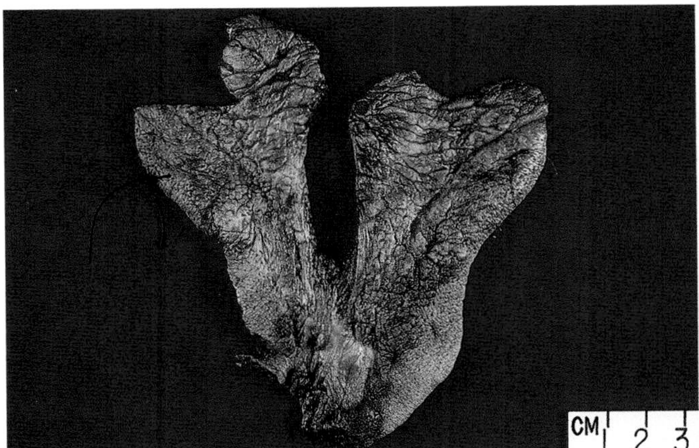

Fig. 19.9 Skinning vulvectomy specimen performed for vulvar intraepithelial neoplasia (VIN).

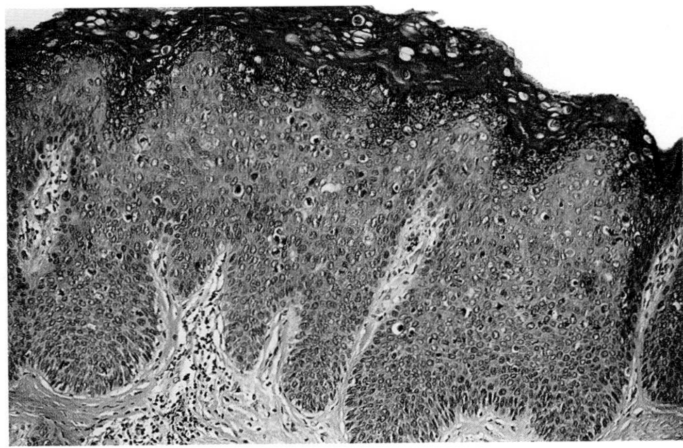

Fig. 19.10 Typical microscopic appearance of VIN III. This form is traditionally known as Bowen disease.

2 *Variant, simplex,* or *differentiated* type.[81,90] This type is consistently negative for HPV, arises in elderly women, is frequently associated with squamous hyperplasia and lichen sclerosus, and is related to invasive squamous cell carcinoma of keratinizing type.[77] Microscopically, it is characterized by maturation, variable degrees of hyperplasia, keratinization, and parabasal atypia. It shows strong staining of the basal and suprabasal epithelial layers for Ki-67 (MIB-1), is negative for p16, and shows a variable pattern of P53 overexpression and mutations.[86,93,103,108]

Low-grade VIN (VIN I) has been traditionally thought to be associated with low-risk viral types; however, recent studies have shown that a significant number of cases contain high-risk HPV types (although not HPV-16).[99]

Clonality studies have shown that low-grade lesions (including bowenoid papulosis) tend to be polyclonal, whereas high-grade lesions (including classic Bowen disease) are usually clonal.[83,106] Alas, clonality has also been detected in keratosis (squamous hyperplasia) without atypia.[101]

The importance of VIN resides in its putative role as a precursor of invasive squamous cell carcinoma,[105] particularly in view of the fact that its incidence is on the increase, especially among young women.[84] The evidence for a causal relationship is very strong, with several studies showing a parallel increase in the incidence of two conditions and a heightening of the risk with increased degrees of VIN.[85] It has been stated that, if left untreated, VIN III will progress into invasive carcinoma in approximately 10% of cases, but the rate of transformation varies widely among the different series.[100] The therapy of VIN depends on the age of the patient and the size, configuration, and distribution of the lesions.[100] Localized lesions can be treated by wide local excision or skinning vulvectomy.[79] A relationship has been found between positive margins and local recurrence.[80] Interesting results have been obtained with the topical application of imiquimod, an immune-response modulator. In one recent study, many of the lesions partially regressed and some showed a complete response.[104]

The most exciting and promising development in the field is the vaccination against HPV-16 for VIN. The preliminary results are very encouraging.[87,88]

Invasive squamous cell carcinoma

General features

Squamous cell carcinoma accounts for approximately 95% of the malignant tumors of this organ. The mean age at presentation is between 60 and 74 years.[115] Risk factors include number of lifetime sexual partners, cigarette smoking, immunodeficiency, and genital granulomatous disease.[111–113] Vulvar carcinoma is frequently associated with malignant tumors elsewhere in the lower genital tract, notably the uterine cervix.[116] This has led to the hypothesis that the epithelium of the entire lower genital tract (cervix, vagina, vulva, and perianal area) reacts as a single tissue field to certain carcinogenic stimuli, particularly HPV infection.[119,120]

On the basis of epidemiologic and virologic studies, and as discussed in the preceding section, it has been proposed that there are two types of vulvar carcinoma: the most common occurring in older women, not related to HPV, microscopically typical keratinizing squamous cell carcinomas, and associated with keratosis (epithelial hyperplasia); and the other occurring in younger women, frequently HPV-positive, often with a basaloid or warty histology, and associated with VIN (see p. 1403).[109,110,114,117,118,121,122]

Morphologic, histochemical, immunohistochemical, and molecular genetic features

Invasive squamous cell carcinoma of the vulva arises most commonly on the labia majora but may be found on the labia minora or in the region of the clitoris[123,124] (Fig. 19.11). Microscopically, most cases have a well-differentiated appearance, although those located in the clitoris tend to be more anaplastic (Fig. 19.12A,B). VIN and keratosis are often present at the margins.[129]

The immunohistochemical features of vulvar squamous cell carcinoma are not distinctive. Cytogenetically, loss in 3p and 4p and gain in 3q have been found with increased frequency.[125] The pattern seems to be similar in HPV-positive and HPV-negative cases,[127] and between the invasive component and the adjacent VIN when the latter is present.[126] At the molecular level, aberrations in the expression pattern of several cell cycle-associated proteins have been noted.[130]

Inactivating mutations of *TP53* and *CDKN2A* are found in 75% and 50% of cases, respectively.[128]

Spread and metastases

Regional lymph node metastases occur in approximately 20% of cases.[133] Tumors of the labia spread first to inguinal lymph nodes, whereas those located in the clitoris may metastasize directly into the deep nodes. It should be noted that ulceration and inflammation in vulvar carcinoma often lead to reactive enlargement of inguinal lymph nodes, which may be confused clinically with metastatic disease.

Lately, the technique of sentinel lymph node biopsy has been introduced as a staging criterion and therapeutic guide for vulvar carcinoma.[131] Preliminary results suggest that the procedure is highly accurate in predicting the inguinofemoral lymph node status of those patients.[132] Regauer[134] recommends scoring the sentinel nodes as positive even when only individual CK-positive cells are identified, a significant departure from the policy followed with sentinel nodes at other sites.

Therapy

The usual treatment of invasive carcinoma is radical vulvectomy with bilateral radical inguinal lymph node dissection.[136] Iliac lymphadenectomy and pelvic exenteration are reserved for advanced cases.[139] Conversely, early cases can be treated with a more conservative approach in the form of wide local excision;[137] it has been shown that leaving a 1 cm tumor-free surgical margin results in a high rate of local control.[138] Alternative methods include radiation therapy (either alone or together with chemotherapy[140]) and the combination of wide local excision and radiation therapy.[135,141]

Prognosis

The overall 5-year survival rate in patients treated for vulvar squamous cell carcinoma has been in the 50–75% range in most large series.[145,149,157]

1 *Stage*. The most important prognostic factors are included in the staging system and are represented by *tumor diameter, depth of invasion,* and *lymph node status*.[145,147,149,150,152,155] The latter is by far the most significant parameter.[144,159]
2 *Extracapsular nodal spread*. In cases with involved nodes, the presence of extracapsular spread and large size of the metastatic focus are poor prognostic indicators.[148,156]

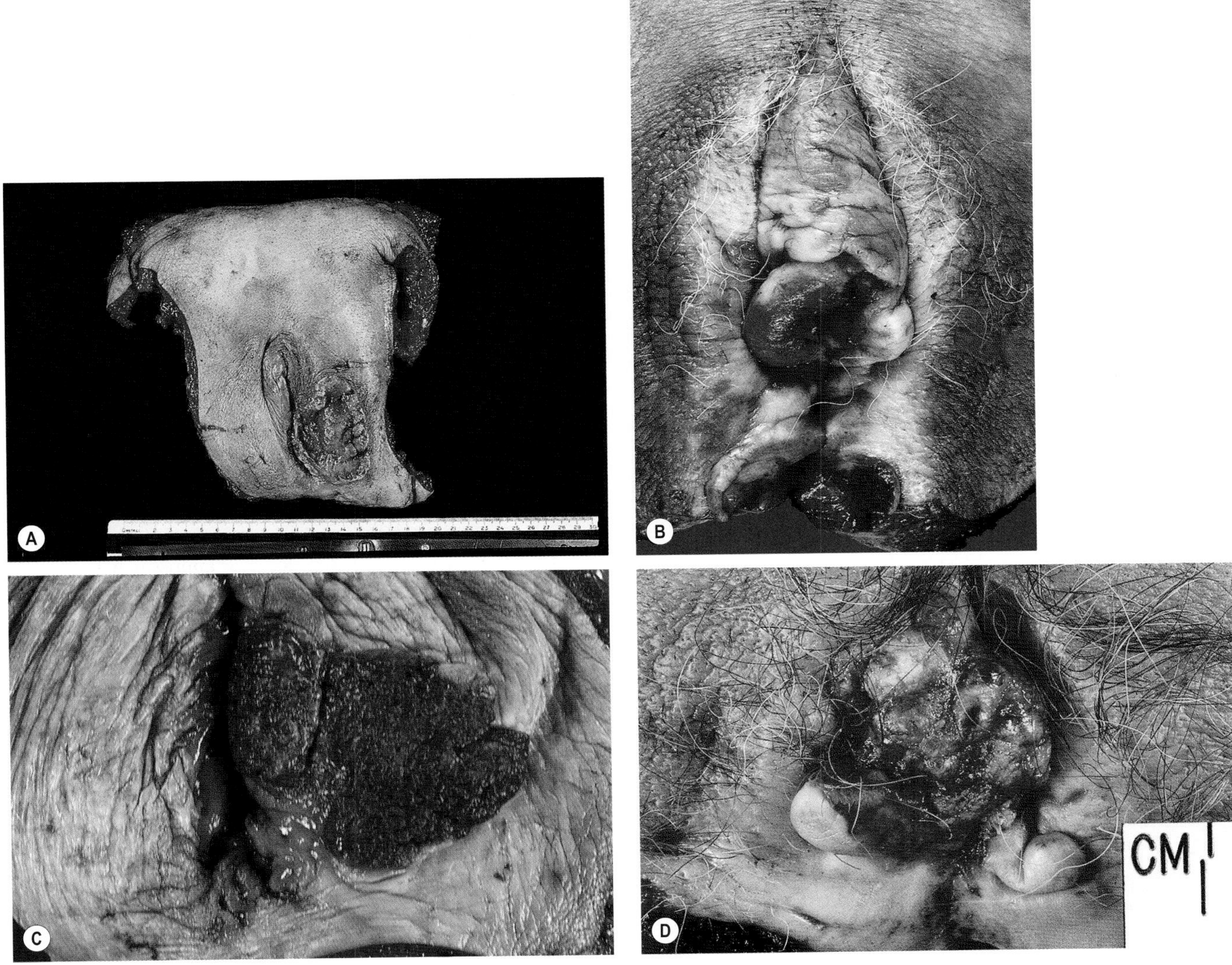

Fig. 19.11 Gross appearance of invasive squamous cell carcinoma of vulva: **A**, tumor of labium majus; **B**, tumor of clitoris; **C**, tumor involving both labia; **D**, huge tumor mass involving all vulvar structures.

3 *Infiltrative margins.* The presence of this feature in the primary tumor correlates with the incidence of nodal metastases.[143,158]
4 *Vascular invasion.* The same comment applies to this parameter.[143,158]
5 *Degree of differentiation.* A well-differentiated cytologic appearance of the cancer has been associated with a significantly better prognosis in some series.[146,151]
6 *Status of adjacent skin.* The presence of a keratotic skin with VIN-type changes at the edge of the invasive tumor is said to be a good prognostic sign.[146,151]
7 *Stromal response.* The observation has been made that carcinomas associated with a prominent fibromyxoid stromal response are associated with an older age group, poorer survival rate, and more extensive lymph node metastases.[142]
8 *P53 protein overexpression.* Diffuse immunohistochemical expression with this marker is associated with decreased survival.[153,154]

Microinvasive carcinoma

The term **microinvasive carcinoma** has been applied to vulvar carcinomas in which the depth of penetration is less than 5 mm (Fig. 19.13). Some authors have suggested that inguinal lymphadenectomy be foregone in these patients because of the low incidence of lymph node metastases.[168] However, enough exceptions have been reported to cast serious doubts on the wisdom of this recommendation[162,164] and on the very use and definition of the term.[160,161,163,166,169] Perhaps the only invasive carcinomas for which conservative surgery is indicated are those that are both well differentiated and very superficial (3 mm or less).

The point has been made that the presence of eosinophils in VIN may represent a clue to the presence of early invasion, which, therefore, should be searched for with particular care in those areas.[167] Additional help may be obtained from the evaluation of slides double-stained for keratin and a basement membrane component (collagen IV or laminin).[165]

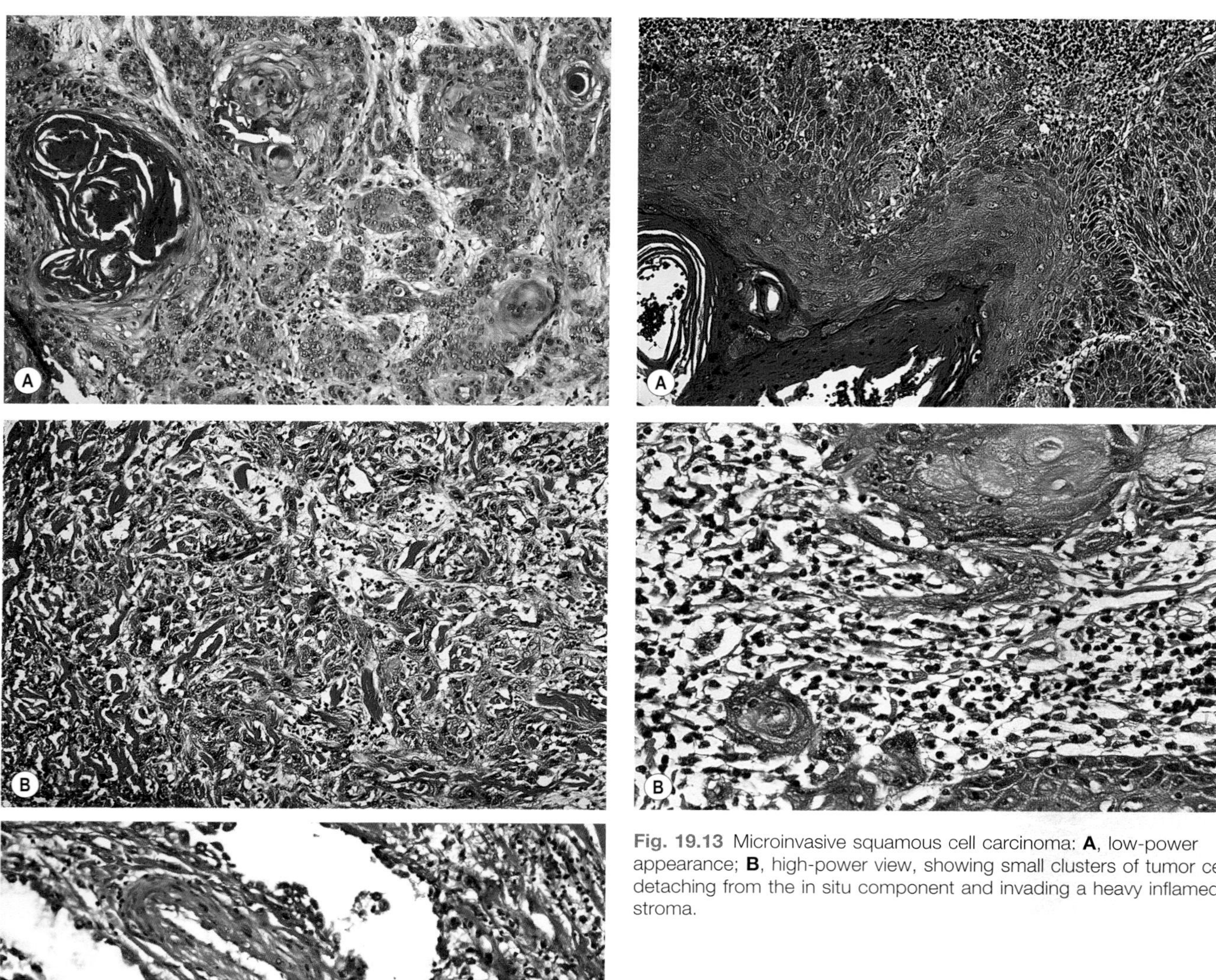

Fig. 19.12 Microscopic appearance of invasive squamous cell carcinoma of vulva: **A**, well-differentiated tumor; **B**, poorly differentiated tumor; **C**, acantholytic variety, resulting in pseudoglandular formations.

Fig. 19.13 Microinvasive squamous cell carcinoma: **A**, low-power appearance; **B**, high-power view, showing small clusters of tumor cells detaching from the in situ component and invading a heavy inflamed stroma.

Other microscopic types

Verrucous carcinoma is a reasonably distinctive type of squamous cell carcinoma of the vulva, similar to its more common counterpart in the upper aerodigestive tract. It may grow to huge dimensions, has a typical exophytic appearance, and infiltrates locally (Figs 19.14 and 19.15). Metastases are practically nonexistent,[175,176] and therefore inguinal lymphadenectomy is not indicated.

The differential diagnosis of verrucous carcinoma includes condyloma acuminatum and conventional squamous cell carcinoma. It is distinguished from the former by its generally larger size and the presence of club-shaped fingers of epithelium invading the underlying stroma in a well-circumscribed ('pushing') fashion.[180] The distinction from squamous cell carcinoma rests entirely on two criteria, which often go together: the presence in the latter of cytologic atypia and/or a clearly infiltrative pattern of growth. The occurrence of either of these features removes the lesion from the verrucous carcinoma category and puts it into the squamous cell category. Immunohistochemically, staining for keratin is more uniform and homogeneous in verrucous carcinoma than in squamous cell carcinoma.[173] Tumors having the overall appearance of verrucous carcinoma but exhibiting focal squamous cell carcinoma features as previously defined are designated by some authors as *hybrid carcinomas*.

Warty carcinoma should not be used as a synonym for verrucous carcinoma, despite the fact that the gross appearance of the latter has sometimes been described as 'warty'. The term warty carcinoma, if used at all, should be reserved for the squamous cell carcinomas in which the tumor cells display marked pleomorphism, enlargement, atypia, and multinucleation. These features are often

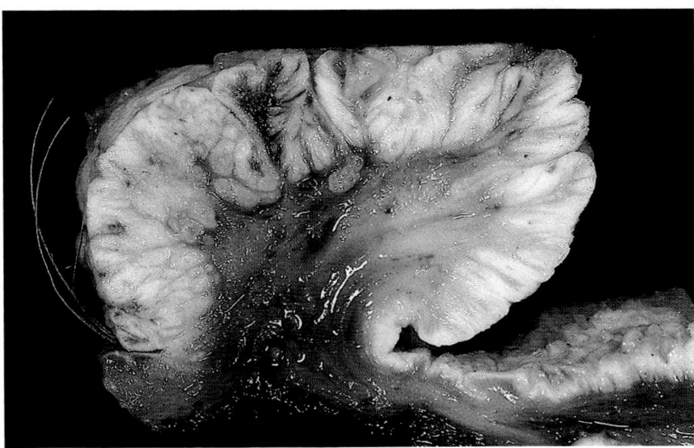

Fig. 19.14 Cut surface of verrucous carcinoma of vulva. *(Courtesy of Dr Pedro J Grases Galofré; from Grases Galofré PJ. Patología ginecológica. Bases para el diagnóstico morfológico. Barcelona, 2002, Masson)*

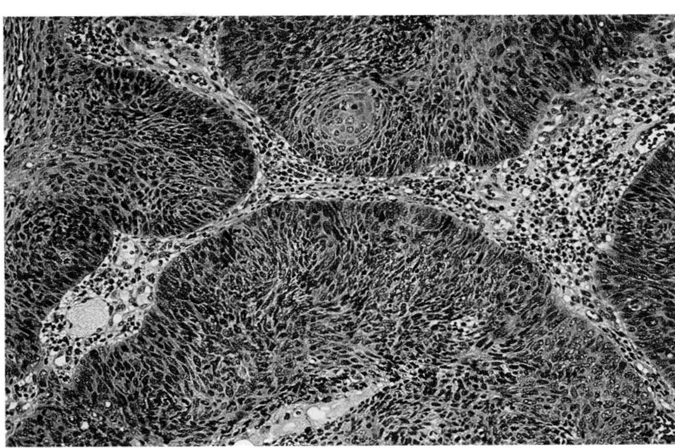

Fig. 19.16 Basaloid squamous cell carcinoma of vulva showing peripheral palisading and deep basophilic staining pattern.

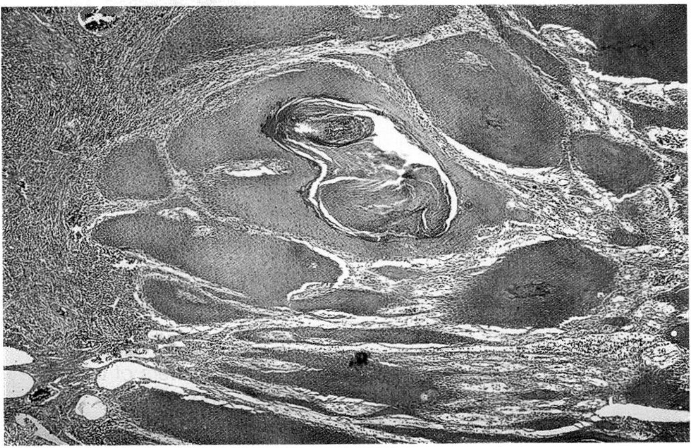

Fig. 19.15 Bulbous pegs of well-differentiated squamous cells infiltrate the stroma in vulvar verrucous carcinoma.

associated with koilocytotic atypia in the adjacent epithelium. HPV DNA is often detected in these tumors.[177]

Basaloid (squamous cell) carcinoma has an appearance analogous to its counterpart in the upper aerodigestive tract.[178] Peripheral palisading is prominent; in some cases there is a well-developed adenoid cyst-like appearance (Fig. 19.16). These features suggest an early differentiation toward adnexal glandular structures and establish a link with basaloid tumors of other sites.[170,179]

Adenoid (pseudoglandular, pseudoangiosarcomatous, acantholytic) squamous cell carcinoma has an appearance similar to that seen in its much more common homonym arising in sun-exposed areas on the basis of actinic keratosis, a factor that one assumes is not likely to play a significant pathogenetic role at this site. The common denominator is the deletion of cell adhesion molecules, with resulting detachment of the tumor cells from their neighbors[174] (see Fig. 19.12C).

Carcinosarcoma (sarcomatoid carcinoma) has been reported in the vulva, the sarcoma-like component showing smooth muscle differentiation.[171]

Lymphoepithelioma-like carcinoma has been described in the vulvar region, but the single reported case was negative for Epstein–Barr virus (EBV).[172]

Paget disease

Paget disease is a malignant tumor of the vulva that could be viewed either as a sweat gland carcinoma arising primarily from the intraepidermal portion of the glands (acrosyringium)[203] or as a carcinoma of multipotential (adnexal stem cells) residing in the infundibulosebaeous unit of the hair follicles and other adnexal structures that differentiate along glandular (sweat gland) lines,[210] the latter explanation being the most likely. A variation in the theme incriminates a population of CK7-positive clear cells associated with the openings of the ducts of the mammary-like glands of the vulva known as Toker cells.[217]

Clinically, Paget disease presents as a crusting, elevated scaling erythematous rash in the labia majora, labia minora, and/or perineal skin of adult and elderly patients (Fig. 19.17). Microscopically, the epidermis contains large pale tumor cells that form solid nests, glandular spaces, or a continuous layer along the epidermal basement membrane and also in pilosebaceous structures and sweat ducts (Fig. 19.18). A cleft often develops between the row of malignant cells and the overlying keratinocytes, resulting in a low-power appearance sometimes reminiscent of an acantholytic suprabasal bulla. Paget disease can also be misinterpreted as malignant melanoma. It should be noted that the presence of melanin granules in some tumor cells *does not* rule out the diagnosis of Paget disease. Histochemically, some or all of the tumor cells contain acidic mucin, as evidenced by their positivity for Mayer mucicarmine and aldehyde fuchsin stains.[195] Immunohistochemically, these mucins are positive for MUC1 and MUC5AC, the latter in striking contrast with Paget disease of the breast.[201,218] They are also reactive for HGM-45, a marker associated with gastric surface mucous cells.[200] Vulvar Paget disease also expresses pankeratin, epithelial membrane antigen (EMA), carcinoembryonic antigen (CEA), B72.3, and GCDF-15 (a marker of apocrine differentiation)[199,206,207,214,215] (Fig. 19.19). S-100 protein is positive in one-third of the cases, and HMB-45 is negative.[191,209] There is also negativity for CDX-2, in contrast to a subset of cases of perianal Paget disease.[219] Vulvar Paget disease lacks estrogen and progesterone receptors, but it frequently expresses androgen receptor.[187,189]

Regarding the keratins, the usual profile of vulvar Paget disease is CK7+/CK20–.[190,213] If it is instead CK20+ (and GCDFP-15 negative), the possibility of an internal malignancy (especially of urothelial nature) should be suspected.[190,216] Confirmation of the latter can be obtained with uroplakin-III immunostains.[184] The ultrastructural

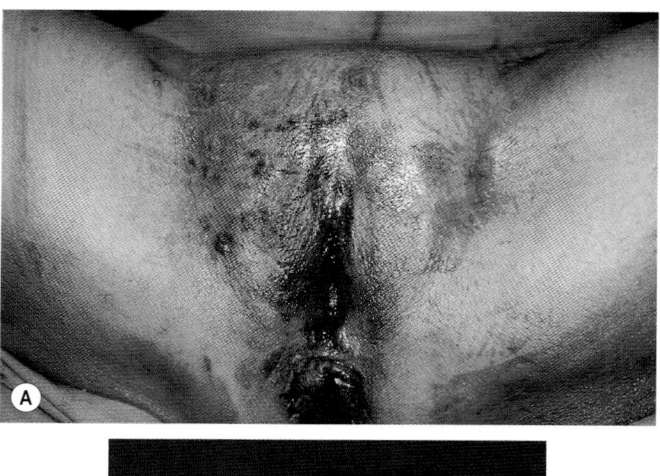

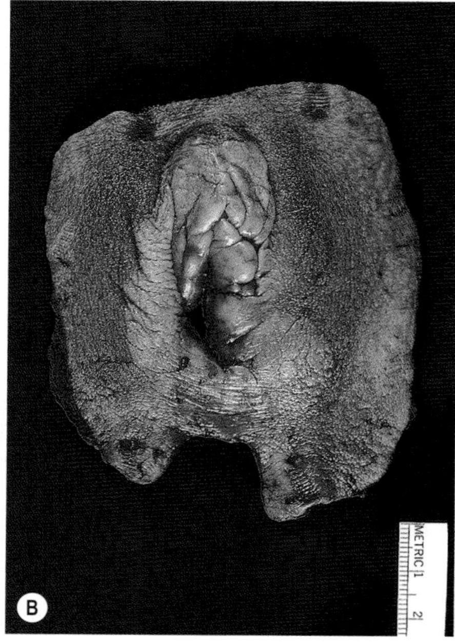

Fig. 19.17 **A** and **B**, Clinical and gross appearance of vulvar Paget disease. In both cases the disease is very extensive.

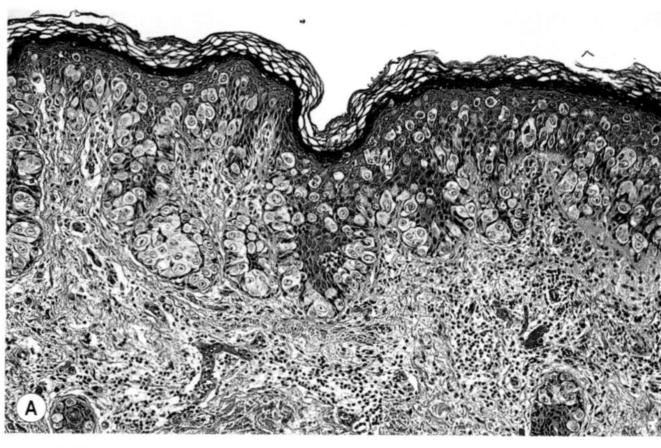

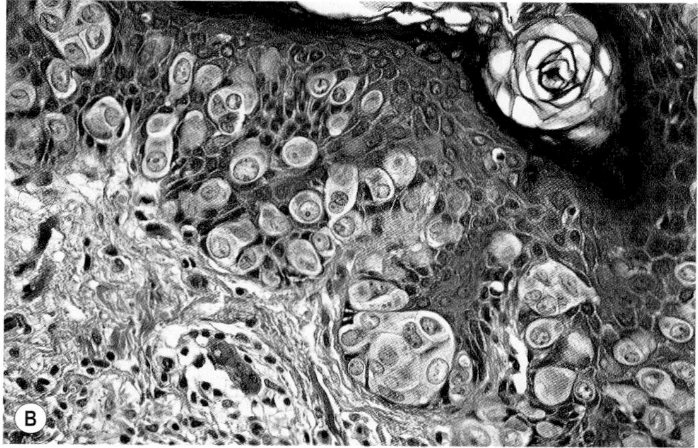

Fig. 19.18 **A** and **B**, Low- and medium-power appearances of vulvar Paget disease. The large clear tumor cells are distinct from the malpighian layer.

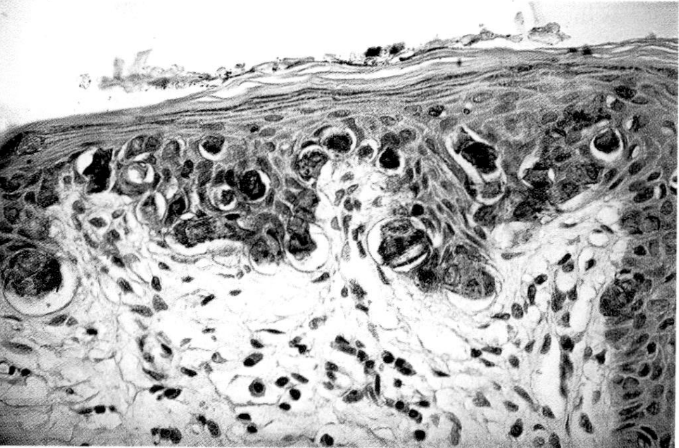

Fig. 19.19 Strong EMA immunoreactivity in cells of Paget disease.

features are indicative of glandular rather than keratinocytic or melanocytic differentiation.[211] Overexpression of HER2 oncoprotein is a constant finding,[208] whereas overexpression of the *RAS* oncogene product p21 has been found in about half the cases.[198,205]

As already indicated, Paget disease of the vulva differs in several respects from Paget disease of the breast. The latter is nearly always associated with an underlying carcinoma, which may be intraductal or invasive, and the intraepidermal malignant cells are more often than not mucin-negative. In contrast, the majority of the cases (about 90%) of vulvar Paget disease are not associated with an invasive underlying carcinoma[212] and are usually (although not always) positive for mucin stains, as previously recorded.[181,196,197] The incidence of underlying invasive carcinoma in vulvar Paget disease ranges from zero to 30% depending on the series,[186,188,202] with some of the invasive cases being in the microinvasive or minimally invasive (>1 mm) category.[185] It has been claimed that stromal invasion in Paget disease is correlated with P53 overexpression.[220] Occasionally, Paget disease is seen in association with VIN, in keeping with its presumed origin from multipotential epidermal basal cells.[194] These cases should be distinguished from the reactive keratinocytic proliferation that sometimes accompanies Paget disease – not always an easy task.[183]

If no invasive component is found in the resected specimen, the prognosis is good. Metastases do not occur under these circumstances, although local recurrence is common (about 30%), sometimes in the form of invasive carcinoma.[185,193,212] Therefore, excision should include a margin of normal skin and the underlying subcutaneous tissue. Unfortunately, the microscopic extent of the disease is often greater than that suspected from clinical examination, and this should be taken into account at the time of surgery.[192] Frozen sections are useful to determine the status of the margins;[182] however, this is only minimally related to the incidence of local recurrence.[185] In some instances local recurrence has been seen in the vulvar split-thickness skin graft.[204] Cases of Paget disease with an invasive component beyond the microinvasive stage have a high incidence of nodal involvement.[185]

Other epithelial tumors

Hidradenoma papilliferum is a benign vulvar tumor that usually presents as a small, well-circumscribed nodule covered by normal skin. Occasionally, it ulcerates through the skin and clinically may simulate carcinoma. Microscopically, it has a complex papillary glandular pattern, with stratification and some degree of pleomorphism and mitotic activity, sometimes brisk.[243] A myoepithelial layer is always apparent (Fig. 19.20). Traditionally, this tumor has been regarded as of sweat gland derivation. However, its close morphologic and immunohistochemical similarity with intraductal papilloma of breast and nipple adenoma suggests an origin from ectopic mammary tissue (see p. 1400). All acceptable examples of this tumor have behaved in a benign fashion.[233,245] However, a case of intraductal carcinoma of mammary-type apocrine epithelium has been reported arising from this tumor.[236]

Benign lesions of epidermal or skin adnexal type occur in the vulva. These include *verruca vulgaris,*[221] *syringoma*[223] (Fig. 19.21), *chondroid syringoma* (benign mixed tumor),[241] *myoepithelioma,*[234] *pigmented apocrine hamartoma,*[226] *adenolipoma,*[235] *benign pilar tumor,*[222] *other trichogenic tumors,*[239] *warty dyskeratoma,*[229] and *inverted follicular keratosis.*[242] Although not necessarily a benign skin adnexal tumor, we thought of mentioning here also the occasional occurrence of vulvar *keratoacanthoma.*[225,240]

Basal cell carcinoma of the vulva usually presents as a nodular mass in the labia majora of elderly patients; it may grow very large and ulcerate.[228,237] Its microscopic appearance and behavior are the same as those of basal cell carcinomas elsewhere in the skin; solid, keratotic, and adenoid types have been described (Fig. 19.22). The differential diagnosis includes basaloid carcinoma (see later section) and the basaloid changes sometimes seen as a component of Bowen disease and invasive squamous cell carcinoma. It should be remembered that, as elsewhere in the skin, basal cell carcinoma may exhibit abrupt squamous differentiation of possible follicular type, a change that does not affect the natural history of the lesion; such tumors should not be referred to as basosquamous carcinomas.

The incidence of nodal metastases in vulvar basal cell carcinoma is extremely low and is largely restricted to the deeply invasive lesions.[237]

Merkel cell carcinoma has been reported in the vulva, sometimes in association with Bowen disease.[224,227] Its behavior has been very aggressive.[232]

Sweat gland carcinoma of the vulva, exclusive of Paget disease, is exceptional; it may present with a variety of morphologic patterns and should be distinguished from metastatic adenocarcinoma.[244] A case has been described showing *mucinous and neuroendocrine*

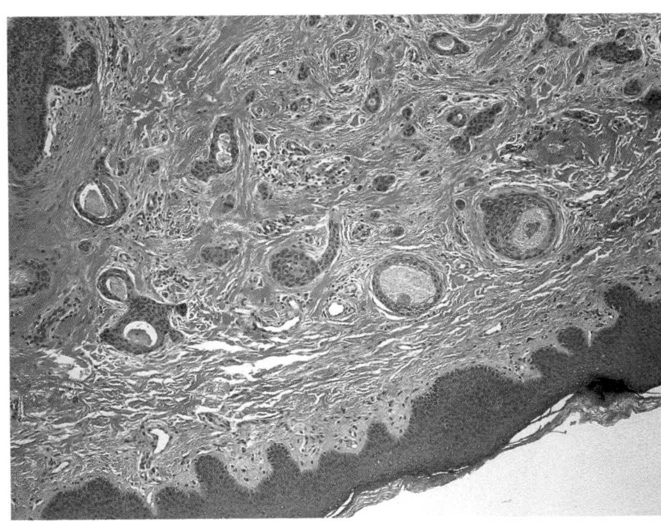

Fig. 19.21 Syringoma of vulva. The tadpole-shaped structures are characteristic.

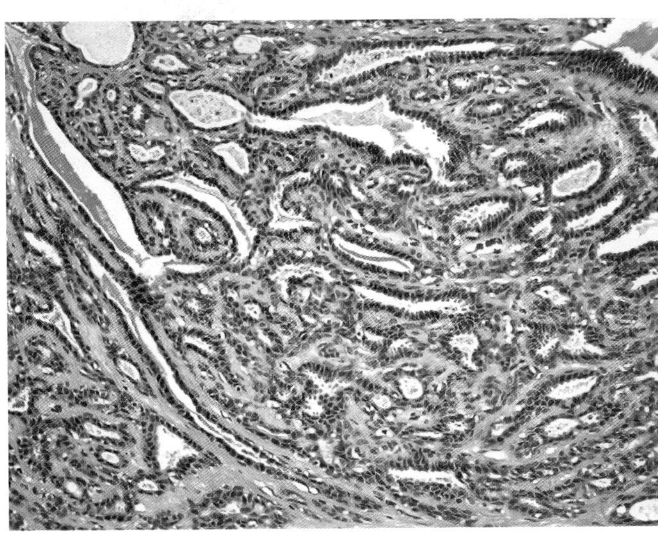

Fig. 19.20 Hidradenoma papilliferum of vulva. This tumor probably arises from ectopic breast tissue.

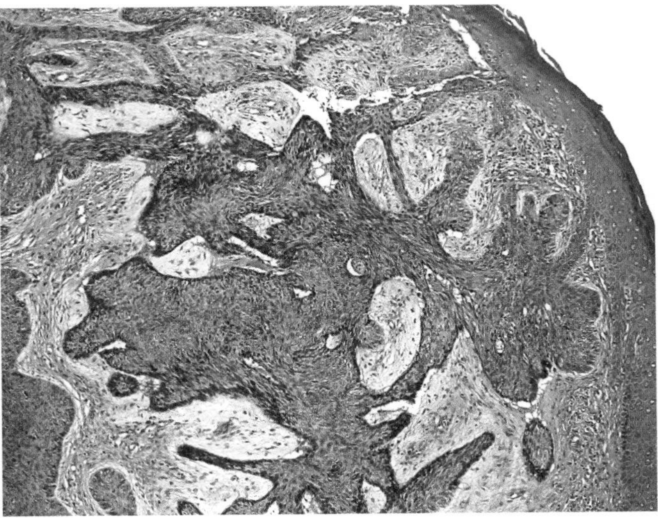

Fig. 19.22 Basal cell carcinoma of vulva. It is important to distinguish this tumor from squamous cell carcinoma, especially the basaloid variant of the latter.

features,[238] another with features of *malignant myoepithelioma*,[231] and another resembling *polymorphous low-grade adenocarcinoma* of salivary glands[246] (see also under Bartholin gland).

Sebaceous carcinoma can occur in the vulva; its appearance is similar to that of its more common counterpart in the head and neck region.[230]

Melanocytic tumors

Melanocytic nevi occur in the vulva, particularly in the labia majora. Those seen in adults are nearly always of intradermal or compound type. Sometimes, a prominent junctional component is seen in nevi of younger women, in which the enlarged junctional nests vary in size, shape, and position, and may lead to an overdiagnosis of malignant melanoma.[248,263] The term *(atypical) genital nevus* is sometimes employed for this microscopically troublesome lesion, which may exhibit a striking degree of cytologic and architectural atypia.[249,251]

Melanoma is the second most common malignant tumor of the vulva, following squamous cell carcinoma and representing roughly 10% of all malignant tumors at this site.[254,257] The large majority of the patients are older than 50 years at the time of diagnosis, a fact of great importance in the differential diagnosis with genital nevus.[260,261] Most lesions are advanced (Clark level III or IV) at the time of diagnosis[265] (Fig. 19.23). The microscopic appearance is similar to that of cutaneous melanoma (see Chapter 4) (Fig. 19.24A). An important differential diagnosis is with Paget disease, a situation complicated by the fact that on occasion the two tumors coexist.[252] Sometimes the melanoma is formed of spindle cells growing in fascicles and simulating sarcoma (Fig. 19.24B).

The usual treatment is radical vulvectomy with bilateral inguinal lymph node dissection, but small lesions with depths of ≤1.75 mm may be treated with wide local excision.[250,253,256] The overall 5-year survival rate is approximately 35%.[247,259] Lymph node status, level or thickness of the primary tumor, and ulceration are the most important prognostic parameters.[255,258,259,262,268] There is some suggestion that the DNA ploidy pattern may also provide prognostic information.[266] Vulvar melanomas are not associated with genital-type HPV (HPV-16), but epidermodysplasia verruciformis-type HPV (HPV-38) and cutaneous type HPV (HPV-3) have been detected in some cases.[264]

Malignant blue nevus of the vulva leading to ovarian metastases has been recorded.[267]

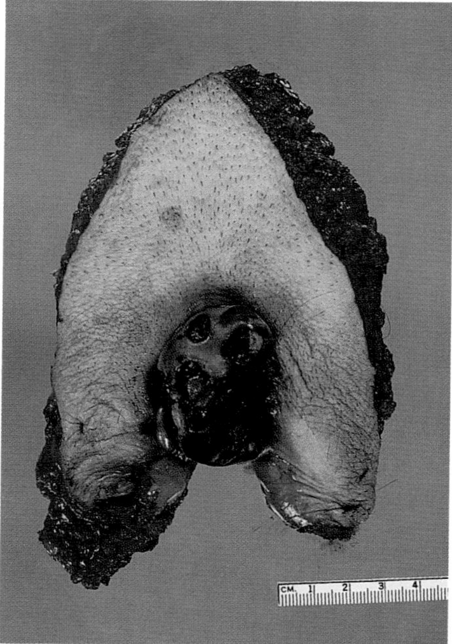

Fig. 19.23 Gross appearance of vulvar malignant melanoma. The tumor is large, polypoid, deeply pigmented, and ulcerated.

Aggressive angiomyxoma and related lesions

Aggressive angiomyxoma is a soft tissue neoplasm that usually arises within the perineum. It often presents as a vulvar mass and

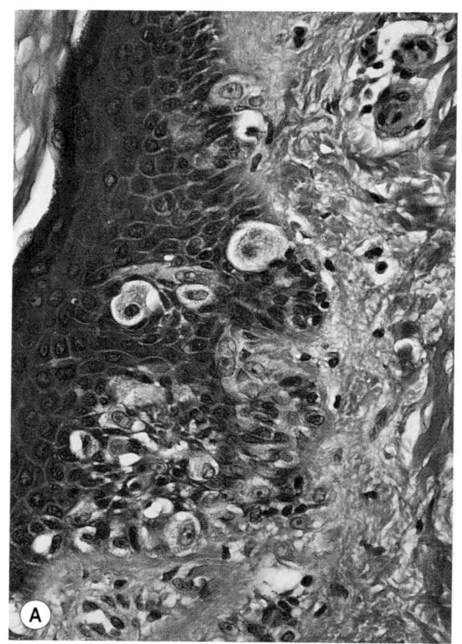

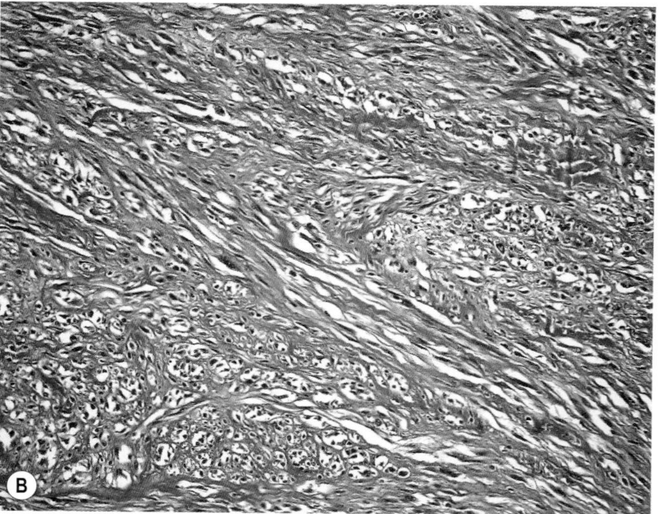

Fig. 19.24 Malignant melanoma of vulva: **A**, superficially spreading type, showing typical intraepidermal growth of pagetoid cells; **B**, melanoma growing in the form of fascicles of spindle cells and simulating a mesenchymal neoplasm.

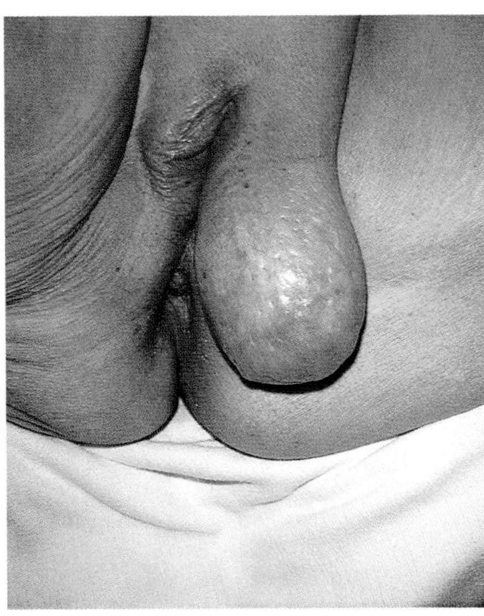

Fig. 19.25 Aggressive angiomyxoma protruding in a polypoid fashion through one of the labia.

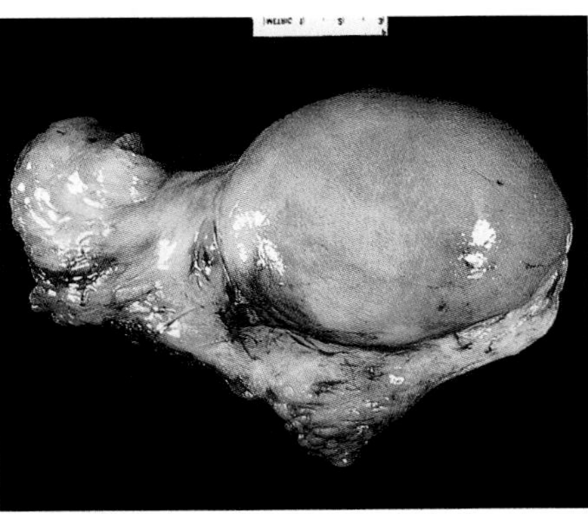

Fig. 19.26 Cut surface of vulvar aggressive angiomyxoma. The tumor is soft, gelatinous, and encapsulated.

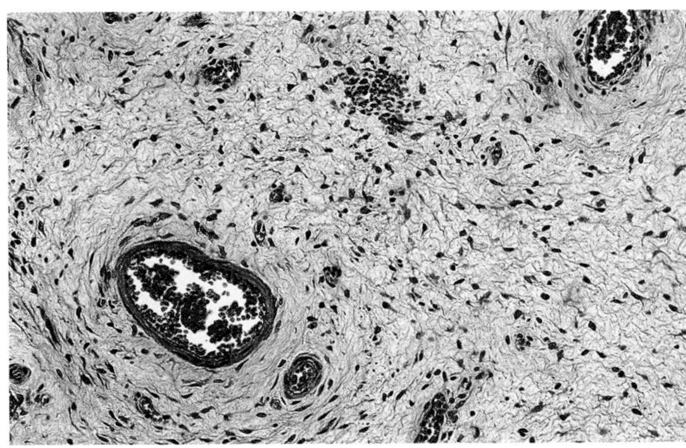

Fig. 19.27 Microscopic appearance of aggressive angiomyxoma. The lesion is hypocellular and features large-sized vessels.

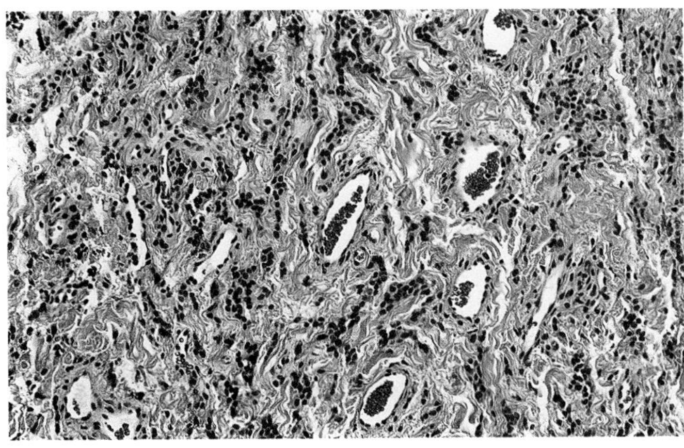

Fig. 19.28 Vulvar angiomyofibroblastoma. Rows of small oval cells are separated by fibrous strands.

clinically simulates a Bartholin gland cyst[270,296] (Fig. 19.25). Most patients are in the second or third decade of life, but cases have also been reported in children.[274,300] A similar tumor has been described in the scrotal region in males.[280]

Grossly, the appearance is edematous and ill defined (Fig. 19.26). Microscopically, a hypocellular stroma devoid of atypicality or mitotic activity is seen intermingling with sizable vessels having dilated lumina and frequent hyaline thickening of the adventitia (Fig. 19.27). This tumor is distinguished from the more common and innocuous fibroepithelial polyp described below because of its larger size, deeper location, and lack of bizarre stromal cells. The differential diagnosis also includes angiomyofibroblastoma, cellular angiofibroma, and massive vulvar edema (see below). The ultrastructural and immunohistochemical features of aggressive angiomyxoma are those of primitive mesenchymal cells focally exhibiting myoid traits.[284,295] Stains for acidic mucins are only weakly positive, suggesting that the stroma is more edematous than myxoid. Immunohistochemically, there is positivity for desmin (less so in the male counterpart of this lesion), smooth muscle actin (about half of the cases), CD34 (about half) and estrogen and progesterone receptors (100%, irrespective of gender).[285,293] A fourth of the cases also show keratin AE1/AE3 positivity.[298] Some cases analyzed cytogenetically have shown a chromosomal translocation involving the region 12q14–15,[282] where the high mobility group AT-hook 2 gene *HMGA2* is located, resulting in overexpression of this molecule.[287,292] Another case had a t(5;8)(p15;q22) translocation.[297]

Recurrence in the ischiorectal and retroperitoneal spaces is common, probably because of the difficulties encountered in achieving a complete surgical excision.[273] In addition, two typical cases have been reported in association with lung metastases.[271,294]

Angiomyofibroblastoma is a benign vulvar tumor characterized by alternating hypercellular and hypocellular areas admixed with small blood vessels.[275,276,299] Spindle and plump stromal cells aggregate around the vessels (Fig. 19.28). These cells are immunoreactive for vimentin, desmin, and hormone receptors, but usually not for actin or keratin.[283,288] There may be a component of mature adipose tissue; when abundant, the tumor is referred to as the *lipomatous variant*.[272] If the vessels are not prominent, the term *myofibroblastoma* (without the 'angio') has been used. The behavior is benign, with an extremely low rate of local recurrence, but a case with sarcomatous transformation ('angiomyofibrosarcoma') has

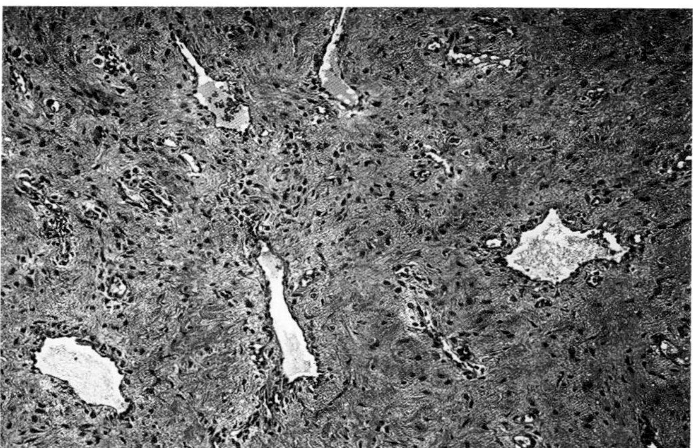

Fig. 19.29 Angiofibroma of vulva. The microscopic appearance is reminiscent of nasopharyngeal angiofibroma.
(Slide courtesy of Dr Robert E Scully, Boston, MA)

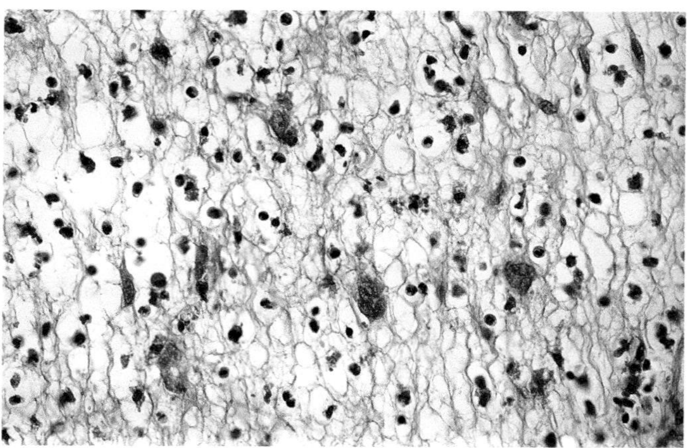

Fig. 19.30 Vulvar polyp containing reactive stromal cells, some of which are multinucleated.

been reported.[289] A relationship between angiomyofibroblastoma and tamoxifen therapy has been suggested.[277]

The typical example of angiomyofibroblastoma differs from aggressive angiomyxoma by virtue of its circumscribed borders, higher cellularity, abundance of blood vessels, plump stromal cells, minimal stromal mucin, and rarity of red blood cell extravasation.[275,279] However, enough common features and transitions occur between it and aggressive angiomyxoma to suggest that they are closely related entities.[269,278,291,295]

Cellular angiofibroma has well-circumscribed margins, like angiomyofibroblastoma. Microscopically, it is composed of uniform, bland, spindle mesenchymal cells accompanied by numerous thick-walled vessels and inconspicuous islands of mature fat (Fig. 19.29).[281] The tumor is cellular and can be mitotically active.[290] Once again, it is hard to escape from the suspicion that this tumor is histogenetically related to the others described in this section, their common denominator being an origin from the specialized hormone-receptor-positive mesenchymal tissue within the lower female genital tract.[285,286]

Other tumors and tumorlike conditions

Asymmetric labium majus enlargement in the pre- and early pubertal age may clinically mimic a neoplasm.[364] It tends to regress spontaneously and probably represents an asymmetric physiologic enlargement in response to the hormonal surges of that tumultuous period, as an example of the phenomenon that in my student days used to be called the 'uneven tissue response' (in Spanish '*respuesta hística despareja*', which sounds even more impressive).

Massive vulvar edema may be seen secondarily to obesity and immobilization.[330] It is similar if not identical to the condition described as *vulvar hypertrophy with lymphedema*.[362] It can simulate aggressive angiomyxoma, but the clinical features should alert the gynecologist and the pathologist to the correct diagnosis.

Fibroepithelial polyp is a superficially located lesion composed of a loose myxoid stroma covered by normal squamous epithelium. Bizarre, stellate, frequently multinucleated cells may be present[301,312,347] (Fig. 19.30). Some lesions are moderately hypercellular. The combination of hypercellularity and bizarre tumor cells may result in overdiagnosis.[343] As in other sites where this lesion occurs, desmin immunoreactivity may be present.[334]

Prepubertal vulvar fibroma presents at a median age of 8 years. It is grossly ill-defined and is microscopically composed of bland spindle-shaped cells in a variably collagenous to edematous or myxoid stroma lacking atypia and mitotic activity. It may recur locally after excision.[321]

Smooth muscle tumors of both benign and malignant types occur.[340] The leiomyomas include a myxoid variety that can simulate aggressive angiomyxoma,[335] and the leiomyosarcomas include epithelioid and myxoid variants.[337,356] Nielsen et al.[340] evaluated the tumors on the basis of size (≥5 cm), infiltrative margins, mitoses (≥5/10 HPF), and moderate to severe cytologic atypia. Tumors that had three or all four of these features were regarded as leiomyosarcomas, tumors that had none or one of the features were called leiomyomas, and tumors that had two features were designated atypical leiomyomas.

Nonepithelial tumors and tumorlike conditions of many other types have been described in the vulva and its surroundings, most of them of soft tissue type.[339,345] They include *endometriosis*, *varices*,[305] *hemangioma* and *hemangiomatosis* (sometimes as a component of Maffucci syndrome),[313] *lymphangioma* (which may clinically simulate warts),[333] *angiokeratoma*,[331] *epithelioid hemangioendothelioma*,[355] *glomus tumor*[323,354] and *glomangiomyoma*,[306] *angiosarcoma*[342] (including the *post-radiation epithelioid type*),[316] *hemangiopericytoma/solitary fibrous tumor*[354] (Fig. 19.31), benign and malignant *granular cell tumors* (some with accompanying pseudoepitheliomatous hyperplasia)[349,351,367] (Fig. 19.32), *schwannoma*,[320] *neurofibroma(tosis)*,[314,319] *malignant peripheral nerve sheath tumor*,[358,359] *sclerosing lipogranuloma*,[324] *yolk sac tumor*,[310] *rhabdomyosarcoma* [317,318] (usually occurring in children and belonging to the embryonal/botryoid variety), *benign lymphoid hyperplasia*,[325] *verruciform xanthoma*,[352] *Langerhans cell histiocytosis*,[303,332,348] *nodular fasciitis*,[346] *postoperative spindle cell nodule*,[327] so-called *malignant fibrous histiocytoma*,[357] *dermatofibrosarcoma protuberans*[304,307,311] (including cases with fibrosarcomatous transformation[315]), *Ewing sarcoma/PNET*,[363] *synovial sarcoma*[341] (including the monophasic type[366]), *fibromatosis/desmoid tumor* (sometimes associated with pregnancy),[302,338] *atypical lipomatous tumor*,[344] a lesion resembling *lipoblastoma*,[326] *malignant lymphoma*,[322,361] *paraganglioma*,[308] *alveolar soft part sarcoma*,[353] *epithelioid sarcoma*,[360] and *angiomatoid fibrous histiocytoma*.

Epithelioid sarcoma is of importance because of its relatively high frequency at this site and the fact that it tends to run a

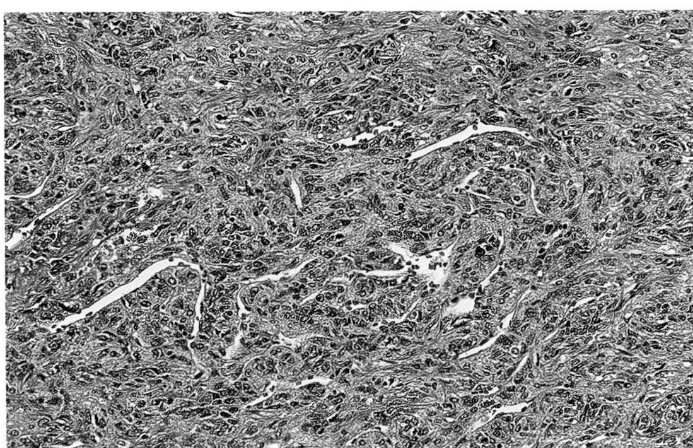

Fig. 19.31 A rare example of hemangiopericytoma/solitary fibrous tumor involving soft tissues of vulva.

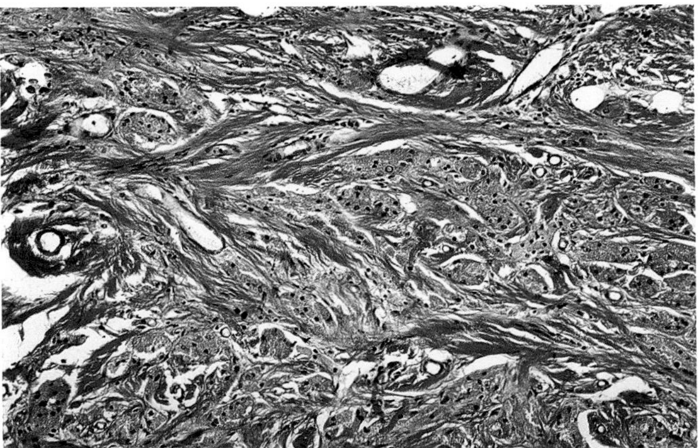

Fig. 19.32 Granular cell tumor of vulva.

more aggressive course here than in its usual location in the distal extremities. This may at least partially result from the fact that this tumor, when located in the vulva, often exhibits rhabdoid features, known to be associated with an aggressive course.[365] As a matter of fact, it may be difficult to decide whether to designate a vulvar tumor with these features as an epithelioid sarcoma or as a malignant rhabdoid tumor.[328,350] The term proximal-type epithelioid sarcoma has been employed for this particular situation, of which the vulva is a prime example (see Chapter 25).

Metastases to the vulva usually originate from the cervix (almost 50%), endometrium, kidney, or gastrointestinal tract.[309] Most are expressions of generalized disease.[329] The labium majus is the most common location.[336]

Lesions of Bartholin glands and related structures

Cysts and abscesses of Bartholin glands are the result of chronic bacterial inflammation, especially from gonorrhea.[391] The lining of the cyst, which is usually of transitional or squamous type, can be destroyed partially or totally by the inflammatory infiltrate. The nature of the cyst can be established by the presence of residual mucinous glands in the fibrotic and inflamed connective tissue that

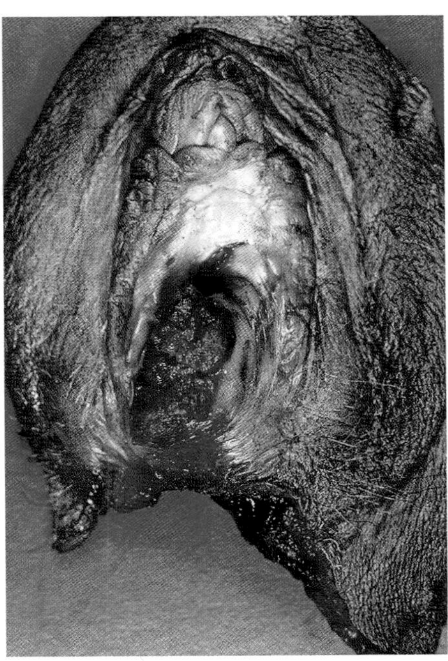

Fig. 19.33 Large carcinoma arising from Bartholin gland.

forms the cyst wall. The secretion product is a nonsulfated sialomucin.[387] Sometimes, extravasation of this mucus into the stroma may induce changes similar to those seen in 'mucocele' of the oral cavity.[378] The cyst may be treated by excision or marsupialization.[368] Exceptionally, the inflammatory infiltrate is found to have the features of *malakoplakia*.[386]

Mucous cysts of the *vulvar vestibule* are usually solitary and lined by mucin-producing columnar cells.[379]

Benign tumors and tumorlike conditions of this area include adenoma of minor vestibular glands (which may well represent focal hyperplastic changes secondary to trauma and inflammation), nodular hyperplasia, adenoma,[369] adenomyoma,[381] mucinous cystadenoma,[372] and papilloma.[375]

Carcinomas of Bartholin gland[373,382,390] may take the form of squamous cell carcinoma (the most common) (Fig. 19.33), adenocarcinoma,[385] urothelial (transitional cell) carcinoma (Fig. 19.34), salivary gland-type basal cell and epithelial–myoepithelial adenocarcinoma,[376,383] small cell (neuroendocrine) carcinoma,[380] and adenoid cystic carcinoma (including the tubular variety)[374,384,388] (Fig. 19.35). Lymph node metastases are common. HPV is often found in the squamous cell carcinoma type,[377] as well as in the transitional cell carcinoma type.[389] The overall survival rate is in the neighborhood of 60%.[370,371]

Lesions of the female urethra

Urethral caruncle has the appearance of a small raspberry protruding from the meatus; it bleeds easily and may become infected. It occurs only in the female urethra and is not a true neoplasm but rather a reactive polypoid lesion. Microscopically, chronic inflammatory cells, dilated vessels, and hyperplastic epithelium are seen in varying proportions. Mistaken diagnoses of malignancy can result from overinterpretation of islands of reactive epithelium or scattered bizarre stromal or lymphoid cells.[420] There is a tendency for these lesions to recur following excision, probably because of persistence of the original inciting factors.

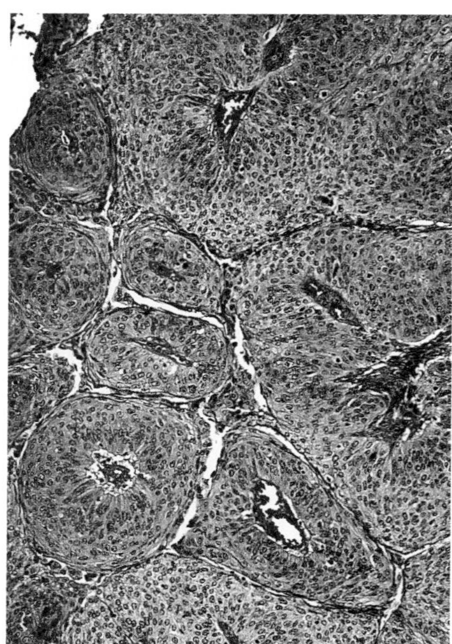

Fig. 19.34 Bartholin gland carcinoma of urothelial type.

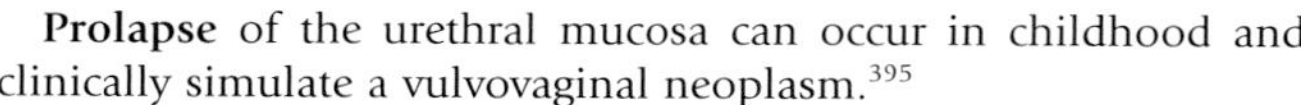

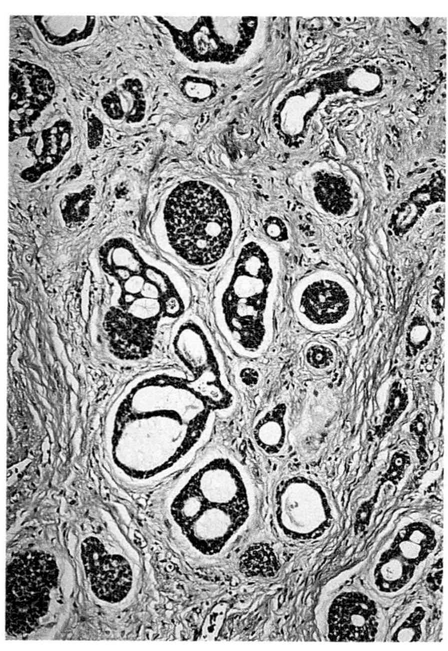

Fig. 19.35 Bartholin gland carcinoma of adenoid cystic type.

Prolapse of the urethral mucosa can occur in childhood and clinically simulate a vulvovaginal neoplasm.[395]

So-called **nephrogenic (mesonephric) adenoma** has been traditionally regarded as a metaplastic change resulting from inflammation rather than a true neoplasm. It is microscopically similar to the more common lesions located in the bladder neck.[398,409] Similarly, an occurrence in the urethra of mucinous epithelium of *colonic* type can also be explained on a metaplastic basis, although a congenital origin is also possible.[401]

Villous adenoma has been reported in the urethra in association with tubulovillous adenoma and adenocarcinoma of the rectum.[406]

Urethral carcinoma occurs in elderly patients and presents with bleeding or dysuria.[394,402] The majority of the cases arise from the meatus, at the junction of the transitional and squamous epithelium. In a series of 35 cases, 19 were anterior (vulvourethral), 4 were posterior (vesicourethral), and 12 involved the entire urethra.[414]

Microscopically, most urethral carcinomas are of squamous cell type.[392,407] Other types include urothelial (transitional cell) carcinoma, columnar/mucinous adenocarcinoma,[405] signet ring adenocarcinoma,[416] and clear cell (mesonephroid) adenocarcinoma.[412,419] Interestingly, nearly half of the carcinomas reported as arising in urethral diverticula have been adenocarcinomas of either conventional or clear cell type.[396,397] Some of the urethral adenocarcinomas have been associated with adenomatous hyperplasia of the periurethral glands.[393] HPV has been detected by PCR techniques in a high proportion of urethral carcinomas.[418]

The prognosis of urethral carcinoma is relatively poor, except when the disease is limited to the anterior portion of the urethra.[404] In one large series, the 5-, 10-, and 15-year actuarial survival rates were 41%, 31%, and 22%, respectively.[399] The usual treatment is radiation therapy,[399,413,417] but, depending on their size and location, they can also be treated by surgery alone or surgery plus irradiation.[400,408]

Leiomyoma of the urethra, although extremely unusual, is the most common type of benign mesenchymal tumor at this site.[415]

Melanoma of the urethra is a highly aggressive neoplasm that is treated by total urethrectomy with bilateral inguinal lymph node dissection.[403,411]

Malignant lymphoma can exceptionally present as a urethral tumor.[410]

Metastatic tumors in the urethra usually originate in other portions of the female genital tract, particularly endometrium.[407]

References

NORMAL ANATOMY

1 McLean JM. Anatomy and physiology of the vulvar area. In Ridley CM (ed.): The vulva. New York, 1988, Churchill Livingstone.

2 Rorat E, Ferenczy A, Richart RM. Human Bartholin gland, duct, and duct cyst. Arch Pathol 1975, **99**: 367–374.

3 van der Putte SC. Anogenital 'sweat' glands. Histology and pathology of a gland that may mimic mammary glands. Am J Dermatopathol 1991, **13**: 557–567.

4 Wilkinson EJ, Hardt NS. Vulva. In Mills SE (ed.): Histology for pathologists, ed. 3. Philadelphia, 2007, Lippincott Williams and Wilkins, pp. 983–998.

ECTOPIC BREAST AND RELATED LESIONS

5 Abbott JJ, Ahmed I. Adenocarcinoma of mammary-like glands of the vulva: report of a case and review of the literature. Am J Dermatopathol 2006, **28**: 127–133.

6 Burger RA, Marcuse PM. Fibroadenoma of the vulva. Am J Clin Pathol 1954, **24**: 965–968.

7 Chulia MT, Paya A, Niveiro M, Ceballos S, Aranda FI. Phyllodes tumor in ectopic breast tissue of the vulva. Int J Surg Pathol 2001, **9**: 81–83.

8 Chung-Park M, Zheng Liu C, Giampoli EJ, Emery JD, Shalodi A. Mucinous adenocarcinoma of ectopic breast tissue of the vulva. Arch Pathol Lab Med 2002, **126**: 1216–1218.

9 Di Bonito L, Patriarca S, Falconieri G. Aggressive 'breast-like' adenocarcinoma of vulva. Pathol Res Pract 1992, **188**: 211–214.

10 Guerry RL, Pratt-Thomas HR. Carcinoma of supernumerary breast of vulva with bilateral mammary cancer. Cancer 1976, **38**: 2570–2574.

11 Kazakov DV, Hügel H, Vanecek T, Michal M. Unusual hyperplasia of anogenital mammary-like glands. Am J Dermatopathol 2006, **28**: 134–137.

12 Kazakov DV, Belousova IE, Sima R, Michal M. Mammary type tubulolobular carcinoma of the anogenital area: report of a case of a unique tumor presumably originating in anogenital mammarylike glands. Am J Surg Pathol 2006, **30**: 1193–1196.

13 Kazakov DV, Spagnolo DV, Stewart CJ, Thompson J, Agaimy A, Magro G, Bisceglia M, Vazmitel M, Kacerovska D, Kutzner H, Mukensnabl P, Michal M. Fibroadenoma and phyllodes tumors of anogenital mammary-like glands: a series of 13 neoplasms in 12 cases, including mammary-type juvenile fibroadenoma, fibroadenoma with lactation changes, and neurofibromatosis-associated pseudoangiomatous stromal hyperplasia with multinucleated giant cells. Am J Surg Pathol 2010, **34**: 95–103.

14 Rose PG, Roman LD, Reale FR, Tak WK, Hunter RE. Primary adenocarcinoma of the breast arising in the vulva. Obstet Gynecol 1990, **76**: 537–539.

15 Simon KE, Dutcher JP, Runowicz CD, Wiernik PH. Adenocarcinoma arising in vulvar breast tissue. Cancer 1988, **62**: 2234–2238.

16 Sington JD, Manek S, Hollowood K. Fibroadenoma of the mammary-like glands of the vulva. Histopathology 2002, **41**: 563–565.

17 Tbakhi A, Cowan DF, Kumar D, Kyle D. Recurring phyllodes tumor in aberrant breast tissue of the vulva. Am J Surg Pathol 1993, **17**: 946–950.

18 van der Putte SC. Mammary-like glands of the vulva and their disorders. Int J Gynecol Pathol 1994, **13**: 150–160.

INFLAMMATORY DISEASES

19 Alexander LJ, Shields TL. Squamous cell carcinoma of the vulva secondary to granuloma inguinale. Arch Dermatol 1953, **67**: 395–402.

20 Andreani SM, Ratnasingham K, Dang HH, Gravante G, Giordano P. Crohn's disease of the vulva. Int J Surg 2010, **8**: 2–5.

21 Barnes R, Masood S, Lammert N, Young RH. Extragenital granuloma inguinale mimicking a soft-tissue neoplasm. A case report and review of the literature. Hum Pathol 1990, **21**: 559–561.

22 Bassa AG, Hoosen AA, Moodley J, Bramdev A. Granuloma inguinale (donovanosis) in women. An analysis of 61 cases from Durban, South Africa. Sex Transm Dis 1993, **20**: 164–167.

23 Chadha S, Gianotten WL, Drogendijk AC, Schultz WC, Blindeman LA, van der Meijden WI. Histopathologic features of vulvar vestibulitis. Int J Gynecol Pathol 1998, **17**: 7–11.

24 Douglas CPL. Lymphogranuloma venereum and granuloma inguinale of the vulva. J Obstet Gynaecol Br Commonw 1962, **69**: 871–880.

25 Guerrieri C, Ohlsson E, Rydén G, Westermark P. Vulvitis granulomatosa. A cryptogenic chronic inflammatory hypertrophy of vulvar labia related to cheilitis granulomatosa and Crohn's disease. Int J Gynecol Pathol 1995, **14**: 352–359.

26 Haidopoulos D, Rodalakis A, Stefanidis K, Blachos G, Sotiropoulou M, Diakomanolis E. Behçet's disease: part of the differential diagnosis of the ulcerative vulva. Clin Exp Obstet Gynecol 2002, **29**: 219–221.

27 Koteen H. Lymphogranuloma venereum. Medicine (Baltimore) 1945, **24**: 1–69.

28 Kremer M, Nussenson E, Steinfeld M, Zuckerman P. Crohn's disease of the vulva. Am J Gastroenterol 1984, **79**: 376–378.

29 Lavery HA, Pinkerton JHM, Sloan J. Crohn's disease of the vulva. Two further cases. Br J Dermatol 1985, **113**: 359–363.

30 Mabey D, Peeling RW. Lymphogranuloma venereum. Sex Transm Infect 2002, **78**: 90–92.

31 O'Farrell N. Donovanosis. Sex Transm Infect 2002, **78**: 452–457.

32 Oriel JD. Infective conditions of the vulva. In Ridley CM, Neill SM (eds): The vulva, ed. 2. Oxford, 1999, Blackwell Science, pp. 71–120.

33 Prayson RA, Stoler MH, Hart WR. Vulvar vestibulitis. A histopathologic study of 36 cases, including human papillomavirus in situ hybridization analysis. Am J Surg Pathol 1995, **19**: 154–160.

34 Rainey R. The association of lymphogranuloma inguinale and cancer. Surgery 1954, **35**: 221–235.

35 Ramdial PK, Kharsany AB, Reddy R, Chetty R. Transepithelial elimination of cutaneous vulval granuloma inguinale. J Cutan Pathol 2000, **27**: 493–499.

36 Roberts DB. Necrotizing fascitis of the vulva. Am J Obstet Gynecol 1987, **157**: 568–571.

37 Sakane T, Takeno M, Suzuki N, Inaba G. Behçet's disease. N Engl J Med 1999, **341**: 1284–1291.

38 Velho PE, Souza EM, Belda Junior W. Donovanosis. Braz J Infect Dis 2008, **12**: 521–525.

39 Vettraino IM, Merritt DF. Crohn's disease of the vulva. Am J Dermatopathol 1995, **17**: 410–413.

40 White JA. Manifestations and management of lymphogranuloma venereum. Curr Opin Infect Dis 2009, **22**: 57–66.

SO-CALLED 'CHRONIC VULVAR DYSTROPHIES'

41 Ambros RA, Malfetano JH, Carlson JA, Mihm MC. Non-neoplastic epithelial alterations of the vulva: recognition assessment and comparisons of terminologies used among the various specialities. Mod Pathol 1997, **10**: 401–408.

42 Carlson JA, Ambros R, Malfetano J, Ross J, Grabowski R, Lamb P, Figge H, Mihm MC. Vulvar lichen sclerosus and squamous cell carcinoma: a cohort, case control, and investigational study with historical perspective; implications for chronic inflammation and sclerosis in the development of neoplasia. Hum Pathol 1998, **29**: 932–948.

43 Carlson JA, Lamb P, Malfetano J, Ambros RA, Mihm MC. Clinicopathologic comparison of vulvar and extragenital lichen sclerosus: histologic variants, evolving lesions, and etiology of 141 cases. Mod Pathol 1998, **11**: 844–854.

44 Fung MA, LeBoit PE. Light microscopic criteria for the diagnosis of early vulvar lichen sclerosus: a comparison with lichen planus. Am J Surg Pathol 1998, **22**: 473–478.

45 Hart WR, Norris JH, Helwig EB. Relation of lichen sclerosus et atrophicus of the vulva to development of carcinoma. Obstet Gynecol 1975, **45**: 369–377.

46 Janovski NA, Ames S. Lichen sclerosus et atrophicus of the vulva. A poorly understood disease entity. Obstet Gynecol 1963, **22**: 697–708.

47 Kim YT, Thomas NF, Kessis TD, Wilkinson EJ, Hedrick L, Cho KR. p53 mutations and clonality in vulvar carcinomas and squamous hyperplasias: evidence suggesting that squamous hyperplasias do not serve as direct precursors of human papillomavirus-negative vulvar carcinomas. Hum Pathol 1996, **27**: 389–395.

48 Kiryu H, Ackerman AB. A critique of current classification of vulvar diseases. Am J Dermatopathol 1990, **12**: 377–392.

49 Laseano EF, Montes LF,Mazzini MA, Lichen sclerosus et atrophicus in childhood. Report of 6 cases.Obstet Gynecol 1964, **24**: 872–877.

50 Lawrence WD. Non-neoplastic epithelial disorders of the vulva (vulvar dystrophies). Historical and current perspectives. Pathol Annu 1993, **28**(Pt 2): 23–51.

51 Lee ES, Allen D, Scurry J. Pseudoepitheliomatous hyperplasia in lichen sclerosus of the vulva. Int J Gynecol Pathol 2002, **22**: 57–62.

52 Nascimento AF, Granter SR, Cviko A, Yuan L, Hecht JL, Crum CP. Vulvar acanthosis with altered differentiation: a precursor to verrucous carcinoma? Am J Surg Pathol 2004, **28**: 638–643.

53 Regauer S, Liegl B, Reich O. Early vulvar lichen sclerosus: a histopathological challenge. Histopathology 2005, **47**: 340–347.

54 Regauer S, Reich O, Beham-Schmid C. Monoclonal gamma-T-cell receptor rearrangement in vulvar lichen sclerosus and squamous cell carcinomas. Am J Pathol 2002, **160**: 1035–1045.

55 Rodke G, Friedrich EG Jr, Wilkinson EJ. Malignant potential of mixed vulvar dystrophy (lichen sclerosus associated with squamous cell hyperplasia). J Reprod Med 1988, **33**: 545–550.

56 Scurry J, Whitehead J, Healey M. Histology of lichen sclerosus varies according to site and proximity to carcinoma. Am J Dermatopathol 2002, **23**: 413–418.

57 Wallace HJ. Lichen sclerosus et atrophicus. Trans St John's Hosp Dermatol Soc 1971, **57**: 9–30.

HUMAN PAPILLOMA VIRUS AND VULVAR PATHOLOGY

58 de Koning MN, Quint WG, Pirog EC. Prevalence of mucosal and cutaneous human papillomaviruses in different histologic subtypes of vulvar carcinoma. Mod Pathol 2008, **21**: 334–344.

59 Santos M, Landolfi S, Olivella A, Lloveras B, Klaustermeier J, Suárez H, Alòs L, Puig-Tintoré LM, Campo E, Ordi J. p16 overexpression identifies HPV-positive vulvar squamous cell carcinomas. Am J Surg Pathol 2006, **30**: 1347–1356.

60 Sawchuk WS. Vulvar manifestations of human papillomavirus infection. Dermatol Clin 1992, **10**: 405–414.

CONDYLOMA AND SEBORRHEIC KERATOSIS

61 Crum CP, Fu YS, Levine RU, Richart RM, Townsend DE, Fenoglio CM. Intraepithelial squamous lesions of the vulva. Biologic and histologic criteria for the distinction of condylomas from vulvar intraepithelial neoplasia. Am J Obstet Gynecol 1982, **144**: 77–83.

62 Ferenczy A. Laser treatment of patients with condylomata and squamous carcinoma precursors of the lower female genital tract. CA Cancer J Clin 1987, **37**: 334–347.

63 Hongwei B, Cviko A, Granter S, Yuan L, Betensky RA, Crum CP. Immunophenotypic and viral (human papillomavirus) correlates of vulvar seborrheic keratosis. Hum Pathol 2003, **34**: 559–564.

64 McLachlin CM, Kozakewich H, Craighill M, O'Connell B, Crum CP. Histologic correlates of vulvar human papillomavirus infection in children and young adults. Am J Surg Pathol 1994, **18**: 728–735.

65 McLachlin CM, Mutter GL, Crum CP. Multinucleated atypia of the vulva. Report of a distinct entity not associated with human papillomavirus. Am J Surg Pathol 1994, **18**: 1233–1239.

66 McMillan A, Bishop PE, Fletcher S. An immunohistological study of condylomata acuminata. Histopathology 1990, **17**: 45–52.

67 Nucci MR, Genest DR, Tate JE, Sparks CK, Crum CP. Pseudobowenoid change of the vulva: a histologic variant of untreated condyloma acuminatum. Mod Pathol 1996, **9**: 375–379.

68 Nuovo GJ, O'Connell M, Blanco JS, Levine RU, Silverstein SJ. Correlation of histology and human papillomavirus DNA detection in condyloma acuminatum and condyloma-like vulvar lesions. Am J Surg Pathol 1989, **13**: 700–706.

69 Pirog EC, Chen YT, Isacson C. MIB-1 immunostaining is a beneficial adjunct test for accurate diagnosis of vulvar condyloma acuminatum. Am J Surg Pathol 2000, **24**: 1393–1399.

70 Quinn TR, Young RH. Epidermolytic hyperkeratosis in the lower female genital tract: an uncommon simulant of mucocutaneous papillomavirus infection – a report of two cases. Int J Gynecol Pathol 1997, **16**: 163–168.

71 Shevchuk MM, Richart RM. DNA content of condyloma acuminatum. Cancer 1982, **49**: 489–492.

72 Wade TR, Ackerman AB. The effects of resin of podophyllin on condyloma acuminatum. Am J Dermatopathol 1984, **6**: 109–122.

SQUAMOUS INTRAEPITHELIAL LESIONS

73 Abell MR, Gosling JRG. Intraepithelial and infiltrating carcinoma of the vulva. Bowen's type. Cancer 1961, **14**: 318–329.

74 Armes JE, Lourie R, Bowlay G, Tabrizi S. Pagetoid squamous cell carcinoma in situ of the vulva: comparison with extramammary Paget disease and nonpagetoid squamous cell neoplasia. Int J Gynecol Pathol 2008, **27**: 118–124.

75 Berger BW, Hori Y. Multicentric Bowen's disease of the genitalia. Spontaneous regression of lesions. Arch Dermatol 1978, **114**: 1698–1699.

76 Bergeron C, Neghashfar Z, Canaan C, Shah K, Fu Y, Ferenczy A. Human papillomavirus type 16 in intraepithelial neoplasia (bowenoid papulosis) and coexistent invasive carcinoma of the vulva. Int J Gynecol Pathol 1987, **6**: 1–11.

77 Chiesa-Vottero A, Dvoretsky PM, Hart WR. Histopathologic study of thin vulvar squamous cell carcinomas and associated cutaneous lesions: a correlative study of 48 tumors in 44 patients with analysis of adjacent vulvar intraepithelial neoplasia types and lichen sclerosus. Am J Surg Pathol 2006, **30**: 310–318.

78 Crum CP, Liskow A, Petras P, Keng WC, Frick HC II. Vulvar intraepithelial neoplasia (severe atypia and carcinoma in situ). A clinicopathologic analysis of 41 cases. Cancer 1984, **54**: 1429–1434.

79 Forney JP, Morrow CP, Townsend DE, DiSaia PJ. Management of carcinoma in situ of the vulva. Am J Obstet Gynecol 1977, **127**: 801–806.

80 Friedrich EG Jr, Wilkinson EJ, Fu YS. Carcinoma in situ of the vulva. A continuing challenge. Am J Obstet Gynecol 1980, **136**: 830–843.

81 Hart WR. Vulvar intraepithelial neoplasia: historical aspects and current status. Int J Gynecol Pathol 2001, **20**: 16–30.

82 Husseinzadeh N, Newman NJ, Wesseler TA. Vulvar intraepithelial neoplasia. A clinicopathological study of carcinoma in situ of the vulva. Gynecol Oncol 1989, **33**: 157–163.

83 Inagaki H, Nonaka M, Eimoto T. Bowenoid papulosis showing polyclonal nature. Diagn Mol Pathol 1999, **7**: 122–126.

84 Jones RW, Rowan DM, Stewart AQ. Vulvar intraepithelial neoplasia: aspects of the natural history and outcome in 405 women. Obstet Gynecol 2005, **106**: 1319–1326.

85 Joura EA, Losch A, Haider-Angeler MG, Breitenecker G, Leodolter S. Trends in vulvar neoplasia. Increasing incidence of vulvar intraepithelial neoplasia and squamous cell carcinoma of the vulva in young women. J Reprod Med 2000, **45**: 613–615.

86 Kaefner HK, Tate JE, McLachlin CM, Crum CP. Vulvar intraepithelial neoplasia. Morphological phenotype, papillomavirus DNA, and coexisting invasive carcinoma. Hum Pathol 1995, **26**: 147–154.

87 Kenter GG, Welters MJ, Valentijn AR, Lowik MJ, Berends-van der Meer DM, Vloon AP, Essahsah F, Fathers LM, Offringa R, Drijfhout JW, Wafelman AR, Oostendorp J, Fleuren GJ, van der Burg SH, Melief CJ. Vaccination against HPV-16 oncoproteins for vulvar intraepithelial neoplasia. N Engl J Med 2009, **361**: 1838–1847.

88 Kenter GG, van der Burg S, Melief CJM. Vaccination against HPV-16 for vulvar intraepithelial neoplasia. N Engl J Med 2010, **362**: 655–656.

89 Kimura A. Condylomata acuminata with pigmented papular lesions. Dermatologica 1980, **160**: 390–397.

90 Mulvany NJ, Allen DG. Differentiated intraepithelial neoplasia of the vulva. Int J Gynecol Pathol 2008, **27**: 125–135.

91 Park JS, Jones RW, McLean MR, Currie JL, Woodruff JD, Shah DV, Kurman RJ. Possible etiologic heterogeneity of vulvar intraepithelial neoplasia. A correlation of pathologic characteristics with human papillomavirus detection by in situ hybridization and polymerase chain reaction. Cancer 1991, **67**: 1599–1607.

92 Patterson JW, Kao GF, Graham JH, Helwig EB. Bowenoid papulosis. A clinicopathologic study with ultrastructural observations. Cancer 1986, **57**: 823–836.

93 Pinto AP, Miron A, Yassin Y, Monte N, Woo TYC, Mehra KK, Medeiros F, Crum CP. Differentiated vulvar intraepithelial neoplasia contains *Tp53* mutations and is genetically linked to vulvar squamous cell carcinoma. Mod Pathol 2010, **23**: 404–412.

94 Prat J. Pathology of vulvar intraepithelial lesions and early invasive carcinoma. Hum Pathol 1991, **22**: 877–883.

95 Raju RR, Goldblum JR, Hart WR. Pagetoid squamous cell carcinoma in situ (pagetoid Bowen disease) of the external genitalia. Int J Gynecol Pathol 2003, **22**: 127–135.

96 Santos M, Montagut C, Mellado B, García A, Ramón y Cajal S, Cardesa A, Puig-Tintoré LM, Ordi J. Immunohistochemical staining for p16 and p53 in premalignant and malignant epithelial lesions of the vulva. Int J Gynecol Pathol 2004, **23**: 206–214.

97 Shatz P, Bergeron C, Wilkinson EJ, Arseneau J, Ferenczy A. Vulvar intraepithelial neoplasia and skin appendage involvement. Obstet Gynecol 1989, **74**: 769–774.

98 Skapa P, Zamecnik J, Hamsikova E, Salakova M, Smahelova J, Jandova K, Robova H, Rob L, Tachezy R. Human papillomavirus (HPV) profiles of vulvar lesions: possible implications for the classification of vulvar squamous cell carcinoma precursors and for the efficacy of prophylactic HPV vaccination. Am J Surg Pathol 2007, **31**: 1834–1843.

99 Srodon M, Stoler MH, Baber GB, Kurman RJ. The distribution of low and high-risk HPV types in vulvar and vaginal intraepithelial neoplasia (VIN and VaIN). Am J Surg Pathol 2006, **30**: 1513–1518.

100 Sykes P, Smith N, McCormick P, Frizelle FA. High-grade vulval intraepithelial neoplasia (VIN 3): a retrospective analysis of patient characteristics, management outcome and relationship to squamous cell carcinoma of the vulva 1989–1999. Aust N Z J Obstet Gynaecol 2002, **42**: 69–74.

101 Tate J, Mutter G, Boynton K, Crum C. Monoclonal origin of vulvar intraepithelial neoplasia and some vulvar hyperplasia. Am J Pathol 1997, **150**: 315–322.

102 Ulbright TM, Stehman FB, Roth LM, Ehrlich CE, Ransburg RC. Bowenoid dysplasia of the vulva. Cancer 1982, **50**: 2910–2919.

103 van der Avoort IA, van der Laak JA, Paffen A, Grefte JM, Massuger LF, de Wilde PC, de Hullu JA, Bulten J. MIB1 expression in basal cell layer: a diagnostic tool to identify premalignancies of the vulva. Mod Pathol 2007, **20**: 770–778.

104 van Seters M, van Beurden M, ten Kate FJ, Beckmann I, Ewing PC, Eijkemans MJ, Kagie MJ, Meijer CJ, Aaronson NK, Kleinjan A, Heijmans-Antonissen C, Zijlstra FJ, Burger MP, Helmerhorst TJ. Treatment of vulvar intraepithelial neoplasia with topical imiquimod. N Engl J Med 2008, **358**: 1465–1473.

105 van Seters M, van Beurden M, de Craen AJ. Is the assumed natural history of vulvar intraepithelial neoplasia III based on enough evidence? A systematic review of 3322 published patients. Gynecol Oncol 2005, **97**: 645–651.

106 Wada H, Enomoto T, Yoshino K, Ozaki K, Kurachi H, Nomura T, Murata Y, Kim N, Weinrich S, Lea-Chou E, Lopez-Uribe D, Shroyer KR. Immunohistochemical localization of telomerase hTERT protein and analysis of clonality in multifocal vulvar intraepithelial neoplasia. Am J Clin Pathol 2000, **114**: 371–379.

107 Walts AE, Koeffler HP, Said JW. Localization of p53 protein and human papillomavirus in anogenital squamous lesions. Immunohistochemical and in situ hybridization studies in benign, dysplastic, and malignant epithelia. Hum Pathol 1993, **24**: 1238–1242.

108 Yang B, Hart WR. Vulvar intraepithelial neoplasia of the simplex (differentiated) type: a clinicopathologic study including analysis of HPV and p53 expression. Am J Surg Pathol 2000, **24**: 429–441.

INVASIVE SQUAMOUS CELL CARCINOMA

GENERAL FEATURES

109 Andersen WA, Franquemont DW, Williams J, Taylor PT, Crum CP. Vulvar squamous cell carcinoma and papillomaviruses. Two separate entities? Am J Obstet Gynecol 1991, **165**: 329–335.

110 Bloss JD, Liao SY, Wilczynski SP, Macri C, Walker J, Peake M, Berman ML. Clinical and histologic features of vulvar carcinomas analyzed for human papillomavirus status. Evidence that squamous cell carcinoma of the vulva has more than one etiology. Hum Pathol 1991, **22**: 711–718.

111 Brinton LA, Nasca PC, Mallin K, Baptiste MS, Wilbanks GD, Richart RM. Case-control study of cancer of the vulva. Obstet Gynecol 1990, **75**: 859–866.

112 Carter J, Carlson J, Fowler J, Hartenbach E, Adcock L, Carson L, Twiggs LB. Invasive vulvar tumors in young women. A disease of the immunosuppressed? Gynecol Oncol 1993, **51**: 307–310.

113 Crum CP. Carcinoma of the vulva. Epidemiology and pathogenesis. Obstet Gynecol 1992, **79**: 448–454.

114 Fox H, Wells M. Recent advances in the pathology of the vulva. Histopathology 2003, **42**: 209–216.

115 Hopkins MP, Nemunaitis-Keller J. Carcinoma of the vulva. Obstet Gynecol Clin North Am 2001, **28**: 791–804.

116 Jimerson GK, Merrill JA. Multicentric squamous malignancy involving both cervix and vulva. Cancer 1970, **26**: 150–153.

117 Kim YT, Thomas NF, Kessis TD, Wilkinson EJ, Hedrick L, Cho KR. p53 mutations and clonality in vulvar carcinomas and squamous hyperplasias: evidence suggesting that squamous hyperplasias do not serve as direct precursors of human papillomavirus-negative vulvar carcinomas. Hum Pathol 1996, **27**: 389–395.

118 Kurman RJ, Trimble CL, Shah KV. Human papillomavirus and the pathogenesis of vulvar carcinoma. Curr Opin Obstet Gynecol 1992, **4**: 582–585.

119 Mitchell MF, Prasad CJ, Silva EG, Rutledge FN, McArthur MC, Crum CP. Second genital primary squamous neoplasms in vulvar carcinoma. Viral and histopathologic correlates. Obstet Gynecol 1993, **81**: 13–18.

120 Sherman KJ, Daling JR, Chu J, McKnight B, Weiss NS. Multiple primary tumours in women with vulvar neoplasms. A case-control study. Br J Cancer 1988, **57**: 423–427.

121 Toki T, Kurman RJ, Park JS, Kessis T, Daniel RW, Shah KV. Probable non-papillomavirus etiology of squamous cell carcinoma of the vulva in older women. A clinicopathologic study using in situ hybridization and polymerase chain reaction. Int J Gynecol Pathol 1991, **10**: 107–125.

122 van der Avoort IA, Shirango H, Hoevenaars BM, Grefte JM, de Hullu JA, de Wilde PC, Bulten J, Melchers WJ, Massuger LF. Vulvar squamous cell carcinoma is a multifactorial disease following two separate and independent pathways. Int J Gynecol Pathol 2006, **25**: 22–29.

MORPHOLOGIC, HISTOCHEMICAL, IMMUNOHISTOCHEMICAL, AND MOLECULAR GENETIC FEATURES

123 Czernobilsky B, Gat A, Evron R, Dgani R, Ben-Hur H, Lifschitz-Mercer B. Carcinoma of the clitoris. A histologic study with cytokeratin profile. Int J Gynecol Pathol 1995, **14**: 274–278.

124 Dvoretsky PM, Bonfiglio TA. The pathology of vulvar squamous cell carcinoma and verrucous carcinoma. Pathol Annu 1986, **21**(Pt 2): 23–45.

125 Jee KJ, Kim YT, Kim KR, Kim HS, Yan A, Knuutila S. Loss in 3p and 4p and gain 3q are concomitant aberrations in squamous cell carcinoma of the vulva. Mod Pathol 2001, **14**: 377–381.

126 Lin MC, Mutter GL, Trivijisilp P, Boynton KA, Sun D, Crum CP. Patterns of allelic loss (LOH) in vulvar squamous carcinomas and adjacent non-invasive epithelia. Am J Pathol 1998, **152**: 1313–1318.

127 Pinto AP, Lin MC, Mutter GL, Sun D, Villa LL, Crum CP. Allelic loss in human papillomavirus-positive and -negative vulvar squamous cell carcinoma. Am J Pathol 1999, **154**: 1009–1015.

128 Soufir N, Queille S, Liboutet M, Thibaudeau O, Bachelier F, Delestaing G, Balloy BC, Breuer J, Janin A, Dubertret L, Vilmer C, Basset-Seguin N. Inactivation of the CDKN2A and the p53 tumour suppressor genes in external genital carcinomas and their precursors. Br J Dermatol 2007, **156**: 448–453.

129 Zaino RJ, Husseinzadeh N, Nahhas W, Mortel R. Epithelial alterations in proximity to invasive squamous carcinoma of the vulva. Int J Gynecol Pathol 1982, **1**: 173–184.

130 Zamparelli A, Mascuillo V, Bovicelli A, Santini D, Ferrandina G, Minimo C, Terzano P, Costa S, Cinti C, Ceccarelli C, Mancuso S, Scambia G, Bovicelli L, Giordano A. Expression of cell-cycle-associated proteins pRB2/p 130 and p27kip1 in vulvar squamous cell carcinomas. Hum Pathol 2001, **32**: 4–9.

SPREAD AND METASTASES

131 Cady B. Sentinel lymph node procedure in squamous cell carcinoma of the vulva. J Clin Oncol 2000, **18**: 2795–2797.

132 de Hullu JA, Hollema H, Piers DA, Herheijen RH, Van Diest PJ, Mourits MJ, Aalders JG, van der Zee AG. Sentinel lymph node procedure is highly accurate in squamous cell carcinoma of the vulva. J Clin Oncol 2000, **18**: 2811–2816.

133 Figge DC, Tamimi HK, Greer BE. Lymphatic spread in carcinoma of the vulva. Am J Obstet Gynecol 1985, **152**: 387–394.

134 Regauer S. Histopathological work-up and interpretation of sentinel lymph nodes removed for vulvar squamous cell carcinoma. Lab Invest 2009, **89**(Suppl 1): 233A.

THERAPY

135 Coleman RL, Santoso JT. Vulvar carcinoma. Curr Treat Options Oncol 2000, **1**: 177–190.

136 Creasman WT, Phillips JL, Menck HR. The National Cancer Data Base Report on early stage invasive vulvar carcinoma. The American College of Surgeons Commission on Cancer and the American Cancer Society. Cancer 1997, **80**: 505–513.

137 Hacker NF, Van der Velden J. Conservative management of early vulvar cancer. Cancer 1993, **71**: 1673–1677.

138 Heaps JM, Fu YS, Montz FJ, Hacker NF, Berek JS. Surgical-pathologic variables predictive of local recurrence in squamous cell carcinoma of the vulva. Gynecol Oncol 1990, **38**: 309–314.

139 Hopkins MP, Morley GW. Pelvic exenteration for the treatment of vulvar cancer. Cancer 1992, **70**: 2835–2838.

140 Moore DH. Chemotherapy and radiation therapy in the treatment of squamous cell carcinoma of the vulva: are two therapies better than one? Gynecol Oncol 2009, **113**: 379–383.

141 Perez CA, Grigsby PW, Galakatos A, Swanson R, Camel HM, Kao MS, Lockett MA. Radiation therapy in management of carcinoma of the vulva with emphasis on conservation therapy. Cancer 1993, **71**: 3707–3716.

PROGNOSIS

142 Ambros RA, Melfetano JH, Mihm MC. Clinicopathologic features of vulvar squamous cell carcinomas exhibiting prominent fibromyxoid stromal response. Int J Gynecol Pathol 1996, **15**: 137–145.

143 Binder SW, Huang I, Fu YS, Hacker NF, Berek JS. Risk factors for the development of lymph node metastasis in vulvar squamous cell carcinoma. Gynecol Oncol 1990, **37**: 9–16.

144 Blecharz P, Karolewski K, Bieda T, Klimek M, Pudelek J, Kojs E, Zur K, Dzialak P, Urbanski K. Prognostic factors in patients with carcinoma of the vulva – our own experience and literature review. Eur J Gynaecol Oncol 2008, **29**: 260–263.

145 Donaldson ES, Powell DE, Hanson MB, van Nagell JR. Prognostic parameters in invasive vulvar cancer. Gynecol Oncol 1981, **11**: 184–190.

146 Gosling JRG, Abell MR, Prolette BM, Loughrin TD. Infiltrative squamous cell (epidermoid) carcinoma of vulva. Cancer 1961, **14**: 330–343.

147 Heaps JM, Fu YS, Montz FJ, Hacker NF, Berek JS. Surgical-pathologic variables predictive of local recurrence in squamous cell carcinoma of the vulva. Gynecol Oncol 1990, **38**: 309–314.

148 Homesley HD. Lymph node findings and outcome in squamous cell carcinoma of the vulva [editorial]. Cancer 1994, **74**: 2399–2402.

149 Homesley HD, Bundy BN, Sedlis A, Yordan E, Berek JS, Jahsan A, Mortel R. Assessment of current International Federation of Gynecology and Obstetrics staging of vulvar carcinoma relative to prognostic factors for survival (a Gynecologic Oncology Group study). Am J Obstet Gynecol 1991, **164**: 997–1003.

150 Homesley HD, Bundy BN, Sedlis A, Yordan E, Berek JS, Jahsan A, Mortel R. Prognostic factors for groin node metastasis in squamous cell carcinoma of the vulva (a Gynecologic Oncology Group study). Gynecol Oncol 1993, **49**: 279–283.

151 Husseinzadeh N, Wesseler T, Schneider D, Schellhas H, Nahhas W. Prognostic factors and the significance of cytologic grading in invasive squamous cell carcinoma of the vulva. A clinicopathologic study. Gynecol Oncol 1990, **36**: 192–199.

152 Husseinzadeh N, Zaino R, Nahhas WA, Mortel R. The significance of histologic findings in predicting nodal metastases in invasive squamous cell carcinoma of the vulva. Gynecol Oncol 1983, **16**: 105–111.

153 Kagie MJ, Kenter GG, Tollenaar RA, Hermans J, Trimbos JB, Fleuren GJ. p53 protein overexpression, a frequent observation in squamous cell carcinoma of the vulva and in various synchronous vulvar epithelia, has no value as a prognostic parameter. Int J Gynecol Pathol 1997, **16**: 124–130.

154 Kojiro S, Growdon WB, Orezzoli JP, Borger S, Rueda BR, Boisvert SL, Iafrate AJ, Oliva E. Expression of p16, p53 and EGFR in squamous cell carcinoma (SCC) of the vulva: a study of 96 cases. Lab Invest 2009, **89**(Suppl 1): 221A.

155 Kunschner A, Kanbour AI, David B. Early vulvar carcinoma. Am J Obstet Gynecol 1978, **132**: 599–606.

156 Paladini D, Cross P, Lopes A, Monaghan JM. Prognostic significance of lymph node variables in squamous cell carcinoma of the vulva. Cancer 1994, **74**: 2491–2496.

157 Perez CA, Grigsby PW, Galakatos A, Swanson R, Camel HM, Kao MS, Lockett MA. Radiation therapy in management of carcinoma of the vulva with emphasis on conservation therapy. Cancer 1993, **71**: 3707–3716.

158 Ross MJ, Ehrmann RL. Histologic prognosticators in stage I squamous cell carcinoma of the vulva. Obstet Gynecol 1987, **70**: 774–784.

159 Woelber L, Mahner S, Voelker K, Eulenburg CZ, Gieseking F, Choschzick M, Jaenicke F, Schwarz J. Clinicopathological prognostic factors and patterns of recurrence in vulvar cancer. Anticancer Res 2009, **29**: 545–552.

MICROINVASIVE CARCINOMA

160 Buckley CH, Butler EB, Fox H. Vulvar intraepithelial neoplasia and microinvasive carcinoma of the vulva. J Clin Pathol 1984, **37**: 1201–1211.

161 Buscerna J, Woodruff JD, Parmley TH, Genadry R. Carcinoma in situ of the vulva. Obstet Gynecol 1980, **55**: 225–230.

162 Dipaola GR, Gomez-Rueda N, Arrighi L. Relevance of microinvasion of carcinoma of the vulva. Obstet Gynecol 1975, **45**: 647–649.

163 Dvoretsky PM, Bonfiglio TA, Helmkamp BF, Ramsey G, Chuang C, Beecham JB. The pathology of superficially invasive, thin vulvar squamous cell carcinoma. Int J Gynecol Pathol 1984, **3**: 331–342.

164 Nakao CY, Nolan JF, DiSaia PJ, Futoran R. Microinvasive epidermoid carcinoma of the vulva with an unexpected natural history. Am J Obstet Gynecol 1974, **120**: 1122–1123.

165 Rush D, Hyjek E, Baergen RN, Ellenson LH, Pirog EC. Detection of microinvasion in vulvar and cervical intraepithelial neoplasia using double immunostaining for cytokeratin and basement membrane components. Arch Pathol Lab Med 2005, **129**: 747–753.

166 Sedlis A, Homesley H, Bundy BN, Marshall R, Yordan E, Hacker N, Lee JH, Whitney C. Positive groin lymph nodes in superficial squamous cell vulvar cancer. A gynecologic oncology group study. Am J Obstet Gynecol 1987, **156**: 1159–1164.

167 Spiegel GW. Eosinophils as a marker for invasion in vulvar squamous neoplastic lesions. Int J Gynecol Pathol 2002, **21**: 108–116.

168 Wharton JT, Gallager S, Rutledge FN. Microinvasive carcinoma of the vulva. Am J Obstet Gynecol 1974, **118**: 159–162.

169 Wilkinson EJ, Rico MJ, Pierson KK. Microinvasive carcinoma of the vulva. Int J Gynecol Pathol 1982, **1**: 29–39.

OTHER MICROSCOPIC TYPES

170 Abell MR. Adenocystic (pseudoadenomatous) basal cell carcinoma of vestibular glands of vulva. Am J Obstet Gynecol 1963, **86**: 470–482.

171 Adam P, Zettl A, Zollner U, Dietl J, Müller-Hermelink HK, Eck M. Metastasizing vulvar carcinosarcoma with squamous carcinomatous and leiomyosarcomatous differentiation: genetic evidence of clonal origin. Hum Pathol 2005, **36**: 1143–1147.

172 Axelsen SM, Stamp IM. Lymphoepithelioma-like carcinoma of the vulvar region. Histopathology 1995, **27**: 281–283.

173 Brisigotti M, Moreno A, Murcia C, Matias-Guiu X, Prat J. Verrucous carcinoma of the vulva. A clinicopathologic and immunohistochemical study of five cases. Int J Gynecol Pathol 1989, **8**: 1–7.

174 Horn LC, Liebert UG, Edelmann J, Höckel M, Einenkel J. Adenoid squamous carcinoma (pseudoangiosarcomatous carcinoma) of the vulva: a rare but highly aggressive variant of squamous cell carcinoma – report of a case and review of the literature. Int J Gynecol Pathol 2008, **27**: 288–291.

175 Japaze H, Van Dinh T, Woodruff JD. Verrucous carcinoma of the vulva. Study of 24 cases. Obstet Gynecol 1982, **60**: 462–466.

176 Kraus FT, Perez-Mesa C. Verrucous carcinoma. Clinical and pathologic study of 105 cases involving oral cavity, larynx and genitalia. Cancer 1966, **19**: 26–38.

177 Kurman RJ, Toki T, Schiffman MH. Basaloid and warty carcinomas of the vulva. Distinctive types of squamous cell carcinoma frequently associated with human papillomaviruses. Am J Surg Pathol 1993, **17**: 133–145.

178 Lasser A, Cornog JL, Morris JM. Adenoid squamous cell carcinoma of the vulva. Cancer 1974, **33**: 224–227.

179 Merino MJ, LiVolsi VA, Schwartz PE, Rudnicki J. Adenoid basal cell carcinoma of the vulva. Int J Gynecol Pathol 1982, **1**: 299–306.

180 Partridge EE, Murad T, Shingleton HM, Austin JM, Hatch KD. Verrucous lesions of the female genitalia. I. Giant condylomata. Am J Obstet Gynecol 1980, **137**: 412–418.

PAGET DISEASE

181 Alguacil-Garcia A, O'Connor R. Mucin-negative biopsy in extra-mammary Paget's disease. A diagnostic problem. Histopathology 1989, **15**: 429–431.

182 Bergen S, Di Saia PJ, Liao SY, Berman ML. Conservative management of extramammary Paget's disease of the vulva. Gynecol Oncol 1989, **33**: 151–156.

183 Brainard J, Hart WR. Proliferative epidermal lesions associated with anogenital Paget's disease. Am J Surg Pathol 2000, **24**: 543–552.

184 Brown HM, Wilkinson EJ. Uroplakin-III to distinguish primary vulvar Paget disease from Paget disease secondary to urothelial carcinoma. Hum Pathol 2002, **33**: 545–548.

185 Crawford D, Nimmo M, Clement PB, Thomson T, Benedet JL, Miller D, Gilks CB. Prognostic factors in Paget's disease of the vulva: a study of 21 cases. Int J Gynecol Pathol 1999, **18**: 351–359.

186 Curtin JP, Rubin SC, Jones WB, Hoskins WJ, Lewis JL Jr. Paget's disease of the vulva. Gynecol Oncol 1990, **39**: 374–377.

187 Diaz de Leon E, Carcangiu ML, Prieto VG, McCue PA, Burchette JL, To G, Norris BA, Kovatich AJ, Sanchez RL, Krigman HR, Gatalica Z. Extramammary Paget's disease is characterized by the consistent lack of estrogen and progesterone receptors but frequently expresses androgen receptor. Am J Clin Pathol 2000, **113**: 572–575.

188 Fenn ME, Morley GW, Abell MR. Paget's disease of vulva. Obstet Gynecol 1971, **38**: 660–670.

189 Fujimoto A, Takata M, Hatta N, Takehara K. Expression of structurally unaltered androgen receptor in extramammary Paget's disease. Lab Invest 2000, **80**: 1465–1471.

190 Goldblum JR, Hart WR. Vulvar Paget's disease: a clinicopathologic and immunohistochemical study of 19 cases. Am J Surg Pathol 1997, **21**: 1178–1187.

191 Guarner J, Cohen C, De Rose PB. Histogenesis of extramammary and mammary Paget cells. An immunohistochemical study. Am J Dermatopathol 1989, **11**: 313–318.

192 Gunn RA, Gallager HS. Vulvar Paget's disease. A topographic study. Cancer 1980, **46**: 590–594.

193 Hart WR, Millman JB. Progression of intraepithelial Paget's disease of the vulva to invasive carcinoma. Cancer 1977, **40**: 2333–2337.

194 Hawley IC, Husain F, Pryse-Davies J. Extramammary Paget's disease of the vulva with dermal invasion and vulval intra-epithelial neoplasia. Histopathology 1991, **18**: 374–376.

195 Helm KF, Goellner JR, Peters MS. Immunohistochemical stains in extramammary Paget's disease. Am J Dermatopathol 1992, **14**: 402–407.

196 Helwig EB, Graham JH. Anogenital (extramammary) Paget's disease. A clinicopathological study. Cancer 1963, **16**: 387–403.

197 Jones RE Jr, Austin C, Ackerman AB. Extramammary Paget's disease. A critical reexamination. Am J Dermatopathol 1979, **1**: 101–132.

198 Keatings L, Sinclair J, Wright C, Corbett IP, Watchorn C, Hennessy C, Angus B, Lennard T, Horne CH. *c-erb*B-2 oncoprotein expression in mammary and extramammary Paget's disease. An immunohistochemical study. Histopathology 1990, **17**: 243–247.

199 Kohler S, Smoller BR. Gross cystic disease fluid protein-15 reactivity in extramammary Paget's disease with and without associated internal malignancy. Am J Dermatopathol 1996, **18**: 118–123.

200 Kondo Y, Kashima K, Daa T, Fujiwara S, Nakayama I, Yokoyama S. The ectopic expression of gastric mucin in extramammary and mammary Paget's disease. Am J Surg Pathol 2002, **26**: 617–623.

201 Kuan SF, Montag AG, Hart J, Krausz T, Recant W. Differential expression of mucin genes in mammary and extramammary Paget's disease. Am J Surg Pathol 2001, **25**: 1469–1477.

202 Lee SC, Roth LM, Ehrlich C, Hall JA. Extramammary Paget's disease of the vulva. A clinicopathologic study of 13 cases. Cancer 1977, **39**: 2540–2549.

203 Liegl B, Leibl S, Gogg-Kamerer M, Tessaro B, Horn LC, Moinfar F. Mammary and extramammary Paget's disease: an immunohistochemical study of 83 cases. Histopathology 2007, **50**: 439–447.

204 Misas JE, Larson JE, Podezaski E, Manetta A, Mortel R. Recurrent Paget disease of the vulva in a split-thickness graft. Obstet Gynecol 1990, **76**: 543–544.

205 Mori O, Hachisuka H, Nakano S, Sasai Y, Shiku H. Expression of *ras* p21 in mammary and extramammary Paget's disease. Arch Pathol Lab Med 1990, **114**: 858–861.

206 Nadji M, Morales AR, Girtanner RE, Ziegels-Weissman J, Penneys NS. Paget's disease of the skin. A unifying concept of histogenesis. Cancer 1982, **50**: 2203–2206.

207 Olson DJ, Fujimura M, Swanson P, Okagaki T. Immunohistochemical features of Paget's disease of the vulva with and without adenocarcinoma. Int J Gynecol Pathol 1991, **10**: 285–295.

208 Perrotto J, Abbott JJ, Ceilley RI, Ahmed I. The role of immunohistochemistry in discriminating primary from secondary extramammary Paget disease. Am J Dermatopathol 2010, **32**: 137–143.

209 Reed W, Oppedal BR, Eeg Larsen T. Immunohistology is valuable in distinguishing between Paget's disease, Bowen's disease and superficial spreading malignant melanoma. Histopathology 1990, **16**: 583–588.

210 Regauer S. Extramammary Paget's disease – a proliferation of adnexal origin? Histopathology 2006, **48**: 723–729.

211 Roth LM, Lee SC, Ehrlich CE. Paget's disease of the vulva. A histogenetic study of five cases including ultrastructural observations and review of the literature. Am J Surg Pathol 1977, **1**: 193–206.

212 Shaco-Levy R, Bean SM, Vollmer RT, Papalas JA, Bentley RC, Selim MA, Robboy SJ. Paget disease of the vulva: a histologic study of 56 cases correlating pathologic features and disease course. Int J Gynecol Pathol 2010, **29**: 69–78.

213 Smith KJ, Tuur S, Corvette D, Lupton BP, Skelton HG. Cytokeratin 7 staining in mammary and extramammary Paget's disease. Mod Pathol 1997, **10**: 1069–1074.

214 Urabe A, Matsukuma A, Shimizu N, Nishimura M, Wada H, Hori Y. Extramammary Paget's disease. Comparative histopathologic studies of intraductal carcinoma of the breast and apocrine adenocarcinoma. J Cutan Pathol 1990, **17**: 257–265.

215 Watanabe S, Ohnishi T, Takahashi H, Ishibashi Y. A comparative study of cytokeratin expression in Paget cells located at various sites. Cancer 1993, **72**: 3323–3330.

216 Wilkinson EJ, Brown HM. Vulvar Paget disease of urothelial origin: a report of three cases and a proposed classification of vulvar Paget disease. Hum Pathol 2002, **33**: 549–554.

217 Willman JH, Golitz LE, Fitzpatrick JE. Vulvar clear cells of Toker: precursors of extramammary Paget's disease. Am J Dermatopathol 2005, **27**: 185–188.

218 Yoshii N, Kitajima S, Yonezawa S, Matsukita S, Setoyama M, Kanzaki T. Expression of mucin core proteins in extramammary Paget's disease. Pathol Int 2002, **52**: 390–399.

219 Zeng HA, Cartun R, Ricci A Jr. Potential diagnostic utility of CDX-2 immunophenotyping in extramammary Paget's disease. Appl Immunohistochem Mol Morphol 2005, **13**: 342–346.

220 Zhang C, Xhang P, Sung J, Lawrence WD. Overexpression of p53 is correlated with stromal invasion in extramammary Paget's disease of the vulva. Hum Pathol 2003, **34**: 880–885.

OTHER EPITHELIAL TUMORS

221 Aguilera-Barrantes I, Magro C, Nuovo GJ. Verruca vulgaris of the vulva in children and adults: a nonvenereal type of vulvar wart. Am J Surg Pathol 2007, **31**: 529–535.

222 Avinoach I, Zirkin HJ, Glezerman M. Proliferating trichilemmal tumor of the vulva. Case report and review of the literature. Int J Gynecol Pathol 1989, **8**: 163–168.

223 Carneiro SJC, Gardner HL, Knox JM. Syringoma. Three cases with vulvar involvement. Obstet Gynecol 1972, **39**: 95–99.

224 Chen KTK. Merkel's cell (neuroendocrine) carcinoma of the vulva. Cancer 1994, **73**: 2186–2191.

225 Chen W, Koenig C. Vulvar keratoacanthoma: a report of two cases. Int J Gynecol Pathol 2004, **23**: 284–286.

226 Chen KT. Pigmented apocrine hamartoma of the vulva: a report of two cases. Int J Gynecol Pathol 2005, **24**: 85–87.

227 Copeland LJ, Cleary K, Sneige N, Edwards CL. Neuroendocrine (Merkel cell) carcinoma of the vulva. A case report and review of the literature. Gynecol Oncol 1985, **22**: 367–378.

228 Cruz-Jimenez PR, Abell MR. Cutaneous basal cell carcinoma of vulva. Cancer 1975, **36**: 1860–1868.

229 Duray PH, Merino MJ, Axiotis C. Warty dyskeratoma of the vulva. Int J Gynecol Pathol 1983, **2**: 286–293.

230 Escalonilla P, Grilli R, Canamero M, Soriano ML, Farina MDC, Manzarbeitia F, Sainz R, Matsukura T, Requena L. Sebaceous carcinoma of the vulva. Am J Dermatopathol 1999, **21**: 468–472.

231 Hinze P, Feyler S, Berndt J, Knolle J, Katenkamp D. Malignant myoepithelioma of the vulva resembling a rhabdoid tumour. Histopathology 1999, **35**: 50–54.

232 Loret de Mola JR, Hudock PA, Steinetz C, Jacobs G, Macfee M, Abdul-Karim FW. Merkel cell carcinoma of the vulva. Gynecol Oncol 1993, **51**: 272–276.

233 Meeker JH, Neubecker RD, Helwig EF. Hidradenoma papilliferum. Am J Clin Pathol 1962, **37**: 182–195.

234 Meenakshi M, McCluggage WG. Myoepithelial neoplasms involving the vulva and vagina: report of 4 cases. Hum Pathol 2009, **40**: 1747–1753.

235 Pantanowitz L, Henneberry JM, Otis CN, Zakhary M. Adenolipoma of the external female genitalia. Int J Gynecol Pathol 2008, **27**: 297–300.

236 Pelosi G, Martignoni G, Bonetti F. Intraductal carcinoma of mammary-type apocrine epithelium arising within a papillary hydradenoma of the vulva. Report of a case and review of the literature. Arch Pathol Lab Med 1991, **115**: 1249–1254.

237 Perrone T, Twiggs LB, Adcock LL, Dehner LP. Vulvar basal cell carcinoma. An infrequently metastasizing neoplasm. Int J Gynecol Pathol 1987, **6**: 152–165.

238 Rahilly MA, Beattie GJ, Lessells AM. Mucinous eccrine carcinoma of the vulva with neuroendocrine differentiation. Histopathology 1995, **27**: 82–86.

239 Regauer S, Nogales FF. Vulvar trichogenic tumors: a comparative study with vulvar basal cell carcinoma. Am J Surg Pathol 2005, **29**: 479–484.

240 Rhatigan RM, Nuss RC. Keratoacanthoma of the vulva. Gynecol Oncol 1985, **21**: 118–123.

241 Rorat E, Wallach RC. Mixed tumors of the vulva. Clinical outcome and pathology. Int J Gynecol Pathol 1984, **3**: 323–328.

242 Roth LM, Look KY. Inverted follicular keratosis of the vulvar skin: a lesion that can be confused with squamous cell carcinoma. Int J Gynecol Pathol 2001, **19**: 369–373.

243 Sington J, Chandrapala R, Manek S, Hollowood K. Mitotic count is not predictive of clinical behavior in hidradenoma papilliferum of the vulva: a clinicopathologic study of 19 cases. Am J Dermatopathol 2006, **28**: 322–326.

244 Wick MR, Goellner JR, Wolfe JT III, Su WPD. Vulvar sweat gland carcinomas. Arch Pathol Lab Med 1985, **109**: 43–47.

245 Woodworth H Jr, Dockerty MB, Wilson RB, Pratt JH. Papillary hidradenoma of the vulva. A clinicopathologic study of 69 cases. Am J Obstet Gynecol 1971, **110**: 501–508.

246 Young S, Leon M, Talerman A, Teresi M, Emmadi R. Polymorphous low-grade adenocarcinoma of the vulva and vagina: a tumor resembling adenoid cystic carcinoma. Int J Surg Pathol 2003, **11**: 43–49.

MELANOCYTIC TUMORS

247 Bradgate MG, Rollason TP, McConkey CC, Powell J. Malignant melanoma of the vulva. A clinicopathological study of 50 women. Br J Obstet Gynaecol 1990, **97**: 124–133.

248 Christensen WN, Friedman KJ, Woodruff JD, Hood AF. Histologic characteristics of vulvar nevocellular nevi. J Cutan Pathol 1987, **14**: 87–91.

249 Clark WH Jr, Hood AF, Tucker MA, Jampel RM. Atypical melanocytic nevi of the genital type with a discussion of reciprocal parenchymal–stromal interactions in the biology of neoplasia. Hum Pathol 1998, **29**: S1–S24.

250 Dunton CJ, Kautzky M, Hanau C. Malignant melanoma of the vulva: a review. Obstet Gynecol Surv 1995, **50**: 739–746.

251 Gleason BC, Hirsch MS, Nucci MR, Schmidt BA, Zembowicz A, Mihm MC Jr, McKee PH, Brenn T. Atypical genital nevi. A clinicopathologic analysis of 56 cases. Am J Surg Pathol 2008, **32**: 51–57.

252 Hill SJ, Berkowitz R, Granter SR, Hirsch MS. Pagetoid lesions of the vulva: a collision between malignant melanoma and extramammary Paget disease. Int J Gynecol Pathol 2008, **27**: 292–296.

253 Irvin WP Jr, Legallo RL, Stoler MH, Rice LW, Taylor PT Jr, Anderson WA. Vulvar melanoma: a retrospective analysis and literature review. Gynecol Oncol 2001, **83**: 457–465.

254 Jaramillo BA, Ganjei P, Averette HE, Sevin B-U, Lovecchio JL. Malignant melanoma of the vulva. Obstet Gynecol 1985, **66**: 398–401.

255 Johnson TL, Kumar NB, White CD, Morley GW. Prognostic features of vulvar melanoma. A clinicopathologic analysis. Int J Gynecol Pathol 1986, **5**: 110–118.

256 Look KY, Roth LM, Sutton GP. Vulvar melanoma reconsidered. Cancer 1993, **72**: 143–146.

257 Panizzon RG. Vulvar melanoma. Semin Dermatol 1996, **15**: 67–70.

258 Podratz KC, Symmonds RE, Taylor WF, Williams TJ. Carcinoma of the vulva. Analysis of treatment and survival. Obstet Gynecol 1983, **61**: 63–74.

259 Raber G, Mempel V, Jackisch C, Hudeiker M, Heinecke A, Kurzl R, Glaubita M, Rompel R, Schneider HP. Malignant melanoma of the vulva: report of 89 patients. Cancer 1996, **78**: 2353–2358.

260 Ragnarsson-Olding B, Johansson H, Rutqvist LE, Ringborg U. Malignant melanoma of the vulva and vagina. Trends in incidence, age distribution, and long-term survival among 245 consecutive cases in Sweden 1960–1984. Cancer 1993, **71**: 1893–1897.

261 Ragnarsson-Olding BK, Kanter-Lewensohn LR, Lagerlof B, Nilsson BR, Ringborg UK. Malignant melanoma of the vulva in a nationwide, 25-year study of 219 Swedish females: clinical observations and histopathologic features. Cancer 1999, **86**: 1273–1284.

262 Ragnarsson-Olding BK, Nilsson BR, Kanter-Lewensohn LR, Lagerlof B, Ringborg UK. Malignant melanoma of the vulva in a nationwide, 25-year study of 219 Swedish females: predictors of survival. Cancer 1999, **86**: 1285–1293.

263 Rock B. Pigmented lesions of the vulva. Dermatol Clin 1992, **10**: 361–370.

264 Rohwedder A, Slominski A, Wolff M, Kredentser D, Carlson JA. Epidermodysplasia verruciformis and cutaneous human papillomavirus DNA, but not genital human papillomavirus DNAs, are frequently detected in vulvar and vaginal melanoma. Am J Dermatopathol 2007, **29**: 13–17.

265 Ronan SG, Eng AM, Briele HA, Walker MJ, Das Gupta TK. Malignant melanoma of the female genitalia. J Am Acad Dermatol 1990, **22**: 428–435.

266 Scheistroen M, Trope C, Koern J, Pettersen EO, Abeler VM, Kristensen GB. Malignant melanoma of the vulva. Evaluation of prognostic factors with emphasis on DNA ploidy in 75 patients. Cancer 1995, **75**: 72–80.

267 Spatz A, Zimmermann U, Bachollet B, Pautier P, Michel G, Duvillard P. Malignant blue nevus of the vulva with late ovarian metastasis. Am J Dermatopathol 1998, **20**: 408–412.

268 Tasseron EW, van der Esch EP, Hart AA, Brutel de la Riviere G, Aartsen EJ. A clinicopathological study of 30 melanomas of the vulva. Gynecol Oncol 1992, **46**: 170–175.

AGRESSIVE ANGIOMYXOMA AND RELATED LESIONS

269 Alameda F, Munné A, Baró T, Iglesias M, Condom E, Lloreta-Trull J, Serrano S. Vulvar angiomyxoma, aggressive angiomyxoma, and angiomyofibroblastoma: an immunohistochemical and ultrastructural study. Ultrastruct Pathol 2006, **30**: 193–205.

270 Bégin LR, Clement PB, Kirk ME, Jothy S, McCaughey WTE, Ferenczy A. Aggressive angiomyxoma of pelvic soft parts. A clinicopathologic study of nine cases. Hum Pathol 1985, **16**: 621–628.

271 Blandamura S, Cruz J, Vergara LF, Puerto IM, Ninfo V. Aggressive angiomyxoma: a second case of metastasis with patient's death. Hum Pathol 2003, **34**: 1072–1074.

272 Cao D, Srodon M, Montgomery EA, Kurman RJ. Lipomatous variant of angiomyofibroblastoma: report of two cases and review of the literature. Int J Gynecol Pathol 2005, **24**: 196–200.

273 Fetsch JF, Laskin WB, Lefkowitz M, Kindblom LG, Meis-Kindblom JM. Aggressive angiomyxoma: a clinicopathologic study of 29 female patients. Cancer 1996, **78**: 79–90.

274 Fetsch JF, Laskin WB, Tavassoli FA. Superficial angiomyxoma (cutaneous myxoma): a clinicopathologic study of 17 cases arising in the genital region. Int J Gynecol Pathol 1998, **16**: 325–334.

275 Fletcher CD, Tsang WY, Fisher C, Lee KC, Chan JK. Angiomyofibroblastoma of the vulva. A benign neoplasm distinct from aggressive angiomyxoma. Am J Surg Pathol 1992, **16**: 373–382.

276 Fukunaga M, Nomura K, Matsumoto K, Doi K, Endo Y, Ushigome S. Vulval angiomyofibroblastoma. Clinicopathologic analysis of six cases. Am J Clin Pathol 1997, **107**: 45–51.

277 Ganesan R, McCluggage WG, Hirschowitz L, Rollason TP. Superficial myofibroblastoma of the lower female genital tract: report of a series including tumours with a vulval location. Histopathology 2005, **46**: 137–143.

278 Granter SR, Nucci MR, Fletcher CD. Aggressive angiomyxoma: reappraisal of its relationship to angiomyofibroblastoma in a series of 16 cases. Histopathology 1997, **30**: 3–10.

279 Hisaoka M, Kouho H, Aoki T, Daimaru Y, Hashimoto H. Angiomyofibroblastoma of the vulva. A clinicopathologic study of seven cases. Pathol Int 1995, **45**: 487–492.

280 Iezzoni JC, Fechner RE, Wong LS, Rosai J. Aggressive angiomyxoma in males. A report of four cases. Am J Clin Pathol 1995, **104**: 391–396.

281 Iwasa Y, Fletcher CD. Cellular angiofibroma: clinicopathologic and immunohistochemical analysis of 51 cases. Am J Surg Pathol 2004, **28**: 1426–1435.

282 Kazmierczak B, Wanschura S, Meyer-Bolte K, Caselitz J, Meister P, Bartnitzke S, Van de Ven W, Bullerdiek J. Cytogenetic and molecular analysis of an aggressive angiomyxoma. Am J Pathol 1995, **147**: 580–585.

283 Laskin WB, Fetsch JF, Tavassoli FA. Angiomyofibroblastoma of the female genital tract: analysis of 17 cases including a lipomatous variant. Hum Pathol 1997, **28**: 1046–1055.

284 Martinez MA, Ballestin C, Carabias E, Lois CG. Aggressive angiomyxoma: an ultrastructural study of four cases. Ultrastruct Pathol 2003, **27**: 227–233.

285 McCluggage WG, Ganesan R, Hirschowitz L, Rollason TP. Cellular angiofibroma and related fibromatous lesions of the vulva: report of a series of cases with a morphological spectrum wider than previously described. Histopathology 2004, **45**: 360–368.

286 McCluggage WG. Recent developments in vulvovaginal pathology. Histopathology 2009, **54**: 156–173.

287 Micci F, Panagopoulos I, Bjerkehagen B, Heim S. Deregulation of HMGA2 in an aggressive angiomyxoma with t(11;12)(q23;q15). Virchows Arch 2006, **448**: 838–842.

288 Nielsen GP, Rosenberg AE, Young RH, Dickersin GR, Clement PB, Scully RE. Angiomyofibroblastoma of the vulva and vagina. Mod Pathol 1996, **9**: 284–291.

289 Nielsen GP, Young RH, Dickersin GR, Rosenberg AE. Angiomyofibroblastoma of the vulva with sarcomatous transformation ('angiomyofibrosarcoma'). Am J Surg Pathol 1997, **21**: 1104–1108.

290 Nucci MR, Granter SR, Fletcher CD. Cellular angiofibroma: a benign neoplasm distinct from angiomyofibroblastoma and spindle cell lipoma. Am J Surg Pathol 1997, **21**: 636–644.

291 Ockner DM, Sayadi H, Swanson PE, Ritter JH, Wick MR. Genital angiomyofibroblastoma. Comparison with aggressive angiomyxoma and other myxoid neoplasms of skin and soft tissue. Am J Clin Pathol 1997, **107**: 36–44.

292 Rabban JT, Dal Cin P, Oliva E. HMGA2 rearrangement in a case of vulvar aggressive angiomyxoma. Int J Gynecol Pathol 2006, **25**: 403–407.

293 Rotmensch EJ, Kasznica J, Hamid MA. Immunohistochemical analysis of hormone receptors and proliferating cell nuclear antigen in aggressive angiomyxoma of the vulva. Int J Gynaecol Obstet 1993, **41**: 171–179.

294 Siassi R, Papadopoulos T, Matzel KE. Metastasizing aggressive angiomyxoma [letter to the editor]. N Engl J Med 1999, **341**: 1772.

295 Skalova A, Michal M, Husek K, Zamecnik M, Leivo I. Aggressive angiomyxoma of the pelvioperineal region. Immunohistological and ultrastructural study of seven cases. Am J Dermatopathol 1993, **15**: 446–451.

296 Steeper TA, Rosai J. Aggressive angiomyxoma of the female pelvis and perineum. Report of nine cases of a distinctive type of gynecologic soft tissue neoplasm. Am J Surg Pathol 1983, **7**: 463–475.

297 Tsuji T, Yoshinaga M, Inomoto Y, Taguchi S, Douchi T. Aggressive angiomyxoma of the vulva with a sole t(5;8)(p15;q22) chromosome change. Int J Gynecol Pathol 2007, **26**: 494–496.

298 van Roggen JF, van Unnik JA, Briaire-de Bruijn IH, Hogendoorn PC. Aggressive angiomyxoma: a clinicopathological and immunohistochemical study of 11 cases with long-term follow-up. Virchows Arch 2005, **446**: 157–163.

299 Vasquez MD, Ro JY, Park YW, Tornos CS, Ordonez NG, Ayala AG. Angiomyofibroblastoma: a clinicopathologic study of eight cases and review of the literature. Int J Surg Pathol 1999, **7**: 161–170.

300 White J, Chan YF. Aggressive angiomyxoma of the vulva in an 11-year-old girl. Pediatr Pathol 1994, **14**: 27–37.

OTHER TUMORS AND TUMORLIKE CONDITIONS

301 Abdul-Karim FW, Cohen RE. Atypical stromal cells of lower female genital tract. Histopathology 1990, **17**: 249–253.

302 Allen MV, Novotny DB. Desmoid tumor of the vulva associated with pregnancy. Arch Pathol Lab Med 1997, **121**: 512–514.

303 Axiotis CA, Merino MJ, Duray PH. Langerhans cell histiocytosis of the female genital tract. Cancer 1991, **67**: 1650–1660.

304 Barnhill DR, Boling R, Nobles W, Crooks L, Burke T. Vulvar dermatofibrosarcoma protuberans. Gynecol Oncol 1988, **30**: 149–152.

305 Bell D, Kane PB, Liang S, Conway C, Tornos C. Vulvar varices: an uncommon entity in surgical pathology. Int J Gynecol Pathol 2007, **26**: 99–101.

306 Blandamura S, Florea G, Brotto M, Salmaso R, Castellan L. Periurethral glomangiomyoma in women: case report and review of the literature [letter]. Histopathology 2000, **36**: 571–572.

307 Bock JE, Andreasson B, Thorn A, Holck S. Dermatofibrosarcoma protuberans of the vulva. Gynecol Oncol 1985, **20**: 129–135.

308 Colgan TJ, Dardick I, O'Connell G. Paraganglioma of the vulva. Int J Gynecol Pathol 1991, **10**: 203–208.

309 Dehner LP. Metastatic and secondary tumors of the vulva. Obstet Gynecol 1973, **42**: 47–57.

310 Dudley AG, Young RH, Lawrence WD, Scully RE. Endodermal sinus tumor of the vulva in an infant. Obstet Gynecol 1983, **61**: 76S–78S.

311 Edelweiss M, Malpica A. Dermatofibrosarcoma protuberans of the vulva: a clinicopathologic and immunohistochemical study of 13 cases. Am J Surg Pathol 2010, **34**: 393–400.

312 Elliott GB, Elliott JDA. Superficial stromal reactions of lower genital tract. Arch Pathol 1973, **95**: 100–101.

313 Fernández-Aguilar S, Fayt I, Noël JC. Spindle cell vulvar hemangiomatosis associated with enchondromatosis: a rare variant of Maffucci's syndrome. Int J Gynecol Pathol 2004, **23**: 68–70.

314 Gersell DJ, Fulling KH. Localized neurofibromatosis of the female genitourinary tract. Am J Surg Pathol 1989, **13**: 873–878.

315 Ghorbani RP, Malpica A, Ayala AG. Dermatofibrosarcoma protuberans of the vulva: clinicopathologic and immununohistochemical analysis of four cases, one with fibrosarcomatous change, and review of the literature. Int J Gynecol Pathol 1999, **18**: 366–373.

316 Guirguis A, Kanbour-Shakir A, Kelley J. Epithelioid angiosarcoma of the mons after chemoradiation for vulvar cancer. Int J Gynecol Pathol 2007, **26**: 265–268.

317 Hays DM, Raney RB Jr, Lawrence W Jr, Gehan EA, Soule EH, Tefft M, Maurer HM. Rhabdomyosarcoma of the female urogenital tract. J Pediatr Surg 1981, **16**: 828–834.

318 Hays DM, Shimada H, Raney RB Jr, Tefft M, Newton W, Crist WM, Lawrence W Jr, Ragab A, Beltangady M, Maurer HM. Clinical staging and treatment results in rhabdomyosarcoma of the female genital tract among children and adolescents. Cancer 1988, **61**: 1893–1903.

319 Hood AF, Lumadue J. Benign vulvar tumors. Dermatol Clin 1992, **10**: 371–385.

320 Huang HJ, Yamabe T, Tagawa H. A solitary neurilemmoma of the clitoris. Gynecol Oncol 1983, **15**: 103–110.

321 Iwasa Y, Fletcher CD. Distinctive prepubertal vulval fibroma: a hitherto unrecognized mesenchymal tumor of prepubertal girls: analysis of 11 cases. Am J Surg Pathol 2004, **28**: 1601–1608.

322 Kaplan MA, Jacobson JO, Ferry JA, Harris NL. T-cell lymphoma of the vulva in a renal allograft recipient with associated hemophagocytosis. Am J Surg Pathol 1993, **17**: 842–849.

323 Katz VL, Askin FB, Bosch BD. Glomus tumor of the vulva. A case report. Obstet Gynecol 1986, **67**: 43S–45S.

324 Kempson RL, Sherman AI. Sclerosing lipogranuloma of the vulva. Report of a case. Obstet Gynecol 1968, **101**: 854–856.

325 Kernen JA, Morgan ML. Benign lymphoid hamartoma of the vulva. Report of a case. Obstet Gynecol 1970, **35**: 290–292.

326 Lae ME, Pereira PF, Keeney GL, Nascimento AG. Lipoblastoma-like tumour of the vulva: report of three cases of a distinctive mesenchymal neoplasm of adipocytic differentiation. Histopathology 2002, **40**: 505–509.

327 Manson CM, Hirsch PJ, Coyne JD. Post-operative spindle cell nodule of the vulva. Histopathology 1995, **26**: 571–574.

328 Matias C, Nunes JF, Vicente LF, Almeida MO. Primary malignant rhabdoid tumour of the vulva. Histopathology 1990, **17**: 576–578.

329 Mazur MT, Hsueh S, Gersell DJ. Metastases to the female genital tract. Analysis of 325 cases. Cancer 1984, **53**: 1978–1984.

330 McCluggage WG, Nielsen GP, Young RH. Massive vulval edema secondary to obesity and immobilization: a potential mimic of aggressive angiomyxoma. Int J Gynecol Pathol 2008, **27**: 447–452.

331 McNeely TB. Angiokeratoma of the clitoris. Arch Pathol Lab Med 1992, **116**: 880–881.

332 Meehan SA, Smoller BR. Cutaneous Langerhans cell histiocytosis of the genitalia in the elderly: a report of three cases. J Cutan Pathol 1998, **25**: 370–374.

333 Mu XC, Tran TA, Dupree M, Carslon JA. Acquired vulvar lymphangioma mimicking genital warts. A case report and review of the literature. J Cutan Pathol 1999, **26**: 150–154.

334 Mucitelli DR, Charles EZ, Kraus FT. Vulvovaginal polyps. Histologic appearance, ultrastructure, immunocytochemical characteristics, and clinicopathologic correlations. Int J Gynecol Pathol 1990, **9**: 20–40.

335 Nemoto T, Shinoda M, Komatsuzaki K, Hara T, Kojima M, Ogihara T. Myxoid leiomyoma of the vulva mimicking aggressive angiomyxoma. Pathol Int 1994, **44**: 454–459.

336 Neto AG, Deavers MT, Silva EG, Malpica A. Metastatic tumors of the vulva. A clinicopathologic study of 66 cases. Am J Surg Pathol 2003, **27**: 799–804.

337 Newman PL, Fletcher CD. Smooth muscle tumours of the external genitalia. Clinicopathological analysis of a series. Histopathology 1991, **18**: 523–529.

338 Nielsen GP, Young RH. Fibromatosis of soft tissue type involving the female genital tract: a report of two cases. Int J Gynecol Pathol 1998, **16**: 383–386.

339 Nielsen GP, Young RH. Mesenchymal tumors and tumor-like lesions of the female genital tract: a selective review with emphasis on recently described entities. Int J Gynecol Pathol 2001, **20**: 105–127.

340 Nielsen GP, Rosenberg AE, Koerner FC, Young RH, Scully RE. Smooth-muscle tumors of the vulva: a clinicopathological study of 25 cases and review of the literature. Am J Surg Pathol 1996, **20**: 779–793.

341 Nielsen GP, Shaw PA, Rosenberg AE, Dickersin GR, Young RH, Scully RE. Synovial sarcoma of the vulva: a report of two cases. Mod Pathol 1997, **9**: 970–974.

342 Nirenberg A, Ostor AG, Slavin J, Riley CB, Rome RM. Primary vulvar sarcomas. Int J Gynecol Pathol 1995, **14**: 55–62.

343 Nucci MR, Young RH, Fletcher CD. Cellular pseudosarcomatous fibroepithelial stromal polyps of the lower female genital tract: an underrecognized lesion often misdiagnosed as sarcoma. Am J Surg Pathol 2000, **24**: 231–240.

344 Nucci MR, Fletcher CD. Liposarcoma (atypical lipomatous tumors) of the vulva: a clinicopathologic study of six cases. Int J Gynecol Pathol 1998, **17**: 17–23.

345 Nucci MR, Fletcher CD. Vulvovaginal soft tissue tumors: update and review. Histopathology 2000, **36**: 97–108.

346 O'Connell JX, Young RH, Nielsen GP, Rosenberg AE, Bainbridge TC, Clement PB. Nodular fasciitis of the vulva: study of six cases and literature review. Int J Gynecol Pathol 1997, **16**: 117–123.

347 Ostor AG, Fortune DW, Riley CB. Fibroepithelial polyps with atypical stromal cells (pseudosarcoma botryoides) of vulva and vagina. A report of 13 cases. Int J Gynecol Pathol 1988, **7**: 351–360.

348 Padula A, Medeiros LJ, Silva EG, Deavers MT. Isolated vulvar Langerhans cell histiocytosis: report of two cases. Int J Gynecol Pathol 2004, **23**: 278–283.

349 Papalas JA, Shaco-Levy R, Robboy SJ, Selim MA. Isolated and synchronous vulvar granular cell tumors: a clinicopathologic study of 17 cases in 13 patients. Int J Gynecol Pathol 2010, **29**: 173–180.

350 Perrone T, Swanson PE, Twiggs L, Ulbright TM, Dehner LP. Malignant rhabdoid tumor of the vulva. Is distinction from epithelioid sarcoma possible? A pathologic and immunohistochemical study. Am J Surg Pathol 1989, **13**: 848–858.

351 Robertson AJ, McIntosh W, Lamont P, Guthrie W. Malignant granular cell tumour (myoblastoma) of the vulva. Report of a case and review of the literature. Histopathology 1981, **5**: 69–79.

352 Santa Cruz J, Martin SA. Verruciform xanthoma of the vulva. Am J Clin Pathol 1979, **71**: 224–228.

353 Shen J-T, D'Ablaing G, Morro CP. Alveolar soft part sarcoma of the vulva. Report of first case and review of literature. Gynecol Oncol 1982, **13**: 120–128.

354 Sonobe H, Ro JY, Ramos M, Diaz I, Mackay B, Ordóñez NG, Ayala AG. Glomus tumor of the female external genitalia. A report of two cases. Int J Gynecol Pathol 1994, **13**: 359–364.

355 Strayer SA, Yum MN, Sutton GP. Epithelioid hemangioendothelioma of the clitoris. A case report with immunohistochemical and ultrastructural findings. Int J Gynecol Pathol 1992, **11**: 234–239.

356 Tavassoli FA, Norris HJ. Smooth muscle tumors of the vulva. Obstet Gynecol 1979, **53**: 213–217.

357 Taylor RN, Bottles K, Miller TR, Braga CA. Malignant fibrous histiocytoma of the vulva. Obstet Gynecol 1985, **66**: 145–148.

358 Terada KY, Schmidt RW, Roberts JA. Malignant schwannoma of the vulva. A case report. J Reprod Med 1988, **33**: 969–972.

359 Thomas WJ, Bevan HE, Hooper DG, Downey EJ. Malignant schwannoma of the clitoris in a 1-year-old child. Cancer 1989, **63**: 2216–2219.

360 Ulbright TM, Brokaw SA, Stehman FB, Roth LM. Epithelioid sarcoma of the vulva. Evidence suggesting a more aggressive behavior than extra-genital epithelioid sarcoma. Cancer 1983, **52**: 1462–1469.

361 Vang R, Medeiros LJ, Malpica A, Levenback C, Deavers M. Non-Hodgkin's lymphoma involving the vulva. Int J Gynecol Pathol 2000, **19**: 236–242.

362 Vang R, Connelly JH, Hammill HA, Shannon RL. Vulvar hypertrophy with lymphedema: a mimicker of aggressive angiomyxoma. Arch Pathol Lab Med 2000, **124**: 1697–1699.

363 Vang R, Taubenberger JK, Mannion CM, Bijwaard K, Malpica A, Ordonez NG, Tavassoli FA, Silver SA. Primary vulvar and vaginal extraosseous Ewing's sarcoma/peripheral neuroectodermal tumor: diagnostic confirmation with CD99 immunostaining and reverse transcriptase-polymerase chain reaction. Int J Gynecol Pathol 2000, **19**: 103–109.

364 Vargas SO, Kozakewich HP, Boyd TK, Ecklund K, Fishman SJ, Laufer MR, Perez-Atayde AR. Childhood asymmetric labium majus enlargement: mimicking a neoplasm. Am J Surg Pathol 2005, **29**: 1007–1016.

365 Weissmann D, Amenta PS, Kantor GR. Vulvar epithelioid sarcoma metastatic to the scalp. A case report and review of the literature. Am J Dermatopathol 1990, **12**: 462–468.

366 White BE, Kaplan A, Lopez-Terrada DH, Ro JY, Benjamin RS, Ayala AG. Monophasic synovial sarcoma arising in the vulva: a case report and review of the literature. Arch Pathol Lab Med 2008, **132**: 698–702.

367 Wolber RA, Talerman A, Wilkinson EJ, Clement PB. Vulvar granular cell tumors with pseudocarcinomatous hyperplasia. A comparative analysis with well-differentiated squamous carcinoma. Int J Gynecol Pathol 1991, **10**: 59–66.

LESIONS OF BARTHOLIN GLANDS AND RELATED STRUCTURES

368 Andersen G, Christensen S, Detlefsen GU, Kern-Hansen P. Treatment of Bartholin's abscess. Marsupialization versus incision, curettage and suture under antibiotic cover. A randomized trial with a 6-months follow-up. Acta Obstet Gynecol Scand 1992, **71**: 59–62.

369 Axe S, Parmley T, Woodruff JD, Hlopak B. Adenomas in minor vestibular glands. Obstet Gynecol 1986, **68**: 16–18.

370 Balat O, Edwards CL, Delclos L. Advanced primary carcinoma of the Bartholin gland: report of 18 patients. Eur J Gynecol Oncol 2001, **22**: 46–49.

371 Cardosi RJ, Speights A, Fiorica JV, Grendys EC Jr, Hakam A, Hoffman MS. Bartholin's gland carcinoma: a 15-year experience. Gynecol Oncol 2001, **82**: 247–251.

372 Chapman GW Jr, Hassan N, Page D, Mostoufi-Zadeh M, Leyman D. Mucinous cystadenoma of Bartholin's gland. A case report. J Reprod Med 1987, **32**: 939–941.

373 Copeland LJ, Sneige N, Gershenson DM, McGuffee VB, Abdul-Karim F, Rutledge FN. Bartholin gland carcinoma. Obstet Gynecol 1986, **67**: 794–801.

374 Copeland LJ, Sneige N, Gershenson DM, Saul PB, Stringer CA, Seski JC. Adenoid cystic carcinoma of Bartholin gland. Obstet Gynecol 1986, **67**: 115–120.

375 Enghardt MH, Valente PT, Day DH. Papilloma of Bartholin's gland duct cyst. First report of a case. Int J Gynecol Pathol 1993, **12**: 86–92.

376 Felix A, Nunes JF, Soares J. Salivary gland-type basal cell adenocarcinoma of presumed Bartholin's gland origin: a case report. Int J Gynecol Pathol 2002, **21**: 194–197.

377 Felix JC, Cote RJ, Kramer EE, Saigo P, Goldman GH. Carcinomas of Bartholin's gland. Histogenesis and the etiological role of human papillomavirus. Am J Pathol 1993, **142**: 925–933.

378 Freedman SR, Goldman RL. Mucocele-like changes in Bartholin's glands. Hum Pathol 1978, **9**: 111–114.

379 Friedrich EG Jr, Wilkinson EJ. Mucous cysts of the vulvar vestibule. Obstet Gynecol 1973, **42**: 407–414.

380 Jones MA, Mann EW, Caldwell CL, Tarraza HM, Dickersin GR, Young RH. Small cell neuroendocrine carcinoma of Bartholin's gland. Am J Clin Pathol 1990, **94**: 439–442.

381 Koenig C, Tavassoli FA. Nodular hyperplasia, adenoma, and adenomyoma of Bartholin's gland. Int J Gynecol Pathol 1998, **17**: 289–294.

382 Leuchter RS, Hacker NF, Voet RL, Berek JS, Townsend DE, Lagasse LD. Primary carcinoma of the Bartholin gland. A report of 14 cases and review of the literature. Obstet Gynecol 1982, **60**: 361–368.

383 McCluggage WG, Aydin NE, Wong NA, Cooper K. Low-grade epithelial–myoepithelial carcinoma of Bartholin gland: report of 2 cases of a distinctive neoplasm arising in the vulvovaginal region. Int J Gynecol Pathol 2009, **28**: 286–291.

384 Milchgrub S, Wiley EL, Vuitch F, Albores-Saavedra J. The tubular variant of adenoid cystic carcinoma of the Bartholin's gland. Am J Clin Pathol 1994, **101**: 204–208.

385 Mossler JA, Woodard BH, Addison A, McArty KS. Adenocarcinoma of Bartholin's gland. Arch Pathol Lab Med 1980, **104**: 523–526.

386 Paquin ML, Davis JR, Weiner S. Malacoplakia of Bartholin's gland. Arch Pathol Lab Med 1986, **110**: 757–758.

387 Rorat E, Ferenczy A, Richart RM. Human Bartholin gland, duct and duct cyst. Histochemical and ultrastructural study. Arch Pathol 1975, **99**: 367–374.

388 Rosenberg P, Simonsen E, Risberg B. Adenoid cystic carcinoma of Bartholin's gland. A report of five new cases treated with surgery and radiotherapy. Gynecol Oncol 1989, **34**: 145–147.

389 Scinicariello F, Rady P, Hannigan E, Dinh TV, Tyring SK. Human papillomavirus type 16 found in primary transitional cell carcinoma of the Bartholin's gland and in a lymph node metastasis. Gynecol Oncol 1992, **47**: 263–266.

390 Wheelock JB, Goplerud DR, Dunn LJ, Oates JF III. Primary carcinoma of the Bartholin gland. A report of ten cases. Obstet Gynecol 1984, **63**: 820–824.

391 Wilkinson EJ. Pathology of the vulva and vagina. In Wilkerson EJ (ed.): Contemporary issues in surgical pathology, **vol. 9**. New York, 1986, Churchill Livingstone.

LESIONS OF THE FEMALE URETHRA

392 Amin MB, Young RH. Primary carcinomas of the urethra. Semin Diagn Pathol 1997, **14**: 147–160.

393 Baxendine-Jones JA, Wedderburn AW, Smart CJ, Theaker JM. Primary adenocarcinoma of the female urethra associated with adenomatous hyperplasia of the periurethral glands. J Urol Pathol 1998, **9**: 233–239.

394 Benson RC, Tunca JC, Buchler DA, Uehling DT. Primary carcinoma of the female urethra. Gynecol Oncol 1982, **14**: 313–318.

395 Capraro VJ, Bayonet-Rivera NP, Magoss I. Vulvar tumor in children due to prolapse of urethral mucosa. Am J Obstet Gynecol 1970, **108**: 572–575.

396 Clayton M, Siami P, Guinan P. Urethral diverticular carcinoma. Cancer 1992, **70**: 665–670.

397 Evans KJ, McCarthy MP, Sands JP. Adenocarcinoma of a female urethral diverticulum. Case report and review of the literature. J Urol 1981, **126**: 124–126.

398 Furusato M, Takaki K, Joh K, Suzuki M, Chiba S, Nakata Y, Kakimoto S, Aizawa S, Ishikawa E. Nephrogenic adenoma in female urethra. Acta Pathol Jpn 1983, **33**: 1009–1015.

399 Garden AS, Zagars GK, Delclos L. Primary carcinoma of the female urethra. Results of radiation therapy. Cancer 1993, **71**: 3102–3108.

400 Grigsby PW, Corn BW. Localized urethral tumors in women. Indications for conservative versus exenterative therapies. J Urol 1992, **147**: 1516–1520.

401 Jarvi OH, Marin S, de Boer WGRM. Further studies of intestinal heterotopia in urethral caruncle. Acta Pathol Microbiol Immunol Scand (A) 1984, **92**: 469–474.

402 Johnson DE, O'Connell JR. Primary carcinoma of female urethra. Urology 1983, **21**: 42–44.

403 Kim CJ, Pak K, Hamaguchi A, Ishida A, Arai Y, Konishi T, Okada Y, Tomoyoshi T. Primary malignant melanoma of the female urethra. Cancer 1993, **71**: 448–451.

404 Mayer R, Fowler JE Jr, Clayton M. Localized urethral cancer in women. Cancer 1987, **60**: 1548–1551.

405 Meis JM, Ayala AG, Johnson DE. Adenocarcinoma of the urethra in women. A clinicopathologic study. Cancer 1987, **60**: 1038–1052.

406 Morgan DR, Dixon MF, Harnden P. Villous adenoma of urethra associated with tubulovillous adenoma and adenocarcinoma of rectum. Histopathology 1998, **32**: 87–89.

407 Mostofi FK, David CJ Jr, Sesterhenn IA. Carcinoma of the male and female urethra. Urol Clin North Am 1992, **19**: 347–358.

408 Narayan P, Konety B. Surgical treatment of female urethral carcinoma. Urol Clin North Am 1992, **19**: 373–382.

409 Odze R, Begin LR. Tubular adenomatous metaplasia (nephrogenic adenoma) of the female urethra. Int J Gynecol Pathol 1989, **8**: 374–380.

410 Ohsawa M, Mishima K, Suzuki A, Hagino K, Doi J, Aozasa K. Malignant lymphoma of the urethra. Report of a case with detection of Epstein–Barr virus genome in the tumor cells. Histopathology 1994, **24**: 525–529.

411 Oliva E, Quinn TR, Amin MB, Eble JN, Epstein JI, Srigley JR, Young RH. Primary malignant melanoma of the urethra: a clinicopathologic analysis of 15 cases. Am J Surg Pathol 2000, **24**: 785–796.

412 Oliva E, Young RH. Clear cell adenocarcinoma of the urethra: a clinicopathologic analysis of 19 cases. Mod Pathol 1997, **9**: 513–520.

413 Prempee T, Amornmarn R, Patanaphan V. Radiation therapy in primary carcinoma of the female urethra. Part II. An update on results. Cancer 1984, **54**: 729–733.

414 Rogers RE, Burns B. Carcinoma of the female urethra. Obstet Gynecol 1969, **33**: 54–57.

415 Saad AG, Kaouk JH, Kaspar HG, Khauli RB. Leiomyoma of the urethra: report of three cases of a rare entity. Int J Surg Pathol 2003, **11**: 123–126.

416 Suzuki K, Morita T, Tokue A. Primary signet ring cell carcinoma of female urethra. Int J Urol 2001, **8**: 509–512.

417 Wegnaupt K, Gerstner GJ, Kucera H. Radiation therapy for primary carcinoma of the female urethra. A survey over 25 years. Gynecol Oncol 1984, **17**: 58–63.

418 Wiener JS, Walther PJ. A high association of oncogenic human papillomaviruses with carcinomas of the female urethra. Polymerase chain reaction-based analysis of multiple histological types. J Urol 1994, **151**: 49–53.

419 Young RH, Scully RE. Clear cell adenocarcinoma of the bladder and urethra. A report of three cases and review of the literature. Am J Surg Pathol 1985, **9**: 816–826.

420 Young RH, Oliva E, Saenz Garcia JA, Bhan AK, Clement PB. Urethral caruncle with atypical stromal cells simulating lymphoma or sarcoma – a distinctive pseudoneoplastic lesion of females: a report of six cases. Am J Surg Pathol 1996, **20**: 1190–1195.

Vagina

CHAPTER CONTENTS

Normal anatomy

The vagina is a tubular structure derived from the paired müllerian ducts that extend from the vestibule of the vulva to the uterus.[5,6] It is composed of three main layers: mucosa, muscularis, and adventitia. The mucosa is composed of stratified squamous epithelium resting on loose connective tissue stroma. The squamous epithelium can be divided, as in the exocervix, into three main zones: basal, intermediate, and superficial.[3] This epithelium is responsive to steroid hormones, its appearance depending on the age of the individual and the time of the menstrual cycle.[5]

The subepithelial stroma or lamina propria contains elastic fibers and a rich venous and lymphatic network. Polygonal to stellate stromal cells – some multinucleated – may be present. These cells are immunoreactive for desmin and hormone receptors but not for actin.

The wolffian (mesonephric) duct in the vagina is represented by *Gartner's duct*,[6] which runs deeply along the lateral vaginal walls. Microscopically, this usually appears in the form of a small single duct, sometimes surrounded by a cluster of small glands, all of them lined by a simple cuboidal epithelium. The presence of inspissated eosinophilic secretion in the lumen is a characteristic feature of these remnants.

Ectopic tissues exceptionally found in the vagina include *prostatic glands*[4] and *sebaceous glands*.[1]

The lymphatic drainage of the vagina is rather complex. The vessels in the upper anterior wall join those of the cervix and terminate in the medial chain of the external iliac nodes (interiliac nodes). Those in the posterior vagina drain into deep pelvic, rectal, and aortic nodes. Some of those of the lower vagina (including the hymenal portion) go to the interiliac nodes; others traverse the paravesical spaces and drain into the inferior gluteal nodes. Finally, the vessels that anastomose with those from the vulva drain to the femoral nodes.[2,3]

Adenosis and related lesions

Adenosis (gland cell prosoplasia) of the vagina was originally described as a partial or complete conversion of the vaginal mucosa from squamous to endocervical-type glandular epithelium[20] (Fig. 19.36), but the concept was later expanded to embrace the presence of any müllerian-type glandular epithelium in the vagina. Sandberg[19] found occult vaginal adenosis in 9 (41%) of 22 vaginas from postpubertal girls obtained at autopsy but in none of 13 prepubertal patients. Kurman and Scully[13] obtained similar results, suggesting that vaginal adenosis can arise on a congenital basis but that steroid hormones probably play a stimulatory role in their development. Excess mucous discharge is the most common complaint in symptomatic cases. Grossly, adenosis appears as red granular spots or patches that do not stain with Lugol solution. Microscopically, the glands may be mucin-secreting and similar to those of the endocervix (most commonly) or have a lining resembling tubal or endometrial mucosa[10] (Fig. 19.37).

Depending on the relative amounts of these components, a *mucinous (endocervical)* and a *tuboendometrial* form of vaginal adenosis have been described. Exceptionally, intestinal metaplasia is encountered.[14] The glandular-type epithelium of vaginal adenosis may be in the lamina propria or it may line the surface of the vagina. As a result, it can be identified in cytologic smears, which represent a useful means for the detection of this disorder. Chronic inflammation and squamous metaplasia (mature, immature, or atypical) are common accompanying features (Fig. 19.38). The latter, which is poor in cytoplasmic glycogen, can obliterate the glandular lumen and appear as a peg continuous with the surface, a feature that may be misinterpreted as vaginal intraepithelial neoplasia (VaIN) or even as squamous cell carcinoma.[16] One should be aware, however, that lesions with the features of VaIN can superimpose themselves on foci of adenosis; the identifying features are the same as those described for similar lesions in the chapter on the uterine cervix.

Sometimes the squamous metaplasia is so extensive that the only evidence of a preexisting adenosis is found in the form of rare intercellular pools or intracellular droplets of mucin, as shown by mucicarmine or other mucin stains. It has been suggested that, as

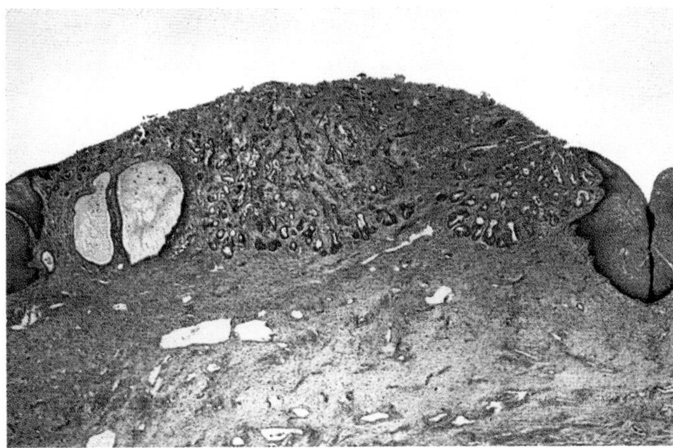

Fig. 19.36 Whole-mount view showing a sharply delimited portion of vagina covered by glandular epithelium in vaginal adenosis.

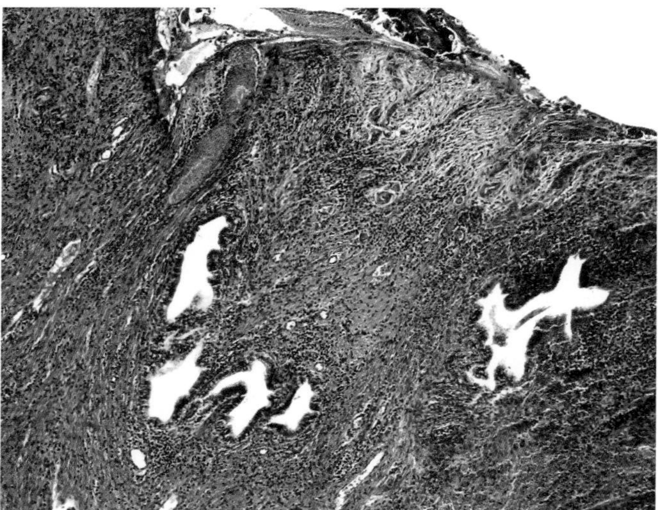

Fig. 19.37 Vaginal adenosis of tuboendometrial type beneath an ulcerated surface. Other areas of this specimen showed adenocarcinoma arising from the adenosis.

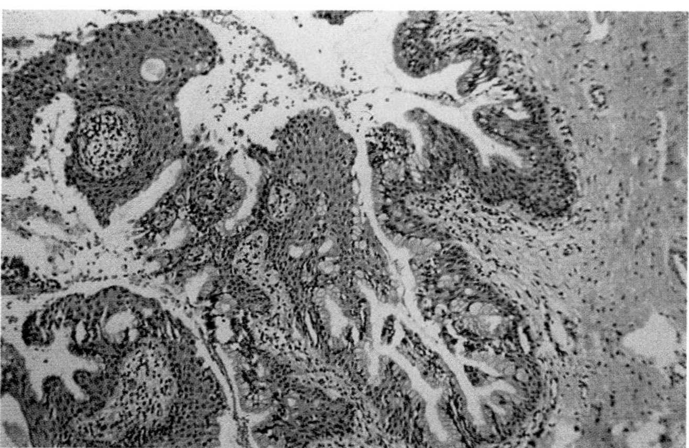

Fig. 19.38 Extensive squamous metaplasia in vaginal adenosis.

these women grow older, vaginal adenosis regresses by the process of squamous metaplasia.[17]

Microglandular hyperplasia can develop within lesions of vaginal adenosis following the use of oral contraceptives; it is important not to confuse this benign lesion with clear cell adenocarcinoma.[18]

A causal relationship between vaginal adenosis and exposure in utero to diethylstilbestrol (DES) was unraveled by the brilliant work of Arthur Herbst and Robert Scully. The reported incidence of adenosis in the exposed population has varied from 35% to more than 90% in the different series.[7] It has been shown that the incidence of vaginal adenosis and related colposcopic abnormalities is close to 100% if the drug is begun during or before the eighth week of pregnancy and only 6% if it is begun during the fifteenth week or later.[21] The microscopic features of adenosis in women exposed in utero to DES are identical to those seen in unexposed women.[8,15]

Transverse ridges and other structural anomalies are also related to DES administration.[11,12] They are found in the upper vagina or cervix in about one-fourth of the exposed population and have been described as cockscomb cervix, rims, collars, hoods, and

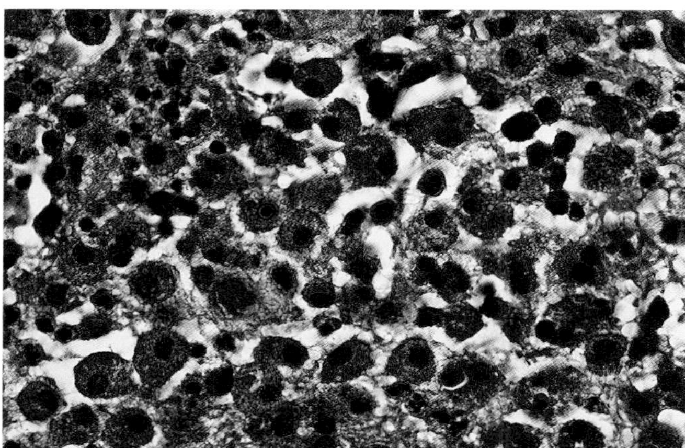

Fig. 19.39 Malakoplakia of vagina. This periodic acid–Schiff stain shows numerous histiocytes containing particulate material in their cytoplasm.

pseudopolyps. Microscopically, the ridge is composed of a core of fibrous tissue lined by mucinous epithelium, metaplastic squamous epithelium, or, rarely, tubal or endometrial epithelium. Although both vaginal adenosis and clear cell carcinoma are related to DES exposure (see p. 1426), it seems that the potential for the development of carcinoma from adenosis is exceedingly small.

DES-related lesions featuring immature squamous metaplasia, atypical metaplasia, and VaIN I usually revert to normal following biopsy or therapy; lesions in the VaIN II or III categories (usually characterized by an aneuploid DNA pattern by microspectrophotometry) tend to persist and recur after biopsy or therapy.[9]

Other non-neoplastic lesions

The adult vagina is impervious to most bacterial infections. However, the overgrowth of facultative and anaerobic bacterial flora may result in a condition known as *bacterial vaginosis*. Microscopically, the most important finding is the presence of squamous cells covered with coccobacilli ('clue cells').[29] The Papanicolaou (Pap) smear is a pretty specific but not very sensitive method for the detection of this condition.[33] Indolent infections caused by *Trichomonas vaginalis* and *Candida albicans* are relatively common, especially during pregnancy.[31] **Lymphogranuloma venereum** can involve the vagina during the late stage of the disease and result in stricture. **Xanthogranulomatous reactions**[32] and **malakoplakia**[23] may occur as a result of unusual bacterial infections and lead to pseudotumor formation or strictures (Fig. 19.39). The use of *tampons* can result in gross vaginal ulcers.[24]

Occasionally, following vaginal hysterectomy, the **tubal fimbria** may become entrapped in the healing vaginal apex, a finding that must not be confused with a neoplastic process.[22] The clinical presentation is that of a mass grossly resembling 'granulation tissue' at the vaginal apex, usually appearing within 6 months following a hysterectomy.[30] Occasionally, the tubal prolapse is associated with an exuberant stromal response with an angiomyofibroblastic appearance, a feature which adds to the diagnostic difficulty.[28]

Endometriosis and the related condition known as **endocervicosis** occur in the vagina, but less commonly than in other portions of the genital tract.[27] Most cases are seen in connection with episiotomy scars.

Cysts of the vagina can be of several different types.[25] The most common is the *epithelial inclusion cyst*, lined by squamous

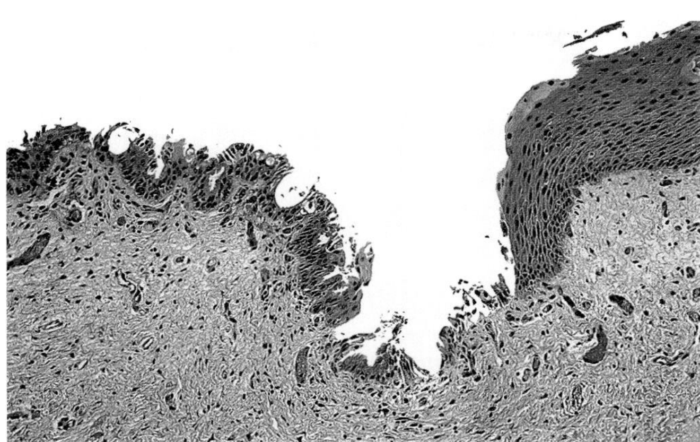

Fig. 19.40 Vaginal cyst lined by müllerian epithelium connecting with surface squamous epithelium.

epithelium and sometimes resulting from surgery or trauma. Another common type is characterized by a simple lining of mucin-secreting, tall columnar, nonciliated epithelium of endocervical type, sometimes associated with focal squamous metaplasia; this has been designated *müllerian cyst* and can be found anywhere in the vagina (Fig. 19.40). *Mesonephric* (*Gartner duct*) *cyst* is rare; it is located in the anterolateral or lateral vaginal wall and is lined by low cuboidal epithelial cells, sometimes ciliated, that do not secrete mucin. Other rare cystic lesions of the vagina include *urothelial cysts* (located in the suburethral portion and probably arising from paraurethral glands and Skene ducts), *emphysematous vaginitis*,[25,26] and the already mentioned *endometriosis*.

Benign epithelial tumors

Intramural papilloma having a branching configuration and a lining of a single layer of cuboidal cells has been rarely described in children. It may present in the surface as polyps or intramurally. It is sometimes referred to as *mesonephric papilloma*, but ultrastructural studies suggest that the lesion is instead of müllerian derivation (hence the newly proposed term *benign müllerian papilloma*).[40,44] *Papillary müllerian cystadenofibroma* of the vagina is probably a histogenetically closely related tumor.[38]

Squamous papilloma may be seen in the adult vagina but less commonly than in the cervix. Many of the cases are probably of viral (HPV) etiology.

Tubulovillous adenoma of the vagina, morphologically similar to its colorectal counterpart, has been described.[35]

Benign mixed tumor (spindle cell epithelioma) is usually located in or near the hymenal ring. It is composed of small stromal-type spindle cells intermixed with mature squamous cells and glands lined by mucinous epithelium[36,42] (Fig. 19.41). Ultrastructural and immunohistochemical studies support an epithelial nature.[34] There is also immunoreactivity for CD34, BCL2, CD99, h-caldesmon and CD10.[41,43] The lesion is benign, but it may recur locally.[34,45]

Tubulosquamous polyp is a newly described distinctive vaginal lesion characterized microscopically by the presence of well-circumscribed expansile nests of epithelial cells embedded in a hypocellular fibrous stroma. The epithelial component is generally of both squamous and glandular type, the former predominating.[39] Prostatic-type tissue can sometimes be found within this polyp.[37]

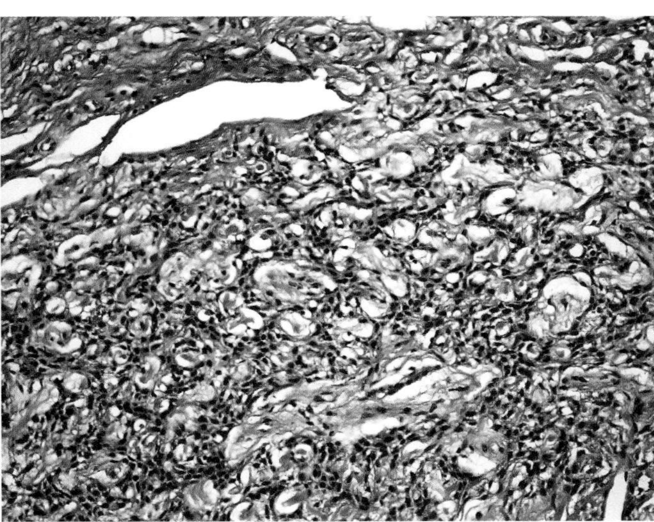

Fig. 19.41 So-called 'benign mixed tumor of vagina'. The plexiform pattern of growth seen in this field is characteristic of the entity.

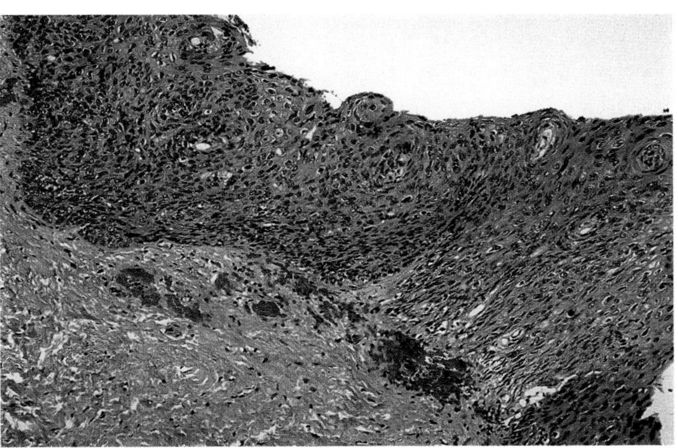

Fig. 19.42 Vaginal intraepithelial neoplasia (VaIN) III. This is the type traditionally known as in situ squamous cell carcinoma.

Squamous intraepithelial lesions

Atypical squamous epithelial lesions of the vagina have been designated as *vaginal intraepithelial neoplasia* (VaIN), borrowing the terminology from the analogous lesions in the cervix (CIN)[52] (Fig. 19.42). It should be noted that the vaginal lesions usually arise from native squamous epithelium, in contrast to most cervical cases, which originate from *metaplastic* squamous epithelium. VaIN is multifocal in about one-half of cases and very frequently associated with concomitant, subsequent, or prior (in situ or invasive) neoplasms of the lower genital tract.[46,48,50] The upper third of the vagina is the most common site, in which case the vaginal and cervical lesions may be confluent.[51] The HPV distribution in VaIN suggests that this condition is more closely related to CIN than to VIN.[53] The type of treatment depends largely on the extent of the disease and may consist of local excision, partial or total vaginectomy, CO_2 laser therapy, or administration of topical 5-fluorouracil.[47–49]

It is important not to overdiagnose transitional cell metaplasia as VaIN, the criteria for the differential diagnosis being the same as for the uterine cervix.[54]

Invasive squamous cell carcinoma

Primary carcinoma of the vagina is much less common than carcinoma of the vulva or cervix.[56,66,73] It is largely a disease of the elderly. HPV has been incriminated as a possible causative agent, as it has been for microscopically similar tumors of cervix and vulva.[62,65,67]

Since most carcinomas involving the vagina represent direct extension from cervical carcinomas, only vaginal tumors that spare the uterine cervix are regarded as primary. Those involving both areas are classified as cervical carcinomas with vaginal extension, regardless of the relative proportion of involvement.

Up to 20% of the patients successfully treated for CIN or invasive squamous cell carcinoma of the cervix will have abnormal cytologic smears from the vagina, and some will develop a similar tumor in the vagina at a later date.[68] The latter event seems to be more common in those patients who were treated by irradiation alone than in those who had only surgery, and the average interval is 5 or 6 years.[57,68] Therefore, patients who had cervical carcinoma should have follow-up examinations for the rest of their lives, with special attention to the possibility of a vaginal recurrence of the cervical tumor or a new primary vaginal carcinoma. The area for biopsy may be detected by colposcopy, Schiller test, or multiple smears taken from all sectors of the vagina.[63] Vaginal carcinoma can also develop following hysterectomy for benign disease; therefore regular Pap tests are still indicated after this operation.[55]

Most primary vaginal carcinomas are grossly nodular or ulcerative[82] (Fig. 19.43). The upper third and the anterior or lateral walls are the most common sites of origin.[78] A few cases have arisen in surgically constructed neovaginas.[76,80]

Microscopically, approximately 95% of vaginal carcinomas are conventional squamous cell carcinomas of varying degrees of differentiation, their morphologic appearance duplicating that of their more common cervical and vulvar counterparts (Fig. 19.44).

Vaginal carcinoma is usually treated by a combination of external and intracavitary radiation;[64,75,79] local excision can be employed for small tumors[69] and radical surgery for selected cases located in the upper vaginal third or posterior wall.[59,61] The overall 5-year survival rate is between 40% and 50%.[61,74,77] The prognosis is closely related to the stage of the disease[69,71] and is similar whether the patient has a previously treated cervical carcinoma or not.[70] In the series from the National Cancer Data Base, the relative 5-year survival was 96% for stage 0, 73% for stage I, 58% for stage II, and 36% for stages III and IV.[58] Most recurrences occur within 1 year of therapy and carry an ominous prognosis. Upper lesions tend to recur locally, whereas lower lesions are more commonly associated with pelvic sidewall and distal recurrence.[81]

The existence of *microinvasive* (*superficially or minimally invasive*) *carcinoma* as a distinct clinical entity in the vagina has been proposed, but the concept faces the same theoretic and practical difficulties for a precise definition as in the vulva (see p. 1405).[72] As in the case of the grossly invasive tumors, some of the reported examples have followed treatment for cervical carcinoma.[60]

Clear cell (adeno)carcinoma

Clear cell (adeno)carcinoma is also known as mesonephroid (adeno)carcinoma, both terms being preferable to the older designation, *mesonephric carcinoma*.[90,93] It characteristically occurs in the anterior or lateral wall of the upper vagina or in the uterine cervix of children, adolescents, and young adults. The average age at the time of diagnosis is 17 years. It is extremely rare before the age of 12 and after the age of 30 years, but there is a second smaller peak at age 70 years.[86] In two-thirds of the patients, there is a history of prenatal exposure to diethylstilbestrol (DES) or related nonsteroid estrogens.[91,94,101] However, the risk of carcinoma in the exposed population is low: it has been estimated to be 1 in 1000.[87,94] It has been found to be higher for those patients whose mothers began therapy before the twelfth week of pregnancy.[88]

Steroid estrogens do not seem to be associated with this complication. Most patients present with vaginal bleeding or discharge, but 16% of those studied by Herbst et al.[89] were asymptomatic. There is a very common association with vaginal adenosis, cervical ectropion, and occasional coexistence of transverse vaginal or cervical ridges. These features strongly suggest the existence of a DES-related disturbance in the development of the lower müllerian tract. Grossly, the larger tumors may involve most of the vagina. The majority are polypoid and nodular; others are flat or ulcerated, with an indurated or granular surface.[97] Most of the tumors are only superficially invasive at the time of diagnosis.

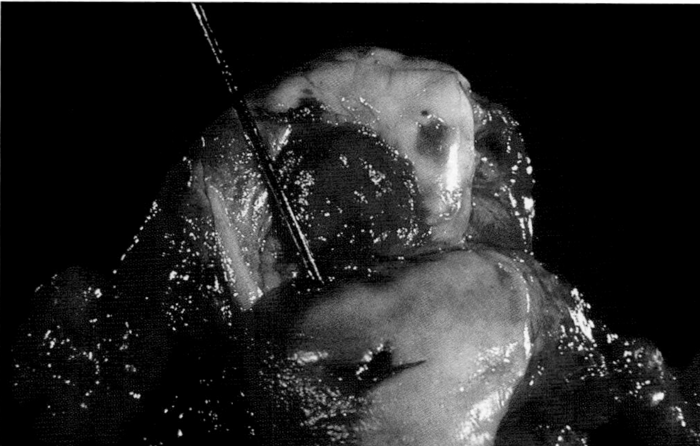

Fig. 19.43 Invasive squamous cell carcinoma resulting in a large ulcerated mass.

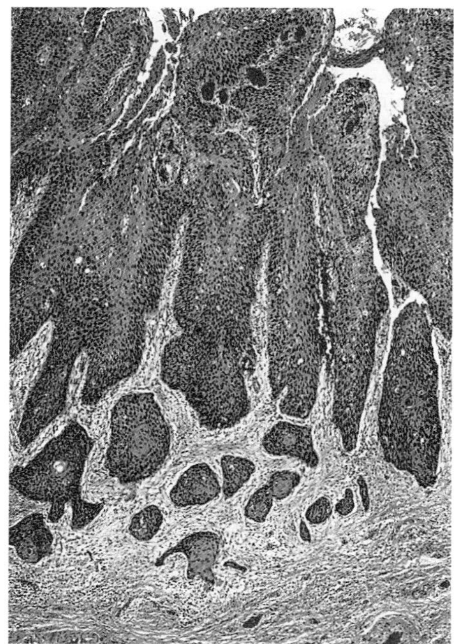

Fig. 19.44 Well-differentiated squamous cell carcinoma of vagina invading the superficial stroma.

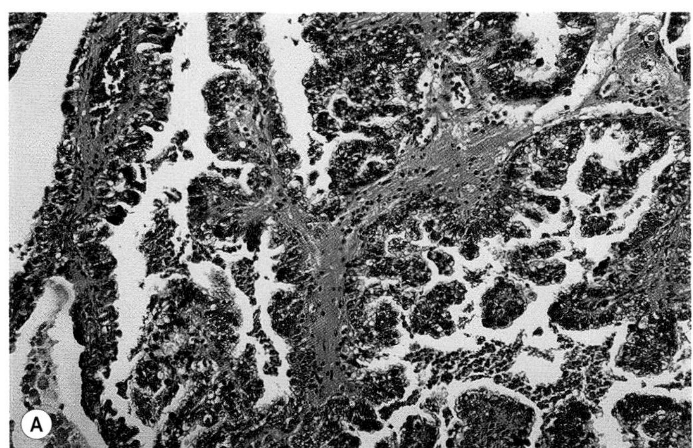

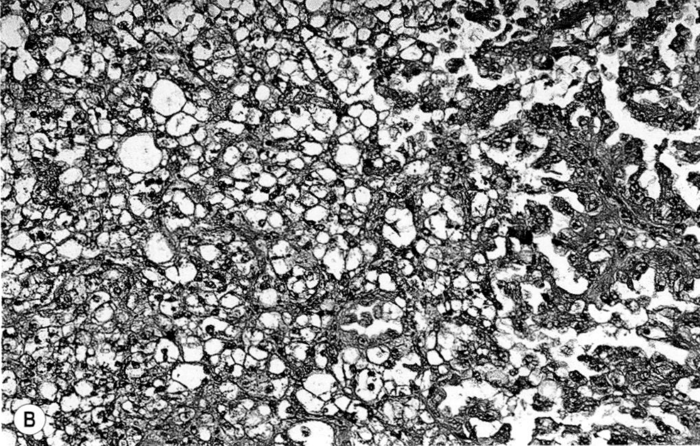

Fig. 19.45 Clear cell carcinoma of vagina. **A**, Papillary pattern; **B**, Prominent clear cell features.

Microscopically, there are tubules and cysts lined by clear cells alternating with more solid areas and papillary formations[95] (Fig. 19.45). Mitotic figures are variable but usually scanty. The tumor cells have an abundant clear cytoplasm because of the presence of glycogen and sometimes fat. Intracytoplasmic mucin is either absent or scanty. Hobnail-shaped cells are frequently seen protruding into the glandular lumen. These cells can be detected by cytologic examination,[85,99] but about one-fourth of patients will have a negative vaginal smear. The microscopic differential diagnosis needs to be made primarily with microglandular hyperplasia, which can occur in areas of vaginal adenosis, and the Arias-Stella reaction related to pregnancy or progestational agents. It is of interest that whereas the lesions of vaginal adenosis are usually strongly positive for mucin stain, this is almost never the case for the cells of clear cell adenocarcinoma. The explanation given is that this tumor tends to arise from the tuboendometrial rather than the mucinous form of adenosis; support for this interpretation comes from a study showing tuboendometrial epithelium in 95% of clear cell adenocarcinomas (usually in greater concentrations at the margin of the tumor) and the presence of atypical changes in 80% of them.[98]

The immunohistochemical profile of these tumors is characterized by consistent positivity for CK7, CAM 5.2, 34βE12, CEA, CD15, vimentin, BCL2, and CA-125; variable positivity for estrogen receptors and HER2/*neu*; and negativity for CK20 and progesterone receptors.[100]

Ultrastructurally, the appearance of clear cell carcinoma is very similar regardless of the architectural or cytologic features as seen by light microscopy and is comparable to the clear cell carcinomas of the endometrium and ovary seen in older women.[84]

At the genetic molecular level, there is widespread instability in these tumors, as manifested by somatic mutation of microsatellite repeats.[83]

The prognosis is relatively good. Small, asymptomatic tumors usually are cured by surgery. Tumors that are large, that are close to the resection margins, or that have penetrated more than 3 mm into the wall tend to recur locally.[96] Metastases occur to pelvic lymph nodes (and sometimes those in the supraclavicular region) and lungs. In the series of Herbst et al.,[89] 24% of the patients developed persistent or recurrent disease, and 16% have died. The recurrences can occur very late after the treatment of the primary tumor.[92]

Other carcinoma types

Verrucous carcinoma is an extremely well-differentiated variant of squamous cell carcinoma. Like its vulvar and cervical counterparts, it invades locally but is practically never associated with lymph node metastases. The local spread can be quite extensive and reach the rectum and coccyx.[123] It should be distinguished from condyloma acuminatum, which may rarely involve the vagina; the criteria are the same as those described in the section on the vulva. HPV has been demonstrated in some cases of vaginal verrucous carcinoma.[119]

Endometrioid adenocarcinoma is the second most common type of primary adenocarcinoma of the vagina. Most cases are located at the vaginal apex.[131] It is thought to arise in most cases on the basis of vaginal endometriosis.[111] The presence of the latter is important in supporting a primary vaginal tumor as opposed to secondary spread from the endometrium. Endometriosis is also the presumed origin for most cases of adenocarcinomas located in the rectovaginal septum and having no mucosal involvement of either the vagina or rectum; this supposition is based on the fact that endometriosis is sometimes detected together with or preceding the carcinoma,[110] and because of the well-known predilection of this condition for the rectovaginal septum.[136]

Mesonephric (wolffian) adenocarcinoma is an exceptionally rare tumor located paravaginally, along the course of the wolffian-derived ducts of Gartner.[102,112]

Sarcomatoid carcinoma (carcinosarcoma) of the vagina probably comprises at least two different entities. The first, in which the epithelial component is of squamous type, can be seen as the equivalent to the homonymous tumor in the upper aerodigestive tract[124,132] (Fig. 19.46). The other, in which the epithelium is glandular, retiform or tubular, is probably of mesonephric (wolffian) origin;[129] indeed, it has been called *malignant mixed mesonephric tumor*.[102] We suspect that some of the tumors reported as synovial sarcoma, 'synovioid' and malignant mixed müllerian tumor of vagina probably belong to one or another of these two categories[120,121,128,133] (although true synovial sarcomas of the vagina do exist, see below).

Mucinous adenocarcinoma of vagina has been described in middle-aged and elderly patients, occasionally arising on the basis of endocervicosis.[117] Its microscopic features are indistinguishable from those of its more common endocervical counterpart.[107] In a few reported cases, the appearance has been reminiscent of enteric epithelium.[108,135]

Small cell (neuroendocrine) carcinoma can occur in the vagina, either in a pure form or associated with squamous or glandular elements.[104,113,114,118] One case has been reported in a background of atypical adenosis.[122] As in other sites where this tumor type occurs, there is usually electron microscopic and immunohistochemical

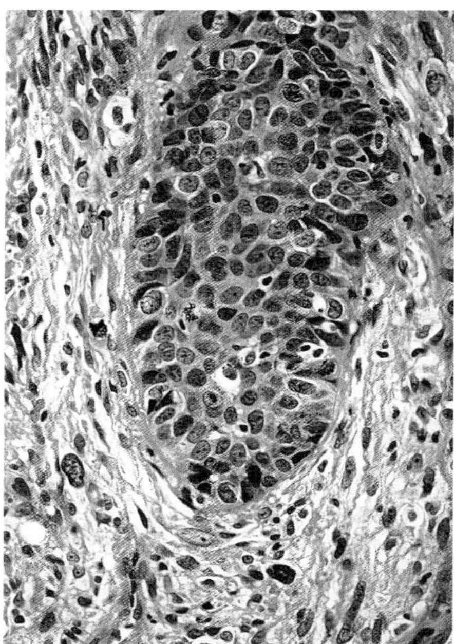

Fig. 19.46 Spindle cell (sarcomatoid) carcinoma of vagina. Elongated cells with a mesenchymal-like appearance surround a well-defined nest having a clearcut epithelial appearance.

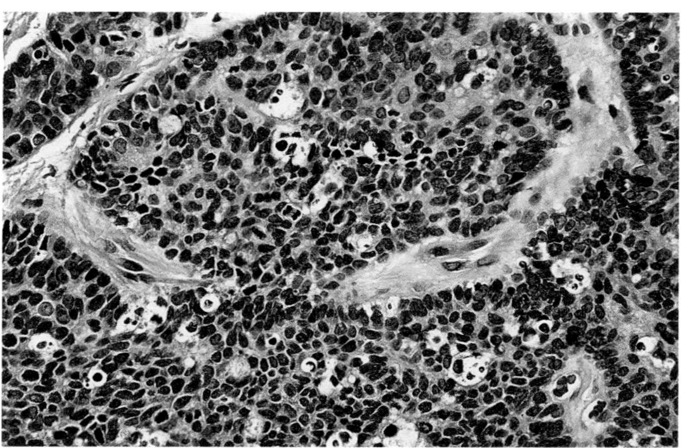

Fig. 19.47 Basaloid carcinoma of vagina.

evidence of neuroendocrine differentiation.[109,127,134] Most cases have been treated by a combination of radiation therapy and chemotherapy.[113] A case of neuroendocrine carcinoma of the vagina with a *Merkel cell* phenotype has also been reported.[105]

Other carcinoma types that have been described in the vagina are *urothelial (transitional cell) carcinoma*[103] (including a pagetoid form[130] and a variant described as *papillary squamotransitional*[126]), *serous (papillary) adenocarcinoma,*[125] *lymphoepithelioma-like carcinoma*[106,116] and *basaloid carcinoma*[115] (Fig. 19.47).

Mesenchymal tumors and tumorlike conditions

Fibroepithelial polyps may be seen in adult women (especially during pregnancy) or in neonates.[159,165] They are probably not true neoplasms but rather manifestations of hormone-induced localized hyperplasia of the loose subepithelial connective tissue zone;[138] others may represent the end stage of granulation tissue[150] (Fig. 19.48). Microscopically, they are formed of a central fibrovascular core and a covering of normal-appearing squamous epithelium (Fig. 19.49). Sometimes the stroma is markedly edematous;[138] in other instances it is hypercellular and/or contains scattered highly atypical stromal cells of stellate shape[137,145,160,168] (Fig. 19.50). These stromal cells are immunoreactive for vimentin, desmin, and steroid receptors but usually not for actin.[151,161] The clinical appearance, nuclear atypia, and desmin immunoreactivity may lead to a mistaken diagnosis of botryoid rhabdomyosarcoma or other types of malignant tumor.[165,167] The slow pace of growth at the clinical level and the fact that a cambium layer, epithelial invasion, and cross striations are absent are among the distinguishing features.

Aggressive angiomyxoma can present as a protruding intravaginal mass and extend through the paravaginal soft tissue.[176] This entity is more fully described on page 1410.

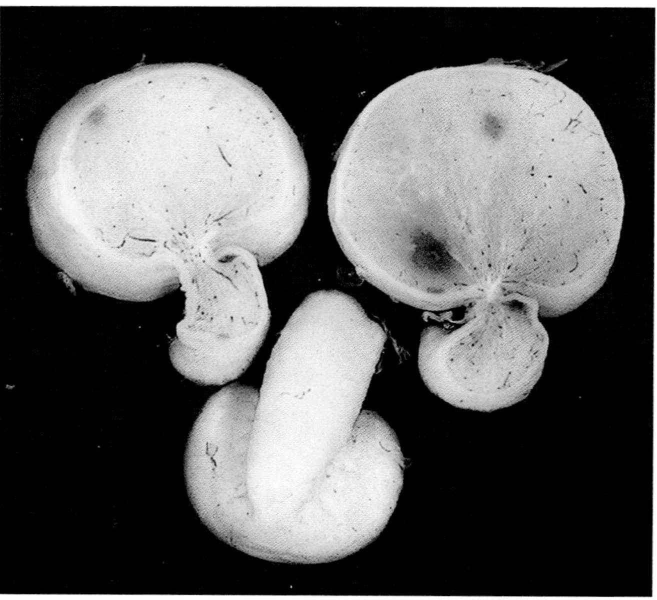

Fig. 19.48 Curious mushroom-like appearance of vaginal fibroepithelial polyp.
(Courtesy of Dr Pedro J Grases Galofré; from Grases Galofré PJ. Patología ginecológica. Bases para el diagnóstico morfológico. Barcelona, 2002, Masson)

Angiomyofibroblastoma, superficial myofibroblastoma, and **solitary fibrous tumor** are other types of benign mesenchymal neoplasms of fibroblastic/myofibroblastic nature that have been reported in the vagina.[157,164,178] The angiomyofibroblastoma has an appearance identical to that of its vulvar counterpart, and the superficial myofibroblastoma represents a minor variation on the theme of benign polypoid tumors of the hormonally responsive mesenchymal cells of the region.[166]

Postoperative spindle cell nodule is a pseudosarcomatous vaginal lesion that occurs a few weeks following hysterectomy or some other surgical procedure in the region and which presents as a small friable reddish mass in the vaginal vault.[172,180] Microscopically, it shows ulceration, granulation tissue, and a very hypercellular spindle cell proliferation characterized by a fascicular pattern of growth, many mitotic figures, and numerous extravasated red blood cells, resulting in a Kaposi sarcoma-like appearance[172]

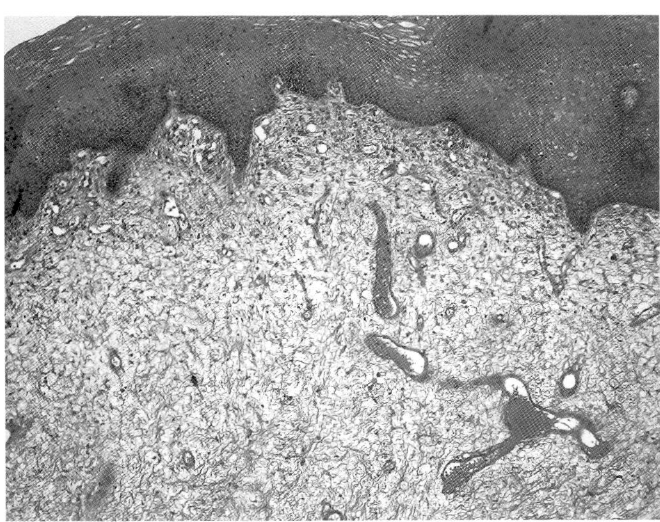

Fig. 19.49 Fibroepithelial polyp of vagina showing loose fibrovascular stroma covered by slightly thickened but otherwise unremarkable squamous epithelium.

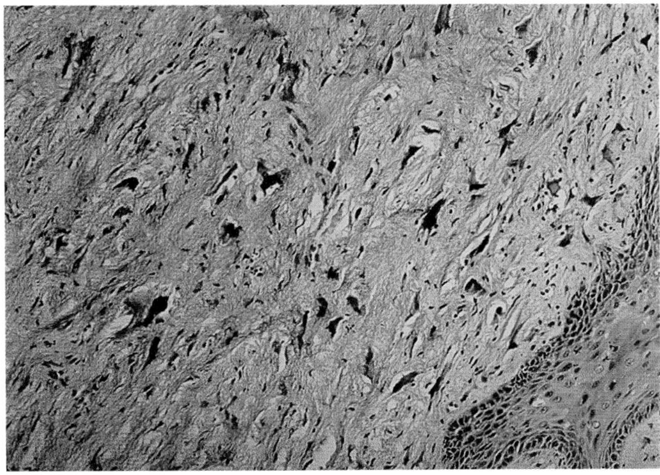

Fig. 19.50 Atypical benign stromal cells in a vaginal polyp.

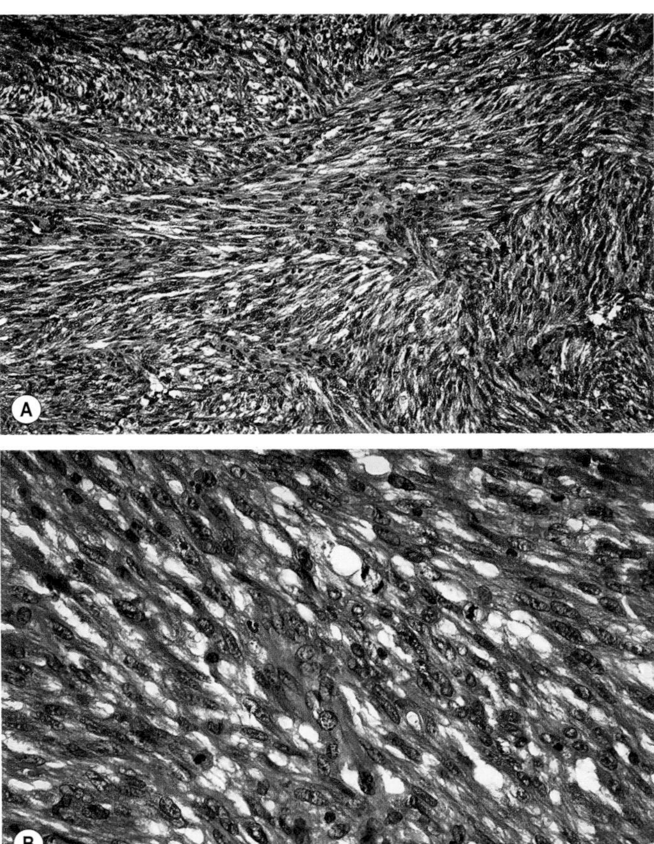

Fig. 19.51 **A** and **B**, Medium- and high-power views of postoperative spindle cell nodule. The lesion is extremely cellular and mitotically active, but there is little pleomorphism.

(Fig. 19.51). It can also be confused with sarcoma (particularly leiomyosarcoma) and sarcomatoid carcinoma. Immunohistochemically, there may be reactivity for low molecular weight keratin, which may contribute to the misinterpretation of the lesion. Clues to its recognition are the distinctly fascicular pattern, the Kaposi sarcoma-like areas, the absence of pleomorphism, the fact that the mitoses – although abundant – are all typical, and, most important, the history of a recent operation in the area.

Leiomyoma is the most common benign mesenchymal tumor of the vagina.[166,177] The patients are adults, and any region of the vagina can be affected. A peculiar case has been seen containing paraganglioma-like tissue within.[162]

Leiomyosarcoma can attain a large size and ulcerate.[146] The majority of the cases manifest their malignancy only through local recurrence. The criteria of malignancy used by Tavassoli and Norris[177] were the presence of moderate to marked atypia and five or more mitotic figures per 10 high-power fields. Poorly differentiated tumors are associated with a high mortality rate.[173]

Rhabdomyoma presents as a polypoid mass.[141] All of the reported cases have occurred in adult patients, an important differential point with botryoid rhabdomyosarcoma, discussed below. Microscopically, the lesion consists of interweaving and haphazardly oriented bundles of spindle- to strap-shaped cells, some with cross striations[149] (Fig. 19.52). Mitoses are scanty or absent, and there is no concentration of neoplastic cells beneath the epithelium.

Other benign mesenchymal tumors that have been reported in the vagina are *hemangioma, hemangiopericytoma,*[156] *glomus tumor,*[175] *benign 'triton' tumor,*[139] *angiomyolipoma,*[144] *(cellular) schwannoma,*[147] and *neurofibroma.*[148]

Botryoid rhabdomyosarcoma (sarcoma botryoides) is a rare polypoid invasive tumor that usually arises from the anterior vaginal wall[153] (Fig. 19.53). Approximately 90% of cases occur in girls under 5 years of age, with close to two-thirds appearing during the first 2 years. Grossly, it presents as a conglomerate of soft polypoid masses resembling a bunch of grapes – hence its name.

Microscopically, a myxoid stroma is seen containing undifferentiated round or spindle cells (Fig. 19.54). Some of these cells contain a bright eosinophilic granular cytoplasm suggestive of rhabdomyoblastic differentiation. Their racquet- or strap-shaped form mimics that of the cells seen during normal muscle embryogenesis. Cross striations may or may not be present. An important diagnostic feature is the crowding of the tumor cells around blood vessels and, most important, beneath the squamous epithelium. The latter results in a distinctive subepithelial dense zone (the 'cambium layer'

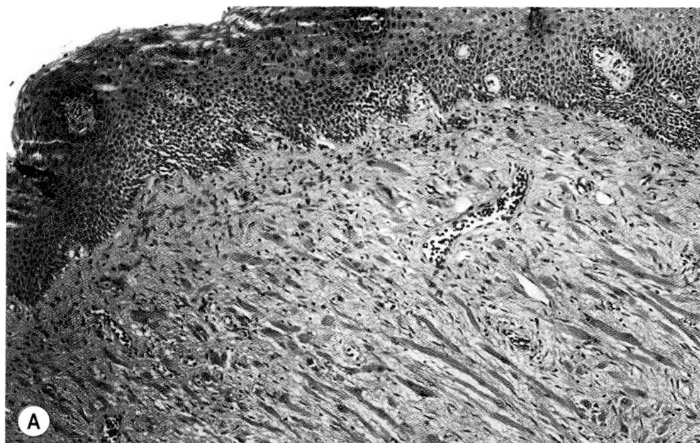

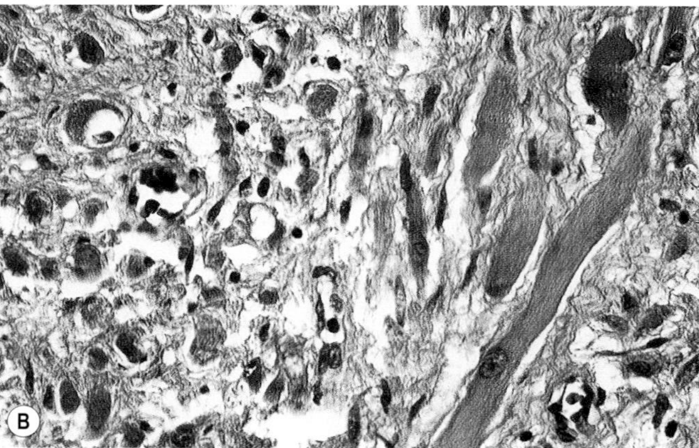

Fig. 19.52 **A** and **B**, Vaginal rhabdomyoma composed of bundles of mature skeletal muscle cells scattered in the stroma beneath normal squamous epithelium.

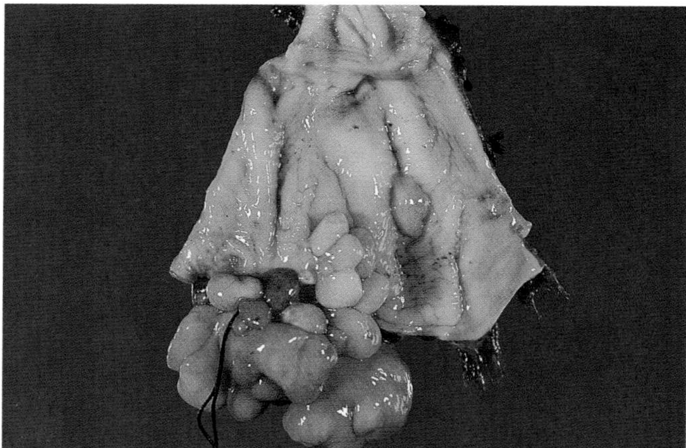

Fig. 19.53 Botryoid rhabdomyosarcoma of vagina. The grape-like configuration of this lesion is characteristic.

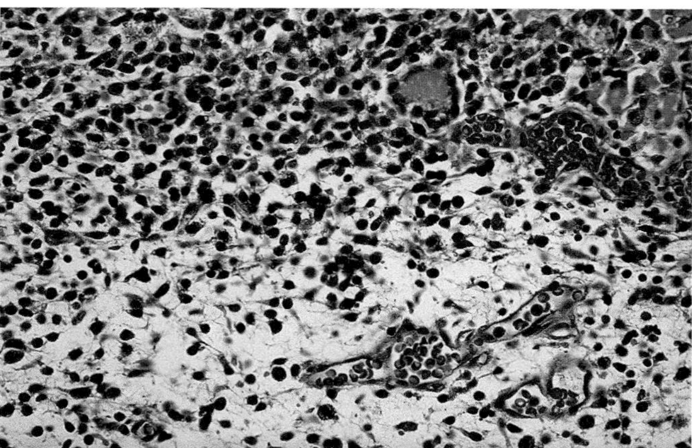

Fig. 19.54 Microscopic appearance of botryoid rhabdomyosarcoma. The differential diagnosis is that of small round cell tumors.

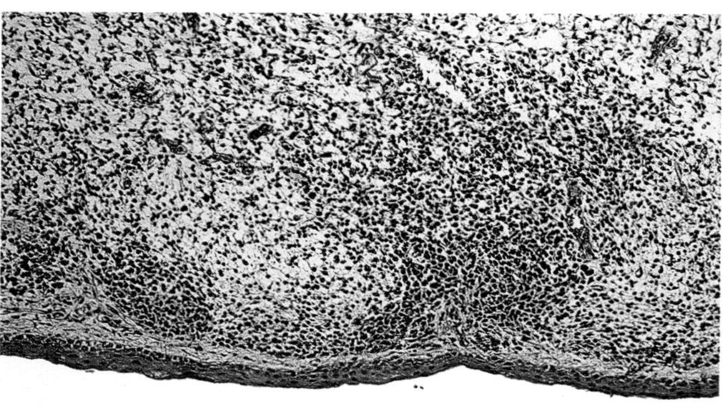

Fig. 19.55 So-called 'cambium layer' beneath non-neoplastic epithelium in botryoid rhabdomyosarcoma.

of Nicholson) (Fig. 19.55). Invasion of the overlying epithelium can be seen. Foci of neoplastic cartilage may be found; these tend to occur in older patients and/or in tumors located higher in the vagina or cervix, and they are said to be associated with a better prognosis. Botryoid tumors are currently regarded as a variation in the growth pattern of embryonal rhabdomyosarcoma, due to their location immediately beneath an expansile epithelial lining. They cause death more often by direct extension than by distant metastases.[158] Of the 15 autopsied cases reviewed by Hilgers et al.,[155] the tumor was confined to the pelvis in about half.

The treatment of this tumor, traditionally consisting of radical surgery,[154,174] is now primarily based on chemotherapy, which can be combined with radiation therapy and/or surgery depending on the circumstances.[152]

Other primary sarcomas that have been reported in the vagina are *stromal sarcoma* of endometrial type,[170] *malignant peripheral nerve sheath tumor,*[170] *angiosarcoma*[171] (sometimes arising as a complication of radiation therapy[142]), *alveolar soft part sarcoma,*[140,143,163] synovial sarcoma,[169] and Ewing sarcoma/PNET.[179]

Melanocytic tumors

Melanoma can occur as a primary vaginal tumor in elderly patients.[183,188,190,191] It presents as a soft polypoid mass, blue or black, frequently ulcerated[192] (Fig. 19.56). Most cases are located in the lower one-third and in the anterolateral aspect.[181] Microscopically, the appearance is similar to that of the cutaneous melanomas, although they tend to show greater anaplasia and pleomorphism

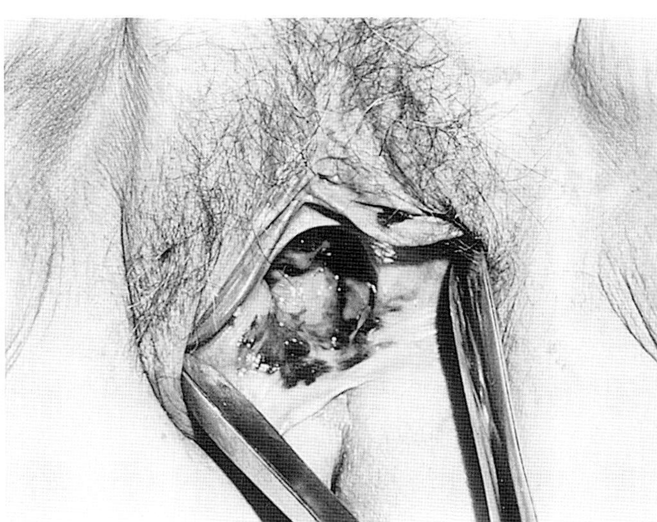

Fig. 19.56 Malignant melanoma of vagina.
*(From Norris HJ, Taylor HB. Melanomas of the vagina. Am J Clin Pathol 1966, **46:** 420–426)*

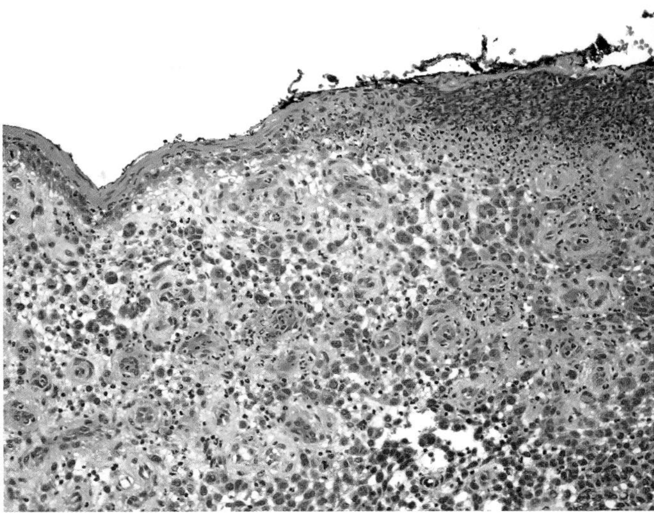

Fig. 19.57 Malignant melanoma of vagina. The tumor has an undifferentiated appearance, is largely amelanotic, and has an ulcerated surface.

(Fig. 19.57). An intraepithelial component of lentiginous appearance should be looked for to substantiate a local origin, although this feature can be destroyed by the tumor ulceration. The prognosis is extremely poor.[184,185,187] The melanocytes that have been identified in 3% of normal vaginas[189] most likely represent the cell of origin of this neoplasm, sometimes through a preceding stage of melanosis or atypical melanocytic hyperplasia.[182,186]

Blue nevus of the ordinary type can present as a primary vaginal lesion.[193]

Other primary tumors

Yolk sac tumor (endodermal sinus tumor) typically affects infants under 2 years of age and is more commonly located in either the posterior wall or the fornices.[197,211] Clinically, it can simulate botryoid rhabdomyosarcoma.[203] Microscopically, the most important differential diagnosis is with clear cell (adeno)carcinoma, a tumor with which it has been confused in the past. Immunohistochemically, reactivity for SALL4 and alpha-fetoprotein favors yolk sac tumor, and reactivity for Leu-M1 favors clear cell carcinoma.[212] In early series, most patients with vaginal yolk sac tumor died with generalized metastases,[206] but the combination of surgical excision and multidrug chemotherapy (sometimes with the addition of radiation therapy) has resulted in many long-term cures.[201,208]

Malignant lymphoma can affect the vagina secondarily or sometimes as the only site of involvement; nearly all cases are of non-Hodgkin type.[196,199,207] The largest group is represented by diffuse large B-cell lymphomas.[210] A case has been reported in association with malakoplakia.[209] Vaginal involvement can also occur in *acute granulocytic leukemia* (granulocytic sarcoma).[199]

Other primary tumors of the vagina or paravaginal region, all exceptionally rare, are *Brenner tumor*,[194,195] *female adnexal tumor of probable wolffian origin*,[198] *PEComa*,[200] *myoepithelioma*,[205] and *gastrointestinal stromal tumor* (presenting in the vaginal wall or in the rectovaginal septum).[202,204]

Metastatic tumors

Metastatic carcinoma to the vagina arises most commonly in the uterine cervix and endometrium, followed by the ovary, large bowel, and kidney.[214,215,217] Some cases represent direct extension, and others are distant metastases. The metastases from endometrial adenocarcinoma are often submucosal and located in the upper third of the organ. The routine practice of preoperative radiation therapy for uterine adenocarcinomas associated with uterine enlargement has reduced their frequency.

Other tumors that can metastasize to vagina are melanoma[213] and malignant trophoblastic neoplasms, including epithelioid trophoblastic tumor.[216]

References

NORMAL ANATOMY

1 Belousova IE, Kazakov DV, Michal M. Ectopic sebaceous glands in the vagina. Int J Gynecol Pathol 2005, **24**: 193–195.

2 Hafez ESE, Evans TN (eds): The human vagina. New York, 1978, North-Holland.

3 Krantz KE. The gross and microscopic anatomy of the human vagina. Ann N Y Acad Sci 1959, **83**: 89–104.

4 McCluggage WG, Ganesan R, Hirschowitz L, Miller K, Rollason TP. Ectopic prostatic tissue in the uterine cervix and vagina: report of a series with a detailed immunohistochemical analysis. Am J Surg Pathol 2006, **30**: 209–215.

5 Robboy SJ, Bently RC. Vagina. In Mills SE (ed.): Histology for pathologists, ed. 3. Philadelphia, 2007, Lippincott Williams and Wilkins, pp. 999–1010.

6 Ulfelder H, Robboy SJ. The embryological development of the human vagina. Am J Obstet Gynecol 1976, **126**: 769–776.

ADENOSIS AND RELATED LESIONS

7 Antonioli DA, Burke L. Vaginal adenosis. Analysis of 325 biopsy specimens from 100 patients. Am J Clin Pathol 1975, **64**: 625–638.

8 Chattopadhyay I, Cruickshan DJ, Packer M. Non diethylstilbesterol induced vaginal adenosis – a case series and review of literature. Eur J Gynecol Oncol 2001, **22**: 260–262.

9 Fu YS, Reagan JW, Richart RM, Townsend DE. Nuclear DNA and histologic studies of genital lesions in diethylstilbestrol-exposed progeny. I. Intraepithelial squamous abnormalities. Am J Clin Pathol 1979, **72**: 503–520.

10 Hart WR, Townsend DE, Aldrich JO, Henderson BE, Roy M, Benton B. Histopathologic spectrum of vaginal adenosis and related changes in stilbestrol-exposed females. Cancer 1976, **37**: 763–775.

11 Herbst AL, Poskanzer DC, Robboy SJ, Friedlander L, Scully RE. Prenatal exposure to stilbestrol. A prospective comparison of exposed female offspring with unexposed controls. N Engl J Med 1975, **292**: 334–339.

12 Jefferies JA, Robboy SJ, O'Brien PC, Bergstralh EJ, Labarthe DR, Barnes AB, Noller KL, Hatab PA, Kaufman RH, Townsend DE. Structural anomalies of the cervix and vagina in women enrolled in the Diethylstilbestrol Adenosis (DESAD) Project. Am J Obstet Gynecol 1984, **148**: 59–66.

13 Kurman RJ, Scully RE. The incidence and histogenesis of vaginal adenosis. An autopsy study. Hum Pathol 1974, **5**: 265–276.

14 Merchant WJ, Gale J. Intestinal metaplasia in stilboestrol-induced vaginal adenosis. Histopathology 1993, **23**: 373–376.

15 Robboy SJ, Hill EC, Sandberg EC, Czernobilsky B. Vaginal adenosis in women born prior to the diethylstilbestrol era. Hum Pathol 1986, **17**: 488–492.

16 Robboy SJ, Scully RE, Welch WR, Herbst AL. Intrauterine diethylstilbestrol exposure and its consequences. Pathologic characteristics of vaginal adenosis, clear cell adenocarcinoma, and related lesions. Arch Pathol Lab Med 1977, **101**: 1–5.

17 Robboy SJ, Szyfelbein WM, Goellner JR, Kaufman RH, Taft PD, Richard RM, Gaffey TA, Prat J, Virata R, Hatab PA, McGorray SP, Noller KL, Townsend D, Lobarthe D, Barnes AB. Dysplasia and cytologic findings in 4589 young women enrolled in the Diethylstilbestrol Adenosis (DESAD) Project. Am J Obstet Gynecol 1981, **140**: 579–586.

18 Robboy SJ, Welch WR. Microglandular hyperplasia in vaginal adenosis associated with oral contraceptives and prenatal diethylstilbestrol exposure. Obstet Gynecol 1977, **49**: 430–434.

19 Sandberg EC. The incidence of distribution of occult vaginal adenosis. Trans Pac Coast Obstet Gynecol Soc 1967, **35**: 36–48.

20 Siders DB, Parrott MH, Abell MR. Gland cell prosoplasia (adenosis) of vagina. Am J Obstet Gynecol 1965, **91**: 190–203.

21 Sonek M, Bibbo M, Wied GL. Colposcopic findings in offspring of DES-treated mothers as related to onset of therapy. J Reprod Med 1976, **16**: 65–71.

OTHER NON-NEOPLASTIC LESIONS

22 Bilodeau B. Intravaginal prolapse of the fallopian tube following vaginal hysterectomy. Am J Obstet Gynecol 1982, **143**: 970–971.

23 Chalvardjan A, Picard L, Shaw R, Davey R, Cairns JD. Malacoplakia of the female genital tract. Am J Obstet Gynecol 1980, **138**: 391–394.

24 Danielson RW. Vaginal ulcers caused by tampons. Am J Obstet Gynecol 1983, **146**: 547–548.

25 Deppisch LM. Cysts of the vagina. Classification and clinical correlations. Obstet Gynecol 1975, **45**: 632–637.

26 Kramer K, Tobón H. Vaginitis emphysematosa. Arch Pathol Lab Med 1987, **111**: 746–749.

27 Martinka M, Allaire C, Clement PB. Endocervicosis presenting as a painful vaginal mass: a case report. Int J Gynecol Pathol 2002, **18**: 274–276.

28 Michal M, Rokyta Z, Mejchar B, Pelikan K, Kummel M, Mukensnabl P. Prolapse of the fallopian tube after hysterectomy associated with exuberant angiomyofibroblastic stroma response: a diagnostic pitfall. Virchows Arch 2000, **437**: 436–439.

29 Robboy SJ, Welch WR. Selected topics in the pathology of the vagina. Hum Pathol 1991, **22**: 868–878.

30 Silverberg SG, Frable WJ. Prolapse of fallopian tube into vaginal vault after hysterectomy. Histopathology, cytopathology, and differential diagnosis. Arch Pathol 1974, **97**: 100–103.

31 Sobel JD. Vaginal infections in adult women. Med Clin North Am 1990, **74**: 1573–1602.

32 Strate SM, Taylor WE, Forney JP, Silva FG. Xanthogranulomatous pseudotumor of the vagina. Evidence of a local response to an unusual bacterium (mucoid *Escherichia coli*). Am J Clin Pathol 1983, **79**: 637–643.

33 Tokyol C, Aktepe OC, Cevrio lu AS, Altindi M, Dilek FH. Bacterial vaginosis: comparison of Pap smear and microbiological test results. Mod Pathol 2004, **17**: 857–860.

BENIGN EPITHELIAL TUMORS

34 Branton PA, Tavassoli FA. Spindle cell epithelioma, the so-called mixed tumor of the vagina. A clinicopathologic, immunohistochemical, and ultrastructural analysis of 28 cases. Am J Surg Pathol 1993, **17**: 509–515.

35 Fox H, Wells M, Harris M, McWilliam LJ, Anderson GS. Enteric tumours of the lower female genital tract. A report of three cases. Histopathology 1988, **12**: 167–176.

36 Fukunaga M, Endo Y, Ishikawa E, Ushigome S. Mixed tumor of the vagina. Histopathology 1997, **28**: 457–461.

37 Kazakov DV, Stewart CJ, Kacerovska D, Leake R, Kreuzberg B, Chudacek Z, Hora M, Michal M. Prostatic-type tissue in the lower female genital tract: a morphologic spectrum, including vaginal tubulosquamous polyp, adenomyomatous hyperplasia of paraurethral Skene glands (female prostate), and ectopic lesion in the vulva. Am J Surg Pathol 2010, **34**: 950–955.

38 Kerner H, Munichor M. Papillary mullerian cystadenofibroma of the vagina. Histopathology 1997, **30**: 84–86.

39 McCluggage WG, Young RH. Tubulo-squamous polyp: a report of ten cases of a distinctive hitherto uncharacterized vaginal polyp. Am J Surg Pathol 2007, **31**: 1013–1019.

40 Mierau GW, Lovell MA, Wyatt-Ashmead J, Goin L. Benign müllerian papilloma of childhood. Ultrastruct Pathol 2005, **29**: 209–216.

41 Oliva E, Gonzalez L, Dionigi A, Young RH. Mixed tumors of the vagina: an immunohistochemical study of 13 cases with emphasis on the cell of origin and potential aid in differential diagnosis. Mod Pathol 2004, **17**: 1243–1250.

42 Sirota RL, Dickersin GR, Scully RE. Mixed tumors of the vagina. Am J Surg Pathol 1981, **5**: 413–422.

43 Skelton H, Smith KJ. Spindle cell epitheliomas of the vagina shows immunohistochemical staining supporting its origin from a primitive/progenitor cell population. Arch Pathol Lab Med 2001, **125**: 547–550.

44 Ulbright TM, Alexander RW, Kraus FT. Intramural papilloma of the vagina. Evidence of müllerian histogenesis. Cancer 1981, **48**: 2260–2266.

45 Wright RG, Buntine DW, Forbes KL. Recurrent benign mixed tumor of the vagina. Gynecol Oncol 1991, **40**: 84–86.

SQUAMOUS INTRAEPITHELIAL LESIONS

46 Aho M, Vesterinen E, Meyer B, Purola E, Paavonen J. Natural history of vaginal intraepithelial neoplasia. Cancer 1991, **68**: 195–197.

47 Audet-Lapointe P, Body G, Vauclair R, Drouin P, Ayoub J. Vaginal intraepithelial neoplasia. Gynecol Oncol 1990, **36**: 232–239.

48 Benedet JL, Sanders BH. Carcinoma in situ of the vagina. Am J Obstet Gynecol 1984, **148**: 695–700.

49 Caglar H, Hertzog RW, Hreshchyshyn MM. Topical 5-fluorouracil treatment of vaginal intraepithelial neoplasia. Obstet Gynecol 1981, **58**: 580–583.

50 Kanbour AI, Klionsky B, Murphy AI. Carcinoma of the vagina following cervical cancer. Cancer 1974, **34**: 1838–1841.

51 Nwabineli NJ, Monaghan JM. Vaginal epithelial abnormalities in patients with CIN. Clinical and pathological features and management. Br J Obstet Gynaecol 1991, **98**: 25–29.

52 Sherman ME, Paull G. Vaginal intraepithelial neoplasia. Reproducibility of pathologic diagnosis and correlation of smears and biopsies. Acta Cytol 1993, **37**: 699–704.

53 Srodon M, Stoler MH, Baber GB, Kurman RJ. The distribution of low and high-risk HPV types in vulvar and vaginal intraepithelial neoplasia (VIN and VaIN). Am J Surg Pathol 2006, **30**: 1513–1518.

54 Weir MM, Bell DA, Young RH. Transitional cell metaplasia of the uterine cervix and vagina: an underrecognized lesion that may be confused with high-grade dysplasia: a report of 59 cases. Am J Surg Pathol 1997, **21**: 510–517.

INVASIVE SQUAMOUS CELL CARCINOMA

55 Bell J, Sevin B-U, Averette H, Nadji M. Vaginal cancer after hysterectomy for benign disease. Value of cytologic screening. Obstet Gynecol 1984, **64**: 699–702.

56 Benedet JL. Vaginal malignancy. Curr Opin Obstet Gynecol 1991, **3**: 73–77.

57 Choo YC, Anderson DG. Neoplasms of the vagina following cervical carcinoma. Gynecol Oncol 1982, **14**: 125–132.

58 Creasman WT, Phillips JL, Menck HR. The National Cancer Data Base Report on cancer in the vagina. Cancer 1998, **83**: 1033–1040.

59 Davis KP, Stanhope CR, Garton GR, Atkinson EJ, O'Brien PC. Invasive vaginal carcinoma. Analysis of early-stage disease. Gynecol Oncol 1991, **42**: 131–136.

60 Eddy GL, Singh KP, Gansler TS. Superficially invasive carcinoma of the vagina following treatment for cervical cancer. A report of six cases. Gynecol Oncol 1990, **36**: 376–379.

61 Houghton CRS, Iversen T. Squamous cell carcinoma of the vagina. A clinical study of the location of the tumor. Gynecol Oncol 1982, **13**: 365–372.

62 Ikenberg H, Runge M, Goppinger A, Pfeiderer A. Human papillomavirus DNA in invasive carcinoma of the vagina. Obstet Gynecol 1990, **76**: 432–438.

63 Kanbour AI, Klionsky B, Murphy AI. Carcinoma of the vagina following cervical cancer. Cancer 1974, **34**: 1838–1841.

64 Kucera H, Vavra N. Radiation management of primary carcinoma of the vagina. Clinical and histopathological variables associated with survival. Gynecol Oncol 1991, **40**: 12–16.

65 Macnab JCM, Walkinshaw SA, Cordiner JW, Clements JB. Human papillomavirus in clinically and histologically normal tissue of patients with genital cancer. N Engl J Med 1986, **315**: 1052–1058.

66 Manetta A, Gutrecht EL, Berman ML, Di Saia PJ. Primary invasive carcinoma of the vagina. Obstet Gynecol 1990, **76**: 639–642.

67 Merino MJ. Vaginal cancer. The role of infectious and environmental factors. Am J Obstet Gynecol 1991, **165**: 1255–1262.

68 Murad TM, Durant JR, Maddox WA, Dowling EA. The pathologic behavior of primary vaginal carcinoma and its relationship to cervical cancer. Cancer 1975, **35**: 787–794.

69 Perez CA, Arneson AN, Dehner LP, Galakatos A. Radiation therapy in carcinoma of the vagina. Obstet Gynecol 1974, **44**: 862–872.

70 Perez CA, Arneson AN, Galakatos A, Samanth HK. Malignant tumors of the vagina. Cancer 1973, **31**: 36–44.

71 Peters WA III, Kumar NB, Morley GW. Carcinoma of the vagina. Factors influencing treatment outcome. Cancer 1985, **55**: 892–897.

72 Peters WA III, Kumar NB, Morley GW. Microinvasive carcinoma of the vagina. A distinct clinical entity? Am J Obstet Gynecol 1985, **153**: 505–507.

73 Piura B, Rabinovich A, Cohen Y, Glezerman M. Primary squamous cell carcinoma of the vagina: report of four cases and review of the literature. Eur J Gynecol Oncol 1998, **19**: 60–63.

74 Prempree T, Viravathana T, Slawson RG, Wizenberg MJ, Cuccia CA. Radiation management of primary carcinoma of the vagina. Cancer 1977, **40**: 109–118.

75 Reddy S, Lee MS, Graham JE, Yordan EL, Phillips R, Saxena VS, Hendrickson FR, Wilbanks GD. Radiation therapy in primary carcinoma of the vagina. Gynecol Oncol 1987, **26**: 19–24.

76 Rotmensch J, Rosenshein N, Dillon M, Murphy A, Woodruff JD. Carcinoma arising in the neovagina. Case report and review of the literature. Obstet Gynecol 1983, **61**: 534–538.

77 Rubin SC, Young J, Mikuta JJ. Squamous carcinoma of the vagina. Treatment complications and long-term follow-up. Gynecol Oncol 1985, **20**: 346–353.

78 Rutledge F. Cancer of the vagina. Am J Obstet Gynecol 1967, **97**: 635–655.

79 Spirtos NM, Doshi BP, Kapp DS, Teng N. Radiation therapy for primary squamous cell carcinoma of the vagina. Stanford University experience. Gynecol Oncol 1989, **35**: 20–26.

80 Steiner E, Woernle F, Kuhn W, Beckmann K, Schmidt M, Pilch H, Knapstein PG. Carcinoma of the neovagina: case report and review of the literature. Gynecol Oncol 2002, **84**: 171–175.

81 Tarraza MH Jr, Muntz H, Decain M, Granai OC, Fuller A Jr. Patterns of recurrence of primary carcinoma of the vagina. Eur J Gynaecol Oncol 1991, **12**: 89–92.

82 Whelton J, Kottmeier HL. Primary carcinoma of the vagina. A study of a Radiumhemmet series of 145 cases. Acta Obstet Gynecol Scand 1962, **41**: 22–40.

CLEAR CELL (ADENO)CARCINOMA

83 Boyd J, Takahashi H, Waggoner SE, Jones LA, Hajek RA, Wharton JT, Liu FS, Fujino T, Barrett JC, McLachlan JA. Molecular genetic analysis of clear cell adenocarcinomas of the vagina and cervix associated and unassociated with diethylstilbestrol exposure in utero. Cancer 1996, **77**: 507–513.

84 Dickersin GR, Welch WR, Erlandson R, Robboy SJ. Ultrastructure of 16 cases of clear cell adenocarcinoma of the vagina and cervix in young women. Cancer 1980, **45**: 1615–1624.

85 Hanselaar AG, Boss EA, Massuger LF, Bernheim JL. Cytologic examination to detect clear cell adenocarcinoma of the vagina or cervix. Gynecol Oncol 1999, **75**: 338–344.

86 Hanselaar A, van Loosbroek M, Schuurbiers O, Helmerhosrt T, Bulten J, Bernheim J. Clear cell adenocarcinoma of the vagina and cervix: an update of the Central Netherlands Registry showing twin age incidence peaks. Cancer 1997, **79**: 2229–2236.

87 Herbst AL, Anderson D. Clear cell adenocarcinoma of the vagina and cervix secondary to intrauterine exposure to diethylstilbestrol. Semin Surg Oncol 1990, **6**: 343–346.

88 Herbst AL, Anderson S, Hubby MM, Haenszel WM, Kaufmann RH, Noller KL. Risk factors for the development of diethylstilbestrol-associated clear cell adenocarcinoma. A case-control study. Am J Obstet Gynecol 1986, **154**: 814–822.

89 Herbst AL, Robboy SJ, Scully RE, Poskanzer DC. Clear-cell adenocarcinoma of the vagina and cervix in girls. Analysis of 170 registry cases. Am J Obstet Gynecol 1974, **119**: 713–724.

90 Herbst AL, Scully RE. Adenocarcinoma of the vagina in adolescence. A report of 7 cases including 6 clear-cell carcinomas (so-called mesonephromas). Cancer 1970, **25**: 745–757.

91 Herbst AL, Ulfelder H, Poskanzer DC. Adenocarcinoma of the vagina. Association of maternal stilbestrol therapy with tumor appearance in young women. N Engl J Med 1971, **284**: 878–881.

92 Jones WB, Tan LK, Lewis JL Jr. Late recurrence of clear cell adenocarcinoma of the vagina and cervix. A report of three cases. Gynecol Oncol 1993, **51**: 266–271.

93 Matias-Guiu X, Lerma E, Prat J. Clear cell tumors of the female genital tract. Semin Diagn Pathol 1998, **14**: 233–239.

94 Melnick S, Cole P, Anderson D, Herbst A. Rates and risks of diethylstilbestrol-related clear-cell adenocarcinoma of the vagina and cervix. An update. N Engl J Med 1987, **316**: 514–516.

95 Nordqvist SRB, Fidler WJ Jr, Woodruff JM, Lewis JL. Clear cell adenocarcinoma of the cervix and vagina. A clinicopathologic study of 21 cases with and without a history of maternal ingestion of estrogens. Cancer 1976, **37**: 858–871.

96 Robboy SJ, Herbst AL, Scully RE. Clear-cell adenocarcinoma of the vagina and cervix in young females. Analysis of 37 tumors that persisted or recurred after primary therapy. Cancer 1974, **34**: 606–614.

97 Robboy SJ, Scully RE, Welch WR, Herbst AL. Intrauterine diethylstilbestrol exposure and its consequences. Pathologic characteristics of vaginal adenosis, clear cell adenocarcinoma, and related lesions. Arch Pathol Lab Med 1977, **101**: 1–5.

98 Robboy SJ, Young RH, Welch WR, Truslow GV, Prat J, Herbst AL, Scully RE. Atypical vaginal adenosis and cervical ectropion. Association with clear cell adenocarcinoma in diethylstilbestrol-exposed offspring. Cancer 1984, **54**: 869–875.

99 Taft PD, Robboy SJ, Herbst AL, Scully RE. Cytology of clear-cell adenocarcinoma of the genital tract in young females. Report of 95 cases from the registry. Acta Cytol (Baltimore) 1974, **18**: 279–290.

100 Vang R, Whitaker BP, Farhood AI, Silva EG, Ro JY, Deavers MT. Immunohistochemical analysis of clear cell carcinoma of the gynaecologic tract. Int J Gynecol Pathol 2001, **20**: 252–259.

101 Welch WR, Prat J, Robboy SJ, Herbst AL. Pathology of prenatal diethylstilbestrol exposure. Pathol Annu 1978, **13(Pt 1)**: 201–216.

OTHER CARCINOMA TYPES

102 Bagué S, Rodríguez IM, Prat J. Malignant mesonephric tumors of the female genital tract: a clinicopathologic study of 9 cases. Am J Surg Pathol 2004, **28**: 601–607.

103 Bass PS, Birch B, Smart C, Theaker JM, Wells M. Low-grade transitional cell carcinoma of the vagina. An unusual cause of vaginal bleeding. Histopathology 1994, **24**: 581–583.

104 Chafe W. Neuroepithelial small cell carcinoma of the vagina. Cancer 1989, **64**: 1948–1951.

105 Coleman NM, Smith-Zagone MJ, Tanyi J, Anderson ML, Coleman RL, Dyson SW, Reed JA. Primary neuroendocrine carcinoma of the vagina with Merkel cell carcinoma phenotype. Am J Surg Pathol 2006, **30**: 405–410.

106 Dietl J, Horny HP, Kaiserling E. Lymphoepithelioma-like carcinoma of the vagina. A case report with special reference to the immunophenotype of the tumor cells and tumor-infiltrating lymphoreticular cells. Int J Gynecol Pathol 1994, **13**: 186–189.

107 Ebrahim S, Daponte A, Smith TH, Tiltman A, Guidozzi F. Primary mucinous adenocarcinomas of the vagina. Gynecol Oncol 2001, **80**: 89–92.

108 Fox A, Wells M, Harris M, McWilliam LJ, Anderson GS. Enteric tumours of the lower female genital tract. A report of three cases. Histopathology 1988, **12**: 167–176.

109 Fukushima M, Twiggs LB, Okagaki T. Mixed intestinal adenocarcinoma. Argentaffin carcinoma of the vagina. Gynecol Oncol 1986, **23**: 387–394.

110 Granai CO, Walters MD, Safaii H, Jelen I, Madoc-Jones H, Moukhtar M. Malignant transformation of vaginal endometriosis. Obstet Gynecol 1984, **64**: 592–595.

111 Haskel S, Chen SS, Spiegel G. Vaginal endometrioid adenocarcinoma arising in vaginal endometriosis. A case report and literature review. Gynecol Oncol 1989, **34**: 232–236.

112 Hinchey WW, Silva EG, Guarda LA, Ordonez NG, Wharton JT. Paravaginal Wolffian duct (mesonephros) adenocarcinoma. A light and electron microscopic study. Am J Clin Pathol 1983, **80**: 539–544.

113 Hopkins MP, Kumar NB, Lichter AS, Peters WA, Morley GW. Small cell carcinoma of the vagina with neuroendocrine features. A report of three cases. J Reprod Med 1989, **34**: 486–491.

114 Kaminski JM, Anderson PR, Han AC, Mitra RK, Rosenblum NG, Edelson MI. Primary small cell carcinoma of the vagina. Gynecol Oncol 2003, **88**: 451–455.

115 Li H, Heller DS, Sama J, Bolanowski PJ, Anderson J. Basaloid squamous cell carcinoma of the vagina metastasizing to the lung. A case report. J Reprod Med 2000, **45**: 841–843.

116 McCluggage WG. Lymphoepithelioma-like carcinoma of the vagina. J Clin Pathol 2001, **54**: 964–965.

117 McCluggage WG, Price JH, Dobbs SP. Primary adenocarcinoma of the vagina arising in endocervicosis. Int J Gynecol Pathol 2001, **20**: 399–402.

118 Miliauskas JR, Leong AS. Small cell (neuroendocrine) carcinoma of the vagina. Histopathology 1992, **21**: 371–374.

119 Okagaki T, Clark BA, Zachow KR, Twiggs LB, Ostrow RS, Pass F, Faras AJ. Presence of human papillomavirus in verrucous carcinoma (Ackerman) of the vagina. Immunocytochemical, ultrastructural, and DNA hybridization studies. Arch Pathol Lab Med 1984, **108**: 567–570.

120 Okagaki T, Ishida T, Hilgers RD. A malignant tumor of the vagina resembling synovial sarcoma. A light and electron microscopic study. Cancer 1976, **37**: 2306–2320.

121 Peters WA III, Kumar NB, Anderson WA, Morley GW. Primary sarcoma of the adult vagina. A clinicopathologic study. Obstet Gynecol 1985, **63**: 699–704.

122 Prasad CJ, Ray JA, Kessler S. Primary small cell carcinoma of the vagina arising in a background of atypical adenosis. Cancer 1992, **70**: 2484–2487.

123 Ramzy I, Smout MS, Collins JA. Verrucous carcinoma of the vagina. Am J Clin Pathol 1976, **65**: 644–653.

124 Raptis S, Haber G, Ferenczy A. Vaginal squamous cell carcinoma with sarcomatoid spindle cell features. Gynecol Oncol 1993, **49**: 100–106.

125 Riva C, Fabbri A, Facco C, Tibiletti MG, Guglielmin P, Capella C. Primary serous papillary adenocarcinomas of the vagina: a case report. Int J Gynecol Pathol 1998, **16**: 286–290.

126 Rose PG, Stoler MH, Abdul-Karin FW. Papillary squamotransitional cell carcinoma of the vagina. Int J Gynecol Pathol 1998, **17**: 372–375.

127 Rusthoven JJ, Daya D. Small-cell carcinoma of the vagina. A clinicopathologic study. Arch Pathol Lab Med 1990, **114**: 728–731.

128 Sebenik M, Yan Z, Khalbuss WE, Mittal K. Malignant mixed mullerian tumor of the vagina: case report with review of the literature, immunohistochemical study, and evaluation for human papilloma virus. Hum Pathol 2007, **38**: 1282–1288.

129 Shevchuk MM, Fenoglio CM, Lattes R, Frick HC II, Richart RM. Malignant mixed tumor of the vagina probably arising in mesonephric rests. Cancer 1978, **42**: 214–233.

130 Singer G, Hohl MK, Hering F, Anabitarte M. Transitional cell carcinoma of the vagina with pagetoid spread pattern. Hum Pathol 1998, **29**: 299–301.

131 Staats PN, Clement PB, Young RH. Primary endometrioid adenocarcinoma of the vagina: a clinicopathologic study of 18 cases. Am J Surg Pathol 2007, **31**: 1490–1501.

132 Steeper TA, Piscioli F, Rosai J. Squamous cell carcinoma with sarcoma-like stroma of the female genital tract. Clinicopathologic study of four cases. Cancer 1983, **52**: 890–898.

133 Takehara M, Hayakawa O, Itoh E, Sagae S, Suzuki Kudo R. A case of a malignant mixed tumor in the vagina. J Obstet Gynaecol Res 1998, **24**: 7–11.

134 Ulich TR, Liao S-Y, Layfield L, Romansky S, Cheng L, Lewin KJ. Endocrine and tumor differentiation markers in poorly differentiated small-cell carcinoids of the cervix and vagina. Arch Pathol Lab Med 1986, **110**: 1054–1057.

135 Yaghsezian H, Palazzo JP, Finkel GC, Carlson JA Jr, Talerman A. Primary vaginal adenocarcinoma of the intestinal type associated with adenosis. Gynecol Oncol 1992, **45**: 62–65.

136 Young EE, Gamble CH. Primary adenocarcinoma of the rectovaginal septum arising from endometriosis. Report of a case. Cancer 1969, **24**: 597–601.

MESENCHYMAL TUMORS AND TUMORLIKE CONDITIONS

137 Abdul-Karim FW, Cohen RE. Atypical stromal cells of lower female genital tract. Histopathology 1990, **17**: 249–253.

138 al-Nafussi AI, Rebello G, Hughes D, Blessing K. Benign vaginal polyp. A histological, histochemical and immunohistochemical study of 20 polyps with comparison to normal vaginal subepithelial layer. Histopathology 1992, **20**: 145–150.

139 Azzopardi JG, Eusebi V, Tison V, Betts CM. Neurofibroma with rhabdomyomatous differentiation. Benign 'triton' tumour of the vagina. Histopathology 1983, **7**: 561–572.

140 Carinelli SG, Giudici MN, Brioschi D, Cefis F. Alveolar soft part sarcoma of the vagina. Tumori 1990, **76**: 77–80.

141 Chabrel CM, Beilby JOW. Vaginal rhabdomyoma. Histopathology 1980, **4**: 645–651.

142 Chan WW, Sen Gupta SK. Postirradiation angiosarcoma of the vaginal vault. Arch Pathol Lab Med 1991, **115**: 527–528.

143 Chapman GW, Genda J, Williams T. Alveolar soft-part sarcoma of the vagina. Gynecol Oncol 1984, **18**: 125–129.

144 Chen KT. Angiomyolipoma of the vagina. Gynecol Oncol 1990, **37**: 302–304.

145 Chirayil SJ, Tobon H. Polyps of the vagina. A clinico-pathologic study of 18 cases. Cancer 1981, **47**: 2904–2907.

146 Ciaravino G, Kapp DS, Vela AM, Fulton RS, Lum BL, Teng NN, Roberts JA. Primary leiomyosarcoma of the vagina. A case report and literature review. Int J Gynecol Cancer 2000, **10**: 340–347.

147 Ellison DW, MacKenzie IZ, McGee JO. Cellular schwannoma of the vagina. Gynecol Oncol 1992, **46**: 119–121.

148 Gersell DJ, Fulling KH. Localized neurofibromatosis of the female genitourinary tract. Am J Surg Pathol 1989, **13**: 873–878.

149 Gold JH, Bossen EH. Benign vaginal rhabdomyoma. A light and electron microscopic study. Cancer 1976, **37**: 2283–2294.

150 Halvorsen TB, Johannesen E. Fibroepithelial polyps of the vagina. Are they old granulation tissue polyps? J Clin Pathol 1992, **45**: 235–240.

151 Hartmann CA, Sperling M, Stein H. So-called fibroepithelial polyps of the vagina exhibiting an unusual but uniform antigen profile characterized by expression of desmin and steroid hormone receptors but no muscle-specific actin or macrophage markers. Am J Clin Pathol 1990, **93**: 604–608.

152 Hays DM, Shimada H, Raney RB Jr, Tefft M, Newton W, Crist WM, Lawrence W Jr, Ragab A, Beltangady M, Maurer HM. Clinical staging and treatment results in rhabdomyosarcoma of the female genital tract among children and adolescents. Cancer 1988, **61**: 1893–1903.

153 Hays DM, Shimada H, Raney RB Jr, Tefft M, Newton W, Crist WM, Lawrence W Jr, Ragab A, Maurer HM. Sarcomas of the vagina and uterus. The Intergroup Rhabdomyosarcoma Study. J Pediatr Surg 1985, **20**: 718–724.

154 Hilgers RD. Pelvic exenteration for vaginal embryonal rhabdomyosarcoma. A review. Obstet Gynecol 1975, **45**: 175–180.

155 Hilgers R, Malkasian GD Jr, Soule EH. Embryonal rhabdomyosarcoma (botryoid type) of the vagina. A clinicopathologic review. Am J Obstet Gynecol 1970, **107**: 484–502.

156 Hiura M, Nogawa T, Nagai N, Yorishima M, Fujiwara A. Vaginal hemangiopericytoma. A light microscopic and ultrastructural study. Gynecol Oncol 1985, **21**: 376–384.

157 Laskin WB, Fetsch JF, Tavassoli FA. Superficial cervicovaginal myofibroblastoma: fourteen cases of a distinctive mesenchymal tumor arising from the specialised subepithelial stroma of the lower female genital tract. Hum Pathol 2001, **32**: 715–725.

158 Leuschner I, Harms D, Mattke A, Koscielniak E, Treuner J. Rhabdomyosarcoma of the urinary bladder and vagina: a clinicopathologic study with emphasis on recurrent disease: a report from the Kiel Pediatric Tumor Registry and the German CWS study. Am J Surg Pathol 2001, **25**: 856–864.

159 McCluggage WG. A review and update of morphologically bland vulvovaginal mesenchymal lesions. Int J Gynecol Pathol 2005, **24**: 26–38.

160 Miettinen M, Wahlstrom T, Vesterinen E, Saksela E. Vaginal polyps with pseudosarcomatous features. A clinicopathologic study of seven cases. Cancer 1983, **51**: 1148–1151.

161 Mucitelli DR, Charles EZ, Kraus FT. Vulvovaginal polyps. Histologic appearance, ultrastructure, immunocytochemical characteristics, and clinicopathologic correlations. Int J Gynecol Pathol 1990, **9**: 20–40.

162 Naidoo P. Vaginal leiomyoma with heterologous paragangliomatous elements. Int J Surg Pathol 2001, **8**: 359–365.

163 Nielsen GP, Oliva E, Young RH, Rosenberg AE, Dickersin GR, Scully RE. Alveolar soft-part sarcoma of the female genital tract. A report of nine cases and review of the literature. Int J Gynecol Pathol 1995, **14**: 283–292.

164 Nielsen GP, Rosenberg AE, Young RH, Dickersin GR, Clement PB, Scully RE. Angiomyofibroblastoma of the vulva and vagina. Mod Pathol 1996, **9**: 284–291.

165 Norris HJ, Taylor HB. Polyps of the vagina. Cancer 1966, **19**: 227–232.

166 Nucci MR, Fletcher CD. Vulvovaginal soft tissue tumors: update and review. Histopathology 2000, **36**: 97–108.

167 Nucci MR, Young RH, Fletcher CD. Cellular pseudosarcomatous fibroepithelial stromal polyps of the lower female genital tract: an underrecognized lesion often misdiagnosed as sarcoma. Am J Surg Pathol 2000, **24**: 231–240.

168 Ostor AG, Fortune DW, Riley CB. Fibroepithelial polyps with atypical stromal cells (pseudosarcoma botryoides) of vulva and vagina. A report of 13 cases. Int J Gynecol Pathol 1988, **7**: 351–360.

169 Pelosi G, Luzzatto F, Landoni F, Staffa N, Maggioni A, Braidotti P, Cabras A, Aiello A, Del Curto B, Viale G. Poorly differentiated synovial sarcoma of the vagina: first reported case with immunohistochemical, molecular and ultrastructural data. Histopathology 2007, **50**: 808–810.

170 Peters WA III, Kumar NB, Anderson WA, Morley GW. Primary sarcoma of the adult vagina. A clinicopathologic study. Obstet Gynecol 1985, **63**: 699–704.

171 Prempree T, Tang C-K, Hatef A, Forster S. Angiosarcoma of the vagina. A clinicopathologic report. A reappraisal of the radiation treatment of angiosarcomas of the female genital tract. Cancer 1983, **51**: 618–622.

172 Proppe KH, Scully RE, Rosai J. Postoperative spindle cell nodules of genitourinary tract resembling sarcomas. A report of eight cases. Am J Surg Pathol 1984, **8**: 101–108.

173 Rastogi BL, Bergman B, Angervall L. Primary leiomyosarcoma of the vagina. A study of five cases. Gynecol Oncol 1984, **18**: 77–86.

174 Rutledge F, Sullivan MP. Sarcoma botryoides. Ann N Y Acad Sci 1967, **142**: 694–708.

175 Spitzer M, Molho L, Seltzer VL, Lipper S. Vaginal glomus tumor. Case presentation and ultrastructural findings. Obstet Gynecol 1985, **66**: 86S–88S.

176 Steeper TA, Rosai J. Aggressive angiomyxoma of the female pelvis and perineum. Report of nine cases of a distinctive type of gynecologic soft tissue neoplasm. Am J Surg Pathol 1983, **7**: 463–475.

177 Tavassoli FA, Norris HJ. Smooth muscle tumors of the vagina. Obstet Gynecol 1979, **53**: 689–693.

178 Vadmal MS, Pellegrini AE. Solitary fibrous tumor of the vagina. Am J Dermatopathol 2000, **22**: 83–86.

179 Vang R, Taubenberger JK, Mannion CM, BiJwaard K, Malpica A, Ordonez NG, Tavassoli FA, Silver SA. Primary vulvar and vaginal extraosseous Ewing's sarcoma/peripheral neuroectodermal tumor: diagnostic confirmation with CD99 immunostaining and reverse transcriptase-polymerase chain reaction. Int J Gynecol Pathol 2000, **19**: 103–109.

180 Young RH, Clement PB. Pseudoneoplastic lesions of the lower female genital tract. Pathol Annu 1989, **24**(Pt 2): 189–226.

MELANOCYTIC TUMORS

181 Borazjani G, Prem KA, Okagaki T, Twiggs LB, Adcock LL. Primary malignant melanoma of the vagina. A clinicopathological analysis of 10 cases. Gynecol Oncol 1990, **37**: 264–267.

182 Bottles K, Lacey CG, Miller TR. Atypical melanocytic hyperplasia of the vagina. Gynecol Oncol 1984, **19**: 226–230.

183 Chung AF, Casey MJ, Flannery JT, Woodruff JM, Lewis JL Jr. Malignant melanoma of the vagina. Report of 19 cases. Obstet Gynecol 1980, **55**: 720–727.

184 Gupta D, Neto AG, Deavers MT, Silva EG, Malpica A. Metastatic melanoma of the vagina: clinicopathologic and immunohistochemical study of three cases and literature review. Int J Gynecol Pathol 2003, **22**: 136–140.

185 Hasumi K, Sakamoto G, Sugano H, Kasuga T, Masubuchi K. Primary malignant melanoma of the vagina. Study of four autopsy cases with ultrastructural findings. Cancer 1978, **42**: 2675–2686.

186 Kerley SW, Blute ML, Keeney GL. Multifocal malignant melanoma arising in vesicovaginal melanosis. Arch Pathol Lab Med 1991, **115**: 950–952.

187 Morrow CP, DiSaia PJ. Malignant melanoma of the female genitalia. A clinical analysis. Obstet Gynecol Surv 1976, **31**: 233–271.

188 Neven P, Shepherd JH, Masotina A, Fisher C, Lowe DG. Malignant melanoma of the vulva and vagina: a report of 23 cases presenting in 10-year period. Int J Gynecol Cancer 1994, **4**: 379–383.

189 Nigogosyan G, De La Pava S, Pickren JW. Melanoblasts in the vaginal mucosa. Origin for primary malignant melanoma. Cancer 1964, **17**: 912–913.

190 Norris HJ, Taylor HB. Melanomas of the vagina. Am J Clin Pathol 1966, **46**: 420–426.

191 Ragnarsson-Olding B, Johansson H, Rutqvist LE, Ringborg U. Malignant melanoma of the vulva and vagina. Trends in incidence, age distribution, and long-term survival among 245 consecutive cases in Sweden 1960–1984. Cancer 1993, **71**: 1893–1897.

192 Schmidt M, Honig A, Schwab M, Adam P, Dietl J. Primary vaginal melanoma: a case report and literature review. Eur J Gynaecol Oncol 2008, **29**: 285–288.

193 Tobon H, Murphy AI. Benign blue nevus of the vagina. Cancer 1977, **40**: 3174–3176.

OTHER PRIMARY TUMORS

194 Ben-Izhak O, Munichor M, Malkin L, Kerner H. Brenner tumor of the vagina. Int J Gynecol Pathol 1998, **17**: 79–82.

195 Chen KTK. Brenner tumor of the vagina. Diagn Gynecol Obstet 1981, **3**: 255–258.

196 Chorlton I, Karnei RF Jr, Norris HJ. Primary malignant reticuloendothelial disease involving the vagina, cervix, and corpus uteri. Obstet Gynecol 1974, **44**: 735–748.

197 Copeland LJ, Sneige N, Ordonex NG, Hancock KC, Gershenson DM, Saul PB, Kavanagh JJ. Endodermal sinus tumor of the vagina and cervix. Cancer 1985, **55**: 2558–2565.

198 Daya D, Murphy J, Simon G. Paravaginal female adnexal tumor of probable wolffian origin. Am J Clin Pathol 1994, **101**: 275–278.

199 Harris NL, Scully RE. Malignant lymphoma and granulocytic sarcoma of the uterus and vagina. A clinicopathologic analysis of 27 cases. Cancer 1984, **53**: 2530–2545.

200 Kalyanasundaram K, Parameswaran A, Mani R. Perivascular epithelioid tumor of urinary bladder and vagina. Ann Diagn Pathol 2005, **9**: 275–278.

201 Kohorn EI, McIntosh S, Lytton B, Knowlton AH, Merino M. Endodermal sinus tumor of the infant vagina. Gynecol Oncol 1985, **20**: 196–203.

202 Lam MM, Corless CL, Goldblum JR, Heinrich MC, Downs-Kelly E, Rubin BP. Extragastrointestinal stromal tumors presenting as vulvovaginal/rectovaginal septal masses: a diagnostic pitfall. Int J Gynecol Pathol 2006, **25**: 288–292.

203 Lopes LF, Chazan R, Sredni ST, de Camargo B. Endodermal sinus tumor of the vagina in children. Med Pediatr Oncol 1999, **32**: 377–381.

204 McCluggage WG. Recent developments in vulvovaginal pathology. Histopathology 2009, **54**: 156–173.

205 Meenakshi M, McCluggage WG. Myoepithelial neoplasms involving the vulva and vagina: report of 4 cases. Hum Pathol 2009, **40**: 1747–1753.

206 Norris HJ, Bagley GP, Taylor HB. Carcinoma of the infant vagina. A distinctive tumor. Arch Pathol 1970, **90**: 473–479.

207 Perren T, Farrant M, McCarthy K, Harper P, Wiltshaw E. Lymphomas of the cervix and upper vagina. A report of five cases and a review of the literature. Gynecol Oncol 1992, **44**: 87–95.

208 Rutledge F, Sullivan MP. Sarcoma botryoides. Ann N Y Acad Sci 1967, **142**: 694–708.

209 Skinnider BF, Clement PB, MacPherson N, Gascoyne RD, Viswanatha DS. Primary non-Hodgkin's lymphoma and malakoplakia of the vagina: a case report. Hum Pathol 1999, **30**: 871–874.

210 Vang R, Medeiros LJ, Silva EG, Gershenson DM, Deavers M. Non-Hodgkin's lymphoma involving the vagina: a clinicopathologic analysis of 14 patients. Am J Surg Pathol 2000, **24**: 719–725.

211 Young RH, Scully RE. Endodermal sinus tumor of the vagina. A report of nine cases and review of the literature. Gynecol Oncol 1984, **18**: 380–392.

212 Zirker TA, Silva EG, Morris M, Ordonez NG. Immunohistochemical differentiation of clear-cell carcinoma of the female genital tract and endodermal sinus tumor with the use of alpha-fetoprotein and Leu-M1. Am J Clin Pathol 1989, **91**: 511–514.

METASTATIC TUMORS

213 Gupta D, Malpica A, Deavers MT, Silva EG. Vaginal melanoma: a clinicopathologic and immunohistochemical study of 26 cases. Am J Surg Pathol 2002, **26**: 1450–1457.

214 Mazur MT, Hsueh S, Gersell DJ. Metastases to the female genital tract. Analysis of 325 cases. Cancer 1984, **53**: 1978–1984.

215 Nerdrum TA. Vaginal metastasis of hypernephroma. Report of three cases. Acta Obstet Gynecol Scand 1966, **45**: 515–524.

216 Ohira S, Yamazaki T, Hatano H, Harada O, Toki T, Konishi I. Epithelioid trophoblastic tumor metastatic to the vagina: an immunohistochemical and ultrastructural study. Int J Gynecol Pathol 2001, **19**: 381–386.

217 Stander RW. Vaginal metastases following treatment of endometrial carcinoma. Am J Obstet Gynecol 1956, **71**: 776–779.

Uterus – cervix

CHAPTER CONTENTS

Normal anatomy

The cervix is the lower portion of the uterus which connects this organ to the vagina through the endocervical canal. It is divided into a portion that protrudes into the vagina (*portio vaginalis*) and one that lies above the vaginal vault (*supravaginal portion*). The outer surface of the portio vaginalis is known as the exocervix or ectocervix, and the portion related to the endocervical canal corresponds to the endocervix. The opening of the endocervical canal onto the exocervix is known as the *external os*, whereas the grossly indistinct upper limit of the endocervical canal is designated the *internal os*.[4]

Most of the exocervix is covered by nonkeratinizing squamous epithelium that in child-bearing age is composed of three layers: basal cell, midzone (stratum spongiosum), and superficial. The portion of the midzone immediately above the basal layer, referred to as the *suprabasal layer*, is well demonstrated with silver stains; according to some authors, the real 'stem cells' of the cervical squamous mucosa are located in this layer rather than in the basal layer.[13] The morphologic appearance of the various layers varies with age; in the postmenopausal period the cells are atrophic and exhibit a high nucleocytoplasmic ratio. These changes should not be misinterpreted as evidence of cervical intraepithelial neoplasia (CIN).

Histochemically, the cells above the basal layer show variable amounts of glycogen, readily appreciated in sections with a periodic acid–Schiff (PAS) stain and clinically by the application of the iodine (Lugol or Schiller) test. Immunohistochemically, the cells of the basal layer are positive for low molecular weight keratin and tissue polypeptide antigen (TPA) but not for high molecular weight (epidermal type) keratin or for involucrin.[5,6,10–12] The latter two markers become positive in the cells above the basal layer. Basal cells are also immunoreactive for estrogen receptors.[7]

The glandular mucosa of the endocervix is formed by a layer of columnar mucus-secreting cells, the histochemical reactivity for the mucin depending on the time of the menstrual cycle.[3] These cells rest on a normally inconspicuous layer of subcolumnar 'reserve' cells, which are also positive for TPA.[5] These 'reserve' cells (in particular, those located at or near the squamocolumnar junction) are primarily involved in the processes of squamous metaplasia, CIN, and carcinoma. The glandular epithelium is immunoreactive for estrogen receptors.[7] In addition to lining the surface, it invaginates into the stroma to produce elongated clefts (usually less than 5 mm deep but sometimes as deep as 1 cm or more), usually referred to as endocervical glands.

The area where the squamous and glandular epithelia meet is known as the *squamocolumnar junction* (Fig. 19.58). It should be noted that this junction is not located in the anatomic external os but rather in the adjacent exocervix, a fact that renders it easily accessible to the colposcope. The portion of endocervical mucosa covering the exocervix is sometimes referred to as *ectropion* and, inaccurately, as *erosion*. This is a very unstable region, in which replacement of one epithelium for another repeatedly occurs, a

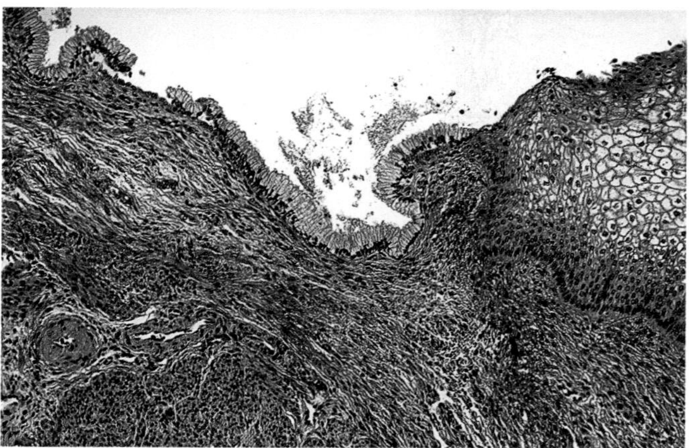

Fig. 19.58 Transition zone of uterine cervix between exocervical squamous cells and endocervical mucin-producing glandular epithelium.

process that Robert Meyer allegorically referred to as 'the fight of the epithelia'. Today, this area is more prosaically known as the *transformation zone*.

Scattered endocrine cells are found in both the normal endocervix and exocervix,[2,9] and melanocytes are occasionally detected along the exocervical basal layer.[8]

The stroma of the cervix is mainly made up of fibrous tissue admixed with elastic fibers and scattered smooth muscle fibers. It has a dominant CD34 immunophenotype, whereas the endometrial stroma has a dominant CD10 phenotype, a difference which may be helpful in determining the site of tumor involvement.[1]

Remnants and ectopias

Mesonephric rests are remnants of the wolffian ducts that are found surrounded by the endocervical stroma in about a third of women. They are composed of tubules lined by a single row of cuboidal cells; they typically contain an inspissated deeply eosinophilic secretion in the lumen (Fig. 19.59). They are immunoreactive for PAX2, a fact potentially useful for their distinction from endocervical adenocarcinoma and other glandular proliferations of the cervix.[16]

Ectopic tissues sometimes found in the cervix include *cutaneous adnexa* (sebaceous glands and hair follicles),[18] *prostatic tissue* (sometimes referred to as 'female prostate'),[14,15,17] and *mature cartilage islands*.[19] The latter (which may be metaplastic rather than ectopic) should not be confused with the cartilaginous component of a mixed müllerian tumor or a botryoid rhabdomyosarcoma.

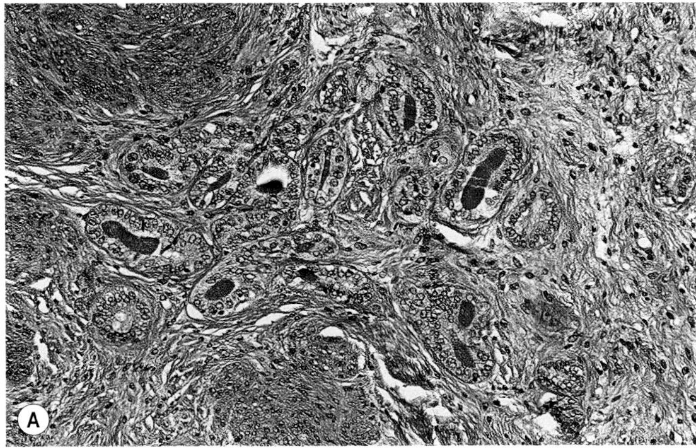

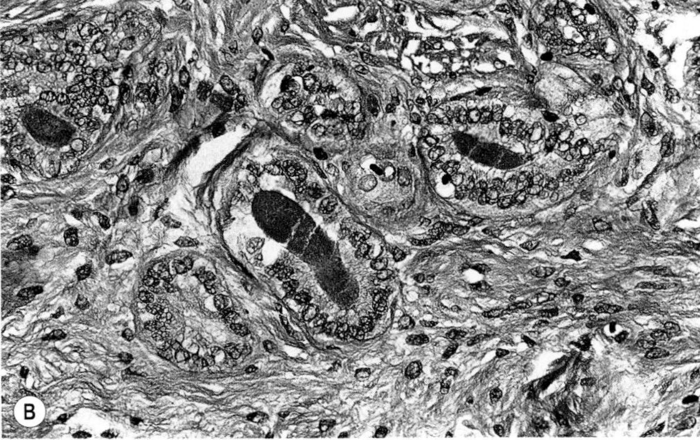

Fig. 19.59 A and **B**, Florid mesonephric rests in endocervix. Note the eosinophilic inspissated secretion in the glandular lumen, an important diagnostic clue.

Squamous and other metaplasias

Various types of metaplastic change of the cervical epithelium occur, their appearance being related to the type of mucosa affected. Squamous metaplasia, by far the most common (to the point that some regard it as a normal finding) is centered on the transformation zone; transitional metaplasia involves the exocervical squamous epithelium; and tubal, tuboendometrial, and intestinal metaplasia affect the glandular epithelium of the endocervix.

The term **squamous metaplasia** is used to designate the focal or extensive replacement of the mucus-secreting glandular epithelium by stratified squamous epithelium, which, in its late stage, is morphologically indistinguishable from the epithelium normally lining the exocervical portion (Fig. 19.60). The pathogenesis of this process, also known as *prosoplasia*, has been a subject of a heated controversy over the years. It is now generally agreed that it most commonly arises on the basis of proliferation and metaplasia of reserve cells. It is possible that in other instances it results from direct ingrowth of mature native squamous epithelium into the endocervical mucosa from the exocervix, possibly as a healing mechanism of a true cervical erosion.[29] Strictly speaking, the latter is not a metaplastic process but rather one of 'squamous epithelialization'. However, it is common usage to employ the term squamous metaplasia regardless of the presumed mechanism for the change.

Some degree of squamous metaplasia is present in almost every uterine cervix during the child-bearing years. Most commonly, the process involves only the superficial epithelium and is recognized by the presence of squamous epithelium overlying endocervical glands. In other instances, it affects the glandular component as well, resulting in a complex microscopic appearance that can

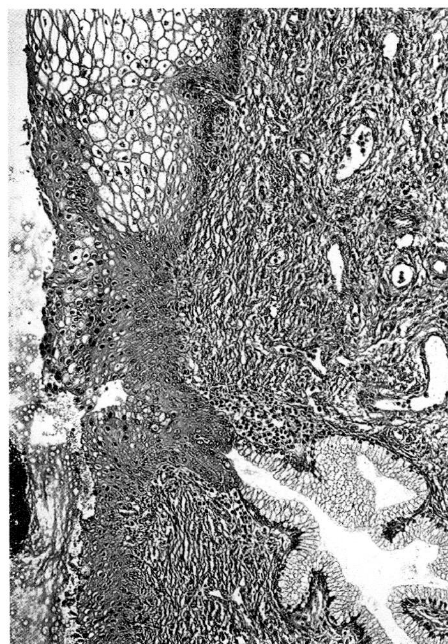

Fig. 19.60 Squamous metaplasia of endocervix involving surface epithelium and glandular openings.

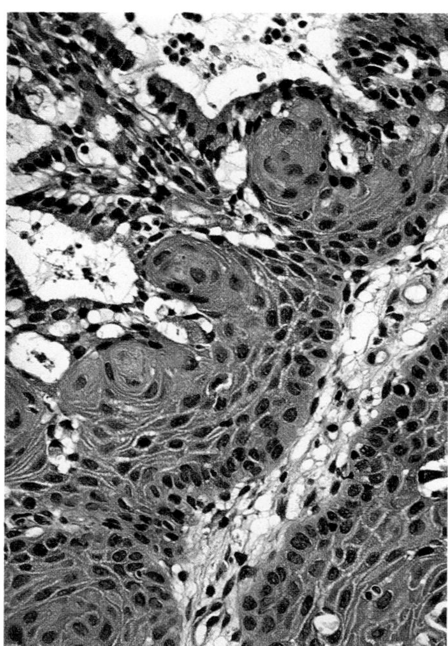

Fig. 19.61 Complex pattern resulting from cervical squamous metaplasia. It may result in an overdiagnosis of squamous cell carcinoma.

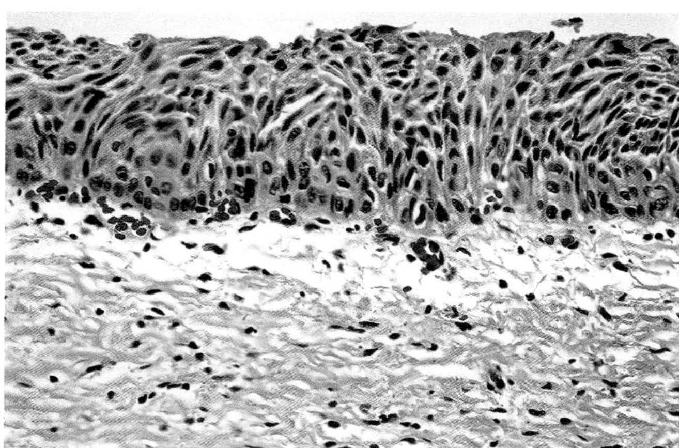

Fig. 19.62 Typical appearance of cervical intraepithelial neoplasia (CIN) III (carcinoma in situ).

be confused with invasive carcinoma by the inexperienced (Fig. 19.61).

Ultrastructural and immunohistochemical markers of squamous epithelium appear *pari passu* with the morphologic changes.[25,42] Variations on this theme, probably representing various stages within a continuum, have been described as *reserve cell hyperplasia* and as *immature, intermediate,* and *mature squamous metaplasia.*[21] A further nuance is *atypical immature metaplasia,* a lesion combining the features of immature metaplasia with some degree of cytologic atypia.[21,26,40] Immunohistochemical and clonality analysis suggest that the latter entity is part of the morphologic spectrum of CIN.[23,33,38]

All of the above changes are characterized by a flat architecture, and are, therefore, different from the condyloma and other papillary processes described on page 1402, including so-called 'papillary immature metaplasia (immature condyloma)'.

Although most cervical carcinomas arise in areas of the cervix that some time in the past had been involved by squamous metaplasia, the latter process has no premalignant connotations per se. Actually, it is so common and insignificant that, unless quite extensive and/or involving the glandular component, we tend to ignore it altogether in our pathology reports.

A somewhat different appearance is seen often in the cervix of prolapsed uteri. The clinical appearance is usually referred to as 'leukoplakic'. Microscopically, the process involves mainly the exocervical portion and is characterized by the appearance of granular and horny layers in the epithelium. This process, which is also unrelated to carcinoma, is best designated as *keratosis*. Sometimes this epithelium contains scattered large pale cells, a change that has been dignified by the term *pagetoid dyskeratosis*.[45]

Transitional metaplasia is seen in the exocervix of older women and it is often associated with atrophy. It morphologically resembles transitional (urothelial) epithelium, and it involves the entire thickness of the mucosa. The nuclei are oval and devoid of atypical features. Their long axes, which are arranged perpendicularly to the surface, often exhibit longitudinal grooves[24,47] (Fig. 19.62). Immunohistochemically, there is positivity for CK13, CK17, and CK18, as in the normal urothelium, but not for CK20.[27] Its phenotypic profile is very similar to that of senile atrophy.[41] This condition has proved controversial, inasmuch as some authorities regard it as nothing less than an atrophic form of CIN.[34] However, the sum of morphologic, cell kinetics, and follow-up data do not support this alternative interpretation.[31,37]

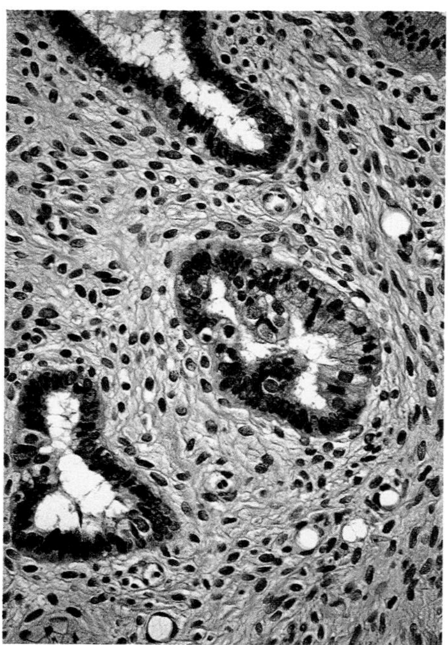

Fig. 19.63 Tubal metaplasia of endocervix. Some of the lining cells are ciliated.

Tubal metaplasia is diagnosed when a specimen from the endocervix (usually from the upper portion) is found to contain all three cell types found in the normal fallopian tube (i.e., ciliated, secretory, and intercalated)[30,44] (Fig. 19.63). In many instances, the

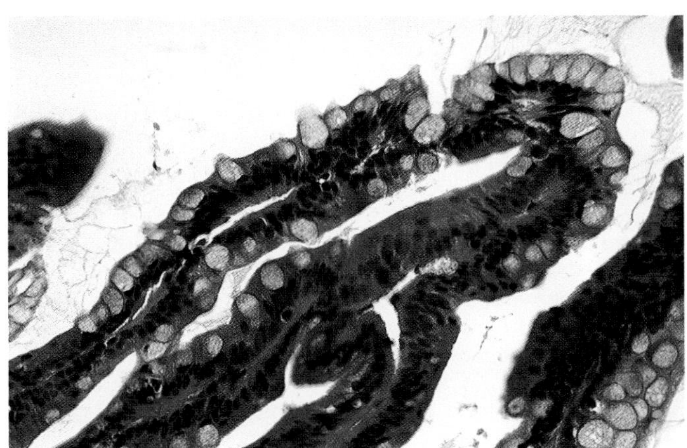

Fig. 19.64 Intestinal metaplasia of cervix. There are numerous goblet cells. This is a very unusual finding.

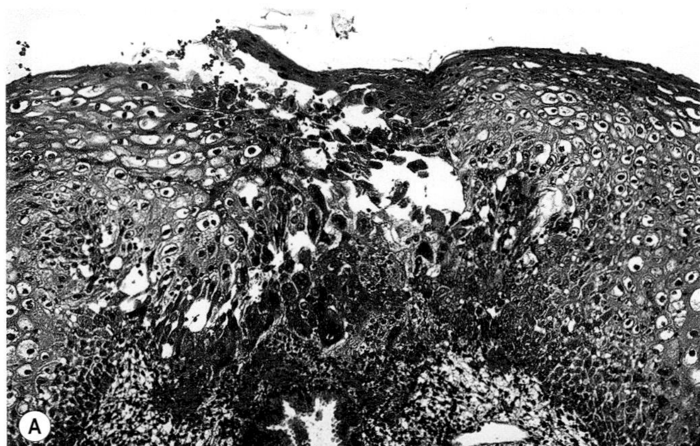

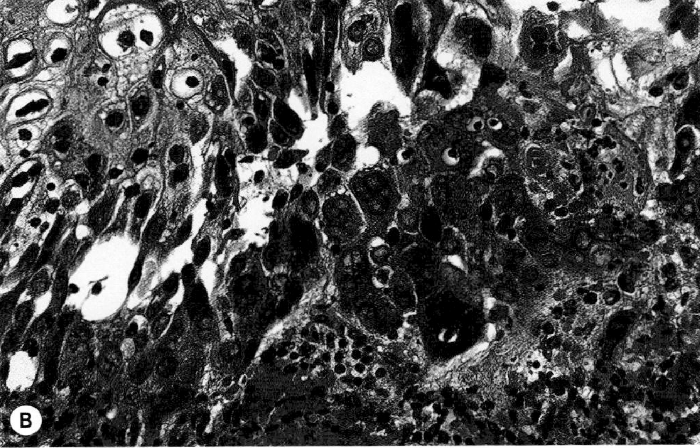

Fig. 19.65 A and B, Low- and high-power appearance of herpes simplex infection of cervix. Multinucleated epithelial cells and intranuclear inclusions are evident in the high-power view.

appearance of the metaplastic epithelium combines features of tubal and endometrial mucosa, in which case the term *tuboendometrial* (*tuboendometrioid*) *metaplasia* is employed.[20,36,48] Diagnostic difficulties may result from the fact that these glands may be deeply seated, irregularly shaped, cystically dilated, and/or accompanied by a hypercellular, edematous, or myxoid stroma.[39] The condition can be identified in cytologic preparations.[22]

Combined staining for MIB-1(Ki-67) and P16^{INK4a} is said to be of help in the differential diagnosis from in-situ and invasive endocervical adenocarcinoma.[36,43] Tubal metaplasia is often found after conization, and it has therefore been suggested that it represents aberrant differentiation following injury.[28] A *pseudoinvasive* form of the condition has been described in women with a history of in utero diethylstilbestrol (DES) exposure, suggesting that it may be a form of DES-related adenosis.[46]

Intestinal metaplasia is a much rarer condition, which may be accompanied by extravasation of mucin into the stroma[49] (Fig. 19.64).

Atypical oxyphilic (eosinophilic) metaplasia is characterized by the presence of large cuboidal or polygonal epithelial cells with dense eosinophilic, focally vacuolated cytoplasm and variable nuclear atypia in the endocervical glands.[32,35] The nature of this condition remains controversial, some observers favoring the interpretation that it is a combination of metaplasia and CIN.[35]

Inflammatory lesions

Chronic cervicitis is an extremely common condition in adult females, at least at the microscopic level. It affects preferentially the squamocolumnar junction and endocervix, and it may be accompanied by hyperemia, edema, fibrosis, and metaplastic changes in the epithelium. The etiology is variable.[64] In most cases the disease is asymptomatic, but it is of importance because it may lead to endometritis, salpingitis, and 'pelvic inflammatory disease' through ascending intraluminal spread, chorioamnionitis, and other complications during pregnancy, and it may also play a role in the initiation or promotion of cervical neoplasia.

Herpes simplex infection of the cervix is now recognized as a relatively common occurrence. The microscopic appearance at the time of biopsy is usually that of an intense nonspecific inflammation with ulceration (Fig. 19.65A). Only rarely are diagnostic multinucleated squamous cells with intranuclear inclusions encountered[63] (Fig. 19.65B). The diagnosis can be confirmed by immunocytochemical demonstration of the viral antigen.[50,61]

***Chlamydia trachomatis* infection** is now recognized as the most common venereal disease in the Western world. The microscopic appearance in the cervix is that of a chronic nonspecific inflammation, with reactive epithelial atypia and sometimes prominent formation of lymphoid follicles.[59,67] The organisms are not visible in routine histologic slides and only with difficulty in cytologic preparations, but they can be detected by immunocytochemical techniques.[67] Culture isolation is regarded as the standard for diagnosis of active infection. Chlamydial cervicitis can be associated with CIN, but there is no evidence of a causal relationship.[62]

Syphilis can affect the cervix, usually in the form of a primary chancre.[66]

Amebiasis may produce a polypoid and ulcerated mass in the cervix clinically simulating carcinoma, and it may also engraft itself upon a preexisting cervical carcinoma.[51,57]

Actinomycosis of the cervix occurs, but it needs to be distinguished from the more common pseudoactinomycotic radiate granules that may form around microorganisms or biologically inert substances.[55]

Bilharziasis (schistosomiasis), common in Africa and Central America, can involve any portion of the female genital tract, including the cervix.[54]

Malakoplakia occurs rarely in the cervix, sometimes in association with disease in the uterine corpus, renal pelvis, or kidney.[56]

Ceroid granuloma of the type more commonly seen in the gallbladder has, exceptionally, been found to involve the cervix.[52,65]

Localized arteritis of the cervix has been described, accompanied by inflammation and ulceration, and apparently restricted to this anatomic site.[58,60] The cervix can also be involved in cases of **Wegener granulomatosis.**[53]

Non-neoplastic glandular lesions

Endocervical polyps are not true neoplasms but probably the result of chronic inflammatory changes ('chronic polypoid cervicitis'). They are usually small but may reach several centimeters in diameter. Microscopically, dilated endocervical glands are seen in an edematous, inflamed, and fibrotic stroma. The surface epithelium usually shows squamous metaplasia. Interestingly, the foci of squamous metaplasia are often immunoreactive for p16, a possible source of overdiagnosis.[71] CIN can develop from these polyps but not more so than in the cervix as a whole. Occasionally, the configuration of these polyps is that of a branching papillary structure, in which case the term *papillary endocervicitis* is employed[99] (Fig. 19.66). This lesion is to be distinguished from so-called 'superficial cervicovaginal myofibroblastoma', which is equally benign and perhaps histogenetically related.[83] Exceptionally, cells with the morphology of signet ring cells are seen beneath an ulcerated endocervical polyp; they are probably the result of ischemia and should not be overdiagnosed as signet ring cell carcinoma.[89]

Nabothian cysts are thought to develop from blockage of the endocervical glands secondarily to inflammation and associated changes; they appear grossly as cystic spaces filled with mucoid material and microscopically as cystically dilated glands lined by a flattened epithelium, sometimes focally absent. Occasionally they extend deeply into the cervical wall, a phenomenon that should not be mistaken for malignancy.[69]

Tunnel clusters, as originally described by Fluhmann, are the result of localized proliferation of endocervical glands (clefts), with side channels growing out from them. This may be accompanied by dilation resulting from the accumulation of inspissated, deeply eosinophilic secretion in the lumen[93] (Fig. 19.67). Tunnel clusters have been divided into *type A* (*noncystic*) and *type B* (*cystic*). Sometimes the former are accompanied by a florid glandular proliferation and a certain degree of atypia. However, they retain a lobular configuration and mitotic activity is practically nil.[77] Interestingly, type A tunnel clusters have been found to secrete gastric-type mucins.[81]

Microglandular hyperplasia of the endocervical epithelium was originally described in women using oral contraceptive drugs and, less frequently, during pregnancy.[82,97] However, it can also be seen in the absence of these conditions and even in postmenopausal patients.[68] As a matter of fact, the very relationship between microglandular hyperplasia and oral contraception or other hormonal perturbations has been questioned.[73] Microscopically, the typical case is characterized by a complex proliferation of small glands lined by flat epithelial cells with little or no atypia (Fig. 19.68). The condition usually evolves into squamous metaplasia, resulting in a complex microscopic picture that may be confused with carcinoma. Additional features that may lead to overdiagnosis include areas of solid proliferation, pseudoinfiltrative pattern, signet ring cells, focal atypia, and occasional mitotic figures[100] (Fig. 19.69). The intervening stroma invariably shows chronic inflammation. There is usually no immunocytochemical reactivity for carcinoembryonic antigen (CEA), a useful feature in the differential diagnosis with endocervical adenocarcinoma.[96]

The **Arias-Stella reaction,** as seen during pregnancy, can involve the endocervical glands. The nuclear abnormalities are similar to those seen more commonly in the endometrial mucosa and should not be confused with malignancy.[70,86,90] The microscopic appearance is quite variable, and includes cells with vacuolated clear cytoplasm, intraglandular tufts, hobnail cells, oxyphilic cytoplasm, filiform papillae, nuclear pseudoinclusions, and cribriform intraglandular growth.[88] In contrast to clear cell carcinoma, the Arias-Stella reaction does not form a mass lesion, lacks a desmoplastic stromal response, and does not have an infiltrative pattern.[88]

Atypical reactive proliferation of the endocervical mucosal surface can be seen following endometrial sampling for endometrial carcinoma or other diseases. It shows nuclear stratification, short micropapillary processes, squamous metaplasia, hobnail cells, and mild cytologic atypia, i.e., many of the features that are associated with microglandular hyperplasia. It should not be

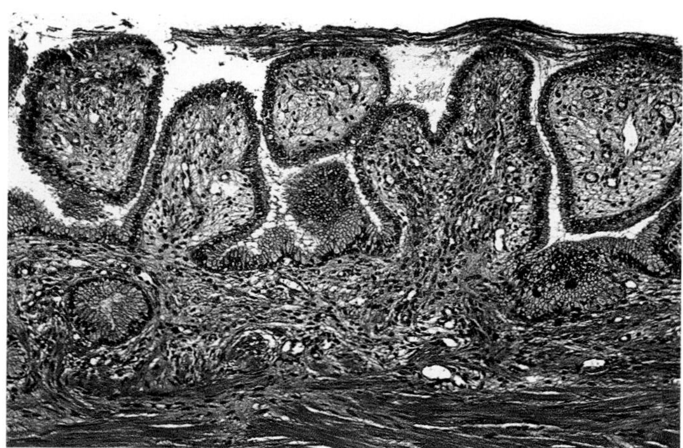

Fig. 19.66 Chronic endocervicitis resulting in a papillary configuration at the surface. This pattern is sometimes referred to as papillary endocervicitis.

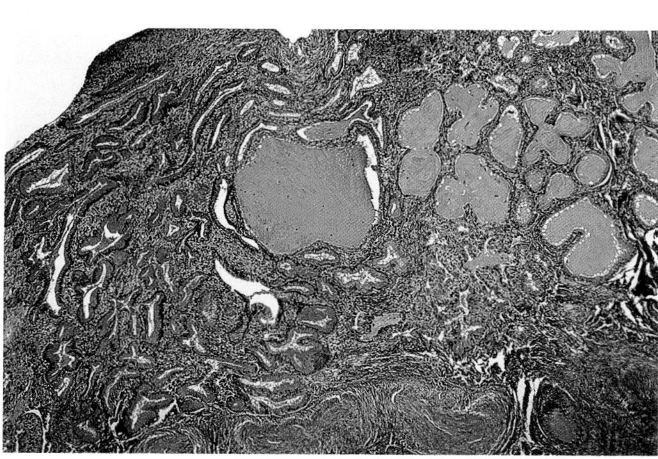

Fig. 19.67 Cervical tunnel clusters of predominantly cystic type.

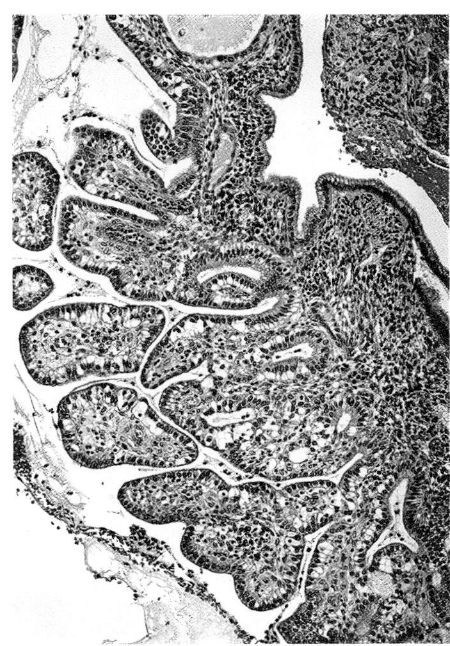

Fig. 19.68 Microglandular adenosis of cervix. The papillary configuration seen here is common in this condition.

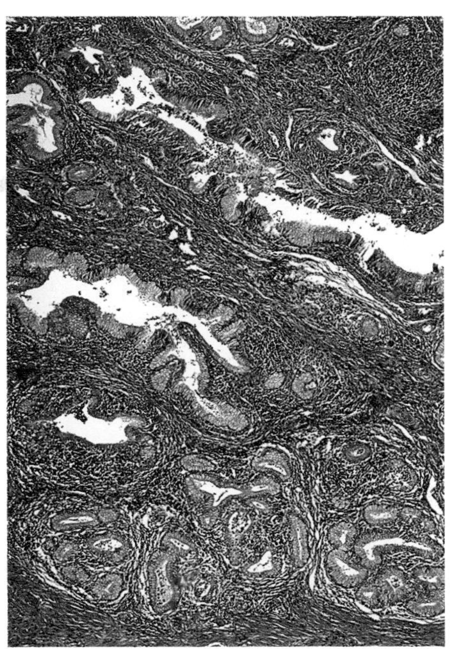

Fig. 19.70 Diffuse laminar endocervical hyperplasia. The glands are medium sized, evenly spaced, and well differentiated.

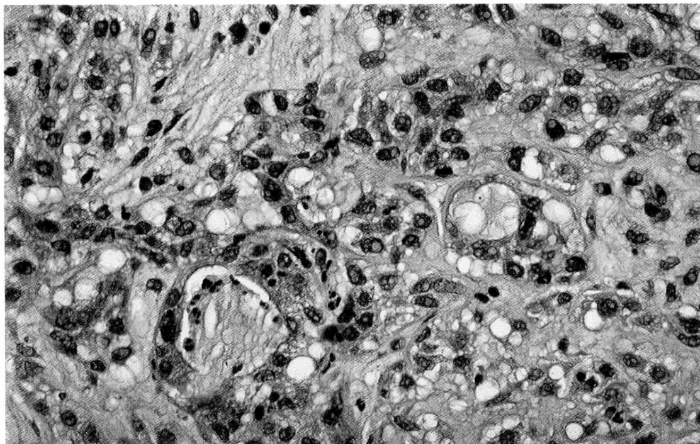

Fig. 19.69 Predominantly solid form of microglandular adenosis. This variety is particularly likely to be overdiagnosed as a malignant process.

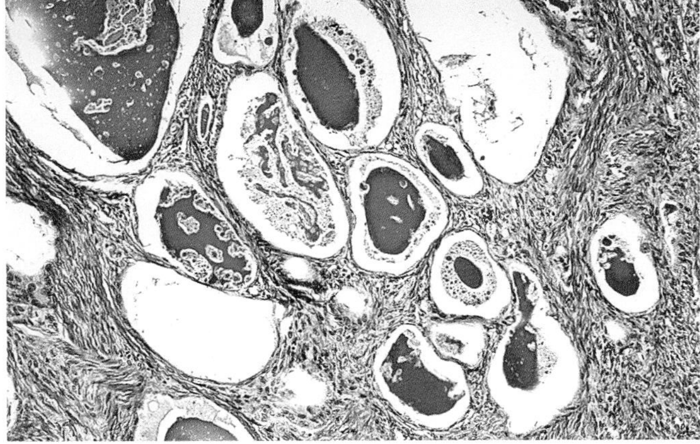

Fig. 19.71 Mesonephric glands embedded within the stroma of the uterine cervix exhibiting cystic dilation. The presence of a dense eosinophilic secretion is characteristic.

interpreted as endocervical involvement by an endometrial carcinoma.[92]

Diffuse laminar endocervical glandular hyperplasia (DLEGH) is a non-neoplastic condition characterized by a proliferation of medium-sized, evenly spaced, well-differentiated glands within the inner third of the cervical wall, sharply separated from the underlying stroma, and often accompanied by chronic inflammation[78] (Fig. 19.70); it should not be confused with adenoma malignum, from which it is distinguishable because of the fact that stromal infiltration, desmoplastic stromal response, and cytologic atypia are absent.[86]

Lobular endocervical glandular hyperplasia (LEGH) is characterized by a distinctly lobular proliferation of small to medium-sized glands, often centered around a larger central gland.[87] The mucin secreted by some of these lesions is of gastric type.[80] In contrast to adenoma malignum, LEGH lacks irregular stromal infiltration, desmoplastic stromal response, and significant cytologic atypia. Interestingly, the phenotype of this process is similar to that of pyloric glands.[84] Nevertheless, a possible pathogenetic relationship between the two conditions (and with other mucinous adenocarcinomas of the cervix) has been suggested on the basis of some immunohistochemical and molecular genetic similarities,[79,85] as well as their occasional association.[80,98]

Mesonephric duct rests (already mentioned on p. 1437) can undergo cystic dilation or be affected by florid and even atypical hyperplastic changes[74,76,94] (Fig. 19.71). This hyperplasia may have

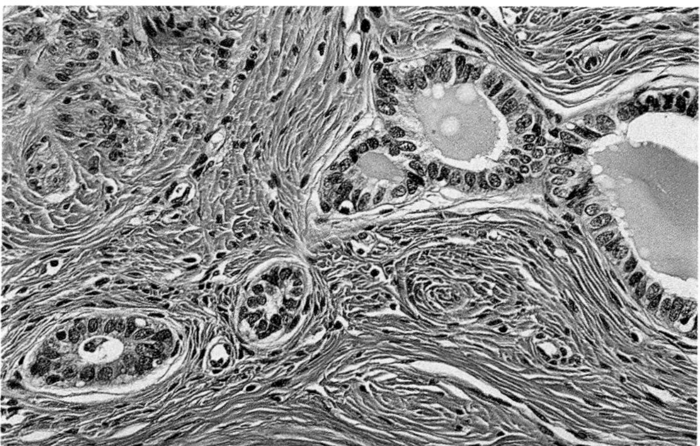

Fig. 19.72 Hyperplastic mesonephric rests with mild atypia.

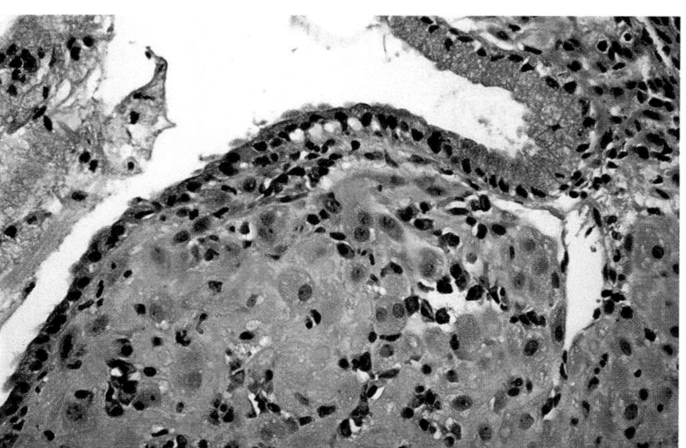

Fig. 19.73 Focus of ectopic cervical decidual reaction.

a lobular, diffuse, or ductal pattern[72] (Fig. 19.72). Rare malignant tumors arising from these structures also occur (see p. 1456). Mesonephric remnants are also rarely involved by CIN.[91]

It is doubtful whether the rare benign polypoid lesion found in the cervix and vagina of young children and described as *mesonephric papilloma* is related to these remnants.[75,95] Microscopically, it is a superficially located lesion composed of delicate connective tissue stalks covered by a layer of cuboidal cells and is probably of müllerian derivation (see also under Vagina).

Non-neoplastic stromal lesions (including endometriosis and related processes)

Multinucleated stromal giant cells can be present beneath the cervical epithelium and be mistaken for a malignancy. They are often accompanied by edema and may result in a vaguely polypoid-appearing lesion.[103,106] These cells are of a reactive fibroblastic/myofibroblastic nature and analogous to those seen in other sites covered by mucosal membranes, such as vulva, vagina, anus, oral cavity, and nasal cavity.[101,109]

Decidual reaction in the cervix during pregnancy usually presents as multiple, small, yellowish or red elevations of the cervical mucosa. They are soft and friable and bleed easily with trauma. Rarely, they develop into fungating masses difficult to distinguish grossly from carcinoma.[104] Microscopically, the decidual cells are characterized by abundant pale granular cytoplasm and bland nuclei (Fig. 19.73). Immunostains for keratin are negative.

Placental site nodule appears as a well-defined hyalinized lesion located immediately beneath the mucosa.[113] It is composed of intermediate trophoblasts exhibiting cytoplasmic vacuolization.[110,115] Some nuclear atypia may be present. This lesion can be confused with carcinoma and with neoplastic cartilage. Immunohistochemically, the trophoblastic cells are reactive for keratin (another factor that may lead to a mistaken diagnosis of malignancy) but also for human placental lactogen (see p. 1645).

Endometriosis of the cervix presents as blue or reddish nodules and may result in abnormal uterine bleeding. Both endometrial glands and stroma are needed to establish the diagnosis. However, the proportion of the two components may vary greatly from case to case. On occasion, the process is composed almost exclusively of endometrial stroma ('stromal endometriosis') and may be confused with a neoplasm.[105] Another source of confusion arises when the endometriosis is superficial, in which case it may be overinterpreted as endocervical glandular dysplasia or adenocarcinoma in situ, one of the reasons being that it may be mitotically active.[102] It differs from tuboendometrial metaplasia of the endocervix because of the concomitant presence of endometrial-type stroma, however scarce. A lesion with an appearance resembling a miniature uterus in the cervix ('uterus-like mass') has been interpreted as a form of superficial endometriosis with florid smooth muscle metaplasia.[108] A bizarre variation on the theme is represented by **endocervicosis**, which can present as a deep-seated cervical mass simulating endocervical adenocarcinoma.[114]

Necrobiotic granulomas resembling tuberculosis or rheumatoid nodules have been seen following cervical surgery.[107] They are probably histologically and pathogenetically analogous to those described postoperatively in the prostate (see Chapter 18).

Florid mesenchymal reactions can develop from the cervical stroma as a result of various surgical interventions and lead to confusion with sarcoma.[111] Some of these have a nodular fasciitis-like appearance and may be looked upon as the genitourinary equivalent of this soft tissue lesion.

Myxoid changes of probable degenerative nature can sometimes be seen in the cervical stroma (and in the myometrium) in the absence of any other pathology.[112]

Human papilloma virus (HPV) and the lower female genital tract

HPV has been linked to many types of cervical disease, ranging from the relatively innocuous condyloma acuminatum (see p. 1443) to the sometimes fatal invasive squamous cell carcinoma.[129,150,169] Notably, cervical cancer is unique among human cancers by being the first found to be virtually solely attributable to the effects of an infectious agent.[171] HPV comprises a family of DNA viruses, of which more than 60 types have been characterized, the most common being types 6 and 11. It can be detected by electron microscopy (as intranuclear crystalline and occasionally filamentous inclusions), but its specific identification depends on immunohistochemical or molecular virologic analysis with in situ or Southern blot hybridization.[132,141,156,160,179] The latter test is currently regarded as the 'gold standard' for the detection of HPV. The main competitor is the Hybrid Capture HPV test, a signal-amplified hybridization

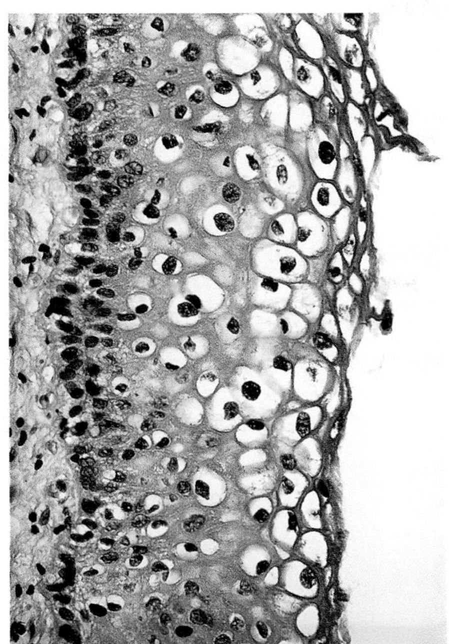

Fig. 19.74 Koilocytotic changes in cervical squamous epithelium. These are diagnostic of HPV infection.

microplate-based array designed to detect close to 20 HPV genotypes using two probe cocktails for high-risk and low-risk groups, respectively (see below).[140]

HPV infection of the cervix is transmitted venereally, and it has a predilection for the metaplastic squamous epithelium. It may remain dormant for long periods or become productive, with release of infectious virus in the terminally differentiated squamous epithelium.

The morphologic hallmark of HPV infection of the cervical squamous epithelium (as first described by two Finnish workers, Esco Purola and Eeva Savia) is *koilocytosis*, also known as *koilocytotic atypia* (two terms coined by Leopold Koss and Grace Durfee). This change is thought to be related to expression of the viral E4 protein and the disruption that this causes in the cytoplasmic keratin matrix. The koilocyte is a superficial or intermediate mature squamous cell characterized by a sharply outlined perinuclear vacuolation, dense- and irregular-staining peripheral cytoplasm, and an enlarged nucleus with an undulating (raisin- or prune-like) nuclear membrane and a rope-like chromatin pattern[146] (Fig. 19.74). Binucleation and multinucleation can occur.[161] It is important that these nuclear changes – which may be accompanied by either a diploid or polyploid nuclear DNA distribution[173] – be present somewhere in the lesion for the diagnosis of koilocytosis (and, by inference, HPV infection) to be made, or else other forms of cytoplasmic clearing (notably those related to glycogen accumulation) will be mistakenly included in this category.[151,174] This is particularly the case for the condition known as *postmenopausal squamous atypia*, in which perinuclear halos can be very prominent.[142] Indeed, there is evidence that the overdiagnosis of HPV infection on the basis of the microscopic appearance of cervical biopsies is frequently made.[116] This is not to imply that HPV infection does not occur in the absence of koilocytosis, because it certainly does. Sometimes, the only abnormality seen in HPV-infected cells is nuclear enlargement, and occasionally there are no detectable changes at all.[126,157,178]

The most difficult and clinically significant problem that these HPV-induced cervical lesions pose is in relation to the differential diagnosis, coexistence, and possible causation of CIN and invasive carcinoma.[118,119,128,135,177] It seems obvious, in retrospect, that many cases diagnosed in the past as mild or moderate dysplasia (CIN I and II) would now be reported as HPV-induced koilocytotic atypia.[121] It has also become apparent that HPV-associated lesions are often seen together with (or preceding those of) CIN or, sometimes, invasive cervical carcinoma.[153,158] Actually, the high frequency of this association on a worldwide basis,[122] the topographic continuity between the two processes,[164] and the respective age distributions of the affected populations[130] all suggest an underlying dependence and perhaps a continuum between the two.[139,168] This concordance is not apparent between cervical carcinoma and other infections of the cervix.[123] The association between HPV and cervical neoplasia is particularly strong for squamous cell tumors, but it has also been documented for both in situ and invasive adenocarcinoma[127,133,134,147] and for adenosquamous carcinoma.[144] The HPV proteins E6 and E7 are thought to play an important role in this process by their interaction with the P53 protein and the RB-susceptibility gene product, respectively.[125,159,169]

Following the realization that koilocytotic atypia equals HPV infection, an attitude took hold in some quarters that the presence of this change in a cervical biopsy was indicative of a benign process. This is not necessarily the case. These biopsies should be evaluated according to the standard criteria applied to CIN. The added presence of the HPV-associated component should be mentioned in the diagnosis but should not modify the diagnostic or clinical approach toward them.[143]

The features in a cervical biopsy exhibiting the signs of HPV infection that indicate the additional presence of CIN are the presence of atypia along the basal layers, a disorderly pattern of maturation, and abnormal mitotic figures.[176,180] A definite association exists between high-degree atypia (CIN III), an aneuploid DNA pattern, P53 overexpression, and the presence of HPV type 16.[131,136,137,170] Along similar lines, the presence of the HPV-16 genome has been documented in most invasive cervical carcinomas and in histologically normal neighboring epithelium.[149]

Currently, HPVs are divided into major categories depending on their level of association with CIN and invasive squamous cell carcinoma. The 'high-risk' ('carcinogenic') types are primarily 16 and 18, but also 31, 33, 35, 39, 45, 51, 52, 56, 58, 59, 68, 73, and 82. HPV types 26, 53, and 66 have been classified as 'probably high-risk', and HPV types 6, 11, 40, 42, 43, 44, 54, 61, 70, 72, 81, and CP6108 are included in the 'low-risk category'.[155] In a recent massive evaluation of the distribution of HPV types in invasive cervical carcinoma, HPV types 16, 18, 31, 33, and 45 were found the most common types all around the world, accounting for 85% of all the cases.[148] There is a statistically significant association between HPV genotype and histologic type: HPV-16 is closely associated with keratinizing carcinoma, while nonkeratinizing cancers are more heterogeneous.[181] Typing of the viral strain is now being used together with cytology for cervical screening,[138,167] and there is great hope that the various HPV vaccines currently being tried will have a considerable impact on the incidence of the disease.[124,145,166] It is of interest that the probability of finding direct evidence of HPV infection in cervical squamous intraepithelial lesions decreases proportionally to the degree of atypia, reaching low levels in CIN III.[120,163] These findings have been explained by postulating that an intact squamous epithelium is needed for virus replication.

It should be mentioned here that Epstein–Barr virus (EBV), often present in cervical carcinoma and once thought to be of importance in its genesis, is not currently believed to play a causative role.[165]

Condyloma acuminatum is a grossly polypoid lesion characterized microscopically by papillomatosis, acanthosis, koilocytosis, and a variable degree of inflammatory infiltration of the stroma. An

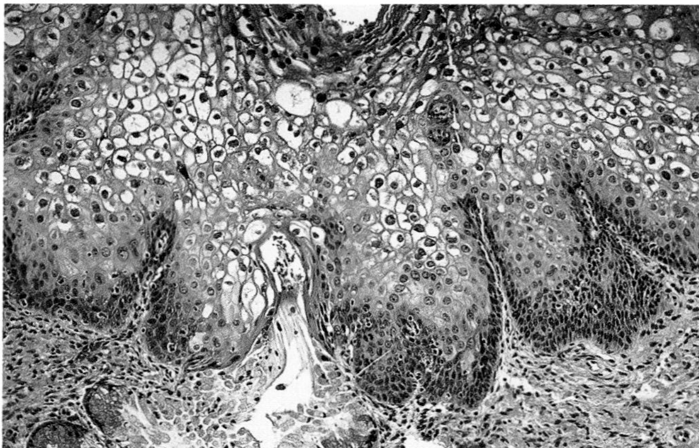

Fig. 19.75 HPV-induced cervical lesion characterized by acanthosis, papillomatosis, and koilocytotic changes.

undulating appearance of the epithelium is a characteristic feature on low-power examination. A mild degree of atypia in the squamous component is common and need not be mentioned; if more severe, it should be evaluated and graded as for the flat squamous intraepithelial lesions (i.e., condyloma with CIN II or III).

Condyloma acuminatum is an HPV-induced lesion (see p. 1442); HPV-6 and HPV-11 are found in 70–90% of the cases, but occasionally other types – such as HPV-16 – are encountered. When the latter is the case, high-grade cytologic atypia is often found.

Other morphologic manifestations of HPV infection of the cervix (which are actually much more common than condyloma acuminatum) include lesions variously described as *flat, spiked,* and *inverted condyloma* and *warty atypia.*[175] Many HPV infections are clinically inapparent. Microscopically, these clinically different lesions share the following features: relatively normal basal cell layer, expanded or hyperplastic parabasal cell layer, orderly maturation, mitotic activity (but few or no abnormal mitoses), and koilocytosis (Fig. 19.75). The proliferation rate of condyloma is higher than that of inflamed or metaplastic cervical squamous epithelium,[154] and is particularly elevated in the presence of high-risk HPV types.[152]

Immature condyloma (papillary immature metaplasia) is the name given to a lesion with a cellular composition similar to immature squamous metaplasia (see p. 1402) but having a filiform papillary configuration.[172] It is believed to be produced by HPV-6 or -11 infection.

Squamous papilloma is a polypoid lesion composed of a fibrovascular stalk covered by mature squamous epithelium. It has also been designated as fibroepithelial papilloma, fibroepithelioma, and ectocervical polyp. Microscopically, the lack of an arborizing pattern and – most important – the absence of koilocytotic changes distinguish this lesion from condyloma acuminatum. The nature of this process is not clear; in at least some instances, squamous papilloma probably represents condyloma in which the recognizable morphologic changes of HPV infection have subsided. The differential diagnosis also includes the papillary form of CIN (in which case the atypical changes present in the epithelium of the polypoid lesion are also seen in the adjacent flat epithelium),[162] verrucous carcinoma (see p. 1451), and well-differentiated squamous cell carcinoma (see p. 1447).

Inverted transitional cell (urothelial) papilloma, similar to its more common bladder counterpart, has been described in the cervix.[117] It is probably not related to HPV and is included here only because it enters into the differential diagnosis with the other polypoid benign lesions of this region.

Tumors

Cervical intraepithelial neoplasia (CIN)

The terminology of cervical intraepithelial lesions composed of squamous epithelium and thought to represent the precursors of invasive carcinoma has evolved over the years and continues changing today. The concept is of great practical and historical importance, since it represents the main model on which the theory of the existence of morphologically identifiable precursor lesions of cancer has been built (a general model that, one should add, has found strong support from molecular studies).[253] The basic premises are the following:

1. Nearly all invasive cervical carcinomas are preceded by a stage in which the abnormal cells are confined to the epithelium (intraepithelial stage).[212]
2. These intraepithelial lesions share many of the cytologic features of the invasive stage, mainly manifested by enlargement, irregularities, and hyperchromasia of the nuclei; increase in mitotic activity; and alteration of the maturation pattern. There is also a diminution or absence of cytoplasmic glycogen, this being the reason for the decrease or lack of staining in the iodine (Lugol or Schiller) test.
3. A continuous range of morphologic abnormalities exists among these lesions, which provide a rough indication of the likelihood with which they will evolve into invasive carcinoma if left untreated.[235] These morphologic abnormalities correlate with immunohistochemical cytogenetic, DNA ploidy, cell proliferation, and molecular changes.[195,198,226,257,260] For instance, autoradiographic studies have shown a continuum in the proportion of cells in DNA synthesis, their number paralleling the degree of atypia.[249] Low-grade lesions usually have a euploid or polyploid pattern, whereas high-grade lesions are generally aneuploid.[188,238,245] A similar relationship has been found among morphologic aberrations and proliferating cell nuclear antigen (PCNA),[230,254] nucleolar organizer region,[218,261] and aberrant expression of various keratins,[255,256] P53 protein,[183,204,242] P16^{INK4a} expression,[182,214] and *RAS* oncogene.[250] The available evidence suggests the existence of a sequence of events that in some cases leads to progression to a full-blown invasive malignancy but in others stops at a given stage or possibly regresses altogether. The often held assumption that the most severe forms will *inevitably* lead to invasive carcinoma is unproven and probably unprovable.[219,232] The milder forms are particularly unstable and tend to regress spontaneously[201,247] (although perhaps not as often if they have marked cytologic atypia[236]). In one oft-quoted study, follow-up evaluation after conservative therapy showed regression in 62% of the cases, persistence in 22%, and progression to a more severe lesion in 16%.[233] The more severe lesions regress less frequently and may persist for long periods. In a classic study, Petersen[239] studied the course of 127 untreated patients with such severe lesions. Invasive carcinoma had developed in 11% at the end of 3 years, in 22% at the end of 5 years, and in 33% at the end of 9 years.
4. In the large majority of cases, the process does not affect the native squamous epithelium of the exocervix but rather areas of squamous metaplasia located at the transformation zone and in its endocervical side.[210] It practically always involves

the surface epithelium, as well as the glandular elements, but by definition shows no stromal invasion. It often ends abruptly, and its extent is highly variable. Occasionally it seems to consist of only a minute focus on the epithelial surface or in an endocervical polyp removable by a simple biopsy or polypectomy;[192] more commonly, it involves large areas of the cervix. Extension up the endocervical canal is particularly common,[206] but it may also grow along the portio and upper vagina[200,243,259] or extend into mesonephric remnants.[252] In exceptional instances, it has been seen to extend into the vagina to the introitus or into the endometrial cavity and even the fallopian tubes.[215,240,251] Sometimes, the intraepithelial change as seen in a cervical biopsy represents only the peripheral manifestation of a more proximally located invasive carcinoma that is diagnosed only by endocervical curettage.

5 The microscopic criteria for the diagnosis of these lesions should be the same regardless of the circumstances. This is true if they are found in the pregnant woman; such changes do not routinely regress postpartum, despite early statements to the contrary. It is also true if they are found following treatment of invasive squamous cell carcinoma with radiation therapy, a change found in approximately one-fourth of the patients and sometimes referred to as **postirradiation atypia or dysplasia**.[224] The available evidence suggests that this is not merely a reaction of a previously normal epithelium to the radiation but rather the expression of a basically abnormal mucosa. Indeed, postirradiation dysplasia appearing within 3 years after treatment is associated with poor prognosis.[264]

6 In a small minority of cases, CIN coexists with adenocarcinoma in situ. That percentage seems to be much higher in cases of CIN with low P53 and RB protein expression.[223]

All of the previously listed basic tenets have been accepted, the current controversy centering on the number of recognizable steps within that range (2, 3, or 4) and the best terminology to use for them (Figs 19.76–19.80).

The classic approach, unchallenged for half a century, has been that of designating these lesions as either dysplasia or carcinoma in situ. The term *dysplasia* was used when the atypical cytologic features mentioned were accompanied by a partial retention of the normal maturation pattern and a preservation of the organization of the basal layer.[193,203] By contrast, the term *carcinoma in situ* was employed when there was no differentiation at any level (despite some occasional flattening of the surface cells) and the basal cell was disorganized.[217,221,244] Dysplasia was further subdivided into mild, moderate, and severe, depending on the severity of the changes. Carcinoma in

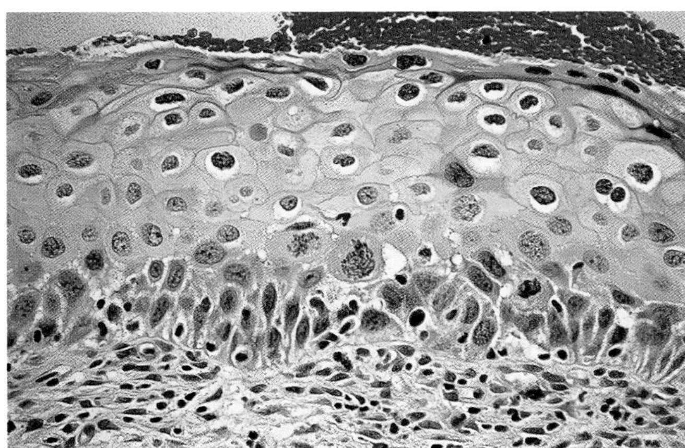

Fig. 19.77 CIN I accompanied by koilocytotic atypia.

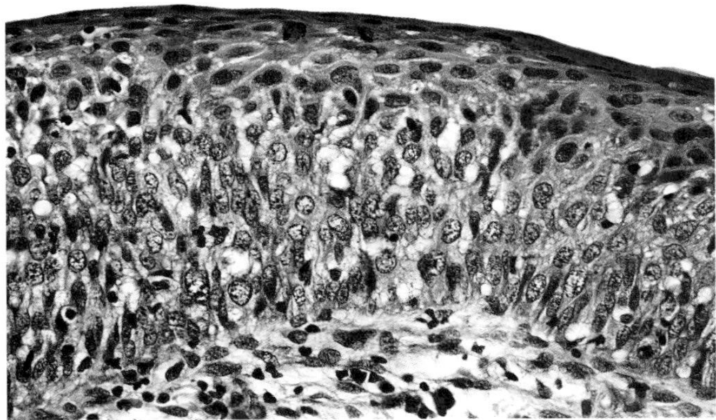

Fig. 19.78 CIN II (moderate dysplasia). There is proliferation and atypia in the lower two-thirds, but some surface maturation is still apparent.

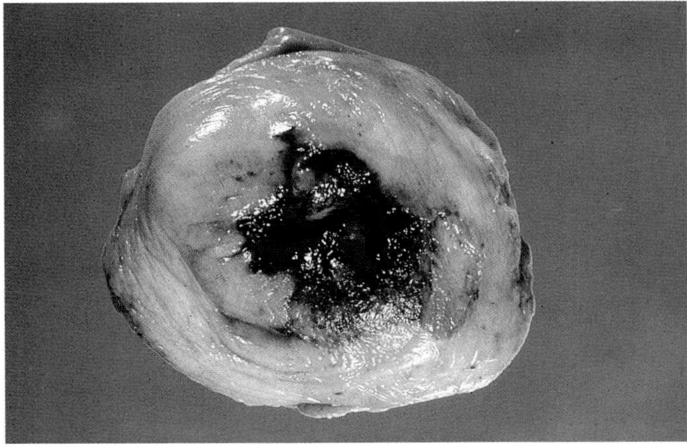

Fig. 19.76 Gross appearance of carcinoma in situ (CIN III) extensively involving the uterine cervix.
(Courtesy of Dr Hector Rodriguez-Martinez, Mexico City)

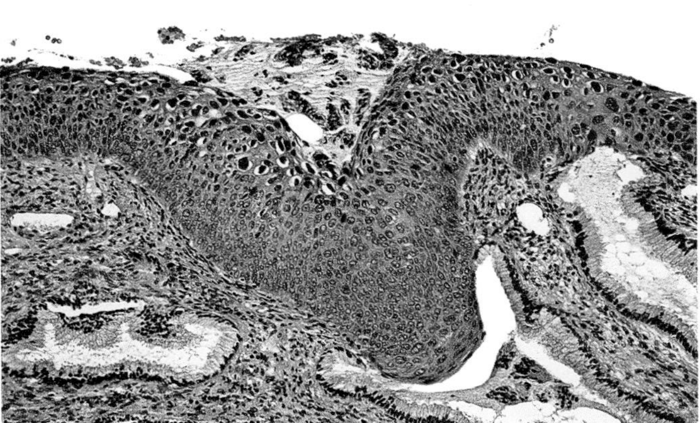

Fig. 19.79 Extensive involvement by CIN III of surface epithelium and glands of endocervix.

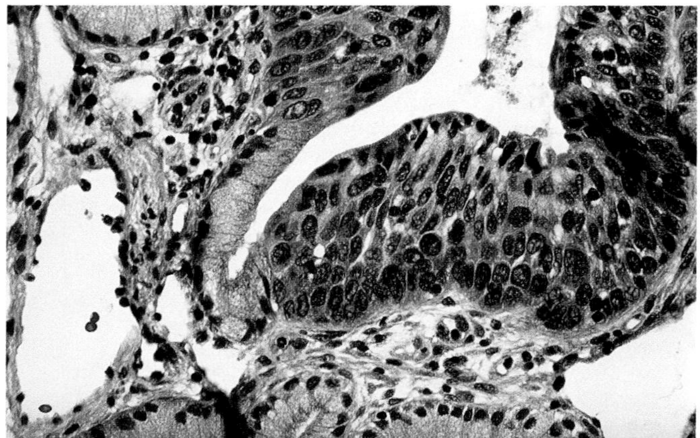

Fig. 19.80 Partial replacement of endocervical glandular epithelium by CIN III.

situ was further subdivided by some authors into parabasal cell (51%), keratinizing cell (37%), pleomorphic cell (3%), and small cell (1.5%) types.[262]

Most of the seminal studies documenting the relationship between these changes and the development of invasive carcinoma have been done using this terminology, which, however, came under attack on the grounds that it implies a significant biologic difference between dysplasia and carcinoma in situ that probably does not exist and also because it may lead to a radically different approach to therapy (i.e., follow-up with cytologic studies in the case of dysplasia as opposed to surgical therapy for carcinoma in situ), which does not seem justified.[253] That the difference between severe dysplasia and carcinoma in situ is based on rather subtle and subjective criteria, and that these criteria vary according to the individual pathologist and institution, has been repeatedly proved.[205,208,211]

In the hope of eliminating at least some of these problems, the alternative term *cervical intraepithelial neoplasia* (CIN) was proposed, with a subdivision into four grades, later cut down to three: CIN I as the equivalent of mild dysplasia, CIN II of moderate dysplasia, and CIN III of severe dysplasia and carcinoma in situ.[245] When it seemed as if this terminology was finally on its way to replacing that of dysplasia/carcinoma in situ,[189,194,207,258] a new one was proposed, referred to as the Bethesda classification.[213,234] In this scheme, which was originally designed for cervical cytologic specimens (see p. 1444) but which some authors would like to see applied also to histologic samples,[197] the preferred generic term is *squamous intraepithelial lesion* (SIL), with a subdivision into low and high grades. The low-grade lesion corresponds to CIN I (as well as some HPV-induced lesions that do not qualify as CIN; see p. 1433), whereas the high-grade lesion corresponds to CIN II and III.

One of the rationales for this new approach is the problem represented by the difficulty often encountered in distinguishing CIN I from HPV-related flat condylomatous changes and the overdiagnosis of CIN that can occur as a result.[184] A suggested way to deal with this problem within the context of the CIN terminology is to designate those doubtful cases as either 'borderline CIN'[202] or 'CIN with HPV-related changes'.[246] Whichever scheme is ultimately chosen, one hopes that it will be applied to both cytologic and histologic specimens.

At a practical level, and regardless of the terminology used, these lesions can be safely treated by conization, electrodiathermy, cryosurgery, laser, or the more recent loop electrosurgical excision, all of them done under colposcopic guidance, assuming that a proper cytologic follow-up can be assured.[196,220,227,229,231,263] In most series, conization has resulted in control of even the most severe forms in over 90% of the patients.[216,222] In making the final decision regarding the timing and type of therapy for this group of lesions, the microscopic diagnosis is only one of the factors to be considered, albeit a very important one. The extension of the lesion, age of the patient, parity, and the desire to have more children all have to be considered. Both the surface and the possible depth of involvement also have to be taken into account. Anderson and Hartley[185] calculated that destruction of tissue to a depth of 2.92 mm would eradicate all involved glands in 95% of the patients, whereas destruction to a depth of 3.8 mm would eradicate 99.7%. Whether all patients with low-grade CIN require therapy remains a contentious issue.[248]

The pathologic report of a cervical biopsy specimen containing this group of lesions should include the degree of abnormality according to the agreed terminology for that institution, the presence or absence of endocervical gland involvement, and the presence or absence of HPV-related or any other associated changes. The report on a conization specimen should also include the status of the surgical margins, of which the endocervical one is the most important. Positive margins and glandular involvement by CIN II or CIN III are independent predictors of residual or recurrent disease.[199,225,237] but that may not be the case for low-grade CIN (CIN I).[191]On a positive note, it could be mentioned that the intra- and interobserver agreement in the evaluation of CIN among experienced gynecologic pathologists has increased substantially in recent times,[190] especially when combined with immunostaining for P16^{INK4a} or using the ProEx C immunocytochemical assay (targeting the expression of topoisomerase II-alpha and minichromosome maintenance protein-2).[186,209,241]

Once the pathologist has made the diagnosis of CIN in a cervical biopsy, it is the responsibility of the gynecologist to determine the presence or absence of invasive carcinoma, especially in the case of the high-grade lesions. Thorough cervical sampling and the proper sectioning of tissue should establish whether or not invasive carcinoma exists. If the latter is found, conventional methods of therapy may be instituted. Whenever the therapy is conservative, long-term follow-up (longer than 5 years) with periodic cytologic examination is imperative. In one series, patients with continuing abnormal cytology after initial treatment of CIN III were found to be 25 times more likely to develop invasive carcinomas than women with normal follow-up cytology.[228]

In addition to HPV-related koilocytotic atypia, the differential diagnosis of CIN includes florid squamous metaplasia and transitional metaplasia (see p. 1437). It should also be mentioned that the iodine test, used to delineate the extent of cervical disease prior to conization, can induce shrinkage, cytoplasmic eosinophilia and vacuolization, and pyknosis in the epithelial cells (particularly when they are abnormal to begin with).[187]

Microinvasive squamous cell carcinoma

Invasive squamous cell carcinomas in which the depth of stromal invasion is minimal (5 mm or less) have been segregated from the others and designated as 'microinvasive carcinoma', 'superficially invasive carcinoma', or 'carcinoma with early stromal invasion'[271,281,283,284] (Fig. 19.81). This corresponds rather closely to stage IA carcinoma in the FIGO system, defined as a lesion with a maximum depth of invasion of 5 mm and a maximum horizontal spread of 7 mm.[267,290]

Regardless of the terminology used, there is justification for the separation since the natural history of the lesion is quite different from that of ordinary invasive carcinoma and more akin to that of high-grade CIN/carcinoma in situ.[266,277,285] Accordingly, the

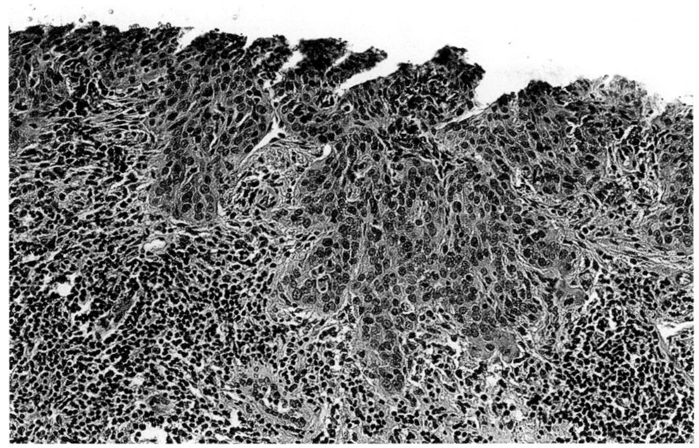

Fig. 19.81 Low-power appearance of microinvasive squamous cell carcinoma of cervix.

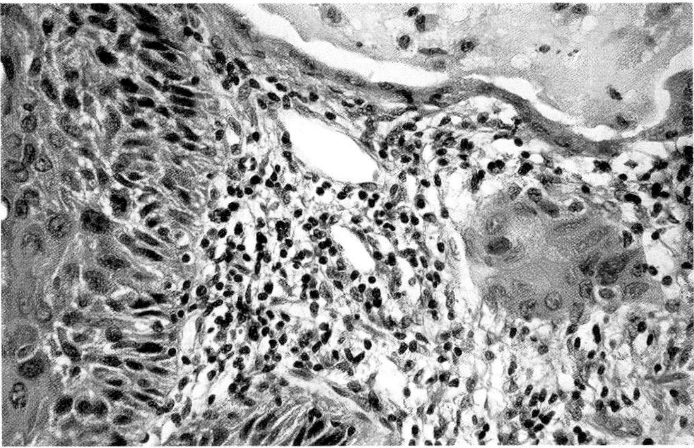

Fig. 19.82 Small focus of invasion in CIN. Note the greater degree of squamous differentiation in the microinvasive component.

treatment can be generally conservative, although it needs to be individualized.[267,269,272,282,293] The area of microinvasion practically always originates from a focus of CIN. The majority of the tumors are located in the anterior lip of the cervix.[284] The common occurrence of pleomorphism, cellular differentiation, presence of conspicuous nucleoli, and individual cell keratinization in the areas of microinvasion has been emphasized[284] (Fig. 19.82). Since these features are rarely seen together in CIN, their presence in an apparently intraepidermal cervical lesion should stimulate the search for areas of incipient invasion.[274] Another feature that should raise the suspicion of beginning stromal invasion is the presence of a desmoplastic stroma rich in acid mucosubstances and characterized by metachromatic staining properties.[275] In the area of invasion, there is a breach of the basement membrane, a feature traditionally evaluated with reticulin stains and now also with immunostains for basement membrane components such as type IV collagen, laminin, or fibronectin, either by themselves or in a cocktail also including keratin.[278,286,289,292]

A comprehensive review of the literature by Benson and Norris[265] revealed that the overall risk for lymph node metastasis in microinvasive carcinoma is approximately 1%. This excellent prognosis also applies to the subset of tumors showing lymphatic invasion and/or a confluent pattern of stromal growth, as long as their depth of invasion does not exceed 5 mm.[273,279,280,287,288] A further refinement and possible modification of the definition of microinvasive carcinoma was introduced by Hasumi et al.[276] These authors found that one (0.9%) of 106 patients with invasion up to 3 mm had lymph node metastases, whereas four (13.19%) of 29 patients with invasion of 3.1–5 mm had nodal metastases; on the basis of these findings, they recommend conservative surgery (as for CIN) for the first group and aggressive therapy (as for invasive carcinoma) for the second. This article and others have led to an ongoing controversy about the exact definition of the term, most authors currently favoring a 3 mm cutoff point, a criterion now included in the FIGO staging system (see Chapter 19).[270,276,291,294] There is evidence suggesting that tumor volume may be a more reliable criterion for the definition of microinvasive carcinoma and the prediction of likelihood of nodal metastases.[268]

Invasive squamous cell carcinoma

General features

Invasive squamous cell carcinoma of the cervix is still the most common malignant tumor of the female genital tract in most countries and the most frequent neoplasm among women in many of them.[295,306] In the United States, the incidence rate has decreased during the last half century among both blacks and whites, presumably as a result of the widespread use of cervical cytologic screening programs, which have counteracted increases anticipated from changes in risk factor prevalence.[297,306] The tumor appears most often in the older age groups but also occurs, with increased *relative* frequency, in young white females.[301] Evidence exists supporting the association of early marriage, multiparity, and low economic level with a high incidence of cervical carcinoma.[296,302] The single most important factor is probably age at first intercourse.[299,302] This tumor has a low incidence in Jewish women and is practically nonexistent in nuns.

In recent years, the crucial role of HPV in the pathogenesis of virtually all cervical squamous cell carcinomas has become obvious (see p. 1442). As a matter of fact, and as already mentioned, cervical cancer is unique among human cancers by being the first found to be directly attributable to the effects of an infectious agent. This extraordinary discovery, for which Harald zur Hausen was deservedly awarded the Nobel Prize in 2008, brings with it the potential of global cervical cancer prevention.[310] However, the fact that of the many women infected with high-risk types of HPV only a few will develop cervical carcinoma suggests that some cofactors must be present.[298] Perhaps other viruses play that role in some cases.

EBV is known to be statistically associated with cervical carcinoma, although currently it is not believed to be causally related.[307,308,312] Human T-cell leukemia virus (HTLV-1) and human immunodeficiency virus (HIV), when present, adversely affect the prognosis of patients with cervical carcinoma and may be associated with a rapidly progressive clinical course, but there is no conclusive evidence for a direct oncogenic effect for them.[303,304,308,311,312]

Host immune response factors contribute to the persistence of HPV infection and progression to cervical neoplasia (CIN and invasive carcinoma). Genes in the human leukocyte antigen (HLA) region of chromosome 6 are associated with increased susceptibility to the transforming properties of high-risk HPV. Impaired immune function, such as immunosuppressant therapy in organ transplantation recipients and HIV infection, is associated with a 5- to 10-fold increased risk of cervical neoplasia.[305]

The possible relationship of oral contraceptives and other hormones (including diethylstilbestrol exposure in utero) to cervical carcinoma remains controversial.[306]

Squamous cell carcinoma can be associated with microscopically similar tumors in the lower and upper genital tracts. In some of these cases, the same clonal pattern has been demonstrated, consistent with a cervical origin of the tumor followed by migration to other areas.[300]

Morphologic features

Grossly, cervical carcinoma may be polypoid or deeply infiltrative (Fig. 19.83). The bulky carcinomas that grow out of the cervix are less likely to invade surrounding structures than are the infiltrating ones.

Some tumors are either clinically inapparent or simply missed by the examiner, and are first discovered on pathologic examination of a uterus removed for a benign condition.[320] Still others develop in the cervical stump left from a supracervical hysterectomy, an operation that (for this very reason) is performed only exceptionally at present.[322]

Microscopically, three major categories of cervical squamous cell carcinoma exist, although admixtures and intermediate forms abound: *large cell nonkeratinizing* (Fig. 19.84), *keratinizing*, and *small cell*.[314,317,324] The latter should be distinguished from small cell neuroendocrine carcinoma, a tumor morphologically similar to small cell carcinoma of the lung and exhibiting features of neuroendocrine differentiation; electron microscopy and immunohistochemistry may be necessary for this purpose (see p. 1456).

The better differentiated forms of keratinizing squamous cell carcinoma differ from the others by their apparent lack of relationship with HPV or CIN; these rare tumors tend to be large and locally aggressive.[323]

Some cervical squamous cell carcinomas have a distinctly papillary pattern of growth; these need to be distinguished from verrucous and warty carcinoma.[316]

Other squamous cell carcinomas are accompanied by acantholysis, which may result in a pseudoglandular pattern.[313] Amyloid deposition in the stroma has been documented in some other cases.[319,327] On occasion, cervical squamous cell carcinoma is found to be associated with intense infiltration by mature eosinophils, with or without accompanying peripheral blood eosinophilia; production of eosinotactic and eosinopoietic substances by the tumor cells has been suggested as the pathogenetic mechanism.[315,321]

Mucicarmine stains will demonstrate the presence of scattered droplets of cytoplasmic mucin in a minority of cases having the morphologic features of squamous cell carcinoma in routinely stained sections, a finding analogous to that sometimes encountered in carcinomas of the lung and other sites.[326] These tumors have been variously referred to as mucoepidermoid carcinoma (a misleading term), adenosquamous carcinoma (less objectionable but not ideal), and squamous (cell) carcinoma with mucin secretion.[318] Whatever term one may wish to employ, it is important to regard this tumor as a morphologic variation on the theme of squamous cell carcinoma rather than as an adenocarcinoma (see p. 1452). Indeed, its behavior seems to be the same as that of the squamous cell carcinoma lacking mucin secretion, and therefore the utility of mucin stains in these circumstances is very limited.[326]

The exceptional occurrence of sebaceous differentiation in cervical carcinoma has also been documented.[325]

Immunohistochemical and molecular genetic features

Immunohistochemically, squamous cell carcinomas of the cervix express keratins (nearly 100% of the cases), CEA (90%),[328] p63 (a homolog of p53 preferentially expressed in basal and immature cervical squamous epithelium),[337] and blood group antigens.[336] The range of keratins found in the tumor varies somewhat depending on the subtype, but it is very wide.[335] There may also be reactivity

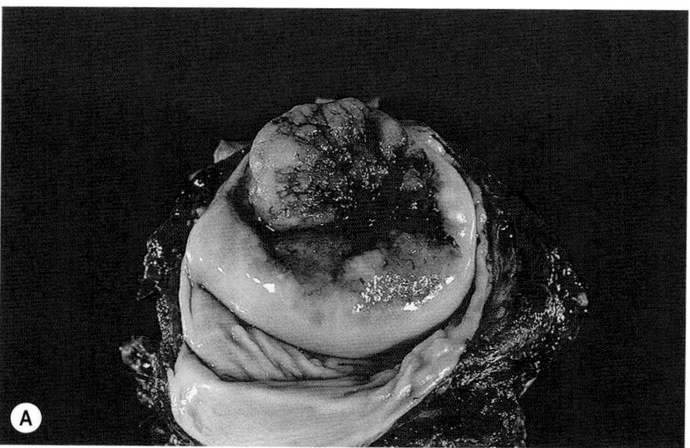

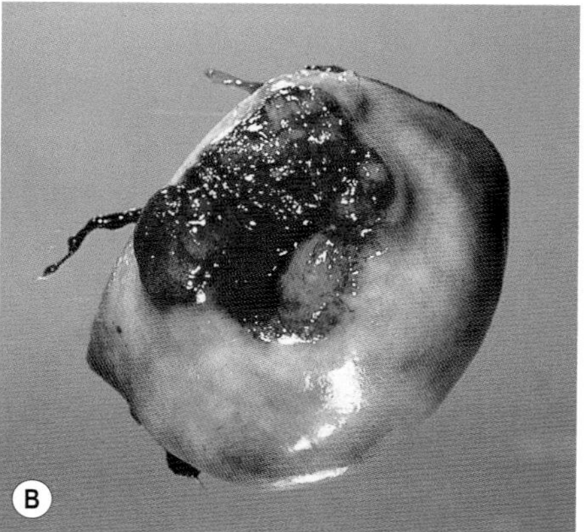

Fig. 19.83 **A** and **B**, Gross appearance of invasive squamous cell carcinoma of cervix.

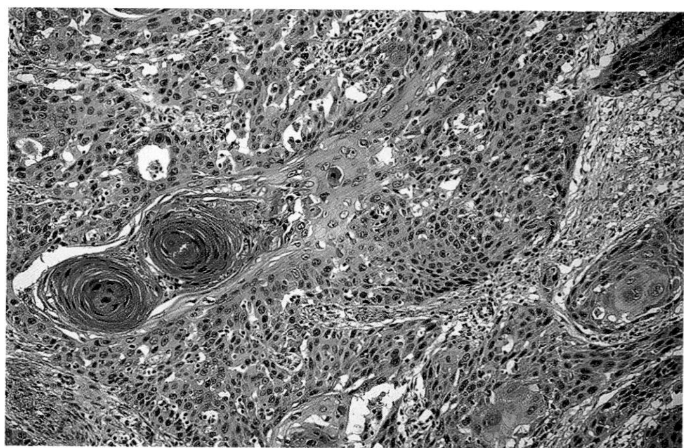

Fig. 19.84 Microscopic appearance of invasive squamous cell carcinoma of cervix of the usual type.

for cathepsin B (although not as frequently as in adenocarcinoma),[332] for β-human chorionic gonadotrophin (β-hCG),[330] and for parathyroid hormone-related gene (although these tumors rarely give rise to hypercalcemia).[329]

In contrast to the situation in many other human malignancies, the *TP53* gene is rarely mutated in cervical squamous cell carcinoma; this is also true for the biologically related *MDM2* gene.[331] Despite the lack of mutation in *TP53*, the function of the latter gene is inactivated due to the effect of HPV-associated E6 protein, which binds to P53 protein, causing its rapid degradation.[334] The *RB* gene function is similarly inactivated due to binding of HPV-associated E7 protein with RB protein.[334]

Aneuploidy has been the rule in DNA studies of cervical squamous cell carcinoma, but there is often considerable heterogeneity within the same lesion.[333]

Spread and metastases

Cervical carcinoma spreads characteristically by direct extension to the vagina, corpus (endometrium and myometrial wall), parametrium, lower urinary tract, and uterosacral ligaments[339,344] (Fig. 19.85).

Lymph node metastases are also common. The pattern of involvement generally proceeds in a sequential fashion. The first station is represented by the paracervical, hypogastric, obturator, and external iliac groups and the second by the sacral, common iliac, aortic, and inguinal groups.[340] The incidence of nodal involvement is directly related to the stage of the disease. Hematogenous metastases were rare in older series, but, with better control of the local lesion, they have increased in frequency.[344] Lungs (9%) and bones (4%) are the most common sites.[338,342,343] Ovarian metastases are less common than with endometrial adenocarcinoma, but they do occur.[346]

The differential diagnosis between primary pulmonary squamous cell carcinoma and a pulmonary metastasis from a cervical carcinoma, which can be very difficult on morphologic grounds, is greatly aided by the detection in the latter of HPV by HPV DNA in-situ hybridization, HPV RNA reverse transcription in-situ PCR, or immunostaining for P16.[341,345]

Treatment

Invasive carcinomas of the cervix can be treated by surgery, irradiation, chemotherapy, or a combination of these modalities.[350,357,362] The choice depends on the extent of the tumor, the general condition of the patient, and the expertise available at the institution where the patient is treated. Early lesions can be treated just as effectively with hysterectomy or intracavitary radium;[349,351] for stage IIa lesions, irradiation alone and a combination of irradiation and surgery have yielded equivalent results in randomized studies.[360] Early lesions can also be treated conservatively with radical vaginal trachelectomy, a fertility-preserving procedure where the cervix is excised at the level of the upper endocervix or lower uterine segment along with a vaginal cuff and parametria. In specimens obtained through this procedure, it is recommended to sample by intraoperative frozen section the entire endocervical/lower uterine segment.[352] If an occult invasive cervical carcinoma is found in a specimen from a simple hysterectomy done for another reason, additional therapy is indicated, usually in the form of a radical reoperation.[355]

Lack of prompt response (within 1–3 months) to radiation therapy is a predictor of likely recurrence and an indicator that adjuvant chemotherapy should be considered.[353] The latter has also been tried to increase the number of operable patients and as a postoperative measure, with some encouraging preliminary results.[354]

In cases of postirradiation relapse of cervical carcinoma, pelvic exenteration should be seriously considered because a considerable number of the patients will have the persistent tumor confined to the pelvis.[358] This operation removes all pelvic viscera and lateral pelvic lymph node-bearing tissue. At laparotomy, the surgeon should examine the upper abdomen carefully, particularly the periaortic area, for evidence of spread outside the pelvis. Any suspicious lymph nodes or liver nodules should be submitted to the pathologist for frozen section before the operative procedure is begun. Gross appraisal of enlarged extrapelvic nodes is unreliable, whereas frozen section examination is a highly accurate procedure.[347] The study of the surgical specimen should include a careful examination of the lymph nodes, the lateral edges of the resection, and the local extent of the tumor. Microscopically, the nodes, vessels, and adjacent organs should be examined for evidence of tumor. The finding of greater prognostic relevance in the pathologic evaluation of pelvic exenteration specimens is the presence or absence of lymph node metastases.[361]

Other indications for pelvic exenteration are locally invasive carcinoma of the rectum, severe pelvic irradiation necrosis, and recurrent carcinoma of the endometrium. The 5-year survival rate for patients undergoing this formidable procedure for postirradiation persistence of carcinoma of the cervix is notably high considering the circumstances; it was approximately 25% in early series[348,356] and has reached the remarkable figure of 73% at one institution.[359]

The microscopic examination of postradiochemotherapy specimens can be difficult due to the extent of regressive changes, manifested in the tumor cells by cytoplasmic eosinophilia, vacuolization, and foamy degeneration. The prognostically most important feature to look for in these specimens is tumor embolism.[363]

Prognosis

The prognosis of cervical carcinoma is related to the following parameters:

1. *Clinical stage*. As for most other human malignancies, this is the most important prognostic determinator.[364]
2. *Nodal status*. This is another crucial predictor, which is incorporated into the staging scheme.[374,382]
3. *Size* of the largest involved node[376] and *number* of positive nodes.[377]
4. *Size of the primary tumor*, as determined by measurement of the tumor's greatest diameter[379,386] or by volumetric techniques.[367]
5. *Depth of invasion*.[375,388,392]
6. *Endometrial extension*. The presence of this feature decreases the survival rate by a factor of 10–20%.[385]
7. *Parametrial involvement*, as detected microscopically.[378]
8. *Blood vessel invasion*.[366,383,391,400]
9. *Microscopic grade*. Whether the degree of tumor differentiation as evaluated in routinely stained sections correlates with survival independently from staging remains a controversial issue.[393,394] If a correlation exists, it must be minimal indeed, whether one uses the Reagan–Ng or the Broders' method of grading.[395,400]
10. *Microscopic type*. A similar comment applies to this parameter, which is roughly related to microscopic grade. Some authors have found a better prognosis with the large cell nonkeratinizing type and a worse prognosis with the small cell type,[399] but others have found no correlation between microscopic classification and prognosis.[369,370]
11. *Tumor-associated tissue eosinophilia* (*TATE*). Presence of numerous mature eosinophils in the inflammatory infiltrate

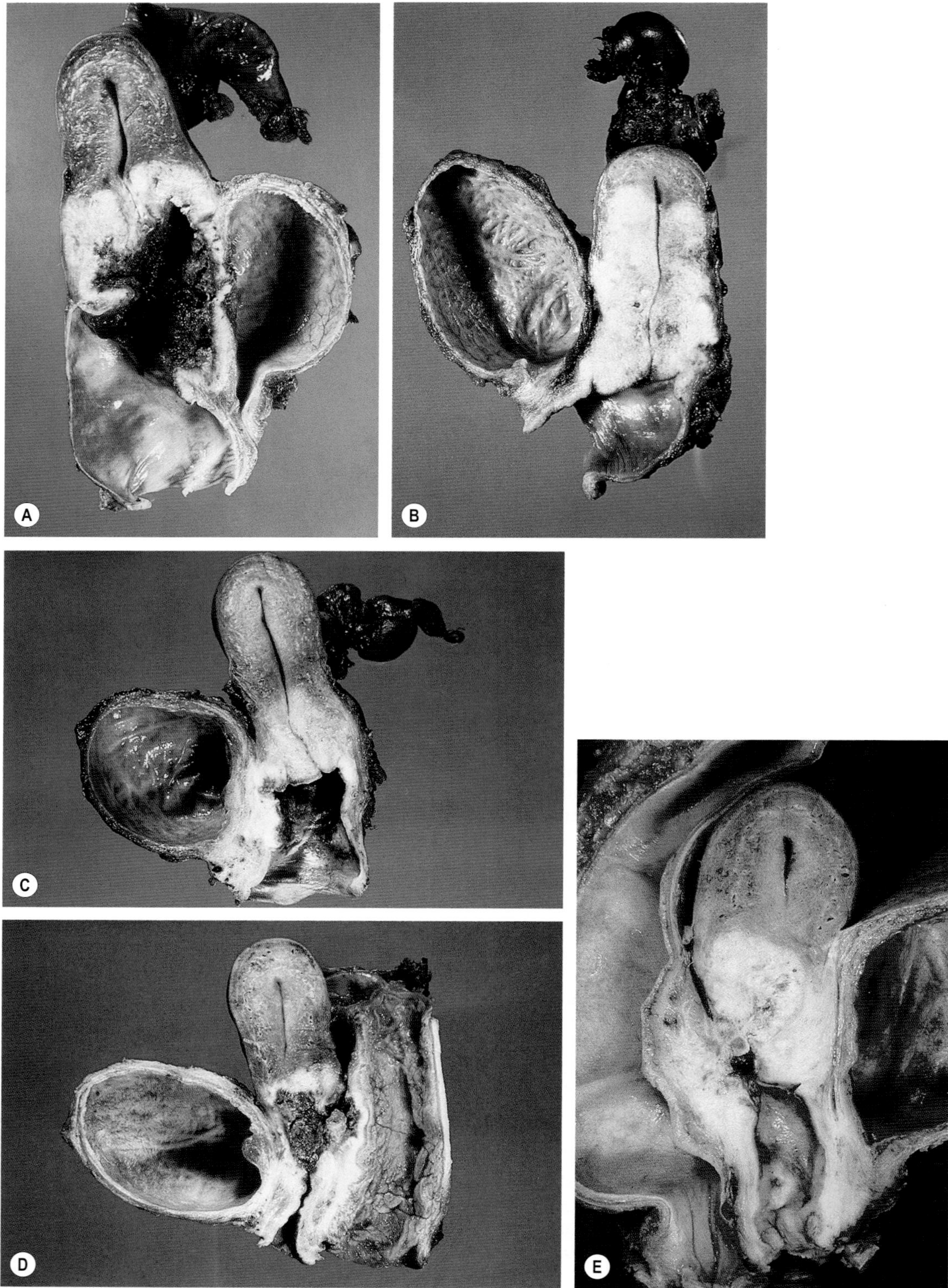

Fig. 19.85 Patterns of spread of squamous cell carcinoma of cervix as seen in pelvic exenteration specimens: **A**, large ulcerated tumor involving uterine isthmus and vagina; **B**, massive extension into uterine corpus; **C**, extension into bladder; **D**, extension into bladder and rectum; **E**, extension into rectal wall, with impingement into rectal mucosa.
(A–D, Courtesy of Dr Hector Rodriguez-Martinez, Mexico City, Mexico)

of cervical carcinoma has been associated with an improved survival in one study[365] and a worse survival in another.[398] At other sites this feature is generally regarded as a good prognostic sign.

12 *Keratin profile* as evaluated immunohistochemically. No predictive value seems to be attached to this parameter.[397]
13 *Cell proliferation index*. High S-phase rates as determined by flow cytometry are correlated to both a poorly differentiated histologic appearance and decreased short-term survival.[396]
14 *Angiogenesis*. There is no evidence of a correlation between microvessel density and prognosis.[389]
15 *HPV*. It has been claimed that HPV is a major determinant of the course of cervical cancer.[372] In one series, the 5-year disease-free survival was 100% for patients with intermediate risk HPV, 58% for patients with HPV-16-positive tumors, and 38% for patients with HPV-18-positive tumors.[380] It has been further claimed that lack of detection of HPV in the tumor cells is a poor prognostic sign.[387]
16 *Others*. Stromal infiltration by S-100 protein-positive Langerhans cells,[381] allelic loss on chromosome 1,[368] and expression of HER2/*neu*,[371,384] *RAS* oncogene,[390] and Tn antigen (a precursor of MN blood group antigen)[373] have all been found to relate to an unfavorable outcome.

It remains to be determined how many of these parameters will prove to have independent prognostic value.

Other microscopic types

Verrucous carcinoma is a highly differentiated variant of squamous cell carcinoma with a polypoid pattern of growth, an extremely well-differentiated cytologic appearance, and a capacity for local invasion but not for metastatic spread. Some cases have been found to extend into the endometrial cavity.[415] Verrucous carcinoma should be distinguished both from condyloma acuminatum and from ordinary squamous cell carcinoma with a prominent papillary pattern of growth.[401,412] The general gross and microscopic features of this tumor are described in Chapter 4.

Spindle cell carcinoma (sarcomatoid carcinoma; squamous cell carcinoma with sarcoma-like stroma; carcinosarcoma) is morphologically analogous to the homonymous tumor in the upper aerodigestive tract.[414] It may contain osteoclast-like giant cells,[411] and there is often evidence of HPV infection.[405] The recognizable epithelial component of this tumor, when present, is of squamous type; this is in contrast with the malignant mixed müllerian tumor, in which that component is usually glandular (see p. 1505). It is advisable to keep these tumors (both of which can occur in the cervix) in separate categories, although both of them probably represent carcinomas with a sarcoma-like component (see also Vagina chapter).

Basaloid (squamous cell) carcinoma is characterized by prominent peripheral palisading, an infiltrative growth pattern, and minimal stromal reaction[403] (Fig. 19.86). The behavior of this tumor is aggressive, as is also the case with the homonymous neoplasm in the upper aerodigestive tract. It is, therefore, very important to clearly separate this tumor from the adenoid cystic carcinomas and adenoid basal carcinomas discussed on page 1409.[404]

Lymphoepithelioma-like carcinoma resembles its more common counterpart in the upper respiratory tract by virtue of the large size of the tumor cells, vesicular nuclei with prominent nucleoli, syncytial appearance, and heavy lymphocytic infiltration.[406,410,417] Some cases have been found to secrete β-hCG, as is also occasionally the case with conventional squamous cell carcinoma.[402] The possible association of this tumor with either EBV or HPV remains controversial.[409,413,416] This tumor type shows considerable overlap with the *circumscribed* type of cervical carcinoma described by Japanese authors (Fig. 19.87).[407]

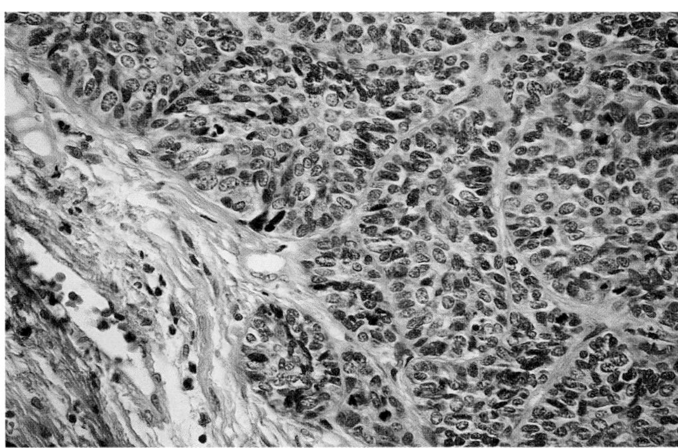

Fig. 19.86 Basaloid squamous cell carcinoma of uterine cervix. The tumor grows in the form of well-defined nests showing peripheral palisading.

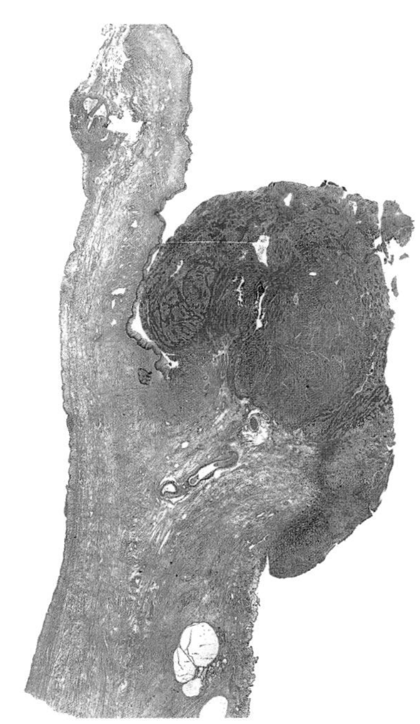

Fig. 19.87 Whole-mount appearance of well-circumscribed cervical carcinoma with a polypoid pattern of growth. Stromal invasion is minimal.

Transitional cell (urothelial) carcinoma having an appearance similar to the homonymous tumor located in the bladder or ovary can occur in the cervix. It needs to be distinguished from *inverted transitional cell papilloma*, which has also been reported in this location. It also needs to be differentiated from papillary squamous cell carcinoma (see p. 1404). The latter is not always an easy task, since the transitional-like and squamous-like areas of these tumors often blend with each other. The term *papillary squamotransitional cell carcinoma* has been proposed for the tumors having an obvious hybrid composition.[408]

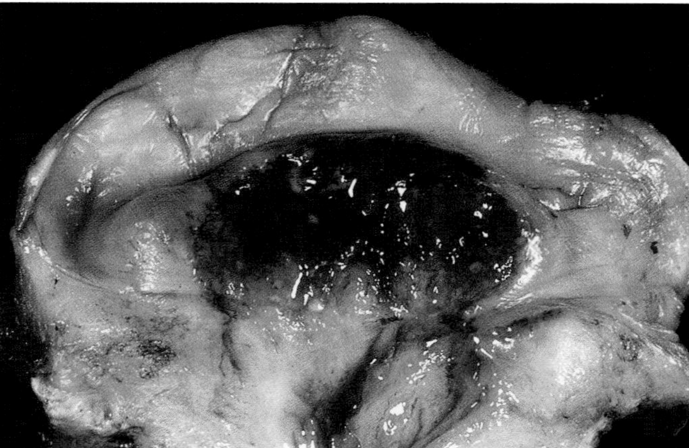

Fig. 19.88 Gross appearance of endocervical adenocarcinoma.

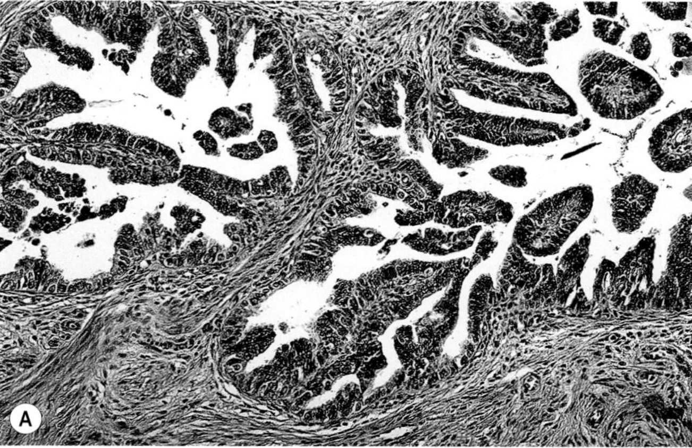

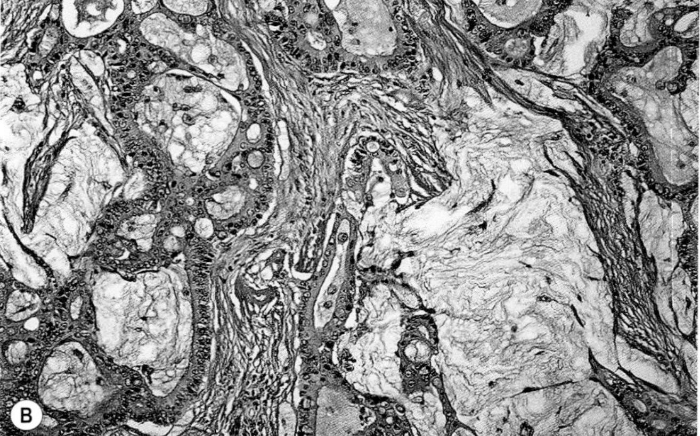

Fig. 19.89 Microscopic appearance of conventional (**A**) and mucinous (**B**) adenocarcinoma of cervix.

Adenocarcinoma

Morphologic and other features

Primary adenocarcinomas make up 5–15% of all carcinomas of the cervix. This percentage is higher in Jewish women,[436] and it has been suggested that its relative incidence is on the rise in the general population, particularly in young women.[455,460,462,465,473] An association has been found between the long-term use of oral contraceptives and the development of endocervical neoplasia in young patients,[432,472] but this has been contested by others.[440]

Because of their topography, they are more difficult to diagnose on Pap smears than cervical squamous cell carcinomas.[441] The tumor presents no distinguishing gross characteristics (Fig. 19.88). Microscopically, the most common pattern is that of a well-differentiated glandular pattern with mucin secretion, some of which can leak into the stroma[446,458,476–478] (Fig. 19.89). However, the degree of differentiation varies, and poorly differentiated forms exist. In addition to the mucin-secreting appearance, which recapitulates the histology of the normal endocervix, cervical carcinomas can have an endometrioid or a serous (papillary) appearance; these are discussed in the section dealing with Variants (see p. 1453).

Histochemically, Alcian blue and mucicarmine-positive material is found intracellularly in nearly all cases of conventional cervical adenocarcinoma.[466] The staining pattern is different from that of normal endocervical glands but similar to that of in-situ adenocarcinoma.[434] Among the mucins, there is positivity for MUC1 in nearly 100%, MUC2 in 40%, MUC4 in 75%. and MUC5AC 'in most'.[420] Keratins, EMA, and CEA are consistently expressed, whereas vimentin is not.[423–425,448] Another marker that is generally present is P16^{INK4a}, which links this tumor to HPV infection.[457,475] Estrogen and progesterone receptors are expressed in only one-fourth of the cases.[431] Overexpression of P53 is frequent.[422,453] Markers common to gastric, intestinal, and pancreatobiliary epithelial cells (such as M1 and cathepsin E) are commonly present.[468] About one-fourth of endocervical adenocarcinomas are positive for CDX2, CK20, or both; this profile correlates usually but not always with intestinal differentiation.[461,467] Cervical adenocarcinomas have also been shown to contain argyrophilic (presumably neuroendocrine) cells,[449] a variety of peptide hormones,[471] mammaglobin (although not as commonly as endometrial adenocarcinoma[459]) and the enzyme amylase.[435] Basement membrane, as investigated immunohistochemically with type IV collagen or laminin, may be present around the tumor cells even in invasive tumors, but usually in a discontinuous fashion.[470,474]

HPV infection (particularly by types 16 and 18) is found in most endocervical adenocarcinomas.[430,469] The few negative tumors tend to be nonmucinous and occur in older women.[469]

Cervical carcinoma spreads directly to endometrium and vagina, and metastasizes to the regional nodes, with a distribution pattern similar to that of cervical squamous cell carcinoma (see above). It can also metastasize to the ovaries, especially when extending to the lower uterine segment.[463] It is possible that some of the reported cases of combined endocervical adenocarcinoma and ovarian mucinous adenocarcinoma (and occasionally even tubal adenocarcinoma)[439,450] represent metastases of the cervical tumor to these organs.[429]

The preferred therapies for cervical adenocarcinoma are radiation alone or a combination of radiation and surgery.[427,433,437] The incidence of residual tumor in the hysterectomy specimens after intracavitary treatment is much higher than for squamous cell carcinoma.[444] The prognosis depends on the clinical stage, amount of tumor (as determined by tumor volume), microscopic grade, and nodal status.[419,428,438,442,445,454] In most series, the overall prognosis has been less favorable than for the squamous cell counterpart.[438,447,456] There is not much difference among the various histologic subtypes,[418] although the endometrioid variety is said to behave slightly better.[464] The presence of nodal metastases is an ominous prognostic sign.[421] Increased serum levels of CA-125 and overexpression of HER2/*neu* and nm23-H1 proteins have also been found to represent poor prognostic factors,[426,443,452] whereas expression of P21 has been associated with a favorable outcome.[451]

Differential diagnosis with endometrial adenocarcinoma

The differential diagnosis between endocervical and endometrial adenocarcinoma can be very difficult, whether the tumor has a conventional mucin-secreting pattern or whether it belongs to one of the variants mentioned later in this chapter.[480,486] Features that favor a primary endocervical origin are the following:

1. Presence of in-situ adenocarcinoma in the cervical glands.
2. Diffuse and abundant intracellular mucin and CEA, since these two markers tend to be present only focally and luminally in endometrial tumors.[482,483,485]
3. Negativity for vimentin.[481]
4. Negativity or only weak positivity for estrogen or progesterone receptors.[483,484]
5. Presence of HPV by in situ hybridization.[484]
6. Immunoreactivity for p16.[479]

Markers of no utility for this purpose are CK7, CK20, 34βE12, and EMA.[481,483]

In situ and microinvasive adenocarcinoma

The documentation of the existence of an in-situ stage of cervical carcinoma has lagged behind that of squamous cell carcinoma, but is now widely accepted.[500,507] Instances of glandular dysplasia have also been described,[498,499,501,502,509,518] with the ensuing proposal to group the dysplastic and the in-situ adenocarcinomatous lesions under the term 'cervical intraepithelial glandular neoplasia',[493,515] a concept that remains controversial.[494,497] Some of the in-situ lesions have been shown to precede the development of invasive adenocarcinoma, just as squamous carcinoma in situ (CIN III) precedes invasive carcinoma of the same type.[489] Cytologic atypia (manifested by nuclear hyperchromasia and pleomorphism) and increased mitotic figures are the two most important identifying features (Fig. 19.90). The presence of numerous apoptotic bodies is another diagnostic clue.[488] The changes can be very subtle and limited to the endocervical surface.[517]

The mucins secreted by the in-situ malignant glands may be similar to those of the normal endocervical mucosa or may resemble the pattern of intestinal goblet cells.[493] The latter, which is referred to as intestinal-type cervical adenocarcinoma in situ, shows consistent expression of CDX2.[506] Most in-situ cervical adenocarcinomas are positive for CEA, less than half for keratin, and one-tenth for secretory component, those figures being lower than for the invasive tumors.[496] The cell proliferative index (as measured by MIB-1) is increased, there is an abnormal expression of cell cycle-related molecules, and the expression of hormone receptors is either decreased or absent.[503]

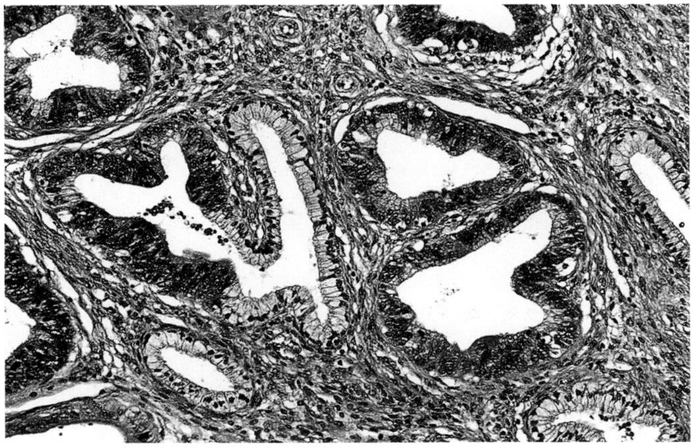

Fig. 19.90 Adenocarcinoma in situ with partial preservation of endocervical glands.

An important differential diagnosis of in-situ cervical adenocarcinoma is with tubal or tubal–endometrial metaplasia, further complicated by the fact that a tubal type of in-situ endocervical adenocarcinoma has been described.[512] Immunohistochemically, the carcinoma tends to be negative for vimentin, diffusely positive for P16^{INK4a}, generally negative for BCL2, and usually exhibits a high proliferative index with MIB-1.[490,505] The generally strong positivity for P16^{INK4a} supports a strong association of in-situ cervical adenocarcinoma with HPV infection.[511]

Almost half of the invasive cervical adenocarcinomas and approximately 75% of their in-situ counterparts have an associated CIN of the conventional squamous type of the overlying epithelium.[492,504,514]

Conization is the treatment of choice for in situ adenocarcinoma of the cervix.[487] The circumferential extent of tumor is a marker of residual/recurrent disease, and it is therefore important to include this information in the pathology report.[495,510]

Microinvasive cervical adenocarcinoma has been defined along lines similar to those previously agreed upon for microinvasive squamous cell carcinoma. Terms such as 'early stage' and 'early invasive' have also been used.[501,508,513] The usual criterion used for its recognition is the presence in an in-situ adenocarcinoma of a focus of stromal invasion not exceeding 5 mm in depth.[501,508] The suggestion has been made that close proximity of neoplastic glands to thick-wall blood vessels (as defined by the distance from the closest gland to a thick-wall vessel being less or equal to the thickness of the vessel wall) is a clue to the presence of stromal invasion.[516] The treatment of microinvasive carcinoma is dependent upon the horizontal extent and whether vascular invasion is present or absent.[518] In view of the generally indolent behavior of this tumor, a conservative type of surgery is advisable for most cases.[491]

Morphologic variants of cervical adenocarcinoma

Endometrioid adenocarcinoma of cervix closely resembles its endometrial and ovarian counterparts. It can be extremely well differentiated,[529,598] and can be seen in association with a synchronous or metachronous endometrioid carcinoma in the ovary or uterine corpus.[552,560] The incidence of this tumor type seems to be on the rise.[520] The differential diagnosis includes endometrioid adenocarcinoma of the endometrium, which can be accompanied by a very deceptive pattern of cervical spread.[592]

Serous (papillary) carcinoma is analogous in appearance to the homonymous uterine and ovarian neoplasm, including the common occurrence of psammoma bodies.[587,600]

Adenoma malignum (minimal deviation adenocarcinoma) is a type of cervical adenocarcinoma so well differentiated structurally and cytologically that it can be diagnosed only as malignant because of the presence of distorted glands with irregular outlines deeply positioned in the cervix and the fact that a portion of the infiltrating tumor is associated with a stromal response[539,557,559,575] (Fig. 19.91). In addition, about half of the cases have small foci with a less well differentiated appearance. Vascular and perineurial invasion may be present. The mucin produced is predominantly of neutral type.[548] Ultrastructurally, some authors claim to have identified gastric phenotypes among the tumor cells,[551] a fact that has been supported histochemically.[594] A minor component of argyrophilic cells can be detected in most of the cases.[539] The fact that these tumors, like the more obvious adenocarcinomas, are CEA positive is of importance

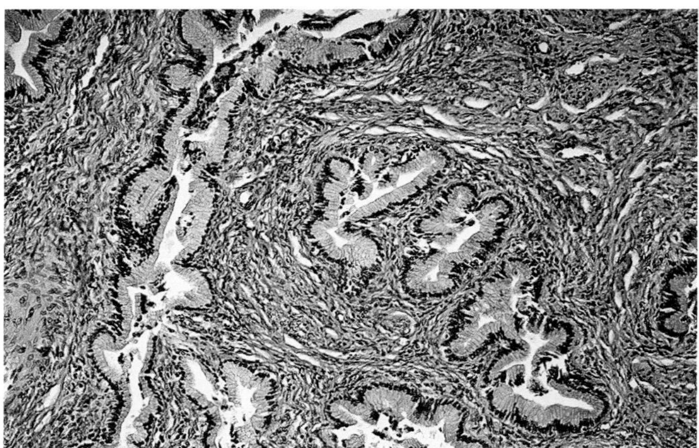

Fig. 19.91 So-called 'adenoma malignum' (minimal deviation adenocarcinoma) of cervix.

in the differential diagnosis with benign lesions such as microglandular hyperplasia.[573,589] Parenthetically, there is no convincing evidence that adenoma malignum and conventional cervical adenocarcinoma are causally related to microglandular hyperplasia.[555] The differential diagnosis also includes endocervical-type *cervical adenomyoma*,[540] and the condition known as *florid deep glands*,[530] in which atypia, architectural disarray, and desmoplastic stromal reaction are lacking. Recently, HIK1083 has been introduced as a putative new marker for adenoma malignum.[572]

Adenoma malignum usually lacks evidence of high-risk HPV and *TP53* mutations.[595]

Adenoma malignum constitutes approximately 1% of all endocervical adenocarcinomas. Some cases are associated with the Peutz–Jeghers syndrome,[539,599] and mutations of the *STK11* gene (a tumor suppressor gene responsible for this syndrome and located at 19p13.3) have been found in over half of the cases of this tumor type.[564]

Villoglandular (papillary) adenocarcinoma presents as an exophytic polypoid lesion with papillae lined by endocervical, endometrial, or intestinal-type epithelium showing only mild atypia (Fig. 19.92). The appearance of the superficial portion is similar to that of colorectal villous adenoma.[546] Most cases are associated with adenocarcinoma in situ and/or CIN,[556] and there is usually evidence of HPV infection.[554] The prognosis is excellent,[597] but only if strict architectural and cytologic criteria (bland appearance of the nuclei) are applied.[549]

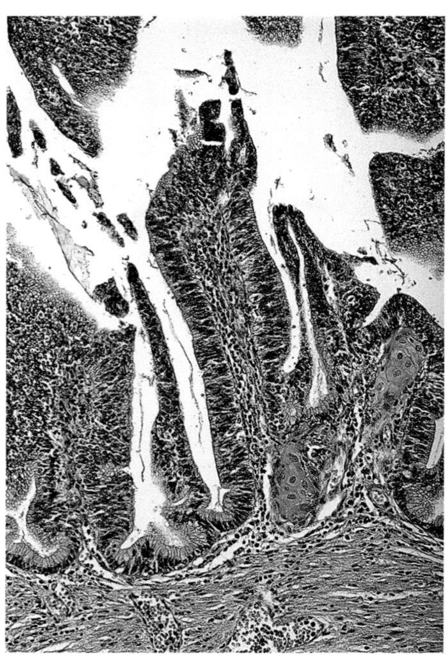

Fig. 19.92 Villoglandular variant of endocervical adenocarcinoma. The architecture is reminiscent of colorectal villous adenoma.

Adenosquamous (mixed) carcinoma combines the patterns of adenocarcinoma with a well-defined squamous component[524] (Figs 19.93 and 19.94). This tumor type seems to be particularly common during pregnancy. It is likely that the cell of origin of adenosquamous carcinomas and most adenocarcinomas of the cervix is the same as for the ordinary squamous cell carcinoma (i.e., the subcolumnar reserve cell).[525,563,579]

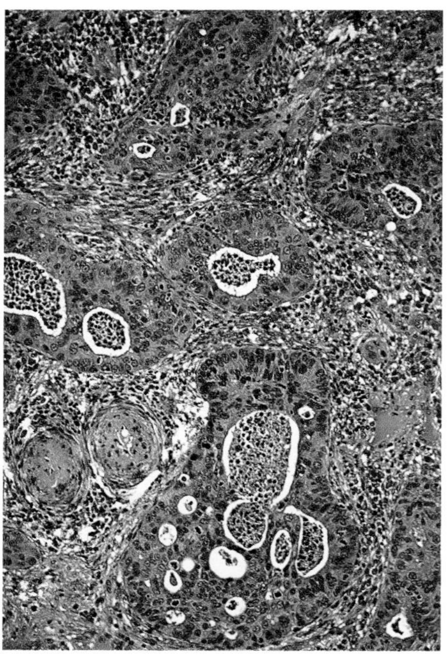

Fig. 19.93 Adenosquamous carcinoma of cervix.

Adenosquamous carcinoma as previously defined should be distinguished from squamous cell carcinoma without glandular formations but with histochemically demonstrable intracellular mucin (see p. 1448).[593]

Adenosquamous carcinomas have been shown in some series to have a worse overall prognosis than pure squamous cell carcinoma or adenocarcinoma, at least in advanced-stage lesions.[532] This is probably due to the fact that most of them are poorly differentiated tumors,[537] as supported by the greater proportion of high-ploidy stem cells found in these lesions when subjected to DNA analysis.[536] However, when compared grade by grade and stage by stage with adenocarcinomas and squamous cell carcinomas, no prognostic differences are found.[528,545]

Auersperg et al.[521] have shown that most cervical carcinomas that appear undifferentiated at the light microscopic level still exhibit traits of squamous and/or glandular differentiation at the ultrastructural level.

Glassy cell carcinoma has been described as a distinct type of poorly differentiated adenosquamous carcinoma.[541] It occurs

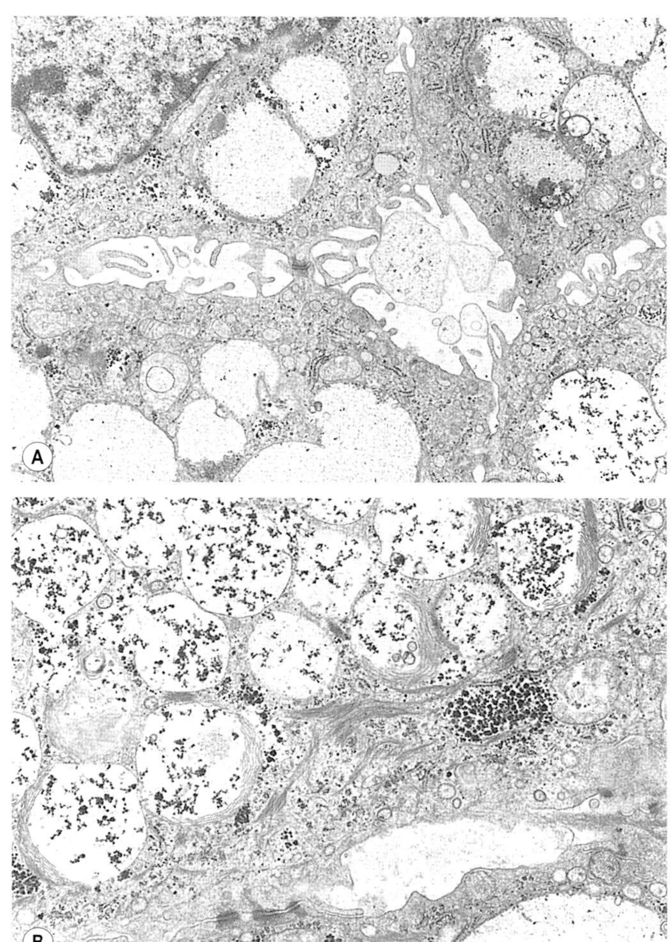

Fig. 19.94 **A** and **B**, Ultrastructural appearance of adenosquamous carcinoma of cervix. **A**, Large mucous secretory vacuoles, true lumen formation, and scattered glycogen may be noted in tumor cells. **B**, Note the presence of tonofilaments in addition to secretory products.

in a younger age group (mean age, 41 years) than other cervical neoplasms and often has been associated with pregnancy. The tumor cells have a moderate amount of cytoplasm with a ground glass or finely granular appearance, a prominent eosinophilic and PAS-positive cell membrane, and large nuclei with prominent nucleoli.

Mitoses are numerous. A prominent inflammatory infiltrate, often rich in eosinophils, is regularly seen in the adjacent stroma, and this may be accompanied by peripheral blood eosinophilia.

In pure cases of glassy cell carcinoma, glandular or squamous differentiation is absent, although it can be consistently detected by ultrastructural examination.[596] Other cases show an admixture with mucin-producing adenocarcinoma and/or clear-cut squamous foci, raising the question whether it is justified to regard glassy cell carcinoma as a distinct entity.[527,568] The immunohistochemical keratin profile is similar to that of reserve cells or immature squamous cells of cervix.[561] The prognosis is poor, a fact probably related to its poorly differentiated nature.[567,576]

Mucinous carcinoma of the endocervix remains an ill-defined concept. Its immunophenotype can be of gastric or intestinal type, including immunoreactivity for CDX2, CK7, p16, and a new marker known as HIK1083.[562,582,583] This tumor type is said to run a more aggressive clinical course than the usual type of endocervical adenocarcinoma.[562]

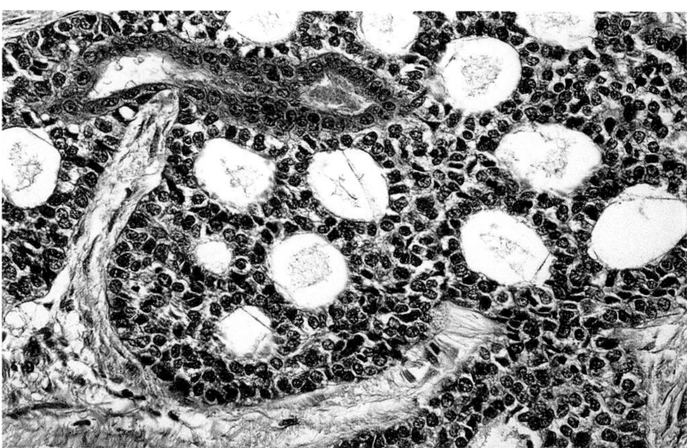

Fig. 19.95 Adenoid cystic carcinoma of cervix with a typical cribriform pattern of growth.

Adenoid cystic carcinoma is a specific variant of cervical adenocarcinoma that tends to occur in elderly multigravid black women[538] and that is associated with a particularly poor prognosis.[535,550] The morphologic appearance is similar to that of the homonymous tumors of salivary glands (Fig. 19.95). Like the former, it may be cribriform (the most common pattern) or grow in a predominantly solid fashion.[519]

Adenoid basal carcinoma (tumor; epithelioma) should be distinguished both from adenoid cystic carcinoma and from basaloid (squamous cell) carcinoma (see p. 1409). Although it shares many phenotypic features with adenoid cystic carcinoma,[542] it is a very low-grade lesion, in contrast with the two neoplasms with which it can be confused. It is usually discovered incidentally, it does not produce a mass lesion, and – when pure – it does not result in metastases.[523,534] The consistent presence of HPV-16 has been documented.[553] The lesion blends with the process that has been called *adenoid basal hyperplasia*. Brainard and Hart[523] have proposed grouping these two conditions under the term *adenoid basal epithelioma* to emphasize their indolent nature. Alas, adenoid basal carcinoma can be found associated with a high-grade component having basaloid, pure squamous, adenoid cystic, or small cell neuroendocrine features. When that happens, an aggressive behavior ensues.[577]

Clear cell carcinoma (formerly called *mesonephric carcinoma*) of the cervix is of müllerian rather than of mesonephric origin.[569] The presence of in-situ changes in the area of the squamocolumnar junction in some of the cases[581] and the electron microscopic features[531] seem to provide conclusive evidence for this interpretation. Glands lined by large cells with abundant clear cytoplasm are characteristic[533] (Fig. 19.96). 'Hobnail' cells are common, as are intraglandular papillary projections. Grossly, the tumor is usually exophytic. This is the most common form of cervical carcinoma in young females, although it occurs in all age groups,[574] and it shows a second peak at age 70 years.[544] The prognosis is relatively good. In the 13 cases studied by Hart and Norris,[547] the actuarial survival rate was 55% at 5 years and 40% at 10 years. The relationship with intrauterine diethylstilbestrol exposure and other features of this tumor are the same as for the analogous vaginal neoplasms.[543,578,585] It is also evident, however, that morphologically identical cases occur in the absence of exposure to this hormone, particularly in older women.[558]

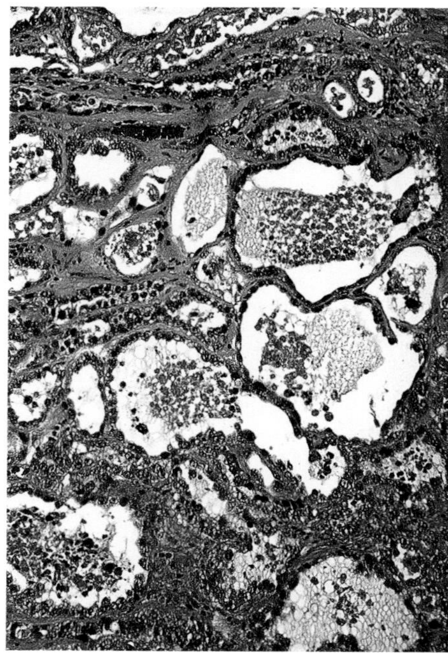

Fig. 19.96 Clear cell adenocarcinoma of cervix showing tubular, microcystic, and tubulocystic features.

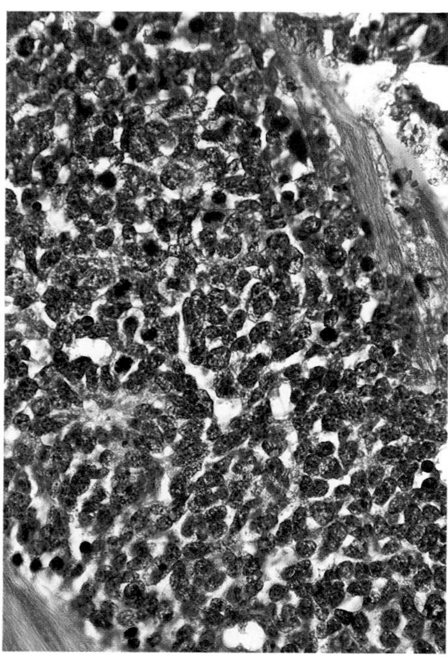

Fig. 19.98 High-grade small cell neuroendocrine carcinoma of cervix.

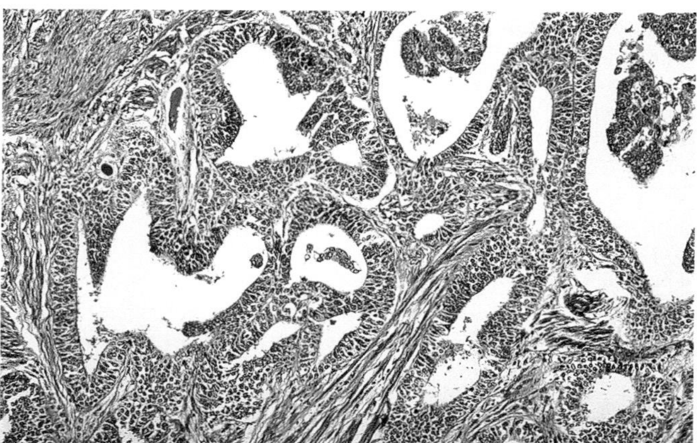

Fig. 19.97 Mesonephric gland carcinoma of cervix.

Mesonephric (adeno)carcinoma is a very rare tumor. Most of the cases that have been reported as such in the past probably represent müllerian-type adenocarcinomas or yolk sac tumors. True mesonephric carcinomas are often found adjacent to mesonephric hyperplasia (sometimes florid and atypical) and may exhibit a variety of patterns, such as ductal (resembling endometrioid adenocarcinoma), small tubular, retiform, solid, sex-cord-like, and spindle[526,565,580] (Fig. 19.97). The immunohistochemical profile is similar to that of mesonephric rests, and includes positivity for CD10 and calretinin,[571] two interesting but not entirely specific findings.[588] Tumors in which the epithelial component is admixed with either a homologous or a heterologous sarcoma-like component are referred to as **malignant mixed mesonephric tumors**.[522]

Other variants of endocervical adenocarcinoma, all of them exceedingly rare, are a microcystic type,[591] a signet ring type,[570,590] a small intestinal (enteric) type,[566,584] and a type with choriocarcinomatous and hepatoid differentiation.[586]

Neuroendocrine carcinoma

A small number of cervical carcinomas exhibit clearcut evidence of neuroendocrine differentiation, as detected by ultrastructural, histochemical, and/or immunohistochemical criteria. These tumors have been variously called (atypical) carcinoid tumor, argyrophil cell carcinoma, (extrapulmonary) small cell carcinoma, (neuro)endocrine carcinoma, and carcinoma with (neuro)endocrine differentiation, the choice in terminology depending on the degree of differentiation of the tumor, the extent of endocrine features present, and the observer's bias[617,632] (Fig. 19.98). It is probably preferable to use terms similar to those employed at other sites for morphologically similar tumors, i.e., typical carcinoid tumor (almost nonexistent in the cervix), atypical carcinoid tumor, small cell neuroendocrine carcinoma, and large cell neuroendocrine carcinoma.[602,609,611,622] Another analogy with other sites worth mentioning is that sometimes one finds neuroendocrine markers in cervical carcinomas of conventional type, a fact that should not result in a change of their designation.[608]

The age distribution of neuroendocrine carcinomas of the cervix is the same as for squamous cell carcinoma. They also show a similar association with HPV.[601,624,631] The carcinoid syndrome is invariably absent, but some cases have been seen in association with Cushing syndrome,[621] and with inappropriate secretion of antidiuretic hormone (ADH).[618] In contrast to squamous cell carcinoma, CIN changes in the adjacent epithelium are extremely rare.[605,631] A possible precursor lesion in the form of endocrine cell hyperplasia of the cervix has been identified.[607]

The better differentiated members of this group have an organoid arrangement, with trabecular, insular, glandular, and spindle patterns of growth. Most cases are pure, but others are combined with

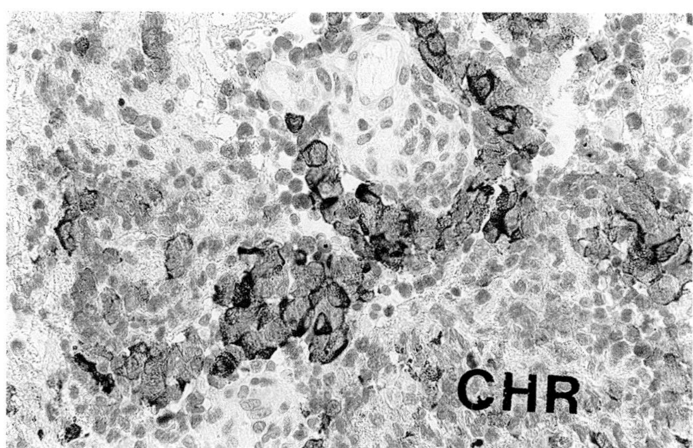

Fig. 19.99 Strong focal immunoreactivity for chromogranin in neuroendocrine carcinoma of cervix.

squamous cell carcinoma[630] or adenocarcinoma.[616,627,629] Some of these combined tumors have been referred to as amphicrine carcinomas[612] or mixed small cell carcinomas.[614]

Argyrophilic (but not argentaffin) granules can be demonstrated in many of the cases, particularly the better differentiated ones. Amyloid may be deposited in the stroma. Ultrastructurally, a variable number of dense-core secretory granules are found in all but the most undifferentiated types. Immunohistochemically, positivity may be found for neuron-specific enolase, CD56,[604] chromogranin (but only in the better differentiated examples), synaptophysin, 5-hydroxytryptamine (serotonin), other generic neuroendocrine markers,[633,634] and a variety of peptide hormones[635] (Fig. 19.99). They also commonly express keratin (befitting their epithelial nature), CEA,[635] TTF-1 (a potentially misleading finding),[625] and p16, the latter suggesting an HPV participation in the genesis of these tumors, further confirmed at the molecular level.[615,619,636] Some examples are immunoreactive for CK20 and P63.[625] There is frequent loss of heterozygosity at 3p and 11p,[623,624] and loss of RB protein expression.[613]

The large majority of these cervical neoplasms are histologically and clinically aggressive. The treatment, especially for high-grade lesions, usually consists of a combination of surgery, radiation therapy, and chemotherapy.[628] The prognosis is generally poor.[601] A definite relationship exists between degree of microscopic differentiation and clinical behavior, the outcome being particularly bleak for the small cell carcinomas.[610,620,626] Naturally, there is also a close relationship between clinical stage and prognosis.[606] Both small cell and large cell (neuro)endocrine carcinomas with a polypoid shape or arising in polyps may be associated with a more favorable prognosis.[603]

Cytology

The broadest and most successful application of clinical cytology has been in the diagnosis of invasive carcinoma of the uterine cervix and precursor lesions through the technique. It was first described by Aureli Babès, a Rumanian pathologist, further developed by George Papanicolaou at Cornell University, and is universally known as the Pap test[654,663] (Fig. 19.100). Today, it is widely used both as a screening test in asymptomatic populations and in the follow-up of patients with cervical carcinomas treated by either conservative surgery or irradiation.[647,657]

Mass cytologic screening has shifted the presentation of cervical carcinoma from the clinical to the preclinical stage. This is an established fact, the statement that the incidence of cervical carcinoma was already declining prior to the introduction of this diagnostic method notwithstanding. Incidentally, the accuracy of the latter statement has been disputed.[645] Following mass screening, there has been a reduction of 38–57% in the overall incidence of invasive carcinoma and a reduction of 67% in the incidence of clinically evident carcinoma (stages Ib–IV).[640,646] Whereas in the prescreening era invasive carcinoma contributed approximately 80% of all diagnosed cases, at the present time it makes up less than 20% of the cases, the remaining being carcinomas in the intraepithelial (CIN) stage.[645] This has resulted in an increased cure rate for the screened population and an increase in the survival times for patients with invasive carcinoma.[642,645,646] In an often quoted article, Christopherson and Scott[641] reported a 70% decrease in mortality from carcinoma of the uterine cervix between 1970/1971 and 1955/1956 in women younger than 60 years of age.

The diagnostic accuracy of cervical cytology is high, as was already amply demonstrated in several large studies done in the 1960s.[658,673] However, in the evaluation of some remarkably high figures, one cannot escape the suspicion that they might have been influenced by the fact that the same person diagnosed the cytology specimen and the cervical biopsy. To avoid subconscious bias, it is better for these two functions to be performed by two different individuals. Seybolt[664] demonstrated this fact by distributing 25 problem cases to eight authorities in cytopathology and requesting them to interpret the cytology slides independently of the histology. There was no universal agreement in any case, and in some instances the disagreements were quite disparate. The conclusion from this survey was that it is not always possible to determine the exact histologic change in the cervix on the basis of the cytology smear. However, a more important demonstration was that if a cervical abnormality was present, this was detected by cytologic examination in the large majority of the cases.

Careful attention to technical factors is essential to achieve good results. The smear should be promptly fixed and carefully stained. Air-dried smears are grossly inadequate in this regard. Even if squamous cells can be rehydrated, they never exhibit the fine structural details of wet-fixed material; glandular cells are even more distorted. It is also highly desirable that the specimen be secured by a trained individual. Self-made samples, obtained with a pipette, are not nearly so satisfactory. Invasive carcinoma is detected at almost the same rate as with the material obtained by the physician, but the accuracy is considerably lower. Furthermore, the percentage of unsatisfactory specimens approaches 20%.[653] It is also important for the detection of early carcinoma that an endocervical sample obtained by the use of a special brush[651] be examined in addition to the ordinary specimen from the exocervix and vaginal pool.

Special techniques are also applicable to cytology smears, including immunohistochemistry, in situ hybridization, and DNA cytometry.[643] For instance, it has been shown that MIB-1 staining of cervical smears improves the diagnostic accuracy of cervical low-grade intraepithelial lesions.[659,675] Immunostaining for P16 in cervical smears is also of value in detection of high-grade squamous intraepithelial lesions.[662]

The terminology used in cervicovaginal cytology has evolved over the course of years, sometimes adapting names from the histopathology lexicon but more often devising some of its own. Papanicolaou's original system had five 'classes' of increasing atypia. Although this nomenclature fulfilled a very important role in the establishment of the technique, it was eventually abandoned

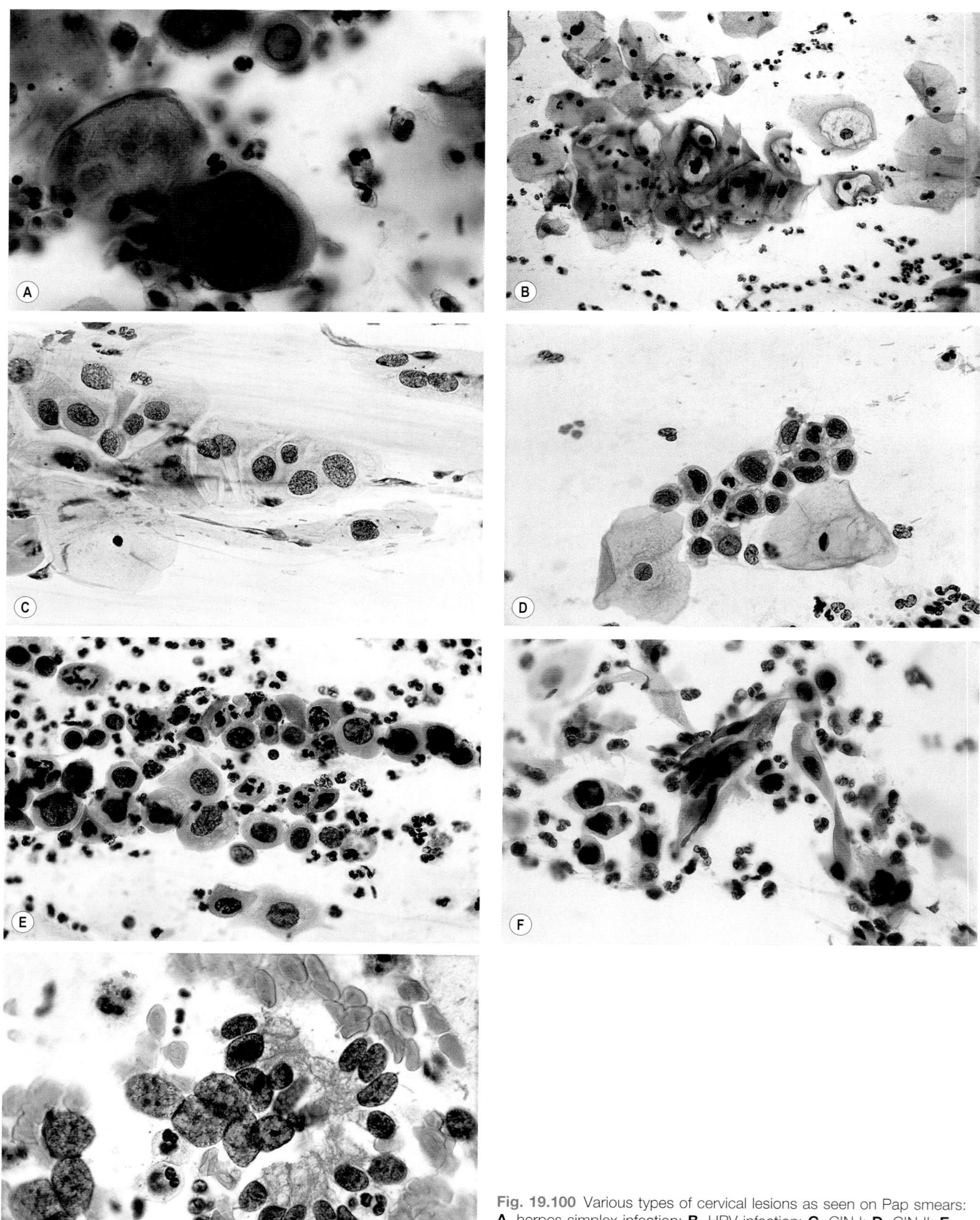

Fig. 19.100 Various types of cervical lesions as seen on Pap smears: **A**, herpes simplex infection; **B**, HPV infection; **C**, CIN I; **D**, CIN II; **E**, CIN III; **F**, invasive squamous cell carcinoma; **G**, adenocarcinoma. *(Courtesy of L. Alasio, Milan, Italy)*

because of the vagueness of the information provided. A 'class III' smear, for instance, could represent anything from a moderate dysplasia to an invasive carcinoma. Therefore, it was progressively replaced in the 1960s by the nomenclature then in vogue among histopathologists (i.e., negative, benign atypia, dysplasia (mild, moderate, or severe), carcinoma in situ, and invasive carcinoma).[664,665] During the 1970s, many institutions switched to the CIN system for both cytologic and histologic specimens (see p. 1444). In 1988, a proposal was made at a meeting in Bethesda to classify squamous intraepithelial lesions (SIL) in the following categories: (1) atypical squamous cells of undetermined significance (ASCUS); (2) low-grade SIL; (3) high-grade SIL; and (4) squamous cell carcinoma.[656,668,672] In this scheme, low-grade SIL corresponds to HPV-associated cellular changes, mild dysplasia, and CIN I, whereas high-grade SIL corresponds to moderate and severe dysplasia, carcinoma in situ, and CIN II and III. The rationale for grouping HPV-related changes (koilocytosis) and CIN I within the low-grade SIL group is based on the many similarities that exist between the lesions, which makes their separation difficult. A similar reasoning lies behind the decision to combine CIN II and III lesions in the category of high-grade SIL. The term 'atypical squamous cells of undetermined significance' (ASCUS) was proposed at the same meeting for cases in which the findings do not fulfill the criteria for either benign reactive change or SIL; as such, it has a more restricted meaning than the traditional terms 'atypia' and 'inflammatory atypia'.

The system has been criticized on several grounds, one of them being the claim that it leads to overtreatment of many individuals whose smears are placed in the low-grade SIL category.[639,649] Partly as a response to these criticisms, the system was revised in 2001 in order to facilitate triage of women for more intensive screening only when a strong suspicion of a high-grade lesion is present.[667,669] The current categories are the following:

1. Atypical squamous cells:
   a. Of unknown significance (ASC-US)
   b. Cannot exclude high-grade squamous intraepithelial lesion (ASC-H)
2. Low-grade squamous intraepithelial lesion (LGSIL)
3. High-grade squamous intraepithelial lesion (HGSIL).

The recommendation is for women with ASC-US to be managed using a program of two repeat cytology tests, immediate colposcopy, or DNA testing for high-risk types of HPV.[674]

The great success of the Pap test has led to overexpectations on the part of clinicians and the public at large and the unreasonable demand that every case of carcinoma be detected with it. One should not forget that it is and will remain a *screening* test and that – as such – it will inevitably be associated with a 'false-negative rate'.[660,670] The reasons include inadequacy of the sample, insufficient time devoted to screening, human fatigue, and inadequate interpretation by the screener and/or pathologist.[655,661,666] Of these, the latter represents only a minor fraction of all cases, as has been repeatedly demonstrated.[663,666]

The areas of innovation in cervical cancer screening consist of the technologies of liquid based-cytology (ThinPrep; AutoCyte), computer assisted screening (AutoPap; PapNet), and molecular testing for high-risk HPV[637,638,644,648,671] (see p. 1442 and Chapter 3). It has been argued that because HPV testing is more sensitive for the detection of cervical precancer and cancer than cervical cytology, it can substitute the latter or be used as first-line in a cervical screening program.[652] An even more sophisticated technique recently applied to cytologic specimens is the detection of genomic amplification of the human telomerase gene (*TERC*) as an independent screening test for HSIL.[650]

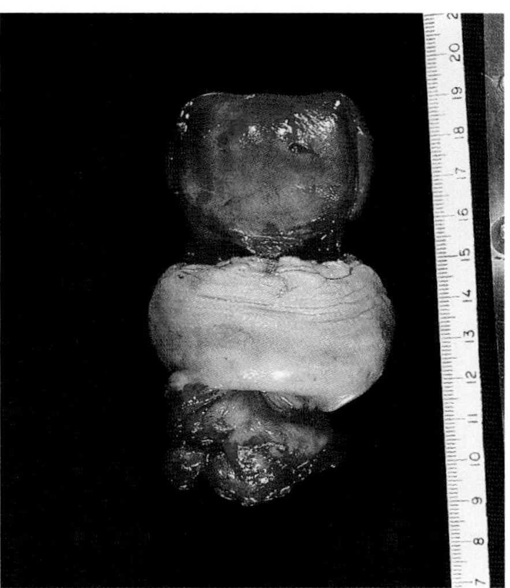

Fig. 19.101 Botryoid rhabdomyosarcoma of cervix protruding in the form of grapelike masses.

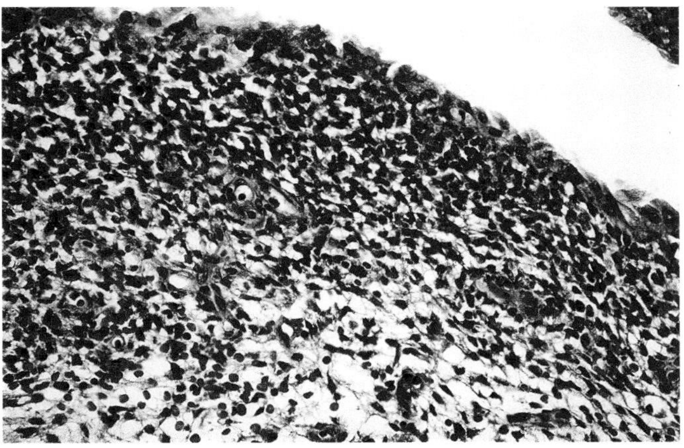

Fig. 19.102 Cambium layer beneath cervical epithelium in botryoid rhabdomyosarcoma of cervix.

Other tumors and tumorlike conditions

Carcinomas of one type or another comprise approximately 99% of all primary cervical malignancies. The remaining 1% is made up of a large variety of neoplasms.

Botryoid rhabdomyosarcoma (a variant of embryonal rhabdomyosarcoma) presents in children and adolescents as a myxoid polypoid mass covered by attenuated epithelium[685,690,721] (Figs 19.101 and 19.102). The appearance is generally similar to that of the homonymous vaginal tumor. However, some of the cervical cases occurring in older patients have been seen to contain cartilage and to be associated with a better prognosis[692] (Fig. 19.103). **Alveolar rhabdomyosarcoma** has also been reported.[735]

Mixed müllerian tumors also present as polypoid masses but generally occur in much older patients, the average age in one series being 65 years.[689] Some tumors look identical to their more common uterine counterparts, but in others the recognizable epithelial component has an adenoid basal or squamous appearance.[689,725] When

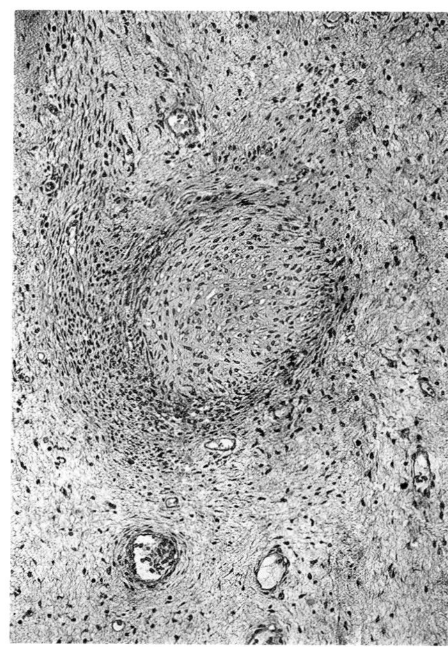

Fig. 19.103 Cartilage formation in botryoid rhabdomyosarcoma. This feature is more commonly seen in cervical than in vaginal examples of this tumor type.

the latter is the case, the appearance blends with that of spindle cell (sarcomatoid) carcinoma.

Müllerian adenosarcoma[699,712] and **stromal sarcoma** of endometrial type also occur in the cervix (Fig. 19.104), the former sometimes featuring foci of ovarian sex-cord-like structures;[708] this includes the better differentiated and presumably benign variant of this tumor originally described as *papillary adenofibroma*.[677,749]

Smooth muscle tumors, both benign and malignant, also occur in the cervix (Fig. 19.105).[742] The diagnostic criteria are the same as for those in the uterine corpus, but the ratio may be slightly different (comparatively more leiomyosarcomas are found in the cervix). Some of the reported leiomyosarcomas have been of the myxoid variety,[698] and others have had a xanthomatous appearance.[704]

Other primary cervical tumors and tumorlike conditions include *teratoma*,[706,714] *glial polyp* (*glial heterotopia, glioma*) of probable fetal origin,[739] and *ganglioneuroma*;[722] *yolk sac* (*endodermal sinus*) *tumor* (closely simulating the clinical appearance of botryoid rhabdomyosarcoma);[691] *choriocarcinoma*;[719] *sebaceous carcinoma*;[746] *extrarenal Wilms tumor*;[682] *traumatic* (*amputation*) *neuroma*[681] (some occurring postpartum);[743] *neurofibroma*;[701] *schwannoma*[705] (including the pigmented variety);[741] *malignant peripheral nerve sheath tumor*;[683,713] *solitary fibrous tumor*;[734] *pigmented neuroectodermal tumor of infancy*;[740] *melanosis* (sometimes developing after cryotherapy for CIN);[693,709,747] *blue nevus*[730,744,750] (Fig. 19.106); *cellular blue nevus*; *malignant melanoma*[687,717] (including the desmoplastic variety[711] and a type simulating malignant peripheral nerve sheath tumor[733]); *benign mesenchymoma*;[745] *hemangioma*[715] (Fig. 19.107); *glomus tumor*;[679] *angiosarcoma*;[688] *osteosarcoma*;[684] *alveolar soft part sarcoma*[697,729,737] (some extremely small[732] and some confirmed with the TFE3 stain[736]); and *Ewing sarcoma/PNET*[686,724] (sometimes combined with other components[694]).

Malignant lymphomas of the cervix present with vaginal bleeding and a subepithelial mass without obvious ulceration.[718] Most

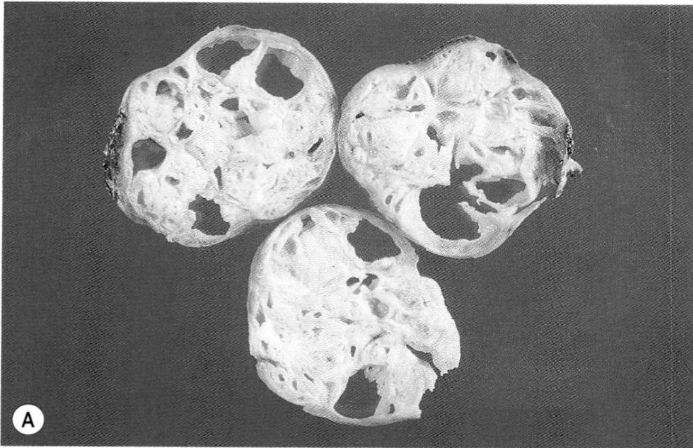

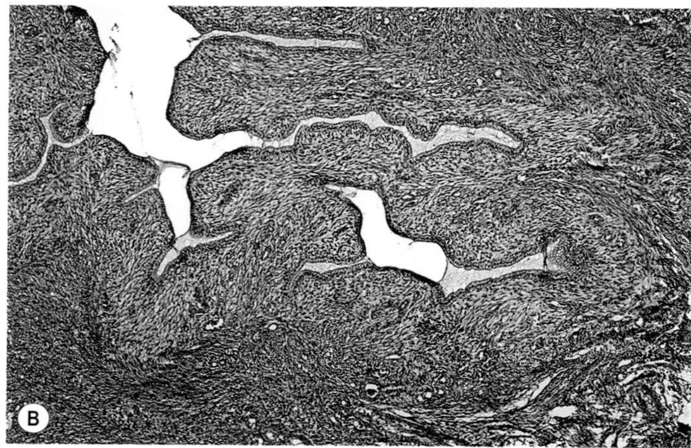

Fig. 19.104 **A** and **B**, Müllerian adenosarcoma of cervix. **A**, Gross appearance. This tumor was extremely well differentiated and qualified as an adenofibroma. **B**, Microscopic appearance of another case. The appearance is reminiscent of phylloides tumor of breast.
*(**A**, Courtesy of Dr Juan José Segura, San José, Costa Rica)*

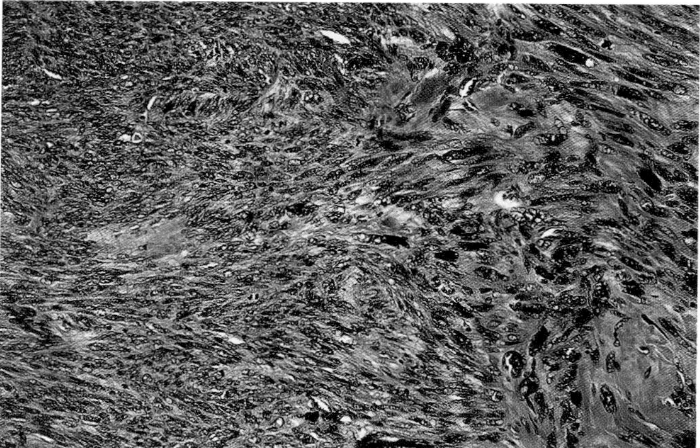

Fig. 19.105 Poorly differentiated leiomyosarcoma of cervix.

are diffuse large B-cell lymphomas and many are accompanied by extensive fibrosis[680,695,696,707,716,731] (Fig. 19.108). An important differential diagnosis is with **lymphoma-like lesions** resulting from focally florid lymphoid proliferation associated with chronic cervicitis or as an expression of infectious mononucleosis;[723,748] these are identified by the polymorphic nature of the infiltrate (including

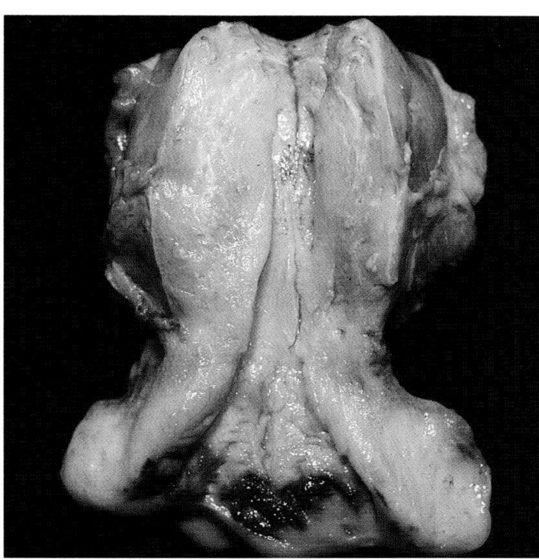

Fig. 19.106 Gross appearance of blue nevus of cervix. *(Courtesy of Dr Luis Spitale, Córdoba, Argentina)*

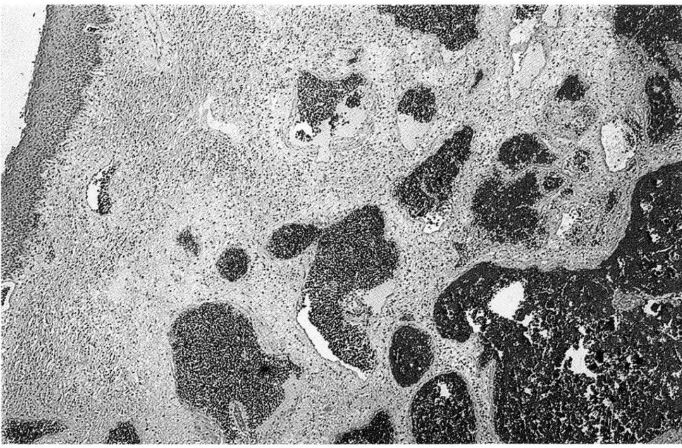

Fig. 19.107 Cavernous hemangioma of cervix, a most unusual occurrence.

mature plasma cells, small lymphocytes, and neutrophils), surface ulceration, and minimal or no sclerosis. Despite the occasional detection of clonality in some cases, the disease has so far followed a benign clinical course.[702] *Granulocytic sarcoma (chloroma)*,[676,700,738] *Hodgkin lymphoma, inflammatory pseudotumor*,[678] localized *amyloidosis*,[703] and *Rosai–Dorfman disease* (sinus histiocytosis with massive lymphadenopathy)[728] can also present initially as a cervical mass.

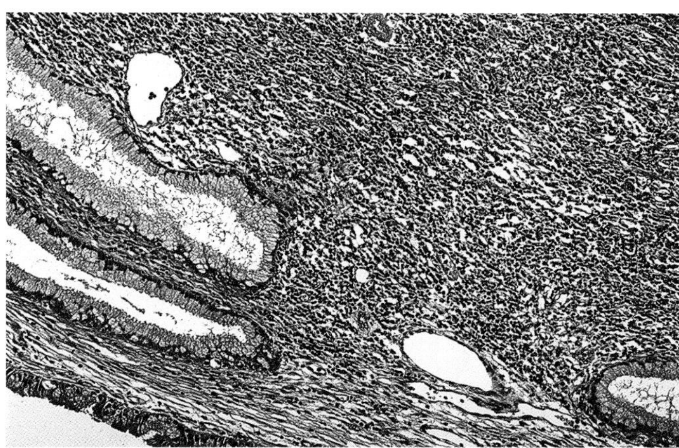

Fig. 19.108 Diffuse large cell lymphoma of cervix growing between normal endocervical glands.

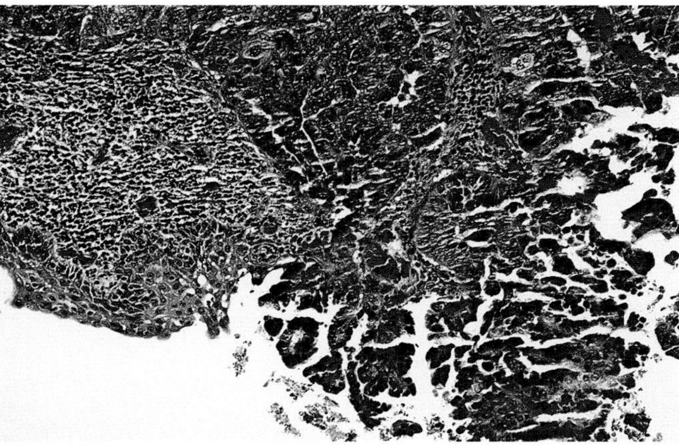

Fig. 19.109 Serous papillary carcinoma of ovary metastatic to cervix.

Metastatic carcinomas to the cervix (excluding direct invasion from endometrial carcinoma) can originate from genital or extragenital organs; the most common sites are the ovary, large bowel, stomach, breast, and kidney[710,720] (Fig. 19.109). Some of them simulate clinically and pathologically the appearance of primary cervical carcinoma, including invasive and in situ cervical adenocarcinoma.[726] Knowledge of the clinical findings may make this mistake avoidable.

An exceptional event is represented by a coating of the endocervical (and endometrial) mucosa by metastatic mucinous tumor of the appendix, a phenomenon somewhat analogous to that seen in pseudomyxoma peritonei and pseudomyxoma ovarii.[727]

References

NORMAL ANATOMY

1 Barroeta JE, Pasha TL, Acs G, Zhang PJ. Immunoprofile of endocervical and endometrial stromal cells and its potential application in localization of tumor involvement. Int J Gynecol Pathol 2007, **26**: 76–82.

2 Fetissof F, Serres G, Arbeille B, de Muret A, Sam-Giao M, Lansac J. Argyrophilic cells and ectocervical epithelium. Int J Gynecol Pathol 1991, **10**: 177–190.

3 Gilks CB, Reid PE, Clement PB, Owen DA. Histochemical changes in cervical mucus-secreting epithelium during the normal menstrual cycle. Fertil Steril 1989, **5**: 286–291.

4 Hendrickson MR, Atkins KA, Kempson RL. Ulterus and fallopian tubes. In Mills SE (ed.): Histology for pathologists, ed. 3. Philadelphia, 2007, Lippincott Williams and Wilkins, pp. 1011–1062.

5 Loning T, Kuhler C, Caselitz J, Stegner HE. Keratin and tissue polypeptide antigen profiles of the cervical mucosa. Int J Gynecol Pathol 1983, **2**: 105–112.

6 Malecha MJ, Miettinen M. Patterns of keratin subsets in normal and abnormal uterine cervical tissues. An immunohistochemical study. Int J Gynecol Pathol 1992, **11**: 24–29.

7 Nonogaki H, Fujii S, Konishi I, Nanbu Y, Ozaki S, Ishikawa Y, Mori T. Estrogen receptor localization in normal and neoplastic epithelium of the uterine cervix. Cancer 1990, **66**: 2620–2627.

8 Osamura RY, Watanabe K, Oh M. Melanin-containing cells in the uterine cervix. Histochemical and electron-microscopic studies of two cases. Am J Clin Pathol 1980, **74**: 239–242.

9 Remadi S, MacGee W, Mégevand E, Chappuis P, Redard M, Seemayer TA. Resident neuroendocrine cells in the normal ectoendocervical epithelium: an immunohistochemical study of 100 cases using a microwave heating technique. Int J Surg Pathol 1997, **5**: 19–24.

10 Smedts F, Ramaekers F, Troyanovsky S, Pruszczynski M, Robben H, Lane B, Leigh I, Plantema F, Vooijs P. Basal-cell keratins in cervical reserve cells and a comparison to their expression in cervical intraepithelial neoplasia. Am J Pathol 1992, **140**: 601–612.

11 Warhol MJ, Antonioli DA, Pinkus GS, Burke L, Rice RH. Immunoperoxidase staining for involucrin. A potential diagnostic aid in cervicovaginal pathology. Hum Pathol 1982, **13**: 1095–1099.

12 Whittaker JR, Samy AM, Sunter JP, Sinha DP, Monaghan JM. Cytokeratin expression in cervical epithelium. An immunohistological study of normal, wart virus-infected and neoplastic tissue. Histopathology 1989, **14**: 151–160.

13 Zwillenberg LO. At 40 years of the 'Golden Chain'. Which are the stem cells in ectocervical epithelium? Gynecol Obstet Invest 1999, **46**: 247–251.

REMNANTS AND ECTOPIAS

14 McCluggage WG, Ganesan R, Hirschowitz L, Miller K, Rollason TP. Ectopic prostatic tissue in the uterine cervix and vagina: report of a series with a detailed immunohistochemical analysis. Am J Surg Pathol 2006, **30**: 209–215.

15 Nucci MR, Ferry JA, Young PR. Ectopic prostatic tissue in the uterine cervix: a report of four cases and review of ectopic prostatic tissue. Am J Surg Pathol 2000, **24**: 1224–1230.

16 Rabban JT, McAlhany S, Lerwill MF, Grenert JP, Zaloudek CJ. PAX2 distinguishes benign mesonephric and mullerian glandular lesions of the cervix from endocervical adenocarcinoma, including minimal deviation adenocarcinoma. Am J Surg Pathol 2010, **34**: 137–146.

17 Rath-Wolfson L, Koren R, Amiel A, Pardo J, Gal R. The 'female prostrate' in cervix uteri: a case report. Appl Immunhistochem 1998, **6**: 50–53.

18 Robledo M, Vazquez J, Contreras-Mejuto F, Lopez-Garcia G. Sebaceous glands and hair follicles in the cervix uteri. Histopathology 1992, **21**: 278–279.

19 Roth E, Taylor HB. Heterotopic cartilage in the uterus. Obstet Gynecol 1966, **27**: 838–844.

SQUAMOUS AND OTHER METAPLASIAS

20 al-Nafussi A, Rahilly M. The prevalence of tubo-endometrial metaplasia and adenomatoid proliferation. Histopathology 1993, **22**: 177–179.

21 Crum CP, Egawa K, Fu YS, Lancaster WD, Barron B, Levine RU, Fenoglio CM, Richart RM. Atypical immature metaplasia (AIM). A subset of human papilloma virus infection of the cervix. Cancer 1983, **51**: 2214–2219.

22 Ducatman BS, Wang HH, Jonasson JG, Hogan CL, Antonioli DA. Tubal metaplasia. A cytologic study with comparison to other neoplastic and non-neoplastic conditions of the endocervix. Diagn Cytopathol 1993, **9**: 95–103.

23 Duggan MA, Akbari M, Magliocco AM. Atypical immature cervical metaplasia: immunoprofiling and longitudinal outcome. Hum Pathol 2006, **37**: 1473–1481.

24 Egan AJM, Russell P. Transitional (urothelial) cell metaplasia of the uterine cervix: morphological assessment of 31 cases. Int J Gynecol Pathol 1997, **16**: 89–98.

25 Feldman D, Romney SL, Edgcomb J, Valentine T. Ultrastructure of normal, metaplastic, and abnormal human uterine cervix. Use of montages to study the topographical relationship of epithelial cells. Am J Obstet Gynecol 1984, **150**: 573–688.

26 Geng L, Connolly DC, Isaacson C, Ronnett BM, Cho KR. Atypical immature metaplasia (AIM) of the cervix: is it related to high-grade squamous intraepithelial lesion (HSIL)? Hum Pathol 1999, **30**: 345–351.

27 Harnden P, Kennedy W, Andrew AC, Southgate J. Immunophenotype of transitional metaplasia of the uterine cervix. Int J Gynecol Pathol 1999, **18**: 125–129.

28 Ismail SM. Cone biopsy causes cervical endometriosis and tubo-endometrioid metaplasia. Histopathology 1991, **18**: 107–114.

29 Johnson LD, Easterday CL, Gore H, Hertig AT. Histogenesis of carcinoma in situ of the uterine cervix. A preliminary report of the origin of carcinoma in situ in subcylindrical cell anaplasia. Cancer 1964, **17**: 213–229.

30 Jonasson JG, Wang HH, Antonioli DA, Ducatman BS. Tubal metaplasia of the uterine cervix. A prevalence study in patients with gynecologic pathologic findings. Int J Gynecol Pathol 1992, **11**: 89–95.

31 Jones MA. Transitional cell metaplasia and neoplasia in the female genital tract: an update. Adv Anat Pathol 1999, **5**: 106–113.

32 Jones MA, Young RH. Atypical oxyphilic metaplasia of the endocervical epithelium: a report of six cases. Int J Gynecol Pathol 1997, **16**: 99–102.

33 Kong CS, Balzer BL, Troxell ML, Patterson BK, Longacre TA. p16^{INK4A} immunohistochemistry is superior to HPV in situ hybridization for the detection of high-risk HPV in atypical squamous metaplasia. Am J Surg Pathol 2007, **31**: 33–43.

34 Koss LG. Transitional cell metaplasia of cervix: a misnomer. Am J Surg Pathol 1998, **22**: 774–776.

35 Ma L, Fisk JM, Zhang RR, Ulukus EC, Crum CP, Zheng W. Eosinophilic dysplasia of the cervix: a newly recognized variant of cervical squamous intraepithelial neoplasia. Am J Surg Pathol 2004, **28**: 1474–1484.

36 McCluggage WG, Maxwell P, McBride HA, Hamilton PW, Bharucha H. Monoclonal antibodies Ki-67 and M1B1 in the distinction of tuboendometrial metaplasia from endocervical adenocarcinoma and adenocarcinoma in situ in formalin-fixed material. Int J Gynecol Pathol 1995, **14**: 209–216.

37 Mittal K, Mesia A, Demopoulos RI. MIB-1 expression is useful in distinguishing dysplasia from atrophy in elderly women. Int J Gynecol Pathol 1999, **18**: 122–124.

38 Miyatake T, Ueda Y, Yoshino K, Shroyer KR, Kanao H, Sun H, Nakashima R, Kimura T, Wakasa T, Enomoto T. Clonality analysis and human papillomavirus infection in squamous metaplasia and atypical immature metaplasia of uterine cervix: is atypical immature metaplasia a precursor to cervical intraepithelial neoplasia 3? Int J Gynecol Pathol 2007, **26**: 180–187.

39 Oliva E, Clement PB, Young RH. Tubal and tubo-endometrioid metaplasia of the uterine cervix. Unemphasized features that may cause problems in differential diagnosis – a report of 25 cases. Am J Clin Pathol 1995, **103**: 618–623.

40 Park JJ, Genest DR, Sun D, Crum CP. Atypical immature metaplastic-like proliferations of the cervix: diagnostic reproducibility and viral (HPV) correlates. Hum Pathol 1999, **30**: 1161–1165.

41 Park SH, Lee YH, Kim KR. The immunoexpressions of biomarkers (p16, Ki67, and PreEx^{TM}C) are beneficial for the differential diagnosis of transitional cell metaplasia from high grade cervical intraepithelial neoplasia of the uterine cervix in perimenopausal and postmenopausal women. Lab Invest 2009, **89**(Suppl 1): 231A.

42 Puts JJG, Moesker O, Kenemans P, Vooijs GP, Ramaekers FCS. Expression of cytokeratins in early neoplastic epithelial lesions of the uterine cervix. Int J Gynecol Pathol 1985, **4**: 300–313.

43 Samarawardana PN, Shroyer KR. Co-localization of p16^{INK4a} and MIB-1 distinguishes high grade premalignant lesions from tuboendometrial metaplasia in cervical mucosa. Lab Invest 2009, **89**(Suppl 1): 235A.

44 Suh KS, Silverberg SG. Tubal metaplasia of the uterine cervix. Int J Gynecol Pathol 1990, **9**: 122–128.

45 Val-Bernal JF, Pinto J, Garijo MF, Gomez MS. Pagetoid dyskeratosis of the cervix: an incidental histologic finding in uterine prolapse. Am J Surg Pathol 2000, **24**: 1518–1523.

46 Vang R, Vinh TN, Burks RT, Barner R, Kurman RJ, Ronnett BM. Pseudoinfiltrative tubal metaplasia of the endocervix: a potential form of in utero diethylstilbestrol exposure-related adenosis simulating minimal deviation adenocarcinoma. Int J Gynecol Pathol 2005, **24**: 391–398.

47 Weir MM, Bell DA, Young RH. Transitional cell metaplasia of the uterine cervix and vagina: an underrecognized lesion that may be confused with high-grade dysplasia: a report of 59 cases. Am J Surg Pathol 1997, **21**: 510–517.

48 Yeh IT, Bronner M, Li Volsi VA. Endometrial metaplasia of the uterine endocervix. Arch Pathol Lab Med 1993, **117**: 734–735.

49 Young RH, Clement PB. Pseudoneoplastic glandular lesions of the uterine cervix. Semin Diagn Pathol 1991, **8**: 234–249.

INFLAMMATORY LESIONS

50 Adams RL, Springall DR, Levene MM. The immunocytochemical detection of herpes simplex virus in cervical smears. A valuable technique for routine use. J Pathol 1984, **143**: 241–247.

51 Albores-Saavedra J, Rosas-Uribe A, Altramirano-Dimas M, Brandt H. Cancer with superimposed amebiasis. Am J Clin Pathol 1968, **49**: 677–682.

52 al Nafussi AI, Hughes D, Rebello G. Ceroid granuloma of the uterine cervix. Histopathology 1992, **21**: 282–284.

53 Bean SM, Conner MG. Wegener's granulomatosis of the uterine cervix: a case report and review of the literature. Int J Gynecol Pathol 2007, **26**: 95–98.

54 Berry A. A cytopathological and histopathological study of bilharziasis of the female genital tract. J Pathol Bacteriol 1966, **91**: 325–338.

55 Bhagavan BS, Ruffier J, Shinn B. Pseudoactinomycotic radiate granules in the lower female genital tract. Relationship to the Splendore–Hoeppli phenomenon. Hum Pathol 1982, **13**: 898–904.

56 Chen KTK, Hendricks EJ. Malakoplakia of the female genital tract. Obstet Gynecol 1985, **65**: 84S–87S.

57 Cohen C. Three cases of amoebiasis of the cervix uteri. J Obstet Gynaecol Br Commonw 1973, **80**: 476–479.

58 Crow J, McWhinney N. Isolated arteritis of the cervix uteri. Br J Obstet Gynaecol 1979, **86**: 393–398.

59 Kiviat NB, Paavonen JA, Wolner-Hanssen P, Critchlow CW, Stamm WE, Douglas J, Eschenbach DA, Corey LA, Holmes KK. Histopathology of endocervical infection caused by *Chlamydia trachomatis*, herpes simplex virus, *Trichomonas vaginalis*, and *Neisseria gonorrhoeae*. Hum Pathol 1990, **21**: 831–837.

60 Marrogi AJ, Gersell DJ, Kraus FT. Localized asymptomatic giant cell arteritis of the female genital tract. Int J Gynecol Pathol 1991, **10**: 51–58.

61 Marsella RC, Buckner SB, Bratthauer GL, O'Connor DM, O'Leary TJ. Identification of genital herpes simplex virus infection by immunoperoxidase staining. Appl Immunohistochem 1995, **3**: 184–189.

62 Mitao M, Reumann W, Winkler B, Richart RM, Fujiwara A, Crum CP. Chlamydial cervicitis and cervical intraepithelial neoplasia. An immunohistochemical analysis. Gynecol Oncol 1984, **19**: 90–97.

63 Naib ZM, Nahmias AJ, Josey WE. Cytology and histopathology of cervical herpes simplex infection. Cancer 1966, **19**: 1026–1031.

64 Paavonen J, Critchlow CW, DeRouen T, Stevens CE, Kiviat N, Brunham RC, Staam WE, Kuo CC, Hyde KE, Corey L, Eschenbach DA, Holmes KK. Etiology of cervical inflammation. Am J Obstet Gynecol 1986, **154**: 556–564.

65 Pikarsky E, Maly B, Maly A. Ceroid granuloma of the uterine cervix. Int J Gynecol Pathol 2002, **21**: 191–193.

66 Tchertkoff V, Ober WB. Primary chancre of cervix uteri. N Y State J Med 1966, **66**: 1921–1924.

67 Winkler B, Crum CP. *Chlamydia trachomatis* infection of the female genital tract. Pathogenetic and clinicopathologic correlations. Pathol Annu 1987, **22**(Pt 1): 193–223.

NON-NEOPLASTIC GLANDULAR LESIONS

68 Chumas JC, Nelson B, Mann WJ, Chalas E, Kaplan CG. Microglandular hyperplasia of the uterine cervix. Obstet Gynecol 1985, **66**: 406–409.

69 Clement PB, Young RH. Deep nabothian cysts of the uterine cervix. A possible source of confusion with minimal-deviation adenocarcinoma (adenoma malignum). Int J Gynecol Pathol 1989, **8**: 340–348.

70 Cove H. The Arias-Stella reaction occurring in the endocervix in pregnancy. Recognition and comparison with an adenocarcinoma of the cervix. Am J Surg Pathol 1979, **3**: 567–568.

71 Dube V, Nofech-Mozes S, Ismiil N, Saad RS, Ghorab Z, Khalifa MA. p16 immunohistochemical expression in squamous metaplasia of endocervical polyps. Lab Invest 2009, **89**(Suppl 1): 212A.

72 Ferry JA, Scully RE. Mesonephric remnants, hyperplasia, and neoplasia in the uterine cervix. A study of 49 cases. Am J Surg Pathol 1990, **14**: 1100–1111.

73 Greeley C, Schroeder S, Silverberg SG. Microglandular hyperplasia of the cervix. A true 'pill' lesion? Int J Gynecol Pathol 1995, **14**: 50–54.

74 Inai K, Arihiro K, Tokuoka S, Katsube Y, Fujiwara A. Mesonephric duct hyperplasia of the uterus. Report of two cases and three other cases of mesonephric duct remnant with findings of mucin histochemistry and lectin binding immunohistochemistry. Acta Pathol Jpn 1989, **39**: 457–464.

75 Janovski NA, Kasdon EJ. Benign mesonephric papillary and polypoid tumors of the cervix in childhood. J Pediatr 1963, **63**: 211–216.

76 Jones MA, Andrews J, Tarraza HM. Mesonephric remnant hyperplasia of the cervix. A clinicopathologic analysis of 14 cases. Gynecol Oncol 1993, **49**: 41–47.

77 Jones MA, Young RH. Endocervical type A (noncystic) tunnel clusters with cytologic atypia: a report of 14 cases. Am J Surg Pathol 1996, **20**: 1312–1318.

78 Jones MA, Young RH, Scully RE. Diffuse laminar endocervical glandular hyperplasia. A benign lesion often confused with adenoma malignum (minimal deviation adenocarcinoma). Am J Surg Pathol 1991, **15**: 1123–1129.

79 Kawauchi S, Kusuda T, Liu XP, Suehiro Y, Kaku T, Mikami Y, Takeshita M, Nakao M, Chochi Y, Sasaki K. Is lobular endocervical glandular hyperplasia a cancerous precursor of minimal deviation adenocarcinoma?: a comparative molecular-genetic and immunohistochemical study. Am J Surg Pathol 2008, **32**: 1807–1815.

80 Kondo T, Hashi A, Murata S, Nakazawa T, Yuminamochi T, Nara M, Hoshi K, Katoh R. Endocervical adenocarcinomas associated with lobular endocervical glandular hyperplasia: a report of four cases with histochemical and immunohistochemical analyses. Mod Pathol 2005, **18**: 1199–1210.

81 Kondo T, Hashi A, Murata SI, Fischer SE, Nara M, Nakazawa T, Yuminamochi T, Hoshi K, Katoh R. Gastric mucin is expressed in a subset of endocervical tunnel clusters: type A tunnel clusters of gastric phenotype. Histopathology 2007, **50**: 843–850.

82 Kyriakos M, Kempson RL, Konikov NF. A clinical and pathologic study of endocervical lesions associated with oral contraceptives. Cancer 1968, **22**: 99–110.

83 Laskin WB, Fetsch JF, Tavassoli FA. Superficial cervicovaginal myofibroblastoma: fourteen cases of a distinctive mesenchymal tumor arising from a specialized subepithelial stroma of the lower female genital tract. Hum Pathol 2001, **32**: 715–725.

84 Mikami Y, Hata S, Melamed J, Fujiwara K, Manabe T. Lobular endocervical glandular hyperplasia is a metaplastic process with a pyloric gland phenotype. Histopathology 2001, **39**: 364–372.

85 Mikami Y, Hata S, Melamed J, Fujiwara K, Manabe T. Lobular endocervical glandular hyperplasia is a metaplastic process with a pyloric gland phenotype. Histopathology 2001, **39**: 364–372.

86 Nucci MR. Tumor-like glandular lesions of the uterine cervix. Int J Gynecol Pathol 2002, **21**: 347–359.

87 Nucci MR, Clement PB, Young RH. Lobular endocervical glandular hyperplasia, not otherwise specified: a clinicopathologic analysis of thirteen cases of a distinctive pseudoneoplastic lesion and comparison with fourteen cases of adenoma malignum. Am J Surg Pathol 1999, **23**: 886–891.

88 Nucci MR, Young RH. Arias-Stella reaction of the endocervix: a report of 18 cases with emphasis on its varied histology and differential diagnosis. Am J Surg Pathol 2004, **28**: 608–612.

89 Ragazzi M, Carbonara C, Rosai J. Nonneoplastic signet-ring cells in the gallbladder and uterine cervix. A potential source of overdiagnosis. Hum Pathol 2009, **40**: 326–331.

90 Rhatigan RM. Endocervical gland atypia secondary to Arias-Stella change. Arch Pathol Lab Med 1992, **116**: 943–946.

91 Samaratunga H, Beresford A, Davison A. Squamous cell carcinoma in situ involving mesonephric remnants. A potential diagnostic pitfall. Am J Surg Pathol 1994, **18**: 1265–1269.

92 Scott M, Lyness RW, McCluggage WG. Atypical reactive proliferation of endocervix: a common lesion associated with endometrial carcinoma and likely related to prior endometrial sampling. Mod Pathol 2006, **19**: 470–474.

93 Segal GH, Hart WR. Cystic endocervical tunnel clusters. A clinicopathologic study of 29 cases of so-called adenomatous hyperplasia. Am J Surg Pathol 1990, **14**: 895–903.

94 Seidman JD, Tavassoli FA. Mesonephric hyperplasia of the uterine cervix. A clinicopathologic study of 51 cases. Int J Gynecol Pathol 1995, **14**: 293–299.

95 Selzer I, Nelson HM. Benign papilloma (polypoid tumor) of the cervix uteri in children. Report of 2 cases. Am J Obstet Gynecol 1962, **84**: 165–169.

96 Speers WC, Picaso LG, Silverberg SG. Immunohistochemical localization of carcinoembryonic antigen in microglandular hyperplasia and adenocarcinoma of the endocervix. Am J Clin Pathol 1983, **79**: 105–107.

97 Taylor HB, Irey NS, Norris HJ. Atypical endocervical hyperplasia in women taking oral contraceptives. JAMA 1967, **202**: 637–639.

98 Tsuda H, Mikami Y, Kaku T, Hasegawa T, Akiyama F, Ohishi Y, Sasajima Y, Kasamatsu T. Reproducible and clinically meaningful differential diagnosis is possible between lobular endocervical glandular hyperplasia and 'adenoma malignum' based on common histopathological criteria. Pathol Int 2005, **55**: 412–418.

99 Young RH, Clement PB. Pseudoneoplastic glandular lesions of the uterine cervix. Semin Diagn Pathol 1991, **8**: 234–249.

100 Young RH, Scully RE. Atypical forms of microglandular hyperplasia of the cervix simulating carcinoma. A report of five cases and review of the literature. Am J Surg Pathol 1989, **13**: 50–56.

NON-NEOPLASTIC STROMAL LESIONS (INCLUDING ENDOMETRIOSIS AND RELATED PROCESSES)

101 Abdul-Karim FW, Cohen RE. Atypical stromal cells of lower female genital tract. Histopathology 1990, **17**: 249–253.

102 Baker PM, Clement PB, Bell DA, Young RH. Superficial endometriosis of the uterine cervix: a report of 20 cases of a process that may be confused with endocervical glandular dysplasia or adenocarcinoma in situ. Int J Gynecol Pathol 2002, **18**: 198–205.

103 Clement PB. Multinucleated stromal giant cells of the uterine cervix. Arch Pathol Lab Med 1985, **109**: 200–202.

104 Clement PB, Young RH, Scully RE. Nontrophoblastic pathology of the female genital tract and peritoneum associated with pregnancy. Semin Diagn Pathol 1989, **6**: 372–406.

105 Clement PB, Young RH, Scully RE. Stromal endometriosis of the uterine cervix. A variant of endometriosis that may simulate a sarcoma. Am J Surg Pathol 1990, **14**: 449–455.

106 Elliott GB, Elliott JDA. Superficial stromal reactions of lower genital tract. Arch Pathol 1973, **95**: 100–101.

107 Evans CS, Goldman RL, Klein HZ, Kohout ND. Necrobiotic granulomas of the uterine cervix. A probable postoperative reaction. Am J Surg Pathol 1984, **8**: 841–844.

108 Fukunaga M. Uterus-like mass in the uterine cervix: superficial cervical endometriosis with florid smooth muscle metaplasia? Virchows Arch 2001, **438**: 302–305.

109 Hariri J, Ingemanssen JL. Multinucleated stromal giant cells of the uterine cervix. Int J Gynecol Pathol 1993, **12**: 228–234.

110 Huettner PC, Gersell DJ. Placental site nodule. A clinicopathologic study of 38 cases. Int J Gynecol Pathol 1994, **13**: 191–198.

111 Kay S, Schneider V. Reactive spindle cell nodule of the endocervix simulating uterine sarcoma. Int J Gynecol Pathol 1985, **4**: 255–257.

112 McCluggage WG, Young RH. Myxoid change of the myometrium and cervical stroma: description of a hitherto unreported non-neoplastic phenomenon with discussion of myxoid uterine lesions. Int J Gynecol Pathol 2010, **29**: 351–357.

113 Van Dorpe J, Moerman P. Placental site nodule of the uterine cervix. Histopathology 1997, **29**: 379–382.

114 Young RH, Clement PB. Endocervicosis involving the uterine cervix: a report of four cases of a benign process that may be confused with deeply invasive endocervical adenocarcinoma. Int J Gynecol Pathol 2001, **19**: 322–328.

115 Young RH, Kurman RJ, Scully RE. Placental site nodules and plaques. A clinicopathologic analysis of 20 cases. Am J Surg Pathol 1990, **14**: 1001–1009.

HUMAN PAPILLOMA VIRUS (HPV) AND THE LOWER FEMALE GENITAL TRACT

116 Abadi MA, Ho GY, Burk RD, Romney SL, Kadish AS. Stringent criteria for histological diagnosis of koilocytosis fail to eliminate overdiagnosis of human papillomavirus infection and cervical intraepithelial neoplasia Grade 1. Hum Pathol 1998, **29**: 54–59.

117 Albores-Saavedra J, Young RH. Transitional cell neoplasms (carcinomas and inverted papillomas) of the uterine cervix. A report of four cases. Am J Surg Pathol 1995, **19**: 1138–1145.

118 Ambros RA, Kurman RJ. Current concepts in the relationship of human papillomavirus infection to the pathogenesis and classification of precancerous squamous lesions of the uterine cervix. Semin Diagn Pathol 1990, **7**: 158–172.

119 Arends MJ, Wyllie AH, Bird CC. Papillomaviruses and human cancer. Hum Pathol 1990, **21**: 686–698.

120 Bergeron C, Barrasso R, Beaudenon S, Flamant P, Croissant O, Orth G. Human papillomaviruses associated with cervical intraepithelial neoplasia. Great diversity and distinct distribution in low- and high-grade lesions. Am J Surg Pathol 1992, **16**: 641–649.

121 Binder MA, Cates GW, Emson HE, Valnicek SJ, MacLachlan TB, Schmidt EW, Popkin DR, Ferenczy A. The changing concepts of condyloma. A retrospective study of colposcopically directed cervical biopsies. Am J Obstet Gynecol 1985, **151**: 213–219.

122 Bosch FX, Manos MM, Muñoz N, Sherman M, Jansen AM, Peto J, Schiffman MH, Moreno V, Kurman R, Shah KV. International Biological Study on Cervical Cancer (IBSCC) Study Group: Prevalence of human papillomavirus in cervical cancer. A worldwide perspective. J Natl Cancer Inst 1995, **87**: 796–802.

123 Boyle CA, Lowell DM, Kelsey JL, Li Volsi VA, Boyle KE. Cervical intraepithelial neoplasia among women with papillomavirus infection compared to women with *Trichomonas* infection. Cancer 1989, **64**: 168–172.

124 Cain JM, Howett MK. Preventing cervical cancer. Science 2000, **288**: 1753–1794.

125 Chen JJ, Reid CE, Band V, Androphy EJ. Interaction of papillomavirus E6 oncoproteins with a putative calcium-binding protein. Science 1995, **269**: 529–531.

126 Colgan TJ, Percy ME, Suri M, Shier RM, Andrews DF, Lickrish GM. Human papillomavirus infection of morphologically normal cervical epithelium adjacent to squamous dysplasia and invasive carcinoma. Hum Pathol 1989, **20**: 316–319.

127 Cooper K, Herrington CS, Lo ES, Evans MF, McGee JO. Integration of human papillomavirus types 16 and 18 in cervical adenocarcinoma. J Clin Pathol 1992, **45**: 382–384.

128 Crum C. Genital papillomaviruses and related neoplasms. Causation, diagnosis and classification (Bethesda). Mod Pathol 1994, **7**: 138–145.

129 Crum CP. Contemporary theories of cervical carcinogenesis: the virus, the host, and the stem cell. Mod Pathol 2000, **13**: 243–251.

130 Crum CP, Egawa K, Barron B, Fenoglio CM, Levine RU, Richart RM. Human papilloma virus infection (condyloma) of the cervix and cervical intraepithelial neoplasia. A histopathologic and statistical analysis. Gynecol Oncol 1983, **15**: 88–94.

131 Crum CP, Ikenberg H, Richart RM, Gissman L. Human papilloma virus type 16 and early cervical neoplasia. N Engl J Med 1984, **310**: 880–883.

132 Delvenne P, Fontaine M, Delvenne C, Nikkels A, Boniver J. Detection of human papillomaviruses in paraffin-embedded biopsies of cervical intraepithelial lesions. Analysis by immunohistochemistry, in situ hybridization, and the polymerase chain reaction. Mod Pathol 1994, **7**: 113–119.

133 Duggan MA, Benoit JL, McGregor SE, Inoue M, Nation JG, Stuart GCE. Adenocarcinoma in situ of the endocervix. Human papillomavirus determination by dot blot hybridization and polymerase chain reaction amplification. Int J Gynecol Pathol 1994, **13**: 143–149.

134 Farnsworth A, Laverty C, Stoler MH. Human papillomavirus messenger RNA expression in adenocarcinoma in situ of the uterine cervix. Int J Gynecol Pathol 1989, **8**: 321–330.

135 Franco EL, Rohan TE, Villa LL. Epidemiologic evidence and human papillomavirus infection as a necessary cause of cervical cancer. J Natl Cancer Inst 1999, **91**: 506–511.

136 Franquemont DW, Ward BE, Andersen WA, Crum CP. Prediction of 'high-risk' cervical papillomavirus infection by biopsy morphology. Am J Clin Pathol 1989, **92**: 577–582.

137 Genest DR, Stein L, Cibas E, Sheets E, Zitz JC, Crum CP. A binary (Bethesda) system for classifying cervical cancer precursors. Criteria, reproducibility, and viral correlates. Hum Pathol 1993, **24**: 730–736.

138 Graf A, Cheung AL, Hauser-Kronberger C, Dandachi N, Tubbs RR, Dietze O, Hacker GW. Clinical relevance of HPV 16/18 testing methods in cervical squamous cell carcinoma. Appl Immunohistochem Mol Morphol 2000, **8**: 300–309.

139 Ho GYF, Burk RD, Klein S, Kadish AS, Chang CJ, Palan P, Basu J, Tachezy R, Lewis R, Romney S. Persistent cervical dysplasia. J Natl Cancer Inst 1995, **87**: 1365–1371.

140 Jenkins D. Diagnosing human papillomaviruses: recent advances. Curr Opin Infect Dis 2001, **14**: 53–62.

141 Johnson TL, Kim W, Plieth DA, Sarkar FH. Detection of HPV 16/18 DNA in cervical adenocarcinoma using polymerase chain reaction (PCR) methodology. Mod Pathol 1992, **5**: 35–40.

142 Jovanovic AS, McLachlin CM, Shen L, Welch WR, Crum CP. Postmenopausal squamous atypia. A spectrum including 'pseudo-koilocytosis.' Mod Pathol 1995, **8**: 408–412.

143 Kaufman R, Koss LG, Kurman RJ, Meisels A, Okagaki T, Patten SF, Reid R, Richart RM, Wied GL. Statement of caution in the interpretation of papilloma virus-associated lesions of the epithelium of uterine cervix. Am J Obstet Gynecol 1983, **146**: 125.

144 Kenny MB, Unger ER, Chenggis ML, Costa MJ. In situ hybridization for human papillomavirus DNA in uterine adenosquamous carcinoma with glassy cell features ('glassy cell carcinoma'). Am J Clin Pathol 1992, **98**: 180–187.

145 Koutsky LA, Ault KA, Wheeler CM, Brown DR, Barr E, Alvarez FB, Chiacchierini LM, Jansen KU. A controlled trial of human papillomavirus type 16 vaccine. N Engl J Med 2002, **347**: 1645–1651.

146 Lee KR, Minter LJ, Crum CP. Koilocytotic atypia in Papanicolaou smears: reproducibility and biopsy correlations. Cancer 1997, **81**: 10–15.

147 Leminen A, Paavonen J, Vesterinen E, Wahlstrom T, Rantala I, Lehtinen M. Human papillomavirus types 16 and 18 in adenocarcinoma of the uterine cervix. Am J Clin Pathol 1991, **95**: 647–652.

148 Lloveras B, Clavero O, Alejo M, Ordi J, de Sanjose S, Klaustermeier J, Quint W, Brunsveld JP, Guimera N, Alemany L, Garland S, Nessa A, Qiao YL, Grce M, Clavel C, Lombardi L, Ferrara A, Bhatla N, Jain A, Mariani L, Sasawaga T, Menendez C, Banjo K, Domingo EJ, Chou CY, Chichareon S, Usubutun A, Oliva E, Wright TC, Garcia V, Sanchez G, Munoz N, Bosch FX. The distribution of HPV types in invasive cervical carcinoma. Analysis of 9760 cases. Lab Invest 2009, **89**(Suppl 1): 225A. (See also Lancet Oncol 2010, **11**: 1048–1056.)

149 Macnab JCM, Walkinshaw SA, Cordiner JW, Clements JB. Human papilloma virus in clinically and histologically normal tissue of patients with genital cancer. N Engl J Med 1986, **315**: 1052–1058.

150 Milde-Langosch K, Riethdorf S, Loning T. Association of human papillomavirus infection with carcinoma of the cervix uteri and its precursor lesions: theoretical and practical implications. Virchows Arch 2000, **437**: 227–233.

151 Mittal KR, Chan W, Demopoulos RI. Sensitivity and specificity of various morphological features of cervical condylomas. An in situ hybridization study. Arch Pathol Lab Med 1990, **114**: 1038–1041.

152 Mittal K, Demopoulos RI, Tata M. A comparison of proliferative activity and atypical mitoses in cervical condylomas with various HPV types. Int J Gynecol Pathol 1998, **17**: 24–28.

153 Mittal KR, Miller HK, Lowell DM. Koilocytosis preceding squamous cell carcinoma in situ of uterine cervix. Am J Clin Pathol 1987, **87**: 243–245.

154 Mittal K, Palazzo J. Cervical condylomas show higher proliferation than do inflamed or metaplastic cervical squamous epithelium. Mod Pathol 1998, **11**: 780–783.

155 Munoz N, Bosch Z, de Sanjose S, Herrero R, Castellsagué X, Shah KV, Snijders PJF, Meijer CJ. Epidemiologic classification of human papillomavirus types associated with cervical cancer. N Engl J Med 2003, **348**: 518–527.

156 Nagai N, Nuovo G, Freidman D, Crum CP. Detection of papillomavirus nucleic acids in genital precancers with the in situ hybridization technique. Int J Gynecol Pathol 1987, **6**: 366–379.

157 Nuovo GJ. Human papillomavirus DNA in genital tract lesions histologically negative for condylomata. Analysis by in situ, Southern blot hybridization and the polymerase chain reaction. Am J Surg Pathol 1990, **14**: 643–651.

158 Nyeem R, Wilkinson EJ, Grover LJ. Condylomata acuminata of the cervix. Histopathology and association with cervical neoplasia. Int J Gynecol Pathol 1982, **1**: 246–257.

159 Paquette RL, Lee YY, Wilczynski SP, Karmakar A, Kizaki M, Miller CW, Koeffler HP. Mutations of p53 and human papillomavirus infection in cervical carcinoma. Cancer 1993, **72**: 1272–1280.

160 Poljak M, Seme K, Gale N. Detection of human papillomaviruses in tissue specimens. Adv Anat Pathol 1999, **5**: 216–234.

161 Prasad CJ, Sheets E, Selig AM, McArthur MC, Crum CP. The binucleate squamous cell. Histologic spectrum and relationship to low-grade squamous intraepithelial lesions. Mod Pathol 1993, **6**: 313–317.

162 Qizilbash AH. Papillary squamous tumors of the uterine cervix. A clinical and pathologic study of 21 cases. Am J Clin Pathol 1974, **61**: 508–520.

163 Richart RM, Nuovo GJ. Human papillomavirus DNA in situ hybridization may be used for the quality control of genital tract biopsies. Obstet Gynecol 1990, **75**: 223–226.

164 Saito K, Saito A, Fu YS, Smotkin D, Gupta J, Shah K. Topographic study of cervical condyloma and intraepithelial neoplasia. Cancer 1987, **59**: 2064–2070.

165 Sasagawa T, Shimakage M, Nakamura M, Sakaike J, Ishikawa H, Inoue M. Epstein–Barr virus (EBV) genes expression in cervical intraepithelial neoplasia and invasive cervical cancer: a comparative study with human papillomavirus (HPV) infection. Hum Pathol 2000, **31**: 318–326.

166 Saslow D, Castle PE, Cox JT, Davey DD, Einstein MH, Ferris DG, Goldie SJ, Harper DM, Kinney W, Moscicki A-B, Noller KL, Wheeler CM, Ades T, Andrews KS, Doroshenk MK, Kahn KG, Schmidt C, Shafey O, Smith RA, Partridge EE (for the Gynecologic Cancer Advisory Group), Garcia F. American Cancer Society Guideline for human papillomavirus (HPV) vaccine use to prevent cervical cancer and its precursors. CA Cancer J Clin 2007, **57**: 7–28.

167 Sawaya GF, Brown AD, Washington AE, Garber AM. Clinical practice. Current approaches to cervical-cancer screening. N Engl J Med 2001, **344**: 1603–1607.

168 Schiffman MH, Bauer HM, Hoover RN, Glass AG, Cadell DM, Rush BB, Scott DR, Sherman ME, Kurman RJ, Wacholder S, et al. Epidemiologic evidence showing that human papillomavirus infection causes most cervical intraepithelial neoplasia. J Natl Cancer Inst 1993, **85**: 958–964.

169 Stoler MH. Human papillomaviruses and cervical neoplasia: a model for carcinogenesis. Int J Gynecol Pathol 2000, **19**: 16–28.

170 ter Harmsel B, van Belkum A, Quint W, Pronk A, Kuijpers J, Ramaekers F, Tandon A, Smedts F. p53 and human papilloma virus type 16 in cervical intraepithelial neoplasia and carcinoma. Int J Gynecol Pathol 1995, **14**: 125–133.

171 Thomison J 3rd, Thomas LK, Shroyer KR. Human papillomavirus: molecular and cytologic/histologic aspects related to cervical intraepithelial neoplasia and carcinoma. Hum Pathol 2008, **39**: 154–166.

172 Trivijitslip P, Mosher R, Sheets EE, Sun D, Crum CP. Papillary immature metaplasia (immature condyloma) of the cervix: a clinicopathologic analysis and comparison with papillary squamous carcinoma. Hum Pathol 1998, **29**: 641–648.

173 Vallejos H, Delmistro AD, Kleinhaus S, Braunstein JD, Halwer M, Koss LG. Characterization of human papilloma virus types in condylomata acuminata in children by in situ hybridization. Lab Invest 1987, **56**: 611–615.

174 Ward BE, Burkett B, Petersen C, Nuckols ML, Brennan C, Birch LM, Crum CP. Cytologic correlates of cervical papillomavirus infection. Int J Gynecol Pathol 1990, **9**: 297–305.

175 Willett GD, Kurman RJ, Reid R, Greenberg M, Jenson AB, Lorincz AT. Correlation of the histologic appearance of intraepithelial neoplasia of the cervix with human papillomavirus types. Emphasis on low grade lesions including so-called flat condyloma. Int J Gynecol Pathol 1989, **8**: 18–25.

176 Winkler B, Crum CP, Fujii T, Ferenczy A, Boon M, Braun L, Lancaster WD, Richart RM. Koilocytotic lesions of the cervix. The relationship of mitotic abnormalities to the presence of papillomavirus antigens and nuclear DNA content. Cancer 1984, **53**: 1081–1087.

177 Wright TC Jr, Richart RM. Role of human papillomavirus in the pathogenesis of genital tract warts and cancer. Gynecol Oncol 1990, **37**: 151–164.

178 Yang GC, Demopoulos RI, Chan W, Mittal KR. Superficial nuclear enlargement without koilocytosis as an expression of human papillomavirus infection of the uterine cervix: an in situ hybridization study. Int J Gynecol Pathol 1992, **1**: 283–287.

179 Zehbe I, Rylander E, Edlund K, Wadell G, Wilander E. Detection of human papillomavirus in cervical intraepithelial neoplasia, using in situ hybridisation and various polymerase chain reaction techniques. Virchows Arch 1996, **428**: 151–157.

180 Ziol M, Di Tomaso C, Biaggi A, Tepper M, Piquet P, Carbillon L, Uzan M, Guettier C. Virological and biological characteristics of cervical intraepithelial neoplasia grade I with marked koilocytotic atypia. Hum Pathol 1998, **29**: 1068–1073.

181 Zuna RE, Dunn ST, Johnson JJ, Zhang RR, Bane BA, Walker JL, Gold MA, McMeekin DS, Allen RA. HPV genotypes and cervical carcinoma: analysis of 163 cases in a US population. Lab Invest 2009, **89**(Suppl 1): 243A.

TUMORS

CERVICAL INTRAEPITHELIAL NEOPLASIA (CIN)

182 Agoff SN, Lin P, Morihara J, Mao C, Kiviat NB, Koutsky LA. P16[INK4a] expression correlates with degree of cervical neoplasia: a comparison with Ki-67 expression and detection of high-risk HPV types. Mod Pathol 2003, **16**: 665–673.

183 Akasofu M, Oda Y. Immunohistochemical detection of p53 in cervical epithelial lesions with or without infection of human papillomavirus types 16 and 18. Virchows Arch 1995, **425**: 593–602.

184 Al-Nafussi AI, Colquhoun MK. Mild cervical intraepithelial neoplasia (CIN 1). A histological overdiagnosis. Histopathology 1990, **17**: 557–561.

185 Anderson MC, Hartley RB. Cervical crypt involvement by intraepithelial neoplasia. Obstet Gynecol 1980, **55**: 546–550.

186 Badr RE, Walts AE, Chung F, Bose S. BD ProEx C: a sensitive and specific marker of HPV-associated squamous lesions of the cervix. Am J Surg Pathol 2008, **32**: 899–906.

187 Benda JA, Lamoreaux J, Johnson SR. Artifact associated with the use of strong iodine solution (Lugol's) in cone biopsies. Am J Surg Pathol 1987, **11**: 367–374.

188 Bibbo M, Dytch HE, Alenghat E, Bartels PH, Wied GL. DNA ploidy profiles as prognostic indicators in CIN lesions. Am J Clin Pathol 1989, **92**: 261–265.

189 Buckley CH, Butler EB, Fox H. Cervical intraepithelial neoplasia. J Clin Pathol 1982, **35**: 1–13.

190 Cai B, Ronnett BM, Stoler M, Ferenczy A, Kurman RJ, Sadow D, Alvarez F, Pearson J, Sings HL, Barr E, Liaw KL. Longitudinal evaluation of interobserver and intraobserver agreement of cervical intraepithelial neoplasia diagnosis among an experienced panel of gynecologic pathologists. Am J Surg Pathol 2007, **31**: 1854–1860.

191 Cardoza-Favarato G, Fadare O. High-grade squamous intraepithelial lesion (CIN 2 and 3) excised with negative margins by loop electrosurgical excision procedure: the significance of CIN 1 at the margins of excision. Hum Pathol 2007, **38**: 781–786.

192 Chin N, Platt AB, Nuovo GJ. Squamous intraepithelial lesions arising in benign endocervical polyps: a report of 9 cases with correlation to the Pap smears, HPV analysis, and immunoprofile. Int J Gynecol Pathol 2008, **27**: 582–590.

193 Christopherson WM. Dysplasia, carcinoma in situ, and microinvasive carcinoma of the uterine cervix. Hum Pathol 1977, **8**: 489–501.

194 Christopherson WM, Gray LA Sr. Dysplasia and preclinical carcinoma of the uterine cervix. Diagnosis and management. Semin Oncol 1982, **9**: 265–279.

195 Cooper K, Haffajee Z, Taylor L. Bcl-2 immunoreactivity, human papillomavirus DNA, and cervical intraepithelial neoplasia. Mod Pathol 1999, **12**: 612–617.

196 Coppleson M, Pixley E, Reid B. Colposcopy. A scientific and practical approach to the cervix in health and disease. Springfield, IL, 1971, Charles C Thomas.

197 Crum CP. Symposium part 1: should the Bethesda system terminology be used in diagnostic surgical pathology? Int J Gynecol Pathol 2002, **22**: 5–12.

198 de Boer CJ, van Dorst E, van Krieken H, Jansen-van Rhijn CM, Warnaar SO, Fleuren GJ, Litvinov SV. Changing roles of cadherins and catenins during progression of squamous intraepithelial lesions in the uterine cervix. Am J Pathol 1999, **155**: 505–515.

199 Demopoulos RI, Horowitz LF, Vamvakas EC. Endocervical gland involvement by cervical intraepithelial neoplasia grade III. Predictive value for residual and/or recurrent disease. Cancer 1991, **68**: 1932–1936.

200 Foote FW Jr, Stewart FW. The anatomical distribution of intraepithelial epidermoid carcinomas of the cervix. Cancer 1948, **1**: 431–440.

201 Fox CH. Biologic behavior of dysplasia and carcinoma in situ. Am J Obstet Gynecol 1967, **99**: 960–974.

202 Fox H, Buckley CH. Current problems in the pathology of intra-epithelial lesions of the uterine cervix. Histopathology 1990, **17**: 1–6.

203 Fu YS, Reagan JW, Richart RM. Definition of precursors. Gynecol Oncol 1981, **12**: S220–S231.

204 Giannoudis A, Herrington CS. Differential expression of p53 and p21 in low grade cervical squamous intraepithelial lesions infected with low, intermediate, and high risk human papillomaviruses. Cancer 2000, **89**: 1300–1307.

205 Govan ADT, Haines RM, Langley FA, Taylor CW, Woodcock AS. Changes in the epithelium of the cervix uteri. J Obstet Gynaecol Br Commonw 1968, **73**: 883–896.

206 Gusberg SB, Moore DB. The clinical pattern of intraepithelial carcinoma of the cervix and its pathologic background. Obstet Gynecol 1953, **2**: 1–14.

207 Heatley MK. How should we grade CIN? Histopathology 2002, **40**: 377–390.

208 Holmquist ND, McMahan CA, Williams OD. Variability in classification of carcinoma in situ of the uterine cervix. Arch Pathol 1967, **84**: 334–345.

209 Horn LC, Reichert A, Oster A, Arndal SF, Trunk MJ, Ridder R, Rassmussen OF, Bjelkenkrantz K, Christiansen P, Eck M, Lorey T, Skovlund VR, Ruediger T, Schneider V, Schmidt D. Immunostaining for p16INK4a used as a conjunctive tool improves interobserver agreement of the histologic diagnosis of cervical intraepithelial neoplasia. Am J Surg Pathol 2008, **32**: 502–512.

210 Howard L, Erickson CC, Stoddard LD. A study of the incidence and histogenesis of endocervical metaplasia and intraepithelial carcinoma. Cancer 1951, **4**: 1210–1223.

211 Ismail SM, Colclough AB, Dinnen JS, Eakins D, Evans DM, Gradwell E, O'Sullivan JP, Summerell JM, Newcombe R. Reporting cervical intra-epithelial neoplasia (CIN). Intra- and interpathologist variation and factors associated with disagreement. Histopathology 1990, **16**: 371–376.

212 Johnson LD, Nickerson RJ, Easterday CL, Stuart RS, Hertig AT. Epidemiologic evidence for the spectrum of change from dysplasia through carcinoma in situ to invasive cancer. Cancer 1968, **22**: 901–914.

213 Joste NE, Rushing L, Granados R, Zitz JC, Genest DR, Crum CP, Cibas ES. Bethesda classification of cervicovaginal smears: reproducibility and viral correlates. Hum Pathol 1996, **27**: 581–585.

214 Kalof AN, Evans MF, Simmons-Arnold L, Beatty BG, Cooper K. p16INK4A immunoexpression and HPV in situ hybridization signal patterns: potential markers of high-grade cervical intraepithelial neoplasia. Am J Surg Pathol 2005, **29**: 674–679.

215 Kanbour AI, Stock RJ. Squamous cell carcinoma in situ of the endometrium and fallopian tube as superficial extension of invasive cervical carcinoma. Cancer 1978, **42**: 570–580.

216 Killackey MA, Jones WB, Lewis JL. Diagnostic conization of the cervix. Review of 460 consecutive cases. Obstet Gynecol 1986, **67**: 766–770.

217 Klavins JV. Intra-epithelial carcinoma with differentiated surface cells and dysplasia. Definition and separation of these lesions. Acta Cytol (Baltimore) 1963, **7**: 351–356.

218 Kobayashi I, Matsuo K, Ishibashi Y, Kanda S, Sakai H. The proliferative activity in dysplasia and carcinoma in situ of the uterine cervix analyzed by proliferating cell nuclear antigen immunostaining and silver-binding argyrophilic nucleolar organizer region staining. Hum Pathol 1994, **25**: 198–202.

219 Kolstad P, Klein V. Long-term follow-up of 1121 cases of carcinoma in situ. Obstet Gynecol 1976, **48**: 125–129.

220 Kolstad P, Stafl A. Atlas of colposcopy. Baltimore, 1972, University Park Press.

221 Kraus FT. Gynecologic pathology. St Louis, 1967, C.V. Mosby, p. 174.

222 Kreiger JS, McCormack LJ. Graded treatment for in situ carcinoma of the uterine cervix. Am J Obstet Gynecol 1968, **101**: 171–182.

223 Kruse AJ, Skaland I, Munk AC, Janssen E, Gudlaugsson E, Baak JP. Low p53 and retinoblastoma protein expression in cervical intraepithelial neoplasia grade 3 lesions is associated with coexistent adenocarcinoma in situ. Hum Pathol 2008, **39**: 573–578.

224 Lesack D, Wahab I, Gilks CB. Radiation-induced atypia of endocervical epithelium: a histological, immunohistochemical and cytometric study. Int J Gynecol Pathol 1997, **15**: 242–247.

225 Livasy CA, Maygarden SJ, Rajaratnam CT, Novotny DB. Predictors of recurrent dysplasia after a cervical loop electrocautery excision procedure for CIN-3: a study of margin, endocervical gland, and quadrant involvement. Mod Pathol 1999, **12**: 233–238.

226 Lopez-Ferrer A, Alameda F, Barranco C, Garrido M, de Bolòs C. MUC4 expression is increased in dysplastic cervical disorders. Hum Pathol 2001, **32**: 1197–1202.

227 Matseoane S, Williams SB, Navarro C, Hedriana H, Mushayandebvu T. Diagnostic value of conization of the uterine cervix in the management of cervical neoplasia: a review of 756 consecutive patients. Gynecol Oncol 1992, **47**: 287–291.

228 McIndoe WA, McLean MR, Jones RW, Mullins PR. The invasive potential of carcinoma in situ of the cervix. Obstet Gynecol 1984, **64**: 451–458.

229 McIndoe GA, Robson MS, Tidy JA, Mason WP, Anderson MC. Laser excision rather than vaporization. The treatment of choice for cervical intraepithelial neoplasia. Obstet Gynecol 1989, **74**: 165–168.

230 Mittal KR, Demopoulos RI, Goswami S. Proliferating cell nuclear antigen (cyclin) expression in normal and abnormal cervical squamous epithelia. Am J Surg Pathol 1993, **17**: 117–122.

231 Montz FJ, Holschneider CH, Thompson LD. Large-loop excision of the transformation zone. Effect on the pathologic interpretation of resection margins. Obstet Gynecol 1993, **81**: 976–982.

232 Murphy WM, Coleman SA. The long-term course of carcinoma in situ of the uterine cervix. Cancer 1976, **38**: 957–963.

233 Nasiell K, Roger V, Nasiell M. Behavior of mild cervical dysplasia during long-term follow-up. Obstet Gynecol 1986, **67**: 665–669.

234 National Cancer Institute Workshop. The 1988 Bethesda System for reporting cervical/vaginal cytologic diagnoses. JAMA 1988, **262**: 931–932.

235 Ostor AG. Natural history of cervical intraepithelial neoplasia. A critical review. Int J Gynecol Pathol 1993, **12**: 186–192.

236 Park K, Ellenson LH, Pirog EC. Low-grade squamous intraepithelial lesions of the cervix with marked cytological atypia – clinical follow-up and human papillomavirus genotyping. Int J Gynecol Pathol 2007, **26**: 457–462.

237 Paterson-Brown S, Chappatte OA, Clark SK, Wright A, Maxwell P, Taub NA, Raju KS. The significance of cone biopsy resection margins. Gynecol Oncol 1992, **46**: 182–185.

238 Perticarari S, Presani G, Michelutti A, Facca MC, Alberico S, Mandruzzato GP. Flow cytometric analysis of DNA content in cervical lesions. Pathol Res Pract 1989, **185**: 686–688.

239 Petersen O. Spontaneous course of cervical precancerous conditions. Am J Obstet Gynecol 1956, **72**: 1063–1071.

240 Pins MR, Young RH, Crum CP, Leach IH, Scully RE. Cervical squamous cell carcinoma in situ with intraepithelial extension to the upper genital tract and invasion of tubes and ovaries: report of a case with human papilloma virus analysis. Int J Gynecol Pathol 1998, **16**: 272–278.

241 Pinto AP, Schlecht NF, Woo TY, Crum CP, Cibas ES. Biomarker (ProEx C, p16(INK4A), and MiB-1) distinction of high-grade squamous intraepithelial lesion from its mimics. Mod Pathol 2008, **21**: 1067–1074.

242 Pollanen R, Soini Y, Vahakangas K, Paakko P, Lehto VP. Aberrant p53 protein expression in cervical intra-epithelial neoplasia. Histopathology 1993, **23**: 471–474.

243 Przybora LA, Plutowa A. Histological topography of carcinoma in situ of the cervix uteri. Cancer 1959, **12**: 263–277.

244 Reagan JW, Seidemann IL, Saracusa Y. Cellular morphology of carcinoma in situ and dysplasia or atypical hyperplasia of the uterine cervix. Cancer 1953, **6**: 224–235.

245 Richart RM. Cervical intraepithelial neoplasia. Pathol Annu 1973, **8**: 301–328.

246 Richart RM. A modified terminology for cervical intraepithelial neoplasia. Obstet Gynecol 1990, **75**: 131–133.

247 Richart RM, Barron BA. A follow-up study of patients with cervical dysplasia. Am J Obstet Gynecol 1969, **105**: 386–393.

248 Richart RM, Wright TC Jr. Controversies in the management of low-grade cervical intraepithelial neoplasia. Cancer 1993, **71**: 1413–1421.

249 Rubio CA, Lagerlöf B. Autoradiographic studies of dysplasia and carcinoma in situ in cervical cones. Acta Pathol Microbiol Scand (A) 1974, **82**: 411–418.

250 Sagae S, Kudo R, Kuzumaki N, Hisada T, Mugikura Y, Nihei T, Takeda T, Hashimoto M. Ras oncogene expression and progression in intraepithelial neoplasia of the uterine cervix. Cancer 1990, **66**: 295–301.

251 Salm R. Superficial intra-uterine spread of intra-epithelial cervical carcinoma. J Pathol 1969, **97**: 719–723.

252 Samaratunga H, Beresford A, Davison A. Squamous cell carcinoma in situ involving mesonephric remnants. A potential diagnostic pitfall. Am J Surg Pathol 1994, **18**: 1265–1269.

253 Sherman ME, Kurman RJ. Intraepithelial carcinoma of the cervix: reflections on half a

century of progress. Cancer 1998, **83**: 2243–2246.

254 Shurbaji MS, Brooks SK, Thurmond TS. Proliferating cell nuclear antigen immunoreactivity in cervical intraepithelial neoplasia and benign cervical epithelium. Am J Clin Pathol 1993, **100**: 22–26.

255 Smedts F, Ramaekers F, Leube RE, Keijser K, Link M, Vooijs P. Expression of keratins 1, 6, 15, 16, and 20 in normal cervical epithelium, squamous metaplasia, cervical intraepithelial neoplasia, and cervical carcinoma. Am J Pathol 1993, **142**: 403–412.

256 Smedts F, Ramaekers F, Robben H, Pruszczynski M, van Muijen G, Lane B, Leigh I, Vooijs P. Changing patterns of keratin expression during progression of cervical intraepithelial neoplasia. Am J Pathol 1990, **136**: 657–668.

257 Southern SA, McDicken IW, Herrington CS. Loss of cytokeratin 14 expression is related to human papillomavirus type and lesion grade in squamous intraepithelial lesions of the cervix. Hum Pathol 2002, **32**: 1351–1355.

258 Suprun HZ, Schwartz J, Spira H. Cervical intraepithelial neoplasia and associated condylomatous lesions. A preliminary report on 4,764 women from northern Israel. Acta Cytol (Baltimore) 1985, **29**: 334–340.

259 Takeuchi A, McKay DB. The area of the cervix involved by carcinoma in situ and anaplasia (atypical hyperplasia). Obstet Gynecol 1960, **15**: 134–145.

260 Tendler A, Kaufman HL, Kadish AS. Increased carcinoembryonic antigen expression in cervical intraepithelial neoplasia grade 3 and cervical squamous cell carcinoma. Hum Pathol 2000, **31**: 1357–1362.

261 Thickett KM, Griffin NR, Griffiths AP, Wells M. A study of nucleolar organizer regions in cervical intraepithelial neoplasia and human papillomavirus infection. Int J Gynecol Pathol 1989, **8**: 331–339.

262 Tweeddale DN, Roddick JW. Histologic types of squamous-cell carcinoma in situ of the cervix. Obstet Gynecol 1969, **33**: 35–40.

263 Walton LA, Edelman DA, Fowler WC Jr, Photropulos GJ. Cryosurgery for the treatment of cervical intraepithelial neoplasm during the reproductive years. Obstet Gynecol 1980, **55**: 353–357.

264 Wentz WB, Reagan JW. Clinical significance of postirradiation dysplasia of the uterine cervix. Am J Obstet Gynecol 1970, **106**: 812–817.

MICROINVASIVE SQUAMOUS CELL CARCINOMA

265 Benson WL, Norris HJ. A critical review of the frequency of lymph node metastasis and death from microinvasive carcinoma of the cervix. Obstet Gynecol 1977, **49**: 632–638.

266 Brudenell M, Cox BS, Taylor CW. The management of dysplasia, carcinoma in situ and microcarcinoma of the cervix. J Obstet Gynaecol Br Commonw 1973, **80**: 673–679.

267 Burghardt E, Girardi F, Lahousen M, Pickel H, Tamussino K. Microinvasive carcinoma of the uterine cervix (International Federation of Gynecology and Obstetrics Stage IA). Cancer 1991, **67**: 1037–1045.

268 Burke TW. Factors affecting recurrence and survival in stage I carcinoma of the uterine cervix. Oncology (Huntingt) 1992, **6**: 111–119.

269 Christopherson WM, Gray LA, Parker JE. Microinvasive carcinoma of the uterine cervix. A long-term follow-up study of eighty cases. Cancer 1976, **38**: 629–632.

270 Clement PB, Scully RE. Carcinoma of the cervix. Histologic types. Semin Oncol 1982, **9**: 251–264.

271 Copeland LJ, Silva EG, Gershenson DM, Morris M, Young DC, Wharton JT. Superficially invasive squamous cell carcinoma of the cervix. Gynecol Oncol 1992, **45**: 307–312.

272 Creasman WT, Fetter BF, Clarke-Pearson DL, Kaufmann L, Parker RT. Management of stage IA carcinoma of cervix. Am J Obstet Gynecol 1985, **153**: 164–172.

273 Fennell RH. Review. Microinvasive carcinoma of the uterine cervix. Obstet Gynecol Surv 1978, **33**: 406–411.

274 Genadry R, Olson J, Parmley T, Woodruff JD. The morphology of the earliest invasive cell in low genital tract epidermoid neoplasia. Obstet Gynecol 1978, **51**: 718–722.

275 Hartveit F, Sandstad E. Stromal metachromasia. A marker for areas of infiltrating tumour growth? Histopathology 1982, **6**: 423–428.

276 Hasumi K, Sakamoto A, Sugano H. Microinvasive carcinoma of the uterine cervix. Cancer 1980, **45**: 928–931.

277 Jones WB, Mercer GO, Lewis JL Jr, Rubin SC, Hoskins WJ. Early invasive carcinoma of the cervix. Gynecol Oncol 1993, **51**: 26–32.

278 Kudo R, Sato T, Mizuuchi H. Ultrastructural and immunohistochemical study of infiltration in microinvasive carcinoma of the uterine cervix. Gynecol Oncol 1990, **36**: 23–29.

279 Langley FA, Crompton AC. Epithelial abnormalities of the cervix uteri. New York, 1973, Springer-Verlag.

280 Lehman MH Jr, Benson WL, Kurman RJ, Park RC. Microinvasive carcinoma of the cervix. Obstet Gynecol 1976, **48**: 571–578.

281 Margulis RR, Ely CW Jr, Ladd JE. Diagnosis and management of stage IA (microinvasive) carcinoma of cervix. Obstet Gynecol 1967, **29**: 529–538.

282 Morris M, Mitchell MF, Silva EG, Copeland LJ, Gershenson DM. Cervical conization as definitive therapy for early invasive squamous carcinoma of the cervix. Gynecol Oncol 1993, **51**: 193–196.

283 Mussey E, Soule EH, Welch JS. Microinvasive carcinoma of the cervix. Am J Obstet Gynecol 1969, **104**: 738–744.

284 Ng ABP, Reagan JW. Microinvasive carcinoma of the uterine cervix. Am J Clin Pathol 1969, **52**: 511–529.

285 Ostor AG. Studies on 200 cases of early squamous cell carcinoma of the cervix. Int J Gynecol Pathol 1993, **12**: 193–207.

286 Richards CJ, Furness PN. Basement membrane continuity in benign, premalignant and malignant epithelial conditions of the uterine cervix. Histopathology 1990, **16**: 47–52.

287 Roche WD, Norris HJ. Microinvasive carcinoma of the cervix. The significance of lymphatic invasion and confluent patterns of stromal growth. Cancer 1975, **36**: 180–186.

288 Rubio CA, Söderberg G, Einhorn N. Histological and follow-up studies in cases of micro-invasive carcinoma of the uterine cervix. Acta Pathol Microbiol Scand (A) 1974, **82**: 397–410.

289 Rush D, Hyjek E, Baergen RN, Ellenson LH, Pirog EC. Detection of microinvasion in vulvar and cervical intraepithelial neoplasia using double immunostaining for cytokeratin and basement membrane components. Arch Pathol Lab Med 2005, **129**: 747–753.

290 Sevin BU, Nadji M, Averette HE, Hilsenbeck S, Smith D, Lampe B. Microinvasive carcinoma of the cervix. Cancer 1992, **70**: 2121–2128.

291 Simon NL, Gore H, Shingleton HM, Soong S-J, Orr JW, Hatch KD. Study of superficially invasive carcinoma of the cervix. Obstet Gynecol 1986, **68**: 19–24.

292 Stewart CJ, McNicol AM. Distribution of type IV collagen immunoreactivity to assess questionable early stromal invasion. J Clin Pathol 1992, **45**: 9–15.

293 Ueki M, Okamoto Y, Misaki O, Seiki Y, Kitsuki K, Ueda M, Sugimoto O. Conservative therapy for microinvasive carcinoma of the uterine cervix. Gynecol Oncol 1994, **53**: 109–113.

294 van Nagell JR, Greenwell N, Powell DF, Donaldson ES, Hanson MB, Gay EC. Microinvasive carcinoma of the cervix. Am J Obstet Gynecol 1983, **145**: 981–991.

INVASIVE SQUAMOUS CELL CARCINOMA

General features

295 Cannistra SA, Niloff JM. Cancer of the uterine cervix. N Engl J Med 1996, **334**: 1030–1038.

296 Devesa SS. Descriptive epidemiology of cancer of the uterine cervix. Obstet Gynecol 1984, **63**: 605–612.

297 Devesa SS, Young JL Jr, Brinton LA, Fraumeni JF Jr. Recent trends in cervix uteri cancer. Cancer 1989, **64**: 2184–2190.

298 Hawes SE, Kiviat NB. Are genital infections and inflammation cofactors in the pathogenesis of invasive cervical cancer? J Nat Cancer Inst 2002, **94**: 1592–1593.

299 Herrero R, Brinton LA, Reeves WC, Brenes MM, Tenorio F, de Britton RC, Gaitan E, Garcia M, Rawls WE. Sexual behavior, venereal diseases, hygiene practices, and invasive cervical cancer in a high-risk population. Cancer 1990, **65**: 380–386.

300 Kushima M, Fujii H, Murakami K, Ota H, Matsumoto T, Motoyama T, Kiyokawa T, Ishikura H. Simultaneous squamous cell carcinomas of the uterine cervix and upper genital tract: loss heterozygosity analysis demonstrates clonal neoplasms of cervical origin. Int J Gynecol Pathol 2001, **20**: 353–358.

301 Larsen NS. Invasive cervical cancer rising in young white females. J Natl Cancer Inst 1994, **86**: 6–7.

302 La Vecchia C, Franceschi S, Decarli A, Fasoli M, Gentile A, Parazzini F, Regallo M. Sexual factors, venereal diseases, and the risk of intraepithelial and invasive cervical neoplasia. Cancer 1986, **58**: 935–941.

303 Maiman M, Fruchter RG, Serur E, Remy JC, Feuer G, Boyce J. Human immunodeficiency virus infection and cervical neoplasia. Gynecol Oncol 1990, **38**: 377–382.

304 Miyazaki K, Yamaguchi K, Tohya T, Ohba T, Takatsuki K, Okamura H. Human T-cell leukemia virus type I infection as an oncogenic and prognostic risk factor in cervical and vaginal carcinoma. Obstet Gynecol 1991, **77**: 107–110.

305 Pfeifer JD. Molecular genetic testing in surgical pathology. Philadelphia, 2006, Lippincott Williams and Wilkins.

306 Piver MS. Invasive cervical cancer in the 1990s. Semin Surg Oncol 1990, **6**: 359–363.

307 Rapp F, Jenkins FJ. Genital cancer and viruses. Gynecol Oncol 1981, **12**: S25–S41.

308 Rellihan MA, Dooley DP, Burke TW, Berkland ME, Longfield RN. Rapidly progressing cervical cancer in a patient with human immunodeficiency virus infection. Gynecol Oncol 1990, **36**: 435–438.

309 Sasagawa T, Shimakage M, Nakamura M, Sakaike J, Ishikawa H, Inoue M. Epstein–Barr virus (EBV) genes expression in cervical intraepithelial neoplasia and invasive cervical cancer: a comparative study with human papillomavirus (HPV) infection. Hum Pathol 2000, **31**: 318–326.

310 Schiffman M, Castle PE. The promise of global cervical-cancer prevention. N Engl J Med 2005, **353**: 2101–2104.

311 Schwartz LB, Carcangiu ML, Bradham L, Schwartz PE. Rapidly progressive squamous cell carcinoma of the cervix coexisting with human immunodeficiency virus infection: clinical opinion. Gynecol Oncol 1991, **41**: 255–258.

312 Wong KY, Collins RJ, Srivastava G, Pittaluga S, Cheung AN, Wong LC. Epstein–Barr virus in carcinoma of the cervix. Int J Gynecol Pathol 1993, **12**: 224–227.

Morphologic features

313 Aho HJ, Talve L, Maenpaa J. Acantholytic squamous cell carcinoma of the uterine cervix with amyloid deposition. Int J Gynecol Pathol 1992, **11**: 150–155.

314 Benda JA. Pathology of cervical carcinoma and its prognostic implications. Semin Oncol 1994, **21**: 3–11.

315 Bostrom SG, Hart WR. Carcinomas of the cervix with intense stromal eosinophilia. Cancer 1981, **47**: 2887–2893.

316 Brinck U, Jakob C, Bau O, Fuzesi L. Papillary squamous cell carcinoma of the uterine cervix: report of three cases and a review of its classification. Int J Gynecol Pathol 2000, **19**: 231–235.

317 Clement PB, Scully RE. Carcinoma of the cervix. Histologic types. Semin Oncol 1982, **9**: 251–264.

318 Colgan TJ, Auger M, McLaughlin JR. Histopathologic classification of cervical carcinomas and recognition of mucin-secreting squamous carcinomas. Int J Gynecol Pathol 1993, **12**: 64–69.

319 Gondo T, Ishihara T, Kawano H, Uchino F, Takahashi M, Iwata T, Matsumoto N, Yokota T. Localized amyloidosis in squamous cell carcinoma of uterine cervix. Electron microscopic features of nodular and star-like amyloid deposits. Virchows Arch [A] 1993, **422**: 225–231.

320 Heller PB, Barnhill Dr, Mayer AR, Fontaine TP, Hoskins WJ, Park RC. Cervical carcinoma found incidentally in a uterus removed for benign indications. Obstet Gynecol 1986, **67**: 187–190.

321 Kapp DS, LiVolsi VA. Intense eosinophilic stromal infiltration in carcinoma of the uterine cervix. A clinicopathologic study of 14 cases. Gynecol Oncol 1983, **16**: 19–30.

322 Miller BE, Copeland LJ, Hamberger AD, Gershenson DM, Saul PB, Herson J, Rutledge FN. Carcinoma of the cervical stump. Gynecol Oncol 1984, **18**: 100–108.

323 Morrison C, Catania F, Wakely P, Nuovo GJ. Highly differentiated keratinising squamous cell cancer of the cervix: a rare, locally aggressive tumor not associated with human papillomavirus or squamous intraepithelial lesions. Am J Surg Pathol 2001, **25**: 1310–1315.

324 Ng ABP, Atkin NB. Histological cell type and DNA value in the prognosis of squamous cell cancer of uterine cervix. Br J Cancer 1973, **28**: 322–331.

325 Rizzardi C, Perin T, Schneider M, Rossi D, Brollo A, Melato M, Canzonieri V. Carcinoma of the uterine cervix with squamous and sebaceous differentiation. Int J Gynecol Pathol 2009, **28**: 292–295.

326 Samlal RA, Ten Kate FJ, Hart AA, Lammes FB. Do mucin-secreting squamous cell carcinomas of the uterine cervix metastasise more frequently to pelvic lymph nodes? A case-control study. Int J Gynecol Pathol 1998, **17**: 201–204.

327 Tsang WY, Chan JK. Amyloid-producing squamous cell carcinoma of the uterine cervix. Arch Pathol Lab Med 1993, **117**: 199–201.

Immunohistochemical and molecular genetic features

328 Bychkov V, Rothman M, Bardawil WA. Immunocytochemical localization of carcinoembryonic antigen (CEA), alpha-fetoprotein (AFP), and human chorionic gonadotropin (HCG) in cervical neoplasia. Am J Clin Pathol 1983, **79**: 414–420.

329 Dunne FP, Rollason T, Ratcliff WA, Marshall T, Heath DA. Parathyroid hormone-related protein gene expression in invasive cervical tumors. Cancer 1994, **74**: 83–89.

330 Hameed A, Miller DS, Muller CY, Coleman RL, Albores-Saavedra J. Frequent expression of beta-human chorionic gonadotropin (beta-hCG) in squamous cell carcinoma of the cervix. Int J Gynecol Pathol 1999, **18**: 381–386.

331 Kessis TD, Slebos RJ, Han SM, Shah K, Bosch XF, Munoz N, Hedrick L, Cho KR. p53 gene mutations and MDM2 amplification are uncommon in primary carcinomas of the uterine cervix. Am J Pathol 1993, **143**: 1398–1405.

332 Mitchell KM, Hale RJ, Buckley CH, Fox H, Smith D. Cathepsin-D expression in cervical carcinoma and its prognostic significance. Virchows Arch [A] 1993, **422**: 357–360.

333 Nguyen HN, Sevin BU, Averette HE, Ramos R, Ganjei P, Perras J. Evidence of tumor heterogeneity in cervical cancers and lymph node metastases as determined by flow cytometry. Cancer 1993, **71**: 2543–2550.

334 Pfeifer JD. Molecular genetic testing in surgical pathology. Philadelphia, 2006, Lippincott Williams and Wilkins.

335 Smedts F, Ramaekers F, Link M, Lauerova L, Troyanovsky S, Schijf C, Voojis GP. Detection of keratin subtypes in routinely processed cervical tissue. Implications for tumour classification and the study of cervix cancer aetiology. Virchows Arch 1994, **425**: 145–155.

336 To ACW, Soong S-J, Shingleton HM, Gore H, Wilkerson JA, Hatch KD, Phillips D, Dollar JR. Immunohistochemistry of the blood group A, B, H isoantigens and Oxford Ca antigen as prognostic markers for stage IB squamous cell carcinoma of the cervix. Cancer 1986, **58**: 2435–2439.

337 Wang TY, Chen BF, Yang YC, Chen H, Wang Y, Cviko A, Quade BJ, Sun D, Yang A, McKeon FD, Crum CP. Histologic and immunophenotypic classification of cervical carcinomas by expression of the p53 homologue p63: a study of 250 cases. Hum Pathol 2001, **32**: 479–486.

Spread and metastases

338 Barmeir E, Langer O, Levy JI, Nissenbaum M, DeMoor NG, Blumenthal NJ. Unusual skeletal metastases in carcinoma of the cervix. Gynecol Oncol 1985, **20**: 307–316.

339 Benedetti-Panici P, Maneschi F, D'Andrea G, Cutillo G, Rabitti C, Congiu M, Coronetta F, Capelli A. Early cervical carcinoma: the natural history of lymph node involvement redefined on the basis of thorough parametrectomy and giant section study. Cancer 2000, **88**: 2267–2274.

340 Henriksen E. The lymphatic spread of carcinoma of the cervix and the body of the uterus. Am J Obstet Gynecol 1949, **58**: 924–942.

341 Plaza JA, Ramirez NC, Nuovo GJ. Utility of HPV analysis for evaluation of possible metastatic disease in women with cervical cancer. Int J Gynecol Pathol 2004, **23**: 7–12.

342 Ratanatharathorn V, Powers WE, Steverson N, Han I, Ahmad K, Grimm J. Bone metastasis from cervical cancer. Cancer 1994, **73**: 2372–2379.

343 Tellis CJ, Beechler CR. Pulmonary metastasis of carcinoma of the cervix. A retrospective study. Cancer 1982, **49**: 1705–1709.

344 Uqmakli A, Bonney WA Jr, Palladino A. The nonlymphatic metastases of carcinoma of the uterine cervix. A prospective analysis based on laparotomy. Cancer 1978, **41**: 1027–1033.

345 Wang CW, Wu TI, Yu CT, Wu YC, Teng YH, Chin SY, Lai CH, Chen TC. Usefulness of p16 for differentiating primary pulmonary squamous cell carcinoma from cervical squamous cell carcinoma metastatic to the lung. Am J Clin Pathol 2009, **131**: 715–722.

346 Young RH, Gersell DJ, Roth LM, Scully RE. Ovarian metastases from cervical carcinomas other than pure adenocarcinomas. A report of 12 cases. Cancer 1993, **71**: 407–418.

Treatment

347 Bjornsson BL, Nelson BE, Reale FR, Rose PG. Accuracy of frozen section for lymph node metastasis in patients undergoing radical hysterectomy for carcinoma of the cervix. Gynecol Oncol 1993, **51**: 50–53.

348 Bricker EM, Butcher HR Jr, Lawler WH Jr, McAfee CA. Surgical treatment of advanced and recurrent cancer of the pelvic viscera. An evaluation of ten years' experience. Ann Surg 1960, **152**: 388–402.

349 Hamberger AD, Fletcher GH, Wharton JT. Results of treatment of early stage I carcinoma of the uterine cervix with intracavitary radium alone. Cancer 1978, **41**: 980–985.

350 Holtz DO, Dunton C. Traditional management of invasive cervical cancer. Obstet Gynecol Clin North Am 2002, **29**: 645–657.

351 Hopkins MP, Morley GW. Radical hysterectomy versus radiation therapy for stage IB squamous cell cancer of the cervix. Cancer 1991, **68**: 272–277.

352 Ismiil N, Ghorab Z, Covens A, Nofech-Mozes S, Saad R, Dube V, Khalifa MA. Intraoperative margin assessment of the radical vaginal trachelectomy specimen. Gynecol Oncol 2009, **113**: 42–46.

353 Jacobs AJ, Faris C, Perez CA, Kao MS, Galakatos A, Camel HM. Short-term persistence of carcinoma of the uterine cervix after radiation. An indicator of long-term prognosis. Cancer 1986, **57**: 944–950.

354 Jones WB. New approaches to high-risk cervical cancer. Advanced cervical cancer. Cancer 1993, **71**: 1451–1459.

355 Kinney WK, Egorshin EV, Ballard DJ, Podratz KC. Long-term survival and sequelae after surgical management of invasive cervical carcinoma diagnosed at the time of simple hysterectomy. Gynecol Oncol 1992, **44**: 24–27.

356 Kiselow M, Butcher HR, Bricker EM. Results of the radical surgical treatment of advanced pelvic cancer. Ann Surg 1967, **166**: 428–437.

357 Morgan LS, Nelson JH. Surgical treatment of early cervical cancer. Semin Oncol 1982, **9**: 312–330.

358 Morley GW. Pelvic exenterative therapy and the treatment of recurrent carcinoma of the cervix. Semin Oncol 1982, **9**: 331–340.

359 Morley GW, Hopkins MP, Lindenauer SM, Roberts JA. Pelvic exenteration, University of Michigan. 100 patients at 5 years. Obstet Gynecol 1989, **74**: 934–943.

360 Perez CA, Camel HM, Kao MS, Hederman MA. Randomized study of preoperative radiation and surgery or irradiation alone in the

treatment of stage IB and IIA carcinoma of the uterine cervix. Final report. Gynecol Oncol 1987, **27**: 129–140.

361 Perez-Mesa C, Spjut HJ. Persistent postirradiation carcinoma of cervix uteri. A pathologic study of 83 pelvic exenteration specimens. Arch Pathol 1963, **75**: 462–474.

362 Thar TL, Million RR, Daly JW. Radiation treatment of carcinoma of the cervix. Semin Oncol 1982, **9**: 299–311.

363 Zannoni GF, Vellone VG, Carbone A. Morphological effects of radiochemotherapy on cervical carcinoma: a morphological study of 50 cases of hysterectomy specimens after neoadjuvant treatment. Int J Gynecol Pathol 2008, **27**: 274–281.

Prognosis

364 Baltzer J, Lohe KJ. What's new in prognosis of uterine cancer? Pathol Res Pract 1984, **178**: 635–641.

365 Bethwaite PB, Holloway LJ, Yeong ML, Thornton A. Effect of tumour associated tissue eosinophilia on survival of women with stage IB carcinoma of the uterine cervix. J Clin Pathol 1993, **46**: 1016–1020.

366 Boyce JG, Fruchter RG, Nicastri AD, DeRegt RH, Ambiavagar PC, Reinis M, Macasaet M, Rotman M. Vascular invasion in stage I carcinoma of the cervix. Cancer 1984, **53**: 1175–1180.

367 Burghardt E, Baltzer J, Tulusan AH, Haas J. Results of surgical treatment of 1028 cervical cancers studied with volumetry. Cancer 1992, **70**: 648–655.

368 Cheung TH, Chung TKJ, Poon CS, Hampton GM, Wand VW, Wong YF. Allelic loss on chromosome 1 is associated with tumor progression of cervical carcinoma. Cancer 1999, **86**: 1294–1298.

369 Goellner JR. Carcinoma of the cervix. Clinicopathologic correlation of 196 cases. Am J Clin Pathol 1976, **66**: 775–785.

370 Gunderson LL, Weems WS, Hebertson RM, Plenk HP. Correlation of histopathology with clinical results following radiation therapy for carcinoma of the cervix. Am J Roentgenol Radium Ther Nucl Med 1974, **120**: 74–87.

371 Hale RJ, Buckley CH, Fox H, Williams J. Prognostic value of c-*erb*B-2 expression in uterine cervical carcinoma. J Clin Pathol 1992, **45**: 594–596.

372 Herrington CS, Wells M. Can HPV typing predict the behaviour of cervical epithelial neoplasia? Histopathology 1997, **31**: 301–303.

373 Hirao T, Sakamoto Y, Kamada M, Hamada S, Aono T. Tn antigen, a marker of potential for metastasis of uterine cervix cancer cells. Cancer 1993, **72**: 154–159.

374 Hopkins MP, Morley GW. Prognostic factors in advanced stage squamous cell cancer of the cervix. Cancer 1993, **72**: 2389–2393.

375 Inoue T. Prognostic significance of the depth of invasion relating to nodal metastases, parametrial extension, and cell types. A study of 628 cases with stage IB, IIA, and IIB cervical carcinoma. Cancer 1984, **54**: 3035–3042.

376 Inoue T, Chihara T, Morita K. The prognostic significance of the size of the largest nodes in metastatic carcinoma from the uterine cervix. Gynecol Oncol 1984, **19**: 187–193.

377 Inoue T, Morita K. The prognostic significance of number of positive nodes in cervical carcinoma stages IB, IIA, and IIB. Cancer 1990, **65**: 1923–1927.

378 Inoue T, Okumura M. Prognostic significance of parametrial extension in patients with cervical carcinoma stages IB, IIA, and IIB. A study of 628 cases treated by radical hysterectomy and lymphadenectomy with or without postoperative irradiation. Cancer 1984, **54**: 1714–1719.

379 Kamura T, Tsukamoto N, Tsuruchi N, Saito T, Matsuyama T, Akazawa K, Nakano H. Multivariate analysis of the histopathologic prognostic factors of cervical cancer in patients undergoing radical hysterectomy. Cancer 1992, **69**: 181–186.

380 Lombard I, Vincent-Salomon A, Validire P, Zafrani B, de la Rochefordiere A, Clough K, Favre M, Pouillart P, Sastre-Garau X. Human papillomavirus genotype as a major determinant of the course of cervical cancer. J Clin Oncol 1998, **16**: 2613–2619.

381 Nakano T, Oka K, Takahashi T, Morita S, Arai T. Roles of Langerhans' cells and T-lymphocytes infiltrating cancer tissues in patients treated by radiation therapy for cervical cancer. Cancer 1992, **70**: 2839–2844.

382 Noguchi H, Shiozawa I, Sakai Y, Yamazaki T, Fukuta T. Pelvic lymph node metastasis of uterine cervical cancer. Gynecol Oncol 1987, **27**: 150–158.

383 Obermair A, Wanner C, Bilgi S, Speiser P, Reisenberger K, Kaider A, Kainz C, Leodolter S, Breitenecker G, Gitsch G. The influence of vascular space involvement on the prognosis of patients with stage IB cervical carcinoma: correlation of results from hematoxylin and eosin staining with results from immunostaining for factor VIII-related antigen. Cancer 1998, **82**: 689–696.

384 Oka K, Nakano T, Arai T. c-*erb*B-2 Oncoprotein expression is associated withpoor prognosis in squamous cell carcinoma of the cervix. Cancer 1994, **73**: 664–671.

385 Perez CA, Camel HM, Askin F, Breaux S. Endometrial extension of carcinoma of the uterine cervix. A prognostic factor that may modify staging. Cancer 1981, **48**: 170–180.

386 Perez CA, Grigsby PW, Nene SM, Camel HM, Galakatos A, Kao MS, Lockett MA. Effect of tumor size on the prognosis of carcinoma of the uterine cervix treated with irradiation alone. Cancer 1992, **69**: 2796–2806.

387 Riou G, Favre M, Jeannel D, Bourhis J, Le Doussal V, Orth G. Association between poor prognosis in early-stage invasive cervical carcinomas and non-detection of HPV DNA. Lancet 1990, **335**: 1171–1174.

388 Robert ME, Fu YS. Squamous cell carcinoma of the uterine cervix – a review with emphasis on prognostic factors and unusual variants. Semin Diagn Pathol 1990, **7**: 173–189.

389 Rutgers JL, Mattox TF, Vargas MP. Angiogenesis in uterine cervical squamous cell carcinoma. Int J Gynecol Pathol 1995, **14**: 114–118.

390 Sagae S, Kuzumaki N, Hisada T, Mugikura Y, Kudo R, Hashimoto M. *ras* Oncogene expression and prognosis of invasive squamous cell carcinomas of the uterine cervix. Cancer 1989, **63**: 1577–1582.

391 Sakuragi N, Takeda N, Hareyama H, Fujimoto T, Todo Y, Okamoto K, Takeda M, Wada S, Yamamoto R, Fujimoto S. A multivariate analysis of blood vessel invasion as predictor of ovarian and lymph node metastases in patients with cervical carcinoma. Cancer 2000, **88**: 2578–2583.

392 Samlal RA, van der Velden J, Ten Kate FJ, Schilthuis MS, Hart AA, Lamnes FB. Surgical pathology factors that predict recurrence in stage IB and IIA cervical carcinoma patients with negative pelvic lymph nodes. Cancer 1997, **80**: 1234–1240.

393 Smiley LM, Burke TW, Silva EG, Morris M, Gershenson DM, Wharton JT. Prognostic factors in stage IB squamous cervical cancer patients with low risk for recurrence. Obstet Gynecol 1991, **77**: 271–275.

394 Stendahl U, Eklund G, Willen R. Prognosis of invasive squamous cell carcinoma of the uterine cervix. A comparative study of the predictive values of clinical staging IB-III and a histopathologic malignancy grading system. Int J Gynecol Pathol 1983, **2**: 42–54.

395 Stock RJ, Zaino R, Bundy BN, Askin FB, Woodward J, Fetter B, Paulson JA, DiSaia PJ, Stehman FB. Evaluation and comparison of histopathologic grading systems of epithelial carcinoma of the uterine cervix; Gynecologic Oncology Group studies. Int J Gynecol Pathol 1994, **13**: 99–108.

396 Strang P. Cytogenetic and cytometric analyses in squamous cell carcinoma of the uterine cervix. Int J Gynecol Pathol 1989, **8**: 54–63.

397 van Bommel PF, Kenemans P, Helmerhorst TJ, Gallee MP, Ivanyi D. Expression of cytokeratin 10, 13, and involucrin as prognostic factors in low stage squamous cell carcinoma of the uterine cervix. Cancer 1994, **74**: 2314–2320.

398 van Driel WJ, Hogendoorn PC, Jansen FW, Zwinderman AH, Trimbos JB, Fleuren GJ. Tumor-associated eosinophilic infiltrate of cervical cancer is indicative for a less effective immune response. Hum Pathol 1996, **27**: 904–911.

399 Wentz WB, Lewis GC Jr. Correlation of histologic morphology and survival in cervical cancer following radiation therapy. Obstet Gynecol 1965, **26**: 228–232.

400 Zaino RJ, Ward S, Delgado G, Bundy B, Gore H, Fetter G, Ganjei P, Frauenhoffer E. Histopathologic predictors of the behavior of surgically treated stage IB squamous cell carcinoma of the cervix. A Gynecologic Oncology Group study. Cancer 1992, **69**: 1750–1758.

Other microscopic types

401 Brinck U, Jakob C, Bau O, Fuzesi L. Papillary squamous cell carcinoma of the uterine cervix: report of three cases and a review of its classification. Int J Gynecol Pathol 2000, **19**: 231–235.

402 Coleman RL, Lindberg G, Muller CY, Miller DS, Hameed A. Ectopic production and localization of beta-human chorionic gonadatropin in lymphoepithelioma-like carcinoma of the cervix: a case report. Int J Gynecol Pathol 2000, **19**: 179–182.

403 Daroca PJ Jr, Dhorandhar HN. Basaloid carcinoma of uterine cervix. Am J Surg Pathol 1980, **4**: 235–239.

404 Grayson W, Cooper K. A reappraisal of 'basaloid carcinoma' of the cervix, and the differential diagnosis of basaloid cervical neoplasms. Adv Anat Pathol 2002, **9**: 290–300.

405 Grayson W, Taylor LF, Cooper K. Carcinosarcoma of the uterine cervix: a report of eight cases with immunohistochemical analysis and evaluation of human papillomavirus status. Am J Surg Pathol 2001, **25**: 338–347.

406 Halpin TF, Hunter RE, Cohen MB. Lymphoepithelioma of the uterine cervix. Gynecol Oncol 1989, **34**: 101–105.

407 Hasumi K, Sugano H, Sakamoto G, Masubuchi K, Kubo H. Circumscribed carcinoma of the uterine cervix, with marked lymphocytic infiltration. Cancer 1977, **39**: 2503–2507.

408 Koenig C, Turnicky RP, Kankam CF, Tavassoli FA. Papillary squamotransitional cell carcinoma of the cervix: a report of 32 cases. Am J Surg Pathol 1997, **21**: 915–921.

409 Matorell MA, Julian JM, Calabuig C, Garcia-Garcia JA, Perez-Valles A. Lymphoepithelioma-like carcinoma of the uterine cervix. Arch Pathol Lab Med 2002, **126**: 1501–1505.

410 Mills SE, Austin MB, Randall ME. Lymphoepithelioma-like carcinoma of the uterine cervix. A distinctive, undifferentiated carcinoma with inflammatory stroma. Am J Surg Pathol 1985, **9**: 883–889.

411 Pang LC. Sarcomatoid squamous cell carcinoma of the uterine cervix with osteoclast-like giant cells: report of two cases. Int J Gynecol Pathol 1998, **17**: 174–177.

412 Randall ME, Andersen WA, Mills SE, Kim JAC. Papillary squamous cell carcinoma of the uterine cervix. A clinicopathologic study of nine cases. Int J Gynecol Pathol 1986, **5**: 1–10.

413 Song JS, Choi J, Lee YH, Kim KR. Lymphoepithelioma-like carcinomas in the uterine cervix and endometrium: a clinicopathologic study of 6 cases with evaluation of Epstein–Barr virus and human papilloma virus genomes. Lab Invest 2009, **89**(Suppl 1): 238A.

414 Steeper TA, Piscioli F, Rosai J. Squamous cell carcinoma with sarcoma-like stroma of the female genital tract. Cancer 1983, **52**: 890–898.

415 Tiltman AJ, Atad J. Verrucous carcinoma of the cervix with endometrial involvement. Int J Gynecol Pathol 1982, **1**: 221–226.

416 Tseng CJ, Pao CC, Tseng LH, Chang CT, Lai CH, Soong YK, Hsueh S, Jyu-Jen H. Lymphoepithelioma-like carcinoma of the uterine cervix: association with Epstein–Barr virus and human papillomavirus. Cancer 1997, **80**: 91–97.

417 Weinberg E, Hoisington S, Eastman AY, Rice DK, Malfetano J, Ross JS. Uterine cervical lymphoepithelial-like carcinoma. Absence of Epstein–Barr virus genomes. Am J Clin Pathol 1993, **99**: 195–199.

ADENOCARCINOMA

Morphologic and other features

418 Alfsen GC, Thorensen S, Kristensen GB, Skovlund E, Abeler VM. Histopathological subtyping of cervical adenocarcinoma reveals increasing incidence rates of endometrioid tumors in all age groups: a population based study with review of all nonsquamous cervical carcinomas in Norway from 1966 to 1970, 1976 to 1980, and 1986 to 1990. Cancer 2000, **89**: 1291–1299.

419 Angel C, Du Beshter B, Lin JY. Clinical presentation and management of stage I cervical adenocarcinoma. A 25 year experience. Gynecol Oncol 1992, **44**: 71–78.

420 Baker AC, Eltoum I, Curry RO, Stockard CR, Manne U, Grizzle WE, Chhieng D. Mucinous expression in benign and neoplastic glandular lesions of the uterine cervix. Arch Pathol Lab Med 2006, **130**: 1510–1515.

421 Berek JS, Hacker NF, Fu Y-S, Sokale JR, Leuchter RC, Lagasse LD. Adenocarcinoma of the uterine cervix. Histologic variables associated with lymph node metastasis and survival. Obstet Gynecol 1985, **65**: 46–52.

422 Cina SJ, Richardson MS, Austin RM, Kurman RJ. Immunohistochemical staining for Ki-67 antigen, carcinoembryonic antigen, and p53 in the differential diagnosis of glandular lesions of the cervix. Mod Pathol 1997, **10**: 176–180.

423 Cohen C, Shulman G, Budgeon LR. Endocervical and endometrial adenocarcinoma. An immunoperoxidase and histochemical study. Am J Surg Pathol 1982, **6**: 151–157.

424 Cooper P, Russell G, Wilson B. Adenocarcinoma of the endocervix. A histochemical study. Histopathology 1987, **11**: 1321–1330.

425 Dabbs DJ, Geisinger KR, Norris HT. Intermediate filaments in endometrial and endocervical carcinomas. The diagnostic utility of vimentin patterns. Am J Surg Pathol 1986, **10**: 568–576.

426 Duk JM, De Bruijn HW, Groenier KH, Fleuren GJ, Aalders JG. Adenocarcinoma of the uterine cervix. Prognostic significance of pretreatment serum CA 125, squamous cell carcinoma antigen, and carcinoembryonic antigen levels in relation to clinical and histopathologic tumor characteristics. Cancer 1990, **65**: 1830–1837.

427 Eifel PJ, Burke TW, Delclos L, Wharton JT, Oswald MJ. Early stage I adenocarcinoma of the uterine cervix. Treatment results in patients with tumors less than or equal to 4 cm in diameter. Gynecol Oncol 1991, **41**: 199–205.

428 Eifel PJ, Morris M, Oswald MJ, Wharton JT, Delclos L. Adenocarcinoma of the uterine cervix. Prognosis and patterns of failure in 367 cases. Cancer 1990, **65**: 2507–2514.

429 Elishaev E, Gilks CB, Miller D, Srodon M, Kurman RJ, Ronnett BM. Synchronous and metachronous endocervical and ovarian neoplasms: evidence supporting interpretation of the ovarian neoplasms as metastatic endocervical adenocarcinomas simulating primary ovarian surface epithelial neoplasms. Am J Surg Pathol 2005, **29**: 281–294.

430 Ferguson AW, Svoboda-Newman SM, Frank TS. Analysis of human papillomavirus infection and molecular alterations in adenocarcinoma of the cervix. Mod Pathol 1998, **11**: 11–18.

431 Fujiwara H, Tortolero-Luna G, Mitchell MF, Koulos JP, Wright TC. Adenocarcinoma of the cervix: expression and clinical significance of estrogen and progesterone receptors. Cancer 1997, **79**: 505–512.

432 Gallup DG, Abell MR. Invasive adenocarcinoma of the uterine cervix. Obstet Gynecol 1977, **49**: 596–603.

433 Greer BE, Figge DC, Tamimi HK, Cain JM. Stage IB adenocarcinoma of the cervix treated by radical hysterectomy and pelvic lymph node dissection. Am J Obstet Gynecol 1989, **160**: 1509–1513.

434 Griffin NR, Wells M. Characterisation of complex carbohydrates in cervical glandular intraepithelial neoplasia and invasive adenocarcinoma. Int J Gynecol Pathol 1994, **13**: 319–329.

435 Griffin NR, Wells M, Fox H. Modulation of the antigenicity of amylase in cervical glandular atypia, adenocarcinoma in situ and invasive adenocarcinoma. Histopathology 1989, **15**: 267–279.

436 Gusberg SB, Corscaden JA. The pathology and treatment of adenocarcinoma of the cervix. Cancer 1951, **4**: 1066–1072.

437 Hopkins MP, Schmidt RW, Roberts JA, Morley GW. The prognosis and treatment of stage I adenocarcinoma of the cervix. Obstet Gynecol 1988, **72**: 915–921.

438 Hopkins MP, Sutton P, Roberts JA. Prognostic features and treatment of endocervical adenocarcinoma of the cervix. Gynecol Oncol 1987, **27**: 69–75.

439 Jackson-York GL, Ramzy I. Synchronous papillary mucinous adenocarcinoma of the endocervix and fallopian tubes. Int J Gynecol Pathol 1992, **11**: 63–67.

440 Jones MW, Silverberg SG. Cervical adenocarcinoma in young women. Possible relationship to microglandular hyperplasia and use of oral contraceptives. Obstet Gynecol 1989, **73**: 984–989.

441 Kalir T, Simsir A, Demopoulos HB, Demopoulos RI. Obstacles to the early detection of endocervical adenocarcinoma. Int J Gynecol Pathol 2005, **24**: 399–403.

442 Kaspar HG, Dinh TV, Doherty MG, Hannigan EV, Kumar D. Clinical implications of tumor volume measurement in stage I adenocarcinoma of the cervix. Obstet Gynecol 1993, **81**: 296–300.

443 Kihana T, Tsuda H, Teshima S, Nomoto K, Tsugane S, Sonoda T, Matsuura S, Hirohashi S. Prognostic significance of the overexpression of c-*erb*B-2 protein in adenocarcinoma of the uterine cervix. Cancer 1994, **73**: 148–153.

444 Kjorstad KE, Bond B. Stage IB adenocarcinoma of the cervix. Metastatic potential and patterns of dissemination. Am J Obstet Gynecol 1984, **150**: 297–299.

445 Kleine W, Rau K, Schwoeorer D, Pfleiderer A. Prognosis of the adenocarcinoma of the cervix uteri: a comparative study. Gynecol Oncol 1989, **35**: 145–149.

446 Konishi I, Fujii S, Nanbu Y, Nonogaki H, Mori T. Mucin leakage into the cervical stroma may increase lymph node metastasis in mucin-producing cervical adenocarcinomas. Cancer 1990, **65**: 229–237.

447 Korhonen MO. Adenocarcinoma of the uterine cervix. Prognosis and prognostic significance of histology. Cancer 1984, **53**: 1760–1763.

448 Kudo R, Sasano H, Koizumi M, Orenstein JM, Silverberg SG. Immunohistochemical comparison of new monoclonal antibody 1C5 and carcinoembryonic antigen in the differential diagnosis of adenocarcinoma of the uterine cervix. Int J Gynecol Pathol 1990, **9**: 325–336.

449 Lee SJ, Rollason TP. Argyrophilic cells in cervical intraepithelial glandular neoplasia. Int J Gynecol Pathol 1994, **13**: 131–132.

450 LiVolsi VA, Merino MJ, Schwartz PE. Coexistent endocervical adenocarcinoma and mucinous adenocarcinoma of ovary. A clinicopathologic study of four cases. Int J Gynecol Pathol 1983, **1**: 391–402.

451 Lu X, Toki T, Konishi I, Nikaido T, Fujii S. Expression of p21WAF1/CIP1 in adenocarcinoma of the uterine cervix: a possible immunohistochemical marker of a favorable prognosis. Cancer 1998, **82**: 2409–2417.

452 Mandai M, Konishi I, Koshiyama M, Komatsu T, Yamamoto S, Nanbu K, Mori T, Fukumoto M. Altered expression of nm23-H1 and c-*erb*B-2 proteins have prognostic significance in adenocarcinoma but not in squamous cell carcinoma of the uterine cervix. Cancer 1995, **75**: 2523–2529.

453 McCluggage WG, McBride HA, Maxwell P, Bharucha H. Immunohistochemical detection of p53 and bcl-2 proteins in neoplastic and non-neoplastic endocervical glandular lesions. Int J Gynecol Pathol 1997, **16**: 22–27.

454 Matthews CM, Burke TW, Tornos C, Eifel PJ, Atkinson EN, Stringer CA, Morris M, Silva EG. Stage I cervical adenocarcinoma. Prognostic evaluation of surgically treated patients. Gynecol Oncol 1993, **49**: 19–23.

455 Miller BE, Flax SD, Arheart K, Photopulos G. The presentation of adenocarcinoma of the uterine cervix. Cancer 1993, **72**: 1281–1285.

456 Moberg PJ, Einhorn N, Silfversward C, Soderberg G. Adenocarcinoma of the uterine cervix. Cancer 1986, **57**: 407–410.

457 Negri G, Egarter-Vigl E, Kasal A, Romano F, Haitel A, Mian C. P16 INK4a is a useful marker for the diagnosis of adenocarcinoma of the cervix uteri and its precursors: an immunohistochemical study with immunocytochemical correlations. Am J Surg Pathol 2003, **27**: 187–193.

458 Nguyen GK, Daya D. Cervical adenocarcinoma and related lesions. Cytodiagnostic criteria and pitfalls. Pathol Annu 1993, **28**(Pt 2): 53–75.

459 Onuma K, Dabbs DJ, Bhargava R. Mammaglobin expression in the female genital tract: immunohistochemical analysis in benign

and neoplastic endocervix and endometrium. Int J Gynecol Pathol 2008, **27**: 418–425.

460 Parazzini F, La Vecchia C. Epidemiology of adenocarcinoma of the cervix. Gynecol Oncol 1990, **39**: 40–46.

461 Park KJ, Bramlage MP, Ellenson LH, Pirog EC. Immunoprofile of adenocarcinomas of the endometrium, endocervix, and ovary with mucinous differentiation. Appl Immunohistochem Mol Morphol 2009, **17**: 8–11.

462 Reagan JW. Cellular pathology and uterine cancer. Ward Burdick Award Address. Am J Clin Pathol 1974, **62**: 150–164.

463 Ronnett BM, Yemelyanova AV, Vang R, Gilks CB, Miller D, Gravitt PE, Kurman RJ. Endocervical adenocarcinomas with ovarian metastases: analysis of 29 cases with emphasis on minimally invasive cervical tumors and the ability of the metastases to simulate primary ovarian neoplasms. Am J Surg Pathol 2008, **32**: 1835–1853.

464 Saigo PE, Cain JM, Kim WS, Gaynor JJ, Johnson K, Lewis JL. Prognostic factors in adenocarcinoma of the uterine cervix. Cancer 1986, **57**: 1584–1593.

465 Shorrock K, Johnson J, Johnson IR. Epidemiological changes in cervical carcinoma with particular reference to mucin-secreting subtypes. Histopathology 1990, **17**: 53–57.

466 Sorvari TE. A histochemical study of epithelial mucosubstances in endometrial and cervical adenocarcinomas. With reference to normal endometrium and cervical mucosa. Acta Pathol Microbiol Scand 1969, **207**(Suppl): 1–85.

467 Sullivan LM, Smolkin ME, Frierson HF Jr, Galgano MT. Comprehensive evaluation of CDX2 in invasive cervical adenocarcinomas: immunopositivity in the absence of overt colorectal morphology. Am J Surg Pathol 2008, **32**: 1608–1612.

468 Tenti P, Romagnoli S, Silini E, Zappatore R, Giunta P, Stella G, Carnevali L. Cervical adenocarcinomas express markers common to gastric, intestinal, and pancreatobiliary epithelial cells. Pathol Res Pract 1994, **190**: 342–349.

469 Tenti P, Romagnoli S, Silini E, Zappatore R, Spinillo A, Giunta P, Cappelini A, Vesentini N, Zara C, Carnevali L. Human papillomavirus types 16 and 18 infection in infiltrating adenocarcinomas of the cervix. PCR analysis of 138 cases and correlation with histologic type and grade. Am J Clin Pathol 1996, **106**: 52–56.

470 Toki N, Kaku T, Tsukamoto N, Matsumura M, Saito T, Kamura T, Matsuyama T, Nakano H. Distribution of basement membrane antigens in the uterine cervical adenocarcinomas. An immunohistochemical study. Gynecol Oncol 1990, **38**: 17–21.

471 Ueda G, Yamasaki M, Inoue M, Tanaka Y, Hiramatsu K, Inoue Y, Abe Y. Immunohistochemical demonstration of peptide hormones in cervical adenocarcinomas with argyrophil cells. Int J Gynecol Pathol 1984, **2**: 373–379.

472 Valente PT, Hanjani P. Endocervical neoplasia in long-term users of oral contraceptives. Clinical and pathologic observations. Obstet Gynecol 1986, **67**: 695–704.

473 Vesterinen E, Forss M, Nieminen U. Increase of cervical adenocarcinoma. A report of 520 cases of cervical carcinoma including 112 tumors with glandular elements. Gynecol Oncol 1990, **33**: 49–53.

474 Yavner DL, Dwyer IM, Hancock WW, Ehrmann RL. Basement membrane of cervical adenocarcinoma. An immunoperoxidase study of laminin and type IV collagen. Obstet Gynecol 1990, **76**: 1014–1019.

475 Yemelyanova A, Ji H, Shih IeM, Wang TL, Wu LS, Ronnett BM. Utility of p16 expression for distinction of uterine serous carcinomas from endometrial endometrioid and endocervical adenocarcinomas: immunohistochemical analysis of 201 cases. Am J Surg Pathol 2009, **33**: 1504–1514.

476 Young RH, Clement PB. Endocervical adenocarcinoma and its variants: their morphology and differential diagnosis. Histopathology 2002, **41**: 185–207.

477 Young RH, Scully RE. Invasive adenocarcinoma and related tumors of the uterine cervix. Semin Diagn Pathol 1990, **7**: 205–227.

478 Zaino RJ. Glandular lesions of the uterine cervix. Mod Pathol 2000, **13**: 261–274.

Differential diagnosis with endometrial adenocarcinoma

479 Ansari-Lari MA, Staebler A, Zaino RJ, Shah KV, Ronnett BM. Distinction of endocervical and endometrial adenocarcinomas: immunohistochemical p16 expression correlated with human papillomavirus (HPV) DNA detection. Am J Surg Pathol 2004, **28**: 160–167.

480 Caron C, Tetu B, Laberge P, Bellemare G, Raymond PE. Endocervical involvement by endometrial carcinoma on fractional curettage. A clinicopathological study of 37 cases. Mod Pathol 1991, **4**: 644–647.

481 Castrilon DH, Lee KR, Nucci MR. Distinction between endometrial and endocervical adenocarcinoma: an immunohistochemical study. Int J Gynecol Pathol 2002, **21**: 4–10.

482 Cohen C, Shulman G, Budgeon LR. Endocervical and endometrial adenocarcinoma. An immunoperoxidase and histochemical study. Am J Surg Pathol 1982, **6**: 151–157.

483 McCluggage WG, Sumathi VP, McBride HA, Patterson A. A panel of immunohistochemical stains, including carcinoembryonic antigen, vimentin, and estrogen receptor, aids the distinction between primary endometrial and endocervical adenocarcinomas. Int J Gynecol Pathol 2002, **21**: 11–15.

484 Staebler A, Sherman ME, Zaino RJ, Ronnett BM. Hormone receptor immunohistochemistry and human papillomavirus in situ hybridisation are useful for distinguishing endocervical and endometrial adenocarcinomas. Am J Surg Pathol 2002, **26**: 998–1006.

485 Tamimi HR, Gown AM, Kim-Deobald J, Figge DC, Greer BE, Cain JM. The utility of immunocytochemistry in invasive adenocarcinoma of the cervix. Am J Obstet Gynecol 1992, **166**: 1655–1661.

486 Zaino RJ. The fruits of our labours: distinguishing endometrial from endocervical adenocarcinoma. Int J Gynecol Pathol 2002, **21**: 1–3.

In situ and microinvasive adenocarcinoma

487 Andersen ES, Arffmann E. Adenocarcinoma in situ of the uterine cervix. A clinico-pathologic study of 36 cases. Gynecol Oncol 1989, **35**: 1–7.

488 Biscotti CV, Hart WR. Apoptotic bodies: a consistent morphologic feature of endocervical adenocarcinoma in situ. Am J Surg Pathol 1998, **22**: 434–439.

489 Boon ME, Baak JPA, Kurver PJH, Overdiep SH, Verdonk GW. Adenocarcinoma in situ of the cervix. An underdiagnosed lesion. Cancer 1981, **48**: 768–773.

490 Cameron RI, Maxwell P, Jenkins D, McCluggage WG. Immunohistochemical staining with MIB1, bcl2, and p16 assists in the distinction of cervical glandular intraepithelial neoplasia from tubo-endometrial metaplasia, endometriosis and microglandular hyperplasia. Histopathology 2002, **41**: 313–321.

491 Ceballos KM, Shaw D, Daya D. Microinvasive cervical adenocarcinoma (FIGO stage 1A tumors): results of surgical staging and outcome analysis. Am J Surg Pathol 2006, **30**: 370–374.

492 Colgan TJ, Lickrish GM. The topography and invasive potential of cervical adenocarcinoma in situ, with and without associated dysplasia. Gynecol Oncol 1990, **36**: 246–249.

493 Gloor E, Hurlimann J. Cervical intraepithelial glandular neoplasia (adenocarcinoma in situ and glandular dysplasia). A correlative study of 23 cases with histologic grading, histochemical analysis of mucins, and immunohistochemical determination of the affinity for four lectins. Cancer 1986, **58**: 1272–1280.

494 Goldstein NS, Ahmad E, Hussain M, Hankin RC, Perez-Reyes N. Endocervical glandular atypia. Does a preneoplastic lesion of adenocarcinoma in situ exist? Am J Clin Pathol 1998, **110**: 200–209.

495 Goldstein NS, Mani A. The status and distance of cone biopsy margins as a predictor of excision adequacy for endocervical adenocarcinoma in situ. Am J Clin Pathol 1998, **109**: 727–732.

496 Hurlimann J, Gloor E. Adenocarcinoma in situ and invasive adenocarcinoma of the uterine cervix. An immunohistologic study with antibodies specific for several epithelial markers. Cancer 1984, **54**: 103–109.

497 Ioffe OB, Sagae S, Moritani S, Dahmoush L, Chen TT, Silverberg SG. Should pathologists diagnose endocervical preneoplastic lesions 'less than' adenocarcinoma in situ? Int J Gynecol Pathol 2002, **22**: 18–21.

498 Jaworski RC. Endocervical glandular dysplasia, adenocarcinoma in situ, and early invasive (microinvasive) adenocarcinoma of the uterine cervix. Semin Diagn Pathol 1990, **7**: 190–204.

499 Jaworski RC, Pacey NF, Greenberg ML, Osborn RA. The histologic diagnosis of adenocarcinoma in situ and related lesions of the cervix uteri. Adenocarcinoma in situ. Cancer 1988, **61**: 1171–1181.

500 Jones MW, Silverberg SG. Cervical adenocarcinoma in young women. Possible relationship to microglandular hyperplasia and use of oral contraceptives. Obstet Gynecol 1989, **73**: 984–989.

501 Lee KR, Flynn CE. Early invasive adenocarcinoma of the cervix. Cancer 2000, **89**: 1048–1055.

502 Lee KR, Sun D, Crum CP. Endocervical intraepithelial glandular atypia (dysplasia): a histopathologic, human papillomavirus, and MIB-1 analysis of 25 cases. Hum Pathol 2000, **31**: 656–664.

503 Lu X, Shiozawa T, Nakayama K, Toki T, Nikaido T, Fujii S. Abnormal expression of sex steroid receptors and cell cycle-related molecules in adenocarcinoma in situ of the uterine cervix. Int J Gynecol Pathol 1999, **18**: 109–114.

504 Maier RC, Norris HJ. Coexistence of cervical intraepithelial neoplasia with primary adenocarcinoma of the endocervix. Obstet Gynecol 1980, **56**: 361–364.

505 Marques T, Andrade LA, Vassallo J. Endocervical tubal metaplasia and adenocarcinoma in situ: role of immunohistochemistry for carcinoembryonic antigen and vimentin in differential diagnosis. Histopathology 1996, **28**: 549–550.

506 McCluggage WG, Shah R, Connolly LE, McBride HA. Intestinal-type cervical adenocarcinoma in situ and adenocarcinoma exhibit a partial enteric immunophenotype with consistent expression of CDX2. Int J Gynecol Pathol 2008, **27**: 92–100.

507 Muntz HG, Bell DA, Lage JM, Goff BA, Feldman S, Rice LW. Adenocarcinoma in situ of the uterine cervix. Obstet Gynecol 1992, **80**: 935–939.

508 Ostor AG. Early invasive adenocarcinoma of the uterine cervix. Int J Gynecol Pathol 2000, **19**: 29–38.

509 Park KJ, Soslow RA. Current concepts in cervical pathology. Arch Pathol Lab Med 2009, **133**: 729–738.

510 Plotkin A, Khalifa MA, Ismiil N, Saad RS, Dube V, Ghorab Z, Nofech-Mozes S. The circumferential extent of disease should be reported in vervical adenocarcinoma in situ (AIS) excised by LEEP and cone biopsies. Lab Invest 2009, **89**(Suppl 1): 232A.

511 Riethdorf L, Riethdorf S, Lee KR, Cviko A, Loning T, Crum CP. Human papillomavirus, expression of p16INK4A, and early endocervical glandular neoplasia. Hum Pathol 2002, **33**: 899–904.

512 Schlesinger C, Silverberg SG. Endocervical adenocarcinoma in situ of tubal type and its relation to atypical tubal metaplasia. Int J Gynecol Pathol 1999, **18**: 1–4.

513 Teshima S, Shimosato Y, Kishi K, Kasamatsu T, Ohmi K, Uei Y. Early stage adenocarcinoma of the uterine cervix. Histopathologic analysis with consideration of histogenesis. Cancer 1985, **56**: 167–172.

514 Weisbrot IM, Stabinsky C, Davis AM. Adenocarcinoma in situ of the uterine cervix. Cancer 1972, **29**: 225–233.

515 Wells M, Brown LJR. Glandular lesions of the uterine cervix. The present state of our knowledge. Histopathology 1986, **10**: 777–792.

516 Wheeler DT, Kurman RJ. The relationship of glands to thick-wall blood vessels as a marker of invasion in endocervical adenocarcinoma. Int J Gynecol Pathol 2005, **24**: 125–130.

517 Witkiewicz A, Lee KR, Brodsky G, Cviko A, Brodsky J, Crum CP. Superficial (early) endocervical adenocarcinoma in situ: a study of 12 cases and comparison to conventional AIS. Am J Surg Pathol 2005, **29**: 1609–1614.

518 Zaino RJ. Adenocarcinoma in situ, glandular dysplasia, and early invasive adenocarcinoma of the uterine cervix. Int J Gynecol Pathol 2002, **21**: 314–326.

Morphologic variants of cervical adenocarcinoma

519 Albores-Saavedra J, Manivel C, Mora A, Vuitch F, Milchgrub S, Gould E. The solid variant of adenoid cystic carcinoma of the cervix. Int J Gynecol Pathol 1992, **11**: 2–10.

520 Alfsen GC, Kristensen GB, Skovlund E, Pettersen EO, Abeler VM. Histologic subtype has minor importance for overall survival in patients with adenocarcinoma of the uterine cervix: a population-based study of prognostic factors in 505 patients with nonsquamous cell carcinomas of the cervix. Cancer 2001, **92**: 2471–2483.

521 Auersperg N, Erber H, Worth A. Histologic variation among poorly differentiated invasive carcinomas of the human uterine cervix. J Natl Cancer Inst 1973, **51**: 1461–1477.

522 Bagué S, Rodríguez IM, Prat J. Malignant mesonephric tumors of the female genital tract: a clinicopathologic study of 9 cases. Am J Surg Pathol 2004, **28**: 601–607.

523 Brainard JA, Hart WR. Adenoid basal epitheliomas of the uterine cervix: a reevaluation of distinctive cervical basaloid lesions currently classified as adenoid basal carcinoma and adenoid basal hyperplasia. Am J Surg Pathol 1998, **22**: 965–975.

524 Choo YC, Naylor B. Coexistent squamous cell carcinoma and adenocarcinoma of the uterine cervix. Gynecol Oncol 1984, **17**: 168–174.

525 Christopherson WM, Nealon N, Gray LA Sr. Noninvasive precursor lesions of adenocarcinoma and mixed adenosquamous carcinoma of the cervix uteri. Cancer 1979, **44**: 975–983.

526 Clement PB, Young RH, Keh P, Östör AG, Scully RE. Malignant mesonephric neoplasms of the uterine cervix. A report of eight cases, including four with a malignant spindle cell component. Am J Surg Pathol 1995, **19**: 1158–1171.

527 Costa MJ, Kenny MB, Hewan-Lowe K, Judd R. Glassy cell features in adenosquamous carcinoma of the uterine cervix. Histologic, ultrastructural, immunohistochemical, and clinical findings. Am J Clin Pathol 1991, **96**: 520–528.

528 Costa MJ, Kenny MB, Judd R. Adenocarcinoma and adenosquamous carcinoma of the uterine cervix. Histologic and immunohistochemical features with clinical correlation. Int J Surg Pathol 1994, **1**: 181–190.

529 Costa MJ, McIlnay KR, Trelford J. Cervical carcinoma with glandular differentiation. Histological evaluation predicts disease recurrence in clinical Stage I or II patients. Hum Pathol 1995, **26**: 829–837.

530 Daya D, Young RH. Florid deep glands of the uterine cervix. Another mimic of adenoma malignum. Am J Clin Pathol 1995, **103**: 614–617.

531 Dickersin GR, Welch WR, Erlandson R, Robboy SJ. Ultrastructure of 16 cases of clear cell adenocarcinoma of the vagina and cervix in young women. Cancer 1980, **45**: 1615–1624.

532 Farley JH, Hickey KW, Carlson JW, Rose GS, Kost ER, Harrison TA. Adenosquamous histology predicts a poor outcome for patients with advanced-stage, but not early-stage, cervical carcinoma. Cancer 2003, **97**: 2196–2202.

533 Fawcett KJ, Dockerty MB, Hunt AB. Mesonephric carcinoma of the cervix uteri. Clinical and pathologic study. Am J Obstet Gynecol 1966, **95**: 1068–1079.

534 Ferry JA, Scully RE. 'Adenoid cystic' carcinoma and adenoid basal carcinoma of the uterine cervix. A study of 28 cases. Am J Surg Pathol 1988, **12**: 134–144.

535 Fowler WC Jr, Miles PA, Surwit EA, Edelman DA, Walton LA, Photopulos GJ. Adenoid cystic carcinoma of the cervix. Obstet Gynecol 1978, **52**: 337–342.

536 Fu YS, Reagan JW, Fu AS, Janiga KE. Adenocarcinoma and mixed carcinoma of the uterine cervix. II. Prognostic value of nuclear DNA analysis. Cancer 1982, **49**: 2571–2577.

537 Fu YS, Reagan JW, Hsiu JG, Storaasli JP, Wentz WB. Adenocarcinoma and mixed carcinoma of the uterine cervix. Cancer 1982, **49**: 2560–2570.

538 Gallager HS, Simpson CB, Ayala AG. Adenoid cystic carcinoma of the uterine cervix. Report of 4 cases. Cancer 1971, **27**: 1398–1402.

539 Gilks CB, Young RH, Aguirre P, De Lellis RA, Scully RE. Adenoma malignum (minimal deviation adenocarcinoma) of the uterine cervix. A clinicopathological and immunohistochemical analysis of 26 cases. Am J Surg Pathol 1989, **13**: 717–729.

540 Gilks CB, Young RH, Clement PB, Hart WR, Scully RE. Adenomyomas of the uterine cervix of endocervical type: a report of ten cases of a benign cervical tumor that may be confused with adenoma malignum [corrected]. Mod Pathol 1996, **9**: 220–224.

541 Glücksmann A, Cherry CP. Incidence, histology, and response to radiation of mixed carcinomas (adenocanthomas) of the uterine cervix. Cancer 1956, **9**: 971–979.

542 Grayson W, Taylor LF, Cooper K. Adenoid cystic and adenoid basal carcinoma of the uterine cervix: comparative morphologic, mucin, and immunohistochemical profile of two rare neoplasms of putative 'reserve cell' origin. Am J Surg Pathol 1999, **23**: 448–458.

543 Hanselaar AG, Van Leusen ND, De Wilde PC, Vooijs GP. Clear cell adenocarcinoma of the vagina and cervix. A report of the Central Netherlands Registry with emphasis on early detection and prognosis. Cancer 1991, **67**: 1971–1978.

544 Hanselaar A, van Loosbroek M, Schuurbiers O, Helmerhorst T, Bulten J, Bernheim J. Clear cell adenocarcinoma of the vagina and cervix: an update of the central Netherlands registry showing twin age incidence peaks. Cancer 1997, **79**: 2229–2236.

545 Harrison TA, Sevin BU, Koechli O, Nguyen HN, Averette HE, Penalver M, Donato DM, Nadji M. Adenosquamous carcinoma of the cervix. Prognosis in early stage disease treated by radical hysterectomy. Gynecol Oncol 1993, **50**: 310–315.

546 Hart WR. Symposium Part II: special types of adenocarcinoma of the uterine cervix. Int J Gynecol Pathol 2002, **21**: 327–346.

547 Hart WR, Norris HJ. Mesonephric adenocarcinomas of the cervix. Cancer 1972, **29**: 106–113.

548 Hayashi I, Tsuda H, Shimoda T. Reappraisal of orthodox histochemistry for the diagnosis of minimal deviation adenocarcinoma of the cervix. Am J Surg Pathol 2000, **24**: 559–562.

549 Heatley MK. Villoglandular adenocarcinoma of the uterine cervix – a systematic review of the literature. Histopathology 2007, **51**: 268–269.

550 Hoskins WJ, Averette HE, Ng ABP, Yon JL. Adenoid cystic carcinoma of the cervix uteri. Report of six cases and review of literature. Gynecol Oncol 1979, **7**: 371–384.

551 Ishii K, Hidaka E, Katsuyama T, Ota H, Shiozawa T, Tzuchiya S. Ultrastructural features of adenoma malignum of the uterine cervix: demonstration of gastric phenotypes. Ultrastruct Pathol 2000, **23**: 375–381.

552 Jiang L, Malpica A, Deavers MT, Guo M, Villa LL, Nuovo G, Merino MJ, Silva EG. Endometrial endometrioid adenocarcinoma of the uterine corpus involving the cervix: some cases probably represent independent primaries. Int J Gynecol Pathol 2010, **29**: 146–156.

553 Jones MW, Kounelis S, Papadaki H, Bakker A, Swalsky PA, Finkelstein SD. The origin and molecular characterization of adenoid basal carcinoma of the uterine cervix. Int J Gynecol Pathol 1998, **16**: 301–306.

554 Jones MW, Kounelis S, Papadaki H, Bakker A, Swalsky PA, Woods J, Finkelstein SD. Well-differentiated villoglandular adenocarcinoma of the uterine cervix: oncogene/tumor suppressor gene alterations and human papillomavirus genotyping. Int J Gynecol Pathol 2000, **124**: 110–117.

555 Jones MW, Silverberg SG. Cervical adenocarcinoma in young women. Possible relationship to microglandular hyperplasia and use of oral contraceptives. Obstet Gynecol 1989, **73**: 984–989.

556 Jones MW, Silverberg SG, Kurman RJ. Well-differentiated villoglandular adenocarcinoma of the uterine cervix. A

clinicopathological study of 24 cases. Int J Gynecol Pathol 1993, **12**: 1–7.

557 Kaku T, Enjoji M. Extremely well-differentiated adenocarcinoma ('adenoma malignum') of the cervix. Int J Gynecol Pathol 1983, **2**: 28–41.

558 Kaminski PF, Maier RC. Clear cell adenocarcinoma of the cervix unrelated to diethylstilbestrol exposure. Obstet Gynecol 1983, **62**: 720–727.

559 Kaminski PF, Norris HJ. Minimal deviation carcinoma (adenoma malignum) of the cervix. Int J Gynecol Pathol 1983, **2**: 141–152.

560 Kaminski PF, Norris HJ. Coexistence of ovarian neoplasms and endocervical adenocarcinoma. Obstet Gynecol 1984, **64**: 553–556.

561 Kato N, Katayama Y, Kaimori M, Motoyama T. Glassy cell carcinoma of the uterine cervix: histochemical, immunohistochemical, and molecular genetic observations. Int J Gynecol Pathol 2002, **21**: 134–140.

562 Kojima A, Mikami Y, Sudo T, Yamaguchi S, Kusanagi Y, Ito M, Nishimura R. Gastric morphology and immunophenotype predict poor outcome in mucinous adenocarcinoma of the uterine cervix. Am J Surg Pathol 2007, **31**: 664–672.

563 Kudo R, Sagae S, Hayakawa O, Ito E, Horimoto E, Hashimoto M. Morphology of adenocarcinoma in situ and microinvasive adenocarcinoma of the uterine cervix. A cytologic and ultrastructural study. Acta Cytol 1991, **35**: 109–116.

564 Kuragaki C, Enomoto T, Ueno Y, Sun H, Fujita M, Nakashima R, Ueda Y, Wada H, Murata Y, Toki T, Konishi I, Fujii S. Mutations in the STK11 gene characterize minimal deviation adenocarcinoma of the uterine cervix. Lab Invest 2003, **83**: 35–45.

565 Lang G, Dallenbach-Hellweg G. The histogenetic origin of cervical mesonephric hyperplasia and mesonephric adenocarcinoma of the uterine cervix studied with immunohistochemical methods. Int J Gynecol Pathol 1990, **9**: 145–157.

566 Lee KR, Trainer TD. Adenocarcinoma of the uterine cervix of small intestinal type containing numerous Paneth cells. Arch Pathol Lab Med 1990, **114**: 731–733.

567 Littman P, Clement PB, Henriksen B, Wang CC, Robboy SJ, Taft PD, Ulfelder H, Scully RE. Glassy cell carcinoma of the cervix. Cancer 1976, **37**: 2238–2246.

568 Maier RC, Norris HJ. Glassy cell carcinoma of the cervix. Obstet Gynecol 1982, **60**: 219–224.

569 Matias-Guiu X, Lerma E, Prat J. Clear cell tumors of the female genital tract. Semin Diagn Pathol 1998, **14**: 233–239.

570 Mayorga M, Garcia-Valtuille A, Fernàndez F, Val-Bernal JF, Cabrera E. Adenocarcinoma of the uterine cervix with massive signet-ring cell differentiation. Int J Surg Pathol 1997, **5**: 95–100.

571 McCluggage WG, Oliva E, Herrington CS, McBride H, Young RH. CD10 and calretinin staining of endocervical glandular lesions, endocervical stroma and endometrioid adendocarcinomas of the uterine corpus: CD10 positivity is characteristic of, but not specific for, mesonephric lesions and is not specific for, endometrial stroma. Histopathology 2003, **43**: 144–150.

572 McCluggage WG. Immunohistochemistry as a diagnostic aid in cervical pathology. Pathology 2007, **39**: 97–111.

573 Michael H, Grawe L, Kraus FT. Minimal deviation endocervical adenocarcinoma. Clinical and histologic features, immunohistochemical staining for carcino-embryonic antigen, and differentiation from confusing benign lesions. Int J Gynecol Pathol 1984, **3**: 261–276.

574 Nordqvist SRB, Fidler WJ Jr, Woodruff JM, Lewis JL Jr. Clear cell adenocarcinoma of the cervix and vagina. A clinicopathologic study of 21 cases with and without a history of maternal ingestion of estrogens. Cancer 1976, **37**: 858–871.

575 Norris HJ, McCauley KM. Unusual forms of adenocarcinoma of the cervix. An update. Pathol Annu 1993, **28**(Pt 1): 73–95.

576 Pak HY, Yokota SB, Paladugu RR, Agliozzo CM. Glassy cell carcinoma of the cervix. Cytologic and clinicopathologic analysis. Cancer 1983, **52**: 307–312.

577 Parwani AV, Smith Sehdev AE, Kurman RJ, Ronnett BM. Cervical adenoid basal tumors comprised of adenoid basal epithelioma associated with various types of invasive carcinoma: clinicopathologic features, human papillomavirus DNA detection, and P16 expression. Hum Pathol 2005, **36**: 82–90.

578 Robboy SJ, Herbst AL, Scully RE. Vaginal and cervical abnormalities related to prenatal exposure to diethylstilbestrol (DES). In Blaustein A (ed.): Pathology of female genital tract. New York, 1977, Springer-Verlag, pp. 87–101.

579 Rollason TP, Cullimore J, Bradgate MG. A suggested columnar cell morphological equivalent of squamous carcinoma in situ with early stromal invasion. Int J Gynecol Pathol 1989, **8**: 230–236.

580 Rosen Y, Dolan TE. Carcinoma of the cervix with cylindromatous features believed to arise in mesonephric duct. Cancer 1975, **36**: 1739–1747.

581 Roth LM, Hornback NB. Clear-cell adenocarcinoma of the cervix in young women. Cancer 1974, **34**: 1761–1768.

582 Saad RS, Ismiil N, Dubé V, Nofech-Mozes S, Khalifa MA. CDX-2 expression is a common event in primary intestinal-type endocervical adenocarcinoma. Am J Clin Pathol 2009, **132**: 531–538.

583 Saad RS, Xu M, Ismiil N, Nofech-Mozes S, Dubé V, Ghorab Z, Khalifa MA. Immunophenotyping of intestinal type of cervical adenocarcinoma. Lab Invest 2009, **89**(Suppl 1): 235A.

584 Savargaonkar PR, Hale RJ, Pope R, Fox H, Buckley CH. Enteric differentiation in cervical adenocarcinomas and its prognostic significance. Histopathology 1993, **23**: 275–277.

585 Scully RE, Robboy SJ, Welch WR. Pathology and pathogenesis of diethylstilbestrol-related disorders of the female genital tract. In Herbst AL (ed.): Intrauterine exposure to diethylstilbestrol in the human. Chicago, IL, 1978, American College of Obstetricians and Gynecologists, pp. 8–22.

586 Shintaku M, Kariya M, Shime H, Ishikura H. Adenocarcinoma of the uterus cervix with choriocarcinomatous and hepatoid differentiation: report of a case. Int J Gynecol Pathol 2000, **19**: 174–178.

587 Shintaku M, Ueda H. Serous papillary adenocarcinoma of the uterine cervix. Histopathology 1993, **22**: 506–507.

588 Silver SA, Devouassoux-Shisheboran M, Mezzetti TP, Tavassoli FA. Mesonephric adenocarcinomas of the uterine cervix: a study of 11 cases with immunohistochemical findings. Am J Surg Pathol 2001, **25**: 379–387.

589 Steeper TA, Wick MR. Minimal deviation adenocarcinoma of the uterine cervix ('adenoma malignum'). An immunohistochemical comparison with microglandular endocervical hyperplasia and conventional endocervical adenocarcinoma. Cancer 1986, **58**: 1131–1138.

590 Suárez-Peñaranda JM, Abdulkader I, Barón-Duarte FJ, González Patiño E, Novo-Domínguez A, Varela-Durán J. Signet-ring cell carcinoma presenting in the uterine cervix: report of a primary and 2 metastatic cases. Int J Gynecol Pathol 2007, **26**: 254–258.

591 Tambouret R, Bell DA, Young RH. Microcystic endocervical adenocarcinomas: a report of eight cases. Am J Surg Pathol 2000, **24**: 369–374.

592 Tambouret R, Clement PB, Young RH. Endometrial endometrioid adenocarcinoma with a deceptive pattern of spread to the uterine cervix. A manifestation of stage IIB endometrial carcinoma liable to be misinterpreted as an independent carcinoma or a benign lesion. Am J Surg Pathol 2003, **27**: 1080–1088.

593 Thelmo WL, Nicastri AD, Fruchter R, Spring H, Di Maio T, Boyce J. Mucoepidermoid carcinoma of uterine cervix stage IB. Long-term follow-up, histochemical and immunohistochemical study. Int J Gynecol Pathol 1990, **9**: 316–324.

594 Toki T, Shiozawa T, Hosaka N, Ishii K, Nikaido T, Fujii S. Minimal deviation adenocarcinoma of the uterine cervix has abnormal expression of sex steroid receptors, CA125, and gastric mucin. Int J Gynecol Pathol 1997, **16**: 111–116.

595 Toki T, Zhai YL, Park JS, Fujii S. Infrequent occurrence of high-risk human papillomavirus and of p53 mutation in minimal deviation adenocarcinoma of the cervix. Int J Gynecol Pathol 2002, **18**: 215–219.

596 Ulbright TM, Gersell DJ. Glassy cell carcinoma of the uterine cervix. A light and electron microscopic study of five cases. Cancer 1983, **51**: 2255–2263.

597 Young RH, Scully RE. Villoglandular papillary adenocarcinoma of the uterine cervix. A clinicopathologic analysis of 13 cases. Cancer 1989, **63**: 1773–1779.

598 Young RH, Scully RE. Minimal-deviation endometrioid adenocarcinoma of the uterine cervix. A report of five cases of distinctive neoplasm that may be misinterpreted as benign. Am J Surg Pathol 1993, **17**: 660–665.

599 Young RH, Welch WR, Dickersin GR, Scully RE. Ovarian sex-cord tumor with annular tubules. Cancer 1982, **50**: 1384–1402.

600 Zhou C, Gilks CB, Hayes M, Clement PB. Papillary serous carcinoma of the uterine cervix: a clinicopathologic study of 17 cases. Am J Surg Pathol 1998, **22**: 113–120.

NEUROENDOCRINE CARCINOMA

601 Abeler VM, Holm R, Nesland JM, Kjorstad KE. Small cell carcinoma of the cervix. A clinicopathologic study of 26 patients. Cancer 1994, **73**: 672–677.

602 Albores-Saavedra J, Gersell D, Gilks B, Henson DE, Lindberg G, Santiago H, Scully RE, Silva E, Sobin LH, Tavassoli FJ, Travis WD, Woodruff JM. Terminology of endocrine tumors of the uterine cervix: results of workshop sponsored by the College of American Pathologists and the National Cancer Institute. Arch Pathol Lab Med 1997, **121**: 34–39.

603 Albores-Saavedra J, Martinez-Benitez B, Luevano E. Small cell carcinomas and large cell neuroendocrine carcinomas of the endometrium and cervix: polypoid tumors and those arising in polyps may have a favorable prognosis. Int J Gynecol Pathol 2008, **27**: 333–339.

604 Albores-Saavedra J, Latif S, Carrick KS, Alvarado-Cabrero I, Fowler MR. CD56 reactivity in small cell carcinoma of the uterine cervix. Int J Gynecol Pathol 2005, **24**: 113–117.

605 Ambros RA, Park JS, Shah KV, Kurman RJ. Evaluation of histologic, morphometric, and immunohistochemical criteria in the differential diagnosis of small cell carcinomas of the cervix with particular reference to human papillomavirus types 16 and 18. Mod Pathol 1991, **4**: 586–593.

606 Chan JK, Loizzi V, Burger RA, Rutgers J, Monk BJ. Prognostic factors in neuroendocrine small cell cervical carcinoma: a multivariate analysis. Cancer 2003, **97**: 568–574.

607 Chan JK, Tsui WM, Tung SY, Ching RC. Endocrine cell hyperplasia of the uterine cervix. A precursor of neuroendocrine carcinoma of the cervix? Am J Clin Pathol 1989, **92**: 825–830.

608 Chavez-Bianco A, Taja-Chayeb L, Cetina L, Chanona-Vilchis G, Trejo-Becerill C, Perez-Cardenaz E, Segura-Pacheco B, Acuna-Gonzales C, Duenas-Gonzales A. Neuroendocrine marker expression in cervical carcinomas of non-small cell type. Int J Gynecol Pathol 2002, **21**: 368–374.

609 Conner MG, Richter H, Moran CA, Hameed A, Albores-Saavedra J. Small cell carcinoma of the cervix: a clinicopathologic and immunohistochemical study of 23 cases. Ann Diagn Pathol 2002, **6**: 345–348.

610 Gersell DJ, Mazoujian G, Mutch DG, Rudloff MA. Small-cell undifferentiated carcinoma of the cervix. A clinicopathologic, ultrastructural, and immunocytochemical study of 15 cases. Am J Surg Pathol 1988, **12**: 684–698.

611 Gilks CB, Young RH, Gersell DJ, Clement PB. Large cell (neuroendocrine) carcinoma of the uterine cervix: a clinicopathologic study of 12 cases. Am J Surg Pathol 1997, **21**: 905–914.

612 Hammar SP, Insalaco SJ, Lee RB, Bockus DE, Remington FL, Yu A. Amphicrine carcinoma of the uterine cervix. Am J Clin Pathol 1992, **97**: 516–522.

613 Herrington CS, Graham D, Southern SA, Bramdev A, Chetty R. Loss of retinoblastoma protein expression is frequent in small cell neuroendocrine carcinoma of the cervix and is unrelated to HPV type. Hum Pathol 1999, **30**: 906–910.

614 Horn LC, Hentschel B, Bilek K, Richter CE, Einenkel J, Leo C. Mixed small cell carcinomas of the uterine cervix: prognostic impact of focal neuroendocrine differentiation but not of Ki-67 labeling index. Ann Diagn Pathol 2006, **10**: 140–143.

615 Horn LC, Lindner K, Szepankiewicz G, Edelmann J, Hentschel B, Tannapfel A, Bilek K, Liebert UG, Richter CE, Einenkel J, Leo C. p16, p14, p53, and cyclin D1 expression and HPV analysis in small cell carcinomas of the uterine cervix. Int J Gynecol Pathol 2006, **25**: 182–186.

616 Husain AN, Gattuso P, Abraham K, Castelli MJ. Synchronous adenocarcinoma and carcinoid of the uterine cervix. Immunohistochemical study of a case and review of literature. Gynecol Oncol 1990, **33**: 125–128.

617 Ibrahim NBN, Briggs JC, Corbishley CM. Extrapulmonary oat cell carcinoma. Cancer 1984, **54**: 1645–1661.

618 Ishibashi-Ueda H, Imakita M, Yutani C, Ohmichi M, Chiba Y, Kubo T, Waki M. Small cell carcinoma of the uterine cervix with syndrome of inappropriate antidiuretic hormone secretion. Mod Pathol 1996, **9**: 397–400.

619 Ishida GM, Kato N, Hayasaka T, Saito M, Kobayashi H, Katayama Y, Sasou S, Yaegashi N, Kurachi H, Motoyama T. Small cell neuroendocrine carcinomas of the uterine cervix: a histological, immunohistochemical, and molecular genetic study. Int J Gynecol Pathol 2004, **23**: 366–372.

620 Johannessen JV, Capella C, Solcia E, Davy M, Sobrinho-Simões M. Endocrine cell carcinoma of the uterine cervix. Diagn Gynecol Obstet 1980, **2**: 127–134.

621 Jones HW III, Plymate S, Gluck FB, Miles PA, Greene JF Jr. Small cell non-keratinizing carcinoma of the cervix associated with ACTH production. Cancer 1976, **38**: 1629–1635.

622 Kawauchi S, Okuda S, Morioka H, Iwasaki F, Fukuma F, Chochi Y, Furuya T, Oga A, Sasaki K. Large cell neuroendocrine carcinoma of the uterine cervix with cytogenetic analysis by comparative genomic hybridization: a case study. Hum Pathol 2005, **36**: 1096–1100.

623 Man YG, Mannion C, Kuhls E, Moinfar F, Bratthauer GL, Albores-Saavedra J, Tavassoli FA. Allelic losses at 3p and 11p are detected in both epithelial and stromal components of cervical small-cell neuroendocrine carcinoma. Appl Immunohistochem Mol Morphol 2001, **9**: 340–345.

624 Mannion C, Park WS, Man YG, Zhuang Z, Albores-Saavedra J, Tavassoli FA. Endocrine tumors of the cervix: morphologic assessment, expression of human papillomavirus, and evaluation for loss of heterozygosity on 1p, 3p, 11q and 17p. Cancer 1998, **83**: 1391–1400.

625 McCluggage WG, Kennedy K, Busam KJ. An immunohistochemical study of cervical neuroendocrine carcinomas: neoplasms that are commonly TTF1 positive and which may express CK20 and P63. Am J Surg Pathol 2010, **34**: 525–532.

626 Miller B, Dockter M, el Torky M, Photopulos G. Small cel carcinoma of the cervix: a clinical and flow-cytometric study. Gynecol Oncol 1991, **42**: 27–33.

627 Mullins JD, Hilliard GD. Cervical carcinoid ('argyrophil cell' carcinoma) associated with an endocervical adenocarcinoma. A light and ultrastructural study. Cancer 1981, **47**: 785–790.

628 Sevin BU, Method MW, Nadji M, Lu Y, Averette HA. Efficacy of radical hysterectomy as treatment for patients with small cell carcinoma of the cervix. Cancer 1996, **77**: 1489–1493.

629 Silva EG, Kott MM, Ordonez NG. Endocrine carcinoma intermediate cell type of the uterine cervix. Cancer 1984, **54**: 1705–1713.

630 Stahl R, Demopoulos RI, Bigelow B. Carcinoid tumor within a squamous cell carcinoma of the cervix. Gynecol Oncol 1981, **11**: 387–392.

631 Stoler MH, Mills SE, Gersell DJ, Walker AN. Small-cell neuroendocrine carcinoma of the cervix. A human papillomavirus type 18-associated cancer. Am J Surg Pathol 1991, **15**: 28–32.

632 Tateishi R, Wada A, Hayakawa K, Hongo J, Ishii S, Terakawa N. Argyrophil cell carcinomas (apudomas) of the uterine cervix. Light and electron microscopic observations of 5 cases. Virchows Arch [A] 1975, **366**: 257–274.

633 Ueda G, Shimizu C, Shimizu H, Saito J, Tanaka Y, Inoue M, Tanizawa O. An immunohistochemical study of small-cell and poorly differentiated carcinomas of the cervix using neuroendocrine markers. Gynecol Oncol 1989, **34**: 164–169.

634 Ueda G, Yamasaki M, Inoue M, Tanaka Y, Inoue Y, Abe Y, Tanizawa O. Immunohistochemical demonstration of HNK-1-defined antigen in gynecologic tumors with argyrophilia. Int J Gynecol Pathol 1986, **5**: 143–150.

635 Ulich TR, Liao S-Y, Layfield L, Romansky S, Cheng L, Lewin KJ. Endocrine and tumor differentiation markers in poorly differentiated small cell carcinoids of the cervix and vagina. Arch Pathol Lab Med 1986, **110**: 1054–1057.

636 Wang HL, Lu DW. Detection of human papillomavirus DNA and expression of p16, Rb, and p53 proteins in small cell carcinomas of the uterine cervix. Am J Surg Pathol 2004, **28**: 901–908.

CYTOLOGY

637 Baldwin P, Laskey R, Coleman N. Translational approaches to improving cervical screening. Nat Rev Cancer 2003, **3**: 217–226.

638 Ball C, Madden JE. Update on cervical cancer screening. Current diagnostic and evidence-based management protocols. Postgrad Med 2003, **113**: 59–70.

639 Bonfiglio TA. Atypical squamous cell of undetermined significance: a continuing controversy. Cancer 2002, **96**: 125–127.

640 Christopherson WM, Mendez WM, Ahuja EM, Lundin FE, Barker JE. Cervix cancer control in Louisville, Kentucky. Cancer 1970, **26**: 29–38.

641 Christopherson WM, Scott MA. Trends in mortality from uterine cancer in relation to mass screening. Acta Cytol (Baltimore) 1977, **21**: 5–9.

642 Cramer DW. The role of cervical cytology in the declining morbidity and mortality of cervical cancer. Cancer 1974, **34**: 2018–2027.

643 Davey DD, Gallion H, Jennings CD. DNA cytometry in postirradiation cervical-vaginal smears. Hum Pathol 1992, **23**: 1027–1031.

644 de Cremoux P, Coste J, Sastre-Garau X, Thioux M, Bouillac C, Labbé S, Cartier I, Ziol M, Dosda A, Le Galès C, Molinié V, Vacher-Lavenu M-C, Cochand-Priollet B, Vielh P, Magdelénat H. Efficiency of the hybrid capture 2 HPV DNA test in cervical cancer screening. Am J Clin Pathol 2003, **120**: 442–499.

645 Dickinson L, Mussey ME, Kurland LT. Evaluation of the effectiveness of cytologic screening for cervical cancer. II. Survival parameters before and after inception of screening. Mayo Clin Proc 1972, **47**: 545–549.

646 Dickinson L, Mussey ME, Soule EH, Kurland LT. Evaluation of the effectiveness of cytologic screening for cervical cancer. I. Incidence and mortality trends in relation to screening. Mayo Clin Proc 1972, **47**: 534–544.

647 Ducatman BS, Wang HH. The PAP smear: controversies in practice. London, 2002, Arnold.

648 Felix JC, Amezcua C. In vitro adjuncts to the pap smear. Obstet Gynecol Clin North Am 2002, **29**: 685–699.

649 Herbst AL. The Bethesda System for cervical/vaginal cytologic diagnoses. A note of caution [editorial]. Obstet Gynecol 1990, **76**: 449–450.

650 Heselmeyer-Haddad K, Janz V, Castle PE, Chaudhri N, White N, Wilber K, Morrison L, Auer G, Burroughs FH, Sherman ME, Ried T. Detection of genomic amplification of the human telomerase gene (TERC) in cytologic specimens as a genetic test for the diagnosis of cervical dysplasia. Am J Pathol 2003, **163**: 1405–1416.

651 Hoffman MS, Sterghos S Jr, Gordy LW, Gunasekaran S, Cavanagh D. Evaluation of the cervical canal with the endocervical brush. Obstet Gynecol 1993, **82**: 573–577.

652 Kinney W, Stoler MH, Castle PE. Special commentary: patient safety and the next generation of HPV DNA tests. Am J Clin Pathol 2010, **134**: 193–199.

653 Klinken L, Koch F, Albrechtsen R. Comparison of pipette and smear methods in population screenings for carcinoma of the uterine cervix. Dan Med Bull 1972, **19**: 138–140.

654 Koss LG. Diagnostic cytology and its histopathologic bases, ed. 3. Philadelphia, 1979, J.B. Lippincott.

655 Koss LG. The Papanicolaou test for cervical cancer detection. A triumph and a tragedy. JAMA 1989, **261**: 737–743.

656 Luff RD. The Bethesda System for reporting cervical/vaginal cytologic diagnoses. Report of the 1991 Bethesda workshop. The Bethesda System Editorial Committee. Hum Pathol 1992, **23**: 719–721.

657 Nguyen GK, Nguyen-Ho P, Husain M, Husain EM. Cervical squamous cell carcinoma and its precursor lesions: cytodiagnostic criteria and pitfalls. Anat Pathol 1998, **1**: 139–164.

658 Patten SF. Diagnostic cytology of the uterine cervix. Baltimore, 1969, Williams and Williams.

659 Pirog EC, Baergen RN, Soslow RA, Tam D, DeMattia AE, Chen YT, Issacson C. Diagnostic accuracy of cervical low-grade squamous intraepithelial lesions is improved with MIB-1 immunostaining. Am J Surg Pathol 2001, **26**: 70–75.

660 Ramzy I, Mody DR. Gynecologic cytology. Practical considerations and limitations. Clin Lab Med 1991, **11**: 271–292.

661 Robertson JH, Woodend B. Negative cytology preceding cervical cancer: causes and prevention. J Clin Pathol 1993, **46**: 700–702.

662 Schledermann D, Andersen BT, Bisgaard K, Dohse M, Ejersbo D, Hoelund B, Horal P, Lindh M, Ryd W. Are adjunctive markers useful in routine cervical cancer screening? Application of p16(INK4a) and HPV-PCR on ThinPrep samples with histological follow-up. Diagn Cytopathol 2008, **36**: 453–459.

663 Schneider V, Henry MR, Jimenez-Ayala M, Turnbull LS, Wright TC, International Consensus Conference on the fight against cervical cancer, IAC Task Force, Chicago, Illinois, USA. Cervical cancer screening, screening errors, and reporting. Acta Cytol 2001, **45**: 493–498.

664 Seybolt JF. Thoughts on 'the numbers game'. Acta Cytol (Baltimore) 1968, **12**: 271–273.

665 Seybolt JF, Johnson WD. Cervical cytodiagnostic problems. A survey. Am J Obstet Gynecol 1971, **109**: 1089–1103.

666 Sherman ME, Kelly D. High-grade squamous intraepithelial lesions and invasive carcinoma following the report of three negative Papanicolaou smears. Screening failures or rapid progression? Mod Pathol 1992, **5**: 337–342.

667 Smith JH. Bethesda 2001. Cytopathology 2002, **13**: 4–10.

668 Solomon D. The Bethesda Sytem for reporting cervical/vaginal cytologic diagnosis. An overview. Int J Gynecol Pathol 1991, **10**: 323–325.

669 Solomon D, Davey D, Kurman R, Moriarty A, O'Connor D, Prey M, Raab S, Sherman M, Wilbur D, Wright T Jr, Young N; Forum Group Members; Bethesda 2001 Workshop. The 2001 Bethesda System: terminology for reporting results of cervical cytology. JAMA 2002, **287**: 2114–2119.

670 Spitzer M. In vitro conventional cytology historical strengths and current limitations. Obstet Gynecol Clin North Am 2002, **29**: 673–683.

671 Stoler MH. Advances in cervical screening technology. Mod Pathol 2000, **13**: 275–284.

672 The Bethesda System for reporting cervical/vaginal cytologic diagnosis: revised after the second National Cancer Institute Workshop, April 29–30, 1991. Acta Cytol 1993, **37**: 115–124.

673 Wied GL, Legorreta G, Mohr D, Rauzy A. Cytology of invasive cervical carcinoma and carcinoma in situ. Ann N Y Acad Sci 1962, **97**: 759–766.

674 Wright TC Jr, Cox JT, Massad LS, Twiggs LB, Wilkinson EJ, ASCCP Sponsored Consensus Conference. 2001 Consensus Guidelines for the management of women with cervical cytological abnormalities. JAMA 2002, **287**: 2120–2129.

675 Zeng Z, Del Priore G, Cohen JM, Mittal K. MIB-1 expression in cervical Papanicolau tests correlates with dysplasia in subsequent cervical biopsies. Appl Immunohistochem Mol Morphol 2002, **10**: 15–19.

OTHER TUMORS AND TUMORLIKE CONDITIONS

676 Abeler V, Kjorstad KE, Langholm R, Marton PF. Granulocytic sarcoma (chloroma) of the uterine cervix. Report of two cases. Int J Gynecol Pathol 1983, **2**: 88–92.

677 Abell MR. Papillary adenofibroma of the uterine cervix. Am J Obstet Gynecol 1971, **110**: 991–993.

678 Abenoza P, Shek Y, Perrone T. Inflammatory pseudotumor of the cervix. Int J Gynecol Pathol 1994, **13**: 80–86.

679 Albores-Saavedra J, Gilcrease M. Glomus tumor of the uterine cervix. Int J Gynecol Pathol 1999, **18**: 69–72.

680 Aozasa K, Saeki K, Ohsawa M, Horiuchi K, Mishima K, Tsujimoto M. Malignant lymphoma of the uterus. Report of seven cases with immunohistochemical study. Cancer 1993, **72**: 1959–1964.

681 Barua R. Post-cone biopsy traumatic neuroma of the uterine cervix. Arch Pathol Lab Med 1989, **113**: 945–947.

682 Bell DA, Shimm DS, Gang DL. Wilms' tumor of the endocervix. Arch Pathol Lab Med 1985, **109**: 371–373.

683 Bernstein HB, Broman JH, Apicelli A, Kredentser DC. Primary malignant schwannoma of the uterine cervix: a case report and literature review. Gynecol Oncol 1999, **74**: 288–292.

684 Bloch T, Roth LM, Stehman FB, Hull MT, Schwenk GR Jr. Osteosarcoma of the uterine cervix associated with hyperplastic and atypical mesonephric rests. Cancer 1988, **62**: 1594–1600.

685 Brand E, Berek JS, Nieberg RK, Hacker NF. Rhabdomyosarcoma of the uterine cervix. Sarcoma botryoides. Cancer 1987, **60**: 1552–1560.

686 Cenacchi G, Pasquinelli G, Montanaro L, Cesaroli S, Vici M, Bisceglia M, Giangaspero F, Martinelli GN, Derenzini M. Primary endocervical extaosseous Ewing's sarcoma/PNET. Int J Gynecol Pathol 1998, **17**: 83–88.

687 Clark KC, Butz WR, Hapke MR. Primary malignant melanoma of the uterine cervix: case report with world literature review. Int J Gynecol Pathol 2002, **18**: 265–273.

688 Clement PB. Miscellaneous primary tumors and metastatic tumors of the uterine cervix. Semin Diagn Pathol 1990, **7**: 228–248.

689 Clement PB, Zubovits JT, Young RH, Scully RE. Malignant mullerian mixed tumors of the uterine cervix: a report of nine cases of a neoplasm with morphology often different from its counterpart in the corpus. Int J Gynecol Pathol 1998, **17**: 211–222.

690 Copeland LJ, Gershenson DM, Saul PB, Sneige N, Stringer CA, Edwards CL. Sarcoma botryoides of the female genital tract. Obstet Gynecol 1985, **66**: 262–266.

691 Copeland LJ, Sneige N, Ordonez NG, Hancock KC, Gershenson DM, Saul PB, Kavanagh JJ. Endodermal sinus tumor of the vagina and cervix. Cancer 1985, **55**: 2558–2565.

692 Daya DA, Scully RE. Sarcoma botryoides of the uterine cervix in young women: a clinicopathological study of 13 cases. Gynecol Oncol 1988, **29**: 290–304.

693 Deppisch LM. Cervical melanosis. Obstet Gynecol 1983, **62**: 525–526.

694 Euscher ED, Deavers MT, Lopez-Terrada D, Lazar AJ, Silva EG, Malpica A. Uterine tumors with neuroectodermal differentiation: a series of 17 cases and review of the literature. Am J Surg Pathol 2008, **32**: 219–228.

695 Ferry JA, Young RH. Malignant lymphoma, pseudolymphoma, and hematopoietic disorders of the female genital tract. Pathol Annu 1991, **26**(Pt 1): 227–263.

696 Ferry JA, Young RH. Malignant lymphoma of the genitourinary tract. Curr Diagn Pathol 1997, **4**: 145–169.

697 Foschini MP, Eusebi V, Tison V. Alveolar soft part sarcoma of the cervix uteri. A case report. Pathol Res Pract 1989, **184**: 354–358.

698 Fraga M, Prieto O, Garcia-Caballero T, Beiras A, Forteza J. Myxoid leiomyosarcoma of the uterine cervix. Histopathology 1994, **25**: 381–383.

699 Gallardo A, Prat J. Mullerian adenosarcoma: a clinicopathologic and immunohistochemical study of 55 cases challenging the existence of adenofibroma. Am J Surg Pathol 2009, **33**: 278–288.

700 Garcia MG, Deavers MT, Knoblock RJ, Chen W, Tsimberidou AM, Manning JT Jr, Medeiros LJ. Myeloid sarcoma involving the gynecologic tract: a report of 11 cases and review of the literature. Am J Clin Pathol 2006, **125**: 783–790.

701 Gersell DJ, Fulling KH. Localized neurofibromatosis of the female genitourinary tract. Am J Surg Pathol 1989, **13**: 873–878.

702 Geyer JT, Ferry JA, Harris NL, Young RH, Longtine JA, Zukerberg LR. Florid reactive lymphoid hyperplasia of the lower female genital tract (lymphoma-like lesions): a benign condition that frequently harbors clonal immunoglobulin heavy chain gene rearrangements. Am J Surg Pathol 2010, **34**: 161–168.

703 Gibbons D, Lindberg GM, Ashfaq R, Saboorian MH. Localized amyloidosis of the uterine cervix. Int J Gynecol Pathol 1998, **17**: 368–371.

704 Grayson W, Fourie J, Tiltman AJ. Xanthomatous leiomyosarcoma of the uterine cervix. Int J Gynecol Pathol 1998, **17**: 89–90.

705 Gwavava NJ, Traub AL. A neurilemmoma of the cervix. Br J Obstet Gynaecol 1980, **87**: 444–446.

706 Hanai J, Tsuji M. Uterine teratoma with lymphoid hyperplasia. Acta Pathol Jpn 1981, **31**: 153–159.

707 Harris NL, Scully RE. Malignant lymphoma and granulocytic sarcoma of the uterus and vagina. A clinicopathologic analysis of 27 cases. Cancer 1984, **53**: 2530–2545.

708 Hirschfield L, Kahn LB, Chen S, Winkler B, Rosenberg S. Müllerian adenosarcoma with ovarian sex cord-like differentiation. Cancer 1986, **57**: 1197–1200.

709 Hytiroglou P, Domingo J. Development of melanosis of uterine cervix after cryotherapy for epithelial dysplasia. A case report and brief review of the literature on pigmented lesions of the cervix. Am J Clin Pathol 1990, **93**: 802–805.

710 Imachi M, Tsukamoto N, Amagase H, Shigematsu T, Amada S, Nakano H. Metastatic adenocarcinoma to the uterine cervix from gastric cancer. A clinicopathologic analysis of 16 cases. Cancer 1993, **71**: 3472–3477.

711 Ishikura H, Kojo T, Ichimura H, Yoshiki T. Desmoplastic malignant melanoma of a uterine cervix: a rare primary malignancy in the uterus mimicking a sarcoma. Histopathology 1998, **33**: 93–94.

712 Jones MW, Lefkowitz M. Adenosarcoma of the uterine cervix. A clinicopathological study of 12 cases. Int J Gynecol Pathol 1995, **14**: 223–229.

713 Keel SB, Clement PB, Prat J, Young RH. Malignant schwannoma of the uterine cervix: a study of three cases. Int J Gynecol Pathol 1998, **17**: 223–230.

714 Khoor A, Fleming MV, Purcell CA, Seidman JD, Ashton AH, Weaver DL. Mature teratoma of the uterine cervix with pulmonary differentiation. Arch Pathol Lab Med 1995, **119**: 848–850.

715 Kondi-Pafiti A, Kairi-Vassilatou E, Spanidou-Carvouni H, Kontongianni K, Dimopoulou K, Goula K. Vascular tumors of the female genital tract: a clinicopathological study of nine cases. Eur J Gynaecol Oncol 2003, **24**: 48–50.

716 Kosari F, Daneshbod Y, Parwaresch R, Krams M, Wacker HH. Lymphomas of the female genital tract: a study of 186 cases and review of the literature. Am J Surg Pathol 2005, **29**: 1512–1520.

717 Kristiansen SB, Anderson R, Cohen DM. Primary malignant melanoma of the cervix and review of the literature. Gynecol Oncol 1992, **47**: 398–403.

718 Lagoo AS, Robboy SJ. Lymphoma of the female genital tract: current status. Int J Gynecol Pathol 2006, **25**: 1–21.

719 Lee JD, Chang TC, Lai YM, Hsueh S, Soong YK. Choriocarcinoma of the cervix. Acta Obstet Gynecol Scand 1992, **71**: 479–481.

720 Lemoine NR, Hall PA. Epithelial tumors metastatic to the uterine cervix. A study of 33 cases and review of the literature. Cancer 1986, **57**: 2002–2005.

721 Loughlin KR, Retik AB, Weinstein HJ, Colodny AH, Shamberger RC, Delorey M, Tarbell N, Cassady JR, Hendren WH. Genitourinary rhabdomyosarcoma in children. Cancer 1989, **63**: 1600–1606.

722 Luevano-Flores E, Sotelo J, Tena-Suck M. Glial polyp (glioma) of the uterine cervix. Report of a case with demonstration of glial fibrillary acidic protein. Gynecol Oncol 1985, **21**: 385–390.

723 Ma J, Shi QL, Zhou XJ, Meng K, Chen JY, Huang WB. Lymphoma-like lesion of the uterine cervix: report of 12 cases of a rare entity. Int J Gynecol Pathol 2007, **26**: 194–198.

724 Malpica A, Moran CA. Primitive neuroectodermal tumor of the cervix: a clinicopathologic and immunohistochemical study of two cases. Ann Diagn Pathol 2002, **6**: 281–287.

725 Mathoulin-Portier MP, Pernault-Llorca F, Labit-Bouvier C, Charafe E, Martin F, Hassoun J, Jacquemier J. Malignant mullerian mixed tumor of the uterine cervix and adenoid cystic component. Int J Gynecol Pathol 1998, **17**: 91–92.

726 McCluggage WG, Hurrell DP, Kennedy K. Metastatic carcinomas in the cervix mimicking primary cervical adenocarcinoma and adenocarcinoma in situ: report of a series of cases. Am J Surg Pathol 2010, **34**: 735–741.

727 Moore WF, Bentley RC, Kim KR, Olatidoye B, Gray SR, Robboy SJ. Goblet-cell mucinous epithelium lining the endometrium and endocervix: evidence of a metastasis from an appendiceal primary tumor through the use of cytokeratin-7 and -20 immunostains. Int J Gynecol Pathol 1998, **17**: 363–367.

728 Murray J, Fox H. Rosai–Dorfman disease of the uterine cervix. Int J Gynecol Pathol 1991, **10**: 209–213.

729 Nielsen GP, Oliva E, Young RH, Rosenberg AE, Dickersin GR, Scully RE. Alveolar soft-part sarcoma of the female genital tract. A report of nine cases and review of the literature. Int J Gynecol Pathol 1995, **14**: 283–292.

730 Patel DS, Bhagavan BS. Blue nevus of the uterine cervix. Hum Pathol 1985, **16**: 79–86.

731 Perren T, Farrant M, McCarthy K, Harper P, Wiltshaw E. Lymphomas of the cervix and upper vagina: a report of five cases and a review of the literature. Gynecol Oncol 1992, **44**: 87–95.

732 Petersson F, Michal M. Minute alveolar soft part sarcoma of the endocervix: the smallest ever published case. Appl Immunohistochem Mol Morphol 2009, **17**: 553–556.

733 Pusceddu S, Bajetta E, Buzzoni R, Carcangiu ML, Platania M, Del Vecchio M, Ditto A. Primary uterine cervix melanoma resembling malignant peripheral nerve sheath tumor: a case report. Int J Gynecol Pathol 2008, **27**: 596–600.

734 Rahimi K, Shaw PA, Chetty R. Solitary fibrous tumor of the uterine cervix. Int J Gynecol Pathol 2010, **29**: 189–192.

735 Rivasi F, Botticelli L, Bettelli SR, Masellis G. Alveolar rhabdomyosarcoma of the uterine cervix. A case report confirmed by FKHR break-apart rearrangement using a fluorescence in situ hybridization probe on paraffin-embedded tissues. Int J Gynecol Pathol 2008, **27**: 442–446.

736 Roma AA, Yang B, Senior ME, Goldblum JR. TFE3 immunoreactivity in alveolar soft part sarcoma of the uterine cervix: case report. Int J Gynecol Pathol 2005, **24**: 131–135.

737 Sahin AA, Silva EG, Ordonez NG. Alveolar soft part sarcoma of the uterine cervix. Mod Pathol 1989, **2**: 676–680.

738 Seo IS, Hull MT, Pak HY. Granulocytic sarcoma of the cervix as a primary manifestation. Case without overt leukemic features for 26 months. Cancer 1977, **40**: 3030–3037.

739 Siddon A, Hui P. Glial heterotopia of the uterine cervix: DNA genotyping confirmation of its fetal origin. Int J Gynecol Pathol 2010, **29**: 394–397.

740 Sobel N, Carcangiu ML. Primary pigmented neuroectodermal tumor of the uterine cervix. Int J Surg Pathol 1994, **2**: 31–36.

741 Terzakis JA, Opher E, Melamed J, Santagada E, Sloan D. Pigmented melanocytic schwannoma of the uterine cervix. Ultrastruct Pathol 1990, **14**: 357–366.

742 Tiltman AJ. Leiomyomas of the uterine cervix: a study of frequency. Int J Gynecol Pathol 1998, **17**: 231–234.

743 Tiltman AJ, Duffield MS. Postpartum microneuromas of the uterine cervix. Histopathology 1996, **28**: 153–156.

744 Uehara T, Izumo T, Kishi K, Takayama S, Kasuga T. Stromal melanocytic foci ('blue nevus') in step sections of the uterine cervix. Acta Pathol Jpn 1991, **41**: 751–756.

745 Volpe R, Canzonieri V, Gloghini A, Carbone A. 'Lipoleiomyoma with metaplastic cartilage' (benign mesenchymoma) of the uterine cervix. Pathol Res Pract 1992, **188**: 799–801.

746 Yamazawa K, Ishikura H, Matsui H, Seki K, Sekiya S. Sebaceous carcinoma of the uterine cervix: a case report. Int J Gynecol Pathol 2002, **22**: 92–94.

747 Yilmaz AG, Chandler P, Hahm GK, O'Toole RV, Niemann TH. Melanosis of the uterine cervix: a report of two cases and discussion of pigmented cervical lesions. Int J Gynecol Pathol 1999, **18**: 73–76.

748 Young RH, Harris NL, Scully RE. Lymphoma-like lesions of the lower female genital tract. A report of 16 cases. Int J Gynecol Pathol 1985, **4**: 289–299.

749 Zaloudek CJ, Norris HJ. Adenofibroma and adenosarcoma of the uterus. Cancer 1981, **48**: 354–366.

750 Zevallos-Giampietri EA, Barrionuevo C. Common blue nevus of the uterine cervix: case report and review. Appl Immunohistochem Mol Morphol 2004, **12**: 79–82.

Uterus – corpus

CHAPTER CONTENTS

Normal anatomy

The adult nulliparous uterus is a hollow, pear-shaped organ that weighs 40–80 g and measures 7–8 cm along its longest axis. It is divided into the *cervix* (discussed in the preceding section of this chapter) and the *corpus*. The portion of the corpus cephalad to a line connecting the insertion of the fallopian tubes is the *fundus*. The two lateral regions of the fundus associated with the intramural portion of the fallopian tubes are referred to as the *cornua*. The portion of the corpus that connects with the cervix is called the *isthmus* or *lower uterine segment*.

The uterine cavity has a triangular shape and a length of approximately 6 cm. It is lined by the endometrial mucosa, which constitutes the inner layer (endometrium) of the organ. It is surrounded by a thick muscular layer (myometrium) and a serosal covering, the latter extending to the point of peritoneal reflection. Two useful clues to distinguish the anterior from the posterior side of a hysterectomy specimen at time of gross examination are: (1) the fact that the point of peritoneal reflection is *lower* on the posterior side; and (2) the fact that the uterine insertion of the fallopian tube is *posterior* to the insertion of the round ligament.[29]

The uterine lymph vessels drain to a rich network of lymph nodes, the main groups being parametrial and paracervical; internal (hypogastric), external, and common iliac; periaortic; and inguinal.

The endometrial mucosa is made up of glands and stroma. It is divided into a deeply seated *basal* layer and a superficial *functional* layer. The basal layer is the equivalent of the reserve cell layer of other epithelia and is responsible for the regeneration of the endometrium following menstruation. It is made up of weakly proliferative glands and spindled stroma. The functional layer is subdivided into two strata, the *compactum* (toward the surface) and the *spongiosum* (close to the basalis). The stroma is mainly composed of endometrial stromal cells (whose appearance changes considerably during the menstrual cycle, see later section) and vessels (of which the spiral arterioles are the most distinctive). Other components include the stromal granulocyte (thought to be a subpopulation of either T lymphocytes or macrophages) and inconstant stromal foamy cells (lipid-containing cells of disputed histogenesis). The immunohistochemical profile of endometrial stromal cells is 'CD10 dominant' in relation to CD34, whereas the reverse is true for the endocervical stroma.[6] This difference, which is unrelated to the cell cycle, may be useful in localizing the anatomic site of involvement in uterine tumors. The phenotypic profile of the endometrial glands will be discussed in connection with the various pathologic conditions that affect that tissue;[15,17] suffice to warn the reader that two markers associated with breast and lung/thyroid – i.e., mammaglobin and thyroid transcription factor-1 (TTF-1), respectively – can be expressed by endometrial cells.[18,23]

During child-bearing age, the normal endometrium undergoes a series of sequential changes in the course of the ovulatory cycle that prepare it to receive the ovum[11] (Fig. 19.110). If the ovum is not fertilized, the proliferative endometrium is cast off by menstruation, and the cycle repeats itself. A normal endometrial cycle is associated with changes in both endometrial glands and stroma that allow the pathologist to diagnose microscopically the phase of the menstrual cycle.[19] In a series of classic articles, Noyes et al.[20–22] set forth specific criteria by which an accurate dating of the endometrium was made possible (Fig. 19.111 and Box 19.1).

In general, the changes are quite uniform throughout the functional endometrium.[20] When this is not the case, the dating should

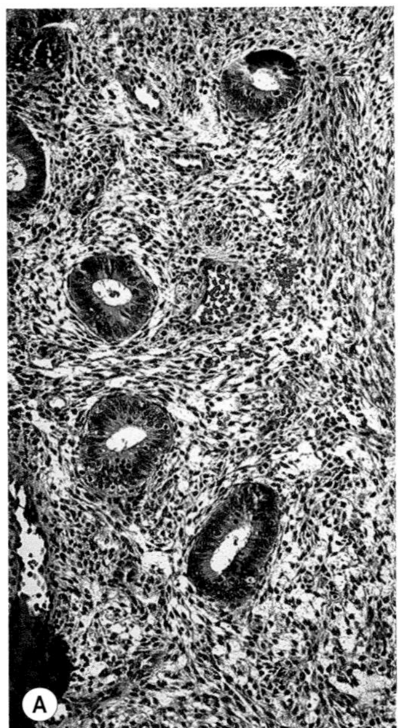
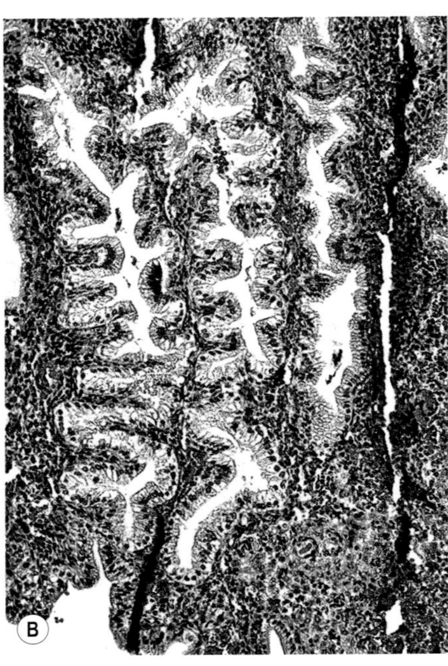

Fig. 19.110 Normal endometrium: **A**, proliferative; **B**, secretory.

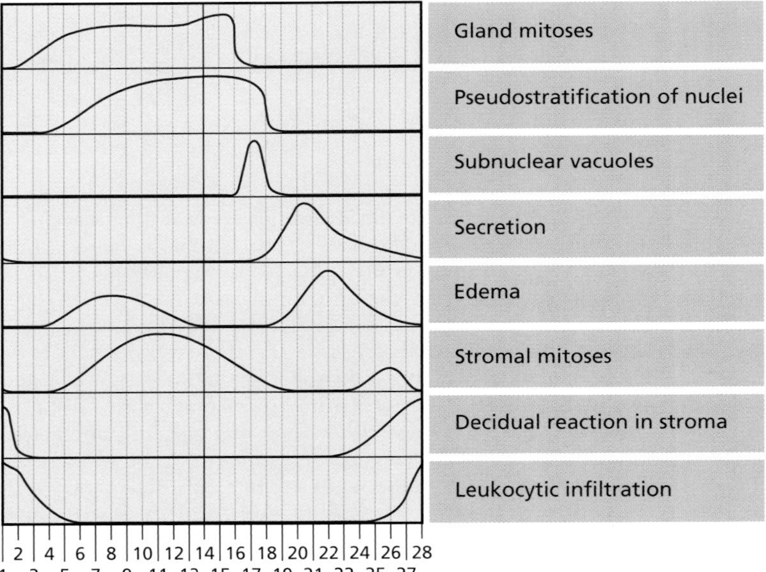

Fig. 19.111 Cyclic changes in endometrium. Approximate relationship of useful microscopic changes.
(After Latour, from the classic article by Noyes RW, Hertig AT, Rock J. Dating the endometrial biopsy. Fertil Steril 1950, ***1:*** *3–25)*

be based on the most advanced area rather than on the average morphologic picture.[21] The surface epithelium is less responsive to the hormonal influences than the glandular epithelium. Radioautographic studies have shown that cell proliferation is highest on the eighth to tenth day in the upper third of the functional layer and that it decreases to nearly zero levels by the nineteenth day.[10] For subnuclear vacuolation to be regarded as evidence of ovulation, it should be present in at least 50% of the functional glands present in the section. A markedly compact stroma may simulate predecidua. One of the earlier signs of the menstrual phase (and also of pathologic crumbling of the stroma) is the presence of nuclear dust at the base of the glandular epithelium.[9] Neutrophils, which are seen in large numbers in areas of tissue degradation (beginning on day 26) are very rare during the other days of the cycle; they should be distinguished from the already mentioned stromal granulocytes, which do not stain for chloroacetate esterase.[24]

The nuclear crowding, squamoid appearance, and focal cytoplasmic acidophilia seen in late menstrual and postcurettage specimens should not be confused with a malignant or other pathologic process. The possibility of overdiagnosis is even greater in the rare instances in which the menstrual endometrium is seen within the lumen of blood vessels.[5] It should be noted that endometrial tissue can also be found in myometrial vessels independently from menstruation.[25]

Box 19.1 Microscopic features for dating endometrium

Proliferative phase

Early (fourth–seventh day) – thin regenerating surface epithelium; straight, short, narrow glands; compact stroma, with some mitotic activity and large nuclei
Mid (eighth–tenth day) – columnar surface epithelium; longer, curving glands; variable amount of stromal edema; numerous mitoses in naked nuclei of stroma
Late (eleventh–fourteenth day) – undulant surface; tortuous glands showing active growth and pseudostratification; moderately dense, actively growing stroma

Secretory phase

36–48 hours after ovulation – no microscopic changes apparent
Sixteenth day – subnuclear vacuolation of epithelium appears
Seventeenth day – orderly row of nuclei with homogenous cytoplasm above them and large vacuoles below
Eighteenth day – vacuoles decrease in size; nuclei approach base of cell
Nineteenth day – few vacuoles; appearance of intraluminal secretion
Twentieth day – peak of acidophilic intraluminal secretion
Twenty-first day – tissue edema appears rather abruptly
Twenty-second day – edema reaches its peak
Twenty-third day – spiral arterioles become prominent
Twenty-fourth day – collections of predecidual cells appear around arterioles
Twenty-fifth day – predecidua appears under surface epithelium
Twenty-sixth day – predecidua appears as solid sheet of well-developed cells; polynuclear cell infiltration appears
Twenty-seventh day – polynuclear infiltration becomes prominent; areas of focal necrosis and hemorrhage begin to appear
Twenty-eighth day – necrosis and hemorrhage prominent

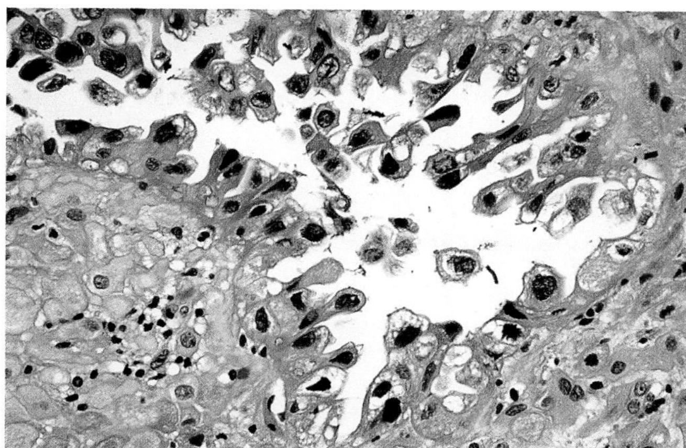

Fig. 19.112 Arias-Stella reaction in endometrial mucosa. This is not to be confused with a malignant condition.

The basal layer of the endometrium is not subject to the influence of progesterone. Therefore, if biopsies are taken in the premenstrual phase for evidence of secretory activity (ovulation) and contain only the basal layer, a proper evaluation cannot be made. Similarly, the mucosa of the lower uterine segment responds only sluggishly to the hormonal stimulations and should be disregarded for dating purposes.[10] This mucosa gradually merges with that of the endocervix; the hybrid endometrial–endocervical appearance of both glands and stroma allows its recognition in dilation and curettage (D&C) specimens.

Biopsies to determine anovulatory cycles are most informative when performed approximately 2 days before the expected onset of menstruation.

The reappearance of glandular secretion and stromal edema once predecidual reaction is established – leading to the simultaneous presence of these three features in an endometrial specimen – is evidence that a fertilized ovum has implanted; this pattern is referred to as *gestational hyperplasia*.[12] An exaggerated expression of this phenomenon is the ***Arias-Stella reaction***, as originally described by the Peruvian pathologist Javier Arias-Stella, as recounted by himself in an inspiring publication.[3] In this condition, secretory or proliferative changes in the endometrial glands are accompanied by prominent nuclear changes, manifested by hyperchromasia and marked enlargement (Fig. 19.112). Normal and abnormal mitoses may also be present.[2] These changes are almost always focal and may also occur in the cervix, endocervical polyps, adenomyosis, and endometriosis.[1] They are more often seen in postabortion curettings (present in 20–70% of cases and persisting for weeks), but they are also seen in normal orthotopic or ectopic pregnancies, hydatidiform mole, choriocarcinoma, and (very rarely) following the administration of exogenous hormones.[4,8,13] In hydatidiform mole and choriocarcinoma, the nuclei of the endometrial cells may attain gigantic sizes. The most important differential diagnosis is with serous and clear cell types of endometrial adenocarcinoma. Immunostains for Ki-67 and p53 are helpful in this regard, both of them being usually negative in the Arias-Stella reaction.[27]

Another interesting pregnancy-related endometrial alteration (often associated with the Arias-Stella reaction) is the focal appearance of optically clear nuclei in the glandular cells, simulating viral inclusions; these are due to the replacement of normal chromatin by a fine filamentous network that is immunoreactive for biotin.[14,26,28]

Exceptionally, an 'idiopathic' decidual reaction is seen in the postmenopausal endometrium in the absence of an exogenous or endogenous source of progesterone excess.[7]

The myometrium has a rich network of vessels in its midportion; this landmark, which can be recognized grossly, has been used to subdivide the uterine wall into subvascular, vascular, and supravascular regions. A peculiar vascular architecture sometimes encountered in the myometrium is that of arteries apparently free-floating within cleft-like spaces, which have been interpreted as venous channels.[16]

Curettage and biopsy

Tissue from the endometrial cavity taken for diagnostic purposes has been traditionally obtained by *dilation* of the cervical canal and *curettage* of the endometrial cavity (D&C). If properly performed, very few endometrial lesions (perhaps only those located deep in a cornu) should escape detection. It has been regarded for a long time as the method of choice for the detection and typing of lesions presumed to be localized, such as polyps and carcinomas.[38] Information about endocervical extension of an endometrial neoplasm can be obtained by performing a *fractional curettage* (i.e., a separate sampling from the endometrial and endocervical cavities during the same procedure). The endocervical specimen should be obtained first so as to minimize contamination from the endometrium. However, even when this precaution is taken, small isolated tumor fragments may be found in endocervical specimens in cases without actual infiltration of the cervix. Therefore, it is our policy to report the presence of endocervical extension of a tumor *only* if cancer and normal endocervical glands are seen *in the same tissue fragment*. Otherwise, we simply record the presence of carcinoma in the material submitted from the endocervix and let the clinician decide whether this is significant on the basis of the findings at the time of curettage.

Endometrial biopsy is a currently preferred alternative to D&C for the evaluation of infertile or dysmenorrheic patients.[30,36] In addition, this procedure (as carried out under hysteroscopic guidance) has become the choice method for the initial approach to patients with suspected endometrial hyperplasia or carcinoma.[32] Kahler et al.,[37] in a pioneer study of 160 patients, demonstrated that, when the endometrial biopsy was performed successfully (137 patients), the tissue obtained was truly representative of the endometrium in all but six, as proved by subsequent D&C or hysterectomy. Furthermore, no endometrial carcinoma was missed when sufficient tissue was obtained. A meta-analysis study with the use of the Pipelle showed a detection rate for endometrial adenocarcinoma of 99.6% in postmenopausal women and 91% in the premenopausal group.[33] Another issue is the accuracy of the grading of endometrial carcinoma done in a biopsy when compared with that seen in the hysterectomy specimen. In one study, the concordance was 45% for grade I, 63.3% for grade II, and 75.6% for grade III, the overall concordance being 64.5%.[40]

Regeneration of the endometrium proceeds very rapidly after biopsy sampling. Complete restoration occurs in 2 or 3 days in most instances.[39] Exceptionally, intrauterine adhesions develop, resulting in amenorrhea and other menstrual abnormalities. This condition, known as *Asherman syndrome*, is seen most often after postpartum or postabortal curettages and is thought to be the result of a subclinical uterine infection.[31,35]

A curious artifact that that be seen in hysteroscopically assessed tissue is *pseudolipomatosis*, a condition analogous to its more common counterpart in the gastrointestinal tract. It results from air or gas entering into the endometrial mucosa and simulating fatty infiltration.[41]

An exceptionally rare occurrence is the failure to find tumor in a hysterectomy specimen following a diagnosis of adenocarcinoma in an endometrial biopsy. This distressing event, which has been referred to as *vanishing endometrial carcinoma* (in analogy to the same phenomenon as described in the prostate) is probably explained by the very minute size of the tumor, most or all of which has been removed by the biopsy procedure.[34]

Effects of hormone administration

Estrogen therapy

Exogenous administration of estrogen preparations exposes the cycling or postmenopausal endometrium to a potent stimulus.[49] Endometrial hyperplasia is present in 15–30% of postmenopausal women receiving estrogen therapy alone, with some of the cases having an atypical pattern.[43,48,50] Furthermore, several case-control population studies have linked the exogenous administration of estrogens to the subsequent appearance of endometrial adenocarcinoma.[42,44] The risk is said to be four to eight times greater in this population.[46,51] The addition of progestin to the medication protects the endometrium and reduces the incidence of hyperplasia and carcinoma.[47]

Fortunately, the large majority of these tumors are well differentiated and superficial and are associated with an excellent prognosis compared with those occurring in postmenopausal women unexposed to exogenous estrogens.[45]

Progestational agents

Owing to the widespread use of progestational agents for therapeutic and contraceptive purposes, a new endometrial morphology has emerged.[54,60] The pathologist should be thoroughly familiar with the variety of changes that the 'pill' and other procedures may induce in the endometrium in order not to confuse them with pathologic conditions. The effect of these agents is exerted on the glands and stroma and differs more according to the regimen used than to the actual drug employed.[59] In the *combined program*, pills of the same mixture, representing a combination of progestogen and estrogen, are taken on consecutive days. They can be administered *continuously* for therapeutic purposes or *cyclically* (for 20 or 21 days with 7-day or 8-day intervals) for contraception or therapy.[54] In the *sequential program*, no longer used, predominantly estrogenic pills were taken for 14 or 16 days followed by progestin-dominant pills for 5 or 6 days. The changes described are those to be expected in a previously normal endometrium.

In the **continuous combined program**, the glands are small, straight, and inactive, with no mitoses or secretion. The stroma is very prominent and edematous, is infiltrated by some neutrophils, and shows striking pseudodecidual changes[52] (Fig. 19.113). The latter, which may appear as fragments of frankly necrotic decidua, are distinguished from the decidua of pregnancy by the completely atrophic glandular pattern. The stromal reaction can be very florid. Foci of endometriosis respond in a similar manner. This must be kept in mind whenever lesions of any pelvic organ are being evaluated microscopically, especially by frozen section.

In the **cyclic combined program**, the glands show little or no evidence of proliferation. There is a short, poorly developed stage of secretory activity, reaching a peak around the fourteenth or fifteenth day, followed by regression of the glands.[61] Pseudodecidual changes appear in the stroma around the twentieth day of the cycle (fifteenth day of treatment). Development of spiral arterioles is inhibited. After prolonged therapy, glandular secretion and stromal pseudodecidual changes become inconspicuous or recede altogether. The stroma acquires an atrophic, fibroblast-like appearance and may form characteristic small polypoid projections covered by atrophic surface epithelium. On very rare occasions, focal glandular changes of the Arias-Stella type may appear in patients taking contraceptive pills. In most cases, discontinuation of the hormones results in a restoration of a normal endometrial pattern in a matter of weeks.

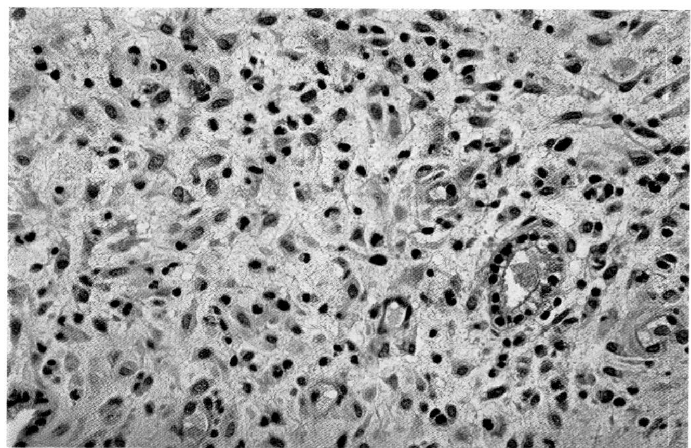

Fig. 19.113 Typical appearance of endometrium after long-term administration of contraceptive pills. The glands are sparse and atrophic, whereas the stroma is prominent and has deciduoid features.

The **sequential program** more nearly parallels the normal cycle and results in a somewhat similar endometrial morphology.[57] The glands show signs of proliferation, followed by tortuosity and the appearance of well-developed secretory changes. The stroma shows inconspicuous pseudodecidual changes. Thus the endometrial morphology on the twenty-sixth day of a cycle induced by sequential therapy (the day after treatment is completed) is roughly analogous to that of the eighteenth or nineteenth day of a normal menstrual cycle. Regressive changes and crumbling of stroma, resulting in withdrawal bleeding, occur soon thereafter.

The sequential program was discontinued in the United States and Canada in 1976 because of several reports suggesting that it promoted the development of endometrial adenocarcinoma.[53,63,64] This complication is probably not the direct result of the hormones being administered sequentially but rather a result of the difference in net estrogenic effect with the combined preparations. Most of these tumors are well differentiated and very superficial, and the prognosis generally has been good.

There are other complications resulting from the prolonged use of contraceptive pills, regardless of the program used. Early studies in England and in the United States have shown an increased incidence of thrombophlebitis and pulmonary embolism.[62,65] Morphologically, the vascular changes are widely distributed and involve arteries and veins. They include thrombi and intimal thickening with endothelial proliferation.[56] With present regimens, the incidence of these complications has decreased substantially.

The **Mirena coil (levonorgestrel)**, increasingly used for the treatment of endometrial hyperplasia, can induce a large variety of alterations in the endometrial mucosa, including pseudodecidualization, mucinous changes, ulceration, inflammatory infiltrates, stromal hyaline nodules, superficial micropapillary changes, infarcted decidua, dystrophic calcification, and others.[55]

Progesterone receptor modulators used in the management of endometriosis and uterine leiomyomas cause only minimal and inconsistent changes in the endometrial mucosa.[58]

Tamoxifen

Tamoxifen is a synthetic anti-estrogen used in the treatment and prophylaxis of breast carcinoma. Not only does it have an anti-estrogenic effect on the endometrium when competing with ovarian estrogen secretion, it also has a paradoxical estrogenic effect in the absence of ovarian estrogen secretion.[68,71,72] It is associated with an increased frequency of proliferative endometrial lesions, including hyperplasias, polyps, and malignant tumors,[67,69] but the latter are not seen often enough to justify routine endometrial biopsies in this population.[66]

According to Kennedy et al.,[70] the most characteristic features of tamoxifen-associated endometrial lesions are polarized glands along the long axis of polyps, a cambium layer, frequent and diverse metaplasias, staghorn glands, small glands, and myxoid degeneration. They felt that none of these features was diagnostic, but that their combined presence strongly suggested tamoxifen exposure. In terms of special studies, tamoxifen-associated endometrial adenocarcinomas are said to be characterized by a lower expression of estrogen receptor-alpha, higher expression of progesterone receptor, and more frequent expression of estrogen receptor-beta than spontaneous tumors.[73]

Endometritis

Acute endometritis is usually seen in association with abortion, the postpartum state, or instrumentation. Gonococcal endometritis is rarely seen by the pathologist because of its very transient nature. Before making a diagnosis of acute endometritis, the pathologist should remember that neutrophils are normally present in the endometrium on days 26, 27, and 28.[108]

Chronic endometritis, characterized by an infiltrate of lymphocytes and plasma cells (often with an additional minor component of eosinophils[74]), may follow pregnancy or abortion, be the result of an intrauterine device (IUD), or be accompanied by mucopurulent cervicitis and/or pelvic inflammatory disease (PID).[106,110] If the diagnosis is suspected clinically, cultures should be taken. The most common symptoms are vaginal bleeding and pelvic pain.[110] It should be emphasized that lymphoid follicles, with or without germinal centers, are a normal occurrence in the functional layers of the endometrial mucosa and, therefore, should not be considered as evidence of chronic endometritis. Actually, some authors believe that they are more common in normal than in abnormal endometria.[113] Therefore, identification of plasma cells constitutes the most important criterion for the diagnosis of chronic endometritis, whether by conventional criteria or – as suggested by some – by immunostaining the sections for immunoglobulins,[86] CD38,[100] VS38,[100] or syndecan-1[77] (Fig. 19.114). As a matter of fact, some authors use the term *chronic plasmacytic endometritis* for this condition.[117] However, it should be kept in mind that scattered plasma cells can be found in the absence of endometritis in women with dysfunctional uterine bleeding and focal stromal breakdown.[92]

The possibility of inflammation should be suspected – and plasma cells searched for – whenever there is an abnormal cyclic pattern, a focal mononuclear infiltrate, inflammatory cells in the glandular lumina, dense stroma, a stellate stromal pattern of proliferation, or foci of necrosis or calcification (Fig. 19.115). Glandular alterations commonly accompany the inflammatory reaction, to the point that endometrial dating becomes impossible. The presence of neutrophils in the endometrial surface is a good predictor of PID, especially if combined with plasma cells in the endometrial stroma.[99]

The myometrium is usually spared in most types of endometritis (sarcoidosis excluded, see below) unless the inflammation is very severe.

Intrauterine devices inserted for the purpose of contraception result in many biologic changes.[85,115] In an old series, only 29% of symptomatic patients and 40% of asymptomatic patients with a

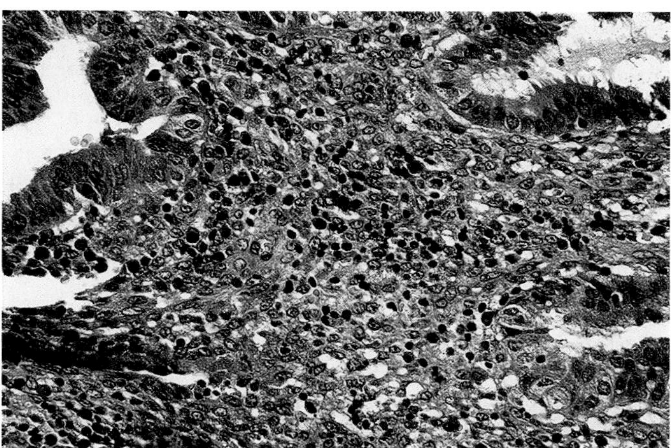

Fig. 19.114 Chronic endometritis showing an inflammatory infiltrate rich in lymphocytes and plasma cells.

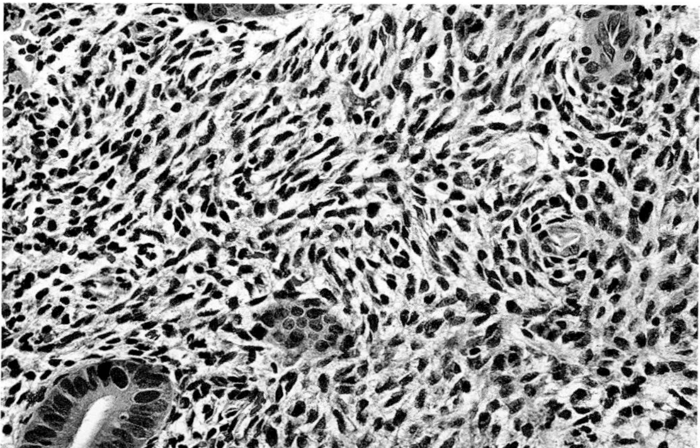

Fig. 19.115 The oval to spindle and occasionally stellate shape of endometrial stromal cells is a clue to the diagnosis of chronic endometritis.

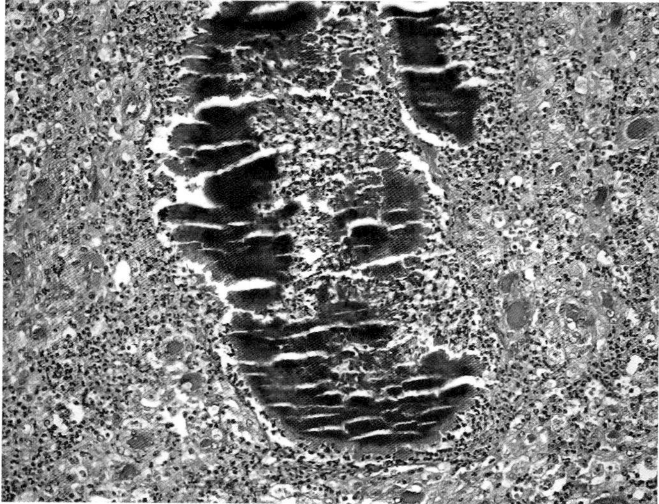

Fig. 19.116 IUD-related uterine actinomycosis. The disease had spread to the pelvic cavity.

polyethylene IUD had a normal endometrial appearance on biopsy.[104] The most common change is focal or extensive chronic endometritis, which may be accompanied by necrosis and squamous metaplasia.[109,112] On occasion, the inflammation spreads through the fallopian tubes to produce PID and sometimes tubo-ovarian abscesses.[119,121] One of the agents involved in the inflammatory process is *Actinomyces*[80,83,103] (Fig. 19.116). The organisms can be detected in microscopic sections or in cytology preparations,[94] but care should be exercised in distinguishing them from pseudo-actinomycotic radiate granules; the latter lack central branching filaments and diphtheroid forms.[81] The changes that can develop following the insertion of the Mirena coil were described in the above section.

Pyometra refers to the accumulation of pus within the endometrial cavity. It is the consequence of the combined effect of obstruction and infection. Whiteley and Hamlett[122] reviewed 35 cases in postmenopausal patients. Only five were secondary to carcinoma; the remaining 30 were the result of benign cervical stricture originating from senile atresia, surgery, or cauterization.

Hematometra is the accumulation of blood within the endometrial cavity, usually as a result of cervical occlusion. This may lead to the disappearance of the endometrial mucosa and its replacement by sheets of lipid-containing histiocytic cells, a process known as *histiocytic* or *xanthogranulomatous endometritis* when diffuse and as *nodular histiocytic hyperplasia* when localized;[82,98] these are not to be confused with the more common histiocytic reaction seen in the stroma of endometrial adenocarcinomas, whether spontaneously or following irradiation.[111]

Sometimes the histiocytes are found to contain a yellowish-brown cytoplasmic pigment, in which case the term *ceroid-containing histiocytic granuloma* has been used.[114]

Endometrial tuberculosis is rare in the United States but still common in other parts of the world. Menstrual disturbances are common. The microscopic diagnosis is based on the demonstration of acid-fast bacilli in tubercles or culture. The presence of plasma cells and leukocytes probably results from secondary infection.[93] Tubercles may be missed unless multiple levels of curettings are examined. Since the granulomas tend to concentrate in the superficial functional layers of the endometrium, it is recommended that the biopsy be taken during the late secretory phase.

Chlamydial infection is now recognized as a major sexually transmitted disease; cases associated with endometritis have been identified through the immunohistochemical demonstration of chlamydial antigens in endometrial epithelial cells[105,123] or by polymerase chain reaction (PCR).[118] These cases are associated with severe acute and/or chronic inflammation. Plasma cells tend to be very numerous; as a matter of fact, it has been proposed that the presence of these cells is linked to *Chlamydia* infection.[107]

Viral infection of the endometrium is probably more common than generally suspected. Cytomegalovirus endometritis and diffuse papillomatosis (condyloma) have both been documented;[87,120] the former can have a granulomatous quality.[90]

Coccidioidomycosis of the uterus has been reported in the United States in a few cases as a localized infection; it probably results from a clinically inapparent and completely resolved primary lung infection.[84,95]

Focal necrotizing endometritis is the name that has been proposed for a patchy necrotizing endometrial process seen in premenopausal women and devoid of plasma cells; it remains to be seen whether this is a bona fide entity.[79]

Postoperative granulomas of the endometrium have been described following endometrial ablation procedures; they may be thought of as the female counterpart of those seen in the prostate or bladder following transurethral resection (TUR).[75,116]

Malakoplakia of the endometrium has been reported, sometimes in a recurrent fashion and occasionally in association with endometrial adenocarcinoma.[102]

Sarcoidosis of the uterus occurs, but it remains a diagnosis of exclusion[96] (Fig. 19.117). In contrast to tuberculosis, the granulomatous reaction usually spreads to the myometrium.[88] Granulomatous endometritis can also follow hysteroscopic resection of the endometrium.[76]

Giant cell arteritis may involve the uterus and other female genital organs of elderly women, either as an isolated finding or as part of a generalized process.[78,89,91] The former event is more frequent than the latter,[91] but sometimes female genital tract disease is the first manifestation of systemic periarteritis nodosa.[101]

Follicular myometritis has been described as a component of inflammatory pelvic disease.[97]

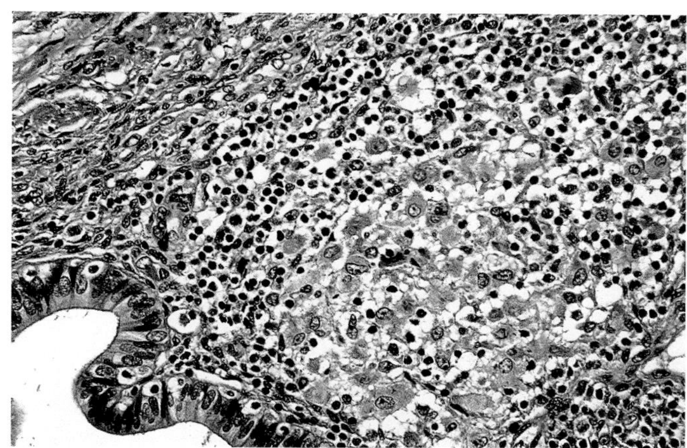

Fig. 19.117 Noncaseating granuloma in endometrial mucosa consistent with sarcoidosis.

Metaplasia

The endometrial glands and stroma are subject to a variety of metaplastic changes, many of them hormonally induced. They are often accompanied by hyperplastic changes in the endometrial glands but can occur independently from them and, therefore, need to be evaluated separately. They should not be regarded by themselves as evidence for the existence of a neoplastic process. At the same time, it should be realized that endometrial metaplasias, like endometrial hyperplasias, tend to be associated with endometrial adenocarcinoma and that they are more common in populations at high risk for the development of endometrial carcinoma (such as those in the United States) than in low-risk populations (such as those in Japan).[137] In additionak, they may show P 53 immunoreactivity, albeit in a weak and heterogeneous fashion.[143] These metaplasias include:

1 **Squamous metaplasia**. This can be encountered in normal or hyperplastic endometrium, sometimes in association with leiomyoma or uterine polyps.[129] Frank keratinization is very rare (*ichthyosis uteri*). A more common finding is the presence of nonkeratinizing squamoid cells occurring either diffusely (adenoacanthosis)[130] or in the form of berry-like aggregates (morules or morular metaplasia)[132] (Fig. 19.118). Most are seen in premenopausal women, in those receiving exogenous hormones, or in association with polycystic ovarian disease.[128,139] This change is distinguished from well-differentiated endometrial adenocarcinoma with squamous metaplasia ('adenoacanthoma') because of the benign appearance of the glandular elements.[134] The morules represent a functionally inert tissue, in the sense of being devoid of sex hormone receptors and having an extremely low proliferation rate.[138] Surprisingly, they are immunoreactive for the intestinal transcription factor CDX2.[136]

2 **Ciliated cell (tubal) metaplasia**. Scattered ciliated cells are normally present in the endometrial mucosa; when markedly increased in number, the appearance resembles that of a fallopian tube, and the term listed above is used[147] (Fig. 19.119). Ciliated cell metaplasia may be seen in an otherwise normal organ but occurs more commonly in the setting of endometrial hyperplasia. Occasionally the condition is associated with atypical nuclear features (*'atypical tubal metaplasia'*), but even under these circumstances it does not seem to constitute a factor of significant risk for the development of endometrial adenocarcinoma.[142]

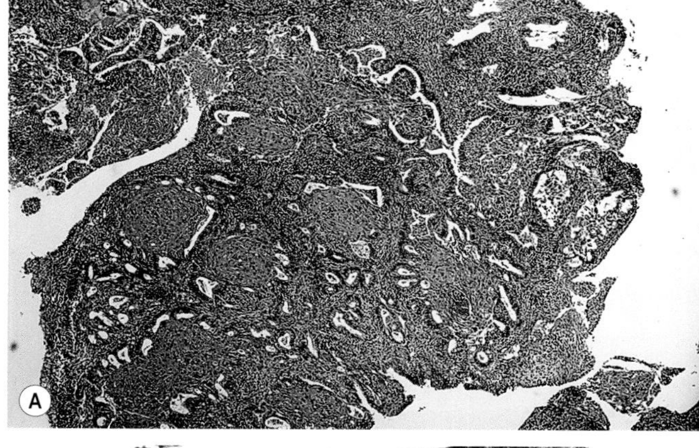

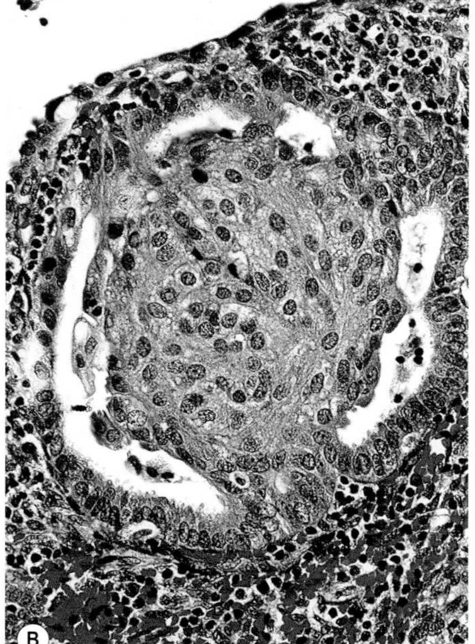

Fig. 19.118 **A** and **B**, Squamous metaplasia of endometrium with morule formation.

3 **Papillary metaplasia** (syncytial papillary hyperplasia, papillary syncytial change). This alteration is characterized by the presence of syncytial to papillary aggregates of eosinophilic cells along the surface epithelium (Fig. 19.120). It is often seen in association with prolonged estrogen stimulation.[144] It has been variously regarded as a metaplastic change, a hyperplastic change, and a retrogressive alteration associated with acute endometrial breakdown,[133,152] the latter view being the one currently favored.[148]

4 **Mucinous metaplasia.** In this condition, the endometrial mucosa reverts to a pattern morphologically, histochemically, and ultrastructurally similar to that of the endocervical mucosa[131,146] (Fig. 19.121). The main differential diagnosis is with the mucinous variant of endometrial adenocarcinoma.[141]

5 **Eosinophilic (oxyphilic; oncocytic) metaplasia**. This is another estrogen-induced lesion, characterized by strong acidophilia of the cytoplasm.[124] It is distinguished from

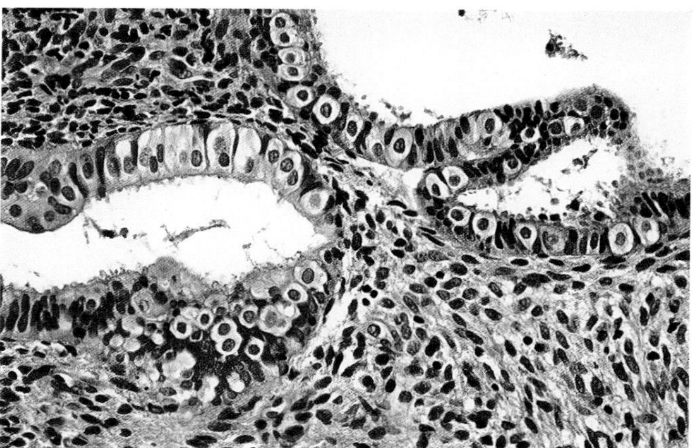

Fig. 19.119 Tubal metaplasia of endometrial mucosa. All three cell types that make up the normal mucosa of the fallopian tube can be recognized.

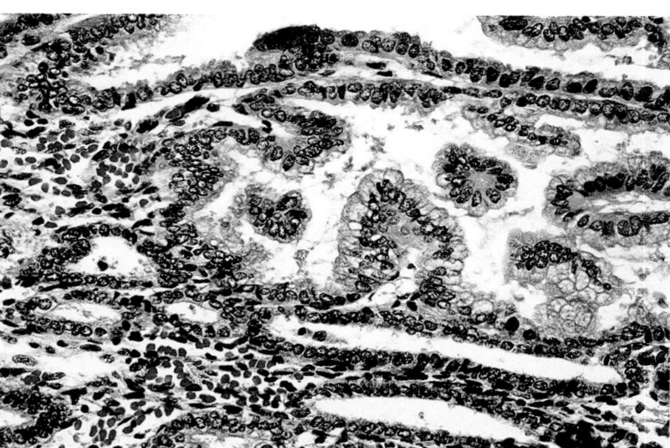

Fig. 19.121 Mucinous metaplasia of endometrium. Note the basal location of the nuclei and the mucin-containing cytoplasm of the columnar cells.

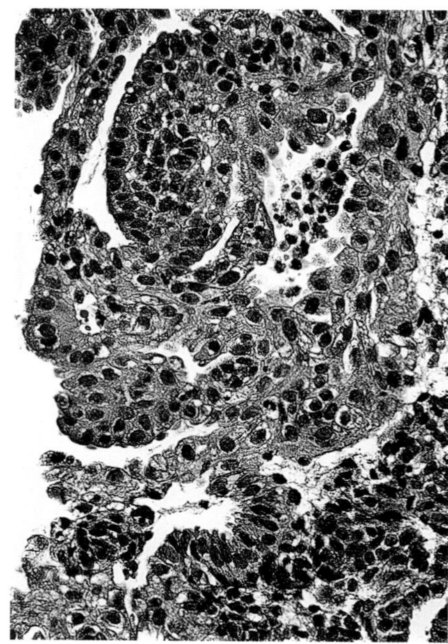

Fig. 19.120 Papillary (syncytial) metaplasia of endometrium.

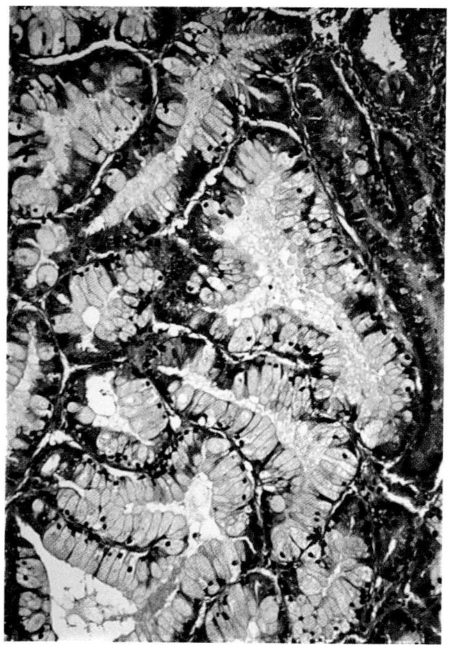

Fig. 19.122 Clear cell metaplasia of endometrium. The cytoplasm has a finely granular quality.

atypical endometrial hyperplasia and the exceptionally rare oncocytic carcinoma by the absence of atypical nuclear features.[134,135,149] It is often associated with mucinous metaplasia and – like the latter – it tends to express MUC5AC.[140] It should be pointed out, however, that expression of gastrointestinal-type mucins is not unusual in the normal or abnormal endometrium (and, of course, in the endocervix).[125]

6 **Hobnail and clear cell (mesonephric or mesonephroid) metaplasia**. In these closely related metaplastic changes, the epithelium is clear, with tall cells having apically located nuclei (Fig. 19.122). The differential diagnosis is with clear cell (mesonephroid) adenocarcinoma.[135]

7 **Intestinal metaplasia**. In this exceptionally rare form, the endometrium resembles intestinal mucosa.[151]

8 **Arias-Stella reaction.** See under Normal anatomy.

9 **Stromal metaplasia**. This includes the formation within the endometrial stroma of islands of smooth muscle,[127] cartilage,[145] and bone.[126] It should be noted that in some instances the presence of cartilage or bone is the result of retained fetal parts.[150]

Adenomyosis and endometriosis

Adenomyosis refers to the presence of islands of endometrial glands and stroma deep within the myometrium, whereas *endometriosis* is the term employed for the occurrence of endometrial tissue outside the uterus.[205] These two disorders are usually regarded as closely related, but their microscopic appearance – and probably their pathogenesis – is somewhat different. Furthermore, they often occur independently of each other. In most cases, adenomyosis is made up of the nonfunctional (basal) layer of the endometrium, is sometimes (and perhaps frequently) connected with the mucosa, and has been viewed by some as representing a *sui generis* form of endometrial diverticulosis. Endometriosis, on the other hand, is composed of the functional layers of the endometrium. As such, it goes through proliferative, secretory, and menstrual stages similar to those of its orthotopic counterpart. However, studies using conventional morphologic techniques, immunohistochemistry, and cell proliferation markers have shown that the endometriotic lesions are consistently more proliferative than the normally located endometrium, both during child-bearing years and in postmenopause.[156,179,204] Accordingly, markers associated with the secretory phase (such as CD44s) tend to be decreased in these lesions.[191] Adenomyosis is rare in postmenopausal women, except for the tamoxifen-associated cases, which tend to show stromal fibrosis, glandular dilation, and various metaplastic changes.[185]

Many pathogenetic theories have been proposed over the years for endometriosis: origin from congenital müllerian or wolffian rests, implantation of endometrium (spontaneous or induced by hysterosalpingography), lymphatic or hematogenous spread, and serosal metaplasia.[181,208] Different pathogenetic routes may be operative depending on the nature and location of the lesion, but a metaplastic change of the secondary müllerian system represented by the pelvic mesothelium is probably the most common and important mechanism.[190] Interestingly, endometriotic cysts have been found to be clonal on evaluation of X-chromosome inactivation and to show loss of heterozygosity.[203,205]

Both endometriosis and adenomyosis may result in pelvic pain, characteristically associated with the menstrual period. Between 30% and 40% of women with endometriosis are infertile, the exact mechanism being still obscure. Exceptionally, adenomyosis may lead to rupture at the time of pregnancy.

Adenomyosis results grossly in an enlarged and globular uterus because of the myometrial hypertrophy that regularly accompanies it.[166,183] This enlargement is often asymmetrical. The diagnosis may be suspected on cut section in the presence of depressed small cystic lesions in obvious but ill-defined bulging zones of muscle hypertrophy (Fig. 19.123). In elderly women, the uterus may appear atrophic despite extensive adenomyosis. Leiomyomas in uteri with adenomyosis may themselves be involved by the process.

Microscopically, the diagnosis of adenomyosis depends on the thresholds used by the individual pathologist, some of which are very liberal indeed.[197] The interphase between endometrium and myometrium is normally an irregular one, without interposition of a submucosal layer; invaginations of the endometrial basal layer into the superficial portions of the myometrium should be regarded as a normal finding. By convention, the diagnosis of adenomyosis should be reserved for those cases in which endometrial glands and stroma are seen in the myometrium at a distance of at least one low-power field from the endometrial–myometrial junction (Fig. 19.124).

Microscopically, the endometrium of adenomyosis usually has a proliferative appearance, consistent with its basal layer nature. When the normally located endometrium is in the secretory phase, this is also true for one-fourth of the foci of adenomyosis.[187] These foci can be involved by any of the diseases affecting the orthotopic endometrium, including hyperplasia and adenocarcinoma.[206] It is important to recognize this phenomenon, lest a case of in situ or superficial endometrial adenocarcinoma associated with similar changes in the foci of adenomyosis be misinterpreted as a deeply invasive malignancy.[172] Involvement of adenomyosis by endometrial adenocarcinoma does not seem to affect outcome,[173] despite

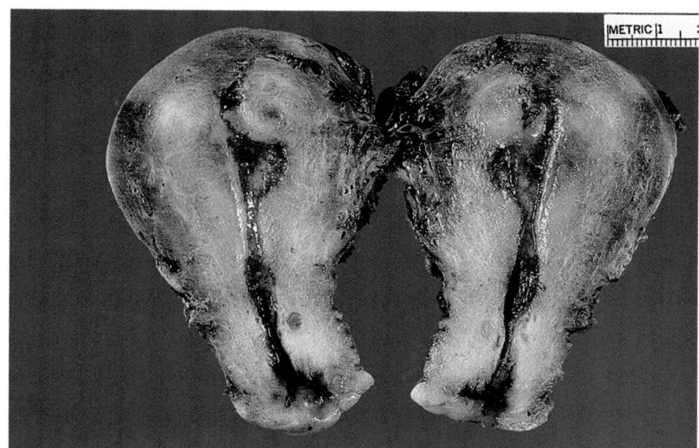

Fig. 19.123 Gross appearance of uterus involved by adenomyosis. The wall is irregularly thickened and contains small hemorrhagic foci.

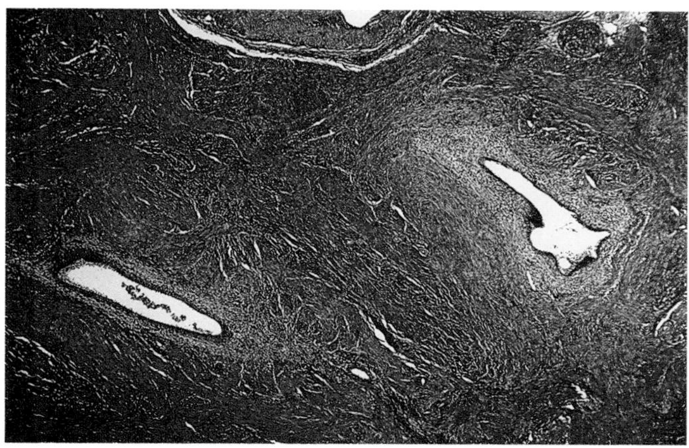

Fig. 19.124 Intramyometrial foci of endometrial glands and stroma in adenomyosis.

the claim that endometrial adenocarcinomas in uteri having foci of adenomyosis are more likely to show true myometrial invasion than the others.[175]

Vascular involvement may be present and should not be overinterpreted as a sign of malignancy.[186]

Some small islands of adenomyosis are made up predominantly of endometrial stroma (*stromal adenomyosis, incomplete adenomyosis* or *adenomyosis with sparse glands*)[157] (Fig. 19.125); however, any sizable intramyometrial focus composed entirely of endometrial stroma is likely to represent an endometrial stromal sarcoma.[171]

Endometriosis, which is thought to occur in 1–7% of women in the United States,[155,159] is a major cause of pelvic pain and subfertility.[170] It can be located in the cervix, vagina, vulva, rectovaginal septum, ovary, fallopian tubes, uterine ligaments, appendix, small and large bowel, bladder and ureters, pelvic peritoneum, hernia sacs, lymph nodes, kidney, and skin, and even within skeletal muscles, peripheral nerves, pleura, lung, and nasal cavity (Figs 19.126 and 19.127). The specific features as they pertain to the various sites are discussed in the respective chapters. Spontaneous cutaneous endometriosis is limited to the umbilicus and inguinal area.[201] In other locations, such as the lower abdominal wall, it practically always arises in surgical scars (particularly those from cesarean sections).

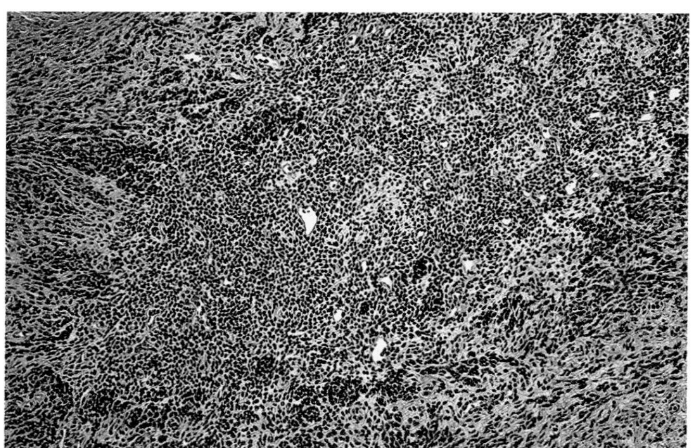

Fig. 19.125 So-called 'stromal adenomyosis'. An ill-defined island of endometrial stroma is deeply embedded within the myometrium.

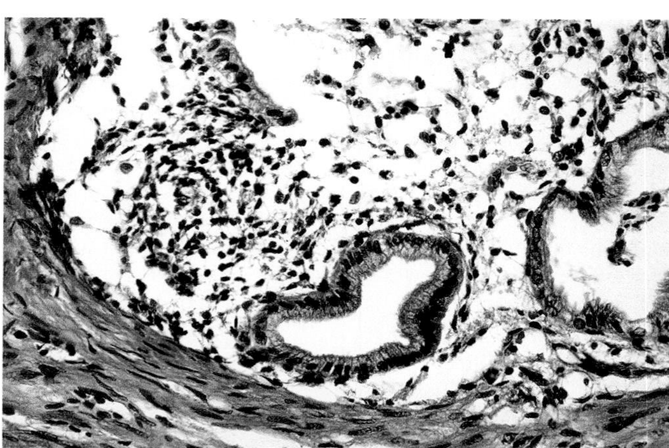

Fig. 19.128 So-called 'endocervicosis'. The stroma has an endometrium-like quality, but the glands are of endocervical type.

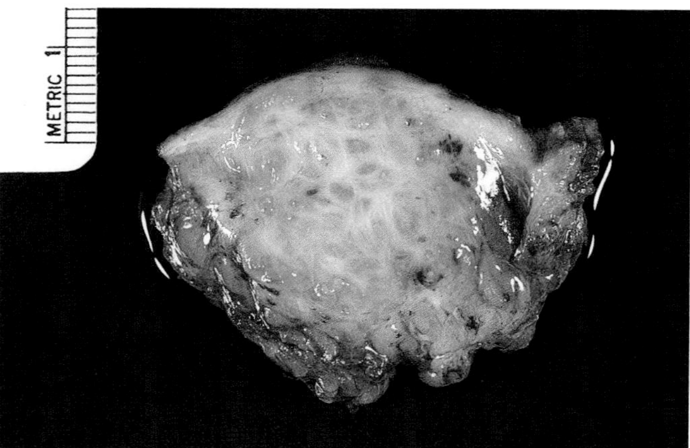

Fig. 19.126 Gross appearance of endometriosis involving the anterior abdominal wall.

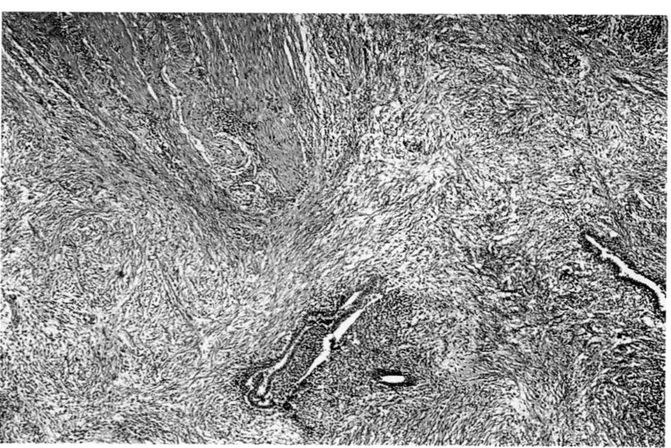

Fig. 19.127 Endometriosis involving the umbilical region.

Grossly, endometriosis appears as bluish cystic nodules, often surrounded by fibrosis. Exceptionally, it may present as multiple polypoid masses grossly simulating a neoplastic process (*polypoid endometriosis* or *endometriotic polyposis*).[188,193] These masses can be located in the colon, ovary, uterine serosa, ureter, fallopian tubes, and several other sites.[193]

Microscopically, endometrial glands and stroma are seen, often embedded in a dense fibrous mass exhibiting signs of fresh and old hemorrhage.[161] The stromal component of endometriosis can undergo smooth muscle metaplasia.[168] Along those lines, it is still being argued whether the nodular lesion resembling a miniature uterus, which can be found in several places within the peritoneal cavity (ovary, small bowel, etc.), is a peculiar variant of endometriosis with smooth muscle metaplasia of the stroma or a malformation of the müllerian ducts.[153,176,198]

Other morphologic variations in the theme of endometriosis, some of which can be of confusing interpretation, include the presence of stromal micronodules, stromal elastosis, prominent myxoid changes, perineurial invasion, and regeneration of the surrounding skeletal muscle.[162,164,165,195] Endometriotic foci can undergo prominent mucinous metaplasia, a change that can result in a mistaken diagnosis of well-differentiated mucinous adenocarcinomas. Such change has been interpreted as a metaplasia toward endocervical-type epithelium and designated as *endocervicosis*[161] (Fig. 19.128).

Although well-documented cases of endometriosis of lymph nodes exist, most cases so designated are made up of glands lined by ciliated or nonciliated cuboidal epithelium unaccompanied by stroma, limited to the capsule or cortical area of the node;[167] as such, they are more reminiscent of fallopian tube than endometrial epithelium and are better designated as *endosalpingiosis*. They have been found in approximately 14% of nodes in females but practically never in males.[177]

Endosalpingiosis is particularly frequent in the pelvic peritoneum in connection with ovarian surface tumors and is discussed on page 1580. It can also present in the form of a florid cystic mass and involve the uterine wall in a transmural fashion.[163,207]

The combination of endometriosis with endocervicosis and/or endosalpingiosis is sometimes referred to as müllerianosis.[199]

Endometriosis, like adenomyosis, is subject to any of the metaplastic, hyperplastic, and atypical changes that may supervene in the orthotopic endometrium.[169,196] More importantly, it may undergo malignant transformation.[174,178] The most common forms are endometrioid and clear cell carcinoma,[154,158,188,202] but endometrial stromal sarcoma and malignant mixed müllerian tumor have also been reported.[160]

Benign and borderline tumors of either serous or endometrioid nature can also develop, both from conventional endometriosis and from endosalpingiosis.[184,189,192,194]

The most common sites for endometriosis-related neoplasms are ovary, pelvic peritoneum, rectovaginal septum, and intestinal wall.[200,202]

The treatment of endometriosis may be hormonal or surgical depending on the circumstances.[180] It is believed that the laparoscopic ablation of minimal and mild endometriosis enhances fecundity in infertile women.[182]

Dysfunctional uterine bleeding and hyperplasia

Normal menstruation is defined as the bleeding from secretory endometrium – associated with an ovulatory cycle – not exceeding a length of 5 days. Any bleeding not fulfilling these criteria is referred to as an **abnormal uterine bleeding**. Some of these are the result of an identifiable lesion, such as endometriosis, submucous myoma, endometrial polyp, or cancer, particularly in the postmenopausal patient. In most series, approximately 5–15% of the cases of postmenopausal bleeding are due to endometrial carcinoma and a similar proportion to endometrial polyps.[238,250] The only finding on D&C in over half of postmenopausal bleeders is an atrophic endometrium;[220] degenerative and other changes in the uterine blood vessels have been suggested as a possible etiology in these cases.[237,240]

Bleeding not associated with an organic cause in women of childbearing age belongs to the large and somewhat nebulous category known as **dysfunctional uterine bleeding**. Examination of specimens obtained on D&C or endometrial biopsy is a continuous source of frustration for the pathologist. Sometimes, provided with minimal clinical information or material taken at an inappropriate moment in the menstrual cycle, one is unable to recognize any abnormality. At most, changes can be detected that only confirm what the gynecologist already knows – i.e., that the patient has an abnormal bleeding. These include the presence of fibrin clumps in the endometrial stroma (a finding not usually present in the normal menstrual endometrium),[251] the identification of fragmented pieces with dense stromal cellularity (a process known as *stromal crumbling*), and the presence of an increased number of apoptotic bodies at the base of the glands (so-called Bernirschke granules).[258]

On the other hand, if a thorough clinical study is available, examination of a correctly timed biopsy can be quite informative.[221,222] Cases of dysfunctional uterine bleeding can be divided into two large categories: those associated with ovulation and the more numerous ones in which ovulation has not occurred. A hybrid group in which ovulatory and anovulatory cycles alternate is frequently seen in premenopausal patients.

In the ovulatory group, bleeding may occur because of an *inadequate proliferative phase*. This is recognized by a disparity between the endometrial pattern observed and that expected from the time of the cycle (for instance, an endometrium chronologically in the fourteenth day, but with a morphologic appearance suggestive of the fourth to seventh day) or by the fact that the morphologic signs of proliferation (such as pseudostratification of nuclei or mitotic activity) are inconspicuous.

Bleeding resulting from an *inadequate secretory phase* (underdeveloped secretory endometrium, luteal phase inadequacy) is recognized by analogous criteria. Traditionally, it has been recommended that the curetting or biopsy should be obtained on the twelfth postovulatory day or 2 days prior to the expected menstruation, but some authors believe that an earlier biopsy taken on the seventh or eighth postovulatory day may be more informative.[219,242] According to Noyes,[249] biopsies should be taken of at least two menstrual cycles, and both the basal temperature shift and the onset of succeeding menses should be used as points of reference to time the length of the secretory phase. The 'date' obtained from the endometrial biopsy should be more than 2 days retarded before the diagnosis of underdeveloped secretory endometrium is entertained. A minor accompanying morphologic change that has been described is the presence of elongated, hyperchromatic nuclei in the glandular cell.[260] Hormone administration often corrects this defect.[227,242]

Another type of defect seen in the ovulatory group of bleeders is known as *irregular shedding of the endometrium*. The term refers to a regularly recurring menorrhagia in which the bleeding phase of the cycle requires 7 days or more for completion, without subsequent prolongation of the cycle. This is due to a lag in the shedding of the secretory endometrium, which is normally completed by the fourth day of menstruation.[239] The tissue should be obtained 5 or more days after the onset of menstrual bleeding, the diagnosis depending on the detection of retained secretory endometrium in addition to fragmented menstrual and/or early proliferative endometrium.

The term *membranous dysmenorrhea* is given to a rare condition characterized by the painful passage of an endometrial cast of the uterus during the first few days of menstruation. This cast has the microscopic appearance of decidua. The disease is thought to result from a hyperprogestational response and may be induced by the administration of high doses of progesterone.[230]

An *anovulatory cycle* can be recognized, at its earliest stage, by finding a proliferative endometrium at a time of the cycle when a secretory pattern would be expected. Most commonly, the prolonged unremitting estrogen stimulation results in **endometrial hyperplasia**. All gradations of this phenomenon occur, ranging from one distinguished only with difficulty from a normal exuberant proliferative endometrium (so-called *disordered proliferative endometrium*) to an atypical one that approaches the appearance of adenocarcinoma.[244] Many classifications of endometrial hyperplasia have been proposed over the years (Box 19.2). The one that is currently preferred and which has been sanctioned by the World Health Organization (WHO) was originally proposed by Kurman and Norris.[235] It takes into account both the architectural and cytologic features, in the sense of dividing the hyperplasias into *simple* and *complex* on the basis of the architecture, and subdividing each into *typical* and *atypical* on the basis of their cytology (Fig. 19.129). The latter criterion is regarded as the most significant. This classification scheme has been criticized on the basis of its complexity and poor reproducibility index.[255,265,266] The alternative proposal is to reduce the four categories to two. The first is endometrial hyperplasia, viewed as a benign lesion, easily treated with hormones, and with a negligible risk for the development of carcinoma; the second (called endometrial neoplasia by one group and endometrial intraepithelial neoplasia by another) is regarded as a premalignant condition with a high risk (approximately 30%) of transformation into an invasive carcinoma.[216,223,243,246,252] The WHO committee that met in 2002 acknowledged the criticisms of the Kurman–Norris scheme, but felt that no other classification system is ready to replace it at present. A particular concern of the panel was that the category of simple atypical hyperplasia was poorly reproducible and of rare occurrence; however, the decision was made to retain it.[245]

Regardless of the classification scheme used, a comment should be made on the significance of *cystic* endometrial glands, in the sense that they are not necessarily diagnostic of hyperplasia. To be sure, they have traditionally been associated with the form of hyperplasia called simplex in the WHO scheme (the old 'swiss cheese'

Box 19.2 Comparison of some proposed classifications of endometrial hyperplasia

Campbell and Barter (1961)[218]

Benign hyperplasia
Atypical hyperplasia, type I
Atypical hyperplasia, type II
Atypical hyperplasia, type III

Beutler, Dockerty, and Randall (1963)[217]

Cystic proliferation
Glandular hyperplasia
Glandular hyperplasia with atypical epithelial proliferation

Gusberg and Kaplan (1963)[231]

Mild adenomatous hyperplasia
Moderate adenomatous hyperplasia
Marked adenomatous hyperplasia

Gore and Hertig (1966)[229]

Cystic hyperplasia
Adenomatous hyperplasia
Anaplasia
Carcinoma in situ

Vellios (1972)[262]

Cystic hyperplasia
Adenomatous hyperplasia
Atypical hyperplasia

Tavassoli and Kraus (1978)[259]

Cystic hyperplasia
Adenomatous hyperplasia
Atypical hyperplasia

Hendrickson and Kempson (1980)[232]

Hyperplasia
- Without atypia
- With mild atypia
- With moderate atypia
- With severe atypia

Kurman and Norris (1986)[235]

Hyperplasia
- Simple
- Complex

Atypical hyperplasia
- Simple
- Complex

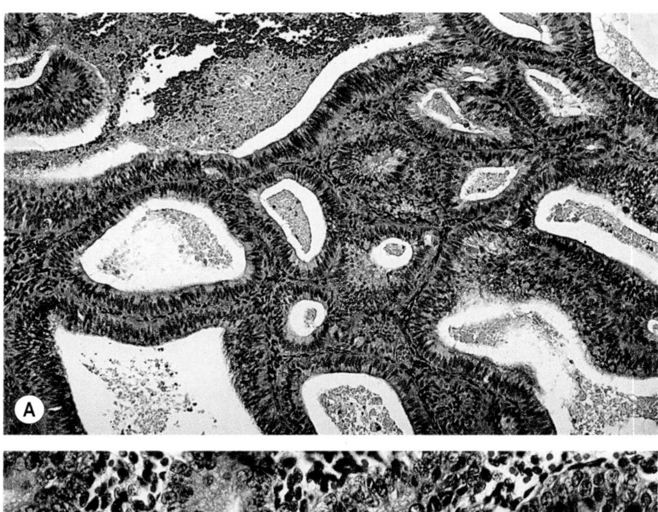

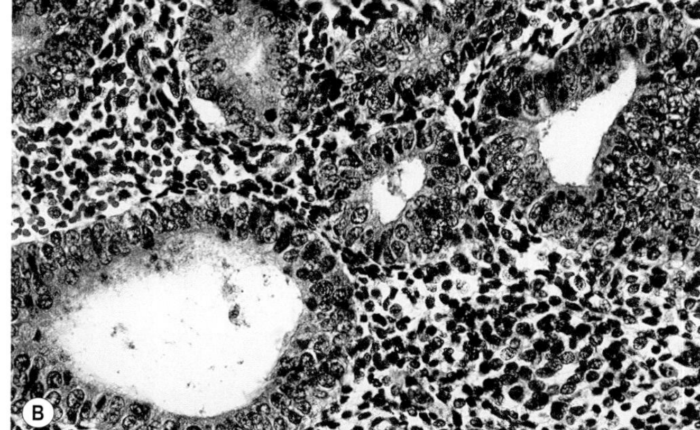

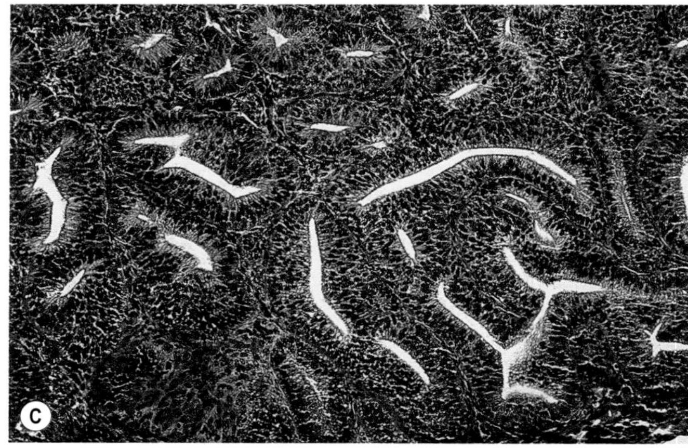

Fig. 19.129 Various types of endometrial hyperplasia: **A**, simple without atypia; **B**, simple with atypia; **C**, complex.

hyperplasia). However, some cystic endometrial glands are not hyperplastic, and some are downright atrophic, as confirmed by MIB-1 staining.[210] The latter condition, known as *cystic endometrial atrophy*, was referred to in the past as 'retrogressive hyperplasia', under the assumption that it represented the end stage of a previous cystic hyperplasia.

Endometrial hyperplasia is most commonly seen during the perimenopausal period. However, it can also be encountered in younger patients, even adolescent ones.[236] Some of these develop as the result of estrogenic stimulation in Stein–Leventhal syndrome and in estrogen-secreting ovarian neoplasms.

The distinction between a case of severe hyperplasia and a well-differentiated adenocarcinoma can be very difficult, largely because of the fact that endometrial hyperplasia and carcinoma represent different points in a disease continuum at the morphologic, ultrastructural, immunocytochemical, and molecular genetic levels.[214,225,228,232,256] Microscopic features favoring carcinoma include marked pleomorphism with loss of polarity, complex ramification of disorderly arranged glands, extensive papillary formations, confluent glandular pattern with a solid or cribriform appearance, and desmoplastic stroma (Table 19.1).[233,234,248,253,254] Fox and Buckley[226] have remarked on the importance of true intraglandular cellular bridges devoid of stromal support and the presence of neutrophils and nuclear debris within glandular lamina. Whether quantitative

Table 19.1 Differential microscopic criteria between endometrial hyperplasia and adenocarcinoma

MICROSCOPIC CRITERIA	ADENOMATOUS HYPERPLASIA	ATYPICAL HYPERPLASIA	ADENOCARCINOMA
Nuclei			
Profiles	Smooth and oval	Irregular	Irregular
Size	Uniform	Large, variable	Large, variable
Nucleoli	Small, round	Large, irregular	Large, irregular, spiculated
Mitoses	Numerous in stroma and glands	Numerous	Variable
Cytoplasm	Abundant, amphophilic	Sometimes scant; may be very abundant, with dense eosinophilia	Scant, pale, amphophilic
Glands			
Lining epithelium	Tall columnar, single layered	Stratification, loss of polarity	Loss of polarity
Profiles	Dilated, irregular, with outpouching and infoldings	Irregular, with intraglandular tufting *but no bridging*	Irregular, with cribriform pattern and intraglandular bridging
Size	Variable	Variable	Variable
Stroma	Usually abundant, cellular	Scant, with crowding	Scant

Adapted from Tavassoli F, Kraus FT. Endometrial lesions in uteri resected for atypical endometrial hyperplasia. Am J Clin Pathol 1978, **70:** 770–779.

morphology (particularly nuclear morphometry), immunohistochemistry, flow cytometry, or other techniques will assist or replace conventional morphology in this difficult problem remains to be seen.[211–213,224,241,247]

In a frequently quoted study, Gore and Hertig[229] designated an endometrial pattern characterized by endometrial glands composed of large cells with abundant eosinophilic cytoplasm as *carcinoma in situ*. Since the assumption that this change inevitably progresses to invasive adenocarcinoma has never been proved and since this alteration has, on occasion, been reversed by hormone manipulations,[257] this and similar patterns[209,257] are now regarded by most as morphologic variants of endometrial hyperplasia with or without associated metaplastic changes.[248,259] Indeed, it is not unusual to see metaplastic changes of various types (squamous, ciliated, clear cell, and others) superimposed on a picture of endometrial hyperplasia. As already stated (see p. 1483), it is important for them to be evaluated separately and for the hyperplasia to be classified independently from them. An endometrium does not necessarily become hyperplastic because it contains a metaplastic change; similarly, a hyperplastic endometrium does not become necessarily malignant because it is accompanied by focal metaplasia of squamous or some other type. Another lesion that is sometimes confused with hyperplasia (and which may actually represent a localized hyperplastic process) is adenomatous polyp, a lesion recognized by its dense fibrotic stroma and thick-walled vessels[264] (see p. 1491).

The term **(atypical) secretory hyperplasia** has been applied to a pattern of architectural abnormalities and cellular atypia within a secretory endometrium, with the atypical glands resembling those seen in the sixteenth to the seventeenth day of the normal cycle.[215,263] This change should be distinguished from the Arias-Stella reaction and from hormonally treated conventional endometrial hyperplasia. The main distinguishing features are increased glandular crowding, architectural irregularity, nuclear atypia, and increased Ki-67 index.[261] The natural history of this condition is not well known. Judging from our experience, it would seem that a conservative therapeutic approach is justified.

Relationship with carcinoma

The relationship between endometrial hyperplasia and carcinoma has been a hotly debated subject.[274,281,282,287] On the basis of the considerable collective experience that has accumulated on the subject, the following statements can be safely made:

1 *Most cases of endometrial carcinoma of the endometrioid type are preceded by a stage of hyperplasia.* This is especially true in the younger woman and/or in cases of the better differentiated tumors, in which this sequence approaches 100%. In the classic series of Hertig and Sommers,[275] published in 1949, *all* patients with endometrial adenocarcinoma who had adequate material from curettage examined 15 years or less before the development of adenocarcinoma had an abnormal endometrial pattern.

2 *Overall, relatively few patients with hyperplasia will subsequently develop cancer.*[276] Rather, the majority of the cases are responsive to progestin treatment.[273] Therefore, the mere presence of hyperplasia is not a basis for hysterectomy.

3 *The more severe the hyperplasia, the more likely it is to be followed by (or to be concurrent with) carcinoma.*[283,286] This is particularly true in regard to the *cytologic* changes, even if these assume even greater significance when coupled with *architectural* changes.[277] In the generally accepted WHO scheme, well-differentiated adenocarcinoma in a background of endometrial hyperplasia is diagnosed when one or more of the following three features are present: (1) a confluent gland pattern; (2) an extensive papillary pattern; (3) a desmoplastic stromal response.[278] The correlation between markedly atypical endometrial hyperplasia and adenocarcinoma has been demonstrated both using conventional morphologic evaluation and morphometric techniques.[268] It has also been stated that GLUT-1 is preferentially expressed in atypical endometrial hyperplasia and adenocarcinoma.[267]

In the case of simple hyperplasia (which is often accompanied by cystic changes), the risk is very small. Thus, in an old series of 544 premenopausal women followed for periods ranging up to 24 years, less than 0.4% developed carcinoma.[279] Conversely, the incidence of carcinoma in women with complex and atypical hyperplasia has been in the neighborhood of 15% and has reached 30% in some series.[269,270,272,277] Tavassoli and Kraus[285] analyzed the pathologic findings in 48 hysterectomy specimens resected usually within 1–6 months after a diagnosis of atypical endometrial hyperplasia (including so-called 'adenocarcinoma in situ') had been made in a curettage specimen. Lesions interpreted as well-differentiated adenocarcinomas were found in 12 instances (25%). In only one case was there myometrial extension, and this measured only 2 mm. Persistent hyperplasia was found in most of the other cases. The authors concluded that, although atypical endometrial hyperplasia poses a threat of carcinoma, this can easily be eliminated by either medical (progestogen therapy) or surgical (hysterectomy) means. The great efficacy of hormonal therapy in controlling most cases of endometrial hyperplasia and in avoiding hysterectomy in surgically high-risk postmenopausal patients has been repeatedly demonstrated.[271,284]

Presence in an endometrial biopsy of endometrial adenocarcinoma in situ within a complex atypical endometrial hyperplasia is associated with an increased incidence of endometrial adenocarcinoma in a subsequent hysterectomy.[280]

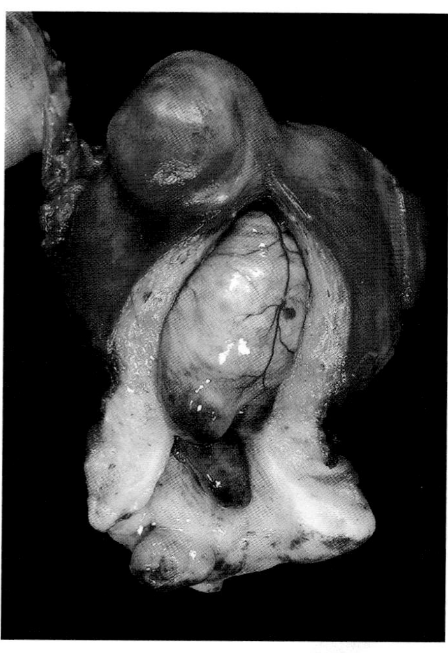

Fig. 19.130 Huge endometrial polyp filling the endometrial cavity. There is also a smaller endocervical polyp and a subserosal leiomyoma.
(Courtesy of Dr Pedro J Grases Galofrè; from Grases Galofrè PJ. Patologia ginecològica. Bases para el diagnòstico morfològico. Barcelona, 2002, Masson)

Tumors

Endometrial polyps

The large majority of endometrial polyps are not true neoplasms but probably represent circumscribed foci of hyperplasia, possibly due to a decreased expression of hormone receptors in the stromal component.[303] Grossly, they protrude into the endometrial cavity and often exhibit secondary changes (Fig. 19.130). The glands usually show some degree of cystic change. They may be lined by an active pseudostratified epithelium containing mitotic figures or, in the postmenopausal patient, by a flat, inactive epithelium (Fig. 19.131).

The glands and stroma of the polyp are unresponsive to progesterone stimulation and retain their integrity throughout the menstrual cycle. In material obtained from D&C, where usually only fragments of the polyp are obtained, the distinction with endometrial hyperplasia is made by examining the stroma. In the latter condition, the stromal cells are active, with large vesicular nuclei and occasional mitotic figures, whereas the stroma of a polyp is composed of spindle (fibroblast-like) cells, contains abundant extracellular connective tissue, and has large blood vessels with thick walls. On occasion, however, the stroma is more cellular and mitotically active, i.e., similar to that of endometrial hyperplasia.[295] Some polypoid lesions exhibit either simple or complex hyperplastic papillary endometrial proliferations, and it is a matter of individual choice whether to regard them as localized forms of endometrial hyperplasia or endometrial polyps with hyperplastic changes.[298] Furthermore, endometrial polyps with a typical appearance often coexist with endometrial hyperplasia. All of these observations point to a shared pathogenesis for these two lesions. In the presence of atypical complex hyperplasia or carcinoma in a polyp, the performance of a hysterectomy should be considered – especially in postmenopausal women – even if the changes appear restricted to the polyp.[304]

Exceptionally, the stroma of endometrial polyps contains scattered atypical (bizarre) cells.[290,310]

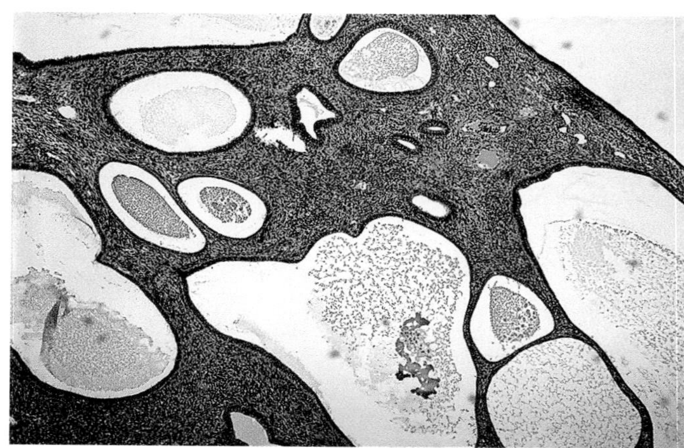

Fig. 19.131 Low-power appearance of endometrial polyp showing cystically dilated glands and a fibrous stroma with thick-walled vessels.

Endometrial polyps occur with increased frequency after tamoxifen exposure. These are characteristically multiple, large, and fibrotic, and may exhibit stromal decidualization and mucinous metaplasia[289,297,307] (Fig. 19.132) (see p. 1481). At the molecular level, they are said to exhibit a higher frequency of *KRAS* mutations.[294]

Rarely, polyps composed of functional endometrium are encountered. The diagnosis is made on the gross features of the lesion rather than on the microscopic pattern of glands and stroma and is, therefore, difficult or even impossible to make on a D&C specimen.

Malignant transformation of endometrial polyps is an exceptional but well-documented occurrence. Some of these cases present

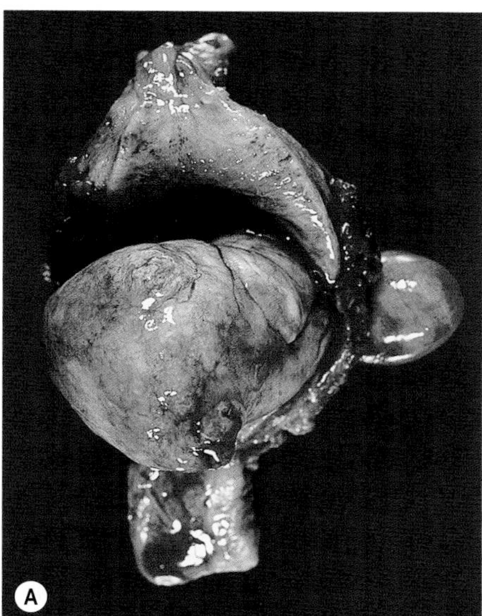

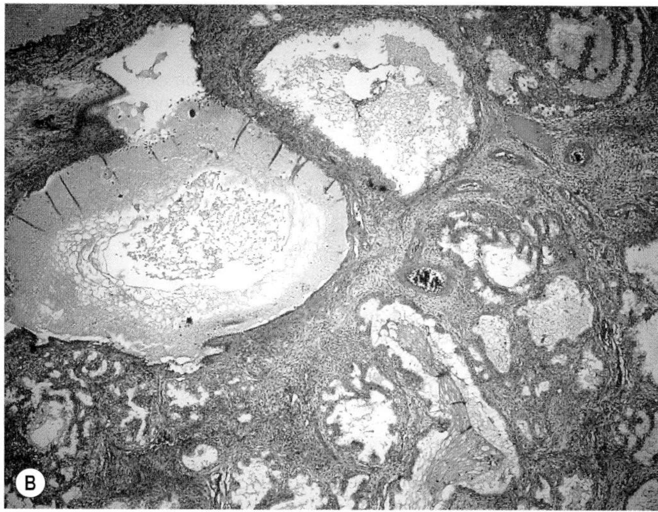

Fig. 19.132 Tamoxifen-related endometrial polyp: **A**, gross appearance; **B**, microscopic appearance.

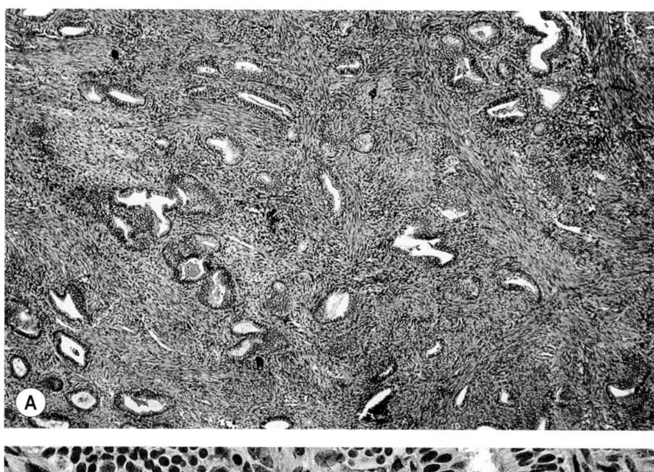

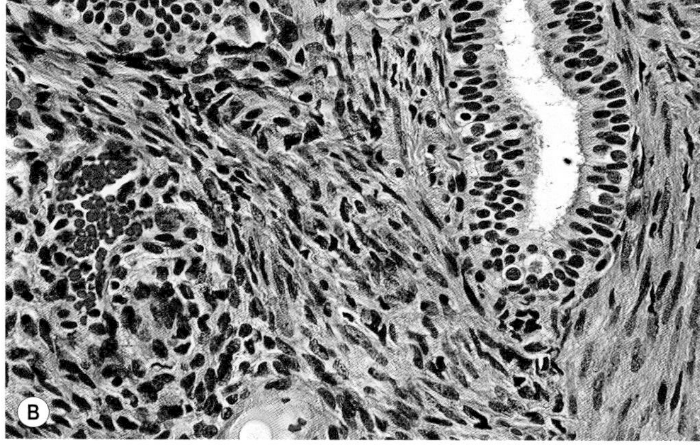

Fig. 19.133 **A** and **B**, Low- and high-power appearance of adenomyomatous polyp.

in the form of in-situ or invasive serous carcinomas[301] (see also p. 1496).

Endometrial polyps having smooth muscle fibers (not connected with blood vessel walls) in addition to the customary glands and stroma are designated as **adenomyomatous polyps** (polypoid adenomyomas).[293] They have a characteristic hard consistency and a grayish color (Fig. 19.133). An important variation on the theme is the **atypical polypoid adenomyoma** (atypical polypoid adenomyofibroma).[296,299,300,309,311] These tend to occur in premenopausal women (average age, 40 years) and present with abnormal uterine bleeding (Fig. 19.134). Some are associated with Turner syndrome.[288] Microscopically, they are identified by the fact that the glands occurring between the endometrial stroma and smooth muscle exhibit varying degrees of hyperplasia and atypia, sometimes approaching the appearance of carcinoma in situ ('of low malignant potential') (Fig. 19.135).[299] The danger is to misdiagnose them as adenocarcinomas with myometrial invasion. CD10 immunostaining is helpful in this differential diagnosis, in that it is negative in the stromal component of polypoid adenomyoma but often positive in the cells immediately surrounding the muscle-invasive glands (so-called fringe-like staining pattern).[305] The behavior is generally benign, but cases have been seen with local recurrences, carcinomatous transformation,[292,308] and coexistent endometrial or ovarian endometrioid carcinoma.[291,302]

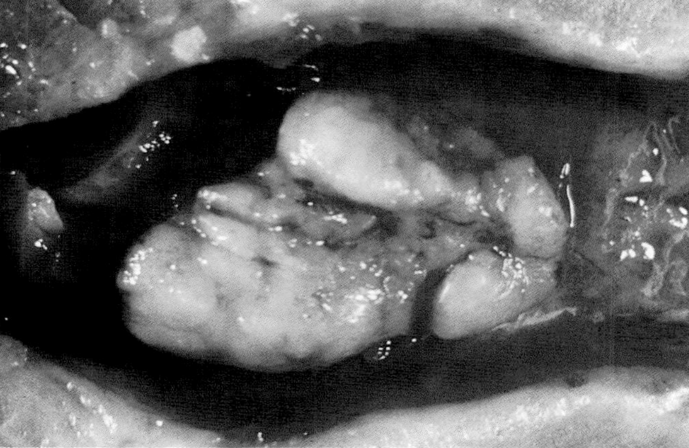

Fig. 19.134 Atypical polypoid adenomyoma. The gross appearance is not substantially different from that of an ordinary polyp.

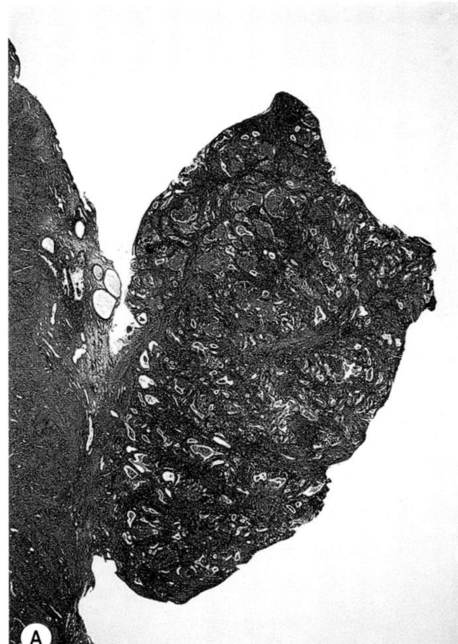
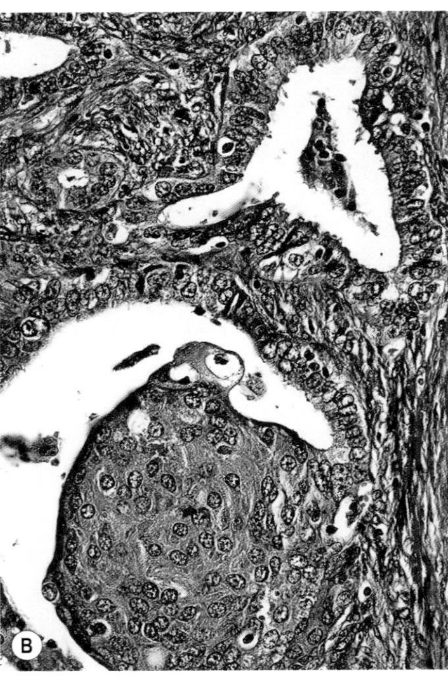

Fig. 19.135 **A** and **B**, Whole-mount and high-power appearance of atypical polypoid adenomyoma. Note the glandular architectural complexity, metaplastic changes, and atypia.

At the molecular level, atypical polypoid leiomyomas share several alterations with complex glandular hyperplasias.[306]

Endometrial carcinoma

General and clinical features

Carcinoma of the endometrium is the most common gynecologic malignancy in developed countries.[340] The highest incidence rates are in the United States and Canada, but in recent years there has been a decline in incidence and mortality. It typically occurs in elderly individuals, 80% of the patients being postmenopausal at the time of diagnosis.[332] However, it can occur in any age group and has even been reported in association with intrauterine pregnancy.[333]Most endometrial adenocarcinomas occurring in women aged 40 years or younger are of endometrioid type, well to moderately differentiated, and early stage disease.[320] Conversely, tumors of elderly patients are more likely to be grade 2 or 3, and to have more advanced disease at the time of diagnosis.[324]

It is currently believed that endometrial carcinomas can be divided in two distinct types on the basis of their pathogenesis: one – by far the more common – occurring as a result of excess estrogenic stimulation and developing against a background of endometrial hyperplasia, and the other developing de novo.[312,316,323,326,337] Patients at high risk for the first category include the obese, diabetic, hypertensive, and infertile; those with failure of ovulation (including Stein–Leventhal syndrome) and dysfunctional bleeding; long-standing estrogen users; breast cancer patients treated with tamoxifen (see below); those with severe degrees of endometrial hyperplasia; and – to a much lesser degree – those with functioning granulosa cell tumors and thecomas.[322,330,335]

In the majority of patients with Stein–Leventhal syndrome, the endometrial pathology is that of hyperplasia and, as such, it will regress with medical therapy.[325] However, a few well-documented cases of carcinoma have been reported; these have almost always been of a well-differentiated nature, and myometrial invasion, if present at all, has been minimal. It has been pointed out that the lesion may be reversible when treated by curettage followed by therapy directed toward reestablishment of ovulation, and a conservative approach to these patients has been recommended.[318] In support of this policy, it has been pointed out that not a single case of well-differentiated adenocarcinoma in a patient with Stein–Leventhal syndrome has been proved to metastasize, recur locally, or cause death. The situation is quite similar regarding the relationship between endometrial pathology and functioning ovarian tumors (see p. 1599).

Gonadal dysgenesis (Turner syndrome) can also be associated with endometrial adenocarcinoma, usually of the well-differentiated type. McCarty et al.[327] found 13 reported cases; 11 patients had received replacement estrogen therapy, usually in high doses and for prolonged periods. It is not clear whether this association represents a complication of long-term estrogen exposure or a rare expression of the Turner phenotype. Interestingly, almost two-thirds of the carcinomas exhibited squamous differentiation.[314]

Hereditary nonpolyposis colorectal carcinoma (HNPCC; Lynch syndrome) patients have an increased incidence of endometrial carcinoma, often presenting at a young age.[321] Many of the tumors have a nonendometrioid histology and are high grade tumors.[313] They often have a Crohn-like lymphoid reaction, lymph vessel permeation, and tumor-infiltrating lymphocytes.[339]

Some cases of endometrial carcinoma, of either endometrioid or papillary serous types, have been seen years after pelvic irradiation for some other condition, but whether these are spontaneous or radiation induced is not clear.[329,331,334]

Patients who receive tamoxifen as long-term treatment for breast carcinoma are at an increased risk for the development of endometrial adenocarcinoma;[315,319] in two reported series a significant number of the cases were high-grade tumors associated with a poor prognosis,[317,328,336] but in others there was a great predominance of low-grade endometrioid adenocarcinomas.[338]

Pathologic features

Grossly, carcinoma of the endometrium may form broad-based polypoid masses or infiltrate diffusely into the myometrium (Fig. 19.136). In general, extensive myometrial invasion is accompanied

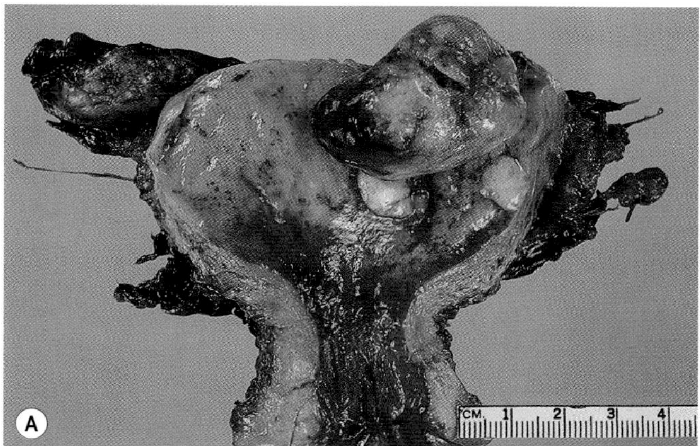

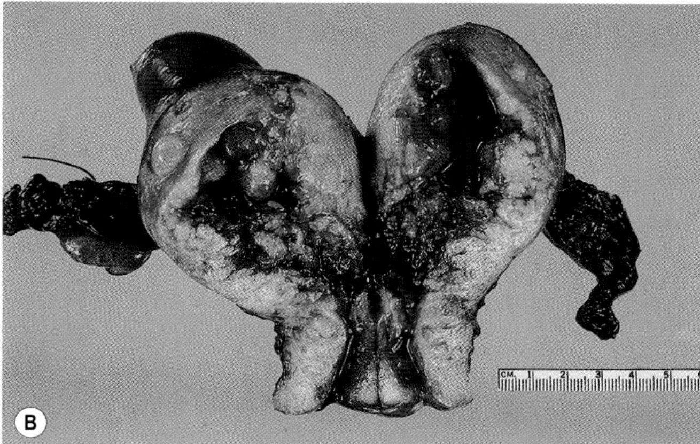

Fig. 19.136 A and **B**, Gross appearances of endometrioid adenocarcinoma. The tumor shown in **A** is polypoid, whereas that depicted in **B** is highly infiltrating.

by clinically detectable uterine enlargement. However, notable exceptions occur; sometimes deep myometrial extension is accompanied by a normal-sized uterus, the pattern of growth resembling that of adenoma malignum of cervix.[362] This pattern has also been described as 'minimal deviation invasive'.[358]

Endometrial carcinoma can develop in any anatomic region of the mucosa. Tumors developing in younger women have a greater tendency to involve the lower uterine segment (isthmus).[350] Parenthetically, tumors thought to have arisen in the isthmus are included among the endometrial rather than the cervical carcinomas.[355] Small carcinomas restricted to a cornu can be missed by a biopsy or even a D&C.

Microscopically, approximately 80% of endometrial malignant epithelial tumors are conventional adenocarcinomas, which are usually divided into well (grade I, 50%), moderately (grade II, 35%), and poorly differentiated (grade III, 15%) tumors (Fig. 19.137A–C). The FIGO three-grade system is primarily based on the growth pattern (relative proportion of glandular and solid areas), but it also makes provisions for nuclear atypia.[372] Alternative two-grade systems (low grade and high grade), mainly based on architectural criteria, have been proposed.[349,360]

The better differentiated tumors closely recapitulate the light and electron microscopic features of the non-neoplastic endometrium,[343,348] hence the term 'endometrioid' that is used for them. Over one-fourth of the endometrioid carcinomas have papillary (villoglandular) foci, either on the surface or in the invasive areas[341,342] (Fig. 19.137D). These tumors should be sharply separated from the much more aggressive papillary serous carcinomas (see p. 1496).[344,345,371] A further variation on the theme is represented by the endometrioid adenocarcinoma containing small nonvillous papillae. These papillae can arise either from an otherwise unremarkable endometrioid carcinoma or from the villous projections of the villoglandular variant of this tumor.[363] It should also be noted that the most superficial portions of endometrial adenocarcinomas can exhibit patterns closely simulating various hyperplastic and metaplastic conditions of the endometrial mucosa.[354] The glandular lumina may contain cell debris similar to that seen in colorectal carcinoma and colloquially known as 'dirty necrosis'. Such debris is associated with high-grade histology, myometrial invasion, and extension into the isthmus.[369]

The stroma of endometrial adenocarcinoma usually has a desmoplastic quality, but occasionally it may be almost completely absent, even in the presence of a diffusely infiltrating tumor.[357] It may contain collections of foamy cells, probably the result of tumor necrosis and a good marker for the presence of carcinoma.[352] However, these cells can also be seen in hyperplasia and in the absence of proliferative epithelial changes. Their immunophenotype corresponds to that of histiocytes rather than endometrial stromal cells.[368] They are fat positive and mucin negative, in contrast to the mucin-positive macrophages sometimes seen in the stroma of benign endometrial polyps.[367]

The non-neoplastic endometrium of a uterus harboring an endometrioid adenocarcinoma is often hyperplastic and only exceptionally exhibits a normal proliferative or secretory pattern; when it does, the assumption has been made that the carcinoma has arisen in a 'progesterone-refractory' mucosal area.[366]

The frequency and extent of myometrial invasion by carcinoma are directly related to the microscopic grade of the tumor.[361] High-grade tumors are also significantly associated with cervical involvement and lymphovascular invasion.[365] Care should be exercised to distinguish true myometrial extension by carcinoma from expansion of the endometrial–myometrial junction and from atypical or malignant changes involving preexisting foci of adenomyosis;[353] the latter condition is recognized by the presence of endometrial stroma around the intramyometrial proliferating glandular foci.[351] It has been proposed that CD10 immunostaining can help in this distinction by highlighting the endometrial stroma associated with the adenomyosis when present.[364] However, a warning has been sounded to the effect that CD10 immunoreactivity can also be found around foci of invasive adenocarcinoma.[370] Extension of the endometrial carcinoma into the cervix occurs in over 10% of cases, usually by direct invasion,[347,359] but allegedly also by implantation following D&C.[346] This extension may be grossly evident or become apparent only on microscopic examination; it may involve the surface only, the fibrous stroma, or both.[356,359] The presence and type of cervical extension – which influences the staging of the tumor – is best detected by fractional curettage; care should be exercised in distinguishing bona fide cervical extension from isolated tumor fragments, or else a high false-positive rate will occur.[356]

The differential diagnosis between endometrial and endocervical carcinoma is discussed on page 1453.

Variants and other microscopic types

Numerous morphologic forms of endometrial adenocarcinoma have been described. Some, such as adenoacanthoma, adenosquamous carcinoma, secretory carcinoma, and ciliated carcinoma, are thought to represent variants of ordinary ('endometrioid') adenocarcinoma. Others, notably papillary serous carcinoma, clear cell

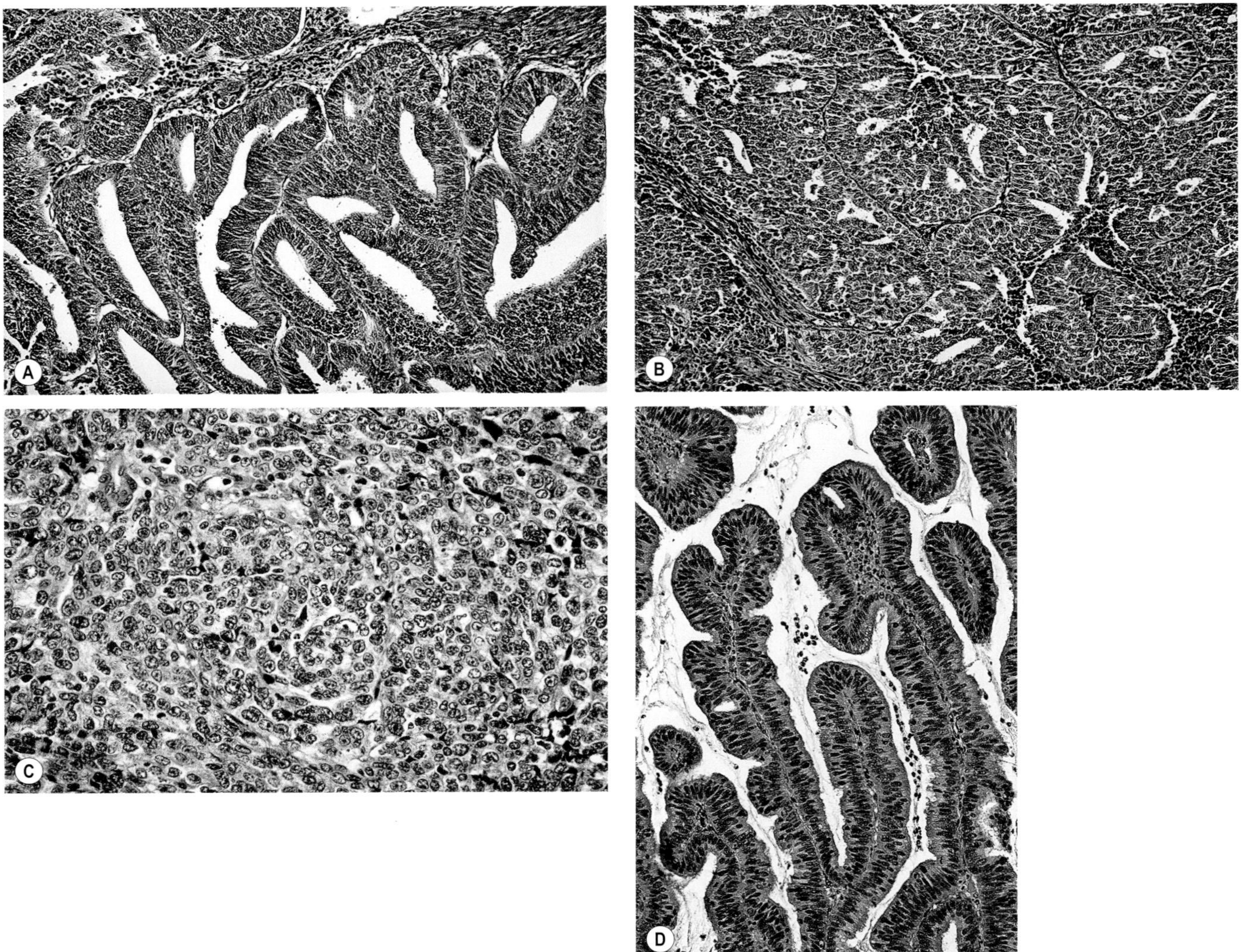

Fig. 19.137 Endometrioid endometrial adenocarcinoma: **A**, well differentiated; **B**, moderately differentiated; **C**, poorly differentiated; **D**, with villoglandular pattern of growth.

carcinoma, and mucinous adenocarcinoma, are regarded as being of nonendometrioid type, although any of them can be seen coexisting with endometrioid adenocarcinoma.

Adenoacanthoma is the term traditionally given to the well-differentiated endometrioid adenocarcinoma containing similarly well-differentiated (benign-appearing) squamous elements derived from metaplasia of the tumor glands (Fig. 19.138). Its natural history closely parallels that of the ordinary adenocarcinoma of a similar degree of differentiation lacking squamous changes.[470]

Adenosquamous (mixed) carcinoma refers to the endometrioid carcinoma containing *malignant-appearing* squamous elements[425] (Fig. 19.139). In some series the incidence of this tumor type has been notably high – up to 30% of all uterine carcinomas and on the rise[425,426] – but this was not our experience or that of others.[376,397] Patients with adenosquamous carcinoma are said to have a worse prognosis than those with adenocarcinoma or adenoacanthoma. However, several studies have shown that, stage by stage and grade by grade, there are no prognostic differences between pure adenocarcinoma, adenoacanthoma, and adenosquamous carcinoma.[443,469] Therefore, it would appear that the bad reputation that the latter tumors have is the result of the fact that most of them are basically high-grade adenocarcinomas, whereas the reverse is true for the adenoacanthomas. In other words, once an endometrial adenocarcinoma is clinically staged and microscopically graded into well-differentiated, intermediate, and poorly differentiated categories, the presence and appearance of a focal squamous component would seem immaterial.[469] Morphologic studies have suggested – and immunocytochemical studies have supported – the notion that adenoacanthoma and adenosquamous carcinoma represent a spectrum of squamous metaplasia in a single tumor type rather than two independent entities.[463]

Glassy cell carcinoma is a special type of adenosquamous carcinoma that has occasionally been reported in the endometrium; its appearance is similar to that of its more common cervical counterpart.[384,396]

Secretory carcinoma is characterized by neoplastic glands having subnuclear vacuolization resembling that of a normal 17-day secretory endometrium and accompanied by a late secretory pattern in the adjacent noninvolved endometrium[454] (Fig. 19.140). This tumor is not believed to be a specific type of endometrial carcinoma but rather the expression of a pattern that may be present diffusely or focally in a well-differentiated endometrioid carcinoma, usually as a result of progesterone stimulation. It should be distinguished from the clear cell carcinoma described below and from endometrioid adenocarcinomas exhibiting other types of clear cell change.[383,412,447]

Ciliated carcinoma is an extremely rare variant of endometrial adenocarcinoma that is composed predominantly of ciliated cells;[398] it needs to be distinguished from the much more common ciliated cell metaplasia (see p. 1483).

Mucinous adenocarcinoma is a tumor subtype characterized by abundant mucin secretion[420] (Fig. 19.141). It is distinguished from mucinous metaplasia by virtue of its architectural and cytologic

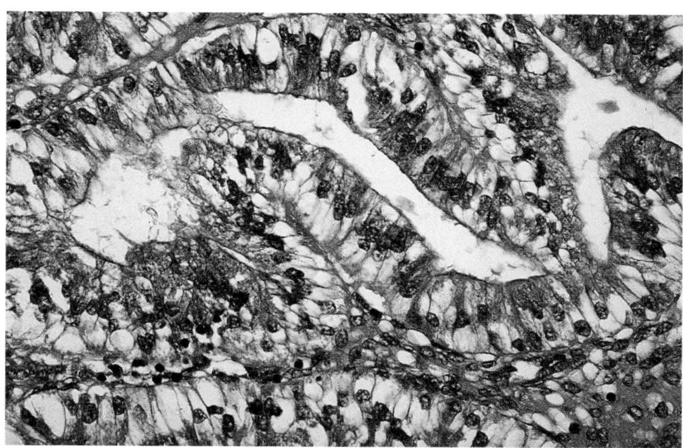

Fig. 19.140 Secretory carcinoma of endometrium. This well-differentiated lesion is a variant of endometrioid adenocarcinoma and is composed of cells with abundant clear to finely granular cytoplasm. It should be distinguished from clear cell carcinoma.

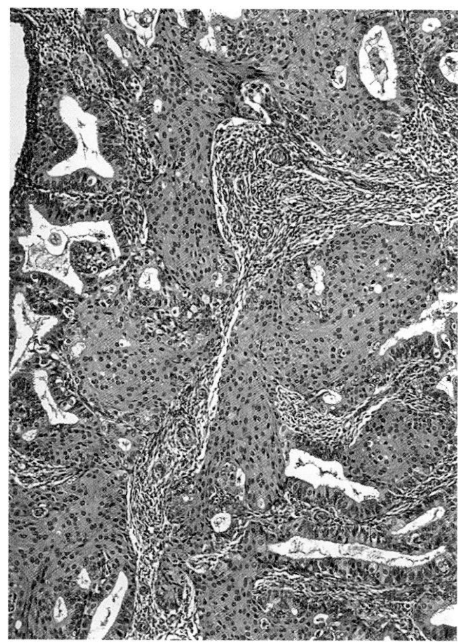

Fig. 19.138 Well-differentiated endometrioid adenocarcinoma with squamous metaplasia (so-called 'adenoacanthoma').

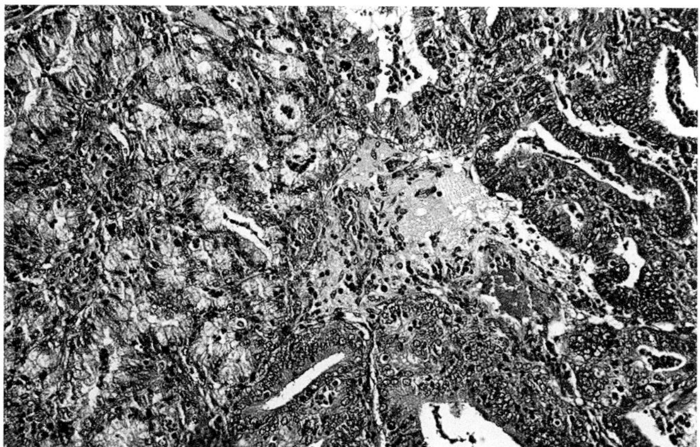

Fig. 19.141 Endometrial adenocarcinoma of mucinous type.

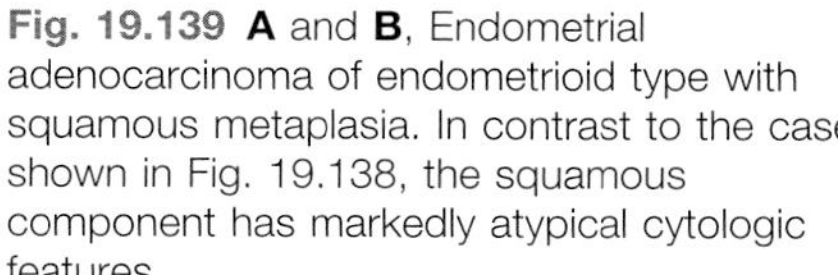

Fig. 19.139 **A** and **B**, Endometrial adenocarcinoma of endometrioid type with squamous metaplasia. In contrast to the case shown in Fig. 19.138, the squamous component has markedly atypical cytologic features.

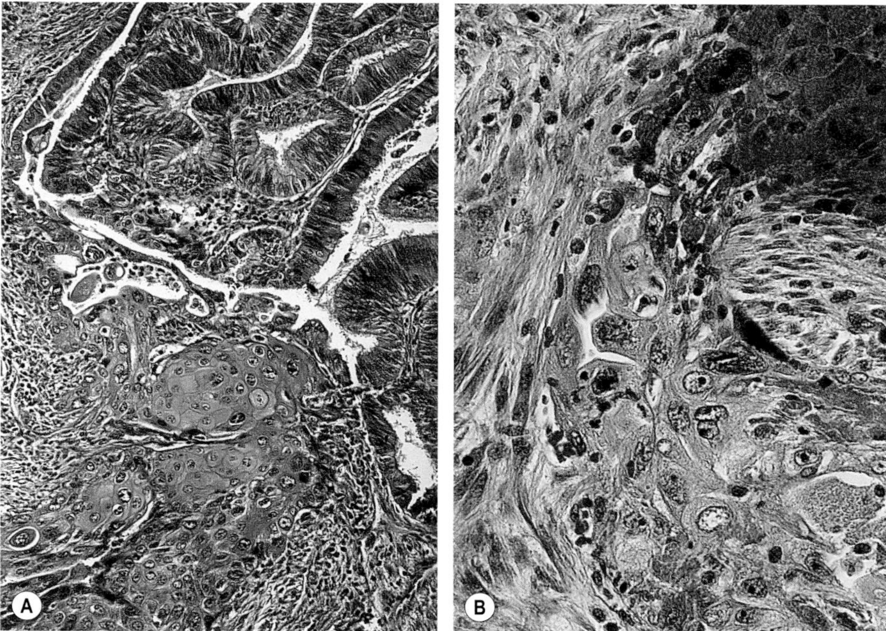

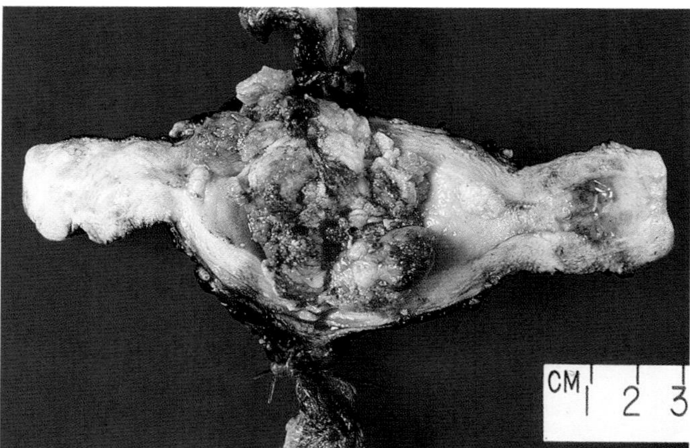

Fig. 19.142 Gross appearance of papillary serous carcinoma of endometrium. The neoplasm fills the endometrial cavity.

atypia, although on occasions the carcinomas exhibit a deceptively bland appearance.[458] It should be noted that scattered foci of mucin positivity are often found in ordinary endometrial adenocarcinoma and that they are not necessarily an indication of endocervical origin.[452] The distinction between endometrial mucinous adenocarcinoma and primary endocervical adenocarcinoma – which is further discussed on page 1453 – cannot be made on the basis of morphologic or histochemical features but rather depends on differential biopsy and fractional curettage.[440] Immunohistochemically, most uterine mucinous adenocarcinomas are reactive for CK7 but not for CK20 or CDX2.[429] However, some of the histochemical features of the mucin produced by a subset of these tumors suggest the existence of enteric differentiation.[416]

On occasion, endometrial adenocarcinomas of mucinous or mixed mucinous–endometrioid type exhibit a conspicuous *microglandular* pattern associated with eosinophilic mucinous intraluminal secretion and prominent acute inflammation, the overall picture simulating the appearance of endocervical microglandular hyperplasia.[468,471]

Papillary serous carcinoma (formerly also known as tubal-type carcinoma) is a highly aggressive form of endometrial adenocarcinoma closely resembling ovarian papillary serous carcinoma[395,399,408] (Fig. 19.142). It is characterized by a complex papillary pattern of growth, a high degree of cytologic atypia (pleomorphism, hyperchromasia, giant nucleoli), numerous mitoses, extensive necrosis, psammoma bodies (30% of the cases), and prominent myometrial invasion (Fig. 19.143). It should be distinguished from the already mentioned (and much more common) endometrial adenocarcinoma with a villoglandular pattern of growth, with which it shares several architectural features[386] (see p. 1493). A key aspect in this regard is the consistently high-grade nature of its cytologic features, which are also apparent on Papanicolaou (Pap) smears.[411] Conversely, papillae may be scanty, the tumor growing predominantly in the form of tubuloglandular structures and raising a differential diagnosis with endometrioid carcinoma.[385] It should be mentioned here that psammoma bodies are not necessarily indicative of a papillary serous-type tumor, since occasionally they are also seen in endometrioid carcinomas.[431]

Uterine papillary serous carcinoma can coexist with endometrioid adenocarcinoma of the uterus or serous carcinoma of the ovary,[380] be confined to an endometrial polyp, or be entirely intramucosal ('minimal serous carcinoma')[380,382,387,403,437,445,446,455,464] (Fig. 19.144). A putative precursor of serous carcinoma has been described under the term *endometrial glandular dysplasia*.[414,472,473]

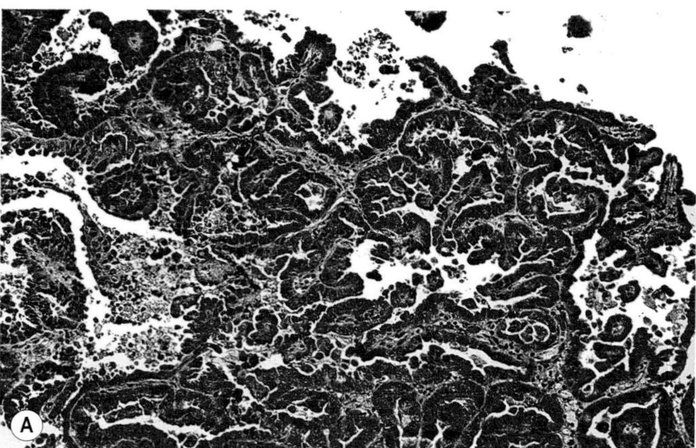

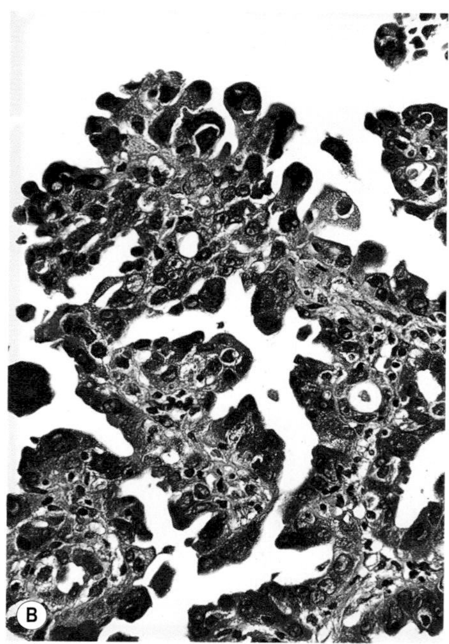

Fig. 19.143 **A** and **B**, Low- and high-power appearance of serous carcinoma. Note the high nuclear grade.

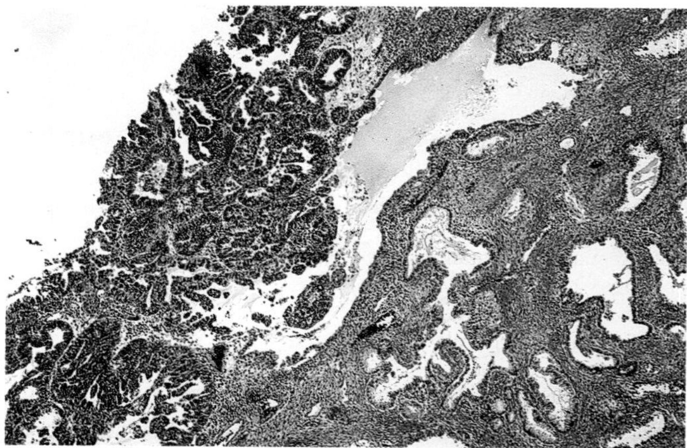

Fig. 19.144 Serous carcinoma limited to the superficial portion of a tamoxifen-related endometrial polyp.

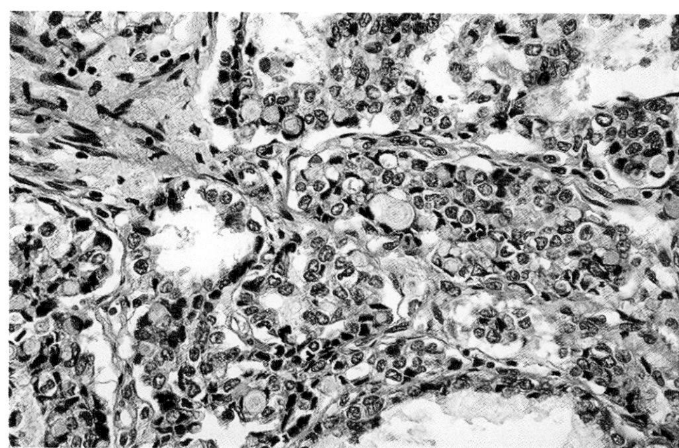

Fig. 19.145 Clear cell carcinoma of endometrium.

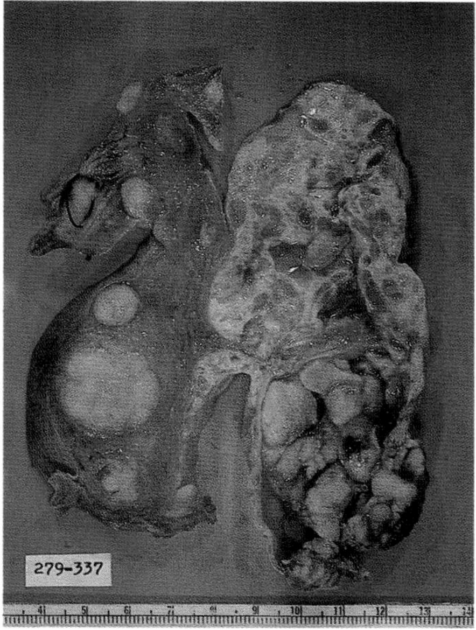

Fig. 19.146 Gross appearance of a clear cell carcinoma involving a large endometrial polyp.
(Courtesy of Dr Juan José Segura, San José, Costa Rica)

Immunohistochemically, strong and diffuse staining for P53 is one of the most characteristic features of serous carcinoma. This is usually associated with patchy p16 expression and lack of hormone receptors.[427,467] In contrast to ovarian serous carcinoma, WT1 is uncommonly positive.[389]

Some cases of uterine serous carcinoma have been described following radiation therapy for carcinoma of the cervix.[430]

Clear cell carcinoma is composed of large clear cells with distinct cellular margins containing variable but usually large amounts of glycogen[412,419] (Fig. 19.145). The papillary formations and 'hobnail' cells found in this variant of adenocarcinoma resemble those seen in the ovarian, cervical, and vaginal tumors that carry the same name. Their presence in superficial endometrial carcinomas, as a focal change in ordinary adenocarcinomas, and, exceptionally, even in benign endometrial polyps[412] and otherwise normal endometria[391] clearly speaks in favor of a müllerian rather than a mesonephric histogenesis (Fig. 19.146). The ultrastructural and immunohistochemical features of this tumor are also supportive of this interpretation.[413,439,441,459] Most patients are postmenopausal, and there seems to be no relationship with intrauterine diethylstilbestrol exposure, as there is for somewhat similar tumors occurring in the vagina and cervix.

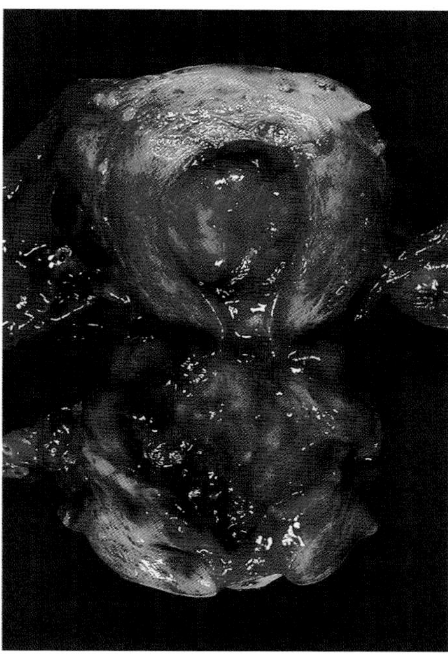

Fig. 19.147 Gross appearance of small cell neuroendocrine carcinoma of endometrium. The tumor is red and fleshy, and has a soft consistency.

Although earlier articles emphasized the similarities that clear cell carcinoma bears with ordinary ('endometrioid') adenocarcinoma,[412,450] the current belief is that it is more closely related to papillary serous carcinoma, both in terms of morphology and natural history.[381,417] A putative precursor lesion has been described, characterized by endometrial cells with clear and/or eosinophilic cytoplasm and varying degrees of nuclear atypia.[390]

Undifferentiated carcinoma is probably the end of the line for endometrial carcinomas of endometrioid, serous, and other microscopic types.[438] It grows in the form of solid sheets of epithelial cells without any signs of differentiation.[374,448] It is important to distinguish it from a grade 3 endometrioid adenocarcinoma because of its worse prognosis.[378] The association of undifferentiated carcinoma with low-grade endometrioid adenocarcinoma is regarded as a form of tumor dedifferentiation.[449] Some of the reported cases of undifferentiated carcinoma have occurred in young women and have pursued a fulminant clinical course.[453]

Small cell (neuroendocrine) carcinoma usually presents grossly as bulky (sometimes polypoid), ill-defined, and invasive tumor (Fig. 19.147). In rare instances it is seen confined to an endometrial polyp.[377] Microscopically, its appearance is similar to that of its more common cervical counterpart (Fig. 19.148). It may be associated with areas of ordinary endometrioid or serous adenocarcinoma or be seen as a component of mixed müllerian tumor[404,432,444] (Fig. 19.149). Immunohistochemically, there is usually reactivity for neuron-specific enolase (NSE) and low molecular weight keratin, and sometimes also for chromogranin and synaptophysin. Dense-core secretory granules can be detected ultrastructurally. The behavior is very aggressive.[460] As in the lung, cervix, and other sites, tumors with similar high-grade neuroendocrine features but composed of cells of intermediate or large size exist, either pure or admixed with

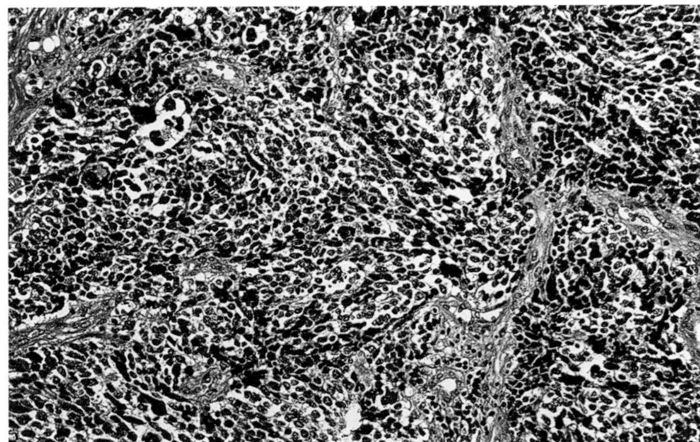

Fig. 19.148 Small cell neuroendocrine carcinoma of endometrium showing a diffuse pattern of growth.

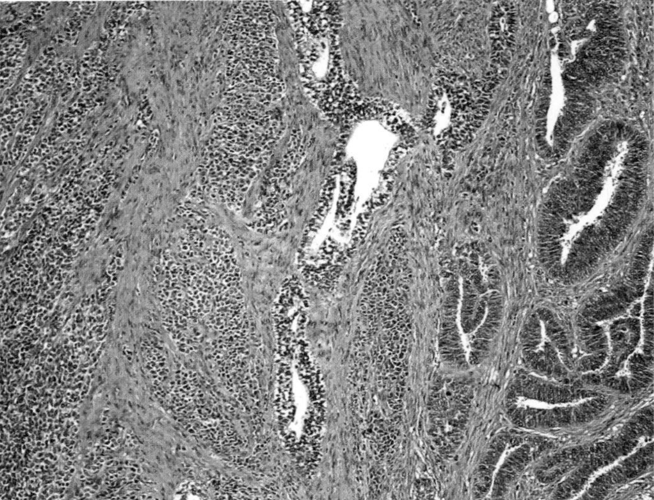

Fig. 19.149 Small cell neuroendocrine carcinoma of endometrium admixed with endometrioid adenocarcinoma. This is a common combination.

endometrioid adenocarcinoma.[374,423] In this context, it should be noted that a minor population of endocrine cells – as detected with argyrophilic stains – is present in 25–50% of otherwise typical endometrial adenocarcinomas.[379,451] Some of these cells have been found to contain chromogranin, NSE, 5-hydroxytryptamine (5-HT; serotonin), somatostatin, adrenocorticotropic hormone (ACTH), and indolamines.[375,406]

Squamous cell carcinoma occurring in the endometrium in a pure form is extremely rare[373,407] and it is, therefore, particularly important to rule out the alternative possibility of extension of a cervical carcinoma.[433] Some cases have developed in elderly patients with pyometra, presumably on the basis of a preexisting endometrial squamous metaplasia.[400] Others have occurred in association with mucinous glands of presumably heterotopic cervical origin.[465] One reported case was associated with *spindle cell* (*sarcomatoid*) changes,[466] and another was of the *verrucous type*.[442]

Giant cell (adeno)carcinoma is a rare pleomorphic form of high-grade endometrial adenocarcinoma featuring poorly cohesive sheets and nests of bizarre multinucleated giant cells.[409,422] It may be combined with better differentiated areas showing endometrioid or clear cell carcinoma features.[436]

Endometrial carcinoma with trophoblastic (choriocarcinomatous) differentiation should be distinguished from the tumor just mentioned and from gestational choriocarcinoma.[410] The multinucleated syncytiotrophoblast-like cells present in the tumor are strongly immunoreactive for human chorionic gonadotropin (hCG).[434] The nontrophoblastic areas are more likely to have a serous than an endometrioid morphology.[401] A related and even rarer phenomenon is that of endometrial carcinoma secreting alpha-fetoprotein.[456]

Oxyphilic cell carcinoma is a rare variant of endometrioid carcinoma characterized by a predominant or exclusive component of large eosinophilic (oxyphilic) cells.[435]

Endometrioid carcinoma with sertoliform (sex cord-like) differentiation similar to that more commonly seen in ovarian endometrioid tumors has been reported.[388,457] This phenomenon is to be distinguished from the uterine tumors resembling ovarian sex-cord tumors (see p. 1503). The term *corded and hyalinized endometrioid carcinoma* has been proposed to indicate its two most characteristic morphologic features.[424]

Transitional cell (urothelial) carcinoma has architectural and cytologic features similar to those of urothelial carcinoma of the lower urinary tract, but it retains a müllerian profile. It is almost always admixed with one or another of the more conventional patterns.[392,415,418] An intriguing association because of their cytologic similarities is that between transitional cell carcinoma of the endometrium and Brenner tumor of the ovary.[394]

Hepatoid adenocarcinoma has been reported as arising from the endometrium, in association with alpha-fetoprotein production.[402]

Signet ring cell adenocarcinoma has been described as a primary uterine tumor.[421] Before making this diagnosis, all attempts should be made to rule out the alternative possibilities of metastasis (particularly from breast and stomach) and of vacuolated decidual cells and stromal histiocytes simulating signet ring cells.[405]

Lymphoepithelioma-like carcinoma looks like its homonym in other sites. The few reported cases have not shown evidence of Epstein–Barr virus infection.[461]

Rhabdoid tumor of the uterus represents, in at least some of the cases, a dedifferentiated form of endometrial adenocarcinoma, as is strongly suggested by its occasional coexistence with a conventional adenocarcinoma appearance.[393]

Mesonephric (adeno)carcinoma of the endometrium, i.e., a tumor truly derived from wolffian remnants and, therefore, unrelated to the clear cell carcinoma described above (which in the past was inaccurately called mesonephric), has been described, presenting as a myometrial mass.[428,462]

Cytology

Unfortunately, the success of mass screening in reducing invasive cervical carcinoma has not had quite the same effect on endometrial carcinoma.[476] The routine Pap smear is not as effective for the detection of this tumor, the positive rate being only 50%.[475] With cervical scrapings, this rate is 60%, and with vaginal pool material it reaches 75%.[483,485] The presence of normal endometrial cells in a cervical cytologic specimen should raise the possibility of endometrial hyperplasia or carcinoma and is an indication for histologic examination of the endometrium.[480] Several cytologic methods have been employed to increase the positive rate, such as endometrial aspiration, tampon smear, endometrial lavage, endometrial brushing, the jet-wash technique, and suction curettage.[474,477–479] Of these, the latter is preferred by many because of its high degree of accuracy and patient acceptance.[477] However, the widespread applicability of any of these methods to mass screening still remains problematic.[481,482,484]

Histochemical and immunohistochemical features

Immunohistochemically, endometrial adenocarcinomas of the conventional (endometrioid) type are positive for keratin (especially keratins 7, 8, 18, and 19),[500,501] vimentin (65% to over 80% of cases),[489,490] PAX8,[510] carcinoembryonic antigen (although less so than cervical carcinomas and generally limited to areas of squamous metaplasia),[512] CA-125,[503] IgA and secretory component,[509] MUC1 (but usually not MUC2 or MUC5AC),[502] *Ulex europaeus*, agglutinin I, and amylase (12% of cases).[511] Coexpression of keratin and vimentin is common.[504] Some tumor cells have also been found to contain glial fibrillary acidic protein.[501]

Estrogen and progesterone receptors are present in most cases of endometrial adenocarcinoma.[487,493,505] Endometrioid carcinoma shows the highest degree of positivity for both receptors, followed by papillary serous carcinoma and clear cell carcinoma.[491] High-grade adenosquamous carcinomas are consistently negative.[497] In endometrioid carcinoma and most of its variants, the presence of hormone receptors correlates with FIGO stage, FIGO grade, and nuclear grade.[496] Degrees of estrogen and progesterone receptor positivity are often similar.[488] Overexpression of HER2/*neu* is present in approximately 20% of endometrial carcinomas.[506] Expression of CD117 (c-kit), as evaluated immunohistochemically, has been found in about half of the adenocarcinomas, while it is present in over 90% of normal proliferative endometria.[492] GLUT-1, a facilitative glucose transporter, is aberrantly expressed in most atypical hyperplasias and adenocarcinomas (especially of the serous type[495]), but allegedly not in normal endometrium or in simple or complex hyperplasias without atypia.[513] Expression of the cell adhesion molecules β-catenin and E-cadherin is related to histiotype, in the sense that both tend to be present in endometrioid carcinoma and absent in papillary serous carcinoma.[507] Conversely, the oncofetal protein IMP3 is related to serous rather than endometrioid carcinoma.[516]

A finding of diagnostic significance is that WT1, which is nearly always positive in papillary serous tumor of the ovary and its metastases, is generally negative in papillary serous tumor of the endometrium,[486,494,498] as well as in other types of primary endometrial carcinoma.[514] Another marker of alleged diagnostic utility in this context is IMP3 (or the combination of IMP3+/PTEN+) as an indicator of serous carcinoma.[499] A potential pitfall is represented by TTF-1, a marker classically associated with lung and thyroid carcinoma but which can be also be expressed in endometrial (and endocervical) adenocarcinoma.[508,515]

Molecular genetic features

The major genetic abnormalities that have been detected in endometrioid adenocarcinomas are microsatellite instability (28% of cases) and mutations in the *PTEN* gene (one-third to one-half of cases), the *PIK3CA* gene (36–39% of cases), the *KRAS* gene (26% of cases), and the *CTNNB1* (β-catenin) gene (13–22% of cases), whereas nonendometrioid carcinomas (notably the papillary serous type) often have *TP53* mutations (>90% of cases) and loss of heterozygosity on several chromosomes.[517,520,523,528,529,535–537] An inverse relation has been found between P53 overexpression and hormone receptor status.[522,525] These differences have been interpreted as probably indicative of different pathogenetic mechanisms for the two major types of endometrial neoplasia.[519,524,526,533]

Other genetic abnormalities that have been documented in endometrial adenocarcinoma include decreased expression of P21 (WAF1/CIP1, a nuclear protein that binds to cyclin-dependent kinase complexes),[530] decreased expression of β1C integrin (member of a group of ubiquitous cell adhesion molecules involved in maintaining normal tissue morphology[527]), overexpression of COX-2 in the poorly differentiated forms,[521] loss of expression of DCC,[531] downregulation of Rb2/p130,[534] and high telomerase activity in the high-grade tumors.[518]

DNA aneuploidy is present in approximately one-fourth of the cases; positive tumors tend to be of advanced surgical stage and higher microscopic grade, associated with deeper myometrial invasion, and accompanied by lymph node metastases. As expected, aneuploidy is the rule in papillary serous carcinoma.[532]

Spread and metastases

The two obvious sites of direct spread of endometrial carcinoma are the myometrium and the cervix, both of these having important prognostic connotations[553] (see p. 1501). For staging purposes, myometrial invasion is divided into two stages: up to 50% of the myometrial thickness or greater. This apparently straightforward determination is actually fraught with many potential inaccuracies.[538] The arcuate vascular plexus of the myometrium has been used as a guideline for this measurement, in the sense that carcinomatous infiltration into or through this plexus can be taken as surrogate evidence that the tumor has invaded over 50% of the myometrium.[554] A particularly difficult situation arises if there is coexistent adenomyosis. On the one hand, involvement of adenomyosis foci by carcinoma can be overinterpreted as deep myometrial invasion; on the other, it has been claimed that involvement of adenomyosis by carcinoma is an indicator of the likely presence of true myometrial invasion elsewhere in the myometrium.[544]

Invasion of the endocervix by endometrial carcinoma is common. This prognostically important feature should be distinguished from the atypical reactive endocervical proliferation that may accompany a uterus affected by endometrial carcinoma, possibly related to prior endometrial sampling.[550]

Lymphovascular invasion is the most important route of spread of endometrial cancer. A warning here is in order. We are referring to the artifact known as *vascular pseudoinvasion* sometimes seen in laparoscopic hysterectomy specimens and characterized by conspicuous tumor fragments in the lumen of thick-walled vessels in the outer myometrium or in ectatic vessels anywhere in the myometrium. These tumor fragments are detached from the vascular wall, lack an inflammatory perivascular infiltrate, and are accompanied by tumor fragments in myometrial clefts. The artifactual nature of this finding seems well established, but the mechanism of production and the identity of the guilty party (surgeon or pathologist) have not.[543,546,548]

The most common sites of extrauterine spread in endometrial adenocarcinoma of the endometrioid type are the pelvic and para-aortic lymph nodes and the ovaries (see next section). Nodal metastases occur in approximately 5–25% of clinically stage I tumors and are more likely to occur in invasive high-grade tumors (even if such tumors are superficial), in large sized and/or deeply invasive tumors regardless of grade, in tumors with cervical extension, and in tumors with vascular invasion.[540,542,549]

Papillary serous carcinoma has a particular propensity for lymph vessel permeation. Involvement of peritoneal surfaces (particularly in the pelvis) occurs early in the disease, and can be present even at the intraepithelial stage.[552] In these cases, molecular analysis has shown that the disease is clonal, suggesting origin at a single site with secondary early spread.[539,547,553]

An additional route of spread of endometrial carcinoma is transtubal,[551] but another warning is in order. On occasion, the keratin present in endometrial carcinoma with squamous metaplasia desquamates into the uterine cavity and from there travels via the fallopian tube to produce implants in the peritoneal surface, leading to the formation of foreign body granulomas.[541] This finding should not be regarded as evidence of metastatic disease *in the absence of viable neoplastic cells.* Follow-up data on these patients suggest that these keratin granulomas have no prognostic significance and that they should be distinguished from viable tumor implants.[545]

The most common sites of recurrence of endometrial carcinoma are the vaginal vault and pelvis. Papillary serous carcinoma characteristically spreads throughout the abdominal cavity in a fashion similar to that of ovarian serous carcinoma. Metastases of this tumor in the bladder can simulate a primary neoplasm of this organ.[555]

Distant metastases of endometrial carcinoma are more common in the lung, liver, bone, central nervous system, and skin. The latter tend to occur in the head and neck region, particularly the scalp.

Coexistent uterine and other genital tract carcinomas

Approximately 8% of endometrial carcinomas are accompanied by a simultaneous **ovarian carcinoma.** When they are of similar microscopic types – which is usually the case – it becomes difficult to decide whether there are two independent tumors or whether one of the sites represents a metastasis.[563] Features favoring a metastatic nature for the ovarian tumor include the following: smaller size, bilateral involvement, multinodular pattern of growth, presence of associated surface implants, and prominent lymphatic or vascular invasion within the ovarian stroma.[560] Immunohistochemical and DNA flow cytometric studies have proved of only limited value in this context.[560] On the other hand, molecular studies done for the evaluation of clonality (loss of heterozygosity, *PTEN* mutations, microsatellite instability) have provided more pertinent information.[562] The results of these combined evaluations seem to indicate that both situations occur but that – at least in the case of endometrioid tumors – there is a greater number of independent primary uterine and ovarian neoplasms than of endometrial tumors metastasizing to the ovary.[557–559,561]

Endometrioid carcinomas have been described involving simultaneously the uterine corpus and the fallopian tube. In about half of them the fallopian tube tumors were located in the distal or fimbriated end, and some of the tumors were in situ.[556]

Treatment

The usual treatment of endometrial carcinoma is total abdominal hysterectomy with bilateral salpingo-oophorectomy. Whenever feasible, this should be supplemented by surgical staging (including biopsies of pelvic and para-aortic lymph nodes) if any of the following is present: greater than 50% myometrial invasion, grade III tumor, cervical involvement, extrauterine spread, unfavorable histologic component (serous, clear cell, or undifferentiated), or palpably enlarged nodes.[574] Radiation therapy, which until recently was administered routinely in conjunction with surgery (either preoperatively or postoperatively), is no longer favored, except for patients with poor prognostic factors that put them at a high risk of recurrence.[575] Tumor sterilization by radiation, as determined by histopathologic study of the hysterectomy specimen, was often obtained for tumors limited to the endometrium but only rarely for tumors invading the myometrium.[573] Postradiation recurrent tumors tend to show decreased expression of hormone receptors and increased expression of P53.[571] Progestational agents, although usually not curative, occasionally induce striking temporary regressions in the primary tumor as well as in the metastases.[565,567] Well-differentiated lesions are more likely to respond and sometimes to regress completely; this is in keeping with the fact that, as already indicated, an association exists between microscopic degree of differentiation and presence of estrogen and progesterone receptors. Well-differentiated carcinomas treated with progestins show a decreased gland-to-stroma ratio, decreased glandular cellularity, decreased or absent mitotic activity, loss of cytologic atypia, and a variety of cytoplasmic changes, including mucinous, secretory, squamous, and eosinophilic metaplasia.[577]

The treatment of papillary serous carcinoma consists of hysterectomy with bilateral salpingo-oophorectomy, omentectomy, and surgical staging, the latter including peritoneal cytology and pelvic and para-aortic lymph node sampling. This is usually followed by adjuvant therapy, except for the minimally invasive tumors.[566,568–570,576]

Tumor relapse may appear in the form of local recrudescence (50%), distant metastases (28%), or both (21%); the median interval is between 1 and 2 years.[564] Local recurrences can be treated successfully with aggressive radiation therapy.[572]

Prognosis

Factors of prognostic importance in endometrial adenocarcinoma are the following:

1 *Tumor stage,* as defined by the FIGO system.[586,587,610,631] This refers to the surgical stage, since the clinical stage frequently underestimates the extent of disease.[628] The surgical staging includes a search for intraperitoneal microscopic tumor dissemination, as evaluated on cytologic preparations, supplemented if necessary with immunohistochemistry.[584]
2 Level of *infiltration* of the myometrial wall, as incorporated into the staging system. Tumors with invasion of over one-half of the myometrium fare worse than those invading less than one-half.[590,596,599,601] Among the latter (stage IB tumors), there is no significant difference between those that invade up to one-third and those that invade greater than one-third but less than one-half.[578]
3 *Microscopic grade* of differentiation, as defined by the FIGO system.[599,611,619,626] As already stated, originally this system was primarily based on architectural rather than nuclear features, except for the papillary serous and clear cell types, which are by definition high-grade tumors.[630] The addition of a nuclear parameter to the FIGO system has improved its prognostic significance.[582] A relationship exists between microscopic grade and level of invasion (well-differentiated tumors being more superficial), but there is also a correlation between grade and survival within a given stage.[608] High grade tumors have a poor prognosis regardless of the histologic subtype to which they belong.[620]
4 *Cervical extension.* This is associated with a somewhat worse prognosis, regardless of the nature or extent of the change.[594,606]
5 *Estrogen dependence.* As a group, tumors associated with – and probably resulting from – chronic estrogenic stimulation have a better prognosis than the others. This includes most tumors in young patients (<40 years) and those associated with Stein–Leventhal syndrome, functioning ovarian tumors, and exogenous estrogen administration.[583,605,617] Along the same lines, adenocarcinomas associated with hyperplasia in the residual endometrium have a better prognosis than those lacking this feature.[583]
6 *Microscopic type.* Among the various morphologic variants, the papillary serous type and clear cell types are the most

aggressive, with a definite tendency for upper abdominal spread for the former.[615] Adenosquamous carcinomas are also highly malignant, but this is probably only a reflection of the fact that they are poorly differentiated tumors. Conversely, the excellent prognosis associated with grade I endometrioid adenocarcinoma, adenoacanthoma, and secretory carcinoma probably relates to their well-differentiated nature.[590,624,629]

7 *Lymph vessel invasion*. Tumor permeation of lymph vessels is a poor prognostic sign,[598,609] particularly if severe (diffuse or multifocal).[597]
8 *Blood vessel invasion*. The presence of blood vessel invasion is an important prognostic factor in stage I adenocarcinoma;[603,609,621] this feature has often been found to be associated with perivascular lymphocytic infiltration.[579]
9 *Hormone receptor status*. Multivariate analyses have shown that the estrogen receptor status (whether measured biochemically or immunohistochemically) is a significant predictor of recurrence and survival.[589,592,595]
10 *P53 overexpression*. This parameter has been found to be associated with tumor type, grade, and stage.[581,616,618]
11 *HER2*/neu *expression*. Intense overexpression of this oncogene is said to be associated with a poor overall survival.[600]
12 *Epidermal growth factor receptor*. Expression of this marker is said to correlate with a high microscopic grade and a shorter survival rate.[612]
13 *DNA ploidy*. Aneuploid tumors are associated with high microscopic grade, high clinical stage, and poor prognosis; it has been claimed that tumor aneuploidy has independent prognostic value.[580,588,602,607,627] In some studies, it has proved to be one of the most important predictors of outcome, together with age and tumor stage.[613]
14 *Cell proliferation*. The degree of tumor cell proliferation, as determined by S-phase fraction, was found in one series to be a strong predictor of outcome.[622] High mitotic rate has also been found to be a sign of aggressiveness in stage I grade I adenocarcinomas.[625]
15 *RB gene*. It has been claimed that the presence of decreased levels of pRb2/p130 is associated with an increased risk of recurrence and tumor death, independently of tumor stage and ploidy status.[623]
16 *Angiogenesis*. In one study, vessel density was found to be an independent prognostic factor in endometrial carcinoma.[604]
17 *Others*. Parameters said to be indicative of favorable outcome are vimentin positivity,[591] S100A1 immunoexpression,[593] Langerhans cell infiltration,[591] low expression of p170 (a cell cycle-related antigen),[585] and absence of *hMLH1* (a mismatch repair gene).[614]

Endometrial stromal tumors

Tumors composed of endometrial stroma tend to occur in middle-aged women (average age, 45 years) and often present with vaginal bleeding.[657]

Microscopically, they are composed of uniform, predominantly oval small cells closely resembling those of the endometrial stroma, individually enveloped by reticulin fibers, which characteristically encircle small vessels that resemble spiral arterioles (Fig. 19.150). In the past, the prominent vascularization sometimes resulted in a mistaken diagnosis of hemangiopericytoma. Other commonly encountered features in endometrial stromal sarcomas include foci of hyalinization and scattered foamy cells.[699] Morphologic variations (other than those described in greater detail below) include the presence of a prominent fibrous or myxoid component,[692] adipose metaplasia,[638] a component of epithelioid cells with

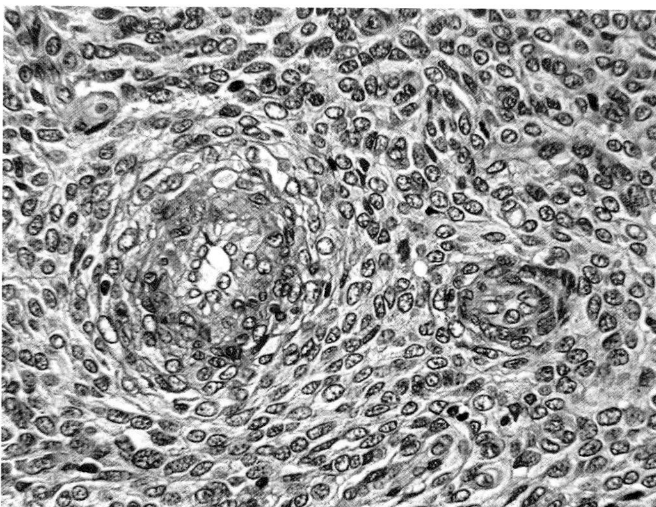

Fig. 19.150 Typical microscopic appearance of endometrial stromal tumor, showing bland oval cells arranged concentrically around spiral arterioles.

abundant eosinophilic cytoplasm,[690] of scattered tumor cells with 'symplasmic' nuclei,[638,697] and of papillary/pseudopapillary formations.[679]

The similarities of the tumor cells to normal endometrial stromal cells are also evident ultrastructurally and phenotypically;[634,652] these cells contain estrogen and progesterone receptors, and the tumors respond to administration of progestins.[696,703] Their immunohistochemical profile is variable. Reactivity for vimentin and CD10 is almost the rule, positivity for actin, WT1 and epidermal growth factor receptor is common, reactivity for keratin (especially CK19) and desmin is focal and inconstant, and negativity for S-100 protein is universal.[633,640,651,656,659,681,682,700]

Three markers of importance in the identification and differential diagnosis of these tumors are CD10 (consistently positive), h-caldesmon, and HDAC8 (consistently negative, in contrast to smooth muscle tumors, see below).[643,650,677,686,695]

Endometrial stromal tumors have been divided according to the type of margins into: (1) a benign category (endometrial stromal nodule) having pushing margins; and (2) a malignant category (endometrial stromal sarcoma) having infiltrating margins.[666,685,689]

Endometrial stromal nodules appear grossly as solitary sharply circumscribed masses of soft consistency and a characteristic yellow-to-orange color (Fig. 19.151). They do not invade veins, lymphatics, or the myometrium. The prognosis is excellent; recurrence did not occur in any of the 60 cases studied by Tavassoli and Norris,[702] even when some irregularities in the margin, high mitotic counts, or glandular foci were present. Cases in which the irregularities at the margins are pronounced but which lack the typical, usually extensive infiltration of the endometrial stromal sarcomas listed below have been referred to as *endometrial stromal tumors with limited infiltration*.[653] Their behavior seems to be as favorable as that of the conventional stromal nodules. Genetically, endometrial stromal nodule is characterized by t(7;17), which results in *JAZF1–JJAZ1* fusion.[648,672]

Endometrial stromal sarcomas, traditionally designated *endolymphatic stromal myosis*, infiltrate the myometrium and have a particular tendency to permeate lymph vessels (Figs 19.152 and 19.153). The latter feature sometimes can be detected grossly by the presence of yellowish, ropy, or ball-like masses filling dilated channels. They may also present as polypoid masses (Fig. 19.154). The

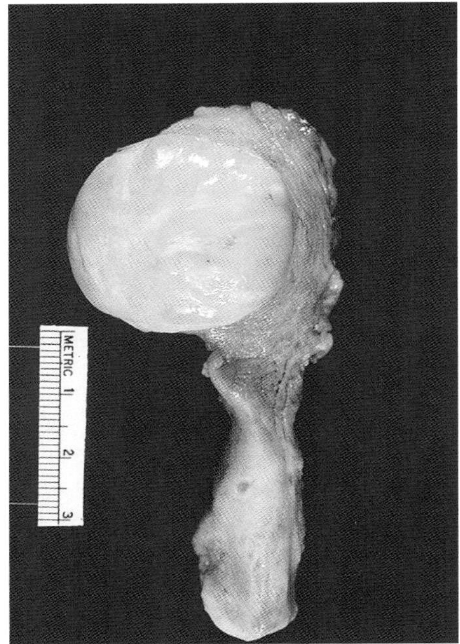

Fig. 19.151 Endometrial stromal nodule. The lesion is characteristically well circumscribed and has a yellow color.

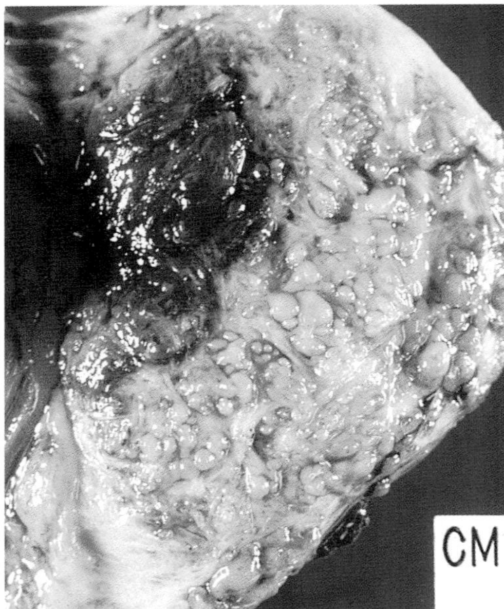

Fig. 19.152 Low-grade endometrial stromal sarcoma showing diffuse permeation of the myometrium in the form of small nodules bulging on the cut surface.

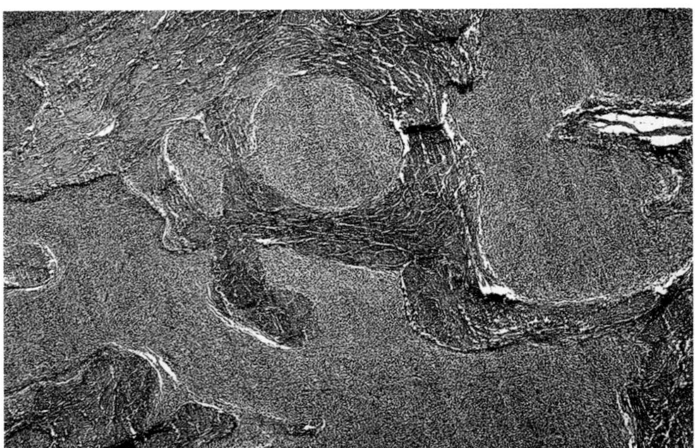

Fig. 19.153 Typical low-power appearance of endometrial stromal sarcoma.

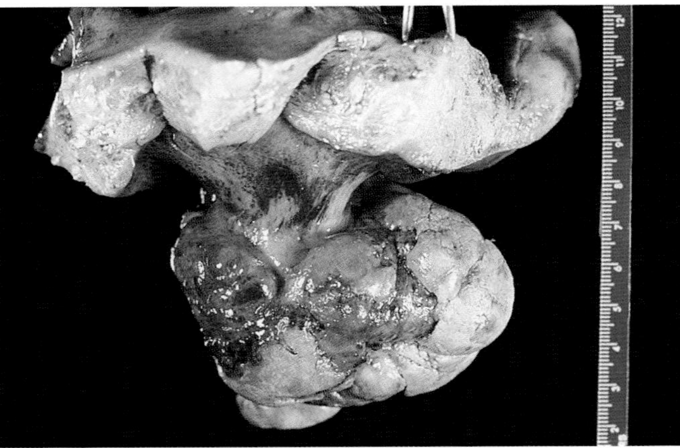

Fig. 19.154 Low-grade endometrial stromal sarcoma presenting as a huge polypoid mass within the endometrial cavity. This pattern of growth is unusual in this tumor type.

local invasion may extend into the broad ligament, tubes, and ovaries. Their low-power appearance is very distinctive, in the sense of showing extensive myometrial permeation by sharply defined tumor islands with pointed edges, somewhat reminiscent of those seen (in an altogether different context) in thymoma.

The proposal had been made to subdivide endometrial stromal sarcoma into low-grade and high-grade types on the basis of their mitotic count (<10 versus ≥10 mitoses/10 high-power fields (HPF), respectively), after a substantial difference in outcome between the two groups was noted.[685] However, more recent and larger series have not supported such a sharp distinction, the tendency at present being to designate the whole group as endometrial stromal sarcoma, to regard mitotic activity as one of the morphologic factors to evaluate for prognostic purposes, and to reserve the term high-grade endometrial sarcoma for an altogether different tumor, although exceptionally one will evolve into the other.[687]

Thus defined, the natural history of endometrial stromal sarcoma is characterized by slow clinical progression, repeated local recurrences (in the pelvis, ovary, intestinal wall, other intra-abdominal sites, and anterior abdominal wall), and occasional metastases[632] (Figs 19.155 and 19.156). A remarkable case has been described involving the placenta.[665]

Size of the tumor, extrauterine extension, and mitotic activity are important prognostic features. Stromal neoplasms less than 4 cm in diameter practically never recur, and tumors confined to the uterus at the time of the initial surgery very rarely do so, regardless of the category to which they belong. As already indicated, there is a relationship between mitotic activity and outcome, but this does not seem to be as significant as previously believed.[642] DNA ploidy analysis is also thought to have prognostic significance.[636,654,661]

A particularly interesting and difficult issue concerns the relationship and differential diagnosis between endometrial stromal tumors and smooth muscle tumors (not too surprising considering their histogenetic closeness), as already hinted at by the fact that even in non-neoplastic conditions one can see foci of smooth muscle 'metaplasia' in the endometrial stroma and foci of endometrial stroma (not connected to adenomyosis) in the myometrium. Regarding the differential diagnosis, which is mainly with the epithelioid cellular variant of smooth muscle tumors, features that favor a diagnosis of endometrial stromal tumor are: multinodular pattern of growth, spiral-type arterioles (some with hyalinized walls), lack or inconspicuousness of large thick-walled vessels and cleft-like spaces, immunoreactivity for CD10, and lack of reactivity for h-caldesmon, desmin, and oxytocin receptor.[643,653,676,686,691] Genetically, about 50% of cases show t(7;17) with *JAZF1–JJAZ1* fusion (identical to that seen in endometrial stromal nodule, but differ in showing concurrent silencing of the unrearranged *JJAZ1* allele), and about 6% of

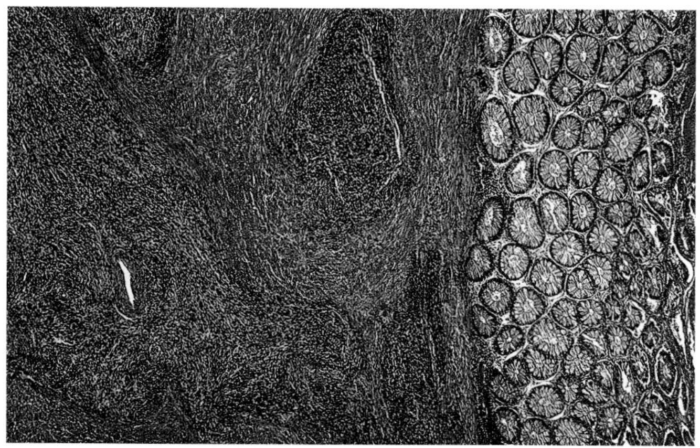

Fig. 19.155 Endometrial stromal sarcoma metastatic to wall of large bowel.

cases show t(6;7) with *JAZF1–PHF1* fusion.[648,672] These genetic findings may be utilized to aid in the diagnosis of endometrial stromal sarcoma by using fluorescent in situ hybridization (FISH) or reverse transcriptase-polymerase chain reaction (RT-PCR).

A related issue concerns the fact that a certain number of mesenchymal uterine tumors show features of *both* endometrial stromal and smooth muscle differentiation. If the latter is present in the form of an inconspicuous focus in the midst of an otherwise typical endometrial stromal tumor, it can be ignored for diagnostic purposes.[705] If sizable (one-third or more of the tumor mass), the neoplasm is referred to as **combined smooth muscle–stromal tumor**;[688,702] this is probably equivalent to the (*nodular*) *stromomyoma* of the older literature.[694,701] The areas featuring the smooth muscle component often show collagen deposition with a characteristic 'starburst' pattern. Behaviorally, these tumors seem to be closer to endometrial stromal than to smooth muscle tumors, and – on the whole – very indolent.[688] A further variation on the theme is represented by the exceptional case exhibiting both smooth and skeletal muscle differentiation; it is important not to confuse this lesion with a malignant mixed müllerian tumor.[638,675]

Epithelial-like formations may appear in endometrial stromal tumors in the form of solid masses, glandular structures, or anastomosing cords. Some of these formations have been likened to those of ovarian sex-cord neoplasms (particularly granulosa cell tumors) and the tumors containing them have been referred to as **uterine tumors resembling ovarian sex-cord tumors (UTROSCT)**[644,646] (Fig. 19.157A). Some cases feature an epithelial retiform component resembling rete ovarii.[684] Their immunohistochemical and ultrastructural profile has varied considerably in the reported series, ranging from myogenous to epithelial.[674] However, at least some of the cases have shown a phenotype consistent indeed with a sex-cord line of differentiation, including reactivity for inhibin, CD99, and melan-A.[637,647,662,668] Uterine tumors in which these structures predominate to almost the exclusion of others (Type II UTROSCT)

Fig. 19.156 **A** and **B**, Low- and high-power appearance of endometrial stromal sarcoma metastatic to lung. This lesion may be misdiagnosed as spindle carcinoid tumor, hemangiopericytoma, or solitary fibrous tumor.

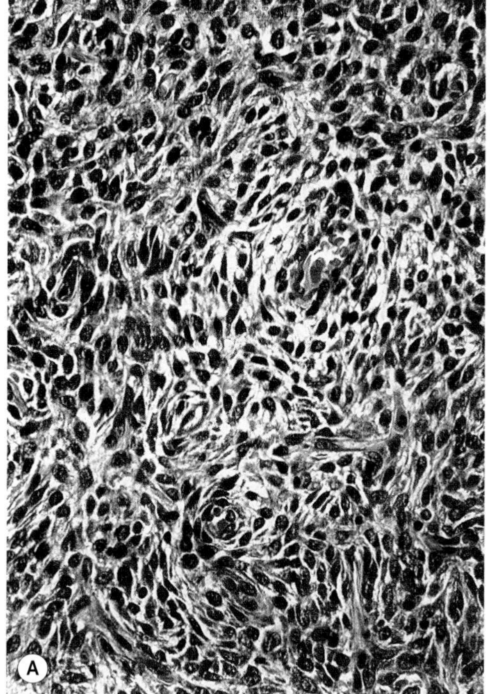

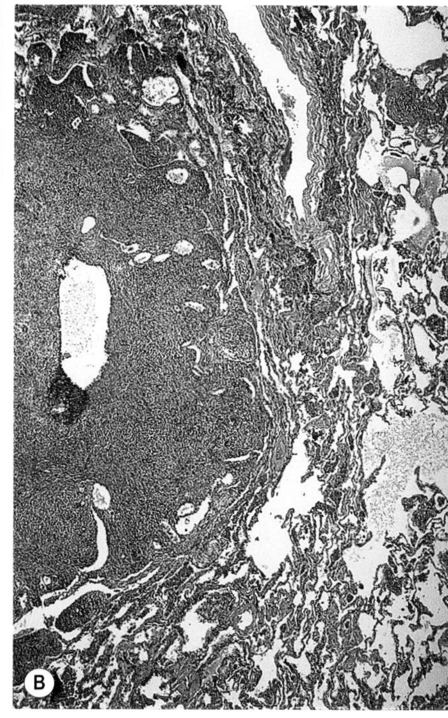

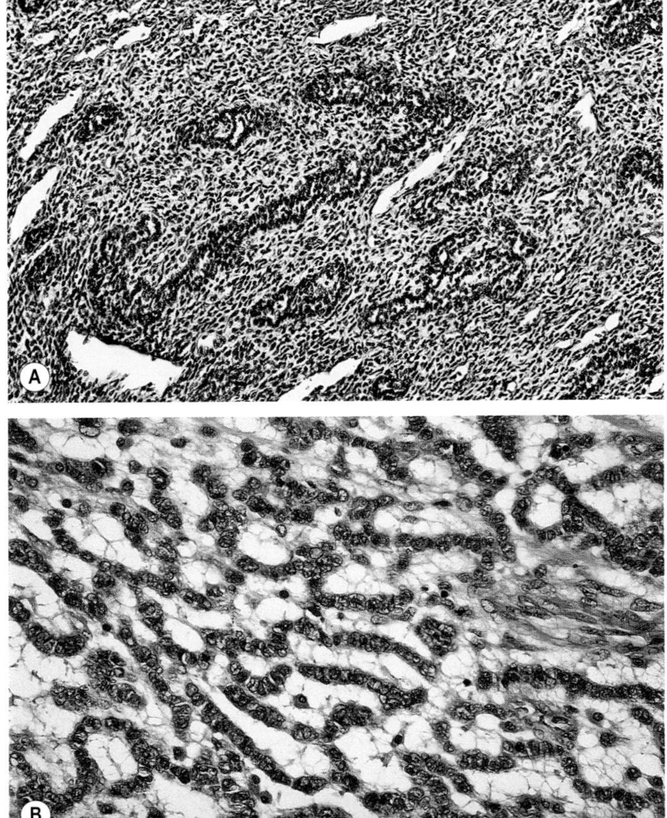

Fig. 19.157 **A**, Endometrial stromal sarcoma with structures resembling ovarian sex cord tumors. **B**, So-called 'plexiform tumor' of the uterus. This lesion is probably related to endometrial stromal neoplasms, but its histogenesis is still controversial.

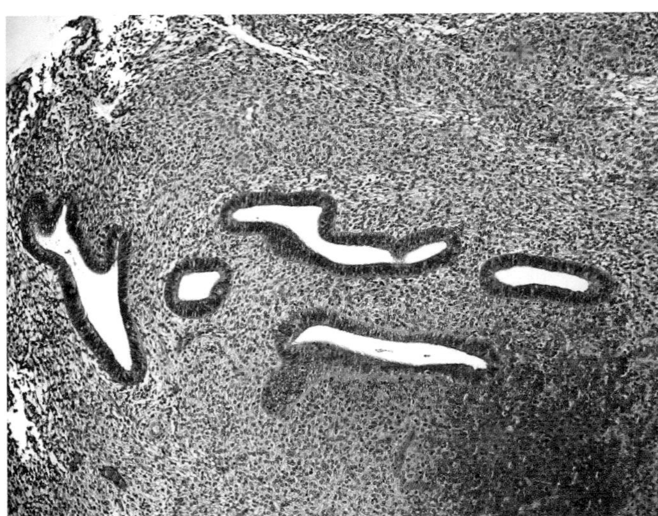

Fig. 19.158 Peritoneal metastasis from endometrial stromal sarcoma accompanied by benign endometrioid glands.

have generally behaved in a benign fashion,[644] but occasional metastasizing examples are on record.[641]

The uterine neoplasm known as **plexiform tumor** or **tumorlet**, and variously claimed to be of endometrial stromal,[671] myofibroblastic,[658] and smooth muscle derivation,[660,664] is a closely related variation, and it is, therefore, not surprising that similar histogenetic arguments have been raised (Fig. 19.157B). The ultrastructural[660] and immunohistochemical evidence (including actin and desmin positivity[639,671]) points toward a sex-cord-like nature with myoid features.[683] This lesion is always an incidental finding; it usually measures less than 1 cm and its behavior is always benign.

A different type of epithelium-like formation that can be seen in endometrial stromal tumor is represented by **endometrioid glandular foci** having a benign, atypical, or carcinomatous appearance[645,678] (Fig. 19.158).

Exceptionally, an endometrial stromal tumor may be seen in a uterus that also contains an endometrial adenocarcinoma. As a matter of fact, the two tumors can collide with each other.[670] It is important not to misinterpret this phenomenon as a malignant mixed müllerian tumor.

Tumors with the appearance of endometrial stromal neoplasms may be found in the cervix,[680] ovary (see p. 1605), pelvis, and retroperitoneum.[704] Some of these are seen in association with endometriosis, from which presumably they have arisen.[698] These extrauterine tumors may have any of the morphologic features and variations described in connection with the uterine neoplasms, including ovarian sex cord-like structures and endometrioid glandular proliferation.[673]

A note of caution is in order. Before making a diagnosis of primary extrauterine endometrial stromal tumor, one should make an effort to rule out a metastasis from a uterine lesion, knowing that these metastases are often solitary and that they can occur years or decades after the excision of the original tumor, which (to complicate things further) might have been misdiagnosed as a peculiar-looking smooth muscle tumor.[635,667] We have seen many such cases in several locations, mainly lung but also intestinal wall, retroperitoneum, and even deep soft tissues of extremity, in which diagnoses of hemangiopericytoma, monophasic synovial sarcoma, solitary fibrous tumor, lymphangioleiomyomatosis, and mesenchymal cystic hamartoma were made.[663] Clues to the diagnosis are the multinodularity as seen on very low power, the uniformly bland appearance of the oval tumor cells, the presence of spiral arteriole-like vessels, and the deposition of coarse collagen fibers among the tumor cells.[689] Immunohistochemical reactivity for estrogen and progesterone receptors and for CD10 will provide confirmatory evidence. The best protection against missing this diagnosis is simply to think about the entity when it occurs in an unexpected place, a situation to which Dr Lauren V. Ackerman used to refer as 'the man from Istanbul'.[693]

Poorly differentiated endometrial (stromal) sarcoma, also known as 'undifferentiated endometrial sarcoma', shows a marked degree of nuclear pleomorphism and atypicality, and lacks the vascular pattern and other distinctive features of endometrial stromal sarcoma (Fig. 19.159). It is an altogether different neoplasm, which behaves in a very aggressive manner and which may actually have a closer relationship to malignant mixed müllerian tumor, the sarcoma-like component of which it greatly resembles.[649,655,657,669,706]

Malignant mixed müllerian tumor (carcinosarcoma)

Malignant mixed müllerian tumors (MMMTs) are practically always seen in postmenopausal patients, although exceptions

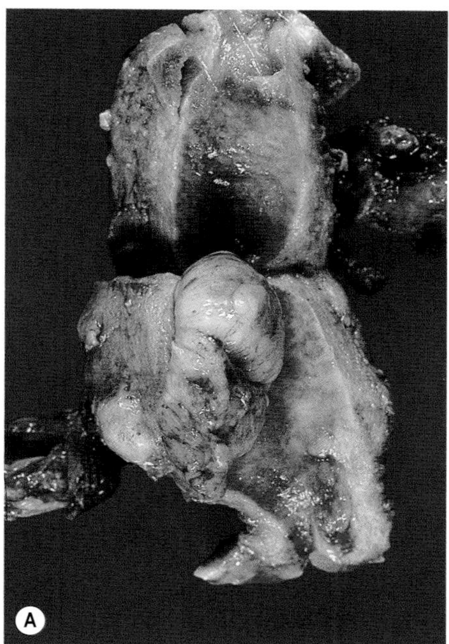

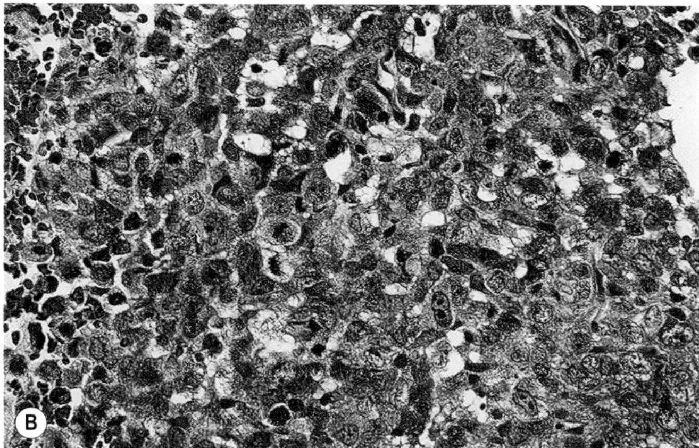

Fig. 19.159 **A** and **B**, Gross and microscopic appearance of high-grade endometrial sarcoma.

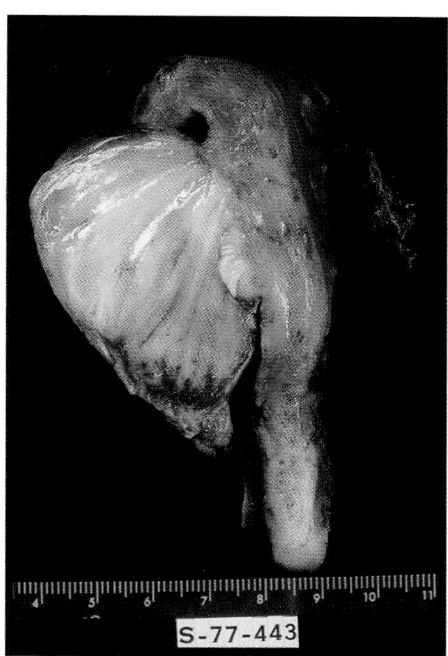

Fig. 19.160 Malignant mixed müllerian tumor of uterus resulting in a huge polypoid mass.

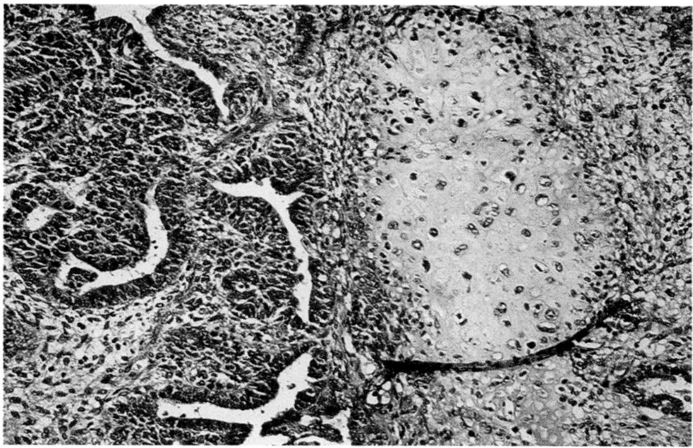

Fig. 19.161 Glandular and mesenchymal components of malignant mixed müllerian tumor. Heterologous elements in the form of cartilage are present.

occur.[711] They present with uterine bleeding and enlargement. Their most common location is the posterior uterine wall in the region of the fundus.[708,734,736] Grossly, they present as large, soft, polypoid growths involving the endometrium and myometrium, sometimes protruding from the cervix (Fig. 19.160). Foci of necrosis and hemorrhage are common.

Microscopically, the distinctive feature of MMMTs is the *admixture of carcinomatous and sarcoma-like elements*, resulting in a characteristic biphasic appearance. The carcinomatous component is usually of glandular type, whether endometrioid, clear cell, or papillary serous (particularly the latter).[741] As a rule, it has a poorly differentiated appearance and is of a high-grade nature; therefore, a careful search for stromal elements should be carried out whenever such patterns are found in an endometrial biopsy, particularly if accompanied by extensive necrosis and hemorrhage. Squamous cell, undifferentiated, and primitive neuroectodermal patterns may also be seen.[725,747] Cases have also been described with melanocytic[707] and yolk sac differentiation.[740]

The appearance of the sarcomatous component is the basis for the time-honored division of these neoplasms into a *homologous* and a *heterologous* variety. In the former, the malignant stroma is composed either of round cells resembling those of the endometrial stroma or of spindle cells resembling leiomyosarcoma or fibrosarcoma. In the latter, specific heterologous mesenchymal elements (such as skeletal muscle, cartilage, bone, or adipose tissue) are also present (Fig. 19.161). Identification of cross striations, or of skeletal muscle markers by immunocytochemistry, is required to document the presence of a rhabdomyosarcomatous component (Fig. 19.162). In some cases this component is so prominent as to overgrow the epithelial elements and to mimic a pure rhabdomyosarcoma.[716] Conversely, the sarcoma-like component may be so

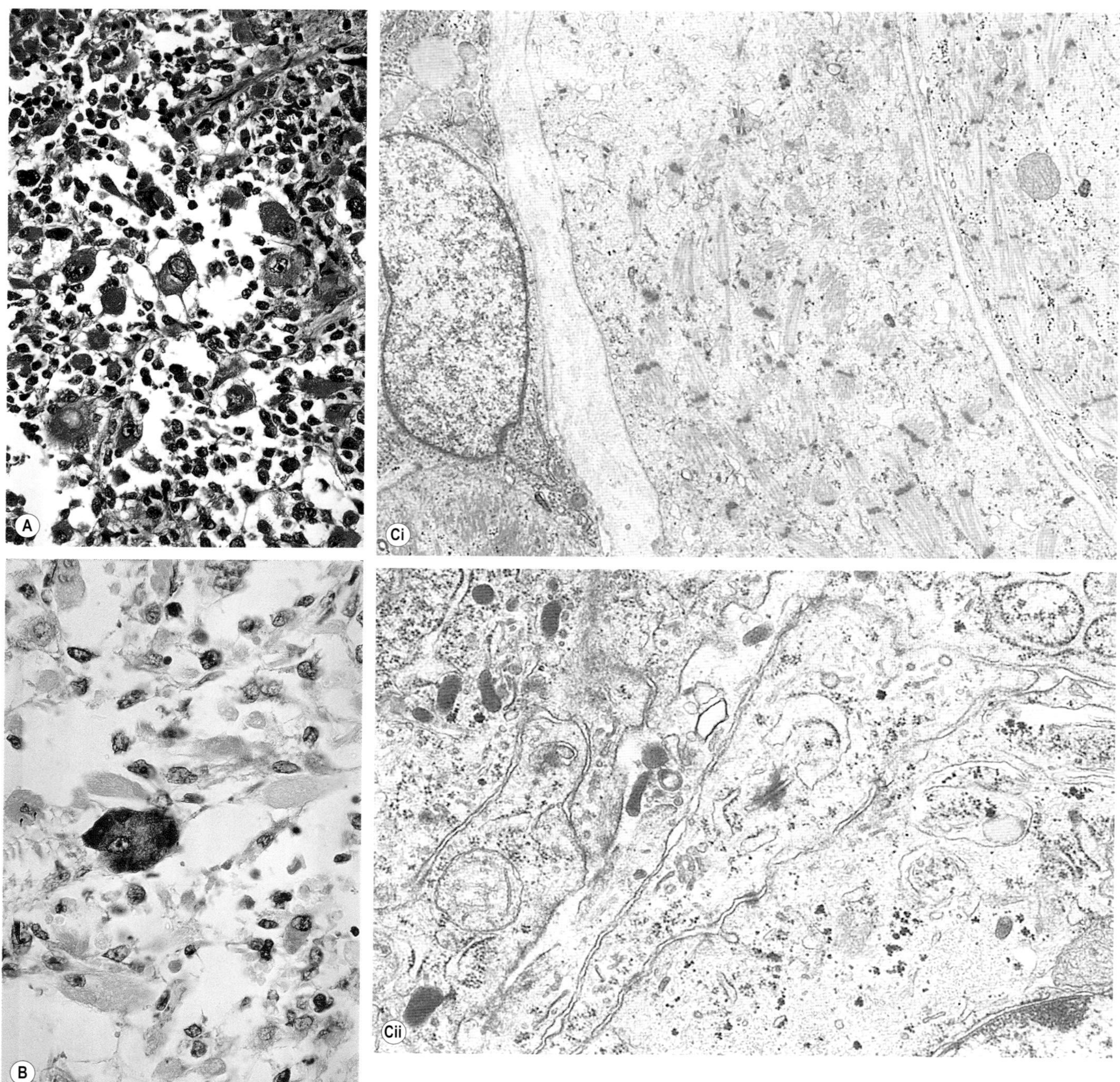

Fig. 19.162 Skeletal muscle elements in malignant mixed müllerian tumor, seen on H&E stain (**A**) and following immunostaining for myoglobin (**B**). **C**, Malignant mixed müllerian tumor. **C(i)**: Area of rhabdomyosarcomatous differentiation. Note Z-band formation. **C(ii)**: Area showing epithelial differentiation; paranuclear microfilaments similar to those of endometrioid endometrial carcinoma are present.

inconspicuous in such a specimen as to be missed altogether, the lesion being misdiagnosed as an ordinary adenocarcinoma. This is particularly the case for the peritoneal metastases, in which the sarcoma-like component is often scanty or altogether absent. Since the epithelial elements can form papillae, be accompanied by psammoma bodies, and have all the other features of papillary serous carcinoma, a confusion with metastatic ovarian carcinoma may occur. Parenthetically, cases have been reported of coexistent uterine MMMT and ovarian serous adenocarcinoma.[729] Exceptionally, a rhabdoid component is present.[733]

The fact that the epithelial component of an MMMT is the one showing the greatest capability for invasion and metastases – also indirectly indicated by its greater microvessel density when compared with the sarcoma-like component[718,748] – suggests that these tumors should be primarily regarded as carcinomas rather than sarcomas, employing a reasoning analogous to that currently accepted for carcinomas with sarcoma-like stroma of the upper aerodigestive tract and other sites.[709,741,744] Immunohistochemical and ultrastructural studies support this view: keratin is always detectable in the epithelial areas, but is also present in the sarcomatous component in over half of the cases;[724] by electron microscopy, hybrid epithelial/stromal cells coexist with those having purely epithelial or stromal features.[714,731] An additional supportive finding is the concordant pattern of P53 staining and type of mutation in the carcinomatous and sarcomatous areas, which would be difficult to explain if these tumors were biclonal.[713,728,730] Other markers that have been encountered in MMMTs are CD10 (in the sarcoma-like component)[732] and HER2/*neu*.[712]

MMMTs are easily distinguished from teratomas by their occurrence in an older age group and by the absence of skin appendages, glia, thyroid, and other tissues; however, as already noted, they may exceptionally contain neuroectodermal elements.[725] They should also be clearly separated from botryoid rhabdomyosarcoma (sarcoma botryoides). The latter term should be reserved for the tumor of childhood or adolescence arising from the cervix or vagina that exhibits skeletal muscle differentiation but lacks a carcinomatous component.

MMMTs are highly aggressive neoplasms, perhaps more so than even the higher grades and the more unfavorable variants of endometrial carcinoma.[723] Extension into the pelvis, lymphatic and vascular permeation, and distant lymph-borne and blood-borne metastases are all common. If the tumor has extended to the serosa of the uterus or beyond at the time of surgery, the prognosis is very poor. The only patients with a significant chance of cure are those in whom the tumor is restricted to the inner half of the myometrium at the time of surgery.[721] This determination implies a thorough sampling of the hysterectomy specimen by the pathologist. Unfortunately, over one-half of these patients will harbor occult metastatic disease.[719,746]

In several series, tumors having only homologous stromal elements have been found to have a better prognosis than those with heterologous elements.[721,734,736,738] It should be pointed out, however, that the difference between the two is generally small, in some series absent altogether, and far outweighed by the stage of the disease.[710,722,743] Taking everything into account, we need to conclude once again that staging remains the most important predictor of prognosis.[726] Abdominal hysterectomy with bilateral salpingo-oophorectomy and pelvic lymphadenectomy is the treatment of choice, usually followed by adjuvant therapy. The response to radiation therapy and chemotherapy has been generally poor, although some encouraging reports have appeared.[727] The most common sites of recurrent disease are lung and abdominal cavity.[742]

Norris and Taylor[735] made the disturbing observation that 30% of patients with heterologous MMMTs and 13% of those with homologous tumors that they studied had a history of previous irradiation to the pelvic area, usually given for some benign disorder. The median interval between irradiation and the time of diagnosis of the tumor was 16.4 years, both in their series and in that of Doss et al.[717] Postirradiation uterine sarcomas tend to occur in a younger age group and spread earlier to the pelvis than comparable tumors not related to irradiation.[720,745]

MMMTs and other sarcoma-like malignant uterine tumors have also been seen in association with chronic estrogenic stimulation (ovarian thecoma, polycystic ovarian disease, and prolonged estrogen therapy).[737]

MMMTs can arise in extrauterine locations, the most common sites being ovary and pelvic structures. Their morphologic and immunohistochemical features are similar to those of their more common uterine counterparts.[715,739]

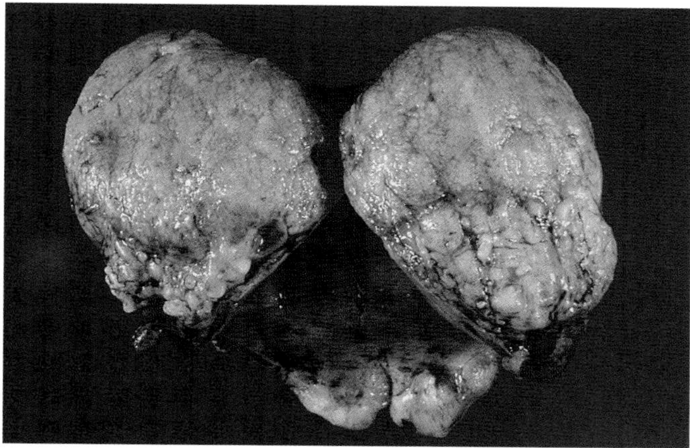

Fig. 19.163 Müllerian adenosarcoma. The tumor shows a lesser degree of necrosis and hemorrhage than the usual malignant mixed müllerian tumor.

Müllerian adenosarcoma and related tumors

Müllerian adenosarcoma is a distinctive type of uterine tumor, traditionally regarded as a low-grade variant of MMMT.[751,754,763] Like the latter, it usually presents in elderly individuals as a bulky polypoid growth filling the endometrial cavity, less commonly as an intramural nodule (Fig. 19.163). Microscopically, it is also composed of an admixture of epithelial and stromal elements. Its distinguishing feature is the fact that the epithelial (glandular) component appears benign, giving to the lesion a sometimes striking similarity to phylloides tumor of the breast (Fig. 19.164). The stromal elements usually resemble endometrial stroma by light and electron microscopic examination.[759,764] As a rule, they do not appear as bizarre and undifferentiated as in the classic MMMT, although multinucleated giant cells and heterologous elements occur in approximately 20% of cases. The latter are usually of skeletal muscle type, but peculiar components such as angiosarcoma have also been observed.[749,765] Extensive areas of stromal fibrosis may result in a deceptively benign appearance.[754]

We view müllerian adenosarcomas not as a type of MMMT but rather as a variant of endometrial stromal sarcoma having the capacity to induce the formation and/or proliferation of glands. Support for this interpretation comes from several pieces of evidence: (1) their extremely similar immunohistochemical profile;[770] (2) the fact that smooth muscle metaplasia and sex cord-like differentiation (two well-known features of endometrial stromal sarcomas) have occasionally been found in them;[753,757,761] and (3) the occurrence of cases in which a typical adenosarcoma is overgrown by a pure sarcoma having a higher grade and exhibiting a greater mitotic rate than the sarcomatous component of the associated adenosarcoma (Fig. 19.165). This latter development is analogous to that well known to occur in phylloides tumor of the breast, a fact that strengthens the analogy between the two entities. These *müllerian adenosarcomas with sarcomatous overgrowth* behave in an aggressive fashion and are often associated with postoperative recurrence or metastases and a fatal outcome.[750,763]

Cases of müllerian adenosarcoma have been reported in association with tamoxifen therapy.[756] Also of interest is the report of a cluster of cases of uterine müllerian adenosarcomas with sarcomatous overgrowth that was detected years ago in the Washington, DC, metropolitan area.[768]

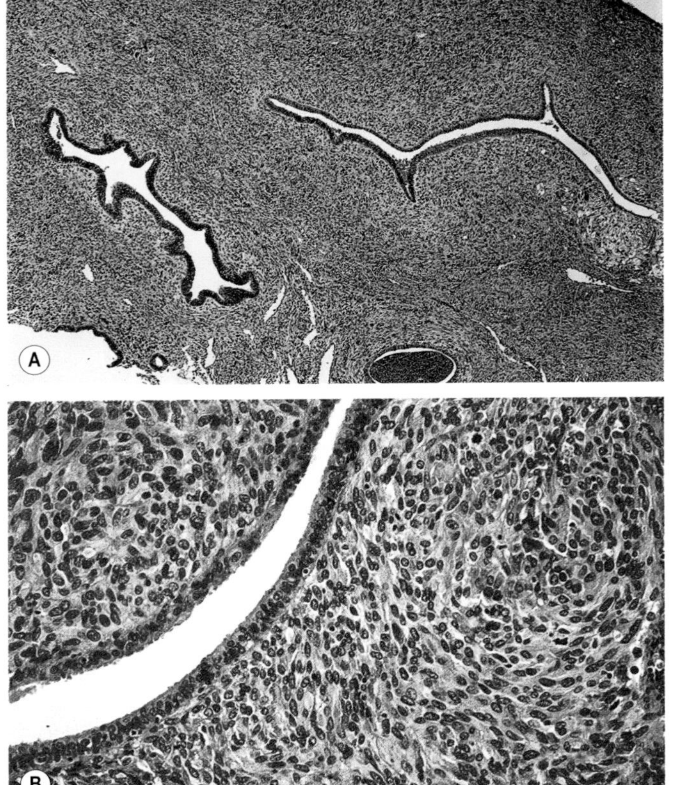

Fig. 19.164 **A** and **B**, Low- and high-power view of müllerian adenosarcoma. The resemblance to phylloides tumor of breast is obvious.

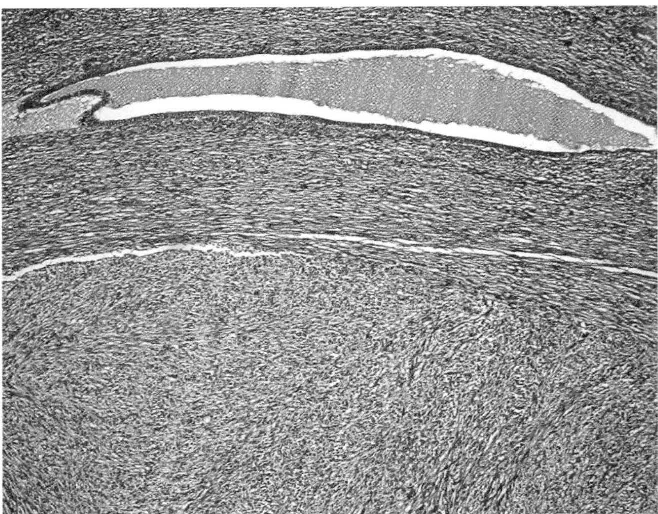

Fig. 19.165 Müllerian adenosarcoma (top) with sarcomatous overgrowth (bottom).

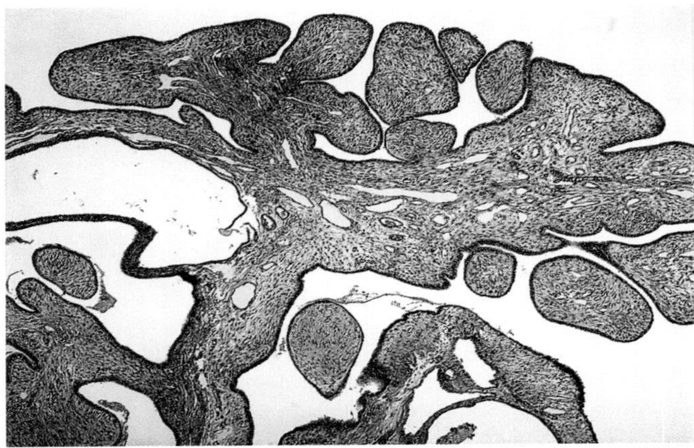

Fig. 19.166 Papillary adenofibroma of uterus. This lesion represents the lower end of the müllerian adenosarcoma spectrum.

Uterine adenofibroma and the related conditions papillary adenofibroma, papillary cystadenofibroma, lipoadenofibroma, and adenomyomatosis[760,762,769,772,773] have been traditionally regarded as the benign counterparts of müllerian adenosarcoma, but the dividing line between the two groups is anything but sharp.[758] (Fig. 19.166). As a matter of fact, tumors with the characteristic features of uterine adenofibroma have occasionally been found to invade myometrium and pelvic veins.[755] The problems in separating them are analogous to those encountered in trying to separate benign from malignant phylloides tumors of the breast. Criteria found to be useful in distinguishing müllerian adenosarcomas from müllerian adenofibromas include two or more stromal mitoses per 10 HPF, marked stromal cellularity, and significant stromal cell atypia.[751] Cases have been reported of papillary adenofibroma involved by adenocarcinoma.[766]

Like MMMTs and endometrial stromal sarcomas, müllerian adenosarcomas can arise outside the uterine corpus. Cases have been described in the cervix, ovary, round and broad ligaments, and pelvic wall.[752,771]

A tumor purported to be the morphologic counterpart of müllerian adenosarcoma – i.e., composed of malignant epithelium and benign stroma – has been reported under terms such as *müllerian carcinofibroma* or *carcinomesenchymoma*.[767] The analogy is ingenious but probably unwarranted.

Leiomyoma

Leiomyomas of the uterus are extremely common neoplasms. The overall incidence is between 4% and 11%, but it rises to nearly 40% in women over the age of 50 years. Clinically apparent lesions are less common in parous than nulliparous women and premenopausal than postmenopausal women.[801] They are known to shrink after menopause; this is associated both with fibrosis and with a reduction in the size of the individual tumor cells.[779,780] The normal myometrium of leiomyoma-containing uteri expresses higher levels of estrogen receptors, a fact that may be related to their pathogenesis.[804] Leiomyomas are much more common in black women, in whom they have a tendency to be very numerous (Fig. 19.167).

Many of these tumors are small and go undetected; a systematic and meticulous study of 100 consecutive hysterectomy specimens revealed leiomyomas in 77 of them, 84% of the tumors being multicentric.[778]

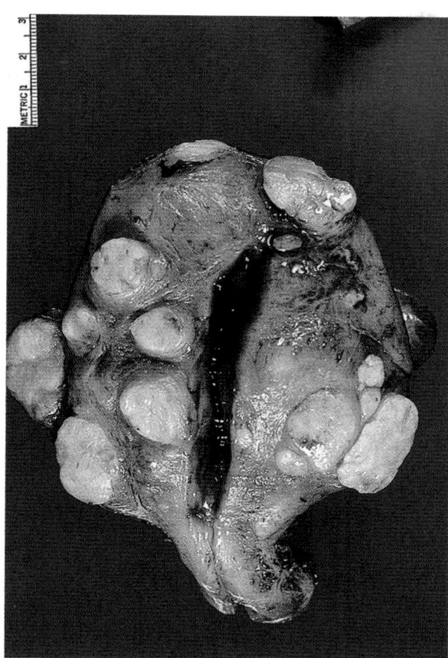

Fig. 19.167 Multiple uterine leiomyomas.

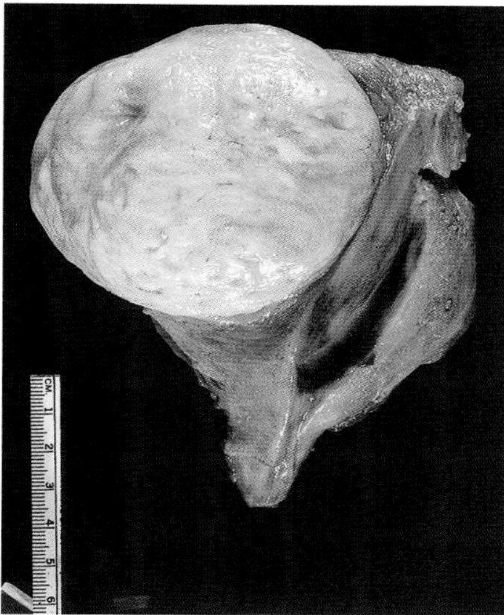

Fig. 19.168 Large uterine leiomyoma with intramural and subserous involvement.

These tumors occur subserosally, intramurally, or submucosally (Fig. 19.168) and produce symptoms referable to their size and location. The conventional teaching (which, like most conventional teachings, is only partially true) is that the submucous tumors produce metrorrhagia (because of endometrial ulceration), the intramural ones result in menorrhagia (because they interfere with myometrial contraction), and the subserosal ones usually remain asymptomatic. They may become large enough to block the ureters, interfere with pregnancy, or cause inflammatory complications. In rare instances, uterine leiomyomas have been associated with polycythemia, which regressed after the tumor was excised ('myomatous erythrocytosis syndrome').[798] These tumors, which are usually very large, have been shown to be the source of erythropoietin.[803]

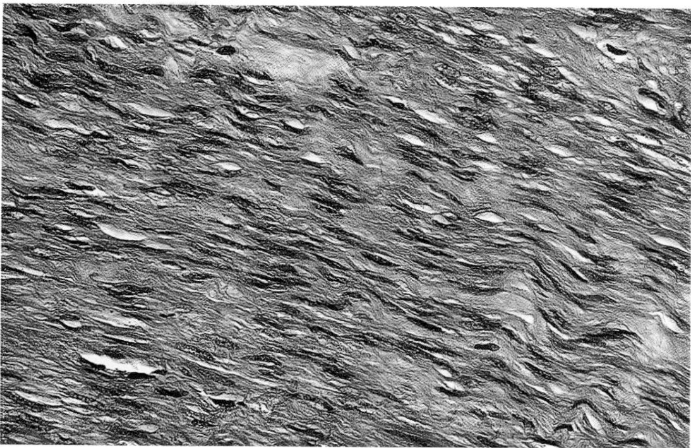

Fig. 19.169 Elongated spindle cells with fibrillary acidophilic cytoplasm in the usual type of uterine leiomyoma.

Submucosal tumors often result in secondary endometrial changes that range from gland distortion to atrophy and ulceration. They may fill the endometrial cavity and emerge from the cervical canal as polypoid growths ('myoma nascens'). Under these circumstances, their surface is usually ulcerated and infected, the gross appearance thus simulating that of a malignant neoplasm.

It is difficult to make a diagnosis of leiomyoma when only a few small fragments of smooth muscle are present in a curettage specimen. Unless these fragments show an obvious increase in cellularity or definite hyaline changes, one is unable in most instances to decide whether they originated in a submucosal leiomyoma or whether they represent normal superficial myometrium curetted out by a vigorous operator.

Grossly, the cut surface of a typical leiomyoma has a raw silk appearance. Microscopically, the tumor is formed by interlacing bundles of smooth muscle cells separated by a greater or lesser amount of well-vascularized connective tissue (Fig. 19.169). Ultrastructurally, the features are those of smooth muscle cells with varying degrees of differentiation.[789] Exceptionally, the tumors may contain skeletal muscle-like cells (which, however, lack cross striations and are myogenin negative; see also under Leiomyoma variants) and rhabdoid cells.[802] The stroma may contain a scattering of lymphocytes. Mast cells are often conspicuous, in contrast with leiomyomas of other sites.[791,795] On average, they are more numerous in cellular and bizarre leiomyomas than in either ordinary leiomyomas or leiomyosarcomas.[800]

Cytogenetic alterations are common in uterine leiomyomas. The most consistent are rearrangements of 6p (involving the *HMGA1* gene), del(7q), +12 (involving the *HMGA2* gene), and t(12;14) (involving the *HMGA2* gene).[781,785,792,799] These have led to the discovery that disruptions or dysregulations of the high-mobility proteins HMGA1 and HMGA2 contribute to the development of these tumors.[788,793]

The treatment of uterine leiomyomas (including that of most of the many variants listed later) varies depending on the size and number of lesions, the age of the patient, and her desire to have children. Most asymptomatic leiomyomas need not be excised. Malignant transformation is such a rare event in these tumors that for practical purposes it can be disregarded.[797] Symptomatic neoplasms can be treated by hysterectomy or, in the case of patients who desire to become pregnant, by myomectomy.[775] Medical therapy includes administration of gonadotropin-releasing hormone analogs, such as leuprolide acetate depot. This may result in a decrease in the size of the leiomyoma – probably as a result of ischemic injury and cellular atrophy[782] – but it does not result in significant pleomorphism or increased mitotic activity.[776,783,784,805] The decrease in cell size and increase in collagenization have also been documented at the ultrastructural level.[787] Other authors have reported tumor infiltration by lymphocytes of predominantly T-cell type[774,790] and vasculitis.[796] Immunohistochemically, leuprolide-treated leiomyomas show a decrease in cell proliferation indices and in hormone receptor expression.[806]

Another treatment modality for uterine leiomyoma is arterial embolization with tris-acryl gelatin microspheres.[807] This results in massive necrosis, sometimes accompanied by calcification, thrombosis, and a foreign body-type reaction to the injected material.[777,794] Infarct-type necrosis has also been observed in uterine leiomyomas of women treated with tranexamic acid, an antifibrinolytic agent.[786]

Leiomyoma variants

Many variations on the basic theme previously described exist. Most of these are the result of secondary changes and are detectable in approximately 65% of cases. These include hyaline degeneration (63%), myxoid changes (19%), calcification (8%), cystic changes (4%), and fatty metamorphosis (3%). There is no relation between symptomatology and the presence of these changes.[862]

Red degeneration (present in 3% of cases) can result in abdominal pain, vomiting, and fever. This change is characterized grossly by a bulging surface and a homogeneous dark red appearance, and microscopically by extensive coagulative necrosis. It is often associated with pregnancy or the use of contraceptive drugs (Fig. 19.170).

Apoplectic leiomyoma is pathogenetically related to red degeneration. It is seen in patients taking birth-control pills and is characterized by stellate zones of recent hemorrhage within nodules of hypercellular smooth muscle, with few or no mitotic figures.[855] Many variations on this basic theme exist, some of which can simulate malignancy.[844]

Hydropic degeneration is characterized by the accumulation of edema fluid, often associated with collagen deposition. It may have a diffuse, perinodular, or other patterns[820,821] (Figs 19.171 and 19.172). The appearance may simulate intravenous leiomyomatosis or myxoid leiomyosarcoma.[820] Regarding the latter, leiomyomas with hydropic degeneration have a delicate filigree pattern rather than thick fascicles, and the extracellular material is edema fluid rather than mucopolysaccharides.

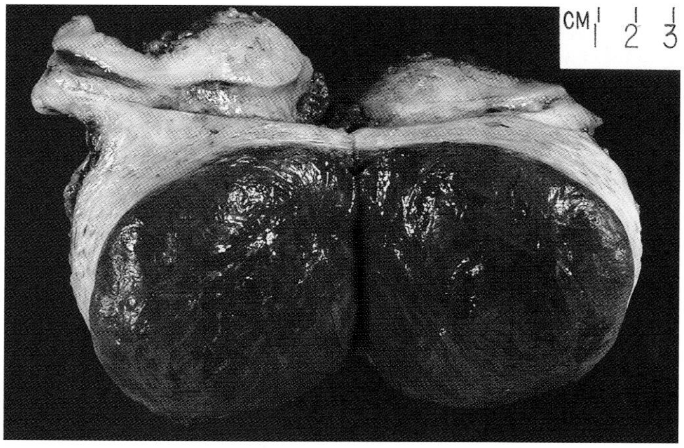

Fig. 19.170 This uterine leiomyoma has undergone massive so-called red degeneration.

Myxoid leiomyoma must be distinguished from both hydropic degeneration and myxoid leiomyosarcoma. The latter is identified because of the presence of destructive myometrial invasion and the conventional features of malignancy.[843]

Leiomyoma with lymphoid infiltration may simulate a malignant lymphoma because of the massiveness of the inflammatory component, which is made up of small lymphocytes, immunoblasts, and plasma cells.[813] Germinal centers may be present. The surrounding myometrium is relatively unaffected.[830,833] A variation on the theme is represented by the leiomyomas with a heavy infiltration by eosinophils.[874] Some of these leiomyomas with infiltration by inflammatory cells had been treated with leuprolide.

Cellular leiomyoma is a term reserved for those tumors having increased cellularity but no coagulative necrosis, atypia, or an excessive number of mitotic figures (Fig. 19.173). Their natural history seems to be the same as for the ordinary leiomyoma. The differential diagnosis includes leiomyosarcoma and endometrial stromal neoplasms.[861] At the cytogenetic level, cellular leiomyoma has been

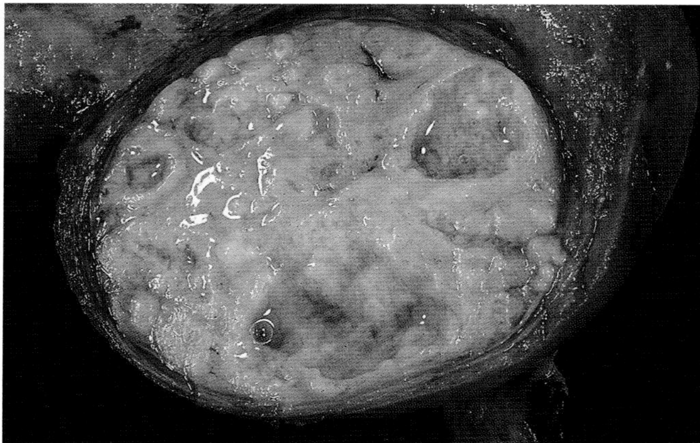

Fig. 19.171 Leiomyoma with edematous (hydropic) changes leading to the formation of cystic cavities.
(Courtesy of Dr Pedro J Grases Galofré; from Grases Galofré PJ. Patología ginecológica. Bases para el diagnóstico morfológico. Barcelona, 2002, Masson)

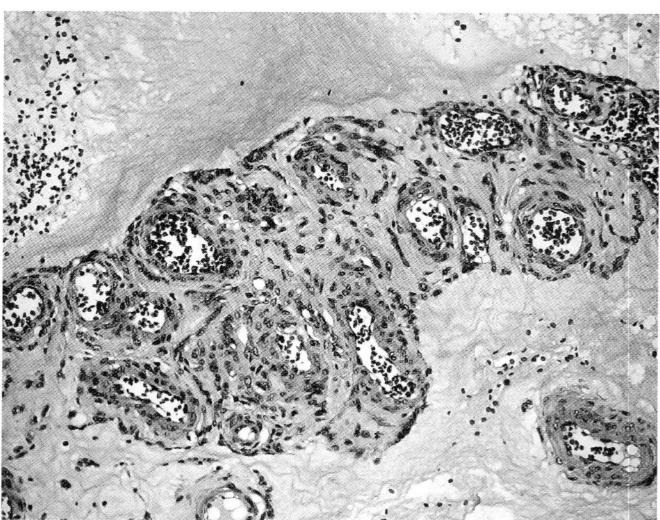

Fig. 19.172 So-called 'perinodular hydropic degeneration' in uterine leiomyoma.

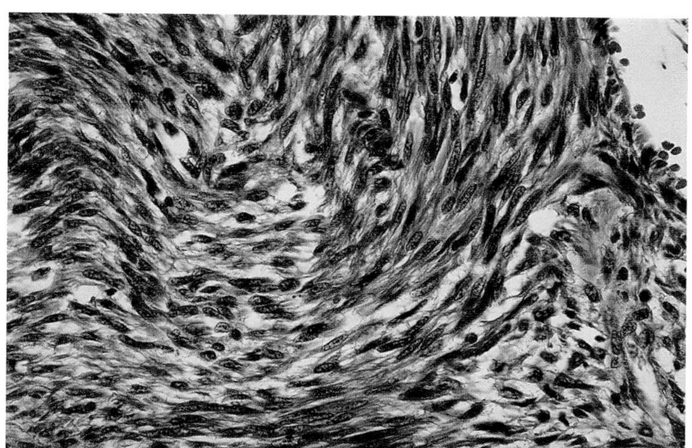

Fig. 19.173 Cellular leiomyoma. There is no pleomorphism, undue mitotic activity, or necrosis.

found to be accompanied by loss of almost the entire short arm of chromosome 1.[825]

Atypical, bizarre, symplasmic (symplastic), or pleomorphic leiomyoma contains bizarre tumor cells with variation in size and shape, hyperchromatic nuclei, and multinucleated forms but no coagulative necrosis or increased mitotic activity (Fig. 19.174).[827] Rarely, the entire tumor is composed of such cells. It may occur spontaneously but is often seen in patients taking progestin compounds.[829,864] The usual assumption has been that the symplasmic cells represent a degenerative phenomenon, but they have been shown to be actively proliferating.[872]

Mitotically active leiomyoma refers to tumors having from 5 to 15 mitotic figures per 10 HPF but lacking coagulative necrosis or cytologic atypia[860,865] (Fig. 19.175). They are discussed in more detail on page 1516.

Granular cell change may exceptionally develop in uterine leiomyoma. We have seen a case of multiple small myometrial tumors exhibiting this alteration. Ultrastructural study left no doubt as to the smooth muscle nature of the tumors on one hand, and the presence of lysosome-like granular cell changes on the other.

Leiomyolipoma (lipoleiomyoma) contains an admixture of smooth muscle and mature adipose tissue[838,863,866,875] (Fig. 19.176). It is believed that some of these tumors and the even rarer **lipomas** result from adipose metaplasia in leiomyomas.[863,871] The differential diagnosis includes adipose tissue-rich angiomyolipomas (PEComas), which are HMB-45 positive (see below).[809] Cases have been reported of liposarcomas developing from lipomyolipomas.[849] A further variation on the theme is the **adenolipoleiomyoma**, a tumor of obscure histogenesis which can exhibit an aggressive behavior.[847,870]

Palisaded leiomyoma is characterized by a degree of nuclear palisading such as to simulate a schwannoma.[818]

Epithelioid (clear cell) leiomyoma (benign leiomyoblastoma) is partially or totally composed of rounded or polygonal cells, its appearance being similar to that of its more common counterpart in the gastrointestinal tract (Fig. 19.177). However, in contrast with the latter, which has been subsumed in the gastrointestinal stromal tumor (GIST) concept, it is negative for CD117. Mixtures of epithelioid, clear cell, and plexiform patterns occur frequently enough to suggest that they represent variants of a single entity.[837,842] A transition to typical smooth muscle is sometimes observed. Ultrastructural studies have also provided support for the smooth muscle derivation of this peculiar neoplasm, as well as for several other types of myometrial tumors of unusual appearance.[826,851,852,876] Morphologically similar tumors occur in the round ligament.[810]

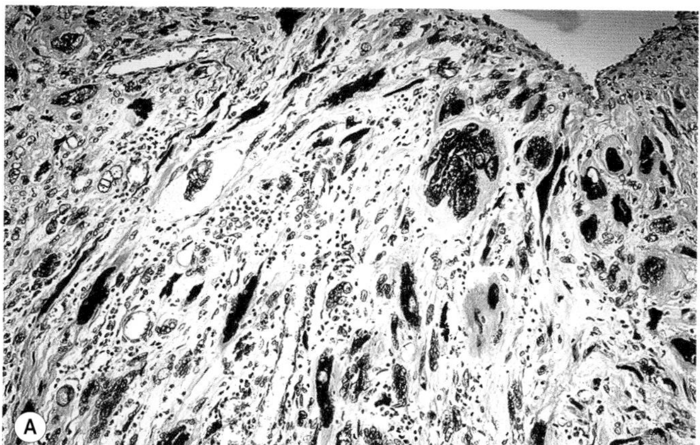

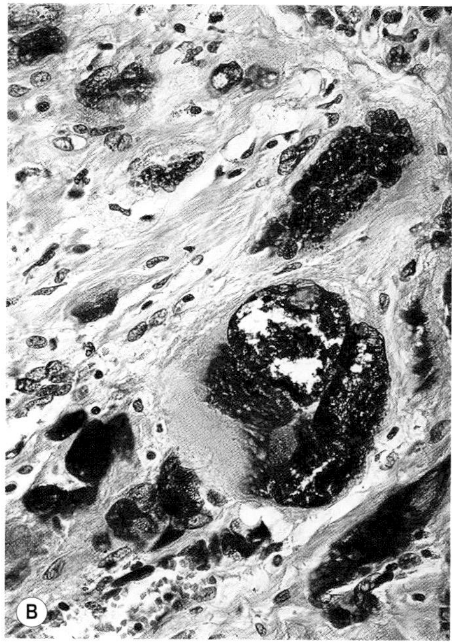

Fig. 19.174 **A** and **B**, Two views of bizarre leiomyoma. The size of some of the tumor cell nuclei makes them almost visible to the naked eye.

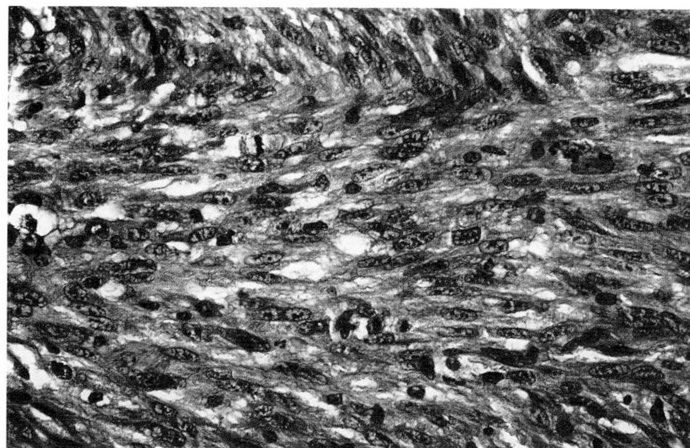

Fig. 19.175 Mitotically active leiomyoma. There is also hypercellularity but no pleomorphism or necrosis.

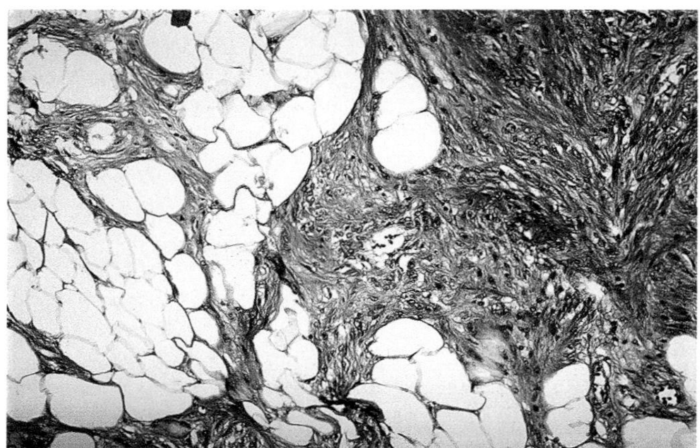

Fig. 19.176 Admixture of mature smooth muscle and adipose tissue in leiomyolipoma.

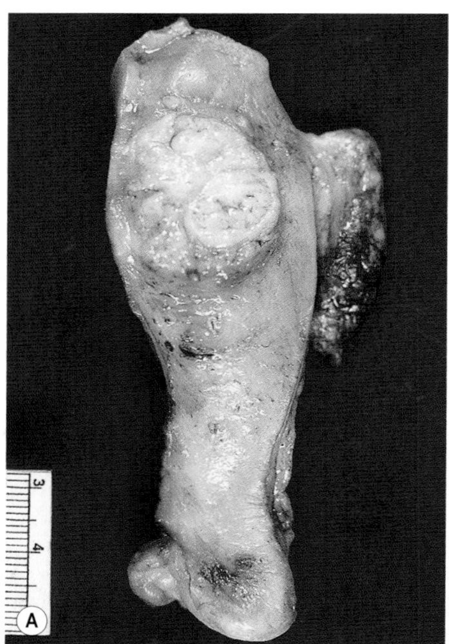

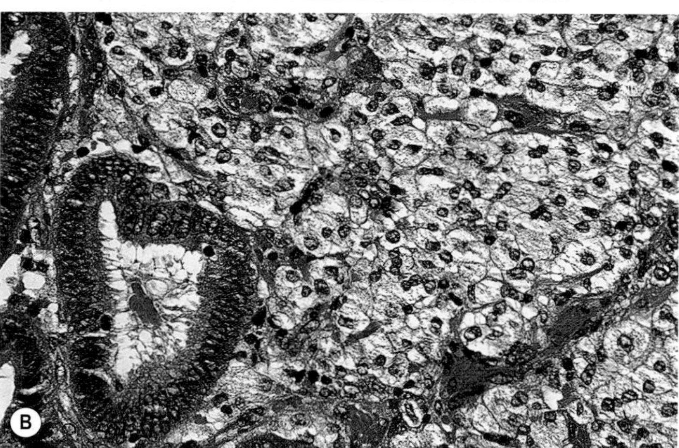

Fig. 19.177 Clear cell leiomyoma (benign leiomyoblastoma): **A**, gross appearance; **B**, microscopic appearance. The tumor cells have a round shape and an artifactually clear cytoplasm.

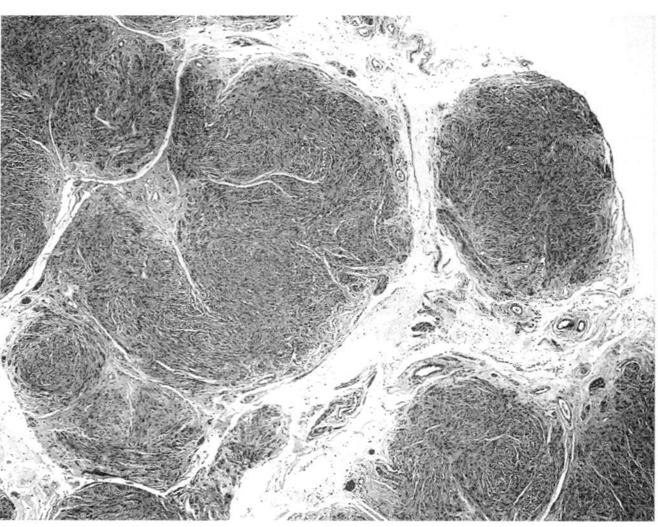

Fig. 19.178 Micronodular microscopic appearance of uterine leiomyoma having the gross appearance of so-called 'cotyledonoid dissecting type'.

Cotyledonoid dissecting leiomyoma is so designated because its gross appearance resembles that of placental tissue. The tumor is exophytic, bulky, and extends from the uterine wall into the broad ligament and pelvic cavity.[816,869] Microscopically, the appearance is that of a leiomyoma with extensive degenerative changes (Fig. 19.178). Despite its dissecting pattern, it lacks vascular invasion and is of benign nature. Variations exist of leiomyomas that are cotyledonoid but not dissecting,[868] and dissecting but not cotyledonoid.[832,867] Believe it or not, there is also a cotyledonoid hydropic intravenous leiomyomatosis.[840]

Parasitic leiomyoma is the term given to the uterine leiomyoma that has become separate from the uterus and has acquired vascular connections with the omentum, pelvic wall, or other intra-abdominal sites, such as the cecal wall. The low-lying retroperitoneal smooth muscle tumors occurring in females and behaving in a benign fashion probably belong to this category, in the sense of being composed of myometrium-type smooth muscle, whether they actually arise from the myometrial wall or not.[812]

Leiomyoma with skeletal muscle differentiation has been reported as an exceptional event.[831,850]

Angioleiomyoma (vascular leiomyoma) is a variant of uterine leiomyoma characterized by a swirling of the spindle cells around myometrial vessels, similar to that seen in the homonymous tumor of soft tissues. This tumor is thought to arise not from the parenchymal myometrial cells (as all other uterine leiomyomas are presumed to), but rather from the smooth muscle cells of the vessel walls.[848] We have seen a variation of the theme in which those cells have a distinct glomoid appearance (*glomangiomyoma*).

Diffuse leiomyomatosis is the term given to involvement of almost the entire myometrium by innumerable, ill-defined leiomyomas, many of microscopic size.[819,853] A clonality analysis done in a case of this condition supports the interpretation that these minute leiomyomas are independent tumors.[811] This extremely rare condition, which is probably analogous to so-called *seedling leiomyomas*,[824] should be distinguished from the nebulous *primary myometrial hypertrophy* or *myometrial hyperplasia*, defined as a uterus weighing over 120 g in the absence of any mass-like myometrial lesion,[822,846] and of which an atypical variant (*'myometrial dysplasia'*) has been recently described.[823]

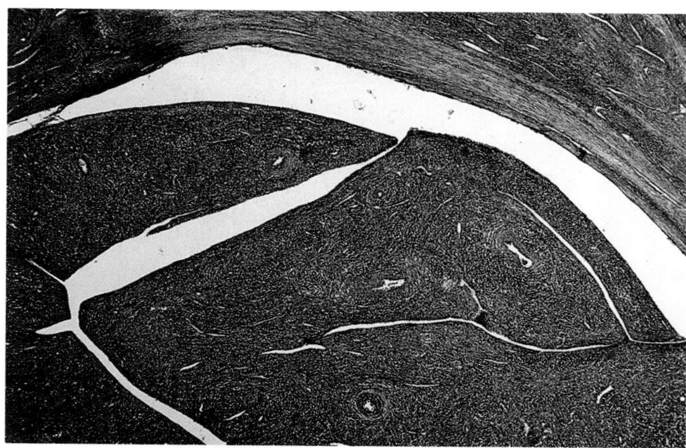

Fig. 19.179 Large plugs of mature smooth muscle filling the vascular lumina in intravenous leiomyomatosis.

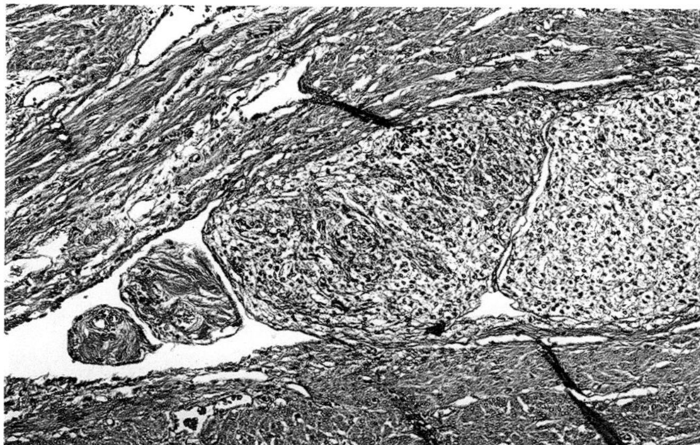

Fig. 19.180 Intravenous leiomyomatosis composed of clear smooth muscle cells.

Intravenous leiomyomatosis is an extremely rare condition characterized by the growth of mature smooth muscle inside the lumen of uterine and pelvic veins[835,857] (Figs 19.179 and 19.180). It is often associated with typical uterine leiomyomas, and it may arise from them.[856] The clinical and gross features are similar to those of the form of endometrial stromal sarcoma, but grossly apparent involvement of veins is more prominent. At the microscopic level, intravenous leiomyomatosis is composed of elongated smooth muscle cells, whereas endometrial stromal sarcoma is made up of round or oval endometrial stromal cells. The two processes may well be histogenetically related in view of the already discussed occurrence of occasional hybrids (combined muscle–stromal tumors) and the close kinship between the endometrial stroma and the myometrial smooth muscle. Mitotic figures are rare or absent. The vessel permeation often extends to vessels in the broad ligament and in uterine and iliac veins; from there, it can proceed along the vena cava and even reach the right atrium.[815] However, distant metastases are exceptionally rare, and the long-term prognosis is excellent.[854] Cases have been described in which the microscopic appearance of the intravenous masses was that of lipoleiomyomas,[814] and others in which the intravenous leiomyomatosis was associated with a benign metastasizing leiomyoma in the lung.[845]

Benign metastasizing leiomyoma is the name given to the uterine tumor having the typical features of a leiomyoma (sometimes on the cellular side but invariably lacking coagulative necrosis, increased mitotic activity, and significant atypia) which is accompanied by nodules in the lung, regional lymph nodes, or other sites having a similar appearance and presumably representing metastases from it.[808] The extrauterine nodules may be just as bland-looking as the original uterine tumor or show features of leiomyosarcoma or smooth muscle tumor of uncertain, unknown, or undetermined malignant potential (STUMP).[828] The interval between hysterectomy and the appearance of the lung nodules is, on average, 15 years. The nodules tend to be multiple, and they have an average size of approximately 2 cm. The patients tend to be younger than those with conventional leiomyosarcoma, and the clinical course is much more indolent, with a median survival of 94 months after the excision of the 'metastases'.[841] Some of these occurrences may be explained on the basis of inadequate sampling of the original tumor, but the fact that in many instances the extrauterine foci have a microscopic appearance that is just as bland suggests that this cannot be the explanation for the entire category. Parenthetically, the similarities with ordinary leiomyomas also apply to their hormone receptor profile (high) and proliferative activity (low), the only difference being perhaps their tendency to overexpress P53[839,841] and the apparently frequent deletion of the long arm of chromosomes 19 and 22.[858] Another possibility that has been advanced is that the extrauterine foci represent independent neoplasms.[817] However, the fact that they have been found to be clonally related speaks in favor of metastasis from a uterine neoplasm.[859,873]

Although this occurrence is unsettling, it is entirely credible. Other examples of tumors that generally behave in a benign fashion but once in a great while result in metastases having the same 'benign' appearance certainly exist, benign mixed tumor of the salivary gland being a prime example. We simply have to accept the fact that tumors do not need to have the conventional morphologic attributes of malignancy to be able to metastasize. As to whether the particular neoplasm discussed in this section should be called a metastasizing leiomyoma or a low-grade leiomyosarcoma mimicking a leiomyoma depends on whether one wishes to designate tumors according to their morphology (in which case it would be a leiomyoma) or their behavior (in which case it would be a leiomyosarcoma). In this regard, it may be opportune to quote here Julian Huxley – the famous biologist, zoologist, humanist, and popular writer – who, in his lecture on 'Biological aspects of cancer', given at the Sloan-Kettering Institute in 1955, stated when discussing the policy for designating lesions solely on the basis of their morphology: "This seems a regrettable example of specialist scholasticism. Cancer (malignancy) must be defined operatively in terms of what the tumor cells do, not what they look like; otherwise the term ceases to have biological meaning."[836]

One is also reminded of the comment made by Allen Graham, surgeon/pathologist at the Cleveland Clinic, as far back as 1924 in an analogous context involving the thyroid gland, when reflecting on "the academically irreconcilable conflict between a purely morphological and a biological interpretation of the term *carcinoma*", and when concluding that "terms such as *metastasizing adenoma*… are confusing, misleading, inaccurate, serve no useful purpose, and should be eliminated".[834] Almost a century has gone by and the 'irreconcilable conflict' remains.

Leiomyosarcoma

Clinical and gross features

Leiomyosarcomas occur in an older average age group than leiomyomas (median age, 54 years), although they can also occur in younger patients. Some of the epidemiologic findings in patients with leiomyosarcoma parallel those from studies in endometrial carcinoma and suggest a role for unopposed estrogen stimulation.[878] The time-honored assumption that most leiomyosarcomas arise from preexisting leiomyomas is probably incorrect, as supported by the fact that the majority of them are solitary and unaccompanied by other leiomyomas.[879] Some leiomyosarcomas are grossly similar to ordinary leiomyomas, but the majority are soft or fleshy, with necrotic or hemorrhagic areas and signs of invasiveness[877] (Fig. 19.181).

Microscopic features

Microscopically, typical leiomyosarcomas are hypercellular, with nuclear atypia and pleomorphism, mitotically active (with some of the mitoses being atypical), and with areas of necrosis (Fig. 19.182).[881] Alas, not all leiomyosarcomas will exhibit simultaneously all of these features, whereas some leiomyomas can display one or several of them.[880] The relative importance of these criteria for the differential diagnosis between leiomyoma and leiomyosarcoma is the subject of a special section below.

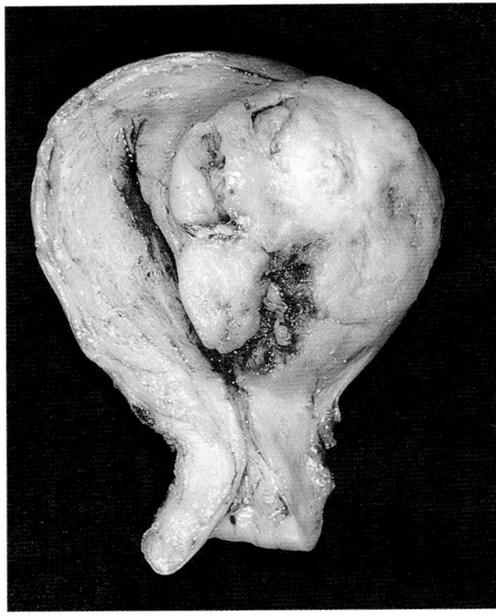

Fig. 19.181 Leiomyosarcoma resulting in a large intramural and submucous mass. There are foci of hemorrhage and necrosis.

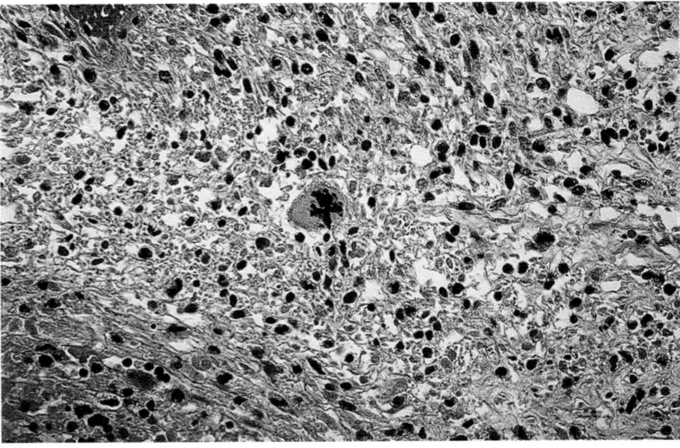

Fig. 19.182 Leiomyosarcoma showing hypercellularity, pleomorphism, atypical mitoses, and necrosis.

Electron microscopic, immunohistochemical, and molecular genetic features

Ultrastructurally and immunohistochemically, the features of leiomyosarcoma are those of smooth muscle cells.[883,887] There is consistent immunoreactivity for smooth and common muscle actin, desmin, calponin, h-caldesmon, and vimentin.[893] There is also common reactivity for low molecular weight keratin (as identified with CAM 5.2) and epithelial membrane antigen,[884] a feature that may lead to a mistaken interpretation, particularly if the tumor cells have an epithelioid appearance.[892] Estrogen and progesterone receptors are expressed, although with a lesser degree of intensity than in leiomyomas.[888,894] Another molecule consistently expressed by these tumors is oxytocin receptor, in a fashion similar to that seen in leiomyomas and in contrast with endometrial stromal tumors.[886] It has been claimed that leiomyosarcomas are accompanied by loss of the cell adhesion molecule CD44, which is present in normal myometrium and in leiomyomas.[890] The immunohistochemical profile of uterine leiomyosarcomas is somewhat different from that of extrauterine leiomyosarcomas (except for those in the pelvic region), probably due at least in part to the estrogen dependency of the former.[891]

At the molecular genetic level, there is no evidence of progression from leiomyoma to leiomyosarcoma.[882] Leiomyosarocmas are characterized by complex karyotypes comparable to their soft tissue counterparts. Breakpoint clusters have been mapped to 1q32 and 10q22.[882] In contrast to leiomyoma, there is commonly *TP53* mutation, which results in overexpression of P53.[885,889,894]

Leiomyosarcoma variants

Epithelioid (clear cell) leiomyosarcoma (malignant leiomyoblastoma) resembles microscopically the gastrointestinal tumors that used to carry this designation, most of which are currently included in the GIST category.[895,898,900] In contrast to the latter, they are usually negative for CD117. The main differential diagnosis is with their benign counterpart, i.e., epithelioid (clear cell) leiomyoma. General criteria apply (see below), such as larger size, infiltrating margins, mitotic activity, and presence of necrosis, and also absence of hyalinization.[898,898,900] The differential diagnosis also includes endometrial stromal tumors and metastatic carcinoma.[901]

Myxoid leiomyosarcoma can arise in the uterine wall, broad ligament, and other pelvic sites.[897] Grossly, it has a gelatinous appearance and deceptively well circumscribed borders. Microscopically, however, it is invasive. The stroma is highly myxoid and the tumor cells are arranged as bundles of typical smooth muscle cells alternating with nondescript mesenchymal cells (Fig. 19.183). The main differential diagnosis (an important one) is with leiomyoma with hydropic degeneration (see p. 1510). In the past, it was frequent to see myxoid leiomyosarcomas underdiagnosed as leiomyomas; at present, the reverse is more likely to occur. Regarding this differential, it is important to point out that the mitotic count criteria used for the usual leiomyosarcoma (see below) do not apply, in the sense that myxoid leiomyosarcomas tend to recur and metastasize whether mitoses are scanty (which is the usual situation) or numerous.[897,899]

Leiomyosarcoma with osteoclast-like giant cells occurs more frequently in the uterus than in any of the other places where malignant smooth muscle tumors can develop (Fig. 19.184). The smooth muscle nature of the tumor cells – as confirmed immuno-

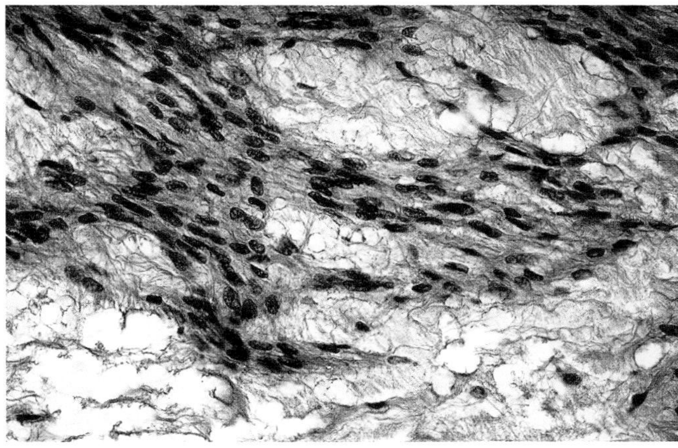

Fig. 19.183 Uterine myxoid leiomyosarcoma.
(Courtesy of Dr Robert E Scully, Boston)

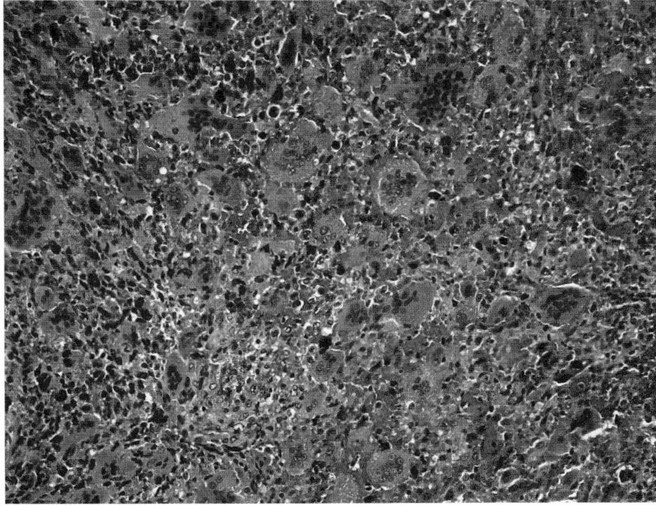

Fig. 19.184 Malignant giant cell tumor of uterus. This is regarded as a variant of leiomyosarcoma with osteoclast-like giant cells.

histochemically – distinguishes this entity from so-called 'malignant giant cell tumor'.[903]

Intravenous leiomyosarcomatosis, an exceptionally rare condition, can be viewed as the malignant counterpart of intravenous leiomyomatosis.[896]

Leiomyosarcoma with skeletal muscle differentiation is a vanishingly rare phenomenon similar to that sometimes seen in endometrial stromal sarcoma.[902]

Spread, metastases, treatment, and prognosis

Uterine leiomyosarcoma usually spreads within the pelvis and in the form of distant metastases to the lung, bone, and other sites.[907] Lymph node metastases are exceptional. The standard treatment is total abdominal hysterectomy with bilateral salpingo-oophorectomy. Prognostic factors include the following:

1 *Tumor stage.* Extension outside the confines of the uterus is a finding of ominous prognosis.[909] In one series of 20 patients in whom this occurred, there were no survivors beyond 29 months.[905]
2 *Tumor size.* This is a significant prognostic factors for tumors confined to the uterus.[904]
3 *Microscopic grade.* No consistent correlation has been found between survival and the histologic grade of the tumor. Specifically, the grading system used for sarcomas of the somatic soft tissue is not applicable.[908]
4 *DNA ploidy.* There is some evidence that the DNA ploidy pattern as determined by flow cytometry may be of prognostic significance.[906,910]

Relationship between morphology and behavior of uterine smooth muscle tumors

The majority of uterine smooth muscle tumors are readily classifiable into benign or malignant.[923,934] There are some lesions, however, for which that placement is very difficult, sometimes excruciatingly so.[931] The morphologic reasons for this, which at the same time represent the main criteria upon which to base a decision, are the following:

1 *Necrosis.* Two patterns of necrosis have been identified in smooth muscle tumors, respectively named coagulative and hyalin (hyaline). In the former there is an abrupt transition between the necrotic and the viable cells. On low power, the typical appearance is that of a cuff of preserved tumor cells around large vessels surrounded by large expanses of necrotic tumor. On high power, two of the classic morphologic forms of nuclear necrosis (pyknosis and karyorrhexis) are evident. In hyaline necrosis, there is a distinct zonal pattern reminiscent of an evolving infarct: a center of 'bland' necrosis (i.e., one in which nuclear debris is difficult to see), a periphery of granulation tissue, and a layer of hyalinized collagen in between. Coagulative necrosis, as above defined, is currently regarded as the most important prognostic predictor in these tumors. Because of the very fact that necrosis (or, rather, a particular type of necrosis) has acquired such a well-deserved significance in this area, it may be worthwhile to discuss it in some detail, beginning with the somewhat questionable nature of the terms chosen, as emerges from the scholarly review on cell death by Majno and Joris.[924] In it, the authors point out that the term coagulation necrosis was first introduced by Conheim in 1877, influenced by the work of Weigert, for the lesion that we call today white infarct, under the mistaken notion that the process was due to a combination of necrosis and a coagulum of fibrin. Therefore, if the term coagulation (or coagulative) necrosis were to be used at all it should be as a synonym for white (anemic) infarct, not in opposition to it. As for 'hyaline' necrosis, it is not much better, since 'hyaline' refers to any homogeneous eosinophilic material, whether extracellular or intracellular (as in Mallory's alcoholic hyaline). Furthermore, in the situation in question, it is applied to the collagen that is deposited at the granulation tissue front of an infarct and is, therefore, dependent upon the stage of the latter. In fact, it would seem that the key morphologic difference between the two forms of necrosis is that the first shows prominent hematoxyphilic nuclear debris (karyorrhectic and pyknotic nuclei) whereas in the second the appearance is more homogeneous ('bland') because the nuclear remnants are difficult to see (karyolysis). It has been suggested that the name of the former be changed to 'tumor cell necrosis',[916] but this is not much of an improvement, since in both types it is largely the tumor cell that is undergoing necrosis.

Semantics aside, the observation made by Bell et al.[912] is of the greatest diagnostic significance and may turn out to have a sound biological basis, since karyorrhectic and pyknotic nuclei are generally a feature of death by apoptosis, whereas karyolytic nuclei are a feature of ischemic and other forms of accidental death (what Majno calls death by murder or oncosis).[924]

2 *Mitotic activity.* This remains another important criterion despite the admittedly imprecise fashion in which it is measured in terms of lack of standardization and poor reproducibility,[914,929,930] in the sense of being influenced by the thickness of the slide, microscope magnification factor, size of tumor cells, proportion of tumor cells to stroma, and observer criteria.[913] Regarding the latter, a common mistake among neophytes is to count the pyknotic nuclei often seen scattered around in smooth muscle tumors (whether from lymphocytes, mast cells, or smooth muscle cells) as mitotic figures. Another theoretical source of variation is the interval between excision and fixation, but this seems not to be important. The best way to eliminate most of these sources of inaccuracy would be to express the number of mitoses as a percentage of the tumor cell population, as has routinely been done when counting thymidine-labeled nuclei or proliferative (Ki-67) index. Another potential improvement would be to use mitosis markers such as PHH3 at the immunohistochemical level.[915] When using current methodology, some practical measures can be taken to improve accuracy. One is to scan the sections for the *most active area*, do the mitotic count in 10 *consecutive fields* in that area, and repeat the procedure a minimum of *four times.* Another obvious measure is to sample the tumor adequately. Kempson[914] recommends a total of *at least 10 sections or one section for each centimeter of diameter, whichever is greater.* The section should have a real thickness as close as possible to the 5 μm indicated in the microtome setting. 'High power field' (HPF) usually means the combination of a 10× eyepiece and a 40× objective. If the operator is using a 15× eyepiece and/or a 63× objective, adjustments should be made. The criteria for identifying mitotic figures should be strict. The members of the Multicenter Morphometric Mammary Carcinoma Project proposed the following:[933]
   1 The nuclear membrane must be absent, so cells must have passed the prophase.
   2 Clear, hairy extensions of nuclear material (condensed chromosomes) must be present, and clotted (beginning metaphase), in a plane (metaphase/anaphase), or in separate clots (telophase). Regular extensions with an empty central zone favor a nonmitosis.
   3 Two parallel, clearly separate chromosome clots are to be counted as if they are separate mitoses, however obvious it is that only one mitotic figure is concerned. This is in view of future automated mitotic figure recognition with image analysis.

3 *Atypia.* This refers to the combination of pleomorphism (meaning marked differences in size and shape) and nuclear hyperchromasia, and should already be evident on low-power examination. It is classified as focal or extensive, and graded (acknowledging the subjectivity of the exercise) as mild, moderate, or severe.

4 *Cellularity.* The term is self-explanatory, and the determination just as subjective. This is one of the least important parameters in this exercise.

5 *Tumor borders,* i.e., the relationship of the tumor with the surrounding myometrium.

The evaluation of these criteria, alone and in combination, allows a fairly accurate *but not infallible* prediction of tumor behavior. The points worth stressing are the following:

1 The weight of the morphologic factors is coagulative necrosis, high mitotic activity, pleomorphism, and cellularity, in this order of significance.

2 Tumors that are hypercellular but lack the other criteria are to be regarded as benign cellular leiomyomas (see p. 1510).

3 Tumors with atypia (even if marked and diffuse) should not be regarded as malignant if they lack coagulative necrosis and mitotic activity. Rather, they belong to the category variously called *atypical, bizarre, symplasmic,* or *pleomorphic* if the change is focal, and to a *borderline category* if it is extensive.

4 Tumors with increased mitotic activity (up to 15 mitoses per 10 HPF) but lacking coagulative necrosis and atypia are to be regarded as *mitotically active leiomyomas* (see p. 1511).

5 Tumors with coagulative necrosis and diffuse atypia and/or increased mitotic activity (>10 per 10 HPF) should be regarded as leiomyosarcomas.

6 Tumors with coagulative necrosis but neither atypia nor increased mitotic activity should be placed in a *'borderline'* category (see below).

7 Tumors with diffuse moderate-to-severe atypia *and* more than 10 mitoses per 10 HPF should be called leiomyosarcoma even if they lack coagulative necrosis.

These recommendations are primarily based on the careful and painstaking work done by Richard Kempson and the changing members of his team (Bari, Hendrikson, Zaloudek, Bell, Longacre, and others) over a 35-year period.[912,916,918,919,923] This is shown in a simplified form for the benefit of the reader in Table 19.2, the arrangement being slightly different from that presented in the original articles. Another difference is the fact that the 'STUMP' category has been retained because it was felt by us and others[917] that it best expresses the fact that in some uterine smooth muscle tumors it is simply impossible with current tools to predict their behavior with certainty. The best proof of this statement is the existence of a tumor type having *none* of the morphologic features that identify it as a leiomyosarcoma but which spreads to distant organs (benign metastasizing leiomyoma, see p. 1513). In our opinion, one would serve the patient and the clinician better (and would also be closer to expressing the truth) by doing away with the traditional binary classification of these tumors into benign and malignant, i.e., leiomyoma versus leiomyosarcoma (which is improved only slightly by the addition of a borderline category), and by switching to a nomenclature that would simply identify these neoplasms as smooth muscle tumors, followed by an estimation (ideally expressed in percentages) of the probability of the tumor recurring or metastasizing, based on a careful evaluation of all the parameters discussed in this section and any others that may be found of help in this regard. Until and unless such a radical change in nosology takes place, and as long as we subject ourselves to the current manicheist approach, the above recommendations will have to do.

Two additional comments are in order. These considerations have been devised for the conventional type of uterine smooth muscle tumor, and cannot be applied unchanged to the variants. For instance, myxoid leiomyosarcoma is to be diagnosed as such even if in most cases it lacks coagulative necrosis, increased mitotic activity, and severe atypia.

The other comment applies to the hope that the abundant information that is being obtained regarding the phenotypic and genotypic features of these tumors will provide assistance to the pathologist in terms of an accurate prognostic assessment and a precise therapeutic recommendation.[920] Some claims are already

Table 19.2 Criteria and diagnostic terms for uterine smooth muscle tumors (freely adapted from the work of Richard Kempson and his co-workers)

COAGULATIVE NECROSIS	MITOTIC COUNT PER 10 HPF	ATYPIA		DIAGNOSIS
Present	Greater than 10	Moderate to severe (focal or diffuse)		Leiomyosarcoma
		None to mild		Leiomyosarcoma
	Equal to or less than 10	Moderate to severe (focal or diffuse)		Leiomyosarcoma
		None to mild		STUMP[a]
Absent	Greater than 10	Moderate to severe	Diffuse	Leiomyosarcoma
			Focal	STUMP[b]
		None to mild		Mitotically active leiomyoma (up to 15 mitoses/10 HPF are allowed)
	Equal to or less than 10	Moderate to severe	Diffuse	STUMP[c]
			Focal	Leiomyoma[d]
		None to mild		Leiomyoma

[a]Of the three tumors here placed in the STUMP category, this is the one most likely to behave in a malignant fashion. Actually, it is regarded as a probable leiomyosarcoma in Kempson's scheme. The alternative possibility of an infarction in a leiomyoma due to torsion or other factors should be considered.
[b]In Kempson's scheme, this is designated as STUMP if the mitotic activity is higher than 15.
[c]This is referred to as 'atypical leiomyoma with low risk of recurrence' in Kempson's scheme.
[d]This is designated as 'leiomyoma with limited experience' in Kempson's scheme.

being made along these lines, in the sense that the following features are usually present in leiomyosarcomas but rare or absent in leiomyomas: loss of heterozygosity for chromosome 10,[927] presence of galectin-3 and its binding site,[928] low levels of estrogen and progesterone receptors,[935] loss of CD44,[926] lack of gamma smooth muscle isoactin gene expression,[932] and expression of p16.[911,921,925] The latter marker seems particularly promising.[922]

As exciting as all these propositions are, it is fair to say that the decision whether to place a uterine smooth muscle tumor into a given prognostic category – no matter how designated – remains for now largely dependent on the time-honored morphologic criteria.

Smooth muscle tumors and PEComas

A very interesting problem is posed by the recent description of uterine neoplasms having a morphologic appearance consistent with smooth muscle tumors but featuring perivascular epithelioid and/or clear cells, sometimes prominent hyalinization, and HMB-45 immunoreactivity.[938,943,947] The controversy that has ensued is whether these tumors should be regarded as variants of epithelioid smooth muscle tumors or as members of the perivascular epithelioid clear cell/angiomyolipoma/PEComa family.[944,947] Some of these tumors have been associated with pelvic lymphangiomyomatosis and/or have developed in patients with tuberous sclerosis, and therefore their link with the PEComa family stands on solid grounds.[939,941,942,948] The situation is not so clear for uterine neoplasms that have the morphologic and immunohistochemical features of smooth muscle and endometrial stromal tumors (usually malignant) and that would surely have been diagnosed as such, were it not for the fact that they exhibit, in addition to muscle or endometrial stromal markers (including the occasional presence of sex cord-like structures[937]), positivity for HMB-45 and related markers, such as Mart-1 (Melan-A).[940,946] Perhaps it is wise to withhold judgment on the issue until additional information is obtained. For the time being, it would seem prudent to diagnose them as smooth muscle tumors, place them in the appropriate category (spindle or epithelioid; benign, STUMP, or malignant), and add a note to the report to the effect that the tumor morphology and the HMB-45 immunoreactivity suggest a histogenetic relationship with the family of tumors currently designated as PEComas.[945] Parenthetically, this conundrum is not exclusive of the uterus. Similar findings and controversies have arisen with analogous tumors located in the renal capsule (see Chapter 17).

From a practical standpoint, it is worth noting that these tumors can be locally aggressive and to metastasize.[936]

Recurrence and/or metastases are strongly associated with tumor size, mitotic activity, and necrosis.[938]

Other tumors and tumorlike conditions

Postoperative spindle cell nodules similar to those occurring in the vagina have been observed in the endometrium.[958]

Idiopathic granulomas similar to those more commonly seen in the ovary (and known there as idiopathic ovarian cortical granulomas) have been occasionally seen in the uterus. Most of them were multiple and located in the myometrium.[986]

Extramedullary hematopoiesis can occur in the uterus in the absence of any hematologic disorder or systemic disease (but see Granulocytic (myeloid) sarcoma below).[1013] Most of the reported cases have been located in endometrial polyps or leiomyomas and have been associated with chronic anemia.[977]

Myxoid changes can occur in the myometrium in the absence of any other pathology.[992]

Adenomatoid tumors identical to those more commonly seen in the fallopian tube are sometimes found in the uterine wall, usually beneath the serosa and close to the cornua.[999,1024] Exceptionally, they will be apparent in a curetting specimen. These tumors are usually small (mean diameter, 2 cm) and characterized microscopically by adenoid, angiomatoid, solid, and cystic patterns occurring singly or in combination[1003,1006] (Fig. 19.185). The most cystic examples can simulate lymphangiomas. They are often accompanied by smooth

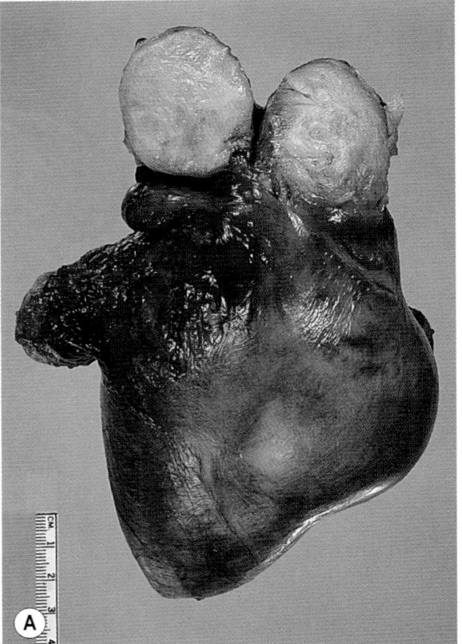

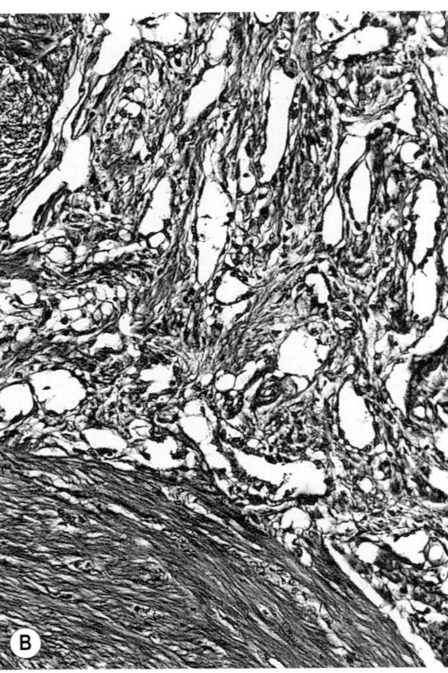

Fig. 19.185 **A** and **B**, Adenomatoid tumor of uterus. **A**, Gross appearance. The location at one of the cornua is characteristic. **B**, Microscopic appearance showing tubular formations lined by flattened mesothelial cells.

muscle hypertrophy and can be confused with leiomyomas. Their mesothelial nature has been established on the basis of ultrastructural and immunohistochemical findings (including calretinin, thrombomodulin, WT1, and D2-40)[991,1002,1010,1012,1016,1018] and is also supported by its occasional coexistence with other lesions of reputed mesothelial derivation, such as so-called benign multicystic mesothelioma.[954]

Arteriovenous fistula in the wall of the uterus may produce large pulsating masses. The vascular connections are demonstrable by angiography.[990]

Benign mesenchymal tumors other than those already described are extremely rare. They include *hemangioma* of the endometrium,[983] *solitary fibrous tumor* (some associated with hypoglycemia),[1023,1028] and *lipoma*. The latter may result, at least in some instances, from adipose metaplasia of leiomyomas.[1005,1008]

Sarcomas of types other than those already described can arise in the uterus. They include *chondrosarcoma*,[957] *osteosarcoma*,[963] *rhabdomyosarcoma*,[967,968,1001,1004] *malignant peripheral nerve sheath tumor*,[961] *angiosarcoma*,[953,995,1011] so-called *malignant fibrous histiocytoma*,[956] *malignant mesenchymoma* (one arising in a leiomyoma),[962] *alveolar soft part sarcoma*,[976] GIST,[1022] so-called *rhabdoid sarcoma*,[949] *Ewing sarcoma/PNET*,[960,980,1027] and *tumors with neuroectodermal differentiation* but lacking the *EWSR1* gene rearrangement[966,971] (Fig. 19.186). Some of these sarcomas have developed following radiation therapy for cervical carcinoma or other malignancies.[997] Some of the angiosarcomas have been of epithelioid type, immunoreactive for keratin, and apparently arising within leiomyomas[1019] (Fig. 19.187).

Before making a diagnosis of uterine sarcoma (particularly if the tumor is very pleomorphic and/or with heterologous elements), the more likely possibility of an MMMT with predominance of the sarcoma-like component should be ruled out with thorough sampling.[965]

Malignant lymphomas can present initially in the endometrium (including an endometrial polyp[1009]), myometrium, or both.[970,978,989,1026] The patients typically complain of bleeding and a mass. Most tumors are of diffuse large B-cell type.[951,987,1026] Cases of low-grade B-cell lymphoma (including marginal zone B-cell

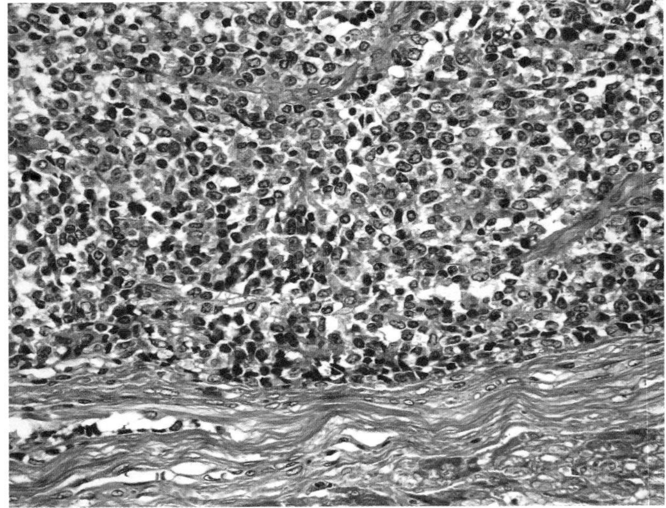

Fig. 19.186 Ewing sarcoma/primitive neuroectodermal tumor presenting as a uterine mass, a most unusual occurrence.

lymphoma)[979,1025] (Fig. 19.188), T-cell lymphoma,[993] Hodgkin lymphoma,[982] angiotropic lymphoma,[959] and intravascular large B-cell lymphoma[1017] with primary uterine involvement have also been described. Malignant lymphomas should be distinguished from florid but reactive lymphoid proliferations involving the endometrium (lymphoma-like lesion),[974,1029] massive lymphoid infiltration of leiomyomas (see above), and *inflammatory pseudotumor/inflammatory myofibroblastic tumor*.[975,1007] In these benign conditions, the large lymphoid cells are usually accompanied by plasma cells, small lymphocytes, and/or neutrophils.[969] **Granulocytic (myeloid) sarcoma** and **plasmacytoma/myeloma** can also involve the uterus, occasionally as the first manifestation of the disease.[972,978,1000,1014]

Other exceptionally rare primary uterine tumors include **Brenner tumor**[952] (microscopically identical to its ovarian counterpart and

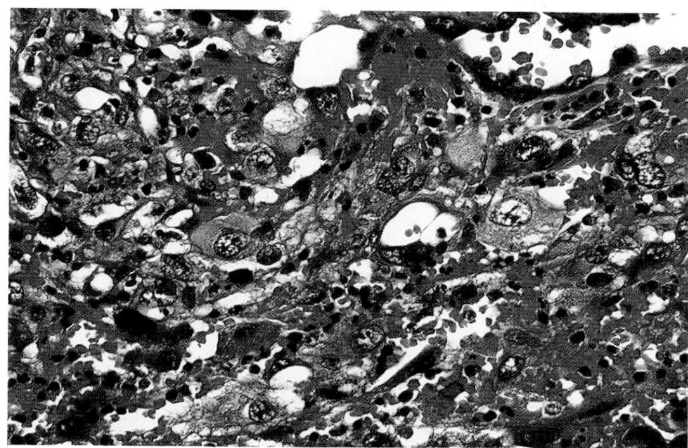

Fig. 19.187 Epithelioid angiosarcoma arising within a uterine leiomyoma.

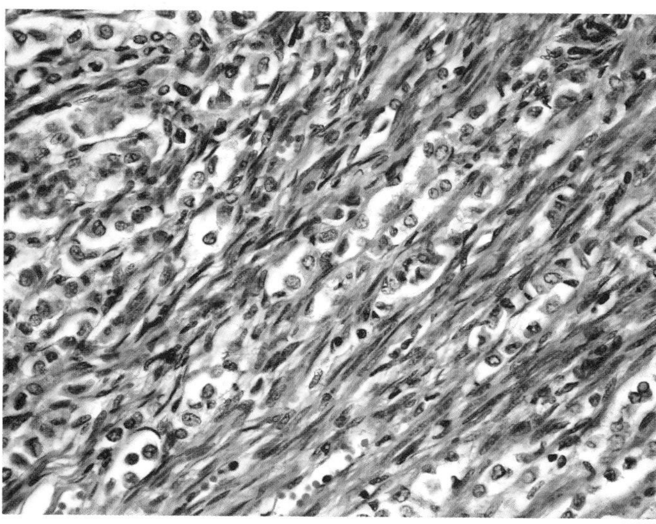

Fig. 19.189 Lobular breast carcinoma metastatic to myometrium. Note the Indian file pattern of growth.

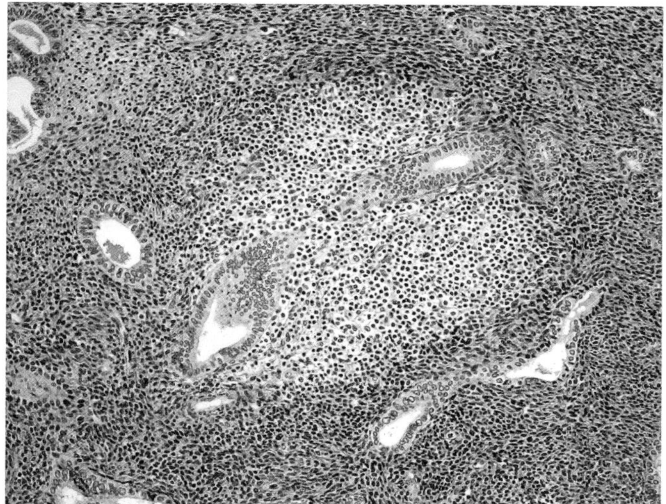

Fig. 19.188 Low-grade marginal zone-type malignant lymphoma involving uterine mucosa.

sometimes having a polypoid configuration),[950] **extrarenal Wilms tumor** (with or without teratoid features),[973,998] **desmoplastic small cell tumor** (personal observation), **glioma,**[1030] **carcinoid tumor,**[955] **paraganglioma**[1031] (including a pigmented variant[1020]), and **yolk sac (endodermal sinus) tumor.**[985]

Metastatic carcinoma from extrapelvic sites may metastasize to the uterus and cause uterine bleeding as the presenting symptom. The breast, gastrointestinal tract, kidney, and skin (melanoma) are the most frequent primary sites.[988,994,1015] The myometrium is more often involved than the endometrium (Fig. 19.189) and sometimes the leiomyomas present contain metastatic tumor; however, it is not rare for the malignancy to be present in material from endometrial curettings, especially in cases of lobular carcinoma of the breast,[1021] and also with neuroendocrine carcinomas and other neoplasms.[984] Exceptionally, a well-differentiated mucinous neoplasm of the appendix will coat the endometrial surface in a pseudomyxomatous fashion.[996] On occasion, a metastatic breast lobular carcinoma has been seen involving a tamoxifen-associated endometrial polyp,[981] and a melanoma has been seen to metastasize into a uterine adenomyoma.[964]

References

NORMAL ANATOMY

1 Arias-Stella J. Atypical endometrial changes produced by chorionic tissue. Hum Pathol 1972, **3**: 450–453.

2 Arias-Stella J Jr, Arias-Velasquez A, Arias-Stella J. Normal and abnormal mitoses in the atypical endometrial change associated with chorionic tissue effect. Am J Surg Pathol 1994, **18**: 694–701.

3 Arias-Stella J. Historia de un descubrimiento cientifico en un pais en desarrollo. Universidad Peruana Cayetano Heredia, 2009, Lima, Peru.

4 Azzopardi JC, Zayid I. Synthetic progestogen-oestrogen therapy and uterine changes. J Clin Pathol 1967, **20**: 731–738.

5 Banks ER, Mills SE, Frierson HF Jr. Uterine intravascular menstrual endometrium simulating malignancy. Am J Surg Pathol 1991, **15**: 407–412.

6 Barroeta JE, Pasha TL, Acs G, Zhang PJ. Immunoprofile of endocervical and endometrial stromal cells and its potential application in localization of tumor involvement. Int J Gynecol Pathol 2007, **26**: 76–82.

7 Clement PB, Scully RE. Idiopathic postmenopausal decidual reaction of the endometrium. A clinicopathologic analysis of four cases. Int J Gynecol Pathol 1988, **7**: 152–161.

8 Dallenbach-Hellweg G, Poulsen HE. Atlas of endometrial histopathology, ed. 2. Berlin, 1996, Springer, p. 225.

9 Ehrmann RL. Histologic dating of the endometrium. J Reprod Med 1969, **3**: 179–200.

10 Ferenczy A, Bertrand G, Gelfand MM. Proliferation kinetics of human endometrium during the normal menstrual cycle. Am J Obstet Gynecol 1979, **133**: 859–867.

11 Hendrickson MR, Atkins KA, Kempson RL. Uterus and fallopian tubes. In Mills SE (ed.): Histology for pathologists, ed. 3. Philadelphia, 2007, Lippincott Williams and Wilkins, 2007, pp. 1011–1062.

12 Hertig AT. Gestational hyperplasia of the endometrium. A morphologic correlation of ova, endometrium, and corpora lutea during early pregnancy. Lab Invest 1964, **13**: 1153–1191.

13 Huettner PC, Gersell DJ. Arias-Stella reaction in nonpregnant women. A clinicopathologic study of nine cases. Int Gynecol Pathol 1994, **13**: 241–247.

14 Mazur MT, Hendrickson MR, Kempson RL. Optically clear nuclei. An alteration of endometrial epithelium in the presence of trophoblast. Am J Surg Pathol 1983, **7**: 415–423.

15 McCluggage WG. Immunohistochemical and functional biomarkers of value in female genital tract lesions. Int J Gynecol Pathol 2006, **25**: 101–120.

16 Merchant S, Malpica A, Deavers MT, Czapar C, Gershenson D, Silva EG. Vessels within vessels in the myometrium. Am J Surg Pathol 2002, **26**: 232–236.

17 Mittal K, Soslow R, McCluggage WG. Application of immunohistochemistry to gynecologic pathology. Arch Pathol Lab Med 2008, **132**: 402–423.

18 Niu HL, Pasha TL, Pawel BR, LiVolsi VA, Zhang PJ. Thyroid transcription factor-1 expression in normal gynecologic tissues and its potential significance. Int J Gynecol Pathol 2009, **28**: 301–307.

19 Norris HJ, Hertig AT, Abell MR. The uterus. Baltimore, 1973, Williams and Wilkins.

20 Noyes RW. Uniformity of secretory endometrium. Study of multiple sections from 100 uteri removed at operation. Fertil Steril 1956, **7**: 103–109.

21 Noyes RW, Haman JO. Accuracy of endometrial dating. Fertil Steril 1954, **4**: 504–517.

22 Noyes RW, Hertig AT, Rock J. Dating the endometrial biopsy. Fertil Steril 1950, **1**: 3–25.

23 Onuma K, Dabbs DJ, Bhargava R. Mammaglobin expression in the female genital tract: immunohistochemical analysis in benign and neoplastic endocervix and endometrium. Int J Gynecol Pathol 2008, **27**: 418–425.

24 Poropatich C, Rojas M, Silverberg SG. Polymorphonuclear leukocytes in the endometrium during the normal menstrual cycle. Int J Gynecol Pathol 1987, **6**: 230–234.

25 Sahin AA, Silva EG, Landon G, Ordonez NG, Gershenson DM. Endometrial tissue in myometrial vessels not associated with menstruation. Int J Gynecol Pathol 1989, **8**: 139–146.

26 Sickel JZ, di Sant'Agnese PA. Anomalous immunostaining of 'optically clear' nuclei in gestational endometrium. A potential pitfall in the diagnosis of pregnancy-related herpesvirus infection. Arch Pathol Lab Med 1994, **118**: 831–833.

27 Vang R, Barner R, Wheeler DT, Strauss BL. Immunohistochemical staining for Ki-67 and p53 helps distinguish endometrial Arias-Stella reaction from high-grade carcinoma, including clear cell carcinoma. Int J Gynecol Pathol 2004, **23**: 223–233.

28 Yokoyama S, Kashima K, Inoue S, Daa T, Nakayama I, Moriuchi A. Biotin-containing intranuclear inclusions in endometrial glands during gestation and puerperium. Am J Clin Pathol 1993, **99**: 13–17.

29 Young ES, Diaz-Arrastia C, Castro CY. The hysterectomy. Ann Diagn Pathol. 2005, **9**: 202–208.

CURETTAGE AND BIOPSY

30 Baitlon D, Hadley JO. Endometrial biopsy. Pathologic findings in 3600 biopsies from selected patients. Am J Clin Pathol 1975, **63**: 9–15.

31 Carmichael DE. Asherman's syndrome. Obstet Gynecol 1970, **36**: 922–928.

32 Chambers JT, Chambers SK. Endometrial sampling. When? Where? Why? With what? Clin Obstet Gynecol 1992, **35**: 28–39.

33 Dijkhuizen FP, Mol BW, Brolmann HA, Heintz AP. The accuracy of endometrial sampling in the diagnosis of patients with endometrial carcinoma and hyperplasia: a meta-analysis. Cancer 2000, **89**: 1765–1772.

34 Dubé V, Macdonald D, Allingham-Hawkins DJ, Kamel-Reid S, Colgan TJ. Vanishing endometrial carcinoma. Int J Gynecol Pathol 2007, **26**: 271–277.

35 Foix A, Bruno RO, Davison T, Lema B. The pathology of postcurettage intrauterine adhesions. Am J Obstet Gynecol 1966, **96**: 1027–1033.

36 Hofmeister FJ, Vondrak B, Barbo DM. The value of the endometrial biopsy. A study of 14,655 office endometrial biopsies. Am J Obstet Gynecol 1966, **95**: 91–98.

37 Kahler VL, Creasy RK, Morris JA. Value of the endometrial biopsy. Obstet Gynecol 1969, **34**: 91–95.

38 Lampe B, Kürzl R, Hantschmann P. Reliability of tumor typing of endometrial carcinoma in prehysterectomy curettage. Int J Gynecol Pathol 1995, **14**: 2–6.

39 McLennan CE. Endometrial regeneration after curettage. Am J Obstet Gynecol 1969, **104**: 185–194.

40 Mitchard J, Hirschowitz L. Concordance of FIGO grade of endometrial adenocarcinomas in biopsy and hysterectomy specimens. Histopathology 2003, **42**: 372–378.

41 Unger ZM, Gonzalez JL, Hanissian PD, Schned AR. Pseudolipomatosis in hysteroscopically resected tissues from the gynecologic tract: pathologic description and frequency. Am J Surg Pathol 2009, **33**: 1187–1190.

EFFECTS OF HORMONE ADMINISTRATION

ESTROGEN THERAPY

42 Antunes CM, Strolley PD, Rosenshein NB, Davies JL, Tonascia JA, Brown C, Burnett L, Rutledge A, Pokempner M, Garcia R. Endometrial cancer and estrogen use. Report of a large case-control study. N Engl J Med 1979, **300**: 9–13.

43 Deligdisch L. Hormonal pathology of the endometrium. Mod Pathol 2000, **13**: 285–294.

44 Gordon J, Reagan JW, Finkle WD, Ziel HK. Estrogen and endometrial carcinoma. An independent pathology review supporting original risk estimate. N Engl J Med 1977, **297**: 570–571.

45 Silverberg SG, Mullen D, Faraci JA, Makowski EL, Miller A, Finch JL, Sutherland JV. Endometrial carcinoma. Clinical–pathologic comparison of cases in post-menopausal women receiving and not receiving exogenous estrogens. Cancer 1980, **45**: 3018–3026.

46 Smith DC, Prentice R, Thompson DJ, Herrmann WL. Association of exogenous estrogen and endometrial carcinoma. N Engl J Med 1975, **293**: 1164–1166.

47 Studd JWW, Thom MH, Paterson MEL, Wade-Evans T. The prevention and treatment of endometrial pathology in postmenopausal women receiving exogenous estrogens. In Pasetto N, Paoletti R, Ambrus JL (eds): The menopause and postmenopause. Lancaster, 1980, MTP Press, pp. 127–139.

48 Whitehead MI, King RJB, McQueen J, Campbell S. Endometrial histology and biochemistry in climacteric women during oestrogen and oestrogen/progestogen therapy. J R Soc Med 1979, **72**: 322–327.

49 Whitehead MI, Townsend PT, Pryse-Davies J, Ryder TA, King RJB. Effects of estrogens and progestins on the biochemistry and morphology of the post-menopausal endometrium. N Engl J Med 1981, **305**: 1599–1605.

50 Wright TC, Holinka CF, Ferenczy A, Gatsonis CA, Mutter GL, Nicosia S, Richart RM. Estradiol-induced hyperplasia in endometrial biopsies from women on hormone replacement therapy. Am J Surg Pathol 2002, **26**: 1269–1275.

51 Ziel HK, Finkle WD. Increased risk of endometrial carcinoma among users of conjugated estrogens. N Engl J Med 1975, **293**: 1167–1170.

PROGESTATIONAL AGENTS

52 Azzopardi JG, Zayid I. Synthetic progestogen–oestrogen therapy and uterine changes. J Clin Pathol 1967, **20**: 731–738.

53 Cohen CJ, Deppe G. Endometrial carcinoma and oral contraceptive agents. Obstet Gynecol 1977, **49**: 390–392.

54 Deligdisch L. Effects of hormone therapy on the endometrium. Mod Pathol 1993, **6**: 94–106.

55 Hejmadi RK, Chaudhri S, Ganesan R, Rollason TP. Morphologic changes in the endometrium associated with the use of the mirena coil: a retrospective study of 106 cases. Int J Surg Pathol 2007, **15**: 148–154.

56 Irey NS, Manion WC, Taylor HB. Vascular lesions in women taking oral contraceptives. Arch Pathol 1970, **89**: 1–8.

57 Maqueo M, Becerra C, Munguia H, Goldzieher JW. Endometrial histology and vaginal cytology during oral contraception with sequential estrogen and progestin. Am J Obstet Gynecol 1964, **90**: 396–400.

58 Mutter GL, Bergeron C, Deligdisch L, Ferenczy A, Glant M, Merino M, Williams AR, Blithe DL. The spectrum of endometrial pathology induced by progesterone receptor modulators. Mod Pathol 2008, **21**: 591–598.

59 Ober WB. Synthetic progestogen-oestrogen preparations and endometrial morphology. J Clin Pathol 1966, **19**: 138–147.

60 Ober WB. Effects of oral and intrauterine administration of contraceptives on the uterus. Hum Pathol 1977, **8**: 513–527.

61 Rice-Wray E, Aranda-Rosell A, Maqueo M, Goldzieher JW. Comparison of the long-term endometrial effects of synthetic progestins used in fertility control. Am J Obstet Gynecol 1963, **87**: 429–433.

62 Sartwell PE, Masi AT, Arthes FG, Greene GR, Smith HE. Thromboembolism and oral contraceptives. An epidemiological case-control study. Am J Epidemiol 1969, **90**: 365–380.

63 Silverberg SG, Makowski EL. Endometrial carcinoma in young women taking oral contraceptive agents. Obstet Gynecol 1975, **46**: 503–506.

64 Silverberg SG, Makowski EL, Roche WD. Endometrial carcinoma in women under 40 years of age. Comparison of cases in oral contraceptive users and non-users. Cancer 1977, **39**: 592–598.

65 Vessey MP, Doll R. Investigation of relation between use of oral contraceptives and thromboembolic disease. A further report. Br Med J 1969, **2**: 651–657.

TAMOXIFEN

66 Barakat RR, Goóewski TA, Almadrones L, Saigo PE, Venkatram E, Hudis C, Hoskins WJ. Effect of adjuvant tamoxifen on the

endometrium in women with breast cancer: a prospective study using office endometrial biopsy. J Clin Oncol 2000, **18**: 3459–3463.

67 Carcangiu ML. Uterine pathology in tamoxifen-treated patients with breast cancer. Anat Pathol 1998, **2**: 53–70.

68 Hachisuga T, Hideshima T, Kawarabayashi T, Eguchi F, Emoto M, Shirakusa T. Expression of steroid receptors, Ki-67, and epidermal growth factor receptor in tamoxifen-treated endometrium. Int J Gynecol Pathol 1999, **18**: 297–303.

69 Ismail SM. Endometrial pathology associated with prolonged tamoxifen therapy: a review. Adv Anat Pathol 1996, **3**: 266–271.

70 Kennedy MM, Baigrie CF, Manek S. Tamoxifen and the endometrium: review of 102 cases and comparison with HRT-related and non-HRT related endometrial pathology. Int J Gynecol Pathol 1999, **18**: 130–137.

71 Leslie KK, Walter SA, Torkko K, Stephens JK, Thompson C, Singh M. Effect of tamoxifen on endometrial histology, hormone receptors, and cervical cytology: a prospective study with follow-up. Appl Immunohistochem Mol Morphol 2007, **15**: 284–293.

72 Seidman JD, Kurman RJ. Tamoxifen and the endometrium. Int J Gynecol Pathol 1999, **18**: 293–296.

73 Wilder JD, Shahin S, Khattar N, Wilder DM, Yin J, Rushing RS, Beaven R, Kaetzel C, van Nagell Jr, Kryscio RJ, Lele SM. Tamoxifen-associated malignant endometrial tumors: pathologic features and expression of hormone receptors estrogen-alpha, estrogen-beta, and progesterone: a case controlled study [abstract]. Mod Pathol 2003, **16**: 214a.

ENDOMETRITIS

74 Adegboyega PA, Pei Y, McLarty J. Relationship between eosinophils and chronic endometritis. Hum Pathol 2010, **41**: 33–37.

75 Almoujahed MO, Briski LE, Prysak M, Johnson LB, Khatib R. Uterine granulomas. Clinical and pathologic features. Am J Clin Pathol 2002, **117**: 771–775.

76 Ashworth MT, Moss CI, Kenyon WE. Granulomatous endometritis following hysteroscopic resection of the endometrium. Histopathology 1991, **18**: 185–187.

77 Bayer-Garner IB, Nickell JA, Korourian S. Routine syndecan-1 immunohistochemistry aids in the diagnosis of chronic endometritis. Arch Pathol Lab Med 2004, **128**: 1000–1003.

78 Bell DA, Mondschein M, Scully RE. Giant cell arteritis of the female genital tract. A report of three cases. Am J Surg Pathol 1986, **10**: 696–701.

79 Bennett AE, Rathore S, Rhatigan RM. Focal necrotizing endometritis: a clinicopathologic study of 15 cases. Int J Gynecol Pathol 2002, **18**: 220–225.

80 Bhagavan BS, Gupta PK. Genital actinomyosis and intrauterine contraceptive devices. Cytopathologic diagnosis and clinical significance. Hum Pathol 1978, **9**: 567–578.

81 Bhagavan BS, Ruffier J, Shinn B. Pseudoactinomycotic radiate granules in the lower female genital tract. Relationship to the Splendore–Hoeppli phenomenon. Hum Pathol 1982, **13**: 898–904.

82 Buckley CH, Fox H. Histiocytic endometritis. Histopathology 1980, **4**: 105–110.

83 Burkman R, Schlesselman S, McCaffrey L, Gupta PK, Spence M. The relationship of genital tract *Actinomyces* and the development of pelvic inflammatory disease. Am J Obstet Gynecol 1982, **143**: 585–589.

84 Bylund DJ, Nanfro JJ, Marsh WL. Coccidioidomycosis of the female genital tract. Arch Pathol Lab Med 1986, **110**: 232–235.

85 Corfman PA, Segal SJ. Biologic effects of intrauterine devices. Am J Obstet Gynecol 1968, **100**: 448–459.

86 Crum CP, Egawa K, Fenoglio CM, Richart RM. Chronic endometritis. The role of immunohistochemistry in the detection of plasma cells. Am J Obstet Gynecol 1983, **147**: 812–815.

87 Dehner LP, Askin FB. Cytomegalovirus endometritis. Obstet Gynecol 1975, **45**: 211–214.

88 Di Carlo FJ Jr, Di Carlo JP, Robboy SJ, Lyons MM. Sarcoidosis of the uterus. Arch Pathol Lab Med 1989, **113**: 941–943.

89 Francke ML, Mihaescu A, Chaubert P. Isolated necrotizing arteritis of the female genital tract: a clinicopathologic and immunohistochemical study of 11 cases. Int J Gynecol Pathol 1998, **17**: 193–200.

90 Frank TS, Himebaugh KS, Wilson MD. Granulomatous endometritis associated with histologically occult cytomegalovirus in a healthy patient. Am J Surg Pathol 1992, **16**: 716–720.

91 Ganesan R, Ferryman SR, Meier L, Rollason TP. Vasculitis of the female genital tract with clinicopathologic correlation: a study of 46 cases with follow-up. Int J Gynecol Pathol 2000, **19**: 258–265.

92 Gilmore H, Fleischhacker D, Hecht JL. Diagnosis of chronic endometritis in biopsies with stromal breakdown. Hum Pathol 2007, **38**: 581–584.

93 Govan ADT. Tuberculous endometritis. J Pathol Bacteriol 1962, **83**: 363–372.

94 Gupta PK. Intrauterine contraceptive devices. Vaginal cytology, pathologic changes and clinical implications. Acta Cytol (Baltimore) 1982, **26**: 571–613.

95 Hart WR, Prins RP, Tsai JC. Isolated coccidioidomycosis of the uterus. Hum Pathol 1976, **7**: 235–239.

96 Ho K-L. Sarcoidosis of the uterus. Hum Pathol 1978, **10**: 219–222.

97 Ismail SM. Follicular myometritis. A previously undescribed component of pelvic inflammatory disease. Histopathology 1990, **16**: 91–93.

98 Kim KR, Lee YH, Ro JY. Nodular histocytic hyperplasia of the endometrium. Int J Gyncol Pathol 2002, **21**: 141–146.

99 Kiviat NB, Wolner-Hanssen P, Eschenbach DA, Wasserheit JN, Paavonen JA, Bell TA, Critchlow CW, Stamm WE, Moore DE, Holmes KK. Endometrial histopathology in patients with culture-proved upper genital tract infection and laparoscopically diagnosed acute salpingitis. Am J Surg Pathol 1990, **14**: 167–175.

100 Leong AS, Vinyuvat S, Leong FW, Suthipintawong C. Anti-CD38 and VS38 antibodies for the detection of plasma cells in the diagnosis of chronic endometritis. Appl Immunohistochem 1997, **5**: 189–193.

101 Lombard CM, Moore MH, Seifer DB. Diagnosis of systemic polyarteritis nodosa following total abdominal hysterectomy and bilateral salpingo-oophorectomy. A case report. Int J Gynecol Pathol 1986, **5**: 63–68.

102 Molnar JJ, Poliak A. Recurrent endometrial malakoplakia. Am J Clin Pathol 1983, **80**: 762–764.

103 Müller-Holzner E, Ruth NR, Abfalter E, Schröcksnadel H, Dapunt O, Martin-Sances L, Nogales FF. IUD-associated pelvic actinomycosis. A report of five cases. Int J Gynecol Pathol 1995, **14**: 70–74.

104 Ober WB, Sobrero AJ, Kurman R, Gold S. Endometrial morphology and polyethylene intrauterine devices. A study of 200 endometrial biopsies. Obstet Gynecol 1968, **32**: 782–793.

105 Paavonen J, Aine R, Teisala K, Heinonen PK, Punnonen R. Comparison of endometrial biopsy and peritoneal fluid cytologic testing with laparoscopy in the diagnosis of acute pelvic inflammatory disease. Am J Obstet Gynecol 1985, **151**: 645–650.

106 Paavonen J, Kiviat N, Brunham RC, Stevens CE, Kuo C-C, Stamm WE, Miettinen A, Soules M, Eschenbach DA, Holmes KK. Prevalence and manifestations of endometritis among women with cervicitis. Am J Obstet Gynecol 1985, **152**: 280–286.

107 Paukku M, Puolakkainen M, Paavonen T, Paavonen J. Plasma cell endometritis is associated with *Chlamydia trachomatis* infection. Am J Clin Pathol 1999, **112**: 211–215.

108 Poropatich C, Rojas M, Silverberg SG. Polymorphonuclear leukocytes in the endometrium during the normal menstrual cycle. Int J Gynecol Pathol 1987, **6**: 230–234.

109 Risse EKJ, Beerthuizen RJCM, Vooijs GP. Cytologic and histologic findings in women using an IUD. Obstet Gynecol 1981, **58**: 569–573.

110 Rotterdam H. Chronic endometritis. A clinicopathologic study. Pathol Annu 1978, **13**(Pt 2): 209–231.

111 Russack V, Lammers RJ. Xanthogranulomatous endometritis. Report of six cases and a proposed mechanism of development. Arch Pathol Lab Med 1990, **114**: 929–932.

112 Schmidt WA. IUDs, inflammation, and infection. Assessment after two decades of IUD use. Hum Pathol 1982, **13**: 878–881.

113 Sen DK, Fox H. The lymphoid tissue of the endometrium. Gynaecologia (Basel) 1967, **163**: 371–378.

114 Shintaku M, Sasaki M, Baba Y. Ceroid-containing histiocytic granuloma of the endometrium. Histopathology 1991, **18**: 169–172.

115 Silverberg SG, Haukkamaa M, Arko H, Nilsson CG, Luukkainen T. Endometrial morphology during long-term use of levonorgestrel-releasing intrauterine devices. Int J Gynecol Pathol 1986, **5**: 235–241.

116 Silvernagel SW, Harshbarger KE, Shevlin DW. Postoperative granulomas of the endometrium: histological features after endometrial ablation. Ann Diagn Pathol 1999, **1**: 82–90.

117 Smith M, Hagerty KA, Skipper B, Bocklage T. Chronic endometritis: a combined histopathologic and clinical review of cases from 2002 to 2007. Int J Gynecol Pathol 2010, **29**: 44–50.

118 Stern RA, Svoboda-Newman SM, Frank TS. Analysis of chronic endometritis for *Chlamydia trachomatis* by polymerase chain reaction. Hum Pathol 1996, **27**: 1085–1088.

119 Taylor ES, McMillan JH, Greer BE, Droegemueller W, Thompson HE. The intrauterine device and tubo-ovarian abscess. Am J Obstet Gynecol 1975, **123**: 338–347.

120 Venkataseshan VS, Woo TH. Diffuse viral papillomatosis (condyloma) of the uterine cavity. Int J Gynecol Pathol 1985, **4**: 370–377.

121 Westrom L, Bengtsson LP, Mardh P. The risk of pelvic inflammatory disease in women using intrauterine contraceptive devices as compared to non-users. Lancet 1976, **2**: 221–224.

122 Whiteley PF, Hamlett JD. Pyometra – a reappraisal. Am J Obstet Gynecol 1971, **109**: 108–112.

123 Winkler B, Reumann W, Mitao M, Gallo L, Richart RM, Crum CP. Chlamydial endometritis. A histological and immunohistochemical analysis. Am J Surg Pathol 1984, **8**: 771–778.

METAPLASIA

124 Abell MR. Endometrial biopsy. Normal and abnormal diagnostic characteristics. In Gold JJ (ed.): Gynecologic endocrinology. New York, 1975, Harper and Row, pp. 156–190.

125 Axelson G, Nassar A, Giorgadze T. Gastrointestinal mucin expression in glandular epithelia of the uterus. Lab Invest 2009, **89**(Suppl 1): 206A–207A.

126 Bhatia NN, Hoshiko MG. Uterine osseous metaplasia. Obstet Gynecol 1982, **60**: 256–259.

127 Bird CC, Willis RA. The production of smooth muscle by the endometrial stroma of the adult human uterus. J Pathol Bacteriol 1965, **90**: 75–81.

128 Blaustein A. Morular metaplasia misdiagnosed as adenoacanthoma in young women with polycystic ovarian disease. Am J Surg Pathol 1982, **6**: 223–228.

129 Bomze EJ, Friedman NB. Squamous metaplasia and adenoacanthosis of the endometrium. Obstet Gynecol 1967, **30**: 619–625.

130 Crum CP, Richart RM, Fenoglio CM. Adenoacanthosis of the endometrium. A clinicopathologic study in premenopausal women. Am J Surg Pathol 1981, **5**: 15–20.

131 Demopoulos RI, Greco MA. Mucinous metaplasia of the endometrium. Ultrastructural and histochemical characteristics. Int J Gynecol Pathol 1983, **1**: 383–390.

132 Dutra FR. Intraglandular morules of the endometrium. Am J Clin Pathol 1959, **31**: 60–65.

133 Gersell DJ. Endometrial papillary syncytial change. Another perspective. Am J Clin Pathol 1993, **99**: 656–657.

134 Hendrickson MR, Kempson RL. Surgical pathology of the uterine corpus. In Bennington JL (ed.): Major problems in pathology, vol. 12. Philadelphia, 1980, W.B. Saunders, pp. 418–438.

135 Hendrickson MR, Kempson RL. Endometrial epithelial metaplasias. Proliferations frequently misdiagnosed as adenocarcinoma. Report of 89 cases and proposed classification. Am J Surg Pathol 1980, **4**: 525–542.

136 Houghton O, Connolly LE, McCluggage WG. Morules in endometrioid proliferations of the uterus and ovary consistently express the intestinal transcription factor CDX2. Histopathology 2008, **53**: 156–165.

137 Kaku T, Silverberg SG, Tsukamoto N, Tsuruchi N, Kamura T, Saito T, Nakano H. Association of endometrial epithelial metaplasias with endometrial carcinoma and hyperplasia in Japanese and American women. Int J Gynecol Pathol 1993, **12**: 297–300.

138 Lin MC, Lomo L, Baak JP, Eng C, Ince TA, Crum CP, Mutter GL. Squamous morules are functionally inert elements of premalignant endometrial neoplasia. Mod Pathol 2009, **22**: 167–174.

139 Miranda MC, Mazur MT. Endometrial squamous metaplasia. An unusual response to progestin therapy of hyperplasia. Arch Pathol Lab Med 1995, **119**: 458–460.

140 Moritani S, Kushima R, Ichihara S, Okabe H, Hattori T, Kobayashi TK, Silverberg SG. Eosinophilic cell change of the endometrium: a possible relationship to mucinous differentiation. Mod Pathol 2005, **18**: 1243–1248.

141 Nucci MR, Prasad CJ, Crum CP, Mutter GL. Mucinous endometrial epithelial proliferations: a morphologic spectrum of changes with diverse clinical significance. Mod Pathol 2000, **12**: 1137–1142.

142 Peng SL, Simon RA, Quddus MR, Zhang C, Lawrence WD, Sung CJ. Atypical tubal metaplasia in endometrial samplings is not associated with increased risk of developing hyperplasia or carcinoma: a long term follow-up study of 63 cases. Lab Invest 2009, **89**(Suppl 1): 231A.

143 Quddus MR, Sung CJ, Zheng W, Lauchlan SC. P53 immunoreactivity in endometrial metaplasia with dysfunctional uterine bleeding. Histopathology 1999, **35**: 44–49.

144 Rorat E, Wallach RC. Papillary metaplasia of the endometrium. Clinical and histopathologic considerations. Obstet Gynecol 1984, **64**: 90S–92S.

145 Roth E, Taylor HB. Heterotopic cartilage in the uterus. Obstet Gynecol 1966, **27**: 838–844.

146 Salm R. Mucin production of the normal and abnormal endometrium. Arch Pathol 1962, **73**: 30–39.

147 Schueller EF. Ciliated epithelia of the human uterine mucosa. Obstet Gynecol 1968, **31**: 215–223.

148 Shah SS, Mazur MT. Endometrial eosinophilic syncytial change related to breakdown: immunohistochemical evidence suggests a regressive process. Int J Gynecol Pathol 2008, **27**: 534–538.

149 Silver SA, Cheung AN, Tavassoli FA. Oncocytic metaplasia and carcinoma of the endometrium: an immunohistochemical and ultrastructural study. Int J Gynecol Pathol 1999, **18**: 12–19.

150 Tyagi SP, Saxena K, Rizvi R, Langley FA. Foetal remnants in the uterus and their relation to other uterine heterotopia. Histopathology 1979, **3**: 339–345.

151 Wells M, Tiltman A. Intestinal metaplasia of the endometrium. Histopathology 1989, **15**: 431–433.

152 Zaman SS, Mazur MT. Endometrial papillary syncytial change. A nonspecific alteration associated with active breakdown. Am J Clin Pathol 1993, **99**: 741–745.

ADENOMYOSIS AND ENDOMETRIOSIS

153 Ahmed AA, Swan RW, Owen A, Kraus FT, Patrick F. Uterus-like mass arising in broad ligament: a metaplasia or mullerian duct anomaly? Int J Gynecol Pathol 1998, **16**: 279–281.

154 Ahn GH, Scully RE. Clear cell carcinoma of the inguinal region arising from endometriosis. Cancer 1991, **67**: 116–120.

155 Barbieri RL. Etiology and epidemiology of endometriosis. Am J Obstet Gynecol 1990, **162**: 565–567.

156 Bergqvist A, Ljungberg O, Myhre E. Human endometrium and endometriotic tissue obtained simultaneously. A comparative histological study. Int J Gynecol Pathol 1984, **3**: 135–145.

157 Black M, Ali R, Stringer A, Deavers MT, Malpica A, Silva EG. Uterine adenomyosis, complete and incomplete [abstract]. Mod Pathol 2003, **16**: 182a.

158 Brooks JJ, Wheeler JE. Malignancy arising in extragonadal endometriosis. A case report and summary of the world literature. Cancer 1977, **40**: 3065–3073.

159 Bulun SE. Endometriosis. N Engl J Med 2009, **360**: 268–279.

160 Chumas JC, Thanning L, Mann WJ. Malignant mixed müllerian tumor arising in extragenital endometriosis. Report of a case and review of the literature. Gynecol Oncol 1986, **23**: 227–233.

161 Clement PB. Pathology of endometriosis. Pathol Annu 1990, **25**(Pt 1): 245–295.

162 Clement PB, Granai CO, Young RH, Scully RE. Endometriosis with myxoid change. A case simulating pseudomyxoma peritonei. Am J Surg Pathol 1994, **18**: 849–853.

163 Clement PB, Young RH. Florid cystic endosalpingiosis with tumor-like manifestations: a report of four cases including the first reported cases of transmural endosalpingiosis of the uterus. Am J Surg Pathol 1999, **23**: 166–175.

164 Clement PB, Young RH. Two previously unemphasized features of endometriosis: micronodular stromal endometriosis and endometriosis with stromal elastosis. Int J Surg Pathol 2001, **8**: 223–227.

165 Colella R, Mameli MG, Bellezza G, Sordo RD, Cavaliere A, Sidoni A. Endometriosis-associated skeletal muscle regeneration: a hitherto undescribed entity and a potential diagnostic pitfall. Am J Surg Pathol 2010, **34**: 10–17.

166 Emge LA. The elusive adenomyosis of the uterus. Its historical past and its present stage of recognition. Am J Obstet Gynecol 1962, **83**: 1541–1563.

167 Ferguson BR, Bennington JL, Haber SL. Histochemistry of mucosubstances and histology of mixed müllerian pelvic lymph node glandular inclusions. Evidence for histogenesis by müllerian metaplasia of coelomic epithelium. Obstet Gynecol 1969, **33**: 617–625.

168 Fukunaga M. Smooth muscle metaplasia in ovarian endometriosis. Histopathology 2000, **36**: 348–352.

169 Fukunaga M, Ushigome S. Epithelial metaplastic changes in ovarian endometriosis. Mod Pathol 1998, **11**: 784–788.

170 Giudice LC. Endometriosis. N Engl J Med 2010, **362**: 2389–2398.

171 Goldblum JR, Clement PB, Hart WR. Adenomyosis with sparse glands. A potential mimic of low-grade endometrial stromal. Am J Clin Pathol 1995, **103**: 218–223.

172 Hall JB, Young RH, Nelson JH. The prognostic significance of adenomyosis in endometrial carcinoma. Gynecol Oncol 1984, **17**: 32–40.

173 Hanley K, Dustin S, Stoler M, Atkins K. The significance of adenomyosis involved by tumor in otherwise low stage endometrioid adenocarcinomas. Int J Gynecol Pathol 2010, **29**: 445–451.

174 Heaps JM, Nieberg RK, Berek JS. Malignant neoplasms arising in endometriosis. Obstet Gynecol 1990, **75**: 1023–1028.

175 Ismiil ND, Rasty G, Ghorab Z, Nofech-Mozes S, Bernardini M, Thomas G, Ackerman I, Covens A, Khalifa MA. Adenomyosis is

associated with myometrial invasion by FIGO 1 endometrial adenocarcinoma. Int J Gynecol Pathol 2007, **26**: 278–283.

176 Jung WY, Shin BK, Kim I. Uterine adenomyoma with uterus-like features: a report of two cases. Int J Surg Pathol 2002, **10**: 163–166.

177 Karp LA, Czernobilsky B. Glandular inclusions in pelvic and abdominal paraaortic lymph nodes. Am J Clin Pathol 1969, **52**: 212–218.

178 Leiman G. Carcinoma ex endometriosis: the jury is still out. Adv Anat Pathol 1996, **3**: 362–366.

179 Li SF, Nakayama K, Masuzawa H, Fujii S. The number of proliferating cell nuclear antigen positive cells in endometriotic lesions differs from that in the endometrium. Analysis of PCNA positive cells during the menstrual cycle and in post-menopause. Virchows Arch [A] 1993, **423**: 257–263.

180 Lu PY, Ory SJ. Endometriosis. Current management. Mayo Clin Proc 1995, **70**: 453–463.

181 Mai KT, Yazdi HM, Perkins DG, Parks W. Development of endometriosis from embryonic duct remnants. Hum Pathol 1998, **29**: 319–322.

182 Marcoux S, Maheux R, Berube S. Laparoscopic surgery in infertile women with minimal or mild endometriosis. Canadian Collaborative Group on Endometriosis. N Engl J Med 1997, **337**: 217–222.

183 Mathur BBL, Shah BS, Bhende YM. Adenomyosis uteri. Am J Obstet Gynecol 1962, **84**: 1820–1829.

184 McCluggage WG, Bryson C, Lamki H, Boyle DD. Benign, borderline, and malignant endometrioid neoplasia arising in endometriosis in association with tamoxifen therapy. Int J Gynecol Pathol 2000, **19**: 276–279.

185 McCluggage WG, Desai V, Manek S. Tamoxifen associated postmenopausal adenomyosis exhibits stromal fibrosis, glandular dilatation and epithelial metaplasia. Histopathology 2000, **37**: 340–346.

186 Meenakshi M, McCluggage WG. Vascular involvement in adenomyosis: report of a large series of a common phenomenon with observations on the pathogenesis of adenomyosis. Int J Gynecol Pathol 2010, **29**: 117–121.

187 Molitor JJ. Adenomyosis. A clinical and pathological appraisal. Am J Obstet Gynecol 1971, **110**: 275–284.

188 Mostoufizadeh M, Scully RE. Malignant tumors arising in endometriosis. Clin Obstet Gynecol 1980, **23**: 951–963.

189 Nagai Y, Kishimoto T, Nikaido T, Nishihara K, Matsumoto T, Suzuki C, Ogishima T, Kuwahara Y, Hurukata Y, Mizunuma M, Nakata Y, Ishikura H. Squamous predominance in mixed-epithelial papillary cystadenomas of borderline malignancy of Mullerian type arising in endometriotic cysts: a study of four cases. Am J Surg Pathol 2003, **27**: 242–247.

190 Nakayama K, Masuzawa H, Li SF, Yoshikawa F, Toki T, Nikaido T, Silverberg SG, Fujii S. Immunohistochemical analysis of the peritoneum adjacent to endometriotic lesions using antibodies for Ber-EP4 antigen, estrogen receptors, and progesterone receptors. Implication of peritoneal metaplasia in the pathogenesis of endometriosis. Int J Gynecol Pathol 1994, **13**: 348–358.

191 Nothnick WB, Fan F, Iczkowski KA, Ashwell R, Thomas P, Tawfik OW. CD44s expression is reduced in endometriotic lesions compared to eutopic endometrium in women with endometriosis. Int J Gynecol Pathol 2001, **20**: 140–146.

192 Nuovo M, Bayani E, Gerold T, Leong M, Mir R. Endometrioid cystadenofibroma developing in juxtahepatic endometriosis: a case report. Int J Surg Pathol 1998, **6**: 109–112.

193 Parker RL, Dadmanesh F, Young RH, Clement PB. Polypoid endometriosis: a clinicopathologic analysis of 24 cases and a review of the literature. Am J Surg Pathol 2004, **28**: 285–297.

194 Prade M, Spatz A, Bentledy R, Duvillard P, Bognel C, Robboy SJ. Borderline and malignant serous tumor arising in pelvic lymph nodes. Evidence of origin in benign glandular inclusions. Int J Gynecol Pathol 1995, **14**: 87–91.

195 Roth LM. Endometriosis with perineural involvement. Am J Clin Pathol 1973, **59**: 807–809.

196 Seidman JD. Prognostic importance of hyperplasia and atypia in endometriosis. Int J Gynecol Pathol 1996, **15**: 1–9.

197 Seidman JD, Kjerulff KH. Pathologic findings from the Maryland Women's Health Study: practice patterns in the diagnosis of adenomyosis. Int J Gynecol Pathol 1997, **15**: 217–221.

198 Shutter J. Uterus-like ovarian mass presenting near menarche. Int J Gynecol Pathol 2005, **24**: 382–384.

199 Sinkre P, Hoang MP, Albores-Saavedra J. Mullerianosis of inguinal lymph nodes: report of a case. Int J Gynecol Pathol 2002, **21**: 60–64.

200 Slavin RE, Krum R, Van Dinh T. Endometriosis-associated intestinal tumors: a clinical and pathologic study of 6 cases and review of the literature. Hum Pathol 2000, **31**: 456–463.

201 Steck WD, Helwig EB. Cutaneous endometriosis. JAMA 1965, **191**: 167–170.

202 Stern RC, Dash R, Bentley RC, Snyder MJ, Haney AF, Robboy SJ. Malignancy in endometriosis: frequency and comparison of ovarian and extraovarian types. Int J Gynecol Pathol 2001, **20**: 133–139.

203 Tamura M, Fukaya T, Murakami T, Uehara S, Yajima A. Analysis of clonality in human endometriotic cysts based on evaluation of X chromosome inactivation in archival formalin-fixed, paraffin-embedded tissue. Lab Invest 1998, **78**: 213–218.

204 Toki T, Horiuchi A, Li SF, Nakayama K, Silverberg SG, Fujii S. Proliferative activity of postmenopausal endometriosis: a histopathologic and immunocytochemical study. Int J Gynecol Pathol 1996, **15**: 45–53.

205 Wells M. Recent advances in endometriosis with emphasis on pathogenesis, molecular pathology, and neoplastic transformation. Int J Gynecol Pathol 2004, **23**: 316–320.

206 Winkelman J, Robinson R. Adenocarcinoma of endometrium involving adenomyosis. Report of an unusual case and review of the literature. Cancer 1966, **19**: 901–908.

207 Youssef AH, Ganesan R, Rollason TP. Florid cystic endosalpingiosis of the uterus. Histopathology 2006, **49**: 546–548.

208 Zheng W, Li N, Wang J, Ulukus EC, Ulukus M, Arici A, Liang SX. Initial endometriosis showing direct morphologic evidence of metaplasia in the pathogenesis of ovarian endometriosis. Int J Gynecol Pathol 2005, **24**: 164–172.

DYSFUNCTIONAL UTERINE BLEEDING AND HYPERPLASIA

209 Abell MR. Adenocarcinoma (gland-cell carcinoma) in situ of endometrium. Pathol Res Pract 1982, **174**: 221–236.

210 Ambros RA. Simple hyperplasia of the endometrium: an evaluation of proliferative activity by Ki-67 immunostaining. Int J Gynecol Pathol 2000, **19**: 206–211.

211 Ausems EWMA, van der Kamp J-K, Baak JPA. Nuclear morphometry in the determination of the prognosis of marked atypical endometrial hyperplasia. Int J Gynecol Pathol 1985, **4**: 180–185.

212 Baak JPA, Kurver PHJ, Diegenbach PC, Delemarre JFM, Brekelmans ECM, Nieuwlaat JE. Discrimination of hyperplasia and carcinoma of the endometrium by quantitative microscopy – a feasibility study. Histopathology 1981, **5**: 61–68.

213 Baak JP, Wisse-Brekelmans EC, Fleege JC, van der Putten HW, Bezemer PD. Assessment of the risk on endometrial cancer in hyperplasia, by means of morphological and morphometrical features. Pathol Res Pract 1992, **188**: 856–859.

214 Baloglu H, Cannizzaro LA, Jones J, Koss LG. Atypical endometrial hyperplasia shares genomic abnormalities with endometrioid carcinoma by comparative genomic hybridisation. Hum Pathol 2001, **32**: 615–622.

215 Bell CD, Ostrezega E. The significance of secretory features and coincident hyperplastic changes in endometrial biopsy specimens. Hum Pathol 1987, **18**: 830–838.

216 Bergeron C, Nogales FF, Masseroli M, Abeler V, Duvillard P, Muller-Holzner E, Pickartz H, Wells M. A multicentric European study testing the reproductivity of the WHO classification of endometrial hyperplasia with a proposal of a simplified working classification for biopsy and curettage specimens. Am J Surg Pathol 1999, **23**: 1102–1108.

217 Beutler HK, Dockerty MB, Randall L. Precancerous lesions of the endometrium. Am J Obstet Gynecol 1963, **86**: 433–443.

218 Campbell PE, Barter RA. The significance of atypical endometrial hyperplasia. J Obstet Gynaecol Br Commonw 1961, **68**: 668–672.

219 Castelbaum AJ, Wheeler J, Coutifaris CB, Mastroianni L Jr, Lessey BA. Timing of the endometrial biopsy may be critical for the accurate diagnosis of luteal phase deficiency. Fertil Steril 1994, **61**: 443–447.

220 Choo YC, Mak KC, Hsu C, Wong TS, Ma HK. Postmenopausal uterine bleeding of nonorganic cause. Obstet Gynecol 1985, **66**: 225–228.

221 Dallenbach-Hellweg G. The endometrium of infertility. Pathol Res Pract 1984, **178**: 527–537.

222 Dallenbach-Hellweg G. Histopathology of the endometrium (English translation by FD Dallenbach), ed. 3. New York, 1985, Springer-Verlag.

223 Dietel M. The histological diagnosis of endometrial hyperplasia: is there a need to simplify? Virchows Arch 2001, **439**: 604–608.

224 Feichter GE, Hoffken H, Heep J, Haag D, Heberling D, Brandt H, Rummel H, Goerttler KL. DNA-flow-cytometric measurements on the normal, atrophic, hyperplastic and neoplastic human endometrium. Virchows Arch [A] 1982, **398**: 53–65.

225 Fenoglio CM, Crum CP, Ferenczy A. Endometrial hyperplasia and carcinoma. Are ultrastructural, biochemical and immunocytochemical studies useful in distinguishing between them? Pathol Res Pract 1982, **174**: 257–284.

226 Fox H, Buckley CH. The endometrial hyperplasias and their relationship to endometrial neoplasia. Histopathology 1982, **6**: 493–510.

227 Gillam JS. Study of the inadequate secretion phase endometrium. Fertil Steril 1955, **6**: 18–36.

228 Gordon MD, Ireland K. Pathology of hyperplasia and carcinoma of the endometrium. Semin Oncol 1994, **21**: 64–70.

229 Gore H, Hertig AT. Carcinoma in situ of the endometrium. Am J Obstet Gynecol 1966, **94**: 135–155.

230 Greenblatt RB, Hammond DO, Clark SL. Membranous dysmenorrhea. Studies in etiology and treatment. Am J Obstet Gynecol 1954, **68**: 835–844.

231 Gusberg SB, Kaplan AL. Precursors of corpus cancer. IV. Adenomatous hyperplasia as stage 0 carcinoma of the endometrium. Am J Obstet Gynecol 1963, **87**: 662–667.

232 Hendrickson MR, Kempson RL. Surgical pathology of the uterine corpus. In Bennington JL (ed.): Major problems in pathology, vol. 12. Philadelphia, 1980, W.B. Saunders, pp. 285–318.

233 Hendrickson MR, Ross JC, Kempson RL. Toward the development of morphologic criteria for well-differentiated adenocarcinoma of the endometrium. Am J Surg Pathol 1983, **7**: 819–838.

234 Kurman RJ, Norris HJ. Evaluation of criteria for distinguishing atypical endometrial hyperplasia from well-differentiated carcinoma. Cancer 1982, **49**: 2547–2559.

235 Kurman RJ, Norris HJ. Endometrium. In Henson DE, Albores-Saavedra J (eds): The pathology of incipient neoplasia. Philadelphia, 1986, W.B. Saunders, pp. 265–277.

236 Lee KR, Scully RE. Complex endometrial hyperplasia and carcinoma in adolescents and young women 15 to 20 years of age. A report of 10 cases. Int J Gynecol Pathol 1989, **8**: 201–213.

237 Loghavi S, Silva EG. Abnormal myometrial vasculature explains some cases of menorrhagia. Lab Invest 2009, **89**(Suppl 1): 225A.

238 McElin TW, Bird CC, Reeves BD, Scott RC. Diagnostic dilation and curettage. A 20-year survey. Obstet Gynecol 1969, **33**: 807–812.

239 McLennan CE, Rydell AH. Extent of endometrial shedding during normal menstruation. Obstet Gynecol 1965, **26**: 605–621.

240 Meyer WC, Malkasian GD, Dockerty MB, Decker DG. Postmenopausal bleeding from atrophic endometrium. Obstet Gynecol 1971, **38**: 731–738.

241 Michael H, Kotylo PA, Mohr M, Roth LM. DNA ploidy, cell cycle kinetics, and low versus high grade atypia in endometrial hyperplasia. Am J Clin Pathol 1996, **106**: 22–28.

242 Moszkowski E, Woodruff JD, Jones GES. The inadequate luteal phase. Am J Obstet Gynecol 1962, **83**: 363–372.

243 Mutter GL. Endometrial intraepithelial neoplasia (EIN): will it bring order to chaos? The Endometrial Collaborative Group. Gynecol Oncol 2000, **76**: 287–290.

244 Mutter GL. Histopathology of genetically defined endometrial precancers. Int J Gynecol Pathol 2001, **19**: 301–309.

245 Mutter GL, Nogales F, Kurman R, Silverberg S, Tavassoli F. Endometrial cancer. In Tavassoli FA, Stratton MR (eds): WHO classification of tumors: pathology and genetics, tumors of the breast and female genital organs. Lyon, 2002, IARC Press.

246 Mutter GL, Zaino RJ, Baak JP, Bentley RC, Robboy SJ. Benign endometrial hyperplasia sequence and endometrial intraepithelial neoplasia. Int J Gynecol Pathol 2007, **26**: 103–114.

247 Norris HJ, Becker RL, Mikel UV. A comparative morphometric and cytophotometric study of endometrial hyperplasia, atypical hyperplasia, and endometrial carcinoma. Hum Pathol 1989, **20**: 219–223.

248 Norris HJ, Tavassoli FA, Kurman RJ. Endometrial hyperplasia and carcinoma. Diagnostic considerations. Am J Surg Pathol 1983, **7**: 839–847.

249 Noyes RW. The underdeveloped secretory endometrium. Am J Obstet Gynecol 1962, **83**: 363–372.

250 Pacheco JC, Kempers RD. Etiology of postmenopausal bleeding. Obstet Gynecol 1968, **32**: 40–46.

251 Picoff RC, Luginbuhl WH. Fibrin in the endometrial stroma. Its relation to uterine bleeding. Am J Obstet Gynecol 1964, **88**: 642–646.

252 Sherman ME, Ronnett BM, Ioffe OB, Richesson DA, Rush BB, Glass AG, Chatterjee N, Duggan MA, Lacey JV Jr. Reproducibility of biopsy diagnoses of endometrial hyperplasia: evidence supporting a simplified classification. Int J Gynecol Pathol 2008, **27**: 318–325.

253 Silverberg SG. Hyperplasia and carcinoma of the endometrium. Semin Diagn Pathol 1988, **5**: 135–153.

254 Silverberg SG. Problems in the differential diagnosis of endometrial hyperplasia and carcinoma. Mod Pathol 2000, **13**: 309–327.

255 Skov BG, Broholm H, Engel U, Franzmann MB, Nielsen AL, Lauritzen AF, Skov T. Comparison of the reproducibility of the WHO classifications of 1975 and 1994 of endometrial hyperplasia. Int J Gynecol Pathol 1997, **16**: 33–37.

256 Söderström K-O. Lectin binding to human endometrial hyperplasias and adenocarcinoma. Int J Gynecol Pathol 1987, **6**: 356–365.

257 Sommers SC. Defining the pathology of endometrial hyperplasia, dysplasia and carcinoma. Pathol Res Pract 1982, **174**: 175–197.

258 Stewart CJ, Campbell-Brown M, Critchley HO, Farquharson MA. Endometrial apoptosis in patients with dysfunctional uterine bleeding. Histopathology 1999, **34**: 99–105.

259 Tavassoli F, Kraus FT. Endometrial lesions in uteri resected for atypical endometrial hyperplasia. Am J Clin Pathol 1978, **70**: 770–779.

260 Thornburgh I, Anderson MC. The endometrial deficient secretory phase. Histopathology 1997, **30**: 11–15.

261 Truskinovsky AM, Lifschitz-Mercer B, Czernobilsky B. Hyperplasia and carcinoma, with or without secretory changes, in secretory endometrium: a diagnostic challenge. Lab Invest 2009, **89**(Suppl 1): 239A.

262 Vellios F. Endometrial hyperplasias, precursors of endometrial carcinoma. Pathol Annu 1972, **7**: 201–229.

263 Welch WR, Scully RE. Precancerous lesions of the endometrium. Hum Pathol 1977, **8**: 503–512.

264 Winkler B, Alvarez S, Richart RM, Crum CP. Pitfalls in the diagnosis of endometrial neoplasia. Obstet Gynecol 1984, **64**: 185–194.

265 Zaino RJ. Endometrial hyperplasia: is it time for a quantum leap to a new classification? Int J Gynecol Pathol 2001, **19**: 314–321.

266 Zaino RJ, Kauderer J, Trimble CL, Silverberg SG, Curtin JP, Lim PC, Gallup DG. Reproducibility of the diagnosis of atypical endometrial hyperplasia: a Gynecologic Oncology Group study. Cancer 2006, **106**: 804–811.

RELATIONSHIP WITH CARCINOMA

267 Ashton-Sager A, Paulino AF, Afify AM. GLUT-1 is preferentially expressed in atypical endometrial hyperplasia and endometrial adenocarcinoma. Appl Immunohistochem Mol Morphol 2006, **14**: 187–192.

268 Baak JP, Wisse-Brekelmans EC, Fleege JC, van der Putten HW, Bezemer PD. Assessment of the risk on endometrial cancer in hyperplasia, by means of morphological and morphometrical features. Pathol Res Pract 1992, **188**: 856–859.

269 Chamlian LD, Taylor HB. Endometrial hyperplasia in young women. Obstet Gynecol 1970, **36**: 659–666.

270 Dietel M. The histological diagnosis of endometrial hyperplasia: is there a need to simplify? Virchows Arch 2001, **439**: 604–608.

271 Gal D. Hormonal therapy for lesions of the endometrium. Semin Oncol 1986, **13**: 33–36.

272 Gusberg SB, Kaplan AL. Precursors of corpus cancer. IV. Adenomatous hyperplasia as stage 0 carcinoma of the endometrium. Am J Obstet Gynecol 1963, **87**: 662–667.

273 Hardesty J, Xie QM, Casey MJ, Bewtra C. Factors affecting treatment response of endometrial hyperplasia. Lab Invest 2009, **89**(Suppl 1): 217A.

274 Henson DE, Albores-Saavedra J. Pathology of incipient neoplasia, ed. 3. New York, 2001, Oxford University Press, p. 839.

275 Hertig AT, Sommers SC. Genesis of endometrial carcinoma. I. Study of prior biopsies. Cancer 1949, **2**: 946–956.

276 Horn LC, Meinel A, Handzel R, Einenkel J. Histopathology of endometrial hyperplasia and endometrial carcinoma: an update. Ann Diagn Pathol 2007, **11**: 297–311.

277 Kurman RJ, Kaminski PF, Norris HJ. The behavior of endometrial hyperplasia. A long-term study of 'untreated' hyperplasia in 170 patients. Cancer 1985, **56**: 403–412.

278 Mazur MT. Endometrial hyperplasia/adenocarcinoma. a conventional approach. Ann Diagn Pathol 2005, **9**: 174–181.

279 McBride JM. Pre-menopausal cystic hyperplasia and endometrial carcinoma. J Obstet Gynaecol Br Emp 1959, **66**: 288–296.

280 Mittal K, Sebenik M, Irwin C, Yan Z, Popiolek D, Curtin J, Palazzo J. Presence of endometrial adenocarcinoma in situ in complex atypical endometrial hyperplasia is associated with increased incidence of endometrial carcinoma in subsequent hysterectomy. Mod Pathol 2009, **22**: 37–42.

281 Scully RE. Definition of precursors in gynecologic cancer. Cancer 1981, **48**: 531–537.

282 Silverberg SG. Hyperplasia and carcinoma of the endometrium. Semin Diagn Pathol 1988, **5**: 135–153.

283 Sivridis E, Giatromanolaki A. Prognostic aspects on endometrial hyperplasia and neoplasia. Virchows Arch 2001, **439**: 118–126.

284 Steiner G, Kistner RW, Craig JM. Histological effects of progestins on hyperplasia and carcinoma in situ of the endometrium – further observations. Metabolism 1965, **14**: 356–386.

285 Tavassoli F, Kraus FT. Endometrial lesions in uteri resected for atypical endometrial hyperplasia. Am J Clin Pathol 1978, **70**: 770–779.

286 Trimble CL, Kauderer J, Zaino R, Silverberg S, Lim PC, Burke JJ 2nd, Alberts D, Curtin J. Concurrent endometrial carcinoma in women with a biopsy diagnosis of atypical endometrial hyperplasia: a Gynecologic Oncology Group study. Cancer 2006, **106**: 812–819.

287 Vellios F. Endometrial hyperplasias, precursors of endometrial carcinoma. Pathol Annu 1972, **7**: 201–229.

TUMORS

ENDOMETRIAL POLYPS

288 Clement PB, Young RH. Atypical polypoid adenomyoma of the uterus associated with Turner's syndrome. A report of three cases, including a review of 'estrogen-associated' endometrial neoplasms and neoplasms associated with Turner's syndrome. Int J Gynecol Pathol 1987, **6**: 104–113.

289 Corley D, Rowe J, Curtis MT, Hogan WM, Noumoff JS, Livolsi VA. Postmenopausal bleeding from unusual endometrial polyps in women on chronic tamoxifen therapy. Obstet Gynecol 1992, **79**: 111–116.

290 Creagh TM, Krausz T, Flanagan AM. Atypical stromal cells in a hyperplastic endometrial polyp. Histopathology 1995, **27**: 386–387.

291 Duggan MA, Rowlands C, Kneafsey PD, Nation JG, Stuart GCE. Uterine atypical polypoid adenomyoma and ovarian endometrioid carcinoma. Metastatic disease or dual primaries? Int J Gynecol Pathol 1995, **14**: 81–86.

292 Fukunaga M, Endo Y, Ushigome S, Ishikawa E. Atypical polypoid adenomyomas of the uterus. Histopathology 1995, **27**: 35–42.

293 Gilks CB, Clement PB, Hart WR, Young RH. Uterine adenomyomas excluding atypical polypoid adenomyomas and adenomyomas of endocervical type: a clinicopathologic study of 30 cases of an underemphasized lesion that may cause diagnostic problems with brief consideration of adenomyomas of other female genital tract sites. Int J Gynecol Pathol 2000, **19**: 195–205.

294 Hachisuga T, Miyakawa T, Tsujioka H, Horiuchi S, Emoto M, Kawarabayashi T. *K-ras* mutation in tamoxifen-related endometrial polyps. Cancer 2003, **98**: 1890–1897.

295 Hattab EM, Allam-Nandyala P, Rhatigan RM. The stromal component of large endometrial polyps. Int J Gynecol Pathol 1999, **18**: 332–337.

296 Heatley MK. Atypical polypoid adenomyoma: a systematic review of the English literature. Histopathology 2006, **48**: 609–610.

297 Kennedy MM, Baigrie CF, Manek S. Tamoxifen and the endometrium: review of 102 cases and comparison with HRT-related and non-HRT related endometrial pathology. Int J Gynecol Pathol 1999, **18**: 130–137.

298 Lehman MB, Hart WR. Simple and complex hyperplastic papillary proliferations of the endometrium: a clinicopathologic study of nine cases of apparently localized papillary lesions with fibrovascular stromal cores and epithelial metaplasia. Am J Surg Pathol 2001, **25**: 1347–1354.

299 Longacre TA, Chung MH, Rouse RV, Hendrickson MR. Atypical polypoid adenomyofibromas (atypical polypoid adenomyomas) of the uterus: a clinicopathologic study of 55 cases. Am J Surg Pathol 1996, **20**: 1–20.

300 Mazur MT. Atypical polypoid adenomyomas of the endometrium. Am J Surg Pathol 1981, **5**: 473–482.

301 McCluggage WG, Sumathi VP, McManus DT. Uterine serous carcinoma and endometrial intraepithelial carcinoma arising in endometrial polyps: report of 5 cases, including 2 associated with tamoxifen therapy. Hum Pathol 2003, **34**: 939–943.

302 Mittal KR, Peng XC, Wallach RC, Demopoulos RI. Coexistent atypical polypoid adenomyoma and endometrial adenocarcinoma. Hum Pathol 1995, **26**: 574–575.

303 Mittal K, Schwartz L, Goswami S, Demopoulos R. Estrogen and progesterone receptor expression in endometrial polyps. Int J Gynecol Pathol 1996, **15**: 345–347.

304 Mittal K, Da Costa D. Endometrial hyperplasia and carcinoma in endometrial polyps: clinicopathologic and follow-up findings. Int J Gynecol Pathol 2008, **27**: 45–48.

305 Ohishi Y, Kaku T, Kobayashi H, Aishima S, Umekita Y, Wake N, Tsuneyoshi M. CD10 immunostaining distinguishes atypical polypoid adenomyofibroma (atypical polypoid adenomyoma) from endometrial carcinoma invading the myometrium. Hum Pathol 2008, **39**: 1446–1453.

306 Ota S, Catasus L, Matius-Guiu X, Bussaglia E, Lagarda H, Pons C, Munoz J, Kamura T, Prat J. Molecular pathology of atypical polypoid adenomyoma of the uterus. Hum Pathol 2003, **34**: 784–788.

307 Schlesinger C, Kamoi S, Ascher SM, Kendell M, Lage JM, Silverberg SG. Endometrial polyps: a comparison study of patients receiving tamoxifen with two control groups. Int J Gynecol Pathol 1998, **17**: 302–311.

308 Staros EB, Shilkitus WF. Atypical polypoid adenomyoma with carcinomatous transformation. A case report. Surg Pathol 1991, **4**: 157–166.

309 Tahlan A, Nanda A, Mohan H. Uterine adenomyoma: a clinicopathologic review of 26 cases and a review of the literature. Int J Gynecol Pathol 2006, **25**: 361–365.

310 Tai LH, Tavassoli FA. Endometrial polyps with atypical (bizarre) stromal cells. Am J Surg Pathol 2002, **26**: 505–509.

311 Young RH, Treger T, Scully RE. Atypical polypoid adenomyoma of the uterus. A report of 27 cases. Am J Clin Pathol 1986, **86**: 139–145.

ENDOMETRIAL CARCINOMA

General and clinical features

312 Beckner ME, Mori T, Silverberg SG. Endometrial carcinoma. Nontumor factors in prognosis. Int J Gynecol Pathol 1985, **4**: 131–145.

313 Carcangiu ML, Radice P, Casalini P, Bertario L, Merola M, Sala P. Lynch syndrome – related endometrial carcinomas show a high frequency of nonendometrioid types and of high FIGO grade endometrioid types. Int J Surg Pathol 2010, **18**: 21–26.

314 Clement PB, Young RH. Atypical polypoid adenomyoma of the uterus associated with Turner's syndrome. A report of three cases, including a review of 'estrogen-associated' endometrial neoplasms and neoplasms associated with Turner's syndrome. Int J Gynecol Pathol 1987, **6**: 104–113.

315 Dallenbach-Hellweg G, Hahn U. Mucinous and clear cell adenocarcinomas of the endometrium in patients receiving antiestrogens (tamoxifen) and gestagens. Int J Gynecol Pathol 1995, **14**: 7–15.

316 Deligdisch L, Cohen CJ. Histologic correlates and virulence implications of endometrial carcinoma associated with adenomatous hyperplasia. Cancer 1985, **56**: 1452–1455.

317 Deligdisch L, Kalir T, Cohen CJ, de Latour M, Le Bouedec G, Penault-Llorca F. Endometrial histopathology in 700 patients treated with tamoxifen for breast cancer. Gynecol Oncol 2000, **78**: 181–186.

318 Fechner RE, Kaufman RH. Endometrial adenocarcinoma in Stein–Leventhal syndrome. Cancer 1974, **34**: 444–452.

319 Fisher B, Costantino JP, Redmond CK, Fisher ER, Wickerham DL, Cronin WM. Endometrial cancer in tamoxifen-treated breast cancer patients. Findings from the National Surgical Adjuvant Breast and Bowel Project (NSABP) B-14. J Natl Cancer Inst 1994, **86**: 527–537.

320 Garg K, Shih K, Barakat R, Zhou Q, Iasonos A, Soslow RA. Endometrial carcinomas in women aged 40 years and younger: tumors associated with loss of DNA mismatch repair proteins comprise a distinct clinicopathologic subset. Am J Surg Pathol 2009, **33**: 1869–1877.

321 Garg K, Soslow RA. Lynch syndrome (hereditary non-polyposis colorectal cancer) and endometrial carcinoma. J Clin Pathol 2009, **62**: 679–684.

322 Geisler HE, Huber CP, Rogers S. Carcinoma of the endometrium in premenopausal women. Am J Obstet Gynecol 1969, **104**: 657–663.

323 Gusberg SB. The changing nature of endometrial cancer. N Engl J Med 1980, **302**: 709–732.

324 Hafezi S, Nofech-Mozes S, Ismiil N, Dube V, Saad RS, Ghorab Z, Kalifa MA. Endometrioid endometrial adenocarcinoma (EEA) in elderly women: a clinic-pathologic study. Lab Invest 2009, **89**(Suppl 1): 216A.

325 Kaufman RH, Abbott JP, Wall JA. The endometrium before and after wedge resection of the ovaries in the Stein–Leventhal syndrome. Am J Obstet Gynecol 1959, **77**: 1271–1285.

326 Kurman RJ, McConnell TG. Precursors of endometrial and ovarian carcinoma. Virchows Arch 2010, **456**: 1–12.

327 McCarty KS Jr, Barton TK, Peete CH Jr, Creasman WT. Gonadal dysgenesis with adenocarcinoma of the endometrium. An electron microscopic and steroid receptor analyses with a review of the literature. Cancer 1978, **42**: 512–520.

328 Magriples U, Naftolin F, Schwartz PE, Carcangiu ML. High-grade endometrial carcinoma in tamoxifen-treated breast cancer patients. J Clin Oncol 1993, **11**: 485–490.

329 Parkash V, Carcangiu ML. Uterine papillary serous carcinoma after radiation therapy for carcinoma of the cervix. Cancer 1992, **69**: 496–501.

330 Robboy SJ, Miller AW III, Kurman RJ. The pathologic features and behavior of endometrial carcinoma associated with exogenous estrogen administration. Pathol Res Pract 1982, **174**: 237–256.

331 Rodriguez J, Hart WR. Endometrial cancers occurring 10 or more years after pelvic irradiation for carcinoma. Int J Gynecol Pathol 1982, **1**: 135–144.

332 Rose PG. Endometrial carcinoma. N Engl J Med 1996, **335**: 640–649.

333 Schammel DP, Mittal KR, Kaplan K, Deligdisch L, Tavassoli FA. Endometrial adenocarcinoma associated with intrauterine pregnancy: a report of five cases and a review of the literature. Int J Gynecol Pathol 1998, **17**: 327–335.

334 Seidman JD, Kumar D, Cosin JA, Winter WE 3rd, Cargill C, Boice CR. Carcinomas of the female genital tract occurring after pelvic irradiation: a report of 15 cases. Int J Gynecol Pathol 2006, **25**: 293–297.

335 Shapiro S, Kelly JP, Rosenberg L, Kaufman DW, Helmrich SP, Rosenshein NB, Lewis JL, Knapp RC, Stolley PD, Schottenfeld D. Risk of localized and widespread endometrial cancer in relation to recent and discontinued use of conjugated estrogens. N Engl J Med 1985, **313**: 969–972.

336 Silva EG, Tornos CS, Follen-Mitchell M. Malignant neoplasms of the uterine corpus in patients treated for breast carcinoma. The effects of tamoxifen. Int J Gynecol Pathol 1994, **13**: 248–258.

337 Silverberg SG. The endometrium. Arch Pathol Lab Med 2007, **131**: 372–382.

338 Turbiner J, Moreno-Bueno G, Dahiya S, Sánchez-Estevez C, Hardisson D, Prat J, Oliva E, Palacios J. Clinicopathological and molecular analysis of endometrial carcinoma associated with tamoxifen. Mod Pathol 2008, **21**: 925–936.

339 van den Bos M, van den Hoven M, Jongejan E, van der Leij F, Michels M, Schakenraad S, Aben K, Hoogerbrugge N, Ligtenberg M, van Krieken JH. More differences between HNPCC-related and sporadic carcinomas from the endometrium as compared to the colon. Am J Surg Pathol 2004, **28**: 706–711.

340 Voigt LF, Weiss NS. Epidemiology of endometrial cancer. Cancer Treat Res 1989, **49**: 1–21.

Pathologic features

341 Ambros RA, Ballouk F, Malfetano JH, Ross JS. Significance of papillary (villoglandular) differentiation in endometrioid carcinoma of the uterus. Am J Surg Pathol 1994, **18**: 569–575.

342 Chen JL, Trost DC, Wilkinson EJ. Endometrial papillary adenocarcinomas. Two clinicopathological types. Int J Gynecol Pathol 1985, **4**: 279–288.

343 Clement PB. Pathology of the uterine corpus. Hum Pathol 1991, **22**: 776–791.

344 Clement PB, Young RH. Endometrioid carcinomas of the uterine corpus: a review of its pathology with emphasis on recent advances and problematic aspects. Adv Anat Pathol 2002, **9**: 145–184.

345 Esteller M, Garcia A, Martinez-Palones JM, Xercavins J, Reventos J. Clinicopathologic features and genetic alterations in endometrioid carcinoma of the uterus with villoglandular differentiation. Am J Clin Pathol 1999, **111**: 336–342.

346 Fanning J, Alvarez PM, Tsukada Y, Piver MS. Cervical implantation metastasis by endometrial adenocarcinoma. Cancer 1991, **68**: 1335–1339.

347 Frauenhoffer EE, Zaino RJ, Wolff TV, Whitney CE. Value of endocervical curettage in the staging of endometrial carcinoma. Int J Gynecol Pathol 1987, **6**: 195–202.

348 Gospel C. Ultrastructure of endometrial carcinoma. Review of fourteen cases. Cancer 1971, **28**: 745–754.

349 Guan H, Arabi H, Hayek K, Bandyopadhyay S, Fathallah L, Feng JN, Ali-Fehmi R. A binary grading system for endometrial carcinoma compared with existing grading systems. Lab Invest 2009, **89**(Suppl 1): 216A.

350 Hachisuga T, Fukuda K, Iwasaka T, Hirakawa T, Kawarabayashi T, Tsuneyoshi M. Endometrial adenocarcinomas of the uterine corpus in women younger than 50 years of age can be divided into two distinct clinical and pathologic entities based on anatomic location. Cancer 2001, **92**: 2578–2584.

351 Hall JB, Young RH, Nelson JH. The prognostic significance of adenomyosis in endometrial carcinoma. Gynecol Oncol 1984, **17**: 32–40.

352 Isaacson PG, Pilot LM Jr, Gooselaw JG. Foam cells in the stroma in carcinoma of the endometrium. Obstet Gynecol 1964, **23**: 9–11.

353 Jacques SM, Lawrence WD. Endometrial adenocarcinoma with variable-level myometrial involvement limited to adenomyosis. A clinicopathologic study of 23 cases. Gynecol Oncol 1990, **37**: 401–407.

354 Jacques SM, Qureshi F, Lawrence WD. Surface epithelial changes in endometrial adenocarcinoma. Diagnostic pitfalls in curettage specimens. Int J Gynecol Pathol 1995, **14**: 191–197.

355 Jacques SM, Qureshi F, Ramirez NC, Malviya VK, Lawrence WD. Tumors of uterine isthmus: clinicopathologic features and immunohistochemical characterization of p53 expression and hormone receptors. Int J Gynecol Pathol 1997, **16**: 38–44.

356 Kadar NRD, Kohorn EI, LiVolsi VA, Kapp DS. Histologic variants of cervical involvement by endometrial carcinoma. Obstet Gynecol 1982, **59**: 85–93.

357 Kalyanasundaram K, Ganesan R, Perunovic B, McCluggage WG. Diffusely infiltrating endometrial carcinomas with no stromal response: report of a series, including cases with cervical and ovarian involvement and emphasis on the potential for misdiagnosis. Int J Surg Pathol 2010, **18**: 138–143.

358 Landry D, Mai KT, Senterman MK, Perkins DG, Yazdi HM, Veinot JP, Thomas J. Endometrioid adenocarcinoma of the uterus with a minimal deviation invasive pattern. Histopathology 2002, **42**: 77–82.

359 Larson DM, Copeland LJ, Gallagher HS, Gershenson DM, Freedman RS, Wharton JT, Kline RC. Nature of cervical involvement in endometrial carcinoma. Cancer 1987, **59**: 959–962.

360 Lax SF, Kurman RJ, Pizer ES, Wu L, Ronnett BM. A binary architectural grading system for uterine endometrial endometrioid carcinoma has superior reproducibility compared with FIGO grading and identifies subsets of advance-stage tumors with favourable and unfavourable prognosis. Am J Surg Pathol 2000, **24**: 1201–1208.

361 Longacre TA, Chung MH, Jensen DN, Hendrickson MR. Proposed criteria for the diagnosis of well-differentiated endometrial carcinoma. A diagnostic test for myoinvasion. Am J Surg Pathol 1995, **19**: 371–406.

362 Longacre TA, Hendrickson MR. Diffusely infiltrative endometrial adenocarcinoma: an adenoma malignum pattern of myoinvasion. Am J Surg Pathol 1999, **23**: 69–78.

363 Murray SK, Young RH, Scully RE. Uterine endometrioid carcinoma with small nonvillous papillae: an analysis of 26 cases of a favourable-prognosis tumor to be distinguished from serous carcinoma. Int J Surg Pathol 2001, **8**: 279–289.

364 Nascimento AF, Hirsch MS, Cviko A, Quade BJ, Nucci MR. The role of CD10 staining in distinguishing invasive endometrial adenocarcinoma from adenocarcinoma involving adenomyosis. Mod Pathol 2003, **16**: 22–27.

365 Nofech-Mozes S, Ghorab Z, Ismiil N, Ackerman I, Thomas G, Barbera L, Covens A, Khalifa MA. Endometrial endometrioid adenocarcinoma: a pathologic analysis of 827 consecutive cases. Am J Clin Pathol 2008, **129**: 110–114.

366 Risberg B, Grontoft O, Westholm B. Origin of carcinoma in secretory endometrium – a study using a whole-organ sectioning technique. Gynecol Oncol 1983, **15**: 32–41.

367 Salm R. Macrophages in endometrial lesions. J Pathol Bacteriol 1962, **83**: 405–409.

368 Silver SA, Sherman ME. Morphologic and immunophenotypic characterization of foam cells in endometrial lesions. Int J Gynecol Pathol 1998, **17**: 140–145.

369 Simon RA, Peng SL, Sung CJ, Lawrence WD, Zhang C. Glandular intraluminal debris in endometrioid adencarcinoma of the endometrium correlates with tumor grade and stage: a clinicopathologic study of 115 cases. Lab Invest 2009, **89**(Suppl 1): 237A.

370 Srodon M, Klein WM, Kurman RJ. CD10 immunostaining does not distinguish endometrial carcinoma invading myometrium from carcinoma involving adenomyosis. Am J Surg Pathol 2003, **27**: 786–789.

371 Zaino RJ, Kurman RJ, Brunetto VL, Morrow CP, Bentley RC, Cappellari JO, Bitterman P. Villoglandular adenocarcinoma of the endometrium: a clinicopathologic study of 61 cases: a Gynecologic Oncology Group Study. Am J Surg Pathol 1998, **22**: 1379–1385.

372 Zaino RJ, Kurman RJ, Diana KL, Morrow CP. The utility of the revised International Federation of Gynecology and Obstetrics histologic grading of endometrial adenocarcinoma using a defined nuclear grading system. A Gynecologic Oncology Group study. Cancer 1995, **75**: 81–86.

Variants and other microscopic types

373 Abeler V, Kjorstad KE. Endometrial squamous cell carcinoma. Report of three cases and review of the literature. Gynecol Oncol 1990, **36**: 321–326.

374 Abeler VM, Kjorstad KE, Nesland JM. Undifferentiated carcinoma of the endometrium. A histopathologic and clinical study of 31 cases. Cancer 1991, **68**: 98–105.

375 Aguirre P, Scully RE, Wolfe HJ, DeLellis RA. Endometrial carcinoma with argyrophil cells. A histochemical and immunohistochemical analysis. Hum Pathol 1984, **15**: 210–217.

376 Alberhasky RC, Connelly PJ, Christopherson WM. Carcinoma of the endometrium. IV. Mixed adenosquamous carcinoma. A clinical–pathological study of 68 cases with long-term follow-up. Am J Clin Pathol 1982, **77**: 655–664.

377 Albores-Saavedra J, Martinez-Benitez B, Luevano E. Small cell carcinomas and large cell neuroendocrine carcinomas of the endometrium and cervix: polypoid tumors and those arising in polyps may have a favorable prognosis. Int J Gynecol Pathol 2008, **27**: 333–339.

378 Altrabulsi B, Malpica A, Deavers MT, Bodurka DC, Broaddus R, Silva EG. Undifferentiated carcinoma of the endometrium. Am J Surg Pathol 2005, **29**: 1316–1321.

379 Bannatyne P, Russell P, Wills EJ. Argyrophilia and endometrial carcinoma. Int J Gynecol Pathol 1983, **2**: 235–254.

380 Carcangiu ML, Chambers JT. Uterine papillary serous carcinoma. A study on 108 cases with emphasis on the prognostic significance of associated endometrioid carcinoma, absence of invasion, and concomitant ovarian carcinoma. Gynecol Oncol 1992, **47**: 298–305.

381 Carcangiu ML, Chambers JT. Early pathologic stage clear cell carcinoma and uterine papillary serous carcinoma of the endometrium. Comparison of clinicopathologic features and survival. Int J Gynecol Pathol 1995, **14**: 30–38.

382 Carcangiu ML, Tan LK, Chambers JT. Stage 1A uterine serous carcinoma: a study of 13 cases. Am J Surg Pathol 1998, **21**: 1507–1514.

383 Christopherson WM, Alberhasky RC, Connelly PJ. Carcinoma of the endometrium. I. A clinicopathologic study of clear cell carcinoma and secretory carcinoma. Cancer 1982, **49**: 1511–1523.

384 Christopherson WM, Alberhasky RC, Connelly PJ. Glassy cell carcinoma of the endometrium. Hum Pathol 1982, **13**: 418–421.

385 Darvishian F, Hummer AJ, Thaler HT, Bhargava R, Linkov I, Asher M, Soslow RA. Serous endometrial cancers that mimic endometrioid adenocarcinomas: a clinicopathologic and immunohistochemical study of a group of problematic cases. Am J Surg Pathol 2004, **28**: 1568–1578.

386 Deligdisch L, Gil J, Heller D, Cohen CJ. Two types of endometrial papillary neoplasm. A morphometric study. Pathol Res Pract 1992, **188**: 473–477.

387 Dotto J, Tavassoli FA. Serous intraepithelial carcinoma arising in an endometrial polyp: a proposal for modification of terminology. Int J Surg Pathol 2008, **16**: 8–10.

388 Eichhorn JH, Young RH, Clement PB. Sertoliform endometrial adenocarcinoma: a study of four cases. Int J Gynecol Pathol 1996, **15**: 119–126.

389 Euscher ED, Malpica A, Deavers MT, Silva EG. Differential expression of WT-1 in serous carcinomas in the peritoneum with or without associated serous carcinoma in endometrial polyps. Am J Surg Pathol 2005, **29**: 1074–1078.

390 Fadare O, Liang SX, Ulukus EC, Chambers SK, Zheng W. Precursors of endometrial clear cell carcinoma. Am J Surg Pathol 2006, **30**: 1519–1530.

391 Fechner RE. Endometrium with pattern of mesonephroma. Report of a case. Obstet Gynecol 1968, **31**: 485–490.

392 Fukunaga M, Ushigome S. Transitional cell carcinoma of the endometrium. Histopathology 1998, **32**: 284–286.

393 Gaertner EM, Farley JH, Taylor RR, Silver SA. Collision of uterine rhaboid tumor and endometrial adenocarcinoma: a case report and review of the literature. Int J Gynecol Pathol 1999, **18**: 396–401.

394 Giordano G, D'Adda T, Gnetti L, Merisio C, Raboni S. Transitional cell carcinoma of the endometrium associated with benign ovarian Brenner tumor: a case report with immunohistochemistry molecular analysis and a review of the literature. Int J Gynecol Pathol 2007, **26**: 298–304.

395 Gitsch G, Friedlander ML, Wain GV, Hacker NF. Uterine papillary serous carcinoma. A clinical study. Cancer 1995, **75**: 2239–2243.

396 Hachisuga T, Sugimori H, Kaku T, Matsukuma K, Tsukamoto N, Nakano H. Glassy cell carcinoma of the endometrium. Gynecol Oncol 1990, **36**: 134–138.

397 Haqqani MT, Fox H. Adenosquamous carcinoma of the endometrium. J Clin Pathol 1976, **29**: 959–966.

398 Hendrickson MR, Kempson RL. Ciliated carcinoma – a variant of endometrial adenocarcinoma. A report of 10 cases. Int J Gynecol Pathol 1983, **2**: 1–12.

399 Hendrickson M, Ross J, Eifel P, Martinez A, Kempson R. Uterine papillary serous carcinoma. A highly malignant form of endometrial adenocarcinoma. Am J Surg Pathol 1982, **6**: 93–108.

400 Hopkin ID, Harlow RA, Stevens PJ. Squamous carcinoma of the body of the uterus. Br J Cancer 1970, **24**: 71–76.

401 Horn LC, Hänel C, Bartholdt E, Dietel J. Mixed serous carcinoma of the endometrium with trophoblastic differentiation: analysis of the p53 tumor suppressor gene suggests stem cell origin. Ann Diagn Pathol 2008, **12**: 1–3.

402 Hoshida Y, Nagakawa T, Mano S, Taguchi K, Aozasa K. Hepatoid adenocarcinoma of the endometrium associated with alpha-fetoprotein production. Int J Gynecol Pathol 1997, **15**: 266–269.

403 Hui P, Kelly M, O'Malley DM, Tavassoli F, Schwartz PE. Minimal uterine serous carcinoma: a clinicopathological study of 40 cases. Mod Pathol 2005, **18**: 75–82.

404 Huntsman DG, Clement PB, Gilks CB, Scully RE. Small-cell carcinoma of the endometrium. A clinicopathological study of sixteen cases. Am J Surg Pathol 1994, **18**: 364–375.

405 Iezzoni GC, Mills SE. Nonneoplastic endometrial signet-ring cells. Vacuolated decidual cells and stromal histiocytes mimicking adenocarcinoma. Am J Clin Pathol 2001, **115**: 249–255.

406 Inoue M, DeLellis RA, Scully RE. Immunohistochemical demonstration of chromogranin in endometrial carcinomas with argyrophil cells. Hum Pathol 1986, **17**: 841–847.

407 Jeffers MD, McDonald GS, McGuinness EP. Primary squamous cell carcinoma of the endometrium. Histopathology 1991, **19**: 177–179.

408 Jeffrey JF, Krepart GV, Lotocki RJ. Papillary serous adenocarcinoma of the endometrium. Obstet Gynecol 1986, **67**: 670–674.

409 Jones MA, Young RH, Scully RE. Endometrial adenocarcinoma with a component of giant cell carcinoma. Int J Gynecol Pathol 1991, **10**: 260–270.

410 Kalir T, Seijo L, Deligdisch L, Cohen C. Endometrial adenocarcinoma with choriocarcinomatous differentiation in an elderly virginal woman. Int J Gynecol Pathol 1995, **14**: 266–269.

411 Kuebler DL, Nikrui N, Bell DA. Cytologic features of endometrial papillary serous carcinoma. Acta Cytol 1989, **33**: 120–126.

412 Kurman RJ, Scully RE. Clear cell carcinoma of the endometrium. An analysis of 21 cases. Cancer 1976, **37**: 872–882.

413 Lax SF, Pizer ES, Ronnett BM, Kurman RJ. Clear cell carcinoma of the endometrium is characterized by a distinctive profile of p53, Ki-67, estrogen, and progesterone receptor expression. Hum Pathol 1998, **29**: 551–558.

414 Liang SX, Chambers SK, Cheng L, Zhang S, Zhou Y, Zheng W. Endometrial glandular dysplasia: a putative precursor lesion of uterine papillary serous carcinoma. Part II: molecular features. Int J Surg Pathol 2004, **12**: 319–331.

415 Lininger RA, Ashfaq F, Albores-Saavedra J, Tavassoli FA. Transitional cell carcinoma of the endometrium and endometrial carcinoma with transitional cell differentiation. Cancer 1997, **79**: 1933–1943.

416 McCluggage WG, Roberts N, Bharucha H. Enteric differentiation in endometrial adenocarcinomas. A mucin histochemical study. Int J Gynecol Pathol 1995, **14**: 255–260.

417 Malpica A, Tornos C, Burke TW, Silva EG. Low-stage clear-cell carcinoma of the endometrium. Am J Surg Pathol 1995, **19**: 769–774.

418 Mariño-Enríquez A, González-Rocha T, Burgos E, Stolnicu S, Mendiola M, Nogales FF, Hardisson D. Transitional cell carcinoma of the endometrium and endometrial carcinoma with transitional cell differentiation: a clinicopathologic study of 5 cases and review of the literature. Hum Pathol 2008, **39**: 1606–1613.

419 Matias-Guiu X, Lerma E, Prat J. Clear cell tumors of the female genital tract. Semin Diagn Pathol 1998, **14**: 233–239.

420 Melhem MF, Tobon H. Mucinous adenocarcinoma of the endometrium. A clinico-pathological review of 18 cases. Int J Gynecol Pathol 1987, **6**: 347–355.

421 Mooney EE, Robboy SJ, Hammond CB, Berchuck A, Bentley RC. Signet-ring cell carcinoma of the endometrium: a primary tumor masquerading as a metastasis. Int J Gynecol Pathol 1997, **16**: 169–172.

422 Mulligan AM, Plotkin A, Rouzbahman M, Soslow RA, Gilks CB, Clarke BA. Endometrial giant cell carcinoma: a case series and review of the spectrum of endometrial neoplasms containing giant cells. Am J Surg Pathol 2010, **34**: 1132–1138.

423 Mulvany NJ, Allen DG. Combined large cell neuroendocrine and endometrioid carcinoma of the endometrium. Int J Gynecol Pathol 2008, **27**: 49–57.

424 Murray SK, Clement PB, Young RH. Endometrioid carcinomas of the uterine corpus with sex cord-like formations, hyalinization, and other unusual morphologic features: a report of 31 cases of a neoplasm that may be confused with carcinosarcoma and other uterine neoplasms. Am J Surg Pathol 2005, **29**: 157–166.

425 Ng ABP. Mixed carcinoma of the endometrium. Am J Obstet Gynecol 1968, **102**: 506–515.

426 Ng ABP, Reagan JW, Storassli JP, Wentz WB. Mixed adenosquamous carcinoma of the endometrium. Am J Clin Pathol 1973, **59**: 765–781.

427 Nofech-Mozes S, Khalifa MA, Ismiil N, Saad RS, Hanna WM, Covens A, Ghorab Z. Immunophenotyping of serous carcinoma of the female genital tract. Mod Pathol 2008, **21**: 1147–1155.

428 Ordi J, Nogales FF, Palacin A, Marquez M, Pahisa J, Vanrell JA, Cardesa A. Mesonephric adenocarcinoma of the uterine corpus: CD10 expression as evidence of mesonephric differentiation. Am J Surg Pathol 2001, **25**: 1540–1545.

429 Park KJ, Bramlage MP, Ellenson LH, Pirog EC. Immunoprofile of adenocarcinomas of the endometrium, endocervix, and ovary with mucinous differentiation. Appl Immunohistochem Mol Morphol 2009, **17**: 8–11.

430 Parkash V, Carcangiu ML. Uterine papillary serous carcinoma after radiation therapy for carcinoma of the cervix. Cancer 1992, **69**: 496–501.

431 Parkash V, Carcangiu ML. Endometrioid endometrial adenocarcinoma with psammoma bodies. Am J Surg Pathol 1997, **21**: 399–406.

432 Paz RA, Frigerio B, Sundblad AS, Eusebi V. Small-cell (oat cell) carcinoma of the endometrium. Arch Pathol Lab Med 1985, **109**: 270–272.

433 Peison B, Benisch B, Fox H. Invasive keratinising squamous cell carcinoma of the endometrium as extension of invasive cervical squamous cell carcinoma. Int J Surg Pathol 1997, **4**: 189–192.

434 Pesce C, Merino MJ, Chambers JT, Nogales F. Endometrial carcinoma with trophoblastic differentiation. An aggressive form of uterine cancer. Cancer 1991, **68**: 1799–1802.

435 Pitman MB, Young RH, Clement PB, Dickersin GR, Scully RE. Endometrioid carcinoma of the ovary and endometrium, oxyphilic cell type. A report of nine cases. Int J Gynecol Pathol 1994, **13**: 290–301.

436 Plotkin A, Rasty G, Rouzbahman M, Gilks CB, Clarke BA. Endometrial giant cell adenocarcinoma. Lab Invest 2009, **89**(Suppl 1): 232A.

437 Rabban JT, Zaloudek CJ. Minimal uterine serous carcinoma: current concepts in diagnosis and prognosis. Pathology 2007, **39**: 125–133.

438 Roh MH, Yassin Y, Miron A, Crum CP, Hirsch MS. High grade serous and endometrioid carcinoma: a convergence of two pathways in pelvic cancer differentiation. Lab Invest 2009, **89**(Suppl 1): 234A.

439 Rorat E, Ferenczy A, Richart RM. The ultrastructure of clear cell adenocarcinoma of endometrium. Cancer 1974, **33**: 880–887.

440 Ross JC, Eifel PJ, Cox RS, Kempson RL, Hendrickson MR. Primary mucinous adenocarcinoma of the endometrium. A clinicopathologic and histochemical study. Am J Surg Pathol 1983, **7**: 715–729.

441 Roth LM. Clear-cell adenocarcinoma of the female genital tract. A light and electron microscopic study. Cancer 1974, **33**: 990–1001.

442 Ryder DE. Verrucous carcinoma of the endometrium – a unique neoplasm with long survival. Obstet Gynecol 1982, **59**: 78S–80S.

443 Salazar OM, DePapp EW, Bonfiglio TA, Feldstein ML, Rubin P, Rudolph JH. Adenosquamous carcinoma of the endometrium. An entity with an inherent poor prognosis? Cancer 1977, **40**: 119–130.

444 Shaco-Levy R, Manor E, Piura B, Ariel I. An unusual composite endometrial tumor combining papillary serous carcinoma and small cell carcinoma. Am J Surg Pathol 2004, **28**: 1103–1106.

445 Sherman ME, Bitterman P, Rosenshein NB, Delgado G, Kurman RJ. Uterine serous carcinoma. A morphologically diverse neoplasm with unifying clinicopathologic features. Am J Surg Pathol 1992, **16**: 600–610.

446 Silva EG, Jenkins R. Serous carcinoma in endometrial polyps. Mod Pathol 1990, **3**: 120–128.

447 Silva EG, Young RH. Endometrioid neoplasms with clear cells: a report of 21 cases in which the alteration is not of typical secretory type. Am J Surg Pathol 2007, **31**: 1203–1208.

448 Silva EG, Deavers MT, Malpica A. Undifferentiated carcinoma of the endometrium: a review. Pathology 2007, **39**: 134–138.

449 Silva EG, Deavers MT, Bodurka DC, Malpica A. Association of low-grade endometrioid carcinoma of the uterus and ovary with undifferentiated carcinoma: a new type of dedifferentiated carcinoma? Int J Gynecol Pathol 2006, **25**: 52–58.

450 Silverberg SG, DeGiorgi LS. Clear cell carcinoma of the endometrium. Cancer 1973, **31**: 1127–1140.

451 Sivridis E, Buckley CH, Fox H. Argyrophil cells in normal, hyperplastic, and neoplastic endometrium. J Clin Pathol 1984, **37**: 378–381.

452 Sorvari TE. A histochemical study of epithelial mucosubstances in endometrial and cervical adenocarcinomas. With reference to normal endometrium and cervical mucosa. Acta Pathol Microbiol Scand 1969, **207**(Suppl): 56–60.

453 Tafe LJ, Garg K, Chew I, Tornos C, Soslow RA. Endometrial and ovarian carcinomas with undifferentiated components: clinically aggressive and frequently underrecognized neoplasms. Mod Pathol 2010, **23**: 781–789.

454 Tobon H, Watkins GJ. Secretory adenocarcinoma of the endometrium. Int J Gynecol Pathol 1985, **4**: 328–335.

455 Trahan S, Têtu B, Raymond PE. Serous papillary carcinoma of the endometrium arising from endometrial polyps: a clinical, histological, and immunohistochemical study of 13 cases. Hum Pathol 2005, **36**: 1316–1321.

456 Tran TA, Ortiz HB, Holloway RW, Bigsby GE, Finkler NJ. Alpha-fetoprotein-producing serous carcinoma of the uterus metastasizing to the ovaries, mimicking primary ovarian yolk sac tumor: a case report and review of the literature. Int J Gynecol Pathol 2007, **26**: 66–70.

457 Usadi RS, Bentley RC. Endometrioid carcinoma of the endometrium with sertoliform differentiation. Int J Gynecol Pathol 1995, **14**: 360–364.

458 Vang R, Tavassoli FA. Proliferative mucinous lesions of the endometrium: analysis of existing criteria for diagnosing carcinoma in biopsies and curettings. Int J Surg Pathol 2003, **11**: 261–270.

459 Vang R, Whitaker BP, Farhood AI, Silva EG, Ro RJ, Deavers MT. Immunohistochemical analysis of clear cell carcinoma of the gynecologic tract. Int J Gynecol Pathol 2001, **20**: 252–259.

460 van Hoeven KH, Hudock JA, Woodruff JM, Suhrland MJ. Small cell neuroendocrine carcinoma of the endometrium. Int J Gynecol Pathol 1995, **14**: 21–29.

461 Vargas MP, Merino MJ. Lymphoepithelio-malike carcinoma: an usual variant of endometrial cancer; a report of two cases. Int J Gynecol Pathol 1998, **17**: 272–276.

462 Wani Y, Notohara K, Tsukayama C. Mesonephric adenocarcinoma of the uterine corpus: a case report and review of the literature. Int J Gynecol Pathol 2008, **27**: 346–352.

463 Warhol MJ, Rice RH, Pinkus GS, Robboy SJ. Evaluation of squamous epithelium in adenoacanthoma and adenosquamous carcinoma of the endometrium. Immunoperoxidase analysis of involucrin and keratin localization. Int J Gynecol Pathol 1984, **3**: 82–91.

464 Wheeler DT, Bell KA, Kurman RJ, Sherman ME. Minimal uterine serous carcinoma: diagnosis and clinicopathologic correlation. Am J Surg Pathol 2000, **24**: 797–806.

465 Yamamoto Y, Izumi K, Otsuka H, Kishi Y, Mimura T, Okitsu O. Primary squamous cell carcinoma of the endometrium. A case report and a suggestion of new histogenesis. Int J Gynecol Pathol 1995, **14**: 75–80.

466 Yamashina M, Kobara TY. Primary squamous cell carcinoma with its spindle cell variant in the endometrium. A case report and review of literature. Cancer 1986, **57**: 340–345.

467 Yemelyanova A, Ji H, Shih IeM, Wang TL, Wu LS, Ronnett BM. Utility of p16 expression for distinction of uterine serous carcinomas from endometrial endometrioid and endocervical adenocarcinomas: immunohistochemical analysis of 201 cases. Am J Surg Pathol 2009, **33**: 1504–1514.

468 Young RH, Scully RE. Uterine carcinomas simulating microglandular hyperplasia. A report of six cases. Am J Surg Pathol 1994, **16**: 1092–1097.

469 Zaino RJ, Kurman RJ. Squamous differentiation in carcinoma of the endometrium. A critical appraisal of adenoacanthoma and adenosquamous carcinoma. Semin Diagn Pathol 1988, **5**: 154–171.

470 Zaino RJ, Kurman R, Herbold D, Gliedman J, Bundy BN, Voet R, Advani H. The significance of squamous differentiation in endometrial carcinoma. Data from a Gynecologic Oncology Group study. Cancer 1991, **68**: 2293–2302.

471 Zaloudek C, Hayashi GM, Ryan IP, Powell CB, Miller TR. Microglandular adenocarcinoma of the endometrium: a form of mucinous adenocarcinoma that may be confused with microglandular hyperplasia of the cervix. Int J Gynecol Pathol 1997, **16**: 52–59.

472 Zheng W, Liang SX, Yu H, Rutherford T, Chambers SK, Schwartz PE. Endometrial glandular dysplasia: a newly defined precursor lesion of uterine papillary serous carcinoma. Part I: morphologic features. Int J Surg Pathol 2004, **12**: 207–223.

473 Zheng W, Liang SX, Yi X, Ulukus EC, Davis JR, Chambers SK. Occurrence of endometrial glandular dysplasia precedes uterine papillary serous carcinoma. Int J Gynecol Pathol 2007, **26**: 38–52.

Cytology

474 Bibbo M, Shanklin DR, Wied L. Endometrial cytology on jet wash material. J Reprod Med 1972, **8**: 90–96.

475 Burk JR, Lehman HF, Wolf FS. Inadequacy of Papanicolaou smears in the detection of endometrial cancer. N Engl J Med 1974, **291**: 191–192.

476 Christopherson WM, Mendez WM, Ahuja EM, Lundin FE, Parker JE. Cervix cancer control in Louisville, Kentucky. Cancer 1970, **26**: 29–38.

477 Gusberg SB, Milano C. Detection of endometrial carcinoma and its precursors. Cancer 1981, **47**: 1173–1175.

478 Hibbard LT, Schwinn CP. Diagnosis of endometrial jet washings. Am J Obstet Gynecol 1971, **111**: 1039–1042.

479 Isaacs JH, Wilmoite RW. Aspiration cytology of the endometrium. Office and hospital sampling procedures. Am J Obstet Gynecol 1974, **118**: 679–687.

480 Ng ABP, Reagan JW, Hawliczek CT, Wentz BW. Significance of endometrial cells in the detection of endometrial carcinoma and its precursors. Acta Cytol (Baltimore) 1974, **18**: 356–361.

481 Reagan JW. Can screening for endometrial cancer be justified? [editorial]. Acta Cytol (Baltimore) 1980, **24**: 87–89.

482 Reagan JW. Cytologic aspects of endometrial neoplasia. Acta Cytol 1980, **24**: 488–489.

483 Reagan JW, Ng ABP. The cells of uterine adenocarcinoma. Baltimore, 1965, Williams and Wilkins.

484 Rodrigues MA, Rubin A, Koss LG, Harris J. Evaluation of endometrial jet wash technique (Gravlee) in 303 patients in a community hospital. Obstet Gynecol 1974, **43**: 392–399.

485 Vuopala S. Diagnostic accuracy and clinical applicability of cytological and histological methods for investigating endometrial carcinoma. Acta Obstet Gynecol Scand 1977, **70**(Suppl): 1–72.

Histochemical and immunohistochemical features

486 Al-Hussaini M, Stockman A, Foster H, McCluggage WG. WT-1 assists in distinguishing ovarian from uterine serous carcinoma and in distinguishing between serous and endometrioid ovarian carcinoma. Histopathology 2004, **44**: 109–115.

487 Brustein S, Fruchter R, Greene GL, Pertschuk LP. Immunocytochemical assay of progesterone receptors in paraffin-embedded specimens of endometrial carcinoma and hyperplasia. A preliminary evaluation. Mod Pathol 1989, **2**: 449–455.

488 Carcangiu ML, Chambers JT, Voynick IM, Pirro M, Schwartz PE. Immunohistochemical evaluation of estrogen and progesterone receptor content in 183 patients with endometrial carcinoma. Part I. Clinical and histologic correlations. Am J Clin Pathol 1990, **94**: 247–254.

489 Dabbs DJ, Geisinger KR, Norris HT. Intermediate filaments in endometrial and endocervical carcinomas. The diagnostic utility of vimentin patterns. Am J Surg Pathol 1986, **10**: 568–576.

490 Dabbs DJ, Sturtz K, Zaino RJ. The immunohistochemical discrimination of endometrioid adenocarcinomas. Hum Pathol 1996, **27**: 172–177.

491 Demopoulos RI, Mesia AF, Mittal K, Vamvakas E. Immunohistochemical comparison of uterine papillary serous and papillary endometrioid carcinoma: clues to pathogenesis. Int J Gynecol Pathol 2002, **18**: 233–237.

492 Elmore LW, Domson K, Moore BS, Kornstein M, Burks RT. Expression of c-kit (CD117) in benign and malignant human endometrial epithelium. Arch Pathol Lab Med 2001, **125**: 146–151.

493 Geisinger KR, Marshall RB, Kute TE, Homesley HD. Correlation of female sex steroid hormone receptors with histologic and ultrastructural differentiation in adenocarcinoma of the endometrium. Cancer 1986, **58**: 1506–1517.

494 Goldstein NS, Uzieblo A. WT1 immunoreactivity in uterine papillary serous carcinomas is different from ovarian serous carcinomas. Am J Clin Pathol 2002, **117**: 541–545.

495 Idrees MT, Schlosshauer P, Li G, Burstein DE. GLUT1 and p63 expression in endometrial intraepithelial and uterine serous papillary carcinoma. Histopathology 2006, **49**: 75–81.

496 Kounelis S, Kapranos N, Kouri E, Coppola D, Papadaki H, Jones MW. Immunohistochemical profile of endometrial adenocarcinoma: a study of 61 cases and review of the literature. Mod Pathol 2000, **13**: 379–388.

497 Lax SF, Pizer ES, Ronnett BM, Kurman RJ. Comparison of estrogen and progesterone receptor, Ki-67, and p53 immunoreactivity in uterine endometrioid carcinoma and endometrioid carcinoma with squamous, mucinous, secretory, and ciliated cell differentiaton. Hum Pathol 1998, **29**: 924–931.

498 McCluggage WG. WT1 is of value in ascertaining the site of origin of serous carcinomas within the female genital tract. Int J Gynecol Pathol 2004, **23**: 97–99.

499 Mhawech-Fauceglia P, Herrmann FR, Rai H, Tchabo N, Lele S, Izevbaye I, Odunsi K, Cheney RT. IMP3 distinguishes uterine serous carcinoma from endometrial endometrioid adenocarcinoma. Am J Clin Pathol 2010, **133**: 899–908.

500 Moll R, Levy R, Czernobilsky B, Hohlweg-Majert P, Dallenbach-Hellweg G, Franke WW. Cytokeratins of normal epithelia and some neoplasms of the female genital tract. Lab Invest 1983, **49**: 599–610.

501 Moll R, Pitz S, Levy R, Weikel W, Franke WW, Czernobilsky B. Complexity of expression of intermediate filament proteins, including glial filament protein, in endometrial and ovarian adenocarcinomas. Hum Pathol 1991, **22**: 989–1001.

502 Morrison C, Merati K, Marsh WL Jr, De Lott L, Cohn DE, Young G, Frankel WL. The mucin expression profile of endometrial carcinoma and correlation with clinical–pathologic parameters. Appl Immunohistochem Mol Morphol 2007, **15**: 426–431.

503 Podczaski E, Kaminski PF, Zaino R. CA 125 and CA 19-9 immunolocalization in normal, hyperplastic, and carcinomatous endometrium. Cancer 1993, **71**: 2551–2556.

504 Puts JJG, Moesker O, Aldeweireldt J, Vooijs GP, Ramaekers FCS. Application of antibodies to intermediate filament proteins in simple and complex tumors of the female genital tract. Int J Gynecol Pathol 1987, **6**: 257–274.

505 Reid-Nicholson M, Iyengar P, Hummer AJ, Linkov I, Asher M, Soslow RA. Immunophenotypic diversity of endometrial adenocarcinomas: implications for differential diagnosis. Mod Pathol 2006, **19**: 1091–1100.

506 Rolitsky CD, Theil KS, McGaughy VR, Copeland LJ, Niemann TH. HER-2/neu amplification and overexpression in endometrial carcinoma. Int J Gynecol Pathol 1999, **18**: 138–143.

507 Schlosshauer PW, Ellenson LH, Soslow RA. Beta-catenin and E-cadherin expression patterns in high-grade endometrial carcinoma are associated with histological subtype. Mod Pathol 2002, **15**: 1032–1037.

508 Siami K, McCluggage WG, Ordonez NG, Euscher ED, Malpica A, Sneige N, Silva EG, Deavers MT. Thyroid transcription factor-1 expression in endometrial and endocervical adenocarcinomas. Am J Surg Pathol 2007, **31**: 1759–1763.

509 Takeda A, Matsuyama M, Kuzuya K, Chihara T, Ariyoshi Y, Suchi T, Kato K. Secretory component and IgA in endometrial adenocarcinomas. An immunohistochemical study. Acta Pathol Jpn 1983, **33**: 725–732.

510 Tong GX, Devaraj K, Hamele-Bena D, Yu WM, Turk A, Chen X, Wright JD, Greenebaum E. PAX8: a marker for carcinoma of Müllerian origin in serous effusions. Diagn Cytopathol 2010, Jul 6. [Epub ahead of print]

511 Ueda G, Yamasaki M, Inoue M, Tanaka Y, Inoue Y, Nishino T, Ogawa M. Immunohistochemical demonstration of amylase in endometrial carcinomas. Int J Gynecol Pathol 1986, **5**: 47–51.

512 Ueda S, Tsubura A, Izumi H, Sasaki M, Morii S. Immunohistochemical studies on carcinoembryonic antigen in adenocarcinomas of the uterus. Acta Pathol Jpn 1983, **33**: 59–69.

513 Wang BY, Kalir T, Sabo E, Sherman DE, Cohen C, Burstein DE. Immunohistochemical staining of GLUT1 in benign, hyperplastic, and malignant endometrial epithelia. Cancer 2000, **88**: 2774–2781.

514 Zhang PJ, Williams E, Pasha T, Acs G. WT1 is expressed in serous, but not in endometrioid, clear cell or mucinous carcinomas of the peritoneum, fallopian tube, ovaries and endometrium [abstract]. Mod Pathol 2003, **16**: 216a. (See also Int J Gynecol Pathol 2004, **23**: 110–118).

515 Zhang PJ, Gao HG, Pasha TL, Litzky L, Livolsi VA. TTF-1 expression in ovarian and uterine epithelial neoplasia and its potential significance, an immunohistochemical assessment with multiple monoclonal antibodies and different secondary detection systems. Int J Gynecol Pathol 2009, **28**: 10–18.

516 Zheng W, Yi X, Fadare O, Liang SX, Martel M, Schwartz PE, Jiang Z. The oncofetal protein IMP3: a novel biomarker for endometrial serous carcinoma. Am J Surg Pathol 2008, **32**: 304–315.

Molecular genetic features

517 Ali IU. Gatekeeper for endometrium: the PTEN tumor suppressor gene. J Nat Cancer Inst 2000, **92**: 861–863.

518 Bonatz G, Frahm SO, Klapper W, Helfenstein A, Heidorn K, Jonat W, Krupp G, Parwaresch R, Rudolph P. High telomerase activity is associated with cell cycle deregulation and rapid progression in endometrioid adenocarcinoma of the uterus. Hum Pathol 2001, **32**: 605–614.

519 Burton JL, Wells M. Recent advances in the histopathology and molecular pathology of carcinoma of the endometrium. Histopathology 1998, **33**: 297–303.

520 Bussaglia E, del Rio E, Matias-Guiu X, Prat J. PTEN mutations in endometrial carcinomas: a molecular and clinicopathologic analysis of 38 cases. Hum Pathol 2000, **31**: 312–317.

521 Cao QJ, Einstein MH, Anderson PS, Runowicz CD, Balan R, Jones JG. Expression of COX-2, Ki-67, cyclin D1, and P21 in endometrioid carcinomas. Int J Gynecol Pathol 2002, **21**: 147–154.

522 Fernando SSE, Wu X, Perera LS. P53 Overexpression and steroid hormone receptor status in endometrial carcinoma. Int J Surg Pathol 2000, **8**: 213–222.

523 Hayes MP, Pirog EC, Ellenson LH. Molecular gynecologic pathology. In Tubbs RR, Stoler MH (eds): Cell and tissue based molecular pathology. Philadelphia, 2009, Churchill Livingstone, pp. 393–410.

524 Hendrick Ellenson L. The molecular biology of endometrial tumorigenesis: does it have a message? Int J Gynecol Pathol 2000, **19**: 314–321.

525 Koshiyama M, Konishi I, Wang DP, Mandai M, Komatsu T, Yamamoto S, Nanbu K, Naito MF, Mori T. Immunohistochemical analysis of p53 protein over-expression in endometrial carcinomas. Inverse correlation with sex steroid receptor status. Virchows Arch [A] 1993, **423**: 265–271.

526 Koul A, Willen R, Bendhal PO, Nilbert M, Borg A. Distinct sites of gene alterations in endometrial carcinoma implicate alternate modes of tumorigenesis. Cancer 2002, **94**: 2369–2379.

527 Lovecchio M, Maiorano E, Vacca RA, Loverro G, Fanelli M, Resta L, Stefanelli S, Selvaggi L, Marra E, Perlino E. β1C integrin expression in human endometrial proliferative diseases. Am J Pathol 2003, **163**: 2453–2553.

528 Machin P, Catasus L, Pons C, Munoz J, Matias-Guiu X, Prat J. CTNNB1 mutations and beta-catenin expression in endometrial carcinoma. Hum Pathol 2002, **33**: 206–212.

529 Matias-Guiu X, Catasus L, Bussaglia E, Lagarda H, Garcia A, Pons C, Munoz J, Arguelles R, Machin P, Prat J. Molecular pathology of endometrial hyperplasia and carcinoma. Hum Pathol 2001, **32**: 569–577.

530 Palazzo JP, Mercer WE, Kovatich AJ, McHugh M. Immunohistochemical localization of p21 (WAF1/CIP1) in normal, hyperplastic, and neoplastic uterine tissues. Hum Pathol 1997, **28**: 60–66.

531 Ronnett BM, Burks RT, Cho KR, Hedrick L. DCC genetic alterations and expression in endometrial carcinoma. Mod Pathol 1997, **10**: 38–46.

532 Sasano H, Comeford J, Wilkinson DS, Schwartz A, Garrett CT. Serous papillary adenocarcinoma of the endometrium. Analysis of proto-oncogene amplification, flow cytometry, estrogen and progesterone receptors, and immunohistochemistry. Cancer 1990, **65**: 1545–1551.

533 Sherman ME. Theories of endometrial carcinogenesis: a multidisciplinary approach. Mod Pathol 2000, **13**: 295–308.

534 Susini T, Massi D, Paglierani M, Masciullo V, Scambia G, Giordano A, Amunni G, Massi G, Taddei GL. Expression of the retinoblastoma-related gene Rb2/p130 is downregulated in atypical endometrial hyperplasia and adenocarcinoma. Hum Pathol 2001, **32**: 360–367.

535 Tashiro H, Lax SF, Gaudin PB, Isacson C, Cho KR, Hedrick L. Microsatellite instability is uncommon in uterine serous carcinoma. Am J Pathol 1997, **150**: 75–79.

536 Tritz D, Pieretti M, Turner S, Powell D. Loss of heterozygosity in usual and special variant carcinomas of the endometrium. Hum Pathol 1997, **28**: 607–612.

537 Watanabe Y, Nakajima H, Nozaki K, Ueda H, Obata K, Hoshiai H, Noda K. Clinicopathologic and immunohistochemical features and microsatellite status of endometrial cancer of the uterine isthmus. Int J Gynecol Pathol 2001, **20**: 368–373.

Spread and metastases

538 Ali A, Black D, Soslow RA. Difficulties in assessing the depth of myometrial invasion in endometrial carcinoma. Int J Gynecol Pathol 2007, **26**: 115–123.

539 Baergen RN, Warren CD, Isaacson C, Ellenson LH. Early uterine serous carcinoma: clonal origin of extrauterine disease. Int J Gynecol Pathol 2001, **20**: 214–219.

540 Boronow RC, Morrow CP, Creasman WT, Disaia PJ, Silverberg SG, Miller A, Blessing JA. Surgical staging in endometrial cancer. Clinical–pathologic findings of a prospective study. Obstet Gynecol 1984, **63**: 825–832.

541 Chen KTK, Kostich ND, Rosai J. Peritoneal foreign body granulomas to keratin in uterine adenoacanthoma. Arch Pathol Lab Med 1978, **102**: 174–177.

542 Creasman WI, Morrow CP, Bundy BN, Homesley HD, Graham JE, Heller PB. Surgical pathologic spread patterns of endometrial cancer. Cancer 1987, **60**: 2035–2041.

543 Folkins AK, Nevadunsky NS, Saleemuddin A, Jarboe EA, Muto MG, Feltmate CM, Crum CP, Hirsch MS. Evaluation of vascular space involvement in endometrial adenocarcinomas: laparoscopic vs abdominal hysterectomies. Mod Pathol 2010, **23**: 1073–1079.

544 Ismiil N, Rasty G, Ghorab Z, Nofech-Mozes S, Bernardini M, Ackerman I, Thomas G, Covens A, Khalifa MA. Adenomyosis involved by endometrial adenocarcinoma is a significant risk factor for deep myometrial invasion. Ann Diagn Pathol 2007, **11**: 252–257.

545 Kim KR, Scully RE. Peritoneal keratin granulomas with carcinomas of endometrium and ovary and atypical polypoid adenomyoma of endometrium. A clinicopathological analysis of 22 cases. Am J Surg Pathol 1990, **14**: 925–932.

546 Kitahara S, Walsh C, Frumovitz M, Malpica A, Silva EG. Vascular pseudoinvasion in laparoscopic hysterectomy specimens for endometrial carcinoma: a grossing artifact? Am J Surg Pathol 2009, **33**: 298–303.

547 Kupryjanczyk J, Thor AD, Beauchamp R, Poremba C, Scully RE, Yandell DW. Ovarian, peritoneal, and endometrial serous carcinoma: clonal origin of multifocal disease. Mod Pathol 1996, **9**: 166–173.

548 Logani S, Herdman AV, Little JV, Moller KA. Vascular 'pseudo invasion' in laparoscopic hysterectomy specimens: a diagnostic pitfall. Am J Surg Pathol 2008, **32**: 560–565.

549 Schink JC, Rademaker AW, Miller DS, Lurain JR. Tumor size in endometrial cancer. Cancer 1991, **67**: 2791–2794.

550 Scott M, Lyness RW, McCluggage WG. Atypical reactive proliferation of endocervix: a common lesion associated with endometrial carcinoma and likely related to prior endometrial sampling. Mod Pathol 2006, **19**: 470–474.

551 Snyder MJ, Bentley R, Robboy SJ. Transtubal spread of serous adenocarcinoma of the endometrium: an underrecognized mechanism of metastasis. Int J Gynecol Pathol 2006, **25**: 155–160.

552 Soslow RA, Pirog E, Isaacson C. Endometrial intraepithelial carcinoma with associated peritoneal carcinomatosis. Am J Surg Pathol 2000, **24**: 726–732.

553 Tambouret R, Clement PB, Young RH. Endometrial endometrioid adenocarcinoma with a deceptive pattern of spread to the uterine cervix. A manifestation of stage IIB endometrial carcinoma liable to be misinterpreted as an independent carcinoma or a benign lesion. Am J Surg Pathol 2003, **27**: 1080–1088.

554 Williams JW, Hirschowitz L. Assessment of uterine wall thickness and position of the vascular plexus in the deep myometrium: implications for the measurement of depth of myometrial invasion of endometrial carcinomas. Int J Gynecol Pathol 2006, **25**: 59–64.

555 Young RH, Johnston WH. Serous adenocarcinoma of the uterus metastatic to the urinary bladder mimicking primary bladder neoplasia. A report of a case. Am J Surg Pathol 1990, **14**: 877–880.

Coexistent uterine and other genital tract carcinomas

556 Culton LK, Deavers MT, Silva EG, Liu J, Malpica A. Endometrioid carcinoma simultaneously involving the uterus and the fallopian tube: a clinicopathologic study of 13 cases. Am J Surg Pathol 2006, **30**: 844–849.

557 Emmert-Buck MR, Chuaqui R, Zhuang Z, Nogales F, Liotta LA, Merino MJ. Molecular analysis of synchronous uterine and ovarian endometrioid tumors. Int J Gynecol Pathol 1997, **16**: 143–148.

558 Fujii H, Matsumoto T, Yoshida M, Furugen Y, Takagaki T, Iwabuchi K, Nakata Y, Takagi Y, Moriya Y, Ohtsuji N, Ohtsuji M, Hirose S, Shirai T. Genetics of synchronous uterine and ovarian endometrioid carcinoma: combined analyses of loss of heterozygosity, PTEN mutations, and microsatellite instability. Hum Pathol 2002, **33**: 421–428.

559 Fujita M, Endomoto T, Wada H, Inoue M, Okudaira Y, Shroyer KR. Application of clonal analysis. Differential diagnosis for synchronous primary ovarian and endometrial cancers and metastatic cancer. Am J Clin Pathol 1996, **105**: 350–359.

560 Prat J, Matias-Guiu X, Barreto J. Simultaneous carcinoma involving the endometrium and the ovary. A clinicopathologic, immunohistochemical, and DNA flow cytometric study of 18 cases. Cancer 1991, **68**: 2455–2459.

561 Press MF. Are synchronous uterine and ovarian carcinomas independent primary tumors? Adv Anat Pathol 1997, **4**: 370–372.

562 Ricci R, Komminoth P, Bannwart F, Torhorst J, Wight E, Heitz PU, Caduff RF. PTEN as a molecular marker to distinguish metastatic from primary synchronous endometrioid carcinomas of the ovary and uterus. Diagn Mol Pathol 2003, **12**: 71–78.

563 Singh N. Synchronous tumours of the female genital tract. Histopathology 2010, **56**: 277–285.

Treatment

564 Aalders JG, Abeler V, Kolstad P. Recurrent adenocarcinoma of the endometrium. A clinical and histopathological study of 379 patients. Gynecol Oncol 1984, **17**: 85–103.

565 Baekelandt M. Hormonal treatment of endometrial carcinoma. Expert Rev Anticancer Ther 2002, **2**: 106–112.

566 Frank AH, Tseng PC, Haffty BG, Papadopoulos DP, Kacinski BM, Dowling SW, Carcangiu ML, Kohorn EI, Chambers JT, Chambers SK, et al. Adjuvant whole-abdominal radiation therapy in uterine papillary serous carcinoma. Cancer 1991, **68**: 1516–1519.

567 Kim YB, Holschneider CH, Ghosh K, Nieberg RK, Montz FJ. Progestin alone as primary treatment of endometrial carcinoma in premenopausal women: report of seven cases and review of the literature. Cancer 1997, **79**: 320–327.

568 Levine DA, Hoskins WJ. Update in the management of endometrial cancer. Cancer J 2002, **8**: S31–S40.

569 Lim P, Al Kushi A, Gilks B, Wong F, Aquino-Parsons C. Early stage uterine papillary serous carcinoma of the endometrium: effect of adjuvant whole abdominal radiotherapy and pathologic parameters and outcome. Cancer 2001, **91**: 752–757.

570 Price FV, Chambers SK, Carcangiu ML, Kohorn EI, Schwartz PE, Chambers JT. Intravenous cisplatin, doxorubicin, and cyclophosphamide in the treatment of uterine papillary serous carcinoma (UPSC). Gynecol Oncol 1993, **51**: 383–389.

571 Santacana M, Pallares J, Lopez S, Yeramian A, Dolcet X, Oliva E, Matias-Guiu X. Immunohistochemical features of post-radiation recurrences of endometrioid carcinomas of the endometrium. Lab Invest 2009, **89**(Suppl 1): 236A.

572 Sears JD, Greven KM, Hoen HM, Randall ME. Prognostic factors and treatment outcome for patients with locally recurrent endometrial cancer. Cancer 1994, **74**: 1303–1308.

573 Silverberg SG, DeGiorgi LS. Histopathologic analysis of preoperative radiation therapy in endometrial carcinoma. Am J Obstet Gynecol 1974, **119**: 698–704.

574 Sonoda Y. Optimal therapy and management of endometrial cancer. Expert Rev Anticancer Ther 2003, **3**: 37–47.

575 Tewari KS, DiSaia PJ. Radiation therapy for gynecologic cancer. J Obstet Gynaecol Res 2003, **28**: 123–140.

576 Trope C, Kristensen GB, Abeler VM. Clear-cell and papillary serous cancer: treatment options. Best Pract Res Clin Obstet Gynaecol 2001, **15**: 433–446.

577 Wheeler DT, Bristow RE, Kurman RJ. Histologic alterations in endometrial hyperplasia and well-differentiated carcinoma treated with progestins. Am J Surg Pathol 2007, **31**: 988–998.

Prognosis

578 Alektiar KM, McKee A, Lin O, Vankatraman E, Zelefsky MJ, Mychalczak BR, McKee B, Hiskins WJ, Barakat RR. The significance of the amount of myometrial invasion in patients with stage IB endometrial carcinoma. Cancer 2002, **95**: 316–321.

579 Ambros RA, Kurman RJ. Combined assessment of vascular and myometrial invasion as a model to predict prognosis in stage I endometrioid adenocarcinoma of the uterine corpus. Cancer 1992, **69**: 1424–1431.

580 Ambros RA, Kurman RJ. Identification of patients with stage I uterine endometrioid adenocarcinoma at high risk of recurrence by DNA ploidy, myometrial invasion, and vascular invasion. Gynecol Oncol 1992, **45**: 235–239.

581 Ambros RA, Vigna PA, Figge J, Kallakury BV, Mastrangelo A, Eastman AY, Malfetano J, Figge HL, Ross JS. Observations on tumor and metastatic suppressor gene status in endometrial carcinoma with particular emphasis on p53. Cancer 1994, **73**: 1686–1692.

582 Ayhan A, Taskiran C, Yuce K, Kucukali T. The prognostic value of nuclear grading and the revised FIGO grading of endometrial adenocarcinoma. Int J Gynecol Pathol 2002, **22**: 71–74.

583 Beckner ME, Mori T, Silverberg SG. Endometrial carcinoma. Nontumor factors in prognosis. Int J Gynecol Pathol 1985, **4**: 131–145.

584 Benevolo M, Mariani L, Vocaturo G, Vasselli S, Natali PG, Mottolese M. Independent prognostic value of peritoneal immunocytodiagnosis in endometrial carcinoma. Am J Surg Pathol 2000, **24**: 241–247.

585 Bonatz G, Luttes J, Hamann S, Mettler L, Jonat W, Parwaresch R. Immunohistochemical assessment of p170 provides prognostic information in endometrial carcinoma. Histopathology 1999, **34**: 43–50.

586 Boronow RC. Advances in diagnosis, staging, and management of cervical and endometrial cancer, stages I and II. Cancer 1990, **65**: 648–659.

587 Boronow RC, Morrow CP, Creasman WT, DiSaia PJ, Silverberg SG, Miller A, Blessing JA. Surgical staging in endometrial cancer. Clinical–pathologic findings of a prospective study. Obstet Gynecol 1984, **63**: 825–832.

588 Britton LC, Wilson TO, Gaffey TA, Cha SS, Wieand HS, Podratz KC. DNA ploidy in endometrial carcinoma. Major objective prognostic factor. Mayo Clin Proc 1990, **65**: 643–650.

589 Chambers JT, Carcangiu ML, Voynick IM, Schwartz PE. Immunohistochemical evaluation of estrogen and progesterone receptor content in 183 patients with endometrial carcinoma. Part II. Correlation between biochemical and immunohistochemical methods and survival. Am J Clin Pathol 1990, **94**: 255–260.

590 Christopherson WM, Connelly PJ, Alberhasky RC. Carcinoma of the endometrium. V. An analysis of prognosticators in patients with favorable subtypes and stage I disease. Cancer 1983, **51**: 1705–1709.

591 Coppola D, Fu L, Nicosia SV, Kounelis S, Jones M. Prognostic significance of p53, bcl-2, vimentin, and S100 protein-positive Langerhans cells in endometrial carcinoma. Hum Pathol 1998, **29**: 455–462.

592 Creasman WT. Prognostic significance of hormone receptors in endometrial cancer. Cancer 1993, **71**: 1467–1470.

593 DeRycke MS, Andersen JD, Harrington KM, Pambuccian SE, Kalloger SE, Boylan KL, Argenta PA, Skubitz AP. S100A1 expression in ovarian and endometrial endometrioid carcinomas is a prognostic indicator of relapse-free survival. Am J Clin Pathol 2009, **132**: 846–856.

594 Fanning J, Alvarez PM, Tsukada Y, Piver MS. Prognostic significance of the extent of cervical involvement by endometrial cancer. Gynecol Oncol 1991, **40**: 46–47.

595 Gehrig PA, Van Le L, Olatidoye B, Geradts J. Estrogen receptor status, determined by immunohistochemistry, as a predictor of the recurrence of stage I endometrial carcinoma. Cancer 2000, **86**: 2083–2089.

596 Greven KM, Lanciano RM, Corn B, Case D, Randall ME. Pathologic stage III endometrial carcinoma. Prognostic factors and patterns of recurrence. Cancer 1993, **71**: 3697–3702.

597 Hachisuga T, Kaku T, Fukuda K, Eguchi F, Emoto M, Kamura T, Iwasaka T, Kawarabayashi T, Sugimori H, Mori M. The grading in lymphovascular space invasion in endometrial carcinoma. Cancer 2000, **86**: 2090–2097.

598 Hanson MB, Van Nagell JR, Powell DE, Donaldson ES, Gallion H, Merhige M, Pavlik EJ. The prognostic significance of lymph-vascular space invasion in stage I endometrial cancer. Cancer 1985, **55**: 1753–1757.

599 Hendrickson M, Ross J, Eifel PJ, Cox RS, Martinez A, Kempson R. Adenocarcinoma of the endometrium. Analysis of 256 cases with carcinoma limited to the uterine corpus. Pathology review and analysis of prognostic variables. Gynecol Oncol 1982, **13**: 373–392.

600 Hetzel DJ, Wilson TO, Keeney GL, Roche PC, Cha SS, Podratz KC. HER-2/neu expression. A major prognostic factor in endometrial cancer. Gynecol Oncol 1992, **47**: 179–185.

601 Homesley HD, Zaino R. Endometrial cancer. Prognostic factors. Semin Oncol 1994, **21**: 71–78.

602 Ikeda M, Watanabe Y, Nanjoh T, Noda K. Evaluation of DNA ploidy in endometrial cancer. Gynecol Oncol 1993, **50**: 25–29.

603 Inoue Y, Obata K, Abe K, Ohmura G, Doh K, Yoshioka T, Hoshiai H, Noda K. The prognostic significance of vascular invasion by endometrial carcinoma. Cancer 1996, **78**: 1447–1451.

604 Kaku T, Kamura T, Kinukawa N, Kobayashi H, Sakai K, Tsuruchi N, Saito T, Kawauchi S, Tsuneyoshi M, Nakano H. Angiogenesis in endometrial carcinoma. Cancer 1997, **80**: 741–747.

605 Kempson RL, Pokorny GE. Adenocarcinoma of the endometrium in women aged forty and younger. Cancer 1968, **21**: 650–662.

606 Larson DM, Copeland LJ, Gallagher HS, Gershenson DM, Freedman RS, Wharton JT, Kline RC. Nature of cervical involvement in endometrial carcinoma. Cancer 1987, **59**: 959–962.

607 Lukes AS, Kohler MF, Pieper CF, Kerns BJ, Bentley R, Rodriguez GC, Soper JT, Clarke-Pearson DL, Bast RC Jr, Berchuck A. Multivariable analysis of DNA ploidy, p53, and HER-2/neu as prognostic factors in endometrial cancer. Cancer 1994, **73**: 2380–2385.

608 Malkasian GD Jr. Carcinoma of the endometrium. Effect of stage and grade on survival. Cancer 1978, **41**: 996–1001.

609 Mannelqvist M, Stefansson I, Salvesen HB, Akslen LA. Importance of tumour cell invasion in blood and lymphatic vasculature among patients with endometrial carcinoma. Histopathology 2009, **54**: 174–183.

610 Mikuta JJ. International Federation of Gynecology and Obstetrics staging of endometrial cancer 1988. Cancer 1993, **71**: 1460–1463.

611 Ng ABP, Reagan JW. Incidence and prognosis of endometrial carcinoma by histologic grade and extent. Obstet Gynecol 1970, **35**: 437–443.

612 Niikura H, Sasano H, Matsunaga G, Watanabe K, Ito K, Sato S, Yajima A. Prognostic value of epidermal growth factor receptor expression in endometrioid endometrial carcinoma. Hum Pathol 1995, **26**: 892–896.

613 Nordstrom B, Strang P, Lindgren A, Bergstrom R, Tribukait B. Carcinoma of the endometrium: do the nuclear grade and DNA ploidy provide more prognostic information than do the FIGO and WHO classifications? Int J Gynecol Pathol 1997, **15**: 191–201.

614 Peiro G, Diebold J, Mayr D, Baretton GB, Kimming R, Schmidt M, Lohrs U. Prognostic relevance of hMLH1, hMSH2, and BAX protein expression in endometrial carcinoma. Mod Pathol 2001, **14**: 777–783.

615 Prat J. Prognostic parameters of endometrial carcinoma. Hum Pathol 2004, **35**: 649–662.

616 Reinartz JJ, George E, Lindgren BR, Niehans GA. Expression of p53, transforming growth factor alpha, epidermal growth factor receptor, and *c-erbB-2* in endometrial carcinoma and correlation with survival and known predictors of survival. Hum Pathol 1994, **25**: 1075–1083.

617 Robboy SJ, Miller AW III, Kurman RJ. The pathologic features and behavior of endometrial carcinoma associated with exogenous estrogen administration. Pathol Res Pract 1982, **174**: 237–256.

618 Sasano H, Watanabe K, Ito K, Sato S, Yajima A. New concepts in the diagnosis and prognosis of endometrial carcinoma. Pathol Annu 1995, **29**(Pt 2): 31–49.

619 Sidawy MK, Silverberg SG. Endometrial carcinoma. Pathologic factors of therapeutic and prognostic significance. Pathol Annu 1992, **27**: 153–185.

620 Soslow RA, Bissonnette JP, Wilton A, Ferguson SE, Alektiar KM, Duska LR, Oliva E. Clinicopathologic analysis of 187 high-grade endometrial carcinomas of different histologic subtypes: similar outcomes belie distinctive biologic differences. Am J Surg Pathol 2007, **31**: 979–987.

621 Stefansson IM, Salvesen HB, Immervoll H, Akslen LA. Prognostic impact of histological grade and vascular invasion compared with tumour cell proliferation in endometrial carcinoma of endometrioid type. Histopathology 2004, **44**: 472–479.

622 Stendahl U, Strang P, Wagenius G, Bergstrom R, Tribukait B. Prognostic significance of proliferation in endometrial adenocarcinomas. A multivariate analysis of clinical and flow cytometric variables. Int J Gynecol Pathol 1991, **10**: 271–284.

623 Susini T, Baldi F, Howard CM, Baldi A, Taddei G, Massi D, Rapi S, Savino L, Massi G, Giordano A. Expression of the retinoblastoma-related gene Rb2/p130 correlates with clinical outcome in endometrial cancer. J Clin Oncol 1998, **16**: 1085–1093.

624 Tobon H, Watkins GJ. Secretory adenocarcinoma of the endometrium. Int J Gynecol Pathol 1985, **4**: 328–335.

625 Tornos C, Silva EG, el-Naggar A, Burke TW. Aggressive stage I grade I endometrial carcinoma. Cancer 1992, **70**: 790–798.

626 Zaino RJ. Pathologic indicators of prognosis in endometrial adenocarcinoma. Selected aspects emphasizing the GOG experience. Gynecologic Oncology Group. Pathol Annu 1995, **30**(Pt 1): 1–28.

627 Zaino RJ, Davis AT, Ohlsson-Wilhelm BM, Brunetto VL. DNA content is an independent prognostic indicator in endometrial adenocarcinoma: a Gynecologic Oncology Group study. Int J Gynecol Pathol 1998, **17**: 312–319.

628 Zaino RJ, Kurman RJ, Diana KL, Morrow CP. Pathologic models to predict outcome for women with endometrial adenocarcinoma: the importance of the distinction between surgical stage and clinical stage – a Gynecologic Oncology Group study. Cancer 1996, **77**: 1115–1121.

629 Zaino RJ, Kurman R, Herbold D, Gliedman J, Bundy BN, Voet R, Advani H. The significance of squamous differentiation in endometrial carcinoma. Data from a Gynecologic Oncology Group study. Cancer 1991, **68**: 2293–2302.

630 Zaino RJ, Silverberg SG, Norris HJ, Bundy BN, Morrow CP, Okagaki T. The prognostic value of nuclear versus architectural grading in endometrial adenocarcinoma. A Gynecologic Oncology Group study. Int J Gynecol Pathol 1994, **13**: 29–36.

631 Zaino RJ. FIGO staging of endometrial adenocarcinoma: a critical review and proposal. Int J Gynecol Pathol 2009, **28**: 1–9.

ENDOMETRIAL STROMAL TUMORS

632 Abrams J, Talcott J, Corson JM. Pulmonary metastases in patients with low-grade endometrial stromal sarcoma. Clinicopathologic findings with immunohistochemical characterization. Am J Surg Pathol 1989, **13**: 133–140.

633 Adegboyega PA, Qiu S. Immunohistochemical profiling of cytokeratin expression by endometrial stroma sarcoma. Hum Pathol 2008, **39**: 1459–1464.

634 Akhtar M, Kim PY, Young I. Ultrastructure of endometrial stromal sarcoma. Cancer 1975, **35**: 406–412.

635 Aubry MC, Myers JL, Colby TV, Leslie KO, Tazelaar HD. Endometrial stromal sarcoma metastatic to the lung: a detailed analysis of 16 patients. Am J Surg Pathol 2002, **26**: 440–449.

636 August CZ, Bauer KD, Lurain J, Murad T. Neoplasms of endometrial stroma. Histopathologic and flow cytometric analysis with clinical correlation. Hum Pathol 1989, **20**: 232–237.

637 Baker RJ, Hildebrandt RH, Rouse RV, Hendrickson MR, Longacre TA. Inhibin and CD99 (MIC2) expression in uterine stromal neoplasms with sex-cord-like elements. Hum Pathol 1999, **30**: 671–679.

638 Baker PM, Moch H, Oliva E. Unusual morphologic features of endometrial stromal tumors: a report of 2 cases. Am J Surg Pathol 2005, **29**: 1394–1398.

639 Balaton AJ, Vuong PN, Vaury P, Baviera EE. Plexiform tumorlet of the uterus. Immunohistological evidence for a smooth muscle origin. Histopathology 1986, **10**: 749–754.

640 Bhargava R, Shia J, Hummer AJ, Thaler HT, Tornos C, Soslow RA. Distinction of endometrial stromal sarcomas from 'hemangiopericytomatous' tumors using a panel of immunohistochemical stains. Mod Pathol 2005, **18**: 40–47.

641 Biermann K, Heukamp LC, Büttner R, Zhou H. Uterine tumor resembling an ovarian sex cord tumor associated with metastasis. Int J Gynecol Pathol 2008, **27**: 58–60.

642 Chang KL, Crabtree GS, Lim-Tan SK, Kempson RL, Hendrickson MR. Primary uterine endometrial stromal neoplasms. A clinicopathologic study of 117 cases. Am J Surg Pathol 1994, **14**: 415–438.

643 Chu PG, Arber DA, Weiss LM, Chang KL. Utility of CD10 in distinguishing between endometrial stromal sarcoma and uterine smooth muscle tumors: an immunohistochemical comparison of 34 cases. Mod Pathol 2001, **14**: 465–471.

644 Clement PB, Scully RE. Uterine tumors resembling ovarian sex-cord tumors. A clinicopathologic analysis of fourteen cases. Am J Clin Pathol 1976, **66**: 512–525.

645 Clement PB, Scully RE. Endometrial stromal sarcomas of the uterus with extensive endometrioid glandular differentiation. A report of three cases that caused problems in differential diagnosis. Int J Gynecol Pathol 1992, **11**: 163–173.

646 Czernobilsky B. Uterine tumors resembling ovarian sex cord tumors: an update. Int J Gynecol Pathol 2008, **27**: 229–235.

647 Czernobilsky B, Mamet Y, David MB, Atlas I, Gitstein G, Lifschitz-Mercer B. Uterine retiform Sertoli–Leydig cell tumor: report of a case providing additional evidence that uterine tumors resembling ovarian sex cord tumors have a histologic and immunohistochemical phenotype of genuine sex cord tumors. Int J Gynecol Pathol 2005, **24**: 335–340.

648 Dal Cin P. Cytogenetics of mesenchymal tumors of the female genital tract. Surg Pathol Clin 2009, **2**: 813–821.

649 De Fusco PA, Gaffey TA, Malkasian GD Jr, Long HJ, Cha SS. Endometrial stromal sarcoma. Review of Mayo Clinic experience, 1945–1980. Gynecol Oncol 1989, **35**: 8–14.

650 deLeval L, Waltregny D, Boniver J, Young RH, Castronovo V, Oliva E. Use of histone deacetylase 8 (HDAC8), a new marker of smooth muscle differentiation, in the classification of mesenchymal tumors of the uterus. Am J Surg Pathol 2006, **30**: 319–327.

651 Devaney K, Tavassoli FA. Immunohistochemistry as a diagnostic aid in the interpretation of unusual mesenchymal tumors of the uterus. Mod Pathol 1991, **4**: 225–231.

652 Dickersin GR, Scully RE. Role of electron microscopy in metastatic endometrial stromal tumors. Ultrastruct Pathol 1993, **17**: 377–403.

653 Dionigi A, Oliva E, Clement PB, Young RH. Endometrial stromal nodules and endometrial stromal tumors with limited infiltration: a clinicopathologic study of 50 cases. Am J Surg Pathol 2002, **26**: 567–581.

654 el-Naggar AK, Abdul-Karim FW, Silva EG, McLemore D, Garnsey L. Uterine stromal neoplasms. A clinicopathologic and DNA flow cytometric correlation. Hum Pathol 1991, **22**: 897–903.

655 Evans HL. Endometrial stromal sarcoma and poorly differentiated endometrial sarcoma. Cancer 1982, **50**: 2170–2182.

656 Farhood AI, Abrams J. Immunohistochemistry of endometrial stromal sarcoma. Hum Pathol 1991, **22**: 224–230.

657 Fekete PS, Vellios F. The clinical and histologic spectrum of endometrial stromal neoplasms. A report of 41 cases. Int J Gynecol Pathol 1984, **3**: 198–212.

658 Fisher ER, Paulson JD, Gregorio RM. The myofibroblastic nature of the uterine plexiform tumor. Arch Pathol Lab Med 1978, **102**: 477–480.

659 Franquemont DW, Frierson HF Jr, Mills SE. An immunohistochemical study of normal endometrial stroma and endometrial stromal neoplasms. Evidence for smooth muscle differentiation. Am J Surg Pathol 1991, **15**: 861–870.

660 Goodhue WW, Susin M, Kramer EE. Smooth muscle origin of uterine plexiform tumors. Ultrastructural and histochemical evidence. Arch Pathol 1974, **97**: 263–268.

661 Hitchcock CL, Norris HJ. Flow cytometric analysis of endometrial stromal sarcoma. Am J Clin Pathol 1992, **97**: 267–271.

662 Irving JA, Carinelli S, Prat J. Uterine tumors resembling ovarian sex cord tumors are polyphenotypic neoplasms with true sex cord differentiation. Mod Pathol 2006, **19**: 17–24.

663 Itoh T, Mochizuki M, Kumazaki S, Ishihara T, Fukayama M. Cystic pulmonary metastases of endometrial stromal sarcoma of the uterus, mimicking lymphangiomyomatosis: a case report with immunohistochemistry of HMB45. Pathol Int 1997, **47**: 725–729.

664 Kaminski PF, Tavassoli FA. Plexiform tumorlet. A clinical and pathologic study of 15 cases with ultrastructural observations. Int J Gynecol Pathol 1984, **3**: 124–134.

665 Katsanis WA, O'Connor DM, Gibb RK, Bendon RW. Endometrial stromal sarcoma involving the placenta. Ann Diagn Pathol 1999, **2**: 301–305.

666 Kempson RL, Hendrickson MR. Smooth muscle, endometrial stromal, and mixed Mullerian tumors of the uterus. Mod Pathol 2000, **13**: 328–342.

667 Kolda TF, Ro JY, Ordonez NG, Tornos C, Park YW, Hyman WJ, Ayala AG. Endometrial stromal sarcoma presenting as extrauterine metastases: a morphologic and immunohistochemical approach to diagnosis. Int J Surg Pathol 1997, **5**: 105–110.

668 Krishnamurthy S, Jungbluth AA, Busam KJ, Rosai J. Uterine tumors resembling ovarian sex-cord tumors have an immunophenotype consistent with true sex-cord differentiation. Am J Surg Pathol 1998, **22**: 1078–1082.

669 Kurihara S, Oda Y, Ohishi Y, Iwasa A, Takahira T, Kaneki E, Kobayashi H, Wake N, Tsuneyoshi M. Endometrial stromal sarcomas and related high-grade sarcomas: immunohistochemical and molecular genetic study of 31 cases. Am J Surg Pathol 2008, **32**: 1228–1238.

670 Lam KY, Khoo US, Cheung A. Collision of endometrioid carcinoma and stromal sarcoma of the uterus: a report of two cases. Int J Gynecol Pathol 1999, **18**: 77–81.

671 Larbig GG, Clemmer JJ, Koss LG, Foote FW. Plexiform tumorlets of endometrial stromal origin. Am J Clin Pathol 1965, **44**: 32–35.

672 Lee CH, Ali R, Gilks CB. Molecular genetics of mesenchymal tumors of the female genital tract. Surg Pathol Clin 2009, **2**: 823–834.

673 Levine PH, Abou-Nassar S, Mittal K. Extrauterine low-grade endometrial stromal sarcoma with florid endometrioid glandular

differentiation. Int J Gynecol Pathol 2001, **20**: 395–398.

674 Lillemoe TJ, Perrone T, Norris HJ, Dehner LP. Myogenous phenotype of epithelial-like areas in endometrial stromal sarcomas. Arch Pathol Lab Med 1991, **115**: 215–219.

675 Lloreta J, Prat J. Ultrastructure of an endometrial stromal nodule with skeletal muscle. Ultrastruct Pathol 1993, **17**: 405–410.

676 Loddenkemper C, Mechsner S, Foss H-D, Dallenbach FE, Anagnostopoulos I, Ebert AD, Stein H. Use of oxytocin receptor expression in distinguishing between uterine smooth muscle tumors and endometrial stromal sarcoma. Am J Surg Pathol 2003, **27**: 1458–1462.

677 McCluggage WG, Sumathi VP, Maxwell P. CD10 is a sensitive and diagnostically useful immunohistochemical marker of normal endometrial stroma and of endometrial stromal neoplasms. Histopathology 2001, **39**: 273–278.

678 McCluggage WG, Ganesan R, Herrington CS. Endometrial stromal sarcomas with extensive endometrioid glandular differentiation: report of a series with emphasis on the potential for misdiagnosis and discussion of the differential diagnosis. Histopathology 2009, **54**: 365–373.

679 McCluggage WG, Young RH. Endometrial stromal sarcomas with true papillae and pseudopapillae. Int J Gynecol Pathol 2008, **27**: 555–561.

680 Mazur MT, Askin FB. Endolymphatic stromal myosis. Unique presentation and ultrastructural study. Cancer 1978, **42**: 2661–2667.

681 Moinfar F, Gogg-Kamerer M, Sommersacher A, Regitnig P, Man YG, Zatloukal K, Denk H, Tavassoli FA. Endometrial stromal sarcomas frequently express epidermal growth factor receptor (EGFR, HER-1): potential basis for a new therapeutic approach. Am J Surg Pathol 2005, **29**: 485–489.

682 Moinfar F, Regitnig P, Tabrizi AD, Denk H, Tavassoli FA. Expression of androgen receptors in benign and malignant endometrial stromal neoplasms. Virchows Arch 2004, **444**: 410–414.

683 Nogales FF, Nicolae A, García-Galvis OF, Aneiros-Fernández J, Salas-Molina J, Stolnicu S. Uterine and extrauterine plexiform tumourlets are sex-cord-like tumours with myoid features. Histopathology 2009, **54**: 497–500.

684 Nogales FF, Stolnicu S, Harilal KR, Mooney E, García-Galvis OF. Retiform uterine tumours resembling ovarian sex cord tumours. A comparative immunohistochemical study with retiform structures of the female genital tract. Histopathology 2009, **54**: 471–477.

685 Norris HJ, Taylor HB. Mesenchymal tumors of the uterus. I, A clinical and pathological study of 53 endometrial stromal tumors. Cancer 1966, **19**: 755–766.

686 Nucci MR, O'Connell JT, Heuttner PC, Cviko A, Sun D, Quade BJ. H-Caldesmon expression effectively distinguishes endometrial stromal tumors from uterine smooth muscle tumors. Am J Surg Pathol 2001, **25**: 455–463.

687 Ohta Y, Suzuki T, Omatsu M, Hamatani S, Shiokawa A, Kushima M, Ota H. Transition from low-grade endometrial stromal sarcoma to high-grade endometrial stromal sarcoma. Int J Gynecol Pathol 2010, **29**: 374–377.

688 Oliva E, Clement PB, Young RH, Scully RE. Mixed endometrial stromal and smooth muscle tumors of the uterus: a clinicopathologic study of 15 cases. Am J Surg Pathol 1998, **22**: 997–1005.

689 Oliva E, Clement PB, Young RH. Endometrial stromal tumors: an update on a group of tumors with a protean phenotype. Adv Anat Pathol 2000, **7**: 257–281.

690 Oliva E, Clement PB, Young RH. Epithelioid endometrial and endometrioid stromal tumors: a report of four cases emphasising their distinction from epithelioid smooth muscle tumors and other oxyphilic uterine and extrauterine tumors. Int J Gynecol Pathol 2002, **21**: 48–55.

691 Oliva E, Young RH, Amin MB, Clement PB. An immunohistochemical analysis of endometrial stromal and smooth muscle tumors of the uterus: a study of 54 cases emphasizing the importance of using a panel because of overlap in immunoreactivity for individual antibodies. Am J Surg Pathol 2002, **26**: 403–412.

692 Oliva E, Young RH, Clement PB, Scully RE. Myxoid and fibrous endometrial stromal tumors of the uterus: a report of 10 cases. Int J Gynecol Pathol 1999, **18**: 310–319.

693 Rosai J, Lauren V Dr. Lauren V. Ackerman and his man from Istanbul. Semin Diagn Pathol 2003; **20**: 247–248.

694 Roth LM, Senteny GE. Stromomyoma of the uterus. Ultrastruct Pathol 1985, **9**: 137–143.

695 Rush DS, Tan J, Baergen RN, Soslow RA. h-Caldesmon, a novel smooth muscle-specific antibody, distinguishes between cellular leiomyoma and endometrial stromal sarcoma. Am J Surg Pathol 2001, **25**: 253–258.

696 Sabini G, Chumas JC, Mann WJ. Steroid hormone receptors in endometrial stromal sarcomas. A biochemical and immunohistochemical study. Am J Clin Pathol 1992, **97**: 381–386.

697 Shah R, McCluggage WG. Symplastic atypia in neoplastic and non-neoplastic endometrial stroma: report of 3 cases with a review of atypical symplastic cells within the female genital tract. Int J Gynecol Pathol 2009, **28**: 334–337.

698 Shiraki M, Otis CN, Powell JL. Endometrial stromal sarcoma arising from ovarian and extraovarian endometriosis – report of two cases and review of the literature. Surg Pathol 1991, **4**: 333–343.

699 Suarez Vilela D, Izquierdo Garcia FM. Foam cells and histiocytes in endometrial stromal tumours. Histopathology 1998, **32**: 568–569.

700 Sumathi VP, Al-Hussaini M, Connolly LE, Fullerton L, McCluggage WG. Endometrial stromal neoplasms are immunoreactive with WT-1 antibody. Int J Gynecol Pathol 2004, **23**: 241–247.

701 Tang C-K, Toker C, Ances IG. Stromomyoma of the uterus. Cancer 1979, **43**: 308–316.

702 Tavassoli FA, Norris HJ. Mesenchymal tumours of the uterus. VII. A clinicopathological study of 60 endometrial stromal nodules. Histopathology 1981, **5**: 1–10.

703 Tsukamoto N, Kamura T, Matsukuma K, Imachi M, Uchino H, Saito T, Ono M. Endolymphatic stromal myosis. A case with positive estrogen and progesterone receptors and good response to progestins. Gynecol Oncol 1985, **20**: 120–128.

704 Ulbright TM, Kraus FT. Endometrial stromal tumors of extra-uterine tissue. Am J Clin Pathol 1981, **76**: 371–377.

705 Yilmaz A, Rush DS, Soslow RA. Endometrial stromal sarcomas with unusual histologic features: a report of 24 primary and metastatic tumors emphasizing fibroblastic and smooth muscle differentiation. Am J Surg Pathol 2002, **26**: 1142–1150.

706 Yoonessi M, Hart WR. Endometrial stromal sarcomas. Cancer 1977, **40**: 898–906.

MALIGNANT MIXED MÜLLERIAN TUMOR (CARCINOSARCOMA)

707 Amant F, Moerman P, Davel GH, De Vos R, Vergote I, Lindeque BG, de Jonge E. Uterine carcinosarcoma with melanocytic differentiation. Int J Gynecol Pathol 2001, **20**: 186–190.

708 Barwick KW, LiVolsi VA. Malignant mixed müllerian tumors of the uterus. Am J Surg Pathol 1979, **3**: 125–135.

709 Bitterman P, Chun B, Kurman RJ. The significance of epithelial differentiation in mixed mesodermal tumors of the uterus. A clinicopathologic and immunohistochemical study. Am J Surg Pathol 1990, **4**: 317–328.

710 Chuang JT, Van Velden DJJ, Graham JB. Carcinosarcoma and mixed mesodermal tumor of the uterine corpus. Review of 49 cases. Obstet Gynecol 1970, **35**: 769–780.

711 Chumas JC, Mann WJ, Tseng L. Malignant mixed müllerian tumor of the endometrium in a young woman with polycystic ovaries. Cancer 1983, **52**: 1478–1481.

712 Costa MJ, Walls J. Epidermal growth factor receptor and c-erbB-2 oncoprotein expression in female genital tract carcinosarcomas (malignant mixed Mullerian tumors): clinicopathologic study of 82 cases. Cancer 1996, **77**: 533–542.

713 Costa MJ, Vogelsan J, Young LJ. p53 gene mutation in female genital tract carcinosarcomas (malignant mixed müllerian tumors). A clinicopathologic study of 74 cases. Mod Pathol 1994, **7**: 619–627.

714 de Brito PA, Silverberg SG, Orenstein JM. Carcinosarcoma (malignant mixed müllerian [mesodermal] tumor) of the female genital tract. Immunohistochemical and ultrastructural analysis of 28 cases. Hum Pathol 1993, **24**: 132–142.

715 Dellers EA, Valente PT, Edmonds PR, Balsara G. Extrauterine mixed mesodermal tumors. An immunohistochemical study. Arch Pathol Lab Med 1991, **115**: 918–920.

716 Donner LR. Uterine carcinosarcoma with complete sarcomatous overgrowth mimicking pure embryonal rhabdomyosarcoma. Int J Gynecol Pathol 2002, **22**: 89–91.

717 Doss LL, Llorens AS, Henriquez EM. Carcinosarcoma of the uterus. A 40-year experience from the state of Missouri. Gynecol Oncol 1984, **18**: 43–53.

718 Emoto M, Iwasaki H, Ishiguro M, Kikuchi M, Horiuchi S, Saito T, Tsukamoto N, Kawarabayashi T. Angiogenesis in carcinosarcomas of the uterus: differences in the microvessel density and expression of vascular endothelial growth factor between the epithelial and mesenchymal elements. Hum Pathol 1999, **30**: 1232–1241.

719 Euscher ED, Malpica A. Histology and pattern of recurrence in uterine malignant mixed mullerian tumor. Lab Invest 2009, **89**(Suppl 1): 213A.

720 Fehr PE, Prem KA. Malignancy of the uterine corpus following irradiation therapy for squamous cell carcinoma of the cervix. Am J Obstet Gynecol 1974, **119**: 685–692.

721 Ferguson SE, Tornos C, Hummer A, Barakat RR, Soslow RA. Prognostic features of surgical stage I uterine carcinosarcoma. Am J Surg Pathol 2007, **31**: 1653–1661.

722 Gagne E, Tetu B, Blondeau L, Raymond PE, Blais R. Morphologic prognostic factors of malignant mixed müllerian tumor of the uterus. A clinicopathologic study of 58 cases. Mod Pathol 1989, **2**: 433–438.

723 George E, Lillemoe TJ, Twiggs LB, Perrone T. Malignant mixed müllerian tumor versus high-grade endometrial carcinoma and aggressive variants of endometrial carcinoma. A comparative analysis of survival. Int J Gynecol Pathol 1995, **14**: 39–44.

724 George E, Manivel JC, Dehner LP, Wick MR. Malignant mixed müllerian tumors. An immunohistochemical study of 47 cases, with histogenetic considerations and clinical correlation. Hum Pathol 1991, **22**: 215–223.

725 Gersell DJ, Duncan DA, Fulling KH. Malignant mixed müllerian tumor of the uterus with neuroectodermal differentiation. Int J Gynecol Pathol 1989, **8**: 169–178.

726 Iwasa Y, Haga H, Konishi I, Kobashi Y, Higuchi K, Katsuyama E, Minamiguchi S, Yamabe H. Prognostic factors in uterine carcinosarcoma: a clinicopathologic study of 25 patients. Cancer 1998, **82**: 512–519.

727 Kohorn EI, Schwartz PE, Chambers JT, Peschel RE, Kapp DS, Merino M. Adjuvant therapy in mixed müllerian tumors of the uterus. Gynecol Oncol 1986, **23**: 212–221.

728 Kounelis S, Jones MW, Papadaki H, Bakker A, Swalsky P, Finkelstein SD. Carcinosarcomas (malignant mixed mullerian tumors) of the female genital tract: comparative molecular analysis of epithelial and mesenchymal components. Hum Pathol 1998, **29**: 82–87.

729 Krigman HR, Coogan AC, Marks JR. Simultaneous endometrial malignant mixed mesodermal tumor and ovarian serous adenocarcinoma. Arch Pathol Lab Med 1995, **119**: 99–103.

730 Mayall P, Rutty K, Campbell F, Goddard H. p53 immunostaining suggests that uterine carcinosarcomas are monoclonal. Histopathology 1994, **24**: 211–214.

731 Meis JM, Lawrence WD. The immunohistochemical profile of malignant mixed müllerian tumor. Overlap with endometrial adenocarcinoma. Am J Clin Pathol 1990, **94**: 1–7.

732 Mikami Y, Hata S, Kiyokawa T, Minabe T. Expression of CD10 in malignant mullerian mixed tumors and adenosarcomas: an immunohistochemical study. Mod Pathol 2002, **15**: 923–930.

733 Mount SL, Lee KR, Taatjes DJ. Carcinosarcoma (malignant mixed müllerian tumor) of the uterus with a rhabdoid tumor component. An immunohistochemical, ultrastructural, and immunoelectron microscopic case study. Am J Clin Pathol 1995, **103**: 235–239.

734 Norris HJ, Roth E, Taylor HB. Mesenchymal tumors of the uterus. II. A clinical and pathologic study of 31 mixed mesodermal tumors. Obstet Gynecol 1966, **28**: 57–63.

735 Norris HJ, Taylor HB. Postirradiation sarcomas of the uterus. Obstet Gynecol 1965, **26**: 689–694.

736 Norris NJ, Taylor HB. Mesenchymal tumors of the uterus. III. A clinical and pathologic study of 31 carcinosarcomas. Cancer 1966, **19**: 1459–1465.

737 Press MF, Scully RE. Endometrial 'sarcomas' complicating ovarian thecoma, polycystic ovarian disease and estrogen therapy. Gynecol Oncol 1985, **21**: 135–154.

738 Schaepman-van Geuns EJ. Mixed tumors and carcinosarcomas of the uterus evaluated five years after treatment. Cancer 1970, **25**: 72–77.

739 Shen DH, Khoo US, Xue WC, Ngan HY, Wang JL, Liu VW, Chan YK, Cheung AN. Primary peritoneal malignant mixed mullerian tumors: a clinicopathologic immunohistochemical, and genetic study. Cancer 2001, **91**: 1052–1060.

740 Shokeir MO, Noel SM, Clement PB. Malignant Müllerian mixed tumor of the uterus with a prominent alpha-fetoprotein-producing component of yolk sac tumor. Mod Pathol 1996, **9**: 647–651.

741 Silverberg SG, Major FJ, Blessing JA, Fetter B, Askin FB, Liao SY, Miller A. Carcinosarcoma (malignant mixed mesodermal tumor) of the uterus. A Gynecologic Oncology Group pathologic study of 203 cases. Int J Gynecol Pathol 1990, **9**: 1–19.

742 Spanos WJ, Peters LJ, Oswald MJ. Patterns of recurrence in malignant mixed müllerian tumor of the uterus. Cancer 1986, **57**: 155–159.

743 Spanos WJ, Wharton JT, Gomez L, Fletcher GH, Oswald MJ. Malignant mixed müllerian tumors of the uterus. Cancer 1984, **53**: 311–316.

744 Sreenan JJ, Hart WR. Carcinosarcomas of the female genital tract. A pathologic study of 29 metastatic tumors – further evidence for the dominant role of the epithelial component and the conversion theory of histogenesis. Am J Surg Pathol 1995, **19**: 666–674.

745 Varela-Duran J, Nochomovitz LE, Prem KA, Dehner LP. Postirradiation mixed müllerian tumors of the uterus. A comparative clinicopathologic study. Cancer 1980, **45**: 1625–1631.

746 Yamada SD, Burger RA, Brewster WR, Anton D, Kohler MF, Monk BJ. Pathologic variables and adjuvant therapy as predictor of recurrence and survival for patients with surgically evaluated carcinosarcoma of the uterus. Cancer 2000, **88**: 2782–2786.

747 Yorokoglu K, Aktas S, Gore O, Ozen E. Malignant mixed mullerian tumor of the uterus with prominent neuroectodermal differentiation: a case report. Int J Surg Pathol 1998, **6**: 155–158.

748 Yoshida Y, Kurokawa T, Fukuno N, Kishikawa Y, Kamitani N, Kotsuj F. Markers of apoptosis and angiogenesis indicate that carcinomatous components play an important role in the malignant behaviour of uterine carcinosarcoma. Hum Pathol 2001, **31**: 1448–1454.

MÜLLERIAN ADENOSARCOMA AND RELATED TUMORS

749 Chen KTK. Rhabdomyosarcomatous uterine adenosarcoma. Int J Gynecol Pathol 1985, **4**: 146–152.

750 Clement PB. Müllerian adenosarcomas of the uterus with sarcomatous overgrowth. A clinicopathological analysis of 10 cases. Am J Surg Pathol 1989, **13**: 28–38.

751 Clement PB, Scully RE. Müllerian adenosarcoma of the uterus. A clinicopathologic analysis of ten cases of a distinctive type of müllerian mixed tumor. Cancer 1974, **34**: 1138–1149.

752 Clement PB, Scully RE. Extrauterine mesodermal (müllerian) adenosarcoma. A clinicopathologic analysis of five cases. Am J Clin Pathol 1978, **69**: 276–283.

753 Clement PB, Scully RE. Müllerian adenosarcomas of the uterus with sex cord-like elements. A clinicopathologic analysis of eight cases. Am J Clin Pathol 1989, **91**: 664–672.

754 Clement PB, Scully RE. Müllerian adenosarcoma of the uterus. A clinicopathologic analysis of 100 cases with a review of the literature. Hum Pathol 1990, **21**: 363–381.

755 Clement PB, Scully RE. Müllerian adenofibroma of the uterus with invasion of myometrium and pelvic veins. Int J Gynecol Pathol 1990, **9**: 363–371.

756 Clement PB, Oliva E, Young RH. Mullerian adenosarcoma of the uterine corpus associated with tamoxifen therapy: a report of six cases and a review of tamoxifen-associated endometrial lesions. Int J Gynecol Pathol 1997, **15**: 222–229.

757 Fehmian C, Jones J, Kress Y, Abadi M. Adenosarcoma of the uterus with extensive smooth muscle differentiation: ultrastructural study and review of the literature. Ultrastruct Pathol 1997, **21**: 73–90.

758 Gallardo A, Prat J. Mullerian adenosarcoma: a clinicopathologic and immunohistochemical study of 55 cases challenging the existence of adenofibroma. Am J Surg Pathol 2009, **33**: 278–288.

759 Gloor E. Müllerian adenosarcoma of the uterus. Am J Surg Pathol 1979, **3**: 203–209.

760 Grimalt M, Arguelles M, Ferenczy A. Papillary cyst-adenofibroma of endometrium. A histochemical and ultrastructural study. Cancer 1975, **36**: 137–144.

761 Hirschfield L, Kahn LB, Chen S, Winkler B, Rosenberg S. Müllerian adenosarcoma with ovarian sex cord-like differentiation. A light and electron-microscopic study. Cancer 1986, **57**: 1197–1200.

762 Horie Y, Ikawa S, Kadowaki K, Minagawa Y, Kigawa J, Terakawa N. Lipoadenofibroma of the uterine corpus. Report of a new variant of adenofibroma (benign müllerian mixed tumor). Arch Pathol Lab Med 1995, **119**: 274–276.

763 Kaku T, Silverberg SG, Major FJ, Miller A, Fetter B, Brady MF. Adenosarcoma of the uterus. A Gynecologic Oncology Group clinicopathologic study of 31 cases. Int J Gynecol Pathol 1992, **11**: 75–88.

764 Katzenstein AA, Askin FB, Feldman PS. Müllerian adenosarcoma of the uterus. An ultrastructural study of four cases. Cancer 1977, **40**: 2233–2242.

765 Lack EE, Bitterman P, Sundeen JT. Müllerian adenosarcoma of the uterus with pure angiosarcoma. Case report. Hum Pathol 1991, **22**: 1289–1291.

766 Miller KN, McClure SP. Papillary adenofibroma of the uterus. Report of a case involved by adenocarcinoma and review of the literature. Am J Clin Pathol 1992, **97**: 806–809.

767 Peters WM, Wells MJ, Bryce FC. Müllerian clear cell carcinofibroma of the uterine corpus. Histopathology 1984, **8**: 1069–1078.

768 Seidman JD, Wasserman CS, Aye LM, MacKoul PJ, O'Leary TJ. Cluster of uterine mullerian adenosarcoma in the Washington, DC metropolitan area with high incidence of sarcomatous overgrowth. Am J Surg Pathol 1999, **23**: 809–814.

769 Silverberg SG. Adenomyomatosis of endometrium and endocervix. A hamartoma? Am J Clin Pathol 1975, **64**: 192–199.

770 Soslow RA, Ali A, Oliva E. Mullerian adenosarcomas: an immunophenotypic analysis of 35 cases. Am J Surg Pathol 2008, **32**: 1013–1021.

771 Valdez VA, Planas AT, Lopez VF, Goldberg M, Herrera NE. Adenosarcoma of uterus and ovary. A clinicopathologic study of two cases. Cancer 1979, **43**: 1439–1447.

772 Vellios F, Ng ABP, Reagan JW. Papillary adenofibroma of the uterus. A benign mesodermal mixed tumor of müllerian origin. Am J Clin Pathol 1973, **60**: 543–551.

773 Zaloudek CJ, Norris HJ. Adenofibroma and adenosarcoma of the uterus. A clinicopathologic study of 35 cases. Cancer 1981, **48**: 354–366.

LEIOMYOMA

774 Bardsley V, Cooper P, Peat DS. Massive lymphocytic infiltration of uterine leiomyomas associated with GnRH agonist treatment. Histopathology 1998, **33**: 80–82.

775 Brown JM, Malkasian GD Jr, Symmonds RE. Abdominal myomectomy. Am J Obstet Gynecol 1967, **99**: 126–129.

776 Colgan TJ, Pendergast S, Le Blanc M. The histopathology of uterine leiomyomas following treatment with gonadotropin-releasing hormone analogues. Hum Pathol 1993, **24**: 1073–1077.

777 Colgan TJ, Pron G, Mocarski EJM, Bennett JD, Asch MR, Common A. Pathologic features of uteri and leiomyomas following uterine artery embolization for leiomyomas. Am J Surg Pathol 2003, **27**: 167–177.

778 Cramer SF, Patel A. The frequency of uterine leiomyomas. Am J Clin Pathol 1990, **94**: 435–438.

779 Cramer SF, Horiszny J, Patel A, Sigrist S. The relation of fibrous degeneration to menopausal status in small uterine leiomyomas with evidence for postmenopausal origin of seeding myomas. Mod Pathol 1997, **9**: 774–780.

780 Cramer SF, Marchetti C, Freedman J, Padela A. Relationships of myoma cell size and menopausal status in small uterine leiomyomas. Arch Pathol Lab Med 2000, **124**: 1448–1453.

781 Dal Cin P. Cytogenetics of mesenchymal tumors of the female genital tract. Surg Pathol Clin 2009, **2**: 813–821.

782 Demopoulus RI, Jones KY, Mittal KR, Vamvakas EC. Histology of leiomyomata in patients treated with leuprolide acetate. Int J Gynecol Pathol 1997, **16**: 131–137.

783 Friedman AJ, Hoffman DI, Comite F, Browneller RW, Miller JD. Treatment of leiomyomata uteri with leuprolide acetate depot. A double-blind, placebo-controlled, multicenter study. The Leuprolide Study Group. Obstet Gynecol 1991, **77**: 720–725.

784 Gutmann JN, Thornton KL, Diamond MP, Carcangiu ML. Evaluation of leuprolide acetate treatment on histopathology of uterine myomata. Fertil Steril 1994, **61**: 622–626.

785 Hu J, Surti U. Subgroups of uterine leiomyomas based on cytogenetic analysis. Hum Pathol 1991, **22**: 1009–1016.

786 Ip PP, Lam KW, Cheung CL, Yeung MC, Pun TC, Chan QK, Cheung AN. Tranexamic acid-associated necrosis and intralesional thrombosis of uterine leiomyomas: a clinicopathologic study of 147 cases emphasizing the importance of drug-induced necrosis and early infarcts in leiomyomas. Am J Surg Pathol 2007, **31**: 1215–1224.

787 Kalir T, Goldstein M, Dottino P, Brodman M, Gordon R, Deligdisch L, Wu H, Gil J. Morphometric and electron-microscopic analyses of the effects of gonadotropin-releasing hormone agonists on uterine leiomyomas. Arch Pathol Lab Med 1998, **122**: 442–446.

788 Klotzbucher M, Wasserfall A, Fuhrmann U. Misexpresson of wild-type and truncated isoforms of the high-mobility group I proteins HMBI-C and HMGI(Y) in uterine leiomyomas. Am J Pathol 1999, **155**: 1535–1542.

789 Konishi I, Fujii S, Ban C, Okuda Y, Okamura H, Tojo S. Ultrastructural study of minute uterine leiomyomas. Int J Gynecol Pathol 1983, **2**: 113–120.

790 Laforga JB, Aranda FI. Uterine leiomyomas with T-cell infiltration associated with GnRH agonist goserelin. Histopathology 1999, **34**: 471–472.

791 Lascano EF. Mast cells in human tumors. Cancer 1958, **11**: 1110–1114.

792 Lee CH, Ali R, Gilks CB. Molecular genetics of mesenchymal tumors of the female genital tract. Surg Pathol Clin 2009, **2**: 823–834.

793 Ligon AH, Morton CC. Genetics of uterine leiomyomata. Genes Chromosomes Cancer 2000, **28**: 235–245.

794 McCluggage WG, Ellis PK, McClure N, Walker WJ, Jackson PA, Manek S. Pathologic features of uterine leiomyomas following uterine artery embolization. Int J Gynecol Pathol 2000, **19**: 342–347.

795 Maluf HM, Gersell DJ. Uterine leiomyomas with high content of mast cells. Arch Pathol Lab Med 1994, **118**: 712–714.

796 McClean G, McCluggage WG. Unusual morphologic features of uterine leiomyomas treated with gonadotropin-releasing hormone agonists: massive lymphoid infiltration and vasculitis. Int J Surg Pathol 2003, **11**: 339–344.

797 Mittal K, Popiolek D, Demopoulos RI. Uterine myxoid leiomyosarcoma within a leiomyoma. Hum Pathol 2000, **31**: 398–400.

798 Nedwich A, Frumin A, Meranze DR. Erythrocytosis associated with uterine myomas. Am J Obstet Gynecol 1962, **84**: 174–178.

799 Nilbert M, Heim S, Mandahl N, Flodérus UM, Willén H, Mitelman F. Karyotypic rearrangements in 20 uterine leiomyomas. Cytogenet Cell Genet 1988, **49**: 300–304.

800 Orii A, Mori A, Zhai YL, Toki T, Nikaido T, Fujii S. Mast cells in smooth muscle tumors of the uterus. Int J Gynecol Pathol 1998, **17**: 336–342.

801 Parazzini F, La Vecchia C, Negri E, Cecchetti G, Fedele L. Epidemiologic characteristics of women with uterine fibroids. A case-control study. Obstet Gynecol 1988, **72**: 853–857.

802 Parker RL, Young RH, Clement PB. Skeletal muscle-like and rhabdoid cells in uterine leiomyomas. Int J Gynecol Pathol 2005, **24**: 319–325.

803 Pollio F, Staibano S, Mansueto G, De Rosa G, Persico F, De Falco M, Di Lieto A. Erythropoietin and erythropoietin receptor system in a large uterine myoma of a patient with myomatous erythrocytosis syndrome: possible relationship with the pathogenesis of unusual tumor size. Hum Pathol 2005, **36**: 120–127.

804 Richards PA, Tiltman AJ. Anatomical variation of the oestrogen receptor in the non-neoplastic myometrium of fibromyomatous uteri. Virchows Arch 1996, **428**: 347–351.

805 Sreenan JJ, Prayson RA, Biscotti CV, Thornton MH, Easley KA, Hart WR. Histopathologic findings in 107 uterine leiomyomas treated with leuprolide acetate compared with 126 controls. Am J Surg Pathol 1996, **20**: 427–432.

806 Vu K, Greenspan DL, Wu TC, Zacur HA, Kurman RJ. Cellular proliferation, estrogen receptor, progesterone receptor, and bcl-2 expression in GnRH agonist-treated uterine leiomyomas. Hum Pathol 1998, **29**: 359–363.

807 Weichert W, Denkert C, Gauruder-Burmester A, Kurzeja R, Hamm B, Dietel M, Kroencke TJ. Uterine arterial embolization with tris-acryl gelatin microspheres: a histopathologic evaluation. Am J Surg Pathol 2005, **29**: 955–961.

Leiomyoma variants

808 Abell MR, Littler ER. Benign metastasizing uterine leiomyoma. Multiple lymph nodal metastases. Cancer 1975, **36**: 2206–2213.

809 Aung T, Goto M, Nomoto M, Kitajima S, Douchi T, Yoshinaga M, Yonezawa S. Uterine lipoleiomyoma: a histopathological review of 17 cases. Pathol Int 2004, **54**: 751–758.

810 Bakotic BW, Cabello-Inchausti B, Willis IH, Suster S. Clear-cell epithelioid leiomyoma of the round ligament. Mod Pathol 1999, **12**: 912–918.

811 Baschinsky DY, Isa A, Niemann TH, Prior TW, Lucas JG, Frankel WL. Diffuse leiomyomatosis of the uterus: a case report with clonality analysis. Hum Pathol 2000, **31**: 1429–1432.

812 Billings SD, Folpe AL, Weiss SW. Do leiomyomas of deep soft tissue exist? An analysis of highly differentiated smooth muscle tumors of deep soft tissue supporting two distinct subtypes. Am J Surg Pathol 2001, **25**: 1134–1142.

813 Botsis D, Koliopoulos C, Kondi-Pafitis A, Creatsas G. Frequency, histological, and immunohistochemical properties of massive inflammatory lymphocytic infiltration of leiomyomas of the uterus: an entity causing diagnostic difficulties. Int J Gynecol Pathol 2005, **24**: 326–329.

814 Brescia RJ, Tazelaar HD, Hobbs J, Miller AW. Intravascular lipoleiomyomatosis. A report of two cases. Hum Pathol 1989, **20**: 252–256.

815 Canzonieri V, D'Amore ES, Bartoloni G, Piazza M, Blandamura S, Carbone A. Leiomyomatosis with vascular invasion. A unified pathogenesis regarding leiomyoma with vascular microinvasion, benign metastasizing leiomyoma and intravenous leiomyomatosis. Virchows Arch 1994, **425**: 541–545.

816 Cheuk W, Chan JK, Liu JY. Cotyledonoid leiomyoma: a benign uterine tumor with alarming gross appearance. Arch Pathol Lab Med 2002, **126**: 210–213.

817 Cho KR, Woodruff JD, Epstein JI. Leiomyoma of the uterus with multiple extrauterine smooth muscle tumors: a case report suggesting multifocal origin. Hum Pathol 1989, **20**: 80–82.

818 Clement PB. The pathology of uterine smooth muscle tumors and mixed endometrial stromal-smooth muscle tumors: a selective review with emphasis on recent advances. Int J Gynecol Pathol 2000, **19**: 39–55.

819 Clement PB, Young RH. Diffuse leiomyomatosis of the uterus. A report of four cases. Int J Gynecol Pathol 1987, **6**: 322–330.

820 Clement PB, Young RH, Scully RE. Diffuse, perinodular, and other patterns of hydropic degeneration within and adjacent to uterine leiomyomas. Problems in differential diagnosis. Am J Surg Pathol 1992, **16**: 26–32.

821 Coad JE, Sulaiman RA, Das K, Staley N. Perinodular hydropic degeneration of a uterine leiomyoma: a diagnostic challenge. Hum Pathol 1997, **28**: 249–251.

822 Cramer SF, Patel A. Myometrial hyperplasia. Proposed criteria for a discrete morphological entity. Mod Pathol 1995, **8**: 71–77.

823 Cramer SF, Newcomb PM, Bonfiglio TA. Myometrial dysplasia (atypical myometrial hyperplasia). Hum Pathol 2007, **38**: 652–655.

824 Cramer SF, Mann L, Calianese E, Daley J, Williamson K. Association of seedling myomas with myometrial hyperplasia. Hum Pathol 2009, **40**: 218–225.

825 Dal Cin P, Christacos N, Morton CC, Quade BJ. Cellular leiomyoma: a genetically distinct entity among benign uterine tumors [abstract]. Mod Pathol 2003, **16**: 187a.

826 Dickersin GR, Selig MK, Park YN. The many faces of smooth muscle neoplasms in a gynecological sampling: an ultrastructural study. Ultrastruct Pathol 1997, **21**: 109–134.

827 Downes KA, Hart WR. Bizarre leiomyomas of the uterus: a comprehensive pathologic study of 24 cases with long-term follow-up. Am J Surg Pathol 1997, **21**: 1261–1270.

828 Esteban JM, Allen WM, Schaerf RH. Benign metastasising leiomyoma of the uterus: histologic and immunohistochemical characterization of primary and metastatic lesions. Arch Pathol Lab Med 1999, **123**: 960–962.

829 Fechner RE. Atypical leiomyomas and synthetic progestin therapy. Am J Clin Pathol 1968, **49**: 697–703.

830 Ferry JA, Harris NL, Scully RE. Uterine leiomyomas with lymphoid infiltration simulating lymphoma. A report of seven cases. Int J Gynecol Pathol 1989, **8**: 263–270.

831 Fornelli A, Pasquinelli G, Eusebi V. Leiomyoma of the uterus showing skeletal muscle differentiation: a case report. Hum Pathol 1999, **30**: 356–359.

832 Fukunaga M, Ushigome S. Dissecting leiomyoma of the uterus with extrauterine extension. Histopathology 1998, **32**: 160–164.

833 Gilks CB, Taylor GP, Clement PB. Inflammatory pseudotumor of the uterus. Int J Gynecol Pathol 1987, **6**: 275–286.

834 Graham A. Malignant epithelial tumors of the thyroid; with special reference to invasion of blood vessels. Surg Gynecol Obstet 1924, **39**: 781–790.

835 Harper RS, Scully RE. Intravenous leiomyomatosis of the uterus. Am J Clin Pathol 1965, **4**: 45–51.

836 Huxley J. Biological aspects of cancer. New York, 1958, Harcourt, Brace, p. 14.

837 Hyde KE, Geisinger KR, Marshall RB, Jones TL. The clear-cell variant of uterine epithelioid leiomyoma. An immunohistologic and ultrastructural study. Arch Pathol Lab Med 1989, **113**: 551–553.

838 Jacobs DS, Cohen H, Johnson JS. Lipoleiomyomas of the uterus. Am J Clin Pathol 1965, **44**: 45–51.

839 Jautzke G, Muller-Ruchholtz E, Thalmann U. Immunohistological detection of estrogen and progesterone receptors in multiple and well differentiated leiomyomatous lung tumors in women with uterine leiomyomas (so-called benign metastasising leiomyomas). A report on 5 cases. Pathol Res Pract 1997, **192**: 215–223.

840 Jordan LB, Al-Nafussi A, Beattie G. Cotyledonoid hydropic intravenous leiomyomatosis: a new variant leiomyoma. Histopathology 2002, **40**: 245–252.

841 Kayser K, Zink S, Schneider T, Dienemann H, Andre S, Kaltner H, Schuring MP, Zick Y, Gabius HJ. Benign metastasising leiomyoma of the uterus: documentation of clinical, immunohistochemical and lectin-histochemical data of ten cases. Virchows Arch 2000, **437**: 284–292.

842 Kurman RJ, Norris HJ. Mesenchymal tumors of the uterus. VI. Epithelioid smooth muscle tumors including leiomyoblastoma and clear-cell leiomyoma. A clinical and pathologic analysis of 26 cases. Cancer 1976, **37**: 1853–1865.

843 Lamb CA, Young RH. Myxoid leiomyomas of the uterus: a report of 14 cases. Lab Invest 2009, **89**(Suppl 1): 223A.

844 Lamb CA, Young RH. Apoplectic change in uterine leiomyomas: an analysis of 70 cases highlighting previously underemphasized aspects. Lab Invest 2009, **89**(Suppl 1): 223A.

845 Lee HJ, Choi J, Kim KR. Pulmonary benign metastasizing leiomyoma associated with intravenous leiomyomatosis of the uterus: clinical behavior and genomic changes supporting a transportation theory. Int J Gynecol Pathol 2008, **27**: 340–345.

846 Lemis PL, Lee ABH, Easler RE. Myometrial hypertrophy. A clinical pathologic study and review of the literature. Am J Obstet Gynecol 1962, **84**: 1032–1041.

847 McCluggage WG, Hamal P, Traub AI, Walsh MY. Uterine adenolipoleimioma: a rare hamartomatous lesion. Int J Gynecol Pathol 2000, **19**: 183–185.

848 McCluggage WG, Boyde A. Uterine angioleiomyomas: a report of 3 cases of a distinctive benign leiomyoma variant. Int J Surg Pathol 2007, **15**: 262–265.

849 McDonald AG, Cin PD, Ganguly A, Campbell S, Imai Y, Rosenberg AE, Oliva E. Liposarcoma arising in uterine lipoleiomyoma: a report of three cases. Lab Invest 2009, **89**(Suppl 1): 228A.

850 Martin-Reay DG, Christ ML, La Pata RE. Uterine leiomyoma with skeletal-muscle differentiation. Report of a case. Am J Clin Pathol 1991, **96**: 344–347.

851 Mazur MT. Clear cell leiomyoma (leiomyoblastoma) of the uterus. Ultrastructural observations. Ultrastruct Pathol 1986, **10**: 249–255.

852 Mazur MT, Kraus FT. Histogenesis of morphologic variations in tumors of the uterine wall. Am J Surg Pathol 1980, **4**: 59–74.

853 Mulvany NJ, Ostör AG, Ross I. Diffuse leiomyomatosis of the uterus. Histopathology 1995, **27**: 175–179.

854 Mulvany NJ, Slavin JL, Ostor AG, Fortune DW. Intravenous leiomyomatosis of the uterus. A clinicopathologic study of 22 cases. Int J Gynecol Pathol 1994, **13**: 1–9.

855 Myles JL, Hart HR. Apoplectic leiomyomas of the uterus. Am J Surg Pathol 1985, **9**: 798–805.

856 Nogales FF, Novano N, Martinez de Victoria JM, Contreras F, Redondo C, Herraiz MA, Seco MA, Velasco A. Uterine intravascular leiomyomatosis. An update and report of seven cases. Int J Gynecol Pathol 1987, **6**: 331–339.

857 Norris HJ, Parmley T. Mesenchymal tumors of the uterus. V. Intravenous leiomyomatosis. A clinical and pathologic study of 14 cases. Cancer 1975, **36**: 2164–2178.

858 Nucci MR, Drapkin R, Dal Cin P, Fletcher CD, Fletcher JA. Distinctive cytogenetic profile in benign metastasizing leiomyoma: pathogenetic implications. Am J Surg Pathol 2007, **31**: 737–743.

859 Patton KT, Cheng L, Papavero V, Blum MG, Yeldandi AV, Adley BP, Luan C, Diaz LK, Hui P, Yang XJ. Benign metastasizing leiomyoma: clonality, telomere length and clinicopathologic analysis. Mod Pathol 2006, **19**: 130–140.

860 O'Connor DM, Norris HJ. Mitotically active leiomyomas of the uterus. Hum Pathol 1990, **21**: 223–227.

861 Oliva E, Young RH, Clement PB, Bhan AK, Scully RE. Cellular benign mesenchymal tumors of the uterus. A comparative morphologic and immunohistochemical analysis of 33 highly cellular leiomyomas and six endometrial stromal nodules, two frequently confused tumors. Am J Surg Pathol 1995, **19**: 769–774.

862 Persaud V, Arjoon PD. Uterine leiomyoma. Incidence of degenerative change and a correlation of associated symptoms. Obstet Gynecol 1970, **35**: 432–436.

863 Pounder DJ. Fatty tumours of the uterus. J Clin Pathol 1982, **35**: 1380–1383.

864 Prakash S, Scully RE. Sarcoma-like pseudopregnancy. Changes in uterine leiomyomas. Report of a case resulting from prolonged norethindrone therapy. Obstet Gynecol 1964, **24**: 106–110.

865 Prayson RA, Hart WR. Mitotically active leiomyomas of the uterus. Am J Clin Pathol 1992, **97**: 14–20.

866 Resta L, Maiorano E, Piscitelli D, Botticella MA. Lipomatous tumors of the uterus. Clinico-pathological features of 10 cases with immunocytochemical study of histogenesis. Pathol Res Pract 1994, **190**: 378–383.

867 Roth LM, Reed RJ. Dissecting leiomyomas of the uterus other than cotyledonoid dissecting leiomyomas: a report of eight cases. Am J Surg Pathol 1999, **23**: 1032–1039.

868 Roth LM, Reed RJ. Cotyledonoid leiomyoma of the uterus: report of a case. Int J Gynecol Pathol 2000, **19**: 272–275.

869 Roth LM, Reed RJ, Sternberg WH. Cotyledonoid dissecting leiomyoma of the uterus: the Sternberg tumor. Am J Surg Pathol 1996, **20**: 1455–1461.

870 Shaco-Levy R, Piura B. Uterine adenolipoleiomyoma: a tumor with potential of aggressive behavior. Int J Gynecol Pathol 2008, **27**: 252–257.

871 Shintaku M. Lipoleiomyomatous tumors of the uterus: a heterogeneous group? Histopathological study of five cases. Pathol Int 1997, **46**: 498–502.

872 Sun X, Mittal K. MIB-1 (Ki-67), estrogen receptor, progesterone receptor, and p53 expression in atypical cells in uterine symplastic leiomyomas. Int J Gynecol Pathol 2009, **29**: 51–54.

873 Tietze L, Gunther K, Horbe A, Pawlik C, Klosterhalfen B, Handt S, Merkelbach-Bruse S. Benign metastasising leiomyoma: a cytogenetically balanced but clonal disease. Hum Pathol 2000, **31**: 126–128.

874 Vang R, Medeiros LJ, Samoszuk M, Deavers MT. Uterine leiomyomas with eosinophils: a clinicopathologic study of 3 cases. Int J Gynecol Pathol 2001, **20**: 239–243.

875 Wang X, Kumar D, Seidman JD. Uterine lipoleiomyomas: a clinicopathologic study of 50 cases. Int J Gynecol Pathol 2006, **25**: 239–242.

876 Watanabe K, Ogura G, Suzuki T. Leiomyoblastoma of the uterus: an immunohistochemical and electron microscopic study of distinctive tumors with immature smooth muscle cell differentiation mimicking fetal uterine myocytes. Histopathology 2001, **42**: 379–386.

LEIOMYOSARCOMA

Clinical and gross features

877 Christopherson WM, Williamson EO, Gray LA. Leiomyosarcoma of the uterus. Cancer 1972, **29**: 70–75.

878 Schwartz SM, Weiss NS, Daling JR, Gammon MD, Liff JM, Watt J, Lynch CF, Newcomb PA, Armstrong BK, Thompson WD. Exogenous sex hormone use, correlates of endogenous hormone levels, and the incidence of histologic types of sarcoma of the uterus. Cancer 1996, **77**: 717–724.

879 Taylor HB, Norris HJ. Mesenchymal tumors of the uterus. IV. Diagnosis and prognosis of leiomyosarcomas. Arch Pathol 1966, **82**: 40–44.

Microscopic features

880 Downes KA, Hart WR. Bizarre leiomyomas of the uterus: a comprehensive pathologic study of 24 cases with long-term follow-up. Am J Surg Pathol 1997, **21**: 1261–1270.

881 Moinfar F, Azodi M, Tavassoli FA. Uterine sarcomas. Pathology 2007, **39**: 55–71.

Electron microscopic, immunohistochemical, and molecular genetic features

882 Dal Cin P. Cytogenetics of mesenchymal tumors of the female genital tract. Surg Pathol Clin 2009, **2**: 813–821.

883 Dickersin GR, Selig MK, Park YN. The many faces of smooth muscle neoplasms in a gynaecological sampling: an ultrastructural study. Ultrastruct Pathol 1997, **21**: 109–134.

884 Iwata J, Fletcher CM. Immunohistochemical detection of cytokeratin and epithelial membrane antigen in leiomyosarcoma: a systematic study of 100 cases. Pathol Int 2000, **50**: 7–14.

885 Lee CH, Ali R, Gilks CB. Molecular genetics of mesenchymal tumors of the female genital tract. Surg Pathol Clin 2009, **2**: 823–834.

886 Loddenkemper C, Mechsner S, Foss H-D, Dallenbach FE, Anagnostopoulos I, Ebert AD, Stein H. Use of oxytocin receptor expression in distinguishing between uterine smooth muscle tumors and endometrial stromal sarcoma. Am J Surg Pathol 2003, **27**: 1458–1462.

887 Marshall RJ, Braye SG. Alpha-1-antitrypsin, alpha-1-antichymotrypsin, actin, and myosin in uterine sarcomas. Int J Gynecol Pathol 1985, **4**: 346–354.

888 Mittal K, Iovine RI. MIB-1 (Ki-67), p53, estrogen receptor, and progesterone receptor expression in uterine smooth muscle tumors. Hum Pathol 2001, **32**: 984–987.

889 Niemann TH, Raab SS, Lenel JC, Rodgers JR, Robinson RA. p53 protein over-expression in smooth muscle tumors of the uterus. Hum Pathol 1995, **26**: 375–379.

890 Poncelet C, Walker F, Modelenat P, Bringuier AF, Scoazec JY, Feldmann G, Darai E. Expression of CD44 standard and isoforms V3 and V6 in uterine smooth muscle tumors: a possible diagnostic tool for the diagnosis of leiomyosarcoma. Hum Pathol 2001, **32**: 1190–1196.

891 Rao UN, Finkelstein SD, Jones MW. Comparative immunohistochemical and molecular analysis of uterine and extrauterine leiomyosarcomas. Mod Pathol 1999, **12**: 1001–1009.

892 Rizeq MN, van de Rijn M, Hendrickson MR, Rouse RV. A comparative immunohisto-chemical study of uterine smooth muscle neoplasms with emphasis on the epithelioid variant. Hum Pathol 1994, **25**: 671–677.

893 Watanabe K, Tajino T, Sekiguchi M, Suzuki T. h-caldesmon as a specific marker for smooth muscle tumors. Comparison with other smooth muscle markers in bone tumors. Am J Clin Pathol 2000, **113**: 663–668.

894 Zhai YL, Kobayashi Y, Mori A, Orii A, Nikaido T, Konishi I, Fujii S. Expression of steroid receptors, Ki-67, and p53 in uterine leiomyosarcoma. Int J Gynecol Pathol 1999, **18**: 20–28.

Leiomyosarcoma variants

895 Buscema J, Carpenter SE, Rosenshein NB, Woodruff JD. Epithelioid leiomyosarcoma of the uterus. Cancer 1986, **7**: 1192–1196.

896 Coard KC, Fletcher HM. Leiomyosarcoma of the uterus with a florid intravascular component ('intravenous leiomyosarcomatosis'). Int J Gynecol Pathol 2002, **21**: 182–185.

897 King E, Dickersin GR, Scully RE. Myxoid leiomyosarcoma of the uterus. Am J Surg Pathol 1982, **6**: 589–598.

898 Kurman RJ, Norris HJ. Mesenchymal tumors of the uterus. VI. Epithelioid smooth muscle tumors including leiomyoblastoma and clear cell leiomyoma. A clinical and pathologic analysis of 26 cases. Cancer 1976, **37**: 1853–1865.

899 Pounder DJ, Iyer PV. Uterine leiomyosarcoma with myxoid stroma. Arch Pathol Lab Med 1985, **109**: 762–764.

900 Prayson RA, Goldblum JR, Hart WR. Epithelioid smooth-muscle tumors of the uterus: a clinicopathologic study of 18 patients. Am J Surg Pathol 1997, **21**: 383–391.

901 Seidman JD, Yetter RA, Papadimitriou JC. Epithelioid component of uterine leiomyosarcoma simulating metastatic carcinoma. Arch Pathol Lab Med 1992, **116**: 287–290.

902 Shintaku M, Sekiyama K. Leiomyosarcoma of the uterus with focal rhabdomyosarcomatous differentiation. Int J Gynecol Pathol 2004, **23**: 188–192.

903 Watanabe K, Hiraki H, Ohishi M, Mashiko K, Saginoya H, Suzuki T. Uterine leiomyosarcoma with osteoclast-like giant cells. Histopathological and cytological observations. Pathol Int 1997, **46**: 656–660.

Spread, metastases, treatment, and prognosis

904 Abeler VM, Røyne O, Thoresen S, Danielsen HE, Nesland JM, Kristensen GB. Uterine sarcomas in Norway. A histopathological and prognostic survey of a total population from 1970 to 2000 including 419 patients. Histopathology 2009, **54**: 355–364.

905 Bartsich EG, Bowe ET, Moore JG. Leiomyosarcoma of the uterus. A 50-year review of 42 cases. Obstet Gynecol 1968, **32**: 101–106.

906 Jeffers MD, Oakes SJ, Richmond JA, Macauley EM. Proliferation, ploidy and prognosis in uterine smooth muscle tumours. Histopathology 1997, **29**: 217–223.

907 Lucas DR, Kolodziej P, Gross ML, Mott MP, Budev H, Zalupski MM, Ryan JR. Metastatic uterine leiomyosarcoma to bone: a clinicopathologic study. Int J Surg Pathol 1997, **4**: 159–168.

908 Pautier P, Genestie C, Rey A, Morice P, Roche B, Lhommé C, Haie-Meder C, Duvillard P. Analysis of clinicopathologic prognostic factors for 157 uterine sarcomas and evaluation of a grading score validated for soft tissue sarcoma. Cancer 2000, **88**: 1425–1431.

909 Salazar OM, Bonfiglio TA, Patten SF, Keller BE, Feldstein M, Dunne ME, Rudolph J. Uterine sarcomas. Natural history, treatment and prognosis. Cancer 1978, **42**: 1152–1160.

910 Tsushima K, Stanhope CR, Gaffey TA, Lieber MM. Uterine leiomyosarcomas and benign smooth muscle tumors. Usefulness of nuclear DNA patterns studied by flow cytometry. Mayo Clin Proc 1988, **63**: 248–255.

RELATIONSHIP BETWEEN MORPHOLOGY AND BEHAVIOR OF UTERINE SMOOTH MUSCLE TUMORS

911 Atkins KA, Arronte N, Darus CJ, Rice LW. The use of p16 in enhancing the histologic classification of uterine smooth muscle tumors. Am J Surg Pathol 2008, **32**: 98–102.

912 Bell SW, Kempson RL, Hendrickson MR. Problematic uterine smooth muscle neoplasms. A clinicopathologic study of 213 cases. Am J Surg Pathol 1994, **18**: 535–558.

913 Donhuijsen K. Mitosis counts. Reproducibility and significance in grading of malignancy. Hum Pathol 1986, **17**: 1122–1125.

914 Editorials. Mitosis counting – I. (Scully RE et al) Mitosis counting – II. (Kempson RL) Mitosis counting – III. (Norris HJ). Hum Pathol 1976, **7**: 481–484.

915 Evason KJ, Rabban JT. The mitosis marker anti-phosphohistone h3 (phh3) distinguishers bizarre leiomyoma from leiomyosarcoma and predicts behavior in uterine smooth muscle tumors. Lab Invest 2009, **89**(Suppl 1): 213A.

916 Hart WR. Problematic uterine smooth muscle neoplasms. Am J Surg Pathol 1997, **21**: 252–255.

917 Ip PP, Cheung AN, Clement PB. Uterine smooth muscle tumors of uncertain malignant potential (STUMP): a clinicopathologic analysis of 16 cases. Am J Surg Pathol 2009, **33**: 992–1005.

918 Kempson RL, Bari W. Uterine sarcomas. Classification, diagnosis, and prognosis. Hum Pathol 1970, **1**: 331–349.

919 Kempson RL, Hendrickson MR. Smooth muscle, endometrial stromal, and mixed Mullerian tumors of the uterus. Mod Pathol 2000, **13**: 328–342.

920 Layfield LJ, Liu K, Dodge R, Barsky SH. Uterine smooth muscle tumors: utility of classification by proliferation, ploidy, and prognostic markers versus traditional histopathology. Arch Pathol Lab Med 2000, **124**: 221–227.

921 Lee CH, Turbin DA, Sung YC, Espinosa I, Montgomery K, van de Rijn M, Gilks CB. A panel of antibodies to determine site of origin and malignancy in smooth muscle tumors. Mod Pathol 2009, **22**: 1519–1531.

922 Lee CH, Sung V, Montgomery K, van de Rijn M, Gilks CB. Immunohistochemical profiling of 312 gynecologic and soft tissue smooth muscle tumors. Lab Invest 2009, **89**(Suppl 1): 223A–224A.

923 Longacre TA, Hendrickson MR, Kempson RL. Predicting clinical outcome for uterine smooth muscle neoplasms with a reasonable degree of certainty. Adv Anat Pathol 1997, **4**: 95–104.

924 Majno G, Joris I. Apoptosis, oncosis, and necrosis. Am J Pathol 1995, **146**: 3–15.

925 O'Neill CJ, McBride HA, Connolly LE, McCluggage WG. Uterine leiomyosarcomas are characterized by high p16, p53 and MIB1 expression in comparison with usual leiomyomas, leiomyoma variants and smooth muscle tumours of uncertain malignant potential. Histopathology 2007, **50**: 851–858.

926 Poncelet C, Walker F, Modelenat P, Bringuier AF, Scoazec JY, Feldman G, Darai E. Expression of CD44 standard and isoforms V3 and V6 in uterine smooth muscle tumors: a possible diagnostic tool for the diagnosis of leiomyosarcoma. Hum Pathol 2001, **32**: 1190–1196.

927 Quade BJ, Pinto AP, Howard DR, Petters III WA, Crum CP. Frequent loss of heterozygosity for chromosome 10 in uterine leiomyosarcoma in contrast to leiomyoma. Am J Pathol 1999, **154**: 945–950.

928 Schwarz G, Remmelink M, Decaestecker C, Gielen I, Budel V, Burchert M, Darro F, Danguy A, Gabius HJ, Salmon I, Kiss R. Galectin fingerprinting in tumor diagnosis. Differential expression of galectin-3 and galectin-3 binding sites, but not galectin-1, in benign vs malignant uterine smooth muscle tumors. Am J Clin Pathol 1999, **111**: 623–631.

929 Silverberg SG. Reproducibility of the mitosis count in the histologic diagnosis of smooth muscle tumors of the uterus. Hum Pathol 1976, **7**: 451–454.

930 Thunnissen FBJM, Ambergen AW, Koss M, Travis WD, O'Leary TJ, Ellis IO. Mitotic counting in surgical pathology: sampling bias, heterogeneity and statistical uncertainty. Histopathology 2001, **39**: 1–8.

931 Toledo G, Oliva E. Smooth muscle tumors of the uterus: a practical approach. Arch Pathol Lab Med 2008, **132**: 595–605.

932 Trzyna W, McHugh M, McCue P, McHugh KM. Molecular determination of the malignant potential of smooth muscle neoplasms. Cancer 1997, **80**: 211–217.

933 van Diest PJ, Baak JP, Matze-Cok P, Wisse-Brekelmans EC, van Galen CM, Kurver PH, Bellot SM, Fijnheer J, van Gorp LH, Kwee WS, et al. Reproducibility of mitosis counting in 2,469 breast cancer specimens; results from the Multicenter Morphometric Mammary Carcinoma Project. Hum Pathol 1992, **23**: 603–607.

934 Wilkinson N, Rollason TP. Recent advances in the pathology of smooth muscle tumors of the uterus. Histopathology 2001, **39**: 331–341.

935 Zhai YL, Kobayashi Y, Mori A, Orii A, Nikaido T, Konishi I, Fujii S. Expression of steroid receptors, Ki-67, and p53 in uterine leiomyosarcoma. Int J Gynecol Pathol 1999, **18**: 20–28.

SMOOTH MUSCLE TUMORS AND PECOMAS

936 Bosincu L, Rocca PC, Martignoni G, Nogales FF, Longa L, Maccioni A, Massarelli G. Perivascular epithelioid cell (PEC) tumors of the uterus: a clinicopathologic study of two cases with aggressive features. Mod Pathol 2005, **18**: 1336–1342.

937 Carvalho FM, Carvalho JP, Maluf FC, Bacchi CE. A new morphological variant of uterine PEComas with sex-cord-like pattern and *WT1* expression: more doubts about the existence of uterine PEComas. Ann Diagn Pathol 2010, **14**: 129–132.

938 Folpe AL, Mentzel T, Lehr HA, Fisher C, Balzer BL, Weiss SW. Perivascular epithelioid cell neoplasms of soft tissue and gynecologic origin: a clinicopathologic study of 26 cases and review of the literature. Am J Surg Pathol 2005, **29**: 1558–1575.

939 Gyure KA, Hart WR, Kennedy AW. Lymphangiomyomatosis of the uterus associated with tuberous sclerosis and malignant neoplasia of the female genital tract. A report of two cases. Int J Gynecol Pathol 1995, **14**: 344–351.

940 Hurrell DP, McCluggage WG. Uterine leiomyosarcoma with HMB45+ clear cell areas: report of two cases. Histopathology 2005, **47**: 540–542.

941 Jameson CF. Angiomyoma of the uterus in a patient with tuberous sclerosis. Histopathology 1990, **16**: 202–203.

942 Liang SX, Pearl M, Liu J, Hwang S, Tornos C. 'Malignant' uterine perivascular epithelioid cell tumor, pelvic lymph node lymphangioleiomyomatosis, and gynecological pecomatosis in a patient with tuberous sclerosis: a case report and review of the literature. Int J Gynecol Pathol 2008, **27**: 86–90.

943 Michal M, Zamecnik M. Hyalinized uterine mesenchymal neoplasms with HMB-45-positive epithelioid cells: epithelioid leiomyomas or angiomyolipomas? Report of four cases. Int J Surg Pathol 2000, **8**: 323–328.

944 Ruco LP, Pilozzi E, Wedard BM, Marzullo A, D'Andrea V, de Antoni E, Silvestrini G, Bonetti F. Epithelioid lymphangioleiomyomatosis-like tumour of the uterus in a patient without tuberous sclerosis: a lesion mimicking epithelioid leiomyosarcoma. Histopathology 1998, **33**: 91–93.

945 Silva EG, Deavers MT, Bodurka DC, Malpica A. Uterine epithelioid leiomyosarcomas with clear cells: reactivity with HMB-45 and the concept of PEComa. Am J Surg Pathol 2004, **28**: 244–249.

946 Simpson KW, Albores-Saavedra J. HMB-45 reactivity in conventional uterine leiomyosarcomas. Am J Surg Pathol 2007, **31**: 95–98.

947 Vang R, Kempson RL. Perivascular epithelioid cell tumor ('PE Coma') of the uterus: a subset of HMB-45 positive epithelioid mesenchymal neoplasms with an uncertain relationship to pure smooth muscle tumors. Am J Surg Pathol 2001, **26**: 1–13.

948 Yavuz E, Cakr C, Tuzlal S, Ahskal B, Topuz S, Ilhan R. Uterine perivascular epithelioid cell tumor coexisting with pulmonary lymphangioleiomyomatosis and renal angiomyolipoma: a case report. Appl Immunohistochem Mol Morphol 2008, **16**: 405–409.

OTHER TUMORS AND TUMORLIKE CONDITIONS

949 Al-Hussaini M, Hirschowitz L, McCluggage WG. Uterine neoplasms composed of rhabdoid cells do not exhibit loss of INI1 immunoreactivity and are not related to childhood malignant rhabdoid tumor. Int J Gynecol Pathol 2008, **27**: 236–242.

950 Angeles-Angeles A, Gutierrez-Villalobos LG, Lome-Maldonado C, Jimenez-Moreno A. Polypoid brenner tumor of the uterus. Int J Gynecol Pathol 2002, **21**: 86–87.

951 Aozasa K, Saeki K, Ohsawa M, Horiuchi K, Mishima K, Tsujimoto M. Malignant lymphoma of the uterus. Report of seven cases with immunohistochemical study. Cancer 1993, **72**: 1959–1964.

952 Arhelger RB, Bocian JJ. Brenner tumor of the uterus. Cancer 1976, **38**: 1741–1743.

953 Cardinale L, Mirra M, Galli C, Goldblum JR, Pizzolitto S, Falconieri G. Angiosarcoma of the uterus: report of 2 new cases with deviant clinicopathologic features and review of the literature. Ann Diagn Pathol 2008, **12**: 217–221.

954 Chan JKC, Fong MH. Composite multicystic mesothelioma and adenomatoid tumour of the uterus: different morphological manifestations of the same process? Histopathology 1997, **29**: 375–377.

955 Chetty R, Clark SP, Bhathal PS. Carcinoid tumor of the uterine corpus. Virchows Arch A Pathol Anat Histopathol 1993, **422**: 93–95.

956 Chou S-T, Fortune D, Beischer NA, McLeish G, Castles LA, McKelvie BA, Planner RS. Primary malignant fibrous histiocytoma of the uterus – ultrastructural and immunocytochemical studies of two cases. Pathology 1985, **17**: 36–40.

957 Clement PB. Chondrosarcoma of the uterus. Report of a case and review of the literature. Hum Pathol 1978, **9**: 726–732.

958 Clement PB. Postoperative spindle-cell nodule of the endometrium. Arch Pathol Lab Med 1988, **112**: 566–568.

959 Davey DD, Munn R, Smith LW, Cibull ML. Angiotropic lymphoma. Presentation in uterine vessels with cytogenetic studies. Arch Pathol Lab Med 1990, **114**: 879–882.

960 Daya D, Lukka H, Clement PB. Primitive neuroectodermal tumors of the uterus. A report of four cases. Hum Pathol 1992, **23**: 1120–1129.

961 de A Focchi GR, Cuatrecasas M, Prat J. Malignant peripheral nerve sheath tumor of the uterine corpus: a case report. Int J Gynecol Pathol 2007, **26**: 437–440.

962 den Bakker MA, Hegt VN, Sleddens HB, Nuijten AS, Dinjens WN. Malignant mesenchymona of the uterus, arising in a leiomyoma. Histopathology 2002, **40**: 65–70.

963 De Young B, Bitterman P, Lack EE. Primary osteosarcoma of the uterus. Report of a case with immunohistochemical study. Mod Pathol 1992, **5**: 212–215.

964 Di Tommaso L, Rahal D, Bresciani G, Roncalli M. Cutaneous melanoma metastatic to uterine adenomyoma: report of a case. Int J Surg Pathol 2005, **13**: 223–225.

965 Donner LR. Uterine carcinosarcoma with complete sarcomatous overgrowth mimicking pure embryonal rhabdomyosarcoma. Int J Gynecol Pathol 2002, **22**: 89–91.

966 Euscher ED, Deavers MT, Lopez-Terrada D, Lazar AJ, Silva EG, Malpica A. Uterine tumors with neuroectodermal differentiation: a series of 17 cases and review of the literature. Am J Surg Pathol 2008, **32**: 219–228.

967 Fadare O, Bonvicino A, Martel M, Renshaw IL, Azodi M, Parkash V. Pleomorphic rhabdomyosarcoma of the uterine corpus: a clinicopathologic study of 4 cases and a review of the literature. Int J Gynecol Pathol 2010, **29**: 122–134.

968 Ferguson SE, Gerald W, Barakat RR, Chi DS, Soslow RA. Clinicopathologic features of rhabdomyosarcoma of gynecologic origin in adults. Am J Surg Pathol 2007, **31**: 382–389.

969 Ferry JA, Young RH. Malignant lymphoma, pseudolymphoma, and hematopoietic disorders of the female genital tract. Pathol Annu 1991, **26**: 227–263.

970 Ferry JA, Young RH. Malignant lymphoma of the genitourinary tract. Curr Diagn Pathol 1997, **4**: 145–169.

971 Fraggetta F, Magro G, Vasquez E. Primitive neuroectodermal tumor of the uterus with focal cartilaginous differentiation. Histopathology 1997, **30**: 483–485.

972 Garcia MG, Deavers MT, Knoblock RJ, Chen W, Tsimberidou AM, Manning JT Jr, Medeiros LJ. Myeloid sarcoma involving the gynecologic tract: a report of 11 cases and review of the literature. Am J Clin Pathol 2006, **125**: 783–790.

973 García-Galvis OF, Stolnicu S, Muñoz E, Aneiros-Fernández J, Alaggio R, Nogales FF. Adult extrarenal Wilms tumor of the uterus with teratoid features. Hum Pathol 2009, **40**: 418–424.

974 Geyer JT, Ferry JA, Harris NL, Young RH, Longtine JA, Zukerberg LR. Florid reactive lymphoid hyperplasia of the lower female genital tract (lymphoma-like lesion): a benign condition that frequently harbors clonal immunoglobulin heavy chain gene rearrangements. Am J Surg Pathol 2010, **34**: 161–168.

975 Gilks CB, Taylor GP, Clement PB. Inflammatory pseudotumor of the uterus. Int J Gynecol Pathol 1987, **6**: 275–286.

976 Gray GF, Glick AD, Kurtin PJ, Jones HW III. Alveolar soft part sarcoma of the uterus. Hum Pathol 1986, **17**: 297–300.

977 Gru AA, Hassan A, Pfeifer JD, Huettner PC. Uterine extramedullary hematopoiesis: what is the clinical significance? Int J Gynecol Pathol 2010, **29**: 366–373.

978 Harris NL, Scully RE. Malignant lymphoma and granulocytic sarcoma of the uterus and vagina. Cancer 1984, **53**: 2530–2545.

979 Heeren JH, Croonen AM, Pijnenborg JM. Primary extranodal marginal zone B-cell lymphoma of the female genital tract: a case report and literature review. Int J Gynecol Pathol 2008, **27**: 243–246.

980 Hendrickson MR, Scheithauer BW. Primitive neuroectodermal tumor of the endometrium. Report of two cases, one with electron microscopic observations. Int J Gynecol Pathol 1986, **5**: 249–259.

981 Houghton JP, Ioffe OB, Silverberg SG, McGrady B, McCluggage WG. Metastatic breast lobular carcinoma involving tamoxifen-associated endometrial polyps: report of two cases and review of tamoxifen-associated polypoid uterine lesions. Mod Pathol 2003, **16**: 395–398.

982 Hung LHY, Kurtz DM. Hodgkin's disease of the endometrium. Arch Pathol Lab Med 1985, **109**: 952–953.

983 Johnson C, Reid-Nicholson M, Deligdisch L, Grinblat S, Natarajan S. Capillary hemangioma of the endometrium: a case report and review of the literature. Arch Pathol Lab Med 2005, **129**: 1326–1329.

984 Jordan CD, Andrews SJ, Memoli VA. Well-differentiated pulmonary neuroendocrine carcinoma metastatic to the endometrium: a case report. Mod Pathol 1997, **9**: 1066–1070.

985 Joseph MG, Fellows FG, Hearn SA. Primary endodermal sinus tumor of the endometrium. A clinicopathologic, immunocytochemical, and ultrastructural study. Cancer 1990, **65**: 297–302.

986 Kelly P, McCluggage WG. Idiopathic uterine granulomas: report of a series with morphological similarities to idiopathic ovarian cortical granulomas. Int J Gynecol Pathol 2006, **25**: 243–246.

987 Kosari F, Daneshbod Y, Parwaresch R, Krams M, Wacker HH. Lymphomas of the female genital tract: a study of 186 cases and review of the literature. Am J Surg Pathol 2005, **29**: 1512–1520.

988 Kumar NB, Hart WR. Metastases to the uterine corpus from extragenital cancers. Cancer 1982, **50**: 2163–2169.

989 Lagoo AS, Robboy SJ. Lymphoma of the female genital tract: current status. Int J Gynecol Pathol 2006, **25**: 1–21.

990 Liggins GC. Uterine arteriovenous fistula. Obstet Gynecol 1964, **23**: 214–217.

991 McAlhany SJ, Rabban JT. Expression of D2-40, a marker of mesothelial and lymphatic endothelial differentiation, in adenomatoid tumors: a potential diagnostic pitfall in distinguishing from lymphatic tumors. Lab Invest 2009, **89**(Suppl 1): 227A.

992 McCluggage WG, Young RH. Myxoid change of the myometrium and cervical stroma: description of a hitherto unreported non-neoplastic phenomenon with discussion of myxoid uterine lesions. Int J Gynecol Pathol 2010, **29**: 351–357.

993 Masunaga A, Abe M, Tsuji E, Suzuki U, Ohgida T, Toyama M, Nakamura H, Mori S, Sugawara I, Itoyama S. Primary uterine T-cell lymphoma. Int J Gynecol Pathol 1998, **17**: 376–379.

994 Mazur MT, Hsueh S, Gersell DJ. Metastases to the female genital tract. Cancer 1984, **53**: 1978–1984.

995 Milne DS, Hinshaw K, Malcolm AJ, Hilton P. Primary angiosarcoma of the uterus. A case report. Histopathology 1994, **16**: 203–205.

996 Moore WF, Bentley RC, Kim KR, Olatidoye B, Gray SR, Robboy SJ. Goblet-cell mucinous epithelium lining the endometrium and endocervix: evidence of a metastasis from an appendiceal primary tumor through the use of cytokeratin-7 and -20 immunostains. Int J Gynecol Pathol 1998, **17**: 363–367.

997 Morrel B, Mulder AF, Chadha S, Tjokrowardojo AJ, Wijnen JA. Angiosarcoma of the uterus following radiotherapy for squamous cell carcinoma of the cervix. Eur J Obstet Gynecol Reprod Biol 1993, **49**: 193–197.

998 Muc RS, Grayson W, Grobbelaar JJ. Adult extrarenal Wilms tumor occurring in the uterus. Arch Pathol Lab Med 2001, **125**: 1081–1083.

999 Nogales FF, Isaac A, Hardisson D, Bosincu L, Palacios J, Ordi J, Mendoza E, Manzarbetia F, Olivera H, O'Valle F, Krasevic M, Marquez M. Adenomatoid tumors of the uterus: an analysis of 60 cases. Int J Gynecol Pathol 2002, **21**: 34–40.

1000 Oliva E, Ferry JA, Young RH, Prat J, Srigley JR, Scully RE. Granulocytic sarcoma of the female genital tract: a clinicopathologic study of 11 cases. Am J Surg Pathol 1997, **21**: 1156–1165.

1001 Ordi J, Stamatakos MD, Tavassoli FA. Pure pleomorphic rhabdomyosarcomas of the uterus. Int J Gynecol Pathol 1998, **16**: 369–377.

1002 Otis CN. Uterine adenomatoid tumors: immunohistochemical characteristics with emphasis on Ber-EP4 immunoreactivity and distinction from adenocarcinoma. Int J Gynecol Pathol 1996, **15**: 146–151.

1003 Palacios J, Suarez Manrique A, Ruiz Villaespesa A, Burgos Lizaldez E, Gamallo Amat C. Cystic adenomatoid tumor of the uterus. Int J Gynecol Pathol 1991, **10**: 296–301.

1004 Podczaski E, Sees J, Kaminski P, Sorosky J, Larson JE, De Geest K, Zaino RJ, Mortel R. Rhabdomyosarcoma of the uterus in a postmenopausal patient. Gynecol Oncol 1990, **37**: 439–442.

1005 Pounder DJ. Fatty tumours of the uterus. J Clin Pathol 1982, **35**: 1380–1383.

1006 Quigley JC, Hart WR. Adenomatoid tumors of the uterus. Am J Clin Pathol 1981, **76**: 627–635.

1007 Rabban JT, Zaloudek CJ, Shekitka KM, Tavassoli FA. Inflammatory myofibroblastic tumor of the uterus: a clinicopathologic study of 6 cases emphasizing distinction from aggressive mesenchymal tumors. Am J Surg Pathol 2005, **29**: 1348–1355.

1008 Resta L, Maiorano E, Piscitelli D, Botticella MA. Lipomatous tumors of the uterus. Clinico-pathological features of 10 cases with immunocytochemical study of histogenesis. Pathol Res Pract 1994, **190**: 378–383.

1009 Rittenbach J, Cao JD, Weiss LM, Rowsell EH, Chick W, Wang J. Primary diffuse large B-cell lymphoma of the uterus presenting solely as an endometrial polyp. Int J Gynecol Pathol 2005, **24**: 347–351.

1010 Sangoi AR, McKenney JK, Schwartz EJ, Rouse RV, Longacre TA. Adenomatoid tumors of the female and male genital tracts: a clinicopathological and immunohistochemical study of 44 cases. Mod Pathol 2009, **22**: 1228–1235.

1011 Schammel DP, Tavassoli FA. Uterine angiosarcomas: a morphologic and immunohistochemcial study of four cases. Am J Surg Pathol 1998, **22**: 246–250.

1012 Shintaku M, Sasaki M, Honda T. Thrombomodulin immunoreactivity in adenomatoid tumour of the uterus. Histopathology 1997, **28**: 375–377.

1013 Sirgi KE, Swanson PE, Gersell DJ. Extramedullary hematopoiesis in the endometrium. Report of four cases and review of the literature. Am J Clin Pathol 1994, **101**: 643–646.

1014 Smith NL, Baird DB, Strausbauch PH. Endometrial involvement by multiple myeloma. Int J Gynecol Pathol 1997, **16**: 173–175.

1015 Stemmermann GN. Extrapelvic carcinoma metastatic to the uterus. Am J Obstet Gynecol 1961, **82**: 1261–1266.

1016 Stephenson TJ, Mill PM. Adenomatoid tumours. An immunohistochemical and ultrastructural appraisal of their histogenesis. J Pathol 1986, **148**: 327–335.

1017 Sur M, Ross C, Moens F, Daya D. Intravascular large B-cell lymphoma of the uterus: a diagnostic challenge. Int J Gynecol Pathol 2005, **24**: 201–203.

1018 Suzuki T, Yoshida Y, Kaku T, Kikuchi K, Mori M. Adenomatoid tumor of the uterus. Ultrastructural, histochemical, and immunohistochemical analysis. Arch Pathol Lab Med 1985, **109**: 1049–1051.

1019 Tallini G, Price FV, Carcangiu ML. Epithelioid angiosarcoma arising in uterine leiomyomas. Am J Clin Pathol 1993, **100**: 514–518.

1020 Tavassoli FA. Melanotic paraganglioma of the uterus. Cancer 1986, **58**: 942–948.

1021 Taxy JB, Trujillo YP. Breast cancer metastatic to the uterus. Clinical manifestations of a rare event. Arch Pathol Lab Med 1994, **118**: 819–821.

1022 Terada T. Gastrointestinal stromal tumor of the uterus: a case report with genetic analyses of c-kit and PDGFRA genes. Int J Gynecol Pathol 2009, **28**: 29–34.

1023 Thaung C, Shanks J, Eyden B, Fitzmaurice R. Solitary fibrous tumour of the uterus. Histopathology 2006, **49**: 199–201.

1024 Tiltman AJ. Adenomatoid tumours of the uterus. Histopathology 1980, **4**: 437–443.

1025 van de Rijn M, Kamel OW, Chang PP, Lee A, Warnke RA, Salhany KE. Primary low-grade endometrial B-cell lymphoma. Am J Surg Pathol 1997, **21**: 187–194.

1026 Vang R, Medeiros LJ, Ha CS, Deavers S. Non-Hodgkin's lymphoma involving the uterus: a clinicopathologic analysis of 26 cases. Mod Pathol 2000, **13**: 19–28.

1027 Varghese L, Arnesen M, Boente M. Primitive neuroectodermal tumor of the uterus: a case report and review of literature. Int J Gynecol Pathol 2006, **25**: 373–377.

1028 Wakami K, Tateyama H, Kawashima H, Matsuno T, Kamiya Y, Jin-No Y, Kimura G, Eimoto T. Solitary fibrous tumor of the uterus producing high-molecular-weight insulin-like growth factor II and associated with hypoglycemia. Int J Gynecol Pathol 2005, **24**: 79–84.

1029 Young RH, Harris NL, Scully RE. Lymphoma-like lesions of the lower female genital tract. A report of 16 cases. Int J Gynecol Pathol 1985, **4**: 289–299.

1030 Young RH, Kleinman GM, Scully RE. Glioma of the uterus. Am J Surg Pathol 1981, **5**: 695–699.

1031 Young TW, Thrasher TV. Nonchromaffin paraganglioma of the uterus. Arch Pathol Lab Med 1982, **106**: 608–609.

Fallopian tube (including broad and round ligaments)

CHAPTER CONTENTS

Normal anatomy

The **fallopian tube** or salpinx is a tubular hollow structure measuring 11–12 cm in length that runs throughout the apex of the broad ligament and spans the distance between the uterine cornus and the ovary. It is divided into four segments: *intramural* (inside the uterine wall), *isthmus* (2–3 cm, thick-walled), *ampulla* (a thin-walled expanded area), and *infundibulum* (a trumpet-shaped ending that opens into the peritoneal cavity through the ostium and is fringed by the *fimbriae*). One of the latter structures, known as the *ovarian fimbria*, attaches the tube to the ovary.

The inner aspect of the tube is lined by mucosa arranged in the shape of longitudinal, branching folds (known as *plicae*), which merge with the fimbriae. There is good correlation between the microscopic features of this mucosa and its salpingoscopic appearance.[4] Microscopically, the epithelium is composed of three distinct cell types: *secretory*, *ciliated*, and *intercalated* (*peg*).[3] Amylase is secreted by the epithelium, and its presence can be demonstrated immunohistochemically.[1] The tubal epithelium also expresses the follicle-stimulating hormone (FSH) receptor, similarly to the surface epithelium of the ovary.[8] Endocrine cells have been found only exceptionally. A low degree of proliferative activity takes place normally in the tubal epithelium, apparently not synchronized with the menstrual cycle. At the time of menstruation, as well as a few days postpartum, the tubal mucosa may be normally infiltrated by neutrophils, probably as a reaction to blood and necrotic debris (*'physiologic salpingitis'*). It is accompanied by negative cultures and should not be confused with a bacterial or other infectious salpingitis.[6,7]

The muscular wall (*myosalpinx*) is composed of an inner circular layer and an outer longitudinal layer; the isthmus near the uterotubal junction also possesses an inner longitudinal layer.

The lymphatics of the fallopian tube leave the tubal wall within the mesosalpinx, where they join efferent lymphatics from the ovary and uterus and follow the ovarian vessels to terminate in the aortic lymph nodes. Other lymphatics course within the broad ligament and drain into the interiliac nodes; a separate lymphatic channel from the ampulla of the tube follows the broad ligament to terminate in the superior gluteal lymph nodes.

The **broad ligament** is the peritoneal fold that supports the uterus on either side, extending from this organ to the pelvic wall. It comprises the mesovarium, mesometrium, and mesosalpinx. The broad ligament and the adjacent areas contain a variety of tubular structures related to the müllerian and wolffian systems that may give rise to grossly evident cysts.[5] Most of these are lined by müllerian-type epithelium and have been variously referred to – depending on their specific location and presumed histogenesis – as *parovarian cyst, paratubal cyst* (*hydatid of Morgagni*), *subserosal müllerian cyst, Kobelt cyst* (*appendix vesiculosa*), *paroöphoron cyst, epoöphoron cyst*, and *rete ovarii cyst*[2] (see p. 1559). *Walthard cell nests*, which can also be cystic, are of a different (probably mesothelial) nature; they are discussed on page 1554.

The **round ligament** is a fibrous cord attached to the superior lateral border of the uterus that passes over the external iliac vessels and the inguinal ligament to leave the abdominal cavity through the deep inguinal ring. From there, it follows the inguinal canal to anchor itself in the labium majus. It serves to orient the uterus by the fact that its insertion is *anterior* to that of the fallopian tube.

Inflammation

Bacterial infection of the fallopian tube is a common disease, and its incidence keeps increasing. It may follow invasive procedures (such as curettage or the insertion of intrauterine devices[10]), and it commonly accompanies endometriosis,[29] but in most cases it is due to an ascending infection, often sexually transmitted[31] (Fig. 19.190). The inflammation may result in fusion of tubal plicae and obliteration of the ostium (Fig. 19.191A). Obstruction of the fimbriated end and, less commonly, of the intramural or isthmic portion leads to infertility.[16] Microscopically, the trapped epithelial spaces produce a complicated gland-like pattern that can simulate malignancy[11] (Fig. 19.191B).

The lumen is often distended and filled with secretions or pus (**pyosalpinx**) (Fig. 19.192). Massive intraluminal hemorrhage may lead to the formation of **hematosalpinx**, a rare condition that needs to be distinguished from the much more common form secondary

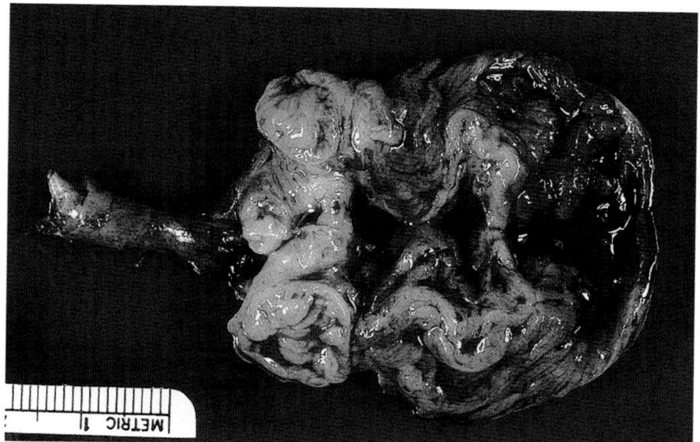

Fig. 19.190 Gross appearance of chronic salpingitis with superimposed acute changes.

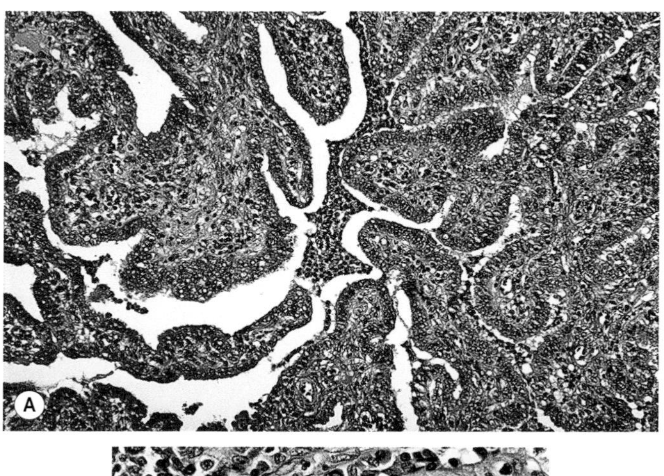

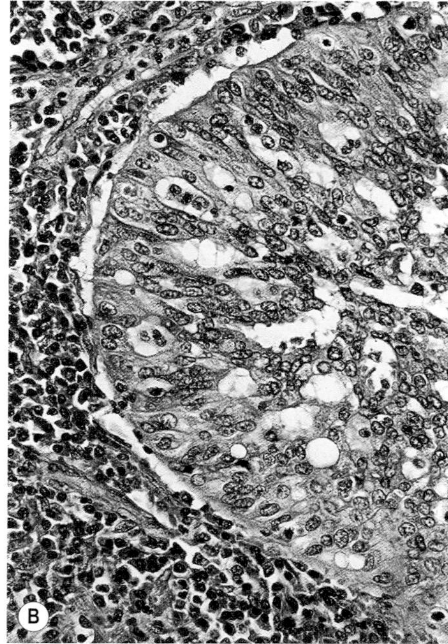

Fig. 19.191 Chronic salpingitis: **A**, blunting of villi due to heavy inflammatory infiltrate; **B**, marked secondary reactive hyperplasia of the mucosa, which may simulate a malignant process.

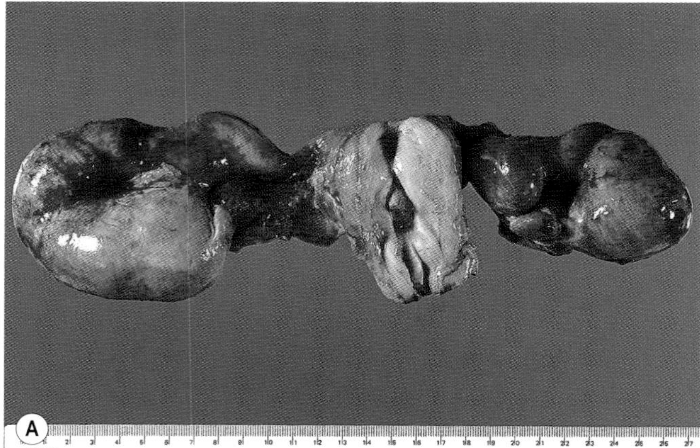

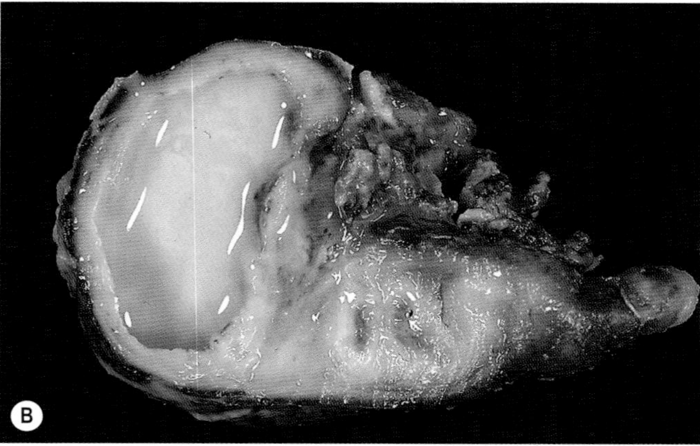

Fig. 19.192 **A** and **B**, Outer aspect and cut surface of pyosalpinx. (*A, Courtesy of Dr RA Cooke, Brisbane, Australia; from Cooke RA, Stewart B. Colour atlas of anatomical pathology. Edinburgh, 2004, Churchill Livingstone; B, Courtesy of Dr Pedro J Grases Galofrè; from Grases Galofrè PJ. Patologia ginecològica. Bases para el diagnòstico morfològico. Barcelona, 2002, Masson*)

to ruptured tubal pregnancy. In chronic inflammatory cases, the tubal wall is markedly fibrotic, and serosal adhesions are prominent. The inflammatory exudate often spreads to the ovary, resulting in the formation of a **tubo-ovarian abscess** and obliteration of the pelvic anatomic relationships (Fig. 19.193). The rupture of such an abscess may lead to localized or generalized peritonitis and requires prompt surgical intervention.[23,27] **Hydrosalpinx** is generally regarded as the end stage of a purulent salpingitis in which pus has been reabsorbed and replaced by a transudate of plasma.[12] The external gross appearance has been likened to that of a retort (Fig. 19.194). Exceptionally, the involvement is limited to the intramural portion of the tube. The wall is thin and fibrotic, with atrophy or even disappearance of the smooth muscle wall. The epithelium is flat and focally absent.

Pelvic inflammatory disease (PID) is the generic term used for inflammatory processes of this region in which the fallopian tube is the epicenter and presumably the source of the inflammation.[22,26,33] Eschenbach et al.[15] recovered *Neisseria gonorrhoeae* from 91 of 204 cases of acute PID in patients with cervical gonococcal infections. Chlamydial infection is also common, accounting for over 20% and perhaps as many as half of the cases.[32,34] This etiology should be suspected in cases of chronic salpingitis accompanied by marked lymphofollicular hyperplasia.[32] Polymicrobial

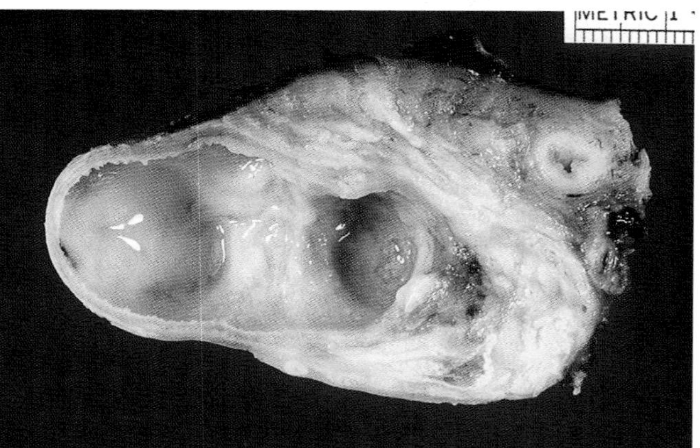

Fig. 19.193 Fusion of fallopian tube and ovary into a tubo-ovarian abscess.

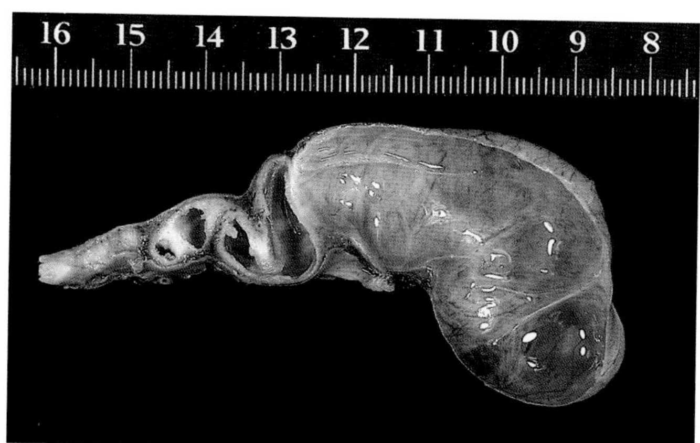

Fig. 19.194 Gross appearance of hydrosalpinx showing the typical retort-type appearance.
(Courtesy of Dr Pedro J Grases Galofré; from Grases Galofré PJ. Patología ginecológica. Bases para el diagnóstico morfológico. Barcelona, 2002, Masson)

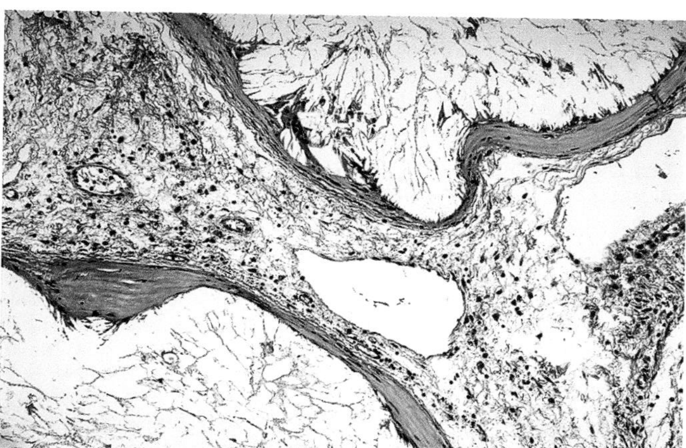

Fig. 19.196 Granulomatous reaction to contrast material injected into the fallopian tube.

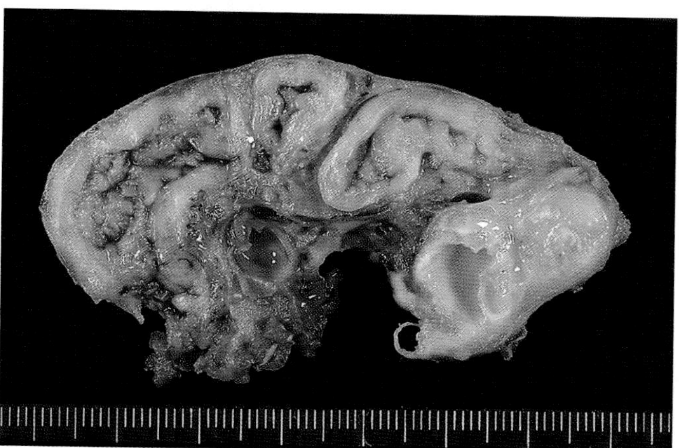

Fig. 19.195 Large caseating nodules in tuberculous salpingitis.
(Courtesy of Dr Pedro J Grases Galofré; from Grases Galofré PJ. Patología ginecológica. Bases para el diagnóstico morfológico. Barcelona, 2002, Masson)

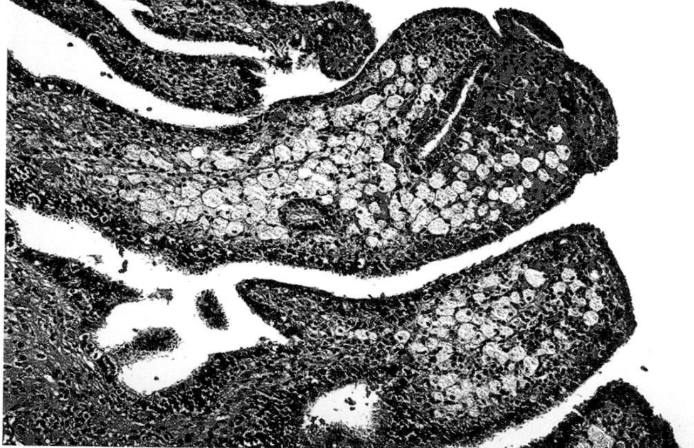

Fig. 19.197 Xanthogranulomatous salpingitis.

tuboperitoneal infection (resulting from *Bacteroides fragilis*, peptostreptococci, peptococci, and other organisms) is responsible for most others. In established tubo-ovarian abscesses, the most common agents recovered are coliform organisms. *N. gonorrhoeae* was isolated only once in a series of 93 case studies by Mickal et al.[23] This finding, however, does not rule out its role as a possible initiating factor before superinfection has occurred, in view of the fact that isolation of *N. gonorrhoeae* is inversely proportional to the number of episodes of salpingitis.[30]

Tuberculosis of the tube develops by the hematogenous route. Most patients are young, and infertility is common.[17,20] In advanced cases, both tubes are replaced by caseous tuberculous masses (Fig. 19.195). There is often extreme adenomatous proliferation of the tubal mucosa in association with granulomatous inflammation, and this may lead to a mistaken diagnosis of carcinoma. The endometrium is concomitantly involved in approximately 80% of cases.[24]

Granulomatous inflammation of the tubes can also be produced by *Schistosoma, Oxyuris vermicularis, Actinomyces, Coccidioides immitis*, and other organisms.[14] *Sarcoidosis* and *Crohn disease* may be accompanied by tubal involvement.

Foreign bodies introduced for diagnostic or therapeutic measures can induce a bizarre granulomatous response (Fig. 19.196). Reaction to the *lipiodol* that used to be introduced in the Rubin test may be so proliferative as to resemble a neoplasm. The push of a uterine sound may drive lubricant into the tube, causing *lipoid granulomas*.[13]

Xanthogranulomatous (pseudoxanthomatous) salpingitis is characterized by an expansion of the tubal plicae by an infiltrate of foamy histiocytes (Fig. 19.197). The distinction some authors make between xanthogranulomatous and pseudoxanthomatous salpingitis is probably unwarranted.[21] Some cases may be due to endometriosis, and, therefore, the term 'salpingitis' may be inaccurate.[18] Accordingly, some authors refer to it as *pseudoxanthomatous salpingiosis*.[28]

Giant cell arteritis is occasionally found in the tubes, ovaries, and uterus of postmenopausal patients, either as an isolated finding (most frequently) or as a manifestation of a generalized immune-mediated disease.[9,19,25]

Torsion

Torsion of the fallopian tube and ovary is usually secondary to inflammation or tumor, but occasionally it develops in a previously normal organ, the appearance at surgery being that of a hemorrhagic infarct. This phenomenon can occur in adults[37] as well as in infants and children.[36,38] In children, torsion of the normal adnexa is about one-third as common as torsion of an ovarian cyst or tumor.[35] If the operation (which can be carried out laparoscopically) is done early enough, untwisting of the adnexa may lead to full recovery. Nonoperated cases may resolve spontaneously or result in a necrotic and calcified mass, which may later detach from the uterus. It has been suggested that this complication, when occurring in previously normal adnexa, is due to the fact that the infundibulopelvic ligament extends along the edge of the ovarian ligament so that the tube and ovary hang on a very narrow stalk.

Tubal pregnancy

The incidence of tubal pregnancy (eccyesis) has increased markedly in recent times.[40] It is often the consequence of chronic salpingitis, which leads to inflammatory destruction of the lining folds and retention of the ovum.[48,56] Congenital tubal abnormalities, functional tubal disturbances, and salpingitis isthmica nodosa are responsible for a minority of the cases.[48,51] A history of infertility is associated with an increased risk of tubal pregnancy,[61] whereas induced abortion has no apparent effect on a woman's risk of tubal pregnancy in subsequent pregnancies.[49] High levels of trophinin, tastin, and bystin (three molecules thought to be involved in human embryo implantation) are expressed at high levels in trophoblast and fallopian tube epithelia in cases of tubal pregnancy, a fact of possible pathogenetic significance.[53]

In tubal pregnancy the gestational sac is completely made up of tubal tissue, with no participation from the ovarian or intraligamentary tissues. Following implantation of the ovum in the tubal epithelium (usually in the ampullo-isthmic or midtubal portion), chorionic villi and extravillous (intermediate) trophoblasts can grow predominantly intraluminally[59] or penetrate into the wall, just as they do in the uterus,[48,57] except that the wall here is much thinner. Trophoblastic invasion of muscle and vessels is a common finding of no clinical significance. Hydropic changes and polar trophoblastic proliferation can occur; they should not be overdiagnosed as hydatidiform mole.[42] Changes resembling atherosclerosis may be seen in tubal arteries at the site of implantation, analogous to those occurring in the uterus in orthotopic pregnancy.[41] The fallopian tube epithelium may undergo clear cell hyperplasia.[60] Although a few tubal pregnancies have gone to term,[44] the usual outcome is abortion. The maternal vessels rupture into the gestational sac and cause hematosalpinx (Fig. 19.198). In the presence of a large hematosalpinx, it may be difficult to identify the products of gestation; numerous blocks *from the intratubal blood clot* should be taken for this purpose. Tubal rupture can occur (usually near the end of the second month) because of destruction of the tubal wall by the invading trophoblast, and this may result in severe intra-abdominal hemorrhage. This rupture may result in a brisk reactive proliferation of the mesothelium, with formation of papillae and psammoma bodies. These changes should be recognized as reactive and not misinterpreted as metastases or implants from an ovarian serous neoplasm. The necrotic trophoblastic tissue may be retained for a long time and appear as hyalinized ghost outlines of chorionic villi.[50] On occasion, the appearance of these retained tissues corresponds to that of so-called *placental site nodule*, as described in the uterine corpus.[43,54]

The usual treatment for tubal pregnancy is salpingectomy, which in most instances can be done laparoscopically.[47,52] It is possible to conserve the homolateral ovary in approximately 80% of cases. Segmental tubal resection may be appropriate in selected cases; some of these individuals may develop recurrent tubal pregnancy, which is more related to the preexisting disease than to the operation.[58] Conservative laparoscopic procedures for tubal ectopic pregnancy can result in extratubal trophoblastic implants accompanied by persistent beta human chorionic gonadotropin (β-hCG) postoperative serum titers.[46] Exceptionally, omental deposits of fetal parts are seen as a sequel of salpingectomy for ruptured ectopic pregnancy.[45]

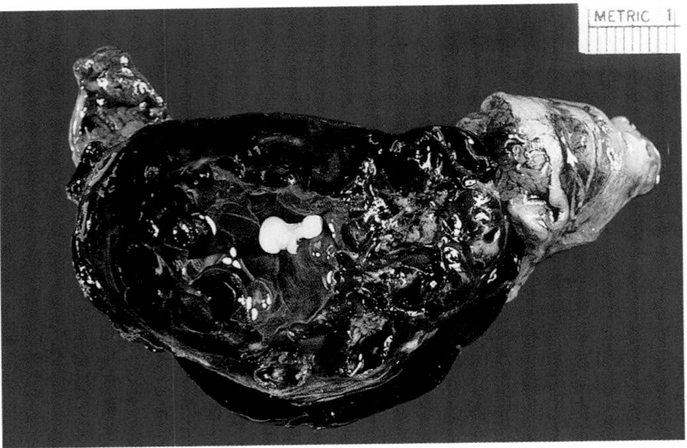

Fig. 19.198 Ruptured tubal pregnancy with marked hemorrhage (hematosalpinx). The tiny embryo is identifiable in the center of the clot.

Uterine curettings in the presence of a *viable* tubal pregnancy show gestational hyperplasia, sometimes associated with the Arias-Stella reaction. The key feature in the differential diagnosis between ectopic pregnancy and missed or incomplete abortion is the absence of fetal parts, chorionic villi, or trophoblastic cells in the latter (except for the extraordinarily rare occurrence of simultaneous intrauterine and ectopic pregnancy). Enlarged hyalinized spiral arteries and a fibrinoid matrix are not seen in the endometrium in cases of ectopic pregnancy, and, therefore, their presence is a strong indicator of intrauterine implantation.[55]

When trophoblastic elements are not obvious in routinely stained sections from the curettings, further search can be made with immunocytochemical stains for hCG, human placental lactogen (hPL), and keratin.[39,55] If none is found and a tubal mass is present, laparoscopy or laparotomy under the presumptive diagnosis of tubal pregnancy is indicated. Death of the embryo or fetus often results in expulsion of the endometrial decidual cast, regeneration of the epithelium, and reestablishment of the cyclic pattern. Therefore, the presence of a proliferative, secretory, or menstrual endometrium in a patient with an adnexal mass does not rule out the possibility of an ectopic pregnancy.

Other non-neoplastic processes

Walthard cell nests are small, glistening, round collections of flat to cuboidal cells with the appearance of urothelium located on the tubal serosa,[80] sometimes accompanied by cystic changes. They are probably of mesothelial rather than müllerian or wolffian nature.[80] They should not be mistaken for serosal implants in patients with ovarian neoplasms.

Paratubal cysts, traditionally known as *hydatids of Morgagni*, are commonly seen as small round cysts attached by a pedicle to the fimbriated end of the tube. Their wall is paper-thin and their content is clear. Occasionally, they attain a large size and may undergo torsion.[82] Most are lined by tubal columnar epithelium containing both ciliated and secretory cells, sometimes projecting in a papillary fashion into the lumen and covered by a thin layer of smooth muscle.[64] Their appearance is consistent with origin from müllerian-type structures. Other paratubal cysts, lined by flat cells and surrounded by a thin fibrous wall, are regarded as of mesothelial origin.[77]

Endometriosis frequently involves the tube in the form of nodules located in the wall or serosa.[78] In this context, it should be mentioned that the most common manifestation of ectopic endometrium in the tube is focal replacement of tubal epithelium by uterine mucosa;[73] however, it is questionable whether this abnormality should be equated with conventional tubal endometriosis.

Cases have also been reported of the pathogenetically related *müllerianosis* (endometriosis plus endosalpingiosis plus endocervicosis) in the mesosalpinx.[68]

Endosalpingiosis is a term originally coined to describe the direct spread of tubal epithelium beyond the anatomic confines of the tube. Thus defined, its most common location is the ovarian surface close to the fimbriae, suggesting that it may be secondary to extension of tubal epithelium over the inflammatory adhesions. Sometimes these changes are seen following surgical interventions, such as vaginal hysterectomy. Following the report of Burmeister et al.,[65] the term is more commonly used for a process of different pathogenesis, usually located in the peritoneum but also lymph node and other sites in the pelvis, probably representing a proliferative disorder of the mesothelium and subjacent tissue in which small cystic structures lined by an epithelium of tubal appearance form. Since this disorder is often associated with ovarian serous tumors, it is discussed in more detail in the next section of this chapter.

Decidual reaction of the tubal mucosa is a common finding in specimens of tubal ligation obtained at the time of cesarean section; it appears as small nodular collections of decidual cells covered by a flattened, sometimes inflamed epithelium (Fig. 19.199). Similar changes have been documented following hormonal therapy.[71]

Arias-Stella reaction can occur in the fallopian tube epithelium in association with either orthotopic or tubal pregnancy.[70]

Salpingitis isthmica nodosa is a usually bilateral lesion that presents grossly as a well-delimited nodular enlargement of the isthmic portion of the tube.[67] Microscopically, cystically dilated gland-like formations are seen surrounded by hypertrophic muscle (Fig. 19.200). Radiographic and tridimensional reconstructive studies have shown that the cystic formations are connected to the lumen of the tube. Although classically regarded as the result of inflammation (hence its name), convincing evidence has been presented that its pathogenesis is analogous to that of uterine adenomyosis.[63] It is accompanied by infertility in approximately one-half of patients, and it may also lead to ectopic pregnancy.[69]

Tubal sterilization procedures can lead to a sequence of morphologic alterations, which include proximal luminal dilation, plical attenuation, chronic inflammation with pseudopolyp formation, and plical thickening in the distal segment.[74] The appearance varies depending on the length of time that has elapsed from the sterilization procedure.[79]

Metaplastic changes of several types can develop in the fallopian tube mucosa. *Transitional cell* (*urothelial*) *metaplasia* is usually located in the fimbriae, where it may mimic carcinoma in situ. It is distinguished from it because of the uniformity in cell size and shape, low nucleocytoplasmic ratio, lack of nuclear atypia, presence of nuclear grooves, lack of mitoses, and absence of P53 expression or increased staining for MIB-1.[66,72] *Eosinophilic metaplasia* (sometimes accompanied by mucinous changes) presenting as a sharply outlined papillary lesion is occasionally encountered in tubes removed in the immediate postpartum period[62,75] (Fig. 19.201). Their behavior is benign. We favor the interpretation that this lesion, which has been called *metaplastic papillary tumor*, is of non-neoplastic nature. *Mucinous changes*, probably of metaplastic nature, have also been described in fallopian tubes in association with appendiceal and ovarian mucinous tumors.[83]

Papillary endothelial hyperplasia can develop in tubal vessels and simulate an angiosarcoma; as in other sites, it is the expression of organization and recanalization of thrombi.[76]

Fallopian tube prolapse into the vaginal apex following vaginal hysterectomy can simulate the microscopic appearance of an aggressive angiomyxoma.[81]

Proliferative epithelial lesions

Proliferative epithelial lesions may be found during the microscopic examination of a specimen from tubal ligation or salpingectomy. They may show one or more of the following features: nuclear crowding, stratification, loss of polarity, mild to moderate atypia, occasional mitoses, acidophilic metaplasia, and papillary formations[88,94,95] (Fig. 19.202). Mild degrees of this change are extremely common; in one study, they were found in 83% of all tubes examined.[97] More severe forms of this process, which are rare, have been

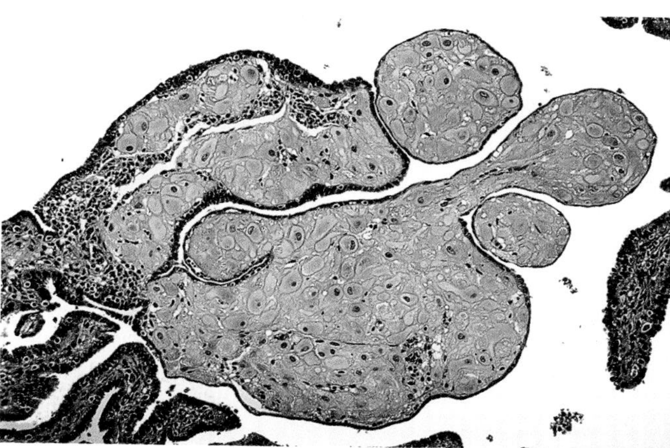

Fig. 19.199 Ectopic decidual reaction in the fallopian tube. This is a very common finding during pregnancy.

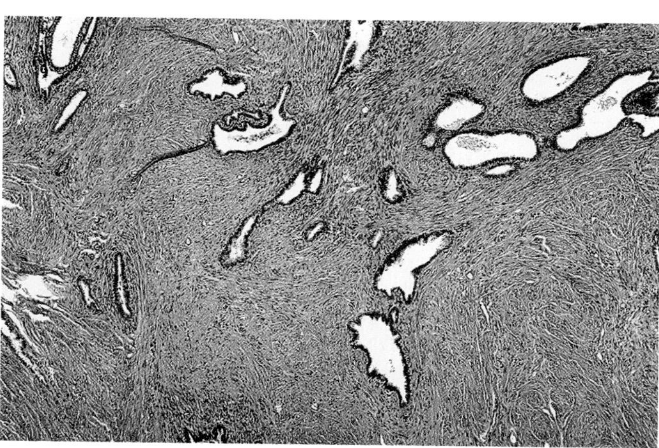

Fig. 19.200 Low-power view of salpingitis isthmica nodosa.

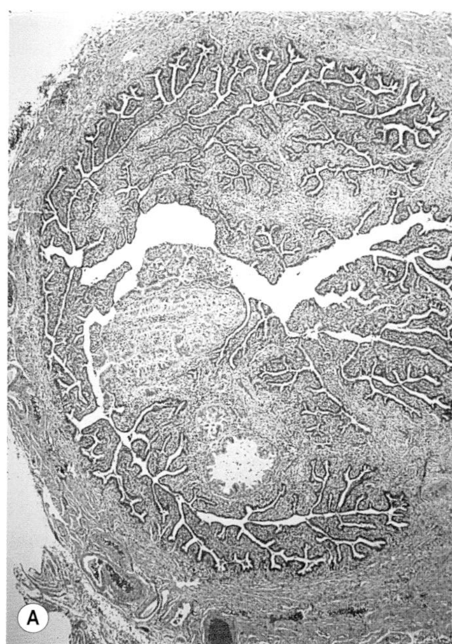

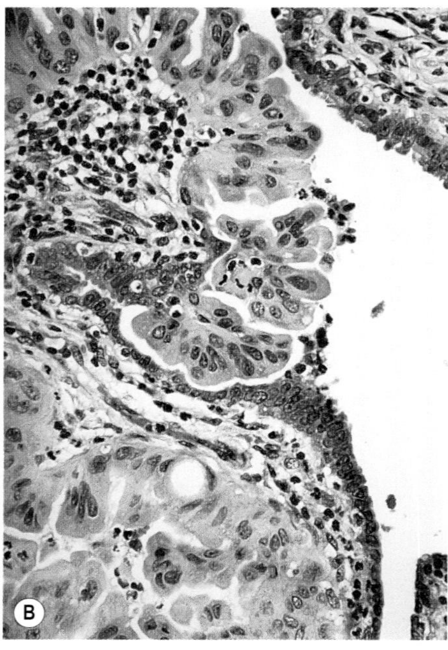

Fig. 19.201 **A** and **B**, So-called metaplastic papillary tumor of fallopian tube. This lesion, which occurred in a pregnant woman, is characterized by a papillary proliferation of acidophilic epithelium. This process is probably of non-neoplastic nature.

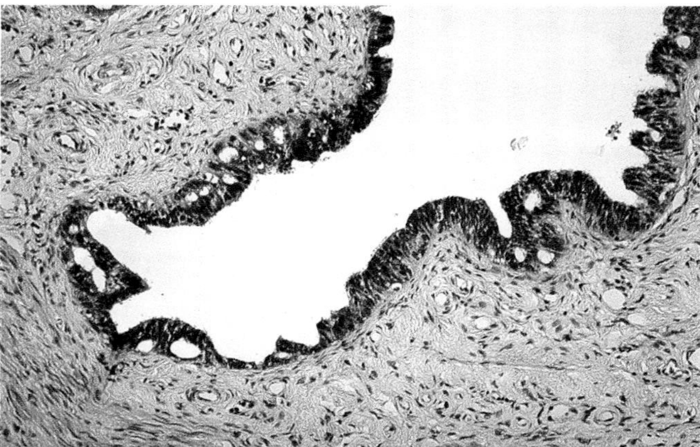

Fig. 19.202 Hyperplasia of the tubal epithelium in a patient with a borderline serous tumor of the homolateral ovary.

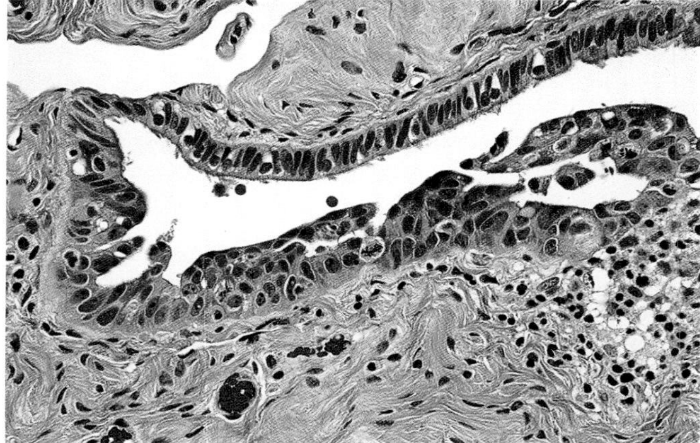

Fig. 19.203 Carcinoma in situ of the tubal epithelium. The ovary was uninvolved.

designated as *adenomatous hyperplasia, atypical hyperplasia, carcinoma in situ*, and *intraepithelial carcinoma*, and regarded as possible precursors of tubal (as well as ovarian) carcinoma[90,94] (Fig. 19.203). The diagnosis of atypical hyperplasia requires the presence of moderate to severe nuclear atypia, whereas the diagnosis of carcinoma in situ implies the presence of cells with 'cytologically malignant nuclei' and abnormal mitotic figures.[97]

Some of the above changes have been found in association with other lesions or situations, such as salpingitis, exogenous or endogenous estrogen stimulation (including tamoxifen administration), and borderline serous tumors of the ovary.[87,91,92,96,97] A particularly interesting subset is that of the proliferative lesions found in tubes of women with *BRCA1/BRCA2* mutations who underwent prophylactic oophorectomy with salpingectomy.[93] In one such study involving 26 women, there were two atypical hyperplasias and two carcinomas in situ of the tube, all of them occurring in *BRCA1* carriers.[85] In an updated study from the same group in which the number of cases studied had risen to 50, there were now three tubal carcinomas in situ and one invasive tubal carcinoma,[85] an incidence which is clearly higher than in controls. These findings, which are similar to those of other authors,[84,89] indicate that ovarian surgical prophylaxis in these patients should be accompanied by removal of the tubes, and stress the need of thoroughly evaluating the specimens at the microscopic level.[86]

Carcinoma

Traditionally, primary carcinoma of the fallopian tube has been regarded as very rare, accounting for approximately 1% of primary genital tract malignancies.[119] However, several recent studies following a standardized grossing protocol and including a larger number of early stages have shown that it reaches approximately 15% of all adnexal tumors.[127] The interesting possibility that a high percentage of ovarian and 'primary peritoneal' serous carcinomas may originate in the tubal fimbriae is discussed on page 1562.[102,116,120]

Most patients with tubal carcinoma are postmenopausal, and the preoperative diagnosis is rarely correct. Nulliparity is common in this population. Tubal carcinoma may be bilateral, but more often the contralateral tube is either normal or the site of a hydrosalpinx. There is often a history and/or morphologic evidence of coexisting or preceding salpingitis, a fact of possible pathogenetic significance.[106] Atypical vaginal bleeding is the most common form of presentation.[110] The classic triad of the disease, represented by pain, vaginal discharge, and a palpable adnexal mass, occurs in less than half of cases. Exceptionally, the initial presentation is in the form of a lymph node metastasis.[108] Cervicovaginal cytology is positive in only a minority of patients,[112] but an endometrial smear will reveal malignant cells in a high percentage of cases.[122] Grossly, the tube is enlarged and has fibrous adhesions, the outer appearance resembling that of chronic salpingitis. The fimbriated end of the tube may be open or closed, a fact of possible prognostic significance (see below) that should be noted in the report. Some tumors arise in the fimbriated portion of the organ and are, therefore, directly exposed to the peritoneal cavity even if they do not invade the tubal wall.[98,130] The cut surface shows a solid or papillary tumor filling the lumen (Fig. 19.204). Microscopically, all the major types of carcinoma known to occur in the ovary (including their variants) have been reported in the tube. The most common type is serous (papillary)[123] (Fig. 19.205). Other reported types are endometrioid (the second most common type, including spindle cell, oxyphilic, adenoacanthomatous, adenosquamous, and squamous types), mucinous, seromucinous, clear cell, transitional cell and hepatoid.[99,101,105,109,111,114,124–126,128] The endometrioid carcinomas typically present as intraluminal masses and may simulate microscopically the so-called 'female adnexal tumor of probable wolffian origin',[104] As in other sites in the female genital tract, serous carcinoma of the fallopian tube often expresses WT1.

Traditionally, a carcinoma extensively involving both endometrium and tube was classified as an endometrial tumor, and one extensively involving both ovary and tube was regarded as an ovarian neoplasm, but these assumptions have been greatly challenged lately, as already indicated (see p. 1500).[102,116,120] In most of the reported cases of anatomically discontinuous endometrioid carcinomas involving simultaneously the tube and the uterus, the former were unilateral and located at the fimbrial end.[103]

The prognosis of tubal carcinoma depends more on staging than histologic grade.[99] The staging system currently used is adapted from the FIGO staging system for ovarian carcinoma.

Involvement of the tubal serosa, of the ovary or corpus uteri, or of other pelvic and abdominal structures is a common finding and indicates a poor prognosis.[100,121] Five-year survival rates are as high as 77% for stage I lesions, approximately 40% for stage II, and approximately 20% for stage III.[107,113,115,117,118] Absence of closure of the fimbriated end of the tube is another unfavorable prognostic sign.[99] Among stage I tumors, features of prognostic significance include the presence or absence of invasion of the tubal wall, depth of invasion when present, and the location of the tumor within the tube (fimbrial is worse than nonfimbrial).[98,99] The initial tumor recurrence is intra-abdominal in over 80% of cases, its pattern of spread mirroring that of ovarian carcinoma.

Borderline epithelial neoplasms have also been described in the fallopian tube. As in the ovary, they can be of serous, endometrioid, or mucinous type.[99,129]

Other tumors

Adenomatoid tumor is a benign, usually small lesion that may be found within the wall of the tube or beneath the uterine serosa near a cornu.[149] The gross and microscopic features are identical to those of its epididymal counterpart (see Chapter 18). The ill-defined, seemingly infiltrating margins may lead to a mistaken diagnosis of carcinoma.[154] A marked degree of smooth muscle hyperplasia may be present and obscure the true nature of the lesion (Fig. 19.206). There is now agreement on the basis of ultrastructural and immunohistochemical findings (the latter including positivity for calretinin, WT1, CK5/6, and D2-40[149,150]) that this entity is of mesothelial (rather than wolffian, müllerian, or endothelial) derivation and that it represents a unique variant of benign mesothelioma largely restricted to the genital region,[142,148] as originally postulated by Pierre Masson. However, the alternative of at least some of these lesions representing examples of nodular mesothelial hyperplasia of a reactive nature should be considered.

Papillary cystadenoma of the mesosalpinx has been seen in patients with von Hippel–Lindau disease.[133] Allelic deletions of the *VHL* gene have been detected in these cases.[152]

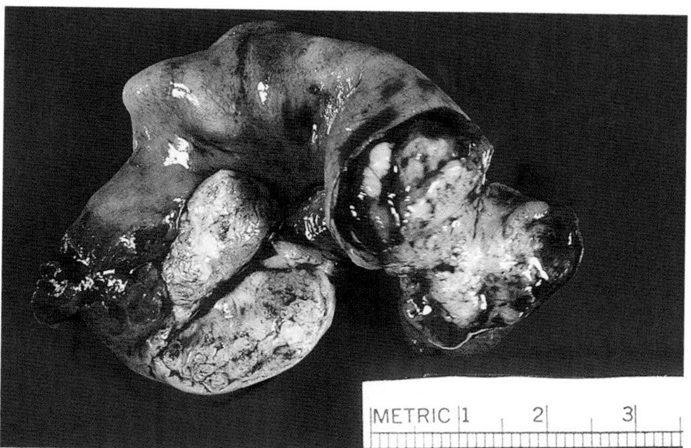

Fig. 19.204 Fallopian tube adenocarcinoma filling and distending the lumen of the organ.

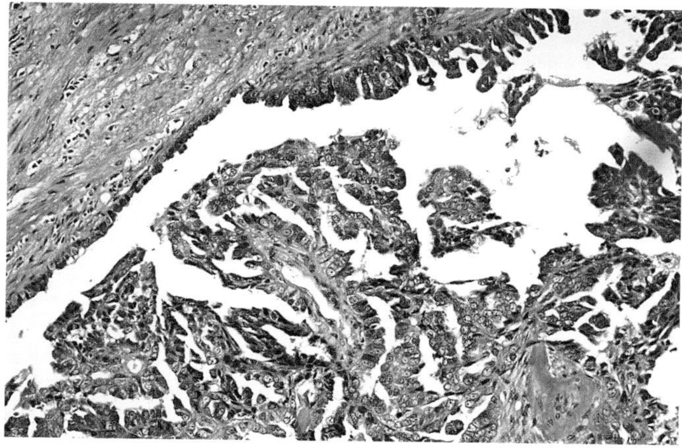

Fig. 19.205 High-power view showing the complex papillary architecture that is characteristic of adenocarcinomas of the fallopian tube.

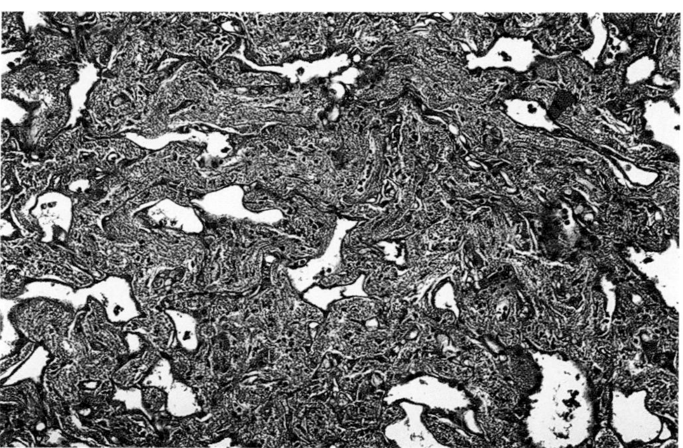

Fig. 19.206 Adenomatoid tumor of fallopian tube accompanied by smooth muscle hyperplasia.

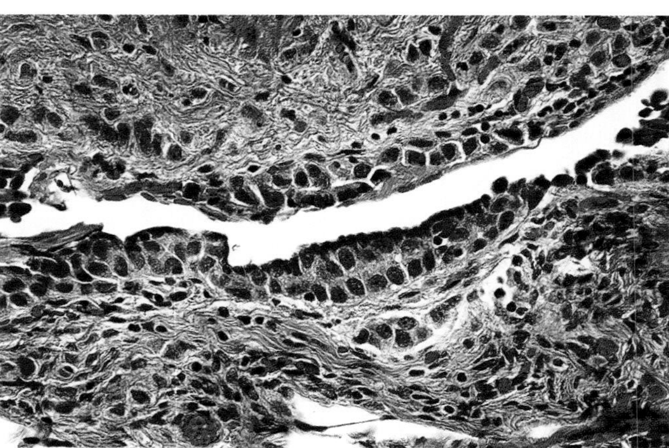

Fig. 19.208 Metastatic lobular carcinoma of breast growing beneath tubal epithelium.

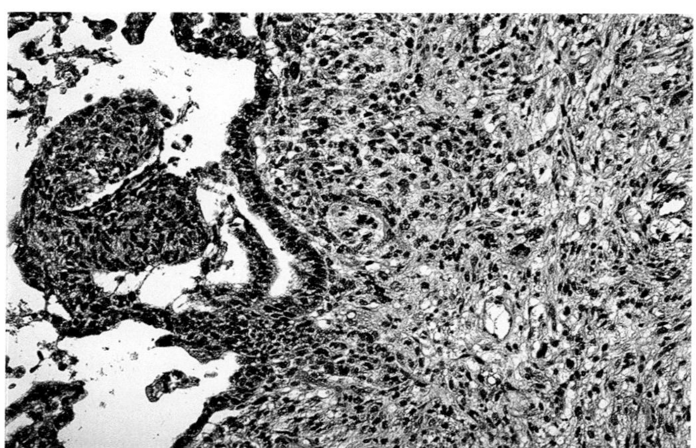

Fig. 19.207 Malignant mixed müllerian tumor of fallopian tube, showing the typical biphasic pattern.

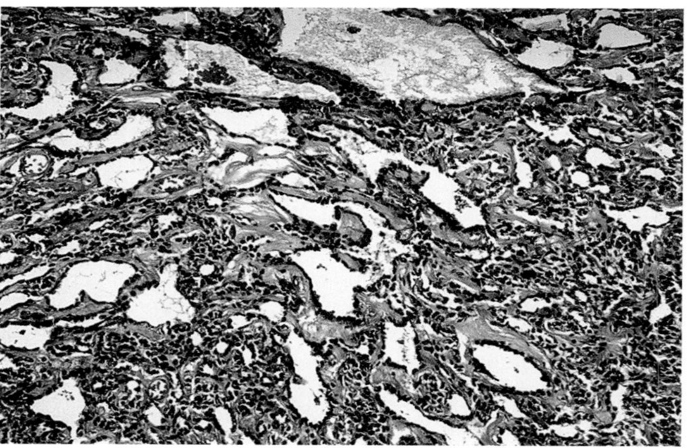

Fig. 19.209 Wolffian adnexal tumor of the broad ligament. The sieve-like low-power appearance is characteristic.

Mucinous lesions of the fallopian tubes comprise a wide variety of processes, which include mucinous metaplasia (see above), mucinous cystadenoma, 'mucinous borderline tumor', and mucinous adenocarcinoma. Some of these lesions have occurred in patients with Peutz–Jeghers syndrome, others in association with in situ or invasive adenocarcinoma of other portions of the female genital tract (such as endocervix), and still others in conjunction with mucinous neoplasms of the appendix.[140,151] It is possible that the latter are tubal metastases or implants of appendiceal primaries.

Approximately 50 cases of tubal **teratomas** have been published, nearly all cystic and benign;[138] one of them contained a *carcinoid tumor* and another was entirely composed of mature thyroid tissue (*struma salpingis*).[137] Other reported benign tubal tumors, all very rare, are **leiomyoma, hemangioma, adenofibroma,**[131,132,141] **sex-cord tumor with annular tubules** (associated with endometriosis),[136] and **papilloma.**[135] The latter should be distinguished from the more common papillary hyperplasia associated with inflammation and hyperestrinism.

Malignant tumors other than carcinoma include **malignant mixed müllerian tumor (carcinosarcoma)**[133,139,141,143,146] (some bilateral[153]) (Fig. 19.207), **leiomyosarcoma, gestational choriocarcinoma,**[147] and **synovial sarcoma.**[145] The first three tumor types resemble, grossly and microscopically, their more common uterine counterparts; tubal extension from the latter should always be considered in the differential diagnosis. Tubal involvement by **malignant lymphoma** is always the expression of systemic disease. **Secondary tubal invasion** by carcinoma of the ovary and uterus is a much more common event than primary tubal carcinoma. Most **metastases** to the tube also originate from genital organs, with very few exceptions[144] (Fig. 19.208).

Tumors and tumorlike conditions of broad and round ligaments

The **round and broad ligaments** are only rarely the site of primary disease.[160,166] **Striated muscle heteroplasia** is an inconsequential incidental finding, thought to represent aberrant persistence of gubernacular rhabdomyoblasts.[161]

Cystic formations derived from müllerian or mesonephric (wolffian) rests can be found in or around the broad ligament; they have been mentioned on page 1544.

Female adnexal tumor of probable wolffian origin (wolffian adnexal tumor) is a distinctive lesion originally described in the broad ligament and subsequently also recognized in the ovary (see p. 1604). In its most typical form, it is seen within the leaves of the broad ligament or hanging on a pedicle from it or the fallopian tube. Grossly, it is predominantly solid. Microscopically, it is composed of epithelial cells growing in diffuse, trabecular, and tubular patterns (Fig. 19.209). Mitotic activity and capsular invasion may be present, but the prognosis is generally good.[162,164] As the name indicates, the tumor is thought to be of wolffian (mesonephric) derivation. Therefore, it could have been designated as mesonephric, but it was feared that such a terminology might have induced confusion with the many lesions in the female genital tract that in the past have been called mesonephric but which have no relation with the mesonephric system.

Other tumors and tumorlike conditions that can be found in the broad ligament unassociated with either uterine or ovarian disease are *endometriosis* (including the possibly related condition known as uterus-like mass);[155] *borderline serous tumors;*[157] *serous, endometrioid, clear cell,* and *mucinous carcinomas;*[156,158] *papillary cystadenomas* and other neoplasms associated with von Hippel–Lindau disease;[163,165] *ependymoma;*[159] *smooth muscle tumors;* and other types of *mesenchymal neoplasm.* Some of the carcinomas of this region are thought to arise from foci of endometriosis.[158]

References

NORMAL ANATOMY

1 Bruns DE, Mills SE, Savory J. Amylase in fallopian tube and serous ovarian neoplasms. Immunohistochemical localization. Arch Pathol Lab Med 1982, **106**: 17–20.

2 Gardner GH, Greene RR, Peckham B. Normal and cystic structures of the broad ligament. Am J Obstet Gynecol 1948, **55**: 917–939.

3 Hendrickson MR, Atkins KA, Kempson RL. Uterus and fallopian tubes. In Mills SE (ed.): Histology for pathologists, ed. 3. Philadelphia, 2007, Lippincott Williams and Wilkins, pp. 1011–1062.

4 Hershlag A, Seifer DB, Carcangiu ML, Patton DL, Diamond MP, De Cherney AH. Salpingoscopy. Light microscopic and electron microscopic correlations (published erratum appears in Obstet Gynecol 1991 May; 77: 809–810). Obstet Gynecol 1991, **77**: 399–405.

5 Hunt JL, Lynn AA. Histologic features of surgically removed fallopian tubes. Arch Pathol Lab Med 2002, **126**: 951–955.

6 Nassberg S, McKay DG, Hertig AT. Physiologic salpingitis. Am J Obstet Gynecol 1954, **67**: 130–137.

7 Rubin A, Czernobilsky B. Tubal ligation. A bacteriologic, histologic and clinical study. Obstet Gynecol 1970, **36**: 199–203.

8 Zheng W, Magid MS, Kramer EE, Chen YT. Follicle-stimulating hormone receptor is expressed in human ovarian surface epithelium and fallopian tube. Am J Pathol 1996, **148**: 47–53.

INFLAMMATION

9 Bell DA, Mondschein M, Scully RE. Giant cell arteritis of the female genital tract. A report of three cases. Am J Surg Pathol 1986, **10**: 696–701.

10 Charonis G, Larsson PG. Prolonged use of intrauterine contraceptive device as a risk factor for tubo-ovarian abscess. Acta Obstet Gynecol Scand 2009, **88**: 680–684.

11 Cheung ANY, Young RH, Scully RE. Pseudocarcinomatous hyperplasia of the fallopian tube associated with salpingitis. A report of 14 cases. Am J Surg Pathol 1994, **18**: 1125–1130.

12 David A, Garcia C-S, Czernobilsky B. Human hydrosalpinx. Histologic study and chemical composition of fluid. Am J Obstet Gynecol 1969, **105**: 400–411.

13 Elliott GB, Brody H, Elliott KA. Implications of 'lipoid salpingitis'. Fertil Steril 1965, **16**: 541–548.

14 Erthan Y, Zekioglu O, Ozdemir N, Sen S. Unilateral salpingitis due to enterobious vermicularis. Int J Gynecol Pathol 2000, **19**: 188–189.

15 Eschenbach DA, Buchanan TM, Pollock HM, Forsyth PS, Alexander ER, Lin JS, Wang SP, Wentworth BB, McCormack WM, Holmes KK. Polymicrobial etiology of acute pelvic inflammatory disease. N Engl J Med 1975, **29**: 166–171.

16 Fortier KJ, Haney AF. The pathologic spectrum of uterotubal junction obstruction. Obstet Gynecol 1985, **65**: 93–98.

17 Francis WAJ. Female genital tuberculosis. A review of 135 cases. J Obstet Gynaecol Br Commonw 1964, **71**: 418–428.

18 Furuya M, Murakami T, Sato O, Kikuchi K, Tanaka S, Shimizu M, Yoshiki T. Pseudoxanthomatous salpingitis of the fallopian tube: a report of four cases and a literature review. Int J Gynecol Pathol 2002, **21**: 56–59.

19 Ganesan R, Ferryman SR, Meier L, Rollason TP. Vasculitis of the female genital tract with clinicopathologic correlation: a study of 46 cases with follow-up. Int J Gynecol Pathol 2000, **19**: 258–265.

20 Henderson DN, Harkins JL, Stitt JF. Pelvic tuberculosis. Am J Obstet Gynecol 1966, **94**: 630–633.

21 Kostopoulou E, Daponte A, Kallitsaris A, Papamichali R, Kalodimos G, Messinis IE, Koukoulis G. Xanthogranulomatous salpingitis: report of three cases and comparison with a case of pseudoxanthomatous salpingitis. Clin Exp Obstet Gynecol 2008, **35**: 291–294.

22 McCormack WM. Pelvic inflammatory disease. N Engl J Med 1994, **330**: 115–119.

23 Mickal A, Sellmann AH, Beebe JL. Ruptured tuboovarian abscess. Am J Obstet Gynecol 1968, **100**: 432–436.

24 Nogales-Ortiz F, Tarancón I, Nogales FF Jr. The pathology of female genital tuberculosis. Obstet Gynecol 1979, **53**: 422–428.

25 Onuma K, Chu CT, Dabbs GJ. Asymptomatic giant-cell (temporal) arteritis involving the bilateral adnexa: case report and literature review. Int J Gynecol Pathol 2007, **26**: 352–355.

26 Paavonen J. Pelvic inflammatory disease. From diagnosis to prevention. Dermatol Clin 1998, **16**: 747–756.

27 Pedowitz R, Bloomfield RD. Ruptured adnexal abscess (tuboovarian) with generalized peritonitis. Am J Obstet Gynecol 1964, **88**: 721–729.

28 Seidman JD, Oberer S, Bitterman P, Aisner SC. Pathogenesis of pseudoxanthomatous salpingiosis. Mod Pathol 1993, **6**: 53–55.

29 Seidman JD, Sherman ME, Bell KA, Katabuchi H, O'Leary TJ, Kurman RJ. Salpingitis, salpingoliths, and serous tumors of the ovaries: is there a connection? Int J Gynecol Pathol 2002, **21**: 101–107.

30 Sweet RL, Draper DL, Hadley WK. Etiology of acute salpingitis. Influence of episode number and duration of symptoms. Obstet Gynecol 1981, **58**: 62–68.

31 Thor AD, Young RH, Clement PB. Pathology of the fallopian tube, broad ligament, peritoneum, and pelvic soft tissues. Hum Pathol 1991, **22**: 856–867.

32 Wallace TM, Hart WR. Acute chlamydial salpingitis with ascites and adnexal mass simulating a malignant neoplasm. Int J Gynecol Pathol 1991, **10**: 394–401.

33 Washington AE, Aral SO, Wolner-Hanssen P, Grimes DA, Holmes KK. Assessing risk for pelvic inflammatory disease and its sequelae. JAMA 1991, **266**: 2581–2586.

34 Winkler B, Reumann W, Mitao M, Gallo L, Richart RM, Crum CP. Immunoperoxidase localization of chlamydial antigens in acute salpingiris. Am J Obstet Gynecol 1985, **152**: 275–278.

TORSION

35 Breech LL, Hillard PJ. Adnexal torsion in pediatric and adolescent girls. Curr Opin Obstet Gynecol 2005, **17**: 483–489.

36 Grosfeld JL. Torsion of normal ovary in the first two years of life. Am J Surg 1969, **117**: 726–727.

37 Hansen OH. Isolated torsion of the fallopian tube. Acta Obstet Gynecol Scand 1970, **49**: 3–6.

38 James DF, Barber HRK, Graber EA. Torsion of normal uterine adnexa in children. Report of three cases. Obstet Gynecol 1970, **35**: 226–230.

TUBAL PREGNANCY

39 Angel E, Davis JR, Nagle RB. Immunohistochemical demonstration of placental hormones in the diagnosis of uterine versus ectopic pregnancy. Am J Clin Pathol 1985, **84**: 705–709.

40 Barnhart KT. Ectopic pregnancy. N Engl J Med 2009, **361**: 379–387.

41 Blaustein A, Shenker L. Vascular lesions of the uterine tube in ectopic pregnancy. Obstet Gynecol 1967, **30**: 551–555.

42 Burton JL, Lidbury EA, Gillespie AM, Tidy JA, Smith O, Lawry J, Hancock BW, Wells M. Over-diagnosis of hydatidiform mole in early tubal ectopic pregnancy. Histopathology 2001, **38**: 409–417.

43 Campello TR, Fittipaldi H, O'Valle F, Carvia RE, Nogales FF. Extrauterine (tubal) placental site nodule. Histopathology 1998, **32**: 562–565.

44 Chokroverty M, Caballes RL, Gear PE. An unruptured tubal pregnancy at term. Arch Pathol Lab Med 1986, **110**: 250–251.

45 Deheragoda MG, Baithun S. Omental deposits of fetal parts as a sequal to salpingectomy for ruptured ectopic pregnancy. Histopathology 2006, 49: 426.

46 Doss BJ, Jacques SM, Qureshi F, Ramirez NC, Lawrence WD. Extratubal secondary trophoblastic implants: clinicopathologic correlation and review of the literature. Hum Pathol 1998, **29**: 184–187.

47 Goldrath MH, Platt LD. Treatment of ectopic tubal pregnancies by laparoscopy. J Am Assoc Gynecol Laparosc 2002, **9**: 409–413.

48 Green LK, Kott ML. Histopathologic findings in ectopic tubal pregnancy. Int J Gynecol 1989, **8**: 255–262.

49 Holt VL, Daling JR, Voigt LF, McKnight B, Stergachis A, Chu J, Weiss NS. Induced abortion and the risk of subsequent ectopic pregnancy. Am J Public Health 1989, **79**: 1234–1238.

50 Jacques SM, Qureshi F, Ramirez NC, Lawrence WD. Retained trophoblastic tissue in fallopian tubes: a consequence of unsuspected ectopic pregnancies. Int J Gynecol Pathol 1998, **16**: 219–224.

51 Majmudar B, Henderson PH, Semple E. Salpingitis isthmica nodosa. A high-risk for tubal pregnancy. Obstet Gynecol 1983, **62**: 73–78.

52 Mohamed H, Maiti S, Phillips G. Laparoscopic management of ectopic pregnancy: a 5-year experience. J Obstet Gynaecol 2002, **22**: 411–414.

53 Nakyama J, Aoki D, Suga T, Akama TO, Ishizone S, Yamaguchi H, Imakawa K, Nadano D, Fazleabas AT, Katsuyama T, Nozawa S, Fukuda MN. Implantation-dependent expression of trophinin by maternal fallopian tube epithelia during tubal pregnancies: possible role of human chorionic gonadotrophin on ectopic pregnancy. Am J Pathol 2003, **163**: 2211–2219.

54 Nayar R, Snell J, Silverberg SG, Lage JM. Placental site nodule occurring in a fallopian tube. Hum Pathol 1997, **27**: 1243–1245.

55 O'Connor DM, Kurman RJ. Intermediate trophoblast in uterine curettings in the diagnosis of ectopic pregnancy. Obstet Gynecol 1988, **72**: 665–670.

56 Pauerstein CJ, Croxatto HB, Eddy CA, Ramzy I, Walters MD. Anatomy and pathology of tubal pregnancy. Obstet Gynecol 1986, **67**: 301–308.

57 Randall S, Buckley CH, Fox H. Placentation in the fallopian tube. Int J Gynecol Pathol 1987, **6**: 132–139.

58 Stock RJ. Histopathology of fallopian tubes with recurrent tubal pregnancy. Obstet Gynecol 1990, **75**: 9–14.

59 Stock RJ. Tubal pregnancy. Associated histopathology. Obstet Gynecol Clin North Am 1991, **18**: 73–94.

60 Tziortziotis DV, Bouros AC, Ziogas VS, Young RH. Clear cell hyperplasia of the fallopian tube epithelium associated with ectopic pregnancy: report of a case. Int J Gynecol Pathol 1997, **16**: 79–80.

61 Yang CP, Chow WH, Daling JR, Weiss NS, Moore DE. Does prior infertility increase the risk of tubal pregnancy? Fertil Steril 1987, **48**: 62–66.

OTHER NON-NEOPLASTIC PROCESSES

62 Bartnik J, Powell WS, Moriber-Katz S, Amenta PS. Metaplastic papillary tumor of the fallopian tube. Case report, immunohistochemical features, and review of the literature. Arch Pathol Lab Med 1989, **113**: 545–547.

63 Benjamin CL, Beaver DC. Pathogenesis of salpingitis isthmica nodosa. Am J Clin Pathol 1951, **21**: 212–222.

64 Bransilver BR, Ferenczy A, Richart RM. Female genital tract remnants. An ultrastructural comparison of hydatid of Morgagni and mesonephric ducts and tubules. Arch Pathol 1973, **96**: 255–261.

65 Burmeister RE, Fechner RE, Franklin RR. Endosalpingiosis of the peritoneum. Obstet Gynecol 1969, **34**: 310–318.

66 Egan AJM, Russell P. Transitional (urothelial) cell metaplasia of the fallopian tube mucosa: morphological assessment of three cases. Int J Gynecol Pathol 1996, **15**: 72–76.

67 Jenkins CS, Williams SR, Schmidt GE. Salpingitis isthmica nodosa: a review of the literature, discussion of clinical significance, and consideration of patient management. Fertil Steril 1993, **60**: 599–607.

68 Lim S, Kim JY, Park K, Kim BR, Ahn G. Mullerianosis of the mesosalpinx: a case report. Int J Gynecol Pathol 2003, **22**: 209–212.

69 Majmudar B, Henderson PH, Semple E. Salpingitis isthmica nodosa. A high-risk for tubal pregnancy. Obstet Gynecol 1983, **62**: 73–78.

70 Milchgrub S, Sandstad J. Arias-Stella reaction in fallopian tube epithelium. A light and electron microscopic study with a review of the literature. Am J Clin Pathol 1991, **95**: 892–895.

71 Mills SE, Fechner RE. Stromal and epithelial changes in the fallopian tube following hormonal therapy. Hum Pathol 1980, **11**: 583–584.

72 Rabban JT, Crawford B, Chen LM, Powell CB, Zaloudek CJ. Transitional cell metaplasia of fallopian tube fimbriae: a potential mimic of early tubal carcinoma in risk reduction salpingo-oophorectomies from women with BRCA mutations. Am J Surg Pathol 2009, **33**: 111–119.

73 Rubin IC, Lisa JR, Trinidad S. Further observations of ectopic endometrium of fallopian tube. Surg Gynecol Obstet 1956, **103**: 469–474.

74 Rubin A, Czernobilsky B. Tubal ligation. A bacteriologic, histologic and clinical study. Obstet Gynecol 1970, **36**: 199–203.

75 Saffos RO, Rhatigan RM, Scully RE. Metaplastic papillary tumor of the fallopian tube – a distinctive lesion of pregnancy. Am J Clin Pathol 1980, **74**: 232–236.

76 Safneck JR, Alguacil-Garcia A, Paraskevas M. Papillary endothelial hyperplasia of adnexal vasculature. Histopathology 1996, **28**: 157–161.

77 Samaha M, Woodruff JD. Paratubal cysts. Frequency, histogenesis, and associated clinical features. Obstet Gynecol 1985, **65**: 691–694.

78 Sheldon RS, Wilson RB, Dockerty MB. Serosal endometriosis of fallopian tubes. Am J Obstet Gynecol 1967, **99**: 882–884.

79 Stock RJ. Histopathologic changes in fallopian tubes subsequent to sterilization procedures. Int J Gynecol Pathol 1983, **2**: 13–27.

80 Teoh TB. The structure and development of Walthard nests. J Pathol Bacteriol 1953, **66**: 433–439.

81 Varnholt H, Otis CN, Nucci MR, Johari VP. Fallopian tube prolapse mimicking aggressive angiomyxoma. Int J Gynecol Pathol 2005, **24**: 292–294.

82 Wittich AC. Hydatid of Morgagni with torsion diagnosed during cesarean delivery. A case report. J Reprod Med 2002, **47**: 680–682.

83 Wong AK, Seidman JD, Barbuto DA, McPhaul LW, Silva EG. Mucinous metaplasia of the fallopian tube: a diagnostic pitfall mimicking metastasis. Int J Gynecol Pathol 2011, **30**: 36–40.

PROLIFERATIVE EPITHELIAL LESIONS

84 Aziz S, Kuperstein G, Rosen B, Cole D, Nedelcu R, McLaughlin J, Narod SA. A genetic epidemiological study of carcinoma of the fallopian tube. Gynecol Oncol 2001, **80**: 341–345.

85 Carcangiu ML, Peissel B, Pasini B, Spatti G, Radice P, Manoukian S. Incidental carcinomas in prophylactic specimens in BRCA1 and BRCA2 germ-line mutation carriers, with emphasis on fallopian tube lesions: report of 6 cases and review of the literature. Am J Surg Pathol 2006, **30**: 1222–1230.

86 Carcangiu ML, Radice P, Manoukian S, Spatti G, Gobbo M, Pensotti V, Crucianelli R, Pasini B. Atypical epithelial proliferation in fallopian tubes in prophylactic salpingo-oophorectomy specimens from BRCA1 and BRCA2 germline mutation carriers. Int J Gynecol Pathol 2004, **23**: 35–40.

87 Colgan TJ. Challenges in the early diagnosis and staging of fallopian-tube carcinomas associated with BRCA mutations. Int J Gynecol Pathol 2003, **22**: 109–120.

88 Moore SW, Enterline HT. Significance of proliferative epithelial lesions of the uterine tube. Obstet Gynecol 1975, **45**: 385–390.

89 Paley PJ, Swisher EM, Garcia RL, Agoff SN, Greer BE, Peters KL, Goff BA. Occult cancer of the fallopian tube in BRCA-1 germline mutation carriers at prophylactic oophorectomy: a case for recommending hysterectomy at surgical prophylaxis. Gynecol Oncol 2001, **80**: 176–180.

90 Pickel H, Reich O, Tamussino K. Bilateral atypical hyperplasia of the fallopian tube associated with tamoxifen: a report of two cases. Int J Gynecol Pathol 1998, **17**: 284–285.

91 Piek JM, van Diest PJ, Zweemer RP, Jansen JW, Poort-Keesom RJ, Menko FH, Gille JJ, Jongsma AP, Pals G, Kenemans P, Verheijen RH. Dysplastic changes in prophylactically removed fallopian tubes of women predisposed to developing ovarian cancer. J Pathol 2001, **195**: 451–456.

92 Robey SS, Silva EG. Epithelial hyperplasia of the fallopian tube. Its association with serous borderline tumors of the ovary. Int J Gynecol Pathol 1989, **8**: 214–220.

93 Shaw PA, Rouzbahman M, Pizer ES, Pintilie ES, Begley H. Candidate serous cancer precursors in fallopian tube epithelium of BRCA1/2 mutation carriers. Mod Pathol 2009, **22**: 1133–1138.

94 Stern J, Buscema J, Parmley T, Woodruff JD, Rosenshein NB. Atypical epithelial proliferations in the fallopian tube. Am J Obstet Gynecol 1981, **140**: 309–312.

95 Woodruff JD, Pauerstein CJ. The fallopian tube. Structure, function, pathology, and management. Baltimore, 1969, Williams and Wilkins.

96 Yanai-Inbar I, Silverberg SG. Mucosal epithelial proliferation of the fallopian tube: prevalence, clinical associations, and optimal strategy for histopathologic assessment. Int J Gynecol Pathol 2000, **19**: 139–144.

97 Yanai-Inbar I, Siriaunkgul S, Silverberg SG. Mucosal epithelial proliferation of the fallopian tube. A particular association with

ovarian serous tumor of low malignant potential? Int J Gynecol Pathol 1995, **14**: 107–113.

CARCINOMA

98 Alvarado-Cabrero I, Navani SS,Young RH, Scully RE. Tumors of the fimbriated end of the fallopian tube: a clinicopathologic analysis of 20 cases, including nine carcinomas. Int J Gynecol Pathol 1997, **16**: 189–196.

99 Alvarado-Cabrero I, Young RH, Vamvakas EC, Scully RE. Carcinoma of the fallopian tube: a clinicopathological study of 105 cases with observations on staging and prognostic factors. Gynecol Oncol 1999, **72**: 367–379.

100 Baekelandt M, Jorunn Nesbakken A, Kristensen GB, Tropè CG, Abeler VM. Carcinoma of the fallopian tube. Cancer 2000, **89**: 2076–2084.

101 Cheung A, So K, Ngan H, Wong L. Primary squamous cell carcinoma of fallopian tube. Int J Gynecol Pathol 1994, **13**: 92–95.

102 Crum CP, Drapkin R, Kindelberger D, Medeiros F, Miron A, Lee Y. Lessons from BRCA: the tubal fimbria emerges as an origin for pelvic serous cancer. Clin Med Res 2007, **5**: 35–44.

103 Culton LK, Deavers MT, Silva EG, Liu J, Malpica A. Endometrioid carcinoma simultaneously involving the uterus and the fallopian tube: a clinicopathologic study of 13 cases. Am J Surg Pathol 2006, **30**: 844–849.

104 Daya D, Young RH, Scully RE. Endometrioid carcinoma of the fallopian tube resembling an adnexal tumor of probable wolffian origin. A report of six cases. Int J Gynecol Pathol 1992, **11**: 122–130.

105 De la Torre FJ, Rojo F, Garcia A. Clear cells carcinoma of fallopian tubes associated with tubal endometriosis. Case report and review. Arch Gynecol Obstet 2002, **266**: 172–174.

106 Demopoulos RI, Aronov R, Mesia A. Clues to the pathogenesis of fallopian tube carcinoma: a morphological and immunohistochemical case control study. Int J Gynecol Pathol 2001, **20**: 128–132.

107 Eddy GL, Copeland LJ, Gershenson DM, Atkinson EN, Wharton JT, Rutledge FN. Fallopian tube carcinoma. Obstet Gynecol 1984, **64**: 546–552.

108 Euscher ED, Silva EG, Deavers MT, Elishaev E, Gershenson DM, Malpica A. Serous carcinoma of the ovary, fallopian tube, or peritoneum presenting as lymphadenopathy. Am J Surg Pathol 2004, **28**: 1217–1223.

109 Fukunaga M, Fujiwara Y, Naito Z. Hepatoid carcinoma with serous component of the fallopian tube: a case report with immunohistochemical and ultrastructural studies. Int J Gynecol Pathol 2006, **25**: 233–237.

110 Hirai Y, Kaku S, Teshima H, Shimizu Y, Chen JT, Hamada T, Fujimoto I, Yamauchi K, Sakamoto A, Hasumi K, et al. Clinical study of primary carcinoma of the fallopian tube. Experience with 15 cases. Gynecol Oncol 1989, **34**: 20–26.

111 Koshiyama M, Konishi I, Yoshida M, Wang D-P, Mandal M, Mori T, Fuji S. Transitional cell carcinoma of the fallopian tube. A light and electron microscopic study. Int J Gynecol Pathol 1994, **13**: 175–180.

112 Lehto L. Cytology of the human fallopian tube. Acta Obstet Gynecol Scand 1963, **42**(Suppl 14): 1–95.

113 McMurray EH, Jacobs AJ, Perez CA, Camel HM, Kao M-S, Galakatos A. Carcinoma of the fallopian tube. Management and sites of failure. Cancer 1986, **58**: 2070–2075.

114 Navani SS, Alvarado-Cabrero I, Young RH, Scully RE. Endometrioid carcinoma of the fallopian tube: a clinicopathologic analysis of 26 cases. Gynecol Oncol 1996, **63**: 371–378.

115 Podratz KC, Podczaski ES, Gaffey TA, O'Brien PC, Schray MF, Malkasian GD. Primary carcinoma of the fallopian tube. Am J Obstet Gynecol 1986, **154**: 1319–1326.

116 Przybycin CG, Kurman RJ, Ronnett BM, Shih IeM, Vang R. Are all pelvic (nonuterine) serous carcinomas of tubal origin? Am J Surg Pathol 2010 **34**: 1407–1416.

117 Roberts JA, Lifshitz S. Primary adenocarcinoma of the fallopian tube. Gynecol Oncol 1982, **13**: 301–308.

118 Rose PG, Piver MS, Tsukada Y. Fallopian tube cancer. The Roswell Park experience. Cancer 1990, **66**: 2661–2667.

119 Rosenblatt KA, Weiss NS, Schwartz SM. Incidence of malignant fallopian tube tumors. Gynecol Oncol 1989, **35**: 236–239.

120 Salvador S, Gilks B, Köbel M, Huntsman D, Rosen B, Miller C. The fallopian tube: primary site of most pelvic high-grade serous carcinomas. Int J Gynecol Cancer 2009, **19**: 58–64.

121 Schiller HM, Silverberg SG. Staging and prognosis in primary carcinoma of the fallopian tube. Cancer 1971, **28**: 389–395.

122 Takashina T, Ito E, Kudo R. Cytologic diagnosis of primary tubal cancer. Acta Cytol (Baltimore) 1984, **29**: 367–372.

123 Talamo TS, Bender BL, Ellis LD, Scioscia EA. Adenocarcinoma of the fallopian tube. An ultrastructural study. Virchows Arch [A] 1982, **397**: 363–368.

124 Thor AD, Young RH, Clement PB. Pathology of the fallopian tube, broad ligament, peritoneum, and pelvic soft tissues. Hum Pathol 1991, **22**: 856–867.

125 Uehira K, Hashimoto H, Tsuneyoshi M, Enjoji M. Transitional cell carcinoma pattern in primary carcinoma of the fallopian tube. Cancer 1993, **72**: 2447–2456.

126 Voet RL, Lifshitz S. Primary clear cell adenocarcinoma of the fallopian tube. Light microscopic and ultrastructural findings. Int J Gynecol Pathol 1982, **1**: 292–298.

127 Wilcox R, Gwin K, Montag A. The incidence of fallopian tube primaries reaches 15% of all adnexal tumors when standardized grossing protocols are followed. Lab Invest 2009, **89**(Suppl 1): 241A.

128 Young RH. Neoplasms of the fallopian tube and broad ligament: a selective survey including historical perspective and emphasising recent developments. Pathology 2007, **39**: 112–124.

129 Zheng W, Wolf S, Kramer EE, Cox KA, Hoda SA. Borderline papillary serous tumor of the fallopian tube. Am J Surg Pathol 1996, **20**: 30–35.

OTHER TUMORS

130 Alvarado-Cabrero I, Navani SS,Young RH, Scully RE. Tumors of the fimbriated end of the fallopian tube: a clinicopathologic analysis of 20 cases, including nine carcinomas. Int J Gynecol Pathol 1997, **16**: 189–196.

131 Bossuyt V, Medeiros F, Drapkin R, Folkins AK, Crum CP, Nucci MR. Adenofibroma of the fimbria: a common entity that is indistinguishable from ovarian adenofibroma. Int J Gynecol Pathol 2008, **27**: 390–397.

132 Carlson J, Ackerman B, Wheeler J. Malignant mixed mullerian tumor of the fallopian tube. Cancer 1993, **71**: 187–192.

133 Gersell DJ, King TC. Papillary cystadenoma of the mesosalpinx in von Hippel-Lindau disease. Am J Surg Pathol 1988, **12**: 145–149.

134 Gisser SD. Obstructing fallopian tube papilloma. Int J Gynecol Pathol 1986, **5**: 179–182.

135 Griffith LM, Carcangiu ML. Sex cord tumor with annular tubules associated with endometriosis of the fallopian tube. Am J Clin Pathol 1991, **96**: 259–262.

136 Hoda SA, Huvos AG. Struma salpingis associated with struma ovarii. Am J Surg Pathol 1993, **17**: 1187–1189.

137 Horn T, Jao W, Keh PC. Benign cystic teratoma of the fallopian tube [letter to the Editor]. Arch Pathol Lab Med 1983, **107**: 48.

138 Imachi M, Tsukamoto N, Shigematsu T, Watanabe T, Uehira K, Amada S, Umezu T, Nakano H. Malignant mixed Mullerian tumor of the fallopian tube. Report of two cases and review of literature. Gynecol Oncol 1992, **47**: 114–124.

139 Jackson-York GL, Ramzy I. Synchronous papillary mucinous adenocarcinoma of the endocervix and fallopian tubes. Int J Gynecol Pathol 1991, **10**: 394–401.

140 Kanbour AI, Burgess F, Salazar H. Intramural adenofibroma of the fallopian tube light and electron microscopy. Cancer 1973, **31**: 1433–1439.

141 Li S, Zimmerman RL, LiVolsi VA. Mixed malignant germ cell tumor of the fallopian tube. Int J Gynecol Pathol 1999, **18**: 183–185.

142 Mackay B, Bennington JL, Skoglund RW. The adenomatoid tumor. Fine structural evidence for a mesothelial origin. Cancer 1971, **27**: 109–115.

143 Manes JL, Taylor HB. Carcinosarcoma and mixed müllerian tumors of the fallopian tube. Report of four cases. Cancer 1976, **38**: 1687–1693.

144 Mazur MT, Hsueh S, Gersell DJ. Metastases to the female genital tract. Analysis of 325 cases. Cancer 1984, **53**: 1978–1984.

145 Mitsuhashi A, Nagai Y, Suzuka K, Yamazawa K, Nojima T, Nikaido T, Ishikura H, Matsui H, Shozu M. Primary synovial sarcoma in fallopian tube: case report and literature review. Int J Gynecol Pathol 2007, **26**: 34–37.

146 Muntz HG, Rutgers JL, Tarraza HM, Fuller AF Jr. Carcinosarcomas and mixed Mullerian tumors of the fallopian tube. Gynecol Oncol 1989, **34**: 109–115.

147 Riggs JA, Wainer AS, Hahn GA, Farell MD. Extrauterine tubal choriocarcinoma. Am J Obstet Gynecol 1964, **88**: 637–641.

148 Salazar H, Kanbour A, Burgess F. Ultrastructure and observations on the histogenesis of mesotheliomas 'adenomatoid tumors' of the female genital tract. Cancer 1972, **29**: 141–152.

149 Sangoi AR, McKenney JK, Schwartz EJ, Rouse RV, Longacre TA. Adenomatoid tumors of the female and male genital tracts: a clinicopathological and immunohistochemical study of 44 cases. Mod Pathol 2009, **22**: 1228–1235

150 Schwartz EJ, Longacre TA. Adenomatoid tumors of the female and male genital tracts express WT1. Int J Gynecol Pathol 2004, **23**: 123–128.

151 Seidman JD. Mucinous lesions of the fallopian tube. A report of seven cases. Am J Surg Pathol 1994, **18**: 1205–1212.

152 Shen T, Zhuang Z, Gersell DJ, Tavassoli FA. Allelic deletion of VHL gene detected in papillary tumors of the broad ligament, epididymis, and retroperitoneum in von Hippel-Lindau disease patients. Int J Surg Pathol 2001, **8**: 207–212.

153 van Dijk CM, Kooijman CD, van Lindert AC. Malignant mixed mullerian tumor of the fallopian tube. Histopathology 1990, **16**: 300–302.

154 Youngs LA, Taylor HB. Adenomatoid tumors of the uterus and fallopian tube. Am J Clin Pathol 1967, **48**: 537–545.

TUMORS AND TUMORLIKE CONDITIONS OF BROAD AND ROUND LIGAMENTS

155 Ahmed AA, Swan RW, Owen A, Kraus FT, Patrick F. Uterus-like mass arising in the broad ligament: a metaplasia or mullerian duct anomaly? Int J Gynecol Pathol 1998, **16**: 279–281.

156 Altaras MM, Jaffe R, Corduba M, Holtzinger M, Bahary C. Primary paraovarian cystadenocarcinoma. Clinical and management aspects and literature review. Gynecol Oncol 1990, **38**: 268–272.

157 Aslani M, Ahn GH, Scully RE. Serous papillary cystadenoma of borderline malignancy of broad ligament. A report of 25 cases. Int J Gynecol Pathol 1988, **7**: 131–138.

158 Aslani M, Scully RE. Primary carcinoma of the broad ligament. Report of four cases and review of the literature. Cancer 1989, **64**: 1540–1545.

159 Bell DA, Woodruff JM, Scully RE. Ependymoma of the broad ligament. A report of two cases. Am J Surg Pathol 1984, **8**: 203–209.

160 Gardner GH, Greene RR, Peckham B. Tumors of the broad ligament. Am J Obstet Gynecol 1957, **73**: 536–555.

161 Honore LH, Manickavel V. Striated muscle heteroplasia in the uterine round ligament. A report of 30 cases. Arch Pathol Lab Med 1991, **115**: 223–225.

162 Kariminejad MH, Scully RE. Female adnexal tumor of probable wolffian origin. A distinctive pathologic entity. Cancer 1973, **31**: 671–677.

163 Korn WT, Schatzki SC, Di Sciullo AJ, Scully RE. Papillary cystadenoma of the broad ligament in von Hippel–Lindau disease. Am J Obstet Gynecol 1990, **163**: 596–598.

164 Rahilly MA, Williams AR, Krausz T, al Nafussi A. Female adnexal tumour of probable Wolffian origin. A clinicopathological and immunohistochemical study of three cases. Histopathology 1995, **26**: 69–74.

165 Werness BA, Guccion JG. Tumor of the broad ligament in von Hippel–Lindau disease of probable mullerian origin. Int J Gynecol Pathol 1998, **16**: 282–285.

166 Young RH. Neoplasms of the fallopian tube and broad ligament: a selective survey including historical perspective and emphasising recent developments. Pathology 2007, **39**: 112–124.

Ovary

CHAPTER CONTENTS

Normal anatomy

The ovaries are paired pelvic organs located on the sides of the uterus close to the lateral pelvic wall, behind the broad ligament and anterior to the rectum. They are connected to the broad ligament by the mesovarium (a double fold of peritoneum), to the uterine cornu by the ovarian (or utero-ovarian) ligament, and to the lateral pelvic wall by the infundibulopelvic (or suspensory) ligament. During the reproductive period, their average size is 4 × 2 × 1 cm, and their average weight is 5–8 g; after menopause, they shrink to one half or less of this size.

The ovarian lymph vessels drain to large trunks that form a plexus at the hilus, from which they travel through the mesovarium to drain into the para-aortic nodes; others drain into the internal iliac, external iliac, interaortic, common iliac, and inguinal nodes.

The ovary is covered by a single layer of modified mesothelium variously known as *surface, coelomic,* or *germinal epithelium.* This epithelium is immunoreactive for keratin, epithelial membrane antigen (EMA), Ber-EP4, CA-125, desmoplakin, vimentin, estrogen and progesterone receptors, epidermal growth factor, and follicle-stimulating hormone.[3,14] The close embryologic and functional relationship of this structure with the lining epithelium of the müllerian ducts (i.e., the progenitor of the tubal, endometrial, and endocervical mucosa) probably explains the marked similarities among these tissues and the tumors arising from them. Indeed, the entire pelvic and lower abdominal mesothelium and the subjacent mesenchyme of females are referred to as the *secondary müllerian system.* Epithelial inclusions glands/cysts are commonly found in the cortex. Interestingly, although the ovarian surface epithelium is negative for PAX8, the lining cells of the epithelial inclusion glands are typically PAX8 positive.[2]

The *ovarian stroma* is divided into a cortical and a medullary region, but the boundaries between them are indistinct. It is composed mainly of spindle-shaped stromal cells resembling fibroblasts, typically arranged in whorls or a storiform pattern. The cells may contain cytoplasmic lipid and are surrounded by a dense network of reticulin fibers. Some of these cells have myoid ('myofibroblastic') features and exhibit immunoreactivity for smooth muscle actin and desmin.[4,9] Foci of smooth muscle hyperplasia may be found, most often in perimenopausal or postmenopausal women.[5] Metaplastic bone formation can also occur.[7] Other cells that may be found in the ovarian stroma are luteinized stromal cells (singly or in small nests, mainly in the medulla), so-called 'enzymatically active' stromal cells, decidual cells, bundles of smooth muscle, nests of cells resembling endometrial stromal cells, mature fat cells, and neuroendocrine cells.[1,3,6]

The life cycle of the *ovarian follicle* includes primordial, maturing (primary, secondary, tertiary, and graafian), and atretic forms, together with corpora lutea and corpora albicantia for those that have reached full maturation. Primordial follicles contain germ cells that have originated from the yolk sac endoderm and migrated into the ovary, where they develop into oogonia and oocytes.[3] These remain arrested at the dictyate stage of mitotic prophase at the time of birth, entering an interphase period at the time of follicular maturation prior to ovulation. The maturing follicle is composed of the oocyte, the granulosa layer, and the two theca layers. *Granulosa cells* lack a reticulum around them and are immunoreactive for vimentin, keratin, and desmoplakin. They feature small rosettelike formations known as Call–Exner bodies, which contain at their center a deeply eosinophilic filamentous material consisting of excess basal lamina. Whether the granulosa cells derive from the ovarian stroma or from the *sex cords* (structures that first appear beneath the surface epithelium of the gonadal anlage and later converge toward the hilus of the gland) is still unresolved. The stroma-derived *theca cells* form an internal layer (which is typically luteinized) and an external layer (which is very cellular and can simulate a neoplastic process when cut tangentially). Internal theca cells are an important site of sex steroid production, as determined indirectly by the immunohistochemical detection of enzymes involved in steroid hormone biosynthesis.[10,11]

The mature *corpus luteum* is a 1.5–2.5 cm round yellow structure with lobulated outlines and a cystic center. Both the granulosa and the theca cells that form it show prominent luteinization. Morphologic criteria for the dating of the corpus luteum have been established.[12] The corpus luteum of pregnancy is characterized by its larger size, bright yellow color, prominent central cavity, and the presence of hyaline droplets and calcification.[3]

At the ovarian hilus, there are clusters of cells analogous to testicular Leydig cells known as *ovarian hilus cells*. They are closely associated with large hilar veins and lymph vessels and may form nodular protrusions within their lumina. They also exhibit an intimate relationship with the nonmedullated nerves of the region.[3,8] They may contain Reinke crystalloids, lipids, and lipochrome pigment. Hyperplasia of these cells is found following the administration of chorionic gonadotropin, in pregnancy, and in the presence of choriocarcinoma.[3]

The *rete ovarii*, present in the ovarian hilus, represents the ovarian counterpart of the rete testis. It consists of a network of clefts, tubules, cysts, and papillae lined by an epithelium of variable height and surrounded by a cuff of spindle cell stroma. This epithelium is immunoreactive for keratin and CA-125.[13]

Walthard cell nests may be cystic or solid. They are located in the mesovarium, in the adjacent mesosalpinx, or within the ovarian hilus, and have a lining of urothelial appearance (sometimes mucin-producing) which is probably of mesothelial nature.

The previous description mainly pertains to the fully developed ovary in women of child-bearing age. The many modifications exhibited by the prepubertal and postmenopausal ovary are beyond the scope of this chapter. It should be mentioned, however, that prominent cystic follicles are normally seen during the first few months of life and at puberty, and that the shrunken postmenopausal ovary ('ovarium gyratum') has thick-walled medullary and hilar vessels (which should not be mistaken for hemangiomas). These atrophic ovaries may also contain clinically inconsequential granulomas and hyaline scars.[3]

The immunohistochemical profiles of the various cell components of the ovary are discussed in connection with the tumors of the respective structures.

Gonadal dysgenesis

Patients with gonadal dysgenesis have abnormally developed gonads and infantile sexual development. The conditions mentioned here are mainly those associated with an abnormal sex chromosome constitution ('abnormalities in sex determination'), to be distinguished from those such as male and female pseudohermaphroditism, persistent müllerian duct syndrome (due to a defect in the müllerian inhibiting substance system), and end-organ defects[27] ('abnormalities in genital differentiation').[23,29]

Sometimes, gonadal tissue is biopsied or removed in the course of evaluation of these malformations.[30,31]

Klinefelter syndrome is usually characterized by the karyotype 47,XXY, and is further discussed in Chapter 18.

In patients with **gonadal dysgenesis**, either '**pure**' (with a 46,XX or 46,XY karyotype) or associated with the somatic features of **Turner syndrome** (with a 45,XO karyotype), both gonads are represented by a streak of fibrous tissue that vaguely resembles ovarian stroma (Fig. 19.210).[19,32,33] These patients do not seem to have an increased incidence of gonadal tumors,[34] but various types of nongonadal neoplasm (such as atypical polypoid adenomyoma of uterus, leukemia, and soft tissue tumors) have been reported in patients with the syndrome.[16,24] Also, several cases of Turner syndrome have been reported in association with endometrial adenocarcinoma; in some of these, prolonged estrogen therapy had been administered.[22]

In **mixed gonadal dysgenesis** (usually characterized by a 45,X/46,XY or 46,XY phenotype), one gonad is represented by a streak gonad or a streak testis and a contralateral testis (that is typically cryptorchid) or bilateral streak testis.[15] Individuals with this condition are particularly prone to the development of gonadoblastomas, a complication prevented by early removal of the gonads[28] (see p. 1604). The tumors may totally obliterate the testicular elements and thus lead to an incorrect typing of the dysgenesis.

True hermaphrodites may have ovotestes containing both ova and immature seminiferous tubules or other combinations of ovary and testis[17,20,21] (Fig. 19.211). The most common karyotypes are 46,XX (60%), 46,XY (12%), and mosaic (28%). Multiple tumors can occur in these gonads.[26]

The familial syndrome of **testicular feminization** is the most common type of male pseudohermaphroditism. It occurs in individuals with a normal male chromosome constitution with an end-organ defect (androgen insensibility). It is characterized by the presence of several well-developed female secondary sex characteristics. These patients consult a gynecologist because of amenorrhea or sterility. They are found to have a vagina, no uterus, and bilateral cryptorchid testes. The latter often contain nodular masses of immature tubules that should not be confused with Sertoli–Leydig cell tumor[18,25] (Fig. 19.212). The syndrome is of further clinical importance because of the eventual occurrence of malignant tumors in the cryptorchid testes of approximately 9% of these patients. For this reason, the testes should be removed after puberty and

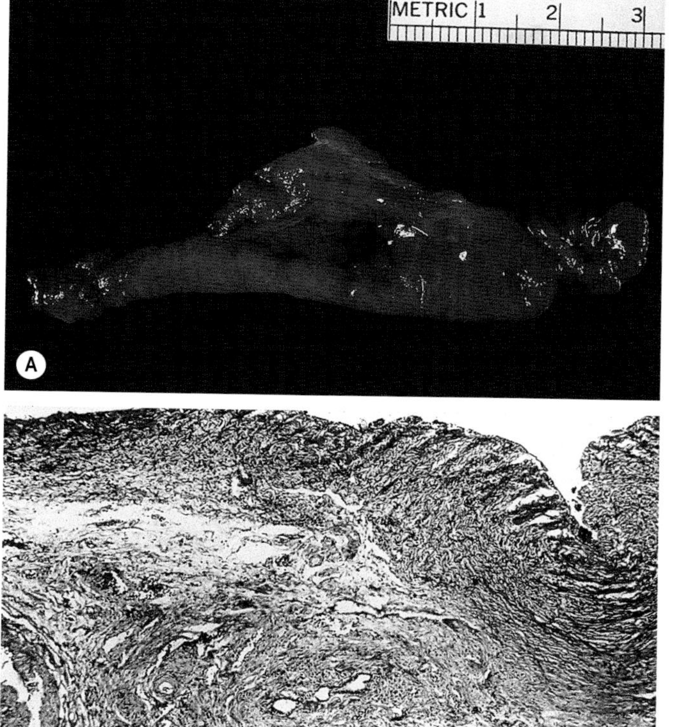

Fig. 19.210 Streak gonad in Turner syndrome: **A**, gross appearance; **B**, microscopic appearance.

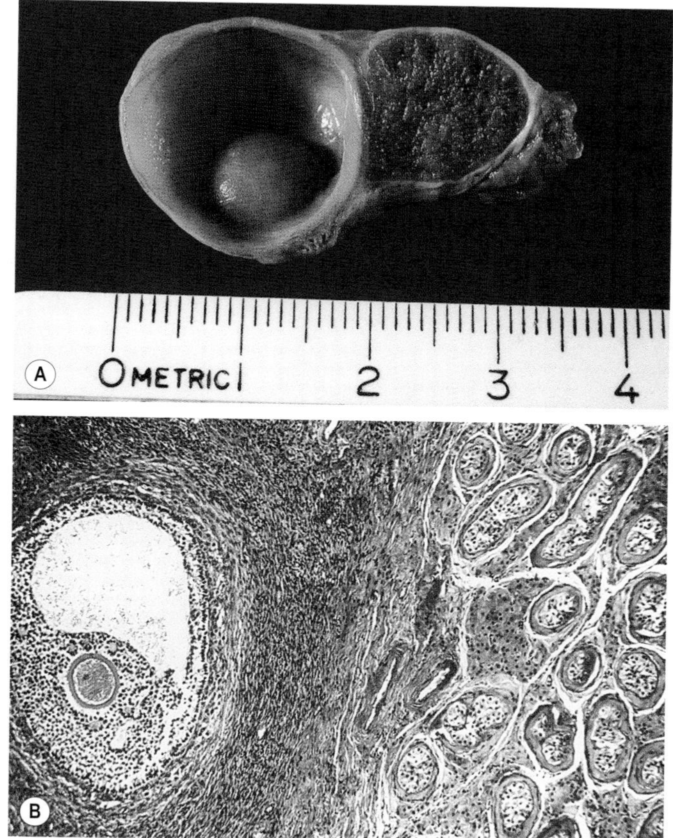

Fig. 19.211 **A** and **B**, Ovotestis in true hermaphroditism. **A**, Gross appearance. The testicular component is represented by the solid nodule, whereas the ovarian component has a largely cystic appearance. **B**, Microscopic appearance of the two components.

supplemental estrogen therapy given. A classification of disorders of sexual development is presented in Table 19.3.

Cysts, stromal hyperplasia, and other non-neoplastic lesions

Ovarian diseases of surgical importance can be broadly divided into non-neoplastic cysts, inflammations, and neoplasms. Non-neoplastic cysts are unfortunately too commonly seen as surgical specimens. It has been said that if the ovaries were located externally, their removal would probably be undertaken with more hesitation. The general surgeon exploring the abdomen may find a mildly cystic or nodular ovary in an otherwise normal abdominal cavity and remove it with the hope that a pathologic process will be found to justify the patient's symptoms and the surgery. More often than not, the microscopic diagnosis will be that of 'cystic follicle' or 'mature corpus luteum', but then it will be too late to replace the organ. Realizing that the ovary is normally a partially cystic structure and that the risk of carcinoma developing in these cystic structures is negligible should help avoid many of these excisions.

Inclusion cysts ('germinal inclusion cysts') are common in older women; they are generally small and multiple and have no clinical significance. Most of them probably arise from invaginations of the surface epithelium, with subsequent loss of the connection with the

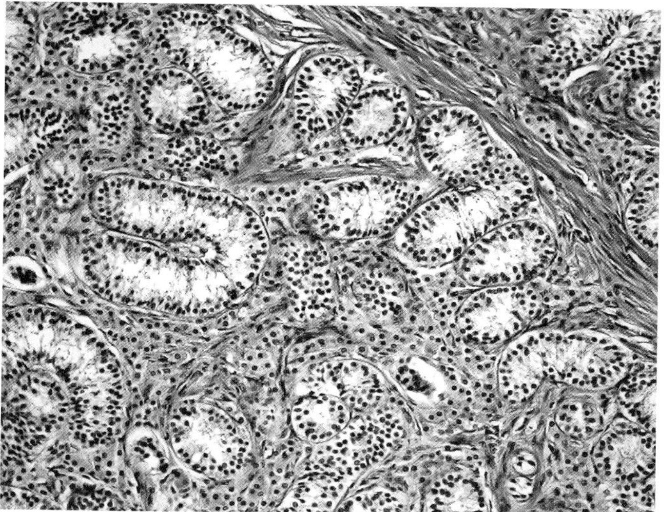

Fig. 19.212 Immature testicular tubules in testicular feminization syndrome.

Table 19.3 Disorders of sexual development[a]

SYNDROME	GONAD	DUCTS	EXTERNAL GENITALIA	PUBERTY	BARR	CHROMOSOMES	FSH	HORMONES 17-KS	ESTROGEN	REMARKS
Klinefelter	Testis with hyalinized sclerotic tubules and clumped Leydig cells	Male	Male	Normal penis with small testes; partial androgen lack	'True' are chromatin positive, a few are 2+ or 3+	All chromatin positive have 2 Xs and a Y in at least some cells. Chromatin negative are 46,YY	↑↑	N or ↑	N	Affects 1:400 newborn males
Turner	Streak gonad with whorled stroma	Female	Female	No pubertal development; rare cases show mild virilization	50% chromatin negative	Second sex chromosome missing or abnormal in some or all of the cells	↑↑	↓	↓	1:7000 newborns, more common in abortuses; short stature
True hermaphrodite	Ovary and testis	All have uterus, most have tubes too, a few have vasa	Ambiguous but 80% favor the male	80% have gynecomastia, 50% menstruate	80% chromatin positive	60% are 46,XX in blood cells only; Y present in most of the others	N	N	N	
Mixed gonadal dysgenesis	Streak plus testis or tumor	Female; vas found occasionally	Vary from female (often with clitoromegaly) to male with hypospadias to normal male	Virilization, sometimes complete; breast development only with tumors	Chromatin negative	Almost all are mosaics including XO stem; many have Y-bearing stem as well	↑	N	?	
Dysgenetic male pseudo-hermaphroditism	Dysgenetic testis	Mixed male and/ or female	Variable virilized	Rarely patients may be fertile	Chromatin negative	Some are XO/XY	↑	N	?	
Familial male pseudo-hermaphroditism that ranges from testicular feminization to	Immature infertile testis	No uterus, ± rudimentary vas	Female with short, blind vagina	Breasts develop but sexual hair is missing	Chromatin negative	46,XY	↑ or N	↑ or N	N	Sex-linked recessive or sex-limited autosomal dominant
Reifenstein syndrome	Infertile testis	Male	Male with hypospadias ± cleft scrotum	Androgen lack is evident in incomplete virilization	Chromatin negative	46,XY	↑ or N	↑ or N	?	
Female pseudo-hermaphroditism										
1. Congenital adrenal hyperplasia	Ovary	Female	Variably virilized	Amenorrhea with virilization	Chromatin positive	46,XX	N	↑↑	N	Autosomal recessive
2. Nonadrenal	Ovary	Female	Variably virilized	Normal	Chromatin positive	46,XX	N	N	N	Consider maternal exposure to progestins or androgens

[a]The summaries under the several headings are necessarily brief; the text should be consulted for details, qualifications, and crucial exceptions.
↑, Increased; ↑↑, markedly increased; ↓, decreased; N, normal.
From Federman DD. Abnormal sexual development. A genetic and endocrine approach to differential diagnosis. Philadelphia, 1967, W.B. Saunders.

surface[39] (Fig. 19.213A). Microscopically, they are lined by a flattened, cuboidal, or columnar epithelium; tubal metaplasia is frequent (Fig. 19.213B). Psammoma bodies may be seen in their lumen or in the adjacent stroma.

Follicular cysts form by distention of developing or atretic follicles and usually do not exceed 10 cm in diameter (Fig. 19.214). It has been proposed that cystic follicular structures be designated as (normal) *cystic follicles* when measuring less than 2.5 cm and as *follicular cysts* when exceeding this diameter. The latter may occur at any age from infancy to menopause and are asymptomatic in the majority of cases. Occasionally, twisting of the pedicle occurs, with the resulting hemorrhagic infarct. In children, the cysts may be seen in conjunction with precocious puberty.[35,75] During reproductive life, they may be associated with endometrial hyperplasia and metrorrhagia.[62] The cyst fluid may contain estrogens.

The cyst wall is lined by theca, with or without an inner granulosa layer (Fig. 19.215). The theca layer is frequently luteinized. The granulosa layer may be luteinized after puberty but not before. **Multiple luteinized follicular cysts** (theca–lutein cysts; hyperreactio luteinalis) are common in cases of hydatidiform mole and choriocarcinoma but also have been seen in twin pregnancies and, exceptionally, in uncomplicated single pregnancies[76] (Fig. 19.216). **Large solitary luteinized follicular cyst** is a rare lesion presenting during pregnancy and puerperium, unaccompanied by endocrine abnormalities. The median diameter of this type of cyst is 25 cm.[43] Marked focal atypia is often seen in the luteinized cells of this lesion.[42]

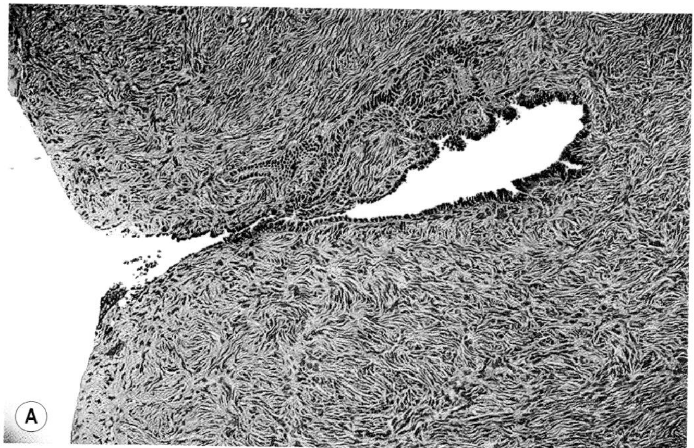

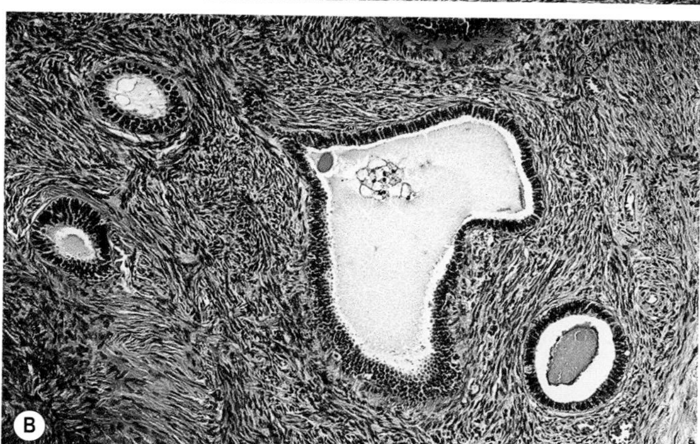

Fig. 19.213 **A** and **B**, Ovarian inclusion cysts. **A**, Cyst being formed through invagination of the surface epithelium. **B**, Multiple inclusion cysts within ovarian cortex. The lining is similar to that of the surface epithelium but tends to be taller and more prominent.

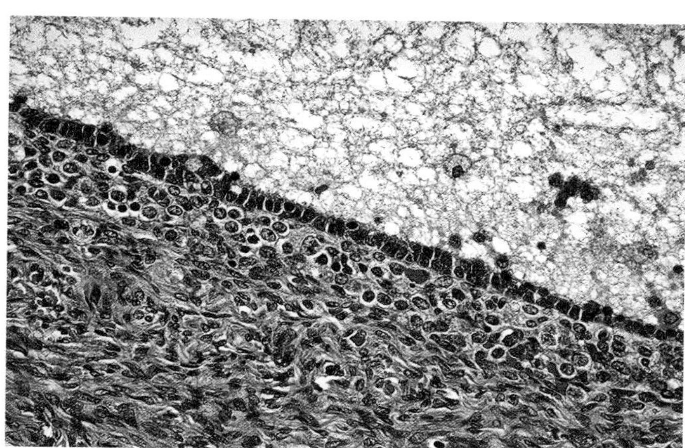

Fig. 19.215 Microscopic appearance of follicular cyst. A single layer of granulosa cells is resting on a thick theca layer.

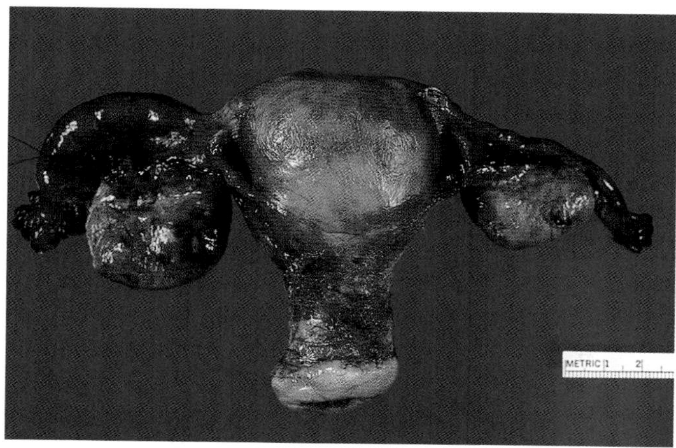

Fig. 19.214 Outer appearance of bilateral ovarian follicular cysts.

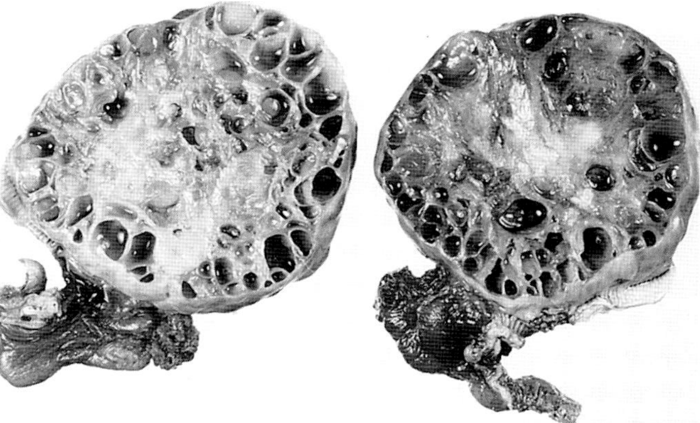

Fig. 19.216 Marked bilateral ovarian enlargement due to multiple theca–lutein cysts associated with normal pregnancy. The changes were misinterpreted as representing neoplasms and both ovaries were excised.

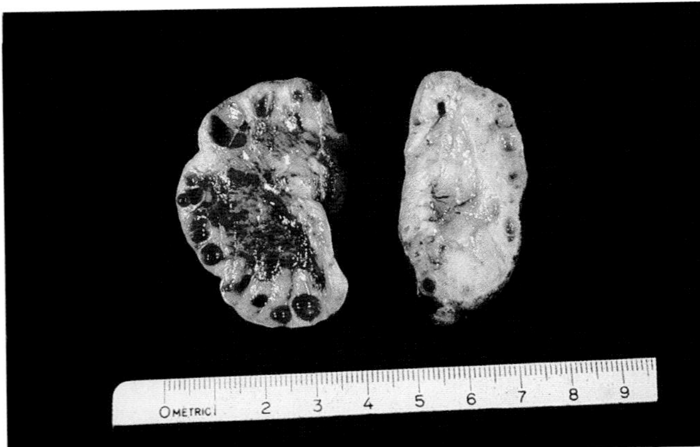

Fig. 19.217 Outer aspect and cut surface of ovary in a patient with Stein–Leventhal syndrome. Note the numerous follicular cysts beneath the ovarian surface and the absence of corpus luteum.

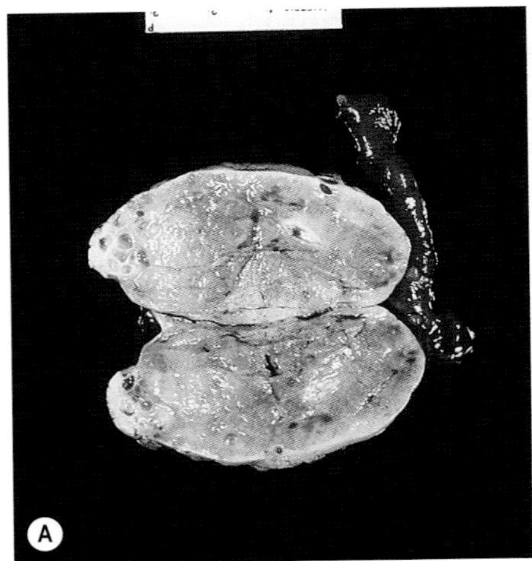

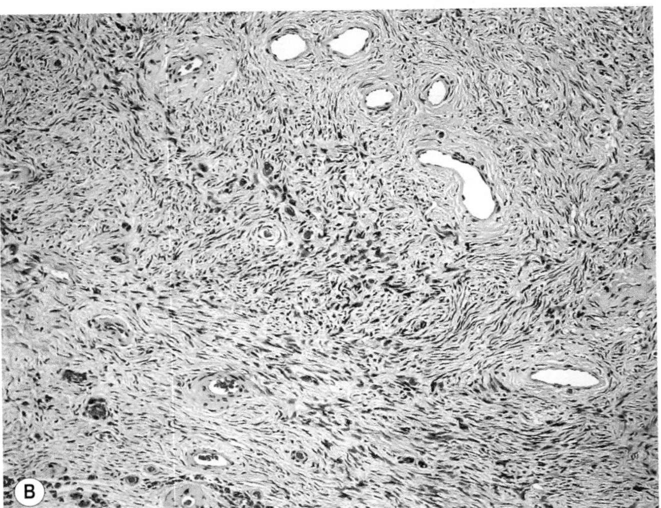

Fig. 19.218 A and **B**, Ovarian stromal hyperplasia. **A**, Gross appearance. The cut surface is solid and has a yellowish hue. **B**, Microscopic appearance. The ovarian stroma is hypercellular and slightly pleomorphic.

Polycystic (sclerocystic) ovaries are characterized by multiple follicular cysts or cystic follicles with varying degrees of luteinization of the theca interna, covered by a dense fibrous capsule[73] (Fig. 19.217). Various clinical syndromes may develop in patients with polycystic ovaries, including Stein–Leventhal syndrome (characterized by amenorrhea and sterility), so-called 'metropathia hemorrhagica' (typically accompanied by endometrial hyperplasia), and frank virilism. These syndromes tend to overlap considerably, as do the pathologic findings.[49] The pathogenesis of Stein–Leventhal syndrome is poorly understood,[53,61] the issue being complicated by the fact that there is no consensus on its definition.[37] Some authors have proposed that it is a genetic disease, based on the occasional familial clustering and the apparently aberrant biochemical and molecular phenotype of the ovarian stromal cells in culture.[57] These patients have 'masculinizing' pituitary and ovarian responses to stimulation by the specific gonadotropin-releasing hormone agonist nafarelin, suggesting that the regulation of the ovarian 17-hydroxylase and C-17,20-lyase activities is abnormal.[38] Dysregulation of 11β-hydroxysteroid dehydrogenase, causing increased oxidation of cortisol to cortisone, has also been documented.[69]

In general, the ovaries of patients with Stein–Leventhal syndrome have the features of polycystic ovaries just described. Corpora lutea and corpora albicantia are almost always absent. Residua of atretic follicles should not be misinterpreted as corpora albicantia. Rarely, typical polycystic ovaries associated with the clinical features of the Stein–Leventhal syndrome have been found associated with congenital adrenal hyperplasia and ovarian neoplasms.[58,60,78] Polycystic ovaries have also been observed in association with primary hypothyroidism.[59]

Most patients with Stein–Leventhal syndrome will respond favorably, with restoration of the menstrual cycle, to medical treatment with cortisone or clomiphene citrate.[61] Recently, metformin (an oral hypoglycemic agent) has been advocated because of the frequent association of polycystic ovaries with hyperinsulinemia.[36] Wedge resection of the ovary, regarded for many years as the standard therapy for this condition, is rarely if ever carried out nowadays. The endometrium of patients with Stein–Leventhal syndrome is usually hyperplastic, sometimes markedly so. Exceptionally, an endometrial carcinoma develops against this background, the tumor being typically well-differentiated and superficial.[45,72]

Stromal hyperplasia is characterized by a diffuse or nodular proliferation of plump ovarian cortical stromal cells encroaching on the medulla.[40] Patchy luteinization of these cells may be present; when extensive, terms such as *(stromal) hyperthecosis, diffuse thecomatosis*, or *stromal luteinization* have been employed (Fig. 19.218). Stromal luteomas and thecomas may develop against this background (see p. 1596). Hyperthecosis may be associated with estrogenic or androgenic effects, obesity, hypertension, and an abnormal glucose tolerance test or even frank diabetes. The onset of symptoms may be abrupt, thus simulating a virilizing ovarian tumor. Immunohistochemical studies have shown androgen production by the luteinized stromal cells, suggesting that estrogenic effects in these cases are mediated through peripheral aromatization of these androgens.[71]

The boundaries between polycystic disease and stromal hyperplasia are ill-defined[54,73] (Fig. 19.219). However, typical stromal hyperplasia lacks cysts and is usually more refractory to therapy.

Corpus luteum cysts are single and usually less than 6 cm in diameter. They may develop at the end of the menstrual cycle or may occur in pregnancy (Fig. 19.220). The cyst wall is composed of luteinized granulosa and theca cell layers. Hyaline bodies and foci of calcification may be found in the cysts associated with

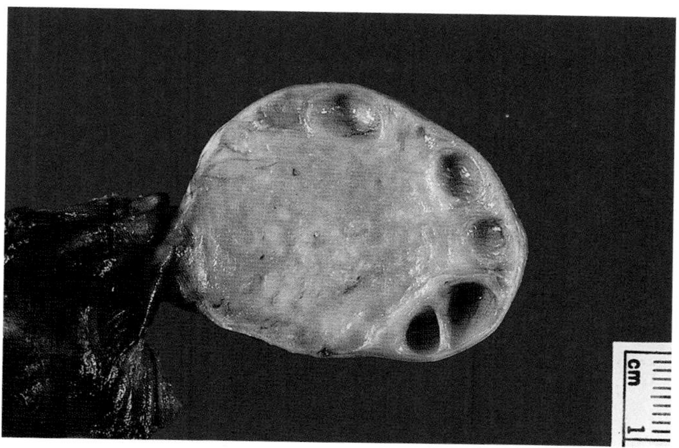

Fig. 19.219 Ovary showing a combination of multiple follicular cysts and stromal hyperplasia, providing support for a pathogenetic link between the two processes.

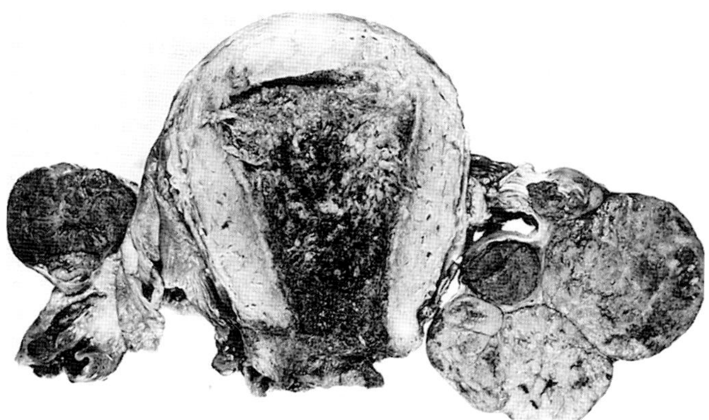

Fig. 19.221 Bilateral pregnancy luteomas in a 29-year-old woman that were discovered incidentally at the time of cesarean section performed for cord prolapse. The tumors bled excessively on manipulation by the surgeon and had to be removed.

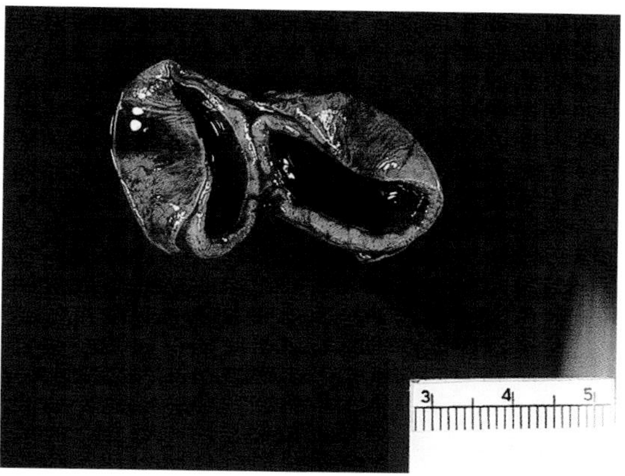

Fig. 19.220 Gross appearance of corpus luteum cyst. The luminal content is typically hemorrhagic.

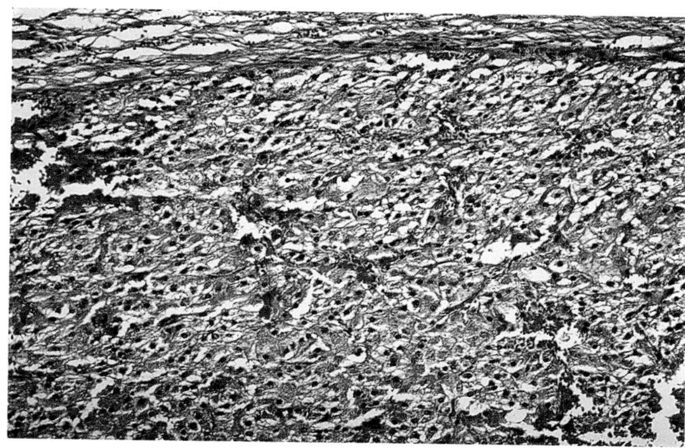

Fig. 19.222 Solid growth pattern of pregnancy luteoma.

pregnancy. The fluid content is often bloody. If the cyst ruptures, hemorrhage into the peritoneal cavity occurs (sometimes over 500 ml), and an erroneous diagnosis of ruptured ectopic pregnancy may be made.[50] It should be remembered that the corpus luteum is normally a cystic structure. The arbitrary diameter of 2.5 cm has been proposed to distinguish the (normal) *cystic corpus luteum* from a *corpus luteum cyst*, in a manner analogous to that employed for follicle-related cystic formations.

Ectopic decidual reaction can occur in the ovary during pregnancy and occasionally even in the absence of current or recent pregnancy. A functioning corpus luteum that has undergone destruction is present in most instances.[67]

So-called **luteomas of pregnancy** are yellow or orange solid nodules that may reach sizable proportions[42] (Fig. 19.221). They have been typically encountered during cesarean section in multiparous women, sometimes accompanied by a mild degree of virilization.[47,66] If these cysts are left undisturbed, they will regress after delivery.[74] Microscopically, the lesions are composed of masses of uniform theca–lutein cells (Fig. 19.222). Occasionally, there is an associated granulosa cell proliferation.[68] Ultrastructurally, the proliferating cells exhibit abundant smooth endoplasmic reticulum, dispersed Golgi apparatus, and tubular cristae in the mitochondria, in keeping with their function as steroid hormone-producing cells.[46] All of the reported lesions have been benign. It is reasonable to regard them as nodular hyperplasias of theca–lutein cells rather than true neoplasms.[66] If pregnancy luteoma is correctly identified by frozen section biopsy, no further surgery is necessary.

Developmental cysts derived from wolffian (mesonephric) and müllerian (paramesonephric) remnants are common in the region of the ovarian hilus. These are discussed on page 1554. Suffice it to say here that, according to some authors, it is possible to distinguish these two types of tissue – and sometimes the cysts derived from them – on microscopic grounds.[48] Wolffian structures are lined by cuboidal, predominantly nonciliated epithelium resting on a well-developed basement membrane; müllerian formations are lined by generally taller, ciliated and nonciliated epithelium with larger nuclei and resting on an inconspicuous basement membrane. Both may have a smooth muscle coat. According to these criteria and some ultrastructural differences,[41] **hydatids of Morgagni** (pedunculated cysts at the fimbriated end of the fallopian tube) are believed to be of müllerian origin, whereas most **parovarian** and **paratubal cysts** (in the tubo-ovarian ligament) and **Gartner duct cysts** (in the vaginal wall) are thought to arise from wolffian remnants.

Cysts of the rete ovarii are characterized by a hilar position, an epithelial lining of variable height that is usually nonciliated, crevices along the inner surfaces, and a fibromuscular wall that

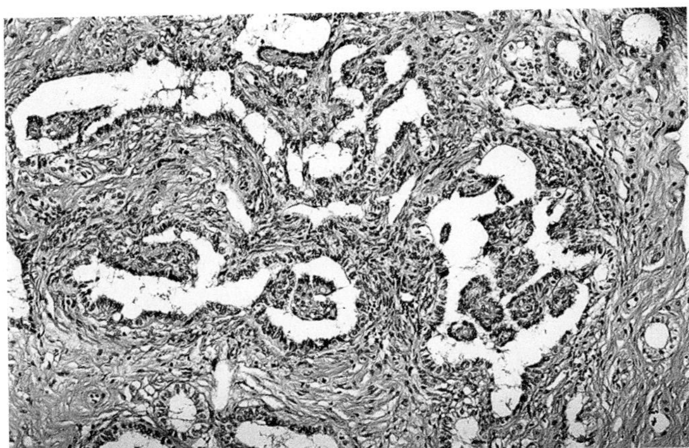

Fig. 19.223 Benign hyperplastic changes in rete ovarii. This alteration is of no clinical significance.

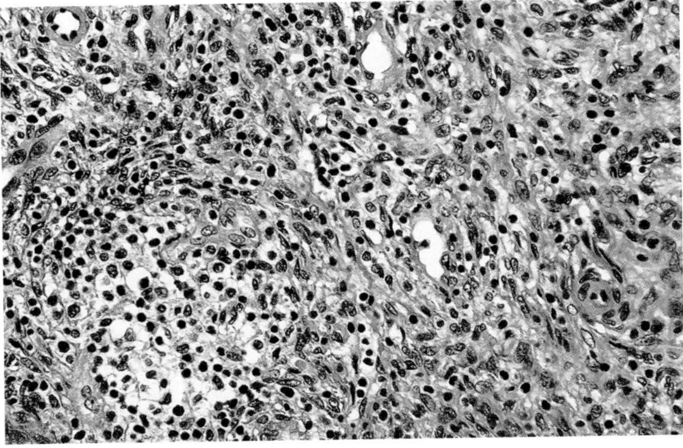

Fig. 19.224 Lymphocytic and plasmacytic infiltrate of ovary in oophoritis. This process is thought to have an autoimmune basis.

often contains hyperplastic hilus cells.[70] The rete ovarii may also be the site of benign proliferative lesions that have been variously reported as adenomatous hyperplasia[51] and adenoma[65] (see p. 1554) (Fig. 19.223).

Epidermoid cysts, exceptionally rare, are thought to be related to Walthard cell nests, but some may well represent mature monodermal teratomas.[44,64,77] (see also p. 1590).

Squamous metaplasia of the ovarian surface epithelium accompanied by subjacent fibrosis has been described in patients on long-term peritoneal dialysis.[52]

Amyloidosis can exceptionally present in the form of bilateral ovarian masses.[63]

Supernumerary ovaries are extremely rare.[55] Most of the reported cases have measured less than 1 cm. They should be distinguished from **accessory ovaries**, which are small portions of ovarian tissue situated near – and sometimes connected to – the normally placed organ.[56]

Inflammation

Nonspecific inflammation of the ovary usually spreads from the endometrium and is practically always associated with tubal involvement. A large, loculated cystic mass filled with pus or secretion is often the result, the ovarian stroma forming part of the cystic wall (tubo-ovarian abscess or cyst). Exceptionally, a solid mass rich in foamy macrophages develops in long-standing cases (*'xanthogranulomatous oophoritis'*).[82,88]

Granulomatous infections such as tuberculosis occur in the ovary. Invariably this is hematogenous in origin and often also involves the tube and endometrium. In time, the infection may subside and leave a large tubo-ovarian cystic mass. Other infectious agents responsible for granulomatous oophoritis are *Actinomyces* (particularly common after the introduction of intrauterine devices), *Schistosoma*, and *Enterobius vermicularis*. Rarely, *sarcoidosis* and *Crohn disease* involve the ovary, the latter as a result of direct extension from the bowel. *Foreign body granulomas* can occur in the ovarian surface secondarily to talc, cornstarch, carbon pigment (at the site of fulguration surgery),[89] other foreign materials,[87] and keratin; the latter may originate from a ruptured ovarian cystic teratoma or may have spilled through the fallopian tube from an endometrial adenoacanthoma.[85] *Palisading granulomas* of unknown etiology have also been reported, most of them in patients with previous pelvic surgery.[83]

Autoimmune oophoritis is a poorly understood disorder characterized microscopically by lymphocytic and plasma cell infiltration in relation to developing follicles but not primordial follicles[81,90] (Fig. 19.224). It results in primary ovarian failure with either primary or secondary amenorrhea.[79] Many of the reported cases have been associated with adrenal failure (Addison disease), hypothyroidism, or both conditions.[79,84]

Eosinophilic perifolliculitis is characterized by a predominantly eosinophilic infiltrate around the follicles; it is not clear how this rare disorder relates to autoimmune oophoritis.[86]

Giant cell arteritis occasionally involves the ovary of elderly women; it may occur as an isolated finding (most frequently) or as a component of generalized giant cell arteritis.[80]

Endometriosis

The ovary is the most common site of endometriosis, as defined by the presence of endometrial glands *and* stroma outside the uterus (see p. 1484).[103] Several pathogenetic mechanisms have been suggested,[107] an interesting recent finding along these lines being the clonal nature of the epithelial cells in this condition.[100] Ovarian endometriosis is usually associated with infertility, and it remains active during the child-bearing years.[96,109] Pain associated with the menstrual cycle is the most common symptom; infrequently, the disease is complicated by massive ascites or perforation into the peritoneal cavity.[106] Grossly, it usually presents as small, slightly raised, blueberry-like spots on the ovarian surface, often accompanied by fibrous adhesions. In cases with extensive involvement, the entire ovary may be converted into a 'chocolate cyst' as a result of repeated hemorrhages (Fig. 19.225). Microscopically, the typical lesions are composed of endometrial glands, endometrial stroma, and fresh and old (hemosiderin-containing) hemorrhagic foci (Fig. 19.226).[92] The endometrial stroma is responsible for the bleeding; it has cells with a 'naked nucleus' surrounded by reticulin and typical spiral arterioles, in conjunction with old and recent hemorrhage. Unfortunately, this diagnostic combination of findings is not always present. The more advanced the endometrial lesion, the more difficult the diagnosis and the greater the number of sections required to make it. Not infrequently, the repeated hemorrhages have totally destroyed the endometrial tissue, the cyst being lined by several layers of hemosiderin-laden macrophages. Under these circumstances, the most the pathologist can do is to report the case as a hemorrhagic cyst and comment that the changes are 'consistent' with those of endometriosis. Sometimes, the lesion is entirely composed of *necrotic pseudoxanthomatous nodules*, to be distinguished from infectious granulomas and necrotic neoplasms[94] (Fig. 19.227). Other morphologic variations of endometriosis include the formation of Liesegang rings,[105] stromal elastosis,[93] and smooth muscle hyperplasia,[97] the latter sometimes resulting in the formation of uterus-like masses (see p. 1486).[104]

The ectopic endometrial tissue of endometriosis is subject to most of the influences that affect the intrauterine endometrium. Consequently, it may be the site of reactive atypia (sometimes referred to as 'atypical endometriosis'),[91,95,99,101] hyperplasia and metaplasia[98] (Fig. 19.228), and malignancy, of which endometrioid carcinoma is the most common form[108] (see p. 1570). Interestingly, p53 is absent in the epithelial cells of benign uncomplicated endometriotic cysts but present in about one-half of the carcinomas arising from them as well as in the adjacent, morphologically non-neoplastic epithelium.[102]

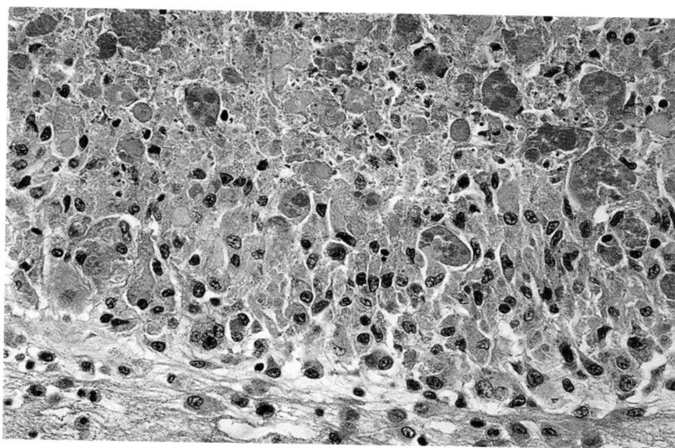

Fig. 19.227 Necrotic nodule surrounded by histiocytes in pelvic endometriosis.

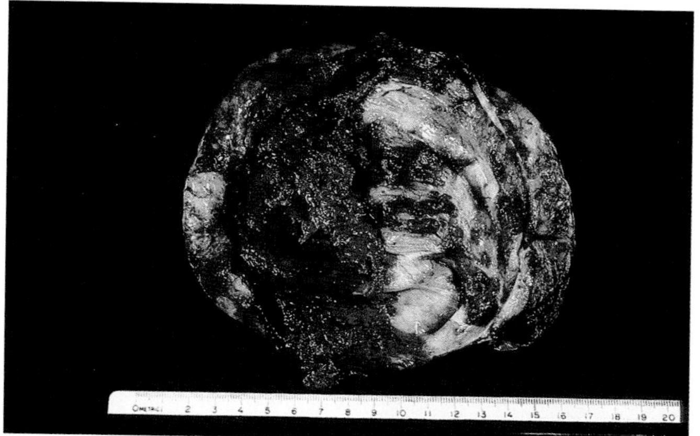

Fig. 19.225 Inner surface of cyst in a case of ovarian endometriosis. The color is typically brown.

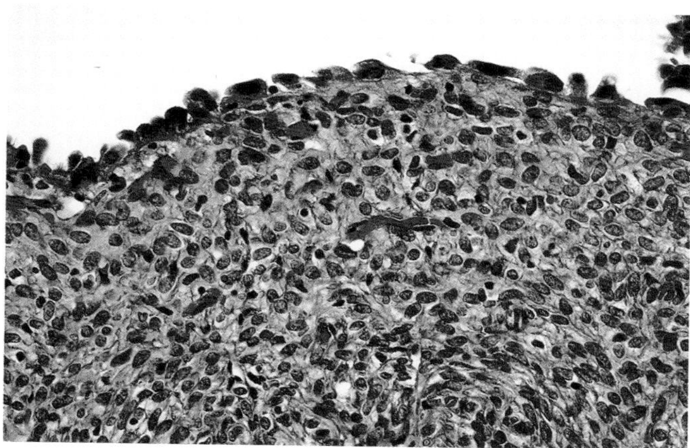

Fig. 19.228 Reactive changes in the lining of an ovarian endometriotic cyst. This change is sometimes referred to as 'atypical endometriosis'.

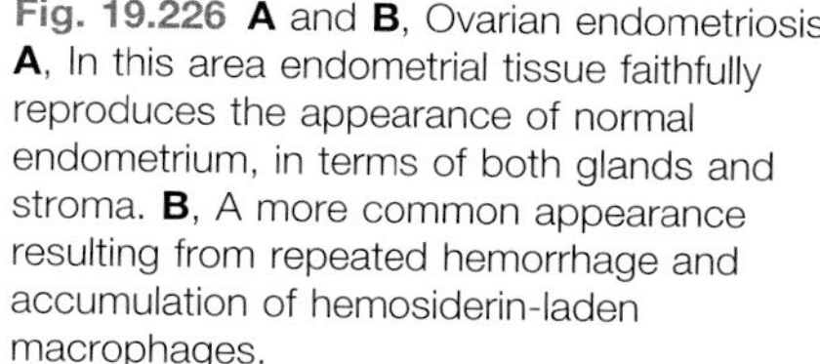

Fig. 19.226 **A** and **B**, Ovarian endometriosis. **A**, In this area endometrial tissue faithfully reproduces the appearance of normal endometrium, in terms of both glands and stroma. **B**, A more common appearance resulting from repeated hemorrhage and accumulation of hemosiderin-laden macrophages.

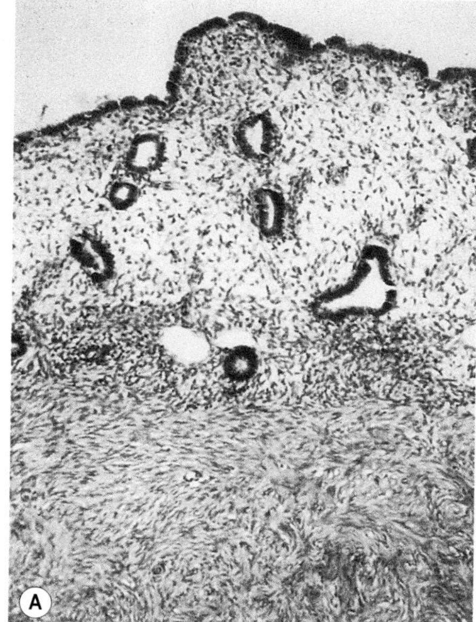

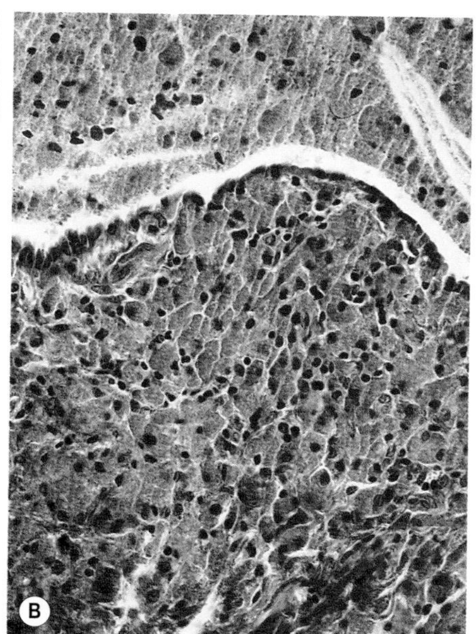

Ovarian biopsy

Ovarian biopsy obtained by either laparotomy or surgical culdoscopy used to be carried out for the evaluation of selected patients with amenorrhea and sterility resulting from anovulation. The specimen, which roughly corresponded to about one-fifth of the organ, was evaluated for the presence and quantity of follicles, evidence of ovulation (corpora lutea and albicantia), and the character of the stroma.[113,114]

Mori[110] attempted to correlate the morphologic findings in the ovarian biopsy with a series of endocrinologic analyses. He found that the ovaries of patients with hypergonadotropic ovarian failure contained no follicles, whereas in those of patients with normogonadotropic or hypogonadotropic ovarian failure, many developing follicles were present. The results were somewhat different in the series of 19 patients reported by Russell et al.,[112] all of whom had premature (before 35 years of age) hypergonadotropic ovarian failure. There were 14 cases classified as premature menopause, characterized by the absence of primordial follicles; three designated as 'resistant ovary syndrome', having primordial follicles but little or no follicular development; and two cases of chronic – presumably autoimmune – oophoritis, characterized by a granulomatous reaction centered in the theca of the developing follicles.

Nowadays, ovarian biopsies are rarely if ever performed in infertile women with a normal karyotype. The reasons for this reluctance are the realization that they do not provide additional significant data and may actually provide misleading information (i.e., cases with no oocytes in the biopsy in which the patients eventually become pregnant), and the fact that affected patients generally require estrogen replacement regardless of the results of the biopsy.[111] Ovarian biopsy can, however, be useful to identify patients with premature ovarian failure when the ovarian reserve is likely to be altered.[115]

Tumors

Classification

The classification of ovarian tumors is primarily morphologic but is intended to reflect current concepts of embryogenesis and histogenesis of this complex organ.[116–122] Since many of these concepts are still controversial, it should be viewed as a working compromise, subject to changes and improvements. It is based on the premise that the ovary contains four major types of tissue, all of which can give rise to a variety of neoplasms, often combined:

1 Surface, coelomic, or germinal epithelium
2 Germ cells
3 Sex cords
4 Ovarian stroma, specialized and nonspecific.

Surface epithelial tumors

Surface epithelial tumors, numerically the most important group of neoplasms, have traditionally been thought to derive from the epithelium that normally lines the outer aspect of the ovary, variously referred to as *surface, coelomic, or germinal*.[125] This epithelium is continuous with the mesothelium that covers the peritoneal cavity, representing a modification of it and sharing with it a common origin and many morphologic features.[126] Some authors have gone as far as suggesting that ovarian tumors arising from this structure should be regarded as mesotheliomas, a proposal that has not met with acceptance, since clearcut immunohistochemical (expression of hormone receptors and many other markers),[124,128,141] ultrastructural,[142] and biologic differences between ovarian surface epithelium and extraovarian peritoneal mesothelium exist.[124,128,130] Furthermore, ovarian epithelial tumors differ significantly as a group from peritoneal mesotheliomas on morphologic and behavioral grounds, these differences being highlighted by two rare but notable occurrences: the ovarian tumor with a bona fide mesotheliomatous appearance[123] and the existence of intra-abdominal extraovarian malignancies having more resemblance to ovarian carcinomas than to peritoneal mesotheliomas (see p. 1579 and Chapter 26).

The ovarian surface epithelium, when involved in metaplastic or neoplastic conditions, often undergoes a 'müllerian differentiation'; as a result, it may produce any of the adult structures formed by the müllerian ducts, including tubal, endometrial, and endocervical mucosa, singly or in combination.[132,145] This plasticity is also evident at the immunohistochemical level.[150]

It has been suggested that the majority of surface tumors of the ovary arise not from the outer epithelium itself, but rather from the portion of this epithelium that has invaginated to produce surface epithelial glands and cysts. This is supported by some immunohistochemical similarities,[140] the overexpression of P53,[135] and the occasional finding of atypical proliferation (dysplasia) or carcinoma in situ in these structures.[134,147] Ovarian endometriosis may also give rise to these tumors, but this is probably true for only a small minority of them, even if they are of endometrioid type.

Yet another proposed origin of some ovarian epithelial tumors (particularly of the serous type), which is being hotly discussed at present, is the epithelium of the tubal fimbriae and related primary or secondary müllerian epithelium surrounding the ovary.[129,136,143,146] Features that have been advanced to support this alternative are the expression of PAX2,[149] the occasional coexistence of a dominant ovarian mass with serous tubal intraepithelial carcinoma,[144] and the fact that the fimbriae are the most common site of early serous carcinoma in women with *BRAC* mutations.[137]

Surface epithelial ovarian tumors are classified according to the following parameters:

1 Cell type: serous, mucinous, endometrioid, etc.
2 Pattern of growth: cystic, solid, surface
3 Amount of fibrous stroma
4 Atypia and invasiveness: benign, borderline, and malignant.

On the basis of these criteria, the various types discussed in the subsequent sections have been identified. In addition, various groupings of these individual tumor types have been proposed, with potential biologic and therapeutic implications.[148] One such scheme (slightly modified), is that proposed by Gilks:[133]

1 High-grade serous, high-grade endometrioid, and undifferentiated carcinomas, and carcinosarcomas/malignant mixed müllerian tumors
2 Low-grade serous carcinomas and serous borderline tumors (including the seromucinous tumors)
3 Mucinous carcinomas and mucinous borderline tumors of intestinal type
4 Low-grade endometrioid carcinomas and endometrioid borderline tumors
5 Clear cell carcinomas
6 Transitional cell carcinomas.

Another attractive scheme recently proposed by Kurman et al.[138,139] is the following:

- *Type I tumors*: slow growing, generally confined to the ovary at the time of diagnosis, and developing from well-established precursor lesions known as 'borderline tumors'. They comprise low-grade micropapillary serous carcinoma, mucinous, endometrioid, and clear cell carcinomas, and malignant Brenner tumor.

- *Type II tumors*: rapidly growing, highly aggressive neoplasms for which well-defined precursor lesions have not been identified. These include high-grade serous carcinoma, undifferentiated carcinoma, and malignant mixed müllerian tumor.

The corollary of this proposal is that types I and II tumors develop independently, although exceptions occur.[131]

Thorough sampling is essential to carry out these important determinations. It has been suggested that one block should be taken for every 1–2 cm of maximum tumor diameter.[127] The selection of the site of sampling is actually more important than the total number of blocks: solid foci, areas adjacent to the ovarian surface, and the base of the papillary formations need to be studied with particular care.

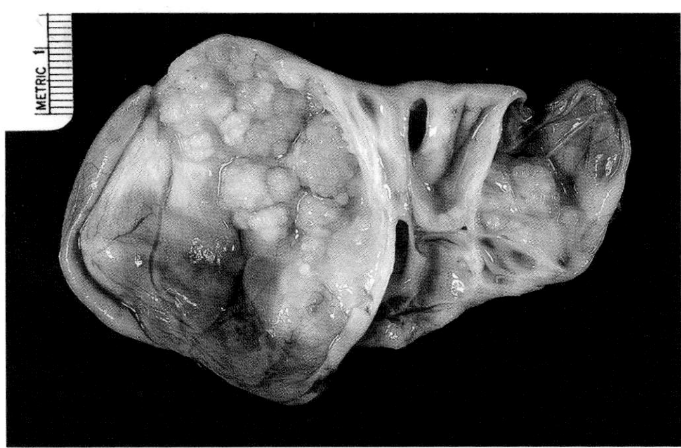

Fig. 19.230 Inner aspect of serous cystadenoma showing papillary structures protruding within.

Serous tumors

Serous tumors make up about one-fourth of all ovarian tumors. Most cases occur in adults. Approximately 30–50% are bilateral; molecular studies in these cases support the theory of a clonal origin.[226] Grossly, the better differentiated tumors consist of cystic masses, usually unilocular, containing a clear but sometimes viscous fluid (Fig. 19.229). Papillary formations are often present, most of them protruding into the cavity but some occasionally occur on the outer surface (Fig. 19.230). The more malignant tumors tend to be solid and invasive, with areas of necrosis and hemorrhage (Fig. 19.231).

Microscopically, cuboidal to columnar cells are seen lining the wall of the cysts and the papillae in the better differentiated tumors (Fig. 19.232). They are similar to normal tubal epithelium at both a light and electron microscopic level.[176] Hobnail cells can be present, not to be taken as evidence of the presence of a clear cell carcinoma component.[213] In approximately 30% of cases, calcific concretions with concentric laminations (psammoma bodies) are present. Ultrastructural studies suggest that the formation of these psammoma bodies is initiated intracellularly in association with autophagocytosis.[177]

A morphologic spectrum of proliferation exists in these tumors. At one end is the benign **serous cystadenoma**, in which the cysts and the papillae (if present, in which case the tumor is called *serous papillary cystadenoma*) are lined by a single layer of cells, without

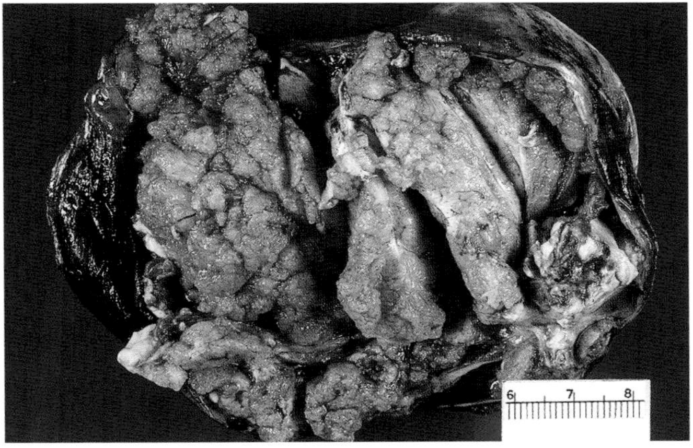

Fig. 19.231 Serous cystadenocarcinoma. The tumor is predominantly solid, with necrotic and hemorrhagic areas.

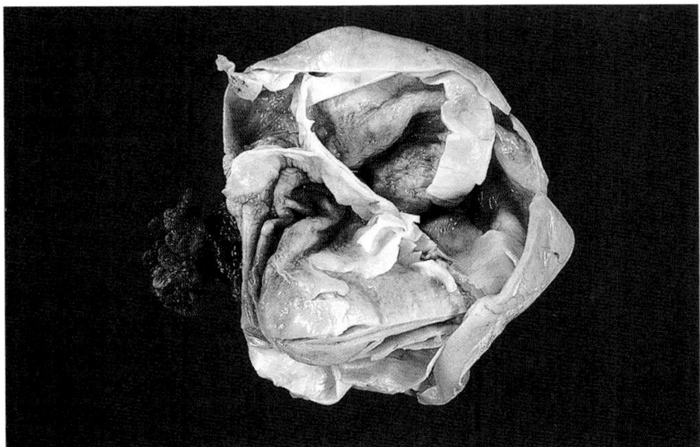

Fig. 19.229 Smooth outer and inner surfaces of the cystic formations in a case of ovarian serous cystadenoma.

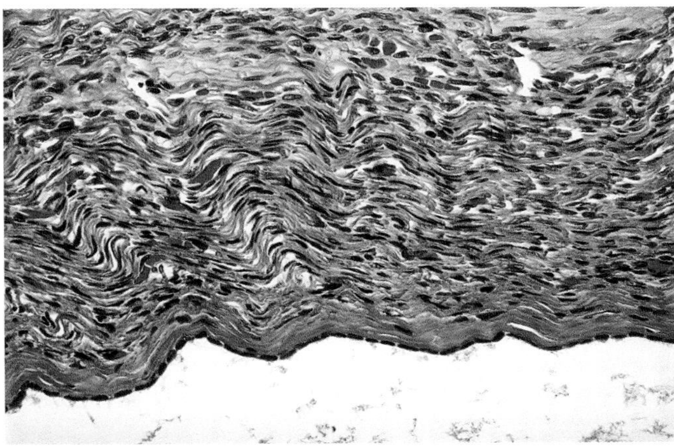

Fig. 19.232 Single layer of bland-looking epithelial cells lining one of the cystic structures of a serous cystadenoma.

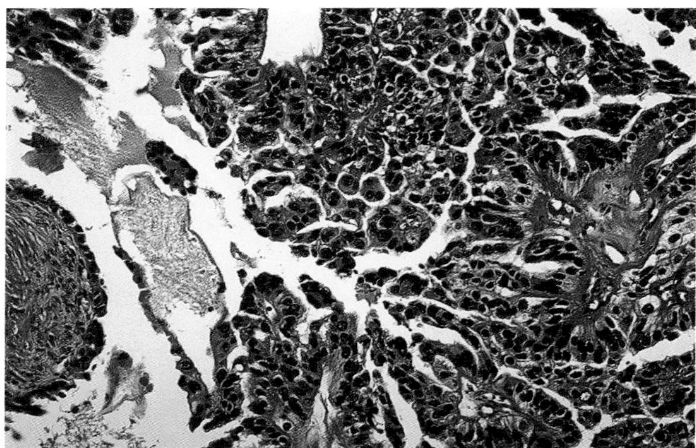

Fig. 19.233 Serous cystadenocarcinoma. The tumor has a complex papillary architecture and a high nuclear grade.

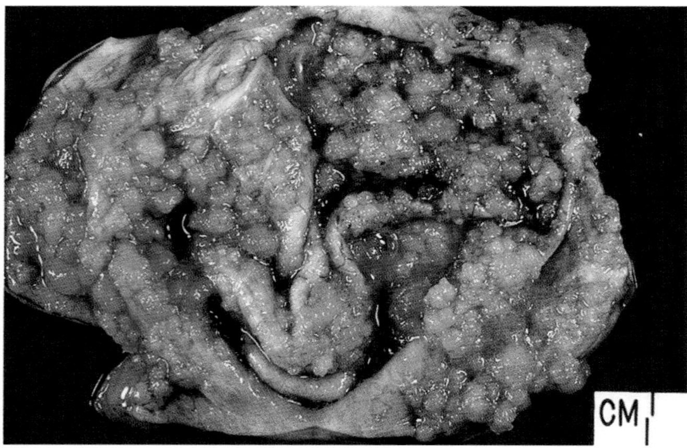

Fig. 19.234 Inner aspect of an ovarian borderline serous neoplasm. Numerous papillary projections facing the lumen can be appreciated.

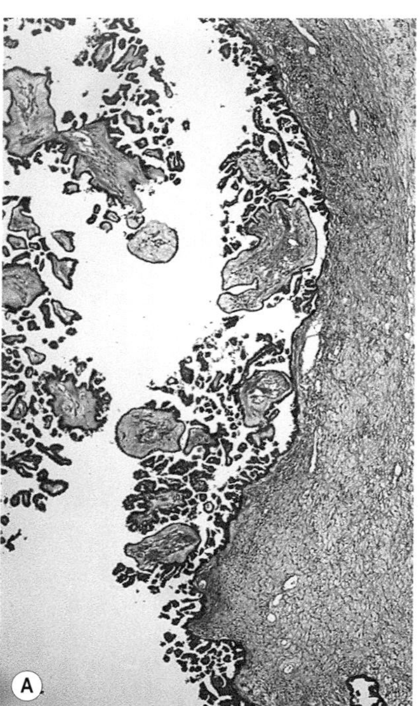

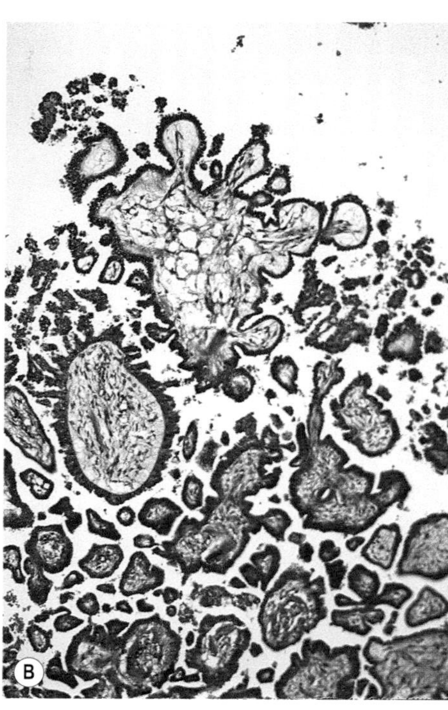

Fig. 19.235 Low- and medium-power appearance of ovarian borderline serous neoplasm. The growth is entirely exophytic.

atypia, architectural complexity, or invasion (see Fig. 19.232). At the other end are the **serous (papillary) adenocarcinoma** and the variant **serous (papillary) cystadenocarcinoma**, characterized by nuclear atypia, high mitotic activity, stratification, glandular complexity, branching papillary fronds, and *stromal invasion* (Fig. 19.233). In between are tumors showing some or all of the features associated with carcinoma but *lacking* definite stromal invasion, i.e., irregular or destructive stromal infiltration by small glands or sheets of cells[166,237] (Figs 19.234 and 19.235) (but see below). These tumors – known as **borderline, indeterminate, intermediate, of low malignant potential**, or **possibly malignant** – make up approximately 15% of all serous tumors.[156,173,185,199,227] It is important to separate them from the obviously invasive tumors because of their vastly better prognosis.[193] The outcome is even more favorable (as a matter of fact, no different from that of cystadenoma) when the 'borderline' features are present only focally in an otherwise benign tumor (*'cystadenomas with focally proliferative areas'*).[193] It should be pointed out that the decision as to whether an ovarian serous neoplasm is of malignant or borderline nature should be made purely on the basis of the morphologic features of the primary tumor, regardless of whether or not peritoneal lesions, lymph node metastases, or even lung deposits exist.[217,234] Allegedly, there are differences in nuclear features between these two tumor types that can be appreciated in a more consistent and reproducible fashion by the use of computerized interactive morphometric analysis.[187,197]

The additional proposal has been made that tumors should still be placed into the borderline category even if they show foci of stromal microinvasion, as long as they are otherwise typical of that category. The microinvasive foci may appear as individual cells, as clusters of cells with abundant eosinophilic cytoplasm ('eosinophilic metaplastic cells'), as small confluent nests with a

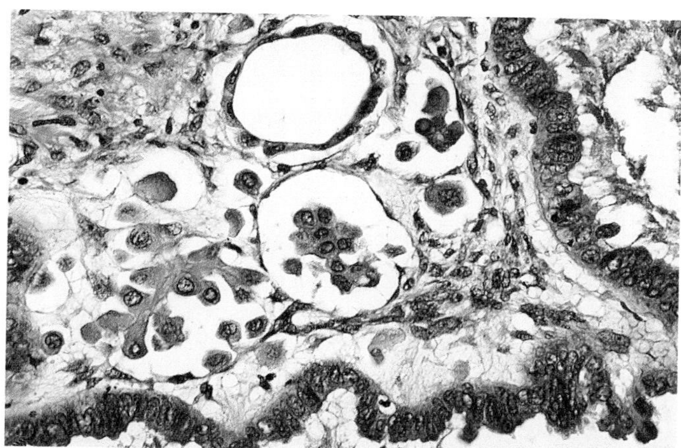

Fig. 19.236 Borderline serous neoplasm with foci of microinvasion represented by clusters of cells with abundant eosinophilic cytoplasm.

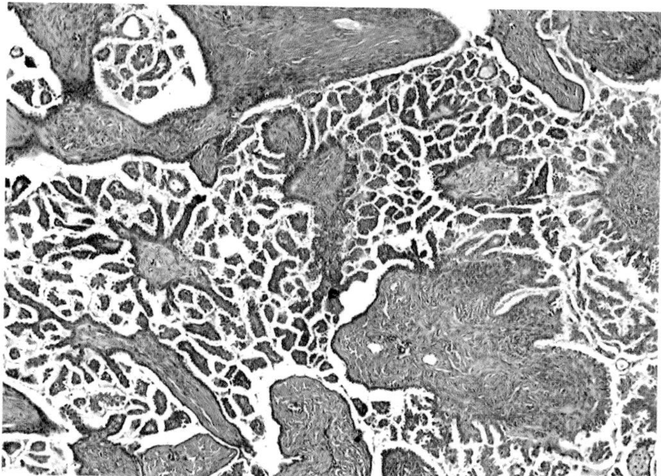

Fig. 19.237 Ovarian serous tumor with a micropapillary pattern of growth.

cribriform pattern, as micropapillae, and as macropapillae.[206,242] This is accompanied in about half of the cases with lymphovascular invasion.[219] These tumors seem to have a prognosis not significantly different from that of the usual noninvasive serous borderline tumor[157,211] (Fig. 19.236). This is a different phenomenon from the presence in a borderline tumor of focal areas having the typical appearance of serous carcinoma; the latter behave as aggressive neoplasms, with a prognosis similar to that of pure serous carcinoma.[194,201,229]

An interesting development has occurred in recent years concerning the serous cystadenoma–borderline tumor–(cyst)adenocarcinoma paradigm. It relates to the proposal by Kurman and his group of adding a fourth category to this scheme, which they have termed **micropapillary serous carcinoma** and placed in between the second and third existing categories.[159,224] These tumors are characterized by a filigree pattern of highly complex micropapillae arising from large bulbous papillary structures (Fig. 19.237). These micropapillae are covered by round to cuboidal cells with a high nucleocytoplasmic ratio, which can also be recognized on cytologic preparations.[154] Sometimes this is associated with a cribriform pattern of growth. This proposal has generated a great deal of controversy, which seems to be centered on the choice of terms (i.e., regarding the lesion as a 'carcinoma', which implies removing it from the borderline category) rather than on the morphologic observation itself, which rests on solid grounds,[178] and for which there is some molecular genetic backing.[232] To this writer, this saga is a perfect example of how a significant and clinically useful piece of information can suffer because of the world of semantic boundaries in which we move, in particular our dogged determination to rigidly divide tumors into benign and malignant categories. To put the matter in perspective, there was a time – not too long ago – when only two types of ovarian serous tumor were recognized: cystadenoma (benign) and (cyst)adenocarcinoma (malignant). Sometime in the 1950s, and after much discussion, a third category – that of borderline tumors – was added.[223] This meant progress at the clinical level, because a group had been carved out that had a natural history of its own, different from either of the two previously recognized entities. It also meant progress at the conceptual level, because it sent the message that tumors do not have to be either benign or malignant but that there is a spectrum of behavior among them. Now we have the proposal to add yet another category, having a set of morphologic (and, most significantly, clinical) features that set it apart from the conventional borderline tumor on one hand and the serous carcinoma on the other. This, again, means progress, and Kurman's team ought to be complimented for the achievement. It is unfortunate, however, that they felt the need to revert to classic terminology to name their entity, which they regarded as the 'malignant' type of borderline tumor, as opposed to the conventional borderline neoplasm, which they viewed as 'benign'. As far as the most important issue (i.e., the biologic validity of their observation) is concerned, there is immunohistochemical support for it in terms of P53 overexpression, and general agreement that Kurman's micropapillary serous tumor is associated with higher rates of recurrence of invasive carcinoma and (in some series) tumor deaths.[171,174,225,230] Another point worth making is that – prognostically speaking – the presence and type (noninvasive versus invasive) of peritoneal implants are more important than whether the primary ovarian tumor is of conventional or micropapillary type, and – if the latter – whether it is noninvasive or invasive.[203,215,216,231]

Going back to the general discussion of serous tumors, it ought to be mentioned that squamous metaplasia is exceptional in them, in contrast to endometrioid tumors; however, well-documented cases of this occurrence are on record.[238]

In some serous neoplasms, the fibroblastic stromal component is unduly prominent, appearing grossly as solid, white, nodular foci in an otherwise typical cystic neoplasm. These, too, can be separated into *benign* (**adenofibroma** and **cystadenofibroma**), *borderline*, and *malignant* (**adenofibrocarcinoma** and **cystadenofibrocarcinoma**) types[167,168] (Fig. 19.238). The benign type occurs much more frequently than the others. The borderline category of this neoplasm is extremely rare; none of the reported cases has developed a recurrence following excision of the neoplasm.[191] Exceptionally, osseous metaplasia develops in these stroma-rich tumors.[158] In other instances, the stroma is partially luteinized and of a functioning nature.[241] An unexpected association has been found between benign and malignant ovarian adenofibromatous tumors with breast cancer and thyroid disorders.[228]

Other serous neoplasms grow exophytically on the surface of the ovary, with little if any involvement of the underlying organ, the normal shape of which is maintained. These are referred to as **surface papillomas** when benign, **borderline surface papillary tumors** when intermediate, and **serous surface papillary (adeno)carcinomas** when malignant. Most of the latter are bilateral, highly aggressive, and usually associated with peritoneal spread at the time of surgery[182,210,240] (Figs 19.239 and 19.240).

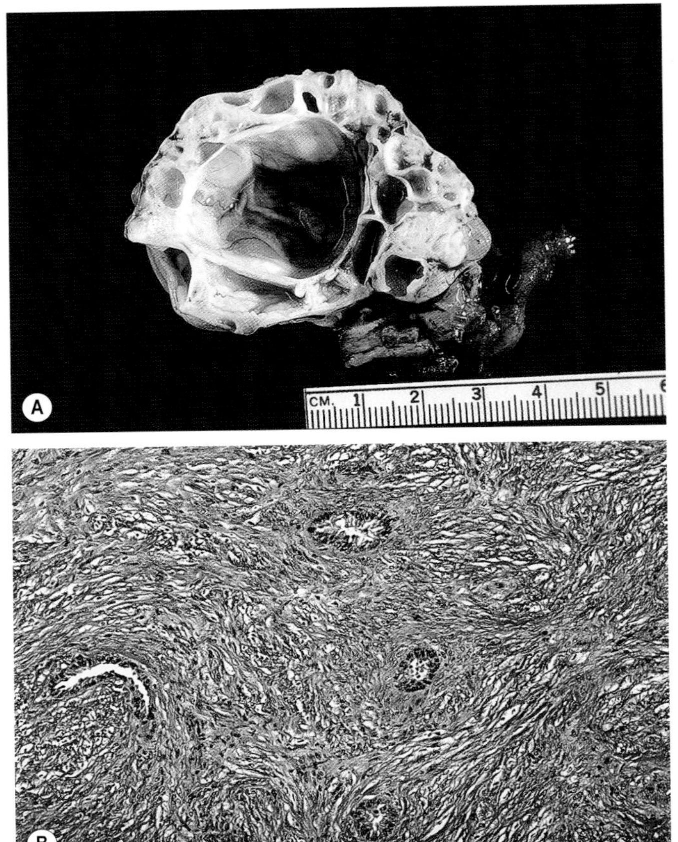

Fig. 19.238 **A** and **B**, Ovarian serous cystadenofibroma: **A**, gross appearance; **B**, microscopic appearance. The well-differentiated glands are embedded within a dense stroma.

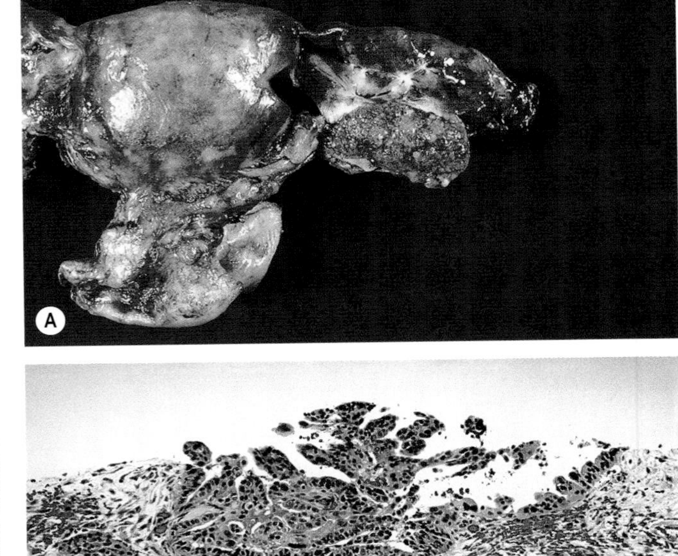

Fig. 19.240 **A** and **B**, Serous surface papillary carcinoma. **A**, Gross appearance. The ovary, which has a papillomatous outer surface, is only minimally enlarged. **B**, Microscopic appearance. There is hardly any infiltration of the stroma.

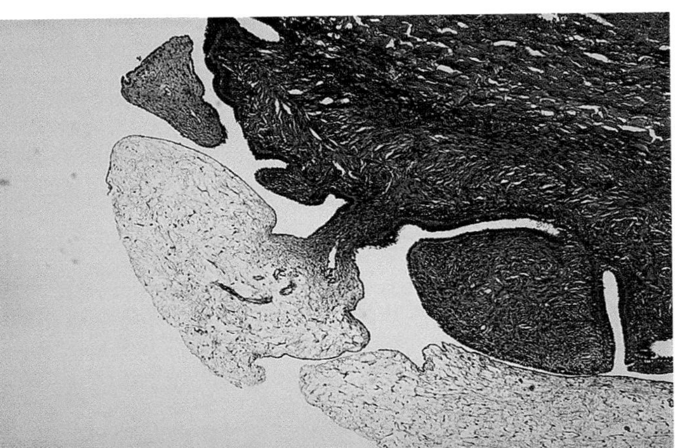

Fig. 19.239 Serous cystadenofibroma. The papillary structures protruding within the lumen have a prominent stromal component.

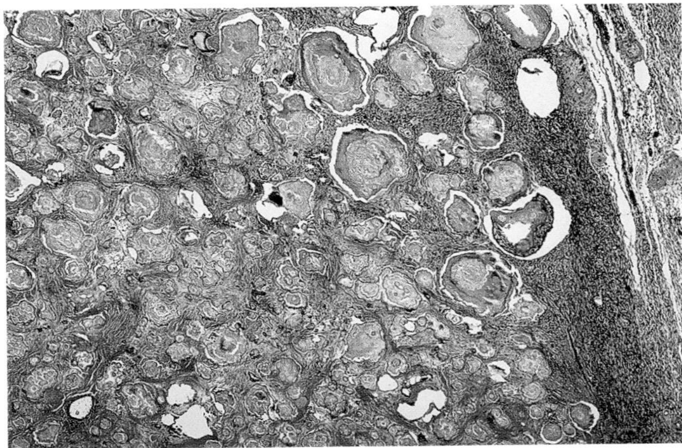

Fig. 19.241 So-called 'serous psammocarcinoma'. Innumerable psammoma bodies are present, and the cellularity is very scanty.

A somewhat different type of tumor predominantly involving the ovarian surface is so-called **serous psammocarcinoma**, a rare variant of serous carcinoma characterized by massive psammoma body formation and low-grade cytologic features (Fig. 19.241); the behavior of these tumors more closely resembles that of borderline serous tumors than of serous carcinomas.[179]

Exceptionally, a mural nodule with the features of a sarcomatoid carcinoma is seen protruding within the cystic portion of a serous borderline tumor, in a fashion analogous to that of its much more common counterpart among mucinous tumors.[155]

Ultrastructurally, cilia are often found in the benign and borderline tumors, but usually not in the carcinomas.[233]

Immunohistochemically, the typical keratin profile of serous tumors is CK7+/CK20−.[162] They also express CK8, 18, and 19, EMA, B72.3,[160,183,209] S-100 protein (particularly borderline tumors),[202] vimentin (erratically),[207] glial fibrillary acidic protein (GFAP) (occasionally),[209] HLA and Ia histocompatibility antigens,[188] the β-subunit of human chorionic gonadotropin (hCG) (in a minority of cases),[208] and receptors for estrogens, progesterone, and androgens (in over half the cases).[164,184] A small minority (around 10%) of serous tumors stain for calretinin and/or inhibin, a potentially confusing finding in the differential diagnosis with sex cord–stromal tumors.[163]

WT1 stains diffusely most ovarian serous carcinomas, as it does mesothelioma of peritoneum and other sites.[186] It stains to a lesser extent ovarian endometrioid carcinoma, and is usually negative in ovarian mucinous carcinoma.[181,225] Significantly, it does not stain uterine papillary serous carcinoma.[153,180] Thus, WT1 is of value in ascertaining the site of origin of serous carcinomas within the female genital tract.[151,205] In addition, along with other types of ovarian epithelial tumor, PAX8 is commonly positive in serous tumors of the ovary.[200,212]

The expression of cadherins and catenins is said to be related to the degree of tumor differentiation, in the sense that it is lower in the carcinomas.[169,170,175] In addition, it has been claimed that mucinous tumors express N-cadherin whereas serous and endometrioid tumors do not.[214]

Serous tumors contain glycoconjugates that result in a pattern of lectin binding different from that of mucinous tumors.[221] Interestingly, one-fourth of the serous and endometrioid tumors (but *not* the mucinous tumors) produce amylase, which can be demonstrated in the tumor cells (by immunohistochemistry), in the cyst fluid, and sometimes in the peripheral blood.[236,239]

Various monoclonal antibodies have been produced against epithelial (mainly serous) ovarian tumors, such as CA-125 and SMO47.[165,196,204]

Other markers that have been detected in ovarian serous tumors, some of them quite unexpectedly, include glycodelin (a glycoprotein with immunosuppressive and contraceptive properties),[190] osteopontin,[235] fibulin-1 (an extracellular matrix protein),[218] Coxsackie-adenovirus receptor,[195] retinoid acid receptor-α protein,[192] GLUT-1 (a facilitative glucose transporter, supposedly only in malignant tumors),[189] MUC5AC,[152] and TTF-1 (an important potential pitfall).[198,243]

Important *negative* markers of serous tumors are CK20 and cytoplasmic carcinoembryonic antigen (CEA), in contrast to primary and metastatic mucinous tumors.[162,165]

A continuous basement membrane (as detected immunohistochemically with antibodies to laminin or type IV collagen) is present in benign cystadenomas and borderline tumors without microinvasion; disruption of this structure occurs in areas of microinvasion (in the borderline tumors) or frank invasion (in the cystadenocarcinomas).[161,172]

The stromal component of these tumors has been shown to express several molecules involved in steroid hormone metabolism, such as 17β-hydroxysteroid dehydrogenase (an estrogen-metabolizing enzyme) and adrenal-4-binding protein (a transcription factor that regulates the expression of steroidogenic enzymes.[220,222]

The molecular genetic abnormalities of these tumors are discussed on page 1578.

Mucinous tumors

Mucinous neoplasms are less common than serous neoplasms and are bilateral in only 10–20% of cases.[304] As in the case of their serous counterparts, ovarian mucinous tumors have been divided into *benign* **(mucinous cystadenoma)**, *borderline*, and *malignant* **(mucinous adenocarcinoma** and **cystadenocarcinoma)**. Grossly, they tend to grow larger than the serous types and are partially or completely cystic, often multiloculated. A fluid to viscous material of mucoid nature is present in the lumen (Figs 19.242–19.244). In the past, these tumors have been designated as *pseudomucinous*

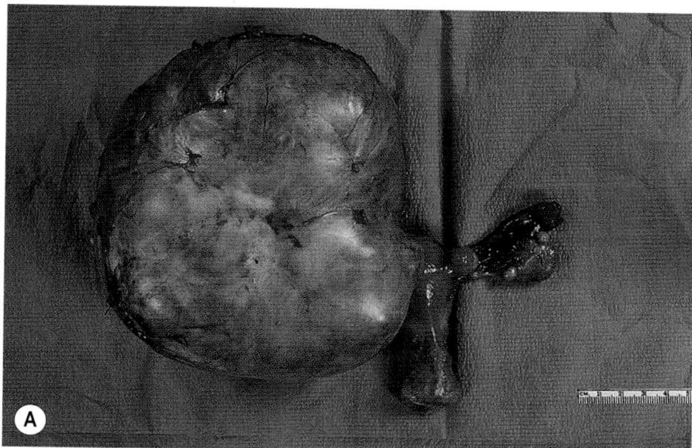

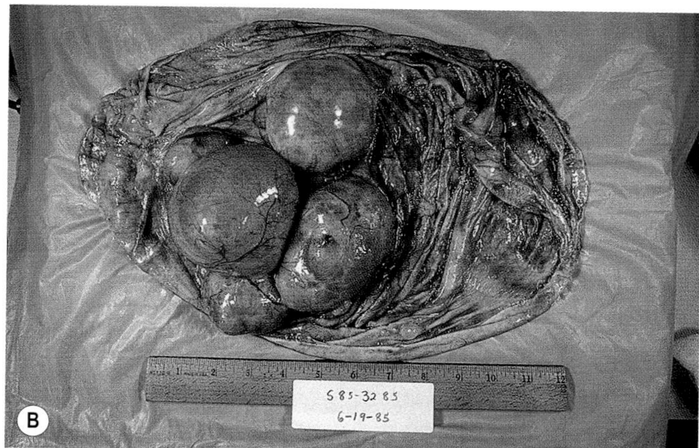

Fig. 19.242 **A** and **B**, Outer and inner aspect of mucinous cystadenoma.

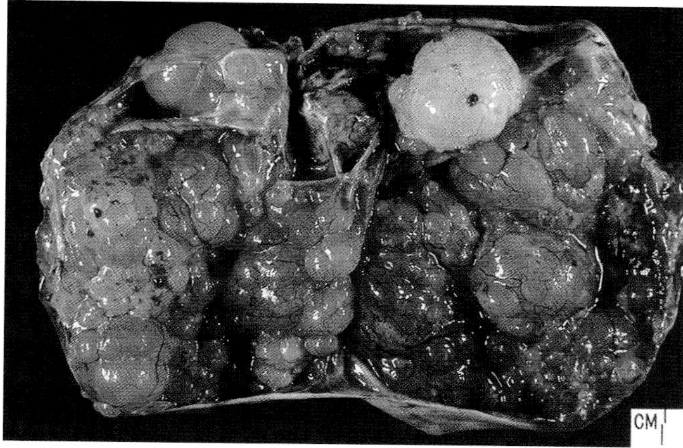

Fig. 19.243 Gross appearance of a mucinous ovarian neoplasm that had borderline features at the microscopic level.

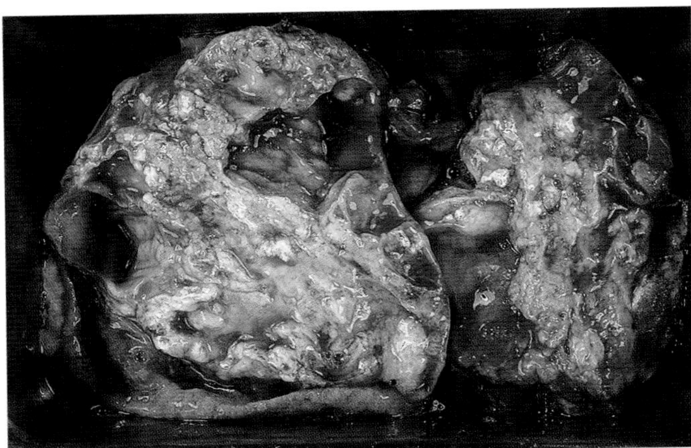

Fig. 19.244 Gross appearance of mucinous cystadenocarcinoma. The neoplasm is predominantly solid, but some mucin-containing cystic spaces can still be appreciated.

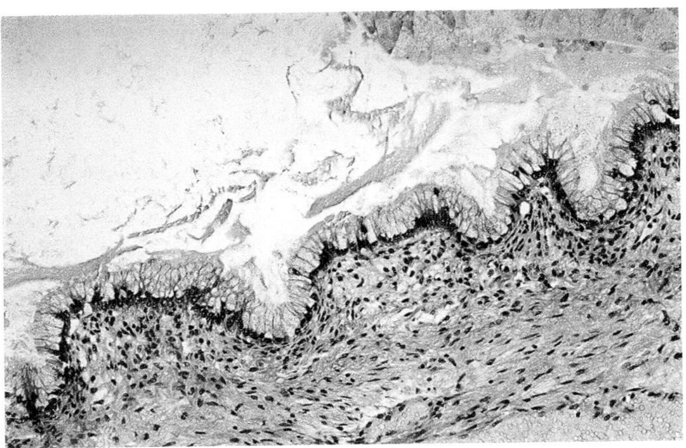

Fig. 19.245 Lining of mucinous cystadenoma. Goblet cells are evident. This subtype, which is by far the most common, is referred to as intestinal.

because the behavior of the luminal content toward acetic acid was allegedly different from that of 'true' mucin; however, since the material secreted by the tumor cells has all the histochemical features of an epithelial mucosubstance, the designation of *mucinous* is wholly appropriate.[288]

Microscopically, ovarian mucinous tumors (particularly those of a borderline nature, see below) have been divided into two major types, a distinction that is not always easy (particularly with the carcinomas, in which it is rarely attempted), but which is backed by ultrastructural, histochemical, and immunohistochemical data.[258,276]

The first and most common type is referred to as *intestinal*, and is characterized by an epithelial lining with a 'picket fence' appearance, goblet cells, Paneth cells, endocrine cells, the secretion of gastrointestinal and pancreatobiliary type mucin,[292] and the production of intestinal enzymes such as lipase, trypsin, amylase, and sucrase[293,298] (Fig. 19.245). The endocrine cells, which are more common in the borderline category, are argyrophil and sometimes argentaffin.[266] 5-Hydroxytryptamine (serotonin, 5-HT), ACTH, gastrin, somatostatin, and other peptide hormones have been

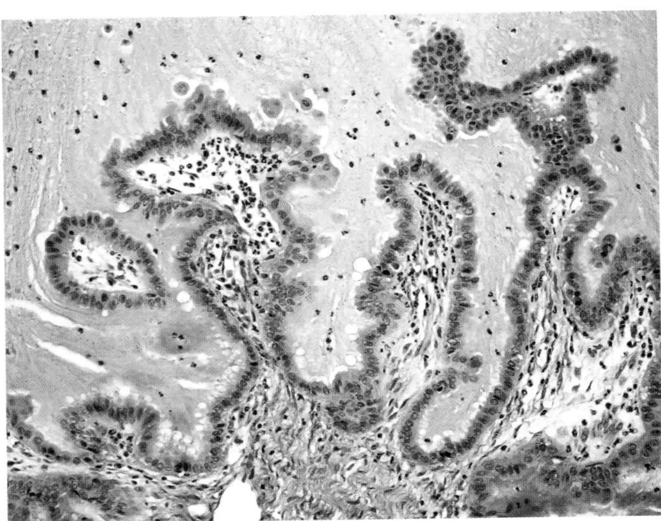

Fig. 19.246 In this instance, the lining of mucinous cystadenoma resembles endocervical epithelium.

detected immunohistochemically in them.[245,271,290,295] There is usually no clinical evidence of hormone excess, but cases associated with Zollinger–Ellison syndrome have been described.[249] Exceptionally, there is a focal component of signet ring cells, which may lead to a mistaken diagnosis of Krukenberg tumor.[272]

The second type of mucinous ovarian neoplasm, referred to as *endocervical* or *müllerian*, is characterized by a papillary architecture similar to that of serous tumor but with a lining of tall nonciliated cells with basally located nuclei and abundant intracellular mucin, which resembles endocervical epithelium both at the light and electron microscopic level[255] (Fig. 19.246). It has been pointed out that the endocervical-type tumors share more morphologic and immunohistochemical features with the serous (or even endometrioid) than the intestinal-type mucinous tumors, and that they should therefore be designated as seromucinous.[260,290,291,302]

Occasionally, mucinous tumors of the intestinal type have been found in association with carcinoid tumors in the same ovary.[285] On the basis of these findings, some authors (including the legendary Robert Meyer) have postulated a monodermal teratomatous derivation for these tumors; most morphologic and genetic evidence, however, favors a metaplastic origin from the müllerian epithelium.[244,256] Indeed, some tumors of the endocervical type have been found to coexist with endocervical adenocarcinoma,[270,307] and sometimes with endometriosis.[267] The stroma can be hypercellular, particularly in the area immediately beneath the neoplastic epithelium; on occasion, it may show signs of luteinization and be accompanied by hormonal manifestations.[261,273]

The *malignant* type of mucinous tumor is characterized by cell atypia, increased layering of cells, greater complexity of the glands and papillae (budding, bridging, appearance of solid foci), and areas of stromal invasion[259,305] (Fig. 19.247). Since the latter may be present in only a small area of the tumor, thorough sampling for microscopic examination is essential.

The existence and clinical significance of a *borderline* category in the mucinous tumors has proved more difficult to define than for their serous counterparts, to the point that some authors have proposed dropping as a specific category.[253,294] One of the problems is that stromal invasion is difficult to evaluate in cases with a complex interaction of glands and stroma. Hart and Norris[257] proposed the following rules for the distinction between borderline and

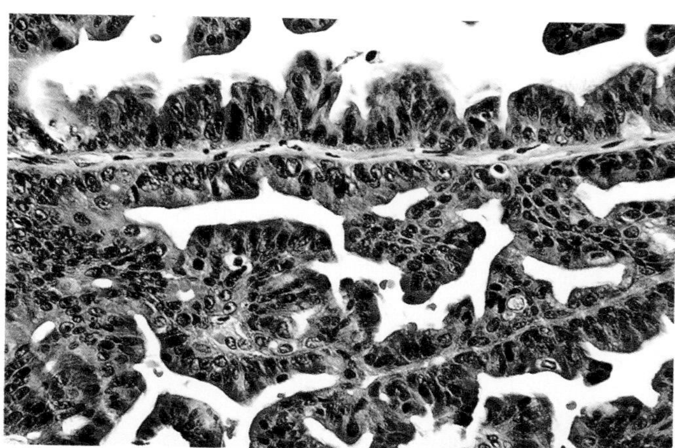

Fig. 19.247 Complex architecture and obvious nuclear atypia in mucinous cystadenocarcinoma.

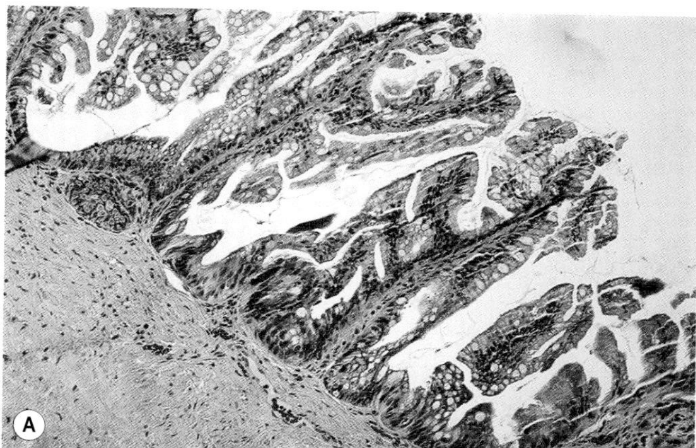

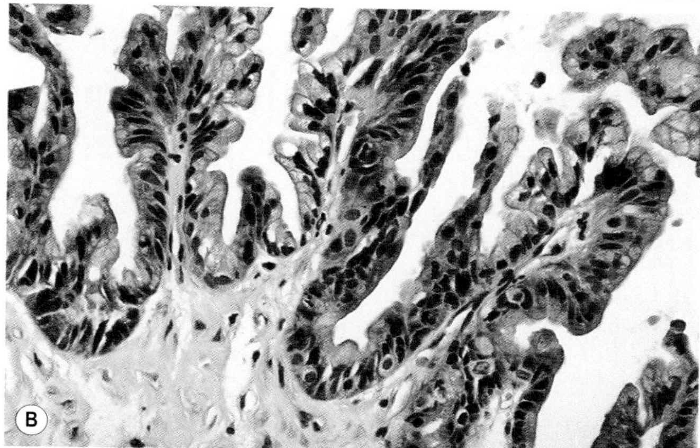

Fig. 19.248 **A** and **B**, Mucinous ovarian neoplasm of borderline type. It has been proposed that borderline tumors showing prominent atypia (**B**) be designated as focal intraepithelial carcinoma.

malignant mucinous tumors: if there is unquestionable invasion, the tumor is classified as a carcinoma; if invasion is uncertain, the tumor is classified as borderline when the atypical epithelium is less than four cells in thickness; and as carcinoma when it is four cells or greater. Some independent studies have confirmed the prognostic utility of this arbitrary and biologically questionable criterion,[251] but others have not.[303] Recently, the proposal has been made to subdivide the mucinous borderline tumors of intestinal type into those with epithelial atypia and those with focal intraepithelial carcinoma[268] (Fig. 19.248). Clinically, their outcome is usually equally favorable, but occasional patients in the latter group have experienced a fatal recurrence.[268,286] Mucinous carcinomas have also been divided into expansile and infiltrative subtypes, some of the latter being microinvasive only.[268,297] Microinvasion is usually associated with an excellent prognosis.[264,268,277]

Some authors have suggested that intestinal-type mucinous tumors be divided into conventional, atypical proliferative, and those with intraepithelial, microinvasive (<5 mm), and invasive (≥5 mm) carcinoma.[284] In a somewhat parallel scheme, it has been proposed that endocervical-like mucinous borderline ovarian tumors be divided into conventional, with intraepithelial carcinoma (13%), and with stromal microinvasion (23% of the cases).[287]

Regarding microinvasion in ovarian mucinous tumors, it should be noted that this event can be simulated by mucin extravasation into the stroma, which is actually nothing more than a mucocele-like change.[265]

There is a subgroup of mucinous tumors in which the stromal component is particularly prominent. These have been designated *mucinous adenofibroma* or *cystadenofibroma* if benign, and *mucinous adenocarcinofibroma* and *cystadenocarcinofibroma* if malignant (Fig. 19.249). The benign ones are sometimes misinterpreted as malignant and even as metastatic because of the irregularly shaped gland in a desmoplastic stroma,[248] or as microinvasive because of the presence of micronests of endocrine cells.[262]

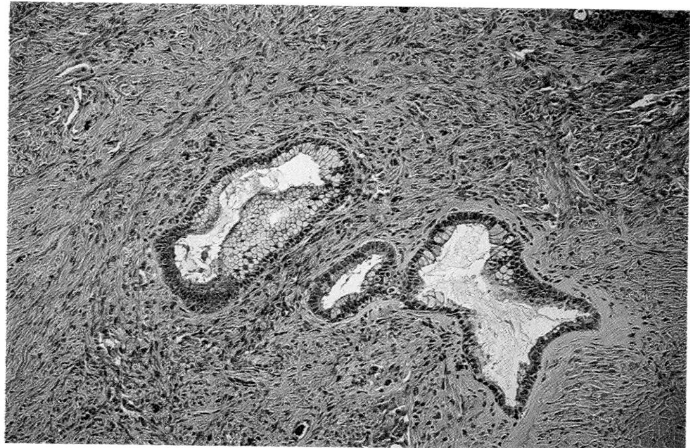

Fig. 19.249 Mucinous adenofibroma showing small glands lined by mucin-producing epithelial cells embedded in a dense fibrous stroma.

Exceptionally, ovarian mucinous tumors have been found to contain foci of: (1) *sarcoma-like nodules*, with a configuration and cytologic composition similar to those of giant cell tumor of soft parts,[281] characterized by a lack of reactivity for keratin;[274] (2) *sarcoma*, usually spindle shaped, sometimes with heterologous features,[280,300] and also unreactive for keratin; and (3) *anaplastic carcinoma*, with pleomorphic round to spindle cells that are immunoreactive for keratin.[275,282] The distinction between the latter two lesions is very tenuous, both on microscopic and histogenetic grounds (as it is in the pancreas or thyroid under similar circumstances), and both are associated with a poor prognosis unless they present as stage I lesions.[283] Actually, we favor the interpretation that the sarcoma-like nodules themselves are not a reactive phenomenon,[247] but rather are of neoplastic nature and related histogenetically to the other two processes, a possibility also expressed by others[254] and supported by the occasional overlap and coexistence of these various lesions.[283] However, it is important to consider the sarcoma-like nodules separately because of their better prognosis.[246,247,281,282] On occasion, the appearance of the mural nodule is that of a benign leiomyomatous growth.[269]

Immunohistochemically, the tumor cells of ovarian mucinous tumors express CEA (more so the intestinal types and/or malignant tumors),[252] keratin, EMA (particularly if malignant),[289] MUC5AC (a gastrin mucin gene), DPC4 (a nuclear transcription factor inactivated in about half of pancreatic adenocarcinomas),[263] hepatocyte nuclear factor 1,[299] and hepatocyte nuclear factor 4 alpha.[296] Importantly, the intestinal-type tumors express markers of gastrointestinal type differentiation (CK20 and CDX2),[250,263,279,301] whereas the endocervical (seromucinous)-type tumors express müllerian-type markers (such as hormone receptors, CA-125 and mesothelin).[302] In contrast to other types of ovarian epithelial tumor, PAX8 is usually negative.[278]

Mucinous cystadenocarcinomas tend to implant on and locally invade neighboring tissues such as the bowel, abdominal wall, and bladder. Metastases to distant areas are infrequent. Sometimes, mucinous tumors involving the ovary are accompanied by extensive deposits of intra-abdominal mucin (pseudomyxoma peritonei). The prevailing opinion at present is that the large majority of these tumors are metastatic to the ovary and peritoneal cavity from an appendiceal origin, and they are, therefore, discussed on page 1607 and Chapter 11. Use of a simple algorithmic approach has been advocated for the distinction between primary and metastatic mucinous tumors of the ovary, heavily relying in size and laterality.[306]

Endometrioid tumors

Endometrioid carcinoma comprises 10–25% of all primary ovarian carcinomas.[325] Coexistent endometriosis can be demonstrated in 10–20% of cases,[327] and some of the tumors can be seen actually arising from these endometriotic foci. However, the identification of endometriosis is not a prerequisite for the diagnosis of endometrioid carcinoma, inasmuch as the majority of these tumors are thought to originate de novo from the ovarian surface epithelium or related müllerian-type epithelium. The occasional admixture of endometrioid with serous and/or mucinous patterns would seem to support this interpretation.

Grossly, endometrioid carcinoma may present as a cystic or solid mass (Fig. 19.250). The content tends to be hemorrhagic rather than serous or mucinous. Visible papillary formations are usually absent or inconspicuous. Microscopically, the tumors resemble greatly the appearance of the ordinary type of endometrial adenocarcinoma – hence their name[313,314] (Fig. 19.251). Most are well differentiated, with or without papillary formations. Half of the tumors have foci of squamous metaplasia, some of these having been reported in the past as adenoacanthomas[323] (Fig. 19.252). Morules can also be present, some of them expressing CDX2 and β-catenin (nuclear translocation).[320] In contrast to serous tumors, psammoma bodies are exceptional. Approximately 10% of endometrioid carcinomas have a component of non-neoplastic luteinized stromal cells.

As in uterine adenoacanthomas, the keratin produced by these ovarian neoplasms can result in the formation of peritoneal keratin granulomas.[322] It seems likely that at least some of the reported cases of primary **squamous cell carcinomas** of the ovary represent the extreme expression of this metaplastic tendency of endometrioid carcinoma.[326,331,339,343] Parenthetically, the other large category of ovarian squamous cell carcinoma is that associated with benign cystic teratomas (dermoid cysts).[332]

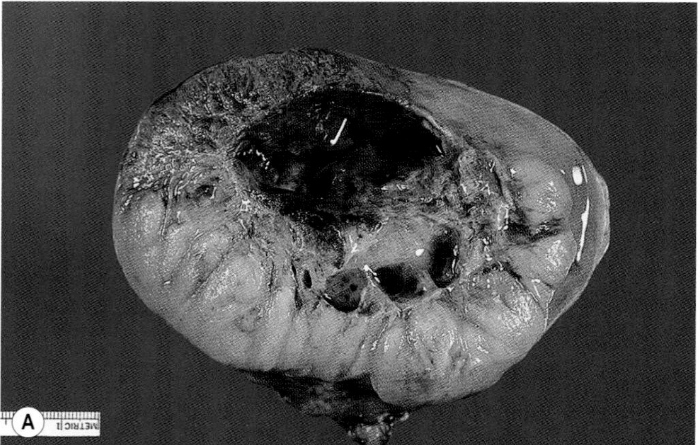

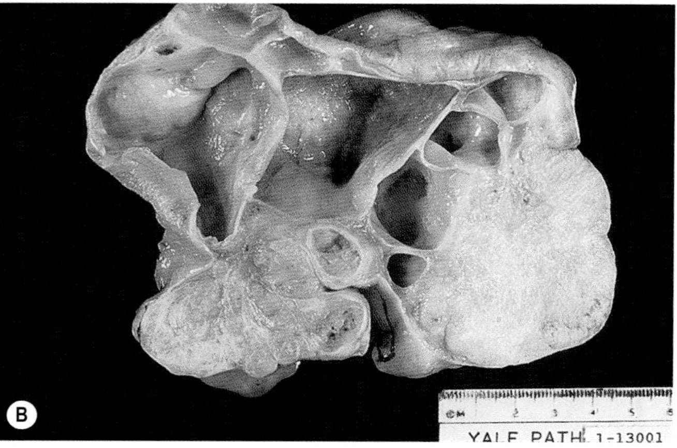

Fig. 19.250 **A** and **B**, Gross appearances of ovarian endometrioid carcinoma. Both tumors show a combination of solid and cystic appearances.

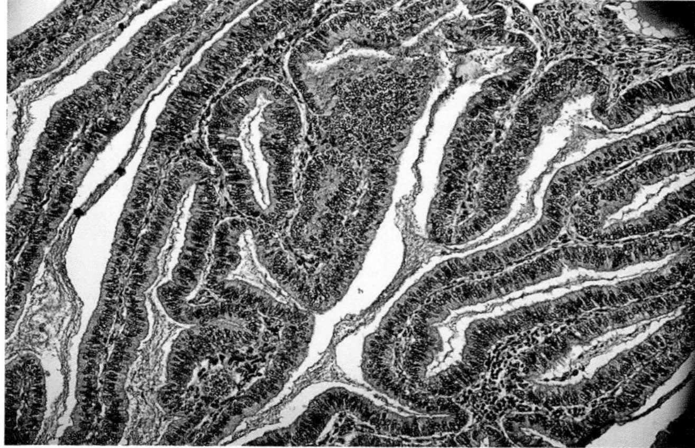

Fig. 19.251 Well-differentiated endometrioid carcinoma of ovary with focally villous architecture.

Histochemically, mucin may be found within the glandular lumina and in the apical border of the tumor cells but not in the cytoplasm. Scattered argyrophil cells are seen in almost half of cases.[341]

Immunohistochemically, the tumor cells are positive for keratin, EMA, vimentin and PAX8, whereas CEA is usually

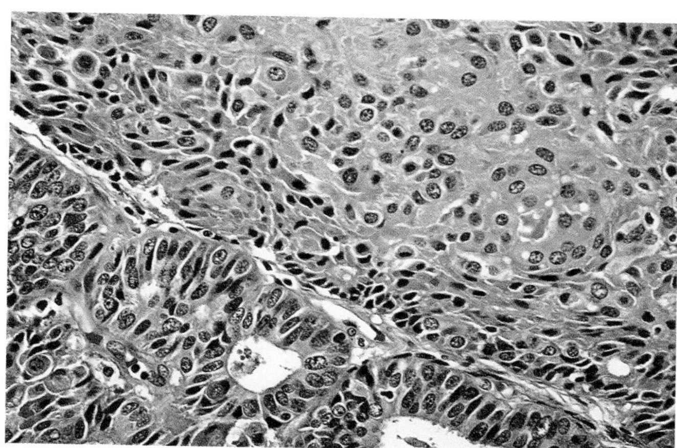

Fig. 19.252 Well-differentiated endometrioid ovarian carcinoma with extensive squamous metaplasia (so-called 'adenoacanthoma').

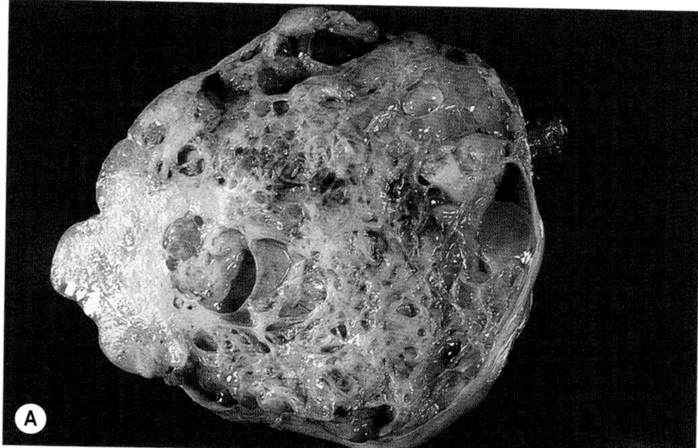

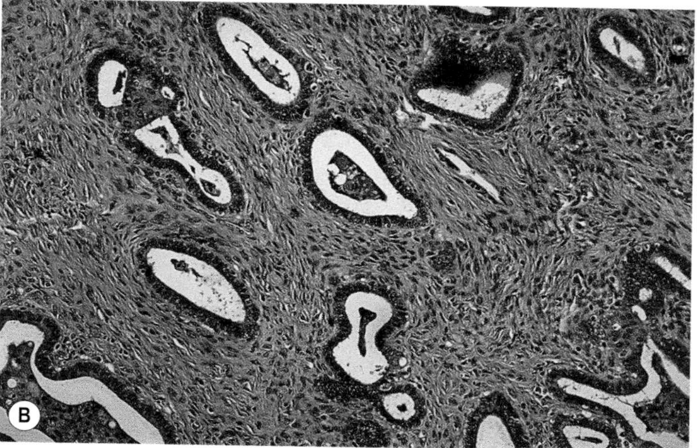

Fig. 19.253 **A** and **B**, Gross and microscopic appearance of endometrioid (cyst)adenofibroma.

negative or weak.[315] There can also be positivity for CA19-9 and hPL.[312,319]

Ultrastructurally, the two most distinctive features (also shared with endometrial adenocarcinoma) are paranuclear collections of microfilaments and nucleoli with a 'mesh basket' appearance.

At the molecular level, there are several differences with endometrioid carcinoma of the uterus despite their morphologic similarities, suggesting a different genetic pathway for their formation.[311] Mutations leading to β-catenin deregulation are found in nearly half of ovarian endometrioid adenocarcinomas.[347] Recently it has been shown that many endometrioid and clear cell carcinomas (i.e., ovarian tumors classically related to endometriosis) have mutations of *ARID1A*, a tumor suppressor gene, in stark contrast with serous carcinomas.[342]

In some endometrioid carcinomas, the neoplastic glands are small and tubular or solid and elongated, simulating the pattern of sex cord–stromal tumors, particularly of Sertoli–Leydig cell type.[336,345] These are referred to either as sertoliform variants of endometrioid carcinoma or as endometrioid carcinoma resembling sex cord–stromal tumors.[330] Features that favor a diagnosis of endometrioid carcinoma in such cases are the older age of the patients, the usual absence of endocrine manifestations, and the occurrence elsewhere in the tumor of larger tubular glands, foci of squamous metaplasia, luminal mucin accumulation, adenofibromatous components, immunoreactivity for keratin (including CK7), and negativity for inhibin.[308,318] Other endometrioid carcinomas simulate the appearance of granulosa cell tumors, from which they can be distinguished (if needed) on immunohistochemical grounds.[317]

Other morphologic variations of endometrioid carcinoma include presence of yolk sac elements,[328,337] tumors composed of ciliated cells,[316] tumors composed of oxyphilic (oncocytic) epithelium,[333,344] and tumors containing foci of collagenous spherulosis that simulate squamous metaplasia.[340] Endometrioid carcinomas containing foci of hepatoid differentiation have also been described.[338]

Benign, atypical (proliferating), and borderline types of endometrioid ovarian tumors exist, in addition to the malignant ones.[309,310,321,335] Most of these have a prominent stromal component and have been traditionally included with the adenofibromas or cystadenofibromas, depending on the degree of cystic change (Figs 19.253 and 19.254). Sometimes, benign and malignant areas coexist in the same case.[321,334] In the atypical category, the epithelial changes are equivalent to those of atypical endometrial hyperplasia; in the borderline category, they are akin to well-differentiated endometrial adenocarcinoma *without stromal invasion*.[309,329] Cytologic atypia and presence of microinvasion do not appear to affect the prognosis, in the sense that oophorectomy is generally curative for all of these forms.[310]

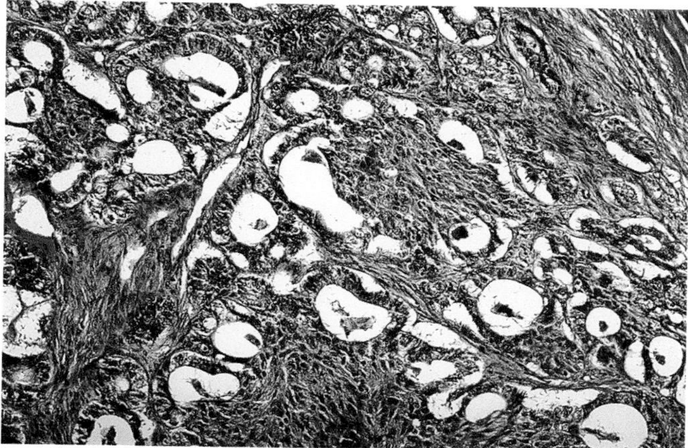

Fig. 19.254 Ovarian endometrioid neoplasm with borderline microscopic features mainly manifested by architectural complexity.

Table 19.4 Differential characteristics of serous, mucinous, and endometrioid carcinomas

CHARACTERISTIC	SEROUS	MUCINOUS	ENDOMETRIOID
Relative frequency	60–80%	5–15%	10–25%
Bilaterality	30–50%	10–20%	15–30%
Size	Moderate	Often huge	Moderate
Usual character of fluid	Clear	Slimy, viscous	Hemorrhagic
Coexistent endometrial hyperplasia or carcinoma	Exceptional	Exceptional	15–30%
Epithelium	Cuboidal	Columnar, with basally located nucleus	Columnar, with centrally located nucleus
Mucin	Only in luminal border	Often abundant, intracytoplasmic	Only in luminal border
Squamous metaplasia	Exceptional	Exceptional	50%
Cilia	Frequent	Absent	Rare
Psammoma bodies	30%	Exceptional	Exceptional

As a group, endometrioid carcinoma has a prognosis twice as good as that of serous or mucinous carcinoma.[324] However, this seems to be mainly a function of the fact that many of these tumors are stage I and well differentiated. When these various tumor types are evaluated stage for stage, the outcome is not significantly different.[313]

Some patients with endometrioid carcinoma of the ovary have either endometrial hyperplasia or a synchronous endometrial adenocarcinoma, often well differentiated and superficial and sometimes exhibiting squamous metaplasia (so-called 'adenoacanthoma').[346] There is a wide disparity in the reported incidence of the latter occurrence (largely because of different diagnostic criteria), with most series ranging from 15% to 30%.[314,346] This is discussed further on page 1581.

The most important differences among serous, mucinous, and endometrioid carcinomas are listed in Table 19.4.

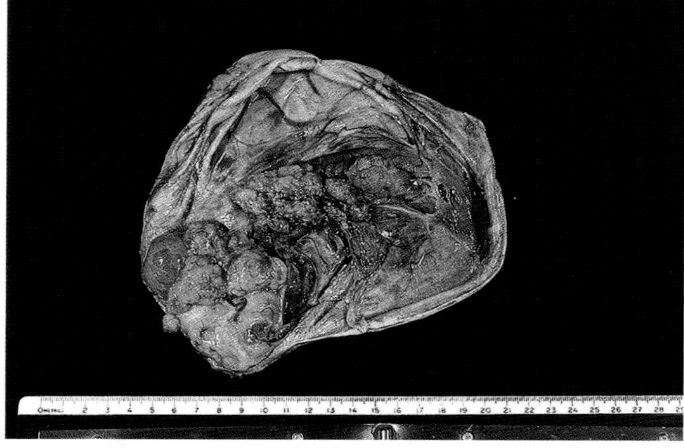

Fig. 19.255 Gross appearance of clear cell carcinoma of ovary. The tumor is predominantly cystic, but it contains several mural nodules.

Clear cell (mesonephroid) tumors

Clear cell (mesonephroid) adenocarcinoma is a distinctive ovarian tumor with a grossly spongy, often cystic appearance (Fig. 19.255), which microscopically can grow in tubular–cystic, papillary, and solid-sheet fashions[363,365] (Fig. 19.256). The cores of the papillae often exhibit prominent hyalinization (Fig. 19.257). Stroma-rich variants of clear cell carcinoma are known as *clear cell adenocarcinofibroma* and *cystadenocarcinofibroma*, depending on whether they are predominantly solid or cystic. In contrast to serous carcinomas, the papillae of clear cell carcinoma have a nonhierarchically branched pattern and lack epithelial stratification.[352]

The tumor cells are large. Some of the nuclei protrude into the lumina, resulting in a 'hobnail' configuration (Fig. 19.258). Their cytoplasm is clear; it often contains glycogen, mucin, and fat, and it may exhibit periodic acid–Schiff (PAS)-positive, diastase-resistant hyaline globules, which are negative for alpha-fetoprotein.[358] In some of the tumor cells, the cytoplasm may appear oxyphilic rather than clear[378,379] (Fig. 19.259). Immunohistochemically, the tumor cells are always reactive for keratin (CK7, CK5/6, CAM 5.2, 34βE12), EMA, CEA, CD15 (Leu-M1), Ber-EP4, vimentin, PAX8, BCL2, P53, and CA-125; variably reactive for estrogen and progesterone receptors, HER2/*neu* and alpha-fetoprotein (the latter not in relation to

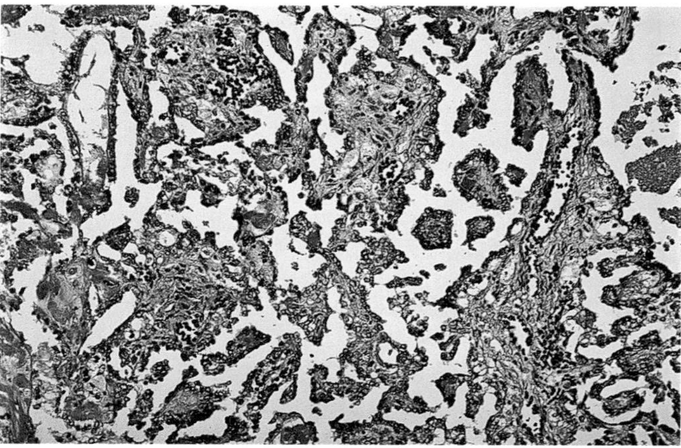

Fig. 19.256 A highly papillary configuration is seen in this low-power view of ovarian clear cell carcinoma.

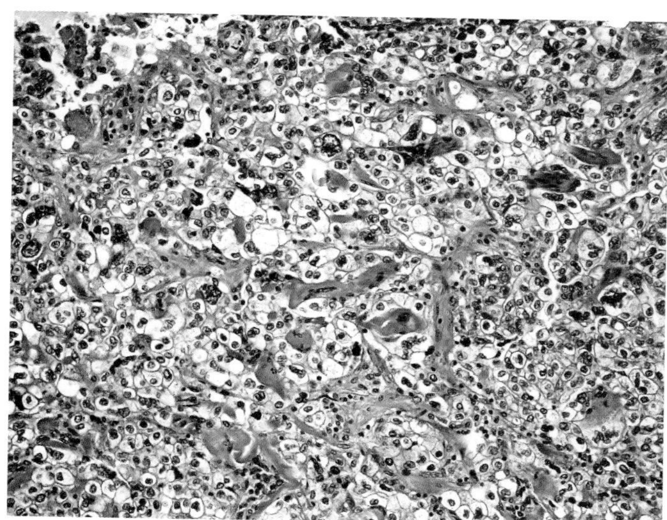

Fig. 19.257 Clear cell carcinoma of ovary showing short papillae with hyalinized cores lined by highly atypical cells.

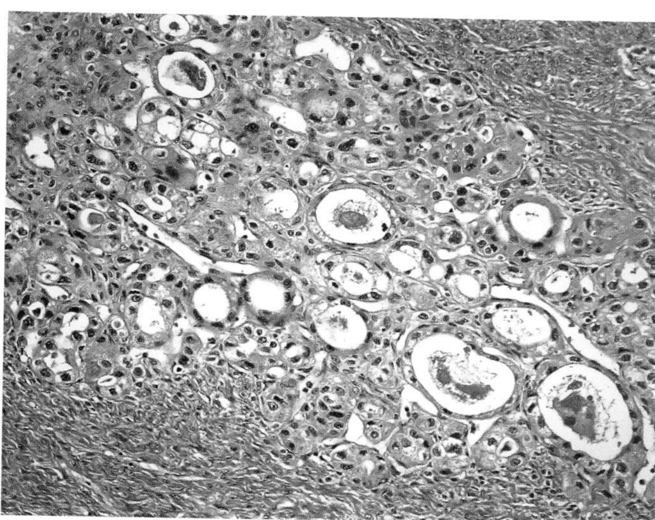

Fig. 19.259 Oxyphilic variant of clear cell carcinoma. Some of the tumor cells have a hybrid appearance.

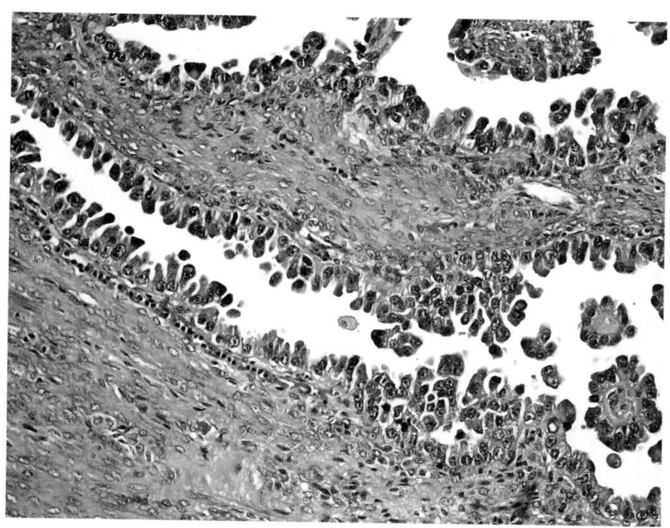

Fig. 19.258 Clear cell carcinoma of ovary. Note the high nuclear grade and the hobnail configuration.

the hyaline bodies); and negative for CK20.[366,375,382] The hormone receptor pattern is peculiar in the sense that there is much greater expression of estrogen receptor (ER) than progesterone receptor (PR), and that the former is exclusively of the beta rather than the alpha type.[354] Two additional markers of ovarian clear cell carcinoma and its benign counterparts (see below) are hepatocyte nuclear factor-1β (HNF-1β, a transcription factor involved with liver differentiation[356,377]) and the oncofetal protein IMP3.[380]

At the molecular level, it has been claimed that clear cell carcinomas have an expression pattern of cell cycle regulatory molecules that is unique among ovarian adenocarcinomas[374] (see also preceding section concerning *ARID1A* mutations).

Clear cell adenocarcinoma was included in Schiller's original description of mesonephroma and regarded as of mesonephric rest derivation;[371] however, overwhelming evidence has been brought forward to indicate that it is of surface epithelial type and specifically related to endometrioid carcinoma, of which it should be regarded a variant.[372,373] This interpretation is supported by the high association with pelvic endometriosis, the origin in some cases from endometriotic cysts, the frequent admixture with typical endometrioid carcinoma, and the ultrastructural similarities with müllerian endometrioid epithelium.[348,372] At the electron microscopic level, the cytoplasmic clearing is seen to be largely due to the accumulation of glycogen,[360] and the stromal hyalinization to the accumulation of basal lamina material.[361,364]

Patients with clear cell adenocarcinoma are usually in the fifth or sixth decade. The incidence of bilaterality is less than 10%, and the 5-year survival rate ranges from 37% to 47%.[350,351,367] Stage for stage, their prognosis is similar to that of patients with other epithelial ovarian carcinomas.[348,350,357] They are thought to be less responsive to chemotherapy than other types of ovarian carcinoma.

Benign and **borderline** (low malignant potential) ovarian clear cell tumors are very rare. They can be 'pure' or be associated with obviously malignant clear cell carcinomas.[376] Their growth pattern may be that of a cystadenoma, an adenofibroma, or a cystadenofibroma.[381] The borderline tumors are identified because of moderate to marked degrees of epithelial proliferation and atypia in the absence of recognizable stromal invasion[369] (Fig. 19.260).

The differential diagnosis of ovarian clear cell carcinoma includes:

- *Metastatic renal cell carcinoma*, which is negative for keratin 34βE12 and positive for CD10, whereas primary clear cell ovarian carcinoma usually (but not always) shows the opposite results.[368]
- *Ovarian yolk sac tumor* (as above commented), which is characteristically positive for OCT3/4 and SALL4.[349] It is also positive for glypican-3,[353] but this is also true for about 40% of clear cell carcinomas.[362]
- *Ovarian serous carcinoma*, as a result of the fact that clear cell carcinomas can have a highly papillary pattern of growth,[370] and that serous carcinomas can contain clear cells.[355] An immunohistochemical panel consisting of WT1, estrogen receptor, and HNF-1β is useful in making the distinction.[359]

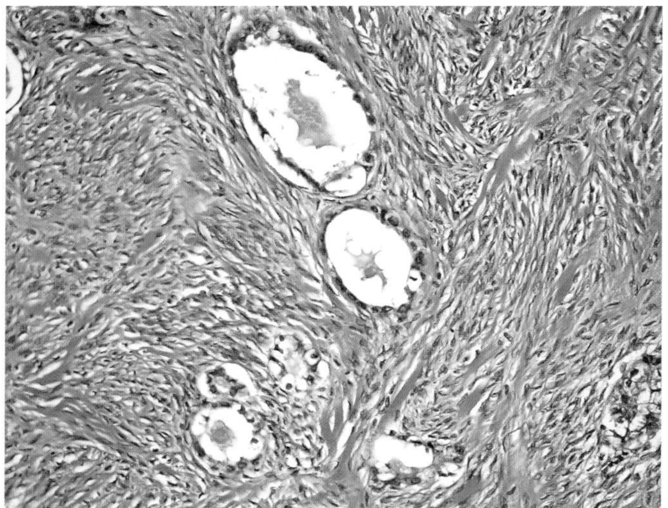

Fig. 19.260 Clear cell adenofibroma with mild to moderate nuclear atypia. These tumors are placed in a borderline or low malignant potential category.

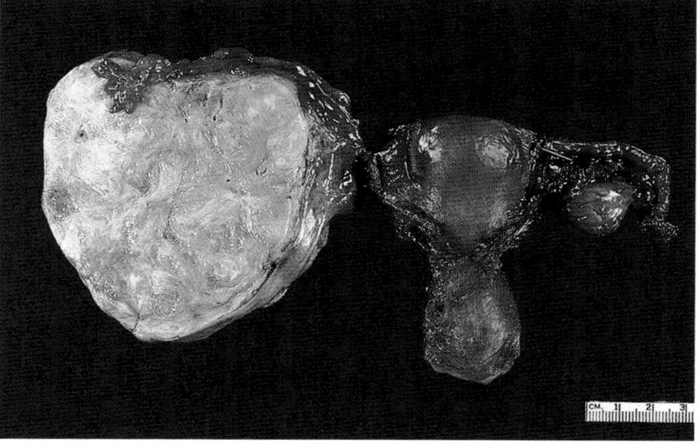

Fig. 19.261 Large Brenner tumor involving the right ovary. The gross appearance of this neoplasm is very similar to that of fibrothecoma.

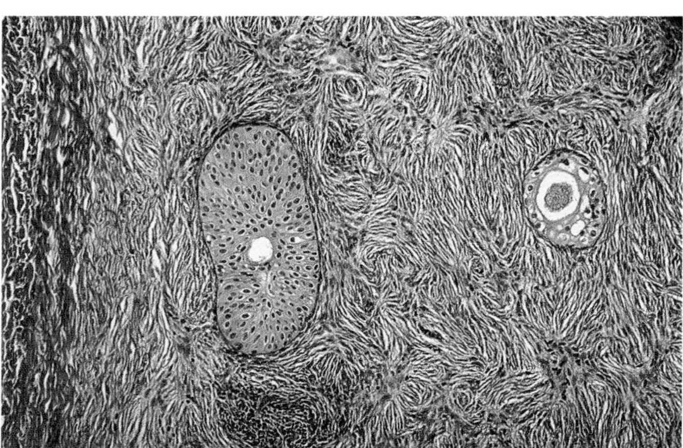

Fig. 19.262 Brenner tumor of ovary showing solid and cystic epithelial cells embedded within fibrous tissue.

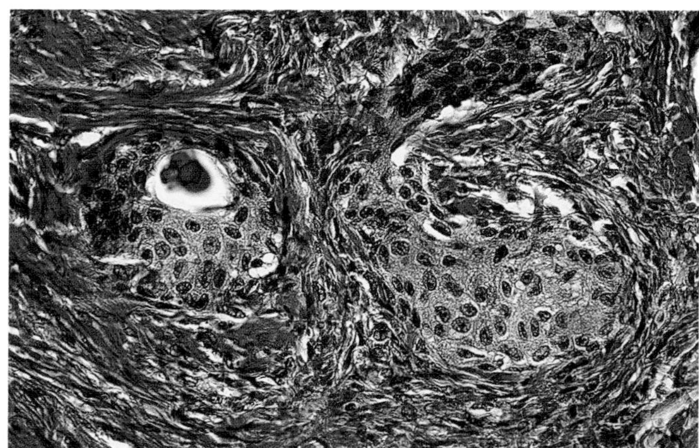

Fig. 19.263 The epithelial nests of Brenner tumor are composed of cells with oval nuclei, many of which exhibit longitudinal grooves.

Brenner tumor and transitional cell carcinoma

Brenner tumors constitute between 1% and 2% of all ovarian neoplasms.[413] The average age at presentation is approximately 50 years, about 70% of the patients being over 40 years of age. Some cases are accompanied by signs of hyperestrinism, such as uterine bleeding from endometrial hyperplasia in the postmenopausal woman.[396] The rate of growth is slow, and ascites is rare. Grossly, these tumors vary greatly in size; they are usually unilateral, firm, and white or yellowish white (Fig. 19.261). They closely resemble fibromas or thecomas, except for the frequent presence of small cystic areas filled with opaque, viscous, yellowish-brown fluid. Microscopically, they consist of solid and cystic nests of epithelial cells resembling transitional epithelium (urothelium) surrounded by an abundant stromal component of dense, fibroblastic nature (Fig. 19.262). The epithelial cells have sharply defined outlines; those lining the cysts may be flattened, cuboidal, or columnar. The nuclei of the tumor cells are oval, with a small but distinct nucleolus and longitudinal grooves similar to those seen in granulosa cell tumors (Fig. 19.263). The cytoplasm is clear and immunoreactive for keratin, EMA, and CEA (the latter also present in the lumen of the cysts).[389] It may contain glycogen, mucin, and lipid.[396,407,412] The latter is found in larger amounts in the stromal cells in the cases accompanied by hyperestrinism. Scattered argyrophilic cells are present in about one-third of cases; they are positive for chromogranin and 5-HT, have dense-core granules at the ultrastructural level, and are similar to those seen in normal urothelium.[383,388] Steroidogenic enzymes as detected immunohistochemically are usually absent.[408]

Sometimes the cystic formations within the tumor are unduly prominent and accompanied by florid mucinous changes (a lesion analogous to cystitis glandularis); Roth et al.[404] refer to this pattern as *metaplastic* Brenner tumor as long as papillary fronds and nuclear atypia are absent. If the latter two features are present (the pattern thus resembling that of a low-grade (grades I or II) transitional carcinoma of the urinary bladder), they designate it as a *proliferating* Brenner tumor[395,404] (Fig. 19.264). When this pattern is associated with a greater degree of atypia (equivalent to a grade III transitional cell carcinoma) but stromal invasion cannot be demonstrated, the terms *borderline* or *low malignant potential* have been suggested.[404] Typical, metaplastic, proliferating, and borderline Brenner tumors have been found to follow a benign clinical course after

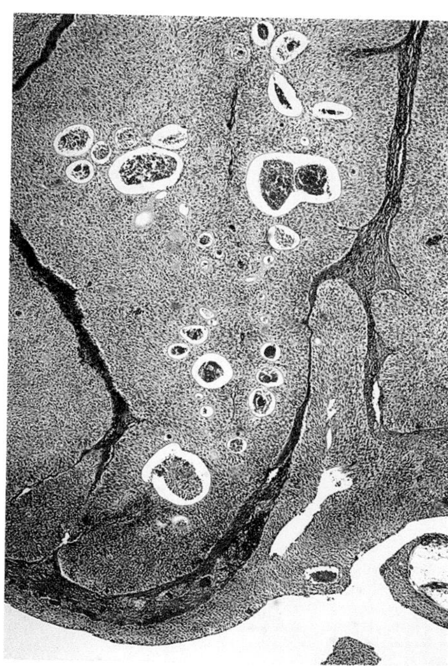

Fig. 19.264 Highly proliferating (borderline) Brenner tumor.

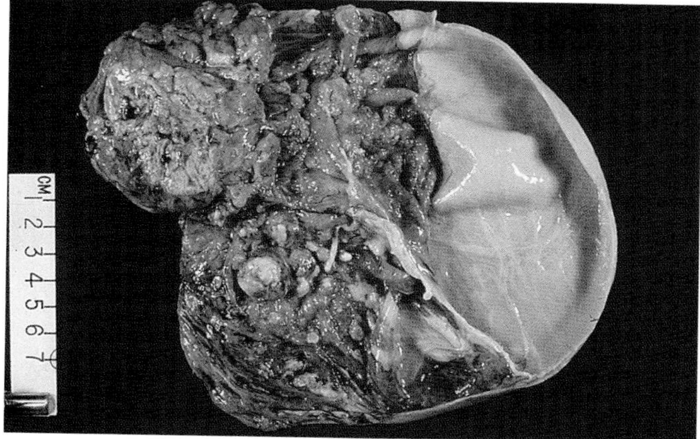

Fig. 19.265 Borderline Brenner tumor showing solid area with papillary formations, associated with a large cystic space.

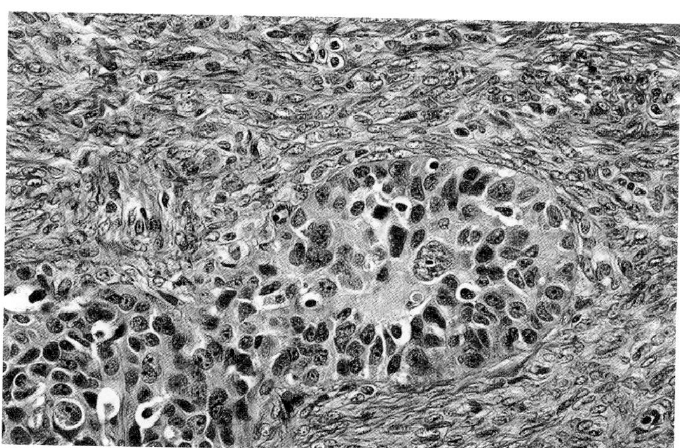

Fig. 19.266 Malignant Brenner tumor. The nuclear atypia is evident. Other areas of the tumor had the typical appearance of Brenner tumor.

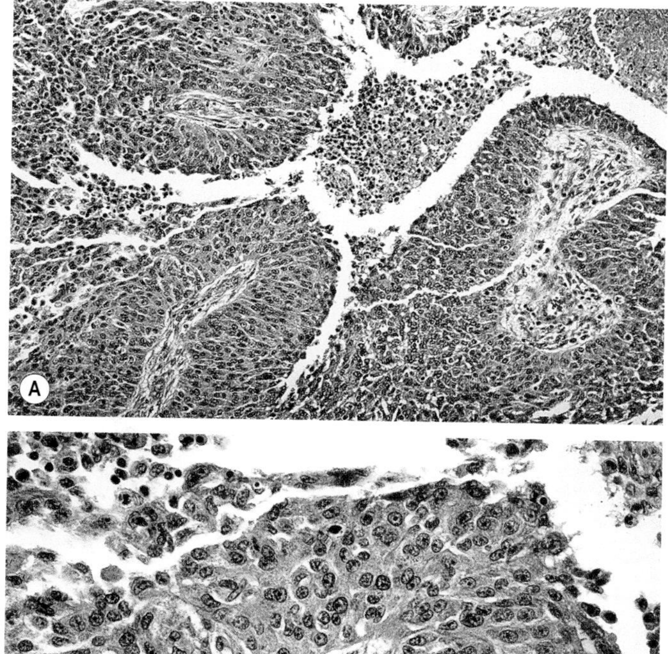

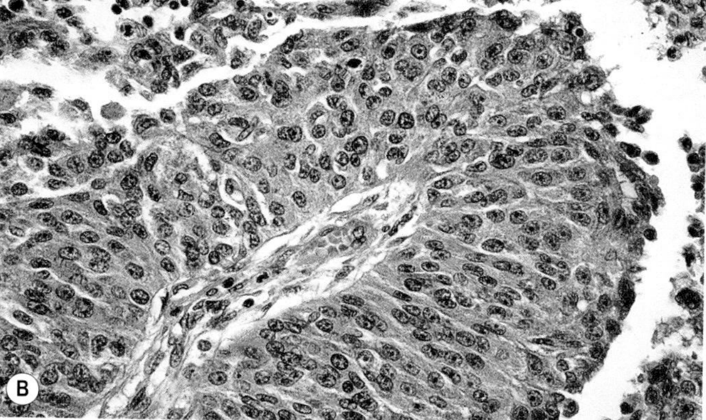

Fig. 19.267 **A** and **B**, Low- and high-power views of transitional cell carcinoma of ovary.

oophorectomy. The latter three types are sometimes grouped under the term *intermediate Brenner tumor.*[405] Cytologically malignant neoplasms associated with *stromal invasion* are referred to as *malignant Brenner tumors* (Fig. 19.265). Some of these cases have been bilateral.[390,395,410] They are recognized mainly because of their association with a typical benign, metaplastic, proliferating, or borderline component.[403] The appearance may be that of a transitional cell, squamous, glandular, or undifferentiated carcinoma, or an admixture of these[403] (Fig. 19.266).

Austin and Norris[384] pointed out that malignant Brenner tumors with an associated benign component have a better prognosis than morphologically similar tumors in which such a component was absent. They refer to the latter as **transitional cell carcinomas** (non-Brenner type)[406] (Fig. 19.267). Features that have been found useful in the identification of this tumor are 'punched out' microspaces, large cystic spaces, and large blunt papillae.[387] The claim that a transitional cell pattern in high-grade ovarian carcinoma is an indicator of favorable response to chemotherapy[402] has not been confirmed in other series, which have shown that – stage for stage – transitional cell carcinoma is not prognostically different from serous carcinoma.[385,392]

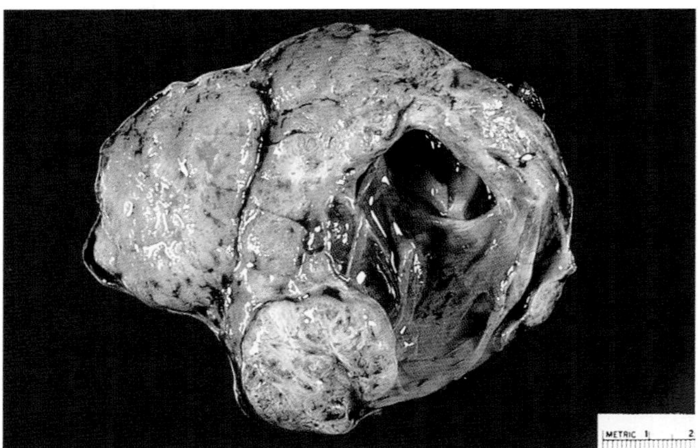

Fig. 19.268 Brenner tumor with typical solid appearance coexisting with mucinous cystadenoma. This is a well-recognized combination.

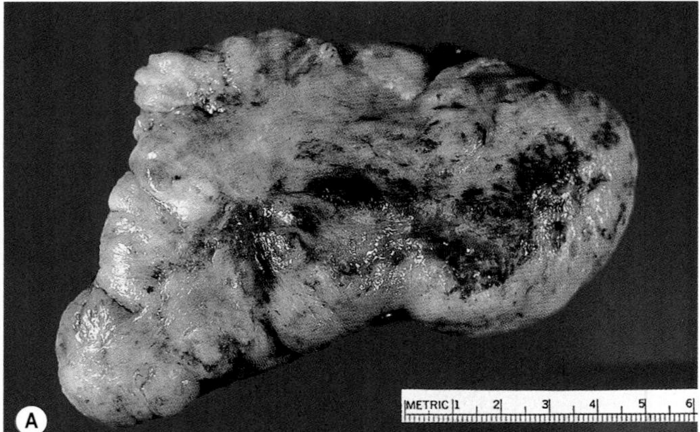

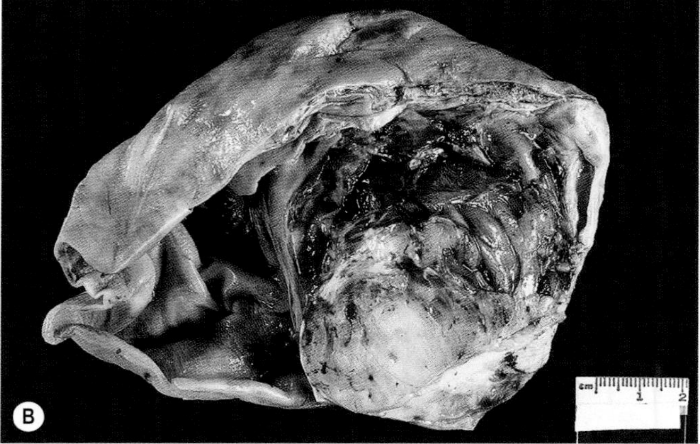

Fig. 19.269 **A** and **B**, Gross appearances of malignant mixed müllerian tumor of ovary. The neoplasms are large, variegated, solid and cystic, with hemorrhagic and necrotic areas.

Brenner tumors show a strong association with mucinous tumors[409] (Fig. 19.268) and are sometimes seen together with struma ovarii.[397] They have also been found to coexist with transitional cell (urothelial) tumors of the urinary bladder.[415,416] About one-fourth of the transitional cell carcinomas are a component of mixed carcinomas, the serous type being the most common representative.[387]

Most authors currently favor for Brenner tumor an origin from surface ovarian epithelium or the cysts derived from them, through a process of metaplasia.[411] The continuity that has been demonstrated between the epithelial nests of Brenner tumor and the ovarian surface supports this concept, which is currently preferred over the alternatives of an origin from Walthard cell nests (microscopically similar but usually located in the mesosalpinx rather than the ovary), granulosa cells, rete ovarii, or germ cells. Whether this metaplasia is truly along transitional cell (urothelial) lines remains controversial. Some authors have found no immunohistochemical similarities between bladder urothelial tumors and either Brenner tumors or ovarian transitional cell carcinoma.[394,399,400,414] Others have found an analogy by way of uroplakins and CK20, but surprisingly only in Brenner tumor and not in ovarian transitional cell carcinoma.[398,401] Another interesting finding relates to the phenotypic differences between Brenner tumors (whether benign, borderline or malignant) and transitional cell carcinomas, suggesting different tumorigenic pathways.[386,393]

Brenner tumors have exceptionally been seen to occur in accessory ovaries[391] or in other female genital tract sites, including vagina (see pp. 1431 and 1518).

Malignant mixed müllerian tumor and müllerian adenosarcoma

Malignant mixed müllerian tumor (MMMT) of the ovary resembles grossly and microscopically in every respect its more common uterine counterpart (Fig. 19.269). Thus a *homologous* variety (with nonspecific malignant stroma; also called *carcinosarcoma*) and a *heterologous* variety (with malignant heterologous elements) occur.[425] The carcinomatous component may be of serous, endometrioid, squamous, or clear cell (mesonephroid) type. The sarcoma-like elements may have the appearance of chondrosarcoma (the most common), osteosarcoma, rhabdomyosarcoma, or angiosarcoma (Fig. 19.270). Hyaline droplets containing α_1-antitrypsin are often present in the cytoplasm of the tumor cells.[424] Although some response to chemotherapy has been noted,[432] the overall prognosis is extremely poor,[423] with some outstanding exceptions.[422] The most reliable prognostic criterion is the initial tumor stage.[417,419,420,431] Unfortunately, most tumors have already extended outside the ovary at the time of surgery.[428] The most important differential diagnosis is with immature (malignant) teratoma. Almost all MMMTs are seen in postmenopausal patients (often with a history of low parity), whereas immature teratomas are typically tumors of children and adolescents. Furthermore, the former usually lack the neural and other germ cell elements of teratomas. However, cases of MMMT featuring prominent neuroectodermal differentiation have been described, their appearance being reminiscent of teratoid carcinosarcoma of the upper respiratory tract.[426,430,433]

Müllerian adenosarcoma, more commonly seen in the endometrium and cervix, also can occur in the ovary.[418,421,427,429] The morphologic appearance and behavior are again similar to those of its uterine counterpart, including the occurrence of sex cordlike elements, sarcomatous overgrowth, and heterologous elements.[427] The subject has already been discussed in this chapter (see Uterus – corpus), in which it was pointed out that müllerian adenosarcoma is probably more closely related to endometrial stromal sarcoma than to MMMT.

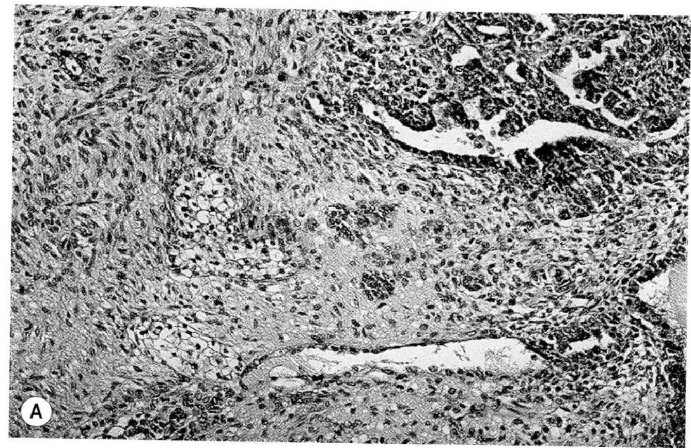

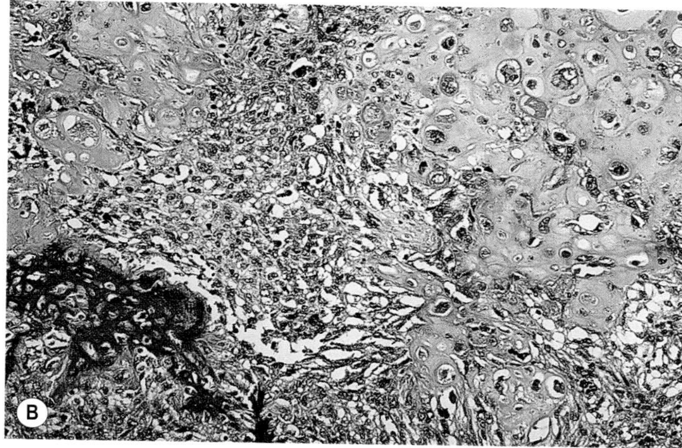

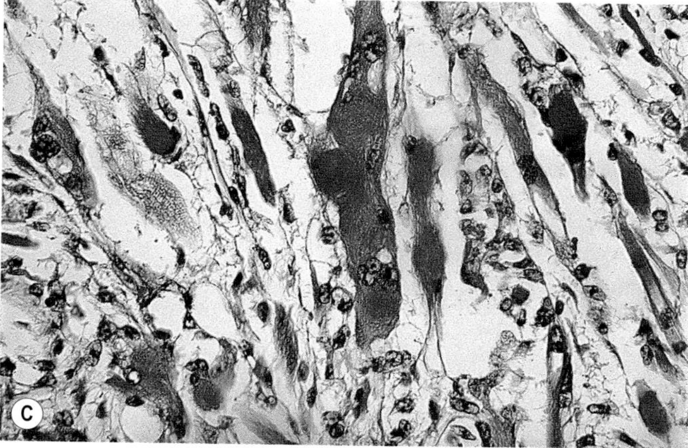

Fig. 19.270 A–C, Malignant mixed müllerian tumor of ovary. The tumor shown in **A** is of the so-called 'homologous type', whereas the others exhibit heterologous foci in the form of bone and cartilage (**B**) or skeletal muscle (**C**).

Adenoid cystic and basaloid carcinomas

Exceptionally, surface epithelial carcinomas of the ovary show a pattern resembling that of salivary gland carcinomas of adenoid cystic type or that of cutaneous basal cell carcinomas.[434–436] These may be seen in pure form or in association with conventional serous, endometrioid, or clear cell patterns. The tumors with an adenoid cystic carcinoma-like appearance are more aggressive than the basaloid neoplasms.[434]

Mixed and other epithelial tumors

As important as the distinctions made in the previous sections are, the fact that ovarian tumors exist with mixed, hybrid, or intermediate features should be recognized.[441] In general, the less differentiated the tumor, the more difficult it is to place it in a specific category in regard to cell type; some must simply remain in an *undifferentiated* or *unclassified* category.[442] It also needs to be acknowledged that the distinction between serous and endometrioid tumors is subject to considerable individual observer variability.[438,439]

Che et al.[437] reported on a peculiar subtype of mixed epithelial tumor with a predominant microcystic growth pattern and signet ring cells, which can be easily confused with a metastatic tumor. There have also been reports of *lymphoepithelioma-like carcinoma* apparently primary in the ovary.[440]

Ovarian carcinoma – overview

General and clinical features

Ovarian carcinoma accounts for the greatest number of deaths from malignancies of the female genital tract and is the fifth leading cause of cancer fatalities in women.[444,456] The incidence remains constant. It is predominantly a disease of older white women of northern European extraction, but it is seen in all ages and ethnic groups.[443,453,461,469] Pregnancy (especially if before age 25 years) and use of oral contraceptives are associated with a diminished risk.[448,450,460,465] A cohort of infertile women treated with clomiphene has been found to be at an increased risk for borderline and invasive ovarian tumors.[462]

Familial predisposition has been noted in approximately 5–10% of cases.[449,452,455,457] The risk for developing ovarian cancer is increased fourfold in women with an affected first-degree relative. The majority of the familial ovarian cancers are due to mutation in the *BRCA1* gene (located in the long arm of chromosome 17) or the *BRCA2* gene (located in the long arm of chromosome 13).[468] It has been calculated that mutations in *BRCA1* occur in approximately 5% of women in whom ovarian cancer is diagnosed before the age of 70 years.[464] Prophylactic salpingo-oophorectomy reduces considerably the risk of gynecologic cancer (and possibly also that of breast cancer) and is, therefore, being performed in an increasing number of these individuals.[451,459] The more than occasional finding in these specimens of incidental tumors in the ovary and other sites provides strong support for this practice.[446,458] Most of the ovarian cancers developing in carriers of the *BRCA1* mutation are of the serous type, but endometrioid and other types can also occur.[463,466] There is a conspicuous absence of borderline and mucinous tumors in this population.[467] Some of the ovarian cancers do not fit easily into the conventional types; some have an admixture of papillary, cribriform, gyriform, and morular patterns of growth, whereas others exhibit a combination of clear cell and squamoid features.[445]

Other familial syndromes associated with an increased risk of ovarian carcinoma are *Lynch type II syndrome* (due to mutations of DNA mismatch repair genes) and *hereditary site-specific ovarian cancer syndrome* (which may also be related to *BRCA1* mutations).

It has been speculated that the rapid cycles of cell division associated with wound repair at the time of follicular rupture may contribute to the development of ovarian carcinoma.[447] A related suggestion is that ovarian inflammation, whether physiologic (related to follicular rupture) or pathologic (as in endometriosis or pelvic inflammatory disease), may possibly contribute to the development of ovarian cancer.[454]

Clinically, ovarian carcinomas usually present with lower abdominal pain, abdominal enlargement (usually due to the presence of ascites) and signs of increased pressure on neighboring organs.

Ovarian tumors in children

Germ cell tumors are the most common tumors in children, accounting for 60–70% of all ovarian tumors in this age group.[472,473,479] Whereas mature cystic teratomas predominate, the proportion of malignant germ cell tumors (especially immature teratomas, yolk sac tumors, and dysgerminomas) is much greater than in adults.[470,471,475–477]

Sex cord–stromal tumors constitute 10–25% of cases and are largely represented by the juvenile form of granulosa cell tumor and fibrothecomas.[480] Tumors of surface epithelium represent only 15–20% of ovarian tumors in children, and the vast majority are benign.[474] Indubitable cases of carcinoma occur, particularly of the mucinous type; however, some cases reported as serous carcinomas actually represent yolk sac tumors or retiform Sertoli–Leydig cell tumors with a prominent papillary component. It has been estimated that only 3% of ovarian carcinomas develop in patients younger than 20 years of age.

As in adults, primary malignant ovarian tumors in children need to be distinguished from metastatic neoplasms. The latter include neuroblastoma, adrenal gland carcinoma, rhabdomyosarcoma, Ewing sarcoma/PNET, and intra-abdominal desmoplastic small cell tumor.[478]

'Early', 'occult', and in situ carcinoma

The concept of carcinoma in situ or ovarian intraepithelial neoplasia distinct from the borderline tumors has only recently gained some acceptance[485] (Fig. 19.271). As in other organs, one of the criteria for its recognition is its occurrence in the remainder of an ovary affected by a primary invasive carcinoma[488] or in the contralateral ovary.[487,490] Bell and Scully[482] studied 14 'early de novo' carcinomas detected as microscopic findings in grossly normal ovaries. All were unilateral, and four were multifocal. Most cases involved the superficial cortex only. The large majority were of serous type. Severe atypia of the noncarcinomatous surface epithelium or its inclusion cysts were present in three cases. In six of the cases, tumor spread developed, indicating an aggressive behavior despite their minute dimensions.

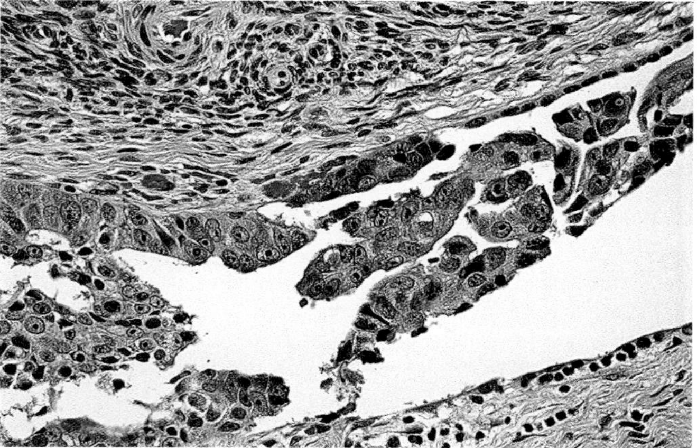

Fig. 19.271 Carcinoma in situ limited to a microscopic focus on the ovarian surface.

Microscopic evaluation of prophylactic oophorectomy specimens in patients with *BRCA1* and *BRCA2* mutations has documented an increased incidence of atypical proliferative epithelial lesions, including in situ carcinoma.[486,489] The rate of the latter has ranged from 13% to 23% in the various series,[481,483,484] and it has been higher in *BRCA1* than in *BRCA2* patients.

Molecular genetic features

Cytogenetically, ovarian carcinomas contain complex numerical and structural anomalies. These include, among others, losses in chromosomes X, 22, 18, 17, 14, 13, 12, and 8; gains in chromosomes 12 and 8; and rearrangements of 1, 3, 6, 11, and 19.[510,513,517] The loci most commonly affected are 19p+ (about half of the cases),[509] the short arm of chromosome 11,[503] and 17q (particularly with the serous tumors).[497] Trisomy 12 is sometimes the only chromosome abnormality found in benign and borderline serous tumors.[518]

Telomerase activity is found in virtually all carcinomas and borderline tumors but not in cystadenomas. Oncogenes reported to be amplified are *HER2/neu*, cyclin D1, cyclin A, *P21*, and *MDM2*.[491–496,499,508,512] In addition, the epidermal growth factor receptor (EGFR) and the M-CSF receptor are expressed along with the respective ligands (peptide growth factors) in some cases.[491,500,501]

Loss of *DAB2* (a candidate tumor suppressor gene) occurs in approximately 80% of ovarian carcinomas; it has also been detected in dysplastic lesions of the ovarian surface epithelium.[516]

Mutations of *TP53* leading to overexpression of the protein product occur in approximately 30% of the cases overall, the prevalence being directly related to tumor grade and stage.[493,504,507] They are particularly common in serous carcinomas (two-thirds of cases), and probably represent early events in the genesis of these tumors.[506]

Mutations of *KRAS* are more common in mucinous than in serous or endometrioid carcinomas.[494,495] Among the serous tumors, they have been found by one group in about half of borderline serous tumors and micropapillary serous tumors with or without microinvasion, but not in high-grade conventional serous carcinomas, suggesting the existence of two different tumorigenic pathways.[511]

Up to 40% of endometrioid carcinomas exhibit deregulation of the Wnt signaling pathway, with nuclear accumulation of β-catenin, usually due to mutations in the β-catenin gene *CTNNB1*, and less commonly inactivating mutation of the *APC* gene.[515]

Amplification and overexpression of the *LMYC* proto-oncogene has recently been found to be a common feature of ovarian carcinoma.[514]

Loss of heterozygosity at the *RB1* locus has been found in approximately 20% of cases; it is more common in the carcinomas than in the borderline tumors, and in the serous than the other types.[498]

Mutations of *DCC*, *BRCA1*, and *BRCA2* are rare in sporadic serous carcinomas.[502]

DNA ploidy analyses have shown that benign and borderline tumors are usually diploid, whereas a majority of the invasive carcinomas are aneuploid.[505]

Spread and metastases

The most common sites of involvement of ovarian serous carcinoma are the contralateral ovary, peritoneal cavity (further discussed in the next section), para-aortic and pelvic lymph nodes, and liver. With intra-abdominal spread, there are often ascites and involvement of the omentum.[531] Invasion of the intestinal wall may result in obstruction.[521] Ureteral involvement is usually associated with hydronephrosis. An umbilical metastasis ('Sister Joseph's nodule') may be the first manifestation of the disease.[519,527] Lung and pleura are the most common sites of extra-abdominal spread.[524] Most lung metastases have a subpleural location. Metastases can also occur in unusual sites, such as the breast.[525]

The spread of borderline serous tumors is mainly in the form of invasive or noninvasive peritoneal implants (see below), but they can also involve lymph nodes of the neck and other sites,[520] lung, pleura, mediastinum (sometimes associated with multilocular thymic cyst) and breast.[520,523,526,528–530] Occasionally cervical lymph node involvement is the first sign of the disease.[522,532]

The sites of involvement of metastatic mucinous and endometrioid ovarian carcinoma are similar to those of the serous tumors, but there is less tendency to early and widespread peritoneal involvement.

Peritoneal lesions and the müllerian system

A variety of proliferative epithelial lesions involving the peritoneum have phenotypic features indicative of müllerian differentiation. Theoretically, they could develop through two different mechanisms: (1) spread from an ovarian (or, less commonly, endometrial or tubal) source; and (2) autochthonous origin from the so-called 'secondary müllerian system', i.e., the pelvic and lower abdominal mesothelium and the subjacent mesenchyme of females. The two most important manifestations of this process are designated respectively as implants and endosalpingiosis, the assumption being that the first is an example of the former phenomenon, and the second of the latter.

Implants. One of the most common patterns of spread of ovarian carcinoma – particularly the serous type – is in the form of tumor deposits on the peritoneal surfaces (Fig. 19.272). Sites of early peritoneal spread are the lateral gutters and diaphragmatic surface (predominantly on the right side), omentum, and pelvic peritoneum, including the serosa of the uterine corpus, the fallopian tube,[546] and the ovarian surface itself ('autoimplants').[565] Involvement of abdominal viscera (bowel, liver, spleen) is generally by direct spread from the underlying peritoneum. There is a tendency for concentration of tumor nodules close to the primary tumor, so the pelvic peritoneum, sigmoid colon, cecum, and terminal ileum are most frequently involved. Sometimes, the entire peritoneal cavity is covered by implants measuring less than 1 cm in diameter and grossly simulating miliary tuberculosis.

Peritoneal implants are present in 16–47% of borderline serous tumors and are associated with a mortality rate of 13–30%.[537] Although traditionally designated as 'implants', it is possible and indeed likely that some arise in situ from the peritoneal mesothelium.[555] The large majority of ovarian borderline neoplasms associated with peritoneal implants have an exophytic pattern of growth on the ovarian surface, which provides them with direct contact with the peritoneal cavity.[566,568] The microscopic appearance of these implants is similar to that of the ovarian tumor and is, therefore, characterized by tufting, stratification, cytologic atypia, and psammoma bodies[535,562] (Fig. 19.273). They can be predominantly cystic or papillary. Some have been known to regress spontaneously, sometimes leaving a shower of psammoma bodies behind. Indeed, it has been suggested that salpingoliths (round calcific structures on the serosa of the fallopian tubes) may have a similar pathogenesis, at least in some instances.[569] Infiltration of underlying tissues and marked cytologic atypia are associated with a high probability of disease progression.[560] Accordingly, these implants have been divided into *noninvasive* and *invasive*. Noninvasive implants are further subdivided into *epithelial* and *desmoplastic*. The epithelial implants may be exophytic or buried within invaginations beneath the peritoneal surface; they are characterized by a papillary pattern of growth, mild to moderate atypia, and lack of inflammation or stromal reaction. In desmoplastic noninvasive implants, the epithelial component is more irregular, the cells have a more abundant acidophilic cytoplasm, and – most importantly – there is inflammation (occasionally severe) and a brisk stromal reaction with a

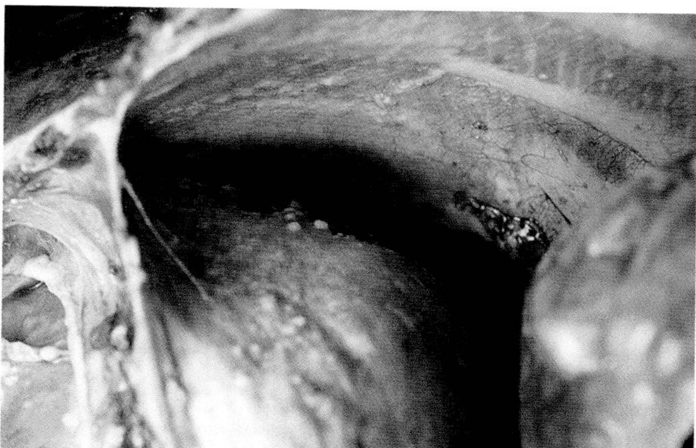

Fig. 19.272 Gross appearance of peritoneal implants from ovarian serous neoplasm.

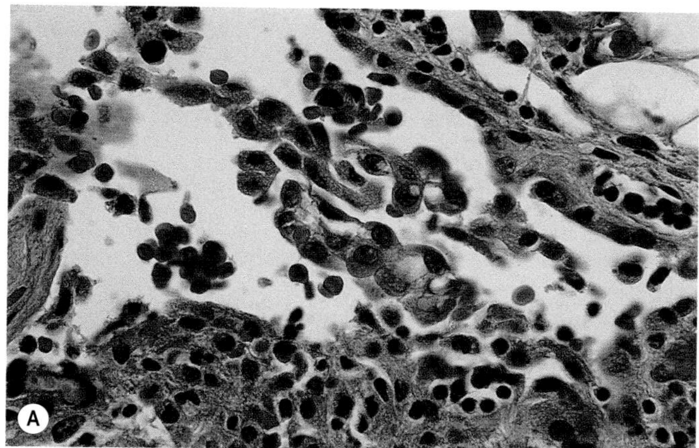

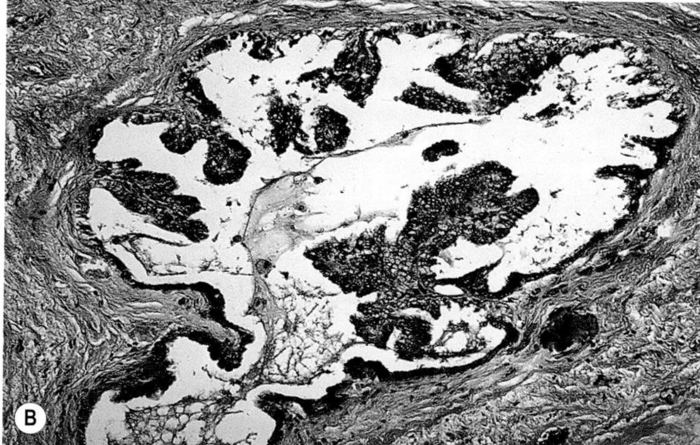

Fig. 19.273 **A** and **B**, Microscopic appearance of peritoneal implants of epithelial (noninvasive, nondesmoplastic) type.

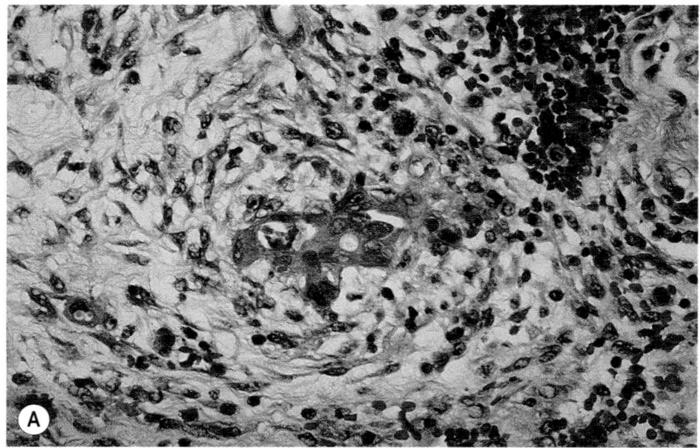

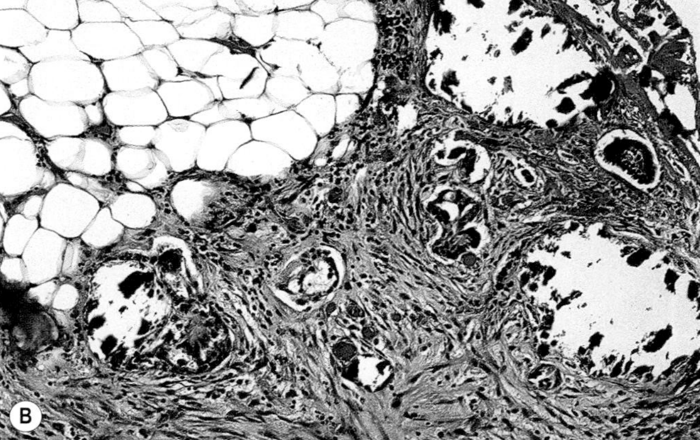

Fig. 19.274 Peritoneal implants of desmoplastic (**A**) and invasive (**B**) types.

granulation tissue-like appearance (Fig. 19.274A). Invasive implants show haphazard 'destructive' infiltration of the stroma (Fig. 19.274B). As a general rule, psammoma bodies are less numerous than in noninvasive implants. The nuclear atypia is not necessarily more pronounced (but see below). Some implants of either noninvasive or invasive type are composed of papillary cores within clear spaces lined by mesothelial cells or tumor cells, resulting in a glomeruloid appearance.[557] Stains for elastic tissue (to identify the peritoneal elastic lamina) are only of limited value in determining whether peritoneal implants are invasive or not.[570]

Peritoneal implants should be distinguished from endosalpingiosis (as described later) and from florid mesothelial hyperplasia, of a type similar to that most commonly seen in hernia sacs and around ruptured tubal pregnancies.[541]

Occasionally, one or multiple peritoneal nodules with features of ovarian serous borderline or malignant tumors can be seen in the presence of minimal or no ovarian involvement.[552] The malignant-appearing lesions have generally been regarded as ovarian carcinomas with widespread metastases if the ovary was affected, however focally and superficially (see discussion of serous surface papillary carcinomas on p. 1565), and as **extraovarian (peritoneal) papillary serous carcinomas** in the absence of ovarian abnormalities.[544,554,559] Their immunohistochemical and ultrastructural profile and their natural history are closer to ovarian serous carcinoma than to diffuse peritoneal mesothelioma;[571,573] they should, therefore, be viewed as *carcinomas* composed of cells analogous to those of the similarly named ovarian tumors. Notably, some of these tumors have developed after prophylactic oophorectomy in women with a family history of ovarian carcinoma.[564]

The immunohistochemical distinction between this tumor type and conventional peritoneal mesothelioma is not as sharp as it is between pleural mesothelioma and lung adenocarcinoma, and therefore the criteria employed in the latter instance are not necessarily applicable to the peritoneal situation. This predicament, which is not generally appreciated, has a very simple explanation: whereas in the thoracic cavity one is dealing with two totally unrelated tissue types (mesothelium and endodermally derived lung epithelium), in the abdomen one is dealing with a proliferation of mesothelial origin that in one instance manifests its potential to differentiate along müllerian lines. There are, however, some markers that are more likely to be positive in one or the other. Thus, B72.3, CEA, Ber-EP4, PAX8, placental alkaline phosphatase (PLAP), and hormone receptors are more likely to be expressed by serous carcinoma, whereas calretinin, thrombomodulin, and CK5/6 are more likely to be seen in conventional mesothelioma.[534,540,551,553] Immunohistochemically, reactive mesothelial cells are more likely to be reactive for calretinin than implants, whereas the reverse is true for Ber-EP4, B72.3, Leu-M1, and PAX8.[550]

The **borderline tumors**, which have also been designated as *peritoneal serous micropapillomatosis of low malignant potential*,[539] have a natural history equivalent to that of their ovarian counterpart (i.e., characterized by a good long-term prognosis).[536,572] Morphologically, these tumors resemble the noninvasive implants of ovarian serous borderline tumors. Cases of primary peritoneal serous psammocarcinomas have also been reported, their morphology and natural history being equivalent in all regards to those of their ovarian counterparts.[572]

Before leaving the subject, one ought to mention the reverse situation, which is much more unusual, i.e., that of an ovarian-based tumor having the morphologic and immunohistochemical features of a conventional mesothelioma.[533,542]

Endosalpingiosis. The term *endosalpingiosis*, originally coined for an inflammatory condition of the fallopian tube characterized by attachment of the fimbria to the ovarian surface followed by spread of the fallopian tube epithelium over the adjacent ovary (see p. 1541), is now applied to the presence beneath the peritoneal surface of glands and tubules (sometimes containing papillae and psammoma bodies), lined by cuboidal to low columnar cells, which are sometimes ciliated. Some resemble the endosalpingian mucosa, hence the name (Fig. 19.275). They are thought to be the result of müllerian differentiation or metaplasia of the coelomic mesothelium. Endosalpingiosis is generally seen in association with ovarian serous tumors, usually of borderline type (alone or in conjunction with implants),[543,545] but it may occur in the absence of ovarian abnormalities.[574] Exceptionally, it has been seen in association with lymphangioleiomyomatosis in retroperitoneal lymph nodes.[561] The vanishingly rare müllerian cysts that have been reported in the omentum, mesentery, and retroperitoneum are probably related to endosalpingiosis.[556,574]

Implants or endosalpingiosis? The distinction between these two abnormalities is not always sharp morphologically, and the belief that the first represents a secondary deposit from an ovarian lesion whereas the second is primary at the site is simply an assumption, which may or may not be correct. As a matter of fact, it has been suggested that most lesions designated endosalpingiosis of lymph nodes on morphologic grounds may be 'bland-appearing' manifestations of metastatic tumor.[563] Molecular studies have provided conflicting results, in the sense of favoring multicentric origin in some instances and a clonal nature in others.[549,554,558,567]

Because of this pathogenetic uncertainty, which is, however, counterbalanced by the well-established prognostic significance of

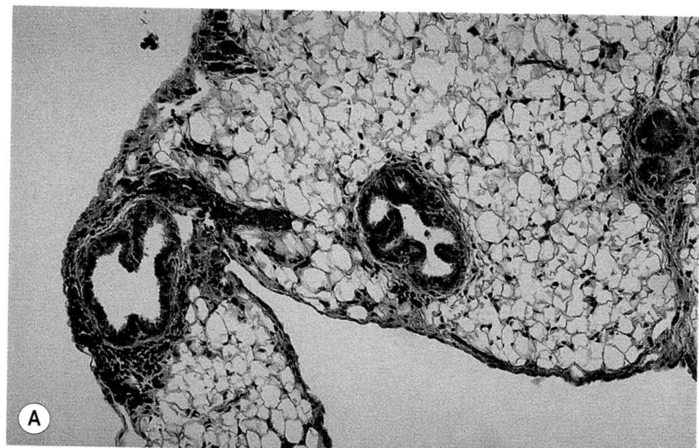

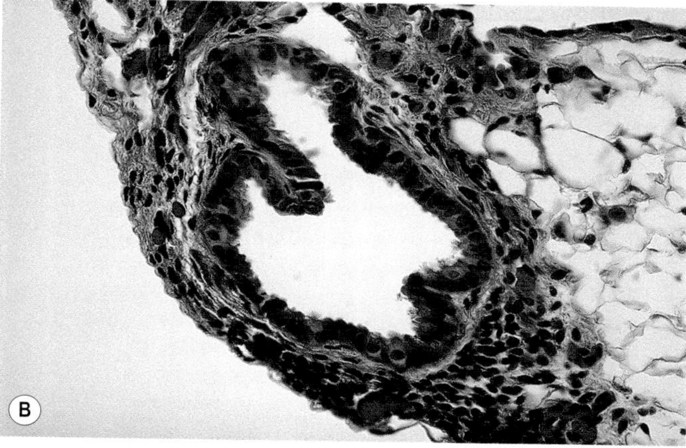

Fig. 19.275 **A** and **B**, Low- and high-power views of peritoneal endosalpingiosis.

the various forms of peritoneal disease, it may be preferable to use a terminology that is pathogenetically noncommittal but which provides the clinician with clinically important information, on the basis of largely architectural criteria. Regardless of whether there is an ovarian component or not, or whether the disease being evaluated is on the peritoneal surface or in a lymph node, one should be able to recognize these main categories:

1 Lesions that are cytologically benign, noninvasive, and nondesmoplastic. These include so-called 'endosalpingiosis' and noninvasive nondesmoplastic ('epithelial') implants. Most of these patients do well and should be treated conservatively, but a small percentage will develop progressive disease.[548]
2 Lesions that lack nuclear atypia and stromal invasion, but which are associated with a prominent desmoplastic response ('desmoplastic' implants). These patients seem to do similarly to those in the first category.[548]
3 Lesions accompanied by 'destructive' stromal invasion, whether they display nuclear atypia or not ('invasive' implants). These tend to behave in an aggressive fashion.[547]
4 Lesions lacking stromal invasion but exhibiting a micropapillary architecture and/or solid epithelial nests surrounded by clefts. This category is controversial, but the authors who proposed these criteria believe that the behavior of this lesion is as aggressive as those in the third category.[538]

Coexistence with uterine carcinoma

The simultaneous presence of carcinoma in the ovary and uterus is an uncommon but well-recognized event.[580] The two tumors may have a similar appearance (usually endometrioid but sometimes papillary serous, clear cell, or mucinous) or be of different histologic types.[576] Theoretically, this phenomenon could be the result of: (1) metastasis from an endometrial carcinoma into the ovary; (2) two independent primary tumors; or (3) metastasis from an ovarian carcinoma to the endometrium.[579] All three events probably occur, the third being by far the least common. A distinction between the first two possibilities is often difficult and may be impossible to make. The criteria used for this distinction and the information that has been recently obtained in this regard from the application of molecular genetic techniques are discussed under Uterus – corpus (see p. 1499). Briefly, ovarian metastasis from an endometrial tumor should be favored in the presence of multiplicity, bilaterality, and/or very small size of the ovarian tumor, involvement of the tubal lumen, and presence of deep myometrial invasion and/or vascular invasion in the uterine tumor.[576] Most neoplasms with an endometrioid appearance in both sites are probably independent neoplasms, and their prognosis is excellent; most of those with histologies other than endometrioid probably represent a single primary tumor with metastases, and their prognosis is correspondingly poor.[576,581] At the immunohistochemical level, a panel of ER+, WT1+, P53+, and IMP3– favors an ovarian origin.[583]

Sometimes, the uterine tumor involves the cervix rather than the corpus; interestingly, a high proportion of these cervical tumors are of endometrioid type.[578] The lesion should be regarded as an ovarian metastasis from a cervical primary if there is bilateral ovarian involvement and extensive extracervical disease, if the microscopic type is one unusual for an ovarian primary (such as squamous cell carcinoma or small cell carcinoma), or if there is evidence of HPV (such as immunoreactivity for p16 or positivity for HPV DNA by in-situ hybridization).[575,577,582]

The association between ovarian and uterine neoplasms is also discussed in connection with the specific histologic types.

Cytology

The main role of diagnostic cytology in ovarian carcinoma is the identification of malignant cells in the peritoneal cavity. The value of peritoneal washing cytology to detect the microscopic spread of ovarian carcinoma has been acknowledged by the fact that the FIGO staging system incorporates the results of the washing in its scheme.[591] This technique is useful during the initial surgical staging and also in the course of second-look operations for the evaluation of therapy effect. Serous and endometrioid carcinomas are more often positive than carcinomas of other types, and high-grade tumors more than low-grade tumors.[590] Specifically, a high positive rate is related to advanced stage of disease, involvement of the ovarian surface, a moderate to large amount of fluid, and non-bloody serous ascites.[589]

Patients with positive fluids have a worse prognosis than others, but at least some of the difference is related to the stage of the disease; analysis of a large number of patients with stage I and II tumors is needed to determine the prognostic significance of a positive cytology independently of other prognostic factors.[587,590]

The interpretation of peritoneal washings can be made difficult by the admixture of reactive mesothelial cells and problems in distinguishing borderline from malignant tumors,[585] including those in the macropapillary category.[584,585,588]

Another potential use of cytology is in the aspiration of ovarian cysts; the procedure is fairly accurate but of limited practical value.[586]

Therapy

The primary form of therapy of surface epithelial tumors is surgical.[593,598,603] Benign tumors are cured by a conservative operation in the form of unilateral salpingo-oophorectomy. Although in the case of occasional small benign tumors (some surface papillomas and cystadenofibromas) the uninvolved portion of the ovary can be preserved, the majority require the excision of the entire gonad. Most borderline tumors in young females can also be treated conservatively with safety, the results following salpingo-oophorectomy being equivalent to those seen following more extensive procedures.[611,613] As a matter of fact, some cases have been treated with cystectomy only, the overall outcome being excellent; however, presence of tumor at the margin is a strong predictor of tumor recurrence.[601]

Carcinomas require bilateral salpingo-oophorectomy with total abdominal hysterectomy and omentectomy, with the possible exception of grade I mucinous cystadenocarcinoma, for which a conservative approach has been suggested by some authors in selected young patients.[612] The role of pelvic lymphadenectomy (as opposed to lymph node sampling) remains controversial.[595]

It is important to examine carefully the peritoneal cavity during the course of the operation and to biopsy selected sites to properly stage the disease for future therapy.[614] This surgical staging, which also applies to borderline tumors, should include sampling from pelvic and abdominal peritoneal surfaces, diaphragm, omentum, and lymph nodes (pelvic and para-aortic).[600,602] If ascitic fluid is present, it should be examined cytologically; if not, peritoneal washings should be taken.[594] Adjuvant therapy (radiation therapy and/or chemotherapy) is said to be particularly important for high-grade stage I tumors, for tumors accompanied by positive ascitic fluid, and for minimal stage III disease.[597,608,615] The standard chemotherapy for newly diagnosed ovarian cancer is a platinum–taxane combination.[592]

In some institutions, 'second-look' operations were done as a standard procedure for patients with ovarian carcinomas treated with surgery and chemotherapy who are clinically free of disease, to determine prognosis and decide whether chemotherapy should be continued, discontinued, or changed. However, the practical value of this procedure has been questioned on the grounds that the subgroup of patients whose condition can be salvaged by a second-line therapy is small (approximately 8%) and that an effective salvage therapy still remains to be identified.[599,606]

The second-look operation includes direct visual inspection of the abdominal cavity, cytologic examination of peritoneal washings, and multiple biopsies of peritoneum, omentum, and lymph nodes. Residual tumor has been found pathologically in over 40% of patients in most series.[605,607,610] This tends to be found in the same site as the initial tumor.[609] The microscopic interpretation can be complicated by the presence of mesothelial hyperplasia, psammoma bodies without accompanying epithelium, foreign body giant cell reaction, focal fibroblastic proliferation, fat necrosis, and other changes.[596] Immunohistochemical staining for CEA, CD15, and other markers can be helpful in the differential diagnosis.[604]

Prognosis

The overall prognosis of ovarian carcinoma remains poor, a direct result of its rapid growth rate and the lack of early symptoms. The overall survival rate is approximately 35% at 5 years, 28% at 10 years, and 15% at 25 years.[641] Factors known to influence prognosis are listed below:

1. *Age*. As a group, younger patients have a better outcome. This is at least partially due to the fact that there is a higher percentage of borderline, well-differentiated, and stage I tumors in this group.[617,664]
2. *BRCA1 mutations and family history*. It seems that the ovarian cancers developing in patients with *BRCA1* mutations have a significantly more favorable clinical course,[618,645,649] although the statement has been challenged.[632] In patients without *BRCA1* mutations, the prognosis is not significantly different whether there is a family history of breast cancer or not.[621]
3. Presence and extent of *tumor spread* beyond the ovary, as expressed by the *clinical staging*.[655] For the carcinomas (as opposed to the borderline tumors, see later section), this is the most important prognostic determinator.
4. *Ascites*. This clinical finding constitutes, by itself, an unfavorable prognostic sign.[616,624]
5. *Borderline tumors versus carcinomas*. This is a distinction of utmost significance for prognostic purposes.[647,654] The incidence of recurrence is nearly zero for borderline mucinous and endometrioid tumors and approximately 20% for borderline serous or seromucinous tumors.[619] The prognosis in borderline tumors is still very good even in the presence of microinvasion, involvement of the peritoneal cavity in the form of noninvasive implants, or tumor recrudescence in the abdominal cavity. In one series, the survival was 99% for stage I tumors and an astonishing 92% for advanced stage disease.[638] Because of these figures, some authors have questioned whether it is justified to keep labeling these tumors as of low-grade malignant potential or even borderline.[638] The answer is probably 'yes' because of the fact that metastases to lymph nodes and other sites (however they may be called) are seen, that recurrences are not uncommon, and that persistent disease as well as deaths occur.[640] The particular situation of micropapillary serous tumors within this scheme is discussed on page 1580. The semantic controversy notwithstanding, there is agreement that this pattern is associated with a higher recurrence rate than the conventional borderline tumor.
6. *Tumor grade and type*. Among the carcinomas, tumor grade correlates closely with survival.[641,662,663] The problem is that the grading system has varied among published reports, and in some studies it has not been specified at all.[643,659] The standard system is the one recommended by the World Health Organization. Silverberg proposed an alternative system, modeled on the Nottingham grading scheme for breast carcinoma, designed to be applied to all invasive carcinomas of the ovary.[651,660] Yet another attempt to grading is the two-tier system proposed by Malpica et al.[642] for serous carcinoma, which shows a good correlation with the WHO and Silverberg's schemes. The microscopic type (serous, mucinous, endometrioid, or other) is of less significance in this regard, particularly among the lesser differentiated tumors.[641] However, as a group, endometrioid carcinomas do better when pure than when mixed with papillary serous or undifferentiated components.[634,665] Silverberg[660] made the important point that grading is less valuable than typing in predicting survival but better at predicting tumor responsiveness to chemotherapy and even as a guide as to which agents should be used. It follows that both grade and type should be specified in the pathology report.[655]
7. *Psammoma bodies*. Serous tumors containing numerous such structures have a better prognosis,[661] the extreme example being psammocarcinoma, which does not behave significantly differently from a borderline tumor. This may be related to the fact that most of these tumors are well differentiated.

8 *Rupture of tumor capsule.* There is no convincing evidence that this occasional intraoperative complication has any influence on survival rates.[616,656]
9 *DNA ploidy.* DNA analysis with flow cytometry (using either fresh tissue or paraffin-embedded material) has proved a strong prognostic indicator among the ovarian carcinomas, in the sense that aneuploid tumors belong to a higher grade and behave in a much more aggressive fashion than the diploid tumors.[628,629,648] Correlation has also been found between tumor DNA ploidy and response to chemotherapy.[620] The value of flow cytometry is very limited in the evaluation of borderline tumors.[623]
10 *CA-125.* This serum marker has been found of great value in the initial evaluation of these patients (particularly in stage II and beyond) and in the follow-up of recurrent disease.[650,657] It is believed to be an independent prognostic factor.[657]
11 *P53.* Overexpression of P53 has been claimed to be a marker of poor prognosis in most but not all studies.[627,631,639,658]
12 *Tumor angiogenesis.* Increased peritumoral vessel density is believed to be a marker of poor prognosis.[636,653]
13 *Intratumoral T cells.* It has been claimed that the presence of tumor-infiltrating T cells correlates with improved outcome in advanced ovarian cancer.[666]
14 *Other markers.* Overexpression of HER2/*neu*,[644] EGFR,[626] fatty acid synthase (OA-519),[630] *nm23* (purported to be a metastasis suppressor gene),[652] P-glycoprotein (responsible for multidrug resistance),[633] various components of the cell cycle,[622,646] CD24,[637] S100A1,[625] and ezrin[635] have all been found to be associated with aggressive behavior in ovarian carcinoma, but their value as independent prognostic factors needs to be established.

Germ cell tumors

Germ cell tumors constitute approximately 20% of all ovarian neoplasms. Most of them are seen in children and young adults. Approximately 95% of these tumors are benign cystic teratomas; the younger the patient, the more likely the germ cell tumor will be malignant.[671,675]

Significant advances have been made in recent years in the understanding of these tumors,[677,678] many of them fueled by the description of new immunohistochemical markers having a high degree of specificity for germ cell tumors in general and for some of the individual types.[667,670,672]

In the sections that follow, the tumors are discussed as individual types; however, it should be recognized that a combination of various elements occurs in approximately 8% of cases. These are referred to as *mixed germ cell tumors;*[669,674] the most common combination is that of dysgerminoma with yolk sac tumor, but many others occur,[679] including some with a predominance of the polyembryoma component.[673]

One of the greatest achievements in oncology is represented by the therapy of malignant germ cell tumors. Chemotherapeutic regimens consisting of a combination of bleomycin, etoposide, and cisplatin have resulted in overall disease-free survival rates greater than 95%.[668,676]

Dysgerminoma

Dysgerminoma constitutes less than 1% of all ovarian tumors and approximately 5% of malignant ones.[688] Most patients are young. In Santesson's series of nearly 300 cases, 81% were under 30 years of age and 44% were under 20 years of age.[701] Dysgerminoma made up 6% of 188 childhood ovarian neoplasms collected by Abell et al.[680] Approximately 5% of dysgerminomas arise in abnormal gonads: pure or mixed gonadal dysgenesis (from a gonadoblastoma, see p. 1604) or testicular feminization (androgen insensitivity) syndrome. Exceptionally, the tumor is associated with hypercalcemia.[690]

Dysgerminoma is somewhat more common on the right side and is bilateral in 15% of cases.[701] It is often large (it may reach over 1000 g) and encapsulated, with a smooth, often bosselated surface (Fig. 19.276). The cut surface is solid and gray; foci of hemorrhage and necrosis can occur, but they are not as common or prominent as in other malignant germ cell tumors (Fig. 19.277). Microscopically, the tumor cells usually group themselves in well-defined nests separated by fibrous strands infiltrated by lymphocytes (most of which are of T-cell type[689]) (Fig. 19.278). Occasionally, a pseudotubular, alveolar, or cordlike arrangement may be seen (the latter particularly at the tumor periphery), which may be quite confusing[682] (Fig. 19.279). Focal necrosis, hyaline changes in vessels, germinal centers, and granulomatous foci may be present. The individual tumor cells are uniform and have large 'squared-off' nuclei, *one or more prominent elongated nucleoli,* and abundant clear to finely granular cytoplasm that contains glycogen and sometimes fine droplets of fat. The cell membrane is prominent.

Immunohistochemically, the tumor cells are consistently reactive for PLAP and CD117, variably for keratin (erratically and focally),

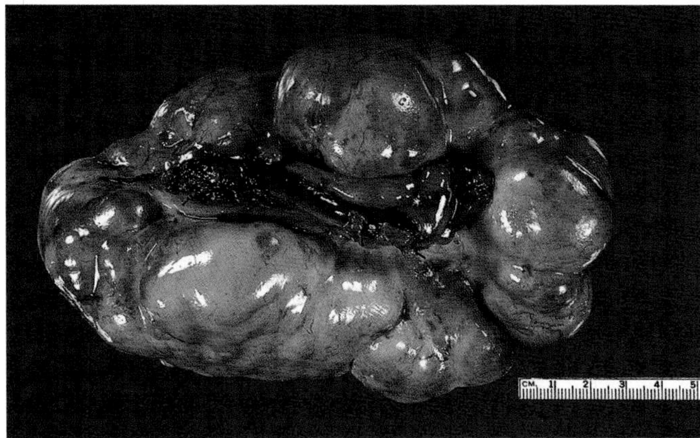

Fig. 19.276 Typical lobulated outer aspect of ovarian dysgerminoma.

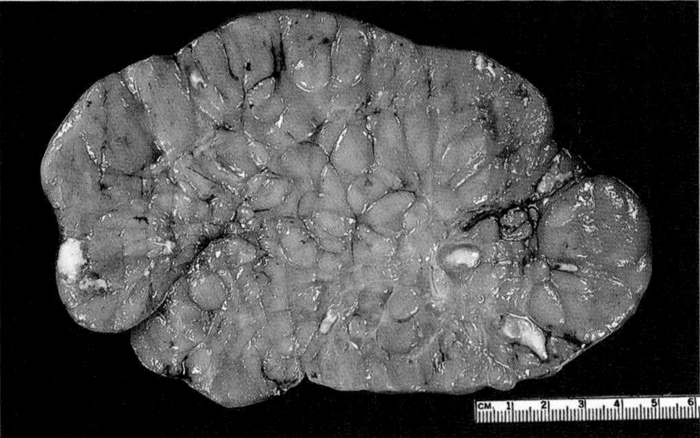

Fig. 19.277 Cut surface of ovarian dysgerminoma. The multinodular solid quality and the tan color are characteristic features.

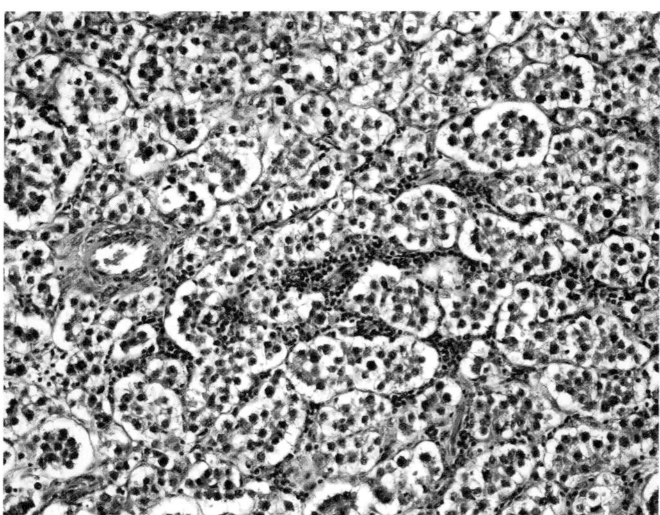

Fig. 19.278 Typical nesting appearance of ovarian dysgerminoma. The septa contain numerous inflammatory cells.

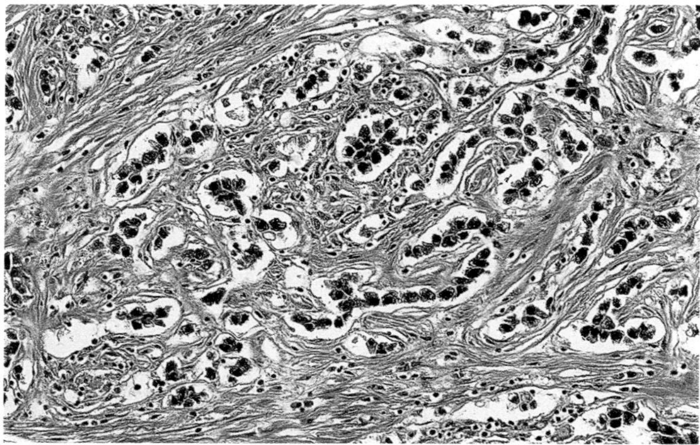

Fig. 19.279 The thin trabecular pattern that dysgerminomas sometimes exhibit may be the source of diagnostic errors.

and sometimes for GFAP and desmin, but not for CD30.[683,687,697,702] A more recent and very promising marker is OCT4, a transcription factor involved in the regulation of pluripotency during embryonic development, which also stains the germ cell component of gonadoblastoma.[686] SALL4, another germ cell tumor marker, is also typically positive.[685]

The microscopic pattern, ultrastructural appearance, immunohistochemical and cytogenetic profiles, clinical behavior, and probable histogenesis (from indifferent or primordial germ cells) of ovarian dysgerminoma are the same as for classic seminoma of the testis.[691,693,695] It differs from the latter with respect to site, type, and frequency of *KIT* point mutations.[700] Like testicular seminoma, ovarian dysgerminoma may exhibit signs of early differentiation toward other types of germ cell elements. These include:

1 Scattered hCG-positive syncytiotrophoblastic cells, often in close proximity to blood vessels or to hemorrhagic foci[703] (Fig. 19.280). This change, seen in approximately 3% of all dysgerminomas, may be accompanied by serum elevation of hCG and tissue immunoreactivity for this marker.

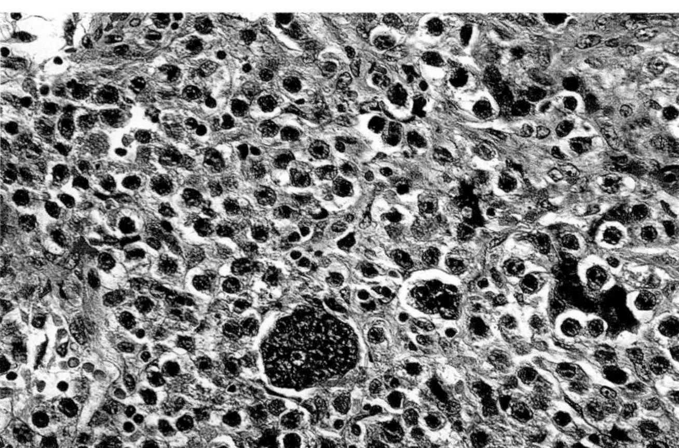

Fig. 19.280 Isolated multinucleated cells of trophoblastic type in ovarian dysgerminoma.

2 'Early carcinomatous differentiation' accompanied by increased mitotic activity (over 30 mitoses per 10 high-power fields), a change sometimes designated – by analogy with its testicular counterpart – *anaplastic dysgerminoma*.[694] This change may be accompanied by increased immunoreactivity for keratin, although – as already noted – positivity for this marker is not unusual in the ordinary dysgerminoma.[697]
3 Abortive yolk sac elements, accompanied by serum elevation of alpha-fetoprotein and tissue immunoreactivity for this marker[699] (Fig. 19.281).

As with the equivalent testicular examples, it is not clear whether any of these changes alters the prognosis of dysgerminoma, and it is, therefore, important to distinguish them from the dysgerminoma admixed with choriocarcinoma, embryonal carcinoma, or yolk sac tumor, a phenomenon that occurs in approximately 10% of cases and that affects prognosis significantly.

Metastases of dysgerminoma occur more commonly in the contralateral ovary, retroperitoneal nodes, and peritoneal cavity, the latter being associated with a decreased survival rate.

The survival rate of pure dysgerminoma is 95%. The initial treatment of unilateral dysgerminoma is oophorectomy. Until recently, radiation therapy was also recommended, since dysgerminoma is an extremely radiosensitive neoplasm. In some institutions this was carried out in all cases, whereas in others it was reserved for the unfavorable ones (i.e., tumors larger than 10 cm and/or if ruptured during removal).[684,688,696] At present, multidrug chemotherapy is regarded as the method of choice for this tumor following its conservative (unilateral) surgical removal.[681,692,698]

Yolk sac tumor (endodermal sinus tumor) and embryonal carcinoma

The history of these two germ cell neoplasms of the ovary is replete with confusing, contradictory, and sometimes erroneous statements as to their origin, relationship, and natural history. Yolk sac tumor was included in Schiller's original description of mesonephroma,[734] together with the ovarian tumor presently designated as clear cell carcinoma.[737] Once it was realized that the latter has a different histogenesis, morphologic appearance, and natural history, the analogy became no longer tenable. The next generation of articles on the subject clearly separated these two neoplasms but used more or less interchangeably the terms *yolk sac tumor* and *embryonal carcinoma*. Since both of these neoplasms are of germ cell derivation,

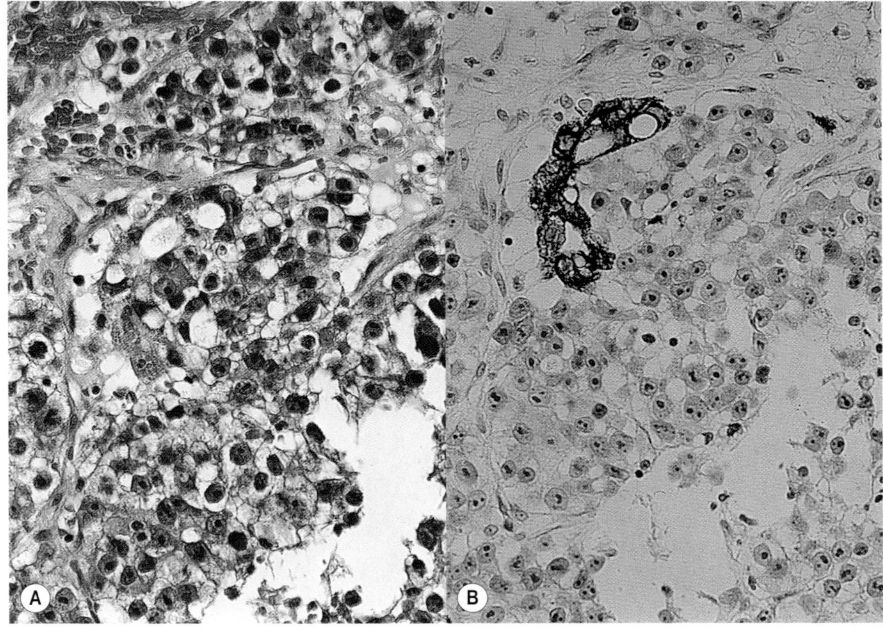

Fig. 19.281 **A** and **B**, Ovarian dysgerminoma with early yolk sac differentiation. **A**, H&E appearance. The foci of early yolk sac differentiation are represented by the small gland-like structures near the center. **B**, This formation is strongly immunoreactive for keratin, in contrast with the rest of the neoplasm.
(Courtesy of Dr Vinita Parash, New Haven, CT)

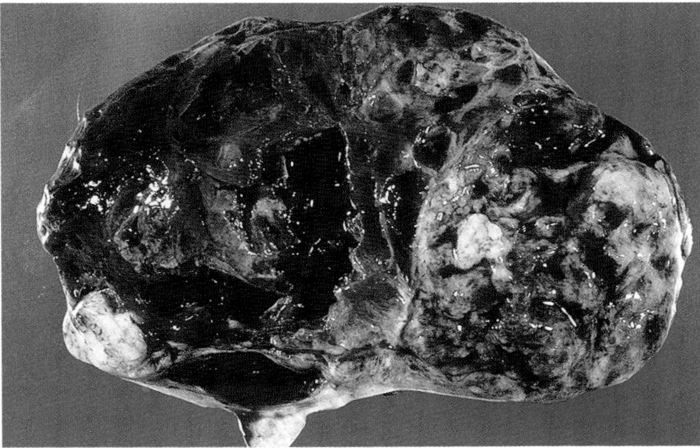

Fig. 19.282 Gross appearance of yolk sac tumor. The cut surface is remarkably heterogeneous due to extensive hemorrhage, necrosis, and cystic degeneration.

share many morphologic features, and are closely related histogenetically, this is not entirely inappropriate.[722] However, enough differences exist between the two to justify their separation.

Yolk sac tumor (endodermal sinus tumor) is generally a neoplasm of children and young adults (median age, 19 years), although it has also been described in the elderly.[730] In the series of Kurman and Norris,[720] 23% of the patients were prepubertal at the time of diagnosis. None of the patients presented with precocious puberty, amenorrhea, or hirsutism. Vaginal bleeding occurred in only 1%. The serum alpha-fetoprotein level was invariably elevated, whereas the chorionic gonadotropin levels were normal, resulting in consistently negative pregnancy tests. Grossly, the tumors had an average diameter of 15 cm, a smooth and glistening external surface, and a variegated cut surface, partially cystic and often containing large foci of hemorrhage and necrosis (Fig. 19.282). A component of benign cystic teratoma was identified in 10 of the 71 cases.

Exceptionally, a yolk sac tumor will be found in the pelvis (in close proximity to the uterus), omentum, or mesentery, unattached to the ovary.[708,716,731]

Microscopically, the appearance of yolk sac tumors is very variable.[713] There are reticular or microcystic areas formed by a loose meshwork lined by flat or cuboidal cells (Fig. 19.283), rounded or festooning pseudopapillary processes with central vessels (Schiller–Duval bodies), and solid 'undifferentiated' areas. The mesenchyme-like component of these tumors has pluripotential properties; it usually presents in the form of spindle cells in a well-vascularized myxoid background, but it exhibits keratin immunoreactivity as a sign of early epithelial differentiation and may contain heterologous elements such as skeletal muscle.[723]

Intracytoplasmic and extracellular PAS-positive hyaline droplets are nearly always present. Their chemical composition is heterogeneous; they usually stain for alpha-fetoprotein, but they may also contain α_1-antitrypsin and basement membrane components (type IV collagen and laminin).[705] Yolk sac tumor also stains for pankeratin, but not for keratin 7 or EMA (in contrast with endometrioid and clear cell ovarian carcinoma), or for WT1 (in contrast with serous ovarian carcinoma).[733] They also exhibit positivity for SALL4 and glypican 3,[740] a property they share with testicular and extragonadal yolk sac tumors.[739] However, OCT4 is typically negative. DNA ploidy studies have shown that yolk sac tumors are almost invariably aneuploid.[719]

A fourth of the yolk sac tumors have vesicular structures with eccentric constrictions surrounded by a dense spindle cell stroma; this has been referred to as a *polyvesicular vitelline pattern* and is said to be associated with a good prognosis when present in a pure form.[727] Others show a scattered hCG-positive syncytiotrophoblast component. Still others exhibit evidence of differentiation toward hepatic, intestinal, and parietal yolk sac structures[709] (Fig. 19.284). The latter are recognized by the presence of thick layers of intercellular basement membrane.[738] The *hepatoid* component, which can predominate almost to the exclusion of the others, is composed of masses, nests, and broad bands of large polyhedral cells with occasional glandular formations and numerous hyaline bodies. Their immunohistochemical profile is similar to that of hepatocellular

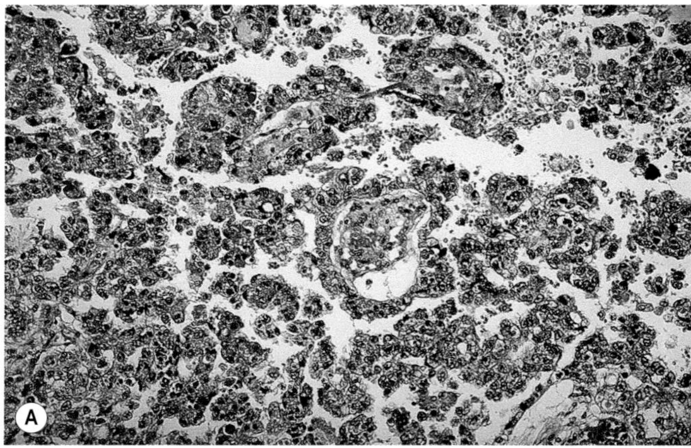

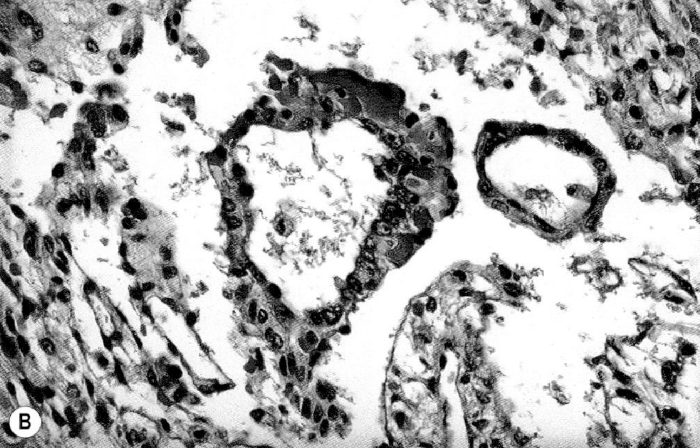

Fig. 19.283 **A** and **B**, Low- and high-power views of ovarian yolk sac tumor. Numerous hyaline globules are seen in the cytoplasm of the tumor cells lining the papillae (**B**).

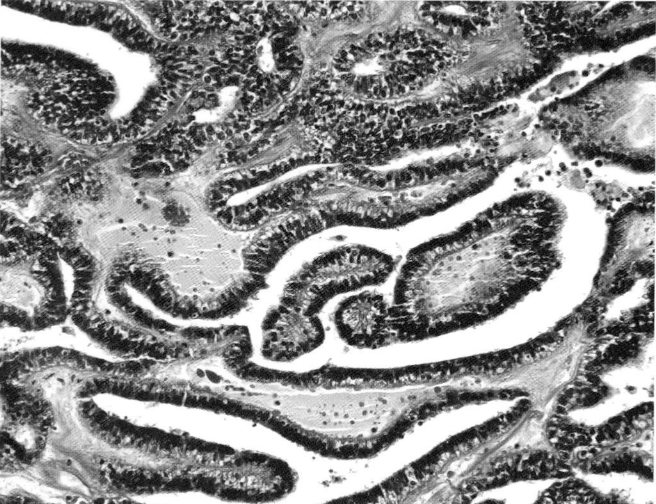

Fig. 19.284 Yolk sac tumor with endometrioid features.

carcinoma, including reactivity for α_1-antitrypsin and a canalicular pattern with polyclonal CEA.[711,732] These hepatoid yolk sac tumors are to be distinguished from *hepatoid ovarian carcinomas,* rare tumors of probable surface epithelial origin[714] (Fig. 19.285). In some yolk sac tumors, the presence of *glandular* formations may simulate the

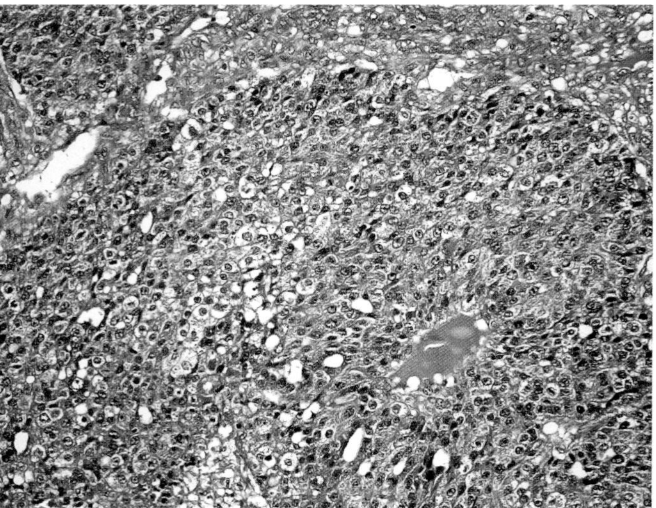

Fig. 19.285 Hepatoid carcinoma of ovary. This tumor, which greatly resembles hepatocellular carcinoma, should be distinguished from yolk sac tumor with hepatoid differentiation.

appearance of endometrioid carcinoma.[707] An exceptional event in ovarian yolk sac tumor is the presence of mucinous carcinoid tumor as a manifestation of endodermal differentiation.[729]

Areas of luteinized stromal cells may be present and may sometimes be responsible for virilization.

Teilum's brilliant hypothesis that this tumor recapitulates normal yolk sac elements[737] has been amply confirmed by histochemical and ultrastructural studies,[725,726,728] including the detection of GATA-4, a transcription factor that regulates the differentiation and function of murine yolk sac endoderm.[735]

In the series of Kurman and Norris,[720] written about 35 years ago, the actuarial survival at 3 years was only 13%; although 71% of the patients were thought to have stage I tumors, subclinical metastases were present in 84%. The introduction of multidrug chemotherapy has dramatically improved survival rates.[712] As usual, clinical stage is the most important prognostic indicator.[718,724] Serial determinations of serum alpha-fetoprotein are useful in monitoring the tumor course.[717,736]

Embryonal carcinoma also occurs in a young age group (median age, 15 years). In one series, 47% of the patients were prepubertal at the time of diagnosis, and 43% of them presented with precocious puberty.[721] Vaginal bleeding was recorded in 33%, amenorrhea in 7%, and hirsutism in 7%. Serum alpha-fetoprotein levels are often (but not always) elevated, whereas chorionic gonadotropin levels are invariably high, to a level that results in consistently positive pregnancy tests.

Grossly, the median diameter of these neoplasms is 17 cm. Their external surface is smooth and glistening, and their cut surface is predominantly solid and variegated, with extensive areas of necrosis and hemorrhage (Fig. 19.286). Microscopically, this tumor has a similar appearance to the embryonal carcinoma of the adult testis. As such, it is composed of solid sheets and nests of large primitive cells, occasionally forming papillae and abortive glandular structures (Fig. 19.286). Syncytiotrophoblast-like tumor cells are frequently seen scattered among the smaller cells; these are immunoreactive for hCG. Embryonal carcinoma shows immunoreactivity for pan-keratin, CD30, OCT4, and SALL4, and variable focal staining for alpha-fetoprotein.[706] In the Kurman and Norris series,[721] the prognosis was somewhat better than for yolk sac tumor, but

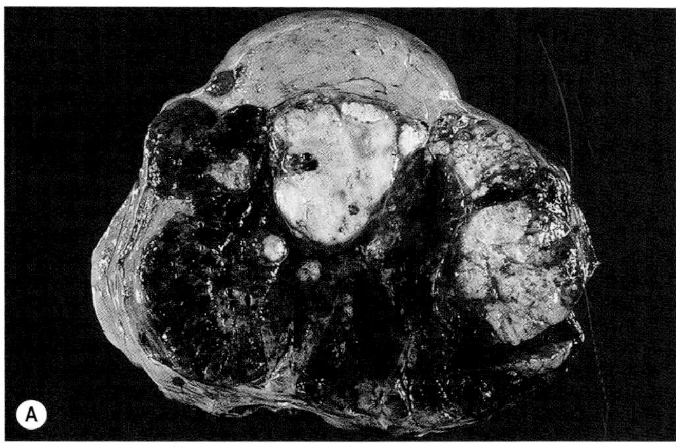

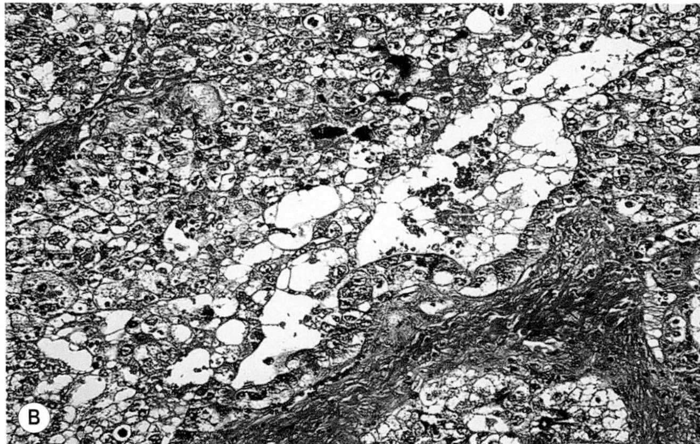

Fig. 19.286 **A** and **B**, Gross and microscopic appearance of embryonal carcinoma of ovary.

current multidrug chemotherapeutic regimens have erased these differences.[704,710]

Embryonal carcinomas largely composed of embryoid bodies are referred to as *polyembryomas*.[715]

Choriocarcinoma

Most choriocarcinomas involving the ovary represent metastases from uterine tumors. The exceedingly rare primary ovarian choriocarcinomas can develop from an ovarian pregnancy (gestational type, which is the most common) or as a form of germ cell neoplasm (nongestational).[744] The latter can be pure or, more frequently, a component of a mixed germ cell tumor. It has also been seen in association with mature cystic teratoma of the contralateral ovary.[745] Microscopically, they show the typical admixture of syncytial and cytotrophoblastic elements in a necrotic and hemorrhagic background. Immunohistochemical reactivity for hCG is the rule; in addition, keratin 7 is said to represent a marker for a subset of trophoblastic cells in these tumors.[742] LK26 (a folate-binding protein) is also consistently expressed, but this can also be found in other ovarian malignancies.[743]

Ovarian choriocarcinomas of either gestational or nongestational type should be distinguished from the exceptionally rare ovarian carcinomas of surface epithelial origin exhibiting choriocarcinomatous differentiation, a phenomenon analogous to that sometimes seen in carcinomas of the lung, breast, endometrium, and other sites.[746]

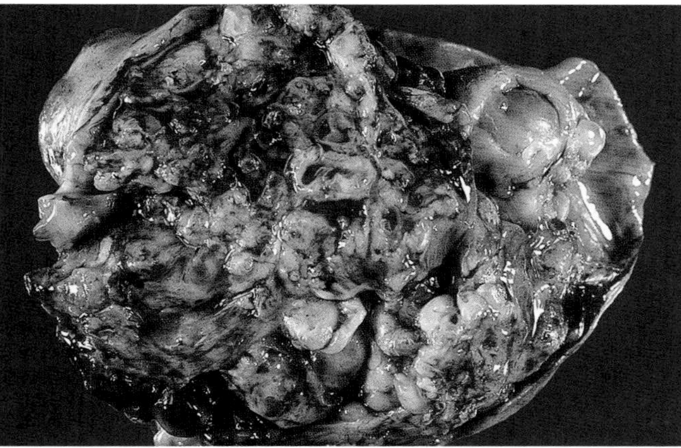

Fig. 19.287 Gross appearance of ovarian immature teratoma.

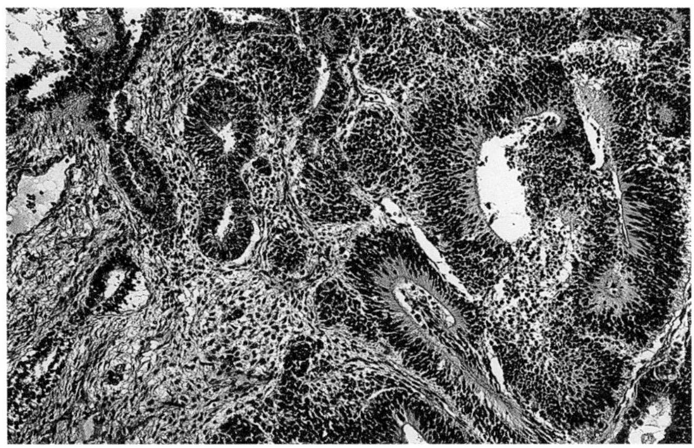

Fig. 19.288 Ovarian immature teratoma with predominance of primitive neuroepithelial elements.

Ovarian gestational choriocarcinomas have a better prognosis than their nongestational counterparts.[747] Among the latter, pure choriocarcinomas are often lethal; conversely, good survival rates have been obtained with the mixed types.[741]

Immature (malignant) teratoma

Immature teratoma is the currently preferred term for the malignant ovarian teratoma usually seen in children and adolescents and composed of a mixture of embryonal and adult tissues derived from all three germ layers, regardless of its gross appearance (Fig. 19.287). Any type of tissue may be represented. The main component is usually neuroepithelial, but mesodermal elements are also common[763] (Fig. 19.288). Some tumors are predominantly composed of endodermal derivatives, including esophagus, liver, and intestinal structures.[765]

Staining for GFAP is helpful in the identification of mature and immature glial tissue.[771] It should be noted, however, that GFAP is also detectable in chondrocytes.[767] Another marker of both immature and mature neural tissue is represented by the long-chain polysialic acid moiety of the neural cell adhesion molecule.[762]

Grossly, immature teratoma may be solid throughout, solid with multiple minute cysts, or predominantly cystic. The prognosis depends a great deal on the nature and amount of the immature component.[750] It is best when the latter is predominantly made up of neuroepithelial tissue. Norris et al.[766] have shown that the size and stage of the teratomas were related to survival but that it was the microscopic grade of the primary tumor that best determined the likelihood of extraovarian spread: similarly, the grade of the metastases correlated best with the subsequent course. Their grading system, which others have shown to correlate with various types of karyotypic abnormality,[756] is the following:

Grade I Abundance of mature tissues, intermixed with loose mesenchymal tissue with occasional mitoses; immature cartilage; tooth anlage

Grade II Fewer mature tissues; rare foci of neuroepithelium with common mitoses, *not exceeding* three low-magnification (×40) fields in any one slide

Grade III Few or no mature tissues; numerous neuroepithelial elements, merging with a cellular stroma *occupying* four or more low-magnification fields.

Obviously, a thorough tumor sampling is necessary for this grading system to be accurate. As an alternative to the above grading scheme, the amount of immature neuroepithelial tissue may also be expressed as an estimated percentage of all the tissue examined microscopically.[768,771]

It is important to separate from this group the teratomas that also have yolk sac or embryonal carcinoma patterns.[750,755] On occasion, an ovarian immature teratoma can be predominantly or exclusively composed of one type of tissue.

Neoplasms with an exclusive or almost exclusive malignant neuroectodermal composition are designated **malignant neuroectodermal tumor** and are generally regarded as a form of monodermal teratoma.[748,760] A variation on the theme is the ovarian **ependymoma**, in which this neuroectodermal component is made up entirely of primitive ependymal structures.[754,759,760] Other teratomas have a prominent component of renal (metanephrogenic),[764] retinal anlage,[758] or skeletal muscle (rhabdomyosarcomatous) nature.[772]

A sometimes confusing pattern seen in teratomas, usually in connection with the neuroectodermal component, is the presence of florid vascular proliferation,[749] a phenomenon possibly due to the secretion of angiogenic factors by the tumor cells and which has also been recorded at other sites.[752]

Another peculiar morphologic change sometimes encountered in these tumors is membranous fat necrosis, perhaps secondary to torsion and ischemia.[769]

The treatment of immature teratoma consists of surgery plus multidrug chemotherapy;[751,757,761] sometimes, only mature tissue is found in metastatic sites following chemotherapy, a sign of excellent prognosis.[770] It is interesting, however, that the abnormal karyotype of the original immature teratoma is maintained in the area of chemotherapy-induced maturation.[753]

Mature solid teratoma

Mature solid teratoma has a predominantly solid gross appearance, but multiple small cystic areas also are present. Because of this, some authors prefer the descriptively more accurate designation of *polycystic*. By definition, the tumor should be *composed entirely of adult tissues* derived from all three germ layers.[774,775]

Clearly, extensive sampling is needed to separate this tumor from a grade I immature teratoma. The two tumors are closely related, and the distinction is somewhat subjective; as a matter of fact, some authors refer to mature solid teratoma as grade 0 immature teratoma.

This rare neoplasm occurs in young women, predominantly in the second decade. The prognosis is excellent, even if peritoneal implants (also mature and for the most part glial in composition) are present[773] (see p. 1589).

Mature cystic teratoma

Mature cystic teratomas make up almost 20% of all ovarian neoplasms. They constitute the most common ovarian tumor in childhood.[787] They are unilateral in 88% of cases and provoke only symptoms relating to the mass. Occasionally, however, they are accompanied by hemolytic anemia,[784,803] or virilization.[780,796] Grossly, they are usually multiloculated. The cystic content is greasy, largely composed of keratin, sebum, and hairs (Fig. 19.289). Teeth are often present[786] (Fig. 19.290). Sometimes the tumor contains an imperfectly formed mandible or even a partial human body-like structure (homunculus); the latter are referred to as *fetiform teratomas*.[799] The teeth tend to be located in a well-defined nipple-like structure covered with hair, known as *Rokitansky's protuberance*. This structure should be selected for microscopic examination (even if decalcification may be required) because it will exhibit the greatest variety of tissue types.

In a classic microscopic study, Blackwell et al.[779] found ectodermal derivatives in 100% of the tumors, mesodermal structures in 93%, and endodermal derivatives in 71%. The cystic cavities

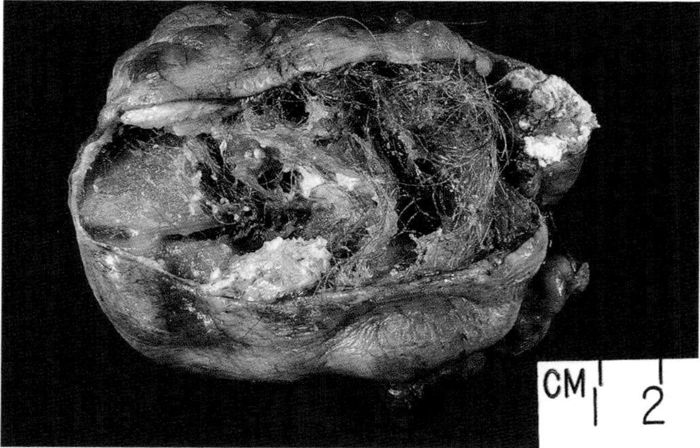

Fig. 19.289 Admixture of sebum and hair within the cavity of an ovarian mature cystic teratoma.

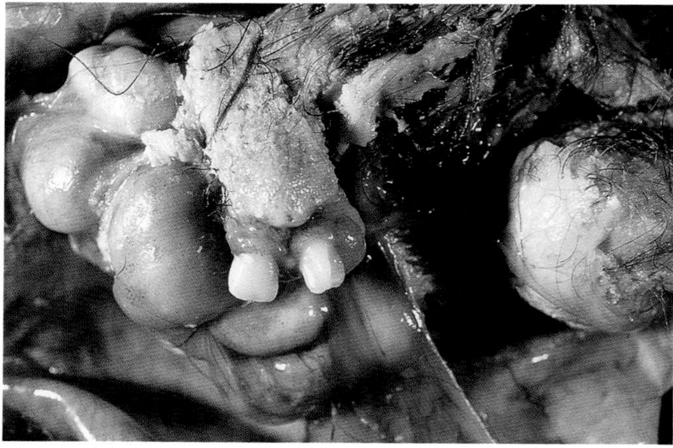

Fig. 19.290 Well-developed teeth in ovarian mature cystic teratoma.

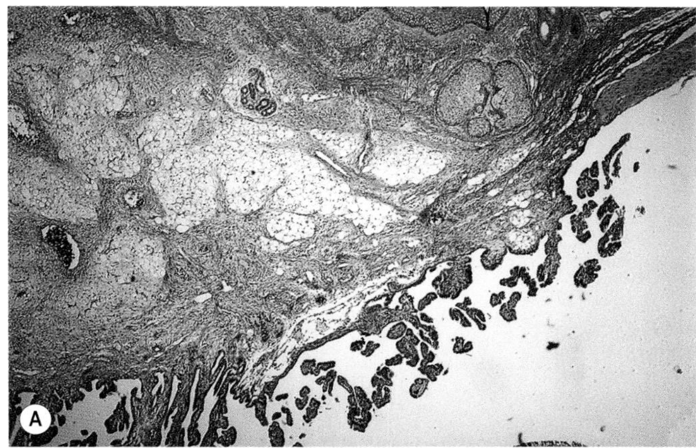

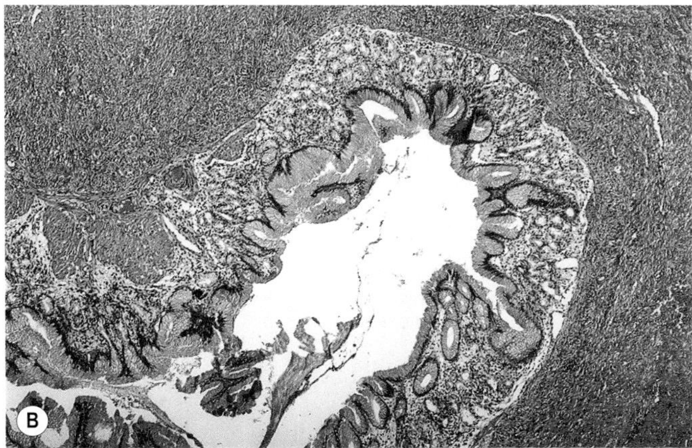

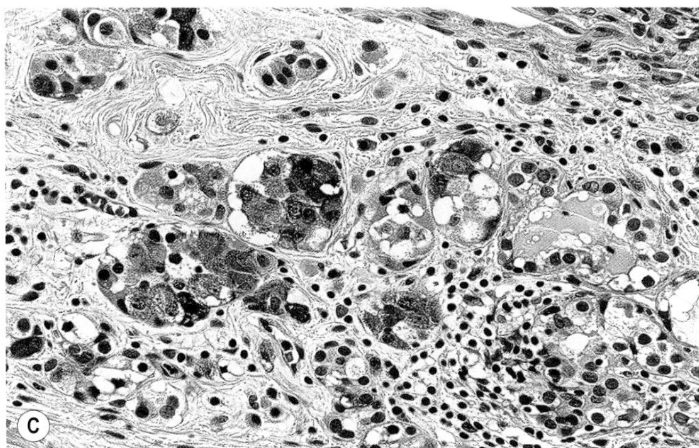

Fig. 19.291 Various tissue components of mature cystic teratoma of ovary: **A**, skin adnexa, glial tissue, and choroid plexus; **B**, gastric mucosa of pyloric type; **C**, anterior pituitary gland.

are lined by mature epidermis. Skin appendages and neural (particularly glial) tissue are extremely common. The latter may feature meningothelial proliferations and Wagner–Meissner corpuscles, and be accompanied by florid vascular proliferation.[783,788] Other common tissue types present are cartilage, respiratory tissue, and gastrointestinal tract tissue (Fig. 19.291). The gastric mucosa can be very well developed anatomically, to the point of containing interstitial cells of Cajal;[777] sometimes it is complicated by peptic ulcer formation.[807] Other tissues include thyroid (10% of cases), various types of melanin-containing tissue (particularly in black patients),[794] anterior pituitary,[797] various types of neuroendocrine cells,[782] prostate,[798,809] pancreas, and cavernous blood vessels.

Because of the usual predominance of skin and skin adnexal structures, and also on historical grounds, some authors still prefer the old term dermoid cyst for ovarian mature cystic teratoma. Time-honored considerations aside, we feel that this term is pathogenetically not very informative and that it does not do justice to the plethora of other tissue types that can be present in these tumors.

By definition, all of the components present in mature cystic teratomas should appear histologically mature. However, on occasions one sees microscopic foci of immature (to be distinguished from malignant, see below) tissue in them. The behavior of these tumors, which should also be distinguished from immature teratomas, is usually benign.[812] Along these lines, it could be mentioned that the phenotype of the morphologically mature epidermal lining of the cysts of this tumor may appear immature at the immunohistochemical level in the sense of resembling stratified nonkeratinizing and metaplastic squamous epithelium.[785]

A female nuclear sex chromatin pattern is present in all cases; chromosomal analyses have shown a 46,XX pattern.[804] Linder et al.[795] have elegantly shown by chromosome-banding studies that these tumors are of parthenogenetic origin and probably arise from a single germ cell after the first meiotic division. Riley and Sutton[805] have proposed a possible mechanism to account for the fact that most ovarian germ cell tumors are benign, whereas most of the testicular ones are malignant, based on the different development of the germ cells in the male and in the female.

Other studies have described a heterozygous genotype in a substantial number of cases, suggesting an origin either from premeiotic germ cells or from somatic cells. However, a microdissection-based analysis supported the basically homozygous nature of the truly teratomatous tissue.[810]

Some authors have raised the possibility of fusion of ova as a mechanism of formation of teratoma, a theory that has received some support from the finding that biovularity and coalescence of primary follicles are more common in ovaries harboring teratomas than in the controls.[801]

Mature cystic teratomas may coexist with mucinous cystadenoma, Brenner tumor, and fibrothecoma.[781,800]

On occasion, teratomas rupture into the abdominal cavity; when this occurs, the keratin and sebum present in the lumen may provoke a prominent foreign body reaction that can look like metastatic cancer to the surgeon, who may be incredulous when the surgical pathologist goes back to him with a benign diagnosis (but not incredulous enough to accept a risky bet about it)[776,778] (Fig. 19.292).

In other instances, mature ovarian teratomas of either the cystic or solid variety – as well as immature teratomas – may be accompanied by peritoneal nodules exclusively composed of mature glial and neuronal tissue, a condition known as *gliomatosis peritonei*[790,791,806,811] (Fig. 19.293). These nodules appear grossly as miliary grayish-white nodules in the peritoneal surface or omentum and may be accompanied by fibrosis and chronic inflammation. This is a benign process, as long as the glial tissue is entirely mature and unaccompanied by other teratomatous elements[789,802,808] (Fig. 19.294). Traditionally, it has been regarded as the manifestation of implants of glial tissue from the teratoma. However, genetic analysis suggests that this tissue is derived from nonteratomatous cells, and that it may represent a metaplastic change in submesothelial cells.[793]

Another teratoma-related process is peritoneal 'melanosis', which can also follow the rupture of a cystic teratoma.[792]

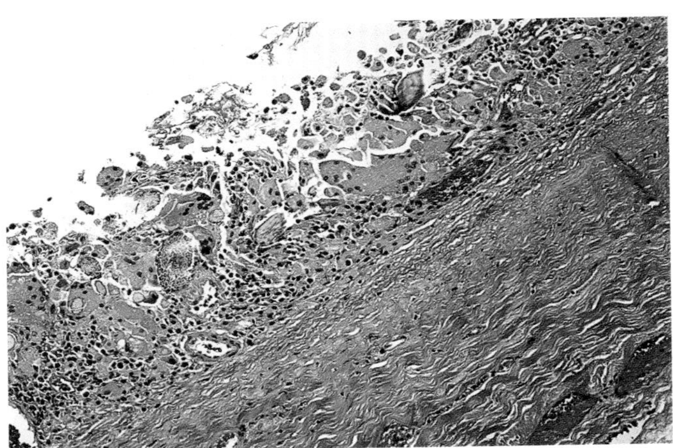

Fig. 19.292 Exuberant foreign body-type giant cell response to contents of ruptured ovarian mature cystic teratoma. These changes may simulate grossly the appearance of tuberculous peritonitis or metastatic carcinoma.

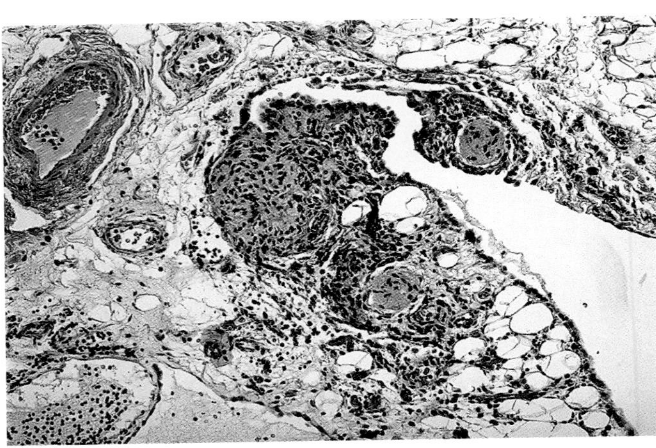

Fig. 19.294 Peritoneal implants secondary to immature ovarian teratoma. When the appearance of the implants is immature, as shown here, the prognosis is more guarded than in gliomatosis peritonei (compare with Fig. 19.293).

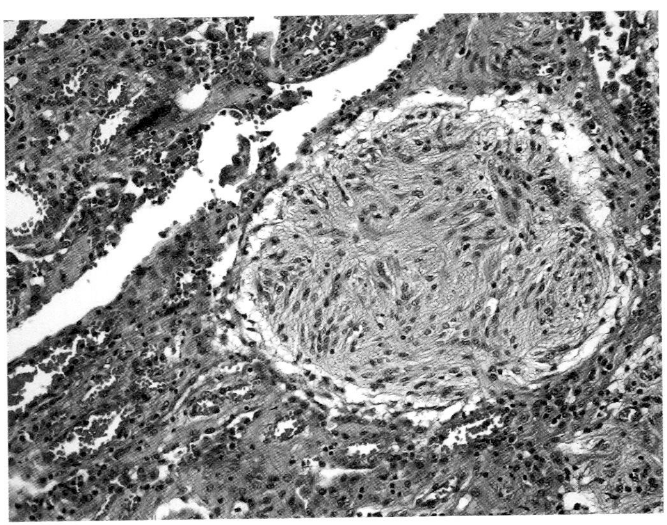

Fig. 19.293 Peritoneal implant of mature glial tissue in ovarian teratoma (so-called 'gliomatosis peritonei').

'Somatic-type' tumors developing in mature cystic teratoma

Emergence of a benign or a malignant neoplasm with somatic-type features is an uncommon event in mature cystic teratoma, occurring in approximately 2% of all cases.

The most common malignant change in cystic teratoma is squamous cell carcinoma (possibly arising from metaplastic columnar epithelium[820]), followed by carcinoid tumor and adenocarcinoma.[814,817,822,827] Other types include malignant melanoma,[815,835] Paget disease,[831] sarcomas of various types, carcinosarcoma, glioblastoma multiforme,[837] central-type neurocytoma,[818] and neuroblastoma/PNET.[821,828] This malignant transformation is accompanied by complex chromosomal aberrations.[830] An interesting twist is the occurrence of mucinous borderline tumors and adenocarcinomas similar to appendiceal neoplasms and resulting in pseudomyxoma peritonei.[819,829,833]

Benign tumors have also been described, such as blue nevus,[823,834] sebaceous adenoma,[813] sweat gland tumors,[825] glomus tumor,[832] epithelioid (histiocytoid) hemangioma,[824] and various types of pituitary adenoma.[826,836]

It ought to be pointed out that although all of these tumors have a morphologic appearance and behavior comparable in all respects to the homonymous somatic tumors, in all likelihood they arise from the germ cell elements of the teratoma and, therefore, are of germ cell nature themselves from a genotypic standpoint. This possibility is supported by the finding on microdissection-based analysis that the tumors have a homozygous genotype identical to that of the teratoma.[816] The occurrence of these tumors provides an excellent demonstration that it is the phenotype rather than the histogenesis that basically determines the biologic properties and clinical behavior of tumors. I am told that David Page, in an effort to drive this important point home in his usual forceful style, has a sign hanging in the Surgical Pathology sign-out area that reads "It is the phenotype, stupid!"

Epidermoid cyst

The rare **epidermoid cyst** of the ovary possibly arises from epithelial cell nests, of the type encountered in Brenner tumors.[838] It is distinguished from mature cystic teratoma on thorough sampling by the absence of skin adnexa and other tissues. It is discussed here not only in the light of this differential diagnosis, but also because of the distinct possibility that some of these lesions were mature cystic teratomas in which the skin adnexal components were either missed or absent.

Struma ovarii

Struma ovarii is the expression of the dominant growth of thyroid tissue in a teratoma, sometimes to the exclusion of other components[852] (Fig. 19.295). Grossly, the mass has the color and consistency of thyroid tissue, but it is often cystic (Fig. 19.296). These cystic changes can be very prominent and obscure the diagnosis.[850,851] The thyroid nature of the lesion has been fully documented with biologic and immunohistochemical studies for TTF-1 and thyroid hormones.[842] The tissue may show any of the pathologic changes seen in a normally placed gland, including diffuse or

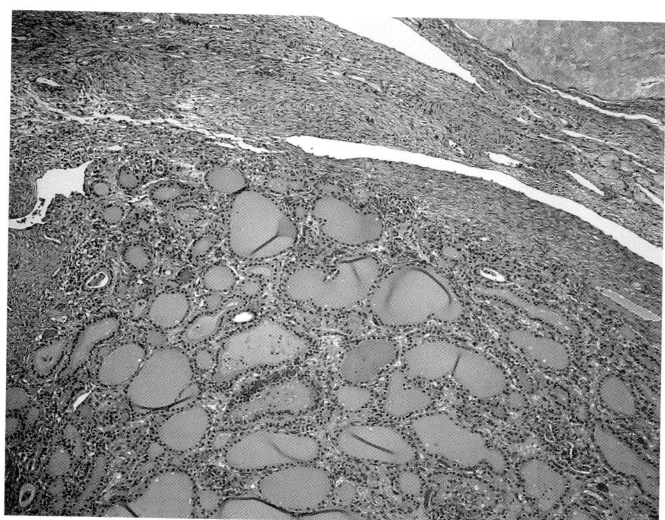

Fig. 19.295 So-called 'struma ovarii'. The thyroid tissue, which has a microscopically unremarkable appearance, is sharply delimited from the ovarian stroma.

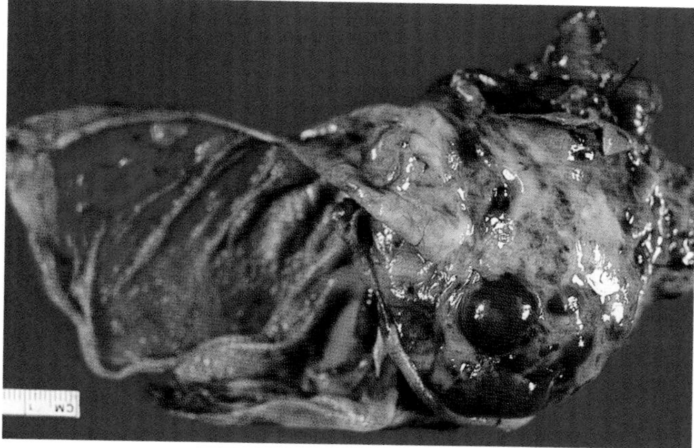

Fig. 19.296 Gross appearance of struma ovarii. The thyroid tissue is represented by the solid areas.

nodular hyperplasia (which may lead to hyperthyroidism[846]), thyroiditis, papillary carcinoma (including the follicular and microcarcinoma variants,[839] and featuring either *RAS* or *BRAF* mutation),[840,848] follicular carcinoma (sometimes resulting in peritoneal spread, so-called peritoneal strumosis[841,844]), and malignant lymphoma.[842,849] Some of the carcinomas are extremely well-differentiated,[841,845,847] whereas others have a predominantly solid or trabecular pattern.[851]

We have seen a case of follicular variant of papillary carcinoma developing in struma ovarii that contained numerous intraluminal crystalloids, and a similar case has been reported.[843]

Struma ovarii can be seen combined with mucinous cystadenoma, Brenner tumor, or carcinoid tumor. The latter combination, known as strumal carcinoid, is discussed in the following section.

Carcinoid tumor and strumal carcinoid

Carcinoid tumor can be seen in the ovary as a metastasis of a primary tumor located in the gastrointestinal tract or elsewhere,[866] as a component of adult cystic teratoma, or as a primary pure

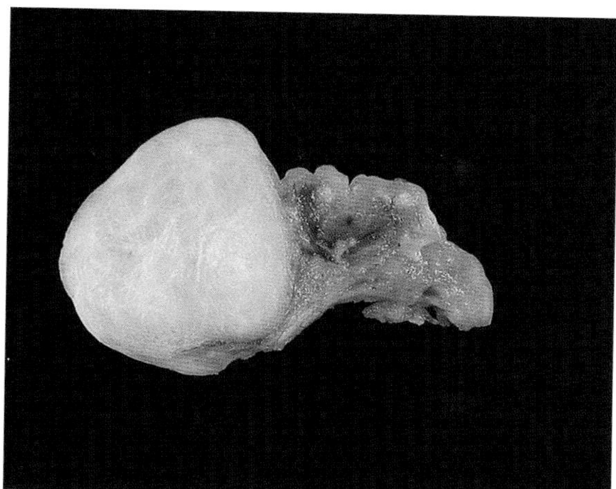

Fig. 19.297 Cut surface of carcinoid tumor of ovary showing typical solid appearance and white to yellowish color.

neoplasm of this organ. Approximately one-third of the latter are associated with the carcinoid syndrome, even in the absence of liver metastases;[865] the larger the tumor, the more likely that the carcinoid syndrome will develop. Some cases present with severe constipation, presumably because of secretion of peptide YY.[861] Small tumors arising in cystic teratomas are nearly always asymptomatic. The large majority of primary ovarian carcinoid tumors are unilateral, but in 16% of cases the contralateral ovary is involved by a cystic teratoma or a mucinous neoplasm.[864] In contrast, most metastatic carcinoid tumors to the ovary are bilateral and associated with peritoneal metastases. The prognosis in primary ovarian carcinoid tumors (whether pure or as a component of cystic teratoma) is very good, whereas metastatic carcinoids have a poor outcome.

Grossly, pure primary carcinoid tumors have a mean diameter of 10 cm; their external surface is smooth or bosselated, and the cut surface is predominantly solid, firm, tan to yellow, and homogeneous (Fig. 19.297). Microscopically, the appearance is similar to that of carcinoid tumors elsewhere, in that they recapitulate the various patterns of this well-differentiated neuroendocrine tumor as seen in various sites. Thus, there are tumors with an *insular* pattern of growth similar to those seen in the appendix and small bowel, tumors with a *trabecular* appearance similar to those seen in the rectum (Fig. 19.298), and tumors with a *mucinous* (goblet cell) appearance similar to those seen primarily in the appendix.[854,867,868] The similarities also apply to the occasional presence of pleomorphic forms,[856] to their histochemical features (argentaffinity or argyrophilia depending on the type), and to the consistent presence of neurosecretory granules at the electron microscopic level.[868]

Neuron-specific enolase (NSE), chromogranin, 5-HT, and a large variety of peptide hormones (including peptide YY) have been demonstrated immunohistochemically, particularly in tumors of the trabecular type.[861,872]

It is not possible to separate primary from metastatic carcinoid tumors on morphologic grounds; however, if the ovarian carcinoid is admixed with areas of teratoma, the chances are overwhelming that it is of primary origin. Conversely, tumors with goblet cell carcinoid-like features and signet ring patterns (traditionally known as goblet cell carcinoid tumors, see Chapter 11) are likely to be metastases from the appendix.[859] A potential pitfall should be mentioned here: both primary ovarian carcinoid tumors and those metastatic from the gastrointestinal tract may express CDX2.[863]

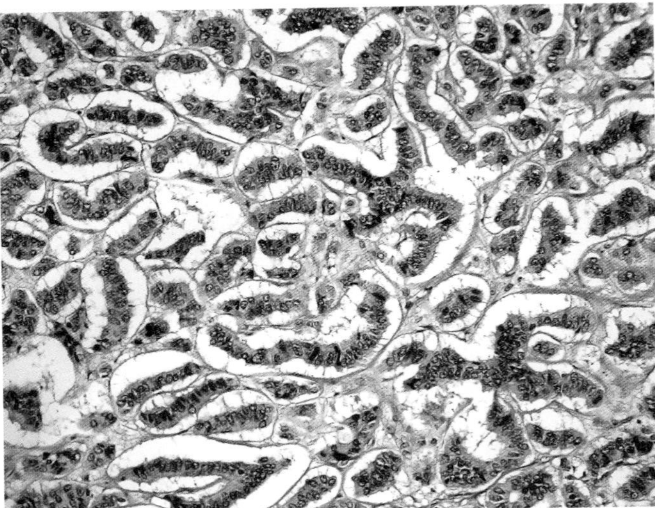

Fig. 19.298 Primary ovarian carcinoid tumor with a trabecular pattern of growth. There is a great resemblance to carcinoid tumors of lung and rectum.

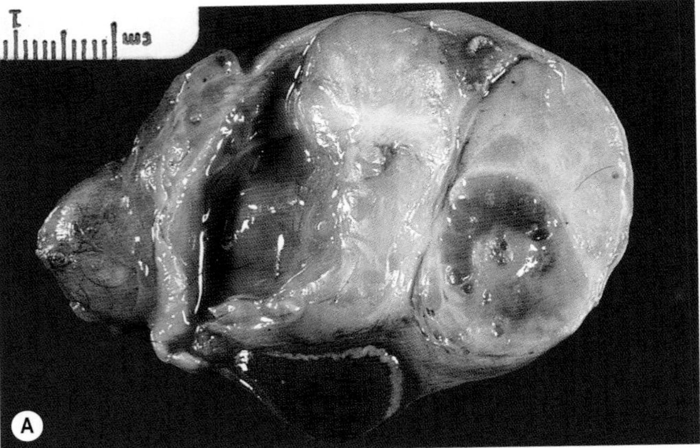

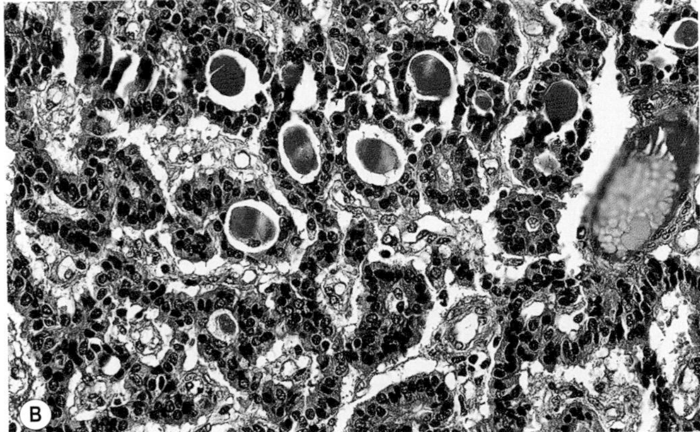

Fig. 19.299 A, Gross appearance of strumal carcinoid showing a variegated appearance resulting from the admixture of carcinoid tumor and struma ovarii. B, Microscopic appearance, showing intimate admixture of thyroid follicles and carcinoid trabecula.

Excision of a primary ovarian carcinoid of insular or trabecular type is usually curative. As in the appendix, the behavior of the mucinous type is more aggressive, particularly if the tumor contains a clearcut carcinomatous component.[854]

Strumal carcinoid is an ovarian neoplasm combining the features of carcinoid tumor and struma ovarii[874] (Fig. 19.299). There was some question about the thyroidal nature of the latter element on the basis of ultrastructural studies, but the immunohistochemical demonstration of thyroglobulin and TTF-1,[858,876] and the occasional occurrence of thyroid-type papillary microcarcinomas[862] have settled the issue. The interesting suggestion has been made that the carcinoid-like component represents a medullary carcinoma arising from thyroid C cells,[853] but the morphologic appearance and immunohistochemical profile of the tumor are more akin to those of a trabecular carcinoid of hindgut derivation;[871,873] specifically, calcitonin and amyloid are only rarely demonstrable.[857] It is of interest that these tumors also exhibit immunoreactivity for prostatic acid phosphatase in the carcinoid component, as further evidence of their similarity to rectal (hindgut-type) carcinoids.[870] The occasional occurrence of severe constipation, presumably due to secretion of peptide YY,[869] and of carcinoid heart disease[855] also link it with pure ovarian carcinoid tumor. Exceptionally, the carcinoid component is of mucinous type.[860]

Other teratomatous elements are found in over 50% of the cases of strumal carcinoid.[865] This lesion has also been observed in association with multiple endocrine neoplasia type 2a.[875]

Sex cord–stromal tumors

Sex cord–stromal tumors, which comprise approximately 5% of all ovarian neoplasms, are tumors that differentiate in the direction of sex cords and/or the specialized ovarian stroma.[909] This includes female-type cells (granulosa and theca cells), male-type cells (Sertoli and Leydig cells), and indifferent elements.[883,908,910] These various elements can occur in combination[906] and exhibit a wide range of differentiation, which often seems to recapitulate the patterns produced during embryogenesis of both the ovary and testis, as proposed many years ago by Gunnar Teilum.[905] Secondary changes, such as luteinization, may also develop. As a result, a wide array of tumor types may be seen, some of which do not fit easily into a rigid classification system. In general, a relationship exists between the morphologic appearance of the tumor and the presence and type of clinically evident hormonal activity.[900,902,904] However, there may be no demonstrable endocrine effects, and rare examples of hormonal effects opposite to those expected from the morphologic features also occur.[884,891] Along similar lines, there is general agreement between the cytoarchitectural features of the tumor and the presence of various steroid hormones, hormone precursors, and related enzymes, as demonstrated by immunohistochemical techniques.[881,903] However, it is important to emphasize that the classification of ovarian neoplasms is primarily based on their morphologic appearance, rather than on the presence or type of steroid hormones as determined immunohistochemically. The latter is plagued with so many conceptual and technical difficulties when evaluated in formalin-fixed, paraffin-embedded material (hormone loss from organic solvents, tissue diffusion of the lipid-soluble hormones, hormone-binding to receptors, etc.) as to make it unwise to classify an ovarian tumor as belonging to the sex cord–stromal category solely on this basis.

Recently, a number of nonsteroid immunohistochemical markers have become available that are of considerable assistance in the identification of these tumors.[893,907]

Inhibin has emerged as one of the most useful.[901] The α-subunit of the molecule seems to have a greater degree of specificity than the βA-subunit.[880,887] It stains all types of sex cord–stromal tumors, the sex cordlike elements of other gynecologic neoplasms, and most trophoblastic tumors.[892,898] It is also useful for the identification of steroid hormone-secreting cells in the non-neoplastic stroma component of epithelial, germ cell, and other types of ovarian tumor.[890] It is also said to stain some carcinomas at other sites,[894] but this seems to be due at least in part to endogenous biotin.[888] It should be also pointed out that negativity for inhibin does not rule out a diagnosis of sex cord–stromal tumor (following the general rule that a negative stain never rules out anything).

Molecules functionally related to inhibin that also stain sex cord–stromal tumors are activin (a molecule biochemically similar to inhibin but with an opposite function, and composed of two βA-subunits), müllerian inhibiting substance (anti-müllerian hormone), and relaxin-like factor.[877,893,896,899]

Calretinin is more sensitive but less specific than inhibin, in the sense that it often stains sex cord–stromal tumors that are inhibin negative, such as fibromas.[879,897] However, it also stains a good number of surface epithelial neoplasms.

A103, an antibody directed against the melanocytic marker Melan-A (Mart-1), has been found consistently to stain sex cord–stromal tumors and other types of steroid-producing cells, such as those of ovarian lipid cell tumor and adrenal cortical neoplasms.[878]

CD99 (O13; MIC2), a marker generally used for Ewing sarcoma/PNET, also frequently (and somewhat unexpectedly) stains this family of neoplasms.[885,896]

CD56 has been proposed as a sensitive marker for ovarian sex cord–stromal tumors,[895] but other studies have challenged this claim.[886]

SF-1 (*steroidogenic factor 1*), the most recent addition to the list, seems to be the most sensitive sex cord–stromal marker.[911]

Before going into the specific subtypes, it should be mentioned that WT1, present in normal granulosa cells, is expressed by a majority of ovarian sex cord–stromal tumors.[882,886]

Sex cord–stromal tumors of ovarian type are exceptionally encountered in extraovarian locations, such as the broad ligament.[889]

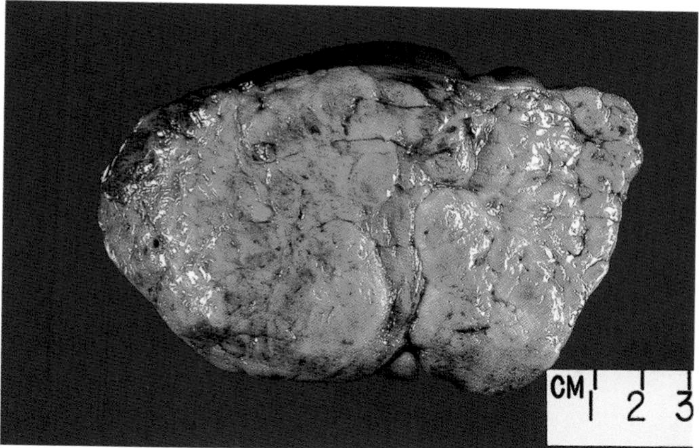

Fig. 19.300 Granulosa cell tumor with solid cut surface.

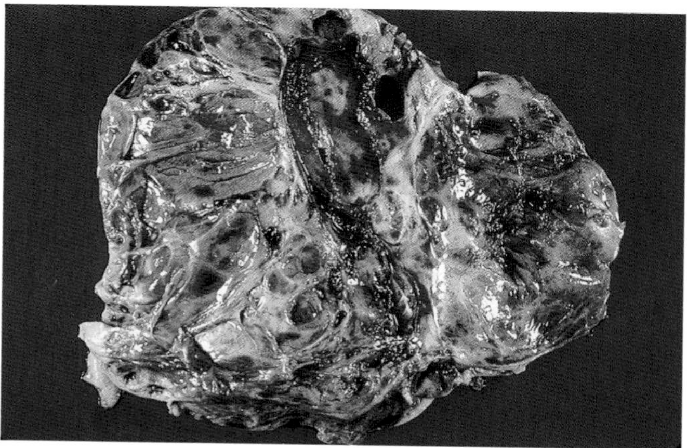

Fig. 19.301 Granulosa cell tumor showing admixture of solid and cystic areas.

Granulosa cell tumor

Granulosa cell tumor is a sex cord–stromal ovarian neoplasm showing differentiation toward follicular granulosa cells. Whether it actually arises from granulosa cells in preexisting follicles or from the specialized ovarian stroma is debatable. Two distinct types exist, known respectively as adult and juvenile.

Adult granulosa cell tumor is usually diagnosed during child-bearing age, but it can occur after menopause and sometimes (despite its name) even before puberty. Three-fourths of cases are associated with hyperestrinism; the excessive production of estrogens can lead to isosexual precocious puberty in children[932] and to metrorrhagia in adults, including postmenopausal patients.[919] Some of the cases are hormonally inactive at the clinical level, and a very few are androgenic.[914,939]

Grossly, adult granulosa cell tumors have a smooth, lobulated outline and a predominantly solid cut surface (Fig. 19.300). The color is usually gray, but it may be yellow in areas of luteinization (Fig. 19.301). Cysts filled with straw-colored or mucoid fluid may be present (Fig. 19.302). Sometimes the cysts are so prominent as to simulate grossly the appearance of a cystadenoma (Fig. 19.303). Interestingly, a disproportionate number of androgenic granulosa cell tumors are large and cystic, either unilocular or multilocular.[939,942] The microscopic appearance of granulosa cell tumors is extremely variable, even within the same neoplasm. Patterns of

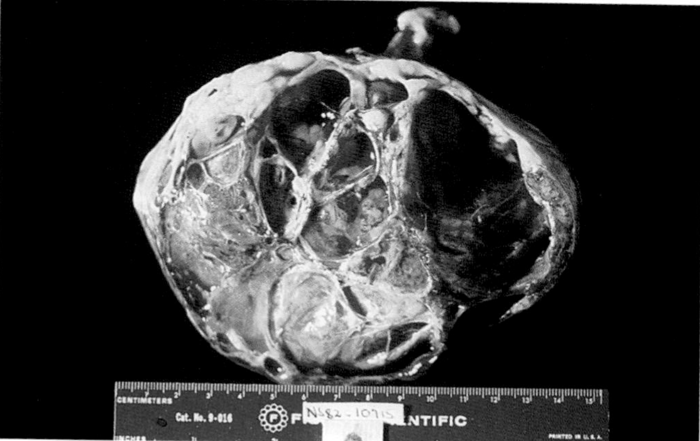

Fig. 19.302 Predominantly cystic granulosa cell tumor.

growth include microfollicular (with Call–Exner bodies), macrofollicular, trabecular, insular, watered-silk, solid, pseudopapillary, and diffuse (sarcomatoid)[928,948] (Fig. 19.304). A theca cell component may also be present. Focal luteinization of either the granulosa or the theca cell component may occur;[958] it is particularly prominent in those tumors associated with pregnancy, together with edema

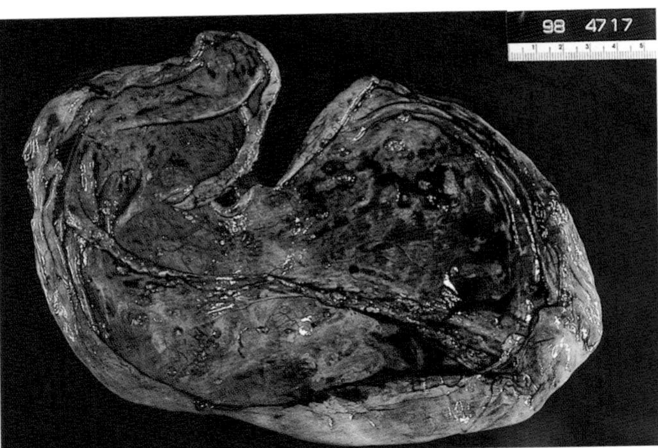

Fig. 19.303 Granulosa cell tumor with an entirely cystic gross appearance.

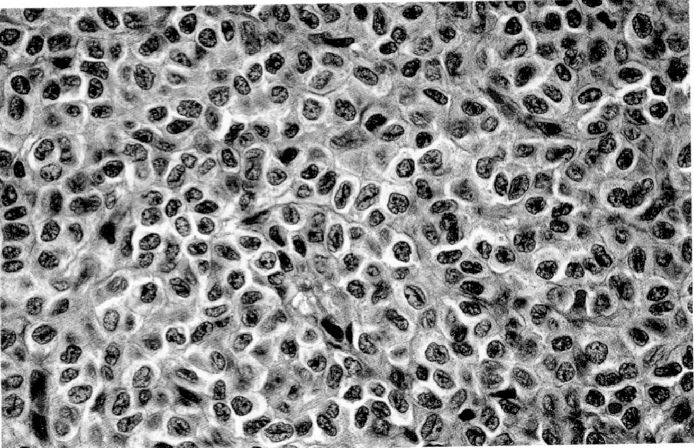

Fig. 19.305 Coffee-bean nuclei in adult type of ovarian granulosa cell tumor.

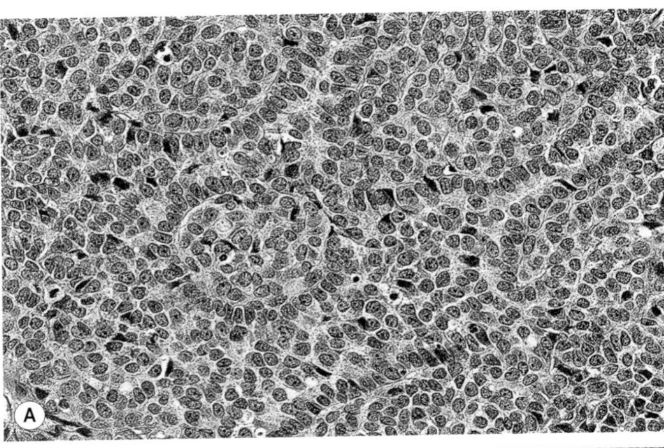

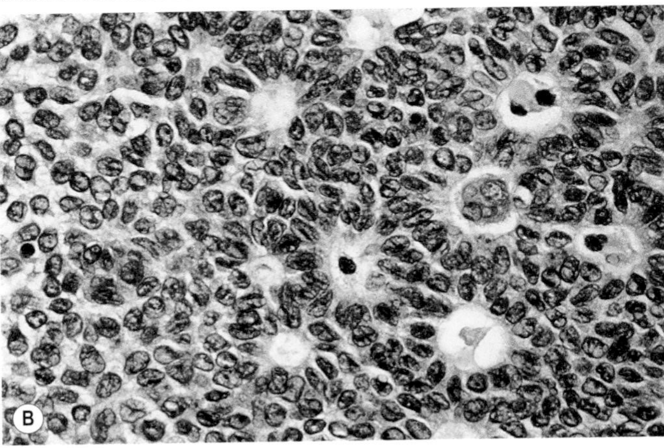

Fig. 19.304 A and **B**, Microscopic appearance of granulosa cell tumor. Call-Exner bodies are seen in **B**.

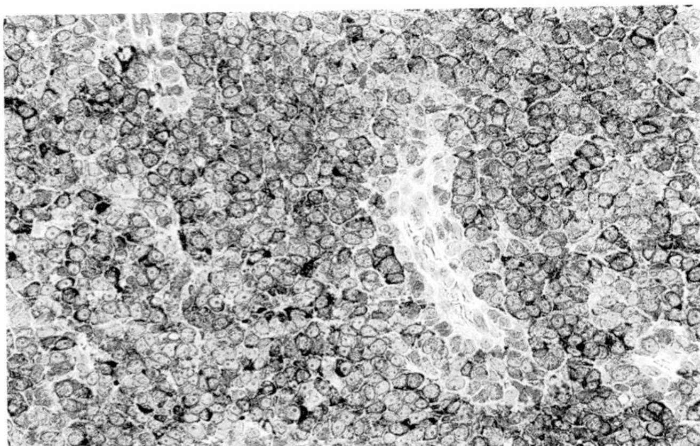

Fig. 19.306 Strong immunoreactivity for inhibin in granulosa cell tumor.

and disorderly arrangement.[957] An important diagnostic feature is the presence of folds or grooves in the nuclei, resulting in a 'coffee-bean' appearance[941] (Fig. 19.305). Occasionally, bizarre nuclei and multinucleated giant cells (some of the 'floret' type) are seen; this change is not a sign of malignancy but rather of a degenerative nature.[960] Cases of granulosa cell tumor have been reported exhibiting hepatocytic differentiation[912,940] and others associated with mucinous cystadenoma.[935]

Traditionally, secretion of steroid hormones has been related to theca cells rather than granulosa cells, both in normal follicles and tumors; however, immunohistochemical studies have shown steroid production in both cell types, with a predominance of estradiol in the granulosa cells and progesterone in luteinized theca cells.[931] Other consistent immunohistochemical markers of granulosa cell tumors include vimentin, desmoplakin (desmosomal plaque protein), inhibin, calretinin, follicle regulatory proteins, A103, and SF-1 (see preceding section)[918,919,933,934,937,944] (Fig. 19.306). Keratin is present in one-third to one-half of cases; it has a typical dot-like distribution and consists mainly of CK8 and CK18 types.[943] Smooth muscle actin is seen in nearly all cases, but desmin less commonly so.[946] Approximately 50% of cases are reactive for S-100 protein, whereas none is immunoreactive for EMA.[917]Estrogen and progesterone receptors are frequently expressed.[921] The peptide hormone inhibin and follicle regulatory proteins, two substances normally produced by ovarian granulosa cells, have been found to be elevated in the serum of patients with granulosa cell tumor.[922] Curiously, granulosa cell tumors have also been found to be often immunoreactive for CD99 (O13; MIC2), a marker associated with Ewing sarcoma/PNET (see Chapter 25).[933]

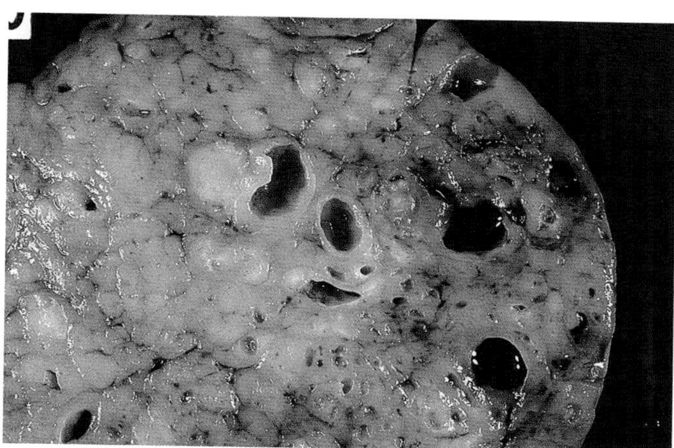

Fig. 19.307 Gross appearance of juvenile granulosa cell tumor.

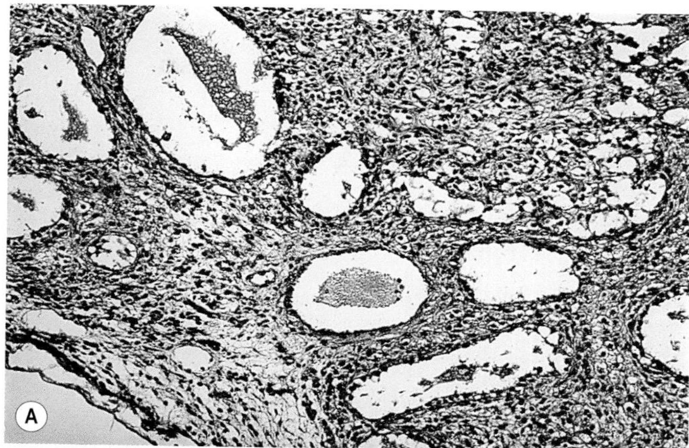

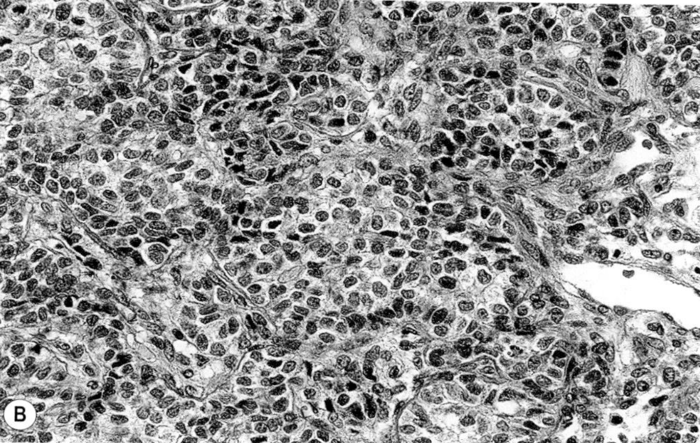

Fig. 19.308 **A** and **B**, Juvenile granulosa cell tumor. The follicle-like spaces seen on low-power examination (**A**) are a common feature of this neoplasm. On high power (**B**) the tumor cells are seen to lack the coffee-bean nuclei seen in the adult type.

Ultrastructurally, the neoplastic granulosa cells have abundant intermediate filaments and specialized cell junctions, some of the latter having the appearance of typical desmosomes.[918] Cytogenetically, there is consistent trisomy for chromosome 12.[923,926] Strangely, in some cases with bizarre nuclei, the only foci showing trisomy 12 by FISH are those in which the bizarre nuclei are present.[925] Other recurrent karyotypic aberrations of this tumor are trisomy 14 and monosomy 22.[936] Recently, it has been shown that almost all cases of adult granulosa cell tumor show somatic mutation in the *FOXL2* gene (402C→G).[930,949] Flow cytometry studies have shown that the large majority of adult granulosa cell tumors are diploid or near-diploid; evidence that DNA ploidy analysis has independent prognostic value remains controversial.[915,920,927,950,954]

Juvenile granulosa cell tumor is diagnosed in nearly 80% of cases during the first two decades of life, most patients presenting with isosexual precocity (Fig. 19.307). A few cases have been associated with enchondromatosis (Ollier disease)[952] or Maffucci syndrome.[953] Typical morphologic features of this subtype include diffuse or macrofollicular patterns of growth (the former predominating), mucin-positive intrafollicular secretion, larger tumor cells with extensive luteinization, paucity of nuclear grooves, presence of a thecal component, nuclear atypia, and variable but often high mitotic activity[945,956,962] (Fig. 19.308). Like their adult counterpart, they may exhibit pseudopapillary features.[928] They also show consistent trisomy for chromosome 12.[947]

DNA ploidy analysis has shown a greater percentage of aneuploidy in juvenile granulosa cell tumors than in the adult variety; however, the prognostic value of this determination still needs to be demonstrated.[929,951]

The differential diagnosis of granulosa cell tumor (particularly of the adult variety) includes poorly differentiated (predominantly solid) carcinoma of surface epithelial origin, carcinoid tumor, and the very rare tumors of endometrial stromal type[961] (see p. 1605). The nuclear features are of crucial importance in this regard. Some early series describing a poor prognosis for granulosa cell tumors are probably contaminated with solid ovarian carcinomas of surface origin. Strong and widespread positivity for keratin should point toward the direction of carcinoma in a controversial case, especially if this positivity is diffuse cytoplasmic rather than dot-like. The differential diagnosis also includes the *ovarian granulosa cell proliferations of pregnancy*; this change is usually microscopic, multiple, and associated with atretic follicles.[916]

The prognosis of granulosa cell tumors is largely dependent on the clinical staging.[938] It also depends on size, tumor rupture, and presence of nuclear atypia.[938,959] As a group, juvenile granulosa cell tumors behave more aggressively than their adult counterparts, and are more likely to produce distant metastases. The effect of the histologic pattern of the adult form on prognosis is not clearcut. Some authors have claimed that tumors with follicular or trabecular patterns have a better prognosis than those with a sarcomatoid pattern, but most studies have failed to demonstrate a convincing relationship.[913] In the series of Norris and Taylor,[941] 12 of 187 patients had persistent tumor after surgery, and 10 died as a result. Most deaths occurred more than 5 years after the original diagnosis and treatment, indicating that 5-year survival figures are not accurate predictors of permanent cure.[924] The granulosa cell origin of a metastatic tumor should be suspected in the presence of a combination of microcystic and trabecular formations, especially if accompanied by Call–Exner bodies and grooved nuclei. Obviously, it is also essential to consider the possibility, otherwise one is likely to confuse it with a transitional cell carcinoma or something else.[955]

Thecoma, fibroma, and related tumors

Fibroma and thecoma are closely related tumors, one often merging with the other, and therefore the term *fibrothecoma* is quite appropriate when referring to the entire group.

Thecoma presents after menopause in 65% of patients. It is usually unilateral and varies considerably in size. It has a

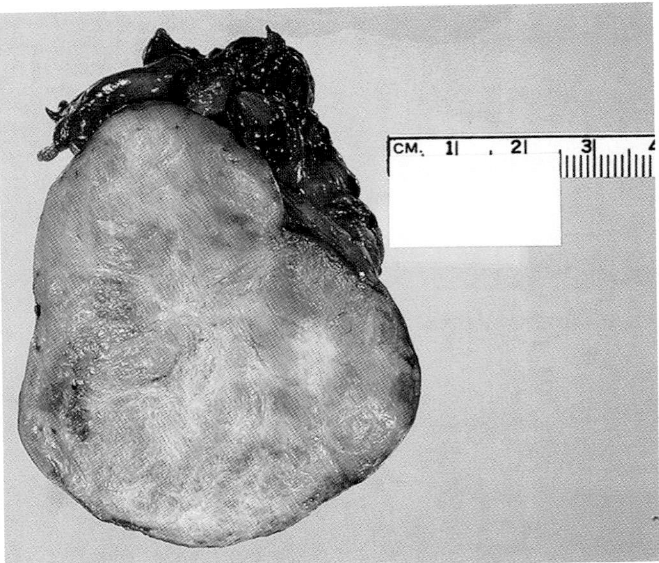

Fig. 19.309 Cut surface of thecoma showing a predominance of yellow areas alternating with whitish foci.

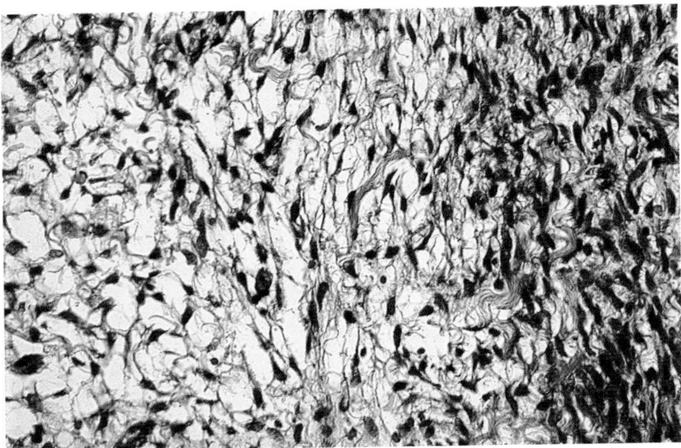

Fig. 19.310 Bland microscopic appearance of thecoma, with some variability in cellularity.

well-defined capsule and a firm consistency. The cut surface is largely or entirely solid, but cysts may be present. It has a yellow color, an important feature in the differential diagnosis with fibroma (Fig. 19.309). Microscopically, it is composed of fascicles of spindle cells with centrally placed nuclei and a moderate amount of pale cytoplasm (Fig. 19.310). The intervening tissue may show considerable collagen deposition and focal hyaline plaque formation. The degree of cellularity varies considerably. Some tumors in young women are heavily calcified.[1001]

With oil red O, the cells of thecoma show abundant intracytoplasmic neutral fat, and silver stains usually demonstrate reticulin fibers surrounding individual cells (as opposed to granulosa cell tumor, in which the reticulin surrounds clusters of cells). However, islands may occur in the thecoma that are devoid of reticulin, especially in areas of luteinization. Immunohistochemical localization of estradiol is usually limited to a small number of tumor cells.[969]

Thecomas may be associated with prominent stromal hyperplasia, particularly in postmenopausal patients. In such cases, transitions may be seen from focal stromal hyperplasia through diffuse thecomatosis (hyperthecosis) to thecoma, suggesting a pathogenetic continuum. It is likely that the small tumors designated as **stromal luteomas**[970,987] are yet another manifestation of this spectrum.

Sometimes, ovarian tumors otherwise typical of thecoma contain cells with the features of steroid hormone-secreting cells (lutein, Leydig, and adrenal cortical).[1004] This tumor has generally been designated as **luteinized thecoma**,[984] whereas the terms *stromal–Leydig cell tumor* or *Leydig cell-containing thecoma* are reserved for the rare examples in which Reinke crystalloids are identified in the cytoplasm of these cells.[990,991,1004] These variants tend to occur in younger women and may have an androgenic rather than estrogenic effect on the host.

Thecomas are typically associated with estrogenic manifestations, although some (particularly those containing steroid cells, as just indicated) may be androgenic. They are nearly always benign, but a few malignant examples have been documented.[998] Some ovarian tumors with the overall appearance of luteinized thecomas have been found to be associated with a peculiar form of *sclerosing peritonitis*.[964,972,999] The alternative possibility has been raised that these lesions are of non-neoplastic nature and that they represent a form of thecomatosis.[989]

Fibromas are common ovarian tumors, usually unilateral, which occur almost invariably after puberty.[968] They are solid, lobulated, firm, uniformly white, and usually not accompanied by adhesions (Fig. 19.311). The average diameter is 6 cm. Myxoid changes may be seen, sometimes resulting in cystic degeneration. Grossly, fibromas need to be distinguished mainly from thecoma, Brenner tumor, and Krukenberg tumor.

Microscopically, fibromas are composed of closely packed spindle stromal cells arranged in a 'feather-stitched' or storiform pattern (Fig. 19.312). Hyaline bands, edema, and hyaline globules may be present.[977] Some fibromas occur in young women with the basal cell nevus (Gorlin) syndrome; these are calcified, usually bilateral, and often multinodular.[982] In an oft-quoted paper, it was proposed that fibromas exhibiting a great deal of cellularity be referred to as *cellular fibromas* if their mitotic activity did not exceed 3 per 10 high-power fields, whereas mitotically more active tumors were regarded as *fibrosarcomas*[981] (see p. 1605) (Figs 19.313 and 19.314). In a recent review of the issue, a modification of this scheme was proposed, in the sense of designating the mitotically active tumors as fibrosarcomas when exhibiting moderate to severe atypia, and as *mitotically active cellular fibromas* those with a bland cytology.[971] Differences between ovarian fibroma and fibrocarcinoma have also been described at the DNA ploidy, genetic, and cell proliferation levels.[996]

Some otherwise typical fibromas have a minor component of sex cord elements.[1002]

Cytogenetically, both thecomas and fibromas have been found to exhibit trisomy of chromosome 12 in a minority of the tumor cells.[980,992] Loss of heterozygosity at both the *PTCH* gene (implicated in Gorlin syndrome) and the *STK11* gene (implicated in Peutz–Jeghers syndrome) is relatively frequent in cellular fibromas.[997]

Ovarian fibroma (especially if large) can be associated with ascites, sometimes in combination with right-sided pleural effusion (Meigs syndrome).[986,1000] This may lead to a mistaken impression of inoperable ovarian neoplasm, but removal of the tumor leads to

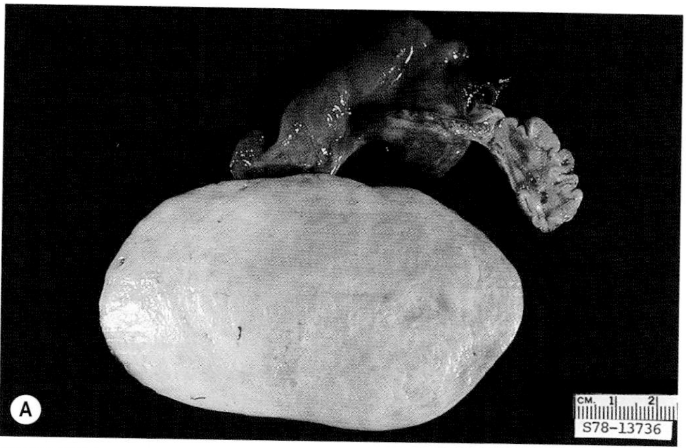

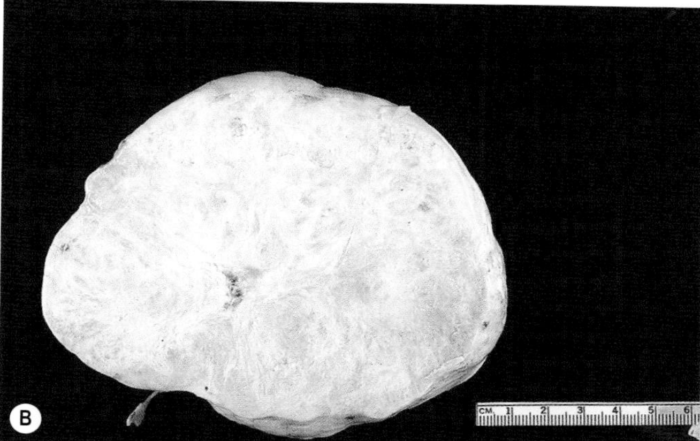

Fig. 19.311 A and **B**, Outer aspect and cut surface of ovarian fibroma. The white color contrasts with the yellow hue of thecoma (compare with Fig. 19.309).

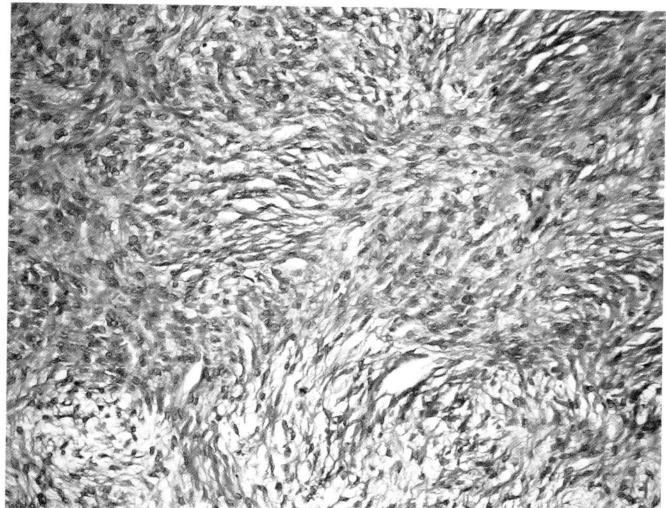

Fig. 19.312 Ovarian fibroma showing, bland nuclear features, and a suggestion of a storiform pattern of growth.

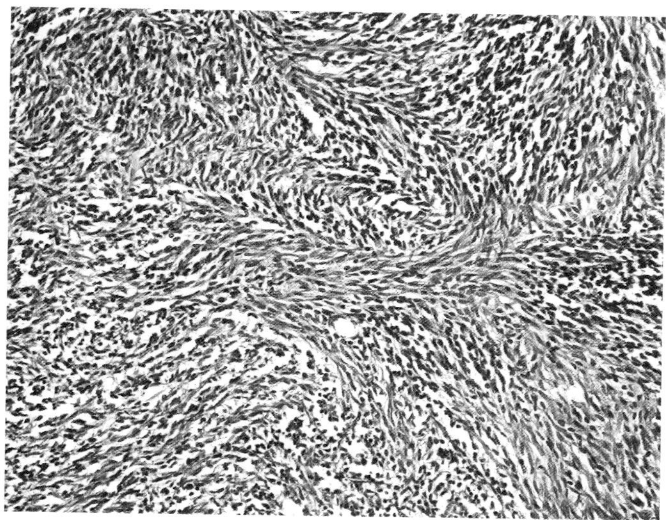

Fig. 19.313 Cellular fibroma. The tumor is hypercellular, but pleomorphism and mitotic activity are minimal.

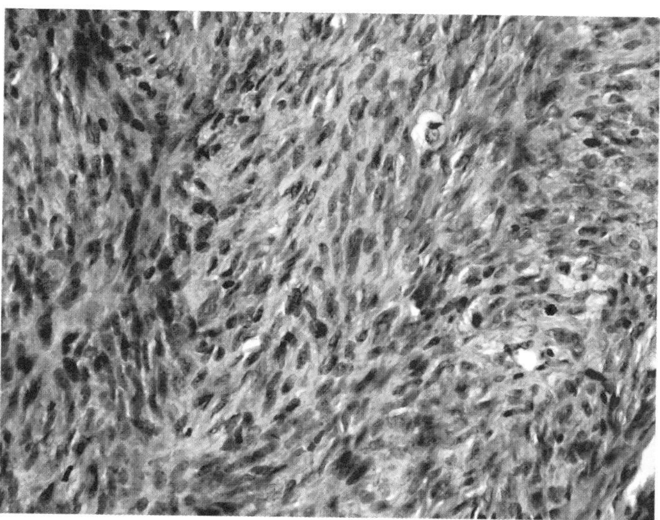

Fig. 19.314 Fibrosarcoma of ovary. Hypercellularity, nuclear hyperchromasia, and brisk mitotic activity are present. The latter is the most important feature in the differential diagnosis with cellular fibroma.

the disappearance of these manifestations. The mechanism for the pleural effusion is said to be related to intrathoracic negative pressure and transdiaphragmatic passage of fluid through peritoneal 'pores' or lymphatics. Meigs syndrome can also occur in association with other ovarian tumors.[976]

Fibromas are benign, and oophorectomy is curative. However, cellular fibromas may recur or be associated with peritoneal implants.[981]

Sclerosing stromal tumor is a benign ovarian neoplasm that shares many features with fibroma and thecoma. However, it occurs in a younger age group, has a less homogeneous gross appearance (Fig. 19.315), and is characterized microscopically by a lobular

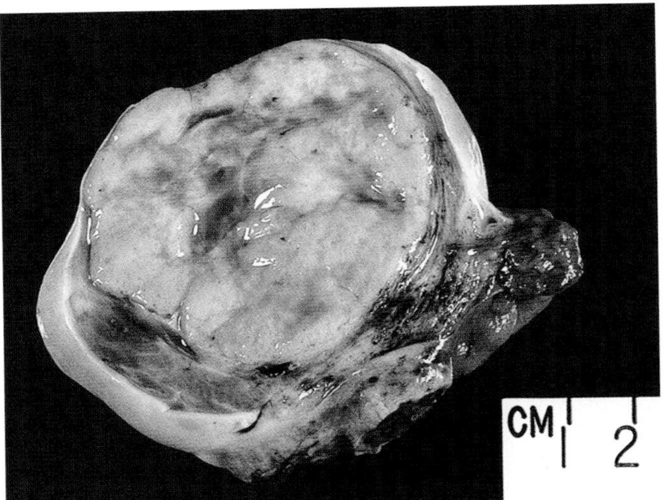

Fig. 19.315 Multinodular quality of cut surface of sclerosing stromal tumor.

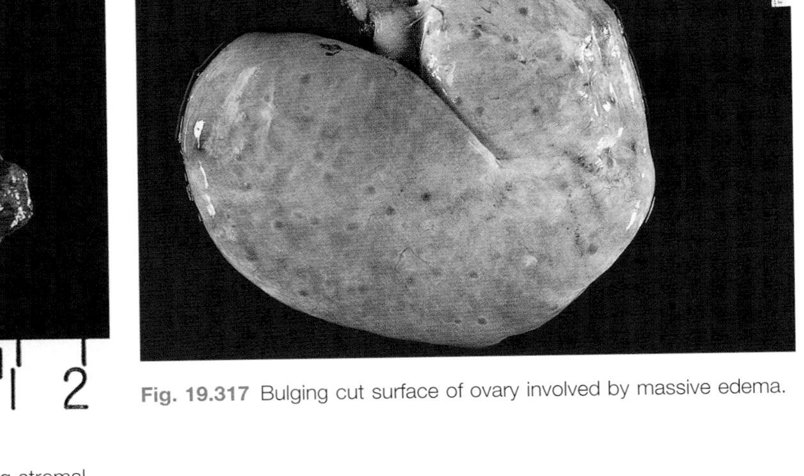

Fig. 19.317 Bulging cut surface of ovary involved by massive edema.

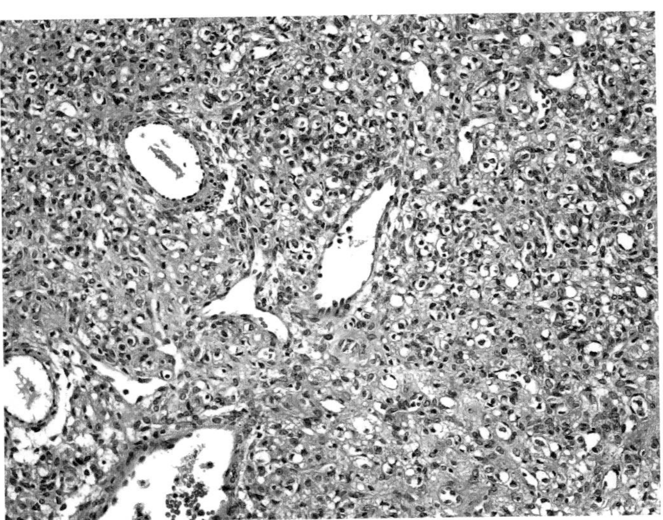

Fig. 19.316 Sclerosing stromal tumor of ovary. The hemangiopericytoma-like foci and the alternation of hypo- and hypercellular areas are important diagnostic clues.

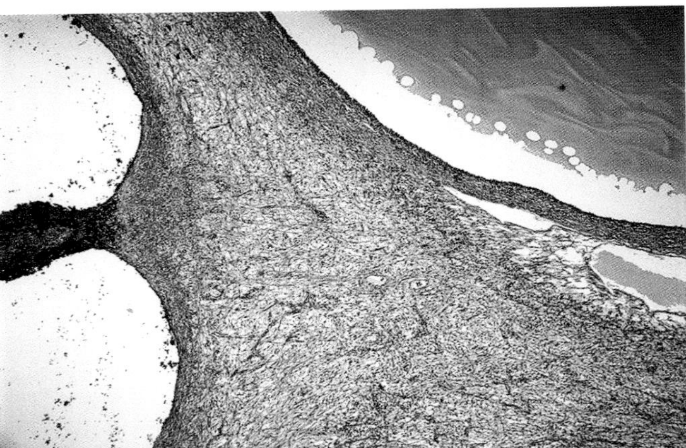

Fig. 19.318 Massive edema of ovary typically surrounding dilated follicles.

pattern of growth, interlobular fibrosis, marked vascularity, and the presence of a dual cell population: collagen-producing spindle cells and lipid-containing round or oval cells (Fig. 19.316). Some of the latter may have a signet ring appearance and thus simulate a Krukenberg tumor[963] (see also p. 1607). Endocrine manifestations are rarely present, and *ligandin* (a probable indicator of steroidogenesis) has been demonstrated immunohistochemically.[994] The tumor cells are also immunoreactive for smooth muscle actin and sometimes for desmin.[985,995] Evidence of differentiation along smooth muscle lines is also seen at the ultrastructural level.[988] Cytogenetically, this tumor shares the tendency for trisomy 12 that is also a feature of fibrothecomas.[974]

Massive edema of the ovary is probably not a neoplasm but is discussed here because of its gross similarities with fibroma. Most patients present with pain, abdominal mass, and/or menstrual irregularities; virilization, precocious puberty, and Meigs syndrome have also been described.[975,983] Partial torsion of the meso-ovarium with interference in the venous and lymphatic drainage has been suggested as the pathogenetic mechanism.[983] The cut surface has been described as watery (Fig. 19.317). Microscopically, there is marked edema of the stroma surrounding follicles and other structures (Fig. 19.318).[979] Clusters of luteinized cells are often present.[973]

Fibromatosis is the term proposed by Young and Scully[1003] for a disorder that they believe is possibly related to massive edema. The patients usually present because of menstrual irregularities. Grossly, the ovaries show a firm, white, cut surface. Microscopically, a diffuse proliferation of spindle cells separated by dense collagen is seen surrounding normal follicular structures. Luteinized cells may be present. The fact that some cases of massive ovarian edema are accompanied by small cellular foci of fibromatosis lends support to their interpretation. The term *fibromatosis*, although descriptively correct, should not be equated with the similarly named lesion of soft tissues, which under exceptional circumstances can involve the ovary.[978]

Myxoma of ovary presents as a solid and cystic mass, some of the cysts being occasionally filled with blood. Microscopically, scattered cells with fibroblastic/myofibroblastic features are seen in a well-vascularized myxoid background.[967,993] Some authors regard this as a distinct type of ovarian neoplasm, whereas others view it as part of the spectrum of differentiation in the fibrothecoma group.[965,966]

Endometrial abnormalities associated with granulosa cell tumor, thecoma, and related tumors

The endometrium of patients with granulosa cell tumors or thecomas exhibits various degrees of hyperplasia in about a fourth of cases,[1007] even when the ovarian tumors are of minute size. In the remaining cases, the endometrium shows a normal proliferative or secretory pattern, and it may even be atrophic. Some of the hyperplasias are so florid as to closely resemble the appearance of an endometrial adenocarcinoma. This fact is at the heart of the controversy as to how often an endometrial adenocarcinoma occurs in the setting of these ovarian neoplasms. The quoted incidence varies from 3% to 21%,[1005,1007] this wide range strongly suggesting the lack of uniform diagnostic criteria. Some of the lesions are undoubtedly hyperplasias, proved by the fact that they have been found to regress following excision of the ovarian tumors. The bona fide carcinomas are nearly always well differentiated and superficial, and this explains the excellent prognosis associated with them. Cases of endometrial adenocarcinoma have also been reported in association with ovarian sclerosing stromal tumor.[1006]

Rarely thecomas have been found to be associated with endometrial sarcomas of one type or another.[1008]

Small cell carcinoma

There are two types of primary ovarian carcinoma composed of small cells, designated as hypercalcemic and pulmonary type, respectively.

Hypercalcemic-type small cell carcinoma, which is by far the most common, is a high-grade ovarian malignancy that may be confused with granulosa cell tumor.[1013,1024,1027] It occurs in young females (average age, 23 years) and is nearly always bilateral. Some familial cases have been reported.[1020] The tumor is associated with hypercalcemia in two-thirds of cases, which disappears following removal of the tumor.[1012] Grossly, the tumor is large and solid, with areas of necrosis and hemorrhage (Fig. 19.319). Microscopically, a diffuse proliferation of small, closely packed cells of carcinomatous appearance with scant cytoplasm and small nuclei is seen (Fig. 19.320). Clusters of larger and more pleomorphic cells may be present, some of them resembling luteinized cells.[1014] Cytoplasmic hyaline globules may also be seen. Tumors containing a large number of these cells have been referred to, tongue-in-cheek, as the large cell variant of small cell carcinoma. There may also be islands, cords, trabeculae, mucinous glands, and *follicle-like structures*. The latter are an important clue to the diagnosis.

The tumor cells usually express keratin, vimentin, EMA, WT1, P53 and laminin, but not B72.3, S-100 protein, chromogranin (disputed), inhibin, CD117, or OCT4.[1009,1010,1021,1023,1025] The combination of WT1 and EMA positivity associated with alpha-inhibin negativity is particularly suggestive of the diagnosis.[1021] Immunoreactivity has apparently been found for human parathyroid hormone-related protein, but the correlation between the degree of staining and the serum calcium level is poor.[1022] Ultrastructurally, the cells have a poorly differentiated appearance, with relatively abundant dilated rough endoplasmic reticulum and specialized cell junctions; neurosecretory-type granules are generally absent.[1014,1015] Most surprisingly, this tumor has been found to have a diploid DNA pattern.[1016]

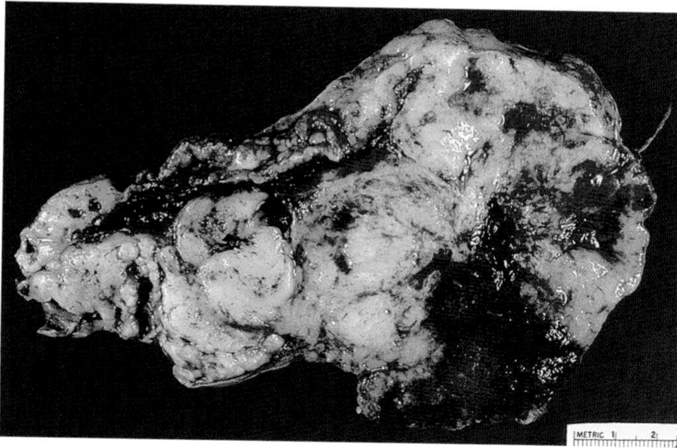

Fig. 19.319 Solid cut surface with hemorrhagic foci in ovarian small cell carcinoma of hypercalcemic type.

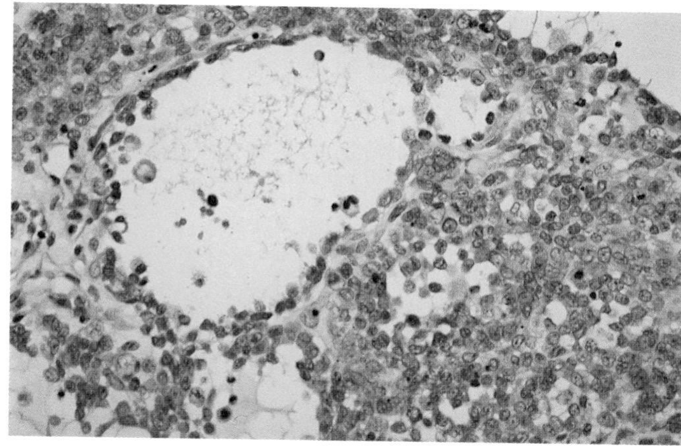
Fig. 19.320 Small cell carcinoma, hypercalcemic type. The presence of follicle-like formations is an important diagnostic feature.

The prognosis is very poor because of frequent extraovarian spread. The histogenesis remains obscure, the messages provided by the various techniques being mixed. The keratin and EMA positivity, the negativity for inhibin, and the finding of *KRAS* mutations[1023] suggest an epithelial origin;[1015] the association with a paraneoplastic syndrome and the reported reactivity for chromogranin[1009] point toward a neuroendocrine tumor; and the age distribution and presence of follicle-like formations are more in keeping with sex cord–stromal derivation.

Pulmonary-type small cell carcinoma resembles in all regards the homonymous lung tumor[1018] (Fig. 19.321). It may be pure or

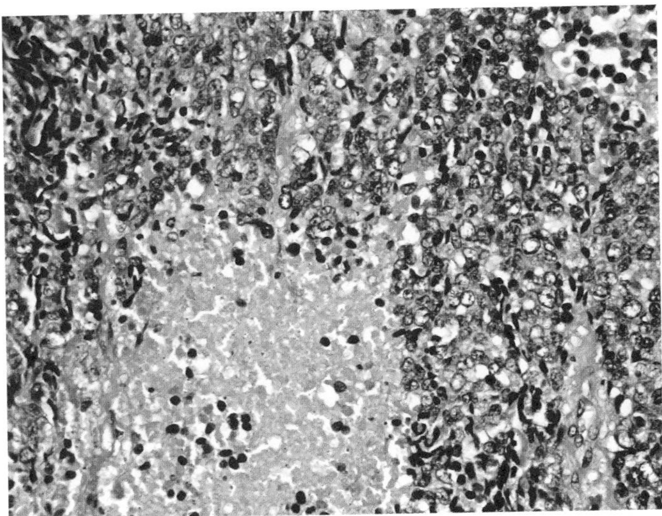

Fig. 19.321 Small cell carcinoma of pulmonary type. The sharply outlined foci of necrosis are a common feature of this tumor, which has a microscopic appearance very similar to its pulmonary counterpart.

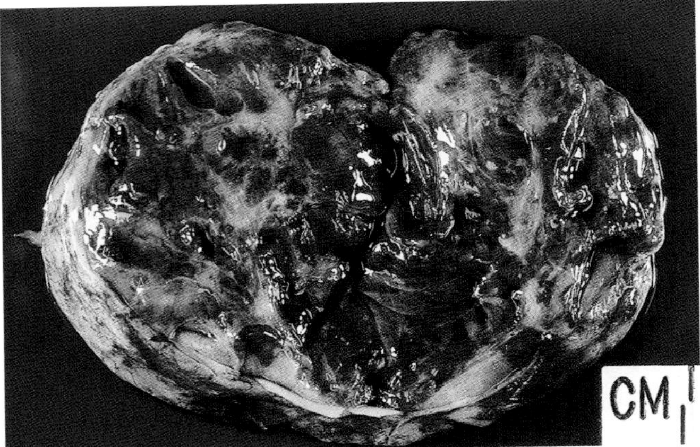

Fig. 19.322 Variegated appearance of cut surface of ovarian Sertoli–Leydig cell tumor.

associated with endometrioid carcinoma or other patterns. Immunohistochemically, there is reactivity for keratin, EMA, NSE, and (rarely) for chromogranin and Leu7 (CD57). Ultrastructurally, neurosecretory-type granules can be identified.[1015] In contrast to the hypercalcemic type, the DNA pattern is often aneuploid.[1018] The prognosis is poor.

As in other organs, there are in the ovary high-grade neuroendocrine carcinomas that have a morphology other than the small cell carcinoma just described.[1026] Some of these have been described as **large cell neuroendocrine carcinoma** and have been seen in association with surface epithelial adenocarcinomas.[1011,1017,1019]

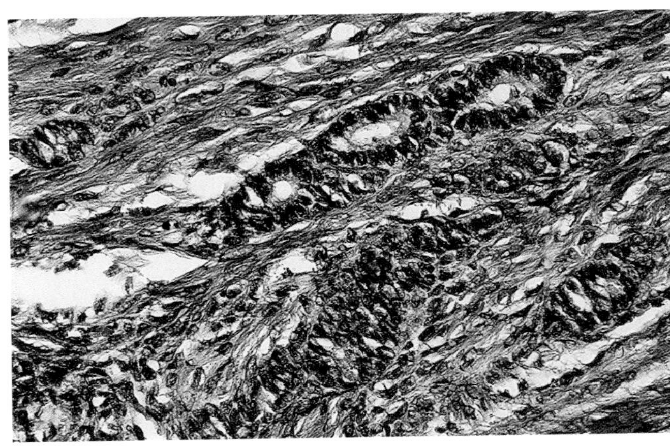

Fig. 19.323 Well-differentiated (Meyer type I) Sertoli–Leydig cell tumor.

Sertoli–Leydig cell tumor

As the name indicates, Sertoli–Leydig cell tumors are composed of a mixture in variable proportions of cells morphologically resembling male Sertoli and Leydig cells. This term replaces the old designations arrhenoblastoma and androblastoma, and should be regarded as synonymous with Sertoli–stromal cell tumor. Pure Sertoli cell tumors are also included in this group, but pure Leydig cell tumors are included with the lipid cell tumors.[1032] Meyer[1038,1054] championed the concept that male-directed cells persisting from the primitive testis-like structure that develops during embryogenesis in the ovarian medulla near the hilus are the origin of this tumor. However, the ultrastructural and immunohistochemical features plus the lack of the *SRY* gene (sex-determining region Y gene) indicate a close histogenetic relationship with granulosa cells.[1034,1035] The interesting point has been made that the only neoplastic component of this tumor may be represented by the Sertoli cells, as the Leydig cell component has been shown to be polyclonal when assessed for loss of heterozygosity with PCR techniques.[1039]

Sertoli–Leydig cell tumors are uncommon, comprising less than 0.1% of ovarian neoplasms. Grossly they are predominantly solid, but cystic areas may also be present (Fig. 19.322).

The microscopic pattern is extremely variable. Several major categories have been described, which may coexist in the same tumor:

1. *Well-differentiated* (*Meyer type I*) (11%). Composed of tubules lined by Sertoli-like cells separated by variable numbers of Leydig-like cells[1061] (Fig. 19.323). Sometimes those tubules have a hollow 'pseudoendometrioid' appearance, the tumor thus simulating a borderline or malignant endometrioid neoplasm.[1037] The opposite phenomenon – i.e., endometrioid adenocarcinoma simulating Sertoli-Leydig cell tumor – also occurs (and is actually more common), immunohistochemical evaluation being sometimes necessary to solve the issue.[1064]
2. *Intermediate* (*Meyer type II*) (54%). Characterized by the formation of cords, sheets, and aggregates of Sertoli-like cells, separated by spindle stromal cells and recognizable Leydig cells (Fig. 19.324).
3. *Poorly differentiated* (*sarcomatoid; undifferentiated; Meyer type III*) (13%). Composed of masses of spindle-shaped cells arranged in a 'sarcomatoid' pattern (Fig. 19.325).

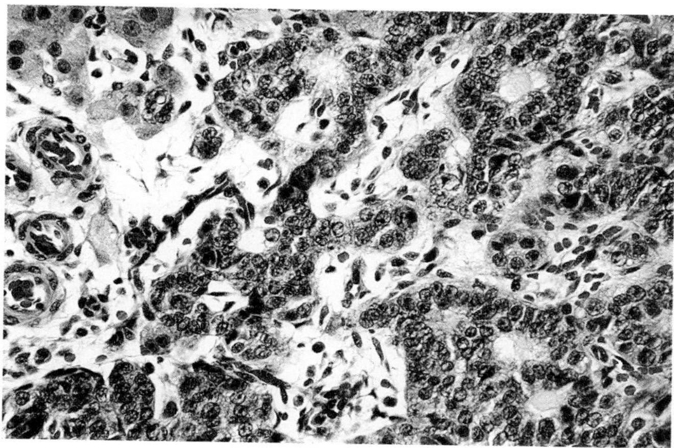

Fig. 19.324 Intermediate (Meyer type II) Sertoli–Leydig cell tumor.

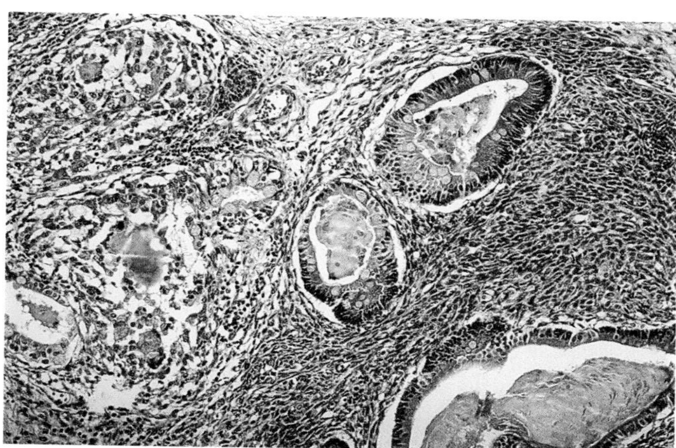

Fig. 19.326 Sertoli–Leydig cell tumor with heterologous elements represented by well-differentiated mucin-secreting glands.

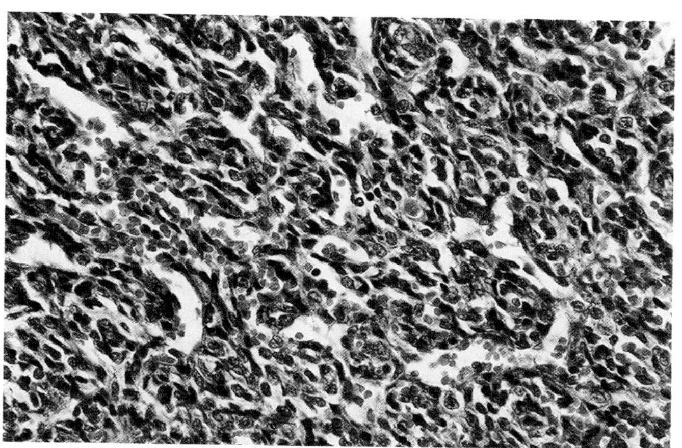

Fig. 19.325 Poorly differentiated (Meyer type III) Sertoli–Leydig cell tumor.

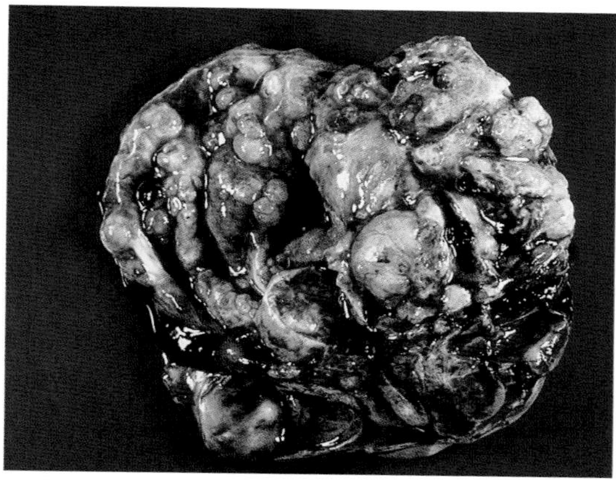

Fig. 19.327 Gross appearance of Sertoli–Leydig cell tumor of the retiform variant.

4 *Pure Sertoli cell tumors* (*tubular androblastoma*). Essentially identical to well-differentiated Sertoli–Leydig cell tumors but lacking Leydig cells and primitive stromal elements.[1043,1060] Abundant lipid may be present in the cytoplasm. The microscopic pattern can be tubular or follicle-like (so-called *folliculoma lipidique*).[1062] Amyloid-like material can be present, and cytoplasmic crystalline structures have been found by electron microscopy.[1052] Some Sertoli cell tumors are composed of cells with oxyphilic cytoplasm.[1031]

5 *With heterologous elements* (*teratoid androblastoma*) (22%). Associated with tissues such as mucinous epithelium of gastrointestinal type, liver,[1056] skeletal muscle, or cartilage[1044,1046] (Fig. 19.326). The epithelial component of this neoplasm contains a variety of endocrine cells[1028] and can give rise to microscopic carcinoid tumors.[1049,1057]

6 *Retiform* (15%). In this category, typical elements of Sertoli–Leydig cell tumors coexist with formations resembling the rete of the ovary or testis (Figs 19.327 and 19.328). These appear as irregular cleft-like spaces lined by low cuboidal cells; blunt papillae with hyalinized or edematous cores are often present. Sometimes the retiform formations predominate almost to the exclusion of the Sertoli–Leydig cell component[1047,1058] (Fig. 19.329). In other instances there is a hepatocytic component in the tumor, which may be difficult to distinguish without immunostains from Leydig cells.[1041]

As in the case of granulosa cell tumor, the cells of a few Sertoli–Leydig cell tumors may contain bizarre and/or multiple nuclei, a change of no apparent prognostic significance.[1059]

Immunohistochemically, testosterone and estradiol are found in both Sertoli and Leydig cells and less frequently in primitive stromal cells.[1036] The areas of Sertoli cell differentiation stain for keratin and Sox-9[1065] (but not for EMA, PLAP, CEA, CA19-9, CA-125, or S-100 protein), whereas the gonadal stromal component is strongly positive for inhibin.[1040] WT1 is usually positive in both components.[1066] Knowledge of this profile is useful in the differential diagnosis between Sertoli–Leydig cell tumors with

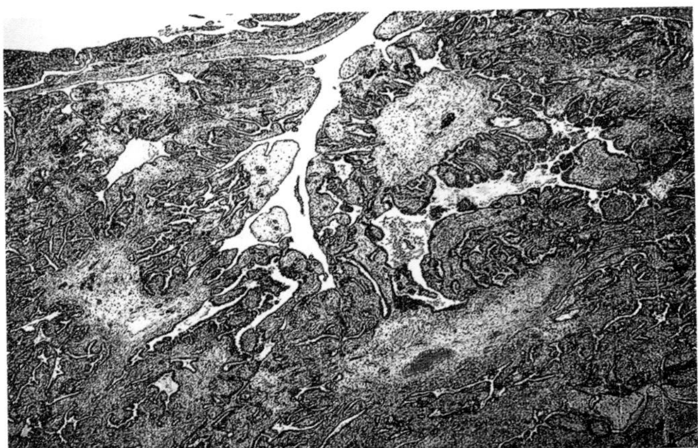

Fig. 19.328 Retiform variant of Sertoli–Leydig cell tumor as seen on low-power examination. The retiform areas are represented by the micropapillary foci.

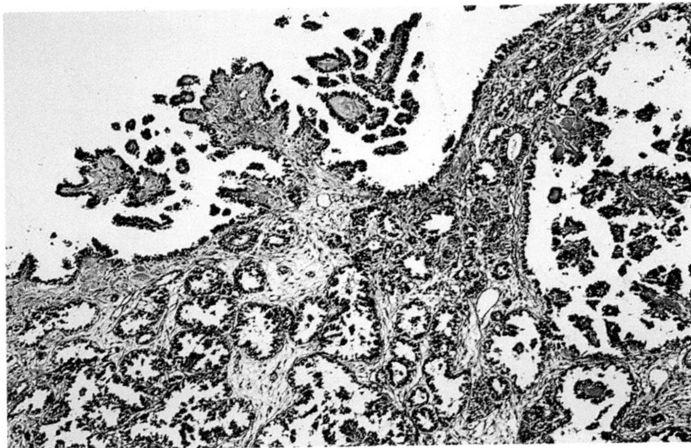

Fig. 19.329 When the retiform type of Sertoli–Leydig cell tumor is made up predominantly or exclusively of retiform elements without conventional foci of Sertoli–Leydig cells, as seen here, the diagnosis can be easily missed.

heterologous elements (in which this profile is maintained) and carcinosarcoma.[1030]

Most Sertoli–Leydig cell tumors are seen in young patients (average age, 25 years) and are relatively rare after menopause. Some are diagnosed during pregnancy.[1055] These tend to exhibit prominent intercellular edema.[1054] Bilateral involvement is seen in less than 2% of cases. Cases have been reported in association with mature cystic teratoma.[1050] Nearly half of the cases are accompanied by signs of androgen excess. This is manifested first by *defeminization* (amenorrhea, breast atrophy, loss of subcutaneous tissue deposits) and later by *masculinization* (clitoral hypertrophy, deepening of the voice, hirsutism). Usually prompt return of feminine characteristics follows excision of the tumor, but the manifestations of masculinization disappear more slowly. Urinary 17-ketosteroids are frequently normal, but elevations have been recorded. Tumor tissue incubated with progesterone or pregnenolone causes a synthesis of various hormones (androstenedione, 17-hydroxyprogesterone, testosterone), but the final aromatizing reaction to estrogens does not occur.[1048,1051]

Some Sertoli–Leydig cell tumors do not have demonstrable endocrine effect, whereas others are accompanied by secretion of estrogen or progesterone. The latter is often the case for pure Sertoli cell tumors.[1053] It is opportune to mention again that the diagnosis of these neoplasms should be based on their morphologic appearance rather than on the nature of their hormonal manifestations; terms such as 'feminizing mesenchymoma' should be avoided. Curiously, some cases of Sertoli–Leydig cell tumor have been associated with serum elevation of alpha-fetoprotein;[1029,1033,1042] this marker has been detected immunohistochemically in areas of hepatocytic differentiation[1056] and in the more conventional Leydig and Sertoli cell-like component.[1034]

The prognosis of Sertoli–Leydig cell tumor, which is usually good, correlates with the stage and degree of differentiation of the tumor.[1045,1063] The overall incidence of clinical malignancy in one large series was 18%; all the well-differentiated tumors were benign, but 11% of those with intermediate differentiation, 59% of those with poor differentiation, and 19% of those with heterologous elements were malignant.[1056] In one series of 28 cases of pure Sertoli cell tumor, there were two recurrences.[1052] Conservative surgery is indicated in young women for Sertoli–Leydig cell tumors grossly confined to the ovary.[1062,1063]

Lipid (lipoid, steroid) cell tumor

A small group of ovarian tumors is composed entirely of cells with morphologic features indicative of steroid hormone secretion. These are manifested by an abundant eosinophilic or vacuolated cytoplasm that is often positive for fat stains and that, at the ultrastructural level, is shown to contain well-developed smooth endoplasmic reticulum and mitochondria with tubulovesicular cristae.[1069] Normal steroid hormone-secreting cells can be of lutein (thecal or stromal), Leydig (hilus), and adrenal cortical type.[1072] Theoretically, these tumors could arise from any of these sources. In the few cases in which Reinke crystalloids are found, the tumor can be categorized as Leydig or hilus cell tumor.[1071,1072,1074] In a few others, an ectopic adrenal origin has been suggested on the basis of their hormonal profile (presence of Cushing syndrome)[1078] and the fact that adrenal cortical rests can be found in the hilus of the ovary and the broad ligament (although not within the adult ovary itself). In the majority of the cases, however, the exact origin of this tumor remains undecided; the descriptive terms **lipid, lipoid**, and – more recently – **steroid cell tumor** have therefore been proposed for the entire group, with the added designations *Leydig cell type* or *adrenal cortical type* whenever indicated.[1077,1078] None of these terms is ideal. 'Lipid' and 'lipoid' have been criticized on the grounds that the tumor cells may not always contain neutral fat, and the term 'steroid cell' has been objected to because of the fact that nearly all of the sex cord–stromal tumors have the capability to secrete steroid hormones. In any event, any of these three designations is preferable to the old terms *luteoma, hypernephroma*, or *masculinovoblastoma*.

Enzymatic conversion studies performed on freshly excised tumors have demonstrated that a variety of androgenic hormones are produced by these tumors in vitro;[1075] occasionally, large amounts of adrenal corticoids have been found.

Lipid cell tumors are usually unilateral and are composed of yellow or yellowish-brown nodules separated by fibrous trabeculae (Fig. 19.330). Microscopically, they are characterized by masses of large rounded or polyhedral cells with the morphologic and ultrastructural features previously described for their normal counterparts (Fig. 19.331). Immunohistochemically, there is reactivity for vimentin in three-fourths of cases, for keratin in one-half,

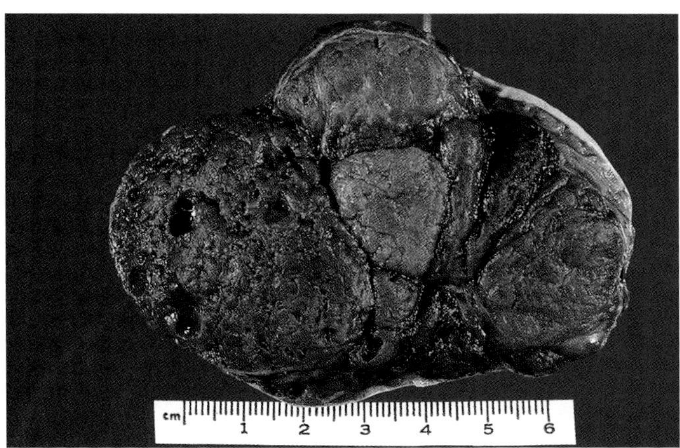

Fig. 19.330 Cut surface of ovarian lipid cell tumor. The deep brown color is reminiscent of a renal or thyroid oncocytoma.

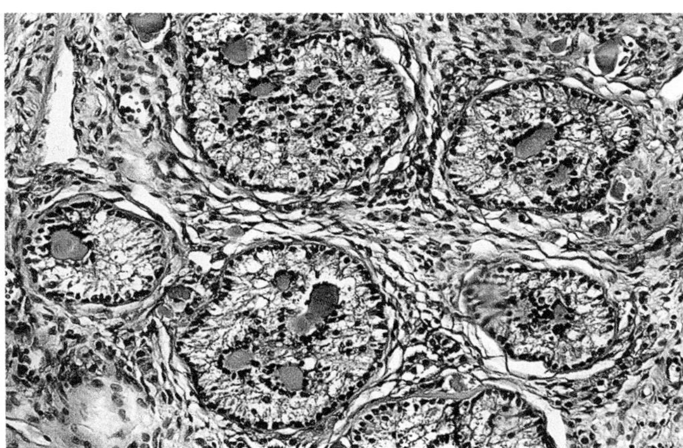

Fig. 19.332 Sex cord tumor with annular tubules. The patient was affected by Peutz–Jeghers syndrome.

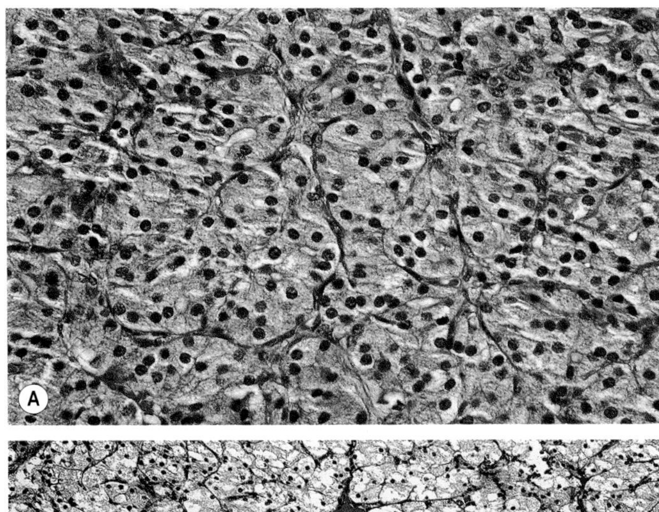

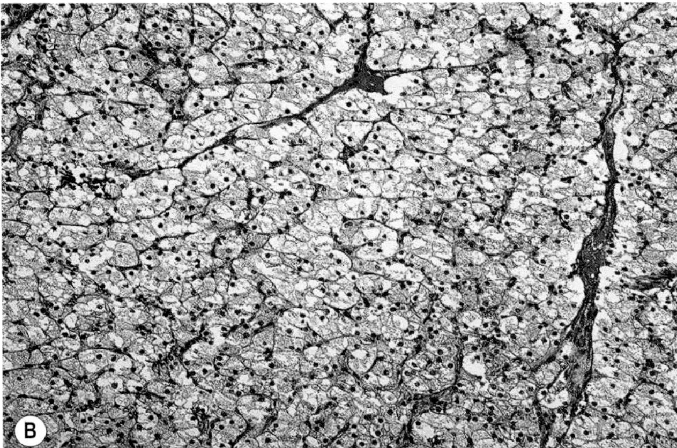

Fig. 19.331 Two cases of lipid cell tumor showing acidophilic (**A**) and clear (**B**) appearances of the cytoplasmic of the tumor cells.

and for actin in about one-third.[1076] There is also consistent reactivity for inhibin and A103/Mart-1.[1070]

This neoplasm can occur at any age.[1077] Most are associated with a virilizing syndrome (with defeminization and amenorrhea) and – as already indicated – a few cases meet the criteria for Cushing syndrome.[1078] Some of the tumors are biologically inactive, at least at the clinical level, and others are associated with estrogenic or progestogenic manifestations. A few cases have been associated with endometrioid carcinoma.[1068] The incidence of clinical malignancy is approximately 25%.[1067,1077] Malignant tumors tend to be larger (7 cm in diameter or greater), with foci of necrosis and hemorrhage, and to exhibit nuclear atypia and mitotic activity.[1067,1077] Tumors containing Reinke crystalloids are almost invariably benign.[1071,1077] The malignant tumors can lead to peritoneal implants.[1077]

Lipid cell tumors should be distinguished from lesions in which proliferation of steroid hormone-producing cells occurs as a secondary event. These include stromal luteoma (although the position of this lesion in the scheme of ovarian neoplasms remains controversial), luteinized granulosa cell tumor (particularly the juvenile type), fibrothecoma, stromal–Leydig cell tumor, and the non-neoplastic proliferation of steroid cells that may be seen at the periphery of other tumors, such as struma ovarii, strumal carcinoid, surface epithelial tumors, and metastatic carcinoma.[1073]

Other types

Gynandroblastoma is the term used for the sex cord–stromal tumor composed of a mixture *in similar amounts* of clearly identifiable granulosa–theca cell and Sertoli–Leydig cell elements.[1087] When thus defined, this entity is extremely rare, to the point that some authors doubt its existence. On occasion the granulosa cell component is of the juvenile rather than the adult type.[1082,1094] Reported cases of this entity have been accompanied by androgenic, estrogenic, or no hormonal effects.[1095,1096] Examples of late recurrence following excision are on record.[1083]

Sex cord tumor with annular tubules is a distinctive ovarian tumor that is associated in one-third of the cases with the Peutz–Jeghers syndrome.[1089,1098] This lesion combines features suggestive of a granulosa cell tumor with a pattern of growth reminiscent of Sertoli cells.[1080] Its morphologic hallmark is the presence of simple and complex annular tubules containing eosinophilic hyaline bodies, often calcified (Fig. 19.332). The appearance is similar to that of gonadoblastoma, from which it differs because of the clinical/genetic background and the presence of a germ cell component in the latter.

The ambiguous or biphasic nature of the tumor cells is also apparent on ultrastructural examination: features consistent with granulosa cell or nonspecialized ovarian stroma[1084,1090] alternate with features indicative of Sertoli cell differentiation, notably the presence of Charcot–Bottcher filaments.[1079] Symptoms suggestive of hyperestrinism have been described in approximately 50% of cases. Tumors associated with the Peutz–Jeghers syndrome are typically multifocal, bilateral, small (or even microscopic), calcified, and usually benign, although exceptions occur.[1093] Those unassociated with the syndrome are unilateral, often large, and clinically malignant in approximately 22% of cases.[1088,1107]

It should be mentioned here that Peutz–Jeghers syndrome can be associated with other neoplasms of the female genital tract, such as other sex cord–stromal ovarian tumors,[1105] mucinous ovarian tumors, and well-differentiated adenocarcinoma (adenoma malignum) of the cervix.

Wolffian adnexal tumor is the abbreviated designation for the tumor entity first named *ovarian tumor of probable wolffian origin*. It was originally described as occurring in the broad ligament[1092] and subsequently in the retroperitoneum[1102] and the ovary itself.[1097,1106] It is thought to be of wolffian (mesonephric) derivation, the first term being chosen to avoid confusion with tumors formerly regarded as of mesonephric nature (such as clear cell carcinoma) and now included in other categories. If this interpretation is correct, these neoplasms are *not* of sex cord–stromal nature, but they are discussed here because of their resemblance to them and the fact that their exact histogenesis is still arguable. Grossly, they may be either solid or solid and cystic. Microscopically, epithelial cells are seen growing in the form of cystic structures, solid or hollow tubules, and diffuse sheets (Fig. 19.333). The sieve-like appearance on low-power examination is a useful diagnostic feature. Conversely, the presence of a predominant spindle cell component can be confusing.[1086] PAS-positive basement membranes are prominent around the epithelial aggregates. These tumors lack stromal cells of steroid hormone-secreting type and are unaccompanied by hormonal manifestations. Mucin stains are negative. Immunohistochemically, the tumor is positive for keratin (CK7 but not CK20), androgen receptor (three-fourths of cases), estrogen and progesterone receptors (one-fourth), inhibin (over half), calretinin (almost all), and vimentin (always). It is negative for CEA. This profile is consistent with but not diagnostic of wolffian derivation.[1085,1103] The behavior is generally benign, but a few have recurred or metastasized.[1081,1100,1106]

Signet ring stromal tumor of the ovary is a very rare type but of great practical importance because of the fact that it can be easily mistaken for Krukenberg tumor. Some of the examples may be variants of sclerosing stromal tumor (see p. 1597). The tumor cells are negative for keratin, PAS, and mucin. Their behavior is benign.[1104]

Microcystic stromal tumor is the latest addition to the group of sex cord–stromal ovarian neoplasms.[1091] It is usually unilateral and nonfunctioning. Microscopically, its most distinctive feature is the presence of small round to oval cystic spaces, in areas coalescing to form larger irregular channels, combined with lobulated cellular masses with intervening fibrous or fibrohyaline stroma.

Sex cord–stromal tumor, indeterminate or unclassified type, is a justifiable designation for ovarian tumors in which the cytologic and/or architectural features are consistent with a sex cord–stromal origin but which cannot be assigned to any specific category. These tumors comprise approximately 10% of cases. Their behavior is similar to that of granulosa cell tumor and Sertoli–Leydig cell tumor, with a generally favorable prognosis when confined to the ovaries.[1099,1101]

Germ cell–sex cord–stromal tumors

The most distinctive member of the group of tumors composed of a combination of germ cells and sex cord–stromal cells is **gonadoblastoma**, also known as *dysgenetic gonadoma* and included among the *gonocytomas* in Teter's elaborate classification.[1126] This tumor occurs practically always in sexually abnormal individuals, most commonly affected by gonadal dysgenesis and carrying the Y chromosome (i.e., XY gonadal dysgenesis and XO-XY mosaicism but not XX gonadal dysgenesis). The testis-specific protein Y-encoded gene is the putative gene for the gonadoblastoma locus on the Y chromosome.[1115]

The risk of neoplasia in these dysgenetic gonads is estimated to be 25%. However, gonadoblastomas have also been documented in phenotypically and chromosomally normal females, even during pregnancy.[1118,1120] They have also been seen in association with ataxia–telangiectasia.[1108] It is often impossible to determine the nature of the gonad bearing the tumor. In some cases it has been identified as a streak and in others as a cryptorchid testis, but never as a normal ovary.

Approximately 36% of the tumors are bilateral. They are usually small, and many become apparent only on microscopic examination[1123] (Fig. 19.334). The key microscopic feature is the admixture of primitive germ cells (resembling those of dysgerminoma) with sex cord–stromal cells resembling morphologically and immunohistochemically immature Sertoli and granulosa cells[1111,1112,1123] (Fig. 19.335). Steroid hormone-producing cells may

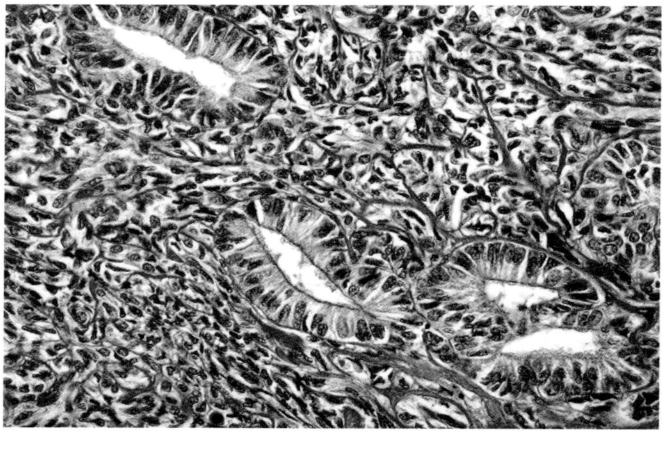

Fig. 19.333 Wolffian adnexal tumor of ovary. Elongated glandular structures are admixed with solid foci composed of oval to spindle cells.

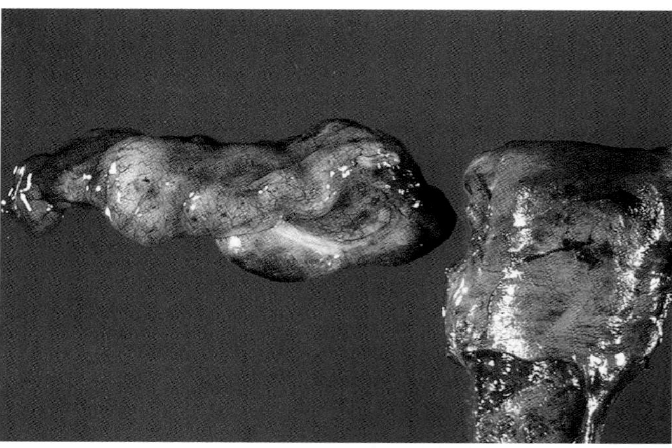

Fig. 19.334 Streak gonad microscopically shown to contain gonadoblastoma. The tumor was barely apparent grossly.

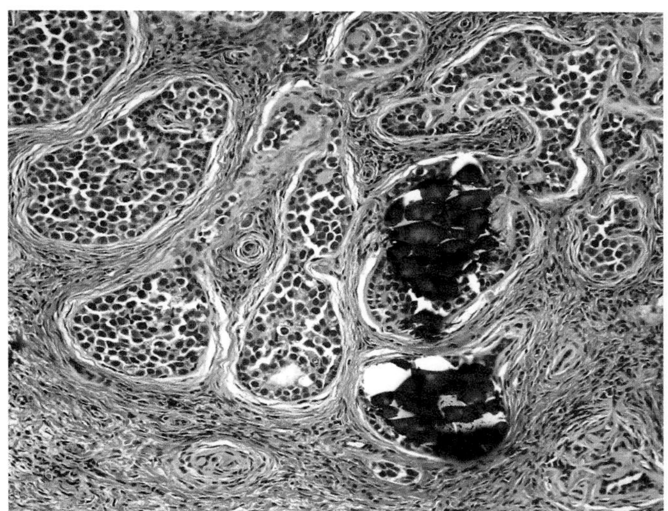

Fig. 19.335 Ovarian gonadoblastoma. Note the sharply outlined tumor nests and the heavy calcification.

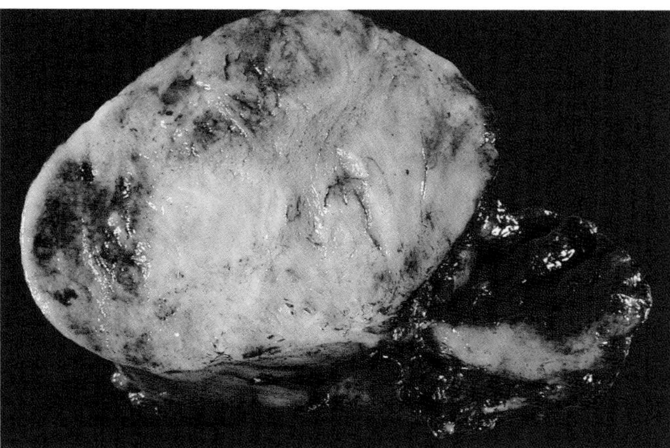

Fig. 19.336 Malignant lymphoma of Burkitt type with massive ovarian involvement.

also be present, especially after puberty; their capacity for steroidogenesis has been demonstrated by their in vitro production of androgens and estrogens.[1116] Hyalinization and calcification are common. The hyaline material reacts strongly with anti-laminin antibodies, indicating basement membrane deposition.[1121] When abundant, this material can become obvious on plain abdominal roentgenograms.

An interesting analogy has been made between gonadoblastoma and intratubular germ cell neoplasia of the testis on the basis of the morphology and the immunohistochemical profile, the implication being that gonadoblastoma is an in-situ germ cell malignancy arising in a dysgenetic gonad.[1113]

The germ cell component of gonadoblastoma may overgrow the stromal elements and result in the formation of a dysgerminoma or, exceptionally, another type of germ cell tumor.[1109,1110] Only under these circumstances is the tumor endowed with a malignant potential. Much more unusual is the overgrowth of the sex cord–stromal component, which may acquire the features of a Sertoli cell tumor.[1119]

Microscopic structures resembling gonadoblastoma and sex cord tumor with annular tubules are sometimes found incidentally in the ovaries of *normal* infants and children in association with follicular cysts; it has been suggested that they represent the precursor of these tumors.[1122]

Rare *germ cell–sex cord–stromal tumors* not fulfilling the diagnostic criteria for gonadoblastoma have been described in genetically normal females,[1124,1125] some of them containing retiform structures.[1127] The germ cell component of these tumors – like that of gonadoblastomas – is positive for PLAP, OCT4, and CD117.[1117] These tumors can be hormonally active and clinically malignant.[1114] Like gonadoblastoma, they can be accompanied by dysgerminoma or other germ cell tumors.

Tumors not specific to ovary

Malignant lymphoma and leukemia

Secondary ovarian involvement by generalized lymphoma or leukemia is well recognized.[1129,1130] Much more rarely, malignant lymphoma involves the ovaries as the primary manifestation of the disease[1128,1130,1132,1136,1138] (Fig. 19.336). This is also true for *granulocytic leukemia* (*granulocytic sarcoma*).[1134,1137]

Nearly all ovarian lymphomas are of non-Hodgkin type.[1133] In children, Burkitt lymphomas predominate; in adults, most are diffuse large B-cell lymphomas.[1133,1140] Immunophenotypically, practically all cases are of B-cell nature.[1131,1133] In the series of Osborne and Robboy,[1135] 55% were bilateral, and 64% also involved extragonadal sites (usually the omentum, fallopian tubes, or lymph nodes); only 9 of their 42 patients survived more than 5 years, and 2 subsequently died of lymphoma.

Exceptionally, ovarian lymphoma has been found to coexist with a borderline serous tumor.[1139]

Sarcoma

Primary sarcomas of the ovary are extremely rare. They need to be distinguished from undifferentiated carcinomas, malignant mixed müllerian tumors, 'sarcomatoid' forms of sex cord–stromal tumors, Krukenberg tumors associated with brisk stromal reaction, and cellular fibromas.

Fibrosarcomas are separated from cellular fibromas mainly on the basis of their mitotic activity (4 or more per 10 high-power fields) plus atypia, and possibly their different cytogenetic makeup (see p. 1596) (see Fig. 19.313). They tend to be large, solid, and accompanied by adhesions. The clinical course is aggressive.[1154] One case has been diagnosed in the context of the nevus–basal cell carcinoma syndrome.[1146]

Endometrial (endometrioid) stromal sarcomas can present as primary ovarian neoplasms; they closely simulate the pattern of growth of the diffuse type of granulosa tumor,[1163] but are recognized because of the presence of plump oval cells arranged around vessels of the spiral arteriole type.[1158] Immunohistochemically, they are reactive for CD10 but generally negative for inhibin.

Müllerian adenosarcoma is discussed on page 1576, although it is probably more closely related to endometrial stromal sarcoma than to malignant mixed müllerian tumor.

Other sarcomas of the adult ovary, all exceptionally rare, are *leiomyosarcoma*[1147,1148] (some of the myxoid type and some in patients with the nevoid basal cell carcinoma syndrome),[1151,1157] *chondrosarcoma,*[1161] *osteosarcoma,*[1141,1143,1155] *malignant peripheral nerve sheath tumor,*[1160] *angiosarcoma,*[1153] *rhabdomyosarcoma,*[1142] *low-grade fibromyxoid sarcoma,*[1162] and *Ewing sarcoma/PNET.*[1144,1145] The rhabdomyosarcomas are usually of the embryonal type, but they can also be of the alveolar variety;[1149] a case has been reported in association with clear cell carcinoma.[1156] The angiosarcomas show a wide morphologic spectrum and can be associated with mature cystic teratoma.[1150,1152]

The treatment of ovarian sarcoma is surgical excision ('cytoreduction') followed by chemotherapy, which usually includes platinum.[1159]

Other primary tumors

Hemangiomas of the ovary are usually small, found incidentally, unilateral, and cavernous in type.[1164] Rarely, they are bilateral and/or associated with hemangiomas elsewhere in the body. Ovarian hemangiomas should be distinguished from lipid cell tumors having a prominent vascular component and from the florid non-neoplastic vascular proliferation that sometimes accompanies the primitive neuroectodermal component of ovarian germ cell tumors.[1166] Other types of vascular tumors that have been reported in the ovary are *infantile hemangioendothelioma,*[1181] *lymphangioma* (which can be bilateral),[1169] and *glomus tumor.*[1173,1183] *Leiomyomas* can exceptionally develop in the ovary, usually in association with uterine leiomyomas;[1168] some are mitotically active and need to be distinguished from leiomyosarcomas.[1172,1175,1180] The criteria for making this distinction are similar to those employed for their infinitely more common uterine counterparts (and just as frustrating).[1176]

Isolated examples of *ovarian myofibroblastoma,*[1182] *epithelioid angiomyolipoma/PEComa,*[1165] *nephroblastoma* (Wilms tumor),[1174] *desmoplastic small cell tumor,*[1170] *pheochromocytoma/paraganglioma,*[1171,1177] and *hydatidiform mole*[1184] have also been described. *Adenomatoid tumor* can occur in an intra- or juxta-ovarian location; it can simulate the appearance of yolk sac tumor,[1185] and it can be predominantly composed of oxyphilic cells.[1179]

The great majority of cases of *melanoma* involving the ovary are metastatic, but cases thought to be primary in the ovary have been described, the most convincing examples being those arising within a mature cystic teratoma or a struma ovarii.[1178]

Lately, a most peculiar tumor type has been added to the list: pancreatic-type solid and pseudopapillary neoplasm (see also Chapter 15).[1167]

Metastatic tumors

The ovary is a common site of involvement for metastases.[1196,1224,1225,1259] Approximately 7% of lesions presenting clinically as primary ovarian tumors are of metastatic origin. Over half are bilateral. The most common sources are stomach, large bowel, appendix, breast, uterus (corpus and cervix[1234]), lung,[1208,1254] and skin (melanoma).[1200,1239,1247,1258] The difficult situation resulting from the simultaneous presence of carcinoma in ovary and uterus is discussed on page 1581. At the time when therapeutic oophorectomies were done in patients with breast carcinoma, it was not unusual to find small and sometimes microscopic (occult) metastases. Their pattern of growth could be either diffuse (with Indian file formations, suggestive of a lobular nature) or glandular, more in keeping with a ductal type.[1201] Immunoreactivity for GCDFP-15 is the rule, a fact of importance in the differential diagnosis with primary ovarian carcinoma, which is generally negative.[1226] The reverse is true for WT1, CA-125 and PAX8, which tend to be positive in the latter and negative in the former.[1227,1238]

Adenocarcinomas of the large bowel are particularly important because of their relatively high frequency and their ability to simulate primary ovarian carcinomas, mainly of the mucinous and endometrioid types but sometimes also of the clear cell and secretory types[1194,1205,1239,1252] (Fig. 19.337). The primary tumors are usually advanced (Dukes stage B or C), but sometimes are small and clinically occult.[1213] The ovarian metastases tend to be cystic, well differentiated, mucin-producing, and associated with necrosis and hemorrhage. In some cases (particularly those of cecal origin), the ovarian metastases are associated with luteinization of the surrounding stroma, which may lead to masculinization and other endocrine changes.[1235]

Features favoring metastasis from large bowel are bilaterality, surface involvement by tumor cells, infiltrative or nodular pattern

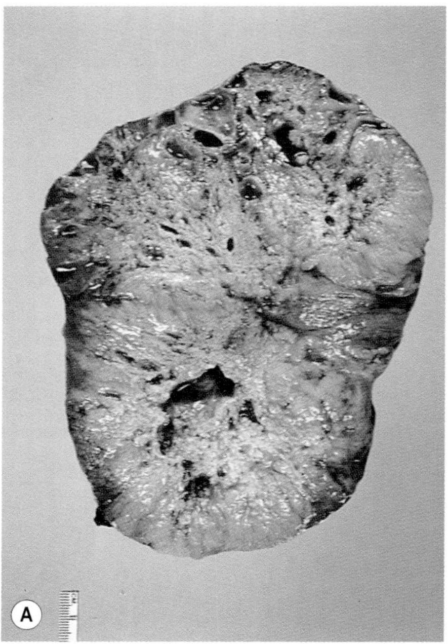

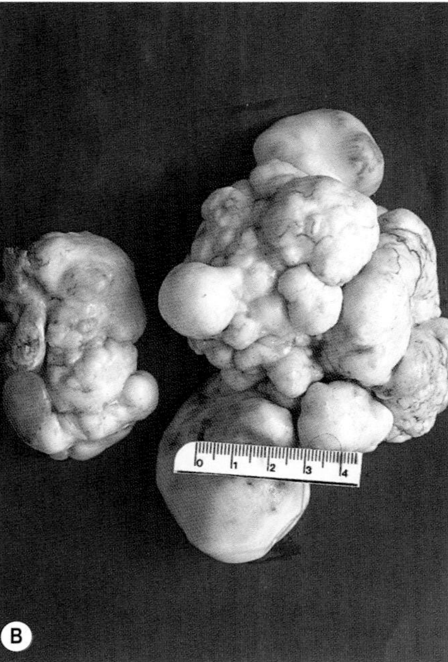

Fig. 19.337 A and **B**, Colonic carcinoma metastatic to ovary. This occurrence may be misdiagnosed as a primary ovarian tumor both grossly and microscopically.

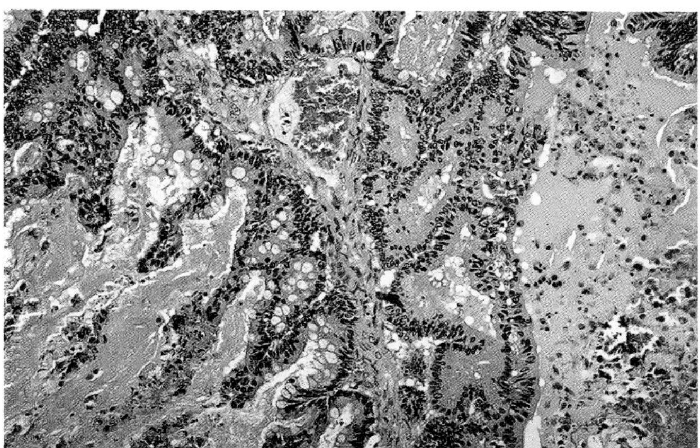

Fig. 19.338 Large bowel adenocarcinoma metastatic to ovary.

of invasion, ovarian hilar involvement, single cell invasion, signet ring cells, garland and cribriform growth pattern, 'dirty' necrosis, segmental destruction of glands, lack of squamous metaplasia, and vascular invasion[1194,1219,1220,1236] (Fig. 19.338). Features favoring a primary ovarian tumor are an expansile (pushing) pattern of invasion, a complex papillary architecture, size over 10 cm, a smooth external surface, and the presence of benign- and borderline-appearing foci.[1220] This combination of primarily architectural features should allow the differential diagnosis to be made in the large majority of cases with the hematoxylin–eosin sections. Unfortunately, exceptions to each and everyone of these criteria exist.[1222] Immunohistochemical stains can be of great assistance, although they also fall short of being pathognomonic. Metastatic large bowel carcinoma is characteristically CK7–/CK20+, CEA+, CA-125–, MUC2+, and often MUC5AC–. By contrast, primary ovarian mucinous carcinomas are nearly always CK7+, variably CK20+ (often only focally), CEA–, CA-125+, and MUC5AC+.[1188,1195,1197,1218] Hormone receptors are of no help, being negative in both metastatic carcinoma from the colon and the usual type of primary ovarian mucinous carcinoma.[1241] It would seem that CK7 is the most discriminating marker in this situation,[1189] although a serious competitor for this role is the intestinal marker CDX2.[1203] Two other discriminators are β-catenin (which stains the nuclei in over 80% of metastatic colorectal carcinomas but less than 10% of primary ovarian mucinous carcinomas[1192]) and guanylyl cyclase C.[1190] It has been stated that combined positivity for CDX2, β-catenin (nuclear staining), and P504S is virtually diagnostic of metastasis from a colorectal primary.[1223] At the cytogenetic level, 13q gain is a marker of colorectal carcinoma.[1197]

It should be realized that these distinctions apply specifically to the large bowel. Ovarian metastases from gastric, biliary, or pancreatic primaries have different phenotypic features[1186,1211,1229,1242] (Fig. 19.339). The peculiar situation concerning the relationship of ovarian mucinous tumors and pseudomyxoma peritonei has been discussed in Chapter 11. Briefly, the current consensus – based on a combination of clinical, morphologic, immunohistochemical, and molecular observations – is that the overwhelming majority of these tumors are primary appendiceal neoplasms that have implanted on the peritoneal surface and on the ovaries.[1233,1237] However, that may not be true for all cases, in the sense that in some instances the molecular evidence favors two separate primary lesions.[1193] It is also not true for the rare appendiceal-type ovarian mucinous adenocarcinomas arising from benign cystic teratomas.[1232]

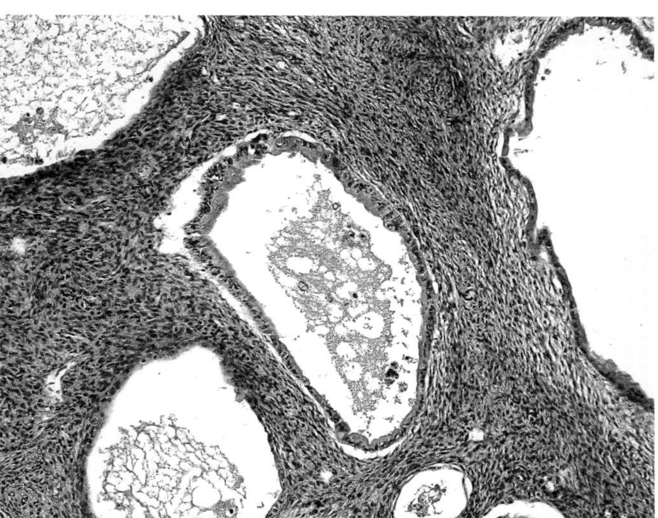

Fig. 19.339 Ovarian metastasis from pancreatic adenocarcinoma. As in the primary tumor, this ovarian metastasis shows the disparity between the extremely well-differentiated architecture and the high degree of nuclear atypia that is characteristic of pancreatobiliary neoplasms.

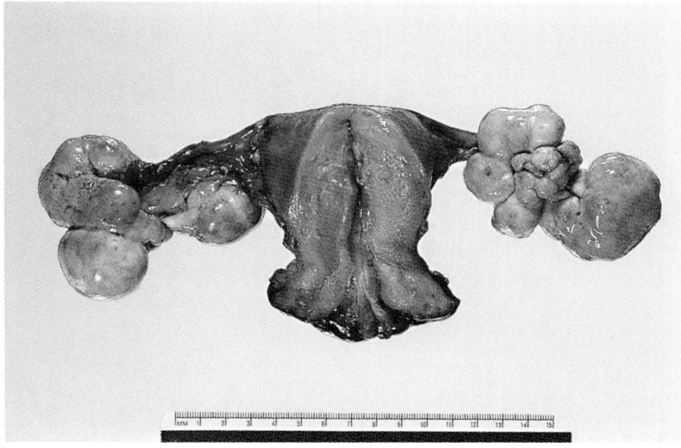

Fig. 19.340 Typical gross appearance of Krukenberg tumors of ovary. The involvement is bilateral and the tumors are characterized by a multinodular outer appearance.
(Courtesy of Dr RA Cooke, Brisbane, Australia; from Cooke RA, Stewart B. Colour atlas of anatomical pathology. Edinburgh, 2004, Churchill Livingstone)

Metastatic carcinoid tumors to the ovary are discussed on page 1591. Small cell (neuroendocrine) carcinomas from the lung, gastrointestinal tract, thymus, and other sites can metastasize to the ovary; these should be distinguished from both the hypercalcemic and the pulmonary type of primary ovarian small cell carcinoma,[1198] the latter being a more difficult task (see p. 1599).

The eponym **Krukenberg tumor** is used to designate an ovarian neoplasm, usually bilateral and nearly always of metastatic origin, characterized grossly by moderate solid multinodular enlargement of the ovaries and microscopically by a diffuse infiltration by signet ring cells containing abundant neutral and acidic (sialo) mucins[1187,1216,1245,1246] (Figs 19.340 and 19.341). Tumor emboli are found in over half of the cases.[1206] Marked stromal proliferation with a storiform pattern of growth and a variable degree of

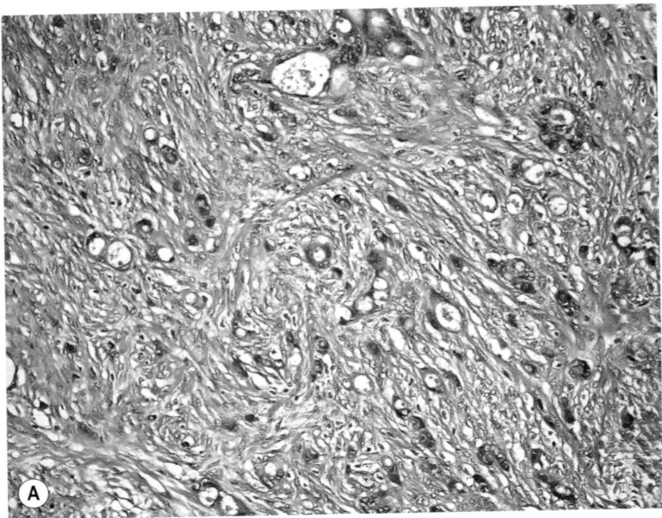

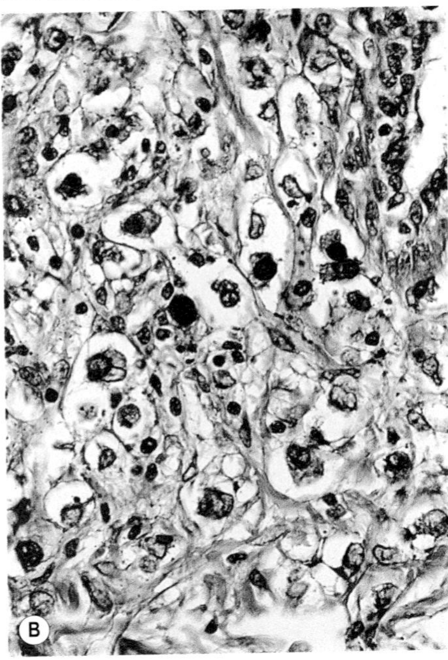

Fig. 19.341 **A** and **B**, Krukenberg tumor of ovary. **A**, Microscopic appearance. Numerous signet ring cells are present in a highly fibrous stroma, either individually or in small nests. **B**, Presence of intracellular mucin evidenced by Meyer mucicarmine stain.

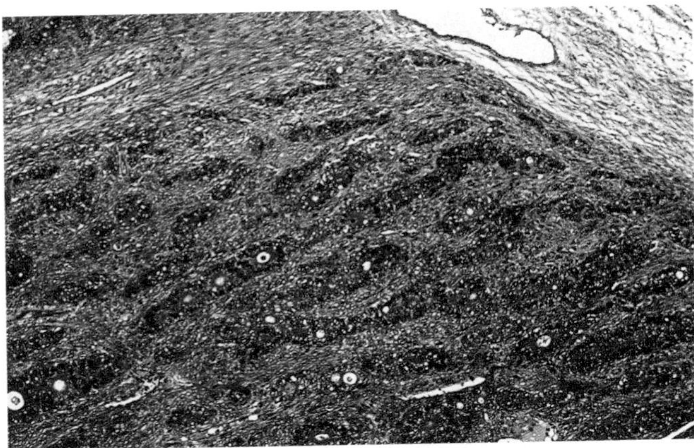

Fig. 19.342 Tubular variant of Krukenberg cell tumor.

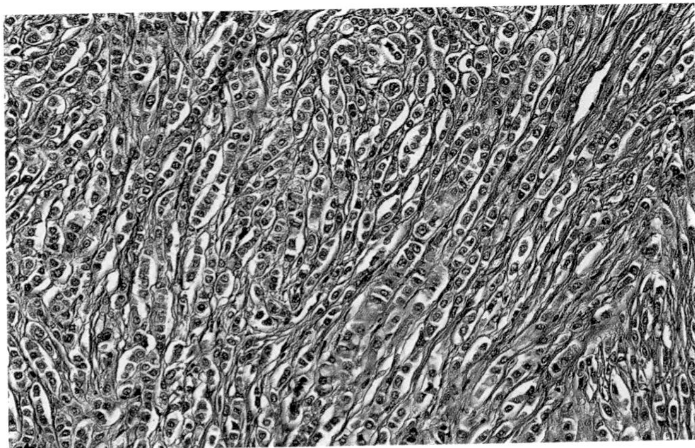

Fig. 19.343 Ovarian metastasis of mammary lobular carcinoma. There is prominent Indian filing.

luteinization are common and may obscure the diagnosis.[1246] Another difficult problem is represented by the variant of this tumor referred to as *tubular*, in which a prominent tubular pattern, stromal luteinization, and occasional associated virilization may lead to a mistaken diagnosis of Sertoli–Leydig cell tumor[1191] (Fig. 19.342); the presence of typical mucin-positive signet ring cells should point toward the correct diagnosis.

Most examples of Krukenberg tumors occur after the age of 40 years, but younger patients can also be affected. In the latter instance, a mistaken diagnosis of granulosa cell tumor or lipid cell tumor is often made.

The usual primary sources of Krukenberg tumor are stomach, large bowel, appendix, and breast[1206,1217,1243] (Fig. 19.343). Of these, diffuse gastric carcinoma ('linitis plastica') used to be the most common, but at present there is a preponderance of cases originating from the breast, at least in the United States. The ovarian deposits can be accompanied by retroperitoneal lymph node metastases and peritoneal implants. A rarer phenomenon is ovarian metastasis from gastric carcinoma of the intestinal type.[1221]

Exceptionally, an extraovarian primary tumor is not found at autopsy in a patient harboring a Krukenberg tumor. In such an instance, the lesion is assumed to be primary in the ovary.[1212] Before such an occurrence is accepted, a meticulous gross and microscopic study of the gastrointestinal tract, breast, and other organs should be carried out.[1206] In the only case that we were almost ready to accept as primary Krukenberg tumor of the ovaries, a random section through a grossly unremarkable gastric antrum revealed diffuse infiltration by signet ring cells. It should be emphasized here that the diagnosis of Krukenberg tumor requires the histochemical identification of intracytoplasmic mucin, and the immunohistochemical detection of epithelial markers, inasmuch as signet ring cells are occasionally seen in other ovarian conditions.[1231]

Other tumors that can metastasize to the ovary and give rise to difficult diagnostic problems are pancreatobiliary ductal adenocarcinoma (which can simulate primary ovarian mucinous tumors and which can arise in the pancreas, gallbladder or extra- or intrahepatic bile ducts),[1214,1215,1250,1256] pancreatic acinar cell carcinoma,[1240] renal cell carcinoma (which mimics ovarian clear cell adenocarcinoma),[1207,1251] carcinoma of the renal pelvis,[1210] thyroid carcinoma

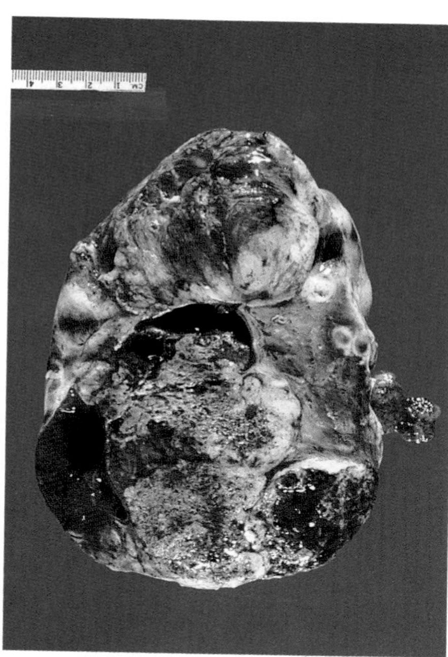

Fig. 19.344 Gross appearance of ovarian metastasis of a malignant melanoma.

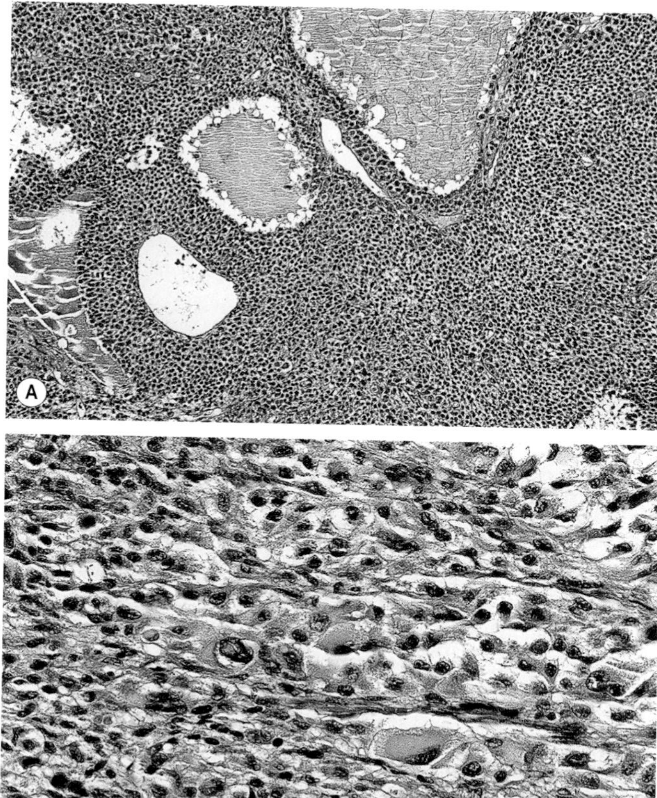

Fig. 19.345 **A** and **B**, Low- and high-power appearances of ovarian metastasis from malignant melanoma. The follicle-like formations seen in **A** may result in a misdiagnosis of juvenile granulosa cell tumor or hypercalcemic-type small cell tumor.

(which can be confused with struma ovarii),[1253] hepatocellular carcinoma and hepatoblastoma (not to be mistaken for hepatoid yolk sac tumor or hepatoid carcinoma, all of which are Hep-Par1-positive[1230]),[1202,1249] intra-abdominal desmoplastic small cell tumor (of which the ovary can be the only manifestation, see p. 1578),[1248,1260] and a variety of sarcomas, including rhabdomyosarcoma,[1255] leiomyosarcoma, osteosarcoma,[1199] gastrointestinal stromal tumor (GIST),[1209]soft tissue-type clear cell sarcoma,[1228] and chordoma.[1257,1259,1261] We have also seen three cases of ovarian metastases from malignant thymoma.

Malignant melanomas are usually easy to recognize because of their pigmentation, nodular pattern of growth, and cytologic features; however, some can be confused with primary ovarian tumors (particularly juvenile granulosa cell tumor and the hypercalcemic type of small cell carcinoma) because of their tendency to form follicle-like spaces[1258] (Figs 19.344 and 19.345). Positivity for S-100 protein, Mart-1 (Melan-A), and HMB-45 should remove whatever doubts may remain after examination of hematoxylin–eosin-stained sections.[1204] Metastatic melanoma should be distinguished from the much rarer primary ovarian melanoma (see p. 1591)

Not surprisingly, carcinoma metastatic to the ovary is generally associated with a very poor prognosis. Factors influencing survival in these patients are the site of the primary tumor, degree of differentiation, menstrual status, and type of treatment.[1244]

References

NORMAL ANATOMY

1 Boss JH, Scully RE, Wegner KH, Cohen RB. Structural variations in the adult ovary. Clinical significance. Obstet Gynecol 1965, **25**: 747–764.

2 Bowen NJ, Logani S, Dickerson EB, Kapa LB, Akhtar M, Benigno BB, McDonald JF. Emerging roles for PAX8 in ovarian cancer and endosalpingeal development. Gynecol Oncol 2007, **104**: 331–337.

3 Clement PB. Ovary. In Mills SE (ed.): Histology for pathologists, ed. 3. Philadelphia, 2007, Lippincott Williams and Wilkins, pp. 1063–1094.

4 Czernobilsky B, Shezen E, Lifschitz-Mercer B, Fogel M, Luzon A, Jacob N, Skalli O, Gabbiani G. Alpha smooth muscle actin (alpha-SM actin) in normal human ovaries, in ovarian stromal hyperplasia and in ovarian neoplasms. Virchows Arch [Cell Pathol] 1989, **57**: 55–61.

5 Doss BJ, Wanek SM, Jacques SM, Qureshi F, Ramirez NC, Lawrence WD. Ovarian smooth muscle metaplasia: an uncommon and possibly underrecognized entity. Int J Gynecol Pathol 1999, **18**: 58–62.

6 Fetissof F, Dubois MP, Heitz PU, Lansac J, Arbeille-Brassart B, Jobard P. Endocrine cells in the female genital tract. Int J Gynecol Pathol 1986, **5**: 75–87.

7 Habib C, Cao QJ, Otis CN, Pantanowitz L. Characterization of bone tissue in the ovary. Lab Invest 2009, **89**(Suppl 1): 216A.

8 Laffargue P, Benkoël L, Laffargue F, Casanova P, Chamlian A. Ultrastructural and enzyme histochemical study of ovarian hilar cells in women and their relationships with sympathetic nerves. Hum Pathol 1978, **9**: 649–659.

9 Lastarria D, Sachdev RK, Babury RA, Yu HM, Nuovo GJ. Immunohistochemical analysis for desmin in normal and neoplastic ovarian stromal tissue. Arch Pathol Lab Med 1990, **114**: 502–505.

10 Sasano H, Sasano N. What's new in the localization of sex steroids in the human ovary and its tumors? Pathol Res Pract 1989, **185**: 942–948.

11 Sasano H, Okamoto M, Mason JI, Simpson ER, Mendelson CR, Sasano N, Silverberg SG. Immunolocalization of aromatase, 17 alpha-hydroxylase and side-chain cleavage cytochromes P-450 in the human ovary. J Reprod Fertil 1989, **85**: 163–169.

12 Visfeldt J, Starup J. Dating of the human corpus luteum of menstruation using histological parameters. Acta Pathol Microbiol Scand (A) 1974, **82**: 137–144.

13 Woolnough E, Russo L, Khan MS, Heatley MK. An immunohistochemical study of the rete ovarii and epoophoron. Pathology 2000, **32**: 77–83.

14 Zheng W, Magid MS, Kramer EE, Chen YT. Follicle-stimulating hormone receptor is expressed in human ovarian surface epithelium and fallopian tube. Am J Pathol 1996, **148**: 47–53.

GONADAL DYSGENESIS

15 Calabrese F, Valente M. Mixed gonadal dysgenesis: histological and ultrastructural finding in two cases. Int J Gynecol Pathol 1996, **15**: 270–277.

16 Clement PB, Young RH. Atypical polypoid adenomyoma of the uterus associated with Turner's syndrome. A report of three cases, including a review of 'estrogen-associated' endometrial neoplasms and neoplasms associated with Turner's syndrome. Int J Gynecol Pathol 1987, **6**: 104–113.

17 Federman DD. Abnormal sexual development. A genetic and endocrine approach to differential diagnosis. Philadelphia, 1967, W.B. Saunders.

18 Ferenczy A, Richart RM. The fine structure of the gonads in the complete form of testicular feminization syndrome. Am J Obstet Gynecol 1972, **113**: 399–409.

19 Jones HW, Ferguson-Smith MA, Heller RH. The pathology and cytogenetics of gonadal agenesis. Am J Obstet Gynecol 1963, **87**: 578–600.

20 Jones HW, Ferguson-Smith MA, Heller RH. Pathologic and cytogenetic findings in true hermaphroditism. Report of 6 cases and review of 23 cases from the literature. Obstet Gynecol 1965, **25**: 435–447.

21 Kim KR, Kwon Y, Young Joung J, Kim KS, Ayala AG, Ro JY. True hermaphroditism and mixed gonadal dysgenesis in young children: a clinicopathologic study of 10 cases. Mod Pathol 2002, **15**: 1013–1019.

22 McCarty KS Jr, Barton TK, Peete CH Jr, Creasman WT. Gonadal dysgenesis with adenocarcinoma of the endometrium. An electron microscopic and steroid receptor analyses with a review of the literature. Cancer 1978, **42**: 512–520.

23 MacLaughlin DT, Donahoe PK. Sex determination and differentiation. N Engl J Med 2004, **350**: 367–378.

24 Males JL, Lain KC. Epithelioid sarcoma in XO/XX Turner's syndrome. Arch Pathol 1972, **94**: 214–216.

25 Neubecker RD, Theiss EA. Sertoli cell adenomas in patients with testicular feminization. Am J Clin Pathol 1962, **38**: 52–59.

26 Radhakrishnan S, Sivaraman L, Natarajan PS. True hermaphrodite with multiple gonadal neoplasms. Report of a case with cytogenetic study. Cancer 1978, **42**: 2726–2732.

27 Robboy SJ, Bentley RC, Russell P. Embryology of the female genital tract and disorders of abnormal sexual development. In Kurman RJ (ed.): Blaustein's pathology of the female genital tract, ed. 5. New York, 2002, Springer-Verlag, pp. 3–36.

28 Robboy SJ, Miller T, Donahoe PK, Jahre C, Welch WR, Haseltine FP, Miller WA, Atkins L, Crawford JD. Dysgenesis of testicular and streak gonads in the syndrome of mixed gonadal dysgenesis. Perspective derived from a clinicopathologic analysis of twenty-one cases. Hum Pathol 1982, **13**: 700–716.

29 Robboy SJ, Jaubert F. Neoplasms and pathology of sexual developmental disorders (intersex). Pathology 2007, **39**: 147–163.

30 Rutgers JL. Advances in the pathology of intersex conditions. Hum Pathol 1991, **22**: 884–891.

31 Scully RE. Gonadal pathology of genetically determined diseases. Monogr Pathol 1991, **33**: 257–285.

32 Sohval AR. The syndrome of pure gonadal dysgenesis. Am J Med 1965, **38**: 615–625.

33 Sybert VP, McCauley E. Turner's syndrome. N Engl J Med 2004, **351**: 1227–1238.

34 Taylor H, Barter RH, Jacobson CB. Neoplasms of dysgenetic gonads. Am J Obstet Gynecol 1966, **96**: 816–823.

CYSTS, STROMAL HYPERPLASIA, AND OTHER NON-NEOPLASTIC LESIONS

35 Adelman S, Benson CD, Hertzler JH. Surgical lesions of the ovary in infancy and childhood. Surg Gynecol Obstet 1975, **141**: 219–222.

36 Awartani KA, Cheung AP. Metformin and polycystic ovary syndrome: a literature review. J Obstet Gynaecol Can 2002, **24**: 393–401.

37 Balen A, Michelmore K. What is polycystic ovary syndrome? Are national views important? Hum Reprod 2002, **17**: 2219–2227.

38 Barnes RB, Rosenfield RL, Burstein S, Ehrmann DA. Pituitary–ovarian responses to nafarelin testing in the polycystic ovary syndrome. N Engl J Med 1989, **320**: 559–565.

39 Blaustein A. Surface cells and inclusion cysts in fetal ovaries. Gynecol Oncol 1981, **12**: 222–233.

40 Boss JH, Scully RE, Wegner KH, Cohen RB. Structural variations in the adult ovary – clinical significance. Obstet Gynecol 1965, **25**: 747–764.

41 Bransilver BR, Ferenczy A, Richart RM. Female genital tract remnants. An ultrastructural comparison of hydatid of Morgagni and mesonephric ducts and tubules. Arch Pathol 1973, **96**: 255–261.

42 Clement PB. Tumor-like lesions of the ovary associated with pregnancy. Int J Gynecol Pathol 1993, **12**: 108–115.

43 Clement PB, Scully RE. Large solitary luteinized follicle cyst of pregnancy and puerperium. A clinicopathological analysis of eight cases. Am J Surg Pathol 1980, **4**: 431–438.

44 Fan LD, Zhang HY, Zhang XS. Ovarian epidermoid cyst: report of eight cases. Int J Gynecol Pathol 1996, **15**: 69–71.

45 Fechner RE, Kaufman RH. Endometrial adenocarcinoma in Stein–Leventhal syndrome. Cancer 1974, **34**: 444–452.

46 Garcia-Bunuel R, Brandes D. Luteoma of pregnancy. Ultrastructural features. Hum Pathol 1976, **7**: 205–214.

47 Garcia-Bunuel R, Berek JS, Woodruff JD. Luteomas of pregnancy. Obstet Gynecol 1975, **45**: 407–414.

48 Gardner GH, Greene RR, Peckham B. Normal and cystic structures of broad ligament. Am J Obstet Gynecol 1948, **55**: 917–939.

49 Goldzieher JW, Green JA. The polycystic ovary. I. Clinical and histologic features. J Clin Endocrinol 1962, **22**: 325–338.

50 Hallatt JG, Steele CH Jr, Snyder M. Ruptured corpus luteum with hemoperitoneum. A study of 173 surgical cases. Am J Obstet Gynecol 1984, **149**: 5–9.

51 Heatley MK. Adenomatous hyperplasia of the rete ovarii. Histopathology 2000, **36**: 383–384.

52 Hosfield EM, Rabban JT, Chen LM, Zaloudek CJ. Squamous metaplasia of the ovarian surface epithelium and subsurface fibrosis: distinctive pathologic findings in the ovaries and fallopian tubes of patients on peritoneal dialysis. Int J Gynecol Pathol 2008, **27**: 465–474.

53 Insler V, Lunenfeld B. Pathophysiology of polycystic ovarian disease. New insights. Hum Reprod 1991, **6**: 1025–1029.

54 Judd HL, Scully RE, Herbst AL, Yen SSC, Ingersol FM, Kliman B. Familial hyperthecosis. Comparison of endocrinologic and histologic findings with polycystic ovarian disease. Am J Obstet Gynecol 1973, **117**: 976–982.

55 Kamiyama K, Moromizato H, Toma T, Kinjo T, Iwamasa T. Two cases of supernumerary ovary: one with large fibroma with Meig's syndrome and the other with endometriosis and cystic change. Pathol Res Pract 2001, **197**: 847–851.

56 Lee B, Gore BZ. A case of supernumerary ovary. Obstet Gynecol 1984, **64**: 738–740.

57 Legro RS, Strauss JF. Molecular progress in infertility: polycystic ovary syndrome. Fertil Steril 2002, **78**: 569–576.

58 Leventhal ML. Functional and morphologic studies of the ovaries and suprarenal glands in the Stein–Leventhal syndrome. Am J Obstet Gynecol 1962, **84**: 154–164.

59 Lindsay AN, Voorhess ML, MacGillivray MH. Multicystic ovaries in primary hypothyroidism. Obstet Gynecol 1983, **61**: 433–437.

60 Lucis OJ, Hobkirk R, Hollenberg CH, MacDonald SA, Blahey P. Polycystic ovaries associated with congenital adrenal hyperplasia. Can Med Assoc J 1966, **94**: 1–7.

61 McKenna TJ. Pathogenesis and treatment of polycystic ovary syndrome. N Engl J Med 1988, **318**: 558–562.

62 Morris JM, Scully RE. Endocrine pathology of the ovary. St Louis, 1958, C.V. Mosby.

63 Mount SL, Eltabbakh GH, Hardin NJ. Beta-2 microglobulin amyloidosis presenting as bilateral ovarian masses: a case report and review of the literature. Am J Surg Pathol 2001, **26**: 130–133.

64 Nogales FF, Silverberg SG. Epidermoid cysts of the ovary. A report of five cases with histogenetic considerations and ultrastructural findings. Am J Obstet Gynecol 1976, **124**: 523–528.

65 Nogales FF, Carvia RE, Donne C, Campello TR, Vidal M, Martin A. Adenomas of the rete ovarii. Hum Pathol 1998, **28**: 1428–1433.

66 Norris HJ, Taylor HB. Nodular theca-lutein hyperplasia of pregnancy (so-called 'pregnancy luteoma'). Am J Clin Pathol 1967, **47**: 557–566.

67 Ober WB, Grady HG, Schoenbucher AK. Ectopic ovarian decidua without pregnancy. Am J Pathol 1957, **33**: 199–217.

68 Piana S, Nogales FF, Corrado S, Cardinale L, Gusolfino D, Rivasi F. Pregnancy luteoma with granulosa cell proliferation: an unusual hyperplastic lesion arising in pregnancy and mimicking an ovarian neoplasia. Pathol Res Pract 1999, **195**: 859–863.

69 Rodin A, Thakkar H, Taylor N, Clayton R. Hyperandrogenism in polycystic ovary syndrome. Evidence of dysregulation of 11β-hydroxysteroid dehydrogenase. N Engl J Med 1994, **330**: 460–465.

70 Rutgers JL, Scully RE. Cysts (cystadenomas) and tumors of the rete ovarii. Int J Gynecol Pathol 1988, **7**: 330–342.

71 Sasano H, Fukunaga M, Rojas M, Silverberg SG. Hyperthecosis of the ovary. Clinicopathologic study of 19 cases with immunohistochemical analysis of steroidogenic enzymes. Int J Gynecol Pathol 1989, **8**: 311–320.

72 Smyczek-Gargya B, Geppert M. Endometrial cancer associated with polycystic ovaries in young women. Pathol Res Pract 1992, **188**: 946–948.

73 Sommers SC. Polycystic ovaries revisited. In Fenoglio CM, Wolfe M (eds): Progress in surgical pathology. New York, 1980, Masson, pp. 221–232.

74 Sternberg WH, Barclay DL. Luteoma of pregnancy. Am J Obstet Gynecol 1966, **95**: 165–184.

75 Towne BH, Mahour GH, Woolley MM, Isaacs H. Ovarian cysts and tumors in infancy and childhood. J Pediatr Surg 1975, **10**: 311–320.

76 Wajda KJ, Lucas JG, Marsh WL Jr. Hyperreactio luteinalis. Benign disorder masquerading as an ovarian neoplasm. Arch Pathol Lab Med 1989, **113**: 921–925.

77 Young RH, Prat J, Scully RE. Epidermoid cyst of the ovary. A report of three cases with comments on histogenesis: Am J Clin Pathol 1980, **73**: 272–276.

78 Zourlas PA, Jones HW Jr. Stein–Leventhal syndrome with masculinizing ovarian tumors. Report of 3 cases. Obstet Gynecol 1969, **34**: 861–866.

INFLAMMATION

79 Bannatyne P, Russell P, Shearman RP. Autoimmune oophoritis. A clinicopathologic assessment of 12 cases. Int J Gynecol Pathol 1990, **9**: 191–207.

80 Francke ML, Mihaescu A, Chaubert P. Isolated necrotizing arteritis of the female genital tract: a clinicopathologic and immunohistochemical study of 11 Cases. Int J Gynecol Pathol 1998, **17**: 193–200.

81 Gloor E, Hurlimann J. Autoimmune oophoritis. Am J Clin Pathol 1984, **81**: 105–109.

82 Gray Y, Libbey P. Xanthogranulomatous salpingitis and oophoritis: a case report and review of the literature. Arch Pathol Lab Med 2001, **125**: 260–263.

83 Herbold DR, Frable WJ, Kraus FT. Isolated noninfectious granulomas of the ovary. Int J Gynecol Pathol 1984, **2**: 380–391.

84 Irvine WJ, Barnes EW. Addison's disease and autoimmune ovarian failure. J Reprod Fertil 1974, **21**(Suppl): 1–31.

85 Kim KR, Scully RE. Peritoneal keratin granulomas with carcinomas of endometrium and ovary and atypical polypoid adenomyoma of endometrium: a clinicopathological analysis of 22 cases. Am J Surg Pathol 1990, **14**: 925–932.

86 Lewis J. Eosinophilic perifolliculitis. A variant of autoimmune oophoritis. Int J Gynecol Pathol 1993, **12**: 360–364.

87 Mostafa SAM, Bargeron CB, Flower RW, Rosenshein NB, Parmley TH, Woodruff JD. Foreign body granulomas in normal ovaries. Obstet Gynecol 1985, **66**: 701–702.

88 Pace EH, Voet RL, Melancon JT. Xanthogranulomatous oophoritis. An inflammatory pseudotumor of the ovary. Int J Gynecol Pathol 1984, **3**: 398–402.

89 Tatum ET, Beattie JF, Bryson K. Postoperative carbon pigment granuloma: a report of eight cases involving the ovary. Hum Pathol 1996, **27**: 1008–1011.

90 Tung KS, Teuscher C. Mechanisms of autoimmune disease in the testis and ovary. Hum Reprod Update 1995, **1**: 35–50.

ENDOMETRIOSIS

91 Ballouk F, Ross JS, Wolf BC. Ovarian endometriotic cysts. An analysis of cytologic atypia and DNA ploidy patterns. Am J Clin Pathol 1994, **102**: 415–419.

92 Clement PB. Pathology of endometriosis. Pathol Annu 1990, **25**: 245–295.

93 Clement PB, Young RH. Two previously unemphasized features of endometriosis: micronodular stromal endometriosis and endometriosis with stromal elastosis. Int J Surg Pathol 2001, **8**: 223–227.

94 Clement PB, Young RH, Scully RE. Necrotic pseudoxanthomatous nodules of ovary and peritoneum in endometriosis. Am J Surg Pathol 1988, **12**: 390–397.

95 Czernobilsky B, Morris WJ. A histologic study of ovarian endometriosis with emphasis on hyperplastic and atypical changes. Obstet Gynecol 1979, **53**: 318–323.

96 Devereux WP. Endometriosis. Long-term observation with particular reference to incidence of pregnancy. Obstet Gynecol 1963, **22**: 444–450.

97 Fukunaga M. Smooth muscle metaplasia in ovarian endometriosis. Histopathology 2000, **36**: 348–352.

98 Fukunaga M, Ushigome S. Epithelial metaplastic changes in ovarian endometriosis. Mod Pathol 1998, **11**: 784–788.

99 Fukunaga M, Nomura K, Ishikawa E, Ushigome S. Ovarian atypical endometriosis. Its close association with malignant epithelial tumors. Histopathology 1997, **30**: 249–255.

100 Jimbo H, Hitomi Y, Yoshikawa H, Yano T, Momoeda M, Sakamoto A, Tsutsumi O, Taketani Y, Esumi H. Evidence for monoclonal expansion of epithelial cells in ovarian endometrial cysts. Am J Pathol 1997, **150**: 1173–1178.

101 La Grenade A, Silverberg SG. Ovarian tumors associated with atypical endometriosis. Hum Pathol 1988, **19**: 1080–1084.

102 Nezhat F, Cohen C, Rahaman J, Gretz H, Cole P, Kalir T. Comparative immunohistochemical studies of bcl-2 and p53 proteins in benign and malignant ovarian endometriotic cyst. Cancer 2002, **94**: 2935–2940.

103 Olive DL, Schwartz LB. Endometriosis. N Engl J Med 1993, **328**: 1759–1769.

104 Pai SA, Desai SB, Borges AM. Uteruslike masses of the ovary associated with breast cancer and raised serum CA 125. Am J Surg Pathol 1998, **22**: 333–337.

105 Perotta PL, Ginsburg FW, Siderides CI, Parkash V. Liesegang rings and endometriosis. Int J Gynecol Pathol 1998, **17**: 358–362.

106 Pratt JH, Shamblin WR. Spontaneous rupture of endometrial cysts of the ovary presenting as an acute abdominal emergency. Am J Obstet Gynecol 1970, **108**: 56–62.

107 Scurry J, Whitehead J, Healey M. Classification of ovarian endometriotic cysts. Int J Gynecol Pathol 2001, **20**: 147–154.

108 Stern RC, Dash R, Bentley RC, Snyder MJ, Haney AF, Robboy SJ. Malignancy in endometriosis: frequency and comparison of ovarian and extraovarian types. Int J Gynecol Pathol 2001, **20**: 133–139.

109 Young RH, Scully RE. Ovarian pathology of infertility. Monogr Pathol 1991, **33**: 104–139.

OVARIAN BIOPSY

110 Mori T. Histological and histochemical studies of human anovulatory ovaries correlated with endocrinological analysis. Acta Obstet Gynaecol Jpn 1969, **16**: 156–164.

111 Reber RW, Erickson GF, Coulam CB. Premature ovarian failure. In Gondos B, Riddick DH (eds): Pathology of infertility; clinical correlations in the male and female. New York, 1987, Thieme, pp. 123–141.

112 Russell P, Bannatyne P, Shearman RP, Fraser IS, Corbett P. Premature hypergonadotropic ovarian failure. Clinicopathological study of 19 cases. Int J Gynecol Pathol 1982, **1**: 185–201.

113 Steele SJ, Beilbui JOW, Papadaki L. Visualization and biopsy of the ovary in the investigation of amenorrhea. Obstet Gynecol 1970, **36**: 899–902.

114 Stevenson CS. The ovaries in infertile women. A clinical and pathologic study of 81 women having ovarian surgery at laparotomy. Fertil Steril 1970, **21**: 411–425.

115 Vital-Reyes V, Chhieng D, Rodríguez-Burford C, Téllez-Velasco S, Grizzle W, Chavarría-Olarte ME, Reyes-Fuentes A. Ovarian biopsy in infertile patients with ovarian dysfunction. Int J Gynecol Pathol 2006, **25**: 90–94.

TUMORS

CLASSIFICATION

116 Fox H, Langley FA. Tumours of the ovary. London, 1976, Heinemann.

117 Gillman J. The development of the gonads in man, with a consideration of the role of fetal endocrines and the histogenesis of ovarian tumors. Contrib Embryol 1948, **32**: 83–131 (Carnegie Institute of Washington).

118 Godwin AK, Testa JR, Hamilton TC. The biology of ovarian cancer development. Cancer 1993, **71**(Suppl 2): 530–536.

119 Scully RE, Young RH, Clement PB. Tumors of the ovary, maldeveloped gonads, fallopian tube, and broad ligament. Atlas of tumor pathology, series 3, fascicle 23. Washington, DC, 1998, Armed Forces Institute of Pathology, p. 527.

120 Teilum G. Special tumors of ovary and testis and related extragonadal lesions: comparative pathology and histological identification, ed. 2. Copenhagen, 1976, Lippincott, p. 513.

121 Van Wagenen G, Simpson ME. Embryology of the ovary and testis. *Homo sapiens* and *Macaca mulatta*. New Haven, 1965, Yale University Press.

122 Witschi E. Migration of the germ cells of human embryos from the yolk sac to the primitive gonadal folds. Contrib Embryol 1948, **32**: 69–80 (Carnegie Institute of Washington).

SURFACE EPITHELIAL TUMORS

123 Addis BJ, Fox H. Papillary mesothelioma of ovary. Histopathology 1983, **7**: 287–298.

124 Barnetson RJ, Burnett RA, Downie I, Harper CM, Roberts F. Immunohistochemical analysis of peritoneal mesothelioma and primary and secondary serous carcinoma of the peritoneum: antibodies to estrogen and progesterone receptors are useful. Am J Clin Pathol 2006, **125**: 67–76.

125 Bell DA. Ovarian surface epithelial–stromal tumors. Hum Pathol 1991, **22**: 750–762.

126 Blaustein A. Peritoneal mesothelium and ovarian surface cells – shared characteristics. Int J Gynecol Pathol 1984, **3**: 361–375.

127 Colgan TJ, Norris HJ. Ovarian epithelial tumors of low malignant potential. A review. Int J Gynecol Pathol 1983, **1**: 367–382.

128 Comin CE, Saieva C, Messerini L. h-caldesmon, calretinin, estrogen receptor, and Ber-EP4: a useful combination of immunohistochemical markers for differentiating epithelioid peritoneal mesothelioma from serous papillary carcinoma of the ovary. Am J Surg Pathol 2007, **31**: 1139–1148.

129 Crum CP, Drapkin R, Kindelberger D, Medeiros F, Miron A, Lee Y. Lessons from BRCA: the tubal fimbria emerges as an origin for pelvic serous cancer. Clin Med Res 2007, **5**: 35–44.

130 Davidson B, Risberg B, Berner A, Bedrossian CW, Reich R. The biological differences between ovarian serous carcinoma and diffuse peritoneal malignant mesothelioma. Semin Diagn Pathol 2006, **23**: 35–43.

131 Dehari R, Kurman RJ, Logani S, Shih IeM. The development of high-grade serous carcinoma from atypical proliferative (borderline) serous tumors and low-grade micropapillary serous carcinoma: a morphologic and molecular genetic analysis. Am J Surg Pathol 2007, **31**: 1007–1012.

132 Feeley KM, Wells M. Precursor lesions of ovarian epithelial malignancy. Histopathology 2001, **38**: 87–95.

133 Gilks CB. Subclassification of ovarian surface epithelial tumors based on correlation of histologic and molecular pathologic data. Int J Gynecol Pathol 2004, **23**: 200–205.

134 Gusberg SB, Deligdisch L. Ovarian dysplasia. A study of identical twins. Cancer 1984, **54**: 1–4.

135 Hutson R, Ramsdale J, Wells M. p53 protein expression in putative precursor lesions of epithelioid ovarian cancer. Histopathology 1995, **27**: 367–371.

136 Jarboe EA, Folkins AK, Drapkin R, Ince TA, Agoston ES, Crum CP. Tubal and ovarian pathways to pelvic epithelial cancer: a pathological perspective. Histopathology 2008, **53**: 127–138.

137 Jarboe E, Folkins A, Nucci MR, Kindelberger D, Drapkin R, Miron A, Lee Y, Crum CP. Serous carcinogenesis in the fallopian tube: a descriptive classification. Int J Gynecol Pathol 2008, **27**: 1–9.

138 Kurman RJ, Shih IeM. The origin and pathogenesis of epithelial ovarian cancer: a proposed unifying theory. Am J Surg Pathol 2010, **34**: 433–443.

139 Kurman RJ, Shih IeM. Pathogenesis of ovarian cancer: lessons from morphology and molecular biology and their clinical implications. Int J Gynecol Pathol 2008, **27**: 151–160.

140 Nouwen EJ, Pollet DE, Schelstraete JB, Eerdekens MW, Hansch C, Van de Voorde A, De Broe ME. Human placental alkaline phosphatase in benign and malignant ovarian neoplasia. Cancer Res 1985, **45**: 892–902.

141 Ordóñez NG. Value of estrogen and progesterone receptor immunostaining in distinguishing between peritoneal mesotheliomas and serous carcinomas. Hum Pathol 2005, **36**: 1163–1167.

142 Ordóñez NG. The diagnostic utility of immunohistochemistry and electron microscopy in distinguishing between peritoneal mesotheliomas and serous carcinomas: a comparative study. Mod Pathol 2006, **19**: 34–48.

143 Przybycin CG, Kurman RJ, Ronnett BM, Shih IeM, Vang R. Are all pelvic (nonuterine) serous carcinomas of tubal origin? Am J Surg Pathol 2010 **34**: 1407–1416.

144 Roh MH, Kindelberger D, Crum CP. Serous tubal intraepithelial carcinoma and the dominant ovarian mass: clues to serous tumor origin? Am J Surg Pathol 2009, **33**: 376–383.

145 Russell P. Common epithelial tumours of the ovary – a new look. Pathology 1985, **17**: 555–557.

146 Salvador S, Gilks B, Köbel M, Huntsman D, Rosen B, Miller C. The fallopian tube: primary site of most pelvic high-grade serous carcinomas. Int J Gynecol Cancer 2009, **19**: 58–64.

147 Scully RE. Ovary. In Henson DE, Albores-Saavedra J (eds): The pathology of incipient neoplasia. Philadelphia, 1986, W.B. Saunders, pp. 279–293.

148 Soslow RA. Histologic subtypes of ovarian carcinoma: an overview. Int J Gynecol Pathol 2008, **27**: 161–174.

149 Tong GX, Chiriboga L, Hamele-Bena D, Borczuk AC. Expression of PAX2 in papillary serous carcinoma of the ovary: immunohistochemical evidence of fallopian tube or secondary Müllerian system origin? Mod Pathol 2007, **20**: 856–863.

150 van Niekerk CC, Boerman OC, Ramaekers FC, Poels LG. Marker profile of different phases in the transition of normal human ovarian epithelium to ovarian carcinomas. Am J Pathol 1991, **138**: 455–463.

Serous tumors

151 Acs G, Pasha T, Zhang PJ. WT1 is differentially expressed in serous, endometrioid, clear cell, and mucinous carcinomas of the peritoneum, fallopian tube, ovary, and endometrium. Int J Gynecol Pathol 2004, **23**: 110–118.

152 Albarracin CT, Jafri J, Montag AG, Hart J, Kuan SF. Differential expression of MUC2 and MUC5AC mucin genes in primary ovarian and metastatic colonic carcinoma. Hum Pathol 2000, **31**: 672–677.

153 Al-Hussaini M, Stockman A, Foster H, McCluggage WG. WT-1 assists in distinguishing ovarian from uterine serous carcinoma and in distinguishing between serous and endometrioid ovarian carcinoma. Histopathology 2004, **44**: 109–115.

154 Alli PM, Ali SZ. Micropapillary serous carcinoma of the ovary: cytomorphologic characteristics in peritoneal/pelvic washing. Cancer 2002, **96**: 135–139.

155 Andrews TD, Dutton PM, Beattie G, Al-Nafussi A. Sarcomatoid carcinoma arising within a serous borderline ovarian tumour: a case report and practical approach to differential diagnosis. Histopathology 2008, **52**: 233–238.

156 Bell DA, Longacre TA, Prat J, Kohn EC, Soslow RA, Ellenson LH, Malpica A, Stoler MH, Kurman RJ. Serous borderline (low malignant potential, atypical proliferative) ovarian tumors: workshop perspectives. Hum Pathol 2004, **35**: 934–948.

157 Bell DA, Scully RE. Ovarian serous borderline tumors with stromal microinvasion. A report of 21 cases. Hum Pathol 1990, **21**: 397–403.

158 Bosscher J, Barnhill D, O'Connor D, Doering D, Nash J, Park R. Osseous metaplasia in ovarian papillary serous cystadenocarcinoma. Gynecol Oncol 1990, **39**: 228–231.

159 Burks RT, Sherman ME, Kurman RJ. Micropapillary serous carcinoma of the ovary: a distinctive low-grade carcinoma related to serous borderline tumors. Am J Surg Pathol 1996, **20**: 1319–1330.

160 Cajigas HE, Fariza E, Scully RE, Thor AD. Enhancement of tumor-associated glycoprotein-72 antigen expression in hormone-related ovarian serous borderline tumors. Cancer 1991, **68**: 348–354.

161 Campo E, Merino MJ, Tavassoli FA, Charonis AS, Stetler-Stevenson WG, Liotta LA. Evaluation of basement membrane components and the 72 kDa type IV collagenase in serous tumors of the ovary. Am J Surg Pathol 1992, **16**: 500–507.

162 Cathro HP, Stoler MH. Expression of cytokeratins 7 and 20 in ovarian neoplasia. Am J Clin Pathol 2002, **117**: 944–951.

163 Cathro HP, Stoler MH. The utility of calretinin, inhibin, and WT1 immunohistochemical staining in the differential diagnosis of ovarian tumors. Hum Pathol 2005, **36**: 195–201.

164 Chadha S, Rao BR, Slotman BJ, van Vroonhoven CC, van der Kwast TH. An immunohistochemical evaluation of androgen and progesterone receptors in ovarian tumors. Hum Pathol 1993, **24**: 90–95.

165 Charpin C, Bhan AK, Zurawski VR Jr, Scully RE. Carcinoembryonic antigen (CEA) and carbohydrate determinant 19-9 (CA 19-9) localization in 121 primary and metastatic ovarian tumors. An immunohistochemical study with the use of monoclonal antibodies. Int J Gynecol Pathol 1982, **1**: 231–245.

166 Colgan TJ, Norris HJ. Ovarian epithelial tumors of low malignant potential A review. Int J Gynecol Pathol 1983, **1**: 367–382.

167 Compton HL, Finck FM. Serous adenofibroma and cystadenofibroma of the ovary. Obstet Gynecol 1970, **36**: 636–645.

168 Czernobilsky B, Bornstein R, Lancet M. Cystadenofibroma of the ovary. A clinicopathologic study of 34 cases and comparison with serous cystadenoma. Cancer 1974, **34**: 1971–1981.

169 Daraï E, Scoazec JY, Walker-Combrouze F, Milka-Cabanne N, Feldmann F, Madelenat P, Potet F. Expression of cadherins in benign, borderline, and malignant ovarian epithelial tumors: a clinicopathologic study of 60 cases. Hum Pathol 1997, **28**: 922–928.

170 Davies BR, Worsley SD, Ponder BA. Expression of E-cadherin, α-catenin and β-catenin in normal ovarian surface epithelium and epithelial ovarian cancers. Histopathology 1998, **32**: 69–80.

171 Deavers MT, Gershenson DM, Tortolero-Luna G, Malpica A, Lu KH, Silva EG. Micropapillary and cribriform patterns in ovarian serous tumors of low malignant potential: a study of 99 advanced stage cases. Am J Surg Pathol 2002, **26**: 1129–1141.

172 De Nictolis M, Garbisa S, Lucarini G, Goteri G, Masiero L, Ciavattini A, Garzetti GG, Stetler-Stevenson WG, Fabbris G, Biagini G, Prat J. 72-kilodalton type IV collagenase, and Ki67 antigen in serous tumors of the ovary: a clinicopathologic, immunohistochemical, and serological study. Int J Gynecol Pathol 1996, **15**: 102–109.

173 Dietel M, Hauptmann S. Serous tumors of low malignant potential of the ovary. 1 Diagnostic pathology. Virchows Arch 2000, **436**: 403–412.

174 Eichhorn JH, Bell DA, Young RH, Scully RE. Ovarian serous borderline tumors with micropapillary and cribriform patterns: a study of 40 cases and comparison with 44 cases without these patterns. Am J Surg Pathol 1999, **23**: 397–409.

175 Faleiro-Rodrigues C, Macedo-Pinto I, Pereira D, Ferreira VM, Lopes CS. Association of E-cadherin and beta-catenin immunoexpression with clinicopathologic features in primary ovarian carcinomas. Hum Pathol 2004, **35**: 663–669.

176 Fenoglio CM. Ultrastructural features of the common epithelial tumors of the ovary. Ultrastruct Pathol 1980, **1**: 419–444.

177 Ferenczy A, Talens M, Zoghby M, Hussain SS. Ultrastructural studies on the morphogenesis of psammoma bodies in ovarian serous neoplasia. Cancer 1977, **39**: 2451–2459.

178 Gershenson DM. Is micropapillary serous carcinoma for real? Cancer 2002, **95**: 677–680.

179 Gilks CB, Bell DA, Scully RE. Serous psammocarcinoma of the ovary and peritoneum. Int J Gynecol Pathol 1990, **9**: 110–121.

180 Goldstein NS, Uzieblo A. WT1 immunoreactivity in uterine papillary serous carcinomas is different from ovarian serous carcinomas. Am J Clin Pathol 2002, **117**: 541–545.

181 Goldstein NS, Bassi D, Uzieblo A. WT1 is an integral component of an antibody panel to distinguish pancreaticobiliary and some ovarian epithelial neoplasms. Am J Clin Pathol 2001, **116**: 246–252.

182 Gooneratne S, Sassone M, Blaustein A, Talerman A. Serous surface papillary carcinoma of the ovary. A clinicopathologic study of 16 cases. Int J Gynecol Pathol 1982, **1**: 258–269.

183 Hanselaar AG, Vooijs GP, Mayall B, Ras-Zeijlmans GJ, Chadha-Ajwani S. Epithelial markers to detect occult microinvasion in serous ovarian tumors. Int J Gynecol Pathol 1993, **12**: 20–27.

184 Harding M, Cowan S, Hole D, Cassidy-L, Kitchener H, Davis J, Leake R. Estrogen and progesterone receptors in ovarian cancer. Cancer 1990, **65**: 486–491.

185 Hart WR. Borderline epithelial tumors of the ovary. Mod Pathol 2005, **18**(Suppl 2): S33–S50.

186 Hwang H, Quenneville L, Yaziji H, Gown AM. Wilms tumor gene product: sensitive and contextually specific marker of serous carcinomas of ovarian surface epithelial origin. Appl Immunohistochem Mol Morphol 2004, **12**: 122–126.

187 Hytiroglou P, Harpaz N, Heller DS, Zhiyuan L, Deligdisch L, Gil J. Differential diagnosis of borderline and invasive serous cystadenocarcinomas of the ovary by computerized interactive morphometric analysis of nuclear features. Cancer 1992, **69**: 988–992.

188 Kabawat SE, Bast RC Jr, Welch WR, Knapp RC, Bhan AK. Expression of major histocompatibility antigens and nature of inflammatory cellular infiltrate in ovarian neoplasms. Int J Cancer 1983, **32**: 547–554.

189 Kalir T, Wang BY, Goldfischer M, Haber RS, Reder I, Demopoulos R, Cohen CJ, Burstein DE. Immunohistochemical staining of GLUT1 in benign, borderline, and malignant ovarian epithelia. Cancer 2002, **94**: 1078–1082.

190 Kamarainen M, Leivo I, Koistinen R, Julkunen M, Karvonen U, Rutanen EM, Speppala M. Normal human ovary and ovarian tumors express glycodelin, a glycoprotein with immunosuppressive and contraceptive properties. Am J Pathol 1996, **148**: 1435–1443.

191 Kao GF, Norris HJ. Cystadenofibromas of the ovary with epithelial atypia. Am J Surg Pathol 1978, **2**: 357–363.

192 Katsetos CD, Stadnicka I, Boyd JC, Ehya H, Zheng S, Soprano CM, Cooper HS, Patchefsky AS, Soprano DR, Soprano KJ. Cellular distribution of retinoid acid receptor-alpha protein in serous adenocarcinomas of ovarian, tubal and peritoneal origin. Comparison with estrogen receptor status. Am J Pathol 1998, **153**: 469–480.

193 Katzenstein AL, Mazur MT, Morgan TE, Kao MS. Proliferative serous tumors of the ovary. Histologic features and prognosis. Am J Surg Pathol 1978, **2**: 339–355.

194 Kennedy AW, Hart WR. Ovarian papillary serous tumors of low malignant potential (serous borderline tumors): a long term follow-up study, including patients with microinvasion, lymph node metastasis, and transformation to invasive serous carcinoma. Cancer 1996, **78**: 278–286.

195 Khuu H, Conner M, Vanderkwaak T, Shultz J, Gomez-Navarro J, Alvarez RD, Curiel DT, Siegal GP. Detection of coxsackie-adenovirus receptor (CAR) immunoreactivity in ovarian tumors of epithelial derivation. Appl Immunohistochem 1999, **7**: 266–270.

196 Koelma IA, Nap M, Rodenburg GJ, Fleuren GJ. The value of tumour marker CA 125 in surgical pathology. Histopathology 1987, **11**: 287–294.

197 Komitowski D, Janson C, Szamaborski J, Czernobilsky B. Quantitative nuclear morphology in the diagnosis of ovarian tumors of low malignant potential (borderline). Cancer 1989, **64**: 905–910.

198 Kubba LA, McCluggage WG, Liu J, Malpica A, Euscher ED, Silva EG, Deavers MT. Thyroid transcription factor-1 expression in ovarian epithelial neoplasms. Mod Pathol 2008, **21**: 485–490.

199 Kurman RJ, Seidman JD, Shih IeM. Serous borderline tumours of the ovary. Histopathology 2005, **47**: 310–315.

200 Laury AR, Hornick JL, Perets R, Krane JF, Corson J, Drapkin R, Hirsch MS. PAX8 reliably distinguishes ovarian serous tumors from malignant mesothelioma. Am J Surg Pathol 2010, **34**: 627–635.

201 Lee KR, Castrillon DH, Nucci MR. Pathologic findings in eight cases of ovarian serous borderline tumors, three with foci of serous carcinoma, that preceded death or morbidity from invasive carcinoma. Int J Gynecol Pathol 2001, **20**: 329–334.

202 Lin M, Hanai J, Wada A, Ozaki M, Nasu K, Okamoto S, Matsumoto K. S-100 protein in ovarian tumors. A comparative immunohistochemical study of 135 cases. Acta Pathol Jpn 1991, **41**: 233–239.

203 Longacre T, Tazelaar H, Kempson R, Hendrickson M. Serous tumors of low malignant potential: Stanford update. Mod Pathol 2003, **16**: 199a.

204 McCluggage WG, Maxwell P, Veenstra H, Fick CE, Laeng RH, Tiltman AJ. Monoclonal antibody SMO47 as an immunohistochemical marker of ovarian adenocarcinoma. Histopathology 2001, **38**: 542–549.

205 McCluggage WG. WT1 is of value in ascertaining the site of origin of serous carcinomas within the female genital tract. Int J Gynecol Pathol 2004, **23**: 97–99.

206 McKenney JK, Balzer BL, Longacre TA. Patterns of stromal invasion in ovarian serous tumors of low malignant potential (borderline tumors): a reevaluation of the concept of stromal microinvasion. Am J Surg Pathol 2006, **30**: 1209–1221.

207 Miettinen M, Lehto V-P, Virtanen I. Expression of intermediate filaments in normal ovaries and ovarian epithelial, sex cord-stromal, and germinal tumors. Int J Gynecol Pathol 1983, **2**: 64–71.

208 Mohabeer J, Buckley CH, Fox H. An immunohistochemical study of the incidence and significance of human chorionic gonadotrophin synthesis by epithelial ovarian neoplasms. Gynecol Oncol 1983, **16**: 78–84.

209 Moll R, Pitz S, Levy R, Weikel W, Franke WW, Czernobilsky B. Complexity of expression of intermediate filament proteins, including glial filament protein, in endometrial and ovarian adenocarcinomas. Hum Pathol 1991, **22**: 989–1001.

210 Mulhollan TJ, Silva EG, Tornos C, Guerrieri C, Fromm GL, Gershenson D. Ovarian involvement by serous surface papillary carcinoma. Int J Gynecol Pathol 1994, **13**: 120–126.

211 Nayar R, Siriaunkgul S, Robbins KM, McGowan L, Ginzan S, Silverberg SG. Microinvasion of low malignant potential tumors of the ovary. Hum Pathol 1996, **27**: 521–527.

212 Nonaka D, Chiriboga L, Soslow RA. Expression of pax8 as a useful marker in distinguishing ovarian carcinomas from mammary carcinomas. Am J Surg Pathol 2008, **32**: 1566–1571.

213 Ohishi Y, Oda Y, Kurihara S, Kaku T, Yasunaga M, Nishimura I, Okuma E, Kobayashi H, Wake N, Tsuneyoshi M. Hobnail-like cells in serous borderline tumor do not represent concomitant incipient clear cell neoplasms. Hum Pathol 2009, **40**: 1168–1175.

214 Peralta Soler A, Knudsen KA, Jaurand MC, Johnson KR, Wheelock MJ, Klein-Szanto AJ, Salazar H. The differential expression of n-cadherin and e-caderin distinguishes pleural mesotheliomas from lung adenocarcinomas. Hum Pathol 1996, **26**: 1363–1369.

215 Prat J. Ovarian tumors of borderline malignancy (tumors of low malignant potential): a critical appraisal. Adv Anat Pathol 1999, **6**: 247–274.

216 Prat J, de Nictolis M. Serous borderline tumors of the ovary: a long-term follow-up study of 137 cases, including 18 with a micropapillary pattern and 20 with microinvasion. Am J Surg Pathol 2002, **26**: 1111–1128.

217 Rice LW, Berkowitz RS, Mark SD, Yavner DL, Lage JM. Epithelial ovarian tumors of borderline malignancy. Gynecol Oncol 1990, **39**: 195–198.

218 Roger P, Pujol P, Lucas A, Baldet P, Rochefort H. Increased immunostaining of fibulin-1, an estrogen-regulated protein in the stroma of human ovarian epithelial tumors. Am J Pathol 1998, **153**: 1579–1588.

219 Sangoi AR, McKenney JK, Dadras SS, Longacre TA. Lymphatic vascular invasion in ovarian serous tumors of low malignant potential with stromal microinvasion: a case control study. Am J Surg Pathol 2008, **32**: 261–268.

220 Sasano H, Kaga K, Sato S, Yajima A, Nagura H. Adrenal 4-binding protein in common epithelial and metastatic tumors of the ovary. Hum Pathol 1996, **27**: 595–598.

221 Sasano H, Saito Y, Nagura H, Kudo R, Rojas M, Silverberg SG. Lectin histochemistry in mucinous and serous ovarian neoplasms. Int J Gynecol 1991, **10**: 252–259.

222 Sasano H, Suzuki T, Niikura H, Kaga K, Sato S, Yajima A, Rainey WE, Nagura H. 17 Beta-hydroxysteroid dehydrogenase in common epithelial ovarian tumors. Mod Pathol 1996, **9**: 386–391.

223 Scully RE. One pathologist's reminiscences of the 20th century and random thoughts about the 21st: reflections at the millennium. Int J Surg Pathol 2002, **10**: 8–13.

224 Seidman JD, Kurman RJ. Subclassification of serous borderline tumors of the ovary into benign and malignant types: a clinicopathologic study of 65 advanced stage cases. Am J Surg Pathol 1996, **20**: 1331–1345.

225 Shimizu M, Toki T, Takagi Y, Konishi L, Fujii S. Immunohistochemical detection of the Wilms' tumor gene (WT1) in epithelial ovarian tumors. Int J Gynecol Pathol 2000, **19**: 158–163.

226 Sieben NL, Kolkman-Uljee SM, Flanagan AM, Le Cessie S, Cleton-Jansen AM, Cornelisse CJ, Fleuren GJ. Molecular genetic evidence for monoclonal origin of bilateral ovarian serous borderline tumors. Am J Pathol 2003, **162**: 1095–1101.

227 Silva EG, Kurman RJ, Russell P, Scully RE. Symposium: ovarian tumors of borderline malignancy. Int J Gynecol Pathol 1996, **15**: 281–307.

228 Silva EG, Tornos C, Malpica A, Deavers MT, Tortolero-Luna G, Gershenson DM. The association of benign and malignant ovarian adenofibromas with breast cancer and thyroid disorders. Int J Surg Pathol 2002, **10**: 33–39.

229 Silva EG, Tornos CS, Malpica A, Gershenson DM. Ovarian serous neoplasms of low malignant potential associated with focal areas of serous carcinoma. Mod Pathol 1997, **10**: 663–667.

230 Slomovitz BM, Caputo TA, Gretz HF, Economs K, Tortoriello DV, Schlosshauer PW, Baergen RN, Isacson C, Soslow RA. A comparative analysis of 57 serous borderline tumor with and without a non-invasive micropapillary component. Am J Surg Pathol 2002, **26**: 592–600.

231 Smith Sehdev AE, Sehdev PS, Kurman RJ. Noninvasive and invasive micropapillary (low-grade) serous carcinoma of the ovary. A clinicopathologic analysis of 135 cases. Am J Surg Pathol 2003, **27**: 725–736.

232 Staebler A, Heselmeyer-Haddad K, Bell K, Riopel M, Periman E, Ried T, Kurman RJ. Micropapillary serous carcinoma of the ovary has distinct patterns of chromosomal imbalances by comparative genomic hybridisation compared with atypical proliferative serous tumors and serous carcinomas. Hum Pathol 2002, **33**: 47–59.

233 Suo Z, Karbovo E, Trope CG, Metodiev K, Nesland JM. Papillary serous carcinoma of the ovary: an ultrastructural and immunohistochemical study. Ultrastruct Pathol 2004, **28**: 141–147.

234 Tan LK, Flynn SD, Carcangiu ML. Ovarian serous borderline tumors with lymph node involvement. Clinicopathologic and DNA content study of seven cases and review of the literature. Am J Surg Pathol 1994, **18**: 904–912.

235 Tiniakos DG, Yu H, Liapis H. Osteopontin expression in ovarian carcinomas and tumors of low malignant potential (LMP). Hum Pathol 1998, **29**: 1250–1254.

236 Ueda G, Yamasaki M, Inoue M, Tanaka Y, Abe Y, Ogawa M. Immunohistochemical study of amylase in common epithelial tumors of the ovary. Int J Gynecol Pathol 1985, **4**: 240–244.

237 Ulbright TM, Roth LM. Common epithelial tumors of the ovary. Proliferating and of low malignant potential. Semin Diagn Pathol 1985, **2**: 2–15.

238 Ulbright TM, Roth LM, Sutton GP. Papillary serous carcinoma of the ovary with squamous differentiation. Int J Gynecol Pathol 1990, **9**: 86–94.

239 Van Kley H, Cramer S, Bruns DE. Serous ovarian neoplastic amylase (SONA). A potentially useful marker for serous ovarian tumors. Cancer 1981, **48**: 1444–1449.

240 White PF, Merino MJ, Barwick KW. Serous surface papillary carcinoma of the ovary. A clinical, pathologic, ultrastructural, and immunohistochemical study of 11 cases. Pathol Annu 1985, **20**(Pt 1): 403–418.

241 Yasuda M, Itoh J, Hirasawa T, Hirazono K, Shinozuka T, Sasano H, Osamura RY. Serous borderline ovarian tumor with functioning stroma in a postmenopausal women: immunohistochemical analysis of steroidogenic pathway. Int J Gynecol Pathol 1998, **17**: 75–78.

242 Yemelyanova A, Mao TL, Nakayama N, Shih IeM, Kurman RJ. Low-grade serous carcinoma of the ovary displaying a macropapillary pattern of invasion. Am J Surg Pathol 2008, **32**: 1800–1806.

243 Zhang PJ, Gao HG, Pasha TL, Litzky L, LiVolsi VA. TTF-1 expression in ovarian and uterine epithelial neoplasia and its potential significance, an immunohistochemical assessment with multiple monoclonal antibodies and different secondary detection systems. Int J Gynecol Pathol 2009, **28**: 10–18.

Mucinous tumors

244 Adamiak A, Schrader I, Senz J, Gilks CB, Huntsman DG. Confirmation of the germ cell origin of ovarian tumors using a standard panel of microsatellite markers. Lab Invest 2009, **89**(Suppl 1): 205A.

245 Aguirre P, Scully RE, Dayal Y, DeLellis RA. Mucinous tumors of the ovary with argyrophil cells. An immunohistochemical analysis. Am J Surg Pathol 1984, **8**: 345–356.

246 Baergen RN, Rutgers JL. Mural nodules in common epithelial tumors of the ovary. Int J Gynecol Pathol 1994, **13**: 62–72.

247 Baguè S, Rodriguez IM, Prat J. Sarcoma-like mural nodules in mucinous cystic tumors of the ovary revisited: a clinicopathologic analysis of 10 additional cases. Am J Surg Pathol 2002, **26**: 1467–1476.

248 Bell DA. Mucinous adenofibromas of the ovary. A report of 10 cases. Am J Surg Pathol 1991, **15**: 227–232.

249 Bhagavan BS, Slavin RE, Goldberg J, Rao RN. Ectopic gastrinoma and Zollinger–Ellison syndrome. Hum Pathol 1986, **17**: 584–592.

250 Cathro HP, Stoler MH. Expression of cytokeratins 7 and 20 in ovarian neoplasia. Am J Clin Pathol 2002, **117**: 944–951.

251 Chaitin BA, Gershenson DM, Evans HL. Mucinous tumors of the ovary. A clinicopathologic study of 70 cases. Cancer 1985, **55**: 1958–1962.

252 Charpin C, Bhan AK, Zurawski VR, Scully RE. Carcinoembryonic antigen (CEA) and carbohydrate determinant 19-9 (CA 19-9) localization in 121 primary and metastatic ovarian tumors. An immunohistochemical study with the use of monoclonal antibodies. Int J Gynecol Pathol 1982, **1**: 231–245.

253 Chiesa AG, Deavers MT, Veras E, Silva EG, Gershenson D, Malpica A. Ovarian intestinal type mucinous borderline tumors: are we ready for a nomenclature change? Int J Gynecol Pathol 2010, **29**: 108–112.

254 Czernobilsky B, Dgani R, Roth LM. Ovarian mucinous cystadenocarcinoma with mural nodule of carcinomatous derivation. A light and electron microscopic study. Cancer 1983, **51**: 141–148.

255 Dubé V, Roy M, Plante M, Renaud MC, Têtu B. Mucinous ovarian tumors of Mullerian-type: an analysis of 17 cases including borderline tumors and intraepithelial, microinvasive, and invasive carcinomas. Int J Gynecol Pathol 2005, **24**: 138–146.

256 Fenoglio CM, Ferenczy A, Richart RM. Mucinous tumors of the ovary. Ultrastructural studies of mucinous cystadenomas with histogenetic considerations. Cancer 1975, **36**: 1709–1722.

257 Hart WR, Norris HJ. Borderline and malignant mucinous tumors of the ovary. Cancer 1973, **31**: 1031–1045.

258 Hart WR. Mucinous tumors of the ovary: a review. Int J Gynecol Pathol 2005, **24**: 4–25.

259 Hoerl HD, Hart WR. Primary ovarian mucinous cystadenocarcinomas: a clinicopathologic study of 49 cases with long-term follow-up. Am J Surg Pathol 1998, **22**: 1449–1462.

260 Hwang JE, Choi J, Paik Y-A, Lee YH, Shim JY, Kim K-R. Endocervical-like (mullerian-type) mucinous borderline tumors of the ovary; are they mucinous tumors? Lab Invest 2009, **89**(Suppl 1): 218A.

261 Ishikura H, Sasano H. Histopathologic and immunohistochemical study of steroidogenic cells in the stroma of ovarian tumors. Int J Gynecol Pathol 1998, **17**: 261–265.

262 Ishikura H, Shibata M, Yoshiki T. Endocrine cell micronests in an ovarian mucinous cystadenofibroma: a mimic of microinvasion. Int J Gynecol Pathol 1999, **18**: 392–395.

263 Ji H, Isacson C, Seidman JD, Kurman RJ, Ronnett BM. Cytokeratins 7 and 20, Dpc4, and MUC5AC in the distinction of metastatic mucinous carcinomas in the ovary from primary ovarian mucinous tumors: Dpc4 assists in identifying metastatic pancreatic carcinomas. Int J Gynecol Pathol 2002, **21**: 391–400.

264 Khunamornpong S, Russell P, Dalrymple JC. Proliferating (LMP) mucinous tumors of the ovaries with microinvasion: morphologic assessment of 13 Cases. Int J Gynecol Pathol 2002, **18**: 238–246.

265 Kim KR, Lee HI, Lee SK, Ro JY, Robboy SJ. Is stromal microinvasion in primary mucinous ovarian tumors with 'mucin granuloma' true invasion? Am J Surg Pathol 2007, **31**: 546–554.

266 Klemi PJ. Pathology of mucinous ovarian cystadenomas. I. Argyrophil and argentaffin cells and epithelial mucosubstances. Acta Pathol Microbiol Scand (A) 1978, **86**: 465–470.

267 Lee KR, Nucci MR. Ovarian mucinous and mixed epithelial carcinoma of mullerian (endocervical-like) type: A clinicopathologic analysis of four cases of an uncommon variant associated with endometriosis. Int J Gynecol Pathol 2002, **22**: 42–51.

268 Lee KR, Scully RE. Mucinous tumors of the ovary: a clinicopathologic study of 196 borderline tumors (of intestinal type) and carcinomas, including an evaluation of 11 cases with 'pseudomyxoma peritonei'. Am J Surg Pathol 2000, **24**: 1447–1464.

269 Lifschitz-Mercer B, Dgani R, Jacob N, Fogel M, Czernobilsky B. Ovarian mucinous cystadenoma with leiomyomatous mural nodule. Int J Gynecol Pathol 1990, **9**: 80–85.

270 LiVolsi VA, Merino MJ, Schwartz PE. Coexistent endocervical adenocarcinoma and mucinous adenocarcinoma of ovary. A clinicopathologic study of four cases. Int J Gynecol Pathol 1983, **1**: 391–402.

271 Louwerens JK, Schaberg A, Bosman FT. Neuroendocrine cells in cystic mucinous tumours of the ovary. Histopathology 1983, **7**: 389–398.

272 McCluggage WG, Young RH. Primary ovarian mucinous tumors with signet ring cells: report of 3 cases with discussion of so-called primary Krukenberg tumor. Am J Surg Pathol 2008, **32**: 1373–1379.

273 Matias-Guiu X, Prat J. Ovarian tumors with functioning stroma. An immunohistochemical study of 100 cases with human chorionic gonadotropin monoclonal and polyclonal antibodies. Cancer 1990, **65**: 2001–2005.

274 Matias-Guiu X, Aranda I, Prat J. Immunohistochemical study of sarcoma-like mural nodules in a mucinous cystadenocarcinoma of the ovary. Virchows Arch [A] 1991, **419**: 89–92.

275 Nichols GE, Mills SE, Ulbright TM, Czernobilsky B, Roth LM. Spindle cell mural nodules in cystic ovarian mucinous tumors. A clinicopathologic and immunohistochemical study of five cases. Am J Surg Pathol 1991, **15**: 1055–1062.

276 Nomura K, Aizawa S. Clinicopathologic and mucin histochemical analysis of 90 cases of ovarian mucinous borderline tumors of intestinal and mullerian types. Pathol Int 1997, **46**: 575–580.

277 Nomura K, Aizawa S. Noninvasive, microinvasive and invasive mucinous carcinomas of the ovary: a clinicopathologic analysis of 40 cases. Cancer 2000, **89**: 1541–1546.

278 Nonaka D, Chiriboga L, Soslow RA. Expression of pax8 as a useful marker in distinguishing ovarian carcinomas from mammary carcinomas. Am J Surg Pathol 2008, **32**: 1566–1571.

279 Park KJ, Bramlage MP, Ellenson LH, Pirog EC. Immunoprofile of adenocarcinomas of the endometrium, endocervix, and ovary with mucinous differentiation. Appl Immunohistochem Mol Morphol 2009, **17**: 8–11.

280 Prat J, Scully RE. Sarcomas in ovarian mucinous tumors. A report of two cases. Cancer 1979, **44**: 1327–1331.

281 Prat J, Scully RE. Ovarian mucinous tumors with sarcoma-like nodules. A report of seven cases. Cancer 1979, **44**: 1332–1344.

282 Prat J, Young RH, Scully RE. Ovarian mucinous tumors with foci of anaplastic carcinoma. Cancer 1982, **50**: 300–304.

283 Provenza C, Young RH, Prat J. Anaplastic carcinoma in mucinous ovarian tumors: a clinicopathologic study of 34 cases emphasizing the crucial impact of stage on prognosis, their histologic spectrum, and overlap with sarcomalike mural nodules. Am J Surg Pathol 2008, **32**: 383–389.

284 Riopel MA, Ronnett BM, Kurman RJ. Evaluation of diagnostic criteria and behavior of ovarian intestinal-type mucinous tumors: atypical proliferative (borderline) tumors and intraepithelial, microinvasive, invasive, and metastatic carcinoma. Am J Surg Pathol 1999, **23**: 617–635.

285 Robboy SJ. Insular carcinoid of ovary associated with malignant mucinous tumors. Cancer 1984, **54**: 2273–2276.

286 Rodriguez IM, Prat J. Mucinous tumors of the ovary: a clinicopathologic analysis of 75 borderline tumors (of intestinal type) and carcinomas. Am J Surg Pathol 2002, **26**: 139–152.

287 Rodriguez IM, Irving JA, Prat J. Endocervical-like mucinous borderline tumors of the ovary: a clinicopathologic analysis of 31 cases. Am J Surg Pathol 2004, **28**: 1311–1318.

288 Rutgers JL, Baergen RN. Mucin histochemistry of ovarian borderline tumors of mucinous and mixed-epithelial types. Mod Pathol 1994, **7**: 825–828.

289 Rutgers JL, Bell DA. Immunohistochemical characterization of ovarian borderline tumors of intestinal and mullerian types. Mod Pathol 1992, **5**: 367–371.

290 Sasaki E, Sasano N, Kimura N, Andoh N, Yajima A. Demonstration of neuroendocrine cells in ovarian mucinous tumors. Int J Gynecol Pathol 1989, **8**: 189–200.

291 Shappell HW, Riopel MA, Smith Sehdev AE, Ronnett BM, Kurman RJ. Diagnostic criteria and behavior of ovarian seromucinous (endocervical-type mucinous and mixed cell-type) tumors: atypical proliferative (borderline) tumors, intraepithelial, microinvasive, and invasive carcinomas. Am J Surg Pathol 2002, **26**: 1529–1541.

292 Shiohara S, Shiozawa T, Shimizu M, Toki T, Ishii K, Nikaido T, Fujii S. Histochemical analysis of estrogen and progesterone receptors and gastric-type mucin in mucinous ovarian tumors with reference to their pathogenesis. Cancer 1997, **80**: 908–916.

293 Shiozawa T, Tsukahara Y, Ishii K, Ota H, Nakayama J, Katsuyama T. Histochemical demonstration of gastrointestinal mucins in ovarian mucinous cystadenoma. Acta Pathol Jpn 1992, **42**: 104–110.

294 Siriaunkgul S, Robbins KM, McGowan L, Silverberg SG. Ovarian mucinous tumors of low malignant potential. A clinicopathologic study of 54 tumors of intestinal and Mullerian type. Int J Gynecol Pathol 1995, **14**: 198–208.

295 Sporrong B, Alumets J, Clase L, Falkmer S, Hakanson R, Ljungberg O, Sundler F. Neurohormonal peptide immunoreactive cells in mucinous cystadenomas and cystadenocarcinomas of the ovary. Virchows Arch [A] 1981, **392**: 271–280.

296 Sugai M, Umezu H, Yamamoto T, Jiang S, Iwanari H, Tanaka T, Hamakubo T, Kodama T, Naito M. Expression of hepatocyte nuclear factor 4 alpha in primary ovarian mucinous tumors. Pathol Int 2008, **58**: 681–686.

297 Tabrizi AD, Kalloger SE, Köbel M, Cipollone J, Roskelley CD, Mehl E, Gilks CB. Primary ovarian mucinous carcinoma of intestinal type: significance of pattern of invasion and immunohistochemical expression profile in a series of 31 cases. Int J Gynecol Pathol 2010, **29**: 99–107.

298 Tenti P, Aguzzi A, Riva C, Usellini L, Zappatore R, Bara J, Samloff M, Solcia E. Ovarian mucinous tumors frequently express markers of gastric, intestinal, and pancreatobiliary epithelial cells. Cancer 1992, **69**: 2131–2142.

299 Tsuchiya A, Sakamoto M, Yasuda J, Chuma M, Ohta T, Ohki M, Yasugi T, Taketani Y, Hirohashi S. Expression profiling in ovarian clear cell carcinoma: identification of hepatocyte nuclear factor-1 as a molecular marker and a possible molecular target for therapy of ovarian clear cell carcinoma. Am J Pathol 2003, **163**: 2503–2512.

300 Tsujimura T, Kawano K. Rhabdomyosarcoma coexistent with ovarian mucinous cystadenocarcinoma. A case report. Int J Gynecol Pathol 1992, **11**: 58–62.

301 Vang R, Gown AM, Wu LS, Barry TS, Wheeler DT, Yemelyanova A, Seidman JD, Ronnett BM. Immunohistochemical expression of CDX2 in primary ovarian mucinous tumors and metastatic mucinous carcinomas involving the ovary: comparison with CK20 and correlation with coordinate expression of CK7. Mod Pathol 2006, **19**: 1421–1428.

302 Vang R, Gown AM, Barry TS, Wheeler DT, Ronnett BM. Ovarian atypical proliferative (borderline) mucinous tumors: gastrointestinal and seromucinous (endocervical-like) types are immunophenotypically distinctive. Int J Gynecol Pathol 2006, **25**: 83–89.

303 Watkin W, Silva EG, Gershenson DM. Mucinous carcinoma of the ovary. Pathologic prognostic factors. Cancer 1992, **69**: 208–212.

304 Werness BA, DiCioccio RA, River MS. Identical, unique p53 mutations in a primary ovarian mucinous adenocarcinoma and a synchronous contralateral ovarian mucinous tumor of low malignant potential suggest a common clonal origin. Hum Pathol 1997, **28**: 626–630.

305 Woodruff JD, Perry H, Genadry R, Parmley T. Mucinous cystadenocarcinoma of the ovary. Obstet Gynecol 1978, **51**: 483–489.

306 Yemelyanova AV, Vang R, Judson K, Wu LS, Ronnett BM. Distinction of primary and metastatic mucinous tumors involving the ovary: analysis of size and laterality data by primary site with reevaluation of an algorithm for tumor classification. Am J Surg Pathol 2008, **32**: 128–138.

307 Young RH, Scully RE. Mucinous ovarian tumors associated with mucinous adenocarcinomas of the cervix. A clinicopathological analysis of 16 cases. Int J Gynecol Pathol 1988, **7**: 99–111.

Endometrioid tumors

308 Aguirre P, Thor AD, Scully RE. Ovarian endometrioid carcinomas resembling sex cord-stromal tumors. An immunohistochemical study. Int J Gynecol Pathol 1989, **8**: 364–373.

309 Bell DA, Scully RE. Atypical and borderline endometrioid adenofibromas of the ovary. A report of 27 cases. Am J Surg Pathol 1985, **9**: 205–214.

310 Bell KA, Kurman RJ. A clinicopathologic analysis of atypical proliferative (borderline) tumors and well-differentiated endometrioid adenocarcinomas of the ovary. Am J Surg Pathol 2000, **24**: 1465–1479.

311 Caduff RF, Svoboda-Newman SM, Bartos RE, Ferguson AW, Frank TS. Comparative analysis of histologic homologues of endometrial and ovarian carcinoma. Am J Surg Pathol 1998, **22**: 319–326.

312 Casper S, van Nagell JR Jr, Powell DF, Dubilier LD, Donaldson ES, Hanson MB, Pavlik EJ. Immunohistochemical localization of tumor markers in epithelial ovarian cancer. Am J Obstet Gynecol 1984, **149**: 154–158.

313 Czernobilsky B. Endometrioid neoplasia of the ovary. A reappraisal. Int J Gynecol Pathol 1982, **1**: 203–210.

314 Czernobilsky B, Silverman BB, Mikuta JJ. Endometrioid carcinoma of the ovary. A clinicopathologic study of 75 cases. Cancer 1970, **26**: 1141–1152.

315 Dabbs DJ, Sturtz K, Zaino RJ. The immunohistochemical discrimination of endometrioid adenocarcinomas. Hum Pathol 1996, **27**: 172–177.

316 Eichhorn JH, Scully RE. Endometrioid ciliated-cell tumors of the ovary: a report of five cases. Int J Gynecol Pathol 1997, **15**: 248–256.

317 Fujibayashi M, Aiba M, Iizuka E, Igarashi A, Muraoka M, Takagi K. Granulosa cell tumor-like variant of endometrioid carcinoma of the ovary exhibiting nuclear clearing with biotin activity: a subtype showing close macroscopic, cytologic, and histologic similarity to adult granulosa cell tumor. Arch Pathol Lab Med 2005, **129**: 1288–1294.

318 Guerrieri C, Franlund B, Malmstrom H, Boeryd B. Ovarian endometrioid carcinomas simulating sex cord–stromal tumors: a study using inhibin and cytokeratin 7. Int J Gynecol Pathol 1998, **17**: 266–271.

319 Helle M, Helin H, Ashorn P, Putkinen EL, Krohn K, Wahlstrom T. The expression of CEA, CA 19-9 and HMFG antigens in ovarian clear-cell and endometrioid carcinomas. Pathol Res Pract 1992, **188**: 74–77.

320 Houghton O, Connolly LE, McCluggage WG. Morules in endometrioid proliferations of the uterus and ovary consistently express the intestinal transcription factor CDX2. Histopathology 2008, **53**: 156–165.

321 Hughesdon PE. Benign endometrioid tumours of the ovary and the müllerian concept of ovarian epithelial tumours. Histopathology 1984, **8**: 977–990.

322 Kim KR, Scully RE. Peritoneal keratin granulomas with carcinomas of endometrium and ovary and atypical polypoid adenomyoma of endometrium. A clinicopathological analysis of 22 cases. Am J Surg Pathol 1990, **14**: 925–932.

323 Kistner RW, Hertig AT. Primary adenoacanthoma of the ovary. Cancer 1952, **5**: 1134–1145.

324 Klemi PJ, Gronroos M. Endometrioid carcinoma of the ovary. Obstet Gynecol 1979, **53**: 572–579.

325 Kline RC, Wharton JT, Atkinson EN, Burke TW, Gershenson DM, Edwards CL. Endometrioid carcinoma of the ovary. Retrospective review of 145 cases. Gynecol Oncol 1990, **39**: 337–346.

326 Macko MB, Johnson LA. Primary squamous ovarian carcinoma. A case report and review of the literature. Cancer 1983, **52**: 1117–1119.

327 Mostoufizadeh M, Scully RE. Malignant tumors arising in endometriosis. Clin Obstet Gynecol 1980, **23**: 951–963.

328 Nogales FF, Carvia RE, Bergeron C, Alvaro T, Fulwood HR. Ovarian endometrioid tumors with yolk sac tumor component, an unusual form of ovarian neoplasm: analysis of six cases. Am J Surg Pathol 1996, **20**: 1056–1066.

329 Norris HJ. Proliferative endometrioid tumors and endometrioid tumors of low malignant potential of the ovary. Int J Gynecol Pathol 1993, **12**: 134–140.

330 Ordi J, Schammel DP, Rasekh L, Tavassoli FA. Sertoliform endometrioid carcinomas of the ovary: a clinicopathologic and immunohistochemical study of 13 cases. Mod Pathol 1999, **12**: 933–940.

331 Park JY, Song JS, Choi G, Kim JH, Nam JH. Pure primary squamous cell carcinoma of the ovary: a report of two cases and review of the literature. Int J Gynecol Pathol 2010, **29**: 328–334.

332 Pins MR, Young RH, Daly WJ, Scully RE. Primary squamous cell carcinoma of the ovary: report of 37 cases. Am J Surg Pathol 1996, **20**: 823–833.

333 Pitman MB, Young RH, Clement PB, Dickersin GR, Scully RE. Endometrioid carcinoma of the ovary and endometrium, oxyphilic cell type. A report of nine cases. Int J Gynecol Pathol 1994, **13**: 290–301.

334 Roth LM, Czernobilsky B, Langley FA. Ovarian endometrioid adenofibromatous and cystadenofibromatous tumors. Benign, proliferating, and malignant. Cancer 1981, **48**: 1838–1845.

335 Roth LM, Emerson RE, Ulbright TM. Ovarian endometrioid tumors of low malignant potential. A clinicopathologic study of 30 cases with comparison to well-differentiated endometrioid adenocarcinoma. Am J Surg Pathol 2003, **27**: 1253–1259.

336 Roth LM, Liban E, Czernobilsky B. Ovarian endometrioid tumors mimicking Sertoli and Sertoli–Leydig cell tumors. Sertoliform variant of endometrioid carcinoma. Cancer 1984, **50**: 1322–1331.

337 Rutgers JL, Young RH, Scully RE. Ovarian yolk sac tumor arising from an endometrioid carcinoma. Hum Pathol 1987, **18**: 1296–1299.

338 Stolnicu S, Preda O, Dohan M, Puscasiu L, García-Galvis OF, Nogales FF. Pseudoglandular hepatoid differentiation in endometrioid carcinoma of the ovary simulates oxyphilic cell change. Int J Gynecol Pathol 2008, **27**: 521–525.

339 Tetu B, Silva EG, Gershenson DM. Squamous cell carcinoma of the ovary. Arch Pathol Lab Med 1987, **111**: 864–866.

340 Treilleux I, Godeneche J, Duvillard P, Clement-Chassagne C, Suignard Y, Bailly C. Collagenous spherulosis mimicking keratinizing squamous metaplasia in a borderline endometrioid tumor of the ovary. Histopathology 1999, **35**: 271–276.

341 Ueda G, Yamasaki M, Inoue M, Tanaka Y, Hiramatsu K, Inoue Y, Saito J, Nishino T, Kurachi K. Argyrophil cells in the endometrioid carcinoma of the ovary. Cancer 1984, **54**: 1569–1573.

342 Wiegand KC, Shah SP, Al-Agha OM, Zhao Y, Tse K, Zeng T, Senz J, McConechy MK, Anglesio MS, Kalloger SE, Yang W, Heravi-Moussavi A, Giuliany R, Chow C, Fee J, Zayed A, Prentice L, Melnyk N, Turashvili G, Delaney AD, Madore J, Yip S, McPherson AW, Ha G, Bell L, Fereday S, Tam A, Galletta L, Tonin PN, Provencher D, Miller D, Jones SJM, Moore RA, Morin GB, Oloumi A, Boyd N, Aparicio SA, Shih IeM, Mes-Masson AM, Bowtell DD, Hirst M, Gilks B, Marra MA, Huntsman DG. *ARID1A* mutations in endometriosis-associated ovarian carcinomas. N Engl J Med 2010, **363**: 1532–1543.

343 Yetman TJ, Dudzinski MR. Primary squamous carcinoma of the ovary. A case report and review of the literature. Gynecol Oncol 1989, **34**: 240–243.

344 Young RH, Scully RE. Oxyphilic tumors of the female and male genital tracts. Semin Diagn Pathol 1999, **16**: 146–161.

345 Young RH, Prat J, Scully RE. Ovarian endometrioid carcinomas resembling sex cord–stromal tumors. A clinicopathological analysis of 13 cases. Am J Surg Pathol 1982, **6**: 513–522.

346 Zaino RJ, Unger ER, Whitney C. Synchronous carcinomas of the uterine corpus and ovary. Gynecol Oncol 1984, **19**: 329–335.

347 Zhai Y, Wu R, Schwartz DR, Darrah D, Reed H, Kollings FT, Nieman MR, Fearon ER, Cho KE. Role of beta-caterin/T-cell factor-regulated genes in ovarian endometrioid adenocarcinomas. Am J Pathol 2002, **160**: 1229–1238.

Clear cell (mesonephroid) tumors

348 Brescia RJ, Dubin N, Demopoulos RI. Endometrioid and clear cell carcinoma of the ovary. Factors affecting survival. Int J Gynecol Pathol 1989, **8**: 132–138.

349 Cao D, Guo S, Allan RW, West AM, Molberg KH, Peng Y. SALL4 is a novel sensitive and specific marker of ovarian primitive germ cell tumors and distinguishes yolk sac tumor from clear cell carcinoma. Lab Invest 2009, **89**(Suppl 1): 208A.

350 Crozier MA, Copeland LJ, Silva EG, Gershenson DM, Stringer CA. Clear cell carcinoma of the ovary. A study of 59 cases. Gynecol Oncol 1989, **35**: 199–203.

351 Czernobilsky B, Silverman BB, Enterline HT. Clear cell carcinoma of the ovary. A clinicopathologic analysis of pure and mixed forms and comparison with endometroid carcinoma. Cancer 1970, **25**: 762–772.

352 DeLair D, Olvia E, Köbel M, Macias A, Gilks CB, Soslow RA. Morphologic spectrum of immunohistochemically characterized clear cell carcinoma of the ovary: a study of 155 cases. Am J Surg Pathol 2011, **35**: 36–44.

353 Esheba GE, Pate LL, Longacre TA. Oncofetal protein glypican-3 distinguishes yolk sac tumor from clear cell carcinoma of the ovary. Am J Surg Pathol 2008, **32**: 600–607.

354 Fujimura M, Hidaka T, Kataoka K, Yamakawa Y, Akada S, Teranishi A, Saito S. Absence of estrogen receptor-(alpha) expression in human ovarian clear cell adenocarcinoma compared with ovarian serous, endometrioid, and mucinous adenocarcinoma. Am J Surg Pathol 2001, **25**: 667–672.

355 Han G, Gilks CB, Leung S, Ewanowich CA, Irving JA, Longacre TA, Soslow RA. Mixed ovarian epithelial carcinomas with clear cell and serous components are variants of high-grade serous carcinoma: an interobserver correlative and immunohistochemical study of 32 cases. Am J Surg Pathol 2008, **32**: 955–964.

356 Kato N, Sasou S, Motoyama T. Expression of hepatocyte nuclear factor-1beta (HNF-1beta) in clear cell tumors and endometriosis of the ovary. Mod Pathol 2006, **19**: 83–89.

357 Kennedy AW, Biscotti CV, Hart WR, Tuason LJ. Histologic correlates of progression-free interval and survival in ovarian clear cell adenocarcinoma. Gynecol Oncol 1993, **50**: 334–338.

358 Klemi PJ, Meurman L, Gronroos M, Talerman A. Clear cell (mesonephroid) tumors of the ovary with characteristics resembling endodermal sinus tumor. Int J Gynecol Pathol 1982, **1**: 95–100.

359 Köbel M, Kalloger SE, Carrick J, Huntsman D, Asad H, Oliva E, Ewanowich CA, Soslow RA, Gilks CB. A limited panel of immunomarkers can reliably distinguish between clear cell and high-grade serous carcinoma of the ovary. Am J Surg Pathol 2009, **33**: 14–21.

360 Kwon TJ, Ro JY, Mackay B. Clear-cell carcinoma: an ultrastructural study of 57 tumors from various sites. Ultrastruct Pathol 1997, **20**: 519–527.

361 Kwon TJ, Ro JY, Tornos C, Ordonez NG. Reduplicated basal lamina in clear-cell carcinoma of the ovary: an immunohistochemical and electron microscopic study. Ultrastruct Pathol 1997, **20**: 529–536.

362 Maeda D, Ota S, Takazawa Y, Aburatani H, Nakagawa S, Yano T, Taketani Y, Kodama T, Fukayama M. Glypican-3 expression in clear cell adenocarcinoma of the ovary. Mod Pathol 2009, **22**: 824–832.

363 Matias-Guiu X, Lerma E, Prat J. Clear cell tumors of the female genital tract. Semin Diagn Pathol 1998, **14**: 233–239.

364 Mikami Y, Hata S, Melamed J, Moriya T, Manabe T. Basement membrane material in ovarian clear cell carcinoma: correlation with growth pattern and nuclear grade. Int J Gynecol Pathol 1999, **18**: 52–57.

365 Montag AG, Jenison EL, Griffiths CT, Welch WR, Lavin PT, Knapp RC. Ovarian clear cell carcinoma. A clinicopathologic analysis of 44 cases. Int J Gynecol Pathol 1989, **8**: 85–96.

366 Nolan LP, Heatley MK. The value of immunohistochemistry in distinguishing between clear cell carcinoma of the kidney and ovary. Int J Gynecol Pathol 2001, **20**: 155–159.

367 Norris HJ, Robinowitz M. Ovarian adenocarcinoma of mesonephric type. Cancer 1971, **28**: 1074–1081.

368 Ohta Y, Suzuki T, Shiokawa A, Mitsuya T, Ota H. Expression of CD10 and cytokeratins in ovarian and renal clear cell carcinoma. Int J Gynecol Pathol 2005, **24**: 239–245.

369 Roth LM, Langley FA, Fox H, Wheeler JE, Czernobilsky B. Ovarian clear cell adenofibromatous tumors. Benign, of low malignant potential, and associated with invasive clear cell carcinoma. Cancer 1984, **53**: 1156–1163.

370 Sangoi AR, Soslow RA, Teng NN, Longacre TA. Ovarian clear cell carcinoma with papillary features: a potential mimic of serous tumor of low malignant potential. Am J Surg Pathol 2008, **32**: 269–274.

371 Schiller W. Mesonephroma ovarii. Am J Cancer 1939, **35**: 1–21.

372 Scully RE, Barlow JF. Mesonephroma of the ovary. Tumor of müllerian nature related to the endometrioid carcinoma. Cancer 1967, **20**: 1405–1417.

373 Shevchuk MM, Winkler-Monsanto B, Fenoglio CM, Richart RM. Clear cell carcinoma of the ovary. A clinicopathologic study with review of the literature. Cancer 1981, **47**: 1344–1351.

374 Shimizu M, Nikaido T, Toki T, Shiozawa T, Fujii S. Clear cell carcinoma has an expression pattern of cell cycle regulatory molecules that is unique among ovarian adenocarcinomas. Cancer 1999, **85**: 669–677.

375 Vang R, Whitaker BP, Farhood AI, Silva EG, Ro JY, Deavers MT. Immunohistochemical analysis of clear cell carcinoma of the gynecologic tract. Int J Gynecol Pathol 2001, **20**: 252–259.

376 Yamamoto S, Tsuda H, Yoshikawa T, Kudoh K, Kita T, Furuya K, Tamai S, Matsubara O. Clear cell adenocarcinoma associated with clear cell adenofibromatous components: a subgroup of ovarian clear cell adenocarcinoma with distinct clinicopathologic characteristics. Am J Surg Pathol 2007, **31**: 999–1006.

377 Yamamoto S, Tsuda H, Aida S, Shimazaki H, Tamai S, Matsubara O. Immunohistochemical detection of hepatocyte nuclear factor 1beta in ovarian and endometrial clear-cell adenocarcinomas and nonneoplastic endometrium. Hum Pathol 2007, **38**: 1074–1080.

378 Young RH, Scully RE. Oxyphilic tumors of the female and male genital tracts. Semin Diagn Pathol 1999, **16**: 146–161.

379 Young RH, Scully RE. Oxyphilic clear cell carcinoma of the ovary. A report of nine cases. Am J Surg Pathol 1987, **11**: 661–667.

380 Zhao F, Zheng W, Ip PPC, Siu MSK, Tam K-F, Cheung ANY. The oncofetal protein IMP3 is differentially expressed in clear cell carcinoma of ovary. Lab Invest 2009, **89**(Suppl 1): 242A.

381 Zhao C, Barner R, Kurman R, Stamatakos M, Vang R. Clinicopathologic analysis of ovarian clear cell carcinoma: comparison of cases with and without adenofibromatous components and implications for pathogenesis. Lab Invest 2009, **89**(Suppl 1): 242A.

382 Zirker TA, Silva EG, Morris M, Ordonez NG. Immunohistochemical differentiation of clear-cell carcinoma of the female genital tract and endodermal sinus tumor with the use of alpha-fetoprotein and Leu-M1. Am J Clin Pathol 1989, **91**: 511–514.

Brenner tumor and transitional cell carcinoma

383 Aguirre P, Scully RE, Wolfe HJ, DeLellis RA. Argyrophil cells in Brenner tumors. Histochemical and immunohistochemical analysis. Int J Gynecol Pathol 1986, **5**: 223–234.

384 Austin RM, Norris HJ. Malignant Brenner tumor and transitional cell carcinoma of the ovary. A comparison. Int J Gynecol Pathol 1987, **6**: 29–39.

385 Costa MJ, Hansen C, Dickerman A, Scudder SA. Clinicopathologic significance of transitional cell carcinoma pattern in nonlocalized ovarian epithelial tumors (stages 2–4). Am J Clin Pathol 1998, **109**: 173–180.

386 Cuatrecasas M, Catasus L, Palacios J, Prat J. Transitional cell tumors of the ovary: a comparative clinicopathologic, immunohistochemical, and molecular genetic analysis of Brenner tumors and transitional cell carcinomas. Am J Surg Pathol 2009, **33**: 556–567.

387 Eichhorn JH, Young RH. Transitional cell carcinoma of the ovary: a morphologic study of 100 cases with emphasis on differential diagnosis. Am J Surg Pathol 2004, **28**: 453–463.

388 Euscher ED, Malpica A. Neuroendocrine cells as a component of ovarian Brenner tumor: the source rare ovarian carcinoid tumors associated with these neoplasms. Lab Invest 2009, **89**(Suppl 1): 212A–213A.

389 Ganjei P, Nadji M, Penneys NS, Averette HE, Morales AR. Immunoreactive prekeratin in Brenner tumors of the ovary. Int J Gynecol Pathol 1983, **1**: 353–358.

390 Hallgrimsson J, Scully RE. Borderline and malignant Brenner tumors of the ovary. A report of 15 cases. Acta Pathol Microbiol Scand 1972, **233**(Suppl): 56–66.

391 Heller DS, Harpaz N, Breakstone B. Neoplasms arising in ectopic ovaries. A case of Brenner tumor in an accessory ovary. Int J Gynecol Pathol 1990, **9**: 185–189.

392 Hollingsworth HC, Steinberg SM, Silverberg SG, Merino MJ. Advanced stage transitional cell carcinoma of the ovary. Hum Pathol 1997, **27**: 1267–1272.

393 Liao XY, Xue WC, Shen DH, Ngan HY, Siu MK, Cheung AN. p63 expression in ovarian tumours: a marker for Brenner tumours but not transitional cell carcinomas. Histopathology 2007, **51**: 477–483.

394 Logani S, Oliva E, Amin MB, Folpe AL, Cohen C, Young RH. Immunoprofile of ovarian tumors with putative transitional cell (urothelial) differentiation using novel urothelial markers. Am J Surg Pathol 2003, **27**: 1434–1441.

395 Miles PA, Norris HJ. Proliferative and malignant Brenner tumors of the ovary. Cancer 1972, **30**: 174–186.

396 Ming SC, Goldman H. Hormonal activity of Brenner tumors in postmenopausal women. Am J Obstet Gynecol 1962, **83**: 666–673.

397 Moon S, Waxman M. Mixed ovarian tumor composed of Brenner and thyroid elements. Cancer 1976, **38**: 1997–2001.

398 Ogawa K, Johansson SL, Cohen SM. Immunohistochemical analysis of uroplakins, urothelial specific proteins, in ovarian Brenner tumors, normal tissues, and benign and neoplastic lesions of the female genital tract. Am J Pathol 1999, **155**: 1047–1050.

399 Ordonez NG. Transitional cell carcinoma of the ovary and bladder are immunophenotypically different. Histopathology 2000, **36**: 433–438.

400 Ordonez NG, Mackay B. Brenner tumor of the ovary: a comparative immunohistochemical and ultrastructural study with transitional cell carcinoma of the bladder. Ultrastruct Pathol 2000, **24**: 157–167.

401 Riedel I, Czernobilsky B, Lifschitiz-Mercer B, Roth LM, Wu XR, Sun TT, Moll R. Brenner tumors but not transitional cell carcinomas of the ovary show urothelial differentiation: immunohistochemical staining of urothelial markers, including cytokeratins and uroplakins. Virchows Arch 2001, **438**: 181–191.

402 Robey SS, Silva EG, Gershenson DM, McLemore D, el-Naggar A, Ordonez NG. Transitional cell carcinoma in high-grade high-stage ovarian carcinoma. An indicator of favorable response to chemotherapy. Cancer 1989, **63**: 839–847.

403 Roth LM, Czernobilsky B. Ovarian Brenner tumors. II. Malignant. Cancer 1985, **56**: 592–601.

404 Roth LM, Dallenbach-Hellweg G, Czernobilsky B. Ovarian Brenner tumors. I. Metaplastic, proliferating, and of low malignant potential. Cancer 1985, **56**: 582–591.

405 Roth LM, Gersell DJ, Ulbright TM. Ovarian Brenner tumors and transitional cell carcinoma. Recent developments. Int J Gynecol Pathol 1993, **12**: 128–133.

406 Roth LM, Gersell DJ, Ulbright TM. Transitional cell carcinoma and other transitional cell tumors of the ovary. Anat Pathol 1998, **1**: 179–191.

407 Santini D, Gelli MC, Mazzoleni G, Ricci M, Severi B, Pasquinelli G, Pelusi G, Martinelli G. Brenner tumor of the ovary. A correlative histologic, histochemical, immunohistochemical, and ultrastructural investigation. Hum Pathol 1989, **20**: 787–795.

408 Sasano H, Wargotz ES, Silverberg SG, Mason JI, Simpson ER. Brenner tumor of the ovary. Immunoanalysis of steroidogenic enzymes in 23 cases. Hum Pathol 1989, **20**: 1103–1107.

409 Seidman JD, Khedmati F. Exploring the histogenesis of ovarian mucinous and transitional cell (Brenner) neoplasms and their relationship with Walthard cell nests: a study of 120 tumors. Arch Pathol Lab Med 2008, **132**: 1753–1760.

410 Seldenrijk CA, Willig AP, Baak JPA, Kuhnel R, Rao BR, Burger CW, van der Harten JJ, Dijkhuizen GH, Meijer CJLM. Malignant Brenner tumor. A histologic, morphometrical, immunohistochemical, and ultrastructural study. Cancer 1986, 58: 754–760.

411 Shevchuk MM, Fenoglio CM, Richart RM. Histogenesis of Brenner tumors. I. Histology and ultrastructure. Cancer 1980, **46**: 2607–2616.

412 Shevchuk MM, Fenoglio CM, Richart RM. Histogenesis of Brenner tumors. II. Histochemistry and CEA. Cancer 1980, **46**: 2617–2622.

413 Silverberg SG. Brenner tumor of the ovary. A clinicopathologic study of 60 tumors in 54 women. Cancer 1971, **28**: 588–596.

414 Soslow RA, Rouse RV, Hendrickson MR, Silva EG, Longacre TA. Transitional cell neoplasms of the ovary and urinary bladder: a comparative immunohistochemical analysis. Int J Gynecol Pathol 1997, **15**: 257–265.

415 Svenes KB, Eide J. Proliferative Brenner tumor or ovarian metastases? A case report. Cancer 1984, **53**: 2692–2697.

416 Young RH, Scully RE. Urothelial and ovarian carcinomas of identical cell types. Problems in interpretation. A report of three cases and review of the literature. Int J Gynecol Pathol 1988, **7**: 197–211.

Malignant mixed müllerian tumor and müllerian adenosarcoma

417 Ariyoshi K, Kawauchi S, Kaku T, Nakano H, Tsuneyoshi M. Prognostic factors in ovarian carcinosarcoma: a clinicopathological and immunohistochemical analysis of 23 cases. Histopathology 2000, **37**: 427–436.

418 Balzer BL, Hendrickson MR. Extrauterine müllerian adenosarcomas: a clinicopathologic study of 24 cases. Mod Pathol 2003, **16**: 181a.

419 Barwick KW, LiVolsi VA. Malignant mixed mesodermal tumors of the ovary. A clinicopathologic assessment of 12 cases. Am J Surg Pathol 1980, **4**: 37–42.

420 Boucher D, Tetu B. Morphologic prognostic factors of malignant mixed mullerian tumors of the ovary. A clinicopathologic study of 15 cases. Int J Gynecol Pathol 1994, **13**: 22–28.

421 Clement PB, Scully RE. Extrauterine mesodermal (müllerian) adenosarcoma. A clinicopathologic analysis of five cases. Am J Clin Pathol 1978, **69**: 276–283.

422 Dass KK, Biscoti CV, Webster K, Saxton JP. Malignant mixed mullerian tumors of the ovary. An analysis of two long-term survivors. Am J Clin Oncol 1993, **16**: 346–349.

423 Dehner LP, Norris HJ, Taylor HB. Carcinosarcomas and mixed mesodermal tumors of the ovary. Cancer 1971, **27**: 207–216.

424 Dictor M. Ovarian malignant mixed mesodermal tumor. The occurrence of hyaline droplets containing alpha-1-antitrypsin. Hum Pathol 1982, **13**: 930–933.

425 Dictor M. Malignant mixed mesodermal tumor of the ovary. A report of 22 cases. Obstet Gynecol 1985, **65**: 720–724.

426 Ehrmann RL, Weidner N, Welch WR, Gleiberman I. Malignant mixed mullerian tumor of the ovary with prominent neuroectodermal differentiation (teratoid carcinosarcoma). Int J Gynecol Pathol 1990, **9**: 272–282.

427 Eichhorn JH, Young RH, Clement PB, Scully RE. Mesodermal (Mullerian) adenosarcoma of the ovary: a clinicopathologic analysis of 40 cases and a review of the literature. Am J Surg Pathol 2002, **26**: 1243–1258.

428 Fenn ME, Abell MR. Carcinosarcoma of the ovary. Am J Obstet Gynecol 1971, **110**: 1066–1074.

429 Fukunaga M, Nomura K, Endo Y, Ushigome S, Aizawa S. Ovarian adenosarcoma. Histopathology 1997, 30: 283–287.

430 García-Galvis OF, Cabrera-Ozoria C, Fernández JA, Stolnicu S, Nogales FF. Malignant Müllerian mixed tumor of the ovary associated with yolk sac tumor, neuroepithelial and trophoblastic differentiation (teratoid carcinosarcoma). Int J Gynecol Pathol 2008, **27**: 515–520.

431 Morrow CP, d'Ablaing G, Brady LW, Blessing JA, Hreshchyshyn MM. A clinical and pathologic study of 30 cases of malignant mixed müllerian epithelial and mesenchymal ovarian tumors. A gynecologic oncology group study. Gynecol Oncol 1984, **18**: 278–292.

432 Plaxe SC, Dottino PR, Goodman HM, Deligdisch L, Idelson M, Cohen CJ. Clinical features of advanced ovarian mixed mesodermal tumors and treatment with doxorubicin- and *cis*-platinum-based chemotherapy. Gynecol Oncol 1990, **37**: 244–249.

433 Tanimoto A, Arima N, Hayashi R, Hamada T, Matsuki Y, Sasaguri Y. Teratoid carcinosarcoma of the ovary with prominent neuroectodermal differentiation. Pathol Int 2002, **51**: 829–832.

Adenoid cystic and basaloid carcinomas

434 Eichhorn JH, Scully RE. 'Adenoid cystic' and basaloid carcinomas of the ovary. Evidence for a surface epithelial lineage. A report of 12 cases. Mod Pathol 1995, **8**: 731–740.

435 Feczko JD, Jentz LD, Roth LM. Adenoid cystic ovarian carcinoma compared with other adenoid cystic carcinomas of the female genital tract. Mod Pathol 1996, **9**: 413–417.

436 Zamecnik M, Michal M, Curik R. Adenoid cystic carcinoma of the ovary. Arch Pathol Lab Med 2000, **124**: 1529–1531.

Mixed and other epithelial tumors

437 Che M, Tornos C, Deavers MT, Malpica A, Gershenson DM, Silva EG. Ovarian mixed-epithelial carcinomas with a microcystic pattern and signet-ring cells. Int J Gynecol Pathol 2001, **20**: 323–328.

438 Cramer SF, Roth LM, Mills SE, Ulbright TM, Gersell DJ, Nunez CA, Kraus FT. Sources of variability in classifying common ovarian cancers using the World Health Organization classification. Application of the pathtracking method. Pathol Annu 1993, **28**(Pt 2): 243–286.

439 Cramer SF, Roth LM, Ulbright TM, Mazur MT, Nunez CA, Gersell DJ, Mills SE, Kraus FT. Evaluation of the reproducibility of the World Health Organization classification of common ovarian cancers. With emphasis on methodology. Arch Pathol Lab Med 1987, **111**: 819–829.

440 Lee S, Park SY, Hong EK, Ro JY. Lymphoepithelioma-like carcinoma of the ovary: a case report and review of the literature. Arch Pathol Lab Med 2007, **131**: 1715–1718.

441 Rutgers JL, Scully RE. Ovarian mixed-epithelial papillary cystadenomas of borderline malignancy of Müllerian type. A clinicopathologic analysis. Cancer 1988, **61**: 546–554.

442 Silva EG, Tornos C, Bailey MA, Morris M. Undifferentiated carcinoma of the ovary. Arch Pathol Lab Med 1991, **115**: 377–381.

OVARIAN CARCINOMA – OVERVIEW

General and clinical features

443 Cannistra SA. Cancer of the ovary. N Engl J Med 1993, **329**: 1550–1559.

444 Cannistra SA. Cancer of the ovary. N Engl J Med 2004, **351**: 2519–2529.

445 Carcangiu ML, Radice P, Spatti G, Manoukian S, Pasini B. Histopathology of ovarian tumors in women with BRCA1 and 2 mutations [abstract]. Mod Pathol 2003, **16**: 184a.

446 Carcangiu ML, Peissel B, Pasini B, Spatti G, Radice P, Manoukian S. Incidental carcinomas in prophylactic specimens in BRCA1 and BRCA2 germ-line mutation carriers, with emphasis on fallopian tube lesions: report of 6 cases and review of the literature. Am J Surg Pathol 2006, **30**: 1222–1230.

447 Godwin AK, Testa JR, Hamilton TC. The biology of ovarian cancer development. Cancer 1993, **71**(Suppl 2): 530–536.

448 Greene MH, Clark JW, Blayney DW. The epidemiology of ovarian cancer. Semin Oncol 1984, **11**: 209–226.

449 Greggi S, Genuardi M, Benedetti-Panici P, Cento R, Scambia G, Neri G, Mancuso S. Analysis of 138 consecutive ovarian cancer patients. Incidence and characteristics of familial cases. Gynecol Oncol 1990, **39**: 300–304.

450 Harlow BL, Weiss NS, Roth GJ, Chu J, Daling JR. Case-control study of borderline ovarian tumors. Reproductive history and exposure to exogenous female hormones. Cancer Res 1988, **48**: 5849–5852.

451 Kauff ND, Satagopan JM, Robson ME, Scheuber L, Hensley M, Hudis CA, Ellis NA, Boyd J, Borgen PI, Barakat RR, Norton L, Offit K. Risk-reducing salpingo-oophorectomy in women with a BRCA1 or BRAC2 mutation. N Engl J Med 2002, **346**: 1609–1615.

452 Lynch HT, Watson P, Bewtra C, Conway TA, Hippee CR, Kaur P, Lynch JF, Ponder BA. Hereditary ovarian cancer. Heterogeneity in age at diagnosis. Cancer 1991, **67**: 1460–1466.

453 Markman M, Lewis JL Jr, Saigo P, Hakes T, Jones W, Rubin S, Reichman B, Barakat R, Curtin J, Almadrones L, et al. Epithelial ovarian cancer in the elderly. The Memorial Sloan-Kettering Cancer Center experience. Cancer 1993, **71**: 634–637.

454 Ness RB, Cottreau C. Possible role of ovarian epithelial inflammation in ovarian cancer. J Natl Cancer Inst 1999, **91**: 1459–1467.

455 Piver MS, Baker TR, Jishi MF, Sandecki AM, Tsukada Y, Natarajan N, Mettlin CJ, Blake CA. Familial ovarian cancer. A report of 658 families from the Gilda Radner Familial Ovarian Cancer Registry, 1981–1991. Cancer 1993, **71**: 582–588.

456 Piver MS, Baker TR, Piedmonte M, Sandecki AM. Epidemiology and etiology of ovarian cancer. Semin Oncol 1991, **18**: 177–185.

457 Prat J, Ribé A, Gallardo A. Hereditary ovarian cancer. Hum Pathol 2005, **36**: 861–870.

458 Rabban JT, Barnes M, Chen LM, Powell CB, Crawford B, Zaloudek CJ. Ovarian pathology in risk-reducing salpingo-oophorectomies from women with BRCA mutations, emphasizing the differential diagnosis of occult primary and metastatic carcinoma. Am J Surg Pathol 2009, **33**: 1125–1136.

459 Rebbeck TR, Lynch HT, Neuhausen SL, Narod, SA van't Veer L, Garber JE, Evans G, Isaacs C, Daly MB, Matloff E, Olopade OI, Weber BL. Prophylactic oophorectomy in carriers of BRCA1 or BRCA2 mutations. N Engl J Med 2002, **34**: 1616–1622.

460 Richardson GS, Scully RE, Nikrui N, Nelson JH. Common epithelial cancer of the ovary. N Engl J Med 1985, **312**: 415–424, 474–483.

461 Rodriguez M, Nguyen HN, Averette HE, Steren AJ, Penalver MA, Harrison T, Sevin BU. National survey of ovarian carcinoma. XII. Epithelial ovarian malignancies in women less than or equal to 25 years of age. Cancer 1994, **73**: 1245–1250.

462 Rossing MA, Daling JR, Weiss NS, Moore DE, Self SG. Ovarian tumors in a cohort of infertile women. N Engl J Med 1994, **331**: 771–776.

463 Shaw PA, McLaughlin JR, Zweemer RP, Narod SA, Risch H, Verheijen RHM, Ryan A, Menko FH, Kenemans P, Jacobs IJ. Histopathologic features of genetically determined ovarian cancer. Int J Gynecol Pathol 2002, **21**: 407–411.

464 Stratton JF, Gayther SA, Russell P, Dearden J, Gore M, Blake P, Easton D, Ponder BA. Contribution of BRCA1 mutations to ovarian cancer. N Engl J Med 1997, **336**: 1125–1130.

465 Weiss NS. Measuring the separate effects of low parity and its antecedents on the incidence of ovarian cancer. Am J Epidemiol 1988, **128**: 451–455.

466 Werness BA, Ramus SJ, Whittemore AS, Garlinghouse-Jones K, Oakley-Girvan I, Dicioccio RA, Tsukada Y, Ponder BA, Piver MS. Histopathology of familial ovarian tumors in women from families with and without germline BRCA1 mutations. Hum Pathol 2000, **31**: 1420–1424.

467 Werness BA, Ramus SJ, DiCioccio RA, Whittemore AS, Garlinghouse-Jones K, Oakley-Girvan I, Tsukada Y, Harrington P, Gayther SA, Ponder BA, Piver MS. Histopathology, FIGO stage, and BRCA mutation status of ovarian cancers from the Gilda Radner Familial Ovarian Cancer Registry. Int J Gynecol Pathol 2004, **23**: 29–34.

468 Wooster R, Weber BL. Breast and ovarian cancer. N Engl J Med 2003, **348**: 2339–2347.

469 Yancik R. Ovarian cancer. Age contrasts in incidence, histology, disease stage at diagnosis, and mortality. Cancer 1993, **71**: 517–523.

Ovarian tumors in children

470 Breen JL, Neubecker RD. Ovarian malignancy in children with special reference to the germ cell tumors. Ann N Y Acad Sci 1967, **142**: 658–674.

471 Ein SH, Darte JMM, Stephens CA. Cystic and solid ovarian tumors in children. A 44-year review. J Pediatr Surg 1970, **5**: 148–156.

472 Hawkins EP. Germ cell tumors. Am J Clin Pathol 1998, **109**: S82–S88.

473 Lack EE, Young RH, Scully RE. Pathology of ovarian neoplasms in childhood and adolescence. Pathol Annu 1992, **27**(Pt 2): 281–356.

474 Morris HB, La Vecchia C, Draper GJ. Malignant epithelial tumors of the ovary in childhood. A clinicopathological study of 13 cases in Great Britain 1962–1978. Gynecol Oncol 1984, **19**: 290–297.

475 Morris HB, La Vecchia C, Draper GJ. Endodermal sinus tumor and embryonal carcinoma of the ovary in children. Gynecol Obstet 1985, **21**: 7–17.

476 Norris HJ, Jensen RD. Relative frequency of ovarian neoplasms in children and adolescents. Cancer 1972, **30**: 713–719.

477 Wollner N, Exelby PR, Woodruff JM, Cham WC, Murphy L, Lewis JL. Malignant ovarian tumors in childhood. Prognosis in relation to initial therapy. Cancer 1976, **37**: 1953–1964.

478 Young RH, Kozakewich HP, Scully RE. Metastatic ovarian tumors in children. A report of 14 cases and review of the literature. Int J Gynecol Pathol 1993, **12**: 8–19.

479 Young RH. Ovarian tumors of the young. Int J Surg Pathol 2010, **18**(Suppl): 155S–161S.

480 Zaloudek C, Norris HJ. Granulosa tumors of the ovary in children. A clinical and pathologic study of 32 cases. Am J Surg Pathol 1982, **6**: 513–522.

'Early', 'occult', and in situ carcinoma

481 Agoff SN, Mendelin JE, Grieco VS, Garcia RL. Unexpected gynecologic neoplasms in patients with proven or suspected BRCA-1 or -2 mutations: implications for gross examination, cytology, and clinical follow-up. Am J Surg Pathol 2002, **26**: 171–178.

482 Bell DA, Scully RE. Early de novo ovarian carcinoma. A study of fourteen cases. Cancer 1994, **73**: 1859–1864.

483 Carcangiu ML, Peissel B, Pasini B, Spatti G, Radice P, Manoukian S. Incidental carcinomas in prophylactic specimens in BRCA1 and BRCA2 germ-line mutation carriers, with emphasis on fallopian tube lesions: report of 6 cases and review of the literature. Am J Surg Pathol 2006, **30**: 1222–1230.

484 Colgan TJ, Murphy J, Cole DE, Narod S, Rosen B. Occult carcinoma in prophylactic oophorectomy specimens: prevalence and association with BRCA germline mutation status. Am J Surg Pathol 2001, **25**: 1283–1289.

485 Fox H. Pathology of early malignant change in the ovary. Int J Gynecol Pathol 1993, **12**: 153–155.

486 Lu KH, Garber JE, Cramer DW, Welch WR, Niloff J, Schrag D, Berkowitz RS, Muto MG. Occult ovarian tumors in women with BRCA1 or BRCA2 mutations undergoing prophylactic oophorectomy. J Clin Oncol 2000, **18**: 2728–2732.

487 Mittal KR, Zeleniuch-Jacquotte A, Cooper JL, Demopoulos RI. Contralateral ovary in unilateral ovarian carcinoma. A search for preneoplastic lesions. Int J Gynecol Pathol 1993, **12**: 59–63.

488 Plaxe SC, Deligdisch L, Dottino PR, Cohen CJ. Ovarian intraepithelial neoplasia demonstrated in patients with stage I ovarian carcinoma. Gynecol Oncol 1990, **38**: 367–372.

489 Salazar H, Godwin AK, Daly MB, Laub PB, Hogan WM, Rosenblum N, Boente MP, Lynch HT, Hamilton TC. Microscopic benign and invasive malignant neoplasms and a cancer-prone phenotype in prophylactic oophorectomies. J Natl Cancer Inst 1997, **88**: 1810–1820.

490 Sherman ME, Lee JS, Burks RT, Struewing JP, Kurman RJ, Hartge P. Histopathologic features of ovaries at increased risk for carcinoma: a case-control analysis. Int J Gynecol Pathol 1999, **18**: 151–157.

Molecular genetic features

491 Berchuck A, Kohler MF, Boente MP, Rodriguez GC, Whitaker RS, Bast RC Jr. Growth regulation and transformation of ovarian epithelium. Cancer 1993, **71**: 545–551.

492 Bosari S, Viale G, Radaelli U, Bossi P, Bonoldi E, Coggi G. p53 accumulation in ovarian carcinomas and its prognostic implications. Hum Pathol 1993, **24**: 1175–1179.

493 Caduff RF, Svoboda-Newman SM, Ferguson AW, Johnston CM, Frank TS. Comparison of mutations of Ki-RAS and p53 immunoreactivity in borderline and malignant epithelial ovarian tumors. Am J Surg Pathol 1999, **23**: 323–328.

494 Cuatrecasas M, Erill N, Musulen E, Costa I, Matias-Guiu X, Prat J. K-ras mutations in nonmucinous ovarian epithelial tumors: a molecular analysis and clinicopathologic study of 144 patients. Cancer 1998, **82**: 1088–1095.

495 Cuatrecasas M, Villanueva A, Matias-Guiu X, Prat J. K-ras mutations in mucinous ovarian tumors: a clinicopathologic and molecular study of 95 cases. Cancer 1997, **79**: 1581–1586.

496 Frank TS, Bartos RE, Haefner HK, Roberts JA, Wilson MD, Hubbell GP. Loss of heterozygosity and overexpression of the p53 gene in ovarian carcinoma. Mod Pathol 1994, **7**: 3–8.

497 Garcia A, Bussaglia E, Machin P, Matias-Guiu X, Prat J. Loss of heterozygosity on chromosome 17q in epithelial ovarian tumors: association with carcinomas with serous differentiation. Int J Gynecol Pathol 2000, **19**: 152–157.

498 Gras E, Pons C, Machin P, Matias-Guiu X, Prat J. Loss of heterozygosity at the RB-1, locus and pRB immunostaining in epithelial ovarian tumors: a molecular, immunohistochemical, and clinicopathologic study. Int J Gynecol Pathol 2001, **20**: 335–340.

499 Hauptmann S, Dietel M. Serous tumors of low malignant potential of the ovary-molecular pathology: part 2. Virchows Arch 2001, **438**: 539–551.

500 Huettner PC, Weinberg DS, Lage JM. Assessment of proliferative activity in ovarian neoplasms by flow and static cytometry. Correlation with prognostic features. Am J Pathol 1992, **141**: 699–706.

501 Kacinski BM, Carter D, Mittal K, Yee LD, Scata KA, Donofrio L, Chambers SK, Wang KI, Yang-Feng T, Rohrschneider LR, et al. Ovarian adenocarcinomas express fms-complementary transcripts and fms antigen, often with coexpression of CSF-1. Am J Pathol 1990, **137**: 135–147.

502 Karbova E, Davidson B, Metodiev K, Thopé CG, Nesland JM. Adenomatous polyposis coli (APC) protein expression in primary and metastatic serous ovarian carcinoma. Int J Surg Pathol 2002, **10**: 175–180.

503 Kiechle-Schwarz M, Bauknecht T, Wienker T, Walz L, Pfleiderer A. Loss of constitutional heterozygosity on chromosome 11p in human ovarian cancer. Positive correlation with grade of differentiation. Cancer 1993, **72**: 2423–2432.

504 Kmet LM, Cook LS, Magliocco AM. A review of p53 expression and mutation in human benign, low malignant potential, and invasive epithelial ovarian tumors. Cancer 2003, **97**: 389–404.

505 Lage JM, Weinberg DS, Huettner PC, Mark SD. Flow cytometric analysis of nuclear DNA content in ovarian tumors. Association of ploidy with tumor type, histologic grade, and clinical stage. Cancer 1992, **69**: 2668–2675.

506 Leitao MM, Soslow RA, Baergen RN, Olvera N, Arroyo C, Boyd J. Mutation and expression of the TP53 gene in early stage epithelial ovarian carcinoma. Gynecol Oncol 2004, **93**: 301–306.

507 Otis CN, Krebs PA, Quezado MM, Alburquerque A, Bryant B, San Jaun X, Kleiner D, Sobel ME, Merino MJ. Loss of heterozygosity in P53, BRCA1, and estrogen receptors genes and correlation to expression of P53 protein in ovarian epithelial tumors of different cell types and biological behavior. Hum Pathol 2000, **31**: 233–238.

508 Palazzo JP, Monzon F, Burke M, Hyslop T, Dunton C, Barusevicius A, Capuzzi D, Kovatich J. Overexpression of p21WAF1/CIP1 and MDM2 characterize serous borderline ovarian tumors. Hum Pathol 2000, **31**: 698–704.

509 Pejovic T, Heim S, Mandahl N, Baldetorp B, Elmfors B, Flodérus U-M, Furgyik S, Göran H, Himmelmann A, Willén H, Mitelman F. Chromosome aberrations in 35 primary ovarian carcinomas. Genes Chromosom Cancer 1992, **4**: 58–68.

510 Persons DL, Hartmann LC, Herath JF, Borell TJ, Cliby WA, Keeney GL, Jenkins RB. Interphase molecular cytogenetic analysis of epithelial ovarian carcinomas. Am J Pathol 1993, **142**: 733–741.

511 Singer G, Kurman RJ, Chang HW, Cho SK, Shih IeM. Diverse tumorigenic pathways in ovarian serous carcinoma. Am J Pathol 2002, **160**: 1223–1228.

512 Slamon DJ, Godolphin W, Jones LA, Holt JA, Wong SG, Keith DE, Levin WJ, Stuart SG, Udove J, Ullrich A, et al. Studies of the HER-2/*neu* proto-oncogene in human breast and ovarian cancer. Science 1989, **244**: 707–712.

513 Tanyi J, Tory K, Amo-Takyi BK, Fuzesi L. Frequent loss of chromosome 12 in human epithelial ovarian tumors: a chromosomal in situ hybridization study. Int J Gynecol Pathol 1998, **17**: 106–112.

514 Wu R, Lin L, Beer DG, Ellenson LH, Lamb BJ, Rouillard J-M, Kuick R, Hanash S, Schwartz DR, Fearon ER, Cho KR. Amplification and overexpression of the L-MYC proto-oncogene in ovarian carcinomas. Am J Pathol 2003, **162**: 1603–1610.

515 Wu R, Zhai Y, Fearon ER, Cho KR. Diverse mechanisms of beta-catenin deregulation in ovarian endometrioid adenocarcinomas. Cancer Res 2001, **61**: 8247–8255.

516 Yang DH, Smith ER, Cohen C, Wu H Patriotis C, Godwin AK, Hamilton TC, Xu XX. Molecular events associated with dysplastic morphologic transformation and initiation of ovarian tumorigenicity. Cancer 2002, **94**: 2380–2392.

517 Yang-Feng TL, Han H, Chen KC, Li SB, Claus EB, Carcangiu ML, Chambers SK, Chambers JT, Schwartz PE. Allelic loss in ovarian cancer. Int J Cancer 1993, **54**: 546–551.

518 Yang-Feng TL, Li SB, Leung WY, Carcangiu ML, Schwartz PE. Trisomy 12 and K-*ras*-2 amplification in human ovarian tumors. Int J Cancer 1991, **48**: 678–681.

Spread and metastases

519 Brustman L, Seltzer V. Sister Joseph's nodule. Seven cases of umbilical metastases from gynecologic malignancies. Gynecol Oncol 1984, **19**: 155–162.

520 Djordjevic B, Malpica A. Lymph node involvement in ovarian serous tumors of low malignant potential: a clinicopathologic study of thirty-six cases. Am J Surg Pathol 2010, **34**: 1–9.

521 Dvoretsky PM, Richards KA, Bonfiglio TA. The pathology and biologic behavior of ovarian cancer. An autopsy review. Pathol Annu 1989, **24**(Pt 1): 1–24.

522 Euscher ED, Silva EG, Deavers MT, Elishaev E, Gershenson DM, Malpica A. Serous carcinoma of the ovary, fallopian tube, or peritoneum presenting as lymphadenopathy. Am J Surg Pathol 2004, **28**: 1217–1223.

523 Gilks CB, Alkushi A, Yue JJ, Lanvin D, Ehlen TG, Miller DM. Advanced-stage serous borderline tumors of the ovary: a clinicopathological study of 49 cases. Int J Gynecol Pathol 2002, **22**: 29–36.

524 Kerr VE, Cadman E. Pulmonary metastases in ovarian cancer. Analysis of 357 patients. Cancer 1985, **56**: 1209–1213.

525 Loredo DS, Powell JL, Reed WP, Rosenbaum JM. Ovarian carcinoma metastatic to breast. A case report and review of the literature. Gynecol Oncol 1990, **37**: 432–436.

526 McKenney JK, Balzer BL, Longacre TA. Lymph node involvement in ovarian serous tumors of low malignant potential (borderline tumors): pathology, prognosis, and proposed classification. Am J Surg Pathol 2006, **30**: 614–624.

527 Majmudar B, Wiskind AK, Croft BN, Dudley AG. The Sister (Mary) Joseph nodule. Its significance in gynecology. Gynecol Oncol 1991, **40**: 152–159.

528 Malpica A, Deavers MT, Gershenson D, Tortolero-Luna G, Silva EG. Serous tumors involving extra-abdominal/extra-pelvic sites after the diagnosis of an ovarian serous neoplasm of low malignant potential. Am J Surg Pathol 2001, **25**: 988–996.

529 Moran CA, Suster S, Silva EG. Low-grade serous carcinoma of the ovary metastatic to the anterior mediastinum simulating multilocular thymic cysts: a clinicopathologic and immunohistochemical study of 3 cases. Am J Surg Pathol 2005, **29**: 496–499.

530 Recine MA, Deavers MT, Middleton LP, Silva EG, Malpica A. Serous carcinoma of the ovary and peritoneum with metastases to the breast and axillary lymph nodes: a potential pitfall. Am J Surg Pathol 2004, **28**: 1646–1651.

531 Steinberg JJ, Demopoulos RI, Bigelow B. The evaluation of the omentum in ovarian cancer. Gynecol Oncol 1986, **24**: 327–330.

532 Verbruggen MB, Verheijen RH, van de Goot FR, van Beurden M, Dorsman JC, van Diest PJ. Serous borderline tumor of the ovary presenting with cervical lymph node involvement: a report of 3 cases. Am J Surg Pathol 2006, **30**: 739–743.

Peritoneal lesions and the müllerian system

533 Attanoos RL, Gibbs AR. Primary malignant gonadal mesotheliomas and asbestos. Histopathology 2000, **37**: 150–159.

534 Attanoos RL, Webb RL, Dojcinov SD, Gibbs AR. Value of mesothelial and epithelial antibodies in distinguishing diffuse peritoneal mesothelioma in females from serous papillary carcinoma of the ovary and peritoneum. Histopathology 2002, **40**: 237–244.

535 Bell DA, Scully RE. Benign and borderline serous lesions of the peritoneum in women. Pathol Annu 1989, **24**: 1–21.

536 Bell DA, Scully RE. Serous borderline tumors of the peritoneum. Am J Surg Pathol 1990, **14**: 230–239.

537 Bell DA, Weinstock MA, Scully RE. Peritoneal implants of ovarian serous borderline tumors. Histologic features and prognosis. Cancer 1988, **62**: 2212–2222.

538 Bell KA, Smith Sehdev AE, Kurman RJ. Refined diagnostic criteria for implants associated with ovarian atypical proliferative serous tumors (borderline) and micropapillary serous carcinoma. Am J Surg Pathol 2001, **25**: 419–432.

539 Biscotti CV, Hart WR. Peritoneal serous micropapillomatosis of low malignant potential (serous borderline tumors of the peritoneum). A clinicopathologic study of 17 cases. Am J Surg Pathol 1992, **16**: 467–475.

540 Bollinger DJ, Wick MR, Dehner LP, Mills SE, Swanson PE, Clarke RE. Peritoneal malignant mesothelioma versus serous-papillary adenocarcinoma. A histochemical and immunohistochemical comparison. Am J Surg Pathol 1989, **13**: 659–670.

541 Clement PB, Young RH. Florid mesothelial hyperplasia associated with ovarian tumors. A potential source of error in tumor diagnosis and staging. Int J Gynecol Pathol 1993, **12**: 51–58.

542 Clement PB, Young RH, Scully RE. Malignant mesotheliomas presenting as ovarian masses: a report of nine cases, including two primary ovarian mesotheliomas. Am J Surg Pathol 1996, **20**: 1067–1080.

543 Clement-Kruzel S, Malpica A, Djordjevic B. Endosalpingiosis in ovarian serous tumors of low malignant potential. Lab Invest 2009, **89**(Suppl 1): 210A.

544 Dalrymple JC, Bannatyne P, Russell P, Solomon HJ, Tattersall MH, Atkinson K, Carter J, Duval P, Elliott P, Friedlander M, et al. Extraovarian peritoneal serous papillary carcinoma. A clinicopathologic study of 31 cases. Cancer 1989, **64**: 110–115.

545 Djordjevic B, Clement-Kruzel S, Atkinson NE, Malpica A. Nodal endosalpingiosis in ovarian serous tumors of low malignant potential with lymph node involvement: a case for a precursor lesion. Am J Surg Pathol 2010, **34**: 1442–1448.

546 Gershenson DM, Silva EG. Serous ovarian tumors of low malignant potential with peritoneal implants. Cancer 1990, **65**: 578–585.

547 Gershenson DM, Silva EG, Levy L, Burke TW, Wolf JK, Tornos C. Ovarian serous borderline tumors with invasive peritoneal implants. Cancer 1998, **82**: 1096–1103.

548 Gershenson DM, Silva EG, Tortolero-Luna G, Levenback C, Morris M, Tornos C. Serous borderline tumors of the ovary with noninvasive peritoneal implants. Cancer 1998, **83**: 2157–2163.

549 Gu J, Roth LM, Younger C, Michael H, Abdul-Karim FW, Zhang S, Ulbright TM, Eble JN, Cheng L. Molecular evidence for the independent origin of extra-ovarian papillary serous tumors of low malignant potential. J Natl Cancer Inst 2001, **93**: 1147–1152.

550 Gupta S, Bhan AK, Bell DA. Can the implants of serous borderline tumors of the ovary be distinguished from mesothelial proliferations by use of immunohistochemistry? [abstract]. Mod Pathol 2003, **16**: 190a.

551 Halperin R, Zehavi S, Hadas E, Habler L, Bukovsky I, Schneider D. Immunohistochemical comparison of primary ovarian serous papillary carcinoma. Int J Gynecol Pathol 2001, **20**: 341–345.

552 Hutton RL, Dalton SR. Primary peritoneal serous borderline tumors. Arch Pathol Lab Med 2007, **131**: 138–144.

553 Khoury N, Raju U, Crissman JD, Zarbo RJ, Greenwald KA. A comparative immunohistochemical study of peritoneal and ovarian serous tumors, and mesotheliomas. Hum Pathol 1990, **21**: 811–819.

554 Kupryjanczyk J, Thor AD, Beauchamp R, Poremba C, Scully RE, Yandell DW. Ovarian, peritoneal, and endometrial serous carcinoma: clonal origin of multifocal disease. Mod Pathol 1996, **9**: 166–173.

555 Lauchlan SC. Non-invasive ovarian carcinoma. Int J Gynecol Pathol 1990, **9**: 158–169.

556 Lee J, Song SY, Park CS, Kim B. Mullerian cysts of the mesentery and retroperitoneum: a case report and literature review. Pathol Int 1999, **48**: 902–906.

557 Lee ES, Leong AS, Kim IS, Kim YS, Lee JH, Cho HY. Glomeruloid peritoneal implants in ovarian serous borderline tumours – distinction between invasive and non-invasive implants and pathogenesis. Histopathology 2009, **55**: 505–513.

558 Li S, Han H, Resnik E, Carcangiu ML, Schwartz PE, Yang-Feng TL. Advanced ovarian carcinoma. Molecular evidence of unifocal origin. Gynecol Oncol 1993, **51**: 21–25.

559 McCaughey WTE. Papillary peritoneal neoplasms in females. Pathol Annu 1985, **20**(Pt 2): 387–404.

560 McCaughey WTE, Kirk ME, Lester W, Dardick I. Peritoneal epithelial lesions associated with proliferative serous tumours of ovary. Histopathology 1984, **8**: 195–208.

561 Matsui K, Travis WD, Gonzalez R, Terzian JA, Rosai J, Moss J, Ferrans VJ. Association of lymphangioleiomyomatosis (LAM) with endosalpingiosis in the retroperitoneal lymph nodes: report of two cases. Int J Surg Pathol 2001, **9**: 155–162.

562 Michael H, Roth LM. Invasive and noninvasive implants in ovarian serous tumors of low malignant potential. Cancer 1986, **57**: 1240–1247.

563 Moore WF, Bentley RC, Berchuck A, Robboy SJ. Some Mullerian inclusion cysts in lymph nodes may sometimes be metastases from serous borderline tumors of the ovary. Am J Surg Pathol 2000, **24**: 710–718.

564 Piver MS, Jishi MF, Tsukada Y, Nava G. Primary peritoneal carcinoma after prophylactic oophorectomy in women with a family history of ovarian cancer. A report of the Gilda Radner Familial Ovarian Cancer Registry. Cancer 1993, **71**: 2751–2755.

565 Rollins SE, Young RH, Bell DA. Autoimplants in serous borderline tumors of the ovary: a clinicopathologic study of 30 cases of a process to be distinguished from serous adenocarcinoma. Am J Surg Pathol 2006, **30**: 457–462.

566 Rothacker D, Möbius G. Varieties of serous surface papillary carcinoma of the peritoneum in Northern Germany. A thirty-year autopsy study. Int J Gynecol Pathol 1995, **14**: 310–318.

567 Schorge JO, Muto MG, Welch WR, Bandera CA, Rubin SC, Bell DA, Berkowitz RS, Mok SC. Molecular evidence for multifocal papillary serous carcinoma of the peritoneum in patients with germline BRCA1 mutations. J Natl Cancer Inst 1998, **90**: 841–845.

568 Segal GH, Hart WR. Ovarian serous tumors of low malignant potential (serous borderline tumors). The relationship of exophytic surface tumor to peritoneal 'implants'. Am J Surg Pathol 1992, **16**: 577–583.

569 Seidman JD, Sherman ME, Bell KA, Katabunchi H, O'Leary TJ, Kurman RJ. Salpingitis, salpingoliths, and serous tumors of the ovaries: is there a connection? Int J Gynecol Pathol 2002, **21**: 101–107.

570 Stewart CJ, Brennan BA, Crook ML, Russell P. Value of elastin staining in the assessment of peritoneal implants associated with ovarian serous borderline tumours. Histopathology 2007, **51**: 313–321.

571 Warhol MJ, Hunter NJ, Corson JM. An ultrastructural comparison of mesotheliomas and adenocarcinomas of the ovary and endometrium. Int J Gynecol Pathol 1982, **1**: 125–134.

572 Weir MM, Bell DA, Young RH. Grade 1 peritoneal serous carcinomas: a report of 14 cases and comparison with 7 peritoneal serous psammocarcinomas and 19 peritoneal serous borderline tumors. Am J Surg Pathol 1998, **22**: 849–862.

573 Wick MR, Mills SE, Dehner LP, Bollinger DJ, Fechner RE. Serous papillary carcinomas arising from the peritoneum and ovaries. A clinicopathologic and immunohistochemical comparison. Int J Gynecol Pathol 1989, **8**: 179–188.

574 Zinsser KR, Wheeler JE. Endosalpingiosis in the omentum. A study of autopsy and surgical material. Am J Surg Pathol 1982, **6**: 109–117.

Coexistence with uterine carcinoma

575 Aguilera-Barrantes I, Euscher ED, Malpica A. Metastatic endocervical adenocarcinoma in the ovary: the MD Anderson experience. Lab Invest 2009, **89**(Suppl 1): 205A.

576 Eifel P, Hendrickson M, Ross J, Ballon S, Martinez A, Kempson R. Simultaneous presentation of carcinoma involving the ovary and the uterine corpus. Cancer 1982, **50**: 163–170.

577 Elishaev E, Gilks CB, Miller D, Srodon M, Kurman RJ, Ronnett BM. Synchronous and metachronous endocervical and ovarian neoplasms: evidence supporting interpretation of the ovarian neoplasms as metastatic endocervical adenocarcinomas simulating primary ovarian surface epithelial neoplasms. Am J Surg Pathol 2005, **29**: 281–294.

578 Kaminski PF, Norris HJ. Coexistence of ovarian neoplasms and endocervical adenocarcinoma. Obstet Gynecol 1984, **64**: 553–556.

579 Press MF. Are synchronous uterine and ovarian carcinomas independent primary tumors? Adv Anat Pathol 1997, **4**: 370–372.

580 Robboy SJ, Datto MB. Synchronous endometrial and ovarian tumors: metastatic disease or independent primaries? Hum Pathol 2005, **36**: 597–599.

581 Ulbright TM, Roth LM. Metastatic and independent cancers of the endometrium and ovary. A clinicopathologic study of 34 cases. Hum Pathol 1985, **16**: 28–34.

582 Young RH, Gersell DJ, Roth LM, Scully RE. Ovarian metastases from cervical carcinomas other than pure adenocarcinomas. A report of 12 cases. Cancer 1993, **71**: 407–418.

583 Zhang Y, Garcia MT, Koru-Sengul T, Ganjei-Azar P. A panel of immunohistochemical markers to distinguish ovarian from uterine serous papillary carcinomas. Lab Invest 2009, **89**(Suppl 1): 242A.

Cytology

584 Alli PM, Ali SZ. Micropapillary serous carcinoma of the ovary: cytomorphologic characteristics in peritoneal/pelvic washing. Cancer 2002, **96**: 135–139.

585 Covell JL, Carry JB, Feldman PS. Peritoneal washings in ovarian tumors. Potential sources of error in cytologic diagnosis. Acta Cytol (Baltimore) 1984, **29**: 310–316.

586 Ganjei P, Dickinson B, Harrison TA, Nassiri M, Lu Y. Aspiration cytology of neoplastic and non-neoplastic ovarian cysts: is it acute? Int J Gynecol Pathol 1996, **15**: 94–101.

587 Schwartz PE, Zheng W. Neoadjuvant chemotherapy for advanced ovarian cancer: the role of cytology in pretreatment diagnosis. Gynecol Oncol 2003, **90**: 644–650.

588 Stewart CJ, Kennedy JH. Peritoneal fluid cytology in serous borderline tumors of the ovary. Cytopathology 1998, **9**: 38–45.

589 Yoshimura S, Scully RE, Bell DA, Taft PD. Correlation of ascitic fluid cytology with histologic findings before and after treatment of ovarian cancer. Am J Obstet Gynecol 1984, **148**: 716–721.

590 Yoshimura S, Scully RE, Taft PD, Herrington JB. Peritoneal fluid cytology in patients with ovarian cancer. Gynecol Oncol 1984, **17**: 161–167.

591 Ziselman EM, Harkavy SE, Hogan M, West W, Atkinson B. Peritoneal washing cytology. Uses and diagnostic criteria in gynecologic neoplasms. Acta Cytol (Baltimore) 1983, **28**: 105–110.

Therapy

592 Armstrong DK, Bundy B, Wenzel L, Huang HQ, Baergen R, Lele S, Copeland LJ, Walker JL, Burger RA; Gynecologic Oncology Group. Intraperitoneal cisplatin and paclitaxel in ovarian cancer. N Engl J Med 2006, **354**: 34–43.

593 Averette HE, Donato DM. Ovarian carcinoma. Advances in diagnosis, staging, and treatment. Cancer 1990, **65**: 703–708.

594 Barber HRK. Ovarian cancer. Diagnosis and management. Am J Obstet Gynecol 1984, **150**: 910–916.

595 Burghardt E, Pickel H, Lahousen M, Stettner H. Pelvic lymphadenectomy in operative treatment of ovarian cancer. Am J Obstet Gynecol 1986, **155**: 315–319.

596 Coffin CM, Adcock LL, Dehner LP. The second-look operation for ovarian neoplasms. A study of 85 cases emphasizing cytologic and histologic problems. Int J Gynecol Pathol 1985, **4**: 97–109.

597 Dembo AJ. Radiotherapeutic management of ovarian cancer. Semin Oncol 1984, **11**: 238–250.

598 Fields AL, Runowicz CD. Current therapies in ovarian cancer. Cancer Invest 2003, **21**: 148–156.

599 Friedman JB, Weiss NS. Second thoughts about second-look laparotomy in advanced ovarian cancer. N Engl J Med 1990, **322**: 1079–1082.

600 Helewa ME, Krepart GV, Lotocki R. Staging laparotomy in early epithelial ovarian carcinoma. Am J Obstet Gynecol 1986, **154**: 282–286.

601 Lim-Tan SK, Cajigas HE, Scully RE. Ovarian cystectomy for serous borderline tumors. A follow-up study of 35 cases. Obstet Gynecol 1988, **72**: 775–781.

602 Lin PS, Gershenson DM, Bevers MW, Lucas KR, Burke TW, Silva EG. The current status of surgical staging of ovarian serous borderline tumors. Cancer 1999, **85**: 905–911.

603 McGuire WP. Primary treatment of epithelial ovarian malignancies. Cancer 1993, **71**: 1541–1550.

604 Manivel JC, Wick MR, Coffin CM, Dehner LP. Immunohistochemistry in the differential diagnosis in the second-look operation for ovarian carcinomas. Int J Gynecol Pathol 1989, **8**: 103–113.

605 Miller DS, Ballon SC, Teng NNH, Seifer DB, Soriero OM. A critical reassessment of second-look laparotomy in epithelial ovarian carcinoma. Cancer 1986, **57**: 530–535.

606 Miller DS, Spirtos NM, Ballon SC, Cox RS, Soriero OM, Teng NN. Critical reassessment of second-look exploratory laparotomy for epithelial ovarian carcinoma. Minimal diagnostic and therapeutic value in patients with persistent cancer. Cancer 1992, **69**: 502–510.

607 Podratz KC, Malkasian GD, Hilton JF, Harris EA, Gaffey TA. Second-look laparotomy in ovarian cancer. Evaluation of pathologic variables. Am J Obstet Gynecol 1985, **152**: 230–238.

608 Richardson GS, Scully RE, Nikrui N, Nelson JH. Common epithelial cancer of the ovary. N Engl J Med 1985, **312**: 415–424, 474–483.

609 Silva EG, Tornos C, Zhuang Z, Merino MJ, Gershenson DM. Tumor recurrence in stage I ovarian serous neoplasms of low malignant potential. Int J Gynecol Pathol 1998, **17**: 1–6.

610 Smirz LR, Stehman FB, Ulbright TM, Sutton GP, Ehrlich CE. Second-look laparotomy after chemotherapy in the management of ovarian malignancy. Am J Obstet Gynecol 1985, **152**: 661–668.

611 Tazelaar HD, Bostwick DG, Ballon SC, Hendrickson MR, Kempson RL. Conservative treatment of borderline ovarian tumors. Obstet Gynecol 1985, **66**: 417–422.

612 Thigpen JT, Lambuth BW, Vance RB. Management of stage I and II ovarian carcinoma. Semin Oncol 1991, **18**: 596–602.

613 Tropé C, Davidson B, Paulsen T, Abeler VM, Kaern J. Diagnosis and treatment of borderline ovarian neoplasms: 'the state of the art'. Eur J Gynaecol Oncol 2009, **30**: 471–482.

614 Young RC. Initial therapy for early ovarian carcinoma. Cancer 1987, **60**: 2042–2049.

615 Young RC, Walton LA, Ellenberg SS, Homesley HD, Wilbanks GD, Decker DG, Miller A, Park R, Major F Jr. Adjuvant therapy in stage I and stage II epithelial ovarian cancer. Results of two prospective randomized trials. N Engl J Med 1990, **322**: 1021–1027.

Prognosis

616 Ahmed FY, Wiltshaw E, Hern RPA, Nicol B, Shepherd J, Blake P, Fisher C. Gore ME. Natural history and prognosis of untreated stage I epithelial ovarian carcinoma. J Clin Oncol 1996, **14**: 2968–2975.

617 Beller U, Bigelow B, Beckman EM, Brown B, Demopoulos RI. Epithelial carcinoma of the ovary in the reproductive years. Clinical and morphological characterization. Gynecol Oncol 1983, **15**: 422–427.

618 Ben David Y, Chetrit A, Hirsh-Yechezkel G, Friedman E, Beck BD, Beller U, Ben-Baruch G, Fishman A, Levavi H, Lubin F, Menczer J, Piura B, Struewing JP, Modan B; National Israeli Study of Ovarian Cancer. Effect of BRCA mutations on the length of survival in epithelial ovarian tumors. J Clin Oncol 2002, **20**: 463–466.

619 Bostwick DG, Tazelaar HD, Ballon SC, Hendrickson MR, Kempson RL. Ovarian epithelial tumors of borderline malignancy. A clinical and pathologic study of 109 cases. Cancer 1986, **58**: 2052–2065.

620 Brescia RJ, Barakat RA, Beller U, Frederickson G, Suhrland MJ, Dubin N, Demopoulos RI. The prognostic significance of nuclear DNA content in malignant epithelial tumors of the ovary. Cancer 1990, **65**: 141–147.

621 Chu CS, Morgan MA, Randall TC, Bandera CA, Rubin SC. Survival of BRCA1 negative ovarian cancer patients based on family history. Gynecol Oncol 2001, **83**: 109–114.

622 Costa MJ, Hansen CL, Walls JE, Scudder SA. Immunohistochemical makers of cell control applied to ovarian and primary peritoneal surface epithelial neoplasms: p21$^{WAF/CIP1}$ predicts survival and good response to platinin-based chemotherapy. Hum Pathol 1999, **30**: 640–647.

623 Demirel D, Laucirica R, Fishman A, Ownes RG, Grey MM, Kaplan AL, Ramzy I. Ovarian tumors of low malignant potential: correlation of DNA index and S-phase fraction with histopathologic grade and clinical outcome. Cancer 1996, **77**: 1494–1500.

624 Demopoulos RI, Bigelow B, Blaustein A, Chait J, Gutman E, Dubin N. Characterization and survival of patients with serous cystadenocarcinoma of the ovaries. Obstet Gynecol 1984, **64**: 557–563.

625 DeRycke MS, Andersen JD, Harrington KM, Pambuccian SE, Kalloger SE, Boylan KL, Argenta PA, Skubitz AP. S100A1 expression in ovarian and endometrial endometrioid carcinomas is a prognostic indicator of relapse-free survival. Am J Clin Pathol 2009, **132**: 846–856.

626 Djordjevic B, Rosen DG, Liu J. Overexpression of EGFR is a poor prognostic indicator in ovarian cancer. Lab Invest 2009, **89**(Suppl 1): 12A.

627 Eltabbakh GH, Belinson JL, Kennedy AW, Biscotti CV, Casey G, Tubbs RR, Blumenson LE. p53 overexpression is not an independent prognostic factor for patients with primary ovarian epithelial cancer. Cancer 1997, **80**: 892–898.

628 Erhardt K, Auer G, Bjorkholm E, Forsslund G, Moberger B, Silfversward C, Wicksell G, Zetterberg A. Combined morphologic and cytochemical grading of serous ovarian tumors. Am J Obstet Gynecol 1985, **151**: 356–361.

629 Feichter GE, Kuhn W, Czernobilsky B, Muller A, Heep J, Abel U, Haag D, Kaufmann M, Rummel HH, Kubli F, Goerttler K. DNA flow cytometry of ovarian tumors with correlation to histopathology. Int J Gynecol Pathol 1985, **4**: 336–345.

630 Gansler TS, Hardman III W, Hunt DA, Schaffel S, Hennigar RA. Increased expression of fatty acid synthase (OA-519) in ovarian neoplasms predicts shorter survival. Hum Pathol 1997, **28**: 686–692.

631 Hartmann LC, Podratz KC, Keeney GL, Kamel NA, Edmonson JH, Grill JP, Su JQ, Katzmann JA, Roche PC. Prognostic significance of p53 immunostaining in epithelial ovarian cancer. J Clin Oncol 1994, **12**: 64–69.

632 Jóhannsson OT, Ranstam J, Borg A, Oisson H. Survival of BRCA1 breast and ovarian cancer patients: a population-based study from southern Sweden. J Clin Oncol 1998, **16**: 397–404.

633 Khalifa MA, Abdoh AA, Mannel RS, Walker JL, Angros LH, Min KW. P-Glycoprotein as a prognostic indicator in pre- and postchemotherapy ovarian adenocarcinoma. Int J Gynecol Pathol 1997, **16**: 69–75.

634 Köbel M, Kalloger SE, Santos JL, Huntsman DG, Gilks CB, Swenerton KD. Tumor type and substage predict survival in stage I and II ovarian carcinoma: insights and implications. Gynecol Oncol 2010, **116**: 50–56.

635 Köbel M, Gradhand E, Zeng K, Schmitt WD, Kriese K, Lantzsch T, Wolters M, Dittmer J, Strauss HG, Thomssen C, Hauptmann S. Ezrin promotes ovarian carcinoma cell invasion and its retained expression predicts poor prognosis in ovarian carcinoma. Int J Gynecol Pathol 2006, **25**: 121–130.

636 Kohn EC. Angiogenesis in ovarian carcinoma: a formidable biomarker. Cancer 1998, **80**: 2219–2221.

637 Kristiansen G, Denkert C, Scluns K, Dahl E, Pilarsky C, Haupmann S. CD24 is expressed in ovarian cancer and is a new independent prognostic marker of patient survival. Am J Pathol 2002, **161**: 1215–1221.

638 Kurman RJ, Trimble CL. The behavior of serous tumors of low malignant potential. Are they ever malignant? Int J Gynecol Pathol 1993, **12**: 120–127.

639 Levesque MA, Katsaros D, Yu H, Zola P, Sismondi P, Giardina G, Diamandis EP. Mutant p53 protein overexpression is associated with poor outcome in patients with well or moderately differentiated ovarian carcinoma. Cancer 1995, **75**: 1327–1338.

640 Longacre TA, McKenney JK, Tazelaar HD, Kempson RL, Hendrickson MR. Ovarian serous tumors of low malignant potential (borderline tumors): outcome-based study of 276 patients with long-term (> or =5-year) follow-up. Am J Surg Pathol 2005, **29**: 707–723.

641 Malkasian GD, Melton LJ, O'Brien PC, Greene MH. Prognostic significance of histologic classification and grading of epithelial malignancies of the ovary. Am J Obstet Gynecol 1984, **149**: 274–284.

642 Malpica A, Deavers MT, Lu K, Bodurka DC, Atkinson EN, Gershenson DM, Silva EG. Grading ovarian serous carcinoma using a two-tier system. Am J Surg Pathol 2004, **28**: 496–504.

643 Mayr D, Diebold J. Grading of ovarian carcinomas. Int J Gynecol Pathol 2001, **19**: 348–353.

644 Meden H, Marx D, Rath W, Kron M, Fattahi-Meibodi A, Hinney B, Kuhn W, Schauer A. Overexpression of the oncogene c-*erb*B2 in primary ovarian cancer. Evaluation of the prognostic value in a Cox proportional hazards multiple regression. Int J Gynecol Pathol 1994, **13**: 45–53.

645 Narod SA, Boyd J. Current understanding of the epidemiology and clinical implications of BRCA1 and BRCA2 mutations for ovarian cancer. Curr Opin Obstet Gynecol 2002, **14**: 19–26.

646 Newcomb EW, Sosnow M, Demopoulos RI, Zeleniuch-Jacquotte A, Sorich J, Speyer JL. Expression of the cell cycle inhibitor p27^{KIP1} is a new prognostic marker associated with survival in epithelial ovarian tumors. Am J Pathol 1999, **154**: 119–125.

647 Nikrui N. Survey of clinical behavior of patients with borderline epithelial tumors of the ovary. Gynecol Pathol 1981, **12**: 107–119.

648 Rodenburg CJ, Cornelisse CJ, Heintz PAM, Hermans J, Fleuren GJ. Tumor ploidy as a major prognostic factor in advanced ovarian cancer. Cancer 1987, **59**: 317–323.

649 Rubin SC, Benjamin I, Behbakht K, Takahasi H, Morgan MA, LiVolsi VA, Berchuck A, Muto MG, Garber JE, Weber BL, Lynch HT, Boyd J. Clinical and pathological features of ovarian cancer in women with germ-line mutations of BRCA1. N Engl J Med 1996, **335**: 1413–1416.

650 Saksela E. Prognostic markers in epithelial ovarian cancer. Int J Gynecol Pathol 1993, **12**: 156–161.

651 Sato Y, Shimamoto T, Amanda S, Asada Y, Hayashi T. Prognostic value of histologic grading of ovarian carcinomas. Int J Gynecol Pathol 2002, **22**: 52–56.

652 Scambia G, Ferrandina G, Marone M, Benedetti Panici P, Giannitelli C, Piantelli M, Leone A, Mancuso S. nm23 in ovarian cancer: correlation with clinical outcome and other clinicopathologic and biochemical prognostic parameters. J Clin Oncol 1996, **14**: 334–342.

653 Schoell WM, Pieber D, Reich O, Lahousen M, Janicek M, Gurcer F, Winter R. Tumor angiogenesis as a prognostic factor in ovarian carcinoma: qualification of endothelial immunoreactivity by image analysis. Cancer 1998, **80**: 2257–2262.

654 Seidman JD, Kurman RJ. Ovarian serous borderline tumors: a critical review of the literature with emphasis on prognostic indicators. Hum Pathol 2000, **31**: 539–557.

655 Seidman JD, Yemelyanova AV, Khedmati F, Bidus MA, Dainty L, Boice CR, Cosin JA. Prognostic factors for stage I ovarian carcinoma. Int J Gynecol Pathol 2010, **29**: 1–7.

656 Sevelda P, Dittrich C, Salzer H. Prognostic value of the rupture of the capsule in stage I epithelial ovarian carcinoma. Gynecol Oncol 1989, **35**: 321–322.

657 Sevelda P, Schemper M, Spona J. CA 125 as an independent prognostic factor for survival in patients with epithelial ovarian cancer. Am J Obstet Gynecol 1989, **161**: 1213–1216.

658 Shahin MS, Hughes JH, Sood AK, Buller RE. The prognostic significance of p53 tumor suppressor gene alterations in ovarian carcinoma. Cancer 2000, **89**: 2006–2017.

659 Shimizu Y, Kamoi S, Amada S, Akiyama F, Silverberg SG. Toward the development of a universal grading system for ovarian epithelial carcinoma: testing of a proposed system in a series of 461 patients with uniform treatment and follow-up. Cancer 1998, **82**: 893–901.

660 Silverberg SG. Histopathologic grading of ovarian carcinoma: a review and proposal. Int J Gynecol Pathol 2000, **19**: 7–15.

661 Sorbe B, Frankendal BO. Prognostic importance of psammoma bodies in adenocarcinomas of the ovaries. Gynecol Oncol 1982, **14**: 6–14.

662 Sorbe B, Frankendal BO, Veress B. Importance of histologic grading in the prognosis of epithelial ovarian carcinoma. Obstet Gynecol 1982, **59**: 576–582.

663 Swenerton KD, Hislop TG, Spinelli J, LeRiche JC, Yang N, Boyes DA. Ovarian carcinoma. A multivariate analysis of prognostic factors. Obstet Gynecol 1985, **65**: 264–270.

664 Thigpen T, Brady MF, Omura GA, Creasman WT, McGuire WP, Hoskins WJ, Williams S. Age as a prognostic factor in ovarian carcinoma. The Gynecologic Oncology Group experience. Cancer 1993, **71**: 606–614.

665 Tornos C, Silva EG, Khorana SM, Burke TW. High-stage endometrioid carcinoma of the ovary. Prognostic significance of pure versus mixed histologic types. Am J Surg Pathol 1994, **18**: 687–693.

666 Zhang L, Conejo-Garcia JR, Katsaros D, Gimotty PA, Massobrio M, Regnani G, Makrigiannakis A, Gray H, Schlienger K, Liebman MN, Rubin SC, Coukos G. Intratumoral T cells, recurrence, and survival in epithelial ovarian cancer. N Engl J Med 2003, **348**: 203–213.

GERM CELL TUMORS

667 Chang MC, Vargas SO, Hornick JL, Hirsch MS, Crum CP, Nucci MR. Embryonic stem cell transcription factors and D2-40 (podoplanin) as diagnostic immunohistochemical markers in ovarian germ cell tumors. Int J Gynecol Pathol 2009, **28**: 347–355.

668 Gershenson DM. Update on malignant ovarian germ cell tumors. Cancer 1993, **71**: 1581–1590.

669 Gershenson DM, Del Junco G, Copeland LJ, Rutledge FN. Mixed germ cell tumors of the ovary. Obstet Gynecol 1984, **64**: 200–206.

670 Hart AH, Hartley L, Parker K, Ibrahim M, Looijenga LH, Pauchnik M, Chow CW, Robb L. The pluripotency homeobox gene NANOG is expressed in human germ cell tumors. Cancer 2005, **104**: 2092–2098.

671 Hawkins EP. Germ cell tumors. Am J Clin Pathol 1998, **109**: S82–S88.

672 Iczkowski KA, Butler SL, Shanks JH, Hossain D, Schall A, Meiers I, Zhou M, Torkko KC, Kim SJ, MacLennan GT. Trials of new germ cell immunohistochemical stains in 93 extragonadal and metastatic germ cell tumors. Hum Pathol 2008, **39**: 275–281.

673 Jondle DM, Shahin MS, Sorosky J, Benda JA. Ovarian mixed germ cell tumor with predominance of polyembryoma: a case report with literature review. Int J Gynecol Pathol 2002, **21**: 78–81.

674 Kurman RJ, Norris HJ. Malignant mixed germ cell tumors of the ovary. A clinical and pathologic analysis of 30 cases. Obstet Gynecol 1976, **48**: 579–589.

675 Kurman RJ, Norris HJ. Malignant germ cell tumors of the ovary. Hum Pathol 1977, **8**: 551–564.

676 Pfleiderer A. Therapy of ovarian malignant germ cell tumors and granulosa tumors. Int J Gynecol Pathol 1993, **12**: 162–165.

677 Roth LM, Talerman A. Recent advances in the pathology and classification of ovarian germ cell tumors. Int J Gynecol Pathol 2006, **25**: 305–320.

678 Ulbright TM. Germ cell tumors of the gonads: a selective review emphasizing problems in differential diagnosis, newly appreciated, and controversial issues. Mod Pathol 2005, **18**(Suppl 2): S61–S79.

679 Young RH. New and unusual aspects of ovarian germ cell tumors. Am J Surg Pathol 1993, **17**: 1210–1224.

Dysgerminoma

680 Abell MR, Johnson VJ, Holtz F. Ovarian neoplasms in childhood and adolescence. Am J Obstet Gynecol 1965, **92**: 1059–1081.

681 Abu-Rustum NR, Aghajanian C. Management of malignant germ cell tumors of the ovary. Semin Oncol 1998, **25**: 235–242.

682 Asadourian LA, Taylor HB. Dysgerminoma. An analysis of 105 cases. Obstet Gynecol 1969, **33**: 370–379.

683 Beckstead JH. Alkaline phosphatase histochemistry in human germ cell neoplasms. Am J Surg Pathol 1983, **7**: 341–349.

684 Bjorkholm E, Lundell M, Gyftodimos A, Silfversward C. Dysgerminoma. The Radiumhemmet series 1927–1984. Cancer 1990, **65**: 38–44.

685 Cao D, Guo S, Allan RW, Molberg KH, Peng Y. SALL4 is a novel sensitive and specific marker of ovarian primitive germ cell tumors and is particularly useful in distinguishing yolk sac tumor from clear cell carcinoma. Am J Surg Pathol 2009, **33**: 894–904.

686 Cheng L, Thomas A, Roth LM, Zheng W, Michael H, Karim FW. OCT4: a novel biomarker for dysgerminoma of the ovary. Am J Surg Pathol 2004, **28**: 1341–1346.

687 Cossu-Rocca P, Jones TD, Roth LM, Eble JN, Zheng W, Karim FW, Cheng L. Cytokeratin and CD30 expression in dysgerminoma. Hum Pathol 2006, **37**: 1015–1021.

688 Creasman WT, Fetter BF, Hammond CB, Parker RT. Germ cell malignancies of the ovary. Obstet Gynecol 1979, **53**: 226–230.

689 Dietl J, Horny HP, Ruck P, Kaiserling E. Dysgerminoma of the ovary. An immunohistochemical study of tumor-infiltrating lymphoreticular cells and tumor cells. Cancer 1993, **71**: 2562–2568.

690 Fleischhacker DS, Young RH. Dysgerminoma of the ovary associated with hypercalcemia. Gynecol Oncol 1994, **52**: 87–90.

691 Freel JH, Cassir JF, Pierce VK, Woodruff J, Lewis JL Jr. Dysgerminoma of the ovary. Cancer 1979, **43**: 798–805.

692 Gershenson DM. Update on malignant ovarian germ cell tumors. Cancer 1993, **71**: 1581–1590.

693 Gibas Z, Talerman A. Analysis of chromosome aneuploidy in ovarian dysgerminoma by flow cytometry and fluorescence in situ hybridization. Diagn Mol Pathol 1993, **2**: 50–56.

694 Gillespie JJ, Arnold LK. Anaplastic dysgerminoma. Cancer 1978, **42**: 1886–1889.

695 Gondos B. Comparative studies of normal and neoplastic ovarian germ cells. II. Ultrastructure and pathogenesis of dysgerminoma. Int J Gynecol Pathol 1987, **6**: 124–131.

696 Krepart G, Smith JP, Rutledge F, Delclos L. The treatment for dysgerminoma of the ovary. Cancer 1978, **41**: 986–990.

697 Lifshitz-Mercer B, Walt H, Kushnir I, Jacob N, Diener PA, Moll R, Czernobilsky B. Differentiation potential of ovarian dysgerminoma. An immunohistochemical study of 15 cases. Hum Pathol 1995, **26**: 62–66.

698 Low JJ, Perrin LC, Crandon AJ, Hacker NF. Conservative surgery to preserve ovarian function in patients with malignant ovarian germ cell tumors: a review of 74 cases. Cancer 2000, **89**: 391–398.

699 Parkash V, Carcangiu ML. Transformation of ovarian dysgerminoma to yolk sac tumor. Evidence for a histogenetic continuum. Mod Pathol 1995, **8**: 881–887.

700 Przgodzki RM, Moran C, Hubbs AE, Malpica A, O'Leary T. Ovarian dysgerminoma: evidence of unique single and multiple KIT mutations [abstract]. Mod Pathol 2003, **16**: 206a.

701 Santesson L. Clinical and pathological survey of ovarian tumors treated at the Radiumhemmet. Acta Radiol (Stockh) 1947, **28**: 643–668.

702 Sever M, Jones TD, Roth LM, Karim FW, Zheng W, Michael H, Hattab EM, Emerson RE, Baldridge LA, Cheng L. Expression of CD117 (c-kit) receptor in dysgerminoma of the ovary: diagnostic and therapeutic implications. Mod Pathol 2005, **18**: 1411–1416.

703 Zaloudek CJ, Tavassoli FA, Norris HJ. Dysgerminoma with syncytiotrophoblastic giant cells. A histologically and clinically distinctive subtype of dysgerminoma. Am J Surg Pathol 1981, **5**: 361–367.

Yolk sac tumor (endodermal sinus tumor) and embryonal carcinoma

704 Abu-Rustum NR, Aghajanian C. Management of malignant germ cell tumors of the ovary. Semin Oncol 1998, **25**: 235–242.

705 Barsky SH, Hannah JB. Extracellular hyaline bodies are basement membrane accumulations. Am J Clin Pathol 1987, **87**: 455–460.

706 Cheng L, Zhang S, Talerman A, Roth LM. Morphologic, immunohistochemical, and fluorescence in situ hybridization study of ovarian embryonal carcinoma with comparison to solid variant of yolk sac tumor and immature teratoma. Hum Pathol 2010, **41**: 716–723.

707 Clement PB, Young RH, Scully RE. Endometrioid-like variant of ovarian yolk sac tumor. A clinicopathological analysis of eight cases. Am J Surg Pathol 1987, **11**: 767–778.

708 Clement PB, Young RH, Scully RE. Extraovarian pelvic yolk sac tumors. Cancer 1988, **62**: 620–626.

709 Cohen MB, Friend DS, Molnar JJ. Gonadal endodermal sinus (yolk sac) tumor with pure intestinal differentiation. A new histologic type. Pathol Res Pract 1987, **182**: 609–616.

710 Creasman WT, Soper JT. Assessment of the contemporary management of germ cell malignancies of the ovary. Am J Obstet Gynecol 1985, **153**: 828–834.

711 Devouassoux-Shisheboran M, Schammel DP, Tavassoli FA. Ovarian hepatoid yolk sac tumors: morphological, immunohistochemical and ultrastructural features. Histopathology 1999, **34**: 462–469.

712 Gershenson DM, Del Junco G, Herson J, Rutledge FN. Endodermal sinus tumor of the ovary. The M.D. Anderson experience. Obstet Gynecol 1983, **61**: 194–202.

713 Gonzalez-Crussi F. The human yolk sac and yolk sac (endodermal sinus) tumors. A review. Persp Pediatr Pathol 1979, **5**: 179–215.

714 Ishikura H, Scully RE. Hepatoid carcinoma of the ovary. A newly described tumor. Cancer 1987, **60**: 2775–2784.

715 Jondle DM, Shahin MS, Sorosky J, Benda JA. Ovarian mixed germ cell tumor with predominance of polyembryoma: a case report with literature review. Int J Gynecol Pathol 2002, **21**: 78–81.

716 Jones MA, Clement PB, Young RH. Primary yolk sac tumors of the mesentery. A report of two cases. Am J Clin Pathol 1994, **101**: 42–47.

717 Kawai M, Furuhashi Y, Kano T, Misawa T, Nakashima N, Hattori S, Okamoto Y, Kobayashi I, Ohta M, Arii Y, et al. Alpha-fetoprotein in malignant germ cell tumors of the ovary. Gynecol Oncol 1990, **39**: 160–166.

718 Kawai M, Kano T, Furuhashi Y, Mizuno K, Nakashima N, Hattori SE, Kazeto S, Iida S, Ohta M, Arii Y, et al. Prognostic factors in yolk sac tumors of the ovary. A clinicopathologic analysis of 29 cases. Cancer 1991, **67**: 184–192.

719 Kommoss F, Bibbo M, Talerman A. Nuclear deoxyribonucleic acid content (ploidy) of endodermal sinus (yolk sac) tumor. Lab Invest 1990, **62**: 223–231.

720 Kurman RJ, Norris HJ. Endodermal sinus tumor of the ovary. A clinical and pathologic analysis of 71 cases. Cancer 1976, **38**: 2404–2419.

721 Kurman RJ, Norris HJ. Embryonal carcinoma of the ovary. A clinicopathologic entity distinct from endodermal sinus tumor resembling embryonal carcinoma of the adult testis. Cancer 1976, **38**: 2420–2433.

722 Langley FA, Govan ADT, Anderson MC, Gowing NFC, Woodcock AS, Harilal KR. Yolk sac and allied tumours of the ovary. Histopathology 1981, **5**: 389–401.

723 Michael H, Ulbright TM, Brodhecker CA. The pluripotential nature of the mesenchyme-like component of yolk sac tumor. Arch Pathol Lab Med 1989, **113**: 1115–1119.

724 Nawa A, Obata N, Kikkawa F, Kawai M, Nagasaka T, Goto S, Nishimori K, Nakashima N. Prognostic factors of patients with yolk sac tumors of the ovary. Am J Obstet Gynecol 2001, **184**: 1182–1188.

725 Nogales FF. Embryologic clues to human yolk sac tumors. A review. Int J Gynecol Pathol 1993, **12**: 101–107.

726 Nogales FF, Beltran E, Pavcovich M, Bustos M. Ectopic somatic endoderm in secondary human yolk sac. Hum Pathol 1992, **23**: 921–924.

727 Nogales FF Jr, Matilla A, Nogales-Ortiz F, Galera-Davidson HL. Yolk sac tumors with pure and mixed polyvesicular vitelline patterns. Hum Pathol 1978, **9**: 553–566.

728 Nogales-Fernandez G, Silverberg SG, Bloustein PA, Martinez-Hernandez A, Pierce GB. Yolk sac carcinoma (endodermal sinus tumor). Ultrastructure and histogenesis of gonadal and extragonadal tumors in comparison with normal human yolk sac. Cancer 1977, **39**: 1462–1474.

729 Nogales FF, Buriticá C, Regauer S, González T. Mucinous carcinoid as an unusual manifestation of endodermal differentiation in ovarian yolk sac tumors. Am J Surg Pathol 2005, **29**: 1247–1251.

730 Oh C, Kendler A, Hernandez E. Ovarian endodermal sinus tumor in a postmenopausal woman. Gynecol Oncol 2001, **82**: 392–394.

731 Park NH, Ryu SY, Park IA, Kang SB, Lee HP. Primary endodermal sinus tumor of the omentum. Gynecol Oncol 1999, **72**: 427–430.

732 Prat J, Bhan AK, Dickersin GR, Robboy SJ, Scully RE. Hepatoid yolk sac tumor of the ovary (endodermal sinus tumor with hepatoid differentiation). A light microscopic, ultrastructural and immunohistochemical study of seven cases. Cancer 1982, **50**: 2355–2368.

733 Ramalingam P, Malpica A, Silva EG, Gershenson DM, Liu JL, Deavers MT. The use of cytokeratin 7 and EMA in differentiating ovarian yolk sac tumors from endometrioid and clear cell carcinomas. Am J Surg Pathol 2004, **28**: 1499–1505.

734 Schiller W. Mesonephroma ovarii. Am J Cancer 1939, **35**: 1–21.

735 Siltanen S, Anttonen M, Heikkila P, Narita N, Laitinen M, Ritvos O, Wilson DB, Heikinheimo M. Transcription factor GATA-4 is expressed in pediatric yolk sac tumors. Am J Pathol 1999, **155**: 1823–1829.

736 Talerman A, Haije WG, Baggerman L. Serum alphafetoprotein (AFP) in diagnosis and management of endodermal sinus (yolk sac) tumor and mixed germ cell tumor of the ovary. Cancer 1978, **41**: 272–278.

737 Teilum G. Endodermal sinus tumors of the ovary and testis. Comparative morphogenesis of the so-called mesonephroma ovarii (Schiller) and extraembryonic (yolk sac-allantoic) structures of the rat's placenta. Cancer 1959, **12**: 1092–1105.

738 Ulbright TM, Roth LM, Brodhecker CA. Yolk sac differentiation in germ cell tumors. A morphologic study of 50 cases with emphasis on hepatic, enteric, and parietal yolk sac features. Am J Surg Pathol 1986, **10**: 151–164.

739 Wang F, Liu A, Peng Y, Rakheja D, Wei L, Xue D, Allan RW, Molberg KH, Li J, Cao D. Diagnostic utility of SALL4 in extragonadal yolk sac tumors: an immunohistochemical study of 59 cases with comparison to placental-like alkaline phosphatase, alpha-fetoprotein, and glypican-3. Am J Surg Pathol 2009, **33**: 1529–1539.

740 Zynger DL, McCallum JC, Luan C, Chou PM, Yang XJ. Glypican 3 has a higher sensitivity than alpha-fetoprotein for testicular and ovarian yolk sac tumour: immunohistochemical investigation with analysis of histological growth patterns. Histopathology 2010, **56**: 750–757.

Choriocarcinoma

741 Axe SR, Klein VR, Woodruff JD. Choriocarcinoma of the ovary. Obstet Gynecol 1985, **66**: 111–114.

742 Damjanov I, Osborn M, Miettinen M. Keratin 7 is a marker for a subset of trophoblastic cells in human germ cell tumors. Arch Pathol Lab Med 1990, **114**: 81–83.

743 Garin-Chesa P, Campbell I, Saigo PE, Lewis JL Jr, Old LJ, Rettig WJ. Trophoblast and ovarian cancer antigen LK26. Sensitivity and specificity in immunopathology and molecular identification as a folate-binding protein. Am J Pathol 1993, **142**: 557–567.

744 Gerbie MV, Brewer JI, Tamini H. Primary choriocarcinoma of the ovary. Obstet Gynecol 1975, **46**: 720–723.

745 Goswami D, Sharma K, Zutshi V, Tempe A, Nigam S. Nongestational pure ovarian choriocarcinoma with contralateral teratoma. Gynecol Oncol 2001, **80**: 262–266.

746 Oliva E, Andrada E, Pezzica E, Prat J. Ovarian carcinomas with choriocarcinomatous differentiation. Cancer 1993, **72**: 2441–2446.

747 Vance RP, Geisinger KR. Pure nongestational choriocarcinoma of the ovary. Report of a case. Cancer 1985, **56**: 2321–2325.

Immature (malignant) teratoma

748 Aguirre P, Scully RE. Malignant neuroectodermal tumor of the ovary, a distinctive form of monodermal teratoma. Report of five cases. Am J Surg Pathol 1982, **6**: 283–292.

749 Baker PM, Rosai J, Young RH. Ovarian teratomas with florid benign vascular proliferation: a distinctive finding associated with the neural component of teratomas that may be confused with a vascular neoplasm. Int J Gynecol Pathol 2002, **21**: 16–21.

750 Beilby JOW, Parkinson C. Features of prognostic significance in solid ovarian teratoma. Cancer 1975, **36**: 2147–2159.

751 Culine S, Lhomme C, Kattan J, Michel G, Duvillard P, Droz JP. Pure malignant immature teratoma of the ovary: the role of chemotherapy and second-look surgery. Int J Gynecol Cancer 1995, **5**: 432–437.

752 Gaudin PB, Rosai J. Florid vascular proliferation associated with neural and neuroendocrine neoplasms. A diagnostic clue and potential pitfall. Am J Surg Pathol 1995, **19**: 642–652.

753 Gibas Z, Talerman A, Faruqi S, Carlson J, Noumoff J. Cytogenetic analysis of an immature teratoma of the ovary and its metastasis after chemotherapy-induced maturation. Int J Gynecol Pathol 1993, **12**: 276–280.

754 Guerrieri C, Jarlsfelt I. Ependymoma of the ovary. A case report with immunohistochemical, ultrastructural, and DNA cytometric findings, as well as histogenetic considerations. Am J Surg Pathol 1993, **17**: 623–632.

755 Heifetz SA, Cushing B, Giller R, Shuster JJ, Stolar CJ, Vinocur CD, Hawkins EP. Immature teratomas in children: pathologic considerations: a report from the combined pediatric oncology group / children's cancer group. Am J Surg Pathol 1998, **22**: 1115–1124.

756 Ihara T, Ohama K, Satoh H, Fujii TV, Nomura K, Fujiwara A. Histologic grade and karyotype of immature teratoma of the ovary. Cancer 1984, **54**: 2988–2994.

757 Kawai M, Kano T, Furuhashi Y, Iwata M, Nakashima N, Imai N, Kuzuya K, Hayashi H, Ohta M, Arii Y, et al. Immature teratoma of the ovary. Gynecol Oncol 1991, **40**: 133–137.

758 King ME, Micha JP, Allen SL, Mouradian JA, Chaganti RSK. Immature teratoma of the ovary with predominant malignant retinal anlage component. A parthenogenically derived tumor. Am J Surg Pathol 1985, **9**: 221–231.

759 Kleinman GM, Young RH, Scully RE. Ependymoma of the ovary. Report of three cases. Hum Pathol 1984, **15**: 632–638.

760 Kleinman GM, Young RH, Scully RE. Primary neuroectodermal tumors of the ovary. A report of 25 cases. Am J Surg Pathol 1993, **17**: 764–778.

761 Koulos JP, Hoffman JS, Steinhoff MM. Immature teratoma of the ovary. Gynecol Oncol 1989, **34**: 46–49.

762 Metzman RA, Warhol MJ, Gee B, Roth J. Polysialic acid as a marker of both immature and mature neural tissue in human teratomas. Mod Pathol 1991, **4**: 491–497.

763 Nogales FF Jr, Favara BE, Major FJ, Silverberg SG. Immature teratoma of the ovary with a neural component ('solid' teratoma). Hum Pathol 1976, **7**: 625–642.

764 Nogales FF Jr, Ortega I, Rivera F, Armas JR. Metanephrogenic tissue in immature ovarian teratoma. Am J Surg Pathol 1980, **4**: 297–299.

765 Nogales FF, Ruiz Avila I, Concha A, del Moral E. Immature endodermal teratoma of the ovary. Embryologic correlations and immunohistochemistry. Hum Pathol 1993, **24**: 364–370.

766 Norris HJ, Zirkin HJ, Benson WL. Immature (malignant) teratoma of the ovary. A clinical and pathologic study of 58 cases. Cancer 1976, **37**: 2359–2372.

767 Notohara K, Hsueh CL, Awai M. Glial fibrillary acidic protein immunoreactivity of chondrocytes in immature and mature teratomas. Acta Pathol Jpn 1990, **40**: 335–342.

768 O'Connor DM, Norris HJ. The influence of grade on the outcome of stage I ovarian immature (malignant) teratomas and the reproducibility of grading. Int J Gynecol Pathol 1994, **13**: 283–289.

769 Ramdial PK, Bagratee JS. Membranous fat necrosis in mature cystic teratomas of the ovary. Int J Gynecol Pathol 1998, **17**: 120–122.

770 Schwartz PE, Merino MJ, LiVolsi VA. Immature ovarian teratomas. Maturation following chemotherapy. Am J Diagn Gynecol Obstet 1979, **1**: 361–366.

771 Steeper TA, Mukai K. Solid ovarian teratomas. An immunocytochemical study of thirteen cases with clinicopathologic correlation. Pathol Annu 1984, **19**(Pt 1): 81–92.

772 Yanai H, Matsuura H, Kawasaki M, Takada Y, Tabuchi Y, Yoshino T. Immature teratoma of the ovary with a minor rhabdomyosarcomatous component and fatal rhabdomyosarcomatous metastases: the first case in a child. Int J Gynecol Pathol 2002, **21**: 82–85.

Mature solid teratoma

773 Benirschke K, Easterday C, Abramson D. Malignant solid teratoma of the ovary. Report of three cases. Obstet Gynecol 1960, **15**: 512–521.

774 Peterson WF. Solid, histologically benign teratomas of the ovary. A report of four cases and review of the literature. Am J Obstet Gynecol 1956, **72**: 1094–1102.

775 Thurlbeck WM, Scully RE. Solid teratoma of the ovary. A clinicopathological analysis of 9 cases. Cancer 1960, **13**: 804–811.

Mature cystic teratoma

776 Ackerman LV. Autobiographical notes. In Rosai J (ed.): Guiding the surgeon's hand. The history of American surgical pathology. Washington, DC, 1997, The American Registry of Pathology/Armed Forces Institute of Pathology, p. 284.

777 Agaimy A, Lindner M, Wuensch PH. Interstitial cells of Cajal (ICC) in mature cystic teratoma of the ovary. Histopathology 2006, **48**: 208–209.

778 Auer EA, Dockerty MB, Mayo CW. Ruptured dermoid cyst of the ovary simulating abdominal carcinomatosis. Mayo Clin Proc 1951, **26**: 489–497.

779 Blackwell WJ, Dockerty MB, Masson JC, Mussey RD. Dermoid cysts of the ovary. Their clinical and pathologic significance. Am J Obstet Gynecol 1946, **51**: 151–172.

780 Boman F, Vantyghem MC, Querleu D, Sasano H. Virilizing ovarian dermoid cyst with peripheral steroid cells: a case study with immunohistochemical study of steroidogenesis. Int J Gynecol Pathol 1999, **18**: 174–177.

781 Burg J, Kommoss F, Bittinger F, Moll R, Kirkpatrick CJ. Mature cystic teratoma of the ovary with struma and benign Brenner tumor: a case report with immunohistochemical characterization. Int J Gynecol Pathol 2002, **21**: 74–77.

782 Calame J, Bosman FT, Schaberg A, Louwerens JWK. Immunocytochemical localization of neuroendocrine hormones and oncofetal antigens in ovarian teratomas. Int J Gynecol Pathol 1984, **3**: 92–100.

783 Chen E, Fletcher CDM, Nucci MR. Meningothelial proliferations in mature cystic teratoma of the ovary: evidence for the common presence of cranially derived tissues paralleling anterior embryonic plate development. An analysis of 25 consecutive cases. Am J Surg Pathol 2010, **34**: 1014–1018.

784 Cobo F, Pereira A, Nomdedeu B, Gallart T, Ordi J, Torne A, Monserrat E, Rozman C. Ovarian dermoid cyst-associated autoimmune hemolytic anemia. A case report with emphasis on pathogenic mechanisms. Am J Clin Pathol 1996, **105**: 567–571.

785 Czernobilsky B, Lifschitz-Mercer B, Luzon A, Jacob N, Ben-Hur H, Gorbacz S, Fogel M. Cytokeratin patterns in the epidermis of human ovarian mature cystic teratomas. Hum Pathol 1989, **20**: 185–192.

786 Dick HM, Honoré LH. Dental structures in benign ovarian cystic teratomas (dermoid cysts). A study of ten cases with a review of the literature. Oral Surg 1985, **60**: 299–307.

787 Ein SH, Darte JMM, Stephens CA. Cystic and solid ovarian tumors in children. A 44-year review. J Pediatr Surg 1970, **5**: 148–156.

788 Fellegara G, Young RH, Kuhn E, Rosai J. Ovarian mature cystic teratoma with florid vascular proliferation and Wagner–Meissner-like corpuscles. Int J Surg Pathol 2008, **16**: 320–323.

789 Fortt RW, Mathie IK. Gliomatosis peritonei caused by ovarian teratoma. J Clin Pathol 1969, **22**: 348–353.

790 Harms D, Janig U, Gobel U. Gliomatosis peritonei in childhood and adolescence. Clinicopathological study of 13 cases including immunohistochemical findings. Pathol Res Pract 1989, **184**: 422–430.

791 Huang AY, Bolen AW, Zaloudek CJ. Neuronal elements within gliomatosis peritonei: immunohistochemical evidence of an under-recognized feature. Lab Invest 2009, **89**(Suppl 1): 218A.

792 Jaworski RC, Boable R, Greg J, Cocks P. Peritoneal 'melanosis' associated with a ruptured ovarian dermoid cyst: report of a case with electron-probe energy dispersive X-ray analysis. Int J Gynecol Pathol 2001, **20**: 386–389.

793 Kwan MY, Kalle W, Lau GT, Chan JK. Is gliomatosis peritonei derived from the associated ovarian teratoma? Hum Pathol 2004, **35**: 685–688.

794 Lewis MG. Melanin-pigmented components in ovarian teratomas in Ugandan Africans. J Pathol Bacteriol 1968, **95**: 405–409.

795 Linder D, McCaw BK, Hecht F. Parthenogenic origin of benign ovarian teratomas. N Engl J Med 1975, **292**: 63–66.

796 López-Beltrán A, Calañas AS, Jimena P, Escudero AL, Campello TR, Muñoz-Torres M, Escobar-Jiménez F, Carvia RE, Nogales FF. Virilizing mature ovarian cystic teratomas. Virchows Arch 1997, **431**: 149–151.

797 McKeel DW Jr, Askin FB. Ectopic hypophyseal hormonal cells in benign cystic teratoma of the ovary. Light microscopic histochemical dye staining and immunoperoxidase cytochemistry. Arch Pathol Lab Med 1978, **102**: 122–128.

798 McLachlin CM, Srigley JR. Prostatic tissue in mature cystic teratomas of the ovary. Am J Surg Pathol 1992, **16**: 780–784.

799 Miyake J, Ireland K. Ovarian mature teratoma with homunculus coexisting with an intrauterine pregnancy. Arch Pathol Lab Med 1986, **110**: 1192–1194.

800 Morimitsu Y, Nakashima O, Kage M, Kojiro M, Kawano K, Koga T. Coexistence of mature teratoma and thecoma in an ovary. A report of two cases. Acta Pathol Jpn 1991, **41**: 922–926.

801 Muretto P, Chilosi M, Rabitti C, Tommasoni S, Colato C. Biovularity and 'coalescence of primary follicles' in ovaries with mature teratomas. Int J Surg Pathol 2001, **9**: 121–126.

802 Nielsen SNJ, Scheithauer BW, Gaffey TA. Gliomatosis peritonei. Cancer 1985, **56**: 2499–2503.

803 Payne D, Muss HB, Homesley HD, Jobson VW, Baird FG. Autoimmune hemolytic anemia and ovarian dermoid cysts. Case report and review of the literature. Cancer 1981, **48**: 721–724.

804 Rashad MH, Fathalla MF, Kerr MG. Sex chromatin and chromosome analysis in ovarian teratomas. Am J Obstet Gynecol 1966, **96**: 461–465.

805 Riley PA, Sutton PM. Why are ovarian teratomas benign whilst teratomas of the testis are malignant? Lancet 1975, **1**: 1360–1362.

806 Robboy SJ, Scully RE. Ovarian teratoma with glial implants on the peritoneum. An analysis of 12 cases. Hum Pathol 1970, **1**: 644–653.

807 Sahin AA, Ro JY, Chen J, Ayala AG. Spindle cell nodule and peptic ulcer arising in a fully developed gastric wall in a mature cystic teratoma. Arch Pathol Lab Med 1990, **114**: 529–531.

808 Truong LD, Jurco S III, McGavran MH. Gliomatosis peritonei. Report of two cases and review of literature. Am J Surg Pathol 1982, **6**: 443–449.

809 Vadmal M, Hadju SI. Prostatic tissue in benign cystic ovarian teratomas. Hum Pathol 1996, **27**: 428–429.

810 Vortmeyer AO, Devouassoux-Shisheboran M, Li G, Mohr V, Tavassoli F, Zhuang Z. Microdissection-based analysis of mature ovarian teratoma. Am J Pathol 1999, **154**: 987–991.

811 Wheeler JE. Extraovarian teratoma with peritoneal gliomatosis. Hum Pathol 1978, **9**: 232–234.

812 Yanai-Inbar I, Scully RE. Relation of ovarian dermoid cysts and immature teratomas. An analysis of 350 cases of immature teratoma and 10 cases of dermoid cyst with microscopic foci of immature tissue. Int J Gynecol Pathol 1987, **6**: 203–212.

'Somatic-type' tumors developing in mature cystic teratoma

813 Chumas JC, Scully RE. Sebaceous tumors arising in ovarian dermoid cysts. Int J Gynecol Pathol 1991, **10**: 356–363.

814 Climie ARW, Heath LP. Malignant degeneration of benign cystic teratomas of the ovary. Review of the literature and report of a chondrosarcoma and carcinoid tumor. Cancer 1968, **22**: 824–832.

815 Davis GL. Malignant melanoma arising in mature ovarian cystic teratoma (dermoid cyst). Report of two cases and literature analysis. Int J Gynecol Pathol 1997, **15**: 356–362.

816 Devouassoux-Shisheboran M, Vortmeyer AO, Silver SA, Zhuang Z, Tavassoli FA. Teratomatous genotype detected in malignancies of a non-germ cell phenotype. Lab Invest 2000, **80**: 81–86.

817 Hirakawa T, Tsuneyoshi M, Enjoji M. Squamous cell carcinoma arising in mature cystic teratoma of the ovary. Clinicopathologic and topographic analysis. Am J Surg Pathol 1989, **13**: 397–405.

818 Hirschowitz L, Ansari A, Cahill DJ, Bamford DS, Love S. Central neurocytoma arising within a mature cystic teratoma of the ovary. Int J Gynecol Pathol 1997, **16**: 176–179.

819 Hwang JH, So KA, Modi G, Lee JK, Lee NW, Lee KW, Kim I. Borderline-like mucinous tumor arising in mature cystic teratoma of the ovary associated with pseudomyxoma peritonei. Int J Gynecol Pathol 2009, **28**: 376–380.

820 Iwasa A, Oda Y, Kaneki E, Ohishi Y, Kurihara S, Yamada T, Hirakawa T, Wake N, Tsuneyoshi M. Squamous cell carcinoma arising in mature cystic teratoma of the ovary: an immunohistochemical analysis of its tumorigenesis. Histopathology 2007, **51**: 98–104.

821 Kanbour-Shakir A, Sawaday J, Kanbour AI, Kunschner A, Stock RJ. Primitive neuroectodermal tumor arising in an ovarian mature cystic teratoma. Immunohistochemical and electron microscopic studies. Int J Gynecol Pathol 1993, **12**: 270–275.

822 Kelley RR, Scully RE. Cancer developing in dermoid cysts of the ovary. Cancer 1961, **14**: 989–1000.

823 Kudo M. The nature of 'blue nevus' in cystic teratomas of the ovary. An ultrastructural evidence for Schwann cell origin. Acta Pathol Jpn 1985, **35**: 693–698.

824 Madison JF, Cooper PH. A histiocytoid (epithelioid) vascular tumor of the ovary. Occurrence within a benign cystic teratoma. Mod Pathol 1989, **2**: 55–58.

825 Morimitsu Y, Nakashima O, Nakashima Y, Kojiro M, Shimokobe T. Apocrine adenocarcinoma arising in cystic teratoma of the ovary. Arch Pathol Lab Med 1993, **117**: 647–649.

826 Palmer PE, Bogojavlensky S, Bhan AK, Scully RE. Prolactinoma in wall of ovarian dermoid cyst with hyperprolactinemia. Obstet Gynecol 1990, **75**: 540–543.

827 Peterson WF. Malignant degeneration of benign cystic teratomas of the ovary. A collective review of the literature. Obstet Gynecol Survey 1957, **12**: 793–830.

828 Reid H, van der Walt JD, Fox H. Neuroblastoma arising in a mature cystic teratoma of the ovary. J Clin Pathol 1983, **36**: 68–73.

829 Ronnett BM, Seidman JD. Mucinous tumors arising in ovarian mature cystic teratomas. Am J Surg Pathol 2003, **27**: 650–657.

830 Shen DH, Khoo US, Xue WC, Cheung AN. Ovarian mature cystic teratoma with malignant transformation: an interphase cytogenetic study. Int J Gynecol Pathol 1998, **17**: 351–357.

831 Shimizu S, Kobayashi H, Suchi T, Torii Y, Narita K, Aoki S. Extramammary Paget's disease arising in mature cystic teratoma of the ovary. Am J Surg Pathol 1991, **15**: 1002–1006.

832 Silver SA, Tavassoli FA. Glomus tumor arising in a mature teratoma of the ovary: report of a case simulating a metastasis from cervical squamous carcinoma. Arch Pathol Lab Med 2000, **124**: 1373–1375.

833 Stewart CJ, Junckerstorff R, Tsukamoto T. Ovarian mucinous tumor arising in mature cystic teratoma associated with pseudomyxoma peritonei: a case with possible respiratory epithelial differentiation. Int J Gynecol Pathol 2008, **27**: 41–43.

834 Tsang P, Berman L, Kasznica J. Adnexal tumor and a pigmented nevoid lesion in a benign cystic ovarian teratoma. Arch Pathol Lab Med 1993, **117**: 846–847.

835 Ueda Y, Kimura A, Kawahara E, Kitagawa H, Nakanishi I. Malignant melanoma arising in a dermoid cyst of the ovary. Cancer 1991, **67**: 3141–3145.

836 Waugh MS, Soler AP, Robboy SJ. Silent corticotroph cell pituitary adenoma in a struma ovarii. Int J Gynecol Pathol 2007, **26**: 26–29.

837 Yadav A, Lellouch-Tubiana A, Fournet JC, Quazza JE, Kalifa C, Sainte-Rose C, Jaubert F. Glioblastoma multiforme in a mature ovarian teratoma with recurring brain tumors. Histopathology 1999, **35**: 170–173.

Epidermoid cyst

838 Young RH, Prat J, Scully RE. Epidermoid cyst of the ovary. A report of three cases with comments on histogenesis. Am J Clin Pathol 1980, **73**: 272–276.

Struma ovarii

839 Boutross-Tadross O, Saleh R, Asa SL. Follicular variant papillary thyroid carcinoma arising in struma ovarii. Endocr Pathol 2007, **18**: 182–186.

840 Coyne C, Nikiforov YE. RAS mutation-positive follicular variant of papillary thyroid carcinoma arising in a struma ovarii. Endocr Pathol 2010, **21**: 144–147.

841 Garg K, Soslow RA, Rivera M, Tuttle MR, Ghossein RA. Histologically bland 'extremely well differentiated' thyroid carcinomas arising in struma ovarii can recur and metastasize. Int J Gynecol Pathol 2009, **28**: 222–230.

842 Hasleton PS, Kelehan P, Wittaker JS, Turner L, Burslem RW. Benign and malignant struma ovarii. Arch Pathol Lab Med 1978, **102**: 180–184.

843 Ro JY, Sahin AA, el-Naggar AK, Ordonez NG, Mackay B, Llamas LL, Ayala AG. Intraluminal crystalloids in struma ovarii. Immunohistochemical, DNA flow cytometric, and ultrastructural study. Arch Pathol Lab Med 1991, **115**: 145–149.

844 Roth LM, Karseladze AI. Highly differentiated follicular carcinoma arising from struma ovarii: a report of 3 cases, a review of the literature, and a reassessment of so-called peritoneal strumosis. Int J Gynecol Pathol 2008, **27**: 213–222.

845 Roth LM, Miller AW 3rd, Talerman A. Typical thyroid-type carcinoma arising in struma ovarii: a report of 4 cases and review of the literature. Int J Gynecol Pathol 2008, **27**: 496–506.

846 Roth LM, Talerman A. The enigma of struma ovarii. Pathology 2007, **39**: 139–146.

847 Roth LM, Talerman A, Wadsley J, Karseladze AI. Risk factors in thyroid-type carcinoma arising in ovarian struma: a report of 15 cases with comparison to ordinary struma ovarii. Histopathology 2010, **57**: 147–167.

848 Schmidt J, Derr V, Heinrich MC, Crum CP, Fletcher JA, Corless CL, Nosé V. BRAF in papillary thyroid carcinoma of ovary (struma ovarii). Am J Surg Pathol 2007, **31**: 1337–1343.

849 Seifer DB, Weiss LM, Kempson RL. Malignant lymphoma arising within thyroid tissue in a mature cystic teratoma. Cancer 1986, **58**: 2459–2461.

850 Szyfelbein WM, Young RH, Scully RE. Cystic struma ovarii. A frequently unrecognized tumor. A report of 20 cases. Am J Surg Pathol 1994, **18**: 785–788.

851 Szyfelbein WM, Young RH, Scully RE. Struma ovarii simulating ovarian tumors of other types. A report of 30 cases. Am J Surg Pathol 1995, **19**: 21–29.

852 Talerman A, Roth LM. Recent advances in the pathology and classification of gonadal neoplasms composed of germ cells and sex cord derivatives. Int J Gynecol Pathol 2007, **26**: 313–321.

Carcinoid tumor and strumal carcinoid

853 Arhelger RB, Kelly B. Strumal carcinoid. Report of a case with electron microscopical observations. Arch Pathol 1974, **97**: 323–325.

854 Baker PM, Oliva E, Young RH, Talerman A, Scully RE. Ovarian mucinous carcinoids including some with a carcinomatous component: a report of 17 cases. Am J Surg Pathol 2001, **25**: 557–568.

855 Brunaud L, Antunes L, Sebbag H, Bresler L, Villemot JP, Boissel P. Ovarian strumal carcinoid tumor responsible for carcinoid heart disease. Eur J Obstet Gynecol Reprod Biol 2001, **98**: 124–126.

856 Czernobilsky B, Segal M, Dgani R. Primary ovarian carcinoid with marked heterogeneity of microscopic features. Cancer 1984, **54**: 585–589.

857 Dayal Y, Tashjian H Jr, Wolfe HJ. Immunocytochemical localization of calcitonin-producing cells in a strumal carcinoid with amyloid stroma. Cancer 1979, **43**: 1331–1338.

858 Hamazaki S, Okino T, Tsukayama C, Okada S. Expression of thyroid transcription factor-1 in strumal carcinoid and struma ovarii: an immunohistochemical study. Pathol Int 2002, **52**: 458–462.

859 Hristov AC, Young RH, Vang R, Yemelyanova AV, Seidman JD, Ronnett BM. Ovarian metastases of appendiceal tumors with goblet cell carcinoidlike and signet ring cell patterns: a report of 30 cases. Am J Surg Pathol 2007, **31**: 1502–1511.

860 Matias-Guiu X, Forteza J, Prat J. Mixed strumal and mucinous carcinoid tumor of the ovary. Int J Gynecol Pathol 1995, **14**: 179–183.

861 Motoyama T, Katayama Y, Watanabe H, Okazaki E, Shibuya H. Functioning ovarian carcinoids induce severe constipation. Cancer 1992, **70**: 513–518.

862 Pelosi G, Sonzogni A, Rosai J. Thyroid-type papillary microcarcinoma in ovarian strumal carcinoid. Int J Surg Pathol 2008, **16**: 435–437.

863 Rabban JT, Lerwill MF, McCluggage WG, Grenert JP, Zaloudek CJ. Primary ovarian carcinoid tumors may express CDX-2: a

potential pitfall in distinction from metastatic intestinal carcinoid tumors involving the ovary. Int J Gynecol Pathol 2009, **28**: 41–48.

864 Robboy SJ, Norris HJ, Scully RE. Insular carcinoid primary in ovary – a clinicopathologic analysis of 48 cases. Cancer 1975, **36**: 406–420.

865 Robboy SJ, Scully RE. Strumal carcinoid of the ovary. An analysis of 50 cases of a distinctive tumor composed of thyroid tissue and carcinoid. Cancer 1980, **46**: 2019–2034.

866 Robboy SJ, Scully RE, Norris HJ. Carcinoid metastatic to ovary. A clinicopathologic analysis of 35 cases. Cancer 1974, **33**: 798–811.

867 Robboy SJ, Scully RE, Norris HJ. Primary trabecular carcinoid of the ovary. Obstet Gynecol 1977, **49**: 202–207.

868 Serratoni FT, Robboy SJ. Ultrastructure of primary and metastatic ovarian carcinoids. Analysis of 11 cases. Cancer 1975, **36**: 157–160.

869 Shigeta H, Taga M, Kurogi K, Kitamura H, Motoyama T, Gorai I. Ovarian strumal carcinoid with severe constipation: immunohistochemical and mRNA analyses of peptide YY. Hum Pathol 1999, **30**: 242–246.

870 Sidhu J, Sanchez RL. Prostatic acid phosphatase in strumal carcinoids of the ovary. An immunohistochemical study. Cancer 1993, **72**: 1673–1678.

871 Snyder RR, Tavassoli FA. Ovarian strumal carcinoid. Immunohistochemical, ultrastructural, and clinicopathologic observations. Int J Gynecol Pathol 1986, **3**: 187–201.

872 Sporrong B, Falkmer S, Robboy SJ, Alumets J, Hakanson R, Ljungber O, Sundler F. Neurohormonal peptides in ovarian carcinoids. An immunohistochemical study of 81 primary carcinoids and of intraovarian metastases from six mid-gut carcinoids. Cancer 1982, **49**: 68–74.

873 Stagno PA, Petras RE, Hart WR. Strumal carcinoids of the ovary. An immunohistologic and ultrastructural study. Arch Pathol Lab Med 1987, **111**: 440–446.

874 Talerman A. Carcinoid tumors of the ovary. J Cancer Res Clin Oncol 1984, **107**: 125–135.

875 Tamsen A, Mazur MT. Ovarian strumal carcinoid in association with multiple endocrine neoplasia, type IIA. Arch Pathol Lab Med 1992, **116**: 200–203.

876 Ulbright TM, Roth LM, Ehrlich CE. Ovarian strumal carcinoid. An immunocytochemical and ultrastructural study of two cases. Am J Clin Pathol 1982, **77**: 622–631.

SEX CORD–STROMAL TUMORS

877 Bamberger AM, Ivell R, Balvers M, Kelp B, Bamberger CM, Riethdorf L, Loning T. Relaxin-like factor (RLF): a new specific marker for Leydig cells in the ovary. Int J Gynecol Pathol 1999, **18**: 163–168.

878 Busam KJ, Iversen K, Coplan KA, Old LJ, Stockert E, Chen YT, McGregor D, Jungbluth A. Immunoreactivity for A103, and antibody to Melan-A (Mart-1), in adrenocortical and other steroid tumors. Am J Surg Pathol 1998, **22**: 57–63.

879 Cao QJ, Jones JG, Li M. Expression of calretinin in human ovary, testis and ovarian sex cord–stromal tumors. Int J Gynecol Pathol 2001, **20**: 346–352.

880 Choi YL, Kim HS, Ahn G. Immunoexpression of inhibin alfa subunit, inhibin/activin beta A subunit and CD99 in ovarian tumors. Arch Pathol Lab Med 2000, **124**: 563–569.

881 Costa MJ, Morris R, Sasano H. Sex steroid biosynthesis enzymes in ovarian sex-cord stromal tumors. Int J Gynecol Pathol 1994, **13**: 109–119.

882 Deavers MT, Malpica A, Liu J, Broaddus R, Silva EG. Ovarian sex cord–stromal tumors: an immunohistochemical study including a comparison of calretinin and inhibin. Mod Pathol 2003, **16**: 584–590.

883 Fox H. Sex cord–stromal tumours of the ovary. J Pathol 1985, **145**: 127–148.

884 Freeman DA. Steroid hormone-producing tumors of the adrenal, ovary, and testes. Endocrinol Metab Clin North Am 1991, **20**: 751–766.

885 Gordon MD, Corles C, Renshaw AA, Beckstead J. CD99, Keratin, and vimentin staining of sex cord–stromal tumors, normal ovary, and testis. Mod Pathol 1998, **11**: 769–773.

886 He H, Luthringer DJ, Hui P, Lau SK, Weiss LM, Chu PG. Expression of CD56 and WT1 in ovarian stroma and ovarian stromal tumors. Am J Surg Pathol 2008, **32**: 884–890.

887 Iczkowski KA, Bostwick DG, Roche PC, Cheville JC. Inhibin A is a sensitive and specific marker for testicular sex cord–stromal tumors. Mod Pathol 1998, **11**: 774–779.

888 Iezzoni JC, Mills SE, Pelkey TJ, Stoler MH. Inhibin is not an immunohistochemical marker for hepatocellular carcinoma. An example of the potential pitfall diagnostic immunohistochemistry caused by endogenous biotin. Am J Clin Pathol 1999, **111**: 229–234.

889 Keitoku M, Konishi I, Nanbu K, Yamamoto S, Mandai M, Kataoka N, Oishi T, Mori T. Extraovarian sex cord–stromal tumor: case report and review of the literature. Int J Gynecol Pathol 1997, **16**: 180–185.

890 Kommoss F, Oliva E, Bhan AK, Young RH, Scully RE. Inhibin expression in ovarian tumors and tumor-like lesions: an immunohistochemical study. Mod Pathol 1998, **11**: 656–664.

891 Lobo RA. Ovarian hyperandrogenism and androgen-producing tumors. Endocrinol Metab Clin North Am 1991, **20**: 773–805.

892 McCluggage WG. Value of inhibin staining in gynecological pathology. Int J Gynecol Pathol 2001, **20**: 79–85.

893 McCluggage WG. Recent advances in immunohistochemistry in gynecological pathology. Histopathology 2002, **40**: 309–326.

894 McCluggage WG, Maxwell P. Adenocarcinomas of various sites may exhibit immunoreactivity with anti-inhibin antibodies. Histopathology 1999, **35**: 216–220.

895 McCluggage WG, McKenna M, McBride HA. CD56 is a sensitive and diagnostically useful immunohistochemical marker of ovarian sex cord–stromal tumors. Int J Gynecol Pathol 2007, **26**: 322–327.

896 Matias-Guiu X, Pons C, Prat J. Mullerian inhibiting substance, alpha-inhibin, and CD99 expression in sex cord stromal tumors and endometrioid ovarian carcinomas resembling sex cord–stromal tumors. Hum Pathol 1998, **29**: 840–845.

897 Movahedi-Lankarani S, Kurman RJ. Calretinin, a more sensitive but less specific marker than alpha-inhibin for ovarian sex cord–stromal neoplasms: an immunohistochemical study of 215 cases. Am J Surg Pathol 2002, **26**: 1477–1483.

898 Pelkey TJ, Frierson HF Jr, Mills SE, Stoler MH. Detection of the alpha-subunit of inhibin in trophoblastic neoplasia. Hum Pathol 1999, **30**: 26–31.

899 Rey R, Sabourin JC, Venara M, Long WQ, Jaubert F, Zeller WP, Duvillard P, Chemes H, Bidart JM. Anti-Mullerian hormone is a specific marker of Sertoli-and granulosa-cell origin in gonadal tumors. Hum Pathol 2000, **31**: 1202–1208.

900 Roth LM, Billings SD. Hormonally functional ovarian neoplasms. Endocrine Pathol 2002, **11**: 1–17.

901 Roth LM. Recent advances in the pathology and classification of ovarian sex cord–stromal tumors. Int J Gynecol Pathol 2006, **25**: 199–215.

902 Sasano H. Functional pathology of human ovarian steroidogenesis. Normal cycling ovary and steroid-producing neoplasms. Endocr Pathol 1994, **5**: 81–89.

903 Sasano H, Okamoto M, Mason JI, Simpson ER, Mendelson CR, Sasano N, Silverberg SG. Immunohistochemical studies of steroidogenic enzymes (aromatase, 17 alpha-hydroxylase and cholesterol side-chain cleavage cytochromes P-450) in sex cord–stromal tumors of the ovary. Hum Pathol 1989, **20**: 452–457.

904 Tavassoli FA. Ovarian tumors with functioning manifestations. Endocr Pathol 1994, **5**: 137–148.

905 Teilum G. Estrogen-producing Sertoli cell tumors (androblastoma tubular lipoides) of the human testis and ovary. Homologous ovarian and testicular tumors. J Clin Endocrinol 1949, **9**: 301–318.

906 Vang R, Herrmann ME, Tavassoli FA. Comparative immunohistochemical analysis of granulosa and sertoli components in ovarian sex cord–stromal tumors with mixed differentiation: potential implications for derivation of sertoli differentiation in ovarian tumors. Int J Gynecol Pathol 2004, **23**: 151–161.

907 Yaziji H, Gown AM. Immunohistochemical analysis of gynecologic tumors. Int J Gynecol Pathol 2000, **20**: 64–78.

908 Young RH, Scully RE. Ovarian sex cord–stromal tumors. Recent progress. Int J Gynecol Pathol 1982, **1**: 101–123.

909 Young RH, Scully RE. Ovarian sex cord–stromal tumors. Problems in differential diagnosis. Pathol Annu 1988, **23**(Pt 1): 273–296.

910 Young RH. Sex cord–stromal tumors of the ovary and testis: their similarities and differences with consideration of selected problems. Mod Pathol 2005, **18**(Suppl 2): S81–S98.

911 Zhao C, Vinh TN, McManus K, Dabbs D, Barner R, Vang R. Identification of the most sensitive and robust immunohistochemical markers in different categories of ovarian sex cord–stromal tumors. Am J Surg Pathol 2009, **33**: 354–366.

Granulosa cell tumor

912 Ahmed E, Young RH, Scully RE. Adult granulosa cell tumor of the ovary with foci of hepatic cell differentiation: a report of four cases and comparison with two cases of granulosa cell tumor with Leydig cells. Am J Surg Pathol 1999, **23**: 1089–1093.

913 Bjorkholm E, Silfversward C. Prognostic factors in granulosa-cell tumors. Gynecol Oncol 1981, **11**: 261–274.

914 Castro CY, Malpica A, Hearne RH, Silva EG, Castro CV. Androgenic adult granulosa cell tumor in a 13-year-old prepubertal patient: a case report and review of the literature. Int J Gynecol Pathol 2000, **19**: 266–271.

915 Chadha S, Cornelisse CJ, Schaberg A. Flow cytometric DNA ploidy analysis of ovarian granulosa cell tumors. Gynecol Oncol 1990, **36**: 240–245.

916 Clement PB, Young RH, Scully RE. Ovarian granulosa cell proliferations of pregnancy. A report of nine cases. Hum Pathol 1988, **19**: 657–662.

917 Costa MJ, De Rose PB, Roth LM, Brescia RJ, Zaloudek CJ, Cohen C. Immunohistochemical phenotype of ovarian granulosa cell tumors. Absence of epithelial membrane antigen has diagnostic value. Hum Pathol 1994, **25**: 60–66.

918 Czernobilsky B, Moll R, Leppien G, Schweikhart G, Franke WW. Desmosomal plaque-associated vimentin filaments in human ovarian granulosa cell tumors of various histologic patterns. Am J Pathol 1987, **126**: 476–486.

919 Evans AT III, Gaffey TA, Malkasian GD Jr, Annegers JF. Clinicopathologic review of 118 granulosa and 82 theca cell tumors. Obstet Gynecol 1980, **55**: 231–238.

920 Evans MP, Webb MJ, Gaffey TA, Katzmann JA, Suman VJ, Hu TC. DNA ploidy of ovarian granulosa cell tumors. Lack of correlation between DNA index or proliferative index and outcome in 40 patients. Cancer 1995, **75**: 2295–2298.

921 Farinola MA, Gown AM, Judson K, Ronnett BM, Barry TS, Movahedi-Lankarani S, Vang R. Estrogen receptor alpha and progesterone receptor expression in ovarian adult granulosa cell tumors and Sertoli–Leydig cell tumors. Int J Gynecol Pathol 2007, **26**: 375–382.

922 Flemming P, Wellmann A, Maschjek H, Lang H, Georgii A. Monoclonal antibodies against inhibin represent key markers of adult granulosa cell tumors of the ovary even in their metastases. A report of three cases with late metastasis, being previously misinterpreted as hemangiopericytoma. Am J Surg Pathol 1995, **19**: 927–933.

923 Fletcher JA, Gibas Z, Donovan K, Perez-Atayde A, Genest D, Morton CC, Lage JM. Ovarian granulosa-stromal cell tumors are characterized by trisomy 12. Am J Pathol 1991, **138**: 515–520.

924 Fox H, Agrawal K, Langley FA. A clinicopathologic study of 92 cases of granulosa cell tumor of the ovary with special reference to the factors influencing prognosis. Cancer 1975, **35**: 231–241.

925 Gaffey MJ, Frierson HF Jr, Iezzoni JC, Mills SE, Clement PB, Gersell DJ, Shashi V, von Kap-Herr C, Young RH. Ovarian granulosa cell tumors with bizarre nuclei: an immunohistochemical analysis with fluorescence in situ hybridization documenting trisomy 12 in bizarre component. Mod Pathol 1996, **9**: 308–315.

926 Halperin D, Visscher DW, Wallis T, Lawrence WD. Evaluation of chromosome 12 copy number in ovarian granulosa cell tumors using interphase cytogenetics. Int J Gynecol Pathol 1995, **14**: 319–323.

927 Hitchcock CL, Norris HJ, Khalifa MA, Wargotz ES. Flow cytometric analysis of granulosa tumors. Cancer 1989, **64**: 2127–2132.

928 Irving JA, Young RH. Granulosa cell tumors of the ovary with a pseudopapillary pattern: a study of 14 cases of an unusual morphologic variant emphasizing their distinction from transitional cell neoplasms and other papillary ovarian tumors. Am J Surg Pathol 2008, **32**: 581–586.

929 Jacoby AF, Young RH, Colvin RB, Flotte TJ, Preffer F, Scully RE, Swymer CM, Bell DA. DNA content in juvenile granulosa cell tumors of the ovary. A study of early-and advanced-stage disease. Gynecol Oncol 1992, **46**: 97–103.

930 Jamieson S, Butzow R, Andersson N, Alexiadis M, Unkila-Kallio L, Heikinheimo M, Fuller PJ, Anttonen M. The FOXL2 C134W mutation is characteristic of adult granulosa cell tumors of the ovary. Mod Pathol 2010, **23**: 1477–1485.

931 Kurman RJ, Goebelsmann U, Taylor CR. Steroid localization in granulosatheca tumors of the ovary. Cancer 1979, **43**: 2377–2384.

932 Lack EE, Perez-Atayde AR, Murthy ASK, Goldstein DP, Crigler JF, Vawter GF. Granulosa theca cell tumors in premenarchal girls. A clinical and pathologic study of ten cases. Cancer 1981, **48**: 1846–1854.

933 Loo KT, Leung AKF, Chan JKC. Immunohistochemical staining of ovarian granulosa cell tumours with MIC2 antibody. Histopathology 1995, **27**: 388–390.

934 McCluggage WG, Maxwell P, Sloan JM. Immunohistochemical staining of ovarian granulosa cell tumors with monoclonal antibody against inhibin. Hum Pathol 1997, **28**: 1034–1038.

935 McKenna M, Kenny B, Dorman G, McCluggage WG. Combined adult granulosa cell tumor and mucinous cystadenoma of the ovary: granulosa cell tumor with heterologous mucinous elements. Int J Gynecol Pathol 2005, **24**: 224-227.

936 Mayr D, Kaltz-Wittman C, Arbogast S, Amann G, Aust DE, Diebold J. Characteristic pattern of genetic aberrations in ovarian granulosa cell tumors. Mod Pathol 2002, **15**: 951–957.

937 Miettinen M, Wahlstrom T, Virtanen I, Talerman A, Astengo-Osuna C. Cellular differentiation in ovarian sex cord–stromal and germ-cell tumors studied with antibodies to intermediate-filament proteins. Am J Surg Pathol 1985, **9**: 640–651.

938 Miller BE, Barron BA, Wan JY, Delmore JE, Silva EG. Prognostic factors in adult granulosa cell tumor of the ovary. Cancer 1997, **79**: 1951–1955.

939 Nakashima N, Young RH, Scully RE. Androgenic granulosa cell tumors of the ovary. A clinicopathologic analysis of 17 cases and review of the literature. Arch Pathol Lab Med 1984, **108**: 786–791.

940 Nogales FF, Concha A, Plata C, Ruiz-Avila I. Granulosa cell tumor of the ovary with diffuse true hepatic differentation simulating stromal luteinization. Am J Surg Pathol 1993, **17**: 85–90.

941 Norris HJ, Taylor HB. Prognosis of granulosa-theca tumors of the ovary. Cancer 1968, **21**: 255–263.

942 Norris HJ, Taylor HB. Virilization associated with cystic granulosa tumors. Obstet Gynecol 1969, **34**: 629–635.

943 Otis CN, Powell JL, Barbuto D, Carcangiu ML. Intermediate filamentous proteins in adult granulosa cell tumors. An immunohistochemical study of 25 cases. Am J Surg Pathol 1992, **16**: 962–968.

944 Rodgers KE, Marks JF, Ellefson DD, Yanagihara DL, Tonetta SA, Vasilev SA, Morrow CP, Montz FJ, di Zerega GS. Follicle regulatory protein. A novel marker for granulosa cell cancer patients. Gynecol Oncol 1990, **37**: 381–387.

945 Roth LM, Nicholas TR, Ehrlich CE. Juvenile granulosa cell tumor. A clinicopathologic study of three cases with ultrastructural observations. Cancer 1979, **44**: 2194–2205.

946 Santini D, Ceccarelli C, Leone O, Pasquinelli G, Piana S, Marabini A, Martinelli GN. Smooth muscle differentiation in normal human ovaries, ovarian stromal hyperplasia and ovarian granulosa-stromal cells tumors. Mod Pathol 1995, **8**: 25–30.

947 Schofield DE, Fletcher JA. Trisomy 12 in pediatric granulosa-stromal cell tumors. Demonstration by a modified method of fluorescence in situ hybridization on paraffin-embedded material. Am J Pathol 1992, **141**: 1265–1269.

948 Scully RE. Ovarian tumors. A review. Am J Pathol 1977, **87**: 686–720.

949 Shah SP, Kobel M, Senz J, Morin RD, Clarke BA, Wiegand KC, Leung G, Zayed A, Mehl E, Kalloger SE, Sun M, Giuliany R, Yorida E, Jones S, Varhol R, Swenerton KD, Miller D, Clement PB, Crane C, Madore J, Provencher D, Leung P, DeFazio A, Khattra J, Turashvili G, Zhao Y, Zeng T, Glover JN, Vanderhyden B, Zhao C, Parkinson CA, Jimenez-Linan M, Bowtell DD, Mes-Masson AM, Brenton JD, Aparicio SA, Boyd N, Hirst M, Gilks CB, Marra M, Huntsman DG. Mutation of FOXL2 in granulosa-cell tumors of the ovary. N Engl J Med 2009, **360**: 2719–2729.

950 Suh KS, Silverberg SG, Rhame JG, Wilkinson DS. Granulosa cell tumor of the ovary. Histopathologic and flow cytometric analysis with clinical correlation. Arch Pathol Lab Med 1990, **114**: 496–501.

951 Swanson SA, Norris HJ, Kelsten ML, Wheeler JE. DNA content of juvenile granulosa tumors determined by flow cytometry. Int J Gynecol Pathol 1990, **9**: 101–109.

952 Tamimi HK, Bolen JW. Enchondromatosis (Ollier's disease) and ovarian juvenile granulosa cell tumor. A case report and review of the literature. Cancer 1984, **53**: 1605–1608.

953 Tanaka Y, Sasaki Y, Nishihira H, Izawa T, Nishi T. Ovarian juvenile granulosa cell tumor associated with Maffucci's syndrome. Am J Clin Pathol 1992, **97**: 523–527.

954 Villella J, Herrmann FR, Kaul S, Lele S, Marchetti D, Natiella J, Odunsi K, Mhawech-Fauceglia P. Clinical and pathological predictive factors in women with adult-type granulosa cell tumor of the ovary. Int J Gynecol Pathol 2007, **26**: 154–159.

955 Voytek TM, Ro JY, El-Naggar AK, Ordonez NG, Tornos C, Welch GR, Ayala AG. Metastatic ovarian granulosa cell tumor to urinary bladder mimicking primary transitional cell carcinoma: a case report with immunohistochemical, electron microscopic, DNA flow cytometry, and interphase cytogenetic studies. J Urol Pathol 1996, **4**: 57–68.

956 Young RH, Dickersin GR, Scully RE. Juvenile granulosa cell tumor of the ovary. A clinicopathologic analysis of 125 cases. Am J Surg Pathol 1984, **8**: 575–596.

957 Young RH, Dudley AG, Scully RE. Granulosa cell, Sertoli–Leydig cell, and unclassified sex cord–stromal tumors associated with pregnancy. A clinico-pathological analysis of thirty-six cases. Gynecol Oncol 1984, **18**: 181–205.

958 Young RH, Oliva E, Scully RE. Luteinized adult granulosa cell tumors of the ovary. A report of four cases. Int J Gynecol Pathol 1994, **13**: 302–310.

959 Young RH, Scully RE. Ovarian sex cord–stromal tumors. Recent progress. Int J Gynecol Pathol 1982, **1**: 101–123.

960 Young RH, Scully RE. Ovarian sex cord–stromal tumors with bizarre nuclei. A clinicopathologic analysis of 17 cases. Int J Gynecol Pathol 1983, **1**: 325–335.

961 Young RH, Scully RE. Ovarian sex cord–stromal tumors. Problems in differential diagnosis. Pathol Annu 1988, **23**(Pt 1): 237–296.

962 Zaloudek C, Norris HJ. Granulosa tumors of the ovary in children. A clinical and pathologic study of 32 cases. Am J Surg Pathol 1982, **6**: 513–522.

Thecoma, fibroma, and related tumors

963 Chalvardjian A, Scully RE. Sclerosing stromal tumors of the ovary. Cancer 1973, **31**: 664–670.

964 Clement PB, Young RH, Hanna W, Scully RE. Sclerosing peritonitis associated with luteinized thecomas of the ovary. A clinicopathological analysis of six cases. Am J Surg Pathol 1994, **18**: 1–13.

965 Costa MJ, Morris R, De Rose PB, Cohen C. Histologic and immunohistochemical evidence for considering ovarian myxoma as a variant of the thecomafibroma group of ovarian stromal tumors. Arch Pathol Lab Med 1993, **117**: 802–808.

966 Costa MJ, Thomas W, Majmudar B, Hewan-Lowe K. Ovarian myxoma. Ultrastructural and immunohistochemical findings. Ultrastruct Pathol 1992, **16**: 429–438.

967 Eichhorn JH, Scully RE. Ovarian myxoma. Clinicopathologic and immunocytologic analysis of five cases and a review of the literature. Int J Gynecol Pathol 1991, **10**: 156–169.

968 Fox H. Sex cord–stromal tumours of the ovary. J Pathol 1985, **145**: 127–148.

969 Gaffney EF, Majmudar B, Hewan-Lowe K. Ultrastructure and immunohistochemical localization of estradiol of three thecomas. Hum Pathol 1984, **15**: 153–160.

970 Hayes MC, Scully RE. Stromal luteoma of the ovary. A clinicopathological analysis of 25 cases. Int J Gynecol Pathol 1987, **6**: 313–321.

971 Irving JA, Alkushi A, Young RH, Clement PB. Cellular fibromas of the ovary: a study of 75 cases including 40 mitotically active tumors emphasizing their distinction from fibrosarcoma. Am J Surg Pathol 2006, **30**: 929–938.

972 Iwasa Y, Minamiguchi S, Konishi I, Onodera H, Zhou J, Yamabe H. Sclerosing peritonitis associated with luteinized thecoma of the ovary. Pathol Int 1996, **46**: 510–514.

973 Kanbour AI, Salazar H, Tobon H. Massive ovarian edema. A non-neoplastic pelvic mass of young women. Arch Pathol Lab Med 1979, **103**: 42–45.

974 Kawauchi S, Tsuji T, Kaku T, Kamura T, Nakano H, Tsuneyoshi M. Sclerosing stromal tumor of the ovary: A clinicopathologic, immunohistochemical, ultrastructural, and cytogenetic analysis with special reference to its vasculature. Am J Surg Pathol 1998, **22**: 83–92.

975 Lacson AG, Alrabeeah A, Gillis DA, Salisbury S, Grantmyre EB. Secondary massive ovarian edema with Meigs' syndrome. Am J Clin Pathol 1989, **91**: 597–603.

976 Meigs JV. Pelvic tumors other than fibromas of the ovary with ascites and hydrothorax. Obstet Gynecol 1954, **3**: 471–486.

977 Michal M, Kacerovska D, Mukensnabl P, Petersson F, Danis D, Adamkov M, Kazakov DV. Ovarian fibromas with heavy deposition of hyaline globules: a diagnostic pitfall. Int J Gynecol Pathol 2009, **28**: 356–361.

978 Nielsen GP, Young RH. Fibromatosis of soft tissue type involving the female genital tract: a report of two cases. Int J Gynecol Pathol 1998, **16**: 383–386.

979 Nogales FF, Martin-Sances L, Mendoza-Garcia E, Salamanca A, Gonzalez-Nunez MA, Pardo Mindan FJ. Massive ovarian oedema. Histopathology 1997, **28**: 229–234.

980 Persons DL, Hartmann LC, Herath JF, Keeney GL, Jenkins RB. Fluorescence in situ hybridization analysis of trisomy 12 in ovarian tumors. Am J Clin Pathol 1994, **102**: 775–779.

981 Prat J, Scully RE. Cellular fibromas and fibrosarcomas of the ovary. A comparative clinicopathologic analysis of seventeen cases. Cancer 1981, **47**: 2663–2670.

982 Raggio M, Kaplan AL, Harberg JF. Recurrent ovarian fibromas with basal cell nevus syndrome (Gorlin syndrome). Obstet Gynecol 1983, **61**: 95S–96S.

983 Roth LM, Deaton RL, Sternberg WH. Massive ovarian edema. A clinicopathologic study of five cases including ultrastructural observations and review of the literature. Am J Surg Pathol 1979, **3**: 11–21.

984 Roth LM, Sternberg WH. Partly luteinized theca cell tumor of the ovary. Cancer 1983, **51**: 1697–1704.

985 Saitoh A, Tsutsumi Y, Osamura RY, Watanabe K. Sclerosing stromal tumor of the ovary. Immunohistochemical and electron-microscopic demonstration of smooth-muscle differentiation. Arch Pathol Lab Med 1989, **113**: 372–376.

986 Samanth KK, Black WC III. Benign ovarian stromal tumors associated with free peritoneal fluid. Am J Obstet Gynecol 1970, **107**: 538–545.

987 Scully RE. Stromal luteoma of the ovary. A distinctive type of lipoid-cell tumor. Cancer 1964, **17**: 769–778.

988 Shaw JA, Dabbs DJ, Geisinger KR. Sclerosing stromal tumor of the ovary. An ultrastructural and immunohistochemical analysis with histogenetic considerations. Ultrastruct Pathol 1992, **16**: 363–377.

989 Staats PN, McCluggage WG, Clement PB, Young RH. Luteinized thecomas (thecomatosis) of the type typically associated with sclerosing peritonitis: a clinical, histopathologic, and immunohistochemical analysis of 27 cases. Am J Surg Pathol 2008, **32**: 1273–1290.

990 Sternberg WH, Roth LM. Ovarian stromal tumors containing Leydig cells. I. Stromal–Leydig cell tumor and non-neoplastic transformation of ovarian stroma to Leydig cells. Cancer 1973, **32**: 940–951.

991 Takeuchi S, Ishihara N, Ohbyashi C, Itoh H, Maruo T. Stromal Leydig cell tumor of the ovary: case report and literature review. Int J Gynecol Pathol 1999, **18**: 178–182.

992 Taruscio D, Carcangiu ML, Ward DC. Detection of trisomy 12 on ovarian sex cord stromal tumors by fluorescence in situ hybridization. Diagn Mol Pathol 1993, **2**: 94–98.

993 Tetu B, Bonenfant JL. Ovarian myxoma. A study of two cases with long-term follow-up. Am J Clin Pathol 1991, **95**: 340–346.

994 Tiltman AJ. Sclerosing stromal tumor of the ovary. Demonstration of ligandin in three cases. Int J Gynecol Pathol 1985, **4**: 362–369.

995 Tiltman AJ, Haffajee Z. Sclerosing stromal tumors, thecomas, and fibromas of the ovary: an immunohistochemical profile. Int J Gynecol Pathol 2002, **18**: 254–258.

996 Tsuji T, Kawauchi S, Utsunomiya T, Nagata Y, Tsuneyoshi M. Fibrosarcoma versus cellular fibroma of the ovary: a comparative study of their proliferative activity and chromosome aberrations using MIB-1 immunostaining, DNA flow cytometry, and fluorescence in situ hybridisation. Am J Surg Pathol 1997, **21**: 52–59.

997 Tsuji T, Catasus L, Prat J. Is loss of heterozygosity at 9q22.3 (PTCH gene) and 19p13.3 (STK11 gene) involved in the pathogenesis of ovarian stromal tumors? Hum Pathol 2005, **36**: 792–796.

998 Waxman M, Vuletin JC, Urcuyo R, Belling CG. Ovarian low-grade stromal sarcoma with thecomatous features. A critical reappraisal of the so-called 'malignant thecoma'. Cancer 1979, **44**: 2206–2217.

999 Werness BA. Luteinized thecoma with sclerosing peritonitis. Arch Pathol Lab Med 1996, **120**: 303–306.

1000 Young RH. Meigs' syndrome: Dr. Richard Cabot's hidden first American case. Int J Surg Pathol 2001, **8**: 165–168.

1001 Young RH, Clement PB, Scully RE. Calcified thecomas in young women. A report of four cases. Int J Gynecol Pathol 1988, **7**: 343–350.

1002 Young RH, Scully RE. Ovarian stromal tumors with minor sex-cord elements. A report of seven cases. Int J Gynecol Pathol 1983, **2**: 227–234.

1003 Young RH, Scully RE. Fibromatosis and massive edema of the ovary, possibly related entities. A report of 14 cases of fibromatosis and 11 cases of massive edema. Int J Gynecol Pathol 1984, **3**: 153–178.

1004 Zhang J, Young RH, Arseneau J, Scully RE. Ovarian stromal tumors containing lutein or Leydig cells (luteinized thecomas and stromal Leydig cell tumors). A clinicopathologic analysis of fifty cases. Int J Gynecol Pathol 1982, **1**: 270–285.

Endometrial abnormalities associated with granulosa cell tumor, thecoma, and related tumors

1005 Gusberg SB, Kardon P. Proliferative endometrial response to theca-granulosa cell tumors. Am J Obstet Gynecol 1971, **111**: 633–643.

1006 Katsube Y, Iwaoki Y, Silverberg SG, Fujiwara A. Sclerosing stromal tumor of the ovary associated with endometrial adenocarcinoma. A case report. Gynecol Oncol 1988, **29**: 392–398.

1007 Norris HJ, Taylor HB. Prognosis of granulosa-theca tumors of the ovary. Cancer 1968, **21**: 255–263.

1008 Press MF, Scully RE. Endometrial 'sarcomas' complicating ovarian thecoma, polycystic ovarian disease and estrogen therapy. Gynecol Oncol 1985, **21**: 135–154.

Small cell carcinoma

1009 Aguirre P, Thor AD, Scully RE. Ovarian small cell carcinoma. Histogenetic considerations based on immunohistochemical and other findings. Am J Clin Pathol 1989, **92**: 140–149.

1010 Carlson JW, Nucci MR, Brodsky J, Crum CP, Hirsch MS. Biomarker-assisted diagnosis of ovarian, cervical and pulmonary small cell carcinomas: the role of TTF-1, WT-1 and HPV analysis. Histopathology 2007, **51**: 305–312.

1011 Chen KTK. Composite large-cell neuroendocrine carcinoma and surface epithelial–stromal neoplasms of the ovary. Int J Surg Pathol 2000, **8**: 169–174.

1012 Clement PB. Selected miscellaneous ovarian lesions: small cell carcinomas, mesothelial lesions, mesenchymal and mixed neoplasms, and non-neoplastic lesions. Mod Pathol 2005, **18**(Suppl 2): S113–S129.

1013 Dickersin GR, Kline IW, Scully RE. Small cell carcinoma of the ovary with hypercalcemia. A report of eleven cases. Cancer 1982, **49**: 188–197.

1014 Dickersin GR, Scully RE. An update on the electron microscopy of small cell carcinoma of the ovary with hypercalcemia. Ultrastruct Pathol 1993, **17**: 411–422.

1015 Dickersin GR, Scully RE. Ovarian small cell tumors: an electron microscopic review. Ultrastruct Pathol 1998, **22**: 199–226.

1016 Eichhorn JH, Bell DA, Young RH, Swymer CM, Flotte TJ, Preffer RI, Scully RE. DNA content and proliferative activity in ovarian small cell carcinomas of the hypercalcemic type. Implications for diagnosis, prognosis, and histogenesis. Am J Clin Pathol 1992, **98**: 579–586.

1017 Eichhorn JH, Lawrence WD, Young RH, Scully RE. Ovarian neuroendocrine carcinomas of non-small-cell type associated with surface epithelial adenocarcinomas: a study of five cases and review of the literature. Int J Gynecol Pathol 1997, **15**: 303–314.

1018 Eichhorn JH, Young RH, Scully RE. Primary ovarian small cell carcinoma of pulmonary type. A clinicopathologic, immunohistologic, and flow cytometric analysis of 11 cases. Am J Surg Pathol 1992, **16**: 926–938.

1019 Jones K, Diaz JA, Donner LR. Neuroendocrine carcinoma arising in an ovarian mucinous cystadenoma. Int J Gynecol Pathol 1996, **15**: 167–170.

1020 Lamovec J, Bracko M, Cerar O. Familial occurrence of small-cell carcinoma of the ovary. Arch Pathol Lab Med 1995, **119**: 551–554.

1021 McCluggage WG, Oliva E, Connolly LE, McBride HA, Young RH. An immunohistochemical analysis of ovarian small cell carcinoma of hypercalcemic type. Int J Gynecol Pathol 2004, **23**: 330–336.

1022 Matias-Guiu X, Prat J, Young RH, Capen CC, Rosol TJ, DeLellis RA, Scully RE. Human parathyroid hormone-related protein in ovarian small cell carcinoma. An immunohistochemical study. Cancer 1994, **73**: 1878–1881.

1023 Riopel MA, Perlman EJ, Seidman JD, Kurman RJ, Sherman ME. Inhibin and epithelial membrane antigen immunohistochemistry assist in the diagnosis of sex cord–stromal tumors and provide clues to the histogenesis of hypercalcemic small cell carcinomas. Int J Gynecol Pathol 1998, **17**: 46–53.

1024 Scully RE. Small cell carcinoma of hypercalcemic type. Int J Gynecol Pathol 1993, **12**: 148–152.

1025 Ulbright TM, Roth LM, Stehman FB, Talerman A, Senekjian EK. Poorly differentiated (small cell) carcinoma of the ovary in young women. Evidence supporting a germ cell origin. Hum Pathol 1987, **18**: 175–184.

1026 Veras E, Deavers MT, Silva EG, Malpica A. Ovarian nonsmall cell neuroendocrine carcinoma: a clinicopathologic and immunohistochemical study of 11 cases. Am J Surg Pathol 2007, **31**: 774–782.

1027 Young RH, Oliva E, Scully RE. Small cell carcinoma of the ovary, hypercalcemic type. A clinicopathological analysis of 150 cases. Am J Surg Pathol 1994, **18**: 1102–1116.

Sertoli–Leydig cell tumor

1028 Aguirre P, Scully RE, DeLellis RA. Ovarian heterologous Sertoli–Leydig cell tumors with gastrointestinal-type epithelium. An immunohistochemical analysis. Arch Pathol Lab Med 1986, **110**: 528–533.

1029 Chadha S, Honnebier WJ, Schaberg A. Raised serum alphafetoprotein in Sertoli–Leydig cell tumor (androblastoma) of ovary. Report of two cases. Int J Gynecol Pathol 1987, **6**: 82–88.

1030 Costa MJ, Morris RJ, Wilson R, Judd R. Utility of immunohistochemistry in distinguishing ovarian Sertoli-stromal cell tumors from carcinosarcomas. Hum Pathol 1992, **23**: 787–797.

1031 Ferry JA, Young RH, Engel G, Scully RE. Oxyphilic Sertoli cell tumor of the ovary. A report of three cases, two in patients with the Peutz–Jeghers syndrome. Int J Gynecol Pathol 1994, **13**: 259–266.

1032 Fox H, Langley FA. Tumours of the ovary. London, 1976, Heinemann, pp. 156–157.

1033 Gagnon S, Tetu B, Silva EG, McCaughey WT. Frequency of alpha-fetoprotein production by Sertoli–Leydig cell tumors of the ovary. An immunohistochemical study of eight cases. Mod Pathol 1989, **2**: 63–67.

1034 Hittmair A, Zelger BG, Obrist P, Dirnhofer S. Ovarian Sertoli–Leydig cell tumor: a SRY gene-independent pathway of pseudomale gonadal differentiation. Hum Pathol 1997, **28**: 1206–1210.

1035 Jenson AB, Fechner RE. Ultrastructure of an intermediate Sertoli–Leydig cell tumor. A histogenetic misnomer. Lab Invest 1969, **21**: 527–535.

1036 Kurman RJ, Ganjei P, Nadji M. Contributions of immunocytochemistry to the diagnosis and study of ovarian neoplasms. Int J Gynecol Pathol 1984, **3**: 3–26.

1037 McCluggage WG, Young RH. Ovarian Sertoli–Leydig cell tumors with pseudoendometrioid tubules (pseudoendometrioid Sertoli–Leydig cell tumors). Am J Surg Pathol 2007, **31**: 592–597.

1038 Meyer R. Tubuläre (testikuläre) und solide Foramen des Andreiblastoma ovarii und ihre Beziehung zur Vermännlickung. Beitr Pathol Anat 1930, **84**: 485–520.

1039 Mooney EE, Man YG, Bratthauer GL, Tavassoli FA. Evidence that Leydig cells in Sertoli–Leydig cell tumors have a reactive rather then a neoplastic profile. Cancer 2000, **86**: 2312–2319.

1040 Mooney EE, Nogales FF, Bergeron C, Tavassoli FA. Retiform Sertoli–Leydig cell tumors: clinical, morphological and immunohistochemical findings. Histopathology 2002, **41**: 110–117.

1041 Mooney EE, Nogales FF, Tavassoli FA. Hepatocytic differentiation in retiform Sertoli–Leydig cell tumors: distinguishing a heterologous element from Leydig cells. Hum Pathol 1999, **30**: 611–617.

1042 Motoyama I, Watanabe H, Gotoh A, Takeuchi S, Tanabe N, Nashimoto I. Ovarian Sertoli–Leydig cell tumor with elevated serum alpha-fetoprotein. Cancer 1989, **63**: 2047–2053.

1043 Oliva E, Alvarez T, Young RH. Sertoli cell tumors of the ovary: a clinicopathologic and immunohistochemical study of 54 cases. Am J Surg Pathol 2005, **29**: 143–156.

1044 Prat J, Young RH, Scully RE. Ovarian Sertoli–Leydig cell tumors with heterologous elements. II. Cartilage and skeletal muscle. A clinicopathologic analysis of twelve cases. Cancer 1982, **50**: 2465–2475.

1045 Roth LM, Anderson MC, Govan ADT, Langley FA, Gowing NFC, Woodcock AS. Sertoli–Leydig cell tumors. A clinicopathologic study of 34 cases. Cancer 1981, **48**: 187–197.

1046 Roth LM, Cleary RE, Rosenfield RL. Sertoli–Leydig cell tumor of the ovary, with an associated mucinous cystadenoma. An ultrastructural and endocrine study. Lab Invest 1974, **31**: 648–657.

1047 Roth LM, Slayton RE, Brady LW, Blessing JA, Johnson G. Retiform differentiation in ovarian Sertoli–Leydig cell tumors. A clinicopathologic study of six cases from a gynecologic oncology group study. Cancer 1985, **55**: 1093–1098.

1048 Savard K, Gut M, Dorfman RI, Gabrilove JL, Soffer LJ. Formation of androgens by human arrhenoblastoma tissue in vitro. J Clin Endocrinol 1961, **21**: 165–174.

1049 Scully RE. Ovarian tumors. A review. Am J Pathol 1977, **87**: 686–720.

1050 Seidman JD, Patterson JA, Bitterman P. Sertoli–Leydig cell tumor associated with a mature cystic teratoma in a single ovary. Mod Pathol 1989, **2**: 687–692.

1051 Stegner H-E, Lisboa BP. Steroid metabolism in an androblastoma (Sertoli–Leydig cell tumor). A histopathological and biochemical study. Int J Gynecol Pathol 1984, **2**: 410–425.

1052 Tavassoli FA, Norris HJ. Sertoli tumors of the ovary. A clinicopathologic study of 28 cases with ultrastructural observations. Cancer 1980, **46**: 2281–2297.

1053 Tracy SL, Askin FB, Reddick RL, Jackson B, Kurman RJ. Progesterone-secreting Sertoli cell tumor of the ovary. Gynecol Oncol 1985, **22**: 85–96.

1054 Young RH. Sertoli–Leydig cell tumors of the ovary. Review with emphasis on historical aspects and unusual variants. Int J Gynecol Pathol 1993, **12**: 141–147.

1055 Young RH, Dudley AG, Scully RE. Granulosa cell, Sertoli–Leydig cell and unclassified sex cord–stromal tumors associated with pregnancy. A clinicopathological analysis of thirty-six cases. Gynecol Oncol 1984, **18**: 181–205.

1056 Young RH, Perez-Atayde AR, Scully RE. Ovarian Sertoli–Leydig cell tumor with retiform and heterologous components. Report of a case with hepatocytic differentiation and elevated serum alpha-fetoprotein. Am J Surg Pathol 1984, **8**: 709–718.

1057 Young RH, Prat J, Scully RE. Ovarian Sertoli–Leydig cell tumors with heterologous elements. I Gastrointestinal epithelium and carcinoid. A clinicopathologic analysis of thirty-six cases. Cancer 1982, **50**: 2448–2456.

1058 Young RH, Scully RE. Ovarian Sertoli–Leydig cell tumors with a retiform pattern. A problem in histopathologic diagnosis. A report of 25 cases. Am J Surg Pathol 1983, **7**: 755–771.

1059 Young RH, Scully RE. Ovarian sex cord–stromal tumors with bizarre nuclei. A clinicopathologic analysis of 17 cases. Int J Gynecol Pathol 1983, **1**: 325–335.

1060 Young RH, Scully RE. Ovarian Sertoli cell tumors. A report of 10 cases. Int J Gynecol Pathol 1984, **2**: 349–363.

1061 Young RH, Scully RE. Well-differentiated ovarian Sertoli–Leydig cell tumors. A clinicopathological analysis of 23 cases. Int J Gynecol 1984, **3**: 277–290.

1062 Young RH, Scully RE. Ovarian Sertoli–Leydig cell tumors. A clinicopathological analysis of 207 cases. Am J Surg Pathol 1985, **9**: 543–569.

1063 Zaloudek C, Norris HJ. Sertoli–Leydig tumors of the ovary. A clinicopathologic study of 64 intermediate and poorly differentiated neoplasms. Am J Surg Pathol 1984, **8**: 405–418.

1064 Zhao C, Bratthauer GL, Barner R, Vang R. Comparative analysis of alternative and traditional immunohistochemical markers for the distinction of ovarian Sertoli cell tumor from endometrioid tumors and carcinoid tumor: a study of 160 cases. Am J Surg Pathol 2007, **31**: 255–266.

1065 Zhao C, Bratthauer GL, Barner R, Vang R. Immunohistochemical analysis of sox9 in ovarian Sertoli cell tumors and other tumors in the differential diagnosis. Int J Gynecol Pathol 2007, **26**: 1–9.

1066 Zhao C, Bratthauer GL, Barner R, Vang R. Diagnostic utility of WT1 immunostaining in ovarian sertoli cell tumor. Am J Surg Pathol 2007, **31**: 1378–1386.

Lipid (lipoid, steroid) cell tumor

1067 Hayes MC, Scully RE. Ovarian steroid cell tumors (not otherwise specified). A clinicopathological analysis of 63 cases. Am J Surg Pathol 1987, **11**: 835–845.

1068 Ichinohasama R, Teshima S, Kishi K, Mukai K, Tsunematsu R, Ishii-Ohba H, Shimosato Y. Leydig cell tumor of the ovary associated with endometrial carcinoma and containing 17 beta-hydroxysteroid dehydrogenase. Int J Gynecol Pathol 1989, **8**: 64–71.

1069 Ishida T, Okagaki T, Tagatz GE, Jacobson ME, Doe RP. Lipid cell tumor of the ovary. An ultrastructural study. Cancer 1977, **40**: 234–243.

1070 Jones MW, Harri R, Dabbs DJ, Carter GJ. Immunohistochemical profile of steroid cell tumor of the ovary: a study of 14 cases and a review of the literature. Int J Gynecol Pathol 2010, **29**: 315–320.

1071 Paraskevas M, Scully RE. Hilus cell tumor of the ovary. A clinicopathological analysis of 12 Reinke crystal-positive and nine crystal-negative cases. Int J Gynecol Pathol 1989, **8**: 299–310.

1072 Roth LM, Sternberg WH. Ovarian stromal tumors containing Leydig cells. II. Pure Leydig cell tumor, nonhilar type. Cancer 1973, **32**: 952–960.

1073 Rutgers JL, Scully RE. Functioning ovarian tumors with peripheral steroid cell proliferation. A report of twenty-four cases. Int J Gynecol Pathol 1986, **5**: 319–337.

1074 Salm R. Ovarian hilus-cell tumours. Their varying presentations. J Pathol 1974, **113**: 117–127.

1075 Sandberg AA, Slaunwhite WR, Jackson JE, Frawley TF. Androgen biosynthesis by an ovarian lipoid cell tumor. J Clin Endocrinol 1962, **22**: 929–934.

1076 Seidman JD, Abbondanzo SL, Bratthauer GL. Lipid cell (steroid cell) tumor of the ovary. Immunophenotype with analysis of potential pitfall due to endogenous biotin-like activity. Int J Gynecol Pathol 1995, **14**: 331–338.

1077 Taylor HB, Norris HJ. Lipid cell tumors of the ovary. Cancer 1967, **20**: 1953–1962.

1078 Young RH, Scully RE. Ovarian steroid cell tumors associated with Cushing's syndrome. A report of three cases. Int J Gynecol Pathol 1987, **6**: 40–48.

Other types

1079 Ahn GH, Chi JG, Lee SK. Ovarian sex cord tumor with annular tubules. Cancer 1986, **57**: 1066–1073.

1080 Anderson MC, Govan ADT, Langley FA, Woodcock AS, Tyagi SP. Ovarian sex cord tumours with annular tubules. Histopathology 1980, **4**: 137–145.

1081 Brescia RJ, Cardoso De Almeida PC, Fuller AF, Dickersin GR, Robboy SJ. Female adnexal tumor of probable wolffian origin with multiple recurrences over 16 years. Cancer 1985, **56**: 1456–1461.

1082 Broshears JR, Roth LM. Gynandroblastoma with elements resembling juvenile granulosa cell tumor. Int J Gynecol Pathol 1998, **16**: 387–391.

1083 Chivukula M, Hunt J, Carter G, Kelley J, Patel M, Kanbour-Shakir A. Recurrent gynandroblastoma of ovary – a case report: a molecular and immunohistochemical analysis. Int J Gynecol Pathol 2007, **26**: 30–33.

1084 Crissman JD, Hart WR. Ovarian sex cord tumors with annular tubules. An ultrastructural study of three cases. Am J Clin Pathol 1981, **75**: 11–17.

1085 Devouassoux-Shisheboran M, Silver SA, Tavassoli FA. Wolffian adnexal tumor, so-called female adnexal tumor of probable wolffian origin (FATWO): immunohistochemical evidence in support of a wolffian origin. Hum Pathol 1999, **30**: 856–863.

1086 Fanghong LI, Szallasi A, Young RH. Wolffian tumor of the ovary with a prominent spindle cell component: report of a case with brief discussion of unusual problems in differential diagnosis, and literature review. Int J Surg Pathol 2008, **16**: 222–225.

1087 Fukunaga M, Endo Y, Ushigome S. Gynandroblastoma of the ovary: a case report with an immunohistochemical and ultrastructural study. Virchows Arch 1997, **430**: 77–82.

1088 Gloor E. Ovarian sex-cord tumor with annular tubules. Clinicopathologic report of two benign and one malignant cases with long follow-ups. Virchows Arch [A] 1979, **384**: 185–193.

1089 Hart WR, Kumar N, Crissman JD. Ovarian neoplasms resembling sex cord tumors with annular tubules. Cancer 1980, **45**: 2352–2363.

1090 Hertel BF, Kempson RL. Ovarian sex cord tumors with annular tubules. An ultrastructural study. Am J Surg Pathol 1977, **1**: 145–153.

1091 Irving JA, Young RH. Microcystic stromal tumor of the ovary: report of 16 cases of a hitherto uncharacterized distinctive ovarian neoplasm. Am J Surg Pathol 2009, **33**: 367–375.

1092 Kariminejad MH, Scully RE. Female adnexal tumor of probable wolffian origin – a distinctive pathological entity. Cancer 1973, **31**: 671–677.

1093 Lele SM, Sawh RN, Zaharopoulos P, Adesokan A, Smith M, Linhart JM, Arrastia CD, Krigman HR. Malignant ovarian sex cord tumor with annular tubules in a patient with Peutz–Jeghers syndrome: a case report. Mod Pathol 2000, **13**: 466–470.

1094 McCluggage WG, Sloan JM, Murnaghan M, White R. Gynandroblastoma of ovary with juvenile granulosa cell component and heterologous intestinal type glands. Histopathology 1997, **29**: 253–257.

1095 Neubecker RD, Breen JL. Gynandroblastoma. A report of five cases, with a discussion of the histogenesis and classification of ovarian tumors. Am J Clin Pathol 1962, **38**: 60–69.

1096 Novak ER. Gynandroblastoma of the ovary. Review of 8 cases from the Ovarian Tumor Registry. Obstet Gynecol 1967, **30**: 709–715.

1097 Rahilly MA, Williams ARW, Krausz T, al Nafussi A. Female adnexal tumour of probable Wolffian origin. A clinicopathological and immunohistochemical study of three cases. Histopathology 1995, **26**: 69–74.

1098 Scully RE. The prolonged gestation, birth, and early life of the sex cord tumor with annular tubules and how it joined a syndrome. Int J Surg Pathol 2001, **8**: 233–238.

1099 Seidman JD. Unclassified ovarian gonadal stromal tumors: a clinicopathologic study of 32 cases. Am J Surg Pathol 1996, **20**: 699–706.

1100 Sheyn I, Mira JL, Bejarano PA, Husseinzadeh N. Metastatic female adnexal tumor of probable Wolffian origin: a case report and review of the literature. Arch Pathol Lab Med 2000, **124**: 431–434.

1101 Simpson JL, Michael H, Roth LM. Unclassified sex cord–stromal tumors of the ovary: a report of eight cases. Arch Pathol Lab Med 1998, **122**: 52–55.

1102 Sivathondan Y, Salm R, Hughesdon PE, Faccini JM. Female adnexal tumour of probably wolffian origin: J Clin Pathol 1979, **32**: 616–624.

1103 Tiltman AJ, Allard U. Female adnexal tumors of probable Wolffian origin: an immunohistochemical study comparing tumors, mesonephric remnants and paramesonephric derivatives. Histopathology 2001, **38**: 237–242.

1104 Vang R, Bagué S, Tavassoli FA, Prat J. Signet-ring stromal tumor of the ovary: clinicopathologic analysis and comparison with Krukenberg tumor. Int J Gynecol Pathol 2004, **23**: 45–51.

1105 Young RH, Dickersin GR, Scully RE. A distinctive ovarian sex cord–stromal tumor causing sexual precocity in the Peutz–Jeghers syndrome. Am J Surg Pathol 1983, **7**: 233–243.

1106 Young RH, Scully RE. Ovarian tumors of probable wolffian origin. A report of 11 cases. Am J Surg Pathol 1983, **7**: 125–135.

1107 Young RH, Welch WR, Dickersin GR, Scully RE. Ovarian sex cord tumor with annular tubules. Review of 74 cases including 27 with Peutz–Jeghers syndrome and four with adenoma malignum of the cervix. Cancer 1982, **50**: 1384–1402.

GERM CELL–SEX CORD–STROMAL TUMORS

1108 Goldsmith CI, Hart WR. Ataxia-telangiectasia with ovarian gonadoblastoma and contralateral dysgerminoma. Cancer 1975, **36**: 1838–1842.

1109 Govan ADT, Woodcock AS, Gowing NFC, Langley FA, Neville AM, Anderson MC. A clinico-pathological study of gonadoblastoma. Br J Obstet Gynecol 1977, **84**: 222–228.

1110 Hart WR, Burkons DM. Germ cell neoplasms arising in gonadoblastomas. Cancer 1979, **43**: 669–678.

1111 Hou-Jensen K, Kempson RL. The ultrastructure of gonadoblastoma and dysgerminoma. Hum Pathol 1974, **5**: 79–91.

1112 Hussong J, Crussi FG, Chou PM. Gonadoblastoma: immunohistochemical localization of Mullerian-inhibiting substance, inhibin, WT-1, and p53. Mod Pathol 1997, **10**: 1101–1105.

1113 Kersemaekers AM, Honecker F, Stoop H, Cools M, Molier M, Wolffenbuttel K, Bokemeyer C, Li Y, Lau YF, Oosterhuis JW, Looijenga LH. Identification of germ cells at risk for neoplastic transformation in gonadoblastoma: an immunohistochemical study for OCT3/4 and TSPY. Hum Pathol 2005, **36**: 512–521.

1114 Lacson AG, Gillis DA, Shawwa A. Malignant mixed germ-cell–sex cord–stromal tumors of the ovary associated with isosexual precocious puberty. Cancer 1988, **61**: 2122–2133.

1115 Li Y, Tabatabai ZL, Lee TL, Hatakeyama S, Ohyama C, Chan WY, Looijenga LH, Lau YF. The Y-encoded TSPY protein: a significant marker potentially plays a role in the pathogenesis of testicular germ cell tumors. Hum Pathol 2007, **38**: 1470–1481.

1116 Mackay AM, Pettigrew N, Symington T, Neville AM. Tumors of dysgenetic gonads (gonadoblastoma). Ultrastructural and steroidogenic aspects. Cancer 1974, **34**: 1108–1125.

1117 Michal M, Vanecek T, Sima R, Mukensnabl P, Hes O, Kazakov DV, Matoska J, Zuntova A, Dvorak V, Talerman A. Mixed germ cell sex cord–stromal tumors of the testis and ovary. Morphological, immunohistochemical, and molecular genetic study of seven cases. Virchows Arch 2006, **448**: 612–622.

1118 Nakashima N, Nagasaka T, Fukata S, Oiwa N, Nara Y, Fukatsu T, Takeuchi J. Ovarian gonadoblastoma with dysgerminoma in a woman with two normal children. Hum Pathol 1989, **20**: 814–816.

1119 Nomura K, Matsui T, Aizawa S. Gonadoblastoma with proliferation resembling sertoli cell tumor. Int J Gynecol Pathol 1999, **18**: 91–93.

1120 Pratt-Thomas HR, Cooper JM. Gonadoblastoma with tubal pregnancy. Am J Clin Pathol 1976, **65**: 121–125.

1121 Roth LM, Eglen DE. Gonadoblastoma. Immunohistochemical and ultrastructural observations. Int J Gynecol Pathol 1989, **8**: 72–81.

1122 Safneck JR, deSa DJ. Structures mimicking sex cord–stromal tumours and gonadoblastomas in the ovaries of normal infants and children. Histopathology 1986, **10**: 909–920.

1123 Scully RE. Gonadoblastoma. A review of 74 cases. Cancer 1970, **25**: 1340–1356.

1124 Talerman A, van der Harten JJ. A mixed germ cell–sex cord–stromal tumor of the ovary associated with isosexual precocious puberty in a normal girl. Cancer 1977, **40**: 889–894.

1125 Talerman A, Roth LM. Recent advances in the pathology and classification of gonadal neoplasms composed of germ cells and sex cord derivatives. Int J Gynecol Pathol 2007, **26**: 313–321.

1126 Teter J. The mixed germ tumours with hormonal activity. Acta Pathol Microbiol Scand (A) 1963, **58**: 306–320.

1127 Tokuoka S, Aoki Y, Hayashi Y, Yokoyama T, Ishii T. A mixed germ cell–sex cord–stromal tumor of the ovary with retiform tubular structure. A case report. Int J Gynecol Pathol 1985, **4**: 161–170.

TUMORS NOT SPECIFIC TO OVARY

Malignant lymphoma and leukemia

1128 Chorlton I, Norris HJ, King FM. Malignant reticuloendothelial disease involving the ovary as a primary manifestation. A series of 19 lymphomas and 1 granulocytic sarcoma. Cancer 1974, **34**: 397–407.

1129 Ferry JA, Young RH. Malignant lymphoma, pseudolymphoma, and hematopoietic disorders of the female genital tract. Pathol Annu 1991, **26**(Pt 1): 227–263.

1130 Ferry JA, Young RH. Malignant lymphoma of the genitourinary tract. Curr Diagn Pathol 1997, **4**: 145–169.

1131 Kosari F, Daneshbod Y, Parwaresch R, Krams M, Wacker HH. Lymphomas of the female genital tract: a study of 186 cases and review of the literature. Am J Surg Pathol 2005, **29**: 1512–1520.

1132 Lagoo AS, Robboy SJ. Lymphoma of the female genital tract: current status. Int J Gynecol Pathol 2006, **25**: 1–21.

1133 Monterroso V, Jaffe ES, Merino MJ, Medeiros LJ. Malignant lymphomas involving the ovary. A clinicopathologic analysis of 39 cases. Am J Surg Pathol 1992, **17**: 154–170.

1134 Oliva E, Ferry JA, Young RH, Prat J, Srigley JR, Scully RE. Granulocytic sarcoma of the female genital tract: a clinicopathologic study of 11 cases. Am J Surg Pathol 1997, **21**: 1156–1165.

1135 Osborne BM, Robboy SJ. Lymphomas or leukemias presenting as ovarian tumors. An analysis of 42 cases. Cancer 1983, **52**: 1933–1943.

1136 Paladugu RR, Bearman RM, Rappaport H. Malignant lymphoma with primary manifestation in the gonad. A clinicopathologic study of 38 patients. Cancer 1980, **45**: 561–571.

1137 Pressler H, Horny HP, Wolf A, Kaiserling E. Isolated granulocytic sarcoma of the ovary. Histologic, electron microscopic, and immunohistochemical findings. Int J Gynecol Pathol 1992, **11**: 68–74.

1138 Rotmensch J, Woodruff JD. Lymphoma of the ovary. Report of twenty new cases and update of previous series. Am J Obstet Gynecol 1982, **143**: 870–875.

1139 Skodras G, Fields V, Kragel PJ. Ovarian lymphoma and serous carcinoma of low malignant potential arising in the same ovary. A case report with literature review of 14 primary ovarian lymphomas. Arch Pathol Lab Med 1994, **118**: 647–650.

1140 Vang R, Medeiros J, Warnke RA, Higgins JP, Deavers MT. Ovarian non-Hodgkin's lymphoma: a clinicopathologic study of eight primary cases. Mod Pathol 2001, **14**: 1093–1099.

Sarcoma

1141 Fadare O, Bossuyt V, Martel M, Parkash V. Primary osteosarcoma of the ovary: a case report and literature review. Int J Gynecol Pathol 2007, **26**: 21–25.

1142 Guerard MJ, Arguelles MA, Ferenczy A. Rhabdomyosarcoma of the ovary. Ultrastructural study of a case and review of literature. Gynecol Oncol 1983, **15**: 325–339.

1143 Hines JF, Compton DM, Stacy CC, Potter ME. Pure primary osteosarcoma of the ovary presenting as an extensively calcified adnexal mass. A case report and review of the literature. Gynecol Oncol 1990, **39**: 259–263.

1144 Kawauchi S, Fukuda T, Miyamoto S, Yoshioka J, Shirahama S, Saito T, Tsukamoto N. Peripheral primitive neuroectodermal tumor of the ovary confirmed by CD99 immunostaining, karyotypic analysis, and RT-PCR for EWS/FLI-1 chimeric mRNA. Am J Surg Pathol 1998, **22**: 1417–1422.

1145 Kojiro S, Quer A, Snuderl M, Daya D, Hayashi T, Bosincu L, Ogawa F, Vu Q, Rosenberg AE, Iafrate AJ, Olivia E. Primitive neuroectodermal tumors (PNETs) of the female genital tract (FGT): a morphologic, immunohistochemical, and molecular study of 18 cases. Lab Invest 2009, **89**(Suppl 1): 222A.

1146 Kraemer BB, Silva EG, Sneige N. Fibrosarcoma of ovary. A new component in the nevoid basal-cell carcinoma syndrome. Am J Surg Pathol 1984, **8**: 231–236.

1147 Lerwill MF, Sung R, Oliva E, Prat J, Young RH. Smooth muscle tumors of the ovary: a clinicopathologic study of 54 cases emphasizing prognostic criteria, histologic variants, and differential diagnosis. Am J Surg Pathol 2004, **28**: 1436–1451.

1148 Nasu M, Inoue J, Matsui M, Minoura S, Matsubara O. Ovarian leiomyosarcoma: an autopsy case report. Pathol Int 2000, **50**: 162–165.

1149 Nielsen GP, Oliva E, Young RH, Rosenberg AE, Prat J, Scully RE. Primary ovarian rhabdomyosarcoma: a report of 13 cases. Int J Gynecol Pathol 1998, **17**: 113–119.

1150 Nielsen GP, Young RH, Prat J, Scully RE. Primary angiosarcoma of the ovary: A report of seven cases and review of the literature. Int J Gynecol Pathol 1998, **16**: 378–382.

1151 Nogales FF, Ayala A, Ruiz-Avila I, Sirvent JJ. Myxoid leiomyosarcoma of the ovary. Analysis of three cases. Hum Pathol 1991, **22**: 1268–1273.

1152 Nucci MR, Krausz T, Lifschitz-Mercer B, Chan JK, Fletcher CD. Angiosarcoma of the ovary: clinicopathologic and immunohistochemical analysis of four cases with a broad morphologic spectrum. Am J Surg Pathol 1998, **22**: 620–630.

1153 Ongkasuwan C, Taylor JE, Tang C-K, Prempree T. Angiosarcomas of the uterus and ovary. Clinicopathologic report. Cancer 1982, **49**: 1469–1475.

1154 Prat J, Scully RE. Cellular fibromas and fibrosarcomas of the ovary. A comparative clinicopathologic analysis of seventeen cases. Cancer 1981, **47**: 2663–2670.

1155 Sakata H, Hirahara T, Ryu A, Sawada T, Yamamoto M, Sakurai I. Primary osteosarcoma of the ovary. A case report. Acta Pathol Jpn 1991, **41**: 311–317.

1156 Sant'Ambrogoio S, Malpica A, Schroeder B, Silva EG. Primary ovarian rhabdomyosarcoma associated with clear cell carcinoma of the ovary: a case report and review of the literature. Int J Gynecol Pathol 2000, **19**: 169–173.

1157 Seracchioli R, Colombo FM, Bagnoli A, Trengia V, Venturoli S. Primary ovarian leiomyosarcoma as a new component in the nevoid basal cell carcinoma syndrome: a case report. Am J Obstet Gynecol 2003, **188**: 1093–1095.

1158 Silverberg SG, Fernandez FN. Endolymphatic stromal myosis of the ovary. A report of three cases and literature review. Gynecol Oncol 1981, **12**: 129–138.

1159 Sood AK, Sorosky JI, Gelder MS, Buller RE, Anderson B, Wilkinson EJ, Benda JA, Morgan LS. Primary ovarian sarcoma: analysis of prognostic variables and the role of surgical cytoreduction. Cancer 1998, **82**: 1731–1737.

1160 Stone GC, Bell DA, Fuller A, Dickersin GR, Scully RE. Malignant schwannoma of the ovary. Report of a case. Cancer 1986, **58**: 1575–1582.

1161 Talerman A, Auerbach WM, Van Meurs AJ. Primary chondrosarcoma of the ovary. Histopathology 1981, **5**: 319–324.

1162 Winfield HL, De Las Casas LE, Greenfield WW, Santin AD, McKenney JK. Low-grade fibromyxoid sarcoma presenting clinically as a primary ovarian neoplasm: a case report. Int J Gynecol Pathol 2007, **26**: 173–176.

1163 Young RH, Prat J, Scully RE. Endometrioid stromal sarcomas of the ovary. A clinicopathologic analysis of 23 cases. Cancer 1984, **53**: 1143–1155.

Other primary tumors

1164 Alvarez M, Cerezo L. Ovarian cavernous hemangioma. Arch Pathol Lab Med 1986, **110**: 77–78.

1165 Anderson AE, Yang X, Young RH. Epithelioid angiomyolipoma of the ovary: a case report and literature review. Int J Gynecol Pathol 2002, **21**: 69–73.

1166 Baker PM, Rosai J, Young RH. Ovarian teratomas with florid benign vascular proliferation: a distinctive finding associated with the neural component of teratomas that may be confused with a vascular neoplasm. Int J Gynecol Pathol 2002, **21**: 16–21.

1167 Deshpande V, Oliva E, Young RH. Solid pseudopapillary neoplasm of the ovary: a report of 3 primary ovarian tumors resembling those of the pancreas. Am J Surg Pathol 2010, **34**: 1514–1520.

1168 Doss BJ, Wanek SM, Jacques SM, Qureshi F, Ramirez NC, Lawrence WD. Ovarian leiomyomas: clinicopathologic features in fifteen cases. Int J Gynecol Pathol 1999, **18**: 63–68.

1169 Evans A, Lytwyn A, Urbach G, Chapman W. Bilateral lymphangiomas of the ovary: an immunohistochemical characterization and review of the literature. Int J Gynecol Pathol 1999, **18**: 87–90.

1170 Fang X, Rodabaugh K, Penetrante R, Wong M, Wagner T, Sait S, Mhawech-Fauceglia P. Desmoplastic small round cell tumor (DSRCT) with ovarian involvement in 2 young women. Appl Immunohistochem Mol Morphol 2008, **16**: 94–99.

1171 Fawcett FJ, Kimbell NKB. Phaeochromocytoma of the ovary. J Obstet Gynaecol Br Commonw 1971, **78**: 458–459.

1172 Friedman HD, Mazur MT. Primary ovarian leiomyosarcoma. An immunohistochemical and ultrastructural study. Arch Pathol Lab Med 1991, **115**: 941–945.

1173 Gokten N, Peterdy G, Philpott T, Maluf HM. Glomus tumor of the ovary: report of a case with immunohistochemical and ultrastructural observations. Int J Gynecol Pathol 2001, **20**: 390–394.

1174 Isaac MA, Vijayalakshmi S, Madhu CS, Bosincu L, Nogales FP. Pure cystic nephroblastoma of the ovary with a review of extrarenal Wilms' tumors. Hum Pathol 2000, **31**: 761–764.

1175 Kandalaft PL, Esteban JM. Bilateral massive ovarian leiomyomata in a young woman. A case report with review of the literature. Mod Pathol 1992, **5**: 586–589.

1176 Lerwill MF, Sung R, Oliva E, Prat J, Young RH. Smooth muscle tumors of the ovary: a clinicopathologic study of 54 cases emphasizing prognostic criteria, histologic variants, and differential diagnosis. Am J Surg Pathol 2004, **28**: 1436–1451.

1177 McCluggage WG, Young RH. Paraganglioma of the ovary: report of three cases of a rare ovarian neoplasm, including two exhibiting inhibin positivity. Am J Surg Pathol 2006, **30**: 600–605.

1178 McCluggage WG, Bissonnette JP, Young RH. Primary malignant melanoma of the ovary: a report of 9 definite or probable cases with emphasis on their morphologic diversity and mimicry of other primary and secondary ovarian neoplasms. Int J Gynecol Pathol 2006, **25**: 321–329.

1179 Phillips V, McCluggage WG, Young RH. Oxyphilic adenomatoid tumor of the ovary: a case report with discussion of the differential diagnosis of ovarian tumors with vacuoles and related spaces. Int J Gynecol Pathol 2007, **26**: 16–20.

1180 Prayson RA, Hart WR. Primary smooth-muscle tumors of the ovary. A clinicopathologic study of four leiomyomas and two mitotically active leiomyomas. Arch Pathol Lab Med 1992, **116**: 1068–1071.

1181 Prus D, Rosenburg AE, Blumenfeld A, Udassin R, Ne'eman Z, Young RH, Ariel I. Infantile hemagioendothlioma of the ovary: a monodermal teratoma or a neoplasm of ovarian somatic cells? Am J Surg Pathol 1997, **21**: 1231–1235.

1182 Rhoades CP, McMahon JT, Goldblum JR. Myofibroblastoma of the ovary: report of a case. Mod Pathol 1999, **12**: 907–911.

1183 Slone SP, Moore GD, Parker LP, Rickard KA, Nixdorf-Miller AS. Glomus tumor of the ovary masquerading as granulosa cell tumor: case report. Int J Gynecol Pathol 2010, **29**: 24–26.

1184 Yenen E, Inanc FA, Babuna C. Primary ovarian hydatidiform mole. Report of a case. Obstet Gynecol 1966, **26**: 721–724.

1185 Young RH, Silva EG, Scully RE. Ovarian and juxtaovarian adenomatoid tumors. A report of six cases. Int J Gynecol Pathol 1991, **10**: 364–371.

Metastatic tumors

1186 Abadeer RA, Malpica A. Metastatic pancreatic adenocarcinoma to the ovary: a clinicopathologic review of twenty nine cases. Lab Invest 2009, **89**(Suppl 1): 204A–205A.

1187 Al-Agha OM, Nicastri AD. An in-depth look at Krukenberg tumor: an overview. Arch Pathol Lab Med 2006, **130**: 1725–1730.

1188 Albarracin CT, Jafri J, Montag AG, Hart J, Kuan SF. Differential expression of MUC2 and MUC5AC mucin genes in primary ovarian and metastatic colonic carcinoma. Hum Pathol 2000, **31**: 672–677.

1189 Berezowski K, Stastny JF, Kornstein MJ. Cytokeratins 7 and 20 and carcinoembryonic antigen in ovarian and colonic carcinoma. Mod Pathol 1996, **9**: 426–429.

1190 Bombonati A, Ciocca V, Palazzo JP, Schulz S, Waldman SA. Guanylyl cyclase C is a specific marker for differentiating primary and metastatic overian mucinous neoplasms. Lab Invest 2009, **89**(Suppl 1): 207A–208A.

1191 Bullon A Jr, Arseneau J, Prat J, Young RH, Scully RE. Tubular Krukenberg tumor. A problem in histopathologic diagnosis. Am J Surg Pathol 1981, **5**: 225–232.

1192 Chou Y-Y, Jeng Y-M, Kao H-L, Chen T-J, Mao T-L, Lin M-C. Differentiation of ovarian mucinous carcinoma and metastatic colorectal adenocarcinoma by immunostaining with β-catenin. Histopathology 2003, **43**: 151–156.

1193 Chuaqui RF, Zhuang Z, Emmert-Buck MR, Bryant BR, Nogales F, Tavassoli FA, Merino MJ. Genetic analysis of synchronous mucinous tumors of the ovary and appendix. Hum Pathol 1996, **27**: 165–171.

1194 Daya D, Nazerali L, Frank GL. Metastatic ovarian carcinoma of large intestinal origin simulating primary ovarian carcinoma. A clinicopathologic study of 25 cases. Am J Clin Pathol 1992, **97**: 751–758.

1195 DeCostanzo DC, Elias JM, Chumas JC. Necrosis in 84 ovarian carcinomas: a morphologic study of primary versus metastatic colonic carcinoma with a selective immunohistochemical analysis of cytokeratin subtypes and carcinoembryonic antigen. Int J Gynecol Pathol 1997, **16**: 245–249.

1196 Demopoulos RI, Touger L, Dubin N. Secondary ovarian carcinoma. A clinical and pathological evaluation. Int J Gynecol Pathol 1987, **6**: 166–175.

1197 Dionigi A, Facco C, Tibiletti MG, Bernasconi B, Riva C, Capella C. Ovarian metastases from colorectal carcinoma. Clinicopathologic profile, immunophenotype, and karyotype analysis. Am J Clin Pathol 2000, **114**: 111–122.

1198 Eichhorn JH, Young RH, Scully RE. Nonpulmonary small cell carcinomas of extragenital origin metastatic to the ovary. Cancer 1993, **71**: 177–186.

1199 Eltabbakh GH, Belinson JL, Biscotti CV. Osteosarcoma metastatic to the ovary: a case report and review of the literature. Int J Gynecol Pathol 1997, **16**: 76–78.

1200 Fitzgibbons PL, Martin SE, Simmons TJ. Malignant melanoma metastatic to the ovary. Am J Surg Pathol 1987, **11**: 959–964.

1201 Gagnon Y, Tetu B. Ovarian metastases of breast carcinoma. A clinicopathologic study of 59 cases. Cancer 1989, **64**: 892–898.

1202 Green LK, Silva EG. Hepatoblastoma in an adult with metastasis to the ovaries. Am J Clin Pathol 1989, **92**: 110–115.

1203 Groisman GM, Meir A, Sabo E. The value of Cdx2 immunostaining in differentiating primary ovarian carcinomas from colonic carcinomas metastatic to the ovaries. Int J Gynecol Pathol 2004, **23**: 52–57.

1204 Gupta D, Deavers MT, Silva EG, Malpica A. Malignanat melanoma involving the ovary: a clinicopathologic and immunohistochemical study of 23 cases. Am J Surg Pathol 2004, **28**: 771–780.

1205 Hart WR. Diagnostic challenge of secondary (metastatic) ovarian tumors simulating primary endometroid and mucinous neoplasms. Pathol Int 2005, **55**: 231–243.

1206 Holtz F, Hart WR. Krukenberg tumors of the ovary. A clinicopathologic analysis of 27 cases. Cancer 1982, **50**: 2438–2447.

1207 Insabato L, De Rosa G, Franco R, D'Onofrio V, Di Vizio D. Ovarian metatasis from renal cell carcinoma: a report of three cases. Int J Surg Pathol 2003, **11**: 309–312.

1208 Irving JA, Young RH. Lung carcinoma metastatic to the ovary: a clinicopathologic study of 32 cases emphasizing their morphologic spectrum and problems in differential diagnosis. Am J Surg Pathol 2005, **29**: 997–1006.

1209 Irving JA, Lerwill MF, Young RH. Gastrointestinal stromal tumors metastatic to the ovary: a report of five cases. Am J Surg Pathol 2005, **29**: 920–926.

1210 Irving JA, Vasques DR, McGuinness TB, Young RH. Krukenberg tumor of renal pelvic origin: report of a case with selected comments on ovarian tumors metastatic from the urinary tract. Int J Gynecol Pathol 2006, **25**: 147–150.

1211 Ji H, Isacson C, Seidman JD, Kurman RJ, Ronnett BM. Cytokeratins 7 and 20, Dpc4, and MUC5AC in the distinction of metastatic mucinous carcinomas in the ovary from primary ovarian mucinous tumors: Dpc4 assists in identifying metastatic pancreatic carcinomas. Int J Gynecol Pathol 2002, **21**: 391–400.

1212 Joshi VV. Primary Krukenberg tumor of ovary. Review of literature and case report. Cancer 1968, **22**: 1199–1207.

1213 Judson K, McCormick C, Vang R, Yemelyanova AV, Wu LS, Bristow RE, Ronnett BM. Women with undiagnosed colorectal adenocarcinomas presenting with ovarian metastases: clinicopathologic features and comparison with women having known colorectal adenocarcinomas and ovarian involvement. Int J Gynecol Pathol 2008, **27**: 182–190.

1214 Khunamornpong S, Lerwill MF, Siriaunkgul S, Suprasert P, Pojchamarnwiputh S, Chiangmai WN, Young RH. Carcinoma of extrahepatic bile ducts and gallbladder metastatic to the ovary: a report of 16 cases. Int J Gynecol Pathol 2008, **27**: 366–379.

1215 Khunamornpong S, Siriaunkgul S, Suprasert P, Pojchamarnwiputh S, Na Chiangmai W, Young RH. Intrahepatic cholangiocarcinoma metastatic to the ovary: a report of 16 cases of an underemphasized form of secondary tumor in the ovary that may mimic primary neoplasia. Am J Surg Pathol 2007, **31**: 1788–1799.

1216 Kiyokawa T, Young RH, Scully RE. Krukenberg tumors of the ovary: a clinicopathologic analysis of 120 cases with emphasis on their variable pathologic manifestations. Am J Surg Pathol 2006, **30**: 277–299.

1217 Klein EA, Rosen MH. Bilateral Krukenberg tumors due to appendiceal mucinous carcinoid. Int J Gynecol Pathol 1996, **15**: 85–88.

1218 Lagendijk JH, Mullink H, Van Diest PJ, Meijer GA, Meijer CJ. Tracing the origin of adenocarcinomas with unknown primary. Using immunohistochemistry: differential diagnosis between colonic and ovarian carcinomas as primary sites. Hum Pathol 1998, **29**: 491–497.

1219 Lash RH, Hart WR. Intestinal adenocarcinomas metastatic to the ovaries. A clinicopathologic evaluation of 22 cases. Am J Surg Pathol 1987, **11**: 114–121.

1220 Lee KR, Young RH. The distinction between primary and metastatic mucinous carcinomas of the ovary: gross and histologic findings in 50 cases. Am J Surg Pathol 2003, **27**: 281–292.

1221 Lerwill MF, Young RH. Ovarian metastases of intestinal-type gastric carcinoma: a clinicopathologic study of 4 cases with contrasting features to those of the Krukenberg tumor. Am J Surg Pathol 2006, **30**: 1382–1388.

1222 Lewis MR, Deavers MT, Silva EG, Malpica A. Ovarian involvement by metastatic colorectal adenocarcinoma: still a diagnostic challenge. Am J Surg Pathol 2006, **30**: 177–184.

1223 Logani S, Oliva E, Arnell PM, Amin MB, Young RH. Use of novel immunohistochemical markers expressed in colonic adenocarcinoma to distinguish primary ovarian tumors from metastatic colorectal carcinoma. Mod Pathol 2005, **18**: 19–25.

1224 McCluggage WG, Wilkinson N. Metastatic neoplasms involving the ovary: a review with an emphasis on morphological and immunohistochemical features. Histopathology 2005, **47**: 231–247.

1225 Mazur MT, Hsueh S, Gersell DJ. Metastases to the female genital tract. Analysis of 325 cases. Cancer 1984, **53**: 1978–1984.

1226 Monteagudo C, Merino MJ, La Porte N, Neumann RD. Value of gross cystic disease fluid protein-15 in distinguishing metastatic breast carcinomas among poorly differentiated neoplasms involving the ovary. Hum Pathol 1991, **22**: 368–372.

1227 Nonaka D, Chiriboga L, Soslow RA. Expression of pax8 as a useful marker in distinguishing ovarian carcinomas from mammary carcinomas. Am J Surg Pathol 2008, **32**: 1566–1571.

1228 Nugent SL, Dim DC, Bridge JA, Ioffe OB. Clear cell sarcoma of soft tissue metastatic to the ovaries: a heretofore unreported occurrence. Int J Gynecol Pathol 2009, **28**: 234–238.

1229 Park SY, Kim HS, Hong EK, Kim WH. Expression of cytokeratins 7 and 20 in primary carcinomas of the stomach and colorectum and their value in the differential diagnosis of metastatic carcinomas of the ovary. Hum Pathol 2002, **33**: 1078–1085.

1230 Pitman MB, Triratanachat S, Young RH, Oliva E. Hepatocyte paraffin 1 antibody does not distinguish primary ovarian tumors with hepatoid differentiation from metastatic hepatocellular carcinoma. Int J Gynecol Pathol 2004, **23**: 58–64.

1231 Ramzy I. Signet-ring stromal tumor of ovary. Histochemical, light, and electron microscopic study. Cancer 1976, **38**: 166–172.

1232 Ronnett BM, Seidman JD. Mucinous tumors arising in ovarian mature cystic teratomas. Am J Surg Pathol 2003, **27**: 650–657.

1233 Ronnett BM, Kurman RJ, Shmookler BM, Sugarbaker PH, Young R. The morphologic spectrum of ovarian metastases of appendiceal: a clinicopathologic immunohistochemical analysis of tumors often misinterpreted as primary ovarian tumors or metastatic tumors from other gastrointestinal sites. Am J Surg Pathol 1997, **21**: 1144–1155.

1234 Ronnett BM, Yemelyanova AV, Vang R, Gilks CB, Miller D, Gravitt PE, Kurman RJ. Endocervical adenocarcinomas with ovarian metastases: analysis of 29 cases with emphasis on minimally invasive cervical tumors and the ability of the metastases to simulate primary ovarian neoplasms. Am J Surg Pathol 2008, **32**: 1835–1853.

1235 Scully RE, Richardson GS. Luteinization of the stroma of metastatic cancer involving the ovary and its endocrine significance. Cancer 1961, **14**: 827–840.

1236 Seidman JD, Kurman RJ, Ronnett BM. Primary and metastatic mucinous adenocarcinomas in the ovaries. Incidence of routine practice with a new approach to improve intraoperative diagnosis. Am J Surg Pathol 2003, **27**: 985–993.

1237 Szych C, Staebler A, Connolly DC, Wu R, Cho KR, Ronnett BM. Molecular genetic evidence supporting the clonality and appendiceal origin of pseudomyxoma peritonei in women. Am J Pathol 1999, **154**: 1849–1855.

1238 Tornos C, Soslow R, Chen S, Akram M, Hummer AJ, Abu-Rustum N, Norton L, Tan LK. Expression of WT1, CA 125, and GCDFP-15 as useful markers in the differential diagnosis of primary ovarian carcinomas versus metastatic breast cancer to the ovary. Am J Surg Pathol 2005, **29**: 1482–1489.

1239 Ulbright TM, Roth LM, Stehman FB. Secondary ovarian neoplasia. A clinicopathologic study of 35 cases. Cancer 1984, **53**: 1164–1174.

1240 Vakiani E, Young RH, Carcangiu ML, Klimstra DS. Acinar cell carcinoma of the pancreas metastatic to the ovary: a report of 4 cases. Am J Surg Pathol 2008, **32**: 1540–1545.

1241 Vang R, Gown AM, Barry TS, Wheeler DT, Ronnett BM. Immunohistochemistry for estrogen and progesterone receptors in the distinction of primary and metastatic mucinous tumors in the ovary: an analysis of 124 cases. Mod Pathol 2006, **19**: 97–105.

1242 Vang R, Gown AM, Barry TS, Wheeler DT, Yemelyanova A, Seidman JD, Ronnett BM. Cytokeratins 7 and 20 in primary and secondary mucinous tumors of the ovary: analysis of coordinate immunohistochemical expression profiles and staining distribution in 179 cases. Am J Surg Pathol 2006, **30**: 1130–1139.

1243 Warren S, Macomber WB. Tumor metastasis. IV. Ovarian metastasis of carcinoma. Arch Pathol 1935, **19**: 75–82.

1244 Webb MJ, Decker DG, Mussey E. Cancer metastatic to the ovary. Factors influencing survival. Obstet Gynecol 1975, **45**: 391–396.

1245 Wong PC, Ferenczy A, Fan L-D, McCaughey E. Krukenberg tumors of the ovary. Ultrastructural, histochemical, and immunohistochemical studies of 15 cases. Cancer 1986, **57**: 751–760.

1246 Woodruff JD, Novak ER. The Krukenberg tumor. Study of 48 cases from the Ovarian Tumor Registry. Obstet Gynecol 1960, **15**: 351–360.

1247 Yazigi R, Sandstad J. Ovarian involvement in extragenital cancer. Gynecol Oncol 1989, **34**: 84–87.

1248 Young RH, Eichhorn JH, Dickersin GR, Scully RE. Ovarian involvement by the intra-abdominal desmoplastic small round cell tumor with divergent differentiation. A report of three cases. Hum Pathol 1992, **23**: 454–464.

1249 Young RH, Gersell DJ, Clement PB, Scully RE. Hepatocellular carcinoma metastatic to the ovary. A report of three cases discovered during life with discussion of the differential diagnosis of hepatoid tumors of the ovary. Hum Pathol 1992, **23**: 574–580.

1250 Young RH, Hart WR. Metastases from carcinomas of the pancreas simulating primary mucinous tumors of the ovary. A report of seven cases. Am J Surg Pathol 1989, **13**: 748–756.

1251 Young RH, Hart WR. Renal cell carcinoma metastatic to the ovary. A report of three cases emphasizing possible confusion with ovarian clear cell adenocarcinoma. Int J Gynecol Pathol 1992, **11**: 96–104.

1252 Young RH, Hart WR. Metastatic intestinal carcinomas simulating primary ovarian clear cell carcinoma and secretory endometrioid carcinoma: clinicopathologic and immunohistochemical study of five cases. Am J Surg Pathol 1998, **22**: 805–815.

1253 Young RH, Jackson A, Wells M. Ovarian metastasis from thyroid carcinoma 12 years after partial thyroidectomy mimicking struma ovarii. Report of a case. Int J Gynecol Pathol 1994, **13**: 181–185.

1254 Young RH, Scully RE. Ovarian metastases from cancer of the lung. Problems in interpretation – a report of seven cases. Gynecol Oncol 1985, **21**: 337–350.

1255 Young RH, Scully RE. Alveolar rhabdomyosarcoma metastatic to the ovary. A report of two cases and a discussion of the differential diagnosis of small cell malignant tumors of the ovary. Cancer 1989, **64**: 899–904.

1256 Young RH, Scully RE. Ovarian metastases from carcinoma of the gallbladder and extrahepatic bile ducts simulating primary tumors of the ovary. A report of six cases. Int J Gynecol Pathol 1990, **9**: 60–72.

1257 Young RH, Scully RE. Sarcomas metastatic to the ovary. A report of 21 cases. Int J Gynecol Pathol 1990, **9**: 231–252.

1258 Young RH, Scully RE. Malignant melanoma metastatic to the ovary. A clinicopathologic analysis of 20 cases. Am J Surg Pathol 1991, **15**: 849–860.

1259 Young RH, Scully RE. Metastatic tumors in the ovary. A problem-oriented approach and review of the recent literature. Semin Diagn Pathol 1991, **8**: 250–276.

1260 Zaloudek C, Miller TR, Stern JL. Desmoplastic small cell tumor of the ovary. A unique polyphenotypic tumor with an unfavorable prognosis. Int J Gynecol Pathol 1995, **14**: 260–265.

1261 Zukerberg LR, Young RH. Chordoma metastatic to the ovary. Arch Pathol Lab Med 1990, **114**: 208–210.

Pregnancy, trophoblastic disease, and placenta

CHAPTER CONTENTS

Normal anatomy

The normal term *placenta* measures 15–20 cm in diameter and 1.5–3 cm in thickness, and weighs 450–600 g. The main components are the umbilical cord, membranes (amnion and chorion), villous parenchyma, and maternal decidual tissue.[5,9,11]

The *umbilical cord* at term measures 55–65 cm in length.[14] It has an outer layer of amniotic epithelium, which becomes stratified at the fetal end. The bulk of the cord is made up of highly mucoid connective tissue known as *Wharton's jelly*. Embedded within its substance are the umbilical vessels, represented by two arteries and a single vein. The arteries have a double-layered muscular wall but no internal elastic lamina. The vein has a larger diameter and a thinner wall, consisting of a single layer of circular smooth muscle, and an internal elastic lamina. The umbilical cord may insert in the placenta in a central or eccentric fashion. Insertion at the margin is referred to as *battledore placenta*. Whereas it is easy to distinguish microscopically the arteries from the vein in the cord itself, this becomes difficult or impossible once those vessels branch into the chorionic plate.

The *placental membranes* consist of the amnion and chorion. The *amnion*, which represents the innermost covering of the amniotic cavity, is lined by a single layer of flat epithelial cells resting on a basement membrane.[3,15] *Squamous metaplasia* is common in them, especially near the insertion of the cord. The *chorion* is composed of a connective tissue membrane that carries the fetal vasculature. Its inner aspect is bounded by the outer layer of the amnion, and the outer aspect is associated with villi that sprout from the surface. The chorion associated with the membrane is referred to as *chorion laeve* and is distinguished from the *chorion frondosum* located in the placenta proper.[11,16] Some of the trophoblast located in the chorion laeve has a characteristic vacuolated appearance.[20]

The *trophoblastic villi* that arise from the trophoectoderm following formation of the blastocyst constitute the functional unit of the placenta. During the first trimester, they are composed of an outer syncytiotrophoblastic layer and an inner cytotrophoblastic layer, which surround a central mesenchymal core containing primitive fibroblasts and scattered macrophages (Hofbauer cells).

The *syncytiotrophoblast* is composed of multinucleated giant cells with abundant acidophilic cytoplasm that is strongly immunoreactive for human chorionic gonadotropin (hCG), keratin, human placental lactogen (hPL; variably, and depending on the gestational age), placental-like alkaline phosphatase (PLAP), pregnancy-specific β_1-glycoprotein (SP1), and inhibin.[7,17] They are negative for epithelial membrane antigen (EMA), HNK1 (CD57), and CD146 (Mel-CAM).[13] The *cytotrophoblast*, which is the progenitor of the syncytiotrophoblast, is made up of mononuclear cells with clear cytoplasm and a well-defined cell membrane, which are negative for all of the above markers except keratin. In the term placenta, the cytotrophoblast is inconspicuous, and the syncytiotrophoblast is clumped in the form of 'syncytial knots'.

The third trophoblastic type is represented by the *intermediate trophoblast*, also known as interstitial extravillous trophoblast and X cells.[10] This type is present in the villi and in the membranes but is particularly numerous in the extravillous region that forms the deepest structural component of the implantation site. The most distinctive immunohistochemical property of these cells is a strong reactivity for hPL. They are also positive for keratin, CD66a (CEACAM1), CD146 (Mel-CAM, a marker for implantation site intermediate trophoblast), HNK1/CD57 (only in the villi), EMA (only in the chorion), and HLA-G (a non-classic major histocompatibility complex class I antigen).[1,19] The proposal has been made that there are three subpopulations of intermediate trophoblastic cells with distinctive morphologic and immunohistochemical features: implantation site type, chorionic type, and villous type.[18] Trophoblastic cells have also been shown to produce and secrete parathyroid hormone-related protein, and this is also true for their neoplastic counterparts.[4] Villous trophoblast shows a membranous pattern of E-cadherin stain and a mixed membranous and granular pattern of β-catenin distribution.[12]

The villous vessels become apparent at 6 weeks. At about 8 weeks they contain only nucleated red blood cells, but by weeks 10–12 the percentage of nucleated cells has dropped to 10%, and after week 12 they are virtually absent.

Decidua is present both in the placental disk (from which, however, it may be denuded during delivery) and on the chorionic side of the membranes. Immunohistochemically, decidual cells are reactive for vimentin, desmin, α_1-antitrypsin, and α_1-antichymotrypsin. On occasion they have also been found to be positive for keratin, PLAP, and β-hCG, a fact to remember when trying to distinguish them from trophoblastic cells.[6] Decidual tissue is thought to contain a special type of dendritic cell (expressing DC-SIGN), which may play a role in the tolerance of the maternal immune system toward the allogeneic embryo.[8]

Gross inspection of a **twin placenta** provides important information with regard to the type of twinning (Figs 19.346 and 19.347). A monochorionic placenta (whether monoamnionic or diamnionic) is indicative of monoygotic twins, whereas dichorionic placentas (whether fused or separated) are compatible with either monozygotic or dizygotic twinning. In a monochorionic placenta, stripping of the amnion reveals a continuous chorionic plate

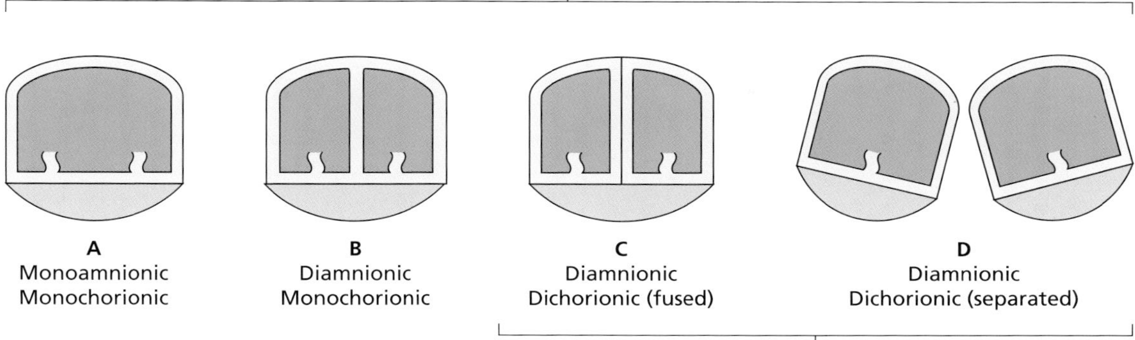

Fig. 19.346 Diagrammatic representation of common variations possible in monochorionic and dichorionic twin placentation. Types A and B of monochorionic twin placenta are seen only with identical twins. Variations C and D are common to both identical and fraternal twins. Hence, identification of dichorionic twin placenta does not distinguish between identical and fraternal twins.
(From Kraus FT. Gynecologic pathology. St Louis, 1967, Mosby)

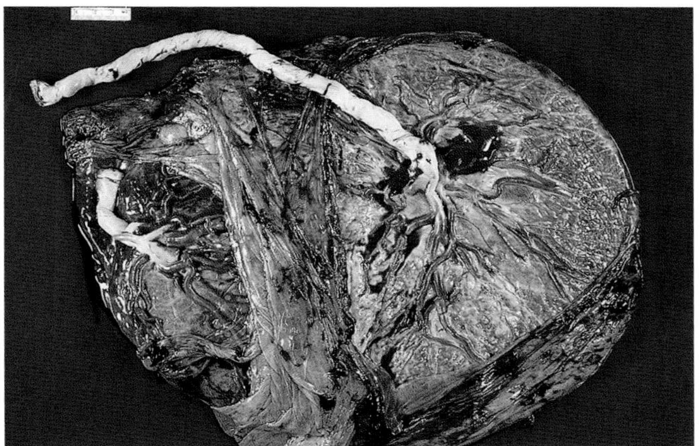

Fig. 19.347 Chorionic ridge at the base of the septum in a dichorionic fused twin placenta.

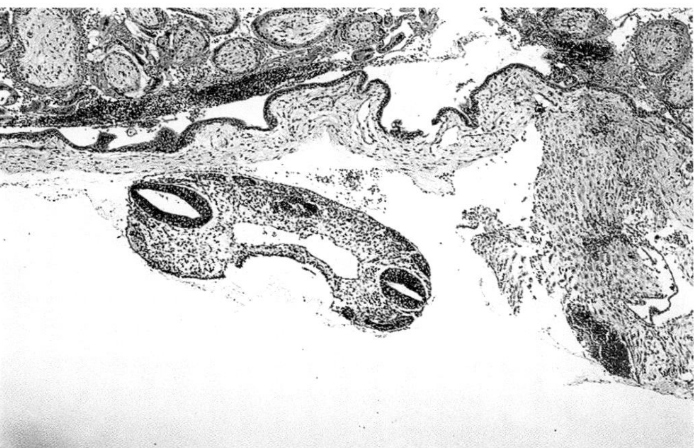

Fig. 19.348 Products of conception represented by small embryo and chorionic villi.

beneath the septum and major vascular anastomoses between the twins. In contrast, dichorionic fused placentas have a rough chorionic ridge at the base of the septum and lack vascular anastomoses.[2]

Abortion

The clinical incidence of spontaneous abortion is approximately 15%, but the real incidence may be as high as 40–80%. The etiologic factors are many. They include infections (particularly rubella, *Campylobacter*, *Listeria*, syphilis, toxoplasmosis, cytomegalovirus and possibly human papilloma virus), mechanical disturbances (uterine leiomyomas, cervical incompetence), endocrine diseases, immunologic mechanisms (autoimmune diseases, ABO incompatibility), and inherited chromosomal abnormalities.[34,50,51,61]

The morphologic confirmation of the occurrence of a pregnancy is one of the most common determinations performed by the pathologist. When fetal parts, gestational sac, or viable chorionic villi are present, the task is easy enough (Fig. 19.348). In the presence of an identifiable fetus, determination should be made whether it is macerated or not and whether it appears normal, grossly disorganized, or focally abnormal.[21,23,37,39,43,47,48,53] There is a good correlation between cytogenetic abnormalities and embryonic growth disorganization leading to early death, usually before the fetal stage (30 mm) is reached.[32,55] Occasionally, only a type of tissue from the embryo survives, such as glial tissue.[56,63] When the gestational sac is identified, a statement should be made as to whether it is intact or ruptured and – in the latter instance – whether it contains a cord stump or not. The chorionic villi may already be apparent grossly to the gynecologist by the simple procedure of examining contents from the curettage in saline solution after rinsing the blood.[40] In other instances, not only are they impossible to identify grossly, but numerous paraffin blocks may be necessary to identify them microscopically.

Sometimes the villi are seen surrounded by the deposition of abundant fibrinoid material, a feature that has been found to be associated with prolonged vaginal bleeding and which is not to be viewed as evidence of maternal thrombophilia or autoimmune disease.[60]

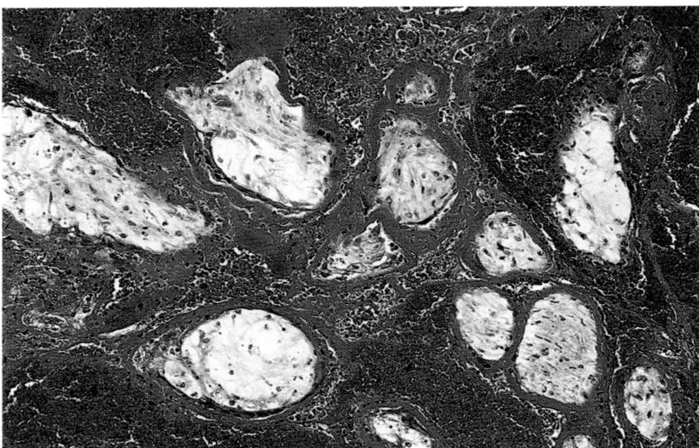

Fig. 19.349 Ghost chorionic villi embedded in a clot.

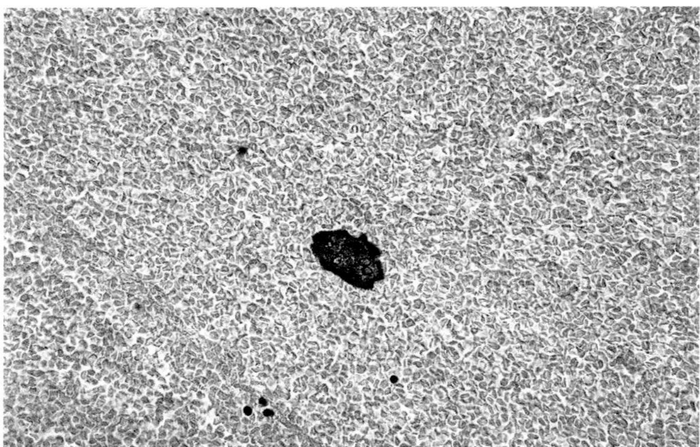

Fig. 19.350 Single syncytiotrophoblast cell strongly immunoreactive to β-hCG despite the presence of advanced necrotic changes.

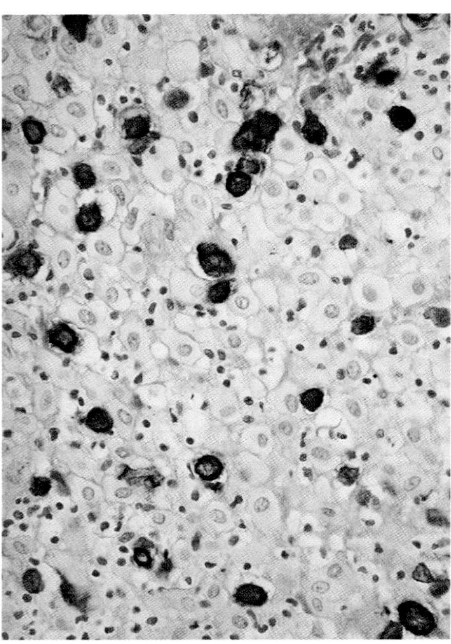

Fig. 19.351 Isolated intermediate trophoblast cells strongly staining for keratin.

Necrotic ('ghost') villi are particularly difficult to recognize, since clumps of fibrin may closely simulate them (Fig. 19.349). The overall configuration and the presence of shadows of stromal cells and trophoblast are the main identifying criteria. In the absence of chorionic villi, a search should be made for trophoblastic cells, whether isolated or in clumps. Care should be exercised not to confuse these trophoblastic cells – particularly those of intermediate type – with decidual cells. Intermediate trophoblastic cells infiltrate the decidua surrounding the blastocyst to form the trophoblastic shell, invade the spiral arterioles of the placental bed, and infiltrate the myometrium beneath the implantation site.[22] They are usually mononuclear, of variable shape (round, polygonal, or spindled), with amphophilic or eosinophilic granular cytoplasm and indistinct cell borders. Their nuclei are round or lobulated, sometimes multiclefted, and frequently hyperchromatic.[59] In contrast, decidual cells have distinct cell borders, pale homogeneous cytoplasm, and round uniform nuclei with fine chromatin.

When it is impossible to determine on the basis of routinely stained sections whether trophoblastic cells of any type are present or not, and this determination is of clinical importance (as in the differential diagnosis between intrauterine and ectopic pregnancy), immunocytochemical stains for hCG, hPL, SP1, and keratin should be employed (Figs 19.350 and 19.351).[25,28,36]

In the absence of fetal parts, villi, or trophoblast (as detected morphologically or immunohistochemically), the diagnosis of intrauterine pregnancy cannot be made with absolute certainty, although enlarged hyalinized spiral arterioles and the presence of a fibrinoid matrix are features suggestive of intrauterine implantation.[43] It should be mentioned that under exceptional circumstances one can find a few villi in the uterine curettage specimen of a patient with an ectopic pregnancy.[33] There are other endometrial patterns that are strongly suggestive that a gestation has occurred, but they do not establish its site (intrauterine versus ectopic) and are not pathognomonic.[26] These include decidual reaction, gestational hyperplasia, and Arias-Stella reaction.[44] The microscopic appearance of the decidua of pregnancy can be closely simulated by the deciduoid changes secondary to the use of oral contraceptives, even if the latter usually lack the dilated vascular channels of true decidua and have a more inactive glandular pattern.

Gestational hyperplasia is characterized by the simultaneous presence in the endometrial mucosa of glandular secretion, stromal edema, and deciduoid changes.[35] The basal glandular cells acquire strong immunoreactivity for S-100 protein.[42] The *Arias-Stella reaction* (discussed earlier in this chapter in the section on Uterus – corpus) is a physiologic response to viable trophoblastic tissue;[44] it characteristically develops during pregnancy, but it may also occur following the use of progestational agents and other exogenous hormones.

In some institutions, frozen sections of curetted endometrial material are requested in an attempt to distinguish intrauterine from ectopic pregnancy. If fetal parts or well-developed chorionic villi are present, the task is easy. However, the identification of trophoblast – particularly of the intermediate type – is difficult enough in formalin-fixed paraffin-embedded material (as previously discussed) to expect for this to be reliably achieved in frozen section material, no matter how experienced the observer. The use of laparoscopy and ultrasonography (particularly after the advent of the vaginal transducer) should obviate the need for this intrinsically unreliable procedure.[45]

Septic abortion is usually caused by coliform organisms or anaerobic streptococci. The pathologist should identify the microorganisms in the tissue sections before making a diagnosis of septic abortion. The presence of neutrophils, even in large numbers, is not necessarily an indication of infection, since it may simply represent an inflammatory reaction to the necrotic decidua and fetal tissues.

Herpes simplex infection has been detected immunohistochemically in material from abortion, suggesting the existence of a latent subclinical infection that has produced transplacental infection of the fetus.[52]

Most patients who have had a miscarriage should undergo a uterine evacuation in order to remove residual trophoblastic tissue. This material should always be examined microscopically in order to rule out early gestational trophoblastic disease.

Hydropic changes may be seen in the chorionic villi of abortion material ('hydropic abortus') and need to be distinguished from those accompanying a complete or a partial mole. In the hydropic abortus, *gross* villous swelling and cistern formation are not seen. More importantly, these villi are typically surrounded by *attenuated* trophoblast. If trophoblastic proliferation is present, it has an orderly, centrifugal, and polar quality and lacks significant nuclear atypia.

Flow cytometric DNA analysis has been applied as an adjunct to this differential diagnosis. A correlation between DNA values, karyotypic abnormalities, and microscopic changes exists, but this is not as close as one might have wished.[27,46,58] As a matter of fact, the degree of interobserver variability and the lack of predictive value of the microscopic evaluation are such as to have led some experts to conclude that a classification of abortion material on morphologic grounds – beyond documenting the fact that a pregnancy has occurred and ruling out gestational trophoblastic disease – is a valueless exercise.[29,57] To be sure, hydropic villi are more likely to have a nondiploid DNA content than nonhydropic ones.[31] However, of the abortuses with a triploid DNA pattern, only half or fewer will show the morphologic features of a partial mole, most of the others being morphologically unremarkable.[31] The differences may be related to the paternal versus maternal (digyny) origin of the extra set of chromosomes.[41] In a correlative cytogenetic–morphologic study of over 1000 spontaneous abortions, the incidence of villous trophoblastic hyperplasia was increased in those with an abnormal karyotype as a group and in the subgroup of trisomy compared with those of a normal karyotype. The highest grades of trophoblastic hyperplasia were more frequent in cases of trisomy of chromosomes 7, 15, 21, and 22.[49]

Immunohistochemically, the trophoblast of hydropic villi is less likely to show overexpression of cyclin E or P53, or high indices of MIB-1 and apoptosis than molar trophoblast, but the differences are not pronounced enough for these stains to be of great diagnostic assistance.[24,38,54,62]

Examination of placental tissue from second-trimester abortions (whether spontaneous, surgically induced, or prostaglandin induced) consistently shows degenerative changes consisting of focal decidual necrosis, intradecidual hemorrhage, and congestion and thrombosis of maternal vessels.[30]

Gestational trophoblastic disease

There is a group of diseases related to normal or abnormal gestation that have as a common denominator the proliferation of trophoblast and that are generically designated as (*gestational*) *trophoblastic disease*. The individual disorders differ remarkably in appearance and clinical significance. The major ones are hydatidiform mole (complete, partial, or invasive), placental site trophoblastic tumor, and choriocarcinoma[67] The pathogenesis of these remains poorly understood, but genomic imprinting is believed to play a key role in the formation of hydatidiform moles.[64–66]

Hydatidiform mole

In hydatidiform moles, the trophoblastic proliferation is associated with swelling of the villi. They are subdivided into complete and partial types, and either type can be invasive.

Complete mole

Complete hydatidiform mole is caused by abnormal gametogenesis and fertilization. The nuclei of the trophoblastic cells in this disease contain only paternal chromosomes and are, therefore, androgenetic in origin, whereas all cytoplasmic DNA is maternally derived.[83,93] In most cases the chromosomal number is normal; 85% of cases are 46,XX and 15% are 46,XY. It has been hypothesized that in the 46,XX cases, the process is fertilization of an 'empty' ovum with no effective genome by a haploid sperm that duplicates without cytokinesis, whereas in the 46,XY cases there might be fertilization of the 'empty' ovum by two haploid sperms with subsequent fusion and replication. This hypothesis is supported by the genetic analysis of molar mitochondrial DNA.[69] In a minority of cases, the DNA pattern is tetraploid, these generally occurring in an older age group.[72]

There is a striking geographic variation in the frequency of complete mole. The incidence of 1 in 2000 deliveries reported in the classic studies by Hertig[87] represents an average for young healthy women in the United States. In South East Asia, the reported incidence is at least four to five times greater.[89,91] Yet higher incidences have been reported from Mexico (1 : 200), the Philippines (1 : 173), India (1 : 160), Taiwan (1 : 125), and Indonesia (1 : 82).[107] Patients with complete mole tend to be older than 30 years of age and more likely to have diets deficient in vitamin A precursors (which may explain some of the geographic differences previously mentioned). The risk is reduced by increased consumption of carotene. A history of previous term birth reduces the risk of molar pregnancy, whereas a history of a previous mole greatly increases the probability of developing another.[91,112,114] 'Repetitive' moles are usually of complete type, but they can be of partial type, or a complete mole may be followed by a partial mole.[110]

Clinically, the uterus involved by a complete mole is disproportionately large for the stage of pregnancy.[68] Serum hCG levels continue to rise after the 14th week, as opposed to the drop typically seen in the course of normal gestation. Evidence of toxemia of pregnancy (hypertension, edema, albuminuria) is frequently found, and this typically occurs during the early stages of the pregnancy. Exceptionally, hyperthyroidism develops as a result of a thyroid stimulator secreted by the molar tissue, perhaps residing in the hCG molecule itself.[75,86,105] At the time of the medical consultation there may be vaginal bleeding, a sign that the mole has begun to abort spontaneously.

Grossly, the complete mole has been typically described as a 'bunch of grapes', with all or nearly all the villi showing hydropic degeneration. The individual vesicles measure anywhere from 1 to 30 mm in diameter, and the total weight is usually over 200 g. In a hysterectomy specimen, these swollen villi are seen to fill and distend the uterus (Fig. 19.352). Characteristically, there are no identifiable embryo, cord, or amniotic membranes. The exceptional cases of bona fide complete mole in which an embryo is present almost invariably represent a twin gestation.[70,116]

Microscopically, the two constant features of a complete mole are *trophoblastic hyperplasia* and *vesicular swelling*, the latter probably

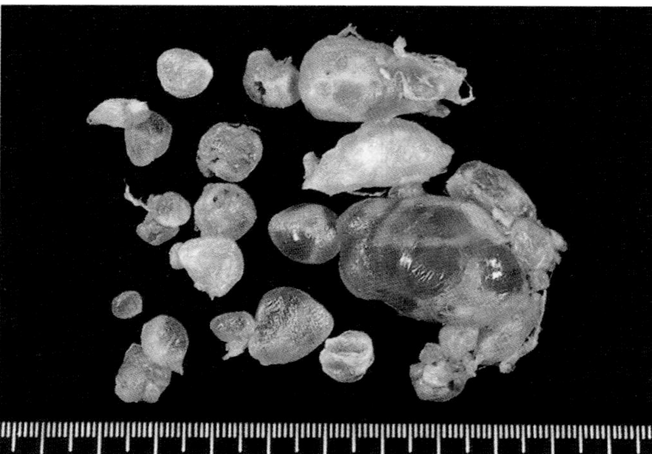

Fig. 19.352 Complete mole. All villi are markedly swollen. *(Courtesy of Dr Pedro J Grases Galofrè; from Grases Galofrè PJ. Patologia ginecològica. Bases para el diagnòstico morfològico. Barcelona, 2002, Masson)*

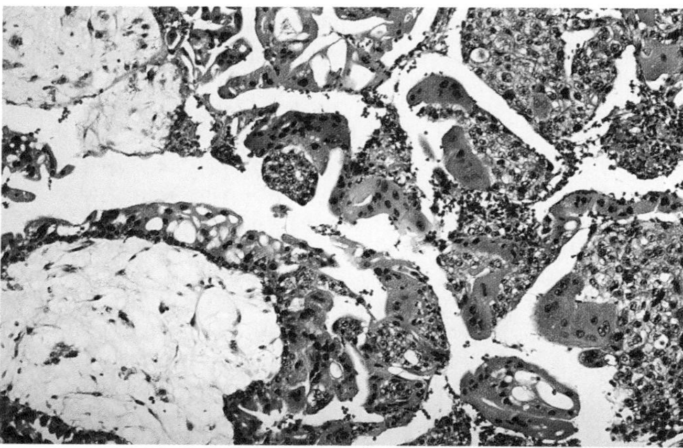

Fig. 19.353 Complete mole showing large villi with stromal edema and marked trophoblastic proliferation.

representing a secondary phenomenon. The severity of the changes varies considerably from case to case and from villus to villus, and may be difficult to appreciate in very early cases, as evidenced by the high degree of inter- and intraobserver variability.[78,82,94] Some of the villi are surrounded by an attenuated layer of degenerating trophoblast. In others, the trophoblast forms large hyperplastic sheets of cells (Fig. 19.353). The distended core of the villus is traversed by widely separated, broken strands of fibrillar material ('cistern' formation). Vessels seem absent or very scanty in hematoxylin–eosin-stained sections, even though they do not seem very diminished in number in CD34-stained preparations.[109] The stromal changes of molar villi, which include stromal mucin and stromal nuclear debris (apoptosis), appear very early and represent a diagnostic clue.[95,96,117] The trophoblastic hyperplasia characteristically has a circumferential but haphazard arrangement around the individual villi, as opposed to the polar proliferation seen in normal first-trimester villi. The plexiform pattern of intermixed syncytiotrophoblast and cytotrophoblast seen in choriocarcinoma does not occur. Trophoblastic hyperplasia with atypia also occurs at the implantation site, to a much greater degree than in hydropic villi of abortion or partial moles.[104]

Ultrastructurally, the molar trophoblast closely resembles that seen during the first trimester of a normal pregnancy.[106]

Immunohistochemically, hCG is widely distributed and PLAP is patchily distributed in the molar syncytiotrophoblast regardless of gestational age, whereas hPL tends to increase with increased gestational age.[73,81] Both the α- and β-subunits of inhibin are evident in the molar syncytiotrophoblast.[98,108] A potentially useful marker for the differential diagnosis of complete mole is $P57^{kip2}$ protein, a cell cycle inhibitor and tumor suppressor encoded by a strongly paternally imprinted gene. It is well expressed in the cytotrophoblast and villous mesenchyme of normal pregnancy, spontaneous abortions, and partial moles, but absent or markedly decreased in complete moles because both copies of the *TP57* gene are of paternal origin, even during the early stage of their development.[74,77,80,92] P53 is expressed in direct relation to the proliferative activity of the trophoblast (mainly cytotrophoblast). Thus the intensity of staining in complete mole is higher than in partial mole and lower than in choriocarcinoma.[101] Interestingly, some staining is also present in the normal trophoblast of early pregnancy and in the hydropic villi of spontaneous abortion.[76,118]

By flow cytometry, 50% of complete moles are diploid, 43% are tetraploid, 3.6% are polyploid, and 1.7% are triploid.[99,100] The claim has been made that the more pronounced the trophoblastic hyperplasia, the higher the chance of the development of a choriocarcinoma. However, the number of exceptions renders this evaluation of little if any practical utility.[90] This is particularly true since the advent of highly sensitive techniques for monitoring serum hCG levels.[79,84] According to Driscoll,[79] molar lesions characterized by the interposition of fibrin-like material at the tumor–host interphase and by the presence of abundant syncytiotrophoblast respond very well to chemotherapy, whereas those having a compact growth of cytotrophoblast with little differentiation tend to be relatively resistant. Heterozygous (dispermic) moles, including dispermic heterozygous XY moles, are associated with a higher incidence of persistent trophoblastic disease than homozygous (monospermic) moles. The proliferation index and DNA ploidy have not been found to be statistically associated with outcome.[99]

The initial therapy of complete mole consists of evacuation of the uterus by curettage.[111] This is followed by sequential quantitative determination of the β-subunit of hCG.[71,88,115] The standard recommendation has been to measure the serum level of hCG at 10, 20, 30, 45, and 60 days after termination of the molar gestation. In approximately 80% of cases, normal levels will be reached by day 60. If there is rising titer between day 45 and day 60 or the level is still elevated by day 60, chemotherapy is administered; this is necessary in approximately 20% of cases.[102] With this approach, the cure rate is close to 100%.[85] Unfortunately, the use of etoposide has been found to be associated with an increased risk of development of second tumors.[113]

Other authors recommend the administration of chemotherapy to those patients who have a plateau of three high values of hCG over a 2-week period after evacuation of the mole (approximately 20–30% of cases). Still others recommend waiting for 4 weeks or even 2 months before initiating chemotherapy, especially if the hCG levels are low.[97]

In a series of 738 patients with mole, spontaneous regression occurred in 81%. Of the remaining patients, 17% developed an invasive mole, and 2% developed choriocarcinoma.[103] The presence of villi or atypical trophoblast following the evacuation of a molar pregnancy indicates 'persistent trophoblastic disease', but the decision of whether to give chemotherapy or not still largely depends on the hCG levels.

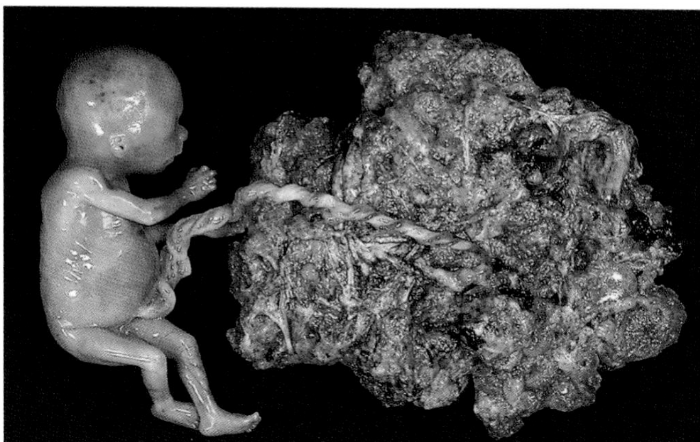

Fig. 19.354 Partial mole with attached fetus. The diagnosis was confirmed by biopsy and flow cytometry. The fetus showed no abnormality and was connected to the mole by a normal umbilical cord.
(Courtesy of Dr Pedro J Grases Galofré; from Grases Galofré PJ. Patología ginecológica. Bases para el diagnóstico morfológico. Barcelona, 2002, Masson)

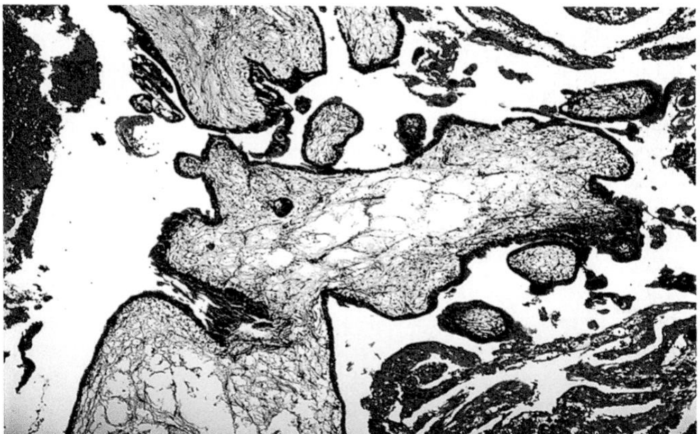

Fig. 19.355 Partial mole showing scalloping of villi and isolated trophoblastic cells embedded in the stroma.

Partial mole

Approximately 15–35% of all moles are of the partial type. In contrast to complete mole, the condition is often associated with the presence of an embryo, although this is usually abnormal ('blighted ovum'). The volume of placental tissue is relatively normal, and the grossly vesicular villi are mixed with normal-appearing ones (Fig. 19.354). The former often show focal edema leading to central 'cisternal' formation and stromal inclusions of trophoblast (Fig. 19.355). Many of the villi have an irregular, scalloped outline and contain vessels with fetal (nucleated) red blood cells. Fibrosis of the villous stroma is common. Trophoblastic proliferation is present, although generally to a lesser degree than in complete mole; cytoplasmic vacuolization of the syncytiotrophoblast is prominent.[123] Immunohistochemically, some differences in localization of hCG and hPL when compared with complete moles have been described,[121] as well as the already mentioned difference in $P57^{kip2}$ staining.

Most partial moles are triploid (69,XXX or 69,XXY) and a few show trisomy 16.[120,138,139] The extra material is of paternal derivation (so-called 'diandric triploidy').[128]

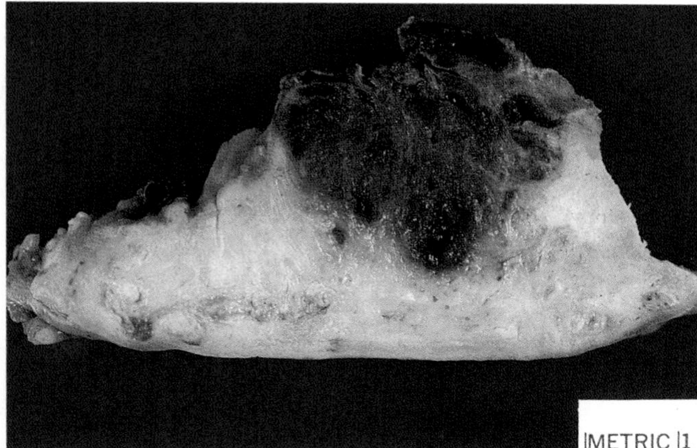

Fig. 19.356 Gross appearance of invasive mole. A hemorrhagic mass has permeated half of the thickness of the myometrial wall.

Because of the generally small size of the lesion, the uterine size is nearly always small or appropriate for the gestational age. Serum hCG levels – although elevated – tend to be relatively low, and the ovarian theca-lutein cysts that commonly accompany complete moles do not occur.[119] The risk for the development of choriocarcinoma following a partial mole is very low, but a few well-documented cases are on record.[127,137] Furthermore, some series document a 5–10% incidence of persistent disease (lower in those evacuated early),[125] indicating that follow-up of these patients is mandatory.[130,132,133] Some of the recurrences have been in the form of invasive mole[126,129,135] and some in the form of lung metastases.[122]

As already pointed out, not all placentas of triploid conceptuses show partial molar transformation; some (perhaps the majority) have a normal morphologic appearance.[124] The triploid fetuses in both groups tend to die at about 8 weeks menstrual age.[136]

Partial moles should be distinguished on one hand from complete moles and on the other from the hydropic villi seen in 15–40% of spontaneous abortions and with rare conditions such as placental stem villous hydrops, mesenchymal dysplasia, and Beckwith–Wiedemann syndrome.[134] In the latter, gross villous swelling and cistern formation are not present. As already stated, the villous trophoblast in spontaneous abortions either is attenuated or – if proliferating – has a polar distribution. Furthermore, trophoblastic atypia is absent or minimal. Flow cytometry studies are of great assistance in the evaluation of this problem.[128,130,131]

Invasive mole

The term *invasive mole* (*chorioadenoma destruens*) refers to a hydatidiform mole (nearly always of the complete type but occasionally of the partial type) in which villi penetrate deeply the myometrium and/or its blood vessels[145,146] (Figs 19.356–19.358). This phenomenon, which occurs in 16% of all complete moles, is an exaggerated expression of the capacity of normal trophoblast for invasion, a necessary property for implantation. Placenta accreta (see p. 1646) is another manifestation of this phenomenon; the common demonstration of microscopic trophoblastic emboli in the lungs after normal pregnancy is yet another.[140]

The myometrial permeation in invasive mole may be extensive and may lead to persistent hemorrhage, but the serosa is usually intact. However, uterine perforation may occur. The vascular invasion may result in trophoblastic nodules in sites outside the uterus,

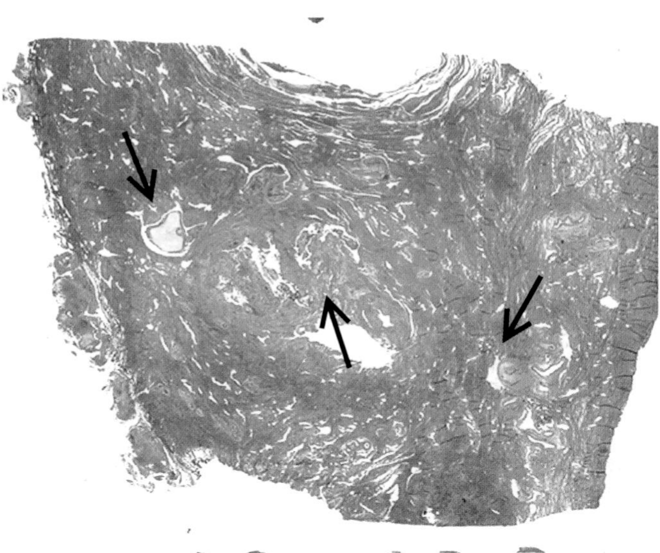

Fig. 19.357 Whole-mount view of invasive mole. Abnormal villi are seen permeating the thickened myometrium (arrows).

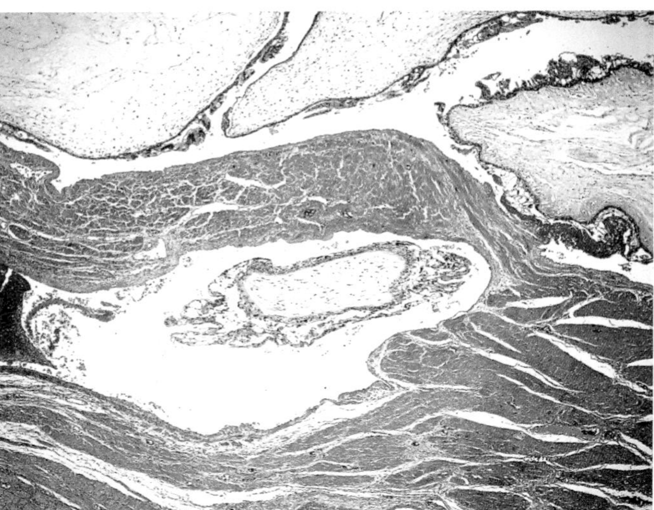

Fig. 19.358 Hydropic villi covered by proliferating trophoblast are seen permeating the myometrium in this invasive mole.

such as the vagina, lung, brain, and spinal cord.[144,147] The lung nodules have a characteristic radiographic appearance;[141,142] they continue to produce hCG and have a similar tendency for hemorrhagic complications. The clinical manifestations depend on the site involved: a sizable mass in the lung may regress spontaneously without ever causing symptoms, whereas a deposit in the brain may produce fatal hemorrhage.[143,149] It should not escape the attention of the reader that an invasive mole has all of the biologic features of a malignant neoplasm except for the fact that it is self-limited. It invades the stroma, it produces tumor emboli, and it metastasizes distantly. This is probably telling us something very important about the neoplastic process, perhaps the fact that the program for the two cardinal properties that characterize it (invasion and metastases) are already present in the normal cell, and that the derepression of this mechanism may be the key to tumor formation.

To return to more pedestrian considerations, it should be mentioned that invasive mole is distinguished from the usual mole by its invasiveness and from choriocarcinoma by the presence of villi, which are also present in the 'metastatic' foci. The degree of trophoblastic proliferation in invasive mole does not differ significantly from that of its ordinary counterpart. Patients with invasive mole are primarily treated with chemotherapy, but hysterectomy may be indicated in some circumstances.[146,148]

Choriocarcinoma

Choriocarcinoma, when untreated, is the most aggressive form of gestational trophoblastic disease. Most cases occur following a complete hydatidiform mole; consequently, this malignant tumor is more common in areas of the world in which hydatidiform mole is prevalent. It has been estimated that 1–2% of complete moles are followed by choriocarcinoma.[152]

Choriocarcinoma can also be preceded by a partial mole (a very unusual event), ectopic pregnancy, nonmolar intrauterine abortion, or term pregnancy.[153,175,180] In the latter instance, which is exceptionally rare, the tumor may appear as one or more masses in an otherwise normal placenta or develop following the delivery.[151,154,170] In addition, cases of 'in-situ' choriocarcinoma arising from the trophoblast of stem villi in the first trimester of pregnancy have been described.[163]

In cases of choriocarcinoma following abortion – whether molar or not – the latent period is almost always less than 1 year, although it can be considerably longer ('latent choriocarcinoma').[159] At the time of the diagnosis of the malignancy, the average age of the patient is 29 years. When reviewing the microscopic sections of a nonmolar abortion in women who subsequently developed choriocarcinoma, it is not unusual to find foci of increased trophoblastic proliferation. These foci, although not diagnostic of trophoblastic disease even in retrospect, suggest the existence of a precursor lesion.

Bagshawe[150] has shown a striking relationship between the incidence and prognosis of choriocarcinoma and the ABO groups of both the woman and her husband. The highest risk is for women of group A married to men of the same group. The relative risk of the two extreme groups was 10.4 : 1. Women married to men of their own ABO group had the highest incidence of spontaneous regression of trophoblast after evacuation of a hydatidiform mole.

Grossly, choriocarcinoma characteristically forms soft, dark red, hemorrhagic, round nodular tumor masses (Fig. 19.359). Microscopically, the tumor is composed of clusters of cytotrophoblast separated by streaming masses of syncytiotrophoblast, resulting in a characteristic dimorphic plexiform pattern[182] (Fig. 19.360). Hemorrhage and necrosis are usually present but have no real diagnostic significance, since they are also commonly found in spontaneous abortions. Villi are characteristically absent; as a matter of fact, their presence is said to rule out the diagnosis of choriocarcinoma no matter how atypical the trophoblastic cells may be.[160] The rationale for this criterion is hard to comprehend. After all, if such choriocarcinomas arise from complete moles, there should be a point in time at which both molar and choriocarcinomatous tissue are simultaneously present. Yet, there is no question that it represents a useful parameter at the practical level.

Immunohistochemically, choriocarcinoma cells are positive for hCG and keratin. There may also be reactivity for hPL, SP1, and CEA.[172] There can be a minor component of intermediate trophoblastic cells immunoreactive for hPL, CD146 (Mel-CAM), HLA-G, and inhibin.

Microscopic grading of choriocarcinoma is of little value. Some attempts at correlating various patterns of growth with prognosis have been recorded;[158,178] of these, the most convincing are those showing an improved prognosis in the presence of an intense

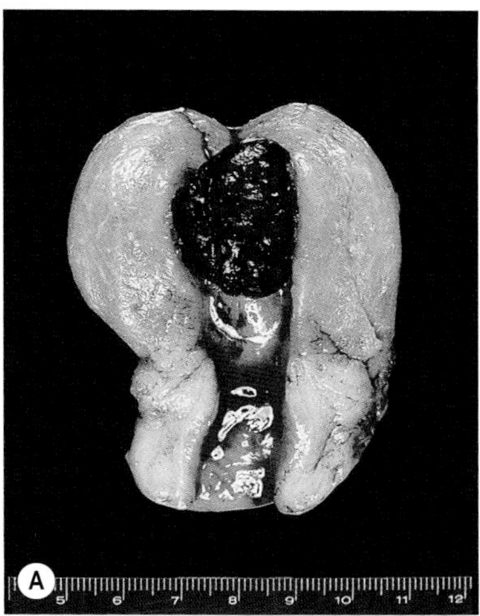

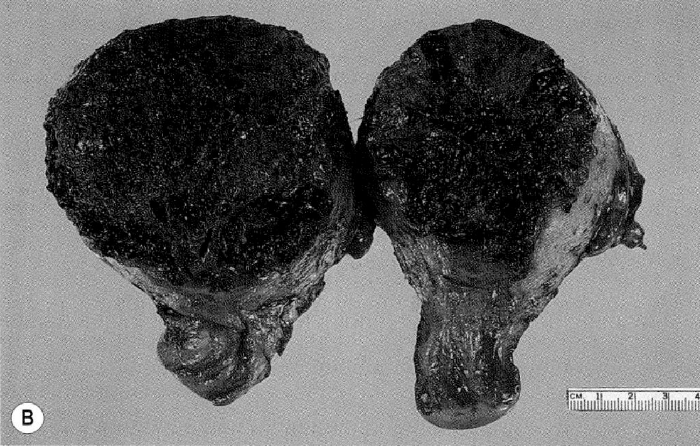

Fig. 19.359 **A** and **B**, Uterine choriocarcinoma showing typical highly hemorrhagic appearance.

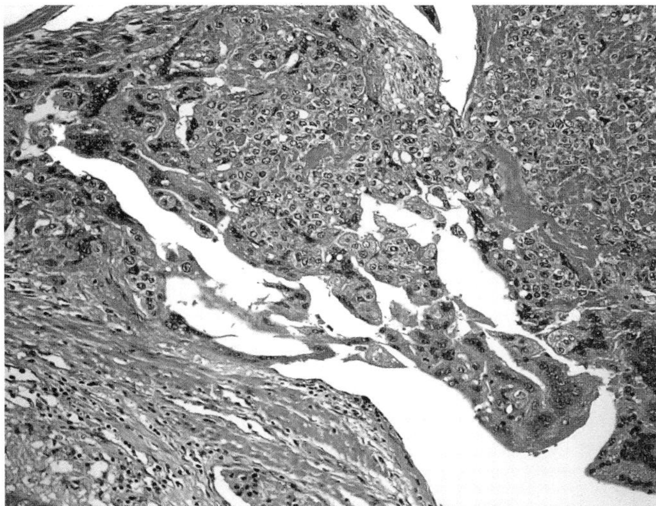

Fig. 19.360 Intimate admixture of syncytiotrophoblast and cytotrophoblast in choriocarcinoma.

inflammatory infiltrate at the interphase between tumor and stroma.[161,164,167,176]

The natural history of untreated choriocarcinoma is characterized by the development of early hematogenous metastases, the most common sites being the lung, brain, liver, kidney, and bowel.[166,174,183] They can be clinically solitary, may occur in the most unusual places, and often present with massive hemorrhage.[165] Interestingly, the fetus is rarely involved, even in cases of widespread metastatic disease.[184] Residual tumor in the uterus of patients dying of disseminated choriocarcinoma may be inconspicuous or altogether absent.[179]

Many of the morphologic changes seen in other organs in patients with choriocarcinoma are the result of increased secretion of hCG and other hormones by the tumor cells. These include hyperplasia of endocervical glands, decidual reaction (both endometrial and ectopic), Arias-Stella phenomenon, bilateral enlargement of the ovaries by theca-lutein cysts ('hyperreactio luteinalis'), and hyperplasia of mammary lobules. The detection of ovarian theca-lutein cysts long after a case of choriocarcinoma has been treated is usually a sign of persistent disease.[169] In the endometrial decidual reaction of patients with choriocarcinoma, the spiral arterioles fail to develop as they do in the normal cycle, the appearance of the mucosa being similar to that seen after the administration of progestogens.[179]

The evolution of the treatment of choriocarcinoma (and of gestational trophoblastic disease in general) is one of the greatest success stories in medical oncology.[181] When treated by surgery alone, the cure rate was only 40% for tumors apparently restricted to the uterus and less than 20% for those accompanied by metastases.[155] With the use of the chemotherapeutic agents methotrexate, actinomycin D, and chlorambucil (a combination usually referred to as MAC), the survival rate is close to 100% for cases restricted to the uterus and approximately 83% for patients with metastatic disease.[168,173] These figures are impressive indeed, although in all fairness it should be pointed out that in most series they apply not just to choriocarcinoma as strictly defined on pathologic terms but to gestational trophoblastic disease (or to 'metastatic' gestational trophoblastic disease) in a more generic sense. Low- and high-risk patient groups have been identified on the basis of location of metastases, hCG, and duration of the disease[177] (Table 19.5 and Box 19.3).

In most cases the uterus can be retained. Hysterectomy is performed in those patients in whom preservation of the reproductive function is not desired and/or who are unresponsive to

Box 19.3 NIH classification of gestational trophoblastic disease

I. Benign GTD
   A. Complete hydatidiform mole
   B. Partial hydatidiform mole
II. Malignant GTD
   A. Nonmetastatic GTD
   B. Metastatic TD
      1. Good prognosis, low risk – absence of any risk factor
      2. Poor prognosis, high risk – presence of any risk factor
         a. Duration >4 months
         b. Pretherapy level of β-hCG in serum >40 000 mIU/mL
         c. Brain or liver metastases
         d. GTD after term gestation
         e. Prior to failed therapy

From SGO handbook. Staging of gynaecologic malignancies. Chicago, 1994, Society of Gynecologic Oncologists.

Table 19.5 World Health Organization Prognostic Index Score for gestational trophoblastic disease

	SCORE[a]			
PROGNOSTIC FACTOR	0	1	2	4
Age (y)	≤39	>39	–	–
Antecedent pregnancy	Hydatidiform mole	Abortion	Term	–
Interval (mo)[b]	4	4–6	7–12	>12
β-hCG (IU/L)	$<10^3$	10^3–10^4	10^4–10^5	$>10^5$
ABO groups (female × male)	–	OxA, AxO	B, AB	–
Largest tumor, including uterine tumor	–	3–5 cm	>5 cm	–
Site of metastases	–	Spleen, kidney	GI tract, liver	Brain
Number of metastases identified	–	1–4	4–8	>8
Prior chemotherapy	–	–	Single drug	Two or more drugs

[a]The total score for a patient is obtained by adding the individual scores for each prognostic factor: low risk, 0–4; intermediate risk, 5–7; high risk ≤8.
[b]Interval is time between end of antecedent pregnancy and start of chemotherapy.
From SGO handbook. Staging of gynecologic malignancies. Chicago, 1994, Society of Gynecologic Oncologists.

chemotherapy alone. Surgery also remains useful in controlling life-threatening hemorrhage from metastatic lesions.[157,171]

The importance of early diagnosis, prompt institution of therapy, and monitoring of the effects of treatment with sequential quantitative determination of hCG production cannot be overemphasized. In regard to the latter, it should be mentioned that hCG secretion is by no means restricted to gestational choriocarcinomas. It can also occur in nongestational choriocarcinoma; other ovarian and testicular germ cell tumors; melanoma; malignant lymphoma; and carcinomas of the esophagus, stomach, pancreas, kidney, liver, lung, urinary bladder, uterus, adrenal gland, breast, and other sites. A feature common to many of these tumors is the presence of tumor giant cells shown to contain hCG by immunocytochemical techniques.[156]

Genetic studies using locus-specific minisatellite probes to identify restriction fragment length polymorphisms in DNA from tumor tissue are useful in distinguishing gestational from nongestational (germ cell) choriocarcinoma and in documenting the tumor derivation from an antecedent complete mole (by establishing the androgenetic nature of the tumor).[162]

Placental site trophoblastic tumor and related lesions of intermediate trophoblast

Placental site trophoblastic tumor is the currently accepted term for a rare form of trophoblastic disease formerly described as *atypical choriocarcinoma* and *trophoblastic pseudotumor*.[195,202,209] About 75% of cases follow a normal pregnancy, with only 5% of the reported patients having had a preceding molar pregnancy.[205] A paternally derived X chromosome and the absence of a Y chromosome may be necessary for its formation, consistent with an origin from the trophectoderm of a female conceptum.[191,192] It presents grossly as a myometrial mass that can be well localized or ill defined (Fig. 19.361A). Hemorrhage is not as conspicuous as in invasive mole or choriocarcinoma. The uterine penetration may be deep, and perforation may result, either spontaneously or following curettage.

Microscopically, large trophoblastic cells with abundant eosinophilic cytoplasm and nuclear pleomorphism are seen invading the myometrium and vessel lumina (Fig. 19.361B). The morphologic, ultrastructural, and immunohistochemical features of these cells correspond to those of intermediate trophoblast.[187,194,198,208] As such, the immunoreactivity for hPL is strong and widespread, whereas that for hCG tends to be focal.[186,196] There is also positivity for keratin, CD66a (CEACAM1), CD146 (Mel-CAM), pregnancy-associated major basic protein, HLA-G, and inhibin.[185,201,206] The DNA pattern, as determined by flow cytometry, is usually diploid,[189,193] and this seems to also be the case in the rare examples with malignant behavior.[207] The MIB-1 (Ki-67) labeling index is higher than in exaggerated placental site reaction but lower than in choriocarcinoma.[203] The *TP53* gene product is highly expressed, together with epidermal growth factor receptor.[199] In contrast, there is no expression of p63, an useful feature in the differential diagnosis with epithelioid trophoblastic tumor (see below).[204]

Although this condition was initially considered to be an exuberant form of syncytial endometritis,[195] additional experience has shown that it is instead a neoplastic process with a 10–20% mortality rate if not treated properly.[197] Some cases have resulted in widespread metastases;[189,200] these have generally shown a high mitotic count in the primary tumor, extensive necrosis, and/or a preponderance of cells with clear cytoplasm.[202]

Serum hCG levels in placental site trophoblastic tumor are usually not as high as in choriocarcinoma and may not accurately reflect the extent of the disease. Sometimes the tumor is totally resistant to chemotherapy.[188,190] A distinctive renal glomerular lesion accompanied by proteinuria and hematuria and characterized by occlusive eosinophilic deposits in the glomerular capillary lumina has been observed in connection with this neoplasm.[210]

The differential diagnosis of placental site trophoblastic tumor includes other gestational trophoblastic diseases, as well as nonneoplastic placental proliferations of intermediate trophoblast. The distinction with choriocarcinoma is made because of a lack of a dimorphic population of cytotrophoblast and syncytiotrophoblast (although scattered multinucleated cells may be present), lack or paucity of hemorrhage, and the presence of an interdigitating pattern of muscle invasion.

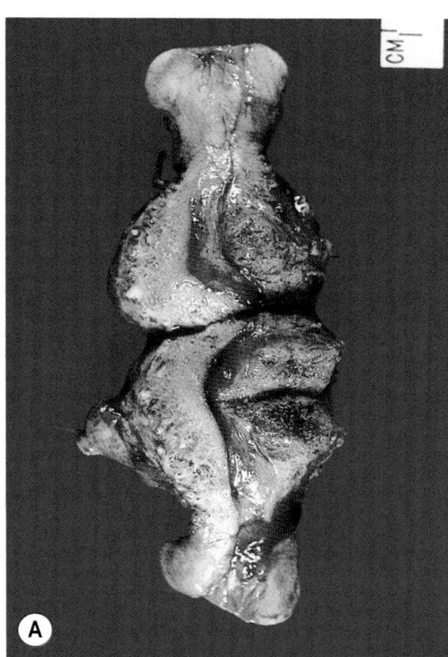

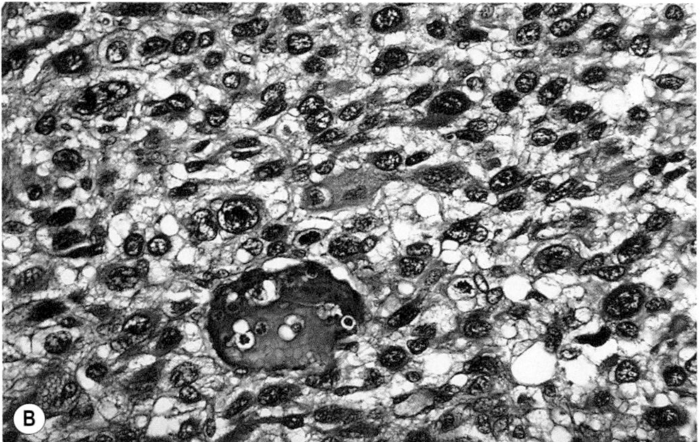

Fig. 19.361 **A** and **B**, Placental site trophoblastic tumor. **A**, Gross appearance. A solid hemorrhagic nodule is seen distending the myometrium and protruding into the endometrial cavity. **B**, Microscopic appearance. Medium-sized cells of intermediate trophoblastic type are seen growing in a diffuse fashion into the myometrium. The biphasic pattern resulting from the admixture of cytotrophoblast and syncytiotrophoblast, which is typical of choriocarcinoma, is absent.

Epithelioid trophoblastic tumor

Epithelioid trophoblastic tumor, the latest entry into the gestational trophoblastic disease family, was originally described as a peculiar change in the metastatic foci of choriocarcinoma surgically excised following chemotherapy,[217] but is now known to also occur *de novo*. Like the other members of the family, it usually occurs in the reproductive age group (although it can be seen after menopause),[211] and it presents with abnormal vaginal bleeding. The primary tumor most commonly occurs in the endomyometrium, but can sometimes be centered in the uterine cervix,[212] develop outside the uterus in places such as the broad ligament,[214] or even present as a primary lung tumor, simulating microscopically squamous and pleomorphic carcinomas of this organ.[215] hCG levels are usually elevated. Grossly, it is solid and cystic, discrete, and hemorrhagic. Microscopically, it is composed of a relatively uniform population of intermediate trophoblastic cells forming nests and solid masses. Necrosis is extensive, and there is a hyaline matrix with a geographic configuration (Fig. 19.362). The appearance closely simulates that of a carcinoma. Immunohistochemically, there is diffuse reactivity for keratin, α-inhibin, EMA, p63, HLA-G, and E-cadherin, but only focal reactivity for hPL, hCG, PLAP, and CD116 (Mel-CAM).[213] Positivity for cyclin E helps in the differential diagnosis with placental site trophoblastic tumor, and lack of reactivity for p16 is useful in the differential diagnosis with cervical and other types of carcinoma.[216] Shih et al.[219] believe that the tumor is composed of chorion laeve-type intermediate trophoblast. Molecular genetic analysis has confirmed its trophoblastic origin by demonstrating a Y-chromosomal locus and/or new (paternal) alleles not present in the adjacent normal uterine tissue.[218] It behaves as a malignant tumor, with metastases to lung and other sites.[219]

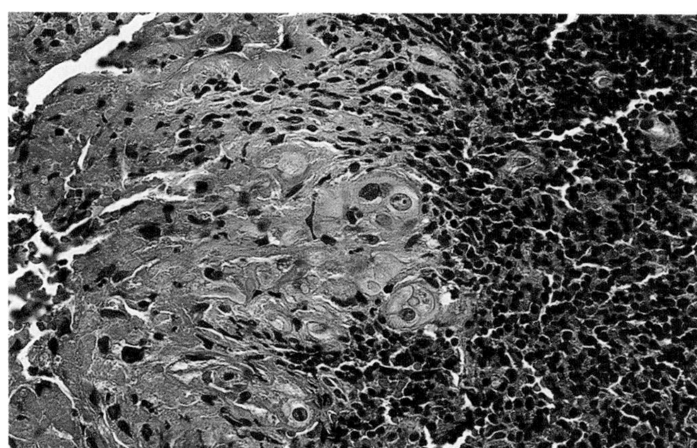

Fig. 19.362 Epithelioid trophoblastic tumor. The microscopic appearance closely simulates carcinoma of either squamous or glassy cell type.

Tumorlike conditions of intermediate trophoblast

Presumably non-neoplastic proliferations of intermediate trophoblast that can create serious problems in the differential diagnosis with malignant trophoblastic tumors are exaggerated placental site reaction, placental site nodule, and placental site plaque.[224]

Exaggerated placental site reaction (EPSR) was called syncytial endometritis in the past, but this was a double misnomer since the lesion is not primarily of inflammatory nature and is not composed of syncytiotrophoblast. As the currently preferred name indicates, it is believed to be the result of excessive but otherwise normal infiltration of the implantation site by intermediate trophoblast (Fig. 19.363). Its distinction from placental site implantation tumor can be difficult because the cytologic and immunohistochemical features are very similar. EPSR is to be favored when the lesion is microscopic in size, lacks mitotic activity, contains a hyaline material between the trophoblastic cells, and is admixed with decidua and villi.

Placental site nodules and plaques appear as single or multiple, mostly well-circumscribed, variably cellular round or flat lesions (nodules and plaques, respectively) that tend to be extensively hyalinized[222,226] (Fig. 19.364). Most cells have abundant amphophilic or acidophilic cytoplasm, irregularly shaped nuclei, and very scanty mitotic activity, but others have a glycogen-rich clear cytoplasm.[225] Mallory bodies (representing abnormal cytoplasmic aggregates of keratin filaments) may be present.[227] These nodules and plaques, which can also occur in the cervix, fallopian tube, and other

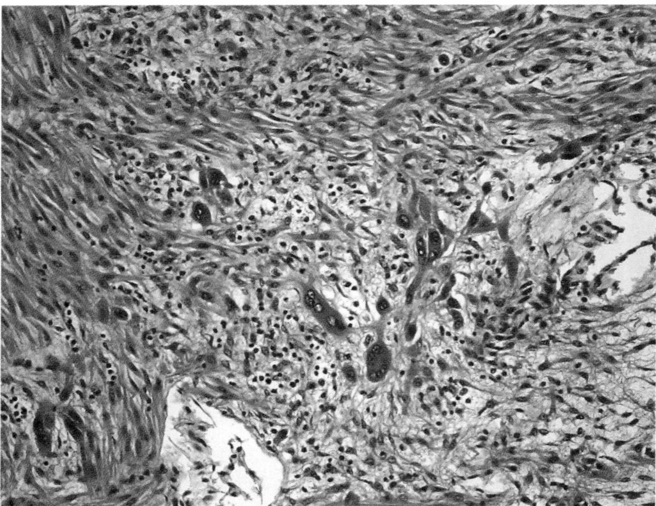

Fig. 19.363 Trophoblastic cells infiltrating the myometrium in a tumorlike fashion in exaggerated placental site reaction.

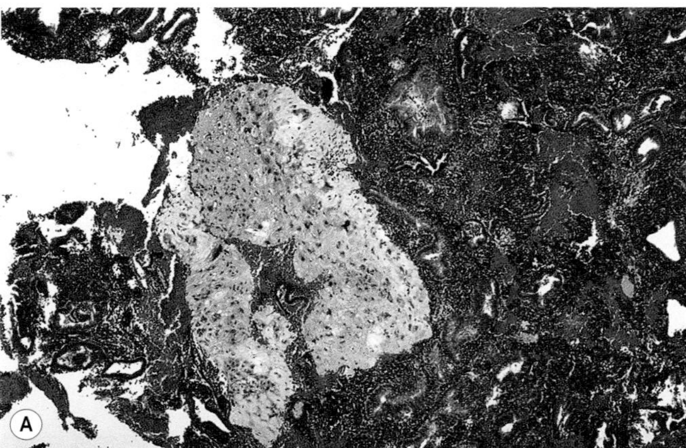

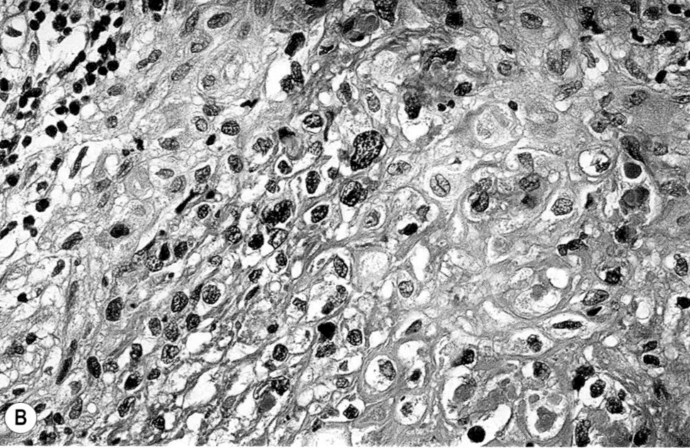

Fig. 19.364 A and **B**, Low- and medium-power appearance of placental site nodule. The appearance is vaguely chondroid and can be easily misinterpreted.

sites,[220,221] are distinguished from placental site trophoblastic tumor because of their smaller size, better circumscription, extensive hyalinization, degenerative appearance, and paucity of mitotic activity.[223,228] It has been pointed out that placental site nodules and plaques closely resemble the intermediate trophoblast of the chorion laeve rather than that at the implantation site. As such, they are diffusely positive for PLAP but only focally positive or negative for hPL and CD146 (Mel-CAM).[225]

The differential diagnosis between placental site trophoblastic tumor and the non-neoplastic proliferations previously mentioned may not be always possible in a curettage specimen. In such cases, subsequent curettings and monitoring of serum levels of hCG and hPL become imperative.

Non-neoplastic lesions of term placenta

The placenta is best examined in the fresh state immediately after delivery.[276,278,286,301] The information obtained from an adequate examination of the placenta can be critical in early neonatal care and in reproductive planning for the family, it can contribute to the understanding of neurologic and other disabilities among surviving children, it can help explain a significant percentage of prenatal and perinatal deaths, and it is of great importance in the resolution of medicolegal cases.[234,237,245,269,279,293,306]

Abnormally large placentas are frequently seen in association with polyhydramnios. They accompany conditions leading to fetal anemia or cardiac failure, such as erythroblastosis fetalis; infections, such as syphilis, toxoplasmosis, or cytomegalovirus; tumors of the placenta and fetus; or fetal renal vein thrombosis.[237,252,275] Histologically, these enlarged placentas retain immature features.

Abnormally small placentas are seen in prematurely born infants and in many growth-retarded ('small for dates') infants. Causes of the latter include maternal vascular disease and fetal malformations,[282,311] but many remain of undetermined etiology.

Placenta accreta refers to a condition in which placental villi adhere to the underlying myometrium, without an intervening layer of decidua[251,265,268] (Fig. 19.365). Morphologic subtypes of this condition are designated as *placenta increta* when the villi invade the myometrium and *placenta percreta* when the villous infiltration extends through the whole thickness of the myometrium.[281] Placenta percreta may result in spontaneous uterine rupture and fatal hemoperitoneum.[243] At the other extreme, mild (microscopic) forms of placenta accreta, which are not uncommon, are detected only through careful sampling of the placental basal plate.[243] The increased amount of implantation site trophoblast detected in placenta accreta may have a role in the pathogenesis of placental ingrowth.[274]

Placenta circummarginata and **placenta circumvallata** are two morphologic variants of extrachorial placenta (i.e., a placenta in which the chorionic plate is smaller than its basal plate). In placenta circummarginata, the transition from the membranous to the villous chorion is flat, whereas in placenta circumvallata the marginal membrane is folded or rolled back on itself. Wentworth[309] examined 895 placentas and found 25.5% to be circummarginate and 6.5% circumvallate. He considered these two malformations of no clinical significance. Others have reported an increased incidence of antepartum bleeding, particularly with circumvallation.[238]

Amnion nodosum is the result of fetal renal agenesis and is associated with oligohydramnios.[230] It presents as small plaques on the amniotic surface, formed by squamous cells and fibrin. Ultrastructural and other studies suggest that amnion nodosum originates from the apposition of desquamated fetal skin elements on the amnion epithelium in the presence of oligohydramnios.[298]

Malformations of umbilical cord of clinical importance include *velamentous insertion* and the *absence of one umbilical artery*[265,268] (Fig. 19.366). The former is seen in 1% of all placentas and may result in massive fetal hemorrhage if located at the cervical opening. The latter, also present in approximately 1% of all cords, is associated

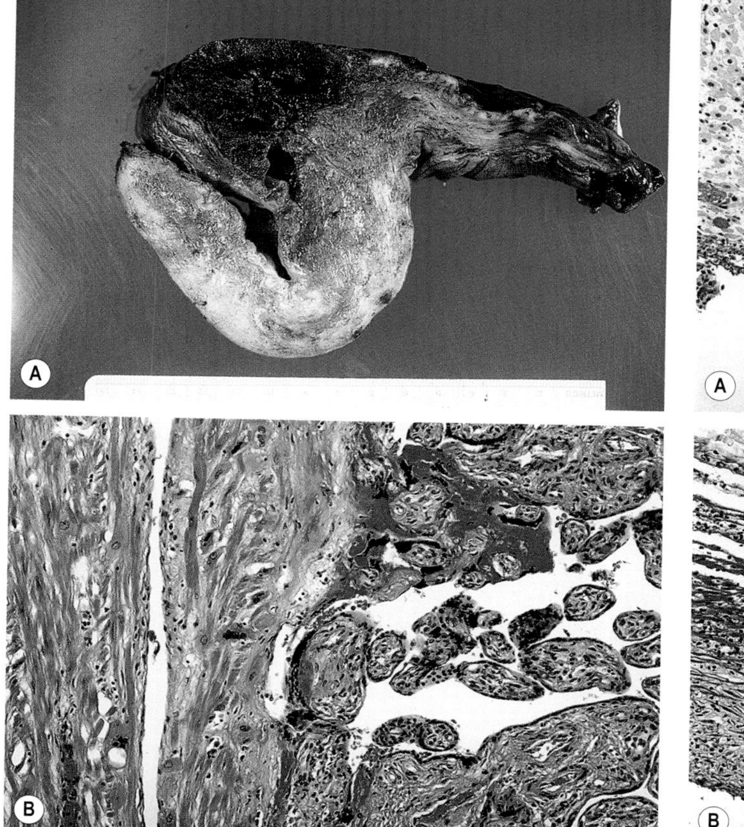

Fig. 19.365 **A** and **B**, Gross and microscopic appearance of placenta accreta. The penetration of the myometrium by chorionic villi is obvious at both levels.

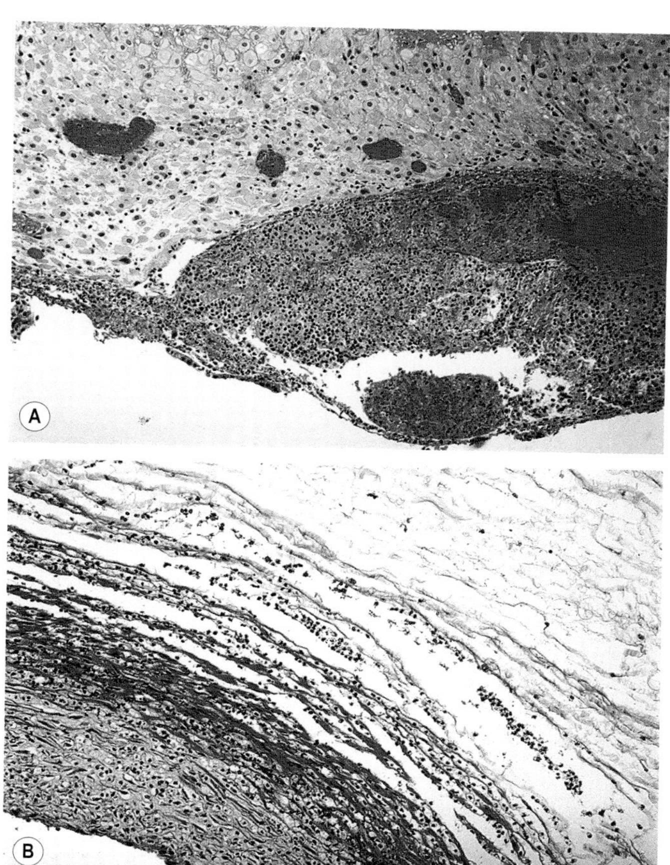

Fig. 19.367 **A** and **B**, Placental inflammation. The specimen shown in **A** shows a concentration of the inflammatory infiltrate on the placental maternal side, whereas the specimen depicted in **B** depicts inflammatory changes centered in umbilical vessels.

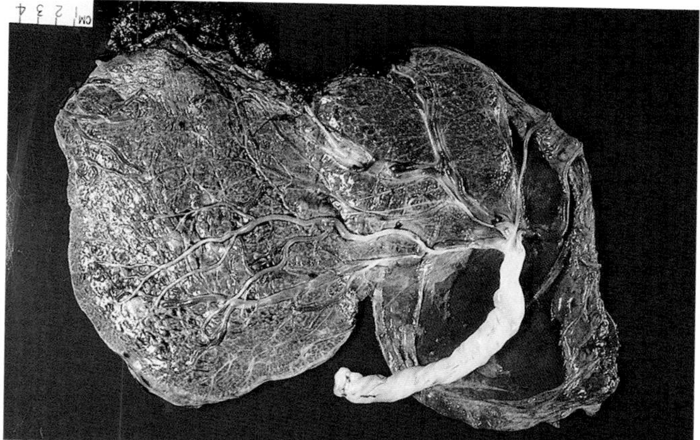

Fig. 19.366 Velamentous insertion of umbilical cord near an accessory placental lobe.

with congenital abnormalities of the infant in 30% of cases.[242,259] These abnormalities may involve the cardiac, renal, skeletal, or other systems. There is also an increased incidence of prematurity (16.5%) and of small size for dates (34%).[242] The absence of one umbilical artery can be detected by gross inspection of the cross section of the cord, but it should always be confirmed microscopically.

Other malformations of the umbilical cord are represented by persistence of embryonic structures.[236] The large majority of these are of no clinical significance and show no particular association with congenital malformations or perinatal complications. Most are located at the fetal end of the cord and are represented by *remnants of the allantoic duct, omphalomesenteric duct,* and *embryonic vessels.*[264]

Infection of the placenta is due most commonly to organisms that ascend from the maternal vaginal tract.[237,240,291] It shows a good correlation with prematurity and sepsis during the first 2 days of life.[294] Overall estimates of its frequency range from 5.4% to 24.4%.[253] It is manifested morphologically by an inflammatory infiltrate of predominantly neutrophilic nature that is contributed by both the maternal and fetal circulation. The former is primarily located in the peripheral membranes and chorionic plate, whereas the latter is concentrated in the umbilical and fetal surface vessels (Fig. 19.367). Grossly, the placental surface may appear cloudy and dull; however, in most cases the inflammation is detectable only microscopically. Infection may also reach the placenta through the maternal bloodstream, leading to inflammatory infiltrates within the villi.[233] These may be of acute, chronic, or granulomatous nature and may be associated with hemorrhagic vasculitis or vascular obliteration.[233,299] It should be mentioned here that fetal anoxia or meconium staining of the membranes *does not* result in inflammatory changes in the placenta.[277]

The most common cause of placental infection acquired from an ascending route is bacterial (including fusobacteria),[232] but

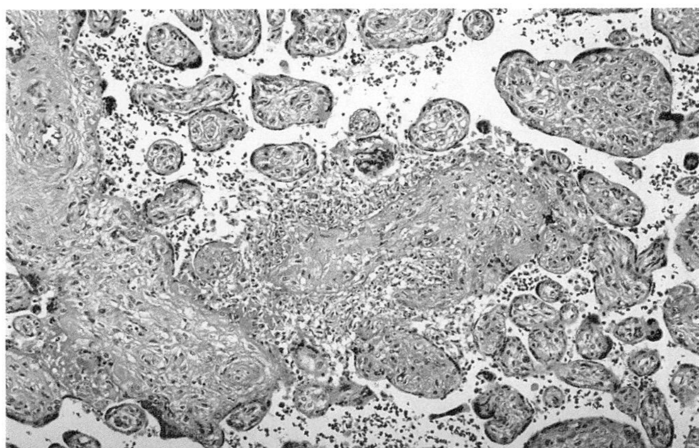

Fig. 19.368 Necrotizing villitis resulting from *Listeria* infection.

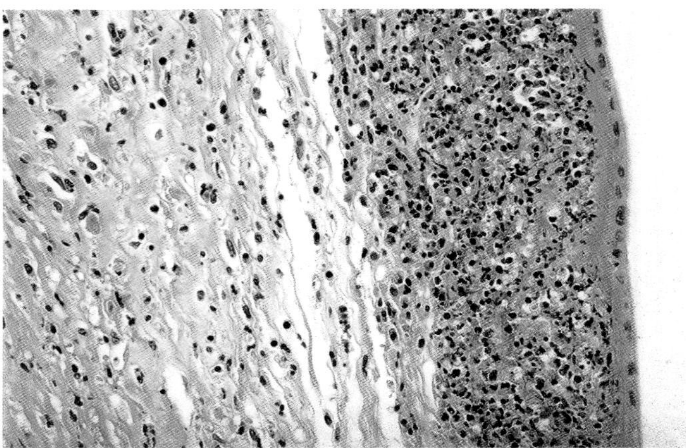

Fig. 19.369 Acute chorioamnionitis.

other vaginal inhabitants such as *herpes virus* or *Candida* may be implicated.[292] Herpetic infection of placental tissues may be accompanied by necrotizing funisitis.[260] The diagnosis of herpetic infection can be confirmed by immunohistochemical stains or in-situ hybridization.[288,303]

The organisms implicated in placentitis acquired through the hematogenous route are numerous.[302] They include cytomegalovirus (CMV), *Listeria*, rubella, syphilis, toxoplasmosis, tuberculosis, coccidioidomycosis, cryptococcosis, malaria, and even psittacosis[261,262,266,267,271,280,289] (Fig. 19.368). In CMV infection, diagnostic viral inclusions are only rarely found.[284,304] However, immunohistochemical staining for CMV antigens is often positive, the infected cells being usually located in the villous stroma.[285] The diagnosis can also be made by detecting CMV genetic material by the polymerase chain reaction (PCR) technique; these studies have shown that approximately 10% of cases of chronic villitis are caused by CMV infection.[287,297] In *syphilis*, the characteristic changes include vascular proliferation, acute or chronic villitis, and relative villous immaturity, manifested by enlarged hypercellular villi; in some instances, acute villitis is also present.[305,307] The diagnosis can be confirmed by performing PCR for *Treponema pallidum* DNA in the placental tissue or by immunostaining for *Treponema*.[255]

Placentas from HIV-infected patients do not have specific gross or microscopic alterations, although there is an increased incidence of chorioamnionitis in them.[300]

Chronic villitis is a nonspecific inflammatory process involving the villi that is morphologically similar to that seen in rubella but unaccompanied by serologic evidence of this infection.[233,295,296] The etiology of this condition, which may be associated with intrauterine growth retardation and occasional unexplained stillbirths, remains unknown; infection by unidentified organisms and abnormal immune reactions have been implicated.[239] It is found in 1–9% of all placentas, depending on the degree of sampling, diagnostic criteria, and patient population studied, and is sometimes seen in subsequent pregnancies of the same individual.[290]

Chronic villitis may be associated with **chronic** chorioamnionitis;[257] in some instances the latter may dominate the microscopic picture[258] (Fig. 19.369). The chorioamnionitis can be graded microscopically into mild, moderate, or severe; its frequency and severity are inversely related to gestational age at preterm birth.[231,263,283,312]

In **chronic intervillositis**, the inflammatory infiltrate is mainly histiocytic and predominantly located in the intervillous space; these rare cases have been found to be associated with poor fetal outcome.[241,263]

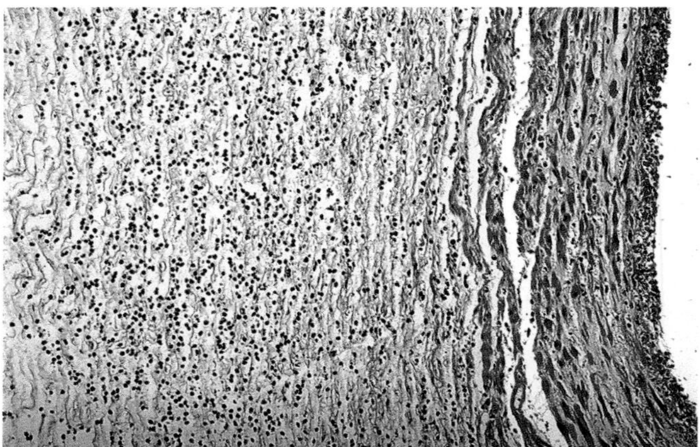

Fig. 19.370 Intense inflammatory infiltrate of the umbilical cord (funisitis).

Acute funisitis, i.e., acute inflammation of the umbilical cord, is a sign of fetal inflammatory response, and therefore its detection is of some clinical importance. The inflammation begins as a discrete multifocal process that eventually coalesces; it is therefore recommended that a section be taken from each third of the umbilical cord.[272] Microscopically, the key feature is umbilical vasculitis (Fig. 19.370). The association with fetal infection is stronger in preterm than in term placentas.[273] Autolysis of umbilical vascular smooth muscle following second trimester fetal death can simulate vasculitis, in that the necrotic cells may be confused with neutrophils.[256]

Placental infarct represents an area of villous necrosis secondary to local obstruction of the *maternal* uteroplacental circulation.[270] Grossly, the fresh infarct is dark red and of firmer consistency than the surrounding tissue. Microscopically, it is characterized by crowding of villi, virtual obliteration of the intervillous space, and marked congestion of the villous vessels. When old, it appears grossly as a hard, white mass of granular appearance and microscopically as a mass of crowded 'ghost' villi (Figs 19.371 and 19.372). True infarcts should be distinguished from hematomas, subchorionic fibrin plaques, foci of intervillous fibrin deposition, and intervillous laminated thrombi.[308] Wigglesworth[311] demonstrated by injection studies that infarcts and hematomas have a lobular distribution, thrombi occur in either the arterial or venous regions of the intervillous space, and perivillous fibrin deposits are predominantly venous lesions.

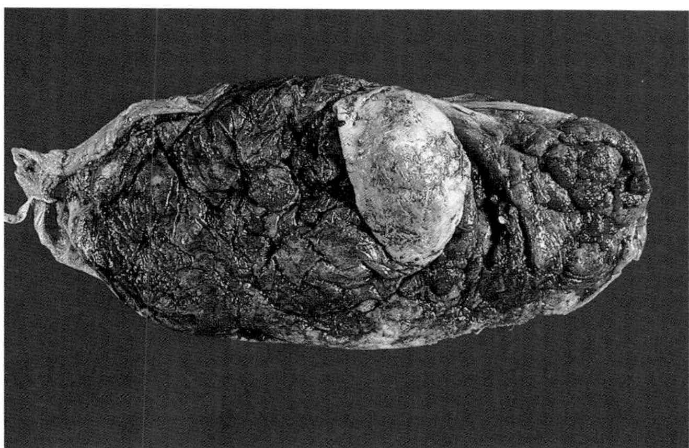

Fig. 19.371 Gross appearance of old placental infarct. The lesion is whitish and had a firm consistency.

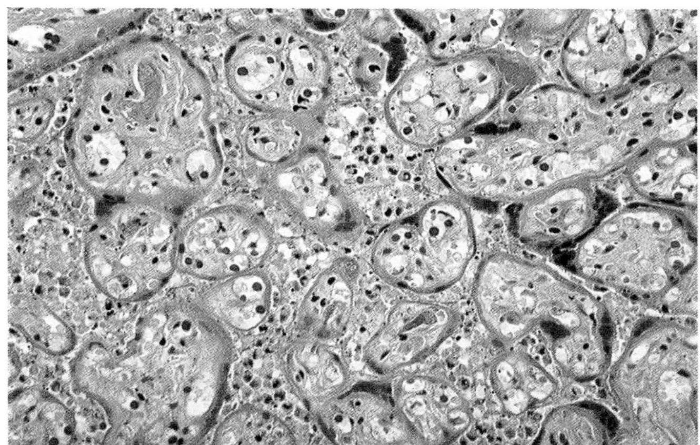

Fig. 19.372 Ghosts of chorionic villi in a long-standing placental infarct.

Minor degrees of infarction are seen in about 25% of placentas from uncomplicated term pregnancies and can, therefore, be regarded as an inconsequential phenomenon. A significant increase in the incidence and severity of infarcts in pregnancies has been found associated with preeclamptic toxemia, essential hypertension, Rh incompatibility, and nontoxic antepartum hemorrhage.[247] However, the fact that more than half of the placentas from pregnancies associated with preeclamptic toxemia show no infarcts indicates that the infarct per se is not necessarily the cause of the clinical manifestations of this disease. In most instances, the infarcts are the result of a retroplacental hematoma (abruptio placentae) or a thrombosed maternal vessel. Extensive placental infarcts are associated with a high incidence of neonatal asphyxia, low birth weight, and intrauterine death.[247]

Thrombosis of fetal arteries should be distinguished from placental infarcts (which, as already stated, are always secondary to occlusion of the maternal uteroplacental circulation).[270,277] The placental changes resulting from thrombosis of fetal arteries appear grossly as roughly triangular or hemispheric pale areas, otherwise indistinguishable from the surrounding normal placenta. They are better seen after formalin fixation. Microscopically, the villi are fibrosed and avascular, except for occasional small, thickened vessels. A thrombosed fetal artery is present at the apex of the lesion. Fox[246] found this lesion in 3.6% of 715 placentas examined. It was particularly frequent in diabetic women, and it did not seem to result in any deleterious effect on the fetus. It should be mentioned here that, in addition to fetal artery thrombosis, placentas of diabetic women often show an increased number of syncytial knots, fibrotic villi, Langhans cells, and foci of villous fibrinoid necrosis.[248–250]

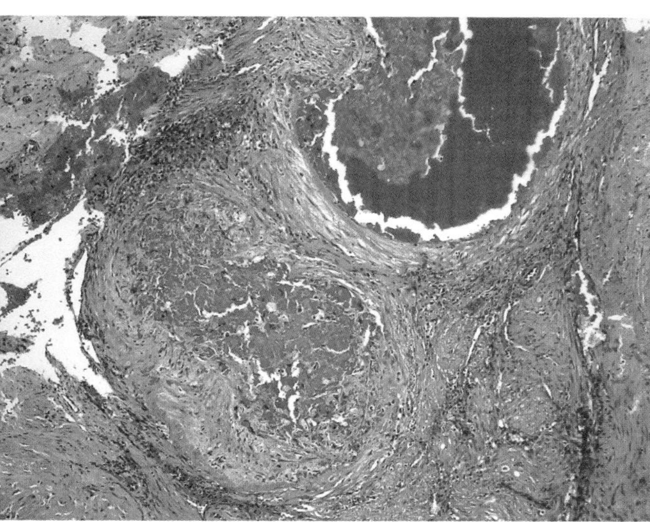

Fig. 19.373 Placental site subinvolution showing thick-walled vessels whose lumen is partially obliterated by organizing thrombi.

Placental iron deposits are normal in the form of granular structures along the trophoblastic basement membrane; their presence in 7.5% or more of the villi is said to be abnormal and to be associated with fetal growth anomalies.[244]

Decidual vascular lesions of a necrotizing or inflammatory nature have been found in patients with lupus erythematosus.[229]

Sickle cell anemia can often be diagnosed by microscopic examination of the placenta, the deformation in the red blood cells developing as a result of the hypoxia created by the separation of the placenta from the uterine wall.[254]

Table 19.6 shows the correlation between morphologic changes in the placenta and a variety of clinical situations.

Placental site subinvolution may result in vaginal bleeding several weeks after delivery of the placenta, even in the absence of retained placental tissue.[310] Curettage specimens from such cases contain large maternal vessels from the placental site partly filled with thrombi (Fig. 19.373). In the normal state, these thrombi become organized and remain as scars in the endometrium or adjacent myometrium. Some differences in deposition of immunoglobulins and complement factors have been detected immunohistochemically between subinvoluted and normal vessels. These have been interpreted as indicating that immunologic factors are necessary for the process of normal involution of uteroplacental arteries and that these may be deficient in subinvoluted vessels.[235]

Tumors and tumorlike conditions of term placenta

Hemangiomas of placenta (chorangiomas) are found in approximately 1 of every 100 term specimens if a careful gross examination is performed.[323] Grossly, they are well circumscribed and purplish red. They may protrude on the fetal surface or be located entirely in the placental substance (Fig. 19.374). Microscopically, they are composed of a network of proliferating capillaries (Fig. 19.375).

Table 19.6 Correlation between morphologic changes in placenta and variety of clinical situations

	NORMAL PREGNANCY	PROLONGED PREGNANCY	PREMATURE ONSET OF LABOR	RH INCOMPATIBILITY	DIABETES	ESSENTIAL HYPERTENSION	TOXEMIA
Infarct	±	±	±	±	+	++	++
Thrombosis of fetal arteries	±	+	±	±	++	±	±
Fibrinoid necrosis of villi	±	–	++	++	++	±	+
Immaturity of villi	±	±	±	++	++	±	±
Senescence of villi	±	++	±	±	±	±	+
Basement membrane thickening of villi	±	+	±	+	+	++	+++
Fibrosis of villi	±	+++	±	±	++	±	±

Based almost entirely on the gross and microscopic examination of placentas by Fox[246–252] and Fox and Langley.[253]

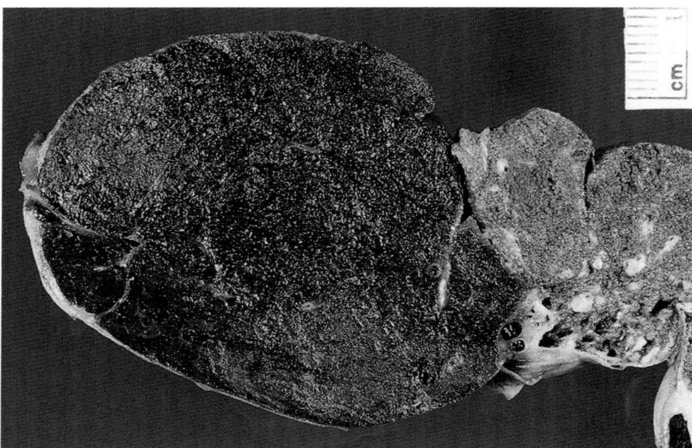

Fig. 19.374 Large placental hemangioma (chorangioma). The tumor is sharply circumscribed and of a deep red color.

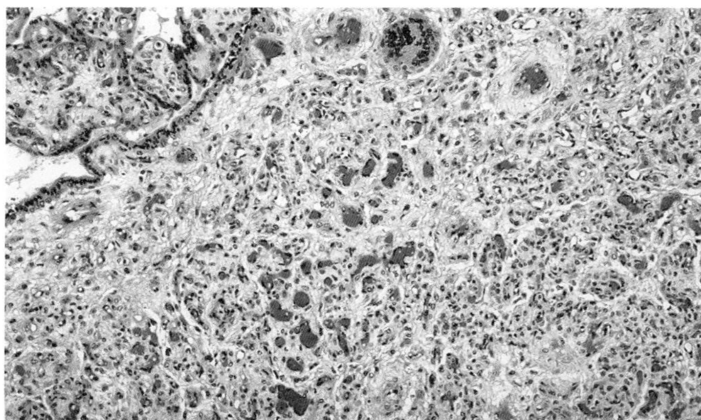

Fig. 19.375 Microscopic appearance of chorangioma. A complex network of capillaries distends the stroma of the placenta.

Mitoses may be present. Degenerative changes are common. Small hemangiomas (which represent the majority of the cases) are almost always asymptomatic, but the larger ones (more than 5 cm) may be associated with hydramnios, hemorrhage, premature delivery, premature placental separation, and placenta previa.[315] These manifestations may result in severe fetal distress and intrauterine death. The left-to-right shunting of blood across the tumor may lead to transient congestive heart failure in the infant.[317] There is apparently no relationship between placental hemangioma and toxemia. A case of placental hemangioma has been seen in association with intraplacental choriocarcinoma.[314]

Immunohistochemically, the tumor cells show focal staining for cytokeratin 18, a finding that has suggested to the authors an origin from blood vessels of the chorionic plate and anchoring villi.[329]

Chorangiosis (villous vascular proliferation) is a condition characterized by an increase in the number of vascular channels per villus, and allegedly associated with neonatal morbidity and mortality.[313] **Chorangiomatosis** is as diffuse as chorangiosis but the vessels have a thicker wall containing actin-positive smooth muscle cells.[333]

Teratoma of the placenta is very rare; its typical location is between the amnion and chorion.[324,327,342]

Hepatocellular adenoma has been reported on several occasions.[318,326,343] An origin from displaced yolk sac elements with hepatocytic differentiation has been suggested.

Heterotopic tissue such as adrenal cortex has also been described.[319]

Umbilical cord tumors are even less common than placental neoplasms. *Hemangiomas* occur, and may lead to nonimmune hydrops fetalis.[338] A few cases of *teratoma*[340] and *angiomyxoma*[344] have also been reported.

Direct extension of uterine tumors into the placenta has been reported in *leiomyoma* and *endometrial stromal sarcoma*.[322,325]

Metastatic tumors of maternal origin can lodge in the placenta and form distinct nodules. This phenomenon has been seen most often with malignant melanoma and malignant lymphoma/leukemia[316,328,332,335,336,339] but can also occur with carcinoma of lung and other organs.[320,337] Associated metastases to the fetus may or may not be present. Awareness of this dramatic event should not obscure the fact that in the large majority of pregnant women with widespread metastatic disease from any source the placenta and fetus are totally spared from the effects of the neoplasia.

An even stranger and rarer phenomenon is that of placental spread from congenital tumors in the fetus; this has been observed with leukemia and neuroblastoma.[330,334]

Giant pigmented nevi of the newborn can be accompanied by clusters of melanocytes in the placenta; this should not be taken as evidence that the tumor is malignant and that it has metastasized.[321,341]

Benign hemangioendothelioma has been seen to involve in a multicentric fashion the fetus and the placenta.[331]

References

NORMAL ANATOMY

1 Bamberger AM, Sudhal S, Wagener C, Loning T. Expression pattern of the adhesion molecule CEACAM1 (C-CAM, CD66a, BGP) in gestational trophoblastic lesions. Int J Gynecol Pathol 2001, **20**: 160–165.

2 Bleisch VR. Diagnosis of monochorionic twin placentation. Am J Clin Pathol 1964, **42**: 277–284.

3 Danforth DM, Hull RW. The microscopic anatomy of the fetal membranes with particular reference to the detailed structure of the amnion. Am J Obstet Gynecol 1958, **75**: 536–550.

4 Deftos LJ, Burton DW, Brandt DW, Pinar H, Rubin LP. Neoplastic hormone-producing cells of the placenta produce and secrete parathyroid hormone-related protein. Studies by immunohistology, immunoassay, and polymerase chain reaction. Lab Invest 1994, **71**: 847–852.

5 Fox H. Pathology of the placenta, ed. 2. London, 1997, W.B. Saunders.

6 Heatley MK, Maxwell P, Toner PG. The immunophenotype of human decidua and extra-uterine decidual reactions. Histopathology 1997, **29**: 437–442.

7 Horne CH, Rankin R, Bremner RD. Pregnancy-specific proteins as markers for gestational trophoblastic disease. Int J Gynecol Pathol 1984, **3**: 27–40.

8 Kämmerer U, Eggert AO, Kapp M, McLellan AD, Geijtenbeek TBH, Dietl J, van Kooyk Y, Kämpgen E. Unique appearance of proliferating antigen-presenting cell expressing DC-SIGN (CD209) in the deciduas of early human pregnancy. Am J Pathol 2003, **162**: 887–896.

9 Kingdom J, Jauniaux E, O'Brien PM, Royal College of Obstetricians and Gynaecologists Study Group. The placenta: basic science and clinical practice. London, 2000, RCOG Press.

10 Kurman RJ, Main CS, Chen H-C. Intermediate trophoblast. A distinctive form of trophoblast with specific morphological, biochemical and functional features. Placenta 1984, **5**: 349–370.

11 Lewis SH, Benirschke K. Placenta. In Mills SE (ed.): Histology for pathologists, ed. 3. Philadelphia, 2007, Lippincott Williams and Wilkins, pp. 1095–1128.

12 Li HW, Cheung AN, Tsao SW, Cheung AL, O WS. Expression of E-cadherin and beta-catenin in trophoblastic tissue in normal and pathological pregnancies. Int J Gynecol Pathol 2002, **22**: 63–70.

13 McCluggage WG. Recent advances in immunohistochemistry in gynaecological pathology. Histopathology 2002, **40**: 309–326.

14 Naeye RL. Umbilical cord length. Clinical significance. J Pediatr 1985, **107**: 278–281.

15 Naeye RL. Disorders of the placenta, fetus, and neonate. Diagnosis and clinical significance. St Louis, 1991, Mosby.

16 Novak RF. A brief review of the anatomy, histology, and ultrastructure of the full-term placenta. Arch Pathol Lab Med 1991, **115**: 654–659.

17 Shih IM, Kurman RJ. Immunohistochemical localization of inhibin-alpha in the placenta and gestational trophoblastic lesions. Int J Gynecol Pathol 1999, **18**: 144–150.

18 Shih IM, Seidman JD, Kurman RJ. Placental site nodule and characterization of distinctive type of intermediate trophoblast. Hum Pathol 1999, **30**: 687–694.

19 Singer G, Kurman RJ, McMaster MT, Shih IM. HLA-G immunoreactivity is specific for intermediate trophoblast in gestational trophoblastic disease and can serve as a useful marker in differential diagnosis. Am J Surg Pathol 2002, **26**: 914–920.

20 Yeh I-T, O'Connor DM, Kurman RJ. Vacuolated cytotrophoblast: a subpopulation of trophoblast in the chorion laeve. Placenta 1989, **10**: 429–438.

ABORTION

21 Abaci F, Aterman K. Changes of the placenta and embryo in early spontaneous abortion. Am J Obstet Gynecol 1968, **102**: 252–263.

22 Al-Tamimi DM. Intermediate trophoblasts: their role in the diagnosis of intrauterine pregnancy. Int J Surg Pathol 1998, **6**: 11–16.

23 Berry CL. The examination of embryonic and fetal material in diagnostic histopathology laboratories. J Clin Pathol 1980, **33**: 317–326.

24 Cheville JC, Robinson RA, Benda JA. P53 expression in placentas with hydropic change and hydatidiform moles. Mod Pathol 1996, **9**: 392–396.

25 Clark RK, Damjanov I. Intermediate filaments of human trophoblast and choriocarcinoma cell lines. Virchows Arch [A] 1985, **407**: 203–208.

26 Clement PB, Young RH, Scully RE. Nontrophoblastic pathology of the female genital tract and peritoneum associated with pregnancy. Semin Diagn Pathol 1989, **6**: 372–406.

27 Conran RM, Hitchcock CL, Popek EJ, Norris HJ, Griffin JL, Geissel A, McCarthy WF. Diagnostic considerations in molar gestations. Hum Pathol 1993, **24**: 41–48.

28 Daya D, Sabet L. The use of cytokeratin as a sensitive and reliable marker for trophoblastic tissue. Am J Clin Pathol 1991, **95**: 137–141.

29 Fox H. Histological classification of tissue from spontaneous abortions. A valueless exercise? Histopathology 1993, **22**: 599–600.

30 Fox H, Herd ME, Harilal KR. Morphological changes in the placenta and decidua after induction of abortion by extra-amniotic prostaglandin. Histopathology 1978, **2**: 145–151.

31 Fukunaga M, Ushigome S, Fukunaga M. Spontaneous abortions and DNA ploidy. An application of flow cytometric DNA analysis in detection of non-diploidy in early abortions. Mod Pathol 1993, **6**: 619–624.

32 Genest DR, Roberts D, Boyd T Bieber FR. Fetoplacental histology as a predictor of karyotype. A controlled study of spontaneous first trimester abortions. Hum Pathol 1995, **26**: 201–209.

33 Gruber K, Gelven PL, Austin RM. Chorionic villi or trophoblastic tissue in uterine samples of four women with ectopic pregnancies. Int J Gynecol Pathol 1997, **16**: 28–32.

34 Hermonat PL, Kechelava S, Lowery CL, Korourian S. Trophoblasts are the preferential target for human papilloma virus infection in spontaneously aborted products of conception. Hum Pathol 1998, **29**: 170–174.

35 Hertig AT. Gestational hyperplasia of endometrium. A morphologic correlation of ova, endometrium, and corpora lutea during pregnancy. Lab Invest 1964, **13**: 1153–1191.

36 Huettner PC, Gersell DJ. Arias-Stella reaction in nonpregnant women. A clinicopathologic study of nine cases. Int J Gynecol Pathol 1994, **13**: 241–247.

37 Jauniaux E, Hustin J. Histological examination of first trimester spontaneous abortions. The impact of materno-embryonic interface features. Histopathology 1992, **21**: 409–414.

38 Kim YT, Cho NH, Ko JH, Yang WI, Kim JW, Choi EK, Lee SH. Expression of cyclin E in placenta with hydropic change and gestational trophoblastic diseases: implications for the malignant transformation of trophoblasts. Cancer 2000, **89**: 673–679.

39 Klatt EC. Pathologic examination of fetal specimens from dilation and evacuation procedures. Am J Clin Pathol 1995, **103**: 415–418.

154 Brewer JI, Mazur MT. Gestational choriocarcinoma. Its origin in the placenta during seemingly normal pregnancy. Am J Surg Pathol 1981, **5**: 267–277.

155 Brewer JI, Smith RT, Pratt GB. Choriocarcinoma. Absolute 5-year survival rates of 122 patients treated by hysterectomy. Am J Obstet Gynecol 1963, **85**: 841–843.

156 Civantos F, Rywlin AM. Carcinomas with trophoblastic differentiation and secretion of chorionic gonadotrophins. Cancer 1972, **29**: 789–798.

157 Clayton LA, Barnard DE, Weed JC Jr, Hammond CB. The role of surgery in the management of gestational trophoblastic disease. Semin Oncol 1982, **9**: 213–220.

158 Deligdisch L, Driscoll SG, Goldstein P. Gestational trophoblastic neoplasms. Morphologic correlates of therapeutic response. Am J Obstet Gynecol 1978, **130**: 801–806.

159 Dyke PC, Fink LM. Latent choriocarcinoma. Cancer 1967, **20**: 150–154.

160 Elston CW, Bagshawe KD. The diagnosis of trophoblastic tumours from uterine curettings. J Clin Pathol 1972, **25**: 111–118.

161 Elston CW, Bagshawe KD. Cellular reaction of trophoblastic tumors. Br J Cancer 1973, **28**: 245–255.

162 Fisher RA, Newlands ES, Jeffreys AJ, Boxer GM, Begent RH, Rustin GJ, Bagshawe KD. Gestational and nongestational trophoblastic tumors distinguished by DNA analysis. Cancer 1992, **69**: 839–845.

163 Fukunaga M, Nomura K, Ushigome S. Choriocarcinoma in situ of a first trimester: report of two cases indicating an origin of trophoblast of a stem villus. Virchows Arch 1996, **429**: 185–188.

164 Greenfield AW. Gestational trophoblastic disease. Prognostic variables and staging. Semin Oncol 1995, **22**: 142–148.

165 Heaton GE, Matthews TH, Christopherson WM. Malignant trophoblastic tumors with massive hemorrhage presenting as liver primary. A report of two cases. Am J Surg Pathol 1986, **10**: 342–347.

166 Ishizuka T, Tomoda Y, Kaseki S, Goto S, Hara T, Kobayashi T. Intracranial metastasis of choriocarcinoma. A clinicopathologic study. Cancer 1983, **52**: 1896–1903.

167 Ito H, Sekine T, Komuro N, Tanaka T, Yokoyama S, Hosokawa T. Histologic stromal reaction of the host with gestational choriocarcinoma and its relation to clinical stage classification and prognosis. Am J Obstet Gynecol 1981, **140**: 781–786.

168 Kaseki S. Prognosis and treatment of trophoblastic diseases. Excerpta Medica (International Congress Series) 1980, **512**: 566–570.

169 Kohorn EI. Theca lutein ovarian cyst may be pathognomonic for trophoblastic neoplasia. Obstet Gynecol 1983, **62**: 80S–81S.

170 Lage J, Roberts DJ. Choriocarcinoma in a term placenta. Pathologic diagnosis of tumor in an asymptomatic patient with metastatic disease. Int J Gynecol Pathol 1993, **12**: 80–85.

171 Lewis J, Ketcham AS, Hertz R. Surgical intervention during chemotherapy of gestational trophoblastic neoplasms. Cancer 1966, **19**: 1517–1522.

172 Lind HM, Haghighi P. Carcinoembryonic antigen staining in choriocarcinoma. Am J Clin Pathol 1986, **86**: 538–540.

173 Lurain JR, Brewer JI, Torok EE, Halpern B. Gestational trophoblastic disease. Treatment results at the Brewer Trophoblastic Disease Center. Obstet Gynecol 1982, **60**: 354–360.

174 Mazur MT, Lurain JR, Brewer JI. Fatal gestational choriocarcinoma. Clinicopathologic study of patients treated at a trophoblastic disease center. Cancer 1982, **50**: 1833–1846.

175 Medeiros F, Callahan MJ, Elvin JA, Dorfman DM, Berkowitz RS, Quade BJ. Intraplacental choriocarcinoma arising in a second trimester placenta with partial hydatidiform mole. Int J Gynecol Pathol 2008, **27**: 247–251.

176 Mogensen B, Olsen S. Cellular reaction to gestational choriocarcinoma and invasive mole. Acta Pathol Microbiol Scand (A) 1973, **81**: 453–456.

177 Mortakis AE, Braga CA. 'Poor prognosis' metastatic gestational trophoblastic disease. The prognostic significance of the scoring system in predicting chemotherapy failures. Obstet Gynecol 1990, **76**: 272–277.

178 Nishikawa Y, Kaseki S, Tomoda Y, Ishizuka T, Asai Y, Susuki T, Ushijima H. Histopathologic classification of uterine choriocarcinoma. Cancer 1985, **55**: 1044–1051.

179 Ober WB, Edgcomb JH, Price EB Jr. The pathology of choriocarcinoma. Ann N Y Acad Sci 1971, **172**: 299–321.

180 Olive DL, Lurain JR, Brewer JI. Choriocarcinoma associated with term gestation. Am J Obstet Gynecol 1984, **148**: 711–716.

181 Ostor A. 'God's first cancer and man's first cure': milestones in gestational trophoblastic disease. Anat Pathol 1998, **1**: 165–178.

182 Redline RW, Abdul-Karim FW. Pathology of gestational trophoblastic disease. Semin Oncol 1995, **22**: 96–108.

183 Soper JT, Mutch DG, Chin N, Clarke-Pearson DL, Hammond CB. Renal metastases of gestational trophoblastic disease. A report of eight cases. Obstet Gynecol 1988, **72**: 796–798.

184 Tsukamoto N, Matsumura M, Matsukuma K, Kamura T, Baba K. Choriocarcinoma in mother and fetus. Gynecol Oncol 1986, **24**: 113–119.

PLACENTAL SITE TROPHOBLASTIC TUMOR AND RELATED LESIONS OF INTERMEDIATE TROPHOBLAST

185 Bamberger AM, Sudhal S, Wagener C, Loning T. Expression pattern of the adhesion molecule CEACAM1 (C-CAM, CD66a, BGP) in gestational trophoblastic lesions. Int J Gynecol Pathol 2001, **20**: 160–165.

186 Berger G, Verbaere J, Feroldi J. Placental site trophoblastic tumor of the uterus. An ultrastructural and immunohistochemical study. Ultrastruct Pathol 1984, **6**: 319–329.

187 Duncan DA, Mazur MT. Trophoblastic tumors. Ultrastructural comparison of choriocarcinoma and placental-site trophoblastic tumor. Hum Pathol 1989, **20**: 370–381.

188 Eckstein RP, Paradinas FJ, Bagshawe KD. Placental site trophoblastic tumour (trophoblastic pseudotumour). A study of four cases requiring hysterectomy including one fatal case. Histopathology 1982, **6**: 211–226.

189 Fukunaga M, Ushigome S. Metastasizing placental site trophoblastic tumor. An immunohistochemical and flow cytometric study of two cases. Am J Surg Pathol 1993, **17**: 1003–1010.

190 Gloor E, Dialdas J, Hurlimann J, Ribolzi J, Barrelet L. Placental site trophoblastic tumor (trophoblastic pseudotumor) of the uterus with metastases and fetal outcome. Clinical and autopsy observations of a case. Am J Surg Pathol 1983, **7**: 483–486.

191 Hui P, Parkash V, Perkins AS, Carcangiu ML. Pathogenesis of placental site trophoblastic tumor may require the presence of a paternally derived X chromosome. Lab Invest 2000, **80**: 965–972.

192 Hui P, Wang HL, Chu P, Yang B, Huang J, Baergen RN, Sklar J, Yang XJ, Soslow RA. Absence of Y chromosome in human placental site trophoblastic tumor. Mod Pathol 2007, **20**: 1055–1060.

193 Kotylo PK, Michael H, Davis TE, Sutton GP, Mark PR, Roth LM. Flow cytometric DNA analysis of placental-site trophoblastic tumors. Int J Gynecol Pathol 1992, **11**: 245–252.

194 Kurman RJ. The morphology, biology, and pathology of intermediate trophoblast. A look back to the present. Hum Pathol 1991, **22**: 847–855.

195 Kurman RJ, Scully RE, Norris HJ. Trophoblastic pseudotumor of the uterus. An exaggerated form of 'syncytial endometritis' simulating a malignant tumor. Cancer 1976, **38**: 1214–1226.

196 Kurman RJ, Young RH, Norris HJ, Main CS, Lawrence WD, Scully RE. Immunocytochemical localization of placental lactogen and chorionic gonadotropin in the normal placenta and trophoblastic tumors, with emphasis on intermediate trophoblast and the placental site trophoblastic tumor. Int J Gynecol Pathol 1984, **3**: 101–121.

197 Lathrop JC, Lauchlan S, Nayak R, Ambler M. Clinical characteristics of placental site trophoblastic tumor (PSTT). Gynecol Oncol 1988, **31**: 32–42.

198 Motoyama T, Ohta T, Ajioka Y, Watanabe H. Neoplastic and non-neoplastic intermediate trophoblasts. An immunohistochemical and ultrastructural study. Pathol Int 1994, **44**: 57–65.

199 Müller-Hocker J, Obernitz N, Johannes A, Löhrs U. p53 gene product and EFG-receptor are highly expressed in placental site trophoblastic tumor. Hum Pathol 1997, **28**: 1302–1306.

200 Orrell JM, Sanders DS. A particularly aggressive placental site trophoblastic tumour. Histopathology 1991, **18**: 559–561.

201 Rhoton-Vlasak A, Wagner JM, Rutgers JL, Baergen RN, Young RH, Roche PC, Plummer TB, Gleich GJ. Placental site trophoblastic tumor: human placental lactogen and pregnancy-associated major basic protein ad immunohistologic markers. Hum Pathol 1998, **29**: 280–288.

202 Scully RE, Young RH. Trophoblastic pseudotumor. A reappraisal. Am J Surg Pathol 1981, **5**: 75–76.

203 Shih IM, Kurman RJ. Ki-67 labeling index in the differential diagnosis of exaggerated placental site, placental site trophoblastic tumor, and choriocarcinoma: a double immunohistochemical staining technique using Ki-67 and MEL-CAM antibodies. Hum Pathol 1998, **29**: 27–33.

204 Shih IM, Kurman RJ. p63 expression is useful in the distinction of epithelioid trophoblastic and placental site trophoblastic tumors by profiling trophoblastic subpopulations. Am J Surg Pathol 2004, **28**: 1177–1183.

205 Silva EG, Tornos C, Lage J, Ordonez NG, Morris M, Kavanagh J. Multiple nodules of intermediate trophoblast following hydatidiform moles. Int J Gynecol Pathol 1993, **12**: 324–332.

206 Singer G, Kurman RJ, McMaster MT, Shih IeM. HLA-G immunoreactivity is specific for intermediate trophoblast in gestational trophoblastic disease and can serve as a useful marker in differential diagnosis. Am J Surg Pathol 2002, **26**: 914–920.

207 Xue WC, Guan XY, Ngam HY, Shen DH, Khoo US, Cheung AN. Malignant placental site trophoblastic tumor: a cytogenetic study using comparative genomic hybridisation and

chromosome in situ hybridisation. Cancer 2002, **94**: 2288–2294.

208 Yeh IT, O'Connor DM, Kurman RJ. Intermediate trophoblast. Further immunocytochemical characterization. Mod Pathol 1990, **3**: 282–287.

209 Young RH, Scully RE. Placental-site trophoblastic tumor. Current status. Clin Obstet Gynecol 1984, **27**: 248–258.

210 Young RH, Scully RE, McCluskey RT. A distinctive glomerular lesion complicating placental site trophoblastic tumor. Report of two cases. Hum Pathol 1985, **16**: 35–42.

Epithelioid trophoblastic tumor

211 Coulson LE, Kong CS, Zaloudek C. Epithelioid trophoblastic tumor of the uterus in postmenpausal women: a case report and review of the literature. Am J Surg Pathol 2000, **24**: 1558–1562.

212 Fadare O, Parkash V, Carcangiu ML, Hui P. Epithelioid trophoblastic tumor: clinicopathological features with an emphasis on uterine cervical involvement. Mod Pathol 2006, **19**: 75–82.

213 Hamazaki S, Nakamoto S, Okino T, Tsukayama C, Mori M, Taguchi K, Okada S. Epithelioid trophoblastic tumor: morphological and immunohistochemical study of three lung lesions. Hum Pathol 1999, **30**: 1321–1327.

214 Kuo KT, Chen MJ, Lin MC. Epithelioid trophoblastic tumor of the broad ligament: a case report and review of the literature. Am J Surg Pathol 2004, **28**: 405–409.

215 Lewin SN, Aghajanian C, Moreira AL, Soslow RA. Extrauterine epithelioid trophoblastic tumors presenting as primary lung carcinomas: morphologic and immunohistochemical features to resolve a diagnostic dilemma. Am J Surg Pathol 2009, **33**: 1809–1814.

216 Mao TL, Seidman JD, Kurman RJ, Shih IeM. Cyclin E and p16 immunoreactivity in epithelioid trophoblastic tumor – an aid in differential diagnosis. Am J Surg Pathol 2006, **30**: 1105–1110.

217 Mazur MT. Metastatic gestational choriocarcinoma. Unusual pathologic variant following therapy. Cancer 1989, **63**: 1370–1377.

218 Oldt RJ III, Kurman RJ, Shih IM. Molecular genetic analysis of placental site trophoblastic tumors and epithelioid trophoblastic tumors confirms their trophoblastic origin. Am J Pathol 2002, **161**: 1033–1037.

219 Shih IM, Kurman RJ. Epithelioid trophoblastic tumor: a neoplasm distinct from choriocarcinoma and placental site trophoblastic tumor simulating carcinoma. Am J Surg Pathol 1998, **22**: 1393–1403.

Tumorlike conditions of intermediate trophoblast

220 Campello TR, Fittipaldi H, O'Valle F, Carvia RE, Nogales FF. Extrauterine (tubal) placental site nodule. Histopathology 1998, **32**: 562–565.

221 El Hag IA, Ramesh K, Kollur SM, Salem M. Extrauterine placental site trophoblastic tumour in association with a lithopedion. Histopathology 2002, **41**: 446–449.

222 Huettner PC, Gersell DJ. Placental site nodules. A clinicopathologic study of 38 cases. Int J Gynecol Pathol 1994, **13**: 191–198.

223 Lee KC, Chan JK. Placental site nodule. Histopathology 1988, **16**: 193–195.

224 Shih IM, Kurman RJ. The pathology of intermediate trophoblastic tumors and tumor-like lesions. Int J Gynecol Pathol 2001, **20**: 31–47.

225 Shih IM, Seidman JD, Kurman RJ. Placental site nodule and characterization of distinctive type of intermediate trophoblast. Hum Pathol 1999, **30**: 687–694.

226 Shitabata PK, Rutgers JL. The placental site nodule. An immunohistochemical study. Hum Pathol 1994, **25**: 1295–1301.

227 Tsang WY, Chum NP, Tang SK, Tse CC, Chan JK. Mallory's bodies in placental site nodule. Arch Pathol Lab Med 1993, **117**: 547–550.

228 Young RH, Kurman RJ, Scully RE. Placental site nodules and plaques. A clinicopathologic analysis of 20 cases. Am J Surg Pathol 1990, 14: 1001–1009.

NON-NEOPLASTIC LESIONS OF TERM PLACENTA

229 Abramowsky CR, Vegas ME, Swinehart G, Gyves MT. Decidual vasculopathy of the placenta in lupus erythematosus. N Engl J Med 1980, **303**: 668–672.

230 Adeniran AJ, Stanek J. Amnion nodosum revisited: clinicopathologic and placental correlations. Arch Pathol Lab Med 2007, **131**: 1829–1833.

231 Altshuler G. Role of the placenta in perinatal pathology (revisited). Pediatr Pathol Lab Med 1996, **16**: 207–233.

232 Altshuler G, Hyde S. Fusobacteria. An important cause of chorioamnionitis. Arch Pathol Lab Med 1985, **109**: 739–743.

233 Altshuler G, Russell P. The human placental villitides. A review of chronic intrauterine infection. Curr Top Pathol 1975, **60**: 63–112.

234 Altshuler G. A conceptual approach to placental pathology and pregnancy outcome. Semin Diagn Pathol 1993, **10**: 204–221.

235 Andrew A, Bulmer JN, Morrison L, Wells M, Buckley CH. Subinvolution of the uteroplacental arteries. An immunohistochemical study. Int J Gynecol Pathol 1993, **12**: 28–33.

236 Baergen RN. Cord abnormalities, structural lesions, and cord 'accidents'. Semin Diagn Pathol 2007, **24**: 23–32.

237 Benirschke K, Kaufmann P. Pathology of the human placenta. New York, 2000, Springer.

238 Benson RC, Fujikura T. Circumvallate and circummarginate placenta. Unimportant clinical entities. Obstet Gynecol 1969, **34**: 799–804.

239 Bjoro K Jr, Myhre E. The role of chronic nonspecific inflammatory lesions of the placenta in intrauterine growth retardation. Acta Pathol Microbiol Immunol Scand (A) 1984, **92**: 133–137.

240 Blanc WA. Pathways of fetal and early neonatal infection. Viral placentitis, bacterial and fungal chorioamnionitis. J Pediatr Surg 1961, **59**: 473–496.

241 Boyd TK, Redline RW. Chronic histiocytic intervillositis: a placental lesion associated with recurrent reproductive loss. Hum Pathol 2000, **31**: 1389–1396.

242 Bryan EM, Kohler HG. The missing umbilical artery. I. Prospective study based on a maternity unit. Arch Dis Child 1974, **49**: 844–852.

243 deRoux SJ, Prendergast NC, Adsay NV. Spontaneous uterine rupture with fatal hemoperitoneum due to placenta accreta percreta: a case report and review of the literature. Int J Gynecol Pathol 1999, **18**: 82–86.

244 Drachenberg CB, Papadimitriou JC. Placental iron deposits: significance in normal and abnormal pregnancies. Hum Pathol 1994, **25**: 379–385.

245 Driscoll SG. Placental examination in a clinical setting. Arch Pathol Lab Med 1991, **115**: 668–671.

246 Fox H. Thrombosis of foetal arteries in the human placenta. J Obstet Gynaecol Br Commonw 1966, **73**: 961–965.

247 Fox H. The significance of placental infarction in perinatal morbidity and mortality. Biol Neonate 1967, **11**: 87–105.

248 Fox H. Fibrinoid necrosis of placental villi. J Obstet Gynaecol Br Commonw 1968, **75**: 448–452.

249 Fox H. Fibrosis of placental villi. J Pathol Bacteriol 1968, **95**: 573–579.

250 Fox H. Pathology of the placenta in maternal diabetes mellitus. Obstet Gynecol 1969, **34**: 792–798.

251 Fox H. Placenta accreta, 1945–1969. Obstet Gynecol Surv 1972, **27**: 475–490.

252 Fox H. Pathology of the placenta, ed. 2. London, 1997, W.B. Saunders.

253 Fox H, Langley FA. Leukocytic infiltration of the placenta and umbilical cord. A clinicopathologic study. Obstet Gynecol 1971, **37**: 451–458.

254 Fujikura T, Froehlich LA. Diagnosis of sickling by placental examination. Geographic differences in incidence. Am J Obstet Gynecol 1968, **100**: 1122–1124.

255 Genest DR, Choi-Hong SR, Tate JE, Qureshi F, Jacques SM, Crum C. Diagnosis of congenital syphilis from placental examination: comparison of histopathology, Steiner stain, and polymerase chain reaction for *Treponema pallidum* DNA. Hum Pathol 1996, **27**: 366–372.

256 Genest DR, Granter S, Pinkus GS. Umbilical cord 'pseudo-vasculitis' following second trimester fetal death: a clinicopathologic and immunohistochemical study of 13 cases. Histopathology 1997, **30**: 563–569.

257 Gersell DJ. Chronic villitis, chronic chorioamnionitis, and maternal floor infarction. Semin Diagn Pathol 1993, **10**: 251–266.

258 Gersell DJ, Phillips NJ, Beckerman K. Chronic chorioamnionitis. A clinicopathologic study of 17 cases. Int J Gynecol Pathol 1991, **10**: 217–229.

259 Heifetz SA. Single umbilical artery. A statistical analysis of 237 autopsy cases and review of the literature. Perspect Pediatr Pathol 1984, **8**: 345–378.

260 Heifetz SA, Bauman M. Necrotizing funisitis and herpes simplex infection of placental and decidual tissues. Study of four cases. Hum Pathol 1994, **25**: 715–722.

261 Hyde SR, Benirschke K. Gestational psittacosis: case report and literature review. Mod Pathol 1997, **10**: 602–607.

262 Ismail MR, Ordi J, Menendez C, Ventura PJ, Aponte JJ, Kahigwa E, Hirt R, Cardesa A, Alonso PL. Placental pathology in malaria: a histological, immunohistochemical and quantitative study. Hum Pathol 2000, **31**: 85–93.

263 Jacques SM, Qureshi F. Chronic intervillositis of the placenta. Arch Pathol Lab Med 1993, **117**: 1032–1035.

264 Jauniaux E, De Munter C, Vanesse M, Wilkin P, Hustin J. Embryonic remnants of the umbilical cord: morphologic and clinical aspects. Hum Pathol 1989, **20**: 458–462.

265 Joshi VV. Handbook of placental pathology. New York, 1984, Igaku-Shoin.

266 Kaplan C. The placenta and viral infections. Semin Diagn Pathol 1993, **10**: 232–250.

267 Kaplan C, Benirschke K, Tarzy B. Placental tuberculosis in early and late pregnancy. Am J Obstet Gynecol 1980, **137**: 858–860.

268 Kaplan CG. Color atlas of gross placental pathology. New York, 1994, Igaku-Shoin.

269 Kaplan C. Placental pathology for the nineties. Pathol Annu 1993, **28**(Pt 1): 15–72.

270 Kaplan CG. Fetal and maternal vascular lesions. Semin Diagn Pathol 2007, **24**: 14–22.

271 Kida M, Abramowsky CR, Santoscoy C. Cryptococcosis of the placenta in a woman with acquired immunodeficiency syndrome. Hum Pathol 1989, **20**: 920–921.

272 Kim CJ, Yoon BH, Kim M, Park JO, Cho SY, Chi JG. Histo-topographic distribution of acute inflammation of the human umbilical cord. Pathol Int 2001, **51**: 861–865.

273 Kim CY, Yoon BH, Park SS, Kim MH, Chi JG. Acute funisitis of preterm but not term placentas is associated with severe fetal inflammatory response. Hum Pathol 2001, **32**: 623–629.

274 Kim KR, Jun SY, Kim JY, Ro JY. Implantation site intermediate trophoblasts in placenta cretas. Mod Pathol 2004, **17**: 1483–1490.

275 Kingdom J, Jauniaux E, O'Brien PM, Royal College of Obstetricians and Gynaecologists Study Group. The placenta: basic science and clinical practice. London, 2000, RCOG Press.

276 Langston C, Kaplan C, Macpherson T, Manci E, Peevy K, Clark B, Murtagh C, Cox S, Glen G. Practice guideline for examination of the placenta: developed by the Placental Pathology Practice Guideline Development Task Force of the College of American Pathologists. Arch Pathol Lab Med 1997, **121**: 449–476.

277 Lauweryns J, Bernat R, Lerut A, Detournay G. Intrauterine pneumonia. An experimental study. Biol Neonate 1978, **22**: 301–318.

278 Lewis SH, Perrin EV. Pathology of the placenta. New York, 1999, Churchill Livingstone.

279 Macpherson T. Fact and fancy. What can we really tell from the placenta? Arch Pathol Lab Med 1991, **115**: 672–681.

280 McCaffree MA, Altshuler G, Benirschke K. Placental coccidioidomycosis without fetal disease. Arch Pathol Lab Med 1978, **102**: 512–514.

281 Morken NH, Henriksen H. Placenta percreta – two cases and review of the literature. Eur J Obstet Gynecol Reprod Biol 2001, **100**: 112–115.

282 Morris ED. Placental insufficiency. Br Med Bull 1968, **24**: 76–79.

283 Mostoufi-zadeh M, Driscoll SG, Biano SA, Kundsin RB. Placental evidence of cytomegalovirus infection of the fetus and neonate. Arch Pathol Lab Med 1984, **108**: 403–406.

284 Mueller-Heubach E, Rubinstein DN, Schwarz SS. Histologic chorioamnionitis and preterm delivery in different patient populations. Obstet Gynecol 1990, **75**: 622–626.

285 Muhlemann K, Miller RK, Metlay L, Menegus MA. Cytomegalovirus infection of the human placenta: an immunocytochemical study. Hum Pathol 1992, **23**: 1234–1237.

286 Naeye RL. Functionally important disorders of the placenta, umbilical cord, and fetal membranes. Hum Pathol 1987, **18**: 680–691.

287 Nakamura Y, Sakuma S, Ohta Y, Kawano K, Hashimoto T. Detection of the human cytomegalovirus gene in placental chronic villitis by polymerase chain reaction. Hum Pathol 1994, **25**: 815–818.

288 Nuovo G. The utility of immunohistochemistry and in situ hybridization in placental pathology. Arch Pathol Lab Med 2006, **130**: 979–983.

289 Qureshi F, Jacques SM, Reyes MP. Placental histopathology in syphilis. Hum Pathol 1993, **24**: 779–784.

290 Redline RW, Abramowsky CR. Clinical and pathologic aspects of recurrent placental villitis. Hum Pathol 1985, **16**: 727–731.

291 Redline RW. Infections and other inflammatory conditions. Semin Diagn Pathol 2007, **24**: 5–13.

292 Robb JA, Benirschke K, Mannino F, Voland J. Intrauterine latent herpes simplex virus infection. II. Latent neonatal infection. Hum Pathol 1986, **17**: 1210–1217.

293 Roberts DJ. Placental pathology, a survival guide. Arch Pathol Lab Med 2008, **132**: 641–651.

294 Russell P. Inflammatory lesions of the human placenta. I. Clinical significance of acute chorioamnionitis. Am J Diagn Gynecol Obstet 1979, **1**: 127–137.

295 Russell P. Inflammatory lesions of the human placenta. II. Villitis of unknown etiology in perspective. Am J Diagn Gynecol Obstet 1979, **1**: 339–346.

296 Russell P, Atkinson K, Krishnan L. Recurrent reproductive failure due to severe placental villitis of unknown etiology. J Reprod Med 1980, **24**: 93–98.

297 Saetta A, Agapitos E, Davaris PS. Determination of CMV placentitis. Diagnostic application of the polymerase chain reaction. Virchows Arch 1998, **432**: 159–162.

298 Salazar H, Kanbour AI. Amnion nodosum. Ultrastructure and histopathogenesis. Arch Pathol 1974, **98**: 39–46.

299 Sander CH, Stevens NG. Hemorrhagic endovasculitis of the placenta. An indepth morphologic appraisal with initial clinical and epidemiologic observations. Pathol Annu 1984, **19**(Pt 1): 37–79.

300 Sander CM. What's new in placental pathology. Pathol Annu 1995, **30**(Pt 1): 59–93.

301 Sander CH. The surgical pathologist examines the placenta. Pathol Annu 1985, **20**(Pt 2): 235–288.

302 Satosar A, Ramirez NC, Bartholomew D, Davis J, Nuovo GJ. Histologic correlates of viral and bacterial infection of the placenta associated with severe morbidity and mortality in the newborn. Hum Pathol 2004, **35**: 536–545.

303 Schwartz DA, Caldwell E. Herpes simplex virus infection of the placenta. The role of molecular pathology in the diagnosis of viral infection of placental-associated tissues. Arch Pathol Lab Med 1991, **115**: 1141–1144.

304 Schwartz DA, Khan R, Stoll B. Characterization of the fetal inflammatory response to cytomegalovirus placentitis. An immunohistochemical study. Arch Pathol Lab Med 1992, **116**: 21–27.

305 Schwartz DA, Larsen SA, Beck-Sague C, Fears M, Rice RJ. Pathology of the umbilical cord in congenital syphilis. Analysis of 25 specimens using histochemistry and immunofluorescent antibody to *Treponema pallidum*. Hum Pathol 1995, **26**: 784–791.

306 Stallmach T, Hebisch G. Placental pathology: its impact on explaining prenatal and perinatal death. Virchows Arch 2004, **445**: 9–16.

307 Walter P, Blot P, Ivanoff B. The placental lesions in congenital syphilis. A study of six cases. Virchows Arch [A] 1982, **397**: 313–326.

308 Wentworth P. Placental infarction and toxemia of pregnancy. Am J Obstet Gynecol 1967, **99**: 318–326.

309 Wentworth P. Circumvallate and circummarginate placentas. Their incidence and clinical significance. Am J Obstet Gynecol 1968, **102**: 44–47.

310 Weydert JA, Benda JA. Subinvolution of the placental site as an anatomic cause of postpartum uterine bleeding: a review. Arch Pathol Lab Med 2006, **130**: 1538–1542.

311 Wigglesworth JS. Vascular anatomy of the human placenta and its significance for placental pathology. J Obstet Gynaecol Br Commonw 1969, **76**: 979–989.

312 Zlatnik FJ, Gellhaus TM, Benda JA, Koontz FP, Burmeister LF. Histologic chorioamnionitis, microbial infection, and prematurity. Obstet Gynecol 1990, **76**: 355–359.

TUMORS AND TUMORLIKE CONDITIONS OF TERM PLACENTA

313 Altshuler G. Chorangiosis. An important placental sign of neonatal morbidity and mortality. Arch Pathol Lab Med 1984, **108**: 71–74.

314 Aonahata M, Masuzawa Y, Tsutsui Y. A case of intraplacental choriocarcinoma associated with placental hemangioma. Pathol Int 1999, **48**: 897–901.

315 Asadourian LA, Taylor HB. Clinical significance of placental hemangiomas. Obstet Gynecol 1968, **31**: 551–555.

316 Baergen RN, Johnson D, Moore T, Benirschke K. Maternal melanoma metastatic to the placenta: a case report and review of the literature. Arch Pathol lab Med 1997, **121**: 508–511.

317 Cash JB, Powell DE. Placental chorioangioma. Presentation of a case with electron-microscopic and immunochemical studies. Am J Surg Pathol 1980, **4**: 87–92.

318 Chen KTK, Ma CK, Kassel SH. Hepatocellular adenoma of the placenta. Am J Surg Pathol 1986, **10**: 436–440.

319 Cox JN, Chavrier F. Heterotopic adrenocortical tissue within a placenta. Placenta 1980, **1**: 131–133.

320 Delerive C, Locquet F, Mallart A, Janin A, Gosselin B. Placental metastasis from maternal bronchial oat cell carcinoma. Arch Pathol Lab Med 1989, **113**: 556–558.

321 Demian SDE, Donnelly WH, Frias JL, Monif GRG. Placental lesions in congenital giant pigmented nevi. Am J Clin Pathol 1974, **61**: 438–442.

322 Ernst LM, Hui P, Parkash V. Intraplacental smooth muscle tumor: a case report. Int J Gynecol Pathol 2001, **20**: 284–288.

323 Fox H. Vascular tumors of the placenta. Obstet Gynecol Surv 1967, **22**: 697–711.

324 Fox H. Pathology of the placenta, ed. 2. London, 1997, W.B. Saunders.

325 Katsanis WA, O'Connor DM, Gibb RK, Bendon RW. Endometrial stromal sarcoma involving the placenta. Ann Diagn Pathol 1999, **2**: 301–305.

326 Khalifa MA, Gersell DJ, Hansen CH, Lage JM. Hepatic (hepatocellular) adenoma of the placenta: a study of four cases. Int J Gynecol Pathol 1998, **17**: 241–244.

327 Kreczy A, Alge A, Menardi G, Gassner I, Gschwendtner A, Mikuz G. Teratoma of the umbilical cord. Case report with review of the literature. Arch Pathol Lab Med 1994, **118**: 934–937.

328 Kurtin PJ, Gaffey TA, Habermann TM. Peripheral T-cell lymphoma involving the placenta. Cancer 1992, **70**: 2963–2968.

329 Lifschitz-Mercer B, Fogel M, Kushnir I, Czernobilsky B. Chorangioma. A cytoskeletal profile. Int J Gynecol Pathol 1989, **8**: 349–356.

330 Lynn AA, Parry SI, Morgan MA, Mennuti MT. Disseminated congenital neuroblastoma involving the placenta. Arch Pathol Lab Med 1997, **121**: 741–744.

331 Marton T, Silhavy M, Csapó Z, Szendo B, Papp Z. Multifocal hemangioendothelioma of the fetus and placenta. Hum Pathol 1997, **28**: 866–869.

332 Meguerian-Bedoyan Z, Lamant L, Hopfner C, Pulford K, Chittal S, Delsol G. Anaplastic large cell lymphoma of maternal origin involving the placenta: case report and literature survey. Am J Surg Pathol 1997, **21**: 1236–1241.

333 Ogino S, Redline RW. Villous capillary lesions of the placenta: distinctions between chorangioma, chorangiomatosis, and chorangiosis. Hum Pathol 2000, **31**: 945–954.

334 Perkins DG, Kopp CM, Haust MD. Placental infiltration in congenital neuroblastoma. A case study with ultrastructure. Histopathology 1980, **4**: 383–389.

335 Potter JF, Schoeneman M. Metastasis of maternal cancer to the placenta and fetus. Cancer 1970, **25**: 380–388.

336 Read EJ Jr, Platzer PB. Placental metastasis from maternal carcinoma of the lung. Obstet Gynecol 1981, **58**: 387–391.

337 Schmitt FC, Zelandi Filho C, Bacchi MM, Castilho ED, Bacchi CE. Adenoid cystic carcinoma of trachea metastatic to the placenta. Hum Pathol 1989, **20**: 193–195.

338 Seifer DB, Ferguson JE II, Behrens CM, Zemel S, Stevenson DK, Ross JC. Nonimmune hydrops fetalis in association with hemangioma of the umbilical cord. Obstet Gynecol 1985, **66**: 283–286.

339 Sheikh SS, Khalifa MA, Marley EF, Bagg A, Lage JM. Acute monocytic leukaemia (FAB M5) involving the placenta associated with delivery of a healthy infant: case report and discussion. Int J Gynecol Pathol 1997, **15**: 363–366.

340 Smith D, Majmudar B. Teratoma of the umbilical cord. Him Pathol 1985, **16**: 190–193.

341 Sotelo-Avila C, Graham M, Hanby DE, Rudolph AJ. Nevus cell aggregates in the placenta. A histochemical and electron microscopic study. Am J Clin Pathol 1988, **89**: 395–400.

342 Unger JL. Placental teratoma. Am J Clin Pathol 1989, **92**: 371–373.

343 Vesoulis Z, Agamanolis D. Benign hepatocellular tumor of the placenta. Am J Surg Pathol 1998, **22**: 355–359.

344 Yavner DL, Redline RW. Angiomyxoma of the umbilical cord with massive cystic degeneration of Wharton's jelly. Arch Pathol Lab Med 1989, **113**: 935–937.

Breast 20

CHAPTER CONTENTS

Normal anatomy

The breast or mammary gland is covered by skin and subcutaneous tissue and rests on the pectoralis muscle, from which it is separated by a fascia. The morphofunctional unit of the organ is the single gland, a complex branching structure that is topographically arranged into *lobes*[40] and which is made up of two major components: the *terminal duct–lobular unit* (*TDLU*) and the *large duct system*.[11] The TDLU is formed by the *lobule* and *terminal ductule* and represents the secretory portion of the gland. It connects with the *subsegmental duct*, which in turn leads to a *segmental duct*, and this to a *collecting* (*lactiferous* or *galactophorous*) *duct*, which empties into the nipple. A fusiform dilation located beneath the nipple between the collecting and the segmental duct is known as the *lactiferous sinus* (Fig. 20.1).

The TDLU is recognized because of its distinctly lobular architecture; the presence of a mantle of specialized, myxoid-appearing hormone-responsive connective tissue; and the absence of elastic fibers. The development of the breast is dependent on the close interaction of these specialized epithelial and mesenchymal tissues.[13] The large ducts have a lesser amount of specialized stroma and are enveloped by a continuous and well-developed layer of elastic tissue.

The entire ductal–lobular epithelial system of the breast is covered by a specialized two-cell-type epithelial lining: the *inner epithelium* with secretory and absorptive functions (often simply called epithelium), and the outer *myoepithelial cells*. These two cell types have distinctive ultrastructural and immunohistochemical features that differ considerably from each other. The most reliable markers for the epithelial cells are the various keratins, epithelial membrane antigens (EMA) – but see later discussion – the related milk fat globule membrane antigen, α-lactalbumin,[10,18] mammaglobin, and GCDFP-15 (Fig. 20.2A). Myoepithelial cells react with other types of keratin (see later discussions), S-100 protein, P-cadherin, smooth muscle actin, calponin, smooth muscle myosin heavy chain, maspin, and caldesmon (the latter only in the ductal portion).[14,17,31,41] They also show nuclear reactivity for p63, a member of the *TP53* gene family[3] (Fig. 20.2B) (not to be equated with the cytoplasmic positivity for this marker that has been found in epithelial cells with secretory changes[7]), and p75NTR (p75 neurotrophin receptor),[29] as well as cell membrane reactivity for CD109.[19] EMA reacts strongly with the apical region of active secretory cells but may be faint or negative in other epithelial cells. Pankeratin antibodies react with both epithelial and myoepithelial cells. The acidic cytokeratins 8, 18, and 19 react with the epithelial cells throughout the system but not with the myoepithelial cells, whereas the reverse is true for cytokeratin 14.[31] Other immunohistochemical features of mammary epithelial cells are discussed in the section on Invasive ductal carcinoma, NOS (see p. 1696).

It has been proposed that the two basic cell lineages of the breast – epithelial and myoepithelial – derive from a common cell that displays the phenotypic features of a committed stem cell. This cell expresses CK5 in the absence of CK8, 18, and 19 and smooth muscle actin.[6]

A sparse population of endocrine cells has been shown in the normal breast with the use of chromogranin stain.[8,34]

The entire glandular epithelial system rests on a continuous basement membrane. This can be demonstrated with reticulin stains, ultrastructurally,[28] or with immunohistochemical reactions for laminin or type IV collagen.[9] Type IV collagenase (an enzyme involved in basement membrane turnover) is strongly expressed in myoepithelial cells and to a lesser degree in epithelial cells of terminal ducts.[27]

The nipple has a very characteristic microscopic appearance. In addition to the large collecting ducts opening into the surface through five to nine orifices arranged as a central and a peripheral group,[25] it contains numerous sebaceous glands that open independently of hair follicles and a dense fibrous stroma in which erectile smooth muscle tissue is embedded. *Montgomery tubercles* are areolar protuberances, usually between 10 and 20 in number, which become prominent during pregnancy; microscopically, they are formed by a collecting (lactiferous) duct associated with a sebaceous apparatus.[37] The epidermis of the nipple and areola resembles that of the skin elsewhere, except for an increase in melanin content in the basal layer and the occasional presence of basally located clear cells known as *Toker cells*, which are related histogenetically to Paget disease[26,39] (see p. 1706). The irregular corrugated appearance of the lactiferous sinus as seen in a tangential cut should not be confused with a pathologic condition. In

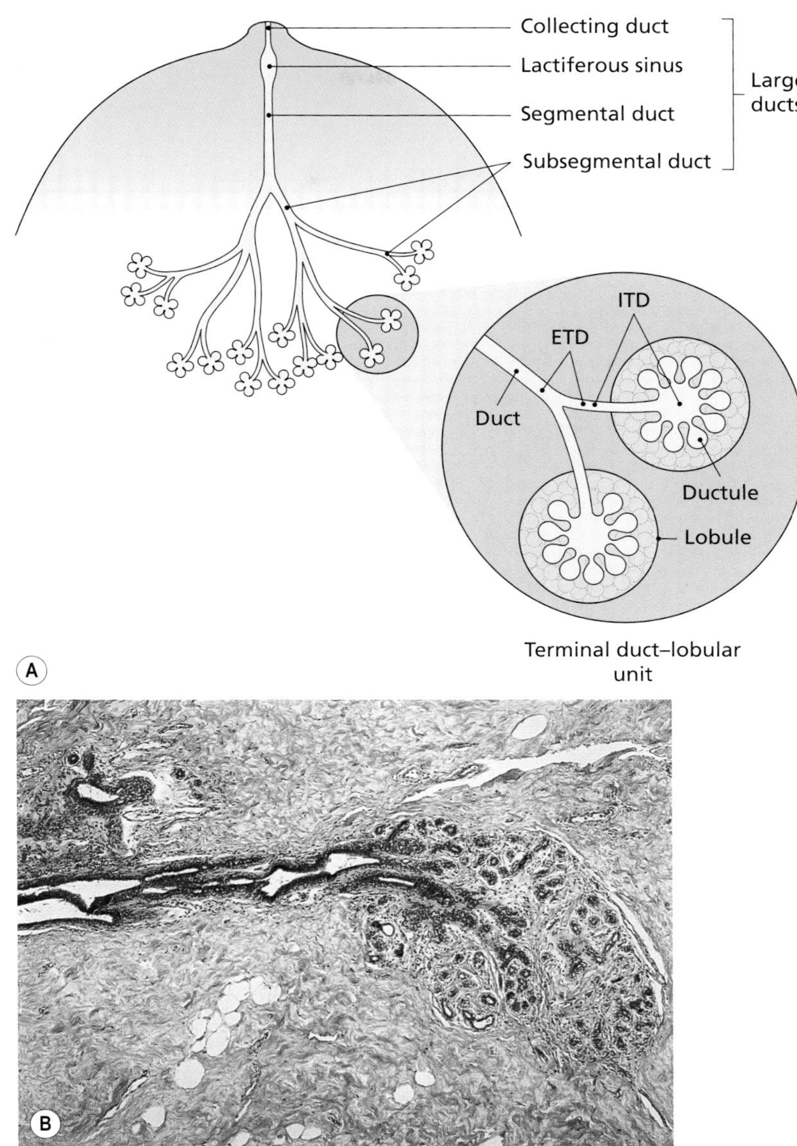

Fig. 20.1 A and **B**, Terminal duct–lobular unit (TDLU). **A**, Diagrammatic representation of this structure. ETD, extralobular terminal duct; ITD, intralobular terminal duct. **B**, Photomicrograph of this unit as seen in a normal adult female.

approximately 17% of individuals, normal breast lobules are present in the nipple region.[32]

Breast tissue responds markedly to hormonal and other influences throughout life, and, as a result, it may display a wide range of 'normal' appearances:[1] the immature and largely resting breast before puberty; the developed breast of reproductive life, which exhibits changes depending on the time of the menstrual cycle;[24,30,42] the actively secreting breast of lactation (Fig. 20.3); and the involuted postmenopausal breast.[12] In the resting breast, cellular proliferation is largely confined to epithelial cells;[21] during pregnancy and lactation, all cell types show a high level of proliferative activity.[5,20,23] Nodularity and spillage of milk into the stroma can occur; exaggerated expressions of these phenomena have been designated *lactating adenoma* and *milk granuloma*, respectively (see p. 1669).[33,36]

Painful engorgement of the breasts occurs not infrequently during the first cycles of contraceptive therapy. This is usually a mild and transient symptom. Microscopically, the only definite mammary change that can be ascribed to the medication is the development of true acini resembling lactating breast.[16]

The process of normal senile involution is more apparent in the TDLU and involves both epithelium and specialized stroma; it may acquire a microcystic quality (*cystic lobular involution*), not to be confused with fibrocystic disease (Fig. 20.4). Deposits of elastic tissue in the stroma (*elastosis*) are found in nearly half of all women over 50 years of age. They may be located diffusely in the stroma, around vessels, and around ducts.[15]

There are two morphologic curiosities of the breast worth knowing about, not because of their clinical significance but because they can simulate other conditions of greater consequence. One is the *pregnancy-like change* seen in one or several lobules in the absence of pregnancy or hormonal manipulation.[22,38] The cells have an abundant vacuolated cytoplasm, the nuclei are large and sometimes apically located (giving the lesion an appearance that resembles the Arias-Stella reaction), and the lumina are dilated (Fig. 20.5A). The pregnancy-like change is thought to be histologically related to so-called *cystic hypersecretory hyperplasia* (see p. 1678) and it has occasionally been found associated (probably coincidentally) with in situ or invasive carcinoma.[35]

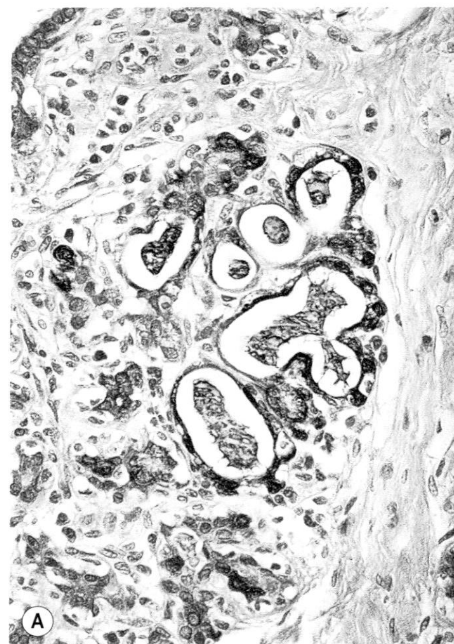
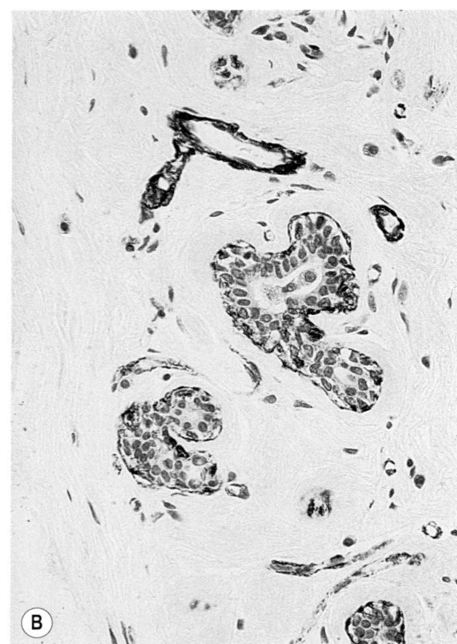

Fig. 20.2 **A** and **B**, Immunocytochemical markers of mammary lobule. **A**, Lactalbumin, showing positivity in secretory epithelium and intraglandular lumina. **B**, Actin, showing positivity in the outer myoepithelial cell component. Smooth muscle cells present in adjacent vessel walls serve as built-in controls.

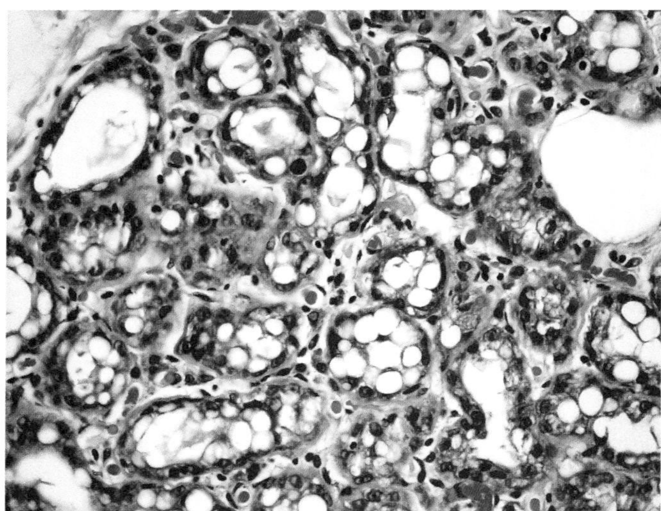

Fig. 20.3 Lactational changes in mammary lobule. There is marked cytoplasmic vacuolization.

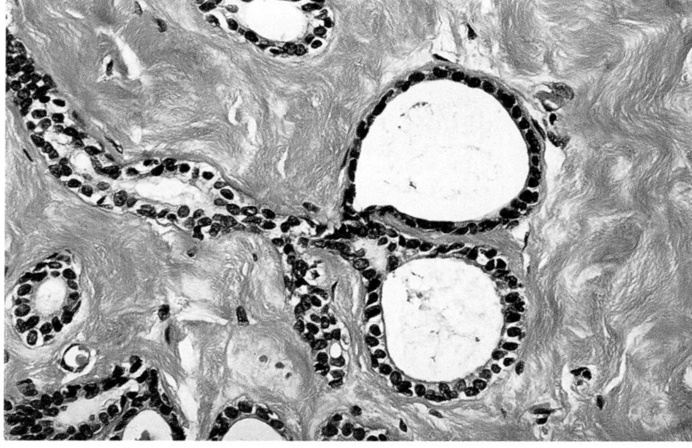

Fig. 20.4 Cystic involution of lobule. This is an age-related change of no clinical significance.

The other process is a *clear cell change* of the ductal or lobular epithelium, in which the cytoplasm acquires a finely granular, finely vacuolated, or totally clear appearance[4,38] (Fig. 20.5B). The mechanism of these two changes, which can occur together, is unknown.

The main importance of the division of the mammary gland unit into two major portions resides in its relation to diseases of this organ. As Wellings et al.[43] convincingly showed and Azzopardi[2] strongly emphasized, the site of origin of fibrocystic disease (including that accompanied by the formation of large cysts), so-called 'ductal hyperplasia' (epitheliosis or papillomatosis), and most carcinomas (including those of so-called 'ductal type') is the TDLU and not the large duct system. The latter is instead the primary site of most single solitary papillomas, duct ectasia, and a few rare types of ductal carcinoma.

Ectopia

The mammary gland is not a sharply demarcated organ; as a result, isolated mammary lobules can sometimes be seen outside the standard anatomic confines of the breast parenchyma, such as in the nipple or in the axilla.[45,48] The latter may explain the occurrence of some seemingly primary breast carcinomas in the axilla.

Ectopic breast tissue has also been reported within axillary lymph nodes and the heart (although with extreme rarity)[44,49,50] and along

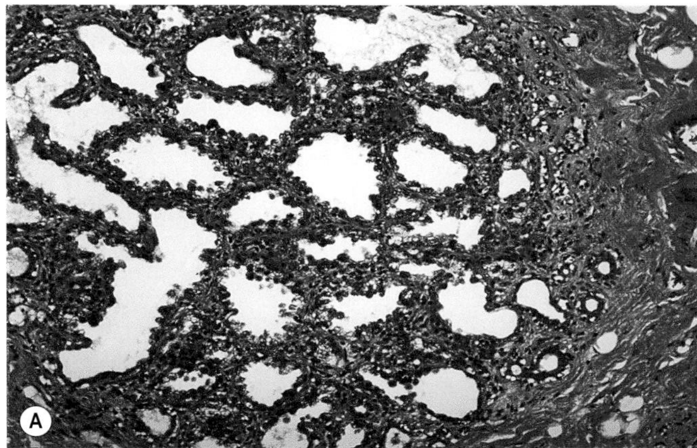

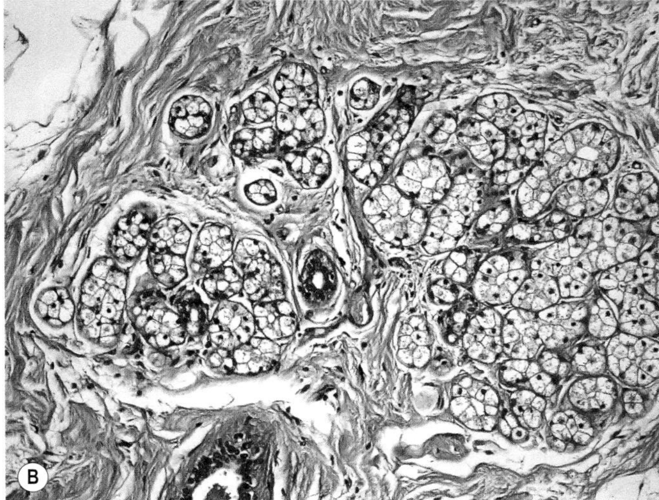

Fig. 20.5 A, Pregnancy-like changes in mammary lobule. **B**, Clear cell changes. These two clinically inconsequential alterations may coexist.

the 'milk line' that runs from the axilla to the inguinal region, the most common sites being the chest wall and the vulva.[46]

Ectopic breast parenchyma is subject to changes similar to those of the orthotopic organ, including lactational changes, benign tumors, and carcinomas.[46] It has been proposed that papillary hidradenoma of the vulva is not a sweat gland neoplasm, as traditionally believed, but an intraductal papilloma arising from ectopic breast parenchyma (see Chapter 19, Vulva). There is certainly a considerable overlap between ectopic breast tissue and breast-like metaplasias of sweat glands, a fact that renders a precise histogenetic identification of some of these lesions almost impossible.[47]

Inflammatory and related lesions

Mammary duct ectasia

Mammary duct ectasia has also been referred to as varicocele tumor, comedomastitis, periductal mastitis, stale milk mastitis, chemical mastitis, granulomatous mastitis, and mastitis obliterans[53] (Fig. 20.6). Most of the cases are seen in premenopausal parous women and probably represent a localized response to different components of stagnant colostrum. As beautifully described and illustrated in the classic article by Haagensen,[51] the disease may produce retraction or inversion of the nipple and thus clinically simulate invasive carcinoma. Nipple discharge is present in 20% of cases. Microscopically, there is dilation of large ducts, with accumulation of fatty detritus in the lumen and fibrous thickening of the wall, which contains an increased amount of elastic fibers.

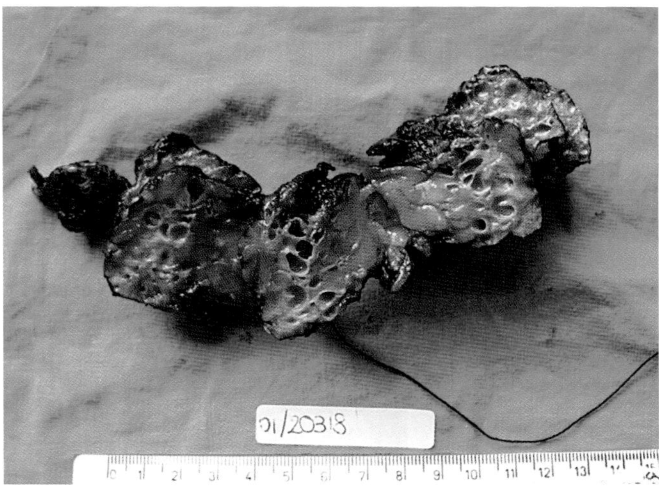

Fig. 20.6 Gross appearance of mammary duct ectasia. Some of the dilated ducts contain a thick dark material.

Calcification is common, producing tubular, annular, and linear shadows on the mammogram. There is usually no accompanying epithelial hyperplasia or apocrine metaplasia. If the luminal material escapes from the duct, a florid inflammatory reaction rich in macrophages and plasma cells may ensue (see p. 1674). It is likely that at least some of the cases categorized in the older literature as *plasma cell mastitis* belong to this category. In advanced stages, fibrous obliteration of the ducts can occur.

Mammary duct ectasia is probably unrelated to fibrocystic disease, although the two may coexist. For the record, the condition is not too uncommon in female dogs, whether sexually intact or spayed.[52]

Fat necrosis

A process with the microscopic features of fat necrosis (i.e., foamy macrophages infiltrating partially necrotic adipose tissue) can be seen in the breast under two disparate circumstances; the distinction between the two has not been made clear in many of the articles on the subject. One is as a secondary and relatively minor event in mammary duct ectasia and – to a lesser extent – fibrocystic disease with large cyst formation. In these cases, the rupture of the dilated or cystic structures leads to extravasation of the luminal content, some degree of tissue necrosis, and a secondary inflammatory reaction in which foamy macrophages can be numerous. In particularly florid cases of this phenomenon the term *xanthogranulomatous mastitis* has been used.[58] Parenthetically, small collections of foamy cells are seen not infrequently within duct lumina or in cohesive masses along duct walls in cases of fibrocystic disease; their immunohistochemical profile is that of histiocytes rather than epithelial cells.[56]

The other circumstance, which perhaps is the only one that deserves to be called fat necrosis, is of the traumatic (either accidental or surgical) type and usually involves the superficial subcutaneous tissue rather than the breast parenchyma itself (Fig. 20.7). A

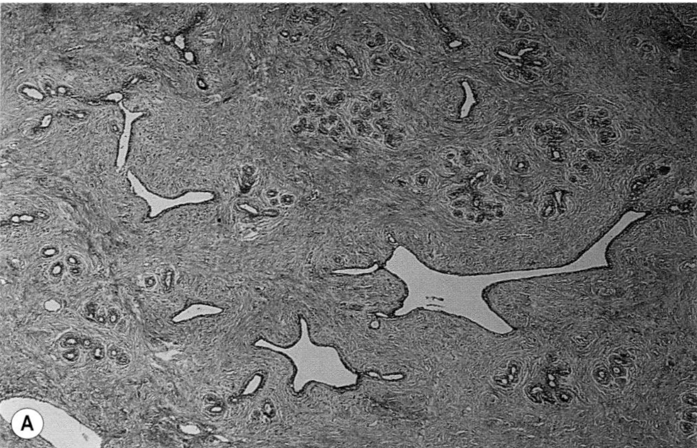
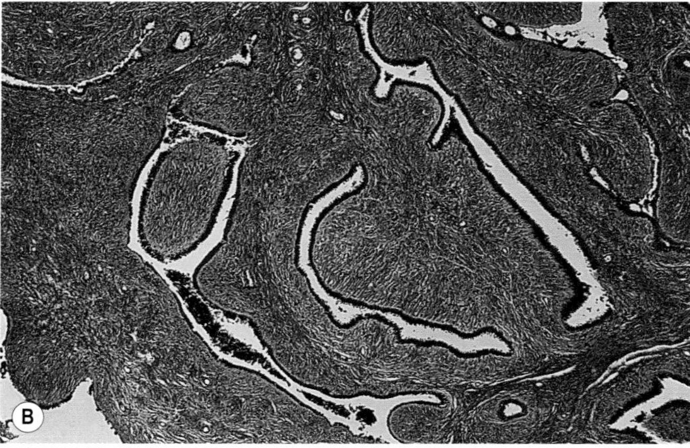

Fig. 20.12 **A** and **B,** Microscopic appearance of fibroadenoma. The tumor shown in **B** has a slightly hypercellular stroma but not to a degree that would justify a diagnosis of phylloides tumor.

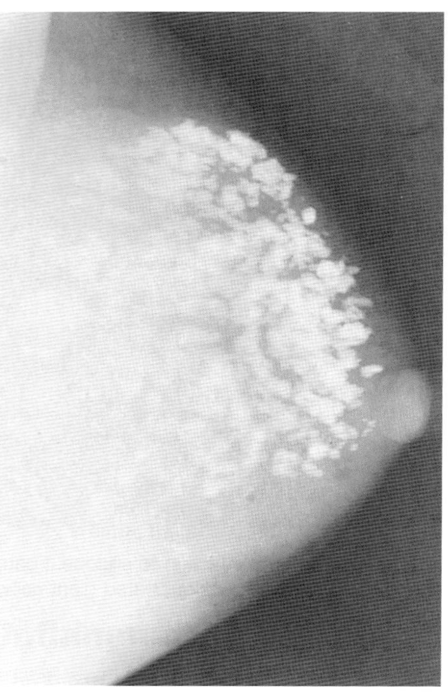

Fig. 20.13 Heavy, coarse calcification in a large breast fibroadenoma as seen in a mammogram.

presumed TDLU origin of the lesion. The cellularity of the stroma varies from case to case, but in any unduly hypercellular lesion the alternative diagnosis of phylloides tumor should be considered (see p. 1723).

Morphologic variations in fibroadenoma are plentiful, some of more significance than others:

1 Hyalinization, calcification, and/or ossification of the stroma. These changes are more commonly seen in older patients and can be appreciated radiographically (Fig. 20.13).
2 Presence in the stroma of multinucleated giant cells of reactive nature, similar to those seen in polypoid lesions of nasal cavity and other sites.[113,124]
3 Presence in the stroma of mature adipose tissue, smooth muscle, or metaplastic cartilage.[123,130,137] Some of the lesions described as hamartoma or choristoma of the breast probably belong to this category[111,127,133] (see p. 1729).
4 Prominent myxoid changes. Most of these fibroadenomas are not otherwise different from the others. However, whenever multiple highly myxoid fibroadenomas are found, the possibility that they are a component of the syndrome that also includes endocrine hyperactivity, cardiac myxoma, cutaneous hyperpigmentation, and other abnormalities (Carney complex) should be investigated. Parenthetically, other breast abnormalities that can be seen in this syndrome are lobular and nodular myxoid changes,[114] and ductal adenoma with tubular features (see p. 1668).
5 Peculiar fibrocellular stroma. Azzopardi[112] has pointed out the existence of a *fibroadenoma variant* in which the stroma is simultaneously highly collagenous and cellular, has a somewhat laminated appearance, and is sometimes accompanied by a mononuclear infiltrate.
6 Hemorrhagic infarct. Fibroadenomas with this complication show grossly a bulging red appearance that can be quite perplexing. This complication is more likely to occur during pregnancy.
7 Ill-defined margins blending with a surrounding breast that shows the features of fibrocystic disease. This form, which has been designated *fibroadenomatosis* or *fibroadenomatoid hyperplasia*, shares the features of fibroadenoma and fibrocystic disease and suggests a pathogenetic link between the two.
8 Apocrine metaplasia. This change is found in approximately 15% of fibroadenomas.[112] In retrospect, it would seem that the change originally described as endocrine neoplasia in fibroadenoma[119] represents a morphologic variation on the theme of apocrine metaplasia; in the cases we have studied, the endocrine-like cells stained strongly for GCDFP-15 but were negative for chromogranin (Fig. 20.14).
9 Sclerosing adenosis. This occurs in less than 10% of cases.[112] Fibroadenomas with cysts, sclerosing adenosis, calcifications, or papillary apocrine changes are sometimes referred to as 'complex'.[126]
10 Squamous metaplasia. This is a rare finding; its presence in abundance should suggest the alternative possibility of phylloides tumor.
11 Lactational changes. These are manifested by an increase in the amount of cytoplasm in the epithelial cells, which appear vacuolated, and by dilation of the glandular lumina by secretion.[131]

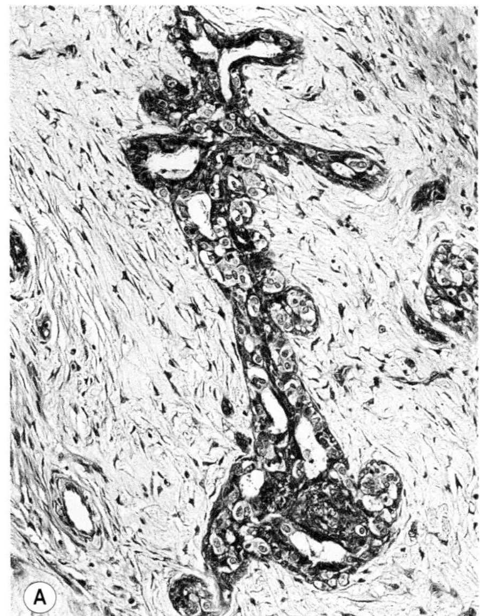

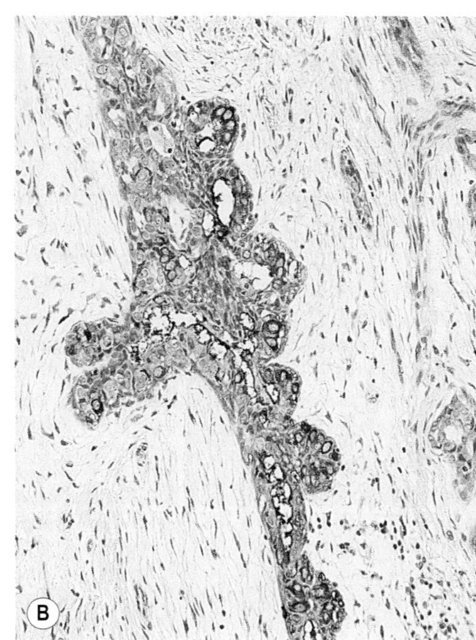

Fig. 20.14 **A** and **B**, Fibroadenoma with apocrine metaplasia. **A**, Hematoxylin–eosin section showing a prominent discontinuous layer of plump eosinophilic cells at the base of the gland. These should not be confused with neuroendocrine cells. **B**, Immunostain for GCDFP-15.

12 Young patients, large tumor size, and hypercellularity. There is a reasonably distinct type of fibroadenoma that tends to occur in adolescents (often in blacks and sometimes involving both breasts), reach a large size (over 10 cm), and show hypercellularity of glands and/or stroma (Fig. 20.15).[117] These attributes can be found independently from each other, but there is clearly a link between them. A plethora of names exists to designate these lesions, depending on which feature predominates or which has impressed the writer the most. There are age-related terms, such as juvenile fibroadenoma;[128,134] size-related terms, such as giant or massive fibroadenoma; and cellularity-related terms, such as fetal or cellular fibroadenoma.[134] When the cellularity is mainly epithelial and very florid, they have also been called *fibroadenomas with atypical epithelial hyperplasia;*[128] when the stroma is prominent, they have been designated *fibroadenomas with stromal cellularity.*[121] It is easy to imagine the difficulty one may encounter in selecting a name for the fibroadenoma that at the same time is very large, is hypercellular, and develops in an adolescent, a not infrequent occurrence. Of course, the choice of term is not very important. What matters is to recognize that the lesion is a fibroadenoma and not to confuse it with virginal hypertrophy or – more cogently – phylloides tumor. The epithelial hypercellularity can be dismissed as clinically inconsequential (unless it has the cytoarchitectural features of carcinoma). The stromal hypercellularity should be evaluated more carefully in terms of degree and atypicality; it is good to remember, however, that it is very rare for phylloides tumors to occur in young patients (although they certainly can).

No differences have been found in the incidence, gross appearance, and microscopic configuration of fibroadenomas removed from patients taking oral contraceptives and those in control cases, except for the occasional formation of acini in the former.[120]

Ultrastructurally, the most interesting feature of fibroadenomas is the constant presence of a multilayered basal lamina around the epithelial and endothelial cells.[115,140] The stromal cells have features

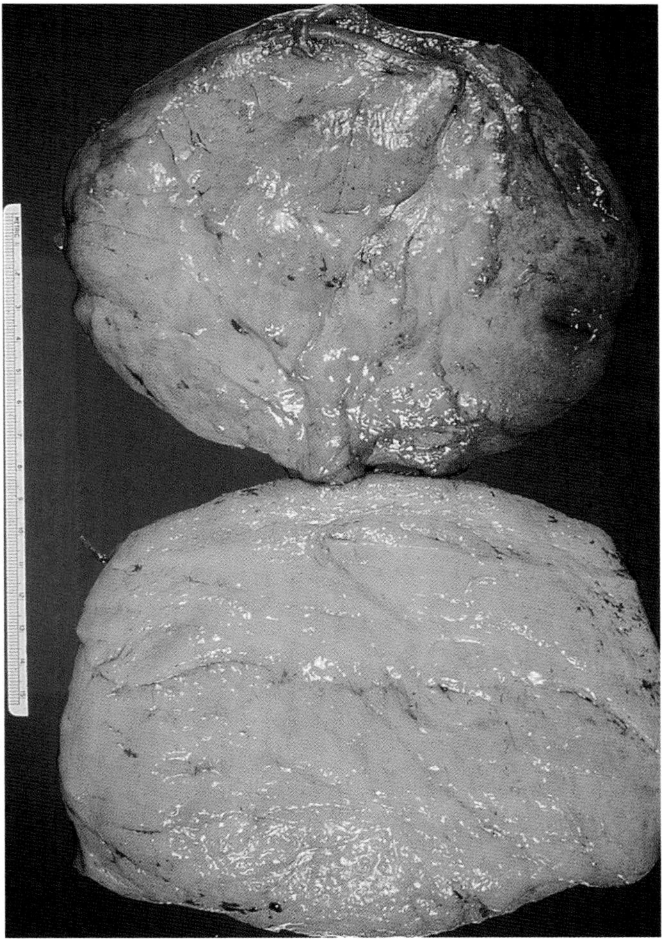

Fig. 20.15 Giant fibroadenoma occurring in an adolescent female.

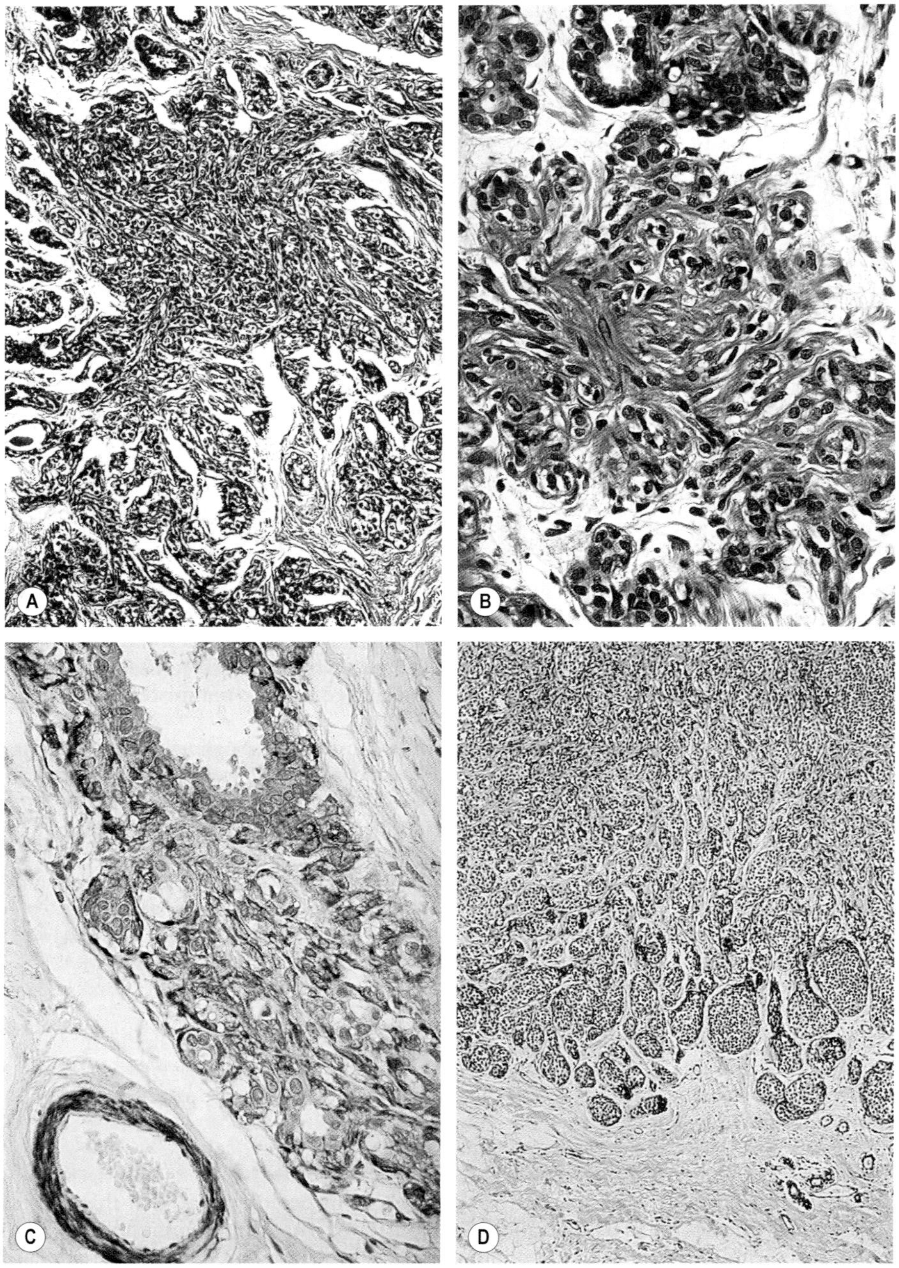

Fig. 20.25 A–D, Sclerosing adenosis. **A**, Low-power view. The lobular configuration of the lesion is obvious. **B**, Medium-power view. Note the spindle shape of the proliferating cells in the center of the lobule and the fibrillary quality of the cytoplasm, indicative of myoepithelial nature. **C**, Immunocytochemical stain for actin showing strong immunoreactivity in the myoepithelial cell component. **D**, Sclerosing adenosis with lobular carcinoma in situ. Note the regularity of the edge and absence of infiltrative features.

*(**D**, Courtesy of Dr Robert E Fechner, Charlottesville, VA)*

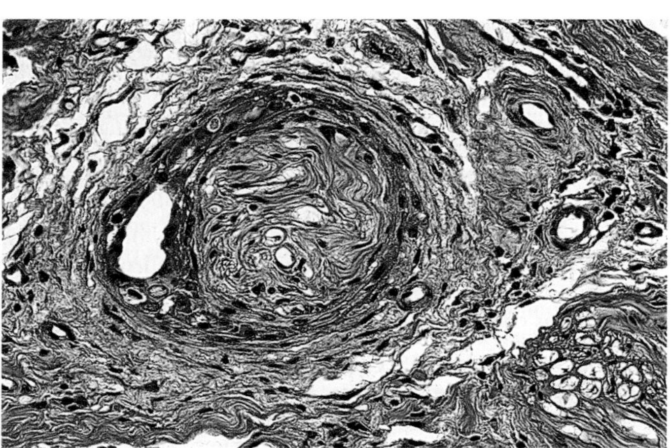

Fig. 20.26 Benign 'perineurial invasion' in a breast lesion that had elsewhere the typical features of sclerosing adenosis.

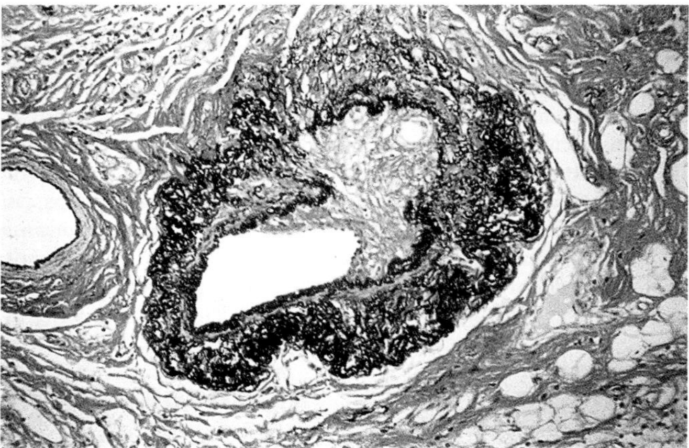

Fig. 20.27 Involvement of the wall of a vessel by sclerosing adenosis, as highlighted by the Verhoeff–van Gieson stain.

(Courtesy of Dr V Eusebi, Bologna, Italy)

latter. Some authors regard nodular adenosis as the early nonsclerotic phase of sclerosing adenosis.

Adenosis tumor is simply a form of nodular or sclerosing adenosis of larger dimensions than usual, which therefore becomes palpable and more tumorlike clinically.[192]

Florid adenosis is a term that has been applied to lesions of nodular or sclerosing adenosis that are unduly cellular and proliferative. Neither of these two forms of adenosis represents a distinct entity.

Microglandular and adenomyoepithelial (apocrine) adenosis

Microglandular adenosis, also known as microglandular hyperplasia, is a rare form of adenosis in which small uniform glands with open lumina containing an eosinophilic secretion are distributed in an irregular fashion within fibrous tissue or fat[194,205,210] (Fig. 20.28). There is no trabecular bar formation. The glands are lined by a single layer of small uniform cuboidal or flat cells with vacuolated or granular cytoplasm, lacking apocrine-type 'snouts'. In contrast to other forms of adenosis, the myoepithelial layer is absent.[194,203] However, there is a thick basement membrane that can be well appreciated immunohistochemically and ultrastructurally.[210] The stroma may be hyalinized but is not cellular or elastotic.

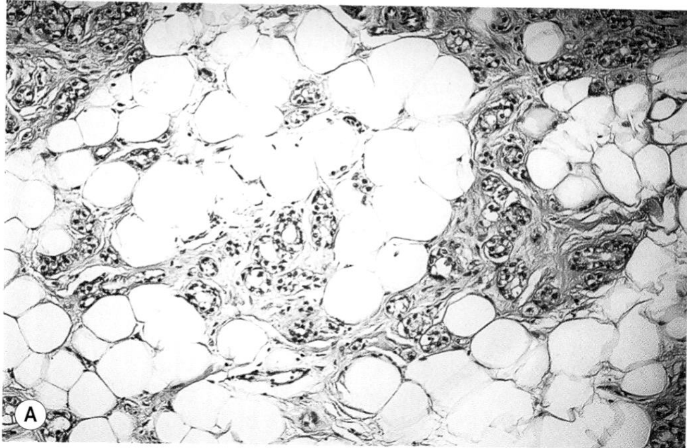

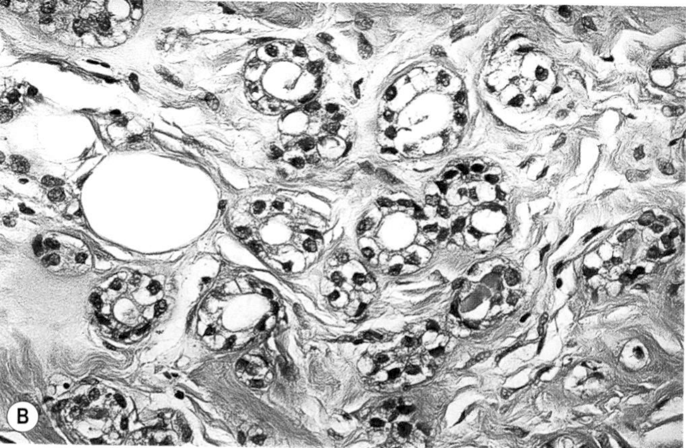

Fig. 20.28 **A** and **B**, Microglandular hyperplasia. **A**, Low-power appearance, showing haphazardly scattered small round glands. **B**, On high power, the glands are open and contain a luminal secretion. The myoepithelial cell layer is not discernible. *(Slide courtesy of Dr J Azzopardi, London)*

The main differential diagnosis of this lesion is with tubular carcinoma.[194] Microglandular adenosis is an indolent condition and should be treated conservatively; however, enough cases have been reported in continuity with carcinoma to suggest that it may evolve into malignancy with a frequency greater than the other forms of adenosis described in this section.[198,201,206,207] Interestingly, a high percentage of these carcinomas in one series have been interpreted as being of the adenoid cystic type.[193] Actually, this frequently occurring spatial relationship with an easily recognizable carcinoma, and the fact that microglandular adenosis is the only benign epithelial breast lesion devoid of myoepithelial cells, makes one wonder whether it may not represent an extremely low-grade form of ductal carcinoma with a very indolent clinical course. At the very least, it should be considered to be a lesion having a significant premalignant potential.[199,201]

Adenomyoepithelial (apocrine) adenosis is a form of adenosis sharing some features with microglandular adenosis, and perhaps representing a variant of it, in which the glands are larger, the lining epithelium is taller and with apocrine metaplasia, and myoepithelial cells are present[196,197,200,209] (Fig. 20.29). The latter can be prominent and sometimes accompanied by nuclear atypia and nucleolar prominence (*atypical apocrine adenosis*). Apocrine adenosis has been found to be a clonal process.[195] It is said to be associated with an increased risk for the development of carcinoma in women over the age of 60 years when accompanied by atypia,[208] but doubts have been expressed about this claim and the very validity of the entity.[204] An interesting aspect of this lesion is that it can give rise to a biphasic breast tumor that has been designated adenomyoepithelioma[196,211] (see p. 1723).

Tubular adenosis is also related to microglandular adenosis, from which it differs by the tubular configuration and the presence of a myoepithelial component. Like microglandular adenosis, it may be accompanied by carcinoma.[202]

Fibrocystic disease

Fibrocystic disease of the breast is an extremely important lesion because of its high frequency; the ability of some of its subtypes to simulate the clinical, radiographic, gross, and microscopic appearance of carcinoma; and the possible relationship of some of its forms to carcinoma.[217] Many other names have been proposed over the years for this disorder, none of which is entirely satisfactory, and some of which are highly objectionable: cystic disease, cystic mastopathy, cystic hyperplasia, mammary dysplasia, Reclus disease, Schimmelbusch disease, mazoplasia, chronic cystic mastitis, benign breast disease, and others. Fibrocystic disease is the name most commonly used in the United States and is likely to remain in use even though it has at least two drawbacks: (1) it overemphasizes the fibrous component of the disorder; and (2) it is linked in the mind of many physicians, patients, and life insurance agents with a precancerous condition, which in most instances it is not. To avoid the potentially serious problems related to the latter situation, a group convened by the College of American Pathologists in 1985 recommended the use of alternative terms such as *fibrocystic changes* or *fibrocystic condition*, followed by specification of the component lesions either in the body of the pathology report or in the diagnosis.[218] The purpose is laudable, but the change in terminology is not necessarily an improvement. There are certainly many 'changes' in this 'condition', but the constellation of these changes clearly fulfills the criteria for a 'disease'. To look at the issue from another angle, if fibrocystic disease of the breast were not a 'disease', nodular hyperplasia of prostate and hyperplasia of thyroid would not qualify either.

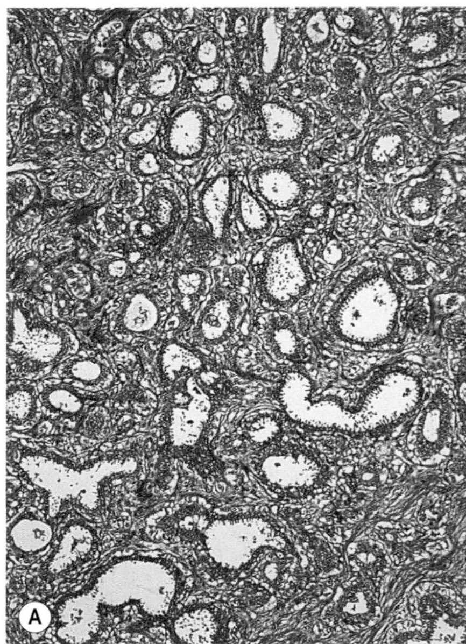
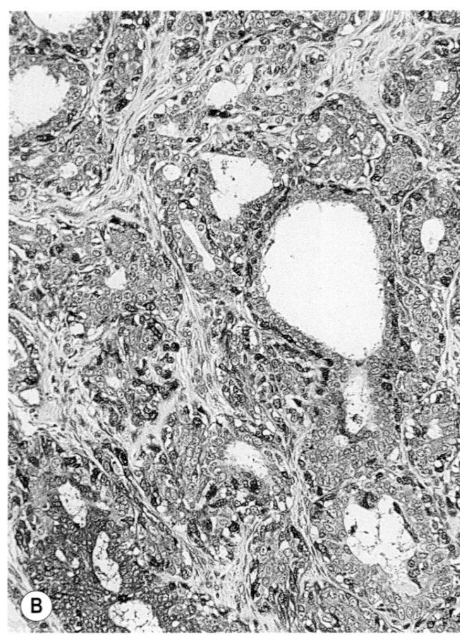

Fig. 20.29 A and **B**, Adenomyoepithelial adenosis. The glands are relatively large, with a wide, open lumen and apocrine metaplasia. The cellular component in between is composed of myoepithelial cells. **B**, S-100 protein stain highlights the prominent myoepithelial component.

Fibrocystic disease is most frequently seen, at least at the clinical level, between the ages of 25 and 45 years. The most proliferative forms of the disease are more common in Anglo-Saxon than in Latin American, American Indian, or Japanese women.[215,231] The real incidence of this disease is difficult to estimate because the diagnosis depends a great deal on the liberality of the individual clinician, radiologist, or pathologist.[220,224,230] Hormones obviously play a role in its development, but the exact pathogenesis remains obscure.[213,221,234] There is no evidence that administration of oral contraceptives increases the degree of epithelial proliferation;[219,222] on the contrary, there are statistical data indicating a lower frequency of fibrocystic disease (at least of those forms without epithelial atypia[223]) among long-term users of contraceptives.[229] Epidemiologic evidence has been presented suggesting a relationship between coffee consumption and the development of fibrocystic disease, but this has not been confirmed in other studies.[212,225]

The process is most often bilateral, but one breast may be much more affected than the other and appear clinically to be the only one involved.

It is important to realize that fibrocystic disease primarily affects the TDLU, although the epithelial hyperplasia can also extend to larger ducts. There is a great degree of variability in the gross and microscopic appearance depending on which manifestation of the disease predominates. The basic morphologic changes are the following:

1 **Cysts.** These can be microscopic or grossly visible, and sometimes reach large proportions. They usually contain a cloudy yellow or clear fluid. Some of these cysts have a bluish cast when seen from the outside ('blue dome cysts' of Bloodgood). Often, numerous small thin-walled cysts are seen in the breast parenchyma surrounding a large cyst. Microscopically, the epithelial lining of most cysts, especially the larger ones, is flattened or altogether absent, the cyst having only a thick fibrous wall. Frequently these cysts rupture and elicit an inflammatory response in the stroma, with abundant foamy macrophages and cholesterol clefts (see discussion following). Azzopardi[214] has remarked that these cysts – no matter how large – arise from the TDLU rather than from ducts.

2 **Apocrine metaplasia.** This is a very common change. It is most often seen in dilated and cystic structures, but it may appear in normal-sized tubules as well. Cysts lined by apocrine-type epithelium containing fluid under pressure are known as *tension cysts*. The appearance of the lining is indistinguishable from the lining of apocrine sweat glands. The individual cells have an abundant granular acidophilic cytoplasm, often with supranuclear vacuoles and yellow–brown pigment, some of which contains iron. The apical portion of the cytoplasm shows the typical 'apocrine snout'. The nucleus is medium sized, and the nucleolus can be very prominent. Periodic acid–Schiff (PAS) stain shows a crescent of coarse glycolipid granules on the luminal side. Immunohistochemical stain for GCDFP-15 shows strong cytoplasmic reactivity, and stain for androgen receptor shows strong nuclear reactivity.[226] Transitional or poorly developed phases of this process exist, which have been termed *partial* or *incomplete* apocrine metaplasia. In some of these cases, the apocrine metaplasia has atypical cytologic features and is accompanied by sclerosis. There is no evidence that patients with *atypical apocrine metaplasia* as thus defined are at an increased risk for the development of carcinoma.[216]

3 **Fibrosis.** This change is often present, but its degree varies markedly. It is probably an event secondary to the rupture of the cysts and it may proceed to hyalinization. The terms *fibrous disease* of the breast and *fibrous mastopathy* have been used by some authors to designate a breast condition in which the main change seems to be a more or less localized stromal fibrosis;[228] it is not clear whether this is related to fibrocystic disease or even whether it represents a distinct clinicopathologic entity, although the latter seems more likely.

4 **Calcification.** This is less common than in duct ectasia or carcinoma; it tends to have a coarse, highly irregular pattern. Chemically, it may be composed of calcium phosphate or calcium oxalate. On mammography, the latter is of an

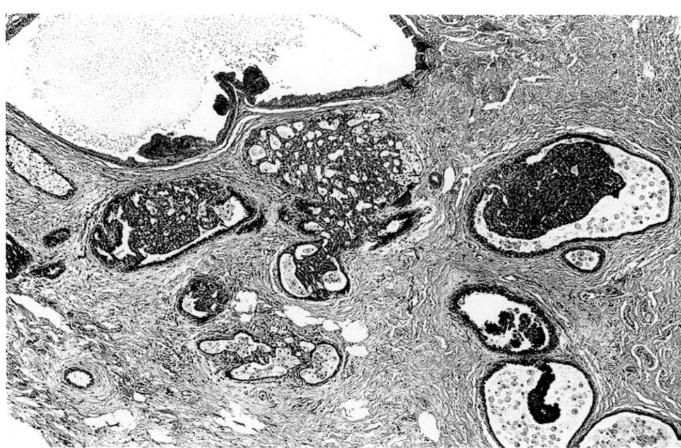

Fig. 20.30 Fibrocystic changes, including cystic dilation, apocrine metaplasia, florid ductal hyperplasia, and fibrosis.

amorphous, low-to-medium density (in contrast to the medium-to-high density of calcium phosphate) and is nearly always associated with benign disease.[235] Calcium phosphate deposition is usually easily detectable on hematoxylin–eosin (H&E) sections and is highlighted by the von Kossa stain, which may be necessary to identify minute foci.[232] However, calcium oxalate crystals can be easily missed with these techniques; they are better seen with polarized lenses (because of their birefringent quality) or after silver nitrate–rubeanic acid with 5% acetic acid pretreatment.[233]

5 **Chronic inflammation.** This is another common but secondary feature of fibrocystic disease. It is not related to infection but rather to the rupture of cysts, with release of secretion in the stroma. Lymphocytes, plasma cells, and foamy histiocytes are the predominant elements. Fibrocystic disease with intense chronic inflammation should not be confused with mammary duct ectasia (see p. 1663).

6 **Epithelial hyperplasia.** This is the most important and troublesome component of fibrocystic disease (Fig. 20.30). It is also the most significant because of its possible relationship to carcinoma and the fact that it is responsible for most difficulties in the differential diagnosis between fibrocystic disease and carcinoma. In most cases it is only of minimal degree, as confirmed by the fact that the degree of cell proliferation as measured by thymidine labeling is generally not significantly higher in fibrocystic disease than in the normal breast.[227] Epithelial hyperplasia is discussed in detail in the next section.

7 **Fibroadenomatoid change.** This is the least common abnormality seen as a component of fibrocystic disease. The stromal proliferation and slit-like epithelial formations result in a picture reminiscent of fibroadenoma but lacking the sharp circumscription of the latter (see p. 1665).

Radial scar and other sclerosing ductal lesions

This is a group of breast lesions characterized by a generally small size, stellate shape, central fibrous and often elastotic core, and variable degree of epithelial distortion and proliferation.[237,253,254,258] They are usually seen within the context of fibrocystic disease and have been variously designated as radial scar, nonencapsulated sclerosing lesion, indurative mastopathy, infiltrating epitheliosis, benign sclerosing ductal proliferation, sclerosing papillary proliferation, scleroelastotic lesion, and sclerosing adenosis with pseudo-infiltration.[244,245,255,257] Some are thought to represent primary proliferative diseases (ductal hyperplasias or even intraductal papillomas) in which the stromal change and epithelial distortion occur as a secondary and often focal event; others are viewed as a primary obliterative disease of the terminal duct (perhaps induced by inflammation) with secondary epithelial proliferation of their branches.[243] Cases exist in which a strong point can be made in favor of one or the other of these postulated mechanisms, such as the otherwise typical ductal hyperplasia (epitheliosis) with a small focus of fibroelastosis or – at the other extreme – the fibroelastotic lesion with almost no epithelial proliferation.[240,243,257] In many lesions, however, it is difficult or impossible to establish with certainty whether the fibrosis or the epithelial proliferation was the primary event. They are therefore described here as a group. On mammography and gross examination, their irregularly stellate shape results in a great resemblance to invasive ductal carcinoma of either conventional or tubular type[248] (Fig. 20.31). Microscopically, the connective tissue center is densely fibrotic, only occasionally cellular (Fig. 20.32). Clumps of basophilic material, strongly reactive for elastic tissue stain, are seen in the walls of obliterated ducts and elsewhere, sometimes in abundance (Fig. 20.33). Embedded within this stroma are small ductular formations that are disorganized but still composed of two cell types; at the periphery of the spokes are larger duct-like structures that may be dilated and/or may exhibit epithelial hyperplastic changes having the features described on page 1677 (Fig. 20.34).

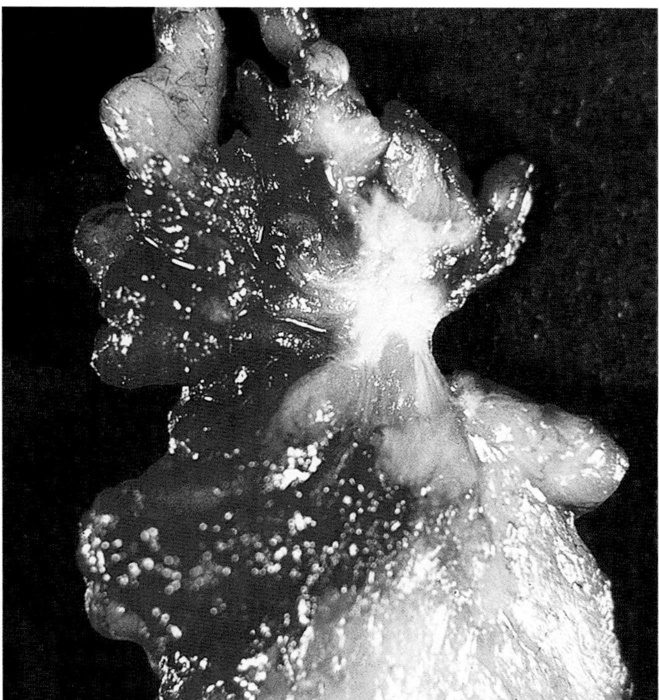

Fig. 20.31 Gross appearance of radial scar.

The most important aspects of the sclerosing ductal lesion are the differential diagnosis and possible relationship with ductal carcinoma (Fig. 20.35). As far as the former problem is concerned, suffice it to say that the diagnostic criteria for the identification of

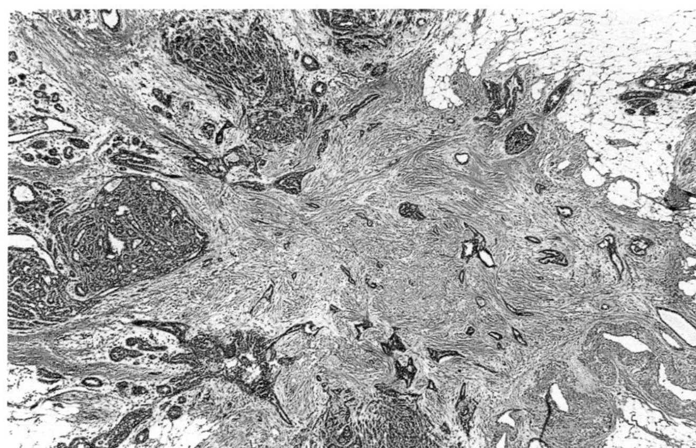

Fig. 20.32 Typical stellate shape of radial scar as seen on low power.

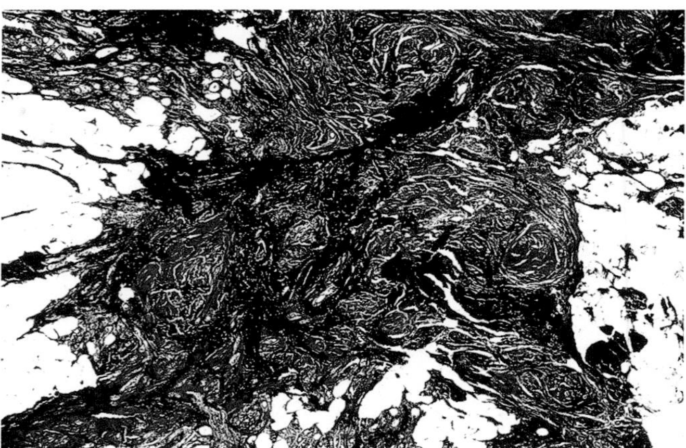

Fig. 20.33 Abundant deposition of elastic tissue in the central portion of a radial scar, as highlighted by the Verhoeff–van Gieson stain.

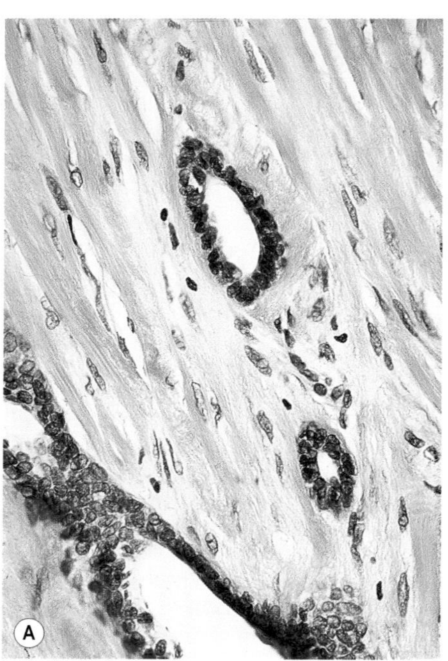

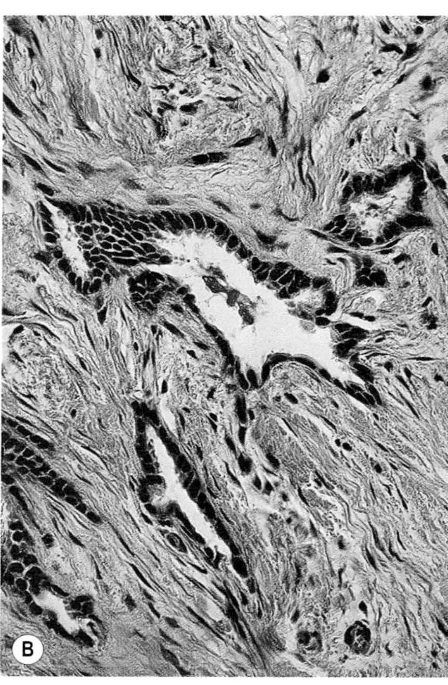

Fig. 20.34 **A**, Benign ductular structures entrapped in radial scar. Note their regular contour and the hypocellular hyaline quality of the stroma. **B**, Tubular carcinoma shown for comparison. Note the angulated shape of the glands and the desmoplastic stroma.

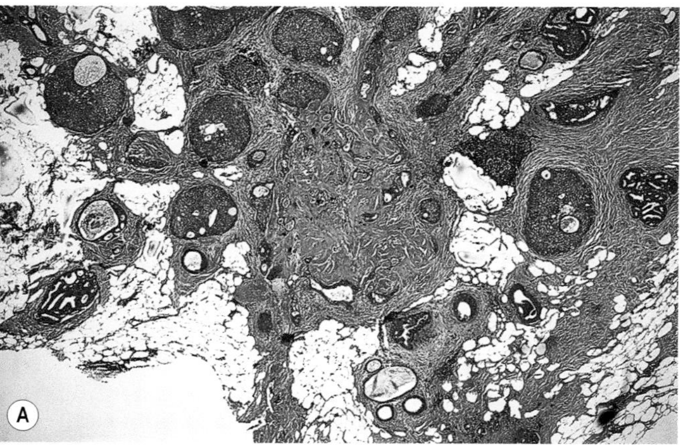

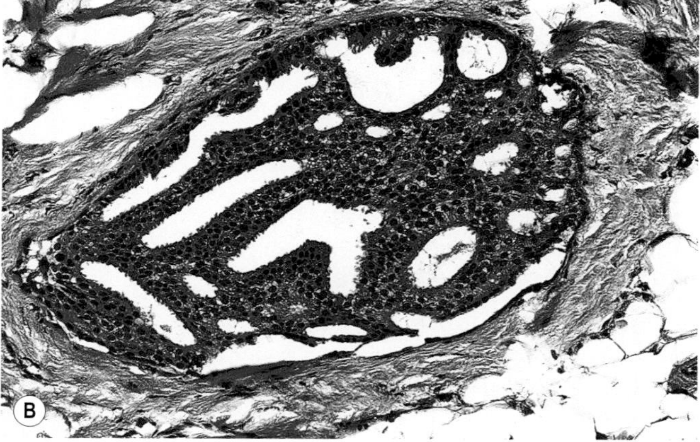

Fig. 20.35 **A** and **B**, Radial scar with associated low-grade intraductal carcinoma.

carcinoma should be the same whether a central scar is present or not. They include the usual cytoarchitectural criteria as seen in H&E-stained sections, as well as the evaluation of myoepithelial cell participation in immunocytochemical preparations.[246,249]

As for the latter problem, the issue is not settled: some authors believe that most tubular carcinomas arise from radial scars; most others do not.[237,250] We have seen enough cases showing continuity between the central elastotic area, the surrounding benign ductal hyperplasia, and foci of tubular carcinoma to favor the interpretation that at least some cases of this type of carcinoma originate on the basis of this sequence, and that the association is particularly frequent if the radial scar is larger than 1 cm.[251] Parenthetically, although most carcinomas involving (and possibly arising from) radial scars are well-differentiated ductal lesions, only a minority are classic tubular carcinomas;[236] some of these carcinomas are of the metaplastic type, with a possible myoepithelial component.[241]

If the radial scar shows no evidence of carcinoma and is totally excised, the general assumption has been that the patient is not at an increased risk of carcinoma.[239,252,256] However, a large-scale study has concluded that women with radial scars have a risk for breast cancer that is almost twice that of women without scars, regardless of the histologic type of benign breast disease.[247] The accepted treatment of mammographically detected radial scar is conservative excision and follow-up.[238,242]

Ductal and lobular hyperplasia

Epithelial hyperplasia of **ductal** type, when florid, has been traditionally designated as papillomatosis, particularly in the United States. Azzopardi[259] has rightly objected to the term on the grounds that in most instances the lesion does not form true papillae. He prefers the term *epitheliosis*, but this has not been widely accepted. Perhaps the more general term *epithelial hyperplasia* is the best compromise, followed by an indication of its degree: *mild* (when made up of three or four epithelial cells in thickness), *moderate to florid* (when more pronounced), and *atypical* (see following discussion). In the most proliferative cases, the entire lumen can be filled by the proliferation. Some forms of hyperplasia have true papillary qualities. The features that we have found most helpful in the identification of the benign nature of the proliferation are the following:

1. Nuclei that are oval (rather than round, except when cut transversely), normochromatic (rather than hyperchromatic), and with slight overlap; small, single, indistinct nucleoli; scanty or no mitotic activity (Fig. 20.36).
2. Cytoplasm that is acidophilic and finely granular rather than pale and homogeneous.
3. Indistinct cytoplasmic borders, so that the nuclei seem to lie in a syncytial mass rather than within sharply outlined cell membranes.
4. Streaming effect, induced by the oval cells being vaguely arranged in parallel bundles (Fig. 20.37).
5. 'Tufts' and 'mounds' projecting into the lumen.
6. Presence of peripheral elongated clefts, bound on one side by a single layer of basally located cells and on the other by a solid intraluminal formation; sometimes this cleft spans almost the entirety of the circumference, with the retracted solid ball of epithelial cells hanging from the wall like the vascular tuft of a renal glomerulus (Fig. 20.38). The intratubular lumina of ductal hyperplasia tend to be irregular in size, shape (elongated rather than round), and location (predominating at the periphery) as opposed to regular in all three parameters as seen in the cribriform pattern of intraductal carcinoma.

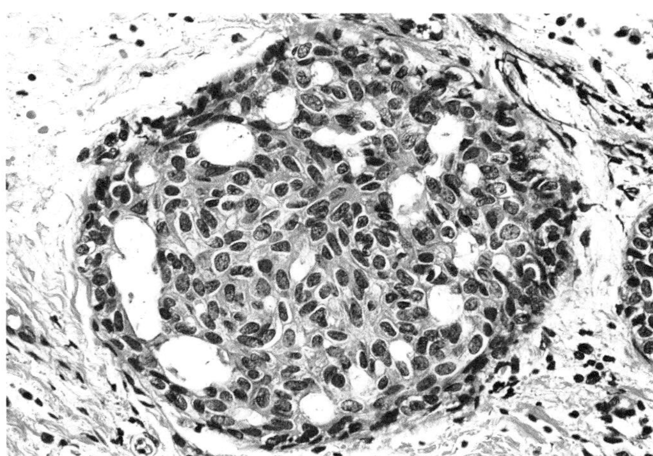

Fig. 20.36 Florid ductal hyperplasia. There is no evidence of necrosis, and individual cells are well supported by their stroma. A prominent cleft has formed between a solid intraluminal proliferation and an outer epithelial row. This feature is usually indicative of a benign condition.

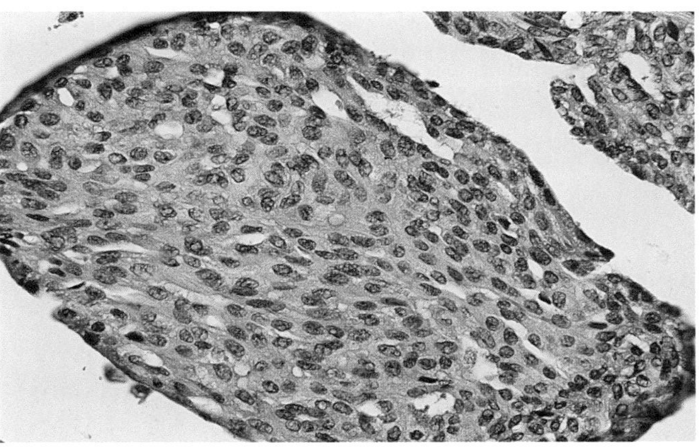

Fig. 20.37 Florid ductal hyperplasia. Note the oval shape of the nuclei and the parallel arrangement, resulting in a 'streaming' effect.

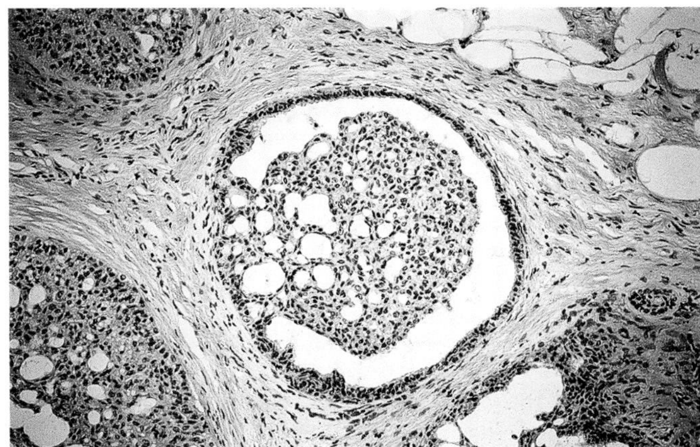

Fig. 20.38 Structure resembling a renal glomerulus in florid ductal hyperplasia.

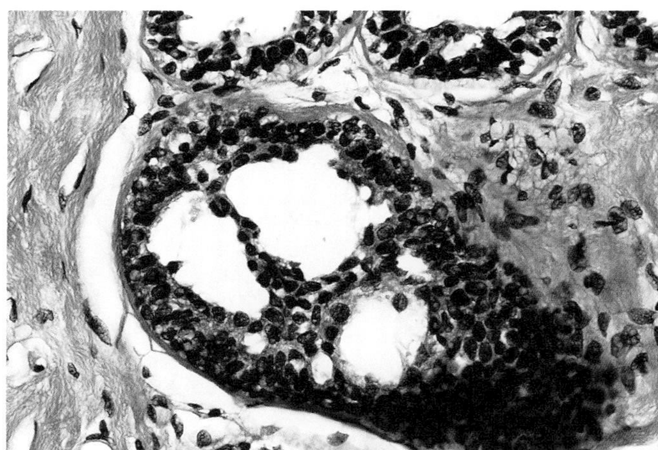

Fig. 20.39 Ductal hyperplasia showing irregularly shaped ridges connecting opposite portions of the wall. Note the fact that the oval nuclei are arranged parallel to the long axis of the ridge.

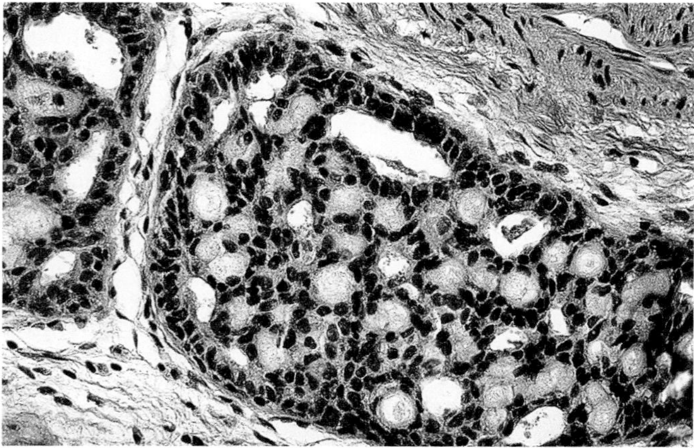

Fig. 20.40 Collagenous spherulosis. The cylinders have a round shape and a homogeneous pink staining quality, consistent with basement membrane material.

7 Presence of irregularly shaped bridges connecting opposite portions of the wall. The cells in these bridges have oval nuclei arranged parallel to the long axis of the bridge (Fig. 20.39). Their appearance is very different from that seen in the rigid trabecular bars and Roman bridges of intraductal carcinoma.
8 Complete or incomplete apocrine metaplasia; cytoplasmic blebbing.
9 Presence of myoepithelial cells, whether scattered or as a continuous row, and clear, acidophilic, or elongated and smooth muscle-like ('myoid').
10 Presence of foamy macrophages, both in the lumen and intimately admixed with the proliferating epithelial cells.[262]
11 Frequent intraluminal or stromal calcification but absence of calcific spherules or psammoma bodies between epithelium and stroma.
12 Absence of necrosis.

As important as these features are, none of them is diagnostic by itself. They need to be weighed against each other, sometimes modified depending on the nature of the case, and occasionally ignored altogether. For instance, very prominent nucleoli and structures reminiscent of Roman bridges are strongly suggestive of intraductal carcinoma under ordinary circumstances but lose much of their significance when occurring in apocrine epithelium. The myoepithelial cell layer may be preserved in intraductal carcinoma. Focal necrosis may be found in benign disease, particularly in nipple adenoma. Furthermore, proliferative benign breast disease and carcinoma can and often do coexist, which means that an area may be diagnostic of intraductal carcinoma even if the immediately surrounding glands show features indicative of benign disease.

Occasionally, one sees in ductal hyperplasia intranuclear round eosinophilic bodies that – when unduly large – may simulate viral inclusions. At the ultrastructural level, these intranuclear *helioid inclusions* appear as single membrane-bound structures containing a laminated or homogeneous electron-dense core with a corona of radiating filaments.[274]

Immunohistochemically, ductal hyperplasia of the usual (including florid) type is characterized by strong immunoreactivity for high molecular weight (HMW) keratin antibody, in particular for keratin 5/6 (which is preferred over 34βE12).[271] This is of importance in the differential diagnosis with atypical ductal hyperplasia and ductal carcinoma in situ (DCIS), of which 90% of cases lack reactivity for HMW keratin.

Rare morphologic variants of ductal hyperplasia have been described.

Collagenous spherulosis is characterized by the presence of intraluminal clusters of generally eosinophilic but sometimes basophilic collagen-rich spherules that seem to arise within the spaces between epithelial and myoepithelial cells.[261,264,270] Ultrastructurally, the spherules show a variable composition of basement membrane material, banded collagen, and mineral deposition[268] (Fig. 20.40). This curious lesion, which may also be seen in salivary gland tumors,[269] can be confused with adenoid cystic carcinoma, signet ring carcinoma, and cribriform ductal carcinoma in situ. It should also be realized that collagenous spherulosis can be associated with intraductal papilloma, sclerosing adenosis, lobular CIS, and atypical ductal hyperplasia.[272] As a matter of fact, the foci of collagenous spherulosis themselves may be involved by lobular CIS.[273]

Cystic hypersecretory hyperplasia (*CHH*) is characterized by the presence of cystically dilated ducts containing a colloid-like material; this lesion should be distinguished from cystic hypersecretory carcinoma, not always an easy task (see p. 1692).[265] CHH can be associated with conventional atypical ductal hyperplasia and ductal carcinoma in situ.[267]

Gynecomastia-like (*gynecomastoid*) *micropapillary hyperplasia* is a most peculiar form of proliferative breast disease of the female breast that resembles the gynecomastia of the male breast.[275]

Thyroid-like breast tumor is yet another bizarre form of ductal proliferation, in which the morphologic features show an uncanny resemblance, both at the architectural and cytologic level, to the tall-cell variant of papillary thyroid carcinoma.[260,263] No *RET* rearrangements or *BRAF* mutations have been found in the few cases so far studied.[260,266] One reported case was associated with metastases in an intramammary lymph node, indicating that this mysterious lesion has malignant potential.[276]

As far as **lobular hyperplasia** is concerned, the term could be used whenever – in the absence of pregnancy, puerperium, or exogenous hormone stimulation – the lobules appear larger and more cellular than usual but do not fulfill the criteria for lobular CIS or even for atypical lobular hyperplasia (ALH). Since the definition of the latter is rather vague itself, it follows that the diagnosis of lobular hyperplasia is of dubious reproducibility and significance.

The special variant of ductal hyperplasia known as juvenile papillomatosis or Swiss cheese disease is discussed on page 1731.

Atypical ductal and lobular hyperplasia

As already mentioned, there is a wide range in the degree of epithelial proliferation in fibrocystic disease. It has been postulated that there is a correlation between the degree of this proliferation and the likelihood of subsequent development of invasive carcinoma, and various attempts have been made to quantify both the degree of the change and the magnitude of the risk.[295] The most ambitious and successful attempts are those of the Page–Dupont team,[281,287,288] who have proposed the terms *atypical ductal hyperplasia* (*ADH*) and *atypical lobular hyperplasia* (*ALH*) for proliferative lesions in which some but not all of the features of intraductal carcinoma or lobular CIS, respectively, are present (Figs 20.41 and 20.42). Using these criteria in a retrospective study, they diagnosed ADH and/or ALH in 3.6% of the cases and concluded that these patients had a risk of invasive breast carcinoma that was four to five times that of the general population (i.e., about half

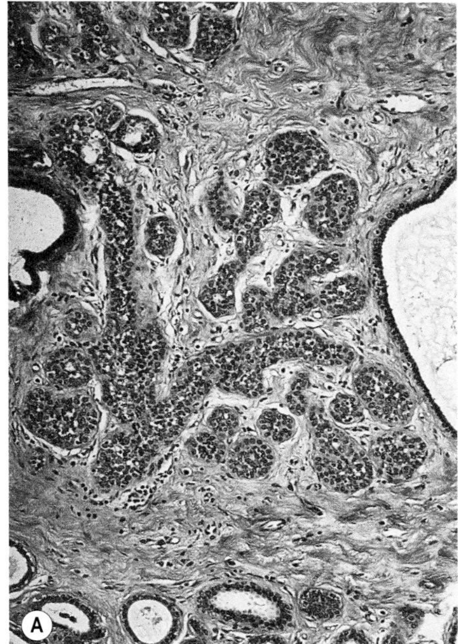

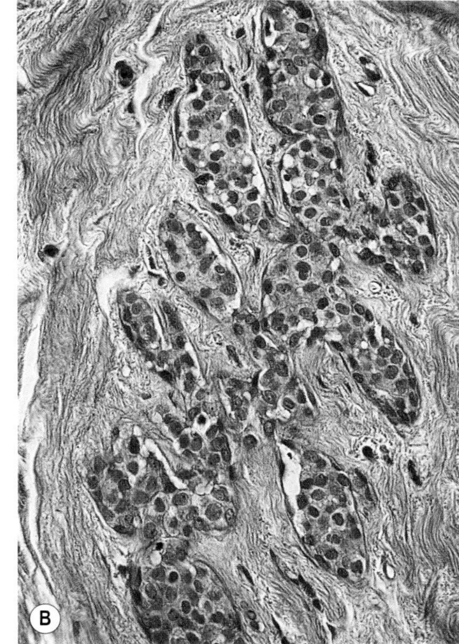

Fig. 20.41 **A** and **B**, Two different breast lesions diagnosed as atypical lobular hyperplasia by four experts in breast pathology. There is lobular enlargement and proliferation, but some lumina are preserved, and there is only minimal distention of individual units.

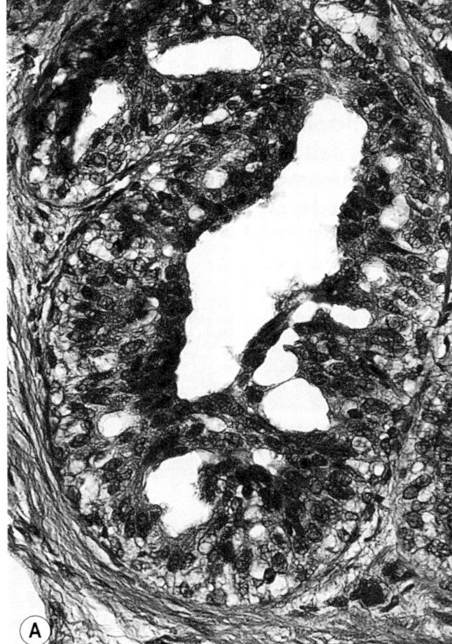

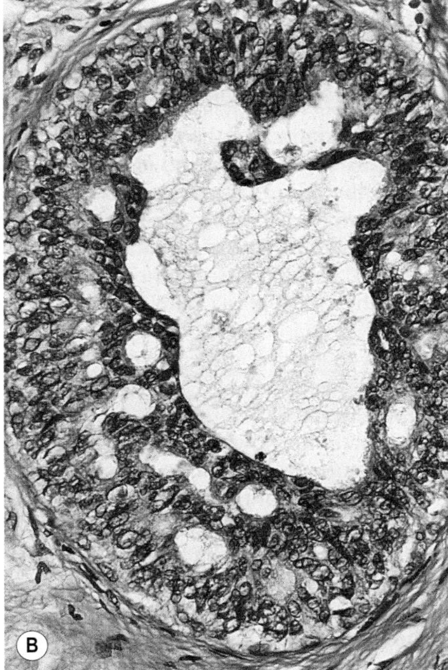

Fig. 20.42 **A** and **B**, Two different breast lesions diagnosed as atypical ductal hyperplasia by two experts in breast pathology. There is marked epithelial proliferation in structures of ductal type associated with atypia, but they were felt not to fulfill criteria for carcinoma in situ.

the prepubertal period are discussed on page 1731. The carcinomas presenting in the elderly do not differ significantly on morphologic or molecular grounds from the others.[343]

Incidence

Breast carcinoma is the most common malignant tumor and the leading cause of carcinoma death in women, with more than 1 000 000 cases occurring worldwide annually.[348] In the United States, approximately 100 000 new cases are diagnosed annually and approximately 30 000 patients die from the disease. The incidence is high in North America and northern Europe (91.4 new cases per 100 000 women/year), intermediate in southern European and Latin American countries, and low in most Asian and African countries (but rising rapidly in recent years with increased affluence of some of these countries). In the United States, there has been a sharp increase in the detection of breast carcinoma, largely due to the widespread use of mammography.[350] Most of these cases have been localized, measuring less than 2 cm in diameter and/or in situ.[345] Until recently, this increase in the number of smaller (and presumably earlier) cases did not translate into an improved survival rate. As a matter of fact, the mortality rate for breast carcinoma changed very little from the 1930s to the early 1990s.[345] However, in some regions of the world (North America, western Europe, and Australia) breast cancer mortality is finally beginning to fall, presumably because of the combined action of earlier diagnosis and improved therapy.[346,349] Unfortunately, this is not true for countries such as Japan, Costa Rica, and Singapore, in which mortality continues to rise.[347]

An interesting figure to be added to the numbers given above is the incidence of clinically occult proliferative disease and carcinoma in reduction mammoplasty specimens. In a study of 516 consecutive cases, Dotto et al.[344] found 92 (18%) usual ductal hyperplasia (UDH), 28 (5%) DIN1, 17 (3%) LIN, and 1 (0.2%) tubular carcinoma. There was not a single case of high-grade DIN or invasive carcinoma.

Risk factors

Several risk factors for the development of breast carcinoma have been established, whereas many others remain questionable.[351] It has been proposed that the common denominator for most of these factors is strong and/or prolonged estrogen stimulation operating on a genetically susceptible background.[366]

1 *Country of birth*. This has already been touched upon in the previous paragraph.
2 *Family history*. Women who have a first-degree relative with breast carcinoma have a risk two or three times that of the general population, a risk further increased if the relative was affected at an early age and/or had bilateral disease.[376] The aspects related to the discovery of the genes responsible for a predisposition to breast carcinoma are discussed in the next section.
3 *Menstrual and reproductive history*. Increased risk is correlated with early menarche, nulliparity, late age at first birth, and late menopause.[365,368] Breast carcinoma is rare in women who have been castrated; oophorectomy before 35 years of age reduces the risk to one-third. Women who have their first child before the age of 18 years have only one-third the risk of those whose first child is delayed until age 30.[378] A reduction in the risk of breast carcinoma among premenopausal women who have lactated has been documented, but no such effect was detected among postmenopausal women.[367] Breast carcinoma risk is increased in postmenopausal women with a hyperandrogenic plasma hormone profile.[363]
4 *Fibrocystic disease and epithelial hyperplasia*. The controversial relationship between these changes and breast carcinoma has been discussed in the preceding section.
5 *Exogenous estrogens*. In some older series, there has been an overall risk increase (2.5-fold),[364,370] whereas in others an increased risk (2- to 9-fold) was observed only in patients with a previous diagnosis of fibrocystic disease.[362] More recently, a large cohort study and a large case-control study have provided strong evidence for a greater increase in breast cancer risk in women using hormone replacement therapy than in those using estrogens alone.[371,372] Even more recently, highly publicized studies have added to the growing body of evidence that recent long-term use of hormone replacement therapy is associated with an increased risk of breast carcinoma, particularly of the lobular type.[355,357] In December 2002, the hormone estrogen was declared a known human carcinogen by the National Toxicology Program.
6 *Contraceptive agents*. The various epidemiologic studies that have been done in this regard have shown no increased risk, or at most a very low increase among young long-term users.[369,371,379] The tumors that have developed in this population have not differed qualitatively from those seen in control cases.[358,359]
7 *Ionizing radiation*. An increased risk of breast carcinoma has been documented with exposure to ionizing radiation, particularly if this exposure occurred at the time of breast development.[360,361,374,375]
8 *Breast augmentation*. Breast carcinomas (mainly of in situ types) are sometimes detected in women who have undergone augmentation mammoplasty.[356] However, the re-analysis of a previously published linkage study has shown that the incidence of breast carcinoma in that cohort was neither higher nor lower than that among the general population.[352,354]
9 *Others*. A peculiar association between breast carcinoma and meningioma has been repeatedly noted.[353] Even more peculiar is that fact that sometimes the breast carcinoma is found to metastasize within the meningioma.

Patients with ataxia–telangiectasia syndrome and with Cowden syndrome have an excess risk of breast cancer.[373,377]

Genetic predisposition

Approximately 5–10% of all breast cancers are familial.[399] An epochal event in the study of breast carcinoma was the discovery of two high-penetrance susceptibility genes which, when affected by germline mutations, are associated with a high life-time risk of development of breast cancer as well as some other cancers, in particular ovarian cancer.[401] Originally, they were thought to be responsible for a high proportion of familial breast carcinomas, but they are now found to be responsible for only about 16% of them.[381,394,399] These are *BRCA1*, located on chromosome 17q21, and *BRCA2*, located on chromosome 13q12.3 (Table 20.1).[383,386,400] Mutations of this gene are present in approximately 2% of Ashkenazi Jews; it has been estimated that the risk for breast carcinoma among carriers is up to 70–80% by the age of 70 years.[392,398] The finding of a positive test for the mutation can lead to an agonizing decision on the part of the affected individual, the main choices being close follow-up and prophylactic mastectomy.[387,390,395,396]

The *BRCA1*-encoded protein has many functions, including homologous recombination DNA repair, cell cycle checkpoint

Table 20.1 Summary of the syndromes associated with hereditary breast cancer

SYNDROME (OMIM)	GENE INVOLVED AND CYTOBAND	CLINICAL FEATURES
Hereditary breast cancer and ovarian cancer syndrome (113705)	*BRCA1* (17q21)	Breast cancer, high risk (50–80%) Ovarian cancer, high risk (40–50%)
Hereditary breast cancer and ovarian cancer syndrome (600185)	*BRCA2* (13q12.3)	Breast cancer, high risk (50–70%) Ovarian cancer, intermediate risk (10%) Prostate cancer Pancreatic cancer Melanoma
CHEK2 mutations (Li–Fraumeni 2 syndrome?)	*CHEK2* (22q 12.1)	Breast cancer, intermediate risk (~twofold) Sarcomas Brain tumors
Other FANC genes (114480, 610355, 607139, 600901, 605882)	*PALB2/FANCN* (16p12) *FANCA* (16q24.3) *FANCE* (6p22–p21) *BRIP1/FANCJ* (17q22)	*PALB2/FANCN* and *BRIP1/FANCJ*: moderate risk of breast cancer development The other FANC genes: low risk of breast cancer development
Familial linitis plastica type gastric cancer and lobular breast carcinomas syndrome (192090)	*CDH1* (16q22.1)	Gastric cancer Lobular breast cancer
Louis–Bar syndrome (208900)	*ATM* (11q22.3)	Lymphoma Cerebellar ataxia Immune deficiency Glioma Medulloblastoma Breast cancer
Li–Fraumeni syndrome (151623)	*TP53* (17p13.1)	High penetrance for breast cancers at young age Risk of soft tissue sarcomas and osteosarcomas, brain tumors, leukemia, and adrenocortical carcinoma
Cowden syndrome (158350)	*PTEN* (10q23.31)	Increased risk of developing neoplasms (breast cancer, thyroid carcinoma, endometrial carcinoma and others) Hamartomatous polyps of the gastrointestinal tract Mucocutaneous lesions
Bannayan–Riley–Rivalcaba syndrome (153480)	*PTEN* (10q23.31)	Breast cancer Meningioma Follicular cell tumors of the thyroid
Peutz–Jeghers syndrome (175200)	*STK11* (19p13.3)	Melanocytic macules of the lips, buccal mucosa, and digits Multiple gastrointestinal hamartomatous polyps Increased risk of various neoplasms (breast, testis, pancreas, and cervix)
Lynch cancer family syndrome II (114400)	*MSH2* (2p22–p21), *MSH3* (5q11–q12), *MSH6* (2p16), *MLH1* (3p21.3), *PMS1* (2q31–q33), *PMS2* (7p22)	Increased risk of endometrial carcinoma and colorectal carcinoma High risk of multiple primary malignant neoplasms, including breast, ovarian, gastrointestinal and genitourinary carcinomas, sarcomas, glioblastoma, and leukemia

FANC, Fanconi anemia.
From Tan DSP, Marchio C, Reis-Filho JS. Hereditary breast cancer: from molecular pathology to tailored therapies. J Clin Pathol 2008, **61:** 1073–1082.

control, ubiquitylation, chromatin remodeling, and DNA decatenation.[389,397,399] The protein encoded by *BRCA2* is involved in DNA repair, cytokinesis, and meiosis.[399] That is, both *BRCA1* and *BRCA2* are essential for accurate repair of DNA double-strand breaks by homologous recombination repair.[399] Loss of such function in the associated cancers is being exploited to develop novel therapies – for example, poly-ADP-ribose polymerase inhibitor (blocking repair of DNA breaks in the tumor cells, which are deficient in DNA repair).[384,385]

Analysis of the breast carcinomas developing in carriers of *BRCA1* mutations has shown a higher percentage of tumors with medullary features, i.e., tumors that tend to be of high grade, mitotically very active, with a syncytial growth pattern, pushing margins, confluent necrosis, negativity for hormone receptors and c-*erb*B-2 ('triple negative'), basal-like gene expression profile, associated with *TP53* mutation.[380,382,384,388,391,393,399] On the other hand, *BRCA2*-associated cancers are a heterogeneous group without a specific morphology or phenotype and commonly positive for hormone receptors.[384,393]

In addition to *BRCA1* and *BRCA2*, several other genes confer a moderate to low risk of development of breast cancer. Hereditary breast cancer can also occur in the setting of multiple cancer syndromes, as summarized in Table 20.1.[399]

Location

The location of breast carcinoma is usually indicated in relation to the breast quadrants. Approximately 50% are in the upper outer quadrant, 15% in the upper inner quadrant, 10% in the lower outer quadrant, 5% in the lower inner quadrant, 17% in the central region (within 1 cm of the areola), and 3% are diffuse (massive or multifocal). The marked difference in the carcinoma frequency depending on the quadrant, surprising at first, becomes easily explainable when one realizes that it matches closely the amount of breast parenchyma in each quadrant.

Several studies have documented the peculiar fact that breast carcinoma is slightly more frequent in the left breast than in the right. In one recent series, the excess for the left side was 13%.[402]

Multicentricity

Multicentricity (as defined by presence of carcinoma in a breast quadrant other than the one containing the dominant mass) was detected by Fisher et al.[407] in 121 (13.4%) of 904 cases of invasive carcinomas; one-third of the smaller foci were invasive and the rest were in situ. Multicentricity was more common in lobular than in ductal carcinomas. As expected, a higher incidence of multicentricity was reported in studies in which whole organ preparations were examined by radiography and light microscopy.[408] Theoretically, multiple breast carcinoma can result from either intramammary spread of a single lesion or from independent events.[405,406] It is probable that both mechanisms operate depending on the case, as suggested by clonal studies.[409–411] If aggregate diameters are used, unifocal and multifocal carcinomas are similar with respect to the frequency of regional lymph node involvement,[404] but a recent study showed that multicentric tumors are associated with a lower survival rate than unicentric tumors of the same aggregate volume.[403]

Bilaterality

The chance that a patient with invasive breast carcinoma will develop a carcinoma in the contralateral breast is about five times that of the general population, and is even higher if there is a family history of breast carcinoma.[412,414,415] In cases of lobular carcinoma, the figure can be as high as 25–50%.

The use of adjuvant chemotherapy significantly decreases the risk of metachronous contralateral breast carcinoma.[413] It is doubtful whether a biopsy of the opposite breast should be taken routinely in patients with breast carcinoma; it seems more logical to limit this practice only to those patients in whom an abnormality is suspected on clinical or mammographic grounds or to those with types of carcinoma for which the incidence of bilaterality is particularly high.[417]

Synchronous bilateral invasive breast carcinomas have a high concordance of histologic features, including the common presence of an extensive in situ component, a feature that favors their independent rather than metastatic nature.[416] When recurrence of a bilateral mammary carcinoma supervenes, it is usually from the ipsilateral tumor.[418]

Diagnosis

Clinical examination

Clinical examination, particularly palpation, is the time-honored method for the detection and evaluation of breast disease. It remains an extremely useful and practical technique, whether carried out by the physician or by the patient herself. However, both its sensitivity and discriminatory power are limited. Only 60% of the tumors detected by mammography are palpable. The clinical impression is incorrect in approximately 15% of the cases thought to be benign and approximately 10% of those thought to be malignant. The clinical evaluation of axillary lymph nodes is also fraught with error. Nodes clinically thought to be positive will be found free of metastases microscopically in 15% of cases.

Mammography

The widespread use of mammography has radically changed the diagnostic approach to breast cancer.[420,423,430] Extremely small tumors (1–2 mm) can be detected with this technique, which relies primarily on the presence of calcification. The incidence of calcification in breast carcinoma is approximately 50–60%, and the incidence in benign breast disease is 20%.[421,431] There are also important qualitative differences in the appearance of the calcification. Mammographic findings in the United States are now universally reported using the Breast Imaging Reporting and Data System (BI-RADS).[419]

It should be kept in mind that a negative mammogram does not rule out the possibility of the presence of carcinoma, since approximately 20% of palpable tumors are not detectable with this technique. The incidence of false positivity is in the neighborhood of 1%.

The proper handling of breast lesions detected by mammography requires close cooperation between radiologist, surgeon, and pathologist.[421,424,433,436] Once the radiologist identifies the abnormal area on mammography, he should provide the surgeon with a 'map' showing the relative position of the suspicious area within the breast. Once the appropriate area is excised, the cephalad and lateral margins should be marked by sutures and an x-ray study taken of the specimen. If no lesion is seen, the surgeon should obtain additional tissue. If the abnormal area is present in the specimen, this can be accurately located by slicing the specimen, identifying the slices with a lead number, taking another x-ray study, and selecting for frozen sections the slice (and the specific area within the slice) containing the abnormal area. The whole procedure takes no more than 15 minutes and is well worth the small delay, otherwise small carcinomas can be entirely missed.[428] The highest yield is obtained from histologic examination of the areas with radiographic calcification and a fibrous parenchyma.[432]

X-ray studies can even be taken of the paraffin blocks to document the fact that the area seen in the mammogram has been embedded (Fig. 20.45). An important source of discrepancy between mammographic and microscopic findings is represented by calcium oxalate crystals, which are easily identified radiographically but often missed on histologic examination.[426]

It should be obvious from the preceding comments that every attempt should be made to identify in the microscopic slide

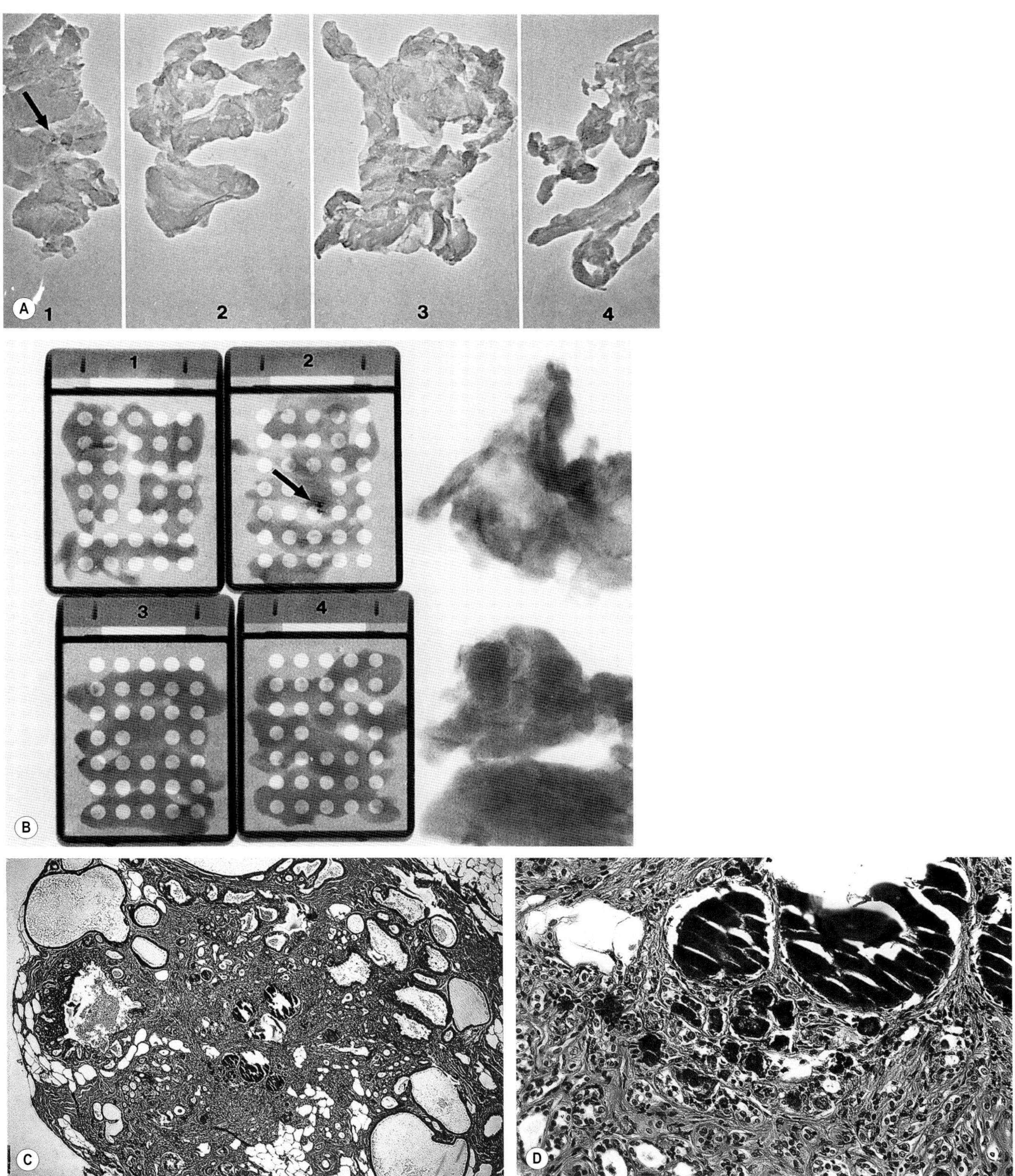

Fig. 20.45 **A–D**, Demonstration of the use of specimen radiography. A mammographically detected breast lesion was excised. **A**, The specimen was sliced into four portions and a radiograph taken. A pattern of calcification identical to that seen in original mammography was detected in slice 1 (arrow). **B**, The portion corresponding to this area of calcification was further divided into four fragments, and all four were embedded in paraffin. A radiograph of the cassettes shows that the suspicious area is in cassette 2 (arrow). The remainder of the slide (two fragments at right) shows no calcification. **C** and **D**, Low- and high-power views of the corresponding microscopic specimen.

the area regarded by the radiologist as 'suspicious' of carcinoma. However, if this is satisfactorily accomplished and the pathologist still fails to find carcinoma, neither he nor the radiologist should be overly surprised. Only 20% of the lesions labeled 'suspicious' mammographically are malignant, and the large majority of these are carcinomas in situ. McDivitt[429] estimated that the chance of the pathologist finding an invasive carcinoma in a biopsy from a nonpalpable lesion that was interpreted 'suspicious' by mammography is less than 2%. On the other hand, 'nonpalpable' should not be viewed as synonymous with inconsequential. In a series of 558 patients with nonpalpable invasive carcinomas detected by mammography and subjected to axillary dissection, 27% had at least one positive node.[435]

Wolfe[438] has divided breasts into four groups on the basis of their mammographic appearance, which he believes correlates with the risk for development of carcinoma. This correlation might well exist, but it is perplexing that, if this is the case, no correlation seems to exist between these four patterns and the types of histologic alteration.[422]

The available information suggests that nuclear magnetic resonance is not likely to replace mammography as the imaging modality of choice, although contrast-enhanced techniques have rendered it more informative and potentially more useful.[434] It is said to be more sensitive for the detection of multicentric carcinoma.[427] Breast ultrasonography has emerged as a valuable examination tool, particularly for determining whether a mass lesion is cystic or solid.[425]

Where adopted for screening purposes, the National Cancer Institute has traditionally recommended for mammography to be done on a biannual basis from the age of 40 years onwards. Great controversy has recently arisen following the revised recommendations from the US Preventive Services Task Force, which calls for mammograms to be done biannually from the ages of 50 to 74.[437]

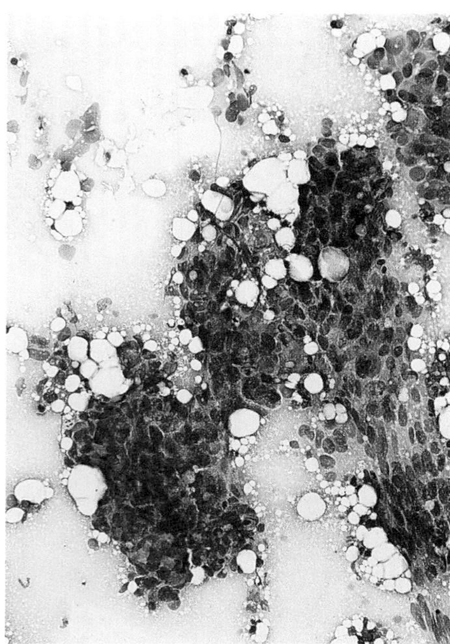

Fig. 20.46 Specimen from a fine needle aspiration (FNA) biopsy performed at Memorial Sloan-Kettering Cancer Center in 1935. This was diagnosed as breast carcinoma and followed by the performance of a mastectomy, which confirmed the cytologic interpretation. *(Courtesy of Dr Maureen Zakowski, Memorial Sloan-Kettering Cancer Center)*

Cytology

The two methods that have been used to obtain cytologic material from breast lesions are aspiration of nipple secretion and aspiration of the lesion with a fine needle.

Nipple secretion aspiration cytology is, in our opinion, of limited use, whether for the diagnosis of a clinically or mammographically detectable breast lesion or for screening purposes. Some carcinomas will undoubtedly be found, but the number of false-positive results is so high as to render this technique of only marginal value. As a matter of fact, its use as a screening procedure may have a deleterious effect because a negative cytologic diagnosis may give a false sense of security and delay recognition of the carcinoma.

The situation with fine needle aspiration (FNA) is quite different, as already shown in the pioneer attempts at Memorial Sloan-Kettering Cancer Center in the 1930s (Fig. 20.46). There is no longer any question that in experienced hands the technique is highly reliable[440,447,452,457] (Fig. 20.47). The average sensitivity is approximately 87%, the specificity close to 100%, the predictive value of a positive diagnosis nearly 100%, and the predictive value of a negative diagnosis between 60% and 90%.[444,451,455,461,464] As expected, most benign lesions misinterpreted cytologically as possibly malignant belong to the fibrocystic disease category with marked epithelial proliferation.[442,446] The cytologic distinction between ADH and intraductal carcinoma has been attempted, both in mammographically detected lesions and to screen women with a family history of breast carcinoma.[439,450,458,460] Since the differential diagnosis between these two conditions is based not only on cytologic but also on architectural criteria as seen on tissue sections, it is not surprising to find that such attempts have not been very successful.[445,458] Along similar lines, it is generally not possible to distinguish between in situ and invasive ductal carcinoma on FNA cytology,[439] although availability of histologic sections prepared from cell blocks of aspirated materials may help in identification of invasion.

The most significant variables in the accuracy of the procedure are size of the lesion and proficiency of the individual performing the aspiration.[441] Material from FNA is also suitable for hormone receptor determination,[453,456] kinetic studies,[454] and oncoprotein expression.[449]

Fine needle aspiration is less than ideal for some types of breast carcinoma. These include those associated with very extensive fibrosis, intraductal carcinoma, tubular and cribriform carcinoma, and, in general, the very small tumors. As Kline et al.[447] wisely pointed out, this technique should be used to supplement, and not to compete with, histologic examination. Most importantly, it should always be remembered that negative or inconclusive cytologic findings are not to be regarded as a definitive diagnosis if there is clinical suspicion of a malignant neoplasm.[443]

The performance of the FNA procedures may lead to mechanical displacement of epithelium, hemorrhage, necrosis, and other changes.[448,462,463] The former is particularly troublesome, because it can mimic stromal and vascular invasion.[459,462] The frequency of this complication is probably related to the type of needle used and the skill of the operator.

Needle core biopsy

In recent years, the use of needle core biopsy (vacuum-assisted and stereotactic/image guided when indicated) for the nonoperative diagnosis of breast carcinoma has been generally favored over the alternative of FNA,[484,488] some strong dissenters notwithstanding.[465] This is based on the fact that core biopsy allows evaluation of both cytologic *and* architectural features, that it may provide a definitive

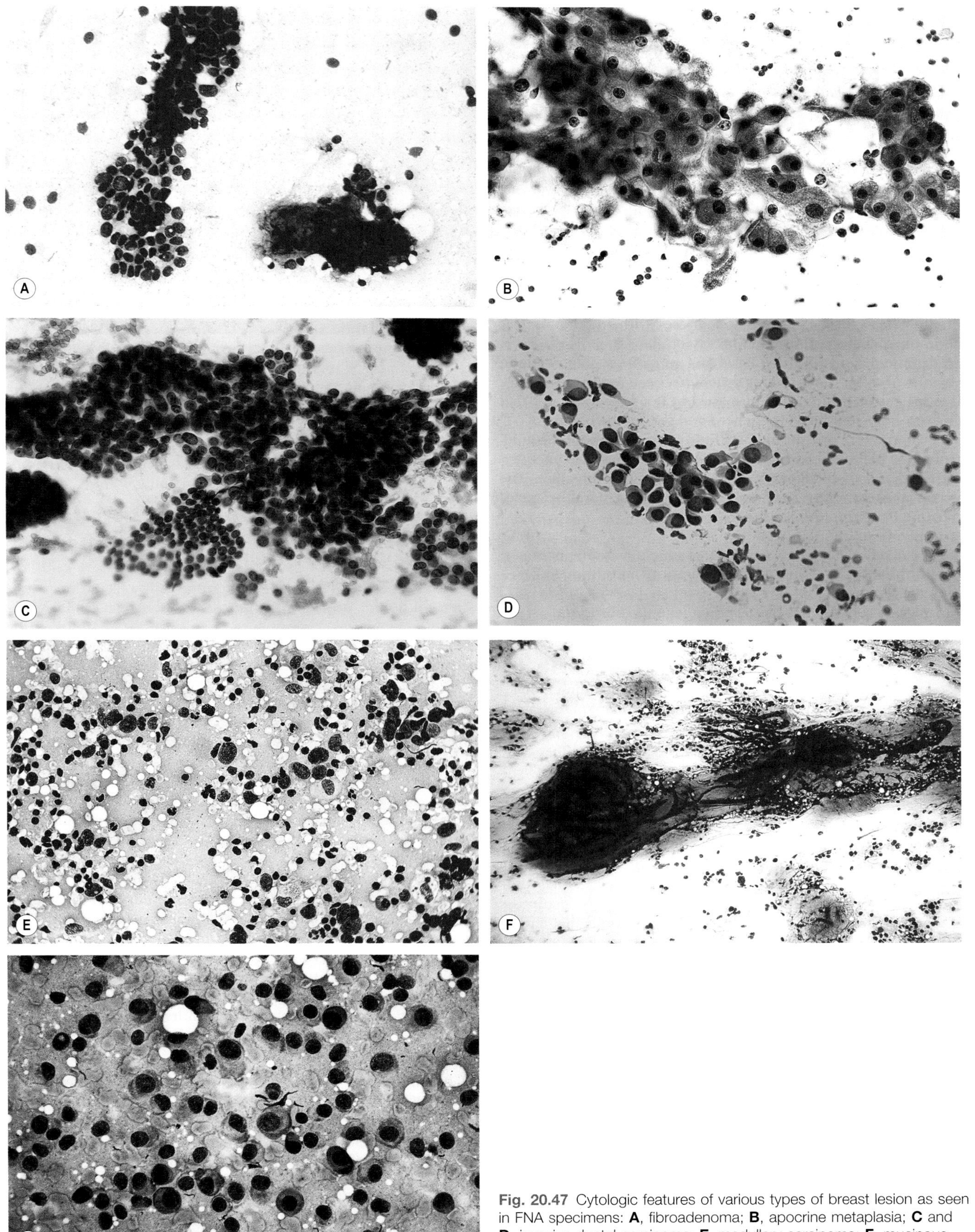

Fig. 20.47 Cytologic features of various types of breast lesion as seen in FNA specimens: **A**, fibroadenoma; **B**, apocrine metaplasia; **C** and **D**, invasive ductal carcinoma; **E**, medullary carcinoma; **F**, mucinous carcinoma; **G**, invasive lobular carcinoma.

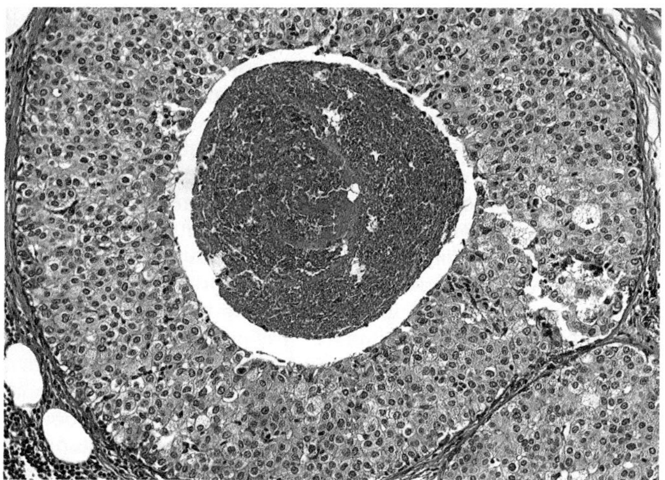

Fig. 20.49 In situ ductal carcinoma with comedo-type necrosis.

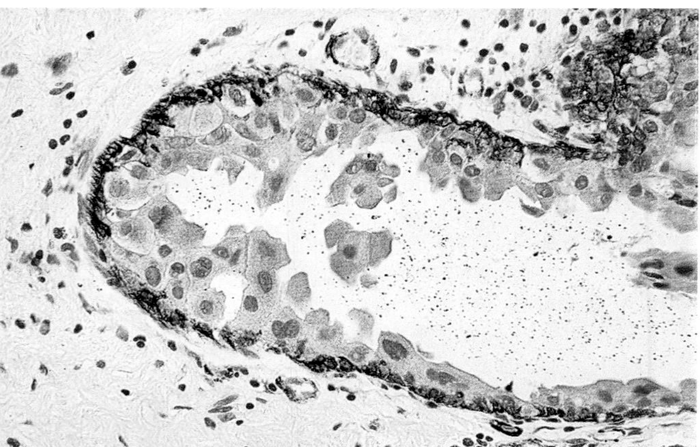

Fig. 20.50 Preservation of a myoepithelial cell layer in high-grade intraductal carcinoma. (Smooth muscle actin immunostain)

Comedocarcinoma

Comedocarcinoma may reach a relatively large size and become palpable. In one series, 28% were over 5 cm in diameter and another 33% were between 2 and 5 cm.[547] Over half of these tumors are centrally located, whereas this is true for less than 20% of invasive tumors.[545,559] The quoted incidence of multicentricity is approximately 33%,[533,541] and the incidence of bilaterality is 10%.[533]

Grossly, the tumor presents as a cluster of thick-walled ducts with normal breast parenchyma between them. When these ducts are compressed, plugs of necrotic tumor reminiscent grossly of those seen in comedones extrude from them, hence the name comedocarcinoma. If the duct walls are not thickened, the tumor may not be apparent grossly. Microscopically, the ducts show a solid growth of large pleomorphic tumor cells accompanied by generally abundant mitotic activity and lacking connective tissue support. Necrosis is always present and constitutes an important diagnostic sign, whether in the form of a large central focus or of individual tumor cells (Fig. 20.49). The mean diameter of the ducts containing necrosis is significantly larger than for those lacking this feature, suggesting the existence of a 'hypoxic compartment' in these tumors.[546] Coarse calcification often supervenes in these necrotic areas, and this can be identified by mammography. Myoepithelial cells usually surround ducts involved by comedocarcinoma[537] (Fig. 20.50). The stroma around the involved ducts shows a characteristic concentric fibrosis accompanied by a mild-to-moderate mononuclear inflammatory reaction, interpreted by some authors as evidence of tumor regression.[535]

Tumors with the classic comedocarcinoma appearance (or the grade 3 DCIS of other classifications) are characterized by aneuploidy, negativity for hormone receptors, metallothionein expression, c-*erb*B-2 overexpression, presence of P-cadherin, and a high frequency of *TP53* mutations.[529–532,538,540,543,544,550,552,553]

Once the diagnosis of comedocarcinoma has been established, two additional important determinations need to be made. The first is the degree of intraductal spread, which in some cases may be very extensive and even reach the nipple, resulting in Paget disease.[548,549] The other is to search for areas of definite stromal invasion and, if these are present, to estimate the relative amounts of in situ and invasive components[557] (Fig. 20.51). The term *extensive intraductal carcinoma* (EIC) has been proposed for tumors in which the intraductal component comprises 25% or more of the area encompassed by the infiltrating tumor and is also present in the surrounding breast tissue.[556] Interestingly, no correlation exists between the size of the tumor and the degree of invasion present in it.[557] Lagios et al.[541] found occult foci of invasion in 21% of their cases. Even if no definite invasion is detected in the sections examined, the possibility always exists with comedocarcinoma – more than with any other form of DCIS – that a minute focus of invasion is present somewhere in the specimen.[534] This may explain the fact that some patients have axillary lymph node metastases in the absence of an identifiable invasive component.[542,554] Another possible explanation is that the comedocarcinomatous areas themselves are actually invasive in a 'pushing' fashion, as suggested by the large size they sometimes attain, the ultrastructural demonstration of basement membrane defects,[551] the prominent fibrosis associated with stromal metachromasia usually found around them,[555] and the fact that neural invasion has been exceptionally demonstrated in them.[539,558] Although we find this hypothesis appealing at the conceptual level, for practical purposes we would advise designating these tumors as invasive only when irregular ('destructive') infiltration of the stroma is detected in them. Rarely, these foci of invasion are accompanied by a granulomatous tissue response.[536]

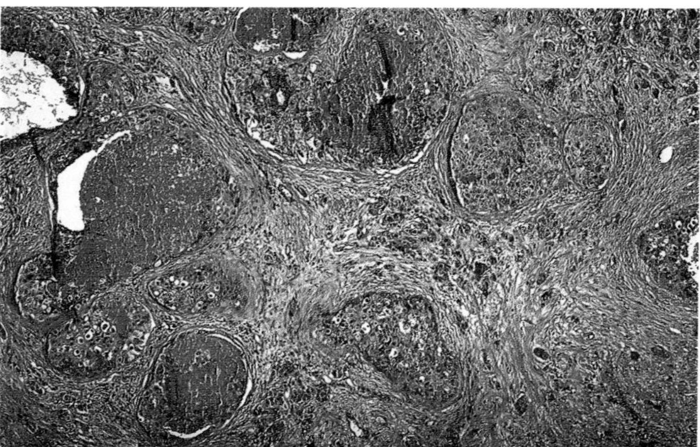

Fig. 20.51 Invasive ductal carcinoma associated with extensive intraductal carcinoma component.

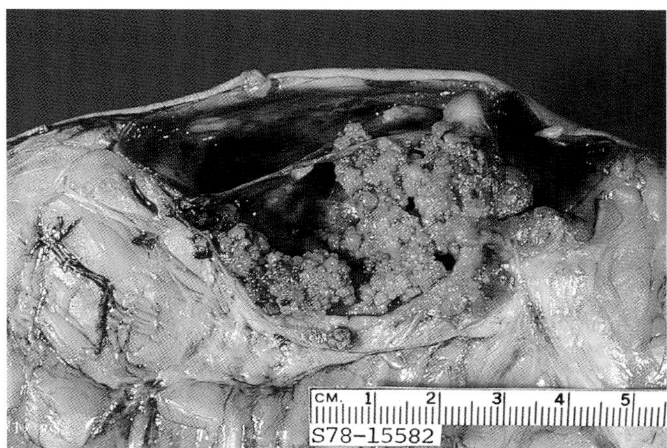

Fig. 20.52 Intracystic carcinoma of the breast. The papillary configuration of the tumor is already grossly evident.

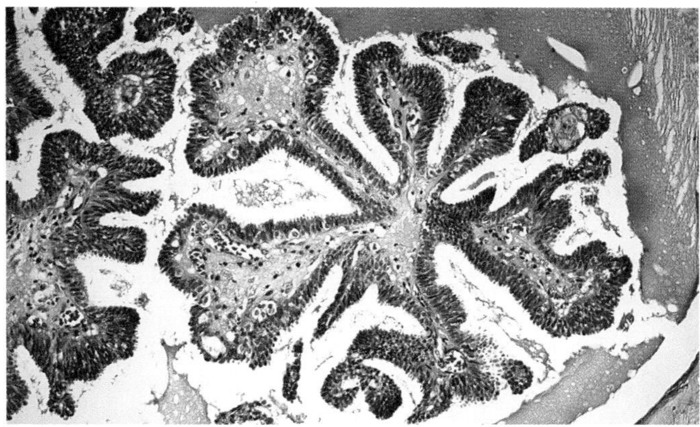

Fig. 20.54 In situ papillary carcinoma. The arborizing nature of this tumor and the stout fibrovascular core are not too different from those of a benign papilloma.

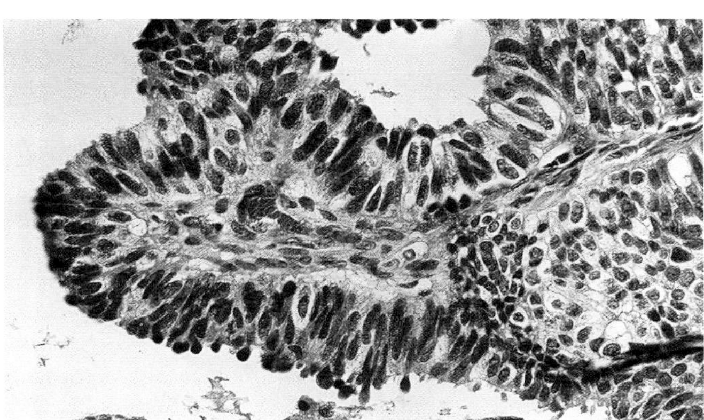

Fig. 20.53 High-power view of an in situ papillary carcinoma. Note the layering of cells, loss of nuclear polarity, marked hyperchromasia, and lack of a myoepithelial cell layer.

(In situ) papillary carcinoma

Papillary carcinoma makes up only a small percentage of breast carcinomas. Grossly, it may present as a well-circumscribed mass, or it may ramify within several ducts to involve an entire breast segment. In the variant known as *intracystic papillary carcinoma*, the tumor appears as a mural nodule within a large cystic space supposedly representing a dilated duct[561,565] (Fig. 20.52). The microscopic criteria for the diagnosis must be strict, because most papillary breast lesions are benign.[566,571] The most important differential features were listed in the classic study by Kraus and Neubecker[564] and further elaborated (and somewhat modified) by Azzopardi.[560] As a group, papillary carcinomas occur in an older age group and are larger than papillomas. Microscopically, features favoring carcinoma are (paradoxically) uniformity in size and shape of the epithelial cells (whether round, oval, or spindle, the latter arranged perpendicularly to the duct axis); presence of one cell type only (i.e., lack of myoepithelial cells); nuclear hyperchromasia and high nucleocytoplasmic ratio; high mitotic activity; lack of apocrine metaplasia, cribriform and trabecular patterns; scanty or absent stroma; and lack of benign proliferative disease in the adjacent breast[560,563,564] (Fig. 20.53).

It should be realized that no feature among those just listed is sufficient in itself to establish the distinction between papilloma and papillary carcinoma. The amount of stroma present could serve as an example of this fact; although scanty or nil in most papillary carcinomas, it may be bulky and well developed in others, prompting a mistaken diagnosis of benignancy (Fig. 20.54). Another diagnostic trap is provided by the presence of scattered large pale eosinophilic cells (known as clear or globoid cells) concentrated in the basilar portion, which can be mistaken for myoepithelial cells[564,567] (Fig. 20.55). Yet another is the so-called *solid variant* of papillary carcinoma (which is different from the solid form of DCIS, see below) and which shares many features with florid ductal hyperplasia. Immunohistochemically, strong and extensive positivity for keratin 5/6 favors the diagnosis of florid ductal hyperplasia over that of DCIS of any type.[569]

It seems likely that most papillary carcinomas arise de novo. In some cases, however, there is convincing morphologic and immunohistochemical evidence for the carcinoma arising inside multiple papillomas.[568] In keeping with their presumed in-situ nature, encapsulated papillary carcinomas are coated by a basement membrane, evidenced with collagen IV or laminin stains.[562]

Papillary carcinoma with invasion is discussed on page 1702.

A very unusual type of papillary carcinoma has been described composed of *transitional-type epithelium*, to be distinguished from the conventional papillary carcinoma and from adnexal-type tumors, such as eccrine acrospiroma (see p. 1722). Another very unusual form is the *encapsulated apocrine papillary carcinoma*, a low-grade lesion with an excellent prognosis.[570]

Other forms

In the *solid* form of DCIS, the glandular lumen is filled by the proliferation of medium-sized cells, which are larger than those of LCIS but smaller and more uniform than those of comedocarcinoma[586] (Fig. 20.56). Azzopardi[573] pointed out the sharp cell edges (as opposed to a 'syncytial' quality) and the pallor of the cytoplasm (as opposed to prominent acidophilia) often exhibited by these cells. In the *cribriform* variety, round regular spaces are formed within the glands; the more regular these spaces are in terms of distribution, size, and shape, the more likely the lesion is to be malignant (Fig. 20.57). These spaces are often associated with two formations of similar pathogenesis, designated by Azzopardi[573] as trabecular bars and Roman bridges, respectively. Trabecular bars are rigid rows of

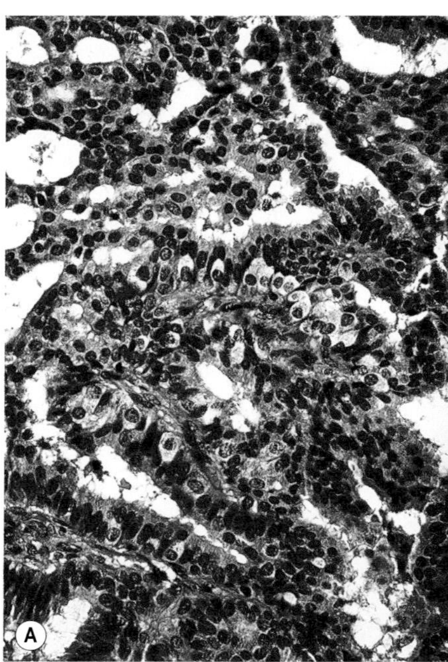

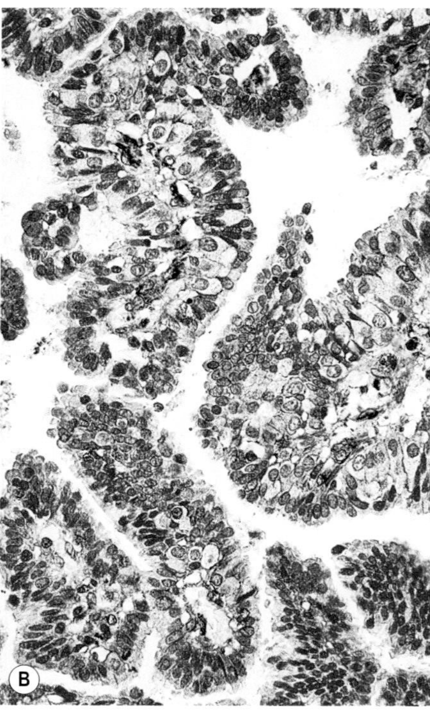

Fig. 20.55 **A** and **B**, Papillary carcinoma with so-called 'globoid' or 'clear cells'. These cells, which are immunoreactive for GCDFP-15, should not be confused with myoepithelial cells. **B**, Negative immunostain for smooth muscle actin.

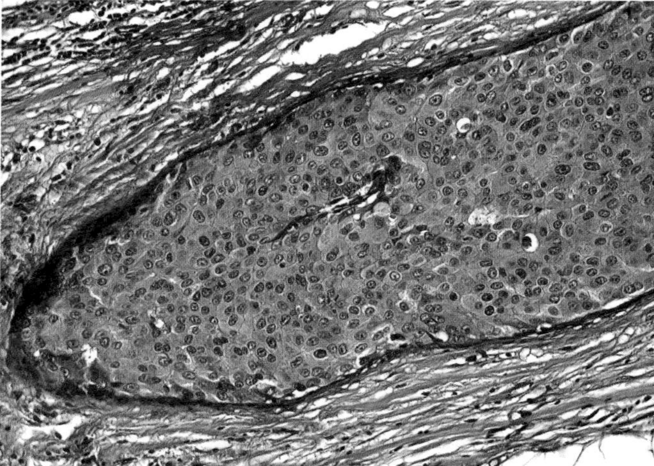

Fig. 20.56 Solid type of in situ ductal carcinoma. There is no necrosis.

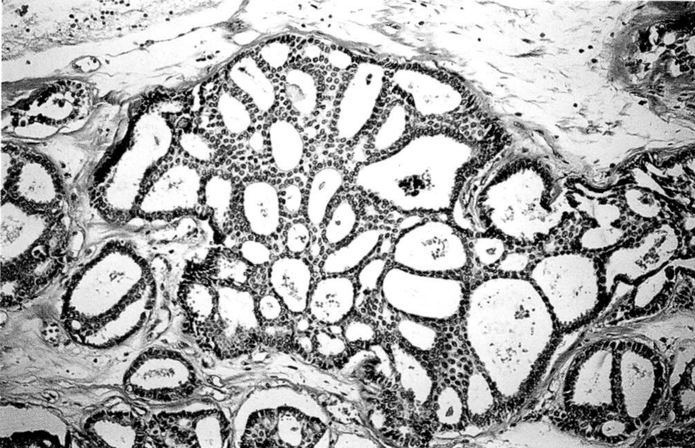

Fig. 20.57 Low-grade in situ ductal carcinoma of cribriform type.

cells with their long axes arranged more or less perpendicular (or at least not parallel) to the long axis of the bar; these should be distinguished from partial detachments of the duct lining (Fig. 20.58). Roman bridges are curvilinear trabecular bars connecting two portions of the epithelial lining. The cribriform pattern of DCIS should not be equated with that of adenoid cystic carcinoma (see p. 1722).

The *micropapillary* variety (more closely connected to the preceding types of DCIS than to conventional papillary carcinoma) shows elongated epithelial projections projecting into the glandular lumen; these lack connective tissue support, may have a space at the base, and often show a bulbous expansion at the tip (Fig. 20.59). This variant is more likely than others to involve multiple quadrants of the breast.[574]

Clinging carcinoma, the more controversial member of this family, shows one or two layers of malignant cells lining a glandular formation with a large empty lumen.[573,591] In the more easily recognizable (high-grade) forms, the tumor cells are large, highly atypical, and associated with individual cell necrosis, features which suggest a link with comedocarcinoma (Fig. 20.60). In other instances, the tumor cells are smaller and more regular; these have been interpreted as being related to the low-grade forms of intraductal carcinoma, particularly the micropapillary variety. Indeed, some authors refer to this as the 'flat' variant of micropapillary in situ carcinoma.

The *cystic hypersecretory* form is a variation of DCIS characterized by cystic formations induced by the abundant secretory material present; although hardly a distinct entity, it deserves mention because of the ease with which it can be confused with a benign process.[581,590,592]

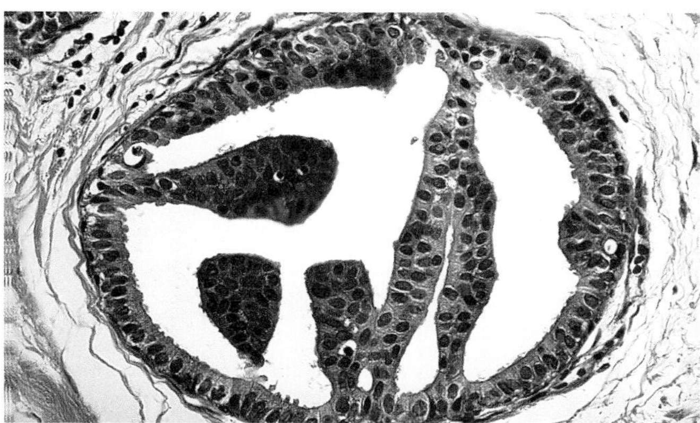

Fig. 20.58 Trabecular bars in intraductal carcinoma. Note the perpendicular arrangement of the nuclei in relation to the long axis of the bars.

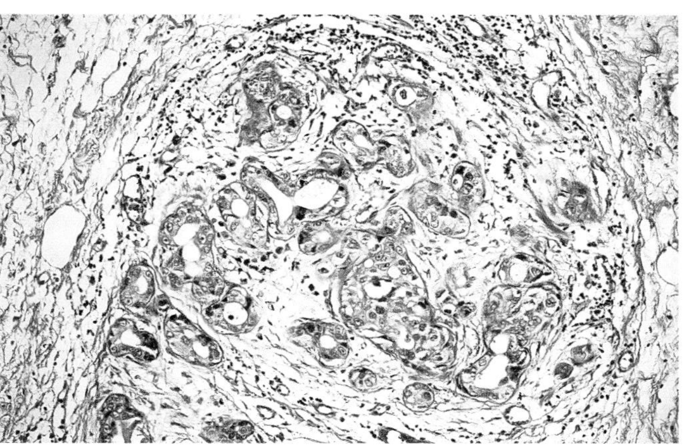

Fig. 20.61 So-called 'lobular cancerization'. The lobule is markedly expanded and composed of relatively large tumor cells with the appearance of ductal-type carcinoma. Typical ductal carcinoma was present elsewhere in the specimen.

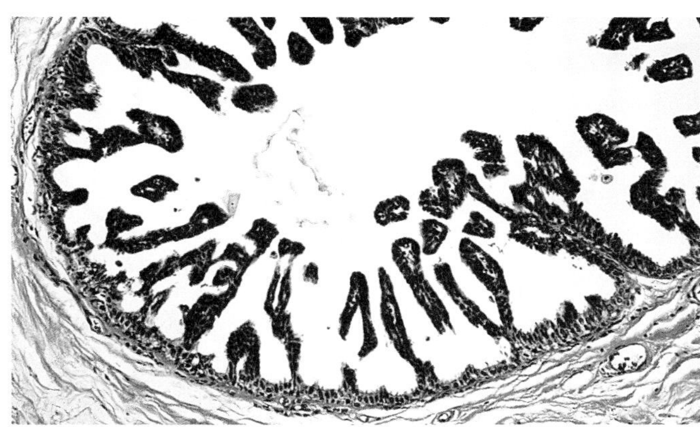

Fig. 20.59 Micropapillary carcinoma of breast. Some of the papillae lack a central fibrovascular core.

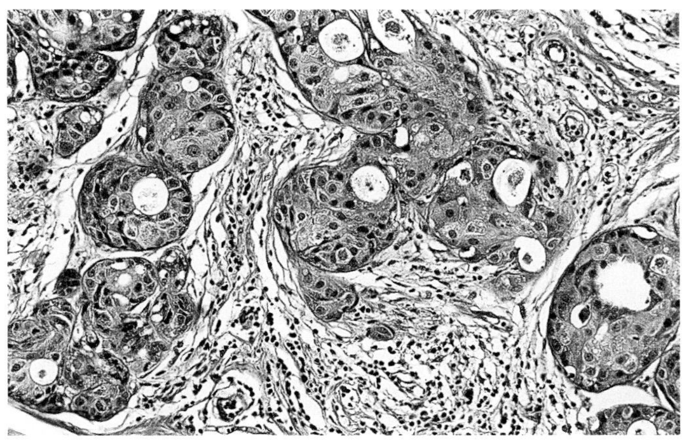

Fig. 20.62 Apocrine variant of in situ ductal carcinoma.

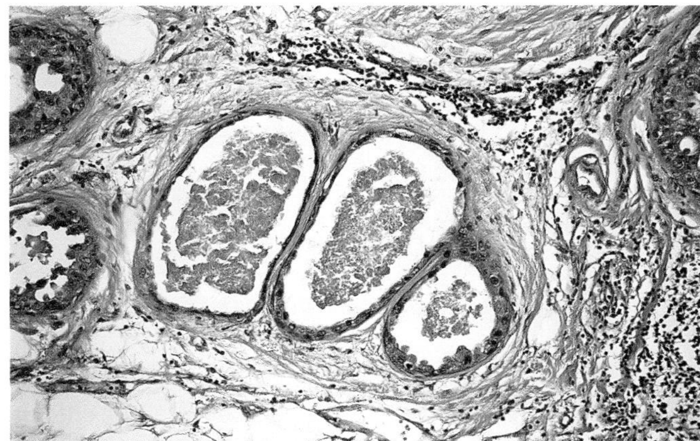

Fig. 20.60 Ductal carcinoma in situ of so-called 'clinging type'. One or two layers of atypical cells line dilated glandular structures containing granular intraluminal material in which ghosts of tumor cells are identified.

Adding to the complexity of the situation is the pattern traditionally known as *lobular cancerization*.[572,579] The term refers to the presence, in a structure easily identifiable as a lobule, of carcinoma with the cytoarchitectural features of DCIS (Fig. 20.61). The change was first described in connection with the high-grade (comedocarcinoma) form, but it was later realized that it could also be seen with the low-grade types. As the name indicates, the original assumption was that this represented a secondary extension into a lobule of a carcinoma of ductal origin, particularly when this was found associated with a conventional DCIS such as comedocarcinoma. This interpretation is probably erroneous. The available evidence suggests that this phenomenon represents instead a variation in the growth pattern of DCIS in which the structure involved is still easily recognizable as belonging to a lobule. Further evidence for the basic unity of these various manifestations comes from the occasional occurrence of DCIS and LCIS in the same TDLU.[589]

Rare additional morphologic variations of DCIS include cases with *signet ring cells*[580] (Fig. 20.62), with *multinucleated giant cells*,[576] with *apocrine-type cytology*,[584,587,594] with *squamous features* (squamous cell carcinoma in situ[582]) and those with evidence of *(neuro)endocrine differentiation*.[577] The latter tumor, known as **(neuro)endocrine**

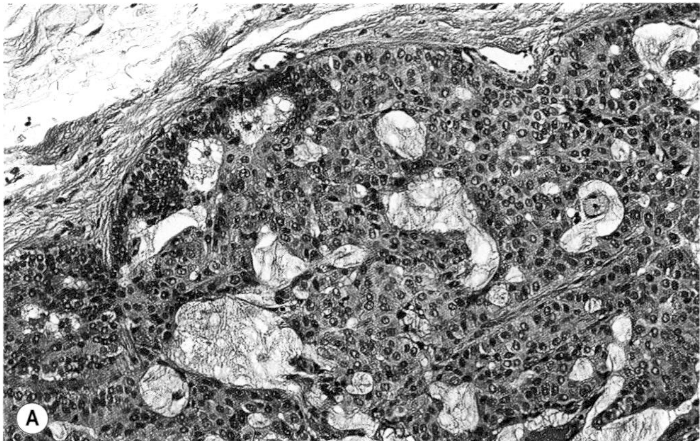

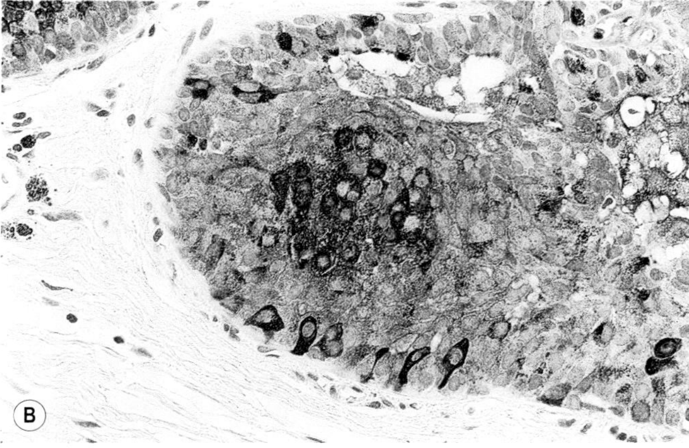

Fig. 20.63 Endocrine-type ductal carcinoma in situ: **A**, hematoxylin–eosin; **B**, chromogranin.

DCIS (E-DCIS), is often accompanied by adjacent intraductal papillomas with pagetoid involvement by the carcinoma.[595] Key features for its recognition include the presence of endocrine-type festoons and rosettes, mucin deposition, bland-looking spindle to ovoid nuclei (an important diagnostic clue[593]), and abundant granular eosinophilic cytoplasm (Fig. 20.63A). The solid islands of tumor in E-DCIS are frequently traversed by delicate fibrovascular septa.[583] Necrosis is usually absent, and neuroendocrine markers such as chromogranin and synaptophysin can be demonstrated[595] (Fig. 20.63B). Sometimes these tumors are accompanied by an invasive component, which is also of neuroendocrine type. This tumor is probably closely related to the lesion that has been described as *spindle cell DCIS*.[578]

A feature of diagnostic importance common to all forms of DCIS (although better developed in the comedocarcinoma type) is the appearance of the luminal content. The presence of nuclear debris, ghosts of dead cell outlines, granular and fragmented products, and inspissated densely stained material should raise suspicion and prompt a thorough search for more diagnostic areas.[573]

Immunohistochemically, two important features of DCIS (particularly in relation to the differential diagnosis with LCIS) are the presence of E-cadherin and the scantiness or absence of HMW keratin (as detected with keratin 5/6 or 34βE12).[575] In addition, the high-grade form of DCIS also shows P-cadherin expression.[588]

The molecular genetic analyses that have been done so far in DCIS and ADH have given confusing and sometimes contradictory results. Suffice it to say that, on the whole, they suggest that genetic alterations may occur very early in breast tumorigenesis, prior to detectable morphologic changes, and that the interaction between epithelium and stroma may play an important role in tumor progression.[585]

Evolution

The assumed implication of the diagnosis of DCIS is that, if left untreated, the lesion will inevitably progress to an invasive carcinoma of similar morphologic features. This is a gross and inaccurate oversimplification of a very complex situation. These are some of the reasonably established facts:

1. The transformation to an invasive phenotype does not occur in all cases, at least during the normal life span of an individual.[609]
2. When such a transformation occurs, the process usually evolves over a period of years if not decades.[609]
3. There is a substantial difference in the frequency with which this phenomenon occurs depending on the type of DCIS: high for comedocarcinoma and low (but still significant) for all the others.[598,600,611,614] This can also be expressed by saying that the risk for the development of invasive carcinoma is directly proportional to the cytologic grade of the tumor.[606]
4. There is a definite relationship between the microscopic type of DCIS and the invasive component, much more so than for LCIS; however, numerous exceptions occur.[603]
5. Not all invasive breast carcinomas go through the sequence just described; some (perhaps the majority) have a very short intraductal stage and become invasive long before being detectable by any technique. It is this very fact that takes some of the value away from screening techniques such as mammography, which are much more likely to detect slow-growing carcinomas with a prolonged in situ stage.

The most informative data on which these conclusions are based derive from retrospective studies on DCIS that were treated by biopsy only.[599,605,608,612] In the series of Page et al.,[608] 7 of 25 patients with DCIS of non-comedocarcinoma type whose cases had been followed for over 3 years developed homolateral invasive breast carcinoma. In an earlier and smaller series by Betsill et al.,[596] invasive carcinoma had developed in 6 of the 10 patients for whom follow-up information was available. In a large series of patients treated with biopsy and local breast irradiation, it was found that comedo-type necrosis and uncertain/involved surgical margins were the best predictors of recurrence.[601,602]

When mastectomy is done within 6 months after the identification of DCIS by biopsy, the incidence of invasive carcinoma in the mastectomy specimen was 6% in one series[610] and 18% in another.[597] Interestingly, residual DCIS was found in 60% of the specimens, a different quadrant being involved in 33% of them.[610] At present, the most common form of treatment of DCIS is local (breast-conserving) surgery with or without irradiation, but there are some patients for whom mastectomy is indicated.[604,607,613]

Lobular carcinoma in situ (LCIS)

Lobular CIS, also known as lobular neoplasia, has no distinguishing features on gross examination and is usually found incidentally in breasts removed for other reasons. It is multicentric in approximately 70% of cases[645] and bilateral in approximately 30–40%.[622] Most cases are found within 5 cm of the nipple from the skin surface in either the outer or inner upper quadrants.[634,636] Residual

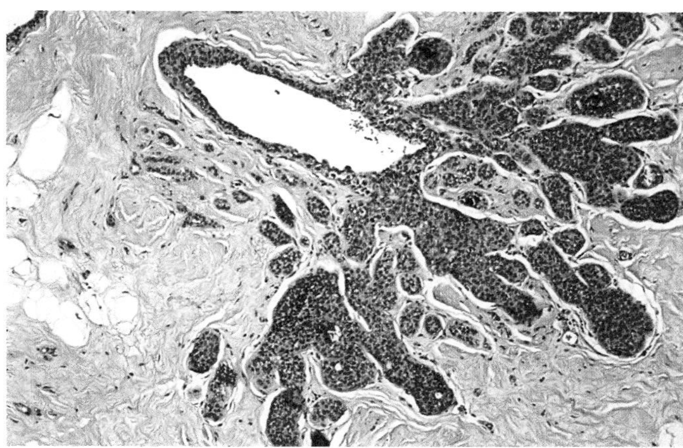

Fig. 20.64 Typical pattern of involvement of terminal duct–lobular unit by lobular carcinoma in situ.

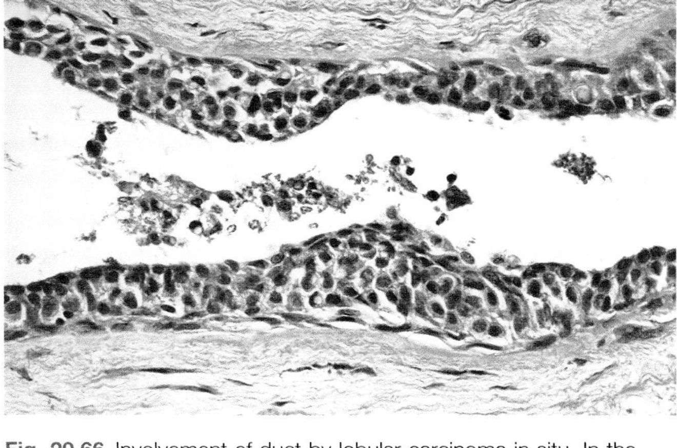

Fig. 20.66 Involvement of duct by lobular carcinoma in situ. In the presence of such change, a thorough search for typical areas of lobular involvement should be undertaken.

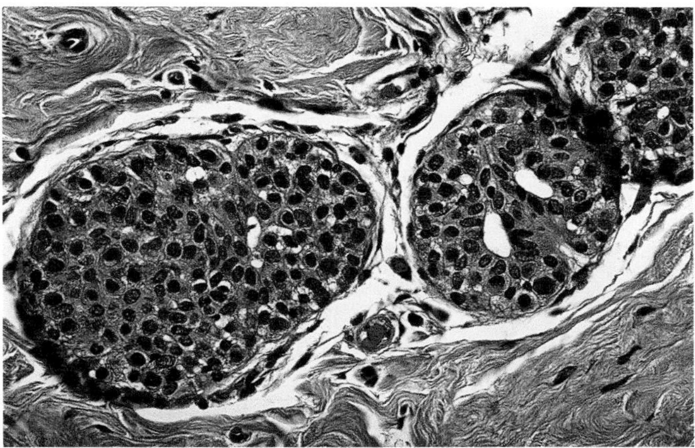

Fig. 20.65 Marked expansion of a lobular unit by lobular carcinoma in situ. A few small spaces are still present in the smaller focus.

tumor foci are found in 60% of breasts removed following a diagnosis of LCIS made from a biopsy specimen.[639]

Microscopically, the lobules are distended and completely filled by relatively uniform, round, small-to-medium-sized cells with round and normochromatic (or only mildly hyperchromatic) nuclei.[632] In the typical case, atypia, pleomorphism, mitotic activity, and necrosis are minimal or absent, and there is some lack of cohesiveness among the tumor cells[641,646] (Figs 20.64 and 20.65). Any of the following minor morphologic variations can occur, singly or in combination: moderate nuclear pleomorphism, larger nuclear size, appreciable mitotic activity, scattered signet ring cells (relatively common), apocrine changes (exceptional), focal necrosis,[626] and variations in the shape of the involved lobules.[620,624,631,639] When the tumor cells are of medium to large size, with moderate to marked pleomorphism, occasional prominent nucleoli, and moderate to abundant cytoplasm, the lesion is referred to as *pleomorphic LCIS*.[643]

In LCIS, the neighboring terminal ducts often exhibit proliferation of cells similar to those involving the lobules. These cells may form a continuous row beneath the secretory epithelium, a pattern that has been referred to as *mural* or *pagetoid* (Fig. 20.66); they can also grow in a solid, cribriform, or micropapillary fashion.[628,645] Occasionally, this change extends to larger (lactiferous) ducts, but Paget disease practically never occurs.[640] The presence of these ductal changes is of histogenetic interest and sometimes the first clue for the existence of typical LCIS nearby, but it does not carry prognostic implications of its own.[617]

LCIS can also be found in fibroadenomas[630] and in foci of sclerosing adenosis[629] or collagenous spherulosis.[642] The diagnosis of LCIS (or whatever equivalent term one might like to use) should be made only in those cases in which the cellular proliferation has resulted in the formation of solid nests that have expanded the lobules, whereas the designation of lobular hyperplasia (preceded by the qualifier 'atypical') is to be given to those lesions accompanied by normal-sized lobules in which central lumina are still identifiable. LCIS should also be distinguished from DCIS, particularly the form traditionally known as lobular cancerization and already discussed on page 1689. The latter is identified by the fact that its cytoarchitectural features are those of one of the forms of DCIS, usually comedocarcinoma. When the latter is the case, there is obvious cellular pleomorphism, atypical nuclear configuration, formation of small lumina, and necrosis.[616,627]

The only conventional special stains of some significance for the evaluation of LCIS are those for mucin, which show positivity in scattered tumor cells in about three-fourths of cases.[618,620] Immunohistochemically, the tumor cells show positivity for keratin, EMA, milk fat globule membrane antigen, and COX-2.[625,637] S-100 protein is demonstrable in 60% of cases.[623] Ultrastructural study or immunohistochemistry for any of the myoepithelial cell markers (see p. 1660) will show residual myoepithelial cells, which may lie flat on the basement membrane, perpendicular to it, or admixed with the tumor cells; the latter do not have myoepithelial features themselves.[621,644] Laminin and collagen type IV can be demonstrated in the underlying basement membrane.

From the point of view of the differential diagnosis with DCIS, the two most important immunohistochemical features of LCIS are the lack of reactivity for E-cadherin and β-catenin, and the positivity for HMW keratin.[635] The latter, demonstrated with 34βE12, often shows a distinctive perinuclear pattern. By contrast, DCIS is consistently positive for E-cadherin and β-catenin, and shows significantly reduced or absent HMW keratin.[615] As expected, the cases with hybrid or intermediate features also show hybrid immunohistochemical features, as manifested by either positivity or negativity for *both* markers.[619,633] The loss of E-cadherin in LCIS is due to gene mutations, which are, however, different from those of the invasive lobular component when present.[638]

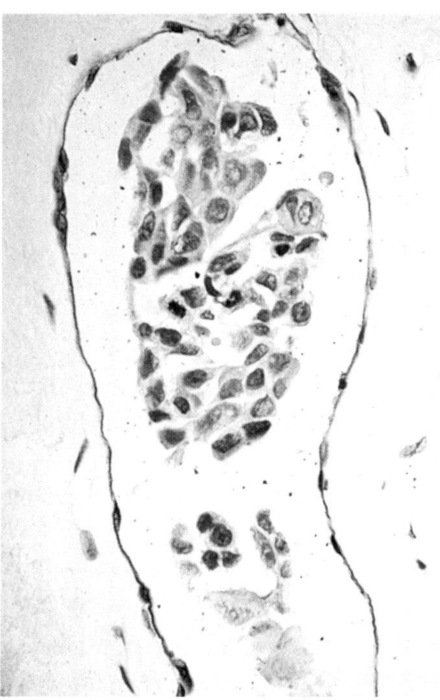

Fig. 20.70 Vascular invasion by breast carcinoma demonstrated by positivity of endothelial cells for *Ulex europaeus* lectin I.

squamous metaplasia) are also immunoreactive for HMW (epidermal-type) keratin.[703] In addition to EMA (which also stains carcinomas of most other sites), the cells of breast carcinoma are reactive for an apparently more organ-specific antigen obtained from milk fat globule membrane.[678] Close to 70% of cases are positive for lactalbumin, another marker almost entirely restricted to mammary epithelium.[671,685]

Two other important breast-related markers are mammaglobin and GCDFP-15, the former being more sensitive but less specific than the latter.[665,690,705]

CEA, B72.3, and BCA-225 are positive in the majority of cases.[684,687,696,698,702] Vimentin may also be expressed,[672] sometimes together with glial fibrillary acidic protein (GFAP).[677] Breast carcinomas can be immunoreactive for S-100 protein, the proportion ranging from 10% to 45% in the various reported series;[673,688] this is a fact to remember in the differential diagnosis of metastatic tumors to axillary nodes, lest a breast carcinoma be mislabeled as metastatic melanoma. Even more treacherous is the fact that some cases may show positivity for HMB-45[667] and TTF-1.[697] An increased expression of the bone matrix proteins osteonectin and osteopontin has been documented, with the added suggestion that this may play a role in the bone homing of breast carcinoma metastases.[664,679] The basement membrane components laminin and collagen IV show a discontinuous linear pattern or are altogether absent, in contrast to the continuous pattern they exhibit in the intraductal lesions.[670,704,706] An increased amount of type V collagen is found in the desmoplastic stroma.[662] Actin and related stains are negative, confirming the absence of myoepithelial cells around the tumor nests. A small number of carcinomas show focal reactivity for human chorionic gonadotrophin (hCG), SP-1 or other placental proteins,[683] chromogranin,[668] or lactoferrin.[669]

The reported increased expression of T and Tn antigens[666,680] and an antigen related to mouse mammary tumor virus[691] have not found confirmation in subsequent studies.

Tubular carcinoma. Tubular carcinoma has also been designated as well-differentiated carcinoma, but the latter term is not advisable because it has also been used for other well-differentiated tumors with different patterns of growth. The average age of the patients is about 50 years.[727] Grossly, tubular carcinoma suggests malignancy by virtue of its poorly circumscribed margins and hard consistency. It is characteristically small, with a mean diameter of about 1 cm.[720,723] Microscopically, it simulates a benign condition (particularly radial scar and microglandular adenosis) because of the well-differentiated nature of the glands, absence of necrosis or mitoses, and scanty pleomorphism.[721] The clues to the diagnosis are the haphazard arrangement of the glands in the stroma with absence of any organoid configuration; frequent invasion of fat at the periphery of the lesion; cellular (but often also elastotic[726]) nature of the stroma; irregular and often angulated contours of the glands; open lumina with basophilic secretion; apocrine-type 'snouts' in the apical cytoplasm; formation of trabecular bars; lack of a myoepithelial cell component (well appreciated in immunostained preparations for p63 and CD10[711]); lack of basement membrane (well seen with an immunostain for type IV collagen); and occurrence in two-thirds or more of the cases of typical DCIS in ducts within or outside the lesion, nearly always of low-grade (micropapillary or cribriform) type[709,715,719,720,727] (Fig. 20.71). Regarding the latter feature, low-grade DCIS and flat epithelial atypia are thought to be precursor lesions of tubular carcinoma.[707,717]

Because of the marked degree of cellular differentiation, it is not unusual for these tumors to be underdiagnosed as fibroadenoma or some other benign process on FNA material.[710] They are better recognized in needle core preparations.

Ultrastructurally, the degree of ductal differentiation is striking, but myoepithelial cells and basement membrane are lacking.[714,716] A high incidence of multicentricity (56%), history of bilateral breast carcinoma (38%), and family history of breast carcinoma (40%) were found by Lagios et al.[718] in a series of 17 tubular carcinomas. At the molecular genetic level, tubular carcinoma shows several differences with invasive ductal carcinoma NOS.[728]

Metastases to axillary nodes occur in approximately 10% of cases,[709,712,720] and the prognosis is excellent.[713] In the series of McDivitt et al.,[720] only 4% of their 135 patients developed recurrent

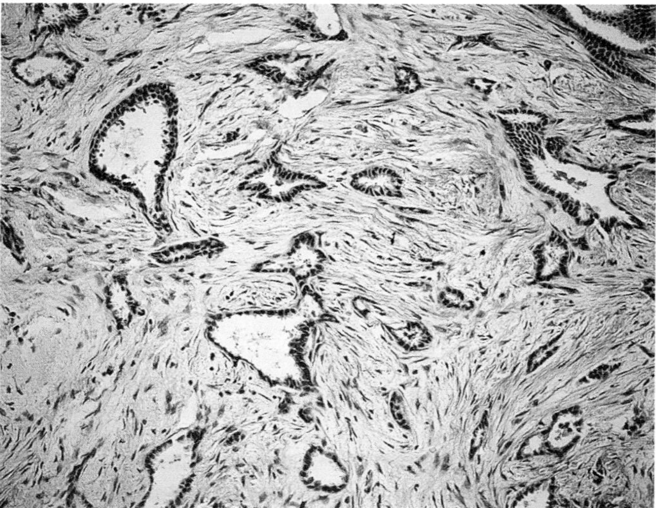

Fig. 20.71 Tubular carcinoma of breast. The angulated shape of the glands and the cellular stroma are characteristic of this lesion.

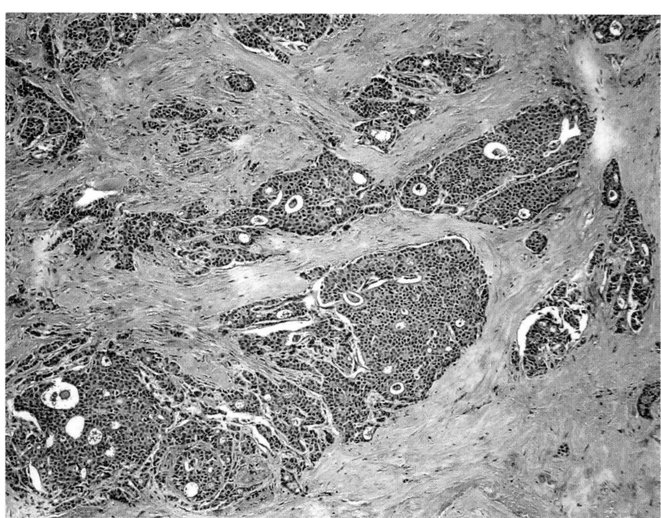

Fig. 20.72 Invasive cribriform carcinoma. Some of the nodules have a predominantly solid appearance.

or metastatic disease during a mean follow-up period of 7.2 years. The recurrence rate after local excision is as high as 50%.[712]

Sometimes, a tubular carcinoma pattern is seen in association with an ordinary invasive ductal carcinoma. The prognosis of these 'mixed' tumors is substantially worse than for pure tubular carcinoma,[708,712,722] although better than for the ordinary invasive ductal carcinoma, at least when the tubular component represents the dominant element.[708,712] It is likely that series of tubular carcinomas in which the incidence of nodal metastases is high include a high proportion of these 'mixed' carcinomas.[724,725]

The tumor type known as tubulolobular carcinoma is discussed on page 1710.

Cribriform carcinoma. Invasive cribriform carcinoma is a rare form of breast malignancy closely related to tubular carcinoma and sharing with it an excellent prognosis.[729,731] As the name indicates, the tumor has a cribriform appearance similar to that seen in the more common in situ counterpart, but it also exhibits stromal invasion (Fig. 20.72). This pattern is often seen in association with tubular formations, the relative proportion of the two elements determining the term used, according to the scheme proposed by Page et al.[729] The most important aspect of this concept is the realization that a breast carcinoma can be cribriform throughout yet invasive; we have seen examples of this tumor extensively invading the breast and beyond and being called in situ tumors simply because they had a cribriform pattern. The proposal has been made for the existence of yet another variation on the theme, in which the tumor has a similar invasive pattern and cytology but a solid configuration (*solid variant* of invasive cribriform carcinoma).[730]

Mucinous carcinoma. Mucinous carcinoma, also known as mucoid, colloid, or gelatinous carcinoma, usually occurs in postmenopausal women.[737,751] Grossly, it is well circumscribed, crepitant to palpation, and formed by a currant jelly-like mass held together by delicate septa (Fig. 20.73). Foci of hemorrhage are frequent. Microscopically, the classic and often quoted description is that of small clusters of tumor cells 'floating in a sea of mucin' (Fig. 20.74). These clusters may be solid, exhibit acinar formations, or form micropapillary structures.[733] The mucin is almost entirely extracellular, and it may be of acid or neutral type.[763] Occasionally, mucinous carcinoma will consist almost entirely of mucin, and a thorough sampling will be necessary to detect the neoplastic

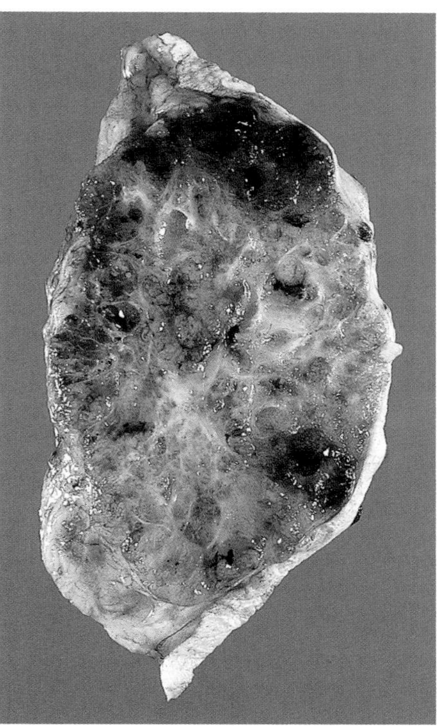

Fig. 20.73 Typical gelatinous gross appearance of pure mucinous carcinoma. Note the sharply circumscribed quality of the tumor. *(Courtesy of Dr RA Cooke, Brisbane, Australia. From Cooke RA, Stewart B. Colour atlas of anatomical pathology. Edinburgh, 2004, Churchill Livingstone)*

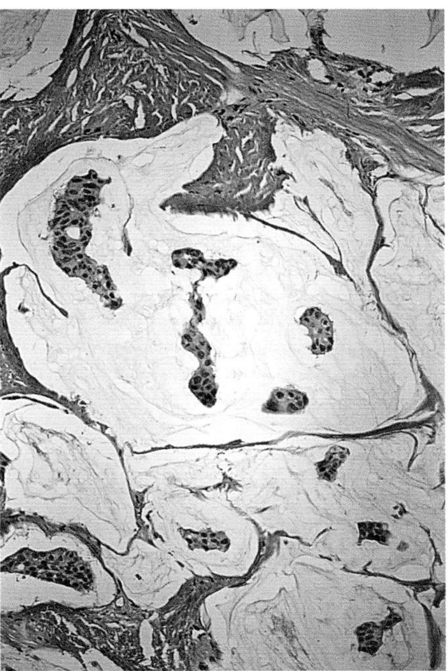

Fig. 20.74 Mucinous carcinoma of the breast. Clusters of well-differentiated tumor cells are seen floating in a sea of mucin.

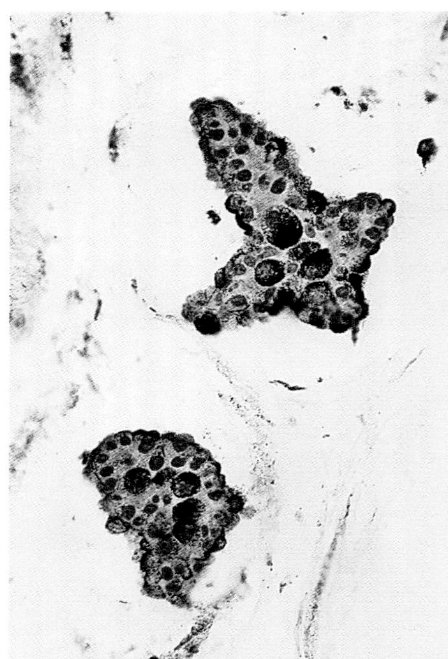

Fig. 20.75 Argyrophilic cells present in another case of mucinous carcinoma of the breast, indicative of neuroendocrine differentiation. (Sevier–Munger stain)

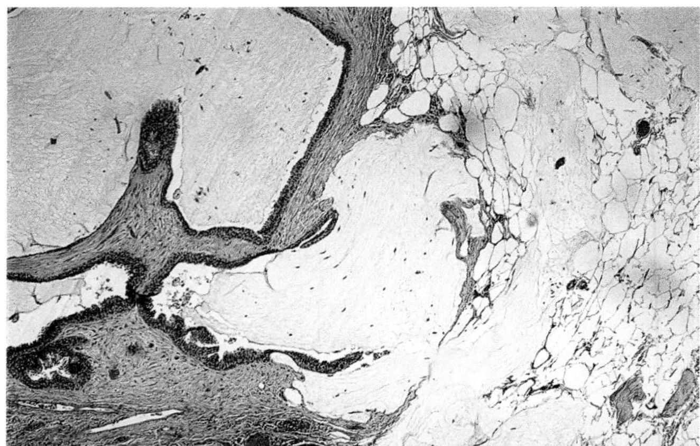

Fig. 20.76 Early form of mucin-producing low-grade carcinoma showing the mechanism of formation of the epithelial strips typically seen floating in the mucin.

epithelium.[757] An easily recognizable in situ component is usually absent or inconspicuous (but see later section). Histochemically, the mucins secreted by this tumor are distinct *O*-acylated forms of sialomucins.[759] Immunohistochemically, there is strong MUC2 cytoplasmic immunoreactivity and decreased MUC1 immunoreactivity compared with ductal carcinoma NOS.[750,752] Both pure and mixed mucinous carcinomas of the breast often express WT1, a potentially diagnostic trap.[741] Hormone receptors are always positive, while c-*erb*B-2 is almost always negative.[748]

Interestingly, about a fourth to nearly half of mucinous carcinomas show features consistent with endocrine differentiation, such as argyrophilia (Fig. 20.75), neuron-specific enolase (NSE) immunoreactivity, and the presence of dense-core secretory granules by ultrastructural examination.[734,743,745,755] This unexpected finding has raised the possibility of a link between mucinous carcinoma and the breast neoplasm originally described as carcinoid tumor (see p. 1703).[743,764] Some authors have suggested the existence of two types of mucinous carcinoma on the basis of the absence or presence of endocrine differentiation, which they have designated as A and B, respectively.[734] Others have found that the variability of morphologic and ultrastructural features within these tumors precludes a sharp segregation,[738,742] or that such segregation has no influence on survival.[760] A recent gene expression profiling study shows that type B mucinous carcinomas and neuroendocrine carcinomas are part of a spectrum of lesions, whereas type A mucinous carcinoma is a discrete entity.[764]

On analysis of the immunohistochemical and array-based comparative genomic hybridization (CGH) profile, pure mucinous carcinomas are homogeneous and cluster together, separately from invasive ductal carcinoma NOS.[748] They less frequently harbor gains of 1q and 16p and losses of 16q and 22q than grade- and ER-matched invasive ductal carcinomas NOS.

It is important for prognostic reasons, and perhaps useful histogenetically, to restrict the term mucinous carcinoma to breast neoplasms exhibiting this feature throughout ('pure' mucinous carcinomas) and to exclude: (1) the 'impure' or 'mixed' tumors in which the mucinous pattern is admixed with an ordinary invasive ductal carcinoma[753,761] (these having a prognosis analogous to the latter, although interestingly the molecular profile of these 'mixed' tumors shows more similarities to pure mucinous carcinomas than invasive ductal carcinomas NOS);[748] and (2) signet ring carcinomas (see p. 1709), even if technically speaking these are also 'mucinous' tumors. Along these lines, it should be pointed out that some degree of mucin production can be identified in over 60% of breast carcinomas. The distinctiveness of signet ring carcinoma resides in the fact that nearly all of it remains within the cell (possibly because of a blockage in secretion), and the uniqueness of mucinous carcinoma is that most of it is extracellular (see later section). In contrast to large bowel and other sites, a combination of these two patterns is very rare in the breast.

Pure mucinous carcinoma is associated with a very low incidence (2–4%) of nodal metastases.[740,751,754] The higher incidence reported in other series is probably attributable to the inclusion of 'mixed' mucinous tumors. Consequently, the pure form of mucinous carcinoma carries an excellent short-term prognosis, particularly when the tumor measures less than 3 cm (or even less than 5 cm) in diameter.[737,751] However, it has been shown that deaths from this tumor can occur 12 years or more after therapy, indicating the need for long-term follow-up.[737,758] As already indicated, several groups found no prognostic difference between the mucinous carcinomas with endocrine-like features and those without,[755] although others claim that the former are associated with favorable histologic and immunohistochemical parameters.[762]

Pure mucinous carcinoma is generally regarded as an invasive type of tumor. We would like to offer an alternative point of view, i.e., that this neoplasm is partially – and sometimes entirely – a form of in situ ductal carcinoma in which some component of the mucin secretion detaches the epithelium from the underlying stroma, breaks it up in strips and nests, and engulfs it (Fig. 20.76). This process may be facilitated by an 'inversion of polarity' of the mucin secretion toward the base of the cell rather than the luminal border, as shown ultrastructurally, which is actually part of a field change.[732,752] The implication is that it is the mucin, rather than the tumor cells, that is 'invading' the stroma, in a fashion analogous to that often seen in mucinous tumors of the appendix. This would explain not only the excellent prognosis of pure mucinous

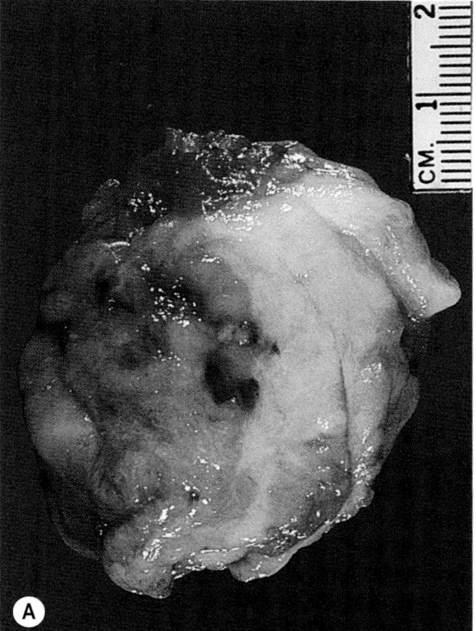

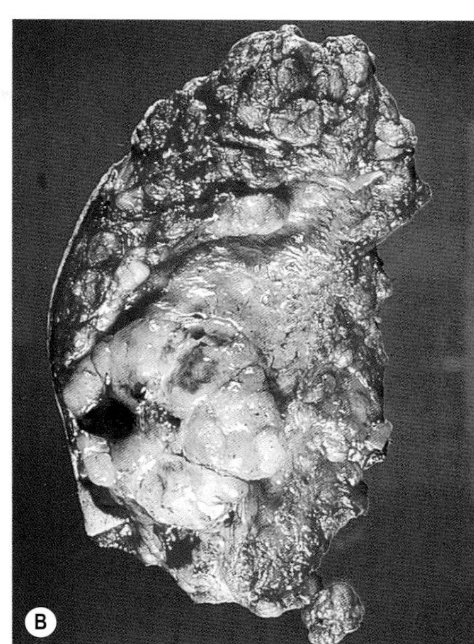

Fig. 20.77 **A** and **B**, Gross appearance of medullary carcinoma. Note the well-circumscribed character and fleshy appearance.

carcinoma but also the seemingly paradoxic fact that nearly all the mucin produced by this tumor is extracellular. Along these lines, it should be pointed out that not all mucin-containing breast nodules represent carcinomas.[736] Papillomas, papillary carcinomas, and ductal hyperplasia of either the florid or atypical type can also be accompanied by focal or sometimes abundant mucin secretion, which may accumulate in large extracellular pools.[747,756] Some of these lesions have been referred to as 'mucocele-like tumors',[757] but we feel that the term should be used in a descriptive rather than diagnostic sense. As in the appendix and other sites, the formation of a 'mucocele' is nearly always the expression of mucin hyperproduction and extravasation by a proliferative epithelial process, which may be hyperplastic or neoplastic, benign or malignant, in situ or invasive.[744] The key determination is the nature of that process, rather than the spectacular, but relatively inconsequential, presence of the 'mucocele'. In practical terms, a thorough sampling is always mandatory.[756] Also, the finding of mucocele-like changes in a core biopsy is an indication for surgical excision, particularly if there is epithelial atypia and/or an associated mass radiographically.[735]

A further variation on the theme is represented by *mucinous cystadenocarcinoma*, an exceptionally rare tumor composed predominantly of tall columnar cells with abundant intracytoplasmic mucin and a multicystic gross quality similar to that of its ovarian counterpart.[739,746,749]

Medullary carcinoma. Medullary carcinoma usually appears in patients under 50 years of age and is said to be particularly common in Japanese women. It is also said to be particularly common in carriers of *BRCA1* mutations.[765,772,790] Grossly, it is well circumscribed and may become large; it can be mistaken clinically and grossly for a fibroadenoma, but it lacks the trabeculation or whorling of the latter. Its cut surface is solid, homogeneous, and gray, sometimes exhibiting small foci of necrosis (Fig. 20.77). Rare examples are partially or predominantly cystic.[777] Microscopically, the borders are always of the 'pushing' type. The pattern of growth is diffuse, with minimal or no glandular differentiation or intraductal growth and absence of mucin secretion. The tumor cells are large and pleomorphic, with large nuclei and prominent nucleoli and numerous mitoses (some of them atypical). The cell borders are

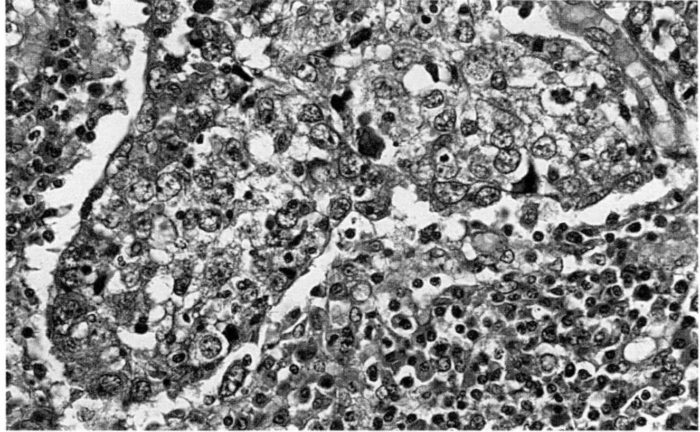

Fig. 20.78 Medullary carcinoma. The large tumor cells grow in a 'syncytial' fashion and are sharply separated from the surrounding stroma, which is heavily infiltrated by lymphocytes and plasma cells.

indistinct, giving the tumor a syncytial or sheet-like appearance somewhat reminiscent of a germ cell tumor of the embryonal carcinoma type. This is accentuated by the fact that the tumor cells located at the periphery of the clusters are more elongated and have a denser, more acidophilic cytoplasm, acquiring a vague resemblance to syncytiotrophoblast. Spindle cell metaplasia, bizarre tumor giant cells, extensive necrosis, and the absence of calcification are other common features.

A constant microscopic component is a prominent lymphoplasmacytic infiltrate at the periphery of the tumor, which is thought to represent a reaction of the host tissues to the neoplasm (Fig. 20.78). Most of the lymphocytes are of the peripheral T-cell type and similar to those seen in ordinary breast carcinoma, except for a possibly greater number of activated cytotoxic/suppressor lymphocytes.[766,774,781,794] The plasma cells are of the IgA-producing type; some of the tumor cells also stain for IgA and for secretory component.[778] Ultrastructurally, the cells of medullary carcinoma do not seem to have distinctive features, despite early statements to the contrary.[776] Immunohistochemically, they share the markers of ordinary invasive ductal carcinoma. They typically express CK7, often vimentin, S-100 protein, and P53, but not CK20.[770,771] They are almost invariably negative for hormone receptors as well as c-*erb*B-2 ('triple negative' phenotype)[779] (see p. 1711).

The claim that medullary carcinomas lack keratin 19, in contrast to ordinary ductal carcinoma, has not been substantiated.[769,791] An interesting feature of medullary carcinoma is the frequent expression of HLA-DR antigen, this being a possible reason for the prominent lymphocytic infiltration.[782,795]

Genetically, medullary carcinoma commonly shows *TP53* gene mutation.[792] Although its gene expression profile is considered to represent part of the basal-like carcinoma spectrum and it shares genetic changes such as 1q and 8q gains and X losses with basal-like carcinomas not otherwise specified, it does show distinct molecular features, including higher numbers of gains and losses on array CGH analysis, as well as recurrent 10p, 9p, and 16q gains, 4p losses, and 1q, 8p, 10p, and 12p amplicons.[792]

Axillary lymph node metastases are common, but they are usually few and limited to the low axillary group. The prognosis for medullary carcinoma is better than for the ordinary invasive ductal carcinoma, a fact already apparent in the early reports on this tumor.[767,787] In the series of Ridolfi et al.,[788] the 10-year survival rate was 84%, as opposed to 63% for ordinary ductal carcinomas. The prognosis was particularly good for tumors that were smaller than 3 cm, and it remained better than for ductal carcinoma even when nodal metastases were present.

The terms *atypical medullary carcinoma* and *invasive ductal carcinoma with medullary features* have been used for tumors that depart somewhat from the foregoing definition, but the delineation of criteria for their recognition remains imprecise.[788,793] We have too often seen the term medullary carcinoma misused for highly cellular breast carcinomas that behaved in a very aggressive fashion, and we caution the reader to use this term only when all the pathologic features necessary for this diagnosis are present.[773,779,786] As a matter of fact, we and others wonder whether medullary carcinoma constitutes a bona fide subtype of breast carcinoma as currently defined.[768,775,789] We are particularly concerned about the lack of precise boundaries between it and the following tumors: the predominantly solid (undifferentiated) form of invasive ductal carcinoma; carcinoma with germ cell-like features, as also seen in the lung, the gastrointestinal tract, and other sites; and so-called 'lymphoepithelioma-like carcinoma'.[780] In regard to the latter, it should be noted that no evidence of EBV participation has been found in medullary carcinoma.[784] Also to be noted is the fact that microsatellite instability, a feature associated with carcinomas with a 'medullary' morphology in large bowel and pancreas, is generally not present in medullary carcinoma of the breast.[783,785]

Invasive papillary carcinoma. Most papillary carcinomas of the breast are entirely or predominantly in situ lesions; these are discussed on page 1691. The invasive component of a papillary carcinoma may also be papillary or have the features of an ordinary ductal-type carcinoma; the prognosis is substantially better for the former.[805] This tumor is said to occur more frequently among whites and postmenopausal women,[800] but, on the whole, it remains a very rare entity. Part of the problem may be that, although the recognition of an ordinary ductal-type carcinoma offers no difficulties, the documentation of invasion in tumors that maintain a well-differentiated pattern may not be as clearcut. For instance, some of the cases reported as intracystic papillary carcinomas[796,802] may well represent invasive papillary carcinomas with a 'pushing' pattern of growth, a possibility supported by a variable loss of myoepithelial cells[797,801] and their occasional association with axillary node metastases.[804,806] This is particularly true for the variant of this tumor known as solid papillary carcinoma.[799,807] The distinctive features of mammary papillary carcinomas can be appreciated on FNA specimens.[798,803]

Invasive micropapillary carcinoma. The recognition of invasive micropapillary carcinoma (IMPCa) as a distinct variant of invasive ductal carcinoma with important prognostic correlates is a relatively recent event, so recent that it was not listed as such in the previous edition of this book.[817] Microscopically, it bears a close similarity with micropapillary carcinoma of other organs, notably endometrium, ovary, and bladder.[815] It is a highly invasive tumor characterized by the formation of pseudopapillary structures lacking a fibrovascular core and by tubular structures free-floating in clear empty spaces. Some of these spaces are lymph vessels, but the majority are newly formed clefts resulting from the inversion of polarity of the secretion by the tumor cells (as evidenced by MUC1 staining), which is directed towards the basal rather than the apical portion.[808,816] The nuclear grade is typically high.[811] Psammoma bodies are present in about one half of the cases.[817] Immunohistochemically, IMPCa is usually positive for estrogen receptors and mammaglobin, and negative for PAX8 and WT1.[812–814] Lymph node metastases are the rule (their frequency being directly related to the presence of lymph vessel permeation[809]), local recurrence is high, and the survival rate is distinctly lower than for conventional invasive ductal carcinoma.[810,817]

Apocrine carcinoma. Apocrine carcinoma is a very rare form of breast malignancy (ranging from 1% to 4% of all cases), at least when defined as composed entirely or predominantly of apocrine-type epithelium.[818,824] The large tumor cells have an abundant acidophilic, somewhat granular cytoplasm, which may contain eosinophilic or golden brown granules that are strongly PAS positive. The nuclei are vesicular and nucleoli are prominent. Glandular differentiation is usually found, the luminal portion of the tumor having a characteristic bulbous expansion ('apocrine snout'). Some of these tumors present as mural nodules within a cyst lined by benign apocrine-type epithelium. Ultrastructurally, the cells of apocrine carcinoma show prominent mitochondria (some with abnormal cristae) and a variable number of large (400–600 nm) membrane-bound vesicles with dense homogeneous osmophilic cores.[823] Immunohistochemically, there is reactivity for GCDFP-15.[821] The gene coding for this marker is located on chromosome 7q and is identical to the gene of the prolactin-inducible protein (PIP); the expression of this gene in apocrine carcinoma has been demonstrated with in situ hybridization techniques.[822,825]

Since apocrine changes in the breast are usually indicative of benignancy (even when the cells exhibit prominent nucleolar enlargement), the diagnosis of apocrine carcinoma should be made only when the architectural features are clearly those of a malignant tumor. It is also important to limit the diagnosis of apocrine carcinoma to malignant tumors in which the apocrine change is widespread, in view of the fact that focal apocrine differentiation (as detected by GCDFP-15) can be detected in close to 10% of ordinary carcinomas.[821] Finally, it should be noted that although apocrine carcinoma is usually a variant of either in situ or invasive ductal carcinoma, apocrine differentiation has also been described in in situ and invasive lobular carcinoma.[820] It has been shown that E-cadherin immunostaining distinguishes the ductal from the lobular lesions, as it does for their non-apocrine counterparts.[819]

Encapsulated apocrine papillary carcinoma is mentioned in page 1691.

Secretory (juvenile) carcinoma. This rare form of breast carcinoma is seen primarily in children, but it can also occur in adults.[829,832,835] Grossly, it is well circumscribed and usually small (Fig. 20.79). The microscopic appearance is distinctive (Fig. 20.80).

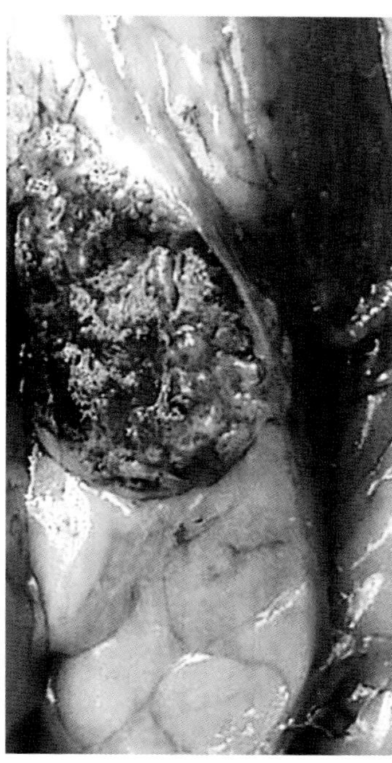

Fig. 20.79 Gross appearance of secretory carcinoma. The tumor is well circumscribed and shows a variegated cut surface.

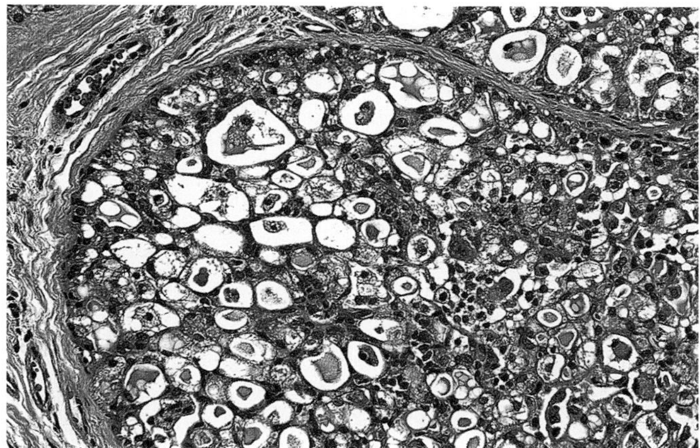

Fig. 20.80 Secretory carcinoma. The small uniform glands are filled by a secretory material.

The margins are of the 'pushing' type, and prominent hyalinization is often present in the central portion. The microscopic appearance is distinctive. Tubuloalveolar and focally papillary formations lined by cells with a vacuolated (sometimes hypernephroid) cytoplasm are seen forming lumina filled by an eosinophilic PAS-positive secretion.[831,833,835] Nucleoli may be prominent, but mitoses are very scanty. Ultrastructurally, the tumor cells contain numerous membrane-bound intracytoplasmic secretory vacuoles.[826]

Immunohistochemically, there is strong reactivity for α-lactalbumin and S-100 protein, accompanied by variable expression of GCDFP-15 and CEA.[830] It has been hypothesized that there may be a histogenetic link between secretory carcinoma and a type of salivary gland tumor traditionally placed among the acinic cell carcinomas, as well as with the newly described acinic cell carcinoma of breast[828] (see p. 1723). This possibility is strongly supported by the fact that a similar molecular genetic abnormality has been found in these tumors.[834] This refers to a recurrent balanced chromosomal translocation, t(12;15)(p13;q25), which leads to fusion of the *ETV6* and *NTRK3* genes.[836]

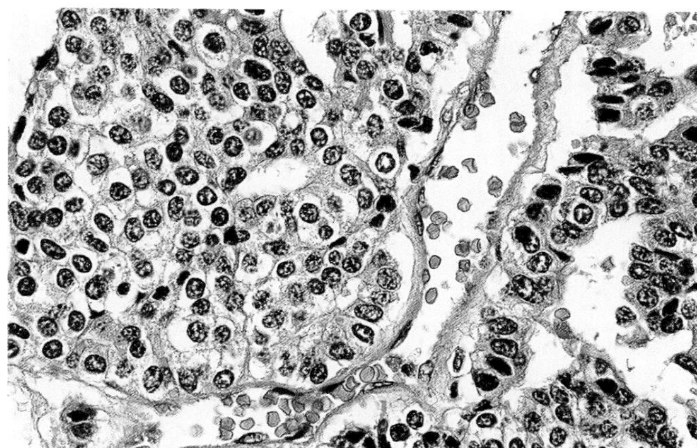

Fig. 20.81 Breast carcinoma with neuroendocrine differentiation.

The overall prognosis is excellent, most series quoting a 5-year survival rate close to 100%.[831] Local recurrences and nodal metastases can develop, sometimes very late in the course of the disease.[829,833,835] Death resulting from disseminated tumor has been recorded only exceptionally.[835] Secretory carcinoma has also been reported to occur in the axillary skin in the absence of a breast primary.[827]

Carcinomas with neuroendocrine features (including so-called 'carcinoid tumor'). The term carcinoid tumor was originally proposed for a type of invasive ductal carcinoma exhibiting features consistent with (neuro)endocrine differentiation.[844] In general, the clinical presentation is no different from that of the ordinary breast carcinoma. Specifically, none of the patients has had carcinoid syndrome, even in the presence of widespread disease. Multicentricity and bilaterality can occur.[844] There are no distinctive gross features.

Microscopically, the tumor cells are small, arranged in solid nests separated by fibrous tissue (Fig. 20.81). Ribbons and rosettelike formations may be seen. Mitoses are generally rare. The presence of an intraductal component and of mucin secretion has been detected in a minority of the cases.[844] The microscopic differential diagnosis includes lobular carcinoma and a metastasis to the breast of a carcinoid tumor located elsewhere.

The tumor cells of carcinoid tumor of the breast are argyrophilic but not argentaffin and are found to contain dense-core secretory granules of various types ultrastructurally[841,844] Fig. 20.82).

The nature of this neoplasm has been controversial from the very first description.[849,862] It has even been suggested – probably erroneously – that the argyrophilia and the dense-core secretory granules are not an indication of neuroendocrine differentiation at all but rather of lactalbumin secretion by the tumor cells.[842] To be sure, not all membrane-bound dense-core cytoplasmic granules are of neurosecretory type.[839] However, the immunohistochemical positivity that has been obtained for chromogranin, synaptophysin, and NSE,[840,854,865,866] and in some instances for specific hormone peptides,[853,860] would seem to verify that these tumors do indeed exhibit signs of endocrine differentiation (Fig. 20.83). Whether this justifies calling them carcinoid tumors is another matter. We believe it does not. It seems to us that they are rather the example of a

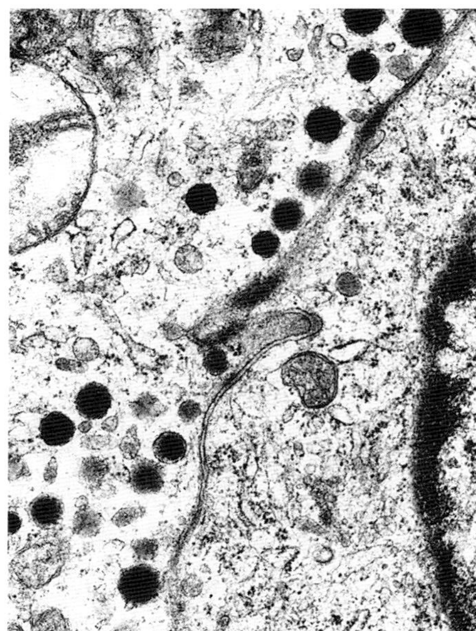

Fig. 20.82 Electron microscopic appearance of breast carcinoma with neuroendocrine differentiation. Primarily ectoplasmic dense-core neurosecretory type granules ranging in size from 140 to 225 nm are seen. (×29 400)
(Courtesy of Dr Robert A Erlandson, Memorial Sloan-Kettering Cancer Center)

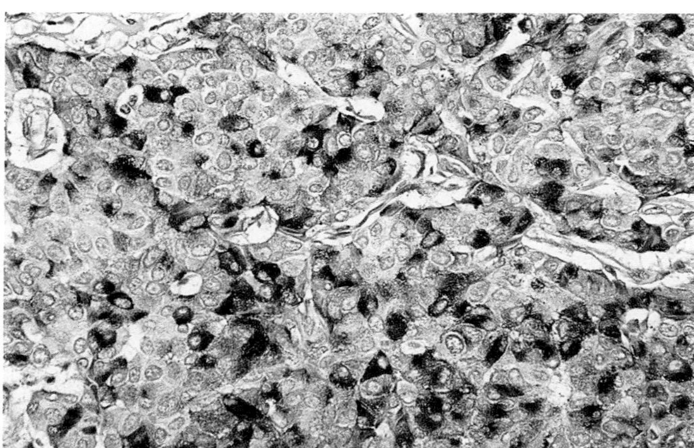

Fig. 20.83 Strong reactivity for chromogranin in breast carcinoma with neuroendocrine differentiation.

phenomenon similar to that described in practically all other organs (i.e., that of a carcinoma arising from primitive epithelial cells with the capacity to differentiate focally or extensively towards an endocrine line).[850] Such carcinomas resemble ordinary ductal-type carcinoma in most other ways: occasional presence of an in situ component, frequent positivity for estrogen receptors, pattern of metastases, expression of apocrine differentiation (especially in aged women), and outcome.[848,851,855,859] Therefore, we like to view and designate this tumor as invasive ductal carcinoma with (neuro)endocrine differentiation or features, a term we prefer to the alternative designation argyrophilic carcinoma.[838,863] According to Azzopardi et al.,[838] this tumor constitutes approximately 5% of all breast carcinomas.

It should be mentioned here that there are breast carcinomas of other morphologic patterns in which (neuro)endocrine features

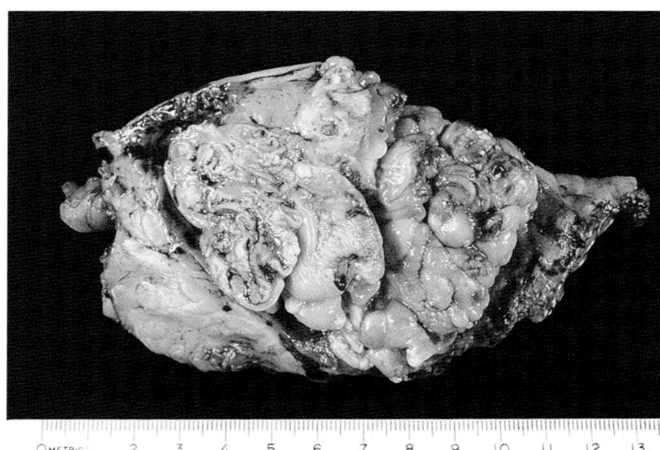

Fig. 20.84 Gross appearance of metaplastic carcinoma. A large, fleshy mass is seen protruding inside a cavity. Microscopically, this tumor showed an admixture of squamous and spindle elements.

have been found.[856] They include the already mentioned mucinous carcinoma[845] (see p. 1700), small cell neuroendocrine carcinoma,[847,857,858,861] invasive ductal-type carcinomas of ordinary type,[852,863] and some types of in situ ductal carcinoma[843,850,864] (see p. 1693). Exceptionally, neuroendocrine carcinoma of either breast or nipple may have Merkel cell-like features.[837,846] Interestingly, carcinoid tumors of the conventional type are virtually nonexistent in the breast. We have seen only one case that had morphologic and histochemical features (argentaffinity) identical to those of classic (insular) carcinoid tumors of midgut derivation; remarkably, it was associated with the presence of argentaffin cells in the adjacent breast epithelium.

Metaplastic carcinoma. Metaplastic carcinoma is a generic term for breast carcinoma of ductal type in which the predominant component of the neoplasm has an appearance other than epithelial and glandular and more in keeping with another cell type.[895,915] As such, the designation is too encompassing and imprecise and should not be used without a qualifier. It includes the following categories, which overlap considerably with each other:

1 A tumor equivalent to the one designated in other sites (notably the upper aerodigestive tract and lung) as *sarcomatoid carcinoma*, carcinoma with sarcoma-like stroma, and carcinosarcoma (Fig. 20.84). Grossly, it tends to be well circumscribed. Microscopically, the sarcoma-like component may resemble so-called malignant fibrous histiocytoma, chondrosarcoma, osteosarcoma, rhabdomyosarcoma, angiosarcoma, or a combination of them.[869,874,884,886,888] There may be a gradual transition from carcinomatous to sarcoma-like elements, or the separation between them can be sharp.[885] When the latter is the case, the term *carcinosarcoma* tends to be used.[906,912] Tumors having overt carcinomas with direct transition to a cartilaginous and/or osseous matrix without an intervening spindle cell zone or osteoclastic giant cells have been referred to as '*matrix-producing carcinomas*',[877,911] but the distinction seems to be of little clinical value and dubious biologic significance.[880,896]

Immunohistochemically, the sarcoma-like elements of these tumors have usually acquired vimentin positivity and other features of a mesenchymal nature ('phenotypic switch') but occasionally still retain epithelial markers,[879,901] a fact best

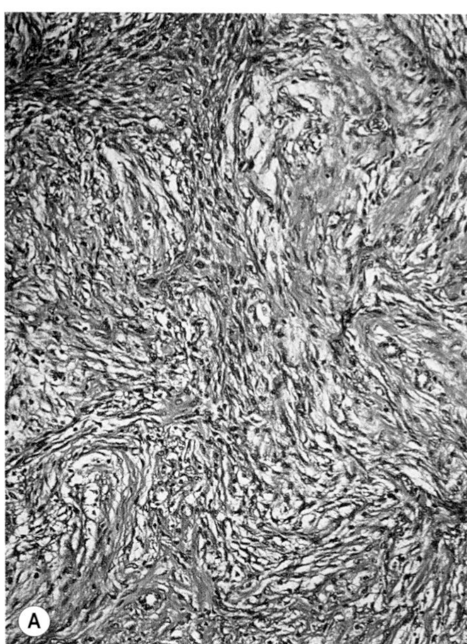
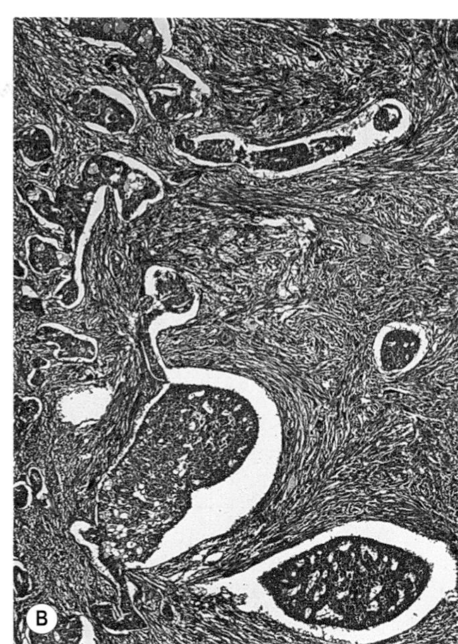

Fig. 20.85 A and **B**, Metaplastic carcinoma. The tumor shown in **A** exhibits a blending of the carcinomatous and sarcoma-like components, whereas that depicted in **B** has a biphasic ('carcinosarcomatous') appearance.

demonstrated by employing wide-spectrum keratin antibodies.[867]

As in other sites, molecular studies support the interpretation that the recognizable epithelial and the sarcoma-like components originate from the same stem cell.[881,908,909,917]

2 *Spindle cell carcinoma*. The overt carcinomatous component of these tumors, when present, may have invasive or in situ ductal features, and it may be entirely squamous.[910] The spindle cell component, which may be deceptively bland, forms abundant fibrocollagenous stroma with feathered, myxoid, angioid, and storiform patterns[872,873,914] (Fig. 20.85). The appearance may closely simulate that of a fibrosarcoma or even fibromatosis.[882,905] Areas of merging between the epithelial and the spindle component are common. The latter foci are usually immunoreactive for keratin and p63.[889,897] Some of these arise in connection with a complex sclerosing lesion or so-called 'adenomyoepithelioma', and contain some of the immunohistochemical markers of myoepithelial cells.[870,876,883,898,904] Whether to call them metaplastic carcinomas or malignant myoepitheliomas seems a matter of personal preference.[878,890]

3 *Carcinoma with osteoclast-like giant cells*.[868,907,913] When these cells appear in conjunction with sarcoma-like elements, the tumor should be regarded as a variant of the first category listed. When they are seen in the stroma of what is otherwise a typical invasive ductal-type carcinoma lacking sarcomatoid foci, the tumor should be placed in a category of its own but closer to ordinary ductal carcinoma. All available evidence suggests that the osteoclast-like elements are of non-neoplastic histiocytic nature and that they form from fusion of mononuclear precursors.[887,891]

4 *Squamous cell carcinoma*. Although technically speaking this represents a form of tumor metaplasia, it differs so substantially from the others that we therefore thought of discussing it separately (see next section).

5 *Others*. A few cases of metaplastic carcinoma with melanocytic differentiation have been reported.[871,900] They are to be distinguished from the more common phenomenon of melanocytic colonization of carcinoma, and from the presence of lipofuscin granules that can simulate melanin.[902] *Choriocarcinomatous features* can be focally present in breast carcinoma.[899] *Pleomorphic carcinoma* is yet another variation of anaplastic breast carcinoma that can resemble sarcoma.[916] This is regarded as a variant of ductal carcinoma and is, therefore, different from pleomorphic lobular carcinoma.[903] As expected, its behavior tends to be rather aggressive.[892] On occasions, the metaplastic changes occur in various directions simultaneously (such as spindle cell, adenoid cystic carcinoma, and melanoma).[893]

The differential diagnosis of these tumor types (particularly the first two categories) includes phylloides tumor and primary breast sarcoma.

On the whole, the behavior of metaplastic carcinoma seems to be more aggressive than that of ordinary invasive ductal-type carcinoma.[873,888,894] The differences in survival among the various subgroups are rather minor, although some authors have suggested a worse prognosis for the 'carcinosarcoma' subgroup. Metastases tend to be hematogenous rather than to lymph nodes, in keeping with the sarcomatous phenotype.[873,875,888] The size of the neoplasm at the time of initial excision is one of the best predictors of survival.[894]

Squamous cell carcinoma and related tumors. Squamous cell carcinoma is an extremely rare variant of breast tumor.[929] Tumors of cutaneous origin and those in which the squamous component is a portion of an otherwise typical phylloides tumor should be excluded. It is also important not to misinterpret the syncytial areas of medullary carcinoma or the partial apocrine changes sometimes seen in other tumors as representing squamous changes.

The gross appearance of squamous cell carcinoma differs little from that of the usual breast carcinomas, although sometimes a large central cyst filled with keratin can be identified. Microscopically, most cases seem to represent instances of squamous metaplasia in ductal carcinoma, indicating that squamous cell carcinoma could be viewed as a special type of metaplastic carcinoma.[927] This view is reinforced by the existence of so-called 'spindle cell carcinoma', in which a well-differentiated squamous component merges with a prominent spindle cell sarcomatoid component[918,925] (see p. 1705). Occasionally, the tumor is accompanied by a prominent myxoid stroma.[924]

Two further variants are *acantholytic squamous cell carcinoma,* in which the lack of cohesiveness of tumor cells results in a pseudovascular or pseudoglandular appearance,[922] and *adenosquamous carcinoma.*[920,926,928,931] Some examples of the latter tumor type have been designated as mucoepidermoid carcinoma,[923] a term that should be avoided except for those tumors having cytoarchitectural features analogous to those of their salivary gland counterparts (see p. 1723).

A high frequency of epidermal growth factor receptor (EGFR) expression has been noted in mammary carcinomas with squamous differentiation, a finding which may have therapeutic implications.[919]

It is difficult to ascertain the prognosis of squamous cell carcinoma in view of the differences in diagnostic criteria from series to series and the rarity of the disease. In the series of Wargotz and Norris,[930] the 5-year disease-specific survival rate was 63%. On the whole, the behavior of this tumor does not seem to be substantially different from that of ordinary ductal-type invasive carcinoma.[918,921] This may not hold true for the acantholytic variant, which seems to be associated with a very aggressive course,[922] or for the low-grade adenosquamous carcinoma, which is said to have a favorable prognosis.[928]

Spread-related variants

Inflammatory carcinoma. The term inflammatory carcinoma was originally used in a clinical context for a type of breast carcinoma in which the entire breast was reddened and warm, with widespread edema of the skin, thus simulating the appearance of mastitis.[938] Pathologic studies in some of those cases revealed the lesion to be an undifferentiated carcinoma with widespread carcinomatosis of the dermal lymphatic vessels (Fig. 20.86). This led to the belief that an 'inflammatory' clinical appearance always corresponded pathologically to dermal lymphatic permeation and vice versa. This assumption is not correct. Patients may have inflammatory carcinoma clinically in the absence of dermal invasion; conversely, widespread permeation of dermal lymphatics can be seen in the absence of the clinical features of inflammatory carcinoma (so-called 'occult' inflammatory carcinoma[939]). From a prognostic standpoint, the presence of dermal lymphatic permeation on microscopic examination is a sign of ominous prognosis, whether the clinical appearance is that of an inflammatory carcinoma or not.[933,935,936,939] The clinical recognition of this entity by an experienced observer is also reliable and associated with a poor prognosis, but ideally it should be accompanied by a skin biopsy showing dermal lymphatic involvement before the tumor is deemed inoperable.[937] Some authors have recommended discarding the term inflammatory carcinoma altogether.[935] The choice of therapy for this neoplasm remains highly controversial.[932,934,940]

Paget disease. Paget disease is the name given to a crusted lesion of the nipple caused by breast carcinoma, as originally described by Sir James Paget in 1874.[962] It is accompanied in nearly all instances by an underlying breast carcinoma of in situ ductal type, with or without associated stromal invasion. In this regard, the presence of Paget disease is only a secondary, albeit dramatic, feature of the tumor. The management and prognosis depend largely on the intraductal versus invasive nature of the underlying carcinoma and on the presence or absence of axillary lymph node involvement, rather than on the presence or appearance of the intraepithelial component in the nipple.[963]

Clinically, these weeping, eczema-like lesions are centered in the nipple (Fig. 20.87). Later they may involve the areola and surrounding epidermis, but they rarely extend more than a few centimeters. If a definite mass can be palpated beneath the diseased nipple, the underlying tumor will have an invasive component in over 90% of cases. Conversely, 66% of cases without a palpable mass are exclusively intraductal.[941]

Microscopically, large clear cells with atypical nuclei are seen within the epidermis, usually concentrated along the basal layer but also permeating the malpighian layer (Fig. 20.88). The cells can be isolated or in clusters, and sometimes they form small glandular structures.[968] In rare instances they have an anaplastic appearance.[964] Occasionally, intracytoplasmic melanin granules are present, a feature that may result in a mistaken diagnosis of malignant melanoma; these granules have probably been transferred from neighboring melanocytes by the process of cytocrinia[942,965] (Fig. 20.89). This phenomenon should be distinguished from the exceptional type of carcinoma with melanocytic differentiation (see

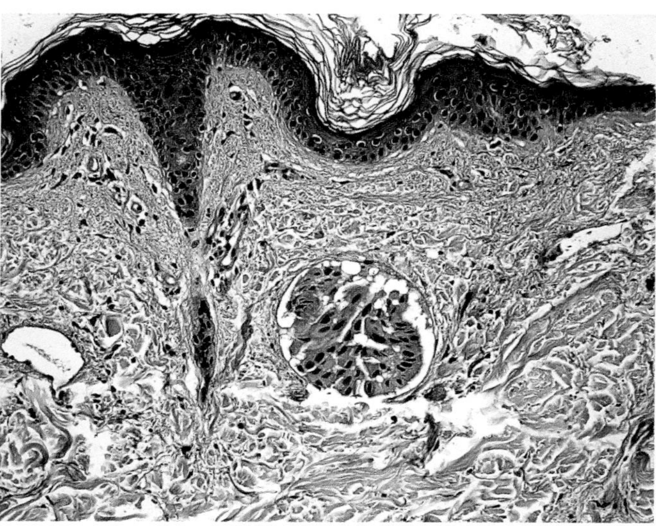

Fig. 20.86 Large tumor embolus in a dermal lymph vessel in a case with the clinical appearance of inflammatory carcinoma.

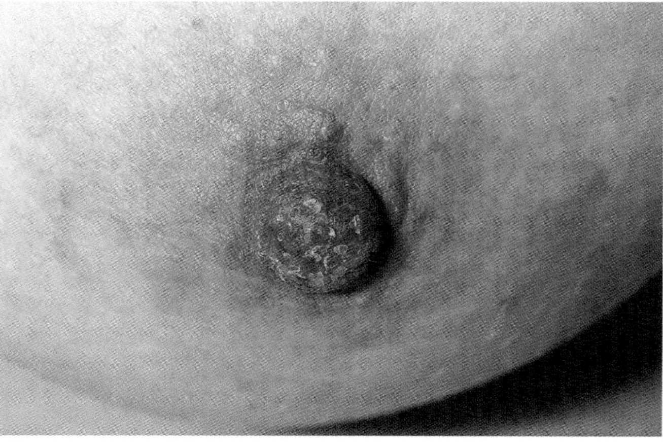

Fig. 20.87 Eczema-like hyperemic and eroded clinical appearance of Paget disease.
(Courtesy of Dr RA Cooke, Brisbane, Australia. From Cooke RA, Stewart B. Colour atlas of anatomical pathology. Edinburgh, 2004, Churchill Livingstone)

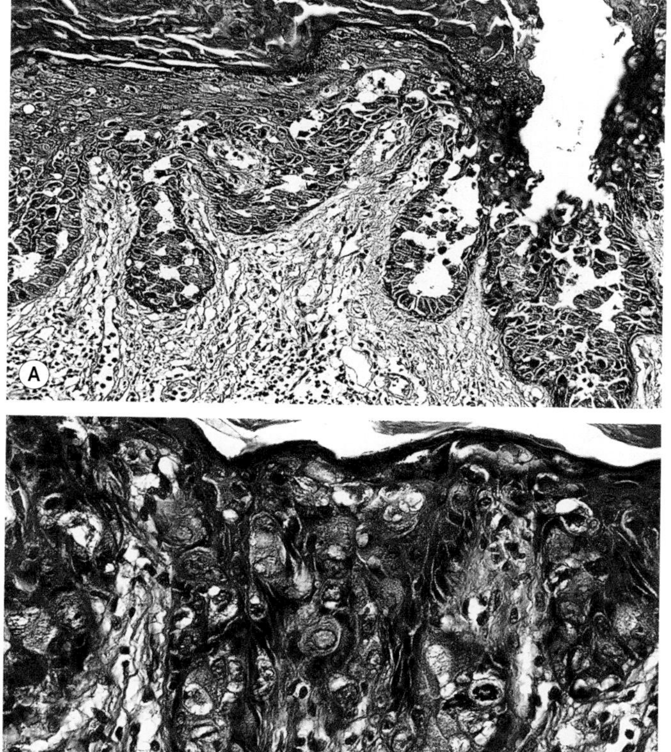

Fig. 20.88 **A** and **B**, Low- and high-power views of Paget disease. The cleft-like separation between the tumor cells and the overlying squamous epithelium is characteristic.

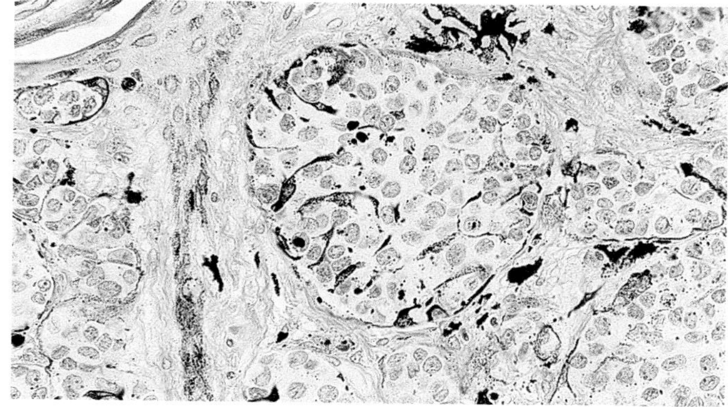

Fig. 20.89 Melanin colonization in breast carcinoma as seen with argentaffin stain.
(Slide prepared by Dr Pierre Masson, University of Montreal, and sent by him to Dr Fred W Stewart, Memorial Sloan-Kettering Cancer Center)

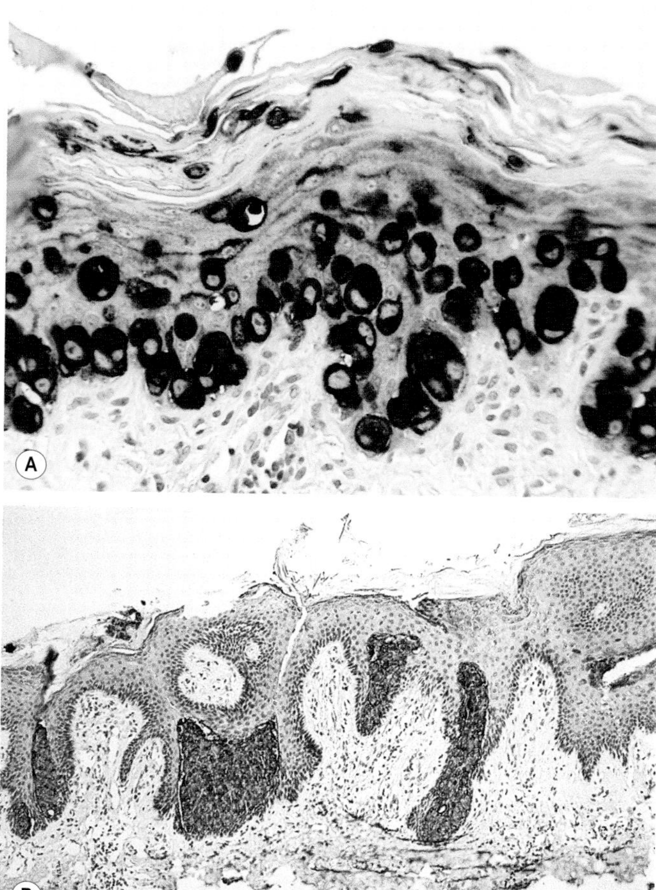

Fig. 20.90 Immunohistochemical demonstration of malignant intraepithelial cells in Paget disease: **A**, EMA immunostain; **B**, HER2/*neu* immunostain.

p. 1705) and from the carcinoma containing cytoplasmic lipofuscin granules mimicking melanin.[967]

The underlying breast carcinoma is practically always of ductal type and is composed of cells similar to those present within the nipple. If enough sections are taken, a connection between the carcinoma within the duct and the Paget disease will be demonstrated in most instances. However, in some cases the underlying tumor is found 2 cm or more from the nipple.[963]

Mucin stains may or may not be positive, in contrast to their almost universal presence in extramammary Paget disease.[959,969] Ultrastructurally, the tumor cells have microvilli and other features indicative of glandular differentiation.[966] Immunohistochemically, they show reactivity for EMA and the related milk fat globule membrane antigen, CEA (at least when using polyclonal antibodies), MUC1, low molecular weight keratin (including CK7), HER2/*neu*, and (in half of the cases) GCDFP-15[943,949,951,953,961,971] (Fig. 20.90). In general, they are negative for high molecular weight keratins, S-100 protein, and involucrin.[951,961]

The main differential diagnosis is with Bowen disease and malignant melanoma. Examples of these disorders located in the nipple have been reported,[972] and there is no reason why they could not involve this structure. We can only say that, in our experience, whenever this differential diagnosis was considered for a lesion of the nipple (because of pigmentation, transepidermal atypia, or any other reason), the definitive diagnosis invariably turned out to be Paget disease.

The heated controversies in the past regarding the glandular versus keratinocytic versus melanocytic origin of Paget disease have subsided. There can no longer be any doubt that Paget cells

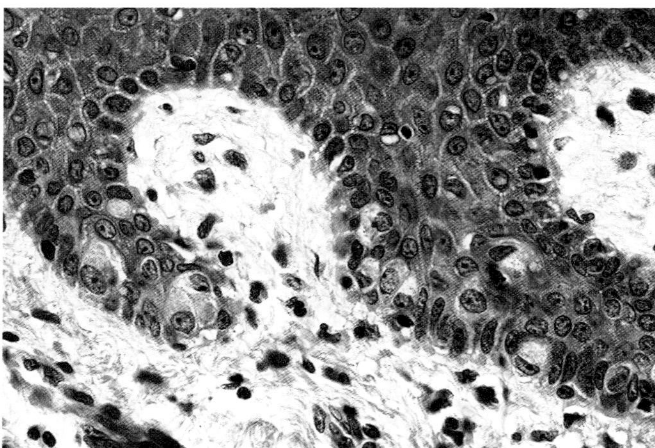

Fig. 20.91 Biopsy of nipple showing scattered clear cells in the basal layer ('Toker cells'). These cells show a mild degree of nuclear atypia and were immunohistochemically similar to the cells of Paget disease.

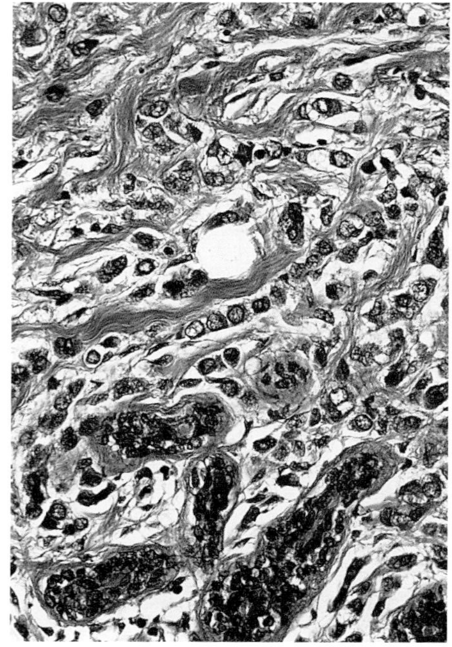

Fig. 20.92 Invasive lobular carcinoma. The tumor cells are small and uniform with round nuclei and grow in an Indian file fashion.

exhibit glandular differentiation.[958] However, a point still unsettled is whether the Paget cells in the nipple have migrated there from deeper ductal structures (possibly as a result of keratinocyte-induced chemotaxis[945]) or whether they represent an in situ malignant transformation either of the intraepidermal portion of the mammary ducts or of basally located multipotential epithelial cells capable of glandular differentiation.[954] The similarities in immunohistochemical profile and oncogene expression (such as HER2/*neu* or *RAS*21) favor the former.[944,948,956,957,973] On the other hand, the existence of rare cases of Paget disease without underlying ductal carcinoma or with very limited in situ carcinoma of the most distal lactiferous ducts suggests that, in some cases, the latter mechanism may be operating.[950,954] In this regard, the observation made by Toker[970] about the presence of clear cells in nipples without clinical evidence of Paget disease and without microscopic evidence of breast carcinoma is of great interest. These cells have some immunohistochemical similarities with Paget cells (positivity for CK7 and EMA, and negativity for p63)[946,953,960] and may exhibit mild nuclear atypical changes, suggesting the possibility of a dysplastic or 'pre-Paget' change[947,952,955] (Fig. 20.91). From a practical standpoint, these cells are distinguished from those of Paget disease because of the lack of eczema-like changes clinically, the absence of clearcut cytologic features of malignancy, and some immunohistochemical differences, such as negativity for CD138 and P53.[946]

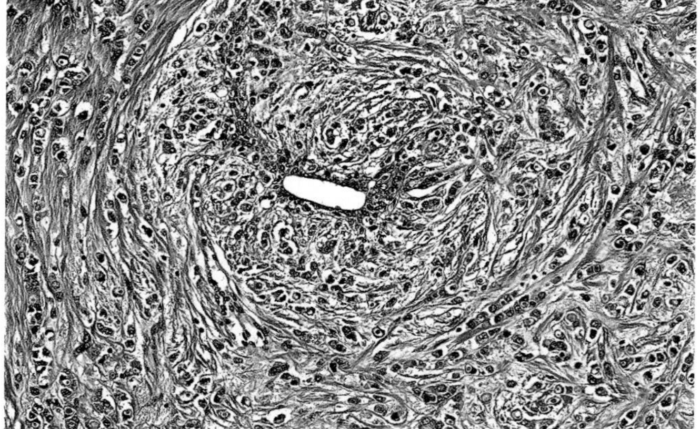

Fig. 20.93 Typical target-like growth of tumor cells around an uninvolved duct in invasive lobular carcinoma.

Invasive lobular carcinoma (ILC)

Classic type. In its most typical form, invasive lobular carcinoma (ILC) is characterized by the presence of small and relatively uniform tumor cells growing singly, in Indian file, and in a concentric ('pagetoid') fashion around lobules involved by in situ lobular neoplasia[977,983] (Figs 20.92–20.94). Most of the breast tumors designated in the past as small cell carcinomas belong to this category. Gland formation is not a feature of classic ILC. The stroma is usually abundant, of dense fibrous type, and containing foci of periductal and perivenous elastosis in virtually every case. A lymphocytic infiltrate may be present, sometimes so intense as to obscure the neoplastic component.

It is currently accepted that the diagnosis of ILC can be made in the presence of these cytoarchitectural features even if an in situ component is absent.[979,985] Conversely, an invasive tumor should not be called ILC simply because it is associated with in situ lobular neoplasia; rather, it should have the features of lobular carcinoma in the invasive component itself in order to deserve this designation.

The histochemical, ultrastructural, and immunohistochemical features of ILC are analogous to those described for its in situ counterpart. This includes the presence of HMW keratin, lack of accumulation of P53, and – most importantly – decrease or absence of E-cadherin[974,978,980,981] (allowing for the anticipated exceptions[984]). To these, p120 catenin has been recently added, supported by the claim that lobular carcinoma shows a characteristic cytoplasmic staining pattern with this marker.[975] While loss of E-cadherin expression is the hallmark of lobular carcinoma, positive immunostaining for E-cadherin does not preclude this diagnosis when the

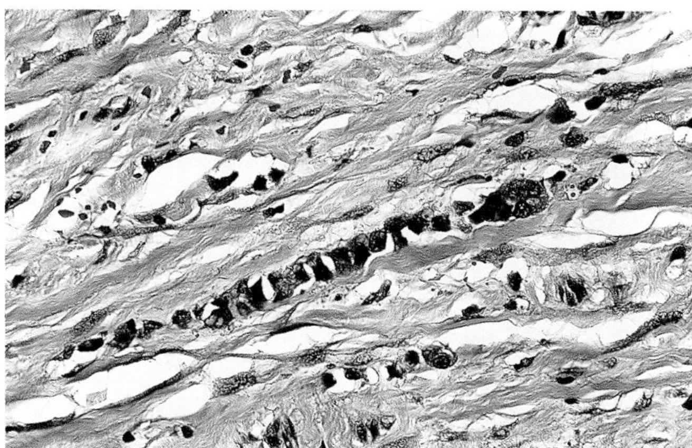

Fig. 20.94 Indian file pattern of growth of invasive lobular carcinoma.

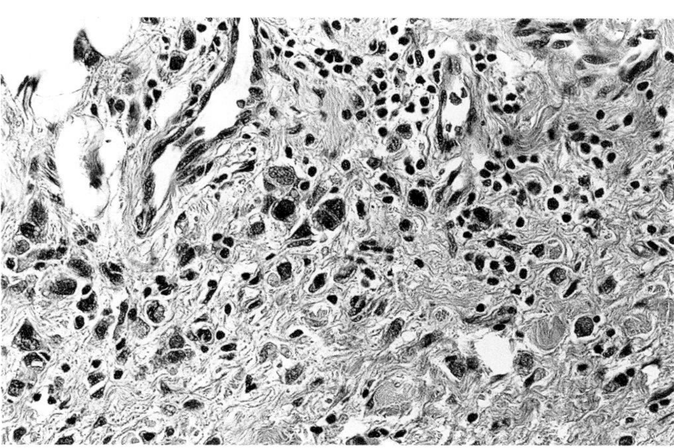

Fig. 20.95 Pleomorphic variant of invasive lobular carcinoma.

morphologic features are compatible.[976] As a matter of fact, up to 16% of cases of invasive lobular carcinomas show immunoreactivity for E-cadherin, but these cases do exhibit abnormal expression of one or more of the catenin complex members, most commonly diffuse cytoplasmic expression of p120 catenin.[984]

The genetic basis for the loss of E-cadherin expression in lobular carcinoma includes: (1) inactivating mutation of the E-cadherin gene *CDH1*, usually attributable to loss of heterozygosity on chromosome 16q or homozygous deletions of *CDH1*; (2) *CDH1* promoter hypermethylation; (3) truncating mutation in *CDH1*; and (4) transcriptional inactivation.[983]

The main differential diagnosis of invasive lobular carcinoma is with invasive ductal carcinoma (IDC). The small size and uniformity of the cells and their lack of cohesiveness are the most important distinguishing features. It should be remarked, however, that in many cases the distinction is difficult and to a large extent subjective, as borne out by the fact that the incidence of ILC ranges from 0.7% to 20% in the published series.[982] Other entities that can be confused with ILC are carcinoma with neuroendocrine features and malignant lymphoma. The latter possibility arises more often when ILC metastasizes to axillary nodes and other sites, particularly the eyelid; we have seen several cases misdiagnosed as large cell malignant lymphoma or malignant histiocytosis because of their diffuse pattern of growth and the histiocyte-like appearance of the tumor cells. Reactions for keratin, EMA, CEA, CD45, and an old-fashioned mucicarmine stain should eliminate any problems not resolved by the examination of the routinely stained slides.

Pleomorphic lobular carcinoma. This form of invasive breast tumor has the pattern of growth of a classic breast carcinoma but exhibits a marked degree of nuclear pleomorphism and abundant cytoplasm[993] (Fig. 20.95). It also frequently shows apocrine differentiation, focal signet ring morphology, lack of hormone receptors, higher expression of P53 and HER2/*neu*, occasional expression of chromogranin, and lack of E-cadherin staining (the latter in keeping with its lobular nature).[986–992]

Histiocytoid carcinoma. Histiocytoid carcinoma is characterized by a diffuse pattern of growth by tumor cells displaying abundant granular, foamy cytoplasm.[997,1000] It may simulate the appearance of a granular cell tumor (myoblastoma), hence the proposed synonym *myoblastoid carcinoma*.[994] This tumor type is currently viewed as a variant of invasive lobular carcinoma exhibiting apocrine differentiation, as evidenced by immunohistochemical reactivity for GCDFP-15 and the demonstration of mRNA for the related prolactin-inducible protein (PIP) by in situ hybridization.[994,1002] In

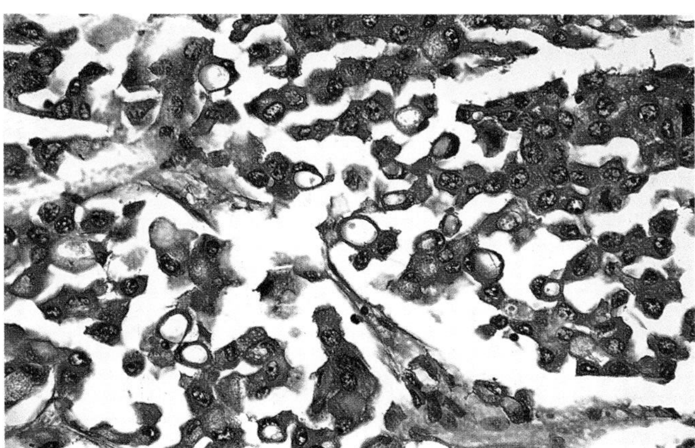

Fig. 20.96 Cytoplasmic vacuolization with nuclear displacement in breast carcinoma due to lipid accumulation.

most cases E-cadherin is absent, as one would expect in a lobular carcinoma-type tumor, but other features are more suggestive of a link with ductal-type tumors.[996] The mucins expressed by this tumor include some 'non-mammary' types, such as MUC2 and MUC5AC.[998]

Histiocytoid carcinoma should also be distinguished from *lipid-rich carcinoma*. The latter is simply a form of breast carcinoma showing lipid accumulation in the cytoplasm of the tumor cells[995,999,1001] (Fig. 20.96).

Signet ring carcinoma. Signet ring carcinoma is a type of breast carcinoma in which a significant number of tumor cells show intracytoplasmic mucin accumulation, resulting in the typical signet ring appearance[1007] (Fig. 20.97). Unfortunately, the term 'significant' is used differently by different people. Some will place a tumor into this category only if the majority of the cells have a signet ring morphology, whereas others would settle for a much smaller number.[1004,1006] In any event, it is important to separate this tumor from mucinous carcinoma (in which the mucin is extracellular) because of their vastly different prognoses. Naturally, one should make room for exceptions. Occasionally the two types have been found to coexist (see p. 1700), and exceptionally the mucin of lobular carcinoma has been seen in an extracellular location.[1012]

Most cases of signet ring carcinoma show cytoarchitectural features (such as small cell size, uniformity, and dissociation) similar

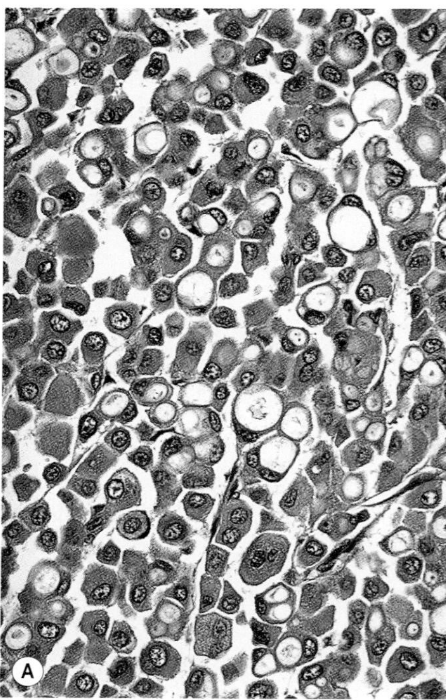

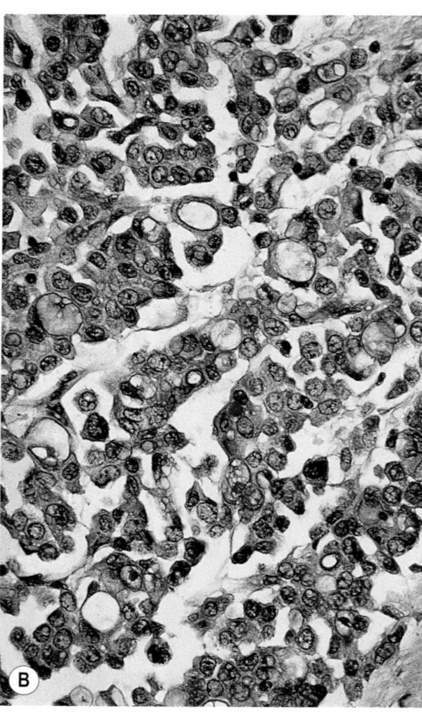

Fig. 20.97 **A** and **B**, Signet ring carcinoma of the breast. This is regarded as a variant of lobular carcinoma. **B**, Alcian blue–PAS stain.

to those of classic ILC and sometimes coexist with it.[1010] Furthermore, it is not rare for in situ or invasive lobular carcinoma to contain scattered signet ring cells.[1011] For these reasons, most cases of signet ring carcinoma are regarded as variants of ILC.[1009,1013] Some, however, are probably more closely related to ductal carcinoma of either invasive[1007] or in situ type.[1005]

The signet ring morphology appears to be the result of deficiency in α-catenin, presumably due to mutations.[1008] Ultrastructurally, it is manifested in its more extreme form by a large membrane-bound vacuole of varying, but usually low, electron density.[1014] As already indicated, this is a different process from that of intracellular lumen formation, which is characterized ultrastructurally by a microvillus-coated cavity and which appears as a bull's-eye on light microscopic examination.

Immunohistochemically, signet ring carcinoma is positive for CK7 and MUC1, and usually negative for E-cadherin.[1003]

Tubulolobular carcinoma. This variant is characterized by the admixture of small tubular formations having a minute or undetectable lumen ('closed' or 'almost closed' tubules) with cords of tumor cells growing in a lobular configuration similar to that of invasive lobular carcinoma.[1016] The in situ component, if present, may be of lobular, ductal or mixed type.[1019] Its immunohistochemical profile is intermediate between those of ductal and lobular carcinoma, in that it shows positivity for both E-cadherin and HMW keratin.[1018,1019] It is associated with a higher incidence of multifocality and positive axillary nodes than pure tubular carcinoma.[1015,1017]

Other types. Some authors restrict their diagnosis of ILC to tumors having the features described for the classic type. Others have expanded considerably the concept and include in this category tumors that traditionally have been placed into the IDC category.[1020,1022,1023] These include most of the tumors just described under the category of invasive lobular carcinoma 'variants'. Furthermore, cases having closely aggregated cells, solid pattern, trabecular pattern, loose alveolar pattern, and spindle cell chains have been accepted as ILC, *as long as the relatively bland and homogeneous cytologic appearance was maintained*. Perhaps the most distinctive of these forms is the *alveolar variant*, in which the tumor cells are arranged in sharply outlined groups separated by fibrous tissue sometimes containing osteoclast-like giant cells.[1024,1025]

The cytologic and/or architectural similarities between these various forms and classic ILC are undeniable. The problem, however, is that the more the concept of ILC is widened, and to some extent diluted, the less distinct the entity becomes and the less significant (or at least the less uniform) its clinical connotations are.[1021]

Mixed ductal and lobular carcinoma

Biphasic carcinomas composed in part of a component with definite features of invasive ductal carcinoma and in part of a component with definite features of invasive lobular carcinoma do occur, but they are very rare. These tumors, of course, should be distinguished from the cases in which two separate neoplasms of different microscopic appearances are present in the same breast. They should also be distinguished from so-called tubulobular carcinoma, which has a reasonably distinct morphologic appearance (see previous section).

Undetermined (unclassified) carcinoma

This category includes all cases of invasive carcinoma in which features of ductal or lobular type are not definite enough to place it into either category. Azzopardi[1026] states that 3–4% of invasive breast carcinomas belong to this category.

Microinvasive breast carcinoma

Once the concept of 'microinvasive carcinoma' was entrenched in the gynecologic literature, especially in connection with cervical squamous cell carcinoma, it was only natural that it would be proposed at other sites, including the breast, and this is exactly what happened. Alas, its application at this site is not as straightforward, one of the reasons being that the mammary epithelium is not separated from the stroma by a sharp, straight line as it is in the cervix.[1032] Be that as it may, the proposal has been made to designate as microinvasive carcinoma any carcinoma in situ of the breast showing one or more areas of stromal invasion not surpassing 1 mm in thickness.[1029] Theoretically, it is applicable to both ductal and lobular lesions, but the term seems to be used more often for the former. It may be single or multiple, the mean number of foci being two.[1031] Immunohistochemical evaluation with myoepithelial and basement membrane markers is useful to confirm the diagnosis.[1029,1033] Problems related to the definition criteria and clinical significance of this finding remain and need to be addressed.[1028,1032] On the whole, it would seem that patients with microinvasive carcinoma are at risk for nodal metastases[1034] but that their survival rate is better than for patients with T1 invasive carcinoma.[1030] Apparently, the risk for metastases is greater if the invasive component is in the form of cell clusters than in the form of a few isolated tumor cells.[1027]

Hormone receptors

A crucial development in the treatment of breast carcinoma has been the realization that the presence of hormone (estrogen and progesterone) receptors in the tumor tissue correlates well with response to hormone therapy and chemotherapy.[1038,1050] As a matter of fact, estrogen receptor status is regarded at present as the most powerful predictive marker in breast cancer management.[1061] Estrogen and progesterone receptors are codependent variables, progesterone receptor (PR) being a weaker predictor of response to endocrine therapy than estrogen receptor (ER).[1057] Traditionally, these hormone receptors were measured by the dextran-coated charcoal and sucrose gradient assay, but this has been replaced by the immunohistochemical method, on the grounds that it offers several important advantages (it does not require fresh tissue, it can be done with minute amounts of tumor, etc.), and that the correlation between the two methods is very good[1039,1049,1054,1070,1074] (Fig. 20.98). Several attempts have been made to semiquantitate the immunohistochemical method by standardizing the technical procedure and reporting, and by using the appropriate controls.[1036,1062,1065,1072,1073] Delay in fixation significantly affects the results, whereas fixation time within reasonable boundaries (between 1 and 9 hours) does not.[1052] Regarding the issue of a proper control, Battifora's team has proposed a very innovative procedure, which they refer to as the Quicgel method.[1066] Although the idea is very ingenious (as we have been accustomed to expect from this group), it may be a little too complex to be widely adopted. At this point, I think it is fair to say that satisfactory standardization of the immunohistochemical method has not yet been achieved. As a matter of fact, an experienced worker in the field has made the provocative statement that this goal is actually beyond the power of the technique.[1059]

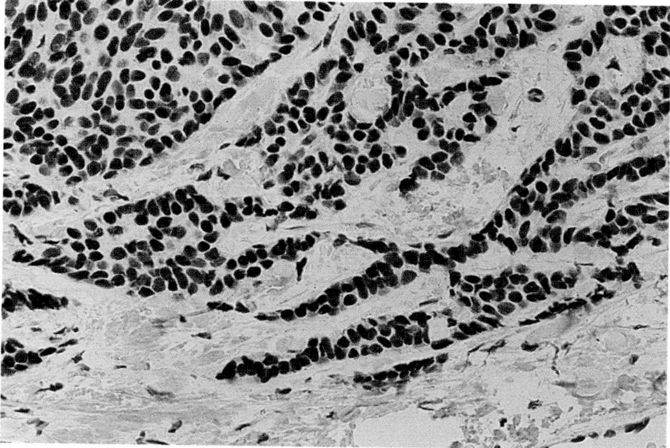

Fig. 20.98 Immunocytochemical stain for estrogen receptors in invasive breast carcinoma. The strong nuclear positivity in tumor cells is shown against a negative cytoplasmic and stromal background.

The two parameters evaluated in immunohistochemical preparations of hormone receptors are the number of tumor cell nuclei stained and the intensity of the reaction. The first is expressed as a percentage of the entire tumor cell nuclei population. The two parameters are sometimes combined into a scoring system, of which three major versions exist (including the popular Allred scoring system).[1049,1064] Although several sophisticated image analysis programs have been devised for this purpose,[1037] in most laboratories these estimations are done visually.

Hormone receptors can also be evaluated in paraffin-embedded breast tissue by the in situ hybridization technique and by PCR.[1044,1047]

About 80% of breast cancers are ER positive, so that an ER-negative rate of 30% or higher suggests that some problems exist with the assay.

Not much correlation exists between the cytoarchitectural type of breast carcinoma and the presence of hormone receptor protein;[1068] specifically, no statistically significant difference has been found between ductal-type and lobular-type tumors. However, as a group, ER-negative breast carcinomas tend to have a grade 3 histology, pushing margins, lymphoid stroma, comedo-type necrosis, and central fibrosis/necrosis.[1063] Most medullary, metaplastic, and apocrine carcinomas are negative, whereas mucinous, tubular and lobular carcinomas have a high rate of positivity.[1056,1058,1069] In ductal carcinoma in situ (DCIS), a predominance of large cells is the best morphologic predictor of ER-negative status.[1042] The positivity in lobular carcinoma in situ is particularly strong, and present in both the glands and the surrounding stroma.[1055] It is very unusual for an ER-negative cancer to turn ER-positive, whereas the reverse is more common, especially if there has been an intervening tamoxifen therapy.

Generally, estrogen receptor concentrations are lower in tumors of premenopausal women than in those of postmenopausal women.[1051,1069] Fisher et al.[1045] found the presence of estrogen receptors to be significantly associated with high nuclear and low histologic grades, absence of tumor necrosis, presence of marked tumor elastosis, and older patient age groups. Hormone receptor positivity also correlates with BCL2 immunoreactivity[1041] and absence of *TP53* mutations,[1043] and correlates inversely with the presence of epidermal growth factor receptors.[1071]

It should be pointed out that most breast carcinoma cells also have receptors for androgens, and that these may be found in the absence of estrogen and progesterone receptors.[1040] As a matter of fact, they seem to be more common in ER-negative tumors.[1035] Tumor types said to have frequent expression of androgen receptors are lobular carcinoma, apocrine carcinoma, and Paget disease.[1053,1060,1067]

The American Society of Clinical Oncology and the College of American Pathologists (ASCO/CAP) have recently jointly published their guideline recommendations for immunohistochemical testing of estrogen and progesterone receptors in breast cancer.[1046,1048] Some of the more salient points of this document are the following:

- The pathologist must report the percentage of cells that are immunoreactive
- Tumors having 1% or higher invasive cancer cells staining are regarded as positive
- The average intensity of the stain must be included (weak, moderate or strong)
- The pathologist must give an interpretation as to whether the sample is positive or negative
- The use of a composite score based on percentage plus intensity (Allred, H, or Quick scores) is optional
- Specimens should be placed in 10% neutral buffered formalin no later than 1 hour (but ideally much sooner) after being removed from the patient
- Fixation time should be at least 6 hours and not longer than 72 hours
- Normal breast cells in the sample can be used as internal positive controls
- Current testing and these guidelines focus only on ER alpha. Although there are data suggesting that high ER beta in the face of an ER alpha-positive tumor is indicative of a greater degree of responsiveness to treatment, the data are too preliminary at this point.

HER2/*neu*

HER2/neu (c-*erb*B-2) is an oncogene that encodes a transmembrane glycoprotein with tyrosine kinase activity known as p185, which belongs to the family of epidermal growth factor receptors.[1086,1098] Its overexpression can be measured by immunohistochemistry or FISH (or its chromogenic equivalent),[1078,1089,1090,1100] and a good correlation exists between these methods[1084,1092,1094,1097] (Fig. 20.99).

A heated controversy has been generated in recent years regarding the relative merits of the two methods, fueled by the availability of trastuzumab (Herceptin) as a therapeutic agent.[1075,1085] Most workers in the field have concluded that the best approach from the point of view of cost effectiveness is to start with the immunohistochemical procedure, which is graded according to the scheme in Table 20.2. If the results are either 3+ or 0, the determination can safely stop there, since the correlation with gene overexpression or lack of it, respectively, as measured by FISH, is nearly 100%. If the immunotest gives instead a result of 1+ or 2+, the performance of FISH is recommended, and the result obtained is regarded as the gold standard.[1080]

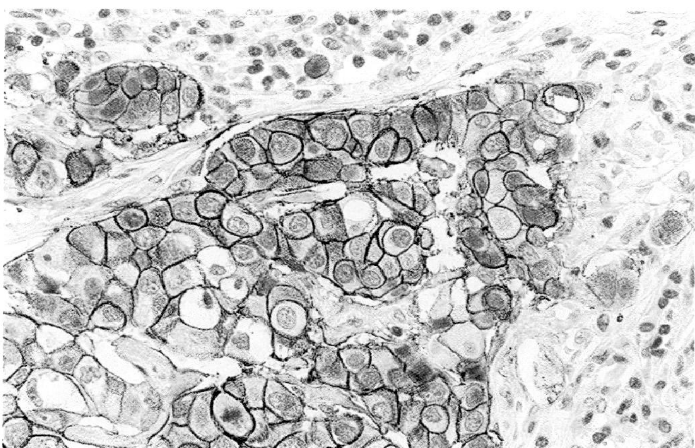

Fig. 20.99 Strong (3+) membrane immunoreactivity for HER2/*neu* in high-grade breast carcinoma.

Overexpression of HER2/*neu* by either technique is a very good predictor of response to trastuzumab, but not a very good predictor of response to chemotherapy or overall survival (see p. 1720).

In terms of relationship with tumor types, HER2/*neu* overexpression is found in nearly all cases of high-grade (comedo-type) DCIS, in 20–30% of invasive ductal carcinomas, and in a smaller percentage of invasive lobular carcinomas.[1081,1082,1087,1095] Conversely, it is typically absent in tubular carcinoma and other grade 1 carcinomas.[1088,1091]

HER2/neu amplification correlates inversely with estrogen and progesterone expression.[1088]

The validity of HER2/*neu* immunohistochemical determination is supported by the fact that there is little intratumoral heterogeneity,[1096] especially in tumors with high-grade amplification.[1077]

Recently, the ASCO/CAP has published their guideline recommendations for HER2/neu testing in breast cancer.[1099] According to this joint document, a *positive* HER2/*neu* result is:

- an immunohistochemical staining of 3+ (uniform, intense membrane staining of >30% of invasive tumor cells), or
- a FISH result of more than six *HER2/neu* gene copies, or
- a FISH ratio (*HER2/neu* gene signals to chromosome 17 signals) of >2.2.

A *negative* HER2/*neu* result is:

- an immunohistochemical staining of 0 or 1+, or
- a FISH result of <4.0 HER2/*neu* copies per nucleus
- a FISH ratio of <1.8.

Before leaving the subject of estrogen/progesterone receptors and HER2/*neu* in breast carcinoma, a few words need to be said about tumors that are negative for all three markers and to which the catchy term **triple negative tumors** has been recently attached.[1083,1093] Leaving aside the fact that it seems odd to define a tumor category exclusively on the basis of negative criteria, one could mention that

Table 20.2 Grading of the immunohistochemical staining for HER2/*neu* overexpression

STAINING PATTERN	SCORE	HER2/*NEU* PROTEIN OVEREXPRESSION ASSESSMENT
No staining is observed or membrane staining is observed in less than 10% of the tumor cells	0	Negative
A faint/barely perceptible membrane staining is detected in more than 10% of the tumor cells. The cells are only stained in part of their membrane	1+	Negative
A weak to moderate complete membrane staining is observed in more than 10% of the tumor cells	2+	Weakly positive
A strong complete membrane staining is observed in more than 30% (formerly 10%) of the tumor cells	3+	Strongly positive

tumors with these features (or lack thereof) overlap considerably with basal-like cancer (another newcomer to the field, more fully discussed in the next section) and breast carcinomas arising in *BRCA1* mutation carriers. However, triple negative cancers are not synonymous with basal-like cancers – only 77% of cases classified by gene expression profiling as basal-like show a triple negative phenotype, while only 72% of cases of triple negative cancers exhibit a basal-like gene expression profile.[1076,1079,1083] Triple negative breast cancers represent a heterogeneous group of tumors, which exhibit the following features: morphologically usually high-grade invasive ductal carcinoma NOS, high degree of aneuploidy, and higher tendency to metastasize to lungs and brain.[1083]

Molecular genetics and molecular classification of breast cancer

Molecular genetics

The development of invasive breast carcinoma involves multiple genetic alterations, similar to other carcinomas of various anatomic sites. The commoner molecular alterations include: (1) growth receptor overexpression (such as HER2/*neu* amplification in 20–25% of cases, EGFR overexpression in 3%, FGFR1 or FGFR2 overexpression in 10–12%); (2) growth factor overexpression (such as FGF1/FGF4 in 20–30%); (3) intracellular signaling molecule alterations (such as *HRAS* mutation in 5–10%); cell cycle regulator alterations (such as *TP53* mutation in 20–60%, *RB* inactivation in 20%, *CCND1* gene amplification in 13–21%); adhesion molecule alterations (such as reduced expression of E-cadherin in 60–70%, reduced expression of P-cadherin in 30%, overexpression of cathepsin D in 20–24%); and others (such as *CMYC* amplification in 5–20%).[1101,1102] In addition, some types of breast carcinoma, such as secretory carcinoma, lobular carcinoma, and adenoid cystic carcinoma, exhibit distinctive genetic changes, as described in the respective sections.

Molecular classification

The pioneering efforts of Perou and colleagues in 2000 to segregate breast cancers into distinct subgroups based on similarities in the gene expression profiles using the microarray platform has been enthusiastically embraced by the medical and scientific community, with the hope that this new approach will provide new insights into the biology of breast cancers and may impact therapeutic strategies.[1106,1111,1113] The grouping has somehow evolved into a molecular classification of breast cancer. Some investigators have predicted that the microarray technology will rule, while conventional pathologic assessment will become obsolete.[1108]

The subtypes of breast cancers recognized by their gene signature include: luminal (type A and B, and questionable type C), HER2/*neu* type, basal-like, and normal breast-like. The last subtype is most likely an artifact rather than a genuine type of breast cancer, resulting from lack or paucity of tumor in the tissue sample used for the microarray analysis. The main features of the molecular subtypes are summarized in Table 20.3.[1105,1106,1111-1113,1116] Among the various subtypes, the basal-like subtype is associated with the worst prognosis.[1113] Since the different subtypes of breast cancers exhibit specific characteristics, they would likely benefit from different approaches of treatment. There are efforts to use immunohistochemistry (such as a panel including antibodies to estrogen receptor, progesterone receptor, HER2/*neu*, cytokeratin 5/6, EGFR, Ki-67) to assign tumors to the various molecular subtypes (Table 20.4),[1103,1104,1112] but discordance is not uncommon, and there are currently no widely agreed criteria to define a positive immunostain for this purpose (such as percentage of positive cells and/or intensity of staining).[1114,1115]

The current molecular classification of breast cancers still has many drawbacks. The molecular subtypes were defined based on a relatively small number of cases, having missed out the less common distinctive types of breast cancer (such as secretory carcinoma).[1116] The basal-like subtype is highly heterogeneous, and encompasses some tumors with a favorable prognosis, such as medullary carcinoma, secretory carcinoma, and adenoid cystic carcinoma, necessitating the creation of a 'low-grade' category of basal-like carcinoma.[1105,1110] It is too simplistic to try to subsume the many different types of breast carcinoma into a few molecular categories, ignoring the known distinctive types with characteristic morphology and biologic features (such as invasive lobular carcinoma and secretory carcinoma). In fact, additional molecular subtypes have since been identified, such as molecular apocrine and claudin-low.[1106,1107] The issues with the standardization of analytic approaches, replication, attaining adequate sample size, and the evaluation of the clinical utility in broader heterogeneous populations by prospective clinical trials still plague the many gene expression profiling studies and their applications in routine diagnosis/prognostication.[1109,1115] Although every published microarray-based system can recognize molecular subtypes with similar survival and can also identify the basal-like subtype fairly consistently, the systems do not reliably assign the same patients to the same molecular groups for the nonbasal-like tumors.[1117]

Despite all the hype surrounding the molecular classification of breast cancers, currently the clinical value of characterizing invasive breast cancers beyond routine histologic type, histologic grade, and ER/PR/HER2 status has not been established. Thus routine assignment of breast cancer cases to a molecular subtype is not a requirement at present, although the practice may change in the near future.[1112]

Spread and metastases

Breast carcinoma spreads by direct invasion, by the lymphatic route, and by the blood vessel route.[1157] Some of these metastases are already present at the time of diagnosis, and others become manifest clinically months, years, or decades after the initial therapy.[1121]

Local invasion can occur in the breast parenchyma itself, nipple, skin, fascia, pectoralis muscle, or other structures of the chest wall. The invasion of the breast stroma can be by direct extension, via intramammary lymph vessels, and possibly via the tissue spaces of so-called 'pseudoangiomatous stromal hyperplasia'.[1128] The degree of local invasion is generally greater in invasive lobular carcinoma and its variants, presumably aided by the lack of E-cadherin in the tumor cells.[1135] The frequency of microscopic invasion in the breast outside the gross confines was evaluated by Rosen et al.[1158] by performing a 'local excision' with a 2 cm gross margin in specimens of radical mastectomy and studying microscopically the remainder of the breast. Of 18 mastectomies for carcinoma measuring less than 1 cm, residual invasive carcinoma was found in 11% and residual in situ carcinoma in an additional 22%. The importance of a thorough pathologic evaluation of local invasion in breast carcinoma and the status of the margins is now greater because of the large number of conservative surgical procedures being performed.[1125,1146]

A somewhat related problem is that of microscopic involvement of the nipple by breast carcinoma, since this structure would obviously be left in place if a local excision of the lump were carried

Table 20.3 Major molecular subtypes of breast cancer determined by gene expression profiling

	MOLECULAR SUBTYPE			
	Luminal A	**Luminal B**	**HER2/*neu***	**Basal-like**[a]
Gene expression pattern	Expression of luminal (low molecular weight) cytokeratins, and high expression of hormone receptors and associated genes	Expression of luminal (low molecular weight) cytokeratins, and moderate to weak expression of hormone receptors and associated genes	High expression of *HER2* and other genes in amplicon on 17q12 Low expression of ER and associated genes	High expression of basal epithelial genes, basal cytokeratins Low expression of ER and associated genes Low expression of HER2/*neu*
Clinical and biologic features	~50% of invasive breast cancers ER/PR positive HER2/*neu* negative	~20% of invasive breast cancers ER/PR positive HER2/*neu* expression variable (positive or negative) Higher proliferation than luminal A Luminal B tends to be higher histologic grade than luminal A	~15% of invasive breast cancers ER/PR negative HER2/*neu* positive (by definition) High proliferation *TP53* mutation common More likely to be high grade and node positive	~15% of invasive breast cancers Most ER/PR and HER2/*neu* negative ('triple negative') High proliferation *TP53* mutation common; *BRCA1* dysfunction (germline, sporadic) Particularly common in African–American women
Histologic correlation	Tubular carcinoma Cribriform carcinoma Low grade invasive ductal carcinoma NOS Classic lobular carcinoma[b]	Invasive ductal carcinoma NOS Micropapillary carcinoma	High grade invasive ductal carcinoma NOS	High grade invasive ductal carcinoma NOS Metaplastic carcinoma Medullary carcinoma
Treatment response and outcome	Respond to endocrine therapy	Respond to endocrine therapy (tamoxifen and aromatase inhibitors) may not be as good as for luminal A	Respond to trastuzumab (Herceptin)	No response to endocrine therapy or trastuzumab (Herceptin)
	Response to chemotherapy variable	Response to chemotherapy variable (greater than luminal A)	Respond to anthracycline-based chemotherapy	Appear to be sensitive to platinum-based chemotherapy and PARP inhibitors
	Good prognosis	Prognosis not as good as for luminal A	Generally poor prognosis	Generally poor prognosis (but not uniformly poor)

PARP, poly(adenosine diphosphate-ribose) polymerase.
[a]There is a low-grade group of basal-like tumors that similarly express basal-type (high molecular weight) cytokeratin and triple negative phenotype, but with low proliferation, e.g., adenoid cystic carcinoma, secretory carcinoma.
[b]While classic lobular carcinoma usually exibits luminal A features, pleomorphic lobular carcinoma often exhibits features of other molecular subtypes.
Modified from Schnitt SJ. Will molecular classification replace traditional breast pathology? Int J Surg Pathol 2010, **18:** 162S–166S; and Correa Geyer F, Reis-Filho JS. Microarray-based gene expression profiling as a clinical tool for breast cancer management: are we there yet? Int J Surg Pathol 2009, **17:** 285–302.

out. Nipple invasion has been found in 23–31% of all clinically detectable invasive carcinomas; the large majority are seen in tumors located less than 2.5 cm from the nipple.[1143,1152,1166]

Local recurrence following mastectomy appears as superficial nodules in or near the surgical scar or as subcutaneous parasternal nodules. Their malignant nature should always be documented by biopsy because the condition can be closely simulated by foreign body granulomas and infectious processes. Although women with local recurrences have an increased risk of distant metastases,[1134] these seem to represent partially independent events that occur at different times.[1165]

Tumor recurrence following local excision often develops in the same breast segment, a fact that has led some authors to recommend a primary excision technique that removes en bloc the tumor mass and the associated duct system.[1141]

The two lymph node stations typically involved with metastatic breast carcinoma are the axilla and the internal mammary region, with the supraclavicular area representing an extension of the former. It should be remembered that it is not too unusual to also find lymph nodes within the substance of the mammary gland ('intramammary lymph nodes').[1159] Axillary node metastases are present in 40–50% of clinically detectable cases and are divided

Table 20.4 Use of immunohistochemistry as surrogate marker for the molecular subtypes of breast cancer

	MOLECULAR SUBTYPE			
Immunoprofile	**Luminal A**	**Luminal B**	**HER2/*neu***	**Basal-like**
ER, PR	ER and/or PR+	ER and/or PR+	ER–, PR–	ER–, PR–
HER2 and others	HER2– Low Ki-67 (<14%)	HER2+ or HER2– Ki-67 ≥14%	HER2+	HER2– CK5/6 and/or EGFR+

EGFR, epidermal growth factor receptor.

Modified from Schnitt SJ. Will molecular classification replace traditional breast pathology? Int J Surg Pathol 2010, **18:** 162S–166S; Cheang MC et al. Basal-like breast cancer defined by five biomarkers has superior prognostic value than triple-negative phenotype. Clin Cancer Res 2008, **14:** 1368–1376; and Cheang MC et al. Ki67 index, HER2 status, and prognosis of patients with luminal B breast cancer. J Natl Cancer Inst. 2009, **101:** 736–750.

into levels according to their topographic relation with the insertion of the pectoralis minor muscle: low or proximal, medium, and high or distal. When extensive, they are clinically detectable, but the margin of error with clinical palpation is high. Careful dissection of the submitted nodes by the pathologist is of extreme importance. The yield of nodes will increase if they are searched for after the axilla is cleared with an organic solvent,[1142] but most workers have not found this necessary for a proper search.

Supraclavicular lymph node involvement is present in close to 20% of patients with axillary lymph node involvement but is almost zero in cases with negative axillae.[1164]

The second major lymph node drainage area is to the internal mammary chain, which lies at the anterior ends of the intercostal spaces by the side of the internal thoracic artery. The overall incidence of metastatic involvement of this chain in clinically detectable breast carcinoma is approximately 22%.[1130] It is less than 1% for tumors in the outer half of the breast and negative axillary nodes, approximately 20% for tumors in the inner half and negative axillary nodes, approximately 30% in tumors of the outer half and positive axillary nodes, and over 50% for tumors in the inner half and positive axillary nodes. Rarely, a metastatic lymph node will appear entirely necrotic and may simulate an infectious process; immunostains for keratin and EMA may be useful to detect the necrotic tumor cells.[1160]

Distant metastases are seen most commonly in the skeletal system, lung and pleura, liver, ovary, adrenal gland, and central nervous system (including leptomeninges and eyes)[1123,1144,1149] (Fig. 20.100). Carcinomatous meningitis is a particularly devastating pattern of spread.[1140] Diffuse metastasis to spleen is very rare, but it can occur and cause idiopathic thrombocytopenic purpura.[1127] Invasive lobular carcinoma (including the signet ring variant) has a particular tendency to metastasize to the abdominal cavity, particularly to the gastrointestinal tract, ovaries, and serosal surfaces[1124,1132,1148] (Fig. 20.101). These metastases usually express estrogen receptors and feature loss of E-cadherin.[1163] A peculiar recipient for metastatic breast carcinoma is meningioma.[1150]

Some morphologic features of the primary tumor correlate with the preferential sites of distant metastases. Thus, presence of fibrotic foci is associated with bone metastases; tumor necrosis and negativity for estrogen and progesterone receptors for lung metastases; and N3 state for liver metastases.[1137] Brain metastases are more likely with tumors that are ER-negative, which express CK5/6, and which overexpress HER2/*neu* or EGFR.[1138]

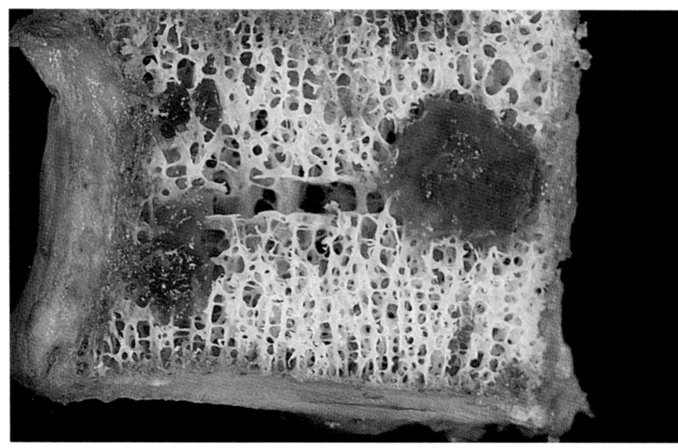

Fig. 20.100 Breast carcinoma metastatic to vertebra. The normal bone marrow has been flushed out by placing a thin slice of tissue under a strong jet of water.

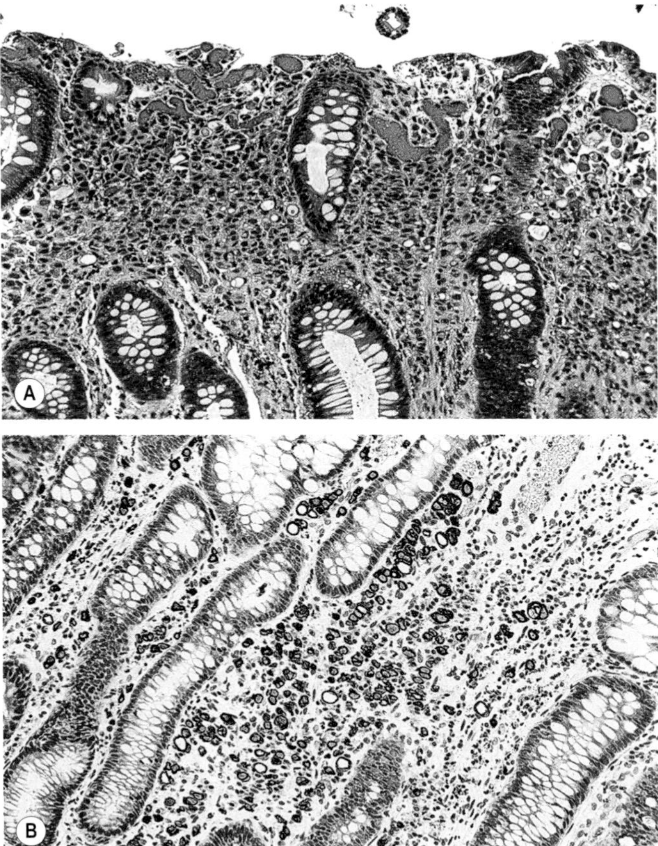

Fig. 20.101 **A** and **B**, Metastasis of mammary lobular carcinoma to lamina propria of large bowel mucosa. **B**, Keratin 7 immunostain.

effective for breast cancers that are HER2 positive (score 3 by immunohistochemistry or *HER2* amplified by molecular studies). Although originally used only for patients with metastatic disease, the drug is increasingly used as an adjuvant for early-stage breast cancer as well.[1217]

The value of poly(adenosine diphosphate-ribose) polymerase inhibitor (PARP inhibitor) for treatment of breast cancers with specific DNA repair defects, including those arising in carriers of *BRCA1* or *BRCA2* mutation and basal-type breast cancers, requires further studies for confirmation.[1223]

Effects of therapy on the tumor and on normal breast

Radiation therapy of breast carcinoma may result in bizarre nuclear changes, formation of giant tumor cells, naked nuclei, and abnormal mitotic figures. Extensive tumor necrosis may develop, which is later surrounded by a thick fibrous wall. It is important to remember that morphologic viability is not necessarily equivalent to biologic viability (i.e., the capacity of the tumor cell to replicate). In the non-neoplastic breast, the most characteristic irradiation effect is atypia of epithelial cells in the terminal ductules, associated with lobular sclerosis and atrophy.[1258,1264] These postradiation changes can persist for years.[1257] Cases of *pseudosclerodermatous panniculitis* after irradiation have been reported.[1267]

Hormonal therapy of responsive tumors leads to prominent stromal fibrosis and hyalinization, an increase in the amount of elastic tissue, and degenerative changes in the tumor cells. The latter are manifested by cytoplasmic vacuolization, rupture of cell membranes, nuclear aberrations, and eventual necrosis. These changes may occur both in the primary tumor and in the metastases, and can be very patchy, in the sense of showing morphologically unaffected cells lying side by side with highly altered cells.

Chemotherapy can also induce striking morphologic changes in the tumor cells, including a degree of vacuolization such as to simulate histiocytes[1253,1256,1265,1266] (Fig. 20.104). It also results in atrophy of the TDLU, with occasional atypia.[1255] However, in most instances it does not affect the histologic grading of the carcinoma.[1254] The microscopic features of the tumor correlate poorly with response to chemotherapy.[1268] In some cases the residual tumor is represented exclusively or predominantly by lymphatic emboli ('pure' and 'predominantly pure intralymphatic carcinoma'), a prognostically unfavorable feature.[1261]

Guidelines have been published detailing the gross examination, sampling, and reporting of breast carcinomas after neoadjuvant therapy.[1259,1260,1262,1263]

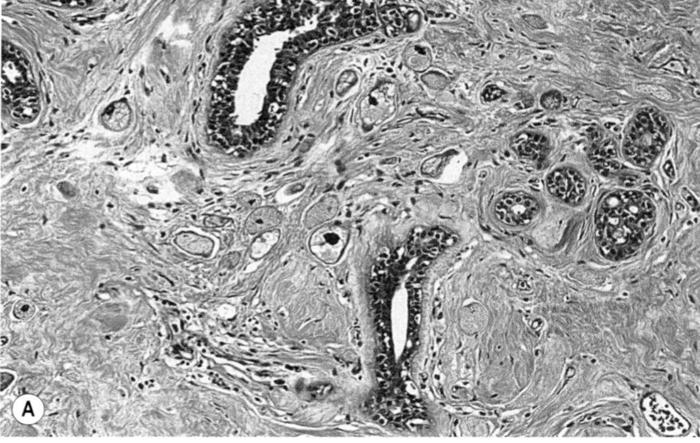

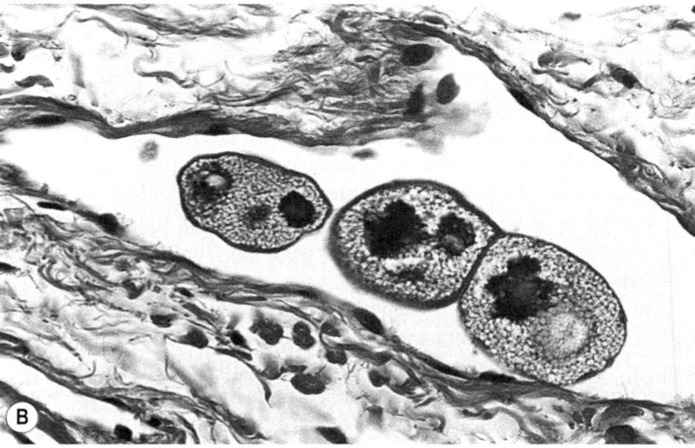

Fig. 20.104 **A** and **B**, Striking vacuolization of breast carcinoma cells induced by chemotherapy. The appearance simulates that of histiocytes. The tumor cells shown in **B** are located within a blood vessel.

(Courtesy of Dr Maria J Merino, Bethesda, MD)

Prognosis

The prognosis of breast carcinoma is related to a huge number of clinical and pathologic factors.[1324–1326,1330,1374,1381,1409,1428,1429,1458] These are listed not according to their relative importance but rather following the order in which they have been discussed in the preceding text.

1. **Patient's age.** Women who are younger than 50 years of age at the time of diagnosis have the best prognosis. Relative survival declines after the age of 50 years and is particularly low in older women.[1272] As far as very young women (≤35 years of age) are concerned, some studies have shown a prognosis similar to that in older patients,[1410] whereas others have shown a significantly higher risk for recurrence and distant metastases,[1385] related to the fact that these patients tend to have higher grade tumors.[1290,1304]
2. **BRCA1 status.** Early studies suggested that breast carcinomas developing in *BRCA1* mutation carriers are associated with a worse overall survival if they have not received adjuvant therapy,[1339,1408] but a recent large study of Israeli women carriers of *BRCA1* and *BRCA2* mutations showed that their breast cancer-specific death rates were similar to those of noncarriers.[1406]
3. **BRCA1 protein expression.** It has been recently claimed that absent or reduced nuclear BRCA1 expression as measured immunohistochemically is associated with several microscopic unfavorable features and a shorter disease-free interval, whereas cytoplasmic expression of this marker seems associated with the development of tumor recurrence.[1402]
4. **Pregnancy and oral contraceptives.** There is general agreement that carcinoma of the breast manifesting during pregnancy or lactation is generally an aggressive tumor with low expression of hormone receptors and high expression of HER2/*neu*,[1405] and that it is associated with an overall poorer prognosis, the 5-year survival rate in most series ranging from 15% to 35%.[1393] However, it has been found that this difference does not reach statistical significance when evaluated stage by stage.[1333,1394]

No convincing evidence has been found that prior use of oral contraceptive agents has an effect on the evolution or survival of breast carcinoma.[1415]

5 **Early diagnosis.** The relative 5-, 8-, and 10-year survival rates for asymptomatic breast carcinomas detected in a large screening project (BCDDP) were 88%, 83%, and 79%, respectively.[1424] These figures are much higher than those for the clinically detectable carcinoma and relate to the fact that the tumors were small in most cases, were usually devoid of axillary metastases, and included a high percentage of microscopically favorable types.

6 **Presence or absence of invasiveness.** Needless to say, this is the single most important prognostic determinator in breast carcinoma. For all practical purposes, in situ carcinomas are 100% curable with mastectomy. In tumors of ductal type that have both an in situ and an invasive component, a relationship exists between the proportion of the invasive component and the probability of nodal metastases. The amount of in situ component correlates with the incidence of multicentricity and, indirectly, with the probability of occult invasion.[1362,1366] It should be noted, however, that sometimes in situ ductal malignancies of the comedocarcinoma type can be associated with metastases in the absence of detectable invasion (see p. 1690).

7 **Size.** The diameter of the primary tumor shows a good correlation with the incidence of nodal metastases and with survival rate.[1301,1417] As a matter of fact – and despite earlier expressions of skepticism[1323] – this easily, quickly, and cheaply determined parameter has been found to be one of the strongest predictors of dissemination and rate of relapse in node-negative breast carcinomas.[1399] It should be noted that in tumors having both an in situ and an invasive component, the size of the latter is a better predictor than is the total tumor size.[1425] It has also been pointed out that size determination has a greater prognostic significance when measured microscopically than grossly.[1270] Size is one of the two criteria for the definition of *minimal breast carcinoma*, which includes all in situ carcinomas regardless of size and invasive carcinomas of 1 cm or less in diameter. Saigo and Rosen[1420] studied 111 patients with invasive breast carcinoma of 1 cm or less in diameter associated with negative nodes who were treated with a minimum of a modified radical mastectomy and followed for at least 10 years: 75% were alive with no evidence of disease, 4% were alive with recurrent carcinoma, 6% had died of disease, and 15% had died of other causes.

8 **Site.** No relationship has been found in most studies between prognosis and the quadrant location of the primary tumor. However, in one recent large study it was found that medial location of the tumor was associated with a higher (about 50%) risk of systemic relapse and tumor death when compared with lateral location.[1371] For a discussion on the relationship between tumor multicentricity and prognosis, see page 1684.

9 **Cytoarchitectural type.** There is no significant prognostic difference between ordinary invasive ductal and invasive lobular carcinoma.[1421] Morphologic variants of invasive ductal carcinoma with a more favorable prognosis are tubular carcinoma, cribriform carcinoma, medullary carcinoma (when strictly defined), pure mucinous carcinoma, papillary carcinoma, adenoid cystic carcinoma, and secretory (juvenile) carcinoma.[1313,1359,1389] A variant of lobular (and sometimes ductal) carcinoma associated with an extremely bad prognosis is signet ring carcinoma. The prognosis of inflammatory carcinoma (as defined microscopically, see p. 1706) is also particularly ominous. Tumors that have been said to be more aggressive than ordinary ductal carcinoma but that actually show little difference in survival rates are squamous cell carcinoma, metaplastic carcinoma, and carcinomas with neuroendocrine features (including so-called 'carcinoid tumor').[1378] The prognostic significance of these and other varieties is further discussed in the section on microscopic types.

10 **Microscopic grade.** The two most widely used systems over the years for the microscopic grading of invasive breast carcinoma have been those of Bloom and Richardson[1293] and Black,[1292] the first based mainly on architectural features (extent of tubular formation) and the second on the degree of nuclear atypia. These are usually estimated by visual microscopic examination of routinely stained sections, although various attempts at quantitating these changes (particularly the nuclear aberrations) by computer-assisted analysis have been made.[1279,1280,1395,1442] Since both architecture and cytology have been found to correlate with prognosis, the sensible proposal has been made to use them in conjunction.[1312,1365,1417] Elston has been the most vocal champion of this approach, which is usually referred to as the Nottingham modification of the Bloom–Richardson system and which also incorporates the evaluation of mitotic activity.[1319,1332] In this scheme, the grade is obtained by adding up the scores for tubule formation, nuclear pleomorphism, and mitotic count, each of which is given 1, 2, or 3 points. This is translated into the final grade by formulae outlined in Box 20.1 and Tables 20.5 and 20.6.

The utility of this and related grading systems has been convincingly and repeatedly proved[1330,1334,1345,1430] to the point that incorporation of this information into the routine pathology report has become a requirement.[1391] This is reinforced by the fact that an acceptable degree of

Box 20.1 Microscopic grading of breast carcinoma: Nottingham modification of the Bloom–Richardson system

Tubule formation

1 point: Tubular formations in >75% of the tumor
2 points: Tubular formations in 10–75% of the tumor
3 points: Tubular formations in <10% of the tumor
Note: For scoring tubule formations, the overall appearance of the tumor has to be taken into consideration.

Nuclear pleomorphism

1 point: Nuclei with minimal variation in size and shape
2 points: Nuclei with moderate variation in size and shape
3 points: Nuclei with marked variation in size and shape
Note: The tumor areas having cells with greatest atypia should be evaluated.

Mitotic count

1, 2, or 3 points, according to Table 20.5
Note: Mitotic figures are to be counted only at the periphery of the tumor. Counting should begin in the most mitotically active area; 10 high-power fields (APF) are to be counted in the same area (but not necessarily contiguous). The fields should be filled with as much tumor as possible; poorly preserved areas are to be avoided. Cells in the prophase should be ignored.

Table 20.5 Assignment of points for mitotic counts according to the field area, using several microscopes

	LEITZ ORTHOLUX	MICROSCOPE NIKON LABOPHOT	LEITZ DIAPLAN
Objective	×25	×40	×40
Field diameter (mm)	0.59	0.44	0.63
Field area (mm^2)	0.274	0.152	0.312
Mitotic count			
1 point	0–9	0–5	0–11
2 points	10–19	6–10	12–22
3 points	>20	>11	>23

Table 20.6 Final grading score

SUM OF POINTS	FINAL GRADE
3–5	I
6–7	II
8–9	III

interobserver reproducibility has been achieved.[1310,1332,1407] The system was largely conceived for invasive ductal carcinoma NOS, but it can also be applied to the special types of ductal carcinoma and to lobular carcinoma.[1281]

As far as carcinoma in situ is concerned, there is also a close relationship between the microscopic grade and the likelihood of local recurrence.[1306]

11 **Type of margins.** Tumors with 'pushing' margins have a better prognosis than tumors with infiltrating margins. This applies not only to medullary carcinoma, but also to other types of well-circumscribed neoplasms.[1302,1348,1360]

12 **Tumor necrosis.** Spontaneous tumor necrosis is associated with an increased incidence of lymph node metastases and decreased survival rates,[1287,1302,1336,1376] particularly if very extensive.[1354] This feature is usually associated with tumors of high histologic grade.[1460]

13 **Stromal reaction.** Surprisingly, it has been found that tumors with an absence of inflammatory reaction at the periphery have a lesser degree of nodal metastases and presumably a better prognosis.[1329] Obviously, these considerations do not apply to the specific case of medullary carcinoma.

14 **Microvessel density.** The interesting observation has been made that invasive breast carcinomas having a prominent vascular component in the surrounding stroma behave in a more aggressive fashion than the others.[1448–1450,1452] Accordingly, attempts have been made to quantitate the 'density' of these vessels and to correlate this feature to other parameters, notably prognosis.[1283] The original proponents of this approach have shown rather impressive results, and these have been corroborated by some independent observers.[1296,1314,1335] Others have failed to show significant correlations and have commented on the great difficulties encountered in estimating the surface or volume of the intricate vascular network that surrounds these tumors.[1277,1390,1427] It should be added that microvessel density is a phenomenon independent from intratumoral endothelial cell proliferation,[1445] and that an increase in microvessel density has also been noted in intraductal carcinoma, particularly of the comedo type.[1341]

15 **Elastosis.** It has been claimed that breast carcinomas with no associated elastosis have a lower rate of response to endocrine therapy than those with gross elastosis.[1375] In terms of survival rate, no convincing differences have been found between tumors with and without elastosis.[1295,1338]

16 **Fibrotic focus.** The presence of a scar-like area in the central portion of a breast carcinoma is thought to be a surrogate marker for hypoxia and lymphangiogenesis, and is an unfavorable prognostic sign.[1438]

17 **Keratin staining pattern.** In one study, carcinomas that expressed CK17 and CK5 had a worse clinical outcome than the others.[1439]

18 **CEA staining pattern.** This immunohistochemical feature has not been found to relate to prognosis.[1440]

19 **Expression of mucins.** Among the various mucins expressed in breast cancer (MUC1, MUC2, MUC3, MUC4, MUC5AC, and MUC6), MUC1 and MUC3 are believed to be potential prognostic indicators, MUC1 having the strongest relationship with favorable patient outcome.[1401]

20 **E-cadherin status.** As already stated, loss of E-cadherin is a nearly constant feature of lobular carcinoma, but it does not seem to be correlated with the established prognostic parameters of this tumor type.[1398] Conversely, loss of E-cadherin in invasive non-lobular carcinoma is said to be associated with a reduced disease-free interval and overall survival.[1400]

21 **Vimentin staining pattern.** The claim has been made that vimentin expression is associated with poor prognosis in node-negative ductal carcinomas.[1316]

22 **Stromal CD10 expression.** This immunohistochemically detected feature has been found to be associated with estrogen receptor negativity, higher tumor grade, and decreased survival.[1372]

23 **Cathepsin D.** Despite original claims to the contrary,[1432] assays for neither cathepsin D immunoreactivity in the tumor nor serum levels of this enzyme have proved to have independent prognostic value.[1274,1317,1356,1363,1403,1419]

24 **HER2/*neu*.** As already stated, overexpression of this oncogene as determined either by immunohistochemistry or FISH is an excellent predictor of response to trastuzumab but a weak predictor of response to chemotherapy.[1382] Although it identifies a subset of patients with poor prognosis, particularly when lymph node metastases are present,[1286,1318,1344,1397] it correlates closely with tumor grade[1436] and loses much of its independent prognostic significance in multivariate analysis.[1278,1412]

25 **P53 and nm23.** Accumulation of P53 protein (presumably as a result of gene mutation) and low expression of the nm23 protein have been said to correlate with reduced patient survival.[1282,1284,1285,1349] However, the authors of a large study comprising 440 node-negative patients concluded that the immunohistochemical demonstration of P53 was not a reliable prognostic indicator in this population and that it was not associated with any major epidemiologic risk factor.[1411] This has been confirmed by others.[1404] It has also

been shown that loss of heterozygosity for *TP53* is strongly associated with high histologic and nuclear grade.[1387]

26 **BCL2.** A relationship between BCL2 protein expression and long-term survival in breast carcinoma has been shown.[1350] BCL2 is also correlated with estrogen receptor status.[1315,1355]

27 **MDM2 expression.** Immunohistochemically measured MDM2 expression was found in a study to be an independent negative prognostic marker.[1437]

28 **COX2.** Expression of cyclooxygenase 2 (COX2), a molecule linked to neovascularization and tumor growth, has been found to be associated with poor prognostic markers in one study,[1383] and with poor outcome in ER-negative breast cancer in another.[1455]

29 **Skin invasion.** Breast carcinomas in which invasion of the overlying skin has occurred are associated with a decreased survival rate.[1423] Invasion of dermal lymph vessels as a determinant of the 'inflammatory carcinoma' picture is a particularly ominous prognostic sign.

30 **Nipple invasion.** Involvement of the nipple by carcinoma is associated with a higher incidence of axillary metastases.[1453]

31 **Lymphatic tumor emboli.** The presence of tumor emboli in lymph vessels within the breast is associated with an increased risk of tumor recurrence.[1311,1384,1414] The association seems to be stronger if the lymph vessel nature of the involved spaces is confirmed by performing immunostaining for the endothelial cell marker D2-40.[1275,1379,1459] This to-be-expected finding is counterbalanced by the curious observation that the presence of tumor nests in spaces that look like retraction artifacts are also associated with poor outcome.[1271] It has been further noted that the presence of apoptotic and mitotic figures in the intravascular tumor emboli is a particularly bad prognostic sign.[1343]

32 **Blood vessel emboli.** This finding shows a high correlation with tumor size, histologic grade, tumor type, lymph node status, development of distant metastases, and poor prognosis.[1297,1325,1367,1380,1396]

33 **Paget disease.** The presence or absence of Paget disease in invasive ductal carcinoma is of no prognostic relevance per se.

34 **Estrogen receptors.** Several authors have concluded that patients with ER-positive tumors – whether determined biochemically or immunohistochemically – have a longer disease-free survival than the others. However, the differences in long-term prognosis are minimal and perhaps not statistically significant.[1269,1298,1346]

35 **DNA ploidy.** Despite numerous studies evaluating DNA ploidy with flow cytometry, it is yet unclear whether this parameter adds *independent* information of therapeutic or prognostic value once the size of the tumor, microscopic grading, lymph node status, and hormone-receptor status have been taken into account.[1276,1289,1331,1357,1433,1456]

36 **Cell proliferation.** This parameter, whether measured by the old-fashioned mitotic count,[1291,1314,1361,1364] by MIB-1 (Ki-67) or analogous immunostain,[1377,1418,1446,1451,1454] or by determination of S-phase fraction by flow cytometry,[1457] has emerged as a very important prognostic determinator,[1331,1388,1426,1447] particularly for node-positive cases.[1434] As such, it has been incorporated into the combined grading scheme espoused by Elston (see paragraph 10). Actually, some view it as the most important component of that system.

37 **Cyclin D1.** Overexpression of this marker as detected by immunohistochemistry does not seem to carry independent prognostic connotations.[1443]

38 **Telomerase activity.** The level of this enzyme is associated with the proliferative index of breast carcinoma, but its measurement is not an independent predictor of survival.[1300]

39 **Axillary lymph node metastases.** This is one of the most important prognostic parameters.[1273,1351] Not only is there a sharp difference in survival rates between patients with positive and negative nodes, but the survival rate also depends on the level of axillary node involved (low, medium, or high),[1288] the absolute number (fewer than four versus four or more),[1320,1327,1431] the amount of metastatic tumor,[1352,1413] the presence or absence of extranodal spread,[1328,1340,1368,1373] and the presence or absence of tumor cells in the efferent vessels.[1305,1342] The prognostic significance of 'micrometastases' and of 'isolated tumor cells' (as applied currently to sentinel lymph nodes) remains to be determined, but seems to be minimal.[1303,1309] For prognostic purposes, the best grouping seems to be the following: negative nodes, one to three positive nodes, and four or more positive nodes.

40 **Pattern of lymph node reaction.** It has been suggested that the microscopic appearance of the regional node (lymphoid response and/or sinus histiocytosis) is an indication of the type of host response to the tumor and that it relates to prognosis.[1435] The issue remains controversial; if there is indeed a correlation, it does not seem to be a statistically significant one.[1327,1329]

41 **Internal mammary lymph node metastases.** Survival in patients with involvement of this lymph node group is lower than in those without such involvement, especially if only patients with one to three positive axillary nodes are evaluated.[1386]

42 **Circulating tumor cells.** There is increasing evidence that the presence and level of carcinoma cells in the bloodstream are independent predictors of survival in patients with metastatic breast cancer.[1308]

43 **Local recurrence.** This is a sign of ominous prognosis. In one series of 60 patients with ipsilateral chest wall recurrence and no detectable distant metastases, all patients eventually died of metastatic breast carcinoma.[1337]

44 **Type of therapy.** This is too complex and multifactorial an issue to be properly addressed here. Suffice to say that all available evidence suggests that the outcome in breast carcinoma depends more on the nature of the individual tumor than on the type of therapy performed. There is certainly a striking similarity in survival rates from different centers employing widely disparate therapeutic approaches.[1370] A complicating factor in evaluating therapeutic results is the marked individual variations in the natural life history of the disease, which renders imperative the use of carefully randomized studies. Most of these studies have shown no significant differences in survival among the various groups, which have included the following:[1321,1322,1353]

a For patients with clinically negative axillary nodes:
Radical mastectomy versus total mastectomy with postoperative regional radiation
Total mastectomy alone versus segmentectomy with postoperative regional radiation

b For patients with clinically positive axillary nodes:
Radical mastectomy versus total mastectomy with postoperative regional radiation.

The results of six large prospective randomized clinical trials have clearly demonstrated that the combination of breast conserving surgery and radiation therapy provides survival rates equivalent to those following mastectomy.[1422]

Bloom et al.[1294] provided a good baseline on which to judge the effectiveness of therapy by showing that in a series of 250 *untreated* breast cancers, the 5-year survival rate after diagnosis was 18%.

45 **Surgical margins.** Microscopically positive surgical margins in specimens from conservative breast excisions are associated with a higher risk of ipsilateral tumor recurrence.[1369] Combining radial and shave margins improves the accuracy of this determination.[1347] Another method for determining the true status of the surgical margins at the time of a lumpectomy/segmentectomy, which we find very attractive and which we have used successfully for many years, is to ask the surgeon to take, at the time of the operation, multiple separate 'cavity margins' (from the wall of the residual cavity) and regard them as the 'final margins' that supersede the oriented initial margins from the excised specimen, which are technically very difficult to handle and which are probably the source of many false-positive results.[1299]

46 **Gene expression profiling.** There are many studies reporting the use of microarray analysis to select gene signatures for separating prognostic/predictive groups, and thus will potentially help with selection of therapy.[1307,1358,1392,1416,1441,1444] Two popular commercially available tests are: (1) MammaPrint (70 gene expression analysis by microarray, but fresh or frozen tumor tissue is required); and (2) Oncotype DX (analysis of expression of 16 cancer-related genes and 5 reference genes by reverse transcription quantitative PCR, and paraffin-embedded tissues are used).[1416] It should be noted, however, that almost all the gene signatures are applicable predominantly to hormone receptor-positive tumors.[1307]

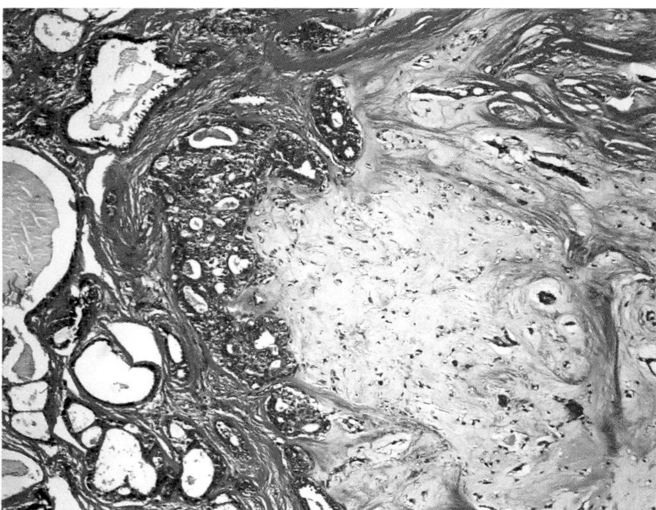

Fig. 20.105 Benign mixed tumor of breast. A prominent myxochondroid stroma is interspersed among the glandular structures.

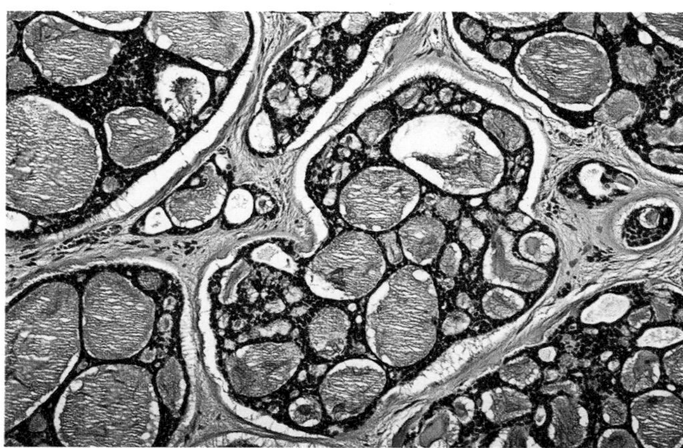

Fig. 20.106 Adenoid cystic carcinoma of breast. The appearance is similar to that of its more common homolog in salivary glands.

Salivary gland and skin adnexal-type tumors (including myoepithelial tumors)

A small proportion of benign and malignant tumors of the breast have an appearance analogous to, or at least reminiscent of, that more commonly seen in salivary glands or skin adnexae, particularly sweat glands.[1533] This should not be too surprising, since the breast is a modified sweat gland and a close analogy exists between sweat gland tumors and salivary gland neoplasms. Some of the malignant tumors in this category share many of the features of ordinary breast carcinoma and could have been discussed in the preceding section. It was arbitrarily chosen to include them here because of the histogenetic link they seem to have (at least at the conceptual level) with benign tumors having an unmistakably salivary gland/skin adnexal-type morphology.

The benign tumors in this category include **eccrine spiradenoma** (which, as in the skin, may undergo malignant transformation),[1479,1512] **syringomatous squamous tumors** (to be distinguished from low-grade mucoepidermoid carcinoma),[1494,1524,1531] **papillary syringocystadenoma**,[1523] dermal-type **cylindroma** (not to be equated with adenoid cystic carcinoma),[1462,1487,1506] **eccrine acrospiroma** (including nodular, solid–cystic, and clear cell hidradenoma; see under adenomyoepithelioma below),[1478,1496] and **benign mixed tumor.** The latter, which is very rare in humans but relatively common in female dogs, has been interpreted by some as a variant of intraductal papilloma,[1521] but its appearance is quite similar to that of benign mixed tumor of salivary glands (pleomorphic adenoma) or of cutaneous sweat glands (chondroid syringoma)[1466,1469,1475] (Fig. 20.105). This tumor can arise in an otherwise normal breast, as single or multiple nodules against a background of ductal hyperplasia, or in association (probably coincidental) with breast carcinoma.[1504]

Adenoid cystic carcinoma is the most important member of the malignant category. It is important not to confuse this very rare neoplasm with the much more common intraductal carcinoma with cribriform pattern (sometimes referred to as pseudoadenoid cystic carcinoma)[1488,1516] or with collagenous spherulosis (see p. 1678). True adenoid cystic carcinoma of the breast shows, as in the salivary glands, two types of cavity formation: true glandular lumina, and the well-known 'cylinders' containing eosinophilic basement membrane material and basophilic mucin[1495,1498] (Fig. 20.106). It may also show foci of sebaceous differentiation, indicating a potential to differentiate into skin adnexal structures.[1527] Perineurial involvement may be present. As in the salivary gland, there are variants with a partially or predominantly solid pattern of growth.[1497,1519] Hormone receptors and HER2/*neu* are typically absent.[1529] They could therefore be viewed as 'triple negative' tumors, although it would be nonsensical to equate them with the mammary carcinomas now bearing that catchy designation.[1486] CD117 is usually expressed, mirroring the pattern of its salivary gland homolog and in contrast with the above-named simulators.[1465,1472] They are also commonly immunoreactive for p63,[1501] but this is also true for collagenous spherulosis.[1510] Like the homologous tumor occurring in the salivary gland, a distinctive chromosomal translocation t(6;9) resulting in *MYB–NFIB* gene fusion is commonly found.[1509]

Axillary lymph node metastases are extremely rare.[1513,1532] Some patients have developed local recurrence or pulmonary metastases many years after initial therapy,[1468,1513] but the prognosis for this tumor as a group is remarkably good.[1463] The relationship between microscopic grading and prognosis is controversial.[1497,1513,1519] As already mentioned (see p. 1673), some cases of adenoid cystic carcinoma are seen in association with microglandular adenosis.[1461]

Acinic cell carcinoma is the newly added member of this family of tumors. As the name indicates, its appearance is highly reminiscent of the homologous tumor in the salivary glands. The similarities extend to the ultrastructural and immunohistochemical features.[1474,1514,1517] (but see under Secretory carcinoma, p. 1702).

Other malignant breast tumors that could be included in this category are **mucoepidermoid carcinoma**[1477] (see below), **polymorphous (low grade) adenocarcinoma,**[1464] **sebaceous carcinoma,**[1491] **apocrine carcinoma** (see p. 1702), **oncocytic carcinoma,**[1473] and **basaloid carcinoma.**[1499]

A more complicated issue is represented by the breast tumors of probable myoepithelial nature.[1484] First, it should be recognized that myoepithelial participation is an integral component of benign proliferative breast diseases (such as sclerosing adenosis, ductal hyperplasia, intraductal papilloma, and nipple adenoma) and that, in some instances, it dominates the histologic picture. Cases of sclerosing adenosis with great predominance of myoepithelial cells and presenting in the form of multifocal microscopic lesions have been designated as **myoepitheliosis.**[1526]

Second, myoepithelial cells are a normal constituent of the ducts and lobules, and therefore one might question whether these neoplasms should be regarded as of salivary or sweat gland type. They are discussed here because the morphologic variations they exhibit and classification problems they elicit are very similar to those they pose in the salivary glands (see Chapter 12). **Adenomyoepithelioma** is a small (average diameter 1 cm), firm, well-circumscribed tumor microscopically composed of cells of polygonal shape and optically clear cytoplasm, arranged in nests that are sometimes centered by gland-forming epithelial cells.[1526] The patterns of growth may be spindle cell (myoid), tubular, or lobulated[1515,1526,1534] (Fig. 20.107). Interestingly, some of these lesions seem to arise on the basis of a peculiar form of adenosis designated as of adenomyoepithelial or apocrine type (see p. 1673). The behavior is generally benign.[1502] In the series of 18 adenomyoepitheliomas reported by Rosen,[1515] two developed local recurrences but there were no instances of metastatic spread. However, isolated instances of metastatic behavior are on record.[1505] It seems likely that some of the cases reported as clear cell hidradenoma[1482] belong to this category (see above). Fully malignant myoepithelial tumors include the **malignant myoepithelioma (myoepithelial carcinoma)** when pure and the **myoepithelial-rich carcinoma** when containing a few ductular structures.[1467,1471] Both forms are cytologically malignant.[1508,1526] Some of these carcinomas (which may be quite undifferentiated and sarcomatoid) arise on the basis of an adenomyoepithelioma, the latter providing the best clue for their recognition.[1470,1490,1503,1520] Intraductal growth may be noted in them,[1525] and they may be multicentric.[1493]

The spindle cell (sarcomatoid) form of this tumor presents as a nonencapsulated cellular spindle cell tumor that grows in a fascicular pattern in the breast stroma.[1500] Its light microscopic appearance resembles very much that of a mesenchymal neoplasm; support for the myoepithelial nature of the few reported cases is largely based on ultrastructural or immunohistochemical observations, and/or the existence of a preceding or coexisting adenomyoepithelioma.[1481,1511,1518] As already mentioned, there is a great deal of similarity between some of the spindle cell forms of metaplastic carcinomas and these spindle malignant myoepitheliomas.

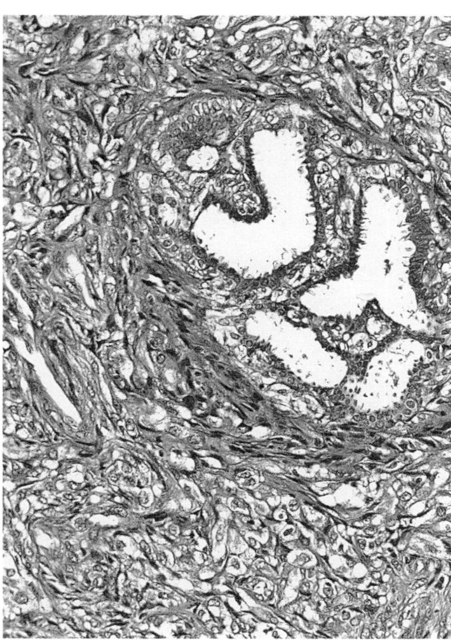

Fig. 20.107 Adenomyoepithelioma. In some areas there is a clear relationship between the secretory and the myoepithelial component (similar to that seen in adenomyoepitheliosis), but in others the spindle myoepithelial cells become the exclusive neoplastic element.

Low-grade adenosquamous carcinoma is a well-differentiated tumor with dual glandular and squamous differentiation. Many of the reported cases have originated from an intraductal papillary tumor.[1480,1530] Local recurrence is common following conservative surgery, but nodal and distant metastases are exceptional.[1530] Whether this neoplasm and the related *low-grade mucoepidermoid carcinoma*[1477,1507] are differentiating in the direction of salivary gland or sweat gland-type structures is not immediately obvious, but the occasional presence of low-grade adenosquamous foci in adenomyoepithelioma supports that interpretation.[1485]

Glycogen-rich (clear cell) carcinoma is composed of large clear cells, which are found to contain abundant glycogen.[1476,1483,1489,1492,1522] The biphasic appearance of adenomyoepithelioma is not apparent. It is possible that some of these tumors are of myoepithelial or apocrine nature, but the evidence for either is not very compelling. These neoplasms are full-blown carcinomas, with a prognosis no better, and perhaps worse, than that of ordinary invasive ductal carcinoma.[1483,1528] Their differential diagnosis includes other breast tumors with clear cytoplasm, including the exceptionally rare clear cell ('sugar') tumor[1476] (see p. 1730).

Stromal tumors and tumorlike conditions

Phylloides tumor

Phylloides tumor (rather than phyllodes tumor) is the term currently preferred for the biphasic neoplasm named cystosarcoma phylloides by Johannes Müller in 1838.[1543,1547,1555] It occurs in the

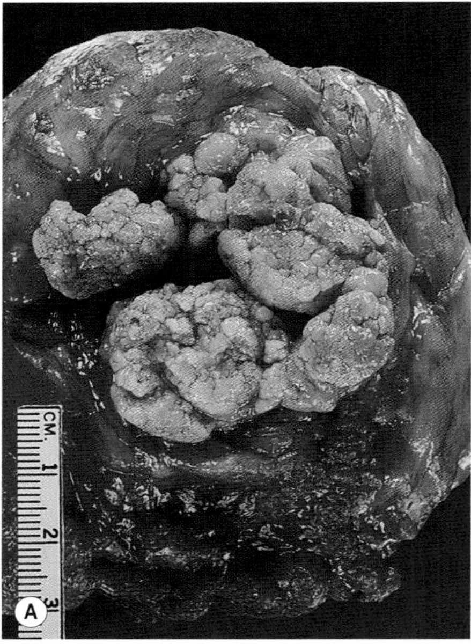

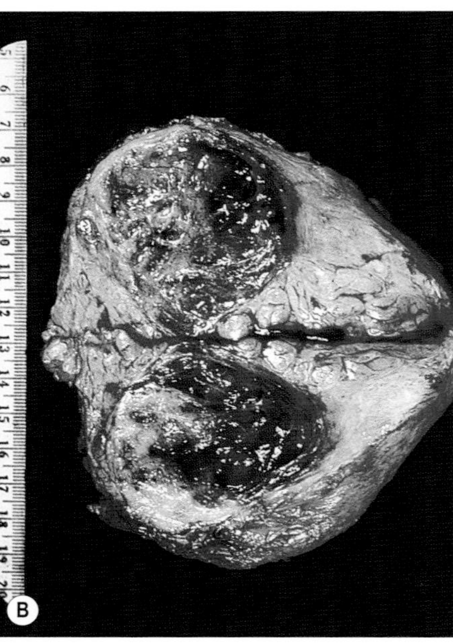

Fig. 20.108 **A** and **B**, Gross appearance of phylloides tumor. The tumor shown in **A** exhibits the typical appearance of the cut surface. The tumor illustrated in **B** has undergone extensive hemorrhagic infarct.

same age group as breast carcinoma, the median age at the time of diagnosis being 45 years.[1537,1561] Very few of the patients are younger than 25 years of age, in striking contrast with the age distribution of fibroadenoma. However, phylloides tumor can certainly occur in young adults and even in adolescents,[1565] and, therefore, the diagnosis cannot be excluded on the basis of age. The interesting observation has been made that phylloides tumors are more common in Hispanics than in other ethnic groups, and that this risk is higher among those Hispanics born in Latin America than those born in the United States.[1537]

Grossly, the typical phylloides tumor is round, relatively well circumscribed, and firm. The nipple may be flattened, but the overlying skin is almost never attached. The cut surface is solid and gray–white and shows the cleft-like spaces that give the tumor its name (Fig. 20.108A). Areas of necrosis, cystic degeneration, and hemorrhage may be present (Fig. 20.108B). Rarely, the entire tumor undergoes hemorrhagic infarct. Many phylloides tumors are large and some reach huge dimensions, but others measure less than 5 cm in diameter. It follows, then, that the diagnosis of phylloides tumor can be neither made nor ruled out by size alone. A lesion with the microscopic appearance of fibroadenoma should still be diagnosed as such even if it reaches 10 cm or more in diameter (see p. 1667).

Microscopically, the two key features of phylloides tumor are stromal hypercellularity and the presence of benign glandular elements as an integral component of the neoplasm[1535] (Fig. 20.109). It is the amount and appearance of the stromal component that determines whether a breast neoplasm should be called a fibroadenoma or a phylloides tumor and, in the latter instance, what the chances are of the tumor behaving clinically in an aggressive fashion. Although a sharp distinction between benign and malignant forms of phylloides tumor is not always possible (particularly on core needle biopsies[1550,1553,1577]), hence the need for a borderline category,[1539] sufficient information is available on the natural history of this neoplasm to allow a statement to be made about the likelihood of metastases (i.e., the risk category) and proper management on the basis of the pathologic features.

Tumors with the configuration of fibroadenomas having a cellular stroma without atypical features concentrated in the periductal

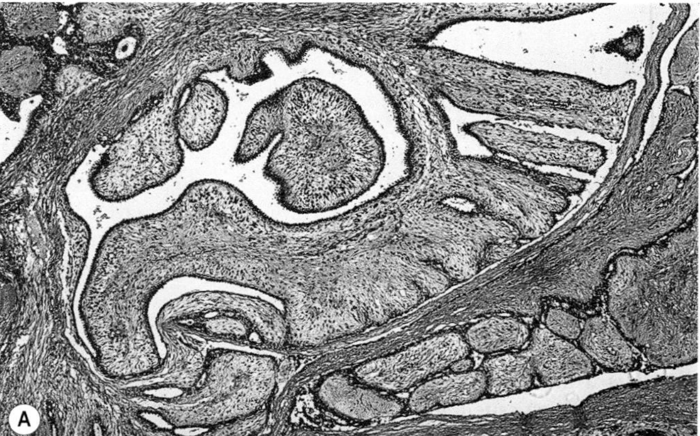

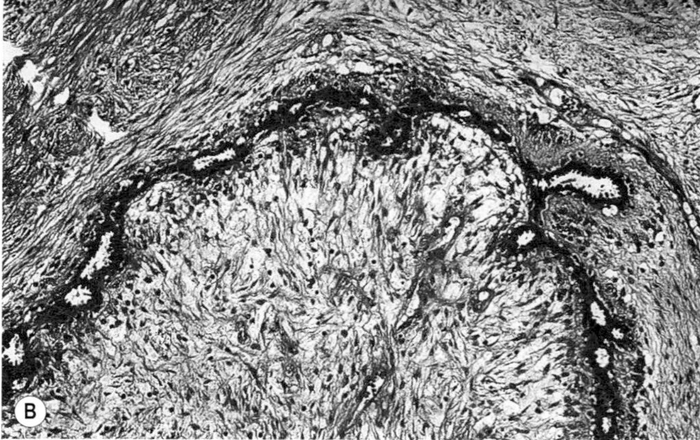

Fig. 20.109 **A** and **B**, Two views of low-grade phylloides tumor, showing cleft-like spaces and concentration of tumor cells beneath the epithelium.

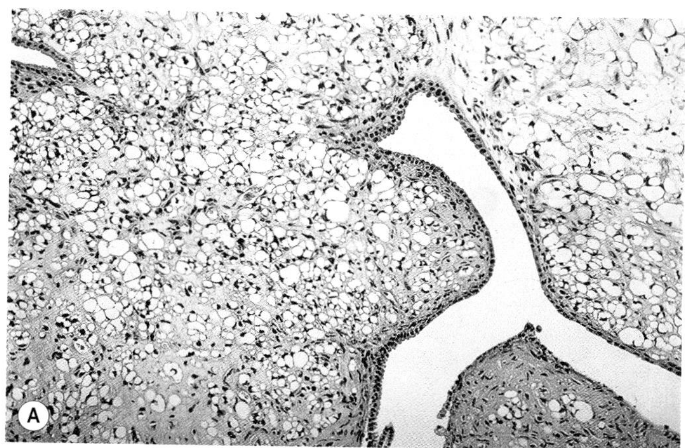

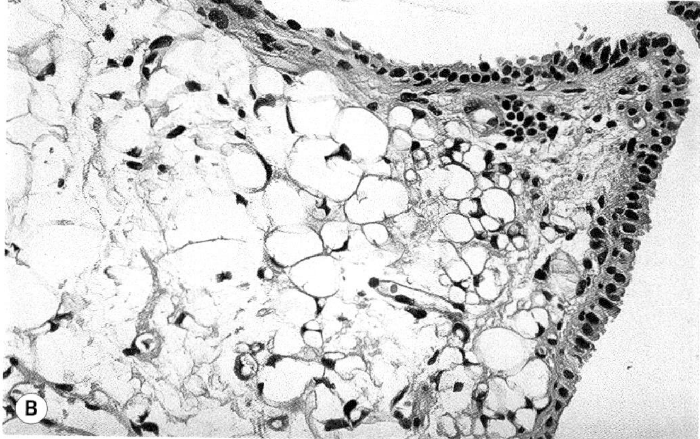

Fig. 20.110 **A** and **B**, Phylloides tumor with adipose tissue differentiation of the neoplastic stromal component.

areas are on the 'benign' end of the spectrum; this stromal component has a fibroblastic appearance, with occasional admixture of mature adipose tissue foci. When the latter are prominent, the term *lipophylloides tumor* has been employed[1569] (Fig. 20.110). Cytologically, malignant phylloides tumors have marked nuclear atypia, numerous mitoses, and loss of the relationship between glands and stroma. An important diagnostic criterion of malignancy is overgrowth of the glands by the sarcomatous stroma so that low-power views of the tumor show only stroma without epithelial elements.[1549,1575] The neoplastic stromal component may be monomorphic or highly pleomorphic, and its appearance may be reminiscent of fibrosarcoma, so-called malignant fibrous histiocytoma, or liposarcoma;[1564] metaplastic cartilage, bone, or, exceptionally, skeletal muscle may be encountered.[1536,1570] Phylloides tumors with stromal elements other than fibromyxoid behave worse than the others. Tumor necrosis is also associated with poor prognosis.[1542]

We view phylloides tumor as a tumor of the specialized mammary stroma with the capacity for epithelial induction.

The epithelial component, although probably not neoplastic, can have a markedly proliferative appearance, as it sometimes also does in fibroadenoma,[1561] a finding of no clinical significance. However, on very rare occasions, the features of carcinoma of either ductal or lobular type will be present in it.[1541,1552,1556,1560,1561]

Ultrastructurally, the features of the tumor cells are largely those of fibroblasts, accompanied by focal myoid differentiation.[1566,1576] Immunohistochemically, there is frequent expression of CD34 and BCL2, similar to other stromal tumors of the breast and in contrast to spindle cell (sarcomatoid) carcinomas, a feature of significance in the differential diagnosis.[1554,1559] CD117 is expressed in about a third of all cases and over half of the malignant ones.[1546,1573] Progesterone receptors are present in nearly all cases and estrogen receptors in about one-third, this profile being similar to that of fibroadenoma.[1574] The presence of these receptors seems to correlate with the microscopic grade of the tumor.[1571] There is overexpression of P53 in a variable number of histologically malignant and borderline cases, but very rarely in those with bland microscopic features.[1557,1572] Cytogenetically, phylloides tumors on the malignant side of the spectrum have a higher complexity of alterations than the others, with a tendency for a near-triploid stem line.[1544]

The behavior of the better-differentiated ('benign') phylloides tumor is characterized by a potential for local recurrence but an extreme rarity of distant metastases.[1551] If an enucleation has been done under the clinical impression of fibroadenoma, the patient can be safely followed for the possibility of recurrence. If the latter develops, or if this type of phylloides tumor is recognized at the time of initial surgery, local excision with a wide margin of normal tissue is the treatment of choice.[1540,1567] Recurrent phylloides tumor, which is the consequence of inadequate excision, may still be cured by wide local excision.[1558]

The cytologically malignant tumors are potentially metastasizing neoplasms, the incidence of metastases ranging from 3% to 12% in the various series. Deposits in the axillary nodes are exceptional. The most common sites of distant involvement are lung and bone, but the central nervous system also can be affected.[1548,1568] The metastases are of stromal elements only, although entrapping of normal structures in the lung may simulate a biphasic composition.

Wide local excision with an adequate margin of normal breast tissue is sufficient therapy for most cytologically malignant phylloides tumors[1567] but if there is any question of invasion of the fascia, the tumor should be removed together with the underlying muscle. There is no need for removal of the axillary nodes, except for the exceptional instances in which they are clinically involved.

For the phylloides tumors that do not fall easily into one of these two extreme categories (the 'borderline' group), the prognostic prediction and therapeutic recommendation have to be made on the basis of size, pushing versus peripheral margins, cellular atypia, and mitotic count.[1561,1563] There is some indication that DNA ploidy and S-phase fraction analysis may be useful adjuncts to the assessment of this tumor.[1545,1562]

The main differential diagnosis of the more malignant-looking phylloides tumors is with other types of sarcoma (largely depending on the presence or absence of a non-neoplastic epithelial component with the right architecture) and with sarcomatoid carcinoma (for which immunohistochemical evaluation may be helpful). The more benign-looking phylloides tumors need to be distinguished mainly from hypercellular fibroadenomas, acknowledging the fact that in some instances this may not be possible at a practical level or justified at a conceptual level. Along these lines, the neoplasm recently described as *periductal stromal tumor* could be viewed as being in between phylloides tumor and stromal sarcoma, in the sense that it contains epithelial structures like those of the former but lacks the phylloides architecture.[1538]

Vascular tumors and tumorlike lesions

Angiosarcoma (malignant hemangioendothelioma) of the breast characteristically occurs in young to middle-aged women.[1610]

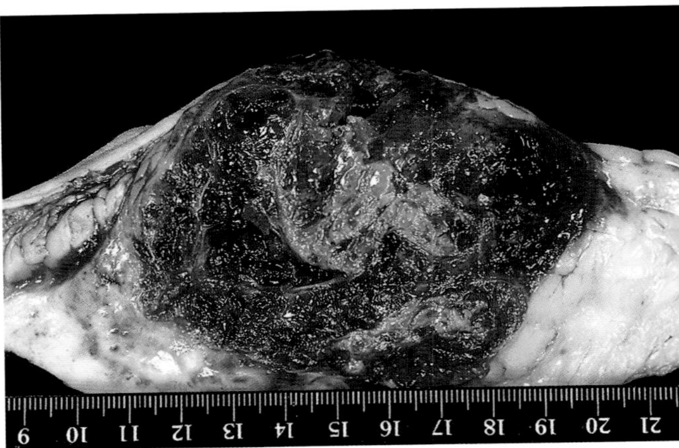

Fig. 20.111 Typical hemorrhagic gross appearance of angiosarcoma of breast.
(Courtesy of Dr Pedro J Grases Galofrè. From Grases Galofrè P. Patologia ginecològica, Bases para el diagnòstico morfològico. Barcelona, 2002, Masson)

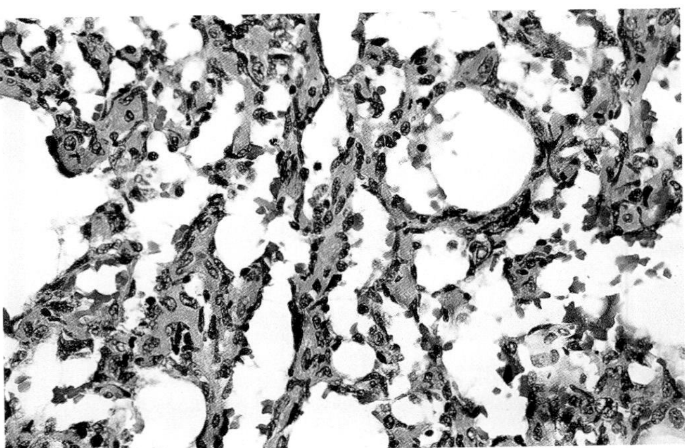

Fig. 20.113 Complex anastomosing vascular pattern in angiosarcoma of breast.

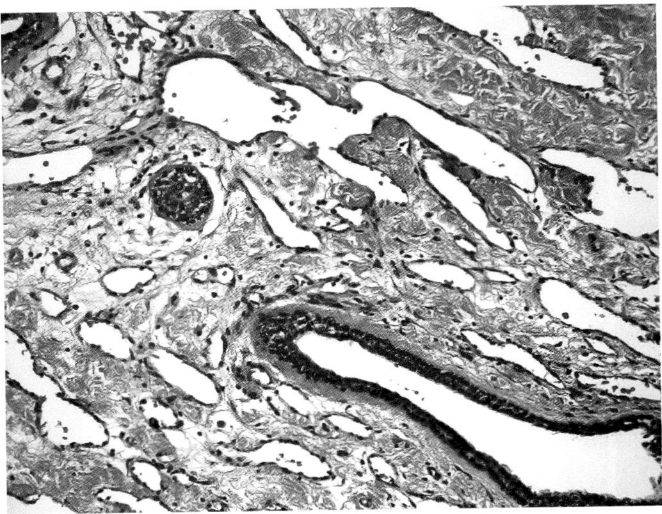

Fig. 20.112 Extremely well-differentiated angiosarcoma of breast.

Mammographically, it presents as a solitary mass that is usually uncalcified.[1591] Grossly, the tumor is soft, spongy, and hemorrhagic (Fig. 20.111). Microscopically, the diagnostic areas are characterized by anastomosing vascular channels lined by atypical endothelial cells (Fig. 20.112). The appearance may vary in the same tumor from that of a highly undifferentiated solid neoplasm to one that is extremely bland cytologically, to the point that some early cases were reported as metastasizing hemangiomas.[1609] However, close examination will usually reveal that even the better differentiated areas exhibit the telltale sign of angiosarcoma (i.e., freely anastomosing vascular channels) (Fig. 20.113). The tumor is thought to be of blood vessel rather than lymph vessel nature and is, therefore, also referred to as hemangiosarcoma. Occasionally, the tumor is of the epithelioid type.[1593] Curiously, some cases of breast angiosarcoma have been found to contain estrogen receptors.[1583] The differential diagnosis of angiosarcoma includes metaplastic carcinoma (see p. 1704), the acantholytic variant of squamous cell carcinoma (see p. 1706), hemangioma (see following discussion), and pseudoangiomatous stromal hyperplasia (see p. 1730). Immunostaining for MIB-1 (Ki-67) is said to be of utility in distinguishing the better differentiated angiosarcomas from the hemangiomas.[1607]

The overall prognosis of angiosarcoma is poor, with most patients developing metastases through the bloodstream.[1609] Donnell et al.[1587] have shown that a good correlation exists between microscopic grade and outcome. In their series, the 5-year disease-free survival was 33%; 10 of their 13 patients with grade I lesions were alive and well. The relationship of grading with prognosis has been confirmed in other series,[1594,1603] but not in a recent one involving 49 patients.[1597]

(Post-mastectomy; post-lymphedema) lymphangiosarcoma was a rare dreadful complication developing in the soft tissues of the upper extremity as a result of long-standing lymphedema following radical mastectomy or, exceptionally, segmental mastectomy[1579] (Stewart–Treves syndrome; see Chapter 25). This is hardly seen at present, but – in a curse-like fashion – it has been replaced by another type of iatrogenic process, this time following radiation therapy for carcinoma of the breast, as described in the following paragraph.

Post-radiation vascular proliferations. Following the administration of radiation therapy to patients with breast carcinoma who have been treated with conservative surgery, the overlying skin can develop a variety of vascular proliferative lesions, which range from lymphangioma-like nodules to full-blown angiosarcomas,[1600] with intermediate forms that have been descriptively named *atypical vascular lesions*, there being considerable overlap among them[1582,1588,1592,1596,1598,1606,1611] (see Chapter 4). The atypical vascular lesions tend to run a benign clinical course, at least on a short term basis, but we found than those featuring capillary lobules tend to evolve into full-blown angiosarcomas, if they are not angiosarcomas already.[1586] In contrast to angiosarcoma of the Stewart–Treves type, the interval between the radiation and the development of the tumor is short and lymphedema is minimal or absent.[1580] Exceptionally, this post-radiation angiosarcoma is located in the breast itself.[1599]

Benign vascular tumors can also develop within the breast parenchyma,[1584,1585] contradicting the old adage that virtually all vascular tumors of the breast are malignant. Although the bland microscopic appearance of some angiosarcomas of this organ

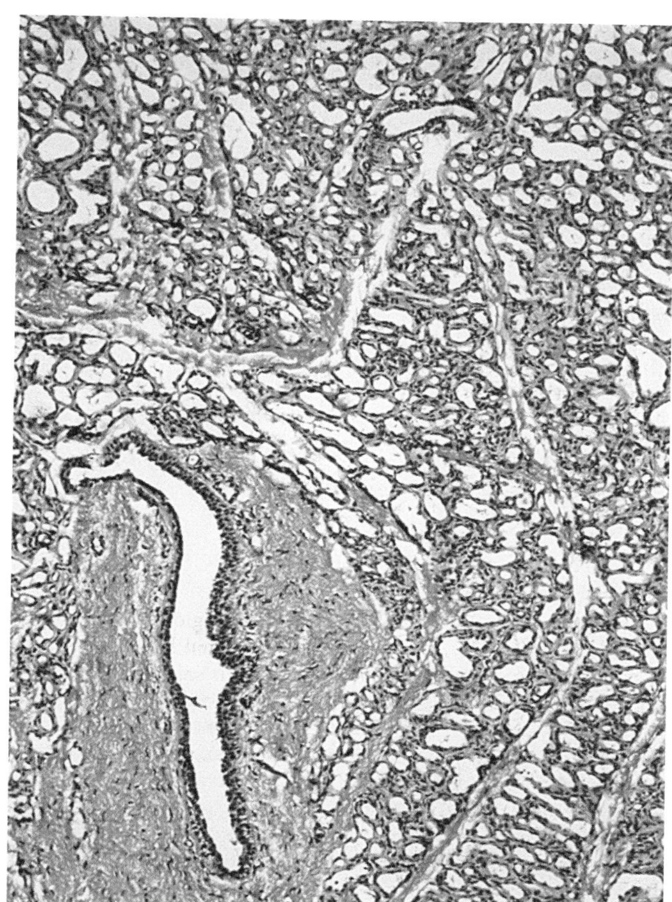

Fig. 20.114 Benign hemangioendothelioma of breast in a child. The appearance is identical to that of the homologous tumor seen more commonly in skin or salivary gland.

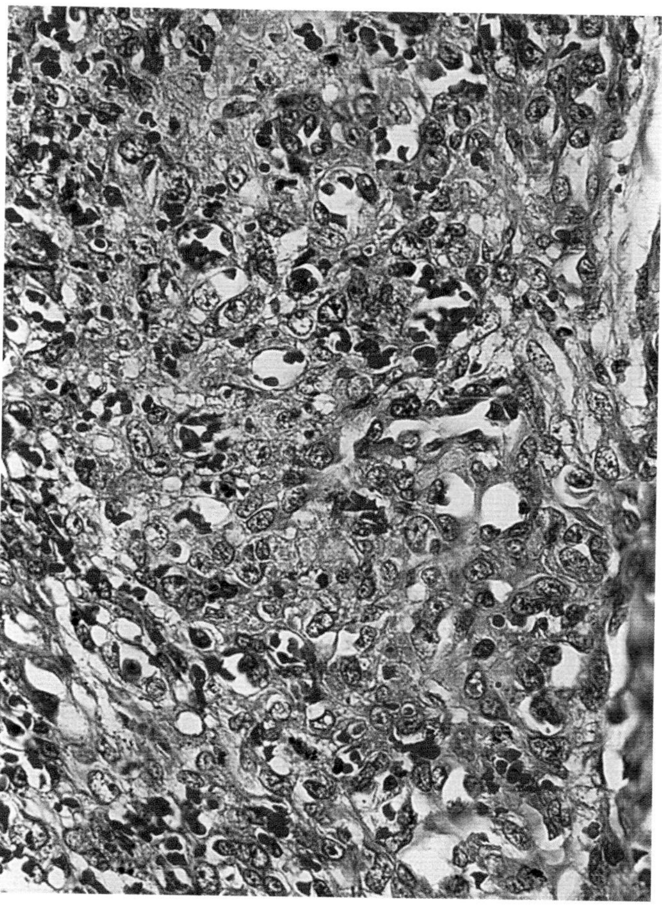

Fig. 20.115 Epithelioid (histiocytoid) hemangioma located within the breast substance.
(Courtesy of Dr Louis P Dehner, St. Louis)

cannot be overemphasized, it is also true that a number of perfectly benign vascular tumors can occur in this area. To begin with, hemangiomas of various types that share the features of those seen elsewhere in the body can develop in the overlying skin and subcutaneous fat. The most likely to be overdiagnosed is *angiolipoma,* because sometimes it can be very cellular and the adipose tissue component can be inconspicuous.[1602,1612] The encapsulation and presence of hyaline thrombi in the vessels are important diagnostic clues (see Chapter 25).

Benign hemangioendothelioma of the breast can occur in children, its microscopic appearance being similar to that of its more common cutaneous counterpart (Fig. 20.114). *Perilobular hemangioma* is usually detected only microscopically; it is characterized by dilated capillary vessels in a perilobular location, without anastomoses or cellular atypia.[1605] Autopsy studies have shown that it is a relatively common lesion, having been found in 11% of all breasts.[1590] Other *hemangiomas* are not located perilobularly; they also tend to be small but can reach a diameter of 2 cm.[1589] There are also *venous hemangiomas.*[1604] A few hemangiomas having a diffuse quality (although without anastomosing channels) have been referred to as *angiomatosis.*[1601] Other benign vascular tumors that can exceptionally involve the breast are *hemangiopericytoma*[1578,1595] and *cystic lymphangioma* (cystic hygroma).[1608] *Epithelioid hemangioma* and *Masson hemangioma* (*intravascular papillary endothelial hyperplasia*) can also be located inside the breast parenchyma[1581,1602] (Fig. 20.115).

Other malignant stromal tumors

Stromal sarcoma is the generic term given to malignant breast tumors thought to arise from the specialized stroma of this organ but lacking an epithelial component with a phylloides pattern[1617,1628] (Fig. 20.116). Grossly, the tumors appear solid, grayish white, and homogeneous. Necrosis may be present. Microscopically, most of them have the features of fibrosarcoma; focal osseous metaplasia can occur. Infiltrative margins and severe atypia indicate a greater tendency for local recurrence and distant metastases.[1628] Many of these sarcomas do not match precisely the appearance of those arising in the usual soft tissue locations, probably owing to the fact that they are composed of a specialized type of stroma. The recently reported cases of CD10-positive mammary sarcomas are examples of this phenomenon.[1625] Having said that, it ought to be acknowledged that tumors with an appearance equivalent to that of various types of sarcomas of somatic soft tissues do exist.[1629] They include *liposarcoma,*[1614,1626] *leiomyosarcoma,*[1613,1618,1619] *rhabdomyosarcoma*[1624] (but most such tumors are metastatic), *fibrosarcoma,*[1622] so-called *malignant fibrous*

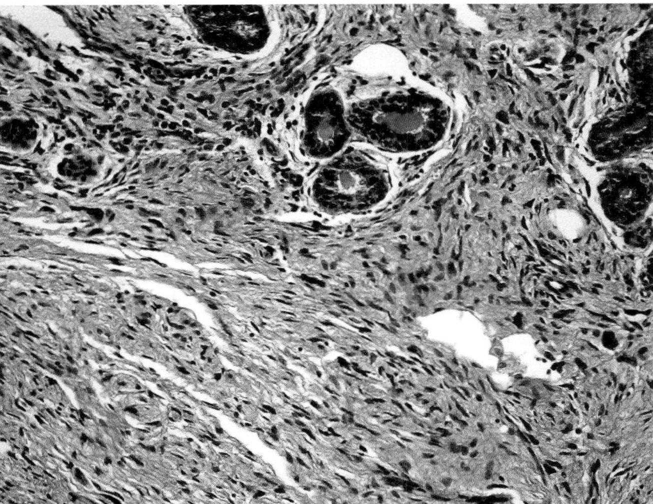

Fig. 20.116 Sarcoma of breast. The entrapped epithelial tissue lacks the features of a phylloides tumor.

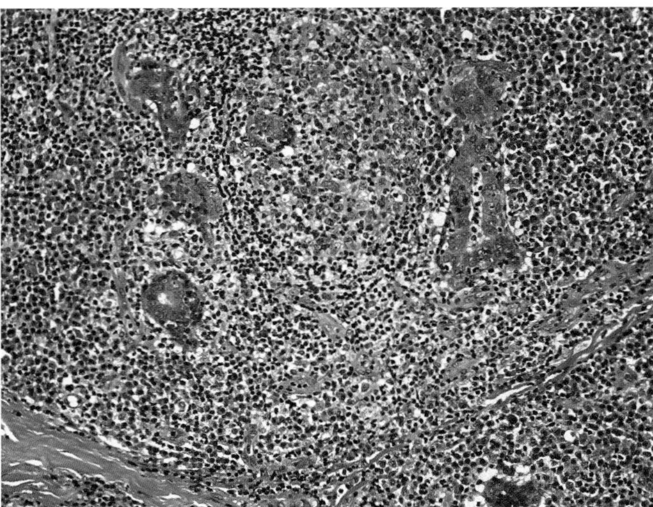

Fig. 20.117 MALT-type malignant lymphoma of breast. Some of the neoplastic lymphocytes infiltrate the glandular structures.

histiocytoma,[1622] *chondrosarcoma,*[1616,1633] *osteosarcoma,*[1615,1621,1632] *follicular dendritic cell sarcoma*[1623,1630] (including a myxoid variant[1620]), the related *interdigitating dendritic cell tumor,*[1634] *alveolar soft part sarcoma,*[1635] and *Ewing sarcoma/PNET.*[1631] *Rhabdoid tumor* also occurs, but we suspect that at least some of the reported cases are undifferentiated carcinomas with a rhabdoid phenotype.[1627]

Lymphoid tumors and tumorlike conditions

Malignant lymphoma can present as a primary mammary neoplasm or involve the breast as part of a systemic process.[1647,1648,1663–1665] A few cases have been reported associated with (and perhaps arising from) lymphocytic lobulitis,[1662] and several cases have been observed surrounding a silicone breast prosthesis (see below).[1646] Grossly, the tumor is soft and grayish white. It is not accompanied by skin retraction or nipple discharge. For some peculiar reason, the right breast is affected more commonly than the left. Multiple nodules are sometimes encountered. The involvement is bilateral in one of every four patients. In adult patients, primary lymphomas of the breast are nearly always of non-Hodgkin type and are usually composed of B cells,[1653,1657] although examples of T-cell lymphoma are also on record.[1637,1652] The B-cell lymphomas can be composed of either large or small cells[1636,1638] and usually show a nongerminal center phenotype.[1668] Most of them fit the category of MALT-type lymphomas[1641,1649,1655] (Fig. 20.117). This includes the tendency to surround and invade the wall and lumina of the epithelial structures, resulting in the so-called 'lymphoepithelial lesion'. Immunohistochemical studies have shown that nearly all of these cases lack evidence of follicular center cell or mantle cell differentiation.[1638,1639] The targetoid pattern sometimes seen around the ducts may simulate the appearance of invasive lobular carcinoma; in such cases, stains for CD45, CD20, and keratin should solve the diagnostic dilemma. The survival of patients with breast lymphoma is related to stage and microscopic type.[1636,1645]

Pseudolymphoma has been described in the breast. As in other organs, its position in relation to MALT-type lymphoma has become fuzzy. Some cases seem clearly reactive on morphologic and immunohistochemical grounds, perhaps representing an exuberant local reaction to injury.[1650,1656,1659] Some cases represent part of the spectrum of IgG4-related sclerosing disease.[1644] Cases have been reported in the nipple, often positive for *Borrelia burgdorferi* detected by PCR or serology.[1640] Other cases, instead, are composed of a monotonous small lymphocytic population and not easily separable from low-grade lymphomas. In some instances, the noncommittal diagnosis of *small lymphocytic proliferation* may be the best approach, followed by a recommendation for no further therapy if no systemic evidence of lymphoma is encountered. As far as the term pseudolymphoma is concerned, it is probably better to avoid it altogether, in the breast and elsewhere.

Burkitt lymphoma in African children has resulted in involvement of the breast, with the formation of huge bilateral masses. Bilateral Burkitt-type lymphoma has also been seen in young women during pregnancy.[1639]

Hodgkin lymphoma primary in the breast is exceptional. Most cases of Hodgkin lymphoma involving the breast represent secondary involvement in stage IV disease.

Plasmacytoma has been seen presenting as a primary breast mass, sometimes associated with a serum monoclonal protein.[1654]

Intravascular lymphoma can involve the breast and bear an uncanny resemblance to high-grade ductal carcinoma in situ, as this writer learned the hard way at a seminar in which he participated many years ago.

Anaplastic large cell lymphoma can also involve the breast.[1658] Notably, the majority of the reported cases have developed around a breast prosthesis ('seroma-associated').[1661] They are CD30 positive and ALK negative, and are associated with an indolent clinical course and excellent prognosis.[1651,1667] Seroma-associated anaplastic large cell lymphoma is probably a distinct entity, very different from systemic ALK-negative anaplastic large cell lymphoma.

Myelocytic leukemia of either acute or chronic type can present as a localized mass (granulocytic or myeloid sarcoma) in the breast and be microscopically confused with large cell lymphoma[1643,1660] (Fig. 20.118). The most important clue to the diagnosis in H&E sections is the presence of eosinophilic myelocytes and metamyelocytes, identified by their round or slightly indented nucleus and bright eosinophilic cytoplasmic granules. The diagnosis can be

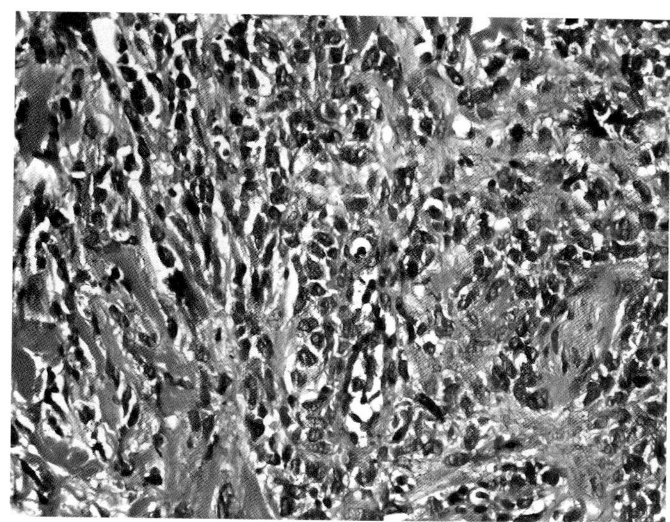

Fig. 20.118 Granulocytic sarcoma of breast. It is easy to misdiagnose this lesion as a large cell lymphoma.

confirmed by performing the Leder chloroacetate esterase stain or immunostains for myeloperoxidase or CD117.[1666]

Myeloid metaplasia (extramedullary hematopoiesis) can exceptionally present in the form of a mass lesion in the breast in patients with idiopathic myelofibrosis.[1642]

Other primary tumors and tumorlike conditions

Basal cell carcinomas, squamous cell carcinomas, keratinous cysts, and **sweat gland tumors** may arise in the skin of the nipple or other sites in the breast, but they are not to be considered primary breast tumors.[1684,1697]

Hamartoma has already been mentioned (see p. 1666). The definition of this entity – if it is an entity at all – remains unsatisfactory. Its identification is said to depend on the combination of clinical, radiologic, and pathologic criteria.[1677,1685] Morphologically, lesions that have been thought to be hamartomas on mammography may exhibit a wide diversity of appearances, the common denominator being the admixture of epithelial and stromal elements, the latter including fat[1683,1691,1699,1709] (Figs 20.119 and 20.120). A reproducible morphologic or immunohistochemical distinction of this process from circumscribed fibrocystic disease and fibroadenoma has yet to be achieved.[1695] *Myoid hamartoma*[1682] (which can contain epithelioid cells[1692]) (Fig. 20.121) and *chondrolipoma* (a benign lesion composed of an admixture of fat, cartilage, and sometimes bone)[1700,1703,1705] are two other processes straddling the fence between malformation and benign neoplasia.

Granular cell tumor is important because of its ability to simulate grossly the appearance of invasive carcinoma.[1680,1686,1698] It is usually small, but it may reach a size of 10 cm or more. On section, it is firm, homogeneous, and white or grayish yellow. As a rule, it is not attached to the overlying skin, but it may be fixed to the underlying fascia. The microscopic appearance is described in Chapter 25. The behavior is benign, and the treatment is local excision[1679] (see also below).

Myofibroblastoma is a benign mesenchymal tumor originally described in the male breast but also occurring in the female organ.[1673] This is described in detail on page 1732.

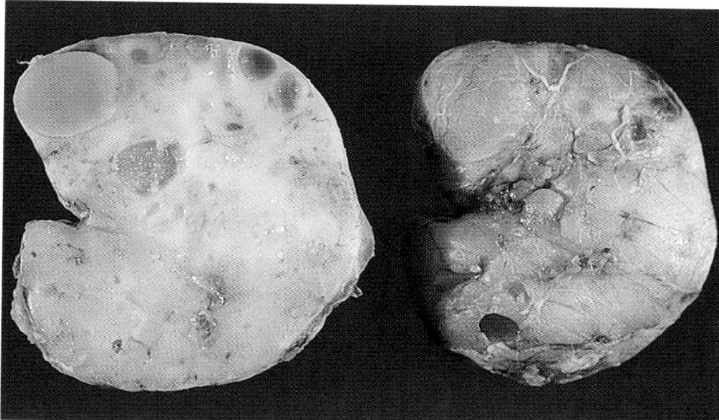

Fig. 20.119 Gross appearance of so-called 'hamartoma'. There is a combination of cystic dilation of ducts, fibrosis, and entrapment of adipose tissue. This lesion is more distinctive and impressive grossly than microscopically.

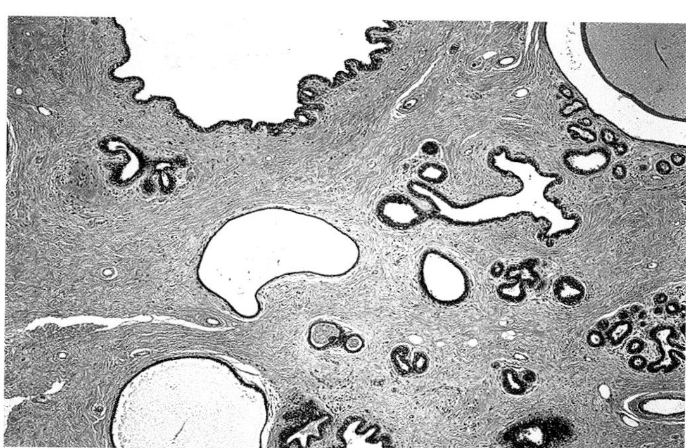

Fig. 20.120 Glandular epithelium and fibrous stroma with distorted arrangement in hamartoma of breast.

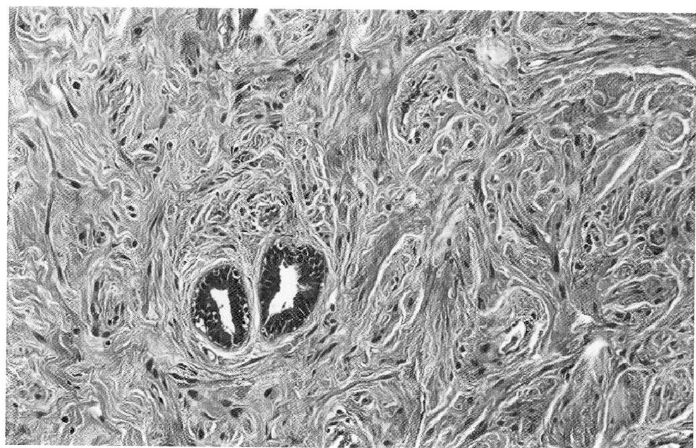

Fig. 20.121 So-called 'myoid hamartoma'.

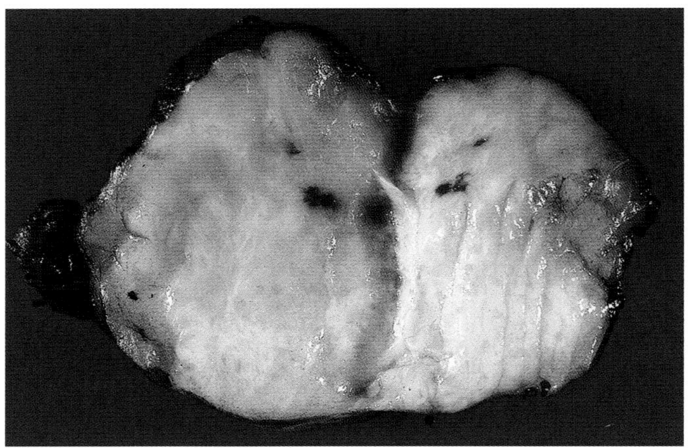

Fig. 20.122 Gross appearance of fibromatosis involving breast. The mass is solid and ill defined.

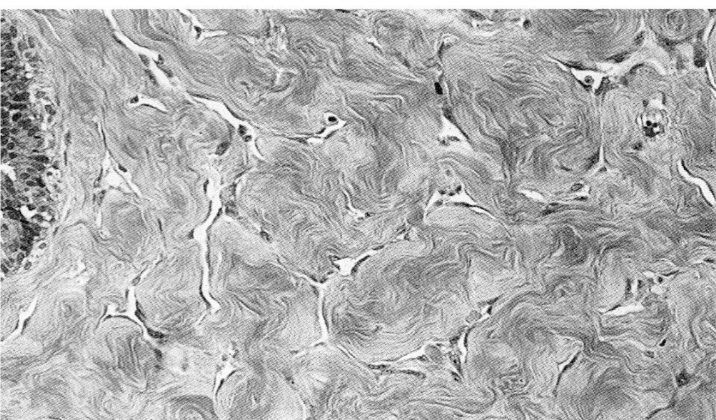

Fig. 20.123 Pseudoangiomatous stromal hyperplasia. Thin channels lined by spindle cells are seen scattered within a hyalinized stroma.

Solitary fibrous tumor has been reported in the breast.[1689] Its morphologic and immunohistochemical features blend with those of spindle cell lipoma and myofibroblastoma.

Leiomyoma usually involves the nipple and is often painful;[1708] occasionally, it is seen within the breast substance.[1688] Some have been reported as having epithelioid features and granular changes.[1714]

Benign peripheral nerve tumors of both *schwannoma*[1678] and *perineurioma*[1676] types have been described. *Traumatic neuromas with granular cell changes* have been observed in mastectomy scars.[1717]

Clear cell ('sugar') tumor (a neoplasm of HMB45-positive epithelioid smooth muscle cells, now generically designated as PEComa) has been reported in the breast.[1693] **Nodular fasciitis** is rarely seen within the breast, its appearance and behavior being similar to those of its more common soft tissue counterpart.

Fibromatosis (extra-abdominal desmoid tumor) can also be found within the substance of the breast (Fig. 20.122). It shares with its homolog in the somatic soft tissue a tendency for infiltration, local aggressiveness, and local recurrence.[1716] This is also true at the molecular level, in the sense that they have a similar spectrum of *CTNNB1* (β-catenin) and *APC* gene alterations.[1669] A significant number of the reported cases of mammary fibromatosis have occurred in or around the capsule of a grossly intact implant, raising the possibility of a pathogenetic relationship.[1671] Parenthetically, the lymph nodes draining a breast with a silicone implant may show clusters of foamy macrophages and fragments of foreign material consistent with silicone and polyurethane.[1701]

Cases of mammary fibromatosis occurring during child-bearing age are, in general, more cellular than those seen after menopause,[1687] in the sense of being infiltrative, aggressive, and prone to local recurrence.[1716] A type of fibromatosis containing eosinophilic inclusions identical to those seen in infantile digital fibromatosis has been identified.[1710] Parenthetically, similar inclusions have been identified in the stromal component of fibroepithelial lesions having a phylloides tumor-like appearance.[1675,1696] Fibromatosis should be distinguished from the low-grade form of metaplastic carcinoma (see p. 1704).

Pseudoangiomatous stromal hyperplasia (PASH) is characterized by a proliferation of stromal spindle cells of fibroblastic/myofibroblastic nature associated with the formation of probably artifactual clefts that simulate vascular channels[1720] (Fig. 20.123). In the more cellular areas the pseudoangiomatous pattern may be absent.[1711] The spindle cells are immunoreactive for vimentin and CD34, and negative for FVIII-related antigen, *Ulex*, and CD31. In addition, they show intense positivity for progesterone receptors. The latter finding suggests that PASH represents a localized form of stromal overgrowth with a hormonal (primarily progestogenic) pathogenesis.[1670] It has been proposed that the stromal proliferation present in PASH is composed of CD34-positive cells similar to those seen in gynecomastoid lesions and in the stroma of fibroadenoma, and that there is a close relationship among these disorders.[1672] Indeed, in one series, PASH-type changes were associated with gynecomastia-like alterations.[1690] As already indicated (p. 1713), breast carcinoma cells can grow along these pseudoangiomatous spaces.[1681]

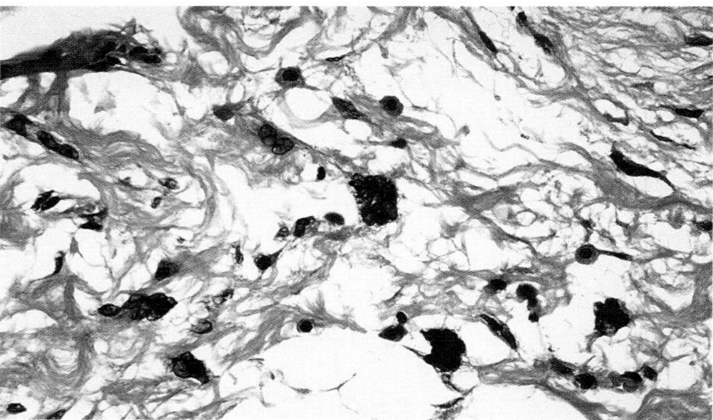

Fig. 20.124 Bizarre multinucleated cells in mammary stroma. This non-neoplastic change is analogous to that more often seen in the stroma of the upper aerodigestive tract and in the genital tract.

Multinucleated giant cells of reactive appearance are sometimes found incidentally in the normal mammary stroma or in the stroma of fibroadenomas;[1674,1715] they are of no clinical significance and are probably analogous to those seen in non-neoplastic polypoid stromal lesions located beneath mucosal membranes, such as the nasal cavity, oral cavity, anus, and lower female genital tract[1715,1718] (Fig. 20.124).

Inflammatory pseudotumor (inflammatory myofibroblastic tumor) may involve the breast, its microscopic features being analogous to those seen in other, more common sites.[1702]

Amyloidosis can appear as a solitary nodule within the breast parenchyma (so-called 'amyloid tumor').[1704,1713]

Rosai–Dorfman disease and **Erdheim-Chester disease**[1712] can also present under exceptional circumstances as breast masses, the former either as an isolated event or as a component of systemic disease.[1694,1707]

Juvenile xanthogranuloma can affect the breast of children and, exceptionally, of adult patients.[1719]

Nodular mucinosis presents as a circumscribed area of myxoid stromal change in the breast.[1706] It should be distinguished from the various epithelial proliferative lesions resulting in a mucocele-like appearance (see p. 1701).

Metastatic tumors

Metastatic malignant tumors rarely affect the breast except when widely disseminated.[1722] They typically appear as superficial, well-defined multinodular masses. Malignant melanoma and carcinoma of the lung, ovary, kidney, and stomach are the most common sources.[1724,1731] Most of the lung tumors are of the small cell neuroendocrine type. Breast metastases have also been documented from better differentiated neuroendocrine tumors, such as bronchial or small bowel carcinoid tumor,[1728] pancreatic (neuro)endocrine tumor, thyroid medullary carcinoma, and even carcinoid tumor arising from a tailgut cyst.[1725,1726,1729,1730] A certain predilection for neuroendocrine carcinoma to metastasize to the breast seems to emerge from these figures.

One should not forget in this listing the metastases from contralateral breast carcinoma, which is not an infrequent finding in autopsy series.[1722] Azzopardi[1721] has made the interesting observation that the presence of elastosis has not been documented in association with metastatic disease of the breast.

Metastatic carcinomas to the breast can simulate primary malignant tumors of this organ; exceptionally, they greatly mimic the appearance of DCIS.[1723]

In children, the most common malignant tumor to metastasize to the breast (hematolymphoid malignancies excluded) is rhabdomyosarcoma, particularly of the alveolar type.[1727]

Breast diseases in children and adolescents

The most common breast 'mass' for which clinical consultation is sought in this age group is actually not a pathologic condition at all but rather precocious, sometimes predominantly unilateral, breast development.[1732] Should such a 'mass' be removed, no development of the breast will occur.[1741]

Fibroadenoma is the most common pathologic condition of the breast between puberty and 20 years of age, but is exceptional before puberty.[1734]

Virginal hypertrophy (gigantomastia; macromastia) may result in massive unilateral or bilateral enlargement.[1732] Microscopically, it is characterized by a combined proliferation of ducts and stroma with little, if any, lobular participation[1736] (Fig. 20.125).

Pseudoangiomatous stromal hyperplasia (PASH) is generally a disorder of adult life, but cases have been documented in adolescents and children (including a 3-year-old boy!).[1740]

Fibrocystic disease of the conventional type is practically never seen in this age group. However, highly proliferative epithelial lesions can develop. Some of them have the appearance of intraductal papillomas.[1735,1737] Others resemble duct hyperplasia (epitheliosis) of the adult breast, with or without associated sclerosis and ductular distortion.[1737] Wilson et al.[1743] studied 74 patients with a process they termed *papillary duct hyperplasia*, which they distinguish from the juvenile papillomatosis described later. They found that 28% of the patients had a family history for breast carcinoma but that none of them had developed carcinoma at the time of the last follow-up.

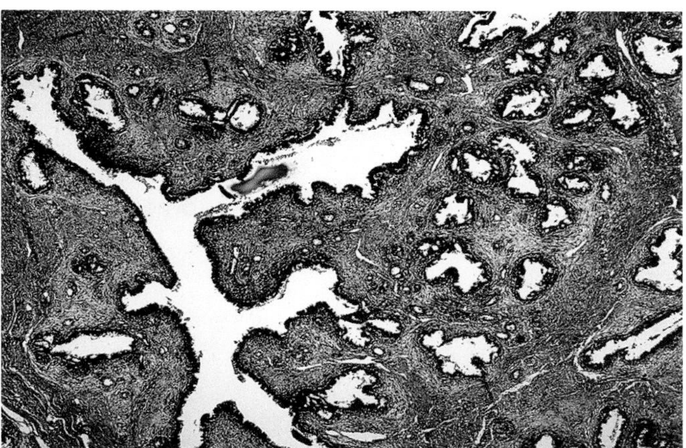

Fig. 20.125 So-called 'virginal hypertrophy' of breast, showing proliferative changes in epithelium and stroma.

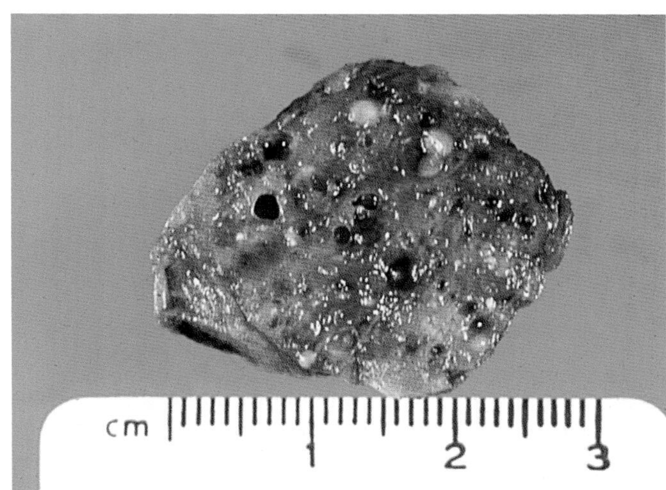

Fig. 20.126 Juvenile papillomatosis (Swiss cheese disease). The gross appearance is that of clustered cystic formations.

Juvenile papillomatosis (Swiss cheese disease) is a probably related but morphologically somewhat distinct form of ductal-type hyperplasia usually seen in young individuals (average age 19 years) but occurring in a wide age range (10–44 years). Clinically, the localized, multinodular masses simulate the appearance of fibroadenoma. Grossly, the clustering of the cystic formations results in a cut surface appearance reminiscent of Swiss cheese – hence the alternative designation for this entity (Fig. 20.126). Microscopically, there is florid epithelial hyperplasia (sometimes with marked atypia and/or focal necrosis), cysts with or without apocrine metaplasia, duct stasis, and sclerosing adenosis[1735,1738] (Fig. 20.127). A family history of breast carcinoma is reported in 58% of cases, and 10% of the patients subsequently develop breast carcinoma.[1739,1742]

Carcinoma of the infantile breast is very rare. Most cases are of the so-called 'secretory (juvenile) type' and are discussed on page 1702. A few tumors have the appearance of ordinary invasive ductal carcinomas.

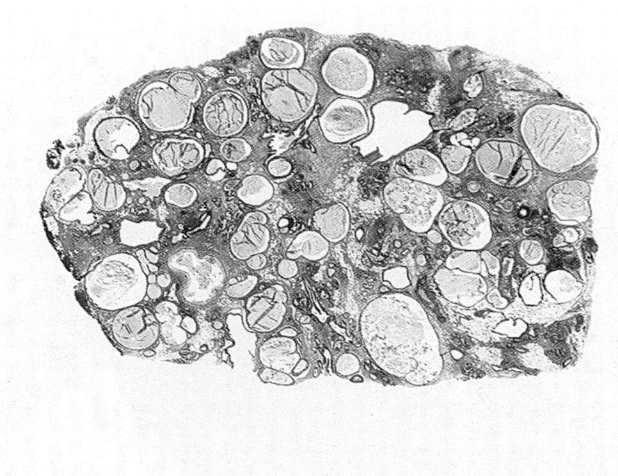

Fig. 20.127 Juvenile papillomatosis (Swiss cheese disease). Whole-mount view showing variously sized cystic formations, alternating with solid epithelial proliferations.

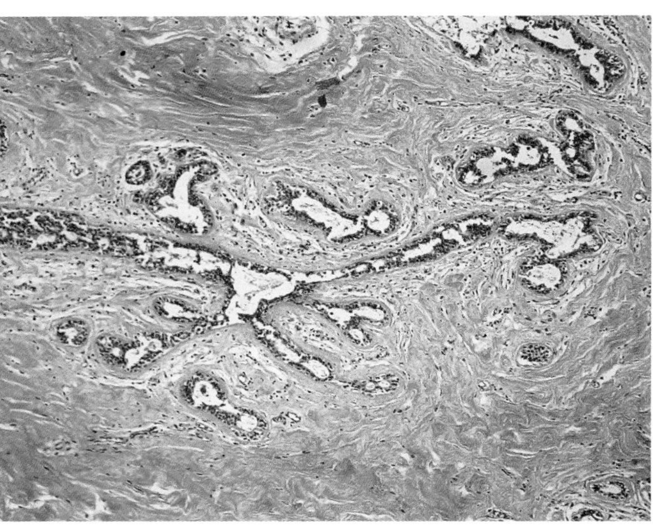

Fig. 20.128 Epithelial proliferation surrounded by a hypocellular myxoid halo in gynecomastia.

In the presence of a high-grade malignant round cell tumor of the breast in a child or adolescent, the possibility should be considered that it may be a solid variant of alveolar rhabdomyosarcoma, whether primary or metastatic.[1733]

Breast diseases in males

Gynecomastia

Gynecomastia is defined as the enlargement of the male breast resulting from hypertrophy and hyperplasia of both glandular and stromal components. It may result from numerous causes, which share a background of relative increase in estrogenic activity (whether endogenous or exogenous), decrease in androgenic activity, or both.[1745,1758] Development of gynecomastia before 25 years of age is usually related to hormonal pubertal changes, whereas development in later years may be caused by hormonally active tumors (Leydig cell tumor of testis, hCG-secreting germ cell tumors, lung carcinoma, or others), cirrhosis, or medications (digitalis, reserpine, phenytoin, and others).[1746] Cases have also been reported in type 1 neurofibromatosis.[1747] Clinical gynecomastia developing in diabetic patients may have the features of diabetic or lymphocytic mastitis, as seen in females[1751] (see p. 1664). Many cases remain idiopathic.

Clinically, gynecomastia is usually centered below the nipple, an important point in the differential diagnosis with carcinoma, which tends to be located eccentrically.[1745] It may be unilateral (at least at the clinical level, the left breast being more commonly involved than the right) or bilateral. It has been noted that pubertal and hormone-induced gynecomastias tend to be bilateral, whereas idiopathic and nonhormonal drug-induced gynecomastias are usually unilateral.[1756]

The gross appearance is characteristic. The mass is oval, disk shaped, of elastic consistency, and with well-circumscribed borders. Microscopically, the ducts show a variable and sometimes very prominent degree of epithelial hyperplasia and are surrounded by a prominent swollen stroma, which results in a typical 'halo' effect[1756] (Fig. 20.128). This stroma contains large amounts of acid mucopolysaccharides (mainly hyaluronic acid) of a type similar to that seen in fibroadenoma of the female breast.[1748] The immunophenotype parallels that of normal breast stroma.[1752] There may be pseudoangiomatous stromal hyperplasia (PASH) and focal squamous metaplasia, and formation of lobules may be observed.[1745,1749] Exceptionally, a population of clear or globoid cells immunoreactive for GCDFP-15 may be present.[1750]

The microscopic changes are related to the duration of the gynecomastia. Cases of short duration tend to have a prominent hyperplastic epithelial component (with high Ki-67 index[1754]) and stromal edema, whereas those of long duration have prominent stromal fibrosis.[1744] In rare cases, the intraductal epithelial hyperplasia is so extreme as to simulate carcinoma. In others, the proliferation has fibroadenoma-like qualities.[1755]

The possible relationship between gynecomastia and carcinoma is discussed below.

The seemingly paradoxical fact that, sometimes, changes morphologically similar to those of gynecomastia can be seen in the female breast has already been mentioned (see p. 1678).[1753,1757] Tongue-in-cheek, one could say that these are cases in which a female breast resembles a male breast that resembles a female breast.

Myofibroblastoma

Myofibroblastoma is the most commonly used term for a benign stromal neoplasm first described by Toker et al.[1775] as benign spindle cell tumor, and also known as myogenic stromal tumor.[1761] Originally thought to involve primarily the male breast, it is now known to occur in the female breast with a higher frequency, and is discussed in this section only on historical grounds.[1776]

Grossly, it is well circumscribed and usually small, although on occasion it can reach a large size.[1759,1760] Microscopically, uniform, bland-looking spindle cells are haphazardly arranged in fascicles separated by broad bands of hyalinized collagen[1771] (Fig. 20.129). The appearance is very reminiscent of both solitary fibrous tumor and spindle cell lipoma,[1762] the suggestion having been made that there is a close histogenetic link between these neoplasms.[1764,1765,1767]

Focally, there may be smooth muscle, cartilaginous or adipose metaplasia.[1763,1774] Ultrastructurally, the features are those of

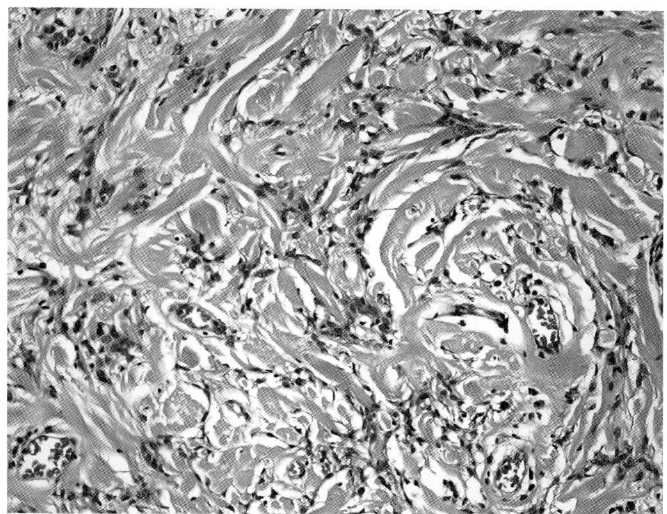

Fig. 20.129 Myofibroblastoma of male breast. The microscopic appearance is very reminiscent of solitary fibrous tumor.

fibroblasts and myoid cells (i.e., myofibroblast-like), and immunoreactivity for desmin and caldesmon has been encountered in some cases.[1768,1776] Although estrogen and progesterone receptors are strongly expressed,[1766] the suggestion has been made that the lesion may be pathogenetically related to androgens.[1772]

A variation on the theme is represented by the *epithelioid*[1770] and the *deciduoid* myofibroblastoma;[1769] cases of the former have been reported against a background of gynecomastia.[1773]

Carcinoma

In the United States, only 1% of all breast carcinomas occur in males, but in some Arab countries the incidence rises to nearly 10%.[1786,1787] An increased incidence of breast carcinoma is seen in patients with Klinefelter syndrome.[1803] Familial cases have also been recorded.[1785,1796] An important and not entirely resolved issue is that of the possible relationship between gynecomastia and breast carcinoma. In one series, microscopic changes consistent with gynecomastia were found in 40% of breast carcinoma cases.[1793] Furthermore, cases of primary breast carcinoma have occurred in patients with prostatic carcinoma treated with estrogens.[1799] Finally, countries in which the incidence of gynecomastia is high also have a high incidence of breast carcinoma. All these data would seem to point toward a pathogenetic link between the two entities.

Clinically, most breast carcinomas present in elderly individuals as breast nodules, with or without associated nipple abnormalities.[1778,1784] Nipple discharge in an adult male, especially if bloody, should arouse a strong suspicion of carcinoma. Skin involvement by fixation and Paget disease are much more common in males. As in females, nipple involvement can simulate malignant melanoma.[1806]

Grossly, microscopically, and immunohistochemically, carcinomas of the male breast are very similar to those seen in females.[1782,1786] As such, they can be in situ or invasive, and low grade or high grade,[1781,1794] but with a higher percentage of high-grade tumors.[1797] All of the microscopic types identified in the female breast have been encountered in males, including tumors with neuroendocrine features.[1800] The incidence of invasive papillary carcinoma seems to be a little higher than in females.[1780] The least common of the major

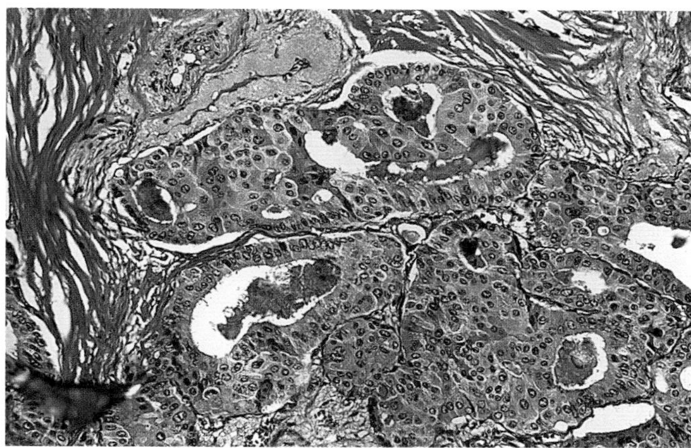

Fig. 20.130 Carcinoma of the male breast composed of well-differentiated tumor cells with abundant granular cytoplasm having oncocytic features.

categories is invasive lobular carcinoma, only a few cases having been observed.[1789,1803,1804] Other very unusual types include adenomyoepithelioma[1807] and oncocytic carcinoma[1783] (Fig. 20.130). Prolactin receptor expression has been detected in about 60% of breast carcinomas in males (and in a lower percentage in cases of gynecomastia).[1788]

The tumors can be identified by fine needle aspiration, the most important differential diagnosis using this modality being gynecomastia.[1779] The incidence of positivity for estrogen receptors is higher than in females.[1792,1797]

The overall survival rate is lower than for breast carcinoma,[1777,1791,1798,1802] but, as is often the case, the differences tend to disappear when the tumors are compared stage by stage.[1790,1810] Indeed, the prognosis of breast cancer in males, like that in females, is heavily influenced by clinical stage and microscopic grade.[1805,1808] It also correlates with mitotic activity, DNA ploidy, and P53 status.[1795,1801,1809]

Other lesions

Mammary duct ectasia[1824] and **sclerosing adenosis**[1813] can occur in the male breast. Fibrocystic disease, fibroadenoma (sometimes bilateral), phylloides tumor, PASH, and nodular fasciitis have also been reported but are vanishingly rare.[1811,1819,1822,1823]

Nipple adenoma and **intraductal papilloma** have been seen on several occasions, in one instance following estrogen therapy for prostatic carcinoma.[1817,1821,1825] There are also reports of **leiomyosarcoma** of the nipple[1818] and **neurofibromatosis** in a child whose condition simulated gynecomastia.[1820]

Metastatic carcinoma to the male breast often originates from the prostate, is often bilateral, and is almost always seen following estrogen therapy.[1812] As such, it occurs against a background of gynecomastia. Some of these cases have been confused with primary breast carcinoma. Immunohistochemical stains for PSA and prostatic acid phosphatase are helpful in the differential diagnosis.[1816] The matter is complicated by the fact that the normal mammary duct epithelium of males and the hyperplastic epithelium of gynecomastia is often immunoreactive for PSA (but not for prostatic acid phosphatase). Male breast carcinoma is negative for both markers.[1815]

The most common type of nonepithelial tumor to metastasize to the male breast is malignant melanoma.[1814]

References

NORMAL ANATOMY

1 Anderson TJ. Normal breast: myths, realities, and prospects. Mod Pathol 1998, **11**: 115–119.

2 Azzopardi JG. Problems in breast pathology. In Bennington JL (consulting ed.): Major problems in pathology, vol. 11. Philadelphia, 1979, W.B. Saunders.

3 Barbareschi M, Pecciarini L, Cangi MG, Macri E, Rizzo A, Viale G, Doglioni C. p63, a p53 homologue, is a selective nuclear marker of myoepithelial cells of the human breast. Am J Surg Pathol 2001, **25**: 1054–1060.

4 Barwick KW, Kashgarian M, Rosen PP. 'Clear-cell' change within duct and lobular epithelium of the human breast. Pathol Annu 1982, **17**: 319–328.

5 Battersby S, Anderson TJ. Histological changes in breast tissue that characterize recent pregnancy. Histopathology 1989, **15**: 415–419.

6 Bocker W, Moll R, Poremba C, Holland R, Van Diest PJ, Dervan P, Burger H, Wai D, Diallo RI, Brandt B, Herbst H, Schmidt A, Lerch MM, Buchwallow IB. Common adult stem cells in the human breast give rise to glandular and myoepithelial cell lineages: a new cell biological concept. Lab Invest 2002, **82**: 737–746.

7 Bratthauer GL, Saenger JS, Strauss BL. Antibodies targeting p63 react specifically in the cytoplasm of breast epithelial cells exhibiting secretory differentiation. Histopathology 2005, **47**: 611–616.

8 Bussolati G, Gugliotta P, Sapino A, Eusebi V, Lloyd RV. Chromogranin reactive endocrine cells in argyrophilic carcinomas ('carcinoids') and normal tissue of the breast. Am J Pathol 1985, **120**: 186–192.

9 Charpin C, Lissitzky JC, Jacquemier J, Lavaut MN, Kopp F, Pourreau-Schneider N, Martin PM, Toga M. Immunohistochemical detection of laminin in 98 human breast carcinomas. A light and electron microscopic study. Hum Pathol 1986, **17**: 355–365.

10 Clayton F, Ordóñez NG, Hanssen GM, Hanssen H. Immunoperoxidase localization of lactalbumin in malignant breast neoplasms. Arch Pathol Lab Med 1982, **106**: 268–270.

11 Collins LC, Schnitt SJ. Breast. In Mills SE (ed.): Histology for pathologists, ed. 3. Philadelphia, 2007, Lippincott Williams & Wilkins, pp. 57–74.

12 Cowan DF, Herbert TA. Involution of the breast in women aged 50 to 104 years. A histological study of 102 cases. Surg Pathol 1989, **2**: 323–334.

13 Cunha GR. Role of mesenchymal–epithelial interactions in normal and abnormal development of the mammary gland and prostate. Cancer 1994, **74**: 1030–1044.

14 Egan MJ, Newman J, Crocker J, Collard M. Immunohistochemical localization of S100 protein in benign and malignant conditions of the breast. Arch Pathol Lab Med 1987, **111**: 28–31.

15 Farahmand S, Cowan DF. Elastosis in the normal aging breast. A histopathologic study of 140 cases. Arch Pathol Lab Med 1991, **115**: 1241–1246.

16 Fechner RE. The surgical pathology of the reproductive system and breast during oral contraceptive therapy. Pathol Annu 1971, **6**: 299–319.

17 Foschini MP, Scarpellini F, Grown AM, Eusebi V. Differential expression of myoepithelial markers in salivary, sweat and mammary glands. Int J Surg Pathol 2000, **8**: 29–37.

18 Greenwalt DE, Johnson VG, Kuhajda FP, Eggleston JC, Mather IH. Localization of a membrane glycoprotein in benign fibrocystic disease and infiltrating duct carcinomas of the human breast with the use of a monoclonal antibody to guinea pig milk fat globule membrane. Am J Pathol 1985, **118**: 351–359.

19 Hasegawa M, Hagiwara S, Sato T, Jijiwa M, Murakumo Y, Maeda M, Moritani S, Ichihara S, Takahashi M. CD109, a new marker for myoepithelial cells of mammary, salivary, and lacrimal glands and prostate basal cells. Pathol Int 2007, **57**: 245–250.

20 Joshi K, Ellis JTB, Hughes CM, Monaghan P, Neville AM. Cellular proliferation in the rat mammary gland during pregnancy and lactation. Lab Invest 1986, **54**: 52–62.

21 Joshi K, Smith JA, Perusinghe N, Monoghan P. Cell proliferation in the human mammary epithelium. Differential contribution by epithelial and myoepithelial cells. Am J Pathol 1986, **124**: 199–206.

22 Kiaer HW, Andersen JA. Focal pregnancy-like changes in the breast. Acta Pathol Microbiol Scand (A) 1977, **85**: 931–941.

23 Larsen BL, Smith VR (eds). Lactation. A comprehensive treatise. New York, 1974, Academic Press.

24 Longacre TA, Bartow SA. A correlative morphologic study of human breast and endometrium in the menstrual cycle. Am J Surg Pathol 1986, **10**: 382–393.

25 Love SM, Barsky SH. Anatomy of the nipple and breast ducts revisited. Cancer 2004, **101**: 1947–1957.

26 Marucci G, Betts CM, Golouh R, Peterse JL, Foschini MP, Eusebi V. Toker cells are probably precursors of Paget cells carcinoma: a morphological and ultrastructural description. Virchows Arch 2002, **441**: 117–123.

27 Monteagudo C, Merino MJ, San-Juan J, Liotta LA, Stetler-Stevenson WG. Immunohistochemical distribution of type IV collagenase in normal, benign, and malignant breast tissue. Am J Pathol 1990, **136**: 585–592.

28 Ozzello L. Epithelial–stromal junction of normal and dysplastic mammary glands. Cancer 1970, **25**: 586–600.

29 Popnikolov NK, Cavone SM, Schultz PM, Garcia FU. Diagnostic utility of p75 neurotrophin receptor (p75NTR) as a marker of breast myoepithelial cells. Mod Pathol 2005, **18**: 1535–1541.

30 Ramakrishnan R, Khan SA, Badve S. Morphological changes in breast tissue with menstrual cycle. Mod Pathol 2002, **15**: 1348–1356.

31 Reis-Filho JS, Milanezi F, Paredes J, Silva P, Pereira EM, Maeda SA, de Carvalho LV, Schmitt FC. Novel and classic myoepithelial/stem cell markers in metaplastic carcinomas of the breast. Appl Immunohistochem Mol Morphol 2003, **11**: 1–8.

32 Rosen PP, Tench W. Lobules in the nipple. Frequency and significance for breast cancer treatment. Pathol Annu 1985, **20**(Pt 2): 317–322.

33 Rytina ER, Coady AT, Millis RR. Milk granuloma. An unusual appearance in lactational breast tissue. Histopathology 1990, **17**: 466–468.

34 Satake T, Matsuyama M. Endocrine cells in a normal breast and non-cancerous breast lesion. Acta Pathol Jpn 1991, **41**: 874–878.

35 Shin SJ, Rosen PP. Carcinoma arising from preexisting pregnancy-like and cystic hypersecretory hyperplasia lesions of the breast: a clinicopathologic study of 9 patients. Am J Surg Pathol 2004, **28**: 789–793.

36 Slavin JL, Billson VR, Ostor AG. Nodular breast lesions during pregnancy and lactation. Histopathology 1993, **22**: 481–485.

37 Smith DM Jr, Peters TG, Donegan WL. Montgomery's areolar tubercle. A light microscopic study. Arch Pathol Lab Med 1982, **106**: 60–63.

38 Tavassoli FA, Yeh IT. Lactational and clear cell changes of the breast in nonlactating, nonpregnant women. Am J Clin Pathol 1987, **87**: 23–29.

39 Toker C. Clear cells of the nipple epidermis. Cancer 1970, **25**: 601–610.

40 Tot T. The theory of the sick breast lobe and the possible consequences. Int J Surg Pathol 2007, **15**: 369–375.

41 Tsubura A, Okada H, Senzaki H, Hatano T, Morii S. Keratin expression in the normal breast and in breast carcinoma. Histopathology 1991, **18**: 517–522.

42 Vogel PM, Georgiade NG, Fetter BF, Vogel FS, McCarty KS Jr. The correlation of histologic changes in the human breast with the menstrual cycle. Am J Pathol 1981, **104**: 23–34.

43 Wellings SR, Jensen HM, Marcum RG. An atlas of subgross pathology of the human breast with special reference to possible precancerous lesions. J Natl Cancer Inst 1975, **55**: 231–273.

ECTOPIA

44 Edlow DW, Carter D. Heterotopic epithelium in axillary lymph nodes. Report of a case and review of the literature. Am J Clin Pathol 1973, **59**: 666–673.

45 Jordan K, Laumann A, Conrad S, Medenica M. Axillary mass in a 20-year-old woman. Diagnosis: axillary accessory breast tissue. Arch Dermatol 2001, **137**: 1367–1372.

46 O'Hara MF, Page DL. Adenomas of the breast and ectopic breast under lactational influences. Hum Pathol 1985, **16**: 707–712.

47 Pfeifer JD, Barr RJ, Wick MR. Ectopic breast tissue and breast-like sweat gland metaplasias: an overlapping spectrum of lesions. J Cutan Pathol 1999, **26**: 190–196.

48 Rosen PP, Tench W. Lobules in the nipple. Frequency and significance for breast cancer treatment. Pathol Annu 1985, **20**(Pt 2): 317–322.

49 Sasaki K, Parwani AV, Demetris AJ, Sasatomi E. Heterotopic breast epithelial inclusion of the heart: report of a case. Am J Surg Pathol 2010, **34**: 1555–1559.

50 Turner DR, Millis RR. Breast tissue inclusions in axillary lymph nodes. Histopathology 1980, **4**: 631–636.

INFLAMMATORY AND RELATED LESIONS

MAMMARY DUCT ECTASIA

51 Haagensen CD. Mammary-duct ectasia. A disease that may simulate carcinoma. Cancer 1951, **4**: 749–761.

52 Miller MA, Kottler SJ, Cohn LA, Johnson GC, Kreeger JM, Pace LV, Ramos-Vara JA, Turk JR, Turnquist SE. Mammary duct ectasia in dogs: 51 cases (1992–1999). J Am Vet Med Assoc 2001, **218**: 1303–1307.

53 Webb AJ. Mammary duct ectasia – periductal mastitis complex. Br J Surg 1995, **82**: 1300–1302.

FAT NECROSIS

54 Clarke D, Curtis JL, Martinez A, Fajardo L, Goffinet D. Fat necrosis of the breast simulating recurrent carcinoma after primary radiotherapy in the management of early stage breast carcinoma. Cancer 1983, **52**: 442–445.

55 Coyne JD, Parkinson D, Baildam AD. Membranous fat necrosis of the breast. Histopathology 1996, **28**: 61–64.

56 Dabbs DJ. Mammary ductal foam cells. Macrophage immunophenotype. Hum Pathol 1993, **24**: 977–981.

57 Kinoshita T, Yashiro N, Yoshigi J, Ihara N, Narita M. Fat necrosis of breast: a potential pitfall in breast MRI. Clin Imaging 2002, **26**: 250–253.

58 Koo JS, Jung W. Xanthogranulomatous mastitis: clinicopathology and pathological implications. Pathol Int 2009, **59**: 234–240.

OTHER INFLAMMATORY DISEASES

59 Allende DS, Booth CN. Wegener's granulomatosis of the breast: a rare entity with daily clinical relevance. Ann Diagn Pathol 2009, **13**: 351–357.

60 Arnaout AH, Shousha S, Metaxas N, Husain OA. Intramammary tuberculous lymphadenitis. Histopathology 1990, **17**: 91–93.

61 Ashton MA, Lefkowitz M, Tavassoli FA. Epithelioid stromal cells in lymphocytic mastitis. A source of confusion with invasive carcinoma. Mod Pathol 1994, **7**: 49–54.

62 Banik S, Bishop PW, Ormerod LP, O'Brien TE. Sarcoidosis of the breast. J Clin Pathol 1986, **39**: 446–448.

63 Bocian JJ, Fahmy RN, Michas CA. A rare case of 'coccidioidoma' of the breast. Arch Pathol Lab Med 1991, **115**: 1064–1067.

64 Catania S, Zurrida S, Veronesi P, Galimberti V, Bono A, Pluchinotta A. Mondor's disease and breast cancer. Cancer 1992, **69**: 2267–2270.

65 Cheuk W, Chan AC, Lam WL, Chow SM, Crowley P, Lloydd R, Campbell I, Thorburn M, Chan JK. IgG4-related sclerosing mastitis: description of a new member of the IgG4-related sclerosing diseases. Am J Surg Pathol 2009, **33**: 1058–1064.

66 Cooper NE. Rheumatoid nodule in the breast. Histopathology 1991, **19**: 193–194.

67 Coyne JD, Baildam AD, Asbury D. Lymphocytic mastopathy associated with ductal carcinoma in situ of the breast. Histopathology 1995, **26**: 579–580.

68 Dener C, Inan A. Breast abscesses in lactating women. World J Surg 2003, **27**: 130–133.

69 Douglas-Jones AG. Lymphocytic lobulitis in breast core biopsy: a peritumoral phenomenon. Histopathology 2006, **48**: 209–212.

70 Eckland DA, Zeigler MG. Abscess in the nonlactating breast. Arch Surg 1973, **107**: 398–401.

71 Ely KA, Tse G, Simpson JF, Clarfeld R, Page DL. Diabetic mastopathy. A clinicopathologic review. Am J Clin Pathol 2000, **113**: 541–545.

72 Farrow JH. Thrombophlebitis of the superficial veins of the breast and anterior chest wall (Mondor's disease). Surg Gynecol Obstet 1955, **101**: 63–68.

73 Fitzgibbons PL, Smiley DF, Kern WH. Sarcoidosis presenting initially as breast mass. Report of two cases. Hum Pathol 1985, **16**: 851–852.

74 Fletcher A, Magrath IM, Riddell RH, Talbot IC. Granulomatous mastitis. A report of seven cases. J Clin Pathol 1982, **35**: 941–945.

75 Fong D, Lann MA, Finlayson C, Page DL, Singh M. Diabetic (lymphocytic) mastopathy with exuberant lymphohistiocytic and granulomatous response: a case report with review of the literature. Am J Surg Pathol 2006, **30**: 1330–1336.

76 Herrmann JB. Thrombophlebitis of breast and contiguous thoracicoabdominal wall (Mondor's disease). NY State J Med 1966, **66**: 3146–3152.

77 Johnson WC, Wallrich R, Helwig EB. Superficial thrombophlebitis of the chest wall. JAMA 1962, **180**: 103–108.

78 Jordan JM, Rowe WT, Allen NB. Wegener's granulomatosis involving the breast. Report of three cases and review of the literature. Am J Med 1987, **83**: 159–164.

79 Kariv R, Sidi Y, Gur H. Systemic vasculitis presenting as a tumorlike lesion. Four case reports and an analysis of 79 reported cases. Medicine (Baltimore) 2000, **79**: 349–359.

80 Kessler EI, Katzav JA. Lobular granulomatous mastitis. Surg Pathol 1990, **3**: 115–120.

81 Khamapirad T, Hennan K, Leonard M Jr, Eltorky M, Qiu S. Granulomatous lobular mastitis: two case reports with focus on radiologic and histopathologic features. Ann Diagn Pathol 2007, **11**: 109–1012.

82 Khanna R, Prasanna GV, Gupta P, Kumar M, Khanna S, Khanna A. Mammary tuberculosis: report on 52 cases. Postgrad Med J 2002, **78**: 422–424.

83 Kinonen C, Gattuso P, Reddy VB. Lupus mastitis: an uncommon complication of systemic or discoid lupus. Am J Surg Pathol 2010, **34**: 901–906.

84 Lammie GA, Bobrow LG, Staunton MD, Levison DA, Page G, Millis RR. Sclerosing lymphocytic lobulitis of the breast. Evidence for an autoimmune pathogenesis. Histopathology 1991, **19**: 13–20.

85 Lower EE, Hawkins HH, Baughman RP. Breast disease in sarcoidosis. Sarcoidosis Vasc Diffuse Lung Dis 2001, **18**: 301–306.

86 Lucey JJ. Spontaneous infarction of the breast. J Clin Pathol 1975, **28**: 937–943.

87 Mayor M, Buron I, De Mora JC, Lazaro TE, Hernandez-Cano N, Rubio FA, Casado M. Mondor's disease. Int J Dermatol 2000, **39**: 922–925.

88 Morgan MC, Weaver MG, Crowe JP, Abdul-Karim FW. Diabetic mastopathy. A clinicopathologic study in palpable and nonpalpable breast lesions. Mod Pathol 1995, **8**: 349–354.

89 Ng WF, Chow LT, Lam PW. Localized polyarteritis nodosa of breast. Report of two cases and a review of the literature. Histopathology 1993, **23**: 535–539.

90 Nigar E, Contractor K, Singhal H, Matin RN. Lupus mastitis – a cause of recurrent breast lumps. Histopathology 2007, **51**: 847–849.

91 Nudelman HL, Kempson RL. Necrosis of the breast. A rare complication of anticoagulant therapy. Am J Surg 1966, **111**: 728–733.

92 Ogura K, Matsumoto T, Aoki Y, Kitabatake T, Fujisawa M, Kojima K. IgG4-related tumour-forming mastitis with histological appearances of granulomatous lobular mastitis: comparison with other types of tumour-forming mastitis. Histopathology 2010, **57**: 39–45.

93 Ojeda H, Sardi A, Totoonchie A. Sarcoidosis of the breast: implications for the general surgeon. Am Surg 2000, **66**: 1144–1148.

94 Osborne BM. Granulomatous mastitis caused by histoplasma and mimicking inflammatory breast carcinoma. Hum Pathol 1989, **20**: 47–52.

95 Passaro ME, Broughan TA, Sebek BA, Esselstyn CB Jr. Lactiferous fistula. J Am Coll Surg 1994, **178**: 29–32.

96 Pugh CM, DeWitty RL. Mondor's disease. J Natl Med Assoc 1996, **88**: 359–363.

97 Rickert RR, Rajan S. Localized breast infarcts associated with pregnancy. Arch Pathol 1974, **97**: 159–161.

98 Robitaille Y, Seemayer TA, Thelmo WL, Cumberlidge MC. Infarction of the mammary region mimicking carcinoma of the breast. Cancer 1974, **33**: 1183–1189.

99 Scholefield JH, Duncan JL, Rogers K. Review of a hospital experience of breast abscesses. Br J Surg 1987, **74**: 469–470.

100 Schwartz IS, Strauchen JA. Lymphocytic mastopathy. An autoimmune disease of the breast? Am J Clin Pathol 1990, **93**: 725–730.

101 Seidman JD, Schnaper LA, Phillips LE. Mastopathy in insulin-requiring diabetes mellitus. Hum Pathol 1994, **25**: 819–824.

102 Shousha S. Diabetic mastopathy: strong CD10+ immunoreactivity of the atypical stromal cells. Histopathology 2008, **52**: 648–650.

103 Symmers WC St. Silicone mastitis in 'topless' waitress and some other varieties of foreign-body mastitis. Br Med J 1968, **3**: 19–22.

104 Tomaszewski JE, Brooks JS, Hicks D, Livolsi VA. Diabetic mastopathy. A distinctive clinicopathologic entity. Hum Pathol 1992, **23**: 780–786.

105 Trueb RM, Scheidegger EP, Pericin M, Singh A, Hoffmann U, Sauva G, Burg G. Periarteritis nodosa presenting as a breast lesion: report of a case and review of the literature. Br J Dermatol 1999, **141**: 1117–1121.

106 Valdez R, Thorson J, Finn WG, Schnitzer B, Kleer CG. Lymphocytic mastitis and diabetic mastopathy: a molecular, immunophenotypic, and clinicopathologic evaluation of 11 cases. Mod Pathol 2003, **16**: 223–228.

107 Vargas MP, Merino MJ. Infarcted myxoid fibroadenoma following fine-needle aspiration. Arch Pathol Lab Med 1996, **120**: 1069–1071.

108 Watt-Boolsen S, Rasmussen NR, Blichert-Toft M. Primary periareolar abscess in the nonlactating breast. Risk of recurrence. Am J Surg 1987, **153**: 571–573.

109 Zen Y, Kasahara Y, Horita K, Miyayama S, Miura S, Kitagawa S, Nakanuma Y. Inflammatory pseudotumor of the breast in a patient with a high serum IgG4 level: histologic similarity to sclerosing pancreatitis. Am J Surg Pathol 2005, **29**: 275–278.

BENIGN PROLIFERATIVE BREAST DISEASE

110 Santen RJ, Mansel R. Benign breast disorders. N Engl J Med 2005, **353**: 275–285.

FIBROADENOMA

111 Arrigoni MG, Dockerty MB, Judd ES. The identification and treatment of mammary hamartoma. Surg Gynecol Obstet 1971, **133**: 577–582.

112 Azzopardi JG. Problems in breast pathology. In Bennington JL (consulting ed.): Major problems in pathology, vol. 11. Philadelphia, 1979, W.B. Saunders.

113 Berean K, Tron VA, Churg A, Clement PB. Mammary fibroadenoma with multinucleated stromal giant cells. Am J Surg Pathol 1986, **10**: 823–827.

114 Carney JA, Toorkey BC. Myxoid fibroadenoma and allied conditions (myxomatosis) of the breast. A heritable disorder with special associations including cardiac and cutaneous myxomas. Am J Surg Pathol 1991, **15**: 713–721.

115 Carstens PHB. Ultrastructure of human fibroadenoma. Arch Pathol 1974, **98**: 23–32.

116 Carter BA, Page DL, Schuyler P, Parl FF, Simpson JF, Jensen RA, Dupont WD. No elevation in long-term breast carcinoma risk for women with fibroadenomas that contain atypical hyperplasia. Cancer 2001, **92**: 30–36.

117 Dehner LP, Hill DA, Deschryver K. Pathology of the breast in children, adolescents, and young adults. Semin Diagn Pathol 1999, **16**: 235–247.

118 Dupont WD, Page DL, Parl FF, Vnencak-Jones CL, Plummer WD Jr, Rados MS, Schuyler PA. Long-term risk of breast cancer in women with fibroadenoma. N Engl J Med 1994, **331**: 10–15.

119 Eusebi V, Azzopardi JG. Lobular endocrine neoplasia in fibroadenoma of the breast. Histopathology 1980, **4**: 413–428.

120 Fechner RE. Fibroadenomas in patients receiving oral contraceptives. A clinical and pathologic study. Am J Clin Pathol 1970, **53**: 857–864.

121 Fekete P, Petrek J, Majmudar B, Someren A, Sandberg W. Fibroadenomas with stromal cellularity. A clinicopathologic study of 21 patients. Arch Pathol Lab Med 1987, **111**: 427–432.

122 Fletcher JA, Pinkus GS, Weidner N, Morton CC. Lineage-restricted clonality in biphasic solid tumors. Am J Pathol 1991, **138**: 1199–1207.

123 Goodman ZD, Taxy JB. Fibroadenomas of the breast with prominent smooth muscle. Am J Surg Pathol 1981, **5**: 99–101.

124 Huo L, Gilcrease MZ. Fibroepithelial lesions of the breast with pleomorphic stromal giant cells: a clinicopathologic study of 4 cases and review of the literature. Ann Diagn Pathol 2009, **13**: 226–232.

125 Kleer CG, Tseng MD, Gutsch DE, Rochford RA, Wu Z, Joynt LK, Helvie MA, Chang T, Van Golen KL, Merajver SD. Detection of Epstein–Barr virus in rapidly growing fibroadenomas of the breast in immunosuppressed hosts. Mod Pathol 2002, **15**: 759–764.

126 Kuijper A, Mommers EC, van der Wall E, van Diest PJ. Histopathology of fibroadenomas of the breast. Am J Clin Pathol 2001, **115**: 736–742.

127 Metcalf JS, Ellis B. Choristoma of the breast. Hum Pathol 1985, **16**: 739–740.

128 Mies C, Rosen PP. Juvenile fibroadenoma with atypical epithelial hyperplasia. Am J Surg Pathol 1987, **11**: 184–190.

129 Moore T, Lee AH. Expression of CD34 and bcl-2 in phyllodes tumors, fibroadenomas and spindle cell lesions of the breast. Histopathology 2001, **38**: 62–67.

130 Oberman HA, Nosanchuk HS, Finger JE. Periductal stromal tumors of breast with adipose metaplasia. Arch Surg 1969, **98**: 384–387.

131 O'Hara MF, Page DL. Adenomas of the breast and ectopic breast under lactational influences. Hum Pathol 1985, **16**: 707–712.

132 Petersson C, Pandis N, Rizou H, Mertens F, Dietrich CU, Adeyinka A, Idvall I, Bondeson L, Georgiou G, Ingvar C, Heim S, Mitelman F. Karyotypic abnormalities in fibroadenomas of the breast. Int J Cancer 1997, **70**: 282–286.

133 Petrik PK. Mammary hamartoma. Am J Surg Pathol 1987, **11**: 234–235.

134 Pike AM, Oberman HA. Juvenile (cellular) adenofibromas. A clinicopathologic study. Am J Surg Pathol 1985, **9**: 730–736.

135 Reddick RL, Shin TK, Sawhney D, Siegal GP. Stromal proliferations of the breast. An ultrastructural and immunohistochemical evaluation of cystosarcoma phyllodes, juvenile fibroadenoma, and fibroadenoma. Hum Pathol 1987, **18**: 45–49.

136 Sapino A, Bosco M, Cassoni P, Castellano I, Arisio R, Cserni G, Dei Tos AP, Fortunati N, Catalano MG, Bussolati G. Estrogen receptor-beta is expressed in stromal cells of fibroadenoma and phyllodes tumors of the breast. Mod Pathol 2006, **19**: 599–606.

137 Shimizu T, Ebihara Y, Serizawa H, Toyoda M, Hirota T. Histopathological study of stromal smooth muscle cells in fibroadenoma of the breast. Pathol Int 1996, **46**: 442–449.

138 Silverman JS, Tamsen A. Mammary fibroadenoma and some phyllodes tumour stroma are composed of CD34+ fibroblasts and factor XIIIa+ dendrophages. Histopathology 1996, **29**: 411–419.

139 Umekita Y, Yoshida H. Immunohistochemical study of hormone receptor and hormone-regulated protein expression in phyllodes tumour: comparison with fibroadenoma. Virchows Arch 1998, **433**: 311–314.

140 Yeh I-T, Francis DJ, Orenstein JM, Silverberg SG. Ultrastructure of cystosarcoma phyllodes and fibroadenoma. A comparative study. Am J Clin Pathol 1985, **84**: 131–136.

MALIGNANT TRANSFORMATION

141 Buzanowski-Konakry K, Harrison EG Jr, Payne WS. Lobular carcinoma arising in fibroadenoma of the breast. Cancer 1975, **35**: 450–456.

142 Curran RC, Dodge OG. Sarcoma of breast, with particular reference to its origin from fibroadenoma. J Clin Pathol 1962, **15**: 1–16.

143 Diaz NM, Palmer JO, McDivitt RW. Carcinoma arising within fibroadenomas of the breast. A clinicopathologic study of 105 patients. Am J Clin Pathol 1991, **95**: 614–622.

144 Fondo EY, Rosen PP, Fracchia AA, Urban JA. The problem of carcinoma developing in a fibroadenoma. Recent experience at Memorial Hospital. Cancer 1979, **43**: 563–567.

145 Goldman RC, Friedman NB. Carcinoma of the breast arising in fibroadenomas with emphasis on lobular carcinoma. A clinicopathologic study. Cancer 1969, **23**: 544–550.

146 McDivitt RW, Stewart FW, Farrow JH. Breast carcinoma arising in solitary fibroadenomas. Surg Gynecol Obstet 1967, **125**: 572–576.

147 Pick PW, Iossifides IA. Occurrence of breast carcinoma within a fibroadenoma. A review. Arch Pathol Lab Med 1984, **108**: 590–594.

ADENOMA

148 Baddoura FK, Judd RL. Apocrine adenoma of the breast. Report of a case with investigation of lectin binding patterns in apocrine breast lesions. Mod Pathol 1990, **3**: 373–376.

149 Carney JA, Toorkey BC. Ductal adenoma of the breast with tubular features. A probable component of the complex of myxomas, spotty pigmentation, endocrine overactivity, and schwannomas. Am J Surg Pathol 1991, **15**: 722–731.

150 Hertel BF, Zaloudek C, Kempson RL. Breast adenomas. Cancer 1976, **37**: 2891–2905.

151 Le Gal Y. Adenomas of the breast. Relationship of adenofibromas to pregnancy and lactation. Am Surg 1961, **27**: 14–22.

152 Morris JA, Kelly JF. Multiple bilateral breast adenomata in identical adolescent Negro twins. Histopathology 1982, **6**: 539–547.

153 O'Hara MF, Page DL. Adenomas of the breast and ectopic breast under lactational influences. Hum Pathol 1985, **16**: 707–712.

INTRADUCTAL PAPILLOMA

154 Ali-Fehmi R, Carolin K, Wallis T, Visscher DW. Clinicopathologic analysis of breast lesions associated with multiple papillomas. Hum Pathol 2003, **34**: 234–239.

155 Azzopardi JG. Problems in breast pathology. In Bennington JL (consulting ed.): Major problems in pathology, vol. 11. Philadelphia, 1979, W.B. Saunders.

156 Azzopardi JG, Salm R. Ductal adenoma of the breast. A lesion which can mimic carcinoma. J Pathol 1984, **144**: 15–23.

157 Collins LC, Schnitt SJ. Papillary lesions of the breast: selected diagnostic and management issues. Histopathology 2008, **52**: 20–29.

158 Egan MJ, Newman J, Crocker J, Collard M. Immunohistochemical localization of S100 protein in benign and malignant conditions of the breast. Arch Pathol Lab Med 1987, **111**: 28–31.

159 Fenoglio C, Lattes R. Sclerosing papillary proliferations in the female breast. A benign lesion often mistaken for carcinoma. Cancer 1974, **33**: 691–700.

160 Ichihara S, Fujimoto T, Hashimoto K, Moritani S, Hasegawa M, Yokoi T. Double immunostaining with p63 and high-molecular-weight cytokeratins distinguishes borderline papillary lesions of the breast. Pathol Int 2007, **57**: 126–132.

161 Jaffer S, Bleiweiss IJ. Intraductal papilloma with 'comedo-like' necrosis, a diagnostic pitfall. Ann Diagn Pathol 2004, **8**: 276–279.

162 Jiao YF, Nakamura S, Oikawa T, Sugai T, Uesugi N. Sebaceous gland metaplasia in intraductal papilloma of the breast. Virchows Arch 2001, **438**: 505–508.

163 Kraus FT, Neubecker RD. The differential diagnosis of papillary tumors of the breast. Cancer 1962, **15**: 444–455.

164 Lammie GA, Millis RR. Ductal adenoma of the breast. A review of fifteen cases. Hum Pathol 1989, **20**: 903–908.

165 Lee KC, Chan JK, Ho LC. Histologic changes in the breast after fine-needle aspiration. Am J Surg Pathol 1994, **18**: 1039–1047.

166 Lewis JT, Hartmann LC, Vierkant RA, Maloney SD, Shane Pankratz V, Allers TM, Frost MH, Visscher DW. An analysis of breast cancer risk in women with single, multiple, and atypical papilloma. Am J Surg Pathol 2006, **30**: 665–672.

167 MacGrogan G, Tavassoli FA. Central atypical papillomas of the breast: a

clinicopathological study of 199 cases. Virchows Arch 2003, **443**: 609–617.

168 Noguchi S, Motomura K, Inaji H, Imaoka S, Koyama H. Clonal analysis of solitary intraductal papilloma of the breast by means of polymerase chain reaction. Am J Pathol 1994, **144**: 1320–1325.

169 Page DL, Salhany KE, Jensen RA, Dupont WD. Subsequent breast carcinoma risk after biopsy with atypia in a breast papilloma. Cancer 1996, **78**: 258–266.

170 Papotti M, Eusebi V, Gugliotta P, Bussolati G. Immunohistochemical analysis of benign and malignant papillary lesions of the breast. Am J Surg Pathol 1983, **7**: 451–461.

171 Papotti M, Gugliotta P, Ghiringhello B, Bussolati G. Association of breast carcinoma and multiple intraductal papillomas. An histological and immunohistochemical investigation. Histopathology 1984, **8**: 963–975.

172 Raju U, Vertes D. Breast papillomas with atypical ductal hyperplasia: a clinicopathological study. Hum Pathol 1996, **27**: 1231–1238.

173 Raju UB, Lee MW, Zarbo RJ, Crissman JD. Papillary neoplasia of the breast. Immunohistochemically defined myoepithelial cells in the diagnosis of benign and malignant papillary breast neoplasms. Mod Pathol 1989, **2**: 569–576.

174 Rosen PP. Arthur Purdy Stout and papilloma of the breast. Comments on the occasion of his 100th birthday. Am J Surg Pathol 1986, **10**(Suppl 1): 100–107.

175 Sapino A, Botta G, Cassoni P, Papotti M, Bussolati G. Multiple papillomas of the breast: morphologic findings and clinical evolution. Anat Pathol 1996, **1**: 205–218.

176 Terada T. Ductal adenoma of the breast: immunohistochemistry of two cases. Pathol Int 2008, **58**: 801–805.

177 Troxell ML, Masek M, Sibley RK. Immunohistochemical staining of papillary breast lesions. Appl Immunohistochem Mol Morphol 2007, **15**: 145–153.

NIPPLE ADENOMA

178 Bhagavan BS, Patchefsky A, Koss LG. Florid subareolar duct papillomatosis (nipple adenoma) and mammary carcinoma. Report of three cases. Hum Pathol 1973, **4**: 289–295.

179 Jones MW, Tavassoli FA. Coexistence of nipple duct adenoma and breast carcinoma. A clinicopathologic study of five cases and review of the literature. Mod Pathol 1995, **8**: 637–642.

180 Myers JL, Mazur MT, Urist MM, Peiper SC. Florid papillomatosis of the nipple. Immunohistochemical and flow cytometric analysis of two cases. Mod Pathol 1990, **3**: 288–293.

181 Perzin KH, Lattes R. Papillary adenoma of the nipple (florid papillomatosis, adenoma, adenomatosis). A clinicopathologic study. Cancer 1972, **29**: 996–1009.

182 Rosen PP, Caicco JA. Florid papillomatosis of the nipple. A study of 51 patients, including nine with mammary carcinoma. Am J Surg Pathol 1986, **10**: 87–101.

183 Taylor HB, Robertson AG. Adenomas of the nipple. Cancer 1966, **18**: 995–1002.

ADENOSIS

BLUNT DUCT ADENOSIS

184 Azzopardi JG. Problems in breast pathology. In Bennington JL (consulting ed.): Major problems in pathology, vol. 11. Philadelphia, 1979, W.B. Saunders.

185 Foote FW, Stewart FW. Comparative studies of cancerous vs. noncancerous breasts. Am Surg 1945, **121**: 6–79.

SCLEROSING ADENOSIS

186 Eusebi V, Azzopardi JG. Vascular infiltration in benign breast disease. J Pathol 1976, **118**: 9–16.

187 Eusebi V, Collina G, Bussolati G. Carcinoma in situ in sclerosing adenosis of the breast. An immunocytochemical study. Semin Diagn Pathol 1989, **6**: 146–152.

188 Fechner RE. Lobular carcinoma in situ in sclerosing adenosis. A potential source of confusion with invasive carcinoma. Am J Surg Pathol 1981, **5**: 233–239.

189 Jensen RA, Page DL, Dupont WD, Rogers LW. Invasive breast cancer risk in women with sclerosing adenosis. Cancer 1989, **64**: 1977–1983.

190 Oberman HA, Markey BA. Noninvasive carcinoma of the breast presenting in adenosis. Mod Pathol 1991, **4**: 31–35.

191 Taylor HB, Norris HJ. Epithelial invasion of nerves in benign diseases of the breast. Cancer 1967, **20**: 2245–2249.

NODULAR ADENOSIS AND RELATED LESIONS

192 Nielsen BB. Adenosis tumour of the breast. A clinicopathological investigation of 27 cases. Histopathology 1987, **11**: 1259–1275.

MICROGLANDULAR AND ADENOMYOEPITHELIAL (APOCRINE) ADENOSIS

193 Acs G, Simpson JF, Bleiweiss IJ, Hugh J, Reynolds C, Olson S, Page DL. Microglandular adenosis with transition into adenoid cystic carcinoma of the breast. Am J Surg Pathol 2003, **27**: 1052–1060.

194 Clement PB, Azzopardi JG. Microglandular adenosis of the breast. A lesion simulating tubular carcinoma. Histopathology 1983, **7**: 169–180.

195 Endoh Y, Tamura G, Katoh N, Motoyama T. Apocrine adenosis of the breast: clonal evidence of neoplasia. Histopathology 2001, **38**: 221–224.

196 Eusebi V, Casedei GP, Bussolati G, Azzopardi JG. Adenomyoepithelioma of the breast with a distinctive type of apocrine adenosis. Histopathology 1987, **11**: 305–315.

197 Eusebi V, Foschini MP, Betts CM, Gherardi G, Millis RR, Bussolati G, Azzopardi JG. Microglandular adenosis, apocrine adenosis, and tubular carcinoma of the breast. An immunohistochemical comparison. Am J Surg Pathol 1993, **17**: 99–109.

198 James B, Cranor M, Rosen PP. Carcinoma of the breast arising in microglandular adenosis. Am J Clin Pathol 1993, **100**: 507–513.

199 Khalifeh IM, Albarracin C, Diaz LK, Symmans FW, Edgerton ME, Hwang RF, Sneige N. Clinical, histopathologic, and immunohistochemical features of microglandular adenosis and transition into in situ and invasive carcinoma. Am J Surg Pathol 2008, **32**: 544–552.

200 Kiaer H, Nielsen B, Paulsen S, Soresen IM, Dyreborg V, Blichert-Toft M. Adenomyoepithelial adenosis and low grade malignant adenomyoepithelioma of the breast. Virchows Arch [A] 1984, **405**: 55–67.

201 Koenig C, Dadmanesh F, Bratthauer GL, Tavassoli FA. Carcinoma arising in microglandular adenosis: an immunohistochemical analysis of 20 intraepithelial and invasive neoplasms. Int J Surg Pathol 2000, **8**: 303–315.

202 Lee K, Chan JK, Gwi E. Tubular adenosis of the breast: a distinctive benign lesion mimicking invasive carcinoma. Am J Surg Pathol 1996, **20**: 46–54.

203 Millis RR, Eusebi V. Microglandular adenosis of the breast. Adv Anat Pathol 1995, **2**: 10–18.

204 Page DL, Simpson JF. What is apocrine adenosis, anyway? Histopathology 2001, **39**: 433–434.

205 Rosen PP. Microglandular adenosis. A benign lesion simulating invasive mammary carcinoma. Am J Surg Pathol 1983, **7**: 137–144.

206 Rosenblum MK, Purrazzella R, Rosen PP. Is microglandular adenosis a precancerous disease? A study of carcinoma arising therein. Am J Surg Pathol 1986, **10**: 237–245.

207 Salarieh A, Sneige N. Breast carcinoma arising in microglandular adenosis: a review of the literature. Arch Pathol Lab Med 2007, **131**: 1397–1399.

208 Seidman JD, Ashton M, Lefkowitz M. Atypical apocrine adenosis of the breast: a clinicopathologic study of 37 patients with 8.7 year follow-up. Cancer 1996, **77**: 2529–2537.

209 Simpson JF, Page DL, Dupont WD. Apocrine adenosis. A mimic of mammary carcinoma. Surg Pathol 1990, **3**: 289–299.

210 Tavassoli FA, Norris NJ. Microglandular adenosis of the breast. A clinicopathologic study of 11 cases with ultrastructural observations. Am J Surg Pathol 1983, **7**: 731–737.

211 Tsuda H, Mukai K, Fukutomi T, Hirohashi S. Malignant progression of adenomyoepithelial adenosis of the breast. Pathol Int 1994, **44**: 475–479.

FIBROCYSTIC DISEASE

212 Allen SS, Froberg DG. The effect of decreased caffeine consumption on benign proliferative breast disease. A randomized clinical trial. Surgery 1987, **101**: 720–730.

213 Angeli A, Bradlow HL, Dogliotti L (eds). Endocrinology of the breast. Basic and clinical aspects. Turin, Italy, September 19–22, 1984. Ann N Y Acad Sci 1986, **464**: 1–640.

214 Azzopardi JG. Problems in breast pathology. In Bennington JL (consulting ed.): Major problems in pathology, vol. 11. Philadelphia, 1979, W.B. Saunders.

215 Bartow SA, Black WC, Waeckerlin RW, Mettler FA. Fibrocystic disease. A continuing enigma. Pathol Annu 1982, **17**(Pt 2): 93–111.

216 Carter DJ, Rosen PP. Atypical apocrine metaplasia in sclerosing lesions of the breast. A study of 51 patients. Mod Pathol 1991, **4**: 1–5.

217 Connolly JL, Schnitt SJ. Benign breast disease. Resolved and unresolved issues. Cancer 1993, **71**: 1187–1189.

218 Consensus Meeting, Oct 3 to 5, 1985, New York, Cancer Committee of the College of American Pathologists: Is 'fibrocystic disease' of the breast precancerous? Arch Pathol Lab Med 1986, **110**: 171–173.

219 Fechner RE. Fibrocystic disease in women receiving oral contraceptive hormones. Cancer 1970, **25**: 1332–1339.

220 Frantz VK, Pickren JW, Melcher GW, Auchincloss H Jr. Incidence of chronic cystic disease in so-called 'normal breast'. Cancer 1951, **4**: 762–783.

221 Golinger RC. Hormones and the pathophysiology of fibrocystic mastopathy. Surg Gynecol Obstet 1978, **146**: 273–285.

222 Hislop TG, Threlfall WJ. Oral contraceptives and benign breast disease. Am J Epidemiol 1984, **120**: 273–280.

223 LiVolsi VA, Stadel BV, Kelsey JL, Holford TR, White C. Fibrocystic breast disease in oral-contraceptive users. A histopathological evaluation of epithelial atypia. N Engl J Med 1978, **299**: 381–385.

224 Love SM, Gelman RS, Silen W. Fibrocystic 'disease' of the breast. A nondisease? N Engl J Med 1982, **307**: 1010–1014.

225 Lubin F, Ron E, Wax Y, Black M, Funaro M, Shitrit A. A case-control study of caffeine and methylxanthines in benign breast disease. JAMA 1985, **253**: 2388–2392.

226 Mazoujian G, Pinkus GS, Davis S, Haagensen DE Jr. Immunohistochemistry of a gross cystic disease fluid protein (GCDFP-15) of the breast. A marker of apocrine epithelium and breast carcinomas with apocrine features. Am J Pathol 1983, **110**: 105–112.

227 Meyer JS, Connor RE. Cell proliferation in fibrocystic disease and post-menopausal breast ducts measured by thymidine labeling. Cancer 1982, **50**: 746–751.

228 Minkowitz S, Hedayati H, Hiller S, Gardner B. Fibrous mastopathy. A clinical histopathologic study. Cancer 1973, **32**: 913–916.

229 Ory H, Cole P, MacMahon B, Hoover R. Oral contraceptives and reduced risk of benign breast diseases. N Engl J Med 1976, **294**: 419–422.

230 Sandison AT. An autopsy study of the adult human breast. With special reference to proliferative epithelial changes of importance in the pathology of the breast. Natl Cancer Inst Monogr 1962, **8**: 1–145.

231 Schuerch C III, Rosen PP, Hirota T, Itabashi M, Yamamoto H, Kinne DW, Beattie EJ Jr. A pathologic study of benign breast disease in Tokyo and New York. Cancer 1982, **50**: 1899–1903.

232 Symonds DA. Use of the von Kossa stain in identifying occult calcifications in breast biopsies. Am J Clin Pathol 1990, **94**: 44–48.

233 Tornos C, Silva E, el-Naggar A, Pritzker KP. Calcium oxalate crystals in breast biopsies. The missing microcalcifications. Am J Surg Pathol 1990, **14**: 961–968.

234 Vorherr H. Fibrocystic breast disease. Pathophysiology, pathomorphology, clinical picture, and management. Am J Obstet Gynecol 1986, **154**: 161–179.

235 Winston JS, Yeh IT, Evers K, Friedman AK. Calcium oxalate is associated with benign breast tissue. Can we avoid biopsy? Am J Clin Pathol 1993, **100**: 488–492.

RADIAL SCAR AND OTHER SCLEROSING DUCTAL LESIONS

236 Alvarado-Cabrero I, Tavassoli FA. Neoplastic and malignant lesions involving or arising in a radial scar: a clinicopathologic analysis of 17 cases. Breast J 2000, **6**: 96–102.

237 Andersen JA, Carter D, Linell F. A symposium on sclerosing duct lesions of the breast. Pathol Annu 1986, **21**(Pt 2): 144–179.

238 Andersen JA, Gram JB. Radial scar in the female breast. A long-term follow-up study of 32 cases. Cancer 1984, **53**: 2557–2560.

239 Consensus Meeting, Oct 3 to 5, 1985, New York, Cancer Committee of the College of American Pathologists: Is 'fibrocystic disease' of the breast precancerous? Arch Pathol Lab Med 1986, **110**: 171–173.

240 Davies JD. Hyperelastosis, obliteration and fibrous plaques in major ducts of the human breast. J Pathol 1973, **110**: 13–26.

241 Denley H, Pinder SE, Tan PH, Sim CS, Brown R, Barker T, Gearty J, Elston CW, Ellis IO. Metaplastic carcinoma of the breast arising within complex sclerosing lesion: a report of five cases. Histopathology 2000, **36**: 203–209.

242 Doyle EM, Banville N, Quinn CM, Flanagan F, O'Doherty A, Hill AD, Kerin MJ, Fitzpatrick P, Kennedy M. Radial scars/complex sclerosing lesions and malignancy in a screening programme: incidence and histological features revisited. Histopathology 2007, **50**: 607–614.

243 Eusebi V, Millis RR. Epitheliosis, infiltrating epitheliosis, and radial scar. Semin Diagn Pathol 2010, **27**: 5–12.

244 Fenoglio C, Lattes R. Sclerosing papillary proliferations in the female breast. A benign lesion often mistaken for carcinoma. Cancer 1974, **33**: 691–700.

245 Fisher ER, Palekar AS, Kotwal N, Lipana N. A non-encapsulated sclerosing lesion of the breast. Am J Clin Pathol 1979, **71**: 240–246.

246 Gottlieb C, Raju U, Greenwald KA. Myoepithelial cells in the differential diagnosis of complex benign and malignant breast lesions. An immunohistochemical study. Mod Pathol 1990, **3**: 135–140.

247 Jacobs TW, Byrne C, Colditz G, Connolly JL, Schnitt SJ. Radial scars in benign breast-biopsy specimens and the risk of breast cancer. N Engl J Med 1999, **340**: 430–436.

248 Keen ME, Murad TM, Cohen MI, Matthies HJ. Benign breast lesions with malignant clinical and mammographic presentations. Hum Pathol 1985, **16**: 1147–1152.

249 Lele SM, Graves K, Galatica Z. Immunohistochemical detection of maspin is a useful adjunct in distinguishing radial sclerosing lesion from tubular carcinoma of the breast. Appl Immunohistochem Mol Morphol 2000, **8**: 32–36.

250 Linell F, Ljungberg O, Andersson I. Breast carcinoma. Aspects of early stages, progression and related problems. Acta Pathol Microbiol Scand [A] 1980, **272**(Suppl): 1–233.

251 Manfrin E, Remo A, Falsirollo F, Reghellin D, Bonetti F. Risk of neoplastic transformation in asymptomatic radial scar. Analysis of 117 cases. Breast Cancer Res Treat 2008, **107**: 371–377.

252 Nielsen M, Christensen L, Andersen J. Radial scars in women with breast cancer. Cancer 1987, **59**: 1019–1025.

253 Nielsen M, Jensen J, Andersen JA. An autopsy study of radial scar in the female breast. Histopathology 1985, **9**: 287–295.

254 Rabban JT, Sgroi DC. Sclerosing lesions of the breast. Semin Diagn Pathol 2004, **21**: 42–47.

255 Rickert RR, Kalisher L, Hutter RVP. Indurative mastopathy. A benign sclerosing lesion of breast with elastosis which may simulate carcinoma. Cancer 1981, **47**: 561–571.

256 Sloane JP, Mayers MM. Carcinoma and atypical hyperplasia in radial scars and complex sclerosing lesions. Importance of lesion size and patient age. Histopathology 1993, **23**: 225–231.

257 Tremblay G, Buell RH, Seemayer TA. Elastosis in benign sclerosing ductal proliferation of the female breast. Am J Surg Pathol 1977, **1**: 155–159.

258 Wellings SR, Alpers CE. Subgross pathologic features and incidence of radial scars in the breast. Hum Pathol 1984, **15**: 475–479.

DUCTAL AND LOBULAR HYPERPLASIA

259 Azzopardi JG. Problems in breast pathology. In Bennington JL (consulting ed.): Major problems in pathology, vol. 11. Philadelphia, 1979, W.B. Saunders.

260 Cameselle-Teijeiro J, Abdulkader I, Barreiro-Morandeira F, Ruiz-Ponte C, Reyes-Santías R, Chavez E, Sobrinho-Simões M. Breast tumor resembling the tall cell variant of papillary thyroid carcinoma: a case report. Int J Surg Pathol 2006, **14**: 79–84.

261 Clement PB, Young RH, Azzopardi JG. Collagenous spherulosis of the breast. Am J Surg Pathol 1987, **11**: 411–417.

262 Damiani S, Cattani MG, Buonamici L, Eusebi V. Mammary foam cells. Characterization by immunohistochemistry and in situ hybridisation. Virchows Arch 1998, **432**: 433–440.

263 Eusebi V, Damiani S, Ellis IO, Azzopardi J, Rosai J. Breast tumor resembling the tall cell variant of papillary thyroid carcinoma: report of five cases. Am J Surg Pathol 2003; **27**: 1114–1118.

264 Grignon DJ, Ro JY, Mackay BN, Ordóñez NG, Ayala AG. Collagenous spherulosis of the breast. Immunohistochemical and ultrastructural studies. Am J Clin Pathol 1989, **91**: 386–392.

265 Guerry P, Erlandson RA, Rosen PP. Cystic hypersecretory hyperplasia and cystic hypersecretory duct carcinoma of the breast. Pathology, therapy, and follow-up of 39 patients. Cancer 1988, **61**: 1611–1620.

266 Hameed O, Perry A, Banerjee R, Zhu X, Pfeifer JD. Papillary carcinoma of the breast lacks evidence of RET rearrangements despite morphological similarities to papillary thyroid carcinoma. Mod Pathol 2009, **22**: 1236–1242.

267 Kasami M, Jensen RA, Simpson JF, Page DL. Lobulocentricity of breast hypersecretory hyperplasia with cytologic atypia: infrequent association with carcinoma in situ. Am J Clin Pathol 2004, **122**: 714–720.

268 Maluf HM, Koerner FC, Dickersin GR. Collagenous spherulosis: an ultrastructural study. Ultrastruct Pathol 1998, **22**: 239–248.

269 Michal M, Skalova A. Collagenous spherulosis. A comment on its histogenesis. Pathol Res Pract 1990, **186**: 365–370.

270 Mooney EE, Kayani N, Tavassoli FA. Spherulosis of the breast. A spectrum of mucinous and collagenous lesions. Arch Pathol Lab Med 1999, **123**: 626–630.

271 Raju U, Crissman JD, Zarbo RJ, Gottlieb C. Epitheliosis of the breast. An immunohistochemical characterization and comparison to malignant intraductal proliferations of the breast. Am J Surg Pathol 1990, **14**: 939–947.

272 Resetkova E, Albarracin C, Sneige N. Collagenous spherulosis of breast: morphologic study of 59 cases and review of the literature. Am J Surg Pathol 2006, **30**: 20–27.

273 Sgroi D, Koerner FC. Involvement of collagenous spherulosis by lobular carcinoma in situ. Potential confusion with cribriform ductal carcinoma in situ. Am J Surg Pathol 1995, **19**: 1366–1370.

274 Tavassoli FA, Majeste RM, Snyder RC. Intranuclear helioid inclusions in mammary intraductal hyperplasias. Ultrastruct Pathol 1991, **15**: 267–279.

275 Tham K, Dupont WD, Page DL, Gray GF, Rogers LW. Micro-papillary hyperplasia with atypical features in female breasts, resembling gynecomastia. Prog Surg Pathol 1989, **10**: 101–110.

276 Tosi AL, Ragazzi M, Asioli S, Del Vecchio M, Cavalieri M, Eusebi LH, Foschini MP. Breast tumor resembling the tall cell variant of papillary thyroid carcinoma: report of 4 cases with evidence of malignant potential. Int J Surg Pathol 2007, **15**: 14–19.

ATYPICAL DUCTAL AND LOBULAR HYPERPLASIA

277 Beck JS. Observer variability in reporting of breast lesions. J Clin Pathol 1985, **38**: 1358–1365.

278 Bodian CA, Perzin KH, Lattes R, Hoffmann P. Reproducibility and validity of pathologic classifications of benign breast disease and implications for clinical applications. Cancer 1993, **71**: 3908–3913.

279 Consensus Meeting. Oct 3 to 5, 1985, New York, Cancer Committee of the College of American Pathologists: Is 'fibrocystic disease' of the breast precancerous? Arch Pathol Lab Med 1986, **110**: 171–173.

280 Crissman JD, Visscher DW, Kubus J. Image cytophotometric DNA analysis of atypical hyperplasias and intraductal carcinomas of the breast. Arch Pathol Lab Med 1990, **114**: 1249–1253.

281 Dupont WD, Page DL. Risk factors for breast cancer in women with proliferative breast disease. N Engl J Med 1985, **312**: 146–151.

282 Fitzgibbons PL, Henson DE, Hutter RV. Benign breast changes and the risk for subsequent breast cancer: an update of the 1985 consensus statement. Cancer Committee of the College of American Pathologists. Arch Pathol Lab Med 1998, **122**: 1053–1055.

283 Ghofrani M, Tapia B, Tavassoli FA. Discrepancies in the diagnosis of intraductal proliferative lesions of the breast and its management implications: results of a multinational survey. Virchows Arch 2006, **449**: 609–616.

284 King EB, Chew KL, Hom JD, Duarte LA, Mayall B, Miller TR, Neuhaus JM, Wrensch MR, Petrakis NL. Characterization by image cytometry of duct epithelial proliferative disease of the breast. Mod Pathol 1991, **4**: 291–296.

285 Ohuchi N, Page DL, Merino MJ, Viglione MJ, Kufe DW, Schlom J. Expression of tumor-associated antigen (DF3) in atypical hyperplasias and in situ carcinomas of the human breast. J Natl Cancer Inst 1987, **79**: 109–117.

286 Page DL. Cancer risk assessment in benign breast biopsies. Hum Pathol 1986, **17**: 871–874.

287 Page DL, Dupont WD, Rogers LW, Rados MS. Atypical hyperplastic lesions of the female breast. A long-term follow-up study. Cancer 1985, **55**: 2698–2708.

288 Page DL, Kidd TE Jr, Dupont WD, Simpson JF, Rogers LW. Lobular neoplasia of the breast: higher risk for subsequent invasive cancer predicted by more extensive disease. Hum Pathol 1991, **22**: 1232–1239.

289 Page DL, Rogers LW. Combined histologic and cytologic criteria for the diagnosis of mammary atypical ductal hyperplasia. Hum Pathol 1992, **23**: 1095–1097.

290 Purcell CA, Norris HJ. Intraductal proliferations of the breast: a review of histologic criteria for atypical intraductal hyperplasia and ductal carcinoma in situ, including apocrine and papillary lesions. Ann Diagn Pathol 1998, **2**: 135–145.

291 Putti TC, Pinder SE, Elston CW, Lee AH, Ellis IO. Breast pathology practice: most common problems in a consultation service. Histopathology 2005, **47**: 445–457.

292 Rosai J. Borderline epithelial lesions of the breast. Am J Surg Pathol 1991, **15**: 209–221.

293 Schnitt SJ, Connolly JL, Tavassoli FA, Fechner RE, Kempson RL, Gelman R, Page DL. Interobserver reproducibility in the diagnosis of ductal proliferative breast lesions using standardized criteria. Am J Surg Pathol 1992, **16**: 1133–1143.

294 Tavassoli FA, Norris HJ. A comparison of the results of long-term follow-up for atypical intraductal hyperplasia and intraductal hyperplasia of the breast. Cancer 1990, **65**: 518–529.

295 Walker R. The pathology of 'precancerous' breast disease. Pathol Annu 1995, **29**(Pt2): 75–97.

296 Yeh IT, Mies C. Application of immunohistochemistry to breast lesions. Arch Pathol Lab Med 2008, **132**: 349–358.

FLAT EPITHELIAL ATYPIA (COLUMNAR CELL LESION)

297 Abdel-Fatah TM, Powe DG, Hodi Z, Lee AH, Reis-Filho JS, Ellis IO. High frequency of coexistence of columnar cell lesions, lobular neoplasia, and low grade ductal carcinoma in situ with invasive tubular carcinoma and invasive lobular carcinoma. Am J Surg Pathol 2007, **31**: 417–426.

298 Brogi E, Oyama T, Koerner FC. Atypical cystic lobules in patients with lobular neoplasia. Int J Surg Pathol 2001, **9**: 201–206.

299 Collins LC, Achacoso NA, Nekhlyudov L, Fletcher SW, Haque R, Quesenberry CP Jr, Alshak NS, Puligandla B, Brodsky GL, Schnitt SJ, Habel LA. Clinical and pathologic features of ductal carcinoma in situ associated with the presence of flat epithelial atypia: an analysis of 543 patients. Mod Pathol 2007, **20**: 1149–1155.

300 Dabbs DJ, Kessinger RL, McManus K, Johnson R. Biology of columnar cell lesions in core biopsies of breast [abstract]. Mod Pathol 2003, **16**: 26a.

301 Dessauvagie BF, Zhao W, Heel-Miller KA, Harvey J, Bentel JM. Characterization of columnar cell lesions of the breast: immunophenotypic analysis of columnar alteration of lobules with prominent apical snouts and secretions. Hum Pathol 2007, **38**: 284–292.

302 Feeley L, Quinn CM. Columnar cell lesions of the breast. Histopathology 2008, **52**: 11–19.

303 Fraser JL, Raza S, Chorny K, Connolly JL, Schnitt SJ. Columnar alteration with prominent apical snouts and secretions: a spectrum of changes frequently present in breast biopsies performed for microcalcifications. Am J Surg Pathol 1998, **22**: 1521–1527.

304 Jhala D, Talley L, Chhieng D, Frost A. Presence of columnar alteration with prominent apical snouts and secretions and relation with biomarker expression in 200 breast cancer patients [abstract]. Mod Pathol 2003, **16**: 34a.

305 Koerner FC, Oyama T, Maluf H. Morphological observations regarding the origins of atypical cystic lobules (low-grade clinging carcinoma of flat type). Virchows Arch 2001, **439**: 523–530.

306 Leibl S, Regitnig P, Moinfar F. Flat epithelial atypia (DIN 1a, atypical columnar change): an underdiagnosed entity very frequently coexisting with lobular neoplasia. Histopathology 2007, **50**: 859–865.

307 Lerwill MF. Flat epithelial atypia of the breast. Arch Pathol Lab Med 2008, **132**: 615–621.

308 Moinfar F. Flat ductal intraepithelial neoplasia of the breast: a review of diagnostic criteria, differential diagnoses, molecular-genetic findings, and clinical relevance – it is time to appreciate the Azzopardi concept! Arch Pathol Lab Med 2009, **133**: 879–892.

309 Moinfar F. Flat ductal intraepithelial neoplasia of the breast: evolution of Azzopardi's 'clinging' concept. Semin Diagn Pathol 2010, **27**: 37–48.

310 Noske A, Pahl S, Fallenberg E, Richter-Ehrenstein C, Buckendahl AC, Weichert W, Schneider A, Dietel M, Denkert C. Flat epithelial atypia is a common subtype of B3 breast lesions and is associated with noninvasive cancer but not with invasive cancer in final excision histology. Hum Pathol 2010, **41**: 522–527.

311 Oyama T, Maluf H, Koerner F. Atypical cystic lobules: an early stage in the formation of low-grade ductal carcinoma in situ. Virchows Arch 1999, **435**: 413–421.

NOMENCLATURE OF PROLIFERATIVE DUCTAL AND LOBULAR LESIONS

312 Azzopardi JG. Problems in breast pathology. In Bennington JL (consulting ed.): Major problems in pathology, vol. 11. Philadelphia, 1979, W.B. Saunders.

313 Bratthauer GL, Tavassoli FA. Lobular intraepithelial neoplasia: previously unexplored aspects assessed in 775 cases and their clinical implications. Virchows Arch 2002, **440**: 134–138.

314 Lopez-Garcia MA, Geyer FC, Lacroix-Triki M, Marchió C, Reis-Filho JS. Breast cancer precursors revisited: molecular features and progression pathways. Histopathology 2010, **57**: 171–192.

315 Rosai J. Borderline epithelial lesions of the breast. Am J Surg Pathol 1991, **15**: 209–221.

316 Tavassoli FA. Ductal carcinoma in situ: introduction of the concept of ductal intraepithelial neoplasia. Mod Pathol 1998, **11**: 140–154.

317 Tavassoli FA, Hoefler H, Rosai J, Holland R, Ellis I, Schnitt S. Intraductal proliferative lesions. Pathology and genetics of tumours of the breast and female genital organs. Lyon, 2003, IARC Press, pp. 14–20.

RELATIONSHIP WITH CARCINOMA AND TREATMENT

318 Aubele MM, Cummings MC, Mattis AE, Zitzelsberger HF, Walch AK, Kremer M, Hofler H, Werner M. Accumulation of chromosomal imbalances from intraductal proliferative lesions to adjacent in situ and invasive ductal breast cancer. Diagn Mol Pathol 2000, **9**: 14–19.

319 Bianchi S, Palli D, Galli M, Zampi G. Benign breast disease and cancer risk. Crit Rev Oncol Hematol 1993, **15**: 221–242.

320 Bodian CA, Perzin KH, Lattes R, Hoffmann P, Abernathy TG. Prognostic significance of benign proliferative breast disease. Cancer 1993, **71**: 3896–3907.

321 Byrne C, Connolly JL, Colditz GA, Schnitt SJ. Biopsy confirmed benign breast disease, postmenopausal use of exogenous female hormones, and breast carcinoma risk. Cancer 2000, **89**: 2046–2052.

424 Gallager HS. Breast specimen radiography. Obligatory, adjuvant and investigative. Am J Clin Pathol 1975, **64**: 749–766.

425 Gisvold JJ. Imaging of the breast. Techniques and results. Mayo Clin Proc 1990, **65**: 56–66.

426 Gonzalez JE, Caldwell RG, Valaitis J. Calcium oxalate crystals in the breast. Pathology and significance. Am J Surg Pathol 1991, **15**: 586–591.

427 Kneeshaw PJ, Turnbull LW, Drew PJ. Current applications and future direction of MR mammography. Br J Cancer 2003, **88**: 4–10.

428 Koehl RH, Snyder RE, Hutter RVP, Foote FW Jr. The incidence and significance of calcifications within operative breast specimens. Am J Clin Pathol 1970, **53**: 3–14.

429 McDivitt RW. Breast carcinoma. Hum Pathol 1978, **9**: 3–21.

430 McLelland R. Screening mammography. Cancer 1991, **67**: 1129–1131.

431 Millis RR, Davis R, Stacey AJ. The detection and significance of calcification in the breasts. A radiological and pathological study. Br J Radiol 1976, **49**: 12–26.

432 Owings DV, Hann L, Schnitt SJ. How thoroughly should needle localization breast biopsies be sampled for microscopic examination? A prospective mammographic/pathologic correlative study. Am J Surg Pathol 1990, **14**: 578–583.

433 Rosen PP, Synder RE, Robbins G. Specimen radiography for nonpalpable breast lesions found by mammography. Procedures and results. Cancer 1974, **34**: 2028–2033.

434 Schnall MD. Breast MR imaging. Radiol Clin North Am 2003, **41**: 43–50.

435 Schwartz GF, Carter DL, Conant EF, Gannon FH, Finkel GC, Feig SA. Mammographically detected breast cancer. Nonpalpable is not a synonym for inconsequential. Cancer 1994, **73**: 1660–1665.

436 Stevens GM, Jamplis RW. Mammographically directed biopsy of nonpalpable breast lesions. Arch Surg 1971, **102**: 292–295.

437 US Preventive Services Task Force. Screening for breast cancer: US Preventive Services Task Force recommendation statement. Ann Intern Med 2009, **151**: 716–726.

438 Wolfe JN. Breast patterns as an index of risk for developing breast cancer. Am J Roentgenol 1976, **126**: 1130–1139.

CYTOLOGY

439 Abendroth CS, Wang HH, Ducatman BS. Comparative features of carcinoma in situ and atypical ductal hyperplasia of the breast on fine-needle aspiration biopsy specimens. Am J Clin Pathol 1991, **96**: 654–659.

440 Arisio R, Cuccorese C, Accinelli G, Mano MP, Bordon R, Fessia L. Role of fine-needle aspiration biopsy in breast lesions: analysis of a series of 4,110 cases. Diagn Cytopathol 1998, **18**: 462–467.

441 Barrows GH, Anderson TJ, Lamb JL, Dixon JM. Fine-needle aspiration of breast cancer. Relationship of clinical factors to cytology results in 689 primary malignancies. Cancer 1986, **58**: 1493–1498.

442 Dawson AE, Mulford DK, Sheils LA. The cytopathology of proliferative breast disease. Am J Clin Pathol 1995, **103**: 438–442.

443 Eisenberg AJ, Hajdu SI, Wilhelmus J, Melamed MR, Kinne D. Preoperative aspiration cytology of breast tumors. Acta Cytol (Baltimore) 1986, **30**: 135–146.

444 Frable WJ. Needle aspiration of the breast. Cancer 1984, **53**: 671–676.

445 Jeffrey PB, Ljung BM. Benign and malignant papillary lesions of the breast. A cytomorphologic study. Am J Clin Pathol 1994, **101**: 500–507.

446 Kline TS. Masquerades of malignancy. A review of 4,241 aspirates from the breast. Acta Cytol (Baltimore) 1981, **25**: 263–266.

447 Kline TS, Joshi LP, Neal HS. Fine-needle aspiration of the breast. Diagnoses and pitfalls. A review of 3545 cases. Cancer 1979, **44**: 1458–1464.

448 Lee KC, Chan JK, Ho LC. Histologic changes in the breast after fine-needle aspiration. Am J Surg Pathol 1994, **18**: 1039–1047.

449 Ljung BM, Chew K, Deng G, Matsumura K, Waldman F, Smith H. Fine needle aspiration techniques for the characterization of breast cancers. Cancer 1994, **74**: 1000–1005.

450 Marshall CJ, Schumann GB, Ward JH, Riding JM, Cannon-Albright L, Skolnick M. Cytologic identification of clinically occult proliferative breast disease in women with a family history of breast cancer. Am J Clin Pathol 1991, **95**: 157–165.

451 Norton LW, Davis JR, Wiens JL, Trego DC, Dunnington GL. Accuracy of aspiration cytology in detecting breast cancer. Surgery 1984, **96**: 806–811.

452 Oertel YC. Fine needle aspiration of the breast. Stoneham, MA, 1987, Butterworths.

453 Reiner A, Spona J, Reiner G, Schemper M, Kolb R, Kwasny W, Függer R, Jakesz R, Holzner JH. Estrogen receptor analysis on biopsies and fine-needle aspirates from human breast carcinoma. Correlation of biochemical and immunohistochemical methods using monoclonal antireceptor antibodies. Am J Pathol 1986, **125**: 443–449.

454 Remvikos Y, Magdelenat H, Zajdela A. DNA flow cytometry applied to fine needle sampling of human breast cancer. Cancer 1988, **61**: 1629–1634.

455 Rosenthal DL. Breast lesions diagnosed by fine needle aspiration. Pathol Res Pract 1986, **181**: 645–656.

456 Silfversward C, Gustafsson J-A, Gustafsson SA, Nordenskjold B, Wallgren A, Wrange O. Estrogen receptor analysis on fine needle aspirates and on histologic biopsies from human breast cancer. Eur J Cancer 1980, **16**: 1351–1357.

457 Sneige N, Singletary SE. Fine-needle aspiration of the breast. Diagnostic problems and approaches to surgical management. Pathol Annu 1994, **29**(Pt 1): 281–301.

458 Sneige N, Staerkel GA. Fine-needle aspiration cytology of ductal hyperplasia with and without atypia and ductal carcinoma in situ. Hum Pathol 1994, **25**: 485–492.

459 Tavassoli FA, Pestaner JP. Pseudoinvasion in intraductal carcinoma. Mod Pathol 1995, **8**: 380–383.

460 Thomas PA, Cangiarella J, Raab SS, Waisman J. Fine needle aspiration biopsy of proliferative breast disease. Mod Pathol 1995, **8**: 130–136.

461 Thomas PA, Vazquez MF, Waisman J. Comparison of fine-needle aspiration and frozen section of palpable mammary lesions. Mod Pathol 1990, **3**: 570–574.

462 Youngson BJ, Cranor M, Rosen PP. Epithelial displacement in surgical breast specimens following needling procedures. Am J Surg Pathol 1994, **18**: 896–903.

463 Youngson BJ, Liberman L, Rosen PP. Displacement of carcinomatous epithelium in surgical breast specimens following stereotaxic core biopsy. Am J Clin Pathol 1995, **103**: 598–602.

464 Wanebo HJ, Feldman PS, Wilhelm MC, Covell JL, Binns RL. Fine needle aspiration cytology in lieu of open biopsy in management of primary breast cancer. Ann Surg 1984, **199**: 569–578.

NEEDLE CORE BIOPSY

465 Ballo MS, Sneige N. Can core needle biopsy replace fine-needle aspiration cytology in the diagnosis of palpable breast carcinoma? A comparative study of 124 women. Cancer 1996, **78**: 773–777.

466 Begum SM, Jara-Lazaro AR, Thike AA, Tse GM, Wong JS, Ho JT, Tan PH. Mucin extravasation in breast core biopsies – clinical significance and outcome correlation. Histopathology 2009, **55**: 609–617

467 Cangiarella J, Guth A, Axelrod D, Darvishian F, Singh B, Simsir A, Roses D, Mercado C. Is surgical excision necessary for the management of atypical lobular hyperplasia and lobular carcinoma in situ diagnosed on core needle biopsy?: a report of 38 cases and review of the literature. Arch Pathol Lab Med 2008, **132**: 979–983.

468 Carder PJ, Garvican J, Haigh I, Liston JC. Needle core biopsy can reliably distinguish between benign and malignant papillary lesions of the breast. Histopathology 2005, **46**: 320–327.

469 Chandrasoma PT. Microcalcification in the breast and the pathologist. Am J Surg Pathol 2002, **26**: 135–136.

470 Chivukula M, Bhargava R, Tseng G, Dabbs DJ. Clinicopathologic implications of 'flat epithelial atypia' in core needle biopsy specimens of the breast. Am J Clin Pathol 2009, **131**: 802–808.

471 Chivukula M, Haynik DM, Brufsky A, Carter G, Dabbs DJ. Pleomorphic lobular carcinoma in situ (PLCIS) on breast core needle biopsies: clinical significance and immunoprofile. Am J Surg Pathol 2008, **32**: 1721–1726.

472 Collins LC, Connolly JL, Page DL, Goulart RA, Pisano ED, Fajardo LL, Berg WA, Caudry DJ, McNeil BJ, Schnitt SJ. Diagnostic agreement in the evaluation of image-guided breast core needle biopsies: results from a randomized clinical trial. Am J Surg Pathol 2004, **28**: 126–131.

473 Davies JD, Nonni A, D'Costa HF. Mammary epidermoid inclusion cysts after wide-core needle biopsies. Histopathology 1997, **31**: 549–551.

474 Elsheikh TM, Silverman JF. Follow-up surgical excision is indicated when breast core needle biopsies show atypical lobular hyperplasia or lobular carcinoma in situ: a correlative study of 33 patients with review of the literature. Am J Surg Pathol 2005, **29**: 534–543.

475 Gao F, Carter G, Tseng G, Chivukula M. Clinical importance of histologic grading of lobular carcinoma in situ in breast core needle biopsy specimens: current issues and controversies. Am J Clin Pathol 2010, **133**: 767–771.

476 Gobbi H, Tse G, Page DL, Olson SJ, Jensen RA, Simpson JF. Reactive spindle cell nodules of the breast after core biopsy or fine needle aspiration. Am J Clin Pathol 2000, **113**: 288–294.

477 Guarda LA, Tran TA. The pathology of breast biopsy site marking devices. Am J Surg Pathol 2005, **29**: 814–819.

478 Hoda SA, Harigopal M, Harris GC, Pinder SE, Lee AHS, Ellis IO. Reporting needle core biopsies of breast carcinomas. Histopathology 2003, **43**: 84–90.

479 Hoda SA, Rosen PP. Practical considerations in the pathologic diagnosis of needle core biopsies of breast. Am J Clin Pathol 2002, **118**: 101–108.

480 Hoda SA, Rosen PP. Practical considerations in the pathologic diagnosis of needle core biopsies of breast. Am J Clin Pathol 2002, **118**: 101–108.

481 Ivan D, Selinko V, Sahin AA, Sneige N, Middleton LP. Accuracy of core needle biopsy diagnosis in assessing papillary breast lesions: histologic predictors of malignancy. Mod Pathol 2004, **17**: 165–171.

482 Jacobs TW, Connolly JL, Schnitt SJ. Nonmalignant lesions in breast core needle biopsy: to excise or not to excise? Am J Surg Pathol 2002, **26**: 1095–1110.

483 Karabakhtsian RG, Johnson R, Sumkin J, Dabbs DJ. The clinical significance of lobular neoplasia on breast core biopsy. Am J Surg Pathol 2007, **31**: 717–723.

484 Kettritz U, Rotter K, Schreer I, Murauer M, Schulz-Wendtland R, Peter D, Heywang-Köbrunner SH. Stereotactic vacuum-assisted breast biopsy in 2874 patients: a multicenter study. Cancer 2004, **100**: 245–251.

485 Koo JS, Jung WH, Kim H. Epithelial displacement into the lymphovascular space can be seen in breast core needle biopsy specimens. Am J Clin Pathol 2010, **133**: 781–787.

486 Kunju LP, Kleer CG. Significance of flat epithelial atypia on mammotome core needle biopsy: should it be excised? Hum Pathol 2007, **38**: 35–41.

487 Lee AH, Denley HE, Pinder SE, Ellis IO, Elston CW, Vujovic P, Macmillan RD, Evans AJ: for the Nottingham Breast Team. Excision biopsy findings of patients with breast needle core biopsies reported as suspicious of malignancy (B4) or lesion of uncertain malignant potential (B3). Histopathology 2003, **42**: 331–336.

488 Litherland JC. Should fine needle aspiration cytology in breast assessment be abandoned? Clin Radiol 2002, **57**: 81–84.

489 Menon S, Porter GJ, Evans AJ, Ellis IO, Elston CW, Hodi Z, Lee AH. The significance of lobular neoplasia on needle core biopsy of the breast. Virchows Arch 2008, **452**: 473–479.

490 Middleton LP, Grant S, Stephens T, Stelling CB, Sniege N, Sahin AA. Lobular carcinoma in situ diagnosed by core needle biopsy: when should it be excised? Mod Pathol 2003, **16**: 120–129.

491 Nagi C, Bleiweiss I, Jaffer S. Epithelial displacement in breast lesions: a papillary phenomenon. Arch Pathol Lab Med 2005, **129**: 1465–1469.

492 Piubello Q, Parisi A, Eccher A, Barbazeni G, Franchini Z, Iannucci A. Flat epithelial atypia on core needle biopsy: which is the right management? Am J Surg Pathol 2009, **33**: 1078–1084.

493 Renshaw AA. Adequate histologic sampling of breast core needle biopsies. Arch Pathol Lab Med 2001, **125**: 1055–1057.

494 Renshaw AA. Predicting invasion in the excision specimen from breast core needle biopsy specimens with only ductal carcinoma in situ. Arch Pathol Lab Med 2002, **126**: 39–41.

495 Renshaw AA, Cartagena N, Schenkman RH, Derhagopian RP, Gould EW. Atypical ductal hyperplasia in breast core needle biopsies. Correlation of size of the lesion, complete removal of the lesion, and the incidence of carcinoma in follow-up biopsies. Am J Clin Pathol 2001, **116**: 92–96.

496 Renshaw AA, Derhagopian RP, Martinez P, Gould EW. Lobular neoplasia in breast core needle biopsy specimens is associated with a low risk of ductal carcinoma in situ or invasive carcinoma on subsequent excision. Am J Clin Pathol 2006, **126**: 310–313.

497 Renshaw AA, Derhagopian RP, Tizol-Blanco DM, Gould EW. Papillomas and atypical papillomas in breast core needle biopsy specimens: risk of carcinoma in subsequent excision. Am J Clin Pathol 2004, **122**: 217–221.

498 Senetta R, Campanino PP, Mariscotti G, Garberoglio S, Daniele L, Pennecchi F, Macrì L, Bosco M, Gandini G, Sapino A. Columnar cell lesions associated with breast calcifications on vacuum-assisted core biopsies: clinical, radiographic, and histological correlations. Mod Pathol 2009, **22**: 762–769.

499 Shah VI, Raju U, Chitale D, Deshpande V, Gregory N, Strand V. False-negative core needle biopsies of the breast: An analysis of clinical, radiologic, and pathologic findings in 27 consecutive cases of missed breast cancer. Cancer 2003, **97**: 1824–1831.

500 Shin SJ, Rosen PP. Excisional biopsy should be performed if lobular carcinoma in situ is seen on needle core biopsy. Arch Pathol Lab Med 2002, **126**: 697–701.

501 Shousha S. Issues in the intrepretation of breast core biopsies. Int J Surg Pathol 2003, **11**: 167–176.

502 Wang J, Simsir A, Mercado C, Cangiarella J. Can core biopsy reliably diagnose mucinous lesions of the breast? Am J Clin Pathol 2007, **127**: 124–127.

503 Youngson BJ, Cranor M, Rosen PP. Epithelial displacement in surgical breast specimens following needling procedures. Am J Surg Pathol 1994, **18**: 896–903.

504 Youngson BJ, Liberman L, Rosen PP. Displacement of carcinomatous epithelium in surgical breast specimens following stereotaxic core biopsy. Am J Clin Pathol 1995, **103**: 598–602.

OPEN BIOPSY AND FROZEN SECTION

505 Bianchi S, Palli D, Ciatto S, Galli M, Giorgi D, Vezzosi V, Rosselli del Turco M, Cataliotti L, Cardona G, Zampi G. Accuracy and reliability of frozen section diagnosis in a series of 672 nonpalpable breast lesions. Am J Clin Pathol 1993, **103**: 199–205.

506 Esteban JM, Zaloudek C, Silverberg SG. Intraoperative diagnosis of breast lesions. Comparison of cytologic with frozen section technics. Am J Clin Pathol 1987, **88**: 681–688.

507 Fechner RE. Frozen section examination of breast biopsies. Practice parameter. Am J Clin Pathol 1995, **103**: 6–7.

508 Ferreiro JA, Gisvold JJ, Bostwick DG. Accuracy of frozen-section diagnosis of mammographically directed breast biopsies. Results of 1,490 consecutive cases. Am J Surg Pathol 1995, **19**: 1267–1271.

509 Laucirica R. Intraoperative assessment of the breast: guidelines and potential pitfalls. Arch Pathol Lab Med 2005, **129**: 1565–1574.

510 Niemann TH, Lucas JG, Marsh WL Jr. To freeze or not to freeze. A comparison of methods for the handling of breast biopsies with no palpable abnormality. Am J Clin Pathol 1996, **106**: 225–228.

511 Oberman HA. A modest proposal [editorial]. Am J Surg Pathol 1992, **16**: 69–70.

512 Recommendations of the Association of Directors of Anatomic and Surgical Pathology. Part I. Immediate management of mammographically detected breast lesions. Hum Pathol 1993, **24**: 689–690.

513 Sauter ER, Hoffman JP, Ottery FD, Kowalyshyn MJ, Litwin S, Eisenberg BL. Is frozen section analysis of reexcision lumpectomy margins worthwhile? Margin analysis in breast reexcisions. Cancer 1994, **73**: 2607–2612.

514 Speights VO Jr. Evaluation of frozen sections in grossly benign breast biopsies. Mod Pathol 1994, **7**: 762–765.

MICROSCOPIC TYPES

515 Andersen JA. Invasive breast carcinoma with lobular involvement. Frequency and location of lobular carcinoma in situ. Acta Pathol Microbiol Scand (A) 1974, **82**: 719–729.

516 Ishige H, Komatsu T, Kondo Y, Sugano I, Horinaka E, Okui K. Lobular involvement in human breast carcinoma. Acta Pathol Jpn 1991, **41**: 227–232.

517 Kerner H, Lichtig C. Lobular cancerization: incidence and differential diagnosis with lobular carcinoma in situ of breast. Histopathology 1986, **10**: 621–629.

518 Wellings SR, Jensen HM, Marcum RG. An atlas of subgross pathology of the human breast with special reference to possible precancerous lesions. J Natl Cancer Inst 1975, **55**: 231–273.

IN SITU CARCINOMA

DUCTAL CARCINOMA IN SITU (DCIS)

519 Badve S, A'Hern RP, Ward AM, Millis RR, Pinder SE, Ellis IO, Gusterson BA, Sloane P. Prediction of local recurrence of ductal carcinoma in situ of the breast using five histological classifications: a comparative study with long follow-up. Hum Pathol 1998, **29**: 915–923.

520 Bellamy CD, McDonald C, Salter DM, Chetty U, Anderson TJ. Noninvasive ductal carcinoma of the breast. The relevance of histologic categorization. Hum Pathol 1993, **24**: 16–23.

520a Collins LC, Achacoso N, Nekhlyudov L, Fletcher SW, Haque R, Quesenberry CP Jr, Puligandla B, Alshak NS, Goldstein LC, Gown AM, Schnitt SJ, Habel LA. Relationship between clinical and pathologic features of ductal carcinoma in situ and patient age: an analysis of 657 patients. Am J Surg Pathol 2009, **33**: 1802–1808.

521 Douglas-Jones AG, Gupta SK, Attanoos RL, Morgan JM, Mansel RE. A critical appraisal of six modern classifications of ductal carcinoma in situ of the breast (DCIS): correlation with grade of associated invasive carcinoma. Histopathology 1996, **29**: 397–409.

522 Ellis IO, Pinder SE, Lee AH, Elston CW. A critical appraisal of existing classification systems of epithelial hyperplasia and in situ neoplasia of the breast with proposals for future methods of categorization: where are we going? Semin Diagn Pathol 1999, **16**: 202–208.

523 Holland R, Hendriks JH. Microcalcifications associated with ductal carcinoma in situ. Mammographic–pathologic correlation. Semin Diagn Pathol 1994, **11**: 181–192.

524 Holland R, Peterse JL, Millis RR, Eusebi V, Faverly D, van de Vijver MJ, Zafrani B. Ductal carcinoma in situ. A proposal for a new classification. Semin Diagn Pathol 1994, **11**: 167–180.

525 Lennington WJ, Jensen RA, Dalton LW, Page DL. Ductal carcinoma in situ of the breast. Heterogeneity of individual lesions. Cancer 1994, **73**: 118–124.

624 Eusebi V, Betts C, Haagensen DE Jr, Gugliotta P, Bussolati G, Azzopardi JG. Apocrine differentiation in lobular carcinoma of the breast. A morphologic, immunologic, and ultrastructural study. Hum Pathol 1984, **15**: 134–140.

625 Eusebi V, Pich A, Macchiorlatti E, Bussolati G. Morpho-functional differentiation in lobular carcinoma of the breast. Histopathology 1977, **1**: 301–314.

626 Fadare O, Dadmanesh F, Alvarado-Cabrero I, Snyder R, Stephen Mitchell J, Tot T, Wang SA, Ghofrani M, Eusebi V, Martel M, Tavassoli FA. Lobular intraepithelial neoplasia [lobular carcinoma in situ] with comedo-type necrosis: a clinicopathologic study of 18 cases. Am J Surg Pathol 2006, **30**: 1445–1453.

627 Fechner RE. Ductal carcinoma involving the lobule of the breast. A source of confusion with lobular carcinoma in situ. Cancer 1971, **28**: 274–281.

628 Fechner RE. Epithelial alterations in the extralobular ducts of breasts with lobular carcinoma. Arch Pathol 1972, **93**: 164–171.

629 Fechner RE. Lobular carcinoma in situ in sclerosing adenosis. A potential source of confusion with invasive carcinoma. Am J Surg Pathol 1981, **5**: 233–239.

630 Fondo EY, Rosen PP, Fracchia AA, Urban JA. The problem of carcinoma developing in a fibroadenoma. Recent experience at Memorial Hospital. Cancer 1979, **43**: 563–567.

631 Haagensen CD, Lane N, Bodian C. Coexisting lobular neoplasia and carcinoma of the breast. Cancer 1983, **51**: 1468–1482.

632 Hanby AM, Hughes TA. In situ and invasive lobular neoplasia of the breast. Histopathology 2008, **52**: 58–66.

633 Jacobs TW, Pliss N, Kouria G, Schnitt SJ. Carcinomas in situ of the breast with indeterminate features: role of E-cadherin staining in categorization. Am J Surg Pathol 2001, **25**: 229–236.

634 Lambird PA, Shelley WM. The spatial distribution of lobular in situ mammary carcinoma. Implications for size and site of breast biopsy. JAMA 1969, **210**: 689–693.

635 Mastracci TL, Tjan S, Bane AL, O'Malley FP, Andrulis IL. E-cadherin alterations in atypical lobular hyperplasia and lobular carcinoma in situ of the breast. Mod Pathol 2005, **18**: 741–751.

636 Newman W. Lobular carcinoma of the female breast. Ann Surg 1966, **164**: 305–314.

637 Perrone G, Zagami M, Santini D, Vincenzi B, Gullotta G, Morini S, Battista C, Guerriero G, Altomare V, Tonini G, Rabitti C. COX-2 expression in lobular in situ neoplasia of the breast: correlation with histopathological grading system according to the Tavassoli classification. Histopathology 2007, **51**: 33–39.

638 Rieger-Christ KM, Pezza JA, Dugan JM, Braasch JW, Hughes KS, Summerhayes IC. Disparate E-cadherin mutations in LCIS and associated invasive breast carcinomas. Mol Pathol 2001, **54**: 91–97.

639 Rosen PP, Lieberman PH, Braun DW Jr, Kosloff C, Adair F. Lobular carcinoma in situ of the breast. Detailed analysis of 99 patients with average follow-up of 24 years. Am J Surg Pathol 1978, **2**: 225–251.

640 Sahoo S, Green I, Rosen PP. Bilateral Paget disease of the nipple associated with lobular carcinoma in situ: application of immunohistochemistry to a rare finding. Arch Pathol Lab Med 2002, **126**: 90–92.

641 Schnitt SJ, Morrow M. Lobular carcinoma in situ: current concepts and controversies. Semin Diagn Pathol 1999, **16**: 209–223.

642 Sgroi D, Koerner FC. Involvement of collagenous spherulosis by lobular carcinoma in situ. Potential confusion with cribriform ductal carcinoma in situ. Am J Surg Pathol 1995, **19**: 1366–1370.

643 Sneige N, Wang J, Baker BA, Krishnamurthy S, Middleton LP. Clinical, histopathologic, and biologic features of pleomorphic lobular (ductal–lobular) carcinoma in situ of the breast: a report of 24 cases. Mod Pathol 2002, **15**: 1044–1050.

644 Tobon H, Price HM. Lobular carcinoma in situ. Some ultrastructural observations. Cancer 1972, **39**: 1082–1091.

645 Warner NE. Lobular carcinoma of the breast. Cancer 1969, **23**: 840–846.

646 Wheeler JE, Enterline HT. Lobular carcinoma of the breast in situ and infiltrating. Pathol Annu 1976, **11**: 161–188.

Evolution

647 Andersen JA. Lobular carcinoma in situ. A long-term follow-up in 52 cases. Acta Pathol Microbiol Scand (A) 1974, **82**: 519–533.

648 Andersen JA. Lobular carcinoma in situ of the breast. An approach to rational treatment. Cancer 1977, **39**: 2597–2602.

649 Fisher ER, Costantino J, Fisher B, Palekar AS, Paik SM, Suarez CM, Wolmark N. Pathologic findings from the National Surgical Adjuvant Breast Project (NSABP) protocol B-17: five-year observations concerning lobular carcinoma in situ. Cancer 1996, **78**: 1403–1416.

650 Fisher ER, Land SR, Fisher B, Mamounas E, Gilarski L, Wolmark N. Pathologic findings from the National Surgical Adjuvant Breast and Bowel Project: twelve-year observations concerning lobular carcinoma in situ. Cancer 2004, **100**: 238–244.

651 Haagensen CD, Lane N, Lattes R, Bodian C. Lobular neoplasia (so-called lobular carcinoma in situ) of the breast. Cancer 1978, **42**: 737–769.

652 Hwang H, Barke LD, Mendelson EB, Susnik B. Atypical lobular hyperplasia and classic lobular carcinoma in situ in core biopsy specimens: routine excision is not necessary. Mod Pathol 2008, **21**: 1208–1216.

653 Li CI, Malone KE, Saltzman BS, Daling JR. Risk of invasive breast carcinoma among women diagnosed with ductal carcinoma in situ and lobular carcinoma in situ, 1988–2001. Cancer 2006, **106**: 2104–2112.

654 Maluf H, Koerner F. Lobular carcinoma in situ and infiltrating ductal carcinoma: frequent presence of DCIS as a precursor lesion. Int J Surg Pathol 2001, **9**: 127–131.

655 Ottesen GL, Graversen HP, Blichert-Toft M, Zedeler K, Andersen JA. Lobular carcinoma in situ of the female breast. Short-term results of a prospective nationwide study. The Danish Breast Cancer Cooperative Group. Am J Surg Pathol 1993, **17**: 14–21.

656 Page DL, Kidd TE Jr, Dupont WD, Simpson JF, Rogers LW. Lobular neoplasia of the breast. Higher risk for subsequent invasive cancer predicted by more extensive disease. Hum Pathol 1991, **22**: 1232–1239.

657 Rosen PP, Lieberman PH, Braun DW Jr, Kosloff C, Adair F. Lobular carcinoma in situ of the breast. Detailed analysis of 99 patients with average follow-up of 24 years. Am J Surg Pathol 1978, **2**: 225–251.

658 Wheeler JE, Enterline HT. Lobular carcinoma of the breast in situ and infiltrating. Pathol Annu 1976, **11**: 161–188.

659 Wheeler JE, Enterline HT, Roseman JM, Tomasulo JP, McIlraine CH, Fitts WT Jr, Kirshenbaum J. Lobular carcinoma in situ of the breast. Long-term follow-up. Cancer 1974, **34**: 554–563.

INVASIVE CARCINOMA

INVASIVE DUCTAL CARCINOMA

Cytoarchitectural variants

660 Berg JW, Hutter RV. Breast cancer. Cancer 1995, **75**: 257–269.

Classic (NOS) invasive ductal carcinoma

661 Azzopardi JG, Laurini RN. Elastosis in breast cancer. Cancer 1974, **33**: 174–183.

662 Barsky SH, Grotendorst GR, Liotta LA. Increased content of type V collagen in desmoplasia of human breast carcinoma. Am J Pathol 1982, **108**: 276–283.

663 Battifora H. Intracytoplasmic lumina in breast carcinoma. A helpful histopathologic feature. Arch Pathol 1975, **99**: 614–617.

664 Bellahcène A, Castronovo V. Increased expression of osteonectin and osteopontin, two bone matrix proteins, in human breast cancer. Am J Pathol 1995, **146**: 95–100.

665 Bhargava R, Beriwal S, Dabbs DJ. Mammaglobin vs GCDFP-15: an immunohistologic validation survey for sensitivity and specificity. Am J Clin Pathol 2007, **127**: 103–113.

666 Bocker W, Klaubert A, Bahnsen J, Schweikhart G, Pollow K, Mitze M, Kreienberg R, Beck T, Stegner H-E. Peanut lectin histochemistry of 120 mammary carcinomas and its relation to tumor type, grading, staging, and receptor status. Virchows Arch [A] 1984, **403**: 149–161.

667 Bonetti F, Colombari R, Manfrin E, Zamboni G, Martignoni G, Mombello A, Chilosi M. Breast carcinoma with positive results for melanoma marker (HMB-45). HMB-45 immunoreactivity in normal and neoplastic breast. Am J Clin Pathol 1989, **92**: 491–495.

668 Bussolati G, Papotti M, Sapino A, Gugliotta P, Ghiringhello B, Azzopardi JG. Endocrine markers in argyrophilic carcinomas of the breast. Am J Surg Pathol 1987, **11**: 248–256.

669 Charpin C, Lachard A, Pourreau-Schneider N, Jacquemier J, Lavaut MN, Andonian C, Martin PM, Toga M. Localization of lactoferrin and nonspecific cross-reacting antigen in human breast carcinomas. An immunohistochemical study using the avidin–biotin–peroxidase complex method. Cancer 1985, **55**: 2612–2617.

670 Charpin C, Lissitzky JC, Jacquemier J, Lavaut MN, Kopp F, Pourreau-Schneider N, Martin PM, Toga M. Immunohistochemical detection of laminin in 98 human breast carcinomas. A light and electron microscopic study. Hum Pathol 1986, **17**: 355–365.

671 Clayton F, Ordóñez NG, Hanssen GM, Hanssen H. Immunoperoxidase localization of lactalbumin in malignant breast neoplasms. Arch Pathol Lab Med 1982, **106**: 268–270.

672 Domagala W, Wozniak L, Lasota J, Weber K, Osborn M. Vimentin is preferentially expressed in high-grade ductal and medullary, but not in lobular breast carcinomas. Am J Pathol 1990, **137**: 1059–1064.

673 Dwarakanath S, Lee AKC, DeLellis RA, Silverman ML, Frasca L, Wolfe HJ. S-100 protein positivity in breast carcinomas. A potential pitfall in diagnostic immunohistochemistry. Hum Pathol 1987, **18**: 1144–1148.

674 Fisher ER. Ultrastructure of the human breast and its disorders. Am J Clin Pathol 1976, **66**: 291–375.

675 Fisher ER, Gregorio RM, Fisher B, with the assistance of Redmond C, Vellios F, Sommers SC, and cooperating investigators. The pathology of invasive breast cancer. A syllabus derived from findings of the National Surgical Adjuvant Breast Project (Protocol No. 4). Cancer 1975, **36**: 1–85.

676 Fisher ER, Palekar AS, Gregorio RM, Redmond C, Fisher B. Pathological findings from the National Surgical Adjuvant Breast Project (Protocol No. 4). IV. Significance of tumor necrosis. Hum Pathol 1978, **9**: 523–530.

677 Gould VE, Koukoulis GK, Jansson DS, Nagle RB, Franke WW, Moll R. Coexpression patterns of vimentin and glial filament protein with cytokeratins in the normal, hyperplastic, and neoplastic breast. Am J Pathol 1990, **137**: 1143–1155.

678 Greenwalt DE, Johnson VG, Kuhajda FP, Eggleston JC, Mather IH. Localization of a membrane glycoprotein in benign fibrocystic disease and infiltrating duct carcinomas of the human breast with the use of a monoclonal antibody to guinea pig milk fat globule-membrane. Am J Pathol 1985, **118**: 351–359.

679 Hirota S, Ito A, Nagoshi J, Takeda M, Kurata A, Takatsuka Y, Kohri K, Nomura S, Kitamura Y. Expression of bone matrix protein messenger ribonucleic acids in human breast cancers. Possible involvement of osteopontin in development of calcifying foci. Lab Invest 1995, **72**: 64–69.

680 Howard DR, Taylor CR. A method for distinguishing benign from malignant breast lesions utilizing antibody present in normal human sera. Cancer 1979, **43**: 2279–2287.

681 Jackson JG, Orr JW. The ducts of carcinomatous breasts, with particular reference to connective-tissue changes. J Pathol Bacteriol 1957, **74**: 265–273.

682 Jarasch E-D, Nagle RB, Kaufmann M, Maurer C, Bocker WJ. Differential diagnosis of benign epithelial proliferations and carcinomas of the breast using antibodies to cytokeratins. Hum Pathol 1988, **19**: 276–289.

683 Kuhajda FP, Bohn H, Mendelsohn G. Pregnancy-specific beta-1 glycoprotein (SP-1) in breast carcinoma. Pathologic and clinical considerations. Cancer 1984, **54**: 1392–1396.

684 Kuhajda FP, Offutt LE, Mendelsohn G. The distribution of carcinoembryonic antigen in breast carcinoma. Diagnostic and prognostic implications. Cancer 1983, **52**: 1257–1264.

685 Lee AK, DeLellis RA, Rosen PP, Herbert-Stanton T, Tallberg K, Garcia C, Wolfe HJ. Alpha-lactalbumin as an immunohistochemical marker for metastatic breast carcinomas. Am J Surg Pathol 1984, **8**: 93–100.

686 Lee AKC, DeLellis RA, Wolfe HJ. Intramammary lymphatic invasion in breast carcinomas. Evaluation using ABH isoantigens as endothelial markers. Am J Surg Pathol 1986, **10**: 589–594.

687 Loy TS, Chapman RK, Diaz-Arias AA, Bulatao IS, Bickel JT. Distribution of BCA-225 in adenocarcinomas. An immunohistochemical study of 446 cases. Am J Clin Pathol 1991, **96**: 326–329.

688 Lunde S, Nesland JM, Holm R, Johannessen JV. Breast carcinomas with protein S-100 immunoreactivity. An immunocytochemical and ultrastructural study. Pathol Res Pract 1987, **182**: 627–631.

689 Martin SA, Perez-Reyes N, Mendelsohn G. Angioinvasion in breast carcinoma. An immunohistochemical study of factor VIII-related antigen. Cancer 1987, **59**: 1918–1922.

690 Mazoujian G, Bodian C, Haagensen DE Jr, Haagensen CD. Expression of GCDFP-15 in breast carcinomas. Relationship to pathologic and clinical factors. Cancer 1989, **63**: 2156–2161.

691 Mesa-Tejada R, Oster MW, Fenoglio CM, Magidson J, Spiegelman S. Diagnosis of primary breast carcinoma through immunohistochemical detection of antigen related to mouse mammary tumor virus in metastatic lesions. A report of two cases. Cancer 1982, **49**: 261–268.

692 Murad TM, Scarpelli DG. The ultrastructure of medullary and scirrhous mammary duct carcinoma. Am J Pathol 1967, **50**: 335–360.

693 Oberman HA. Invasive carcinoma of the breast with granulomatous response. Am J Clin Pathol 1987, **88**: 718–721.

694 Ohtani H, Sasano N. Myofibroblasts and myoepithelial cells in human breast carcinoma. An ultrastructural study. Virchows Arch [A] 1980, **385**: 247–261.

695 Ordóñez NG, Brooks T, Thompson S, Batsakis JG. Use of *Ulex europaeus* agglutinin I in the identification of lymphatic and blood vessel invasion in previously stained microscopic slides. Am J Surg Pathol 1987, **11**: 543–550.

696 Prey MU, Bedrossian CW, Masood S. The value of monoclonal antibody B72.3 for the diagnosis of breast carcinoma. Experience with the first commercially available source. Hum Pathol 1991, **22**: 598–602.

697 Robens J, Goldstein L, Gown AM, Schnitt SJ. Thyroid transcription factor-1 expression in breast carcinomas. Am J Surg Pathol 2010, **34**: 1881–1885.

698 Robertson JF, Ellis IO, Bell J, Todd JH, Robins A, Elston CW, Blamey RW. Carcinoembryonic antigen immunocytochemistry in primary breast cancer. Cancer 1989, **64**: 1638–1645.

699 Rosen PP. Tumor emboli in intramammary lymphatics in breast carcinoma. Pathologic criteria for diagnosis and clinical significance. Pathol Annu 1983, **18**(Pt 2): 215–232.

700 Saigo PE, Rosen PP. The application of immunohistochemical stains to identify endothelial-lined channels in mammary carcinoma. Cancer 1987, **59**: 51–54.

701 Sobrinho-Simões M, Johannessen JV, Gould VE. The diagnostic significance of intracytoplasmic lumina in metastatic neoplasms. Ultrastruct Pathol 1981, **2**: 327–335.

702 Tavassoli FA, Jones MW, Majeste RM, Bratthauer GL, O'Leary TJ. Immunohistochemical staining with monoclonal Ab B72.3 in benign and malignant breast disease. Am J Surg Pathol 1990, **14**: 128–133.

703 Tsubura A, Okada H, Senzaki H, Hatano T, Morii S. Keratin expression in the normal breast and in breast carcinoma. Histopathology 1991, **18**: 517–522.

704 Wetzels RH, Holland R, van Haelst UJ, Lane EB, Leigh IM, Ramaekers FC. Detection of basement membrane components and basal cell keratin 14 in non-invasive and invasive carcinomas of the breast. Am J Pathol 1989, **134**: 571–579.

705 Wick MR, Lillemoe TJ, Copland GT, Swanson PE, Manivel JC, Kiang DT. Gross cystic disease fluid protein-15 as a marker for breast cancer. Immunohistochemical analysis of 690 human neoplasms and comparison with alpha-lactalbumin. Hum Pathol 1989, **20**: 281–287.

706 Willebrand D, Bosman FT, De Goeij AFPM. Patterns of basement membrane deposition in benign and malignant breast tumours. Histopathology 1986, **10**: 1231–1241.

Tubular carcinoma

707 Aulmann S, Elsawaf Z, Penzel R, Schirmacher P, Sinn HP. Invasive tubular carcinoma of the breast frequently is clonally related to flat epithelial atypia and low-grade ductal carcinoma in situ. Am J Surg Pathol 2009, **33**: 1646–1653.

708 Carstens PHB, Greenberg RA, Francis D, Lyon H. Tubular carcinoma of the breast. A long term follow-up. Histopathology 1985, **9**: 271–280.

709 Carstens PHB, Huvos AG, Foote FW Jr, Ashikari R. Tubular carcinoma of the breast. A clinicopathologic study of 35 cases. Am J Clin Pathol 1972, **58**: 231–238.

710 Dawson AE, Logan-Young W, Mulford DK. Aspiration cytology of tubular carcinoma. Diagnostic features with mammographic correlation. Am J Clin Pathol 1994, **101**: 488–492.

711 de Moraes Schenka NG, Schenka AA, de Souza Queiroz L, de Almeida Matsura M, Alvarenga M, Vassallo J. p63 and CD10: reliable markers in discriminating benign sclerosing lesions from tubular carcinoma of the breast? Appl Immunohistochem Mol Morphol 2006, **14**: 71–77.

712 Deos PH, Norris HJ. Well-differentiated (tubular) carcinoma of the breast. A clinicopathologic study of 145 pure and mixed cases. Am J Clin Pathol 1982, **78**: 1–7.

713 Diab SG, Clark GM, Osborne CK, Libby A, Allred DC, Elledge RM. Tumor characteristics and clinical outcome of tubular and mucinous breast carcinomas. J Clin Oncol 1999, **17**: 1442–1448.

714 Erlandson RA, Carstens PHB. Ultrastructure of tubular carcinoma of the breast. Cancer 1972, **29**: 987–995.

715 Flotte TJ, Bell DA, Greco MA. Tubular carcinoma and sclerosing adenosis. The use of basal lamina as a differential feature. Am J Surg Pathol 1980, **4**: 75–77.

716 Jao W, Recant W, Swerdlow MA. Comparative ultrastructure of tubular carcinoma and sclerosing adenosis of the breast. Cancer 1976, **38**: 180–186.

717 Kunju LP, Ding Y, Kleer CG. Tubular carcinoma and grade 1 (well-differentiated) invasive ductal carcinoma: comparison of flat epithelial atypia and other intra-epithelial lesions. Pathol Int 2008, **58**: 620–625.

718 Lagios MD, Rose MR, Margolin FR. Tubular carcinoma of the breast. Association with multicentricity, bilaterality, and family history of mammary carcinoma. Am J Clin Pathol 1980, **73**: 25–30.

719 Lele SM, Graves K, Galatica Z. Immunohistochemical detection of maspin is a useful adjunct in distinguishing radial sclerosing lesion from tubular carcinoma of the breast. Appl Immunohistochem Mol Morphol 2000, **8**: 32–36.

720 McDivitt RW, Boyce W, Gersell D. Tubular carcinoma of the breast. Clinical and pathological observations concerning 135 cases. Am J Surg Pathol 1982, **6**: 401–411.

721 Oberman HA, Fidler WJ Jr. Tubular carcinoma of the breast. Am J Surg Pathol 1979, **3**: 387–395.

722 Parl FF, Richardson LD. The histologic and biologic spectrum of tubular carcinoma of the breast. Hum Pathol 1983, **14**: 694–698.

723 Peters GN, Wolff M, Haagensen CD. Tubular carcinoma of the breast. Clinical pathologic correlations based on 100 cases. Ann Surg 1981, **193**: 138–149.

724 Stalsberg H, Hartmann WH. The delimitation of tubular carcinoma of the breast. Hum Pathol 2000, **31**: 601–607.

725 Taylor HB, Norris HJ. Well-differentiated carcinoma of the breast. Cancer 1970, **25**: 687–692.

726 Tremblay G. Elastosis in tubular carcinoma of the breast. Arch Pathol 1974, **98**: 302–307.

727 van Bogaert L-J. Clinicopathologic hallmarks of mammary tubular carcinoma. Hum Pathol 1982, **13**: 558–562.

728 Waldman FM, Hwang ES, Etzell J, Eng C, de Vries S, Bennington J, Thor A. Genomic alterations in tubular breast carcinomas. Hum Pathol 2001, **32**: 222–226.

Cribriform carcinoma

729 Page DL, Dixon JM, Anderson TJ, Lee D, Stewart HJ. Invasive cribriform carcinoma of the breast. Histopathology 1983, **7**: 525–536.

730 Sanders ME, Page DL, Simpson JF, Edgerton ME, Jensen RA. Solid variant of cribriform carcinoma: a study of 24 cases [abstract]. Mod Pathol 2003, **16**: 45a.

731 Venable JG, Schwartz AM, Silverberg SG. Infiltrating cribriform carcinoma of the breast. A distinctive clinicopathologic entity. Hum Pathol 1990, **21**: 333–338.

Mucinous carcinoma

732 Adsay NV, Merati K, Nassar H, Shia J, Sarkar F, Pierson CR, Cheng JD, Visscher DW, Hruban RH, Klimstra DS. Pathogenesis of colloid (pure mucinous) carcinoma of exocrine organs. Coupling of gel-forming mucin (MUC2) production with altered cell polarity and abnormal cell-stroma interaction may be the key factor in the morphogenesis and idolent behaviour of colloid carcinoma in the breast and pancreas. Am J Surg Pathol 2003, **27**: 571–578.

733 Bal A, Joshi K, Sharma SC, Das A, Verma A, Wig JD. Prognostic significance of micropapillary pattern in pure mucinous carcinoma of the breast. Int J Surg Pathol 2008, **16**: 251–256.

734 Capella C, Eusebi V, Mann B, Azzopardi JG. Endocrine differentiation in mucoid carcinoma of the breast. Histopathology 1980, **4**: 613–630.

735 Carder PJ, Murphy CE, Liston JC. Surgical excision is warranted following a core biopsy diagnosis of mucocoele-like lesion of the breast. Histopathology 2004, **45**: 148–154.

736 Chinyama CN, Davies JD. Mammary mucinous lesions: congeners, prevalence and important pathological associations. Histopathology 1996, **29**: 533–539.

737 Clayton F. Pure mucinous carcinomas of breast. Morphologic features and prognostic correlates. Hum Pathol 1986, **17**: 34–38.

738 Coady AT, Shousha S, Dawson PM, Moss M, James KR, Bull TB. Mucinous carcinoma of the breast. Further characterization of its three subtypes. Histopathology 1989, **15**: 617–626.

739 Coyne JD, Irion L. Mammary mucinous cystadenocarcinoma. Histopathology 2006, **49**: 659–660.

740 Diab SG, Clark GM, Osborne CK, Libby A, Allred DC, Elledge RM. Tumor characteristics and clinical outcome of tubular and mucinous breast carcinomas. J Clin Oncol 1999, **17**: 1442–1448.

741 Domfeh AB, Carley AL, Striebel JM, Karabakhtsian RG, Florea AV, McManus K, Beriwal S, Bhargava R. WT1 immunoreactivity in breast carcinoma: selective expression in pure and mixed mucinous subtypes. Mod Pathol 2008, **21**: 1217–1223.

742 Ferguson DJP, Anderson TJ, Wells CA, Battersby S. An ultrastructural study of mucoid carcinoma of the breast. Variability of cytoplasmic features. Histopathology 1986, **10**: 1219–1230.

743 Fisher ER, Palekar AS, NSABP collaborators. Solid and mucinous varieties of so-called mammary carcinoid tumors. Am J Clin Pathol 1979, **72**: 909–916.

744 Hamele-Bena D, Cranor ML, Rosen PP. Mammary mucocele-like lesions: benign and malignant. Am J Surg Pathol 1996, **20**: 1081–1085.

745 Hull MT, Warfel KA. Mucinous breast carcinomas with abundant intracytoplasmic mucin and neuroendocrine features. Light microscopic, immunohistochemical, and ultrastructural study. Ultrastruct Pathol 1987, **11**: 29–38.

746 Koenig C, Tavassoli FA. Mucinous cystadenocarcinoma of the breast. Am J Surg Pathol 1998, **22**: 698–703.

747 Komaki K, Sakamoto G, Sugano H, Kasumi F, Watanabe S, Nishi M, Morimoto T, Monden Y. The morphologic feature of mucus leakage appearing in low papillary carcinoma of the breast. Hum Pathol 1991, **22**: 231–236.

748 Lacroix-Triki M, Suarez PH, MacKay A, Lambros MB, Natrajan R, Savage K, Geyer FC, Weigelt B, Ashworth A, Reis-Filho JS. Mucinous carcinoma of the breast is genomically distinct from invasive ductal carcinomas of no special type. J Pathol 2010, **222**: 282–298.

749 Lee SH, Chaung CR. Mucinous metaplasia of breast carcinoma with macrocystic transformation resembling ovarian mucinous cystadenocarcinoma in a case of synchronous bilateral infiltrating ductal carcinoma. Pathol Int 2008, **58**: 601–605.

750 Matsukita S, Nomoto M, Kitajima S, Tanaka S, Goto M, Irimura T, Kim YS, Sato E, Yonezawa S. Expression of mucins (MUC1, MUC2, MUC5AC and MUC6) in mucinous carcinoma of the breast: comparison with invasive ductal carcinoma. Histopathology 2003, **42**: 26–36.

751 Norris HJ, Taylor HB. Prognosis of mucinous (gelatinous) carcinoma of the breast. Cancer 1965, **18**: 879–885.

752 O'Connell JT, Shao ZM, Drori E, Basbaum CB, Barsky SH. Altered mucin expression is a field change that accompanies mucinous (colloid) breast carcinoma histogenesis. Hum Pathol 1998, **29**: 1517–1523.

753 Rasmussen BB. Human mucinous breast carcinomas and their lymph node metastases. A histological review of 247 cases. Pathol Res Pract 1985, **180**: 377–382.

754 Rasmussen BB, Rose C, Christensen IB. Prognostic factors in primary mucinous breast carcinoma. Am J Clin Pathol 1987, **87**: 155–160.

755 Rasmussen BB, Rose C, Thorpe SM, Andersen KW, Hou- Jensen K. Argyrophilic cells in 202 human mucinous breast carcinomas. Relation to histopathologic and clinical factors. Am J Clin Pathol 1985, **84**: 737–740.

756 Ro JY, Sneige N, Sahin AA, Silva EG, del Junco GW, Ayala AG. Mucocele-like tumor of the breast associated with atypical ductal hyperplasia or mucinous carcinoma. A clinicopathologic study of seven cases. Arch Pathol Lab Med 1991, **115**: 137–140.

757 Rosen PP. Mucocele-like tumors of the breast. Am J Surg Pathol 1986, **10**: 464–469.

758 Rosen PP, Wang T-Y. Colloid carcinoma of the breast. Analysis of 64 patients with long-term follow-up [abstract]. Am J Clin Pathol 1980, **73**: 304.

759 Saez C, Japon MA, Poveda MA, Segura DI. Mucinous (colloid) adenocarcinomas secrete distinct O-acylated forms of sialomucins: a histochemical study of gastric, colorectal and breast adenocarcinomas. Histopathology 2001, **39**: 554–560.

760 Scopsi L, Andreola S, Pilotti S, Bufalino R, Baldini MT, Testori A, Rilke F. Mucinous carcinoma of the breast. A clinicopathologic, histochemical, and immunocytochemical study with special reference to neuroendocrine differentiation. Am J Surg Pathol 1994, **18**: 702–711.

761 Toikkanen S, Kujari H. Pure and mixed mucinous carcinomas of the breast. A clinicopathologic analysis of 61 cases with long-term follow-up. Hum Pathol 1989, **20**: 758–764.

762 Tse GM, Ma TK, Chu WC, Lam WW, Poon CS, Chan WC. Neuroendocrine differentiation in pure type mammary mucinous carcinoma is associated with favorable histologic and immunohistochemical parameters. Mod Pathol 2004, **17**: 568–572.

763 Walker RA. Mucoid carcinomas of the breast. A study using mucin histochemistry and peanut lectin. Histopathology 1982, **6**: 571–579.

764 Weigelt B, Geyer FC, Horlings HM, Kreike B, Halfwerk H, Reis-Filho JS. Mucinous and neuroendocrine breast carcinomas are transcriptionally distinct from invasive ductal carcinomas of no special type. Mod Pathol 2009, **22**: 1401–1414.

Medullary carcinoma

765 Armes JE, Venter DJ. The pathology of inherited breast cancer. Pathology 2002, **34**: 309–314.

766 Ben-Ezra J, Sheibani K. Antigenic phenotype of the lymphocytic component of medullary carcinoma of the breast. Cancer 1987, **59**: 2037–2041.

767 Bloom HJG, Richardson WW, Fields JR. Host resistance and survival in carcinoma of breasts. A study of 104 cases of medullary carcinoma in a series of 1,411 cases of breast cancer followed for 20 years. Br Med J 1970, **3**: 181–188.

768 Crotty TB. Medullary carcinoma: it is a reproducible and prognostically significant type of mammary carcinoma? Adv Anat Pathol 1996, **3**: 179–184.

769 Dalal P, Shousha S. Keratin 19 in paraffin sections of medullary carcinoma and other benign and malignant breast lesions. Mod Pathol 1995, **8**: 413–416.

770 Dwarakanath S, Lee AKC, DeLellis RA, Silverman ML, Frasca L, Wolfe HJ. S-100 protein positivity in breast carcinomas. A potential pitfall in diagnostic immunohistochemistry. Hum Pathol 1987, **18**: 1144–1148.

771 Eichhorn JH. Medullary carcinoma, provocative now as then. Semin Diagn Pathol 2004, **21**: 65–73.

772 Farshid G, Balleine RL, Cummings M, Waring P; Kathleen Cuningham Consortium for Research into Familial Breast Cancer (kConFab). Morphology of breast cancer as a means of triage of patients for BRCA1 genetic testing. Am J Surg Pathol 2006, **30**: 1357–1366.

773 Flucke U, Flucke MT, Hoy L, Breuer E, Goebbels R, Rhiem K, Schmutzler R, Winzenried H, Braun M, Steiner S, Buettner R, Gevensleben H. Distinguishing medullary carcinoma of the breast from high-grade hormone receptor-negative invasive ductal carcinoma: an immunohistochemical approach. Histopathology 2010, **56**: 852–859.

774 Gaffey MJ, Frierson HF Jr, Mills SE, Boyd JC, Zarbo RJ, Simpson JF, Gross LK, Weiss LM. Medullary carcinoma of the breast. Identification of lymphocyte subpopulations and their significance. Mod Pathol 1993, **6**: 721–728.

775 Gaffey MJ, Mills SE, Frierson HF Jr, Zarbo RJ, Boyd JC, Simpson JF, Weiss LM. Medullary carcinoma of the breast. Interobserver variability in histopathologic diagnosis. Mod Pathol 1995, **8**: 31–38.

776 Harris M, Lessells AM. The ultrastructure of medullary, atypical medullary and non-medullary carcinomas of the breast. Histopathology 1986, **10**: 405–414.

777 Howell LP, Kline TS. Medullary carcinoma of the breast. An unusual cytologic finding in cyst fluid aspirates. Cancer 1990, **65**: 277–282.

778 Hsu S-M, Raine L, Nayak RN. Medullary carcinoma of breast. An immunohistochemical study of its lymphoid stroma. Cancer 1981, **48**: 1368–1376.

779 Jensen ML, Kiaer H, Andersen J, Jensen V, Melsen F. Prognostic comparison of three classifications for medullary carcinomas of the breast. Histopathology 1997, **30**: 523–532.

780 Kumar S, Kumar D. Lymphoepithelioma-like carcinoma of the breast. Mod Pathol 1994, **7**: 129–131.

781 Kuroda H, Tamaru J, Sakamoto G, Ohnisi K, Itoyama S. Immunophenotype of lymphocytic infiltration in medullary carcinoma of the breast. Virchows Arch 2005, **446**: 10–14.

782 Lazzaro B, Anderson AE, Kajdacsy-Balla A, Hessner MJ. Antigenic characterization of medullary carcinoma of the breast: HLA-DR expression in lymph node positive cases. Appl Immunohistochem Mol Morphol 2001, **9**: 234–241.

783 Lee SC, Berg KD, Sherman ME, Griffin CA, Eshleman JR. Microsatellite instability is infrequent in medullary breast cancer. Am J Clin Pathol 2001, **115**: 823–827.

784 Lespagnard L, Cochaux P, Larsimont D, Degeyter M, Velu T, Heimann R. Absence of Epstein–Barr virus in medullary carcinoma of the breast as demonstrated by immunophenotyping, *in situ* hybridization and polymerase chain reaction. Am J Clin Pathol 1995, **103**: 449–452.

785 Osin P, Lu Y-J, Stone J, Crook T, Houlston RS, Gasco M, Gusterson BA, Shipley J. Distinct genetic and epigenetic changes in medullary breast cancer. Int J Surg Pathol 2003, **11**: 153–158.

786 Rapin V, Contesso G, Mouriesse H, Bertin F, LaCombe MJ, Piekarski JD, Travagli JP, Gadenne C, Friedman S. Medullary breast carcinoma. A reevaluation of 95 cases of breast cancer with inflammatory stroma. Cancer 1988, **61**: 2503–2510.

787 Richardson WW. Medullary carcinoma of the breast. A distinctive tumour type with a relatively good prognosis following radical mastectomy. Br J Cancer 1956, **10**: 415–423.

788 Ridolfi RL, Rosen PP, Port A, Kinne D, Miké V. Medullary carcinoma of the breast. A clinicopathologic study with 10 year follow-up. Cancer 1977, **40**: 1365–1385.

789 Rigaud C, Theobald S, Noel P, Badreddine J, Barlier C, Delobelle A, Gentile A, Jacquemier J, Maisongrosse V, Peffault de Latour M, et al. Medullary carcinoma of the breast. A multicenter study of its diagnostic consistency. Arch Pathol Lab Med 1993, **117**: 1005–1008.

790 Shousha S. Medullary carcinoma of the breast and BRCA1 mutation. Histopathology 2000, **37**: 182–185.

791 Tot T. The cytokeratin profile of medullary carcinoma of the breast. Histopathology 2000, **37**: 175–181.

792 Vincent-Salomon A, Gruel N, Lucchesi C, MacGrogan G, Dendale R, Sigal-Zafrani B, Longy M, Raynal V, Pierron G, de Mascarel I, Taris C, Stoppa-Lyonnet D, Pierga JY, Salmon R, Sastre-Garau X, Fourquet A, Delattre O, de Cremoux P, Aurias A. Identification of typical medullary breast carcinoma as a genomic sub-group of basal-like carcinomas, a heterogeneous new molecular entity. Breast Cancer Res 2007, **9**: R24.

793 Wargotz ES, Silverberg SG. Medullary carcinoma of the breast: a clinicopathologic study with appraisal of current diagnostic criteria. Hum Pathol 1988, **19**: 1340–1346.

794 Yakirevich E, Ben Izhak O, Rennert G, Kovacs ZG, Resnick MB. Cytotoxic phenotype of tumor infiltrating lymphocytes in medullary carcinoma of the breast. Mod Pathol 1999, **12**: 1050–1056.

795 Yazawa T, Kamma H, Ogata T. Frequent expression of HLA-DR antigen in medullary carcinoma of the breast. A possible reason for its prominent lymphocytic infiltration and favorable prognosis. Appl Immunohistochem 1993, **1**: 289–296.

Invasive papillary carcinoma

796 Carter D, Orr SL, Merino MJ. Intracystic papillary carcinoma of the breast. After mastectomy, radiotherapy or excisional biopsy alone. Cancer 1983, **52**: 14–19.

797 Collins LC, Carlo VP, Hwang H, Barry TS, Gown AM, Schnitt SJ. Intracystic papillary carcinomas of the breast: a reevaluation using a panel of myoepithelial cell markers. Am J Surg Pathol 2006, **30**: 1002–1007.

798 Corkill ME, Sneige N, Fanning T, el-Naggar A. Fine-needle aspiration cytology and flow cytometry of intracystic papillary carcinoma of breast. Am J Clin Pathol 1990, **94**: 673–680.

799 Coyne JD. Invasive solid papillary breast carcinoma with papillary metastasis. Histopathology 2007, **50**: 515–516.

800 Fisher ER, Palekar AS, Redmond C, Barton B, Fisher B. Pathologic findings from the National Surgical Adjuvant Breast Project (Protocol No. 4). VI. Invasive papillary cancer. Am J Clin Pathol 1980, **73**: 313–322.

801 Hill CB, Yeh IT. Myoepithelial cell staining patterns of papillary breast lesions: from intraductal papillomas to invasive papillary carcinomas. Am J Clin Pathol 2005, **123**: 36–44.

802 Leal C, Costa I, Fonseca D, Lopes P, Bento MJ, Lopes C. Intracystic (encysted) papillary carcinoma of the breast: a clinical, pathological, and immunohistochemical study. Hum Pathol 1998, **29**: 1097–1104.

803 Michael CW, Buschmann B. Can true papillary neoplasms of breast and their mimickers be accurately classified by cytology? Cancer Cytopathol 2002, **96**: 92–100.

804 Mulligan AM, O'Malley FP. Metastatic potential of encapsulated (intracystic) papillary carcinoma of the breast: a report of 2 cases with axillary lymph node micrometastases. Int J Surg Pathol 2007, **15**: 143–147.

805 Nassar H, Qureshi H, Volkanadsay N, Visscher D. Clinicopathologic analysis of solid papillary carcinoma of the breast and associated invasive carcinomas. Am J Surg Pathol 2006, **30**: 501–507.

806 Nicolas MM, Wu Y, Middleton LP, Gilcrease MZ. Loss of myoepithelium is variable in solid papillary carcinoma of the breast. Histopathology 2007, **51**: 657–665.

807 Otsuki Y, Yamada M, Shimizu S, Suwa K, Yoshida M, Tanioka F, Ogawa H, Nasuno H, Serizawa A, Kobayashi H. Solid–papillary carcinoma of the breast: clinicopathological study of 20 cases. Pathol Int 2007, **57**: 421–429.

Invasive micropapillary carcinoma

808 Acs G, Esposito NN, Rakosy Z, Laronga C, Zhang PJ. Invasive ductal carcinomas of the breast showing partial reversed cell polarity are associated with lymphatic tumor spread and may represent part of a spectrum of invasive micropapillary carcinoma. Am J Surg Pathol 2010, **34**: 1637–1646.

809 Acs G, Paragh G, Chuang ST, Laronga C, Zhang PJ. The presence of micropapillary features and retraction artifact in core needle biopsy material predicts lymph node metastasis in breast carcinoma. Am J Surg Pathol 2009, **33**: 202–210.

810 Chen L, Fan Y, Lang RG, Guo XJ, Sun YL, Cui LF, Liu FF, Wei J, Zhang XM, Fu L. Breast carcinoma with micropapillary features: clinicopathologic study and long-term follow-up of 100 cases. Int J Surg Pathol 2008, **16**: 155–163.

811 De la Cruz C, Moriya T, Endoh M, Watanabe M, Takeyama J, Yang M, Oguma M, Sakamoto K, Suzuki T, Hirakawa H, Orita Y, Ohuchi N, Sasano H. Invasive micropapillary carcinoma of the breast: clinicopathological and immunohistochemical study. Pathol Int 2004, **54**: 90–96.

812 Kuroda N, Sugimoto T, Takahashi T, Moriki T, Toi M, Miyazaki E, Hiroi M, Enzan H. Invasive micropapillary carcinoma of the breast: an immunohistochemical study of neoplastic and stromal cells. Int J Surg Pathol 2005, **13**: 51–55.

813 Lee AH, Paish EC, Marchio C, Sapino A, Schmitt FC, Ellis IO, Reis-Filho JS. The expression of Wilms' tumour-1 and Ca125 in invasive micropapillary carcinoma of the breast. Histopathology 2007, **51**: 824–828.

814 Lotan TL, Ye H, Melamed J, Wu XR, Shih IeM, Epstein JI. Immunohistochemical panel to identify the primary site of invasive micropapillary carcinoma. Am J Surg Pathol 2009, **33**: 1037–1041.

815 Moritani S, Ichihara S, Hasegawa M, Endo T, Oiwa M, Yoshikawa K, Sato Y, Aoyama H, Hayashi T, Kushima R. Serous papillary adenocarcinoma of the female genital organs and invasive micropapillary carcinoma of the breast. Are WT1, CA125, and GCDFP-15 useful in differential diagnosis? Hum Pathol 2008, **39**: 666–671.

816 Nassar H, Pansare V, Zhang H, Che M, Sakr W, Ali-Fehmi R, Grignon D, Sarkar F, Cheng J, Adsay V. Pathogenesis of invasive micropapillary carcinoma: role of MUC1 glycoprotein. Mod Pathol 2004, **17**: 1045–1050.

817 Pettinato G, Manivel CJ, Panico L, Sparano L, Petrella G. Invasive micropapillary carcinoma of the breast: clinicopathologic study of 62 cases of a poorly recognized variant with highly aggressive behavior. Am J Clin Pathol 2004, **121**: 857–866.

Apocrine carcinoma

818 Abati AD, Kimmel M, Rosen PP. Apocrine mammary carcinoma. A clinicopathologic study of 72 cases. Am J Clin Pathol 1990, **94**: 371–377.

819 Chen X, Hoda SA, Rosen PP. E-Cadherin immunostain distinguishes apocrine ductal carcinoma from apocrine lobular carcinoma [abstract]. Mod Pathol 2003, **16**: 24a.

820 Eusebi V, Betts C, Haagensen DE Jr, Gugliotta P, Bussolati G, Azzopardi JG. Apocrine differentiation in lobular carcinoma of the breast. A morphologic, immunologic, and ultrastructural study. Hum Pathol 1984, **15**: 134–140.

821 Eusebi V, Millis RR, Cattani MG, Bussolati G, Azzopardi JG. Apocrine carcinoma of the breast. A morphologic and immunocytochemical study. Am J Pathol 1986, **123**: 532–541.

822 Losi L, Lorenzini R, Eusebi V, Bussolati G. Apocrine differentiation in invasive carcinoma of the breast. Comparison of monoclonal and polyclonal gross cystic disease fluid protein-15 antibodies with prolactin-inducible protein mRNA gene expression. Appl Immunohistochem 1995, **3**: 91–98.

823 Mossler JA, Barton TK, Brinkhous AD, McCarty KS, Moylan JA, McCarty KS Jr. Apocrine differentiation in human mammary carcinoma. Cancer 1980, **46**: 2463–2471.

824 O'Malley FP, Bane A. An update on apocrine lesions of the breast. Histopathology 2008, **52**: 3–10.

825 Pagani A, Sapino A, Eusebi V, Bergnolo P, Bussolati G. PIP/GCDFP-15 gene expression and apocrine differentiation in carcinomas of the breast. Virchows Arch [A] 1994, **425**: 459–465.

Secretory (juvenile) carcinoma

826 Akhtar M, Robinson C, Ali MA, Godwin JT. Secretory carcinoma of the breast in adults. Light and electron microscopic study of three cases with review of the literature. Cancer 1983, **51**: 2245–2254.

827 Brandt SM, Swistel AJ, Rosen PP. Secretory carcinoma in the axilla: probable origin from axillary skin appendage glands in a young girl. Am J Surg Pathol 2009, **33**: 950–953.

828 Hirokawa M, Sugihara K, Sai T, Monobe Y, Kudo H, Sano N, Sano T. Secretory carcinoma of the breast: a tumor analogous to salivary gland acinic cell carcinoma? Histopathology 2002, **40**: 223–230.

829 Krausz T, Jenkins D, Grontoft O, Pollock DJ, Azzopardi JG. Secretory carcinoma of the breast in adults. Emphasis on late recurrence and metastasis. Histopathology 1989, **14**: 25–36.

830 Lamovec J, Bracko M. Secretory carcinoma of the breast. Light microscopical, immunohistochemical and flow cytometric study. Mod Pathol 1994, **7**: 475–479.

831 McDivitt RW, Stewart FW. Breast carcinoma in children. JAMA 1966, **195**: 388–390.

832 Oberman HA. Secretory carcinoma of the breast in adults. Am J Surg Pathol 1980, **4**: 465–470.

833 Rosen PP, Cranor ML. Secretory carcinoma of the breast. Arch Pathol Lab Med 1991, **115**: 141–144.

834 Skálová A, Vanecek T, Sima R, Laco J, Weinreb I, Perez-Ordonez B, Starek I, Geierova M, Simpson RH, Passador-Santos F, Ryska A, Leivo I, Kinkor Z, Michal M. Mammary analogue secretory carcinoma of salivary glands, containing the ETV6–NTRK3 fusion gene: a hitherto undescribed salivary gland tumor entity. Am J Surg Pathol 2010, **34**: 599–608.

835 Tavassoli FA, Norris HJ. Secretory carcinoma of the breast. Cancer 1980, **45**: 2404–2413.

836 Tognon C, Knezevich SR, Huntsman D, Roskelley CD, Melnyk N, Mathers JA, Becker L, Carneiro F, MacPherson N, Horsman D, Poremba C, Sorensen PH. Expression of the ETV6–NTRK3 gene fusion as a primary event in human secretory breast carcinoma. Cancer Cell 2002, **2**: 367–376.

Carcinomas with neuroendocrine features (including so-called 'carcinoid tumor')

837 Asioli S, Dorji T, Lorenzini P, Eusebi V. Primary neuroendocrine (Merkel cell) carcinoma of the nipple. Virchows Arch 2002, **440**: 4443–4454.

838 Azzopardi JG, Muretto P, Goddeeris P, Eusebi V, Lauweryns JM. 'Carcinoid' tumours of the breast. The morphological spectrum of argyrophil carcinomas. Histopathology 1982, **6**: 549–569.

839 Battersby S, Dely CJ, Hopkinson HE, Anderson TJ. The nature of breast dense core granules. Chromogranin reactivity. Histopathology 1992, **20**: 107–114.

840 Bussolati G, Papotti M, Sapino A, Gugliotta P, Ghiringhello B, Azzopardi JG. Endocrine markers in argyrophilic carcinomas of the breast. Am J Surg Pathol 1987, **11**: 248–256.

841 Capella C, Usellini L, Papotti M, Macri L, Finzi G, Eusebi V, Bussolati G. Ultrastructural features of neuroendocrine differentiated carcinomas of the breast. Ultrastruct Pathol 1990, **14**: 321–334.

842 Clayton F, Sibley RK, Ordóñez NG, Hanssen G. Argyrophilic breast carcinomas. Evidence of lactational differentiation. Am J Surg Pathol 1982, **6**: 323–333.

843 Cross AS, Azzopardi JG, Krausz T, Van Noorden S, Polak JM. A morphological and immunocytochemical study of a distinctive variant of ductal carcinomas in-situ of the breast. Histopathology 1985, **9**: 21–37.

844 Cubilla AL, Woodruff JM. Primary carcinoid tumor of the breast. A report of eight patients. Am J Surg Pathol 1977, **1**: 283–292.

845 Fisher ER, Palekar AS, NSABP Collaborators. Solid and mucinous varieties of so-called mammary carcinoid tumors. Am J Clin Pathol 1979, **72**: 909–916.

846 Fukunaga M. Neuroendocrine carcinoma of the breast with Merkel cell carcinoma-like features. Pathol Int 1998, **48**: 557–561.

847 Hoang MP, Maitra A, Gazdar AF, Albores-Saavedra J. Primary mammary small-cell carcinoma: a molecular analysis of 2 cases. Hum Pathol 2001, **32**: 753–757.

848 Makretsov N, Gilks B, Coldman AJ, Hayes M, Huntsman D. Tissue microarray analysis of neuroendocrine differentiation and its prognostic significance in breast cancer. Hum Pathol 2003, **34**: 1001–1008.

849 Maluf HM, Koerner FC. Carcinomas of the breast with endocrine differentiation. A review. Virchows Arch 1994, **425**: 449–457.

850 Maluf HM, Koerner FC. Solid papillary carcinoma of the breast. A form of intraductal carcinoma with endocrine differentiation frequently associated with mucinous carcinoma. Am J Surg Pathol 1995, **19**: 1237–1244.

851 Miremadi A, Pinder SE, Lee AH, Bell JA, Paish EC, Wencyk P, Elston CW, Nicholson RI, Blamey RW, Robertson JF, Ellis IO. Neuroendocrine differentiation and prognosis in breast adenocarcinoma. Histopathology 2002, **40**: 215–222.

852 Nesland JM, Holm R, Johannessen JV, Gould VE. Neurone specific enolase immunostaining in the diagnosis of breast carcinomas with neuroendocrine differentiation. Its usefulness and limitations. J Pathol 1986, **148**: 35–43.

853 Nesland JM, Memoli VA, Holm R, Gould VE, Johannessen JV. Breast carcinomas with neuroendocrine differentiation. Ultrastruct Pathol 1985, **8**: 225–240.

854 Pagani A, Papotti M, Hofler H, Weiler R, Winkler H, Bussolati G. Chromogranin A and B gene expression in carcinomas of the breast. Correlation of immunocytochemical, immunoblot, and hybridization analyses. Am J Pathol 1990, **136**: 319–327.

855 Papotti M, Macri L, Finzi G, Capella C, Eusebi V, Bussolati G. Neuroendocrine differentiation in carcinomas of the breast. A study of 51 cases. Semin Diagn Pathol 1989, **6**: 174–188.

856 Righi L, Sapino A, Marchiò C, Papotti M, Bussolati G. Neuroendocrine differentiation in breast cancer: established facts and unresolved problems. Semin Diagn Pathol 2010, **27**: 69–76.

857 Salmo EN, Connolly CE. Primary small cell carcinoma of the breast: report of a case and review of the literature. Histopathology 2001, **38**: 277–278.

858 Samli B, Celik S, Evrensel T, Orhan B, Tasdelen I. Primary neuroendocrine small cell carcinoma of the breast. Arch Pathol Lab Med 2000, **124**: 296–298.

859 Sapino A, Righi L, Cassoni P, Papotti M, Gugliotta P, Bussolati G. Expression of apocrine differentiation markers in neuroendocrine breast carcinomas of aged women. Mod Pathol 2001, **14**: 768–776.

860 Scopsi L, Balslev E, Brunner N, Poulsen HS, Andersen J, Rank F, Larsson LI. Immunoreactive opioid peptides in human breast cancer. Am J Pathol 1989, **134**: 473–479.

861 Shin SJ, DeLellis RA, Ying L, Rosen PP. Small cell carcinoma of the breast: a clinicopathologic and immunohistochemical study of nine patients. Am J Surg Pathol 2000, **24**: 1231–1238.

862 Taxy JB, Tischler AS, Insalaco SJ, Battifora H. 'Carcinoid' tumor of the breast. A variant of conventional breast cancer? Hum Pathol 1981, **12**: 170–179.

863 Toyoshima S. Mammary carcinoma with argyrophil cells. Cancer 1983, **52**: 2129–2138.

864 Tsang WY, Chan JK. Endocrine ductal carcinoma in situ (E-DCIS) of the breast: a form of low-grade DCIS with distinctive clinicopathologic and biologic characteristics. Am J Surg Pathol 1996, **20**: 921–943.

865 Uccini S, Monardo F, Paradiso P, Masciangelo R, Marzullo A, Ruco LP, Baroni CD. Synaptophysin in human breast carcinomas. Histopathology 1991, **18**: 271–273.

866 Wilander E, Påhlman S, Sällström J, Lindgren A. Neuron-specific enolase expression and neuroendocrine differentiation in carcinomas of the breast. Arch Pathol Lab Med 1987, **111**: 830–832.

Metaplastic carcinoma

867 Adem C, Reynolds C, Adlakha H, Roche PC, Nascimento AG. Wide spectrum screening keratin as a marker of metaplastic spindle cell carcinoma of the breast: an immunohistochemical study of 24 patients. Histopathology 2002, **40**: 556–562.

868 Agnantis NT, Rosen PP. Mammary carcinoma with osteoclast-like giant cells. A study of eight cases with follow-up data. Am J Clin Pathol 1979, **72**: 383–389.

869 Banerjee SS, Eyden BP, Wells S, McWilliam LJ, Harris M. Pseudoangiosarcomatous

carcinoma. A clinicopathological study of seven cases. Histopathology 1992, **21**: 13–23.

870 Barsky SH, Shanmugasundaram G, Wu D. Metaplastic carcinoma, matrix-producing type (matrix-producing carcinomas) of the breast exhibit a myoepithelial histogenesis [abstract]. Mod Pathol 2003, **16**: 23a.

871 Bendic A, Bozic M, Durdov MG. Metaplastic breast carcinoma with melanocytic differentiation. Pathol Int 2009, **59**: 676–680.

872 Brogi E. Benign and malignant spindle cell lesions of the breast. Semin Diagn Pathol 2004, **21**: 57–64.

873 Carter MR, Hornick JL, Lester S, Fletcher CD. Spindle cell (sarcomatoid) carcinoma of the breast: a clinicopathologic and immunohistochemical analysis of 29 cases. Am J Surg Pathol 2006, **30**: 300–309.

874 Chhieng C, Cranor M, Lesser ME, Rosen PP. Metaplastic carcinoma of the breast with osteocartilaginous heterologous elements. Am J Surg Pathol 1998, **22**: 188–194.

875 Davis WG, Hennessy B, Babiera G, Hunt K, Valero V, Buchholz TA, Sneige N, Gilcrease MZ. Metaplastic sarcomatoid carcinoma of the breast with absent or minimal overt invasive carcinomatous component: a misnomer. Am J Surg Pathol 2005, **29**: 1456–1463.

876 Denley H, Pinder SE, Tan PH, Sim CS, Brown R, Barker T, Gearty J, Elston CW, Ellis IO. Metaplastic carcinoma of the breast arising within complex sclerosing lesion: a report of five cases. Histopathology 2000, **36**: 203–209.

877 Downs-Kelly E, Nayeemuddin KM, Albarracin C, Wu Y, Hunt KK, Gilcrease MZ. Matrix-producing carcinoma of the breast: an aggressive subtype of metaplastic carcinoma. Am J Surg Pathol 2009, **33**: 534–541.

878 Dunne B, Lee AHS, Pinder SE, Bell JA, Ellis IO. An immunohistochemcial study of metaplastic spindle cell carcinoma, phyllodes tumor and fibromatosis of the breast. Hum Pathol 2003, **34**: 1009–1015.

879 Eusebi V, Cattani MG, Ceccarelli C, Lamovec J. Sarcomatoid carcinomas of the breast. An immunohistochemical study of 14 cases. Progr Surg Pathol 1989, **10**: 83–100.

880 Foschini MP, Dina RE, Eusebi V. Sarcomatoid neoplasms of the breast. Proposed definitions for biphasic and monophasic sarcomatoid mammary carcinomas. Semin Diagn Pathol 1993, **10**: 128–136.

881 Geyer FC, Weigelt B, Natrajan R, Lambros MB, de Biase D, Vatcheva R, Savage K, Mackay A, Ashworth A, Reis-Filho JS. Molecular analysis reveals a genetic basis for the phenotypic diversity of metaplastic breast carcinomas. J Pathol 2010, **220**: 562–573.

882 Gobbi H, Simpson JF, Borowsky A, Jensen RA, Page DL. Metaplastic breast tumors with a dominant fibromatosis-like phenotype have a high risk of local recurrence. Cancer 1999, **85**: 2170–2182.

883 Gobbi H, Simpson JF, Jensen RA, Olson SJ, Page DL. Metaplastic spindle cell breast tumors arising within papillomas, complex sclerosing lesions, and nipple adenomas. Mod Pathol 2003, **16**: 893–901.

884 Gwin K, Wheeler DT, Bossuyt V, Tavassol FA. Breast carcinoma with chondroid differentiation: a clinicopathologic study of 21 triple negative (ER–, PR–, Her2/neu–) cases. Int J Surg Pathol 2010, **18**: 27–35.

885 Harris M, Persaud V. Carcinosarcoma of the breast. J Pathol 1974, **112**: 99–105.

886 Herrington CS, Tarin D, Buley I, Athanasou N. Osteosarcomatous differentiation in carcinoma of the breast. A case of 'metaplastic' carcinoma with osteoclasts and osteoclast-like giant cells. Histopathology 1994, **24**: 282–285.

887 Holland R, van Haelst UJGM. Mammary carcinoma with osteoclast-like giant cells. Additional observations on six cases. Cancer 1984, **53**: 1963–1973.

888 Kaufman MW, Marti JR, Gallager HS, Hoehn JL. Carcinoma of the breast with pseudosarcomatous metaplasia. Cancer 1984, **53**: 1908–1917.

889 Koker MM, Kleer CG. p63 expression in breast cancer: a highly sensitive and specific marker of metaplastic carcinoma. Am J Surg Pathol 2004, **28**: 1506–1512.

890 Leibl S, Gogg-Kammerer M, Sommersacher A, Denk H, Moinfar F. Metaplastic breast carcinomas: are they of myoepithelial differentiation? Immunohistochemical profile of the sarcomatoid subtype using novel myoepithelial markers. Am J Surg Pathol 2005, **29**: 347–353.

891 Nielsen BB, Kiaer HW. Carcinoma of the breast with stromal multinucleated giant cells. Histopathology 1985, **9**: 183–193.

892 Nguyen CV, Falcón-Escobedo R, Hunt KK, Nayeemuddin KM, Lester TR, Harrell RK, Bassett RL Jr, Gilcrease MZ. Pleomorphic ductal carcinoma of the breast: predictors of decreased overall survival. Am J Surg Pathol 2010, **34**: 486–493.

893 Noske A, Schwabe M, Pahl S, Fallenberg E, Richter-Ehrenstein C, Dietel M, Kristiansen G. Report of a metaplastic carcinoma of the breast with multi-directional differentiation: an adenoid cystic carcinoma, a spindle cell carcinoma and melanoma. Virchows Arch 2008, **452**: 575–579.

894 Oberman HA. Metaplastic carcinoma of the breast. A clinicopathologic study of 29 patients. Am J Surg Pathol 1987, **11**: 918–929.

895 Okada N, Hasebe T, Iwasaki M, Tamura N, Akashi-Tanaka S, Hojo T, Shibata T, Sasajima Y, Kanai Y, Kinoshita T. Metaplastic carcinoma of the breast. Hum Pathol 2010, **41**: 960–970.

896 Pitts WC, Rojas VA, Gaffey MJ, Rouse RV, Esteban J, Frierson HF, Kempson RL, Weiss LM. Carcinomas with metaplasia and sarcomas of the breast. Am J Clin Pathol 1991, **95**: 623–632.

897 Raju GC, Wee A. Spindle cell carcinoma of the breast. Histopathology 1990, **16**: 497–499.

898 Reis-Filho JS, Milanezi F, Paredes J, Silva P, Pereira EM, Maeda SA, de Carvalho LV, Schmitt FC. Novel and classic myoepithelial/stem cell markers in metaplastic carcinomas of the breast. Appl Immunohistochem Mol Morphol 2003, **11**: 1–8.

899 Resetkova E, Sahin A, Ayala AG, Sneige N. Breast carcinoma with choriocarcinomatous features. Ann Diagn Pathol 2004, **8**: 74–79.

900 Ruffolo EF, Koerner FC, Maluf HM. Metaplastic carcinoma of the breast with melanocytic differentiation. Mod Pathol 1997, **10**: 592–596.

901 Santeusanio G, Pascal RR, Bisceglia M, Costantino AM, Bosman C. Metaplastic breast carcinoma with epithelial phenotype of pseudosarcomatous components. Arch Pathol Lab Med 1988, **112**: 82–85.

902 Shin SJ, Kanomata N, Rosen PP. Mammary carcinoma with prominent cytoplasmic lipofuscin granules mimicking melanocytic differentiation. Histopathology 2000, **37**: 456–459.

903 Silver SA, Tavassoli FA. Pleomorphic carcinoma of the breast: clinicopathological analysis of 26 cases of an unusual high-grade phenotype of ductal carcinoma. Histopathology 2000, **36**: 505–514.

904 Simpson RH, Cope N, Skalova A, Michal M. Malignant adenomyoepithelioma of the breast with mixed osteogenic, spindle cell, and carcinomatous differentiation. Am J Surg Pathol 1998, **22**: 631–636.

905 Sneige N, Yaziji H, Mandavilli SR, Perez ER, Ordonez NG, Gown AM, Ayala A. Low-grade (fibromatosis-like) spindle cell carcinoma of the breast. Am J Surg Pathol 2001, **25**: 1009–1016.

906 Tavassoli FA. Classification of metaplastic carcinomas of the breast. Pathol Annu 1992, **27**(Pt 2): 89–119.

907 Tavassoli FA, Norris HJ. Breast carcinoma with osteoclastlike giant cells. Arch Pathol Lab Med 1986, **110**: 636–639.

908 Wada H, Enomoto T, Tsjuimoto M, Nomura T, Murata Y, Shroyer KR. Carcinosarcoma of the breast: molecular-biological study for analysis of histogenesis. Hum Pathol 1998, **29**: 1324–1328.

909 Wang X, Mori I, Tang W, Yang Q, Nakamura M, Nakamura K, Sato M, Sakurai T, Kennichi K. Metaplastic carcinoma of the breast: p53 analysis identified the same point mutation in the three histologic components. Mod Pathol 2001, **14**: 1183–1186.

910 Wargotz ES, Deos PH, Norris HJ. Metaplastic carcinomas of the breast. II. Spindle cell carcinoma. Hum Pathol 1989, **20**: 732–740.

911 Wargotz ES, Norris HJ. Metaplastic carcinomas of the breast. I. Matrix-producing carcinoma. Hum Pathol 1989, **20**: 628–635.

912 Wargotz ES, Norris HJ. Metaplastic carcinomas of the breast. III. Carcinosarcoma. Cancer 1989, **64**: 1490–1499.

913 Wargotz ES, Norris HJ. Metaplastic carcinomas of the breast. V. Metaplastic carcinoma with osteoclastic giant cells. Hum Pathol 1990, **21**: 1142–1150.

914 Weidner N. Malignant breast lesions that may mimic benign tumors. Semin Diagn Pathol 1995, **12**: 2–13.

915 Yamaguchi R, Horii R, Maeda I, Suga S, Makita M, Iwase T, Oguchi M, Ito Y, Akiyama F. Clinicopathologic study of 53 metaplastic breast carcinomas: their elements and prognostic implications. Hum Pathol 2010, **41**: 679–685.

916 Zhao J, Lang R, Guo X, Chen L, Gu F, Fan Y, Fu X, Fu L. Clinicopathologic characteristics of pleomorphic carcinoma of the breast. Virchows Arch 2010, **456**: 31–37.

917 Zhuang Z, Lininger RA, Man Y-G, Albuquerque A, Merino MJ, Tavassoli FA. Identical clonality of both components of mammary carcinosarcoma with differential loss of heterozygosity. Mod Pathol 1997, **10**: 354–362.

Squamous cell carcinoma and related tumors

918 Bauer TW, Rostock RA, Eggleston JC, Baral E. Spindle cell carcinoma of the breast. Four cases and review of the literature. Hum Pathol 1984, **15**: 147–152.

919 Bossuyt V, Fadare O, Martel M, Ocal IT, Burtness B, Moinfar F, Leibl S, Tavassoli FA. Remarkably high frequency of EGFR expression in breast carcinomas with squamous differentiation. Int J Surg Pathol 2005, **13**: 319–327.

920 Drudis T, Arroyo C, Van Hoeven K, Cordon-Cardo C, Rosen PP. The pathology of low-grade adenosquamous carcinoma of the breast. An immunohistochemical study. Pathol Annu 1994, **29**(Pt 2): 181–197.

921 Eggers JW, Chesney TM. Squamous cell carcinoma of the breast. A clinicopathologic analysis of eight cases and review of the literature. Hum Pathol 1984, **15**: 526–531.

922 Eusebi V, Lamovec J, Cattani MG, Fedeli F, Millis RR. Acantholytic variant of squamous-cell carcinoma of the breast. Am J Surg Pathol 1986, **10**: 855–861.

923 Fisher ER, Palekar AS, Gregorio RM, Paulson JD. Mucoepidermoid and squamous cell carcinomas of breast with reference to squamous metaplasia and giant cell tumors. Am J Surg Pathol 1983, **7**: 15–27.

924 Foschini MP, Fulcheri E, Baraechini P, Ceccarelli C, Betts CM, Eusebi V. Squamous cell carcinoma with prominent myxoid stroma. Hum Pathol 1990, **21**: 859–865.

925 Gersell DJ, Katzenstein A-LA. Spindle cell carcinoma of the breast. A clinicopathologic and ultrastructural study. Hum Pathol 1981, **12**: 550–561.

926 Ho BC, Tan HW, Lee VK, Tan PH. Preoperative and intraoperative diagnosis of low-grade adenosquamous carcinoma of the breast: potential diagnostic pitfalls. Histopathology 2006, **49**: 603–611.

927 Oberman HA. Metaplastic carcinoma of the breast. A clinicopathologic study of 29 patients. Am J Surg Pathol 1987, **11**: 918–929.

928 Rosen PP, Ernsberger D. Low-grade adenosquamous carcinoma. A variant of metaplastic mammary carcinoma. Am J Surg Pathol 1987, **11**: 351–358.

929 Toikkanen S. Primary squamous cell carcinoma of the breast. Cancer 1981, **48**: 1629–1632.

930 Wargotz ES, Norris HJ. Metaplastic carcinomas of the breast. IV. Squamous cell carcinoma of ductal origin. Cancer 1990, **65**: 272–276.

931 Woodard BH, Brinkhous AD, McCarty KS Sr, McCarty KS Jr. Adenosquamous differentiation in mammary carcinoma. An ultrastructural and steroid receptor study. Arch Pathol Lab Med 1980, **104**: 130–133.

Spread-related variants

Inflammatory carcinoma

932 Buzdar AU, Montague ED, Barker JL, Hortobagyi GN, Blumenschein GR. Management of inflammatory carcinoma of breast with combined modality approach. An update. Cancer 1981, **47**: 2537–2542.

933 Chang S, Parker SL, Pham T, Buzdar AU, Hursting SD. Inflammatory breast carcinoma incidence and survival: the surveillance, epidemiology, and end results program of the National Cancer Institute, 1975–1992. Cancer 1998, **82**: 2366–2372.

934 Chu AM, Wood WC, Doucette JA. Inflammatory breast carcinoma treated by radical radiotherapy. Cancer 1980, **45**: 2730–2737.

935 Ellis DL, Teitelbaum SL. Inflammatory carcinoma of the breast. A pathological definition. Cancer 1974, **33**: 1045–1047.

936 Fields JN, Kuske RR, Perez CA, Fineberg BB, Bartlett N. Prognostic factors in inflammatory breast cancer. Univariate and multivariate analysis. Cancer 1989, **63**: 1225–1232.

937 Lucas FV, Perez-Mesa C. Inflammatory carcinoma of the breast. Cancer 1978, **41**: 1595–1605.

938 Robertson FM, Bondy M, Yang W, Yamauchi H, Wiggins S, Kamrudin S, Krishnamurthy S, Le-Petross H, Bidaut L, Player AN, Barsky SH, Woodward WA, Buchholz T, Lucci A, Ueno N, Cristofanilli M. Inflammatory breast cancer: the disease, the biology, the treatment. CA Cancer J Clin 2010, **60**: 351–375.

939 Saltzstein SL. Clinically occult inflammatory carcinoma of the breast. Cancer 1974, **34**: 382–388.

940 Schafer P, Alberto P, Forni M, Obradovic D, Pipard G, Krauer F. Surgery as part of a combined modality approach for inflammatory breast carcinoma. Cancer 1987, **59**: 1063–1067.

Paget disease

941 Ashikari R, Park K, Huvos AG, Urban JA. Paget's disease of the breast. Cancer 1970, **26**: 680–685.

942 Azzopardi JG, Eusebi V. Melanocyte colonization and pigmentation of breast carcinoma. Histopathology 1977, **1**: 21–30.

943 Bussolati G, Pich A. Mammary and extramammary Paget's disease. An immunocytochemical study. Am J Pathol 1975, **80**: 117–127.

944 Cohen C, Guarner J, De Rose PB. Mammary Paget's disease and associated carcinoma. An immunohistochemical study. Arch Pathol Lab Med 1993, **117**: 291–294.

945 de Potter CR, Eeckhout I, Schelfhout AM, Geerts ML, Roels HJ. Keratinocyte induced chemotaxis in the pathogenesis of Paget's disease of the breast. Histopathology 1994, **24**: 349–356.

946 Di Tommaso L, Franchi G, Destro A, Broglia F, Minuti F, Rahal D, Roncalli M. Toker cells of the breast. Morphological and immunohistochemical characterization of 40 cases. Hum Pathol 2008, **39**: 1295–1300.

947 Fernandez-Flores A. Toker-cell pathology as a unifying concept. Histopathology 2008, **52**: 889–904.

948 Keatings L, Sinclair J, Wright C, Corbett IP, Watchorn C, Hennessy C, Angus B, Lennard T, Horne CH. *c-erb*B-2 oncoprotein expression in mammary and extramammary Paget's disease. An immunohistochemical study. Histopathology 1990, **17**: 243–247.

949 Kirkham N, Berry N, Jones DB, Taylor-Papadimitriou J. Paget's disease of the nipple. Immunohistochemical localization of milk fat globule membrane antigens. Cancer 1985, **55**: 1510–1512.

950 Lagios MD, Westdahl PR, Rose MR, Concannon S. Paget's disease of the nipple. Alternative management in cases without or with minimal extent of underlying breast carcinoma. Cancer 1984, **54**: 545–551.

951 Liegl B, Leibl S, Gogg-Kamerer M, Tessaro B, Horn LC, Moinfar F. Mammary and extramammary Paget's disease: an immunohistochemical study of 83 cases. Histopathology 2007, **50**: 439–447.

952 Liegl B, Moinfar F. 'Toker cells' as origin of Paget's disease: fact or fiction? Histopathology 2008, **52**: 891–892.

953 Lundquist K, Kohler S, Rouse RV. Intraepidermal cytokeratin 7 expression is not restricted to Paget cells but is also seen in Toker cells and Merkel cells. Am J Surg Pathol 1999, **23**: 212–219.

954 Mai KT. Morphological evidence for field effect as a mechanism for tumour spread in mammary Paget's disease. Histopathology 1999, **35**: 567–576.

955 Marucci G, Betts CM, Golouh R, Peterse JL, Foschini MP, Eusebi V. Toker cells are probably precursors of Paget cell carcinoma: a morphological and ultrastructural description. Virchows Arch 2002, **441**: 117–123.

956 Meissner K, Riviere A, Haupt G, Loning T. Study of neu-protein expression in mammary Paget's disease with and without underlying breast carcinoma and in extramammary Paget's disease. Am J Pathol 1990, **137**: 1305–1309.

957 Mori O, Hachisuka H, Nakano S, Sasai Y, Shiku H. Expression of *ras* p21 in mammary and extramammary Paget's disease. Arch Pathol Lab Med 1990, **114**: 858–861.

958 Nagle RB, Lucas DO, McDaniel KM, Clark VA, Schmalzel GM. New evidence linking mammary and extramammary Paget cells to a common cell phenotype. Am J Clin Pathol 1985, **83**: 431–438.

959 Neubecker RD, Bradshaw RP. Mucin, melanin, and glycogen in Paget's disease of the breast. Am J Clin Pathol 1961, **36**: 40–53.

960 Ogawa E, Okuyama R, Egawa T, Nagoshi H, Tagami H, Ikawa S, Aiba S. Ectopic expression of the p53 homologue p63 is linked to squamous metaplasia in extramammary Paget's disease with invasive adenocarcinoma. Histopathology 2009, **54**: 378–381.

961 Ordóñez NG, Awalt H, Mackay B. Mammary and extramammary Paget's disease. An immunocytochemical and ultrastructural study. Cancer 1987, **59**: 1173–1183.

962 Paget J. On disease of the mammary areola preceding cancer of the mammary gland. St Barth Hosp Rep 1874, **10**: 87–89.

963 Paone JF, Baker RR. Pathogenesis and treatment of Paget's disease of the breast. Cancer 1981, **48**: 825–829.

964 Rayne SC, Santa Cruz DJ. Anaplastic Paget's disease. Am J Surg Pathol 1992, **16**: 1085–1091.

965 Rodríguez-Martínex HA, Chávez Mercado L, Rodríguez-Reyes AA, López Vancell D, Pérez Olvera O, Medina Cruz A, Picaso-Hernández RM. Migración de melanocitos epidérmicos dendríticos y colonización de un carcinoma mamario infiltrante. Patologia (Mexico) 2011 (Submitted for publication)

966 Sagebiel RW. Ultrastructural observations on epidermal cells in Paget's disease of the breast. Am J Pathol 1969, **57**: 49–64.

967 Shin SJ, Kanomata N, Rosen PP. Mammary carcinoma with prominent cytoplasmic lipofuscin granules mimicking melanocytic differentiation. Histopathology 2000, **37**: 456–459.

968 Shousha S. Glandular Paget's disease of the nipple. Histopathology 2007, **50**: 812–814.

969 Sitakalin C, Ackerman AB. Mammary and extramammary Paget's disease. Am J Dermatopathol 1985, **7**: 335–340.

970 Toker C. Clear cells of the nipple epidermis. Cancer 1970, **25**: 601–610.

971 Vanstapel M-J, Gatter KC, DeWolf-Peeters C, Millard PR, Desmet VJ, Mason DY. Immunohistochemical study of mammary and extra-mammary Paget's disease. Histopathology 1984, **8**: 1013–1023.

972 Venkataseshan VS, Budd DC, Kim DU, Hutter RVP. Intraepidermal squamous carcinoma (Bowen's disease) of the nipple. Hum Pathol 1994, **25**: 1371–1374.

973 Wolber RA, Dupuis BA, Wick MR. Expression of *c-erb*B-2 oncoprotein in mammary and extramammary Paget's disease. Am J Clin Pathol 1991, **96**: 243–247.

INVASIVE LOBULAR CARCINOMA (ILC)

Classic type

974 Acs G, Lawton TJ, Rebbeck TR, Li Volsi VA, Zhang PJ. Differential expression of E-cadherin in lobular and ductal neoplasms of the breast and its biologic and diagnostic implications. Am J Clin Pathol 2001, **115**: 85–98.

975 Dabbs DJ, Bhargava R, Chivukula M. Lobular versus ductal breast neoplasms: the diagnostic utility of p120 catenin. Am J Surg Pathol 2007, **31**: 427–437.

976 Da Silva L, Parry S, Reid L, Keith P, Waddell N, Kossai M, Clarke C, Lakhani SR, Simpson PT. Aberrant expression of E-cadherin in lobular carcinomas of the breast. Am J Surg Pathol 2008, **32**: 773–783.

977 Di Costanzo D, Rosen PP, Gareen I, Franklin S, Lesser M. Prognosis in infiltrating lobular carcinoma. An analysis of 'classical' and variant tumors. Am J Surg Pathol 1990, **14**: 12–23.

978 Domagala W, Harezga B, Szadowska A, Markiewski M, Weber K, Osborn M. Nuclear p53 protein accumulates preferentially in medullary and high-grade ductal but rarely in lobular breast carcinomas. Am J Pathol 1993, **142**: 669–674.

979 Fechner RE. Infiltrating lobular carcinoma without lobular carcinoma in situ. Cancer 1972, **29**: 1539–1545.

980 Goldstein NS, Bassi D, Watts JC, Layfield LJ, Yaziji H, Gown AM. E-cadherin reactivity of 95 non-invasive ductal and lobular lesions of the breast: implications for the interpretation of problematic lesions. Am J Clin Pathol 2001, **115**: 534–542.

981 Lehr H-A, Folpe A, Yaziji H, Kommoss F, Gown AM. Cytokeratin 8 immunostaining pattern and E-cadherin expression distinguish lobular from ductal breast carcinoma. Am J Clin Pathol 2000, **114**: 190–196.

982 Martinez V, Azzopardi JG. Invasive lobular carcinoma of the breast. Incidence and variants. Histopathology 1979, **3**: 467–488.

983 Rakha EA, Ellis IO. Lobular breast carcinoma and its variants. Semin Diagn Pathol 2010, **27**: 49–61.

984 Rakha EA, Patel A, Powe DG, Benhasouna A, Green AR, Lambros MB, Reis-Filho JS, Ellis IO. Clinical and biological significance of E-cadherin protein expression in invasive lobular carcinoma of the breast. Am J Surg Pathol 2010, **34**: 1472–1479.

985 Silverstein MJ, Lewinsky BS, Waisman JR, Gierson ED, Colburn WJ, Senofsky GM, Gamagami P. Infiltrating lobular carcinoma. Is it different from infiltrating duct carcinoma? Cancer 1994, **73**: 1673–1677.

Pleomorphic lobular carcinoma

986 Chen YY, Hwang ES, Roy R, DeVries S, Anderson J, Wa C, Fitzgibbons PL, Jacobs TW, MacGrogan G, Peterse H, Vincent-Salomon A, Tokuyasu T, Schnitt SJ, Waldman FM. Genetic and phenotypic characteristics of pleomorphic lobular carcinoma in situ of the breast. Am J Surg Pathol 2009, **33**: 1683–1694.

987 Dabbs DJ, Kaplai M, Chivukula M, Kanbour A, Kanbour-Shakir A, Carter GJ. The spectrum of morphomolecular abnormalities of the E-cadherin/catenin complex in pleomorphic lobular carcinoma of the breast. Appl Immunohistochem Mol Morphol 2007, **15**: 260–266.

988 Frolik D, Caduff R, Varga Z. Pleomorphic lobular carcinoma of the breast: its cell kinetics, expression of oncogenes and tumour suppressor genes compared with invasive ductal carcinomas and classification infiltrating lobular carcinomas. Histopathology 2001, **39**: 503–513.

989 Middleton LP, Palacios DM, Bryant BR, Krebs P, Otis CN, Merino MJ. Pleomorphic lobular carcinoma: morphology, immunohistochemistry, and molecular analysis. Am J Surg Pathol 2000, **24**: 1650–1656.

990 Palacios J, Sarrió D, Garcia-Macias MC, Bryant B, Sobel ME, Merino MJ. Frequent E-cadherin gene inactiviation by loss of heterozygosity in pleomorphic lobular carcinoma of the breast. Mod Pathol 2003, **16**: 674–678.

991 Radhi JM. Immunohistochemical analysis of pleomorphic lobular carcinoma: higher expression of p53 and chromogranin and lower expression of ER and PgR. Histopathology 2000, **36**: 156–160.

992 Wahed A, Connelly J, Reese T. E-cadherin expression in pleomorphic lobular carcinoma: an aid to differentiation from ductal carcinoma. Ann Diagn Pathol 2002, **6**: 349–351.

993 Weidner N, Semple JP. Pleomorphic variant of invasive lobular carcinoma of the breast. Hum Pathol 1992, **23**: 1167–1171.

Histiocytoid carcinoma

994 Eusebi V, Foschini MP, Bussolati G, Rosen PP. Myoblastomatoid (histiocytoid) carcinoma of the breast. A type of apocrine carcinoma. Am J Surg Pathol 1995, **19**: 553–562.

995 Fisher ER, Gregorio R, Kim WS, Redmond C. Lipid in invasive cancer of the breast. Am J Clin Pathol 1977, **68**: 558–561.

996 Gupta D, Croitoru CM, Ayala AG, Sahin AA, Middleton LP. E-cadherin immunohistochemical analysis of histiocytoid carcinoma of the breast. Ann Diagn Pathol 2002, **6**: 141–147.

997 Hood CI, Font RL, Zimmerman LE. Metastatic mammary carcinoma in the eyelid with histiocytoid appearance. Cancer 1973, **31**: 793–800.

998 Kasashima S, Kawashima A, Zen Y, Ozaki S, Kobayashi M, Tsujibata A, Minato H. Expression of aberrant mucins in lobular carcinoma with histiocytoid feature of the breast. Virchows Arch 2007, **450**: 397–403.

999 Ramos CV, Taylor HB. Lipid-rich carcinoma of the breast. Cancer 1974, **33**: 812–819.

1000 Shimizu S, Kitamura H, Ito T, Nakamura T, Fujisawa J, Matsukawa H. Histiocytoid breast carcinoma: histological, immunohistochemical, ultrastructural, cytological and clinicopathologic studies. Pathol Int 1998, **48**: 549–556.

1001 van Bogaert LJ, Maldague P. Histologic variants of lipid-secreting carcinoma of the breast. Virchows Arch [A] 1977, **375**: 345–353.

1002 Walford N, ten Velden J. Histiocytoid breast carcinoma. An apocrine variant of lobular carcinoma. Histopathology 1989, **14**: 515–522.

Signet ring carcinoma

1003 Chu PG, Weiss LM. Immunohistochemical characterization of signet-ring cell carcinomas of the stomach, breast, and colon. Am J Clin Pathol 2004, **121**: 884–892.

1004 Eltorky M, Hall JC, Osborne PT, el Zeky F. Signet-ring cell variant of invasive lobular carcinoma of the breast. A clinicopathologic study of 11 cases. Arch Pathol Lab Med 1994, **118**: 245–248.

1005 Fisher ER, Brown R. Intraductal signet ring carcinoma. A hitherto undescribed form of intraductal carcinoma of the breast. Cancer 1985, **55**: 2533–2537.

1006 Frost AR, Terahata S, Yeh IT, Siegel RS, Overmoyer B, Silverberg SG. The significance of signet ring cells in infiltrating lobular carcinoma of the breast. Arch Pathol Lab Med 1995, **119**: 64–68.

1007 Hull MT, Seo IS, Battersby JS, Csicsko JF. Signet-ring cell carcinoma of the breast. A clinicopathologic study of 24 cases. Am J Clin Pathol 1980, **73**: 31–35.

1008 Maeno Y, Moroi S, Nagashima H, Noda T, Shoizaki H, Monden M, Tsukita S, Nagafuchi A. α-catenin-deficient F9 cells differentiate into signet ring cells. Am J Pathol 1999, **154**: 1323–1328.

1009 Martinez V, Azzopardi JG. Invasive lobular carcinoma of the breast. Incidence and variants. Histopathology 1979, **3**: 467–488.

1010 Merino MJ, LiVolsi VA. Signet ring carcinoma of the female breast. A clinicopathologic analysis of 24 cases. Cancer 1981, **48**: 1830–1837.

1011 Quincey C, Raitt N, Bell J, Ellis IO. Intracytoplasmic lumina – a useful diagnostic feature of adenocarcinomas. Histopathology 1991, **19**: 83–87.

1012 Rosa M, Mohammadi A, Masood S. Lobular carcinoma of the breast with extracellular mucin: new variant of mucin-producing carcinomas? Pathol Int 2009, **59**: 405–409.

1013 Steinbrecher JS, Silverberg SG. Signet-ring cell carcinoma of the breast. The mucinous variant of infiltrating lobular carcinoma? Cancer 1976, **37**: 828–840.

1014 Yoshida A, Hatanaka S, Oneda S, Yoshida H. Signet ring cells in breast carcinoma. An immunohistochemical and ultrastructural study. Acta Pathol Jpn 1992, **42**: 523–528.

Tubulolobular carcinoma

1015 Esposito NN, Chivukula M, Dabbs DJ. The ductal phenotypic expression of the E-cadherin/catenin complex in tubulolobular carcinoma of the breast: an immunohistochemical and clinicopathologic study. Mod Pathol 2007, **20**: 130–138.

1016 Fisher ER, Gregorio RM, Redmond C, Fisher B. Tubulolobular invasive breast cancer. A variant of lobular invasive cancer. Hum Pathol 1977, **8**: 679–683.

1017 Green I, McCormick B, Cranor M, Rosen PP. A comparative study of pure tubular and tubulolobular carcinoma of the breast. Am J Surg Pathol 1997, **21**: 653–657.

1018 Kuroda H, Tamaru J, Takeuchi I, Ohnisi K, Sakamoto G, Adachi A, Kaneko K, Itoyama S. Expression of E-cadherin, alpha-catenin, and beta-catenin in tubulolobular carcinoma of the breast. Virchows Arch 2006, **448**: 500–505.

1019 Wheeler DT, Tai LH, Bratthauer GL, Waldner DL, Tavassoli FA. Tubulolobular carcinoma of the breast: an analysis of 27 cases of a tumor with a hybrid morphology and immunoprofile. Am J Surg Pathol 2004, **28**: 1587–1593.

Other types

1020 Azzopardi JG. Problems in breast pathology. In Bennington JL (consulting ed.): Major problems in pathology, vol. 11. Philadelphia, 1979, W.B. Saunders.

1021 Dixon JM, Anderson TJ, Page DL, Lee D, Duffy SW. Infiltrating lobular carcinoma of the breast. Histopathology 1982, **6**: 149–161.

1022 Fechner RE. Histologic variants of infiltrating lobular carcinoma of the breast. Hum Pathol 1975, **6**: 373–378.

1023 Martinez V, Azzopardi JG. Invasive lobular carcinoma of the breast. Incidence and variants. Histopathology 1979, **3**: 467–488.

1024 Pettinato G, Manivel JC, Picone A, Petrella G, Insabato L. Alveolar variant of infiltrating lobular carcinoma of the breast with stromal osteoclast-like giant cells. Pathol Res Pract 1989, **185**: 388–394.

1025 Shousha S, Backhous CM, Alaghband-Zadeh J, Burn I. Alveolar variant of invasive lobular carcinoma of the breast. A tumor rich in estrogen receptors. Am J Clin Pathol 1986, **85**: 1–5.

UNDETERMINED (UNCLASSIFIED) CARCINOMA

1026 Azzopardi JG. Problems in breast pathology. In Bennington JL (consulting ed.): Major problems in pathology, vol. 11. Philadelphia, 1979, W.B. Saunders.

MICROINVASIVE BREAST CARCINOMA

1027 De Mascarel I, MacGrogan G, Mathoulin-Pelissier S, Soubeyran I, Picot V, Coindre JM. Breast ductal carcinoma in situ with microinvasion: a definition supported by a long-term study of 1248 serially sections ductal carcinomas. Cancer 2002, **94**: 2134–2142.

1028 Ellis IO, Lee AH, Elston CW, Pinder SE. Microinvasive carcinoma of the breast: diagnostic criteria and clinical relevance. Histopathology 1999, **35**: 470–472.

1029 Hoda SA, Prasad ML, Moore A, Hoda RS, Giri D, Ellis IO, Lee AH, Elston CW, Pinder SE. Microinvasive carcinoma of the breast: can it be diagnosed reliably and is it clinically significant? Histopathology 1999, **35**: 468–472.

1030 Padmore RF, Fowble B, Hoffman J, Rosser C, Hanlon A, Patchefsky AS. Microinvasive breast carcinoma: clinicopathologic analysis of a single institution experience. Cancer 2000, **88**: 1403–1409.

1031 Prasad ML, Osborne MP, Giri DD, Hoda SA. Microinvasive carcinoma (T1mic) of the breast: clinicopathologic profile of 21 cases. Am J Surg Pathol 2000, **24**: 422–428.

1032 Schnitt SJ. Microinvasive carcinoma of the breast: a diagnosis in search of a definition. Adv Anat Pathol 1998, **5**: 367–372.

1033 Werling RW, Hwang H, Yaziji H, Gown AM. Immunohistochemical distinction of invasive from non-invasive breast lesions: a comparative study of p63 versus calponin and smooth muscle myosin heavy chain. Am J Surg Pathol 2003, **27**: 82–90.

1034 Zavotsky J, Hansen N, Brennan MB, Turner RR, Giuliano AE. Lymph node metastasis from ductal carcinoma in situ with microinvasion. Cancer 1999, **85**: 2439–2443.

HORMONE RECEPTORS

1035 Agoff SN, Swanson PE, Linden H, Hawes SE, Lawton TJ. Androgen receptor expression in estrogen receptor-negative breast cancer. Immunohistochemical, clinical, and prognostic associations. Am J Clin Pathol 2003, **120**: 725–731.

1036 Allred DC, Harvery JM, Berardo M, Clark GM. Prognostic and predictive factors in breast cancer by immunohistochemical analysis. Mod Pathol 1998, **11**: 155–168.

1037 Baddoura FK, Cohen C, Unger ER, De Rose PB, Chenggis M. Image analysis for quantitation of estrogen receptor in formalin-fixed paraffin-embedded sections of breast carcinoma. Mod Pathol 1991, **4**: 91–95.

1038 Barnes DM, Hanby AM. Oestrogen and progesterone receptors in breast cancer: past, present and future. Histopathology 2001, **38**: 271–274.

1039 Battifora H, Mehta P, Ahn C, Esteban J. Estrogen receptor immunohistochemical assay in paraffin-embedded tissue. A better gold standard? Appl Immunohistochem 1993, **1**: 39–45.

1040 Bayer-Garner IB, Smoller B. Androgen receptors: a marker to increase sensitivity for identifying breast cancer in skin metastasis of unknown primary site. Mod Pathol 2000, **13**: 119–122.

1041 Bhargava V, Kell DL, van de Rijn M, Warnke RA. *Bcl*-2 immunoreactivity in breast carcinoma correlates with hormone receptor positivity. Am J Pathol 1994, **145**: 535–540.

1042 Bur ME, Zimarowski MJ, Schnitt SJ, Baker S, Lew R. Estrogen receptor immunohistochemistry in carcinoma in situ of the breast. Cancer 1992, **69**: 1174–1181.

1043 Caleffi M, Teague MW, Jensen RA, Vnencak-Jones CL, Dupont WD, Parl FF. p53 gene mutations and steroid receptor status in breast cancer. Clinicopathologic correlations and prognostic assessment. Cancer 1994, **73**: 2147–2156.

1044 Carmeci C, DeConinck EC, Lawton T, Block DA, Weigel RJ. Analysis of estrogen receptor messenger RNA in breast carcinomas from archival specimens is predictive of tumor biology. Am J Pathol 1997, **150**: 1563–1570.

1045 Fisher ER, Redmond CK, Liu H, Rockette H, Fisher B, and collaborating NSABP investigators. Correlation of estrogen receptor and pathologic characteristics of invasive breast cancer. Cancer 1980, **45**: 349–353.

1046 Fitzgibbons PL, Murphy DA, Hammond ME, Allred DC, Valenstein PN. Recommendations for validating estrogen and progesterone receptor immunohistochemistry assays. Arch Pathol Lab Med 2010, **134**: 930–935.

1047 Graham DM, Jin L, Lloyd RV. Detection of estrogen receptor in paraffin-embedded sections of breast carcinoma by immunohistochemistry and in situ hybridization. Am J Surg Pathol 1991, **15**: 475–485.

1048 Hammond MEH, Hayes DF, Dowsett M, Allred DC, Hagerty KL, Badve S, Fitzgibbons PL, Francis G, Goldstein NS, Hayes M, Hicks DG, Lester S, Love R, Mangu PB, McShane L, Miller K, Osborne CK, Paik S, Perlmutter J, Rhodes A, Sasano H, Schwartz JN, Sweep FCG, Taube S, Torlakovic EE, Valenstein P, Viale G, Visscher D, Wheeler T, Williams RB, Wittliff JL, Wolff AC. American Society of Clinical Oncology/College of American Pathologists guideline recommendations for immunohistochemical testing of estrogen and progesterone receptors in breast cancer. J Clin Oncol 2010, **28**: 2784–2795; Arch Pathol Lab Med 2010, **134**: 907–922.

1049 Harvey JM, Clark GM, Osborne CK, Allred DC. Estrogen receptor status by immunohistochemistry is superior to the ligand-binding assay for predicting response to adjuvant endocrine therapy in breast cancer. J Clin Oncol 1999, **17**: 1474–1481.

1050 Hawkins RA, Roberts MM, Forrest APM. Oestrogen receptors and breast cancer. Current status. Br J Surg 1980, **67**: 162–165.

1051 Honma N, Sakamoto G, Akiyama F, Esaki Y, Sawabe M, Arai T, Hosoi T, Harada N, Younes M, Takubo K. Breast carcinoma in women over the age of 85: distinct histological pattern and androgen, oestrogen, and progesterone receptor status. Histopathology 2003, **41**: 120–127.

1052 Ibarra JA, Rogers LW, Kyshtoobayeva A, Bloom K. Fixation time does not affect the expression of estrogen receptor. Am J Clin Pathol 2010, **133**: 747–755.

1053 Liegl B, Horn LC, Moinfar F. Androgen receptors are frequently expressed in mammary and extramammary Paget's disease. Mod Pathol 2005, **18**: 1283–1288.

1054 MacGrogan F, Soubeyran I, De Mascarel I, Wafflart J, Bonichon F, Durand M, Avril A, Mauriac L, Trojani M, Coindre JM. Immunohistochemical detection of progesterone receptors in breast invasive ductal carcinomas: a correlative study of 942 cases. Appl Immunohistochem 1996, **4**: 219–227.

1055 Middleton LP, Perkins GH, Tucker SL, Sahin AA, Singletary SE. Expression of ERalpha and ERbeta in lobular carcinoma in situ. Histopathology 2007, **50**: 875–880.

1056 Mohammed RH, Lakatua DJ, Haus E, Yasmineh WJ. Estrogen and progesterone receptors in human breast cancer. Correlation with histologic subtype and degree of differentiation. Cancer 1986, **58**: 1076–1081.

1057 Mohsin SK, Weiss H, Havighurst T, Clark GM, Berardo M, Roanh le D, To TV, Qian Z, Love RR, Allred DC. Progesterone receptor by immunohistochemistry and clinical outcome in breast cancer: a validation study. Mod Pathol 2004, **17**: 1545–1554.

1058 Nadji M, Gomez-Fernandez C, Ganjei-Azar P, Morales AR. Immunohistochemistry of estrogen and progesterone receptors reconsidered: experience with 5,993 breast cancers. Am J Clin Pathol 2005, **123**: 21–27.

1059 Nadji M. Quantitative immunohistochemistry of estrogen receptor in breast cancer: 'much ado about nothing!' Appl Immunohistochem Mol Morphol 2008, **16**: 105–107.

1060 Niemeier LA, Dabbs DJ, Beriwal S, Striebel JM, Bhargava R. Androgen receptor in breast cancer: expression in estrogen receptor-positive tumors and in estrogen receptor-negative tumors with apocrine differentiation. Mod Pathol 2010, **23**: 205–212.

1061 Payne SJL, Bowen RL, Jones JL, Wells CA. Predictive markers in breast cancer – the present. Histopathology 2008, **52**: 82–90.

1062 Phillips T, Murray G, Wakamiya K, Askaa J, Huang D, Welcher R, Pii K, Allred DC. Development of standard estrogen and progesterone receptor immunohistochemical assays for selection of patients for antihormonal therapy. Appl Immunohistochem Mol Morphol 2007, **15**: 325–331.

1063 Putti TC, El-Rehim DM, Rakha EA, Paish CE, Lee AH, Pinder SE, Ellis IO. Estrogen receptor-negative breast carcinomas: a review of morphology and immunophenotypical analysis. Mod Pathol 2005, **18**: 26–35.

1064 Regitnig P, Reiner A, Dinges HP, Hofler G, Muller-Holzner E, Lax S, Obrist P, Rudas M, Quehenberger F. Quality assurance for detection of estrogen and progesterone receptors by immunohistochemistry in Austrian pathology laboratories. Virchows Arch 2002, **441**: 328–334.

1065 Rhodes A, Jasani B, Balaton AJ, Barnes DM, Anderson E, Bobrow L, Miller KD. Study of interlaboratory reliability and reproducibility of estrogen and progesterone receptor assays in Europe. Documentation of poor reliability and identification of insufficient microwave antigen retrieval time as a major contributory element of unreliable assays. Am J Clin Pathol 2001, **115**: 44–58.

1066 Riera J, Simpson JF, Tamayo R, Battifora H. Use of cultured cells as a control for quantitative immunocytochemical analysis of estrogen receptor in breast cancer. The Quicgel method. Am J Clin Pathol 1999, **111**: 329–335.

1067 Riva C, Dainese E, Caprara G, Rocca PC, Massarelli G, Tot T, Capella C, Eusebi V. Immunohistochemical study of androgen receptors in breast carcinoma. Evidence of their frequent expression in lobular carcinoma. Virchows Arch 2005, **447**: 695–700.

1068 Scawn R, Shousha S. Morphologic spectrum of estrogen receptor-negative breast carcinoma. Arch Pathol Lab Med 2002, **126**: 325–330.

1069 Silfverswärd C, Gustafsson JÅ, Gustafsson SA, Humla S, Nordenskjöld B, Wallgren A, Wrange Ö. Estrogen receptor concentrations in 269 cases of histologically classified human breast cancer. Cancer 1980, **45**: 2001–2005.

1070 Taylor CR. Paraffin section immunocytochemistry for estrogen receptor: the time has come. Cancer 1996, **77**: 2419–2422.

1071 van Agthoven T, Timmermans M, Foekens JA, Dorssers LC, Henzen-Logmans SC. Differential expression of estrogen, progesterone, and epidermal growth factor receptors in normal, benign, and malignant human breast tissues using dual staining immunohistochemistry. Am J Pathol 1994, **144**: 1238–1246.

1072 Wells CA, Sloane JP, Coleman D, Munt C, Amendoeira I, Apostolikas N, Bellocq JP, Bianchi S, Boecker W, Bussolati G, Connolly CE, Dervan P, Drijkoningen M, Ellis IO, Elston CW, Eusebi V, Faverly D, Heikkila P, Holland R, Jacquemier J, Lacerda M, Martinez-Penuela J, De Miguel C, Peterse JL, Rank F, Reiner A, Saksela E, Sigal-Zafrani B, Sylvan M, Borisch B, Cserni G, Decker T, Kerner H, Kulka J, Regitnig P, Sapino A, Tanous AM, Thorstenson S, Zozaya E; European Working Group for Breast Screening Pathology. Consistency of staining and reporting of oestrogen receptor immunocytochemistry within the European Union – an inter-laboratory study. Virchows Arch 2004, **445**: 119–128.

1073 Yaziji H, Taylor CR, Goldstein NS, Dabbs DJ, Hammond MEH, Hewlett B, Floyd AD, Barry TS, Martin AW, Badve S, Baehner F, Cartun RW, Eisen RN, Swanson PE, Hewitt SM, Vyberg M, Hicks DG; Members of the Standardization Ad-Hoc Consensus Committee. Consensus recommendations on estrogen receptor testing in breast cancer by immunohistochemistry. Appl Immunohistochem Mol Morphol 2008, **16**: 513–520.

1074 Zafrani B, Aubriot MH, Mouret E, De Cremoux P, De Rycke Y, Nicolas A, Boudou E, Vincent-Salomon A, Magdelenat H, Sastre-Garau X. High sensitivity and specificity of immunohistochemistry for the detection of hormone receptors in breast carcinoma: comparison with biochemical determination in a prospective study of 793 cases. Histopathology 2001, **37**: 536–545.

HER2/*NEU*

1075 Barron JJ, Cziraky MJ, Weisman T, Hicks DG. HER2 testing and subsequent trastuzumab treatment for breast cancer in a managed care environment. Oncologist 2009, **14**: 760–768.

1076 Bertucci F, Finetti P, Cervera N, Esterni B, Hermitte F, Viens P, Birnbaum D. How basal are triple-negative breast cancers? Int J Cancer 2008, **123**: 236–240.

1077 Brunelli M, Manfrin E, Martignoni G, Miller K, Remo A, Reghellin D, Bersani S, Gobbo S, Eccher A, Chilosi M, Bonetti F. Genotypic intratumoral heterogeneity in breast carcinoma with HER2/neu amplification: evaluation according to ASCO/CAP criteria. Am J Clin Pathol 2009, **131**: 678–682.

1078 Carbone A, Botti G, Gloghini A, Simone G, Truini M, Curcio MP, Gasparini P, Mangia A, Perin T, Salvi S, Testi A, Verderio P. Delineation of HER2 gene status in breast carcinoma by silver in situ hybridization is reproducible among laboratories and pathologists. J Mol Diagn 2008, **10**: 527–536.

1079 Correa Geyer F, Reis-Filho JS. Microarray-based gene expression profiling as a clinical tool for breast cancer management: are we there yet? Int J Surg Pathol 2009, **17**: 285–302.

1080 Cuadros M, Villegas R. Systematic review of HER2 breast cancer testing. Appl Immunohistochem Mol Morphol 2009, **17**: 1–7.

1081 Dawkins HJ, Robbins PD, Smith KL, Sarna M, Harvey JM, Sterrett GF, Papadimitriou JM. What's new in breast cancer? Molecular perspectives of cancer development and the role of the oncogene *c-erb*B-2 in prognosis and disease. Pathol Res Pract 1993, **189**: 1233–1252.

1082 De Potter CR, Schelfhout A-M. The *neu*-protein and breast cancer. Virchows Archiv 1995, **426**: 107–115.

1083 Foulkes WD, Smith IE, Reis-Filho JS. Triple-negative breast cancer. N Engl J Med 2010, **363**: 1938–1948.

1084 Gupta D, Middleton LP, Whitaker MJ, Abrams J. Comparison of fluorescence and chromogenic in situ hybridisation for detection of HER-2/neu oncogene in breast cancer. Am J Clin Pathol 2003, **119**: 381–387.

1085 Hicks DG, Kulkarni S. HER2+ breast cancer: review of biologic relevance and optimal use of diagnostic tools. Am J Clin Pathol 2008, **129**: 263–273.

1086 Hung MC, Lau YK. Basic science of HER-2/neu: a review. Sem Oncol 1999, **26**(S.12): 51–59.

1087 Kaptain S, Tan LK, Chen B. Her-2/neu and breast cancer. Diagn Mol Pathol 2001, **10**: 139–152.

1088 Lal P, Tan LK, Chen B. Correlation of HER-2 status with estrogen and progesterone receptors and histologic features in 3,655 invasive breast carcinomas. Am J Clin Pathol 2005, **123**: 541–546.

1089 Lewis F, Jackson P, Lane S, Coast G, Hanby AM. Testing for HER2 in breast cancer. Histopathology 2004, **45**: 207–217.

1090 Li-Ning-TE, Ronchetti R, Torres-Cabala C, Merino MJ. Role of chromogenic in situ hybridization (CISH) in the evaluation of HER2 status in breast carcinoma: comparison with immunohistochemistry and FISH. Int J Surg Pathol 2005, **13**: 343–351.

1091 Oakley GJ 3rd, Tubbs RR, Crowe J, Sebek B, Budd GT, Patrick RJ, Procop GW. HER-2 amplification in tubular carcinoma of the breast. Am J Clin Pathol 2006, **126**: 55–58.

1092 Papouchado BG, Myles J, Lloyd RV, Stoler M, Oliveira AM, Downs-Kelly E, Morey A, Bilous M, Nagle R, Prescott N, Wang L, Dragovich L, McElhinny A, Garcia CF, Ranger-Moore J, Free H, Powell W, Loftus M, Pettay J, Gaire F, Roberts C, Dietel M, Roche P, Grogan T, Tubbs R. Silver in situ hybridization (SISH) for determination of *HER2* gene status in breast carcinoma: comparison with FISH and assessment of interobserver reproducibility. Am J Surg Pathol 2010, **34**: 767–776.

1093 Reis-Filho JS, Tutt ANJ. Triple negative tumours: a critical review. Histopathology 2008, **52**: 108–118.

1094 Rhodes A, Jasani B, Anderson E, Dodson AR, Balaton AJ. Evaluation of HER-2/neu immunohistochemical assay sensitivity and scoring in formalin-fixed and paraffin-processed cell lines and breast tumors. A comparative study involving results from laboratories in 21 countries. Am J Clin Pathol 2002, **118**: 408–417.

1095 Rosenthal SR, Weilbaecher KN, Quigley C, Fisher DE. Comparison of HER-2/neu oncogene amplification detected by fluorescence in situ hybridisation in lobular and ductal breast cancer. Appl Immunohistochem Mol Morphol 2002, **10**: 40–46.

1096 Shin SJ, Hyjek E, Early E, Knowles DM. Intratumoral heterogeneity of her-2/neu in invasive mammary carcinomas using fluorescence in-situ hybridization and tissue microarray. Int J Surg Pathol 2006, **14**: 279–284.

1097 Smith KL, Robbins PD, Dawkins HJ, Papadimitriou JM, Redmond SL, Carrello S, Harvey JM, Sterrett GF. *c-erb*B-2 amplification in breast cancer. Detection in formalin-fixed, paraffin-embedded tissue by in situ hybridization. Hum Pathol 1994, **25**: 413–418.

1098 Suo Z, Risberg B, Karlsson MG, Villman K, Skovlund E, Nesland JM. The expression of EGFR family ligands in breast carcinomas. Int J Surg Pathol 2002, **10**: 91–99.

1099 Wolff AC, Hammond MEH, Schwartz JN, Hagerty KL, Allred DC, Cote RJ, Dowsett M, Fitzgibbons PL, Hanna WM, Langer A, McShane LM, Paik S, Pegram MD, Perez EA, Press MF, Rhodes A, Sturgeon C, Taube SE, Tubbs R, Vance GH, van de Vijver M, Wheeler TM, Hayes DF. American Society of Clinical Oncology/College of American Pathologists guideline recommendations for human epidermal growth factor receptor 2 testing in breast cancer. J Clin Oncol 2007, **25**: 118–145.

1100 Zhao J, Wu R, Au A, Marquez A, Yu Y, Shi Z. Determination of HER2 gene amplification by chromogenic in situ hybridization (CISH) in archival breast carcinoma. Mod Pathol 2002, **15**: 657–665.

MOLECULAR GENETICS AND MOLECULAR CLASSIFICATION OF BREAST CANCER

MOLECULAR GENETICS

1101 Arrick BA. Breast cancer. In Mendelsohn J, Howley PM, Israel MA, Gray JW, Thompson CB (eds): The molecular basis of cancer, ed. 3. Philadelphia, 2008, Saunders, pp. 423–429.

1102 Pfeifer JD. Breast. In Pfeifer JD (ed.) Molecular genetic testing in surgical pathology. Philadelphia, 2006, Lippincott Williams & Wilkins, pp. 401–414.

MOLECULAR CLASSIFICATION

1103 Cheang MC, Voduc D, Bajdik C, Leung S, McKinney S, Chia SK, Perou CM, Nielsen TO. Basal-like breast cancer defined by five biomarkers has superior prognostic value than triple-negative phenotype. Clin Cancer Res 2008, **14**: 1368–1376.

1104 Cheang MC, Chia SK, Voduc D, Gao D, Leung S, Snider J, Watson M, Davies S, Bernard PS, Parker JS, Perou CM, Ellis MJ, Nielsen TO. Ki67 index, HER2 status, and prognosis of patients with luminal B breast cancer. J Natl Cancer Inst 2009, **101**: 736–750.

1105 Constantinidou A, Jones RL, Reis-Filho JS. Beyond triple-negative breast cancer: the need to define new subtypes. Expert Rev Anticancer Ther 2010, **10**: 1197–1213.

1106 Correa Geyer F, Reis-Filho JS. Microarray-based gene expression profiling as a clinical tool for breast cancer management: are we there yet? Int J Surg Pathol 2009, **17**: 285–302.

1107 Farmer P, Bonnefoi H, Becette V, Tubiana-Hulin M, Fumoleau P, Larsimont D, Macgrogan G, Bergh J, Cameron D, Goldstein D, Duss S, Nicoulaz AL, Brisken C, Fiche M, Delorenzi M, Iggo R. Identification of molecular apocrine breast tumours by microarray analysis. Oncogene 2005, **24**: 4660–4671.

1108 He YD, Friend SH. Microarrays – the 21st century divining rod? Nat Med 2001, **7**: 658–659.

1109 Kim K, Zakharkin SO, Allison DB. Expectations, validity, and reality in gene expression profiling. J Clin Epidemiol 2010, **63**: 950–959.

1110 Moinfar F. Is 'basal-like' carcinoma of the breast a distinct clinicopathological entity? A critical review with cautionary notes. Pathobiology 2008, **75**: 119–131.

1111 Perou CM, Sorlie T, Eisen MB, van de Rijn M, Jeffrey SS, Rees CA, Pollack JR, Ross DT, Johnsen H, Akslen LA, Fluge O, Pergamenschikov A, Williams C, Zhu SX, Lonning PE, Borresen-Dale AL, Brown PO, Botstein D. Molecular portraits of human breast tumours. Nature 2000, **406**: 747–752.

1112 Schnitt SJ. Will molecular classification replace traditional breast pathology? Int J Surg Pathol 2010, **18**: 162S–166S.

1113 Sorlie T, Perou CM, Tibshirani R, Aas T, Geisler S, Johnsen H, Hastie T, Eisen MB, van de Rijn M, Jeffrey SS, Thorsen T, Quist H, Matese JC, Brown PO, Botstein D, Eystein Lonning P, Borresen-Dale AL. Gene expression patterns of breast carcinomas distinguish tumor subclasses with clinical implications. Proc Natl Acad Sci U S A 2001, **98**: 10869–10874.

1114 Tang P, Skinner KA, Hicks DG. Molecular classification of breast carcinomas by immunohistochemical analysis: are we ready? Diagn Mol Pathol 2009, **18**: 125–132.

1115 Tavassoli FA. Correlation between gene expression profiling-based molecular and morphologic classification of breast cancer. Int J Surg Pathol 2010, **18**: 167S–169S.

1116 Weigelt B, Horlings HM, Kreike B, Hayes MM, Hauptmann M, Wessels LF, de Jong D, Van de Vijver MJ, Van't Veer LJ, Peterse JL. Refinement of breast cancer classification by molecular characterization of histological special types. J Pathol 2008, **216**: 141–150.

1117 Weigelt B, Mackay A, A'Hern R, Natrajan R, Tan DS, Dowsett M, Ashworth A, Reis-Filho JS. Breast cancer molecular profiling with single sample predictors: a retrospective analysis. Lancet Oncol 2010, **11**: 339–349.

SPREAD AND METASTASES

1118 Bitter MA, Fiorito D, Corkill ME, Huffer WE, Stemmer SM, Shpall EJ, Archer PG, Franklin WA. Bone marrow involvement by lobular carcinoma of the breast cannot be identified reliably by routine histological examination alone. Hum Pathol 1994, **25**: 781–788.

1119 Braun S, Pantel K, Muller P, Janni W, Hepp F, Kentenich CR, Gastroph S, Wischnik A, Dimpfl T, Kindermann G, Riethmuller G, Schlimok G. Cytokeratin-positive cells in the bone marrow and survival of patients with stage I, II, or III breast cancer. N Engl J Med 2000, **342**: 525–533.

1120 Braun S, Vogl FD, Naume B, Janni W, Osborne MP, Coombes RC, Schlimok G, Diel IJ, Gerber B, Gebauer G, Pierga JY, Marth C, Oruzio D, Wiedswang G, Solomayer EF, Kundt G, Strobl B, Fehm T, Wong GYC, Bliss J, Vincent-Salomon A, Pantel K. A pooled analysis of bone marrow micrometastasis in breast cancer. N Engl J Med 2005, **353**: 793–802.

1121 Brinkley D, Haybittle JL. The curability of breast cancer. Lancet 1975, **2**: 95–97.

1122 Chaubert P, Hurlimann J. Mammary origin of metastases. Immunohistochemical determination. Arch Pathol Lab Med 1992, **116**: 1181–1188.

1123 Cifuentes N, Pickren JW. Metastases from carcinoma of mammary gland. An autopsy study. J Surg Oncol 1979, **11**: 193–205.

1124 Cohn M, Middleton L, Valero V, Sahin A. Gastrointestinal metastases of carcinoma of the breast [abstract]. Mod Pathol 2003, **16**: 26a.

1125 Connolly JL, Schnitt SJ. Evaluation of breast biopsy specimens in patients considered for treatment by conservative surgery and radiation therapy for early breast cancer. Pathol Annu 1988, **23**(Pt 1): 1–23.

1126 Cote RJ, Rosen PP, Hakes TB, Sedira M, Bazinet M, Kinne DW, Old LJ, Osborne MP. Monoclonal antibodies detect occult breast carcinoma metastases in the bone marrow of patients with early stage disease. Am J Surg Pathol 1988, **12**: 333–340.

1127 Cummings OW, Mazur MT. Breast carcinoma diffusely metastatic to the spleen. A report of two cases presenting as idiopathic thrombocytopenic purpura. Am J Clin Pathol 1992, **97**: 484–489.

1128 Damiani S, Peterse JL, Eusebi V. Malignant neoplasms infiltrating 'pseudoangiomatous' stromal hyperplasia of the breast: an unrecognised pathway of tumour spread. Histopathology 2002, **41**: 208–215.

1129 Datta YH, Adams PT, Drobyski WR, Ethier SP, Terry VH, Roth MS. Sensitive detection of occult breast cancer by the reverse-transcriptase polymerase chain reaction. J Clin Oncol 1994, **12**: 475–482.

1130 Donegan WL. The influence of untreated internal mammary metastases upon the course of mammary cancer. Cancer 1977, **39**: 533–538.

1131 Fisher B, Montague E, Redmond C, Barton B, Borland D, Fisher ER, Deutsch M, Schwarz G, Margolese R, Donegan W, Volk H, Honvolinka C, Gardner B, Cohn I Jr, Lesnick G, Cruz AB, Lawrence W, Nealon T, Butcher H, Lawton R. Comparison of radical mastectomy with alternative treatments for primary breast cancer. A first report of results from a prospective randomized clinical trial. Cancer 1977, **39**: 2827–2839.

1132 Gagnon Y, Tetu B. Ovarian metastases of breast carcinoma: a clinicopathologic study of 59 cases. Cancer 1989, **64**: 892–898.

1133 Gal S, Fidler C, Lo YM, Chin K, Moore J, Harris AL, Wainscoat JS. Detection of mammoglobin mRNA in the plasma of breast cancer patients. Ann N Y Acad Sci 2001, **945**: 192–194.

1134 Gilliland MD, Barton RM, Copeland EM III. The implications of local recurrence of breast cancer as the first site of therapeutic failure. Ann Surg 1983, **197**: 284–287.

1135 Goldstein NS. Does the level of E-cadherin expression correlate with the primary breast carcinoma infiltration pattern and type of systemic metastases? Am J Clin Pathol 2002, **118**: 425–434.

1136 Grunewald K, Haun M, Urbanek M, Fiegl M, Muller-Holzner E, Gunsilus E, Dunser M, Marth C, Gastl G. Mammaglobin gene expression: a superior marker of breast cancer cells in peripheral blood in comparison to epidermal-growth factor receptor and cytokeratin-19. Lab Invest 2000, **80**: 1071–1077.

1137 Hasebe T, Imoto S, Yokose T, Ishii G, Iwasaki M, Wada N. Histopathologic factors significantly associated with initial organ-specific metastasis by invasive ductal carcinoma of the breast: a prospective study. Hum Pathol 2008, **39**: 681–693.

1138 Hicks DG, Short SM, Prescott NL, Tarr SM, Coleman KA, Yoder BJ, Crowe JP, Choueiri TK, Dawson AE, Budd GT, Tubbs RR, Casey G, Weil RJ. Breast cancers with brain metastases are more likely to be estrogen receptor negative, express the basal cytokeratin CK5/6, and overexpress HER2 or EGFR. Am J Surg Pathol 2006, **30**: 1097–1104.

1139 Ingle JN, Tormey DC, Tan HK. The bone marrow examination in breast cancer. Diagnostic considerations and clinical usefulness. Cancer 1978, **41**: 670–674.

1140 Jayson GC, Howell A, Harris M, Morgenstern G, Chang J, Ryder WD. Carcinomatous meningitis in patients with breast cancer. An aggressive disease variant. Cancer 1994, **74**: 3135–3141.

1141 Johnson JE, Page DL, Winfield AC, Reynolds VH, Sawyers JL. Recurrent mammary carcinoma after local excision. A segmental problem. Cancer 1995, **75**: 1612–1618.

1142 Koren R, Kyzer S, Paz A, Veltman V, Klein B, Gal R. Lymph node revealing solution: a new method for detection of minute axillary lymph nodes in breast cancer specimens. Am J Surg Pathol 1997, **21**: 1387–1390.

1143 Lagios MD, Gates EA, Westdahl PR, Richards V, Alpert BS. A guide to the frequency of nipple involvement in breast cancer. A study of 149 consecutive mastectomies using a serial subgross and correlated radiographic technique. Am J Surg 1979, **138**: 135–142.

1144 Lamovec J, Zidar A. Association of leptomeningeal carcinomatosis in carcinoma of the breast with infiltrating lobular carcinoma. An autopsy study. Arch Pathol Lab Med 1991, **115**: 507–510.

1145 Landys K. Prognostic value of bone marrow biopsy in breast cancer. Cancer 1982, **49**: 513–518.

1146 Leong C, Boyages J, Jayasinghe UW, Bilous M, Ung O, Chua B, Salisbury E, Wong AY. Effect of margins on ipsilateral breast tumor recurrence after breast conservation therapy for lymph node-negative breast carcinoma. Cancer 2004, **100**: 1823–1832.

1147 Lyda MH, Tetef M, Carter NH, Ikle D, Weiss LM, Arber DA. Keratin immunohistochemistry detects clinically significant metastasis in bone marrow biopsy specimens in women with lobular breast carcinoma. Am J Surg Pathol 2000, **24**: 1593–1599.

1148 Merino MJ, LiVolsi VA. Signet ring carcinoma of the female breast. A clinicopathologic analysis of 24 cases. Cancer 1981, **48**: 1830–1837.

1149 Merrill CF, Kaufman DI, Dimitrov NV. Breast cancer metastatic to the eye is a common entity. Cancer 1991, **68**: 623–627.

1150 Miller RE. Breast cancer and meningioma. J Surg Oncol 1986, **31**: 182–183.

1151 Monteagudo C, Merino MJ, La Porte N, Neumann RD. Value of gross cystic disease fluid protein-15 in distinguishing metastatic breast carcinomas among poorly differentiated neoplasms involving the ovary. Hum Pathol 1991, **22**: 368–372.

1152 Morimoto T, Komaki K, Inui K, Umemoto A, Yamamoto H, Harada K, Inoue K. Involvement of nipple and areola in early breast cancer. Cancer 1985, **55**: 2459–2463.

1153 Noguchi S, Aihara T, Nakamori S, Motomura K, Inaji H, Imaoka S, Koyama H. The detection of breast carcinoma micrometastases in axillary lymph nodes by means of reverse transcriptase-polymerase chain reaction. Cancer 1994, **74**: 1595–1600.

1154 Nonaka D, Chiriboga L, Soslow RA. Expression of pax8 as a useful marker in distinguishing ovarian carcinomas from mammary carcinomas. Am J Surg Pathol 2008, **32**: 1566–1571.

1155 Ozbas S, Dafydd H, Purushotham AD. Bone marrow micrometastasis in breast cancer. Br J Surg 2003, **90**: 290–301.

1156 Porro G, Menard S, Tagliabue E, Orefice S, Salvadori B, Squicciarini P, Andreola S, Rilke F, Colnaghi MI. Monoclonal antibody detection of carcinoma cells in bone marrow biopsy specimens from breast cancer patients. Cancer 1988, **61**: 2407–2411.

1157 Price JE. The biology of metastatic breast cancer. Cancer 1990, **66**: 1313–1320.

1158 Rosen PP, Fracchia AA, Urban JA, Schattenfeld D, Robbins GF. 'Residual' mammary carcinoma following simulated partial mastectomy. Cancer 1975, **35**: 739–747.

1159 Schmidt WA, Boudoussquie AC, Vetto JT, Pommier RF, Alexander P, Thurmond A, Scanlan RM, Jones MK. Lymph nodes in the human female breast: a review of their detection and significance. Hum Pathol 2001, **32**: 178–187.

1160 Sethi S, Carter D. Breast carcinoma associated with necrotic granulomas in axillary lymph nodes. Ann Diagn Pathol 1998, **2**: 370–376.

1161 Takeda Y, Tsuta K, Shibuki Y, Hoshino T, Tochigi N, Maeshima AM, Asamura H, Sasajima Y, Ito T, Matsuno Y. Analysis of expression patterns of breast cancer-specific markers (mammaglobin and gross cystic disease fluid protein 15) in lung and pleural tumors. Arch Pathol Lab Med 2008, **132**: 239–243.

1162 Tornos C, Soslow R, Chen S, Akram M, Hummer AJ, Abu-Rustum N, Norton L, Tan LK. Expression of WT1, CA 125, and GCDFP-15 as useful markers in the differential diagnosis of primary ovarian carcinomas versus metastatic breast cancer to the ovary. Am J Surg Pathol 2005, **29**: 1482–1489.

1163 van Velthuysen ML, Taal BG, van der Hoeven JJ, Peterse JL. Expression of oestrogen receptor and loss of E-cadherin are diagnostic for gastric metastasis of breast carcinoma. Histopathology 2005, **46**: 153–157.

1164 Veronesi U, Cascinelli N, Bufalino R, Morabito A, Greco M, Galluzzo D, Delle Donne V, DeLellis R, Piotti P, Sacchini V, Conti R, Clemente C. Risk of internal mammary lymph node metastases and its relevance on prognosis of breast cancer patients. Ann Surg 1983, **198**: 681–684.

1165 Veronesi U, Marubini E, Del Vecchio M, Manzari A, Andreola S, Greco M, Luini A, Merson M, Saccozzi R, Rilke F, Salvadori B. Local recurrences and distant metastases after conservative breast cancer treatments: partly independent events. J Natl Cancer Inst 1995, **87**: 19–27.

1166 Wertheim U, Ozzello L. Neoplastic involvement of nipple and skin flap in carcinoma of the breast. Am J Surg Pathol 1980, **4**: 543–549.

OCCULT BREAST CARCINOMA

1167 Ashikari R, Rosen PP, Urban JA, Senoo T. Breast cancer presenting as an axillary mass. Ann Surg 1976, **183**: 415–417.

1168 Ishag MT, Baschinsky DY, Beliava IV, Niemann TH, Marsh WL Jr. Pathologic findings in reduction mammaplasty specimens. Am J Clin Pathol 2003, **120**: 377–380.

1169 Lloyd MS, Nash AG. 'Occult' breast cancer. Ann R Coll Surg Engl 2001, **83**: 420–424.

1170 Merson M, Andreola S, Galimberti V, Bufalino R, Marchini S, Veronesi U. Breast carcinoma presenting as axillary metastases without evidence of a primary tumor. Cancer 1992, **70**: 504–508.

1171 Rosen PP, Kimmel M. Occult breast carcinoma presenting with axillary lymph node metastases. A follow-up study of 48 patients. Hum Pathol 1990, **21**: 518–523.

SENTINEL LYMPH NODE

1172 Allred DC, Elledge RM. Caution concerning micrometastatic breast carcinoma in sentinel lymph nodes. Cancer 1999, **86**: 905–907.

1173 Beach RA, Lawson D, Waldrop SM, Cohen C. Rapid immunohistochemistry for cytokeratin in the intraoperative evaluation of sentinel lymph nodes for metastatic breast carcinoma. Appl Immunohistochem Mol Morphol 2003, **11**: 45–50.

1174 Bold RJ. Standardization of sentinel lymph node biopsy in breast carcinoma. Cancer 2005, **103**: 444–446.

1175 Cao Y, Paner GP, Rajan PB. Sentinel node status and tumor characteristics: a study of 234 invasive breast carcinomas. Arch Pathol Lab Med 2005, **129**: 82–84.

1176 Carter BA, Jensen RA, Simpson JF, Page DL. Benign transport of breast epithelium into axillary lymph nodes after biopsy. Am J Clin Pathol 2000, **113**: 259–265.

1177 Cohen C, Alazraki N, Styblo T, Waldrop SM, Grant SF, Larsen T. Immunohistochemical evaluation of sentinel lymph nodes in breast carcinoma patients. Appl Immunohistochem Mol Morphol 2002, **10**: 296–303.

1178 Corben AD, Nehhozina T, Garg K, Vallejo CE, Brogi E. Endosalpingiosis in axillary lymph nodes: a possible pitfall in the staging of patients with breast carcinoma. Am J Surg Pathol 2010, **34**: 1211–1216.

1179 Creager AJ, Geisinger KR. Intraoperative evaluation of sentinel lymph nodes for breast carcinoma: current methodologies. Adv Anat Pathol 2002, **9**: 233–243.

1180 Cserni G. Evaluation of sentinel lymph nodes in breast cancer. Histopathology 2005, **46**: 697–702.

1181 de Boer M, van Deurzen CH, van Dijck JA, Borm GF, van Diest PJ, Adang EM, Nortier JW, Rutgers EJ, Seynaeve C, Menke-Pluymers MB, Bult P, Tjan-Heijnen VC. Micrometastases or isolated tumor cells and the outcome of breast cancer. N Engl J Med 2009, **361**: 653–663.

1182 Diaz LK, Hunt K, Ames F, Meric F, Kuerer H, Babiera G, Ross M, Singletary E, Middleton LP, Symmans WF, Kirshnamurthy S, Sahin A, Sneige N, Gilcrease MZ. Histologic localization of sentinel lymph node metastases in breast cancer. Am J Surg Pathol 2003, **27**: 385–389.

1183 Diaz NM, Cox CE, Ebert M, Clark JD, Vrcel V, Stowell N, Sharma A, Jakub JW, Cantor A, Centeno BA, Dupont E, Muro-Cacho C, Nicosia S. Benign mechanical transport of breast epithelial cells to sentinel lymph nodes. Am J Surg Pathol 2004, **28**: 1641–1645.

1184 Douglas-Jones AG, Woods V. Molecular assessment of sentinel lymph node in breast cancer management. Histopathology 2009, **55**: 107–113.

1185 Freneaux P, Nos C, Vincent-Salomon A, Genin P, Sigal-Zafrani B, Al Ghuzian A, Birolini MJ, Clough K, Sastre-Garau X. Histological detection of minimal metastatic involvement in axillary sentinel nodes: a rational basis for a sensitive methodology usable in daily practice. Mod Pathol 2002, **15**: 641–646.

1186 Jani AB, Basu A, Heimann R, Hellman S. Sentinel lymph node versus axillary lymph node dissection for early-stage breast carcinoma: a comparison using a utility-adjusted number needed to treat analysis. Cancer 2003, **97**: 359–366.

1187 Johnston EI, Beach RA, Waldrop SM, Lawson D, Cohen C. Rapid intraoperative immunohistochemical evaluation of sentinel lymph nodes for metastatic breast carcinoma. Appl Immunohistochem Mol Morphol 2006, **14**: 57–62.

1188 Jonjic N, Mustac E, Dekanic A, Marijic B, Gaspar B, Kolic I, Coklo M, Sasso F. Predicting sentinel lymph node metastases in infiltrating breast carcinoma with vascular invasion. Int J Surg Pathol 2006, **14**: 306–311.

1189 Krag D, Weaver D, Ashikaga T, Moffat F, Klimberg VS, Shriver C, Feldman S, Kusminsky R, Gadd M, Kuhn J, Harlow S, Beitsch P. The sentinel node in breast: a multicenter validation study. N Engl J Med 1998, **339**: 941–946.

1190 Krogerus LA, Leidenius MH, Toivonen TS, von Smitten KJ. Towards reasonable workload in diagnosis of sentinel lymph nodes: comparison of two frozen section methods. Histopathology 2004, **44**: 29–34.

1191 Leikola JP, Toivonen TS, Krogerus LA, von Smitten KA, Leidenius MH. Rapid immunohistochemistry enhances the intraoperative diagnosis of sentinel lymph node metastases in invasive lobular breast carcinoma. Cancer 2005, **104**: 14–19.

1192 McMasters KM, Giuliano AE, Ross MI, Reintgen DS, Hunt KK, Byrd DR, Klimberg VS, Whitworth PW, Tafra LC, Edwards MJ. Sentinel-lymph-node biopsy for breast cancer – not yet the standard of care. N Engl J Med 1998, **339**: 990–995.

1193 Maiorano E, Massarol GM, Pruneri G, Mastropasqua MG, Zurrida S, Orvieto E, Viale G. Ectopic breast tissue as a possible cause of false-positive axillary sentinel lymph node biopsies. Am J Surg Pathol 2003, **27**: 513–518.

1194 Moore KH, Thaler HT, Tan LK, Borgen PI, Cody HS 3rd. Immunohistochemically detected tumor cells in the sentinel lymph nodes of patients with breast carcinoma: biologic metastasis or procedural artifact? Cancer 2004, **100**: 929–934.

1195 Ouellette RJ, Richard D, Maïcas E. RT-PCR for mammaglobin genes, *MGB1* and *MGB2*, identifies breast cancer micrometastases in sentinel lymph nodes. Am J Clin Pathol 2004, **121**: 637–643.

1196 Piñero A, Giménez J, Merck B, Vázquez C; Grupo de Expertos. [Consensus meeting about sentinel lymph node selective biopsy in breast cancer. Spanish Society of Senology and Breast Pathology]. Rev Esp Patol 2007, **40**: 91–95.

1197 Reintgen D, Giuliano R, Cox CE. Sentinel node biopsy in breast cancer: an overview. Breast J 2000, **6**: 299–305.

1198 Rivera M, Merlin S, Hoda RS, Gopalan A, Hoda SA. Minimal involvement of sentinel lymph node in breast carcinoma: prevailing concepts and challenging problems. Int J Surg Pathol 2004, **12**: 301–306; Viale G. An alternative viewpoint. Int J Surg Pathol 2004, **12**: 307–309.

1199 Sahin AA, Guray M, Hunt KK. Identification and biologic significance of micrometastases in axillary lymph nodes in patients with invasive breast cancer. Arch Pathol Lab Med 2009, **133**: 869–878.

1200 Schwartz GF, Giuliano AE, Veronesi U; Consensus Conference Committee. Proceedings of the consensus conference on the role of sentinel lymph node biopsy in carcinoma of the breast, April 19–22, 2001, Philadelphia, Pennsylvania. Hum Pathol 2002, **33**: 579–589.

1201 Silverberg SG. Sentinel node processing: recommendations for pathologists. Am J Surg Pathol 2002, **26**: 383–385.

1202 Taback B, Hashimoto K, Kuo CT, Chan A, Giuliano AE, Hoon DS. Molecular lymphatic mapping of the sentinel lymph node. Am J Pathol 2002, **161**: 1153–1161.

1203 Turner RR, Ollila DW, Stern S, Giuliano AE. Optimal histopathologic examination of the sentinel lymph node for breast carcinoma staging. Am J Surg Pathol 1999, **23**: 263–267.

1204 van Deurzen CH, de Bruin PC, Koelemij R, Hillegersberg R, van Diest PJ. Isolated tumor cells in breast cancer sentinel lymph nodes: displacement or metastases? An immunohistochemical study. Hum Pathol 2009, **40**: 778–782.

1205 van Deurzen CH, Bult P, de Boer M, Koelemij R, van Hillegersberg R, Tjan-Heijnen VC, Hobbelink MG, de Bruin PC, van Diest PJ. Morphometry of isolated tumor cells in breast cancer sentinel lymph nodes: metastases or displacement? Am J Surg Pathol 2009, **33**: 106–110.

1206 Veronesi U, Paganelli G, Viale G, Galimberti V, Luini A, Zurrida S, Robertson C, Sacchini V, Veronesi P, Orvieto E, de Cicco C, Intra M, Tosi G, Scarpa D. Sentinel lymph node biopsy and axillary dissection in breast cancer: results in a large series. J Natl Cancer Inst 1999, **91**: 368–373.

1207 Viale G, Bosari S, Mazzorol G, Galimberti V, Luini A, Veronesi P, Paganelli G, Bedoni M, Orvieto E. Intraoperative examination of axillary sentinel lymph nodes in breast carcinoma patients. Cancer 1999, **85**: 2433–2438.

1208 Viale G, Zurrida S, Maiorano E, Mazzarol G, Pruneri G, Paganelli G, Maisonneuve P, Veronesi U. Predicting the status of axillary sentinel lymph nodes in 4351 patients with invasive breast carcinoma treated in a single institution. Cancer 2005, **103**: 492–500.

1209 Viale G, Mastropasqua MG, Maiorano E, Mazzarol G. Pathologic examination of the axillary sentinel lymph nodes in patients with early-stage breast carcinoma: current and resolving controversies on the basis of the European Institute of Oncology experience. Virchows Arch 2006, **448**: 241–247.

1210 Weaver DL, Le UP, Dupuis SL, Weaver KA, Harlow SP, Ashikaga T, Krag DN. Metastasis detection in sentinel lymph nodes: comparison of a limited widely spaced (NSABP protocol B-32) and a comprehensive narrowly spaced paraffin block sectioning strategy. Am J Surg Pathol 2009, **33**: 1583–1589.

1211 Weaver DL. Sentinel lymph nodes and breast carcinoma. Which micrometastases are clinically significant? Am J Surg Pathol 2003, **27**: 842–845.

STAGING AND GRADING

1212 Kinne DW. Staging and follow-up of breast cancer patients. Cancer 1991, **67**: 1196–1198.

THERAPY

1213 Ben-David MA, Kleer CG, Paramagul C, Griffith KA, Pierce LJ. Is lobular carcinoma in situ as a component of breast carcinoma a risk factor for local failure after breast-conserving therapy? Results of a matched pair analysis. Cancer 2006, **106**: 28–34.

1214 Bonadonna G, Valagussa P, Brambilla C, Moliterni A, Zambetti M, Ferrari L. Adjuvant and neoadjuvant treatment of breast cancer with chemotherapy and/or endocrine therapy. Semin Oncol 1991, **18**: 515–524.

1215 Bonadonna G, Valagussa P, Moliterni A, Zambetti M, Brambilla C. Adjuvant cyclophosphamide, methotrexate, and fluorouracil in node-positive breast cancer. The results of 20 years of follow-up. N Engl J Med 1995, **332**: 901–906.

1216 Bonadonna G, Veronesi U, Brambilla C, Ferrari L, Luini A, Greco M, Bartoli C, Coopmans de Yoldi G, Zucali R, Rilke F, et al. Primary chemotherapy to avoid mastectomy in tumors with diameters of three centimeters or more. J Natl Cancer Inst 1990, **82**: 1539–1545.

1217 Brufsky A. Trastuzumab-based therapy for patients with HER2-positive breast cancer: from early scientific development to foundation of care. Am J Clin Oncol 2010, **33**: 186–195.

1218 Ceilley E, Jagsi R, Goldberg S, Kachnic L, Powell S, Taghian A. The management of ductal carcinoma in situ in North America and Europe. Results of a survey. Cancer 2004, **101**: 1958–1967.

1219 Coleman RE. High dose chemotherapy: rationale and results in breast carcinoma. Cancer 2000, **88**: 3059–3064.

1220 Connolly JL, Boyages J, Nixon AJ, Peiro G, Gage I, Silver B, Recht A, Harris JR, Schnitt SJ. Predicators of breast recurrence after conservative surgery and radiation therapy for invasive breast cancer. Mod Pathol 1998, **11**: 134–139.

1221 Early Breast Cancer Trialists' Collaborative Group. Tamoxifen for early breast cancer. An overview of the randomised trials. Lancet 1998, **351**: 1451–1467.

1222 Emery J, Spanier SS, Kasnic G Jr, Hardt NS. The synovial structure of breast-implant associated bursae. Mod Pathol 1994, **7**: 728–733.

1223 Fong PC, Boss DS, Yap TA, Tutt A, Wu P, Mergui-Roelvink M, Mortimer P, Swaisland H, Lau A, O'Connor MJ, Ashworth A, Carmichael J, Kaye SB, Schellens JH, de Bono JS. Inhibition of poly(ADP-ribose) polymerase in tumors from BRCA mutation carriers. N Engl J Med 2009, **361**: 123–134.

1224 Frykberg ER, Bland KI. Overview of the biology and management of ductal carcinoma in situ of the breast. Cancer 1994, **74**: 350–361.

1225 Fyles AW, McCready DR, Manchul LA, Trudeau ME, Merante P, Pintilie M, Weir LM, Olivotto IA. Tamoxifen with or without breast irradiation in women 50 years of age or older with early breast cancer. N Engl J Med 2004, **351**: 963–970.

1226 Goldhirsch A, Wood WC, Gelber RD, Coates AS, Thurlimann B, Senn HJ. Meeting highlights: updated international expert consensus on the primary therapy of early breast cancer. J Clin Oncol 2003, **21**: 3357–3365.

1227 Goldstein NS, Kestin L, Vicini F. Factors associated with ipsilateral breast failure and distant metastases in patients with invasive breast carcinoma treated with breast-conserving therapy. Am J Clin Pathol 2003, **120**: 500–527.

1228 Hameed MR, Erlandson R, Rosen PP. Capsular synovial-like hyperplasia around mammary implants similar to detritic synovitis. A morphologic and immunohistochemical study of 15 cases. Am J Surg Pathol 1995, **19**: 433–438.

1229 Hughes KS, Schnaper LA, Berry D, Cirrincione C, McCormick B, Shank B, Wheeler J, Champion LA, Smith TJ, Smith BL, Shapiro C, Muss HB, Winer E, Hudis C, Wood W, Sugarbaker D, Henderson IC, Norton L; Cancer and Leukemia Group B; Radiation Therapy Oncology Group; Eastern Cooperative Oncology Group. Lumpectomy plus tamoxifen with or without irradiation in women 70 years of age or older with early breast cancer. N Engl J Med 2004, **351**: 971–977.

1230 Jacobson JA, Danforth DN, Cowan KH, D'Angelo T, Steinberg SM, Pierce L, Lippman ME, Lichter AS, Glatstein E, Okunieff P. Ten-year results of a comparison of conservation with mastectomy in the treatment of stage I and II breast cancer. New Engl J Med 1995, **332**: 907–911.

1231 Kasper CS. Histologic features of breast capsules reflect surface configuration and composition of silicone bag implants. Am J Clin Pathol 1994, **102**: 655–659.

1232 Kinne DW. Surgical management of stage I and stage II breast cancer. Cancer 1990, **66**: 1373–1377.

1233 Kitchen SB, Paletta CE, Shehadi SI, Bauer WC. Epithelialization of the lining of a breast implant capsule. Possible origins of squamous cell carcinoma associated with a breast implant capsule. Cancer 1994, **73**: 1449–1452.

1234 Liu LW, Truong LD. Morphologic characterization of polyvinyl sponge (Ivalon) breast prosthesis. Arch Pathol Lab Med 1996, **120**: 876–878.

1235 McGuire WP. High-dose chemotherapy and autologous bone marrow or stem cell reconstruction for solid tumors. Curr Probl Cancer 1998, **22**: 135–177.

1236 Mansfield CM, Krishnan L, Komarnicky LT, Ayyangar KM, Kramer CA. A review of the role of radiation therapy in the treatment of patients with breast cancer. Semin Oncol 1991, **18**: 525–535.

1237 Meric F, Mirza NQ, Vlastos G, Buchholz TA, Kuerer HM, Babiera GV, Singletary SE, Ross MI, Ames FC, Feig BW, Krishnamurthy S, Perkins GH, McNeese MD, Strom EA, Valero V, Hunt KK. Positive surgical margins and ipsilateral breast tumor recurrence predict disease-specific survival after breast-conserving therapy. Cancer 2003, **97**: 926–933.

1238 Morrow M, Strom EA, Bassett LW, Dershaw DD, Fowble B, Giuliano A, Harris JR, O'Malley F, Schnitt SJ, Singletary SE, Winchester DP. Standard for breast conservation therapy in the management of invasive breast carcinoma. CA Cancer J Clin 2002, **52**: 277–300.

1239 National Institutes of Health Consensus Development Panel. National Institutes of Health consensus development conference statement: adjuvant therapy for breast cancer, November 1–3, 2000. J Natl Cancer Inst 2001, **93**: 979–989.

1240 Olivotto IA, Bajdik CD, Plenderleith IH, Coppin CM, Gelmon KA, Jackson SM, Ragaz J, Wilson KS, Worth A. Adjuvant systemic therapy and survival after breast cancer. N Engl J Med 1994, **330**: 805–810.

1241 Osborne CK. Tamoxifen in the treatment of breast cancer. N Engl J Med 1998, **339**: 1609–1618.

1242 Park CC, Mitsumori M, Nixon A, Recht A, Connolly J, Gelman R, Silver B, Hetelekidis S, Abner A, Harris YR, Schnitt ST. Outcome at 8 years after breast-conserving surgery and radiation therapy for invasive breast cancer: influence of margin status and systemic therapy on local recurrence. J Clin Oncol 2000, **18**: 1668–1675.

1243 Romond EH, Perez EA, Bryant J, Suman VJ, Geyer CE Jr, Davidson NE, Tan-Chiu E, Martino S, Paik S, Kaufman PA, Swain SM, Pisansky TM, Fehrenbacher L, Kutteh LA, Vogel VG, Visscher DW, Yothers G, Jenkins RB, Brown AM, Dakhil SR, Mamounas EP, Lingle WL, Klein PM, Ingle JN, Wolmark N. Trastuzumab plus adjuvant chemotherapy for operable HER2-positive breast cancer. N Engl J Med 2005, **353**: 1673–1684.

1244 Rosner D, Lane WW. Should all patients with node-negative breast cancer receive adjuvant therapy? Identifying additional subsets of low-risk patients who are highly curable by surgery alone. Cancer 1991, **68**: 1482–1494.

1245 Rosti G, Ferrante P, Ledermann J, Leyvraz S, Ladenstein R, Koscileniak E, Crown J, Dazzi C, Cariello A, Marangolo M. High-dose chemotherapy for solid tumors: results of the EBMT. Crit Rev Oncol Hematol 2002, **41**: 129–140.

1246 Schnitt SJ, Abner A, Gelman R, Connolly JL, Recht A, Duda RB, Eberlein TJ, Mayzel K, Silver B, Harris JR. The relationship between microscopic margins of resection and the risk of local recurrence in patients with breast cancer treated with breast-conserving surgery and radiation therapy. Cancer 1994, **74**: 1746–1751.

1247 Silverstein MJ, Gierson ED, Colburn WJ, Cope LM, Furmanski M, Senofsky GM, Gamagami P, Waisman JR. Can intraductal breast carcinoma be excised completely by local excision? Clinical and pathologic predictors. Cancer 1994, **73**: 2985–2989.

1248 Solin LJ, Recht A, Fourquet A, Kurtz J, Kuske R, McNeese M, McCormick B, Cross MA, Schultz DJ, Bornstein BA, et al. Ten-year results of breast-conserving surgery and definitive irradiation for intraductal carcinoma (ductal carcinoma in situ) of the breast. Cancer 1991, **68**: 2337–2344.

1249 Veronesi U. How important is the assessment of resection margins in conservative surgery for breast cancer? Cancer 1994, **74**: 1660–1661.

1250 Veronesi U, Cascinelli N, Mariani L, Greco M, Saccozzi R, Luini A, Aguiler M, Marubini E. Twenty-year follow-up of a randomized study comparing breast-conserving surgery with radical mastectomy for early breast cancer. N Engl J Med 2002, **347**: 1227–1232.

1251 Voogd AC, van Tienhoven G, Peterse HL, Crommelin MA, Rutgers EJ, van de Velde CJ, van Geel BN, Slot A, Rodrigus PT, Jobsen JJ, Von Meyenfeldt MF, Coebegh JW, for the Dutch Study Group on Local Recurrence after Breast Conservation (BORST). Local recurrence after breast conservation therapy for early stage breast carcinoma. Detection, treatment, and outcome in 266 patients. Cancer 1999, **85**: 437–446.

1252 Wong K, Henderson IC. Management of metastatic breast cancer. World J Surg 1994, **18**: 98–111.

EFFECTS OF THERAPY ON THE TUMOR AND ON NORMAL BREAST

1253 Aktepe F, Kapucuoglu N, Pak I. The effects of chemotherapy on breast cancer tissue in locally advanced breast cancer. Histopathology 1996, **29**: 63–67.

1254 Frierson HF Jr, Fechner RE. Histologic grade of locally advanced infiltrating ductal carcinoma after treatment with induction chemotherapy. Am J Clin Pathol 1994, **102**: 154–157.

1255 Kennedy S, Merino MJ, Swain SM, Lippman ME. The effects of hormonal and chemotherapy on tumoral and nonneoplastic breast tissue. Hum Pathol 1990, **21**: 192–198.

1256 Moll UM, Chumas J. Morphologic effects of neoadjuvant chemotherapy in locally advanced breast cancer. Pathol Res Pract 1997, **193**: 187–196.

1257 Moore GH, Schiller JE, Moore GK. Radiation-induced histopathologic changes of the breast: the effects of time. Am J Surg Pathol 2004, **28**: 47–53.

1258 Oyama T, Maluf H, Koerner F. Pathologic findings after therapeutic irradiation of mammary tissues and carcinomas. Anat Pathol 1998, **3**: 181–193.

1259 Penault-Llorca F, Abrial C, Raoelfils I, Cayre A, Mouret-Reynier MA, Leheurteur M, Durando X, Achard JL, Gimbergues P, Chollet P. Comparison of the prognostic significance of Chevallier and Sataloff's pathologic classifications after neoadjuvant chemotherapy of operable breast cancer. Hum Pathol 2008, **39**: 1221–1228.

1260 Pinder SE, Provenzano E, Earl H, Ellis IO. Laboratory handling and histology reporting of breast specimens from patients who have received neoadjuvant chemotherapy. Histopathology 2007, **50**: 409–417.

1261 Rabban JT, Glidden D, Kwan ML, Chen YY. Pure and predominantly pure intralymphatic breast carcinoma after neoadjuvant chemotherapy: an unusual and adverse pattern of residual disease. Am J Surg Pathol 2009, **33**: 256–263.

1262 Rajan R, Esteva FJ, Symmans WF. Pathologic changes in breast cancer following neoadjuvant chemotherapy: implications for the assessment of response. Clin Breast Cancer 2004, **5**: 235–238.

1263 Sahoo S, Lester SC. Pathology of breast carcinomas after neoadjuvant chemotherapy: an overview with recommendations on specimen processing and reporting. Arch Pathol Lab Med 2009, **133**: 633–642.

1264 Schnitt SJ, Connolly JL, Harris JR, Cohen RB. Radiation-induced changes in the breast. Hum Pathol 1984, **15**: 545–550.

1265 Seno R, Sparano JA, Fineberg SA. Gross and histologic features of locally advanced breast cancer after neoadjuvant chemotherapy. Anat Pathol 1998, **3**: 169–180.

1266 Sharkey FE, Addington SL, Fowler LJ, Page CP, Cruz AB. Effects of preoperative chemotherapy on the morphology of resectable breast carcinoma. Mod Pathol 1996, **9**: 893–900.

1267 Winkelmann RK, Grado GL, Quimby SR, Connolly SM. Pseudosclerodermatous panniculitis after irradiation. An unusual complication of megavoltage treatment of breast carcinoma. Mayo Clin Proc 1993, **68**: 122–127.

1268 Ziegler LD, Connelly JH, Frye D, Smith TL, Hortobagyi GN. Lack of correlation between histologic findings and response to chemotherapy in metastatic breast cancer. Cancer 1991, **68**: 628–633.

PROGNOSIS

1269 Aamdal S, Bormer O, Jorgensen O, Host H, Eliassen G, Kaalhus O, Pihl A. Estrogen receptors and long-term prognosis in breast cancer. Cancer 1984, **53**: 2525–2529.

1270 Abner AL, Collins L, Peiro G, Recht A, Come S, Shulman LN, Silver B, Nixon A, Harris JR, Schnitt SJ, Connolly JL. Correlation of tumor size and axillary lymph node involvement with prognosis in patients with T1 breast carcinoma. Cancer 1998, **83**: 2502–2508.

1271 Acs G, Dumoff KL, Solin LJ, Pasha T, Xu X, Zhang PJ. Extensive retraction artifact correlates with lymphatic invasion and nodal metastasis and predicts poor outcome in early stage breast carcinoma. Am J Surg Pathol 2007, **31**: 129–140.

1272 Adami H-O, Malker B, Holmberg L, Persson I, Stone B. The relation between survival and age at diagnosis in breast cancer. N Engl J Med 1986, **315**: 559–563.

1273 Alderson MR, Hamlin I, Staunton MD. The relative significance of prognostic factors in breast carcinoma. Br J Cancer 1971, **25**: 646–655.

1274 Armas OA, Gerald WL, Lesser ML, Arroyo CD, Norton L, Rosen PP. Immunohistochemical detection of cathepsin D in T2N0M0 breast carcinoma. Am J Surg Pathol 1994, **18**: 158–166.

1275 Arnaout-Alkarain A, Kahn HJ, Narod SA, Sun PA, Marks AN. Significance of lymph vessel invasion identified by the endothelial lymphatic marker D2-40 in node negative breast cancer. Mod Pathol 2007, **20**: 183–191.

1276 Auer G, Eriksson E, Azavedo E, Caspersson T, Wallgren A. Prognostic significance of nuclear DNA content in mammary adenocarcinomas in humans. Cancer Res 1984, **44**: 394–396.

1277 Axelsson K, Ljung B-M, Moore DH II, Thor AD, Chew KL, Edgerton SM, Smith HS, Mayall BH. Tumor angiogenesis as a prognostic assay for invasive ductal breast carcinoma. J Natl Cancer Inst 1995, **87**: 997–1008.

1278 Baak JP, Chin D, van Diest PJ, Ortiz R, Matze-Cok P, Bacus SS. Comparative long-term prognostic value of quantiative HER-2/neu protein expression, DNA ploidy, and morphometric and clinical features in paraffin-embedded invasive breast cancer. Lab Invest 1991, **64**: 215–223.

1279 Baak JPA, Kurver PHJ, de Snoo-Niewlaat AJE, de Graef S, Makkink B, Boon ME. Prognostic indicators in breast cancer. Morphometric methods. Histopathology 1982, **6**: 327–339.

1280 Baak JPA, Van Dop H, Kurver PHJ, Hermans J. The value of morphometry to classic prognosticators in breast cancer. Cancer 1985, **56**: 374–382.

1281 Bane AL, Tjan S, Parkes RK, Andrulis I, O'Malley FP. Invasive lobular carcinoma: to grade or not to grade. Mod Pathol 2005, **18**: 621–628.

1282 Barbareschi M. Prognostic value of the immunohistochemical expression of p53 in breast carcinomas: a review of the literature involving over 9,000 patients. Appl Immunohistochem 1996, **4**: 106–116.

1283 Barbareschi M, Weidner N, Gasparini G, Morelli L, Forti S, Ercher C, Fina P, Caffo O, Leonardi E, Mauri F, Bevilacqua P, Dalla Palma P. Microvessel density quantification in breast carcinomas. Assessment by light microscopy vs. a computer-aided image analysis system. Appl Immunohistochem 1995, **3**: 75–84.

1284 Barnes DM, Dublin EA, Fisher CJ, Levison DA, Millis RR. Immunohistochemical detection of p53 protein in mammary carcinoma. An important new independent indicator of prognosis? Hum Pathol 1993, **24**: 469–476.

1285 Barnes R, Masood S, Barker E, Rosengard AM, Coggin DL, Crowell T, King CR, Porter-Jordan K, Wargotz ES, Liotta LA, et al. Low nm23 protein expression in infiltrating ductal breast carcinomas correlates with reduced patient survival. Am J Pathol 1991, **139**: 245–250.

1378 Miremadi A, Pinder SE, Lee AHS, Bell JA, Paish EC, Wencyk P, Elston CW, Nicholson RI, Blamey RW, Robertson JF, Ellis IO. Neuroendocrine differentiation and prognosis in breast adenocarcinoma. Histopathology 2002, **40**: 215–222.

1379 Mohammed RA, Martin SG, Gill MS, Green AR, Paish EC, Ellis IO. Improved methods of detection of lymphovascular invasion demonstrate that it is the predominant method of vascular invasion in breast cancer and has important clinical consequences. Am J Surg Pathol 2007, **31**: 1825–1833.

1380 Mohammed RA, Ellis IO, Lee AH, Martin SG. Vascular invasion in breast cancer; an overview of recent prognostic developments and molecular pathophysiological mechanisms. Histopathology 2009, **55**: 1–9.

1381 Mori I, Yang Q, Kukudo K. Predictive and prognostic markers for invasive breast cancer. Pathol Int 2002, **52**: 186–194.

1382 Muss HB, Thor AD, Berry DA, Kute T, Liu ET, Koerner F, Cirrincione CT, Budman DR, Wood WC, Barcos M, et al. c-*erb*B-2 expression and response to adjuvant therapy in women with node-positive early breast cancer. N Engl J Med 1994, **330**: 1260–1266.

1383 Nassar A, Radhakrishnan A, Cabrero IA, Cotsonis G, Cohen C. COX-2 expression in invasive breast cancer: correlation with prognostic parameters and outcome. Appl Immunohistochem Mol Morphol 2007, **15**: 255–259.

1384 Nime FA, Rosen PP, Thaler HT, Ashikari R, Urban JA. Prognostic significance of tumor emboli in intramammary lymphatics in patients with mammary carcinoma. Am J Surg Pathol 1977, **1**: 25–30.

1385 Nixon AJ, Neuberg D, Hayes DF, Gelman R, Connolly JL, Schnitt S, Abner A, Recht A, Vicini F, Harris JR. Relationship of patient age to pathologic features of the tumor and prognosis for patients with stage I or II breast cancer. J Clin Oncol 1994, **12**: 888–894.

1386 Noguchi M, Ohta N, Koyasaki N, Taniya T, Miyazaki I, Mizukami Y. Reappraisal of internal mammary node metastases as a prognostic factor in patients with breast cancer. Cancer 1991, **68**: 1918–1925.

1387 Otis CN, Krebs PA, Albuquerque A, Quezado MM, San Juan X, Sobel ME, Merino MJ. Loss of heterozygosity of p53, BRCA1, VHL, and estrogen receptor genes in breast carcinoma: correlation with related protein products and morphologic features. Int J Surg Pathol 2002, **10**: 237–245.

1388 Page DL. Prognosis and breast cancer. Recognition of lethal and favorable prognostic types. Am J Surg Pathol 1991, **15**: 334–349.

1389 Page DL. Special types of invasive breast cancer, with clinical implications. Am J Surg Pathol 2003, **27**: 832–835.

1390 Page DL, Dupont WD. Breast cancer angiogenesis. Through a narrow window. JNCI 1992, **84**: 1850–1851.

1391 Page DL, Ellis IO, Elston CW. Histologic grading of breast cancer. Let's do it [editorial]. Am J Clin Pathol 1995, **103**: 123–124.

1392 Perou CM, Serlie T, Elsen MB, van de Rijn M, Jeffrey SS, Rees CA, Pollack JR, Ross DT, Johnsen H, Akslen LA, Fluge O, Pergamenschikov A, Williams C, Zhu SX, Lenning PE. Molecular portraits of human breast tumors. Nature 2000, **406**: 747–752.

1393 Peters MV. The effect of pregnancy on breast cancer. In Forrest APM, Kunkler PB (eds): Prognostic factors in breast carcinoma. Baltimore, 1968, Williams & Wilkins.

1394 Petrek JA, Dukoff R, Rogatko A. Prognosis of pregnancy-associated breast cancer. Cancer 1991, **67**: 869–872.

1395 Pienta KJ, Coffey DS. Correlation of nuclear morphometry with progression of breast cancer. Cancer 1991, **68**: 2012–2016.

1396 Pinder SE, Ellis IO, Galea M, O'Rouke S, Blamey RW, Elston CW. Pathological prognostic factors in breast cancer. III. Vascular invasion. Relationship with recurrence and survival in a large study with long-term follow-up. Histopathology 1994, **24**: 41–47.

1397 Press MF, Bernstein L, Thomas PA, Meisner LF, Zhou JY, Ma Y, Hung G, Robinson RA, Harris C, El-Naggar A, Slamon DJ, Phillips RN, Ross JS, Wolman SR, Flom KJ. HER-2/neu gene amplification characterized by fluorescence in situ hybridisation: poor prognosis in node-negative breast carcinomas. J Clin Oncol 1997, **15**: 2894–2904.

1398 Qureshi HS, Linden MD, Divine G, Raju UB. E-cadherin status in breast cancer correlates with histologic type but does not correlate with established prognostic parameters. Am J Clin Pathol 2006, **125**: 377–385.

1399 Quiet CA, Ferguson DJ, Weichselbaum RR, Hellman S. Natural history of node-negative breast cancer. A study of 826 patients with long-term follow-up. J Clin Oncol 1995, **13**: 1144–1151.

1400 Rakha EA, Abd El Rehim D, Pinder SE, Lewis SA, Ellis IO. E-cadherin expression in invasive non-lobular carcinoma of the breast and its prognostic significance. Histopathology 2005, **46**: 685–693.

1401 Rakha EA, Boyce RW, Abd El-Rehim D, Kurien T, Green AR, Paish EC, Robertson JF, Ellis IO. Expression of mucins (MUC1, MUC2, MUC3, MUC4, MUC5AC and MUC6) and their prognostic significance in human breast cancer. Mod Pathol 2005, **18**: 1295–1304.

1402 Rakha EA, El-Sheikh SE, Kandil MA, El-Sayed ME, Green AR, Ellis IO. Expression of BRCA1 protein in breast cancer and its prognostic significance. Hum Pathol 2008, **39**: 857–865.

1403 Ravdin PM, Tandon AK, Allred DC, Clark GM, Fuqua SA, Hilsenbeck SH, Chamness GC, Osborne CK. Cathepsin D by Western blotting and immunohistochemistry. Failure to confirm correlations with prognosis in node-negative breast cancer. J Clin Oncol 1994, **12**: 467–474.

1404 Reed W, Hannidal E, Boehler PJ, Gunderson S, Host H, Marthin J. The prognostic value of p53 and c-erb B-2 immunostaining is overrated for patients with lymph node negative breast carcinoma: a multivariate analysis of prognostic factors in 613 patients with a follow-up of 14–30 years. Cancer 2000, **88**: 804–813.

1405 Reed W, Sandstad B, Holm R, Nesland JM. The prognostic impact of hormone receptors and c-erbB-2 in pregnancy-associated breast cancer and their correlation with BRCA1 and cell cycle modulators. Int J Surg Pathol 2003, **11**: 485–488.

1406 Rennert G, Bisland-Naggan S, Barnett-Griness O, Bar-Joseph N, Zhang S, Rennert HS, Narod SA. Clinical outcomes of breast cancer in carriers of *BRCA1* and *BRCA2* mutations. N Engl J Med 2007, **357**: 115–123.

1407 Robbins P, Pinder S, de Klerk N, Dawkins H, Harvey J, Sterrett G, Ellis I, Elston C. Histological grading of breast carcinomas. A study of interobserver agreement. Hum Pathol 1995, **26**: 873–879.

1408 Robson M. Are BRCA1- and BRCA2-associated breast cancers different? Prognosis of BRCA1-associated breast cancer. J Clin Oncol 2000, **18**: 113S–118S.

1409 Rosen PP, Groshen S, Kinne DW, Norton L. Factors influencing prognosis in node-negative breast carcinoma. Analysis of 767 T1N0M0/T2N0M0 patients with long-term follow-up. J Clin Oncol 1993, **11**: 2090–2100.

1410 Rosen PP, Lesser ML, Kinne DW, Beattie EJ. Breast carcinoma in women 35 years of age or younger. Ann Surg 1984, **199**: 133–142.

1411 Rosen PP, Lesser ML, Arroyo CD, Cranor M, Borgen P, Norton L. p53 in node-negative breast carcinoma. An immunohistochemical study of epidemiologic risk factors, histologic features, and prognosis. J Clin Oncol 1995, **13**: 821–830.

1412 Rosen PP, Lesser ML, Arroyo CD, Cranor M, Borgen P, Norton L. Immunohistochemical detection of HER2/*neu* in patients with axillary lymph node-negative breast carcinoma. A study of epidemiologic risk factors, histologic features, and prognosis. Cancer 1995, **75**: 1320–1326.

1413 Rosen PP, Saigo PE, Braun DW, Weathers E, Fracchia AA, Kinne DW. Axillary micro- and macrometastases in breast cancer. Prognostic significance of tumor size. Ann Surg 1981, **196**: 585–591.

1414 Roses DF, Bell DA, Flotte TJ, Taylor R, Ratech H, Dubin N. Pathologic predictors of recurrence in stage 1 (T1N0M0) breast cancer. Am J Clin Pathol 1982, **78**: 817–820.

1415 Rosner D, Lane WW. Oral contraceptive use has no adverse effect on the prognosis of breast cancer. Cancer 1986, **57**: 591–596.

1416 Ross JS. Multigene classifiers, prognostic factors, and predictors of breast cancer clinical outcome. Adv Anat Pathol 2009, **16**: 204–215.

1417 Russo J, Frederick J, Ownby HE, Fine G, Hussain M, Kirckstein HI, Robbins TO, Rosenberg B. Predictors of recurrence and survival of patients with breast cancer. Am J Clin Pathol 1987, **88**: 123–131.

1418 Sahin AA, Ro J, Ro JY, Blick MB, el-Naggar AK, Ordonez NG, Fritsche HA, Smith TL, Hortobagyi GN, Ayala AG. Ki-67 immunostaining in node-negative stage I/II breast carcinoma. Significant correlation with prognosis. Cancer 1991, **68**: 549–557.

1419 Sahin AA, Sneige N, Ordonez NG, Singletary SE, Ro JY, El Naggar AK, Ayala AG. Immunohistochemical assessment of cathepsin D in stages I and II node-negative breast cancer. Appl Immunohistochem 1994, **2**: 15–21.

1420 Saigo P, Rosen PP. Prognostic factors in invasive mammary carcinomas 1.0 cm or less in diameter [abstract]. Am J Clin Pathol 1980, **73**: 303–304.

1421 Santiago RJ, Harris EE, Qin L, Hwang WT, Solin LJ. Similar long-term results of breast-conservation treatment for Stage I and II invasive lobular carcinoma compared with invasive ductal carcinoma of the breast: The University of Pennsylvania experience. Cancer 2005, **103**: 2447–2454.

1422 Schnitt SJ. Risk factors for local recurrence in patients with invasive breast cancer and negative surgical margins of excision: where are we and where are we going? Am J Clin Pathol 2003, **120**: 485–488.

1423 Sears HF, Janus C, Levy W, Hopson R, Creech R, Grotzinger P. Breast cancer without axillary metastases. Are there high-risk biologic subpopulations? Cancer 1982, **50**: 1820–1827.

1424 Seidman H, Gelb SK, Silverberg E, LaVerda N, Lubera JA. Survival experience in the breast cancer detection demonstration project. CA Cancer J Clin 1987, **37**: 258–290.

1425 Seidman JD, Schnaper LA, Aisner SC. Relationship of the size of the invasive component of the primary breast carcinoma to axillary lymph node metastasis. Cancer 1995, **75**: 65–71.

1426 Sigurdsson H, Baldetorp B, Borg A, Dalberg M, Ferno M, Killander D, Olsson H. Indicators of prognosis in node-negative breast cancer. N Engl J Med 1990, **322**: 1045–1053.

1427 Siitonen SM, Haapasalo HK, Rantala IS, Helin HJ, Isola JJ. Comparison of different immunohistochemical methods in the assessment of angiogenesis. Lack of prognostic value in a group of 77 selected node-negative breast carcinomas. Mod Pathol 1995, **8**: 745–752.

1428 Simpson J, Page D. Prognostic value of histopathology in the breast. Semin Oncol 1992, **19**: 254–262.

1429 Simpson JF, Page DL. Status of breast cancer prognostication based on histopathologic data. Am J Clin Pathol 1994, **102**: S3–S8.

1430 Simpson JF, Page DL. Cellular proliferation and prognosis in breast cancer. Statistical purity versus clinical utility. Hum Pathol 1994, **25**: 331–332.

1431 Smith JA III, Gamez-Araujo J, Gallager HS, White EC, McBride CM. Carcinoma of the breast. Analysis of total lymph node involvement versus level of metastasis. Cancer 1977, **39**: 527–532.

1432 Tandon AK, Clark GM, Chammness GC, Chirgwin JM, McGuire WL. Cathepsin D and prognosis in breast cancer. N Engl J Med 1990, **322**: 297–302.

1433 Toikkanen S, Joensuu H, Klemi P. Nuclear DNA content as a prognostic factor in T1-2N0 breast cancer. Am J Clin Pathol 1990, **93**: 471–479.

1434 Treré D, Ceccarelli C, Migaldi M, Santini D, Taffurelli M, Tosti E, Chieco P, Derenzini M. Cell proliferation in breast cancer is a major determinant of clinical outcome in node-positive but not in node-negative patients. Appl Immunohistochem Mol Morphol 2006, **14**: 314–323.

1435 Tsakraklides V, Olson P, Kersey JH, Good RA. Prognostic significance of the regional lymph node histology in cancer of the breast. Cancer 1974, **34**: 1259–1266.

1436 Tsuda H, Hirohashi S, Shimosato Y, Hirota T, Tsugane S, Watanabe S, Terada M, Yamamoto H. Correlation between histologic grade of malignancy and copy number of *c-erb*B-2 gene in breast carcinoma. A retrospective analysis of 176 cases. Cancer 1990, **65**: 1794–1800.

1437 Turbin DA, Cheang MC, Bajdik CD, Gelmon KA, Yorida E, De Luca A, Nielsen TO, Huntsman DG, Gilks CB. MDM2 protein expression is a negative prognostic marker in breast carcinoma. Mod Pathol 2006, **19**: 69–74.

1438 Van den Eynden GG, Colpaert CG, Couvelard A, Pezzella F, Dirix LY, Vermeulen PB, Van Marck EA, Hasebe T. A fibrotic focus is a prognostic factor and a surrogate marker for hypoxia and (lymph)angiogenesis in breast cancer: review of the literature and proposal on the criteria of evaluation. Histopathology 2007, **51**: 440–451.

1439 van de Rijn M, Perou CM, Tibshirani R, Haas P, Kallioniemi O, Kononen J, Torhorst J, Sauter G, Zuber M, Kochli OR, Mross F, Dieterich H, Seitz R, Ross D, Botstein D, Brown P. Expression of cytokeratins 17 and 5 identifies a group of breast carcinomas with poor clinical outcome. Am J Pathol 2002, **161**: 1991–1996.

1440 van der Linden JC, Baak JPA, Lindeman J, Smeulders AWM, Meyer CJLM. Carcinoembryonic antigen expression and peanut agglutinin binding in primary breast cancer and lymph node metastases. Lack of correlation with clinical, histopathological, biochemical and morphometric features. Histopathology 1985, **9**: 1051–1059.

1441 van de Vijver MJ, He YD, van't Veer LJ, Dai H, Hart AA, Voskuil DW, Schreiber GJ, Peterse JL, Roberts C, Marton MJ, Parrish M, Atsma D, Witteveen A, Glas A, Delahaye L, van der Velde T, Bartelink H, Rodenhuis S, Rutgers ET, Friend SH, Bernards R. A gene-expression signature as a predictor of survival in breast cancer. N Engl J Med 2002, **347**: 1999–2009.

1442 van Diest PJ, Baak JP. The morphometric prognostic index is the strongest prognosticator in premenopausal lymph node-negative and lymph node-positive breast cancer patients. Hum Pathol 1991, **22**: 326–330.

1443 van Diest PJ, Michalides RJ, Jannink I, van der Valk P, Peterse HL, de Jong JS, Meijer CJ, Baak JP. Cyclin D1 expression in invasive breast cancer correlations and prognostic value. Am J Pathol 1997, **150**: 705–711.

1444 van't Veer LJ, Dal H, van de Vijver MJ, He YD, Hart AA, Mao M, Peterse HL, van der Kooy K, Marton MJ, Witteveen AT, Schreiber GJ, Kerkhoven RM, Roberts C, Linsley PS, Bernards R, Friend SH. Gene expression profiling predicts clinical outcome of breast cancer. Nature 2002, **415**: 530–536.

1445 Vartanian RK, Weidner N. Correlation of intratumoral endothelial cell proliferation with microvessel density (tumor angiogenesis) and tumor cell proliferation in breast carcinoma. Am J Pathol 1994, **144**: 1188–1194.

1446 Vielh P, Chevillard S, Mosseri V, Donatini B, Magdelenat H. Ki67 index and S-phase fraction in human breast carcinomas. Comparison and correlations with prognostic factors. Am J Clin Pathol 1990, **94**: 681–686.

1447 Visscher DW, Zarbo RJ, Greenawald KA, Crissman JD. Prognostic significance of morphological parameters and flow cytometric DNA analysis in carcinoma of the breast. Pathol Annu 1990, **25**(Pt 1): 171–210.

1448 Weidner N. Tumor angiogenesis. Review of current applications in tumor prognostication. Semin Diagn Pathol 1993, **10**: 302–313.

1449 Weidner N. Intratumor microvessel density as a prognostic factor in cancer. Am J Pathol 1995 **147**: 9–19.

1450 Weidner N, Folkman J, Pozza F, Bevilacqua P, Allred EN, Moore DH, Meli S, Gasparini G. Tumor angiogenesis. A new significant and independent prognostic indicator in early-stage breast carcinoma. J Natl Cancer Inst 1992, **84**: 1875–1887.

1451 Weidner N, Moore DH, Vartanian R. Correlation of Ki-67 antigen expression with mitotic figure index and tumor grade in breast carcinomas using the novel 'paraffin'-reactive MIB1 antibody. Hum Pathol 1994, **25**: 337–342.

1452 Weidner N, Semple JP, Welch WR, Folkman J. Tumor angiogenesis and metastasis – correlation in invasive breast carcinoma. N Engl J Med 1991, **324**: 1–8.

1453 Wertheim U, Ozzello L. Neoplastic involvement of nipple and skin flap in carcinoma of the breast. Am J Surg Pathol 1980, **4**: 543–549.

1454 Wintzer HO, Zipfel I, Schulte-Monting J, Hellerich U, von Kleist S. Ki-67 immunostaining in human breast tumors and its relationship to prognosis. Cancer 1991, **67**: 421–428.

1455 Witton CJ, Hawe SJ, Cooke TG, Bartlett JM. Cyclooxygenase 2 (COX2) expression is associated with poor outcome in ER-negative, but not ER-positive, breast cancer. Histopathology 2004, **45**: 47–54.

1456 Witzig TE, Gonchoroff NJ, Therneau T, Gilbertson DT, Wold LE, Grant C, Grande J, Katzmann JA, Ahmann DL, Ingle JN. DNA content flow cytometry as a prognostic factor for node-positive breast cancer. The role of multiparameter ploidy analysis and specimen sonication. Cancer 1991, **68**: 1781–1788.

1457 Witzig TE, Ingle JN, Cha SS, Schaid DJ, Tabery RL, Wold LE, Grant C, Gonchoroff NJ, Katzmann JA. DNA ploidy and the percentage of cells in S-phase as prognostic factors for women with lymph node negative breast cancer. Cancer 1994, **74**: 1752–1761.

1458 Wold LE, Ingle JN, Pisansky TM, Johnson RE, Donohue JH. Prognostic factors for patients with carcinoma of the breast. Mayo Clin Proc 1995, **70**: 678–679.

1459 Yamauchi C, Hasebe T, Iwasaki M, Imoto S, Wada N, Fukayama M, Ochiai A. Accurate assessment of lymph vessel tumor emboli in invasive ductal carcinoma of the breast according to tumor areas, and their prognostic significance. Hum Pathol 2007, **38**: 247–259.

1460 Yu L, Yang W, Cai X, Shi D, Fan Y, Lu H. Centrally necrotizing carcinoma of the breast: clinicopathological analysis of 33 cases indicating its basal-like phenotype and poor prognosis. Histopathology 2010, **57**: 193–201.

SALIVARY GLAND AND SKIN ADNEXAL-TYPE TUMORS (INCLUDING MYOEPITHELIAL TUMORS)

1461 Acs G, Simpson JF, Bleiweiss IJ, Hugh J, Reynolds C, Olson S, Page DL. Microglandular adenosis with transition into adenoid cystic carcinoma of the breast. Am J Surg Pathol 2003, **27**: 1052–1060.

1462 Albores-Saavedra J, Heard SC, McLaren B, Kamino H, Witkiewicz AK. Cylindroma (dermal analog tumor) of the breast: a comparison with cylindroma of the skin and adenoid cystic carcinoma of the breast. Am J Clin Pathol 2005, **123**: 866–873.

1463 Arpino G, Clark GM, Mohsin S, Bardou VJ, Elledge RM. Adenoid cystic carcinoma of the breast: molecular markers, treatment, and clinical outcome. Cancer 2002, **94**: 2119–2127.

1464 Asioli S, Marucci G, Ficarra G, Stephens M, Foschini MP, Ellis IO, Eusebi V. Polymorphous adenocarcinoma of the breast. Report of three cases. Virchows Arch 2006, **448**: 29–34.

1465 Azoulay S, Laé M, Fréneaux P, Merle S, Al Ghuzlan A, Chnecker C, Rosty C, Klijanienko J, Sigal-Zafrani B, Salmon R, Fourquet A, Sastre-Garau X, Vincent-Salomon A. KIT is highly expressed in adenoid cystic carcinoma of the breast, a basal-like carcinoma associated with a favorable outcome. Mod Pathol 2005, **18**: 1623–1631.

1466 Ballance WA, Ro JY, el-Naggar AK, Grignon DJ, Ayala AG, Romsdahl MG. Pleomorphic adenoma (benign mixed tumor) of the breast. An immunohistochemical, flow cytometric, and ultrastructural study and review of the literature. Am J Clin Pathol 1990, **93**: 795–801.

1467 Buza N, Zekry N, Charpin C, Tavassoli FA. Myoepithelial carcinoma of the breast: a clinicopathological and immunohistochemical study of 15 diagnostically challenging cases. Virchows Arch 2010, **457**: 337–345.

1468 Cavanzo FJ, Taylor HB. Adenoid cystic carcinoma of the breast. An analysis of 21 cases. Cancer 1969, **24**: 740–745.

1469 Chen KT. Pleomorphic adenoma of the breast. Am J Clin Pathol 1990, **93**: 792–794.

1470 Chen PC, Chen CK, Nicastri AD, Wait RB. Myoepithelial carcinoma of the breast with distant metastasis and accompanied by adenomyoepitheliomas. Histopathology 1994, **24**: 543–548.

1471 Coyne JD, Dervan PA, Barr L. High-grade carcinomas of the breast showing patterns of mixed ductal and myoepithelial differentiation (including myoepithelial cell-rich carcinoma of the breast). Histopathology 2004, **44**: 580–584.

1472 Crisi GM, Marconi SA, Makari-Judson G, Goulart RA. Expression of c-kit in adenoid cystic carcinoma of the breast. Am J Clin Pathol 2005, **124**: 733–739.

1473 Damiani S, Eusebi V, Losi L, d'Adda T, Rosai J. Oncocytic carcinoma (malignant oncocytoma) of the breast. Am J Surg Pathol 1998, **22**: 221–230.

1474 Damiani S, Pasquinelli G, Lamovec J, Peterse JL, Eusebi V. Acinic cell carcinoma of the breast: an immunohistochemical and ultrastructural study. Virchows Arch 2000, **437**: 74–81.

1475 Diaz NM, McDivitt RW, Wick MR. Pleomorphic adenoma of the breast. A clinicopathologic and immunohistochemical study of 10 cases. Hum Pathol 1991, **22**: 1206–1214.

1476 Dina R, Eusebi V. Clear cell tumors of the breast. Semin Diagn Pathol 1997, **14**: 175–182.

1477 Di Tommaso L, Foschini MP, Ragazzini T, Magrini E, Fornelli A, Ellis IO, Eusebi V. Mucoepidermoid carcinoma of the breast. Virchows Arch 2004, **444**: 13–19.

1478 Domoto H, Terahata S, Sato K, Tamai S. Nodular hidradenoma of the breast: report of two cases with literature review. Pathol Int 1998, **48**: 907–911.

1479 Draheim JH, Neubecker RD, Sprinz H. An unusual tumor of the breast resembling eccrine spiradenoma. Am J Clin Pathol 1959, **31**: 511–516.

1480 Drudis T, Arroyo C, Van Hoeven K, Cordon-Cardo C, Rosen PP. The pathology of low-grade adenosquamous carcinoma of the breast. An immunohistochemical study. Pathol Annu 1994, **29**(Pt 2): 181–197.

1481 Erlandson RA, Rosen PP. Infiltrating myoepithelioma of the breast. Am J Surg Pathol 1982, **6**: 785–793.

1482 Finck FM, Schwinn CP, Keasby LE. Clear cell hidradenoma of the breast. Cancer 1968, **22**: 125–135.

1483 Fisher ER, Tavares J, Bulatao IS, Sass R, Fisher B, collaborating NSABP investigators. Glycogen-rich, clear cell breast cancer. With comments concerning other clear cell variants. Hum Pathol 1985, **16**: 1085–1090.

1484 Foschini MP, Eusebi V. Carcinomas of the breast showing myoepithelial cell differentiation. A review of the literature. Virchows Arch 1998, **432**: 303–310.

1485 Foschini MP, Pizzicannella G, Peterse JL, Eusebi V. Adenomyoepithelioma of the breast associated with low-grade adenosquamous and sarcomatoid carcinomas. Virchows Archiv 1995, **427**: 243–250.

1486 Foschini MP, Krausz T. Salivary gland-type tumors of the breast: a spectrum of benign and malignant tumors including 'triple negative carcinomas' of low malignant potential. Semin Diagn Pathol 2010, **27**: 77–90.

1487 Gokaslan ST, Carlile B, Dudak M, Albores-Saavedra J. Solitary cylindroma (dermal analog tumor) of the breast: a previously undescribed neoplasm at this site. Am J Surg Pathol 2001, **25**: 823–826.

1488 Harris M. Pseudoadenoid cystic carcinoma of the breast. Arch Pathol Lab Med 1977, **101**: 307–309.

1489 Hayes MMM, Seidman JD, Ashton MA. Glycogen-rich clear cell carcinoma of the breast. A clinicopathologic study of 21 cases. Am J Surg Pathol 1995, **19**: 904–911.

1490 Hermann ME, Bratthauer G, Stamatakos MD, Matusik J, Tavassoli FA. Malignancies arising in adenomyoepithelioma (AME) of breast: clinical outcome and immunohistochemical characterization [abstract]. Mod Pathol 2003, **16**: 33a.

1491 Hisaoka M, Takamatsu Y, Hirano Y, Maeda H, Hamada T. Sebaceous carcinoma of the breast: case report and review of the literature. Virchows Arch 2006, **449**: 484–488.

1492 Hull MT, Warfel KA. Glycogen-rich clear cell carcinomas of the breast. A clinicopathologic and ultrastructural study. Am J Surg Pathol 1986, **10**: 553–559.

1493 Jolicoeur F, Seemayer TA, Gabbiani G, Robidouz A, Gaboury L, Oligny LL, Schurch W. Multifocal, nascent, and invasive myoepithelial carcinoma (malignant myoepithelioma) of the breast: an immunohistochemical and ultrastructural study. Int J Surg Pathol 2002, **10**: 281–291.

1494 Jones MW, Norris HJ, Snyder RC. Infiltrating syringomatous adenoma of the nipple. A clinical and pathological study of 11 cases. Am J Surg Pathol 1989, **13**: 197–201.

1495 Kasami M, Olson SJ, Simpson JF, Page DL. Maintenance of polarity and dual cell population in adenoid cystic carcinoma of the breast: an immunohistochemical study. Histopathology 1998, **32**: 232–238.

1496 Kazakov DV, Vanecek T, Belousova IE, Mukensnabl P, Kollertova D, Michal M. Skin-type hidradenoma of the breast parenchyma with t(11;19) translocation: hidradenoma of the breast. Am J Dermatopathol 2007, **29**: 457–461.

1497 Kleer CG, Oberman HA. Adenoid cystic carcinoma of the breast: value of histologic grading and proliferative activity. Am J Surg Pathol 1998, **22**: 569–575.

1498 Koss LG, Brannan CD, Ashikari R. Histologic and ultrastructural features of adenoid cystic carcinoma of the breast. Cancer 1970, **26**: 1271–1279.

1499 Lamovec J, Falconieri G, Salviato T, Pizzolitto S. Basaloid carcinoma of the breast: a review of 9 cases, with delineation of a possible clinicopathologic entity. Ann Diagn Pathol 2008, **12**: 4–11.

1500 Maiorano E, Ricco R, Virgintino D, Lastilla G. Infiltrating myoepithelioma of the breast. Appl Immunohistochem 1994, **2**: 130–136.

1501 Mastropasqua MG, Maiorano E, Pruneri G, Orvieto E, Mazzarol G, Vento AR, Viale G. Immunoreactivity for c-kit and p63 as an adjunct in the diagnosis of adenoid cystic carcinoma of the breast. Mod Pathol 2005, **18**: 1277–1282.

1502 McLaren BK, Smith J, Schuyler PA, Dupont WD, Page DL. Adenomyoepithelioma: clinical, histologic, and immunohistologic evaluation of a series of related lesions. Am J Surg Pathol 2005, **29**: 1294–1299.

1503 Michal M, Baumruk L, Burger J, Manhalova M. Adenomyoepithelioma of the breast with undifferentiated carcinoma component. Histopathology 1994, **24**: 274–276.

1504 Moran CA, Suster S, Carter D. Benign mixed tumors (pleomorphic adenomas) of the breast. Am J Surg Pathol 1990, **14**: 913–921.

1505 Nadelman CM, Leslie KO, Fishbein MC. 'Benign,' metastasizing adenomyoepithelioma of the breast: a report of 2 cases. Arch Pathol Lab Med 2006, **130**: 1349–1353.

1506 Nonaka D, Rosai J, Spagnolo D, Fiaccavento S, Bisceglia M. Cylindroma of the breast of skin adnexal type: a study of 4 cases. Am J Surg Pathol 2004, **28**: 1070–1075.

1507 Patchefsky AS, Frauenhoffer CM, Krall RA, Cooper HS. Low-grade mucoepidermoid carcinoma of the breast. Arch Pathol Lab Med 1979, **103**: 196–198.

1508 Pauwels C, De Potter C. Adenomyoepithelioma of the breast with features of malignancy. Histopathology 1994, **24**: 94–96.

1509 Persson M, Andren Y, Mark J, Horlings HM, Persson F, Stenman G. Recurrent fusion of MYB and NFIB transcription factor genes in carcinomas of the breast and head and neck. Proc Natl Acad Sci U S A 2009, **106**: 18740–18744.

1510 Rabban JT, Swain RS, Zaloudek CJ, Chase DR, Chen YY. Immunophenotypic overlap between adenoid cystic carcinoma and collagenous spherulosis of the breast: potential diagnostic pitfalls using myoepithelial markers. Mod Pathol 2006, **19**: 1351–1357.

1511 Reis-Filho JS, Milanezi F, Paredes J, Silva P, Periera EM, Maeda SA, De Carvalho LV, Schmitt FC. Novel and classic myoepithelial/stem cell markers in metaplastic carcinoma of the breast. Appl Immunohistochem Mol Morphol 2003, **11**: 1–8.

1512 Ribeiro-Silva A, Shaletich C, Careta RS, Kazava DK, Siqueira MC, Ponton F. Spiradenocarcinoma of the breast arising in a long-standing spiradenoma. Ann Diagn Pathol 2004, **8**: 162–166.

1513 Ro JY, Silva EG, Gallager HS. Adenoid cystic carcinoma of the breast. Hum Pathol 1987, **18**: 1276–1281.

1514 Roncaroli F, Lamovec J, Zidar A, Eusebi V. Acinic cell-like carcinoma of the breast. Virchows Arch 1996, **429**: 69–74.

1515 Rosen PP. Adenomyoepithelioma of the breast. Hum Pathol 1987, **18**: 1232–1237.

1516 Rosen PP. Adenoid cystic carcinoma of the breast. A morphologically heterogeneous neoplasm. Pathol Annu 1989, **24**(Pt 2): 237–254.

1517 Schmitt FC, Ribeiro CA, Alvarenga S, Lopes JM. Primary acinic-like carcinoma of the breast – a variant with good prognosis. Histopathology 2000, **36**: 286–289.

1518 Schürch W, Potvin C. Malignant myoepithelioma (myoepithelial carcinoma) of the breast. An ultrastructural and immunocytochemical study. Ultrastruct Pathol 1985, **8**: 1–11.

1519 Shin SJ, Rosen PP. Solid variant of mammary adenoid cystic carcinoma with basaloid features: a study of nine cases. Am J Surg Pathol 2002, **26**: 413–420.

1520 Simpson RH, Cope H, Skalova A, Michal M. Malignant adenomyoepithelioma of the breast with mixed osteogenic, spindle cell, and carcinomatous differentiation. Am J Surg Pathol 1998, **22**: 631–636.

1521 Smith BH, Taylor HB. The occurrence of bone and cartilage in mammary tumors. Am J Clin Pathol 1969, **51**: 610–618.

1522 Storensen FB, Paulsen SM. Glycogen-rich clear cell carcinoma of the breast. A solid variant with mucus. A light microscopic, immunohistochemical and ultrastructural study of a case. Histopathology 1987, **11**: 857–869.

1523 Subramony C. Bilateral breast tumors resembling syringocystadenoma papilliferum. Am J Clin Pathol 1987, **87**: 656–659.

1524 Suster S, Moran CA, Hurt MA. Syringomatous squamous tumors of the breast. Cancer 1991, **67**: 2350–2355.

1525 Tamai M. Intraductal growth of malignant mammary myoepithelioma. Am J Surg Pathol 1992, **16**: 1116–1125.

1526 Tavassoli FA. Myoepithelial lesions of the breast. Myoepitheliosis, adenomyoepithelioma, and myoepithelial carcinoma. Am J Surg Pathol 1991, **15**: 554–568.

1527 Tavassoli FA, Norris HJ. Mammary adenoid cystic carcinoma with sebaceous differentiation. A morphologic study of the cell types. Arch Pathol Lab Med 1986, **110**: 1045–1053.

1528 Toikkanen S, Joensuu H. Glycogen-rich clear-cell carcinoma of the breast. A clinicopathologic and flow cytometric study. Hum Pathol 1991, **22**: 81–83.

1529 Trendell-Smith NJ, Peston D, Shousha S. Adenoid cystic carcinoma of the breast: a tumor commonly devoid of oestrogen receptors and related proteins. Histopathology 1999, **35**: 241–248.

1530 Van Hoeven KH, Drudis T, Cranor ML, Erlandson RA, Rosen PP. Low-grade adenosquamous carcinoma of the breast. A clinicopathologic study of 32 cases with ultrastructural analysis. Am J Surg Pathol 1993, **17**: 248–258.

1531 Ward BE, Cooper PH, Subramony C. Syringomatous tumor of the nipple. Am J Clin Pathol 1989, **92**: 692–696.

1532 Wells CA, Nicoll S, Ferguson DJP. Adenoid cystic carcinoma of the breast. A case with axillary lymph node metastasis. Histopathology 1986, **10**: 415–424.

1533 Wick MR, Ockner DM, Mills SE, Ritter JH, Swanson PE. Homologous carcinomas in the breast, skin, and salivary glands. A histologic and immunohistochemical comparison of ductal mammary carcinoma, ductal sweat gland carcinoma, and salivary duct carcinoma. Am J Clin Pathol 1998, **109**: 75–84.

1534 Zarbo RJ, Oberman HA. Cellular adenomyoepithelioma of the breast. Am J Surg Pathol 1983, **7**: 863–870.

STROMAL TUMORS AND TUMORLIKE CONDITIONS

PHYLLOIDES TUMOR

1535 Azzopardi JG. Problems in breast pathology. In Bennington JL (consulting ed.): Major problems in pathology. Philadephia, 1979, W.B. Saunders.

1536 Barnes L, Pietruszka M. Rhabdomyosarcoma arising within a cystosarcoma phyllodes. Case report and review of the literature. Am J Surg Pathol 1978, **2**: 423–429.

1537 Bernstein L, Deapen D, Ross RK. The descriptive epidemiology of malignant cystosarcoma phyllodes tumors of the breast. Cancer 1993, **71**: 3020–3024.

1538 Burga AM, Tavassoli FA. Periductal stromal tumor: a rare lesion with low-grade sarcomatous behaviour. Am J Surg Pathol 2003, **27**: 343–348.

1539 Carter BA, Page DL. Phyllodes tumor of the breast: local recurrence versus metastatic capacity. Hum Pathol 2004, **35**: 1051–1052.

1540 Chaney AW, Pollack A, Mcneese MD, Zagars GK, Pisters PW, Pollock RE, Hunt KK. Primary treatment of cystosarcoma phyllodes of the breast. Cancer 2000, **89**: 1502–1511.

1541 Christensen L, Nielsen M, Madsen PM. Cystosarcoma phyllodes. A review of 19 cases with emphasis on the occurrence of associated breast carcinoma. Acta Pathol Microbiol Immunol Scand (A) 1986, **94**: 35–41.

1542 Cohn-Cedermark G, Rutqvist LE, Rosendahl I, Silfversward C. Prognostic factors in cystosarcoma phyllodes. A clinicopathologic study of 77 patients. Cancer 1991, **68**: 2017–2022.

1543 Del Vecchio M, Eusebi V. Tumors of the breast showing dual differentiation: a review. Int J Surg Pathol 2004, **12**: 345–350.

1544 Dietrich CU, Pandis N, Rizou H, Petersen C, Bardi G, Qvist H, Apostolikas N, Bohler PJ, Andersen JA, Idvall I, Mitelman F, Heim S. Cytogenetic findings in phyllodes tumors of the breast: karyotypic complexity differentiates between malignant and benign tumors. Hum Pathol 1997, **28**: 1379–1382.

1545 el-Naggar AK, Ro JY, McLemore D, Garnsy L. DNA content and proliferative activity of cystosarcoma phyllodes of the breast. Potential prognostic significance. Am J Clin Pathol 1990, **93**: 480–485.

1546 Esposito NN, Mohan D, Brufsky A, Lin Y, Kapali M, Dabbs DJ. Phyllodes tumor: a clinicopathologic and immunohistochemical study of 30 cases. Arch Pathol Lab Med 2006, **130**: 1516–1521.

1547 Fiks A. Cystosarcoma phyllodes of the mammary gland – Müller's tumor. For the 180th birthday of Johannes Müller. Virchows Arch [A] 1981, **392**: 1–6.

1548 Grimes MM, Lattes R, Jaretzki A III. Cystosarcoma phyllodes. Report of an unusual case, with death due to intraneural extension to the central nervous system. Cancer 1985, **56**: 1691–1695.

1549 Hart WR, Bauer RC, Oberman HA. Cystosarcoma phyllodes. A clinicopathologic study of twenty-six hypercellular periductal stromal tumors of the breast. Am J Clin Pathol 1978, **70**: 211–216.

1550 Jacobs TW, Chen YY, Guinee DG Jr, Holden JA, Cha I, Bauermeister DE, Hashimoto B, Wolverton D, Hartzog G. Fibroepithelial lesions with cellular stroma on breast core needle biopsy: are there predictors of outcome on surgical excision? Am J Clin Pathol 2005, **124**: 342–354.

1551 Kleer CG, Giordano TJ, Braun T, Oberman H. Pathologic, immunohistochemical, and molecular features of benign and malignant phyllodes tumor of the breast. Mod Pathol 2001, **14**: 185–190.

1552 Knudsen PJT, Ostergaard J. Cystosarcoma phylloides with lobular and ductal carcinoma in situ. Arch Pathol Lab Med 1987, **111**: 873–875.

1553 Lee AH, Hodi Z, Ellis IO, Elston CW. Histological features useful in the distinction of phyllodes tumour and fibroadenoma on needle core biopsy of the breast. Histopathology 2007, **51**: 336–344.

1554 Lee AHS. Recent developments in the histological diagnosis of spindle cell carcinoma, fibromatosis and phyllodes tumour of the breast. Histopathology 2008, **52**: 45–57.

1555 Lerwill MF. Biphasic lesions of the breast. Semin Diagn Pathol 2004, **21**: 48–56.

1556 Macher-Goeppinger S, Marme F, Goeppert B, Penzel R, Schirmacher P, Sinn HP, Aulmann S. Invasive ductal breast cancer within a malignant phyllodes tumor: case report and assessment of clonality. Hum Pathol 2010, **41**: 293–296.

1557 Millar EK, Beretov J, Marr P, Sarris M, Clarke RA, Kersley JH, Lee CS. Malignant phyllodes tumours of the breast display increased stromal p53 protein expression. Histopathology 1999, **34**: 491–496.

1558 Moffat CJC, Pinder SE, Dixon AR, Elston CW, Blarney RW, Ellis IO. Phyllodes tumours of the breast. A clinicopathological review of thirty-two cases. Histopathology 1995, **27**: 205–218.

1559 Moore T, Lee AH. Expression of CD34 and bcl-2 in phyllodes tumors, fibroadenomas and spindle cell lesions of the breast. Histopathology 2001, **38**: 62–67.

1560 Nishimura R, Hasebe T, Imoto S, Mukai K. Malignant phyllodes tumour with a noninvasive ductal carcinoma component. Virchows Arch 1998, **432**: 89–93.

1561 Norris HJ, Taylor HB. Relationship of histologic features to behavior of cystosarcoma phyllodes. Analysis of ninety-four cases. Cancer 1967, **20**: 2090–2099.

1562 Palko MJ, Wang SE, Shackney SE, Cottington EM, Levitt SB, Hartsock RJ. Flow cytometric S fraction as a predictor of clinical outcome in cystosarcoma phyllodes. Arch Pathol Lab Med 1990, **114**: 949–952.

1563 Pietruszka M, Barnes L. Cystosarcoma phyllodes: a clinicopathologic analysis of 42 cases. Cancer 1978, **41**: 1974–1983.

1564 Powell CM, Rosen PP. Adipose differentiation in cystosarcoma phyllodes. A study of 14 cases. Am J Surg Pathol 1994, **18**: 720–727.

1565 Rajan PB, Cranor ML, Rosen PP. Cystosarcoma phyllodes in adolescent girls and young women: a study of 45 patients. Am J Surg Pathol 1998, **22**: 64–69.

1566 Reddick RL, Shin TK, Sawhney D, Siegal GP. Stromal proliferations of the breast. An ultrastructural and immunohistochemical evaluation of cystosarcoma phyllodes, juvenile fibroadenoma, and fibroadenoma. Hum Pathol 1987, **18**: 45–49.

1567 Reinfuss M, Mituś J, Duda K, Stelmach A, Ryś J, Smolak K. The treatment and prognosis of patients with phyllodes tumor of the breast: an analysis of 170 cases. Cancer 1996, **77**: 910–916.

1568 Rhodes RH, Frankel KA, Davis RL, Tatter D. Metastatic cystosarcoma phyllodes. A report of 2 cases presenting with neurological symptoms. Cancer 1978, **41**: 1179–1187.

1569 Rosen PP, Romain K, Liberman L. Mammary cystosarcoma with mature adipose stromal differentiation (lipophyllodes tumor) arising in a lipomatous hamartoma. Arch Pathol Lab Med 1994, **118**: 91–94.

1570 Silver SA, Tavassoli FA. Osteosarcomatous differentiation in phyllodes tumors. Am J Surg Pathol 1999, **23**: 815–821.

1571 Tse GM, Lee CS, Kung FY, Scolyer RA, Law BK, Lau TS, Putti TC. Hormonal receptors expression in epithelial cells of mammary phyllodes tumors correlates with pathologic grade of the tumor. A multicenter study of 143 cases. Am J Clin Pathol 2002, **118**: 522–526.

1572 Tse GM, Putti TC, Kung FY, Scolyer RA, Law BK, Lau TS, Lee CS. Increased p53 protein expression in malignant mammary phyllodes tumors. Mod Pathol 2002, **15**: 734–740.

1573 Tse GM, Putti TC, Lui PC, Lo AW, Scolyer RA, Law BK, Karim R, Lee CS. Increased c-kit (CD117) expression in malignant mammary phyllodes tumors. Mod Pathol 2004, **17**: 827–831.

1574 Umekita Y, Yoshida H. Immunohistochemical study of hormone receptor and hormone-regulated protein expression in phyllodes tumour: comparison with fibroadenoma. Virchows Arch 1998, **433**: 311–314.

1575 Ward RM, Evans HL. Cystosarcoma phyllodes. A clinicopathologic study of 26 cases. Cancer 1986, **58**: 2282–2289.

1576 Yeh I-T, Francis DJ, Orenstein JM, Silverberg SG. Ultrastructure of cystosarcoma phyllodes and fibroadenoma. A comparative study. Am J Clin Pathol 1985, **84**: 131–136.

1577 Yohe S, Yeh IT. 'Missed' diagnoses of phyllodes tumor on breast biopsy: pathologic clues to its recognition. Int J Surg Pathol 2008, **16**: 137–142.

VASCULAR TUMORS AND TUMORLIKE LESIONS

1578 Arias Stella J Jr, Rosen PP. Hemangiopericytoma of the breast. Mod Pathol 1988, **2**: 98–103.

1579 Benda JA, Al-Jurf AS, Benson AB III. Angiosarcoma of the breast following segmental mastectomy complicated by lymphedema. Am J clin Pathol 1987, **87**: 651–655.

1580 Billings SD, McKenney JK, Folpe AL, Hardacre MC, Weiss SW. Cutaneous angiosarcoma following breast-conserving surgery and radiation: an analysis of 27 cases. Am J Surg Pathol 2004, **28**: 781–788.

1581 Branton PA, Lininger R, Tavassoli FA. Papillary endothelial hyperplasia of the breast: the great impostor for angiosarcoma. A clinicopathologic review of 17 cases. Int J Surg Pathol 2003, **11**: 83–87.

1582 Brenn T, Fletcher CD. Postradiation vascular proliferations: an increasing problem. Histopathology 2006, **48**: 106–114.

1583 Brentani MM, Pacheco MM, Oshima CTF, Nagai MA, Lemos LB, Góes JCS. Steroid receptors in breast angiosarcoma. Cancer 1983, **51**: 2105–2111.

1584 Brodie C, Provenzano E. Vascular proliferations of the breast. Histopathology 2008, **52**: 30–44.

1585 Chen KTK. Rare variants of benign vascular tumors of the breast. Surg Pathol 1991, **4**: 309–316.

1586 Di Tommaso L, Rosai J. The capillary lobule: a deceptively benign feature of post-radiation angiosarcoma of the skin: report of three cases. Am J Dermatopathol 2005, **27**: 301–305.

1587 Donnell RM, Rosen PP, Lieberman PH, Kaufman RJ, Kay S, Braun DW Jr, Kinne DW. Angiosarcoma and other vascular tumors of the breast. Pathologic analysis as a guide to prognosis. Am J Surg Pathol 1981, **5**: 629–642.

1588 Fineberg S, Rosen PP. Cutaneous angiosarcoma and atypical vascular lesions of the skin and breast after radiation therapy for breast carcinoma. Am J Clin Pathol 1994, **102**: 757–763.

1589 Jozefczyk MA, Rosen PP. Vascular tumors of the breast. II. Perilobular hemangiomas and hemangiomas. Am J Surg Pathol 1985, **9**: 491–503.

1590 Lesueur GC, Brown RW, Bhathal PS. Incidence of perilobular hemangioma in the female breast. Arch Pathol Lab Med 1983, **107**: 308–310.

1591 Liberman L, Dershaw DD, Kaufman RJ, Rosen PP. Angiosarcoma of the breast. Radiology 1992, **183**: 649–654.

1592 Lucas DR. Angiosarcoma, radiation-associated angiosarcoma, and atypical vascular lesion. Arch Pathol Lab Med 2009, **133**: 1804–1809.

1593 Macias-Martinez V, Murrieta-Tiburcio L, Molina-Cardenas H, Donimguez-Malagon H. Epithelioid angiosarcoma of the breast: clinicopathological, immunohistochemical and ultrastructural study of a case. Am J Surg Pathol 1997, **21**: 599–604.

1594 Merino MJ, Carter D, Berman M. Angiosarcoma of the breast. Am J Surg Pathol 1983, **7**: 53–60.

1595 Mittal KR, Gerald W, True LD. Hemangiopericytoma of the breast. Report of a case with ultrastructural and immunohistochemical findings. Hum Pathol 1986, **17**: 1181–1183.

1596 Monroe AT, Feigenberg SJ, Mendenhall NP. Angiosarcoma after breast-conserving therapy. Cancer 2003, **97**: 1832–1840.

1597 Nascimento AF, Raut CP, Fletcher CD. Primary angiosarcoma of the breast: clinicopathologic analysis of 49 cases, suggesting that grade is not prognostic. Am J Surg Pathol 2008, **32**: 1896–1904.

1598 Otis CN, Peschel R, McKhann C, Merino MJ, Duray PH. The rapid onset of cutaneous angiosarcoma after radiotherapy for breast carcinoma. Cancer 1986, **57**: 2130–2134.

1599 Parham DH, Fisher C. Angiosarcoma of the breast developing post radiotherapy. Histopathology 1997, **31**: 189–195.

1600 Patton KT, Deyrup AT, Weiss SW. Atypical vascular lesions after surgery and radiation of the breast: a clinicopathologic study of 32 cases analyzing histologic heterogeneity and association with angiosarcoma. Am J Surg Pathol 2008, **32**: 943–950.

1601 Rosen PP. Vascular tumors of the breast. III. Angiomatosis. Am J Surg Pathol 1985, **9**: 652–658.

1602 Rosen PP. Vascular tumors of the breast. V. Nonparenchymal hemangiomas of mammary subcutaneous tissues. Am J Surg Pathol 1985, **9**: 723–729.

1603 Rosen PP, Kimmel M, Ernsberger DL. Mammary angiosarcoma. The prognostic significance of tumor differentiation. Cancer 1988, **62**: 2145–2151.

1604 Rosen PP, Jozefczyk MA, Boram LH. Vascular tumors of the breast. IV. The venous hemangioma. Am J Surg Pathol 1985, **9**: 659–665.

1605 Rosen PP, Ridolfi RL. The perilobular hemangioma. A benign microscopic vascular lesion of the breast. Am J Clin Pathol 1977, **68**: 21–23.

1606 Rosso R, Gianelli U, Carnevali L. Acquired progressive lymphangioma of the skin following radiotherapy for breast carcinoma. J Cutan Pathol 1995, **22**: 164–167.

1607 Shin SJ, Lesser M, Rosen PP. Hemangiomas and angiosarcomas of the breast: diagnostic utility of cell cycle markers with emphasis on Ki-67. Arch Pathol Lab Med 2007, **131**: 538–544.

1608 Sieber PR, Sharkey FE. Cystic hygroma of the breast. Arch Pathol Lab Med 1986, 110: 353.

1609 Steingaszner LC, Enzinger FM, Taylor HB. Hemangiosarcoma of the breast. Cancer 1965, **18**: 352–361.

1610 Vorburger SA, Xing Y, Hunt KK, Lakin GE, Benjamin RS, Feig BW, Pisters PW, Ballo MT, Chen L, Trent J 3rd, Burgess M, Patel S, Pollock RE, Cormier JN. Angiosarcoma of the breast. Cancer 2005, **104**: 2682–2688.

1611 Weaver J, Billings SD. Postradiation cutaneous vascular tumors of the breast: a review. Semin Diagn Pathol 2009, **26**: 141–149.

1612 Yu GH, Fishman SJ, Brooks JS. Cellular angiolipoma of the breast. Mod Pathol 1993, **6**: 497–499.

OTHER MALIGNANT STROMAL TUMORS

1613 Arista-Nasr J, Gonzalez-Gomez I, Angeles-Angeles A, Illanes-Baz E, Brandt-Brandt H, Larriva-Sahd J. Primary recurrent leiomyosarcoma of the breast. Case report with ultrastructural and immunohistochemical study and review of the literature. Am J Clin Pathol 1989, **92**: 500–505.

1614 Austin RM, Dupree WB. Liposarcoma of the breast. A clinicopathologic study of 20 cases. Hum Pathol 1986, **17**: 906–913.

1615 Bahrami A, Resetkova E, Ro JY, Ibañez JD, Ayala AG. Primary osteosarcoma of the breast: report of 2 cases. Arch Pathol Lab Med 2007, **131**: 792–795.

1616 Beltaos E, Banerjee TK. Chondrosarcoma of the breast. Report of two cases. Am J Clin Pathol 1979, **71**: 345–349.

1617 Callery CD, Rosen PP, Kinne DW. Sarcoma of the breast. A study of 32 patients with reappraisal of classification and therapy. Ann Surg 1985, **201**: 527–532.

1618 Chen KTK, Kuo T-T, Hoffmann KD. Leiomyosarcoma of the breast. A case of long survival and late hepatic metastasis. Cancer 1981, **47**: 1883–1886.

1619 Falconieri G, della Libera D, Zanconati F, Bittesini L. Leiomyosarcoma of the female breast. Report of two new cases and a review of the literature. Am J Clin Pathol 1997, **108**: 19–25.

1620 Fisher C, Magnusson B, Hardarson S, Smith ME. Myxoid variant of follicular dendritic cell sarcoma arising in the breast. Ann Diagn Pathol 1999, **3**: 92–98.

1621 Going JJ, Lumsden AB, Anderson TJ. A classical osteogenic sarcoma of the breast. Histology, immunohistochemistry and ultrastructure. Histopathology 1986, **10**: 631–641.

1622 Jones MW, Norris HJ, Wargotz ES, Weiss SW. Fibrosarcoma–malignant fibrous histiocytoma of the breast. A clinicopathological study of 32 cases. Am J Surg Pathol 1992, **16**: 667–674.

1623 Kapucuoglu N, Percinel S, Ventura T, Lang R, Al-Daraji W, Eusebi V. Dendritic cell sarcomas/tumours of the breast: report of two cases. Virchows Arch 2009, **454**: 333–339.

1624 Kyriazis AP, Kyriazis AA. Primary rhabdomyosarcoma of the female breast: report of a case and review of the literature. Arch Pathol Lab Med 1998, **122**: 747–749.

1625 Leibl S, Moinfar F. Mammary NOS-type sarcoma with CD10 expression: a rare entity with features of myoepithelial differentiation. Am J Surg Pathol 2006, **30**: 450–456.

1626 Mazaki T, Tanak T, Suenaga Y, Tomioka K, Takayama T. Liposarcoma of the breast: a case report and review of the literature. Int Surg 2002, **87**: 164–170.

1627 Mogotlane L, Chetty R. Infiltrating ductal carcinoma of the breast with rhabdoid phenotype. Int J Surg Pathol 2001, **9**: 237–239.

1628 Norris HJ, Taylor HB. Sarcomas and related mesenchymal tumors of the breast. Cancer 1968, **22**: 22–28.

1629 Pollard SG, Marks PV, Temple LN, Thompson HH. Breast sarcoma. A clinicopathologic review of 25 cases. Cancer 1990, **66**: 941–944.

1630 Pruneri G, Masullo M, Renne G, Taccagni G, Manzotti M, Luini A, Viale G. Follicular dendritic cell sarcoma of the breast. Virchows Arch 2002, **441**: 194–199.

1631 Sezer O, Jugovic D, Blohmer JU, Turzynski A, Thiel G, Langelotz C, Possinger K, Kovar H. CD99 positivity and EWS-FLI1 gene rearrangement identify a breast tumor in 60-year-old patient with attributes of the Ewing family of neoplasms. Diagn Mol Pathol 1999, **8**: 120–124.

1632 Silver SA, Tavassoli FA. Primary osteogenic sarcoma of the breast: a clinicopathologic analysis of 50 cases. Am J Surg Pathol 1998, **22**: 925–933.

1633 Smith BH, Taylor HB. The occurrence of bone and cartilage in mammary tumors. Am J Clin Pathol 1969, **51**: 610–618.

1634 Uluoğlu O, Akyürek N, Uner A, Coşkun U, Ozdemir A, Gökçora N. Interdigitating dendritic cell tumor with breast and cervical lymph-node involvement: a case report and review of the literature. Virchows Arch 2005, **446**: 546–554.

1635 Wu J, Brinker DA, Haas M, Montgomery EA, Argani P. Primary alveolar soft part sarcoma (ASPS) of the breast: report of a deceptive case with xanthomatous features confirmed by TFE3 immunohistochemistry and electron microscopy. Int J Surg Pathol 2005, **13**: 81–85.

LYMPHOID TUMORS AND TUMORLIKE CONDITIONS

1636 Abbondanzo SL, Seidman JD, Lefkowitz M, Tavassoli FA, Krishnan J. Primary diffuse large B-cell lymphoma of the breast. A clinicopathologic study of 31 cases. Pathol Res Pract 1996, **192**: 37–43.

1637 Aguilera NS, Tavassoli FA, Chu WS, Abbondonzo SL. T-cell lymphoma presenting in the breast: a histologic, immunophenotypic and molecular genetic study of four cases. Mod Pathol 2000, **13**: 599–605.

1638 Arber DA, Simpson JF, Weiss LM, Rappaport H. Non-Hodgkin's lymphoma involving the breast. Am J Surg Pathol 1994, **18**: 288–295.

1639 Bobrow LG, Richards MA, Happerfield LC, Diss TC, Isaacson PG, Lammie GA, Millis RR. Breast lymphomas. A clinicopathologic review. Hum Pathol 1993, **24**: 274–278.

1640 Boudova L, Kazakov DV, Sima R, Vanecek T, Torlakovic E, Lamovec J, Kutzner H, Szepe P, Plank L, Bouda J, Hes O, Mukensnabl P, Michal M. Cutaneous lymphoid hyperplasia and other lymphoid infiltrates of the breast nipple: a retrospective clinicopathologic study of fifty-six patients. Am J Dermatopathol 2005, **27**: 375–386.

1641 Brogi E, Harris NL. Lymphomas of the breast: pathology and clinical behaviour. Semin Oncol 1999, **26**: 357–364.

1642 Brooks JJ, Krugman DT, Damjanov I. Myeloid metaplasia presenting as a breast mass. Am J Surg Pathol 1980, **4**: 281–285.

1643 Byrd JC, Edenfield WJ, Shields DJ, Dawson NA. Extramedullary myeloid cell tumors in acute nonlymphocytic leukemia. A clinical review. J Clin Oncol 1995, **13**: 1800–1816.

1644 Cheuk W, Chan AC, Lam WL, Chow SM, Crowley P, Lloydd R, Campbell I, Thorburn M, Chan JK. IgG4-related sclerosing mastitis: description of a new member of the IgG4-related sclerosing diseases. Am J Surg Pathol 2009, **33**: 1058–1064.

1645 Cohen PL, Brooks JJ. Lymphomas of the breast. A clinicopathologic and immunohistochemical study of primary and secondary cases. Cancer 1991, **67**: 1359–1369.

1646 Cook PD, Osborne BM, Connor RL, Strauss JF. Follicular lymphoma adjacent to foreign body granulomatous inflammation and fibrosis surrounding silicone breast prosthesis. Am J Surg Pathol 1995, **19**: 712–717.

1647 Domchek SM, Hecht JL, Fleming MD, Pinkus GS, Cannellos GP. Lymphomas of the breast: primary and secondary involvement. Cancer 2002, **94**: 6–13.

1648 Duncan VE, Reddy VV, Jhala NC, Chhieng DC, Jhala DN. Non-Hodgkin's lymphoma of the breast: a review of 18 primary and secondary cases. Ann Diagn Pathol 2006, **10**: 144–148.

1649 Farinha P, Andre S, Cabecadas J, Soares J. High frequency of MALT lymphoma in a series of 14 cases of primary breast lymphoma. Appl Immunohistochem Mol Morphol 2002, **10**: 115–120.

1650 Fisher ER, Palekar AS, Paulson JD, Golinger R. Pseudolymphoma of breast. Cancer 1979, **44**: 258–263.

1651 Fritzsche FR, Pahl S, Petersen I, Burkhardt M, Dankof A, Dietel M, Kristiansen G. Anaplastic large-cell non-Hodgkin's lymphoma of the breast in periprosthetic localisation 32 years after treatment for primary breast cancer – a case report. Virchows Arch 2006, **449**: 561–564.

1652 Gualco G, Bacchi CE. B-cell and T-cell lymphomas of the breast: clinical–pathological features of 53 cases. Int J Surg Pathol 2008, **16**: 407–413.

1653 Hugh JC, Jackson FI, Hanson J, Poppema S. Primary breast lymphoma. An immunohistologic study of 20 new cases. Cancer 1990, **66**: 2602–2611.

1654 Kirshenbaum G, Rhone DP. Solitary extramedullary plasmacytoma of the breast with serum monoclonal protein. A case report and review of the literature. Am J Clin Pathol 1985, **83**: 230–232.

1655 Koerner FC, Mattia AR. Mammary lymphoid tissue: a unique component of the mucosal immune system. Anat Pathol 1996, **1**: 53–67.

1656 Lin JJ, Farha GJ, Taylor RJ. Pseudolymphoma of the breast. I. In a study of 8,654 consecutive tylectomies and mastectomies. Cancer 1980, **45**: 973–978.

1657 Lin Y, Govindan R, Hess JL. Malignant hematopoietic breast tumors. Am J Clin Pathol 1997, **107**: 177–186.

1658 Miranda RN, Lin L, Talwalkar SS, Manning JT, Medeiros LJ. Anaplastic large cell lymphoma involving the breast: a clinicopathologic study of 6 cases and review of the literature. Arch Pathol Lab Med 2009, **133**: 1383–1390.

1659 Oberman HA. Primary lymphoreticular neoplasms of the breast. Surg Gynecol Obstet 1966, **123**: 1047–1051.

1660 Pascoe HR. Tumors composed of immature granulocytes occurring in the breast in chronic granulocytic leukemia. Cancer 1970, **25**: 697–704.

1661 Roden AC, Macon WR, Keeney GL, Myers JL, Feldman AL, Dogan A. Seroma-associated primary anaplastic large-cell lymphoma adjacent to breast implants: an indolent T-cell lymphoproliferative disorder. Mod Pathol 2008, **21**: 455–463.

1662 Rooney N, Snead D, Goodman S, Webb AJ. Primary breast lymphoma with skin involvement arising in lymphocytic lobulitis. Histopathology 1994, **24**: 81–84.

1663 Schouten JT, Weese JL, Carbone PP. Lymphoma of the breast. Ann Surg 1981, **194**: 749–753.

1664 Talwalkar SS, Miranda RN, Valbuena JR, Routbort MJ, Martin AW, Medeiros LJ. Lymphomas involving the breast: a study of 106 cases comparing localized and disseminated neoplasms. Am J Surg Pathol 2008, **32**: 1299–1309.

1665 Topalovski M, Crisan D, Mattson JC. Lymphoma of the breast: a clinicopathologic study of primary and secondary cases. Arch Pathol Lab Med 1999, **123**: 1208–1218.

1666 Valbuena JR, Admirand JH, Gualco G, Medeiros LJ. Myeloid sarcoma involving the breast. Arch Pathol Lab Med 2005, **129**: 32–38.

1667 Wong AK, Lopategui J, Clancy S, Kulber D, Bose S. Anaplastic large cell lymphoma associated with a breast implant capsule: a case report and review of the literature. Am J Surg Pathol 2008, **32**: 1265–1268.

1668 Yoshida S, Nakamura N, Sasaki Y, Yoshida S, Yasuda M, Sagara H, Ohtake T, Takenoshita S, Abe M. Primary breast diffuse large B-cell lymphoma shows a non-germinal center B-cell phenotype. Mod Pathol 2005, **18**: 398–405.

OTHER PRIMARY TUMORS AND TUMORLIKE CONDITIONS

1669 Abraham SC, Reynolds C, Lee JH, Montgomery EA, Baisden BL, Krasinskas AM, Wu TT. Fibromatosis of the breast and mutations involving the APC/beta-catenin pathway. Hum Pathol 2002, **33**: 39–46.

1670 Anderson C, Ricci A Jr, Pedersen CA, Cartun RW. Immunocytochemical analysis of estrogen and progesterone receptors in benign stromal lesions of the breast. Evidence for hormonal etiology in pseudoangiomatous hyperplasia of mammary stroma. Am J Surg Pathol 1991, **15**: 145–149.

1671 Balzer BL, Weiss SW. Do biomaterials cause implant-associated mesenchymal tumors of the breast? Analysis of 8 new cases and review of the literature. Hum Pathol 2009, **40**: 1564–1570.

1672 Bansal I, Alassi O, Lee MW, Raju U. Stromal proliferations of the breast, a histologic continuum in fibroadenoma, pseudoangiomatous stromal hyperplasia and gynecomastoid lesions: an immunohistochemical study [abstract]. Mod Pathol 2003, 16: 23a.

1673 Begin LR, Mitmaker B, Bahary J-P. Infiltrating myofibroblastoma of the breast. Surg Pathol 1989, **2**: 151–156.

1674 Berean K, Tron VA, Churg A, Clement PB. Mammary fibroadenoma with multinucleated stromal giant cells. Am J Surg Pathol 1986, **10**: 823–827.

1675 Bittesini L, Dei Tos AP, Doglioni C, Della Libera D, Laurino L, Fletcher CD. Fibroepithelial tumor of the breast with digital fibroma-like inclusions in the stromal component. Case report with immunocytochemical and ultrastructural analysis. Am J Surg Pathol 1994, **18**: 296–301.

1676 Carneiro F, Brandao O, Correia AC, Sobrinho-Simoes M. Spindle cell tumor of the breast. Ultrastruct Pathol 1989, **13**: 593–598.

1677 Charpin C, Mathoulin MP, Andrac L, Barberis J, Boulat J, Sarradour B, Bonnier P, Piana L. Reappraisal of breast hamartomas. A morphological study of 41 cases. Pathol Res Pract 1994, **190**: 362–371.

1678 Cohen MB, Fisher PE. Schwann cell tumors of the breast and mammary region. Surg Pathol 1991, **4**: 47–56.

1679 Damiani S, Dina R, Eusebi V. Eosinophilic and granular cell tumors of the breast. Semin Diagn Pathol 1999, **16**: 117–125.

1680 Damiani S, Koerner FC, Dickersin GR, Cook MG, Eusebi V. Granular cell tumour of the breast. Virchows Arch [A] 1992, **420**: 219–226.

1681 Damiani S, Peterse JL, Eusebi V. Malignant neoplasms infiltrating 'pseudoangiomatous' stromal hyperplasia of the breast: an unrecognised pathway of tumour spread. Histopathology 2002, **41**: 208–215.

1682 Daroca PJ Jr, Reed RJ, Love GL, Kraus SD. Myoid hamartomas of the breast. Hum Pathol 1985, **16**: 212–219.

1683 Davies JD, Kulka J, Mumford AD, Armstrong JS, Wells CA. Hamartomas of the breast. Six novel diagnostic features in three-dimensional thick sections. Histopathology 1994, **24**: 161–168.

1684 Davis AB, Patchefsky AS. Basal cell carcinoma of the nipple. Case report and review of the literature. Cancer 1977, **40**: 1780–1781.

1685 Daya D, Trus T, D'Souza TJ, Minuk T, Yemen B. Hamartoma of the breast, an underrecognized breast lesion. A clinicopathologic and radiographic study of 25 cases. Am J Clin Pathol 1995, **103**: 685–689.

1686 DeMay RM, Kay S. Granular cell tumor of the breast. Pathol Annu 1982, **19**(Pt 2): 121–148.

1687 Devouassoux-Shisheboran M, Schammel MD, Man YG, Tavassoli FA. Fibromatosis of the breast: age-correlated morphological features of 33 cases. Arch Pathol Lab Med 2000, **124**: 276–280.

1688 Diaz-Arias AA, Hurt MA, Loy TS, Seeger RM, Bickel JT. Leiomyoma of the breast. Hum Pathol 1989, **20**: 396–399.

1689 Falconieri G, Lamovec J, Mirra M, Pizzolitto S. Solitary fibrous tumor of the mammary gland: a potential pitfall in breast pathology. Ann Diagn Pathol 2004, **8**: 121–125.

1690 Ferreira M, Albarracin CT, Resetkova E. Pseudoangiomatous stromal hyperplasia tumor: a clinical, radiologic and pathologic study of 26 cases. Mod Pathol 2008, **21**: 201–207.

1691 Fisher CJ, Hanby AM, Robinson L, Millis RR. Mammary hamartoma – a review of 35 cases. Histopathology 1992, **20**: 99–106.

1692 Garfein CF, Aulicino MR, Leytin A, Drossman S, Hermann G, Bleiweiss IJ. Epithelioid cells in myoid hamartoma of the breast: a potential diagnostic pitfall for core biopsies. Arch Pathol Lab Med 1996, **120**: 676–680.

1693 Govender D, Sabaratnam RM, Essa AS. Clear cell 'sugar' tumor of the breast: another extrapulmonary site and review of the literature. Am J Surg Pathol 2002, **26**: 670–675.

1694 Green I, Dorfman RF, Rosai J. Breast involvement by extranodal Rosai–Dorfman disease: report of seven cases. Am J Surg Pathol 1997, **21**: 664–668.

1695 Herbert M, Sandbank J, Liokumovich P, Yanai O, Pappo I, Karni T, Segal M. Breast hamartomas: clinicopathological and immunohistochemical studies of 24 cases. Histopathology 2002, **41**: 30–34.

1696 Hiraoka N, Mukai M, Hosoda Y, Hata J. Phyllodes tumor of the breast containing the intracytoplasmic inclusion bodies identical with infantile digital fibromatosis. Am J Surg Pathol 1994, **18**: 506–511.

1697 Ilie B. Neoplasms in skin and subcutis over the breast, simulating breast neoplasms. Case reports and literature review. J Surg Oncol 1986, **31**: 191–198.

1698 Ingram DL, Mossler JA, Snowhite J, Leight GS, McCarty KS Jr. Granular cell tumors of the breast. Steroid receptor analysis and localization of carcinoembryonic antigen, myoglobin, and S100 protein. Arch Pathol Lab Med 1984, **108**: 897–901.

1699 Jones MW, Norris HJ, Wargotz ES. Hamartomas of the breast. Surg Gynecol Obstet 1991, **173**: 54–56.

1700 Kaplan L, Walts AE. Benign chondrolipomatous tumor of the human female breast. Arch Pathol Lab Med 1977, **101**: 149–151.

1701 Katzin WE, Centeno JA, Feng LJ, Kiley M, Mullick FG. Pathology of lymph nodes from patients with breast implants: a histologic and spectroscopic evaluation. Am J Surg Pathol 2005, **29**: 506–511.

1702 Khanafshar E, Phillipson J, Schammel DP, Minobe L, Cymerman J, Weidner N. Inflammatory myofibroblastic tumor of the breast. Ann Diagn Pathol 2005, **9**: 123–129.

1703 Lugo M, Reyes JM, Putong PB. Benign chondrolipomatous tumors of the breast. Arch Pathol Lab Med 1982, **106**: 691–692.

1704 Luo JH, Rotterdam H. Primary amyloid tumor of the breast: a case report and review of the literature. Mod Pathol 1997, **10**: 735–738.

1705 Marsh WL Jr, Lucas JG, Olsen J. Chondrolipoma of the breast. Arch Pathol Lab Med 1989, **113**: 369–371.

1706 Michal M, Ludvikova M, Zamecnik M. Nodular mucinosis of the breast: report of three cases. Pathol Int 1998, **48**: 542–544.

1707 Morkowski JJ, Nguyen CV, Lin P, Farr M, Abraham SC, Gilcrease MZ, Moran CA, Wu Y. Rosai–Dorfman disease confined to the breast. Ann Diagn Pathol 2010, **14**: 81–87.

1708 Nascimento AG, Karas M, Rosen PP, Caron AG. Leiomyoma of the nipple. Am J Surg Pathol 1979, **3**: 151–154.

1709 Oberman HA. Hamartomas and hamartoma variants of the breast. Semin Diagn Pathol 1989, **6**: 135–145.

1710 Pettinato G, Manivel JC, Gould EW, Albores-Saavedra J. Inclusion body fibromatosis of the breast. Two cases with immunohistochemical and ultrastructural findings. Am J Clin Pathol 1994, **101**: 714–718.

1711 Powell CM, Cranor ML, Rosen PP. Pseudoangiomatous stromal hyperplasia (PASH). A mammary stromal tumor with myofibroblastic differentiation. Am J Surg Pathol 1995, **19**: 270–277.

1712 Provenzano E, Barter SJ, Wright PA, Forouhi P, Allibone R, Ellis IO. Erdheim–Chester disease presenting as bilateral clinically malignant breast masses. Am J Surg Pathol 2010, **34**: 584–588.

1713 Rocken C, Kronsbein H, Sletten K, Roessner A, Bassler R. Amyloidosis of the breast. Virchows Arch 2002, **440**: 527–535.

1714 Roncaroli F, Rossi R, Severi B, Martinelli GN, Eusebi V. Epithelioid leiomyoma of the breast with granular cell change. A case report. Hum Pathol 1993, **24**: 1260–1263.

1715 Rosen PP. Multinucleated mammary stromal giant cells. A benign lesion that simulates invasive carcinoma. Cancer 1979, **44**: 1305–1308.

1716 Rosen PP, Ernsberger D. Mammary fibromatosis. A benign spindle-cell tumor with significant risk for local recurrence. Cancer 1989, **63**: 1363–1369.

1717 Rosso R, Scelsi M, Carnevali L. Granular cell traumatic neuroma: a lesion occurring in mastectomy scars. Arch Pathol Lab Med 2000, **124**: 709–711.

1718 Ryska A, Reynolds C, Keeney GL. Benign tumors of the breast with multinucleated stromal giant cells. Immunohistochemical analysis of six cases and review of the literature. Virchows Arch 2001, **439**: 768–775.

1719 Shin SJ, Scamman W, Gopalan A, Rosen PP. Mammary presentation of adult-type 'juvenile' xanthogranuloma. Am J Surg Pathol 2005, **29**: 827–831.

1720 Vuitch MF, Rosen PP, Erlandson RA. Pseudoangiomatous hyperplasia of mammary stroma. Hum Pathol 1986, **17**: 185–191.

METASTATIC TUMORS

1721 Azzopardi JG. Problems in breast pathology. In Bennington JL (consulting ed.): Major problems in pathology, vol. 11. Philadelphia, 1979, W.B. Saunders.

1722 Di Bonito L, Luchi M, Giarelli L, Falconieri G, Viehl P. Metastatic tumors to the female breast. An autopsy study of 12 cases. Pathol Res Pract 1991, **187**: 432–436.

1723 Gupta D, Merino MJ, Farhood A, Middleton LP. Metastases to breast simulating ductal carcinoma in situ: report of two cases and review of the literature. Ann Diagn Pathol 2001, **4**: 15–20.

1724 Hajdu SI, Urban JA. Cancers metastatic to the breast. Cancer 1968, **22**: 1691–1696.

1725 Harrist TJ, Kalisher L. Breast metastasis. An unusual manifestation of a malignant carcinoid tumor. Cancer 1977, **40**: 3102–3106.

1726 Horenstein MG, Erlandson RA, Gonzalez-Cueto DM, Rosai J. Presacral carcinoid tumors: report of three cases and review of the literature. Am J Surg Pathol 1998, **22**: 251–255.

1727 Howarth CB, Caces JN, Pratt CB. Breast metastases in children with rhabdomyosarcoma. Cancer 1980, **46**: 2520–2524.

1728 Mosunjac MB, Kochhar R, Mosunjac MI, Lau SK. Primary small bowel carcinoid tumor with bilateral breast metastases: report of 2 cases with different clinical presentations. Arch Pathol Lab Med 2004, **128**: 292–297.

1729 Treilleux I, Freyer G, Tabone E, Chassagne-Clement C, Bremond A, Bailly C. Pancreatic neuroendocrine carcinoma metastatic to the breast as part of the multiple endocrine neoplasia type 1 syndrome. Endocr Pathol 1997, **8**: 251–258.

1730 Warner TFCS, Seo IS. Bronchial carcinoid appearing as a breast mass. Arch Pathol Lab Med 1980, **104**: 531–534.

1731 Yamasaki H, Saw D, Zdanowitz J, Faltz LL. Ovarian carcinoma metastasis to the breast case report and review of the literature. Am J Surg Pathol 1993, **17**: 193–197.

BREAST DISEASES IN CHILDREN AND ADOLESCENTS

1732 Bauer BS, Jones KM, Talbot CW. Mammary masses in the adolescent female. Surg Gynecol Obstet 1987, **165**: 63–65.

1733 Dehner LP, Hill DA, Deschryver K. Pathology of the breast in children, adolescents, and young adults. Semin Diagn Pathol 1999, **16**: 235–247.

1734 Farrow JH, Ashikari H. Breast lesions in young girls. Surg Clin North Am 1969, **49**: 261–269.

1735 Kiaer HW, Kiaer WW, Linell F, Jacobsen S. Extreme duct papillomatosis of the juvenile

breast. Acta Pathol Microbiol Scand (A) 1979, **87**: 353–359.
1736 Pettinato G, Manivel JC, Kelly DR, Wold LE, Dehner LP. Lesions of the breast in children exclusive of typical fibroadenoma and gynecomastia. A clinipathologic study of 113 cases. Pathol Annu 1989, **24**(Pt 2): 296–328.
1737 Rosen PP. Papillary duct hyperplasia of the breast in children and young adults. Cancer 1985, **56**: 1611–1617.
1738 Rosen PP, Cantrell B, Mullen DL, DePalo A. Juvenile papillomatosis (Swiss cheese disease) of the breast. Am J Surg Pathol 1980, **4**: 3–12.
1739 Rosen PP, Kimmel M. Juvenile papillomatosis of the breast. A follow-up study of 41 patients having biopsies before 1979. Am J Clin Pathol 1990, **93**: 599–603.
1740 Shehata BM, Fishman I, Collings MH, Wang J, Poulik JM, Ricketts RR, Parker PM, Heiss K, Bhatia AM, Worcester HD, Gow KW. Pseudoangiomatous stromal hyperplasia of the breast in pediatric patients: an underrecognized entity. Pediatr Dev Pathol 2009, **12**: 450–454.
1741 Steiner MW. Enlargement of the breast during childhood. Pediatr Clin North Am 1955, **2**: 575–593.
1742 Taffurelli M, Santini D, Martinelli G, Mazzoleni G, Rossati U, Giosa F, Grassigli A, Marrano D. Juvenile papillomatosis of the breast. A multidisciplinary study. Pathol Annu 1991, **26**(Pt 1): 25–35.
1743 Wilson M, Cranor ML, Rosen PP. Papillary duct hyperplasia of the breast in children and young women. Mod Pathol 1993, **6**: 570–574.

BREAST DISEASES IN MALES

GYNECOMASTIA

1744 Andersen JA, Gram JB. Gynecomasty. Histological aspects in a surgical material. Acta Pathol Microbiol Immunol Scand (A) 1982, **90**: 185–190.
1745 Bannayan GA, Hajdu SI. Gynecomastia. Clinicopathologic study of 351 cases. Am J Clin Pathol 1972, **57**: 431–437.
1746 Coen P, Kulin H, Ballantine T, Zaino R, Frauenhoffer E, Boal D, Inkster S, Brodie A, Santen R. An aromatase-producing sex-cord tumor resulting in prepubertal gynecomastia. N Engl J Med 1991, **324**: 317–322.
1747 Damiani S, Eusebi V. Gynecomastia in type-1 neurofibromatosis with features of pseudoangiomatous stromal hyperplasia with giant cells. Report of two cases. Virchows Arch 2001, **438**: 513–516.
1748 Fisher ER, Creed DL. Nature of the periductal stroma in gynecomastia. Lab Invest 1956, **5**: 267–275.
1749 Gottfried MR. Extensive squamous metaplasia in gynecomastia. Arch Pathol Lab Med 1986, **110**: 971–973.
1750 Guillou L, Gebhard S. Gynecomastia with unusual intraductal 'clear cell' changes mimicking pagetoid ductal spread of lobular neoplasia. Path Res Pract 1995, **191**: 156–163.
1751 Hunfeld KP, Bassler R, Kronsbein H. 'Diabetic mastopathy' in the male breast – a special type of gynecomastia. A comparative study of lymphocytic mastitis and gynecomastia. Pathol Res Pract 1997, **193**: 197–205.
1752 Kalekou H, Kostopoulos I, Milias S, Papadimitriou CS. Comparative study of CD34, α-SMA and h-caldesmon expression in the stroma of gynaecomastia and male breast carcinoma. Histopathology 2005, **47**: 74–81.
1753 Kang Y, Wile M, Schinella R. Gynecomastia-like changes of the female breast: a clinicopathologic study of 4 cases. Arch Pathol Lab Med 2001, **125**: 505–509.
1754 Kono S, Kurosumi M, Simooka H, Kawanowa K, Ninomiya J, Takei H, Suemasu K, Kuroda Y. Immunohistochemical study of the relationship between Ki-67 labeling index of proliferating cells of gynecomastia, histological phase and duration of disease. Pathol Int 2006, **56**: 655–658.
1755 Nielsen BB. Fibroadenomatoid hyperplasia of the male breast. Am J Surg Pathol 1990, **14**: 774–777.
1756 Sirtori C, Veronesi U. Gynecomastia. A review of 218 cases. Cancer 1957, **10**: 645–654.
1757 Umlas J. Gynecomastia-like lesions in the female breast. Arch Pathol Lab Med 2000, **124**: 844–847.
1758 Wilson JD, Aiman J, MacDonald PC. The pathogenesis of gynecomastia. Adv Intern Med 1980, **25**: 1–32.

MYOFIBROBLASTOMA

1759 Ali S, Teichberg S, De Risi DC, Urmacher C. Giant myofibroblastoma of the male breast. Am J Surg Pathol 1994, **18**: 1170–1176.
1760 Al-Nafussi A. Spindle cell tumours of the breast: practical approach to diagnosis. Histopathology 1999, **35**: 1–13.
1761 Begin LR. Myogenic stromal tumor of the male breast (so-called myofibroblastoma). Ultrastruct Pathol 1991, **15**: 613–622.
1762 Damiani S, Miettinen M, Peterse JL, Eusebi V. Solitary fibrous tumour (myofibroblastoma) of the breast. Virchows Arch 1994, **425**: 89–92.
1763 Eyden BP, Shanks JH, Iochim E, Ali HH, Christensen L, Howat AJ. Myofibroblastoma of breast: evidence favouring smooth-muscle rather than myofibroblastic differentiation. Ultrastruct Pathol 1999, **23**: 249–258.
1764 McMenamin ME, DeSchryver K, Fletcher CD. Fibrous lesions of the breast: a review. Int J Surg Pathol 2000, **8**: 99–108.
1765 McMenamin ME, Fletcher CD. Mammary-type myofibroblastoma of soft tissue: a tumor closely related to spindle cell lipoma. Am J Surg Pathol 2001, **25**: 1022–1029.
1766 Magro G, Bisceglia M, Michal M. Expression of steroid hormone receptors, their regulated proteins, and bcl-2 protein in myofibroblastoma of the breast. Histopathology 2000, **36**: 515–521.
1767 Magro G, Bisceglia M, Michal M, Eusebi V. Spindle cell lipoma-like tumor, solitary fibrous tumor and myofibroblastoma of the breast: a clinico-pathological analysis of 13 cases in favour of a unifying histogenetic concept. Virchows Arch 2002, **440**: 249–260.
1768 Magro G, Gurrera A, Bisceglia M. H-caldesmon expression in myofibroblastoma of the breast: evidence supporting the distinction from leiomyoma. Histopathology 2003, **42**: 233–238.
1769 Magro G, Gangemi P, Greco P. Deciduoid-like myofibroblastoma of the breast: a potential pitfall of malignancy. Histopathology 2008, **52**: 652–654.
1770 Magro G. Epithelioid-cell myofibroblastoma of the breast: expanding the morphologic spectrum. Am J Surg Pathol 2009, **33**: 1085–1092.
1771 Magro G. Mammary myofibroblastoma: a tumor with a wide morphologic spectrum. Arch Pathol Lab Med 2008, **132**: 1813–1820.
1772 Morgan MB, Pitha JV. Myofibroblastoma of the breast revisited: an etiologic association with androgens? Hum Pathol 1998, **29**: 347–351.
1773 Reis-Filho JS, Faoro LN, Gasparetto EL, Totsugui JT, Schmitt FC. Mammary epithelioid myofibroblastoma arising in bilateral gynecomastia: case report with immunohistochemical profile. Int J Surg Pathol 2001, **9**: 331–334.
1774 Thomas TM, Myint A, Mak CK, Chan JK. Mammary myofibroblastoma with leiomyomatous differentiation. Am J Clin Pathol 1997, **107**: 52–55.
1775 Toker C, Tang C-K, Whitely JF, Berkheiser SW, Rachman R. Benign spindle cell breast tumor. Cancer 1981, **48**: 1615–1622.
1776 Wargotz ES, Weiss SW, Norris HJ. Myofibroblastoma of the breast. Sixteen cases of a distinctive benign mesenchymal tumor. Am J Surg Pathol 1987, **11**: 493–502.

CARCINOMA

1777 Adami HO, Hakulinen T, Ewertz M, Tretli S, Holmberg L, Karjalainen S. The survival pattern in male breast cancer. An analysis of 1429 patients from the Nordic countries. Cancer 1989, **64**: 1177–1182.
1778 Bavafa S, Reyes CV, Choudhury AM. Male breast carcinoma. An updated experience at a Veterans Administration hospital and review of the literature. J Surg Oncol 1983, **24**: 41–45.
1779 Bhagat P, Kline TS. The male breast and malignant neoplasms. Diagnosis by aspiration biopsy cytology. Cancer 1990, **65**: 2338–2341.
1780 Burga AM, Fadare O, Lininger RA, Tavassoli FA. Invasive carcinomas of the male breast: a morphologic study of the distribution of histologic subtypes and metastatic patterns in 778 cases. Virchows Arch 2006, **449**: 507–512.
1781 Camus MG, Joshi MG, Mackarem G, Lee AK, Rossi RL, Munson JL, Buyske J, Barbarisi LJ, Sanders LE, Hughes KS. Ductal carcinoma in situ of the male breast. Cancer 1994, **74**: 1289–1293.
1782 Ciocca V, Bombonati A, Gatalica Z, Di Pasquale M, Milos A, Ruiz-Orrico A, Dreher D, Folch N, Monzon F, Santeusanio G, Perou CM, Bernard PS, Palazzo JP. Cytokeratin profiles of male breast cancers. Histopathology 2006, **49**: 365–370.
1783 Costa MH, Silverberg SG. Oncocytic carcinoma of the male breast. Arch Pathol 1989, **113**: 1396–1398.
1784 Cunha F, Andre S, Soares J. Morphology of male breast carcinoma in the evaluation of prognosis. Pathol Res Pract 1990, **186**: 745–750.
1785 Demeter JG, Waterman NG, Verdi GD. Familial male breast carcinoma. Cancer 1990, **65**: 2342–2343.
1786 Donegan WL. Cancer of the breast in men. CA Cancer J Clin 1991, **41**: 339–354.
1787 El-Gazayerli M, Abdel-Aziz AS. On bilharziasis and male breast cancer in Egypt. A preliminary report and review of the literature. Br J Cancer 1963, **17**: 566–571.
1788 Ferreira M, Mesquita M, Quaresma M, André S. Prolactin receptor expression in gynaecomastia and male breast carcinoma. Histopathology 2008, **53**: 56–61.
1789 Giffler RF, Kay S. Small-cell carcinoma of the male mammary gland. A tumor resembling infiltrating lobular carcinoma. Am J Clin Pathol 1976, **66**: 715–722.

1790 Goss PE, Reid C, Pintilie M, Lim R, Miller N. Male breast carcinoma. A review of 229 patients who presented to the Princess Margaret Hospital during 40 years: 1955–1996. Cancer 1999, **85**: 629–639.

1791 Guinee VF, Olsson H, Moller T, Shallenberger RC, van den Blink JW, Peter Z, Durand M, Dische S, Cleton FJ, Zewuster R, et al. The prognosis of breast cancer in males. A report of 335 cases. Cancer 1993, **71**: 154–161.

1792 Hecht JR, Winchester DJ. Male breast cancer. Am J Clin Pathol 1994, **102**: S25–S30.

1793 Heller KS, Rosen PP, Schottenfeld D, Ashikari R, Kinne DW. Male breast cancer. A clinicopathologic study of 97 cases. Ann Surg 1978, **188**: 60–65.

1794 Hittmair AP, Lininger RA, Tavassoli FA. Ductal carcinoma in situ (DCIS) in the male breast: a morphologic study of 84 cases of pure DCIS and 30 cases of DCIS associated with invasive carcinoma: a preliminary report. Cancer 1998, **83**: 2139–2149.

1795 Joshi MG, Lee AK, Loda M, Camus MG, Petersen C, Heatley GJ, Hughes KS. Male breast carcinoma: an evaluation of prognostic factors contributing to a poorer outcome. Cancer 1996, **77**: 490–498.

1796 Kozak FK, Hall JG, Baird PA. Familial breast cancer in males. A case report and review of the literature. Cancer 1986, **58**: 2736–2739.

1797 Muir D, Kanthan R, Kanthan SC. Male versus female breast cancers: a population-based comparative immunohistochemical analysis. Arch Pathol Lab Med 2003, **127**: 36–41.

1798 Norris HJ, Taylor HB. Carcinoma of the male breast. Cancer 1969, **23**: 1428–1435.

1799 O'Grady WP, McDivitt RW. Breast cancer in a man treated with diethylstilbestrol. Arch Pathol 1969, **88**: 162–165.

1800 Papotti M, Tanda F, Bussolati G, Pugno F, Bosincu L, Massareli G. Argyrophilic neuroendocrine carcinoma of the male breast. Ultrastruct Pathol 1993, **17**: 115–121.

1801 Pich A, Margaria E, Chiusa L, Ponti R, Geuna M. DNA ploidy and p53 expression correlate with survival and cell proliferative activity in male breast carcinoma. Hum Pathol 1996, **27**: 676–682.

1802 Ribeiro GG. Carcinoma of the male breast. A review of 200 cases. Br J Surg 1977, **64**: 381–383.

1803 Sanchez AG, Villanueva AG, Redondo C. Lobular carcinoma of the breast in a patient with Klinefelter's syndrome. A case with bilateral, synchronous, histologically different breast tumors. Cancer 1986, **57**: 1181–1183.

1804 San Miguel P, Sancho M, Enriquez JL, Fernandez J, Gonzalez-Palacios F. Lobular carcinoma of the male breast associated with the use of cimetidine. Virchows Arch 1997, **430**: 261–263.

1805 Spence RAJ, Mackenzie G, Anderson JR, Lyons AR, Bell M. Long-term survival following cancer of the male breast in Northern Ireland. A report of 81 cases. Cancer 1985, **55**: 648–652.

1806 Stretch JR, Denton KJ, Millard PR, Horak E. Paget's disease of the male breast clinically and histopathologically mimicking melanoma. Histopathology 1991, **19**: 470–472.

1807 Tamura G, Monma N, Suzuki Y, Satodate R, Abe H. Adenomyoepithelioma (myoepithelioma) of the breast in a male. Hum Pathol 1993, **24**: 678–681.

1808 Visfeldt J, Scheike O. Male breast cancer. I. Histologic typing and grading of 187 Danish cases. Cancer 1973, **32**: 985–990.

1809 Wang-Rodriguez J, Cross J, Gallagher S, Djahanban M, Armstrong JM, Wiedner N, Shapiro DH. Male breast carcinoma: correlation of ER, PR, Ki-67, Her2-Neu, and p53 with treatment and survival, a study of 65 cases. Mod Pathol 2002, **15**: 853–861.

1810 Wick MR, Sayadi H, Ritter JH, Hill DA, Reddy VB, Gattuso P. Low-stage carcinoma of the male breast. A histologic, immunohistochemical, and flow cytometric comparison with localized female breast carcinoma. Am J Clin Pathol 1999, **111**: 59–69.

OTHER LESIONS

1811 Badve S, Sloane JP. Pseudoangiomatous hyperplasia of male breast. Histopathology 1995, **26**: 463–466.

1812 Benson WR. Carcinoma of the prostate with metastases to breast and testis. Cancer 1957, **10**: 1235–1245.

1813 Bigotti G, Kasznica J. Sclerosing adenosis in the breast of a man with pulmonary oat cell carcinoma. Report of a case. Hum Pathol 1986, **17**: 861–863.

1814 Burga AM, Fadare O, Lininger RA, Tavassoli FA. Invasive carcinomas of the male breast: a morphologic study of the distribution of histologic subtypes and metastatic patterns in 778 cases. Virchows Arch 2006, **449**: 507–512.

1815 Gatalica Z, Norris BA, Kovatich AJ. Immunohistochemical localization of prostatic-specific antigen in ductal epithelium of male breast: potential diagnostic pitfall in patients with gynecomastia. Appl Immunohistochem Mol Morphol 2000, **8**: 158–161.

1816 Green LK, Klima M. The use of immunohistochemistry in metastatic prostatic adenocarcinoma to the breast. Hum Pathol 1991, **22**: 242–246.

1817 Hassan MO, Gogate PA, Al-Kaisi N. Intraductal papilloma of the male breast. An ultrastructural and immunohistochemical study. Ultrastruct Pathol 1994, **18**: 601–610.

1818 Hernandez FJ. Leiomyosarcoma of male breast originating in the nipple. Am J Surg Pathol 1978, **2**: 299–304.

1819 Hilton DA, Jameson JS, Furness PN. A cellular fibroadenoma resembling a benign phyllodes tumour in a young male with gynaecomastia. Histopathology 1991, **18**: 476–477.

1820 Lipper S, Willson CF, Copeland KC. Pseudogynecomastia due to neurofibromatosis. A light microscopic and ultrastructural study. Hum Pathol 1981, **12**: 755–779.

1821 Sara AS, Gottfried MR. Benign papilloma of the male breast following chronic phenothiazine therapy. Am J Clin Pathol 1987, **87**: 649–650.

1822 Shin SJ, Rosen PP. Bilateral presentation of fibroadenoma with digital fibroma-like inclusions in the male breast. Arch Pathol Lab Med 2007, **131**: 1126–1129.

1823 Squillaci S, Tallarigo F, Patarino R, Bisceglia M. Nodular fasciitis of the male breast: a case report. Int J Surg Pathol 2007, **15**: 69–72.

1824 Tedeschi LG, McCarthy PE. Involutional mammary duct ectasia and periductal mastitis in a male. Hum Pathol 1974, **5**: 232–236.

1825 Waldo ED, Sidhu GS, Hu AW. Florid papillomatosis of the male nipple after diethylstilbestrol therapy. Arch Pathol 1975, **99**: 364–366.

21 Lymph nodes

CHAPTER CONTENTS

Normal anatomy

The lymph node is one of the major anatomic components of the immune system.[1,6]

The three major regions of a lymph node are the *cortex*, *paracortex*, and *medulla* (Fig. 21.1A). The cortex is situated beneath the capsule, and represents the compartment where most lymphoid follicles reside. The medulla, close to the hilum, grows in the form of cords. It is rich in lymph sinuses, arteries, and veins but contains only a minor lymphocytic component. Both cortex and medulla represent B zones and are therefore associated with humoral types of immune response.[4] The appearance of the follicles varies according to their state of activity. Primary follicles appear as round aggregates of lymphocytes; secondary follicles appear following antigenic stimulation and are characterized by the presence of germinal centers.[3] The cells present in these formations are B lymphocytes known as follicular center cells (centroblasts and centrocytes or small and large cleaved and noncleaved cells), macrophages, and follicular dendritic cells. The germinal center shows polarization toward the side of antigen stimulation and is surrounded by a mantle of small B lymphocytes[4] (Fig. 21.1B). Proliferated germinal centers are always indicative of humoral antibody production. Under conditions of intense antigenic stimulation, they also can appear within the medullary cords.[5]

The paracortex is the zone situated between the cortex and the medulla, which contains the mobile pool of T lymphocytes responsible for cell-mediated immune responses.[4] A characteristic feature is the presence of postcapillary venules, which are identifiable by their lining of high endothelial cells and the presence of lymphocytes migrating through their cytoplasm. Another cell type present in the paracortex is the interdigitating dendritic cell, a member of the accessory immune system. Expansion of the paracortex is indicative of a cell-mediated immunologic reaction. The number of lymphocytes within the lumen and wall of postcapillary venules gives a rough indication of the degree of lymphocyte recirculation.[2]

Afferent lymph vessels penetrate the nodal capsule to open into the marginal sinus; this communicates with an intricate intranodal sinus network that merges into efferent lymph vessels exiting the

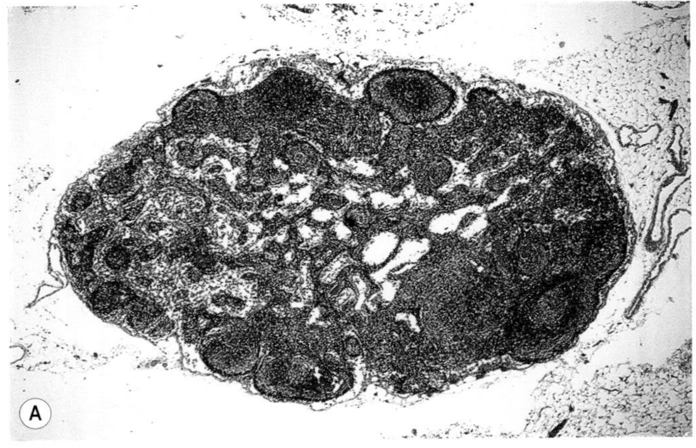

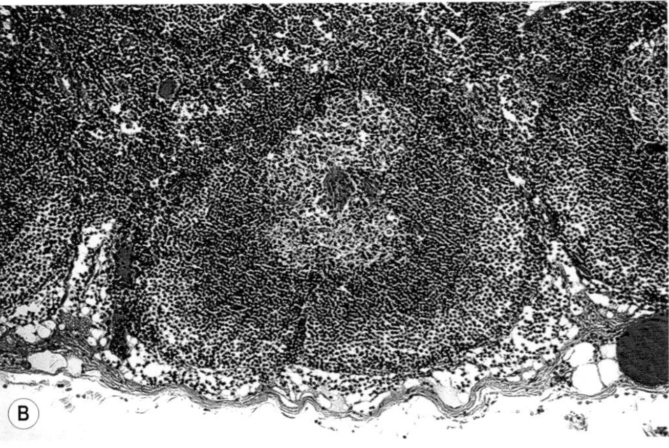

Fig. 21.1 **A** and **B**, Normal lymph node. **A**, The morphologic differences among the various nodal compartments are particularly evident in mesenteric lymph nodes, of which this is an example. **B**, Secondary lymphoid follicle with obvious polarity of the germinal center.

node at the hilum. The endothelial lining of the outer (subcapsular) side of the marginal sinus is nonphagocytic and similar to that of the afferent and efferent vessels; the lining of the intranodal sinuses has strong phagocytic properties (littoral cells or sinus-lining histiocytes). The main arteries and veins pass through the hilum and radiate to the medulla, paracortex, and inner part of the cortex; other blood vessels penetrate the capsule to supply the superficial cortex and a small area surrounding the trabeculae.

The morphologic and phenotypic features of the various populations of lymphoid cells and cells of the accessory immune system are discussed in the next sections and in connection with the respective proliferative pathologic changes affecting these populations.

Lymph node evaluation

The proper examination of a lymph node is a complicated task that may require the performance of a variety of specialized procedures depending on the nature of the case.

Biopsy

Selection of the lymph node to be biopsied is of great importance. In cases of generalized lymphadenopathy, inguinal nodes are to be avoided whenever possible because of a high frequency of nonspecific chronic inflammatory and fibrotic changes. Axillary or cervical nodes are more likely to be informative. Whenever possible, the largest lymph node in the region should be biopsied. Small superficial nodes may show only nonspecific hyperplasia, whereas a deeper node of the same group may show diagnostic features.

The surgeon biopsying intra-abdominal nodes or large cervical or axillary masses should have a frozen section performed to be certain that the tissue is representative – *not* necessarily to obtain a specific diagnosis at this point. This may save a second biopsy.

Adherence to a strict technique for the preparation of lymph nodes in the pathology laboratory is of paramount importance[7–9] (see Appendix E). The specimen should be received fresh in the laboratory immediately after excision, bisected as soon as it is received, and sampled for the appropriate studies. The portion to be embedded in paraffin (which should not exceed 3 mm in thickness) can be placed in 10% buffered formalin and/or a mercury-containing fixative such as B5. As a routine procedure, initial examination of a preparation stained with hematoxylin–eosin is perfectly adequate, followed by whatever additional stains and special techniques the nature of the case may require (which may range from very many to none).[7,10]

A technique that complements the study of tissue sections and that is too often neglected is the examination of touch preparations from the cut surface of the fresh lymph node stained with Giemsa or Wright solution (see Appendix E). This is particularly useful in the evaluation of lymphoma and leukemia, and in the initial triage of the specimen (such as sending tissue for culture if granulomas are seen). For instance, granulocytic leukemia can closely simulate large cell lymphoma in a hematoxylin–eosin-stained section, but an imprint will readily distinguish the two conditions.

Needle biopsy

Core needle biopsy is adequate for the diagnosis of metastatic carcinoma. Although not preferred for the evaluation of primary lymphoid disorders, core biopsies are increasingly used nowadays, putting pressure on the pathologist to render a diagnosis based on limited amounts of tissue. Compression artifact is very common in core biopsies, with the cells appearing smaller and the nuclei appearing darker compared with those seen in excisional biopsies. Very often, more extensive immunohistochemical evaluation is required to maximize the information obtainable from the biopsies.

Fine needle aspiration of lymph nodes is particularly useful for the documentation of metastatic carcinoma (Fig. 21.2). It is used most often in cervical lymph nodes[13] but also in other locations, including intra-abdominal and retroperitoneal regions.[11] The cytologic diagnosis of malignant lymphoma can be made in 50–75% of the cases, the accuracy being greatest in the high-grade lesions[12,14,15] (Fig. 21.2). The technique has been found most useful for the selection of a representative node for biopsy, for the diagnosis of recurrent lymphoma, for staging the extent of the disease, and for monitoring treatment.[17] Hemorrhage, necrosis, and myofibroblastic proliferation may develop along the needle tract; the latter should not be confused with Kaposi sarcoma or other neoplasms.[16]

Bacteriologic examination

If there is a possibility that the node contains an infectious process, an adequate sample of the biopsied lymph node must be sent directly for bacteriologic study or at least be placed in a sterile Petri dish in the refrigerator. If permanent sections show an inflammatory process, the material can then be retrieved and studied bacteriologically (see Appendix E). For some mysterious lesions, this technically trivial step is the one most commonly forgotten.

Electron microscopy

Ultrastructural examination of lymph nodes can be of use in a few specific diseases, such as Langerhans cell histiocytosis and various metastatic tumors. Its role in the evaluation of primary lymphoid disorders is very limited since the advent of immunocytochemical and molecular genetic techniques.[18,19]

Immunophenotyping

Phenotyping of lymphoid disorders has evolved into a highly complex field, as a result of the enormous cellular diversity within the immune system and the huge number (over 1000) of markers that have become available for this purpose.

Rosetting tests with coated or uncoated red blood cells and polyclonal antibodies, which were so useful for the early characterization of lymphomas, have been all but replaced by the use of monoclonal antibodies. These have received a multitude of designations, which are more dependent on the manufacturer's source than the features of the antibody.[20,21] Fortunately, an internationally agreed-upon nomenclature (the CD system, which stands for *cluster designation*) has evolved, and this has allowed for better communication among the various laboratories.[23] Over 250 CD antigens have been identified. Many of these monoclonal antibodies are now applicable to paraffin sections (Table 21.1), whereas others can be employed only in fresh cells (from suspension, cytospin preparations, or frozen section). A detailed discussion of these tests and their optimal use in the differential diagnosis of hematolymphoid disorders is clearly outside the scope of this book.[22]

Immunophenotyping can be performed by flow cytometry (requiring fresh tissue) or on paraffin-embedded materials. Two major advantages of the former are rapid availability of results, and excellent assessment of surface immunoglobulin and hence B-cell clonality. The disadvantages are the need for immediate handling of fresh tissue, and suboptimal architectural–morphologic correlation.

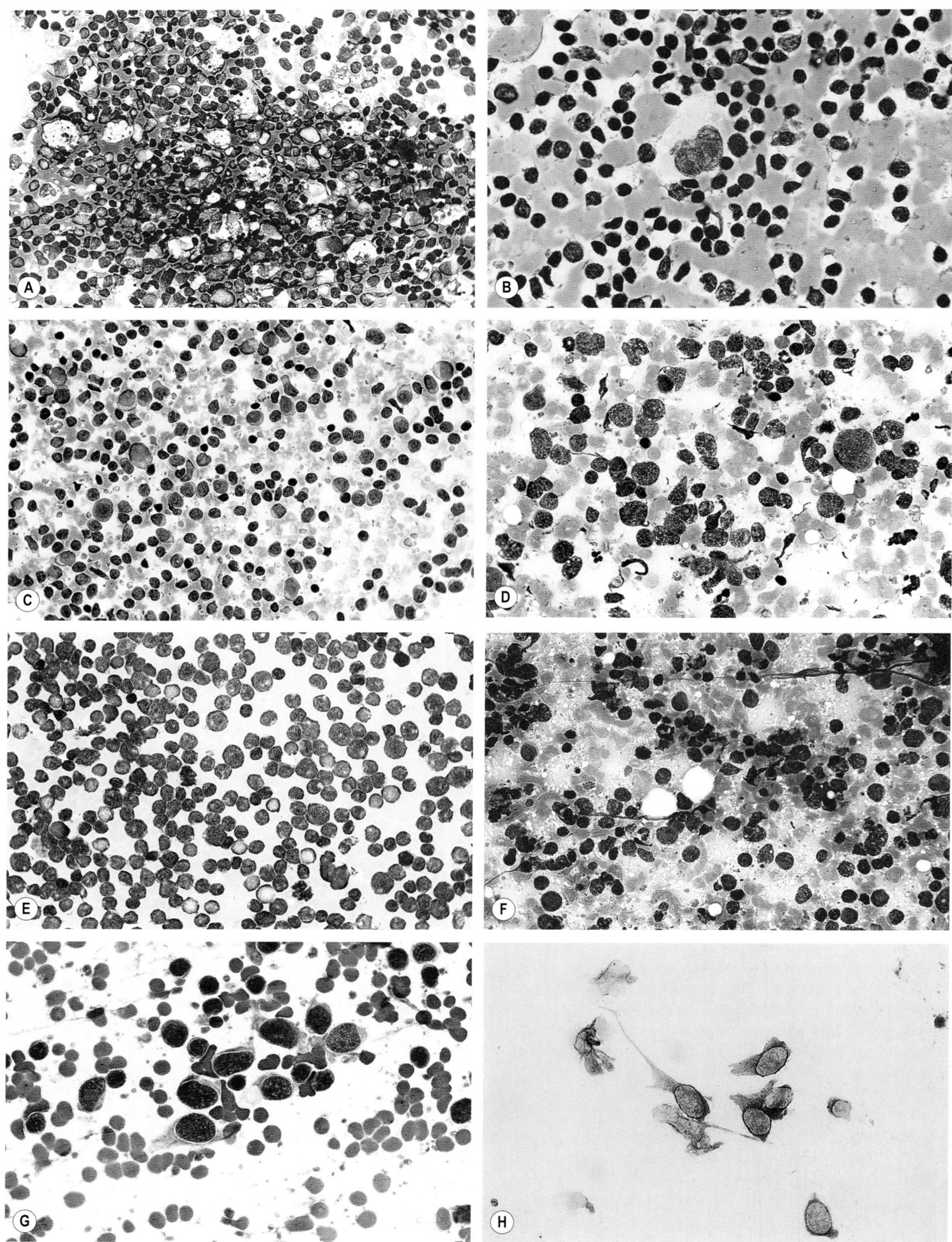

Fig. 21.2 **A–H**, Appearance of various lymph node diseases as seen in fine needle aspiration specimens: **A**, follicular hyperplasia; **B**, Hodgkin lymphoma (Reed–Sternberg cell); **C**, small lymphocytic lymphoma/chronic lymphocytic leukemia; **D**, follicular lymphoma, large cleaved cell type; **E**, lymphoblastic lymphoma; **F**, metastatic pulmonary small cell carcinoma; **G**, metastatic alveolar rhabdomyosarcoma; **H**, same case as **G**, immunostained for desmin.
(Courtesy of L Alasio, Milan, Italy)

Table 21.1 Principal antibodies applicable on paraffin tissue sections

CD ANTIGEN AND/OR ANTIBODY	PREDOMINANT NORMAL CELL REACTIVITY	REACTIVITY IN NEOPLASMS	COMMENT/CAUTION
Leukocytes			
CD45RB Leukocyte common antigen*	B cells and most T cells, macrophages, myeloid cells	Most lymphomas and leukemias	Plasma cell neoplasms and Reed–Sternberg cells usually unreactive; some lymphoblastic and anaplastic large cell lymphomas unreactive
B lymphocytes			
C20 (L26)	B cells, except plasma cells	Most B-cell lymphomas; L&H cells in NLPHL; some Reed–Sternberg cells in ≈20% of classic Hodgkin lymphomas; rare T-cell lymphomas	May not work well in acid-decalcified tissues; plasmablastic and plasma cell neoplasms usually unreactive; some thymomas may stain
Immunoglobulin light chains	B cells and plasma cells	B-cell and plasma cell neoplasms	Diffuse cytoplasmic staining for both light chains seen in macrophages, Reed–Sternberg cells, and degenerated cells (attributed to passive uptake); cytoplasmic Ig often detectable in paraffin sections; surface Ig often requires frozen tissue
CD79a	B cells, including plasma cells	Most B-cell lymphomas; B-cell leukemias from pre-B-cell stage	CD79a is associated with antigen receptor (Ig) on B cells in a similar manner as CD3 on T cells
PAX5 (B-cell specific activator protein)	B cells, except plasma cells	B-cell neoplasms, including B-lymphoblastic neoplasms; L&H cells in NLPHL; Reed–Sternberg cells in classic Hodgkin lymphoma show moderate to weak staining	Plasma cell neoplasms are unreactive
OCT-2	B cells, including plasma cells	B-cell neoplasms, including plasma cell and plasmablastic neoplasms	
BOB.1	B cells, including plasma cells	B-cell neoplasms, including plasma cell and plasmablastic neoplasms	Some T-cell lymphomas can be BOB.1 positive
B lymphocyte differentiation stage			
CD10 (CALLA)	Precursor B cells, follicular center B cells; follicular center T helper cells; granulocytes	Many B-cell and some T-cell lymphoblastic lymphomas/leukemias; follicular lymphoma; Burkitt lymphoma; some large B-cell lymphomas; angioimmunoblastic T-cell lymphoma	Useful in separating follicular from other low-grade B-cell lymphomas; expressed by subset of myeloma; reactive with a variety of nonhematolymphoid neoplasms
BCL6	Follicular center B cells; follicular center T-helper cells; rare subpopulations of T cells	Follicular lymphoma; Burkitt lymphomas; some large B-cell lymphomas; angioimmunoblastic T-cell lymphoma; anaplastic large cell lymphoma	
MUM1	Plasma cells and plasmablasts; subpopulation of BCL6 follicular center B cells; small percentage of activated T cells	Plasma cell and plasmablastic neoplasms; lymphoplasmacytic lymphoma; diffuse large B-cell lymphoma (75% of cases); other B-cell lymphomas (variable); some T-cell lymphomas (variable)	MUM1 may be positive in nonhematolymphoid neoplasms, such as malignant melanoma
CD138 (syndecan 1)	Plasma cells and plasmablasts; some immunoblasts	Plasma cell and plasmablastic neoplasms; some large B-cell lymphomas	CD138 is positive in normal epithelial cells and many nonhematolymphoid neoplasms
CD23	Mantle zone B cells, subset of follicular dendritic cells	CLL/small lymphocytic lymphomas often reactive; follicular lymphoma (some cases); mediastinal large B-cell lymphoma; follicular dendritic cell tumor	Low-affinity Fc receptor for IgE; upregulated by EBV infection

Continued

Table 21.1 Principal antibodies applicable on paraffin tissue sections—cont'd

CD ANTIGEN AND/OR ANTIBODY	PREDOMINANT NORMAL CELL REACTIVITY	REACTIVITY IN NEOPLASMS	COMMENT/CAUTION
T and NK lymphocytes			
Cytoplasmic CD3 (detected by polyclonal or monoclonal antibody)	T cells and NK cells	Most T-cell and NK-cell lymphomas; exceptional cases of B-cell lymphoma can be CD3+	CD3 demonstrable in paraffin sections represents cytoplasmic CD3; this is present in T cells as well as NK cells. Surface CD3, which is typically positive in T cells but negative in NK cells (and their neoplasms), requires fresh or frozen tissue for demonstration, using different antibodies (e.g., OKT3, Leu4)
CD2	T cells, NK cells	Most T-cell and NK-cell lymphomas and leukemias; few myeloid leukemias	CD2 is the sheep erythrocyte receptor
CD5	T cells, weak expression by small B-cell subset	Most T-cell lymphomas and leukemia; chronic lymphocytic leukemia/small lymphocytic lymphoma; mantle cell lymphoma; rare subset of diffuse large B-cell lymphoma	CD5-reactive B cells may be elevated in autoimmune disorders; expression of CD5 by diffuse small B-cell neoplasms useful in diagnosis; CD5 typically negative in NK cells and their neoplasms; CD5 can be expressed in nonhematolymphoid neoplasms, such as thymic carcinoma
CD7	Most T cells, NK cells	Most T-cell and some NK-cell lymphomas and leukemias; some myeloid leukemias	Earliest expressed antigen in T-cell ontogeny and one of the best T-cell markers for lymphoblastic neoplasms; most commonly deleted antigen in peripheral T-cell malignancy, particularly mycosis fungoides
βF1 (T-cell receptor beta chain)	T cells	Many T-cell lymphomas	NK cells and their neoplasms are unreactive
CD56	NK cells, minor subpopulation of T cells	NK-cell lymphomas; some peripheral T-cell lymphomas; some plasma cell neoplasms	Also reacts with neural and neuroendocrine cells and their neoplasms
CD43	T cells, macrophages, Langerhans cells, myeloid cells, minor subset of B cells	Most T-cell lymphomas; some B-cell lymphomas; myeloid leukemias; histiocytic neoplasms; Langerhans cell histiocytosis; some plasma cell neoplasms	Can be exploited for diagnosis of small B-cell lymphoma/leukemia
CD45RO	T cells, some macrophages, myeloid cells	Most T-cell lymphomas, few B-cell lymphomas; myeloid leukemias; histiocytic neoplasms	
T or NK cell subset or differentiation stage			
CD57	Some NK cells; subset of germinal center T cells	T-cell large granular lymphocyte leukemia; rare cases of T-lymphoblastic neoplasm	CD57+ cells often rosette around L&H cells in NLPHL
CD4	Most helper/inducer T cells, many macrophages, many dendritic cells	Many peripheral T-cell lymphomas; histiocytic neoplasms; Langerhans cell histiocytosis	HIV receptor generally predominates
CD8	Most cytotoxic/suppressor T cells, subset of NK cells, splenic sinus lining cells	Minority of peripheral T-cell lymphomas	
Precursor cell marker			
Terminal deoxynucleotidyl transferase (TdT)	Precursor cells in marrow, cortical thymocytes	Most lymphoblastic lymphomas and leukemias of a T or B lineage; some myeloid leukemias	Useful as marker of precursor cell lymphomas/leukemia

Table 21.1 Principal antibodies applicable on paraffin tissue sections—cont'd

CD ANTIGEN AND/OR ANTIBODY	PREDOMINANT NORMAL CELL REACTIVITY	REACTIVITY IN NEOPLASMS	COMMENT/CAUTION
Hodgkin lymphoma-associated			
CD30	Some activated B and T cells, some plasma cells	Reed–Sternberg cells in most cases of classic Hodgkin lymphoma; anaplastic large cell lymphomas; some B- and T-cell lymphomas	Embryonal carcinomas and few other nonhematolymphoid neoplasms reactive
CD15 (Leu-M1)	Granulocytes, some macrophages	Reed–Sternberg cells in most cases of classic Hodgkin lymphoma; large cells in some B- and T-cell lymphomas; histiocytic neoplasms; some myeloid leukemias	Many carcinomas reactive; CMV-infected cells reactive; antibody of IgM isotype and thus may benefit from isotype-specific detection; L&H cells usually unreactive
Accessory cells			
CD68	Macrophages and monocytes; myeloid cells positive with KP1 but not PGM1 antibody	True histiocytic neoplasms; monocytic leukemias; myeloid leukemias positive with KP1	Reactive in granular cell tumors, some melanomas, malignant fibrous histiocytomas, and renal cell carcinomas
CD163	Macrophages except those of germinal centers and splenic white pulp	Histiocytic neoplasms; acute monocytic leukemia	Dendritic cells and their tumors are unreactive
Lysozyme	Macrophages, myeloid cells	Histiocytic neoplasms; many myeloid leukemias	Reactive with many nonhematolymphoid neoplasms
S-100 protein	Langerhans cells, interdigitating (IDRC) and sometimes follicular dendritic cells	Langerhans cell histiocytosis; IDRC tumors; rare T-cell lymphomas; histiocytic neoplasms; Rosai–Dorfman disease	Reactive with many nonhematolymphoid neoplasms
CD1a	Cortical thymocytes, Langerhans cells	Some T-lymphoblastic lymphomas/ leukemias; Langerhans cell histiocytosis	
CD207 (langerin)	Langerhans cells	Langerhans cell histiocytosis	
CD21	Mantle and marginal zone B cells, follicular dendritic cells	Some B-cell lymphomas; follicular dendritic cell tumors	C3d (CR2) complement receptor; receptor for EBV
CD35	Mantle and marginal zone B cells, follicular dendritic cells, some macrophages	Some B-cell lymphomas; follicular dendritic cell tumors; some myeloid leukemias	C3b (CR1) complement receptor
Miscellaneous			
BCL2	Nongerminal center B cells, most T cells, plasma cells	Overexpressed in most follicular lymphomas and some diffuse large B-cell lymphomas; also expressed in many other lymphomas and leukemias	Most useful in differentiating follicular lymphoma from reactive follicular hyperplasia
Cyclin D1	Some histiocytes ; normal lymphoid cells are negative	Mantle cell lymphoma; rare cases of diffuse large B-cell lymphoma; some plasma cell neoplasms; some cases of hairy cell leukemia	Cyclin D1 is expressed in many nonhematolymphoid neoplasms
Anaplastic lymphoma kinase (ALK)	None	ALK+ anaplastic large cell lymphoma; ALK+ large B-cell lymphoma; ALK+ histiocytosis	ALK also positive in some cases of inflammatory myofibroblastic tumor
Myeloperoxidase	Myeloid cells	Myeloid leukemias	Most sensitive and specific marker for myeloid neoplasms

*CMV, cytomegalovirus; CLL, chronic lymphocytic leukemia; EBV, Epstein–Barr virus; NLPHL, nodular lymphocyte predominant Hodgkin lymphoma.
Modified from Warnke RA, Weiss LM, Chan JKC, Cleary ML, Dorfman RF. Tumors of the lymph nodes and spleen. Atlas of tumor pathology, series 3, fascicle 14. Washington, DC, 1995, Armed Forces Institute of Pathology.

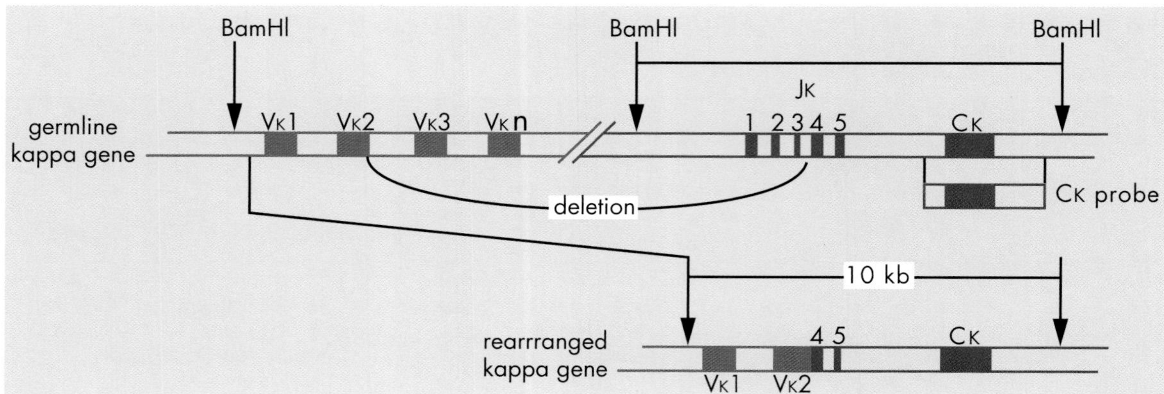

Fig. 21.3 Schematic representation of immunoglobulin gene rearrangement. The germline configuration of the kappa light chain gene (upper line) consists of numerous variable gene segments (V-kappa, 1–n), five joining gene segments (J-kappa, 1–5), and a single constant region gene segment (C-kappa). To assemble a functional light chain gene (lower line), select V and J segments are juxtaposed with each other by deletion of the intervening DNA. The deletion reconfigures restriction enzyme cutting sites upstream of J-kappa, changing the size of the *BamH1* fragment detected with a C-kappa hybridization probe (12 kb germline versus 10 kb rearranged in figure).
(From Warnke RA, Weiss LM, Chan JKC, Cleary ML, Dorfman RF. Tumors of the lymph nodes and spleen. Atlas of tumor pathology, series 3, fascicle 14. Washington, DC, 1995, Armed Forces Institute of Pathology)

Gene rearrangement analysis

Antigen receptor genes code for immunoglobulin and T-cell receptor protein molecules. B cells express immunoglobulins in both a membrane and soluble form, whereas T cells express T-cell receptors, which are membrane-bound molecules. These two kinds of molecules have significant functional and structural similarities and are involved in the specific recognition of antigens by lymphocytes.

Both molecules are multisubunit glycoproteins. Each subunit can be divided roughly into two parts: a constant region and a variable region. Variable regions of two subunits collaborate to form highly specific antigen-binding sites. A given lymphocyte, throughout its lifetime, can express only one type of variable region for each of two (or in the case of T cells, at most three) antigen receptor subunits.

Genetic rearrangements that occur within the genes of these subunits determine which variable region is expressed for a given subunit (Fig. 21.3). During the lifetime of a lymphocyte, rearrangement generally occurs only once per allele or twice for a given gene, as there are two alleles for each gene. The rearrangement can be detected by Southern blot or polymerase chain reaction (PCR).[27,30]

Three general types of application of gene rearrangements to the diagnosis of lymphoid neoplasms exist: (1) for the differential diagnosis between benign and malignant lesions; (2) as markers for B- or T-cell derivation; and (3) as markers for the presence of multiple lymphocytic clones in a single patient (Table 21.2).[26,29,32,33]

Mature B-cell lymphomas almost always show clonal rearrangements of the immunoglobulin genes, although rare cases may show simultaneous rearrangements of T-cell receptor genes.[24] Mature T-cell lymphomas almost always show clonal rearrangements of the T-cell receptor genes, but rare cases may show simultaneous rearrangements of the immunoglobulin genes, an occurrence which is particularly common in angioimmunoblastic T-cell lymphomas (20–30%), probably due to the presence of supervening Epstein–Barr virus (EBV)-associated B-cell proliferation.[28,35] However, precursor lymphoblastic lymphomas frequently show cross-lineage antigen receptor gene rearrangements.[36]

Table 21.2 Commonly encountered gene rearrangement patterns and their interpretation

ANTIGEN RECEPTOR GENE STATUS					
IgH	**Igκ**	**Igλ**	**TCRβ**	**TCRγ**	**Most probable interpretation**
R	R	G	G	G	B-cell neoplasms
R	R	R	G	G	B-cell neoplasms
G	G	G	R	R	T-cell neoplasm
R	G	G	R	R	T-cell neoplasm
G	G	G	G	G	No molecular support for lymphoma

G, germline band; R, rearranged band.
From Warnke RA, Weiss LM, Chan JKC, Cleary ML, Dorfman RF. Tumors of the lymph nodes and spleen. Atlas of tumor pathology, series 3, fascicle 14. Washington, DC, 1995, Armed Forces Institute of Pathology.

Analysis of the immunoglobulin and T-cell receptor gene status in lymphoid proliferations may help in determining clonality, which generally but not invariably indicates a neoplastic process,[25] and in determining lineage, with the caveats of possible cross-lineage gene rearrangements.[24,31] Demonstration of clonal immunoglobulin or T-cell receptor gene rearrangements is most commonly achieved by PCR, which has superseded the much more laborious and demanding Southern blot technique.[34] Although PCR is a highly sensitive technique, being able to demonstrate even minor clonal populations, there can be significant false-negative results due to imperfect annealing of the consensus primers with the target DNA sequences.[24] However, false-negative results can be significantly reduced by using multiple primer pairs against the antigen receptor gene target, such as using the BIO-MED2 primers.[36,37]

Table 21.3 Recurrent chromosomal abnormalities in lymphomas

CHROMOSOMAL ABNORMALITY	MOST FREQUENT TYPES OF LYMPHOMA	ANTIGEN RECEPTOR GENE	ONCOGENE
t(8;14)(q24;q32) t(2;8)(2p12;q24) t(8;22)(q24;q11)	Burkitt lymphoma, and rarely diffuse large B-cell lymphoma	*IGH* *IGκ* *IGλ*	*CMYC* *CMYC* *CMYC*
t(14;18)(q32;q21)	Follicular lymphoma; subset of diffuse large B-cell lymphomas	*IGH*	*BCL2*
t(11;14)(q13;q32)	Mantle cell lymphoma	*IGH*	*CCND1* (cyclin D1)
t(3;v)(q27;v)[a]	Large B-cell lymphoma; small subset of follicular lymphomas	*IGH, IGκ, IGλ*, others	*BCL6*
t(14;v)(q11;v)	T-lymphoblastic lymphoma; adult T-cell leukemia/lymphoma	*TCRα/TCRγ*	Several
t(7;v)(q35;v)	T-lymphoblastic lymphoma	*TCRβ*	Several
t(2;5)(p23;q35)	Anaplastic large cell lymphoma, ALK+	NA	*NPM–ALK* fusion gene
t(11;18)(q21;q21) t(14;18)(q32;q21) t(3;14)(p14.1;q32) t(1;14)(p22;q32)	Extranodal marginal zone lymphoma of mucosa-associated lymphoid tissue	NA *IGH* *IGH* *IGH*	*API2–MALT1* fusion gene *MALT1* *FOXP1* *BCL10*

[a]Variable. NA, not applicable.
Modified from Warnke RA, Weiss LM, Chan JKC, Cleary ML, Dorfman RF. Tumors of the lymph nodes and spleen. Atlas of tumor pathology, series 3, fascicle 14. Washington, DC, 1995, Armed Forces Institute of Pathology.

Cytogenetics and molecular genetics

Chromosomal translocation

Several nonrandom chromosomal translocations have been detected in malignant lymphoma (Table 21.3).[40,42,45–47] Remarkably, most of these translocations are associated with specific lymphoma subtypes even if exceptions occur.

Chromosomal translocation results in fusion of two separate genes, which has one of the following two consequences:[39]

1 Juxtaposition of the regulatory elements of a highly expressed gene in the cell type (e.g., immunoglobulin gene in a B cell) with the coding sequences of a partner gene results in overexpression of the latter, causing increased production of a structurally normal protein; for example, BCL2 protein as a result of t(14;18) causing fusion of *IGH* with *BCL2*.
2 Juxtaposition of the coding sequences of the two involved genes results in gene fusions that code for a novel chimeric protein; for example, t(2;5) leads to production of a protein which is partly encoded by *ALK* and partly encoded by *NPM*.

Chromosomal translocations can be detected by conventional cytogenetics, Southern blot analysis, reverse transcriptase PCR (RT-PCR) and fluorescent in situ hybridization (FISH). Each of these techniques has its own advantages and limitations. However, the FISH technique, either using breakapart probe or dual-fusion probe, generally offers the highest sensitivity.[38,41,43,44]

Chromosome copy change and chromosomal gain or deletion

Increase in copies of entire chromosomes is common in certain lymphoma types, such as trisomy 3 or trisomy 18 in extranodal marginal zone lymphoma, and trisomy 12 in chronic lymphocytic leukemia/small lymphocytic lymphoma.[48,50] Lymphomas can also exhibit deletions or gains of specific regions of chromosome, such as del 6q21–25 in extranodal NK/T-cell lymphoma, del 6q23.3 in marginal zone lymphoma, and gain of 3q26 in mantle cell lymphoma.[49] These chromosomal changes can be demonstrated by conventional cytogenetics, FISH, or single nucleotide polymorphisms (SNP) microarrays.

Gene mutation, amplification, and hypermethylation

Point mutations in specific genes are characteristic of some lymphoma types, including activating mutations of proto-oncogenes, such as point mutations in genes involved in regulation of the nuclear factor kappa B (NFκB) in some cases of diffuse large B-cell lymphoma, and inactivating mutations of tumor suppressor genes, such as *A20* in various lymphoma types.[51,54–56] An inactivating mutation in a tumor suppressor gene is often accompanied by chromosomal/gene deletion in the remaining allele, resulting in complete loss of function of the gene.[54,56] Tumor suppressors genes are alternatively inactivated in some lymphomas through hypermethylation of the gene promoters, such as p16 in mantle cell lymphoma.[53] Gene amplifications are found in some lymphomas, such as *REL* in diffuse large B-cell lymphoma.[52]

DNA ploidy studies

Examination of DNA ploidy by flow cytometry of cell suspensions from fluids or material from fine needle aspiration or from tissue sections has shown a good correlation with the microscopic grades of malignant lymphoma.[57,58,60] Whether it provides prognostic information above and beyond that obtainable from conventional

Table 21.5 Architectural and cytologic features of follicular lymphoma and of reactive follicular hyperplasia as described in a classic and still very pertinent article on the subject

FOLLICULAR LYMPHOMA	REACTIVE FOLLICULAR HYPERPLASIA
Architectural features	
Complete effacement of normal architecture	Preservation of nodal architecture
Even distribution of follicles throughout cortex and medulla	Follicles more prominent in cortical portion of lymph node
Slight or moderate variations in size and shape of follicles	Marked variations in size and shape of follicles with presence of elongated, angulated, and dumbbell-shaped forms
Fading of follicles	Sharply demarcated reaction centers
Massive infiltration of capsule and pericapsular fat with or without formation of neoplastic follicles outside capsule	No, or only moderate, infiltration of capsule and pericapsular fat tissue with inflammatory cells that may be arranged in perivascular focal aggregates (when associated with lymphadenitis)
Condensation of reticulin fibers at periphery of follicles	Little or no alteration of reticular framework
Cytologic features	
Follicles composed of neoplastic cells exhibiting cellular pleomorphism with nuclear irregularities	Centers of follicles (reaction centers) composed of lymphoid cells, histiocytes, and 'reticulum cells', with few or no cellular and nuclear irregularities
Lack of phagocytosis	Active phagocytosis in reaction centers
Relative paucity of mitotic figures usually without significant difference in their number inside and outside the follicles; occurrence of atypical mitoses	Moderate to pronounced mitotic activity in reaction centers; rare or no mitoses outside reaction centers; no atypical mitoses
Similarity of cell type inside and outside follicles	Infiltration of tissue between reaction centers with inflammatory cells (when associated with lymphadenitis)

Slightly modified from Rappaport H, Winter WJ, Hicks EB. Follicular lymphoma. A re-evaluation of its position in the scheme of malignant lymphoma, based on a survey of 253 cases. Cancer 1956, **9:** 792–821.

in involved nodes, or they may appear in the absence of NLPHL in recurrent post-therapy adenopathy done for the latter[84,86,92] (see p. 1811). Indeed, the main differential diagnosis of progressively transformed germinal centers is with NLPHL, which should be suspected if T-cell rosettes are prominent. A thorough search for the atypical cells seen in this condition (see p. 1811) should then be undertaken.[88]

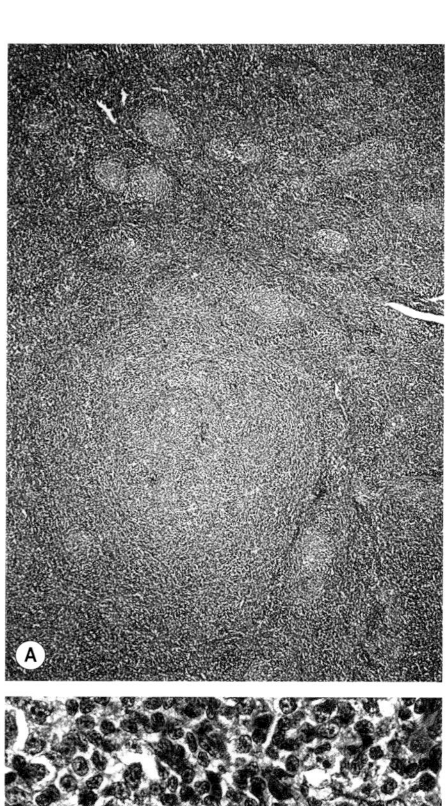

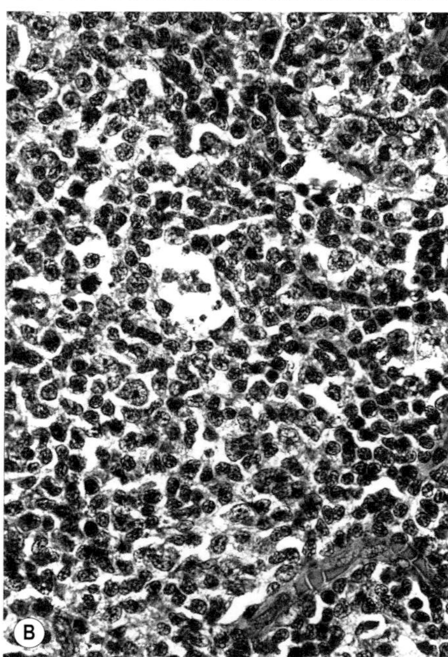

Fig. 21.5 **A** and **B**, Progressively transformed germinal centers. **A**, Low-power view showing that this formation is larger and less well defined than the adjacent hyperplastic follicles. **B**, High-power view showing cytologic composition not too dissimilar from that of ordinary hyperplastic follicles.

Regressively transformed germinal centers are small, practically devoid of lymphoid cells, and composed of follicular dendritic cells, vascular endothelial cells, and hyalinized periodic acid–Schiff (PAS)-positive intercellular material. These abnormal centers have an onion-skin appearance in low-power examination. Regressively transformed germinal centers are particularly prominent and numerous in Castleman disease (see p. 1796). A peculiar form of regressive germinal centers with 'follicular dendritic cells only' has been described in organ transplant recipients.[94]

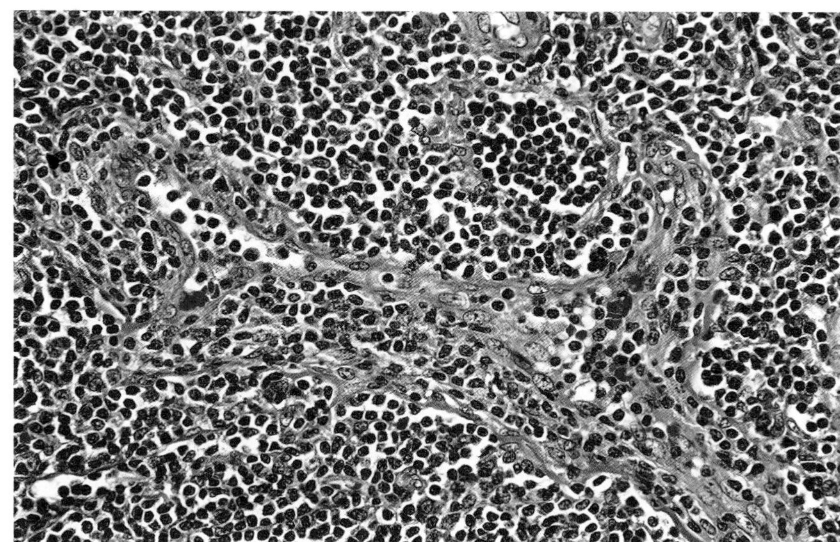

Fig. 21.6 Paracortical hyperplasia, identified by the prominence of postcapillary venules.

Mantle/marginal zone hyperplasia

This pattern of hyperplasia, which blends with the lymphoid subtype of hyaline vascular Castleman disease (see p. 1796), is characterized by a monomorphic proliferation of small lymphoid cells with round nuclei and clear cytoplasm which may be arranged in a nodular, inverse follicular, and/or marginal zone pattern. The main differential diagnosis is with mantle cell lymphoma (see p. 1831). Features in favor of benignancy at the hematoxylin–eosin level are the lack of pericapsular infiltration, preservation of sinuses, scattered reactive follicles, and paracortical nodular hyperplasia.[95] Immunoglobulin gene rearrangement studies may be necessary to settle the issue.

Paracortical hyperplasia

Expansion of the paracortical (interfollicular) region can be nodular or diffuse. The nodular form is characteristic of dermatopathic lymphadenitis (see p. 1800) and of nodal reactions to malignancy.[96] The diffuse form is a feature of viral lymphadenitis (see p. 1793), drug reactions (see p. 1799), and immunoblastic proliferations in general (Fig. 21.6).

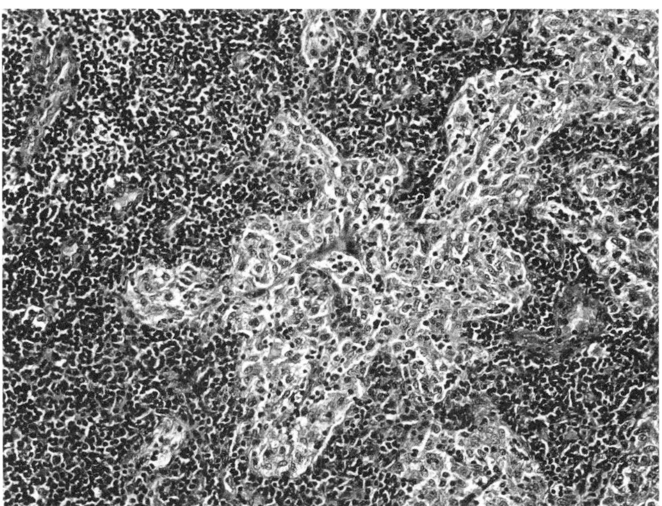

Fig. 21.7 Sinus hyperplasia. The cells present in the sinus represent an admixture of histiocytes and sinus lining cells.

Sinus hyperplasia

The sinuses appear dilated and prominent in various disorders. The most common and least significant is *sinus hyperplasia* (sinus histiocytosis, sinus 'catarrh') seen in nodes draining infectious or neoplastic processes and characterized by an increased number of macrophages in the lumen (Fig. 21.7). Other reactive disorders involving primarily the sinuses are Rosai–Dorfman disease (RDD) (see p. 1801), Langerhans cell histiocytosis (see p. 1803), Whipple disease, vascular transformation of sinuses, and virus-associated hemophagocytic syndrome (see p. 1845).

Granulomatous inflammation

There are a large number of diseases that can result in granulomatous formations in lymph nodes. They include various types of infection, foreign body reactions, aberrant immune reactions, and secondary responses in lymph nodes draining carcinoma[97,102] or in patients with Hodgkin lymphoma and other lymphomas, whether the node is involved by the malignancy or not.[98,99,101] Sometimes the appearance of the granulomas is such that a specific diagnosis can be strongly suggested on the basis of the hematoxylin–eosin-stained slide.[100] Features of importance in this regard are the presence and type of necrosis; presence, number, and size of Langhans giant cells; size, shape, and distribution of the granulomas; and type of associated changes in the intervening tissue. In most cases, however, a combination of clinical, morphologic, and bacteriologic data is necessary to determine the etiology of the granulomas. It is therefore important that any node suspected of harboring a granulomatous process be sampled for bacteriologic analysis in addition to being subjected to the standard microscopic examination.

Other cell types involved in nodal hyperplasia

Monocytoid B cells

Monocytoid B-cell hyperplasia is characterized by the filling of the sinuses by small lymphoid cells with round or angulated nuclei

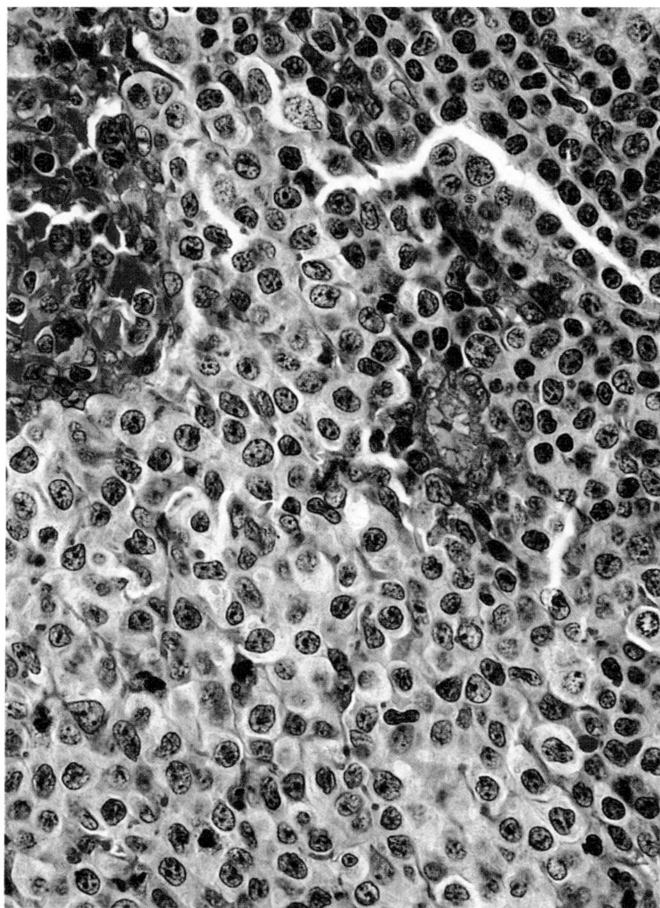

Fig. 21.8 Monocytoid B-cell hyperplasia. These cells are characterized by centrally located nuclei and clear appearance of the cytoplasm.

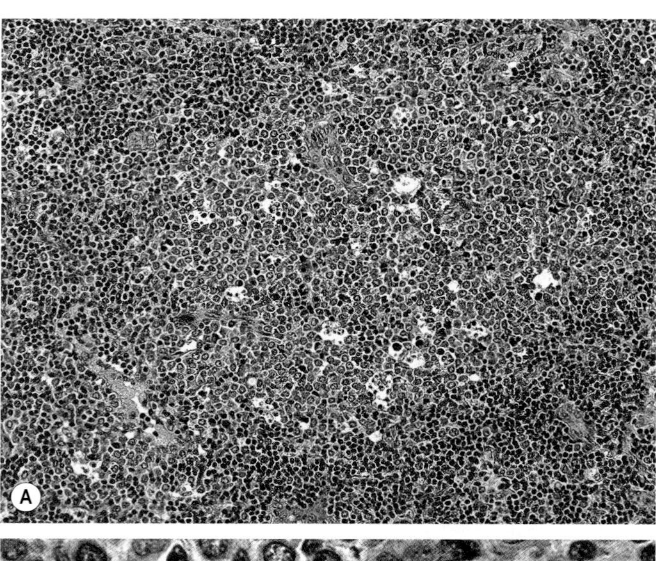

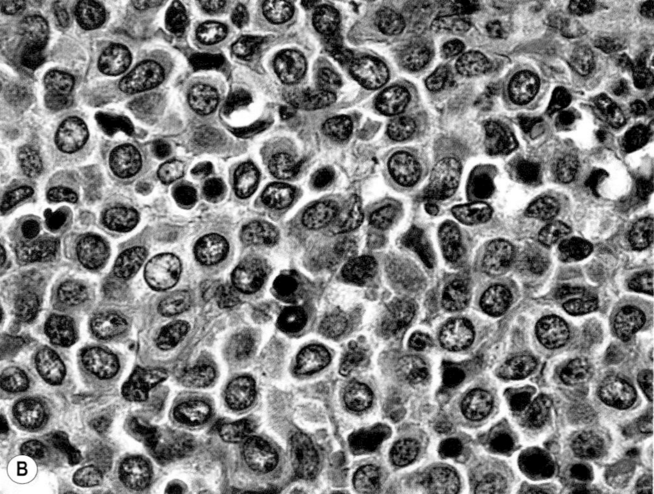

Fig. 21.9 Plasmacytoid monocytes as seen on low (**A**) and high power (**B**).

and clear cytoplasm, sometimes admixed with neutrophils (Fig. 21.8). A variant characterized by the presence of a larger cell component has also been recognized.[106] It was originally described as *immature sinus histiocytosis*, but marker studies have shown that these monocytoid clear cells are of B-cell type.[107,109] This alteration occurs most frequently in toxoplasmosis, but it has also been seen in many other reactive disorders, including cat-scratch disease,[104] infectious mononucleosis, AIDS, and autoimmune disorders;[103] it may also accompany malignant lymphomas, including Hodgkin lymphoma.[105] It should be distinguished from other nodal lesions featuring cells with clear cytoplasm (such as peripheral T-cell lymphomas, hairy cell leukemia, and mastocytosis) and also from a type of malignant lymphoma composed of cells with features of monocytoid B cells (nodal marginal zone B-cell lymphoma) (see p. 1833).[108]

Plasmacytoid dendritic cells

Clusters of cells with plasmacytoid cytoplasm, fine nuclear chromatin pattern, and small nucleoli are sometimes seen in a variety of reactive nodal lesions (Fig. 21.9). Pyknosis and starry-sky pattern may be present.[118] These cells were originally interpreted as T-associated plasma cells and later as a subtype of T cells, but then as macrophages/monocytes (plasmacytoid monocytes), and more recently as a special form of dendritic cells.[110,114,115] They are particularly common in Kikuchi necrotizing lymphadenitis and Castleman disease,[112,113] but they can also be seen in other lymphadenitides.[111] A variety of malignant lymphoma composed of plasmacytoid dendritic cells has also been described[116,117] (see p. 1844).

Polykaryocytes

The term *polykaryocyte* is used for a type of multinucleated giant cell found in lymphoid tissues, of which the Warthin–Finkeldey giant cell of measles is the paradigm. These cells can be found in lymph nodes in association with a variety of reactive and neoplastic disorders. They measure 25–150 μm in diameter and have as many as 60 nuclei arranged in grapevine clusters.[119] Their cytoplasm is very scanty (Fig. 21.10). Although some early studies suggested a T-cell phenotype, more recent evaluations are in keeping with the hypothesis that these cells are multinucleated forms of follicular dendritic cells, a possibility that fits much better their morphologic appearance.[120]

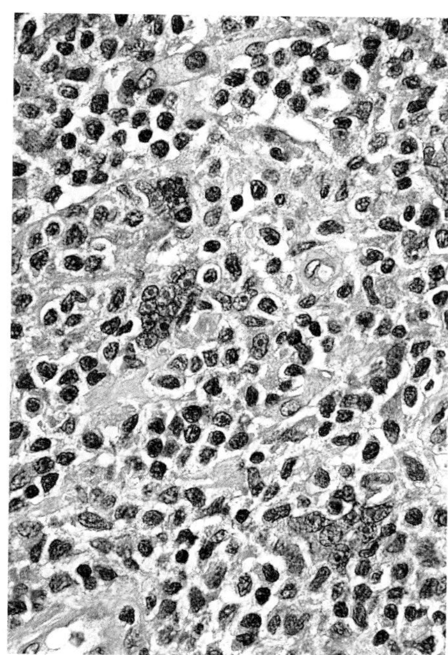

Fig. 21.10 So-called 'polykaryocytes'. These cells are characterized by numerous clustered nuclei.

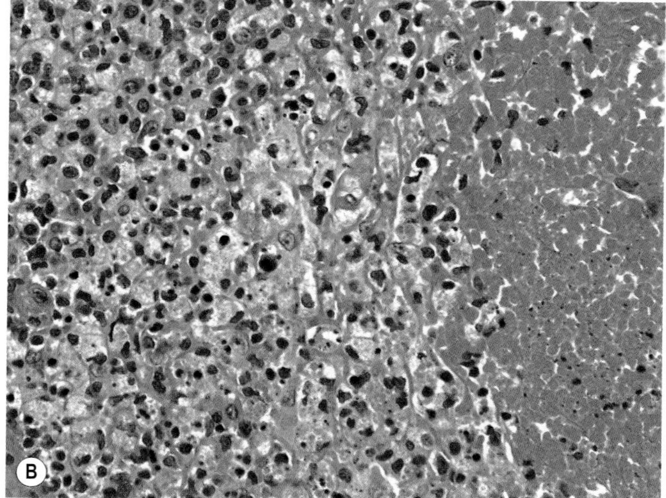

Fig. 21.11 **A** and **B**, Necrotizing lymphadenitis. **A**, Low-power view showing necrotizing change centered in the subcapsular region. **B**, High-power view showing the boundary between an area of karyorrhexis/pyknosis and an area of karyolysis.

Inflammatory/hyperplastic diseases

Acute nonspecific lymphadenitis

The typical case of acute nonspecific lymphadenitis is rarely biopsied. Microscopically, the earliest change is sinus dilation resulting from increased flow of lymph, followed by accumulation of neutrophils, vascular dilation, and edema of the capsule. *Suppurative lymphadenitis* is a feature of staphylococcal infection, mesenteric lymphadenitis (see p. 1789), lymphogranuloma venereum (see p. 1791), and cat-scratch disease (see p. 1790). *Necrotizing features* may be seen in bubonic plague, tularemia, anthrax, typhoid fever, melioidosis, and the entity known as Kikuchi necrotizing lymphadenitis (see next section).

Kikuchi necrotizing lymphadenitis

Kikuchi necrotizing lymphadenitis (Kikuchi lymphadenitis; Kikuchi–Fujimoto disease) is seen most commonly in Japan and other Asian countries,[123] but it also occurs elsewhere, including the United States and Western Europe. Most patients are young women with a persistent, painless cervical lymphadenopathy of modest dimensions that may be accompanied by fever.[121] Microscopically, the affected nodes show focal, well-circumscribed, paracortical necrotizing lesions. There are abundant karyorrhectic debris, scattered fibrin deposits, and collections of mononuclear cells[127] (Fig. 21.11). Special studies have shown that the necrosis is the expression of cytotoxic lymphocyte-mediated apoptotic cell death.[130,142] Plasma cells and neutrophils are very scanty, a feature of diagnostic importance.[137,145] Instead, plasmacytoid dendritic cells and activated T-cells are often numerous.[129,141] When these cells are abundant, the appearance may simulate that of malignant lymphoma.[122,136,144] The main lesional cells include histiocytes (CD68+) that coexpress myeloperoxidase and plasmacytoid dendritic cells (CD68+, CD123+).[133,138] On occasion, a prominent secondary xanthomatous reaction is seen.[135] Ultrastructurally, tubuloreticular structures and intracytoplasmic rodlets similar to those described in lupus erythematosus are often found.[128]

The diagnosis can be made or at least suspected in material from fine needle aspiration because of the prominence of phagocytic histiocytes with peripherally placed ('crescentic') nuclei and medium-sized cells with eccentrically placed nuclei consistent with plasmacytoid dendritic cells.[143]

The evolution is generally benign and self-limited. However, cases have been described with recurrent lymphadenopathy or accompanied by skin lesions.[134,139] Isolated fatal cases are also on record.[125] The etiology is unknown; an early suggestion that *Toxoplasma* may be involved has not been substantiated. Epstein–Barr virus (EBV), human herpesvirus type 6 (HHV6), HHV8, and other viruses have been implicated, but the evidence for their involvement is not conclusive.[126,131,132,140] The most important differential diagnosis is with malignant lymphoma with secondary necrosis. Cases of necrotizing lymphadenitis have been seen following diffuse large

B-cell lymphoma,[146] and changes morphologically consistent with necrotizing lymphadenitis have been reported in cases of stroma-rich Castleman disease[124] and in cases of lupus erythematosus (see p. 1796).

Chronic nonspecific lymphadenitis

The morphologic features and the very concept of chronic lymphadenitis merge with those of hyperplasia (see p. 1780). The general features of chronic lymphadenitis are follicular hyperplasia; prominence of postcapillary venules; increased number of immunoblasts, plasma cells, and histiocytes; and fibrosis. The capsule may appear inflamed and/or fibrotic, and the process may extend into the immediate perinodal tissues. In some cases, one may find an undue predominance in the number of eosinophils, foamy macrophages, and/or mast cells. Terms such as *eosinophilic* or *xanthogranulomatous lymphadenitis* have been sometimes used, depending on the type of the infiltrate.[147] The presence of numerous eosinophils in a lymph node should raise the possibility of Langerhans cell histiocytosis, parasitic infections, Hodgkin lymphoma, autoimmune disorders, and Kimura disease. Eosinophils can also be numerous in epithelioid hemangioma/angiolymphoid hyperplasia with eosinophilia (which may rarely involve lymph nodes), Churg–Strauss disease, and anaplastic large cell lymphoma.[148]

Tuberculosis

Lymph nodes involved by tuberculosis may become adherent to each other and form a large multinodular mass that can be confused clinically with metastatic carcinoma (Fig. 21.12). The most common location of clinically apparent lymphadenopathy is the cervical region ('scrofula'), where a draining sinus that communicates with the skin ('scrofuloderma') may form.[150] Microscopically, the appearance ranges from multiple small epithelioid granulomas reminiscent of sarcoidosis to huge caseous masses surrounded by Langhans giant cells, epithelioid cells, and lymphocytes. Demonstration of the organisms by special stains, cultures, or PCR is necessary to establish the diagnosis.[149]

Atypical mycobacteriosis

Atypical mycobacteria are a common cause of granulomatous lymphadenitis. In the United States, caseating granulomatous disease in a cervical lymph node of a child unaccompanied by pulmonary involvement is more likely to be caused by an atypical mycobacterium. The process typically involves lateral nodes in the midportion of the neck. Drainage may continue for months or years in the absence of specific therapy, and healing may result in scarring and contractures. Microscopically, the host reaction may be indistinguishable from that of tuberculosis, but often the granulomatous response is overshadowed by suppurative changes.[153–155] A nontuberculous mycobacterial etiology should also be suspected if the granulomas are ill-defined (nonpalisading), irregularly shaped, or serpiginous.[151,154] An acid-fast stain should be performed in every granulomatous and suppurative lymphadenitis of unknown etiology, especially if the patient is a child or an HIV-infected individual.[156] The final identification of the organism rests on the cultural or molecular characteristics.

In immunosuppressed patients, mycobacterial infections may result in a florid spindle cell proliferation that can simulate a neoplastic process (*mycobacterial spindle cell pseudotumor*) (see p. 1860).[152]

Sarcoidosis

The enigmatic clinicopathologic entity known as sarcoidosis has a worldwide distribution.[175] Scandinavian countries are particularly affected.[181] In the United States, the disease is 10–15 times more common in blacks than in whites. Practically every organ can be involved, but the ones most commonly affected are lung, lymph nodes, eyes, skin, and liver.[159,162,166] Erythema nodosum often precedes or accompanies the disease. Functional hypoparathyroidism is the rule, although a few cases of sarcoidosis coexisting with primary hyperparathyroidism have also been reported.[161,184] This seems to be due to the secretion of a parathyroid hormone (PTH)-related protein by the cells in the granuloma.[185]

Microscopically, the basic lesion is a small granuloma mainly composed of epithelioid cells, with scattered Langhans giant cells and lymphocytes[179] (Fig. 21.13). As a general rule, the Langhans giant cells are smaller and have fewer nuclei than those typically seen in tuberculosis. Necrosis is either absent or limited to a small

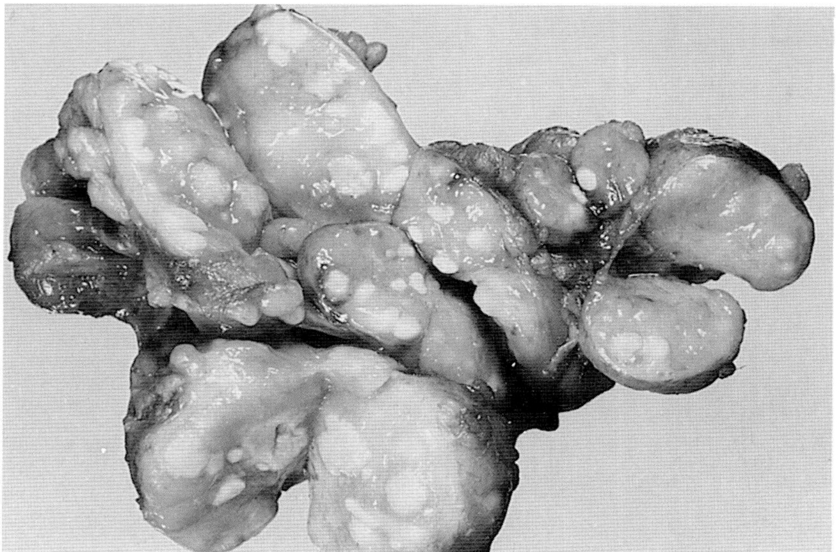

Fig. 21.12 Large adherent tuberculous lymph nodes containing extensive foci of caseation necrosis.

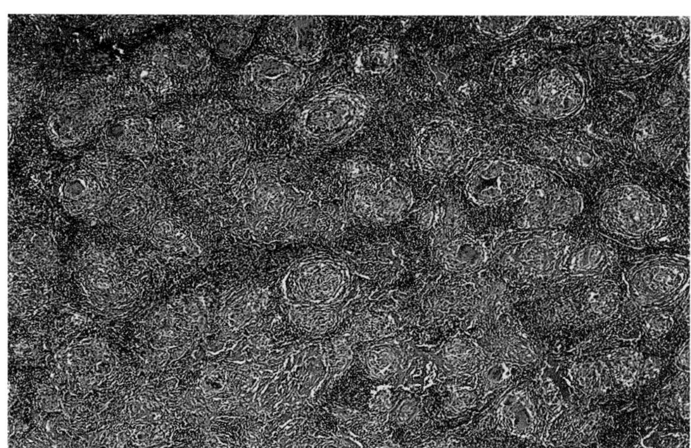

Fig. 21.13 Numerous confluent non-necrotizing granulomas mainly composed of epithelioid cells in a lymph node affected by sarcoidosis.

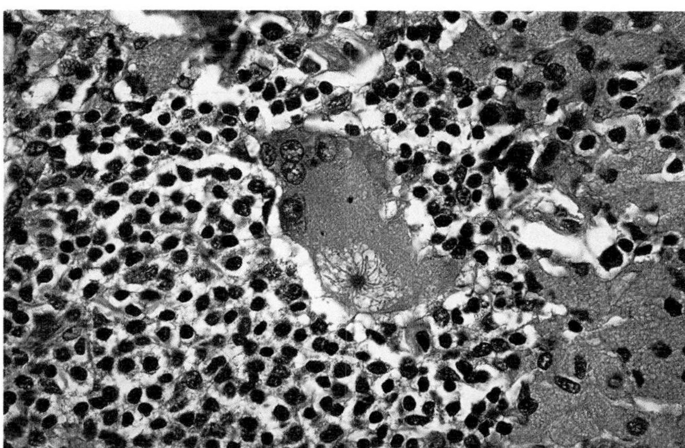

Fig. 21.14 Asteroid body in the cytoplasm of a multinucleated giant cell in sarcoidosis.

Fig. 21.15 Hamazaki–Wesenberg bodies in a lymph node with sarcoidosis, as shown in hematoxylin–eosin (**A**), periodic acid–Schiff (**B**), and Gomori methenamine-silver stains (**C**).

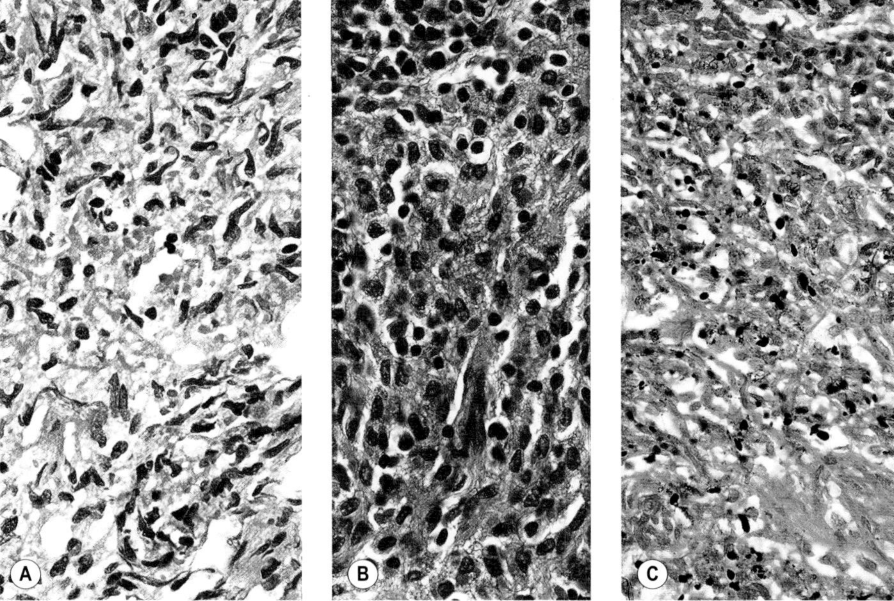

central fibrinoid focus ('hard' granulomas); a 'necrotizing' variant of sarcoidosis exists, but this is usually extranodal. Schaumann bodies, asteroid bodies, and calcium oxalate crystals are sometimes found in the cytoplasm of the giant cells[177] (Figs 21.14 and 21.15). Schaumann bodies are round, have concentric laminations, and contain iron and calcium. Ultrastructurally, asteroid bodies are composed of radiating filamentous arms enveloped by 'myelonoid' membranes.[171] Elemental analysis has shown calcium, phosphorus, silicon, and aluminum in these formations.[171,179] Peculiar PAS-positive inclusions known as Hamazaki–Wesenberg, yellow, or ovoid bodies were claimed to be specific for sarcoidosis, but subsequent histochemical and ultrastructural studies[180] have shown that they have no etiologic or pathogenetic significance. They probably represent large lysosomes containing hemolipofuscin material and are found in a large variety of conditions.[177,182] None of these inclusions is specific for sarcoidosis. As a matter of fact, from a pathologic standpoint the diagnosis of sarcoidosis is always one of exclusion. A noncaseating granulomatous inflammation in the lymph nodes or skin microscopically indistinguishable from sarcoidosis can be seen in tuberculosis, atypical mycobacteriosis (including swimming pool granuloma), fungus diseases, leprosy, syphilis, leishmaniasis, brucellosis, tularemia, chalazion, zirconium granuloma, berylliosis, Crohn disease, Hodgkin lymphoma; in nodes draining a carcinoma; and in several other conditions.[160] Only when all these possibilities have been excluded and the clinical picture is characteristic is there justification in labeling a case as consistent with sarcoidosis.

Most of the lymphocytes present in the sarcoidal granulomas are T cells with the helper phenotype; both these cells and the epithelioid histiocytes exhibit features of proliferation and/or activation, as shown by their immunocytochemical positivity with the Ki-67 antibody and for interleukin-1, respectively.[158,163] Pathogenetically, sarcoidosis is thought to represent a dysfunction of circulating T cells with overactivity of B cells.[170] The association of particular human leukocyte antigens (HLAs) with sarcoidosis suggests a role for HLA-linked immune response genes and disease susceptibility.[167] Specifically, it has been shown that certain types of genetic polymorphism are associated with increased risk of disease or affect disease presentation.[157]

The Kveim test for sarcoidosis is an intradermal reaction that occurs following inoculation with an extract of human spleen involved with the disease. It is positive in 60–85% of patients with sarcoidosis, and the number of false-positive results is small. The test is regarded as positive when a biopsy of the area taken 4–6 weeks after inoculation shows microscopically sarcoid-type granuloma. A trial employing a single test suspension among 2400 subjects in 37 countries on six continents showed a similar level of reactivity and microscopic appearance from country to country, supporting the concept that sarcoidosis is the same disease the world over. The Kveim test is rarely practiced today because of lack of availability of the antigen.

The etiology and pathogenesis of sarcoidosis remain elusive.[178] It is not even clear whether it is a bona fide entity or a pattern of reaction to a variety of agents. Mycobacterial organisms have long been suspected.[164,165] Substances like α-diaminopimelic acid and mycolic acid, which occur in mycobacteria but are foreign to human tissue, have been identified in sarcoid lesions.[174] In several careful microscopic and cultural studies performed on morphologically typical cases of sarcoidosis, acid-fast organisms have been identified in a significant number of cases.[173,183] PCR studies have provided conflicting results, but the number of articles documenting the presence of mycobacterial DNA in a percentage ranging from 33% to 80% of sarcoidal granulomas is becoming difficult to ignore.[168,169,172,176]

Fungal infections

Fungal infections of lymph nodes may present as chronic suppurative lesions, as granulomatous processes, or as a combination of the two. The most important fungal lymphadenitis is *histoplasmosis*, which in addition to the previously mentioned patterns can also result in widespread nodal necrosis and in marked diffuse hyperplasia of sinus histiocytes (Fig. 21.16). Other fungal diseases known to result in lymphadenitis are blastomycosis, paracoccidioidomycosis, coccidioidomycosis, and sporotrichosis.[186] To these, one should add opportunistic infections such as cryptococcosis, aspergillosis, mucormycosis, and candidiasis.

The fungal organisms can usually be demonstrated with Gomori methenamine-silver (GMS) or PAS–Gridley stains, but sometimes their number is so small that they can be detected only in cultures or by molecular testing.

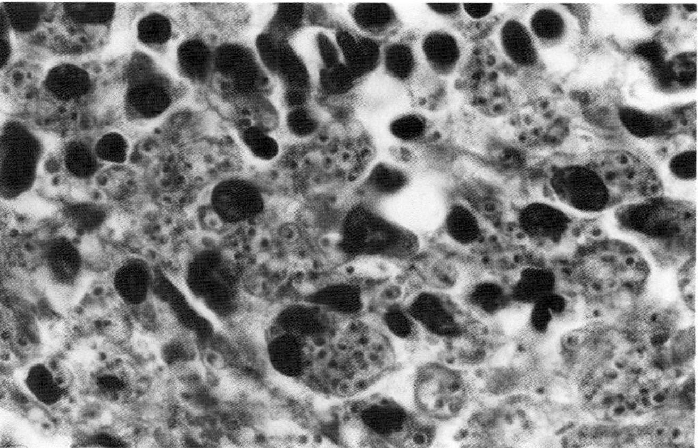

Fig. 21.16 Numerous *Histoplasma* organisms in the cytoplasm of histiocytes.

Toxoplasmosis

Toxoplasmosis, one of the most common parasitic infections of humans and other warm-blooded animals, is caused by the protozoan parasite *Toxoplasma gondii*.[190] Toxoplasmic lymphadenitis (formerly known as Piringer–Kuchinka lymphadenitis), in its most typical form, involves the posterior cervical nodes of young women.[191] On palpation, the nodes are firm and only moderately enlarged. Microscopically, the nodal architecture is rather well preserved. The typical triad of the disease, which, however, is not present in all cases, is constituted by: (1) marked follicular hyperplasia, associated with intense mitotic activity and phagocytosis of nuclear debris; (2) small granulomas composed almost entirely of epithelioid cells, located within the hyperplastic follicles and at the periphery, encroaching on and blurring their margins; and (3) distention of marginal and cortical sinuses by monocytoid B cells (Fig. 21.17). An additional feature is the presence of immunoblasts and plasma cells in the medullary cords.[193] Variations on the theme include presence in the granulomas of necrosis or more than an occasional Langhans giant cell.

It is extremely rare to find *Toxoplasma* organisms by morphologic examination and just as difficult to detect the *Toxoplasma gondii* genome by PCR[187,194] (Fig. 21.18). The latter finding contrasts sharply with the results obtained in toxoplasmic encephalitis and myocarditis.[194] However, the combination of microscopic features described correlates remarkably well with serologic studies. Of 31 cases studied by Dorfman and Remington,[188] the Sabin–Feldman dye test was positive in all, and the IgM immunofluorescent antibody test was positive in 97% of the cases.

If the diagnosis of toxoplasmic lymphadenitis is suspected from the microscopic pattern, it should be confirmed serologically, keeping in mind, however, that these tests may be normal in the early stages of the disease.[189]

The differential diagnosis of toxoplasmosis includes other infectious diseases and the lymphocyte predominant form of Hodgkin lymphoma. In this regard, Miettinen and Franssila[192] have made the interesting point that occurrence of collections of epithelioid cells *within* germinal centers seems to be a nearly specific feature for toxoplasmosis.

Syphilis

Generalized lymphadenopathy is a common finding in secondary syphilis, whereas localized node enlargement can be seen in the primary and tertiary stages of the disease. In secondary syphilis, the changes are those of a florid follicular hyperplasia. In primary syphilis, the combination of changes may result in a mistaken diagnosis of malignant lymphoma. Most of the cases have presented as solitary inguinal lymphadenopathy.[198] There are capsular and pericapsular inflammation and extensive fibrosis, diffuse plasma cell infiltration, proliferation of blood vessels with endothelium swelling and inflammatory infiltration of their wall (phlebitis and endarteritis), and follicular hyperplasia[198] (Fig. 21.19). Rarely, noncaseating granulomas and abscesses are present. Exceptionally, the appearance is that of a nodal inflammatory pseudotumor, the message being that spirochetes should be searched for whenever making that diagnosis in a nodal biopsy, by histochemical or immunohistochemical stain.[196]

The morphologic features of syphilitic infection are not substantially different when occurring in HIV-infected patients[197] and can be identified in most cases by the Warthin–Starry or Levaditi stains, by immunofluorescence techniques applied to imprint preparations, or immunohistochemical staining on paraffin section.[195] The organisms are most frequently found in the wall of blood vessels.

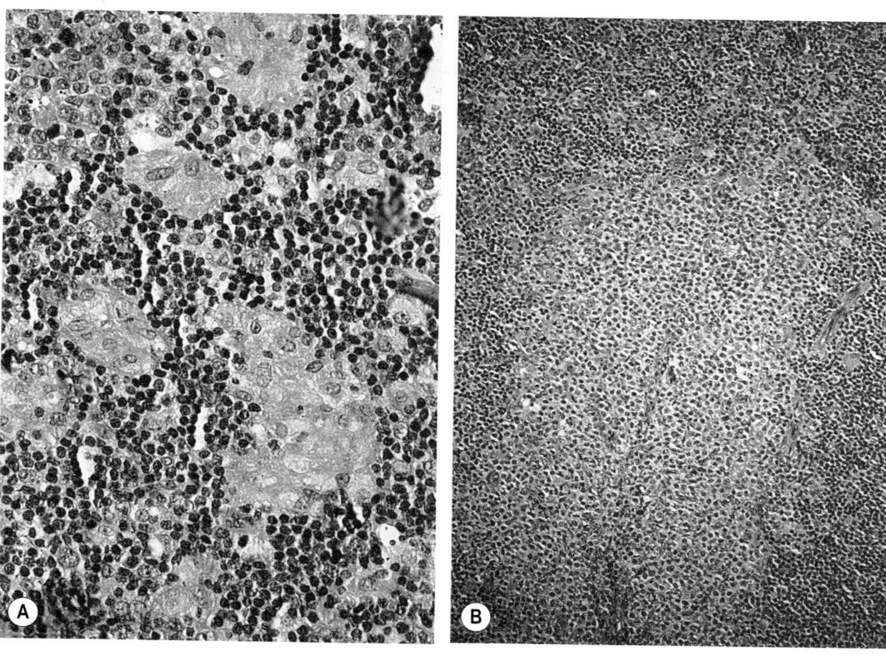

Fig. 21.17 **A** and **B**, Toxoplasmosis of lymph node. **A**, Small noncaseating granulomas composed of epithelioid cells are located at the periphery of a hyperplastic follicle. This picture is almost pathognomonic of this disease. **B**, An area of massive monocytoid B-cell hyperplasia.

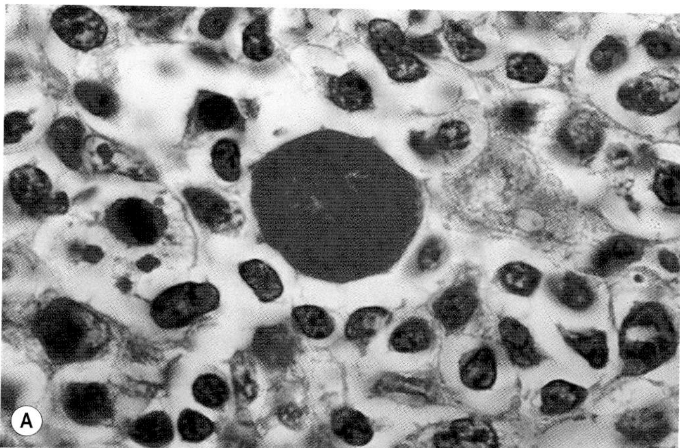

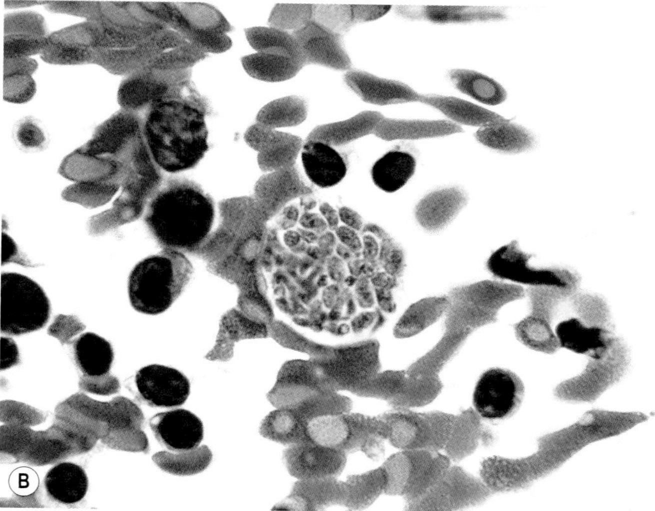

Fig. 21.18 *Toxoplasma* cyst as seen in a microscopic section (**A**) and a touch preparation (**B**). This is a very unusual finding in lymph nodes affected by the disease.

Detection of *Treponema pallidum* is now also feasible in lymph node biopsies and fine needle aspirations by PCR and Southern blotting.[199]

Leprosy

Lymph nodes involved by the lepromatous type of leprosy have a very characteristic microscopic appearance. The main change is the progressive accumulation of large, pale, rounded histiocytes ('lepra' or 'Virchow' cells), without granuloma formation and with minimal or no necrosis (Fig. 21.20). Wade–Fite and Fite–Faraco stains (which are modified Ziehl–Neelsen reactions) demonstrate packing of the cytoplasm by acid-fast organisms, which can also be demonstrated by a fluorescent method,[200] and with the PCR technique.[201]

Mesenteric lymphadenitis

Mesenteric (Masshoff) lymphadenitis is produced by *Yersinia pseudotuberculosis* or *Yersinia enterocolitica*, two gram-negative polymorphic coccoid or ovoid motile organisms.[203–205,207] It is a benign, self-limited disease that can clinically simulate acute appendicitis. Microscopically, there are capsular thickening and edema, increase of immunoblasts and plasma cells in the cortical and paracortical region, dilation of sinuses with accumulation of large lymphocytes within, and germinal center hyperplasia.[202,208] In the lymphadenitis produced by *Yersinia pseudotuberculosis*, small granulomas and abscesses are commonly present, whereas this is unusual in infection caused by *Yersinia enterocolitica*.[208] These nodal changes are accompanied by inflammatory changes of the terminal ileum and cecum. Ideally, the diagnosis should be confirmed with cultures. Too often, the diagnosis of mesenteric lymphadenitis is made on normal or mildly hyperplastic nodes in an attempt to explain why a patient with the clinical picture of acute appendicitis has a normal appendix.

The organism can be identified with PCR techniques. Interestingly, pathogenetic *Yersinia* DNA has been detected in mesenteric lymph nodes in patients with Crohn disease.[206]

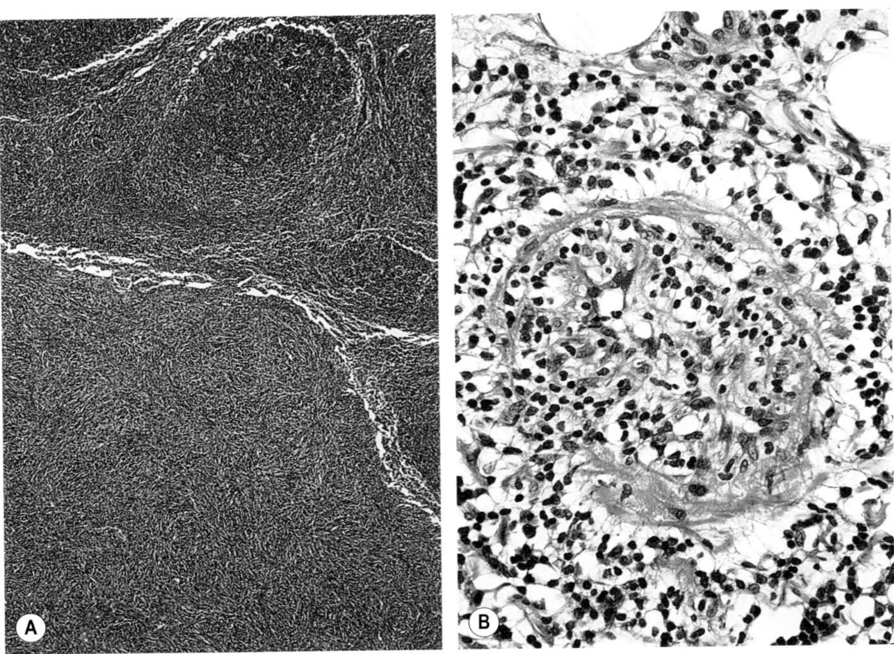

Fig. 21.19 **A** and **B**, Syphilis of lymph node. **A**, Follicular hyperplasia associated with striking pericapsular inflammation and fibrosis. **B**, The prominent vasculitis seen in this field is an important clue to the diagnosis.

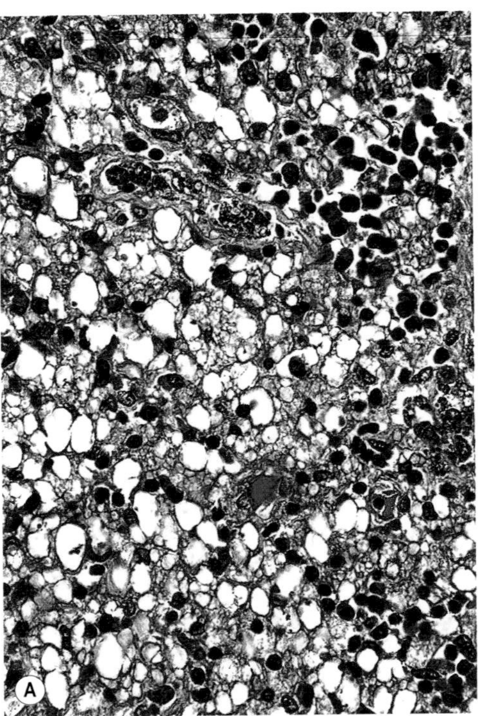

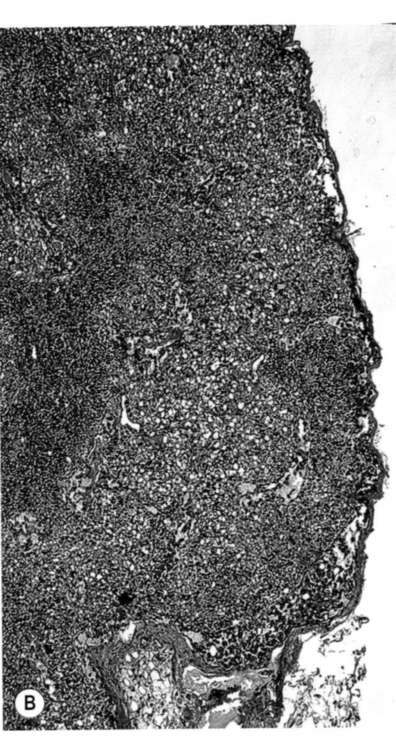

Fig. 21.20 Lymph node involvement by lepromatous leprosy. The sinuses are massively dilated as a result of the accumulation of foamy histiocytes.

Cat-scratch disease

Cat-scratch disease is characterized by a primary cutaneous lesion and enlargement of regional lymph nodes, usually axillary or cervical[210] (Fig. 21.21). The changes in the nodes vary with time. Early lesions have histiocytic proliferation and follicular hyperplasia, intermediate lesions have granulomatous changes, and late lesions have abscesses of various sizes[223] (Fig. 21.22). These abscesses are very suggestive of the diagnosis because of their pattern of central, sometimes stellate necrosis with neutrophils, surrounded by a palisading of histiocytes.[217] However, similar abscesses can be seen in lymphogranuloma venereum. Another common feature of lymph nodes with cat-scratch disease is the packing of sinuses by monocytoid B cells, which, together with the follicular hyperplasia, may simulate toxoplasmosis.[216] However, clusters of perifollicular and intrafollicular epithelioid cells are absent.[213]

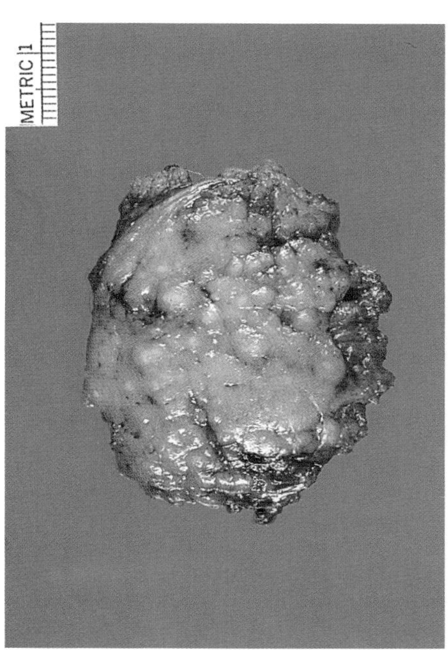

Fig. 21.21 Lymph node involved by cat-scratch disease.

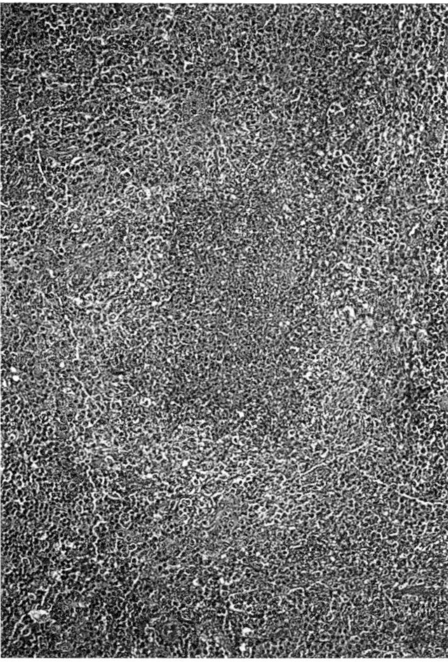

Fig. 21.22 An area of stellate necrosis in a proven case of cat-scratch disease.

The primary lesion is a red papule in the skin at the site of inoculation, usually appearing between 7 and 12 days following contact. It may become pustular or crusted. Microscopically, there are foci of necrosis in the dermis surrounded by a mantle of histiocytes. Multinucleated giant cells, lymphocytes, and eosinophils are also present.[215]

The agent of cat-scratch disease is a coccobacillary pleomorphic extracellular bacterium that can be identified with the Warthin–Starry silver stain, particularly in those cases exhibiting extensive necrosis.[214,218,221] This organism, which has also been detected ultrastructurally,[219] was originally designated *Rochalimaea henselae* and has been renamed *Bartonella henselae*. The diagnosis can be confirmed by serology, immunohistochemistry, or PCR.[209,212,220,222]

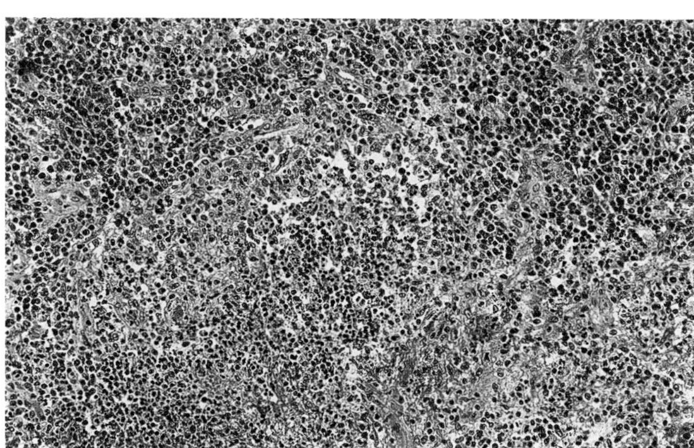

Fig. 21.23 Necrotizing granuloma in a lymph node affected by lymphogranuloma venereum.

Rare complications of the disease include granulomatous conjunctivitis ('oculoglandular syndrome of Parinaud'), thrombocytopenic purpura, and central nervous system manifestations.[211]

Lymphogranuloma venereum

This sexually transmitted disease (not to be confused with granuloma inguinale) is caused by *Chlamydia trachomatis* organisms corresponding to serotypes L1, L2, and L3.[225] The initial lesion is a small (2–3 mm), painless genital vesicle or ulcer which often goes unnoticed and heals in a few days. This is followed by inguinal adenopathy, which can be very prominent. The earliest microscopic change in an affected node is represented by tiny necrotic foci infiltrated by neutrophils. These enlarge and coalesce to form the stellate abscess that represents the most characteristic feature of this disease (Fig. 21.23). In later stages, epithelioid cells, scattered Langhans giant cells, and fibroblasts are seen to line the abscesses' walls. Confluence of these abscesses is common, and cutaneous sinus tracts may develop. The healing stage is represented by nodules with dense fibrous walls surrounding amorphous material.[227]

The microscopic picture just described is not pathognomonic of this disease. Similar changes can occur in cat-scratch disease, atypical mycobacteriosis, and tularemia. Therefore a presumptive diagnosis of lymphogranuloma venereum should be confirmed with the Frei test (a delayed hypersensitivity skin test using purified 'lygranum' chlamydial antigen), complement fixation, immunofluorescence, or molecular testing.[224–226,228]

Tularemia

Tularemia is a bacterial disease produced by *Francisella tularensis*, an extremely virulent pathogen,[229,230,235] which has recently gained notoriety as a potential biowarfare agent.[231,236] In the ulceroglandular form of the disease, prominent lymphadenopathy occurs; this predominates in the axillary region when mammalian vectors are involved and in cervical or inguinal regions with arthropod vectors.[232] A history of handling rabbits suggests the diagnosis in the first instance. The diagnosis is supported by a rise in hemagglutinin titers.[230,233]

Microscopically, the picture in the acute phase is that of an intense lymphadenitis with widespread necrosis, sometimes associated with irregularly shaped microabscesses and granulomas.[231] In the more chronic forms, there is a granulomatous reaction that in some cases may have a frankly tuberculosis-like appearance.[234]

Brucellosis

Brucellosis is caused by *Brucella abortus, melitensis,* or *suis*.[240] In the United States it has evolved from an occupational to a foodborne illness related to consumption of milk and cheese.[237] The most common clinical manifestations are fever, hepatomegaly, and splenomegaly.[238] Lymphadenopathy is uncommon and, when present, usually of modest dimensions. Microscopically, there may be nonspecific follicular hyperplasia and clusters of epithelioid histiocytes sometimes forming large noncaseating granulomas. This is accompanied by a polymorphic infiltrate containing eosinophils, plasma cells, and immunoblasts. When the latter are numerous, the microscopic picture may show a vague resemblance to Hodgkin lymphoma.

A definitive diagnosis can only be made by recovery of the organism with bacteriologic or PCR techniques[239] or the detection of a high agglutination titer.[241]

AIDS-related lymphadenopathy

The lymph node abnormalities in AIDS patients can be of various types. They include mycobacterial and other opportunistic infections (some resulting in spindle cell pseudotumors),[251,258] Kaposi sarcoma, malignant lymphomas of either Hodgkin or non-Hodgkin type, and *florid reactive hyperplasia*.[243,254] The latter change is the most common (Fig. 21.24). It may be accompanied by collections of monocytoid B cells in the sinuses, neutrophils, and features of dermatopathic lymphadenopathy. In many of the cases, the reactive germinal centers show a feature termed *follicle lysis*, characterized by invagination of mantle lymphocytes into the germinal centers. This is associated with disruption of these centers ('moth-eaten appearance') and a distinctive clustering of large follicular center cells,[244,260] resulting in an appearance that has been termed *explosive follicular hyperplasia*. Ultrastructurally, a prominence of follicular dendritic cells exhibiting alterations of their fine processes has been described;[256] it has been suggested also on the basis of immunohistochemically (fascin stain) that the AIDS virus preferentially infects these cells.[255,257] It has been suggested that the polykaryocytes (Warthin–Finkeldey cells) that are sometimes seen in HIV-infected nodes are a multinucleated form of follicular dendritic cell.[253] Immunohistochemically, positive stain for the HIV core protein P24 has been documented within the abnormal germinal centers.[246,252]

This combination of follicular changes is not pathognomonic of AIDS, but the possibility of this disease should be considered and investigated whenever they are found, such as by immunostaining for P24 or by serologic study.[246]

Some lymph nodes in AIDS patients may also show advanced lymphocyte depletion, with or without abnormal (regressively transformed) germinal centers.[244,256]

The interfollicular tissue may show prominent vascular proliferation, the resulting picture acquiring a vague resemblance to Castleman disease. It is important to search in these areas and in the subcapsular region for the earliest signs of development of Kaposi sarcoma.[249] These changes should be distinguished from those of vascular transformation of the sinuses (see p. 1855).

A rough relationship has been found among the pattern of nodal reaction, the cell suspension immunophenotypic data, and the patient's HIV status.[245,259]

The term *chronic lymphadenopathy syndrome* has been defined as an unexplained enlargement of nodes of at least 3 months' duration at two or more extrainguinal sites in an individual at risk for AIDS.[242] The microscopic picture is similar to that described previously.[250] Overall, up to a fourth of the patients have developed AIDS on follow-up, cachexia and weight loss being the clinical signs of this progression.[247,248]

The HIV-associated lymphoproliferative diseases of lymph nodes are discussed on page 1847.

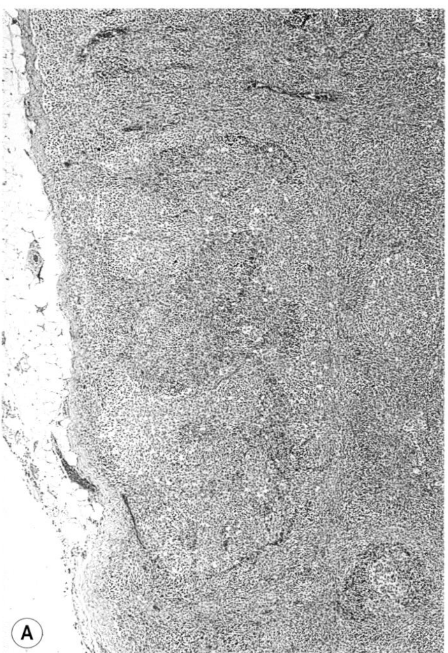

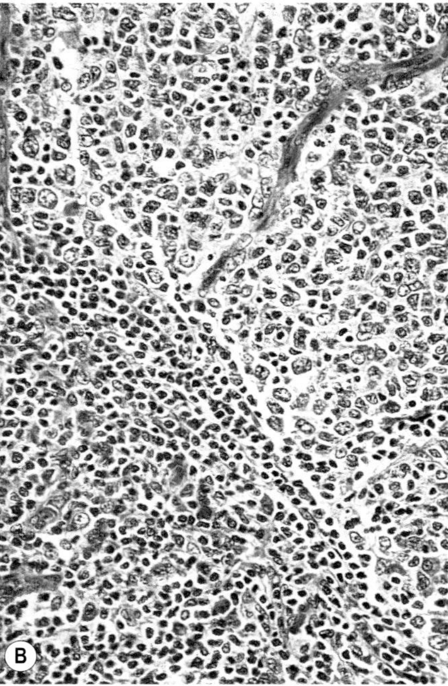

Fig. 21.24 Low-power (**A**) and high-power (**B**) microscopic views of AIDS-related lymphadenopathy. The depicted germinal center shows disruption of its architecture by intrusion of small lymphocytes from the mantle zone. This is a common but not pathognomonic feature of this disease.

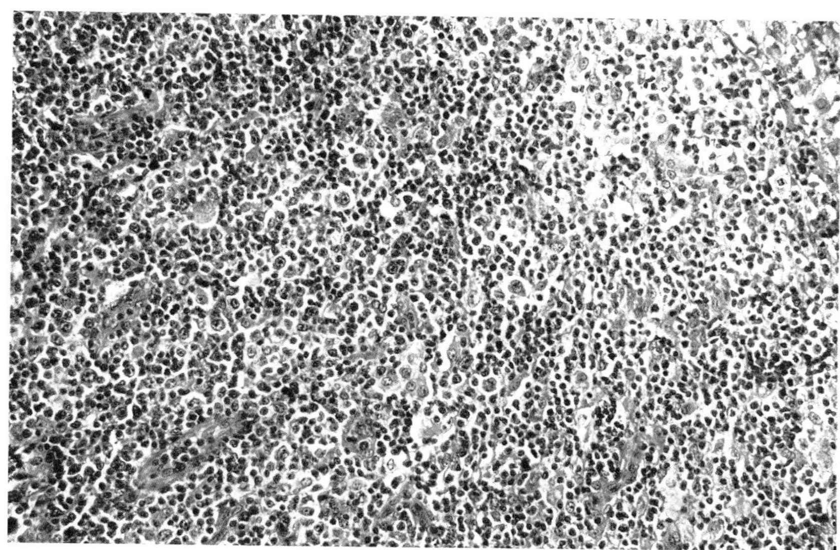

Fig. 21.25 Lymph node involved by infectious mononucleosis. There is a marked effacement of the architecture by a polymorphic lymphoid infiltrate.

Infectious mononucleosis

The etiologic agent of classic infectious mononucleosis is the EBV,[267] but other agents may be involved in atypical cases.[262] It is rare for the pathologist to see a lymph node from a patient with a typical clinical picture because in most instances the presumptive clinical diagnosis is confirmed by examination of the peripheral blood and serologic evaluation without need of a lymph node biopsy.[264] It is in the atypical case, presenting with lymphadenopathy without fever, sore throat, or splenomegaly, that the clinician will perform a lymph node biopsy to rule out the possibility of malignant lymphoma.

Microscopically, nodes and other lymphoid organs affected by infectious mononucleosis can be confused with malignant lymphoma because of the effacement of the architecture; infiltration of the trabecula, capsule, and perinodal fat; and the marked proliferation of immunoblasts, immature plasma cells, and mature plasma cells ('polymorphic B-cell hyperplasia') (Figs 21.25 and 21.26). These features are particularly prominent when the disease develops in transplant recipients or other immunosuppressed patients.[261] Necrosis may also be present; this is usually only focal but in immunodeficient children it may be massive.

Features of importance in the differential diagnosis with lymphoma include the predominantly sinusal distribution of the large lymphoid cells, follicular hyperplasia with marked mitotic activity and phagocytosis (these follicles being usually small), increase in the number of plasma cells, and vascular proliferation.[268] Another important feature is the fact that, although the nodal architecture may appear effaced, the sinusal pattern remains intact or even focally accentuated, a fact appreciated particularly well with reticulin stains. Another supposedly characteristic feature of this disease is the presence in the sinuses of clusters or 'colonies' of lymphocytes in graduated sizes, from the small lymphocyte to the large lymphoid cell or immunoblast.[270] The latter cell usually has only one large vesicular nucleus with a thin nuclear membrane and one or two prominent amphophilic or basophilic nucleoli. A paranuclear 'hof' is often seen. When binucleated, this cell may closely resemble a Reed–Sternberg cell and result in a mistaken diagnosis of Hodgkin lymphoma[265,272] (Fig. 21.26). Immunophenotyping evaluation should resolve the issue in most cases, despite the existence of an overlap that may be providing a pathogenetic insight into the nature and possible relationship of these two disorders.[266] The diagnosis of infectious mononucleosis can be confirmed by in situ hybridization techniques[263,269,271] (Fig. 21.27).

Other viral (including postvaccinial) lymphadenitides

Lymph nodes draining an area of the skin subjected to smallpox vaccination can enlarge and become painful. If removed and examined microscopically, they can be easily confused with lymphoma, especially if the history of vaccination is overlooked. Of 20 cases of postvaccinial lymphadenitis reported by Hartsock,[276] 13 were located in the supraclavicular region on the side of the vaccination. The largest node measured 6 cm in diameter. The interval between the vaccination and the biopsy varied between 1 week and 3 months.

Microscopically, the changes are those of a diffuse or nodular paracortical expansion, with mixed cellular proliferation, consisting of eosinophils, plasma cells, and a large number of immunoblasts. The alterations are accompanied by vascular and sinusal changes and focal discrete necrosis. The most important histologic feature of postvaccinial hyperplasia is the presence of numerous immunoblasts scattered among the lymphocytes and imparting to the lymphoid tissue a mottled appearance (Fig. 21.28). Hartsock[276] noted that follicular hyperplasia was present only in those nodes removed more than 15 days after vaccination. These changes have been reproduced experimentally.[276]

Viral lymphadenitis resulting from *herpes simplex infection* may be localized[279] or generalized.[277] The morphologic features are similar to those of postvaccinial lymphadenitis, particularly in reference to the marked immunoblastic proliferation.[278,280] Intranuclear viral inclusions may be found, especially at the edge of necrotic areas.[273,275,281] The nodal changes seen in herpes zoster lymphadenitis and infectious mononucleosis are of similar nature; the latter are discussed under a separate heading (see preceding section). It is likely that analogous morphologic changes occurring in the absence of these clinical conditions are, in most cases, the result of some unidentified viral infection.

Prominent regional lymphadenopathy also may follow the administration of live attenuated measles virus vaccine.

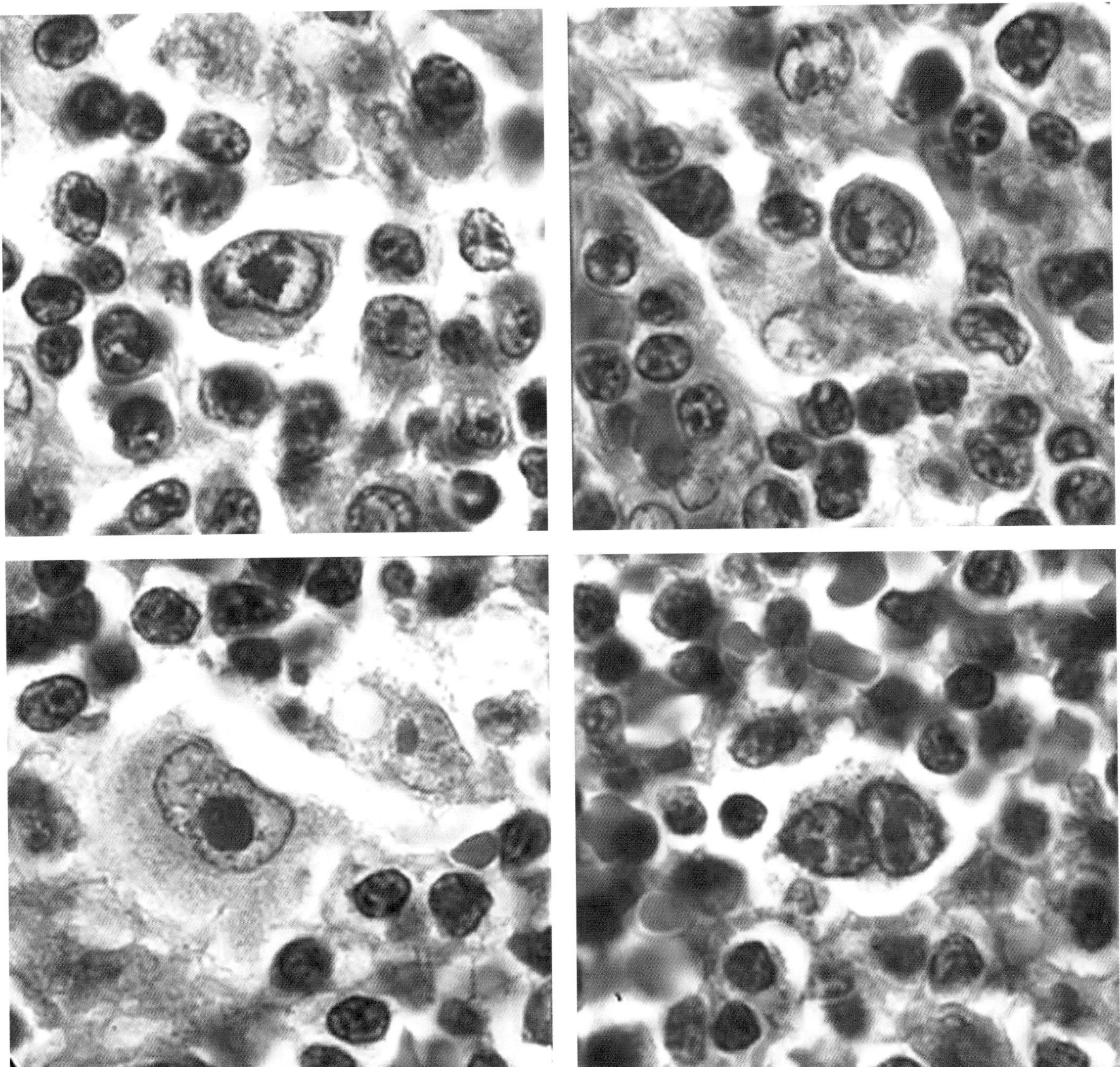

Fig. 21.26 Various types of immunoblast seen in a lymph node involved by infectious mononucleosis. The binucleated form (shown in the fourth image) can simulate Reed–Sternberg cells. Note the basophilic character of the nucleus and the presence of a paranuclear hof.

Microscopically, the typical multinucleated giant cell of Warthin–Finkeldey (polykaryocytes) may be found[274] (see Fig. 11.114).

Mucocutaneous lymph node syndrome

Mucocutaneous lymph node syndrome, also known as Kawasaki syndrome, is a febrile disorder of unknown etiology usually affecting children, originally described in the Japanese literature but having a worldwide distribution.[282] Fever, cervical lymphadenopathy, pharyngeal and conjunctival inflammation, and erythematous skin rashes are the most common clinical symptoms. Sometimes lymphadenopathy represents the dominant manifestation of the disease.[286] Arthritis is present in approximately 40% of the cases. Coronary arteritis may lead to fatal complications. The etiology is unknown, but an infectious agent is suspected.

Microscopically, the affected lymph nodes often show fibrin thrombi in the smaller vessels accompanied by patchy infarcts.[284,285] These changes have been interpreted as the expression of an acute vasculitis. The main differential diagnosis is Kikuchi necrotizing lymphadenitis. Persistent damage to the coronary arteries occurs in approximately one-fourth of untreated children.[283]

Lupus erythematosus

The lymph node changes in lupus erythematosus are generally of a nonspecific nature and consist of moderate follicular hyperplasia associated with increased vascularization and scattered immunoblasts and plasma cells; some of the latter contain PAS-positive cytoplasmic bodies that represent sites of immunoglobulin production.[289] Occasionally, one encounters a peculiar form of necrosis characterized by the deposition of hematoxyphilic material in the stroma, in the sinuses, and on the wall of blood vessels[291] (Fig. 21.29). These have been found to be composed of DNA derived from karyorrhectic nuclear material, presumably from lymphocytes. As a matter of fact, the microscopic appearance of lupus lymphadenitis may be indistinguishable from that of Kikuchi disease[287] (see p. 1785). On occasion the changes are morphologically similar to those of either the hyaline vascular or intermediate types of Castleman disease.[288,289] In other instances, Warthin–Finkeldey-like polykaryocytes have been numerous.[290] The immunophenotype of lupus lymphadenitis is nonspecific.[291]

Rheumatoid arthritis

Most patients with rheumatoid arthritis have generalized lymphadenopathy at some time during their illness.[297] The lymph node enlargement may precede the arthritis and raise the clinical suspicion of lymphoma.

Microscopically, the most important changes are follicular hyperplasia and plasma cell proliferation, with formation of Russell bodies.[296] Vascular proliferation is also a consistent finding. The appearance may be quite similar to that of the plasma cell type of Castleman disease. Small foci of necrosis and clumps of neutrophils are seen in some instances. The capsule is often infiltrated by lymphocytes. Immunohistochemically, the plasma cell proliferation is of polyclonal nature.[293] **Still disease** can also result in an intense hyperplastic change that can vaguely resemble peripheral

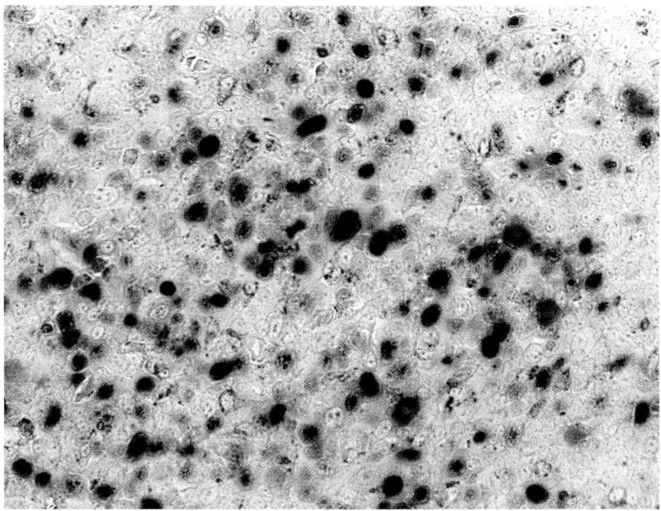

Fig. 21.27 Demonstration of EBER antigen by in situ hybridization in a case of infectious mononucleosis.

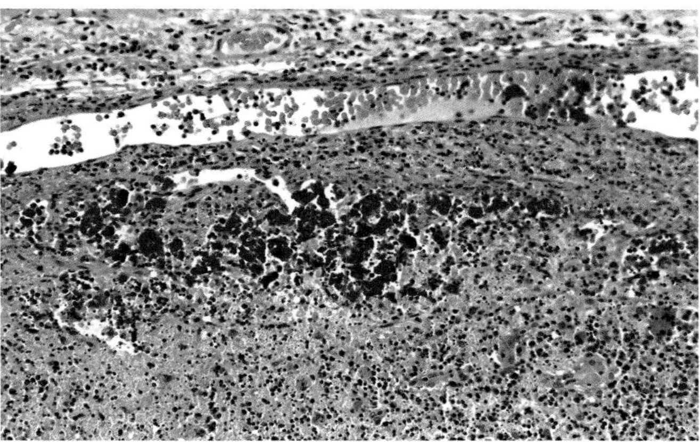

Fig. 21.29 Large accumulations of DNA-containing basophilic material in the subcapsular region of a lymph node in a patient with systemic lupus erythematosus.

Fig. 21.28 Viral lymphadenitis showing scattered immunoblasts resulting in a 'salt-and-pepper' appearance.

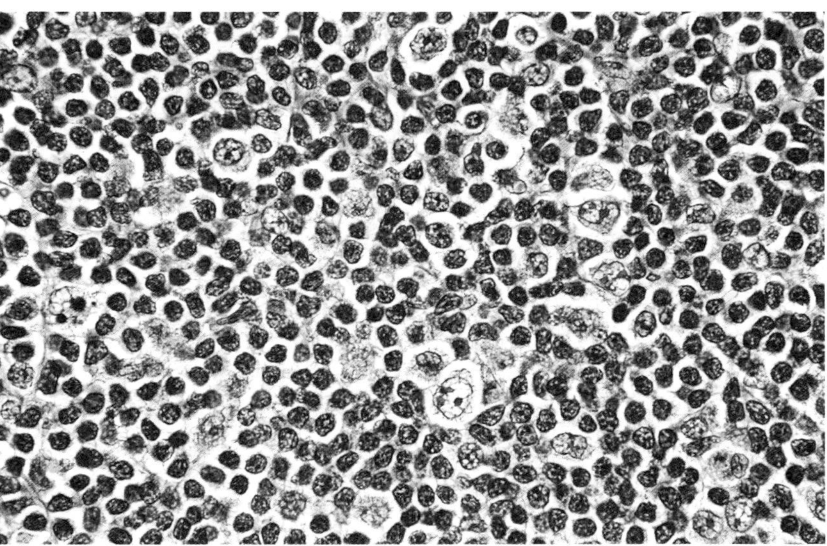

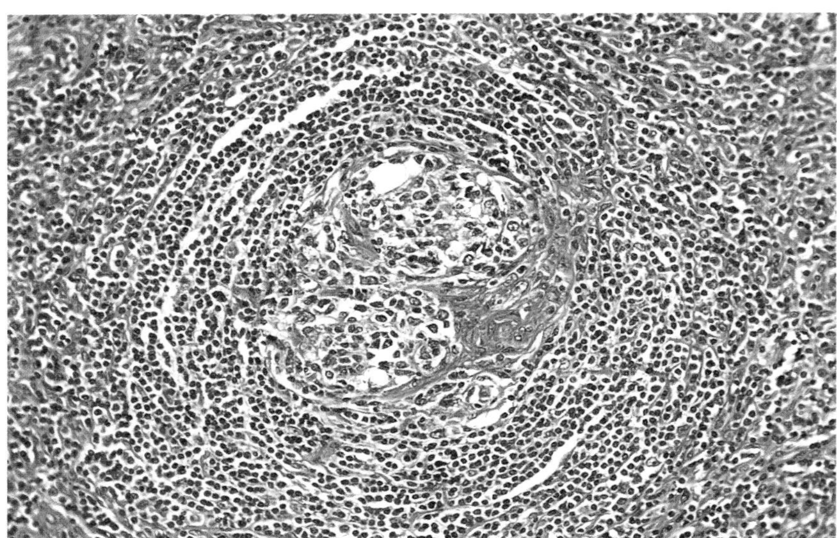

Fig. 21.30 Castleman disease of hyaline vascular type. There is a prominent germinal center showing well-developed changes.

T-cell lymphoma.[294] Other immune-mediated diseases, such as lupus erythematosus, polyarteritis nodosa, and scleroderma, are usually not associated with this type of lymph node abnormality.

Patients with rheumatoid arthritis treated with gold compounds can develop **gold-associated lymphadenopathy**.[298] They are also said to have a slightly increased incidence of malignant lymphomas[292,295] (see p. 1848).

Castleman disease

Castleman disease (giant lymph node hyperplasia) represents a morphologically distinct form of lymph node hyperplasia rather than a neoplasm or a hamartoma. It occurs most commonly in adults but it can also affect children.[346] Microscopically, two major categories have been described.[310,323] The first, designated as *hyaline-vascular type* or angiofollicular, shows large follicles scattered in a mass of lymphoid tissue. The follicles show marked vascular proliferation and hyalinization of their abnormal germinal centers; they have been confused with Hassall corpuscles and with splenic white pulp, prompting in the first case a mistaken diagnosis of thymoma and in the second of ectopic spleen (Fig. 21.30). Their appearance corresponds to that of regressively transformed germinal centers (see p. 1781). Many of the large cells with vesicular nuclei present in the hyaline center are follicular dendritic cells, as evidenced by their strong immunoreactivity for CD21 and CD35.[336] There is a tight concentric layering of lymphocytes at the periphery of the follicles (corresponding to the mantle zone), resulting in an onion-skin appearance. The interfollicular stroma is also prominent, with numerous hyperplastic vessels of the postcapillary venule type and an admixture of plasma cells, eosinophils, immunoblasts, and CD68-positive plasmacytoid dendritic cells.[309,334] Sinuses are characteristically absent. In the variant of the hyaline-vascular type described as the *lymphoid subtype*, the follicles have a marked expansion of the mantle zone and small, relatively inconspicuous germinal centers. This variant of Castleman disease merges with the process known as *mantle zone hyperplasia*, and it is the one more likely to be confused with malignant lymphoma of either follicular or mantle cell type. Immunohistochemically, there is polyclonal immunoglobulin production by plasma cells, and large numbers of suppressor T cells are found in the interfollicular areas. An aberrant phenotype of Ki-B3-negative B lymphocytes has been detected in the mantle zone cells.[332] Strong positivity for factor VIII-related antigen is seen in the endothelium of the interfollicular vessels, but only a weak and focal reaction for this marker is found in the hyalinized vessels located in the center of the follicles.[321]

The second major morphologic category of Castleman disease is known as the *plasma cell type*.[323] It is characterized by a diffuse plasma cell proliferation in the interfollicular tissue, sometimes accompanied by numerous Russell bodies. The hyaline-vascular changes in the follicles are inconspicuous or absent; instead, one often encounters in the center of these follicles a deposition of an amorphous acidophilic material that probably contains fibrin and immune complexes. The overall appearance is reminiscent of that seen in the lymph nodes from patients with rheumatoid arthritis (Fig. 21.31). The abundant expression of interleukin-6 that has been detected in this condition is thought to be responsible for the marked plasma cell infiltration.[319]

From the point of view of clinical presentation, Castleman disease has been divided into a solitary and a multicentric form. The *solitary form* presents as a mass located most commonly in the mediastinum but also described in the neck, lung, axilla, mesentery, broad ligament, retroperitoneum, soft tissues of the extremities (including subcutis and skeletal muscle),[322] nasopharynx, meninges, and several other sites.[315] Grossly, it is round, well-circumscribed, with a solid gray cut surface, and can measure 15 cm or more in diameter (Fig. 21.32). Although this form by definition presents as a single mass, microscopic changes suggesting an early stage of the same process are sometimes seen in adjacent nodes. Microscopically, over 90% of the cases are of the hyaline-vascular type (including the lymphoid subtype), and the remainder are of the plasma cell type. The former is usually asymptomatic, whereas the plasma cell type is often associated with fever, anemia, elevated erythrocyte sedimentation rate, hypergammaglobulinemia, and hypoalbuminemia. The disease reported in the Orient as *idiopathic plasmacytic lymphadenopathy with polyclonal hypergammaglobulinemia* is probably different from the plasma cell type of Castleman disease, but may represent IgG4-related lymphadenopathy in a significant proportion of cases.[306,324] The treatment of solitary Castleman disease is surgical excision, which has been found to result in rapid regression of the associated abnormalities whenever present.[303]

The *multicentric* or *systemic form* is nearly always of the plasma cell type,[330] although occasional examples of the hyaline-vascular type

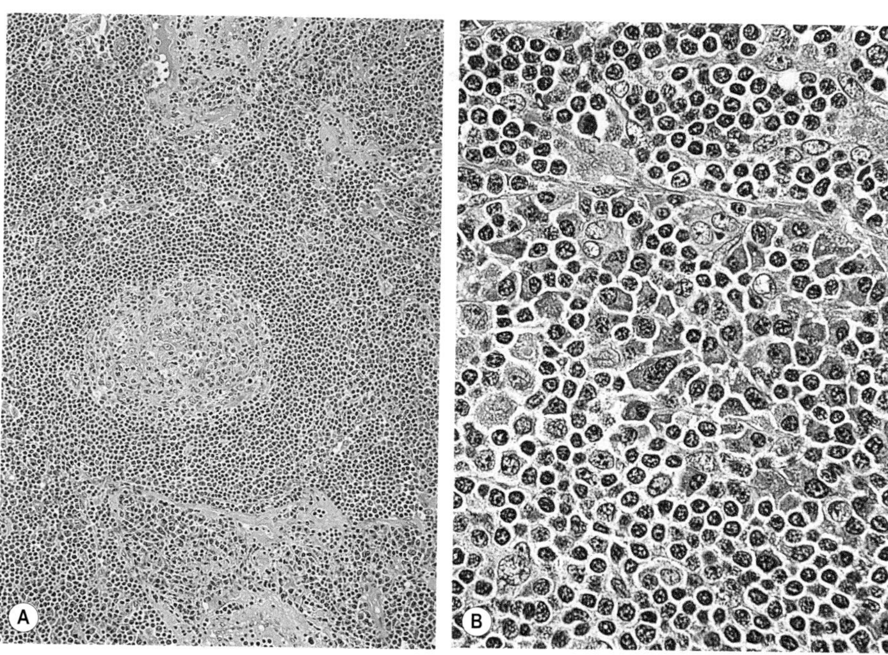
Fig. 21.31 **A** and **B**, Castleman disease of plasma cell type. **A**, Low-power view showing follicular hyperplasia without hyaline vascular changes. **B**, High-power view of the interfollicular region showing a massive infiltration by plasma cells. Some of these plasma cells show multinucleation and mild nuclear atypia.

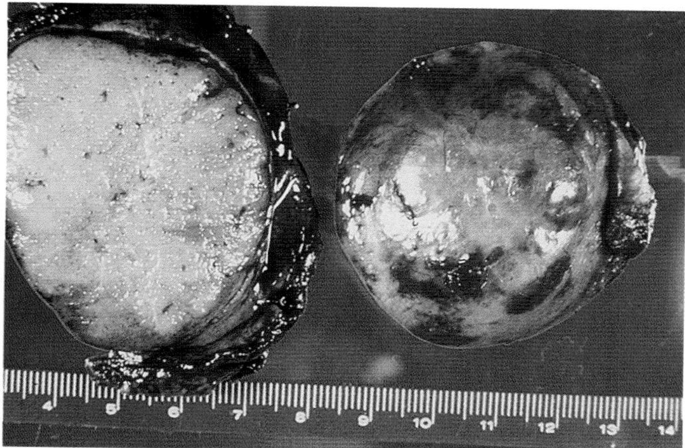
Fig. 21.32 Gross appearance of Castleman disease of the hyaline vascular type.

(involving even the skin) are on record.[345] It presents with generalized lymphadenopathy and may also involve the spleen.[311,312,348] The clinical and laboratory features are similar to those of angioimmunoblastic lymphadenopathy. The etiology is unknown, the two main hypotheses (not mutually exclusive) being abnormal immune response and viral infection.[320] Regarding the latter, a definite link has been documented between HHV8 and a subset of multicentric Castleman disease (this virus being also linked to Kaposi sarcoma and primary effusion sarcoma).[302,308,339] Cases of HHV8+ Castleman disease are said to be characterized morphologically by dissolution of the lymphoid follicles.[301] It has been hypothesized that HHV8 induces the changes of Castleman disease through the production of interleukin-6.[318,331]

Sometimes multicentric Castleman disease is seen in association with the POEMS syndrome, an acronymic designation for polyneuropathy, organomegaly, endocrinopathy, M-protein, and skin changes.[329,333] The latter include a distinctive vascular lesion known as glomeruloid hemangioma.[304] In other instances, Castleman disease has been reported in association with amyloid deposits.[300,338]

The long-term prognosis of systemic Castleman disease is poor; the disease tends to persist for months or years and to result sometimes in renal or pulmonary complications.[341] Furthermore, some of the patients have been found to have Kaposi sarcoma. Indeed, the coexistence of multicentric Castleman disease and Kaposi sarcoma in the same tissue sample is not an uncommon phenomenon.[335] Other cases have developed large cell lymphomas of immunoblastic type. Evidence of clonal rearrangement for immunoglobulin and T-cell receptor genes has been found in cases of systemic Castleman disease together with copies of the EBV genome, no such features having been detected in the solitary form of the disease.[316,317,337,342] This suggests that multicentric Castleman disease is a disorder different from the classic localized type and one that may evolve into a clonal lymphoproliferation. Some authors actually regard it as a lymphoproliferative process rather than a reactive/inflammatory condition.

An important theme of the hyaline-vascular type of Castleman disease is the active participation of a variety of nonlymphoid cellular components. One such component is the dendritic follicular cell, which is prominently present in the hyalinized nodules that characterize the disease and which is thought by some authors to be at the core of the pathogenesis of this disorder[336,344] (Fig. 21.33). These cells can become atypical ('dysplastic') both in the abnormal germinal centers and in the intervening tissue,[344] and can manifest cytogenetic and molecular evidence of clonality[307,340] (Fig. 21.34). Furthermore, they may result in the formation of full-blown follicular dendritic cell tumors (see p. 1850).[305,326] Another type of proliferation involves the vascular and related contractile (myoid) elements that are present in the interfollicular tissue. Cases of Castleman disease in which these elements are unduly prominent have been referred to as *stroma-rich*[309] (Fig. 21.35). Further proliferation of this component results in the formation of *angiomyoid proliferative lesions*,[326] and of lesions that have been referred to as *angiomatous hamartomas*[327] (Fig. 21.36) or *vascular neoplasms*, the latter sometimes having hemangiopericytoma-like features.[305] Finally, cases

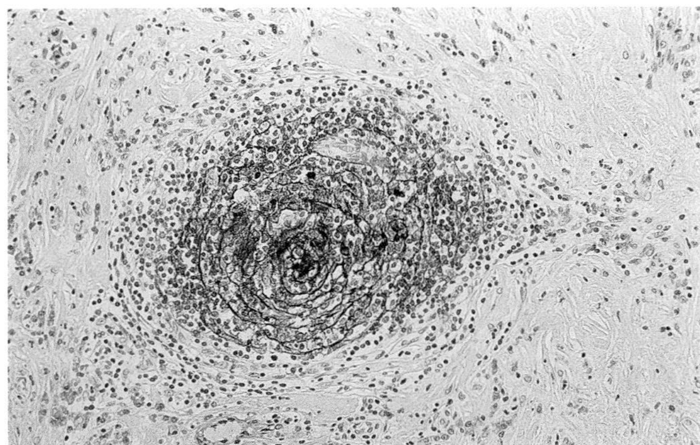

Fig. 21.33 Prominent network of CD21-positive dendritic follicular cells in the abnormal germinal center of Castleman disease.

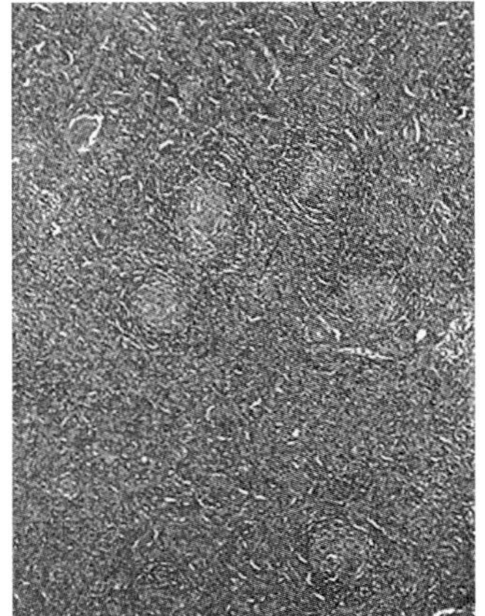

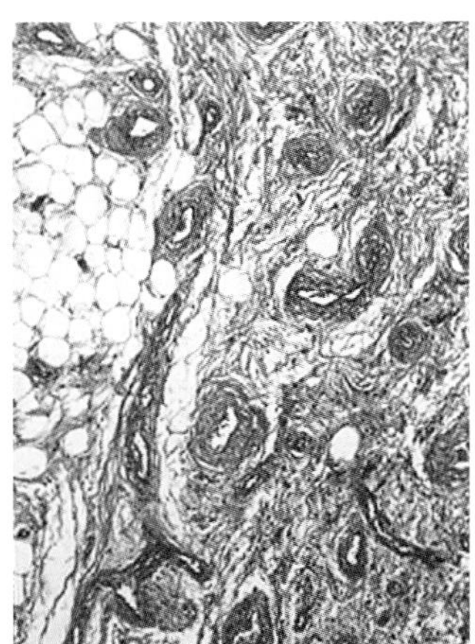

Fig. 21.36 Castleman disease associated with vascular proliferation in the surrounding soft tissues.
(Courtesy of Dr Pietro Muretto, Pesaro, Italy)

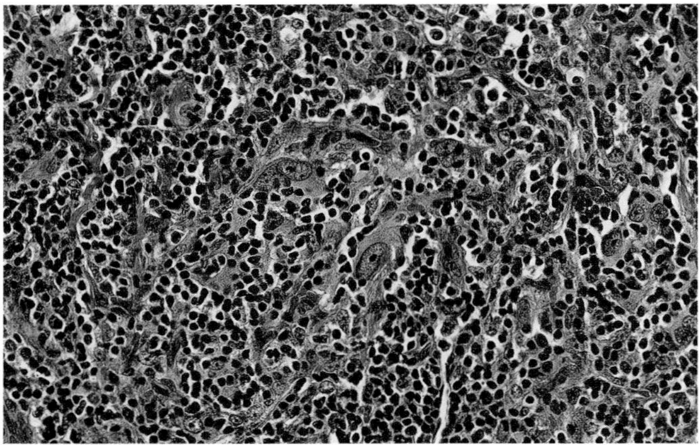

Fig. 21.34 'Dysplasia' of reticular/dendritic cells in Castleman disease. These cells were immunoreactive for desmin.

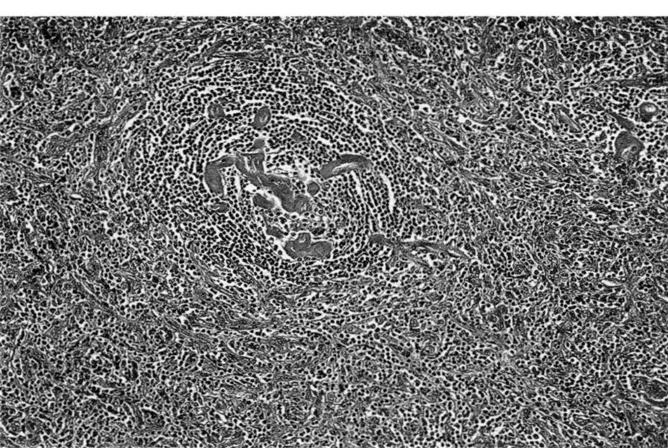

Fig. 21.35 Castleman disease of hyaline vascular type with a prominent stromal component which is richly vascularized ('stroma-rich' variant).

have been described of high-grade spindle cell sarcomas arising in Castleman disease, which have been originally interpreted as of probable vascular nature because of the presence of myoid tumor cells closely apposed to vascular structures[313] (Fig. 21.37). Whether these myoid cells are truly vessel-related or whether they originate from yet another member of the reticulum/dendritic cell family (so-called 'fibroblastic reticulum cells', 'myoid reticulum cells', or 'dychthyocytes') is not clear.

In the light of the above information, one might conclude that the neoplastic potentialities of Castleman disease tend to manifest themselves mainly through the development of lymphoid tumors in the plasma cell type and of dendritic/stromal tumors in the hyaline-vascular type. However, exceptions occur, in the sense that isolated cases of the latter have been accompanied or preceded by plasmacytoma,[314,343] follicular lymphoma,[325,347] and particularly Hodgkin lymphoma.[299,328,349]

Angioimmunoblastic lymphadenopathy

Angioimmunoblastic lymphadenopathy (AILD, immunoblastic lymphadenopathy) is currently regarded by most authors as a form (perhaps the most common) of peripheral T-cell lymphoma.[351] It is discussed here for historical reasons and also because some experts believe that atypical and oligoclonal proliferations may precede the development of lymphoma, and that some cases may actually be reactive or at most preneoplastic.[373] It occurs almost exclusively in adults and elderly individuals and is characterized clinically by fever, anemia (usually hemolytic), polyclonal hypergammaglobulinemia, and generalized lymphadenopathy.[357,358,367] Other common manifestations include hepatomegaly, splenomegaly, constitutional symptoms, and skin rash.[352,359,371] In 27% of the patients studied in the classic series by Lukes and Tindle,[367] the disease occurred abruptly after administration of drugs, particularly penicillin.

Microscopically, the disease is systemic, with lesions in the lymph nodes, spleen, liver, bone marrow, and skin. The lymph node changes are characterized by obliteration of the nodal architecture (with focal preservation of sinuses) by a polymorphic cellular infiltrate and by an extensive proliferation of finely arborizing vessels of the caliber of postcapillary venules (Fig. 21.38). The cellular infiltrate is composed of small lymphocytes, plasma

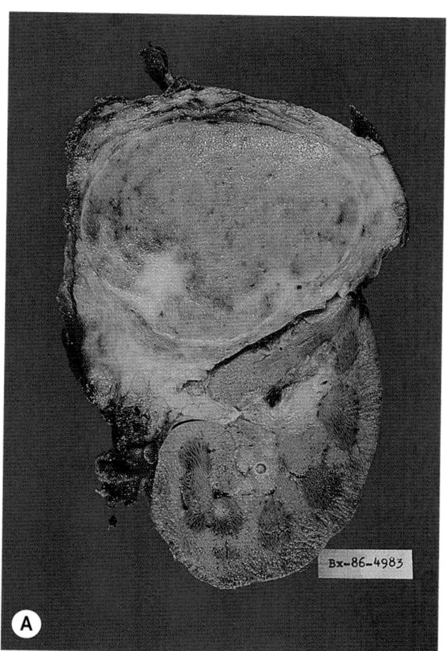

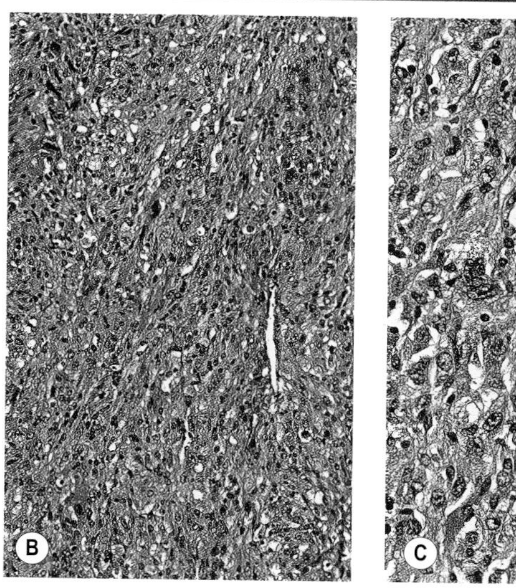

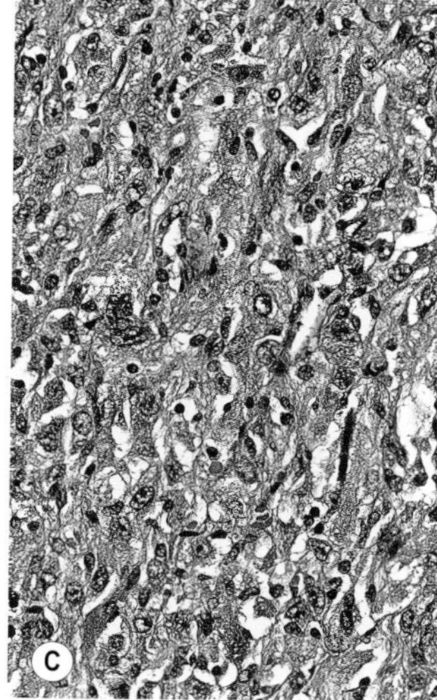

Fig. 21.37 A–C, Castleman disease complicated by the development of sarcoma. **A**, Gross appearance of a case located in the perirenal region. **B**, Microscopic appearance of another case. The tumor has a vaguely hemangiopericytomatous quality. **C**, High-power view.

cells, numerous immunoblasts, frequent and sometimes abundant eosinophils, and, occasionally, multinucleated giant cells. Normal germinal centers are consistently absent; what one may find instead are germinal centers composed of loose aggregates of pale histiocytes, rare immunoblasts, or large epithelioid cells; these are referred to as 'burnt-out germinal centers' and can closely resemble the appearance of granulomas. Only occasionally one finds hyperplastic germinal centers of the conventional type.[370] There may also be a component of proliferating cells of dendritic/reticulum nature, some of them strongly positive for desmin.[360] An amorphous, eosinophilic PAS-positive intercellular material may be found scattered throughout the node. Extension of the infiltrate in the capsule and pericapsular tissue is common. Immunoperoxidase stain reveals a polyclonal pattern of immunoglobulin production. Lymphoid cells positive for EBV are found in over 75% of the cases; most but not all of these cells are of B-cell nature.[369]

The nature of AILD has been controversial since the time of its first description and remains so today. It was originally regarded as a non-neoplastic hyperimmune proliferation of the B-cell system with an exaggerated transformation of lymphocytes into immunoblasts and plasma cells, possibly induced by a primary abnormality of the T-cell system (such as a loss of suppressor T cells).[353,354,364] However, subsequent studies revealed the existence of cases having the AILD pattern but also exhibiting features suggesting the presence of a neoplastic lymphoid component. Thus Nathwani et al.[368] described cases of AILD characterized by the appearance of 'clones' (clusters or islands) of tightly packed immunoblasts, followed by a diffuse replacement of the node by these elements (Fig. 21.39). Several Japanese groups described cases with the AILD pattern that also exhibited cytologic atypia in the small and large lymphoid cells (clear cells and/or convoluted cells).[372] In many of these cases, the existence of a clonal population of T lymphocytes was documented by molecular techniques.[366,374] Although these cases were initially interpreted as AILD-like T-cell lymphomas and an attempt was made to separate them from 'true' AILD, it has become increasingly apparent that a sharp separation among these lesions is impossible. AILD should be viewed as an arbitrarily defined morphologic portion of a spectrum of atypical immunoproliferative disorders (also known as lymphogranulomatosis X in some circles)[362] that range from the probably reactive and reversible to the clearly neoplastic and aggressive. At present, the consensus is that the overwhelming majority of cases belong to the latter category and that they represent a subtype of peripheral T-cell lymphoma. It is further believed that this subtype is characterized by the expression of CD10.

The issue is further complicated by the fact that some cases show a clonal population of B cells *in addition* to a clonal population of T cells.[356] The possible role of a viral agent in the genesis of this disorder has been repeatedly proposed but not yet conclusively demonstrated.[361,363,369]

From a practical standpoint, the presence of atypical lymphoid cells (whether immunoblastic 'clones', clear cells, or small cells with convoluted nuclei) correlates with a more aggressive clinical course.[350,368] In retrospect, we believe that the cases that we described many years ago as 'malignant histiocytosis with cutaneous involvement and eosinophilia'[365] belong to this general category as representatives of the more aggressive and neoplastic type. Similar cases have been described by others.[355]

Drug hypersensitivity

Antiepileptic drugs derived from hydantoin, such as diphenylhydantoin (Dilantin) and mephenytoin (Mesantoin), can result in a hypersensitivity reaction manifested by skin rash, fever, generalized lymphadenopathy (mainly cervical), and peripheral eosinophilia. The reaction, which is quite uncommon, tends to occur within the first few months of therapy. The changes disappear if the drug is discontinued. The nodal enlargement can occur in the absence of some of the other manifestations of the drug reaction.

Microscopically, partial effacement of the architecture by a polymorphic cellular infiltration is seen.[375] Histiocytes, immunoblasts, eosinophils, neutrophils, and plasma cells are all present. Some of the immunoblasts have atypical nuclear features, but Reed–Sternberg cells are absent. Foci of necrosis were noted in the classic article by Salzstein and Ackerman in which this condition was first described.[376] In some of the cases, the microscopic appearance is

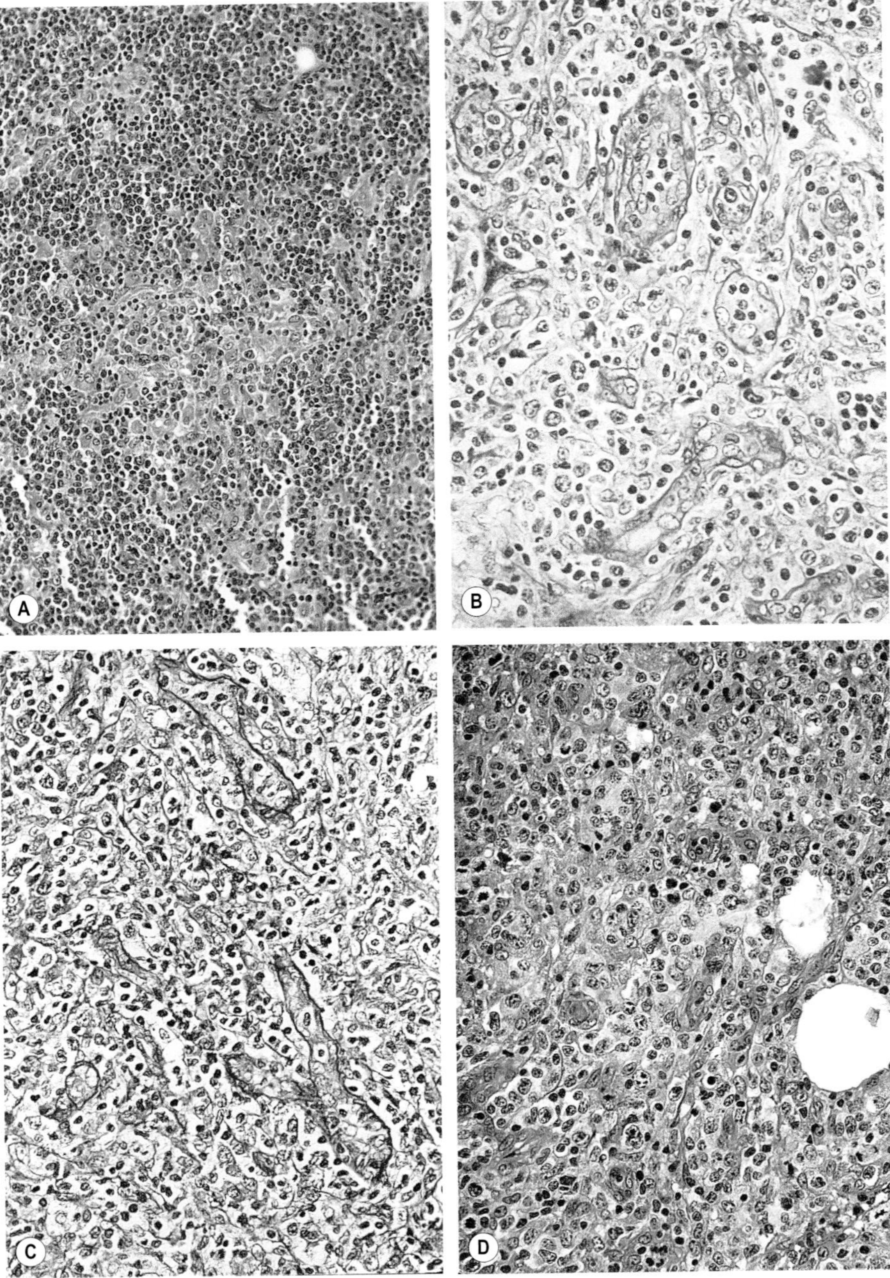

Fig. 21.38 A–D, Lymph node involvement by angioimmunoblastic lymphadenopathy. **A**, Low-power view showing a moderate effacement of the architecture by a polymorphic infiltrate composed of lymphocytes, plasma cells, and histiocytes. There is also marked vascular proliferation. **B** and **C**, The PAS stain highlights the prominence of the postcapillary venules. **D**, Atypical lymphoid cells are present in this polymorphic infiltrate. There are also scattered eosinophils.

indistinguishable from that of AILD. The problem may simply be one of semantics, as one could interpret these cases as examples of the rare nonmalignant type of AILD induced by the anticonvulsant therapy.

Dermatopathic lymphadenitis

Dermatopathic lymphadenitis (lipomelanosis reticularis of Pautrier) is a form of nodal hyperplasia usually secondary to a generalized dermatitis, particularly those with exfoliative features. Pathogenetically, it represents a T-cell response to skin antigens processed and presented by interdigitating dendritic cells. It may occur in any skin disorder in which itching and scratching are prominent; this includes inflammatory dermatoses such as psoriasis and neoplastic diseases such as mycosis fungoides. Rarely, the morphologic changes of dermatopathic lymphadenitis are seen in the absence of clinical skin disease.[379]

Grossly, the lymph node is enlarged, the cut surface bulging, and the color pale yellow. In florid cases, black linear areas are seen in the periphery, representing clumps of melanin pigment and simulating the appearance of malignant melanoma.

Microscopically, the nodal architecture is preserved. The main change is represented by a marked pale widening of the paracortical zone, which stands out prominently on low-power examination[381] (Fig. 21.40). Most of the large nonlymphoid cells occupying this area are thought to be of three types: histiocytes, Langerhans cells, and interdigitating dendritic cells.[377,380] Many of the histiocytes contain phagocytosed melanin and neutral fat in their cytoplasm. Plasma cell infiltration and follicular hyperplasia are often present. A scattering of eosinophils also may be seen.

Nodes affected by dermatopathic lymphadenitis may be confused with Hodgkin lymphoma, mycosis fungoides, monocytic leukemia, or Langerhans cell histiocytosis. The differential diagnosis with mycosis fungoides is of particular concern because of the fact that mycosis fungoides is one of the cutaneous disorders that can be associated with dermatopathic lymphadenitis.[378] Diagnostic assistance can be obtained from immunohistochemistry and molecular pathology. Dermatopathic lymph nodes *that are also involved by mycosis fungoides* may show loss of CD7 and CD62L expression, and sometimes also loss of the pan–T-cell markers CD5, CD3, and CD2.[383] At the molecular level, clonal rearrangements of T-cell receptor genes may be demonstrated.[382]

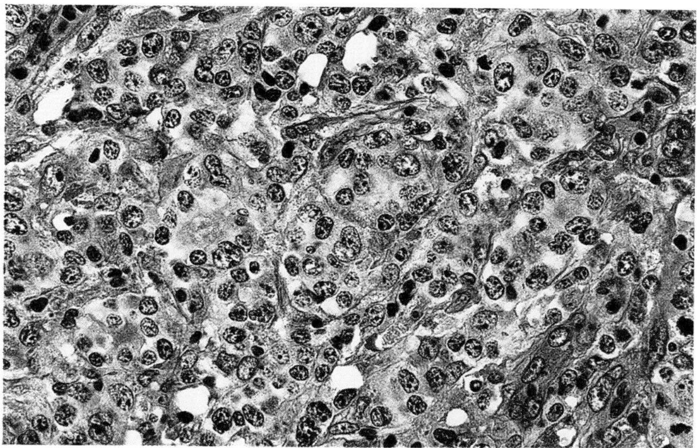

Fig. 21.39 Angioimmunoblastic lymphadenopathy with uniform proliferation of large lymphoid cells of neoplastic appearance.

Rosai–Dorfman disease

Rosai–Dorfman disease (RDD), originally described as sinus histiocytosis with massive lymphadenopathy (SHML), presents in its most typical form as massive, painless, bilateral lymph node enlargement in the neck, associated with fever, leukocytosis, elevated erythrocyte sedimentation rate, and polyclonal hypergammaglobulinemia.[396,425] Most cases occur during the first or second decade of life, but any age group can be affected. A few cases have affected two members of the same family.[411] There is a predisposition for the condition in blacks. Although the disease has a widespread geographic distribution and most of the reported cases have been from the United States and Western Europe, there is a disproportionally high number of cases from Africa and the Caribbean region.[396] Although the cervical region is by far the most common and most prominent site of involvement, other peripheral or central lymph node groups can be affected, with or without cervical disease.

Grossly, the nodes are matted together by prominent perinodal fibrosis. Their cut surface varies from gray to golden yellow, depending on the amount of fat present.

Microscopically, there is a pronounced dilation of the lymph sinuses, resulting in partial or complete architectural effacement (Fig. 21.41). These sinuses are occupied by lymphocytes, plasma cells, and – most notably – by numerous cells of histiocytic appearance with a large vesicular nucleus and abundant clear or lightly eosinophilic cytoplasm that may contain large amounts of neutral lipids. Many of these histiocytes have within their cytoplasm numerous intact lymphocytes, a feature that has been designated as emperipolesis or lymphocytophagocytosis. Although not specific, this is a constant feature of RDD (as least in the lymph node location) and is therefore of great diagnostic significance (Fig. 21.42). Sometimes other cell types are present within the cytoplasm of the histiocytes, such as plasma cells and red blood cells.

The intersinusal tissue exhibits a variable but sometimes impressive number of mature plasma cells, some of which may contain Russell bodies. Capsular and pericapsular inflammation and fibrosis are common, but intranodal fibrosis is minimal or absent. In a minority of cases, small microabscesses or foci of necrosis are

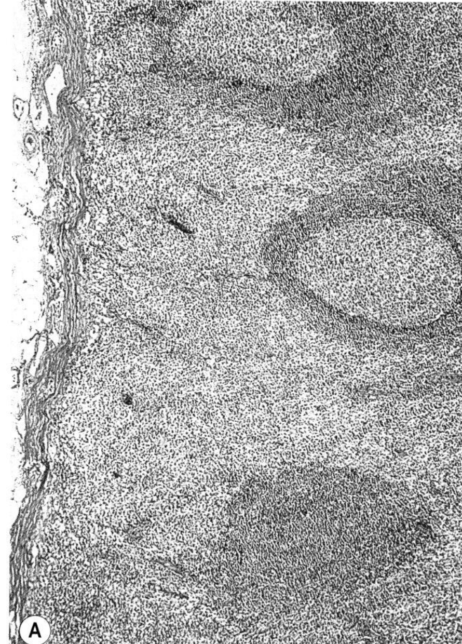

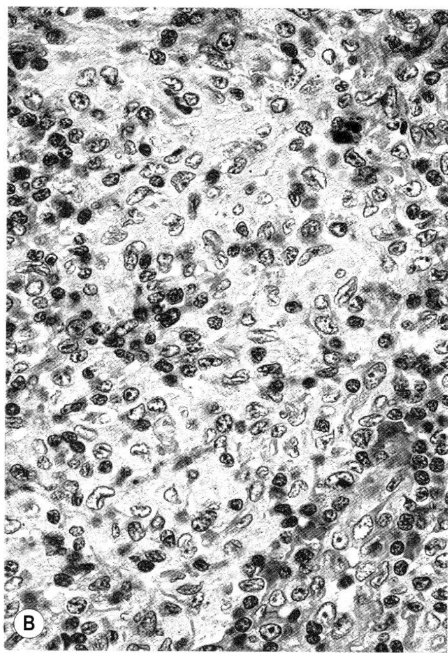

Fig. 21.40 **A** and **B**, Dermatopathic lymphadenitis. **A**, Massive expansion of the paracortical region, resulting in a wide, pale area between the capsule and the lymphoid follicles. **B**, High-power view of the paracortical region showing numerous cells with oval vesicular nuclei, which correspond to an admixture of interdigitating dendritic cells and Langerhans cells.

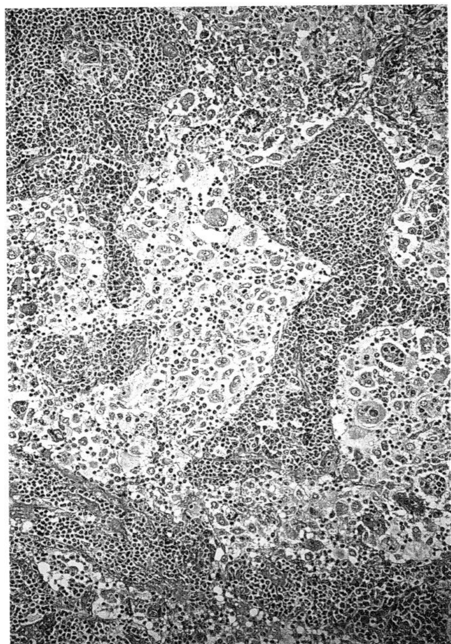

Fig. 21.41 Rosai–Dorfman disease. Low-power view showing massive distension of the sinuses by the histiocytic infiltrate.

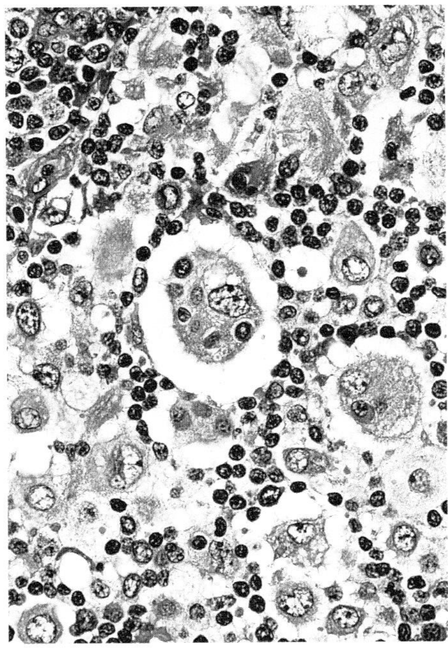

Fig. 21.42 Rosai–Dorfman disease. High-power view showing lymphocytophagocytosis by the sinus histiocytes.

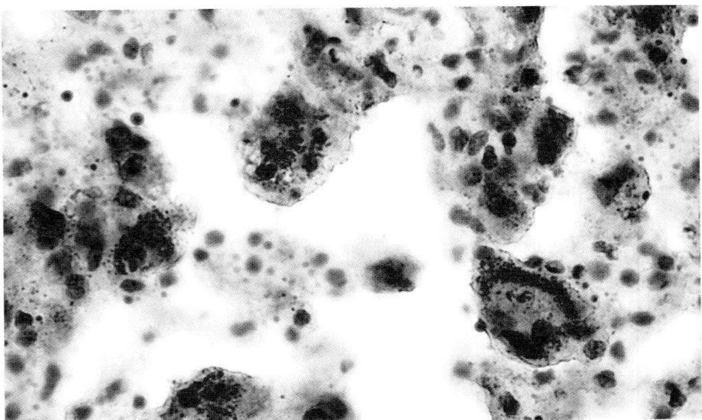

Fig. 21.43 Rosai–Dorfman disease. Oil red O stain showing abundant neutral lipid in the cytoplasm of the histiocytes.

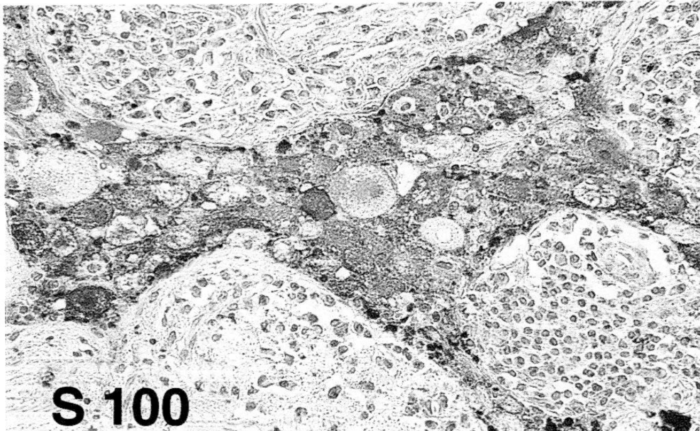

Fig. 21.44 Strong immunoreactivity of the sinus histiocytes for S-100 protein in Rosai–Dorfman disease.

found within the dilated sinuses. Ultrastructurally, the histiocytes located in the sinuses have extensive pseudopodia and lack Birbeck granules; viral particles or other evidence of infection is consistently lacking. The sinus histiocytes contain cytoplasmic fat (Fig. 21.43) and are strongly reactive for S-100 protein[413] and CD68 (Fig. 21.44), but negative for CD1a; some of them are also positive for immunoglobulin, presumably phagocytosed from the surroundings. Their immunohistochemical profile (including the adhesion molecules pattern) suggests that they are monocytes that have been recently recruited from the circulation.[388,391,420,423] The plasma cells show a polyclonal pattern of immunoglobulin expression. The lymphocytes present are an admixture of B and T cells.

In over one-fourth of the cases, RDD involves extranodal sites.[396] This usually occurs in the presence of massive lymphadenopathy, and the disease is therefore easily recognized. However, in some cases these extranodal manifestations represent the predominant or even exclusive manifestation of the disease. Practically all organ systems have been recorded as being the site of the disease. The most common are eyes and ocular adnexa (especially orbit),[394] head and neck region,[432] upper respiratory tract,[393,407] skin and subcutaneous tissue (perhaps more commonly in the Orient),[386,389,405,410,414,428] skeletal system,[430] and central nervous system.[387,397,426] However, the disease has been reported in many other sites, including gastrointestinal tract,[384,406,418] pancreas,[421] salivary glands,[402] genitourinary tract, thyroid,[390] mediastinum,[400] breast,[399,415] and uterine cervix.[416] In some instances, widespread nodal and extranodal dissemination is found.[435] Organs that stand out because of their almost universal sparing by the disorder are lung, spleen, and bone marrow (the latter exclusive of the focal bone lesions mentioned above). The histopathologic features of RDD in extranodal sites are similar to the nodal disease except for the fact that fibrosis tends to be more pronounced and lymphocytophagocytosis less conspicuous.

The etiology of RDD remains unknown, the two most likely possibilities (not mutually exclusive) being infection by a virus or some other microorganism and the manifestation of a subtle undefined immunologic defect. It has been suggested that stimulation of monocytes/macrophages via macrophage colony stimulating factor (M-CSF) leading to immune suppressive macrophages may be the main pathogenetic mechanism.[412] Despite some suggestive early data derived from serologic tests, it is now acknowledged that the histiocytes of this disease are not infected by EBV.[429] HHV6 has been detected in RDD tissues, but this organism is so commonly present in lymphoid tissue that the significance of this finding remains dubious.[408] Molecular studies done on involved tissue have failed to show evidence of clonality, in keeping with their presumed reactive nature. This contrasts with the findings in at least some studies of Langerhans cell histiocytosis, a disease that it otherwise resembles in many clinical, morphologic, and phenotypic aspects,[419,433,434] and with which it can coexist.[431] O'Malley et al.[417] have reported nine such cases and suggested that that two entities can be pathophysiologically related.

RDD is relatively unaffected by therapy, although chemotherapy has proved effective in some cases,[404,422,427] occasionally with allegedly complete and permanent results.[401] In many cases, RDD undergoes quick and complete spontaneous resolution. In others, it follows a protracted clinical course for years or decades. The latter is particularly true in cases with widespread extranodal involvement. In some instances the disease disappears, only to come back years later at another site. Some patients have died as a result of RDD, either because of extensive disease affecting vital organs or because of complications related to the immunologic abnormalities that may be present,[395,398] such as amyloidosis.[424]

The differential diagnosis of RDD includes nonspecific sinus hyperplasia (in which the cells lack emperipolesis and are S-100 protein-negative), Langerhans cell histiocytosis (in which the cells are positive for both S-100 protein and CD1a), leprosy, rhinoscleroma (with which it can apparently coexist[403]), and metastatic malignant melanoma. Perhaps the condition that resembles it most is the sinus histiocytosis induced by cobalt-chromium and titanium that can occur in pelvic lymph nodes after hip replacement.[385]

It should also be noted that focal RDD-like changes can sometimes be seen in lymph nodes involved by other processes, such as Hodgkin[392] or non-Hodgkin lymphoma, a phenomenon analogous to that sometimes seen in Langerhans cell histiocytosis.[409] Similar changes can also occur in lymph nodes involved by autoimmune lymphoproliferative syndrome (see next section).

Autoimmune lymphoproliferative syndrome

Autoimmune lymphoproliferative syndrome (ALPS; Canale-Smith disease) is an inherited disorder due to defects in FAS-mediated apoptosis, and characterized in most instances by lymphadenopathy, splenomegaly, hypergammaglobulinemia, and autoimmune phenomena.[441,443] Most patients present in childhood, but cases of adult onset are on record.[436] Most patients with ALPS have germline, and less commonly somatic, mutations of *FAS* (*TNFRSF6*), *FASL* or *CASPASE* gene.[437] Four subtypes of this condition have been described.[437] A characteristic feature is an increased number of CD3+CD4−CD8− (double negative) alpha/beta T cells.[440]

Microscopically, the main change in the affected lymph nodes is a marked paracortical expansion by a mixed population of small and intermediate-sized lymphocytes and numerous large immunoblasts.[438,439] This expansion can be so extensive as to simulate a lymphoma. In addition, there is often florid follicular hyperplasia, frequently accompanied by focal progressive transformation of germinal centers. A polyclonal plasmacytosis is also common.[439]

An increased incidence of malignant lymphoma has been detected in this population.[442] Interestingly, we have found that as many as 41% of patients with type Ia ALPS had RDD-like changes in their lymph nodes, raising the possibility that RDD may be related to ALPS and possibly represent a forme fruste of it.[440]

Langerhans cell histiocytosis

The terms Langerhans cell histiocytosis (LCH), Langerhans cell granulomatosis, histiocytosis X, differentiated histiocytosis, and eosinophilic granuloma are applied to a specific, although remarkably variable, clinicopathologic entity characterized and defined by the proliferation of Langerhans cells.[457,471,479] These cells are regarded as a distinct type of immune 'accessory' cells that are involved in the capturing of some antigens and their presentation to the lymphoid cells. Contrary to a formerly held belief, these cells are not primarily phagocytic in nature. Their nuclei are highly characteristic: irregular, usually elongated, with prominent grooves and folds that traverse them in all directions. The cytoplasm is abundant and acidophilic, sometimes to the point that an embryonal rhabdomyosarcoma is simulated. Most Langerhans cells are mononuclear, but occasional ones contain several nuclei while still maintaining the aforementioned nuclear and cytoplasmic features. Histochemically, they show weak acid phosphatase and nonspecific esterase activity but considerable leucyl-β-naphthylamidase activity and membrane-bound ATPase activity.[446] They are believed to develop from a lymphoid-committed precursor,[444] a hypothesis supported by the presence of an identical rearrangement of the immunoglobulin heavy chain gene in a case we studied which had both neoplastic Langerhans cells and B lymphocytes.[473]

In paraffin sections, both Langerhans cells and the cells of LCH are reactive for S-100 protein, vimentin, langerin (CD207), fascin (a dendritic cell marker), CD1a, CD74, and HLA-DR in most cases[462,484,490] (Fig. 21.45). They also tend to be positive for peanut agglutinin lectin and the macrophage-associated antigens CD68, cathepsin D, and cathepsin E.[460,483,485] They generally do not express CD45RA, CD45RB, CDw75, α_1-antitrypsin, epithelial membrane

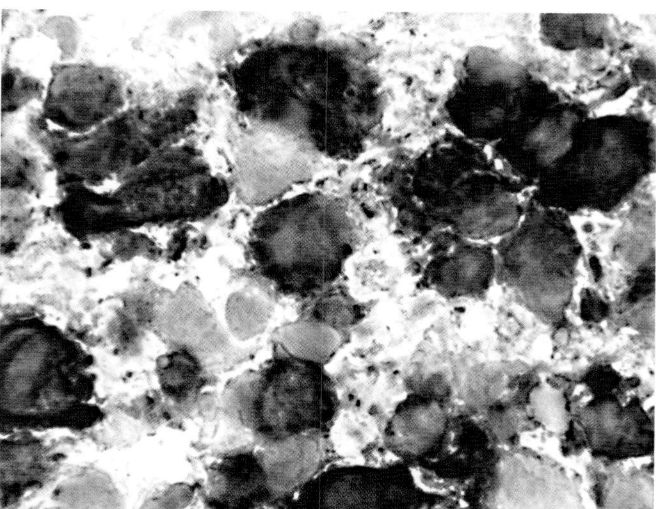

Fig. 21.45 Immunoreactivity of the cells of Langerhans cell histiocytosis for langerin.

Chronic granulomatous disease

Chronic granulomatous disease is the result of a genetically determined enzymatic defect of granulocytes and monocytes.[511,516] These cells ingest microorganisms but are unable to destroy them because of their inability to generate superoxide anion (O_2^-). This is due to a defect in any one of four components of NADPH oxidases, the enzyme responsible for the generation of the antimicrobial oxidants.[516] A pattern of Y-linked inheritance is seen in approximately 65% of the patients and results from mutations in the gene that encodes the g91-phox subunit of the cytochrome b558 component of the oxidase. The remaining 35% of patients inherit the disease in an autosomal recessive manner resulting from mutations in the genes that encode the other three oxidase components.[509,514,517] The traditional laboratory technique for the detection of the disease is the nitro blue tetrazolium test.[508]

The main clinical features are recurrent lymphadenitis, hepatosplenomegaly, skin rash, pulmonary infiltrates, anemia, leukocytosis, and hypergammaglobulinemia.[510,512,515] Microscopically, granulomas with necrotic purulent centers are seen in lymph nodes and other organs. They closely simulate the appearance of cat-scratch disease and lymphogranuloma venereum. Collections of histiocytes containing a lipofuscin-like pigment are also commonly observed and represent an important clue to the diagnosis.[513]

Lipophagic reactions

Accumulation of neutral lipid with formation of foamy macrophages (xanthoma cells) can be seen as an inconsequential secondary event in a variety of inflammatory and neoplastic conditions of lymph nodes, including Langerhans cell histiocytosis, RDD, Erdheim–Chester disease, and Hodgkin lymphoma. There are, in addition, conditions in which the **lipophagic granuloma** is the primary alteration. The lipophagic granuloma is defined as a collection of mononuclear and multinucleated giant cells, both of them exhibiting a cytoplasmic foamy appearance and lacking a significant participation of other cell types. By far the most common situation in which this occurs (so common as to be nearly universal, at least in Western countries) is represented by the incidental microscopic finding in periportal and mesenteric nodes in asymptomatic individuals, probably the result of mineral oil ingestion[522] (Fig. 21.48). Boitnott and Margolis[520] found this change in 78% of a series of 49 autopsied adults. Their chemical and histochemical studies showed that the oil droplets represent deposits of liquid-saturated hydrocarbons. Mineral oil is extensively used in the food processing industry, as a release agent and lubricant in capsules, tablets, bakery products, and dehydrated fruits and vegetables. Lipophagic granulomas of an extensive degree have been reported in association with long-term total parenteral nutrition therapy for short bowel syndrome.[523]

Whipple disease can result in marked enlargement of mesenteric lymph nodes, with formation of numerous lipophagic granulomas. Collections of histiocytes containing a PAS-positive glycoprotein are also present.[521] Under oil immersion and with electron microscopy, the characteristic bacillary bodies can be identified. Collections of PAS-positive histiocytes can also develop in peripheral nodes and may be the first clue to the diagnosis in a patient with gradual weight loss, weakness, and polyarthritis. Steatorrhea, the other classic symptom of the disease, may appear only in a later stage. In the presence of suggestive findings in routinely stained sections, confirmation of the diagnosis can now be obtained by the demonstration of the responsible organism (*Tropheryma whipplei*) by immunofluorescence or PCR.[518,519]

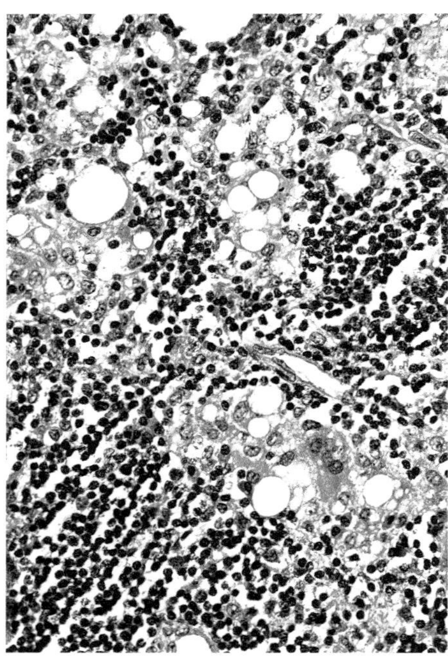

Fig. 21.48 Lymph node containing lipophagic granulomas. The change is manifested by the presence of mononuclear and multinucleated histiocytes located in the sinuses and containing large cytoplasmic vacuoles.

Lymphangiography, a procedure now largely abandoned, induces a lipophagic granulomatous reaction that may persist for several months. The sinuses are markedly distended and lined by histiocytes, many of which are multinucleated. Eosinophils may be present in appreciable numbers in the medullary cords. This is preceded by a predominantly neutrophilic infiltration.[524]

Malignant lymphoma

Malignant lymphoma is the generic term given to tumors of the lymphoid system and specifically of lymphocytes and their precursor cells, whether of T, B, or null phenotypes. Although traditionally tumors presumed to be composed of histiocytes and other cells of the accessory immune system have also been included in the category of malignant lymphoma, it would seem more appropriate to regard them separately for both conceptual and practical reasons. Such tumors undoubtedly exist, and are discussed later in this chapter. One should be aware, however, that the large majority of tumors that were designated in the past as histiocytic lymphomas or reticulum cell sarcomas are in reality of lymphocytic nature and therefore true malignant lymphomas.

Although some overlapping exists, the term *malignant lymphoma* is reserved for those neoplastic processes that initially present as localized lesions and are characterized by the formation of gross tumor nodules. Conversely, neoplastic lymphoid proliferations that are systemic and diffuse from their inception are included among the leukemias (see Chapter 23).

The malignant lymphomas can be divided into two major categories: Hodgkin lymphoma and all the others, which, for lack of a better term, are known collectively as non-Hodgkin lymphomas.[525,527,528,530,531] Both groups are further subdivided into several more or less distinct subcategories, the classification currently in vogue being that proposed by the World Health Organization in 2001 and updated in 2008 (see below). This classification has incorporated a wealth of information gathered from the fields of immunohistochemistry, molecular genetics, genomics, and proteomics. The results have been spectacular, but unfortunately they have resulted in calling into question the role of traditional histologic examination in lymphoma diagnosis. As several of the most accomplished hematopathologists have pointed out in sharp editorials and essays, that role is, and is likely to remain, critical.[526,529]

Hodgkin lymphoma

The disease originally described by Thomas Hodgkin in 1832 and which Samuel Wilks first proposed to be called Hodgkin disease makes one of the richest chapters of history of oncologic pathology.[532,539,540,546] The original color illustrations have become icons,[534] and the original cases, still housed at the pathology museum of Guy's Hospital in London, have been 'exhumed', studied microscopically and immunohistochemically, and the diagnosis has been confirmed (at least in some of the cases) after well over a century of fixation.[544] The interest in this enigmatic disease remains unabated, having been quoted as the paradigm for the emerging science of 'molecular morphology'.[547]

The conventional definition of Hodgkin disease – a very ingrained term that the World Health Organization (WHO) Committee has replaced by that of Hodgkin lymphoma – is that of a type of malignant lymphoma in which Reed–Sternberg cells are present in a 'characteristic background' of reactive inflammatory cells of various types, accompanied by fibrosis of a variable degree. Thus identification of typical Reed–Sternberg cells is necessary for the initial diagnosis of Hodgkin lymphoma (except for NLPHL, see below). As far as the 'characteristic background' or 'appropriate milieu' is concerned, it is highly variable, but it lacks the monomorphic appearance of most other malignant lymphomas (again with the exception of NLPHL). Mature lymphocytes, eosinophils, plasma cells, and histiocytes may all be present in greater or lesser amount, depending on the microscopic type. Many of the Reed–Sternberg cells are surrounded by T lymphocytes arranged in a rosettelike fashion.

The etiology of Hodgkin lymphoma remains unknown, but there is considerable evidence to suggest that the EBV plays an important role.[537,548] Individuals with a history of infectious mononucleosis have an increased incidence of Hodgkin lymphoma;[535,536] patients with Hodgkin lymphoma have an altered antibody pattern to EBV prior to diagnosis;[542] marked phenotypic similarities exist between infectious mononucleosis and Hodgkin lymphoma;[545] and EBV genomes have been identified in Reed–Sternberg cells in up to half of the cases (particularly in the mixed cellularity subtype, in young patients, and/or in developing countries)[533,538,543,549,550] (Fig. 21.49). There is also evidence for a genetic susceptibility factor.[541]

Gross features

Except for the very early stages, lymph nodes involved by Hodgkin lymphoma are enlarged, sometimes massively so. The gross appearance is somewhat dependent on the microscopic subtypes (see later section). The consistency varies from soft to hard depending on the amount of fibrosis. Some degree of nodularity is often appreciated, particularly in the nodular sclerosis form (Fig. 21.50). Foci of necrosis may be present. Except for NLPHL, the cut surface of the node has a more heterogeneous appearance than most non-Hodgkin lymphomas. In advanced cases, several nodes from the same group become matted together, a feature spectacularly demonstrated in the drawing that accompanied Hodgkin's classic article.

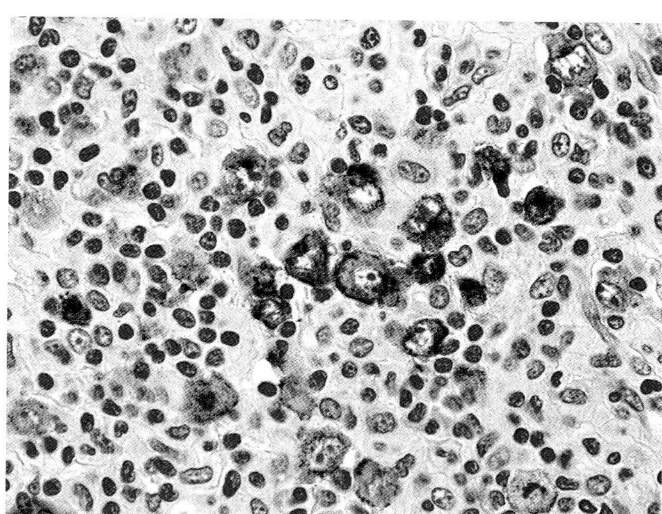

Fig. 21.49 Presence of the EBV genome in a case of Hodgkin lymphoma as demonstrated immunohistochemically by the detection of LMP1 antigen.

Reed–Sternberg cell

The classic Reed–Sternberg cell, as seen in all subtypes of classic Hodgkin lymphoma (but not in NLPHL, see below), is a large cell (20–50 μm in diameter or more) with abundant weakly acidophilic or amphophilic cytoplasm, which may appear homogeneous or granular and which lacks a pale zone in the Golgi area (Fig. 21.51). The nucleus is bilobed or polylobed so that the cell appears binucleated or multinucleated; it is possible that in some cases bona fide binucleation or multinucleation actually occurs (Fig. 21.52). The nuclear membrane is thick and sharply defined. The nuclear pattern is usually vesicular but with some coarse chromatin clumps scattered throughout. There is a very large, variously shaped, but usually rounded, highly acidophilic central nucleolus surrounded by a clear halo. In the most typical example of the Reed–Sternberg cell, the two nuclear lobes face each other ('mirror image'), resulting in the oft-cited 'owl eye' appearance. When multilobation occurs, the appearance has been likened to that of an 'egg basket'. Cells with this set of features but lacking nuclear lobation have been referred to as mononuclear variants of Reed–Sternberg cells or Hodgkin cells. Although their presence should suggest the possibility of Hodgkin lymphoma, they are not diagnostic by themselves. It has been stated that the minimal requirement for a diagnostic Reed–Sternberg cell is a bilobed nucleus in which at least one of the lobes has a prominent acidophilic nucleolus. At the other end of this spectrum is the Reed–Sternberg cell of giant size and highly pleomorphic hyperchromatic nuclei, having an appearance such as to simulate the cells of anaplastic carcinoma or one of the pleomorphic sarcomas. Another type of Reed–Sternberg cell, characterized by a darkly staining and retracted quality, is referred to as the mummified or necrobiotic variant and appears to be the morphologic expression of apoptosis (Fig. 21.52). Additional morphologic variations of Reed–Sternberg cells exist, and these will be discussed with the various types of Hodgkin lymphoma.

The Reed–Sternberg cell of Hodgkin lymphoma needs to be distinguished from other multinucleated cells that may be present in lymph nodes. Megakaryocytes can simulate it closely in hematoxylin–eosin-stained sections, but they can be identified by the presence of a strongly PAS-positive substance in their

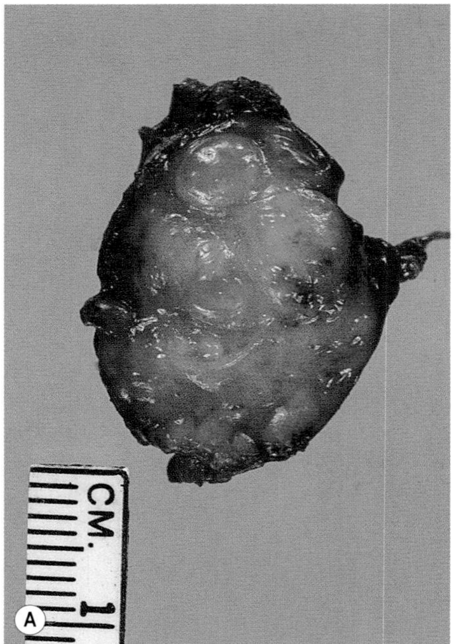

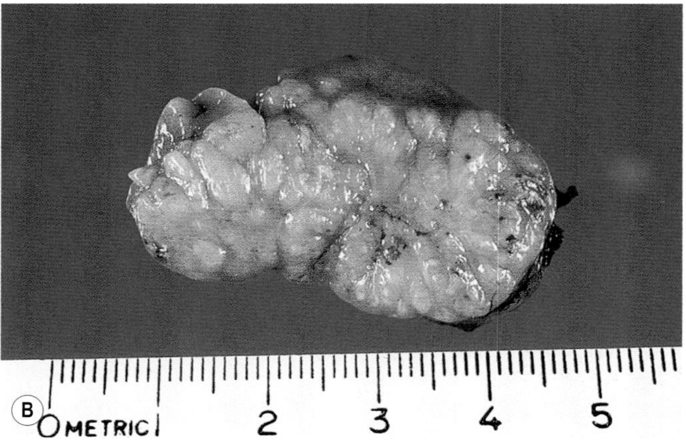

Fig 21.50 Gross appearance of lymph nodes involved by Hodgkin lymphoma. Note nodularity and sclerosis.

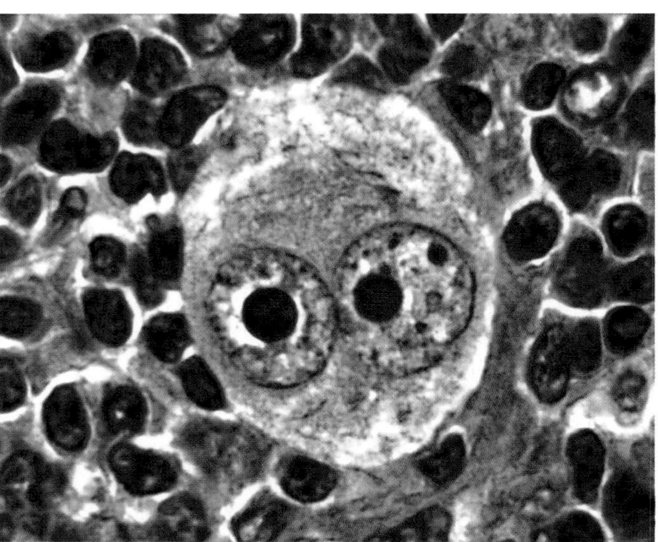

Fig. 21.51 Spectacular example of a Reed–Sternberg cell. *(Courtesy of Dr Fabio Facchetti, Brescia, Italy)*

Table 21.6 Major morphologic differences between the pleomorphic immunoblast (Reed–Sternberg-like cell) of infectious mononucleosis and the Reed–Sternberg cell of Hodgkin lymphoma

FEATURE	IMMUNOBLAST	REED–STERNBERG CELL
Nucleolus		
Staining pattern	Basophilic	Acidophilic
Contours	Irregular	Regular, with clear halo (inclusion-like)
Position	Adjacent to nuclear membrane	More centrally located
Cytoplasm		
Staining pattern	Usually amphophilic	Usually acidophilic
Pyroninophilia	Invariably strong	Variable
Paranuclear hof	Prominent	Inconspicuous
Surrounding cells	Mononuclear immunoblasts and plasmacytoid cells	Lymphocytes and histiocytes

Compiled from data in Dorfman RF, Warnke R. Lymphadenopathy simulating the malignant lymphomas. Hum Pathol 1974, **5:** 519–550.

cytoplasm and their different immunophenotype, which includes positivity for factor VIII-related antigen and CD61. Cells morphologically very similar to Reed–Sternberg cells, representing pleomorphic immunoblasts, can be seen in infectious mononucleosis and other viral diseases.[590] The most important morphologic differences between these two cells are summarized in Table 21.6. Neoplastic cells from a variety of epithelial and mesenchymal tumors also can resemble Reed–Sternberg cells[589] (Fig. 21.53). Finally, some malignant lymphomas of non-Hodgkin type may be accompanied by cells with the appearance of Reed–Sternberg cells, a fact that raises some questions about the very definition of Hodgkin lymphoma and its existence as an entity. In all of these disorders – and especially in the lymphomas – it is of the utmost importance to examine not only the putative Reed–Sternberg cells but also the background in which they are situated. The more cytologically atypical the lymphoid population, the less likely the diagnosis of Hodgkin lymphoma.

The requirement for the presence of classic Reed–Sternberg cells, which is absolute for the initial diagnosis of Hodgkin lymphoma, can be lessened somewhat in subsequent biopsies from patients with documented Hodgkin lymphoma or when the typical immunophenotype can be demonstrated. Under these circumstances, the presence of a polymorphic infiltrate *with atypical mononuclear cells* but not classic Reed–Sternberg cells in a biopsy of bone marrow, liver, or some other organ can be taken as evidence of involvement by Hodgkin lymphoma; however, a note of caution should be

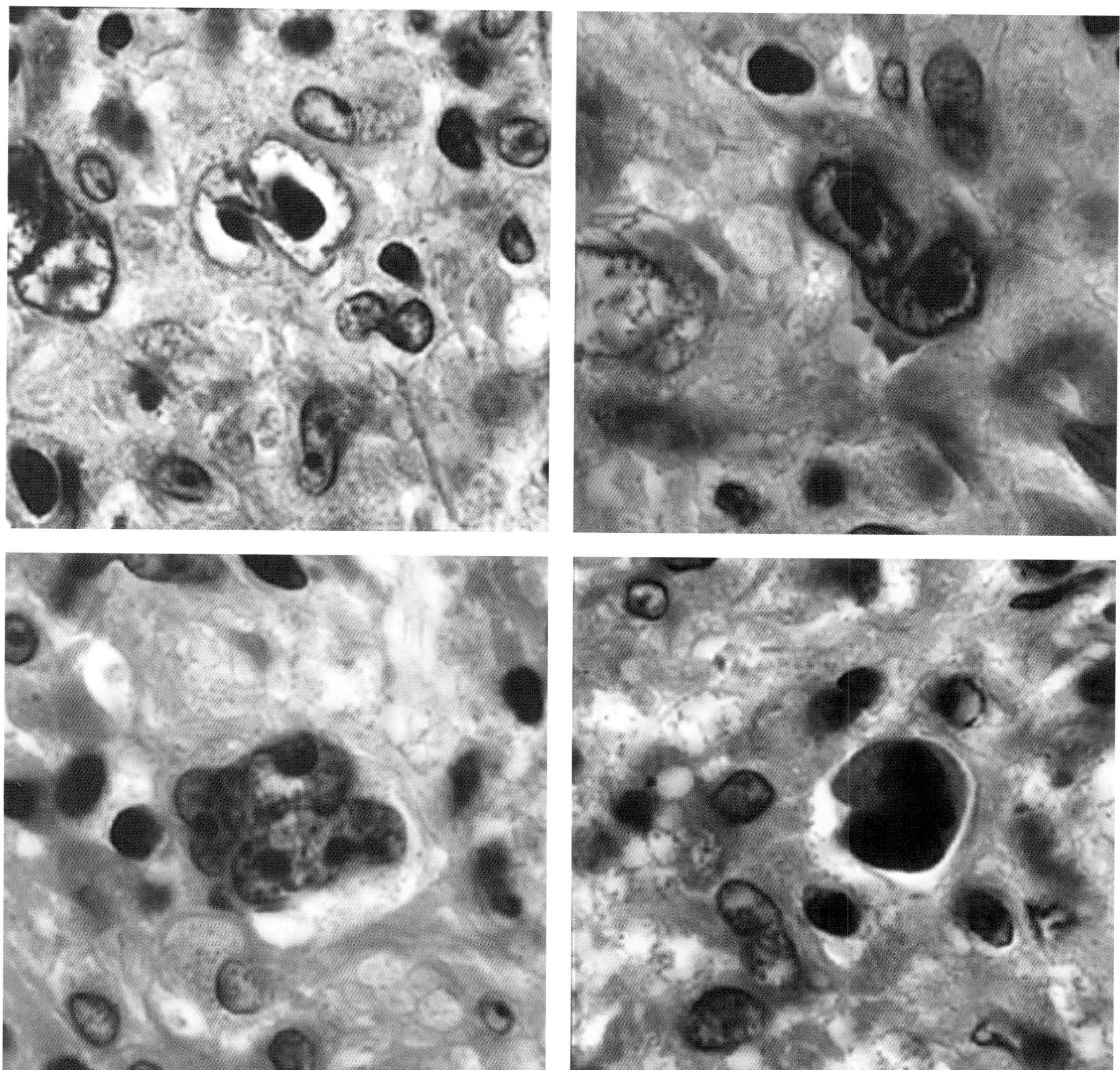

Fig. 21.52 Various appearances of Reed–Sternberg cells. The cell located at the bottom right has a 'mummified' appearance.

interjected. Atypical large lymphoid cells *need* to be present; an infiltrate of eosinophils, lymphocytes, and plasma cells or a collection of epithelioid granulomas is not enough.

The nature of the Reed–Sternberg cell has been one of the most controversial issues in pathology. Practically all the cells present in the normal node (and even some that are not) have been proposed at one time or another as possible progenitors, including B cells, T cells, histiocytes, follicular dendritic cells, and interdigitating dendritic cells, but current evidence indicates that most if not all cases of Hodgkin lymphoma represent neoplasms of B cells (functional B cells for NLPHL, and 'crippled' B cells for classic Hodgkin lymphoma).[570]

The immunocytochemical profile of the Reed–Sternberg cell in classic Hodgkin lymphoma is yet to be totally agreed upon because of the discrepancies among the various laboratories, which may be due to technical factors or to the heterogeneity of the disease, which sometimes manifests itself in sequential biopsies of the same case.[591,593] The most important results in paraffin-embedded material are the following:[551,553–555,557,559,562,564,567,571,581,586,587,596]

- CD15 (Leu-M1): This is expressed in over 80% of the cases; the pattern may be paranuclear (corresponding to the Golgi region), diffuse cytoplasmic, and/or related to the cell membrane.

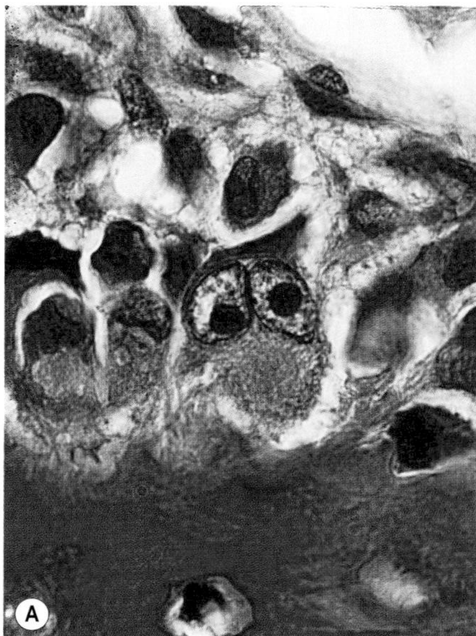

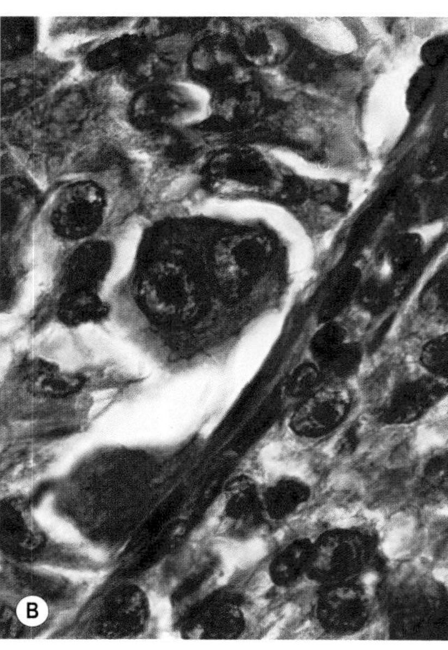

Fig. 21.53 Reed–Sternberg-like cells in malignant melanoma (**A**), and osteoblastoma (**B**).

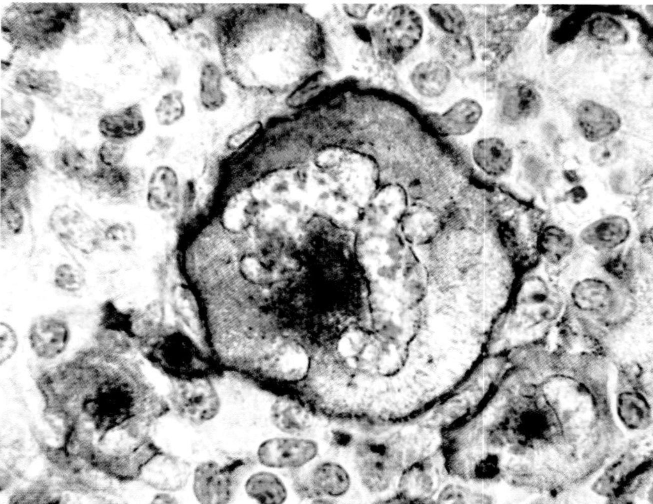

Fig. 21.54 Membrane and Golgi-type immunoreactivity for CD30 in a Reed–Sternberg cell.
(Courtesy of Dr Fabio Facchetti, Brescia, Italy)

- CD30 (Ki-1): As recognized by the monoclonal antibody Ber-H2, this is found in over 90% of the cases (Fig. 21.54).
- CD45 (LCA): This is expressed in less than 10% of the cases.
- CD45RO and CD43 (T-lineage-related antigens): These are expressed in less than 10% of the cases.
- CD20 (L26, B-lineage antigen): This is expressed in 10–20% of the cases, usually in a heterogeneous pattern, i.e. only a fraction of Reed–Sternberg cells are positive and stain with variable intensities.
- PAX5, a B-cell transcription factor, is positive in most cases, supporting the B-lineage of Reed–Sternberg cells. However, the intensity of staining is often weak to moderate compared with normal B cells. This marker is of great help for distinguishing classic Hodgkin lymphoma from anaplastic large cell lymphoma (PAX5 negative).
- CD40 (a protein present in B cells and nerve growth factor receptor): This is expressed in approximately 70%.
- CD74: This is expressed in over 75%.
- Fascin: This is an actin-bundling protein which is normally expressed by dendritic cells.[561,584] This unexpected observation, coupled with the report of a subset of cases of Hodgkin lymphoma in which the Reed–Sternberg cells stained for CD21 (another dendritic follicular cell marker) but not for any B-cell marker, is intriguing and not exactly in line with the prevailing hypothesis about the nature of these cells.[578]
- Restin (an intermediate filament-associated protein): This is present in approximately 80%. The same is true for anaplastic large cell lymphoma but not for other types of non-Hodgkin lymphoma.[559]
- Peanut agglutinin and *Bauhinia purpurea* lectins: They are expressed in over 60% of the cases, in contrast to their near universal absence in non-Hodgkin lymphoma.
- Others, such as CD95 (a member of the superfamily that includes the nerve growth factor and tumor necrosis factors receptors, TNFRs) and its ligand,[579,585] the factor associated to TNFRs,[568] Fas ligand,[592] granzyme B (a serine protease expressed by activated cytotoxic T cells and NK cells),[582] and TARC (a lymphocyte-directed CC chemokine that attracts activated T-helper type 2 cells).[583]

In frozen sections, a large percentage of Reed–Sternberg cells have been found to exhibit reactivity for one or more pan–T cell or pan–B cell antigens, including the framework antigen of the T-cell receptor β chain. They also express polyclonal IgG (probably representing passive uptake via the Fc receptor), HLA-DR, CD25 (the interleukin-2 receptor), and CD71 (the transferrin receptor).[551]

Molecular studies have also given rise to controversial results. Most cases of Hodgkin lymphoma yield a germline configuration for immunoglobulin heavy and light chain genes and the β T-cell receptor genes, but this simply results from a dilution factor by the non-neoplastic cells; indeed, some studies suggest that an increased number of Reed–Sternberg cells and their variants is associated with a detectable increase in clonal rearrangements of either gene.[558,563,572,575,595] In a remarkable experiment, Reed–Sternberg cells were isolated from 12 cases of 'classic' Hodgkin lymphoma (see next section) and found to have rearranged immunoglobulin variable-region heavy-chain (V_H) genes, indicating their origin from B cells. In half of the cases the population of Reed–Sternberg cells was polyclonal, and in the other half it was monoclonal or mixed.[566] Several other workers have provided additional evidence in favor of the interpretation that Reed–Sternberg cells derive from mature B cells at the germinal center stage of differentiation,[552,569,576,577] although some discordant hard-to-explain findings persist.[561,565]

In contrast with anaplastic large cell lymphoma, there is no t(2;5) translocation.[594]

Another controversial issue is the prevalence of t(14;18) in Hodgkin lymphoma, the reported figures ranging from zero to over 30%; perhaps of significance in this regard is the fact that the BCL2 protein (a hallmark of the 14;18 translocation) is never overexpressed, except in those exceptional instances of Hodgkin lymphoma that arise in the setting of follicular lymphoma.[573,574,580,588]

Overexpression of the P53 product as detected immunohistochemically is common in Hodgkin lymphoma, but it does not correlate with gene mutations, which are rare.[556,560]

Microscopic types

For many years, Jackson and Parker's classification of Hodgkin lymphoma into granuloma, paragranuloma, and sarcoma variants[598] was widely used because of its reproducibility and clearcut prognostic implications, the major objection being that too many of the cases (approximately 80%) fell into one of the categories – i.e., Hodgkin granuloma. The concept of a sclerosing type of Hodgkin lymphoma associated with a very good prognosis was first introduced by Smetana and Cohen in 1956[604] and incorporated into a new classification proposed by Lukes et al.[600,601] In this scheme, six categories were included: lymphocytic and/or histiocytic (L&H) nodular, L&H diffuse, nodular sclerosis, mixed cellularity, diffuse fibrosis, and reticular. This classification, somewhat simplified and with some changes in nomenclature (not always for the better), was adopted by the Nomenclature Committee at the Rye Conference on Hodgkin lymphoma.[601] This classification recognized four major types of Hodgkin lymphoma: nodular sclerosis, lymphocyte predominance, lymphocyte depletion, and mixed cellularity. In the REAL/WHO scheme currently in use there has been a further reshuffling of the types into two major categories: the nodular subtype of lymphocyte predominant and the classic, the latter incorporating all other types of the Rye classification.[597,602,603,605] The relationships between these classifications is shown in Table 21.7.

Nodular lymphocyte predominant Hodgkin lymphoma

In **nodular lymphocyte predominant** Hodgkin lymphoma (NLPHL), the predominant cell is a small B lymphocyte, with or without an accompanying population of benign-appearing histiocytes.[627,634] Postcapillary venules with high endothelium may be prominent.[619,631] The lymph node architecture is partially or totally effaced, and the infiltrate has a variously well-developed nodular pattern of growth.[626] The nodularity may be so pronounced as to simulate on low power the appearance of follicular lymphoma; however, the nodules of NLPHL are more irregular in size and staining quality, and the admixture of lymphocytes and epithelioid cells gives them a mottled appearance (Fig. 21.55). A rim of uninvolved or hyperplastic lymphoid tissue may be present. Progressively transformed germinal centers may be seen adjacent to the lesion.[613] Eosinophils, plasma cells, and foci of fibrosis are scanty or absent. Classic Reed–Sternberg cells are absent. One sees instead a variable but usually large number of a type of Reed–Sternberg cell (the L&H cell, LP cell, or 'popcorn' cell) characterized by a folded, multilobed nucleus with smaller nucleoli. These cells are most commonly found within the nodules. If numerous typical Reed–Sternberg cells are found in a node with a lymphocyte predominant background, the case probably belongs in the classic category (lymphocyte-rich subtype). Occasionally, the L&H cells predominate at the margins of the nodules, creating a 'wreath' around them. In others, they may cluster in large confluent sheets resembling diffuse large cell lymphoma.[612]

Poppema et al.[623–625] first proposed that cases of NLPHL (the L&H nodular type of the classification of Lukes et al.[616]) arise from B-cell regions of the node and specifically from progressively transformed germinal centers (see p. 1781). They supported their theory by showing that the L&H cell that is characteristic of this condition is of B-cell lineage, and this has been confirmed by many others.[608–610,615,620,621,625,628,635] L&H cells express the pan-B-cell markers CD19, CD20, CD22, PAX5, CD74, CDw75, and CD45RA (Table 21.8). They are also positive for CD45RB (LCA) but consistently negative for T-cell markers. They commonly express EMA, and generally lack CD30 and CD15 expression. J chain, a protein associated with immunoglobulin synthesis, has been found in these cells, and immunoglobulin heavy or light chains can sometimes be demonstrated.[629,630] Conclusive evidence that NLPHL is a κ light chain-restricted monotypic B-cell neoplasm arising from germinal center cells at the centroblastic stage of differentiation is now

Table 21.7 Comparison between the different classifications of Hodgkin lymphoma proposed over the years

JACKSON AND PARKER (1947)[598]	SMETANA AND COHEN'S ADDITION (1956)[604]	LUKES (1963)[599]	RYE CONFERENCE (1966)[601]	REAL/WHO (2001/2008)[756,769]
Paragranuloma	Paragranuloma	Lymphocytic and histiocytic, nodular Lymphocytic and histiocytic, diffuse	Lymphocyte predominant	Nodular lymphocyte predominant Classic, lymphocyte-rich subtype
Granuloma	Granuloma	Mixed cellularity	Mixed cellularity	Classic, mixed cellularity subtype
	Nodular sclerosis	Nodular sclerosis	Nodular sclerosis	Classic, nodular sclerosis subtype
Sarcoma	Sarcoma	Diffuse fibrosis Reticular	Lymphocyte depletion	Classic, lymphocyte depletion subtype

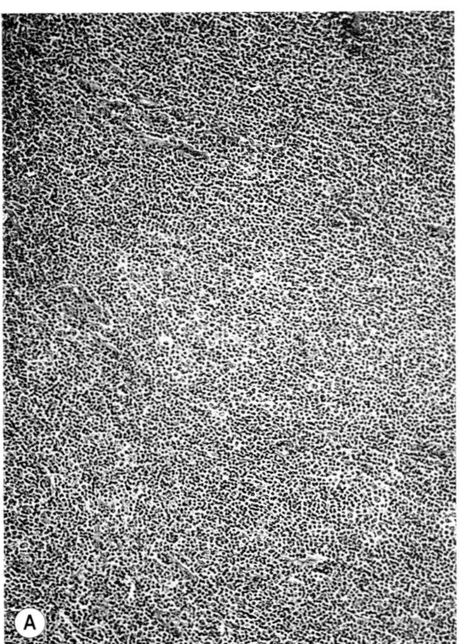
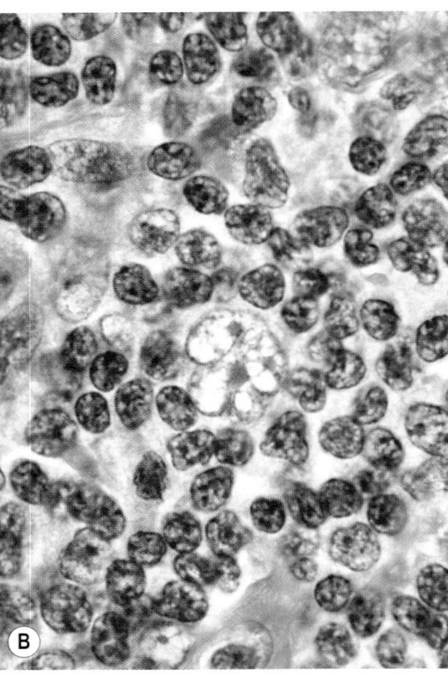

Fig. 21.55 A and **B**, Lymphocyte predominant Hodgkin lymphoma. **A**, Low-power view showing a mottled appearance of the node. **B**, High-power view showing the lymphocytic and/or histiocytic (L&H) type of cell ('popcorn' cell) that is characteristic of this condition.

available.[606,607,617,620,632] The neoplastic cells commonly occur within nodules of small B cells (CD20+); furthermore, the individual neoplastic cells are typically rosetted by T cells which express CD3, BCL6, and CD57.

NLPHL should be sharply separated (also on epidemiologic and clinical grounds) from all other forms of Hodgkin lymphoma (herein designated as classic), even if occasionally the two are seen to coexist.[614,618] Parenthetically, cases have also been described of NLPHL coexisting with T-cell lymphoma.[611]

Further proof of the B-cell nature of this malignancy is derived from the fact that when it undergoes tumor progression in the form of a large B-cell lymphoma, the tumor cells have been found to be clonally related.[622]

The differential diagnosis between NLPHL and T-cell-rich B-cell lymphoma, which is fraught with notable practical and conceptual difficulties, is discussed on page 1837.

As for the Lukes and Collins *diffuse* L&H type of Hodgkin lymphoma (which was part of lymphocyte predominant Hodgkin lymphoma in the Rye classification), it is probable that some cases are examples of NLPHL in which the nodularity is minimal or absent, and that others are examples of the lymphocyte-rich subtype of classic Hodgkin lymphoma.

Classic Hodgkin lymphoma

This category, which subsumes all types of Hodgkin lymphoma except for NLPHL, is regarded as a nosologic entity because of the similar immunophenotype of the tumor cells. The differences consist in sites of involvement, clinical features, growth pattern, presence of fibrosis, composition of cellular background, number and degree of atypia of the tumor cells, and prevalence of EBV infection. These subtypes are nodular sclerosis, mixed cellularity, lymphocyte rich, and lymphocyte depletion.

Nodular sclerosis Hodgkin lymphoma is characterized in its fully developed stage by broad collagen bands separating the lymphoid tissue in well-defined nodules (Fig. 21.56). These fibrous bands, which have a birefringent quality when examined under polarized light, often center around blood vessels. In addition to

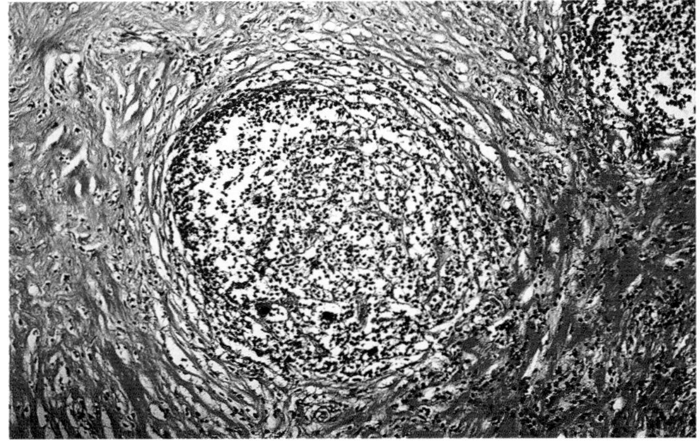

Fig. 21.56 A well-developed case of nodular sclerosis Hodgkin lymphoma. The lymphoid nodule is encased in dense fibrohyaline tissue.

the classic Reed–Sternberg cell, nodular sclerosis Hodgkin lymphoma also displays a variant known as *lacunar* or *cytoplasmic* (Fig. 21.57). This cell type is quite large (40–50 µm in diameter), with an abundant clear cytoplasm and multilobulated nuclei having complicated infoldings and nucleoli of smaller size than those of the classic Reed–Sternberg cell. The 'frail' cytoplasm of these cells is retracted close to the nuclear membrane so that the cell appears to be floating in a 'lacuna'. This is the result of an artifact induced by formalin fixation, inasmuch as it is absent in tissues fixed in B5 or Zenker. In some cases, there is clustering of these lacunar cells, particularly around areas of necrosis. They form sheets and cohesive nests, to the point that a mistaken diagnosis of large cell non-Hodgkin lymphoma, carcinoma, germ cell tumor, or thymoma can be made. Cases of nodular sclerosis Hodgkin lymphoma showing prominence of this feature have been referred to as the *syncytial*, *sarcomatoid*, or *sarcomatous* variant.[647]

Table 21.8 Summary of various types of lymphoma with a diffuse mixed cell population

TYPE	LINEAGE	CLINICAL FEATURES	HISTOLOGIC FEATURES	IMMUNOHISTOCHEMICAL FEATURES	BEHAVIOR
Diffuse follicular lymphoma (diffuse centroblastic–centrocytic)	B	Adults, usually presenting with lymphadenopathy; may have known history of follicular lymphoma or arising *de novo*; disease often at high stage at presentation; extranodal involvement is common	Small cells with angulated (cleaved) or elongated nuclei, fairly condensed chromatin, and scanty cytoplasm; large cells with round or folded nuclei, vesicular chromatin, and multiple distinct nucleoli; neoplastic follicles should be absent; sclerosis common	Pan–B+; CD5-; CD10±; BCL+; may have irregular loose meshworks of follicular dendritic cells	No reliable data in literature on its behavior; some studies suggest that it is low-grade neoplasm, but prognosis is less favorable than for follicular lymphoma
Peripheral T-cell lymphoma	T	Usually adults; nodal or extranodal presentation; disease often at high stage at presentation	Prominent high endothelial venules; continuous spectrum of small, medium-sized, and large lymphoid cells; nuclear irregularities, chromatin pattern often granular; clear cytoplasm commonly seen in some cells; may show rich component of inflammatory cells (such as eosinophils, histiocytes, and epithelioid cells)	Pan–T+ (often with loss of one or more pan–T antigens; usually CD4+, sometimes CD8+, CD4+/CD8+, or CD4–/CD8–)	Generally aggressive neoplasm
Lymphoplasmacytic lymphoma with increased blasts (polymorphic subtype)	B	Usually older adults; nodal or extranodal presentation; may have monoclonal gammopathy (20–40%); disease often disseminated at presentation; occasional cases may have circulating lymphoma cells	Small lymphocytes; lymphoplasmacytoid cells; plasma cells; immunoblasts; rare follicular center cells; Dutcher bodies (nuclear pseudoinclusions of immunoglobulin) may be found; specific lymphoma types should be excluded (e.g., follicular lymphoma, low-grade B-cell lymphoma of MALT)	Pan B+; CD5–; CD10–; CD23–; sIg+, cIg+ (usually IgM type)	Low-grade neoplasm, but prognosis is worse than that of B-SLL/CLL; median survival 55 months; may rarely transform to diffuse large cell lymphoma
T-cell/histiocyte-rich large B-cell lymphoma	B	Older adults, usually presenting with lymphadenopathy; disease often disseminated at presentation	Small lymphocytes with round or irregular nuclei; scattered atypical large cells with round to folded nuclei, distinct nucleoli, and amphophilic cytoplasm; may show rich vascularity and component of inflammatory cells	Large atypical cells: pan–B+; small cells: pan–T+	Aggressive neoplasm; prognosis similar to or worse than conventional diffuse large cell lymphoma
Extranodal marginal zone lymphoma of mucosa-associated lymphoid tissue (MALT)	B	Any age; tumor often localized to mucosal site and/or regional lymph nodes at presentation	Small lymphoid cells with round or irregular nuclei and pale to clear cytoplasm; scattered large blast cells with vesicular nuclei and distinct nucleoli; glandular invasion (lymphoepithelial lesions) common; plasma cells common	Pan–B+; CD5–; CD10–; CD23–	Low-grade neoplasm, with median survival of 8 years; may show late relapse locally or in other mucosal sites; may transform to diffuse large cell lymphoma

CLL, chronic lymphocytic leukemia; MALT, mucosa-associated lymphoid tissue; SLL, small lymphocytic lymphoma.
Modified from Warnke RA, Weiss LM, Chan JKC, Cleary ML, Dorfman RF. Tumors of the lymph nodes and spleen. Atlas of tumor pathology, series 3, fascicle 14. Washington, DC, 1995, Armed Forces Institute of Pathology.

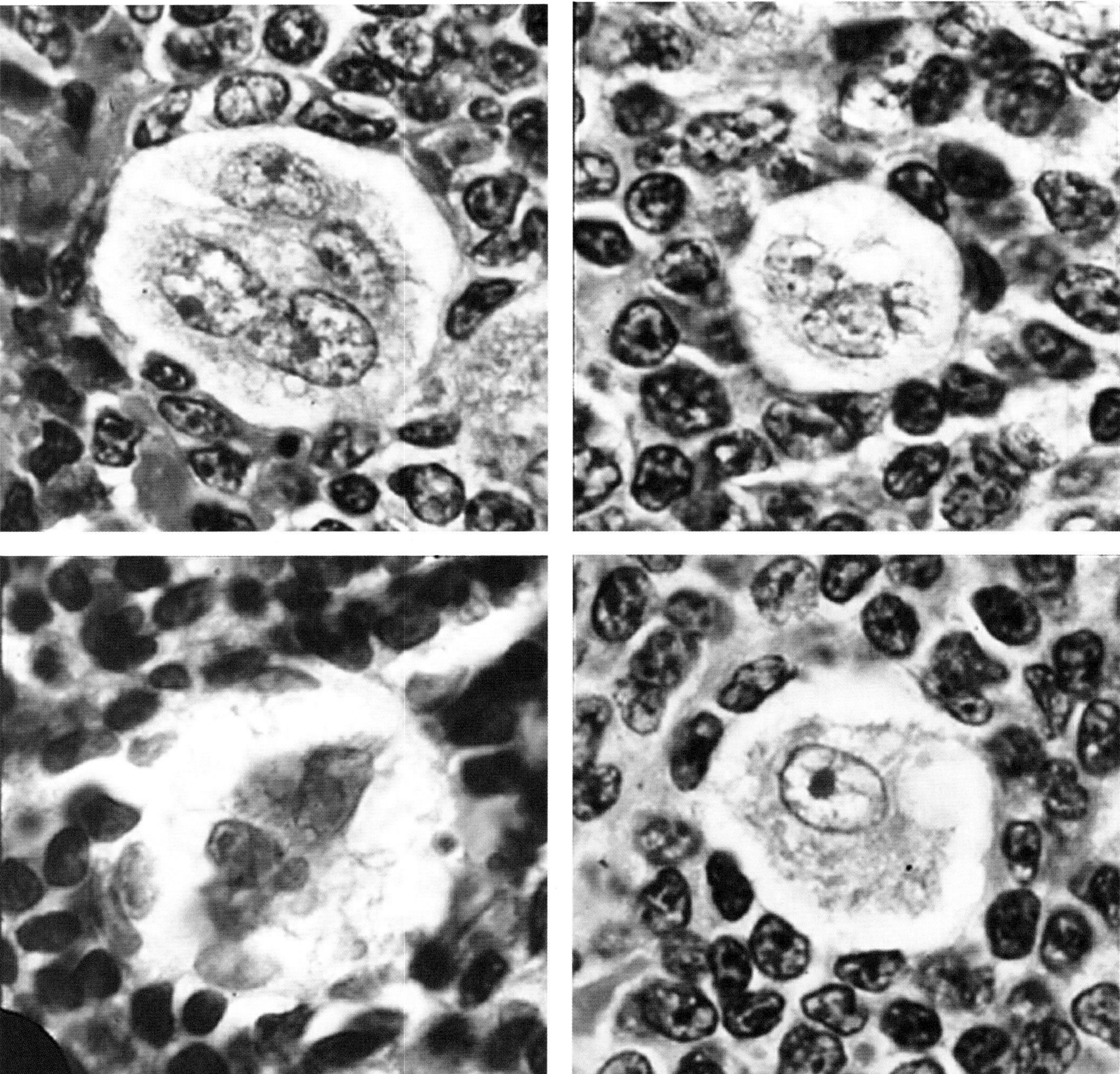

Fig. 21.57 Various appearances of lacunar cells in nodular sclerosis Hodgkin lymphoma.

Some workers regard the lacunar variant of Reed–Sternberg cells as more typical of this type of Hodgkin lymphoma than the fibrosis itself and make the diagnosis of nodular sclerosis Hodgkin lymphoma in the presence of lacunar cells even if fibrosis is totally lacking (so-called *cellular phase*)[647] (Fig. 21.58); however, it should be remarked that lacunar cells are not pathognomonic of this condition. They can also be seen in mixed cellularity Hodgkin lymphoma and even in reactive disorders.[644]

The composition of the non-neoplastic infiltrate varies widely, to the point that some authors have proposed to subdivide nodular sclerosis Hodgkin lymphoma into lymphocyte predominant, mixed cellularity, and lymphocyte depletion categories, and have claimed that this subdivision carries some prognostic implications. Along similar lines, the British National Lymphoma Investigation group has proposed to divide cases of nodular sclerosis Hodgkin lymphoma into two grades. In their scheme, cases are assigned to the allegedly more aggressive grade II if any of these features are present: (1) a 'reticular' or 'pleomorphic' pattern of lymphocytic depletion in over 25% of the cellular nodules; (2) a 'fibrohistiocytic' pattern of lymphocyte depletion in over 80% of the cellular nodules; and (3) the presence of numerous bizarre and highly anaplastic Reed–Sternberg and Hodgkin cells without lymphocyte depletion in over

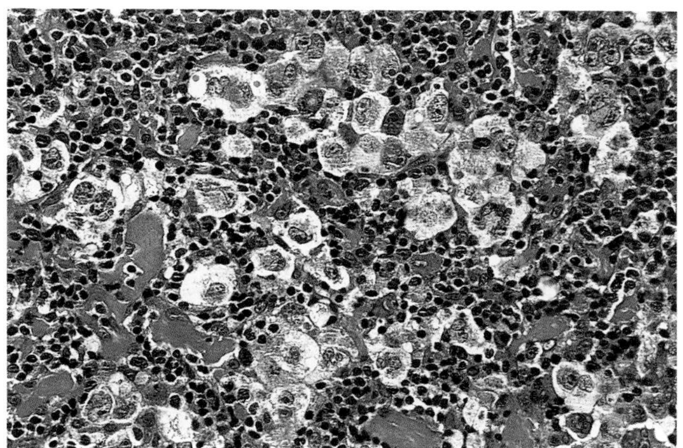

Fig. 21.58 Cellular phase of nodular sclerosis Hodgkin lymphoma. Lacunar cells are plentiful.

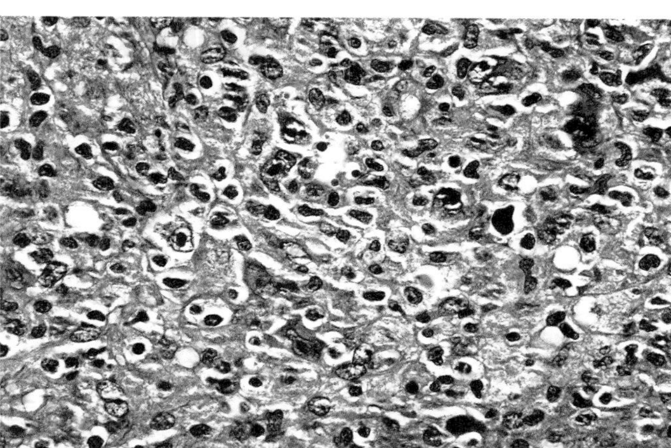

Fig. 21.60 Lymphocyte depletion type of Hodgkin lymphoma. Numerous atypical cells are present in a densely fibrotic stroma. Lymphocytes are scanty.

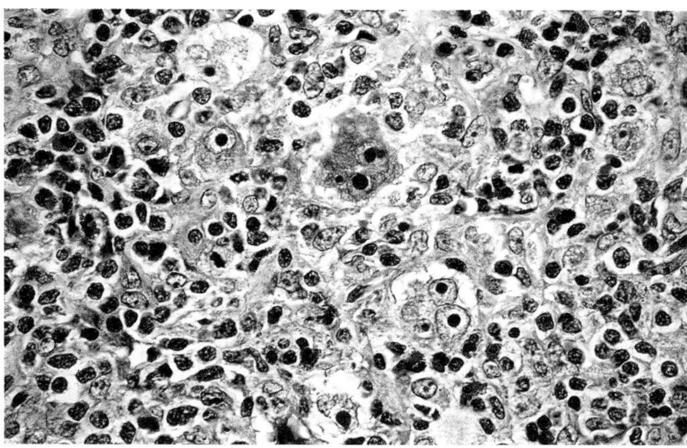

Fig. 21.59 Mixed cellularity Hodgkin lymphoma. Several diagnostic Reed–Sternberg cells are seen admixed with a polymorphic lymphoid infiltrate rich in eosinophils.

25% of the nodules.[643] Grade II lesions include the already mentioned 'syncytial' variant of other authors.

By electron microscopy, nodular sclerosis Hodgkin lymphoma shows abundant collagen fibers together with myofibroblasts;[646] it has been suggested that the latter contribute to the retraction seen in this condition. In regard to the fibrosis, it should be kept in mind that practically all types of Hodgkin lymphoma can exhibit some degree of this change, particularly after therapy. If the pathologist is too liberal in the criteria for diagnosis of the nodular sclerosis variant, the clinical and prognostic connotations associated with it will lose most of their meaning.

In **mixed cellularity** Hodgkin lymphoma, a large number of eosinophils, plasma cells, and atypical mononuclear cells are admixed with classic Reed–Sternberg cells, which tend to be numerous. Focal necrosis may be present, but fibrosis should be minimal or absent (Fig. 21.59). It is somewhat ironic that mixed cellularity Hodgkin lymphoma, which fits more closely the histopathologic picture of the disease as depicted in the classic textbooks, has now almost become a diagnosis of exclusion.

The **lymphocyte-rich** type is characterized by the presence of Reed–Sternberg cells scattered against a nodular (most commonly) or diffuse background, largely composed of small lymphocytes and practically devoid of eosinophils and neutrophils.[645] The main differential diagnosis is with NLPHD, and is primarily based on the presence of cells with the typical morphologic and immunohistochemical features of Reed–Sternberg cells.

The **lymphocyte-depletion** group, which comprises less than 5% of all cases of Hodgkin lymphoma, includes two morphologically different subtypes, designated as 'diffuse fibrosis' and 'reticular' in the original Lukes classification. In the diffuse fibrosis subtype, the number of lymphocytes and other cells progressively decreases as the result of heavy deposition of collagen fibers. The reticular subtype is characterized by a very large number of diagnostic Reed–Sternberg cells (many of them of bizarre configuration) among atypical mononuclear cells and other elements (Fig. 21.60). Areas of necrosis are more common than in other types. The 'reticular' subtype of lymphocyte depletion Hodgkin lymphoma needs to be distinguished from non-Hodgkin lymphoma of large cell type (including the anaplastic CD30+ type) and from the variant of nodular sclerosis Hodgkin lymphoma with aggregates of lacunar cells.[636]

The immunophenotypic profile of the Reed–Sternberg cells in classic Hodgkin lymphoma is described in a preceding section on 'Reed–Sternberg cells'. The background lymphocytes are predominantly T cells.

The histologic subtypes of classic Hodgkin lymphoma remain constant over long follow-up periods in most cases, particularly for the nodular sclerosis form.[648] In patients who had relapses in a site *not included* in the radiation field (and who have not received chemotherapy), the same histologic appearance was often maintained in the relapse biopsies.[638] When change occurs, it usually is toward a histologically more malignant form. It also should be remembered that patients with Hodgkin lymphoma may develop non-Hodgkin lymphoma or leukemia,[639,642] either spontaneously or as a result of therapy. This includes diffuse large B-cell lymphoma[641] and marginal zone B-cell lymphoma. The former includes so-called *mediastinal gray zone lymphoma*, which has been viewed as the pathogenetic missing link between the two diseases.[649]

The microscopic typing of Hodgkin lymphoma should always be made on examination of a biopsy obtained before the institution of treatment. Radiation therapy and chemotherapy result in focal necrosis, fibrosis, and profound nuclear aberrations – features that may render impossible a proper pathologic evaluation. These alterations may be seen in post-therapy biopsy material or at autopsy.[637]

The currently used terminology of Hodgkin lymphoma is far from ideal, in the sense that there is very little relation between the names given and the microscopic picture observed. A case exhibiting lymphocyte predominance or mixed cellularity will be diagnosed as nodular sclerosis if bands of fibrous tissue are present. A case with marked predominance of lymphocytes will be categorized as mixed cellularity if there are numerous Reed–Sternberg cells. In lymphocyte depletion Hodgkin lymphoma, lymphocytes are still the numerically more abundant cells, more so than in the mixed cellularity type.[644]

An interesting alternative approach was tried by Coppleson et al.[640] and consisted of evaluating individually the frequencies of the different cell types. They found that the presence of a large number of lymphocytes was associated with a good prognosis, whereas malignant and mononuclear cells and benign-appearing histiocytes independently influenced the prognosis adversely. Reed–Sternberg cells had no prognostic effect independent of the malignant mononuclear cells, and eosinophils and plasma cells had no prognostic value. However, these authors concluded that the Rye classification of Hodgkin lymphoma (now substituted by the REAL/WHO scheme) furnished more prognostic information than any estimates of individual cell frequencies.

The differential diagnosis between Hodgkin lymphoma and anaplastic large cell lymphoma is discussed on page 1840.

Other microscopic features

There are some microscopic variations on the theme of Hodgkin lymphoma worth mentioning, mainly because lack of knowledge of their occurrence may result in mistaken diagnoses. These mainly apply to classic Hodgkin lymphoma and its subtypes rather than NLPHL.

1 *Foamy macrophages*. Clumps of foamy macrophages resulting in a xanthogranulomatous appearance may be found, particularly in the nodular sclerosis form.[662]
2 *Eosinophils*. In some instances, the intensity of eosinophilic infiltration is massive and accompanied by so-called 'eosinophilic microabscesses'. Such cases may be confused with Langerhans cell histiocytosis, hypersensitivity reaction, or 'allergic granulomatosis'.
3 *Other inflammatory cells*. S-100 protein-positive dendritic cells,[650] mast cells,[652] and monocytoid B cells[656] may be very numerous.
4 *Focal interfollicular involvement*. In the early stages of the disease, only focal involvement of a lymph node may be encountered,[661] often restricted to the paracortical region between florid hyperplastic follicles; this pattern, which has been referred to as *interfollicular Hodgkin lymphoma*, is not regarded as a specific subtype.[653]
5 *Follicular involvement*. Sometimes the nodal involvement by Hodgkin lymphoma is mainly in the germinal centers, the appearance being reminiscent of NLPHL.[655]
6 *Castleman disease-like features*. Cases of Hodgkin lymphoma may be accompanied or preceded by a plasmacytic infiltrate and abnormalities of germinal centers closely resembling those seen in plasma cell type Castleman disease, probably attributable to interleukin-6 secretion by Reed–Sternberg cells (see p. 1796).
7 *Fibrosis*. In cases of nodular sclerosis Hodgkin lymphoma but sometimes also in other types, the amount of fibrosis can be such as to simulate the appearance of one of the inflammatory fibroscleroses (such as sclerosing mediastinitis or retroperitoneal fibrosis).
8 *Spindle cell proliferation*. In rare cases of Hodgkin lymphoma, there is a proliferation of oval to spindle cells of such a degree as to simulate fibrosarcoma, malignant fibrous histiocytoma, or a follicular dendritic cell tumor; such lesions have been referred to as **fibrosarcomatous or fibroblastic Hodgkin lymphoma**. Some of these spindle cells have a degree of nuclear atypia such as to indicate their neoplastic nature and relationship with Reed–Sternberg and Hodgkin cells; indeed, most of these lesions would be included in the grade II category of nodular sclerosis Hodgkin lymphoma proposed by the British National Lymphoma Investigation Group (see p. 1812). Others are of a reactive nature and stromal derivation (i.e., made up of fibroblasts and myofibroblasts).[651]
9 *Noncaseating granulomas*. These formations are sometimes present in nodes and other organs involved by Hodgkin lymphoma. Occasionally they are so numerous as to obscure the diagnostic features of the disease (Fig. 21.61). In other instances, these granulomas may be seen within otherwise uninvolved organs of patients with Hodgkin lymphoma.[654] Their significance is unknown. Perhaps they represent an expression of delayed hypersensitivity. Some seen in the past were reactions to the contrast material used in lymphangiography.[657] Their presence does not indicate involvement of that organ by Hodgkin lymphoma and should therefore not influence the staging criteria. Actually, it has been suggested that, within a given stage, the presence of these granulomas is associated with a better prognosis.[659]
10 *Vascular invasion*. Blood vessel infiltration has been detected microscopically in 6–14% of the cases of Hodgkin lymphoma by the use of elastic tissue stains[660] (Fig. 21.62). This finding is said to be associated with an increased incidence of extranodal organ involvement,[658] but the statement and the very validity of the observation have been questioned.

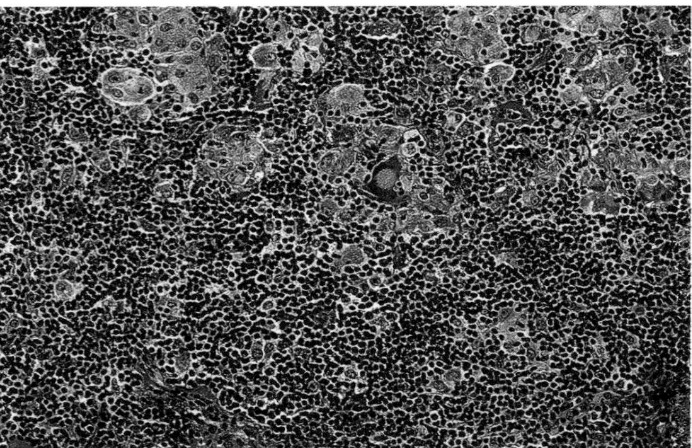

Fig. 21.61 Hodgkin lymphoma accompanied by numerous sarcoid-like granulomas. The presence of this component can obscure the basic nature of the disease.

Molecular genetics

NLPHL

Microdissected neoplastic (L&H/LP) cells exhibit clonal rearrangements of the immunoglobulin genes, which show hypermutation

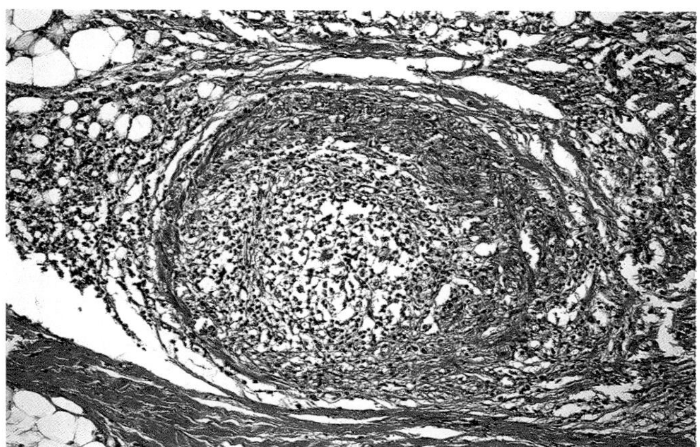

Fig. 21.62 Blood vessel invasion in Hodgkin lymphoma.

and ongoing mutations, compatible with transformed antigen-selected germinal center B cells.[663,664,666,667] The rearranged immunoglobulin genes are functional, and can be transcribed into immunoglobulin mRNA, and further translated to immunoglobulin.[667,669]

Cytogenetic studies reveal complex karyotypes, often in the diploid range, with the commonest abnormalities being gain or partial gain of 1q, loss of chromosome 4q28–q32, and rearrangement involving 3q27 (shown to implicate *BCL6*, which is fused with a variety of partner genes, including the *IGH* gene at 14q32).[668,670,672]

With rare exceptions, NLPHL is not associated with EBV.[665,671]

Classic Hodgkin lymphoma

In almost all cases of classic Hodgkin lymphoma, clonal immunoglobulin gene rearrangements can be demonstrated in microdissected neoplastic (Reed–Sternberg) cells or tissue samples rich in neoplastic cells; only exceptionally are clonal T-cell receptor gene rearrangements present instead.[675,679,684,687] The variable regions of the immunoglobulin genes frequently show hypermutation but not ongoing mutations. Remarkably, immunoglobulin mRNA transcripts are usually absent, which may result from functional defects in immunoglobulin gene regulatory elements or crippling mutations in the immunoglobulin genes.[678,684] That is, the neoplastic cells are compatible with germinal center B cells that have lost the capacity to express a functional antigen receptor, but which differ from their normal counterpart in having been rescued from apoptosis by various mechanisms, such as presence of EBV or aberrant activation of the NFκB pathway.[673,680,681]

Cytogenetic studies of classic Hodgkin lymphoma reveal complex karyotypes, commonly featuring hyperdiploidy or hypertetraploidy.[682,686] Recent FISH studies have shown rearrangements of the immunoglobulin genes in approximately 20% of cases, involving variable partners genes which may include *BCL2*, *BCL3*, *BCL6*, *REL*, *MYC*, and unidentified genes.[685,688]

About 40% of cases of classic Hodgkin lymphoma are associated with EBV, which can be demonstrated by EBV-LMP1 immunohistochemistry or EBV-encoded early RNA (EBER) in-situ hybridization.[676] The association with EBV is stronger at the extremes of age, i.e. children/young adults and elderly adults, and in the mixed cellularity subtype. Of note, the overall frequency of EBV association is much higher in individuals with immunodeficiency (approximately 100%) or from developing countries (80–100%).[674,676,677,683,689]

General and clinical features

Hodgkin lymphoma comprises approximately 20–30% of all malignant lymphomas in the United States and Western Europe but a much lower percentage in Japan and other Oriental countries.[690] There is a wide range in age incidence, which varies according to geographic location. In the United States, there is a bimodal distribution, with a peak at 15–40 years and a second, smaller peak in the seventh decade. In Japan, the peak in young adulthood is absent. In poorly developed countries, there is a high incidence in children, a relatively low incidence in the 15- to 40-year age group, and a third peak later in life.[693,696] There is a male preponderance (approximately 1.5 : 1) in all microscopic types except nodular sclerosis. The disease may present in a variety of ways, the most common (approximately 90% of the cases) being painless enlargement of superficial (usually cervical) lymph nodes. Fever, night sweats, and loss of weight (so-called 'B symptoms') occur in approximately 25% of the cases; their presence influences the clinical staging. Pruritus is also frequent.

Important clinical differences exist related to the microscopic types. The typical patient with NLPHL is a man in his forties with involvement of the high cervical nodes. This microscopic form uncommonly involves the spleen, liver, or bone marrow except when it changes to a more aggressive histologic pattern.[692,698,701]

Nodular sclerosis is by far the most common type of Hodgkin lymphoma in the United States. It characteristically presents in the neck and/or mediastinum of young females.[694]

Lymphocyte depletion Hodgkin lymphoma may present in adults or elderly patients as a febrile illness with pancytopenia or lymphocytopenia, hepatomegaly, abnormal liver function tests, and no peripheral lymphadenopathy,[699] or it may manifest the usual clinical presentation of Hodgkin lymphoma.[695] This form is extremely rare in children, in whom nodular sclerosis and lymphocyte predominance predominate greatly.[700,705]

Mediastinal involvement is the rule in nodular sclerosis, inconstant in mixed cellularity and lymphocyte depletion, and exceptional in NLPHL.[692] The risk of abdominal involvement is greater in patients with B symptoms and in lymphocyte depletion or mixed cellularity types; the lowest risk is for asymptomatic females with nodular sclerosis histology (6%).[703]

The diagnosis of Hodgkin lymphoma should be questioned for any lymphoma involving Waldeyer's ring, the skin, and the gastrointestinal tract, especially if this happens to be the first manifestation of the disease. Most of these cases are examples of non-Hodgkin lymphomas with Reed–Sternberg-like cells.

Patients with Hodgkin lymphoma often have defects in cellular immunity, which leads to an increased susceptibility to some infections.[697] However, a diagnosis of Hodgkin lymphoma should be viewed with suspicion if it presents as a complication of a natural immune deficiency, immunosuppression, or other immune diseases. Although indubitable cases of this association exist (particularly in patients with ataxia–telangiectasia and with HIV infection),[691,704] most of these cases actually represent large cell sarcomas containing binucleated immunoblasts morphologically similar to Reed–Sternberg cells. HIV-associated Hodgkin lymphoma tends to present at a high stage and to run an aggressive clinical course.[702]

Spread

Most cases of Hodgkin lymphoma begin in lymph nodes and spread from there to other lymph node groups and to extranodal sites. Important information has been acquired in regard to the frequency and significance of this spread as a result of an aggressive diagnostic approach, particularly with the use of laparotomy as a routine staging procedure.[707,708]

1 *Direct extension*. The disease may spread to the perinodal tissues, sometimes extensively, and result in a fusion of the involved nodes. In advanced cases, direct invasion of skin, skeletal muscle, and other sites can occur. Mediastinal Hodgkin lymphoma can extend by continuity into the large vessels, lung, and chest wall.[710]
2 *Other lymph node groups*. Most cases of Hodgkin lymphoma spread by involvement of adjacent lymph node groups.[709] This contiguous manner of spread is particularly common in the nodular sclerosis and lymphocyte predominance types.[710] Nodal spread has been evaluated with lymphangiogram, CT scan, and staging laparotomy. When it was carried out with some frequency, lymphangiography had an overall diagnostic accuracy in excess of 90%; it was more effective in detecting involvement below the level of the second lumbar vertebra but inconsistent for nodes situated higher in the periaortic area. Approximately 30% of patients with negative lymphangiograms in whom the para-aortic nodes were left untreated later demonstrated disease below the diaphragm.[706] Of the nodes biopsied at laparotomy during the course of a staging procedure, the most likely to be involved were those located in the splenic hilum and retroperitoneum. Mesenteric nodes are almost always spared.
3 *Spleen*. A spleen weighing 400 g or more is practically always histologically positive. The converse is not true: spleens below this weight are involved in a high proportion of cases. The focal nature of the disease calls for a careful gross examination of this organ. The specimens should be sectioned throughout in thin slices, and every suspicious area should be examined microscopically. If no nodules are detected on gross inspection, the chances of finding Hodgkin lymphoma in random microscopic sections are negligible. Splenic involvement is thought to represent a critical stage in the spread of Hodgkin lymphoma and is an early manifestation of blood vessel dissemination. The approximate number of tumor nodules present in the spleen should be indicated because of their relation to prognosis; specifically, it should be stated whether there are five or more. It is not important to subclassify the disease in the spleen into the specific type.
4 *Liver*. Hepatic disease is almost invariably associated with splenic and retroperitoneal lymph node involvement and with so-called 'B symptoms'. Clinical assessment of liver involvement is quite unreliable. Care should be exercised in distinguishing involvement by Hodgkin lymphoma from benign lymphoid aggregates, some of which may show mild atypia.[711]
5 *Bone marrow*. This is discussed in Chapter 23.
6 *Others*. Practically any other organ can show secondary involvement by Hodgkin lymphoma, such as the lung, skin, gastrointestinal tract, and central nervous system (see respective chapters).

Staging

The current staging classification for Hodgkin lymphoma was established by the Ann Arbor Workshop in 1971 and modified at Cotswolds in 1989[712,714,715] (Box 21.2). Clinical staging refers to all procedures short of laparotomy. It includes physical examination, bone marrow aspiration and biopsy, clinical laboratory evaluation, and numerous radiographic studies. Chest x-ray and thoracic and abdominal CT studies have become the norm, and these are supplemented in some centers by bipedal lymphangiogram and gallium scans. Pathologic staging used to refer to the findings at staging laparotomy during which liver, splenectomy, and biopsies of retroperitoneal lymph nodes, liver, and bone marrow were performed. Although much important information has been obtained from the performance of routine staging laparotomy in patients with Hodgkin lymphoma, the procedure is now used only sparingly, the reasons being the increased diagnostic power of radiographic techniques, the high efficiency of current therapies, and the occurrence of postsurgical complications, particularly in the pediatric population.[713,714]

Box 21.2 Ann Arbor staging classification for Hodgkin lymphoma[a] (as modified at Costwolds)

Stage I

Involvement of a single lymph node region (I) or a single extralymphatic organ or site (Ig)

Stage II

Involvement of two or more lymph node regions on the same side of the diaphragm (II) or localized involvement of an extralymphatic organ or site (IIg)

Stage III

Involvement of lymph node regions on both sides of the diaphragm (III) or localized involvement of an extralymphatic organ or site (IIIg) or spleen (IIIg) or both (IIIse)

Stage IV

Diffuse or disseminated involvement of one or more extralymphatic organs with or without associated lymph node involvement. The organ(s) involved should be identified by a symbol[b]

[a]See also Appendix C.
[b]A, Asymptomatic; B, fever >38°C previous month, sweats previous month, weight loss >10% of body weight previous 6 months; X, bulk (>10 cm for lymph node, >1/3 of internal transverse diameter of thorax at >5/6 on a posteroanterior chest radiograph).
From Warnke RA, Weiss LM, Chan JKC, Cleary ML, Dorfman RF. Tumors of the lymph nodes and spleen. Atlas of tumor pathology, series 3, fascicle 14. Washington, DC, 1995, Armed Forces Institute of Pathology.

Treatment

The treatment of patients with early-stage Hodgkin lymphoma is one of the success stories of modern oncology.[717] The two pillars of therapy are radiation therapy and chemotherapy, the choice being largely dependent on the stage of the disease and the bias of the individual centers.[720,721,723] Increasingly, chemotherapy is adopted as the mainstay of treatment. Bone marrow transplantation is used in selected cases.[716,719]

Successful therapy results in disappearance of the tumor foci, some of which are still detectable on post-therapy biopsy or at autopsy as fibrous nodules.[718] Sometimes Hodgkin lymphoma persists for a long time following therapy, even if it has been controlled on clinical grounds. Of 19 autopsied patients who died after having survived Hodgkin lymphoma for 10 years or more, Strum and Rappaport[722] found residual disease in 16.

Patients treated for Hodgkin lymphoma (particularly those in the pediatric age group) are at an increased risk for the development of a second tumor, including breast carcinoma, soft tissue sarcoma, and malignant mesothelioma.[724,725]

Prognosis

The current overall 5-year survival rate of Hodgkin lymphoma is over 75%.

Many clinical and morphologic parameters have been found to correlate with prognosis.[741] These parameters follow, but only after making the proviso that the spectacular advances in the therapy of this disease have blurred the differences, to the point that most of them are no longer significant.

1 *Clinical stage*. This remains by far the most important prognostic parameter, although the differences between the various stages have greatly diminished. Only stage IV disease and constitutional symptoms continue to present serious therapeutic problems.[736]
2 *Age*. Patients over 50 years of age have a worsened prognosis.[733]
3 *Sex and race*. In some series, males and blacks with nodular sclerosis disease have had a less favorable course than females and whites, respectively.
4 *Pregnancy*. This appears to have no effect on the course of the disease.
5 *Location, number, and size of tumor masses*. A large mediastinal mass (greater than one-third of the maximum intrathoracic diameter), multiple nodules in the spleen, or multiple extranodal sites of involvement are unfavorable prognostic factors. The latter feature relates directly to the staging and is of great prognostic import.[742] There is, however, a substantial difference depending on whether the involvement is at a distance ('metastatic') or whether it represents spread in contiguity from a nodal site. For instance, direct extension from mediastinal nodes of lung or chest wall in nodular sclerosis Hodgkin lymphoma does not result in an appreciable decrease in survival.[737]
6 *Laboratory findings*. Decreased hematocrit, elevated levels of lactate dehydrogenase, increased erythrocyte sedimentation rate, increased β_2-microglobulin, and elevated serum levels of CD30 and soluble CD25 have all been claimed to have a negative impact on survival in high-stage patients.[732,735,738]
7 *Microscopic types*. Traditionally, NLPHL and nodular sclerosis have been the most favorable forms, mixed cellularity has been intermediate, and the lymphocyte depletion form has had the worst prognosis.[729,730] The long-term prognosis of NLPHL is so good that some authors have referred to it as 'the benign form' of Hodgkin lymphoma, and have even doubted that it represents a neoplastic process.[745] It should be said that this favorable prognosis is shared by the lymphocyte-rich form of classic Hodgkin lymphoma.[731] A stark contrast is offered by lymphocyte depletion Hodgkin lymphoma; in the series of Bearman et al.,[728] the median survival was 25.1 months, with only eight (21%) patients surviving 4 years or longer. In general, no prognostic differences have been found between the subtypes of nodular sclerosis or lymphocyte depletion;[743] however, the suggestion has been made that nodular sclerosis cases belonging to what in the UK are called grade II lesions (which include the so-called 'syncytial variant' of other authors) are somewhat more aggressive[734] (see p. 1814).

   It has been pointed out that at least some of the prognostic significance of the various microscopic types depends on the clinical stage, in view of the fact that a definite correlation between the two exists. Thus most NLPHL and nodular sclerosis cases are in stages I and II, whereas most lymphocyte depletion cases are in stages III and IV; however, until relatively recently the prognostic differences among microscopic types were maintained even within staging groups.[737] This is no longer the case. At present, only lymphocyte depletion histology carries an unfavorable significance, and in some series even this difference has been erased.[740]
8 *Noncaseating granulomas*. The presence of these formations may be associated with a slightly better prognosis within a given stage.[739]
9 *Follicular dendritic cells*. Cases with an extensive network of these cells in a follicle-like distribution are said to have a better prognosis than the others.[726,727]
10 *Epstein–Barr virus*. No differences in survival have been found between EBV-positive and EBV-negative cases.
11 *CD15*. It has been claimed that lack of expression of CD15 in cases of classic Hodgkin lymphoma is an independent negative prognostic factor for relapses.[744]

Non-Hodgkin lymphoma

The classification of non-Hodgkin lymphoma that was most widely used until the early 1980s in the United States and many other countries was that proposed by Rappaport in 1966[766] (Table 21.9). This represented a slight modification of the classification that Gall and Rappaport had presented at a seminar of the American Society of Clinical Pathologists held in New Orleans, Louisiana, in 1963. This, in turn, was based on the classification proposed by Gall and Mallory[753] as part of their comprehensive critical study of 618 lymphomas. Rappaport's classification was, of necessity, based entirely on morphologic grounds. Numerous independent clinicopathologic studies have shown its reproducibility, usefulness, and clinical relevance.[747] However, application of the remarkable advances in the fields of immunology, cytogenetics, and molecular pathology in the past 40 years to the study of lymphomas has shown that these can be viewed as clonal expansions of the normal anatomic and functional components of the immune system. Most of them have been studied using immunologic and molecular genetic markers and, as a result, have been 'typed' as to their normal counterparts, from which presumably they arose. This 'functional' approach, championed by Lukes[746,761] in the United States and by Lennert in Germany,[758] incorporated a number of entities and showed that a functional classification of lymphoma was possible to some extent on the basis of morphologic interpretation of routinely stained sections[759,760] (Table 21.9). Independent of this, aggressive clinical investigations coupled with staging laparotomies provided a wealth of new information on the sites of predilection and spread of the lymphomas according to type.[751,754,767] The results obtained with these investigations pointed to some inaccuracies and other deficiencies of Rappaport's classification and the need to revise it, taking into account all these new data.

Five new classifications were proposed,[750,758,762,763] which, needless to say, resulted in a confusing state of affairs for both pathologists and clinicians.

Because there was no clearcut evidence that one classification was significantly superior to the others, the National Cancer Institute sponsored a retrospective study of 1175 cases of non-Hodgkin lymphoma, which were classified according to the different categories by the investigators who proposed them, as well as by a panel of 'control' pathologists.[764,765] Analysis of the data showed that all six classifications were successful in predicting the prognosis in a large number of lymphoma patients and that no classification appeared clearly superior to any other in this respect.[764] It also confirmed that lymphomas with a follicular pattern of growth (a feature consistently identified by all reviewers) had a more favorable prognosis than those with diffuse patterns within the same cytologic subtypes. This was true whether the nodularity was extensive or only partial.

Table 21.9 Major historic classification schemes of non-Hodgkin lymphoma

RAPPAPORT	LUKES AND COLLINS	KIEL
Nodular	Undefined cell type	Low-grade malignancy
Lymphocytic, well differentiated	T-cell type	Lymphocytic
Lymphocytic, poorly differentiated	Small lymphocytic	Chronic lymphocytic leukemia
Mixed (lymphocytic and histiocytic)	Sézary-mycosis fungoides (cerebriform)	Other
Histiocytic	Convoluted lymphocytic	Lymphoplasmacytoid
Diffuse	Immunoblastic sarcoma (T-cell)	Centrocytic
Lymphocytic, well differentiated	Small lymphocytic	Centroblastic-centrocytic
Without plasmacytoid features	B-cell type	Follicular, without sclerosis
With plasmacytoid features	Small lymphocytic	Follicular, with sclerosis
Lymphocytic, poorly differentiated	Plasmacytoid lymphocytic	Follicular and diffuse, without sclerosis
Without plasmacytoid features	Follicular center cell[a]	Follicular and diffuse, with sclerosis
With plasmacytoid features	Small cleaved	Diffuse
Lymphoblastic	Large cleaved	Unclassified
Convoluted	Small noncleaved	High-grade malignancy
Nonconvoluted	Large noncleaved	Centroblastic
Mixed (lymphocytic and histiocytic)	Immunoblastic sarcoma (B-cell)	Lymphoblastic
Histiocytic	Histiocytic	Burkitt type
Without sclerosis	Unclassified	Convoluted cell type
With sclerosis	Composite	Other (unclassified)
Burkitt tumor		Immunoblastic
Undifferentiated		Unclassified
Unclassified		Unclassified
Composite		Composite

INTERNATIONAL FORMULATION[765]

Low grade	Intermediate grade	High grade	Miscellaneous
ML,[b] small lymphocytic	ML, follicular, predominantly large cell	ML, large cell, immunoblastic	Composite
Consistent with chronic lymphocytic leukemia	With diffuse areas	Plasmacytoid	Mycosis fungoides
Plasmacytoid	With sclerosis	Clear cell	Histiocytic
ML, follicular, predominantly small cleaved cell	ML, diffuse, small cleaved cell	Polymorphous	Extramedullary plasmacytoma
With diffuse areas	With sclerosis	With epithelioid cell component	Unclassifiable
With sclerosis	ML, diffuse, mixed (small and large cell)	ML, lymphoblastic	Other
ML, follicular, mixed (small cleaved and large cell)	With sclerosis	Convoluted	
With diffuse areas	With epithelioid cell component	Nonconvoluted	
With sclerosis	ML, diffuse, large cell	ML, small noncleaved cell	
	Cleaved cell	Burkitt	
	Noncleaved cell	With follicular areas	
	With sclerosis		

[a]Subdivided into: (1) follicular, follicular and diffuse, and diffuse; and (2) without sclerosis and with sclerosis.
[b]Malignant lymphoma.

Finally, it confirmed the suspicion that within the 'histiocytic lymphoma' category of Rappaport there was a variety of morphologically recognizable neoplasms with a different natural history. As a result of the analysis of these 1175 cases, the investigators involved in this study proposed a new classification (hiding it under the euphemism 'Working Formulation') of non-Hodgkin malignant lymphomas, based primarily on light microscopic differences as seen in sections stained with hematoxylin–eosin, that showed a good correlation with survival. Ten major types plus a miscellaneous group were identified, and these were subdivided into three major prognostic groups that were of favorable, intermediate, and unfavorable prognosis, respectively.

Although this de facto classification gained some degree of acceptability, it was viewed by many as a compromise rather than a conceptual advance, just as the Rye classification of Hodgkin lymphoma had been seen as a compromise (not necessarily for the better) over the Lukes–Butler classification.[752] It was also pointed out from the very beginning that the Working Formulation did not take into account all the entities that had been recognized at that time. This, plus the continuing advances that have been made in the field, has led to additions and other substantial changes to the scheme.[764,768]

In the mid 1990s, an international group of hematopathologists prepared a list of lymphoid neoplasms that they felt could be recognized with available techniques and which appeared to be clinically distinctive.[749,755] The approach was strictly pragmatic, in the sense that the list included only those categories that appeared reasonably identifiable as such, without attempting to always relate them to normal stages of lymphoid differentiation. This attempt, to which the cute term REAL (Revised European American Lymphoma Classification) was given, has been the model upon which the new WHO classification of tumors of hematopoietic and lymphoid tissues published in 2001[756] and updated in 2008[769] is based (Box 21.3). The scheme and terminology recommended in the latter publication will be followed in the rest of the chapter, fully aware of the high probability that yet another classification will replace it by the time that the next edition of this book is published.[748,757]

As one reflects upon this tortuous history and browses over the current scheme, one cannot help but smile when remembering the caustic comment of Rupert Willis in 1948 to the effect that "nowhere in pathology has a chaos of names so clouded clear concepts as in the subject of lymphoid tumors" and his criticism of the "artificial distinctions ... created by naming tumours merely according to the degree of differentiation attained by their cells".[770] What would he think, one wonders, if he were alive today?

Small lymphocytic lymphoma

Small lymphocytic lymphoma (commonly referred to as 'chronic lymphocytic leukemia/small lymphocytic lymphoma') preferentially occurs in middle-aged and elderly individuals.[778,820] The patients often have few or no symptoms, the evolution is prolonged, and the survival is very good. It is not unusual to find the disease incidentally in lymph node dissections done for carcinoma of one type or another.[835]

The architecture of the node in small lymphocytic lymphoma is massively and monotonously effaced by a population of small round lymphocytes with clumped chromatin, inconspicuous nucleoli, barely visible cytoplasm, and scanty mitotic activity (Figs 21.63 and 21.64). There are also variable numbers of larger cells (prolymphocytes and paraimmunoblasts) with vesicular nuclei and distinct nucleoli, singly or in small aggregates that simulate germinal centers[787,800,822,826] (Fig. 21.65). These formations (known as proliferative centers, growth centers, or pseudofollicles) have an increased number of Ki-67-positive cells.[816] This feature, which is apparently of no prognostic significance,[775] should not lead to confusion with follicular lymphoma or NLPHL. As a matter of fact, the presence of these pseudofollicular formations and of prolymphocytes/paraimmunoblasts corroborates the diagnosis of small lymphocytic lymphoma as opposed to mantle cell lymphoma.

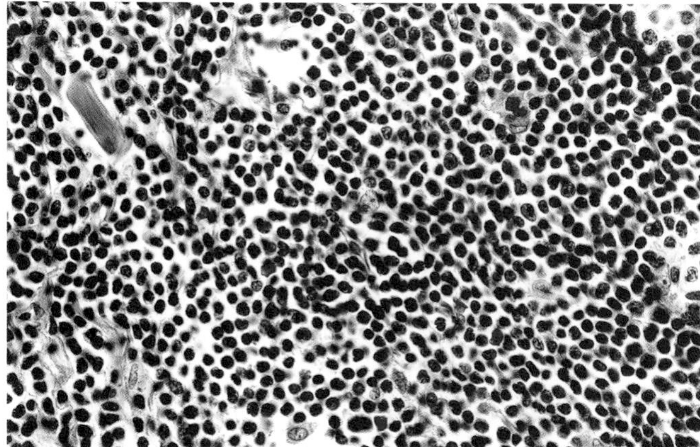

Fig. 21.63 Low-power view of small lymphocytic lymphoma. A monotonous proliferation of small lymphocytes effaces the architecture of the node.

Box 21.3 REAL/WHO 2001/WHO 2008 classification[756,769]

B-cell neoplasms

Precursor B-cell neoplasm

B lymphoblastic leukemia/lymphoma

Mature B-cell neoplasms

Chronic lymphocytic leukemia/small lymphocytic lymphoma
B-cell prolymphocytic leukemia
Lymphoplasmacytic lymphoma
Splenic marginal zone lymphoma
Hairy cell leukemia
Plasma cell neoplasms (plasma cell myeloma/plasmacytoma)
Extranodal marginal zone lymphoma of mucosa-associated lymphoid tissue (MALT-lymphoma)
Nodal marginal zone lymphoma
Follicular lymphoma
Primary cutaneous follicle center lymphoma
Mantle cell lymphoma
Diffuse large B-cell lymphomas (DLBCL)
- DLBCL, not otherwise specified
- T-cell/histiocyte-rich large B-cell lymphoma
- Primary DLBCL of the central nervous system
- Primary cutaneous DLBCL, leg-type
- Epstein–Barr virus + DLBCL of the elderly
- Primary mediastinal (thymic) large B-cell lymphoma
- Intravascular large B-cell lymphoma
- DLBCL associated with chronic inflammation
- Lymphomatoid granulomatosis
- ALK+ large B-cell lymphoma
- Plasmablastic lymphoma
- Large B-cell lymphoma arising in HHV8-associated multicentric Castleman disease
- Primary effusion lymphoma

Burkitt lymphoma
B-cell lymphoma, unclassifiable, with features intermediate between diffuse large B-cell lymphoma and Burkitt lymphoma
B-cell lymphoma, unclassifiable, with features intermediate between diffuse large B-cell lymphoma and classical Hodgkin lymphoma

T-cell and NK-cell neoplasms

Precursor T-cell neoplasms

T lymphoblastic leukemia/lymphoma

Mature T-cell and NK cell neoplasms

T-cell prolymphocytic leukemia
T-cell large granular lymphocytic leukemia
Aggressive NK cell leukemia
Adult T-cell leukemia/lymphoma
Epstein–Barr virus + T-cell lymphoproliferative diseases of childhood
Extranodal NK-/T-cell lymphoma, nasal type
Enteropathy-associated T-cell lymphoma
Hepatosplenic T-cell lymphoma
Subcutaneous panniculitis-like T-cell lymphoma
Mycosis fungoides
Sézary syndrome
Primary cutaneous CD30+ T-cell lymphoproliferative disorders
Primary cutaneous peripheral T-cell lymphomas, rare subtypes
Peripheral T-cell lymphoma, not otherwise specified
Angioimmunoblastic T-cell lymphoma
Anaplastic large cell lymphoma, ALK+
Anaplastic large cell lymphoma, ALK–

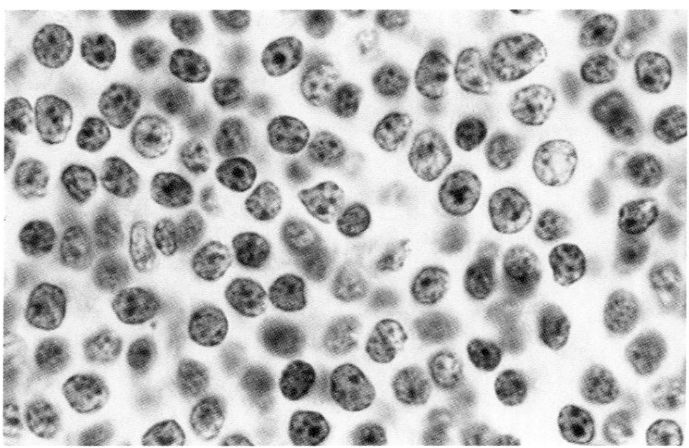

Fig. 21.64 High-power view of small lymphocytic lymphoma. The nuclear contours are regular, the chromatin is clumped, and nucleoli are inconspicuous.

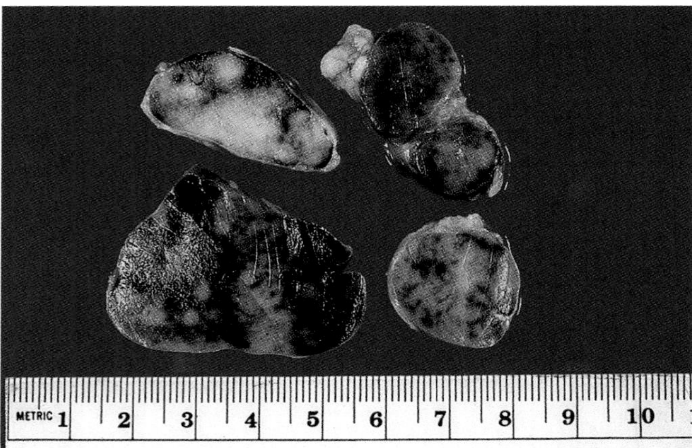

Fig. 21.66 Gross appearance of lymph nodes involved by chronic lymphocytic leukemia with anaplastic transformation (so-called 'Richter syndrome').

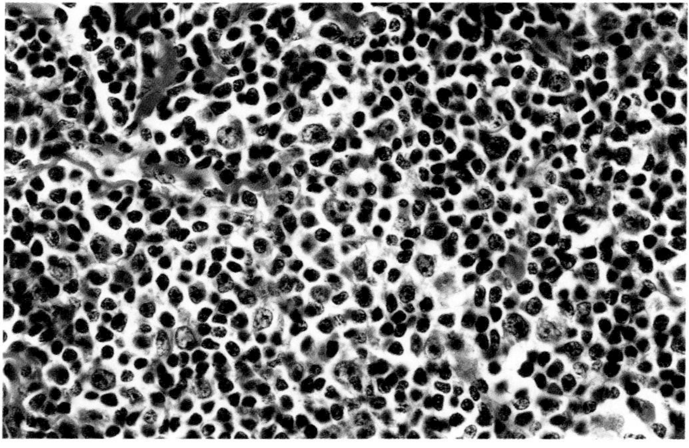

Fig. 21.65 So-called 'growth center' in a lymph node involved by small lymphocytic lymphoma.

The distribution of the disease is usually diffuse, but on occasions it is confined to the marginal zone, the perifollicular regions, or the interfollicular regions surrounding benign lymphoid follicles, the latter pattern being referred to as *interfollicular small lymphocytic lymphoma*.[785,791,795] Some cases show a propensity for invasion of the wall of veins.[810] Extranodal extension is seen in approximately one-third of the cases.[833]

Cases of small lymphocytic lymphomas can be divided into three categories: (1) those with absolute lymphocytosis (i.e., chronic lymphocytic leukemia); (2) those associated with monoclonal gammopathy (50% of which have bone marrow involvement); and (3) those with neither; the latter are often accompanied by hypogammaglobulinemia.[778,780,797,816,822] There are no statistical differences in survival between these three groups and no appreciable morphologic differences between the first and the third groups.[777] In the cases associated with monoclonal gammopathy, some or most of the neoplastic lymphocytes may exhibit morphologic signs of plasmacytoid differentiation (as evidenced by oval shape, lateralization of the nucleus, appearance of a perinuclear halo, and pyroninophilia) and admixture of plasma cells. Effacement of the nodal architecture is generally not as complete as with the usual type. These cases are referred to as *small lymphocytic lymphoma with plasmacytic differentiation* and are discussed further in the section on lymphoma and dysproteinemia.

Immunohistochemically, small lymphocytic lymphomas are always of B-cell type.[831] Monoclonal immunoglobulins, including both IgM and IgD types, are consistently found on their surface. They differ from the B lymphocytes of follicular lymphoma in the intensity and appearance of the reaction (brighter and more clumped in the latter), as well as by their lesser content of complement receptors. They are usually CD20+ (not uncommonly weak), CD5+, CD23+, CD43+, and cyclin D1.[789,808,832] At the molecular level, Ig heavy and light chain genes are rearranged. Cytogenetically, trisomy 12 has been reported in one-third of the cases (said to be associated with a poor prognosis), and abnormalities of 13q in up to one-fourth (said to be associated with a good survival).[805] Cases showing somatic hypermutation of the immunoglobulin gene (with negative staining for ZAP-70 being a surrogate marker) are associated with a favorable prognosis.[799]

There is a rare small lymphoid cell neoplasm of T-lineage which is clinically and pathologically different from small lymphocytic lymphoma, and which therefore should not be classified within this category[783,815] (see Chapter 23). The cells are usually somewhat larger, have numerous azurophilic granules, and contain large amounts of acid phosphatase and β-glucuronidase.

On occasion one sees cases of small lymphocytic lymphoma with typical Reed–Sternberg cells, suggesting a possible transformation to Hodgkin lymphoma; it has been hypothesized that such a transformation may be mediated by the EBV.[819] A development of even greater clinical significance is the transformation of a small lymphocytic lymphoma (or a chronic lymphocytic leukemia) into a 'blastic', 'histiocytic', or large cell neoplasm[774] (Figs 21.66 and 21.67). This occurrence, when developing in the background of chronic lymphocytic leukemia, has been traditionally known as *Richter syndrome*[814,821] and is accompanied by a precipitous decline in the clinical course. Fever, increasing lymphadenopathy, weight loss, and abdominal pain are frequent,[834] sometimes accompanied by hepatomegaly and splenomegaly. The earliest infiltrates may be detected in the lymph nodes or in the bone marrow.[793] Cell surface studies in these cases have shown that the large cells generally possess the same type of immunoglobulin heavy and light chain as the preexisting small lymphocytes, indicating that they represent dedifferentiation of the

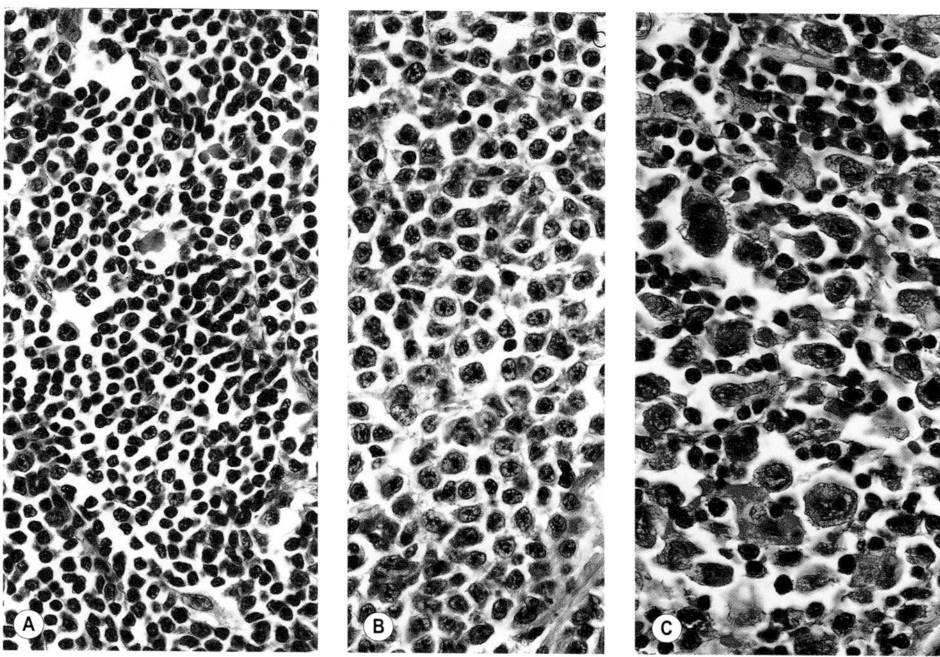

Fig. 21.67 Various morphologic types of lymph node involvement by chronic lymphocytic leukemia: **A**, monotonous infiltrate of small mature lymphocytes; **B**, somewhat immature forms, with slightly larger nuclei and more open chromatin; **C**, large pleomorphic tumor cells (so-called 'Richter syndrome').

original tumor rather than a second neoplasm. However, exceptions to this rule have been reported.[781,830,836]

Lymphoma and dysproteinemia. In view of the fact that most malignant lymphomas arise from B lymphocytes (i.e., cells normally engaged in humoral immune responses) it is not surprising that in some of them the tumor cells express those potentialities by secreting immunoglobulins of one sort or another.[772,807] Ranging in between the typical malignant lymphoma without immunoglobulin abnormalities and the typical plasma cell myeloma with monoclonal peak and Bence Jones proteinuria, all types of morphologic and biochemical hybrids have been encountered.[779] Tumors have been described that secrete completely assembled immunoglobulins of the IgG, IgA, IgM, IgD, or IgE type (with or without concomitant production of isolated light chains), isolated light chains to the almost total exclusion of complete immunoglobulin molecules, and 'heavy chains' (or, more accurately, Fc fragments) of IgG, IgM, or IgA specificity. Some of these immunoglobulins have the physicochemical properties of cryoglobulins and can result in necrotizing vasculitis.[782] This remarkably diverse expression of function has led to the introduction of such names as Waldenström macroglobulinemia, light chain disease, α-chain disease, and Franklin heavy chain disease, and even to the proposal of grouping all immunoglobulin-secreting lymphoid and plasmacytic tumors under the term *immunocytoma*.[786,794,806]

This practice has led to considerable confusion, as happens whenever morphologic and functional parameters are mixed in a common terminology. For instance, the serum picture of macroglobulinemia can be associated with a microscopic picture of small lymphocytic lymphoma, small lymphocytic lymphoma with plasmacytic differentiation, plasma cell myeloma, or large cell lymphoma.[812] It is obvious that by giving a tissue diagnosis 'consistent with macroglobulinemia', the pathologist is not rendering an accurate account of the situation. We believe that these neoplasms should be classified according to conventional morphologic criteria rather than by the biochemical findings in the patient's serum – i.e., a small lymphocytic lymphoma should be designated as such whether it produces macroglobulins, heavy chains, light chains, or no detectable globulins. Five main cytologic patterns are observed in these immunoglobulin-secreting neoplasms:[813]

1. Malignant lymphomas of conventional appearance, usually of small lymphocytic type, indistinguishable from those not associated with immunoglobulin abnormalities.
2. Plasmacytomas, in which most of the tumor cells have the characteristic light and electron microscopic features of plasma cells.[776]
3. Tumors having the overall appearance of a malignant lymphoma of small lymphocytic type but in which a variable proportion of the tumor cells has undergone plasmacytic differentiation, as evidenced light microscopically by lateralization of the nucleus, coarse chromatin clumping, appearance of a perinuclear clear halo, and/or increased basophilic cytoplasm, and ultrastructurally by prominence of the Golgi apparatus and abundance of granular endoplasmic reticulum.[780,797]

   Some of the tumor cells may be PAS positive. Immunoperoxidase stains will often show monoclonal immunoglobulin in the cytoplasm of the plasmacytoid cells much more frequently than in ordinary small lymphocytic lymphomas or chronic lymphocytic leukemias.[823,824] These tumors have been designated as small lymphocytic malignant lymphomas with plasmacytic differentiation, lymphoplasmacytoid lymphomas, or immunocytomas, lymphoplasmacytic type.[773] Their cell marker profile is similar to that of ordinary small lymphocytic lymphomas except for the presence of *cytoplasmic* immunoglobulin in some of the cells and a lesser percentage and degree of reactivity for CD5.[837] Intranuclear immunoglobulin inclusions (Dutcher bodies) can also occur (Fig. 21.68).
4. Large cell lymphomas predominantly or exclusively composed of B immunoblasts and/or plasmablasts. These

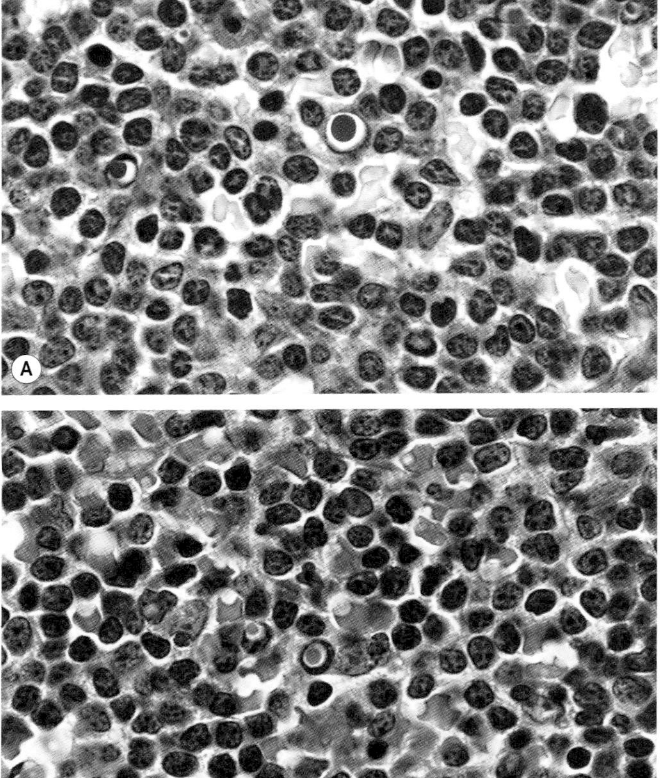

Fig. 21.68 Intranuclear immunoglobulin inclusions (Dutcher bodies) in a lymph node affected by lymphoplasmacytoid lymphoma as seen after hematoxylin–eosin (**A**) and PAS stains (**B**).

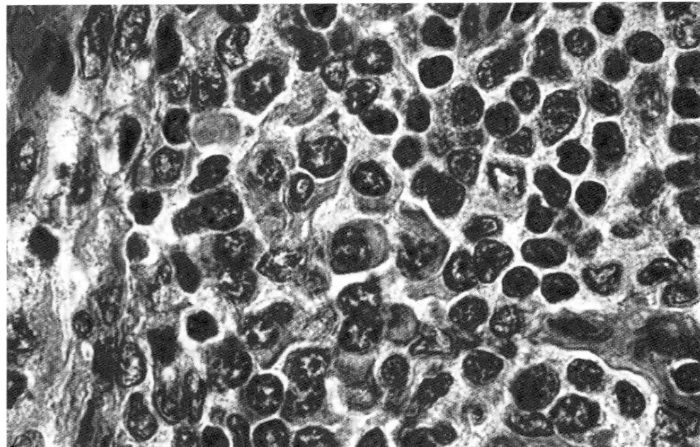

Fig. 21.69 Malignant lymphoma composed of lymphocytes and immature plasmacytoid forms (so-called 'pleomorphic immunocytoma').

cases, once known as immunoblastic sarcomas, are better designated as large cell lymphoma, immunoblastic or plasmablastic type, depending on the appearance of the predominant large cells. Plasmablastic lymphomas in HIV-positive patients are often EBV-associated and run an aggressive clinical course.[788]

5 Lymphomas composed of an admixture of immunoblasts, large plasmacytoid cells (plasmablasts), and mature plasma cells. These cases, which are part of the same spectrum as those listed in the previous paragraph, have sometimes been designated *polymorphic immunocytomas* (Fig. 21.69). Some of the reported cases of primary plasmacytomas of lymph nodes[771,792] belong to this or to one or another of the previous categories. The term *plasmacytoma* of lymph nodes should be restricted to those rare cases having typical bone marrow involvement by plasmacytoma and/or cases in which nearly all of the malignant cells have plasmacytoid features, and in which a lymphocytic component is absent[776,811] (Fig. 21.70).

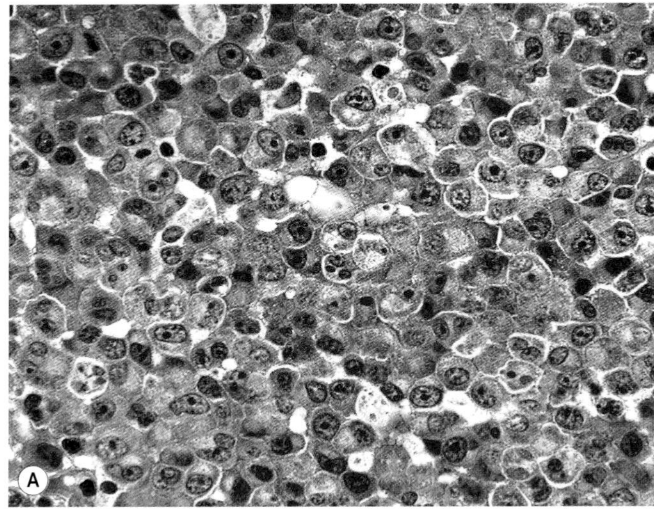

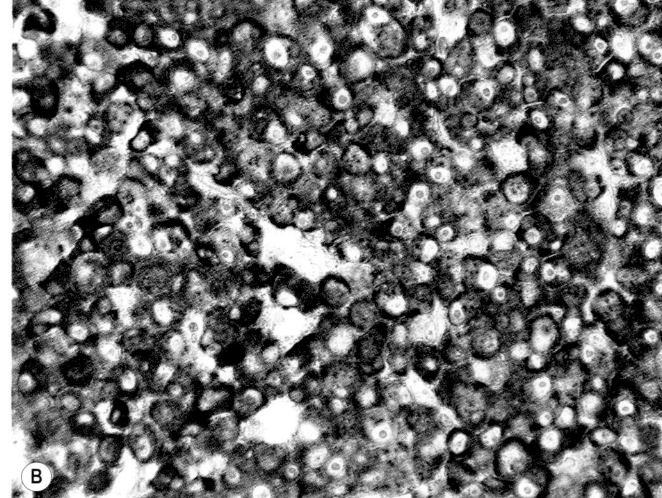

Fig. 21.70 Plasmacytoma of lymph node composed entirely of immature plasma cells (plasmablasts): **A**, hematoxylin–eosin; **B**, lambda immunostain.

Even under these circumstances the disease seems to be immunohistochemically different from other forms of extramedullary plasmacytomas, and almost never progresses to multiple myeloma.[817]

Attempts to correlate the microscopic appearance with the secretory activity of these tumors have been made by several authors. The results have been largely discouraging, although a few more or less distinctive patterns have emerged.[798,804] In general, tumors producing IgM globulin or 'heavy chains' have the anatomic distribution and cytologic appearance of malignant lymphoma, whereas most of those secreting IgG globulin or a light chain are clinically and microscopically classifiable as plasma cell myeloma. Intranuclear and cytoplasmic inclusions are not specific for any type of immunoglobulin.[825] However, those composed of IgM or IgA are often PAS positive because of their high carbohydrate content, whereas those composed of IgG are not.[784,790] The immunoglobulin inclusions may appear as round eosinophilic bodies or crystals.[818] The former may be so abundant and prominent (perhaps resulting from a blockage in secretion) as to displace the nucleus laterally, creating a signet ring effect.[803] Plasmacytomas expressing IgA tend to run an indolent course, with low risk of clinical progression.[829]

A most peculiar variant on the theme is represented by the cases in which the immunoglobulin crystals are massively phagocytosed by histiocytes, resulting in an appearance that may simulate a variety of nonlymphoid diseases, including rhabdomyoma. This bizarre condition has been term *crystal-storing histiocytosis* but it truly represents a dysproteinemia-associated lymphoproliferative process akin to those described in this section. Examples have been reported in the soft tissue (particularly in the head and neck region), lung and other sites, and are discussed in the respective chapters.[796,801,802]

Tumors that have been reported as secreting IgA 'heavy chains' have involved the gastrointestinal tract[828] or, much less commonly, the respiratory tract.[827] The former is discussed in Chapter 11. Production of IgM heavy chains, an exceptionally rare event, occurs in elderly patients who present with chronic lymphocytic leukemia.[809]

Of all the anatomic types of malignant lymphoma, Hodgkin lymphoma and follicular lymphoma are the least likely to be associated with immunoglobulin serum abnormalities. The more obvious the plasmacytic differentiation, the higher the chances of immunoglobulin alterations. However, it should be remembered that even fully differentiated plasma cell tumors may sometimes be associated with complete lack of detectable immunoglobulin production.

Follicular lymphoma

Follicular (nodular) lymphoma is a B-cell neoplasm that recapitulates the architectural and cytologic features of the normal secondary lymphoid follicle.[872] This tumor comprises up to 40% of all adult non-Hodgkin lymphomas in the United States, but in other countries the relative incidence is much lower. Most cases occur in elderly individuals. It is very unusual under 20 years of age and relatively uncommon in blacks.[873] Most of the cases diagnosed in the past as follicular lymphomas in children actually represent NLPHL or reactive follicular hyperplasia. However, well-documented cases of follicular lymphoma in children are on record.[893,910]

Grossly and at low-power examination, the most distinctive feature of these tumors is the nodular pattern of growth (Figs 21.71 and 21.72). Rappaport et al.[894] have carefully outlined in a classic article the differential points between these neoplastic nodules and the reactive follicles of follicular hyperplasia (Figs

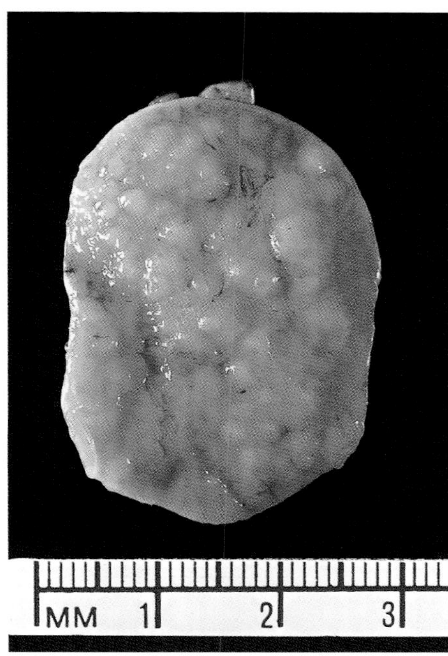

Fig. 21.71 Gross appearance of a lymph node affected by follicular lymphoma. The neoplastic nodules bulge onto the surface.
(Courtesy of Dr RA Cooke, Brisbane, Australia; from Cooke RA, Stewart B. Colour atlas of anatomical pathology. Edinburgh, 2004, Churchill Livingstone)

21.73 and 21.74) (see Table 21.8). With progression of the disease, this distinct nodularity becomes blurred, and eventually most of the proliferation acquires a diffuse pattern. The cytologic composition of the neoplastic nodules is characterized by a mixture in different proportions of small and large lymphoid cells, both of which resemble their normal follicular counterparts.[880] The small cells have scanty cytoplasm and an irregular, elongated cleaved nucleus with prominent indentations and infoldings; the size is similar to or slightly larger than that of normal lymphocytes, the chromatin is coarse, and the nucleolus is inconspicuous (Fig. 21.75). These cells have been variously referred to as germinocytes, centrocytes, poorly differentiated lymphocytes, and small cleaved follicular center cells. The large cells are two or three times the size of normal lymphocytes; they have a distinct rim of cytoplasm and a vesicular nucleus with one or three nucleoli often adjacent to the nuclear membrane. These cells, which have a rapid turnover rate and probably represent the proliferating component of the tumor, have been designated over the years as germinoblasts, centroblasts, histiocytes, large (cleaved or noncleaved) follicular center cells, large lymphoid cells, and lymphoblasts. Some may be binucleated and simulate Reed–Sternberg cells.[884] It ought to be mentioned here that another type of large cell seen in follicular lymphoma is the non-neoplastic follicular dendritic cell, for the very reason that the tumor involves lymphoid follicles; it is recognized because of its finely dispersed chromatin, the lack of identifiable cell boundaries, and the inconspicuousness of the nucleolus. In contrast to their counterparts in benign follicles, these cells show little or no immunoreactivity for fascin.[899]

Immunohistochemically, the follicles of follicular lymphoma (including all its variants) are composed of a monoclonal population of B cells admixed with variable numbers of non-neoplastic small T cells, macrophages, and follicular dendritic cells, corresponding to the cellular composition of a normal germinal

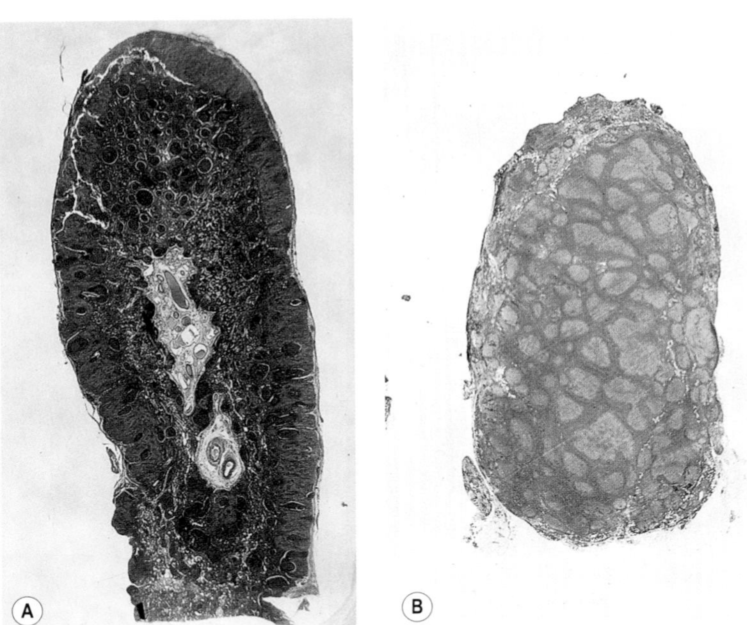

Fig. 21.72 Even distribution of neoplastic follicles in follicular lymphoma (**B**), as opposed to the predominantly cortical distribution typical of follicular hyperplasia (**A**).

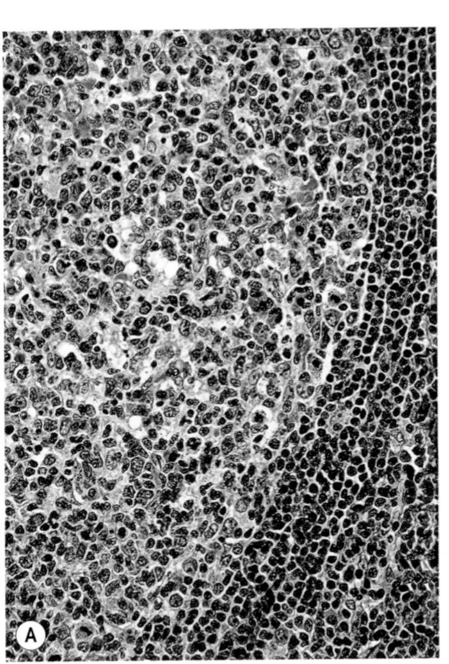

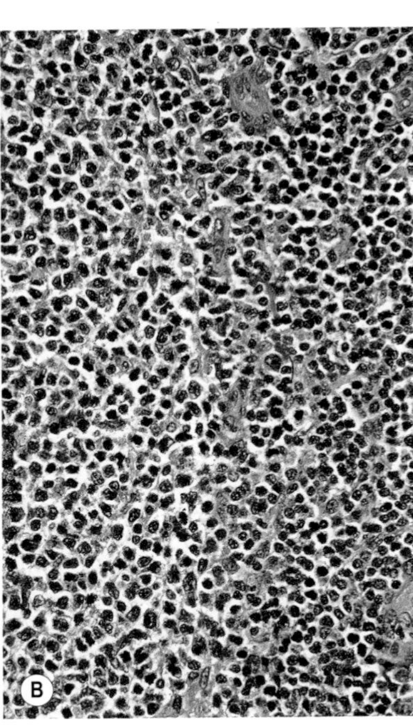

Fig. 21.73 Fuzzy edge of neoplastic nodule of follicular lymphoma (**B**), as opposed to sharp edge bound by the mantle zone in follicular hyperplasia (**A**).

center[901,904] (Figs 21.76 and 21.77). The tumor cells express pan–B-antigens, such as CD19, CD20, CD22, and CD79a, in addition to HLA-DR. They also express surface and/or cytoplasmic immunoglobulins (usually of the IgM type) with light chain restriction. CD10 (CALLA), a germinal center cell marker, is detected in approximately 60–70% of the cases.[911] This marker can aid in distinction from reactive follicular hyperplasia when significant numbers of CD10+ cells are found in the interfollicular zone as an indication of interfollicular invasion. BCL6, another germinal center cell marker, is expressed in most cases. CD5 and CD43 are usually negative.

The BCL2 protein can be identified immunohistochemically in approximately 85% of cases, and is thus one of the most useful markers for the differential diagnosis with reactive follicular hyperplasia (BCL2 negative), although it is important to realize that BCL2 negativity does not totally rule out follicular lymphoma.[861,904,906] Immunostaining for BCL2 cannot be used for distinction of follicular lymphoma from other low-grade B-cell lymphomas, because the latter are commonly BCL2 positive; to deal with such a diagnostic problem, immunostaining for follicular center cell markers such as CD10 and BCL6 is more helpful.[841,846]

Follicular lymphoma shows clonal rearrangements of the immunoglobulin genes, which also feature hypermutations and ongoing somatic mutations, as characteristic of follicle center B cells.[891]

The hallmark genetic alteration of follicular lymphoma is t(14;18)(q32;q21), found in 85% of cases. The chromosomal translocation

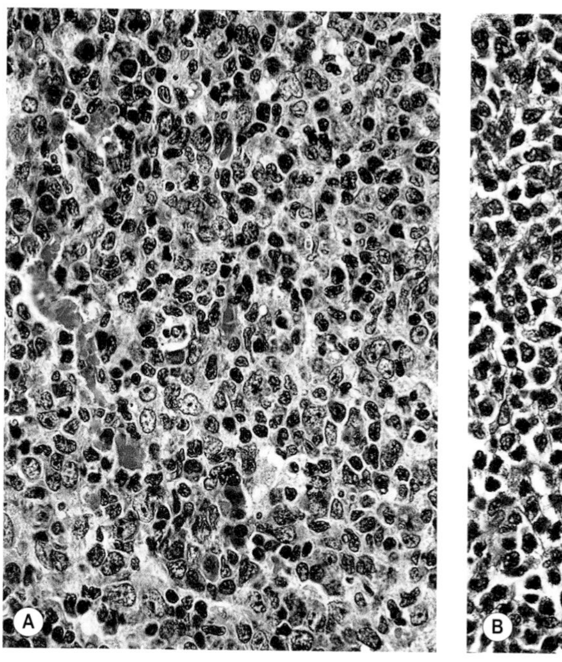

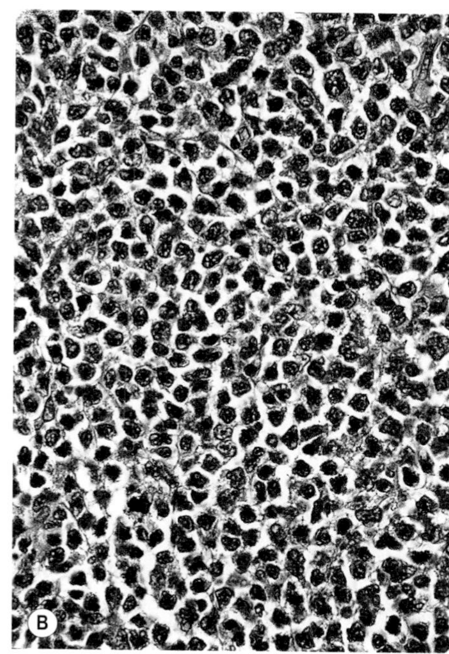

Fig. 21.74 Homogeneous population of small cleaved cells in follicular lymphoma (**B**), as opposed to the polymorphic composition seen in follicular hyperplasia, including the presence of tingible-body macrophages (**A**).

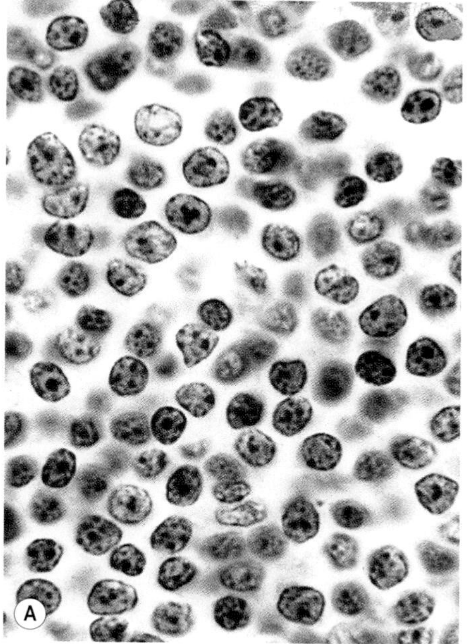

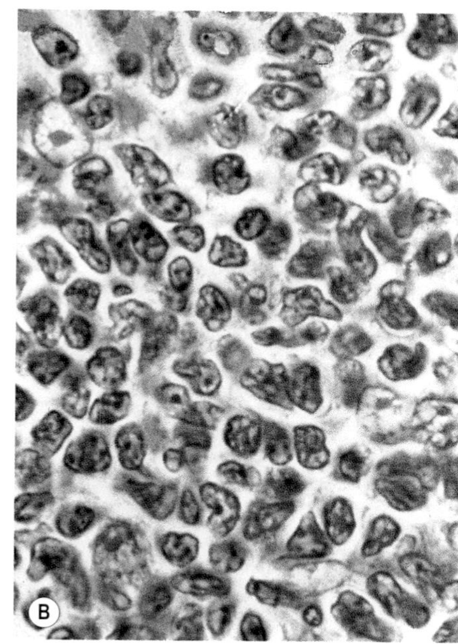

Fig. 21.75 Marked contrast between the cleaved cells of follicular lymphoma (**B**) and the regular mature lymphocytes of small lymphocytic lymphoma (**A**).

juxtaposes *IGH* with the *BCL2* gene, driving overexpression of BCL2 protein, an anti-apoptotic molecule located in the inner mitochondrial membrane whose expression is typically switched off in normal follicle center B cells.[844,869,903] As a result of aberrant BCL2 expression, the neoplastic follicle center cells do not undergo apoptosis. Thus follicular lymphoma results more from cell accumulation than cell proliferation. Although *BCL2* rearrangement is also seen in some cases of diffuse large B-cell lymphoma, demonstration of this molecular alteration provides a good support for a diagnosis of follicular lymphoma in the appropriate context, such as distinction from atypical follicular hyperplasia, marginal zone lymphoma with follicular growth pattern and mantle cell lymphoma. For this purpose, FISH is more sensitive than PCR.[865] Certain types of follicular lymphoma uncommonly or do not exhibit *BCL2* rearrangement, including pediatric follicular lymphoma, primary cutaneous follicle center lymphoma, and grade 3b follicular lymphoma.[850,851,863,883,890,909]

The presence of t(14;18) alone appears to be insufficient for the development of follicular lymphoma, because this is rarely the sole genetic aberration and even healthy subjects commonly harbor low numbers of B lymphocytes with t(14;18).[845,849,867,897,898] Common additional genetic changes include −1p36, +2p15, −6q,

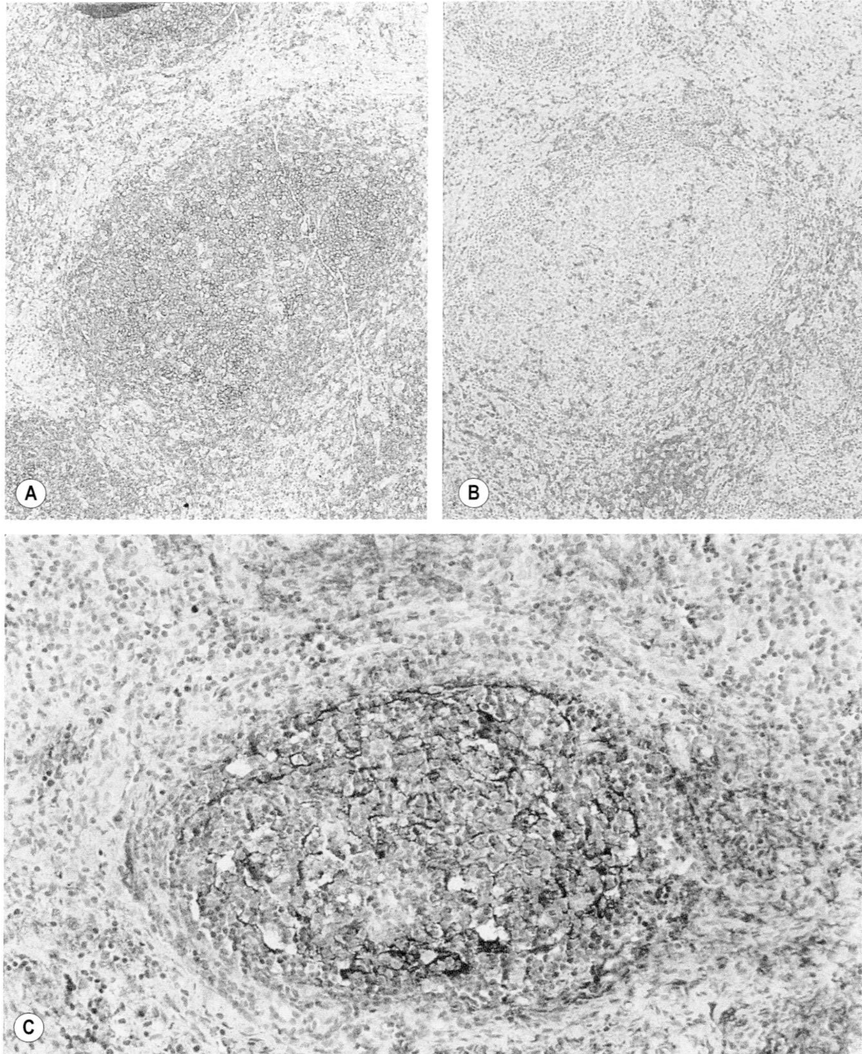

Fig. 21.76 A–C, Follicular lymphoma. **A**, CD20 stain decorates the neoplastic nodule and identifies the cells as of B-cell nature. **B**, CD3 stain shows a rim of non-neoplastic T cells around the follicles. **C**, CD21 stain shows a large number of dendritic follicular cells within the neoplastic follicle.
(Courtesy of Dr Glauco Frizzera, New York, NY, USA)

+7p, +7q, −9p, +12q, −17p, +18q, and +X, with some of them, such as −1p36, −6q, −9p, and +18q, being associated with a worse prognosis.[870,879,898,907]

BCL6 translocation occurs in approximately 10% of the cases, usually mutually exclusive to *BCL2* translocation.[866,871,890] This is correlated with grade 3b histology, high proliferative index, and infrequent expression of CD10 and BCL2.[863,866,878] Follicular lymphomas with del6q23–26 or del17p at presentation are at increased risk of transformation to high-grade B-cell lymphoma.[903] Genetic changes that mediate such a transformation may include *MYC* translocation, *TP53* mutation, *BCL2* mutation, deletions of 9p21 involving P16 and p15, and mutation of the 5′ noncoding region of *BCL6*.[882,885,902]

The gene expression profile of follicular lymphoma recapitulates that of normal germinal center B cells, and furthermore clusters close to resting B cell samples, in keeping with its indolent nature.[840] On microarray analysis, the immune response-1 signature, reflecting presence of a complex infiltrate of T cells and other immune cells, predicts long survival, while immune response-2 signature, reflecting a significant infiltrate of monocytes and dendritic cells, predicts short survival.[857]

Depending on the relative proportion of small and large cells, follicular lymphomas are subdivided into three categories, respectively designated in the WHO classification as follows:

1. Grade 1, with 0–15 centroblasts (large nucleolated cells) per high-power field.
2. Grade 2, with 6–15 centroblasts per high-power field.
3. Grade 3, with more than 15 centroblasts per high-power field. Cases with admixed centrocytes are referred to as grade 3a, while cases with solid sheets of centroblasts are referred to as grade 3b. In the first category, which is the most common, mitotic activity is infrequent. Conversely, the appearance of large cells is often accompanied by a parallel increase in the number of mitoses.

Several important clinical differences exist between these groups.[854,905] Patients with grade 1 follicular lymphoma are often asymptomatic, usually have generalized disease (often involving extranodal sites, such as the liver and bone marrow), and have a good prognosis,[864] to the point that some authors advise against aggressive treatment for them.[847,855,875,881,895,913] Grade 3 tumors are more commonly localized at the time of presentation but run a

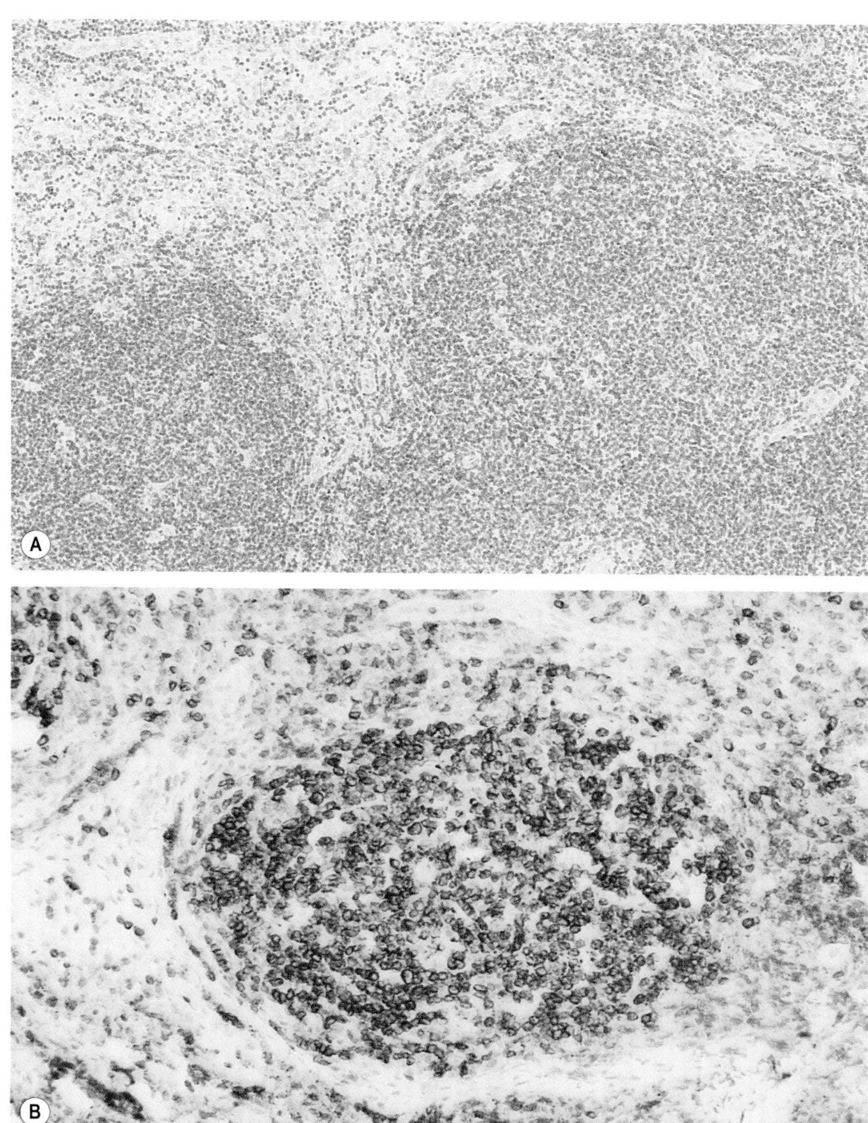

Fig. 21.77 Follicular lymphoma stained for MT2 (**A**) and BCL2 (**B**).
(Courtesy of Dr Glauco Frizzera, New York, NY, USA)

more aggressive clinical course[868,873] and are more likely to lose their nodular pattern of growth and become diffuse. The prognosis of grade 2 tumors is intermediate between these two but closer to grade 1. As a matter of fact, in an early series it was associated with an even longer survival.[843] Because of this fact, the first two categories are sometimes grouped under the term *low-grade follicular lymphoma,* the implication being that the predominantly large cell lymphoma (grade 3) is a high-grade tumor.

Another morphologic parameter that has been evaluated in follicular lymphoma is the relative degree of nodularity. Warnke et al.[908] have shown that among the predominantly small cleaved cell and mixed lymphomas, the survival rate is similar in patients with purely follicular tumors and those with tumors of a follicular and diffuse pattern. However, in the predominantly large cell category (grade 3), patients with tumors of both follicular and diffuse patterns have a worse prognosis than those with tumors of a pure follicular pattern.

The extranodal spread of follicular lymphoma is quite predictable. In the spleen, it tends to affect the B-derived lymphoid follicles located eccentrically in the white pulp. In the liver, the infiltrate is predominantly periportal. The bone marrow infiltrates tend to have a paratrabecular location. In the skin, there is an extensive dermal infiltrate without particular relation to vessels or adnexa.

In some cases of follicular lymphoma (particularly grade 1), malignant cells are found in the peripheral blood; hematologists refer to them by the inelegant term 'buttock' cells because of their prominent nuclear cleft (Fig. 21.78). No prognostic significance has been assigned to this finding.

Specimens from subsequent biopsies or autopsy from patients with grade 1 follicular lymphomas may show a similar microscopic appearance or a progression to grade 2 or 3.[860,892] A more ominous development is represented by the occasional 'blastic' or 'blastoid' transformation of follicular lymphoma, in which the tumor cells resemble those of Burkitt or lymphoblastic lymphoma; this is accompanied by a highly aggressive clinical course.[856,886] The resulting high-grade malignant tumor may also have the morphologic and immunohistochemical features of a CD30+ large cell lymphoma with anaplastic features.[842]

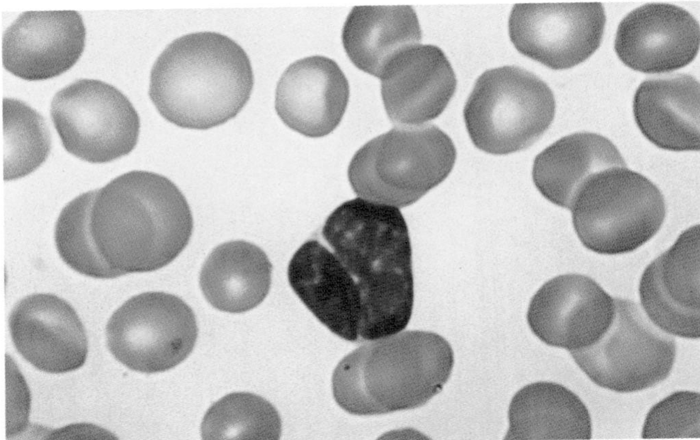

Fig. 21.78 Blood smear from a patient with follicular lymphoma showing a so-called 'notched nucleus cell' or 'buttock cell'.

Several morphologic variations in the theme of follicular lymphoma have been described. They include the following:

1. Presence of fine or coarse bands of fibrosis that accentuate even more the nodular character of the lesion but, in so doing, may induce confusion with carcinoma. This feature is more commonly seen in grade 3 tumors;[848] it is particularly frequent in the retroperitoneum, but it also occurs in the cervical region, mediastinum, and other locations.
2. Presence of monocytoid B cell/marginal zone differentiation. In about 10% of follicular lymphomas, discrete foci of monocytoid B cells are seen, typically appearing on low-power examination as a pale rim around the neoplastic follicles.[874,900] Molecular studies have shown a common clonal origin of the monocytoid B cells from follicle center cells.[838,912] Clinically, this feature is said to be associated with a shorter survival time.[887]
3. Deposition of proteinaceous material in the center of the nodules, similar to that seen in some reactive conditions, particularly the plasma cell variant of Castleman disease (Fig. 21.79). The material is amorphous, acellular, brightly eosinophilic, and PAS positive.[854,896] Ultrastructurally, it is composed of membranous structures, membrane-bound vesicles, and electron-dense bodies.[854] It can appear in both grade 1 and grade 2 follicular lymphomas.[896]
4. Presence of large cytoplasmic eosinophilic globules – presumably immunoglobulins – or a single vacuole that push the nucleus laterally and result in a signet ring effect[876] (Fig. 21.80).
5. Clearcut plasmacytic differentiation in some or many of the neoplastic follicular center cells.[858,874]
6. Presence of cells with cerebriform nuclei (similar to those of T-cell lymphoma)[888] or multilobated nuclei.[853]
7. Permeation of the tumor follicles by small round lymphocytes of presumably mantle zone origin, the appearance simulating that of progressively transformed germinal centers ('floral' variant)[862,889] (Fig. 21.81).
8. Presence of rosettes made up of cytoplasm and cytoplasmic processes of the lymphoid tumor cells and simulating the appearance of a neuroendocrine neoplasm (Fig. 21.82).[859]
9. Presence of hyaline vascular follicles similar to those seen in the vascular-hyaline type of Castleman disease.
10. Inversion of the usual staining pattern as seen on low-power examination so that the neoplastic follicles appear darker

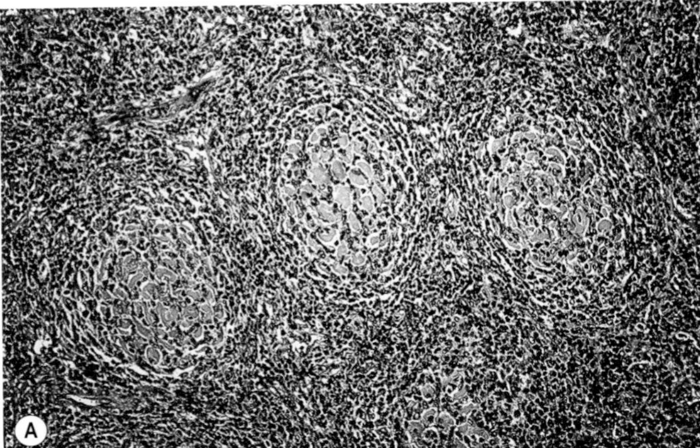

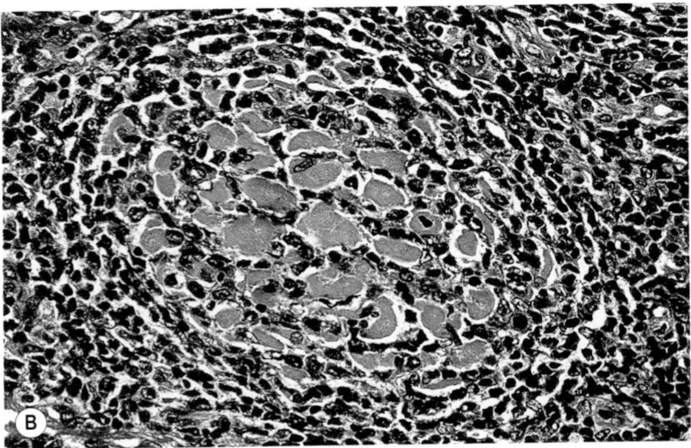

Fig. 21.79 **A** and **B**, Follicular lymphoma with deposition of proteinaceous material among the tumor cells. Ultrastructurally, some of this material was found to be within the cytoplasm of dendritic follicular cells.

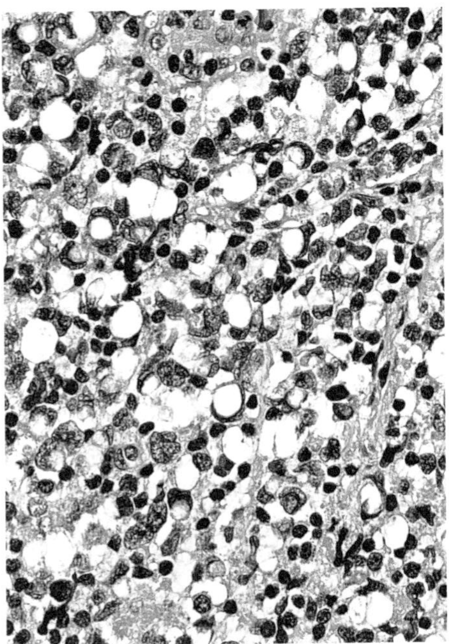

Fig. 21.80 Malignant lymphoma featuring signet ring changes in some of the tumor cells.

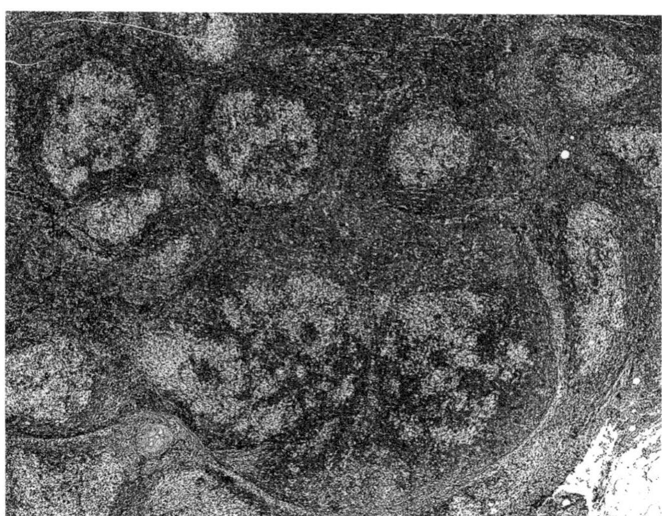

Fig. 21.81 So-called 'floral variant' of follicular lymphoma.

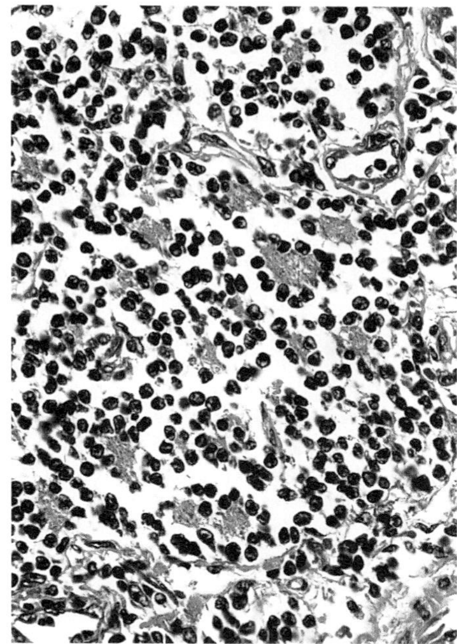

Fig. 21.82 Malignant lymphoma showing rosette formation by some of the lymphoid cells.

than the surrounding lymphoid tissue. This pattern, which is referred to as the 'reverse' or 'inverse' variant of follicular lymphoma, carries no prognostic significance.[852]

11 Prominent epithelioid granulomatous response.[877]

12 Preserved reactive germinal centers in some foci of the involved lymph node. This feature is said to be a strong indicator of limited disease stage.[839]

Mantle cell lymphoma

Mantle cell lymphoma is a low-grade neoplasm also known as intermediate lymphocytic, mantle zone, centrocytic, and diffuse small cleaved cell lymphoma.[923,938,956] It comprises from 3% to 10% of all cases of non-Hodgkin lymphoma. Like follicular lymphoma, it usually occurs in middle-aged and elderly individuals.[926,950] The low-power appearance is largely that of a diffuse lymphoma, although there may be a suggestion of nodularity accentuated by the occasional presence of small germinal center-like structures ('naked' germinal centers) (Fig. 21.83).[962] The neoplastic cells are small, and often show irregular and indented nuclear contours similar to those seen in small cleaved cell follicular lymphoma[960] (Fig. 21.84). On occasion, some of the tumor cells show plasma cell differentiation.[963] In some cases, the tumor cells have larger nuclei with more dispersed chromatin and a higher proliferative fraction ('blastoid' or 'pleomorphic' variant)[928] (Fig. 21.85). Sometimes one form is seen evolving into the other, an event confirmed by clonality studies.[939] The blastoid form of mantle cell lymphoma (and sometimes also the classic form) may be accompanied by blood, bone marrow, and spleen involvement ('mantle cell leukemia').[945,952,953,959]

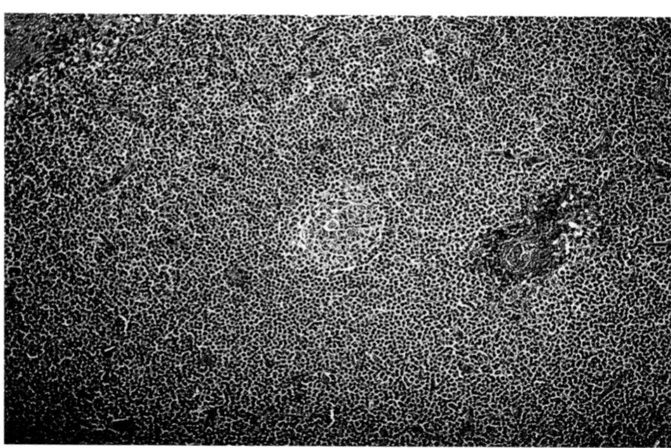

Fig. 21.83 Mantle cell lymphoma surrounding a small residual germinal center.

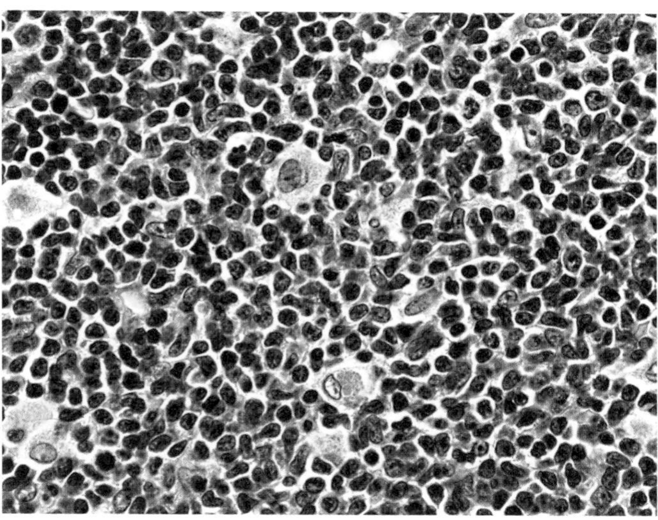

Fig. 21.84 High-power view of mantle cell lymphoma. There are subtle abnormalities of the nuclear contours, the appearance being intermediate between that seen in small cleaved follicular lymphoma and that of small lymphocytic lymphoma.

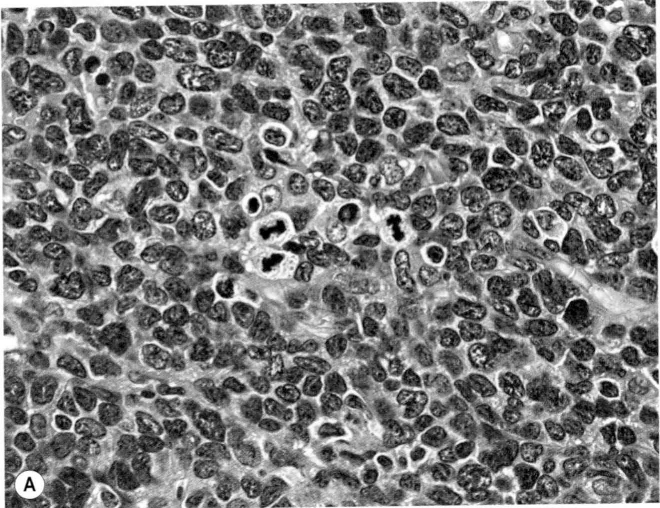

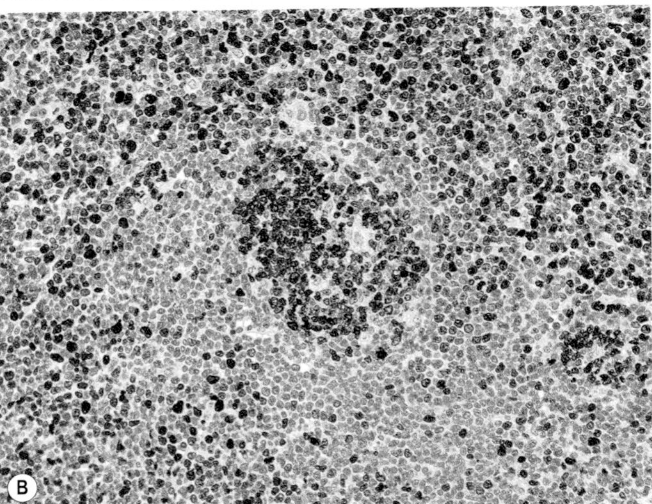

Fig. 21.85 **A** and **B**, So-called 'blastoid variant' of mantle cell lymphoma. **A**, Hematoxylin–eosin-stained section showing high mitotic activity. **B**, A high percentage of the tumor cells show nuclear immunoreactivity for MIB-1.

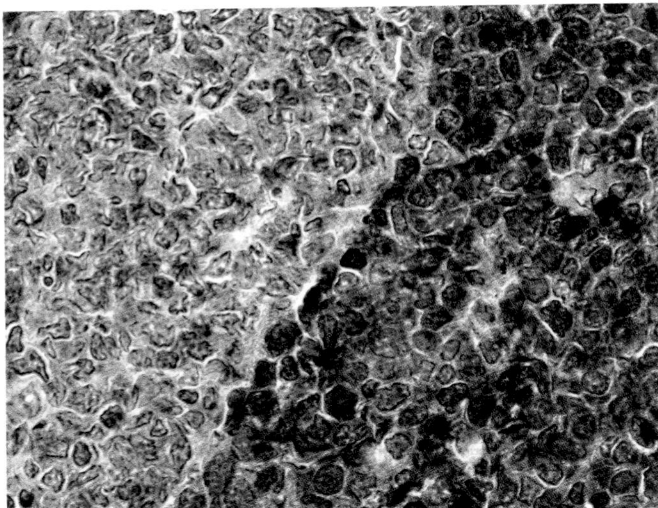

Fig. 21.86 Immunoreactivity for cyclin D1 in mantle zone lymphoma.

Two common morphologic features of mantle cell lymphoma are hyalinized blood vessels and a scattering of epithelioid histiocytes, the former representing an important diagnostic clue and the latter sometimes resulting in a starry sky appearance.[962]

The immunocytochemical profile suggests that mantle cell lymphoma is a distinct type of malignant lymphoma having the features of the lymphocytes of primary follicles and/or the mantle zones of secondary follicles, i.e., naive pregerminal center cells.[955,958] The tumor cells are positive for immunoglobulins (IgM and often also IgD), B-cell-associated antigens, and CD5.[915,919] The general absence of CD23 is useful in distinguishing mantle cell lymphoma from small lymphocytic lymphoma,[927,937] and the presence of CD5 is useful in the differential diagnosis with follicular and marginal zone lymphomas. It should be remarked, however, that CD5 expression is not always present in mantle cell lymphoma[941] and can be present in some diffuse large B-cell lymphomas apparently unrelated to mantle cell lymphoma.[936] As explained below, overexpression of cyclin D1 protein is a constant and nearly specific feature of mantle cell lymphoma, which therefore becomes of great importance in its differential diagnosis[914,944] (Fig. 21.86). Although immunohistochemical demonstration of cyclin D1 has been difficult in the past,[924,944] this has now become easy with the availability of a rabbit monoclonal antibody against cyclin D1.[925]

The immunoglobulin genes are clonally rearranged, and the variable regions are usually nonmutated, suggesting a naive B-cell stage of differentiation.[921,935] Nearly all cases show fusion of *CCND1* (cyclin D1) with the *IGH* gene, which results from t(11;14)(q13;q32) (in approximately 70% of cases) or a cryptic translocation.[940,957] As a consequence, cyclin D1, a cell-cycle protein, is overexpressed, promoting cell proliferation. *CCND1* translocation is practically specific for mantle cell lymphoma, except that it also occurs in some cases of plasma cell myeloma, and thus its demonstration may help confirm a diagnosis of mantle cell lymphoma.[918,929] Fluorescent in situ hybridization gives the highest sensitivity (>95%), and is superior to conventional cytogenetics, Southern blot, or PCR.[917,940]

Additional genetic changes are common in mantle cell lymphoma, such as inactivating mutation of *ATM* (11q22–23), homozygous deletions of *INK4a/ARF* (p16) and *TP53* mutation.[922,942,949] The blastoid/pleomorphic variant is correlated with presence of *TP53* mutation, *MYC* abnormalities, and tetraploidy.[916,931,947,948]

Microarray studies have shown that mantle cell lymphoma exhibits a unique gene expression signature distinct from other lymphoma types, and furthermore confirm the existence of a cyclin D1-negative subset of mantle cell lymphoma (up to 7% of cases).[943,951] At least some cases of the latter subset express cyclin D2 or cyclin D3 instead of cyclin D1.[930,951,961] Based on the expression level of proliferation signature genes, patients can be further stratified into four prognostic groups with median survival times of 0.8, 2.3, 3.3, and 6.7 years, respectively.[951] Use of quantitative RT-PCR to measure the expression of five genes (*RAN, MYC, TNFRSF10B, POLE2, SLC29A2*), applicable to frozen or paraffin-embedded tissue, holds promise as a simpler method for survival prediction that can be performed in the diagnostic laboratory.[932]

Mantle cell lymphoma may be difficult to distinguish from follicular hyperplasia with a prominence of mantle zone cells ('mantle zone hyperplasia') and Castleman disease.[934] Determination of clonality of the infiltrate by immunocytochemical techniques is of importance in this regard. The differential diagnosis also includes grade 1 follicular lymphoma. The fact that centroblasts and immunoblast-like cells are totally absent in mantle cell lymphoma is an important differential feature.

Finally, the blastoid form of mantle cell lymphoma needs to be distinguished from either T- or B-cell lineage lymphoblastic lymphoma.[954]

The median survival of mantle cell lymphoma is approximately 3–5 years. As a group, it is characterized by more widespread disease and a much lower response rate to chemotherapy than follicular lymphoma.[933,944] The blastic variant has a more aggressive clinical course.[920,923] A rare indolent type of mantle cell lymphoma has also been described.[946]

Marginal zone B-cell lymphoma

Marginal zone B-cell lymphoma is the generic term used in the REAL/WHO schemes to designate an increasingly larger family of low-grade B-cell lymphomas comprised of a heterogeneous population of small B cells. The concept represents a grouping of entities that had been described separately, most of them at extranodal sites.[977] There appears to be considerable clinical, morphologic, and immunohistochemical overlap among the three entities (extranodal, nodal, and splenic).[973] Consequently, the proposal has been made that they represent a related family of neoplasms showing morphologic evidence of differentiation into cells of marginal zone type.[984,995] These cells are thought to have the capacity to mature into both monocytoid B cells and plasma cells, and to display tissue-specific homing patterns. A corollary of this proposal is that the various clinical syndromes may be the result of the homing pattern of the specific neoplastic clone.[977] The proposal has been generally accepted, although it has been pointed out that important clinical and molecular genetic differences among the subgroups and even within a given subgroup exist.[965,966,980]

1 *Nodal marginal zone lymphoma (monocytoid B-cell lymphoma)*. This term has been used for a tumor of small to medium-sized lymphocytes with round or slightly indented nuclei and relatively abundant clear cytoplasm, usually located in lymph nodes, hence its alternate designation as nodal.[982] The tumor cells have been regarded as the neoplastic counterpart of the monocytoid B lymphocytes found in lymph node sinuses in toxoplasmosis and other reactive disorders[990] (see p. 1784). Plasmacytoid features are prominent in some cases. The pattern of involvement is predominantly sinusal and interfollicular,[969] but cases have been seen with 'follicular colonization' and with 'floral' features.[975] Clinically, the disease is more common in women, and can be localized or generalized at presentation.[968] Some patients have suffered from autoimmune disorders such as Sjögren disease. In all cases, the possibility of nodal spread from an extranodal marginal zone lymphoma has to be excluded by clinical workup. Histologic transformation to large cell lymphoma has been documented in some cases.

   Little is known about the molecular genetics of nodal marginal zone lymphoma. The distinctive chromosomal translocations of extranodal marginal zone lymphoma are lacking.[976] Similar to extranodal marginal zone lymphoma, some cases exhibit loss of function of *A20*.[983]

2 *Extranodal marginal zone lymphoma of mucosa-associated lymphoid tissue* (usually abbreviated as MALT lymphoma).[979] This is a neoplasm in which the cell population – all of small size – has been described as including small round lymphocytes, monocytoid B cells, cells with slightly irregular nuclei (centrocyte-like), plasmacytoid cells, and plasma cells. Occasional large lymphoid cells may also be seen (Figs 21.87 and 21.88).

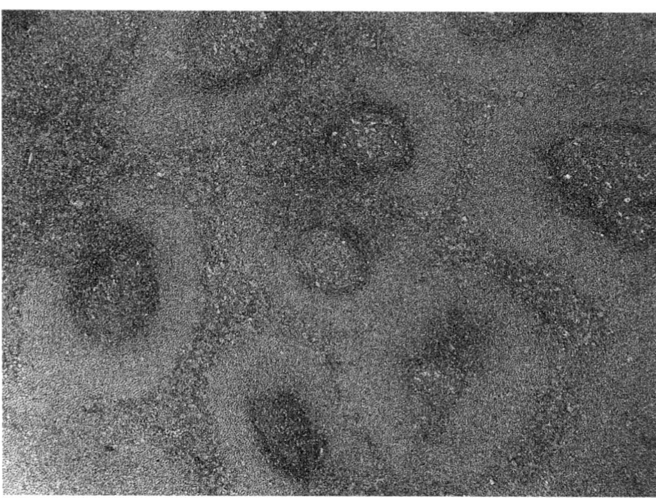

Fig. 21.87 Lymph node involvement by marginal zone B-cell lymphoma. There are numerous residual germinal centers.

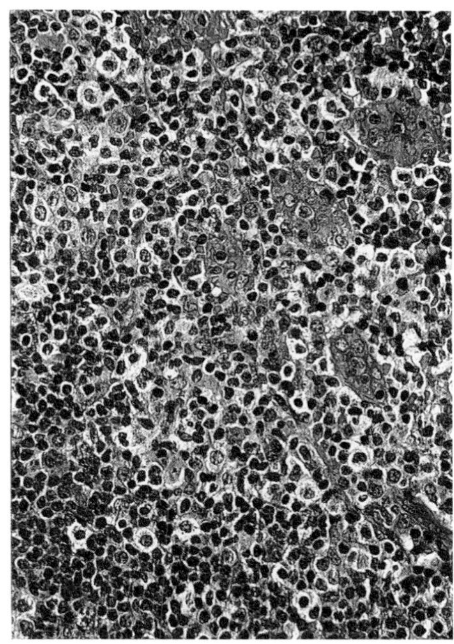

Fig. 21.88 Lymph node involvement by marginal zone B-cell lymphoma. This tumor also affected the thymus gland. *(Courtesy of Dr John Chan, Hong Kong)*

   This tumor was originally described at extranodal sites in relation to mucosae or glandular epithelia, such as gastrointestinal tract, salivary and lacrimal glands, lung, thyroid, conjunctiva, bladder, and skin. It characteristically remains localized for a long time and has a tendency to relapse in the same or other epithelium-containing extranodal sites. It is now believed that many of the extranodal processes described years ago as pseudolymphomas of the lung, stomach, skin, and other sites are examples of this process. Patients may suffer from autoimmune disorders such as Sjögren disease and Hashimoto thyroiditis.

   Immunohistochemically, the cells of MALT lymphoma are B cells with immunoglobulin light chain restriction. There are currently no specific positive cell markers that separate MALT lymphoma from the other low-grade B-cell lymphomas listed at the beginning of this section. However, as a group they usually do not express CD5, CD23, CD10, or cyclin D1.

Extranodal marginal zone lymphoma shows clonal rearrangements of the immunoglobulin genes. The variable region of the immunoglobulin heavy chain gene is hypermutated, supporting a postgerminal center stage of differentiation.[985] There are usually no rearrangements of the *CCND1*, *BCL2*, and *BCL6* genes.

This lymphoma type exhibits distinctive chromosomal translocations including t(11;18)(q21;q21), t(14;18)(q32;q21), t(1;14)(p22;q32), and t(3;14)(q14;q32), involving *API2-MALT1*, *IGH-MALT1*, *BCL10-IGH*, and *FOXP1-IGH* fusion genes, respectively, and being mutually exclusive.[986,987] The relative frequencies of these translocations in the various anatomic sites is highly variable. For example, *API2-MALT1* occurs predominantly in the gastrointestinal tract and lung; *IGH-MALT1* in the salivary gland, ocular adnexa and skin; and *FOXP1-IGH* in the thyroid and ocular adnexa.[987,992,993] *BCL10-IGH* translocation is very rare.[987] Since the chromosomal translocations are specific for extranodal marginal zone lymphoma, their demonstration, such as by FISH or RT-PCR, can aid in diagnosis and classification, with the caveat that such translocations are found in only about 30% of the cases.[987,992,997] The first three forms of chromosomal translocations all produce the same end result of constitutive activation of NF-κB, which transactivates genes such as cytokines and growth factors important for cellular activation, proliferation, and survival.[970,974]

Trisomy 3 and trisomy 18 are found in some cases, being more frequent in the intestine and salivary gland, and mutually exclusive of the chromosomal translocations.[986,987,992,996] Some cases demonstrate loss of function of *A20*, a negative regulator of the NF-κB pathway, by mutation, deletion, or promoter methylation.[967,972,983]

3 *Splenic marginal zone lymphoma*. Cases of lymphoma involving the marginal zone of the spleen have been reported, sometimes in association with bone marrow and peripheral blood involvement.[981,989] The disease is probably related if not identical to that reported under the term 'splenic lymphoma with villous lymphocytes'.

The distinctive chromosomal translocations of extranodal marginal zone lymphoma are not found in splenic marginal zone lymphoma.[976,994] Various chromosomal abnormalities have been reported, with complete or partial trisomy 3q being the commonest but not specific.[964,971,991] On the other hand, deletion or translocation involving 7q32, found in 40% of cases, is a characteristic chromosomal aberration.[964,978,991] Microarray analysis shows that the expression of three genes (*ILF1, SENATAXIN, CD40*) can help distinguish splenic marginal zone lymphoma from other low-grade B-cell lymphomas.[988]

Diffuse mixed (small and large cell) lymphoma

Diffuse mixed lymphoma is not a specific lymphoma type but a heterogeneous category composed of lymphomas of various types that share a mixed composition of large and small lymphoid cells.[998–1000] It includes: (1) the diffuse mixed cell form of follicular lymphoma; (2) peripheral T-cell lymphoma; (3) lymphoplasmacytic lymphoma with an increased number of immunoblasts (also known as polymorphic immunocytoma); (4) T-cell-rich large B-cell lymphoma; and (5) some examples of marginal zone B-cell lymphoma with an admixture of large cells; and probably others. The differential diagnosis among these various entities is based on a combination of clinical, morphologic, and immunohistochemical criteria (see Table 21.9).

Diffuse large B-cell lymphoma

Diffuse large B-cell lymphoma (DLBCL) is the most complex and heterogeneous of all the non-Hodgkin lymphomas.[1061] The term replaces the old histiocytic lymphoma, which in turn replaced the older reticulum cell sarcoma. It is characterized morphologically by large size of the cells, vesicular nuclei with prominent nucleoli, and relatively abundant cytoplasm, and immunophenotypically by expression of B-lineage markers.

As a group, DLBCL occurs both in children and adults, but mostly in the latter.[1062] In comparison with most other types of lymphoma, it has a greater tendency for extranodal presentation and for being localized at the time of presentation. The progression is rapid and the prognosis is poor if untreated. Indeed, it constitutes a high percentage of so-called aggressive lymphomas.[1033,1035] However, excellent responses have been obtained with multidrug chemotherapy, in particular in combination with rituximab (anti-CD20 therapy).[1003,1012,1031] In more than half of the cases, the tumor is limited to one side of the diaphragm (40%, as opposed to 90% for follicular lymphoma).[1010] Involvement of the bone marrow or liver is less common than in follicular or small lymphocytic lymphomas.[1066] Approximately 40% of the cases present in extranodal sites, such as the digestive system, skin, and skeletal system.[1010] When the liver or spleen is involved, it is usually in the form of scattered large tumor masses instead of the multiple smaller nodules or miliary type seen with the group of lymphomas composed of small lymphocytes. The involved nodes are usually markedly enlarged, homogeneous, individualized, and with little or no necrosis (Fig. 21.89).

Microscopically, the pattern of nodal involvement is by definition diffuse. However, it may be complete or partial, and on occasion it may be interfollicular or sinusal (see below). There is commonly extranodal extension, sometimes with accompanying sclerosis. Mitoses are numerous and a starry sky pattern may be present.

On cytologic grounds, a sharp separation used to be made between tumors composed of germinal center (large cleaved and noncleaved; centroblastic) cells and immunoblastic cells, but that distinction is not much stressed at present, one of the reasons being the poor intra- and interobserver reproducibility. Accordingly, some pathologists simply use the term DLBCL without qualifiers. Others prefer to keep subclassifying them whenever possible into the types listed below, the first one being by far the most common.

Centroblastic. This is regarded as the diffuse counterpart of follicular lymphoma of large cell type (grade 3) and is thought to be more aggressive.[1071] It is composed of an admixture in varying proportions of cleaved and noncleaved large cells (Fig. 21.90). When the latter predominate, the distinction with the immunoblastic variant described below becomes particularly difficult. The subtle differences are the lighter-staining and less pyroninophilic cytoplasm, the more peripheral location of the nucleoli, the absence of plasmacytoid differentiation, the presence of scattered small and large cleaved cells, and the presence of a coexisting component of follicular lymphoma.[1041]

Immunoblastic. In this form, the predominant tumor cell has the appearance of an immunoblast: large vesicular nucleus with prominent central nucleolus and thick nuclear membrane, and a deeply staining amphophilic and pyroninophilic cytoplasm with a distinct nuclear hof (Fig. 21.91). Some of the cells are binucleated or multinucleated and simulate Reed–Sternberg cells, and others acquire plasmacytoid features (cartwheel chromatin, larger

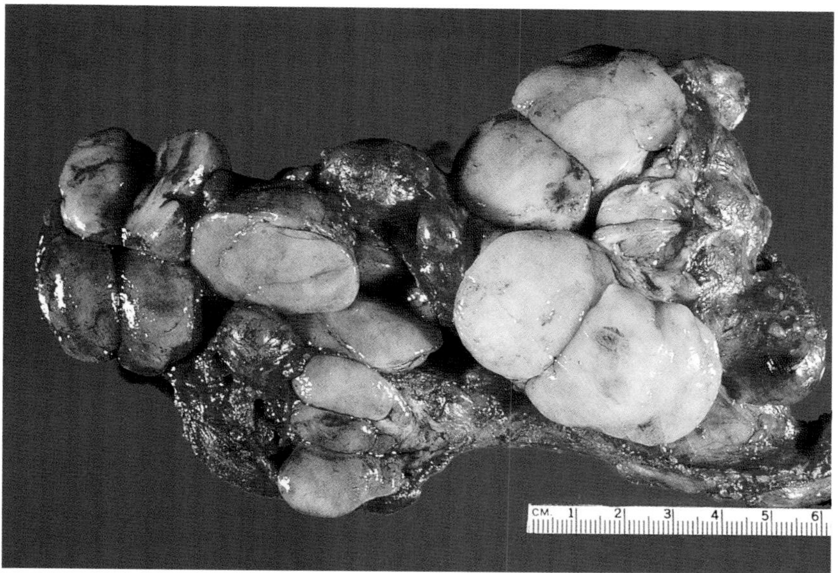

Fig. 21.89 Gross appearance of lymph nodes involved by non-Hodgkin lymphoma of diffuse large B-cell type. The nodes are enlarged and show a homogeneous tan cut surface.

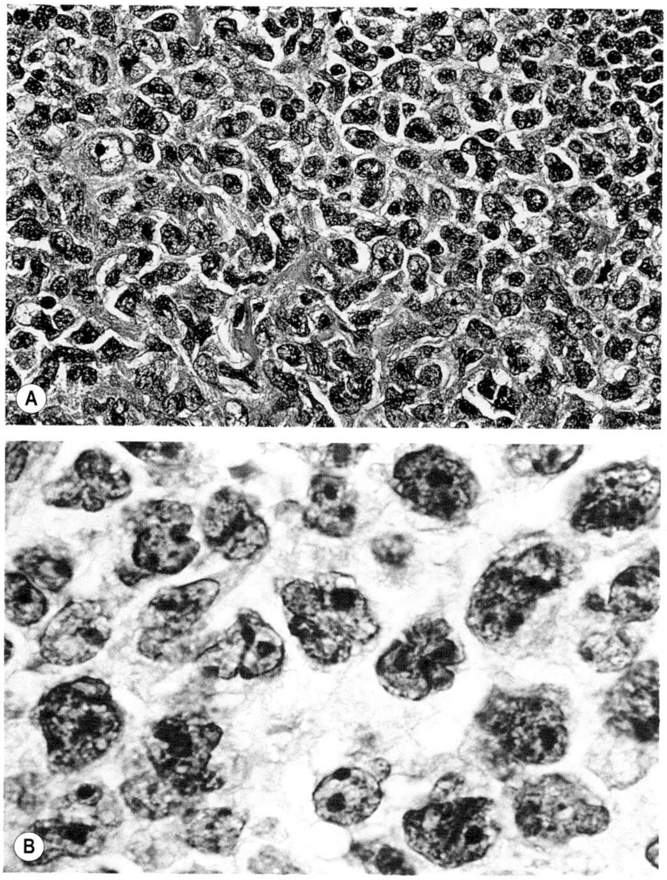

Fig. 21.90 Medium- (**A**) and high-power (**B**) views of diffuse large B-cell lymphoma of large cleaved type.

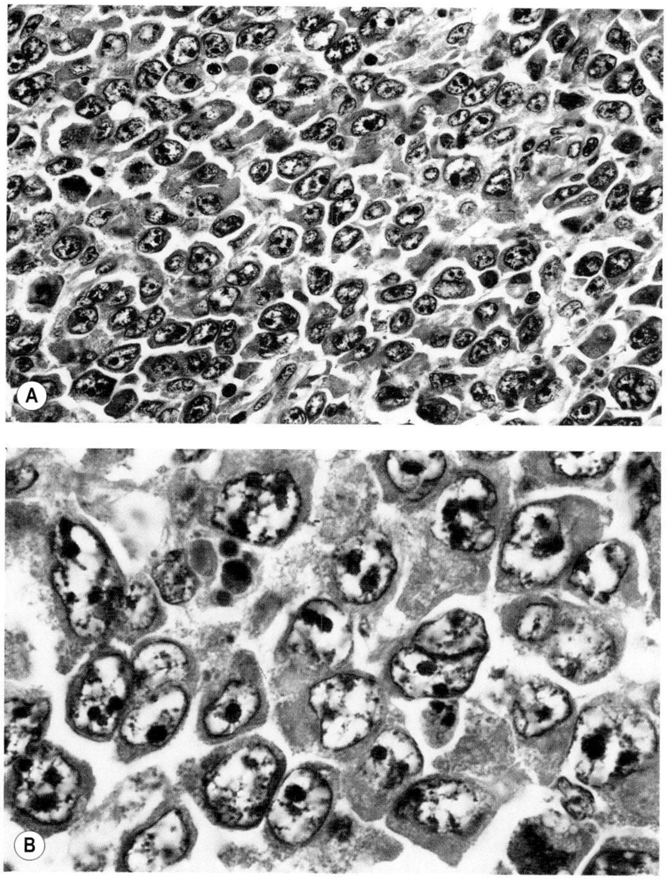

Fig. 21.91 Medium- (**A**) and high-power (**B**) views of diffuse large B-cell lymphoma of immunoblastic type.

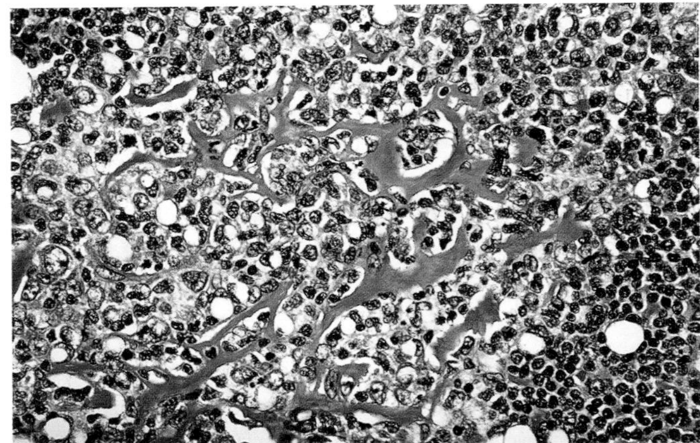

Fig. 21.92 Marked sclerosis and hyalinization in diffuse large B-cell lymphoma.

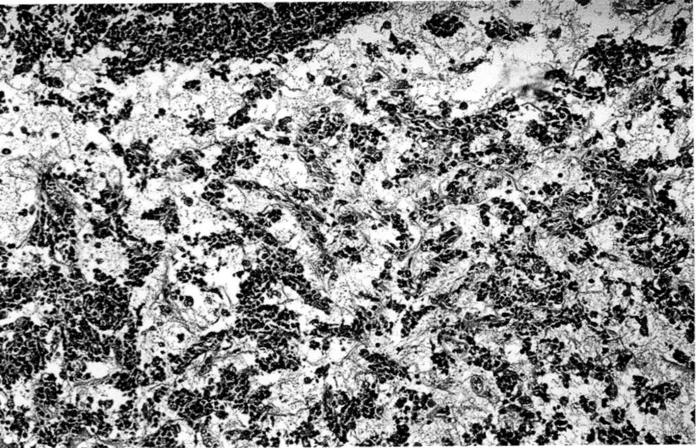

Fig. 21.93 Myxoid stromal change in diffuse large B-cell lymphoma. This is an exceptional occurrence.

perinuclear hof). Immunoperoxidase staining often shows intracytoplasmic immunoglobulin. Immunoblastic lymphoma is the most common subtype of diffuse large B-cell lymphoma arising on the basis of natural immunodeficiency, immunosuppression, immunoproliferative states (such as angioimmunoblastic lymphadenopathy), and other immune-mediated diseases, such as Hashimoto thyroiditis, Sjögren disease, and lupus erythematosus.[1036]

Anaplastic. This rare variant is characterized by the presence of large bizarre tumor cells, some resembling Reed–Sternberg cells, often growing in a cohesive pattern and/or sinusal pattern mimicking carcinoma. Despite the obvious morphologic similarities, this tumor is biologically unrelated to the anaplastic large cell lymphoma (a T-cell neoplasm) discussed on page 1840.

Morphologic variants. Numerous morphologic variations on the theme of DLBCL have been described, some of a cytologic and others of an architectural/topographic nature. Some of them relate to the lymphoma types described above and others do not. Most of these variations do not have an impact on therapy or prognosis, but they are important because they may result in a mistaken diagnosis. They include the following:

1 *Sclerosis*. Diffuse large cell lymphomas can undergo marked sclerosing changes, similar to those seen in follicular lymphomas[1004,1056,1057,1067] (Fig. 21.92). This material is mainly composed of types I, III, and V collagen and fibronectin.[1043] Sclerosis is a particularly common feature in mediastinal (thymic) large B-cell lymphomas (see Chapter 8).
2 *Spindling of tumor cells*. This phenomenon, which is probably related to the aforementioned fibrosis, seems to be more common in large cell lymphomas of mediastinum and bone, but it can be seen in any location, including lymph nodes.[1068] It is thought to be related to the presence of markers characteristic of a germinal center B-cell origin.[1008]
3 Presence of a *myxoid stroma* that can simulate the appearance of myxoid malignant fibrous histiocytoma or myxoid chondrosarcoma[1019,1065] (Fig. 21.93).
4 *Rosette formation*. This peculiar change, originally described in follicular lymphoma, has also been seen in large cell lymphoma. Ultrastructural studies have shown that the material in the center of the rosettes is made up of complex cell prolongations.[1064]
5 *Filiform cell prolongations*. This phenomenon, which is probably related to that described in the previous paragraph, is appreciable in ultrastructural preparations and is similar to that sometimes seen in carcinomas, mesotheliomas, and other neoplasms. Large cell lymphomas exhibiting this spectacular feature have been designated anemone cell, microvillous, filiform cell, villiform cell, and porcupine lymphomas.[1005,1051]
6 *Signet ring features*. This alteration, which is more common in follicular lymphoma, is rarely seen in large cell lymphoma and may simulate metastatic adenocarcinoma.[1073]
7 *Sinusal pattern of spread*, in which the tumor cells are predominantly or entirely confined to the lymph node sinuses (and therefore should be referred to as sinusal rather than sinusoidal) resulting in an appearance closely simulating that of metastatic carcinoma, malignant melanoma, or anaplastic large cell lymphoma[1031,1052] (Fig. 21.94).
8 *Interfollicular pattern of growth*. This is more common in T-cell tumors but has also been described in B-cell neoplasms.
9 *Nuclear multilobation*. Although originally thought to be a feature of T-cell tumors, this alteration is now known to be more common in B-cell neoplasms.[1048,1072]

Immunophenotypically, DLBCL is by definition positive for B-lineage markers (most importantly CD20) and variably immunoglobulin (surface or cytoplasmic).[1011] The follicle center cell markers CD10 and BCL6 are expressed in 40% and 60% of cases, respectively. A proportion of cases express postgerminal center cell or plasma cell-associated markers such as CD38, VS38, and MUM1. About 50% of cases express BCL2 protein. A minority of DLBCLs express CD30, usually in a heterogeneous pattern. CD5 is expressed in 10% of cases. Ki-67 staining usually shows a high proliferation index, with some cases showing an index approaching 100%. An exceptionally rare occurrence is immunoreactivity for cytokeratin, which may lead the unwary to a misdiagnosis of carcinoma.[1032]

DLBCLs show rearrangements of the immunoglobulin genes as expected for a B-lineage neoplasm. The variable region of the immunoglobulin heavy chain gene (*IGH*) is usually hypermutated, with some cases also showing ongoing somatic mutations, indicating a germinal center or postgerminal center stage of B-cell differentiation.[1040]

There are at least two different molecular pathways in the genesis of DLBCL: a transformation pathway and a *de novo* pathway:

1 Approximately 20% of cases of DLBCLs show *BCL2* rearrangement due to t(14;18)(q32;q21), a hallmark of follicular lymphoma.[1020,1023,1074] Such cases may have transformed from a known or occult follicular lymphoma, or may have even directly evolved to DLBCL without a precursor

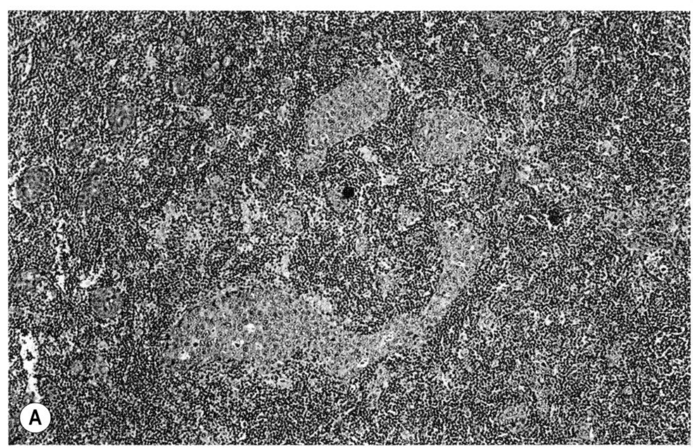

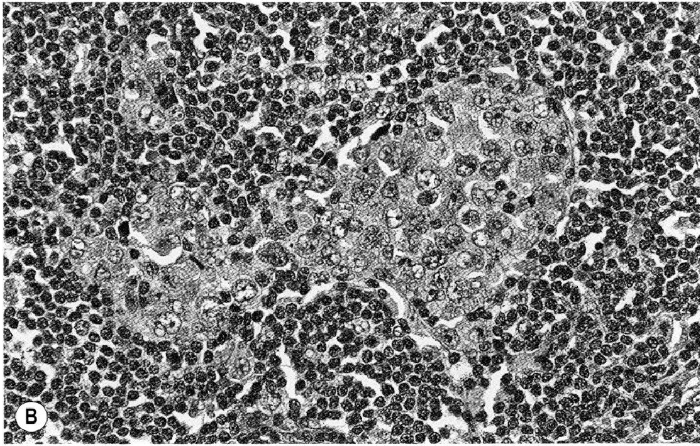

Fig. 21.94 A and **B**, Large B-cell lymphoma with a sinusal pattern of growth that simulates a metastatic tumor.

phase of follicular lymphoma. However, additional genetic alterations are required for the development of DLBCL, such as *TP53* mutation.

2 The *BCL6* gene encodes a transcription factor essential for formation of secondary lymphoid follicles and T-cell-dependent antibody responses, and its aberrant expression plays an important role in the *de novo* pathway of DLBCL formation. In about 35% of cases of DLBCLs, translocation of *BCL6* (3q27) with a variety of partner genes (with *IGH* gene located on 14q32 being the commonest) results in constitutive overexpression of BCL6 protein, causing a sustained proliferative setting in which additional mutations can occur.[1038,1049,1053,1060] This translocation is not specific for DLBCL, but is also found in a subset of follicular lymphomas.[1006,1022] In addition, about 75% of cases of DLBCLs show somatic mutations in the 5′ noncoding regions of the *BCL6* gene, a phenomenon also commonly observed in other germinal center and postgerminal center B-cell lymphomas.[1007,1044] At least some of the mutations result in deregulation of *BCL6* expression.[1069] These mutations, occurring independent of *BCL6* translocation, are generated by the same somatic hypermutation mechanism that targets the variable regions of immunoglobulin genes.[1054,1055]

Gene expression profiling studies can identify two major groups of DLBCLs:[1001,1025,1026,1034,1058,1063] (1) germinal center B-cell-like (GCB) DLBCL that expresses genes characteristic of germinal center B cells, and is correlated with presence of t(14;18) translocation and *C-REL* amplification; and (2) activated B-cell-like (ABC) DLBCL that expresses genes normally induced during in vitro activation of peripheral blood B cells, and is correlated with presence of *BCL6* translocation, *PRDM1/BLIMP1* inactivation, and constitutive activation of NFκB due to somatic mutations in genes encoding the NFκB pathway components, such as *A20/TNFAIP3* and *CARD11*.[1034] The GCB group is associated with a better prognosis than the ABC group, with 5-year overall survival of 60% versus 35% with CHOP or CHOP-like therapy.[1058] However, currently it is not a requirement to distinguish between these two groups of DLBCLs, because reproducible techniques applicable in the diagnostic laboratories are not yet available. A promising marker for the GCB group is *LMO2*, which can be studied by measuring the mRNA level or immunostaining for protein.[1046,1047,1058]

MYC (8q24) translocation is found in up to 10% of DLBCLs.[1027,1029,1030,1042] In contrast to Burkitt lymphoma, the *MYC* gene is usually fused with a nonimmunoglobulin gene, and the karyotype is complex. *MYC* translocation is associated with a highly aggressive behavior.[1024]

There are several types of DLBCL with distinctive clinicopathologic features, listed below.

Primary mediastinal (thymic) large B-cell lymphoma. See Chapter 8.

Intravascular large B-cell lymphoma (angiotropic lymphoma).[1075] This systemic malignant disease, originally regarded as a multicentric malignant transformation of endothelial cells and designated as malignant angioendotheliomatosis, is now known to be a type of malignant lymphoma with a remarkable tropism for blood vessels[1045] (see Chapter 4).

T-cell/histiocyte-rich large B-cell lymphoma. In this type, the neoplastic B-cell population is overshadowed by a reactive population of T cells (Fig. 21.95). There may also be a population of histiocytes, this being the reason why, in the WHO classification, this variant is referred to as *T cell/histiocyte rich*.[1037,1070] The tumor cells may represent less than 10% of the entire cell population. The pattern of growth is predominantly diffuse and there may be a fine interstitial fibrosis. The main differential diagnosis is with NLPHL, with which it shares many phenotypic features,[1059] and which could be legitimately viewed as a special type of T-cell-rich B-cell lymphoma. As a matter of fact, some authors have questioned the validity of separating the two entities.[1014] It would seem, though, that there are enough clinical, morphologic, and molecular genetic differences to keep them apart for the time being. To wit, T-cell/histiocyte-rich large B-cell lymphoma is clinically more aggressive,[1017] has a different pattern of follicular dendritic cell staining,[1016] and is said to have a different genetic pattern on comparative genomic hybridization.[1018]

Primary DLBCL of the central nervous system. See Chapter 28.

Primary cutaneous DLBCL, leg type. This form of DLBCL is composed exclusively of large transformed B cells (with no admixed centrocytes), most commonly arising in the skin of the leg and less commonly in other cutaneous sites (10–15%). The tumor is moderately aggressive. The most common immunophenotype is: pan-B+, CD10−, BCL2+, BCL6+, MUM1+, FOXP1+, and cytoplasmic IgM+.[1028]

DLBCL associated with chronic inflammation. This variant occurs in the context of long-standing chronic inflammation, and shows consistent association with EBV.[1011] Most cases involve body cavities or narrow spaces, with the prototype being pyothorax-associated lymphoma, which involves the pleural cavity of patients with long-standing pyothorax.[1002] Occasional cases are discovered incidentally in surgical specimens, such as splenic cyst, hydrocele sac, and atrial myxoma.[1039]

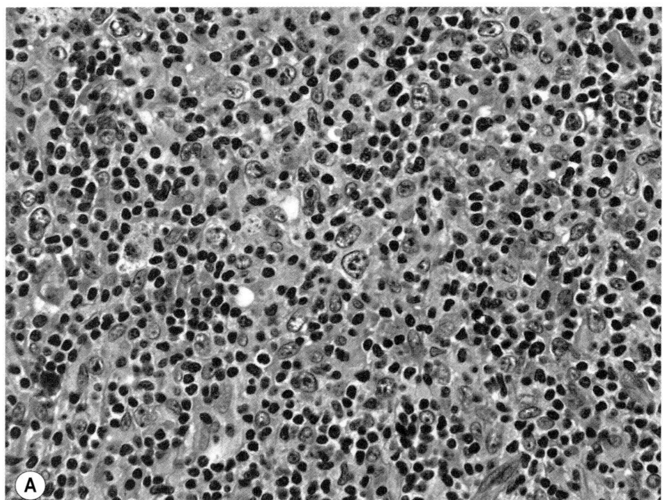

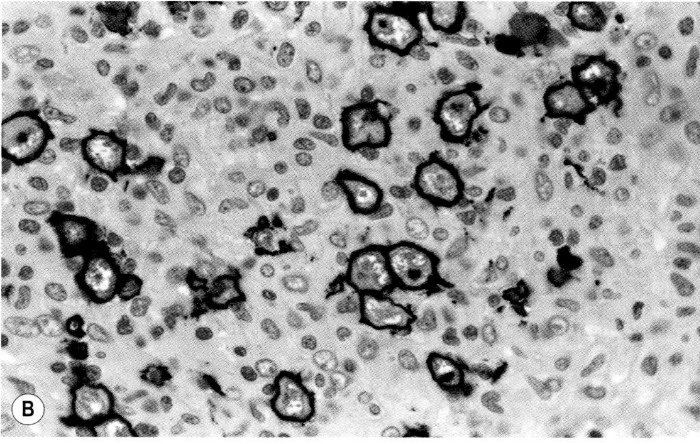

Fig. 21.95 T-cell-rich large B-cell lymphoma: **A**, hematoxylin–eosin; **B**, membrane and Golgi-type immunoreactivity for CD20 in the large tumor cells.

EBV-positive DLBCL of the elderly. This is a type of DLBCL that occurs in adults aged over 50 years, without overt underlying immunodeficiency, and by definition harboring EBV. This is a diagnosis of exclusion, in the sense that a case will not be classified as such if it fits other defined DLBCL entities (such as DLBCL associated with chronic inflammation).

Plasmablastic lymphoma. Plasmablastic lymphoma is a B-cell neoplasm that corresponds to the differentiation stage between a B immunoblast and a plasma cell.[1011] It is an incompletely characterized entity without universal agreement on the minimum diagnostic criteria. Notwithstanding, this is an important type of DLBCL to recognize because it poses significant diagnostic problems (the diagnosis can be difficult because conventional lymphoid markers are not uncommonly all negative) and has therapeutic implications (probably not responsive to rituximab due to lack of CD20 expression). Plasmablastic lymphoma is highly aggressive. It can affect HIV-infected subjects (most commonly oral cavity) or immunocompetent subjects, either involving lymph node or extranodal sites. Conceptually, there are several subgroups with similar morphology and immunophenotype:[1013] (1) ALK+ large B-cell lymphoma; (2) primary effusion lymphoma; and (3) plasmablastic lymphoma, not otherwise specified. However, by convention the first two subgroups (see below) are not labeled as plasmablastic lymphoma. Morphologically, plasmablastic lymphoma comprises large cells with vesicular nuclei, single centrally located prominent nucleolus or multiple peripheral nucleoli, abundant basophilic cytoplasm, and paranuclear hof. The neoplastic population is monomorphic or shows admixed immature plasma cells. The immunophenotype mirrors that of normal plasma cells, being CD45–, CD20–, CD79a+/–, PAX5–, CD38+, VS38c+, CD138+, MUM1+. There is variable expression of cytoplasmic immunoglobulin. EBV is positive in 60–75% of cases, and HHV8 is positive in a small proportion of cases. In practice, it is extremely difficult to distinguish plasmablastic lymphoma from anaplastic/plasmablastic plasmacytoma.

ALK+ large B-cell lymphoma. This is an uncommon form of DLBCL with plasmablastic differentiation and a poor prognosis. The tumor cells have an immunoblastic or plasmablastic appearance, and sinusoidal infiltration is common.[1011] Since they can appear deceptively cohesive, they are not uncommonly misinterpreted as carcinoma cells. The immunophenotype is characteristic of plasmablastic lymphoma, CD30 is negative, and IgA is commonly positive. The commonest molecular alteration is t(2;17)(p23;q23), which fuses the *ALK* gene with the *CLTC* gene.[1015,1021] Since *CLTC* encodes a granule-associated protein, immunostaining for ALK is typically in the form of cytoplasmic granules. Rare cases exhibit t(2;5) with *NPM–ALK* fusion as in ALK+ ALCL, and ALK immunoreactivity is similarly nuclear–cytoplasmic.[1050] EBV and HHV8 are negative.

Primary effusion lymphoma. This is a DLBCL with plasmablastic differentiation, occurring predominantly in patients with AIDS, and showing a strong association with HHV8 and EBV. A solid tissue counterpart also exists[1009] (see Chapter 7).

Peripheral (post-thymic) T-cell and NK-cell lymphomas

Peripheral (post-thymic) T-cell and NK-cell lymphoma is the generic group given to a family of tumors composed of neoplastic lymphocytes with phenotypic and genotypic features of mature T cells or NK cells.[1079,1109] This is an extremely heterogeneous group of lesions, many of them occurring primarily at extranodal sites, and which have received a myriad of designations. Most of them were identified as entities long before their peripheral T-cell or NK-cell nature was ascertained. They include:

- *Mycosis fungoides* and *Sézary syndrome* (see Chapter 4)
- *NK/T-cell lymphoma, nasal type,* which includes most of the cases traditionally diagnosed as lethal midline granuloma[1084,1089] (see Chapter 7)
- *Enteropathy-associated T-cell lymphoma,* which includes most of the cases of intestinal lymphoma arising as a complication of celiac disease (see Chapter 11)
- *Hepatosplenic T-cell lymphoma* (see Chapters 13 and 22)
- *Subcutaneous panniculitis-like T-cell lymphoma* (see Chapter 4)
- *Angioimmunoblastic T-cell lymphoma* has already been discussed with *angioimmunoblastic lymphadenopathy* in the section on reactive/inflammatory conditions (see p. 1798). While angioimmunoblastic T-cell lymphoma expectedly shows clonal rearrangements of the T-cell receptor genes in most cases, it is unique among mature T-cell lymphomas in that up to 40% of cases show simultaneous clonal rearrangements of the immunoglobulin genes, probably attributable to the frequent presence of an EBV-driven B-cell proliferation as a result of the lymphoma-associated immunologic disturbance.[1090,1103] In some patients, the B-cell proliferation can evolve into an overt large B-cell lymphoma.[1076,1111]

Chromosomal alterations in angioimmunoblastic T-cell lymphoma are common but nondistinctive, such as +3, +5, +18, +19, +21, +X, −6q, and −7.[1090,1094,1101,1108] The gene expression profile shows a strong contribution by the admixed follicular dendritic cells, B cells and stromal components, as well as overexpression of genes characteristic of normal follicular helper T cells.[1080,1085,1097]

- The tumor type originally described by Lennert as malignant lymphoma with a constantly high number of epithelioid cells and variously known as *Lennert lymphoma* and *lymphoepithelioid lymphoma*.[1078,1091,1096] It occurs in adults, is often generalized (74% of the patients have stage IV disease at presentation), and the prognosis is poor.[1087,1104] Microscopically, there is effacement of the architecture by a lymphohistiocytic infiltrate, often accompanied by plasma cells and eosinophils and by proliferation of small vessels with plump endothelial cells. The polymorphic nature of the infiltrate and the occasional presence of Reed–Sternberg-like cells often elicit a mistaken diagnosis of Hodgkin lymphoma. The key to the diagnosis resides in the atypical appearance of the small lymphocytes located between the reactive histiocytes (Fig. 21.96). In addition to Hodgkin lymphoma, the differential diagnosis includes angioimmunoblastic lymphadenopathy. Some cases of Lennert lymphoma have been seen to undergo a 'blastic' transformation into a peripheral T-cell lymphoma predominated by large cells.[1088]
- *Adult T-cell leukemia/lymphoma*, an HTLV-1-related pleomorphic T-cell lymphoma occurring in an endemic form in Japan.[1095,1106,1107]
- Miscellaneous peripheral T-cell lymphomas described under the designations of T-cell immunoblastic sarcoma, T-cell lymphoma with multilobated nuclei,[1099] erythrophagocytic T-cell lymphoma,[1092] T-zone lymphoma,[1086] peripheral T-cell lymphoma with perifollicular growth pattern,[1100] and nodal CD8+ cytotoxic T-cell lymphoma[1083,1093] (Fig. 21.97).
- *Anaplastic large cell lymphoma* and its variants (see next section).

Peripheral T-cell and NK-cell lymphomas in general are highly aggressive. Their morphologic features are variable depending on the type, but immunohistochemical studies are always required to confirm their T-cell or NK-cell nature. They are commonly immunoreactive for CD3, CD45RO, CD2, CD5, and CD7, although expression of one or more of these pan–T-cell markers may be lost (so-called aberrant immunophenotype, which is sometimes utilized to support the neoplastic nature of a T-cell proliferation). NK-cell lymphomas are commonly CD2+, CD3+, CD5−, and CD56+. Most cases of peripheral T-cell lymphoma express a CD4+/CD8− mature helper phenotype; approximately 20% express a CD4−/CD8+ cytotoxic/suppressor phenotype, with rare cases having CD4−/CD8− or CD4+/CD8+ phenotypes.

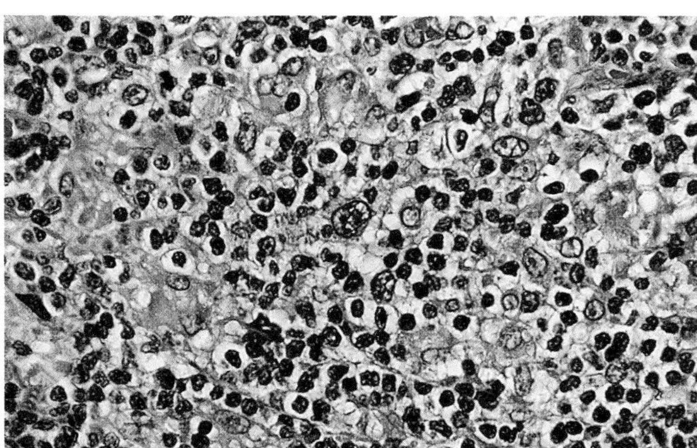

Fig. 21.96 Peripheral T-cell lymphoma with a high content of non-neoplastic histiocytes (so-called 'Lennert lymphoma').

At the molecular level, peripheral T-cell lymphomas exhibit clonal rearrangements of the γ and β T-cell receptor genes, although about 10% of cases may show simultaneous clonal rearrangements of the immunoglobulin heavy chain gene.[1102] Karyotypic aberrations are often complex but nondistinctive. Recurrent chromosomal translocations have been identified in only a minority of cases. t(5;9)(q33;q22), which results in *ITK–SYK* fusion, is associated with a follicular or perifollicular growth pattern, medium-sized or large lymphoma cells with clear cytoplasm, and a germinal center T-helper cell immunophenotype (CD4+, CD10+, BCL6+).[1105] *IRF4/MUM1* translocation, sometimes with the T-cell receptor alpha gene as partner, has been identified in rare cases of peripheral T-cell lymphomas not otherwise specified.[1082]

Peripheral T-cell lymphoma not otherwise specified shows a gene expression profile distinct from that of angioimmunoblastic T-cell lymphoma and anaplastic large cell lymphoma. It shows diverse profiles, indicating that it represents a heterogeneous

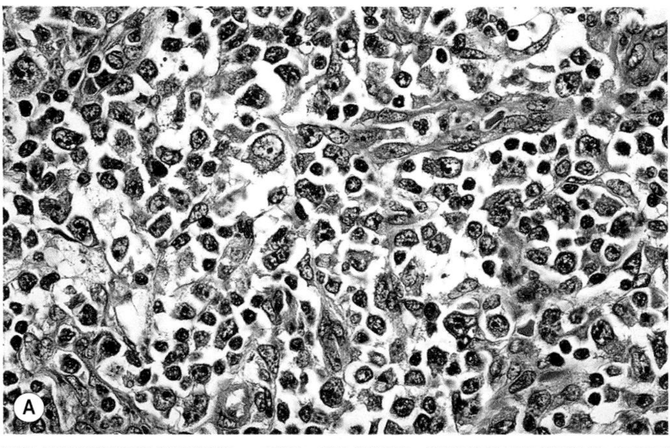

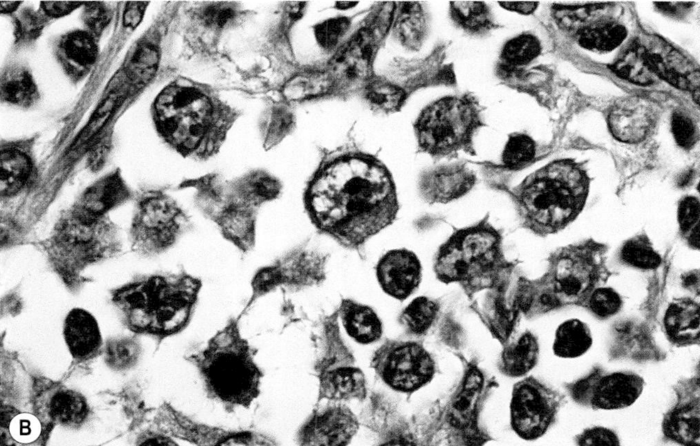

Fig. 21.97 **A** and **B**, Peripheral large T-cell lymphoma in a patient from Japan. Note the polymorphic appearance of the infiltrate and the prominent postcapillary venules.

category.[1077,1085,1098] A proportion of cases (5–11%) show association with EBV, and seem to have a worse prognosis.[1081,1110]

Anaplastic large cell lymphoma

Anaplastic large cell lymphoma (ALCL, also known as Ki-1 lymphoma) is characterized by highly atypical and pleomorphic neoplastic cells with expression of the activation marker CD30.[1112,1124,1142,1143] Although previously a secondary form supervening on other types of lymphoma (such as mycosis fungoides and Hodgkin lymphoma) was recognized in addition to the more common *de novo* (primary) form, currently only the latter is acceptable for the category of ALCL according to the WHO classification. There is also a change from the initial characterization of this entity, in that only cases of T- or null-cell lineage are included in the category of ALCL; cases of B-lineage are simply diagnosed as 'diffuse large B-cell lymphoma, anaplastic variant'.

Clinically, two types of presentation are recognized: a systemic form and a primary cutaneous form (without extracutaneous involvement at the time of presentation).[1116,1120,1127]

Systemic ALCL. The systemic form of ALCL can involve lymph nodes or extranodal sites, such as the bone marrow, bone, respiratory tract, skin, and gastrointestinal tract.[1115,1121,1164] It can occur in children or adults, and is rather aggressive.[1126,1141,1160,1165] Exceptionally, it is accompanied by leukemic manifestations.[1113] Systemic symptoms such as fever can be present. Currently two types are segregated based on ALK expression, owing to differences in clinical features and prognosis. ALK+ ALCL tends to occur in children and young adults, and the outcome is good if appropriate treatment is given. On the other hand, ALK– ALCL tends to occur over a wider age range, especially older adults, and is associated with a poor outcome similar to peripheral T-cell lymphoma not otherwise specified.

Microscopically, the infiltrate has a polymorphic appearance, often with a variable admixture of neutrophils, lymphocytes, and histiocytes, with the highly atypical large lymphoma cells showing marked pleomorphism.[1144] The nuclei of these cells are often horseshoe shaped or multilobed, and nucleoli are prominent. Cells indistinguishable from Reed–Sternberg cells may be seen. The cytoplasm is abundant and eosinophilic. Cohesive growth and preferential sinusal involvement are common (Fig. 21.98). The undue prominence of the latter feature in some cases was one of the reasons for this lesion to be mistakenly placed in the category of malignant histiocytosis. ALCL can also simulate malignant melanoma, undifferentiated carcinoma, and various types of soft tissue sarcoma.[1119]

Several morphologic variants of ALCL (usually ALK+) have been described.

1 *Small cell.* As the name indicates, this shows a predominant population of small to medium-sized cells. A very important clue is the presence of the characteristic large anaplastic cells around blood vessels.[1118,1145] Cases of the small cell variant have been seen to transform into the classic anaplastic large cell form.[1140]
2 *Lymphohistiocytic.* The distinctiveness of this variant results from the presence of a large number of admixed reactive (nonepithelioid) histiocytes[1146,1157,1158] (Fig. 21.99). As for the previous variant, an important diagnostic clue is the clustering of anaplastic tumor cells around vessels.
3 Other morphologic variations of ALCL which do not qualify as bona fide tumor variants are the neutrophil – and/or eosinophil – rich,[1150,1151] sarcomatoid,[1119] giant cell,[1132] signet ring-like,[1131] and hypocellular.[1123]

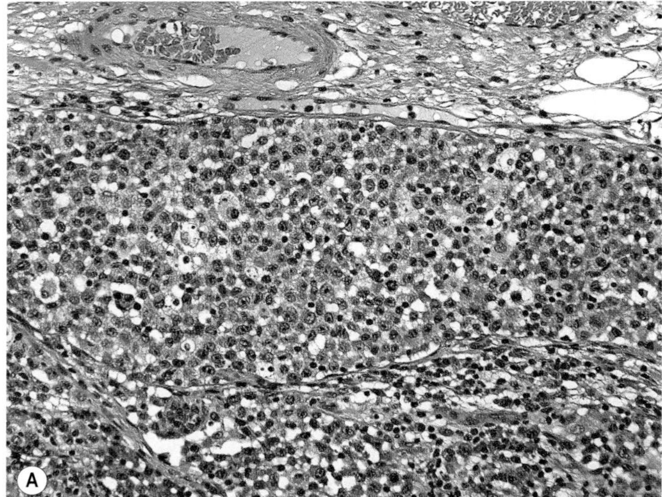

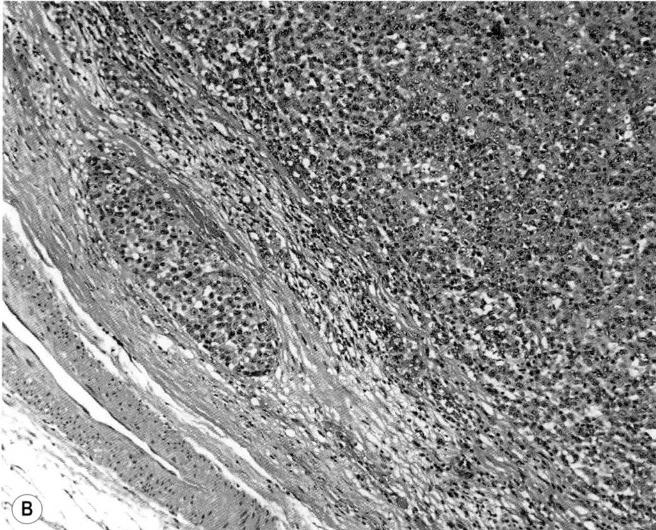

Fig. 21.98 **A** and **B**, Anaplastic large cell lymphoma. **A**, Packing of the peripheral sinus. **B**, Vascular involvement.

Immunohistochemically, the tumor cells of ALCL are by definition CD30+ (Ki-1) positive[1138] (Fig. 21.100). There is also consistent positivity for EMA, interleukin-2 receptor,[1128] clusterin (in a Golgi pattern),[1154] cadherins,[1114,1153] and galectin-3 (a β-galactoside-binding animal lectin).[1147] There is occasional reactivity for keratin.[1137]

There is variable expression of T-lineage markers, and application of a wide panel may be required to have one or two markers staining up. In the so-called null-cell cases, T-lineage markers cannot be demonstrated. B-cell markers are, by definition, absent. The B-cell transcription factor PAX5 is not expressed, and this marker is extremely helpful for distinction of ALCL from classic Hodgkin lymphoma (PAX5+). ALK, by definition, is expressed in ALK+ ALCL, but not in ALK– ALCL (Fig. 21.101).

The T-cell receptor genes are clonally rearranged in approximately 90% of cases of ALK+ ALCL, including cases lacking expression of T-lineage markers.[1129,1163] The hallmark of this lymphoma type is translocation of *ALK* (anaplastic lymphoma kinase gene on 2p23), although this molecular alteration is also found in an uncommon subtype of diffuse large B-cell lymphoma (ALK+ large B-cell

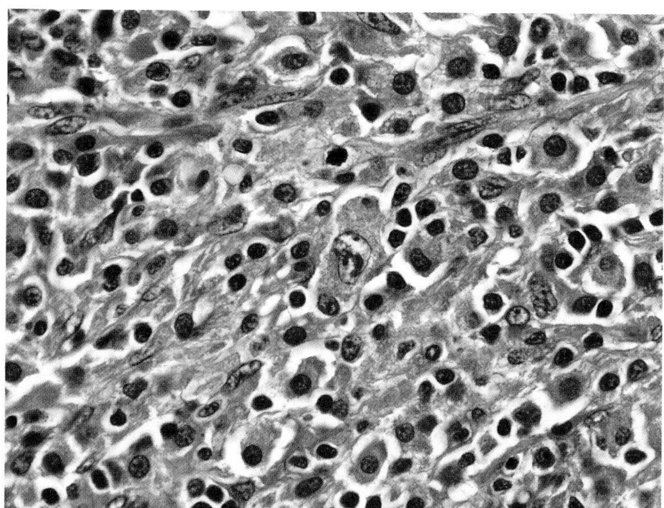

Fig. 21.99 So-called 'lymphohistiocytic variant' of anaplastic large cell lymphoma.

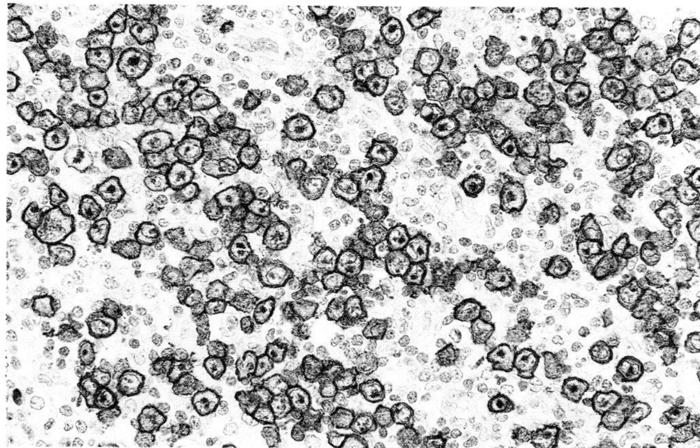

Fig. 21.100 Strong membranous and Golgi-type immunoreactivity for CD30 in anaplastic large cell lymphoma.

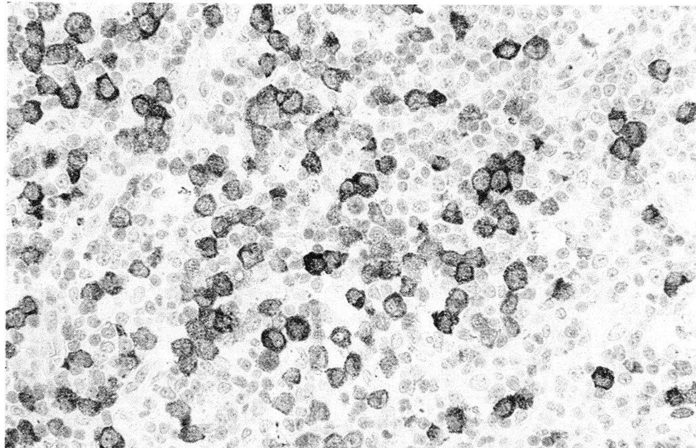

Fig. 21.101 ALK immunoreactivity in anaplastic large cell lymphoma.

lymphoma), ALK+ histiocytosis, inflammatory myofibroblastic tumor and an uncommon subset of pulmonary adenocarcinoma.[1122,1125,1129,1130,1149,1159,1161] The *ALK* gene can be fused with a variety of partner genes, most of which are housekeeping genes.[1162] The translocation results in production of a chimeric protein, in which the ALK domain (a tyrosine kinase receptor) is constitutively activated due to presence of an oligomerization domain at the N-terminus. The commonest partner gene is *NPM* (nucleophosmin gene on 5q35), accounting for 80% of cases. Other partner genes include *TPM3* (tropomyosin-III), *TPM4* (tropomyosin-IV), *TFG* (*TRK* fused gene), *ATIC, CLTL* (clathrin), *MSN* (moesin), *CARS*, and *MYH9*. Interestingly, the subcellular localization of ALK on immunostaining correlates well with the normal distribution of the protein encoded by the partner gene, e.g. nuclear-cytoplasmic staining for nucleophosmin, cytoplasmic staining with subplasmalemmal accentuation for tropomyosin, cell membrane staining for moesin, and cytoplasmic granular staining for clathrin. The partner gene fused with the *ALK* gene does not influence the prognosis of ALK+ anaplastic large cell lymphoma.[1133]

ALCLs with *ALK* translocation have a much more favorable prognosis than ALK– ALCLs.[1129,1133] Gene expression profiling studies have also confirmed that these two types of ALCL represent distinct entities.[1148] EBV is generally negative.[1163]

Primary cutaneous ALCL. The cutaneous form occurs predominantly in adults and has an indolent course, with some of the individual lesions regressing spontaneously.[1117,1136] In retrospect, it should be acknowledged that the cases originally reported as *regressive atypical histiocytosis* and most of the cases diagnosed as malignant histiocytosis belong to this category[1135,1139,1152,1156] (see p. 1845 and Chapter 4). In contrast to systemic ALK+ ALCL, primary cutaneous ALCL does not exhibit *ALK* translocation. Instead, 26–57% of cases show *IRF4/MUM1* translocation, although the partner gene is currently not yet known.[1134,1155]

Lymphoblastic lymphoma

Lymphoblastic lymphoma is seen primarily in children and adolescents, but it also occurs in adults.[1176,1179] It has a distinctive clinical presentation. In approximately half of the cases there is a mediastinal mass in the thymic region (the old Sternberg sarcoma). The clinical course of the untreated disease is extremely aggressive, with rapid multisystem dissemination, leukemic blood picture (acute lymphoblastic leukemia),[1178] and death after a few months.[1172] Grossly, the tumor is whitish and soft and often exhibits foci of hemorrhage and necrosis. Microscopically, there is a diffuse and relatively monomorphic pattern of proliferation, broken only by a focal starry sky appearance in some of the cases. The tumor often extends outside the node or thymus to invade the adipose tissue in a diffuse fashion. Permeation of the wall of blood vessels in a targetoid fashion is another characteristic feature. The neoplastic cells have scanty cytoplasm and a nucleus that has a round contour (instead of the angulated shape typical of follicular lymphoma) but that shows, on close examination, the presence of delicate convolutions resulting from multiple small invaginations of the nuclear membrane (see Chapter 8). Oil-immersion examination of well-prepared, very thin sections is necessary to demonstrate this feature, which may be present in only a small percentage of the tumor cells or sometimes practically absent[1172] (Fig. 21.102). The chromatin is finely stippled, and nucleoli are inconspicuous. Mitotic activity is extremely high. These convoluted cells are similar to the cerebroid cells of mycosis fungoides–Sézary syndrome (as one might assume from their similar names) but differ from the latter because the nuclear membrane is thinner, the chromatin more dispersed, and the invaginations more delicate. Actually, the need for distinction

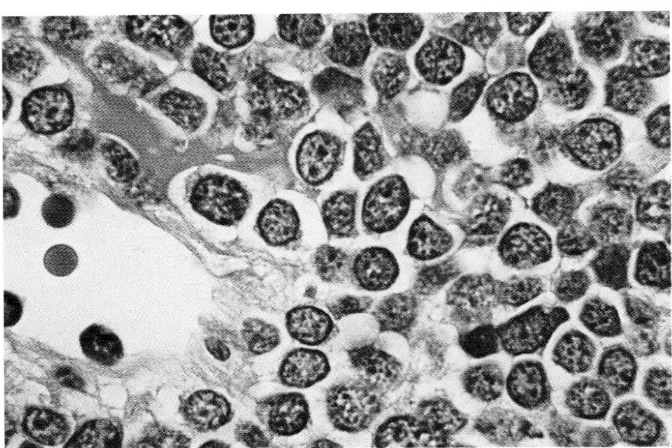

Fig. 21.102 Lymphoblastic lymphoma. In this example the nuclear convolutions are barely evident.

between these two cell types is more theoretical than real because of the fact that the two diseases are vastly different in their clinical presentation.

An *atypical* or *large cell* variant of lymphoblastic lymphoma has been described, which is said to comprise approximately 10% of the cases.[1168]

Remnants of thymus often are found in the mediastinal mass, and this may lead to a mistaken diagnosis of thymoma; in this regard, it should be remembered that thymoma is very infrequent in children and that, when it occurs, it is characterized by a population of small or activated lymphocytes but not convoluted ones. When lymphoblastic lymphoma spreads to lymph nodes, it preferentially involves the paracortical (thymic-dependent) zone.

At the enzyme histochemical level, features of the cells of lymphoblastic lymphoma include the presence of acid phosphatase (focally strong in a paranuclear location, as in normal thymocytes), β-glucuronidase, α-naphthyl acetate esterase,[1177] and terminal deoxynucleotidyl transferase (TdT), a marker of thymocytes.[1167,1169] The latter can also be demonstrated immunohistochemically in paraffin-embedded material.[1173,1180]

Approximately 80–85% of lymphoblastic lymphomas show T-cell markers. Their phenotypes recapitulate those of the various stages of intrathymic T-cell differentiation, i.e., those of the precursor T lymphoblast, hence the choice of the WHO Committee to designate this tumor as precursor T lymphoblastic lymphoma (and as precursor T lymphoblastic leukemia when extensive marrow and peripheral blood involvement are present, an arbitrary distinction).[1175] The immunohistochemical hallmark of lymphoblastic lymphoma is TdT, a marker for precursor lymphoid cells. In approximately 90% of the cases, these tumors express all of the pan-T-antigens, such as CD1, CD2, CD7, cytoplasmic CD3, and CD43. Practically all cases express CD71 (the transferrin receptor antigen), 20% express HLA-DR, and 20% express markers of NK cells, such as CD16 and CD57. Positivity is also consistently encountered for CD99.

In approximately a third of the cases, translocations have been identified involving the alpha and delta T-cell receptor loci at 14q11.2, the beta locus at 7q35, and the gamma locus at 7p14–15 with a variety of partner genes (such as *MYC, TAL1, RBTN1, RBTN2,* and *HOX11*), leading to a dysregulation of transcription of the latter.

In approximately 15–20% of the cases of lymphoblastic lymphoma, the tumor cells express B-cell rather than T-cell markers, such as CD19, CD20, CD21, and CD24.[1181] These tumors are referred to as precursor B lymphoblastic lymphomas (or as precursor B lymphoblastic leukemia if accompanied by extensive bone marrow and peripheral blood involvement) in the WHO classification. These are predominantly extranodal tumors with low propensity for leukemic involvement.[1171] In keeping with their precursor nature, they may express cytoplasmic immunoglobulin but not surface immunoglobulin. Yet other lymphoblastic lymphomas lack both T-cell and B-cell features.[1170]

The differential diagnosis of lymphoblastic lymphoma includes the already mentioned thymoma when in a mediastinal location, as well as Ewing sarcoma/PNET, Burkitt lymphoma, and the blastoid variant of mantle cell lymphoma.[1166,1174,1182,1183]

Burkitt lymphoma

Burkitt lymphoma is a high-grade malignant lymphoma composed of germinal center B cells which can present in three clinical settings:

1 *Endemic.* This occurs in the equatorial strip of Africa and is the most common form of childhood malignancy in this area. The patients characteristically present with jaw and orbital lesions. Involvement of the gastrointestinal tract, ovaries, kidney, and breast are also common.
2 *Sporadic.* This is seen throughout the world. It affects mainly children and adolescents, and has a greater tendency for involvement of the abdominal cavity than the endemic form.[1203]
3 *Immunodeficiency-associated.* This is seen primarily in association with HIV infection and often occurs as the initial manifestation of the disease.[1190,1205]

In all three forms peripheral lymphadenopathy is rare and, when present, usually limited to a single group.[1184,1185] Bone marrow involvement is common in the late stage of the disease, but leukemic manifestations are very rare.[1201,1203]

Microscopically, the pattern of growth of Burkitt lymphoma is usually diffuse, although early cases may show preferential involvement of germinal centers.[1200] The tumor cells are medium sized (10–25 μm) and round. The nuclei are round or oval and have *several* prominent basophilic nucleoli. The chromatin is coarse and the nuclear membrane is rather thick. The cytoplasm is easily identifiable; it is amphophilic in hematoxylin–eosin-stained preparations and strongly pyroninophilic. Fat-containing small vacuoles are present; these are particularly well appreciated in touch preparations. Mitoses are numerous, and a prominent starry sky pattern is the rule, although by no means pathognomonic[1186] (Fig. 21.103). There are also many admixed apoptotic bodies. In well-fixed material, the cytoplasm of individual cells 'squares off', forming acute angles in which the membranes of adjacent cells abut on each other. Occasionally, the tumor is accompanied by a florid granulomatous reaction.[1192] Ultrastructurally, the main features are abundant ribosomes, frequent lipid inclusions, lack of glycogen particles, and presence of nuclear pockets or projections[1187] (Fig. 21.104).

Two morphologic variants of Burkitt lymphoma are recognized. In the form with *plasmacytoid differentiation,* which is more common in HIV-related cases, some tumor cells exhibit eccentric basophilic cytoplasm containing immunoglobulin and a single central nucleolus. In the *atypical* or *pleomorphic* form, the cell size is larger and a distinct pleomorphism is evident.[1199] Most of the cells have a well-defined rim of cytoplasm; their nucleus contains a large, eosinophilic nucleolus. Binucleated and multinucleated cells are common. Phagocytosis of nuclear debris by reactive histiocytes is as common as in the classic form, resulting in a starry sky appearance. The pattern of growth is generally diffuse, but areas of minimal

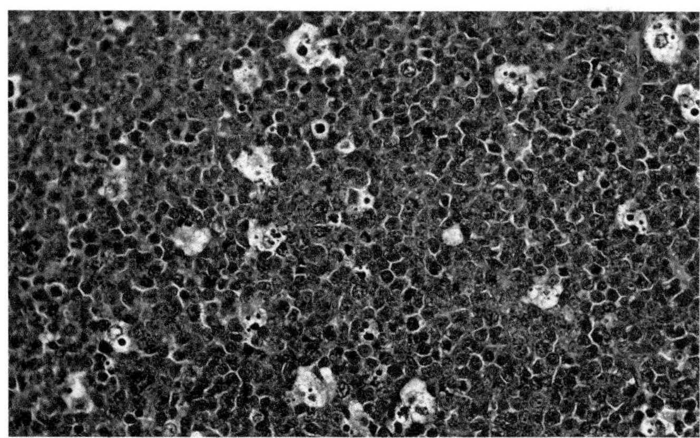

Fig. 21.103 Burkitt lymphoma with characteristic starry sky appearance.

nodularity may be encountered. Clinically, gastrointestinal involvement is less common and bone marrow involvement more frequent than in the classic form. The clinical course is said to be more aggressive[1184,1185,1199] although the response to therapy is similar.[1206] In the 2008 WHO classification, it is recommended that the term 'atypical Burkitt lymphoma' be dropped; a case would be simply classified as 'Burkitt lymphoma' if the immunophenotypic and genotypic features are compatible.

Burkitt lymphomas are of B-cell lineage. They express immunoglobulins (predominantly IgM), invariably associated with heavy and light chain restriction.[1191] B-cell-specific antigens (such as CD19, CD20, and CD22) and B-cell-associated antigens (such as CD24 and HLA-DR) are present. Most cases also express the germinal center cell markers CD10 and BCL6.[1193] They are negative for the activation markers CD25 and CD30. In contrast to lymphoblastic lymphoma, they do not express TdT. The most helpful immunohistochemical profile to aid in diagnosis of Burkitt lymphoma includes

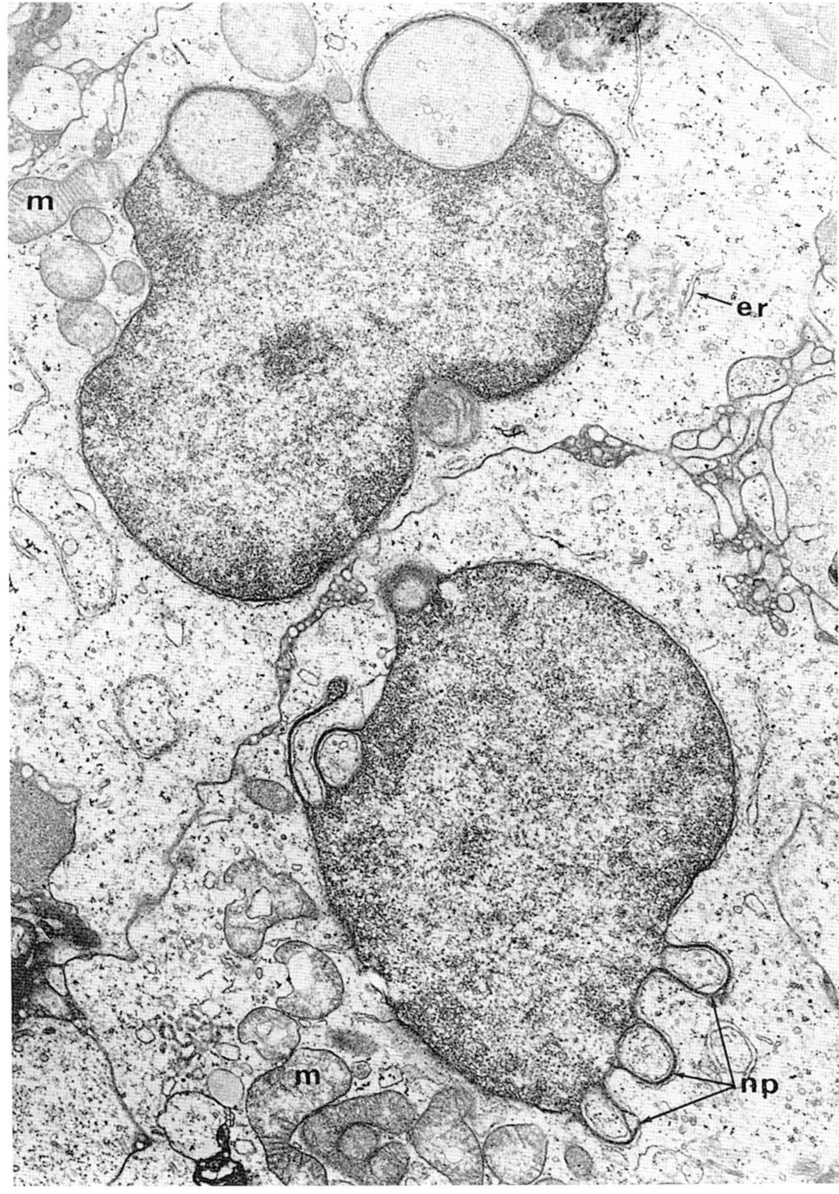

Fig. 21.104 These neoplastic cells from a patient with Burkitt lymphoma have numerous peculiar, though not unique, nuclear projections (np), polar aggregation of mitochondria (m), sparse endoplasmic reticulum (er), and scattered ribosomes.

CD20+, CD10+, BCL2– (although weak staining can be seen in some cases), and a Ki-67 index over 95%.

As expected of a B-lineage neoplasm, Burkitt lymphoma shows clonal rearrangements of the immunoglobulin genes. The hallmark genetic change is t(8;14), t(2;8), or t(8;22), which fuses the *MYC* gene with an immunoglobulin heavy chain, kappa light chain, or lambda light chain gene.[1198] As a result, the *MYC* gene is overexpressed, promoting cell cycle progression and inhibiting differentiation.[1188] However, *MYC* translocation is not entirely specific for Burkitt lymphoma; it can also be observed in transformed follicular lymphomas, rare cases of diffuse large B-cell lymphoma, and the highly lethal 'double-hit' lymphomas (with presence of both *MYC* and *BCL2* translocation).[1195–1197,1202,1204] In contrast to Burkitt lymphoma, the translocation partner of *MYC* in the latter lymphoma types is commonly a gene other than the immunoglobulin gene, and the karyotype is usually more complex.[1195]

Gene expression profiling has recently been shown to be a superior technology for identifying 'true' Burkitt lymphomas (so-called molecular Burkitt lymphomas), some cases of which are missed even by expert hematopathologists.[1189,1195] Nonetheless, this is still a research tool. Currently, if cytogenetic data are not available, FISH studies are most helpful for supporting a diagnosis of Burkitt lymphoma, especially when the morphology is not classic and in adults, to demonstrate presence of *MYC* translocation (preferably confirmed to be with an immunoglobulin gene) together with absence of *BCL2* and *BCL6* translocations.[1194]

There is an association of Burkitt lymphoma with EBV, with frequencies of approximately 100% for the endemic type, 20–30% for the sporadic type, and 25–40% for the immunodeficiency-associated type (Fig. 21.105).[1198] The EBV shows type I latency, i.e., EBER and EBNA1 are expressed, while LMP1 and EBNA2 are negative.

Other non-Hodgkin lymphomas

Types of non-Hodgkin malignancies of the lymphoid system other than those already described include the following:

1. *Leukemias* and *myeloma* (see Chapter 23).
2. *Lymphomatoid granulomatosis* (see Chapter 7).
3. *Hairy cell leukemia*. This entity is fully discussed in Chapter 22. Suffice it to say here that the lymph nodes can be involved by the disease and that this involvement is characterized by diffuse infiltration of the subcapsular sinuses, cortex, and medullary cords by typical small mononuclear cells having nuclei slightly larger than those of lymphocytes, fine chromatin pattern, relatively abundant cytoplasm, and essentially no mitotic activity (Fig. 21.106). Despite the extensiveness of the infiltrate, the nodal architecture is partially preserved.[1207]
4. *Lymphoma of plasmacytoid dendritic cells*. These were formerly known as plasmacytoid T-cell or plasmacytoid monocytic lymphomas.[1208,1209]
5. The various types of primarily extranodal T-cell lymphomas listed on page 1838.

Composite and discordant lymphomas

In general, there is constancy within the various types of malignant lymphoma, so that a patient with a certain type of lymphoma at a given site will have the same type at other sites and will maintain it during the entire evolution of the disease. However, on occasion one encounters two distinct types of lymphoma in the same patient, either sequentially or simultaneously, even in the same lymph node. The occurrence of two different and well-delineated varieties of lymphoma occurring in a single anatomic site or mass is known as *composite lymphoma*, and the occurrence of two different types of lymphoma at separate anatomic sites has been referred to as *discordant lymphoma*.[1215,1228] Some of these combinations may represent the occurrence of two unrelated neoplasms, either spontaneously or as a result of the therapy given for one of them. The majority, however, are probably the result of different biologic and morphologic manifestations of the same lesion, the more malignant one representing the morphologic expression of tumor progression.[1229,1238] Most of these examples of this progression are discussed in connection with the corresponding tumor types, but we thought it would be useful to list the most important manifestations of this phenomenon:

1. Low-grade B-cell lymphoma (small lymphocytic, follicular, or T-cell-rich B-cell lymphoma) that transforms into a diffuse large B-cell lymphoma.[1211,1216,1233,1235,1237,1242]
2. Transformation of mantle cell lymphoma into a higher-grade tumor ('blastic transformation').[1230]
3. Low-grade T-cell lymphoma (such as mycosis fungoides) that transforms into a large T-cell lymphoma (see Chapter 4).[1213,1218,1221,1234,1239]
4. Combination of NLPHL and other lymphomas, particularly diffuse large cell lymphoma.[1220,1222–1224]

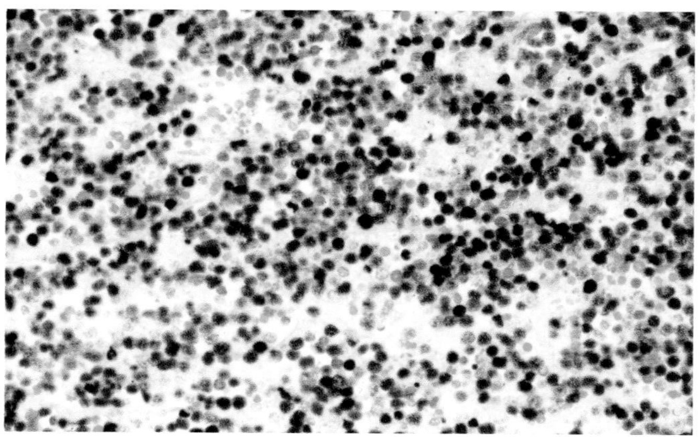

Fig. 21.105 Presence of EBV genome in Burkitt lymphoma, as demonstrated with in situ hybridization for EBER.

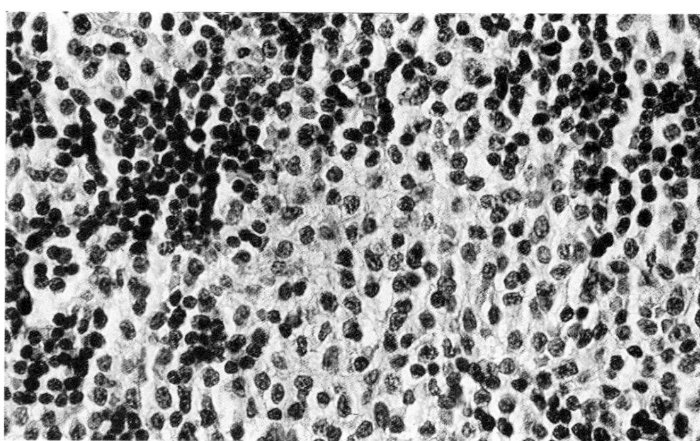

Fig. 21.106 Lymph node involvement by hairy cell leukemia.

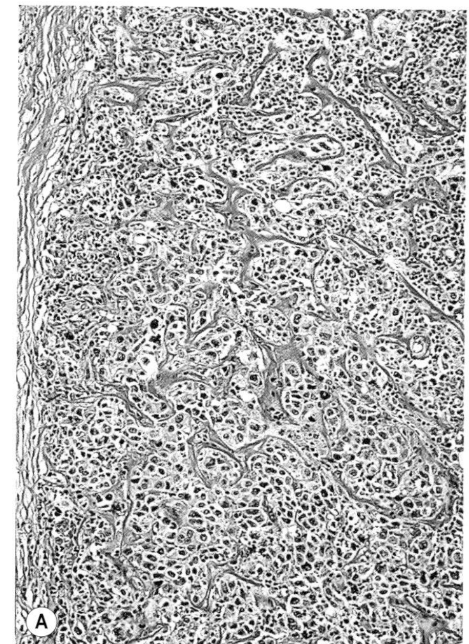

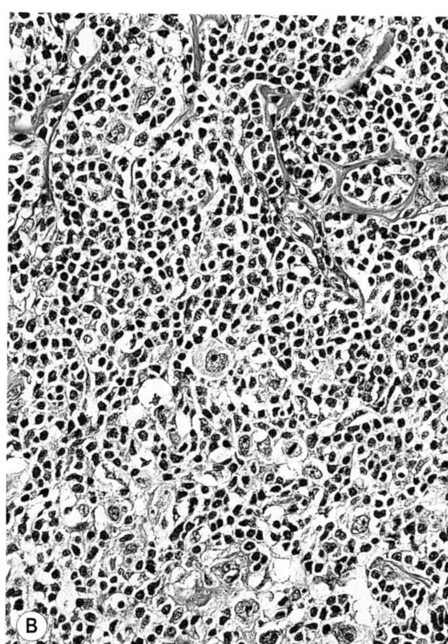

Fig. 21.107 **A** and **B**, Composite lymphoma of mediastinum. **A**, Corresponds to large cell lymphoma with sclerosis (which had a B immunophenotype). **B**, Corresponds to nodular sclerosis Hodgkin lymphoma (which had the typical phenotype of Reed–Sternberg cells).
(Slides contributed by Dr Kiyoshi Mukai, Tokyo, Japan)

5 Combination of 'classic' Hodgkin lymphoma and large B-cell lymphoma (Fig. 21.107).[1217] We have seen this combination several times in the thymic region.[1217,1220,1225] The Hodgkin lymphoma may coexist with, follow, or precede the non-Hodgkin lymphoma.[1227,1240,1241]
6 Combination of classic Hodgkin lymphoma and follicular lymphoma, representing one of the commonest forms of composite lymphoma.
7 Combination of classic Hodgkin lymphoma and peripheral (post-thymic) T-cell lymphoma.[1212,1214,1219,1225] Some of these tumors express CD20.[1231]
8 Combination of classic Hodgkin lymphoma and chronic lymphocytic leukemia.[1236]
9 Combination of classic Hodgkin lymphoma and marginal zone B-cell lymphoma.[1243]
10 Transformation of classic Hodgkin lymphoma into anaplastic large cell lymphoma.[1232]
11 Malignant lymphomas with B- and T-cell neoplastic components.[1210]
12 Combination of small lymphocytic lymphoma and dendritic cell neoplasm.[1226]

So-called 'malignant histiocytosis'

Malignant histiocytosis is no longer regarded as a bona fide entity, but I thought it was useful to discuss in a single section the various clinicopathologic conditions to which the term was applied (with or without a qualifier), with a mention of their place in the current nosologic scheme.

The term malignant histiocytosis was first proposed by Rappaport[1258] for a disease characterized by a systemic, neoplastic proliferation histologically resembling histiocytes and their precursors. Thus defined, the disease was found to affect any age group but with a predilection for children and young adults.[1262,1267] Fever, lymph node enlargement, and constitutional symptoms appeared early in the course of the disease. Hepatomegaly, splenomegaly, and skin involvement also were common.[1244,1260] In some patients, pulmonary symptoms dominated the clinical presentation.[1247] It was typical of the disease for the patient to be acutely ill when first seen by the physician. Common laboratory findings were anemia, leukopenia, and thrombocytopenia.[1264] Microscopically, the distinctive feature in the involved lymph nodes was said to be the proliferation of atypical cells with the appearance of histiocytes within the subcapsular or medullary sinuses and/or within the lymphoid parenchyma (Fig. 21.108). The degree of atypia varied greatly from case to case.[1265] The tumor cells were often found to surround lymphoid follicles in a concentric fashion. A variable number of cells within the infiltrate were seen to exhibit phagocytosis (especially of red blood cells), but it was noted that it was difficult to decide whether this phagocytosis was occurring in neoplastic cells or in accompanying reactive histiocytes. This feature was better demonstrated in bone marrow smears and touch preparations of lymph nodes than in tissue sections.[1263]

Most of the cases were rapidly progressive and fatal, two-thirds of the patients dying within the first months after diagnosis.[1248,1257] At autopsy, widespread organ involvement was found, usually without formation of large tumor masses but rather growing diffusely in the interstitium.

The entity described by Scott and Robb-Smith[1261] as *histiocytic medullary reticulosis* needs to be discussed in this context.[1259,1260] This was originally described clinically as characterized by hepatosplenomegaly, jaundice, and rapidly fatal outcome, and pathologically by prominent erythrophagocytosis by more or less atypical histiocytes. Probably some of these cases were of the same kind as the malignant histiocytosis as just described;[1245] as a matter of fact, some authors used the two terms synonymously.[1264] Other cases might have been examples of the virus-associated hemophagocytic syndrome[1255] (see Chapter 23). Along similar lines, it is possible that so-called 'familial hemophagocytic reticulosis' is a viral infection occurring in families with an immune defect that makes them susceptible to the virus.[1255,1256] Similarly, it is possible that some of the reported cases of lymphoma, leukemia, or myeloproliferative diseases terminating in 'histiocytic medullary

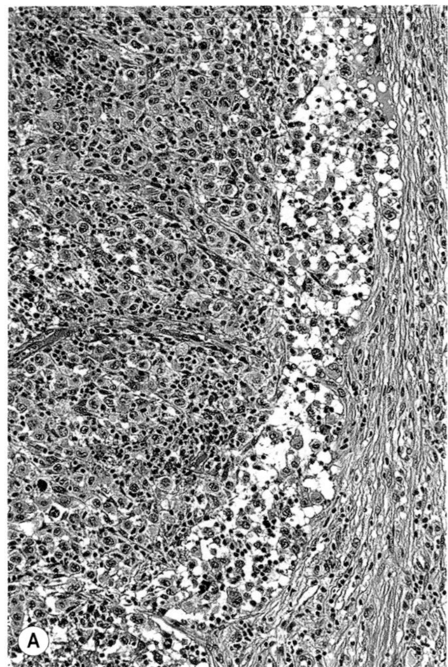
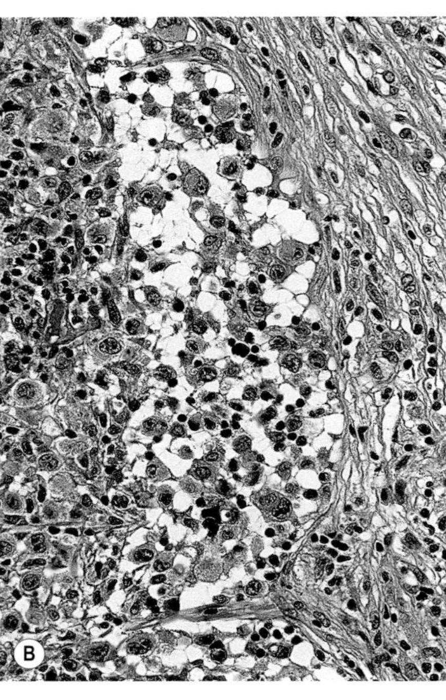

Fig. 21.108 **A** and **B**, Typical peripheral sinus involvement in the disease formerly known as malignant histiocytosis. Most of these cases (including the one depicted here) proved to be anaplastic cell lymphomas.

reticulosis'[1249,1252] represent overwhelming viral infections in a compromised host.

Some of the above considerations apply to the concept of malignant histiocytosis in a more global sense. The original definition of the disease was based on clinicomorphologic criteria; subsequent enzyme histochemical, immunohistochemical, and ultrastructural studies claimed to have found support for the histiocytic nature of the cellular proliferation.[1251,1253,1254] However, cell marker and molecular analysis studies have shown that most cases are actually examples of lymphoma, usually anaplastic large cell (CD30+) lymphoma or peripheral T-cell lymphoma[1246,1266] (with or without a hemophagocytic syndrome component). Malignant histiocytosis of the small bowel has been reinterpreted as a T-cell lymphoma (enteropathy-type, see Chapter 11). In view of these findings, the current view is that 'malignant histiocytosis' is not a single disease entity and that effort should be made to classify each case according to current terminology based on a thorough immunohistochemical and molecular evaluation of the case.[1250]

Lymphoma in immunodeficiency states

An increase in the incidence of malignant lymphoma has been documented in most types of congenital and acquired immunodeficiency.[1287,1301,1309] Chronic antigenic stimulation – possibly by oncogenic viruses – and perhaps loss of antibody feedback inhibition of the lymphoid proliferation may account for the high rate of lymphoid malignancies.[1332] The EBV in particular has been repeatedly implicated.[1314]

1 *Primary immunodeficiencies*. Patients with genetically determined immune deficiencies have an increased incidence of malignant tumors, especially lymphomas.[1287,1307,1336] This includes ataxia–telangiectasia, Wiskott–Aldrich syndrome, X-linked lymphoproliferative syndrome, common variable immunodeficiency, and severe combined immunodeficiency syndrome.[1333]

   Patients with *ataxia–telangiectasia* and *Wiskott–Aldrich syndrome* are particularly prone to this complication, approximately 10% of the reported patients having died from it.[1318] An interesting correlation exists between the type of immune deficiency and the type of lymphoma. In a series from the University of Minnesota, all the lymphomas arising in Wiskott–Aldrich syndrome were of non-Hodgkin type (predominantly large B-cell lymphomas with immunoblastic features) presenting as localized extranodal masses, whereas those arising in patients with ataxia–telangiectasia were of both Hodgkin and non-Hodgkin types, with a more conventional organ distribution. Surprisingly for this age group, half of the cases of Hodgkin lymphoma belonged to the lymphocyte depletion type. These cases are atypical in other regards, leading some authors to question whether they really belong to the Hodgkin lymphoma category.[1339] Most of the non-Hodgkin lymphomas in ataxia–telangiectasia were of the histologic types associated with the 14q+ chromosomal abnormality.[1292] Parenthetically, a gene for ataxia–telangiectasia (*ATM*) that encodes a product similar to PI-3 kinase has been recently cloned.[1305,1334] Also, mutations of the *JAK3* gene have been detected in severe combined immunodeficiency syndrome.[1316]

   The microscopic diagnosis of lymphoma can be extremely difficult in early cases; sometimes the only morphologic diagnosis possible is that of an atypical lymphoproliferative process. The immunologic status of the patient is just as important a predictor of prognosis as the type of lymphoma that has developed.[1276]

   Several members of families affected by the *X-linked lymphoproliferative syndrome* (believed to result from an immunodeficiency to the EBV)[1325] have developed sporadic Burkitt lymphoma, large B-cell lymphoma with immunoblastic features, fatal infectious mononucleosis, or 'plasmacytoma'.

2 *Organ transplant recipients*. The incidence of lymphoma is increased in recipients of all types of organ transplant as a direct or indirect result of the induced immunosuppression.[1326] In renal transplant recipients, this

incidence is in the order of 4–6%.[1290] Skin tumors, malignant lymphomas, Kaposi sarcoma, and cervical carcinoma are the most common neoplasms. The frequency of lymphoma has been estimated to be 350 times higher than in the age-matched general population.[1290,1310,1324] The incidence has been found to be particularly high in adult cardiac transplant patients treated with OKT-3-containing regimens.[1283,1338] In approximately half of the reported cases, the central nervous system is involved, compared with less than 1% in lymphoma patients in general. In 30% of the cases, the allograft is also involved.

Microscopically, most of these lymphomas show marked cytologic polymorphism (small and large follicular center cells and immunoblasts), atypia of the immunoblasts, and extensive necrosis[1299] (Fig. 21.109). The initial infiltrate has polyclonal B-cell features, in keeping with a reactive nature.[1297,1298,1341] The development of lymphoma is signaled by the appearance of a monoclonal component with chromosomal aberrations.[1291] The term 'polymorphic B-cell lymphoma' has been suggested for this tumor type. A transition has been observed from a polyclonal activation of B cells to an oligoclonal B-cell proliferation and finally to a monoclonal B-cell lymphoma[1298,1336,1339] (Fig. 21.110). This separation is clinically relevant.[1281] Immunoglobulin rearrangement studies have shown the existence of a monoclonal population in the early stages of the process, before the malignancy is recognizable morphologically.[1280,1283,1313] Virtually all cases of post-transplant lymphoproliferative disorders harbor the EBV genome.[1327] In most cases, these genomes are clonal, indicating the presence of the EBV in the progenitor B cell that originated the neoplastic population.[1322] In addition to this nearly constant latent activity, there is often also evidence of lytic activity by the virus,[1317] sometimes in a recurrent pattern.[1344]

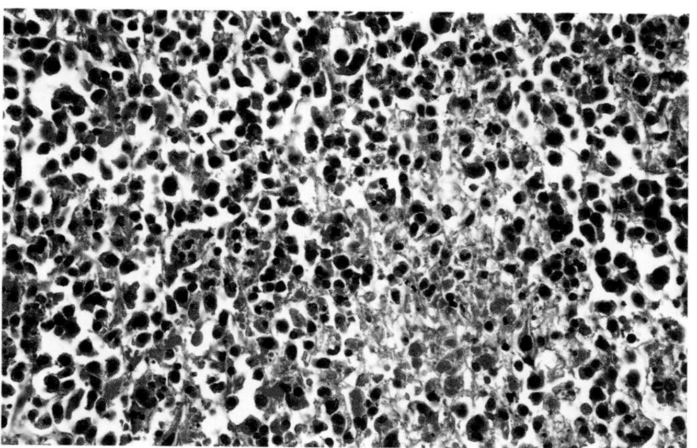

Fig. 21.109 Polymorphic lymphoproliferative process associated with necrosis in lymph node of a renal transplant patient. There was evidence of active EBV infection.

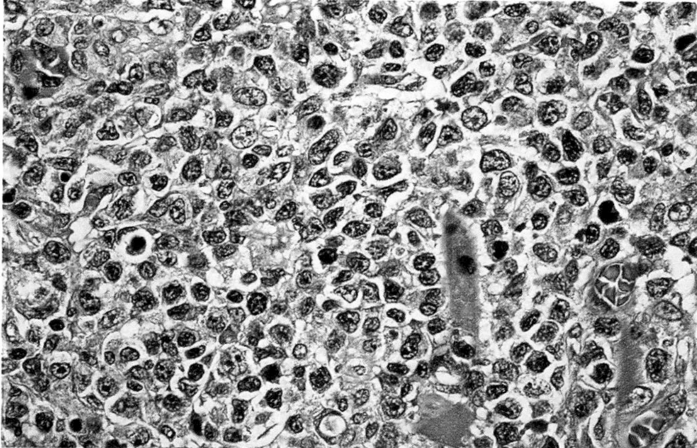

Fig. 21.110 Large B-cell lymphoma in a recipient of a renal transplant.

In contrast to HIV-associated lymphoma, *MYC* rearrangements are uncommon in post-transplant lymphoma. A minority of these tumors have been found to be of T-cell type.[1294,1312] Cases have also been reported of post-transplant lymphomas having the morphologic and immunohistochemical features of Burkitt lymphoma.[1295]

Molecular studies have confirmed the recipient origin of the lymphoma in the transplanted patients.[1343]

The clinical course of post-transplant lymphoma/lymphoproliferative disease is usually very rapid.[1320,1328]

Treatment of post-transplant lymphoproliferative disorders consists of a combination of immunosuppression reduction and standard lymphoma therapy (chemotherapy and radiation).[1271]

3 *HIV*. Patients with HIV infection are at a high risk for developing malignant tumors, principally Kaposi sarcoma and malignant lymphoma,[1275,1286,1293,1302,1308,1331,1342] sometimes in combination.[1289] It has been estimated that approximately 3% of AIDS patients develop non-Hodgkin lymphoma, and that the risk of developing a lymphoma in this population is 60-fold greater than in the normal population. The incidence of lymphoma is highest in hemophiliacs and lowest in individuals born in the Caribbean or Africa who have acquired the disease by heterosexual contact. As a group, the age at diagnosis is younger than in the immunocompetent population.[1285] The majority of the cases present with multiple sites of extranodal involvement, with a high incidence of involvement of the gastrointestinal tract, central nervous system, bone marrow, liver, oral cavity, body cavities, and heart.[1277,1302] Practically all cases are of B-cell lineage and – as such – show clonal immunoglobulin gene rearrangements.[1282,1286,1315] Morphologically, most cases are of Burkitt or large B-cell type, the latter often showing immunoblastic or plasmablastic features (including primary effusion lymphoma).[1279,1284,1329,1337] Cases have also been reported of peripheral T-cell lymphomas with a peculiar component of Touton-like giant cells,[1269] and others having the features of the polymorphic lymphoproliferative disorders seen more often in solid organ transplant recipients.[1319] Some of the lymphomas contain the HHV8 virus and display anaplastic large cell features.[1306]

The molecular and cytogenetic features of Burkitt lymphoma seen in the HIV-positive population are similar to those of sporadic Burkitt lymphoma, especially in regard to rearrangements of the *MYC* gene.[1278,1309] The *BCL2* and T-cell receptor genes are unaffected. Evidence of EBV infection is often present.[1296,1311,1323]

The incidence of Hodgkin lymphoma in HIV-infected patients does not seem to be unduly increased, but the disease presents several differences from that seen in the immunocompetent population.[1274] Almost all cases are clinical stage III or IV at presentation, with frequent involvement of unusual sites such as the liver and skin; spread often occurs in a noncontiguous fashion; there is a predominance of unfavorable histologic subtypes; Reed–Sternberg cells and (especially) their variants are more numerous and more atypical; there is an increased number of nonlymphoid stromal cells; and there is a much higher incidence of EBV genomes in Reed–Sternberg cells (reaching almost 100% in some series).[1270,1272,1300,1330,1340] It has been suggested that the immunomodulatory drugs that are given for these disorders may be pathogenetically involved with the development of these lymphomas.[1303] It has also been pointed out that the demographic, clinical, and prognostic features of Hodgkin lymphoma developing in HIV-infected patients are nearly identical to those of HIV-related non-Hodgkin lymphoma.[1331]

Sometimes, EBV+ B-cell lymphoproliferative disorders similar in all regards to those of immunocompromised individuals are seen in elderly individuals without overt immunodeficiencies of any type.[1321]

4 *Others*. Acquired diseases of the immune system in which an increased incidence of lymphoma has been recorded include rheumatoid arthritis,[1288,1304] Sjögren syndrome,[1335] Hashimoto thyroiditis, and other autoimmune diseases.[1273] As already stated, it is possible that some or perhaps most of the latter represent early or preneoplastic stages of malignant lymphoma.

Cases of EBV+ lymphoproliferative disorders have also been seen in patients with low-grade B-cell neoplasms who had been treated with the immunosuppressive agent fludarabine.[1268]

Lymph node inclusions

Inclusions of various types of benign tissue can occur within lymph nodes.[1358] Lack of awareness of this phenomenon can lead to a mistaken diagnosis of metastatic carcinoma. These include the following:

1 *Salivary gland tissue*. This is an extremely common finding in high cervical nodes, to be regarded as a normal event related to the embryology of the region[1349] (Fig. 21.111). Both ducts and acini are usually present. These inclusions may undergo neoplastic changes. Warthin tumor is the most common type, but many other types have been reported, including benign mixed tumor, monomorphic adenoma, mucoepidermoid carcinoma, and acinic cell carcinoma (see Chapter 12).

2 *Squamous epithelium*. Microscopic cystic structures lined by well-differentiated squamous epithelium are sometimes seen in the upper cervical lesion. They are thought to represent an anomaly related to the aforementioned one, in the sense of being composed of branchial pouch derivatives. The term 'benign lymphoepithelial cyst' is sometimes applied to them (see Chapter 12). We have hypothesized that these formations result from cystic dilation of preexisting epithelial inclusions as the result of their stimulation by the lymphoid component that surrounds them, a pathogenesis that also applies to multilocular thymic cysts, other cystic structures of the head and neck region, and possibly to Warthin tumor itself (see Chapter 9). Similar formations have been described in peripancreatic lymph nodes.[1345] The obvious differential diagnosis is metastatic well-differentiated squamous cell carcinoma, which in the cervical region is notorious for its tendency to undergo marked cystic changes.[1361]

3 *Thyroid follicles*. These can be found in the capsular or subcapsular region of midcervical nodes in the absence of pathologic changes of the thyroid gland. The differential diagnosis with metastatic thyroid carcinoma can be very difficult (see Chapter 9).

4 *Decidual reaction*. During pregnancy, decidual reaction may occur within pelvic nodes and mimic metastatic carcinoma.[1350] The decidual reaction can occur in the stromal cells of endometriosis or in hormonally receptive cells of the region, in a fashion similar to that seen in peritoneal decidual reaction.

5 *Müllerian-type epithelium*. Glandular inclusions lined by cuboidal cells with a müllerian or coelomic appearance are commonly found in the capsule of the pelvic lymph nodes of females and sometimes within the node itself.[1357,1359] Their appearance and pathogenesis are similar to those of the peritoneal lesions generally known as endosalpingiosis (Fig. 21.112). Like the latter, these lymph node inclusions may be difficult to distinguish from metastases originating in low-grade ovarian neoplasms, since they may grow into the peripheral sinuses, form papillae, be accompanied by psammoma bodies, and even proliferate as small sheets of cells.[1352] Some authors have suggested that some of these

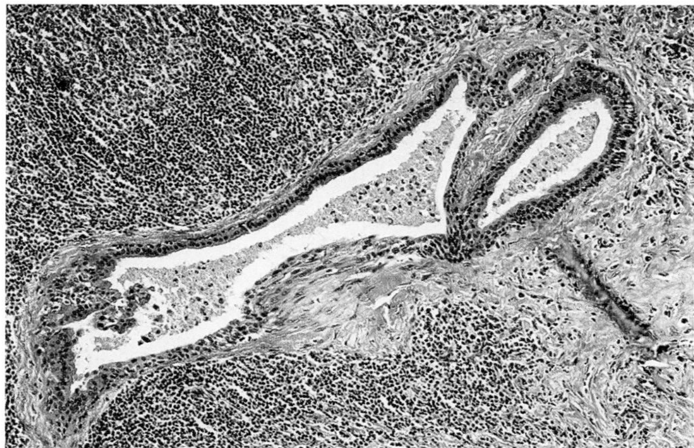

Fig. 21.111 Salivary gland inclusion composed of ductal structures in a high cervical lymph node. This is a very common occurrence.

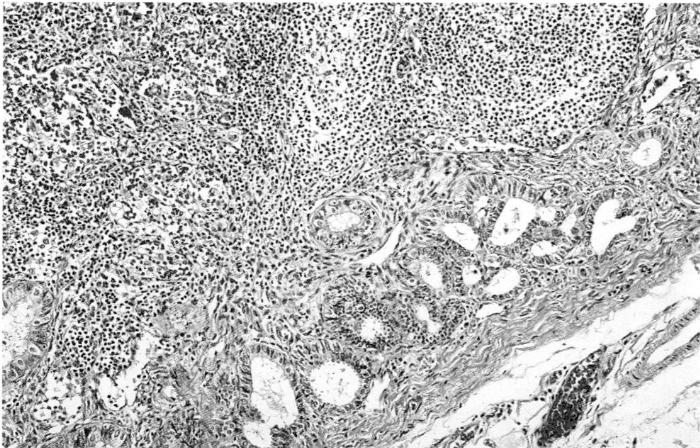

Fig. 21.112 Pelvic lymph node involved by endosalpingiosis. Glands lined by cuboidal cells with a müllerian appearance and lacking atypical figures are present in the capsule of the node.

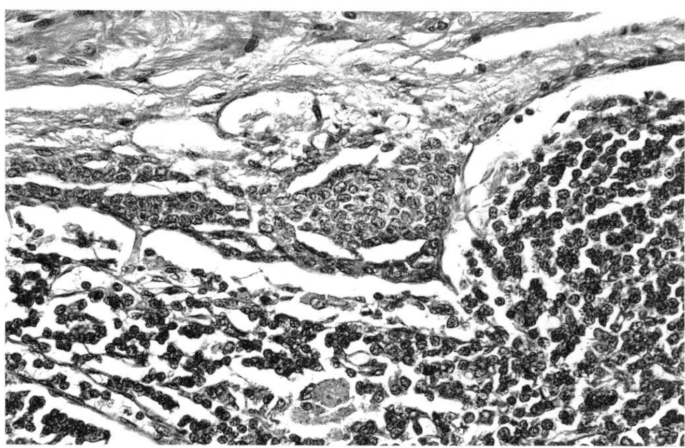

Fig. 21.113 Nevus cells in the capsule of an axillary lymph node. These inconsequential formations should not be mistaken for metastatic melanoma or metastatic carcinoma.

'inclusions' are actually metastases from ovarian serous borderline tumors.[1362] Morphologically similar inclusions have been seen in the mediastinal nodes of males[1358] and axillary nodes of females.

Nodal glandular inclusions of similar appearance but surrounded by endometrial-type stroma occur less frequently and represent *nodal endometriosis*. All of these müllerian-related nodal processes are discussed in more detail in Chapter 19.

6 *Nevus cells*. Clusters of normal-appearing nevus cells are occasionally found in the capsule of lymph nodes, without involvement of the nodal parenchyma (Fig. 21.113). Most of the reported cases have occurred in axillary lymph nodes.[1356] A related lesion is the *blue nevus* that has been reported in the lymph node capsule[1347] (Fig. 21.114). The morphologic features of these formations and their differential diagnosis with metastatic malignant melanoma are discussed in Chapter 4.

7 *Mesothelial cells*. Occasionally, mesothelial cells are found within lymph nodes in the apparent absence of a malignant mesothelioma.[1346,1348,1363] The obvious differential diagnosis is with metastatic malignant mesothelioma from an occult primary in the peritoneal cavity or pleura.[1364] The issue is discussed in more detail in Chapter 7.

8 *Breast tissue*. One of the most unusual forms of ectopia is represented by normal mammary lobules within axillary lymph nodes.[1351,1360,1365] A slightly more common occurrence is the presence in axillary nodes of tubules lined by a single layer of cuboidal cells (sometimes with a hobnail appearance), located in the nodal capsule or immediately beneath. These formations are similar to the müllerian-type epithelial inclusions in pelvic lymph nodes previously described. Since some of these cases occur in patients with breast carcinoma, the distinct possibility exists of mistaking them for metastatic tumor.[1354,1355] We have recently reviewed 17 cases of epithelial inclusions in axillary lymph nodes of females, and classified them into three major groups: those composed exclusively of glandular structures, those made up only of squamous cysts, and those containing both glandular and squamous epithelium.[1353] The issue is further discussed in Chapter 20.

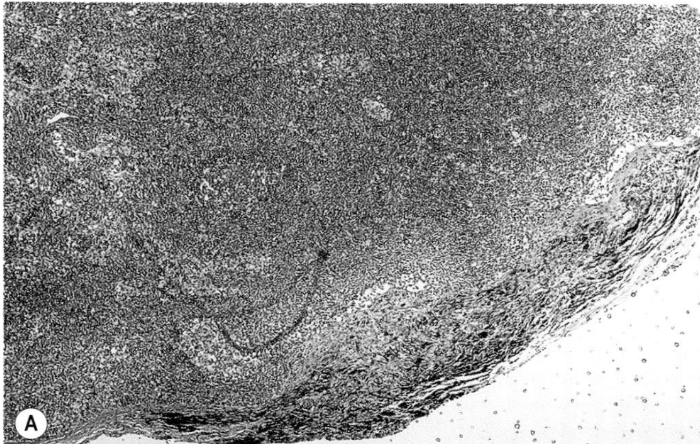

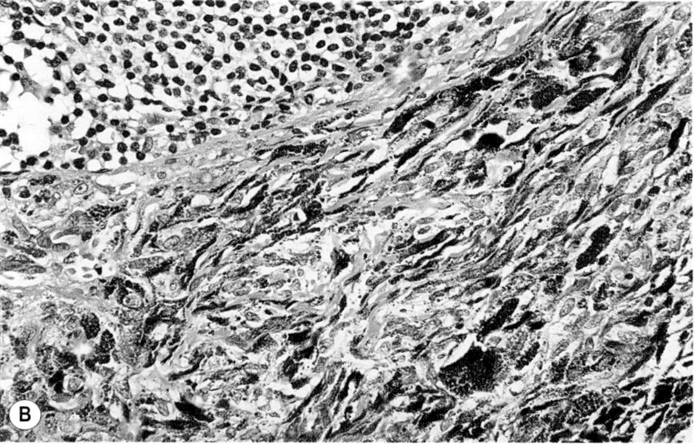

Fig. 21.114 **A** and **B**, Blue nevus involving lymph node capsule.

Other non-neoplastic lesions

Adipose metaplasia of lymph nodes is very common. When extensive, it may lead to the formation of large masses, up to 10 cm or more in diameter. These nodes are sometimes referred to as *lipolymph nodes*; the external iliac and obturator groups are the sites most commonly involved.[1372]

Ectopic thymus sometimes seen in supraclavicular lymph node biopsies should be mentioned here for the sake of differential diagnosis even if it is not a lymph node lesion. The pathologist unaware of this occurrence might easily misinterpret the Hassall corpuscles as islands of metastatic squamous cell carcinoma.

Vasculitis involving lymph nodes may be seen in a large number of disorders: polyarteritis nodosa (having necrotizing qualities and only rarely biopsied), Henoch–Schönlein purpura (leukocytoclastic, also rarely biopsied), Wegener granulomatosis (sometimes accompanied by extensive infarct), systemic lupus erythematosus, drug hypersensitivity (see p. 1799), and mucocutaneous lymph node syndrome (see p. 1794). Some nodes otherwise showing the typical features of angioimmunoblastic lymphadenopathy may also show extensive vasculitis. One should also mention the obliterative vasculitis often seen in syphilitic lymphadenitis (see p. 1788).

Infarction of the lymph nodes presents with painful swelling, usually located in a superficial lymph node chain. Microscopically, there is extensive necrosis of medullary and cortical lymphoid cells, with marked reactive perinodal inflammation and a layer of granulation tissue. A thin rim of viable subcapsular lymphoid tissue may be present.[1369] Thrombosis of veins within the substance and the hilum of the nodes has been suggested as the pathogenesis.[1369] Similar changes can be seen in mesenteric lymph nodes in patients with intestinal volvulus.[1373] Other cases are the result of embolism, arterial occlusion in cases of polyarteritis nodosa and related disorders, or fine needle aspiration;[1370,1375] in these instances, the nodal infarct tends to have a segmental quality. The differential diagnosis of lymph node infarction includes necrotizing lymphadenitis (see p. 1785), mucocutaneous lymph node syndrome (see p. 1794), infectious mononucleosis,[1371] necrotizing granulomatous inflammation, and necrotic malignant tumors. Two types of malignancy that have been occasionally found to undergo extensive and sometimes massive infarct-type necrosis when involving lymph nodes are malignant lymphoma[1368,1374] and metastatic malignant melanoma. Therefore thorough examination of the infarcted node, the extranodal region, and other nodes submitted is mandatory in order to exclude a concomitant or underlying malignancy[1374] (Fig. 21.115A,B). A thorough immunohistochemical study is also in order. We have often been amazed at the degree of preservation of the tumor cells' reactivity in the face of extensive necrotic changes[1376,1378] (Fig. 21.115C). As a general rule, the possibility of an underlying malignancy should be suspected if the infarcted node is markedly enlarged.

Hyaline material sometimes accumulates in the stroma of lymph nodes. This finding is very frequent in those situated in the aorto-iliac region (Fig. 21.116). The material can undergo secondary calcification. Because of its homogeneous eosinophilic appearance, it can be confused with amyloid and has been referred to in the past as *para-amyloid*. It should also be distinguished from the hyaline material deposited in nodes in cases of hemorrhagic spindle cell tumor with amianthoid fibers (see p. 1859). The presence of this hyaline material, which is probably an abnormal type of collagen, has no clinical significance.

Proteinaceous lymphadenopathy is the name given to a lymph node abnormality in which an eosinophilic extracellular material of proteinaceous nature is deposited in lymph nodes. This material simulates the appearance of amyloid but is histochemically and ultrastructurally distinct from it. The few patients that have been described with this obscure abnormality had hypergammaglobulinemia, and the hyaline material itself has been shown to contain precipitated immunoglobulin.[1367]

Foreign material of various types can accumulate in lymph nodes. One example is the *silicone lymphadenopathy* developing as a side effect of mammary augmentation produced by injection of liquid silicone or by placement of a bag-gel prosthesis. Microscopically, a nonbirefringent refractive material is present in the sinuses, together with variously sized vacuoles and multinucleated giant cells[1377] (Fig. 21.117).

Another example is the already mentioned sinus histiocytosis of pelvic lymph nodes, which is induced by the cobalt-chromium and titanium contained in hip prostheses and which closely simulates the appearance of RDD[1366] (Fig. 21.118).

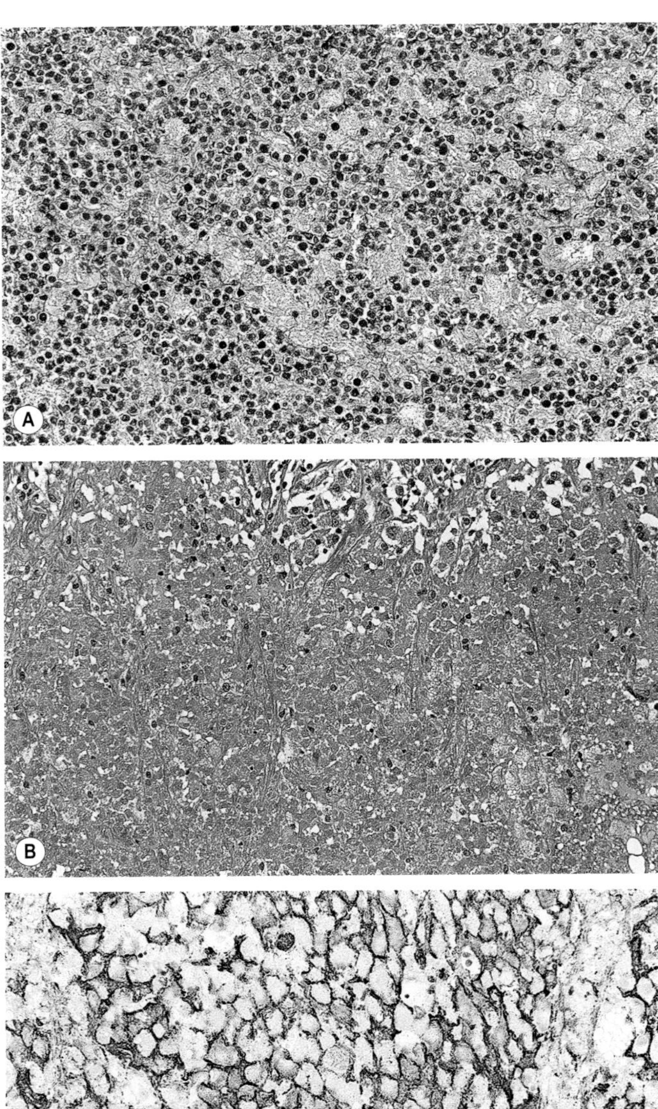

Fig. 21.115 A–C, Large B-cell lymphoma that has undergone massive infarct-type necrosis. **A**, The outlines of the tumor cells can still be discerned. **B**, A totally necrotic area, indistinguishable from that of a 'benign' infarct. **C**, There is a remarkable degree of retained immunoreactivity for CD20 in the necrotic area.

Tumors of the cells of the accessory immune system

The accessory immune system includes two major categories of cells: antigen-presenting cells (dendritic cells) and antigen-processing cells (macrophages).[1381,1397,1421,1452,1455,1457] The dendritic cells belong to the group of nonlymphoid elements traditionally designated by histologists and pathologists as reticulum cells, which have been divided into more or less well-defined subtypes on the basis of location, enzyme histochemical, ultrastructural, and immunohistochemical features. These are:

1 **Follicular dendritic cells.** These are associated with the B zones of the node and specifically with the germinal centers. Ultrastructurally, they have complex cell prolongations joined by complex desmosomes. Immunohistochemically, they exhibit reactivity for CD21, CD35, clusterin, Ki-M4p, Ki-FDRC1p, CNA.42, fascin, Ki-M9, estrogen receptor α, epidermal growth factor receptor, and the low affinity nerve growth factor receptor.[1380,1411,1416,1425,1434,1439,1444]

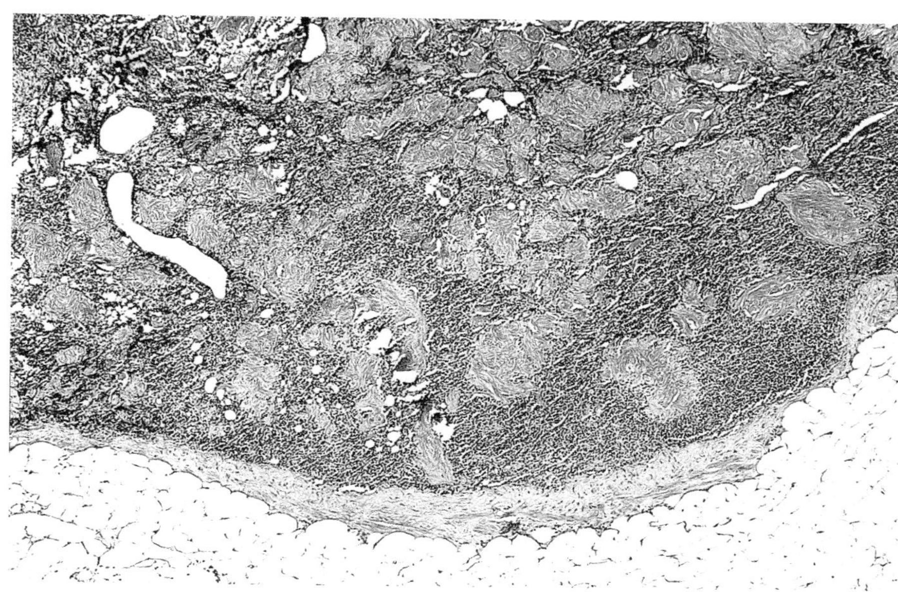

Fig. 21.116 Hyaline deposits in pelvic lymph node. This change is of no clinical significance.

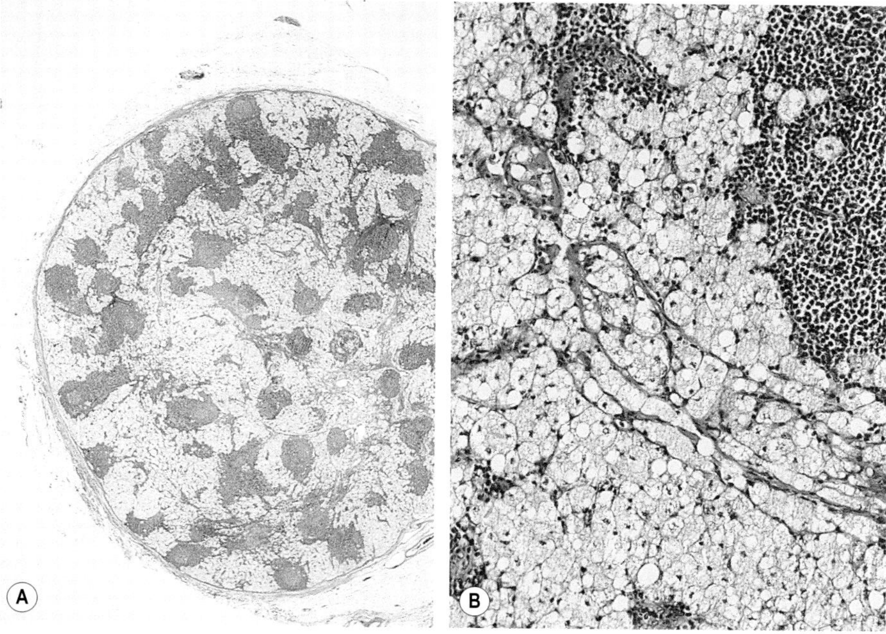

Fig. 21.117 Low-power (**A**) and medium-power (**B**) appearances of silicone lymphadenitis. The sinuses are massively expanded by a histiocytic infiltrate, which simulates the appearance of Rosai–Dorfman disease.

2 **Interdigitating dendritic cells.** These cells are associated with the T zones of the nodes. They also have complex cell prolongations that interdigitate with each other, but desmosomes are absent. Immunohistochemically, they are reactive for S-100 protein.[1412,1427]

3 **Langerhans cells** (see p. 1803). These are characterized by immunoreactivity to S-100 protein, CD1a, and langerin, and the presence of Birbeck granules at the ultrastructural level. They are closely related to the interdigitating dendritic cells.[1409] It has even been suggested that they represent two different morphofunctional manifestations of the same cell. Other closely related cells are indeterminate cells, veiled cells, and dermal dendrocytes.

4 **Fibroblastic reticulum cells.** These are located in the capsule, hilus, and other stroma-rich areas of the node. They have a high content of alkaline phosphatase, exhibit filaments with focal condensations at the ultrastructural level, and probably correspond to the *myoid cells* described by others. A subset of these cells shows immunoreactivity for keratin.[1410] It is not clear whether these cells play a role in the immune reaction or whether they are structural supporting elements.

5 **Macrophages.** These cells are thought to be involved in the processing of antigens through the process of phagocytosis, hence the synonym of phagocytes. They are closely related to circulating monocytes. When the term *histiocyte* is used without a qualifier, the cell usually referred to is the

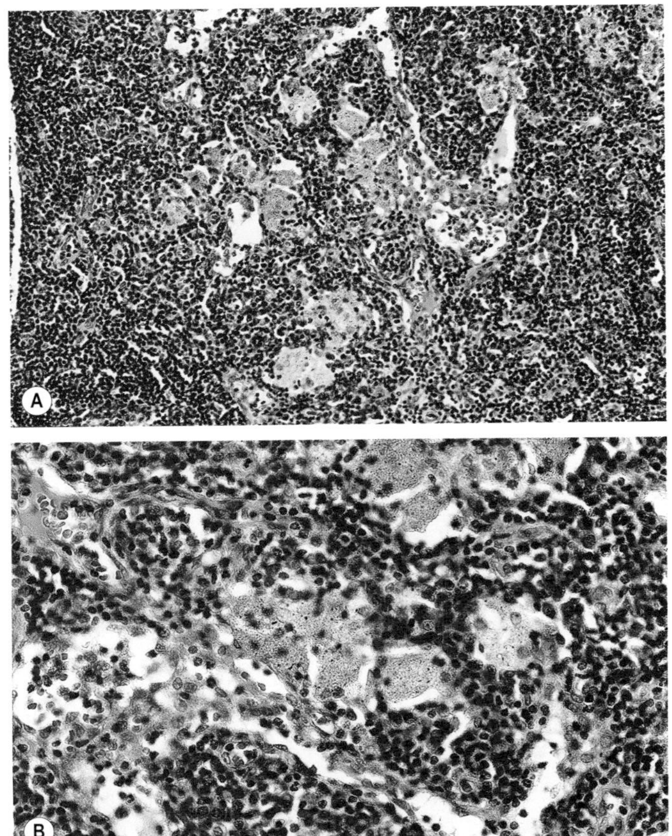

Fig. 21.118 **A** and **B**, Lymph node changes in a patient who had a prosthesis implanted in the joint drained by this node. A fine particulate black material can be appreciated in the high-power view. It is easy to dismiss this material as 'dirt'.

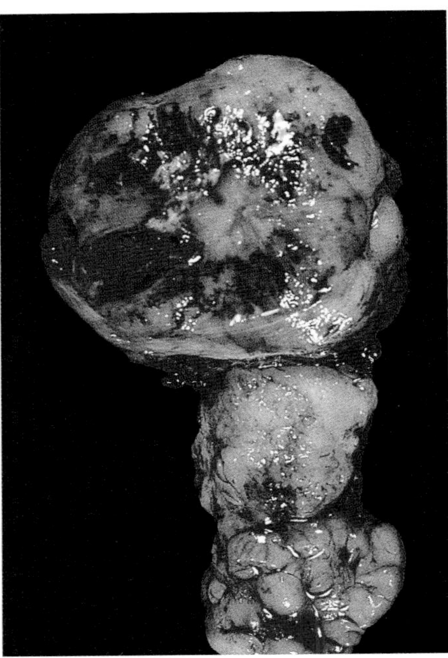

Fig. 21.119 Gross appearance of dendritic follicular tumor.

macrophage. The practice is, however, confusing because the same term has been used by others as a generic designation for *all* the cells of the accessory immune system, and still by others for some members of the antigen-presenting subset (as in Langerhans cell histiocytosis).

6 **Sinus lining cells.** These cells, also known as *littoral cells* (particularly in the spleen), belong generically to the system because they exhibit macrophagic properties. They also have endothelial features, and therefore come as close as any of the cells described in this section to fulfill the criteria for the elaborate reticuloendothelial system concept as proposed many years ago by Aschoff and Kiyono. Some authors believe that there is an interconversion between sinus-lining cells and some of the dendritic cell subtypes. The recently reported immunoreactivity for the dendritic cell marker Ki-M9 supports this interpretation.[1455]

7 **Plasmacytoid dendritic cells.** See page 1784.

Tumors composed of cells having features corresponding to one or another of the cells of this system exist, the saga of their recognition constituting a very interesting chapter in the history of neoplastic hematopathology.

Once upon a time, primary nodal tumors composed of large cells were thought to derive from reticulum cells and were therefore called reticulum cell sarcomas. It was then proposed that such tumors were composed of histiocytes (in the sense of macrophages), and that reticulum cell sarcomas (or, for that matter, reticulum cells) did not exist. Later on, it was realized that the overwhelming majority of these large cell tumors were actually of lymphocytic nature, a concept that became easily accepted once it was found that the small lymphocyte could undergo a transformation into a large cell when stimulated. At that point, it seemed as if neither reticulum cells nor histiocytic sarcomas/lymphomas existed. Then, slowly but surely, reports began to appear showing that tumors composed of cells having the phenotype of dendritic/reticulum or histiocytic/macrophagic cells were real entities, and their occurrence is now no longer doubted. As a matter of fact, in recent years there has been a deluge of case reports of these lesions, some of them more convincing than others. Naturally, this characterization is largely dependent on the degree of specificity of the markers available for the corresponding normal cells.[1435] Reasonably specific markers exist for follicular dendritic cells, and therefore the evidence of the existence of a follicular dendritic cell tumor is pretty solid. The markers for interdigitating dendritic cells and most of the other types are far less specific, and as a consequence the identification of a neoplastic counterpart is on shakier ground. Not surprisingly, tumors sharing markers of two of these subtypes exist.[1422,1426] The existence of occasional cases of combined dendritic cell neoplasms and bona fide malignant lymphomas of one type or another has been rationalized by postulating a transdifferentiation of the lymphoma clone.[1407,1415] Another comment of a general nature pertains to the position of these cells (and the tumors thereof) in a general histogenetic scheme, and specifically whether they should be regarded as members of the lymphoid or the stromal/mesenchymal systems. If the former, the tumors should be regarded as lymphomas; if the latter, as sarcomas. The issue is not completely resolved, but it would seem as if tumors of interdigitating dendritic cells, Langerhans cells, and macrophages are closer to the lymphoid side, whereas tumors of follicular dendritic and fibroblastic dendritic cells have a closer link to the mesenchymal neoplasms.

Follicular dendritic cell tumor (follicular dendritic cell sarcoma; dendritic reticulum cell sarcoma) often presents as a solitary mass in a cervical lymph node[1429] (Fig. 21.119), but can involve other lymph node groups and a large variety of extranodal sites,[1449] including stomach,[1413] small bowel,[1417] large bowel,[1391] omentum,[1458] mesentery,[1430] liver,[1392] nasopharynx,[1382] oral cavity,[1390] tonsil,[1431] soft tissues of head and neck region,[1383] mediastinum,[1398] spleen,[1423] lung,[1447] and breast.[1405,1437] Some cases of follicular dendritic cell tumor have occurred as a complication of the hyaline vascular type of Castleman disease,[1386,1443] and others in connection with inflammatory pseudotumor of the liver,[1446] two conditions characterized by proliferation of follicular dendritic cells. In the latter instance, there has been a constant involvement of EBV.[1392,1395,1448]

Microscopically, follicular dendritic cell tumor is characterized by a proliferation of oval to spindle cells that form fascicles and whorls[1456] (Fig. 21.120). Sometimes there is a suggestion of a storiform or palisading pattern.[1416,1429] In other instances the stroma has a myxoid quality.[1405] The appearance at low power may simulate that of meningioma. The nuclei are generally oval, with a vesicular chromatin pattern, small nucleoli, and scanty mitotic activity. Pseudonuclear inclusions and multinucleated giant cells may be present. A characteristic feature is the presence of small lymphocytes scattered throughout the tumor cells, resulting in a thymoma-like appearance.[1388] The ultrastructural and immunohistochemical features correspond to those of follicular dendritic cells (Fig. 21.121). Markers that are particularly useful for their identification are CD21, CD35, clusterin, Ki-M4P, and Ki-FDRC1p.[1411,1434]

The tumor cells are negative or equivocal for CD45RB and erratically positive for S-100 protein. In frozen sections, they also stain for the follicular dendritic cell marker R4/23, HLA-DR, and the lymphocyte adhesion markers CD11a and CD18[1390] (Fig. 21.122). Although it was thought previously that these tumors do not exhibit clonal rearrangements of the immunoglobulin or the T-cell

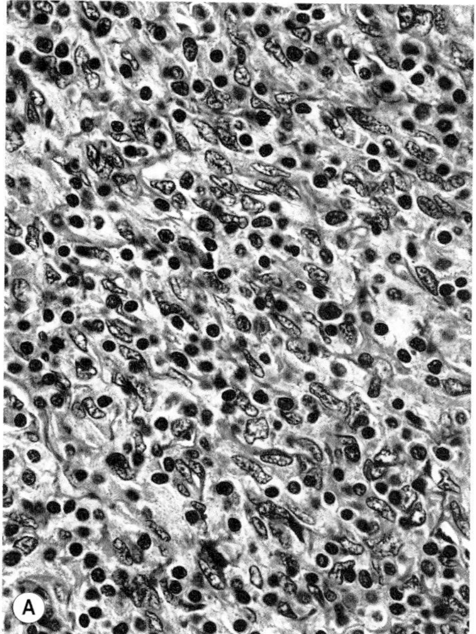

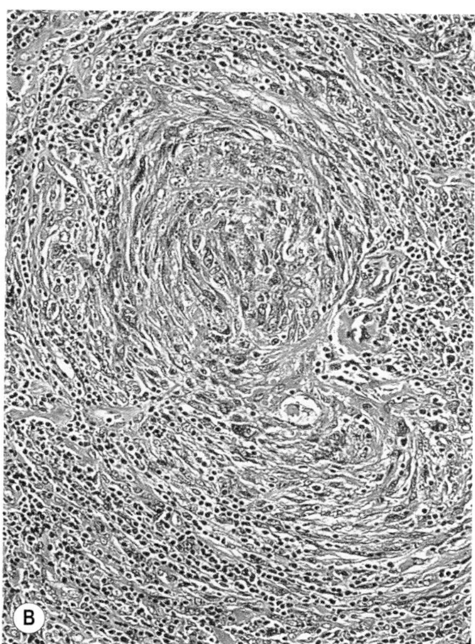

Fig. 21.120 A and **B**, Dendritic follicular cell tumor of lymph node. **A**, The admixture of neoplastic cells with predominantly oval vesicular nuclei and non-neoplastic small lymphocytes results in an appearance reminiscent of thymoma. **B**, Prominent whorling in a case of dendritic follicular cell tumor, engrafted upon Castleman disease.

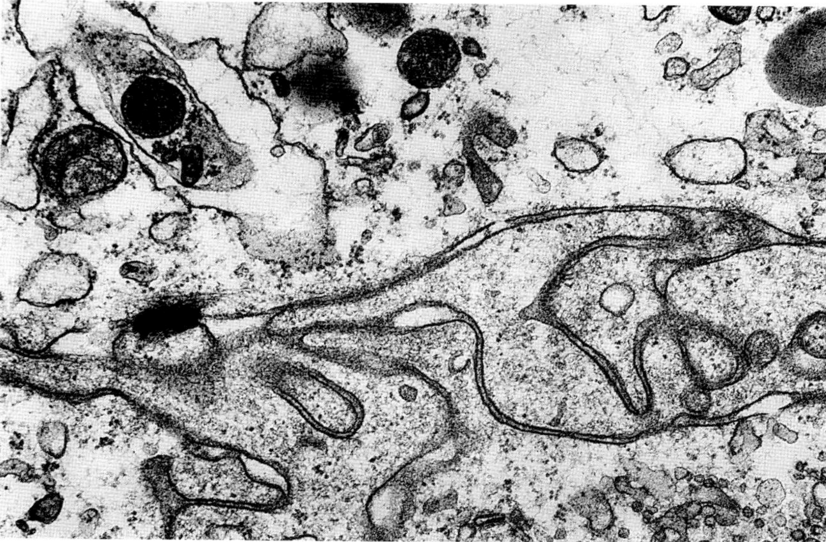

Fig. 21.121 Electron microscopic appearance of dendritic follicular cell tumor. A characteristic feature is the presence of well-developed cytoplasmic prolongations joined by desmosomes.

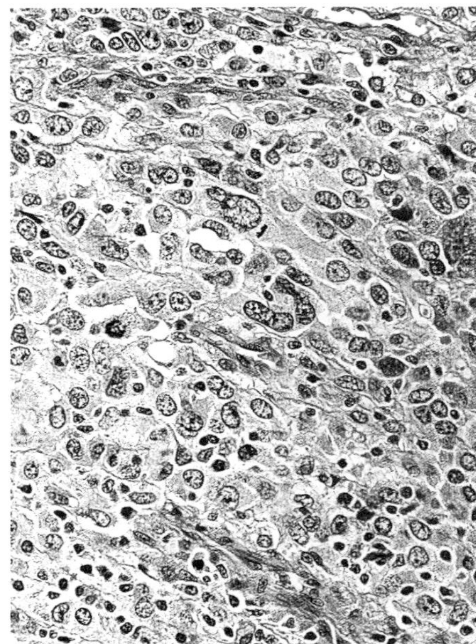

Fig. 21.122 Recurrent dendritic follicular cell tumor. There is a greater degree of pleomorphism than in the original neoplasm.

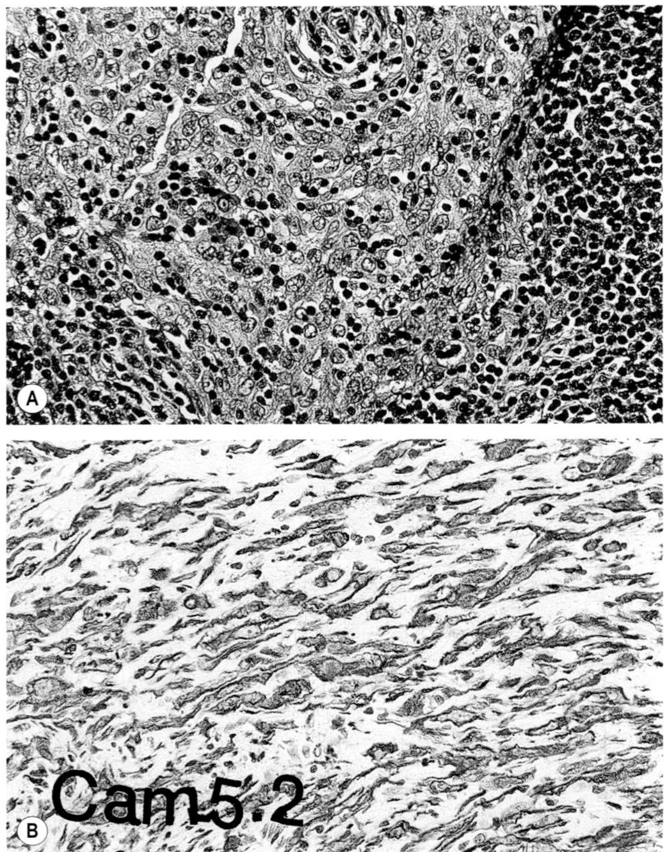

Fig. 21.123 **A** and **B**, Neoplasm interpreted as tumor of keratin-positive reticulum/dendritic cells. **A**, Hematoxylin–eosin. **B**, Immunostain for low molecular weight keratin (CAM 5.2).

receptor genes, it has been shown recently that a proportion of cases indeed exhibit clonal rearrangements of immunoglobulin genes.[1393]

The behavior is that of a malignant tumor, with local recurrence and distant metastases to sites such as the liver and lung.[1433,1434] The pattern of spread resembles that of a soft tissue sarcoma more than that of a malignant lymphoma. Intra-abdominal neoplasms tend to be particularly aggressive.[1389] Recurrent and metastatic lesions may show increased atypia and pleomorphism.[1434]

Interdigitating dendritic cell tumor (interdigitating reticulum cell sarcoma) is even more uncommon, or perhaps not as easily recognized.[1408] Most patients are adults, but it can also occur in the pediatric population.[1436] Most of the reported cases have arisen in lymph nodes,[1403,1410] but instances of extranodal involvement in sites such as skin, bowel, spleen, and testis have been recorded.[1420,1423,1424,1427] The microscopic appearance can be indistinguishable from that of follicular dendritic cell tumor, but there is more tendency to spindling and pleomorphism.[1453,1459] The diagnosis is dependent on the immunohistochemical profile, which unfortunately is not entirely specific. The tumor cells are positive for CD45RB, S-100 protein, and the macrophage marker CD68, but are negative for CD21 and CD35. The behavior seems more aggressive than for follicular dendritic cell tumor. Contrary to earlier belief, a proportion of cases are shown to exhibit clonal rearrangements of the immunoglobulin genes.[1393,1400]

Langerhans cell histiocytosis has been discussed on page 1803. Its neoplastic versus reactive nature is still controversial, but a few cases of **Langerhans cell sarcoma** have been described in which a clearly malignant neoplasm displays the markers of Langerhans cells.[1404] A proportion of cases exhibit clonal immunoglobulin or T-cell receptor gene rearrangement, including cases that occur sporadically and cases that have transdifferentiated from lymphoblastic leukemia/lymphoma or low-grade B-cell lymphoma.[1384,1394,1401]

Other reticulum/dendritic cell tumors. Other recently described tumors which may belong to this family are those thought to arise from fibroblastic reticulum cells (exhibiting immunoreactivity for vimentin, smooth muscle actin, and desmin),[1379] and those which in addition exhibit reactivity for low molecular weight keratin[1387,1445] (Fig. 21.123). The reticulum/dendritic cell nature of these tumors is supported by their ultrastructural features and already suggested by the scattering of non-neoplastic lymphocytes that is a constant feature of this tumor family. It is also possible that at least some of the 'sarcomas' that have been described as a complication of Castleman disease (above and beyond the already mentioned follicular dendritic cell tumors) and some of the so-called inflammatory myofibroblastic tumors may be of reticulum/dendritic cell nature.[1432] Cases of indeterminate cell tumor have also been described.[1441] Finally, evidence has been recently brought forward to suggest the existence of tumors of *plasmacytoid dendritic cells*.[1440]

True histiocytic sarcomas (true histiocytic lymphomas) in the sense of tumors of macrophages, i.e., the antigen-processing cells of the accessory immune system, remain rare and controversial.[1399,1435] The issue is complicated by the fact that – as already mentioned – the majority of neoplasms to which the term 'histiocytic' was applied in the past (such as Rappaport's histiocytic lymphoma, Isaacson's malignant histiocytosis, and Flynn's regressing atypical histiocytosis) have been shown to be of lymphocytic nature in the overwhelming majority of the cases. However, it would seem that tumors of true histiocytes do exist. Their presentation is highly variable, with a high proportion of extranodal involvement in sites such as the spleen, skin, bone, and particularly the gastrointestinal tract.[1396,1406,1418,1428,1450] As in the case of the dendritic cell tumors, some 'true histiocytic sarcomas' have been seen in combination with bona fide malignant lymphoma.[1442] A unique case of histiocytic sarcoma has recently been reported in a patient with autoimmune lymphoproliferative syndrome (ALPS) with associated Rosai–Dorfman disease-like features.[1454]

Microscopically, the tumor cells are large, with irregularly shaped nuclei and abundant, generally acidophilic cytoplasm. Immunohistochemically, the tumor cells lack by definition B-cell- and T-cell-related markers and show reactivity for histiocytic markers, such as CD68, CD163, lysozyme, CD11c, CD13, CD14, CD15, CD32, CD33, and Mac-387.[1414,1419,1438]

Although the presence of immunoglobulin or T-cell receptor gene rearrangement was previously considered to be incompatible with a diagnosis of histiocytic sarcoma, recent studies have shown that clonal immunoglobulin gene rearrangement, and rarely T-cell receptor gene rearrangement, can occur in up to 50% of cases.[1393,1400] This phenomenon is observed in sporadic cases as well as cases that occur subsequent to or concurrent with B- or T-lymphoblastic leukemia/lymphoma or low-grade B-cell lymphoma (especially follicular lymphoma).[1384,1393,1400–1402] In the latter scenario, the histiocytic sarcoma often shares the clonal markers of the previous leukemia/lymphoma, such as immunoglobulin gene rearrangement, *BCL2* rearrangement, and clonal cytogenetic aberrations.[1384,1400]

The nature of the entity called ALK+ histiocytosis remains to be clarified.[1385] It may represent a special form of histiocytic neoplasm occurring predominantly in infancy, characterized by systemic infiltration of large atypical histiocytes, most prominently in the liver. The histiocytic cells are S100+, CD68+, and ALK+.

Vascular tumors and tumorlike conditions

Hemangioma and **lymphangioma** involving nodes usually represent extension by contiguity of primary soft tissue lesions. However, rare cases of primary nodal hemangioma and lymphangioma have been described[1460,1471] (Fig. 21.124).

Epithelioid vascular neoplasms of lymph nodes include epithelioid hemangioma, epithelioid hemangioendothelioma, spindle and epithelioid hemangioendothelioma, and polymorphous hemangioendothelioma.[1462,1465,1479,1481] The differential diagnosis includes: (1) epithelioid hemangioma of soft tissue with a peripheral rim of germinal centers resulting in a nodelike appearance on low power (a much more common occurrence than true nodal epithelioid hemangioma);[1483] (2) Kimura disease (an altogether different process lacking epithelioid endothelial cells; see p. 1805); and (3) bacillary angiomatosis.

Bacillary angiomatosis, which occurs almost exclusively in the setting of immunodeficiency (especially in patients with HIV infection), presents as multiple coalescent intranodal clusters of proliferating vessels. These vessels are lined by plump, somewhat epithelioid endothelial cells (hence the original term epithelioid angiomatosis for this condition). A feature of great diagnostic importance is the presence of abundant eosinophilic to amphophilic, amorphous, or granular material in the interstitium. When stained with the Warthin–Starry technique, this material is shown to be composed of aggregated bacillary organisms that are indistinguishable from those of cat-scratch disease. Another helpful feature is the presence of neutrophils, sometimes forming microabscesses.[1463,1466,1478]

Vascular transformation of sinuses is characterized by a conversion of lymph node sinuses into a complex network of anastomosing endothelial-lined channels (Fig. 21.125).[1472] Fibrosis and

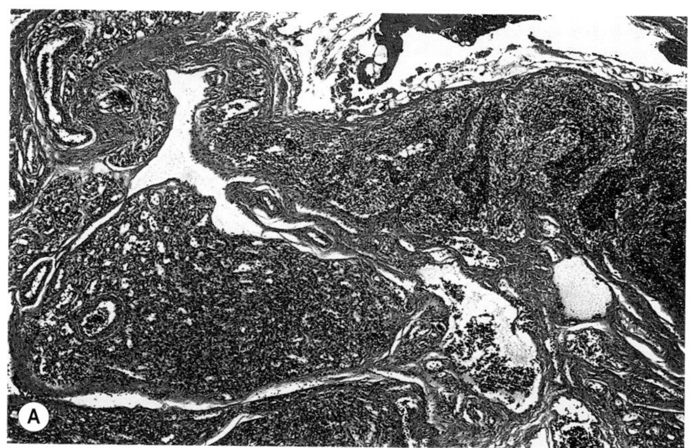

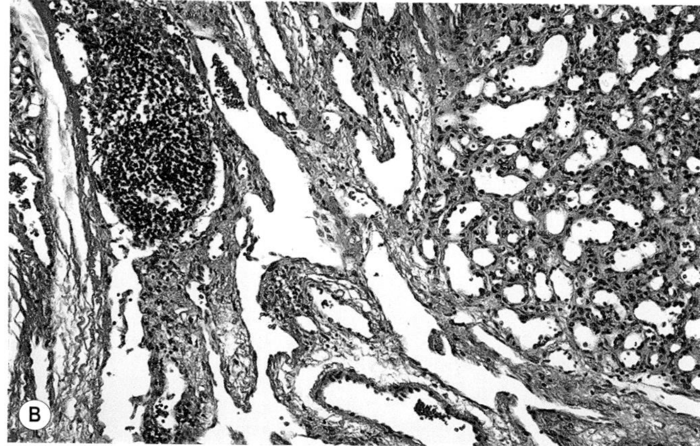

Fig. 21.124 Low-power (**A**) and medium-power (**B**) views of nodal hemangioma.

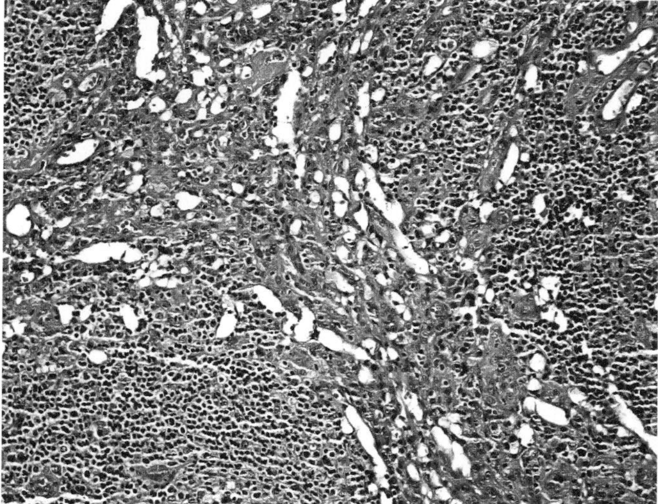

Fig. 21.125 Lymph node involvement by bacillary angiomatosis. An intense vascular proliferation featuring epithelioid endothelial cells is seen in the interfollicular region, accompanied by neutrophils and other inflammatory cells.

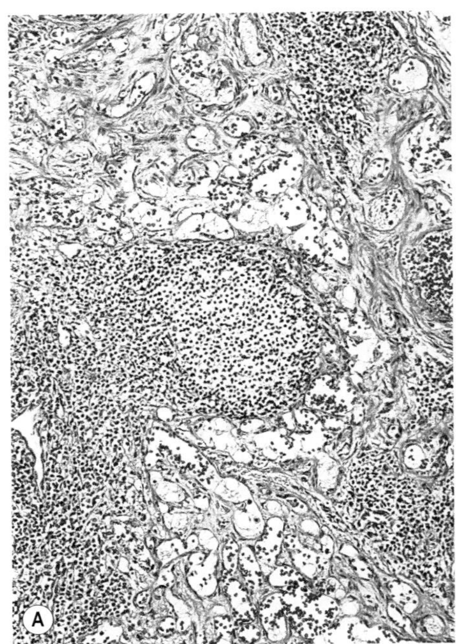
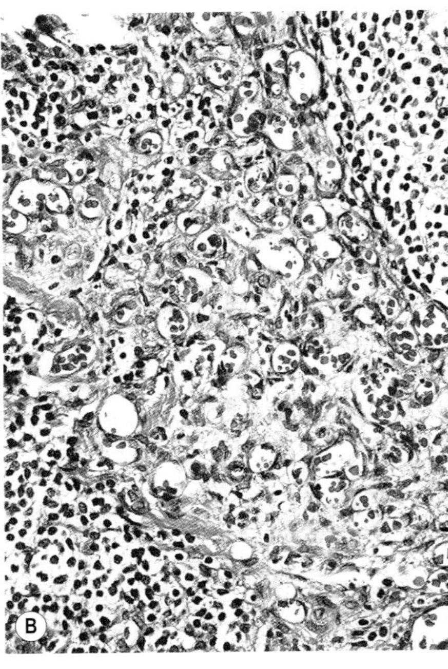

Fig. 21.126 A and **B**, Vascular transformation of lymph nodes. The process involves the sinuses, and it has a reactive appearance.

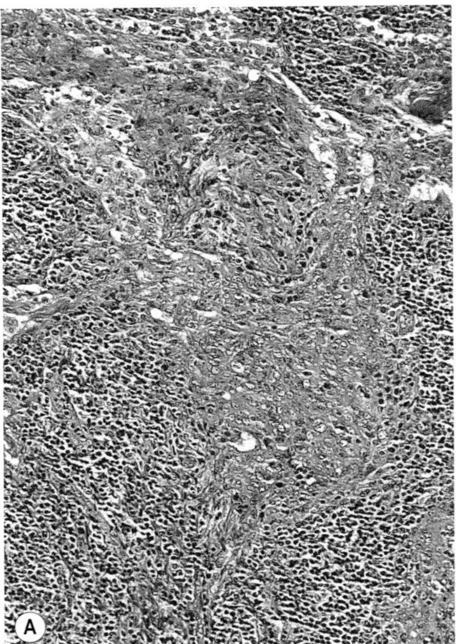
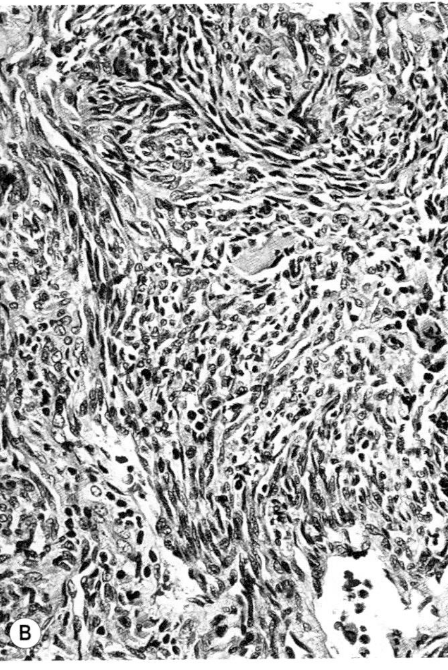

Fig. 21.127 A and **B**, Solid form of vascular transformation of lymph nodes. This process has also been designated as nodal angiomatosis. **A** shows the predominantly sinusal distribution of the lesions. The example shown in **B** occurred in a retroperitoneal lymph node in a patient with renal cell carcinoma.

reactive stromal changes are commonly present.[1477] *Nodal angiomatosis* probably refers to a more cellular form of the same condition[1468,1475] (Fig. 21.126). In the *nodular spindle-cell variant*, spindle-cell nodules composed of interlacing fascicles alternate with the vascular clefts.[1464] This variant is particularly likely to be misdiagnosed as Kaposi sarcoma. It is distinguished from the latter because it is confined to the sinuses (with sparing of the capsule and parenchyma), there is no cellular atypia, the fascicles blend with well-formed vascular channels, fibrosis is common, and PAS-positive hyaline globules are almost invariably absent. We have seen cases of this nodular spindle-cell variant in retroperitoneal lymph nodes draining renal cell carcinomas and have speculated about the possibility of its being the result of secretion of angiogenic factor by the carcinoma cells[1467,1474] (Fig. 21.127). Other cases of vascular transformation may result from proximal obstruction of the efferent vessels; indeed, the process has been reproduced experimentally by complete occlusion of these vessels.[1480]

Angiolipoma (including its cellular variant) is usually located in the soft tissue, but exceptionally it may be centered in a lymph node.[1473]

Kaposi sarcoma of the lymph nodes may be associated with typical skin lesions or develop in their absence.[1476] The latter occurrence is seen mainly in African children, but it also occurs in adults (usually but not always HIV-infected). Microscopically, the involved

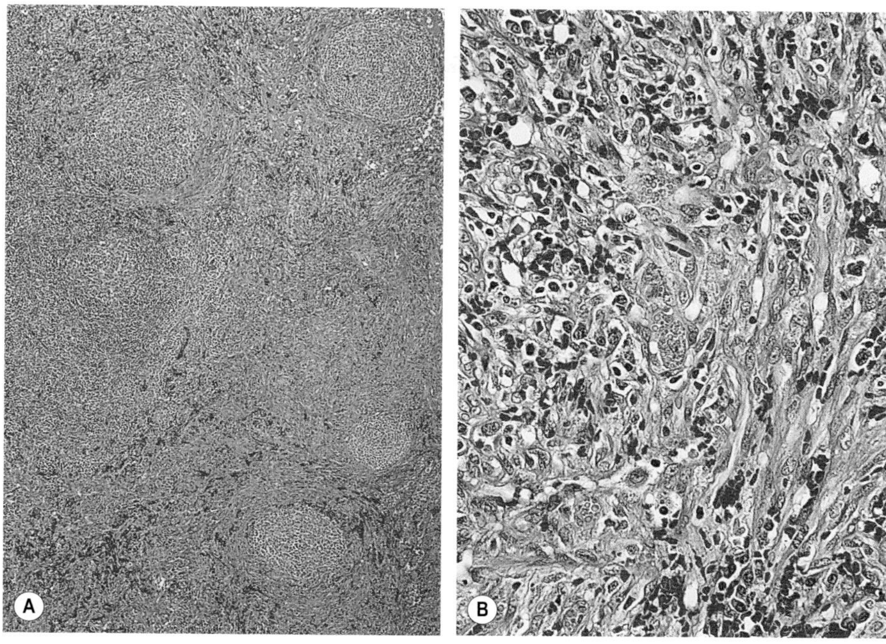

Fig. 21.128 **A** and **B**, Lymph node involvement by Kaposi sarcoma. The infiltrate is predominantly sinusal and is characterized by a proliferation of spindle cells forming slits containing red blood cells.

nodes show proliferation of spindle cells separated by slitlike spaces containing red blood cells[1461] (Fig. 21.128). The earliest changes are seen in the nodal capsule, but eventually there is involvement of the entire node and extension into the perinodal tissues. Cytoplasmic and extracellular hyaline globules that are positive for PAS and PTAH are almost always present.[1470] Recognition of early nodal involvement by Kaposi sarcoma is an extremely difficult task; often, only a diagnosis of 'atypical vascular proliferation suggestive of early Kaposi disease' is possible, although a more definitive diagnosis can be made if immunostaining for HHV8 is positive in the proliferating spindle cells. In well-developed cases, the tumor may grow in a diffuse fashion or as discrete deposits. The spindle-cell lesion is often accompanied by a lymphoid proliferation with a prominent component of plasma cells and immunoblasts. Sometimes, this reactive lymphoid process acquires the features of Castleman disease of the plasma cell type.[1469] In other instances, nodal Kaposi sarcoma coexists with malignant lymphoma or leukemia.[1482]

If a lymph node is involved by a malignant tumor with the morphologic features of **angiosarcoma**, there is a high probability that the tumor is metastatic (Fig. 21.129).

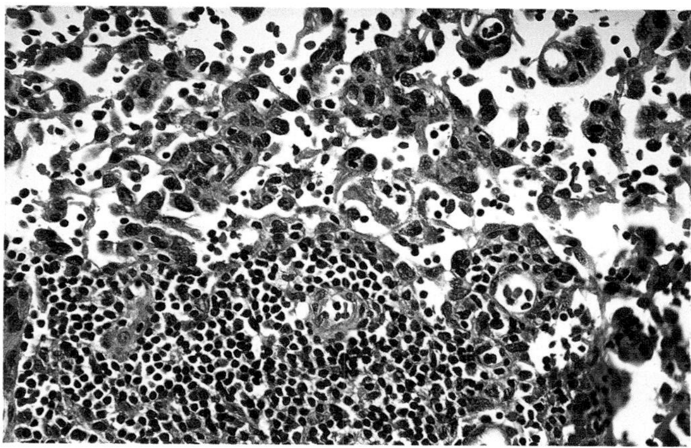

Fig. 21.129 Angiosarcoma of skin of scalp metastatic to a posterior cervical lymph node. The nodal lesion was the first manifestation of the disease.

Other primary tumors and tumorlike conditions

Mastocytosis of the diffuse (systemic) type often involves lymph nodes, resulting in partial or complete effacement of the architecture by a monotonous proliferation of round or polygonal cells[1489,1509] (Fig. 21.130). Clues as to the nature of the proliferation include the regular contours of the round or oval nucleus, the clear or granular cytoplasm, the well-defined cell outlines, admixture of eosinophils, and accompanying sclerosis. Special techniques that allow the identification of mast cells include Giemsa, metachromatic stains (i.e., toluidine blue, polychrome methylene blue), chloroacetate esterase (Leder), and immunohistochemical demonstration of tryptase, CD117, and the adhesion molecule CD44/HCAM[1484,1493,1501–1503,1510,1525] (Fig. 21.131).

It should be remembered that occasional mast cells are normally present in small number in lymph nodes. Their number is increased in some parasitoses, in Waldenström macroglobulinemia, and in several types of lymphadenitis, as documented in an early article by the Lennert group.[1508]

Acute myeloid leukemia can first be seen in a lymph node biopsy and misdiagnosed as malignant lymphoma.[1512] Traditionally, the disease has been referred to as granulocytic sarcoma or chloroma when appearing as a tumor mass in a lymph node or some other location outside the bone marrow. Clues to the diagnosis include a patchy or sinusal type of nodal involvement, sometimes associated with a single-file pattern of infiltration in the capsule; fine granularity of the cytoplasm; and presence of eosinophilic myelocytes. Immunohistochemically, there is reactivity for CD43, lysozyme, myeloperoxidase, CD99, and CD117.[1486,1518] Four phenotypic variants have been described.[1486] *Extramedullary hematopoiesis*

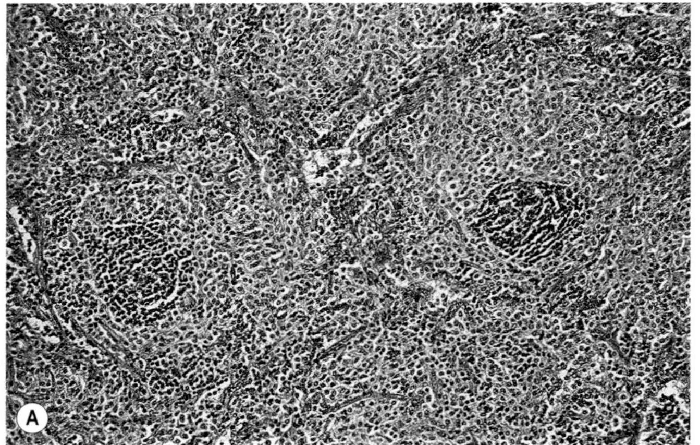

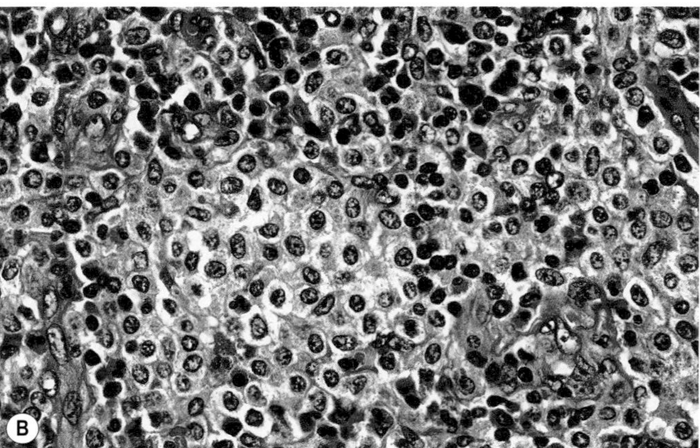

Fig. 21.130 Medium-power (**A**) and high-power (**B**) views of lymph node involvement in systemic mastocytosis. Note the perfectly round shape of the centrally located nuclei, the finely granular cytoplasm, and the well-defined cell membranes.

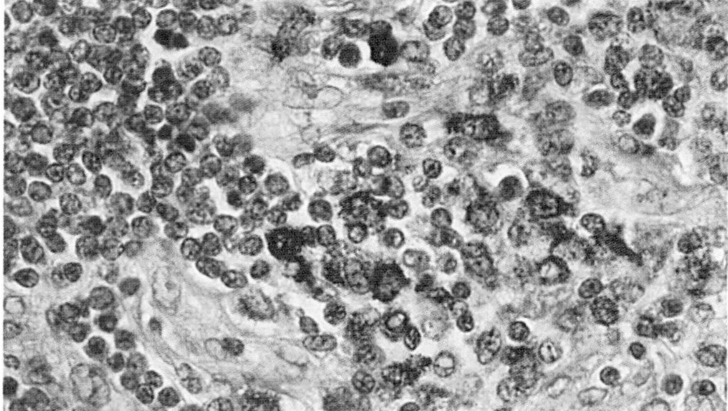

Fig. 21.131 Lymph node involved by systemic mastocytosis. The myeloid precursors stain an intense red color. (Leder chloroacetate esterase.)

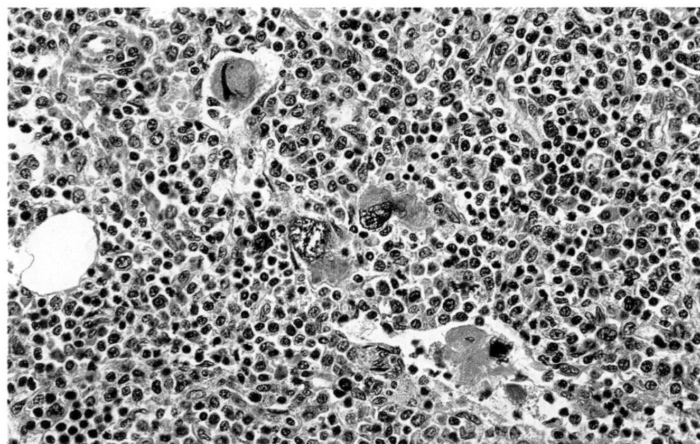

Fig. 21.132 Scattered megakaryocytes in lymph node involved by extramedullary hematopoiesis. These elements should not be confused with Reed–Sternberg cells or carcinoma cells.

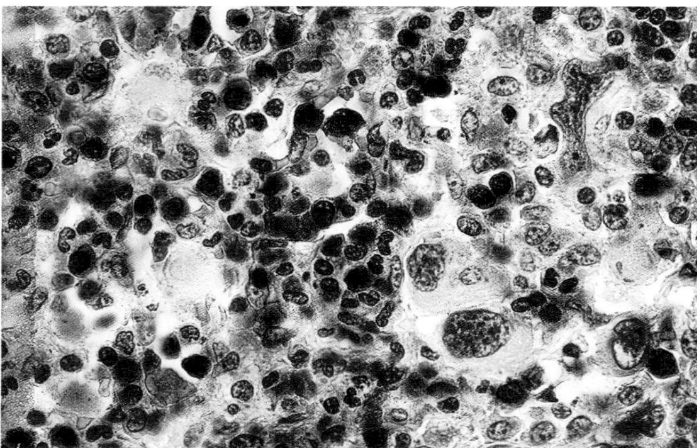

Fig. 21.133 Positivity with Leder (chloroacetate esterase) stain in the myeloid precursors present in lymph node affected by extramedullary hematopoiesis.

accompanied by megakaryocytes can be confused with Hodgkin lymphoma and other malignancies (Fig. 21.132). A Leder chloroacetate stain will reveal the immature myeloid forms (Fig. 21.133).

Smooth muscle proliferations of a primary nature can be seen within lymph nodes in the following situations:

1 *Smooth muscle proliferation in the hilum.* This is often accompanied by fibrosis and prominent vascularity.[1491] It is most common in the inguinal region and is of no clinical significance.
2 *Angiomyolipoma.* The most common location is the retroperitoneal region, usually in conjunction with a renal tumor of the same type (see Chapter 17).[1488] Immunoreactivity for HMB-45 and other melanocyte-related markers is a constant feature of this entity.
3 *Lymphangiomyomatosis.* This is seen exclusively in women, often in association with pulmonary involvement, but sometimes showing pelvic lymph node involvement alone as an incidental finding.[1492] Like the previous entity, to which it is histogenetically related, it exhibits immunoreactivity for HMB-45.
4 *Leiomyomatosis.* This has been reported mainly in intra-abdominal nodes, sometimes in association with uterine leiomyomas or leiomyomatosis peritonealis disseminata.[1500,1511]
5 *Angiomatous hamartoma.* This is a distinctive form of smooth muscle proliferation that seems to occur only in the inguinal

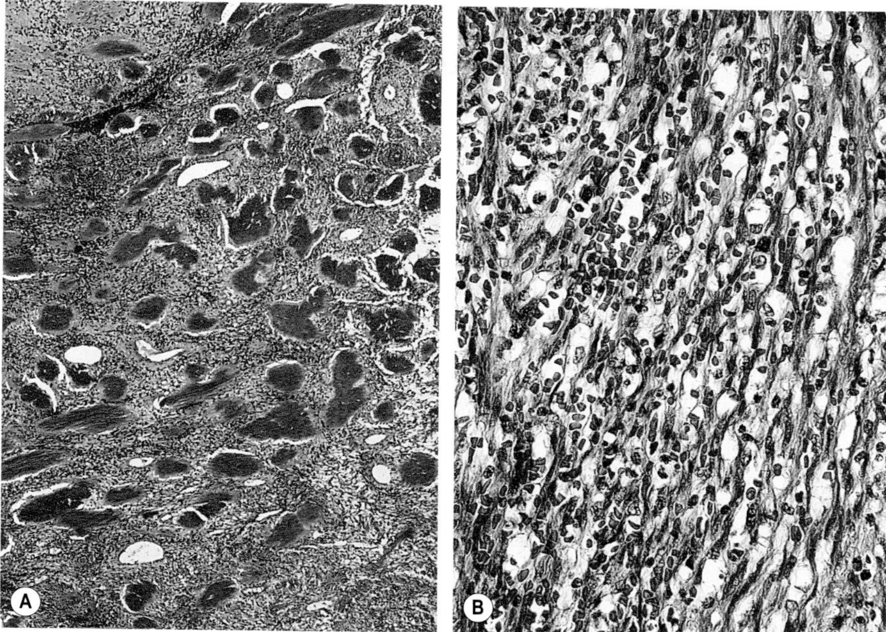

Fig. 21.134 **A** and **B**, Hemorrhagic spindle cell tumor with amianthoid fibers. **A**, Prominent deposition of 'amianthoid' collagen throughout the tumor. **B**, The admixture of neoplastic spindle cells and extravasated red blood cells results in a Kaposi sarcoma-like appearance.

region. It is characterized by a proliferation of thick-walled hilar blood vessels that sometimes extends into the nodal parenchyma.[1490]

6 *Intranodal leiomyoma*. Some of the reported cases have occurred in the setting of HIV infection.[1520]

Hemorrhagic spindle-cell tumor with amianthoid fibers (also known as palisaded myofibroblastoma) is a distinctive benign neoplasm that occurs preferentially in inguinal lymph nodes but that can involve nodes of other sites, such as the neck and mediastinum.[1487,1498,1499,1507,1520,1521,1523] The main microscopic features are the proliferation of bland-looking spindle cells, sometimes in a palisading fashion; extensive foci of recent and old hemorrhage; and giant rosettelike collections of collagen fibers (so-called 'amianthoid fibers')[1513,1519,1522] (Fig. 21.134). The differential diagnosis includes Kaposi sarcoma and intranodal schwannoma. Immunohistochemically, the spindle cells are reactive for vimentin and actin, particularly around the rosettelike formations. The staining qualities and ultrastructural features are more in favor of a smooth muscle than a myofibroblastic derivation.[1524] The behavior has been benign in all reported cases, but there has been an isolated instance of recurrence.[1494]

Inflammatory pseudotumor of lymph nodes may be localized or affect several lymph node groups and may be accompanied by fever, anemia, elevated erythrocyte sedimentation rate, and hypergammaglobulinemia.[1495,1496,1504,1505,1516] Microscopically, the process involves primarily the fibrous stroma of the node, with secondary spread into the lymphoid tissue and perinodal tissues. It is characterized by a storiform pattern of growth, vascular proliferation, and a polymorphic infiltrate composed of fibroblasts, plasma cells, immunoblasts, small lymphocytes, histiocytes, dendritic cells, and neutrophils (Fig. 21.135). Morphologic variations on this basic theme exist, which have been attributed to the stage of the disease at which the biopsy has been taken.[1514] Presence of the EBV genome has been documented in a minority of cases.

Inflammatory pseudotumor of lymph nodes (and spleen) seems to be a different entity from its homonym in the soft tissue, lung, and other sites. The latter group, which can follow an aggressive

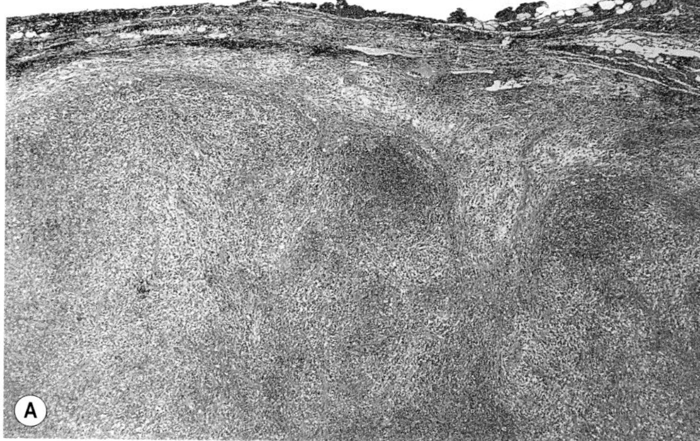

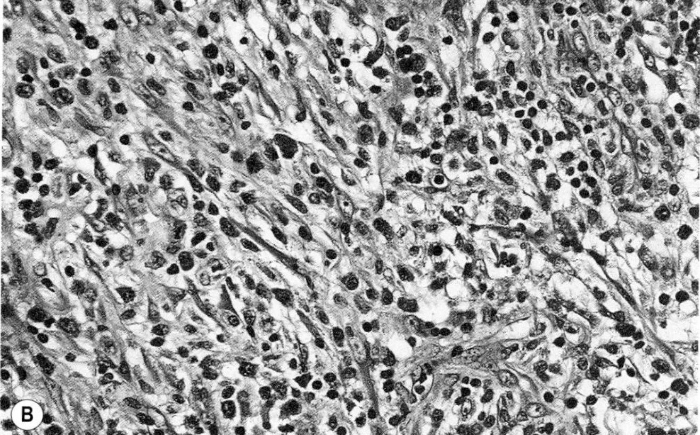

Fig. 21.135 **A** and **B**, Inflammatory pseudotumor of lymph node. **A**, Low-power appearance showing partial effacement of architecture and expansion of the sinusal and perinodal regions by a reactive proliferation. **B**, High-power view showing a polymorphic infiltrate composed of lymphocytes, plasma cells, and myofibroblasts.

clinical course and which is accompanied by a balanced chromosomal translocation involving the *ALK* gene, is now regarded as a neoplastic process and has accordingly been renamed inflammatory myofibroblastic tumor. Conversely, the lymph node condition consistently lacks this genetic aberration and follows a generally favorable course, suggesting that it is truly an inflammatory/reactive process, perhaps related to the group of conditions generically known as inflammatory fibrosclerosis.[1506] A very interesting recent development in this field is the realization that the inflammatory pseudotumor appearance can result from syphilitic infection.[1497] Consideration should also be given to the possibility of the actin- and desmin-positive spindle cells present in this disorder being of fibroblastic reticulum/dendritic cell rather than myofibroblastic type.[1515] Inflammatory pseudotumors of an altogether different type can result from *Mycobacterium avium-intracellulare* infection in immunocompromised individuals (mycobacterial spindle cell pseudotumor) (Fig. 21.136).

Anthracosis and **anthracosilicosis** can result in a pseudoneoplastic appearance because of the presence of a sometimes intense histiocytic proliferation with a focally storiform pattern of growth[1485] (Fig. 21.137).

Solar elastotic material can be found in the subcapsular sinus and parenchyma of lymph nodes, presumably as a result of mechanical transport from the skin.[1517]

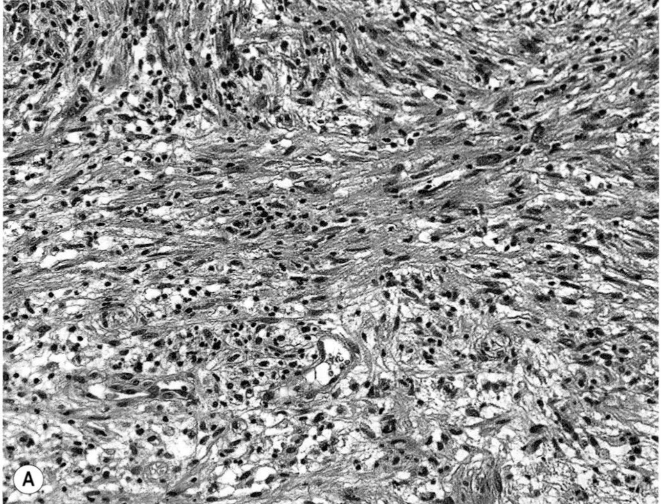

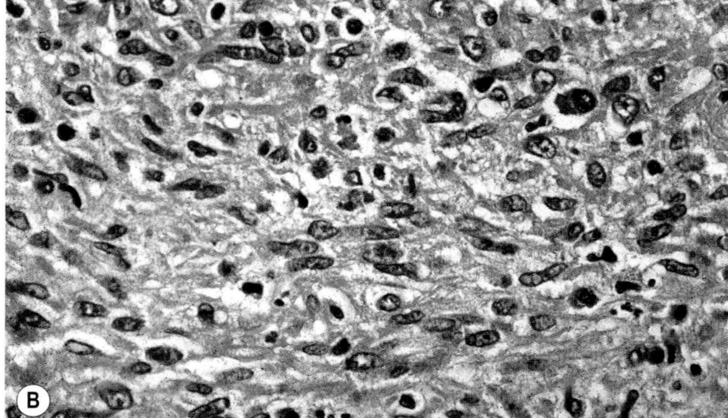

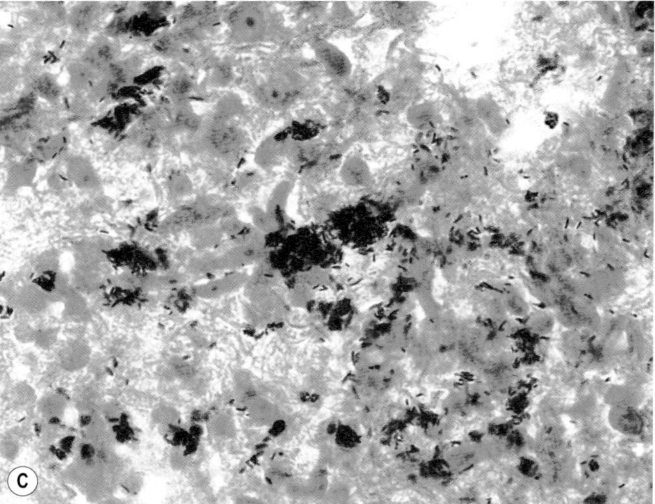

Fig. 21.136 A–C, Inflammatory pseudotumor of lymph node due to *Mycobacterium avium-intracellulare* infection in an HIV-infected patient. **A**, Low-power view, showing spindle cell admixed with lymphocytes. **B**, High-power view. **C**, Acid-fast stain.

Metastatic tumors

Lymph nodes are the most common site of metastatic malignancy, and sometimes constitute the first clinical manifestation of the disease.[1533,1539,1546] The task of the pathologist is to identify the presence of a malignant process in the node, to establish whether it is metastatic or not, and – if metastatic – to provide an estimate of its amount, microscopic type, and possible source. If malignant cells are identified within the efferent lymph vessels and/or extranodal adipose tissue, this should also be noted in the report because of the possible prognostic significance of these findings.

Any malignant tumor can give rise to lymph node metastases, but the incidence varies greatly depending on the tumor type. It is common with carcinomas, malignant melanomas, and germ cell tumors, and rare with sarcomas and central nervous system tumors. It should also be noted that large cell lymphomas primary in an organ (such as stomach or thyroid) sometimes involve the regional nodes in a pattern consistent with metastatic spread (see also p. 1838).

An additional diagnosis to consider in a lymph node involvement by metastatic tumor is that of malignant mesothelioma (Fig. 21.138). We have seen several examples of this tumor type presenting initially with lymphadenopathy in the cervical or inguinal region; most of the primary tumors were located in the peritoneum rather than the pleura, regardless of the location of the nodes.[1545] The differential diagnosis includes reactive benign mesothelial cells in lymph nodes (see p. 1849) (Fig. 21.139).

It is very rare for soft tissue sarcomas to present initially as a lymph node metastasis. The outstanding exception is alveolar rhabdomyosarcoma (particularly the solid variant), which can be confused with malignant lymphoma not only on morphologic grounds but also because it may involve several lymph node groups (so-called 'lymphadenopathic form') (Fig. 21.140). Other sarcomas that have a greater than average tendency to metastasize to regional nodes are embryonal rhabdomyosarcoma, angiosarcoma, epithelioid sarcoma, and synovial sarcoma.

The differential diagnosis between metastatic undifferentiated carcinoma and diffuse large cell lymphoma in routine sections may be difficult or even impossible in some cases. Features favoring lymphoma are presence of focal nodularity within the tumor not induced by fibrosis, and diffuse permeation of walls of veins (as opposed to tumor thrombi) and adipose tissue if an extranodal component is present. Features favoring metastatic tumor are focal nodal involvement, definite nesting, extensive necrosis, predominantly sinusal distribution, and solid tumor plugs in lymphatic vessels. The types of malignant lymphoma most likely to be misdiagnosed as metastatic carcinoma are anaplastic large cell lymphoma, large B-cell lymphoma with sclerosis resulting in prominent nesting, large B-cell lymphoma with a predominantly sinusal pattern of growth, nodular sclerosis Hodgkin lymphoma with concentration of large mononuclear variants of Reed–Sternberg cells around areas of necrosis, and signet ring cell lymphoma. Yet another type is the composite lymphoma made up of follicular small cleaved and diffuse large cell components, the double error consisting in diagnosing the latter component as metastatic carcinoma and the former as follicular hyperplasia.

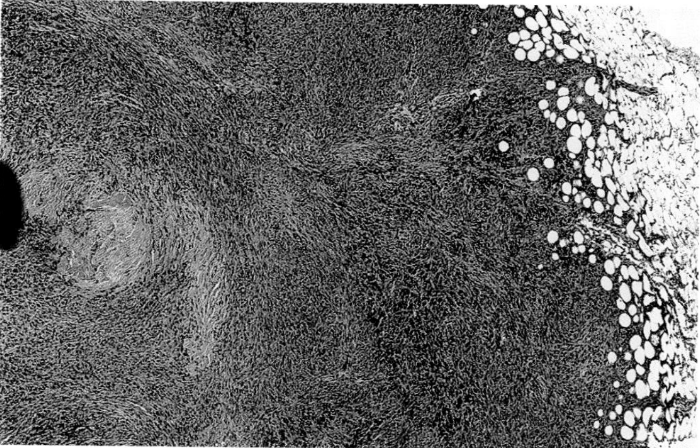

Fig. 21.137 Anthracosilicotic nodules in mediastinal lymph node. When florid, these changes may acquire pseudoneoplastic features.

The metastatic carcinomas that most closely simulate a malignant lymphoid process are nasopharyngeal lymphoepithelial carcinoma and lobular carcinoma of the breast (Figs 21.141 and 21.142). The first may masquerade clinically and pathologically as Hodgkin lymphoma because of its common presentation in a young adult with painless unilateral cervical lymphadenopathy and the presence of a polymorphic population (including eosinophils) on microscopic examination.[1536] The second may be confused with malignant lymphomas of one type or another. This is particularly true of the type composed of small uniform cells with only occasional signet ring formations, which can look remarkably lymphocyte-like (Fig. 21.143). Metastatic small cell neuroendocrine carcinoma from the lung or other sites can be difficult to distinguish from lymphoma; dense nuclear chromatin pattern, nuclear molding, focal areas of necrosis, and hematoxyphilic staining of vessel walls favor a diagnosis of small cell carcinoma. Somewhat similar considerations pertain to the diagnosis of metastatic Merkel cell carcinoma. Metastatic melanoma can closely simulate on cytologic grounds the appearance of large cell lymphoma and plasmacytoma. The balloon cell variety can closely mimic Rosai–Dorfman disease (Fig. 21.144). One should also not forget that metastases can develop in a node already involved by lymphoma or leukemia.

Among the conventional special stains, the two most likely to help in the differential diagnosis between metastatic carcinoma and lymphoma are PAS and mucin stains. In general, positivity for the latter will establish the diagnosis of adenocarcinoma. The presence of abundant glycogen and/or diastase-resistant mucosubstances in the cytoplasm of a large cell tumor on a PAS stain will also rule out, for all practical purposes, a diagnosis of lymphoma. We have found reticulin stains of only limited value in this differential diagnosis. Instead, touch preparations can be of great diagnostic utility by showing clumping of the tumor cells in carcinoma and the absence of clumping in lymphoma. Ultrastructural examination is also

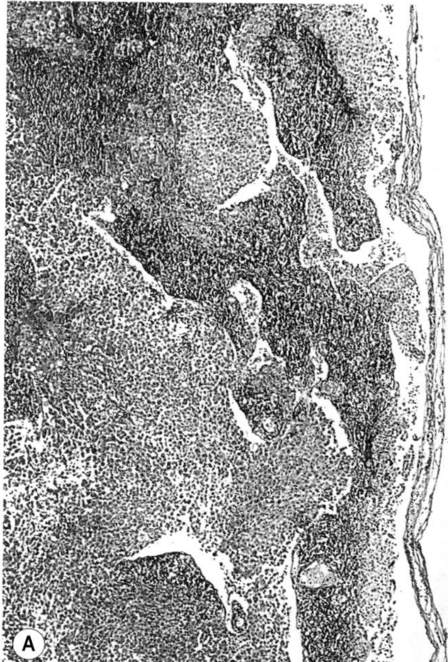

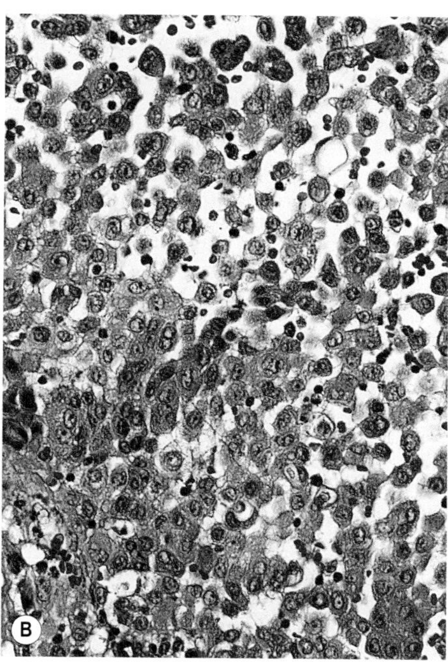

Fig. 21.138 **A** and **B**, Lymph node involved by metastatic mesothelioma. The tumor massively expands the sinuses and is composed of cuboidal cells with a central nucleus and acidophilic cytoplasm. The primary tumor was located in the peritoneal cavity.

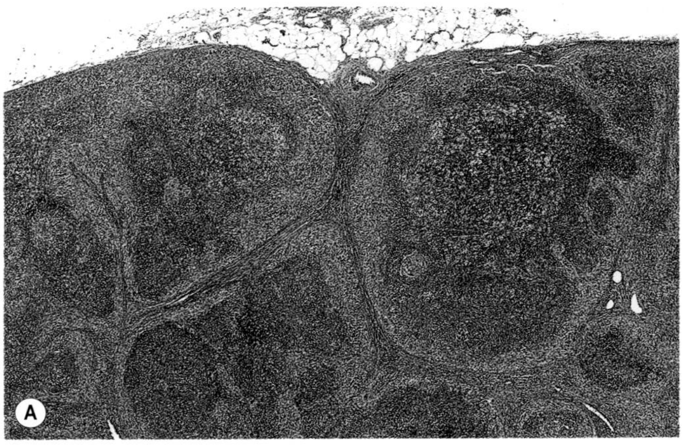

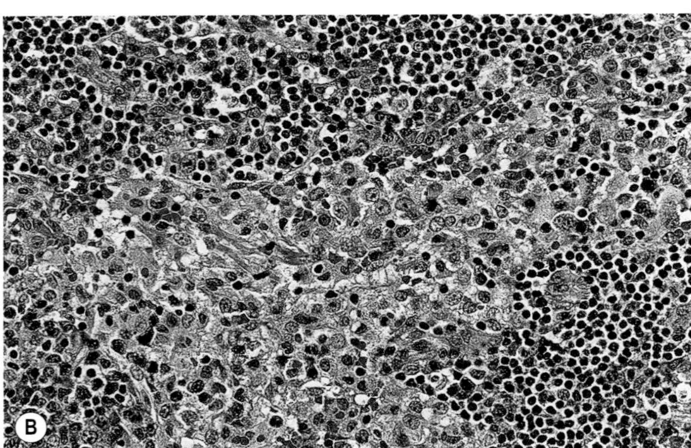

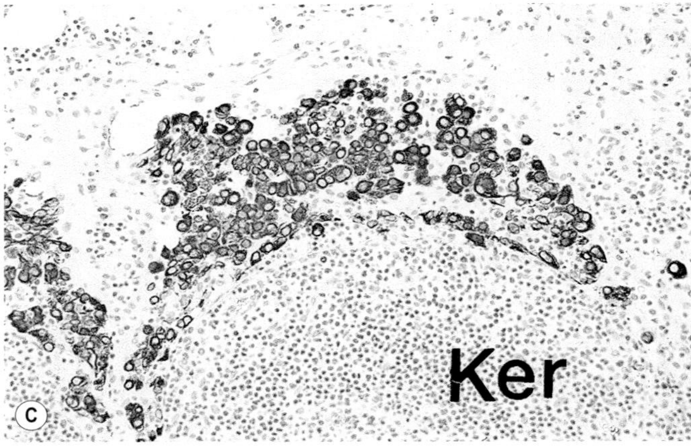

Fig. 21.139 A–C, Hyperplastic mesothelial cells in lymph node. **A**, Sinusal distribution. **B**, Bland cytologic appearance. **C**, Strong immunoreactivity for keratin.

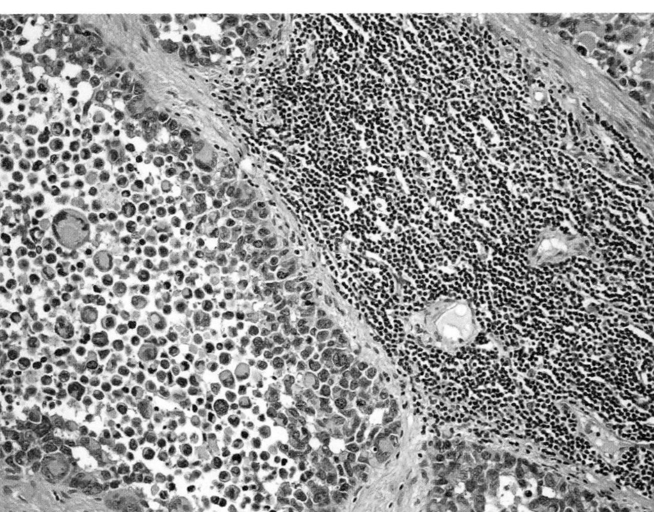

Fig. 21.140 Alveolar rhabdomyosarcoma metastatic to a lymph node. This is a relatively common occurrence in this tumor type and it may be the first clinical manifestation of the disease.

likely to be useful because it will usually demonstrate epithelial features such as complex desmosomes, tonofibrils, and extracellular or intracellular glandular lumina.[1534] However, the special technique that is clearly the top choice for the efficient resolution of this problem is immunocytochemistry. The 'basic kit' with which to approach an obviously malignant tumor involving a lymph node is CD45, keratin, and S-100 protein, as markers for lymphoid, epithelial, and melanocytic cells, respectively. A second line of reagents could include EMA, CEA, CD20, CD3, vimentin, and – depending on the circumstances – GCDFP-15 and lactalbumin (for breast), chromogranin (for endocrine tumors), and PSA/PAP (for prostate). When properly applied and interpreted, the performance of these reactions should solve all but a very small minority of cases.

Nodal metastases of squamous cell carcinoma have a particular tendency to undergo cystic changes. When these are prominent in a node located in the neck, a mistaken diagnosis of branchial cleft cyst may ensue (Figs 21.145 and 21.146).

It is just as important to mention some of the benign conditions of lymph nodes that can mistakenly be interpreted as metastatic carcinoma. They include hyperplastic mesothelial cells,[1527] megakaryocytes,[1540] signet ring sinus histiocytosis,[1538] the related nodal muciphages and mucicarminophilic histiocytosis,[1532,1537] florid anthracosis/anthracosilicosis,[1526] and the various lymph node epithelial inclusions listed on page 1848, without forgetting the banal germinal centers of hyperplastic follicles cut tangentially.

The location of a node involved by metastatic carcinoma gives important clues about the possible site of the primary. The large

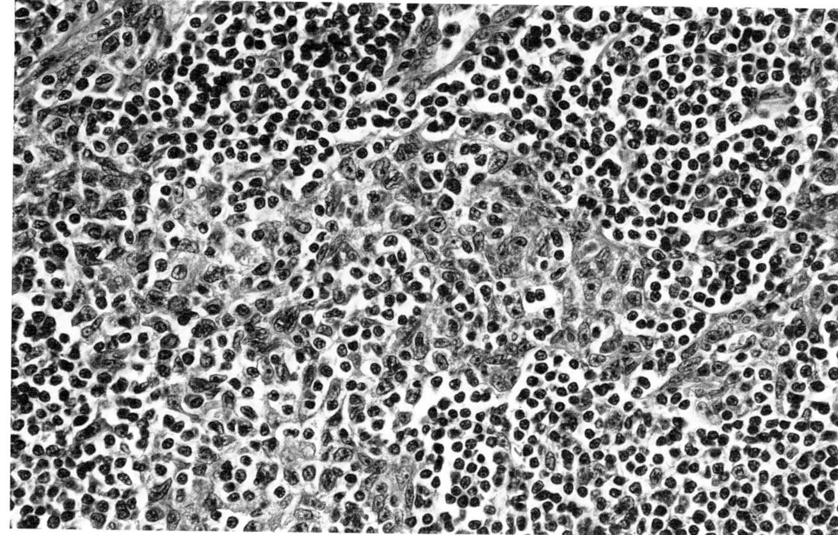

Fig. 21.141 Lymph node involved by metastatic lymphoepithelioma from the nasopharynx. The relatively diffuse pattern of the proliferation may result in a mistaken diagnosis of malignant lymphoma.

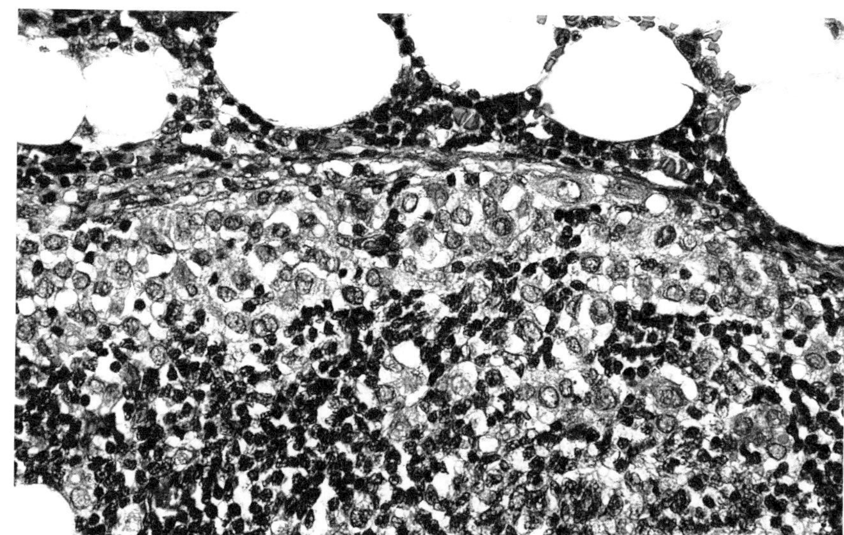

Fig. 21.142 Breast carcinoma of lobular type metastatic to the sinuses of a lymph node. The cytologic appearance may be confused with that of a malignant lymphoma.

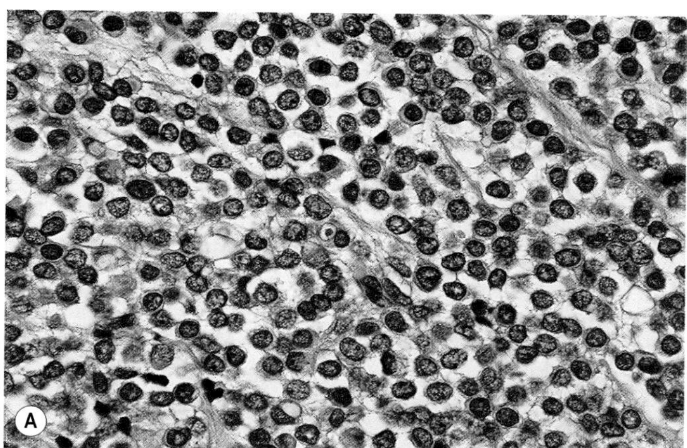

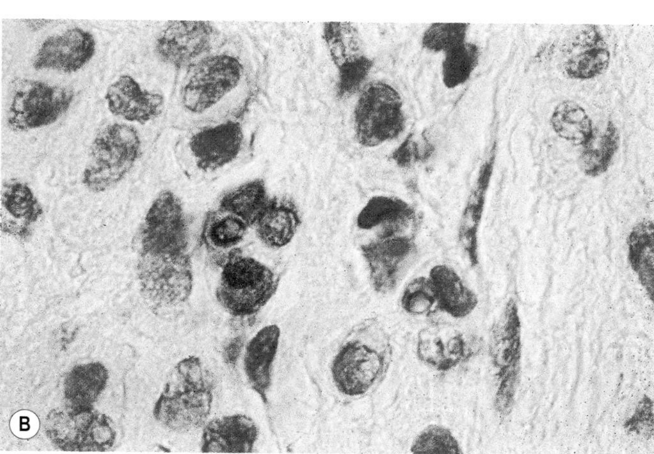

Fig. 21.143 **A** and **B**, Poorly differentiated adenocarcinoma with signet ring features initially misinterpreted as a malignant lymphoma. The mistake may have been partially induced by the fact that the tumor developed in a renal transplant recipient. **A**, Hematoxylin–eosin. **B**, Mucicarmine stain, showing a few droplets of intracytoplasmic mucin.

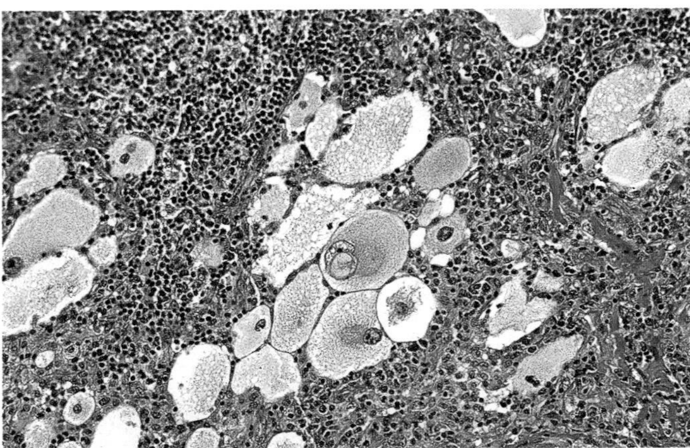

Fig. 21.144 Balloon cell melanoma metastatic to a lymph node and simulating a histiocytic disorder.

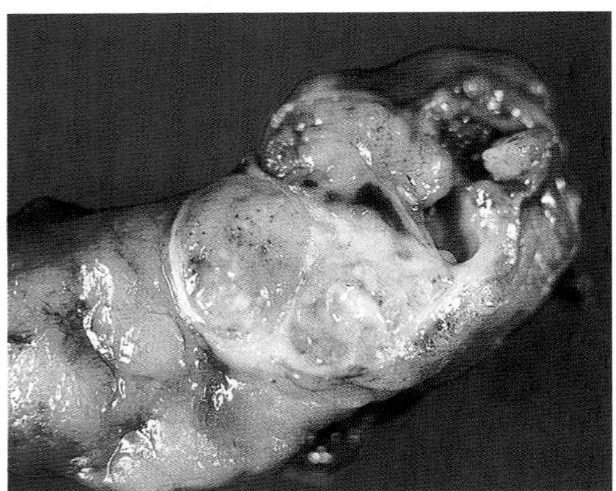

Fig. 21.145 Squamous cell carcinoma metastatic to lymph node. The tumor has undergone partial cystic transformation.

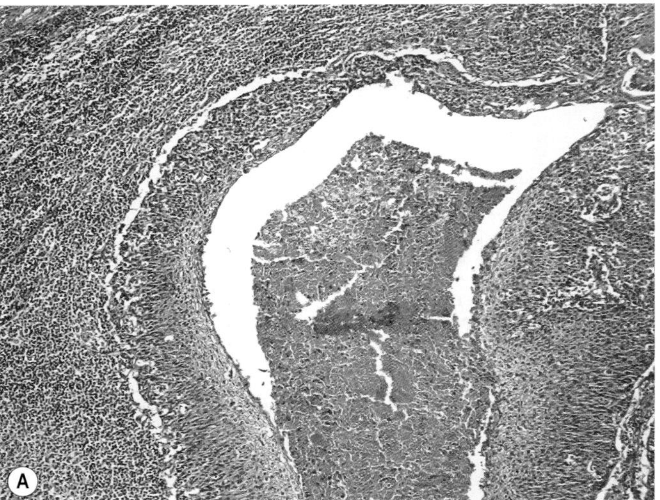

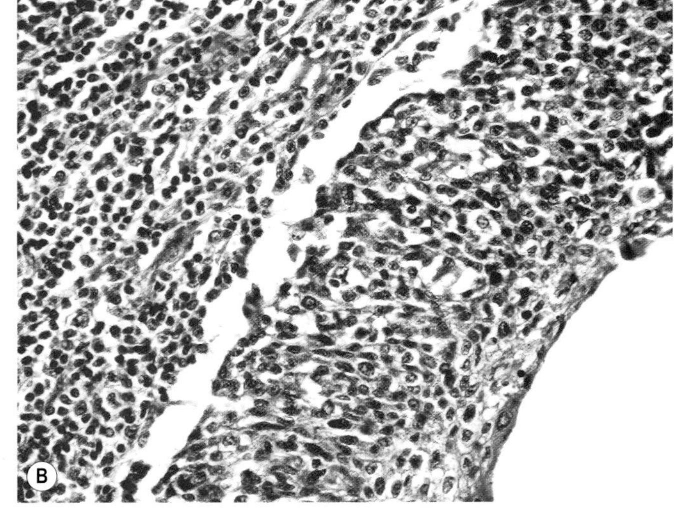

Fig. 21.146 A and **B**, Squamous cell carcinoma metastatic to cervical lymph node. **A**, Medium-power view, showing marked cystic change that may result in a mistaken diagnosis of branchial cleft cyst. **B**, High-power view showing malignant cytologic features involving the entire thickness of the epithelial strip.

majority of tumors metastatic to *upper cervical* lymph nodes originate from the upper aerodigestive tract. Sites well known for harboring small, clinically undetectable primaries in the presence of cervical adenopathy are the nasopharynx and retrotonsillar pillar.[1528,1541,1542] *Midcervical* nodes containing papillary carcinoma are usually examples of metastatic thyroid carcinoma, a possibility that becomes a virtual certainty in the presence of psammoma bodies. However, these papillary tumors may also originate from salivary gland, female genital tract, or thymus (see respective chapters). Squamous cell carcinomas in lymph nodes of this region usually arise in the upper aerodigestive tract, particularly pharynx and larynx.[1544] Most carcinomas metastatic to *supraclavicular* lymph nodes originate in the lung or breast. Other sources of metastases to this nodal group, particularly if located on the left side, are carcinoma of stomach, pancreas, prostate, and testis.[1541,1543] These reach the node through the terminal collecting lymphatic trunks. Supraclavicular nodes involved by intra-abdominal carcinomas are sometimes referred to as Virchow or Troisier nodes.[1529] The large majority of metastatic tumors in *axillary* nodes of adult females are breast carcinoma and malignant melanoma.[1531,1535] Lung carcinoma should also be considered, especially in older patients with a smoking history.[1530] *Inguinal* nodes are often the recipients of carcinomas from the external genital organs (usually evident on clinical examination) or malignant melanomas of the lower extremities, but only rarely from the internal abdominal organs (ovary, uterine cervix, anal canal) and even less commonly from the testis, unless direct extension to the scrotal skin has occurred.[1547]

References

NORMAL ANATOMY

1 Delves PJ, Roitt IM. The immune system. First of two parts. N Engl J Med 2000, **343**: 37–49.

2 Ioachim HL, Medeiros LJ. Ioachim's lymph node pathology, ed. 4. Philadelphia, 2008, Lippincott Williams & Wilkins.

3 Liu YJ, Zhang J, Lane PJ, Chan EY, MacLennan IC. Sites of specific B cell activation in primary and secondary responses to T-cell-dependent and T-cell-independent antigens. Eur J Immunol 1991, **21**: 2951–2962.

4 Stein H, Bonk A, Tolksdorf G, Lennert K, Rodt H, Gerdes J. Immunohistologic analysis of the organization of normal lymphoid tissue and non-Hodgkin's lymphomas. J Histochem Cytochem 1980, **28**: 746–760.

5 Szakal AK, Kosco MH, Tew JG. Microanatomy of lymphoid tissue during humoral immune responses. Structure function relationships. Annu Rev Immunol 1989, **7**: 91–109.

6 van der Valk P, Meijer CJLM. Lymph nodes. In Mills SE (ed.): Histology for pathologists, ed. 3. Philadelphia, 2007, Lippincott Williams & Wilkins, pp. 763–782.

LYMPH NODE EVALUATION

BIOPSY

7 Banks PM. Technical factors in the preparation and evaluation of lymph node biopsies. In Knowles DM (ed.): Neoplastic hematopathology, ed. 2. Philadelphia, 2001, Lippincott Williams & Wilkins, pp. 467–482.

8 Banks PM, Long JC, Howard CA. Preparation of lymph node biopsy specimens. Hum Pathol 1979, **10**: 617–621.

9 Beard C, Nabers K, Bowling MC, Berard CW. Achieving technical excellence in lymph node specimens. An update. Lab Med 1985, **16**: 468–475.

10 Weiss LM, Dorfman RF, Warnke RA. Lymph node work-up. In Fenoglio-Preiser C (ed.): Advances in pathology, vol. 1. Chicago, 1988, Year Book Medical Publishers.

NEEDLE BIOPSY

11 Cafferty LL, Katz RL, Ordonez NG, Carrasco CH, Cabanillas FR. Fine needle aspiration diagnosis of intraabdominal and retroperitoneal lymphomas by a morphologic and immunocytochemical approach. Cancer 1990, **65**: 72–77.

12 Frable WJ, Kardos TF. Fine needle aspiration biopsy. Applications in the diagnosis of lymphoproliferative diseases. Am J Surg Pathol 1988, **12**(Suppl 1): 62–72.

13 Kardos TF, Maygarden SJ, Blumberg AK, Wakely PE Jr, Frable WJ. Fine needle aspiration biopsy in the management of children and young adults with peripheral lymphadenopathy. Cancer 1989, **63**: 703–707.

14 Kern WH. Exfoliative and aspiration cytology of malignant lymphomas. Semin Diagn Pathol 1986, **3**: 211–218.

15 Pitts WC, Weiss LM. Fine needle aspiration biopsy of lymph nodes. Pathol Annu 1988, **23**(Pt 2): 329–360.

16 Tsang WY, Chan JK. Spectrum of morphologic changes in lymph nodes attributable to fine needle aspiration. Hum Pathol 1992, **23**: 562–565.

17 van Heerde P, Go DMDS, Koolman-Schellekens MA, Peterse JL. Cytodiagnosis of non-Hodgkin's lymphoma. A morphological analysis of 215 biopsy proven cases. Virchows Arch [A] 1984, **403**: 213–233.

ELECTRON MICROSCOPY

18 Mackay B. Ultrastructural diagnosis of lymphomas and leukemias. Ultrastruct Pathol 1985, **9**: 209–214.

19 Peiper SC, Kahn LB. Ultrastructural comparison of Hodgkin's and non-Hodgkin's lymphomas. Histopathology 1982, **6**: 93–109.

IMMUNOPHENOTYPING

20 Chu PG, Chang KL, Arber DA, Weiss LM. Immunophenotyping of hematopoietic neoplasms. Semin Diagn Pathol 2000, **17**: 236–256.

21 Frizzera G, Wu D, Inghirami G. The usefulness of immunophenotypic and genotypic studies in the diagnosis and classification of hematopoietic and lymphoid neoplasms. An update. Am J Clin Pathol 1999, **111**: S13–S39.

22 Higgins RA, Blankenship JE, Kinney MC. Application of immunohistochemistry in the diagnosis of non-Hodgkin and Hodgkin lymphoma. Arch Pathol Lab Med 2008, **132**: 441–461.

23 Mason D, André P, Densussan A, Buckley C, Civin C, Clark E, De Haas M, Goyert S, Hadam M, Hart D, Horejsi V, Meuer S, Morrisey J, Schwartz-Albiez R, Shaw S, Simmons D, Ugussioni M, Van Der Schoot E, Vivier E, Zola H. CD antigens 2001. Mod Pathol 2002, **15**: 71–76.

Gene rearrangement analysis

24 Chan JK, Kwong YL. Common misdiagnoses in lymphomas and avoidance strategies. Lancet Oncol 2010, **6**: 579–588.

25 Collins RD. Is clonality equivalent to malignancy: specifically, is immunoglobulin gene rearrangement diagnostic of malignant lymphoma? Hum Pathol 1997, **28**: 757–759.

26 Davis RE, Warnke RA, Dorfman RF, Cleary ML. Utility of molecular genetic analysis for the diagnosis of neoplasia in morphologically and immunophenotypically equivocal hematolymphoid lesions. Cancer 1991, **67**: 2890–2899.

27 Dubeau L, Weinberg K, Jones PA, Nichols PW. Studies on immunoglobulin gene rearrangement in formalin-fixed, paraffin-embedded pathology specimens. Am J Pathol 1988, **130**: 588–594.

28 Feller AC, Griesser H, Schilling CV, Wacker HH, Dallenbach F, Bartels H, Kuse R, Mak TW, Lennert K. Clonal gene rearrangement patterns correlate with immunophenotype and clinical parameters in patients with angioimmunoblastic lymphadenopathy. Am J Pathol 1988, **133**: 549–556.

29 Henni T, Gaulard P, Divine M, Le Couedic JP, Rocha D, Haioun C, Henni Z, Marolleau JP, Pinaudeau Y, Goossens M, et al. Comparison of genetic probe with immunophenotype analysis in lymphoproliferative disorders. A study of 87 cases. Blood 1988, **72**: 1937–1943.

30 Ilyas M, Jalal H, Linton C, Rooney N. The use of the polymerase chain reaction in the diagnosis of B-cell lymphomas from formalin-fixed paraffin-embedded tissue. Histopathology 1995, **26**: 333–338.

31 Jevremovic D, Viswanatha DS. Molecular diagnosis of hematopoietic and lymphoid neoplasms. Hematol Oncol Clin North Am 2009, **23**: 903–933.

32 Kamat D, Laszewski MJ, Kemp JD, Goeken JA, Lutz CT, Platz CE, Dick FR. The diagnostic utility of immunophenotyping and immunogenotyping in the pathologic evaluation of lymphoid proliferations. Mod Pathol 1990, **3**: 105–112.

33 Medeiros LJ, Bagg A, Cossman J. Application of molecular genetics to the diagnosis of hematopoietic neoplasms. In Knowles DM (ed.): Neoplastic hematopathology. Baltimore, 1992, Williams and Wilkins.

34 Sandberg Y, van Gastel-Mol EJ, Verhaaf B, Lam KH, van Dongen JJ, Langerak AW. BIOMED-2 multiplex immunoglobulin/T-cell receptor polymerase chain reaction protocols can reliably replace Southern blot analysis in routine clonality diagnostics. J Mol Diagn 2005, **7**: 495–503.

35 Tan BT, Warnke RA, Arber DA. The frequency of B- and T-cell gene rearrangements and Epstein–Barr virus in T-cell lymphomas: a comparison between angioimmunoblastic T-cell lymphoma and peripheral T-cell lymphoma, unspecified with and without associated B-cell proliferations. J Mol Diagn 2006, **8**: 466–475, quiz 527.

36 van Dongen JJ, Langerak AW, Brüggemann M, Evans PA, Hummel M, Lavender FL, Delabesse E, Davi F, Schuuring E, García-Sanz R, van Krieken JH, Droese J, González D, Bastard C, White HE, Spaargaren M, González M, Parreira A, Smith JL, Morgan GJ, Kneba M, Macintyre EA. Design and standardization of PCR primers and protocols for detection of clonal immunoglobulin and T-cell receptor gene recombinations in suspect lymphoproliferations: report of the BIOMED-2 Concerted Action BMH4-CT98-3936. Leukemia 2003, **17**: 2257–2317.

37 van Krieken JH, Langerak AW, Macintyre EA, Kneba M, Hodges E, Sanz RG, Morgan GJ, Parreira A, Molina TJ, Cabeçadas J, Gaulard P, Jasani B, Garcia JF, Ott M, Hannsmann ML, Berger F, Hummel M, Davi F, Brüggemann M, Lavender FL, Schuuring E, Evans PA, White H, Salles G, Groenen PJ, Gameiro P, Pott Ch, Dongen JJ. Improved reliability of lymphoma diagnostics via PCR-based clonality testing: report of the BIOMED-2 Concerted Action BHM4-CT98-3936. Leukemia 2007, **21**: 201–206.

CYTOGENETICS AND MOLECULAR GENETICS

Chromosomal translocation

38 Belaud-Rotureau MA, Parrens M, Carrere N, Turmo M, Ferrer J, de Mascarel A, Dubus P, Merlio JP. Interphase fluorescence in situ hybridization is more sensitive than BIOMED-2 polymerase chain reaction protocol in detecting IGH-BCL2 rearrangement in both fixed and frozen lymph node with follicular lymphoma. Hum Pathol 2007, **38**: 365–372.

39 Jevremovic D, Viswanatha DS. Molecular diagnosis of hematopoietic and lymphoid neoplasms. Hematol Oncol Clin North Am 2009, **23**: 903–933.

40 LeBeau M. The role of cytogenetics in the diagnosis and classification of hematopoietic neoplasms. In Knowles DM (ed.): Neoplastic hematopathology. Baltimore, 1992, Williams and Wilkins.

41 Medeioros LJ, Carr J. Overview of the role of molecular methods in the diagnosis of malignant lymphomas. Arch Pathol Lab Med 2000, **123**: 1189–1207.

42 Ngan BY, Chen-Levy Z, Weiss LM, Warnke RA, Cleary ML. Expression in non-Hodgkin's lymphoma of the bcl-2 protein associated with the t(14;18) chromosomal translocation. N Engl J Med 1988, **318**: 1638–1644.

43 Sen F, Vega F, Medeiros LJ. Molecular genetic methods in the diagnosis of hematologic neoplasms. Semin Diagn Pathol 2002, **19**: 72–93.

44 Staudt LM. Molecular diagnosis of the hematologic cancers. N Engl J Med 2003, **348**: 1777–1779.

45 Testa JR, Arthur DC. Cytogenetics of leukemia and lymphoma. In Wiernik PH (ed.): Contemporary issues in clinical oncology. Leukemias and lymphomas. New York, 1985, Churchill Livingstone, pp. 155–182.

46 Weiss LM, Warnek RA, Sklar J, Cleary ML. Molecular analysis of the t(14;18) chromosomal translocation in malignant lymphomas. N Engl J Med 1987, **317**: 1185–1189.

47 Yunis JJ, Frizzera G, Olsen MM, McKenna J, Theologides A, Arnesen M. Multiple recurrent genomic defects in follicular lymphoma. A possible model for cancer. N Engl J Med 1987, **316**: 79–84.

Chromosome copy change and chromosomal gain or deletion

48 Streubel B, Simonitsch-Klupp I, Müllauer L, Lamprecht A, Huber D, Siebert R, Stolte M, Trautinger F, Lukas J, Püspök A, Formanek M, Assanasen T, Müller-Hermelink HK, Cerroni L, Raderer M, Chott A. Variable frequencies of MALT lymphoma-associated genetic aberrations in MALT lymphomas of different sites. Leukemia 2004, **18**: 1722–1726.

49 Wong KF, Chan JK, Kwong YL. Identification of del(6)(q21q25) as a recurring chromosomal abnormality in putative NK cell lymphoma/leukaemia. Br J Haematol 1997, **98**: 922–926.

50 Wotherspoon AC, Finn TM, Isaacson PG. Trisomy 3 in low-grade B-cell lymphomas of mucosa-associated lymphoid tissue. Blood 1995, **85**: 2000–2004.

Gene mutation, amplification, and hypermethylation

51 Compagno M, Lim WK, Grunn A, Nandula SV, Brahmachary M, Shen Q, Bertoni F, Ponzoni M, Scandurra M, Califano A, Bhagat G, Chadburn A, Dalla-Favera R, Pasqualucci L. Mutations of multiple genes cause deregulation of NF-kappaB in diffuse large B-cell lymphoma. Nature 2009, **459**: 717–721.

52 Houldsworth J, Mathew S, Rao PH, Dyomina K, Louie DC, Parsa N, Offit K, Chaganti RS. REL proto-oncogene is frequently amplified in extranodal diffuse large cell lymphoma. Blood 1996, **87**: 25–29.

53 Hutter G, Scheubner M, Zimmermann Y, Kalla J, Katzenberger T, Hübler K, Roth S, Hiddemann W, Ott G, Dreyling M. Differential effect of epigenetic alterations and genomic deletions of CDK inhibitors [p16(INK4a), p15(INK4b), p14(ARF)] in mantle cell lymphoma. Genes Chromosomes Cancer 2006, **45**: 203–210.

54 Kato M, Sanada M, Kato I, Sato Y, Takita J, Takeuchi K, Niwa A, Chen Y, Nakazaki K, Nomoto J, Asakura Y, Muto S, Tamura A, Iio M, Akatsuka Y, Hayashi Y, Mori H, Igarashi T, Kurokawa M, Chiba S, Mori S, Ishikawa Y, Okamoto K, Tobinai K, Nakagama H, Nakahata T, Yoshino T, Kobayashi Y, Ogawa S. Frequent inactivation of A20 in B-cell lymphomas. Nature 2009, **459**: 712–716.

55 Lenz G, Davis RE, Ngo VN, Lam L, George TC, Wright GW, Dave SS, Zhao H, Xu W, Rosenwald A, Ott G, Muller-Hermelink HK, Gascoyne RD, Connors JM, Rimsza LM, Campo E, Jaffe ES, Delabie J, Smeland EB, Fisher RI, Chan WC, Staudt LM. Oncogenic CARD11 mutations in human diffuse large B cell lymphoma. Science 2008, **319**: 1676–1679.

56 Novak U, Rinaldi A, Kwee I, Nandula SV, Rancoita PM, Compagno M, Cerri M, Rossi D, Murty VV, Zucca E, Gaidano G, Dalla-Favera R, Pasqualucci L, Bhagat G, Bertoni F. The NF-κB negative regulator TNFAIP3 (A20) is inactivated by somatic mutations and genomic deletions in marginal zone lymphomas. Blood 2009, **113**: 4918–4921.

DNA PLOIDY STUDIES

57 Braylan RC. Flow-cytometric DNA analysis in the diagnosis and prognosis of lymphoma. Am J Clin Pathol 1993, **99**: 374–380.

58 Duque RE. Flow cytometric analysis of lymphomas and acute leukemias. Ann N Y Acad Sci 1993, **677**: 309–325.

59 Duque RE, Andreeff M, Braylan RC, Diamond LW, Peiper SC. Consensus review of the clinical utility of DNA flow cytometry in neoplastic hematopathology. Cytometry 1993, **14**: 492–496.

60 Zander DS, Iturraspe JA, Everett ET, Massey JK, Braylan RC. Flow cytometry. In vitro assessment of its potential application for diagnosis and classification of lymphoid processes in cytologic preparations from fine needle aspirates. Am J Clin Pathol 1994, **101**: 577–586.

Gene expression profiling

61 Alizadeh AA, Eisen MB, Davis RE, Ma C, Lossos IS, Rosenwald A, Boldrick JC, Sabet H, Tran T, Yu X, Powell JI, Yang L, Marti GE, Moore T, Hudson J Jr, Lu L, Lewis DB, Tibshirani R, Sherlock G, Chan WC, Greiner TC, Weelsenburger DD, Armitage JO, Warnke R, Levy R, Wilson W, Grever MR, Byrd JC, Botstein D, Brown PO, Staudt LM. Distinct types of diffuse large B-cell lymphoma identified by gene expression profiling. Nature 2000, **403**: 503–511.

62 Alizadeh AA, Eisen MB, Davis RE, Ma C, Lossos IS, Rosenwald A, Boldrick JC, Sabet H, Tran T, Yu X, Powell JI, Yang L, Marti GE, Moore T, Hudson J Jr, Lu L, Lewis DB, Tibshirani R, Sherlock G, Chan WC, Greiner TC, Weisenburger DD, Armitage JO, Warnke R, Levy R, Wilson W, Grever MR, Byrd JC, Botstein D, Brown PO, Staudt LM. Distinct types of diffuse large B-cell lymphoma identified by gene expression profiling. Nature 2000, **403**: 503–511.

63 Hoefnagel JJ, Dijkman R, Basso K, Jansen PM, Hallermann C, Willemze R, Tensen CP, Vermeer MH. Distinct types of primary cutaneous large B-cell lymphoma identified by gene expression profiling. Blood 2005, **105**: 3671–3678.

64 Klein U, Gloghini A, Gaidano G, Chadburn A, Cesarman E, Dalla-Favera R, Carbone A. Gene expression profile analysis of AIDS-related primary effusion lymphoma (PEL) suggests a plasmablastic derivation and identifies PEL-specific transcripts. Blood 2003, **101**: 4115–4121.

65 Rosenwald A, Wright G, Chan WC, Connors JM, Campo E, Fisher RI, Gascoyne RD, Müller-Hermelink K, Smeland EB, Staudt LM. The use of molecular profiling to predict survival after chemotherapy for diffuse large B-cell lymphoma. N Engl J Med 2002, **346**: 1937–1947.

PRIMARY IMMUNODEFICIENCIES

66 Buckley RH. Primary immunodeficiency disease due to defects in lymphocytes. N Engl J Med 2000, **343**: 1313–1324.

67 Elenitoba-Johnson KS, Jaffe ES. Lymphoproliferative disorders associated with congenital immunodeficiencies. Semin Diagn Pathol 1997, **14**: 35–47.

68 Gitlin D, Janeway CA, Apt L, Craig JM. Agammaglobulinemia. In Lawrence H (ed.): Cellular and humoral aspects of hypersensitivity states. New York, 1959, Paul B Hoeber, pp. 375–441.

69 Heymer B, Niethammer D, Spanel R, Galle J, Kleihauer E, Haferkamp O. Pathomorphology of humoral, cellular and combined primary immunodeficiencies. Virchows Arch [A] 1977, **374**: 87–103.

70 Huber J, Zegers BJ, Schuurman HJ. Pathology of congenital immunodeficiencies. Semin Diagn Pathol 1992, **9**: 31–62.

71 Knowles DM. Immunodeficiency-associated lymphoproliferative disorders. Mod Pathol 1999, **12**: 200–217.

72 Lekstrom-Himes JA, Gallin JI. Immunodeficiency disease caused by defects in phagocytes. N Engl J Med 2000, **343**: 1703–1714.

73 Rosen FS, Cooper MD, Wedgwood RJP. The primary immunodeficiencies. N Engl J Med 1995, **333**: 431–440.

74 Tinguely M, Vonlanthen R, Müller E, Dommann-Scherrer CC, Schneider J, Laissue JA, Borisch B. Hodgkin's disease-like lymphoproliferative disorders in patients with different underlying immunodeficiency states. Mod Pathol 1998, **11**: 307–312.

PATTERNS OF HYPERPLASIA

75 Dorfman RF, Warnke R. Lymphadenopathy simulating the malignant lymphomas. Hum Pathol 1974, **5**: 519–550.

76 Ioachim HL, Medeiros LJ. Ioachim's lymph node pathology, ed. 4. Philadelphia, 2008, Lippincott Williams & Wilkins.

77 Swerdlow SH. Genetic and molecular genetic studies in the diagnosis of atypical lymphoid hyperplasias versus lymphoma. Hum Pathol 2003, **34**: 346–351.

78 van der Valk P, Meijer CJLM. Lymph nodes. In Mills SE (ed.): Histology for pathologists, ed. 3. Philadelphia, 2007, Lippincott Williams & Wilkins, pp. 763–782.

79 Warnke RA, Weiss LM, Chan JKC, Cleary ML, Dorfman RF. Tumors of the lymph nodes and spleen. Atlas of tumor pathology, 3rd series, fascicle 14. Washington, DC, 1995, Armed Forces Institute of Pathology.

FOLLICULAR HYPERPLASIA

80 Kojima M, Nakamura S, Shimizu K, Iijima M, Murayama K, Ohno Y, Itoh H, Sakata N, Masawa N. Reactive lymphoid hyperplasia of the lymph nodes with giant follicles: a clinicopathologic study of 14 Japanese cases, with special reference to Epstein–Barr virus infection. Int J Surg Pathol 2005, **13**: 267–272.

81 Nathwani BN, Winberg CD, Diamond LW, Bearman RM, Kim H. Morphologic criteria for the differentiation of follicular lymphoma from florid reactive hyperplasia. A study of 80 cases. Cancer 1981, **48**: 1794–1806.

82 Rappaport H, Winter WJ, Hicks EB. Follicular lymphoma. A reevaluation of its position in the scheme of malignant lymphoma, based on a survey of 253 cases. Cancer 1956, **9**: 792–821.

83 Ree HJ, Kadin ME, Kikuchi M, Ko YH, Go JH, Suzumiya J, Kim DS. Angioimmunoblastic lymphoma (AILD-type T-cell lymphoma) with hyperplasia germinal centers. Am J Surg Pathol 1998, **22**: 643–655.

Progressively and regressively transformed germinal centers

84 Burns BF, Colby TV, Dorfman RF. Differential diagnostic features of nodular L&H Hodgkin's disease, including progressive transformation of germinal centers. Am J Surg Pathol 1984, **8**: 253–261.

85 Ferry JA, Zukerberg LR, Harris NL. Florid progressive transformation of germinal centers. A syndrome affecting young men, without early progression to nodular lymphocyte predominance Hodgkin's disease. Am J Surg Pathol 1992, **16**: 252–258.

86 Hansmann ML, Fellbaum C, Hui PK, Moubayed P. Progressive transformation of germinal centers with and without association to Hodgkin's disease. Am J Clin Pathol 1990, **93**: 219–226.

87 Kojima M, Nakamura S, Motoori T, Itoh H, Shimizu K, Yamane N, Ohno Y, Ban S, Yoshida K, Hoshi K, Oyama T, Shimano S, Sugihara S, Sakata N, Masawa N. Progressive transformation of germinal centers: a clinicopathologic study of 42 Japanese patients. Int J Surg Pathol 2003, **11**: 101–107.

88 Nguyen PL, Ferry JA, Harris NL. Progressive transformation of germinal centers and nodular lymphocyte predominance Hodgkin's disease, a comparative immunohistochemical study. Am J Surg Pathol 1999, **23**: 27–33.

89 Osborne BM, Butler JJ. Follicular lymphoma mimicking progressive transformation of germinal centers. Am J Clin Pathol 1987, **88**: 264–269.

90 Osborne BM, Butler JJ, Gresik MV. Progressive transformation of germinal centers. Comparison of 23 pediatric patients to the adult population. Mod Pathol 1992, **5**: 135–140.

91 Poppema S, Kaiserling E, Lennert K. Hodgkin's disease with lymphocytic predominance, nodular type (nodular paragranuloma) and progressively transformed germinal centers. A cytohistological study. Histopathology 1979, **3**: 295–308.

92 Poppema S, Kaiserling E, Lennert K. Nodular paragranuloma and progressively transformed germinal centers. Ultrastructural and immunohistologic findings. Virchows Arch [Cell Pathol] 1979, **31**: 211–225.

93 Stein H, Gerdes J, Mason DY. The normal and malignant germinal centre. Clin Hematol 1982, **11**: 531–559.

94 Yamakawa M, Ikeda I, Masuda A, Enomoto H, Ando A, Kasajima T. An unusual regressive germinal center, the 'FDC-only lymphoid follicle', in lymph nodes or organ transplant recipients. Am J Surg Pathol 1999, **23**: 536–545.

MANTLE/MARGINAL ZONE HYPERPLASIA

95 Hunt JP, Chan JA, Samoszuk M, Brynes RK, Hernandez AM, Bass R, Weisenburger DD, Müller-Hermelink K, Nathwani BN. Hyperplasia of mantle/marginal zone B-cells with clear cytoplasm in peripheral lymph nodes. A clinicopathologic study of 35 cases. Am J Clin Pathol 2001, **116**: 550–559.

PARACORTICAL HYPERPLASIA

96 van den Oord JJ, de Wolf-Peeters C, Desmet VJ, Takahashi K, Ohtsuki Y, Akagi T. Nodular alteration of the paracortical area. An in situ immunohistochemical analysis of primary, secondary, and tertiary T-nodules. Am J Pathol 1985, **120**: 55–66.

GRANULOMATOUS INFLAMMATION

97 Gorton G, Linell F. Malignant tumours and sarcoid reactions in regional lymph nodes. Acta Radiol (Stockh) 1957, **47**: 381–392.

98 Hall PA, Kingston J, Stansfeld AG. Extensive necrosis in malignant lymphoma with granulomatous reaction mimicking tuberculosis. Histopathology 1988, **13**: 339–346.

99 Hollingsworth HC, Longo DL, Jaffe ES. Small noncleaved cell lymphoma associated with florid epithelioid granulomatous response. A clinicopathologic study of seven patients. Am J Surg Pathol 1993, **17**: 51–59.

100 Ioachim HL (ed.): Pathology of granulomas. New York, 1983, Raven Press.

101 Kadin ME, Donaldson SS, Dorfman RF. Isolated granulomas in Hodgkin's disease. N Engl J Med 1970, **283**: 859–861.

102 Nadel E, Ackerman LV. Lesions resembling Boeck's sarcoid. Am J Clin Pathol 1952, **20**: 952–957.

OTHER CELL TYPES INVOLVED IN NODAL HYPERPLASIA

Monocytoid B cells

103 Aozasa K, Ohsawa M, Horiuchi K, Saeki K, Katayama S, Matsuzuka F, Yamamura T. The occurrence of monocytoid B lymphocytes in autoimmune disorders. Mod Pathol 1993, **6**: 121–124.

104 Kojima M, Hosomura Y, Itoh H, Johshita T, Ohno Y, Yoshida K, Asano S, Wakasa H, Nakamura S, Suchi T. Monocytoid B lymphocytes and epithelioid cell clusters in abscess-forming granulomatous lymphadenitis. With special reference to cat scratch disease. Acta Pathol Jpn 1991, **41**: 363–368.

105 Ohsawa M, Kanno H, Naka N, Aozasa K. Occurrence of monocytoid B lymphocytes in Hodgkin's disease. Mod Pathol 1994, **7**: 540–543.

106 Plank L, Hansmann ML, Fischer R. The cytological spectrum of the monocytoid B-cell reaction. Recognition of its large cell type. Histopathology 1993, **23**: 425–431.

107 Sheibani K, Fritz RM, Winberg CD, Burke JS, Rappaport H. 'Monocytoid' cells in reactive follicular hyperplasia with and without multifocal histiocytic reactions. An immunohistochemical study of 21 cases including suspected cases of toxoplasmic lymphadenitis. Am J Clin Pathol 1984, **81**: 453–458.

108 Shin SS, Sheibani K. Monocytoid B-cell lymphoma. Am J Clin Pathol 1993, **99**: 421–425.

109 van den Oord JJ, de Wolf-Peeters C, De Vos R, Desmet VJ. Immature sinus histiocytosis. Light- and electron-microscopic features, immunologic phenotype, and relationship with marginal zone lymphocytes. Am J Pathol 1985, **118**: 266–277.

Plasmacytoid dendritic cells

110 Facchetti F, de Wolf-Peeters C, Mason DY, Pulford K, van den Oord JJ, Desmet VJ. Plasmacytoid T-cells. Immunohistochemical evidence for their monocyte/macrophage origin. Am J Pathol 1988, **133**: 15–21.

111 Facchetti F, de Wolf-Peeters C, de Vos R, van den Oord JJ, Pulford KA, Desmet VJ. Plasmacytoid monocytes (so-called plasmacytoid T-cells) in granulomatous lymphadenitis. Hum Pathol 1989, **20**: 588–593.

112 Facchetti F, de Wolf-Peeters C, van den Oord JJ, de Vos R, Desmet VJ. Plasmacytoid monocytes (so-called plasmacytoid T-cells) in Kikuchi's lymphadenitis. An immunohistologic study. Am J Clin Pathol 1989, **92**: 42–50.

113 Hansmann ML, Kikuchi M, Wacker HH, Radzun HJ, Nathwani BN, Hesse K, Parwaresch MR. Immunohistochemical monitoring of plasmacytoid cells in lymph node sections of Kikuchi–Fujimoto disease by a new panmacrophage antibody Ki-MIP. Hum Pathol 1992, **23**: 676–680.

114 Jegalian AG, Facchetti F, Jaffe ES. Plasmacytoid dendritic cells: physiologic roles and pathologic states. Adv Anat Pathol 2009, **16**: 392–404.

115 Koo CH, Mason DY, Miller R, Ben-Ezra J, Sheibani K, Rappaport H. Additional evidence that 'plasmacytoid T-cell lymphoma' associated with chronic myeloproliferative disorders is of macrophage/monocyte origin. Am J Clin Pathol 1990, **93**: 822–827.

116 Müller-Hermelink HK, Stein H, Steinmann G, Lennert K. Malignant lymphoma of plasmacytoid T-cells. Morphologic and immunologic studies characterizing a special type of T-cell. Am J Surg Pathol 1983, **7**: 849–862.

117 Prasthofer EF, Grizzle WE, Prchal JT, Grossi CE. Plasmacytoid T-cell lymphoma associated with chronic myeloproliferative disorder. Am J Surg Pathol 1985, **9**: 380–387.

118 Vollenweider R, Lennert K. Plasmacytoid T-cell clusters in nonspecific lymphadenitis. Virchows Arch [Cell Pathol] 1983, **44**: 1–14.

Polykaryocytes

119 Kjeldsberg CR, Kim H. Polykaryocytes resembling Warthin–Finkeldey giant cells in reactive and neoplastic lymphoid disorders. Hum Pathol 1981, **12**: 267–272.

120 Orenstein JM. The Warthin–Finkeldey-type giant T-cell in HIV infection, what is it? Ultrastruct Pathol 1998, **22**: 293–303.

INFLAMMATORY/HYPERPLASTIC DISEASES

KIKUCHI NECROTIZING LYMPHADENITIS

121 Bosch X, Guilabert A, Miquel R, Campo E. Enigmatic Kikuchi–Fujimoto disease: a comprehensive review. Am J Clin Pathol 2004, **122**: 141–152.

122 Chamulak GA, Brynes RK, Nathwani BN. Kikuchi–Fujimoto disease mimicking malignant lymphoma. Am J Surg Pathol 1990, **14**: 514–523.

123 Chan JKC, Saw D. Histiocytic necrotizing lymphadenitis (Kikuchi's disease). A clinicopathologic study of 9 cases. Pathology 1986, **18**: 22–28.

TULAREMIA

229 Ellis J, Oyston PC, Green M, Titball RW. Tularemia. Clin Microbiol Rev 2002, **15**: 631–646.

230 Evans ME, Gregory DW, Schaffner W, McGee ZA. Tularemia. A 30-year experience with 88 cases. Medicine (Baltimore) 1985, **64**: 251–267.

231 Lamps LW, Havens JM, Sjostedt A, Page DL, Scott MA. Histologic and molecular diagnosis of tularemia: a potential bioterrorism agent endemic to North America. Mod Pathol 2004, **17**: 489–495.

232 Ohara Y, Sato T, Fujita H, Ueno T, Homma M. Clinical manifestations of tularemia in Japan – analysis of 1,355 cases observed between 1924 and 1987. Infection 1991, **19**: 14–17.

233 Sato T, Fujita H, Ohara Y, Homma M. Microagglutination test for early and specific serodiagnosis of tularemia. J Clin Microbiol 1990, **28**: 2372–2374.

234 Sutinen S, Syrjälä H. Histopathology of human lymph node tularemia caused by *Francisella tularensis* var *palaearctica*. Arch Pathol Lab Med 1986, **110**: 42–46.

235 Tarnvik A, Berglund L. Tularaemia. Eur Respir J 2003, **21**: 361–373.

236 Tjaden JA, Lazarus AA, Martin GJ. Bacteria as agents of biowarfare. How to proceed when the worst is suspected. Postgrad Med 2002, **112**: 67–70.

BRUCELLOSIS

237 Chomel BB, De Bess EE, Mangiamele DM, Reilly KF, Farver TB, Sun RK, Barrett LR. Changing trends in the epidemiology of human brucellosis in California from 1973 to 1992. A shift toward foodborne transmission. J Infect Dis 1994, **170**: 1216–1223.

238 Namiduru M, Gungor K, Dikensoy O, Baydar I, Ekinci E, Karaoglan I, Bekir NA. Epidemiological, clinical and laboratory features of brucellosis: a prospective evaluation of 120 adult patients. Int J Clin Pathol 2003, **57**: 20–24.

239 Nimri LF. Diagnosis of recent and relapsed cases of human brucellosis by PCR assay. BMC Infect Dis 2003, **3**: 5.

240 Trujillo IZ, Zavala AN, Caceres JG, Miranda CQ. Brucellosis. Infect Dis Clin North Am 1994, **8**: 225–241.

241 Weed LA, Dahlin DC. Bacteriologic examination of tissues removed for biopsy. Am J Clin Pathol 1950, **20**: 116–132.

AIDS-RELATED LYMPHADENOPATHY

242 Abrams DI. Lymphadenopathy syndrome in male homosexuals. Adv Host Def Mechan 1985, **5**: 75–97.

243 Baroni CD, Uccini S. The lymphadenopathy of HIV infection. Am J Clin Pathol 1993, **99**: 397–401.

244 Burns BF, Wood GS, Dorfman RF. The varied histopathology of lymphadenopathy in the homosexual male. Am J Surg Pathol 1985, **9**: 287–297.

245 Chadburn A, Metroka C, Mouradian J. Progressive lymph node histology and its prognostic value in patients with acquired immunodeficiency syndrome and AIDS-related complex. Hum Pathol 1989, **20**: 579–587.

246 de Paiva GR, Laurent C, Godel A, da Silva NA Jr, March M, Delsol G, Brousset P. Discovery of human immunodeficiency virus infection by immunohistochemistry on lymph node biopsies from patients with unexplained follicular hyperplasia. Am J Surg Pathol 2007, **31**: 1534–1538.

247 Fishbein DB, Kaplan JE, Spira TJ, Miller B, Schonberger LB, Pinsky PF, Getchell JP, Kalyanaraman VS, Braude JS. Unexplained lymphadenopathy in homosexual men. A longitudinal study. JAMA 1985, **254**: 929–935.

248 Groopman JE. Clinical symptomatology of the acquired immunodeficiency syndrome (AIDS) and related disorders. Prog Allergy 1986, **37**: 182–193.

249 Harris NL. Hypervascular follicular hyperplasia and Kaposi's sarcoma in patients at risk for AIDS. N Engl J Med 1984, **310**: 462–463.

250 Ioachim HL, Cronin W, Roy M, Maya M. Persistent lymphadenopathies in people at high risk for HIV infection. Clinicopathologic correlations and long-term follow-up in 79 cases. Am J Clin Pathol 1990, **93**: 208–218.

251 Logani S, Lucas DR, Cheng JD, Iochim HL, Adsay NV. Spindle cell tumors associated with mycobacteria in lymph nodes of HIV-positive patients: 'Kaposi sarcoma with mycobacteria' and 'mycobacterial pseudotumor'. Am J Surg Pathol 1999, **23**: 656–661.

252 O'Hara CJ, Groopman JE, Federman M. The ultrastructural and immunohistochemical demonstration of viral particles in lymph nodes from human immunodeficiency virus-related and nonhuman immunodeficiency virus-related lymphadenopathy syndromes. Hum Pathol 1988, **19**: 545–549.

253 Orenstein JM. The Warthin–Finkeldey-type giant T-cell in HIV infection, what is it? Ultrastruct Pathol 1998, **22**: 293–303.

254 Said JW. AIDS-related lymphadenopathies. Semin Diagn Pathol 1988, **5**: 365–375.

255 Said JW, Pinkus JL, Yamashita J, Mishalani S, Matsumura F, Yamashiro S, Pinkus GS. The role of follicular and interdigitating dendritic cells in HIV-related lymphoid hyperplasia: localization of fascin. Mod Pathol 1997, **10**: 421–427.

256 Schuurman H-J, Kluin PM, Gmelig Meijling FHJ, Van Unnik JAM, Kater L. Lymphocyte status of lymph node and blood in acquired immunodeficiency syndrome (AIDS) and AIDS-related complex disease. J Pathol 1985, **147**: 269–280.

257 Tacchetti C, Favre A, Moresco L, Meszaros P, Luzzi P, Truini M, Rizzo F, Grossi CE, Ciccone E. HIV is trapped and masked in the cytoplasm of lymph node follicular dendritic cells. Am J Pathol 1997, **150**: 533–542.

258 Umlas J, Federman M, Crawford C, O'Hara CJ, Fitzgibbon JS, Modeste A. Spindle cell pseudotumor due to *Mycobacterium avium-intracellulare* in patients with acquired immunodeficiency syndrome (AIDS). Positive staining of mycobacteria for cytoskeleton filaments. Am J Surg Pathol 1991, **15**: 1181–1187.

259 Westermann CD, Hurtubise PE, Linnemann CC, Swerdlow SH. Comparison of histologic nodal reactive patterns, cell suspension immunophenotypic data, and HIV status. Mod Pathol 1990, **3**: 54–60.

260 Wood GS, Garcia CF, Dorfman RF, Warnke RA. The immunohistology of follicle lysis in lymph node biopsies from homosexual men. Blood 1985, **66**: 1092–1097.

INFECTIOUS MONONUCLEOSIS

261 Frizzera G, Hanto DW, Gajl-Peczalska KJ, Rosai J, McKenna RW, Sibley RK, Holahan KP, Lindquist LL. Polymorphic diffuse B-cell hyperplasias and lymphomas in renal transplant recipients. Cancer Res 1981, **41**: 4262–4279.

262 Godshall SE, Kirchner JT. Infectious mononucleosis. Complexities of a common syndrome. Postgrad Med 2000, **107**: 175–186.

263 Gulley ML. Molecular diagnosis of Epstein–Barr virus-related diseases. J Mol Diagn 2001, **3**: 1–10.

264 Luzuriaga K, Sullivan JL. Infectious mononucleosis. N Engl J Med 2010, **362**: 1993–2000.

265 McMahon NJ, Gordon HW, Rosen RB. Reed–Sternberg cells in infectious mononucleosis. Am J Dis Child 1970, **120**: 148–150.

266 Reynolds DJ, Banks PM, Gulley ML. New characterization of infectious mononucleosis and a phenotypic comparison with Hodgkin's disease. Am J Pathol 1995, **146**: 379–388.

267 Rickinson A. Epstein–Barr virus. Virus Res 2002, **82**: 109–113.

268 Salvador AH, Harrison EG, Kyle RA. Lymphadenopathy due to infectious mononucleosis. Its confusion with malignant lymphoma. Cancer 1971, **27**: 1029–1040.

269 Shin SS, Berry GJ, Weiss LM. Infectious mononucleosis. Diagnosis by in situ hybridization in two cases with atypical features. Am J Surg Pathol 1991, **15**: 625–631.

270 Sieracki JC, Fisher ER. Diagnostic problems involving nodal lymphomas. Pathol Annu 1970, **5**: 91–124.

271 Strickler JG, Fedeli F, Horwitz CA, Copenhaver CM, Frizzera G. Infectious mononucleosis in lymphoid tissue. Histopathology, in situ hybridization, and differential diagnosis. Arch Pathol Lab Med 1993, **117**: 269–278.

272 Tindle BH, Parker JW, Lukes RJ. 'Reed–Sternberg cells' in infectious mononucleosis? Am J Clin Pathol 1972, **58**: 607–617.

OTHER VIRAL (INCLUDING POSTVACCINIAL) LYMPHADENITIDES

273 Audouin J, Le Tourneau A, Aubert J-P, Diebold J. Herpes simplex virus lymphadenitis mimicking tumoral relapse in a patient with Hodgkin's disease in remission. Virchows Arch [A] 1985, **408**: 313–321.

274 Dorfman RF, Herweg JC. Live, attenuated measles virus vaccine. Inguinal lymphadenopathy complicating administration. JAMA 1966, **198**: 320–321.

275 Gaffey MJ, Ben-Ezra JM, Weiss LM. Herpes simplex lymphadenitis. Am J Clin Pathol 1991, **95**: 709–714.

276 Hartsock RJ. Postvaccinial lymphadenitis. Hyperplasia of lymphoid tissue that simulates malignant lymphomas. Cancer 1968, **21**: 632–649.

277 Howat AJ, Campbell AR, Stewart DJ. Generalized lymphadenopathy due to herpes simplex virus type I. Histopathology 1991, **19**: 563–564.

278 Lapsley M, Kettle P, Sloan JM. Herpes simplex lymphadenitis. A case report and review of the published work. J Clin Pathol 1984, **37**: 1119–1122.

279 Miliauskas JR, Leong AS. Localized herpes simplex lymphadenitis. Report of three cases and review of the literature. Histopathology 1991, **19**: 355–360.

280 Tamaru J, Mikata A, Horie H, Itoh K, Asai T, Hondo R, Mori S. Herpes simplex lymphadenitis. Report of two cases with review of the literature. Am J Surg Pathol 1990, **14**: 571–577.

281 Witt MD, Torno MS, Sun N, Stein T. Herpes simplex virus lymphadenitis: case report and review of the literature. Clin Infect Dis 2002, **34**: 1–6.

MUCOCUTANEOUS LYMPH NODE SYNDROME

282 Beitz LO, Barron KS. Kawasaki syndrome. Curr Opin Dermatol 1995, **1**: 114–122.

283 Burns JC. Kawasaki disease: the mystery continues. Minerva Pediatr 2002, **54**: 287–294.

284 Giesker DW, Krause PJ, Pastuszak WT, Hine P, Forouhar FA. Lymph node biopsy for early diagnosis in Kawasaki disease. Am J Surg Pathol 1982, **6**: 493–501.

285 Marsh WL, Bishop JW, Koenig HM. Bone marrow and lymph node findings in a fatal case of Kawasaki's disease. Arch Pathol Lab Med 1980, **104**: 563–567.

286 Stamos JK, Corydon K, Donaldson J, Shulman ST. Lymphadenitis as the dominant manifestation of Kawasaki disease. Pediatrics 1994, **93**: 525–528.

LUPUS ERYTHEMATOSUS

287 Hu S, Kuo T-T, Hong H-S. Lupus lymphadenitis simulating Kikuchi's lymphadenitis in patients with systemic lupus erythematosus: a clinicopathological analysis of six cases and review of the literature. Pathol Int 2003, **53**: 221–226.

288 Kojima M, Nakamura S, Itoh H, Yoshida K, Asano S, Yamane N, Komatsumoto S, Ban S, Joshita T, Suchi T. Systemic lupus erythematosus (SLE) lymphadenopathy presenting with histopathologic features of Castleman's disease, a clinicopathologic study of five cases. Pathol Res Pract 1997, **193**: 565–571.

289 Kojima M, Nakamura S, Morishita Y, Itoh H, Yoshida K, Ohno Y, Oyama T, Asano S, Joshita T, Mori S, Suchi T, Masawa N. Reactive follicular hyperplasia in the lymph node lesions from systemic lupus erythematosus patients: a clinicopathological and immunohistological study of 21 cases. Pathol Int 2000, **50**: 304–312.

290 Kubota K, Tamura J, Kurabayashi H, Yanagisawa T, Shirakura T, Mori S. Warthin–Finkeldey-like giant cells in a patient with systemic lupus erythematosus. Hum Pathol 1988, **19**: 1358–1359.

291 Medeiros LJ, Kaynor B, Harris NL. Lupus lymphadenitis. Report of a case with immunohistologic studies on frozen sections. Hum Pathol 1989, **20**: 295–299.

RHEUMATOID ARTHRITIS

292 Kamel OW, van de Rijn M, Le Brun DP, Weiss LM, Warnke RA, Dorfman RF. Lymphoid neoplasms in patients with rheumatoid arthritis and dermatomyositis. Frequency of Epstein–Barr virus and other features associated with immunosuppression. Hum Pathol 1994, **25**: 638–643.

293 Kojima M, Hosomura Y, Itoh H, Johshita T, Yoshida K, Nakamura S, Suchi T. Reactive proliferative lesions in lymph nodes from rheumatoid arthritis patients. A clinicopathological and immunohistological study. Acta Pathol Jpn 1990, **40**: 249–254.

294 Kojima M, Nakamura S, Miyawaki S, Yashiro K, Oyama T, Itoh H, Sakata N, Sugihara S, Masawa N. Lymph node lesion in adult-onset Still's disease resembling peripheral T-cell lymphoma: a report of three cases. Int J Surg Pathol 2002, **10**: 197–202.

295 Kojima M, Itoh H, Shimizu K, Saruki N, Murayama K, Higuchi K, Tamaki Y, Matsumoto M, Hirabayashi K, Igarishi S, Masawa N, Nakamura S. Malignant lymphoma in patients with systemic rheumatic disease (rheumatoid arthritis, systemic lupus erythematosus, systemic sclerosis, and dermatomyositis): a clinicopathologic study of 24 Japanese cases. Int J Surg Pathol 2006, **14**: 43–48.

296 Nosanchuk JS, Schnitzer B. Follicular hyperplasia in lymph nodes from patients with rheumatoid arthritis. A clinicopathologic study. Cancer 1969, **24**: 343–354.

297 Robertson MDJ, Hart FD, White WF, Nuki G, Boardman PL. Rheumatoid lymphadenopathy. Ann Rheum Dis 1968, **27**: 253–260.

298 Rollins SD, Craig JP. Gold-associated lymphadenopathy in a patient with rheumatoid arthritis. Histologic and scanning electron microscopic features. Arch Pathol Lab Med 1991, **115**: 175–177.

CASTLEMAN DISEASE

299 Abdel-Reheim FA, Koss W, Rappaport ES, Arber DA. Coexistence of Hodgkin's disease and giant lymph node hyperplasia of the plasma-cell type (Castleman's disease). Arch Pathol Lab Med 1966, **120**: 91–96.

300 Altiparmak MR, Pamuk GE, Pamuk ON, Dogusoy G. Secondary amyloidosis in Castleman's disease: review of the literature and report of a case. Ann Hematol 2002, **81**: 336–339.

301 Amin HM, Medeiros LJ, Manning JT, Jones D. Dissolution of the lymphoid follicle is a feature of the HHV8+ variant of plasma cell Castleman's disease. Am J Surg Pathol 2002, **27**: 91–100.

302 Ascoli V, Sirianni MC, Mezzaroma I, Mastroianni CM, Vullo V, Andreoni M, Narciso P, Scalzo CC, Nardi F, Pistilli A, Lo Coco F. Human herpesvirus-8 in lymphomatous and nonlymphomatous body cavity effusions developing in Kaposi's sarcoma and multicentric Castleman's disease. Ann Diagn Pathol 2000, **3**: 357–363.

303 Bowne WB, Lewis JJ, Filippa DA, Niesvizky R, Brooks AD, Burt ME, Brennan MF. The management of unicentric and multicentric Castleman's disease. A report of 16 cases and a review of the literature. Cancer 1999, **85**: 706–717.

304 Chan JK, Fletcher CD, Hicklin GA, Rosai J. Glomeruloid hemangioma. A distinctive cutaneous lesion of multicentric Castleman's disease associated with POEMS syndrome. Am J Surg Pathol 1990, **14**: 1036–1046.

305 Chan JK, Tsang WY, Ng CS. Follicular dendritic cell tumor and vascular neoplasm complicating hyaline-vascular Castleman's disease. Am J Surg Pathol 1994, **18**: 517–525.

306 Cheuk W, Yuen HK, Chu SY, Chiu EK, Lam LK, Chan JK. Lymphadenopathy of IgG4-related sclerosing disease. Am J Surg Pathol 2008, **32**: 671–681.

307 Cokelaere K, Debiec-Rychter M, De Wolf-Peeters C, Hagemeijer A, Sciot R. Hyaline vascular Castleman's disease with HMGIC rearrangement in follicular dendritic cells: molecular evidence of mesenchymal tumorigenesis. Am J Surg Pathol 2002, **26**: 662–669.

308 Cronin DM, Warnke RA. Castleman disease: an update on classification and the spectrum of associated lesions. Adv Anat Pathol 2009, **16**: 236–246.

309 Danon AD, Krishnan J, Frizzera G. Morpho-immunophenotypic diversity of Castleman's disease, hyaline-vascular type. With emphasis on a stroma-rich variant and a new pathogenetic hypothesis. Virchows Arch [A] 1993, **423**: 369–382.

310 Frizzera G. Castleman's disease and related disorders. Semin Diagn Pathol 1988, **5**: 346–364.

311 Frizzera G, Banks PM, Massarelli G, Rosai J. A systemic lymphoproliferative disorder with morphologic features of Castleman's disease. Pathological findings in 15 patients. Am J Surg Pathol 1983, **7**: 211–231.

312 Frizzera G, Peterson BA, Bayrd ED, Goldman A. A systemic lymphoproliferative disorder with morphologic features of Castleman's disease. Clinical findings and clinicopathologic correlations in 15 patients. J Clin Oncol 1985, **3**: 1202–1216.

313 Gerald W, Kostianovsky M, Rosai J. Development of vascular neoplasia in Castleman's disease. Report of seven cases. Am J Surg Pathol 1990, **14**: 603–614.

314 Gould SJ, Diss T, Isaacson PG. Multicentric Castleman's disease in association with a solitary plasmacytoma. A case report. Histopathology 1990, **17**: 135–140.

315 Gulati P, Sun NC, Herman BK, Said JW, Cornford ME. Isolated leptomeningeal Castleman's disease with viral particles in the follicular dendritic cells. Arch Pathol Lab Med 1998, **122**: 1026–1029.

316 Hall PA, Donaghy M, Cotter FE, Stansfeld AG, Levison DA. An immunohistological and genotypic study of the plasma cell form of Castleman's disease. Histopathology 1989, **14**: 333–346.

317 Hanson CA, Frizzera G, Patton DF, Peterson BA, McClain KL, Gajl-Peczalska KJ, Kersey JH. Clonal rearrangement for immunoglobulin and T-cell receptor genes in systemic Castleman's disease. Association with Epstein–Barr virus. Am J Pathol 1988, **131**: 84–91.

318 Hengge UR, Ruzicka T, Tyring SK, Stuschke M, Rogendorf M, Schwartz RA, Seeber S. Update on Kaposi's sarcoma and other HHV-8 associated disease. Part 2: Pathogenesis, Castleman's disease, and pleural effusion lymphoma. Lancet Infect Dis 2002, **2**: 344–352.

319 Hsu SM, Waldron JA, Xie SS, Barlogie B. Expression of interleukin-6 in Castleman's disease. Hum Pathol 1993, **24**: 833–839.

320 Isaacson PG. Commentary: Castleman's disease. Histopathology 1989, **14**: 429–432.

321 Jones EL, Crocker J, Gregory J, Guibarra M, Curran RC. Angiofollicular lymph node hyperplasia (Castleman's disease). An immunohistochemical and enzyme-histochemical study of the hyaline-vascular form of lesion. J Pathol 1984, **144**: 131–147.

322 Kazakov DV, Fanburg-Smith JC, Suster S, Neuhauser TS, Palmedo G, Zamecnik M, Kempf W, Michal M. Castleman disease of the subcutis and underlying skeletal muscle: report of 6 cases. Am J Surg Pathol 2004, **28**: 569–577.

323 Keller AR, Hochholzer L, Castleman, B. Hyaline-vascular and plasma-cell types of giant lymph node hyperplasia of mediastinum and other locations. Cancer 1972, **29**: 670–683.

324 Kojima M, Nakamura S, Shimizu K, Itoh H, Yamane Y, Murayama K, Tanaka H, Sugihara S, Shimano S, Sakata N, Masawa N. Clinical implication of idiopathic plasmacytic lymphadenopathy with polyclonal hypergammaglobulinemia. A report of 16 cases. Int J Surg Pathol 2004, **12**: 25–30.

325 Larroche C, Cacoub P, Soulier J, Oksenhendler E, Chauvel JP, Piette JC, Raphael M. Castleman's disease and lymphoma: report of eight cases in HIV-negative patients and literature review. Am J Hematol 2002, **69**: 119–126.

326 Lin O, Frizzera G. Angiomyoid and follicular dendritic cell proliferative lesions in Castleman's disease of hyaline-vascular type: a study of 10 cases. Am J Surg Pathol 1997, **21**: 1295–1306.

327 Madero S, Oñate JM, Garzón A. Giant lymph node hyperplasia in an angiolipomatous mediastinal mass. Arch Pathol Lab Med 1986, **110**: 853–855.

328 Maheswaran PR, Ramsay AD, Norton AJ, Roche WR. Hodgkin's disease presenting with the histological features of Castleman's disease. Histopathology 1991, **18**: 249–253.

329 Mandler RN, Kerrigan DP, Smart J, Kuis W, Villiger P, Lotz M. Castleman's disease in POEMS syndrome with elevated interleukin-6. Cancer 1992, **69**: 2697–2703.

330 Menke DM, Camoriano JK, Banks PM. Angiofollicular lymph node hyperplasia. A comparison of unicentric, multicentric, hyaline vascular, and plasma cell types of disease by morphometric and clinical analysis. Mod Pathol 1992, **5**: 525–530.

331 Menke DM, Chadbum A, Cesarman E, Green E, Berenson J, Said J, Tiemann M, Parwaresch R, Thome SD. Analysis of the human herpesvirus 8 (HHV-8) genome and HHV-8 vIL-6 expression in archival cases of Castleman disease at low risk for HIV infection. Am J Clin Pathol 2002, **117**: 268–275.

332 Menke DM, Tiemann M, Camoriano JK, Chang SF, Madan A, Chow M, Habermann TM, Parwaresch R. Diagnosis of Castleman's disease by identification of an immuno-phenotypically aberrant population of mantle zone B lymphocytes in paraffin-embedded lymph node biopsies. Am J Clin Pathol 1996, **105**: 268–276.

333 Munoz G, Geijo P, Moldenhauer F, Perez-Moro E, Razquin J, Piris MA. Plasmacellular Castleman's disease and POEMS syndrome. Histopathology 1990, **17**: 172–174.

334 Nagai K, Sato I, Shimoyama N. Pathohistological and immunohistochemical studies on Castleman's disease of the lymph node. Virchows Arch [A] 1986, **409**: 287–297.

335 Naresh KN, Rice AJ, Bower M. Lymph nodes involved by multicentric Castleman disease among HIV-positive individuals are often involved by Kaposi sarcoma. Am J Surg Pathol 2008, **32**: 1006–1012.

336 Nguyen DT, Diamond LW, Hansmann ML, Alavaikko MJ, Schroder H, Fellbaum C, Fischer R. Castleman's disease. Differences in follicular dendritic network in the hyaline vascular and plasma cell variants. Histopathology 1994, **24**: 437–443.

337 Ohyashiki JH, Ohyashiki K, Kawakubo K, Serizawa H, Abe K, Mikata A, Toyama K. Molecular genetic, cytogenetic, and immunophenotypic analyses in Castleman's disease of the plasma cell type. Am J Clin Pathol 1994, **101**: 290–295.

338 Ordi J, Grau JM, Junque A, Nomdedeu B, Palacin A, Cardesa A. Secondary (AA) amyloidosis associated with Castleman's disease. Report of two cases and review of the literature. Am J Clin Pathol 1993, **100**: 394–397.

339 Parravicini C, Chandran B, Corbellino M, Berti E, Pauli M, Moore PS, Chang Y. Differential viral protein expression in Kaposi's sarcoma-associated herpesvirus-infected diseases. Kaposi's sarcoma, primary effusion lymphoma, and multicentric Castleman's disease. Am J Pathol 2000, **156**: 743–749.

340 Pauwels P, Dal Cin P, Vlasved LT, Aleva RM, van Erp WF, Jones D. A chromosomal abnormality in hyaline vascular Castleman's disease: evidence for clonal proliferation of dysplastic stromal cells. Am J Surg Pathol 2000, **24**: 882–888.

341 Peterson BA, Frizzera G. Multicentric Castleman's disease. Semin Oncol 1993, **20**: 636–647.

342 Radaszkiewicz T, Hansmann ML, Lennert K. Monoclonality and polyclonality of plasma cells in Castleman's disease of the plasma cell variant. Histopathology 1989, **14**: 11–24.

343 Rolon PG, Audouin J, Diebold J, Rolon PA, Gonzalez A. Multicentric angiofollicular lymph node hyperplasia associated with a solitary osteolytic costal IgG lambda myeloma. POEMS syndrome in a South American (Paraguayan) patient. Pathol Res Pract 1989, **185**: 468–469.

344 Ruco LP, Gearing AJ, Pigott R, Pomponi D, Burgio VL, Cafolla A, Baiocchini A, Baroni CD. Expression of ICAM-1, VCAM-1 and ELAM-1 in angiofollicular lymph node hyperplasia (Castleman's disease). Evidence for dysplasia of follicular dendritic reticulum cells. Histopathology 1991, **19**: 523–528.

345 Skelton HG, Smith KJ. Extranodal multicentric Castleman's disease with cutaneous involvement. Mod Pathol 1998, **11**: 93–98.

346 Smir BN, Greiner TC, Weisenburger DD. Multicentric angiofollicular lymph node hyperplasia in children: a clinicopathologic study of eight patients. Mod Pathol 1997, **9**: 1135–1142.

347 Vasef M, Katzin WE, Mendelsohn G, Reydman M. Report of a case of localized Castleman's disease with progression to malignant lymphoma. Am J Clin Pathol 1992, **98**: 633–636.

348 Weisenburger DD, Nathwani BN, Winberg CD, Rappaport H. Multicentric angiofollicular lymph node hyperplasia. A clinicopathologic study of 16 cases. Hum Pathol 1985, **16**: 162–172.

349 Zarate-Osorno A, Medeiros LJ, Danon AD, Neiman RS. Hodgkin's disease with coexistent Castleman-like histologic features. A report of three cases. Arch Pathol Lab Med 1994, **118**: 270–274.

ANGIOIMMUNOBLASTIC LYMPHADENOPATHY

350 Aozasa K, Ohsawa M, Fujita MQ, Kanayama Y, Tominaga N, Yonezawa T, Matsubuchi T, Hirata M, Uda H, Kanamaru A, et al. Angioimmunoblastic lymphadenopathy. Review of 44 patients with emphasis on prognostic behavior. Cancer 1989, **63**: 1625–1629.

351 Attygalle AD, Kyriakou C, Dupuis J, Grogg KL, Diss TC, Wotherspoon AC, Chuang SS, Cabeçadas J, Isaacson PG, Du MQ, Gaulard P, Dogan A. Histologic evolution of angioimmunoblastic T-cell lymphoma in consecutive biopsies: clinical correlation and insights into natural history and disease progression. Am J Surg Pathol 2007, **31**: 1077–1088.

352 Bernengo MG, Levi L, Zina G. Skin lesions in angioimmunoblastic lymphadenopathy. Histological and immunological studies. Br J Dermatol 1981, **104**: 131–139.

353 Bluming AZ, Cohen HG, Saxon A. Angioimmunoblastic lymphadenopathy with dysproteinemia. A pathogenetic link between physiologic lymphoid proliferation and malignant lymphoma. Am J Med 1979, **67**: 421–428.

354 Cullen MH, Stansfeld AG, Oliver RTD, Lister TA, Malpas JS. Angioimmunoblastic lymphadenopathy. Report of ten cases and review of the literature. Q J Med 1979, **48**: 151–177.

355 Dargent JL, Jacobovitz D, Pradier O, Velu T, Martiat P, Delplace J, Neve P, Diebold J. A case of pleomorphic T-cell lymphoma with a high content of reactive histiocytes presented with hypereosinophilia. Pathol Res Pract 1995, **191**: 463–468.

356 Feller AC, Griesser H, Schilling CV, Wacker HH, Dallenbach F, Bartels H, Kuse R, Mak TW, Lennert K. Clonal gene rearrangement patterns correlate with immunophenotype and clinical parameters in patients with angioimmunoblastic lymphadenopathy. Am J Pathol 1988, **133**: 549–556.

357 Freter CE, Cossman J. Angioimmunoblastic lymphadenopathy with dysproteinemia. Semin Oncol 1993, **20**: 627–635.

358 Frizzera G, Moran EM, Rappaport H. Angio-immunoblastic lymphadenopathy with dysproteinaemia. Lancet 1974, **1**: 1070–1073.

359 Frizzera G, Moran EM, Rappaport H. Angio-immunoblastic lymphadenopathy. Diagnosis and clinical course. Am J Med 1975, **59**: 803–818.

360 Jones D, Jorgensen JL, Shasafaei A, Dorfman DM. Characteristic proliferations of reticular and dendritic cells in angioimmunoblastic lymphoma. Am J Surg Pathol 1998, **22**: 956–964.

361 Khan G, Norton AJ, Slavin G. Epstein–Barr virus in angioimmunoblastic T-cell lymphomas. Histopathology 1993, **22**: 145–149.

362 Knecht H, Schwarze E-W, Lennert K. Histological, immunohistological and autopsy findings in lymphogranulomatosis X (including angioimmunoblastic lymphadenopathy). Virchows Arch [A] 1985, **406**: 105–124.

363 Kon S, Sato T, Onodera K, Satoh M, Kikuchi K, Imai S, Osato T. Detection of Epstein–Barr virus DNA and EBV-determined nuclear antigen in angioimmunoblastic lymphadenopathy with dysproteinemia type T-cell lymphoma. Pathol Res Pract 1993, **189**: 1137–1144.

364 Kosmidis PA, Axelrod AR, Palacas C, Stahl M. Angioimmunoblastic lymphadenopathy. A T-cell deficiency. Cancer 1978, **42**: 447–452.

365 Liao DT, Rosai J, Daneshbod K. Malignant histocytosis with cutaneous involvement and eosinophilia. Am J Clin Pathol 1972, **57**: 438–448.

366 Lorenzen J, Li G, Zhao-Hohn M, Wintzer C, Fischer R, Hansmann ML. Angioimmunoblastic lymphadenopathy type of T-cell lymphoma and angioimmunoblastic lymphadenopathy. A clinicopathological and molecular biological study of 13 Chinese patients using polymerase chain reaction and paraffin-embedded tissues. Virchows Arch 1994, **424**: 593–600.

367 Lukes RJ, Tindle BH. Immunoblastic lymphadenopathy. A hyperimmune entity resembling Hodgkin's disease. N Engl J Med 1975, **292**: 1–8.

368 Nathwani BN, Rappaport H, Moran EM, Pangalis GA, Kim H. Malignant lymphoma arising in angioimmunoblastic lymphadenopathy. Cancer 1978, **41**: 578–606.

369 Ohshima K, Takeo H, Kikuchi M, Kozuru M, Uike N, Masuda Y, Yoneda S, Takeshita M, Shibata T, Akamatsu M. Heterogeneity of Epstein–Barr virus infection in angioimmunoblastic lymphadenopathy type T-cell lymphoma. Histopathology 1994, **25**: 569–580.

370 Ree HJ, Kadin ME, Kikuchi M, Ko YH, Go JH, Suzumiya J, Kim DS. Angioimmunoblastic lymphoma (AILD-type T-cell lymphoma) with hyperplasia germinal centers. Am J Surg Pathol 1998, **22**: 643–655.

371 Seehafer JR, Goldberg NC, Dicken CH, Su WPD. Cutaneous manifestations of angioimmunoblastic lymphadenopathy. Arch Dermatol 1980, **116**: 41–45.

372 Shimoyama M, Minato K, Saito H, Takenaka T, Watanabe S, Nagatani T, Naruto M. Immunoblastic lymphadenopathy (IBL)-like T-cell lymphoma. Jpn J Clin Oncol 1979, 9(Suppl 1): 347–356.

373 Smith JL, Hodges E, Quin CT, McCarthy KP, Wright DH. Frequent T- and B-cell oligoclones in histologically and immunophenotypically characterized angioimmunoblastic lymphadenopathy. Am J Pathol 2000, **156**: 661–669.

374 Weiss LM, Strickler JG, Dorfman RF, Horning SJ, Warnke RA, Sklar J. Clonal T-cell populations in angioimmunoblastic lymphadenopathy and angioimmunoblastic lymphadenopathy-like lymphoma. Am J Pathol 1986, **122**: 392–397.

DRUG HYPERSENSITIVITY

375 Abbondanzo SL, Irey NS, Frizzera G. Dilantin-associated lymphadenopathy. Spectrum of histopathologic patterns. Am J Surg Pathol 1995, **19**: 675–686.

376 Saltzstein SL, Ackerman LV. Lymphadenopathy induced by anticonvulsant drugs clinically and pathologically mimicking malignant lymphomas. Cancer 1959, **12**: 164–182.

DERMATOPATHIC LYMPHADENITIS

377 Asano S, Muramatsu T, Kanno H, Wakasa H. Dermatopathic lymphadenopathy. Electronmicroscopic, enzyme-histochemical and immunohistochemical study. Acta Pathol Jpn 1987, **37**: 887–900.

378 Burke JS, Colby TV. Dermatopathic lymphadenopathy. Comparison of cases associated and unassociated with mycosis fungoides. Am J Surg Pathol 1981, **5**: 343–352.

379 Gould E, Porto R, Albores-Saavedra J, Ibe MJ. Dermatopathic lymphadenitis. The spectrum and significance of its morphologic features. Arch Pathol Lab Med 1988, **112**: 1145–1150.

380 Rausch E, Kaiserling E, Goos M. Langerhans cells and interdigitating reticulum cells in the thymus-dependent region in human dermatopathic lymphadenitis. Virchows Arch [Cell Pathol] 1977, **25**: 327–343.

381 Ree H, Fanger H. Paracortical alteration in lymphadenopathic and tumor-draining lymph nodes. Histologic study. Hum Pathol 1975, **6**: 363–372.

382 Weiss LM, Hu E, Wood GS, Moulds C, Cleary ML, Warnke R, Sklar J. Clonal rearrangements of T-cell receptor genes in mycosis fungoides and dermatopathic lymphadenopathy. N Engl J Med 1985, **313**: 539–544.

383 Weiss LM, Wood GS, Warnke RA. Immunophenotypic differences between dermatopathic lymphadenopathy and lymph node involvement in mycosis fungoides. Am J Pathol 1985, **120**: 179–185.

ROSAI–DORFMAN DISEASE

384 Alatassi H, Ray MB, Galandiuk S, Sahoo S. Rosai–Dorfman disease of the gastrointestinal tract: report of a case and review of the literature. Int J Surg Pathol 2006, **14**: 95–99.

385 Albores-Saavedra J, Vuitch F, Delgado R, Wiley E, Hagler H. Sinus histiocytosis of pelvic lymph nodes after hip replacement. A histiocytic proliferation induced by cobalt-chromium and titanium. Am J Surg Pathol 1994, **18**: 83–90.

386 Al-Daraji W, Anandan A, Klassen-Fischer M, Auerbach A, Marwaha JS, Fanburg-Smith JC. Soft tissue Rosai–Dorfman disease: 29 new lesions in 18 patients, with detection of polyomavirus antigen in 3 abdominal cases. Ann Diagn Pathol 2010, **14**: 309–316.

387 Andriko JA, Morridon A, Colegial CH, Davis BJ, Jones RV. Rosai–Dorfman disease isolated to the central nervous system: a report of 11 cases. Mod Pathol 2001, **14**: 172–178.

388 Bonetti F, Chilosi M, Menestrina F, Scarpa A, Pelicci PG, Amorosi E, Fiore-Donati L, Knowles DM. Immunohistological analysis of Rosai–Dorfman histiocytosis. A disease of S-100 + CD1-histiocytes. Virchows Arch [A] 1987, **411**: 129–135.

389 Brenn T, Calonje E, Granter SR, Leonard N, Grayson W, Fletcher CD, McKee PH. Cutaneous Rosai–Dorfman disease is a distinct clinical entity. Am J Dermatopathol 2002, **24**: 385–391.

390 Cocker RS, Kang J, Kahn LB. Rosai–Dorfman disease. Report of a case presenting as a midline thyroid mass. Arch Pathol Lab Med 2003, **127**: e197–200.

391 Eisen RN, Buckley PJ, Rosai J. Immunophenotypic characterization of sinus histiocytosis with massive lymphadenopathy (Rosai–Dorfman disease). Semin Diagn Pathol 1990, **7**: 74–82.

392 Falk S, Stutte HJ, Frizzera G. Hodgkin's disease and sinus histiocytosis with massive lymphadenopathylike changes. Histopathology 1991, **19**: 221–224.

393 Foucar E, Rosai J, Dorfman RF. Sinus histiocytosis with massive lymphadenopathy. Ear, nose, and throat manifestations. Arch Otolaryngol 1978, **104**: 687–693.

394 Foucar E, Rosai J, Dorfman RF. The ophthalmologic manifestations of sinus histiocytosis with massive lymphadenopathy. Am J Ophthalmol 1979, **87**: 354–367.

395 Foucar E, Rosai J, Dorfman RF. Sinus histiocytosis with massive lymphadenopathy. An analysis of 14 deaths occurring in a patient registry. Cancer 1984, **54**: 1834–1840.

396 Foucar E, Rosai J, Dorfman R. Sinus histiocytosis with massive lymphadenopathy (Rosai–Dorfman disease). Review of the entity. Semin Diagn Pathol 1990, **7**: 19–73.

397 Foucar E, Rosai J, Dorfman RF, Brynes RK. The neurologic manifestations of sinus histiocytosis with massive lymphadenopathy. Neurology 1982, **32**: 365–371.

398 Foucar E, Rosai J, Dorfman RF, Eyman JM. Immunologic abnormalities and their significance in the pathogenesis of sinus histiocytosis with massive lymphadenopathy. Am J Clin Pathol 1984, **82**: 515–525.

399 Green I, Dorfman RF, Rosai J. Breast involvement by extranodal Rosai–Dorfman disease: report of seven cases. Am J Surg Pathol 1997, **21**: 664–668.

400 Hida AI, Yagi S, Obase Y, Nishimura H, Akiyama T, Irei I, Hamazaki S, Oka M, Sadahira Y. Rosai–Dorfman disease presenting as a solitary mediastinal mass. Pathol Int 2009, **59**: 265–268.

401 Jabali Y, Smrcka V, Pradna J. Rosai–Dorfman disease: successful long-term results by combination chemotherapy with prednisone, 6-mercaptopurine, methotrexate, and vinblastine: a case report. Int J Surg Pathol 2005, **13**: 285–289.

402 Juskevicius R, Finley JL. Rosai–Dorfman disease of the parotid gland: cytologic and histopathologic findings with immunohistochemical correlation. Arch Pathol Lab Med 2001, **125**: 1348–1350.

403 Kasper HU, Hegenbarth V, Buhtz P. Rhinoscleroma associated with Rosai–Dorfman reaction of regional lymph nodes. Pathol Int 2004, **54**: 101–104.

404 Komp DM. The treatment of sinus histiocytosis with massive lymphadenopathy (Rosai–Dorfman disease). Semin Diagn Pathol 1990, **7**: 83–86.

405 Kong YY, Kong JC, Shi DR, Lu HF, Zhu XZ, Wang J, Chen ZW. Cutaneous Rosai–Dorfman disease: a clinical and histopathologic study of 25 cases in China. Am J Surg Pathol 2007, **31**: 341–350.

406 Lauwers GY, Perez-Atayde A, Dorfman RF, Rosai J. The digestive system manifestations of Rosai–Dorfman disease (sinus histiocytosis with massive lymphadenopathy): review of 11 cases. Hum Pathol 2000, **31**: 380–385.

407 Leighton SE, Gallimore AP. Extranodal sinus histiocytosis with massive lymphadenopathy affecting the subglottis and trachea. Histopathology 1994, **24**: 393–394.

408 Levine PH, Jahan N, Murari P, Manak M, Jaffe ES. Detection of human herpesvirus 6 in tissues involved by sinus histiocytosis with massive lymphadenopathy (Rosai–Dorfman disease). J Infect Dis 1992, **166**: 291–295.

409 Lu D, Estalilla OC, Manning JT, Medeiros LJ. Sinus histiocytosis with massive lymphadenopathy and malignant lymphoma involving the same lymph node: a report of four cases and review of the literature. Mod Pathol 2000, **13**: 414–419.

410 Lu CI, Kuo TT, Wong WR, Hong HS. Clinical and histopathologic spectrum of cutaneous Rosai–Dorfman disease in Taiwan. J Am Acad Dermatol 2004, **51**: 931–939.

411 Marsh WL Jr, McCarrick JP, Harlan DM. Sinus histiocytosis with massive lymphadenopathy. Occurrence in identical twins with retroperitoneal disease. Arch Pathol Lab Med 1988, **112**: 298–301.

412 Middel P, Hemmerlein B, Fayyazi A, Kaboth U, Radzun HJ. Sinus histiocytosis with massive lymphadenopathy: evidence for its relationship to macrophages and for a cytokine-related disorder. Histopathology 2000, **35**: 525–533.

413 Miettinen M, Paljakka P, Haveri P, Saxén E. Sinus histiocytosis with massive lymphadenopathy. A nodal and extranodal proliferation of S-100 protein positive histiocytes? Am J Clin Pathol 1987, **88**: 270–277.

414 Montgomery EA, Meis JM, Frizzera G. Rosai–Dorfman disease of soft tissue. Am J Surg Pathol 1992, **16**: 122–129.

415 Morkowski JJ, Nguyen CV, Lin P, Farr M, Abraham SC, Gilcrease MZ, Moran CA, Wu Y. Rosai–Dorfman disease confined to the breast. Ann Diagn Pathol 2010, **14**: 81–87.

416 Murray J, Fox H. Rosai–Dorfman disease of the uterine cervix. Int J Gynecol Pathol 1991, **10**: 209–213.

417 O'Malley DP, Duong A, Barry TS, Chen S, Hibbard HK, Ferry JA, Hasserjian RP, Thompson MA, Richardson MS, Jaffe R, Sidhu JS, Banks PM. Co-occurrence of Langerhans cell histiocytosis and Rosai–Dorfman disease: possible relationship of two histiocytic disorders in rare cases. Mod Pathol 2010, **23**: 1616–1623.

418 Osborne BM, Hagemeister FB, Butler JJ. Extranodal gastrointestinal sinus histiocytosis with massive lymphadenopathy. Clinically presenting as a malignant tumor. Am J Surg Pathol 1981, **5**: 603–611.

419 Paulli M, Feller AC, Boveri E, Kindl S, Berti E, Rosso R, Merz H, Facchetti F, Gambini C, Bonetti F, et al. Cathepsin D and E co-expression in sinus histiocytosis with massive lymphadenopathy (Rosai–Dorfman disease) and Langerhans' cell histiocytosis. Further evidences of a phenotypic overlap between these histiocytic disorders. Virchows Arch 1994, **424**: 601–606.

420 Paulli M, Rosso R, Kindl S, Boveri E, Marocolo D, Chioda C, Agostini C, Magrini U, Facchetti F. Immunophenotypic characterization of the cell infiltrate in five cases of sinus histiocytosis with massive lymphadenopathy (Rosai–Dorfman disease). Hum Pathol 1992, **23**: 647–654.

421 Podberezin M, Angeles R, Guzman G, Peace D, Gaitonde S. Primary pancreatic sinus histiocytosis with massive lymphadenopathy (Rosai–Dorfman disease): an unusual extranodal manifestation clinically simulating malignancy. Arch Pathol Lab Med 2010, **134**: 276–278.

422 Pulsoni A, Anghel G, Falcucci P, Matera R, Pescarmona E, Ribersan M, Villiva N, Mandelli F. Treatment of sinus histiocytosis with massive lymphadenopathy (Rosai–Dorfman disease): report of a case and literature review. Am J Hematol 2002, **69**: 67–71.

423 Quaglino P, Tomasini C, Novelli M, Colonna S, Bernengo MG. Immunohistologic findings and adhesion molecule pattern in primary pure cutaneous Rosai–Dorfman disease with xanthomatous features. Am J Dermatopathol 1998, **20**: 393–398.

424 Röcken C, Wieker K, Grote H-J, Müller G, Franke A, Roessner A. Rosai–Dorfman disease and generalized AA amyloidosis: a case report. Hum Pathol 2000, **31**: 621–624.

425 Rosai J, Dorfman RF. Sinus histiocytosis with massive lymphadenopathy. A pseudolymphomatous benign disorder. Analysis of 34 cases. Cancer 1972, **30**: 1174–1188.

426 Song SK, Schwartz IS, Strauchen JA, Huang YP, Sachdev V, Daftary DR, Vas CJ. Meningeal nodules with features of extranodal sinus histiocytosis with massive lymphadenopathy. Am J Surg Pathol 1989, **13**: 406–412.

427 Suarez CR, Zeller WP, Silberman S, Rust G, Messmore H. Sinus histiocytosis with massive lymphadenopathy. Remission with chemotherapy. Am J Pediatr Hematol Oncol 1983, **5**: 235–241.

428 Thawerani H, Sanchez RL, Rosai J, Dorfman RF. The cutaneous manifestations of sinus histiocytosis with massive lymphadenopathy. Arch Dermatol 1978, **114**: 191–197.

429 Tsang WY, Yip TT, Chan JK. The Rosai–Dorfman disease histiocytes are not infected by Epstein–Barr virus. Histopathology 1994, **25**: 88–90.

430 Walker PD, Rosai J, Dorfman RF. The osseous manifestations of sinus histiocytosis with massive lymphadenopathy. Am J Clin Pathol 1981, **75**: 131–139.

431 Wang KH, Cheng CJ, Hu CH, Lee WR. Coexistence of localized Langerhans cell histiocytosis and cutaneous Rosai–Dorfman disease. Br J Dermatol 2002, **147**: 770–774.

432 Wenig BM, Abbondanzo SL, Childers EL, Kapadia SB, Heffner DR. Extranodal sinus histiocytosis with massive lymphadenopathy (Rosai–Dorfman disease) of the head and neck. Hum Pathol 1993, **24**: 483–492.

433 Willman CL, Busque L, Griffith BB, Favara BE, McClain KL, Duncan MH, Gilliland DG. Langerhans-cell histiocytosis (histiocytosis X). A clonal proliferative disease. N Engl J Med 1994, **331**: 154–160.

434 Woda BA, Sullivan JL. Reactive histiocytic disorders. Am J Clin Pathol 1993, **99**: 459–463.

435 Wright DH, Richards DB. Sinus histiocytosis with massive lymphadenopathy (Rosai–Dorfman disease). Report of a case with widespread nodal and extra nodal dissemination. Histopathology 1981, **5**: 697–709.

AUTOIMMUNE LYMPHOPROLIFERATIVE SYNDROME

436 Deutsch M, Tsopanou E, Dourakis SP. The autoimmune lymphoproliferative syndrome (Canale-Smith) in adulthood. Clin Rheumatol 2004, **23**: 43–44.

437 Jackson CE, Puck JM. Autoimmune lymphoproliferative syndrome, a disorder of apoptosis. Curr Opin Pediatr 1999, **11**: 521–527.

438 Kraus MD, Shenoy S, Chatila T, Hess JL. Light microscopic, immunophenotypic, and molecular genetic study of autoimmune lymphoproliferative syndrome caused by fas mutation. Pediatr Dev Pathol 2000, **3**: 101–109.

439 Lim MS, Straus SE, Dale JK, Fleisher TA, Stetler-Stevenson M, Strober W, Sneller MC, Puck JM, Lenardo MJ, Elenitoba-Johnson KSJ, Lin AY, Raffeld M, Jaffe ES. Pathological findings in human autoimmune lymphoproliferative syndrome. Am J Pathol 1998, **153**: 1541–1550.

440 Maric I, Pittaluga S, Dale JK, Niemela JE, Delsol G, Diment J, Rosai J, Raffeld M, Puck JM, Straus SE, Jaffe ES. Histologic features of sinus histiocytosis with massive lymphadenopathy in patients with autoimmune lymphoproliferative syndrome. Am J Surg Pathol 2005, **29**: 903–911.

441 Oliveira JB, Bleesing JJ, Dianzani U, Fleisher TA, Jaffe ES, Lenardo MJ, Rieux-Laucat F, Siegel RM, Su HC, Teachey DT, Rao VK. Revised diagnostic criteria and classification for the autoimmune lymphoproliferative syndrome: report from the 2009 NIH International Workshop. Blood, 2010, **116**: e35–40.

442 Straus SE, Jaffe ES, Puck JM, Dale JK, Elkon KB, Rösen-Wolff A, Peters AM, Sneller MC, Hallahan CW, Wang J, Fischer RE, Jackson CM, Lin AY, Bäumler C, Siegert E, Marx A, Vaishnaw AK, Grodzicky T, Fleisher TA, Lenardo MJ. The development of lymphomas in families with autoimmune lymphoproliferative syndrome with germline Fas mutations and defective lymphocyte apoptosis. Blood 2001, **98**: 194–200.

443 Teachey DT, Seif AE, Grupp SA. Advances in the management and understanding of autoimmune lymphoproliferative syndrome (ALPS). Br J Haematol 2010, **148**: 205–216.

LANGERHANS CELL HISTIOCYTOSIS

444 Anjuère F, Del Hoyo GM, Martin P, Ardavin C. Langerhans' cells develop from a lymphoid-committed precursor. Blood 2000, **96**: 1633–1637.

445 Axiotis CA, Merino MJ, Duray PH. Langerhans cell histiocytosis of the female genital tract. Cancer 1991, **67**: 1650–1660.

446 Beckstead JH, Wood GS, Turner RR. Histiocytosis X cells and Langerhans cells. Enzyme histochemical and immunologic similarities. Hum Pathol 1984, **15**: 826–833.

447 Ben-Ezra J, Bailey A, Azumi N, Delsol G, Stroup R, Sheibani K, Rappaport H. Malignant histiocytosis X. A distinct clinicopathologic entity. Cancer 1991, **68**: 1050–1060.

448 Berg LC, Norelle A, Morgan WA, Washa DM. Cat-scratch disease simulating histiocytosis X. Hum Pathol 1998, **29**: 649–651.

449 Bingham EA, Bridges JM, Kelly AMT, Burrows D, Nevins NC. Letterer–Siwe disease. A study of thirteen cases over a 21-year period. Br J Dermatol 1982, **106**: 205–209.

450 Boulac A, Boullard ML, Geissmann F, Fraitag S, Andry P, Teillac D, Bensussan A, Revuz J, Boumsell L, Wechsler J, Bagot M. CD101 expression by Langerhan's cell histiocytosis cells. Histopathology 2000, **36**: 229–232.

451 Brabencova E, Tazi A, Lorenzato M, Bonay M, Kambouchner M, Emile JF, Hance AJ, Soler P. Langerhan's cells in Langerhan's cell granulomatosis are not actively proliferating cells. Am J Pathol 1998, **152**: 1143–1149.

452 Burns BF, Colby TV, Dorfman RF. Langerhans cell granulomatosis (histiocytosis X) associated with malignant lymphomas. Am J Surg Pathol 1983, **7**: 529–533.

453 Chen W, Wang J, Wang E, Lu Y, Lau SK, Weiss LM, Huang Q. Detection of clonal lymphoid receptor gene rearrangements in Langerhans cell histiocytosis. Am J Surg Pathol 2010, **34**: 1049–1057.

454 Christie LJ, Evans AT, Bray SE, Smith ME, Kernohan NM, Levison DA, Goodlad JR. Lesions resembling Langerhans cell histiocytosis in association with other lymphoproliferative disorders: a reactive or neoplastic phenomenon? Hum Pathol 2006, **37**: 32–39.

455 Edelweiss M, Medeiros LJ, Suster S, Moran CA. Lymph node involvement by Langerhans cell histiocytosis: a clinicopathologic and immunohistochemical study of 20 cases. Hum Pathol 2007, **38**: 1463–1469.

456 Emile J-F, Wechsler J, Brousse N, Boulland ML, Cologon R, Freitag S, Voisin M-C, Gaulard P, Boumsell L, Zafrani E-S. Langerhans' cell histiocytosis. Definitive diagnosis with the use of monoclonal antibody O10 on routinely paraffin-embedded samples. Am J Surg Pathol 1995, **19**: 636–641.

457 Favara BE. Langerhans' cell histiocytosis pathobiology and pathogenesis. Semin Oncol 1991, **18**: 3–7.

458 Gilcrease MZ, Rajan B, Ostrowski ML, Ramzy I, Schwartz MR. Localized thymic Langerhan's cell histiocytosis and its relationship with myasthenia gravis: immunohistochemical, ultrastructural, and cytometric studies. Arch Pathol Lab Med 1997, **121**: 134–138.

459 Giona F, Caruso R, Testi AM, Moleti ML, Malagnino F, Martelli M, Ruco L, Giannetti GP, Annibali S, Mandell F. Langerhan's cell histiocytosis in adults: a clinical and therapeutic analysis of 11 patients from a single institution. Cancer 1997, **80**: 1786–1791.

460 Hage C, Willman CL, Favara BE, Isaacson PG. Langerhans' cell histiocytosis (histiocytosis X). Immunophenotype and growth fraction. Hum Pathol 1993, **24**: 840–845.

461 Hashimoto K, Griffin D, Kohsbaki M. Self-healing reticulohistiocytosis. A clinical, histologic, and ultrastructural study of the fourth case in the literature. Cancer 1982, **49**: 331–337.

462 Herzog KM, Tubbs RR. Langerhan's cell histiocytosis. Adv Anat Pathol 1999, **5**: 347–358.

463 Howarth DM, Gilchrist GS, Mullan BP, Wiseman GA, Edmonson JH, Schomberg PJ. Langerhans cell histiocytosis: diagnosis, natural history, management and outcome. Cancer 1999, **85**: 2278–2290.

464 Kaplan KJ, Goodman ZD, Ishak KG. Liver involvement in Langerhan's cell histiocytosis: a study of nine cases. Mod Pathol 1999, **12**: 370–378.

465 Kenn W, Eck M, Allolio B, Jacob F, Illg A, Marx A, Müller-Hermelink HK, Hahn D. Erdheim–Chester disease: evidence for a disease entity different from Langerhan's cell histiocytosis? Three cases with detailed radiological and immunohistochemical analysis. Hum Pathol 2000, **31**: 734–739.

466 Kjedlsberg CR, Kim H. Eosinophilic granuloma as an incidental finding in malignant lymphoma. Arch Pathol Lab Med 1980, **104**: 137–140.

467 Komp DM. Concepts in staging and clinical studies for treatment of Langerhans' cell histiocytosis. Semin Oncol 1991, **18**: 18–23.

468 Lahey ME. Prognostic factors in histiocytosis X. Am J Pediatr Hematol/Oncol 1981, **3**: 57–65.

469 Lau SK, Chu PG, Weiss LM. Immunohistochemical expression of Langerin in Langerhans cell histiocytosis and non-Langerhans cell histiocytic disorders. Am J Surg Pathol 2008, **32**: 615–619.

470 Leahy MA, Krejci SM, Friednash M, Stockert SS, Wilson H, Huff JC, Weston WL, Brice SL. Human herpesvirus 6 is present in lesions of Langerhans cell histiocytosis. J Invest Dermatol 1993, **101**: 642–645.

471 Lieberman PH, Jones CR, Steinman RM, Erlandson RA, Smith J, Gee T, Huvos A, Garin-Chesa P, Filippa DA, Urmacher C, Gangi MD, Sperber M. Langerhan's cell (eosinophilic) granulomatosis; a clinicopathologic study encompassing 50 years. Am J Surg Pathol 1996, **20**: 519–552.

472 McClain K, Jin H, Gresik V, Favara B. Langerhans cell histiocytosis. Lack of a viral etiology. Am J Hematol 1994, **47**: 16–20.

473 Magni M, Di Nocola M, Carlo-Stella C, Matteucci P, Lavazza C, Grisanti S, Bifulco C, Pilotti S, Papini D, Rosai J, Gianni AM. Identical rearrangement of immunoglobulin heavy chain gene in neoplastic Langerhan's cells and B-lymphocytes: evidence for a common precursor. Leuk Res 2002, **36**: 1131–1133.

474 Meehan SA, Smoller BR. Cutaneous Langerhans' cell histiocytosis of the genitalia in the elderly: a report of three cases. J Cutan Pathol 1998, **25**: 370–374.

475 Mierau GW, Favara BE, Brenman JM. Electron microscopy in histiocytosis X. Ultrastruct Pathol 1982, **3**: 137–142.

476 Motoi M, Helbron D, Kaiserling E, Lennert K. Eosinophilic granuloma of lymph nodes. A variant of histiocytosis X. Histopathology 1980, **4**: 585–606.

477 Murakami I, Gogusev J, Fournet JC, Glorion C, Jaubert F. Detection of molecular cytogenetic aberrations in Langerhans' cell histiocytosis of bone. Hum Pathol 2002, **33**: 555–560.

478 Neumann MP, Frizzera G. The coexistence of Langerhans' cell granulomatosis and malignant lymphoma may take different forms. Report of seven cases with a review of the literature. Hum Pathol 1986, **17**: 1060–1065.

479 Nezelof C, Basset F. From histiocytosis X to Langerhans' cell histiocytosis: a personal account. Int J Surg Pathol 2001, **9**: 137–146.

480 Ornvold K, Nielsen MH, Clausen N. Disseminated histiocytosis X. A clinical and immunohistochemical retrospective study. Acta Pathol Microbiol Immunol Scand (A) 1985, **93**: 311–316.

481 Ornvold K, Ralfkiaer E, Carstensen H. Immunohistochemical study of the abnormal cells in Langerhans cell histiocytosis (histiocytosis X). Virchows Arch [A] 1990, **416**: 403–410.

482 Otis CN, Fischer RA, Johnson N, Kelleher JF, Powell JL. Histiocytosis X of the vulva. A case report and review of the literature. Obstet Gynecol 1990, **75**: 555–558.

483 Paulli M, Feller AC, Boveri E, Kindl S, Berti E, Rosso R, Merz H, Facchetti F, Gambini C, Bonetti F, et al. Cathepsin D and E co-expression in sinus histiocytosis with massive lymphadenopathy (Rosai–Dorfman disease) and Langerhans' cell histiocytosis. Further evidences of a phenotypic overlap between these histiocytic disorders. Virchows Arch 1994, **424**: 601–606.

484 Pinkus GS, Lones MA, Matsumura F, Yamashiro S, Said JW, Pinkus JL. Langerhans cell histiocytosis. Immunohistochemical expression of fascin, a dendritic cell marker. Am J Clin Pathol 2002, **118**: 335–343.

485 Ree HJ, Kadin ME. Peanut agglutinin. A useful marker for histiocytosis X and interdigitating reticulum cells. Cancer 1986, **57**: 282–287.

486 Reid H, Fox H, Whittaker JS. Eosinophilic granuloma of lymph nodes. Histopathology 1977, **1**: 31–37.

487 Richmond I, Eyden BP, Banerjee SS. Intranodal Langerhans' cell histiocytosis associated with malignant melanoma. Histopathology 1995, **26**: 380–382.

488 Risdall RJ, Dehner LP, Duray P, Kobrinsky N, Robison L, Nesbit ME Jr. Histiocytosis X (Langerhans' cell histiocytosis). Prognostic role of histopathology. Arch Pathol Lab Med 1983, **107**: 59–63.

489 Safali M, McCutcheon JM, Wright DH. Langerhans cell histiocytosis of lymph nodes: draining a papillary carcinoma of the thyroid. Histopathology 1997, **30**: 599–603.

490 Santamaria M, Llamas L, Ree HJ, Sheibani K, Ho YS, Su I-J, Hsu S-M. Expression of sialylated leu-M1 antigen in histiocytosis X. Am J Clin Pathol 1988, **89**: 211–219.

491 Sholl LM, Hornick JL, Pinkus JL, Pinkus GS, Padera RF. Immunohistochemical analysis of langerin in Langerhans cell histiocytosis and pulmonary inflammatory and infectious diseases. Am J Surg Pathol 2007, **31**: 947–952.

492 Terracciano L, Kocher T, Cathomas G, Bubendorf L, Lehmann FS. Langerhans' cell histicyotosis of the stomach with atypical morphological features. Pathol Int 1999, **49**: 553–556.

493 Thompson LD, Wenig BM, Adair CF, Smith BC, Heffess CS. Langerhan's cell histiocytosis of the thyroid: a series of seven cases and a review of the literature. Mod Pathol 1996, **9**: 145–149.

494 Vernon ML, Fountain L, Krebs HM, Barbosa LH, Fuccillo DA, Sever JL. Birbeck granules (Langerhans' cell granules) in human lymph nodes. Am J Clin Pathol 1973, **60**: 771–779.

495 Williams JW, Dorfman RF. Lymphadenopathy as the initial manifestation of histiocytosis X. Am J Surg Pathol 1979, **3**: 405–421.

496 Willman CL, Busque L, Griffith BB, Favara BE, McClain KL, Duncan MH, Gilliland DG. Langerhans'-cell histiocytosis (histiocytosis X) – a clonal proliferative disease. N Engl J Med 1994, **331**: 154–160.

497 Wood C, Wood GS, Deneau DG, Oseroff A, Beckstead JH, Malin J. Malignant histiocytosis X. Report of a rapidly fatal case in an elderly man. Cancer 1984, **54**: 347–352.

498 Yousem SA, Colby TV, Chen YY, Chen WG, Weiss LW. Pulmonary Langerhan's cell histiocytosis: molecular analysis of clonality. Am J Surg Pathol 2001, **25**: 630–636.

499 Yu RC, Chu AC. Lack of T-cell receptor gene rearrangements in cells involved in Langerhans' cell histiocytosis. Cancer 1995, **75**: 1162–1166.

KIMURA DISEASE

500 Chan JK, Hui PK, Ng CS, Yuen NW, Kung IT, Gwi E. Epithelioid haemangioma (angiolymphoid hyperplasia with eosinophilia) and Kimura's disease in Chinese. Histopathology 1989, **15**: 557–574.

501 Chen H, Thompson LDR, Aguilera NS, Abbondanzo SL. Kimura disease: a clinicopathologic study of 21 cases. Am J Surg Pathol 2004, **28**: 505–513.

502 Chim CS, Fung A, Shek TW, Liang R, Ho WK, Kwong YL. Analysis of clonality in Kimura's disease. Am J Surg Pathol 2002, **26**: 1083–1086.

503 Googe PB, Harris NL, Mihm MC Jr. Kimura's disease and angiolymphoid hyperplasia with eosinophilia. Two distinct histopathological entities. J Cutan Pathol 1987, **14**: 263–271.

504 Hui PK, Chan JK, Ng CS, Kung IT, Gwi E. Lymphadenopathy of Kimura's disease. Am J Surg Pathol 1989, **13**: 177–186.

505 Kung ITM, Gibson JB, Bannatyne PM. Kimura's disease. A clinico-pathological study of 21 cases and its distinction from angiolymphoid hyperplasia with eosinophilia. Pathology 1984, **16**: 39–44.

506 Kuo TT, Shih LY, Chan HL. Kimura's disease. Involvement of regional lymph nodes and distinction from angiolymphoid hyperplasia with eosinophilia. Am J Surg Pathol 1988, **12**: 843–854.

507 Urabe A, Tsuneyoshi M, Enjoji M. Epithelioid hemangioma versus Kimura's disease. A comparative clinicopathologic study. Am J Surg Pathol 1987, **11**: 758–766.

CHRONIC GRANULOMATOUS DISEASE

508 Baehner RL, Nathan DG. Quantitative nitroblue tetrazolium test in chronic granulomatous disease. N Engl J Med 1968, **278**: 971–976.

509 Curnutte JT. Chronic granulomatous disease: The solving of a clinical riddle at the molecular level. Clin Immunol Immunopathol 1993, **67**: S2–15.

510 Johnston RB Jr. Clinical aspects of chronic granulomatous disease. Curr Opin Hematol 2001, **8**: 17–22.

511 Lakshman R, Finn A. Neutrophil disorders and their management. J Clin Pathol 2001, **54**: 7–19.

512 Lekstrom-Himes JA, Gallin JI. Immunodeficiency disease caused by defects in phagocytes. N Engl J Med 2000, **343**: 1703–1714.

513 Levine S, Smith VV, Malone M, Sebire NJ. Histopathological features of chronic granulomatous disease (CGD) in childhood. Histopathology 2005, **47**: 508–516.

514 Roos D. The genetic basis of chronic granulomatous disease. Immunol Rev 1994, **138**: 121–157.

515 Segal BH, Holland SM. Primary phagocytic disorders of childhood. Pediatr Clin North Am 2000, **47**: 1311–1338.

516 Segal BH, Leto TL, Gallin JL, Malech HL, Holland SM. Genetic, biochemical, and clinical features of chronic granulomatous disease. Medicine (Baltimore) 2000, **79**: 170–200.

517 Umeki S. Mechanisms for the activation/electron transfer of neutrophil NADPH-oxidase complex and molecular pathology of chronic granulomatous disease. Ann Hematol 1994, **68**: 267–277.

LIPOPHAGIC REACTIONS

518 Alkan S, Beals TF, Schnitzer B. Primary diagnosis of Whipple disease manifesting as lymphadenopathy. Use of polymerase chain reaction for detection of *Tropheryma whippelii*. Am J Clin Pathol 2001, **116**: 899–904.

519 Baisden BL, Lepidi H, Raoult D, Argani P, Yardley JH, Dumler JS. Diagnosis of Whipple disease by immunohistochemical analysis. A sensitive and specific method for the detection of *Tropheryma whipplei* (the Whipple bacillus) in paraffin-embedded tissue. Am J Clin Pathol 2002, **118**: 742–748.

520 Boitnott JK, Margolis S. Mineral oil in human tissues. II. Oil droplets in lymph nodes of the porta hepatis. Bull Hopkins Hosp 1966, **118**: 414–422.

521 Fisher ER. Whipple's disease. Pathogenetic considerations. Electron microscopic and histochemical observations. JAMA 1962, **181**: 396–403.

522 Kelsall GR, Blackwell JB. The occurrence and significance of lipophage clusters in lymph nodes and spleen. Pathology 1969, **1**: 211–220.

523 Perez-Jaffe LA, Furth EE, Minda JM, Unger LD, Lawton TJ. Massive macrophage lipid accumulation presenting as hepatosplenomegaly and lymphadenopathy associated with long-term total parenteral nutrition therapy for short bowel syndrome. Hum Pathol 1998, **29**: 651–655.

524 Ravel R. Histopathology of lymph nodes after lymphangiography. Am J Clin Pathol 1966, **46**: 335–355.

MALIGNANT LYMPHOMA

525 Jaffe ES. Surgical pathology of the lymph nodes and related organs, ed. 2. Philadelphia, 1995, W.B. Saunders.

526 Jaffe ES, Harris NL, Stein H, Isaacson PG. Classification of lymphoid neoplasms: the microscope as a tool for disease discovery. Blood 2008, **112**: 4384–4399.

527 Knowles DM. Molecular pathology of acquired immunodeficiency syndrome-related non-Hodgkin's lymphoma. Semin Diagn Pathol 1997, **14**: 67–82.

528 Lennert K, Feller AC. Histopathology of non-Hodgkin's lymphomas, ed. 2. New York, 1992, Springer-Verlag.

529 Nathwani BN, Sasu SJ, Ahsanuddin AN, Hernandez AM, Drachenberg MR. The critical role of histology in an era of genomics and proteomics: a commentary and reflection. Adv Anat Pathol 2007, 14: 375–400.

530 Swerdlow SH, Campo E, Harris NL, Pileri SA, Stein H, Thiele J, Vardiman JW. WHO classification of tumours of haematopoietic and lymphoid tissues, ed. 4. Lyon, 2008, IARC Press.

531 Warnke RA, Weiss LM, Chan JKC, Cleary ML, Dorfman RF. Tumors of the lymph nodes and spleen. Atlas of tumor pathology, 3rd series, fascicle 14. Washington, DC, 1995, Armed Forces Institute of Pathology.

HODGKIN LYMPHOMA

532 Bonadonna G. Historical review of Hodgkin's disease. Br J Haematol 2000, **110**: 504–511.

533 Chang KL, Albujar PF, Chen YY, Johnson RM, Weiss LM. High prevalence of Epstein-Barr virus in the Reed-Sternberg cells of Hodgkin's disease occurring in Peru. Blood 1993, **81**: 496–501.

534 Dawson PJ. The original illustrations of Hodgkin's disease. Ann Diagn Pathol 2000, **3**: 386–393.

535 Gutensohn N, Cole P. Childhood social environment and Hodgkin's disease. N Engl J Med 1981, **304**: 135–140.

536 Hjalgrim H, Askling J, Rostgaard K, Hamilton-Dutoit S, Frisch M, Zhang J-S, Madsen M, Rosdahl N, Konradsen HB, Strom HH, Melbye M. Characteristics of Hodgkin's lymphoma after infectious mononucleosis. N Engl J Med 2003, **349**: 1324–1332.

537 Jaffett RF. Viruses and Hodgkin's disease. Ann Oncol 2002, **13**: 23–29.

538 Jarrett RF, Gallagher A, Jones DB, Alexander FE, Krajewski AS, Kelsey A, Adams J, Angus B, Gledhill S, Wright DH, et al. Detection of Epstein–Barr virus genomes in Hodgkin's disease. Relation to age. J Clin Pathol 1991, **44**: 844–848.

539 Kaplan HS. Hodgkin's disease. Cambridge 1980, **2**: 689.

540 Kass AM, Kass EH. Perfecting the world: the life and times of Dr Thomas Hodgkin 1798–1866. Boston, 1988, Harcourt Brace Jovanovich, 1: 642.

541 Mack TM, Cozen W, Shibata DK, Weiss LM, Nathwani BN, Hernandez AM, Taylor CR, Hamilton AS, Deapen DM, Rappaport EB. Concordance for Hodgkin's disease in identical twins suggesting genetic susceptibility to the young adult form of the disease. N Engl J Med 1995, **332**: 413–418.

542 Mueller N, Evans A, Harris NL, Comstock GW, Jellum E, Magnus K, Orentreich N, Polk BF, Vogelman J. Hodgkin's disease and Epstein–Barr virus. Altered antibody pattern before diagnosis. N Engl J Med 1989, **320**: 689–695.

543 Pallesen G, Hamilton-Dutoit SJ, Rowe M, Young LS. Expression of Epstein–Barr virus latent gene products in tumour cells of Hodgkin's disease. Lancet 1991, **337**: 320–322.

544 Poston RN. Positive Leu-M1 immunohistochemistry and diagnosis of the lymphoma cases described by Hodgkin in 1832. AIMM 1999, **7**: 6–8.

545 Reynolds DJ, Banks PM, Gulley ML. New characterization of infectious mononucleosis and a phenotypic comparison with Hodgkin's disease. Am J Pathol 1995, **146**: 379–388.

546 Taylor CR, Riley CR. Evolving concepts of the nature of Hodgkin's disease: a history. Ann Diagn Pathol 2001, **4**: 337–346.

547 Taylor CR, Riley CR. Molecular morphology of Hodgkin's lymphoma. Appl Immunohistochem Mol Morphol 2001, **9**: 187–202.

548 Thomas RK, Re D, Zander T, Wolf J, Diehl V. Epidemiology and etiology of Hodgkin's lymphoma. Ann Oncol 2002, **13**: 147–152.

549 Weiss LM, Chang KL. Molecular biologic studies of Hodgkin's disease. Semin Diagn Pathol 1992, **9**: 272–278.

550 Weiss LM, Chen YY, Liu XF, Shibata D. Epstein–Barr virus and Hodgkin's disease. A correlative in situ hybridization and polymerase chain reaction study. Am J Pathol 1991, **139**: 1259–1265.

Reed–Sternberg cell

551 Agnarsson BA, Kadin ME. The immunophenotype of Reed–Sternberg cells. A study of 50 cases of Hodgkin's disease using fixed frozen tissues. Cancer 1989, **63**: 2083–2087.

552 Brauninger A, Hansmann ML, Strickler JG, Dummer R, Burg G, Rajewsky K, Küppers R. Identification of common germinal-center B-cell precursors in two patients with both Hodgkin's disease and non-Hodgkin's lymphoma. New Engl J Med 1999, **340**: 1239–1247.

553 Carbone A, Gloghini A, Gruss H-J, Pinto A. CD40 antigen expression on Reed–Sternberg cells. A reliable diagnostic tool for Hodgkin's disease. Am J Pathol 1995, **146**: 780–781.

554 Casey TT, Olson SJ, Cousar JB, Collins RD. Immunophenotypes of Reed–Sternberg cells. A study of 19 cases of Hodgkin's disease in plastic-embedded sections. Blood 1989, **74**: 2624–2628.

555 Chang KL, Curtis CM, Momose H, Lopategui J, Weiss LM. Sensitivity and specificity of *Bauhinia purpurea* as a paraffin section marker for the Reed–Sternberg cells of Hodgkin's disease. Appl Immunohistochem 1993, **1**: 208–212.

556 Chen WG, Chen YY, Kamel OW, Koo CH, Weiss LM. P53 mutations in Hodgkin's disease. Lab Invest 1996, **75**: 519–527.

557 Chittal SM, Caverivière P, Schwarting R, Gerdes J, Al Saati T, Rigal-Huguet F, Stein H, Delsol G. Monoclonal antibodies in the diagnosis of Hodgkin's disease. The search for a rational panel. Am J Surg Pathol 1988, **12**: 9–21.

558 Dallenbach FE, Stein H. Expression of T-cell-receptor β chain in Reed–Sternberg cells. Lancet 1989, **2**: 828–830.

559 Delabie J, Shipman R, Bruggen J, De Strooper B, van Leuven F, Tarcsay L, Cerletti N, Odink K, Diehl V, Bilbe G, et al. Expression of the novel intermediate filament-associated protein restin in Hodgkin's disease and anaplastic large-cell lymphoma. Blood 1992, **80**: 2891–2896.

560 Elenitoba-Johnson KS, Medeiros LJ, Khorsand J, King TC. P53 expression in Reed–Sternberg cells does not correlate with gene mutations in Hodgkin's disease. Am J Clin Pathol 1997, **106**: 728–738.

561 Fan G, Kotylo P, Neiman RS, Braziel RM. Comparison of fascin expression in anaplastic large cell lymphoma and Hodgkin's disease. Am J Clin Pathol 2003, **119**: 199–204.

562 Foss H-D, Hummel M, Gottstein S, Ziemann K, Falini B, Herbst H, Stein H. Frequent expression of IL-7 gene transcripts in tumor cells of classical Hodgkin's disease. Am J Pathol 1995, **146**: 33–39.

563 Griesser H, Feller AC, Mak TW, Lennert K. Clonal rearrangements of T-cell receptor and immunoglobulin genes and immunophenotypic antigen expression in different subclasses of Hodgkin's disease. Int J Cancer 1987, **40**: 157–160.

564 Hsu S-M, Yang K, Jaffe ES. Phenotypic expression of Hodgkin's and Reed–Sternberg cells in Hodgkin's disease. Am J Pathol 1985, **118**: 209–217.

565 Hsu PL, Xie SS, Hsu SM. Absence of T-cell- and B-cell-specific transcription factors TCF-1, GATA-3, and BSAP in Hodgkin's Reed–Sternberg cells. Lab Invest 1997, **74**: 395–405.

566 Hummel M, Ziemann K, Lammert H, Pileri S, Sabattini E, Stein H. Hodgkin's disease with monoclonal and polyclonal populations of Reed–Sternberg cells. N Engl J Med 1995, **333**: 901–906.

567 Hyder DM, Schnitzer B. Utility of Leu M1 monoclonal antibody in the differential diagnosis of Hodgkin's disease. Arch Pathol Lab Med 1986, **110**: 416–419.

568 Izban KF, Ergin M, Martinez RL, Alkan S. Expression of the tumor necrosis factor receptor-associated factors (TRAFs) 1 and 2 is a characteristic feature of Hodgkin's and Reed–Sternberg cells. Mod Pathol 2000, **13**: 1324–1331.

569 Izban KF, Nawrocki JF, Alkan S, Hsi ED. Monoclonal IgH gene rearrangement in microdissected nodules from nodular sclerosis Hodgkin's disease. Am J Clin Pathol 1998, **110**: 599–606.

570 Kadin ME. A reappraisal of the Reed–Sternberg cell. A commentary. Blood Cells 1980, **6**: 525–532.

571 Kadin ME, Muramoto L, Said J. Expression of T-cell antigens on Reed–Sternberg cells in a subset of patients with nodular sclerosing and mixed cellularity Hodgkin's disease. Am J Pathol 1988, **130**: 345–353.

572 Knowles DM, Neri A, Pelicci PG, Burke JS, Wu A, Winberg CD, Sheibani K, Dalla-Favera R. Immunoglobulin and T-cell receptor β-chain gene rearrangement analysis of Hodgkin's disease. Implications for lineage determination and differential diagnosis. Proc Natl Acad Sci U S A 1986, **83**: 7942–7946.

573 Le Brun DP, Ngan BY, Weiss LM, Huie P, Warnke RA, Cleary ML. The bcl-2 oncogene in Hodgkin's disease arising in the setting of follicular non-Hodgkin's lymphoma. Blood 1994, **83**: 223–230.

574 Louie DC, Kant JA, Brooks JJ, Reed JC. Absence of t(14;18) major and minor breakpoints and of Bcl-2 protein overproduction in Reed–Sternberg cells of Hodgkin's disease. Am J Pathol 1991, **139**: 1231–1237.

575 Manzanal AI, Santón A, Acevedo A, Aguilera B, Oliva H, Bellas C. Molecular analysis of the IgH gene in 212 cases of Hodgkin's disease: correlation of IgH clonality with the histologic and the immunocytochemical features. Mod Pathol 1997, **10**: 679–685.

576 Marafioti T, Hummel M, Foss HD, Laumen H, Korbiuhn P, Anagnostopoulos I, Lammert H, Demel G, Theil J, Wirth T, Stein H. Hodgkin's and Reed–Sternberg cell represent an expansion of a single clone originating from a germinal center B-cell with functional immunoglobulin gene rearrangements but defective immnoglobulin transcription. Blood 2000, **95**: 1443–1450.

577 Muschen M, Küppers R, Spieker T, Brauninger A, Rajewsky K, Hansmann ML. Molecular single-cell analysis of Hodgkin's and Reed–Sternberg cells harbouring unmutated immunoglobulin variable region genes. Lab Invest 2001, **81**: 289–295.

578 Nakamura S, Nagahama M, Kagami Y, Yatabe Y, Takeuchi T, Kojima M, Motoori T, Suzuki R, Taji H, Ogura M, Mizoguchi Y, Okamoto M, Suzuki H, Oyama A, Seto M, Morishima Y, Koshikawa T, Takahashi T, Kurita S, Suchi T. Hodgkin's disease expressing follicular dendritic cell marker CD21 without any other B-cell marker; a clinicopathologic study of nine cases. Am J Surg Pathol 1999, **23**: 363–376.

579 Nguyen PL, Harris NL, Ritz J, Robertson MJ. Expression of CD95 antigen and bcl-2 protein in non-Hodgkin's lymphomas and Hodgkin's disease. Am J Pathol 1997, **148**: 847–853.

580 Nolte M, Werner M, Spann W, Schnabel B, von Wasielewski R, Wilkens L, Hubner K, Fischer R, Georgii A. The bcl/2/JH gene rearrangement is undetectable in Hodgkin's lymphomas. Results from the German Hodgkin trial. Virchows Arch 1995, **426**: 37–42.

581 O'Grady JT, Stewart S, Lowrey J, Howie SE, Krajewski AS. CD40 expression in Hodgkin's disease. Am J Pathol 1994, **144**: 21–26.

582 Oudejans JJ, Kummer JA, Jiwa M, Van Der Valk P, Ossenkoppele GJ, Kluin PM, Kluin-Nelemans JC, Meijer CJ. Granzyme B expression in Reed–Sternberg cells of Hodgkin's disease. Am J Pathol 1996, **148**: 233–240.

583 Peh SC, Kim LH, Poppema S. TARC, a CC chemokine, is frequently expressed in classic Hodgkin's lymphoma but not in NLP Hodgkin's lymphoma, T-cell-rich B-cell lymphoma, and most cases of anaplastic large cell lymphoma. Am J Surg Pathol 2001, **25**: 925–929.

584 Pinkus GS, Pinkus JL, Langhoff E, Matsumura F, Yamashiro S, Mosialos G, Said JW. Fascin, a sensitive new marker for Reed–Sternberg cells of Hodgkin's disease. Evidence for a dendritic or B-cell derivation? Am J Pathol 1997, **150**: 543–562.

585 Sakuma I, Yoshino T, Omonishi K, Nishiuchi R, Teramoto N, Yanai H, Kawahara K, Kubonishi I, Matsuo Y, Akagi T. CD95 ligand is expressed in Reed–Sternberg cells of Hogkin's disease. Pathol Int 1999, **49**: 103–109.

586 Sarker AB, Akagi T, Jeon HJ, Miyake K, Murakami I, Yoshino T, Takahashi K, Nose S. *Bauhinia purpurea* – a new paraffin section marker for Reed–Sternberg cells of Hodgkin's disease. A comparison with Leu-M1 (CD15), LN2 (CD74), peanut agglutinin, and Ber-H2 (CD30). Am J Pathol 1992, **141**: 19–23.

587 Schmid C, Pan L, Diss T, Isaacson PG. Expression of B-cell antigens by Hodgkin's and Reed–Sternberg cells. Am J Pathol 1991, **139**: 701–707.

588 Stetler-Stevenson M, Crush-Stanton S, Cossman J. Involvement of the bcl-2 gene in Hodgkin's disease. J Natl Cancer Inst 1990, **82**: 855–858.

589 Strum SB, Park JK, Rappaport H. Observation of cells resembling Sternberg–Reed cells in conditions other than Hodgkin's disease. Cancer 1977, **26**: 176–190.

590 Tindle BH, Parker JW, Lukes RJ. 'Reed–Sternberg cells' in infectious mononucleosis? Am J Clin Pathol 1972, **58**: 607–617.

591 Vasef MA, Alsabeh R, Medeiros LJ, Weiss LM. Immunophenotype of Reed–Sternberg and Hodgkin's cells in sequential biopsy specimens of Hogkin's disease. A paraffin-section immunohistochemical study using the heat-induced epitope retrieval method. Am J Clin Pathol 1997, **108**: 54–59.

592 Verbeke CS, Wenthe U, Grobholz R, Zentgraf H. Fas ligand expression in Hodgkin's lymphoma. Am J Surg Pathol 2001, **25**: 388–394.

593 Watanabe K, Yamashita Y, Nakayama A, Hasegawa Y, Kojima H, Nagasawa T, Mori N. Varied B-cell immunophenotypes of Hodgkin/Reed–Sternberg cells in classic Hodgkin's disease. Histopathology 2000, **36**: 353–361.

594 Weber-Matthiesen K, Deerberg-Wittram J, Rosenwald A, Poetsch M, Grote W, Schlegelberger B. Translocation t(2;5) is not a primary event in Hodgkin's disease: simultaneous immunophenotyping and interphase cytogenetics. Am J Pathol 1996, **149**: 463–468.

595 Weiss LM, Strickler JG, Hu E, Warnke RA, Sklar J. Immunoglobulin gene rearrangements in Hodgkin's disease. Hum Pathol 1986, **17**: 1009–1014.

596 Zukerberg LR, Collins AB, Ferry JA, Harris NL. Coexpression of CD15 and CD20 by Reed–Sternberg cells in Hodgkin's disease. Am J Pathol 1991, **139**: 475–483.

Microscopic types

597 Harris NL. Hodgkin's disease: classification and differential diagnosis. Mod Pathol 1999, **12**: 159–175.

598 Jackson H, Parker F. Hodgkin's disease. 1. General considerations. N Engl J Med 1944, **230**: 1–8.

599 Lukes RJ. Relationship of histologic features to clinical stages in Hodgkin's disease. Am J Roentgenol 1963, **90**: 944–955.

600 Lukes RJ, Butler JJ, Hicks EB. Natural history of Hodgkin's disease as related to its pathologic picture. Cancer 1966, **19**: 317–344.

601 Lukes RJ, Craver LF, Hall TC, Rappaport H, Ruben P. Report of Nomenclature Committee. Cancer Res 1966, **16**: 1311.

602 Mauch PM. Hodgkin's disease. Philadelphia, 1999, Williams and Wilkins.

603 Pileri SA, Ascani S, Leoncini L, Sabattini E, Zinzani PL, Piccaluga P, Pileri A Jr, Giunti M, Falii B, Bolis GB, Stein H. Hodgkin's lymphoma: the pathologist's viewpoint. J Clin Pathol 2002, **55**: 162–176.

604 Smetana HF, Cohen BM. Mortality in relation to histologic type in Hodgkin's disease. Blood 1956, **11**: 211–224.

605 Swerdlow SH, Campo E, Harris NL, Pileri SA, Stein H, Thiele J, Vardiman JW. WHO classification of tumours of haematopoietic and lymphoid tissues, ed. 4. Lyon, 2008, IARC Press.

Nodular lymphocyte predominant Hodgkin lymphoma

606 Brauninger A, Hansmann ML, Strickler JG, Dummer R, Burg G, Rajewsky K, Küppers R. Identification of common germinal-center B-cell precursors in two patients with both Hodgkin's disease and non-Hodgkin's lymphoma. New Engl J Med 1999, **340**: 1239–1247.

607 Brauninger A, Küppers R, Strickler JG, Wacker HH, Rajewsky K, Hansmann ML. Hodgkin's and Reed–Sternberg cells in lymphocyte predominant Hodgkin's disease represent clonal populations of germinal center-derived tumor B-cells. Proc Natl Acad Sci U S A 1997, **94**: 9337–9342.

608 Chittal SM, Alard C, Rossi JF, al Saati T, Le Tourneau A, Diebold J, Delsol G. Further phenotypic evidence that nodular, lymphocyte-predominant Hodgkin's disease is a large B-cell lymphoma in evolution. Am J Surg Pathol 1990, **14**: 1024–1035.

609 Cibull ML, Stein H, Gatter KC, Mason DY. The expression of the CD3 antigen in Hodgkin's disease. Histopathology 1989, **15**: 599–605.

610 Coles FB, Cartun RW, Pastuszak WT. Hodgkin's disease, lymphocyte-predominant type. Immunoreactivity with B-cell antibodies. Mod Pathol 1988, **1**: 274–278.

611 Delabie J, Greiner TC, Chan WC, Weisenberger DD. Concurrent lymphocyte predominance Hodgkin's disease and T-cell lymphoma: a report of three cases. Am J Surg Pathol 1997, **20**: 355–362.

612 Fan Z, Natkunam Y, Bair E, Tibshirani R, Warnke RA. Characterization of variant patterns of nodular lymphocyte predominant Hodgkin lymphoma with immunohistologic and clinical correlation. Am J Surg Pathol 2003, **27**: 1346–1356.

613 Ferry JA, Zukerberg LR, Harris NL. Florid progressive transformation of germinal centers. A syndrome affecting young men, without early progression to nodular lymphocyte predominance Hodgkin's disease. Am J Surg Pathol 1992, **16**: 252–258.

614 Gelb AB, Dorfman RF, Warnke RA. Coexistence of nodular lymphocyte predominance Hodgkin's disease and Hodgkin's disease of the usual type. Am J Surg Pathol 1993, **17**: 364–374.

615 Kamel OW, Gelb AB, Shibuya RB, Warnke RA. Leu 7 (CD57) reactivity distinguishes nodular lymphocyte predominance Hodgkin's disease from nodular sclerosing Hodgkin's disease, T-cell-rich B-cell lymphoma and follicular lymphoma. Am J Pathol 1993, **142**: 541–546.

616 Lukes RJ, Butler JJ, Hicks EB. Natural history of Hodgkin's disease as related to its pathologic picture. Cancer 1966, **19**: 317–344.

617 Marafioti T, Hummel M, Anagnostopoulos I, Foss HD, Falini B, Delsol G, Isaacson PG, Pileri S, Stein H. Origin of nodular lymphocyte-predominant Hodgkin's disease from a clonal expansion of highly mutated germinal-center B-cells. N Engl J Med 1997, **337**: 453–458.

618 Mason DY, Banks PM, Chan J, Cleary ML, Delsol G, de Wolf Peeters C, Falini B, Gatter K, Grogan TM, Harris NL, et al. Nodular lymphocyte predominance Hodgkin's disease. A distinct clinicopathological entity [editorial]. Am J Surg Pathol 1994, **18**: 526–530.

619 Möller P, Lennert K. On the angiostructure of lymph nodes in Hodgkin's disease. An immunohistochemical study using the lectin I of *Ulex europaeus* as endothelial marker. Virchows Arch [A] 1984, **403**: 257–270.

620 Momose H, Chen YY, Ben-Ezra J, Weiss LM. Nodular lymphocyte-predominant Hodgkin's disease. Study of immunoglobulin light chain protein and mRNA expression. Hum Pathol 1992, **23**: 1115–1119.

621 Nicholas DS, Harris S, Wright DH. Lymphocyte predominance Hodgkin's disease – an immunohistochemical study. Histopathology 1990, **16**: 157–165.

622 Ohno T, Huang JZ, Wu G, Park KH, Weisenburger DD, Chan WC. The tumor cells in nodular lymphocyte-predominant Hodgkin's disease are clonally related to the large cell lymphoma occurring in the same individual. Direct demonstration by single cell analysis. Am J Clin Pathol 2001, **116**: 506–511.

623 Poppema S. Lymphocyte-predominance Hodgkin's disease. Semin Diagn Pathol 1992, **9**: 257–264.

624 Poppema S, Kaiserling E, Lennert K. Epidemiology of nodular paragranuloma (Hodgkin's disease with lymphocytic predominance, nodular). J Cancer Res Clin Oncol 1979, **95**: 57–63.

625 Poppema S, Kaiserling E, Lennert K. Hodgkin's disease with lymphocytic pre-dominance, nodular type (nodular paragranuloma) and progressively transformed germinal centers. A cytohistological study. Histopathology 1979, **3**: 295–308.

626 Regula DP Jr, Hoppe RT, Weiss LM. Nodular and diffuse types of lymphocyte predominance Hodgkin's disease. N Engl J Med 1988, **318**: 214–219.

627 Regula DP Jr, Weiss LM, Warnke RA, Dorfman RS. Lymphocyte predominance Hodgkin's disease. A reappraisal based upon histological and immunophenotypical findings in relapsing cases. Histopathology 1987, **11**: 1107–1120.

628 Ruprai AK, Pringle JH, Angel CA, Kind CN, Lauder I. Localization of immunoglobulin light chain mRNA expression in Hodgkin's disease by in situ hybridization. J Pathol 1991, **164**: 37–40.

629 Said JW, Sassoon AF, Shintaku IP, Kurtin PJ, Pinkus GS. Absence of bcl-2 major breakpoint region and JH gene rearrangement in lymphocyte predominance Hodgkin's disease. Results of Southern blot analysis and polymerase chain reaction. Am J Pathol 1991, **138**: 261–264.

630 Schmid C, Sargent C, Isaacson PG. L and H cells of nodular lymphocyte predominant Hodgkin's disease show immunoglobulin light-chain restriction. Am J Pathol 1991, **139**: 1281–1289.

631 Söderström N, Norberg B. Observations regarding the specific postcapillary venules of lymph nodes in malignant lymphomas. Acta Pathol Microbiol Scand (A) 1974, **82**: 71–79.

632 Stoler MH, Nichols GE, Symbula M, Weiss LM. Lymphocyte predominance Hodgkin's disease. Evidence for a kappa light chain-restricted monotypic B-cell neoplasm. Am J Pathol 1995, **146**: 810–818.

633 Swerdlow SH, Campo E, Harris NL, Pileri SA, Stein H, Thiele J, Vardiman JW. WHO classification of tumours of haematopoietic and lymphoid tissues, ed. 4. Lyon, 2008, IARC Press.

634 Trudel MA, Krikorian JG, Neiman RS. Lymphocyte predominance Hodgkin's disease. A clinicopathologic reassessment. Cancer 1987, **59**: 99–106.

635 Von Wasielewski R, Werner M, Fischer R, Hansmann ML, Hubner K, Hasenclever D, Franklin J, Sextro M, Diehl V, Georgii A. Lymphocyte-predominant Hodgkin's disease. An immunohistochemical analysis of 208 reviewed Hodgkin's disease cases from the German Hodgkin's Study Group. Am J Pathol 1997, **150**: 793–803.

Classic Hodgkin lymphoma

636 Benharroch D, Levy A, Gopas J, Sacks M. Lymphocyte-depleted classic Hodgkin lymphoma – a neglected entity? Virchows Arch 2008, **453**: 611–616.

637 Colby TV, Hoppe RT, Warnke RA. Hodgkin's disease at autopsy. 1972–1977. Cancer 1981, **47**: 1852–1862.

638 Colby TV, Warnke RA. The histology of the initial relapse of Hodgkin's disease. Cancer 1980, **45**: 289–292.

639 Coleman CN, Williams CJ, Flint A, Glatstein EJ, Rosenberg SA, Kaplan HS. Hematologic neoplasia in patients treated for Hodgkin's disease. N Engl J Med 1977, **297**: 1249–1252.

640 Coppleson LW, Rappaport H, Strum SB, Rose J. Analysis of the Rye classification of Hodgkin's disease. The prognostic significance of cellular composition. J Natl Cancer Inst 1973, **51**: 379–390.

641 Huang Q, Wilczynski SP, Chang KL, Weiss LM. Composite recurrent Hodgkin lymphoma and diffuse large B-cell lymphoma: one clone, two faces. Am J Clin Pathol 2006, **126**: 222–229.

642 Krikorian JG, Burke JS, Rosenberg SA, Kaplan HS. Occurrence of non-Hodgkin's lymphoma after therapy for Hodgkin's disease. N Engl J Med 1979, **300**: 452–458.

643 MacLennan KA, Bennett MH, Tu A, Hudson BV, Easterling MJ, Hudson GV, Jelliffe AM. Relationship of histopathologic features to survival and relapse in nodular sclerosing Hodgkin's disease. A study of 1659 patients. Cancer 1989, **64**: 1686–1693.

644 Marshall AHE, Matilla A, Pollock DJ. A critique and case study of nodular sclerosing Hodgkin's disease. J Clin Pathol 1976, **29**: 923–930.

645 Nam-Cha SH, Montes-Moreno S, Salcedo MT, Sanjuan J, Garcia JF, Piris MA. Lymphocyte-rich classical Hodgkin's lymphoma: distinctive tumor and microenvironment markers. Mod Pathol 2009, **22**: 1006–1015.

646 Seemayer TA, Lagace R, Schürch W. On the pathogenesis of sclerosis and nodularity in nodular sclerosing Hodgkin's disease. Virchows Arch [A] 1980, **385**: 283–291.

647 Strickler JG, Michie SA, Warnke RA, Dorfman RF. The 'syncytial variant' of nodular sclerosing Hodgkin's disease. Am J Surg Pathol 1986, **10**: 470–477.

648 Strum SB, Rappaport H. Interrelations of the histologic types of Hodgkin's disease. Arch Pathol 1971, **91**: 127–134.

649 Traverse-Glehen A, Pittaluga S, Gaulard P, Sorbara L, Alonso MA, Raffeld M, Jaffe ES. Mediastinal gray zone lymphoma: the missing link between classic Hodgkin's lymphoma and mediastinal large B-cell lymphoma. Am J Surg Pathol 2005, **29**: 1411–1421.

Other microscopic features

650 Alavaikko MJ, Hansmann ML, Nebendahl C, Parwaresch MR, Lennert K. Follicular dendritic cells in Hodgkin's disease. Am J Clin Pathol 1991, **95**: 194–200.

651 Colby TV, Hoppe RT, Warnke RA. Hodgkin's disease. A clinicopathologic study of 659 cases. Cancer 1982, **49**: 1848–1858.

652 Crocker J, Smith PJ. A quantitative study of mast cells in Hodgkin's disease. J Clin Pathol 1984, **37**: 519–522.

653 Doggett RS, Colby TV, Dorfman RF. Interfollicular Hodgkin's disease. Am J Surg Pathol 1983, **7**: 145–149.

654 Kadin ME, Donaldson SS, Dorfman RF. Isolated granulomas in Hodgkin's disease. N Engl J Med 1970, **283**: 859–861.

655 Kansal R, Singleton TP, Ross CW, Finn WG, Padmore RF, Schnitzer B. Follicular Hodgkin's lymphoma: a histopathologic study. Am J Clin Pathol 2002, **117**: 29–35.

656 Mohrmann RL, Nathwani BN, Brynes RK, Sheibani K. Hodgkin's disease occurring in monocytoid B-cell clusters. Am J Clin Pathol 1991, **95**: 802–808.

657 Pak HY, Friedman NB. Pseudosarcoid granulomas in Hodgkin's disease. Hum Pathol 1981, **12**: 832–837.

658 Rappaport H, Strum SB, Hutchison G, Allen LW. Clinical and biological significance of vascular invasion in Hodgkin's disease. Cancer Res 1971, **31**: 1794–1798.

659 Sacks EL, Donaldson SS, Gordon J, Dorfman RF. Epithelioid granulomas associated with Hodgkin's disease. Clinical correlations in 55 previously untreated patients. Cancer 1978, **41**: 562–567.

660 Strum SB, Hutchison GB, Park JK, Rappaport H. Further observations on the biologic

significance of vascular invasion in Hodgkin's disease. Cancer 1971, **27**: 1–6.

661 Strum SB, Rappaport H. Significance of focal involvement of lymph nodes for the diagnosis and staging of Hodgkin's disease. Cancer 1970, **25**: 1314–1319.

662 Variakojis D, Strum SB, Rappaport H. The foamy macrophages in Hodgkin's disease. Arch Pathol 1971, **93**: 453–456.

Molecular genetics

NLPHL

663 Braeuninger A, Küppers R, Strickler JG, Wacker HH, Rajewsky K, Hansmann ML. Hodgkin and Reed–Sternberg cells in lymphocyte predominant Hodgkin disease represent clonal populations of germinal center-derived tumor B cells. Proc Natl Acad Sci U S A 1997, **94**: 9337–9342.

664 Brune V, Tiacci E, Pfeil I, Döring C, Eckerle S, van Noesel CJ, Klapper W, Falini B, von Heydebreck A, Metzler D, Bräuninger A, Hansmann ML, Küppers R. Origin and pathogenesis of nodular lymphocyte-predominant Hodgkin lymphoma as revealed by global gene expression analysis. J Exp Med. 2008, **205**: 2251–2268.

665 Chang KC, Khen NT, Jones D, Su IJ. Epstein–Barr virus is associated with all histological subtypes of Hodgkin lymphoma in Vietnamese children with special emphasis on the entity of lymphocyte predominance subtype. Hum Pathol 2005, **36**: 747–755.

666 Küppers R, Hansmann ML, Rajewsky K. Clonality and germinal centre B-cell derivation of Hodgkin/Reed–Sternberg cells in Hodgkin's disease. Ann Oncol 1998, **9**(Suppl 5): S17–S20.

667 Marafioti T, Hummel M, Anagnostopoulos I, Foss HD, Falini B, Delsol G, Isaacson PG, Pileri S, Stein H. Origin of nodular lymphocyte-predominant Hodgkin's disease from a clonal expansion of highly mutated germinal-center B cells. N Engl J Med 1997, **337**: 453–458.

668 Renne C, Martin-Subero JI, Hansmann ML, Siebert R. Molecular cytogenetic analyses of immunoglobulin loci in nodular lymphocyte predominant Hodgkin's lymphoma reveal a recurrent IGH-BCL6 juxtaposition. J Mol Diagn 2005, **7**: 352–356.

669 Schmid C, Sargent C, Isaacson PG. L and H cells of nodular lymphocyte predominant Hodgkin's disease show immunoglobulin light-chain restriction. Am J Pathol 1991, **139**: 1281–1289.

670 Stamatoullas A, Picquenot JM, Dumesnil C, Ruminy P, Penther D, Bertrand P, Courel MN, Maisonneuve C, François A, Gaulard P, Tilly H, Bastard C. Conventional cytogenetics of nodular lymphocyte-predominant Hodgkin's lymphoma. Leukemia 2007, **21**: 2064–2067.

671 Stein H, Diehl V, Marafioti T, Jox A, Wolf J, Hummel M. The nature of Reed–Sternberg cells, lymphocytic and histiocytic cells and their molecular biology in Hodgkin's disease. In Mauch PM, Armitage JO, Diehl V, Hoppe RT, Weiss LM (eds): Hodgkin's disease. Philadelphia, 1999, Lippincott Williams & Wilkins, pp. 121–137.

672 Wlodarska I, Nooyen P, Maes B, Martin-Subero JI, Siebert R, Pauwels P, De Wolf-Peeters C, Hagemeijer A. Frequent occurrence of BCL6 rearrangements in nodular lymphocyte predominance Hodgkin lymphoma but not in classical Hodgkin lymphoma. Blood 2003, **101**: 706–710.

Classic Hodgkin lymphoma

673 Bechtel D, Kurth J, Unkel C, Küppers R. Transformation of BCR-deficient germinal-center B cells by EBV supports a major role of the virus in the pathogenesis of Hodgkin and posttransplantation lymphomas. Blood 2005, **106**: 4345–4350.

674 Carbone A, Gloghini A, Serraino D, Spina M. HIV-associated Hodgkin lymphoma. Curr Opin HIV AIDS 2009, **4**: 3–10.

675 Chute DJ, Cousar JB, Mahadevan MS, Siegrist KA, Silverman LM, Stoler MH. Detection of immunoglobulin heavy chain gene rearrangements in classic Hodgkin lymphoma using commercially available BIOMED-2 primers. Diagn Mol Pathol 2008, **17**: 65–72.

676 Glaser SL, Lin RJ, Stewart SL, Ambinder RF, Jarrett RF, Brousset P, Pallesen G, Gulley ML, Khan G, O'Grady J, Hummel M, Preciado MV, Knecht H, Chan JK, Claviez A. Epstein–Barr virus-associated Hodgkin's disease: epidemiologic characteristics in international data. Int J Cancer 1997, **70**: 375–382.

677 Glaser SL, Clarke CA, Gulley ML, Craig FE, DiGiuseppe JA, Dorfman RF, Mann RB, Ambinder RF. Population-based patterns of human immunodeficiency virus-related Hodgkin lymphoma in the Greater San Francisco Bay Area, 1988–1998. Cancer 2003, **98**: 300–309.

678 Kanzler H, Küppers R, Hansmann ML, Rajewsky K. Hodgkin and Reed–Sternberg cells in Hodgkin's disease represent the outgrowth of a dominant tumor clone derived from (crippled) germinal center B cells. J Exp Med 1996, **184**: 1495–1505.

679 Küppers R, Rajewsky K, Zhao M, Simons G, Laumann R, Fischer R, Hansmann ML. Hodgkin disease: Hodgkin and Reed-Sternberg cells picked from histological sections show clonal immunoglobulin gene rearrangements and appear to be derived from B cells at various stages of development. Proc Natl Acad Sci U S A 1994, **91**: 10962–10966.

680 Küppers R, Hansmann ML, Rajewsky K. Clonality and germinal centre B-cell derivation of Hodgkin/Reed–Sternberg cells in Hodgkin's disease. Ann Oncol 1998, **9**(Suppl 5): S17–S20.

681 Küppers R, Hansmann ML. The Hodgkin and Reed/Sternberg cell. Int J Biochem Cell Biol 2005, **37**: 511–517.

682 Ladanyi M, Parsa NZ, Offit K, Wachtel MS, Filippa DA, Jhanwar SC. Clonal cytogenetic abnormalities in Hodgkin's disease. Genes Chromosomes Cancer 1991, **3**: 294–299.

683 Leoncini L, Spina D, Nyong'o A, Abinya O, Minacci C, Disanto A, De Luca F, De Vivo A, Sabattini E, Poggi S, Pileri S, Tosi P. Neoplastic cells of Hodgkin's disease show differences in EBV expression between Kenya and Italy. Int J Cancer 1996, **65**: 781–784.

684 Marafioti T, Hummel M, Foss HD, Laumen H, Korbjuhn P, Anagnostopoulos I, Lammert H, Demel G, Theil J, Wirth T, Stein H. Hodgkin and Reed–Sternberg cells represent an expansion of a single clone originating from a germinal center B-cell with functional immunoglobulin gene rearrangements but defective immunoglobulin transcription. Blood 2000, **95**: 1443–1450.

685 Martín-Subero JI, Klapper W, Sotnikova A, Callet-Bauchu E, Harder L, Bastard C, Schmitz R, Grohmann S, Höppner J, Riemke J, Barth TF, Berger F, Bernd HW, Claviez A, Gesk S, Frank GA, Kaplanskaya IB, Möller P, Parwaresch RM, Rüdiger T, Stein H, Küppers R, Hansmann ML, Siebert R; Deutsche Krebshilfe Network Project Molecular Mechanisms in Malignant Lymphomas. Chromosomal breakpoints affecting immunoglobulin loci are recurrent in Hodgkin and Reed–Sternberg cells of classical Hodgkin lymphoma. Cancer Res 2006, **66**: 10332–10338.

686 Schlegelberger B, Weber-Matthiesen K, Himmler A, Bartels H, Sonnen R, Kuse R, Feller AC, Grote W. Cytogenetic findings and results of combined immunophenotyping and karyotyping in Hodgkin's disease. Leukemia 1994, **8**: 72–80.

687 Seitz V, Hummel M, Marafioti T, Anagnostopoulos I, Assaf C, Stein H. Detection of clonal T-cell receptor gamma-chain gene rearrangements in Reed–Sternberg cells of classic Hodgkin disease. Blood 2000, **95**: 3020–3024.

688 Szymanowska N, Klapper W, Gesk S, Küppers R, Martin-Subero JI, Siebert R. BCL2 and BCL3 are recurrent translocation partners of the IGH locus. Cancer Genet Cytogenet 2008, **186**: 110–114.

689 Weinreb M, Day PJ, Niggli F, Powell JE, Raafat F, Hesseling PB, Schneider JW, Hartley PS, Tzortzatou-Stathopoulou F, Khalek ER, Mangoud A, El-Safy UR, Madanat F, Al Sheyyab M, Mpofu C, Revesz T, Rafii R, Tiedemann K, Waters KD, Barrantes JC, Nyongo A, Riyat MS, Mann JR. The role of Epstein–Barr virus in Hodgkin's disease from different geographical areas. Arch Dis Child 1996, **74**: 27–31.

General and clinical features

690 Akazaki K, Wakasa H. Frequency of lymphoreticular tumors and leukemias in Japan. J Natl Cancer Inst 1974, **52**: 339–343.

691 Bellas C, Santon A, Manzanal A, Campo E, Martin C, Acevedo A, Varona C, Forteza J, Morente M, Montalban C. Pathological, immunological, and molecular features of Hodgkin's disease associated with HIV infection: comparison with ordinary Hodgkin's disease. Am J Surg Pathol 1996, **20**: 1520–1524.

692 Bodis S, Kraus MD, Pinkus G, Silver B, Kadin ME, Canellos GP, Shulman LN, Tarbell NJ, Mauch PM. Clinical presentation and outcome in lymphocyte-predominant Hodgkin's disease. J Clin Oncol 1997, **15**: 3060–3066.

693 Correa P, O'Conor GT. Epidemiologic patterns of Hodgkin's disease. Int J Cancer 1971, **8**: 192–201.

694 Cross RM. A clinicopathological study of nodular sclerosing Hodgkin's disease. J Clin Pathol 1968, **21**: 303–310.

695 Greer JP, Kinney MC, Cousar JB, Flexner JM, Dupont WD, Graber SE, Greco FA, Collins RD, Stein RS. Lymphocyte-depleted Hodgkin's disease. Clinicopathologic review of 25 patients. Am J Med 1986, **81**: 208–214.

696 Grufferman S, Delzell E. Epidemiology of Hodgkin's disease. Epidemiol Rev 1984, **6**: 76–106.

697 Levy R, Kaplan HS. Impaired lymphocyte function in untreated Hodgkin's disease. N Engl J Med 1974, **290**: 181–186.

698 Neiman RS. Current problems in the histopathologic diagnosis and classification of Hodgkin's disease. Pathol Annu 1978, **13**(Pt 2): 289–328.

699 Neiman RS, Rosen PJ, Lukes RJ. Lymphocyte-depletion Hodgkin's disease. A clinicopathologic entity. N Engl J Med 1973, **288**: 751–755.

700 Poppema S, Lennert K. Hodgkin's disease in childhood. Histopathologic classification in relation to age and sex. Cancer 1980, **45**: 1443–1447.

701 Siebert JD, Stuckey JH, Kurtin PJ, Banks PM. Extranodal lymphocyte predominance Hodgkin's disease. Clinical and pathologic features. Am J Clin Pathol 1995, **103**: 485–491.

702 Thompson LD, Fisher SI, Chu WS, Nelson A, Abbondanzo SL. HIV-associated Hodgkin lymphoma: a clinicopathologic and immunophenotypic study of 45 cases. Am J Clin Pathol 2004, **121**: 727–738.

703 Trotter MC, Cloud GA, Davis M, Sanford SP, Urist MM, Soong S-J, Halpern NB, Maddox WA, Balch CM. Predicting the risk of abdominal disease in Hodgkin's lymphoma. A multifactorial analysis of staging laparotomy results in 255 patients. Ann Surg 1985, **201**: 465–469.

704 Unger PD, Strauchen JA. Hodgkin's disease in AIDS complex patients. Report of four cases and tissue immunologic marker studies. Cancer 1986, **58**: 821–825.

705 White L, McCourt BA, Isaacs H, Siegel SE, Stowe SM, Higgins GR. Patterns of Hodgkin's disease at diagnosis in young children. Am J Pediatr Hematol Oncol 1983, **5**: 251–257.

Spread

706 Aisenberg AC. Malignant lymphoma. N Engl J Med 1973, **288**: 883–890, 935–941.

707 Glatstein E, Trueblood HW, Enright LP, Rosenberg SA, Kaplan HS. Surgical staging of abdominal involvement in unselected patients with Hodgkin's disease. Radiology 1970, **97**: 425–432.

708 Kadin ME, Glatstein E, Dorfman RF. Clinicopathologic studies of 117 untreated patients subjected to laparotomy for the staging of Hodgkin's disease. Cancer 1971, **27**: 1277–1294.

709 Kaplan HS. Contiguity and progression in Hodgkin's disease. Cancer Res 1971, **31**: 1811–1813.

710 Keller AR, Kaplan HS, Lukes RJ, Rappaport H. Correlation of histopathology with other prognostic indicators in Hodgkin's disease. Cancer 1968, **22**: 487–499.

711 Leslie KO, Colby TV. Hepatic parenchymal lymphoid aggregates in Hodgkin's disease. Hum Pathol 1984, **15**: 808–809.

Staging

712 Carbone PP, Kaplan HS, Musshoff K, Smithers DW, Tubiana M. Report of the committee on Hodgkin's disease staging classification. Cancer Res 1971, **31**: 1860–1861.

713 Hays DM, Ternberg JL, Chen TT, Sullivan MP, Fuller LM, Tefft M, Kung F, Gilchrist G, Fryer C, Heller RN, Wharam M, White L, Jenkins DL, Higgins G, Gehan EA. Complications related to 234 staging laparotomies performed in the Intergroup Hodgkin's Disease in Childhood Study. Surgery 1984, **96**: 471–478.

714 Lacher MJ. Routine staging laparotomy for patients with Hodgkin's disease is no longer necessary. Cancer Invest 1983, **1**: 93–99.

715 Lister TA, Crowther D, Sutcliffe SB, Glatstein E, Canellos GP, Young RC, Rosenberg SA, Coltman CA, Tubiana M. Report of a committee convened to discuss the evaluation and staging of patients with Hodgkin's disease. Cotswolds meeting. J Clin Oncol 1989, **7**: 1630–1636.

Treatment

716 Anderson JE, Litzow MR, Appelbaum FR, Schoch G, Fisher LD, Buckner CD, Petersen FB, Crawford SW, Press OW, Sanders JE, et al. Allogeneic, syngeneic, and autologous marrow transplantation for Hodgkin's disease. The 21-year Seattle experience. J Clin Oncol 1993, **11**: 2342–2350.

717 Armitage JO. Early-stage Hodgkin's lymphoma. N Engl J Med 2010, **363**: 653–662.

718 Colby TV, Hoppe RT, Warnke RA. Hodgkin's disease at autopsy. 1972–1977. Cancer 1981, **47**: 1852–1862.

719 Jones RJ, Piantadosi S, Mann RB, Ambinder RF, Seifter EJ, Vriesendorp HM, Abeloff MD, Burns WH, May WS, Rowley SD, et al. High-dose cytotoxic therapy and bone marrow transplantation for relapsed Hodgkin's disease. J Clin Oncol 1990, **8**: 527–537.

720 Rosenberg SA, Kaplan HS. The evolution and summary results of the Stanford randomized clinical trials of the management of Hodgkin's disease. 1962–1984. Int J Radiat Oncol Biol Phys 1985, **11**: 5–22.

721 Straus DJ. Strategies in the treatment of Hodgkin's disease. Semin Oncol 1985, **13**: 26–34.

722 Strum SB, Rappaport H. The persistence of Hodgkin's disease in long-term survivors. Am J Med 1971, **51**: 222–240.

723 Urba WJ, Longo DL. Hodgkin's disease. N Engl J Med 1992, **326**: 678–687.

724 Weissman LB, Corson JM, Neugut AI, Antman KH. Malignant mesothelioma following treatment for Hodgkin's disease. J Clin Oncol 1996, **14**: 2098–2100.

725 Wolden SL, Lamborn KR, Cleary SF, Tate DJ, Donaldson SS. Second cancers following pediatric Hodgkin's disease. J Clin Oncol 1998, **16**: 535–544.

Prognosis

726 Alavaikko MJ, Blanco G, Aine R, Lehtinen T, Fellbaum C, Taskinen PJ, Sarpola A, Hansmann ML. Follicular dendritic cells have prognostic relevance in Hodgkin's disease. Am J Clin Pathol 1994, **101**: 761–767.

727 Baur AS, Meuge-Moraw C, Michel G, Delacretaz F. Prognostic value of follicular dendritic cells in nodular sclerosing Hodgkin's disease. Histopathology 1998, **32**: 512–520.

728 Bearman RM, Pangalis GA, Rappaport H. Hodgkin's disease, lymphocyte depletion type. A clinicopathologic study of 39 patients. Cancer 1978, **41**: 293–302.

729 Butler JJ. Relationship of histologic findings to survival in Hodgkin's disease. Gann Monogr Cancer Res 1973, **15**: 275–286.

730 Colby TV, Hoppe RT, Warnke RA. Hodgkin's disease. A clinicopathologic study of 659 cases. Cancer 1981, **49**: 1848–1858.

731 Diehl V, Sextro M, Franklin J, Hansmann ML, Harris N, Jaffe E, Poppema S, Harris M, Franssila K, van Krieken J, Marafioti T, Anagnostopoulos I, Stein H. Clinical presentation, course, and prognostic factors in lymphocyte-predominant Hodgkin's disease and lymphocyte-rich classical Hodgkin's disease: report from the European Task Force on Lymphoma Project on Lymphocyte-Predominant Hodgkin's Disease. J Clin Oncol 1999, **17**: 776–783.

732 Dimopoulos MA, Cabanillas F, Lee JJ, Swan F, Fuller L, Allen PK, Hagemeister FB. Prognostic role of serum β2-microglobulin in Hodgkin's disease. J Clin Oncol 1993, **11**: 1108–1111.

733 Eghbali H, Hoerni-Simon G, de Mascarel I, Durand M, Chauvergne J, Hoerni B. Hodgkin's disease in the elderly. A series of 30 patients aged older than 70 years. Cancer 1984, **53**: 2191–2193.

734 Ferry JA, Linggood RM, Convery KM, Efird JT, Eliseo R, Harris NL. Hodgkin disease, nodular sclerosis type. Implications of histologic subclassification. Cancer 1993, **71**: 457–463.

735 Gause A, Roschansky V, Tschiersch A, Smith K, Hasenclever D, Schmits R, Diehl V, Pfreundschuh M. Low serum interleukin-2 receptor levels correlate with a good prognosis in patients with Hodgkin's lymphoma. Ann Oncol 1991, **2**(Suppl): 43–47.

736 Kaplan HS. Hodgkin's disease, ed. 2. Cambridge, MA, 1980, Harvard University Press.

737 Keller AR, Kaplan HS, Lukes RJ, Rappaport H. Correlation of histopathology with other prognostic indicators in Hodgkin's disease. Cancer 1968, **22**: 487–499.

738 Pizzolo G, Vinante F, Chilosi M, Dallenbach F, Josimovic-Alasevic O, Diamantstein T, Stein H. Serum levels of soluble CD30 molecule (Ki-1 antigen) in Hodgkin's disease. Relationship with disease activity and clinical stage. Br J Haematol 1990, **75**: 282–284.

739 Sacks EL, Donaldson SS, Gordon J, Dorfman RF. Epithelioid granulomas associated with Hodgkin's disease. Clinical correlations in 55 previously untreated patients. Cancer 1978, **41**: 562–567.

740 Shankar AG, Ashley S, Radford M, Barrett A, Wright D, Pinkerton CR. Does histology influence outcome in childhood Hodgkin's disease? Results from the United Kingdom Children's Cancer Study Group. J Clin Oncol 1997, **15**: 2622–2630.

741 Straus DJ, Gaynor JJ, Myers J, Merke DP, Caravelli J, Chapman D, Yahalom J, Clarkson BD. Prognostic factors among 185 adults with newly diagnosed advanced Hodgkin's disease treated with alternating potentially noncross-resistant chemotherapy and intermediate-dose radiation therapy. J Clin Oncol 1990, **8**: 1173–1186.

742 Torti FM, Portlock CS, Rosenberg SA, Kaplan HS. Extralymphatic Hodgkin's disease. Prognosis and response to therapy. Am J Med 1981, **70**: 487–492.

743 Trudel MA, Krikorian JG, Neiman RS. Lymphocyte predominance Hodgkin's disease. A clinicopathologic reassessment. Cancer 1987, **59**: 99–106.

744 Von Wasielewski R, Mengel M, Fischer R, Hansmann ML, Hübner K, Franklin J, Tesch H, Paulus U, Werner M, Diehl V, Georgii A. Classical Hodgkin's disease. Clinical impact of the immunophenotype. Am J Pathol 1997, **151**: 1123–1130.

745 Wright CJE. Prospects of cure in lymphocyte-predominant Hodgkin's disease. Am J Clin Pathol 1977, **67**: 507–511.

NON-HODGKIN LYMPHOMA

746 Alavaikko M, Aine R. The Lukes and Collins classification on non-Hodgkin's lymphomas. 1. A histological reappraisal of 301 cases. Acta Pathol Microbiol Immunol Scand (A) 1982, **90**: 241–249.

747 Byrne GE Jr. Rappaport classification of non-Hodgkin's lymphoma. Histologic features and clinical significance. Cancer Treat Rep 1977, **61**: 935–944.

748 Chan JK. The new World Health Organization classification of lymphomas: the past, the present and the future. Hematol Oncol 2001, **19**: 129–150.

749 Chan JKC, Banks PM, Cleary ML, Delsol G, De Wolf-Peeters C, Falini B, Gatter KC, Grogan TM, Harris NL, Isaacson PG, Jaffe ES, Knowles DM, Mason DY, Müller-Hermelink HK, Pileri SA, Piris MA, Ralfkiaer E, Stein H, Warnke RA. A revised European–American classification of lymphoid neoplasms proposed by the International Lymphoma Study Group. A summary version. Am J Clin Pathol 1995, **103**: 543–560.

750 Dorfman RF. Classification of the malignant lymphomas. Am J Surg Pathol 1977, **1**: 167–170.

751 Dorfman RF, Kim H. Relationship of histology to site in the non-Hodgkin's lymphomata. A study based on surgical staging procedures. Br J Cancer 1975, **31**: 217–220.

752 Ersboll J, Schultz HB, Hougaard P, Nissen NI, Hou-Jensen K. Comparison of the working formulation of non-Hodgkin's lymphoma with the Rappaport, Kiel, and Lukes and Collins classifications. Translational value and prognostic significance based on review of 658 patients treated at a single institution. Cancer 1985, **55**: 2442–2458.

753 Gall EA, Mallory TB. Malignant lymphoma. A clinicopathologic survey of 618 cases. Am J Pathol 1942, **18**: 381–429.

754 Goffinet DR, Warnke R, Dunnick NR, Castellino R, Glatstein E, Nelsen TS, Dorfman RF, Rosenberg SA, Kaplan AS. Clinical and surgical (laparotomy) evaluation of patients with non-Hodgkin's lymphomas. Cancer Treat Rep 1977, **61**: 981–992.

755 Harris NL, Jaffe ES, Stein H, Banks PM, Chan JK, Cleary ML, Delsol G, De Wolf-Peeters C, Falini B, Gatter KC, et al. A revised European–American classification of lymphoid neoplasms. A proposal from the International Lymphoma Study Group. Blood 1994, **84**: 1361–1392.

756 Jaffe ES, Harris NL, Stein H, Vardiman JW (eds): World Health Organization classification of tumours. Pathology and genetics of tumours of haematopoietic and lymphoid tissues. Lyon, 2001, IARC Press.

757 Jaffe ES. The 2008 WHO classification of lymphomas: implications for clinical practice and translational research. Hematology Am Soc Hematol Educ Program 2009: 523–531.

758 Lennert K. Classification of non-Hodgkin's lymphomas. In Lennert K, Mohri N, Stein H, Kaiserling E, Müller-Hermelink HK (eds): Malignant lymphomas other than Hodgkin's disease. Histology, cytology, ultrastructure, immunology. Berlin, 1978, Springer-Verlag, pt 3, pp. 83–110.

759 Lennert K, Collins RD, Lukes RJ. Concordance of the Kiel and Lukes–Collins classifications of non-Hodgkin's lymphomas. Histopathology 1983, **7**: 549–559.

760 Lukes RJ, Collins RD. Immunologic characterization of human malignant lymphomas. Cancer 1974, **34**: 1488–1503.

761 Lukes RJ, Parker JW, Taylor CR, Tindle BH, Cramer AD, Lincoln TL. Immunologic approach to non-Hodgkin lymphomas and related leukemias. Analysis of the results of multiparameter studies of 425 cases. Semin Hematol 1978, **15**: 322–351.

762 Nathwani BN. A critical analysis of the classifications of non-Hodgkin's lymphomas. Cancer 1979, **44**: 347–384.

763 Nathwani BN, Kim H, Rappaport H, Solomon J, Fox M. Non-Hodgkin's lymphomas. A clinicopathologic study comparing two classifications. Cancer 1978, **41**: 303–325.

764 NCI Non-Hodgkin's Classification Project Writing Committee. Classification of non-Hodgkin's lymphomas. Reproducibility of major classification systems. Cancer 1985, **55**: 91–95.

765 Non-Hodgkin's Lymphoma Pathologic Classification Project. National Cancer Institute sponsored study of classifications of non-Hodgkin's lymphoma. Summary and description of a working formulation for clinical usage. Cancer 1982, **49**: 2112–2135.

766 Rappaport H. Tumors of the hematopoietic system. In Atlas of tumor pathology, series 3, fascicle 8. Washington, DC, 1966, Armed Forces Institute of Pathology.

767 Rosenberg SA, Dorfman RF, Kaplan HS. A summary of the results of a review of 405 patients with non-Hodgkin's lymphoma at Stanford University. Br J Cancer 1975, **31**: 168–173.

768 Sabattini E, Bacci F, Sagramoso C, Pileri SA. WHO classification of tumours of haematopoietic and lymphoid tissues in 2008: an overview. Pathologica 2010, **102**: 83–87.

769 Swerdlow SH, Campo E, Harris NL, Jaffe ES, Pileri SA, Stein H, Thiele J, Vardiman JW (eds): WHO classification of tumours of haematopoietic and lymphoid tissues, ed. 4. Lyon, 2008, IARC Press.

770 Willis RA. The tumours of lymphoid tissue. In Willis RA: Pathology of tumours. St Louis, 1948, CV Mosby, pp. 760–761.

Small lymphocytic lymphoma

771 Addis BJ, Isaacson P, Billings JA. Plasmacytoma of lymph nodes. Cancer 1980, **46**: 340–346.

772 Alexanian R. Monoclonal gammopathy in lymphoma. Arch Intern Med 1975, **135**: 62–66.

773 Andriko JW, Swerdlow SH, Aguilera NI, Abbondanzo SL. Is lymphoplasmacytic lymphoma/immunocytoma a distinct entity? A clinicopathologic study of 20 cases. Am J Surg Pathol 2001, **25**: 742–751.

774 Armitage JO, Dick FR, Corder MP. Diffuse histocytic lymphoma complicating chronic lymphocytic leukemia. Cancer 1978, **41**: 422–427.

775 Asplund SL, McKenna RW, Howard MS, Kroft SH. Immunophenotype does not correlate with lymph node histology in chronic lymphocytic leukemia/small lymphocytic lymphoma. Am J Surg Pathol 2002, **26**: 624–629.

776 Banerjee SS, Verma S, Shanks JH. Morphological variants of plasma cell tumours. Histopathology 2004, **44**: 2–8.

777 Batata A, Shen B. Relationship between chronic lymphocytic leukemia and small lymphocytic lymphoma. A comparative study of membrane phenotypes in 270 cases. Cancer 1992, **70**: 625–632.

778 Ben-Ezra J, Burke JS, Swartz WG, Brownell MD, Brynes RK, Hill LR, Nathwani BN, Oken MM, Wolf BC, Woodruff R, et al. Small lymphocytic lymphoma. A clinicopathologic analysis of 268 cases. Blood 1989, **73**: 579–587.

779 Berger F, Felman P, Sonet A, Salles G, Bastion Y, Bryon PA, Coiffier B. Non-follicular small B-cell lymphomas. A heterogeneous group of patients with distinct clinical features and outcome. Blood 1994, **83**: 2829–2835.

780 Bonato M, Pittaluga S, Tierens A, Criel A, Verhoef G, Wlodarska I, Vantysel L, Michaux L, Vandekerckhove P, Van Den Berghe H, De Wolf-Peeters C. Lymph node histology in typical and atypical chronic lymphocytic leukemia. Am J Surg Pathol 1998, **22**: 49–56.

781 Brecher M, Banks PM. Hodgkin's disease variant of Richter's syndrome. Report of eight cases. Am J Clin Pathol 1990, **93**: 333–339.

782 Brouet J-C, Clauvel J-P, Danon F, Klein M, Seligmann M. Biologic and clinical significance of cryoglobulins. A report of 86 cases. Am J Med 1974, **57**: 775–788.

783 Brouet J-C, Sasportes M, Flandrin G, Preud'Homme J-L, Seligmann M. Chronic lymphocytic leukaemia of T-cell origin. Immunological and clinical evaluation in eleven patients. Lancet 1975, **2**: 890–893.

784 Brunning RD, Parkin J. Intranuclear inclusions in plasma cells and lymphocytes from patients with monoclonal gammopathies. Am J Clin Pathol 1976, **66**: 10–21.

785 Carbone A, Pinto A, Gloghini A, Volpe R, Zagonel V. B-zone small lymphocytic lymphoma. A morphologic, immunophenotypic, and clinical study with comparison to 'well-differentiated' lymphocytic disorders. Hum Pathol 1992, **23**: 438–448.

786 Cohen RJ, Bohannon RA, Wallterstein RO. Waldenstrom's macroglobulinemia. A study of ten cases. Am J Med 1966, **41**: 274–284.

787 Dick FR, Maca RD. The lymph node in chronic lymphocytic leukemia. Cancer 1978, **41**: 283–292.

788 Dong HY, Scadden DT, de Leval L, Tang Z, Isaacson PG, Harris NL. Plasmablastic lymphoma in HIV-positive patients: an aggressive Epstein–Barr virus-associated extramedullary plasmacytic neoplasm. Am J Surg Pathol 2005, **29**: 1633–1641.

789 Dorfman DM, Pinkus GS. Distinction between small lymphocytic and mantle cell lymphoma by immunoreactivity for CD23. Mod Pathol 1994, **7**: 326–331.

790 Dutcher TF, Fahey JL. The histopathology of the macroglobulinemia of Waldenstrom. J Natl Cancer Inst 1959, **22**: 887–917.

791 Ellison DJ, Nathwani BN, Cho SY, Martin SE. Interfollicular small lymphocytic lymphoma. The diagnostic significance of pseudofollicles. Hum Pathol 1989, **20**: 1108–1118.

792 Fishkin BG, Spiegelberg HL. Cervical lymph node metastasis as the first manifestation of localized extramedullary plasmacytoma. Cancer 1976, **38**: 1641–1644.

793 Foucar C, Rydell RE. Richter's syndrome in chronic lymphocytic leukemia. Cancer 1980, **46**: 118–134.

794 Franklin EC, Lowenstein J, Bigelow B, Meltzer M. Heavy chain disease. A new disorder of serum gamma-globulins. Report of the first case. Am J Med 1964, **37**: 332–350.

795 Gupta D, Lim MS, Medeiros LJ, Elenitoba-Johnson KS. Small lymphocytic lymphoma with perifollicular, marginal zone, or interfollicular distribution. Mod Pathol 2001, **13**: 1161–1166.

796 Harada M, Shimada M, Fukayama M, Kaneko T, Kitazume K, Weiss SW. Crystal-storing histiocytosis associated with lymphoplasmacytic lymphoma mimicking Weber–Christian disease: immunohistochemical, ultrastructural, and gene-rearrangement studies. Hum Pathol 1996, **27**: 84–87.

797 Harris NL, Bhan AK. B-cell neoplasms of the lymphocytic, lymphoplasmacytoid, and plasma cell types. Immunohistologic analysis and clinical correlation. Hum Pathol 1985, **16**: 829–837.

798 Harrison CV. The morphology of the lymph node in the macroglobulinaemia of Waldenstrom. J Clin Pathol 1972, **25**: 12–16.

799 Hsi ED. The leukemias of mature lymphocytes. Hematol Oncol Clin North Am 2009, **23**: 843–871.

800 Inamdar KV, Bueso-Ramos CE. Pathology of chronic lymphocytic leukemia: an update. Ann Diagn Pathol 2007, **11**: 363–389.

801 Jones D, Bhatia VK, Krausz T, Pinkus GS. Crystal-storing histiocytosis: a disorder occurring in plasmacytic tumors expressing immunoglobulin kappa light chain. Hum Pathol 2000, **30**: 1441–1448.

802 Kapadia SB, Enzinger FM, Heffner DK, Hyams VJ, Frizzera G. Crystal-storing histiocytosis associated with lymphoplasmacytic neoplasms: report of three cases mimicking adult rhabdomyoma. Am J Surg Pathol 1993, **17**: 461–467.

803 Kim H, Dorfman RF, Rappaport H. Signet ring cell lymphoma. A rare morphologic and functional expression of nodular (follicular) lymphoma. Am J Surg Pathol 1978, **2**: 119–132.

804 Kim H, Heller P, Rappaport H. Monoclonal gammopathies associated with lymphoproliferative disorders. A morphologic study. Am J Clin Pathol 1973, **59**: 282–294.

805 Knuutila S, Elonen E, Teerenhovi L, Rossi L, Leskinen R, Bloomfield CD, de la Chapelle A. Trisomy 12 in B-cells of patients with B-cell chronic lymphocytic leukemia. N Engl J Med 1986, **314**: 865–869.

806 Kraus MD. Lymphoplasmacytic lymphoma/ Waldenström macroglobulinemia. One disease or three? Am J Clin Pathol 2001, **116**: 799–801.

807 Krauss S, Sokal JE. Paraproteinemia in the lymphomas. Am J Med 1966, **40**: 400–413.

808 Kumar S, Green GA, Teruya-Feldstein J, Raffeld M, Jaffe ES. Use of CD23 (BU38) on paraffin sections in the diagnosis of small lymphocytic lymphoma and mantle cell lymphoma. Mod Pathol 1996, **9**: 925–929.

809 Lee SL, Rosner F, Ruberman W, Glasberg S. µ-Chain disease. Ann Intern Med 1971, **75**: 407–414.

810 Lennert K. Malignant lymphomas other than Hodgkin's disease. Histology. Cytology. Ultrastructure. Immunology. Berlin, 1978, Springer-Verlag.

811 Lin BT, Weiss LM. Primary plasmacytoma of lymph nodes. Hum Pathol 1997, **28**: 1083–1090.

812 Lin P, Bueso-Ramos C, Wilson CS, Mansoor A, Medeiros LJ. Waldenstrom macroglobulinemia involving extramedullary sites. Am J Surg Pathol 2003, **27**: 1104–1113.

813 Lin P, Hao S, Handy BC, Bueso-Ramos CE, Medeiros LJ. Lymphoid neoplasms associated with IgM paraprotein: a study of 382 patients. Am J Clin Pathol 2005, **123**: 200–205.

814 Long JC, Aisenberg AC. Richter's syndrome. A terminal complication of chronic lymphocytic leukemia with distinct clinicopathologic features. Am J Clin Pathol 1975, **63**: 786–795.

815 McKenna RW, Parkin J, Kersey JH, Gajl-Peczalska KJ, Peterson L, Brunning RD. Chronic lymphoproliferative disorder with unusual clinical, morphologic, ultrastructural and membrane surface marker characteristics. Am J Med 1977, **62**: 588–596.

816 Medeiros LJ, Strickler JG, Picker LJ, Gelb AB, Weiss LM, Warnke RA. 'Well-differentiated' lymphocytic neoplasms. Immunologic findings correlated with clinical presentation and morphologic features. Am J Pathol 1987, **129**: 523–535.

817 Menke DM, Horny HP, Griesser H, Tiemann M, Katzmann JA, Kaiserling E, Parwaresch R, Kyle RA. Primary lymph node plasmacytomas (plasmacytic lymphomas). Am J Clin Pathol 2001, **115**: 119–126.

818 Mennemeyer R, Hammar SP, Cathey WJ. Malignant lymphoma with intracytoplasmic IgM crystalline inclusions. N Engl J Med 1974, **291**: 960–963.

819 Momose H, Jaffe ES, Shin SS, Chen YY, Weiss LM. Chronic lymphocytic leukemia/small lymphocytic lymphoma with Reed–Sternberg-like cells and possible transformation to Hodgkin's disease. Mediation by Epstein–Barr virus. Am J Surg Pathol 1992, **16**: 859–867.

820 Morrison WH, Hoppe RT, Weiss LM, Picozzi VJ Jr, Horning SJ. Small lymphocytic lymphoma. J Clin Oncol 1989, **7**: 598–606.

821 Nakamura N, Abe M. Richter syndrome in B-cell chronic lymphocytic leukaemia. Pathol Int 2003, **53**: 195–203.

822 Pangalis GA, Nathwani BN, Rappaport H. Malignant lymphoma, well differentiated lymphocytic. Its relationship with chronic lymphocytic leukemia and macroglobulinemia of Waldenström. Cancer 1977, **39**: 999–1010.

823 Pangalis GA, Nathwani BN, Rappaport H. Detection of cytoplasmic immunoglobulin in well-differentiated lymphoproliferative diseases by the immunoperoxidase method. Cancer 1980, **45**: 1334–1339.

824 Papadimitriou CS, Müller-Hermelink U, Lennert K. Histologic and immunohistochemical findings in the differential diagnosis of chronic lymphocytic leukemia of B-cell type and lymphoplasmacytic/lymphoplasmacytoid lymphoma. Virchows Arch [A] 1979, **384**: 149–158.

825 Peters O, Thielemans C, Steenssens L, De Waele M, Hijmans W, Van Camp B. Intracellular inclusion bodies in 14 patients with B-cell lymphoproliferative disorders. J Clin Pathol 1984, **37**: 45–50.

826 Schmid C, Isaacson PG. Proliferation centres in B-cell malignant lymphoma, lymphocytic (BCLL). An immunophenotypic study. Histopathology 1994, **24**: 445–451.

827 Seligmann M. Immunochemical, clinical, and pathological features of alpha-chain disease. Arch Intern Med 1975, **135**: 78–82.

828 Seligmann M, Danon F, Hurez D, Mihaesco E, Preud'homme J-L. Alpha-chain disease. A new immunoglobulin abnormality. Science 1968, **162**: 1396–1397.

829 Shao H, Xi L, Raffeld M, Pittaluga S, Dunleavy K, Wilson WH, Spector N, Milito C, Morais JC, Jaffe ES. Nodal and extranodal plasmacytomas expressing immunoglobulin A: an indolent lymphoproliferative disorder with a low risk of clinical progression. Am J Surg Pathol 2010, **34**: 1425–1435.

830 Sheibani K, Nathwani BN, Winberg CD, Scott EP, Teplitz RR, Rappaport H. Small lymphocytic lymphoma. Morphologic and immunologic progression. Am J Clin Pathol 1985, **84**: 237–243.

831 Spier CM, Grogan TM, Fielder K, Richter L, Rangel C. Immunophenotypes in 'well-differentiated' lymphoproliferative disorders, with emphasis on small lymphocytic lymphoma. Hum Pathol 1986, **17**: 1126–1136.

832 Sundeen JT, Longo DL, Jaffe ES. CD5 expression in B-cell small lymphocytic malignancies. Correlations with clinical presentation and sites of disease. Am J Surg Pathol 1992, **16**: 130–137.

833 Swerdlow SH. Small B-cell lymphomas of the lymph nodes and spleen: practical insights to diagnosis and pathogenesis. Mod Pathol 1999, **12**: 125–140.

834 Trump DL, Mann RB, Phelps R, Roberts H, Conley CL. Richter's syndrome. Diffuse histiocytic lymphoma in patients with chronic lymphocytic leukemia. A report of five cases and review of the literature. Am J Med 1980, **68**: 539–548.

835 Weir EG, Epstein JI. Incidental small lymphocytic lymphoma/chronic lymphocytic leukemia in pelvic lymph nodes excised at radical prostatectomy. Arch Pathol Lab Med 2003, **127**: 567–570.

836 Williams J, Schned A, Cotelingam JD, Jaffe ES. Chronic lymphocytic leukemia with coexistent Hodgkin's disease. Implications for the origin of the Reed–Sternberg cell. Am J Surg Pathol 1991, **15**: 33–42.

837 Zukerberg LR, Medeiros LJ, Ferry JA, Harris NL. Diffuse low-grade B-cell lymphomas. Four clinically distinct subtypes defined by a combination of morphologic and immunophenotypic features. Am J Clin Pathol 1993, **100**: 373–385.

Follicular lymphoma

838 Abou-Elella A, Shafer MT, Wan XY, Velanker M, Weisenburger DD, Nathwani BN, Gascoyne RD, Greiner TC, Chan WC. Lymphomas with follicular and monocytoid B-cell components: evidence for a common clonal origin from follicle centre cells. Am J Clin Pathol 2000, **114**: 516–522.

839 Adam P, Katzenberger T, Eifert M, Ott MM, Rosenwald A, Müller-Hermelink HK, Ott G. Presence of preserved reactive germinal centers in follicular lymphoma is a strong histopathologic indicator of limited disease stage. Am J Surg Pathol 2005, **29**: 1661–1664.

840 Alizadeh AA, Eisen MB, Davis RE, Ma C, Lossos IS, Rosenwald A, Boldrick JC, Sabet H, Tran T, Yu X, Powell JI, Yang L, Marti GE, Moore T, Hudson J Jr, Lu L, Lewis DB, Tibshirani R, Sherlock G, Chan WC, Greiner TC, Weisenburger DD, Armitage JO, Warnke R, Levy R, Wilson W, Grever MR, Byrd JC, Botstein D, Brown PO, Staudt LM. Distinct types of diffuse large B-cell lymphoma identified by gene expression profiling. Nature 2000, **403**: 503–511.

841 Almasri NM, Iturraspe JA, Braylan RC. CD10 expression in follicular lymphoma and large cell lymphoma is different from that of reactive lymph node follicles. Arch Pathol Lab Med 1998, **122**: 539–544.

842 Alsabeh R, Medeiros LJ, Glackin C, Weiss LM. Transformation of follicular lymphoma into CD30-large cell lymphoma with anaplastic cytologic features. Am J Surg Pathol 1997, **21**: 528–536.

843 Anderson T, Bender RA, Fisher RI, DeVita VT, Chabner BA, Berard CW, Norton L, Young RC. Combination chemotherapy in non-Hodgkin's lymphoma. Results of long-term followup. Cancer Treat Rep 1977, **61**: 1057–1066.

844 Aster JC, Longtine JA. Detection of BCL2 rearrangements in follicular lymphoma. Am J Pathol 2002, **160**: 759–763.

845 Aster JC, Kobayashi Y, Shiota M, Mori S, Sklar J. Detection of the t(14;18) at similar frequencies in hyperplastic lymphoid tissues from American and Japanese patients. Am J Pathol 1992, **141**: 291–299.

846 Barcus ME, Karageorge LS, Veloso YL, Kornstrin MJ. CD10 expression in follicular lymphoma versus reactive follicular hyperplasia: evaluation in paraffin-embedded tissue. Appl Immunohistochem Mol Morphol 2000, **8**: 253–266.

847 Bastion Y, Berger F, Bryon PA, Felman P, Ffrench M, Coiffier B. Follicular lymphomas. Assessment of prognostic factors in 127

patients followed for 10 years. Ann Oncol 1991, **2**: 123–129.

848 Bennett MH. Sclerosis in non-Hodgkin's lymphomata. Br J Cancer 1975, **31**: 44–52.

849 Bentz M, Werner CA, Döhner H, Joos S, Barth TF, Siebert R, Schröder M, Stilgenbauer S, Fischer K, Möller P, Lichter P. High incidence of chromosomal imbalances and gene amplifications in the classical follicular variant of follicle center lymphoma. Blood 1996, **88**: 1437–1444.

850 Bosga-Bouwer AG, van den Berg A, Haralambieva E, de Jong D, Boonstra R, Kluin P, van den Berg E, Poppema S. Molecular, cytogenetic, and immunophenotypic characterization of follicular lymphoma grade 3B; a separate entity or part of the spectrum of diffuse large B-cell lymphoma or follicular lymphoma? Hum Pathol 2006, **37**: 528–533.

851 Cerroni L, Volkenandt M, Rieger E, Soyer HP, Kerl H. bcl-2 protein expression and correlation with the interchromosomal 14;18 translocation in cutaneous lymphomas and pseudolymphomas. J Invest Dermatol 1994, **102**: 231–235.

852 Chan JK, Ng CS, Hui PK. An unusual morphological variant of follicular lymphoma. Report of two cases. Histopathology 1988, **12**: 649–658.

853 Chan JK, Ng CS, Tung S. Multilobated B-cell lymphoma, a variant of centroblastic lymphoma. Report of four cases. Histopathology 1986, **10**: 601–612.

854 Chittal SM, Caverivière P, Voigt J-J, Dumont J, Benévent B, Fauré P, Bordessoule GD, Delsol G. Follicular lymphoma with abundant PAS-positive extracellular material. Immunohistochemical and ultrastructural observations. Am J Surg Pathol 1987, **11**: 618–624.

855 Coiffier B, Bastion Y, Berger F, Felman P, Bryon PA. Prognostic factors in follicular lymphomas. Semin Oncol 1993, **20**: 89–95.

856 Come SE, Jaffe ES, Anderson JC, Mann RB, Johnson BL, DeVita VT, Young RC. Non-Hodgkin's lymphomas in leukemic phase. Clinicopathologic correlations. Am J Med 1980, **69**: 667–674.

857 Dave SS, Wright G, Tan B, Rosenwald A, Gascoyne RD, Chan WC, Fisher RI, Braziel RM, Rimsza LM, Grogan TM, Miller TP, LeBlanc M, Greiner TC, Weisenburger DD, Lynch JC, Vose J, Armitage JO, Smeland EB, Kvaloy S, Holte H, Delabie J, Connors JM, Lansdorp PM, Ouyang Q, Lister TA, Davies AJ, Norton AJ, Muller-Hermelink HK, Ott G, Campo E, Montserrat E, Wilson WH, Jaffe ES, Simon R, Yang L, Powell J, Zhao H, Goldschmidt N, Chiorazzi M, Staudt LM. Prediction of survival in follicular lymphoma based on molecular features of tumor-infiltrating immune cells. N Engl J Med 2004, **351**: 2159–2169.

858 Frizzera G, Anaya JS, Banks PM. Neoplastic plasma cells in follicular lymphomas. Clinical and pathologic findings in six cases. Virchows Arch [A] 1986, **409**: 149–162.

859 Frizzera G, Gajl-Peczalska K, Sibley RK, Rosai J, Cherwitz D, Hurd DD. Rosette formation in malignant lymphoma. Am J Pathol 1985, **119**: 351–356.

860 Garvin AJ, Simon RM, Osborne CK, Merrill J, Young RC, Berard CW. An autopsy study of histologic progression in non-Hodgkin's lymphomas. 192 cases from the National Cancer Institute. Cancer 1983, **52**: 393–398.

861 Gaulard P, d'Agay MF, Peuchmaur M, Brousse N, Gisselbrecht C, Solal-Celigny P, Diebold J, Mason DY. Expression of the bcl-2 gene product in follicular lymphoma. Am J Pathol 1992, **140**: 1089–1095.

862 Goates JJ, Kamel OW, Le Brun DP, Benharroch D, Dorfman RF. Floral variant of follicular lymphoma. Immunological and molecular studies support a neoplastic process. Am J Surg Pathol 1994, **18**: 37–47.

863 Goodlad JR, Batstone PJ, Hamilton DA, Kernohan NM, Levison DA, White JM. BCL2 gene abnormalities define distinct clinical subsets of follicular lymphoma. Histopathology 2006, **49**: 229–241.

864 Goodlad JR, MacPherson S, Jackson R, Batstone P, White J; Scotland and Newcastle Lymphoma Group. Extranodal follicular lymphoma: a clinicopathological and genetic analysis of 15 cases arising at non-cutaneous extranodal sites. Histopathology 2004, **44**: 268–276.

865 Gu K, Chan WC, Hawley RC. Practical detection of t(14;18)(IgH/BCL2) in follicular lymphoma. Arch Pathol Lab Med 2008, **132**: 1355–1361.

866 Gu K, Fu K, Jain S, Liu Z, Iqbal J, Li M, Sanger WG, Weisenburger DD, Greiner TC, Aoun P, Dave BJ, Chan WC. t(14;18)-negative follicular lymphomas are associated with a high frequency of BCL6 rearrangement at the alternative breakpoint region. Mod Pathol 2009, **22**: 1251–1257.

867 Hirt C, Dolken G, Janz S, Rabkin CS. Distribution of t(14;18)-positive, putative lymphoma precursor cells among B-cell subsets in healthy individuals. Br J Haematol 2007, **138**: 349–353.

868 Horning SJ, Weiss LM, Nevitt JB, Warnke RA. Clinical and pathologic features of follicular large cell (nodular histiocytic) lymphoma. Cancer 1987, **59**: 1470–1474.

869 Horsman DE, Gascoyne RD, Coupland RW, Coldman AJ, Adomat SA. Comparison of cytogenetic analysis, southern analysis, and polymerase chain reaction for the detection of t(14;18) in follicular lymphoma. Am J Clin Pathol 1995, **103**: 472–478.

870 Horsman DE, Connors JM, Pantzar T, Gascoyne RD. Analysis of secondary chromosomal alterations in 165 cases of follicular lymphoma with t(14;18). Genes Chromosomes Cancer 2001, **30**: 375–382.

871 Horsman DE, Okamoto I, Ludkovski O, Le N, Harder L, Gesk S, Siebert R, Chhanabhai M, Sehn L, Connors JM, Gascoyne RD. Follicular lymphoma lacking the t(14;18)(q32;q21): identification of two disease subtypes. Br J Haematol 2003, **120**: 424–433.

872 Isaacson PG. Malignant lymphomas with a follicular growth patterns. Histopathology 1996, **28**: 487–495.

873 Jones SE, Fuks Z, Bull M, Kadin ME, Dorfman RF, Kaplan HS, Rosenberg SA, Kim H. Non-Hodgkin's lymphomas. IV. Clinicopathologic correlation in 405 cases. Cancer 1973, **31**: 806–823.

874 Keith TA, Cousar JB, Glick AD, Vogler LB, Collins RD. Plasmacytic differentiation in follicular center cell (FCC) lymphomas. Am J Clin Pathol 1985, **84**: 283–290.

875 Kim H, Dorfman RF. Morphological studies of 84 untreated patients subjected to laparotomy for the staging of non-Hodgkin's lymphomas. Cancer 1974, **33**: 657–674.

876 Kim H, Dorfman RF, Rappaport H. Signet ring cell lymphoma. A rare morphologic and functional expression of nodular (follicular) lymphoma. Am J Surg Pathol 1978, **2**: 119–132.

877 Kojima M, Nakamura S, Ichimura K, Suzuki R, Kagami Y, Kondo E, Motoori T, Hosomura Y, Oyama T, Itoh H, Ban S, Yoshida K, Ohno Y, Shimizu K, Masawa N, Sugihara S. Centroblastic and centroblastic/centrocytic lymphoma associated with a prominent epithelioid granulomatous response: a clinicopathologic study of 50 cases. Mod Pathol 2002, **15**: 750–758.

878 Leich E, Salaverria I, Bea S, Zettl A, Wright G, Moreno V, Gascoyne RD, Chan WC, Braziel RM, Rimsza LM, Weisenburger DD, Delabie J, Jaffe ES, Lister A, Fitzgibbon J, Staudt LM, Hartmann EM, Mueller-Hermelink HK, Campo E, Ott G, Rosenwald A. Follicular lymphomas with and without translocation t(14;18) differ in gene expression profiles and genetic alterations. Blood 2009, **114**: 826–834.

879 Lestou VS, Gascoyne RD, Sehn L, Ludkovski O, Chhanabhai M, Klasa RJ, Husson H, Freedman AS, Connors JM, Horsman DE. Multicolour fluorescence in situ hybridization analysis of t(14;18)-positive follicular lymphoma and correlation with gene expression data and clinical outcome. Br J Haematol 2003, **122**: 745–759.

880 Levine GD, Dorfman RF. Nodular lymphoma. An ultrastructural study of its relationship to germinal centers and a correlation of light and electron microscopic findings. Cancer 1975, **35**: 148–164.

881 Lister TA. The management of follicular lymphoma. Ann Oncol 1991, **2**(Suppl 2): 131–135.

882 Lo Coco F, Gaidano G, Louie DC, Offit K, Chaganti RS, Dalla-Favera R. p53 mutations are associated with histologic transformation of follicular lymphoma. Blood 1993, **82**: 2289–2295.

883 Lorsbach RB, Shay-Seymore D, Moore J, Banks PM, Hasserjian RP, Sandlund JT, Behm FG. Clinicopathologic analysis of follicular lymphoma occurring in children. Blood 2002, **99**: 1959–1964.

884 McKenna RW, Brunning RD. Reed–Sternberg-like cells in nodular lymphoma involving the bone marrow. Am J Clin Pathol 1975, **63**: 779–785.

885 Matolcsy A, Casali P, Warnke RA, Knowles DM. Morphologic transformation of follicular lymphoma is associated with somatic mutation of the translocated Bcl-2 gene. Blood 1996, **88**: 3937–3944.

886 Nathunam Y, Warnke RA, Zehnder JL, Jones CD, Milatovich-Cherry A, Cornbleet PJ. Blastic/blastoid transformation of follicular lymphoma: immunohistologic and molecular analyses of five cases. Am J Surg Pathol 2000, **24**: 525–534.

887 Nathwani BN, Anderson JR, Armitage JO, Cavalli F, Diebold J, Drachenberg MR, Harris NL, MacLennan KA, Müller-Hermelink HK, Ullrich FA, Weisenburger DD. Clinical significance of follicular lymphoma with monocytoid B cells. Hum Pathol 1999, **30**: 263–268.

888 Nathwani BN, Sheibani K, Winberg CD, Burke JS, Rappaport H. Neoplastic B-cells with cerebriform nuclei in follicular lymphomas. Hum Pathol 1985, **16**: 173–180.

889 Osborne BM, Butler JJ. Follicular lymphoma mimicking progressive transformation of germinal centers. Am J Clin Pathol 1987, **88**: 264–269.

890 Ott G, Katzenberger T, Lohr A, Kindelberger S, Rüdiger T, Wilhelm M, Kalla J, Rosenwald A, Müller JG, Ott MM, Müller-Hermelink HK. Cytomorphologic, immunohistochemical, and cytogenetic profiles of follicular lymphoma: 2 types of follicular lymphoma grade 3. Blood 2002, **99**: 3806–3812.

891 Ottensmeier CH, Thompsett AR, Zhu D, Wilkins BS, Sweetenham JW, Stevenson FK. Analysis of VH genes in follicular and diffuse lymphoma shows ongoing somatic mutation and multiple isotype transcripts in early disease with changes during disease progression. Blood 1998, **91**: 4292–4299.

892 Oviatt DL, Cousar JB, Collins RD, Flexner JM, Stein RS. Malignant lymphomas of follicular center cell origin in humans. V. Incidence, clinical features, and prognostic implications of transformation of small cleaved cell nodular lymphoma. Cancer 1984, **53**: 1109–1114.

893 Pinto A, Hutchison RE, Grant LH, Trevenen CL, Berard CW. Follicular lymphomas in pediatric patients. Mod Pathol 1990, **3**: 308–313.

894 Rappaport H, Winter WJ, Hicks EB. Follicular lymphoma. A re-evaluation of its position in the scheme of malignant lymphoma, based on a survey of 253 cases. Cancer 1956, **9**: 792–821.

895 Rohatiner AZ, Lister TA. New approaches to the treatment of follicular lymphoma. Br J Haematol 1991, **79**: 349–354.

896 Rosas-Uribe A, Variakojis D, Rappaport H. Proteinaceous precipitate in nodular (follicular) lymphomas. Cancer 1973, **31**: 534–542.

897 Roulland S, Navarro JM, Grenot P, Milili M, Agopian J, Montpellier B, Gauduchon P, Lebailly P, Schiff C, Nadel B. Follicular lymphoma-like B cells in healthy individuals: a novel intermediate step in early lymphomagenesis. J Exp Med 2006, **203**: 2425–2431.

898 Schwaenen C, Viardot A, Berger H, Barth TF, Bentink S, Döhner H, Enz M, Feller AC, Hansmann ML, Hummel M, Kestler HA,Klapper W, Kreuz M, Lenze D, Loeffler M, Möller P, Müller-Hermelink HK, Ott G, Rosolowski M, Rosenwald A, Ruf S, Siebert R, Spang R, Stein H, Truemper L, Lichter P, Bentz M, Wessendorf S; Molecular Mechanisms in Malignant Lymphomas Network Project of the Deutsche Krebshilfe. Microarray-based genomic profiling reveals novel genomic aberrations in follicular lymphoma which associate with patient survival and gene expression status. Genes Chromosomes Cancer 2009, **48**: 39–54.

899 Said JW, Pinkus JL, Shinataku IP, DeVos S, Matsumura F, Yamashiro S, Pinkus GS. Alterations in fascin-expressing germinal center dendritic cells in neoplastic follicles of B-cell lymphomas. Mod Pathol 1998, **11**: 1–5.

900 Schmid U, Cogliatti SB, Diss TC, Isaacson PG. Monocytoid/marginal zone B-cell differentiation in follicle centre cell lymphoma. Histopathology 1997, **29**: 201–208.

901 Scoazec JY, Berger F, Magaud JP, Brochier J, Coiffier B, Bryon PA. The dendritic reticulum cell pattern in B-cell lymphomas of the small cleaved, mixed, and large cell types. An immunohistochemical study of 48 cases. Hum Pathol 1989, **20**: 124–131.

902 Szereday Z, Csernus B, Nagy M, Laszlo T, Warnke RA, Matolcsy A. Somatic mutation of the 5′ noncoding region of the BCL-6 gene is associated with intraclonal diversity and clonal selection in histological transformation of follicular lymphoma. Am J Pathol 2000, **156**: 1017–1024.

903 Tilly H, Rossi A, Stamatoullas A, Lenormand B, Bigorgne C, Kunlin A, Monconduit M, Bastard C. Prognostic value of chromosomal abnormalities in follicular lymphoma. Blood 1994, **84**: 1043–1049.

904 Utz GL, Swerdlow SH. Distinction of follicular hyperplasia from follicular lymphoma in B5-fixed tissues. Comparison of MT2 and bcl-2 antibodies. Hum Pathol 1993, **24**: 1155–1158.

905 van den Berg HM, Molenaar WM, Poppema S, Halie MR. The heterogeneity of follicular follicle center cell tumors. II. Clinical follow-up of 30 patients. Cancer 1983, **52**: 2264–2268.

906 Veloso JD, Rezuke WN, Cartun RW, Abernathy EC, Pastuszak WT. Immunohistochemical distinction of follicular lymphoma from follicular hyperplasia in formalin-fixed tissues using monoclonal antibodies MT2 and bcl-2. Appl Immunohistochem 1995, **3**: 153–159.

907 Viardot A, Möller P, Högel J, Werner K, Mechtersheimer G, Ho AD, Ott G, Barth TF, Siebert R, Gesk S, Schlegelberger B, Döhner H, Bentz M. Clinicopathologic correlations of genomic gains and losses in follicular lymphoma. J Clin Oncol 2002, **20**: 4523–4530.

908 Warnke RA, Kim H, Fuks D, Dorfman RF. The coexistence of nodular and diffuse patterns in nodular non-Hodgkin's lymphomas. Significance and clinicopathologic correlation. Cancer 1977, **40**: 1229–1233.

909 Willemze R, Jaffe ES, Burg G, Cerroni L, Berti E, Swerdlow SH, Ralfkiaer E, Chimenti S, Diaz-Perez JL, Duncan LM, Grange F,Harris NL, Kempf W, Kerl H, Kurrer M, Knobler R, Pimpinelli N, Sander C, Santucci M, Sterry W, Vermeer MH, Wechsler J,Whittaker S, Meijer CJ. WHO–EORTC classification for cutaneous lymphomas. Blood 2005, **105**: 3768–3785.

910 Winberg CD, Nathwani BN, Bearman RM, Rappaport H. Follicular (nodular) lymphoma during the first two decades of life. A clinicopathologic study of 12 patients. Cancer 1981, **48**: 2223–2235.

911 Wood BL, Bacchi MM, Bacchi CE, Kidd P, Gown AM. Immunocytochemical differentiation of reactive hyperplasia from follicular lymphoma using monoclonal antibodies to cell surface and proliferation-related markers. Diagn Immunohistochem 1994, **2**: 48–53.

912 Yegappan S, Schmitzer B, Hsi ED. Follicular lymphoma with marginal zone differentiation: microdissection demonstrates the t(14;18) in both the follicular and marginal zone components. Mod Pathol 2001, **14**: 191–196.

913 Young RC, Longo DL, Glatstein E, Ihde DC, Jaffe ES, DeVita VT Jr. The treatment of indolent lymphomas. Watchful waiting V aggressive combined modality treatment. Semin Hematol 1988, **25**: 11–16.

Mantle cell lymphoma

914 Aguilera NS, Bijwaard KE, Duncan B, Krafft AE, Chu WS, Abbondanzo SL, Lichy JH, Taubenberger JK. Differential expression of cyclin D1 in mantle cell lymphoma and other non-Hodgkin's lymphomas. Am J Pathol 1998, **153**: 1969–1976.

915 Banks PM, Chan J, Cleary ML, Delsol G, De Wolf Peeters C, Gatter K, Grogan TM, Harris NL, Isaacson PG, Jaffe ES, et al. Mantle cell lymphoma. A proposal for unification of morphologic, immunologic and molecular data. Am J Surg Pathol 1992, **16**: 637–640.

916 Beà S, Ribas M, Hernández JM, Bosch F, Pinyol M, Hernández L, García JL, Flores T, González M, López-Guillermo A, Piris MA, Cardesa A, Montserrat E, Miró R, Campo E. Increased number of chromosomal imbalances and high-level DNA amplifications in mantle cell lymphoma are associated with blastoid variants. Blood 1999, **93**: 4365–4374.

917 Belaud-Rotureau MA, Parrens M, Dubus P, Garroste JC, de Mascarel A, Merlio JP. A comparative analysis of FISH, RT-PCR, PCR, and immunohistochemistry for the diagnosis of mantle cell lymphomas. Mod Pathol 2002, **15**: 517–525.

918 Bergsagel PL, Kuehl WM. Molecular pathogenesis and a consequent classification of multiple myeloma. J Clin Oncol 2005, **23**: 6333–6338.

919 Bookman MA, Lardelli P, Jaffe ES, Duffey PL, Longo DL. Lymphocytic lymphoma of intermediate differentiation. Morphologic, immunophenotypic, and prognostic factors. J Natl Cancer Inst 1990, **82**: 742–748.

920 Bosch F, López-Guillermo A, Campo E, Ribera JM, Conde E, Piris MA, Vallespi T, Woessner S, Montserrat E. Mantle cell lymphoma: presenting features, response to therapy, and prognostic factors. Cancer 1998, **82**: 567–575.

921 Camacho FI, Algara P, Rodríguez A, Ruíz-Ballesteros E, Mollejo M, Martínez N, Martínez-Climent JA, González M, Mateo M, Caleo A, Sánchez-Beato M, Menárguez J, García-Conde J, Solé F, Campo E, Piris MA. Molecular heterogeneity in MCL defined by the use of specific VH genes and the frequency of somatic mutations. Blood 2003, **101**: 4042–4046.

922 Camacho E, Hernández L, Hernández S, Tort F, Bellosillo B, Beà S, Bosch F, Montserrat E, Cardesa A, Fernández PL, Campo E. ATM gene inactivation in mantle cell lymphoma mainly occurs by truncating mutations and missense mutations involving the phosphatidylinositol-3 kinase domain and is associated with increasing numbers of chromosomal imbalances. Blood 2002, **99**: 238–244.

923 Campo E, Raffeld M, Jaffe ES. Mantle-cell lymphoma. Semin Hematol 1999, **36**: 115–127.

924 Chan JK, Miller KD, Munson P, Isaacson PG. Immunostaining of cyclin D1 and the diagnosis of mantle cell lymphoma: is there a reliable method? Histopathology 1999, **34**: 266–270.

925 Cheuk W, Wong KO, Wong CS, Chan JK. Consistent immunostaining for cyclin D1 can be achieved on a routine basis using a newly available rabbit monoclonal antibody. Am J Surg Pathol 2004, **28**: 801–807.

926 Duggan MJ, Weisenburger DD, Ye YL, Bast MA, Pierson JL, Linder J, Armitage JO. Mantle zone lymphoma. A clinicopathologic study of 22 cases. Cancer 1990, **66**: 522–529.

927 Dunphy CH, Wheaton SE, Perkins SL. CD23 expression in transformed small lymphocytic lymphomas/chronic lymphocytic leukemias and blastic transformations of mantle cell lymphoma. Mod Pathol 1997, **10**: 818–822.

928 Ellison DJ, Turner RR, Van Antwerp R, Martin SE, Nathwani BN. High-grade mantle zone lymphoma. Cancer 1987, **60**: 2717–2720.

929 Fonseca R, Bergsagel PL, Drach J, Shaughnessy J, Gutierrez N, Stewart AK, Morgan G, Van Ness B, Chesi M, Minvielle S, Neri A, Barlogie B, Kuehl WM, Liebisch P, Davies F, Chen-Kiang S, Durie BG, Carrasco R, Sezer O, Reiman T, Pilarski L, Avet-Loiseau H; International Myeloma Working Group. International Myeloma Working Group molecular classification of multiple myeloma: spotlight review. Leukemia 2009, **23**: 2210–2221.

930 Fu K, Weisenburger DD, Greiner TC, Dave S, Wright G, Rosenwald A, Chiorazzi M, Iqbal J, Gesk S, Siebert R, De Jong D, Jaffe ES, Wilson

WH, Delabie J, Ott G, Dave BJ, Sanger WG, Smith LM, Rimsza L, Braziel RM, Müller-Hermelink HK, Campo E, Gascoyne RD, Staudt LM, Chan WC; Lymphoma/Leukemia Molecular Profiling Project. Cyclin D1-negative mantle cell lymphoma: a clinicopathologic study based on gene expression profiling. Blood 2005, **106**: 4315–4321.

931 Hao S, Sanger W, Onciu M, Lai R, Schlette EJ, Medeiros LJ. Mantle cell lymphoma with 8q24 chromosomal abnormalities: a report of 5 cases with blastoid features. Mod Pathol 2002, **15**: 1266–1272.

932 Hartmann E, Fernàndez V, Moreno V, Valls J, Hernández L, Bosch F, Abrisqueta P, Klapper W, Dreyling M, Hoster E, Müller-Hermelink HK, Ott G, Rosenwald A, Campo E. Five-gene model to predict survival in mantle-cell lymphoma using frozen or formalin-fixed, paraffin-embedded tissue. J Clin Oncol 2008, **26**: 4966–4972.

933 Hiddemann W, Unterhalt M, Herrmann R, Woltjen HH, Kreuser ED, Trumper L, Reuss-Borst M, Terhardt-Kasten E, Busch M, Neubauer A, Kaiser U, Hanrath RD, Middeke H, Helm G, Freund M, Stein H, Tiemann M, Parwaresch R. Mantle-cell lymphomas have more widespread disease and a slower response to chemotherapy compared with follicle-centre lymphomas: results of a prospective comparative analysis of the German Low-grade Lymphoma Study Group. J Clin Oncol 1998, **16**: 1922–1930.

934 Hunt JP, Chan JA, Samoszuk M, Brynes RK, Hernandez AM, Bass R, Weisenburger DD, Müller-Hermelink K, Nathwani BN. Hyperplasia of mantle/marginal zone B-cells with clear cytoplasm in peripheral lymph nodes. A clinicopathologic study of 35 cases. Am J Clin Pathol 2001, **116**: 550–559.

935 Kienle D, Kröber A, Katzenberger T, Ott G, Leupolt E, Barth TF, Möller P, Benner A, Habermann A, Müller-Hermelink HK, Bentz M, Lichter P, Döhner H, Stilgenbauer S. VH mutation status and VDJ rearrangement structure in mantle cell lymphoma: correlation with genomic aberrations, clinical characteristics, and outcome. Blood 2003, **102**: 3003–3009.

936 Kroft SH, Howard MS, Picker LJ, Ansari MQ, Aquino DB, McKenna RW. De novo CD5+ diffuse large B-cell lymphomas. A heterogeneous group containing an unusual form of splenic lymphoma. Am J Clin Pathol 2000, **114**: 523–533.

937 Kumar S, Green GA, Teruya-Feldstein J, Raffeld M, Jaffe ES. Use of CD23 (BU38) on paraffin sections in the diagnosis of small lymphocytic lymphoma and mantle cell lymphoma. Mod Pathol 1996, **9**: 925–929.

938 Kurtin PJ. Mantle cell lymphoma. Adv Anat Pathol 1999, **5**: 376–398.

939 Laszlo T, Matolcsy A. Blastic transformation of mantle cell lymphoma: genetic evidence for a clonal link between the two stages of the tumour. Histopathology 1999, **35**: 355–359.

940 Li JY, Gaillard F, Moreau A, Harousseau JL, Laboisse C, Milpied N, Bataille R, Avet-Loiseau H. Detection of translocation t(11;14)(q13;q32) in mantle cell lymphoma by fluorescence in situ hybridization. Am J Pathol 1999, **154**: 1449–1452.

941 Liu Z, Dong HY, Gorczyca W, Tsang P, Cohen P, Stephenson CF, Berger CS, Wu CD, Weisberger J. CD5- mantle cell lymphoma. Am J Clin Pathol 2002, **118**: 216–224.

942 Louie DC, Offit K, Jaslow R, Parsa NZ, Murty VV, Schluger A, Chaganti RS. p53 overexpression as a marker of poor prognosis in mantle cell lymphomas with t(11;14)(q13;q32). Blood 1995, **86**: 2892–2899.

943 Martínez N, Camacho FI, Algara P, Rodríguez A, Dopazo A, Ruíz-Ballesteros E, Martín P, Martínez-Climent JA, García-Conde J, Menárguez J, Solano F, Mollejo M, Piris MA. The molecular signature of mantle cell lymphoma reveals multiple signals favoring cell survival. Cancer Res 2003, **63**: 8226–8232.

944 Miranda RN, Briggs RC, Kinney MC, Veno PA, Hammer RD, Cousar JB. Immunohistochemical detection of cyclin D1 using optimized conditions is highly specific for mantle cell lymphoma and hairy cell leukemia. Mod Pathol 2000, **13**: 1308–1314.

945 Monina TJ, Delmer A, Cymbalista F, Le Tourneau A, Perrot JY, Ramond S, Marie JP, Audouin J, Zittoun R, Diebold J. Mantle cell lymphoma, in leukaemic phase with prominent splenomegaly. A report of eight cases with similar clinical presentation and aggressive outcome. Virchows Arch 2001, **437**: 591–598.

946 Nodit L, Bahler DW, Jacobs SA, Locker J, Swerdlow SH. Indolent mantle cell lymphoma with nodal involvement and mutated immunoglobulin heavy chain genes. Hum Pathol 2003, **34**: 1030–1034.

947 Ott G, Kalla J, Ott MM, Schryen B, Katzenberger T, Müller JG, Müller-Hermelink HK. Blastoid variants of mantle cell lymphoma: frequent bcl-1 rearrangements at the major translocation cluster region and tetraploid chromosome clones. Blood 1997, **89**: 1421–1429.

948 Parrens M, Belaud-Rotureau MA, Fitoussi O, Carerre N, Bouabdallah K, Marit G, Dubus P, de Mascarel A, Merlio JP. Blastoid and common variants of mantle cell lymphoma exhibit distinct immunophenotypic and interphase FISH features. Histopathology 2006, **48**: 353–362.

949 Pinyol M, Hernandez L, Cazorla M, Balbín M, Jares P, Fernandez PL, Montserrat E, Cardesa A, Lopez-Otín C, Campo E. Deletions and loss of expression of p16INK4a and p21Waf1 genes are associated with aggressive variants of mantle cell lymphomas. Blood 1997, **89**: 272–280.

950 Pittaluga S, Wlodarska I, Stul MS, Thomas J, Verhoef G, Cassiman JJ, van den Berghe H, De Wolf-Peeters C. Mantle cell lymphoma. A clinicopathological study of 55 cases. Histopathology 1995, **26**: 17–24.

951 Rosenwald A, Wright G, Wiestner A, Chan WC, Connors JM, Campo E, Gascoyne RD, Grogan TM, Müller-Hermelink HK,Smeland EB, Chiorazzi M, Giltnane JM, Hurt EM, Zhao H, Averett L, Henrickson S, Yang L, Powell J, Wilson WH, Jaffe ES, Simon R, Klausner RD, Montserrat E, Bosch F, Greiner TC, Weisenburger DD, Sanger WG, Dave BJ, Lynch JC, Vose J, Armitage JO, Fisher RI, Miller TP, LeBlanc M, Ott G, Kvaloy S, Holte H, Delabie J, Staudt LM. The proliferation gene expression signature is a quantitative integrator of oncogenic events that predicts survival in mantle cell lymphoma. Cancer Cell 2003, **3**: 185–197.

952 Schlette E, Lai R, Onciu M, Doherty D, Bueso-Ramos C, Medeiors LJ. Leukemic mantle cell lymphoma: clinical and pathologic spectrum of twenty-three cases. Mod Pathol 2001, **14**: 1133–1140.

953 Singleton TP, Anderson MM, Ross CW, Schnitzer B. Leukemic phase of mantle cell lymphoma, blastoid variant. Am J Clin Pathol 1999, **111**: 495–500.

954 Soslow RA, Zukerberg LR, Harris NL, Warnke RA. BCL-1 (PRAD-1/cyclin D-1) overexpression distinguishes the blastoid variant of mantle cell lymphoma from B-lineage lymphoblastic lymphoma. Mod Pathol 1997, **10**: 810–817.

955 Strickler JG, Medeiros, LJ, Copenhaver CM, Weiss LM, Warnke RA. Intermediate lymphocytic lymphoma. An immunophenotypic study with comparison to small lymphocytic lymphoma and diffuse small cleaved cell lymphoma. Hum Pathol 1988, **19**: 550–554.

956 Swerdlow SH, Williams ME. From centrocytic to mantle cell lymphoma: a clinicopathologic and molecular review of 3 decades. Hum Pathol 2002, **33**: 7–20.

957 Swerdlow SH, Williams ME. From centrocytic to mantle cell lymphoma: a clinicopathologic and molecular review of 3 decades. Hum Pathol 2002, **33**: 7–20.

958 van den Oord JJ, de Wolf-Peeters C, Pulford KAF, Mason DY, Desmet VJ. Mantle zone lymphoma. Immuno- and enzyme-histochemical studies on the cell of origin. Am J Surg Pathol 1986, **10**: 780–788.

959 Viswanatha DS, Foucar K, Berry BR, Gascoyne RD, Evans L, Leith CP. Blastic mantle cell leukemia: an unusual presentation of blastic mantle cell lymphoma. Mod Pathol 2000, **13**: 825–833.

960 Weisenburger DD, Nathwani BN, Diamond LW, Winberg BD, Rappaport H. Malignant lymphoma, intermediate lymphocytic type. A clinicopathologic study of 42 cases. Cancer 1981, **48**: 1415–1425.

961 Wlodarska I, Dierickx D, Vanhentenrijk V, Van Roosbroeck K, Pospísilová H, Minnei F, Verhoef G, Thomas J, Vandenberghe P,De Wolf-Peeters C. Translocations targeting CCND2, CCND3, and MYCN do occur in t(11;14)-negative mantle cell lymphomas. Blood 2008, **111**: 5683–5690.

962 Yatabe Y, Suzuki R, Matsuno Y, Tobinai KK, Ichinohazama R, Tamaru JI, Mizoguchi Y, Hashimoto Y, Yamaguchi M, Kojima M, Uike N, Okamoto M, Isoda K, Ichimura K, Morishima Y, Seto M, Suchi T, Nakamura S. Morphological spectrum of cyclin D1-positive mantle cell lymphoma: study of 168 cases. Pathol Int 2002, **51**: 747–761.

963 Young KH, Chan WC, Fu K, Iqbal J, Sanger WG, Ratashak A, Greiner TC, Weisenburger DD. Mantle cell lymphoma with plasma cell differentiation. Am J Surg Pathol 2006, **30**: 954–961.

Marginal zone B-cell lymphoma

964 Andersen CL, Gruszka-Westwood A, Atkinson S, Matutes E, Catovsky D, Pedersen RK, Pedersen BB, Pulczynski S, Hokland P, Jacobsen E, Koch J. Recurrent genomic imbalances in B-cell splenic marginal-zone lymphoma revealed by comparative genomic hybridization. Cancer Genet Cytogenet 2005, **156**: 122–128.

965 Burke JS. Are there site-specific differences among the MALT lymphomas – morphologic, clinical? Am J Clin Pathol 1999, **111**: S133–S143.

966 Camacho FI, Algara P, Mollejo M, García JF, Montalbán C, Martínez N, Sánchez-Beato M, Piris MA. Nodal marginal zone lymphoma: a heterogeneous tumor: a comprehensive analysis of a series of 27 cases. Am J Surg Pathol 2003, **27**: 762–771.

967 Chanudet E, Ye H, Ferry J, Bacon CM, Adam P, Müller-Hermelink HK, Radford J, Pileri SA, Ichimura K, Collins VP, Hamoudi RA, Nicholson AG, Wotherspoon AC, Isaacson PG, Du MQ. A20 deletion is associated with copy number gain at the TNFA/B/C locus and occurs preferentially in translocation-negative MALT lymphoma of the ocular adnexa and salivary glands. J Pathol 2009, **217**: 420–430.

968 Cogliatti SB, Lennert K, Hansmann ML, Zwingers TL. Monocytoid B-cell lymphoma. Clinical and prognostic features of 21 patients. J Clin Pathol 1990, **43**: 619–625.

969 Cousar JB, McGinn DL, Glick AD, List AF, Collins RD. Report of an unusual lymphoma arising from parafollicular B lymphocytes (PBLs) or so-called 'monocytoid' lymphocytes. Am J Clin Pathol 1987, **87**: 121–128.

970 Du MQ. MALT lymphoma: recent advances in aetiology and molecular genetics. J Clin Exp Hematop 2007, **47**: 31–42.

971 Hernández JM, García JL, Gutiérrez NC, Mollejo M, Martínez-Climent JA, Flores T, González MB, Piris MA, San Miguel JF. Novel genomic imbalances in B-cell splenic marginal zone lymphomas revealed by comparative genomic hybridization and cytogenetics. Am J Pathol 2001, **158**: 1843–1850.

972 Honma K, Tsuzuki S, Nakagawa M, Tagawa H, Nakamura S, Morishima Y, Seto M. TNFAIP3/A20 functions as a novel tumor suppressor gene in several subtypes of non-Hodgkin lymphomas. Blood 2009, **114**: 2467–2475.

973 Isaacson PG, Spencer J. Monocytoid B-cell lymphomas. Am J Surg Pathol 1990, **14**: 888–891.

974 Isaacson PG, Du MQ. MALT lymphoma: from morphology to molecules. Nat Rev Cancer 2004, **4**: 644–653.

975 Karube K, Ohshima K, Tsuchiya T, Yamaguchi T, Kawano R, Suzumiya J, Harada M, Kikuchi M. A 'floral' variant of nodal marginal zone lymphoma. Hum Pathol 2005, **36**: 202–206.

976 Maes B, Baens M, Marynen P, De Wolf-Peeters C. The product of the t(11;18), an API2-MLT fusion, is an almost exclusive finding in marginal zone cell lymphoma of extranodal MALT-type. Ann Oncol 2000, **11**: 521–526.

977 Maes B, De Wolf-Peeters C. Marginal zone cell lymphoma – an update on recent advances. Histopathology 2002, **40**: 117–126.

978 Mateo M, Mollejo M, Villuendas R, Algara P, Sánchez-Beato M, Martínez P, Piris MA. 7q31-32 allelic loss is a frequent finding in splenic marginal zone lymphoma. Am J Pathol 1999, **154**: 1583–1589.

979 Mori N, Yatabe Y, Asai J. Mucosa-associated lymphoid tissue (MALT) lymphoma. Pathol Int 1995, **45**: 544–551.

980 Nathwani BN, Mohrmann RL, Brynes RK, Taylor CR, Hansmann ML, Sheibani K. Monocytoid B-cell lymphomas. An assessment of diagnostic criteria and a perspective on histogenesis. Hum Pathol 1992, **23**: 1061–1071.

981 Neiman RS, Sullivan AL, Jaffe R. Malignant lymphoma simulating leukemic reticuloendotheliosis. A clinicopathologic study of ten cases. Cancer 1979, **43**: 329–342.

982 Ngan BY, Warnke RA, Wilson M, Takagi K, Cleary ML, Dorfman RF. Monocytoid B-cell lymphoma. A study of 36 cases. Hum Pathol 1991, **22**: 409–421.

983 Novak U, Rinaldi A, Kwee I, Nandula SV, Rancoita PM, Compagno M, Cerri M, Rossi D, Murty VV, Zucca E, Gaidano G, Dalla-Favera R, Pasqualucci L, Bhagat G, Bertoni F. The NF-κB negative regulator TNFAIP3 (A20) is inactivated by somatic mutations and genomic deletions in marginal zone lymphomas. Blood 2009, **113**: 4918–4921.

984 Piris MA, Rivas C, Morente M, Cruz MA, Rubio C, Oliva H. Monocytoid B-cell lymphoma, a tumour related to the marginal zone. Histopathology 1988, **12**: 383–392.

985 Qin Y, Greiner A, Trunk MJ, Schmausser B, Ott MM, Müller-Hermelink HK. Somatic hypermutation in low-grade mucosa-associated lymphoid tissue-type B-cell lymphoma. Blood 1995, **86**: 3528–3534.

986 Raderer M, Wöhrer S, Streubel B, Troch M, Turetschek K, Jäger U, Skrabs C, Gaiger A, Drach J, Puespoek A, Formanek M,Hoffmann M, Hauff W, Chott A. Assessment of disease dissemination in gastric compared with extragastric mucosa-associated lymphoid tissue lymphoma using extensive staging: a single-center experience. J Clin Oncol 2006, **24**: 3136–3141.

987 Remstein ED, Dogan A, Einerson RR, Paternoster SF, Fink SR, Law M, Dewald GW, Kurtin PJ. The incidence and anatomic site specificity of chromosomal translocations in primary extranodal marginal zone B-cell lymphoma of mucosa-associated lymphoid tissue (MALT lymphoma) in North America. Am J Surg Pathol 2006, **30**: 1546–1553.

988 Ruiz-Ballesteros E, Mollejo M, Rodriguez A, Camacho FI, Algara P, Martinez N, Pollán M, Sanchez-Aguilera A, Menarguez J,Campo E, Martinez P, Mateo M, Piris MA. Splenic marginal zone lymphoma: proposal of new diagnostic and prognostic markers identified after tissue and cDNA microarray analysis. Blood 2005, **106**: 1831–1838.

989 Schmid C, Kirkham N, Diss T, Isaacson PG. Splenic marginal zone cell lymphoma. Am J Surg Pathol 1992, **16**: 455–466.

990 Sheibani K, Burke JS, Swartz WG, Nademanee A, Winberg CD. Monocytoid B-cell lymphoma. Clinicopathologic study of 21 cases of a unique type of low-grade lymphoma. Cancer 1988, **62**: 1531–1538.

991 Solé F, Salido M, Espinet B, Garcia JL, Martinez Climent JA, Granada I, Hernández JM, Benet I, Piris MA, Mollejo M, Martinez P, Vallespí T, Domingo A, Serrano S, Woessner S, Florensa L. Splenic marginal zone B-cell lymphomas: two cytogenetic subtypes, one with gain of 3q and the other with loss of 7q. Haematologica 2001, **86**: 71–77.

992 Streubel B, Simonitsch-Klupp I, Müllauer L, Lamprecht A, Huber D, Siebert R, Stolte M, Trautinger F, Lukas J, Püspök A,Formanek M, Assanasen T, Müller-Hermelink HK, Cerroni L, Raderer M, Chott A. Variable frequencies of MALT lymphoma-associated genetic aberrations in MALT lymphomas of different sites. Leukemia 2004, **18**: 1722–1726.

993 Streubel B, Vinatzer U, Lamprecht A, Raderer M, Chott A. T(3;14)(p14.1;q32) involving IGH and FOXP1 is a novel recurrent chromosomal aberration in MALT lymphoma. Leukemia 2005, **19**: 652–658.

994 Streubel B, Lamprecht A, Dierlamm J, Cerroni L, Stolte M, Ott G, Raderer M, Chott A. T(14;18)(q32;q21) involving IGH and MALT1 is a frequent chromosomal aberration in MALT lymphoma. Blood 2003, **101**: 2335–2339.

995 van Krieken JH, von Schilling C, Kluin PM, Lennert K. Splenic marginal zone lymphocytes and related cells in the lymph node. A morphologic and immunohistochemical study. Hum Pathol 1989, **20**: 320–325.

996 Wotherspoon AC, Finn TM, Isaacson PG. Trisomy 3 in low-grade B-cell lymphomas of mucosa-associated lymphoid tissue. Blood 1995, **85**: 2000–2004.

997 Zhang W, Garces J, Dong HY. Detection of the t(11;18) API2/MALT1 translocation associated with gastric MALT lymphoma in routine formalin-fixed, paraffin-embedded small endoscopic biopsy specimens by robust real-time RT-PCR. Am J Clin Pathol 2006, **126**: 931–940.

Diffuse mixed (small and large cell) lymphoma

998 Hu E, Weiss LM, Hoppe RT, Horning SJ. Follicular and diffuse mixed small-cleaved and large-cell lymphoma – a clinicopathologic study. J Clin Oncol 1985, **3**: 1183–1187.

999 Katzin WE, Linden MD, Fishleder AJ, Tubbs RR. Immunophenotypic and genotypic characterization of diffuse mixed non-Hodgkin's lymphomas. Am J Pathol 1989, **135**: 615–621.

1000 Medeiros LJ, Lardelli P, Stetler-Stevenson M, Longo DL, Jaffe ES. Genotypic analysis of diffuse mixed cell lymphomas. Comparison with morphologic and immunophenotypic findings. Am J Clin Pathol 1991, **95**: 547–555.

Diffuse large B-cell lymphoma

1001 Alizadeh AA, Eisen MB, Davis RE, Ma C, Lossos IS, Rosenwald A, Boldrick JC, Sabet H, Tran T, Yu X, Powell JI, Yang L, Marti GE, Moore T, Hudson J Jr, Lu L, Lewis DB, Tibshirani R, Sherlock G, Chan WC, Greiner TC, Weisenburger DD, Armitage JO, Warnke R, Levy R, Wilson W, Grever MR, Byrd JC, Botstein D, Brown PO, Staudt LM. Distinct types of diffuse large B-cell lymphoma identified by gene expression profiling. Nature 2000, **403**: 503–511.

1002 Aozasa K, Takakuwa T, Nakatsuka S. Pyothorax-associated lymphoma: a lymphoma developing in chronic inflammation. Adv Anat Pathol 2005, **12**: 324–331.

1003 Armitage JO. Treatment of non-Hodgkin's lymphoma. N Engl J Med 1993, **328**: 1023–1030.

1004 Bennett MH. Sclerosis in non-Hodgkins's lymphoma. Br J Cancer 1975, **31**: 44–52.

1005 Bernier V, Azar HA. Filiform large-cell lymphomas. An ultrastructural and immunohistochemical study. Am J Surg Pathol 1987, **11**: 387–396.

1006 Bosga-Bouwer AG, Haralambieva E, Booman M, Boonstra R, van den Berg A, Schuuring E, van den Berg E, Kluin P, Poppema S. BCL6 alternative translocation breakpoint cluster region associated with follicular lymphoma grade 3B. Genes Chromosomes Cancer 2005, **44**: 301–304.

1007 Capello D, Vitolo U, Pasqualucci L, Quattrone S, Migliaretti G, Fassone L, Ariatti C, Vivenza D, Gloghini A, Pastore C, Lanza C, Nomdedeu J, Botto B, Freilone R, Buonaiuto D, Zagonel V, Gallo E, Palestro G, Saglio G, Dalla-Favera R, Carbone A, Gaidano G. Distribution and pattern of BCL-6 mutations throughout the spectrum of B-cell neoplasia. Blood 2000, **95**: 651–659.

1008 Carbone A, Gloghini A, Libra M, Gasparotto D, Navolanic PM, Spina M, Tirelli U. A spindle cell variant of diffuse large B-cell lymphoma possesses genotypic and phenotypic markers characteristic of a germinal center B-cell origin. Mod Pathol 2006, **19**: 299–306.

1009 Carbone A, Gloghini A, Vaccher E, Cerri M, Gaidano G, Dalla-Favera R, Tirelli U. Kaposi's sarcoma-associated herpesvirus/human herpesvirus type 8-positive solid lymphomas:

a tissue-based variant of primary effusion lymphoma. J Mol Diagn 2005, **7**: 17–27.

1010 Chabner BA, Johnson RE, Young RC, Canellos GP, Hubbard SP, Johnson SK, DeVita VT Jr. Sequential nonsurgical and surgical staging of non-Hodgkin's lymphoma. Ann Intern Med 1976, **85**: 149–154.

1011 Chan ACL, Chan JKC. Diffuse large B-cell lymphoma. In Jaffe ES, Harris NL, Vardiman J, Campo E, Arber DA (eds): Hematopathology. Philadelphia, 2010, Saunders.

1012 Coiffier B. State-of-the-art therapeutics: diffuse large B-cell lymphoma. J Clin Oncol 2005, **23**: 6387–6393.

1013 Colomo L, Loong F, Rives S, Pittaluga S, Martínez A, López-Guillermo A, Ojanguren J, Romagosa V, Jaffe ES, Campo E. Diffuse large B-cell lymphomas with plasmablastic differentiation represent a heterogeneous group of disease entities. Am J Surg Pathol 2004, **28**: 736–747.

1014 De Jong D, Van Gorp J, Sie-Go D, Van Heerde P. T-cell rich B-cell non-Hodgkin's lymphoma: a progressed form of follicle centre cell lymphoma and lymphocyte predominance Hodgkin's disease. Histopathology 1996, **28**: 15–24.

1015 De Paepe P, Baens M, van Krieken H, Verhasselt B, Stul M, Simons A, Poppe B, Laureys G, Brons P, Vandenberghe P, Speleman F, Praet M, De Wolf-Peeters C, Marynen P, Wlodarska I. ALK activation by the CLTC–ALK fusion is a recurrent event in large B-cell lymphoma. Blood 2003, **102**: 2638–2641.

1016 Fleming MD, Shahsafaei A, Dorfman DM. Absence of dendritic reticulum cell staining is helpful for distinguishing T-cell-rich B-cell lymphoma from lymphocyte predominance Hodgkin's disease. Appl Immunohistochem 1998, **6**: 16–22.

1017 Fraga M, Garcia-Riviero A, Sanchez-Verde L, Forteza J, Piris MA. T-cell/histiocyte-rich large B-cell lymphoma is a disseminated aggressive neoplasm: differential diagnosis from Hodgkin's lymphoma. Histopathology 2002, **41**: 216–229.

1018 Franke S, Wlodarska I, Maes B, Vandenberghe P, Achten R, Hagemeijer A, De Wolf-Peeters C. Comparative genomic hybridization pattern distinguishes T-cell/histiocyte-rich B-cell lymphoma from nodular lymphocyte predominance Hodgkin's lymphoma. Am J Pathol 2002, **161**: 1861–1867.

1019 Fung DT, Chan JK, Tse CC, Sze WM. Myxoid change in malignant lymphoma. Pathogenetic considerations. Arch Pathol Lab Med 1992, **116**: 103–105.

1020 Gascoyne RD, Adomat SA, Krajewski S, Krajewska M, Horsman DE, Tolcher AW, O'Reilly SE, Hoskins P, Coldman AJ, Reed JC, Connors JM. Prognostic significance of Bcl-2 protein expression and Bcl-2 gene rearrangement in diffuse aggressive non-Hodgkin's lymphoma. Blood 1997, **90**: 244–251.

1021 Gascoyne RD, Lamant L, Martin-Subero JI, Lestou VS, Harris NL, Müller-Hermelink HK, Seymour JF, Campbell LJ, Horsman DE, Auvigne I, Espinos E, Siebert R, Delsol G. ALK-positive diffuse large B-cell lymphoma is associated with Clathrin-ALK rearrangements: report of 6 cases. Blood 2003, **102**: 2568–2573.

1022 Gu K, Fu K, Jain S, Liu Z, Iqbal J, Li M, Sanger WG, Weisenburger DD, Greiner TC, Aoun P, Dave BJ, Chan WC. t(14;18)-negative follicular lymphomas are associated with a high frequency of BCL6 rearrangement at the alternative breakpoint region. Mod Pathol 2009, **22**: 1251–1257.

1023 Hill ME, MacLennan KA, Cunningham DC, Vaughan Hudson B, Burke M, Clarke P, Di Stefano F, Anderson L, Vaughan Hudson G, Mason D, Selby P, Linch DC. Prognostic significance of BCL-2 expression and bcl-2 major breakpoint region rearrangement in diffuse large cell non-Hodgkin's lymphoma: a British National Lymphoma Investigation Study. Blood 1996, **88**: 1046–1051.

1024 Hummel M, Bentink S, Berger H, Klapper W, Wessendorf S, Barth TF, Bernd HW, Cogliatti SB, Dierlamm J, Feller AC, Hansmann ML, Haralambieva E, Harder L, Hasenclever D, Kühn M, Lenze D, Lichter P, Martin-Subero JI, Möller P, Müller-Hermelink HK, Ott G, Parwaresch RM, Pott C, Rosenwald A, Rosolowski M, Schwaenen C, Stürzenhofecker B, Szczepanowski M, Trautmann H, Wacker HH, Spang R, Loeffler M, Trümper L, Stein H, Siebert R; Molecular Mechanisms in Malignant Lymphomas Network Project of the Deutsche Krebshilfe. A biologic definition of Burkitt's lymphoma from transcriptional and genomic profiling. N Engl J Med 2006, **354**: 2419–2430.

1025 Iqbal J, Greiner TC, Patel K, Dave BJ, Smith L, Ji J, Wright G, Sanger WG, Pickering DL, Jain S, Horsman DE, Shen Y, Fu K, Weisenburger DD, Hans CP, Campo E, Gascoyne RD, Rosenwald A, Jaffe ES, Delabie J, Rimsza L, Ott G, Müller-Hermelink HK, Connors JM, Vose JM, McKeithan T, Staudt LM, Chan WC; Leukemia/Lymphoma Molecular Profiling Project. Distinctive patterns of BCL6 molecular alterations and their functional consequences in different subgroups of diffuse large B-cell lymphoma. Leukemia 2007, **21**: 2332–2343.

1026 Kato M, Sanada M, Kato I, Sato Y, Takita J, Takeuchi K, Niwa A, Chen Y, Nakazaki K, Nomoto J, Asakura Y, Muto S, Tamura A, Iio M, Akatsuka Y, Hayashi Y, Mori H, Igarashi T, Kurokawa M, Chiba S, Mori S, Ishikawa Y, Okamoto K, Tobinai K, Nakagama H, Nakahata T, Yoshino T, Kobayashi Y, Ogawa S. Frequent inactivation of A20 in B-cell lymphomas. Nature 2009, **459**: 712–716.

1027 Kawasaki C, Ohshim K, Suzumiya J, Kanda M, Tsuchiya T, Tamura K, Kikuchi M. Rearrangements of bcl-1, bcl-2, bcl-6, and c-myc in diffuse large B-cell lymphomas. Leuk Lymphoma 2001, **42**: 1099–1106.

1028 Koens L, Vermeer MH, Willemze R, Jansen PM. IgM expression on paraffin sections distinguishes primary cutaneous large B-cell lymphoma, leg type from primary cutaneous follicle center lymphoma. Am J Surg Pathol 2010, **34**: 1043–1048.

1029 Kramer MH, Hermans J, Wijburg E, Philippo K, Geelen E, van Krieken JH, de Jong D, Maartense E, Schuuring E, Kluin PM. Clinical relevance of BCL2, BCL6, and MYC rearrangements in diffuse large B-cell lymphoma. Blood 1998, **92**: 3152–3162.

1030 Ladanyi M, Offit K, Jhanwar SC, Filippa DA, Chaganti RS. MYC rearrangement and translocations involving band 8q24 in diffuse large cell lymphomas. Blood 1991, **77**: 1057–1063.

1031 Lai R, Medeiros LJ, Dabbagh L, Formenti KS, Coupland RW. Sinusoidal CD30-positive large B-cell lymphoma: a morphologic mimic of anaplastic large cell lymphoma. Mod Pathol 2000, **13**: 223–228.

1032 Lasota J, Hyjek E, Koo CH, Blonski J, Miettinen M. Cytokeratin-positive large-cell lymphomas of B-cell lineage: a study of five phenotypically unusual cases verified by polymerase chain reaction. Am J Surg Pathol 1997, **20**: 346–354.

1033 Lenz G, Staudt LM. Aggressive lymphomas. N Engl J Med 2010, **362**: 1417–1429.

1034 Lenz G, Davis RE, Ngo VN et al. Oncogenic CARD11 mutations in human diffuse large B cell lymphoma. Science 2008, **319**: 1676–1679.

1035 Leoncini L, Delsol G, Gascoyne RD, Harris NL, Pileri SA, Piris MA, Stein H. Aggressive B-cell lymphomas: a review based on the workshop of the XI Meeting of the European Association for Haematopathology. Histopathology 2005, **46**: 241–255.

1036 Lichtenstein A, Levine AM, Lukes RJ, Cramer AD, Taylor CR, Lincoln TL, Feinstein DI. Immunoblastic sarcoma. A clinical description. Cancer 1979, **43**: 343–352.

1037 Lim MS, Beaty M, Sorbara L, Cheng RZ, Pittaluga S, Raffeld M, Jaffe ES. T-cell/histiocyte-rich large B-cell lymphoma: a heterogeneous entity with derivation from germinal center B-cells. Am J Surg Pathol 2002, **26**: 1458–1466.

1038 Lo Coco F, Ye BH, Lista F, Corradini P, Offit K, Knowles DM, Chaganti RS, Dalla-Favera R. Rearrangements of the BCL6 gene in diffuse large cell non-Hodgkin's lymphoma. Blood 1994, **83**: 1757–1759.

1039 Loong F, Chan AC, Ho BC, Chau YP, Lee HY, Cheuk W, Yuen WK, Ng WS, Cheung HL, Chan JK. Diffuse large B-cell lymphoma associated with chronic inflammation as an incidental finding and new clinical scenarios. Mod Pathol 2010, **23**: 493–501.

1040 Lossos IS, Alizadeh AA, Eisen MB, Chan WC, Brown PO, Botstein D, Staudt LM, Levy R. Ongoing immunoglobulin somatic mutation in germinal center B cell-like but not in activated B cell-like diffuse large cell lymphomas. Proc Natl Acad Sci U S A 2000, **97**: 10209–10213.

1041 Lukes RJ, Parker JW, Taylor CR, Tindle BH, Cramer AD, Lincoln TL. Immunologic approach to non-Hodgkin lymphomas and related leukemias. Analysis of the results of multiparameter studies of 425 cases. Semin Hematol 1978, **15**: 322–351.

1042 McClure RF, Remstein ED, Macon WR, Dewald GW, Habermann TM, Hoering A, Kurtin PJ. Adult B-cell lymphomas with Burkitt-like morphology are phenotypically and genotypically heterogeneous with aggressive clinical behavior. Am J Surg Pathol 2005, **29**: 1652–1660.

1043 McCurley TL, Gay RE, Gay S, Glick AD, Haralson MA, Collins RD. The extracellular matrix in 'sclerosing' follicular center cell lymphomas. An immunohistochemical and ultrastructural study. Hum Pathol 1986, **17**: 930–938.

1044 Migliazza A, Martinotti S, Chen W, Fusco C, Ye BH, Knowles DM, Offit K, Chaganti RS, Dalla-Favera R. Frequent somatic hypermutation of the 5′ noncoding region of the BCL6 gene in B-cell lymphoma. Proc Natl Acad Sci U S A 1995, **92**: 12520–12524.

1045 Nakamura S, Suchi T, Koshikawa T, Kitoh K, Koike K, Komatsu H, Iida S, Kagami Y, Ogura M, Katoh E, Kurita S, Suzuki H, Kobashi Y, Yamabe H, Hirabayashi N, Ueda R, Takahashi T. Clinicopathologic study of CD56 (NCAM)-positive angiocentric lymphoma occurring in sites other than the upper and lower respiratory tract. Am J Surg Pathol 1995, **19**: 284–296.

1046 Natkunam Y, Zhao S, Mason DY, Chen J, Taidi B, Jones M, Hammer AS, Hamilton Dutoit S, Lossos IS, Levy R. The oncoprotein LMO2 is expressed in normal germinal-center B cells and in human B-cell lymphomas. Blood 2007, **109**: 1636–1642.

1047 Natkunam Y, Farinha P, Hsi ED, Hans CP, Tibshirani R, Sehn LH, Connors JM, Gratzinger D, Rosado M, Zhao S, Pohlman B, Wongchaowart N, Bast M, Avigdor A, Schiby G, Nagler A, Byrne GE, Levy R, Gascoyne RD, Lossos IS. LMO2 protein expression predicts survival in patients with diffuse large B-cell lymphoma treated with anthracycline-based chemotherapy with and without rituximab. J Clin Oncol 2008, **26**: 447–454.

1048 O'Hara CJ, Said JW, Pinkus GS. Non-Hodgkin's lymphoma, multilobated B-cell type. Report of nine cases with immunohistochemical and immunoultrastructural evidence for a follicular center cell derivation. Hum Pathol 1986, **17**: 593–599.

1049 Ohno H. Pathogenetic role of BCL6 translocation in B-cell non-Hodgkin's lymphoma. Histol Histopathol 2004, **19**: 637–650.

1050 Onciu M, Behm FG, Downing JR, Shurtleff SA, Raimondi SC, Ma Z, Morris SW, Kennedy W, Jones SC, Sandlund JT. ALK-positive plasmablastic B-cell lymphoma with expression of the NPM–ALK fusion transcript: report of 2 cases. Blood 2003, **102**: 2642–2644.

1051 Osborne BM, Mackay B, Butler JJ, Ordonez NG. Large cell lymphoma with microvillus-like projections. An ultrastructural study. Am J Clin Pathol 1983, **79**: 443–450.

1052 Osborne BM, Butler JJ, Mackay B. Sinusoidal large cell ('histiocytic') lymphoma. Cancer 1980, **46**: 2484–2491.

1053 Otsuki T, Yano T, Clark HM, Bastard C, Kerckaert JP, Jaffe ES, Raffeld M. Analysis of LAZ3 (BCL-6) status in B-cell non-Hodgkin's lymphomas: results of rearrangement and gene expression studies and a mutational analysis of coding region sequences. Blood 1995, **85**: 2877–2884.

1054 Pasqualucci L, Migliazza A, Fracchiolla N, William C, Neri A, Baldini L, Chaganti RS, Klein U, Küppers R, Rajewsky K, Dalla-Favera R. BCL-6 mutations in normal germinal center B cells: evidence of somatic hypermutation acting outside Ig loci. Proc Natl Acad Sci U S A 1998, **95**: 11816–11821.

1055 Peng HZ, Du MQ, Koulis A, Aiello A, Dogan A, Pan LX, Isaacson PG. Nonimmunoglobulin gene hypermutation in germinal center B cells. Blood 1999, **93**: 2167–2172.

1056 Ree HJ, Leone LA, Crowley JP. Sclerosis in diffuse histiocytic lymphoma. A clinicopathologic study of 25 cases. Cancer 1982, **49**: 1636–1648.

1057 Rosas-Uribe A, Rappaport H. Malignant lymphoma, histiocytic type with sclerosis (sclerosing reticulum cell sarcoma). Cancer 1972, **29**: 946–953.

1058 Rosenwald A, Wright G, Chan WC, Connors JM, Campo E, Fisher RI, Gascoyne RD, Müller-Hermelink HK, Smeland EB, Giltnane JM, Hurt EM, Zhao H, Averett L, Yang L, Wilson WH, Jaffe ES, Simon R, Klausner RD, Powell J, Duffey PL, Longo DL, Greiner TC, Weisenburger DD, Sanger WG, Dave BJ, Lynch JC, Vose J, Armitage JO, Montserrat E, López-Guillermo A, Grogan TM, Miller TP, LeBlanc M, Ott G, Kvaloy S, Delabie J, Holte H, Krajci P, Stokke T, Staudt LM; Lymphoma/Leukemia Molecular Profiling Project. The use of molecular profiling to predict survival after chemotherapy for diffuse large-B-cell lymphoma. N Engl J Med 2002, **346**: 1937–1947.

1059 Rudiger T, Ott G, Ott MM, Muller-Deubert SM, Müller-Hermelink HK. Differential diagnosis between classic Hodgkin's lymphoma, T-cell-rich B-cell lymphoma, and paragranuloma by paraffin immunohistochemistry. Am J Surg Pathol 1998, **22**: 1184–1191.

1060 Saito M, Gao J, Basso K, Kitagawa Y, Smith PM, Bhagat G, Pernis A, Pasqualucci L, Dalla-Favera R. A signaling pathway mediating downregulation of BCL6 in germinal center B cells is blocked by BCL6 gene alterations in B cell lymphoma. Cancer Cell 2007, **12**: 280–292.

1061 Strauchen JA, Young RC, DeVita VT Jr, Anderson T, Fantone JC, Berard CW. Clinical relevance of the histopathological subclassification of diffuse 'histiocytic' lymphoma. N Engl J Med 1978, **299**: 1382–1387.

1062 Straus DJ, Filippa DA, Lieberman PH, Koziner B, Thaler HT, Clarkson BD. The non-Hodgkin's lymphomas. I. A retrospective clinical and pathologic analysis of 499 cases diagnosed between 1958 and 1969. Cancer 1983, **51**: 101–109.

1063 Tam W, Gomez M, Chadburn A, Lee JW, Chan WC, Knowles DM. Mutational analysis of PRDM1 indicates a tumor-suppressor role in diffuse large B-cell lymphomas. Blood 2006, **107**: 4090–4100.

1064 Tsang WY, Chan JK, Tang SK, Tse CC, Cheung MM. Large cell lymphoma with fibrillary matrix. Histopathology 1992, **20**: 80–82.

1065 Tse CC, Chan JK, Yuen RW, Ng CS. Malignant lymphoma with myxoid stroma. A new pattern in need of recognition. Histopathology 1991, **18**: 31–35.

1066 Veronesi U, Musumeci R, Pizzetti F, Gennari L, Bonadonna G. The value of staging laparotomy in non-Hodgkin's lymphomas (with emphasis on the histiocytic type). Cancer 1974, **33**: 446–459.

1067 Waldron JA Jr, Newcomer LN, Katz ME, Cadman E. Sclerosing variants of follicular center cell lymphomas presenting in the retroperitoneum. Cancer 1983, **52**: 712–720.

1068 Wang J, Sun NCJ, Nozawa Y, Arber DA, Chu P, Chang KL, Weiss LM. Histological and immunohistochemical characterization of extranodal diffuse large-cell lymphomas with prominent spindle cell features. Histopathology 2001, **39**: 476–481.

1069 Wang X, Li Z, Naganuma A, Ye BH. Negative autoregulation of BCL-6 is bypassed by genetic alterations in diffuse large B cell lymphomas. Proc Natl Acad Sci U S A 2002, **99**: 15018–15023.

1070 Wang J, Sun NC, Chen YY, Weiss LM. T-cell/histiocyte-rich large B-cell lymphoma displays a heterogeneity similar to diffuse large B-cell lymphoma: a clinicopathologic, immunohistochemical, and molecular study of 30 cases. Appl Immunohistochem Mol Morphol 2005, **13**: 109–115.

1071 Warnke RA, Kim H, Fuks Z, Dorfman RE. The coexistence of nodular and diffuse patterns in nodular non-Hodgkin's lymphomas. Significance and clinicopathologic correlation. Cancer 1977, **40**: 1229–1233.

1072 Weiss RL, Kjeldsberg CR, Colby TV, Marty J. Multilobated B-cell lymphomas. A study of 7 cases. Hematol Oncol 1985, **3**: 79–86.

1073 Weiss LM, Wood GS, Dorfman RF. T-cell signet-ring cell lymphoma. A histologic, ultrastructural, and immunohistochemical study of two cases. Am J Surg Pathol 1985, **9**: 273–280.

1074 Xu Y, McKenna RW, Doolittle JE, Hladik CL, Kroft SH. The t(14;18) in diffuse large B-cell lymphoma: correlation with germinal center-associated markers and clinical features. Appl Immunohistochem Mol Morphol 2005, **13**: 116–123.

1075 Yegappan S, Coupland R, Arber DA, Wand N, Miocibovic R, Tubbs RR, Hsi ED. Angiotropic lymphoma: an immunophenotypically and clinically heterogeneous lymphoma. Mod Pathol 2001, **14**: 1147–1156.

Peripheral (post-thymic) T-cell and NK-cell lymphomas

1076 Attygalle AD, Kyriakou C, Dupuis J, Grogg KL, Diss TC, Wotherspoon AC, Chuang SS, Cabeçadas J, Isaacson PG, Du MQ, Gaulard P, Dogan A. Histologic evolution of angioimmunoblastic T-cell lymphoma in consecutive biopsies: clinical correlation and insights into natural history and disease progression. Am J Surg Pathol 2007, **31**: 1077–1088.

1077 Ballester B, Ramuz O, Gisselbrecht C, Doucet G, Loï L, Loriod B, Bertucci F, Bouabdallah R, Devilard E, Carbuccia N, Mozziconacci MJ, Birnbaum D, Brousset P, Berger F, Salles G, Brière J, Houlgatte R, Gaulard P, Xerri L. Gene expression profiling identifies molecular subgroups among nodal peripheral T-cell lymphomas. Oncogene 2006, **25**:.1560–1570.

1078 Burke JS, Butler JJ. Malignant lymphoma with a high content of epithelioid histiocytes (Lennert's lymphoma). Am J Clin Pathol 1976, **66**: 1–9.

1079 Cabeçadas JM, Isaacson PG. Phenotyping of T-cell lymphomas in paraffin sections – which antibodies? Histopathology 1991, **19**: 419–424.

1080 de Leval L, Rickman DS, Thielen C, Reynies A, Huang YL, Delsol G, Lamant L, Leroy K, Brière J, Molina T, Berger F, Gisselbrecht C, Xerri L, Gaulard P. The gene expression profile of nodal peripheral T-cell lymphoma demonstrates a molecular link between angioimmunoblastic T-cell lymphoma (AITL) and follicular helper T (TFH) cells. Blood 2007, **109**: 4952–4963.

1081 Dupuis J, Emile JF, Mounier N, Gisselbrecht C, Martin-Garcia N, Petrella T, Bouabdallah R, Berger F, Delmer A, Coiffier B, Reyes F, Gaulard P; Groupe d'Etude des Lymphomes de l'Adulte (GELA). Prognostic significance of Epstein–Barr virus in nodal peripheral T-cell lymphoma, unspecified: a Groupe d'Etude des Lymphomes de l'Adulte (GELA) study. Blood 2006, **108**: 4163–4169.

1082 Feldman AL, Law M, Remstein ED, Macon WR, Erickson LA, Grogg KL, Kurtin PJ, Dogan A. Recurrent translocations involving the IRF4 oncogene locus in peripheral T-cell lymphomas. Leukemia 2009, **23**: 574–580.

1083 Geissinger E, Odenwald T, Lee SS, Bonzheim I, Roth S, Reimer P, Wilhelm M, Müller-Hermelink HK, Rüdiger T. Nodal peripheral T-cell lymphomas and, in particular, their lymphoepithelioid (Lennert's) variant are often derived from CD8(+) cytotoxic T-cells. Virchows Arch 2004, **445**: 334–343.

1084 Ichimura K, Kagami Y, Suzuki R, Kojima M, Yoshino T, Ohshima K, Koike K, Kondo E, Taji H, Ogura M, Morishima Y, Akagi T, Takahashi T, Nakamura S. Phenotypic analysis of peripheral T/NK cell lymphoma: study of 408 Japanese cases with special reference to their anatomical sites. Pathol Int 2003, **53**: 333–344.

1085 Iqbal J, Weisenburger DD, Greiner TC, Vose JM, McKeithan T, Kucuk C, Geng H, Deffenbacher K, Smith L, Dybkaer K, Nakamura S, Seto M, Delabie J, Berger F, Loong F, Au WY, Ko YH, Sng I, Armitage JO, Chan WC; International Peripheral T-Cell Lymphoma Project. Molecular signatures to improve diagnosis in peripheral T-cell lymphoma and prognostication in angioimmunoblastic T-cell lymphoma. Blood 2010, **115**: 1026–1036.

1086 Kazakov DV, Kempf W, Michaelis S, Schmid U, Cogliatti S, Dummer R, Burg G. T-zone lymphoma with cutaneous involvement: a case report and review of the literature. Br J Dermatol 2002, **146**: 1096–1100.

1087 Kim H, Jacobs C, Warnke RA, Dorfman RF. Malignant lymphoma with a high content of epithelioid histiocytes. A distinct clinicopathologic entity and a form of so-called 'Lennert's lymphoma.' Cancer 1978, **41**: 620–635.

1088 Klein MA, Jaffe R, Neiman RS. 'Lennert's lymphoma' with transformation to malignant lymphoma, histiocytic type (immunoblastic sarcoma). Am J Clin Pathol 1977, **68**: 601–605.

1089 Ko YH, Cho EY, Kim JE, Lee SS, Huh JR, Chang HK, Yang WI, Kim CW, Kim SW, Ree HJ. NK and NK-like T-cell lymphoma in extranasal sites: a comparative clinicopathological study according to site and EBV status. Histopathology 2004, **44**: 480–489.

1090 Lachenal F, Berger F, Ghesquières H, Biron P, Hot A, Callet-Bauchu E, Chassagne C, Coiffier B, Durieu I, Rousset H, Salles G. Angioimmunoblastic T-cell lymphoma: clinical and laboratory features at diagnosis in 77 patients. Medicine (Baltimore) 2007, **86**: 282–292.

1091 Lennert K, Mestdagh J. Lymphogranulomatosen mit konstant hohem Epitheloidzellgehalt. Virchows Arch [A] 1968, **344**: 1–20.

1092 Macon WR, Williams ME, Greer JP, Cousar JB. Paracortical nodular T-cell lymphoma. Identification of an unusual variant of peripheral T-cell lymphoma. Am J Surg Pathol 1995, **19**: 297–303.

1093 Mukai HY, Hasegawa Y, Kojima H, Okoshi Y, Takei N, Yamashita Y, Nagasawa T, Mori N. Nodal CD8 positive cytotoxic T-cell lymphoma: a distinct clinicopathological entity. Mod Pathol 2002, **15**: 1131–1139.

1094 Nelson M, Horsman DE, Weisenburger DD, Gascoyne RD, Dave BJ, Loberiza FR, Ludkovski O, Savage KJ, Armitage JO, Sanger WG. Cytogenetic abnormalities and clinical correlations in peripheral T-cell lymphoma. Br J Haematol 2008, **141**: 461–469.

1095 Ohshima K, Suzumiya J, Kikuchi M. The World Health Organization classification of malignant lymphoma: incidence and clinical prognosis in HTLV-1-endemic area of Fukuoka. Pathol Int 2002, **52**: 1–12.

1096 Patsouris E, Noël H, Lennert K. Histological and immunohistological findings in lymphoepithelioid cell lymphoma (Lennert's lymphoma). Am J Surg Pathol 1988, **12**: 341–350.

1097 Piccaluga PP, Agostinelli C, Califano A, Carbone A, Fantoni L, Ferrari S, Gazzola A, Gloghini A, Righi S, Rossi M, Tagliafico E, Zinzani PL, Zupo S, Baccarani M, Pileri SA. Gene expression analysis of angioimmunoblastic lymphoma indicates derivation from T follicular helper cells and vascular endothelial growth factor deregulation. Cancer Res 2007, **67**: 10703–10710.

1098 Piccaluga PP, Agostinelli C, Califano A, Rossi M, Basso K, Zupo S, Went P, Klein U, Zinzani PL, Baccarani M, Dalla Favera R, Pileri SA. Gene expression analysis of peripheral T cell lymphoma, unspecified, reveals distinct profiles and new potential therapeutic targets. J Clin Invest 2007, **117**: 823–834.

1099 Pinkus GS, Said JW, Hargreaves H. Malignant lymphoma, T-cell type. A distinct morphologic variant with large multilobulated nuclei, with a report of four cases. Am J Clin Pathol 1979, **72**: 540–550.

1100 Rudiger T, Ichinohasama R, Ott MM, Muller-Deubert S, Miura I, Ott G, Müller-Hermelink HK. Peripheral T-cell lymphoma with distinct perifollicular growth pattern: a distinct subtype of T-cell lymphoma. Am J Surg Pathol 2000, **24**: 117–122.

1101 Schlegelberger B, Zhang Y, Weber-Matthiesen K, Grote W. Detection of aberrant clones in nearly all cases of angioimmunoblastic lymphadenopathy with dysproteinemia-type T-cell lymphoma by combined interphase and metaphase cytogenetics. Blood 1994, **84**: 2640–2648.

1102 Sheibani K, Wu A, Ben-Ezra J, Stroup R, Rappaport H, Winberg C. Rearrangement of kappa-chain and T-cell receptor b-chain genes in malignant lymphomas of 'T-cell' phenotype. Am J Pathol 1987, **129**: 201–207.

1103 Smith JL, Hodges E, Quin CT, McCarthy KP, Wright DH. Frequent T and B cell oligoclones in histologically and immunophenotypically characterized angioimmunoblastic lymphadenopathy. Am J Pathol 2000, **156**: 661–669.

1104 Spier CM, Lippman SM, Miller TP, Grogan TM. Lennert's lymphoma. A clinicopathologic study with emphasis on phenotype and its relationship to survival. Cancer 1988, **61**: 517–524.

1105 Streubel B, Vinatzer U, Willheim M, Raderer M, Chott A. Novel t(5;9)(q33;q22) fuses ITK to SYK in unspecified peripheral T-cell lymphoma. Leukemia 2006, **20**: 313–318.

1106 Su I-J, Wang CH, Cheng A-L, Chen Y-C, Hsieh H-C, Chen C-J, Tien H-F, Woei-Tsay, Huang S-S, Hu C-Y, Chen P-J, Chen J-Y, Hsu H-C, Chuang S-M, Shen M-C, Kadin ME. Characterization of the spectrum of post-thymic T-cell malignancies in Taiwan. A clinicopathologic study of HTLV-1-positive and HTLV-1-negative cases. Cancer 1988, **61**: 2060–2070.

1107 Tajima K, Kuroishi T. Estimation of rate of incidence of ATL among ATLV (HTLV-I) carriers in Kyushu, Japan. Jpn J Clin Oncol 1985, **15**: 423–430.

1108 Thorns C, Bastian B, Pinkel D, Roydasgupta R, Fridlyand J, Merz H, Krokowski M, Bernd HW, Feller AC. Chromosomal aberrations in angioimmunoblastic T-cell lymphoma and peripheral T-cell lymphoma unspecified: a matrix-based CGH approach. Genes Chromosomes Cancer 2007, **46**: 37–44.

1109 van Krieken JH, Elwood L, Andrade RE, Jaffe ES, Cossman J, Medeiros LJ. Rearrangement of the T-cell receptor delta chain gene in T-cell lymphomas with a mature phenotype. Am J Pathol 1991, **139**: 161–168.

1110 Went P, Agostinelli C, Gallamini A, Piccaluga PP, Ascani S, Sabattini E, Bacci F, Falini B, Motta T, Paulli M, Artusi T, Piccioli M,Zinzani PL, Pileri SA. Marker expression in peripheral T-cell lymphoma: a proposed clinical–pathologic prognostic score. J Clin Oncol 2006, **24**: 2472–2479.

1111 Willenbrock K, Brauninger A, Hansmann ML. Frequent occurrence of B-cell lymphomas in angioimmunoblastic T-cell lymphoma and proliferation of Epstein–Barr virus-infected cells in early cases. Br J Haematol 2007, **138**: 733–739.

Anaplastic large cell lymphoma

1112 Agnarsson BA, Kadin ME. Ki-1 positive large cell lymphoma. A morphologic and immunologic study of 19 cases. Am J Surg Pathol 1988, **12**: 264–274.

1113 Anderson MM, Ross CW, Singleton TP, Sheldon S, Schnitzer B. Ki-1 anaplastic large cell lymphoma with a prominent leukemic phase. Hum Pathol 1996, **27**: 1093–1095.

1114 Ashton-Key M, Cowley GP, Smith MEF. Cadherins in reactive lymph nodes and lymphomas: high expression in anaplastic large cell lymphomas. Histopathology 1996, **28**: 55–59.

1115 Bakshi NA, Ross CW, Finn WG, Valdez R, Ruiz R, Koujok K, Schnitzer B. ALK-positive anaplastic large cell lymphoma with primary bone involvement in children. Am J Clin Pathol 2006, **125**: 57–63.

1116 Banerjee SS, Heald J, Harris M. Twelve cases of Ki-1 positive anaplastic large cell lymphoma of skin. J Clin Pathol 1991, **44**: 119–125.

1117 Beljaards RC, Kaudewitz P, Berti E, Gianotti R, Neumann C, Rosso R, Paulli M, Meijer CJ, Willemze R. Primary cutaneous CD30-positive large cell lymphoma. Definition of a new type of cutaneous lymphoma with a favorable prognosis. A European Multicenter Study of 47 patients. Cancer 1993, **71**: 2097–2104.

1118 Chan JK. The perivascular cuff of large lymphoid cells: a clue to diagnosis of anaplastic large cell lymphoma. Int J Surg Pathol 2000, **8**: 153–156.

1119 Chan JK, Buchanan R, Fletcher CD. Sarcomatoid variant of anaplastic large-cell Ki-1 lymphoma. Am J Surg Pathol 1990, **14**: 983–988.

1120 Chan JK, Ng CS, Hui PK, Leung TW, Lo ES, Lau WH, McGuire LJ. Anaplastic large cell Ki-1 lymphoma. Delineation of two morphological types. Histopathology 1989, **15**: 11–34.

1121 Chan JK, Ng CS, Hui PK, Leung WT, Sin VC, Lam TK, Chick KW, Lam WY. Anaplastic large cell Ki-1 lymphoma of bone. Cancer 1991, **68**: 2186–2191.

1122 Chan JK, Lamant L, Algar E, Delsol G, Tsang WY, Lee KC, Tiedemann K, Chow CW. ALK+ histiocytosis: a novel type of systemic histiocytic proliferative disorder of early infancy. Blood 2008, **112**: 2965–2968.

1123 Cheuk W, Hill RW, Bacchi C, Dias MA, Chan JK. Hypocellular anaplastic large cell lymphoma mimicking inflammatory lesions of lymph nodes. Am J Surg Pathol 2000, **24**: 1537–1543.

1124 Chott A, Kaserer K, Augustin I, Vesely M, Heinz R, Oehlinger W, Hanak H, Radaszkiewicz T. Ki-1 positive large cell lymphoma. A clinicopathologic study of 41 cases. Am J Surg Pathol 1990, **14**: 439–448.

1125 Coffin CM, Patel A, Perkins S, Elenitoba-Johnson KS, Perlman E, Griffin CA. ALK1 and p80 expression and chromosomal rearrangements involving 2p23 in inflammatory myofibroblastic tumor. Mod Pathol 2001, **14**: 569–576.

1126 d'Amore ES, Menin A, Bonoldi E, Bevilacqua P, Cazzavillan S, Donofrio V, Gambini C, Forni M, Gentile A, Magro G, Boldrini R, Pillon M, Rosolen A, Alaggio R. Anaplastic large cell lymphomas: a study of 75 pediatric patients. Pediatr Dev Pathol 2007, **10**: 181–191.

1127 de Bruin PC, Beljaards RC, van Heerde P, Van Der Valk P, Noorduyn LA, Van Krieken JH, Kluin-Nelemans JC, Willemze R, Meijer CJ. Differences in clinical behaviour and immunophenotype between primary cutaneous and primary nodal anaplastic large cell lymphoma of T-cell or null cell phenotype. Histopathology 1993, **23**: 127–135.

1128 Delsol G, Al Saati T, Gatter KC, Gerdes J, Schwarting R, Caveriviere P, Rigal-Huguet F, Robert A, Stein H, Mason DY. Coexpression of epithelial membrane antigen (EMA), Ki-1, and interleukin-2 receptor by anaplastic large cell lymphomas. Diagnostic value in so-called malignant histiocytosis. Am J Pathol 1988, **130**: 59–70.

1129 Delsol G, Campo E, Gascoyne R. ALK-positive large B-cell lymphoma. In Swerdlow SH, Campo E, Harris NL, Jaffe ES, Pileri SA, Stein H, Thiele J, Vardiman JW (eds): WHO classification of tumours of haematopoietic and lymphoid tissues, ed. 4. Lyon, 2008, IARC Press, pp. 254–255.

1130 Delsol G, Falini B, Müller-Hermelink HK, Campo E, Jaffe ES, Gascoyne RD, et al. Anaplastic large cell lymphoma (ALCL), ALK-positive. In Swerdlow SH, Campo E, Harris NL, Jaffe ES, Pileri SA, Stein H, Thiele J, Vardiman JW (eds): WHO classification of tumours of haematopoietic and lymphoid tissues, ed. 4. Lyon, 2008, IARC Press, pp. 312–316.

1131 Falini B, Bigerna B, Fizzotti M, Pulford K, Pileri SA, Delsol G, Carbone A, Paulli M, Magrini U, Menestrina F, Giardini R, Pilotti S, Mezzelani A, Ugolini B, Billi M, Pucciarini A, Pacini R, Pelicci PG, Flenghi L. ALK expression defines a distinct group of T/null lymphomas ('ALK lymphomas') with a wide morphological spectrum. Am J Pathol 1998, **153**: 875–886.

1132 Falini B, Liso A, Pasqualucci L, Flenghi L, Ascani S, Pileri S, Bucciarelli E. CD30+ anaplastic large-cell lymphoma, null type, with signet-ring appearance. Histopathology 1997, **30**: 90–92.

1133 Falini B, Pulford K, Pucciarini A, Carbone A, De Wolf-Peeters C, Cordell J, Fizzotti M, Santucci A, Pelicci PG, Pileri S, Campo E, Ott G, Delsol G, Mason DY. Lymphomas expressing ALK fusion protein(s) other than NPM-ALK. Blood 1999, **94**: 3509–3515.

1134 Feldman AL, Law M, Remstein ED, Macon WR, Erickson LA, Grogg KL, Kurtin PJ, Dogan A. Recurrent translocations involving the IRF4 oncogene locus in peripheral T-cell lymphomas. Leukemia 2009, **23**: 574–580.

1135 Flynn KJ, Dehner LP, Gajl-Peczalska KJ, Dahl MV, Ramsay N, Wang N. Regressing atypical histiocytosis. A cutaneous proliferation of atypical neoplastic histiocytes with unexpectedly indolent biologic behavior. Cancer 1982, **49**: 959–970.

1136 Greer JP, Kinney MC, Collins RD, Salhany KE, Wolff SN, Hainsworth JD, Flexner JM, Stein RS. Clinical features of 31 patients with Ki-1 anaplastic large-cell lymphoma. J Clin Oncol 1991, **9**: 539–547.

1137 Gustmann C, Altmannsberger M, Osborn M, Griesser H, Feller AC. Cytokeratin expression and vimentin content in large cell anaplastic lymphomas and other non-Hodgkin's lymphomas. Am J Pathol 1991, **138**: 1413–1422.

1138 Hansmann ML, Fellbaum C, Bohm A. Large cell anaplastic lymphoma. Evaluation of immunophenotype on paraffin and frozen sections in comparison with ultrastructural features. Virchows Arch [A] 1991, **418**: 427–433.

1139 Headington JT, Roth MS, Schnitzer B. Regressing atypical histiocytosis. A review and critical appraisal. Semin Diagn Pathol 1987, **4**: 28–37.

1140 Hodges KB, Collins RD, Greer JP, Kadin ME, Kiney MC. Transformation of the small cell variant Ki-1+ lymphoma to anaplastic large cell lymphoma: pathologic and clinical features. Am J Surg Pathol 1999, **23**: 49–58.

1141 Kadin ME. Ki-1/CD30+ (anaplastic) large-cell lymphoma. Maturation of a clinicopathologic entity with prospects of effective therapy [editorial]. J Clin Oncol 1994, **12**: 884–887.

1142 Kaudewitz P, Greer JP, Glick AD, Salhany KE, Collins RD. Anaplastic large-cell Ki-1 malignant lymphomas. Recognition, biological and clinical implications. Pathol Annu 1991, **26**(Pt 1): 1–24.

1143 Kaudewitz P, Stein H, Dallenbach F, Eckert F, Bieber K, Burg G, Braun-Falco O. Primary and secondary cutaneous Ki-1+ (CD30+) anaplastic large cell lymphomas. Morphologic, immunohistologic, and clinical characteristics. Am J Pathol 1989, **135**: 359–367.

1144 Kinney MC, Kadin ME. The pathologic and clinical spectrum of anaplastic large cell lymphoma and correlation with ALK gene dysregulation. Am J Clin Pathol 1999, **11**: S56–S67.

1145 Kinney MC, Collins RD, Greer JP, Whitlock JA, Sioutos N, Kadin ME. A small-cell-predominant variant of primary Ki-1 (CD30)+ T-cell lymphoma. Am J Surg Pathol 1993, **17**: 859–868.

1146 Klapper W, Böhm M, Siebert R, Lennert K. Morphological variability of lymphohistiocytic variant of anaplastic large cell lymphoma (former lymphohistiocytic lymphoma according to the Kiel classification). Virchows Arch 2008, **452**: 599–605.

1147 Konstantinov KN, Robbins BA, Liu FT. Galectin-3, a beta-galactoside-binding animal lectin, is a marker of anaplastic large-cell lymphoma. Am J Pathol 1996, **148**: 25–30.

1148 Lamant L, de Reyniès A, Duplantier MM, Rickman DS, Sabourdy F, Giuriato S, Brugières L, Gaulard P, Espinos E, Delsol G. Gene-expression profiling of systemic anaplastic large-cell lymphoma reveals differences based on ALK status and two distinct morphologic ALK+ subtypes. Blood 2007, **109**: 2156–2164.

1149 Laurent C, Do C, Gascoyne RD, Lamant L, Ysebaert L, Laurent G, Delsol G, Brousset P. Anaplastic lymphoma kinase-positive diffuse large B-cell lymphoma: a rare clinicopathologic entity with poor prognosis. J Clin Oncol 2009, **27**: 4211–4216.

1150 McCluggage WG, Walsh MY, Bharucha H. Anaplastic large cell malignant lymphoma with extensive eosinophilic or neutrophilic infiltration. Histopathology 1998, **32**: 110–115.

1151 Mann KP, Hall B, Kamino H, Borowitz MJ, Ratech H. Neutrophil-rich, Ki-1-positive anaplastic large-cell malignant lymphoma. Am J Surg Pathol 1995, **19**: 407–416.

1152 Motley RJ, Jasani B, Ford AM, Poynton CH, Calonje-Daly JE, Holt PJ. Regressing atypical histiocytosis, a regressing cutaneous phase of Ki-1-positive anaplastic large cell lymphoma. Immunocytochemical, nucleic acid, and cytogenetic studies of a new case in view of current opinion. Cancer 1992, **70**: 476–483.

1153 Nascimento AF, Pinkus JL, Pinkus GS, Brigham and Women's Hospital and Harvard Medical School, Boston MA. Clusterin, a marker for anaplastic large cell lymphoma: immunohistochemical profile in hematopoietic and non-hematopoietic malignancies. Mod Pathol 2003, **16**: 246a.

1154 Nascimento AF, Pinkus JL, Pinkus GS. Clusterin, a marker for anaplastic large cell lymphoma immunohistochemical profile in hematopoietic and nonhematopoietic malignant neoplasms. Am J Clin Pathol 2004, **121**: 709–717.

1155 Pham-Ledard A, Prochazkova-Carlotti M, Laharanne E, Vergier B, Jouary T, Beylot-Barry M, Merlio JP. IRF4 gene rearrangements define a subgroup of CD30-positive cutaneous T-cell lymphoma: a study of 54 cases. J Invest Dermatol 2010, **130**: 816–825.

1156 Pileri S, Bocchia M, Baroni CD, Martelli M, Falini B, Sabattini E, Gherlinzoni F, Amadori S, Poggi S, Mazza P, et al. Anaplastic large cell lymphoma (CD30+/Ki-1+). Results of a prospective clinico-pathological study of 69 cases. Br J Haematol 1994, **86**: 513–523.

1157 Pileri S, Falini B, Delsol G, Stein H, Baglioni P, Poggi S, Martelli MF, Rivano MT, Mason DY, Stansfeld AG. Lymphohistiocytic T-cell lymphoma (anaplastic large cell lymphoma CD301/Kil 1 with a high content of reactive histiocytes). Histopathology 1990, **16**: 383–391.

1158 Pileri SA, Pulford K, Mori S, Mason DY, Sabattini E, Roncador G, Piccioli M, Ceccarelli C, Piccaluga PP, Santini D, Leone O, Stein H, Falini B. Frequent expression of the NPM-ALK chimeric fusion protein in anaplastic large-cell lymphoma, lympho-histocytic type. Am J Pathol 1997, **150**: 1207–1211.

1159 Rodig SJ, Mino-Kenudson M, Dacic S, Yeap BY, Shaw A, Barletta JA, Stubbs H, Law K, Lindeman N, Mark E, Janne PA, Lynch T, Johnson BE, Iafrate AJ, Chirieac LR. Unique clinicopathologic features characterize ALK-rearranged lung adenocarcinoma in the western population. Clin Cancer Res 2009, **15**: 5216–5223.

1160 Shulman LN, Frisard B, Antin JH, Wheeler C, Pinkus G, Magauran N, Mauch P, Nobles E, Mashal R, Cancellos G, et al. Primary Ki-1 anaplastic large-cell lymphoma in adults. Clinical characteristics and therapeutic outcome. J Clin Oncol 1993, **11**: 937–942.

1161 Soda M, Choi YL, Enomoto M, Takada S, Yamashita Y, Ishikawa S, Fujiwara S, Watanabe H, Kurashina K, Hatanaka H, Bando M, Ohno S, Ishikawa Y, Aburatani H, Niki T, Sohara Y, Sugiyama Y, Mano H. Identification of the transforming EML4–ALK fusion gene in non-small-cell lung cancer. Nature 2007, **448**: 561–566.

1162 Stein H, Foss HD, Dürkop H, Marafioti T, Delsol G, Pulford K, Pileri S, Falini B. CD30(+) anaplastic large cell lymphoma: a review of its histopathologic, genetic, and clinical features. Blood 2000, **96**: 3681–3695.

1163 Tan BT, Seo K, Warnke RA, Arber DA. The frequency of immunoglobulin heavy chain gene and T-cell receptor gamma-chain gene rearrangements and Epstein–Barr virus in ALK+ and ALK– anaplastic large cell lymphoma and other peripheral T-cell lymphomas. J Mol Diagn 2008, **10**: 502–512.

1164 Wong KF, Chan JK, Ng CS, Chu YC, Lam PW, Yuen HL. Anaplastic large cell Ki-1 lymphoma involving bone marrow. Marrow findings and association with reactive hemophagocytosis. Am J Hematol 1991, **37**: 112–119.

1165 Zinzani P, Bendandi M, Martelli M, Falini B, Sabattini E, Amadori S, Gherlinzoni F, Martelli MF, Mandelli F, Tura S, Pileri SA. Anaplastic large-cell lymphoma: clinical and prognostic evaluation of 90 adult patients. J Clin Oncol 1996, **14**: 955–962.

Lymphoblastic lymphoma

1166 Brownell MD, Sheibani K, Battifora H, Winberg CD, Rappaport H. Distinction between undifferentiated (small noncleaved) and lymphoblastic lymphoma. An immunohistologic study on paraffin-embedded, fixed tissue sections. Am J Surg Pathol 1987, **11**: 779–787.

1167 Donlon JA, Jaffe ES, Braylan RC. Terminal deoxynucleotidyl transferase activity in malignant lymphomas. N Engl J Med 1977, **297**: 461–464.

1168 Griffith RC, Kelly DR, Nathwani BN, Shuster JJ, Murphy SB, Hvizdala E, Sullivan MP, Berard CW. A morphologic study of childhood lymphoma of the lymphoblastic type. The Pediatric Oncology Group experience. Cancer 1987, **59**: 1126–1131.

1169 Jaffe ES, Braylan RC, Frank MM, Green I, Berard CW. Heterogeneity of immunologic markers and surface morphology in childhood lymphoblastic lymphoma. Blood 1976, **48**: 213–222.

1170 Karube K, Ohshima K, Tsuchiya T, Yamaguchi T, Suefuji H, Suzumiya J, Harada M, Kikuchi M. Non-B, non-T neoplasms with lymphoblast morphology. Am J Surg Pathol 2003, **27**: 1366–1374.

1171 Lin P, Jones D, Dorfman DM, Medeiros LJ. Precursor B-cell lymphoblastic lymphoma: a predominantly extranodal tumor with low propensity for leukemic involvement. Am J Surg Pathol 2000, **24**: 1480–1490.

1172 Nathwani BN, Kim H, Rappaport H. Malignant lymphoma, lymphoblastic. Cancer 1976, **38**: 964–983.

1173 Orazi A, Cattoretti G, John K, Neiman RS. Terminal deoxynucleotidyl transferase staining of malignant lymphomas in paraffin sections. Mod Pathol 1994, **7**: 582–586.

1174 Ozdemirli M, Fanburg-Smith JC, Hartmann DP, Azumi N, Miettinen M. Differentiating lymphoblastic lymphoma and Ewing's sarcoma: lymphocyte markers and gene rearrangement. Mod Pathol 2001, **14**: 1175–1182.

1175 Pangalis GA, Nathwani BN, Rappaport H, Rosen RB. Acute lymphoblastic leukemia. The significance of nuclear convolutions. Cancer 1979, **43**: 551–557.

1176 Picozzi VJ Jr, Coleman CN. Lymphoblastic lymphoma. Semin Oncol 1990, **17**: 96–103.

1177 Pinkus GS, Hargreaves HK, McLeod JA, Nadler LM, Rosenthal DS, Said JW. α-Naphthyl acetate esterase activity. A cytochemical marker for T lymphocytes. Correlation with immunologic studies of normal tissues, lymphocytic leukemias, non-Hodgkin's lymphomas, Hodgkin's disease, and other lymphoproliferative disorders. Am J Pathol 1979, **97**: 17–42.

1178 Pui C-H, Relling MV, Pharm D, Downing JR. Acute lymphoblastic leukemia. N Engl Med 2004, **350**: 1535–1548.

1179 Rosen PJ, Feinstein DI, Pattengale PK, Tindle BH, Williams AH, Cain MJ, Bonorris JB, Parker JW, Lukes RJ. Convoluted lymphocytic lymphoma in adults. A clinicopathologic entity. Ann Intern Med 1978, **89**: 319–324.

1180 Said JW, Shintaku IP, Pinkus GS. Immunohistochemical staining for terminal deoxynucleotidyl transferase (TDT). An enhanced method in routinely processed formalin-fixed tissue sections. Am J Clin Pathol 1988, **89**: 649–652.

1181 Sheibani K, Nathwani BN, Winberg CD, Burke JS, Swartz WG, Blayney D, van de Velde S, Hill LR, Rappaport H. Antigenically defined subgroups of lymphoblastic lymphoma. Relationship to clinical presentation and biologic behavior. Cancer 1987, **60**: 183–190.

1182 Soslow RA, Bhargava V, Warnke RA. MIC2, Tdt, bcl-2, and CD34 expression in paraffin-embedded high-grade lymphoma/acute lymphoblastic leukemia distinguishes between distinct clinicopathologic entities. Hum Pathol 1997, **28**: 1158–1165.

1183 Soslow RA, Zukerberg LR, Harris NL, Warnke RA. BCL-1 (PRAD-1/cyclin D-1) overexpresion distinguishes the blastoid variant of mantle cell lymphoma from B-lineage lymphoblastic lymphoma. Mod Pathol 1997, **10**: 810–817.

BURKITT LYMPHOMA

1184 Arseneau JC, Canellos GP, Banks PM, Berard CW, Gralnick HR, DeVita VT Jr. American Burkitt's lymphoma. A clinicopathologic study of 30 cases. I. Clinical factors relating to prolonged survival. Am J Med 1975, **58**: 314–321.

1185 Banks PM, Arseneau JC, Gralnick HR, Cannellos GP, DeVita VT Jr, Berard CW. American Burkitt's lymphoma. A clinicopathologic study of 30 cases. II. Pathologic correlations. Am J Med 1975, **58**: 322–329.

1186 Berard CB, O'Connor GT, Thomas LB, Torloni H. Histopathologic definition of Burkitt's tumor. Bull WHO 1969, **40**: 601–608.

1187 Bernhard W. Fine structure of Burkitt's lymphoma. In Burkitt DP, Wright DH (eds): Burkitt's lymphoma. Edinburgh, 1970, E and S Livingstone, pp. 103–117.

1188 Dang CV. c-Myc target genes involved in cell growth, apoptosis, and metabolism. Mol Cell Biol 1999, **19**: 1–11.

1189 Dave SS, Fu K, Wright GW, Lam LT, Kluin P, Boerma EJ, Greiner TC, Weisenburger DD, Rosenwald A, Ott G, Müller-Hermelink HK, Gascoyne RD, Delabie J, Rimsza LM, Braziel RM, Grogan TM, Campo E, Jaffe ES, Dave BJ, Sanger W, Bast M, Vose JM, Armitage JO, Connors JM, Smeland EB, Kvaloy S, Holte H, Fisher RI, Miller TP, Montserrat E, Wilson WH, Bahl M, Zhao H, Yang L, Powell J, Simon R, Chan WC, Staudt LM; Lymphoma/Leukemia Molecular Profiling Project. Molecular diagnosis of Burkitt's lymphoma. N Engl J Med 2006, **354**: 2431–2442.

1190 Davi F, Delecluse HJ, Guiet P, Gabarre J, Fayon A, Gentilhomme O, Felman P, Bayle C, Berger F, Audouin J, Bryon PA, Diebold J, Raphael M. Burkett-like lymphomas in AIDS patients: characterization within a series of 103 human immunodeficiency virus-associated non-Hodgkin's lymphomas. J Clin Oncol 1999, **16**: 3788–3795.

1191 Garcia CF, Weiss LM, Warnke RA. Small noncleaved cell lymphoma. An immunophenotypic study of 18 cases and comparison with large cell lymphoma. Hum Pathol 1986, **17**: 454–461.

1192 Haralambieva E, Rosati S, van Noesel C, Boers E, van Marwijk Kooy M, Schuuring E, Kluin P. Florid granulomatous reaction in Epstein–Barr virus-positive nonendemic Burkitt lymphomas: report of four cases. Am J Surg Pathol 2004, **28**: 379–383.

1193 Haralambieva E, Boerma EJ, van Imhoff GW, Rosati S, Schuuring E, Müller-Hermelink HK, Kluin PM, Ott G. Clinical, immunophenotypic, and genetic analysis of adult lymphomas with morphologic features of Burkitt lymphoma. Am J Surg Pathol 2005, **29**: 1086–1094.

1194 Haralambieva E, Boerma EJ, van Imhoff GW, Rosati S, Schuuring E, Müller-Hermelink HK, Kluin PM, Ott G. Clinical, immunophenotypic, and genetic analysis of adult lymphomas with morphologic features of Burkitt lymphoma. Am J Surg Pathol 2005, **29**: 1086–1094.

1195 Hummel M, Bentink S, Berger H, Klapper W, Wessendorf S, Barth TF, Bernd HW, Cogliatti SB, Dierlamm J, Feller AC, Hansmann ML, Haralambieva E, Harder L, Hasenclever D, Kühn M, Lenze D, Lichter P, Martin-Subero JI, Möller P, Müller-Hermelink HK, Ott G, Parwaresch RM, Pott C, Rosenwald A, Rosolowski M, Schwaenen C, Stürzenhofecker B, Szczepanowski M, Trautmann H, Wacker HH, Spang R, Loeffler M, Trümper L, Stein H, Siebert R; Molecular Mechanisms in Malignant Lymphomas Network Project of the Deutsche Krebshilfe. A biologic definition of Burkitt's lymphoma from transcriptional and genomic profiling. N Engl J Med 2006, **354**: 2419–2430.

1196 Johnson NA, Savage KJ, Ludkovski O, Ben-Neriah S, Woods R, Steidl C, Dyer MJ, Siebert R, Kuruvilla J, Klasa R, Connors JM, Gascoyne RD, Horsman DE. Lymphomas with concurrent BCL2 and MYC translocations: the critical factors associated with survival. Blood 2009, **114**: 2273–2279.

1197 Klapper W, Stoecklein H, Zeynalova S, Ott G, Kosari F, Rosenwald A, Loeffler M, Trümper L, Pfreundschuh M, Siebert R; German High-Grade Non-Hodgkin's Lymphoma Study Group. Structural aberrations affecting the MYC locus indicate a poor prognosis independent of clinical risk factors in diffuse large B-cell lymphomas treated within randomized trials of the German High-Grade Non-Hodgkin's Lymphoma Study Group (DSHNHL). Leukemia 2008, **22**: 2226–2229.

1198 Leoncini L, Raphael M, Stein H, Harris NL, Jaffe ES, Kluin P. Burkitt lymphoma. In Swerdlow SH, Campo E, Harris NL, Jaffe ES, Pileri SA, Stein H, Thiele J, Vardiman JW (eds): WHO classification of tumours of haematopoietic and lymphoid tissues, ed. 4. Lyon, 2008, IARC Press, pp. 262–264.

1199 Levine AM, Pavlova Z, Pockros AW, Parker JW, Teitelbaum AH, Paganini-Hill A, Powars DR, Lukes RJ, Feinstein DI. Small noncleaved follicular center cell (FCC) lymphoma. Burkitt and non-Burkitt variants in the United States. Cancer 1983, **52**: 1073–1079.

1200 Mann RB, Jaffe ES, Braylan RC, Nanba K, Frank MM, Ziegler JL, Berard CW. Nonendemic Burkitt's lymphoma. A B-cell tumor related to germinal centers. N Engl J Med 1976, **295**: 685–691.

1201 Minerbrook M, Schulman P, Budman DR, Teichberg S, Vinciguerra V, Kardon N, Degnan TJ. Burkitt's leukemia. A re-evaluation. Cancer 1982, **49**: 1444–1448.

1202 Niitsu N, Okamoto M, Miura I, Hirano M. Clinical features and prognosis of de novo diffuse large B-cell lymphoma with t(14;18) and 8q24/c-MYC translocations. Leukemia 2009, **23**: 777–783.

1203 Nkrumah FK, Perkins IV. Burkitt's lymphoma. A clinical study of 100 patients. Cancer 1976, **37**: 671–676.

1204 Savage KJ, Johnson NA, Ben-Neriah S, Connors JM, Sehn LH, Farinha P, Horsman DE, Gascoyne RD. MYC gene rearrangements are associated with a poor prognosis in diffuse large B-cell lymphoma patients treated with R-CHOP chemotherapy. Blood 2009, **114**: 3533–3537.

1205 Spina M, Tirelli U, Zagonel V, Gioghini A, Volpe R, Babare R, Abbruzzese L, Talamini R, Vaccher E, Carbone A. Burkitt's lymphoma in adults with and without human immunodeficiency virus infection: a single-institution clinicopathologic study of 75 patients. Cancer 1998, **82**: 766–774.

1206 Ziegler JL. Treatment results of 54 American patients with Burkitt's lymphoma are similar to the African experience. N Engl J Med 1977, **297**: 75–80.

Other non-Hodgkin lymphomas

1207 Burke JS, Byrne GE Jr, Rappaport H. Hairy cell leukemia (leukemic reticuloendotheliosis). I. A clinical pathologic study of 21 patients. Cancer 1974, **33**: 1399–1410.

1208 Müller-Hermelink HK, Stein H, Steinmann G, Lennert K. Malignant lymphoma of plasmacytoid T-cells. Morphologic and immunologic studies characterizing a special type of T-cell. Am J Surg Pathol 1983, **7**: 849–862.

1209 Prasthofer EF, Grizzle WE, Prchal JT, Grossi CE. Plasmacytoid T-cell lymphoma associated with chronic myeloproliferative disorder. Am J Surg Pathol 1985, **9**: 380–387.

COMPOSITE AND DISCORDANT LYMPHOMAS

1210 Abruzzo LV, Griffith LM, Nandedkar M, Aguilera NS, Taubenberger JK, Raffeld M, Stass SA, Abbondanzo SL, Jaffe ES. Histologically discordant lymphomas with B-cell and T-cell components. Am J Clin Pathol 1997, **108**: 316–323.

1211 Alsabeh R, Medeiros LJ, Glackin C, Weiss LM. Transformation of follicular lymphoma into CD30-large cell lymphoma with anaplastic cytologic features. Am J Surg Pathol 1997, **21**: 528–536.

1212 Brown JR, Weng AP, Freedman AS. Hodgkin disease associated with T-cell non-Hodgkin lymphomas: case reports and review of the literature. Am J Clin Pathol 2004, **121**: 701–708.

1213 Cerroni L, Rieger E, Hodl S, Kerl H. Clinicopathologic and immunologic features associated with transformation of mycosis fungoides to large-cell lymphoma. Am J Surg Pathol 1992, **16**: 543–552.

1214 Chan WC, Griem ML, Grozea PN, Freel RJ, Variakojis D. Mycosis fungoides and Hodgkin's disease occurring in the same patient. Report of three cases. Cancer 1979, **44**: 1408–1413.

1215 Cossman J, Schnitzer B, Deegan MJ. Coexistence of two lymphomas with distinctive histologic, ultrastructural, and immunologic features. Am J Clin Pathol 1978, **70**: 409–415.

1216 Cullen MH, Lister TA, Brearley RI, Shand WS, Stansfield AG. Histological transformation of non-Hodgkin's lymphoma. A prospective study. Cancer 1979, **44**: 645–651.

1217 Damotte D, Le Tourneau A, Audouin J, Duval C, Martin-Bastenaire F, Villain O, Delobelle-Deroide A, Diebold J. Discordant malignant lymphoma synchronous or successive high-grade B lymphoma associated with Hodgkin's disease. A clinicopathologic and immunophenotypic study of 4 cases. Pathol Res Pract 1995, **191**: 8–15.

1218 Dmitrovsky E, Matthews MJ, Bunn PA, Schechter GP, Makuch RW, Winkler CF, Eddy J, Sausville EA, Ihde DC. Cytologic transformation in cutaneous T-cell lymphoma. A clinicopathologic entity associated with poor prognosis. J Clin Oncol 1987, **5**: 208–215.

1219 Donald D, Green JA, White M. Mycosis fungoides associated with nodular sclerosing Hodgkin's disease. A case report. Cancer 1980, **46**: 2505–2508.

1220 Gonzalez CL, Medeiros LJ, Jaffe ES. Composite lymphoma. A clinicopathologic analysis of nine patients with Hodgkin's disease and B-cell non-Hodgkin's lymphoma. Am J Clin Pathol 1991, **96**: 81–89.

1221 Greer JP, Salhany KE, Cousar JB, Fields JP, King LE, Graber SE, Flexner JM, Stein RS, Collins RD. Clinical features associated with transformation of cerebriform T-cell lymphoma to a large cell process. Hematol Oncol 1990, **8**: 215–227.

1222 Grossman DM, Hanson CA, Schnitzer B. Simultaneous lymphocyte predominant Hodgkin's disease and large-cell lymphoma. Am J Surg Pathol 1991, **15**: 668–676.

1223 Hansmann ML, Fellbaum C, Hui PK, Lennert K. Morphological and immunohistochemical investigation of non-Hodgkin's lymphoma combined with Hodgkin's disease. Histopathology 1989, **15**: 35–48.

1224 Hansmann ML, Stein H, Fellbaum C, Hui PK, Parwaresch MR, Lennert K. Nodular paragranuloma can transform into high-grade malignant lymphoma of B type. Hum Pathol 1989, **20**: 1169–1175.

1225 Harris NL. The relationship between Hodgkin's disease and non-Hodgkin's lymphoma. Semin Diagn Pathol 1992, **9**: 304–310.

1226 Harvell JD, Fulton R, Jones CD, Terris DJ, Warnke RA. Composite dendritic cell neoplasm (NOS) and small lymphocytic lymphoma. Appl Immunohistochem Mol Morphol 2000, **8**: 322–328.

1227 Jaffe ES, Zarate-Osorno A, Medeiros LJ. The interrelationship of Hodgkin's disease and non-Hodgkin's lymphomas – lessons learned from composite and sequential malignancies. Semin Diagn Pathol 1992, **9**: 297–303.

1228 Kim H, Hendrickson MR, Dorfman RF. Composite lymphoma. Cancer 1977, **40**: 959–976.

1229 Kroft SH. Lymphoma transformation. Genetic relatedness, stealth lymphomas, and the final frontier. Am J Clin Pathol 2001, **116**: 811–814.

1230 Laszlo T, Matolcsy A. Blastic transformation of mantle cell lymphoma: genetic evidence for a clonal link between the two stages of the tumour. Histopathology 1999, **35**: 355–359.

1231 Mohrmann RL, Arber DA. CD20 positive peripheral T-cell lymphoma: report of a case after nodular sclerosis Hodgkin's disease and review of the literature. Mod Pathol 2001, **13**: 1244–1252.

1232 Mori N, Watanabe K, Yamashita Y, Nakayama A, Yatabe Y, Narita M, Kobayashi T, Hasegawa Y, Kojima H, Nagasawa T. Hodgkin's disease with subsequent transformation to CD30 positive non-Hodgkin's lymphoma in six patients. Cancer 1999, **85**: 970–979.

1233 Said J. Transformation to aggressive B-cell lymphoma. Appl Immuno Mol Morphol 2003, **11**: 199–205.

1234 Salhany KE, Cousar JB, Greer JP, Casey TT, Fields JP, Collins RD. Transformation of cutaneous T-cell lymphoma to large cell lymphoma. A clinicopathologic and immunologic study. Am J Pathol 1988, **132**: 265–277.

1235 Wang Q, Unger PD, Strauchen JA. T-cell-rich B-large-cell lymphoma simulating Hodgkin's disease: report of two cases with transformation to pleomorphic B-large-cell lymphoma. Int J Surg Pathol 1997, **5**: 31–36.

1236 Weisenberg E, Anastasi J, Adeyanju M, Variakojis D, Vardiman JW. Hodgkin's disease associated with chronic lymphocytic leukemia. Eight additional cases, including two of the nodular lymphocyte predominant type. Am J Clin Pathol 1995, **103**: 479–484.

1237 Weiss LM, Warnke RA. Follicular lymphoma with blastic conversion. A report of two cases with confirmation by immunoperoxidase studies on bone marrow sections. Am J Clin Pathol 1985, **83**: 681–686.

1238 Woda BA, Knowles DM II. Nodular lymphocytic lymphoma eventuating into diffuse histiocytic lymphoma. Immunoperoxidase demonstration of monoclonality. Cancer 1979, **43**: 303–307.

1239 Wood GS, Bahler DW, Hoppe RT, Warnke RA, Sklar JL, Levy R. Transformation of mycosis fungoides. T-cell receptor β gene analysis demonstrates a common clonal origin for plaque-type mycosis fungoides and CD30+ large-cell lymphoma. J Invest Dermatol 1993, **101**: 296–300.

1240 Zarate-Osorno A, Medeiros LJ, Kingma DW, Longo DL, Jaffe ES. Hodgkin's disease following non-Hodgkin's lymphoma. A clinicopathologic and immunophenotypic study of nine cases. Am J Surg Pathol 1993, **17**: 123–132.

1241 Zarate-Osorno A, Medeiros LJ, Longo DL, Jaffe ES. Non-Hodgkin's lymphomas arising in patients successfully treated for Hodgkin's disease. A clinical, histologic, and immunophenotypic study of 14 cases. Am J Surg Pathol 1992, **16**: 885–895.

1242 Zelenetz AD, Chen TT, Levy R. Histologic transformation of follicular lymphoma to diffuse lymphoma represents tumor progression by a single malignant B-cell. J Exp Med 1991, **173**: 197–207.

1243 Zettl A, Rüdiger T, Marx A, Müller-Hermelink HK, Ott G. Composite marginal zone B-cell lymphoma and classical Hodgkin's lymphoma: a clinicopathological study of 12 cases. Histopathology 2005, **46**: 217–228.

SO-CALLED 'MALIGNANT HISTIOCYTOSIS'

1244 Aozasa K, Tsujimoto M, Inoue A. Malignant histiocytosis. Report of twenty five cases with pulmonary, renal and/or gastro-intestinal involvement. Histopathology 1985, **9**: 39–49.

1245 Byrne GE Jr, Rappaport H. Malignant histiocytosis. Gann Monogr Cancer Res 1973, **15**: 145–162.

1246 Cattoretti G, Villa A, Vezzoni P, Giardini R, Lombardi L, Rilke F. Malignant histiocytosis. A phenotypic and genotypic investigation. Am J Pathol 1990, **136**: 1009–1019.

1247 Colby TV, Carrington CB, Mark GJ. Pulmonary involvement in malignant histiocytosis. A clinicopathologic spectrum. Am J Surg Pathol 1981, **5**: 61–73.

1248 Ducatman BS, Wick MR, Morgan TW, Banks PM, Pierre RV. Malignant histiocytosis. A clinical, histologic and immunohistochemical study of 20 cases. Hum Pathol 1984, **15**: 368–377.

1249 Griffin JD, Ellman L, Long JC, Dvorak AM. Development of a histiocytic medullary reticulosislike syndrome during the course of acute lymphocytic leukemia. Am J Med 1978, **64**: 851–858.

1250 Hsu SM, Ho YS, Hsu PL. Lymphomas of true histiocytic origin. Expression of different phenotypes in so-called true histiocytic lymphoma and malignant histiocytosis. Am J Pathol 1991, **138**: 1389–1404.

1251 Huhn D, Meister P. Malignant histiocytosis. Morphologic and cytochemical findings. Cancer 1978, **42**: 1341–1349.

1252 Karcher DS, Head DR, Mullins JD. Malignant histiocytosis occurring in patients with acute lymphocytic leukemia. Cancer 1978, **41**: 1967–1973.

1253 Lombardi L, Carbone A, Pilotti S, Rilke F. Malignant histiocytosis. A histological and ultrastructural study of lymph nodes in six cases. Histopathology 1978, **2**: 315–328.

1254 Mendelsohn G, Eggleston JC, Mann RB. Relationship of lysozyme (muramidase) to histiocytic differentiation in malignant histiocytosis. An immunohistochemical study. Cancer 1980, **45**: 273–279.

1255 Ost A, Nilsson-Ardnor S, Henter JI. Autopsy findings in 27 children with haemophagocytic lymphohistiocytosis. Histopathology 1998, **32**: 310–316.

1256 Perry MC, Harrison EG Jr, Burgert EO, Gilchrist GS. Familial erythrophagocytic lymphohistiocytosis. Report of two cases and clinicopathologic review. Cancer 1976, **38**: 209–218.

1257 Pileri S, Mazza P, Rivano MT, Martinelli G, Cavazzini G, Gobbi M, Taruscio D, Lauria F, Tura S. Malignant histiocytosis (true histiocytic lymphoma) clinicopathological study of 25 cases. Histopathology 1985, **9**: 905–920.

1258 Rappaport H. Tumors of the hematopoietic system. In Atlas of tumor pathology, series 3, fascicle 8. Washington, DC, 1966, Armed Forces Institute of Pathology, pp. 91–206.

1259 Reiner AP, Spivak JL. Hematophagic histiocytosis. A report of 23 new patients and a review of the literature. Medicine (Baltimore) 1988, **67**: 369–388.

1260 Robb-Smith AH. Before our time. Half a century of histiocytic medullary reticulosis. A T-cell teaser? Histopathology 1990, **17**: 279–283.

1261 Scott RB, Robb-Smith AH. Histiocytic medullary reticulosis. Lancet 1939, **2**: 194–198.

1262 Sonneveld P, van Lom K, Kappers-Klunne M, Prins ME, Abels J. Clinicopathological diagnosis and treatment of malignant histiocytosis. Br J Haematol 1990, **75**: 511–516.

1263 Takeshita M, Kikuchi M, Ohshima K, Nibu K, Suzumiya J, Hisano S, Miyamoto Y, Okamura T. Bone marrow findings in malignant histiocytosis and/or malignant lymphoma with concurrent hemophagocytic syndrome. Leuk Lymphoma 1993, **12**: 79–89.

1264 Warnke RA, Kim H, Dorfman RF. Malignant histiocytosis (histiocytic medullary reticulosis). I. Clinicopathologic study of 29 cases. Cancer 1975, **35**: 215–230.

1265 Weiss LM, Azzi R, Dorfman RF, Warnke RA. Sinusoidal hematolymphoid malignancy ('malignant histiocytosis') presenting as atypical sinusoidal proliferation. A study of nine cases. Cancer 1986, **58**: 1681–1688.

1266 Wilson MS, Weiss LM, Gatter KC, Mason DY, Dorfman RF, Warnke RA. Malignant histiocytosis. A reassessment of cases previously reported in 1975 based on paraffin section immunophenotyping studies. Cancer 1990, **66**: 530–536.

1267 Zucker JM, Caillaux JM, Vanel D, Gerard-Marchant R. Malignant histiocytosis in childhood. Clinical study and therapeutic results in 22 cases. Cancer 1980, **45**: 2821–2829.

LYMPHOMA IN IMMUNODEFICIENCY STATES

1268 Abruzzo LV, Rosales CM, Medeiros LJ, Vega F, Luthra R, Manning JT, Keating MJ, Jones D. Epstein–Barr virus positive B-cell lymphoproliferative disorders arising in immunodeficient patients previously treated with fludarabine for low-grade B-cell neoplasms. Am J Surg Pathol 2002, **26**: 630–636.

1269 Arber DA, Chang KL, Weiss LM. Peripheral T-cell lymphoma with Toutonlike tumor giant cells associated with HIV infection: report of two cases. Am J Surg Pathol 1999, **23**: 519–522.

1270 Arber DA, Shibata D, Chen YY, Weiss LM. Characterization of the topography of Epstein–Barr virus infection in human immunodeficiency virus-associated lymphoid tissues. Mod Pathol 1992, **5**: 559–566.

1271 Armitage JM, Kormos RL, Stuart RS, Fricker FJ, Griffith BP, Nalesnik M, Hardesty RL, Dummer JS. Posttransplant lymphoproliferative disease in thoracic organ transplant patients. Ten years of cyclosporine-based immunosuppression. J Heart Lung Transplant 1991, **10**: 877–887.

1272 Audouin J, Diebold J, Pallesen G. Frequent expression of Epstein–Barr virus latent membrane protein-1 in tumour cells of Hodgkin's disease in HIV-positive patients. J Pathol 1992, **167**: 381–384.

1273 Banks PM, Witrak GA, Conn DL. Lymphoid neoplasia following connective tissue disease. Mayo Clin Proc 1979, **54**: 104–108.

1274 Bellas C, Santón A, Manzanal A, Campo E, Martin C, Acevedo A, Varona C, Forteza J, Morente M, Montalbán C. Pathological, immunological, and molecular features of Hodgkin's disease associated with HIV infection. Comparison with ordinary Hodgkin's disease. Am J Surg Pathol 1996, **20**: 1520–1524.

1275 Beral V, Peterman T, Berkelman R, Jaffe H. AIDS-associated non-Hodgkin lymphoma. Lancet 1991, **337**: 805–809.

1276 Canioni D, Jabado N, MacIntyre E, Patey N, Emile JF, Brousse N. Lymphoproliferative disorders in children with primary immunodeficiencies: immunological status may be more predictive of the outcome than other criteria. Histopathology 2001, **38**: 146–159.

1277 Carbone A. AIDS-related non-Hodgkin's lymphomas: from pathology and molecular pathogenesis to treatment. Hum Pathol 2002, **33**: 392–404.

1278 Carbone A. Emerging pathways in the development of AIDS-related lymphomas. Lancet Oncol 2003, **4**: 22–29.

1279 Carbone A, Gloghini A, Gaidano G, Cilia AM, Bassi P, Polito P, Vaccher E, Saglio G, Tirelli U. AIDS-related Burkitt's lymphoma. Morphologic and immunophenotypic study of biopsy specimens. Am J Clin Pathol 1995, **103**: 561–567.

1280 Chadburn A, Cesarman E, Knowles DM. Molecular pathology of posttransplantation lymphoproliferative disorders. Semin Diagn Pathol 1997, **14**: 15–26.

1281 Chadburn A, Chen JM, Hsu DT, Frizzera G, Cesarman E, Garrett TJ, Mears JG, Zangwill SD, Addonizio LJ, Michler RE, Knowles DM. The morphologic and molecular genetic categories of posttransplantation lymphoproliferative disorders are clinically relevant. Cancer 1998, **82**: 1978–1987.

1282 Chetty R, Hlatswayo N, Muc R, Sabaratnam R, Gatter K. Plasmablastic lymphoma in HIV+ patients: an expanding spectrum. Histopathology 2003, **42**: 605–609.

1283 Cleary ML, Warnke R, Sklar J. Monoclonality of lymphoproliferative lesions in cardiac-transplant recipients. Clonal analysis based on immunoglobulin-gene rearrangements. N Engl J Med 1984, **310**: 477–482.

1284 Davi F, Delecluse HJ, Guiet P, Gabarre J, Fayon A, Gentilhomme O, Felman P, Bayle C, Berger F, Audouin J, Bryon PA, Diebold J, Raphael M. Burkitt-like lymphomas in AIDS patients: characterization within a series of 103 human immunodeficiency virus-associated non-Hodgkin's lymphomas. J Clin Oncol 1999, **16**: 3788–3795.

1285 Demopoulos BP, Vamvakas E, Ehrlich JE, Demopoulos R. Non-acquired immunodeficiency syndrome-defining malignancies in patients infected with human immunodeficiency virus. Arch Pathol Lab Med 2003, **127**: 589–591.

1286 Di Carlo EF, Amberson JB, Metroka CE, Ballard P, Moore A, Mouradian JA. Malignant lymphomas and the acquired immunodeficiency syndrome. Evaluation of 30 cases using a working formulation. Arch Pathol Lab Med 1986, **110**: 1012–1016.

1287 Elenitoba-Johnson KSJ, Jaffe ES. Lymphoproliferative disorders associated with congenital immunodeficiencies. Semin Diagn Pathol 1997, **14**: 35–47.

1288 Ellman MH, Hurwitz H, Thomas C, Kozloff M. Lymphoma developing in a patient with rheumatoid arthritis taking low dose weekly methotrexate. J Rheumatol 1991, **18**: 1741–1743.

1289 Engels EA, Pittaluga S, Whitby D, Rabkin C, Aoki Y, Jaffe ES, Goedert JJ. Immunoblastic lymphoma in persons with AIDS-associated Kaposi's sarcoma: a role for Kaposi's sarcoma-associated herpevirus. Mod Pathol 2003, **16**: 424–429.

1290 Ferry JA, Jacobson JO, Conti D, Delmonico F, Harris NL. Lymphoproliferative disorders and hematologic malignancies following organ transplantation. Mod Pathol 1989, **2**: 583–592.

1291 Frizzera G, Hanto DW, Gajl-Peczalska KJ, Rosai J, McKenna RW, Sibley RK, Holahan KP, Lindquist LL. Polymorphic diffuse B-cell hyperplasias and lymphomas in renal transplant recipients. Cancer Res 1981, **41**: 4262–4279.

1292 Frizzera G, Rosai J, Dehner LP, Spector BD, Kersey JH. Lymphoreticular disorders in primary immunodeficiencies. New findings based on an up-to-date histologic review of 35 cases. Cancer 1980, **46**: 692–699.

1293 Gail MH, Pluda JM, Rabkin CS, Biggar RJ, Goedert JJ, Horm JW, Sondik EJ, Yarchoan R, Broder S. Projections of the incidence of non-Hodgkin's lymphoma related to acquired immunodeficiency syndrome. J Natl Cancer Inst 1991, **83**: 695–701.

1294 Garvin AJ, Self S, Sahovic EA, Stuart RK, Marchalonis JJ. The occurrence of a peripheral T-cell lymphoma in a chronically immunosuppressed renal transplant patient. Am J Surg Pathol 1988, **12**: 64–70.

1295 Gong JZ, Stenzel TT, Bennett ER, Lagoo AS, Dunphy CH, Moore JO, Rizzieri DA, Tepperberg JH, Papenhausen P, Buckley PJ. Burkitt lymphoma arising in organ transplant recipients. Am J Surg Pathol 2003, **27**: 818–827.

1296 Hamilton-Dutoit SJ, Raphael M, Audouin J, Diebold J, Lisse I, Pedersen C, Oksenhendler E, Marelle L, Pallesen G. In situ demonstration of Epstein–Barr virus small RNAs (EBER 1) in acquired immunodeficiency syndrome-related lymphomas. Correlation with tumor morphology and primary site. Blood 1993, **92**: 610–624.

1297 Hanto DW, Birkenbach M, Frizzera G, Gajl-Peczalska KJ, Simmons RL, Schubach WH. Confirmation of the heterogeneity of posttransplant Epstein–Barr virus-associated B-cell proliferations by immunoglobulin gene rearrangement analyses. Transplantation 1989, **47**: 458–464.

1298 Hanto DW, Frizzera G, Gajl-Peczalska KJ, Sakamoto K, Purtilo DT, Balfour HH Jr, Simmons RL, Najarian JS. Epstein–Barr virus induced B-cell lymphoma after renal transplantation. Acyclovir therapy and transition from polyclonal to monoclonal B-cell proliferation. N Engl J Med 1982, **306**: 913–918.

1299 Harris NL, Ferry JA, Swerdlow SH. Posttransplant lymphoproliferative disorders: a summary of Society for Hematopathology workshop. Semin Diagn Pathol 1997, **14**: 8–14.

1300 Herndier B, Sanchez H, Chang KC, Chen YY, Weiss LM. High prevalence of detection of EBV RNA in the Reed–Sternberg cells of HIV-associated Hodgkin's disease. Am J Pathol 1993, **142**: 1073–1079.

1301 Ioachim HL. Neoplasms associated with immune deficiencies. Pathol Annu 1987, **22**(Pt 2): 177–222.

1302 Ioachim HL, Cooper MC, Hellman GC. Lymphomas in men at high risk for acquired immune deficiency syndrome (AIDS). A study of 21 cases. Cancer 1985, **56**: 2831–2842.

1303 Kamel OW. Iatrogenic lymphoproliferative disorders in non-transplantation settings. Recent results. Cancer Res 2002, **159**: 19–26.

1304 Kamel OW, van de Rijn M, Weiss LM, Del Zoppo GJ, Hench PK, Robbins BA, Montgomery PG, Warnke RA, Dorfman RF. Brief report. Reversible lymphomas associated with Epstein–Barr virus occurring during methotrexate therapy for rheumatoid arthritis and dermatomyositis. N Engl J Med 1993, **328**: 1317–1321.

1305 Kastan M. Ataxia-telangiectasia. Broad implications for a rare disorder. N Engl J Med 1995, **333**: 662–663.

1306 Katano H, Suda T, Morishita Y, Yamamoto K, Hoshino Y, Nakamur K, Tachikawa N, Sata T, Hamaguchi H, Iwamoto A, Mori S. Human herpesvirus 8-associated solid lymphomas that occur in AIDS patients take anaplastic large cell morphology. Mod Pathol 2000, **13**: 77–85.

1307 Kersey JH, Spector BD, Good RA. Primary immunodeficiency disease and cancer. The Immunodeficiency-Cancer Registry. Int J Cancer 1973, **12**: 333–347.

1308 Knowles DM. Acquired immunodeficiency syndrome-related lymphoma. Blood 1992, **80**: 8–20.

1309 Knowles DM. Immunodeficiency-associated lymphoproliferative disorders. Mod Pathol 1999, **12**: 200–217.

1310 Leblond V, Sutton L, Dorent R, Davi F, Bitker M-O, Gabarre J, Charlotte F, Ghoussoub J-J, Fourcase C, Fischer A, Gandjbakhch I, Binet J-L, Raphael M. Lymphoproliferative disorders after organ transplantation. A report of 24 cases observed in a single center. J Clin Oncol 1995, **13**: 961–968.

1311 Liebowitz D. Epstein–Barr virus and a cellular signaling pathway in lymphomas from immunosuppressed patients. N Engl J Med 1998, **338**: 1413–1421.

1312 Lippman SM, Grogan TM, Carry P, Ogden DA, Miller TP. Post-transplantation T-cell lymphoblastic lymphoma. Am J Med 1987, **82**: 814–816.

1313 Locker J, Nalesnik M. Molecular genetic analysis of lymphoid tumors arising after organ transplantation. Am J Pathol 1989, **135**: 977–987.

1314 Louie S, Schwartz RS. Immunodeficiency and the pathogenesis of lymphoma and leukemia. Semin Hematol 1978, **15**: 117–138.

1315 Lowenthal DA, Straus DJ, Campbell SW, Gold JWM, Clarkson BD, Koziner B. AIDS-related lymphoid neoplasia. The Memorial Hospital experience. Cancer 1988, **61**: 2325–2337.

1316 Macchi P, Villa A, Gillani S, Sacco MG, Frattini A, Porta F, Ugazio AG, Johnston JR, Candotti F, O'Shea JJ, Vezzoni P, Notarangelo LD. Mutations of Jak-3 gene in patients with autosomal severe combined immune deficiency (SCID). Nature 1995, **377**: 65–68.

1317 Montone KT, Hodinka RL, Salhany KE, Lavi E, Rostami A, Tomaszewski JE. Identification of Epstein-Barr virus activity in post-transplantation lymphoproliferative disease. Mod Pathol 1996, **9**: 621–630.

1318 Morrell D, Cromartie E, Swift M. Mortality and cancer incidence in 263 patients with ataxia-telangiectasia. J Natl Cancer Inst 1986, **77**: 89–92.

1319 Nador RG, Chadburn A, Gundapa G, Cesarman E, Said JW, Knowles DM. Human immunodeficiency virus (HIV)-associated polymorphic lymphoproliferative disorders. Am J Surg Pathol 2003, **27**: 293–302.

1320 Orazi A, Hromas RA, Neiman RS, Greiner TC, Lee CH, Rubin L, Haskins S, Heerema NA, Gharpure V, Abonour R, Srour EF, Cornetta K. Posttransplantation lymphoproliferative disorders in bone marrow transplant recipients are aggressive diseases with a high incidence of adverse histologic and immunobiologic features. Am J Clin Pathol 1997, **107**: 419–429.

1321 Oyama T, Ichimura K, Suzuki R, Suzumiya J, Ohshima K,Yatabe Y, Yokoi T, Kojima M, Kamiya Y, Taji H, Kagami Y, Ogura M, Saito H, Morishima Y, Nakamura S. Senile EBV+ B-cell lymphoproliferative disorders: a clinicopathologic study of 22 patients. Am J Surg Pathol 2003, **27**: 16–26.

1322 Patton DF, Wilkowski CW, Hanson CA, Shapiro R, Gajl-Peczalska KJ, Filipovich AH, McClain KL. Epstein–Barr virus-determined clonality in posttransplant lymphoproliferative disease. Transplantation 1990, **49**: 1080–1084.

1323 Pedersen C, Gerstoft J, Lundgren JD, Skinhoj P, Bottzauw J, Geisler C, Hamilton-Dutoit SJ, Thorsen S, Lisse I, Ralfkiaer E, et al. HIV-associated lymphoma. Histopathology and association with Epstein–Barr virus genome related to clinical, immunological and prognostic features. Eur J Cancer 1991, **27**: 1416–1423.

1324 Penn I. Tumor incidence in human allograft recipients. Transplant Proc 1979, **11**: 1047–1051.

1325 Purtilo DT, DeFlorio D Jr, Hutt LM, Bhawan J, Yang JP, Otto R, Edwards W. Variable phenotypic expression of an X-linked recessive lymphoproliferative syndrome. N Engl J Med 1977, **297**: 1077–1081.

1326 Ramalingam P, Rybicki L, Smith MD, Abrahams NA, Tubbs RR, Pettay J, Farver CF. Posttransplant lymphoproliferative disorders in lung transplant patients: the Cleveland Clinic experience. Mod Pathol 2002, **15**: 647–656.

1327 Randhawa PS, Jaffe R, Demetris AJ, Nalesnik M, Starzl TE, Chen YY, Weiss LM. The systemic distribution of Epstein–Barr virus genomes in fatal post-transplantation lymphoproliferative disorders. An in situ hybridization study. Am J Pathol 1991, **138**: 1027–1033.

1328 Randhawa PS, Yousem SA, Paradis IL, Dauber JA, Griffith BP, Locker J. The clinical spectrum, pathology, and clonal analysis of Epstein–Barr virus-associated lymphoproliferative disorders in heart-lung transplant recipients. Am J Clin Pathol 1989, **92**: 177–185.

1329 Raphael M, Gentilhomme O, Tulliez M, Byron PA, Diebold J. Histopathologic features of high-grade non-Hodgkin's lymphomas in acquired immunodeficiency syndrome. The French Study Group of Pathology for Human Immunodeficiency Virus-Associated Tumors. Arch Pathol Lab Med 1991, **115**: 15–20.

1330 Ree HJ, Strauchen JA, Khan AA, Gold JE, Crowley JP, Kahn H, Zalusky R. Human immunodeficiency virus-associated Hodgkin's disease. Clinicopathologic studies of 24 cases and preponderance of mixed cellularity type characterized by the occurrence of fibrohistiocytoid stromal cells. Cancer 1991, **67**: 1614–1621.

1331 Said JW. Human immunodeficiency virus-related lymphoid proliferations. Semin Diagn Pathol 1997, **14**: 48–53.

1332 Said JW. Genetic and molecular genetic studies in the diagnosis of immune-related lymphoproliferative disorders. Hum Pathol 2003, **34**: 341–345.

1333 Sander CA, Medeiros LJ, Weiss LM, Yano T, Sneller MC, Jaffe ES. Lymphoproliferative lesions in patients with common variable immunodeficiency syndrome. Am J Surg Pathol 1992, **16**: 1170–1182.

1334 Savitsky K, Bar-Shira A, Gilad S, Rotman G, Ziv Y, Vanagaite L, Tagle DA, Smith S, Uziel T, Sfez S, Ashkenazi M, Pecker I, Frydman M, Harnik R, Patanjali SR, Simmons A, Clines GA, Sartiel A, Gatti RA, Chessa L, Sanal O, Lavin MF, Jaspers NGJ, Taylor AMR, Arlett CF, Miki T, Weissman SM, Lovett M, Collins FS, Shiloh Y. A single ataxia telangiectasia gene with a product similar to PI-3 kinase. Science 1995, **268**: 1749–1753.

1335 Schmid U, Helbron D, Lennert K. Development of malignant lymphoma in myoepithelial sialadenitis (Sjögren's syndrome). Virchows Arch [A] 1982, **395**: 11–43.

1336 Spector BD, Perry GS III, Kersey JH. Genetically determined immunodeficiency diseases (GDID) and malignancy. Report from the Immunodeficiency-Cancer Registry. Clin Immunol Immunopathol 1978, **11**: 12–29.

1337 Spina M, Tirelli U, Zagonel V, Gloghini A, Volpe R, Babare R, Abbruzzese L, Talamini R, Vaccher E, Carbone A. Burkitt's lymphoma in adults with and without human immunodeficiency virus infection: a single-institution clinicopathologic study of 75 patients. Cancer 1998, **82**: 766–774.

1338 Swinnen LJ, Costanzo-Nordin MR, Fisher SG, O'Sullivan EJ, Johnson MR, Heroux AL, Dizikes GJ, Pifarre R, Fisher RI. Increased incidence of lymphoproliferative disorder after immunosuppression with the monoclonal antibody OKT3 in cardiac-transplant recipients. N Engl J Med 1990, **323**: 1723–1728.

1339 Tinguely M, Vonlanthen R, Muller E, Dommann-Scherrer CC, Schneider J, Laissue JA, Borisch B. Hodgkin's disease-like lymphoproliferative disorders in patients with different underlyng immunodeficiency states. Mod Pathol 1998, **11**: 307–312.

1340 Tirelli U, Errante D, Dolcetti R, Gloghini A, Serraino D, Vaccher E, Franceschi S, Boiocchi M, Carbone A. Hodgkin's disease and human immunodefiency virus infection. Clinicopathologic and virologic features of 114 patients from the Italian Cooperative Group on AIDS and Tumors. J Clin Oncol 1995, **13**: 1758–1767.

1341 Tsao L, Hsi ED. The clinicopathologic spectrum of posttransplantation lymphoproliferative disorders. Arch Pathol Lab Med 2007, **131**: 1209–1218.

1342 Wang C-Y, Snow JL, Su WPD. Lymphoma associated with human immunodeficiency virus infection. Mayo Clin Proc 1995, **70**: 665–672.

1343 Wood BL, Sabath D, Broudy VC, Raghu G. The recipient origin of post-transplant lymphoproliferative disorders in pulmonary transplant patients: a report of three cases. Cancer 1996, **78**: 2223–2228.

1344 Wu TT, Swerdlow SH, Locker J, Bahler D, Randhawa P, Yunis EJ, Dickman PS, Nalesnik

MA. Recurrent Epstein–Barr virus-associated lesions in organ transplant recipients. Hum Pathol 1996, **27**: 157–164.

LYMPH NODE INCLUSIONS

1345 Arai T, Kino I, Nakamura S, Ogawa H. Epidermal inclusions in abdominal lymph nodes. Report of two cases studied immunohistochemically. Acta Pathol Jpn 1992, **42**: 126–129.

1346 Argani P, Rosai J. Hyperplastic mesothelial cells in lymph nodes: report of six cases of a benign process that can simulate metastatic involvement by mesothelioma or carcinoma. Hum Pathol 1998, **29**: 339–346.

1347 Azzopardi JG, Ross CMD, Frizzera G. Blue naevi of lymph node capsule. Histopathology 1977, **1**: 451–461.

1348 Brooks JS, Li Volsi VA, Pietra GG. Mesothelial cell inclusions in mediastinal lymph nodes mimicking metastatic carcinoma. Am J Clin Pathol 1990, **93**: 741–748.

1349 Brown RB, Gaillard RA, Turner JA. The significance of aberrant or heterotopic parotid gland tissue in lymph nodes. Ann Surg 1953, **138**: 850–856.

1350 Covell LM, Disciullo AJ, Knapp RC. Decidual change in pelvic lymph nodes in the presence of cervical squamous cell carcinoma during pregnancy. Am J Obstet Gynecol 1977, **127**: 674–676.

1351 Edlow DW, Carter D. Heterotopic epithelium in axillary lymph nodes. Am J Clin Pathol 1973, **59**: 666–673.

1352 Ehrmann RL, Federschneider JM, Knapp RC. Distinguishing lymph node metastases from benign glandular inclusions in low-grade ovarian carcinoma. Am J Obstet Gynecol 1980, **136**: 737–746.

1353 Fellegara G, Carcangiu ML, Rosai J. Benign epithelial inclusions in axillary lymph nodes. Report of 18 cases and review of the literature. Am J Surg Pathol (submitted).

1354 Fisher CJ, Hill S, Millis RR. Benign lymph node inclusions mimicking metastatic carcinoma. J Clin Pathol 1994, **47**: 245–247.

1355 Holdsworth PJ, Hopkinson JM, Leveson SH. Benign axillary epithelial lymph node inclusions – a histological pitfall. Histopathology 1988, **13**: 226–228.

1356 Johnson WT, Helwig EB. Benign nevus cells in the capsule of lymph nodes. Cancer 1969, **23**: 747–753.

1357 Koss LG. Miniature adenoacanthoma arising in an endometriotic cyst in an obturator lymph node. Report of first case. Cancer 1963, **16**: 1369–1372.

1358 Longo S. Benign lymph node inclusions. Hum Pathol 1976, **7**: 349–354.

1359 Maassen V, Hiller K. Glandular inclusions in lymph nodes: Pattern of distribution and metaplastic transformation. Arch Gynecol Obstet 1994, **255**: 1–8.

1360 Maiorano E, Mazzarol GM, Pruneri G, Mastropasqua MG, Zurrida S, Orvieto E, Viale G. Ectopic breast tissue as a possible cause of false-positive axillary sentinel lymph node biopsies. Am J Surg Pathol 2003, **27**: 513–518.

1361 Micheau C, Cachin Y, Caillou B. Cystic metastases in the neck revealing occult carcinoma of the tonsil. A report of six cases. Cancer 1974, **33**: 228–233.

1362 Moore WF, Bentley RC, Berchuck A, Robboy SJ. Some mullerian inclusion cysts in lymph nodes may sometimes be metastases from serous borderline tumors of the ovary. Am J Surg Pathol 2000, **24**: 710–718.

1363 Parkash V, Vidwans M, Carter D. Benign mesothelial cells in mediastinal lymph nodes. Am J Surg Pathol 1999, **23**: 1264–1269.

1364 Sussman J, Rosai J. Lymph node metastasis as the initial manifestation of malignant mesothelioma. Report of six cases. Am J Surg Pathol 1990, **14**: 819–828.

1365 Turner DR, Millis RR. Breast tissue inclusions in axillary lymph nodes. Histopathology 1980, **4**: 631–636.

OTHER NON-NEOPLASTIC LESIONS

1366 Albores-Saavedra J, Vuitch F, Delgado R, Wiley E, Hagler H. Sinus histiocytosis of pelvic lymph nodes after hip replacement. A histiocytic proliferation induced by cobalt-chromium and titanium. Am J Surg Pathol 1994, **18**: 83–90.

1367 Banerjee D, Mills DM, Hearn SA, Meek M, Turner KL. Proteinaceous lymphadenopathy due to monoclonal nonamyloid immunoglobulin deposit disease. Arch Pathol Lab Med 1990, **114**: 34–39.

1368 Cleary KR, Osborne BM, Butler JJ. Lymph node infarction foreshadowing malignant lymphoma. Am J Surg Pathol 1982, **6**: 435–442.

1369 Davies JD, Stansfeld AG. Spontaneous infarction of superficial lymph nodes. J Clin Pathol 1972, **25**: 689–696.

1370 Davies JD, Webb AJ. Segmental lymph-node infarction after fine needle aspiration J Clin Pathol 1982, **35**: 855–857.

1371 Kojima M, Nakamura S, Sugihara S, Sakata N, Masawa N. Lymph node infarction associated with infectious mononucleosis. Int J Surg Pathol 2002, **10**: 223–226.

1372 Magrina JF, Symmonds RE, Dahlin DC. Pelvic 'lipolymph nodes'. A consideration in the differential diagnosis of pelvic masses. Am J Obstet Gynecol 1980, **136**: 727–731.

1373 Mahy NJ, Davies JD. Ischaemic changes in human mesenteric lymph nodes. J Pathol 1984, **144**: 257–267.

1374 Maurer R, Schmid U, Davies JD, Mahy NJ, Stansfeld AG, Lukes RJ. Lymph node infarction and malignant lymphoma. A multicentre survey of European, English and American cases. Histopathology 1986, **10**: 571–588.

1375 Shah KH, Kisilevsky R. Infarction of the lymph nodes. A cause of a palisading macrophage reaction mimicking necrotizing granulomas. Hum Pathol 1978, **9**: 597–599.

1376 Strauchen JA, Miller LK. Lymph node infarction: an immunohistochemical study of 11 cases. Arch Pathol Lab Med 2003, **127**: 60–63.

1377 Truong LD, Cartwright J Jr, Goodman MD, Woznicki D. Silicone lymphadenopathy associated with augmentation mammaplasty. Morphologic features of nine cases. Am J Surg Pathol 1988, **12**: 484–491.

1378 Vega F, Lozano MD, Alcalde J, Pardo-Mindan FJ. Utility of immunophenotypic and immunogenotypic analysis in the study of necrotic lymph nodes. Virchows Arch 1999, **434**: 245–248.

TUMORS OF THE CELLS OF THE ACCESSORY IMMUNE SYSTEM

1379 Andriko JW, Kaldijan EP, Tsokos M, Abbondanzo SL, Jaffe ES. Reticulum cell neoplasms of lymph nodes: a clinicopathologic study of 11 cases with recognition of a new subtype derived from fibroblastic reticular cells. Am J Surg Pathol 1998, **22**: 1048–1058.

1380 Bagdi E, Krenacs L, Krenacs T, Miller K, Isaacson PG. Follicular dendritic cells in reactive and neoplastic lymphoid tissues: a re-evaluation of staining patterns of CD21, CD23, and CD35 antibodies in paraffin sections after wet heat-induced epitope retrieval. Appl Immunohistochem Mol Morphol 2001, **9**: 117–124.

1381 Banchereau J, Steinman RM. Dendritic cells and the control of immunity. Nature 1998, **392**: 245–252.

1382 Beham-Schmid C, Beham A, Jakse R, Aubock L, Hofler G. Extranodal follicular dendritic cell tumour of the nasopharynx. Virchows Arch 1998, **432**: 293–298.

1383 Biddle DA, Ro JY, Yoon GS, Yong YW, Ayala AG, Ordonez NG. Extranodal follicular dendritic cell sarcoma of the head and neck region: three new cases, with a review of the literature. Mod Pathol 2002, **15**: 50–58.

1384 Castro EC, Blazquez C, Boyd J, Correa H, de Chadarevian JP, Felgar RE, Graf N, Levy N, Lowe EJ, Manning JT Jr, Proytcheva MA, Senger C, Shayan K, Sterba J, Werner A, Surti U, Jaffe R. Clinicopathologic features of histiocytic lesions following ALL, with a review of the literature. Pediatr Dev Pathol 2010, **13**: 225–237.

1385 Chan JK, Lamant L, Algar E, Delsol G, Tsang WY, Lee KC, Tiedemann K, Chow CW. ALK+ histiocytosis: a novel type of systemic histiocytic proliferative disorder of early infancy. Blood 2008, **112**: 2965–2968

1386 Chan AC, Chan KW, Chan JK, Au WY, Ho WK, Ng WM. Development of follicular dendritic cell sarcoma in hyaline-vascular Castleman's disease of nasopharynx: tracing its evolution by sequential biopsies. Histopathology 2001, **38**: 510–518.

1387 Chan AC, Serrano-Olmo J, Erlandson RA, Rosai J. Cytokeratin-positive malignant tumors with reticulum cell morphology: a subtype of fibroblastic reticulum cell neoplasms? Am J Surg Pathol 2000, **24**: 107–116.

1388 Chan JK. Proliferative lesions of follicular dendritic cells: an overview, including a detailed account of follicular dendritic cell sarcoma, a neoplasm with many faces and uncommon etiologic association. Adv Anat Pathol 1997, **4**: 387–411.

1389 Chan JK, Fletcher CD, Nayler SJ, Cooper K. Follicular dendritic cell sarcoma: clinicopathologic analysis of 17 cases suggesting a malignant potential higher than currently recognized. Cancer 1997, **79**: 294–313.

1390 Chan JK, Tsang WY, Ng CS, Tang SK, Yu HC, Lee AW. Follicular dendritic cell tumors of the oral cavity. Am J Surg Pathol 1994, **18**: 148–157.

1391 Chang KC, Jin YT, Chen FF, Su IJ. Follicular dendritic cell sarcoma of the colon mimicking stromal tumour. Histopathology 2001, **38**: 25–29.

1392 Chen TC, Kuo TT, NG KF. Follicular dendritic cell tumor of the liver: a clinicopathologic and Epstein–Barr virus study of two cases. Mod Pathol 2001, **14**: 354–360.

1393 Chen W, Lau SK, Fong D, Wang J, Wang E, Arber DA, Weiss LM, Huang Q. High frequency of clonal immunoglobulin receptor gene rearrangements in sporadic histiocytic/dendritic cell sarcomas. Am J Surg Pathol 2009, **33**: 863–873.

1394 Chen W, Wang J, Wang E, Lu Y, Lau SK, Weiss LM, Huang Q. Detection of clonal lymphoid receptor gene rearrangements in Langerhans cell histiocytosis. Am J Surg Pathol 2010, **34**: 1049–1057.

1395 Cheuk W, Chan JK, Shek T, Chang JH, Tsou MH, Yuen NW, Ng WF, Chan AC, Prat J. Inflammatory pseudotumor-like follicular dendritic cell tumor: a distinctive low-grade malignant intra-abdominal neoplasm with consistent Epstein–Barr virus association. Am J Surg Pathol 2001, **25**: 721–731.

1396 Copie-Bergman C, Wotherspoon AC, Norton AJ, Diss TC, Isaacson PG. True histiocytic lymphoma: a morphologic, immunohistochemical, and molecular genetic study of 13 cases. Am J Surg Pathol 1998, **22**: 1386–1392.

1397 Dorfman DM, Shahsafaei A, Chan JKC, Fletcher CD. Dendritic reticulum cell (DRC) sarcomas are immunoreactive for low-affinity nerve growth factor receptor (LNGFR). Further evidence for DRC differentiation. Appl Immunohistochem 1996, **4**: 249–258.

1398 Fassina A, Marino F, Poletti A, Rea F, Pennelli N, Ninfo V. Follicular dendritic cell tumor of the mediastinum. Ann Diagn Pathol 2001, **5**: 361–367.

1399 Favara B, Feller A, Members of WHO Committee on Histocytic/Reticulum Cell Proliferations. Contemporary classification of histiocytic disorders. Reclassification Working Group of the Histiocyte Society. Med Pediatr Oncol 1997, **29**: 157–166.

1400 Feldman AL, Arber DA, Pittaluga S, Martinez A, Burke JS, Raffeld M, Camos M, Warnke R, Jaffe ES. Clonally related follicular lymphomas and histiocytic/dendritic cell sarcomas: evidence for transdifferentiation of the follicular lymphoma clone. Blood 2008, **111**: 5433–5439.

1401 Feldman AL, Berthold F, Arceci RJ, Abramowsky C, Shehata BM, Mann KP, Lauer SJ, Pritchard J, Raffeld M, Jaffe ES. Clonal relationship between precursor T-lymphoblastic leukaemia/lymphoma and Langerhans-cell histiocytosis. Lancet Oncol 2005, **6**: 435–437.

1402 Feldman AL, Minniti C, Santi M, Downing JR, Raffeld M, Jaffe ES. Histiocytic sarcoma after acute lymphoblastic leukaemia: a common clonal origin. Lancet Oncol 2004, **5**: 248–250.

1403 Feltkamp CA, van Heerde P, Feltkamp-Vroom TM, Koudstaal J. A malignant tumor arising from interdigitating cells; light microscopical, ultrastructural, immuno- and enzyme-histochemical characteristics. Virchows Arch [A] 1981, **393**: 183–192.

1404 Ferringer T, Banks PM, Metcalf JS. Langerhans cell sarcoma. Am J Dermatopathol 2006, **28**: 36–39.

1405 Fisher C, Magnusson B, Hardarson S, Smith ME. Myxoid variant of follicular dendritic cell sarcoma arising in the breast. Ann Diagn Pathol 1999, **3**: 92–98.

1406 Franchino C, Reich C, Distenfeld A, Ubriaco A, Knowles DM. A clinicopathologically distinctive primary splenic histiocytic neoplasm. Demonstration of its histiocyte derivation by immunophenotypic and molecular genetic analysis. Am J Surg Pathol 1988, **12**: 398–404.

1407 Fraser CR, Wang W, Gomez M, Zhang T, Mathew S, Furman RR, Knowles DM, Orazi A, Tam W. Transformation of chronic lymphocytic leukemia/small lymphocytic lymphoma to interdigitating dendritic cell sarcoma: evidence for transdifferentiation of the lymphoma clone. Am J Clin Pathol 2009, **132**: 928–939.

1408 Gaertner EM, Tsokos M, Derringer GA, Neuhauser TS, Arciero C, Andriko JA. Interdigitating dendritic cell sarcoma. A report of four cases and review of the literature. Am J Clin Pathol 2001, **115**: 589–597.

1409 Girolomoni G, Caux C, Lebecque S, Dezutter-Dambuyant C, Ricciardi-Castagnoli P. Langerhans cells: still a fundamental paradigm for studying the immunobiology of dendritic cells. Trends Immunol 2002, **23**: 6–8.

1410 Gould VE, Bloom KJ, Franke WW, Warren WH, Moll R. Increased numbers of cytokeratin-positive interstitial reticulum cells (CIRC) in reactive, inflammatory and neoplastic lymphadenopathies. Hyperplasia or induced expression? Virchows Arch 1995, **425**: 617–630.

1411 Grogg KL, Lae ME, Kurtin PJ, Macon WR. Clusterin expression distinguishes follicular dendritic cell tumors from other dendritic cell neoplasms: report of a novel follicular dendritic cell marker and clinicopathologic data on 12 additional follicular dendritic cell tumors and 6 additional interdigitating dendritic cell tumors. Am J Surg Pathol 2004, **28**: 988–998.

1412 Hammar SP, Rudolph RH, Bockus DE, Remington FL. Interdigitating reticulum cell sarcoma with unusual features. Ultrastruct Pathol 1991, **15**: 631–645.

1413 Han JH, Kim SH, Noh SH, Lee YC, Kim HG, Yang WI. Follicular dendritic cell sarcoma presenting as a submucosal tumor of the stomach. Arch Pathol Lab Med 2000, **124**: 1693–1696.

1414 Hanson CA, Jaszcz W, Kersey JH, Astorga MG, Peterson BA, Gajl-Peczalska KJ, Frizzera G. True histiocytic lymphoma. Histopathologic, immunophenotypic and genotypic analysis. Br J Haematol 1989, **73**: 187–198.

1415 Harvell JD, Fulton R, Jones CD, Terris DJ, Warnke RA. Composite dendritic cell neoplasm (NOS) and small lymphocytic lymphoma. Appl Immunohistochem Mol Morphol 2000, **8**: 322–328.

1416 Hollowood K, Pease C, Mackay AM, Fletcher CD. Sarcomatoid tumours of lymph nodes showing follicular dendritic cell differentiation. J Pathol 1991, **163**: 205–216.

1417 Hollowood K, Stamp G, Zouvani J, Fletcher CDM. Extranodal follicular dendritic cell sarcoma of the gastrointestinal tract. Morphologic, immunohistochemical and ultrastructural analysis of two cases. Am J Clin Pathol 1995, **103**: 90–97.

1418 Hornick JL, Jaffe ES, Fletcher CD. Extranodal histiocytic sarcoma: clinicopathologic analysis of 14 cases of a rare epithelioid malignancy. Am J Surg Pathol 2004, **28**: 1133–1144.

1419 Hsu SM, Ho YS, Hsu PL. Lymphomas of true histiocytic origin. Expression of different phenotypes in so-called true histiocytic lymphoma and malignant histiocytosis. Am J Pathol 1991, **138**: 1389–1404.

1420 Hui PK, Feller AC, Kaiserling E, Hesse G, Rodermund OE, Haneke E, Weber L, Lennert K. Skin tumor of T accessory cells (interdigitating reticulum cells) with high content of T lymphocytes. Am J Dermatopathol 1987, **9**: 129–137.

1421 Imal Y, Yamakawa M. Morphology, function and pathology of follicular dendritic cells. Pathol Int 1997, **46**: 807–833.

1422 Jones D, Amin M, Ordonez NG, Glassman AB, Hayes KJ, Medeiros LJ. Reticulum cell sarcoma of lymph node with mixed dendritic and fibroblastic features. Mod Pathol 2001, **14**: 1059–1067.

1423 Kawachi K, Nakatani Y, Inayama Y, Kawano N, Toda N, Misugi K. Interdigitating dendritic cell sarcoma of the spleen: report of a case with a review of the literature. Am J Surg Pathol 2002, **26**: 530–537.

1424 Luk IS, Shek TW, Tang VW, Ng WF. Interdigitating dendritic cell tumor of the testis: a novel testicular spindle cell neoplasm. Am J Surg Pathol 1999, **23**: 1141–1148.

1425 Maeda K, Matsuda M, Suzuki H, Saitoh HA. Immunohistochemical recognition of human follicular dendritic cells (FDCs) in routinely processed paraffin section. J Histochem Cytochem 2002, **50**: 1475–1486.

1426 Masuuaga A, Nakamura H, Katata T, Furubayashi T, Kanayama T, Yamada A, Shiroko Y, Itoyama S. Follicular dendritic cell tumor with histiocytic characteristics and fibroblastic antigen. Pathol Int 1997, **47**: 707–712.

1427 Miettinen M, Fletcher CD, Lasota J. True histiocytic lymphoma of small intestine. Analysis of two S-100 protein-positive cases with features of interdigitating reticulum cell sarcoma. Am J Clin Pathol 1993, **100**: 285–292.

1428 Milchgrub S, Kamel OW, Wiley E, Vuitch F, Cleary ML, Warnke RA. Malignant histiocytic neoplasms of the small intestine. Am J Surg Pathol 1992, **16**: 11–20.

1429 Monda L, Warnke R, Rosai J. A primary lymph node malignancy with features suggestive of dendritic reticulum cell differentiation. A report of 4 cases. Am J Pathol 1986, **122**: 562–572.

1430 Moriki T, Takahashi T, Wada M, Ueda S, Ichien M, Yamane T, Hara H. Follicular dendritic cell tumor of the mesentery. Pathol Res Pract 1998, **193**: 629–639.

1431 Nayler SJ, Verhaart MJ, Cooper K. Follicular dendritic cell tumor of the tonsil. Histopathology 1996, **28**: 89–92.

1432 Nonaka D, Birbe R, Rosai J. So-called inflammatory myofibroblastic tumour: a proliferative lesion of fibroblastic reticulum cells? Histopathology 2005, **46**: 604–613.

1433 Perez-Ordóñez B, Rosai J. Follicular dendritic cell tumor: review of the entity. Semin Diagn Pathol 1998, **15**: 144–154.

1434 Perez-Ordóñez B, Erlandson RA, Rosai J. Dendritic follicular cell tumor. Report of 13 additional cases of a distinctive entity. Am J Surg Pathol 1996, **20**: 944–955.

1435 Pileri SA, Grogan TM, Harris NL, Banks P, Campo E, Chan JK, Favera RD, Delsol G, De Wolf-Peeters C, Falini B, Gascoyne RD, Gaulard P, Gatter KC, Isaacson PG, Jaffe ES, Kluin P, Knowles DM, Mason DY, Mori S, Müller-Hermelink HK, Piris MA, Ralfkiaer E, Stein H, Su IJ, Warnke RA, Weiss LM. Tumors of histiocytes and accessory dendritic cells: an immunohistochemical approach to classification from the International Lymphoma Society Group based on 61 cases. Histopathology 2002, **41**: 1–29.

1436 Pillay K, Solomon R, Daubenton JD, Sinclair-Smith CC. Interdigitating dendritic cell sarcoma: a report of four paediatric cases and review of the literature. Histopathology 2004, **44**: 283–291.

1437 Pruneri G, Masullo M, Renne G, Taccagni G, Manzotti M, Luini A, Viale G. Follicular dendritic cell sarcoma of the breast. Virchows Arch 2002, **441**: 194–199.

1438 Ralfkiaer E, Delsol G, O'Connor NT, Brandtzaeg P, Brousset P, Vejlsgaard GL, Mason DY. Malignant lymphomas of true histiocytic origin. A clinical, histological, immunophenotypic and genotypic study. J Pathol 1990, **160**: 9–17.

1439 Raymond I, Al Saati T, Tkaczuk J, Chittal S, Delsol G. CAN.42, a new monoclonal antibody directed against a fixative-resistant antigen of follicular dendritic reticulum cells. Am J Pathol 1998, **151**: 1577–1585.

1440 Reichard KK, Burks EJ, Foucar MK, Wilson CS, Viswanatha DS, Hozier JC, Larson RS. CD4(+) CD56(+) lineage-negative malignancies are rare tumors of plasmacytoid dendritic cells. Am J Surg Pathol 2005, **29**: 1274–1283.

1441 Rezk SA, Spagnolo DV, Brynes RK, Weiss LM. Indeterminate cell tumor: a rare dendritic neoplasm. Am J Surg Pathol 2008, **32**: 1868–1876. .

1442 Rodilla CM, Acenero JF, Mayor LP, Carmona AA. True histiocytic lymphoma as a second neoplasm in a follicular centroblastic-centrocytic lymphoma. Pathol Res Pract 1997, **193**: 319–322.

1443 Saiz AD, Chan O, Strauchen JA. Follicular dendritic cell tumor in Castleman's disease: a report of two cases. Int J Surg Pathol 1997, **5**: 25–30.

1444 Sapino A, Cassoni P, Ferrero E, Bongiovanni M, Righi L, Fortunati N, Crafa P, Chiarle R, Bussolati G. Estrogen receptor alpha is a novel marker expressed by follicular dendritic cells in lymph nodes and tumor-associated lymphoid infiltrates. Am J Pathol 2003, **163**: 1313–1320.

1445 Schuerfeld K, Lazzi S, de Santi MM, Gozzetti A, Leoncini L, Pileri SA. Cytokeratin-positive intersititial cell neoplasm: a case report and classification issues. Histopathology 2003, **43**: 491–494.

1446 Selves J, Meggetto F, Brousset P, Voigt JJ, Pradere B, Grasset D, Icart J, Mariame B, Knecht H, Delsol G. Inflammatory pseudotumor of the liver: evidence for follicular dendritic reticulum cell proliferation associated with clonal Epstein–Barr virus. Am J Surg Pathol 1996, **20**: 747–753.

1447 Shah RN, Ozden O, Yeldandi A, Peterson LA, Rao S, Laskin WB. Follicular dendritic cell tumor presenting in the lung: a case report. Hum Pathol 2001, **32**: 745–749.

1448 Shek TW, Ho FC, Ng IO, Chan AC, Ma L, Srivastava G. Follicular dendritic cell tumor of the liver: evidence for Epstein–Barr virus-related clonal proliferation of follicular dendritic cells. Am J Surg Pathol 1997, **20**: 313–324.

1449 Shia J, Chen W, Tang LH, Carlson DL, Qin J, Guillem JG, Nobrega J, Wong WD, Klimstra DS. Extranodal follicular dendritic cell sarcoma: clinical, pathologic, and histogenetic characteristics of an underrecognized disease entity. Virchows Arch 2006, **449**: 148–158.

1450 Soria C, Orradre JL, García-Almagro D, Martínez B, Algara P, Piris MA. True histiocytic lymphoma (monocytic sarcoma). Am J Dermatopathol 1992, **14**: 511–517.

1451 Sun X, Chang K-C, Abruzzo LV, Lai R, Younes A, Jones D. Epidermal growth factor receptor expression in follicular dendritic cells: a shared feature of follicular dendritic cell sarcoma and Castleman's disease. Hum Pathol 2003, **34**: 835–840.

1452 Takahashi K, Naito M, Takeya M. Development and heterogeneity of macrophages and their related cells through their differentiation pathways. Pathol Int 1997, **46**: 473–485.

1453 van den Oord JJ, de Wolf-Peeters C, de Vos R, Thomas J, Desmet VJ. Sarcoma arising from interdigitating reticulum cells. Report of a case, studied with light and electron microscopy, and enzyme- and immunohistochemistry. Histopathology 1986, **10**: 509–523.

1454 Venkataraman G, McClain KL, Pittaluga S, Rao VK, Jaffe ES. Development of disseminated histiocytic sarcoma in a patient with autoimmune lymphoproliferative syndrome and associated Rosai–Dorfman disease. Am J Surg Pathol 2010, **34**: 589–594.

1455 Wacker HH, Frahm SO, Heidebrecht HJ, Parwaresch R. Sinus-lining cells of lymph nodes recognized as a dendritic cell type by the new monoclonal antibody Ki-M9. Am J Pathol 1997, **151**: 423–434.

1456 Weiss LM, Berry GJ, Dorfman RF, Banks P, Kaiserling E, Curtis J, Rosai J, Warnke RA. Spindle cell neoplasms of lymph nodes of probable reticulum cell lineage. True reticulum cell sarcoma? Am J Surg Pathol 1990, **14**: 405–414.

1457 Wright-Browne V, McClain KL, Talpaz M, Ordonez N, Estrov Z. Physiology and pathophysiology of dendritic cells. Hum Pathol 1997, **28**: 563–579.

1458 Yamakawa M, Andoh A, Masuda A, Miyauchi S, Kasajima T, Ohmori A, Oguma T, Takasaki K. Follicular dendritic cell sarcoma of the omentum. Virchows Arch 2002, **440**: 660–663.

1459 Yamakawa M, Matsuda M, Imai Y, Arai S, Harada K, Sato T. Lymph node interdigitating cell sarcoma. A case report. Am J Clin Pathol 1992, **97**: 139–146.

VASCULAR TUMORS AND TUMORLIKE CONDITIONS

1460 Almagro UA, Choi H, Rouse TM. Hemangioma in a lymph node. Arch Pathol Lab Med 1985, **109**: 576–578.

1461 Bonzanini M, Togni R, Barabareschi M, Parenti A, Dalla Palma P. Primary Kaposi's sarcoma of intraparotid lymph node. Histopathology 1992, **21**: 489–491.

1462 Chan JK, Frizzera G, Fletcher CD, Rosai J. Primary vascular tumors of lymph nodes other than Kaposi's sarcoma. Analysis of 39 cases and delineation of two new entities. Am J Surg Pathol 1992, **16**: 335–350.

1463 Chan JK, Lewin KJ, Lombard CM, Teitelbaum S, Dorfman RF. Histopathology of bacillary angiomatosis of lymph node. Am J Surg Pathol 1991, **15**: 430–437.

1464 Chan JK, Warnke RA, Dorfman R. Vascular transformation of sinuses in lymph nodes. A study of its morphological spectrum and distinction from Kaposi's sarcoma. Am J Surg Pathol 1991, **15**: 732–743.

1465 Cho NH, Yang WI, Lee WJ. Spindle and epithelioid hemangioendothelioma of the inguinal lymph nodes. Histopathology 1997, **30**: 595–598.

1466 Cockerell CJ, Whitlow MA, Webster GF, Friedman-Kien AE. Epithelioid angiomatosis. A distinct vascular disorder in patients with the acquired immunodeficiency syndrome or AIDS-related complex. Lancet 1987, **2**: 654–656.

1467 Cook PD, Czerniak B, Chan JKC, Mackay B, Ordóñez NG, Ayala AG, Rosai J. Nodular spindle-cell vascular transformation of lymph nodes. A benign process occurring predominantly in retroperitoneal lymph nodes draining carcinomas that can simulate Kaposi's sarcoma or metastatic tumor. Am J Surg Pathol 1995, **19**: 1010–1020.

1468 Fayemi AO, Toker C. Nodal angiomatosis. Arch Pathol 1975, **99**: 170–172.

1469 Frizzera G, Banks PM, Massarelli G, Rosai J. A systemic lymphoproliferative disorder with morphologic features of Castleman's disease. Pathological findings in 15 patients. Am J Surg Pathol 1983, **7**: 211–231.

1470 Fukunaga M, Silverberg SG. Hyaline globules in Kaposi's sarcoma. A light microscopic and immunohistochemical study. Mod Pathol 1991, **4**: 187–190.

1471 Goldstein JED, Bartal N. Hemangioendothelioma of the lymph node. A case report. J Surg Oncol 1985, **23**: 314–317.

1472 Haferkamp O, Rosenau W, Lennert K. Vascular transformation of lymph node sinuses due to venous obstruction. Arch Pathol Lab Med 1971, **92**: 81–83.

1473 Kazakov DV, Hes O, Hora M, Sima R, Michal M. Primary intranodal cellular angiolipoma. Int J Surg Pathol 2005, **13**: 99–101.

1474 Le Jan S, Amy C, Cases A, Monnot C, Lamandé N, Favier J, Philippe J, Sibony M, Gasc J, Corvol P, Germain S. Angiopoietin-like 4 is a proangiogenic factor produced during ischemia and in convential renal cell carcinoma. Am J Pathol 2003, **162**: 1521–1523.

1475 Lott MF, Davies JD. Lymph node hypervascularity. Haemangiomatoid lesions and pan-nodal vasodilatation. J Pathol 1983, **140**: 209–219.

1476 O'Connell KM. Kaposi's sarcoma in lymph nodes. Histological study of lesions from 16 cases in Malawi. J Clin Pathol 1977, **30**: 696–703.

1477 Ostrowski ML, Siddiqui T, Barnes RE, Howton MJ. Vascular transformation of lymph node sinuses. A process displaying a spectrum of histologic features. Arch Pathol Lab Med 1990, **114**: 656–660.

1478 Perez-Piteira J, Ariza A, Mate JL, Ojanguren I, Navas-Palacios JJ. Bacillary angiomatosis. A gross mimicker of malignancy. Histopathology 1995, **26**: 476–478.

1479 Silva EG, Phillips MJ, Langer B, Ordonez NG. Spindle and histiocytoid (epithelioid) hemangioendothelioma. Primary in lymph node. Am J Clin Pathol 1986, **85**: 731–735.

1480 Steinmann G, Földi M, Racz P, Lennert K. Morphologic findings in lymph nodes after occlusion of their efferent lymphatic vessels and veins. Lab Invest 1982, **47**: 43–50.

1481 Tsang WY, Chan JK, Dorfman RF, Rosai J. Vasoproliferative lesions of the lymph node. Pathol Annu 1994, **29**(Pt 1): 63–133.

1482 Weshler Z, Leviatan A, Krasnokuki D, Kopolovitch J. Primary Kaposi's sarcoma in lymph nodes concurrent with chronic lymphatic leukemia. Am J Clin Pathol 1979, **71**: 234–237.

1483 Wright DH, Padley NR, Judd MA. Angiolymphoid hyperplasia with eosinophilia simulating lymphadenopathy. Histopathology 1981, **5**: 127–140.

OTHER PRIMARY TUMORS AND TUMORLIKE CONDITIONS

1484 Arber DA, Tamoyo R, Weiss LM. Paraffin section detection of the c-kit gene product (CD117) in human tissues: value in the diagnosis of mast cell disorders. Hum Pathol 1998, **29**: 498–504.

1485 Argani P, Ghossein R, Rosai J. Anthracotic and anthracosilicotic spindle cell pseudotumors of mediastinal lymph nodes: report of five cases of a reactive lesion that simulates malignancy. Hum Pathol 1998, **29**: 851–855.

1486 Audouin J, Comperat E, Le Tourneau A, Camilleri-Broët S, Adida C, Molina T, Diebold J. Myeloid sarcoma, clinical and morphological criteria useful for diagnosis. Int J Surg Pathol 2003, **11**: 271–282.

1487 Barbareschi M, Mariscotti C, Ferrero S, Pignatiello U. Intranodal haemorrhagic spindle cell tumour. A benign Kaposi-like nodal tumour. Histopathology 1990, **17**: 93–96.

1488 Brecher ME, Gill WB, Straus FH. Angiomyolipoma with regional lymph node involvement and long-term follow-up study. Hum Pathol 1986, **17**: 962–963.

1489 Brunning RD, McKenna RW, Rosai J, Parkin JL, Risdall R. Systemic mastocytosis. Extracutaneous manifestations. Am J Surg Pathol 1983, **7**: 425–438.

1490 Chan JK, Frizzera G, Fletcher CD, Rosai J. Primary vascular tumors of lymph nodes other than Kaposi's sarcoma. Analysis of 39 cases and delineation of two new entities. Am J Surg Pathol 1992, **16**: 335–350.

1491 Channer JL, Davies JD. Smooth muscle proliferation in the hilum of superficial lymph nodes. Virchows Arch [A] 1985, **406**: 261–270.

1492 Corrin B, Liebow AA, Friedman PJ. Pulmonary lymphangiomyomatosis. Am J Pathol 1975, **79**: 348–382.

1493 Craig SS, DeBlois G, Schwartz LB. Mast cells in human keloid, small intestine, and lung by an immunoperoxidase technique using a murine monoclonal antibody against tryptase. Am J Pathol 1986, **124**: 427–435.

1494 Creager AJ, Garwacki CP. Recurrent intranodal palisaded myofibroblastoma with metaplastic bone formation. Arch Pathol Lab Med 1999, **123**: 433–436.

1495 Davis RE, Warnke RA, Dorfman RF. Inflammatory pseudotumor of lymph nodes. Additional observations and evidence for an inflammatory etiology. Am J Surg Pathol 1991, **15**: 744–756.

1496 Facchetti F, De Wolf Peeters C, De Wever I, Frizzera G. Inflammatory pseudotumor of lymph nodes. Immunohistochemical evidence for its fibrohistiocytic nature. Am J Pathol 1990, **137**: 281–289.

1497 Facchetti F, Incardona P, Lonardi S, Fisogni S, Legrenzi L, Chioda C, Ponzoni M, Chiodera PL. Nodal inflammatory pseudotumor caused by luetic infection. Am J Surg Pathol 2009, **33**: 447–453.

1498 Fletcher CD, Stirling RW. Intranodal myofibroblastoma presenting in the submandibular region. Evidence of a broader clinical and histological spectrum. Histopathology 1990, **16**: 287–293.

1499 Hisaoka M, Hashiomoto H, Daimaru Y. Intranodal palisaded myofibroblastoma with so-called amianthoid fibers: a report of two cases with a review of the literature. Pathol Int 1998, **48**: 307–312.

1500 Horie A, Ishii N, Matsumoto M, Hashizume Y, Kawakami M, Sato Y. Leiomyomatosis in the pelvic lymph node and peritoneum. Acta Pathol Jpn 1984, **34**: 813–819.

1501 Horny HP, Menke DM, Kaiserling E. Neoplastic human tissue mast cells express the adhesion molecule CD44/HCAM. Virchows Arch 1996, **429**: 91–94.

1502 Horny HP, Sillaber C, Menke D, Kaiserling E, Wehrmann M, Stehberger B, Chott A, Lechner K, Lennert K, Valent P. Diagnostic value of immunostaining for tryptase in patients with mastocytosis. Am J Surg Pathol 1998, **22**: 1132–1140.

1503 Hudock J, Chatten J, Miettinen M. Immunohistochemical evaluation of myeloid leukemia infiltrates (granulocytic sarcomas) in formaldehyde-fixed, paraffin-embedded tissue. Am J Clin Pathol 1994, **102**: 55–60.

1504 Kemper CA, Davis RE, Deresinski SC, Dorfmann RF. Inflammatory pseudotumor of intra-abdominal lymph nodes manifesting as recurrent fever of unknown origin. A case report. Am J Med 1991, **90**: 519–523.

1505 Kojima M, Nakamura S, Shimizu K, Hosomura Y, Ohno Y, Itoh H, Yamane N, Yoshiba K, Masawa N. Inflammatory pseudotumor of lymph nodes: clinicopathologic and immunohistological study of 11 Japanese cases. Int J Surg Pathol 2001, **9**: 207–214.

1506 Kutok JL, Pinkus GS, Dorfman DM, Fletcher CD. Inflammatory pseudotumor of lymph node and spleen: an entity biologically distinct from inflammatory myofibroblastic tumor. Hum Pathol 2002, **32**: 1382–1387.

1507 Lee JY, Abell E, Shevechik GJ. Solitary spindle cell tumor with myoid differentiation of the lymph node. Arch Pathol Lab Med 1989, **113**: 547–550.

1508 Lennert K, Illert E. Die Häufigkeit der Gewebsmastzellen im Lymphknoten bei verschiedenen Erkrankungen. Frankf Z Pathol 1959, **70**: 121–131.

1509 Lennert K, Parwaresch MR. Mast cells and mast cell neoplasia. A review. Histopathology 1979, **3**: 349–365.

1510 Li WV, Kapadia SB, Sonmez-Alpan E, Swerdlow SH. Immunohistochemical characterization of mast cell disease in paraffin sections using tryptase, CD68, myeloperoxidase, lysozyme, and CD20 antibodies. Mod Pathol 1997, **9**: 982–988.

1511 Mazzoleni G, Salerno A, Santini D, Marabini A, Martinelli G. Leiomyomatosis in pelvic lymph nodes. Histopathology 1992, **21**: 588–589.

1512 Menasce LP, Banerjee SS, Beckett E, Harris M. Extra-medullary myeloid tumour (granulocytic sarcoma) is often misdiagnosed: a study of 26 cases. Histopathology 1999, **34**: 391–398.

1513 Michal M, Chlumska A, Povysilova V. Intranodal 'amianthoid' myofibroblastoma. Report of six cases immunohistochemical and electron microscopical study. Pathol Res Pract 1992, **188**: 199–204.

1514 Moran CA, Suster S, Abbondanzo SL. Inflammatory pseudotumor of lymph nodes: a study of 25 cases with emphasis on morphological heterogeneity. Hum Pathol 1997, **28**: 332–338.

1515 Nonaka D, Birbe R, Rosai J. So-called inflammatory myofibroblastic tumour: a proliferative lesion of fibroblastic reticulum cells? Histopathology 2005, **46**: 604–613.

1516 Perrone T, De Wolf-Peeters C, Frizzera G. Inflammatory pseudotumor of nodal lymph nodes. A distinctive pattern of nodal reaction. Am J Surg Pathol 1988, **12**: 351–361.

1517 Pulitzer MP, Gerami P, Busam K. Solar elastotic material in dermal lymphatics and lymph nodes. Am J Surg Pathol 2010, **34**: 1492–1497.

1518 Roth MJ, Medeiros LJ, Elenitoba-Johnson K, Kuchnio M, Jaffe ES, Stetler-Stevenson M. Extramedullary myeloid cell tumors. An immunohistochemical study of 29 cases using routinely fixed and processed paraffin-embedded tissue sections. Arch Pathol Lab Med 1995, **119**: 790–798.

1519 Skalova A, Michal M, Chlumska A, Leivo I. Collagen composition and ultra-structure of the so-called amianthoid fibres in palisaded myofibroblastoma. Ultrastructural and immunohistochemical study. J Pathol 1992, **167**: 335–340.

1520 Starasoler L, Vuitch F, Albores-Saavedra J. Intranodal leiomyoma. Another distinctive primary spindle cell neoplasm of lymph node. Am J Clin Pathol 1991, **95**: 858–862.

1521 Suster S, Rosai J. Intranodal hemorrhagic spindle-cell tumor with 'amianthoid' fibers. Report of six cases of a distinctive mesenchymal neoplasm of the inguinal region that simulates Kaposi's sarcoma. Am J Surg Pathol 1989, **13**: 347–357.

1522 Tanda F, Massarelli G, Cossu A, Bosincu L, Cossu S, Ibba M. Primary spindle cell tumor of lymph node with 'amianthoid' fibers. A histological, immunohistochemical and ultrastructural study. Ultrastruct Pathol 1993, **17**: 195–205.

1523 Weiss SW, Gnepp DR, Bratthauer GL. Palisaded myofibroblastoma. A benign mesenchymal tumor of lymph node. Am J Surg Pathol 1989, **13**: 341–346.

1524 White JET, Chan YF, Miller MV. Intranodal leiomyoma or myofibroblastoma. An identical lesion? Histopathology 1995, **26**: 188–189.

1525 Yang F, Tran TA, Carlson JA, Hsi ED, Ross CW, Arber DA. Paraffin section immunophenotype of cutaneous and extracutaneous mast cell disease: comparison to other hematopoietic neoplasms. Am J Surg Pathol 2000, **24**: 703–709.

METASTATIC TUMORS

1526 Argani P, Ghossein R, Rosai J. Anthracotic and anthracosilicotic spindle cell pseudotumors of mediastinal lymph nodes: report of five cases of a reactive lesion that simulates malignancy. Hum Pathol 1998, **29**: 851–855.

1527 Argani P, Rosai J. Hyperplastic mesothelial cells in lymph nodes: report of six cases of a benign process that can simulate metastatic involvement by mesothelioma or carcinoma. Hum Pathol 1998, **29**: 339–346.

1528 Batsakis JG. The pathology of head and neck tumors. The occult primary and metastases to the head and neck, part 10. Head Neck Surg 1981, **3**: 409–423.

1529 Cervin JR, Silverman JF, Loggie BW, Geisinger KR. Virchow's node revisited. Analysis with clinicopathologic correlation of 152 fine needle aspiration biopsies of supraclavicular lymph nodes. Arch Pathol Lab Med 1995, **119**: 727–730.

1530 Clary CF, Michel RP, Wang N-S, Hanson RE. Metastatic carcinoma. The lung as the site for the clinically undiagnosed primary. Cancer 1983, **51**: 362–366.

1531 Copeland EM, McBride CM. Axillary metastases from unknown primary sites. Ann Surg 1973, **178**: 25–27.

1532 De Petris G, Siew S. Peritumoral and nodal muciphages. Am J Surg Pathol 1998, **22**: 545–549.

1533 Didlolker MS, Fanous N, Elias EG, et al. Metastatic carcinomas from occult primary tumors. A study of 254 patients. Ann Surg 1977, **186**: 628–630.

1534 Dvorak AM, Monahan RA. Metastatic adenocarcinoma of unknown primary site. Diagnostic electron microscopy to determine the site of tumor origin. Arch Pathol Lab Med 1982, **106**: 21–24.

1535 Feigenberg Z, Zer M, Dintsman M. Axillary metastases from an unknown primary source. Isr J Med Sci 1976, **12**: 1153–1158.

1536 Giffler RF, Gillespie JJ, Ayala AG, Newland JR. Lymphoepithelioma in cervical lymph nodes of children and young adults. Am J Surg Pathol 1977, **1**: 293–302.

1537 Groisman GM, Amar M, Weiner P, Zamir D. Mucicarminophilic histiocytosis (benign signet-ring cells) and hyperplastic mesothelial cells: two mimics of metastatic carcinoma within a single lymph node. Arch Pathol Lab Med 1998, **122**: 282–284.

1538 Guerrero-Medrano J, Delgado R, Albores-Saavedra J. Signet-ring sinus histiocytosis: a reactive disorder that mimics metastatic adenocarcinoma. Cancer 1997, **80**: 277–285.

1539 Haagensen CD, Feind CR, Herter FP, Slanetz CA Jr, Weinberg JA. The lymphatics in cancer. Philadelphia, 1972, W.B. Saunders.

1540 Hoda SA, Resetkova E, Yusuf Y, Cahan A, Rosen PP. Megakaryocytes mimicking metastatic breast carcinoma. Arch Pathol Lab Med 2002, **126**: 618–620.

1541 Lindbergh R. Distribution of cervical lymph node metastases from squamous cell carcinoma of the upper respiratory and digestive tracts. Cancer 1972, **29**: 1446–1449.

1542 Mancuso AA, Hanafee WN. Elusive head and neck carcinomas beneath intact mucosa. Laryngoscope 1983, **93**: 133–139.

1543 Markman M. Metastatic adenocarcinoma of unknown primary site. Analysis of 245 patients seen at the Johns Hopkins Hospital from 1965–1979. Med Pediatr Oncol 1982, **10**: 569–574.

1544 Silverman CL, Marks JE. Metastatic cancer of unknown origin. Epidermoid and undifferentiated carcinomas. Semin Oncol 1982, **9**: 435–441.

1545 Sussman J, Rosai J. Lymph node metastases as the initial manifestation of malignant mesothelioma. Report of six cases. Am J Surg Pathol 1990, **14**: 819–828.

1546 Willis RA. The spread of tumours in the human body, ed. 3. Stoneham, MA, 1973, Butterworth.

1547 Zaren HA, Copeland EM. Inguinal node metastases. Cancer 1978, **41**: 919–923.

Spleen 22

CHAPTER CONTENTS

Normal anatomy

The spleen performs a variety of functions, most of which have been correlated with specific anatomic compartments.[2,4–6,11] The most important are: (1) hematopoiesis (erythrocytes, granulocytes, megakaryocytes, lymphocytes, and macrophages); (2) reservoir (storage or sequestration of platelets and other formed elements); (3) phagocytosis (removal of particulate matter, red blood cell destruction, pitting, and erythroclasis); and (4) immunity (trapping and processing of antigen, 'homing' of lymphocytes, lymphocyte transformation and proliferation, and antibody production).[2,6] The first two functions are not important in normal adult humans.

Anatomically, the spleen is divided into two compartments – white pulp and red pulp – separated by an ill-defined interphase known as the marginal zone.[3,8,10,11] The white pulp is made up of T and B lymphocytes, the former located in the periarteriolar lymphoid sheath and the latter eccentrically to this sheath in the form of primary lymphoid follicles.[7] These lymphoid follicles contain germinal centers, particularly in children.

The red pulp consists of a complex network of venous sinuses and the cords of Billroth. The ring fibers, which demarcate the cordal–sinusoidal relationships in the red pulp, are best appreciated with the periodic acid–Schiff (PAS) stain. The cords contain most of the splenic macrophages, which are responsible for the important phagocytic function of this organ. The sinuses are lined by a particular type of endothelial cell endowed with endothelial and histiocytic markers (known as a littoral cell) and have a discontinuous wall, which allows traffic of blood cells between cords and sinuses.[1,9,12]

Biopsy and fine needle aspiration

Biopsy of the spleen is rarely attempted because of the possibility of hemorrhage and the preconceived notion that the biopsy will not be of diagnostic help. Obviously, the procedure should not be performed on patients with a bleeding tendency. A few authors have used it routinely, either with the Vim–Silverman-type needle to obtain a core of tissue or with a fine needle to obtain an aspirate.[14] These authors claim that morbidity is nil and that in some instances the technique results in a definitive diagnosis that is not easily obtainable by other means. A multicenter study in Italy on ultrasound-guided fine needle aspiration (FNA) of the spleen documented the high yield and low risk of the procedure.[13] The overall accuracy was 91%, and the incidence of major complications was less than 1%. Aspiration cytology and core needle biopsy gave similar diagnostic yields, except for malignant lymphoma, in which core needle biopsy proved superior.

The material obtained by FNA is suitable for flow cytometry immunophenotyping.[15]

Rupture and splenectomy

Blunt trauma to the abdomen and surgical intervention within the abdominal cavity are the two most common factors responsible for rupture of the normal spleen.[36] In most instances, hemoperitoneum is an immediate consequence, leading to an emergency splenectomy. In about 15% of the cases, the rupture is 'delayed' anywhere from 48 hours to several months.[27] Examination of the excised spleen will reveal the ruptured area, which, in many cases, is limited to a deceptively small capsular tear, often in the superior pole and/or hilum. A neutrophilic infiltrate may be seen subcapsularly and along the edges of the tear. Foci of intraparenchymal hemorrhage are often present. Germinal centers with an expanded marginal zone and other signs of lymphoid hyperplasia were found more commonly by Farhi and Ashfaq[24] in ruptured spleens than in control cases, leading them to conclude that immunologically stimulated organs may be more prone to traumatic rupture. If the marginal zone expansion is prominent, the possibility of a splenic marginal zone lymphoma needs to be considered; however, it has been shown that the large majority of ruptured spleens with expanded marginal zones do not contain a clonal B-cell population.[31]

Following traumatic rupture, splenic tissue may implant in the form of encapsulated nodules on the peritoneal surface, abdominal wall (including surgical scars), and even within the pleural cavity, lung parenchyma and brain, a process known as **splenosis**.[17-19,34,38,39] Although some are poorly developed architecturally,[26] others show a full complement of red and white pulp, resulting in an appearance similar to that of accessory spleen.[20] In most cases, the pathogenesis is probably through mechanical implant on the surface, but in the single instance of cerebral splenosis, a hematogenous spread of splenic tissue has to be assumed.[38]

The diseases most commonly associated with spontaneous rupture of the spleen are infectious mononucleosis,[16] malaria, typhoid fever, subacute bacterial endocarditis, peliosis lienis[28,32] (see p. 1907), malignant lymphomas (including those occurring in HIV-infected patients),[25] leukemias, and primary nonlymphoid splenic neoplasms.[41] In every case of ruptured spleen without a history of trauma or in which the trauma seems insignificant, a careful microscopic study should be performed in order to rule out these possibilities. Rupture of the spleen with resulting hemoperitoneum is the most frequent cause of death in infectious mononucleosis. This complication usually occurs from 10 to 21 days after the onset of the disease.[37] In rare cases, 'spontaneous' rupture may occur in an apparently normal spleen, particularly during pregnancy.[21]

Splenectomy performed in adults for traumatic rupture of the spleen usually does not result in any sequelae of significance.[35] Conversely, an increased incidence and severity of infections have been reported following splenectomy in young children.[33] It has been shown that this is the result of a decrease in immunoglobulin production and phagocytic activity during episodes of transient bacteremia.[22,23] Overwhelming infection may occur days to years after removal of the spleen; it begins abruptly, frequently lacks an identifiable focus, and usually progresses rapidly despite appropriate antibiotic therapy, resulting in a mortality of 50–80%.[40] Because of this, an attempt is now made to save splenic function in children by performing repair of the laceration or by partial splenectomy. If a total splenectomy is necessary, spleen autotransplant has been recommended.[40] The patient's immune function is better preserved by any of these measures than by splenectomy alone.[42]

Splenectomy performed in the presence of diffuse splenomegaly or a discrete splenic mass for the purpose of obtaining a diagnosis almost always achieves that purpose. About 75% of the cases prove to be malignant tumors.[30]

Whenever splenectomy is performed for hematologic disorders, a thorough search should be made for accessory spleens in order to excise them if present. A similar precept applies if the operation is done laparoscopically, a procedure that has proved safe and effective for benign splenic diseases.[29]

Congenital anomalies

Accessory (supernumerary) spleen is found in about 10% of individuals. It may be solitary or multiple, usually measures no more than 4 cm in diameter, and has a gross and microscopic appearance similar to that of the parent organ. Its most common location is the hilum of the spleen, and it is sometimes seen in contiguity with the tail of the pancreas. It should be distinguished from lymph nodes (especially when the latter are involved by Castleman disease) and splenosis (see previous section). Accessory spleens may contain epithelial cysts within them (see p. 1903).

Congenital absence of the spleen (asplenia) is associated in more than 80% of the cases with malformations of the heart, nearly always involving the atrioventricular endocardial cushion and the ventricular outflow tracts.[49] Anomalies of the blood vessels, lung, and abdominal viscera also are frequent.[44] In polysplenia, the cardiac anomalies are less severe and the prognosis is therefore more favorable.[51] A hereditary form of splenic hypoplasia has been reported.[46]

Splenic–gonadal fusion occurs in two forms. One is continuous, in which the main spleen is connected by a cord of splenic and fibrous tissue to the gonadal (usually testicular) mesonephric structures; the other is discontinuous, in which discrete masses of splenic tissue are found fused to these same structures[47,48,50] (Fig. 22.1). Of the 52 cases reviewed by Watson,[53] only four were in females. Eleven were associated with other congenital defects, such as peromelus and micrognathia. Various degrees of testicular ectopia and inguinal hernias are common. All of the reported cases have been on the left side.[40]

Cases of splenohepatic and splenorenal fusion have also been recorded,as a well as an isolated case of ectopic prostatic tissue in the spleen.[43,45,52]

Cysts

Pseudocysts (false or secondary cysts) constitute approximately 75% of the nonparasitic cysts of the spleen (Fig. 22.2).[58] Their wall is composed of dense fibrous tissue, often calcified, with no epithelial lining. The content is a mixture of blood and necrotic debris. If the cyst ruptures, massive hemoperitoneum may result. The majority of these cysts are solitary and asymptomatic. Trauma is the most

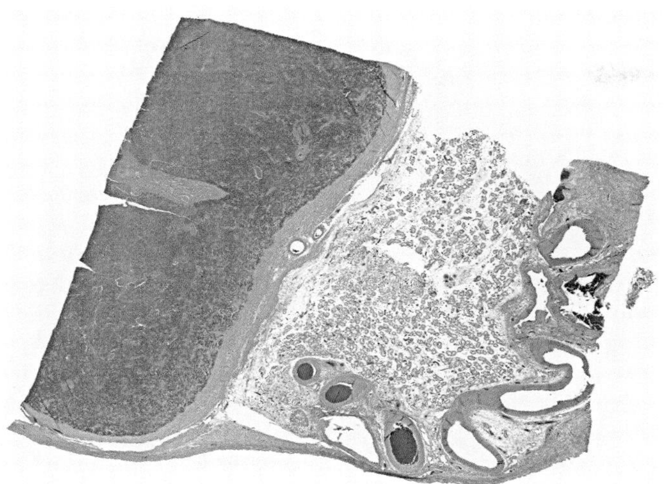

Fig. 22.1 Splenogonadal fusion. Splenic tissue (left) is attached to testicular tissue.

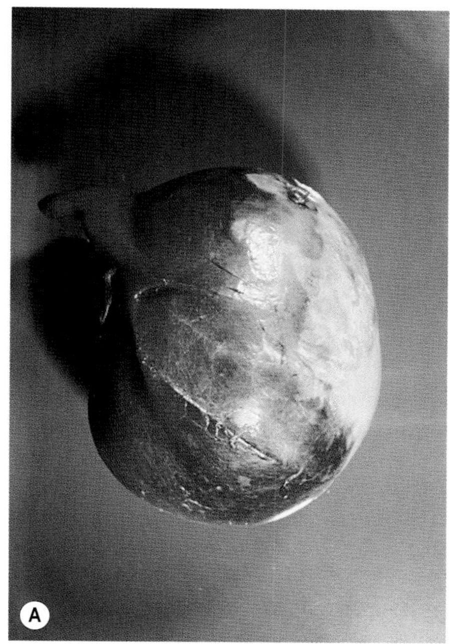

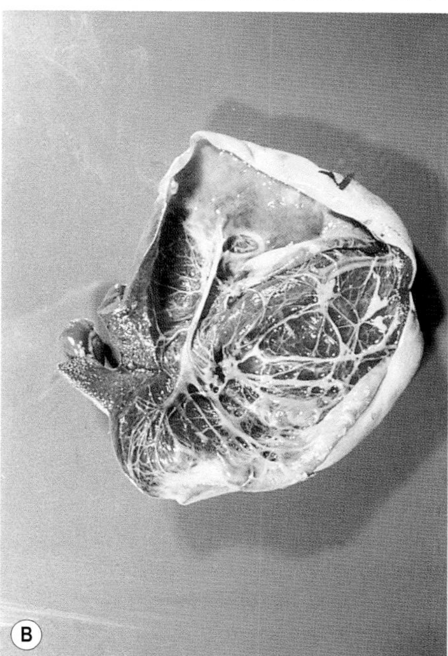

Fig. 22.2 Pseudocyst (false or secondary cyst). **A**, Outer aspect. **B**, Inner surface. Notice the white trabeculation.

likely etiologic factor, although it is possible that some are epithelial cysts of the type described below in which part or all of the lining has been destroyed.

Epithelial (primary) cysts are mainly seen in children or young adults.[54,63,65] They are usually solitary, but can be multiple. Cases have also been described in accessory spleens.[61,64] Grossly, a glistening inner surface with marked trabeculation is often seen (Fig. 22.3A). Microscopically, the wall is lined by columnar, cuboidal (mesothelial-like), or squamous epithelium (Fig. 22.3B). When the latter is the case, the term *epidermoid cyst* is employed.[55] Curiously, the stratified epithelium lining these cysts is immunoreactive for carcinoembryonic antigen (CEA) and CA19-9, and these markers can be elevated in the serum.[59] Skin adnexae are absent. The histogenesis is unknown; embryonic inclusions of epithelial cells from adjacent structures, invagination of capsular surface mesothelium, and a monodermal teratomatous nature have been proposed.[56,62] The immunohistochemical profile of some is in keeping with a teratomatous derivation or origin from fetal squamous epithelium,[60] whereas others have the profile of mesothelial cells (mesothelial cyst)[54] (Fig. 22.4). A case occurring in an intrapancreatic accessory spleen that has the appearance of a lymphoepithelial cyst has been reported by Tateyama.[64] Most cases of epithelial splenic cysts are large and require splenectomy. If enough parenchyma is preserved, the performance of a partial splenectomy should be attempted, particularly in children.

Mucinous epithelial cysts can occur within the spleen in association with pseudomyxoma peritonei; rarely, splenomegaly due to this change is the presenting manifestation of the disease or an indicator of recurrence.[57]

Parasitic cysts resulting from *Echinococcus* infestation can involve the spleen (Fig. 22.5).

Inflammation

Reactive follicular hyperplasia of the spleen can be seen as an acute phenomenon in response to a systemic infection. Morphologically, it is often associated with variable degrees of congestion, diffuse immunoblastic and plasmacytic proliferation, and outpouring of neutrophils in the red pulp (so-called **septic spleen** or **acute septic splenitis**); measles and typhoid fever are the two better known etiologies. It also occurs in a chronic form in a large number of infectious diseases – including AIDS[72,77] – and in immune-mediated diseases, such as idiopathic thrombocytopenic purpura, acquired hemolytic anemia, rheumatoid arthritis (including Felty syndrome),[73] and the systemic form of Castleman disease,[74,88] as well as in hemodialyzed patients.[82]

Diffuse lymphoid hyperplasia with production of immunoblasts and plasma cells can be the result of infection (particularly viral), graft rejection, or a component of so-called angioimmunoblastic lymphadenopathy (see Chapter 21). In infectious mononucleosis, the splenic involvement is mainly in the red pulp.

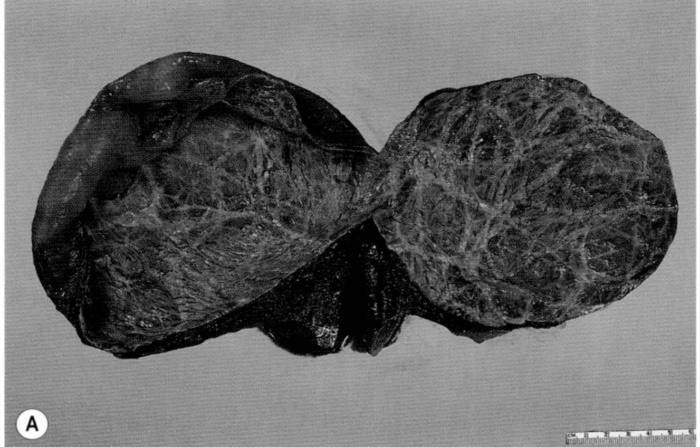

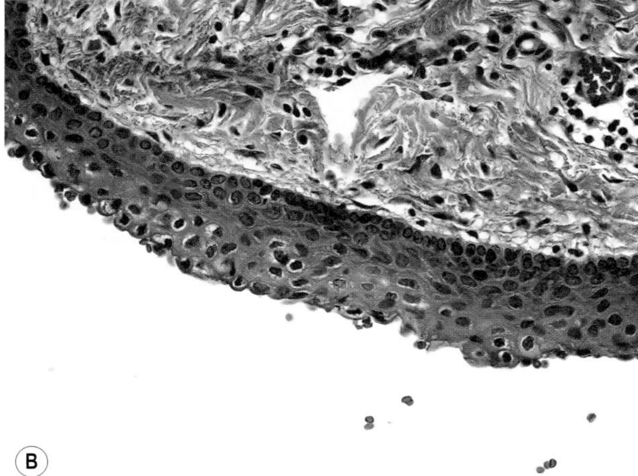

Fig. 22.3 **A**, Epithelial cyst. Grossly, it is very difficult, if not impossible, to distinguish this lesion from a pseudocyst. **B**, Squamous lining of the inner surface.

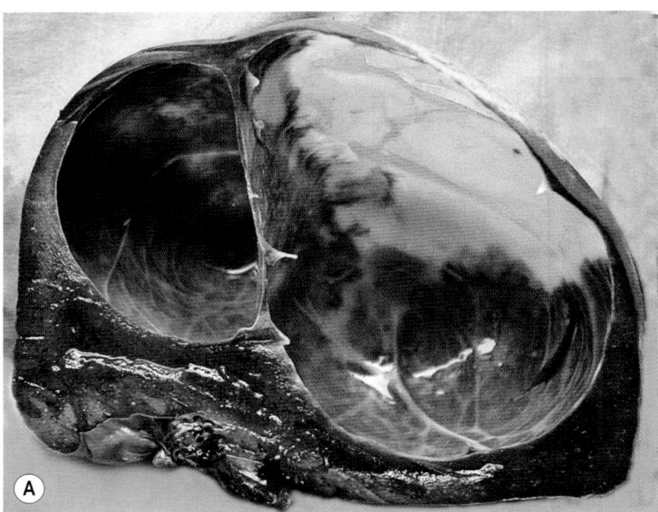

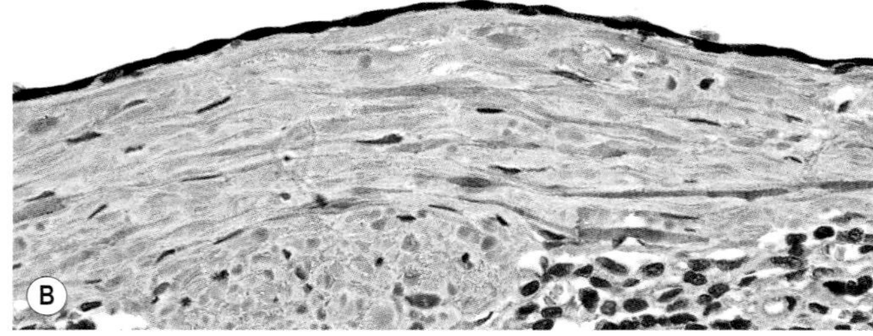

Fig. 22.4 Splenic cyst lined by mesothelial cells. **A**, Gross appearance. **B**, Immunoreactivity of the lining cells for calretinin.

Bagshawe[66] compared the clinical and laboratory features of hypersplenism (see next section) among 46 patients with congestive splenomegaly and 29 with reactive splenomegaly and found no significant differences between them. Massive splenomegaly of a reactive nature is commonly seen in inhabitants of several tropical countries, such as Madagascar, the Democratic Republic of Congo, Nigeria, and New Guinea.[71] Spleens removed for this tropical splenomegaly syndrome are often extremely heavy (mean, 3270 g) and exhibit a uniform dark red, cut surface. Microscopically, there is marked dilation of the sinuses and foci of extramedullary hematopoiesis but no significant fibrosis or hemosiderin deposition.[83] Signs of hypersplenism are the rule. Epidemiologic and therapeutic studies suggest a causal relationship with malaria.[83,85] In this regard, it is interesting that the cases of idiopathic splenomegaly reported by Banti in 1883[78] were from an area of central Italy that at the time was endemic for malaria (see p. 1907).

Abscess of the spleen, an extremely rare condition, can be the result of trauma or metastatic spread of infection from another site[69,70] (Fig. 22.6). Septic abscesses of the spleen secondary to subacute bacterial endocarditis may necessitate surgical intervention.[75]

Granulomatous inflammation is a relatively common finding in splenectomy specimens. The granulomas can be roughly divided into three major types: (1) large active granulomas containing

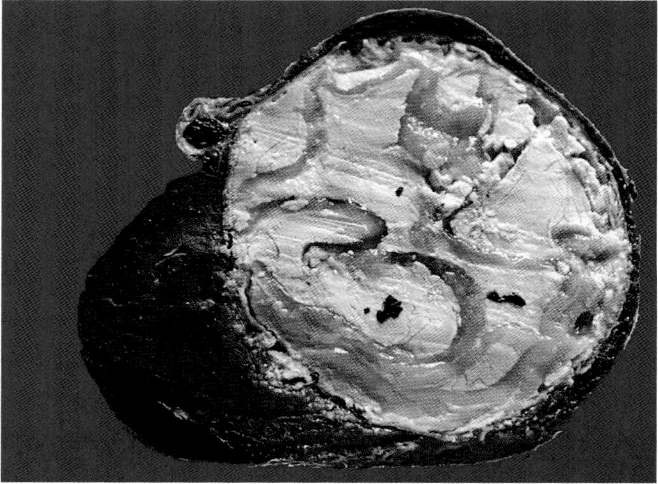

Fig. 22.5 Hydatidosis of spleen.

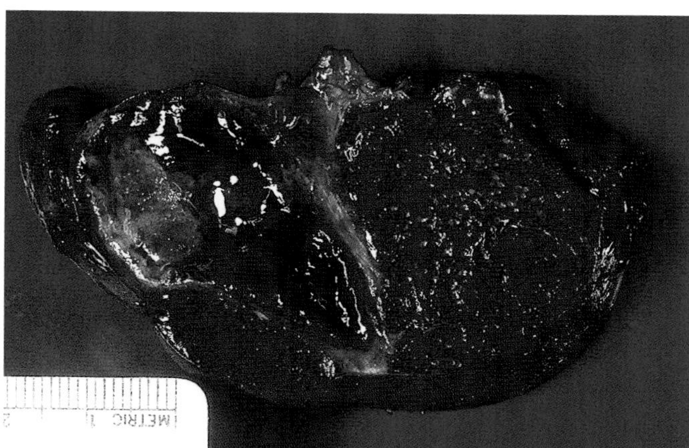

Fig. 22.6 Gross appearance of a thick-walled splenic abscess. The content is partially purulent and partially hemorrhagic.

epithelioid and Langhans-type giant cells, with or without central necrosis; (2) small, widespread, sarcoid-like epithelioid granulomas with scanty giant cells and no necrosis (not to be equated with 'epithelioid' germinal centers);[80] and (3) old inactive granulomas, with fibrosis and calcification. A variant of the first type, characterized by extensive necrotizing changes, has been seen as a complication of leukemia in childhood.[87]

The third type of granuloma, which can be solitary or found scattered throughout the spleen, is particularly common in areas of endemic histoplasmosis.[89] We have evaluated 20 cases of splenectomy done for splenomegaly and/or hypersplenism in which the only major pathologic finding was the presence of active granulomas of either the first or second type.[79] All of the patients were adults. Fever, weight loss, hepatosplenomegaly, and the various manifestations of hypersplenism were the most common symptoms, and these were markedly ameliorated with splenectomy. The splenic granulomas were nearly always the expression of a generalized disease, which also often involved lymph nodes, liver, and bone marrow. Despite the performance of special stains and cultures, the etiology remained unknown in all but three cases. In these, the organisms identified were *Histoplasma capsulatum*, an atypical *Mycobacterium*, and *Sporotrichum schenckii*, respectively (Fig. 22.7). None of the patients developed malignant lymphoma on follow-up.

Sarcoid-like granulomas can be seen in the spleen of patients with Hodgkin lymphoma[76] and, less commonly, non-Hodgkin lymphoma and hairy cell leukemia,[67] with or without involvement of the spleen by tumor. In some cases of non-Hodgkin lymphoma, the numerous granulomas may obscure the underlying lymphoma.[68] It should be emphasized that the presence of splenic granulomas in patients with lymphoma is not an indication per se that the spleen is involved by tumor. Actually, some authors have suggested that in patients with Hodgkin lymphoma, this finding is associated with an improved prognosis.[84] Neiman[81] found sarcoid-like granulomas in 24 of 412 splenectomy specimens; in addition to the conditions previously listed, he found them in chronic uremia and in a single case of IgA deficiency. He pointed out that in all cases the granulomas appeared to arise in the periarteriolar lymphoid sheath, suggesting that they are the result of abnormal or defective processing of antigen presented to the spleen. Granulomas have also been described in spleens affected by infectious mononucleosis.[86]

Perisplenitis presents as thick white fibrous plaques coating the surface. It is a common incidental finding at autopsy (Fig. 22.8).

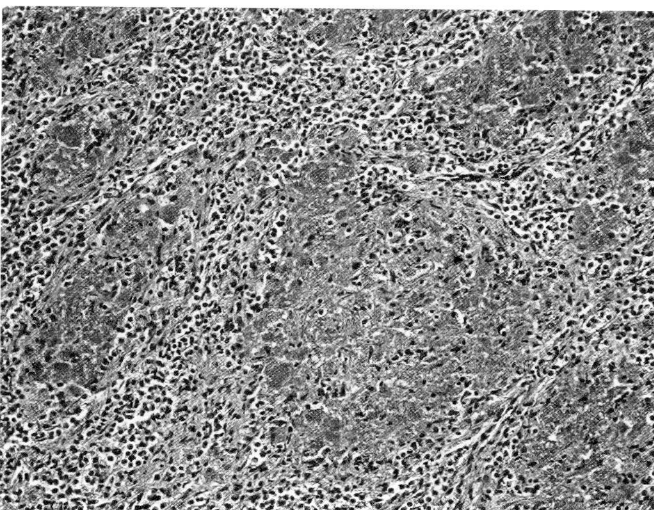

Fig. 22.7 Granulomas of spleen due to *M. avium* in an immunosuppressed patient.

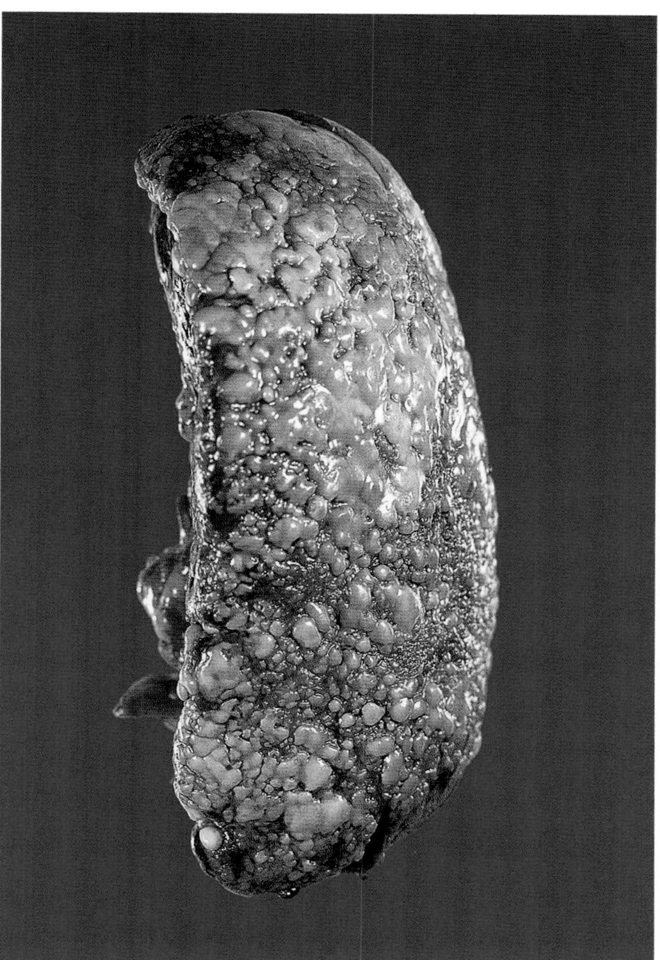

Fig. 22.8 Typical gross appearance of perisplenitis ('sugar-coated' or 'snow-covered' spleen).
(Courtesy of Dr RA Cooke, Brisbane, Australia. From Cooke RA, Stewart B. Colour atlas of anatomical pathology. Edinburgh, 2004, Churchill Livingstone)

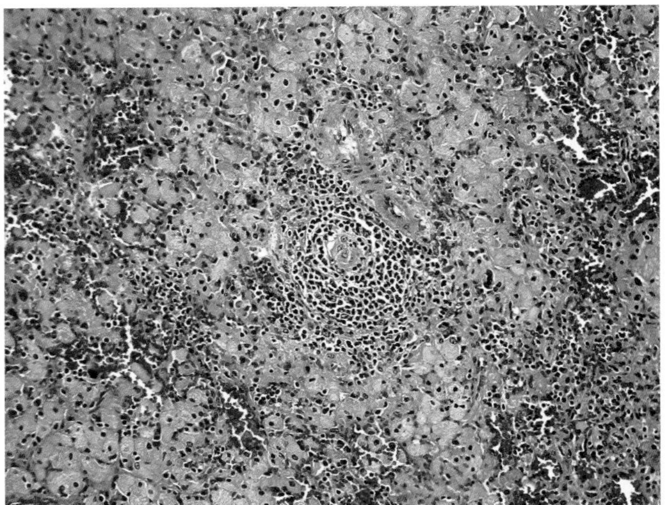

Fig. 22.9 Gaucher disease of spleen. Macrophages with abundant pale acidophilic cytoplasm pack the red pulp.

Hypersplenism

Hypersplenism (dysplenism) is the generic term used for the group of disorders in which the removal of hematopoietic elements by the spleen increases to a pathologic degree.[90,92] Any of the cellular elements of the blood may be affected, singly or in combination. Thus neutropenia, thrombocytopenia, hemolytic anemia, or pancytopenia may all be present. In some conditions, such as spherocytic hemolytic anemia or idiopathic thrombocytopenic purpura, the basic abnormality resides in the blood elements themselves. In others, the hypersplenism results from widening of the splenic cords with an increase in macrophages and/or connective tissue fibers and premature destruction of the normal elements of the blood. Hypersplenism resulting from this mechanism can be seen with congestive splenomegaly, Gaucher disease (Fig. 22.9), malignant lymphoma, leukemia, Langerhans cell histiocytosis, hemangioma, hamartoma, angiosarcoma, and practically any condition involving more or less diffusely the splenic parenchyma and particularly in the red pulp.[93]

A syndrome of hypersplenism developing in uremic hemodialyzed patients has also been recognized.[91] Splenectomy results in a marked improvement; a striking degree of lymphoid hyperplasia is found in the excised spleens.

Thrombocytopenic purpuras

Immune thrombocytopenic purpura (traditionally known as idiopathic thrombocytopenic purpura) is caused by an antiplatelet IgG, which is produced largely in the spleen.[99,106] Occasionally, thrombocytopenic purpura is seen as a manifestation of lupus erythematosus, viral infection, drug hypersensitivity,[94] chronic lymphocytic leukemia,[101] or Hodgkin lymphoma.[108] The antibody-coated platelets have a short life span because they are rapidly removed by the cells of the reticuloendothelial system, particularly in the spleen and liver. There is some evidence that the number of antibody molecules bound to the platelets may determine the main site of removal. Heavily coated platelets are removed by the liver phagocytes, whereas lightly coated platelets pass through the liver but are sequestered in the spleen.

Grossly, the spleen is of normal size or only mildly enlarged;[103] malpighian follicles may be prominent. Microscopically, there is formation of secondary follicles with well-developed germinal centers (containing the platelet antigen CD41),[104] prominence of histiocytes in the red pulp, dilation of sinuses, variable numbers of perivascular plasma cells in the marginal zone, and infiltration with neutrophils of the red pulp.[98] Mild myeloid metaplasia, usually in the form of megakaryocytes, is present in most cases.[97,98,103] The germinal centers, which usually show phagocytosis of nuclear debris and periarterial fibrosis,[95] are no longer prominent in cases previously treated with steroids.[102]

Collections of foamy macrophages containing phospholipid deposits are present in the red pulp in some of the cases.[100,109] They are the result of phagocytosis of platelets and of incompletely degraded membrane-derived phospholipids,[105,112] as supported by the fact that the platelet antigen CD41 has been detected immunohistochemically in them.[104] The phagocytosis of platelets by splenic histiocytes can be better appreciated in touch preparations. It should be noted that the presence of foamy macrophages in the spleen is not pathognomonic of this disorder (see p. 1907).

Splenectomy in idiopathic thrombocytopenic purpura is reserved for patients unresponsive to steroid or immunosuppressive therapy.[96] It achieves sustained remission in 50–80% of the cases.[110] It is difficult to predict its effectiveness in an individual case. However, Chang et al.[98] have shown that patients with prominent secondary follicles have a higher rate of antiplatelet antibody production and exhibit a better initial response, with a great increase in platelets postoperatively.

Thrombotic thrombocytopenic purpura may be accompanied by splenic enlargement.[107] The most important pathologic change is the presence of thrombi in arteries and arterioles without associated inflammation. PAS-positive hyaline subendothelial deposits are present. Other changes include hyperplasia of B cells and germinal centers, periarteriolar concentric fibrosis, hemosiderin-laden macrophages, hemophagocytosis, and extramedullary hematopoiesis.[111]

Hemolytic anemia

Congenital hemolytic anemia (hereditary spherocytosis) is a genetically determined disease in which the red blood cells acquire a spheric shape (spherocytes).[115] The abnormality lies in the cell membrane of the red blood cell. Consistent molecular alterations of spectrin and ankyrin have been detected, resulting in defects in the horizontal interactions that hold the membrane skeleton together, particularly the critical spectrin self-association reaction.[116,119,121,123] As a result, the erythrocytes lack the plasticity of normal red blood cells and become trapped in the interstices of the spleen.[124] The splenic function itself is normal.

Acquired hemolytic anemia can be caused by toxins (bacterial hemolysins), plasma lipid abnormalities, parasites that invade red blood cells, and – most important – immune reactions that result in deposition of immune complexes on red blood cell membranes.[118] About one-half of the cases of immune hemolytic anemias are unassociated with other significant pathologic abnormalities. The remaining cases are seen as a manifestation of a large variety of disease, such as various forms of acute and chronic leukemia, Hodgkin lymphoma, sarcoidosis, lupus erythematosus, tuberculosis, and brucellosis. The Coombs test is the classic method to distinguish between the acquired (positive) and congenital (negative) types of hemolytic anemia. A positive Coombs test consists of agglutination of the patient's washed red blood cells following mixture with antihuman globulin rabbit serum.

Grossly, the spleen of both congenital and acquired hemolytic anemia is fairly firm and deep red, has a thin capsule and no grossly discernible malpighian follicles, and ranges in weight from 100 to 1000 g. In congenital hemolytic anemia, the splenic cords are congested, whereas the sinusoids appear relatively empty because of the presence of ghost red blood cells.[125] The lining cells of the sinuses are prominent, sometimes resulting in a glandlike appearance. Hemosiderin deposition and erythrophagocytosis are present in both conditions but are usually more pronounced in the acquired variety. Ultrastructural studies have shown that the splenic cords are not empty but rather contain red blood cells that have lost their electron density, thus corresponding to the red cell ghosts of light microscopy.[117]

In acquired hemolytic anemia, the congestion may predominate in the cords or sinuses or be equally prominent in both. A high correlation exists between spherocytosis and increased osmotic fragility on one hand and the degree of cord congestion on the other. Foci of extramedullary hematopoiesis may be present. Splenic infarcts are found in one-fourth of the cases.[120]

Hereditary spherocytosis is the hematologic disease that most benefits from splenectomy.[122] The clinical cure rate is almost 100%, although the intrinsic red cell abnormality persists.[114] In acquired hemolytic anemia, splenectomy is usually reserved for cases that cannot be controlled by steroid or immunosuppressive therapy. A sustained remission rate is obtained in about 50% of the cases and an objective improvement is obtained in an additional 25% of the cases. Studies of splenic sequestration using Cr^{51}-tagged red cells give a rough estimation of the benefit to be expected from splenectomy.[113]

Congestive splenomegaly

Congestive splenomegaly is a direct consequence of portal hypertension. It may be caused by cirrhosis (by far the most common pathogenesis); thrombosis of hepatic veins (Budd–Chiari syndrome); thrombosis of the splenic veins; or occlusive thrombosis, cavernous transformation (recanalized thrombosis), sclerosis, or stenosis of the portal vein. Portal vein thrombosis may be the result of inflammation, trauma, or extrinsic pressure by inflammatory or neoplastic tissue.[126] Stenotic or sclerotic changes may be the result of extension into the main portal vein of the physiologic obliterative process that takes place at birth in the umbilical vein and the ductus venosum as they empty into the left portal vein. Cases of portal hypertension accompanied by congestive splenomegaly in which no apparent cause is discernible either in the liver or in the hepatic or portal veins are referred to as **idiopathic portal hypertension**. This condition was originally described by Guido Banti at the University of Florence, Italy, and is generally known as *Banti syndrome*. It has been regarded by many with skepticism, but cases with similar features are still being seen today, particularly in Japan and India.[127,128] The main changes in the liver are capillary dilation, phlebosclerosis, and fibroelastosis in the portal tracts, accompanied by disturbance of the acinar architecture[127] (see also p. 1906).

Congestive splenomegaly may be accompanied by signs of hypersplenism, such as anemia, leukopenia, and/or thrombocytopenia. Grossly, the spleen is large, firm, and dark. Fibrous thickening of the capsule is frequent.[130] Microscopically, there is marked dilation of the veins and sinuses, fibrosis of the red pulp, and accumulation of hemosiderin-containing macrophages (Fig. 22.10). Lymphoid follicles are inconspicuous. Iron incrustation of the connective tissue and sclerosiderotic nodules ('Gamna-Gandy bodies') develop as a result of focal hemorrhages. Because fibrosis is commonly present in advanced cases, the condition is also known as fibrocongestive splenomegaly.

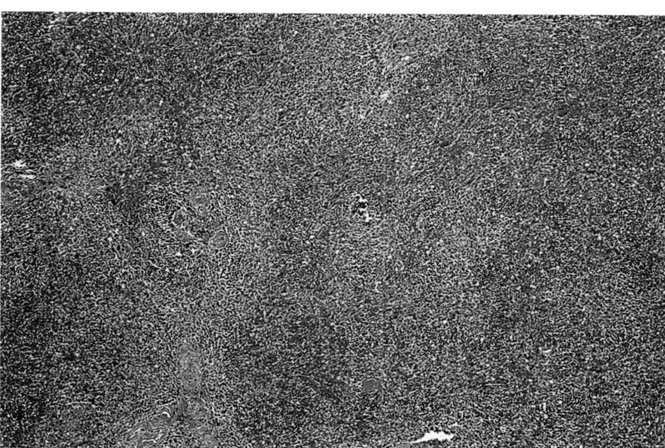

Fig. 22.10 Passive congestion of spleen. The red pulp is massively expanded due to increased content of red blood cells.

Splenectomy without shunt is successful when the coronary vein joins the portal system central to the point of obstruction. Otherwise, shunt is indicated. Various types have been done, including anastomosis of the splenic vein to the renal vein and anastomosis of the portal vein to the vena cava. These operations have been successful as a means of controlling repetitive hemorrhage from esophageal varices but do not seem to prolong life.[129]

Other non-neoplastic disorders

Foamy macrophages can be found in the spleens of patients with idiopathic thrombocytopenic purpura, as already indicated (see p. 1906). They also occur, as an incidental finding without clinical significance, in the malpighian follicles of normal individuals (so-called follicular or mineral oil lipidosis) in association with similar changes in the liver and intra-abdominal lymph nodes.[150] They are much more common in North American than in Latin American or African populations.[132,133] Biochemical studies have demonstrated the presence of saturated hydrocarbons, which imply the ingestion of exogenous mineral oil. The most common source seems to be material related to the packaging and display of foodstuff.[132,140]

Foamy histiocytes have also been described in Gaucher disease, Niemann–Pick disease,[135] Tay–Sachs disease, chronic granulomatous disease, thalassemia,[138] and hyperlipemic stages.[147] Histochemical techniques usually allow for a distinction among these various conditions.[145] It is now accepted that the process originally designated as sea-blue histiocyte syndrome[148] is not a specific entity and that histiocytes with a sea-blue appearance can be present in any of the disorders previously mentioned[143] and also in chronic myelogenous leukemia.

Infarction of the spleen may result from thrombosis of the splenic vein, a phenomenon not always associated with a detectable etiology. Infarct of the spleen is one of the complications of Wegener granulomatosis and may result in rupture of the organ.[137,141,146] Splenic infarcts are also common in cases of massive splenomegaly, regardless of its cause (Fig. 22.11).

Peliosis of the spleen (peliosis lienis) is characterized by widespread, blood-filled cystic spaces. Most reported cases have been associated with peliosis hepatis,[139] but it may occur independently from it.[149] The most common location for the lesions is the parafollicular region.[149] Cases have been reported in which this condition led to splenic rupture[136] and death[149] (see p. 1902). Most cases have occurred in patients with wasting diseases, such as tuberculosis and carcinomatosis, or in patients who have received anabolic–androgenic steroids.[151] They have also been seen in association with chronic leukemia[136] and following liver transplantation.[144]

Radiation injury to the spleen, usually produced in the course of therapy for lymphoma, results in an organ with a wrinkled, thick capsule and parenchymal collapse, with diffuse fibrosis of the red pulp and lymphocyte depletion.[134]

Amyloidosis of the spleen is nearly always an expression of the 'secondary' form of the disease. 'Sago spleen' and 'lardaceous spleen' are the classic descriptions, depending respectively on the follicular versus diffuse locations of the deposits. Exceptional cases of localized splenic amyloid nodules ('amyloid tumor') have also been described.[131] Amyloidosis of the spleen should be distinguished from the common hyaline adventitial thickening of splenic vessels, a change sometimes referred to as para-amyloid and said to be accentuated in AIDS patients.[142]

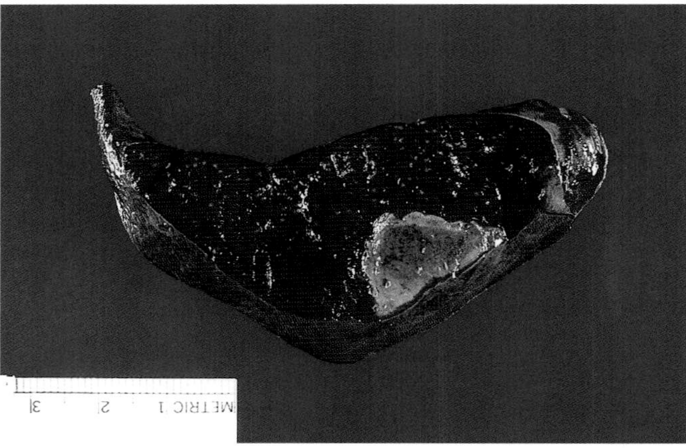

Fig. 22.11 Typical wedge-shaped appearance and 'anemic' quality of splenic infarct. A second smaller infarct is also present.

Hematolymphoid tumors and tumorlike conditions

Non-Hodgkin lymphoma

Malignant lymphoma is by far the most common malignant tumor involving the spleen. Although usually affected as part of a generalized process, in some cases the spleen represents the only detectable site of disease. In either case, splenic involvement by malignant lymphoma may present as an asymptomatic splenomegaly or result in a picture of hypersplenism. Ahmann et al.[152] described four gross patterns of involvement: homogeneous, miliary, multiple masses, and solitary masses, which show some correspondence to the various microscopic types (Fig. 22.12).

Primary splenic lymphoma (defined as restricted to the spleen and hilar lymph nodes) is rare, accounting for less than 1% of all lymphomas. The majority are examples of **large cell lymphoma**, which can present as large modules ('macronodular pattern'), as small nodules ('micronodular pattern'), or as diffuse red pulp infiltration[191] (Fig. 22.12). A subset of this tumor type is represented by *T-cell/histiocyte-rich large B-cell lymphoma*, which typically shows a micronodular pattern of splenic involvement.[164,183]

These patients often present with left-upper-quadrant pain, fever, weight loss, and an elevated erythrocyte sedimentation rate.[173] Some of the cases have been seen in association with HIV infection,[156] and others (particularly in Japan) have occurred in patients with hepatitis C virus infection.[211] Grossly, transgression of the splenic capsule is common, sometimes accompanied by invasion of adjacent structures. Hilar and retroperitoneal lymph nodes are often involved. Immunophenotypically, B-cell neoplasms predominate over T-cell tumors; most are BCL6 positive.[168,191] Morphologic features favoring a B-cell phenotype are multiple discrete nodules in the white pulp, large coalescing nodules, coexistence of small lymphocytic lymphoma, and plasmacytoid features (Fig. 22.13). Features favoring a T-cell phenotype are epithelioid histiocytic reaction, tumor confinement to the periarteriolar lymphoid sheath and marginal zone, and clear cell or polymorphous cytologic features[160,209,213] (Fig. 22.14). Along these lines, it should be mentioned that the cases originally interpreted as a chronic form of malignant histiocytosis with predominant splenic involvement on the basis of phagocytic

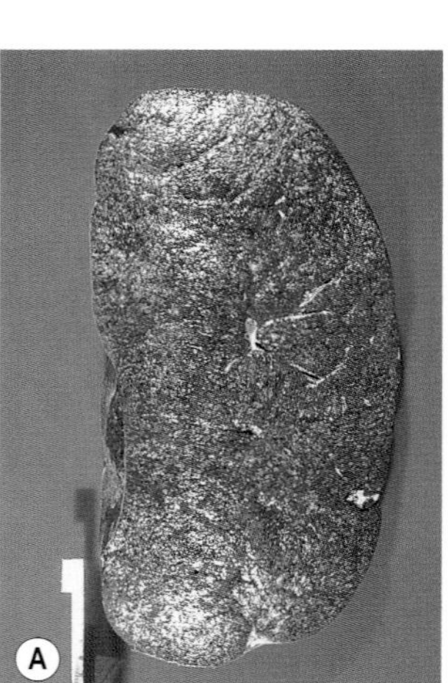

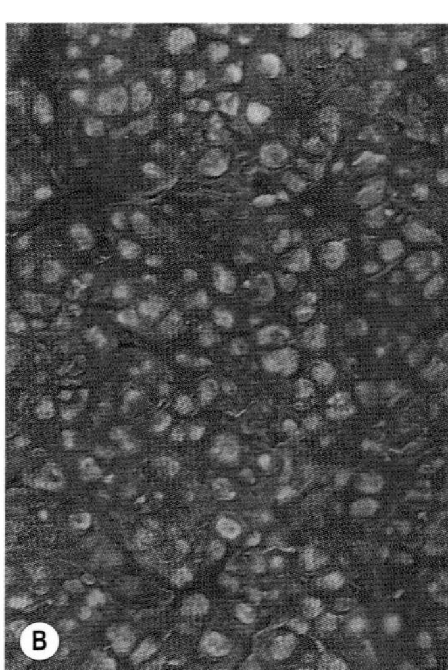

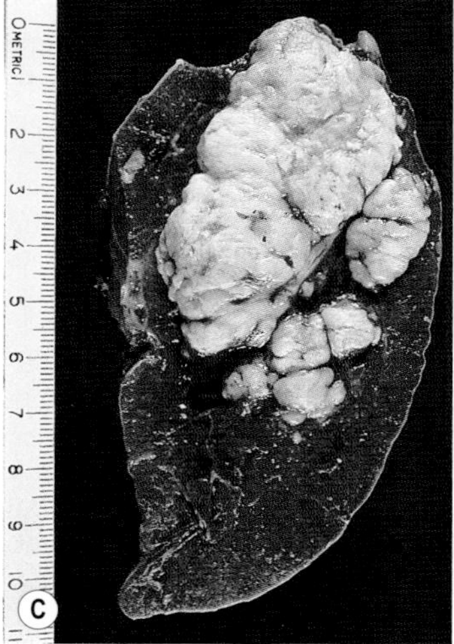

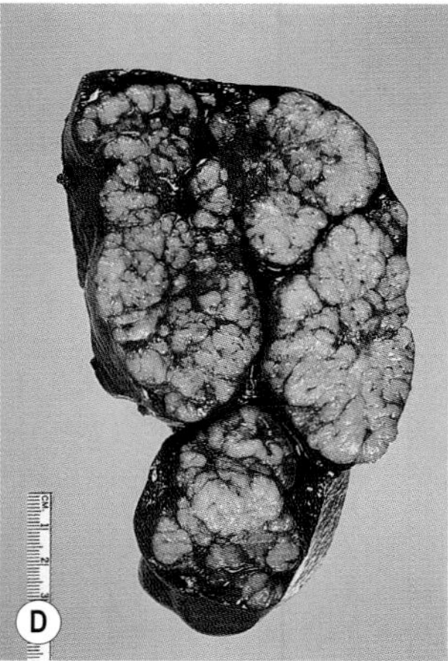

Fig. 22.12 Gross appearances of various types of malignant lymphoma involving the spleen. **A**, Small lymphocytic lymphoma. **B**, Follicular lymphoma. **C** and **D**, Large cell lymphoma.

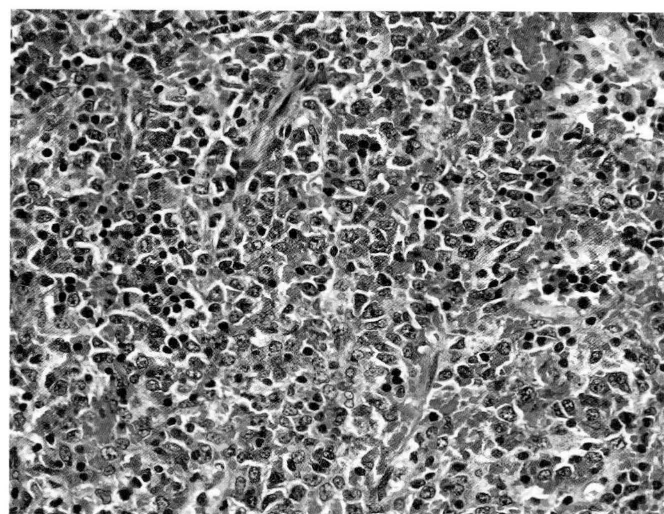

Fig. 22.13 Large B-cell lymphoma of spleen causing diffuse infiltration of the organ.

activity, lysozyme positivity, and clinical evolution probably represent instead variants of large T-cell lymphoma.[158]

Secondary splenic involvement by tumor is particularly common in low-grade lymphomas, most of which are of B-cell type.[210] This includes small lymphocytic lymphoma, the closely related lymphoplasmacytoid and paraimmunoblastic types (Fig. 22.15), mantle cell lymphoma, follicular lymphoma (particularly of the small cell type), and marginal zone B-cell lymphoma.

Splenic small lymphocytic lymphoma usually presents grossly as nodules measuring a few millimeters in diameter ('miliary' nodules) scattered throughout the organ. The low-power appearance is also distinctly nodular because of the preferential involvement of the white pulp.[181] In this regard, it is important to point out that a nodular pattern of growth is common to several types of lymphoproliferative disease of the spleen (including chronic lymphocytic leukemia) and that its presence should not be equated with a diagnosis of follicular lymphoma[157] (Fig. 22.16).

In the early stages, the diagnosis of small lymphocytic lymphoma can be easily missed. Clues to the diagnosis in these cases include prominent enlargement and coalescence of follicles; marked expansion of the mantle zone; germinal centers that are absent, inconspicuous, or overrun by small cells; and presence of clusters of small lymphoid cells protruding beneath the endothelium of trabecular veins[171] (Fig. 22.17). The only other condition in which we have seen the latter change in a prominent degree in an adult has been infectious mononucleosis. We have also seen the subendothelial space occupied by red cell precursors in infants with erythroblastosis fetalis and (together with granulocyte precursors) in adults with myelofibrosis. A helpful hint for the diagnosis of lymphoma is to carefully dissect and examine the lymph nodes in the splenic hilum, since they may show obvious lymphoma when the changes in the spleen are only equivocal.

An 'entity' that exemplifies the difficulties sometimes encountered in the recognition of splenic small lymphocytic lymphoma is so-called *idiopathic nontropical splenomegaly* (see above). Although originally regarded as a benign and probably reactive form of splenomegaly,[162] a follow-up study by the same group showed that half of these cases actually represented malignant lymphoma.[163]

The treatment of malignant lymphoma involving exclusively or preferentially the spleen includes splenectomy, followed by chemotherapy.[195] The prognosis is directly related to the microscopic type and the clinical stage, in the sense that it is distinctly better for small lymphocytic tumors and for stage I and II disease.[152,175] Patients with localized splenic non-Hodgkin lymphoma seem to have the same rate of survival as other stage I non-Hodgkin lymphoma patients.[182]

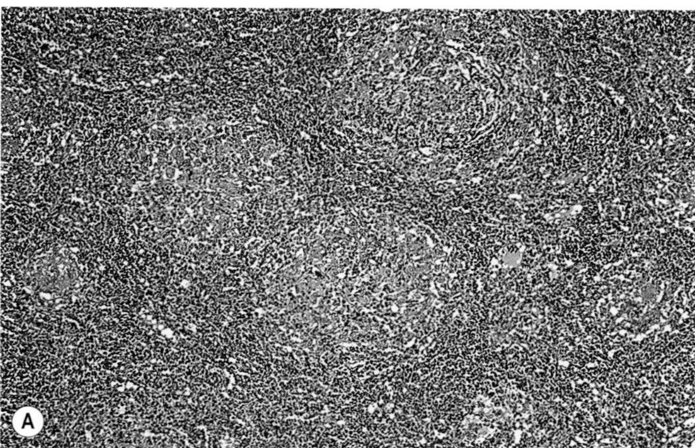

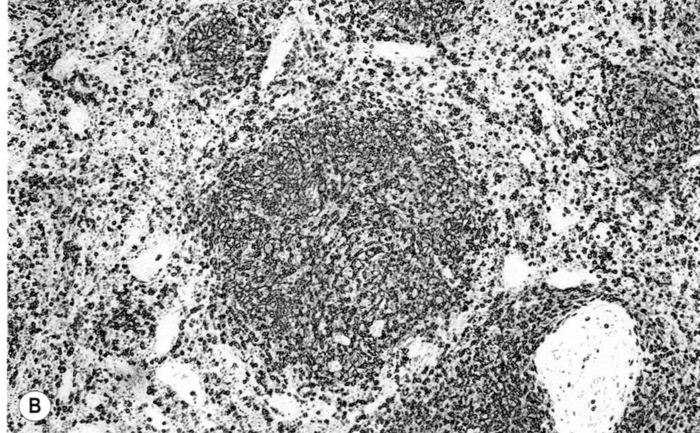

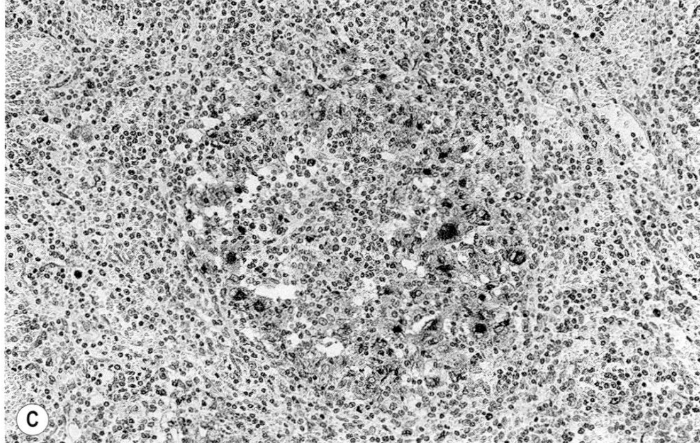

Fig. 22.14 Large T-cell lymphoma of spleen rich in reactive histiocytes. **A**, Low-power appearance. **B**, CD43 immunoreactivity of neoplastic T cells. **C**, Lysozyme positivity of reactive histiocytes.

Follicular lymphoma can be accompanied with prominent architectural abnormalities or with a fair preservation of the splenic architecture, displaying an exclusively intrafollicular growth pattern. In some series they have shown a consistent CD10+/BCL2+

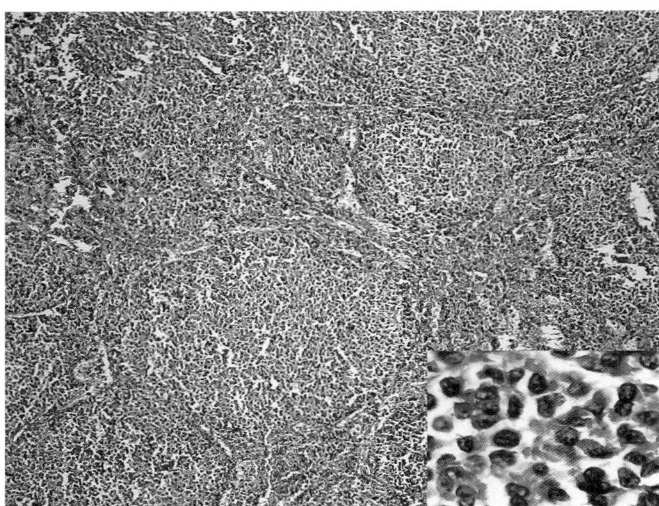

Fig. 22.15 Small lymphocytic lymphoma of spleen, so-called 'paraimmunoblastic' type.

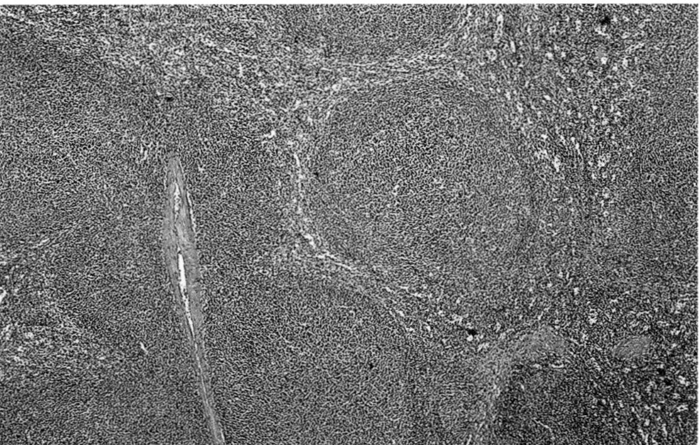

Fig. 22.16 Malignant lymphoma of spleen with a nodular pattern of growth, which in this organ is not limited to follicular lymphoma but can be seen in many types of Hodgkin and non-Hodgkin lymphoma.

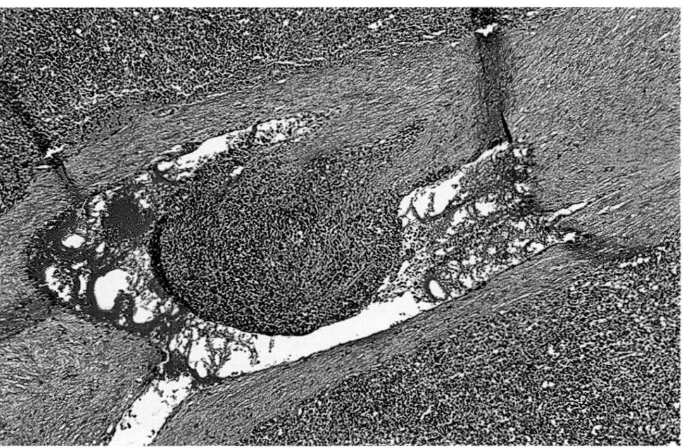

Fig. 22.17 Polypoid growth of malignant lymphoma cells beneath the endothelium of a trabecular vein. This is a useful diagnostic sign.

phenotype,[176] whereas in others the phenotype is heterogeneous, including CD10- and/or BCL2-negative cases.[194]

Two types of malignant lymphoma of the spleen that need to be singled out because of their distinctive features are splenic marginal zone B-cell lymphoma and hepatosplenic T-cell lymphoma.

Splenic marginal zone lymphoma (SMZL) of the spleen usually presents with splenomegaly, anemia, and weight loss.[172,180,207] The bone marrow is involved with an intrasinusoidal component in nearly all cases, and liver involvement is also common.[177] Grossly, the splenic involvement manifests itself through miliary expansion of the white pulp.

Histologically, there are nodular lymphoid infiltrates centered on preexistent germinal centers, which are barely visible.[165] The tumor cells are small lymphocytes, with a component of medium-sized cells with irregular nuclei and pale cytoplasm located towards the periphery of the nodules. Immunohistochemically, the cells express CD20, surface immunoglobulin (usually IgM ± IgD) and BCL2, but not CD5, CD10, CD23, CD11c, or CD43.[193] There is no cyclin D1 protein expression.[204] Various chromosomal abnormalities have been reported, with complete or partial trisomy 3q being the commonest but not specific.[154,174,206] On the other hand, deletion or translocation involving 7q32, found in 40% of cases, is a characteristic chromosomal aberration.[154,186,206] Microarray analysis shows that the expression of three genes (*ILF1*, *SENATAXIN*, *CD40*) can help distinguish SMZL from other low-grade B-cell lymphomas.[202]

Somatic mutation analysis has shown that the tumor cells of SMZL are memory B lymphocytes,[189] but other cases seem to be composed of naive marginal zone B cells.[155] The differential diagnosis of SMZL includes mantle cell lymphoma[190,200] (Fig. 22.18) and follicular lymphoma with preferential involvement of the marginal zone.[153]

Variants of SMZL include cases with predominant red pulp involvement,[192] with plasmacytic differentiation,[212] with an increased number of blasts and a more aggressive clinical course,[184] and with progression to large B-cell lymphoma.[159]

SMZL does not appear to represent the splenic equivalent of MALT lymphoma of other sites, since the distinctive chromosomal translocations of the latter are not found in SMZL.[175,178,187,199,201,205,208] There is marked overlap with *splenic lymphoma with circulating*

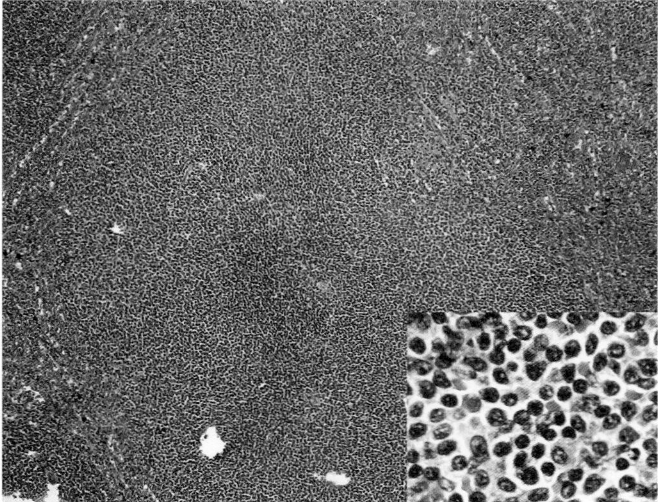

Fig. 22.18 Mantle cell lymphoma. Note the tiny residual germinal center. The inset shows the centrocyte-like appearance of the tumor cells.

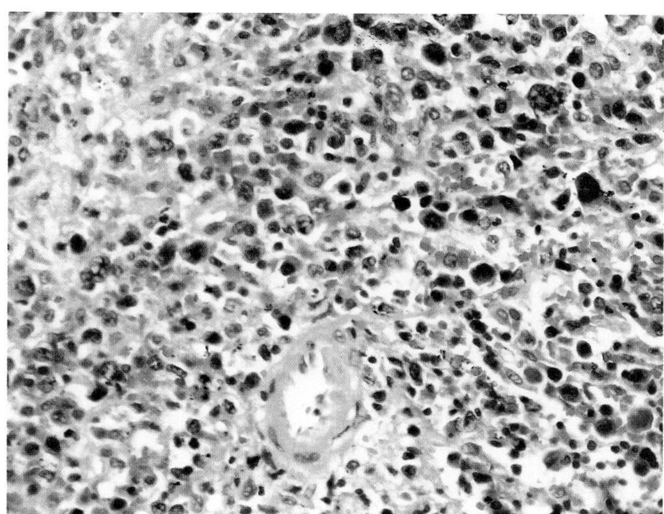

Fig. 22.19 Hepatosplenic T-cell lymphoma. Highly atypical lymphoid cells are present in a polymorphic background.

lymphocytes,[188] which may be a leukemic variant of SMZL[179] or represent a heterogeneous group of low-grade B-cell lymphomas.[167,196,198]

Hepatosplenic T-cell lymphoma, previously known as hepatosplenic gamma-delta T-cell lymphoma, seems to be a distinct clinical entity within the spectrum of peripheral T-cell lymphomas.[161,166,214] It typically presents with hepatosplenomegaly, fever, and weight loss in young males, and carries a poor prognosis. Cases have been described in immunocompromised patients and in association with Epstein–Barr virus (EBV).[170,197,215] Grossly, the spleen is usually very large, with a uniform cut surface in which the malpighian follicles cannot be identified. Microscopically, the neoplastic infiltration involves the cords and sinuses and is composed of medium-sized lymphoid cells with oval or folded nuclei, moderately condensed chromatin, and pale cytoplasm (Fig. 22.19). Tumor involvement of the liver and bone marrow is characterized by an intrasinusoidal distribution.[169]

The main differential diagnosis is with hairy cell leukemia, from which it is distinguished by the absence of blood lakes and its different immunophenotype, which includes positivity for pan-T and cytotoxic markers. The majority of cases express gamma-delta T-cell receptor, but some cases express alpha-beta T-cell receptor.[185,203]

At the molecular level, there is usually clonal rearrangement of the gamma or delta chain of the T-cell receptor gene, and cytogenetically there is an isochromosome 7q.[170]

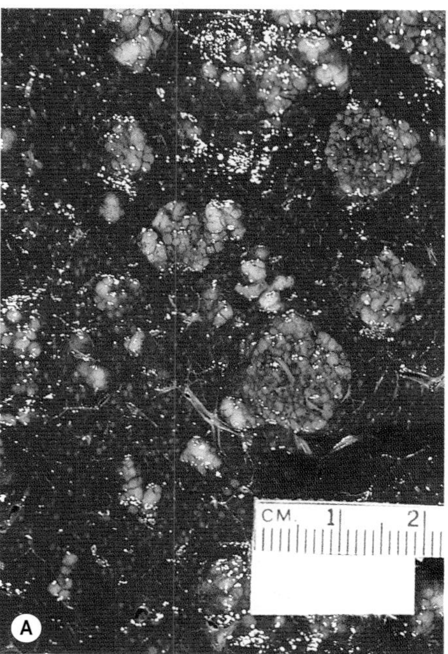

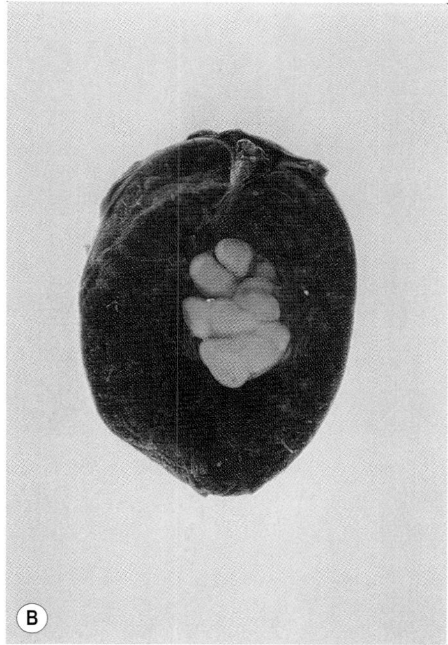

Fig. 22.20 **A** and **B**, Gross appearance of Hodgkin lymphoma involving the spleen.

Hodgkin lymphoma

The spleen is the most common site of extranodal organ involvement by Hodgkin lymphoma, but primary Hodgkin lymphoma of the spleen is extremely rare. The morphologic features of Hodgkin lymphoma in the spleen are discussed in Chapter 21. Grossly the involvement is in the form of one or multiple nodules, sometimes indistinguishable from those of large cell lymphoma (Fig. 22.20). Foci of involvement can be only a few millimeters in size, a fact which calls for a very meticulous gross inspection of the organ. The earliest lesions are located in the periarterial lymphoid sheath or marginal zones of the follicles. By far the most common type is the nodular sclerosis subtype of classic Hodgkin lymphoma, but others may be seen as well, including lymphocyte predominance[217] (Fig. 22.21). Some cases have initially presented with spontaneous splenic rupture.[216] As already mentioned, sarcoid-type granulomas can be seen in spleens of patients with Hodgkin lymphoma and should not be construed by themselves as evidence of splenic involvement by the lymphoma.

Leukemias

Any type of leukemia can involve the spleen, the location being predominantly the red pulp except in chronic lymphocytic

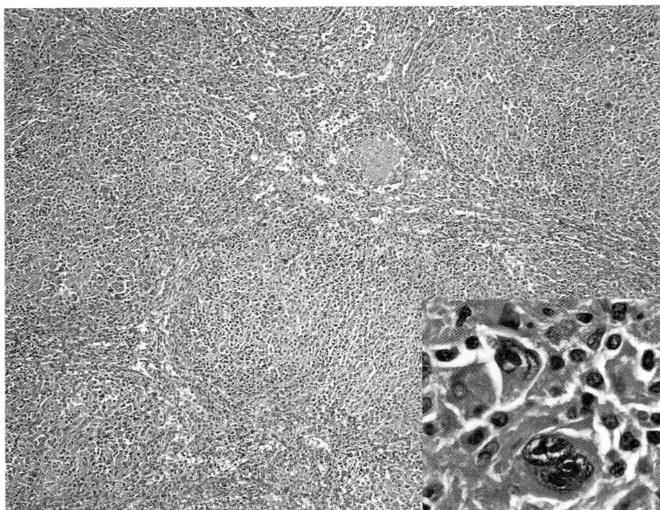

Fig. 22.21 Classic Hodgkin lymphoma of spleen, nodular sclerosis subtype. The inset shows typical Reed–Sternberg cells.

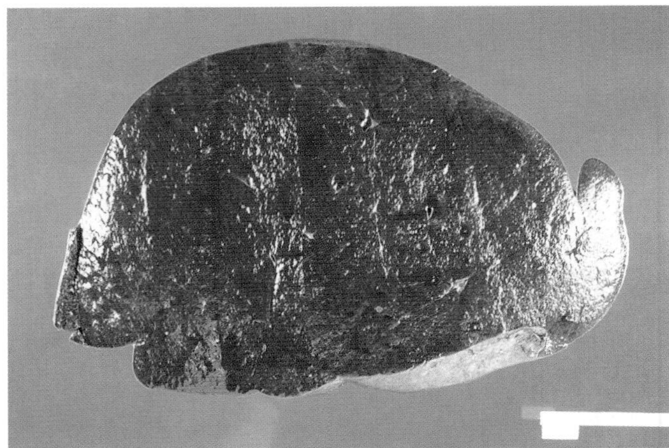

Fig. 22.23 Gross appearance of hairy cell leukemia. Note the diffuse involvement, lack of nodularity, and dark red color.

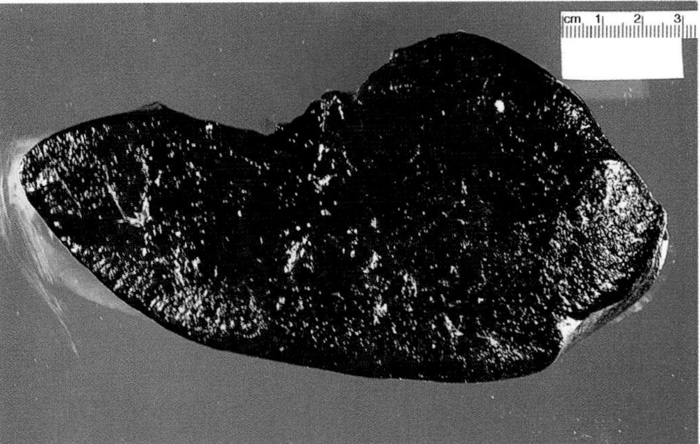

Fig. 22.22 The splenic involvement by chronic lymphocytic leukemia results in marked diffuse enlargement of the organ.

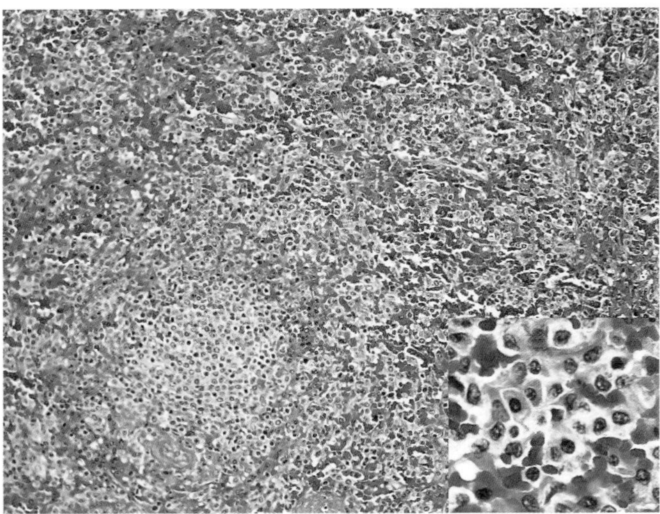

Fig. 22.24 Splenic involvement by hairy cell leukemia. The inset shows the bland monotonous appearance of the infiltrate.

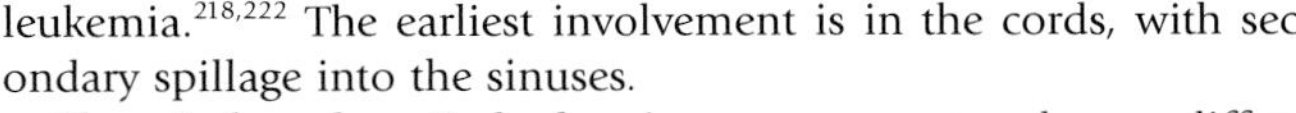

leukemia.[218,222] The earliest involvement is in the cords, with secondary spillage into the sinuses.

Chronic lymphocytic leukemia may appear grossly as a diffuse or miliary enlargement (Fig. 22.22). From a morphologic standpoint, it is not possible to distinguish it from small lymphocytic lymphoma.

Prolymphocytic leukemia shows a similar type of involvement, but the lymphocytes have nuclei that are larger, often indented, and with distinct nucleoli.[231] Massive splenomegaly is the predominant clinical finding. Most cases are of T-cell type. The differential diagnosis includes *T-cell large granular prolymphocytic leukemia.*[234]

Chronic myelogenous leukemia preferentially results grossly in a large, dark red, diffusely involved organ in which malpighian follicles are inconspicuous or absent. Infarcts are common. In rare cases, blastic transformation is first seen in a splenectomy specimen.

Myelodysplasia (defined as a group of bone marrow disorders characterized by dysplastic changes in one or more myeloid cell lines, with or without concurrent increases in myeloblasts in the bone marrow and peripheral blood; see also Chapter 23) may be accompanied by several types of splenic abnormality, including erythrophagocytosis, red pulp plasmacytosis, extramedullary hematopoiesis, and clusters of monocytes, the latter allegedly correlating with an increased risk of disease progression.[230] Clinically, detectable splenomegaly is rare in this condition. This condition should be distinguished from the extramedullary hematopoiesis that is seen in a variety of reactive conditions. It helps in this regard to remember that reactivity for CD34 or CD117 is characteristic of neoplastic myeloid disorders.[233]

Hairy cell leukemia, formerly known as leukemic reticuloendotheliosis, is a specific subtype of indolent B-cell malignancy;[223,240] it is further discussed in Chapter 23. Grossly the spleen shows diffuse and usually marked enlargement without formation of nodules, except in the very early stages of the disease (Fig. 22.23).[227] Microscopically, hairy cell leukemia is a disease of the red pulp, which shows diffuse infiltration by a monotonous population of small mononuclear cells with very scanty mitotic activity and practically no phagocytosis[219,235] (Fig. 22.24). The initial involvement occurs around the fibrous trabeculae. The nuclei of the hairy cells are small, round, or oval, with irregular contours, occasional deep indentations ('coffee beans'), and inconspicuous nucleoli. Rarely, the nuclei have a multilobular appearance simulating those of T-cell lymphoma.[226] The cytoplasm is usually moderate to abundant and lightly stained. Ultrastructurally, prominent cytoplasmic villous projections are evident.[220] The distinctive enzyme histochemical feature of the disease is the presence of tartrate-resistant acid phosphatase (isoenzyme 5); this enzyme can now be demonstrated immunohistochemically.[228] In addition to the above, the usual antigenic phenotype of hairy cells is CD45+, CD45RA+, CD20+, DBA.44+, CD103+, annexin A1+, T-bet+, CDw75+, CD74+, LN3+, CD45RO−, CD43−, CD15−, and CD30−.[224,225,229,238,239] The splenic vasculature is abnormal in the sense of showing an absolute increase in the volume, surface, and length of pulp arterial vessels, as well as enlargement of pulp cords and sinuses.[237] Pools of blood in the red pulp, lined by hairy cells and simulating dilated sinuses or even hemangiomas, are commonly seen and constitute an important diagnostic feature.[232] It has been suggested that this results from the hairy cells adhering to the sinus surface, producing endothelial cell injury and impeding the venous blood flow.[236] In what is perhaps the preceding stage of this process, some of the tumor cells are seen to aggregate in the subendothelial spaces of trabecular veins; sometimes this is the only recognizable site of involvement.[221]

The lymph nodes in the splenic hilum are often involved, the pattern of permeation being interfollicular.

Myelofibrosis

Myelofibrosis (agnogenic myeloid metaplasia) is discussed in Chapter 23. Spleen involvement in the disease is the rule, the average weight being 2 kg.[244] Grossly, the spleen is diffusely dark red and moderately firm, with frequent areas of hemorrhage (Fig. 22.25). Microscopically, the diagnostic feature is the presence in the red pulp of all three hematopoietic cell lines: megakaryocytes, erythroid precursors, and granulocyte precursors. The latter are made evident with Leder chloroacetate esterase stain (Fig. 22.26). The megakaryocytes often have atypical nuclear features and can be confused with Reed–Sternberg cells; in contrast with the latter, their cytoplasm is strongly PAS positive.[242] They are immunohistochemically reactive for factor VIII-related antigen and negative for CD30 and Leu-M1.

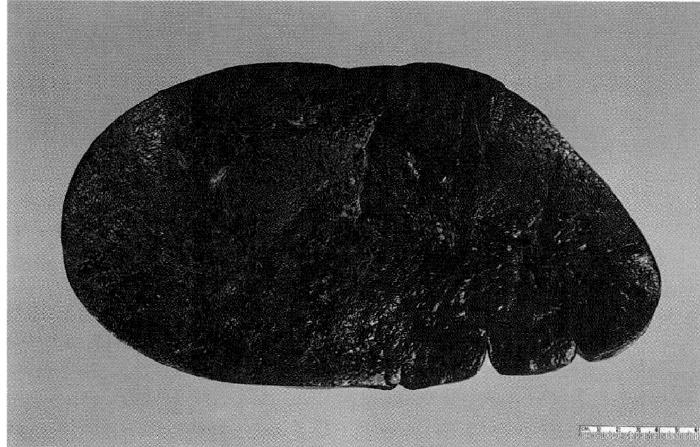

Fig. 22.25 Diffuse involvement of the spleen by myelofibrosis.

It is believed that the hematopoietic cells present in the spleen result from filtration of circulating cells from the peripheral blood rather than arising de novo from splenic stem cells.[243,247]

Other splenic changes in myelofibrosis include congestion, hemosiderosis, and paucity of lymphoid follicles.[245,246]

Splenectomy is sometimes carried out for this disease, especially when thrombocytopenia or hemolytic phenomena are severe. The results are not spectacular, but in some cases a moderate improvement has been noted.

Splenic extramedullary hematopoiesis as seen in myelofibrosis should be distinguished from the rare myelolipomas occurring within or adjacent to the spleen.[241]

Mastocytosis

The general features of systemic mastocytosis are discussed in Chapter 23.[256] The spleen is always involved, and the morphologic changes in it can be very deceptive.[250] Grossly, ill-defined granuloma-like nodules having a fibrotic appearance are scattered throughout the organ. Microscopically, these highly fibrotic foci are often centered by a vessel, an important diagnostic clue.[250,257] The diagnosis depends on the identification of mast cells, which usually appear as pale-staining small clusters embedded in fibrous tissue, accompanied by a variable number of eosinophils, lymphocytes, or histiocytes (Fig. 22.27). The nucleus is centrally located and of regular outline; the cytoplasm is light staining, with a variable degree of

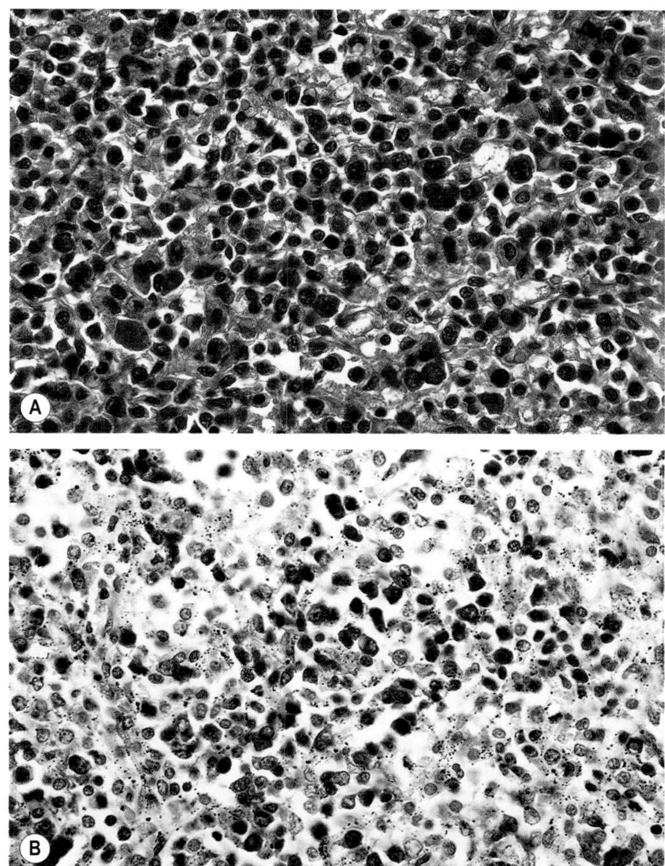

Fig. 22.26 Extramedullary hematopoiesis in spleen, as seen in H&E section (**A**) and with Leder chloroacetate esterase stain (**B**).

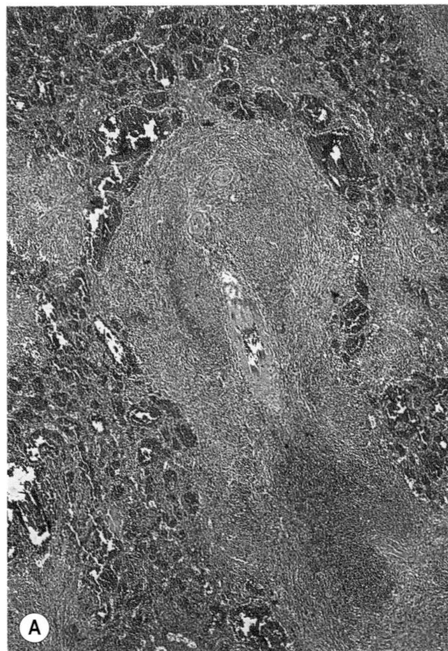

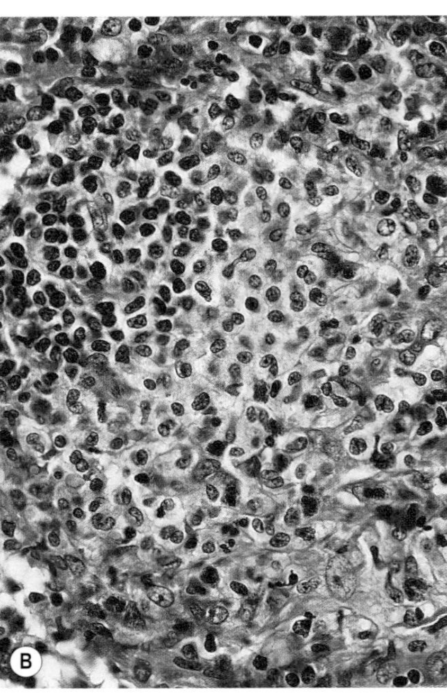

Fig. 22.27 Involvement of the spleen by systemic mastocytosis. **A**, Low-power view showing the perimalpighian and perivascular arrangement of the infiltrate. **B**, High-power view showing clusters of mast cells.

granularity; the cell borders tend to be sharply outlined. Confirmation of the diagnosis is obtained by staining the cytoplasmic granules with metachromatic dyes, with Leder chloroacetate esterase reaction, or by the immunohistochemical demonstration of mast cell tryptase, chymase, carboxypeptidase, CD68, and CD117 (KIT).[249,250,253,258] Conversely, mast cells are only weakly reactive for lysozyme and negative for myeloperoxidase and CD20.[255] Immunoreactivity for CD25 is indicative of systemic disease.[251,252]

Most patients with systemic mastocytosis exhibit the D816V point mutation in the *KIT* gene, involving the tyrosine kinase domain of the transmembrane receptor.[248]

The lymph nodes in the splenic hilum are often involved; the diagnosis may be easier on them than on the spleen. The foci of involvement in the lymph nodes are usually perifollicular and may also show a perivascular distribution. The gastrointestinal tract is also commonly affected.[254]

Other hematolymphoid conditions

Focal lymphoid hyperplasia can present in the spleen as a solitary nodule that may be confused grossly with lymphoma, especially if the patient is known to suffer from that condition. Microscopically, the nodule is formed either by aggregates of reactive germinal centers or by a localized proliferation of lymphocytes, immunoblasts, and plasma cells.[260,261]

Langherhans cell histiocytosis of the spleen is almost always the expression of systemic disease and is therefore rarely seen as a surgical specimen. The red pulp is preferentially affected.[259]

Castleman disease can involve the spleen, although it rarely results in prominent splenomegaly. Most of the reported types have been of the plasma cell type,[264] but a few instances of the hyaline vascular type are also on record (Fig. 22.28).[262] As an aside, it could be mentioned here that the hyaline vascular form of Castleman disease shows a close resemblance to spleen on low-power examination, to the point that it is sometimes misdiagnosed as ectopic or supernumerary spleen when located in places such as mediastinum or retroperitoneum.

Wiskott–Aldrich syndrome, an X-linked hematologic disorder characterized by thrombocytopenia, eczema, and immunodeficiency, is accompanied by a general depletion of the splenic white pulp, with significant reduction of the marginal zone thickness.[263]

Vascular tumors

Hemangioma is the most common primary tumor of the spleen.[265,276,283] It is often of the cavernous variety. Most are less than 2 cm in diameter and present as incidental findings. Rarely, they are large and/or multiple, and they may involve the entire spleen (Fig. 22.29). They may be associated with hemangiomas of other sites (*angiomatosis*). The most common complication is rupture and bleeding.[279] Cases associated with anemia, thrombocytopenia, and consumption coagulopathy (Kasabach–Merritt syndrome) have been reported.[273,289]

Littoral cell angioma varies in size from minute foci to large nodules almost completely replacing the splenic tissue (Fig. 22.30). Microscopically, it is composed of anastomosing vascular channels resembling splenic sinuses (Fig. 22.31). These channels have irregular lumina often featuring papillary projections and cystlike spaces. They are lined by tall endothelial cells, some of which show hemophagocytosis. Immunohistochemically, the neoplastic cells express both endothelial (factor VIII) and histiocytic (KP1/CD68, lysozyme) markers and occasionally also S-100 protein, mirroring the dual differentiation potential of the reticuloendothelial cells (littoral cells) lining the normal sinuses[274] (Fig. 22.32). However, their negativity for CD8 (not known at the time of the original report) has cast some doubts on their proposed littoral cell derivation.[265] An intriguing number of patients have been recorded in which splenic littoral angiomas were associated with carcinomas of internal organs (probably coincidental, but perhaps worth evaluating further).[269]

Other types of splenic hemangioma include *venous hemangioma, capillary hemangioma, benign (infantile) hemangioendothelioma,*[282] and

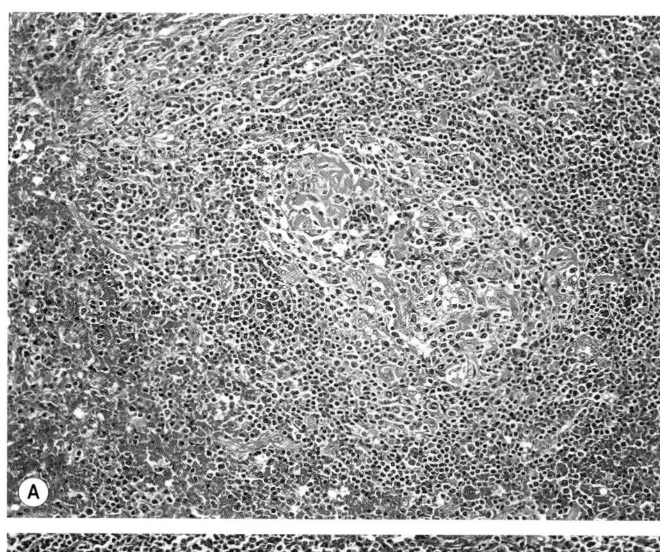

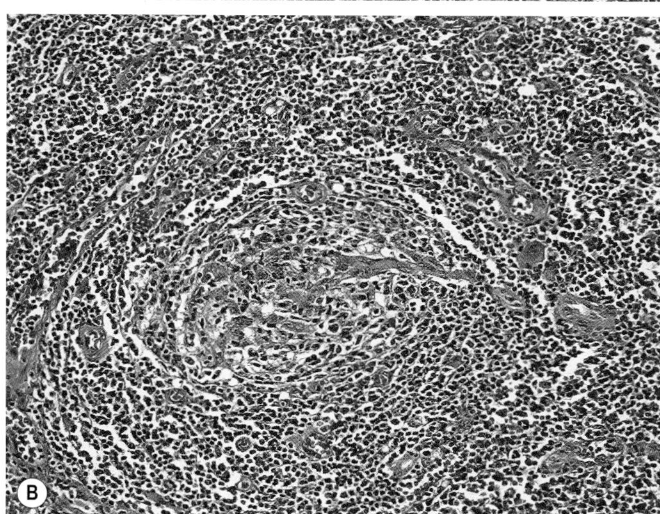

Fig. 22.28 Castleman disease of hyaline-vascular type. **A**, Splenic involvement. **B**, Lymph node involvement in the same case.

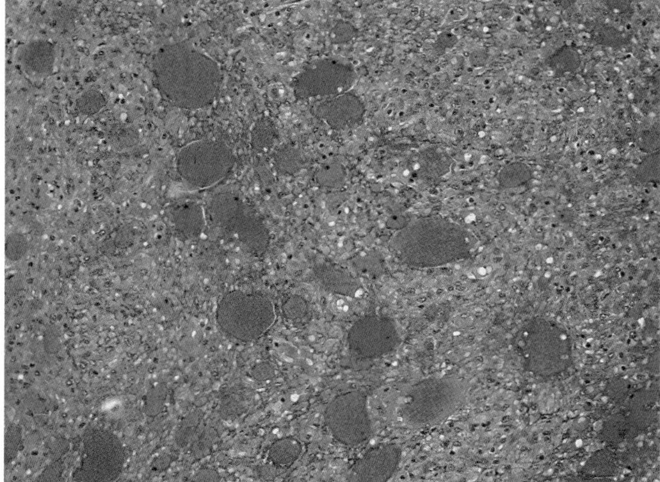

Fig. 22.29 Diffuse involvement of spleen by benign vascular tumor ('angiomatosis').

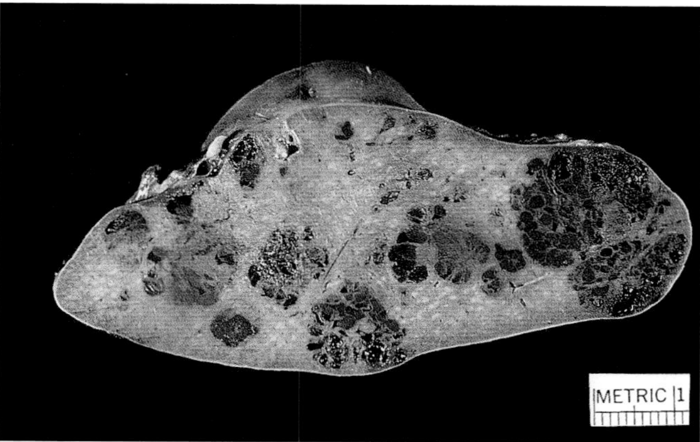

Fig. 22.30 Gross appearance of littoral cell angioma. Numerous hemorrhagic lesions with a lobular configuration are seen.

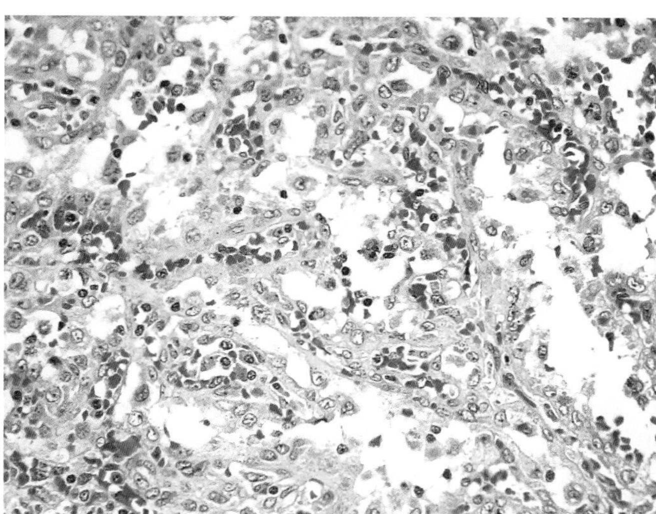

Fig. 22.31 Littoral cell angioma of spleen. The vascular spaces are lined by plump cells with the appearance of sinus lining ('littoral') cells.

diffuse sinusoidal hemangiomatosis (in which the entire spleen is permeated by blood vessels).[265,287]

Lymphangioma tends to be located in the subcapsular region but may involve the entire organ (*diffuse lymphangiomatosis*)[288] (Fig. 22.33). Most cases have been reported in children, sometimes in association with lymphangiomas in other organs.[277] At least some cases originally diagnosed as splenic lymphangioma represent mesothelial cyst instead.[266]

Hemangioendothelioma is the term that has been applied in the spleen (as in many other sites) in a somewhat loose fashion to vascular endothelial neoplasms that are either more cellular and/or are thought to be potentially more aggressive than conventional hemangiomas but are not full-fledged angiosarcomas. Some of these tumors have been described as *epithelioid* (sometimes associated with functional hyposplenism),[270] some as *epithelioid and spindle-cell,*[291] and some as combining endothelial and myoid features (*myoid angioendothelioma*).[280,281] Some of these hemangioendotheliomas have been viewed as 'borderline' (low-grade malignant) counterparts of littoral cell angiomas in view of the presence of combined endothelial and histiocytic markers and the occasional

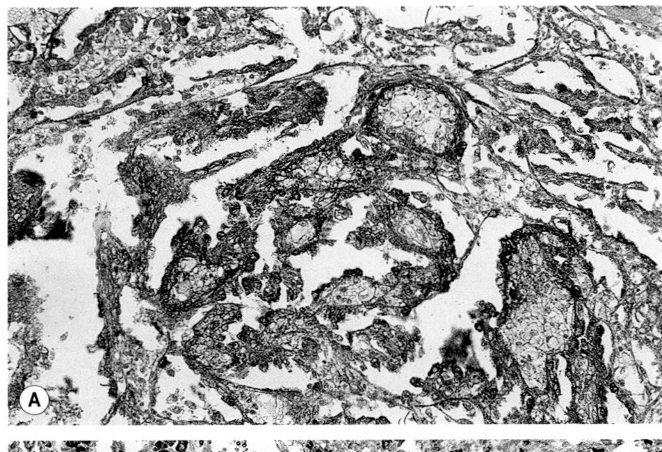

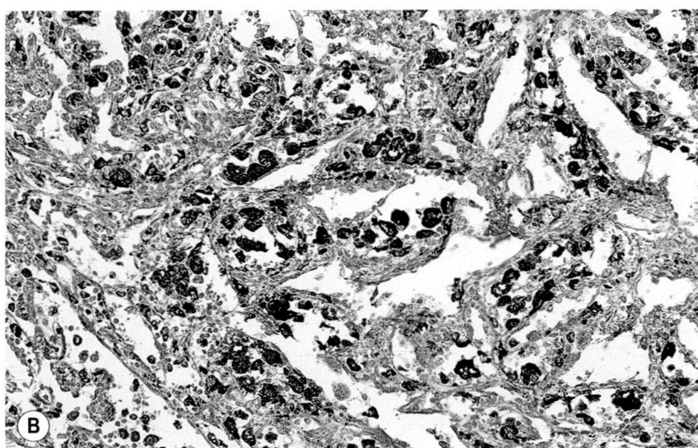

Fig. 22.32 Littoral cell angioma of spleen showing combined expression of endothelial and histiocytic markers. **A**, Factor VIII-related antigen. **B**, Lysozyme.

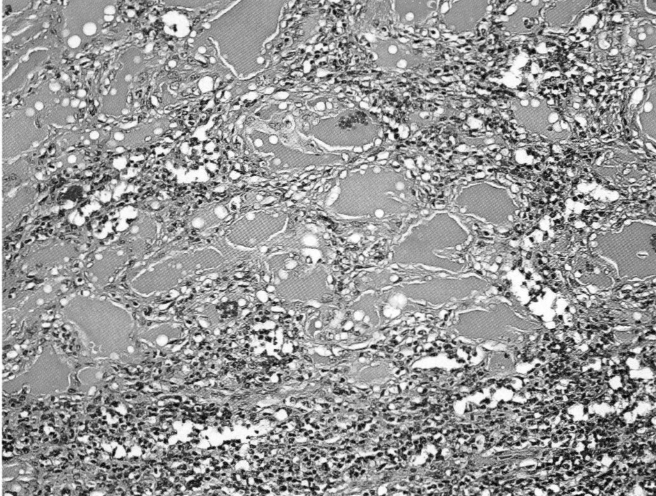

Fig. 22.33 Lymphangioma of spleen.

aggressive behavior.[268,275] As in other sites, it is probably wise never to use in the spleen the term hemangioendothelioma without a qualifier.

Angiosarcoma (malignant hemangioendothelioma) is the most common malignant primary nonlymphoid tumor of the spleen.[290]

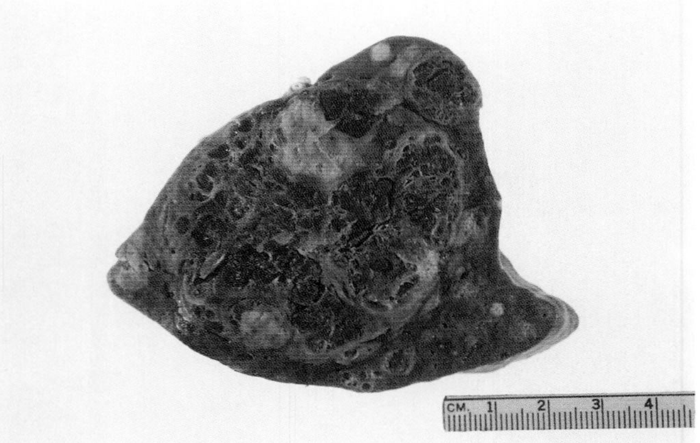

Fig. 22.34 Angiosarcoma of spleen. The tumor is markedly hemorrhagic and necrotic.

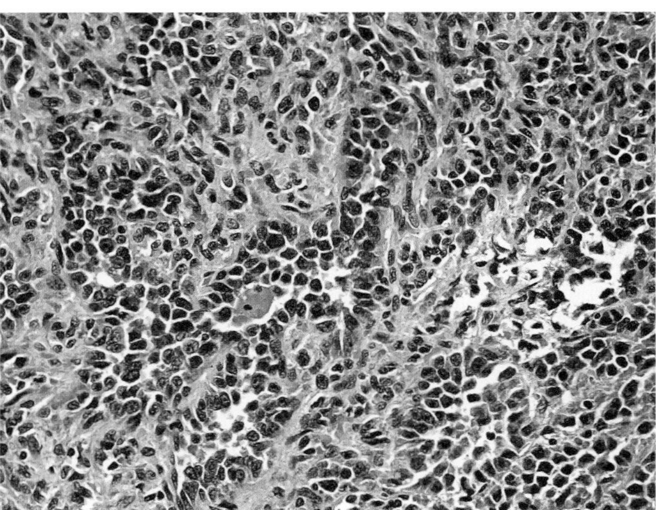

Fig. 22.35 Angiosarcoma of spleen. The tumor cells have markedly hyperchromatic nuclei that protrude into the vascular lumina.

It may present as a well-defined hemorrhagic nodule or involve the spleen diffusely, and may lead to spontaneous rupture of the organ[267,271] (Fig. 22.34). It may also be accompanied by microangiopathic anemia, thrombocytopenia, and consumption coagulopathy.[278] As in other sites, there are cases of angiosarcoma of spleen that have developed many years following the insertion of a foreign body (gauze sponge).[272] Microscopically, the pattern of growth of angiosarcoma may be solid, papillary, or characterized by the classic freely anastomosing vascular channels[285] (Fig. 22.35). Intracytoplasmic hyaline globules are common. Sometimes the tumor cells have an epithelioid appearance (*epithelioid angiosarcoma*).[272] Immunohistochemically, the tumor cells exhibit endothelial markers and often also histiocytic markers.[285] The latter finding supports the littoral cell nature of at least some angiosarcomas and demonstrates that this combined immunohistochemical staining pattern is not limited to a specific tumor type (littoral cell angioma) but rather shared by a spectrum of splenic vascular tumors.[265,286] The clinical course of splenic angiosarcoma is rapid and almost invariably fatal, with widespread metastases occurring frequently.[285]

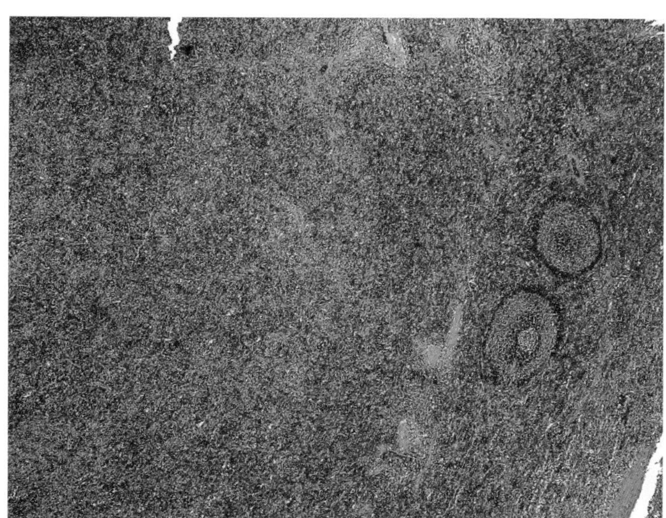

Fig. 22.36 Low-power appearance of splenic hamartoma. The lesion is formed by disorganized red pulp without malpighian follicles. Residual normal spleen is seen on the right.

Hemangiopericytoma is mentioned last in this listing of vascular splenic tumor because of its exceptional rarity[284] and the controversies that exist about its real nature.

Other primary tumors and tumorlike conditions

Hamartoma (splenadenoma or splenoma) is the term used for a nodular lesion of the spleen composed exclusively of red pulp elements, without intervening white pulp[304,316,321,327] (Fig. 22.36). It does not contain follicles or follicular dendritic cells, fibrous trabeculae are scanty, and foci of extramedullary hematopoiesis may be present.[300] Occasionally, it may contain a population of bizarre stromal cells of probable dendritic/reticulum or myoid cell nature, which should not be overdiagnosed as malignant.[295,307] Immunohistochemically, a reverse pattern of factor VIII and CD31 staining when compared with the adjacent normal spleen has been described in splenic hamartoma.[292] This lesion may attain a large size and be accompanied by thrombocytopenia and other signs of hypersplenism.[317]

Sclerosing angiomatoid nodular transformation of the spleen (SANT) is a distinctive splenic process having a striking multinodular quality that can simulate the appearance of granulomas on low-power examination[293,303,311] (Fig. 22.37A). The individual nodules, which have a vaguely lobular architecture, are surrounded by a hyaline shell (Fig. 22.37B). The vessels within the nodules are markedly cellular, to the point that we had initially interpreted them as neoplastic and had named the condition in the previous edition of his book as multinodular hemangioma. Immunostaining reveals three distinct types of vessel: CD34+/CD8−/CD31+ capillaries, CD34−/CD8+/CD31+ sinusoids, and CD34−/CD8−/CD31+ small veins, recapitulating the composition of the normal splenic red pulp (Fig. 22.37C). The internodular stroma consists of variably myxoid to dense fibrous tissue with scattered plump myofibroblasts, plasma cells, lymphocytes, and siderophages. The lesion is almost always solitary and the evolution is benign. Its pathogenesis remains controversial. It shares a number of features with inflammatory pseudotumor,[298] it may contain numerous IgG4-positive plasma cells,[305] and it was found in one instance to be positive for EBV.[324]

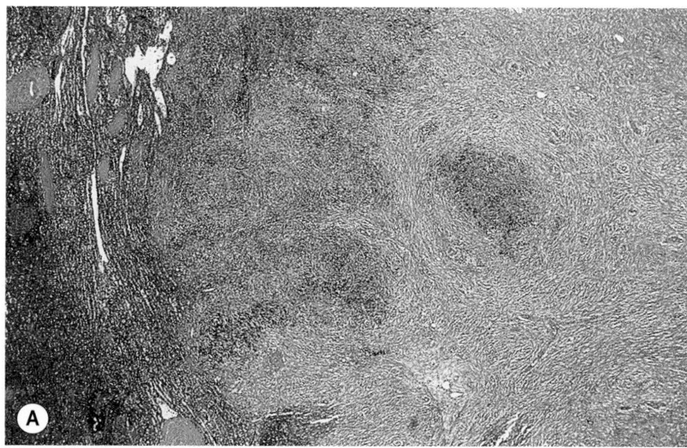

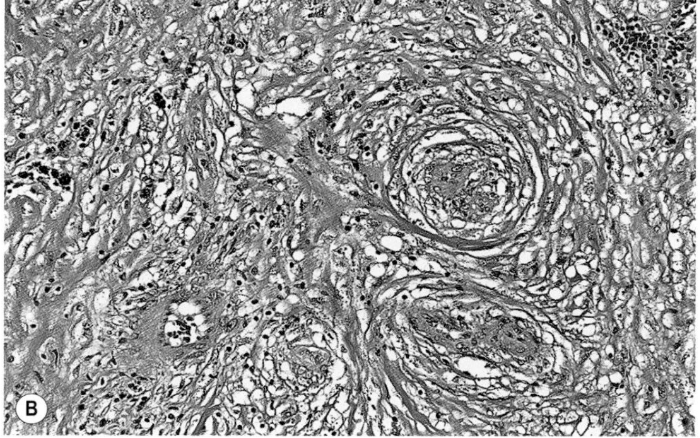

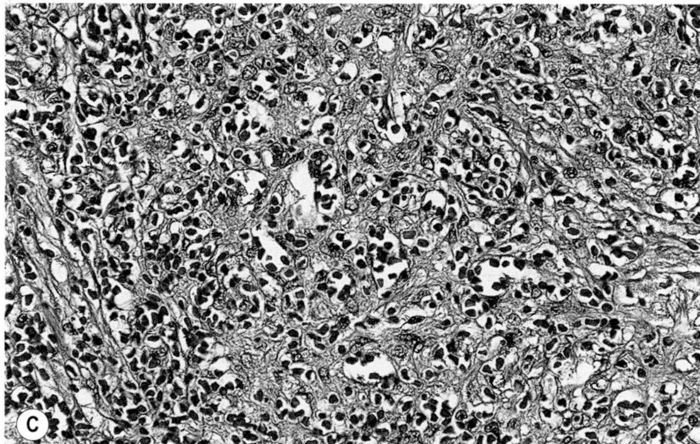

Fig. 22.37 Sclerosing angiomatoid nodular transformation of spleen (SANT). **A**, Low-power appearance showing a distinctly nodular architecture. **B**, Highly hyalinized area simulating an ancient granuloma. **C**, Cellular area of clearly angiomatous nature.

Inflammatory pseudotumor is a supposedly reactive tumor-like condition that may be encountered as an incidental finding at laparotomy or that may present as an asymptomatic splenic mass.[304,312] Grossly, there is a great size range, with some lesions reaching up to 11 cm (Fig. 22.38). The lesions are usually solitary and may be multinodular.[323] Microscopically, there is a variable mixture of lymphocytes, plasma cells, eosinophils, histiocytes, and spindle cells, the latter having an immunophenotype that has been

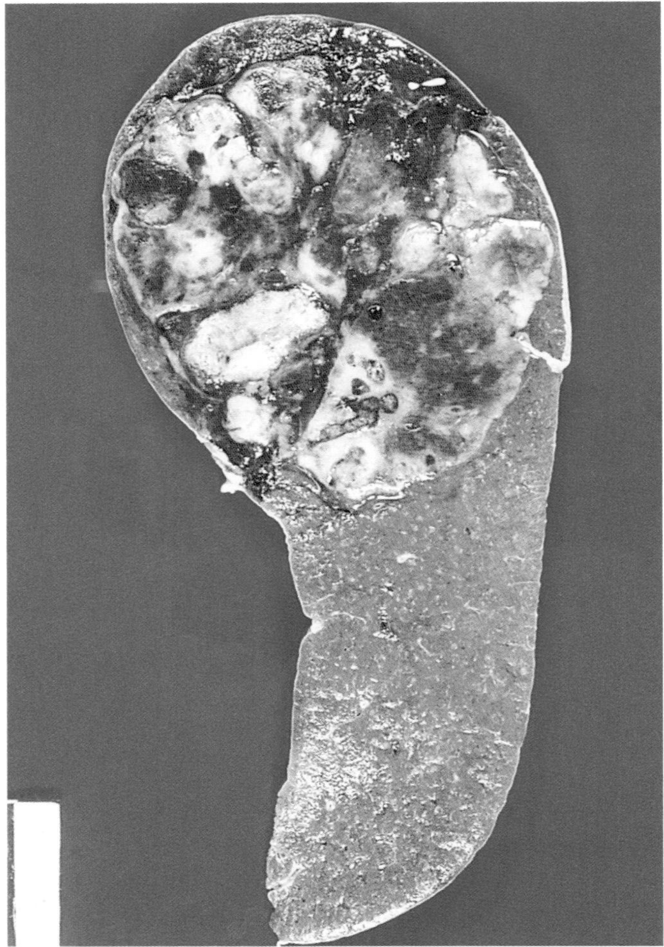

Fig. 22.38 Gross appearance of inflammatory pseudotumor of the spleen. The cut surface has a variegated color resulting from a combination of necrosis, hemorrhage, and cellular infiltration.

interpreted as myofibroblastic, although we think that it is equally compatible (and pathogenetically more appealing) with the fibroblastic (myoid) subtype of dendritic cells (Fig. 22.39). The predominant pattern of growth may be sclerotic, xanthogranulomatous, or plasma cell granuloma-type.[297,319,323] Central coagulative necrosis is often present, usually in association with a neutrophilic infiltrate. Most of the small lymphocytes are of the T-cell type.[323] The evolution following splenectomy is benign.

The exact nature of this disorder is not clear. An analogy has been drawn between this lesion and inflammatory pseudotumor of soft tissue, a lesion now generally regarded as neoplastic and redesignated inflammatory myofibroblastic tumor.[314] However, whereas the latter is characterized by expression of ALK kinase and is unassociated with EBV, inflammatory pseudotumor of the spleen (like its homonym in the liver) is ALK negative and often positive for EBV-encoded RNA with in situ hybridization tests.[296,306,314]

It should also be noted that *splenic spindle cell pseudoneoplastic lesions* can result from mycobacterial infection in immunocompromised patients.[322]

Tumors of dendritic/reticulum cells may present as splenic tumors. Some have exhibited the phenotype of follicular dendritic cells,[296,308,315,318] whereas others have probably arisen from fibroblastic reticulum cells; the latter are distinguished from inflammatory pseudotumor (a sometimes very difficult task) by virtue of the predominance of the spindle cell component with atypical features.[310] A case has been seen in association with large B-cell lymphoma.[308]

Along possibly related lines, cases with the morphologic features of malignant fibrous histiocytoma or large cell lymphoma have been reported in the spleen that had the phenotype of true histiocytes.[302,320,326]

Muscle tumors of the spleen include the *EBV-related smooth muscle neoplasms* seen in the context of AIDS (often occurring in children) and following renal transplantation,[294,309] and an exotic case of primary *rhabdomyosarcoma*.[301]

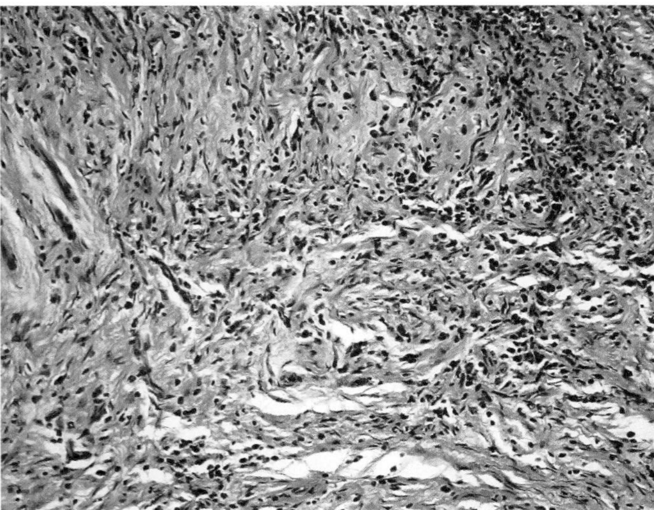

Fig. 22.39 Inflammatory pseudotumor of spleen. Spindle cells of myofibroblastic appearance are admixed with various types of inflammatory cell.

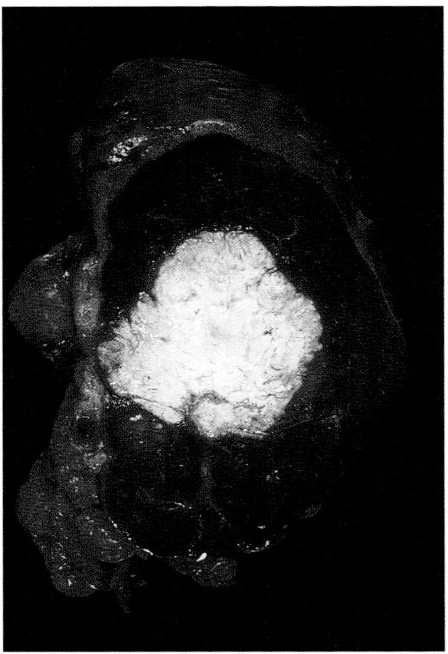

Fig. 22.40 Metastatic endometrial carcinoma to the spleen presenting as a single well-circumscribed nodule.

Lipoma has been reported as a solitary intrasplenic mass.[299]

Carcinosarcoma apparently primary in the spleen has been imaginatively interpreted as an extragenital counterpart of malignant mixed müllerian tumor.[325]

Low grade mucinous cystadenocarcinoma has been reported to arise in the spleen.[313]

Metastatic tumors

Metastatic malignancy of the spleen is a very uncommon clinical problem[338] but a not too unusual finding at autopsy if a thorough examination of the organ is carried out.[328] Malignant melanoma and carcinoma of lung, breast, stomach, large bowel, pancreas, and liver are the most common types.[329] Many others have been encountered, including ileal carcinoid[332,339] (Fig. 22.40). There appears to be an unusual tendency for gynecologic cancers to develop delayed solitary metastasis in the spleen.[333–337] Grossly, splenic metastases can appear as solitary or diffuse nodules, involve the organ diffusely, or be limited to the splenic capsule.[339] Breast carcinoma diffusely metastatic to the spleen may present as idiopathic thrombocytopenic purpura.[330] Occasionally, metastases in the spleen may be accompanied by nodular transformation of the red pulp simulating follicular lymphoma on low-power examination.[331] The metastases can be superimposed on preexistent diseases of the spleen, such as hairy cell leukemia.[340]

References

NORMAL ANATOMY

1 Bishop MB, Lansing LS. The spleen. A correlative overview of normal and pathologic anatomy. Hum Pathol 1982, **13**: 334–342.

2 Enriquez P, Neiman RS. The pathology of the spleen. A functional approach. Chicago, 1976, American Society of Clinical Pathology.

3 Ham AW. The structure of the spleen. In Blaustein A (ed.): The spleen. New York, 1963, McGraw-Hill.

4 Han J, van Krieken JM, Orazi A. Spleen. In Mills SE (ed.): Histology for pathologists, ed. 3. Philadelphia, 2007, Lippincott Williams & Wilkins, pp. 783–798.

5 Kraus MD. Splenic histology and histopathology: an update. Semin Diagn Pathol 2003, **20**: 84–93.

6 Lennert K, Harms D (eds). Die Milz. Berlin, 1970, Springer-Verlag.

7 van Krieken JHJM, te Velde J. Immunohistology of the human spleen. An inventory of the localization of lymphocyte subpopulations. Histopathology 1986, **10**: 285–294.

8 van Krieken JH, te Velde J. Normal histology of the human spleen. Am J Surg Pathol 1988, **12**: 777–785.

9 van Krieken JHJM, te Velde J, Hermans J, Welvaart K. The splenic red pulp. A histomorphometrical study in splenectomy specimens embedded in methylmethacrylate. Histopathology 1985, **9**: 401–416.

10 van Krieken JHJM, te Velde J, Kleiverda K, Leenheers-Binnendijk L, Van de Velde CJH. The human spleen. A histological study in splenectomy specimens embedded in methylmethacrylate. Histopathology 1985, **9**: 571–585.

11 Weiss L. The structure of the normal spleen. Semin Hematol 1965, **2**: 205–228.

12 Weiss L, Tavassoli M. Anatomical hazards to the passage of erythrocytes through the spleen. Semin Hematol 1970, **7**: 372–380.

BIOPSY AND FINE NEEDLE ASPIRATION

13 Civardi G, Vallisa D, Berte R, Giorgio A, Filice C, Caremani M, Caturelli E, Pompili M, De Sio I, Buscarini E, Cavanna L. Ultrasound-guided fine needle biopsy of the spleen: high clinical efficacy and low risk in a multicenter Italian study. Am J Hematol 2001, **67**: 93–99.

14 Soderström N. Cytologie der Milz in Punktaten. In Lennert K, Harms D (eds): Die Milz. Berlin, 1970, Springer-Verlag.

15 Zeppa P, Picardi M, Marino G, Troncone G, Fulciniti F, Vetrani A, Rotoli B, Palombini L. Fine-needle aspiration biopsy and flow cytometry immunophenotyping of lymphoid and myeloproliferative disorders of the spleen. Cancer 2003, **99**: 118–127.

RUPTURE AND SPLENECTOMY

16 Aldrete JS. Spontaneous rupture of the spleen in patients with infectious mononucleosis [editorial]. Mayo Clin Proc 1992, **67**: 910–912.

17 Baack BR, Varsa EW, Burgdorf WH, Blaugrund AC. Splenosis. A report of subcutaneous involvement. Am J Dermatopathol 1990, **12**: 585–588.

18 Boudová L, Kazakov DV, Hes O, Zahálka M, Mukensnabl P, Kocová J, Michal M. Subcutaneous splenosis of the abdominal wall. Am J Dermatopathol 2006, **28**: 208–210.

19 Carr NJ, Turk EP. The histological features of splenosis. Histopathology 1992, **21**: 549–553.

20 Dalton ML Jr, Strange WH, Downs EA. Intrathoracic splenosis. Case report and review of the literature. Am Rev Respir Dis 1971, **103**: 827–830.

21 Debnath D, Valerio D. Atraumatic rupture of the spleen in adults. J R Coll Surg Edinb 2002, **47**: 437–445.

22 Editorial. Infective hazards of splenectomy. Lancet 1976, **1**: 1167–1168.

23 Ellis EF, Smith RT. The role of the spleen in immunity. Pediatrics 1966, **37**: 111–119.

24 Farhi DC, Ashfaq R. Splenic pathology after traumatic injury. Am J Clin Pathol 1996, **105**: 474–478.

25 Fausel R, Sun NC, Klein S. Splenic rupture in a human immunodeficiency virus-infected patient with primary splenic lymphoma. Cancer 1990, **66**: 2414–2416.

26 Fleming CR, Dickson ER, Harrison EG Jr. Splenosis. Autotransplantation of splenic tissue. Am J Med 1976, **61**: 414–419.

27 Foster RP. Delayed haemorrhage from the ruptured spleen. Br J Surg 1970, **57**: 189–192.

28 Gabor S, Back F, Csiffary D. Peliosis lienis. Uncommon cause of rupture of the spleen. Pathol Res Pract 1992, **188**: 380–383.

29 Katkhouda N, Hurwitz MB, Rivera RT, Chandra M, Waldrep DJ, Gugenheim J, Mouiel J. Laparoscopic splenectomy: outcome and efficacy in 103 consecutive patients. Ann Surg 1998, **228**: 568–578.

30 Kraus MD, Fleming MD, Vonderheide RH. The spleen as a diagnostic specimen: a review of 10 years' experience at two tertiary care institutions. Cancer 2001, **91**: 2001–2009.

31 Kroft SH, Singleton TP, Dahiya M, Ross CW, Schnitzer B, Hsi ED. Ruptured spleens with expanded marginal zones do not reveal occult b-cell clones. Mod Pathol 1997, **10**: 1214–1220.

32 Kubosawa H, Konno A, Komatsu T, Ishige H, Kondo Y. Peliosis hepatis. An unusual case involving the spleen and lymph nodes. Acta Pathol Jpn 1989, **39**: 212–215.

33 Nordøy A. The spleenless state in man. In Lennert K, Harms D (eds): Die Milz. Berlin, 1970, Springer-Verlag.

34 O'Connor JV, Brown CC, Thomas JK, Williams J, Walsh E. Thoracic splenosis. Ann Thorac Surg 1998, **66**: 552–553.

35 Pedersen B, Videbaek A. On the late effects of removal of the normal spleen. A follow-up study of 40 persons. Acta Chir Scand 1966, **131**: 89–98.

36 Pratt DB, Andersen RC, Hitchcock CR. Splenic rupture. A review of 114 cases. Minn Med 1971, **54**: 177–184.

37 Rawsthorne GB, Cole TP, Kyle J. Spontaneous rupture of the spleen in infectious mononucleosis. Br J Surg 1970, **57**: 396–398.

38 Rickert CH, Maasjosthusmann U, Probst-Cousin S, August C, Gullotta F. A unique case of cerebral spleen. Am J Surg Pathol 1998, **22**: 894–896.

39 Sarda R, Sproat I, Kurtycz DF, Hafez R. Pulmonary parenchyma splenosis. Diagn Cytopathol 2001, **24**: 352–355.

40 Sherman R. Management of trauma to the spleen. Adv Surg 1984, **17**: 37–71.

41 Stites TB, Ultmann JE. Spontaneous rupture of the spleen in chronic lymphocytic leukemia. Cancer 1966, **19**: 1587–1590.

42 Traub A, Giebink GS, Smith C, Kuni CC, Brekke ML, Edlund D, Perry JF. Splenic reticuloendothelial function after splenectomy, spleen repair, and spleen autotransplantation. N Engl J Med 1987, **317**: 1559–1564.

CONGENITAL ANOMALIES

43 Cotelingam JD, Saito R. Hepatolienal fusion. Case report of an unusual lesion. Hum Pathol 1978, **9**: 234–236.

44 Esterly JR, Oppenheimer EH. Lymphangiectasis and other pulmonary lesions in the asplenia syndrome. Arch Pathol 1970, **90**: 553–560.
45 Gonzalez-Crussi F, Raibley S, Ballantine TVN, Grosfeld JL. Splenorenal fusion. Heterotopia simulating a renal neoplasm. Am J Dis Child 1977, **131**: 994–996.
46 Kevy SV, Tefft M, Vawter GF, Rosen FS. Hereditary splenic hypoplasia. Pediatrics 1968, **42**: 752–757.
47 Meneses MF, Ostrowski ML. Female splenic-gonadal fusion of the discontinuous type. Hum Pathol 1989, **20**: 486–488.
48 Oliva E, Young RH. Paratesticular tumor-like lesions. Semin Diagn Pathol 2000, **17**: 340–358.
49 Putschar WGJ, Manion WC. Congenital absence of the spleen and associated anomalies. Am J Pathol 1956, **26**: 429–470.
50 Putschar WGJ, Manion WC. Splenic-gonadal fusion. Cancer 1956, **32**: 15–34.
51 Rose V, Izukawa T, Moës CAF. Syndromes of asplenia and polysplenia. A review of cardiac and noncardiac malformations in 60 cases with special reference to diagnosis and prognosis. Br Heart J 1975, **37**: 840–852.
52 Vogel U, Negri G, Bultmann B. Ectopic prostatic tissue in the spleen. Virchows Arch 1996, **427**: 543–545.
53 Watson RJ. Splenogonadal fusion. Surgery 1968, **63**: 853–858.

CYSTS

54 Arber DA, Strickler JG, Weiss LM. Splenic mesothelial cysts mimicking lymphangiomas. Am J Surg Pathol 1997, **21**: 334–338.
55 Blank E, Campbell JR. Epidermoid cysts of the spleen. Pediatrics 1973, **51**: 75–84.
56 Bürring K-F. Epithelial (true) splenic cysts. Pathogenesis of the mesothelial and so-called epidermoid cyst of the spleen. Am J Surg Pathol 1988, **12**: 275–281.
57 Du Plessis DG, Louw JA, Wranz PA. Mucinous epithelial cysts of the spleen associated with pseudomyxoma peritonea. Histopathology 1999, **35**: 551–557.
58 Garvin DF, King FM. Cysts and nonlymphomatous tumors of the spleen. Pathol Annu 1981, **16**(Pt 1): 61–80.
59 Higaki K, Jimi A, Watanabe J, Kusaba A, Kojiro M. Epidermoid cyst of the spleen with CA 19-9 or carcinoembryonic antigen productions: a report of three cases. Am J Surg Pathol 1998, **22**: 704–708.
60 Lifschitz-Mercer B, Open M, Kushnir I, Czernobilsky B. Epidermoid cyst of the spleen. A cytokeratin profile with comparison to other squamous epithelia. Virchows Arch 1994, **424**: 213–216.
61 Morohoshi T, Hamamoto T, Kunimura T, Yoshida E, Kanda M, Funo K, Nagayama T, Maeda M, Araki S. Epidermoid cyst derived from an accessory spleen in the pancreas. A case report with literature survey. Acta Pathol Jpn 1991, **41**: 916–921.
62 Ough YD, Nash HR, Wood DA. Mesothelial cysts of the spleen with squamous metaplasia. Am J Clin Pathol 1981, **76**: 666–669.
63 Talerman A, Hart S. Epithelial cysts of the spleen. Br J Surg 1970, **57**: 201–204.
64 Tateyama H, Tada T, Murase T, Fujitake S, Eimoto T. Lymphoepithelial cyst and epidermoid cyst of the accessory spleen in the pancreas. Mod Pathol 1998, **11**: 1171–1177.
65 Tsakraklikes V, Hadley TW. Epidermoid cysts of the spleen. A report of five cases. Arch Pathol 1973, **96**: 251–254.

INFLAMMATION

66 Bagshawe A. A comparative study of hypersplenism in reactive and congestive splenomegaly. Br J Haematol 1970, **19**: 729–737.
67 Bendix-Hansen K, Kristensen IB. Granulomas of spleen and liver in hairy cell leukaemia. Acta Pathol Microbiol Immunol Scand (A) 1984, **92**: 157–160.
68 Braylan RC, Long J, Jaffe ES, Greco FA, Orr SL, Berard CW. Malignant lymphoma obscured by concomitant extensive epithelioid granulomas. Report of three cases with similar clinicopathologic features. Cancer 1977, **39**: 1146–1155.
69 Briggs RD, Davidson AI, Fletcher BRG. Solitary abscesses of the spleen. J R Coll Surg Edinb 1977, **22**: 345–347.
70 Chun CH, Raff MJ, Contreras L, Varghese R, Waterman N, Daffner R, Melo JC. Splenic abscess. Medicine (Baltimore) 1980, **59**: 50–65.
71 Editorial. Tropical splenomegaly syndrome. Lancet 1976, **1**: 1058–1059.
72 Falk S, Muller H, Stutte HJ. The spleen in acquired immunodeficiency syndrome (AIDS). Pathol Res Pract 1988, **183**: 425–433.
73 Fishman D, Isenberg DA. Splenic involvement in rheumatic diseases. Semin Arthritis Rheum 1997, **27**: 141–155.
74 Gaba AR, Stein RS, Sweet DL, Variakojis D. Multicentric giant lymph node hyperplasia. Am J Clin Pathol 1978, **69**: 86–90.
75 Hermann RE, Deltaven KE, Hawk WA. Splenectomy for the diagnosis of splenomegaly. Ann Surg 1968, **168**: 896–900.
76 Kadin ME, Donaldson SS, Dorfman RF. Isolated granulomas in Hodgkin's disease. N Engl J Med 1970, **283**: 859–861.
77 Klatt EC, Meyer PR. Pathology of the spleen in the acquired immunodeficiency syndrome. Arch Pathol Lab Med 1987, **111**: 1050–1053.
78 Klemperer P. The pathologic anatomy of splenomegaly. Am J Clin Pathol 1936, **6**: 99–159.
79 Kuo T, Rosai J. Granulomatous inflammation in splenectomy specimens. Clinicopathologic study of 20 cases. Arch Pathol 1974, **98**: 261–268.
80 Millikin PD. Epithelioid germinal centers in the human spleen. Arch Pathol 1970, **89**: 314–320.
81 Neiman RS. Incidence and importance of splenic sarcoid-like granulomas. Arch Pathol 1977, **101**: 518–521.
82 Neiman RS, Bischel MD, Lukes RJ. Hypersplenism in the uremic hemodialyzed patient. Pathology and proposed pathophysiologic mechanisms. Am J Clin Pathol 1973, **60**: 502–511.
83 Pitney WR. The tropical splenomegaly syndrome. Trans R Soc Trop Med Hyg 1968, **62**: 717–728.
84 Sacks EL, Donaldson SS, Gordon J, Dorfman RF. Epithelioid granulomas asociated with Hodgkin's disease. Clinical conditions in 55 previously untreated patients. Cancer 1978, **41**: 562–567.
85 Sagoe AS. Tropical splenomegaly syndrome. Long-term proguanil therapy correlated with spleen size, serum IgM, and lymphocyte transformation. Br Med J 1970, **3**: 378–382.
86 Thomas DM, Akosa AB, Lampert IA. Granulomatous inflammation of the spleen in infectious mononucleosis. Histopathology 1990, **17**: 265–267.
87 Walker DA, Howat AJ, Shannon RS, Bouch DC, Lilleyman JS. Necrotizing granulomatous splenitis complicating leukemia in childhood. Cancer 1985, **56**: 371–373.
88 Weisenburger DD. Multicentric angiofollicular lymph node hyperplasia. Pathology of the spleen. Am J Surg Pathol 1988, **12**: 176–181.
89 Young JM, Bills RJ, Ulrich E. Discrete splenic calcification in necropsy material. Am J Pathol 1957, **33**: 189–197.

HYPERSPLENISM

90 Bowdler AJ. Splenomegaly and hypersplenism. Clin Haematol 1983, **12**: 467–488.
91 Neiman RS, Bischel MD, Lukes RJ. Hypersplenism in the uremic hemodialyzed patient. Pathology and proposed pathophysiologic mechanisms. Am J Clin Pathol 1973, **60**: 502–511.
92 Peck-Radosavljevic M. Hypersplenism. Eur J Gastroenterol Hepatol 2001, **13**: 317–323.
93 Rappaport H. The pathologic anatomy of the splenic red pulp. In Lennert K, Harms D (eds): Die Milz. Berlin, 1970, Springer-Verlag.

THROMBOCYTOPENIC PURPURAS

94 Baldini M. Idiopathic thrombocytopenic purpura. N Engl J Med 1966, **274**: 1245–1251, 1301–1306, 1360–1367.
95 Berendt HL, Mant MJ, Jewell LD. Periaterial fibrosis in the spleen in idiopathic thrombocytopenic purpura. Arch Pathol Lab Med 1986, **110**: 1152–1154.
96 Bowdler AJ. The role of the spleen and splenectomy in autoimmune hemolytic disease. Semin Hematol 1976, **13**: 335–348.
97 Bowman HE, Pettit VD, Caldwell FT, Smith EB. Morphology of the spleen in idiopathic thrombocytopenic purpura. Lab Invest 1955, **4**: 206–216.
98 Chang CS, Li CY, Cha SS. Chronic idiopathic thrombocytopenic purpura. Splenic pathologic features and their clinical correlation. Arch Pathol Lab Med 1993, **117**: 981–985.
99 Cines DB, Blanchette VA. Immune thrombocytopenic purpura. N Engl J Med 2002, **346**: 995–1008.
100 Cohn J, Tygstrup I. Foamy histiocytosis of the spleen in patients with chronic thrombocytopenia. Scand J Hematol 1976, **16**: 33–37.
101 Ebbe S, Wittels B, Dameshek W. Autoimmune thrombocytopenic purpura ('ITP' type) with chronic lymphocytic leukemia. Blood 1962, **19**: 23–27.
102 Hassan NMR, Neiman RS. The pathology of the spleen in steroid-treated immune thrombocytopenic purpura. Am J Clin Pathol 1985, **84**: 433–438.
103 Hayes MM, Jacobs P, Wood L, Dent DM. Splenic pathology in immune thrombocytopenia. J Clin Pathol 1985, **38**: 985–988.
104 Jiang DY, Li C-Y. Immunohistochemical study of the spleen in chronic immune thrombocytopenic purpura with special reference to hyperplastic follicles and foamy macrophages. Arch Pathol Lab Med 1995, **119**: 533–537.
105 Luk SC, Musclow E, Simon GT. Platelet phagocytosis in the spleen of patients with idiopathic thrombocytopenic purpura (ITP). Histopathology 1980, **4**: 127–136.
106 McMillan R. Chronic idiopathic thrombocytopenic purpura. N Engl J Med 1981, **304**: 1135–1147.
107 Moake JL. Thrombotic thrombocytopenic purpura: the systemic clumping 'plague'. Annu Rev Med 2002, **53**: 75–88.

108 Rudders RA, Aisenberg AC, Schiller AL. Hodgkin's disease presenting as 'idiopathic' thrombocytopenic purpura. Cancer 1972, **30**: 220–230.

109 Saltzstein SL. Phospholipid accumulation in histiocytes of splenic pulp associated with thrombocytopenic purpura. Blood 1961, **18**: 73–88.

110 Sandler SG. The spleen and splenectomy in immune (idiopathic) thrombocytopenic purpura. Semin Hematol 2000, **37**(Suppl 1): 10–12.

111 Saracco SM, Farhi DC. Splenic pathology in thrombotic thrombocytopenic purpura. Am J Surg Pathol 1990, **14**: 223–229.

112 Tavasoli M, McMillan R. Structure of the spleen in idiopathic thrombocytopenic purpura. Am J Clin Pathol 1975, **64**: 180–191.

HEMOLYTIC ANEMIA

113 Amorosi EL. Hypersplenism. Semin Hematol 1965, **2**: 249–285.

114 Crosby WH. Splenectomy in hematologic disorders. N Engl J Med 1972, **286**: 1252–1254.

115 Jacob HS. The defective red blood cell in hereditary spherocytosis. Annu Rev Med 1969, **20**: 41–46.

116 Miraglia del Giudice E, Iolascon A, Pinto L, Nobili B, Perrotta S. Erythrocyte membrane protein alterations underlying clinical heterogeneity in hereditary spherocytosis. Br J Haematol 1994, **88**: 52–55.

117 Molnar Z, Rappaport H. Fine structure of the red pulp of the spleen in hereditary spherocytosis. Blood 1972, **39**: 81–98.

118 Pattern E. Immunohematologic diseases. JAMA 1987, **258**: 2945–2951.

119 Peters LL, Lux SE. Ankyrins. Structure and function in normal cells and hereditary spherocytes. Semin Hematol 1993, **30**: 85–118.

120 Rappaport H, Crosby WH. Autoimmune hemolytic anemia. II. Morphologic observations and clinicopathologic correlation. Am J Pathol 1957, **33**: 429–458.

121 Saad ST, Costa FF, Vicentim DL, Salles TS, Pranke PH. Red cell membrane protein abnormalities in hereditary spherocytosis in Brazil. Br J Haematol 1994, **88**: 295–299.

122 Sandusky WR, Leavell BS, Burton IB. Splenectomy. Indications and results in hematologic disorders. Ann Surg 1964, **159**: 695–710.

123 Tse WT, Lux SE. Red blood cell membrane disorders. Br J Haematol 1999, **104**: 2–13.

124 Weed RI. The importance of erythrocyte deformability. Am J Med 1970, **49**: 147–150.

125 Wiland OK, Smith EB. The morphology of the spleen in congenital hemolytic anemia (hereditary spherocytosis). Am J Clin Pathol 1956, **26**: 619–629.

CONGESTIVE SPLENOMEGALY

126 Bowder AJ. Splenomegaly and hypersplenism. Clin Haematol 1983, **12**: 467–488.

127 Ludwig J, Hashimoto E, Obata H, Baldus WP. Idiopathic portal hypertension. A histopathological study of 26 Japanese cases. Histopathology 1993, **22**: 227–234.

128 Okudaira M, Ohbu M, Okuda K. Idiopathic portal hypertension and its pathology. Semin Liver Dis 2002, **22**: 59–72.

129 Satterfield JV, Mulligan LV, Butcher HR Jr. Bleeding esophageal varices. Arch Surg 1965, **90**: 667–672.

130 Wanless IR, Bernier V. Fibrous thickening of the splenic capsule. A response to chronic splenic congestion. Arch Pathol Lab Med 1983, **107**: 595–599.

OTHER NON-NEOPLASTIC DISORDERS

131 Chen KTK, Flam MS, Workman RD. Amyloid tumor of the spleen. Am J Surg Pathol 1987, **11**: 723–725.

132 Cruickshank B. Follicular (mineral oil) lipidosis. I. Epidemiologic studies of involvement of the spleen. Hum Pathol 1984, **15**: 724–730.

133 Cruickshank B, Thomas MJ. Mineral oil (follicular) lipidosis. II. Histologic studies of spleen, liver, lymph nodes, and bone marrow. Hum Pathol 1984, **15**: 731–737.

134 Dailey MO, Coleman CN, Fajardo LF. Splenic injury caused by therapeutic irradiation. Am J Surg Pathol 1981, **5**: 325–331.

135 Dawson PJ, Dawson G. Adult Niemann–Pick disease with sea-blue histiocytes in the spleen. Hum Pathol 1982, **13**: 1115–1120.

136 Diebold J, Audouin J. Peliosis of the spleen. Report of a case associated with chronic myelomonocytic leukemia, presenting with spontaneous splenic rupture. Am J Surg Pathol 1983, **7**: 197–204.

137 Gal AA, Masor JJ. Splenic involvement in Wegener's granulomatosis. Arch Pathol Lab Med 1996, **120**: 974–977.

138 Gupta PC, Chatterjea JB, Mukherjee AM, Chatterji A. Observations on the foam cell in thalassemia. Blood 1960, **16**: 1039–1044.

139 Lacson A, Berman LD, Neiman RS. Peliosis of the spleen. Am J Clin Pathol 1979, **71**: 586–590.

140 Liber A, Rose HG. Saturated hydrocarbons in follicular lipidosis of the spleen. Arch Pathol 1967, **83**: 116–122.

141 McCain M, Quinet R, Davis W, Serebro L, Zakem J, Nair P, Ishaq S. Splenic rupture as the presenting manifestation of vasculitis. Semin Arthritis Rheum 2002, **31**: 311–316.

142 Markowitz GS, Factor SM, Borczuk AC. Splenic para-amyloid material: a possible vasculopathy of the acquired immunodeficiency syndrome. Hum Pathol 1998, **29**: 371–376.

143 Parker AC, Bain AD, Brydon WG, Harkness RA, Smith AF, Smith II, Boyd DHA. Sea-blue histiocytosis associated with hyperlipidemia. J Clin Pathol 1976, **29**: 634–638.

144 Raghavan R, Alley S, Tawfik O, Webb P, Forster J, Uhl M. Splenic peliosis: a rare complication following liver transplantation. Dig Dis Sci 1999, **44**: 1128–1131.

145 Reidbord HR, Branimir LH, Fisher ER. Splenic lipidoses. Histochemical and ultrastructural differentiation with special reference to the syndrome of the sea-blue histiocyte. Arch Pathol 1972, **93**: 518–524.

146 Rentsch J, McColl G. Splenic infarction in Wegener's granulomatosis. J Rheumatol 2000, **27**: 1553–1555.

147 Rywlin AM, Lopez-Gomez A, Tachimes P, Pardo V. Ceroid histiocytosis of the spleen in hyperlipemia. Relationship to the syndrome of the sea-blue histiocyte. Am J Clin Pathol 1971, **56**: 572–579.

148 Silverstein MN, Ellefson RD, Ahern EJ. The syndrome of the sea-blue histiocyte. N Engl J Med 1970, **282**: 1–4.

149 Tada T, Wakabayashi T, Kishimoto H. Peliosis of the spleen. Am J Clin Pathol 1983, **79**: 708–713.

150 Wanless IR, Geddie WR. Mineral oil lipogranulomata in liver and spleen. A study of 465 autopsies. Arch Pathol Lab Med 1985, **109**: 283–286.

151 Warfel KA, Ellis GH. Peliosis of the spleen. Report of a case and review of the literature. Arch Pathol Lab Med 1982, **106**: 99–100.

HEMATOLYMPHOID TUMORS AND TUMORLIKE CONDITIONS

NON-HODGKIN LYMPHOMA

152 Ahmann DL, Kiely JM, Harrison EG Jr, Payne S. Malignant lymphoma of the spleen. Cancer 1966, **19**: 461–469.

153 Alkan S, Ross CW, Hanson CA, Schnitzer B. Follicular lymphoma with involvement of the splenic marginal zone: a pitfall in the differential diagnosis of splenic marginal zone cell lymphoma. Hum Pathol 1996, **27**: 503–506.

154 Andersen CL, Gruszka-Westwood A, Atkinson S, Matutes E, Catovsky D, Pedersen RK, Pedersen BB, Pulczynski S, Hokland P, Jacobsen E, Koch J. Recurrent genomic imbalances in B-cell splenic marginal-zone lymphoma revealed by comparative genomic hybridization. Cancer Genet Cytogenet 2005, **156**: 122–128.

155 Bahler DW, Pindzola JA, Swerdlow SH. Splenic marginal zone lymphomas appear to originate from different B cell types. Am J Pathol 2002, **161**: 81–88.

156 Bellamy CO, Krajewski AS. Primary splenic large cell anaplastic lymphoma associated with HIV infection. Histopathology 1994, **24**: 481–483.

157 Burke JS. Surgical pathology of the spleen. An approach to the differential diagnosis of splenic lymphomas and leukemias. I. Diseases of the white pulp. Am J Surg Pathol 1981, **5**: 551–563.

158 Burke JS. Surgical pathology of the spleen. An approach to the differential diagnosis of splenic lymphomas and leukemias. II. Diseases of the red pulp. Am J Surg Pathol 1981, **5**: 681–694.

159 Camacho FI, Mollejo M, Mateo MS, Algara P, Navas C, Hernández JM, Santoja C, Solé F, Sánchez-Beato M, Piris MA. Progression to large B-cell lymphoma in splenic marginal zone lymphoma: a description of a series of 12 cases. Am J Surg Pathol 2001, **25**: 1268–1276.

160 Chan JKC. Splenic involvement by peripheral T-cell and NK-cell neoplasms. Semin Diagn Pathol 2003, **20**: 105–120.

161 Chang KL, Arber DA. Hepatosplenic gamma-delta T-cell lymphoma – not just alphabet soup. Adv Anat Pathol 1998, **5**: 21–29.

162 Dacie JV, Brain MC, Harrison CV, Lewis SM, Worlledge SM. Non-tropical idiopathic splenomegaly (primary hypersplenism). A review of ten cases and their relationship to malignant lymphomas. Br J Haematol 1969, **17**: 317–333.

163 Dacie JV, Galton DAG, Gordon-Smith EC, Harrison CV. Non-tropical 'idiopathic splenomegaly'. A follow-up study of ten patients described in 1969. Br J Haematol 1978, **38**: 185–193.

164 Dogan A, Burke JS, Goteri G, Stitson RN, Wotherspoon AC, Isaacson PG. Micronodular T-cell/histiocyte-rich large B-cell lymphoma of the spleen: histology, immunophenotype, and differential diagnosis. Am J Surg Pathol 2003, **27**: 903–911.

165 Dogan A, Isaacson PG. Splenic marginal zone lymphoma. Semin Diagn Pathol 2003, **20**: 121–127.

166 Dommann-Scherrer CC, Baumann Kurer S, Zimmermann DR, Odermatt BF, Dours-Zimmermann MT, Briner J, Heitz PU. Occult hepatosplenic T-lymphoma. Value of genotypic analysis in the differential diagnosis. Virchows Arch 1995, **426**: 629–634.

167 Dufresne SD, Felgar RE, Sargent RL, Surti U, Gollin SM, McPhail ED, Cook JR, Swerdlow SH. Defining the borders of splenic marginal zone lymphoma: a multiparameter study. Hum Pathol 2010, **41**: 540–551.

168 Falk S, Stutte HJ. Primary malignant lymphomas of the spleen. A morphologic and immunohistochemical analysis of 17 cases. Cancer 1990, **66**: 2612–2619.

169 Franco V, Florena AM, Campesio G. Instrasinusoidal bone marrow infiltration: a possible hallmark of splenic lymphoma. Histopathology 1996, **29**: 571–575.

170 François A, Lesesve JF, Stamatoullas A, Comoz F, Lenormand B, Etienne I, Mendel I, Hémet J, Bastard C, Tilly H. Hepatosplenic gamma/delta T-cell lymphoma: a report of two cases in immunocompromised patients, associated with isochromosome 7q. Am J Surg Pathol 1997, **21**: 781–790.

171 Goldberg GM. A study of malignant lymphomas and leukemias. VII. Lymphogenous leukemia and lymphosarcoma involvement of the lymphatic and hemic bed, with reference to differentiating criteria. Cancer 1964, **17**: 277–287.

172 Hammer RD, Glick AD, Greer JP, Collins RD, Cousar JB. Splenic marginal zone lymphoma: a distinct B-cell neoplasm. Am J Surg Pathol 1996, **20**: 613–626.

173 Harris NL, Aisenberg AC, Meyer JE, Ellman L, Elman A. Diffuse large cell (histiocytic) lymphoma of the spleen. Clinical and pathologic characteristics of ten cases. Cancer 1984, **54**: 2460–2467.

174 Hernández JM, García JL, Gutiérrez NC, Mollejo M, Martínez-Climent JA, Flores T, González MB, Piris MA, San Miguel JF. Novel genomic imbalances in B-cell splenic marginal zone lymphomas revealed by comparative genomic hybridization and cytogenetics. Am J Pathol 2001, **158**: 1843–1850.

175 Hollema H, Visser L, Poppema S. Small lymphocytic lymphomas with predominant splenomegaly. A comparison of immunophenotypes with cases of predominant lymphadenopathy. Mod Pathol 1991, **4**: 712–717.

176 Howard MT, Dufresne S, Swerdlow SH, Cook JR. Follicular lymphoma of the spleen: multiparameter analysis of 16 cases. Am J Clin Pathol 2009, **131**: 656–662.

177 Iannitto E, Ambrosetti A, Ammatuna E, Colosio M, Florena AM, Tripodo C, Minardi V, Calvaruso G, Mitra ME, Pizzolo G, Menestrina F, Franco V. Splenic marginal zone lymphoma with or without villous lymphocytes. Hematologic findings and outcomes in a series of 57 patients. Cancer 2004, **101**: 2050–2057.

178 Isaacson PG, Piris MA. Splenic marginal zone lymphoma. Adv Anat Pathol 1997, **4**: 191–201.

179 Isaacson PG, Matutes E, Burke M, Catavsky D. The histopathology of splenic lymphoma with villous lymphocytes. Blood 1994, **84**: 3828–3834.

180 Isaacson PG, Piris MA. Splenic marginal zone lymphoma. Adv Anat Pathol 1997, **4**: 191–201.

181 Kansal R, Ross CW, Singleton TP, Finn WG, Schnitzer B. Histopathologic features of splenic small B-cell lymphomas. Am J Clin Pathol 2003, **120**: 335–347.

182 Kehoe J, Straus DJ. Primary lymphoma of the spleen. Clinical features and outcome after splenectomy. Cancer 1988, **62**: 1433–1438.

183 Li S, Mann KP, Holden JT. T-cell-rich B-cell lymphoma presenting in the spleen: a clinicopathologic analysis of 3 cases. Int J Surg Pathol 2004, **12**: 31–37.

184 Lloret E, Mollejo M, Mateo MS, Villuendas R, Algara P, Martínez P, Piris MA. Splenic marginal zone lymphoma with increased number of blasts: an aggressive variant? Hum Pathol 1999, **30**: 1153–1160.

185 Macon WR, Levy NB, Kurtin PJ, Salhany KE, Elkhalifa MY, Casey TT, Craig FE, Vnencak-Jones CL, Gulley ML, Park JP, Cousar JP. Hepatosplenic alpha beta T-cell lymphomas: a report of 14 cases and comparison with hepatosplenic gamma delta T-cell lymphomas. Am J Surg Pathol 2001, **25**: 285–296.

186 Mateo M, Mollejo M, Villuendas R, Algara P, Sánchez-Beato M, Martínez P, Piris MA. 7q31-32 allelic loss is a frequent finding in splenic marginal zone lymphoma. Am J Pathol 1999, **154**: 1583–1589.

187 Maes B, Baens M, Marynen P, De Wolf-Peeters C. The product of the t(11;18), an API2-MLT fusion, is an almost exclusive finding in marginal zone cell lymphoma of extranodal MALT-type. Ann Oncol 2000, **11**: 521–526.

188 Melo JV, Hedge U, Parreira A, Thompson I, Lampert IA, Catovsky D. Splenic B cell lymphoma with circulating villous lymphocytes. Differential diagnosis of B cell leukaemias with large spleens. J Clin Pathol 1987, **40**: 642–651.

189 Miranda RN, Cousar JB, Hammer RD, Collins RD, Vnencak-Jones CL. Somatic mutation analysis of IgH variable regions reveals that tumor cells of most parafollicular (monocytoid) B-cell lymphoma, splenic marginal zone B-cell lymphoma, and some hairy cell leukaemia are composed of memory B lymphocytes. Hum Pathol 1999, **30**: 306–312.

190 Molina TJ, Delmer A, Cymbalista F, Le Torneau A, Perrot JY, Raymond S, Marie JP, Audouin J, Zittoun R, Diebold J. Mantle cell lymphoma, in leukaemic phase with prominent splenomegaly. A report of eight cases with similar clinical presentation and aggressive outcome. Virchows Arch 2000, **437**: 591–598.

191 Mollejo M, Algara P, Mateo MS, Menárguez J, Pascual E, Fresno MF, Camacho FI, Piris MA. Large B-cell lymphoma presenting in the spleen; identification of different clinicopathologic conditions. Am J Surg Pathol 2003, **27**: 895–902.

192 Mollejo M, Algara P, Mateo MS, Sanchez-Beato M, Lloret E, Medina MT, Piris MA. Splenic small B-cell lymphoma with predominant red pulp involvement: a diffuse variant of splenic marginal zone lymphoma? Histopathology 2002, **40**: 22–30.

193 Mollejo M, Lloret E, Menarguez J, Piris MA, Isaacson PG. Lymph node involvement by splenic marginal zone lymphoma: morphological and immunohistochemical features. Am J Surg Pathol 1997, **21**: 772–780.

194 Mollejo M, Rodríguez-Pinilla MS, Montes-Moreno S, Algara P, Dogan A, Cigudosa JC, Juarez R, Flores T, Forteza J, Arribas A, Piris MA. Splenic follicular lymphoma: clinicopathologic characteristics of a series of 32 cases. Am J Surg Pathol 2009, **33**: 730–738.

195 Morel P, Dupriez B, Gosselin B, Fenaux P, Estienne MH, Facon T, Jouet JP, Bauters F. Role of early splenectomy in malignant lymphomas with prominent splenic involvement (primary lymphomas of the spleen). A study of 59 cases. Cancer 1993, **71**: 207–215.

196 Neiman RS, Orazi A. Histopathologic manifestation of lymphoproliferative and myeloproliferative disorders involving the spleen. In Neoplastic hematopathology, ed. 2. Philadelphia, 2001, Lippincott Williams & Wilkins, pp. 1881–1914.

197 Ohshima K, Haroaka S, Harada N, Kamimura T, Suzumiya J, Kanda M, Kawasaki C, Sugihara M, Kikuchi M. Hepatosplenic gamma delta T-cell lymphoma: relation to Epstein–Barr virus and activated cytotoxic molecules. Histopathology 2000, **36**: 127–135.

198 Papadaki T, Stamatopoulos K, Belessi C, Pouliou E, Parasi A, Douka V, Laoutaris N, Fassas A, Anagnostopoulos A, Anagnostou D. Splenic marginal-zone lymphoma: one or more entities? A histologic, immunohistochemical, and molecular study of 42 cases. Am J Surg Pathol 2007, **31**: 438–446.

199 Pawade J, Wilkins BS, Wright DH. Low-grade B-cell lymphomas of the splenic marginal zone. A clinicopathological and immunohistochemical study of 14 cases. Histopathology 1995, **17**: 129–137.

200 Pittaluga S, Verhoef G, Criel A, Wlodarska I, Dierlamm J, Mecucci C, Van Den Berghe H, De Wold-Peeters C. 'Small' B-cell non-Hodgkin's lymphomas with splenomegaly at presentation are either mantle cell lymphoma or marginal zone cell lymphoma. A study based on histology, cytology, immunohistochemistry, and cytogenetic analysis. Am J Surg Pathol 1996, **20**: 211–223.

201 Rosso R, Neiman RS, Paulli M, Boveri E, Kindl S, Magrini U, Barosi G. Splenic marginal zone cell lymphoma. Report of an indolent variant without massive splenomegaly presumably representing an early phase of the disease. Hum Pathol 1995, **26**: 39–46.

202 Ruiz-Ballesteros E, Mollejo M, Rodriguez A, Camacho FI, Algara P, Martinez N, Pollán M, Sanchez-Aguilera A, Menarguez J, Campo E, Martinez P, Mateo M, Piris MA. Splenic marginal zone lymphoma: proposal of new diagnostic and prognostic markers identified after tissue and cDNA microarray analysis. Blood 2005, **106**: 1831–1838.

203 Salhany KE, Feldman M, Kahn MJ, Peritt D, Schretzenmair RD, Wilson DM, DiPaola RS, Glick AD, Kant JA, Nowell PC, Kamoun M. Hepatosplenic gamma delta T-cell lymphoma: ultrastructural, immunophenotypic, and functional evidence of cytotoxic T lymphocyte differentiation. Hum Pathol 1997, **28**: 674–685.

204 Savilo E, Campo E, Mollejo M, Pinyol M, Piris MA, Zukerberg LR, Yang WI, Koeliker DD, Nguyen PL, Harris NL. Absence of cyclin D1 protein expression in splenic marginal zone lymphoma. Mod Pathol 1998, **11**: 601–606.

205 Schmid C, Kirkham N, Diss T, Isaacson PG. Splenic marginal zone cell lymphoma. Am J Surg Pathol 1992, **16**: 455–466.

206 Solé F, Salido M, Espinet B, Garcia JL, Martinez Climent JA, Granada I, Hernández JM, Benet I, Piris MA, Mollejo M, Martinez P, Vallespí T, Domingo A, Serrano S, Woessner S, Florensa L. Splenic marginal zone B-cell lymphomas: two cytogenetic subtypes, one with gain of 3q and the other with loss of 7q. Haematologica 2001, **86**: 71–77.

207 Spier CM, Kjeldsberg CR, Eyre HJ, Behm FG. Malignant lymphoma with primary presentation in the spleen. A study of 20 patients. Arch Pathol Lab Med 1985, **109**: 1076–1080.

208 Streubel B, Lamprecht A, Dierlamm J, Cerroni L, Stolte M, Ott G, Raderer M, Chott A. T(14;18)(q32;q21) involving IGH and MALT1 is a frequent chromosomal aberration in MALT lymphoma. Blood 2003, **101**: 2335–2339.

209 Stroup RM, Burke JS, Sheibani K, Ben-Ezra J, Brownell M, Winberg CD. Splenic involvement by aggressive malignant lymphomas of B-cell and T-cell types. A morphologic and immunophenotypic study. Cancer 1992, **69**: 413–420.

210 Swerdlow SH. Small B-cell lymphomas of the lymph nodes and spleen: practical insights to diagnosis and pathogenesis. Mod Pathol 1999, **12**: 125–140.

211 Takeshita M, Sakai H, Okamura S, Oshiro Y, Higaki K, Nakashima O, Uike N, Yamamoto I, Kinjo M, Matsubara F. Splenic large B-cell lymphoma in patients with hepatitis C virus infection. Hum Pathol 2005, **36**: 878–885.

212 Van Huyen JP, Molina T, Delmer A, Audouin J, Le Tourneau A, Zittoun R, Bernardou A, Diebold J. Splenic marginal zone lymphoma with or without plasmacytic differentiation. Am J Surg 2000, **24**: 1581–1592.

213 van Krieken JH, Feller AC, te Velde J. The distribution of non-Hodgkin's lymphoma in the lymphoid compartments of the human spleen. Am J Surg Pathol 1989, **13**: 757–765.

214 Wong KF, Chan JK, Matutes E, McCarthy K, Ng CS, Chan CH, Ma SK. Hepatosplenic gamma delta T-cell lymphoma. A distinctive aggressive lymphoma type. Am J Surg Pathol 1995, **19**: 718–726.

215 Wu H, Wasik MA, Przybylski G, Finan J, Haynes B, Moore H, Leonard DG, Montone KT, Naji A, Nowell PC, Kamoun M, O'Tamaszewski JE, Salhany KE. Hepatosplenic gamma-delta T-cell lymphoma as a late-onset post-transplant lymphoproliferative disorder in renal transplant recipients. Am J Clin Pathol 2000, **113**: 487–496.

HODGKIN LYMPHOMA

216 Brissette M, Dhru RD. Hodgkin's disease presenting as spontaneous splenic rupture. Arch Pathol Lab Med 1992, **116**: 1077–1079.

217 Siebert JD, Stuckey JH, Kurtin PJ, Banks PM. Extranodal lymphocyte predominance Hodgkin's disease. Clinical and pathologic features. Am J Clin Pathol 1995, **103**: 485–491.

LEUKEMIAS

218 Burke JS. Surgical pathology of the spleen. An approach to the differential diagnosis of splenic lymphomas and leukemias II. Diseases of the red pulp. Am J Surg Pathol 1981, **5**: 681–694.

219 Burke JS, Byrne GE Jr, Rappaport H. Hairy cell leukemia (leukemic reticuloendotheliosis). I. A clinical pathologic study of 21 patients. Cancer 1974, **33**: 1399–1410.

220 Burke JS, Mackay B, Rappaport H. Hairy cell leukemia II. Ultrastructure of the spleen. Cancer 1976, **37**: 2267–2274.

221 Burke JS, Sheibani K, Winberg CD, Rappaport H. Recognition of hairy cell leukemia in a spleen of normal weight. The contribution of immunohistologic studies. Am J Clin Pathol 1987, **87**: 276–281.

222 Butler JJ. Pathology of the spleen in benign and malignant conditions. Histopathology 1983, **7**: 453–474.

223 Chang KL, Stroup R, Weiss LM. Hairy cell leukemia. Current status. Am J Clin Pathol 1992, **97**: 719–738.

224 Dong HY, Weisberger J, Liu Z, Tugulea S. Immunophenotypic analysis of CD103+ B-lymphoproliferative disorders: hairy cell leukemia and its mimics. Am J Clin Pathol 2009, **131**: 586–595.

225 Falini B, Tiacci E, Liso A, Basso K, Sabattini E, Pacini R, Foa R, Pulsoni A, Dalla Favera R, Pileri S. Simple diagnostic assay for hairy cell leukaemia by immunocytochemical detection of annexin A1 (ANXA1). Lancet 2004, **363**: 1869–1870.

226 Hanson CA, Ward PC, Schnitzer B. A multilobular variant of hairy cell leukemia with morphologic similarities to T-cell lymphoma. Am J Surg Pathol 1989, **13**: 671–679.

227 Hogan SF, Osborne BM, Butler JJ. Unexpected splenic nodules in leukemic patients. Hum Pathol 1989, **20**: 62–68.

228 Hoyer JD, Li CY, Yam LT, Hanson CA, Kurtin PJ. Immunohistochemical demonstration of acid phosphatase isoenzyme 5 (tartrate-resistant) in paraffin sections of hairy cell leukemia and other hematologic disorders. Am J Clin Pathol 1997, **108**: 308–315.

229 Johrens K, Stein H, Anagnostopoulos I. T-bet transcription factor detection facilitates the diagnosis of minimal hairy cell leukemia infiltrates in bone marrow trephines. Am J Surg Pathol 2007, **31**: 1181–1185.

230 Kraus MD, Bartlett NL, Fleming MD, Dorfman DM. Splenic pathology in myelodysplasia: a report of 13 cases with clinical correlation. Am J Surg Pathol 1998, **22**: 1255–1266.

231 Lampert I, Catovsky D, Marsh GW, Child JA, Galton DAG. The histopathology of prolymphocytic leukaemia with particular reference to the spleen. A comparison with chronic lymphocytic leukaemia. Histopathology 1980, **4**: 3–19.

232 Nanba K, Soban EJ, Bowling MC, Berard CW. Splenic pseudosinuses and hepatic angiomatous lesions. Distinctive features of hairy cell leukemia. Am J Clin Pathol 1977, **67**: 415–426.

233 O'Malley DP, Kim YS, Perkins SL, Baldridge L, Juliar BE, Orazi A. Morphologic and immunohistochemical evaluation of splenic hematopoietic proliferations in neoplastic and benign disorders. Mod Pathol 2005, **18**: 1550–1561.

234 Osuji N, Matutes E, Catovsky D, Lampert I, Wotherspoon A. Histopathology of the spleen in T-cell large granular lymphocyte leukemia and T-cell prolymphocytic leukemia: a comparative review. Am J Surg Pathol 2005, **29**: 935–941.

235 Pilon VA, Davey FR, Gordon GB. Splenic alterations in hairy cell leukemia. Arch Pathol Lab Med 1981, **105**: 577–581.

236 Pilon VA, Davey FR, Gordon GB, Jones DB. Splenic alterations in hairy-cell leukemia. II. An electron microscopic study. Cancer 1982, **49**: 1617–1623.

237 Re G, Pileri S, Cau R, Bucchi ML, Casali AM, Cavalli G. Histometry of splenic microvascular architecture in hairy cell leukaemia. Histopathology 1988, **13**: 425–434.

238 Strickler JG, Schmidt CM, Wick MR. Immunophenotype of hairy cell leukemia in paraffin sections. Mod Pathol 1990, **3**: 518–523.

239 Stroup R, Sheibani K. Antigenic phenotypes of hairy cell leukemia and monocytoid B-cell lymphoma. An immunohistochemical evaluation of 66 cases. Hum Pathol 1992, **23**: 172–177.

240 Van Norman AS, Nagorney DM, Martin JK, Phyliky RL, Ilstrup DM. Splenectomy for hairy cell leukemia. A clinical review of 63 patients. Cancer 1986, **57**: 644–648.

MYELOFIBROSIS

241 Cina SJ, Gordon BM, Curry NS. Ectopic adrenal myelolipoma presenting as a splenic mass. Arch Pathol Lab Med 1995, **119**: 561–563.

242 Fisher ER, Hazard JB. Differentiation of megakaryocyte and Reed–Sternberg cell. Lab Invest 1954, **3**: 261–269.

243 O'Keane JC, Wolf BC, Neiman RS. The Pathogenesis of splenic extramedullary hematopoiesis in metastatic carcinoma. Cancer 1989, **63**: 1539–1543.

244 Pitcock JA, Reinhard EH, Justus BW, Mendelsohn RA. A clinical and pathological study of seventy cases of myelofibrosis. Ann Intern Med 1962, **57**: 73–84.

245 Söderström N, Bandmann U, Lundh B. Patho-anatomical features of the spleen and liver. In Videbaek A (ed.): Polycythaemia and myelofibrosis. Clin Haematol 1975, **4**: 309–329.

246 Varki A, Lottenberg R, Griffith R, Reinhard E. The syndrome of idiopathic myelofibrosis. A clinicopathologic review with emphasis on the prognostic variables predicting survival. Medicine (Baltimore) 1983, **62**: 353–371.

247 Wilkins BS, Green A, Wild AE, Jones DB. Extramedullary haemopoiesis in fetal and adult human spleen. A quantitative immunohistological study. Histopathology 1994, **24**: 241–247.

MASTOCYTOSIS

248 Akin C. Molecular diagnosis of mast cell disorders: a paper from the 2005 William Beaumont Hospital Symposium on Molecular Pathology. J Mol Diagn 2006, **8**: 412–419.

249 Arber DA, Rappaport H, Weiss LN. Non-Hodgkin's lymphoproliferative disorders involving the spleen. Mod Pathol 1997, **10**: 18–32.

250 Brunning RD, Parkin JL, McKenna RW, Risdall R, Rosai J. Systemic mastocytosis. Extracutaneous manifestations. Am J Surg Pathol 1983, **7**: 425–438.

251 Hahn HP, Hornick JL. Immunoreactivity for CD25 in gastrointestinal mucosal mast cells is specific for systemic mastocytosis. Am J Surg Pathol 2007, **31**: 1669–1676.

252 Hollmann TJ, Brenn T, Hornick JL. CD25 expression on cutaneous mast cells from adult patients presenting with urticaria pigmentosa is predictive of systemic mastocytosis. Am J Surg Pathol 2008, **32**: 139–145.

253 Horny HP, Sillaber C, Menke D, Kaiserling E, Wehrmann M, Stehberger B, Chott A, Lechner K, Lennert K, Valent P. Diagnostic value of immunostaining for tryptase in patients with mastocytosis. Am J Surg Pathol 1998, **22**: 1132–1140.

254 Kirsch R, Geboes K, Shepherd NA, de Hertogh G, Di Nicola N, Lebel S, Mickys U, Riddell RH. Systemic mastocytosis involving the gastrointestinal tract: clinicopathologic and molecular study of five cases. Mod Pathol 2008, **21**: 1508–1516.

255 Li WV, Kapadia SB, Sonmez-Alpan E, Swerdlow SH. Immunohistochemical characterization of mast cell disease in paraffin sections using tryptase, CD68, myeloperoxidase, lysozyme and CD20 antibodies. Mod Pathol 1996, **9**: 982–988.

256 Patnaik MM, Rindos M, Kouides PA, Tefferi A, Pardanani A. Systemic mastocytosis: a concise clinical and laboratory review. Arch Pathol Lab Med 2007, **131**: 784–791.

257 Travis WD, Li C-Y. Pathology of the Lymph node and spleen in systemic mast cell disease. Mod Pathol 1988, **1**: 4–14.

258 Weidner N, Horan RF, Austen KF. Mast-cell phenotype in indolent forms of mastocytosis. Ultrastructural features, fluorescence detection of avidin binding, and immunofluorescent determination of chymase, tryptase, and carboxypeptidase. Am J Pathol 1992, **140**: 847–857.

OTHER HEMATOLYMPHOID CONDITIONS

259 Burke JS. Surgical pathology of the spleen. An approach to the differential diagnosis of splenic lymphomas and leukemias. II. Diseases of the red pulp. Am J Surg Pathol 1981, **5**: 681–694.

260 Burke JS. Splenic lymphoid hyperplasias versus lymphomas/leukemias. A diagnostic guide. Am J Clin Pathol 1993, **99**: 486–493.

261 Burke JS, Osborne BM. Localized reactive lymphoid hyperplasia of the spleen simulating malignant lymphoma. A report of seven cases. Am J Surg Pathol 1983, **7**: 373–380.

262 Gaba AR, Stein RS, Sweet DL, Variakojis D. Multicentre giant lymph node hyperplasia. Am J Clin Pathol 1978, **69**: 86–90.

263 Vermi W, Blanzouli L, Kraus MD, Grigolato P, Donato F, Loffredo G, Marino CE, Alberti D, Notarangelo LD, Facchetti F. The spleen in the Wiskott–Aldrich syndrome: histopathologic abnormalities of the white pulp correlate with the clinical phenotype of the disease. Am J Surg Pathol 1999, **23**: 182–191.

264 Weisenburger DD. Multicentric angiofollicular lymph node hyperplasia. Pathology of the spleen. Am J Surg Pathol 1988, **12**: 176–181.

VASCULAR TUMORS

265 Arber DA, Strickler JG, Chen YY, Weiss LM. Splenic vascular tumors: a histologic, immunophenotypic and virologic study. Am J Surg Pathol 1997, **21**: 827–835.

266 Arber DA, Strickler JG, Weiss LM. Splenic mesothelial cysts mimicking lymphangiomas. Am J Surg Pathol 1997, **21**: 334–338.

267 Autry JR, Weitzner S. Hemangiosarcoma of spleen with spontaneous rupture. Cancer 1975, **35**: 534–539.

268 Ben-Izhak O, Bejar J, Ben-Eliezer S, Vlodasky E. Splenic littoral cell haemangioendothelioma: a new low-grade variant of malignant littoral cell tumour. Histopathology 2001, **39**: 469–475.

269 Bisceglia M, Sickel JZ, Giangaspero F, Gomes V, Amini M, Michal M. Littoral cell angioma of the spleen: an additional report of four cases with emphasis on the association with visceral organ cancers. Tumori 1998, **84**: 595–599.

270 Budke HL, Breitfeld PP, Neiman RS. Functional hyposplenism due to a primary epithelioid hemangioendothelioma of the spleen. Arch Pathol Lab Med 1995, **119**: 755–757.

271 Chen TK, Bolles J, Gilbert EF. Angiosarcoma of the spleen. Arch Pathol Lab Med 1979, **103**: 122–124.

272 Cokelaere K, Vanvuchelen J, Michielsen P, Sciot R. Epithelioid angiosarcoma of the splenic capsule. Report of a case reiterating the concept of inert foreign body tumorigenesis. Virchows Arch 2001, **438**: 398–403.

273 Defau JP, le Tourneanu A, Audouin J, Delmer A et al. Isolated diffuse haemangiomatosis of the spleen with Kasaback–Merritt like syndrome. Histopathology 1999, **35**: 337–344.

274 Falk S, Stutte HJ, Frizzera G. Littoral cell angioma. A novel splenic vascular lesion demonstrating histiocytic differentiation. Am J Surg Pathol 1991, **15**: 1023–1033.

275 Fernandez S, Cook GW, Arber DA. Metastasizing splenic littoral cell hemangioendothelioma. Am J Surg Pathol 2006, **30**: 1036–1040.

276 Garvin DF, King FM. Cysts and nonlymphomatous tumors of the spleen. Pathol Annu 1981, **16**(Pt 1): 61–80.

277 Hamoudi AB, Vassy LE, Morse TS. Multiple lymphangioendothelioma of the spleen in a 13-year-old girl. Arch Pathol 1975, **99**: 605–606.

278 Hermann GG, Fogh J, Graem N, Hansen OP, Hippe E. Primary hemangiosarcoma of the spleen with angioscintigraphic demonstration of metastases. Cancer 1984, **53**: 1682–1685.

279 Husni EA. The clinical course of splenic hemangioma with emphasis on spontaneous rupture. Arch Surg 1961, **83**: 681–688.

280 Karim RZ, Ma-Wyatt J, Cox M, Scolyer RA. Myoid angioendothelioma of the spleen. Int J Surg Pathol 2004, **12**: 51–56.

281 Karim RZ, Ma-Wyatt J, Cox M, Scolyer RA. Myoid angioendothelioma of the spleen. Int J Surg Pathol 2004, **12**: 51–56.

282 Kaw YT, Duwaji MS, Knisley RE, Esparza AR. Hemangioendothelioma of the spleen. Arch Pathol Lab Med 1992, **116**: 1079–1082.

283 Kutok JL, Fletcher CDM. Splenic vascular tumors. Semin Diagn Pathol 2003, **20**: 128–139.

284 Neill JS, Park HK. Hemangiopericytoma of the spleen. Am J Clin Pathol 1991, **95**: 680–683.

285 Nauhauser TS, Derringer GA, Thompson LD, Fanburg-Smith JC, Miettinen M, Saaristo A, Abbondanzo SL. Splenic angiosarcoma: a clinicopathologic and immunophenotypic study of 28 cases. Mod Pathol 2000, **13**: 978–987.

286 Rosso R, Paulli M, Gianelli U, Boveri E, Stella G, Magrini U. Littoral cell angiosarcoma of the spleen. Case report with immunohistochemical and ultrastructural analysis. Am J Surg Pathol 1995, **19**: 1203–1208.

287 Ruck P, Horny HP, Xiao JC, Bajinski R, Kaiserling E. Diffuse sinusoidal hemangiomatosis of the spleen. A case report with enzyme-histochemical, immunohistochemical, and electron-microscopic findings. Pathol Res Pract 1994, **190**: 708–714.

288 Schmid C, Beham A, Uranus S, Melzer G, Aubock L, Seewann HL, Klimpfinger M. Non-systemic diffuse lymphangiomatosis of spleen and liver. Histopathology 1991, **18**: 478–480.

289 Shanberge JN, Tanaka K, Grouhl MC. Chronic consumption coagulopathy due to hemangiomatous transformation of the spleen. Am J Clin Pathol 1971, **56**: 723–729.

290 Smith VC, Eisenberg BL, McDonald EC. Primary splenic angiosarcoma. Case report and literature review. Cancer 1985, **55**: 1625–1627.

291 Suster S. Epithelioid and spindle-cell hemangioendothelioma of the spleen. Report of a distinctive splenic vascular neoplasm of childhood. Am J Surg Pathol 1992, **16**: 785–792.

OTHER PRIMARY TUMORS AND TUMORLIKE CONDITIONS

292 Ali TZ, Beyer G, Taylor M, Volpe C, Papadimitriou JC. Splenic hamartoma: immunohistochemical and ultrastructural profile of two cases. Int J Surg Pathol 2005, **13**: 103–111.

293 Awamleh AA, Perez-Ordoñez B. Sclerosing angiomatoid nodular transformation of the spleen. Arch Pathol Lab Med 2007, **131**: 974–978.

294 Barbashina V, Heller DS, Hameed M, Albanese E, Goldstein M, Dashefsky B, Dieudonne A, Chakraborty R. Splenic smooth-muscle tumors in children with acquired immunodeficiency syndrome: report of two cases of this unusual location with evidence of an association with Epstein–Barr virus. Virchows Arch 2000, **436**: 138–139.

295 Cheuk W, Lee AK, Arora N, Ben-Arie Y, Chan JK. Splenic hamartoma with bizarre stromal cells. Am J Surg Pathol 2005, **29**: 109–114.

296 Cheuk W, Chan JK, Shek TW, Chang JH, Tsou MH, Yuen NW, Ng WF, Chan AC, Prat J. Inflammatory pseudotumor-like follicular dendritic cell tumor: a distinctive low-grade malignant intra-abdominal neoplasm with consistent Epstein–Barr virus association. Am J Surg Pathol 2001, **25**: 721–731.

297 Cotelingam JD, Jaffe ES. Inflammatory pseudo-tumor of the spleen. Am J Surg Pathol 1984, **8**: 375–380.

298 Diebold J, Le Tourneau A, Marmey B, Prevot S, Müller-Hermelink HK, Sevestre H, Molina T, Billotet C, Gaulard P, Knopf JF, Bendjaballah S, Mangnan-Marai A, Brière J, Fabiani B, Audouin J. Is sclerosing angiomatoid nodular transformation (SANT) of the splenic red pulp identical to inflammatory pseudotumour? Report of 16 cases. Histopathology 2008, **53**: 299–310.

299 Easler RE, Dowlin WM. Primary lipoma of the spleen. Report of a case. Arch Pathol 1969, **88**: 557–559.

300 Falk S, Stutte HJ. Hamartomas of the spleen. A study of 20 biopsy cases. Histopathology 1989, **14**: 603–612.

301 Feakins RM, Norton AJ. Rhabdomyosarcoma of the spleen. Histopathology 1996, **29**: 577–579.

302 Franchino C, Reich C, Distenfeld A, Ubriaco A, Knowles DM. A clinicopathologically distinctive primary splenic histiocytic neoplasm. Demonstration of its histiocytic derivation by immunophenotypic and molecular genetic analysis. Am J Surg Pathol 1988, **12**: 398–404.

303 Koreishi AF, Saenz AJ, Fleming SE, Teruya-Feldstein J. Sclerosing angiomatoid nodular transformation (SANT) of the spleen: a report of 3 cases. Int J Surg Pathol 2009, **17**: 384–389.

304 Krishnan J, Frizzera G. Two splenic lesions in need of clarification: hamartoma and inflammatory pseudotumor. Semin Diagn Pathol 2003, **20**: 94–104.

305 Kuo TT, Chen TC, Lee LY. Sclerosing angiomatoid nodular transformation of the spleen (SANT): clinicopathological study of 10 cases with or without abdominal disseminated calcifying fibrous tumors, and the presence of a significant number of IgG4+ plasma cells. Pathol Int 2009, **59**: 844–850.

306 Kutok JL, Pinkus GS, Dorfman DM, Fletcher CDM. Inflammatory pseudotumor of lymph node and spleen: an entity biologically distinct from inflammatory myofibroblastic tumor. Hum Pathol 2001, **32**: 1382–1387.

307 Laskin WB, Alasadi R, Variakojis D. Splenic hamartoma. Am J Surg Pathol 2005, **29**: 1114–1115.

308 Laurent C, Meggetto F, de Paiva GR, Selves J, Palasse J, Laurent G, Brousset P. Follicular dendritic cell tumor of the spleen associated with diffuse large B-cell lymphoma. Hum Pathol 2008, **39**: 776–780.

309 Le Bail B, Morel D, Merel P, Corneau F, Merlio JP, Carles J, Trillaud H, Bioulac-Sage P. Cystic smooth-muscle tumor of the liver and spleen associated with Epstein–Barr virus after renal transplantation. Am J Surg Pathol 1996, **20**: 1418–1425.

310 Martel M, Sarli D, Colecchia M, Coppa J, Romito R, Schiavo M, Mazzaferro V, Rosai J. Fibroblastic reticular cell tumor of the spleen: report of a case and review of the entity. Hum Pathol 2003, **34**: 954–957.

311 Martel M, Cheuk W, Lombardi L, Lifschitz-Mercer B, Chan JK, Rosai J. Sclerosing angiomatoid nodular transformation (SANT): report of 25 cases of a distinctive benign splenic lesion. Am J Surg Pathol 2004, **28**: 1268–1279.

312 Monforte-Munoz H, Ro JY, Manning JT Jr, Landon G, Del Junco G, Carlson TS, Ayala AG. Inflammatory pseudotumor of the spleen.

Report of two cases with a review of the literature. Am J Clin Pathol 1991, **96**: 491–495.

313 Morinaga S, Ohyama R, Koizumi J. Low-grade mucinous cystadenocarcinoma in the spleen. Am J Surg Pathol 1992, **16**: 903–908.

314 Neuhauser TS, Derringer GA, Thompson LD, Fanburg-Smith JC et al. Splenic inflammatory myofibroblastic tumor (inflammatory pseudotumor): a clinicopathologic and immunophenotypic study of 12 cases. Arch Pathol Lab Med 2001, **125**: 379–385.

315 Perez-Ordonez B, Erlandson RA, Rosai J. Follicular dendritic cell tumor: report of 13 additional cases of a distinctive entity. Am J Surg Pathol 1996, **20**: 944–955.

316 Rappaport H. The pathologic anatomy of the splenic red pulp. In Lennert K, Harms D (eds): Die Milz. Berlin, 1970, Springer-Verlag.

317 Ross CS, Schiller KFR. Hamartoma of spleen associated with thrombocytopenia. J Pathol 1971, **105**: 62–64.

318 Sander B, Middel P, Gunawan B, Schulten HJ, Baum F, Golas MM, Schulze F, Grabbe E, Parwaresch R, Füzesi L. Follicular dendritic cell sarcoma of the spleen. Hum Pathol 2007, **38**: 668–672.

319 Sheahan K, Wolf BC, Neiman RS. Inflammatory pseudotumor of the spleen. A clinicopathology study of three cases. Hum Pathol 1988, **19**: 1024–1029.

320 Sieber SC, Lopez V, Rosai J, Buckley PJ. Primary tumor of spleen with morphologic features of malignant fibrous histiocytoma. Immunohistochemical evidence for a macrophage origin. Am J Surg Pathol 1990, **14**: 1061–1070.

321 Silverman ML, LiVolsi VA. Splenic hamartoma. Am J Clin Pathol 1978, **70**: 224–229.

322 Suster S, Moran CA, Blanco M. Mycobacterial spindle-cell pseudotumor of the spleen. Am J Clin Pathol 1994, **101**: 539–542.

323 Thomas RM, Jaffe ES, Zarate-Osorno A, Medeiros LJ. Inflammatory pseudotumor of the spleen. A clinicopathologic and immunophenotypic study of eight cases. Arch Pathol Lab Med 1993, **117**: 921–926.

324 Weinreb I, Bailey D, Battaglia D, Kennedy M, Perez-Ordoñez B. CD30 and Epstein–Barr virus RNA expression in sclerosing angiomatoid nodular transformation of spleen. Virchows Arch 2007, **451**: 73–79.

325 Westra WH, Anderson BO, Klimstra DS. Carcinosarcoma of the spleen. An extragenital malignant mixed müllerian tumor? Am J Surg Pathol 1994, **18**: 309–315.

326 Wick MR, Scheithauer BW, Smith SL, Beart RW Jr. Primary nonlymphoreticular malignant neoplasms of the spleen. Am J Surg Pathol 1982, **6**: 229–242.

327 Zukerberg LR, Kaynor BL, Silverman ML, Harris NL. Splenic hamartoma and capillary hemangioma are distinct entities. Immunohistochemical analysis of CD8 expression by endothelial cells. Hum Pathol 1991, **22**: 1258–1261.

METASTATIC TUMORS

328 Berge T. Splenic metastases. Frequencies and patterns. Acta Pathol Microbiol Scand (A) 1974, **82**: 499–506.

329 Compérat E, Bardier-Dupas A, Camparo P, Capron F, Charlotte F. Splenic metastases: clinicopathologic presentation, differential diagnosis, and pathogenesis. Arch Pathol Lab Med 2007, **131**: 965–969.

330 Cummings OW, Mazur MT. Breast carcinoma diffusely metastatic to the spleen. A report of two cases presenting as idiopathic thrombocytopenic purpura. Am J Clin Pathol 1992, **97**: 484–489.

331 Fakan F, Michal M. Nodular transformation of splenic red pulp due to carcinomatous infiltration. A diagnostic pitfall. Histopathology 1994, **25**: 175–178.

332 Falk S, Stutte HJ. Splenic metastasis in an ileal carcinoid tumor. Pathol Res Pract 1989, **185**: 238–242.

333 Gilks CB, Acker BD, Clement PB. Recurrent endometrial adenocarcinoma: presentation as a splenic mass mimicking malignant lymphoma. Gynecol Oncol 1989, **33**: 209–211.

334 Giuliani A, Caporale A, Di Bari M, Demoro M, Mingazzini P. Isolated splenic metastasis from endometrial carcinoma. J Exp Clin Cancer Res 1999, **18**: 93–96.

335 Goktolga U, Dede M, Deveci G, Yenen MC, Deveci MS, Dilek S. Solitary splenic metastasis of squamous cell carcinoma of the uterine cervix: a case report and review of the literature. Eur J Gynaecol Oncol 2004, **25**: 742–744.

336 Hadjileontis C, Amplianitis I, Valsamides C, Harisis G, Nepka H, Kafanas A. Solitary splenic metastasis of endometrial carcinoma ten years after hysterectomy. Case report and review of the literature. Eur J Gynaecol Oncol 2004, **25**: 233–235.

337 Jorgensen LN, Chrintz H. Solitary metastatic endometrial carcinoma of the spleen. Acta Obstet Gynecol Scand 1988, **67**: 91–92.

338 Klein B, Stein M, Kuten A, Steiner M, Barshalom D, Robinson E, Gal D. Splenomegaly and solitary spleen metastasis in solid tumors. Cancer 1987, **60**: 100–102.

339 Lam KY, Tang V. Metastatic tumors to the spleen: a 25 year clinicopathologic study. Arch Pathol Lab Med 2000, **124**: 526–530.

340 Sharpe RW, Rector JT, Rushin JM, Garvin DF, Cotelingam JD. Splenic metastasis in hairy cell leukemia. Cancer 1993, **71**: 2222–2226.

Bone marrow

23

Richard D. Brunning M.D. Daniel A. Arber M.D.

CHAPTER CONTENTS

Biopsy procedure and processing of specimen

Trephine biopsy of the bone marrow has wide application in clinical medicine; its greatest utility is in the evaluation of patients with malignant lymphoma, acute leukemias, myeloproliferative neoplasms, myelodysplastic syndromes, metastatic tumor, granulomatous disorders, myelofibrosis, aplastic anemia, and plasma cell dyscrasias.[1,2,4–9] It also serves as the most reliable method for assessing marrow cellularity following the administration of antineoplastic drugs and in assessing the status of engraftment following bone marrow transplantation. Marrow biopsy is also utilized in the investigation of patients with infectious disease and metabolic disorders.

The trephine biopsy should be viewed as one component of the bone marrow specimen that ideally also includes smears and particle crush preparations from aspirated marrow and touch imprint preparations of the core biopsy specimen. In some instances, because of marrow fibrosis, the trephine biopsy specimen will be the only marrow tissue available for examination. Marrow biopsy can usually be done with relatively little discomfort to the patient and is accompanied by very low morbidity when performed by experienced individuals with the biopsy needles presently available.[13] The posterior superior iliac spines are the preferred sites. Bilateral trephine biopsies may be useful in the staging of patients with some types of lymphoma, granulomatous disorders, and metastatic tumor. This approach should be decided on an individual basis, considering both the reason for the procedure and the impact of positive findings for therapy.[4,16,18] In general, severe thrombocytopenia is not a contraindication to marrow biopsy. Whenever a marrow biopsy is performed, careful attention should be directed to preventing hematoma formation by applying an adequate pressure bandage to the biopsy site following the procedure. Prior to performing a biopsy on a patient with a bleeding disorder or on anticoagulants, consultation should be obtained from a physician expert in coagulation disorders.

Considerable discussion has occurred about the relative merits of trephine biopsy of the bone marrow as opposed to sections of particles obtained by aspiration biopsy.[6,7,12,14] Particle sections are of limited value in marrow disorders that are accompanied by fibrosis; these frequently result in inadequately aspirated specimens.[1,2] In addition, assessment of cellularity, determination of the extent of marrow involvement by neoplastic processes, and the relationship of lesions to marrow structures such as bone trabeculae and vasculature can be accurately assessed only in trephine biopsies. Nevertheless, any particles obtained in a marrow aspirate should be processed for histologic examination.

Paraffin embedding is the preferred method for the routine processing of bone marrow biopsies, and the observations described in this chapter are based primarily on examination of specimens prepared in this manner.[10,16] Plastic embedding offers some advantages over the paraffin method, such as excellent cytology and the ability to perform numerous histochemical reactions.[3] However, plastic embedding techniques are more time-consuming than the processing of paraffin-embedded tissue, and with careful attention to technical detail, excellent results can be obtained with specimens processed in paraffin. Additionally, immunohistochemistry with a wide range of antibodies can now be performed with excellent results on most paraffin-embedded specimens.[11]

Myelofibrosis is one of the more vexing problems in bone marrow histopathology because of the wide range of disorders that may cause marrow fibrosis and the usual difficulty in obtaining satisfactory aspirates for cytologic studies.[15] Although marrow fibrosis occurs as a primary disorder, it is usually a secondary phenomenon; the most common causes are metastatic tumor and malignant lymphoma. Fibrosis also occurs relatively frequently in the evolution of chronic myeloproliferative neoplasms, such as chronic myelogenous leukemia and polycythemia vera. In general, fibrosis that occurs as a component of hematopoietic proliferations is characterized initially by the deposition of increased reticulin fibers; metastatic tumors such as breast and prostate are usually characterized by a severe desmoplastic reaction with collagenous fibrosis and possibly osteosclerosis.

In those instances in which the etiology for the marrow fibrosis is not apparent, several techniques may be used in an attempt to determine the cause. Immunohistology, using paraffin-embedded specimens and the several antibodies described in the section on immunohistology, may be particularly helpful in identifying lymphoma or metastatic tumor; antibodies to myeloperoxidase, lysozyme or CD68, both KP-1 and PGM-1, and CD34, are particularly useful for identifying cells of granulocytic or monocytic origin.[17] An additional procedure that may be useful in hematopoietic disorders associated with marrow fibrosis is the preparation of particle crush preparations from trephine biopsy specimens. This approach may necessitate a second biopsy unless the problem of fibrosis is anticipated before the initial procedure. As soon as possible after the trephine specimen is obtained and before it is placed in a fixative, small portions of the biopsy are cut away with a sharp scalpel blade and used for particle crush preparations in the same manner as particles from aspirated specimens. These crush preparations can be used for routine stains, cytochemistry, and immunocytochemistry. Portions of the biopsy specimen obtained in this manner may also be used for cytogenetics, flow cytometry studies, routine electron microscopy, and ultrastructural cytochemistry. However, electron microscopy is less frequently necessary because of the availability of immunohistochemistry.

The use of special stains in bone marrow pathology should be determined following review of the routinely stained biopsy and the patient's clinical history.

Several instruments are available for the bone marrow trephine biopsy procedure. The most satisfactory from the standpoint of safety, ease of performance, and overall quality of specimen obtained is the Jamshidi-type biopsy needle; several such instruments, both reusable and disposable, are commercially available.[13] These instruments are produced in several sizes for both adult and pediatric patients. The 11-gauge needle is the most commonly used for routine procedures in adults and older children. The 8-gauge instruments are preferred by some for lymphoma staging procedures; this size may result in more postbiopsy discomfort. If difficulty is encountered with the 11-gauge needle in obtaining adequate specimens from patients with severe osteoporosis, an 8- or 9-gauge instrument should be used. Numerous modifications of the original instruments are available.

The importance of proper technique in performing the biopsy procedure cannot be overemphasized. Instructions for the use of the biopsy needles are included with the instruments, and some manufacturers provide audiovisual aids that illustrate proper technique. Accurate identification of body landmarks is crucial in obtaining satisfactory specimens; an improperly positioned needle may cause considerable discomfort to the patient and frequently yields an inadequate biopsy specimen. Individuals not acquainted with the biopsy technique are advised to familiarize themselves with the procedure on cadavers.

Optimally, the biopsy specimen should be at least 1.5 cm in length and should be free of distortion caused by crushing or other damage. Crush artifact and the deposition of fibrin in torn biopsies may render accurate interpretation difficult or impossible. In such instances the biopsy should be repeated. Aspiration through the biopsy needle prior to obtaining the trephine biopsy specimen should be discouraged because of the possibility of introducing hemorrhage or other artifact in the biopsy specimen.

Occasionally, in patients undergoing frequent repeat biopsies, a specimen may be obtained from a recently biopsied site. In these instances, the changes will reflect the stage of healing. The presence of granulation tissue in the biopsy may result in misinterpretation of cellularity. The appearance of the marrow biopsy may be inconsistent with the marrow smears, which show recovering or normal hematopoiesis (Fig. 23.1).

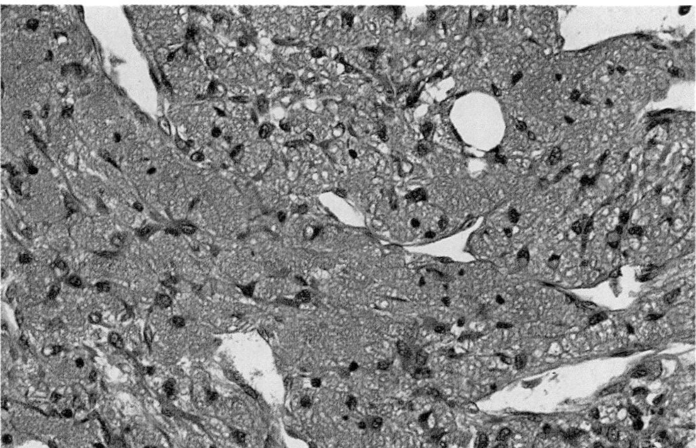

Fig. 23.1 Marrow biopsy obtained at site of a biopsy performed 14 days previously. The marrow space is replaced by granulation tissue.

Imprint preparations should be routinely made from the biopsy specimen immediately after it is removed from the biopsy needle and prior to being placed in a fixative. These can be used for Romanowsky stains and special cytochemical and immunocytochemical procedures. Following the preparation of imprints, the specimen is placed in an appropriate fixative; the most satisfactory are B5, 10% buffered neutral formalin, and AZF (acetic-acid zinc formalin).[16,17] Zenker acetic acid gives excellent cytology but ablates several antigens which may be useful in evaluating neoplastic processes; importantly it and B5 contain mercury which is environmentally hazardous. In laboratories where bone marrow specimens are processed with other tissues, buffered neutral formalin may be the preferred fixative. Because of the environmental concerns and disposal problems, some institutions prohibit the use of mercury-based fixatives. As noted in the section on immunohistochemistry, reactivity with some antibodies may be ablated by some fixatives, and the choice of fixative may be determined by the reason for the biopsy. Following fixation for an appropriate period of time, the biopsy is decalcified. Several decalcification solutions are commercially available. Most biopsy specimens will be adequately decalcified following 45–60 minutes in a rapid decalcifying solution. A discussion of the relative merits and disadvantages of several fixatives and decalcifying agents used for bone marrow biopsies has been published.[17]

The biopsies should be sectioned at 3–4 μm with a sharp knife that is checked frequently for the presence of defects. In those patients being evaluated for the extent of lymphomatous involvement, metastatic tumor, or granulomatous disease, the specimens should be completely sectioned and stepwise serial sections mounted for hematoxylin and eosin staining.[4,18] The remaining ribbons should be numbered and retained in a manner that will facilitate the ready and accurate mounting of additional sections for special stains, immunocytochemical reactions, and molecular studies.[9,17] Most of the stains used for other fixed tissues are also applicable to bone marrow sections. However, tissue processed with acid fixatives such as B5 and Zenker or with acid decalcifiers will yield unsatisfactory results with the chloroacetate esterase stain.

Optimally, when interpreting the trephine biopsy, the pathologist should examine the trephine imprints, bone marrow aspirate, blood smears, and other pathology specimens. Knowledge of the patient's clinical history, hematology profile, immunoelectrophoretic studies, and radiographic findings may be of considerable importance and may greatly facilitate the interpretation of the biopsy specimen.

Immunohistology

As in other areas of pathology, immunohistology is an important resource in the evaluation of proliferative processes involving the marrow.[23] The availability of antibodies reactive in paraffin-embedded tissue and the use of antigen retrieval have been of considerable importance in the application of immunohistology in bone marrow pathology. Although cryostat sections of marrow may be used for immunohistology, the procedure is difficult and is essentially limited to specialized laboratories.[34] In addition, cytologic preservation in cryostat sections is frequently of marginal quality.

Although decalcification with rapid acid decalcifiers may result in ablation of some antigens, an increasing number of antibodies to membrane antigens and cytoplasmic constituents are reactive in paraffin-embedded decalcified marrow biopsies and can be of considerable aid in identifying the lineage of immature cell populations in the marrow; these include antibodies to kappa and lambda light chains, leukocyte common antigen, myeloperoxidase, hemoglobin A, von Willebrand factor (factor VIII-related antigen), CD68, CD20 (L26), CD79a, CD3, CD45, CD34, terminal deoxynucleotidyl transferase (TdT), and tumor-related antigens and proliferation antigens[21,22,24,25,27,28,31–48] (Figs 23.2–23.10). Antibody to PAX5, a B-cell transcription factor present in all stages of B-cell development up to the plasma cell, appears to have application in identifying a wide spectrum of B lymphocytes from precursor B to mature B cells.[44] The commercially available antibody is a monoclonal antibody BSAP, clone 24. It is reactive in both formalin and Zenker fixed tissue. Antibodies to kappa and lambda immunoglobulin light chains are particularly useful for determining the relative proportions of kappa- and lambda-containing cells in immunoproliferative disorders such as multiple myeloma.[39] Reactivity with these antibodies is generally restricted to processes in which the cells contain cytoplasmic immunoglobulin. The technique is not sufficiently sensitive to detect surface immunoglobulin on the lymphocytes in most B lymphoproliferative diseases. Occasionally the lymphocytes in a B-cell lymphocytic lymphoma contain cytoplasmic immunoglobulin that may be detected by this method. The

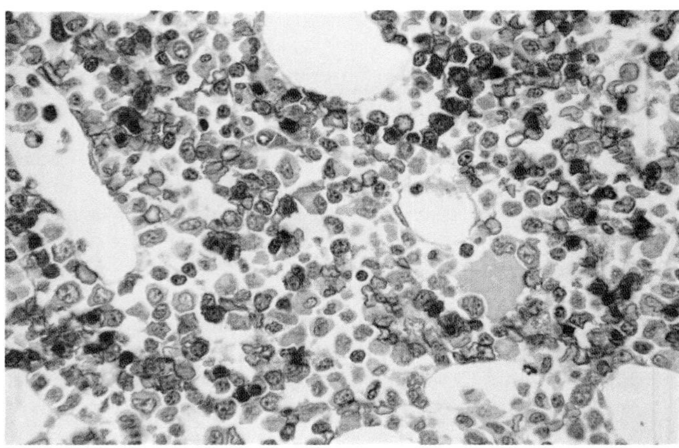

Fig. 23.4 Marrow biopsy from 2-year-old child with congenital neutropenia reacted with antibody to glycophorin A. There are numerous positive erythroid precursors at all stages of maturation. (Immunoperoxidase)

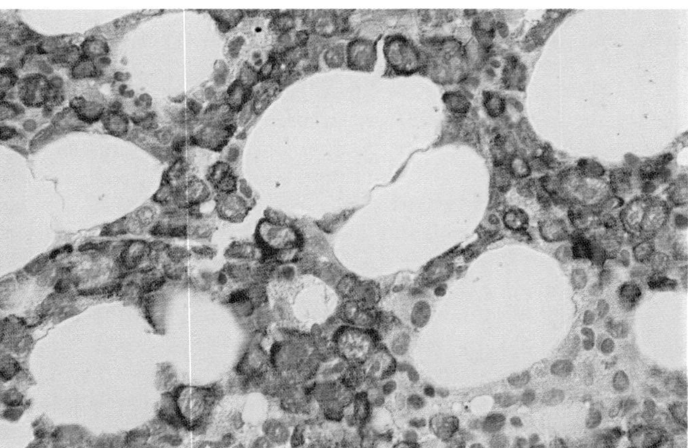

Fig. 23.2 Marrow biopsy from patient with multiple myeloma reacted with polyclonal antibody to lambda light chain; the blastic appearing plasma cells show intense cytoplasmic reaction. (Immunoperoxidase)

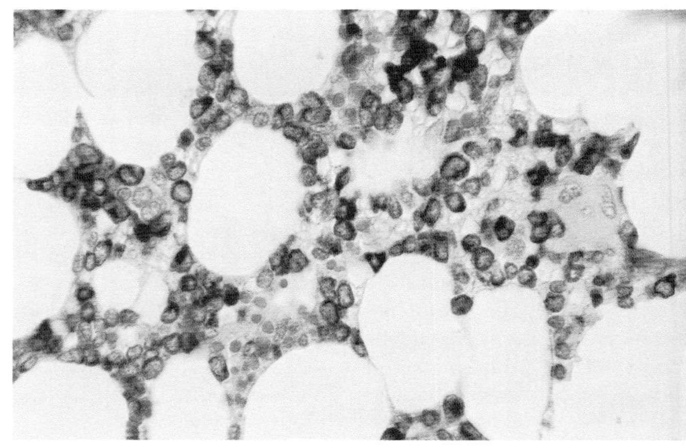

Fig. 23.5 Bone marrow biopsy from a patient with hypocellular acute myeloid leukemia reacted with polyclonal antibody to myeloperoxidase. The predominant myeloblasts and promyelocytes show intense cytoplasmic reactivity. (Immunoperoxidase)

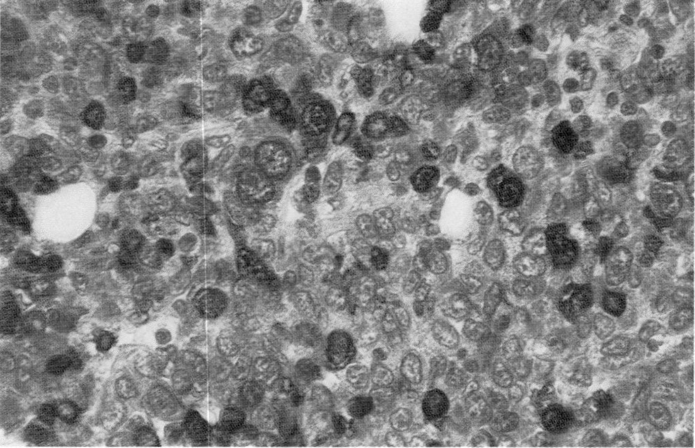

Fig. 23.3 Marrow from patient with acute erythroleukemia reacted with antibody to hemoglobin A; many of the erythroblasts show a positive cytoplasmic reaction. Intensity of reaction varies from very slight to marked. (Immunoperoxidase)

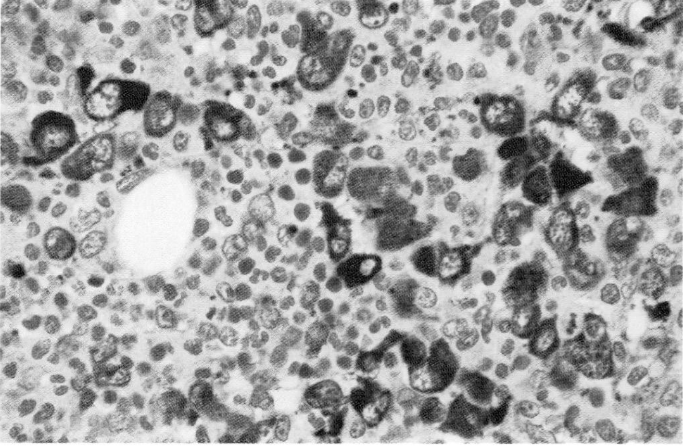

Fig. 23.6 Bone marrow biopsy from a patient with chronic myelogenous leukemia in accelerated phase reacted with polyclonal antibody to factor VIII-related antigen (von Willebrand factor). There are numerous dysplastic megakaryocytes with hypolobulated nuclei which show intense cytoplasmic reactivity. (Immunoperoxidase)

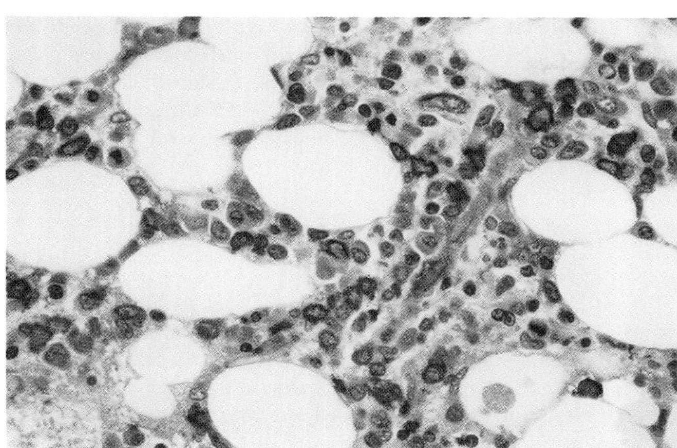

Fig. 23.7 Bone marrow biopsy from an adult male with therapy-related myelodysplastic syndrome and hypocellular marrow reacted with antibody to CD34. The number of positive cells approximates the 18.5% blasts in the marrow smear. (Immunoperoxidase)

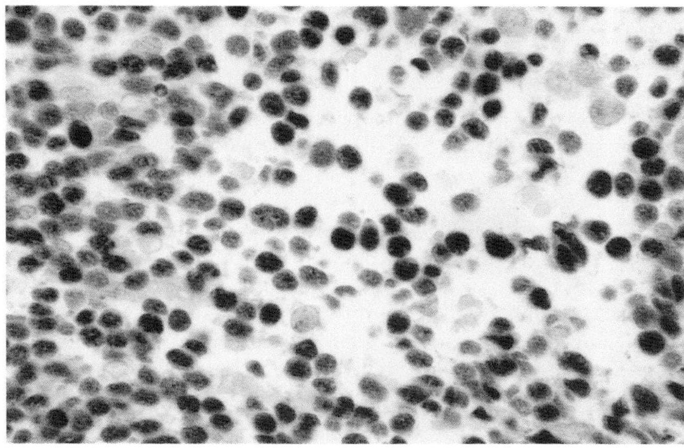

Fig. 23.8 Marrow biopsy from a child with precursor B acute lymphoblastic leukemia reacted with polyclonal antibody to TdT; the lymphoblasts show intense nuclear reactivity. (Immunoperoxidase)

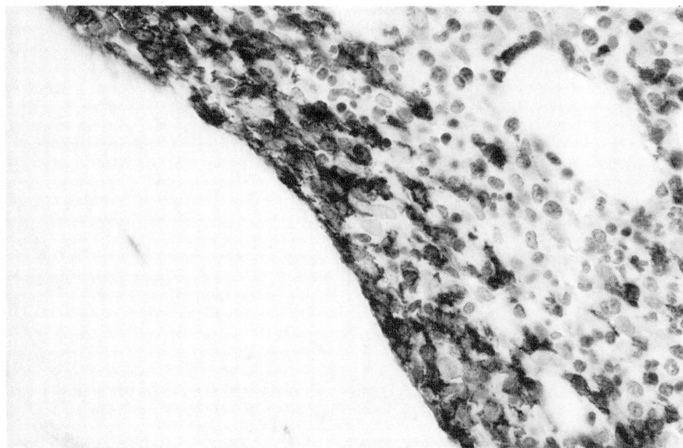

Fig. 23.9 Marrow biopsy from an adult male with recurrent follicular center cell lymphoma reacted with antibody to CD20 (L26). Numerous reacting lymphocytes are present in a paratrabecular location. (Immunoperoxidase)

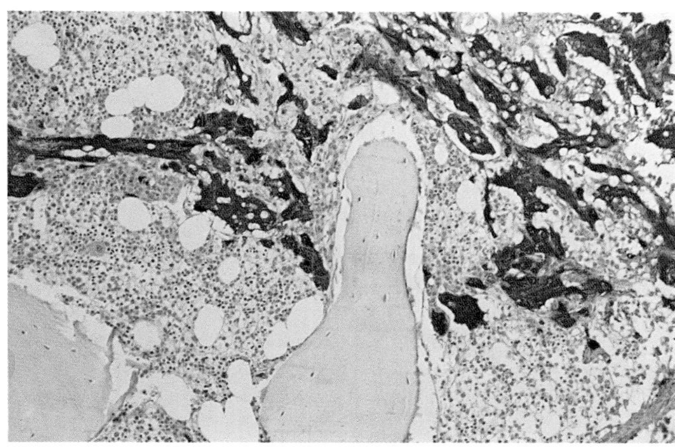

Fig. 23.10 Marrow biopsy from a child with neuroblastoma with ganglion differentiation reacted with antibody to neuron-specific enolase. The tumor cells are intensely reactive. (Immunoperoxidase)

antibodies to lymphocyte antigens are useful in determining the B- or T-cell origin of the lymphoproliferative processes and the extent of marrow involvement (see Fig. 23.9). These antibodies are not determinants of clonality. Polyclonal antibody to myeloperoxidase is a specific and sensitive antibody for cells of neutrophil origin that reacts with the myeloblasts in acute myeloid leukemia[19,20,41] (see Fig. 23.5). Some studies, however, have shown that in immunocytochemical reaction in paraffin-embedded tissue, monoclonal antibodies to myeloperoxidase are more specific. Several panels for the immunocytochemical characterization of acute leukemia have been described.[19,20,24,26,40,45] These generally include antibodies to CD68 (both PGM-1 and KP-1), myeloperoxidase, CD34, lysozyme, lymphocyte antibodies, and TdT.

It is important that the reactivity pattern of all antibodies be determined by each laboratory. The range of reactivity attributed to an antibody by the manufacturer should be confirmed with lesions of known antigenicity. The pattern of reactivity of the antibodies to lymphoid cells is generally based on studies of lymph nodes fixed in B5 or buffered neutral formalin. The same reactivity results may not be applicable to marrow biopsies decalcified with a rapid acid decalcifier; L26, an excellent antibody to CD20, a pan B-cell antigen, works well in bone marrow biopsies decalcified with a rapid acid decalcifier, but may not react in Zenker fixed tissue decalcified in the same manner. The effects of decalcification on antibody reactivity should be determined by subjecting lymph node tissue to the same decalcification procedure employed for bone marrow biopsies.

Most large histopathology laboratories use automated instruments for immunohistochemistry; with careful attention to detail, generally very good results are obtained.

In addition to routine histopathologic studies, the bone marrow specimen is being increasingly utilized for molecular and cytogenetic studies.[29,30] These special techniques should, if possible, be anticipated prior to obtaining the biopsy in order for the specimen to be processed in an appropriate manner. However, not infrequently, the need for these studies is not determined until a biopsy specimen is examined with routine stains. In these instances, it would be appropriate to repeat the biopsy for the necessary specimens. Fixed specimens embedded in paraffin have been used for some of these studies with some measure of success. This may suffice if the reliability of the technique is assured from quality control studies. Decalcified specimens may yield distinctly different results from nondecalcified fixed specimens.

This section is not intended to serve as a complete description of all of the antibodies available for bone marrow immunohistology; the individual antibodies that may be useful will be noted in the discussion of the various disease conditions.

Normocellular bone marrow

Assessment of marrow cellularity must take into account the age of the patient because the amount of hematopoietic tissue in bone marrow from normal individuals varies with age as demonstrated in both histologic and radiologic imaging studies.[49–51] In the first decade, the mean marrow cellularity is 79%; the mean cellularity in the eighth decade is 29%. In the first three decades of life more than half of the marrow is composed of hematopoietic cells. During this period, there is a gradual decrease in the amount of hematopoietic tissue with an increase in fat cells. From the fourth to the seventh decade, there is relative stabilization of the number of hematopoietic cells (Figs 23.11 and 23.12); beginning in the eighth decade, there is a renewed decrease. The increase in adipose tissue results from a decrease in both hematopoietic and bone tissue.[51]

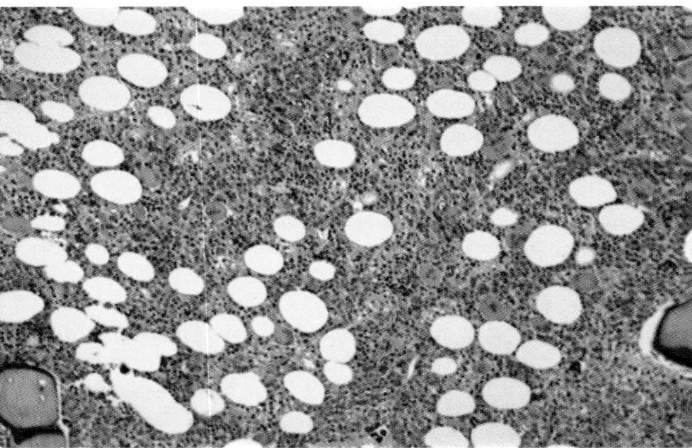

Fig. 23.11 Normocellular bone marrow from 42-year-old man obtained as part of evaluation as potential donor for bone marrow transplant. Hematopoietic cells and adipose tissue are present in approximately equal quantities.

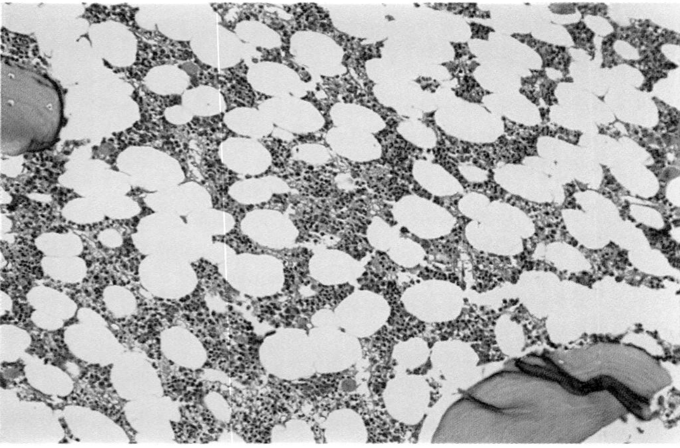

Fig. 23.12 Marrow biopsy from a 70-year-old male being evaluated for metastatic tumor. The marrow is approximately 30–35% cellular, normal for age. There was no evidence of tumor.

The immediate subcortical area of the bone marrow may normally be more hypocellular than the deeper medullary areas. As a result, specimens that contain a substantial amount of subcortical marrow may be inadequate for estimating cellularity. In addition, the immediate paratrabecular areas may be preferentially hypocellular.

Alterations in cellularity

Aplastic anemia

Acquired aplastic anemia has historically been classified as idiopathic or secondary, the latter cases allegedly resulting from exposure to drugs, chemicals, viral infections, or ionizing radiation.[52,62–64,68] Contemporary theories have focused on immunologic mechanisms as the causative factor in the majority of cases.[77,78] These mechanisms involve activation of T-cell subsets which attack marrow stem cells and progenitor cells. In some instances, apparently acquired aplastic anemia is related to inherited genetic mutations.

The biologic mechanisms underlying the occasional evolution of aplastic anemia to paroxysmal nocturnal hemoglobinuria (PNH) is not presently known.[70]

The term 'constitutional aplastic anemia' has been used collectively for all congenital aplastic anemias, familial and nonfamilial, with and without associated abnormalities of body structures. There are several inherited bone marrow failure syndromes which may manifest marrow aplasia or hypoplasia including Fanconi anemia, Shwachman–Diamond syndrome, dyskeratosis congenita, and Diamond–Blackfan anemia.[53,55,57–61,73,74,76]

Fanconi anemia is a syndrome of familial hypoplastic anemia occurring primarily in the first decade of life that is associated with multiple organ malformations, including hypoplasia of the kidneys and absent or hypoplastic thumbs or radii.[55,59–61] An association of hypoplastic bone marrow and pancreatic dysfunction (Shwachman–Diamond syndrome) is a rare disorder occurring in children.[73] Diamond–Blackfan anemia is characterized by erythroid aplasia or hypoplasia manifesting usually in the first year of life.

Selective aplasia or hypoplasia of the megakaryocytes associated with missing radii (TAR syndrome) is a rare disorder. An inherited autosomal dominant hematologic disorder associated with proximal fusion of the radius and ulna has been reported; the hematologic manifestations are somewhat variable and include adult onset of generalized bone marrow failure and amegakaryocytic thrombocytopenia presenting in childhood. The latter presentation has been associated with a mutation in homeobox genes *HOXA11*. The homeobox genes encode regulatory proteins that have a role in skeletal morphogenesis and hematopoiesis.[58,66,76]

In the most severe form of aplastic anemia, the intertrabecular marrow space is occupied predominantly by adipose tissue with scattered lymphocytes, plasma cells, tissue mast cells, and hemosiderin-laden macrophages (Fig. 23.13). In less severe processes, there is an increased amount of fat tissue and scattered small collections of erythroblasts, granulocytes, and megakaryocytes; in some instances, the decrease in megakaryocytes is disproportionate to other cell types. The blood findings in aplastic anemia are characterized by varying degrees of pancytopenia.

Uncommonly, the marrow biopsy in a patient with aplastic anemia contains aggregates of well-differentiated lymphocytes similar to the lesions that occur in a variety of immune disorders; these are described in this chapter as polymorphous lymphoid aggregates. Unusually large aggregates of benign T lymphocytes have been observed in aplastic marrows in patients with invasive malignant thymoma with an associated nonclonal T lymphocytosis in the blood (Fig. 23.14).[75]

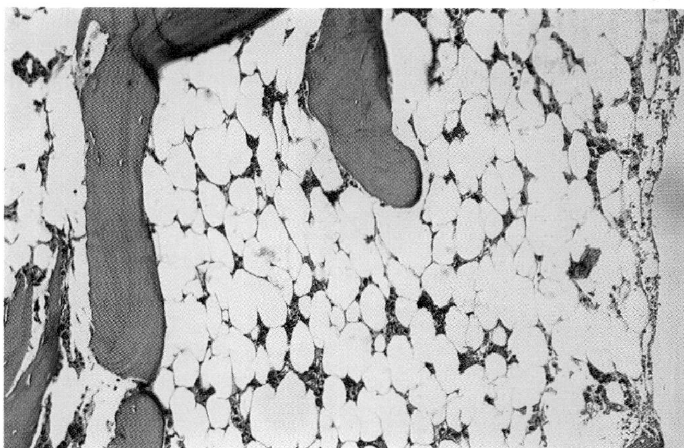

Fig. 23.13 Bone marrow section from a 7-year-old girl with idiopathic acquired aplastic anemia. Hematopoietic cells are almost totally absent. Sinuses and capillaries are prominent. Iron-laden macrophages reflecting increased iron stores from repeated red blood cell transfusions are present.

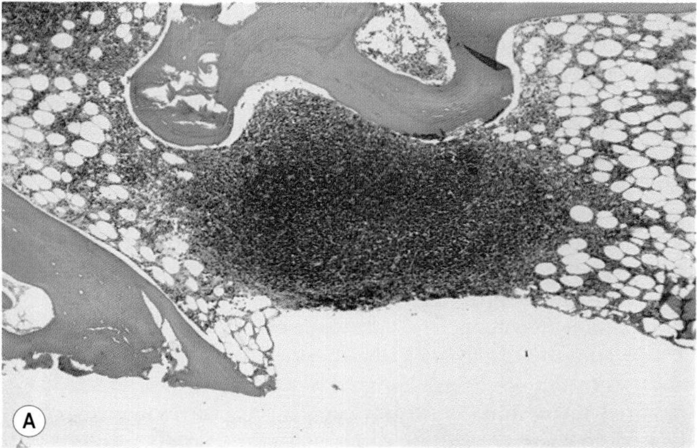

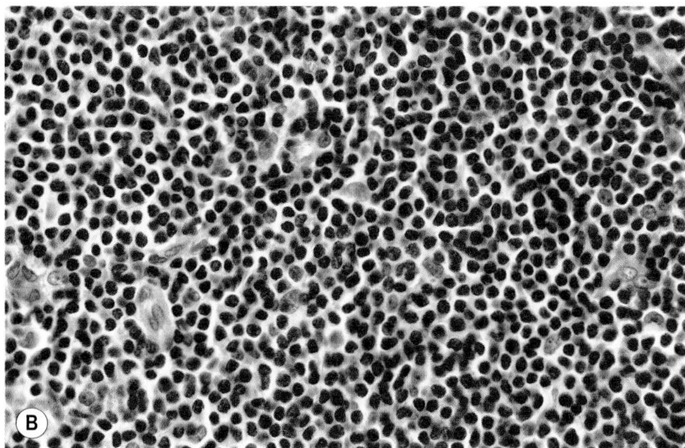

Fig. 23.14 **A,** Marrow biopsy from a 75-year-old male with invasive thymoma and nonclonal T-cell CD3+, CD4+, CD5+, CD8+ lymphocytosis. The markedly hypocellular marrow contains several large aggregates of small lymphocytes as illustrated; the predominant lymphocytes in the marrow specimen had the same phenotype as the blood and were nonclonal by molecular studies. The repeat marrow biopsy following thymectomy showed regression of the lymphocytic aggregates but persistence of hypoplasia. **B**, High magnification of specimen in **A**.

Hypoplastic marrows may be encountered in some newly diagnosed cases of acute leukemia and myelodysplastic syndromes. These can generally be distinguished from true aplastic anemia by the population of blasts and immature granulocytes, in contrast to the mature lymphocytes, plasma cells and tissue mast cells in aplastic/hypoplastic marrows. The use of anti-CD34 is an additional aid in identifying blast cells.[69] However, it is important to note that not all blasts express CD34 and a negative reaction does not exclude a blast population. Concurrent staining for myeloperoxidase should be performed. Cytogenetic studies show distinct clinical outcomes for cytogenetic abnormalities arising in aplastic anemia.[65]

The use of bone marrow transplantation as a therapeutic approach to aplastic anemia in patients who do not respond to immunosuppressive therapy has gained wide acceptance. Evidence of marrow reconstitution usually is present in biopsies obtained 2–3 weeks following transplantation and consists of foci or islands of hematopoietic cells. Sequential marrow biopsies in the subsequent 5- to 10-week period show increasing numbers of erythroid precursors, granulocytes, and megakaryocytes in patients with engraftment. Impending rejection of engraftment may be heralded by a decrease in one myeloid cell line. An association between high mast cell counts in post marrow transplant specimens from patients with aplastic anemia and marrow rejection has been reported, but this has not been a uniform observation.[67,72]

Growth factor therapy, immunosuppressive and antibiotic therapy may alter the morphology of the proliferating engrafted cells, and evidence of dyserythropoiesis and dysgranulopoiesis may be present. At times, agranulocytosis with a 'maturation arrest' of the proliferating neutrophil precursors at the promyelocyte stage may occur as a result of antibiotic or other drug therapy. The use of recombinant granulocyte growth factor may result in a marked shift to immaturity in the developing neutrophils. Selective hypoplasia of myeloid cell lines may occur and is frequently related to specific drug- or virus-related immune mechanisms. Selective erythroid hypoplasia may occur in patients with parvovirus B19 infection and in association with some drugs such as the immunosuppressive drug, mycophenolate mofetil.[54,56,71]

Marrow hyperplasia

Hyperplasia of one or more myeloid cell lines (erythroid, granulocytic–monocytic, megakaryocytic) may be found in several hematopoietic disorders. Several benign hematologic disorders are characterized by hypercellularity; these include cell maturation defects such as the megaloblastic and sideroblastic anemias or disorders with increased rates of destruction or utilization of various cell types in which the hypercellularity is due to compensatory hyperplasia. Hemolytic anemias are generally characterized by a marked erythroid hyperplasia. In immune thrombocytopenia in which there is an increased rate of platelet destruction, the megakaryocytes are normal to increased in number. One of the major problems in evaluation of marrow from patients with benign disorders, such as megaloblastic anemia in which the marrow may be very hypercellular and precursor cells may show striking nuclear changes, is that the proliferating erythroblasts or other myeloid cells may be misinterpreted as a leukemic proliferation; examination of the blood and marrow smears will prevent the possibility of this type of error.

Infrequently, a posterior iliac spine biopsy may contain findings unrelated to the reason for which the biopsy is performed. One such finding is osteitis fibrosa cystica related to secondary hyperparathyroidism in patients with chronic renal disease (Fig. 23.15). It is imperative for pathologists and hematologists to recognize the

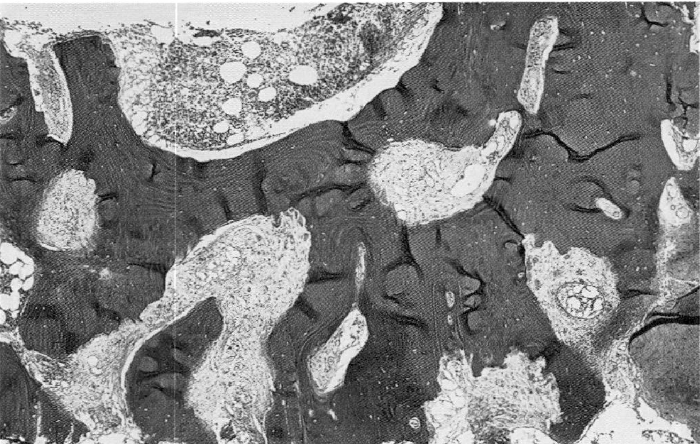

Fig. 23.15 Osteitis fibrosa cystica. Marrow biopsy from posterior iliac spine from a patient with chronic renal disease and secondary hyperparathyroidism. A portion of normal-appearing marrow is at the top. The remainder of this area shows new bone formation, loose marrow fibrosis, and increased osteoblasts and osteoclasts.

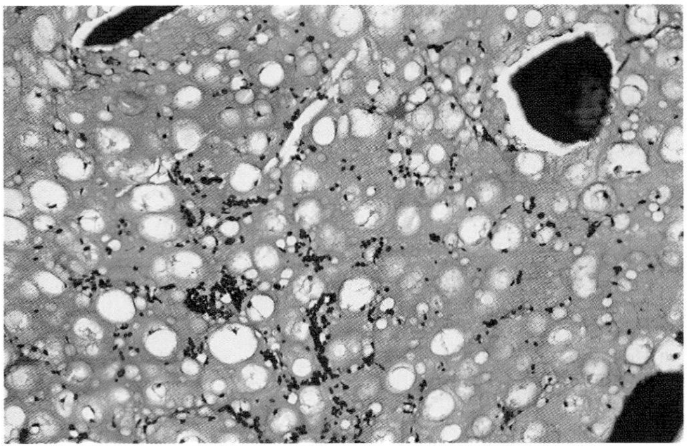

Fig. 23.16 Bone marrow section from a 19-year-old male with anorexia nervosa and severe weight loss showing marked serous degeneration (gelatinous transformation). There is marked reduction in hematopoietic and fat cells with accumulation of an amorphous, eosinophilic substance.

potential for diseases other than hematologic disorders that manifest in marrow biopsies.

Gelatinous transformation (serous degeneration)

Gelatinous (serous) transformation is a degenerative change of the marrow characterized by atrophy of the fat and hematopoietic cells and accumulation of serous fluid in the interstitium.[79,80,82,83] It is an epiphenomenon associated with several disorders which are usually accompanied by extreme malnourishment and weight loss; it is potentially reversible with resolution of the underlying problem and restoration of normal nutritional status. The etiologic bases are somewhat age related: anorexia nervosa, human immunodeficiency virus (HIV) syndrome, and acute febrile illnesses are the most common factors in young individuals; alcoholism and lymphomas in middle age; and carcinomas, lymphomas, and congestive heart failure in older individuals. It may also be observed in the pediatric population.[81,84] The majority of patients are anemic.

The areas of gelatinous transformation in the marrow biopsy may be focal with intervening areas of normal hematopoietic and fat cells, or the entire biopsy may manifest the transformation which appears as a homogeneous lightly eosinophilic appearance in sections stained with hematoxylin and eosin; it is pale pink with periodic acid–Schiff (PAS) and slightly bluish with Giemsa (Fig. 23.16). Bone marrow aspirate smears contain a dense metachromatic, mucoid-appearing material with Giemsa stain.

Osteopetrosis

Osteopetrosis is a rare genetic disorder of osteoclast function and/or development, characterized by impaired bone resorption and increased bone sclerosis.[87,91,92] There are several possible genetic mutations which may result in osteoclast dysfunction or lack of development.[87,88,91] Several classifications have been proposed. Generally two major groups are recognized: autosomal recessive osteopetrosis and autosomal dominant osteopetrosis. A rare sex linked form has also been reported. There is wide variation in the clinical severity of the disease both in the autosomal dominant group (also known as Albers–Schonberg disease, which includes asymptomatic individuals and adults) and the autosomal recessive group. The most severe forms of the disease which occur in young infants are lethal and are usually autosomal recessive.[87] A less severe form of autosomal recessive osteopetrosis is caused by a mutation in the gene encoding CA II (CA 2) resulting in carbonic anhydrase II deficiency; in addition to the osteopetrosis, these patients have renal tubular acidosis and cerebral calcifications. The few X-linked cases have been associated with ectodermal dysplasia, lymphedema, and immune deficiency.[85,87,91,92] The incidence of infantile malignant osteopetrosis is 1 in 300 000 births, except in Costa Rica where it is 3–4 in 100 000 births.

Most cases of osteopetrosis are associated with a failure of osteoclast function resulting in disturbances of intracellular and extracellular pH of the osteoclast resorption compartment which leads to impaired resorption of organic and inorganic bone matrix.[91] In some cases there is a failure of osteoclast development; this autosomal recessive form is associated with a mutation of the *RANKL* gene.[85,87,92] In the severe forms of the disease there is sclerosis of all of the bones. In the less severe forms there is sclerosis of the bones of the skull, pelvis, vertebrae, and phalanges.

The radiographs in osteopetrosis show increased bone density. The increased bone sclerosis results in reduced marrow space and impaired myeloid hematopoiesis, essentially a form of bone marrow failure; this is accompanied by extramedullary hematopoiesis with hepatosplenomegaly and a leukoerythroblastic blood picture. Reduction in the size of the foramina in the skull leads to optic and auditory nerve compression with visual and auditory defects. Although the bones are dense there is increased fragility and propensity for fractures. Dentition problems are also a part of the clinical picture. The only known cure for the infantile malignant form of the disease is allogeneic hematopoietic stem cell transplant (HSCT) which is successful in approximately 50% of cases. Many cases of the autosomal dominant form of osteopetrosis are asymptomatic; the most common clinical manifestation is increased fragility of bone leading to fractures.

Posterior iliac crest biopsy may be performed prior to and following HSCT. The diagnostic features of the disorder include marked thickening of the bone trabeculae and marked reduction in the medullary cavity (Fig. 23.17). There is usually increased connective tissue in the medullary space although this may be difficult to judge because of the overall reduction in the space. The bone

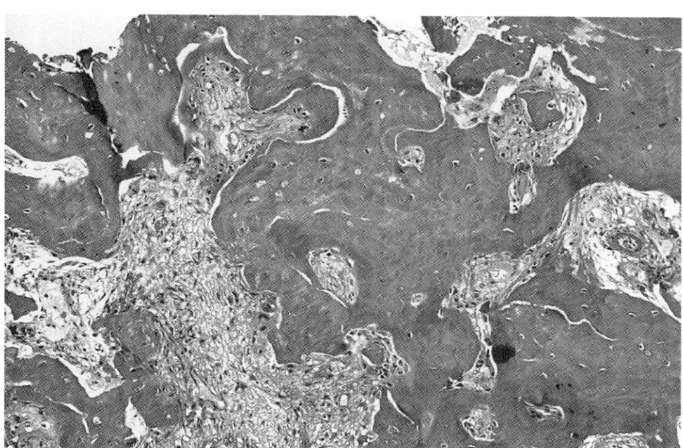

Fig. 23.17 Decalcified posterior iliac spine bone marrow trephine biopsy from an 8-month-old girl with osteopetrosis. Marrow space is markedly reduced as consequence of widely expanded bone structure. Lighter areas in bone structure represent cartilaginous plates. Numerous osteoclasts are present in some areas along the endosteal surface.

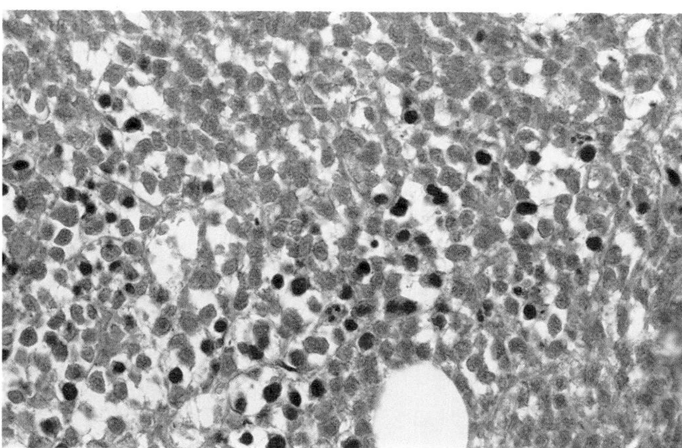

Fig. 23.18 Marrow biopsy from a patient with marrow involvement by Burkitt lymphoma. Most of the lymphoma cells show evidence of karyolysis; a few scattered pyknotic cells are present.

structures contain cartilaginous plates which in nondecalcified specimens show calcium deposition. Osteoclasts are frequently numerous along the endosteal surface. The osteoclasts lack a normal ruffled border.[90] In the small number of cases of failure of osteoclast production associated with a mutation of the *RANKL* gene, there is an absence of osteoclasts.

Following successful allogeneic HSCT there is gradual resorption of the abnormal bone structure, regression of the cartilaginous plates, and expansion of the medullary space with abundant hematopoietic tissue. This is accompanied by regression of splenomegaly and reversal of the leukoerythroblastic blood picture.[86,89]

Bone marrow necrosis

Bone marrow necrosis unrelated to chemotherapy or radiation therapy occurs occasionally in patients with acute leukemia, malignant lymphoma, and metastatic tumor;[93–98] it has also been observed in patients with sickle cell anemia, infectious processes, systemic lupus erythematosus, caisson disease, voluntary starvation, and megaloblastic anemia complicated by infection.[94,95,98] The process may be accompanied by severe and generalized bone pain.

The aspirated marrow specimens from these patients frequently have a gelatinous consistency. The microscopic picture in the trephine section reflects the stage of necrosis; different stages are frequently found in the same biopsy specimen. In the early stages, the nuclei show pyknosis and karyorrhexis, and the cells have a granular appearance; this is followed by karyolysis. In advanced stages, all cell outlines disappear, and the marrow space is replaced by an amorphous, granular, eosinophilic debris. The trabeculae may be involved and show loss of osteocytes. The necrosis may be patchy or involve virtually all of the cells in the biopsy specimen (Fig. 23.18).

Inflammatory disorders

Granulomatous inflammation

The inflammatory diseases that are most readily identified in marrow biopsies are those associated with a granulomatous

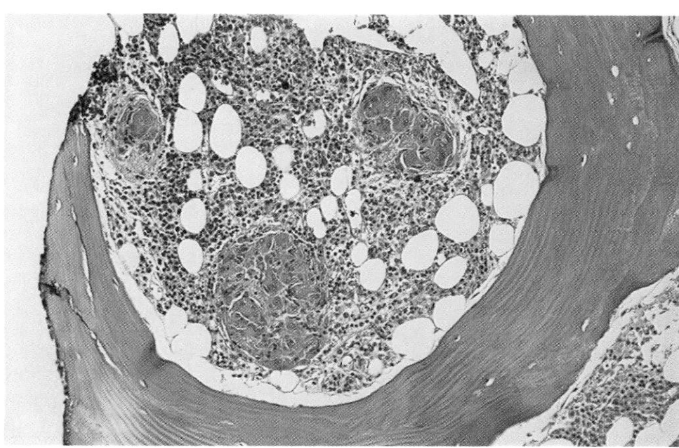

Fig. 23.19 Multiple noncaseating granulomas in marrow biopsy of a 33-year-old male admitted with marked hypercalcemia. Clinical diagnosis of sarcoidosis was established.

reaction; the etiologic bases include fungi, *Mycobacterium tuberculosis*, *Mycobacterium avium-intracellulare*, sarcoidosis, *Mycoplasma pneumoniae*, and viral infections such as Epstein–Barr.[99,102–104,106,109,110,117–122] Marrow granulomas have been observed in patients with cytopenias who are on the antidysrhythmic agent amiodarone.[112,113] Granulomas may also be found in patients with Hodgkin disease and non-Hodgkin lymphomas, with or without marrow involvement by the lymphoma, and in occasional cases of a drug reaction.[100,107,119] Perivascular granulomas may be related to hypersensitivity states. With a combination of studies, including histochemical stains, microbiologic culture, serology, enzyme immunoassay of body fluids, and molecular analysis, the etiologic basis for the granulomas should be established in a very high percentage of cases, approximately 80–90%. In approximately 80% of the cases, the etiologic basis is identified by culture, stain or molecular studies.[106,108,109]

Granulomas in the marrow are similar to those in other sites; the most commonly encountered are composed only of a collection of epithelioid histiocytes that may be surrounded by a rim of well-differentiated lymphocytes. Others may contain large numbers of multinucleated giant cells. The number may range from a single lesion to numerous and confluent granulomas (Figs 23.19–23.21).

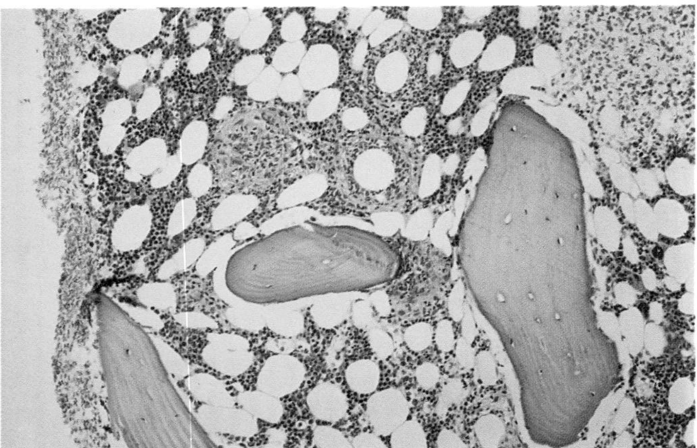

Fig. 23.20 Marrow biopsy with scattered granuloma-like lesions; many of the lesions had a central lumen and were interpreted as 'doughnut' granulomas. No etiologic basis was identified.

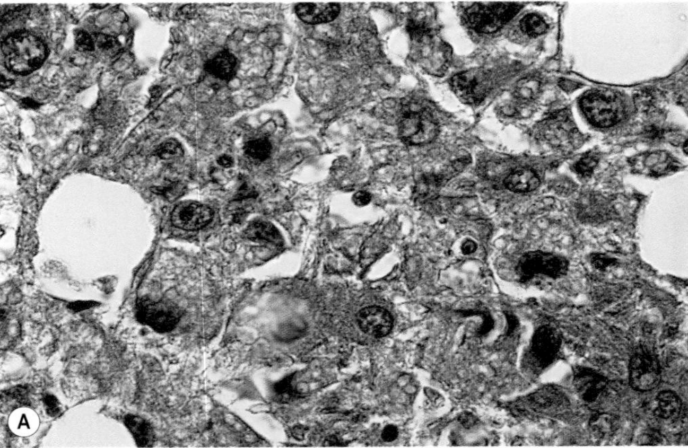

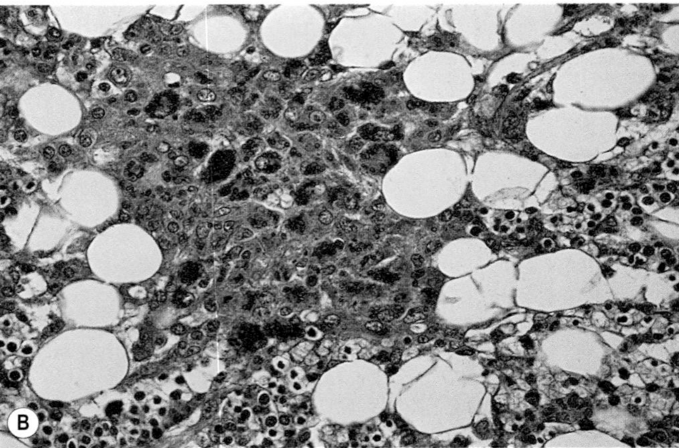

Fig. 23.21 Marrow biopsy from a patient with treated Hodgkin disease. Numerous granulomas contain macrophages with numerous organisms **A** which were intensely PAS positive **B**. Culture studies were positive for histoplasmosis.

An unusual granulomatous lesion referred to as a 'doughnut' or ring granuloma, because of a central clear area or lumen, has been described in the bone marrow of some patients with Q fever.[102,118] The appearance of these lesions, which is similar to those in other organs, such as the liver, varies from what appear to be vascular structures or fat globules encircled by a rim of fibrinoid material, polymorphonuclear leukocytes, and monocytes to a collection of epithelioid histiocytes surrounding a clear space (Fig. 23.20). The vascular-associated granulomas observed in hypersensitivity states are similar in appearance. In addition to Q fever, these lesions may be observed in marrows from patients with a variety of diseases, both neoplastic and non-neoplastic.[117] In one series the most frequent association was with Epstein–Barr virus (EBV) infection.

Cells with prominent intranuclear inclusions may be found in granulomas in the marrow of patients with cytomegalovirus or other viral infection.

Acute parvovirus B19 infection may be associated with marked erythroblast hypoplasia and very immature giant erythroblasts; scattered erythroblasts may contain intranuclear inclusions[124] (Fig. 23.22). Recovery from the erythroid hypoplasia may be marked by a wave of regeneration with a large number of erythroblasts at an early stage of maturation, analogous to the proliferation of promyelocytes and myelocytes that occurs in agranulocytosis. Immunodeficient patients may develop a chronic parvovirus B19 infection; in these cases there may be an erythroid hyperplasia with numerous intranuclear inclusions in the erythroid precursors; the inclusions are most prominent in the basophilic and polychromatic stages of maturation (Fig. 23.22C).[124] The parvovirus B19 relationship to the inclusions may be demonstrated with in situ hybridization studies.

As with other tissues, stains for acid-fast bacilli (AFB) and fungi should be performed in all cases of marrow granulomas. Failure to detect AFB does not exclude infection with *M. tuberculosis*; organisms are found in approximately 25–35% of marrow specimens from patients with documented disease by culture studies.[105,114,115,119] Occasional patients with negative culture studies have AFB stain positive biopsies. The need for culture of a portion of the bone marrow aspirate for AFB and fungi should be anticipated in all patients suspected of having a granulomatous disorder, particularly those with AIDS or patients being investigated for a fever of undetermined etiology.[108,109,121]

Bone marrow biopsies performed on immunosuppressed patients should always be thoroughly examined for opportunistic infections (Figs 23.21, 23.23–23.25). Typical granuloma formation may not be present in the marrows of some patients with disseminated fungal or mycobacterial disease. Marrow biopsies from patients with HIV syndrome may contain scattered macrophages with AFB in the absence of granuloma formation (Fig. 23.25). Uncommonly, *Pneumocystis jirovecii* (formerly *P. carinii*) may be observed in scattered macrophages in sections stained with PAS or methenamine silver (Fig. 23.24). An increased number of macrophages with or without evident phagocytosis is sufficient reason to perform special stains for microorganisms.

The presence of infection-related granulomas in the bone marrow sections may occasionally be accompanied by macrophages containing microorganisms in the Romanowsky-stained bone marrow smears or trephine imprints. The morphology of the organisms in these preparations is usually sufficient to establish a diagnosis.

Lipid granulomas, which have been reported to be the most frequent type of granuloma in bone marrow, are similar to those found in the liver, spleen, and lymph node.[101,116] These granulomas range from 0.2 to 0.8 μm in size and usually are associated with lymphocytic aggregates or sinusoids. The loosely spaced macrophages contain fat vacuoles of varying size. The lesions also contain admixed lymphocytes, plasma cells, and eosinophils; giant cells are found in approximately 5% of cases. Some of these granulomas resemble those found in sarcoidosis.

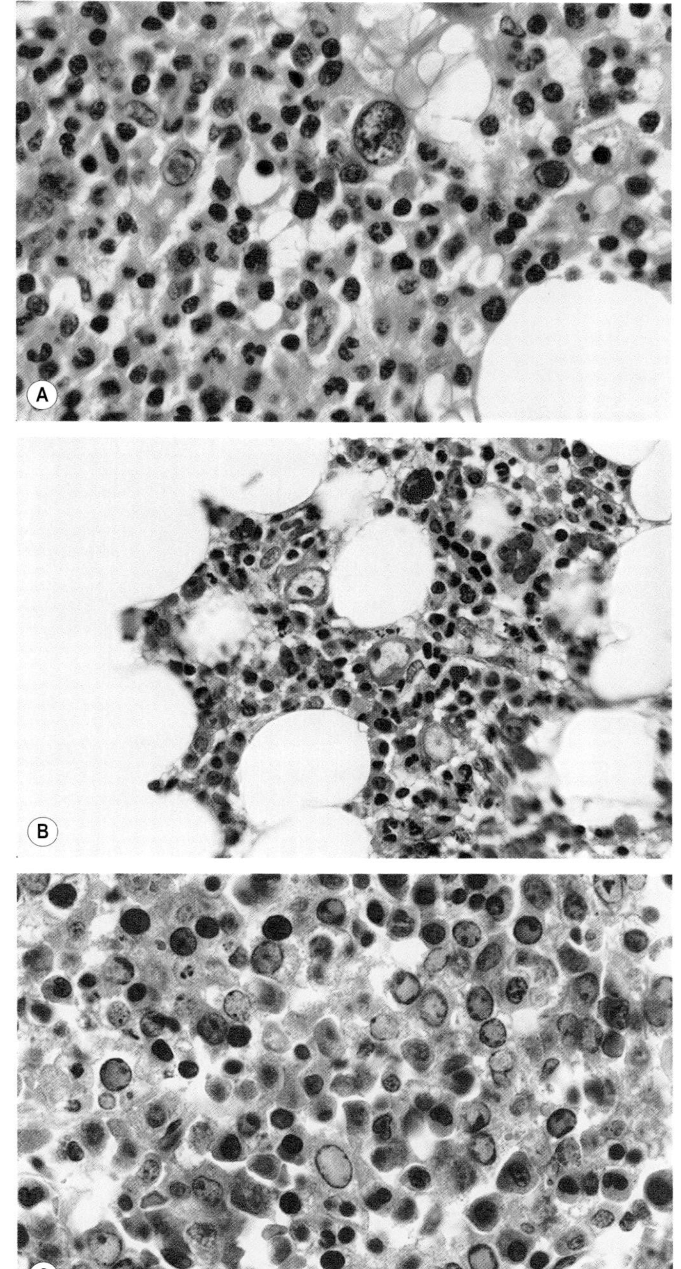

Fig. 23.22 **A**, Pre-transplant marrow biopsy from a 4-year-old child with Hunter syndrome (acid mucopolysaccharides, type II) and erythroid aplasia. Several cells that reacted with antihemoglobin A contained intranuclear inclusions. Giant erythroblasts were present in the marrow smear and biopsy as illustrated and the findings were interpreted as consistent with infection with parvovirus B19. **B**, Marrow biopsy from a 17-year-old being treated for metastatic medulloblastoma; occasional, very large erythroblasts with abundant cytoplasm and very prominent nucleoli were present. These cells and the overall marked erythroid hypoplasia are characteristic findings in parvovirus B19 infection. (Wright–Giemsa) **C**, Marrow biopsy from an adult male with AIDS and concurrent parvovirus B19 infection. There are numerous erythroid precursors at all stages of maturation. Many of the more immature erythroblasts contain prominent intranuclear inclusions.

*(**C** contributed by Dr Robert W McKenna, Dallas, USA)*

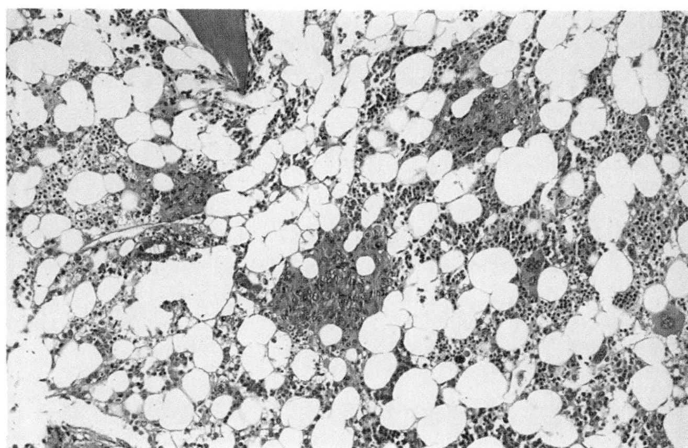

Fig. 23.23 Post-chemotherapy marrow biopsy from patient with marrow involvement by mantle cell lymphoma. Several granulomas containing microorganisms interpreted as cryptococcus are shown. The organisms were positive with Gomori methenamine silver; culture studies were confirmatory of cryptococcus.

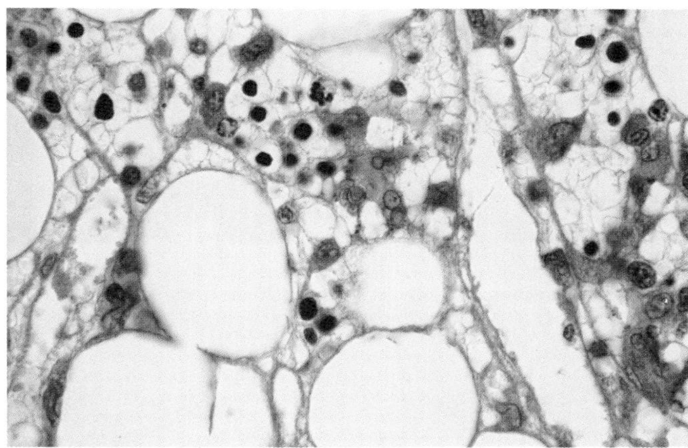

Fig. 23.24 Marrow from a patient with AIDS with scattered *Pneumocystis jirovecii* microorganisms occurring both singly and in small clusters. Microorganisms are not associated with any recognizable tissue response. (PAS)

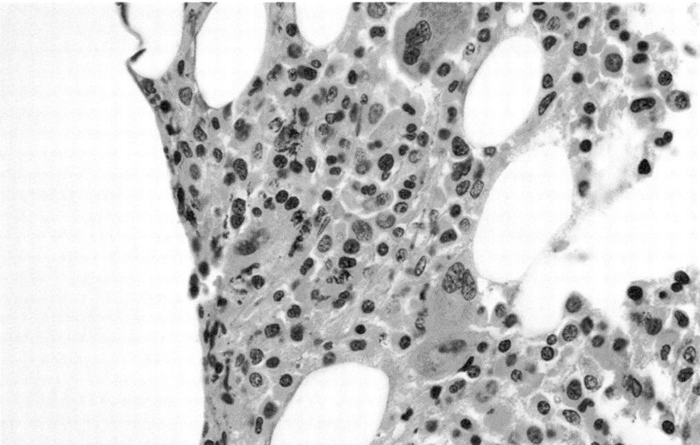

Fig. 23.25 Marrow biopsy from an AIDS patient. No granulomas were identified but numerous macrophages containing acid-fast bacilli were scattered throughout the marrow interstitium, some in perivascular locations as illustrated.

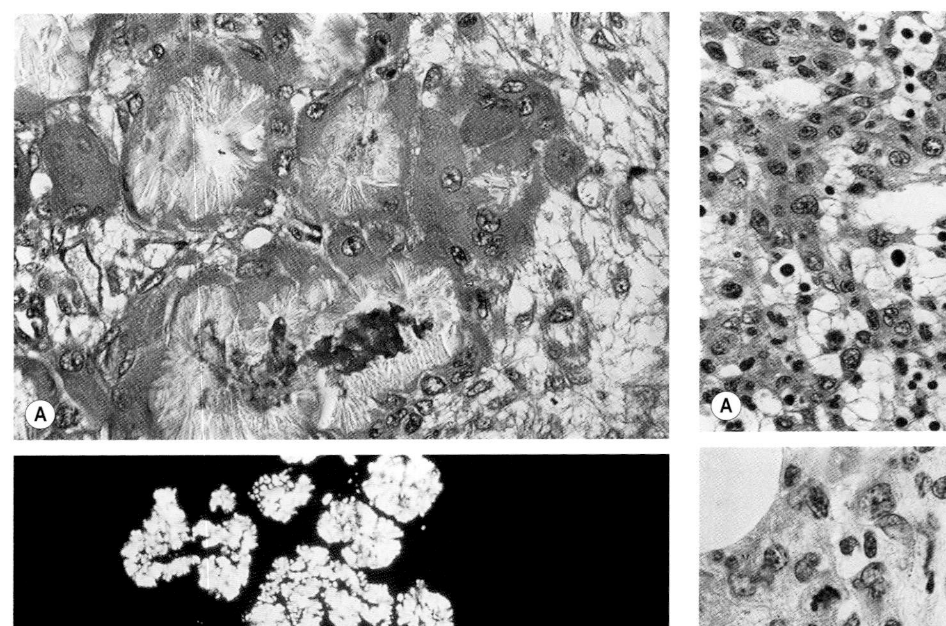

Fig. 23.26 **A**, Section of bone marrow trephine biopsy from a child with primary oxaluria. Calcium oxalate crystals in giant cells form a radial pattern. **B**, Calcium oxalate crystals are doubly refractile in polarized light.

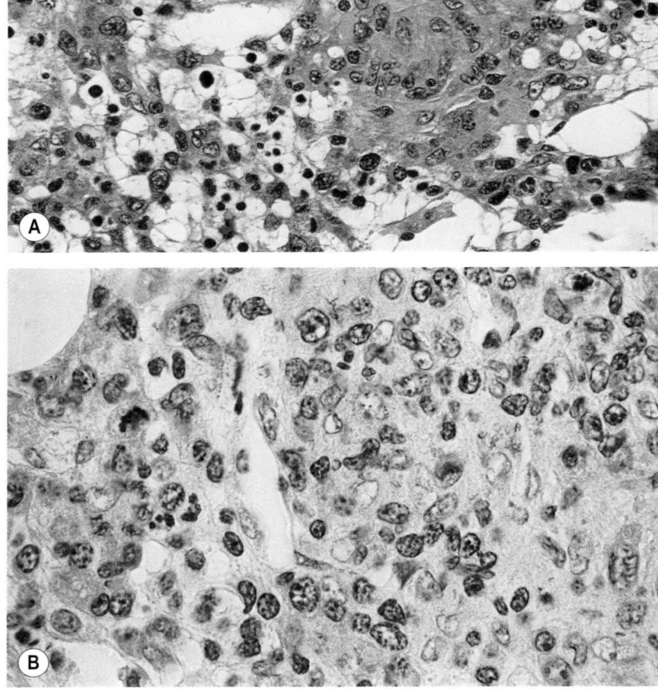

Fig. 23.27 **A**, Marrow biopsy from a patient with AIDS showing granuloma without evident necrosis. **B**, One of the granulomas in **A** showing numerous intracellular acid-fast bacilli. (**B** Fite)

An unusual form of granulomatous reaction can be found in the bone marrow of patients with the genetic disorder of glyoxylate metabolism, primary hyperoxaluria.[111,123] This finding is secondary to the deposition of calcium oxalate crystals. The crystals, which have a slightly yellowish tinge, form a radial pattern, are encircled or engulfed by epithelioid and giant cells, and are doubly refractile with polarized light (Fig. 23.26). Substantial portions of the marrow biopsy may be replaced by these lesions, which are similar to those found in the kidneys and other tissues.

Nonspecific inflammatory reactions

Nonspecific inflammatory alterations may be noted in the marrow from patients with a variety of systemic disorders, including acute infection, malignancy, connective tissue disease, and immune disorders, most notably AIDS. These alterations generally are characterized by changes in both the vascular structures and parenchyma. The terms tumor myelopathy and myelitis have been applied to the nonspecific marrow changes that are observed in a high percentage of patients with malignant lymphoma.[126] These changes include edema of the vessel walls, plasma cell and mast cell proliferations in the adventitia, protein deposits adjacent to the vessels, patchy edema, depressed erythropoiesis, and increased granulopoiesis and megakaryocytopoiesis. Acute necrosis of bone marrow tissue is reported in patients with tuberculosis and typhoid fever.[125]

Human immunodeficiency virus syndrome (HIV, AIDS)

Marrow biopsies from patients with HIV have been generally reported to be hypercellular, although normocellular and hypocellular specimens may be observed; nonspecific findings include marrow damage, increased plasma cells, myelodysplasia, serous degeneration, lymphocytic infiltration, increased reticulin and 'naked' megakaryocytic nuclei.[132,135,138,145–148] The marrow specimen may serve as a vehicle for the rapid diagnosis of febrile illnesses in HIV-infected patients.[135,136,138] Opportunistic organisms including AFB and *P. jirovecii* and fungal organisms may be present, occasionally without granuloma formation (Figs 23.24, 23.25 and 23.27).[129,133,134,140] Immune thrombocytopenia may be observed.[127,137,140]

HIV-infected individuals may develop a persistent parvovirus B19 infection because of ineffective production of IgG parvovirus neutralizing antibodies.[130,131] This may result in chronic anemia and erythroid hyperplasia with all stages of maturation in contrast to the erythroid aplasia which may occur in acute parvovirus B19 infection. The erythroid precursors in these patients may show intranuclear inclusions primarily in the basophilic and polychromatic erythroblasts (Fig. 23.22C).

Negative stains for microorganisms and absence of granulomas do not exclude the possibility of infection by microorganism; a minority of patients with infection by *Mycobacterium avium* complex have demonstrable granulomas or AFB in their marrow biopsies. In addition, although infrequent, marrow with only mild nonspecific changes may contain scattered macrophages with mycobacteria. These macrophages may resemble pseudo-Gaucher cells in hematoxylin–eosin-stained sections. Scattered macrophages containing *P. jirovecii* may also be present in a background of essentially normal appearing or only slightly altered marrow. As a result, it is considered prudent by some observers to routinely stain marrows from HIV patients for AFB and fungi, regardless of the appearance of the marrow with routine stains.

The marrow damage that may be present in HIV patients is characterized principally by a loosely structured, hypocellular interstitium. Areas of fibrinoid necrosis may be present. The changes resemble those found in marrows from patients recovering from chemotherapy with myelotoxic agents and are distinct from serous degeneration, which usually occurs in severely malnourished individuals and which may also be present in marrow biopsies from patients with HIV. Both of these alterations may be accompanied by an increase in plasma cells.

Lymphocytic aggregates of varying size occur in the marrow of a relatively high percentage of patients with HIV.[128,141] These are randomly distributed without any preferential paratrabecular distribution; in some cases the lesions appear to be preferentially perisinusoidal. They are composed primarily of small lymphocytes, some of which may have irregularly shaped nuclei. There are usually associated plasma cells, histiocytes, and increased vascular structures; eosinophils may be increased (Fig. 23.28). Occasional immunoblasts may be noted. This type of lymphocyte proliferation, polymorphous reactive lymphoid hyperplasia, is not unique to patients with HIV and may be observed in marrow biopsies in a wide range of immunologic disorders. Because of the large size and cellular composition, these aggregates may be difficult to distinguish from the lesions of peripheral T-cell lymphoma; the latter lesions are frequently accompanied by numerous epithelioid histiocytes and scattered large transformed cells. In some instances, the distinction between the two processes based on morphologic criteria may not be possible.[141] Peripheral T-cell lymphoma in HIV patients, however, is quite rare, and such a diagnosis should be established with considerable caution and only after review of all pathology specimens.[139] Molecular studies for T-cell receptor rearrangement may be necessary.

Occasionally, marrow specimens from patients with HIV contain benign lymphoid follicles with germinal centers.

In addition to reactive lymphocytic lesions, the marrow biopsies from AIDS patients may exhibit a florid immunocytic reaction. In rare cases, this may be accompanied by a proliferation of immunoblasts and may resemble a neoplastic process because of the degree of replacement of marrow. The use of immunocytochemical reactions with anti-kappa and anti-lambda antibodies can be very useful in demonstrating the polyclonal nature of these lesions. In equivocal cases, immunoglobulin gene rearrangement studies may be necessary for determination of the biology of these processes.

Although it is important to recognize that marrow biopsies from patients with HIV may show a variety of reactive lymphocytic proliferations, it is equally important to appreciate that these patients have an increased incidence of malignant lymphoma, of either non-Hodgkin or Hodgkin type, and the marrow biopsy may be the initial diagnostic specimen.[139,142] The most common HIV-associated lymphomas which may involve the marrow are B-cell lymphomas, including Burkitt lymphoma, diffuse large B-cell lymphoma, and plasmablastic. A single biopsy may contain both reactive lymphocytic lesions and malignant lymphoma. In suspected cases of Hodgkin disease, adherence to established criteria for marrow involvement by Hodgkin disease should be observed.

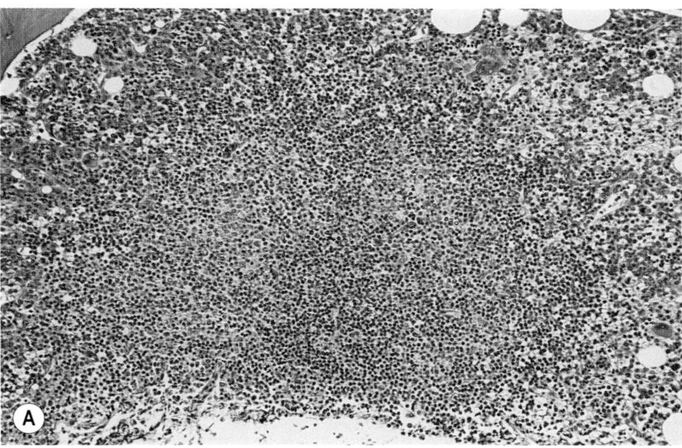

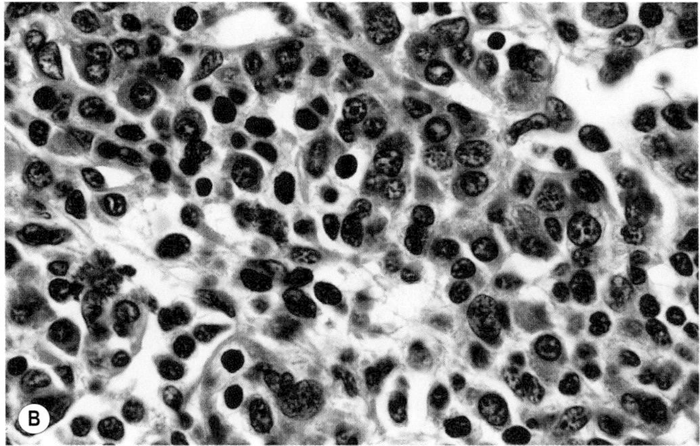

Fig. 23.28 A, One of several lymphocytic–histiocytic aggregates in marrow biopsy from a patient with advanced AIDS. Acid-fast bacilli were also identified in this specimen. **B**, High magnification of specimen in **A** illustrating polycellular characteristics of the lesion.

Patients with HIV who are receiving zidovudine (AZT) may develop evidence of marrow suppression such as anemia and neutropenia. Marrow hypoplasia may be present.[143] Abnormal megakaryocytes with sparse cytoplasm, 'naked' megakaryocyte nuclei, may be numerous; this finding is not specific for AIDS and may be present in other disorders, including the myeloproliferative neoplasms. The incidence of immune thrombocytopenia is increased in individuals with HIV.[144]

Leukemias and related disorders

Acute leukemia

The diagnosis and classification of the acute leukemias are optimally established from examination of Romanowsky-stained blood and bone marrow smears in conjunction with appropriate immunophenotypic, cytogenetic and/or molecular genetic and cytochemical techniques; this approach forms the basis for the 2001 and 2008 World Health Organization (WHO) classifications.[149,153,174,175] Terminology from the French–American–British (FAB) Cooperative Group classification remains in common usage, but this classification system should no longer be used by itself.[158] Chromosome analysis has an important role in the evaluation of cases of acute leukemia, primarily in regard to prognostic significance, and is incorporated into the diagnosis of many categories of acute

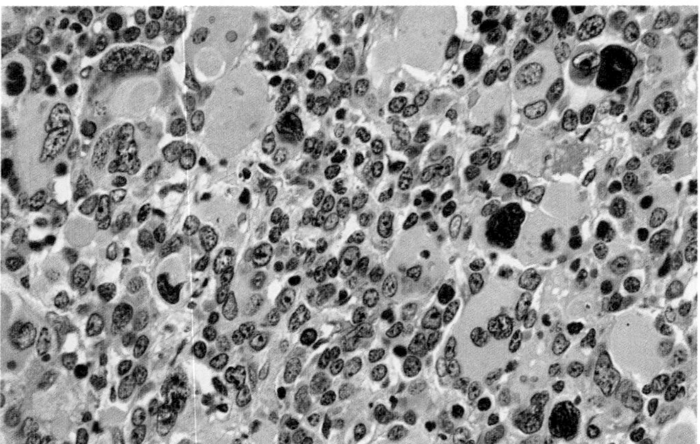

Fig. 23.29 Marrow from a patient with acute megakaryoblastic leukemia (AML-M7). The predominant cell population consists of blasts and numerous megakaryocytes at varying stages of maturation. Mature megakaryocytes have abundant cytoplasm that is uniformly eosinophilic.

leukemia in the 2008 WHO classification.[155,176] The ideal approach to the diagnosis and classification of acute leukemia requires correlation of peripheral blood findings, bone marrow aspirate smear morphology and the bone marrow trephine biopsy.[174] Immunophenotyping and cytogenetic or molecular genetic studies, which are now performed on all cases, are best performed on marrow aspirate material. Although smears and imprint preparations are generally superior to sections in classifying the majority of cases of acute leukemia, there are some types of acute leukemia which are accompanied by fibrosis or with unusual morphologic patterns such as acute megakaryocytic leukemia with an associated t(1;22)(p13;q13) cytogenetic abnormality which occurs in infants in which the bone marrow sections are often more informative than the bone marrow smears (Figs 23.29–23.31). In addition, as noted in the section on immunohistology, the development of antibodies reactive in paraffin-embedded tissue, most notably myeloperoxidase, lysozyme, TdT, and CD34 antibodies, has greatly enhanced the recognition of myeloid leukemia in trephine biopsy sections.[154,166,171]

The 2008 WHO classification of acute leukemia includes general categories of acute myeloid leukemia (AML), precursor lymphoid neoplasms, which include the related acute lymphoblastic leukemias (ALLs) and their corresponding lymphoblastic lymphomas, and acute leukemias of ambiguous lineage. Acute myeloid leukemia (Box 23.1) is further subdivided into AML with recurrent genetic abnormalities, AML with myelodysplasia-related changes, therapy-related myeloid neoplasms, myeloid proliferations of Down syndrome and AML, not otherwise specified.[150–152,157,173] AML with myelodysplasia-related changes may be diagnosed by the presence of: (1) a history of prior myelodysplasia; (2) presence of a myelodysplasia-related cytogenetic abnormality (Table 23.1); or (3) multilineage dysplasia defined as dysplasia in 50% or more of two nonblast cell lines; and the absence of prior cytotoxic chemotherapy for an unrelated disease and absence of one of the cytogenetic abnormalities of AML with recurrent genetic abnormalities. All cases of AML are defined by the presence of 20% or more blast cells in the peripheral blood, except for cases of AML with t(8;21)(q22;q22), AML with inv(16)(p13.1q22) or t(16;16)(p13.1;q22) and acute promyelocytic leukemia with t(15;17)(q22;q12) in which a diagnosis of AML can be made with less than 20% peripheral blood and bone marrow blast cells.

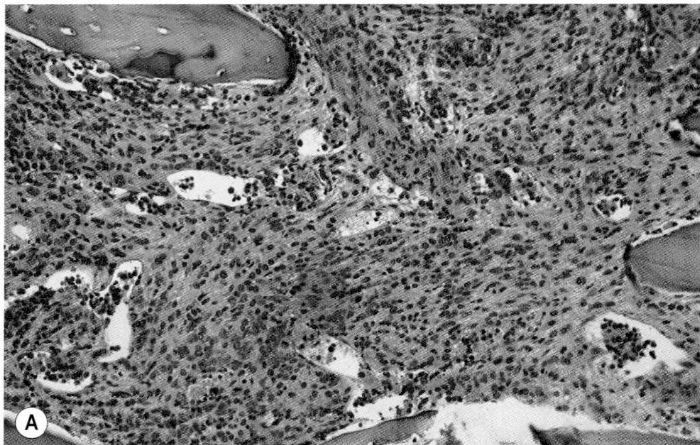

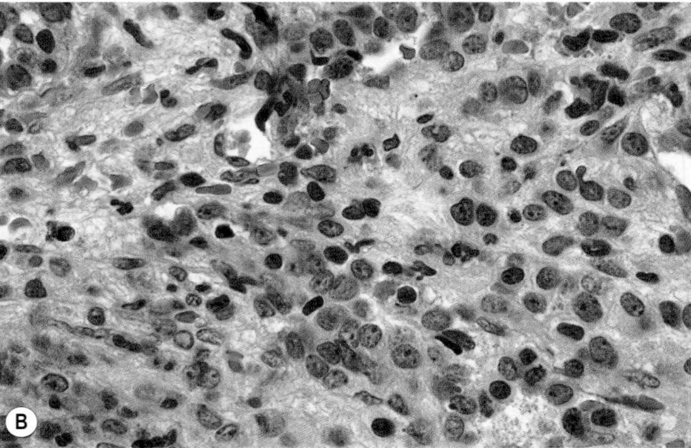

Fig. 23.30 **A**, Marrow biopsy from a 14-month-old child with acute megakaryoblastic leukemia with an associated t(1;22)(p13;q13) cytogenetic abnormality. The blasts frequently have a spindle shape and sometimes form intertwining bundles resembling metastatic tumor. **B**, High magnification of the specimen in **A** showing undifferentiated blasts.

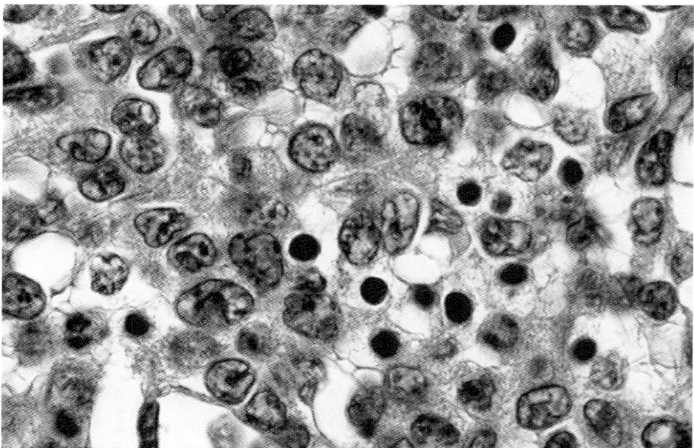

Fig. 23.31 Bone marrow biopsy from an adult female with a mediastinal mass and partial marrow involvement by precursor T-lymphoblastic lymphoma. In this area the lymphoblasts are the predominant cells; some of the lymphoblasts have convoluted nuclei. Scattered erythroid precursors are present.

Box 23.1 2008 WHO classification of acute myeloid leukemia[150–152]

AML with recurrent genetic abnormalities

AML with t(8;21)(q22;q22); *RUNX1-RUNX1T1*
AML with inv(16)(p13.1q22) or t(16;16)(p13;q22); *CBFB-MYH11*
Acute promyelocytic leukemia with t(15;17)(q22;q11.2); *PML-RARA*
AML with t(9;11)(p22;q23); *MLLT3-MLL*
AML with t(6;9)(p23;q34); *DEK-NUP214*
AML with inv(3)(q21q26.2) or t(3;3)(q21;q26.2); *RPN1-EVI1*
AML (megakaryoblastic) with t(1;22)(p13;q13); *RBM15-MKL1*
Provisional entity: AML with mutated *NPM1*
Provisional entity: AML with mutated *CEBPA*

AML with myelodysplasia-related changes

Therapy-related AML, myelodysplastic syndromes and myelodysplastic/myeloproliferative neoplasms

AML not otherwise categorized

AML minimally differentiated
AML without maturation
AML with maturation
Acute myelomonocytic leukemia
Acute monoblastic and monocytic leukemia
Acute erythroid/myeloid leukemia and pure erythroid leukemia
Acute megakaryocytic leukemia
Acute basophilic leukemia
Acute panmyelosis with myelofibrosis

Myeloid proliferations of Down syndrome

Table 23.1 Cytogenetic abnormalities sufficient for a diagnosis of AML with myelodysplasia-related changes when bone marrow or blood blasts are 20% or more[151]

COMPLEX KARYOTYPE (THREE OR MORE UNRELATED ABNORMALITIES)	
Unbalanced abnormalities	**Balanced abnormalities**
−7/del(7q)	t(11;16)(q23;p13.3)[a]
−5/del(5q)	t(3;21)(q26.2;q22.1)[a]
i(17q)/t(17p)	t(1;3)(p26.3;q21.1)
−13/del(13q)	t(2;11)(p21;q23)
del(11q)	t(5;12)(q33;p12)
del(12p)/t(12p)	t(5;7)(q33;q11.2)
del(9q)	t(5;17)(q33;p13)
idic(X)(q13)	t(5;10)(q33;q21)
	t(3;5)(q25;q34)

[a]Must exclude therapy-related disease.

Acute lymphoblastic leukemia (Box 23.2) is subdivided into precursor B- and T-cell types with precursor B-ALL further subgrouped into cases with recurrent genetic abnormalities and B-ALL, not otherwise specified.[161–163] Acute lymphoblastic leukemia is biologically and morphologically identical to lymphoblastic lymphoma

Box 23.2 2008 WHO classification of acute lymphoblastic leukemia[161–163]

- B Lymphoblastic leukemia/lymphoma, not otherwise specified
- B Lymphoblastic leukemia/lymphoma with recurrent genetic abnormalities
  - B Lymphoblastic leukemia/lymphoma with t(9;22)(q34;q11.2); *BCR/ABL1*
  - B Lymphoblastic leukemia/lymphoma with t(v;11q23); *MLL* rearranged
  - B Lymphoblastic leukemia/lymphoma with t(12;21)(p13;q22); *TEL-AML1* (*ETV6-RUNX1*)
  - B Lymphoblastic leukemia/lymphoma with hyperdiploidy
  - B Lymphoblastic leukemia/lymphoma with hypodiploidy (hypodiploid ALL)
  - B Lymphoblastic leukemia/lymphoma with t(5;14)(q31;q32); *IL3-IGH*
  - B Lymphoblastic leukemia/lymphoma with t(1;19)(q23;p13.3); *E2A-PBX1* (*TCF3-PBX1*)
- T Lymphoblastic leukemia/lymphoma

although the clinical presentation varies between the two. For this reason, the two are combined in the WHO classification. While most cases of acute lymphoblastic leukemia are of precursor B lineage, lymphoblastic lymphoma is of precursor T-cell origin in approximately 80% of cases and B-cell precursor type in 20%. Precursor T-cell acute lymphoblastic leukemia has a high incidence of mediastinal mass, occurs in young adults, more frequently in males, and has a predilection for early blood and marrow involvement[156,161–163,168] (see Fig. 23.31). Lymphoblasts of both precursor B or T lineage are TdT positive. The blood and marrow may be involved at the time of initial diagnosis and the designation of a case as lymphoblastic lymphoma or acute lymphoblastic leukemia is arbitrary. The presence of extramedullary tumor masses and evidence of sparing of marrow function as indicated by a normal platelet count, hemoglobin levels greater than 10 g/dL, and a normal number of neutrophils in the blood are more compatible with a diagnosis of lymphoma with marrow involvement as opposed to acute lymphoblastic leukemia. The Children's Cancer Study Group proposed distinguishing leukemia from lymphoblastic lymphoma on the basis of the percentage of lymphoblasts in the marrow.[170] If there are less than 25% lymphoblasts, the case is classified as lymphoma; if there are more than 25% lymphoblasts, the case is classified as leukemia. In the cases of lymphoma, there may be substantial residual normal marrow with the lymphoma cells diffusely scattered in the interstitium. The therapeutic approach in these two fundamentally similar processes is the same. B lymphoblastic lymphoma appears to have lower propensity for blood and marrow involvement than T lymphoblastic lymphoma.[168]

The acute leukemias of ambiguous lineage (Box 23.3) are divided into acute undifferentiated leukemia and mixed phenotype acute leukemias.[160] The latter group also includes specific genetic subtypes.

In the majority of cases of acute leukemia, both myeloid and lymphoblastic, in children and adults, the marrow is markedly hypercellular because of the proliferation of leukemic cells, with replacement of normal hematopoietic cells. In a small minority of patients, particularly older individuals, acute myeloid leukemia and, rarely, acute lymphoblastic leukemia may present with a hypocellular marrow (i.e., hypoplastic or hypocellular acute leukemia).[159,164,167] The marrow biopsies in these patients may, on low magnification, suggest the diagnosis of aplastic anemia (Fig. 23.32).

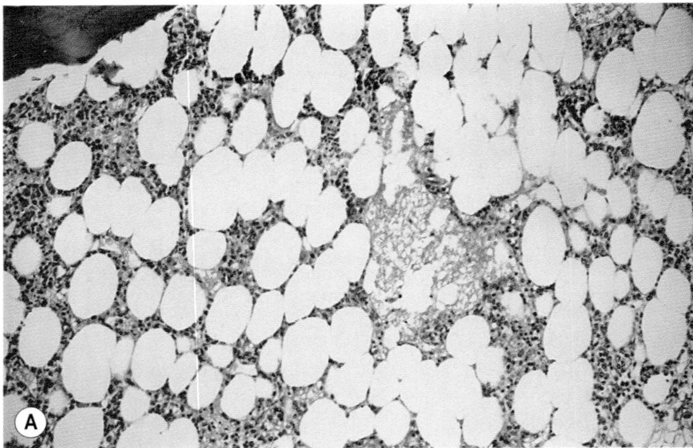

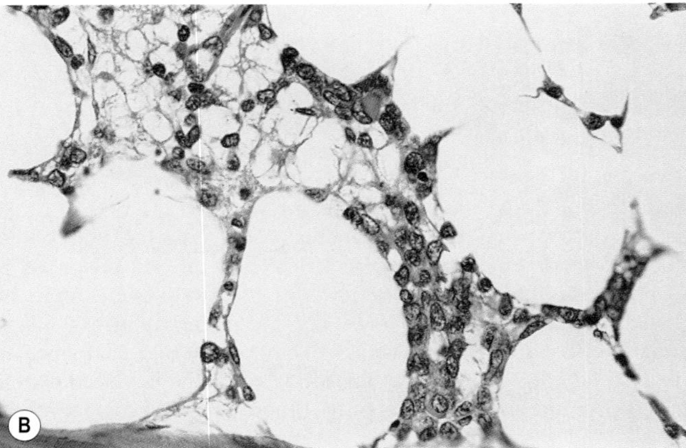

Fig. 23.32 **A**, Marrow section from a 67-year-old male with acute myeloid leukemia with markedly hypocellular marrow. **B**, Higher magnification of the same specimen showing numerous blast cells in the interstitium.

Box 23.3 2008 WHO classification of acute leukemias of ambiguous lineage[160]

- Acute undifferentiated leukemia
- Mixed phenotype acute leukemia with t(9;22)(q34;q11.2); *BCR/ABL1*
- Mixed phenotype acute leukemia with t(v;11q23); *MLL* rearranged
- Mixed phenotype acute leukemia, B/myeloid, not otherwise specified
- Mixed phenotype acute leukemia, T/myeloid, not otherwise specified

In contrast to aplastic anemia, in which the residual cells are well-differentiated lymphocytes and plasma cells, the cell population in the interstitium is principally blasts; some normal cells may be present but are markedly reduced. The diagnosis is confirmed by examination of blood and bone marrow smears and the use of appropriate immunocytochemical reactions, particularly anti-myeloperoxidase, anti-lysozyme, anti-CD117 (*KIT*) and anti-CD34. In rare instances, acute lymphoblastic leukemia in children is preceded by an aplastic or hypocellular phase.

Myelofibrosis with a slight-to-moderate increase in reticulin fibers may be present in the initial or late stages of acute leukemia in a minority of cases; it may occur in both acute lymphoblastic and acute myeloid leukemia.[169] The presence of myelofibrosis in acute leukemia may result in difficult and inadequate marrow aspiration and an erroneous diagnosis of aplastic anemia if trephine biopsy sections are not available. This emphasizes the importance of obtaining adequate marrow biopsies. The long-held view that difficult aspirations in acute leukemia are caused by 'packed' marrows has little basis in fact. The vast majority of hypercellular marrows in acute leukemia are readily aspirated. If aspiration is difficult, it is probably a result of poor biopsy technique or an increase in reticulin fibers.

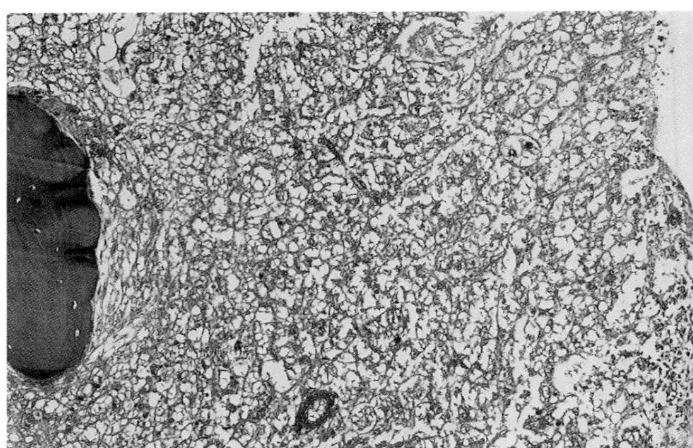

Fig. 23.33 Marrow biopsy 14 days after institution of therapy with daunorubicin and cytosine arabinoside for acute myeloid leukemia. Marrow is markedly hypocellular with dilated sinuses. Interstitial areas contain lightly eosinophilic, proteinaceous debris that represents residue of leukemic cell necrosis.

The trephine biopsy provides the only accurate assessment of marrow cellularity and is of considerable importance in monitoring changes following treatment for leukemia. The rapidity of development and degree of necrosis and aplasia following the institution of therapy will vary with the different chemotherapeutic agents or combination of agents used. In general, the sequence of histopathologic events is marked initially by nuclear karyorrhexis followed by karyolysis; the cells then disintegrate into relatively uniform granular, eosinophilic debris. Subsequently the marrow shows a somewhat irregular, loosely structured appearance with scattered fat cells, vessels, stromal elements, and distended sinusoids (Fig. 23.33). Regeneration of fat cells is followed by regeneration of normal hematopoietic cells in the successfully treated patient. The erythroid cells are usually the first to recover and frequently manifest dyserythropoietic changes as the result of chemotherapeutic drugs.[165] The regeneration of the erythroid cells is followed in sequence by that of the granulocytes and megakaryocytes. This sequence may be altered with different drug regimens and the use of recombinant growth factors. The marrow from patients receiving recombinant granulocyte growth factor may show an early marked increase in neutrophil promyelocytes and myelocytes. In some patients, particularly in the pediatric age group, the post-chemotherapy marrow may contain numerous hematogones which may resemble lymphoblasts. These can usually be distinguished from lymphoblasts by careful morphologic assessment and immunophenotypic characteristics.[172] The bone marrow biopsy can be particularly useful in this differential diagnosis, as leukemic blasts tend to cluster on biopsy sections, while hematogones represent a spectrum of B lymphocyte maturation dispersed throughout the biopsy. The infiltration pattern can be further assessed by immunohistochemical

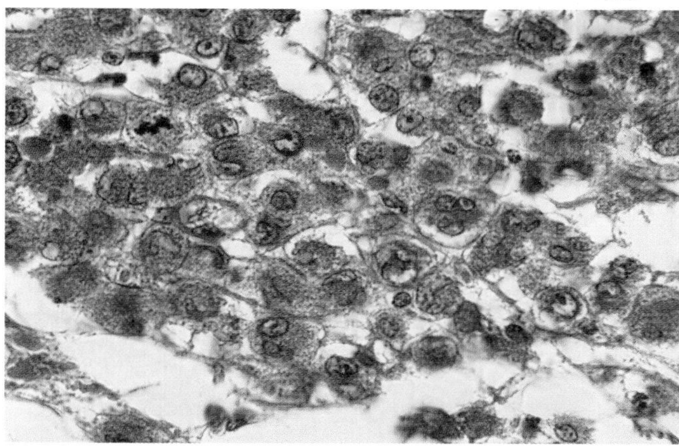

Fig. 23.34 Marrow biopsy from an adult woman with acute promyelocytic leukemia following two courses of chemotherapy which did not include all-*trans*-retinoic acid. Large areas of marrow are replaced by leukemic promyelocytes.

markers for CD34 or TdT to identify the clusters of leukemia cells versus the more scattered B cell progenitors (hematogones).

As noted, the course of events described in the preceding discussion is characteristic of effective therapy. In those patients in whom there has been partial or no response to treatment, the marrow will show varying numbers of leukemic cells. In the totally nonresponsive patient, the findings are essentially those of the pretreatment specimen; scattered isolated areas of necrosis may be present. In a partial response, the areas of residual leukemia will be intermixed with necrotic or regenerating normal marrow cells. In some patients, the areas of residual leukemia may be very small and difficult to distinguish from foci of regenerating normal cells, particularly early erythroblasts and promyelocytes. Careful comparison of suspicious foci with the cytologic pattern in the initial diagnostic biopsy should always be performed. Distinguishing foci of normal regenerative promyelocytes from the foci of leukemic promyelocytes in patients being treated for acute promyelocytic leukemia may be particularly troublesome. Normal promyelocyte regeneration is usually accentuated along the endosteal surface of the bone trabeculae and in perivascular locations. Acute promyelocytic leukemia in marrows with partial response may manifest as large or small focal lesions unrelated to bone trabeculae or vascular structures (Fig. 23.34). The cytoplasm of the leukemic promyelocyte may be more abundant than in normal promyelocytes.

In addition to assessment of the effects of chemotherapy, post-chemotherapy biopsy specimens should always be carefully evaluated for the presence of granulomas or other evidence of infection. In some instances, a focus of microorganisms may be present only as an area of nonspecific necrosis with a few histiocytes. These foci may be very difficult to recognize in a marrow biopsy showing cell necrosis as a result of chemotherapy. Any suspicious lesion should be studied with special stains. Proliferation of histiocytes, with and without hemophagocytosis, may be prominent in infected patients. The histiocytes are widely dispersed throughout the interstitium and in the sinusoids; in some patients this may be a very prominent feature.

Patients being monitored for the effects of chemotherapy will usually have sequential marrow biopsies at relatively short time intervals. If a specimen is from the area of a recent biopsy procedure, there may be evidence of granulation tissue and new bone formation (see Fig. 23.1). The biopsy repair site will usually be relatively well demarcated from the remainder of the biopsy specimen but at times may lead to difficulties in interpretation.

Acute panmyelosis with myelofibrosis (acute myelofibrosis)

Although primary myelofibrosis (chronic idiopathic myelofibrosis or agnogenic myeloid metaplasia) is usually a chronic disorder, an uncommon entity that is characterized by idiopathic marrow fibrosis and a rapid clinical course has been recognized. Several terms have been used for this process, including acute panmyelosis with myelofibrosis, acute myelofibrosis, acute myelosclerosis, malignant myelosclerosis, and acute myelodysplasia with myelofibrosis.[178–181] This entity is distinguished from chronic idiopathic myelofibrosis by abrupt onset, little or no red cell poikilocytosis, absence of or minimal splenomegaly, and a rapid clinical course.[177,182,183] Cases with features of acute panmyelosis with myelofibrosis have also been reported as part of a spectrum of therapy-related leukemia occurring in patients previously treated with chemotherapy, primarily alkylating agents, and/or radiotherapy for a variety of tumors and occasionally benign conditions,[181] and such cases would be classified as therapy-related disease in the 2008 WHO classification.

In acute panmyelosis with myelofibrosis there is hyperplasia of all three myeloid cell lines: erythroblasts, granulocytes, and megakaryocytes (Fig. 23.35). The megakaryocytes, because of their size, developmental characteristics, and tendency to occur in clusters, may be particularly conspicuous; there may be considerable size variation from very small megakaryocytes with nonlobulated nuclei to large cells with bizarre nuclear shapes. The nuclear chromatin is usually finely stippled in contrast to the megakaryocytes in primary myelofibrosis in which the chromatin is more dense. Staining with antibodies for von Willebrand factor (factor VIII-related antigen), CD41, CD61 and CD31 and with PAS may be particularly useful in accentuating the megakaryocytes (Fig. 23.35C). The granulocytes and erythroid cells in acute myelofibrosis are predominantly immature, but some evidence of maturation is usually present. The more immature cells may be difficult to categorize in routinely stained sections. Giemsa-stained sections and sections immunocytochemically reactive with antibodies to myeloperoxidase, CD68 (KP-1 and PGM-1), lysozyme, and hemoglobin or glycophorin A may be of considerable help in distinguishing granulocytes, monocyte precursors, and erythroblasts (see Figs 23.3–23.6). The reticulin stain in acute panmyelosis with myelofibrosis shows an increase in reticulin fibers; the fibers may be dense and confluent (Fig. 23.36). Stains for collagen are usually negative, although an occasional case may show collagen fibrosis.

The relationship of acute panmyelosis with myelofibrosis to acute megakaryoblastic leukemia has been the subject of considerable discussion, and some observers have equated the two disorders. Some cases of acute megakaryoblastic leukemia present with myelofibrosis; however, this is not an invariant finding, and myelofibrosis is not a feature of all cases of acute megakaryoblastic leukemia. In contrast to acute megakaryoblastic leukemia, acute panmyelosis with myelofibrosis is a panmyeloid disorder, and cases with similar features but over 20% marrow megakaryoblasts should be considered as acute megakaryoblastic leukemia. Acute panmyelosis with myelofibrosis is probably a type of myelodysplasia-related acute myeloid leukemia in which myelofibrosis is a prominent feature and cases that meet criteria for acute myeloid leukemia with myelodysplasia-related changes should be diagnosed as such.

Acute myelofibrosis is distinguished from other types of acute myeloid leukemia presenting with marrow fibrosis by the

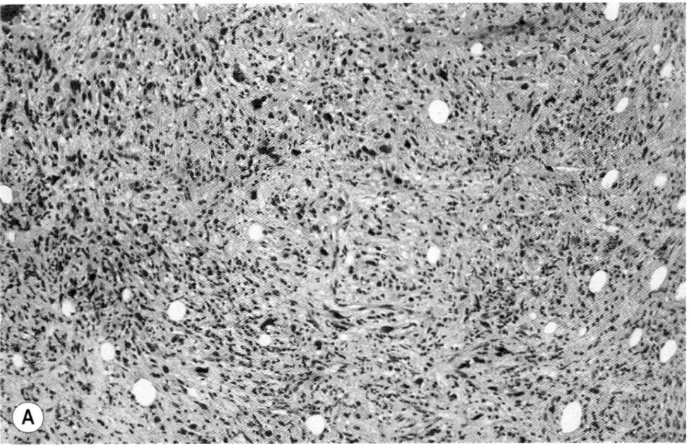

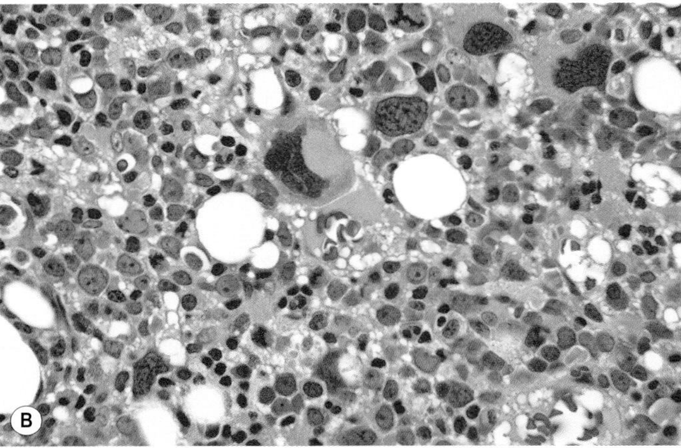

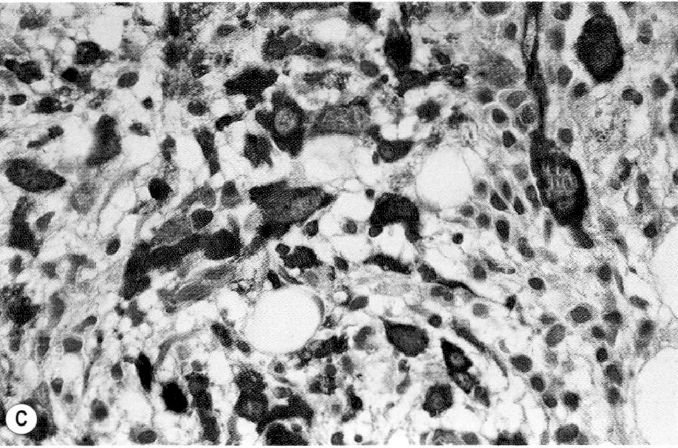

Fig. 23.35 **A**, Bone marrow biopsy from an adult male with acute panmyelosis with myelofibrosis. Marrow is markedly hypercellular as a result of panmyeloid hyperplasia. Megakaryocytes are numerous and vary markedly in size. **B**, High magnification of marrow biopsy from patient with acute panmyelosis with myelofibrosis. There is an increased number of blastic-appearing cells and markedly dysplastic megakaryocytes. **C**, High magnification of the specimen in **A** reacted with antibody to von Willebrand factor (factor VIII-related antigen). (**C**, Immunoperoxidase)

*(**B** contributed by Dr Attillio Orazi, Indianapolis, USA)*

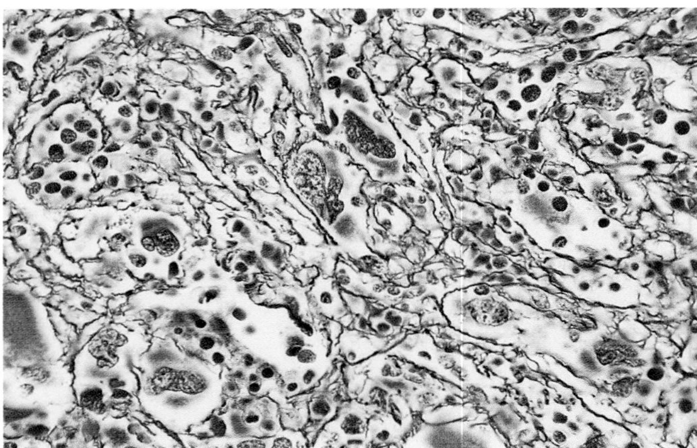

Fig. 23.36 Reticulin stain of biopsy from a case of acute panmyelosis with myelofibrosis showing a moderate to marked increase in coarse reticulin fibers. (Wilder reticulin stain)

predominance of one cell line in most cases of acute leukemia and the essentially panmyeloid proliferation in acute myelofibrosis. This distinction between these entities, however, may not be possible in all instances and the therapeutic importance of the distinction is not completely clear.

Myeloid sarcoma

Myeloid sarcoma (granulocytic sarcoma; extramedullary myeloid tumor) is an unusual variant of myeloid malignancy in which there is an extramedullary tumor mass composed of myeloblasts, with or without mature neutrophils.[188,191–194,196,197,199–201] The tumor may occur as an isolated finding or may be associated with acute myeloid leukemia, chronic myelogenous leukemia, primary myelofibrosis, hypereosinophilic syndrome, and polycythemia vera.[184,185,187,194] An association of myeloid sarcoma and acute myeloid leukemia with the t(8;21) chromosome abnormality has been reported,[199] and appears to be more common in children. These tumors have also been associated with acute myeloid leukemia with abnormalities of chromosome 16. In earlier literature, the term chloroma was used for these lesions because of the green appearance of the freshly cut surface of the tumor. The green color, which is due to the presence of peroxidase in the leukemic cells, is not present in all tumors of this type, and the less specific designation of myeloid sarcoma is preferred. Although tumors of monocytes have not previously been classified with the myeloid sarcomas, they represent a similar process with a similar predilection to leukemic evolution, primarily acute monoblastic leukemia,[190,195] and are now considered in the spectrum of myeloid sarcoma if they create a tumor mass.[197]

The myeloid sarcomas are more frequent in children than adults and are most commonly associated with the subperiosteal bone structures; the most common sites are the skull, paranasal sinuses, sternum, ribs, vertebrae, and pelvis; lymph nodes and skin are also relatively frequently involved. Orbital masses leading to proptosis and spinal canal lesions resulting in neurologic manifestations are two of the clinical presentations associated with these tumors (Fig. 23.37). A high incidence of myeloid sarcomas involving the orbit has been reported in Turkish children with acute myelomonocytic leukemia.[186] Myeloid sarcomas may present as a mediastinal mass and clinically resemble a mediastinal lymphoma.[185]

A myeloid sarcoma may occur simultaneously with a typical blood and bone marrow pattern of acute myeloid leukemia or other

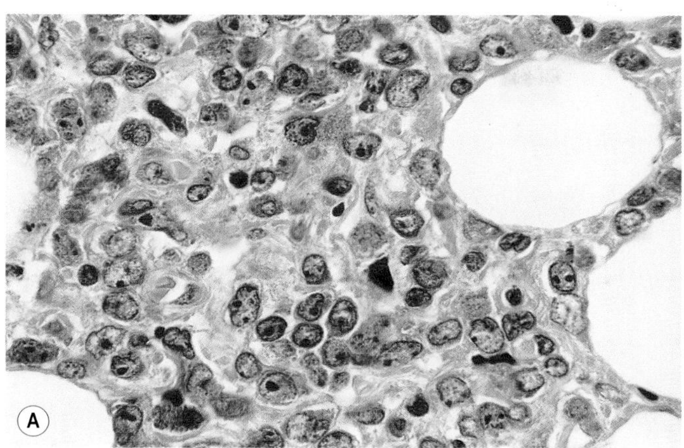

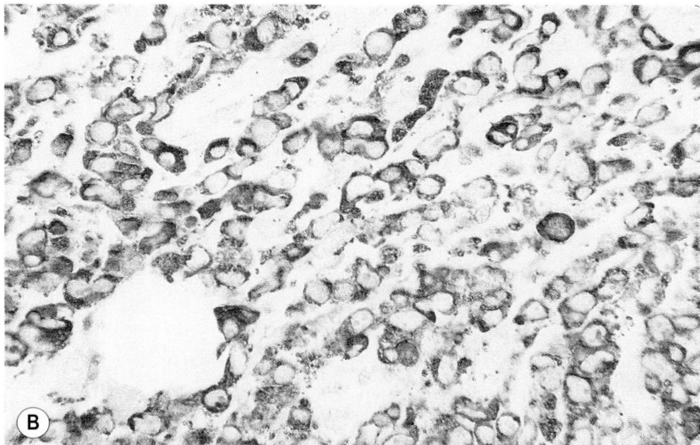

Fig. 23.37 A, Biopsy of orbital myeloid sarcoma from a 6-year-old child who presented with bilateral proptosis. Numerous blasts are present. Cytogenetic studies of this lesion showed t(8;21)(q22;q22) chromosome abnormality. Blood and marrow smears showed acute myeloblastic leukemia with maturation. **B**, The same specimen reacted with antibody to myeloperoxidase. Virtually all blasts are positive. (**B**, Immunoperoxidase)

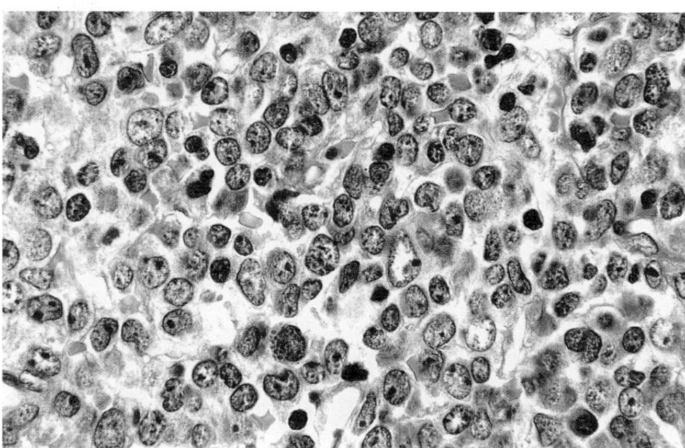

Fig. 23.38 Biopsy of a myeloid sarcoma from subcutaneous tissue of the chest wall of a 49-year-old man. The tumor is composed of poorly differentiated blast cells interpreted as myeloid sarcoma. There is essentially no evidence of differentiation. Blood and marrow showed no evidence of leukemia.

type of myeloproliferative disorder or may antedate leukemia by many months or rarely years.[192] It may be the first evidence of relapse in a patient with acute myeloid leukemia on maintenance chemotherapy and may be the only evidence of recurrence. These tumors may also represent the initial manifestation of a blast crisis of chronic myelogenous leukemia, and an isolated tumor mass or enlarged lymph node in a patient with chronic myelogenous leukemia should be evaluated for this possibility, including cytogenetic studies for the Philadelphia chromosome or molecular studies for evidence of the *BCR/ABL1* fusion gene.[187,194]

Histologically, the tumor is composed of a relatively uniform population of immature cells and may be misdiagnosed as an aggressive malignant lymphoma; this is particularly a problem with those lesions comprised predominantly of blasts. Occasionally, the presence of immature eosinophils and maturing neutrophils may indicate the true nature of the lesion. Attempts at histopathologic classification have generally resulted in three levels of differentiation: blastic, immature, and differentiated.[192,194] The blastic type is composed primarily of myeloblasts with little evidence of maturation to the promyelocyte stage (Fig. 23.38). The myeloblasts have a slight to moderate rim of basophilic cytoplasm, fine nuclear chromatin, and two to four nucleoli. Eosinophil myelocytes are not usually found with this degree of maturation. The immature type with an intermediate degree of differentiation contains principally myeloblasts and promyelocytes; eosinophil myelocytes are usually present. The differentiated type primarily consists of promyelocytes and later stages of maturation. Eosinophil myelocytes are most abundant in this type. Immunocytochemistry using antibodies to myeloperoxidase, lysozyme, CD68 (PG-M1), CD34 and CD117 (*KIT*) are very useful in identification[198] (Fig. 23.37B). The naphthol ASD chloroacetate esterase reaction, which is positive only in neutrophils and mast cells, is also useful for the diagnosis of some of the lesions; however, the reaction is partially ablated by mercury-based fixation and has largely been replaced by immunohistochemical reactions.[189] In the unusual myeloid lesions composed of immature erythroid cells or megakaryocytes, antibodies to hemoglobin A and glycophorin A for red blood cells, and von Willebrand factor (factor VIII-related antigen), CD41, CD61, and CD31 for megakaryocytes may be used. Monocytic lesions react with antibodies to lysozyme and CD68 (KP-1 and PGM-1) and CD163.

Imprint preparations of tumor masses may be particularly useful in identifying the myeloid nature of the cells. Auer rods may be found, and the myeloblasts may show intense staining with the myeloperoxidase cytochemical reaction.

Localized tumor masses occurring in the absence of blood or marrow involvement may respond to local radiation therapy. Eventually the process in the majority of patients will evolve into a form of acute myeloid leukemia or may be associated with additional tumor masses at other sites. The leukemic evolution may be characterized by a gradual increase in myeloblasts in the blood and marrow; frequently, blasts containing Auer rods are identified. Rarely the leukemic cells may be identified in body fluids due to the occurrence of myeloid sarcoma in one of these areas.

In 7 of 16 patients with isolated granulocytic sarcomas reported by Meis et al.,[192] the process did not show a leukemic evolution although 3 of the 7 patients developed granulocytic sarcomas at additional sites and died 2–8 months following initial presentation. The other 4 patients showed no evidence of recurrent disease from 3.5 to 16 years following presentation.

Unlike the myeloid sarcomas that occur in patients with established hematologic disorders, which are usually correctly diagnosed, the predominantly blastic myeloid sarcomas occurring as isolated lesions in the absence of some type of leukemia may be misdiagnosed as a malignant lymphoma or poorly differentiated tumor because of the lack of diagnostic features.[192] In lymph nodes involved by myeloid sarcoma, the germinal centers are frequently preserved; the infiltrate is usually present in the sinuses and occasionally in the paracortical and medullary areas. In other tissues, the cells usually display an infiltrative pattern with the overall architecture remaining intact. The presence of immature eosinophils or cells with lobulated nuclei should evoke suspicion of a myeloid sarcoma.

Myelodysplastic syndromes

The myelodysplastic syndromes are a heterogeneous group of myeloid disorders with varying potential for bone marrow failure and evolution to acute myeloid leukemia.[203,204,209,220] The myelodysplastic syndromes are basically disorders of ineffective myelopoiesis with hyperplastic marrows and cytopenias, dysplastic changes, frequently pancytopenia with or without an increase in blasts. In a minority of cases, the marrow is hypocellular.[208,214] Seven major categories have been proposed in the WHO classification of hematopoietic neoplasms: (1) refractory anemia; (2) idiopathic refractory sideroblastic anemia; (3) refractory cytopenia with multilineage dysplasia with or without ring sideroblasts; (4) refractory anemia with excess blasts-1; (5) refractory anemia with excess blasts-2; (6) myelodysplastic syndrome, unclassified; and (7) the isolated del(5q) syndrome.[204] The classification is based primarily on examination of blood and bone marrow smears. However, marrow section specimens may add important diagnostic information such as foci of blasts, increased fibrosis and megakaryocyte dysplasia.[205,211,213,215,217,220] Marrow sections in the del(5q) syndrome may be particularly informative in demonstrating megakaryocytes with hypolobulated nuclei characteristic of the disorder.[206,212]

The WHO proposal also includes a category of myeloid disorders, referred to as myelodysplastic syndrome/myeloproliferative neoplasms (MDS/MPN), for those myeloid processes which share features of both a myelodysplastic syndrome and a myeloproliferative process.[219] This category includes chronic myelomonocytic leukemia, juvenile myelomonocytic leukemia, atypical chronic myeloid leukemia, and myelodysplastic syndrome/myeloproliferative neoplasm unclassified.[216]

The trephine biopsy has a very important role in the evaluation of MDS and may provide important prognostic information.[204,205,207,208,214,217,220] The cell population in biopsy specimens varies according to the subtype.[204] In sideroblastic anemia, there is generally a marked increase in erythroid precursors, with greatly increased iron accumulation in macrophages. In refractory anemia with excess blasts 1 and 2, the marrow is hypercellular in the majority of patients, with an increase in neutrophil precursors. Chronic myelomonocytic leukemia, which is classified by the WHO as a myelodysplastic/myeloproliferative neoplasm, is characterized by a hypercellular marrow with an increase in both monocytes and neutrophils.[216] In any of these types of myelodysplastic syndrome, the marrow may be hypocellular in a minority of patients (Fig. 23.39).[208,214] This has been associated with an adverse prognosis in some studies.

Increased reticulin fibers may be observed in chronic myelomonocytic leukemia and refractory anemia with excess blasts, but is not usually a prominent feature.[207,211] In approximately 10% of patients there is a marked increase in reticulin fibers (Fig. 23.40). These cases usually satisfy the criteria for refractory anemia with excess blasts. These cases have been associated with an adverse prognosis in some studies.

A finding referred to as abnormal localization of immature precursors (ALIP), characterized by aggregates (3–5 cells) and clusters (>5 cells) of myeloblasts and promyelocytes in central areas of the marrow tissue away from the endosteal surface of the bone trabeculae and vascular structures, has been described in the myelodysplastic syndromes[217] (Fig. 23.41); the finding of three or more ALIP in a bone marrow section has been reported to have predictive value for evolution to leukemia. Apoptosis may be a prominent feature in some cases (Fig. 23.42).

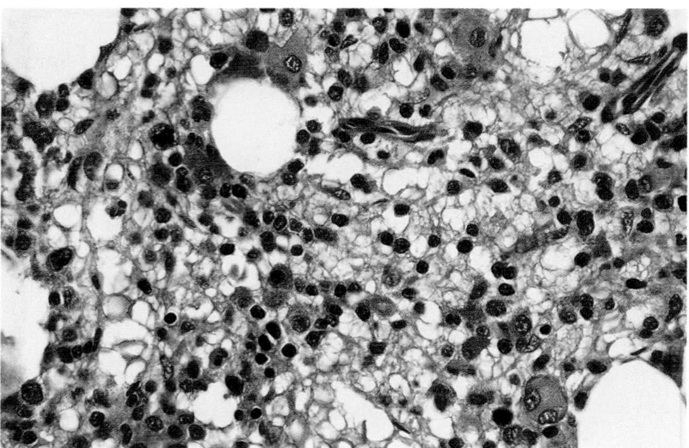

Fig. 23.39 Marrow biopsy from a 2-year-old child with myelodysplastic syndrome associated with isolated monosomy 7 cytogenetic abnormality. Marrow is moderately to markedly hypocellular for age with increased fat and prominent interstitial cell depletion. Small megakaryocytes with hypolobulated nuclei are present.

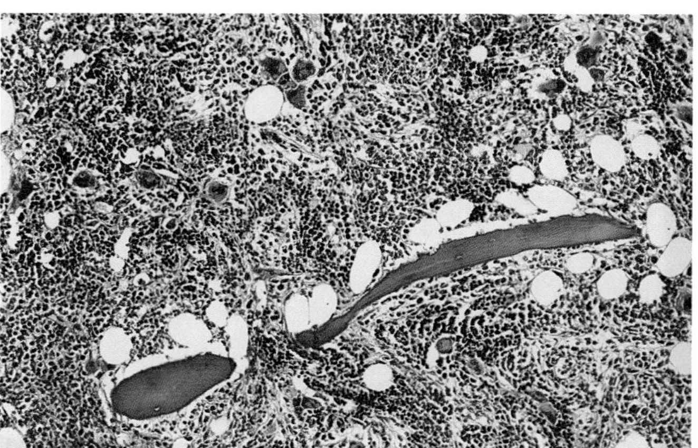

Fig. 23.40 Bone marrow biopsy from an adult male with refractory anemia with excess blasts-2 (RAEB-2) based on presence of 18% marrow blasts and myeloblasts with Auer rods. There is marked fibrosis with numerous megakaryocytes.

Although the precise classification of the myelodysplastic syndromes is based principally on the evaluation of blood and marrow smears, there are some types of myelodysplastic syndrome in which the bone marrow biopsy findings are highly suggestive of a specific classification. The de novo 5q− syndrome is a myelodysplastic syndrome occurring primarily in older women who present with a macrocytic anemia that is often severe, normal to increased platelet count, and usually prolonged survival; the blast percentage in the marrow is less than 5% and less than 1% in the blood.[206,212] The marrow biopsy usually shows increased normal sized to slightly small megakaryocytes, many with hypolobulated nuclei (Fig. 23.43). There is usually no significant dysplasia in the erythroid and

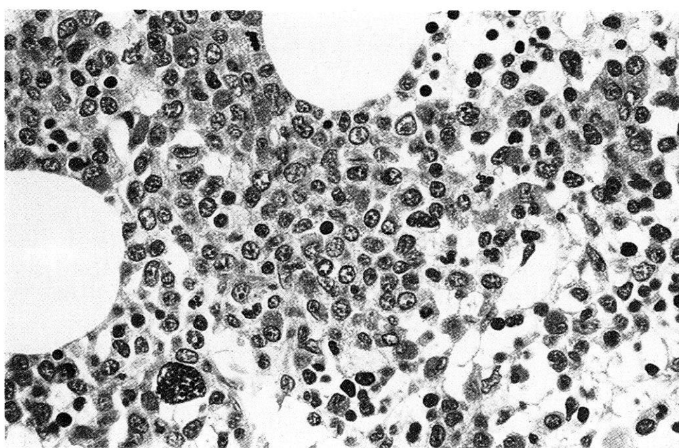

Fig. 23.41 Marrow biopsy from an adult with refractory anemia with excess blasts-2 (RAEB-2). Marrow is hypercellular. There are occasional foci of immature myeloid cells in the central marrow in nonparatrabecular and nonperivascular locations (ALIP).

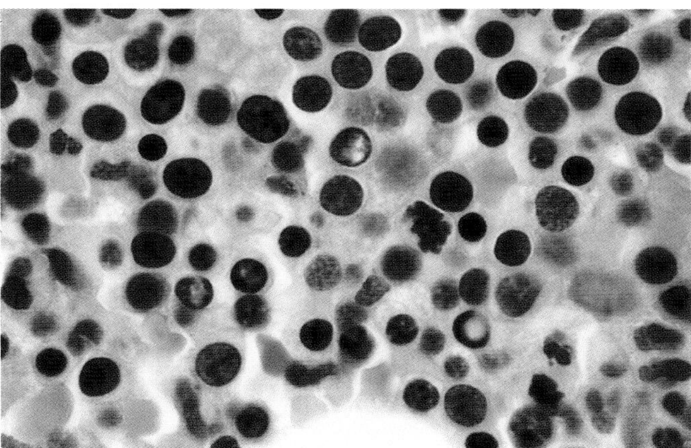

Fig. 23.42 Marrow from a patient with refractory anemia (RA) with marked erythroid hyperplasia and dyserythropoiesis. Several erythroid precursors with apoptotic nuclei are present.

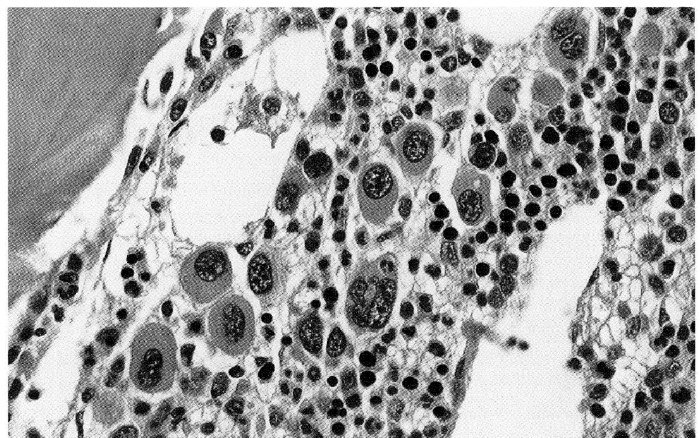

Fig. 23.43 Marrow biopsy from an adult woman with de novo myelodysplastic syndrome associated with an isolated del(5q) (q21;q32) cytogenetic abnormality. There is an increase in megakaryocytes, many of which have hypolobulated nuclei. The majority of megakaryocytes are normal in size; small megakaryocytes are present.

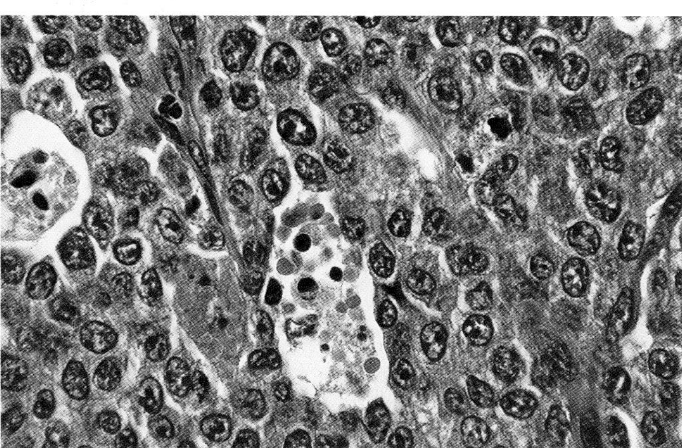

Fig. 23.44 Portion of a myeloid sarcoma presenting as a subcutaneous chest wall mass in an elderly woman with a 1-year history of chronic myelomonocytic leukemia with less than 5% blasts in marrow and blood. The mass consists of a relatively uniform population of blasts; scattered mitotic figures are present. Numerous tingible body macrophages impart a 'starry sky' appearance to the lesion. Many of the blasts reacted with antibody to myeloperoxidase and CD68 (KP-1). Blood and marrow examination at the time of appearance of the chest wall mass was essentially unchanged from the previous year, with less than 5% blasts.

neutrophil series. The presence of an isolated del(5q) cytogenetic abnormality with the described findings characterizes the del(5q) syndrome. Patients with this syndrome may respond favorably to treatment with the thalidomide analog, lenalidomide. Patients with del(5q) and additional cytogenetic abnormalities or blasts in excess of 5% in the marrow may also benefit from lenalidomide.

Increased megakaryocytes may also be observed in association with abnormalities of chromosome 3 at bands q21 and q26. The megakaryocytes in cases with this association are abnormally small, many with hypolobulated nuclei.

Similar to the acute myeloid leukemias and myeloproliferative neoplasms, extramedullary myeloid sarcomas may occur in the course of a myelodysplastic syndrome (Fig. 23.44).

The therapy-related acute leukemias and myelodysplastic syndromes occur in patients who have been treated with chemotherapy, radiation therapy or both for a variety of malignant and nonmalignant conditions. Two major forms have been recognized: alkylating agent/radiation-related type and topoisomerase II inhibitor-related type.[218] The alkylating agent-related type is generally a panmyelopathy which may or may not evolve to acute leukemia; in either instance, AML or MDS, it is a poor prognosis lesion with relatively short survival. The topoisomerase II-related type usually presents as acute leukemia with specific cytogenetic abnormalities, notably abnormalities involving chromosome 11q23. The bone marrow cellularity in the therapy-related myelodysplastic syndromes related to alkylating agents is more variable than with the de novo myelodysplastic syndromes: in approximately 50% of patients the marrow is hypercellular; in 25% normocellular; and in 25% hypocellular.[204] In addition to changes characteristic of a myelodysplastic syndrome, the marrow specimen may show evidence of the initial lesion for which treatment was indicated. Megakaryocyte abnormalities may be particularly prominent in marrow biopsies (Fig. 23.45). Reticulin fibrosis may be marked, and some of these cases have been described as acute myelodysplasia with myelofibrosis when there is a pronounced shift to immature cells.

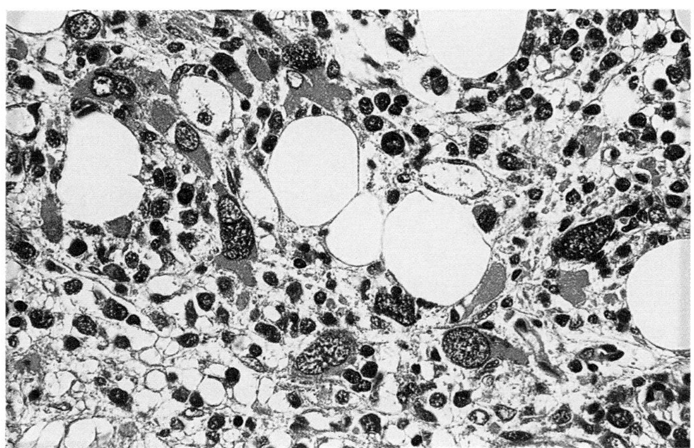

Fig. 23.45 Bone marrow biopsy from a patient with therapy-related myelodysplasia with myelofibrosis. There is predominance of neutrophils and megakaryocytes. Megakaryocytes show marked dysplasia.

Immunohistochemistry may be very useful in evaluating the myelodysplastic syndromes. CD34 may be particularly useful in identifying blast in cases of hypoplastic myelodysplastic syndromes that may resemble aplastic anemia.[207] However, the absence of CD34 reactivity does not exclude blasts since not all myeloblasts are CD34 positive. Anti-myeloperoxidase, anti-CD15, anti-CD117, and anti-lysozyme antibodies are useful for recognizing myeloblasts and monoblasts. Antibodies to von Willebrand factor (factor VIII-related antigen), CD41, CD61, and CD31 may facilitate the recognition of small and abnormal megakaryocytes.

Cytogenetic studies performed on an aspirate specimen have a critical role in the evaluation of the myelodysplastic syndromes, both for determining clonality and for prognostic factors (see Table 23.1).[204,206,210,217]

The 2008 edition of the *WHO Classification of Tumours of the Haematopoietic and Lymphoid Tissues* recognizes a recently described MDS, refractory cytopenia of childhood (RCC) as a provisional entity.[202,219] Although this entity is reported to be the most common subtype of MDS in children, accounting for approximately 50% of MDS, it is very uncommon since MDS accounts for approximately 4% of hematologic malignancies in children. Patients present with persistent cytopenias; there are less than 5% blasts in the bone marrow and less than 2% blasts in the blood. Dysplastic features are present in all cell lineages in the smears. Evaluation of a marrow biopsy is critical for the diagnosis. About 75% of the patients have a markedly hypocellular marrow biopsy, which may have the appearance of aplastic anemia. The distinction may not always be possible on initial examination and repeat biopsies may be necessary.

The disorder occurs in all childhood age groups and both sexes are affected with equal frequency. The evaluation of marrow biopsies is critical to the diagnosis.

The majority of children with RCC have marrows with a cellularity of 5–10%. There are one to several foci of 10 or more immature erythroid precursors with increased mitoses. Megakaryocytes are usually markedly decreased to absent. Rare micromegakaryocytes may be found and are helpful in establishing a diagnosis; anti-von Willebrand factor (factor VIII-related antigen) and CD61 may facilitate their detection. Granulopoiesis is sparsely distributed and left shifted. In the minority of patients with RCC who present with normal or hypercellular marrows there is a slight to moderate increase in erythropoiesis, with a predominance of proerythroblasts with increased mitoses. Granulopoiesis is slightly to moderately decreased with a shift to immaturity. Blasts are less than 5% of the cells. Most cases show a normal karyotype; the most common cytogenetic abnormality when one is present is monosomy 7. The demonstration of a clonal abnormality is extremely helpful in establishing the diagnosis.

As noted, it may be very difficult to distinguish RCC from aplastic anemia and also, as noted, more than one observation may be necessary. In aplastic anemia there is generally no evidence of dysplasia in the smears. The erythropoiesis in the marrow sections is markedly decreased to absent; the several foci characteristic of RCC are usually not found and if one is present it contains fewer than 10 cells which show evidence of maturation. Dysplastic megakaryocytes are not present. Granulocytes are markedly diminished and show normal maturation.

Myeloproliferative neoplasms

Considerable progress has been made in the classification of the myeloproliferative neoplasms since the previous edition of this book. This progress is the result of several discoveries of molecular alterations which may accompany these disorders. These discoveries have had impact on both the classification of these neoplasms as well as the recognition of entities which previously were grouped under a nonspecific morphologic classification.[238]

The discovery of the *JAK2*V617F mutation has been the most significant contribution to the classification of the myeloproliferative neoplasms since the discovery of the Philadelphia chromosome in 1959 and subsequently of its molecular counterpart, the *BCR/ABL1* fusion gene in chronic myelogenous leukemia. The relationship of the *JAK2*V617F mutation to the specific myeloproliferative neoplasms will be noted in the diagnostic criteria for these individual disorders.

Although affecting a much smaller number of patients, the discovery of the genetic abnormalities in the *PDGFRA* and *PDGFRB* genes has important implications for possible therapy with tyrosine kinase inhibitors for a group of diseases previously refractory to most forms of therapy. The recognition of this group of diseases is based on cytogenetic studies, fluorescent in situ hybridization (FISH), and molecular genetic analysis. Most but not all of these patients present with marked eosinophilia.

Chronic myelogenous leukemia

Chronic myelogenous leukemia (CML) is a stem cell disorder arising from fusion of the *ABL1* gene on chromosome 9 with the *BCR* gene on chromosome 22. The altered chromosome 22 is referred to as the Philadelphia chromosome.[225,239] Chronic myelogenous leukemia, *BCR/ABL1* positive, is distinct from other myeloproliferative disorders which are *BCR/ABL1* negative.[237,238] CML usually has three clinical pathologic stages, not always clearly distinguished: chronic, accelerated, and blast. The vast majority of patients present in the chronic phase; uncommonly patients present in an accelerated or blast phase.

The initial presentation in the chronic phase is characterized by marked leukocytosis, thrombocytosis, and basophilia and usually splenomegaly.[239] Atypical presentations such as marked thrombocytosis or basophilia without leukocytosis may occur. The number of myeloblasts in the blood and marrow smears in the chronic phase does not usually exceed 5%. The trephine sections are markedly hypercellular, primarily because of an increase in granulocytes and megakaryocytes.[234,239] Macrophages resembling Gaucher cells, usually occurring singly, may be present in the bone marrow smears and sections; they are more prominent in perivascular locations.

Increased reticulin fibers are present in approximately 30% of cases and megakaryocytes are increased in approximately 40% of cases. Many of the megakaryocytes are small with hypolobulated nuclei. The increase in reticulin fibers correlates with an increase in microvascularity.[228,234]

The chronic phase, usually of 3–4 years' duration, is followed by the accelerated phase of shorter duration, characterized by increasing blasts in the blood and marrow, progressive basophilia, increasing myelofibrosis, and additional cytogenetic changes. The blast phase usually occurs abruptly and may occur without an intermediate accelerated phase; the blasts exceed 20% in the blood or marrow[225,231,239] (Figs 23.46–23.48). Approximately 70% of blast crises are morphologically and immunophenotypically myeloid, and 30% are lymphoblastic. The myeloid type may be characterized by proliferation of any of the myeloid cell lineages, including myeloblasts, erythroblasts, and megakaryoblasts. Immunohistochemical studies may be very useful in identifying the distribution and lineage of blast populations. In some patients, blast transformation may be initially manifest in bone marrow sections as large, irregular, focal collections of blasts. Extramedullary manifestation of blast crisis also occurs, and the diagnosis should be suspected in any patient with CML who develops a tumor mass or lymphadenopathy.

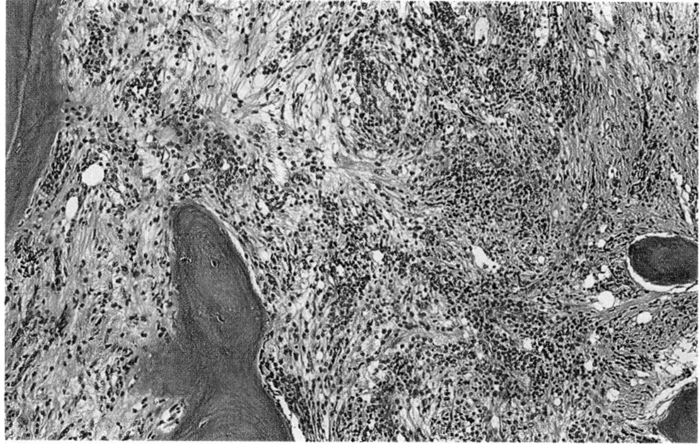

Fig. 23.46 Marrow biopsy from a patient in accelerated phase of chronic myelogenous leukemia. There is marked reticulin fibrosis and small clusters of blasts.

The development of extensive myelofibrosis in patients with CML usually occurs late in the disease and has been associated with a more aggressive clinical course.[222,235,239] Exceptions to this generalization have been reported and myelofibrosis may occur in the early stages of CML with the same prognostic implications as when it occurs late in the disease.[222,223] The myelofibrosis in CML is usually characterized by an increase in reticulin fibers; collagenous fibrosis is not common but may occasionally occur (Fig. 23.46). As noted, the increase in reticulin fibers correlates with an increase in angiogenesis. Reversal of myelofibrosis may occur following bone marrow transplantation and imatinib therapy.[227,230] A positive correlation between the degree of reticulin fibrosis and the number of CD61-positive megakaryocytes has been reported both pre- and post-allogeneic marrow transplant.[233]

The introduction of therapy with the tyrosine kinase inhibitor imatinib mesylate (Gleevec) for CML has been one of the major success stories in the field of leukemia therapy; the agent induces hematologic remission in a high percentage of patients with CML in the chronic phase and accelerated phases of the disease.[221,224,226,229,232] The hematologic remission is accompanied by morphologic normalization or near normalization of the bone marrow in most cases. The normalization of the marrow may occur even with persistence of the Philadelphia chromosome, or evidence of the *BCR/ABL1* fusion gene. The normalization of the marrow usually may lag behind remission of blood findings and may not be complete for several months.[221] Treatment with interferon usually results in a decrease in overall marrow cellularity and an increase in erythroid precursors. There may be a concurrent increase in megakaryocytes and reticulin fibers. Hydroxyurea therapy generally results in a decrease in cellularity and no increase in megakaryocytes or reticulin fibers.[236]

Polycythemia vera

Polycythemia vera (PV) is classified with the myeloproliferative neoplasms; the major diagnostic feature is an increased red blood cell mass, and there is usually splenomegaly and some degree of leukocytosis and thrombocytosis.[264] Precise criteria for the diagnosis of PV have been established by the Polycythemia Vera Study Group (PVSG); these were modified in the 2001 WHO proposal for

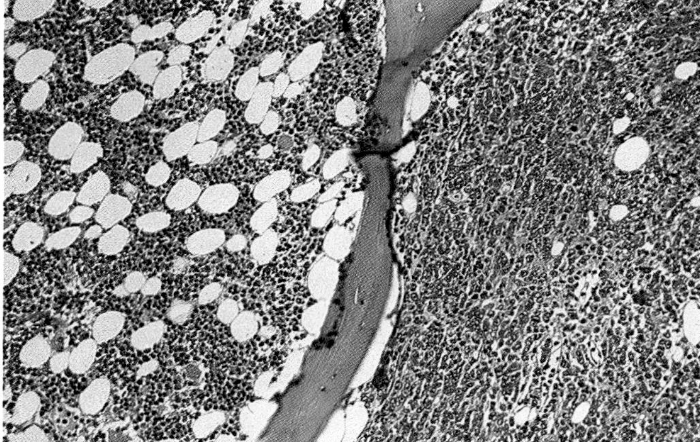

Fig. 23.47 Erythroblastic crisis of chronic myelogenous leukemia. The marrow to the left of the bone trabecula shows the findings of treated chronic phase. The proliferation of primitive erythroblasts to the right of the bone represents a focus of blast transformation.

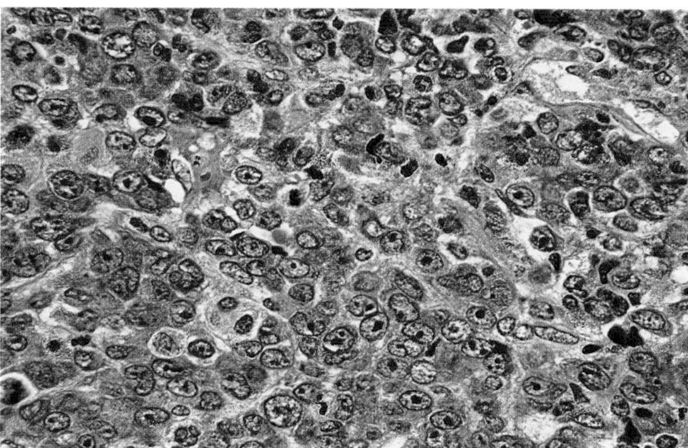

Fig. 23.48 High magnification of marrow biopsy from a patient with erythroblastic transformation of chronic myelogenous leukemia. Cells are large with prominent nucleoli and basophilic cytoplasm.

Box 23.4 2008 WHO diagnostic criteria[a] for polycythemia vera[264]

Major criteria

1. Hemoglobin >18.5 g/dL in men; >16.5 g/dL women or other evidence of increased red blood cell mass.
2. *JAK2*V617F mutation or similar functional mutation such as *JAK2* exon 12 mutation

Minor criteria

1. Hypercellular bone marrow biopsy with features of a panmyelosis.
2. Erythropoietin level below the normal range.
3. Endogenous erythroid colony formation in vitro.

[a]Diagnosis requires both major criteria and one minor criterion, or the first major criterion and two minor criteria.

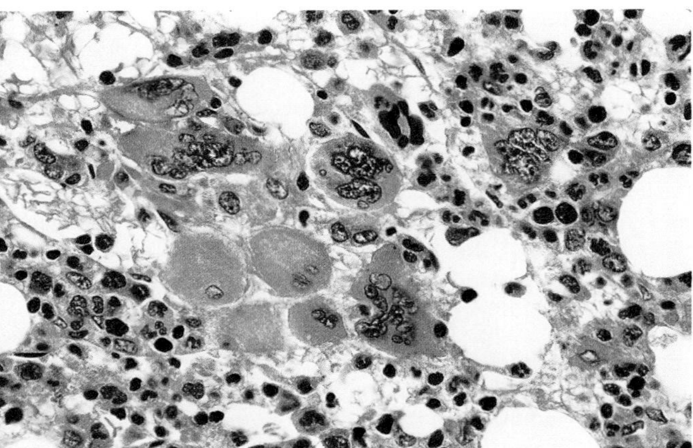

Fig. 23.49 Hyperplastic bone marrow from a patient with polycythemia vera. All cellular elements are increased. Megakaryocytes are prominent and show considerable variation in size; many are unusually large with hyperlobulated nuclei.

the classification of hematopoietic neoplasms. An important addition to the diagnostic criteria for PV in the 2008 WHO classification is the recognition of the Janus 2 kinase gene mutation *JAK2*V617F or similar mutations such as *JAK2* exon 12 mutation (Box 23.4).[244,250,251,260,261,264] The discovery of this mutation has also led to the identification of a marker for familial cases of PV.[259]

Three clinical phases of PV are recognized: (1) prodromal prepolycythemia phase with borderline to slight erythrocytosis; (2) overt polycythemia vera with a significant increase in red blood cell mass; and (3) spent phase or post polycythemia with myelofibrosis.[243,245,249,253,255,257,258,264]

The blood smear in the overt phase shows increased erythrocytes, reflecting the increased red blood cell mass, leukocytosis, and thrombocytosis. The bone marrow is usually markedly hypercellular.[240,241,243,262–264] However, this is not an invariant finding; 13% of the patients enrolled in the National Cancer Institute Polycythemia Vera Study had marrow biopsies with cellularity of less than 60%.[241] The cellularity of the marrows from patients in the study ranged from 37% to 100%, with a mean of 82%. The hypercellularity is due to a panhyperplasia of myeloid cells, principally erythroid precursors and megakaryocytes; the megakaryocytes range in size from small to unusually large, frequently with hyperlobulated nuclei and in clusters.[240,241,262–264] (Fig. 23.49). The clusters may be accentuated in perisinusoidal and paratrabecular locations. Stains for iron usually show decreased or no hemosiderin deposits.[240] A slight increase in reticulin fibers is present at the outset of the disease in 25% of cases; 11% of pretreatment biopsies show a marked increase in reticulin fibers.[240] The increase in reticulin corresponds, in general, to an increase in marrow cellularity and the number of megakaryocytes. An increase in reticulin fibers in pretreatment marrow biopsies is not necessarily indicative of the spent phase of the disease. Similar to other myeloproliferative neoplasms, there is an increase in vascular structures in PV.[246,252]

Approximately 20% of patients with PV have cytogenetic abnormalities; the most frequently detected are +8, del(20q), del(13q), and del(9p). The incidence increases with disease progression.[264]

Polycythemia vera may be difficult to distinguish from the other non-CML myeloproliferative neoplasms based solely on marrow examination. As a result, it is critical to adhere to established diagnostic guidelines when making a diagnosis.[263,264] Although the *JAK2*V617F mutation readily distinguishes PV from other causes of erythrocytosis, the mutation is shared by essential thrombocytosis and primary myelofibrosis, albeit less frequently. Morphology

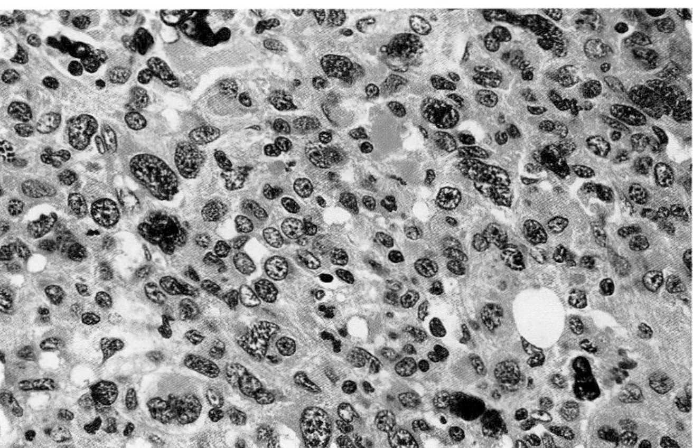

Fig. 23.50 Marrow biopsy from a patient in spent phase of polycythemia vera. Marrow is markedly hypercellular as a result of granulocytic and megakaryocytic hyperplasia. Megakaryocytes show dysplastic features.

continues to have a central role in the diagnosis along with the clinical data.[242,256,262–264]

The evolution of PV to the spent or post-polycythemic phase may be marked by a decrease in red blood cell mass with anemia and the development of myelofibrosis with a marked increase in reticulin fibers, increased angiogenesis, collagenous fibrosis, and clusters of abnormal megakaryocytes; the incidence of this complication varies from 9% to 20%[245,249,253,255–257,264] (Fig. 23.50). This is accompanied by a leukoerythroblastic blood picture and increased red blood cell poikilocytosis with numerous dacryocytes and increasing splenomegaly due to extramedullary hematopoiesis. An additional complication in some patients is the development of acute leukemia and myelodysplasia; the incidence is higher in patients treated with chemotherapy, P^{32}, or radiation as opposed to those treated only with phlebotomy.[247,248,254,265]

Essential thrombocythemia

Essential thrombocythemia (ET) is a myeloproliferative disorder that is closely related to polycythemia vera but lacks the essential

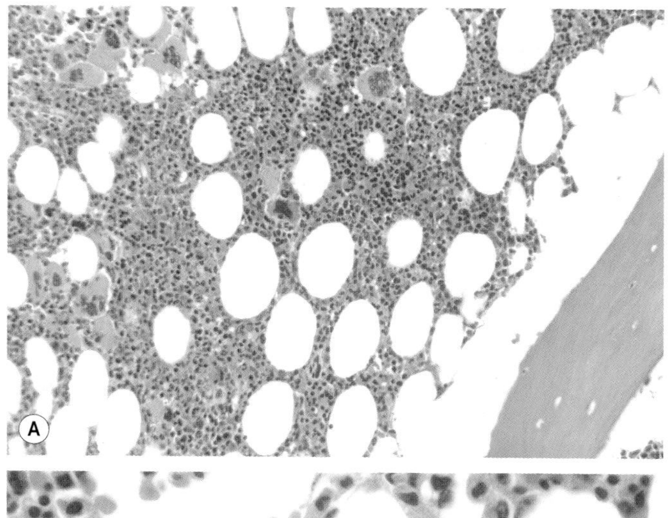

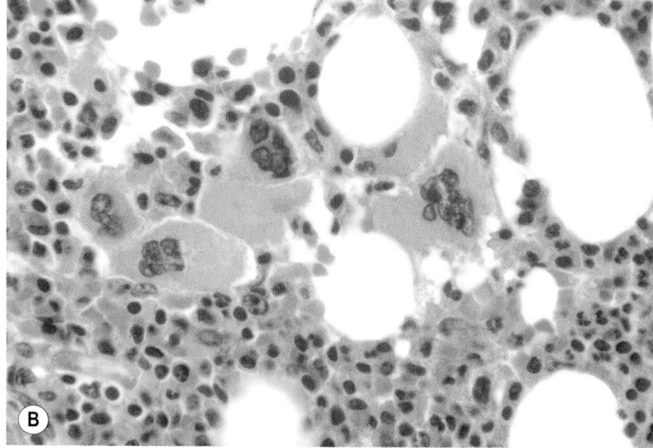

Fig. 23.51 **A**, Marrow biopsy from a patient with essential thrombocythemia. Marrow is normocellular with numerous scattered large megakaryocytes. **B**, High magnification of specimen in **A** showing the very large megakaryocytes, some with hyperlobulated nuclei.

Box 23.5 2008 WHO diagnostic criteria[a] for essential thrombocythemia[274]

1. Sustained platelet count of >450 × 10^9/L.
2. Bone marrow biopsy showing proliferation primarily of mature enlarged megakaryocytes.[b]
3. Not satisfying WHO criteria for any other myeloproliferative neoplasm or other myeloid disorder.
4. *JAK2*V617F mutation or other clonal abnormality or in the absence of *JAK2*V617F, no evidence for a reactive thrombocytosis.

[a]All four criteria should be present.
[b]There should be no evidence of relevant reticulin fibrosis, collagen or leukoerythroblastic blood picture.

Box 23.6 2008 WHO diagnostic criteria[a] for primary myelofibosis[300]

Major criteria

1. Megakaryocyte proliferation with atypia, usually accompanied by increased reticulin fibers and/or collagen; in the absence of significant reticulin fibrosis, the megakaryocyte changes must be accompanied by increased marrow cellularity characterized by granulocytic proliferation and often decreased erythropoiesis.
2. Not satisfying WHO criteria for CML, PV, MDS, or other myeloid disorders
3. Demonstration of *JAK2*V617F or other clonal marker or in the absence of a clonal marker no evidence for a secondary myelofibrosis.

Minor criteria

1. Leukoerythroblastic blood picture.
2. Increased serum lactic dehydrogenase level.
3. Anemia.
4. Splenomegaly.

[a]Diagnosis requires satisfying all three major and two minor criteria.

diagnostic criteria of polycythemia vera, most notably an increase of red blood cell mass.[266,270,273,274] The principal morphologic findings relate to the increased megakaryocytes and thrombocytosis. The marrow is usually normocellular for age but may be hypercellular or hypocellular. The bone marrow findings are principally related to increased and large megakaryocytes with hyperlobulated nuclei (Fig. 23.51).[269] The megakaryocytes occur singly and in clusters. The erythroid and granulocytic cell lines are usually normal. Reticulin is usually normal but may be slightly increased and there may be an associated increase in angiogenesis.[272] There is no specific molecular marker for ET, such as the *BCR/ABL1* fusion gene in CML, but approximately 40–60% of patients with ET have the *JAK2*V617F mutation which may also be present in PV and primary myelofibrosis.[271,274] The WHO criteria for diagnosis of essential thrombocythemia are listed in Box 23.5.

The distinction between essential thrombocytosis and secondary forms of thrombocytosis may be difficult from routine morphologic studies.[272] The clinical history is important in excluding possible causes for a secondary thrombocytosis. Demonstration of the *JAK2*V617F or similar mutation would be definitive in excluding a secondary thrombocytosis.[267,268,270,271]

Essential thrombocythemia is an indolent disease in most patients with survival of 10–15 years. Transformation to acute myeloid leukemia occurs in less than 5% of patients and may be related to chemotherapy.[274]

Primary myelofibrosis

Primary myelofibrosis (chronic idiopathic myelofibrosis, agnogenic myeloid metaplasia) is a clonal myeloproliferative disease of undetermined etiology characterized by myeloid cell proliferation and reactive fibrosis.[279,287,290,295–301,304–306] It occurs primarily in adults; the average age at diagnosis is approximately 60 years.[279,301,303] Rare cases have been reported in the pediatric population.[302] There is some degree of detectable hepatosplenomegaly caused by extramedullary hematopoiesis.

Primary myelofibrosis (PM) may, at times, be confused with chronic myelogenous leukemia or other types of chronic myeloproliferative neoplasms because of occasional similarities in the blood findings; the important differentiating clinical and laboratory findings have been described in detail.[297,300,301] The principal clinical and morphologic features have been described in the 2008 edition of the *WHO Classification of Tumours of Haematopoietic and Lymphoid Tissues*[300] (Box 23.6). The most important distinguishing biologic feature is the presence of the Philadelphia chromosome or molecular evidence of the *BCR/ABL1* fusion gene in the hematopoietic cells in chronic myelogenous leukemia and its absence in the cells from patients with primary myelofibrosis and the possible presence of the *JAK2*V617F mutation in PM.[284,287,288,300] In addition, neutrophil alkaline phosphatase is decreased in approximately 90% of patients with chronic myelogenous leukemia and is normal or increased in the majority of patients with primary myelofibrosis. Marrow fibrosis in chronic myelogenous leukemia is generally a late occurrence, and its onset usually heralds a more aggressive evolution, unlike PM in which marrow fibrosis is present to some extent from inception and is generally associated with a more prolonged clinical course.[281,282] Approximately 30% of patients have a cytogenetic abnormality at presentation; the incidence increases with leukemic progression. The most common abnormalities are del(13q), del(20q), +8, and abnormalities of chromosomes 1, 7, and 9.[293,300]

Primary myelofibrosis is usually characterized by progression from a prefibrotic stage to a fibrotic stage, although biopsies from different sites have been reported to show substantial variation in the degree of fibrosis. Approximately 20–30% of patients with PM present in the prefibrotic stage.[300,301] The marrow in this stage is hypercellular for age; there is an increase in abnormal megakaryocytes and granulocytes (Fig. 23.52). Erythroid precursors may be reduced. The megakaryocytes may form clusters adjacent to sinuses and bone trabeculae. The megakaryocytes vary in size and are frequently very large with abnormal clumping of the chromatin. There is no or minimal increase in reticulin fibers in the prefibrotic stage. Aggregates of well-differentiated lymphocytes may be present. The fibrotic stage is marked by variable degrees of reticulin and/or collagen fibrosis; the marrow varies from hypocellular to hypercellular. Expansion of the bone trabeculae may be present. The density of reticulin fibers may vary substantially in different areas of the biopsy. Sinusoids are usually increased in number and distended, and contain hematopoietic cells. Megakaryocytes may be particularly prominent in the sinusoids (Fig. 23.53). In some cases, the marrow may be almost uniformly densely fibrotic with scattered foci of hematopoietic cells (Fig. 23.54). Scattered abnormal megakaryocytes may be the only recognizable hematopoietic cells. In approximately 40% of the patients with PM, osteosclerotic changes can be demonstrated by radiographic examination, most notably in the bones of the axial skeleton and the proximal portions of the long bones.[304] The relative proportion of hematopoietic cells and fibrous tissue has been generally assumed to vary with the stage of disease, the amount of fibrous connective tissue progressively increasing, with the end stage characterized by marked marrow fibrosis and marked splenomegaly. Studies have been reported that show no correlation between extent of marrow fibrosis and duration of disease and spleen size.[306]

Increase in bone marrow microvascular density evaluated in sections stained with CD34 has been found in a high percentage of cases of primary myelofibrosis.[285,289,291] The increase in microvascular density correlated significantly with spleen size and was a significant independent risk factor for survival in some studies. The degree of increased microvascular density was independent of reticulin fibrosis but correlated positively with hypercellularity and megakaryocyte clumping. Immunohistochemistry with CD105 (endoglin) in PM is reported to show increased microvascular density and positive correlation with marrow fibrosis.[292]

The megakaryocytes in PM, including the prefibrotic phase, show strong expression of nuclear b-fibroblast growth factor (b-FGF) on immunohistochemical staining; an increase has also been observed in PV and ET. This contrasts with CML and a reactive increase in megakaryocytes in which the megakaryocytes show no or weak expression of b-FGF.[280]

Similar to CML, PM may progress to an accelerated phase with increased blasts (Fig. 23.55). These may be present diffusely or

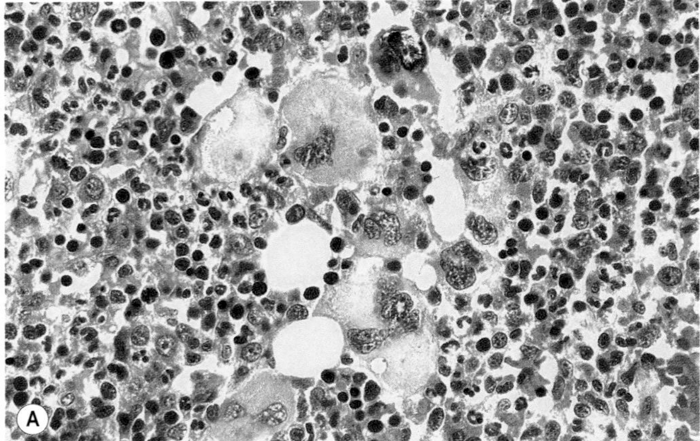

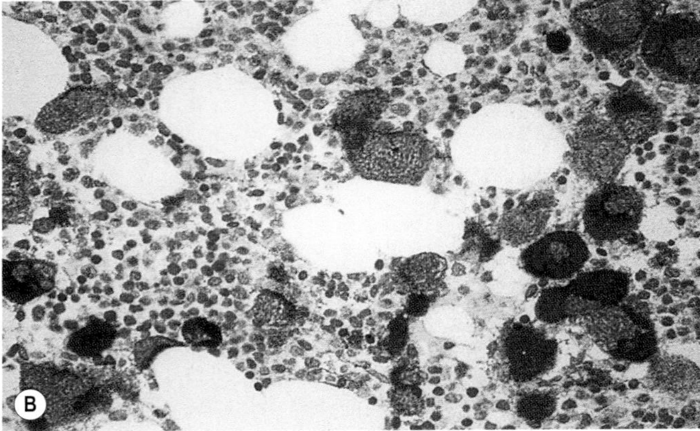

Fig. 23.52 A, Marrow biopsy from the prefibrotic stage of primary myelofibrosis. There is a cluster of megakaryocytes which vary in size. Several are large with marked variation in nucleocytoplasmic ratio. **B**, Bone marrow section from prefibrotic stage of chronic idiopathic myelofibrosis reacted with antibody to CD61. This highlights the megakaryocytes, which vary in size from small to large. The nuclei show markedly abnormal chromatin clumping.
*(**B** contributed by Dr J. Thiele, Cologne, Germany, and reproduced from World Health Organization Classification of Tumours: Pathology and Genetics of Tumours of Haematopoietic and Lymphoid Tissues. Lyon, 2001, IARC Press)*

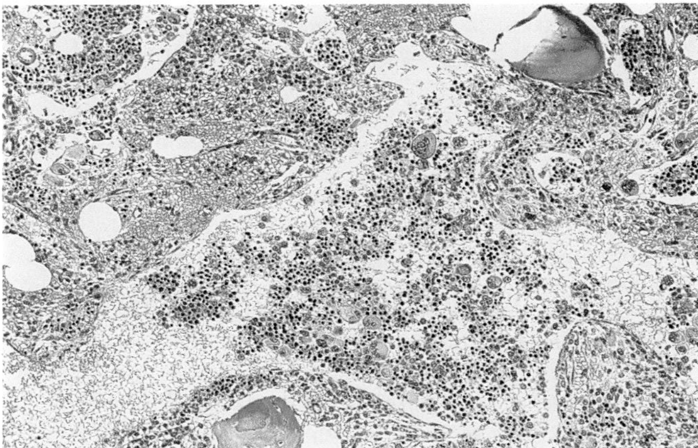

Fig. 23.53 Bone marrow biopsy from a patient with primary myelofibrosis showing prominent intrasinusoidal hematopoiesis. Predominant cells in the sinusoid are erythroid precursors and megakaryocytes.

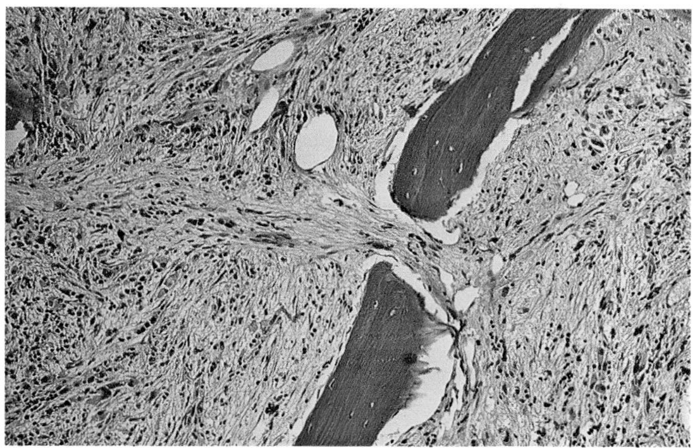

Fig. 23.54 Trephine biopsy from an adult with a 7-year history of primary myelofibrosis (agnogenic myeloid metaplasia). There is extensive marrow fibrosis with marked reduction in hematopoietic tissue.

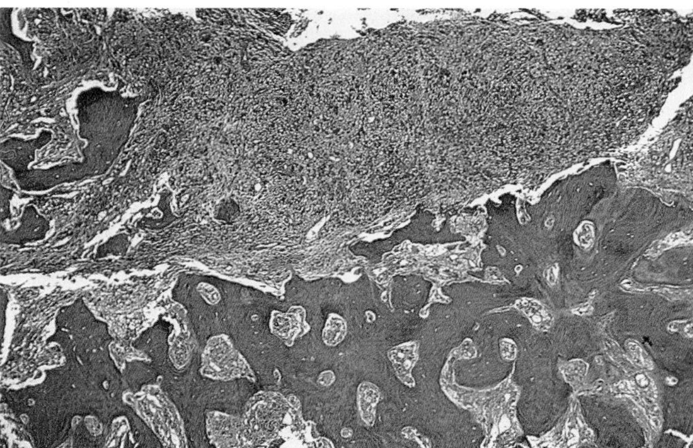

Fig. 23.55 Marrow biopsy from a patient with primary myelofibrosis shows extensive osteosclerosis and a cellular area comprised predominantly of blasts.

uncommonly in focal aggregates. Myeloid sarcomas have been reported in patients with long-standing PM.[278] The lesions occur most frequently in the retroperitoneum, pelvis, mesentery, and pleura; lymph node and skin may also be involved. The tumors are usually composed primarily of hematopoietic cells with varying degrees of stromal reaction. The megakaryocytes may be particularly prominent because of their number and frequently bizarre appearance. Rarely, marked fibrosis may be present.[278] A hyperplasia of hematogones has been reported in the bone marrow of patients with PM following therapy.[286]

The majority of patients with PM have a relatively long clinical course, with an estimated median survival of 3–5 years from the onset of disease.[300] A minor population of patients with this disorder has a more aggressive clinical course with a median survival of approximately 2 years.[277,283] Amyloidosis has been reported as a concurrent condition.[275]

Marrow fibrosis may be an accompaniment of several disorders, both hematologic and nonhematologic, including autoimmune disorders, and a diagnosis of primary myelofibrosis should be based on firm diagnostic criteria.[276,294]

Hematopoietic neoplasms associated with eosinophilia and fusion abnormalities of *PDGFRA* (platelet-derived growth factor receptor α), *PDGFRB* (platelet-derived growth factor receptor β) and *FGFR1* (fibroblast growth factor receptor 1)

PDGFRA *abnormalities*

The most common myeloproliferative neoplasm associated with an abnormality of *PDGFRA* results from a *FIP1L1/PDGFRA* fusion gene. This results from a cryptic deletion on chromosome 4 at band q12.[307,308,311] The deletion also results in the loss of the *CHIC2* gene; this finding serves as a reliable surrogate marker for the *FIP1L1/PDGFRA* fusion.[310,316] There is a marked male predominance in the disorder and the median age is in the late forties. There is usually marked eosinophilia, and cardiac and pulmonary symptoms are frequent. Splenomegaly is common. The serum vitamin B12 level is elevated. The presentation is commonly chronic eosinophilic leukemia (CEL). The bone marrow is hypercellular with markedly increased eosinophils and frequently increased mast cells which are dispersed or in loose nonparatrabecular, nonperivascular clusters; occasionally the mast cells appear in dense bundles virtually indistinguishable morphologically from systemic mastocytosis (Fig. 23.56). The mast cells are highlighted by reaction with mast cell tryptase and are usually CD2−, CD25+. Importantly, this neoplasm is responsive to the tyrosine kinase inhibitor imatinib.[307,308,311–313]

Because of the finding of increased mast cells in the marrow of patients with *FIP1L1/PDGFRA* fusion, there may be cases in which the distinction between CEL and systemic mastocytosis is difficult based solely on the morphologic findings.[317] The definitive distinguishing finding is molecular evidence of the fusion gene. However, there are several clinical and laboratory findings which, viewed in aggregate, may aid in distinguishing the two processes. There is a marked male predominance in CEL; in systemic mastocytosis the sex distribution is more evenly distributed. Patients with systemic mastocytosis commonly have a history of urticaria pigmentosa and gastrointestinal symptoms; patients with CEL uncommonly have these manifestations. The laboratory findings for the two disorders are more distinctive; patients with systemic mastocytosis have much higher serum tryptase levels, a median level of 207 ng/mL compared to a median level of 24 ng/mL in CEL. The median peak absolute eosinophil count is 2187/mm^3 in mastocytosis and 12474/mm^3 in CEL.[314,315] In systemic mastocytosis there are dense aggregates of mast cells in the marrow biopsy whereas in CEL the mast cells are usually dispersed. However, this finding is not always a reliable distinguishing feature (see Fig. 23.56). The molecular studies are definitive.

PDGFRB *abnormalities*

The most frequent myeloproliferative neoplasm associated with rearrangement of the *PDGFRB* gene on chromosome 5q31–33 usually has the morphologic features of chronic myelomonocytic leukemia; eosinophilia is usually but not invariably present.[307] The disease is more common in men, with a median age at presentation in the upper forties and an age range of 8–72 years. Most patients have splenomegaly. Cytogenetic studies show a t(5;12)(q31–33;p12) abnormality and molecular analysis shows an *ETV6/PDGFRB* fusion gene.[309] The bone marrow is hypercellular with increased eosinophils, and there may be an increase in mast cells which may be spindled or fusiform in shape. Other types of myeloid presentation with other fusion genes have been reported. The disorder is responsive to the tyrosine kinase inhibitor imatinib.

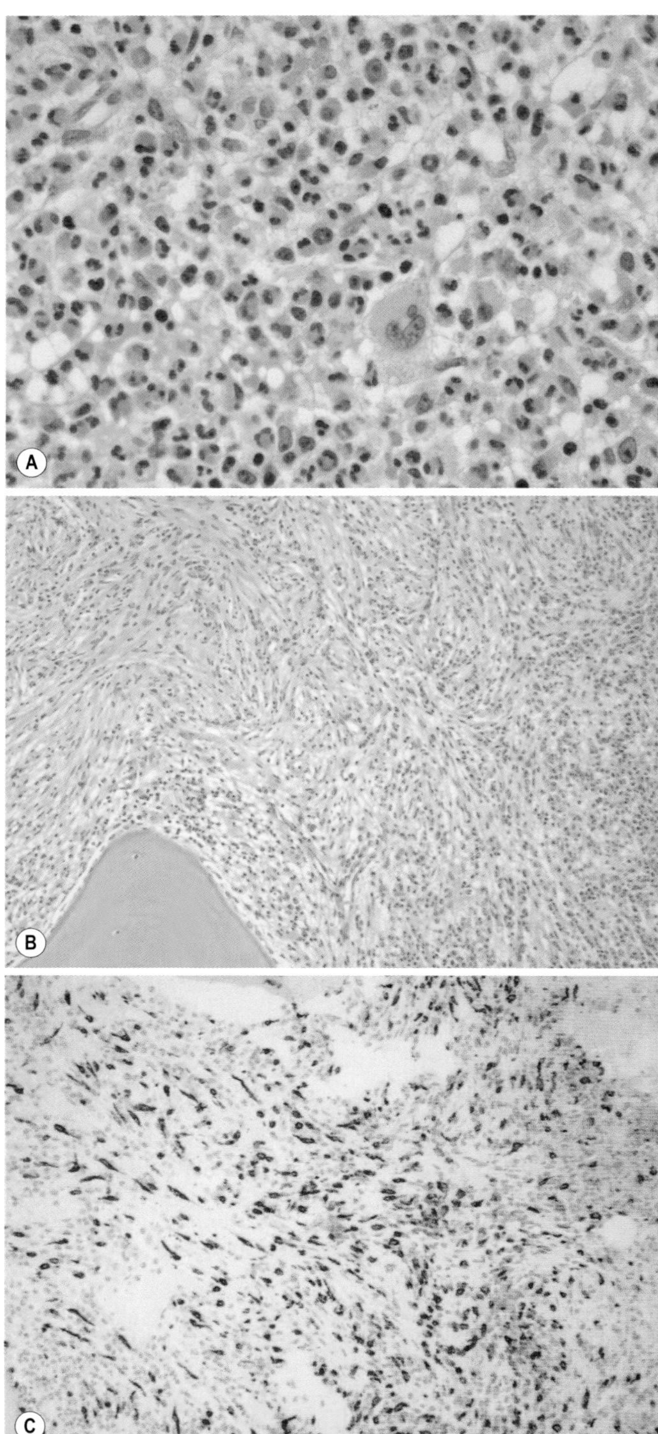

Fig. 23.56 **A**, Bone marrow biopsy from an adult male with a WBC count of 18.6 × 10^9/L with 86% eosinophils. The marrow is markedly hypercellular with a marked increase in mature eosinophils. **B**, Another area of the same biopsy showing an aggregate of intertwining mast cells, most of which are fusiform in shape. The mast cell infiltrate is partly juxtaposed to a bone trabecula. **C**, Mast cell tryptase of the lesion in **B** highlighting the mast cells. Genetic studies showed a deletion of *CHIC2*, a surrogate marker for *PDGFRA/FIP1L1* fusion gene. The patient is in remission 3 years following initiation of therapy with imatinib.

(Contributed by Dr Curt Hanson, Rochester, MD)

FGFR1 *abnormalities*

The hematopoietic neoplasms associated with *FGFR1* rearrangement are somewhat heterogeneous and include myeloproliferative neoplasms, acute myeloid leukemia, T and B lymphoblastic lymphomas/leukemias, and mixed phenotype acute leukemia.[307] There is a wide age range; the median age is 32 years. The associated cytogenetic abnormality is t(8;13)(p11;q12). Patients presenting with a myeloproliferative disorder usually have eosinophilia. The cases presenting with lymphoma usually show eosinophilic infiltration of the lymphoma.

In contrast to the lesions associated with abnormalities of *PDGFRA* and *PDGFRB*, the neoplasms associated with abnormalities of *FGFR1* are not responsive to imatinib and the prognosis is poor.

Systemic mastocytosis

Systemic mastocytosis is a relatively rare disorder characterized by mast cell proliferation in several organs. It usually occurs in combination with urticaria pigmentosa but may present in patients without cutaneous involvement.[318,319] The median age for patients presenting with systemic mastocytosis with urticaria pigmentosa is 45 years; the median age for patients presenting with systemic mastocytosis without urticaria pigmentosa is around 75 years.[318,320,328,335] The clinical symptoms are varied and include diarrhea, weakness, fractures, weight loss, arthralgia, flushing episodes, and bronchospasm.[318,329,331,332] An occasional patient may experience anaphylactoid shock. Slight splenomegaly may be present. Osteoblastic, osteolytic, or concurrent osteoblastic–osteolytic lesions may be found on radiologic examination; generalized osteoporosis may also occur (Fig. 23.57).

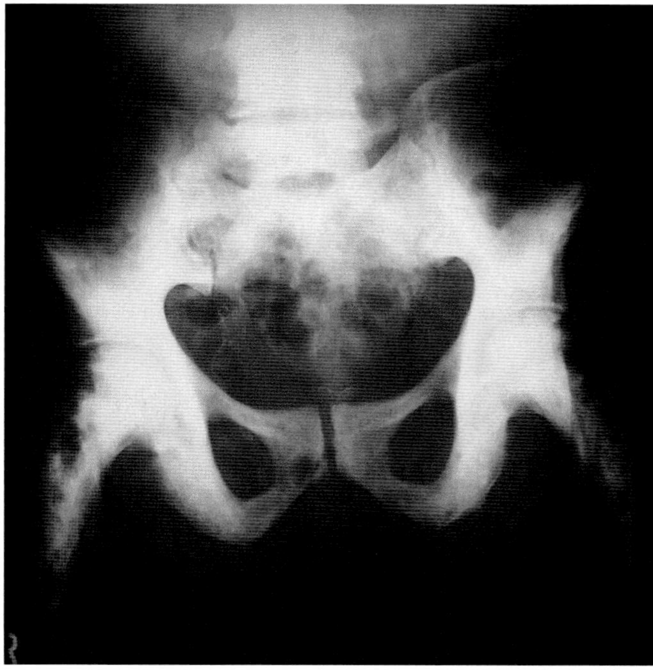

Fig. 23.57 Radiograph of pelvis and upper femurs from a patient with systemic mastocytosis; both osteosclerotic and osteolytic changes are prominent.

Box 23.7 WHO classification of mastocytosis[320,333]

- Cutaneous mastocytosis
- Indolent systemic mastocytosis
- Systemic mastocytosis with associated clonal hematologic disorder
- Aggressive systemic mastocytosis
- Mast cell leukemia
- Mast cell sarcoma
- Extracutaneous mastocytoma

Box 23.8 WHO diagnostic criteria[a] for systemic mastocytosis[320,333]

Major criterion

Multifocal dense infiltrates of mast cells (>15 mast cells) in aggregates detected in sections of bone marrow and/or other extracutaneous organs confirmed by tryptase immunohistochemistry.

Minor criteria

1. In biopsy sections of bone marrow or other extracutaneous organs, more than 25% of the mast cells in the infiltrate are spindle shaped and have atypical morphology, or, of all the mast cells in bone marrow smears, more than 25% are immature or atypical mast cells.
2. Detection of *KIT* point mutations at codon 816 in specimens of bone marrow, blood or other extracutaneous organs.
3. Mast cells in bone marrow, blood or other extracutaneous organs that coexpress CD117 with CD2 and/or CD25.
4. Serum total tryptase of >20 ng/mL unless there is an associated clonal myeloid disorder, in which case this parameter is invalid.

[a]The diagnosis of mastocytosis may be made if the major and one minor criteria are present, or if three of the minor criteria are present.

The WHO classification of mastocytosis, based principally on a consensus classification published in 2001, is shown in Box 23.7.[320,333] The WHO proposes one major and four minor criteria for the diagnosis of systemic mastocytosis, which is the type with bone marrow involvement (Box 23.8).[320] The blood findings in systemic mastocytosis may include eosinophilia, anemia, leukocytosis or leukopenia, thrombocytopenia, and pancytopenia.[323,324]

The bone marrow is the most frequent site of noncutaneous involvement in systemic mastocytosis; lesions may be found as a result of a specific search or may be detected in a biopsy performed for some purpose unrelated to suspected mastocytosis. In the latter instance, when there is no clinical suspicion of the disease, the lesions may be overlooked or misinterpreted because of the difficulty in identifying mast cells in routine sections and because of the changes inherent in the mast cells in this disease; the cells are frequently large, spindled, or have lobulated nuclei and decreased granules that may be much smaller than normal mast cell granules.[320,321,332,333] Smears obtained by bone marrow aspirate may suggest the diagnosis of mastocytosis if large numbers of atypical mast cells are present; however, up to 7% of mast cells have been reported in aspirate preparations in patients without mast cell disease. An increase in mast cells may also be observed in lymphocytic and lymphoplasmacytic lymphomas and hairy cell leukemia.[336] A marked increase in mast cells in the marrow has been observed following the administration of stem cell growth factor. Because systemic mastocytosis may be associated with marked fibrosis, mast cells may not be readily aspirated.

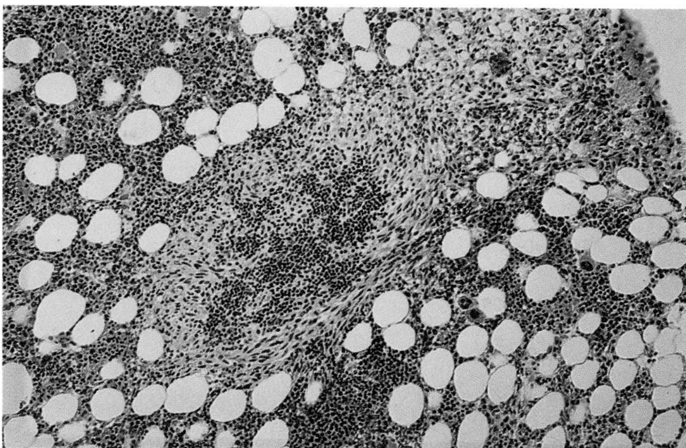

Fig. 23.58 Lesion in bone marrow from a patient with systemic mastocytosis and no evidence of urticaria pigmentosa. A central focus of well-differentiated lymphocytes is surrounded by lighter-staining mast cells.

The marrow lesions may be focal or diffuse. Focal lesions are more common and may be paratrabecular, perivascular, or randomly distributed.[318–321,326,329,331–333,335] The paratrabecular lesions frequently are marked by a margination of the infiltrate along the bone trabeculae or juxtaposition of a lesion to a bone spicule. The perivascular lesions may be associated with prominent medial and adventitial hypertrophy and collagen fibrosis. The focal lesions are variable in appearance but generally can be classified into two primary types based on cell composition: polycellular and monocellular. Both types may be observed in the same specimen. The polycellular lesions are characterized by mast cells, lymphocytes, histiocytes, eosinophils, neutrophils, fibroblasts, and endothelial cells in varying proportions; the eosinophils are frequently more numerous at the margins of the lesion. In some cases the different cell types appear to be randomly distributed; in others, the mast cells occur in a central aggregate and are surrounded by well-differentiated lymphocytes, or the mast cells encircle a focus of lymphocytes (Fig. 23.58). The mast cells in these lesions are frequently atypical and characterized by spindle shape and abundant eosinophilic cytoplasm with very fine granules. In the monomorphic lesions, the cellular composition is predominantly mast cells with only scattered lymphocytes and eosinophils (Fig. 23.59). The mast cells in these lesions may appear as intertwining bundles and vary in shape from round in cross section to spindle shaped in longitudinal cut. The cytoplasm is pale to lightly eosinophilic. The nuclei are round or oval; occasionally the nuclei have a monocytoid configuration. Nucleoli are inconspicuous, and mitotic figures are rare. Some of these lesions may resemble aggregates of histiocytes or granulomas. The marrow exclusive of the mast cell lesions is usually hypercellular or normocellular with a granulocytic hyperplasia.[318,320,329,331–333,335] The diffuse lesions are characterized by the same cell types as the focal lesions. Changes in the bone trabeculae may be present; both widening and erosion of the trabeculae may be observed. Rarely, evidence of new bone formation may be present (Fig. 23.60). Reticulin stains show varying degrees of reticulin fibrosis.

Mast cell leukemia is a very rare variant of mast cell disease. The marrow shows diffuse replacement with immature-appearing mast cells which may be hypogranular and resemble histiocytes. The

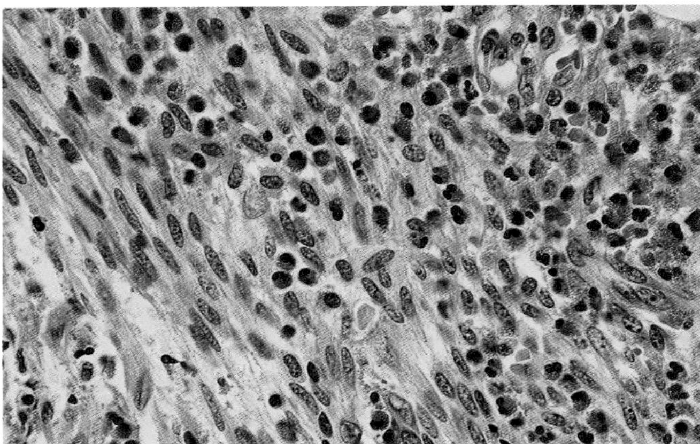

Fig. 23.59 High magnification of a marrow lesion in systemic mastocytosis. The mast cells have a spindle appearance. There are numerous interspersed eosinophils.

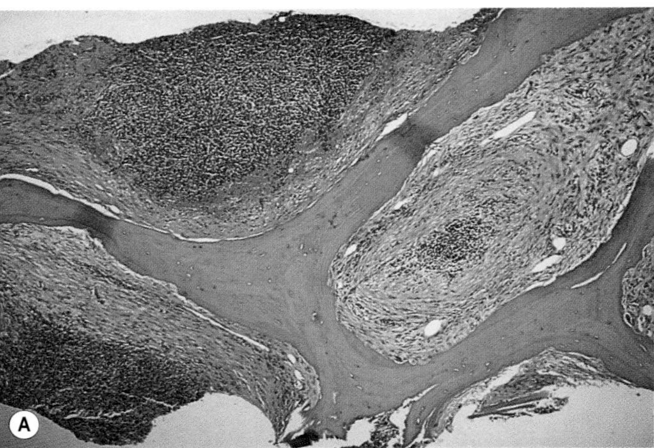

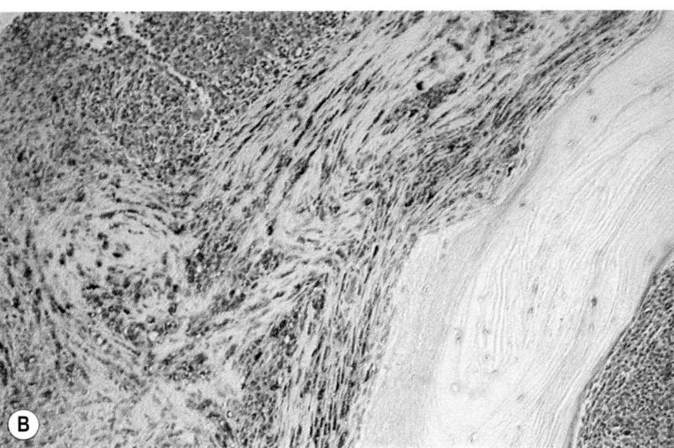

Fig. 23.60 **A**, Marrow biopsy from an adult male with systemic mastocytosis associated with a myeloproliferative disorder and no evidence of urticaria pigmentosa. There is extensive paratrabecular fibrosis and widening of bone trabeculae. The intervening marrow is markedly hypercellular, principally due to myeloid hyperplasia. Radiographic studies showed diffuse osteoblastic changes. **B**, Mast cell tryptase stain of the lesion in **A** showing numerous reactive cells.

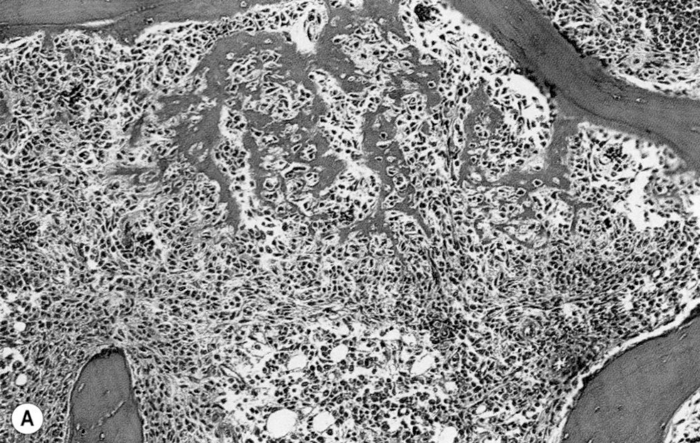

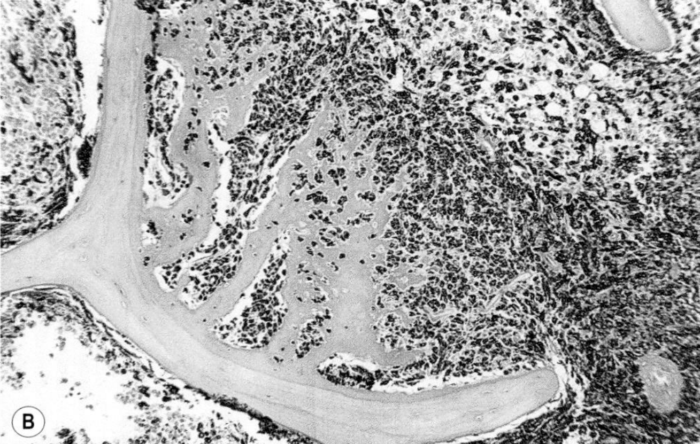

Fig. 23.61 **A**, Bone marrow biopsy from a patient with concurrent acute myeloid leukemia and systemic mastocytosis. Mast cell infiltration in this area of biopsy was associated with new bone formation. No other areas in bilateral biopsies show this finding. This was the patient's first marrow biopsy. **B**, Specimen in **A** reacted with antibody to mast cell tryptase. (**B**, Immunoperoxidase)

disease is usually nonresponsive to therapy and has a very aggressive clinical course.

There is an increased incidence of myeloproliferative disorders in patients with systemic mastocytosis: this is recognized in the WHO classification. The spectrum of disorders includes acute leukemia, myelodysplastic syndromes, and chronic myeloproliferative neoplasms[320,323,324] (Fig. 23.61). Philadelphia chromosome positive chronic myelogenous leukemia, however, is rarely encountered. Lymphoproliferative disorders have also been reported but are considerably less frequent. The chronic myeloproliferative disorder occurring with systemic mastocytosis has more the features of a chronic myelomonocytic leukemia or an unclassified chronic myeloproliferative neoplasm. Caution should be exercised in the diagnosis of a concurrent myeloproliferative process in patients with mastocytosis as it is possible that marked myeloid hyperplasia may occur as the result of cytokines produced by the mast cell proliferation.

A highly specific antibody to human mast cell tryptase that may be used on decalcified and routinely fixed and processed paraffin-embedded specimens is invaluable for identification of mast cell lesions[334] (Figs 23.60 and 23.61B). Other antibodies that react with mast cells include antibodies to α-antitrypsin and α-antichymotrypsin.[332,335,337]

Normal mast cells express CD9, CD45, CD68, and CD117; CD117 is a very sensitive but not specific marker for mast cells.[325]

Mast cells are negative for CD14 and CD15. Neoplastic mast cells also express CD2 and/or CD25. Expression of CD2 and/or CD25 is one of the minor criteria for the diagnosis of mastocytosis in the WHO criteria.[320,322]

Because the mast cells in mastocytosis may be very atypical and possess very abundant cytoplasm without evident granules or have a fibroblastic appearance, there may be considerable difficulty in recognizing the true nature of the cells. Mast cell granules react with both toluidine blue and Giemsa stains. The granules are metachromatic and appear reddish purple. Considerable variability in degree of positivity and number of positive granules may be observed among different cells. The reactivity of the granules can be enhanced in decalcified tissue by treatment of the sections with potassium permanganate followed by oxalic acid before the staining procedure. Zenker and B5 fixatives may interfere with reactivity with both Giemsa and toluidine blue stains. Mast cells also react with chloroacetate esterase in formalin-fixed tissue decalcified with EDTA; this stain may not work satisfactorily in specimens decalcified in rapid acid decalcifier or biopsy specimens processed with acid fixatives such as Zenker or B5. The metachromatic and chloroacetate reactions have been largely supplanted by immunohistochemical studies.

The differential diagnosis of mast cell lesions in the marrow includes angioimmunoblastic T-cell lymphoma, Hodgkin disease, primary myelofibrosis, and granulomatous inflammation. The eosinophilic fibrohistiocytic lesion described by Rywlin and colleagues has many of the histopathologic characteristics of mastocytosis lesions and in most instances is a form of mast cell disease.[327] The primary distinction of mastocytosis from the other disorders is based on the immunohistochemical demonstration of mast cells with antibody to mast cell tryptase. Mast cells may be increased in lymphocytic and lymphoplasmacytic lymphomas and hairy cell leukemia in marrow biopsies but are diffusely scattered among the lymphoma cells and do not form mass lesions.[336]

The treatment of systemic mast cell disease has generally been unsatisfactory with most antineoplastic agents. Fortunately for most patients with indolent systemic mastocytosis, treatment is unnecessary as the disease follows an indolent clinical course. For patients with aggressive systemic mastocytosis or mast cell leukemia, several agents including interferon alpha2b, corticosteroids, and cladribine (2-chlorodeoxyadenosine) have been used with very limited degrees of success.[330,332] Tyrosine kinase inhibitors such as imatinib (Gleevec) have been successful in occasional patients with the wild type of *KIT*. In general, mastocytosis is a disease awaiting a therapeutic breakthrough.

Because of the lack of satisfactory therapy for most patients with mastocytosis, it is important to exclude the possibility of an abnormality of *PDGFRA* or *PDGFRB* in which there may be an increase in marrow mast cells; these disorders may respond to the tyrosine kinase inhibitors with a distinctly more favorable prognosis than mastocytosis without this association. These entities are described in more detail in the section on myeloproliferative neoplasms.

Mature B-cell neoplasms

Mature B-cell neoplasms may involve the bone marrow as primary leukemias or may represent lymphomas secondarily involving the marrow. Lymphomas that frequently involve marrow and blood may present terminology problems because of their close relationship to leukemic processes: these include small B-lymphocytic lymphoma, Burkitt lymphoma, lymphoblastic lymphoma, and adult T-cell leukemia/lymphoma. The designation of these processes as leukemia or lymphoma may be arbitrary.

Chronic lymphocytic leukemia

Chronic lymphocytic leukemia (CLL), as currently defined, is a monoclonal B-cell disorder that is characterized by weak surface immunoglobulin heavy and light chain and CD20 expression, as well as expression of CD5 and CD23.[338,346,348,350–352] Cases previously diagnosed as T-cell CLL[341] are now considered to be other specific T-cell neoplasms involving the blood, including T-cell prolymphocytic leukemia and T-cell large granular lymphocytic leukemia. The diagnosis of B-cell CLL is usually established when there is a persistent absolute lymphocytosis in excess of 10×10^9/L, although the diagnosis can be made when a persistent, monoclonal absolute lymphocyte count exceeding 5×10^9/L is present with a characteristic CLL immunophenotype and in some clinical settings even when the lymphocyte count is less than 5×10^9/L.[346] Chronic lymphocytic leukemia is usually accompanied by some degree of lymphadenopathy and hepatosplenomegaly. The morphology of the proliferating lymphocytes in CLL and small lymphocytic lymphoma is the same and the two disorders are considered by the WHO as different manifestations of the same process.[351,353] The distinction between these two closely related entities is based on arbitrary criteria; if the marrow shows a pattern of infiltration by small lymphocytes, and the absolute lymphocyte count in the blood is less than 5×10^9/L, the diagnosis of small lymphocytic lymphoma is more appropriate. Small lymphocytic lymphoma may progress to blood involvement, but the magnitude of the leukocytosis does not usually reach the levels observed in CLL.

Clinical staging systems based on both laboratory and clinical features have been introduced: the higher the stage, the greater the tumor burden.[339,346,354] The system proposed by Rai et al. includes five stages: 0, lymphocytosis in blood and marrow; I, lymphocytosis and lymphadenopathy; II, lymphocytosis and hepatomegaly and/or splenomegaly; III, lymphocytosis and anemia; and IV, lymphocytosis and thrombocytopenia.[354] The system introduced by Binet has three stages: (A) no anemia, no thrombocytopenia, fewer than three lymphoid areas enlarged (cervical, axillary, and inguinal lymphadenopathy, spleen, liver); (B) no anemia, no thrombocytopenia, more than three lymphoid areas involved; and (C) anemia (Hb <10 g/dL) and/or platelet count $<100 \times 10^9$/L.[339] The higher clinical stages are generally associated with a shorter survival compared to the lower clinical stages. Additionally, high CD38 or ZAP70 expression on the lymphocytes has been reported to be associated with a significantly shorter survival than cases lacking CD38 or ZAP70 expression regardless of clinical stage.[342,343,355] Two factors have been shown to have major prognostic impact on prognosis in CLL: the mutation status of the surface immunoglobulin variable region gene, and the presence and type of genomic aberrations.[343,344] Patients in whom the leukemic cells have apparently traversed the germinal center and undergone somatic mutations of the immunoglobulin variable region gene have a significantly better prognosis than patients in whom the mutation has not occurred (pre-germinal center lymphocytes). There appears to be an inverse relationship in the majority of cases between expression of CD38 and/or ZAP70 on the lymphocytes and the mutation status. CD38 and ZAP70 expression, however, do not always correlate with mutational status[342,355] and is often difficult to measure in a reliable manner by flow cytometry; therefore, determination of the mutation status is considered the most reliable means of assessing this prognostic factor.

The detection of genomic aberrations in the lymphocyte in CLL by fluorescent in situ hybridization has shown significant differences in survival patterns. Patients with 17p, 11q22–23, and 6q deletions appear to have a worse outcome than patients with trisomy 12, normal karyotype, and 13q14 deletion. Patients with 17p– have the shortest survival and patients with 13q– have the longest survival.[344] *TP53* abnormalities (located at 17p) in B-CLL have been associated with an excess of prolymphocytes and poor prognosis,[347] while patients with trisomy 12 often have an atypical or mixed morphology.

Histopathologic staging of B-CLL is based on the pattern of involvement in bone marrow sections.[352,356] Five possible patterns are generally recognized: focal, diffuse, interstitial, focal and interstitial, and focal and diffuse (Fig. 23.62). In small lymphocytic lymphoma, the focal pattern is the most common, whereas in CLL the pattern is usually interstitial, mixed interstitial and focal, or diffuse. Patients with focal, interstitial, or a combination of focal and interstitial involvement are predominantly in low clinical stages. The diffuse or focal and diffuse patterns generally occur in patients with advanced clinical stages. The diffuse pattern of marrow involvement has been found to have adverse prognostic significance in several studies.[349,352,357]

Marrow biopsies from approximately 25% of patients with B-CLL demonstrate a slight increase in reticulin fibers.

In some patients with B-CLL, there is a dedifferentiation or transformation of the proliferating cell type; this usually occurs late in the course of the disease in less than 5% of the patients and has been referred to as 'prolymphocytoid' transformation.[345] This dedifferentiation is distinct from B prolymphocytic leukemia which is a de novo process with different morphologic features. In these patients, the marrow infiltration may contain foci of prolymphocytoid lymphocytes and paraimmunoblasts (Fig. 23.63). The prolymphocytoid lymphocytes have a moderate amount of basophilic to amphophilic cytoplasm, coarsely reticular nuclear chromatin, and relatively prominent single nucleoli. The paraimmunoblasts are larger, with more abundant cytoplasm, more dispersed nuclear chromatin, and frequently a single prominent eosinophilic nucleolus. These foci may be circumscribed by more well-differentiated lymphocytes and are similar to the immature foci or proliferation centers noted in the lymph nodes of some patients with this process[356] (Fig. 23.64). Difficulties may occur in distinguishing foci of transformation in CLL from follicular lymphoma. An important feature in CLL is the residual population of well-differentiated lymphocytes. In most instances, examination of the blood and marrow smears aids considerably in distinguishing these processes, as well as immunophenotyping studies demonstrating aberrant CD5 expression in CLL as opposed to the common expression of CD10 on the B cells of follicular lymphoma. Concurrence of CLL and other B-cell neoplasms, including multiple myeloma and hairy cell leukemia, has been reported.[340]

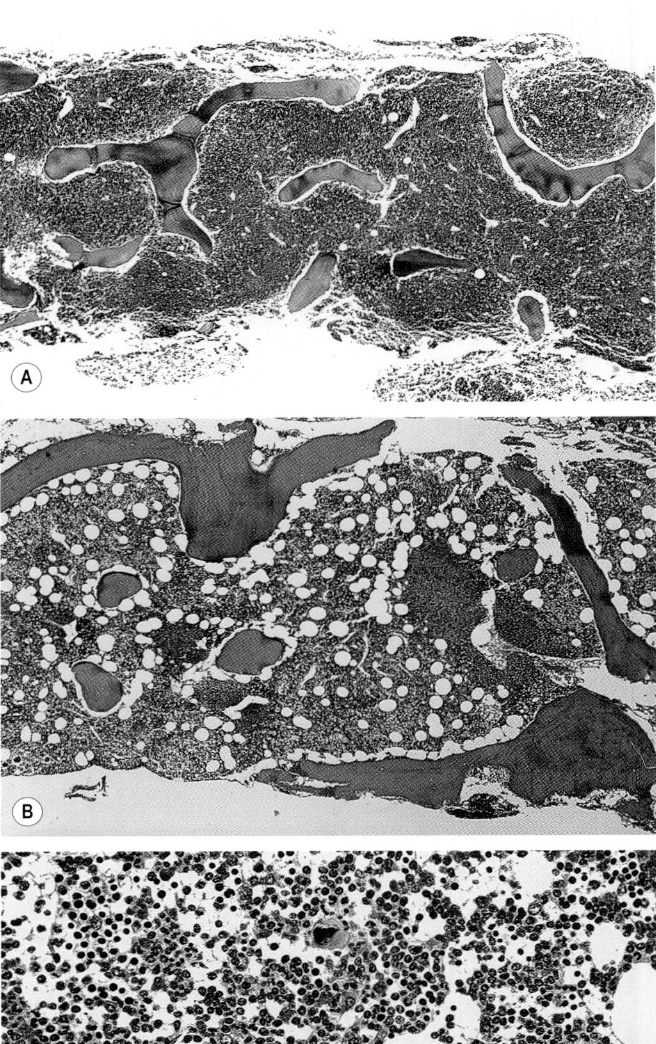

Fig. 23.62 **A**, Marrow biopsy from a patient with CLL showing diffuse pattern of involvement. The small lymphocytes completely replace normal marrow cells. **B**, Marrow biopsy from a patient with CLL with focal involvement. Leukemic cells occur in relatively well-demarcated foci, which are randomly distributed and surrounded by normal-appearing marrow. **C**, Marrow section from a patient with CLL illustrating an interstitial pattern of involvement; overall marrow architecture is preserved.

Richter syndrome

Richter syndrome is the occurrence of an aggressive lymphoma, usually diffuse large B-cell lymphoma, in a patient with a prior history of B-CLL[359,360,362,365,368,370,371] or another low-grade B-cell lymphoproliferative disorder. The reported incidence in B-CLL ranges from less than 1% to 10%.[371] The syndrome is usually characterized by an abrupt change in clinical course with the onset of fever, weight loss, localized adenopathy, dysglobulinemia, and histopathologic evidence of an aggressive lymphoma frequently containing multinucleated giant cells. A Hodgkin type variant has been described,[358] but is less common than diffuse large B cell lymphoma, should show the typical background of classical Hodgkin lymphoma, and should not be confused with cases of CLL with admixed Reed–Sternberg cells.[367] The locus of the lymphomatous process is not restricted to hematopoietic organs.[359] A high incidence of lytic bone lesions has been reported.[371] The bone marrow may be involved by the aggressive lymphoma; evidence of CLL and the supervening lymphoma may be present in the same biopsy specimen (Fig. 23.65). The blood smear usually shows no involvement by the non-CLL cells and there may be lymphocytopenia. This

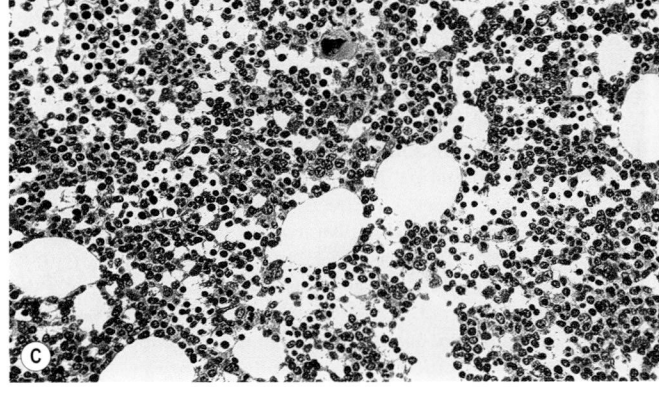

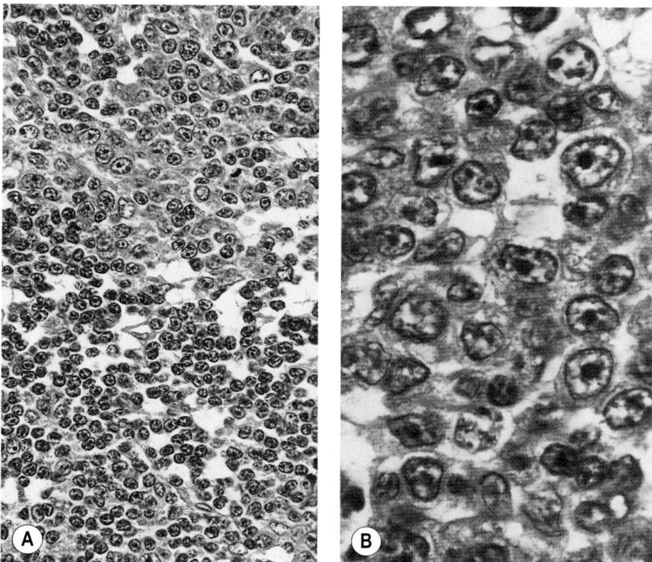

Fig. 23.63 **A**, Marrow biopsy from an adult female with a 4-year history of untreated B-cell chronic lymphocytic leukemia. There are two morphologic populations of lymphocytes; the lower portion of the figure is predominantly small lymphocytes; the upper portion is predominantly prolymphocytoid lymphocytes and paraimmunoblasts. **B**, High magnification of the upper area of the specimen illustrating the prominent prolymphocytoid lymphocytes and paraimmunoblasts with very prominent, usually single, nucleoli.

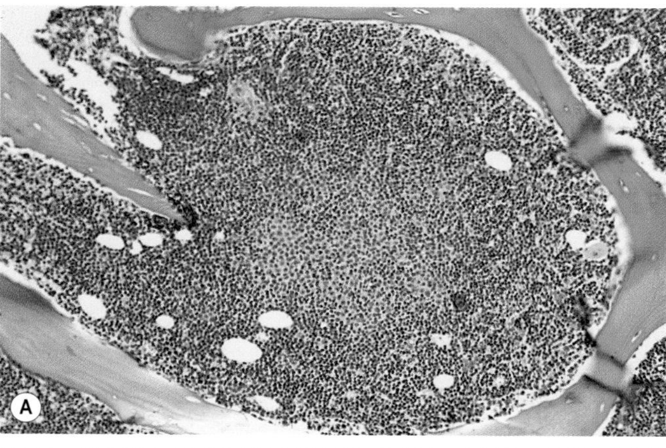

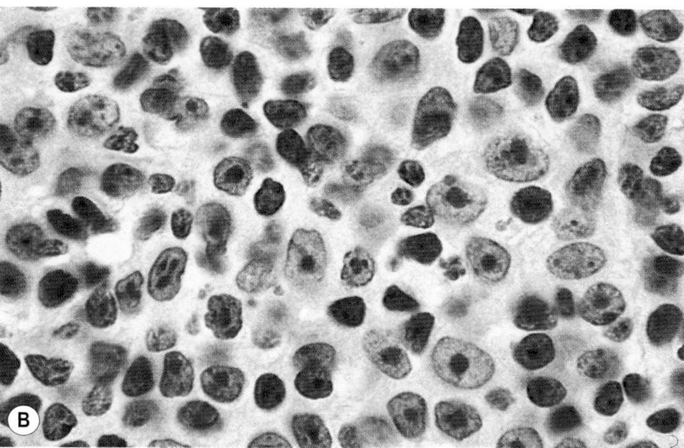

Fig. 23.64 **A**, Marrow biopsy illustrating a proliferation center in a patient with B-CLL. **B**, High magnification of the central portion of the proliferation center with prominent prolymphocytoid lymphocytes and paraimmunoblasts.

transformation is marked by an aggressive clinical course and rapid deterioration. The term Richter transformation has been used to describe a somewhat broader spectrum of pathologic findings in patients with B-CLL who present with a similar clinical evolution.[361]

The biologic events resulting in Richter transformation are not completely understood, but a dedifferentiation or transformation of the well-differentiated lymphocyte has been suggested.[363,369] This theory is supported by evidence in some cases in which an identical clone has been detected in the patient's CLL as in the transformed lymphoma (Fig. 23.66).[364,370] This clonal relation appears to occur more commonly in the unmutated type of CLL, and instances in which the lymphocytes of the CLL and the cells of the second lymphoma are different clones are more commonly associated with mutated type of CLL.[366]

Prolymphocytic leukemia

Prolymphocytic leukemia (PL), initially described by Galton et al.,[376] is a very rare disease that occurs primarily in older individuals and is characterized by a predominant proliferation of lymphocytes referred to as prolymphocytes. The disorder is distinct from chronic lymphocytic leukemia and prolymphocytoid transformation of CLL. Approximately 80% of the initially reported cases of this type of leukemia were of B-cell origin, the remainder of T-cell type.[377] The exact ratio of B- to T-cell prolymphocytic leukemia is difficult to determine because of the low frequency of both disorders and the reclassification of many of the B-cell disorders into other B-cell lymphoma categories. The lymphocyte count in PL of either B or T type is usually moderately to markedly increased; the

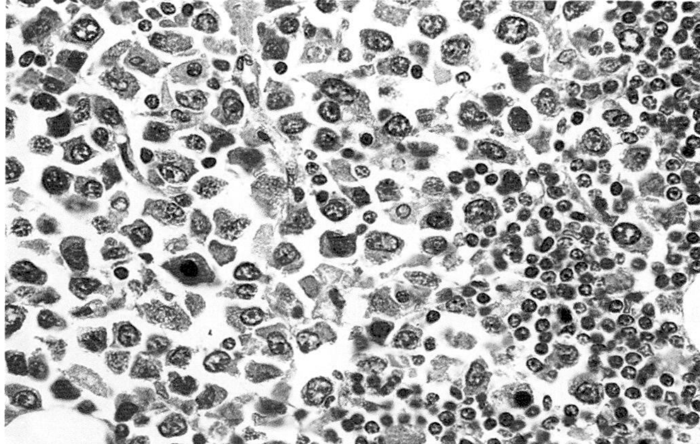

Fig. 23.65 Bone marrow trephine biopsy from a patient with a history of CLL who developed a pleomorphic lymphoma (B-immunoblastic lymphoma) and a clinical picture typical of Richter syndrome. Biopsy contains two distinct cell populations, small lymphocytes, and large pleomorphic cells, some of which are multinucleated.

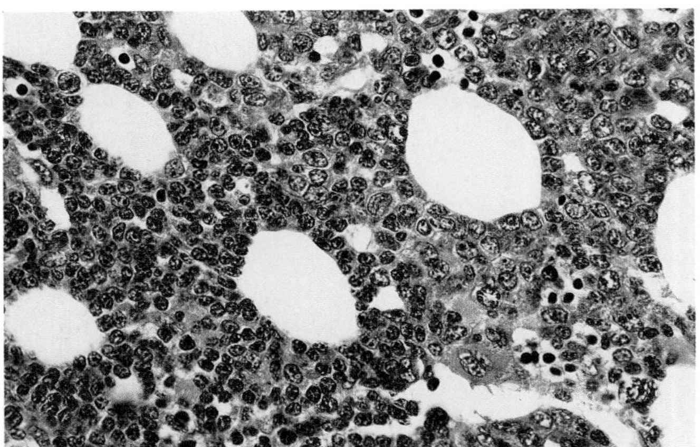

Fig. 23.66 Marrow biopsy from an adult male with a 9-year history of B-CLL. The patient had recent onset of fever, night sweats, myalgia, and axillary, cervical, and inguinal adenopathy prior to this biopsy. A population of small lymphocytes is at lower left. Burkitt lymphoma cells predominate at upper right. Blood and marrow smears contained two lymphocyte populations: small well-differentiated lymphocytes and Burkitt lymphoma cells. Cytogenetic studies of the marrow specimen showed t(8;22)(q24;q11) cytogenetic abnormality.

number of prolymphocytes in the blood usually exceeds 55% of lymphocytes and may be more than 90%.

B-PL is a clonal B-cell disorder that may lack expression of CD5 and/or CD23 and does not include cases of transformed CLL, CLL with increased prolymphocytes, or cases with cyclin D1 expression or evidence of t(11;14)(q13;q32).[374] The patients with B-cell PL usually have massive splenomegaly without prominent peripheral lymphadenopathy.[378,379] The prolymphocytes in B-PL are more uniform in appearance than the prolymphocytoid cells in prolymphocytoid transformation of B-CLL. In B-PL the prolymphocytes are medium to large in size, with a moderate amount of basophilic cytoplasm. There is usually a single prominent nucleolus. The marrow infiltration is usually diffusely interstitial. Mitotic activity is reported as low, although cases with increased mitotic activity have been observed.[372,381] B-PL is usually marked by an aggressive clinical course; occasionally patients have a prolonged survival. The leukemic phase of the blastic variant of mantle cell lymphoma may be characterized by large lymphocytes with prominent nucleoli;[380,382] it can be distinguished from prolymphocytic leukemia by cytogenetic and molecular studies for t(11;14)(q13;q32).[373]

A very uncommon variant of B-CLL intermediate between typical B-CLL and B-PL and referred to as chronic lymphocytic leukemia/prolymphocytic leukemia has been described; it is distinguished by the presence of 11–55% prolymphocytoid lymphocytes in the blood.[378,379] Typical B-CLL has less than 11% prolymphocytes in the blood; B-PL is distinguished by more than 55% prolymphocytes. The degree of splenomegaly in patients with chronic lymphocytic leukemia/prolymphocytic leukemia is disproportionate to the degree of lymphadenopathy. Two major clinical patterns are described in this variant: one is characterized by a course similar to typical CLL and the other by a more rapidly progressive clinical evolution. The distinction of B-CLL/PL from prolymphocytoid transformation of B-CLL may be very difficult unless prior material more typical of CLL is available (which would suggest transformation). Leukemic mantle cell lymphoma may resemble CLL/PL and because of its more aggressive clinical course it is important to exclude the possibility of leukemic mantle cell lymphoma when findings suggest CLL/PL.

T-PL has a somewhat variable presentation. Patients often have hepatosplenomegaly and lymphadenopathy, and 20% have skin lesions. While the absolute lymphocyte count is usually over 100 × 10^9/L, some cases may show only a modest elevation.[375,377] Unlike B-PL, the lymphocytes of T-PL may not have an unusually prominent nucleolus. Such cases are often termed small cell variant of T-PL and this type of T-PL was considered as T-CLL in the past. Marrow infiltration may be modest with very substantial sparing of normal myeloid cells. T-PL is a clonal T-cell disorder that may show weak CD3 expression and is usually CD4 positive. Increased expression of CD52 and T-cell leukemia 1 (TCL-1) is characteristic of the disorder. The majority of cases of T-PL have inv(14)(q11;q32) or t(14;14)(q11;q32).

Hairy cell leukemia

Hairy cell leukemia is a clonal chronic lymphoproliferative disorder of B-cell origin that is manifest primarily in blood, marrow, and spleen. There is a male predominance.[384,391,392,405,409] The age range is 20–80 years with a median of approximately 50 years. The patients generally have cytopenias or pancytopenia and splenomegaly without prominent peripheral lymphadenopathy; there is usually an associated monocytopenia. The majority of patients present with leukopenia and only occasional leukemic cells in the blood. Some 5–10% of patients have white blood cell counts exceeding 10 × 10^9/L; the hairy cells usually comprise the majority of the blood leukocytes in these patients.

The typical hairy cell measures 10–14 μm. The clear to lightly basophilic cytoplasm is variable in amount. The surface of the cell is marked by numerous delicate and broad projections; this finding is particularly striking in specimens examined by phase and electron microscopy.[398] Vacuoles and occasionally delicate azurophilic granules may be identified in the cytoplasm. The nucleus is oval, folded, or indented; the chromatin is coarsely reticular, and nucleoli are inconspicuous.

Aspiration biopsy of the marrow in patients with hairy cell leukemia is unsuccessful in 30–50% of cases because of increased reticulin fibrosis.[392,405] The interstitial pattern of marrow infiltration in trephine sections is virtually diagnostic in most patients.[385,386,408,414] The marrow in the majority of patients is hypercellular; in 10–15% of patients the involved marrow is hypocellular.[400] The involvement may be diffuse or partial; the diffuse type is more common (Fig. 23.67). Leukemic infiltrates in partial involvement are irregular in outline and poorly demarcated from the normal marrow cells. In the very early stages of the disease, partial involvement may take the form of relatively small, indistinctly outlined foci of leukemic cells. In formalin-fixed tissue, there is frequently a halo-like effect or clear area around the nucleus because of the abundant cytoplasm. The cell borders have an interlocking appearance. With some fixatives, such as Zenker, the cytoplasm of the hairy cells is retracted with a resultant loosely structured appearance. The loosely structured appearance and widely spaced nuclei in hairy cell leukemia contrast with the marrow infiltrates in the lymphocytic lymphomas and CLL in which the nuclei of the cells are in close apposition. The nuclear chromatin of the hairy cells is relatively fine. Nucleoli are distinct but not usually prominent and mitotic figures are infrequent. In an occasional case, the hairy cells have a spindled or fusiform appearance and may resemble the marrow lesions in systemic mastocytosis (Fig. 23.68). A morphologic variant with hyperlobulated nuclei resembling T-cell lymphoma has been described.[394] Marrow uninvolved by the leukemic process may be hypocellular or hypercellular. Morphologic subtypes of

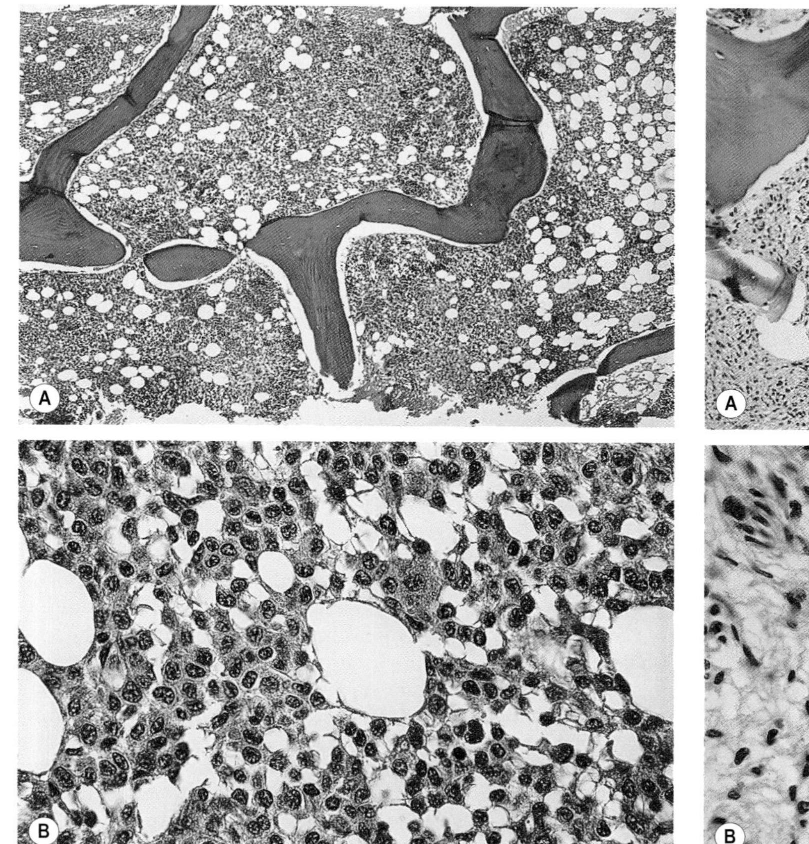

Fig. 23.67 **A**, Bone marrow section from a patient with extensive replacement by hairy cell leukemia; scattered foci of normal hematopoiesis are present. **B**, High magnification of specimen in **A**. Hairy cells are loosely spaced, in contrast to aggregates of lymphocytes in chronic lymphocytic leukemia and small lymphocyte lymphoma. Hairy cells have a relatively abundant, lightly eosinophilic cytoplasm. Many of their nuclei are folded or irregular in outline. Nucleoli are inconspicuous and mitotic figures rare. The halo effect around nuclei, characteristic of formalin-fixed tissue, is not prominent in this specimen fixed with Zenker acetic acid.

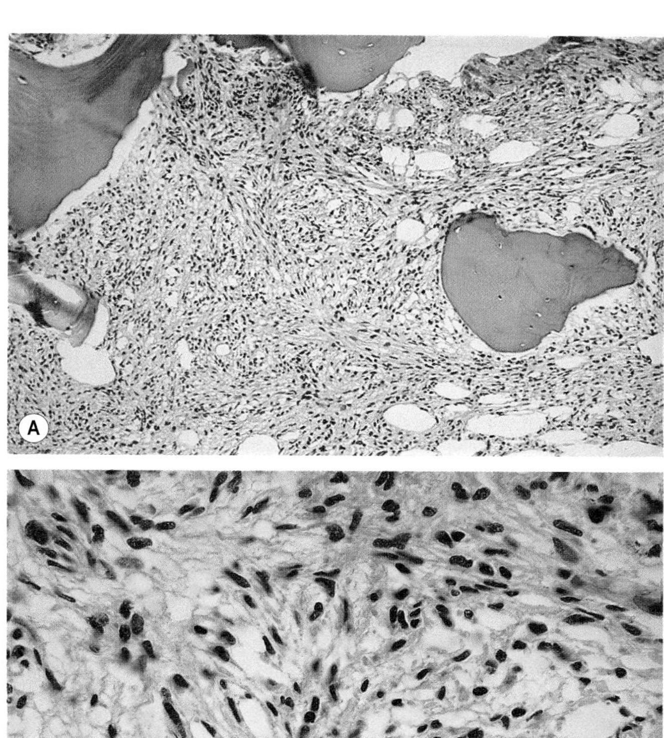

Fig. 23.68 **A**, Marrow biopsy from a patient with the stromal variant of hairy cell leukemia. **B**, High magnification of the biopsy in **A**. Many leukemia cells are elongated or spindle shaped.

hairy cell leukemia based on histopathology have been reported to have prognostic significance.[383] Normal-appearing mast cells may be increased.

Reticulin stain shows increased deposition of thickened reticulin fibers in the areas of the infiltrates; the reticulin fibers often appear to encircle individual cells. The reticulin fibers frequently extend into the adjacent normal-appearing marrow.

Hairy cells express light chain-restricted cytoplasmic and surface immunoglobulin and pan-B-cell antibodies, including CD19, CD20, CD22, DBA44, CD79a, and PAX5, but not CD79b;[391,411] CD20 (L26) and DBA44 are of considerable aid in evaluating the extent of the leukemic infiltrate and in assessing the effects of chemotherapy in paraffin-embedded biopsy sections[393] (Fig. 23.69). In addition, they express CD11c, which is also expressed on myeloid cells, CD25, interleukin-2 receptor, CD103, and annexin A1.[390] They are negative for CD5, a T-cell antigen, and CD23, which are expressed on the lymphocytes in the majority of cases of B-CLL, but a subset of cases express CD10.[388] Hairy cells also contain tartrate-resistant acid phosphatase (TRAP),[396] although this finding alone

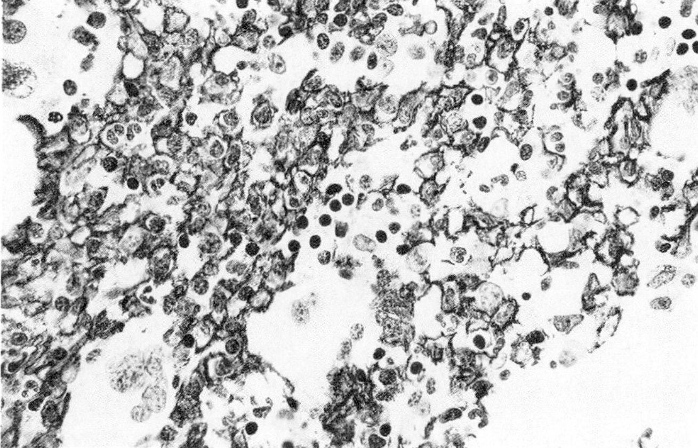

Fig. 23.69 Bone marrow biopsy from a patient with hairy cell leukemia reacted with antibody to CD20 (L26). Reactivity accentuates the leukemic infiltrate. Scattered normal myeloid cells, principally erythroid precursors, are present. (Immunoperoxidase)

by immunohistochemistry is not entirely specific and paraffin section detection of annexin A1 expression on B cells is considered more specific for hairy cell leukemia.[390]

Rarely, hairy cell leukemia may focally involve the skeleton as a painful localized destructive lesion. This usually occurs in a patient with an established diagnosis; more rarely, hairy cell leukemia may present as a localized skeletal lesion as the initial and only manifestation of the disease.[389,395,399,401] These lesions occur principally in the upper portion of the femurs. Although the majority of these localized lesions are osteolytic, osteoblastic lesions may also occur. The localized lesions appear to respond to the purine analogs 2-deoxycoformycin and 2-deoxyadenosine and to radiation.

Treatment of hairy cell leukemia with the purine analogs, often coupled with rituximab or other monoclonal antibodies, results in durable complete or partial remissions in the majority of cases.[407,409,410,413] The bone marrow biopsies from these patients generally show a return to normal marrow hematopoiesis. As noted, the recognition of residual leukemia is facilitated by the use of pan-B-cell monoclonal antibodies reactive in paraffin-embedded biopsies; anti-CD20, DBA44, and T-bet are particularly good antibodies for this purpose.[393,397,412] Treatment with the interferons frequently results in characteristic marrow changes with some evidence of residual leukemia.[404] Approximately 0.25% of cases of hairy cell leukemia develop abdominal lymphadenopathy as demonstrated by CT studies. The incidence is higher in patients who relapse after previously successful therapy or have long-standing disease. The development of abdominal adenopathy may be associated with resistant disease and with the appearance of large hairy cells in both the bone marrow and the enlarged lymph node. This constellation of clinical and morphologic findings has been interpreted as a type of transformation.[403]

Hairy cell leukemia variant

Hairy cell leukemia variant is a lymphoproliferative disorder usually presenting with a marked leukocytosis and was originally restricted to cases with lymphocytes with morphologic characteristics intermediate between hairy cells and prolymphocytes[384,387,402] (Fig. 23.70). In those cases, the cells are large with basophilic cytoplasm with stellate projections and relatively prominent nucleoli. Other morphologic variants, including cases with blastic or convoluted nuclear features, as well as cases showing immunophenotypic variations, are not included in this category which is felt to be biologically distinct from typical hairy cell leukemia.[406] The disease is very rare and occurs primarily in older individuals. In contrast to typical hairy cell leukemia, there is no associated neutropenia and monocytopenia. The cells may be TRAP positive. The cells usually express CD11c but are negative for CD25; they express CD103 and annexin A1 less commonly than typical cases of hairy cell leukemia.[402] The marrow shows a diffuse interstitial pattern of infiltration similar to typical hairy cell leukemia. The pattern of splenic infiltration is similar to hairy cell leukemia, with a predominantly red pulp involvement. Hairy cell leukemia variant, unlike typical hairy cell leukemia, does not respond to interferon alpha or purine analogs, but still has a relatively indolent clinical course.

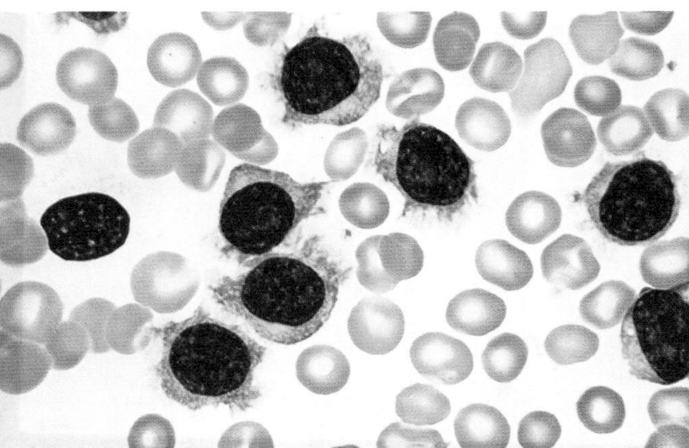

Fig. 23.70 Hairy cell leukemia variant. Several lymphoid cells in the blood smear of an adult male with markedly elevated leukocyte count. The hairy cell variant lymphocytes are large with a moderate amount of basophilic cytoplasm with stellate projections. The nuclei of several cells contain variably prominent nucleoli. (Wright–Giemsa)

Splenic marginal zone lymphoma

Splenic marginal zone lymphoma (SMZL) is a clonal proliferation of small B lymphocytes with clinical and hematologic features that may resemble hairy cell leukemia.[418,423,426,427] When it involves the blood, it often shows morphologic features that have also been described as splenic lymphoma with villous lymphocytes (SLVL). The disease shows no sex predilection and usually occurs in adults over 50 years of age. With blood involvement, there is a slight to moderate lymphocytosis; the leukocyte count is less than 25×10^9/L in the majority of patients. Anemia and thrombocytopenia are present in approximately 50% of cases with blood involvement. Most patients have marked splenomegaly.[418]

The lymphocytes in the blood often have short villous projections that may have a polar distribution. Villi may not be present on all of the lymphoma cells and there may be considerable variation in the appearance of the cells. Some have a distinct but not prominent nucleolus (Fig. 23.71A). Plasmacytoid lymphocytes may be present.

The lymphocytes express moderate to intense surface immunoglobulin and pan-B-lymphocyte markers, including CD19, CD22, and CD24,[423,425] while they are usually negative for CD5, CD10, CD43, BCL6, cyclin D1, and annexin A1. Many cases have a low IgM monoclonal gammopathy.[427] Chromosome 7q31–32 deletion is found in approximately 40% of cases; trisomy 3 is present in 17% of cases.[423] Cases of SMZL do not show evidence of t(14;18) of follicular lymphoma, t(11;14) of mantle cell lymphoma, or translocations of nonsplenic, extranodal marginal zone B-cell lymphomas.

Virtually all patients with SMZL have some degree of marrow involvement. The degree and pattern of marrow involvement vary substantially; the pattern may be focal nonparatrabecular, focal paratrabecular, interstitial, diffuse or intrasinusoidal; there may be a predominance of one pattern in an individual case but mixed patterns are common[415,416,419,420,422,424] (Fig. 23.71B,C). The lymphoma cells may be predominantly small lymphocytes or an admixture of small lymphocytes and scattered large lymphocytes with relatively abundant cytoplasm, slightly dispersed chromatin, and variably prominent nucleoli. Mitotic figures are usually sparse. Some degree of plasma cell proliferation may be present. Occasionally, foci of lymphoma with remnants of germinal centers may be found (Fig. 23.72).

The spleen shows a characteristic biphasic pattern of white pulp B cells, with the central white pulp composed of small cells with scant cytoplasm surrounded by an outer zone of medium-sized cells with irregular nuclei and abundant cytoplasm.[423] Aggregates of clonal B cells often infiltrate into the red pulp.

Patients with SMZL generally have a prolonged clinical course. Splenectomy is frequently beneficial in patients with severe anemia,

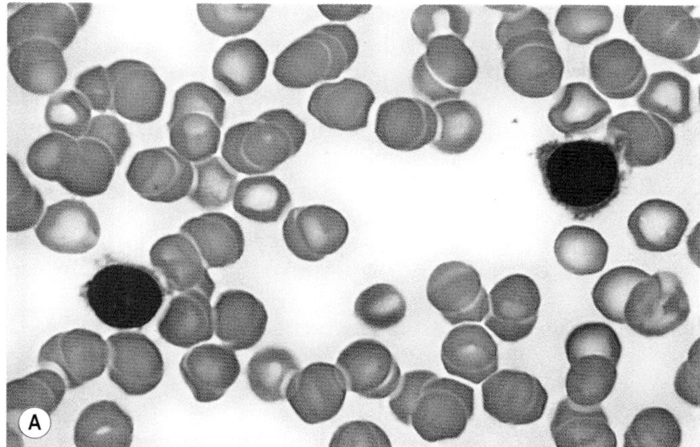

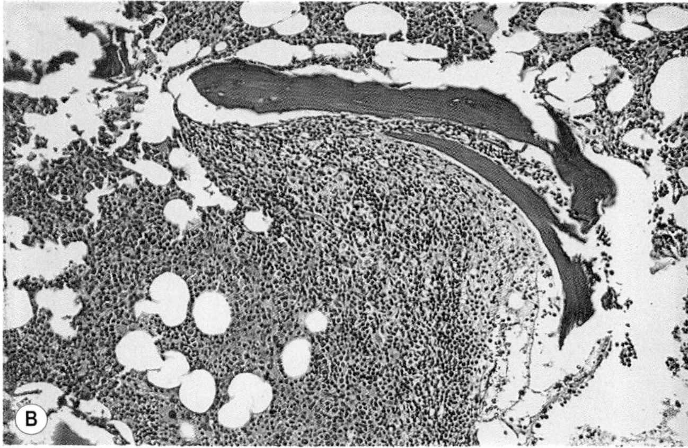

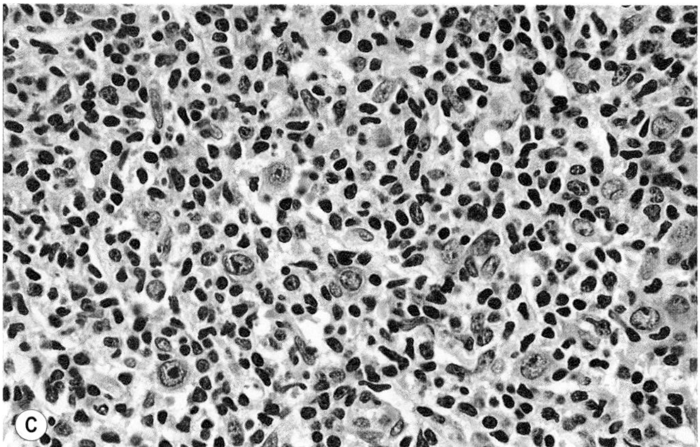

Fig. 23.71 **A**, Lymphocytes in blood smear from an adult male with splenic marginal zone lymphoma (SMZL) with villous lymphocytes. The cytoplasm of two of the lymphocytes has small villous projections. Nuclear chromatin is coarse. There are distinct but not prominent nucleoli. **B**, Bone marrow biopsy from a patient with SMZL showing a paratrabecular, poorly demarcated aggregate of lymphocytes. **C**, High magnification of a lesion from a patient with SMZL showing a predominant population of small lymphocytes with scattered large cells with abundant cytoplasm and prominent nucleoli. (**A**, Wright–Giemsa)

neutropenia, and thrombocytopenia. Rare cases have recurred as diffuse large B-cell lymphoma at other sites.[417]

A small number of patients with SMZL and concurrent hepatitis C infection have undergone remission of the lymphoma with antiviral therapy.[421]

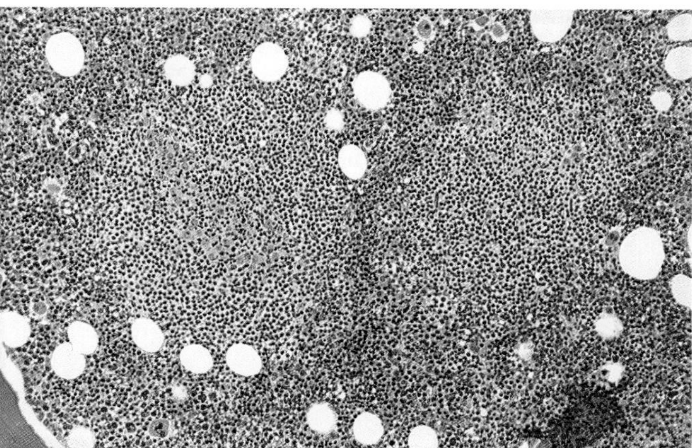

Fig. 23.72 Bone marrow biopsy from a patient with SMZL illustrating two well-circumscribed foci of lymphocytes. The lesion on the left contains a central area suggesting remnants of a germinal center with several centroblast-like cells.

Burkitt lymphoma/leukemia

Burkitt lymphoma presents with marrow involvement in 15–30% of patients.[428,430–432,434] In the WHO classification of hematopoietic tumors, the FAB designation of acute lymphoblastic leukemia L3 has been replaced by combining the leukemic presentation with Burkitt lymphoma, reflecting the fundamental identities of these two different manifestations of the same process.[429,433] A leukemic presentation is frequently associated with Burkitt lymphoma involving the ileocecal region of the small bowel with a t(8;14)(q24;q32) or variant chromosome translocation, (t(2;8)(q11;q24), t(8;22)(q24;q11)) and is TdT negative.[428,431,433] The diagnostic terminology used in these cases should reflect the status of the marrow and blood. If tumor cells are present in the blood and the marrow is diffusely replaced, Burkitt leukemia is an appropriate designation. If few or no tumor cells are present in the blood, and the marrow is partially involved with substantial sparing of normal hematopoiesis, a diagnosis of lymphoma is more appropriate. The therapeutic approach in these two situations is the same. Marrow involvement in Burkitt lymphoma is usually characterized by diffuse infiltration of the interstitium with some preservation of adipose tissue although small focal lesions may occur. The 'starry sky' appearance characteristic of lymph nodes in Burkitt lymphoma is infrequently present in bone marrow biopsies. In contrast to the majority of cases of B-cell precursor ALL in which mitotic figures are sparse, there is prominent mitotic activity in Burkitt lymphoma/leukemia. Burkitt lymphoma is a mature B-cell neoplasm, expressing CD20 and clonal surface immunoglobulin light chains as well as CD10. In contrast to B-ALL, it does not express CD34 or TdT.

Non-Hodgkin lymphoma

B-cell lymphoma

The incidence of marrow involvement in non-Hodgkin lymphoma at the time of initial diagnosis, other than those previously described with a leukemic presentation, varies with the different histopathologic subtypes; the incidence in aggregate for all types ranges from 40% to 55% in most of the larger studies of adults.[445] The incidence is higher in the low-grade lymphomas than in many of the high-grade lymphomas. Approximately 60–70% of the cases of follicular center cell lymphoma have marrow involvement at the time of initial diagnosis, compared to 25–33% for large cell lymphomas. Splenic marginal zone B-cell lymphoma is reported to have a very high incidence of involvement, approximately 80–90%; a similarly high incidence of involvement has been observed in mantle cell lymphoma.[440,441,469,477] Marrow involvement in mucosa-associated lymphoid tissue (MALT) lymphoma was reported in approximately 20% of cases in one study.[473] The incidence of marrow involvement in peripheral T-cell or node-based T-cell lymphoma varies from 30% to 70% in different series.[454,455,458] Blood involvement may occur with all types of lymphoma.[436,440,451,462,463,472]

The extent of lymphomatous infiltration varies considerably; it is less than 30% in more than half of cases with involvement.[435,450,451] In general, the small lymphocytic and follicular center cell lymphomas are characterized by substantial sparing of normal bone marrow.

The pattern of marrow involvement may be diffuse, focal paratrabecular, focal nonparatrabecular, interstitial, intrasinusoidal, and rarely intravascular (Figs 23.73–23.80); uncommonly, marrow lesions of follicular lymphoma are characterized by recapitulation of the neoplastic follicle as found in the lymph node[435,437,442,448,451,452,465,468,474] (Figs 23.76 and 23.77). The diffuse and focal nonparatrabecular patterns may occur with all types of lymphoma of both B- and T-cell type. The focal paratrabecular pattern occurs principally but not exclusively in the follicular center cell lymphomas; follicular lymphomas may also involve the marrow in a focal nonparatrabecular pattern. The marrow biopsies from patients with mantle cell lymphoma and splenic marginal zone B-cell lymphoma may also show both focal paratrabecular and nonparatrabecular lesions.[435,475] The infiltrate in an occasional case of mantle cell lymphoma and splenic marginal zone B-cell lymphoma may contain remnants of benign germinal centers (Fig. 23.78B).[479] Splenic marginal zone B-cell lymphoma and hepatosplenic T-cell lymphoma may occur principally in an intrasinusoidal pattern[457] (Fig. 23.80).

The interstitial pattern of involvement, in which the lymphoma cells infiltrate the interstitium of the marrow with preservation of the overall marrow architecture with some sparing of normal hematopoiesis, may occur with all types of non-Hodgkin lymphoma. The bone marrow in this type of involvement may be deceptively normal in appearance at low magnification and emphasizes the importance of examination of marrow biopsies at high magnification when evaluating for lymphoma involvement

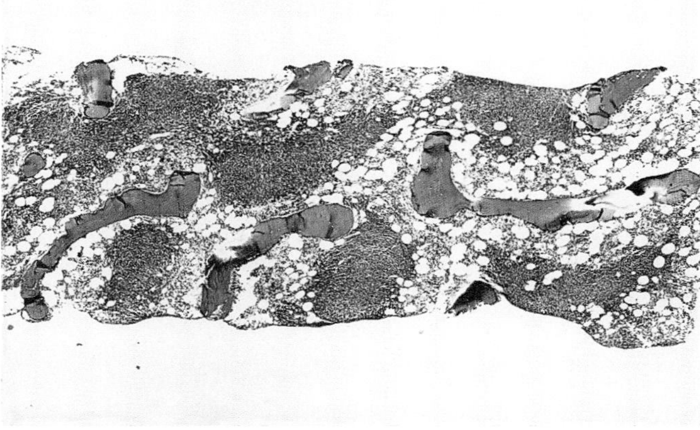

Fig. 23.73 Several focal aggregates of lymphocytes in marrow in a patient with small lymphocytic lymphoma. Foci of lymphocytes vary in size and have irregular, poorly circumscribed outlines.

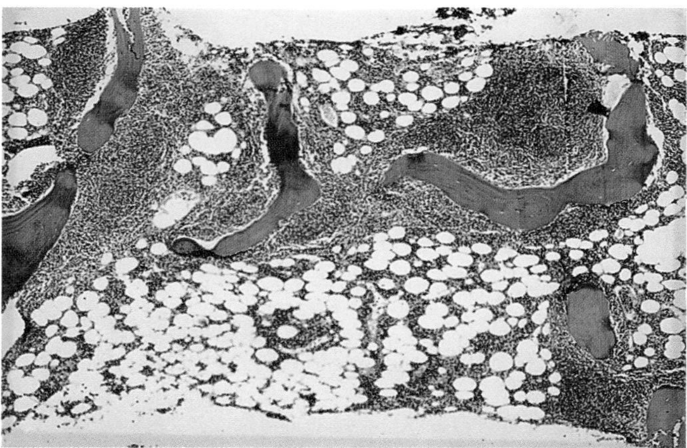

Fig. 23.74 Bone marrow section from a patient with follicular center cell lymphoma illustrating the prominent paratrabecular distribution of the infiltrate.

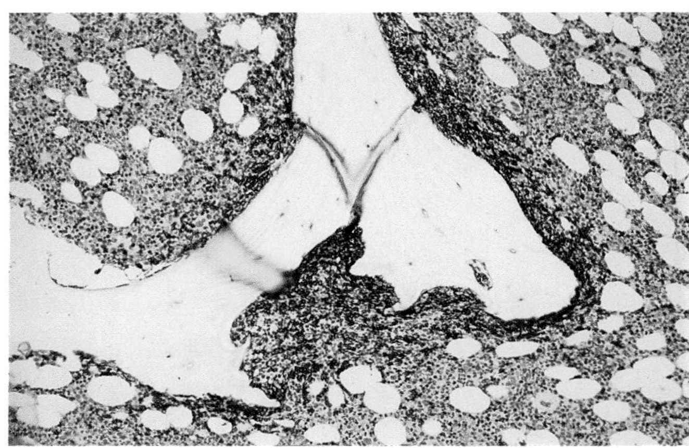

Fig. 23.75 Marrow from a patient with marrow involvement by follicular center cell lymphoma with prominent paratrabecular involvement reacted with antibody to CD20 (L26). The infiltrate is accentuated by CD20 antibody. (Immunoperoxidase)

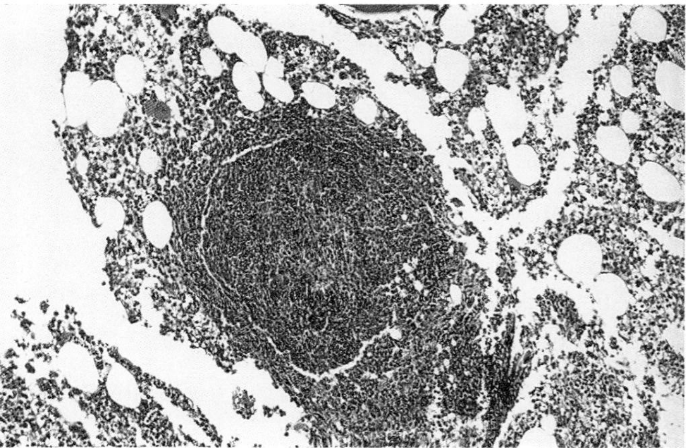

Fig. 23.76 Marrow biopsy from a patient with follicular center cell lymphoma with focal paratrabecular and nonparatrabecular involvement. A few of the nonparatrabecular foci, as illustrated, recapitulate neoplastic follicles. Amorphous eosinophilic proteinaceous debris is deposited in the central portion of the lesion.

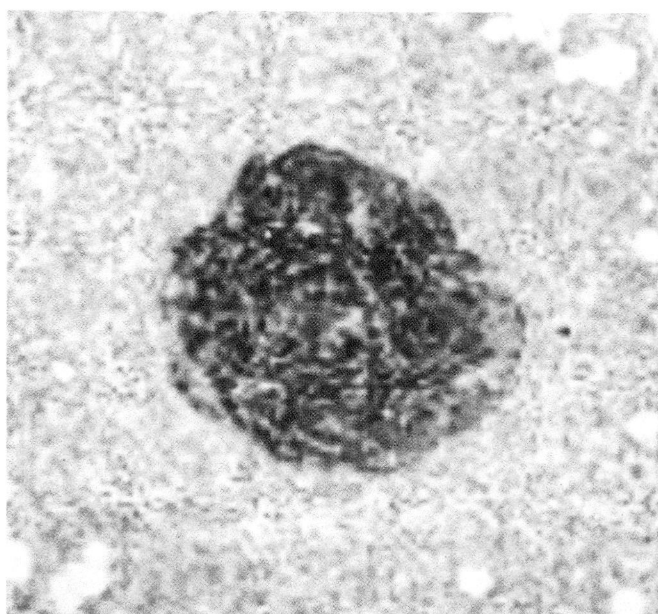

Fig. 23.77 Neoplastic follicle in marrow reacted with antibodies to CD21 and BCL2. The dendritic cells express CD21 and the lymphocytes express CD20. (Immunoperoxidase)
(Reproduced from Am J Clin Pathol ©2002 American Society for Clinical Pathology. Reprinted with permission)

(Fig. 23.79). This pattern of infiltration may be present at the time of initial diagnosis or in patients who have received chemotherapy. Interstitial involvement in the more aggressive lymphomas may be accompanied by considerable depletion of normal hematopoietic cells.

The intrasinusoidal pattern of involvement may be particularly difficult to identify in routinely stained sections, even in well-prepared specimens. The use of immunohistochemistry has been particularly important in recognizing this type of lesion, which appears to occur most frequently with splenic marginal zone B-cell lymphoma and gamma/delta T-cell lymphoma, in which it may be the predominant pattern of involvement (Fig. 23.80). It may be observed in other types of lymphoma, usually combined with other patterns.[457]

The follicular pattern of follicular lymphoma as observed in lymph nodes is uncommonly recapitulated in the marrow lesions (Fig. 23.76).[435,474] Occasionally foci of transformation in B-CLL may mimic follicle formation (see Fig. 23.64). As noted, benign germinal centers may be found in occasional cases of mantle cell lymphoma and splenic marginal zone B-cell lymphoma[479] (Fig. 23.78). In some marrow lesions of follicular lymphoma, the margins of the lymphomatous focus may be composed of transforming cells, imparting a somewhat reverse germinal center character to the lesion. In addition, the paratrabecular lesions may show a zoning phenomenon with a less differentiated population of cells immediately adjacent to the endosteal surface.

The cytopathology of the lesions in the marrow sections usually parallels the cytologic characteristics in the lymph node; this is particularly true for the T-cell lymphomas and Burkitt lymphoma.[438,446] In 20–25% of lymphomas, predominantly follicular, there may be discordance between the predominant cell type in the lymph node and the predominant cell type in the marrow.[435,441,449,452,471] In these cases, the marrow lesions usually consist of small cleaved cells, and the lymph node findings are a

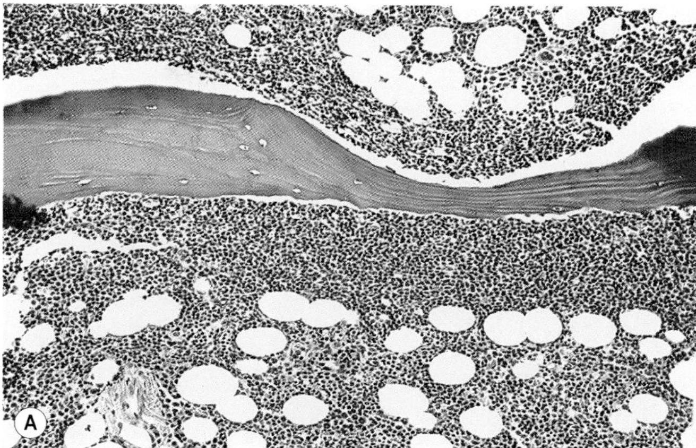

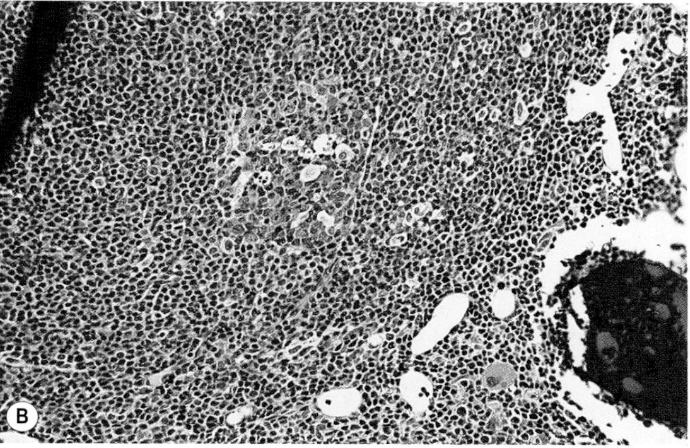

Fig. 23.78 **A**, Bone marrow biopsy from an adult male with extensive blood and marrow involvement by mantle cell lymphoma. Lymphoma cells expressed pan-B-cell markers, CD5, and intense surface immunoglobulin. In some areas, lymphoma marginates along the bone trabecula. **B**, Focus of marrow involvement from the same biopsy showing structure with remnants of germinal center including dendritic histiocytes.

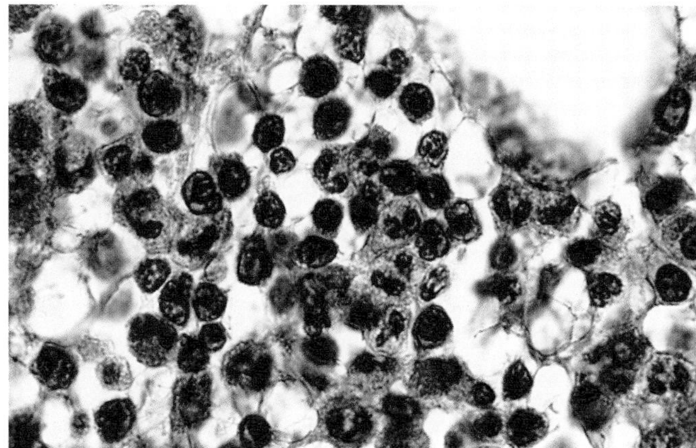

Fig. 23.79 High magnification of a marrow biopsy from a patient being treated for follicular center cell lymphoma. There is an infiltration of the interstitium by a population of small lymphocytes, several of which have irregular and cleaved nuclei.

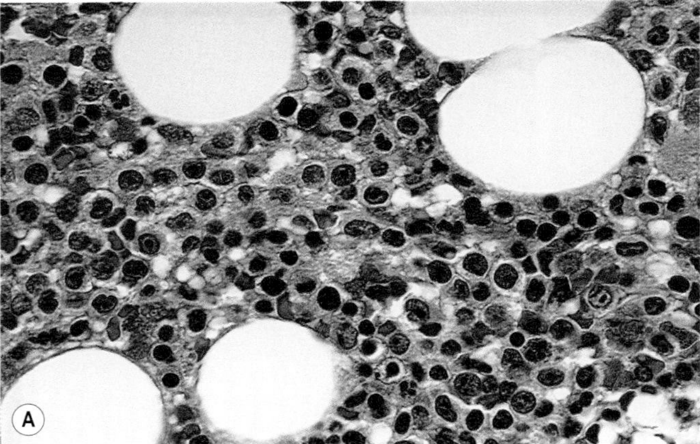

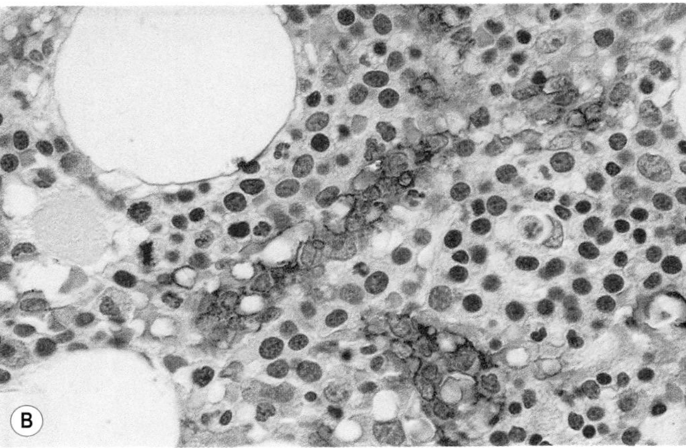

Fig. 23.80 **A**, Bone marrow biopsy from a patient with splenic marginal zone B-cell lymphoma showing a preferential intrasinusoidal localization of the lymphoma cells. **B**, The same specimen as **A** reacted with antibody to CD20 (L26) illustrating the preferential intrasinusoidal location of lymphoma cells. (**B**, Immunoperoxidase)

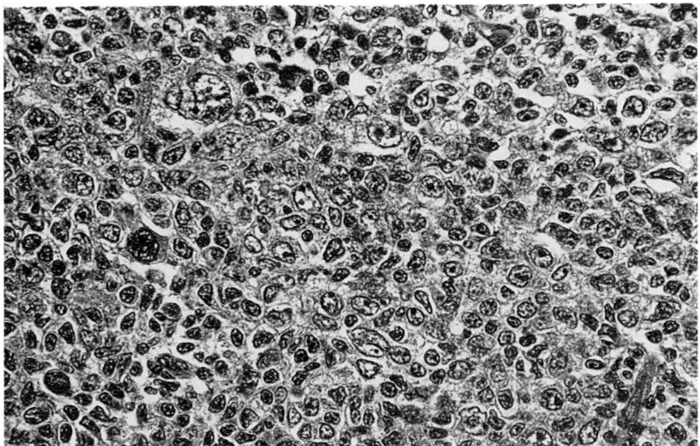

Fig. 23.81 Bone marrow section from a patient with a 6-year history of follicular center cell lymphoma. Cells resembling Reed–Sternberg cells and mononuclear variants are present.

mixed or large cell type; the converse occurs but is less frequent. Those patients with diffuse large cells in the lymph node and small cleaved cells in the bone marrow usually have a high rate of complete remission and a high rate of 5-year survival compared to patients with large cells in the lymph node and bone marrow who have a low rate of complete remission with low 5-year survival.[471] In either instance, the cytologic characteristics in both sites are usually those of follicular center cell lymphoma. Molecular studies of microdissected lesions in 21 cases of discordant lymphoma have shown the same clone in the lymph node and marrow lesions in 44% of the specimens.[461] In two cases different clones were identified and in four cases the marrow lesions were polyclonal. These studies emphasize the importance of critical evaluation of lesions in post-therapy marrow; it cannot be assumed that all lymphocytic infiltrates are residual lymphomas, nor can it be assumed that a small lymphocyte proliferation in the marrow of a patient with large cell lymphoma elsewhere is benign. These caveats are particularly important in those instances where there is discordant morphology following antibody therapy.

Immunohistochemistry with an appropriate panel of antibodies has an important role in the evaluation of marrow biopsies in patients with lymphoma. It has utility in defining the cell type, extent of involvement, and detection of residual disease following therapy.[447,460]

Similar to the findings in lymph nodes, lymphomas of predominantly small lymphocytes in the marrow, B-cell chronic lymphocytic leukemia or B small lymphocytic lymphoma, may show foci of transformation. In occasional cases of follicular cell lymphoma or chronic lymphocytic leukemia, transformed cells resembling Reed–Sternberg cells or Reed–Sternberg mononuclear variants may be present[464,466] (Fig. 23.81).

There is no relationship between a diffuse or follicular pattern in the lymph node and the presence of focal or diffuse lesions in the marrow. Cases in which the lymph node has a diffuse pattern of involvement such as small lymphocytic lymphoma or chronic lymphocytic leukemia may manifest as focal lesions in the marrow. Cases with a follicular pattern in the lymph node may manifest as diffuse marrow involvement. Only rarely is the follicular pattern recapitulated in the marrow.[435,474]

Unusual variants of non-Hodgkin lymphoma involving marrow may lead to diagnostic problems because of the unusual morphology of the lymphoma cells or because of an accompanying proliferation of reactive cells. In anaplastic large cell lymphoma, the lymphoma cells may by virtue of size and nuclear irregularity mimic megakaryocytes. The problem is accentuated when the foci of lymphoma are small and indistinctly demarcated from the surrounding normal marrow tissue or when the lymphoma cells are intermingled with normal marrow cells. In cases of the small cell variant of anaplastic large cell lymphoma, the marrow infiltration may be scattered in the interstitium and difficult to recognize amongst the normal myeloid cells.[458] Despite this, marrow involvement by anaplastic large cell lymphoma can be detected on hematoxylin–eosin-stained sections alone in most cases. Antibody studies, including CD30, may be useful in clarifying the origin of the abnormal cells in equivocal cases.[453,458,478] The lymphoma cells in histiocyte-rich B-cell lymphoma and T-cell-rich B-cell lymphoma may be partially obscured by the nonmalignant cell proliferation.[444] In T-cell/histiocyte-rich B-cell lymphoma, reactions with antibodies to B lymphocytes such as CD20 and histiocytes (CD68) are useful in delineating the two cell populations (Fig. 23.82). The blastic variant of mantle cell lymphoma may resemble acute lymphoblastic leukemia. Reactions for TdT (positive in lymphoblastic lymphoma/leukemia) and cyclin D1 (positive in mantle cell lymphoma) will help to distinguish those two processes.[476]

Post-transplant lymphoma of B-cell type does not commonly involve the marrow; when it does, the degree of infiltrate varies considerably.[456,459] Immunohistochemical reactions for B-cell origin

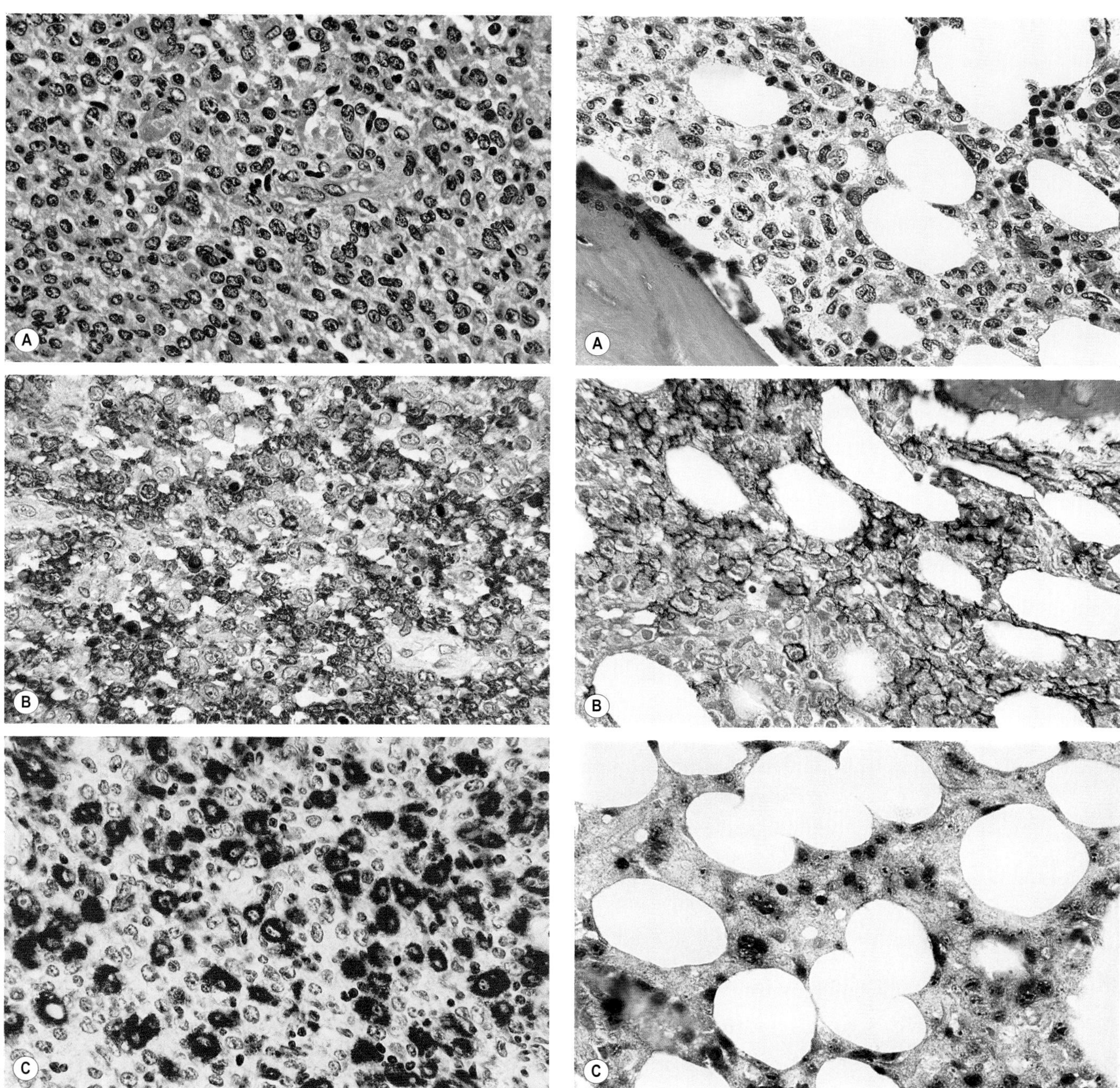

Fig. 23.82 **A**, Marrow from a patient with T-cell/histiocyte-rich B-cell lymphoma. Histiocytes predominate in this area. **B**, The specimen in **A** reacted with antibody to CD20. The numerous lymphocytes are reactive, contrasting with the negative histiocytes. **C**, The marrow biopsy in **A** reacted with antibody to CD68 (KP-1). The numerous positively reacting histiocytes in this area contrast with the negatively reacting lymphoma cells. (**B** and **C**, Immunoperoxidase)

Fig. 23.83 Post-transplant B-cell lymphoma. **A**, The lymphoma cells extensively infiltrate the marrow interstitium in this area; some residual myelopoiesis is present. **B**, The same specimen as **A** reacted with antibody to CD20; large lymphoma cells are positive. **C**, Numerous lymphoma cells are EBER positive. (**B**, Immunoperoxidase; **C**, EBER)

and EBER studies may be very helpful in establishing the diagnosis (Fig. 23.83).

Granulomas may be found in all types of lymphoma in the marrow, with and without marrow involvement.[439]

Other types of lymphoma with marrow involvement may present with blood involvement. Twenty to 40% of the cases of follicular center cell lymphoma with lymphoma in the marrow have lymphoma cells in the blood.[435,463] In some instances, the count may be very high and resemble CLL. The distinction is based on the presence of lymphocytes with cleaved nuclei and the characteristic pattern of focal paratrabecular involvement in small cleaved cell lymphoma. Expression of CD5 and weak surface immunoglobulin on the lymphocytes supports a diagnosis of CLL; lack of CD5 and expression of CD10 and intense surface immunoglobulin are more

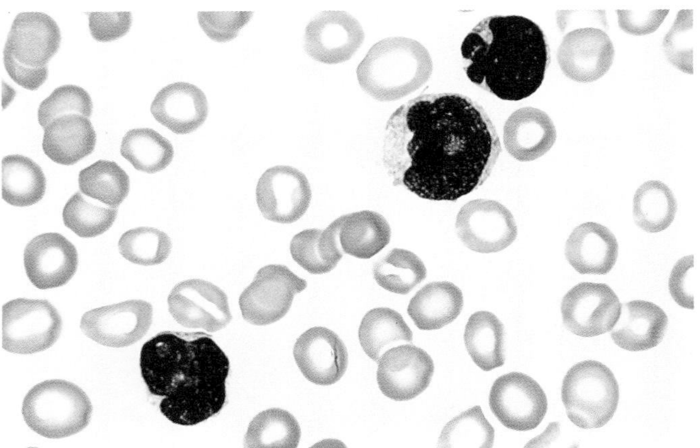

Fig. 23.84 Blood smear from an adult male with leukemic mantle cell lymphoma. The lymphoma cells vary considerably in size, nuclear lobulation, and degree of chromatin clumping. The large cell with a prominent nucleolus resembles a prolymphocyte. The smear is from the same patient as the specimen illustrated in Figure 23.78.

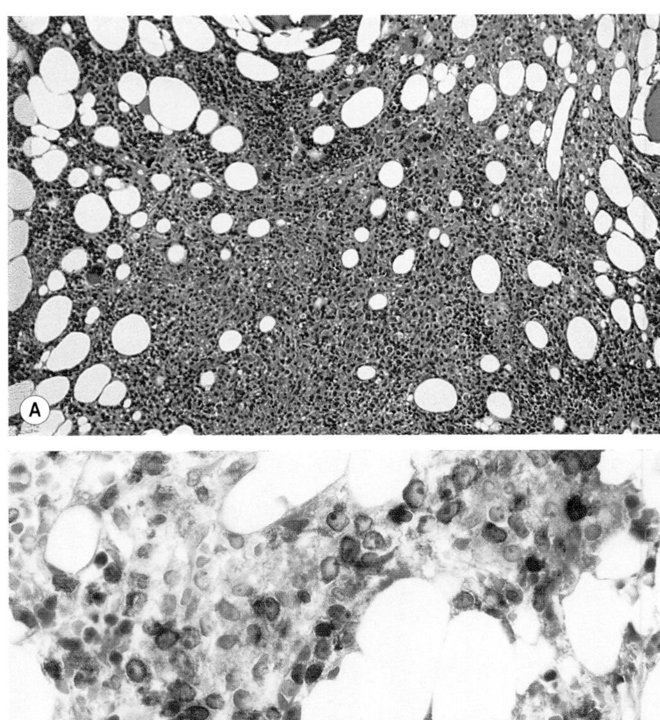

Fig. 23.85 **A**, Marrow section from a patient with partial involvement by peripheral T-cell lymphoma. The lymphoma population is poorly demarcated and infiltrates the interstitium with some preservation of normal architecture. **B**, Margin of the lesion in **A** reacted with antibody to CD3. Numerous large lymphocytes, some with prominent nucleoli, are positive. (**B**, Immunoperoxidase)

compatible with follicular lymphoma.[462,480] The lymph node findings are definitive.

Mantle cell lymphoma may present with marked involvement of the marrow and blood, and blood involvement is present in approximately half of cases with marrow disease.[435] Leukocyte counts of 270×10^9/L have been reported.[443,470,472] The blood findings may resemble CLL, CLL/PL, PLL, and small cleaved cell lymphoma. The lymphoma cells may be quite pleomorphic with variation in size, nucleocytoplasmic ratio, degree of nuclear irregularity, and prominence of nucleoli (Fig. 23.84).[467] The lymphocytes express pan-B-cell antigens, CD5, and strong surface immunoglobulin. The lymphocytes usually do not express CD23 or CD10. The bone marrow involvement may be diffuse or focal; the focal involvement may be paratrabecular or nonparatrabecular. Rarely, naked germinal centers may be observed in the marrow lesions. The lymphoma cells express cyclin D1 by immunohistochemistry and the t(11;14)(q13;q32) chromosome abnormality by fluorescence in situ hybridization. The latter assay is particularly useful on peripheral blood samples.

T- and NK-cell lymphomas/leukemias

Peripheral T-cell lymphoma, not otherwise specified

Peripheral T-cell lymphoma, not otherwise specified (PTCL, NOS) consists of all mature T-cell lymphomas that do not correspond to any of the more specific disease entities in the WHO classification.[486,487] It has such unusual features in bone marrow biopsies as to warrant separate consideration.[481,482,484,485] This type of lymphoma is characterized by a high incidence of marrow involvement at the time of initial diagnosis, ranging from 30% to 70% in some studies. The marrow lesions are diffuse in approximately 60% of involved cases and focal in 40%.[484] The focal lesions are usually randomly distributed in contrast to the preferential paratrabecular involvement in follicular center cell lymphomas; occasional cases present with a focal nonparatrabecular and paratrabecular pattern. The infiltrates vary substantially in size and are usually irregular in configuration with poorly demarcated margins; in many instances the lesions appear to extend almost imperceptibly into adjacent normal marrow (Fig. 23.85). The diffuse lesions are characterized by complete intertrabecular replacement of marrow; in some instances the entire biopsy specimen is replaced (Fig. 23.86). Increased reticulin fibers are present in the area of lymphomatous involvement and frequently extend into the adjacent normal-appearing marrow.

The predominant cytologic pattern in the marrow lesions usually corresponds to the pattern in lymph node or other tissue biopsies and can be heterogeneous, ranging from small cells with irregular nuclei to cases with predominantly large, pleomorphic cells. Mixed and large cell infiltrates are most frequently encountered. In some instances there is a relatively distinct demarcation between large and small cells. Large lymphoid cells with abundant amphophilic cytoplasm and prominent eosinophilic nucleoli, resembling Reed–Sternberg cells and mononuclear Reed–Sternberg variants, may be present. The small- and medium-sized lymphocytes have nuclei with condensed chromatin which vary from regular to irregular in outline. The mixed cell and large cell/immunoblastic types usually have an associated polycellular infiltrate consisting of histiocytes, plasma cells, eosinophils, and neutrophils. Epithelioid histiocytes are frequently noted, either in focal clusters or scattered throughout the lesions. The focal collections frequently have a granulomatous appearance. Increased vascularity may be a prominent feature; the vascular component is

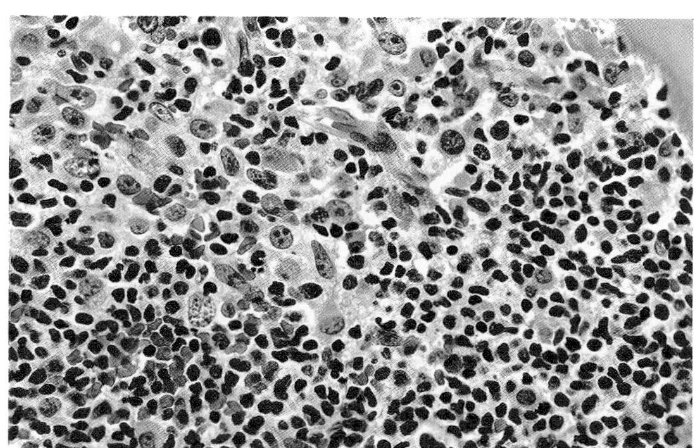

Fig. 23.86 Marrow biopsy from a patient with peripheral T-cell lymphoma, showing extensive diffuse marrow involvement. The predominant cell population consists of small lymphocytes with a focus of large lymphocytes that have prominent nucleoli.

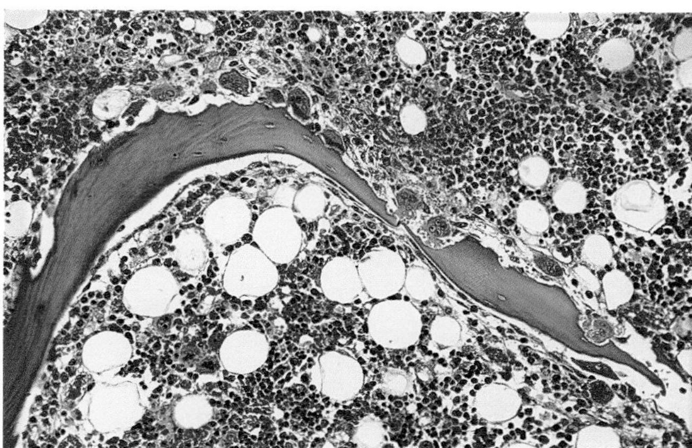

Fig. 23.87 Marrow biopsy from a patient with adult T-cell leukemia and hypercalcemia. Marked osteoclastic activity with bone resorption is present.

primarily an endothelial cell proliferation with straight-lined channels. Immunohistochemical reactions are useful in identifying the atypical cells as T cells.

The differential diagnosis of PTCL, NOS in marrow includes Hodgkin disease, systemic mastocytosis, and polymorphous reactive lymphoid hyperplasia.[482,484] The most difficult problem relates to the last lesion, which may be present in marrow specimens from patients with a wide variety of immunologic disorders, including AIDS. Polymorphous reactive lymphoid hyperplasia has many histopathologic features similar to PTCL, NOS, including a heterogeneous population of lymphocytes with intermixed plasma cells, immunoblasts, eosinophils, endothelial cells, and epithelioid histiocytes. Distinction between the focal lesions of PTCL, NOS and the polymorphous reactive lymphoid lesions may not be possible solely on morphologic features. Markedly atypical cells with prominent nucleoli are more compatible with lymphoma. The size of the lesions is not always a reliable distinguishing feature; reactive lesions may show extensive marrow replacement, particularly in patients with AIDS. The lesions of PTCL, NOS may be relatively small. Molecular genetic studies to detect a clonal T-cell population, supportive of T-cell lymphoma, may be useful in this differential diagnosis.

Hodgkin disease in the marrow may appear similar to the lesions of PTCL, NOS. The presence of classical Reed–Sternberg cells and the lack of atypia in the background lymphocyte population are suggestive of Hodgkin disease. Multinucleated immunoblasts resembling Reed–Sternberg cells may be present in PTCL, NOS; in these instances, review of lymph nodes and other tissue biopsies and immunologic studies are critical in distinguishing PTCL, NOS from Hodgkin disease.

The lesions of systemic mastocytosis may be distinguished from PTCL by the reactivity of mast cells with antibody to mast cell tryptase. The cells of systemic mastocytosis, however, may aberrantly express the T lineage-associated marker CD2, but should not express other T-cell markers, such as CD3, CD5 or CD7.

Genotypic studies to determine T-cell clonality are an important advance in distinguishing PTCL in marrow biopsies or other tissues from the disorders considered in the differential diagnosis.[488] Clonal rearrangement of one of the T-cell receptors is substantial evidence of a malignant process. The determination of clonality may be made on fresh aspirate or trephine biopsy specimens and fixed, paraffin-embedded tissue.[483]

Adult T-cell leukemia/lymphoma

Adult T-cell leukemia/lymphoma is an unusual form of mature (post-thymic) T-cell lymphoma occurring primarily in Japan; it is associated with the human retrovirus HTLV-1.[490,491,492] The highest incidence of this disease is in the Kyushu region of Japan; other endemic areas include the Caribbean basin and parts of western Africa. Sporadic cases are observed in other areas of the world, including the USA. The disease occurs in three principal clinical forms: smoldering, chronic, and acute. There are several histopathologic types including small, medium, and large pleomorphic cell types, large cell anaplastic, and Hodgkin-like. Blood and marrow involvement occurs principally in the acute form. Marrow involvement is characterized by a patchy infiltration of abnormal lymphocytes with lobulated or round nuclei. The distribution may be patchy even in cases with marked leukocytosis. Hypercalcemia is present in 28% of patients at diagnosis and in 50% of patients at some time during the course of the disease. The vast majority of patients with hypercalcemia have bone marrow involvement. However, increased osteoclastic activity may be present in cases with or without marrow involvement by the lymphoma and the findings may be those of osteitis fibrosa generalisata[489,490] (Fig. 23.87).

Sézary syndrome

Sézary syndrome is a lymphoproliferative disorder, usually of CD4-positive T-helper lymphocytes, related to mycosis fungoides and defined by the presence of erythroderma, generalized lymphadenopathy, and neoplastic T cells in the blood, skin, and lymph nodes.[493,495,497–499] The leukocyte count may be normal or markedly elevated with a high percentage of Sézary cells. The Sézary cells, as observed in Romanowsky-stained blood smears, have distinctive features. The nucleus frequently has an unusual configuration that has been characterized as cerebriform (Fig. 23.88A). Cytoplasmic vacuoles, which stain positively with the PAS reaction, may be present in a perinuclear location. Large and small cell variants have been described.[493] Ultrastructurally, the cells show marked nuclear convolutions[494,499] (Fig. 23.88B). Despite the generalized nature of the disorder, the bone marrow sections in the majority of patients are normal. Involved cases usually show a sparse, interstitial infiltrate.[496] Marked marrow infiltration with replacement of normal

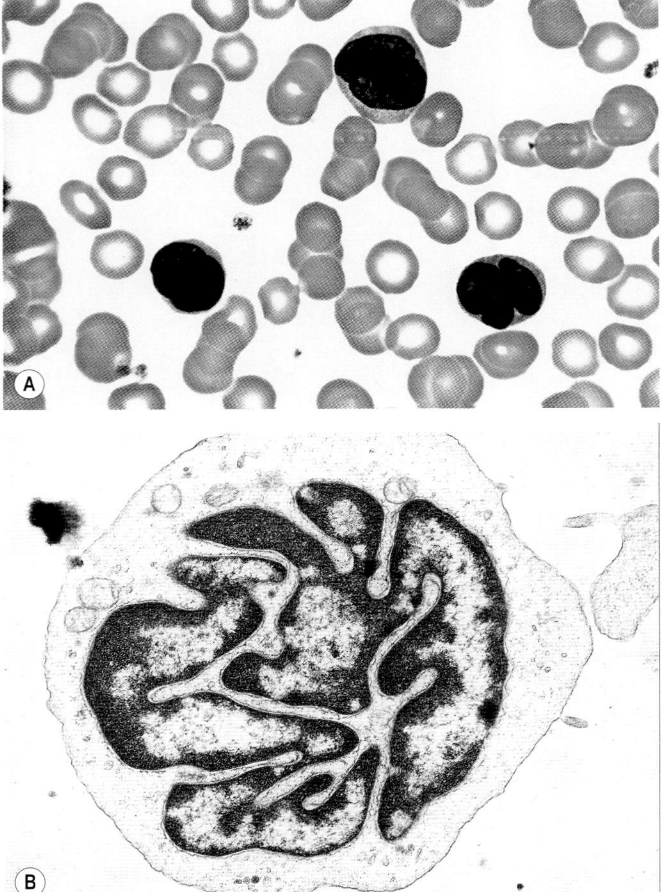

Fig. 23.88 **A**, Three Sézary cells in blood smear. The nucleus in the larger cell in the upper field has delicate folds imparting a 'cerebriform' appearance. The two smaller cells in the lower field have a more condensed chromatin and markedly lobulated nuclei. **B**, Ultrastructure of a Sézary cell; extreme convolution of the nucleus is a characteristic feature (**B**, Uranyl acetate–lead citrate; ×22 000)

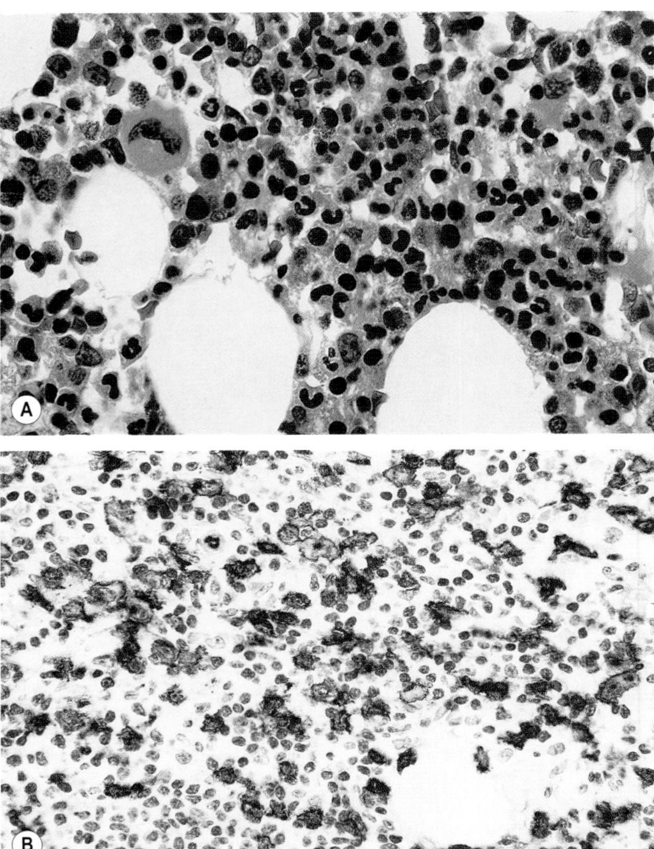

Fig. 23.89 **A**, Bone marrow biopsy from an adult female with large granulated T-cell lymphocytic leukemia. The leukemic lymphocytes are interspersed in the interstitium. **B**, Specimen in **A** reacted with antibody to CD8. There are numerous CD8 positive cells in the interstitium. (**B**, Immunoperoxidase)

hematopoietic cells is very uncommon. Rarely, small aggregates of Sézary cells may be observed.[493]

Large granulated T-cell lymphocytic leukemia

The large granulated lymphocytic leukemias are uncommon lymphoproliferative disorders which consist of two entities: T-cell large granulated lymphocytic leukemia (T-LGL) and NK-cell large granulated lymphocytic leukemia (NK-LGL).[500,503,509–511] The two conditions are morphologically indistinguishable; their distinction is based on immunophenotypic characteristics and clonality studies. The characteristic lymphocytes in the blood in the two disorders are medium to large, with abundant slightly basophilic to pale cytoplasm containing a variable number of coarse azurophilic granules, and are frequently abundant in reactive processes, most notably viral infections and immune reactions. They may also be increased after myocardial infarction. In the leukemic processes the increase in LGLs, which may be modest, is sustained. Immunophenotypic and clonal studies are essential to the diagnosis.

There frequently is severe neutropenia in T-LGL. Approximately 50% of patients have splenomegaly but lymphadenopathy is uncommon. Rheumatoid factor and hypergammaglobulinemia are present in a subset of patients. The lymphocytes in T-LGL characteristically express CD3 and CD8, and are CD4 negative; CD11b, CD56, and CD57 are variably present.[501,502] Occasional cases express CD4 or CD4/CD8. The definitive diagnostic evidence is based on T-cell receptor gene rearrangement studies, which usually show *TCRB* and *TCRG* rearrangements.[500,504,505–508,512]

The marrow involvement in T-LGL, which is usually interstitial, may be very difficult to recognize in routine sections; reactivity with antibody to CD8 is particularly useful in identifying the infiltrates (Fig. 23.89).[500,503,504,508] Approximately 50% of cases also have an intrasinusoidal distribution of the leukemic lymphocytes. Occasional aggregates of lymphocytes may be present and they usually contain an admixture of T and B cells. The T cells in these aggregates are usually CD4 positive and are not part of the leukemic process. The splenic infiltration is principally in the red pulp.

NK-LGL is referred to in the 2008 edition of the *WHO Classification of Tumours of the Haematopoietic and Lymphoid Tissues* as a chronic lymphoproliferative disorder of NK cells and is given provisional status as a distinct entity.[502] NK-LGL is usually an indolent disorder occurring in adults who are usually asymptomatic and without organomegaly. The lymphocytes in the blood are as described for T-LGL. The bone marrow infiltrate is interstitial and intrasinusoidal; the lymphocytes are small with a moderate amount of cytoplasm.

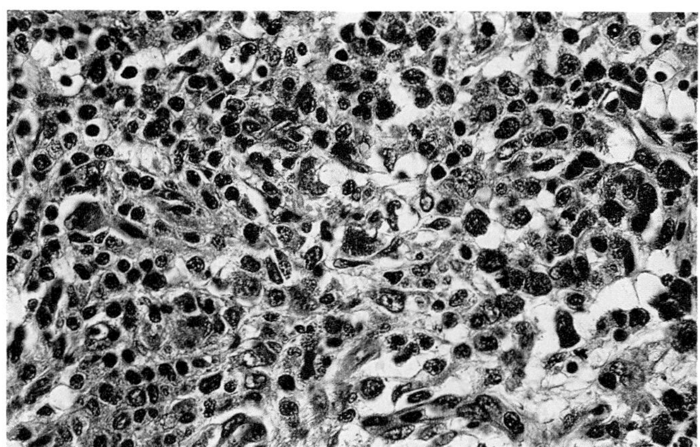

Fig. 23.90 Bone marrow biopsy from a patient with lymph node diagnosis of angioimmunoblastic T-cell lymphoma. Marrow is diffusely involved by the process with a heterogeneous cell population.

The cells are membrane CD3 negative but may contain intracytoplasmic CD3. Other T-cell markers are negative. There is usually weak CD56 positivity and the cytotoxic markers T-cell restricted intracellular antigen 1 (T1A-1), granzyme B, and granzyme M are positive. There is no evidence of T-cell receptor rearrangement on molecular analysis.

Angioimmunoblastic T-cell lymphoma

The reported incidence of marrow involvement in this lesion, originally described as angioimmunoblastic lymphadenopathy, is 50–70%.[513,514,518] The blood may show several abnormalities including reactive lymphocytes, immunoblasts, and eosinophilia.[519,520]

The bone marrow lesions may be diffuse or focal; focal involvement is more common.[515,516] The margins of the focal lesions are usually somewhat indistinct, with poor demarcation from the surrounding hematopoietic tissue. In some cases, confluent multifocal lesions replace extensive areas of normal marrow. The lesions of angioimmunoblastic T-cell lymphoma are somewhat loosely structured and contain varying proportions of lymphocytes, immunoblasts, plasma cells, and histiocytes; neutrophils and eosinophils are also present (Fig. 23.90). Vascular proliferation, endothelial cells, and fibroblasts are frequently identified. Stains for reticulin show a marked increase in reticulin fibers in the involved areas. Collections of epithelioid histiocytes, imparting a granulomatoid appearance to some of the lesions, are reported. The amorphous PAS-positive material found in lymph node biopsies is less frequently encountered in bone marrow lesions. Immunocytochemical reactions with antibodies to kappa and lambda light chains show a polyclonal proliferation of immunoblasts and plasma cells in most cases, but coexisting B cell and clonal plasma cell proliferations may occur with some cases.[517] The neoplastic T cells are of germinal center origin in this lymphoma and often express CD10, CXCL13, and PD1.[516] The uninvolved marrow is frequently hypercellular. The hypercellularity may be a result of panhyperplasia or principally erythroid hyperplasia. The bone marrow and blood smears may contain varying numbers of lymphocytes at varying stages of development, including immunoblasts and mature plasma cells. Reactive lymphocytes and eosinophilia may be observed. Because of the high number of admixed reactive cells in the marrow with this disease, gene rearrangement studies for T-cell clonality are often useful if a prior lymph node or other tissue diagnosis of lymphoma has not been made.[521]

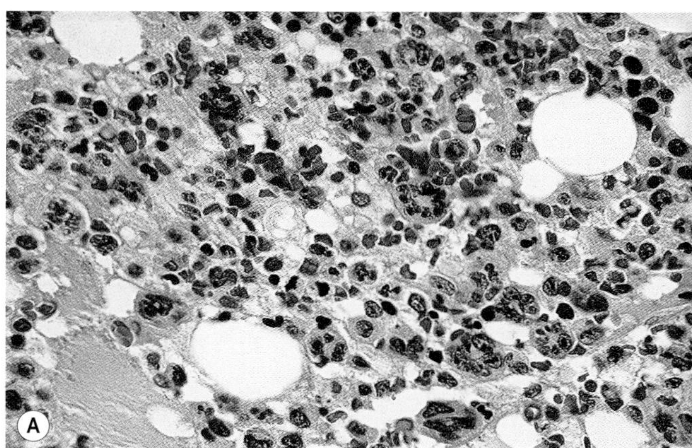

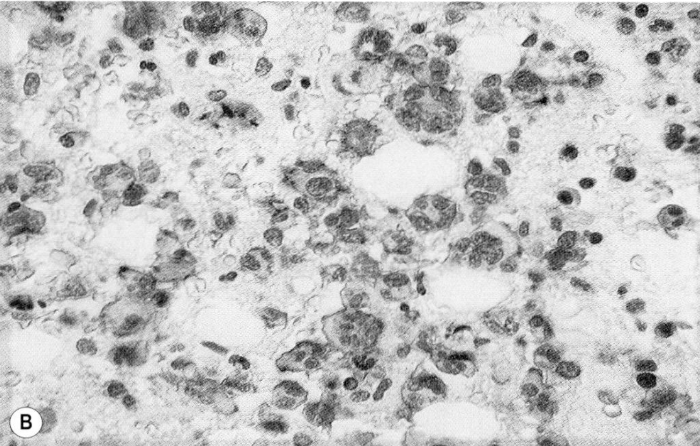

Fig. 23.91 **A**, Area of marrow biopsy from a patient with anaplastic large cell lymphoma, T-cell type. The lymphoma cells are intermixed with normal marrow cells. **B**, Specimen in **A** reacted with antibody to CD30. The lymphoma cells are positive. (**B**, Immunoperoxidase)

The significance of marrow involvement in regard to clinical outcome is unclear. Some, but not all, studies have indicated that patients with marrow involvement have a shorter survival than patients without marrow involvement.[513,520]

Anaplastic large cell lymphoma

The diagnosis of anaplastic large cell lymphoma is now restricted to cases of T- or null-cell type and are subdivided into anaplastic lymphoma kinase (ALK)-positive and ALK-negative types.[523,528] Peripheral blood involvement is rare and is associated with extensive extranodal disease, including marrow involvement.[525] The marrow usually shows massive involvement, but in rare cases the cells may be almost imperceptibly scattered among the normal hematopoietic cells. The interstitium in the cases with marrow involvement may be very loosely structured with cell depletion (Fig. 23.91). The cases with lymphoma cells scattered among the normal hematopoietic cells may be overlooked in routinely stained sections, and immunohistochemical study for CD30 expression will detect these subtle cases[524,529] (Fig. 23.91B).

The small cell variant of anaplastic large cell lymphoma has a high incidence of marrow involvement when evaluated by routine morphology and immunohistochemistry[527] (Fig. 23.92), and appears to be more commonly associated with peripheral blood

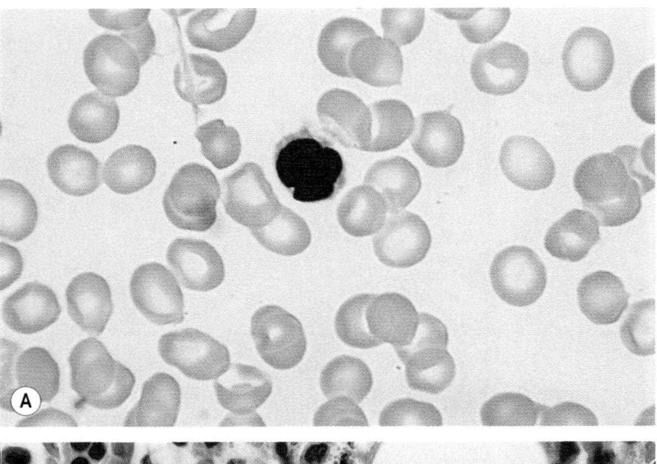

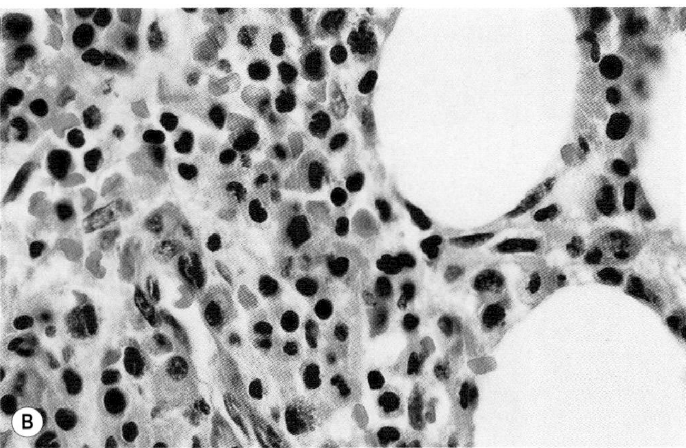

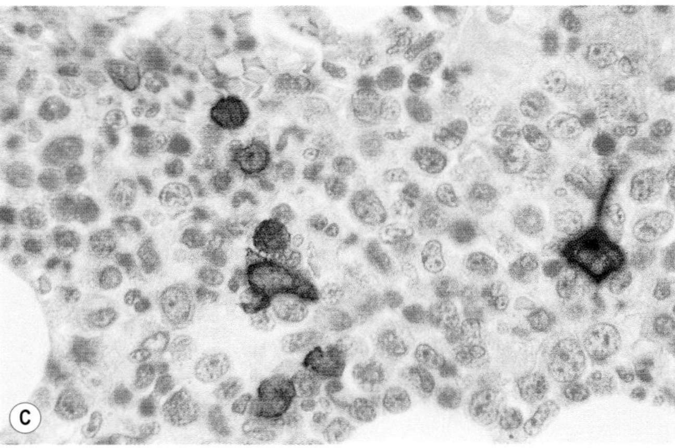

Fig. 23.92 **A**, Lymphoma cell in blood smear from a 17-year-old male with small cell variant of anaplastic large cell lymphoma with associated t(2;5)(p23;p35). The cell has a convoluted nucleus. **B**, Bone marrow section from the same patient. The few lymphoma cells are scattered in the interstitium and difficult to recognize in this H&E stain. **C**, The same specimen as **B** reacted with antibody to CD30, which highlights the small and large lymphoma cells. (**C**, Immunoperoxidase)

involvement. The degree of marrow involvement may be difficult to appreciate in routinely stained sections and immunohistochemistry may be useful in such cases (Fig. 23.92B). Because many cases of anaplastic large cell lymphoma show aberrant expression of the myeloid-associated marker CD13,[522,526] detection of CD30 and T-cell antigens, as well as evidence of a clonal T-cell gene rearrangement, are helpful in the differential diagnosis with acute myeloid leukemia.

Hepatosplenic T-cell lymphoma, post-transplant T-cell lymphoma, and aggressive NK-cell lymphoma

Several uncommon types of T-cell lymphomas and NK-cell lymphomas have been reported in which the marrow is commonly involved. They include hepatosplenic T-cell lymphoma, post-transplant T-cell lymphoma, and aggressive NK-cell lymphoma. These are of relatively rare occurrence and it is difficult to generalize about patterns of involvement.

Hepatosplenic T-cell lymphoma may be marked by an intrasinusoidal pattern but may also show subtle interstitial involvement without the characteristic intrasinusoidal pattern[532,534,536,538] (Fig. 23.93). The lymphoma cells may have blastic features or be very atypical. The lymphoma cells are CD3+, TCRδ1+, TCRαβ–, CD56+/–, CD4–, CD8–/+, and CD5+ in most cases. Immunohistochemistry, particularly anti-CD3, is very important in identifying the extent of disease and the intrasinusoidal pattern of involvement. Cytogenetic studies usually show isochromosome 7, which is frequently associated with trisomy 8 and other abnormalities.[530,533,535]

Post-transplant T-cell lymphoma may be characterized by focal or extensive interstitial marrow involvement (Fig. 23.94). The use of immunohistochemistry may be extraordinarily important in identifying the presence, extent, and nature of these lesions since they may be overlooked in suboptimally prepared specimens. Examination of cytologic preparations, immunophenotyping, cytogenetics, and molecular studies may be important in classifying these lymphomas.

Aggressive NK-cell leukemia is a rare type of leukemia/lymphoma; it occurs most frequently in Asian teenagers and young adults.[531,537] This disorder may represent the leukemic counterpart of extranodal NK/T-cell lymphoma, nasal type.[539] The blood, marrow, liver, and spleen are commonly involved. The leukemia/lymphoma cells are large with ample and pale to slightly basophilic cytoplasm, which may contain fine or coarse azurophilic granules (Fig. 23.95A). The bone marrow infiltrates in biopsy sections may be diffuse, focal, or minimally interstitial. The leukemic cells appear monotonous with regularly shaped nuclei, coarse chromatin, and small nucleoli (Fig. 23.95B). The disease generally follows an aggressive clinical course as the name implies. Bone marrow involvement in the nasal type of NK-cell lymphoma at diagnosis is uncommon.

Benign lymphocytic aggregates

Benign lymphocytic aggregates occur relatively frequently in bone marrow trephine and particle sections. The incidence in biopsy specimens varies from 3% to 47%.[547,548,550] The reported incidence in autopsy specimens is 26–62%. The incidence appears to increase with age and is higher in females than males. The aggregates occur in patients with a wide range of disorders, and the number and size in individual specimens vary considerably. Although lesions up to 1000 μm have been reported, the majority of aggregates are relatively small and well circumscribed.[551] Unusually large aggregates may occur in the marrows of patients with diseases related to the immune system such as AIDS and rheumatoid arthritis. Large and numerous lymphoid aggregates, sometimes with germinal center formation, may be observed in the marrow of patients receiving immunotherapy. These lesions may occasionally be paratrabecular (Fig. 23.96), but paratrabecular aggregates should be viewed with

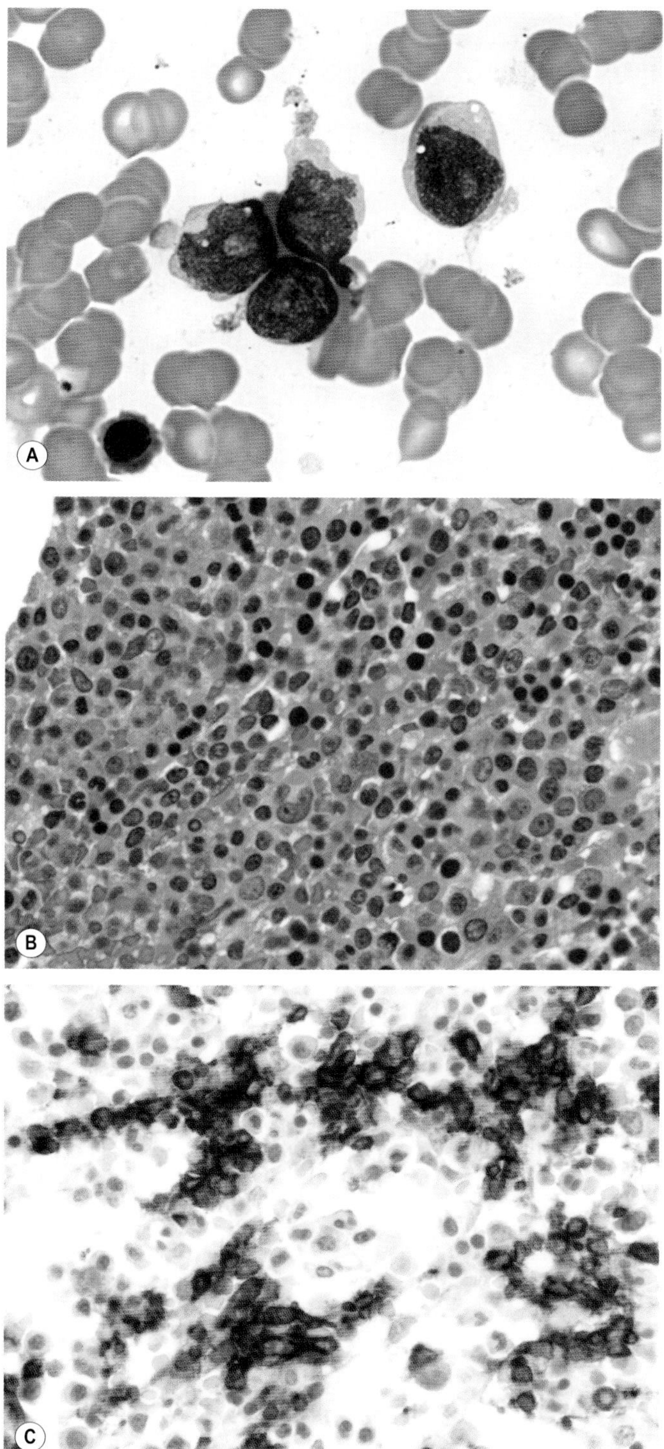

Fig. 23.93 **A**, Bone marrow smear from a 17-year-old male with hepatosplenic gamma/delta T-cell lymphoma. The lymphoma cells vary in appearance and some have blast-like features. **B**, The marrow biopsy is markedly hypercellular, with extensive involvement and both an interstitial and intrasinusoidal pattern. **C,** Specimen in **B** reacted with anti-CD3 which highlights the intrasinusoidal pattern. (**C,** Immunoperoxidase)

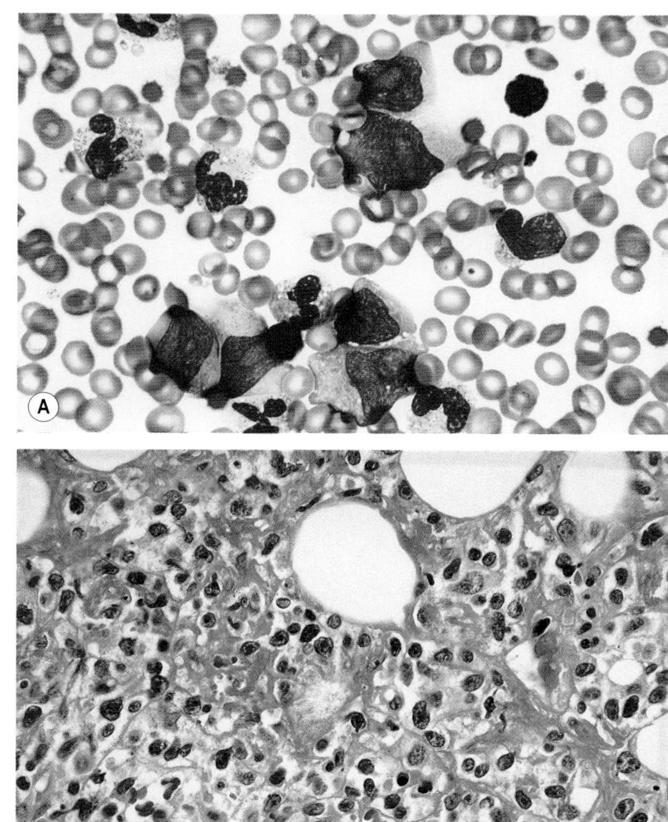

Fig. 23.94 Post-transplant T-cell lymphoma. **A**, Bone marrow smear from a 40-year-old female, 28 and 8 years following renal transplantation. The lymphoma cells, which expressed CD2 and CD3, are large with abundant cytoplasm and very prominent nucleoli. **B**, High magnification of marrow section showing extensive interstitial involvement by noncohesive lymphoma cells. There is substantial depletion of normal hematopoiesis with cellular debris.

a high suspicion for malignancy, particularly follicular lymphoma. The biologic significance of marrow lymphocytic aggregates in the majority of patients is unknown.[546]

The morphologic distinction between benign lymphocytic aggregates and malignant lymphoma, small lymphocytic type, in marrow biopsies from adults may be very difficult on morphology alone, and usually require immunophenotyping studies. Such studies show a T-cell predominance in most reactive lymphoid aggregates and a clonal B-cell predominance with aberrant CD5 expression in small lymphocytic lymphoma. Although general guidelines for making this distinction have been proposed, it is important to recognize that exceptions to these generalizations occur with distressing frequency.[542,552]

Benign aggregates are usually few in number, well circumscribed, loosely structured, and contain histiocytes and plasma cells and frequently mast cells in addition to lymphocytes. The lymphocytes are usually small with generally round nuclei that have condensed chromatin and inconspicuous or no evident nucleoli. Occasional nuclei may have irregular outlines. Vascular structures are frequently present. Germinal centers are uncommon in lymphocytic lesions in the marrow but when present are usually but not always evidence of a benign process. As previously noted, germinal centers may be observed in marrow lesions of mantle cell lymphoma and splenic

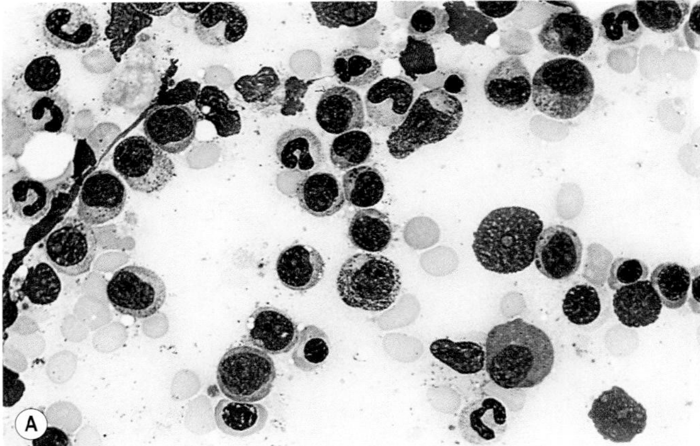

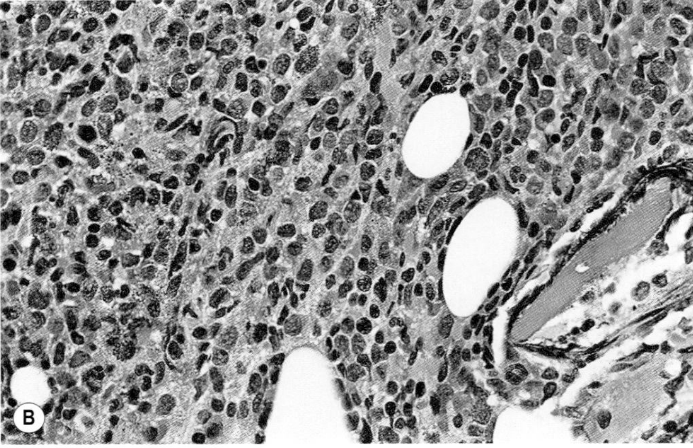

Fig. 23.95 Aggressive NK-cell leukemia. **A**, Bone marrow smear from a patient with aggressive NK-cell leukemia. The lymphoma cells have relatively abundant cytoplasm containing numerous coarse azurophilic granules; the lymphoma cells are distinguished from neutrophil myelocytes by the lack of specific granules. **B**, Marrow biopsy from the patient in **A** showing extensive replacement. The lymphoma cells are relatively uniform in appearance with round nuclei and abundant cytoplasm.
(Slides contributed by Dr John KC Chan, Hong Kong)

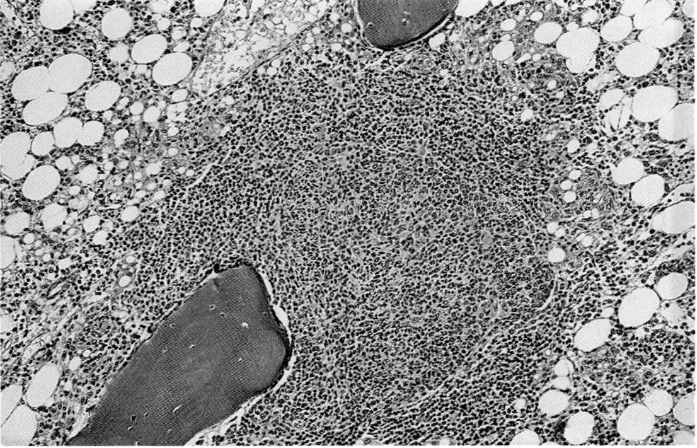

Fig. 23.96 Paratrabecular germinal center formation in marrow of a patient receiving interleukin-2 therapy for metastatic melanoma. Several vacuolated macrophages are present at the margin of the lesion.

marginal zone B-cell lymphoma. A preferential paratrabecular margination of a lymphoid infiltrate, usually associated with reticulin fibrosis, is evidence for a diagnosis of lymphoma. A random distribution of lymphoid aggregates with an occasional aggregate juxtaposed to a trabecula has no diagnostic specificity, since this pattern may occur with benign or malignant lesions. In occasional cases of follicular lymphoma, the follicular pattern in the lymph node is recapitulated in marrow lesions.

A particularly difficult diagnostic problem is the lymphocytic lesion referred to as polymorphous reactive lymphoid hyperplasia (see Fig. 23.28). These lymphoid aggregates are usually focal, poorly circumscribed, and randomly distributed. The lymphocytes are generally well differentiated; the nuclei of some and sometimes of many of the lymphocytes may be irregular. The infiltrate may be predominantly lymphocytes or have associated populations of plasma cells, immunoblasts, eosinophils, endothelial cells, phagocytic histiocytes, and epithelioid histiocytes. This lesion may occur in the marrow in any age group and is frequently associated with immune disorders such as immune cytopenias, collagen vascular disease, and, most notably, AIDS. The aggregates may be very large and in certain instances be virtually indistinguishable from the lesions of PTCL. Lesions of this type in marrow specimens from patients with AIDS are almost invariably reactive. In other instances in which the clinical or other tissue findings are equivocal, immunophenotypic or genotypic studies for clonality may be necessary.

It is important to recognize that benign lymphocytic aggregates may be present in marrow of patients with a prior diagnosis of marrow involvement by lymphoma; lymphoid aggregates in marrow specimens following chemotherapy should be evaluated as critically as those in the initial staging marrow biopsy. Marrow involvement by lymphoma in a patient with no other manifestation of the disease is very uncommon, and the diagnosis in such a situation should be approached with considerable caution and only if supporting immunophenotypic or genotypic evidence of a clonal process is present.

Marrow biopsies containing lymphocytic aggregates from patients treated with rituximab therapy for lymphoma should be carefully evaluated with immunohistochemistry to ascertain if the lymphocytes express the same antigens as the lymphoma cells which were present in the pretreatment specimen. Some loosely structured lesions, both randomly distributed and in paratrabecular locations, may be composed of reactive T cells rather than the B-cell lymphoma; this phenomenon is probably related to the therapeutic effects of the antibody (Fig. 23.97). Because rituximab is directed against CD20, other B-cell markers, such as CD79a and PAX5, are needed to exclude the presence of admixed neoplastic B cells in this setting.[543,544]

The application of antibodies that react with lymphocytes in paraffin-embedded, decalcified specimens often aids in distinguishing benign from malignant lymphocytic aggregates; as noted, this may be particularly critical after chemotherapy or therapy with monoclonal antibodies.[540,549] However, antibodies to B lymphocytes and T lymphocytes do not provide information about clonality. Antibodies to kappa and lambda light chains which may impart evidence of clonality are not sufficiently sensitive in most instances to identify surface immunoglobulins in lymphomas in paraffin-embedded biopsies. Despite this, most reactive marrow lymphocytes are T cells and detection of an increased B-cell population in the marrow in the absence of germinal centers is usually supportive of B-cell lymphoma. One exception is in the setting of autoimmune disease in which B cells may predominate in reactive lymphoid aggregates. The presence of a mixed reactivity pattern (i.e., lymphocyte populations expressing both T and B surface antigens) in marrow lesions has been found to be more consistent with reactive

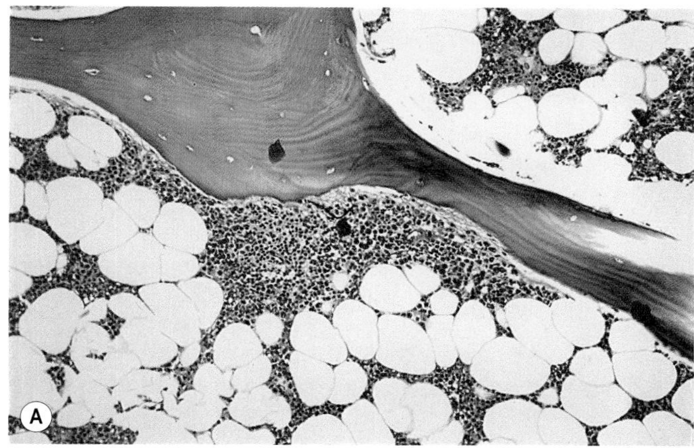

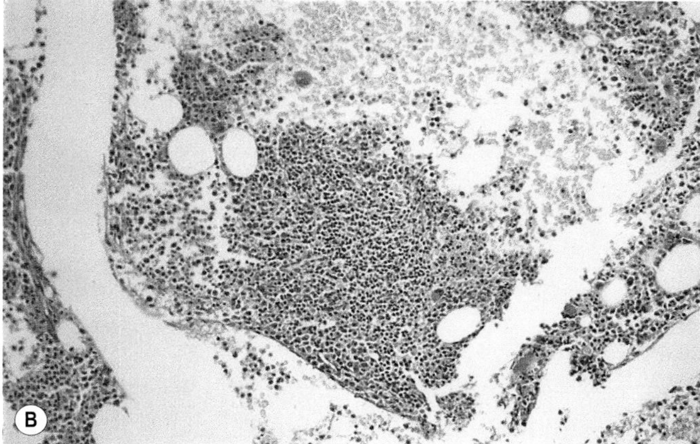

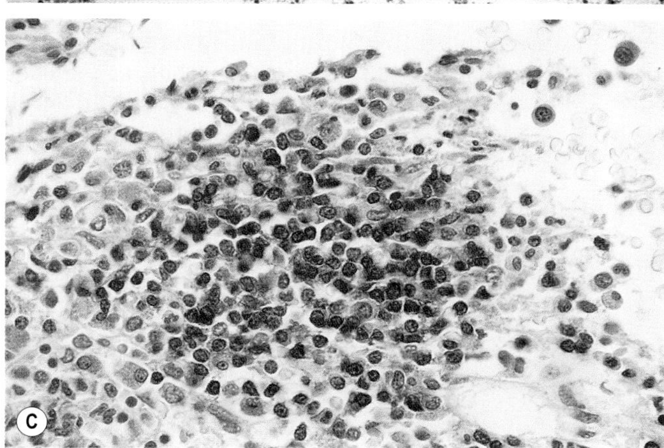

Fig. 23.97 Post rituximab therapy. **A**, One of several paratrabecular and nonparatrabecular lymphocytic aggregates in bone marrow biopsy following rituximab therapy. **B**, Same specimen as **A** reacted with antibody to CD20; the lymphocytes are nonreactive. Similar results were found with antibody to CD79a. **C**, Same specimen as **A** and **B** reacted with antibody to CD3. Most of the lymphocytes are intensely reactive. Similar results were found in other lymphocytic aggregates. (**B** and **C**, Immunoperoxidase)

lesions. A panel of antibodies, including CD10, CD5, CD3, and CD20, has been suggested as useful in distinguishing benign or atypical lymphocytic aggregates in the marrow from lymphoma; most benign aggregates do not express CD10 and CD23. As mentioned, in the setting of anti-CD20 therapy, the addition of other B-cell markers such as CD79a and PAX5 may also be useful. There are exceptions to all generalizations, and caution should be exercised in the interpretation of immunocytochemical reactivity. Careful analysis of both lymph node and bone marrow specimens with the same panel of antibodies is necessary in evaluating marrow biopsies for lymphoma. Genotypic studies should be performed in those instances in which the marrow findings are indeterminate, and a therapeutic decision is contingent on the presence or absence of marrow involvement. Even with this approach, difficulties in distinguishing benign from malignant lesions persist, especially in the setting of autoimmune disease,[545] and continued observation is the most prudent course in some patients. In cases in which the morphologic and immunophenotypic studies are inconclusive, some authors have suggested the terminology 'indeterminate for lymphoma' for staging marrows.[541,542]

Hodgkin lymphoma

The incidence of marrow involvement in Hodgkin lymphoma varies with the histopathologic type: it is approximately 10% in classical Hodgkin mixed cellularity type and approximately 1% in lymphocyte-predominant Hodgkin and lymphocyte-rich classical Hodgkin disease.[565,567,568] Nodular sclerosis has an incidence of approximately 3%.[555,561,568] The overall incidence of bone marrow involvement in patients with stage IV disease is reported to be 32% and varies with the histologic subtype: 3% lymphocyte predominant, 37% nodular sclerosis, 49% mixed cellularity, and 10% unclassified type.[561] The prognosis for patients with stage IV disease does not appear to be adversely affected by bone marrow involvement.

The lymphocyte depletion type of Hodgkin lymphoma, which has a high incidence of marrow involvement, approximately 50%, is an uncommon form of Hodgkin lymphoma.[557,562] Because the clinical presentation in some patients with lymphocyte depletion type disease is characterized by little or no peripheral lymphadenopathy, the initial diagnostic specimen may be the bone marrow biopsy.

The detection of marrow involvement appears in part to be related to the amount of tissue available for examination. Marrow involvement in most instances results from widely disseminated disease, is significantly associated with B symptoms, bulky disease, involvement of lymph nodes both above and below the diaphragm, and is negatively correlated with a large mediastinal mass.[561] Forty to 50% of patients with AIDS who develop Hodgkin lymphoma have marrow involvement; the marrow may be the initial diagnostic specimen and the only site of involvement in this situation.[564]

The histopathologic classification of Hodgkin lymphoma should not be based on examination of involved bone marrow because of different manifestations of the disease in lymph node and bone marrow tissue. Fibrosis is a common finding in Hodgkin lesions in the marrow and is not limited to nodular sclerosis and lymphocyte depletion types.

Definitive histopathologic criteria for the diagnosis of marrow involvement in Hodgkin lymphoma include typical Reed–Sternberg cells in a cellular background characteristic of Hodgkin lymphoma or mononuclear Reed–Sternberg variants in a cellular background typical of Hodgkin lymphoma if typical Reed–Sternberg cells are identified in other specimens[556,559,566] (Fig. 23.98). The presence of atypical cells lacking the features of Reed–Sternberg cells or mononuclear variants in a characteristic Hodgkin environment in a patient with histopathologically proven disease has historically been considered highly suspicious for involvement; however, if the atypical cells express CD30 and CD15, typical immunophenotypic features of classical Hodgkin lymphoma, the

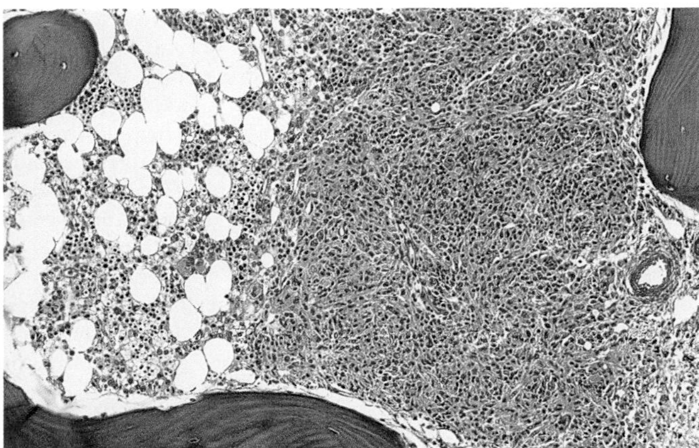

Fig. 23.98 Bone marrow biopsy from a patient with mixed cellularity Hodgkin lymphoma. There is extensive involvement in this area of the biopsy.

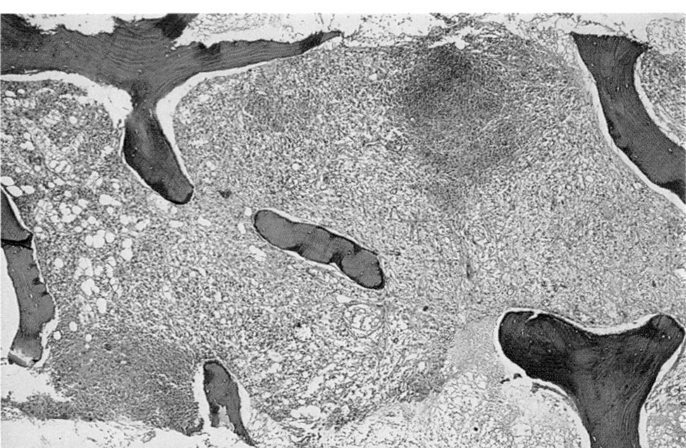

Fig. 23.100 Two foci of Hodgkin lymphoma in a large area of necrotic debris in a post-treatment marrow specimen.

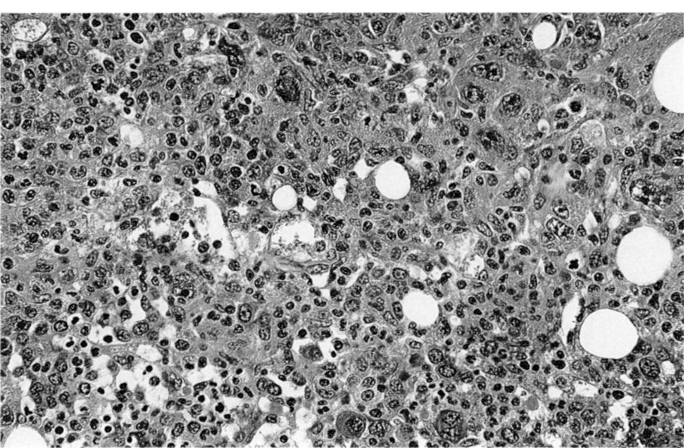

Fig. 23.99 Marrow with several scattered foci of Hodgkin lymphoma. The lesions, which contain several Reed–Sternberg cells, are indistinctly demarcated from normal marrow.

marrow can be considered involved by disease. Foci of fibrosis in the absence of Reed–Sternberg cells or mononuclear variants in a patient with an established diagnosis of Hodgkin lymphoma is not in itself sufficient evidence for a definitive diagnosis of marrow involvement but should be viewed as suspicious. In the latter instance, and when immunophenotyping studies of atypical cells are not conclusive, repeat biopsies should be performed.

Hodgkin lesions in marrow may be diffuse or focal; the extent of involvement ranges from a single, small lesion to complete replacement of multiple biopsy specimens. Diffuse involvement is found in 70–80% of positive marrow biopsies; the Hodgkin tissue in these cases replaces the entire area between trabeculae.[563] Focal lesions are variable in size and may be surrounded by normal hematopoietic tissue or scattered in a hypocellular background (Fig. 23.99); the latter pattern is more frequent following chemotherapy. The focal lesions tend to be polycellular, with a predominant population of small lymphocytes with admixed neutrophils, eosinophils, plasma cells, histiocytes, Reed–Sternberg cells, and mononuclear variants. The diffuse lesions may manifest in several patterns. In the majority of cases, the Hodgkin tissue is hypercellular with a population of cells characteristic of mixed cellularity Hodgkin lymphoma in the lymph node (see Fig. 23.98). In some patients the marrow shows extensive hypocellularity characterized by a generally loose, sparsely cellular connective tissue with scattered, variably sized hypercellular areas containing lymphocytes, histiocytes, Reed–Sternberg cells, and mononuclear variants. Areas of necrosis may be present and are more common in post-therapy specimens than at initial diagnosis (Fig. 23.100). Varying degrees of fibrosis may be present. In some cases, entire biopsy specimens show replacement by dense fibrous connective tissue with few identifiable lymphocytes or histiocytes (Fig. 23.101). In others, scattered islands of cells are interspersed among the collagen fibers: some of these cells show features suggestive of Hodgkin cells; others are too distorted for accurate identification. In some instances the Hodgkin lesions are very hypercellular with a predominant population of Reed–Sternberg cells or mononuclear variants. Various combinations of these patterns may be present in the same biopsy specimen or in different specimens from the same patient. Necrosis and hypocellularity are more common in marrow from treated patients than untreated patients. In marrow involvement with lymphocyte depletion Hodgkin lymphoma, a typical consolidated lesion characterized by an inflammatory cellular infiltrate accompanied by a distinct amorphous deposition of eosinophilic background substance and Reed–Sternberg cells has been described.[557]

The presence of Reed–Sternberg cells or mononuclear variants is of critical importance to the recognition of Hodgkin lymphoma in marrow, and a definitive diagnosis should not be established without their identification in the appropriate cellular milieu. Several serial sections of the marrow biopsies may have to be examined before satisfactory Reed–Sternberg cells or mononuclear variants are detected. It is important not to misinterpret megakaryocytes as forms of Reed–Sternberg cells; this problem can be avoided by strict adherence to the principle of identifying Reed–Sternberg cells or variants only in the appropriate cellular background and by the use of immunohistochemical studies. Reed–Sternberg-like cells may be observed in marrow specimens with involvement by follicular center cell lymphoma, PTCL, and anaplastic large cell lymphoma (see Fig. 23.81); the clinical history, membrane surface marker studies, and characteristic tissue changes of Hodgkin lymphoma should aid in distinguishing these disorders.[560] In classical Hodgkin lymphoma, the Reed–Sternberg cells and mononuclear variants express CD30 and usually express CD15. The cells also show weak nuclear expression of PAX5, may show weak and variable expression of CD20, and are CD45 and CD3 negative. In some instances, in which a T-cell lymphoma such as anaplastic large cell lymphoma

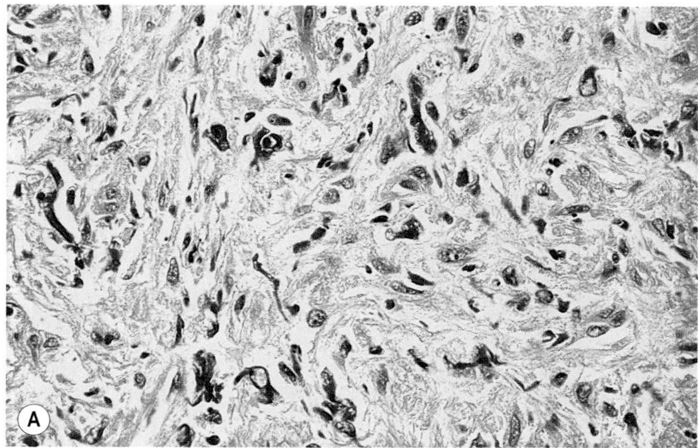

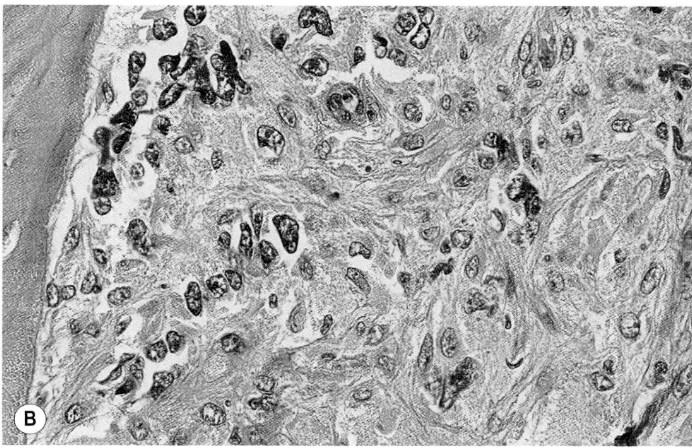

Fig. 23.101 **A**, Marrow biopsy from a patient with Hodgkin lymphoma. The marrow space is completely replaced by dense fibrous connective tissue. Numerous vascular structures and small foci of distorted cells resembling Reed–Sternberg cells and mononuclear variants are present. **B**, Same specimen as **A** showing several focal collections of cells that resemble distorted Reed–Sternberg cells and mononuclear variants.

is in the differential diagnosis, genotypic studies for T-cell clonality may be necessary.

Although marrow involvement by lymphocyte-predominant Hodgkin lymphoma is rare, when present it shows features more similar to histiocyte and T-cell rich large B-cell lymphoma than classical Hodgkin lymphoma, with large atypical cells admixed with T cells and histiocytes, and usually lacking a prominent eosinophil component.[554,567] In contrast to classical Hodgkin lymphoma, the neoplastic cells of lymphocyte-predominant Hodgkin lymphoma are strongly and uniformly CD20 positive and usually CD30 negative.[565,568]

Uninvolved areas of marrow in specimens with involvement by Hodgkin lymphoma may be hypercellular, normocellular, or hypocellular.[569] Nonspecific alterations, including stromal damage, inflammatory cell infiltration, and disturbed hematopoiesis, may be present.[553] These alterations may occur singly or in combination.

Similar to spleen, liver, and lymph nodes, benign granulomatous lesions may be present in bone marrow sections in patients with Hodgkin lymphoma.[563] The marrow is the least likely organ in this group to contain the granulomas, but their presence may lead to diagnostic difficulty. The lack of typical Reed–Sternberg cells or mononuclear variants is an important feature in distinguishing these lesions from Hodgkin lymphoma. The presence of granulomas does not constitute evidence of involvement. Granulomas in post-therapy patients should always be evaluated for the possibility of an infectious agent.[558,563] Benign lymphocytic aggregates may also be present.

Rarely, a patient whose disease is being staged for marrow involvement by Hodgkin lymphoma has a concurrent parvovirus B19 infection. The presence of very large erythroid precursors in the smears or sections may result in confusion with Reed–Sternberg cells and consideration of marrow Hodgkin lymphoma (see Fig. 23.22B). The lack of a characteristic cellular environment and the usually marked erythroid hypoplasia are strong evidence of parvovirus B19 infection. Serologic or molecular studies for parvovirus B19 should be performed in suspected cases.

Histiocytic disorders

Malignant histiocytosis

Malignant histiocytosis is a rare disease that uncommonly involves marrow. As a result, any comments about the characteristics of these lesions in the marrow are based on limited observations. The histiocytic tumors are defined in the 2008 edition of the *WHO Classification of Tumours of the Haematopoietic and Lymphoid Tissues* as 'histiocytic and dendritic cell neoplasms derived from phagocytic and accessory cells which have major roles in the processing and presentation of antigens to lymphocytes'.[571,572] The changing concept of 'malignant histiocytosis', and the recognition that many of the lesions previously classified under this term represent other disorders, mean that prior descriptions of marrow involvement in malignant histiocytosis may no longer be valid.[570,573–579] Generalizations about patterns of marrow involvement must be qualified because of the rare occurrence of the disorder and the even more rare occurrence of marrow involvement. If the morphologic characteristics of a marrow lesion suggest a histiocytic disorder, appropriate cytochemical, immunologic, cytogenetic, and molecular studies should be performed. The diagnosis is essentially one of exclusion. Other poorly differentiated neoplasms of the hematopoietic system may have morphologic features that have been associated with malignant histiocytosis.[579] Cell marker studies for B- and T-cell lineage should be performed to exclude poorly differentiated lymphomas. Poorly differentiated carcinomas and plasmablastic tumors must also be excluded. Since the macrophage is derived from the monocyte system it may be difficult in some instances to distinguish between what is termed malignant histiocytosis and what is monoblastic/monocytic leukemia. The use of one or other of these terms may be arbitrary based on the constellation of clinical and morphologic findings.

In marrow biopsies, the infiltration by malignant histiocytes may be focal or diffuse (Fig. 23.102). Bone marrow involvement may be extremely difficult to recognize in sections that contain only scattered malignant cells. In smear preparations, the cells occur singly or in small groups scattered among the normal hematopoietic cells or, because of their large size, at the edges of the smears. The malignant histiocytes vary in size; cells up to 40–50 μm or larger may be found. The cytoplasm is usually abundant, with evidence of pseudopod formation and fragmentation; it is variably basophilic, occasionally with numerous small, sharply defined vacuoles in some cells. Very small azurophilic granules may be present in the cytoplasm of some of the larger cells. Occasional malignant histiocytes show evidence of phagocytosis; prominent hemophagocytosis is a relatively uncommon finding in unequivocally malignant-appearing cells. The nucleus may be round or

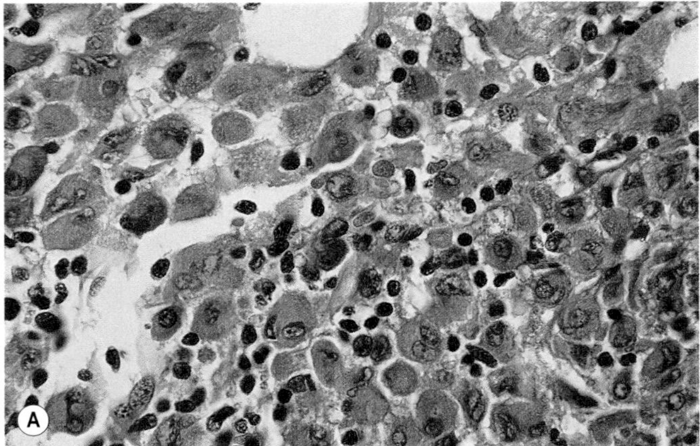

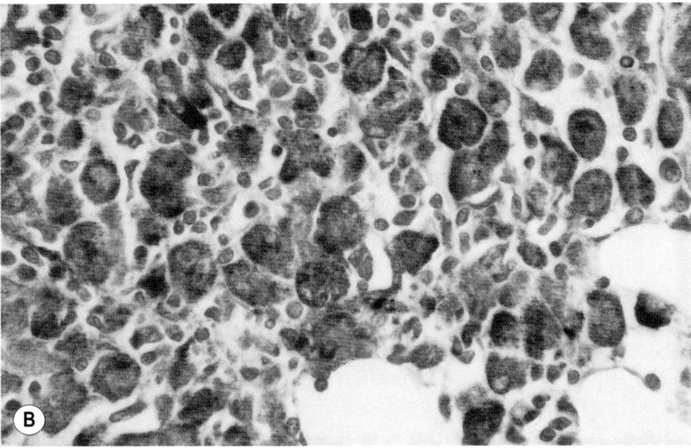

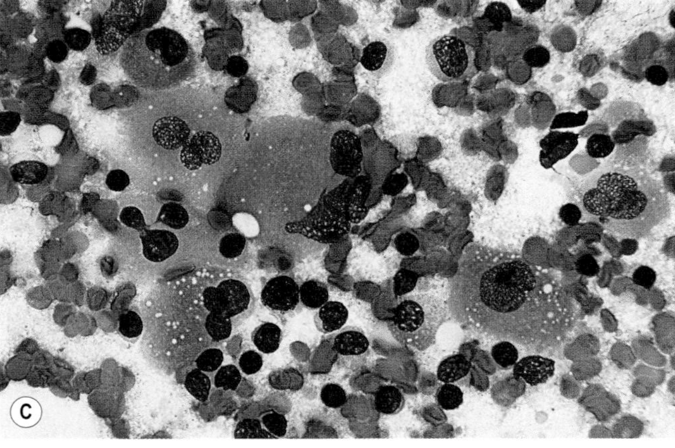

Fig. 23.102 **A**, Marrow biopsy from an adult female with marrow involvement by a histiocytic proliferation with an associated clonal t(9;11)(p21;q23) cytogenetic abnormality. The histiocytes have a somewhat bland appearance with abundant cytoplasm. **B**, The biopsy in **A** reacted with antibody to CD68 (KP-1). **C**, Smear from the specimen in **A** and **B** showing several histiocytes, most of which have lobulated nuclei and abundant cytoplasm. (**B**, Immunoperoxidase)

contorted; the larger cells generally have more contorted nuclei. The chromatin is coarsely reticular. Nucleoli may be very prominent or inconspicuous. Stains for nonspecific esterase and acid phosphatase are positive. The demonstration of nonspecific esterase reactivity in poorly differentiated cells, however, is not sufficient to establish a diagnosis of malignant histiocytosis since this enzyme may be present in other poorly differentiated malignant cells. The malignant histiocyte should be reactive with antibodies to lysozyme and CD68 (KP-1 and PGM-1) and nonreactive to antibodies to T and B lymphocytes (Fig. 23.102B). There may be some degree of reactivity with antibody to S-100 protein. The proliferation of the malignant histiocytes may be accompanied by a proliferation of benign-appearing histiocytes with abundant cytoplasm and prominent hemophagocytosis; this probably results from cytokine stimulation related to the malignant cell proliferation.

Cytogenetic studies may be helpful in identifying a clonal abnormality in the malignant cells, e.g., the presence of an abnormality involving chromosome 11 at band q23 characteristic of monoblastic leukemia.

Hemophagocytic syndromes

The hemophagocytic syndromes are a group of disorders with the unifying morphologic features of a proliferation of phagocytic histiocytes that may be present in all hematopoietic organs. These processes usually have systemic manifestations and may be accompanied by a fulminant clinical course and high mortality.

The hemophagocytic syndromes occur both as genetic and acquired disorders.[586,589,603,610] The genetic disorders include familial hemophagocytic lymphohistiocytosis (FHLH) which is an autosomal recessive disorder and in which the hemophagocytosis is the only manifestation of the disease and the immune deficiency syndromes Chediak–Higashi syndrome, Giscelli syndrome, and X-linked lymphoproliferative syndrome which have additional clinical features. Several genetic defects are involved in FHLH: 13–50% of the patients have mutations in the perforin 1 (*PFR1*) gene which results in impaired perforin production.[595,606] Mutations of the *MUNC13D* gene, which is on chromosome 17q25, occur in 17–30% of cases and result in impaired granule exocytosis.[586,588,606,610]

The acquired hemophagocytic syndromes occur at all ages. Several agents, including viruses and other infectious organisms, and malignant lymphomas have been implicated as causative factors. The viruses most frequently implicated include EBV, cytomegalovirus, adenovirus, and parvovirus B19.[583–587,591–594,596,597,600,605,607,608] The syndrome has also been associated with protozoan infections including *Babesia microti* and *Leishmania*.

The macrophage activation syndrome (MAC) is a subtype of the secondary hemophagocytic syndromes which is a complication of systemic inflammatory diseases in children, particularly juvenile rheumatoid arthritis.[598,599] Similar to other types of these syndromes, it appears to be related to hyperactivation and proliferation of T lymphocytes and macrophages.

The hemophagocytic syndromes are an epiphenomenon in which the underlying mechanism appears to be activation of the immune system including NK cells, cytotoxic T lymphocytes, and the monocyte–macrophage system, which then interact. Defective cytotoxic activity on the part of this system leads to sustained high cytotoxic levels which result in the constellation of the findings in the syndrome.[580,585,591,593,596,597–605,607–611]

The hemophagocytic syndromes frequently have an abrupt onset. Evidence of multisystem disease is usually present, particularly in patients with viral infections.[594,603,608] A high percentage of patients have coagulation abnormalities with disseminated intravascular coagulation. Laboratory studies show elevated triglycerides, ferritin, transaminases, and lactate dehydrogenase. The fibrinogen level is decreased. There are usually cytopenias, frequently pancytopenia.

The marrow smears contain numerous histiocytes, many showing evidence of phagocytosis of erythrocytes and precursors, platelets, and granulocytes. There is frequently an accompanying depression of erythroid precursors, granulocyte precursors, or both;

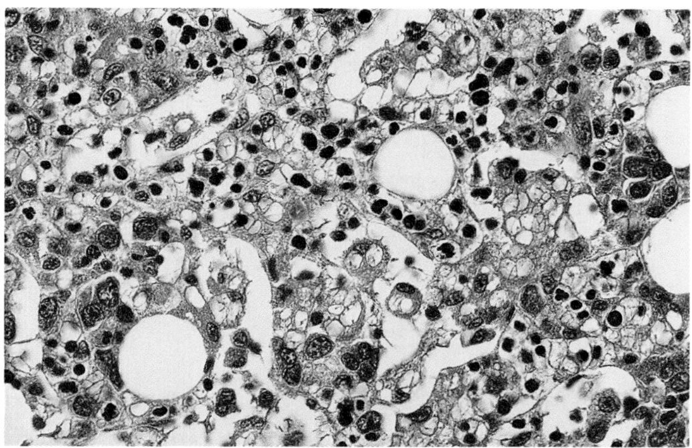

Fig. 23.103 Marrow biopsy from an adult male who developed hemophagocytic syndrome associated with bacterial infection. Numerous histiocytes, some showing hemophagocytosis, are present in sinusoids and interstitium.

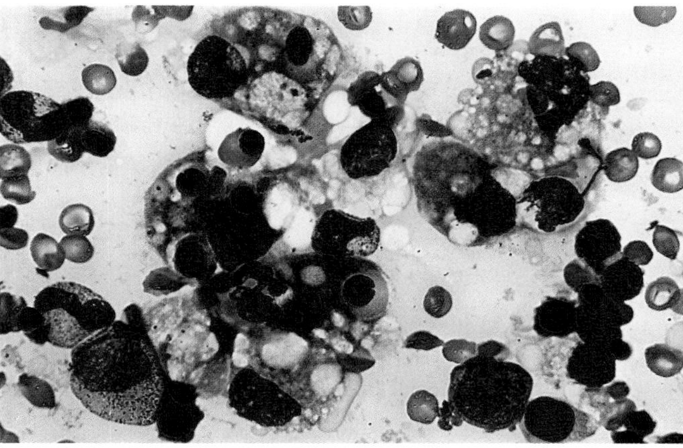

Fig. 23.104 Bone marrow smear from a lupus erythematosus patient with virus-associated hemophagocytic syndrome. Numerous macrophages with ingested red blood cells and erythroblasts are present. (Wright–Giemsa)

megakaryocytes may be normal or increased in number. In biopsy sections, the increased histiocytes are dispersed throughout the interstitium and sinuses; occasional clusters may be present (Fig. 23.103). The evidence of phagocytic activity may be less prominent in sections compared with smear preparations (Fig. 23.104). In addition to the histiocytic proliferation, granulomas may be noted, and areas of cellular necrosis are frequently present. The bone marrow findings may change substantially over a period of days, with fluctuations in the number of granulocyte and erythroid precursors and megakaryocytes. Lymph nodes may show a marked increase in histiocytes in the sinusoidal spaces; evidence of hemophagocytosis may be much less marked than in the bone marrow or there may be marked erythrophagocytosis. The spleen may be markedly enlarged with prominent histiocytic infiltration in the red pulp. Areas of nonsuppurative necrosis have been observed in lymph nodes and spleen.[601]

The mechanism of macrophage activation in the hemophagocytic syndromes is not completely understood but appears to be related to the release of chemokines and cytokines, including macrophage inflammatory protein-1 alpha and interferon gamma.[596] The phenomenon appears to be preceded in some patients by proliferation of activated or neoplastic EBV-infected T lymphocytes that produce tumor necrosis factor alpha (TNF-α).

The EBV or T-cell related hemophagocytic syndromes may be difficult to distinguish morphologically from familial hemophagocytic lymphocytic histiocytosis. The latter disorder appears to be related to mutation of the perforin gene and diminished perforin in cytotoxic T cells and T/NK cells.[595,606] This contrasts with the normal levels of perforin in cytotoxic cells in patients with secondary hemophagocytic syndromes.

The clinicopathologic features of virus-associated hemophagocytic syndrome (VAHS) have been reported in 80% of a group of patients with fatal infectious mononucleosis.[597] The VAHS phase was preceded by features of a viral-like illness. Sequential changes were present in the marrows of these patients; initially there was infiltration by atypical lymphoid cells with areas of necrosis, followed by depletion of normal hematopoietic cells and histiocytic activation with prominent hemophagocytosis; the end stage was marked by marrow aplasia. A similar sequence of histopathologic changes was found in the lymph nodes, spleen, and thymus gland.

Hemophagocytic histiocytosis has been reported as a terminal event in patients with T-cell lymphomas and T/NK-cell lymphomas; uncommonly it is associated with B-cell lymphoma.[585,591,604] The pathologic findings are similar to those in VAHS. The production of macrophage-activating cytokines by the malignant cells has been suggested as a causative mechanism of the histiocyte proliferation. The hemophagocytic syndrome may be associated with other types of lymphoma including anaplastic large cell lymphoma with an associated t(2;5) chromosome abnormality.[583]

The distinction between the hemophagocytic syndrome and 'malignant histiocytosis' may be difficult because of similarities in clinical presentation.[581,582,593,594] The cells in the hemophagocytic syndrome are morphologically distinct; they have a low nucleocytoplasmic ratio and abundant lightly staining cytoplasm containing large vacuoles of varying sizes and phagocytosed cells or cellular products. Nucleoli, when present, are not prominent, and mitotic figures are rare. Although the hemophagocytic histiocyte proliferation may coexist with 'malignant histiocytosis' or a malignant lymphoma, there is no evidence of a transition from the obviously malignant cells to the benign histiocytes.

Serologic studies for viral infection in patients with the picture of a hemophagocytic syndrome may not be reliable because impaired immune function may preclude a detectable antibody response. In these cases, molecular hybridization studies may be useful in documenting an EBV or parvovirus B19 infection.[587,593,594] In addition to studies for a viral infection, it is important that patients with a hemophagocytic process be carefully evaluated for immune suppression and non-Hodgkin lymphoma. Patients with a hemophagocytic syndrome with both an EBV infection and a malignant lymphoproliferative lesion may be observed.

Etoposide appears to be an effective therapy for some patients with the EBV-associated hemophagocytic syndrome.[590]

Langerhans cell histiocytosis

Marrow involvement in Langerhans cell histiocytosis (histiocytosis X) is uncommon and usually associated with the multisystem multifocal form of the disease (Letterer–Siwe disease).[612] The marrow lesions may be focal and small and barely perceptible or confluent and extensive replacing large areas of a biopsy (Fig. 23.105).[613] The small lesions may have a granulomatous appearance. Similar to the lesions in other organs, the Langerhans cells have a low nucleocytoplasmic ratio; the nuclei are grooved, folded

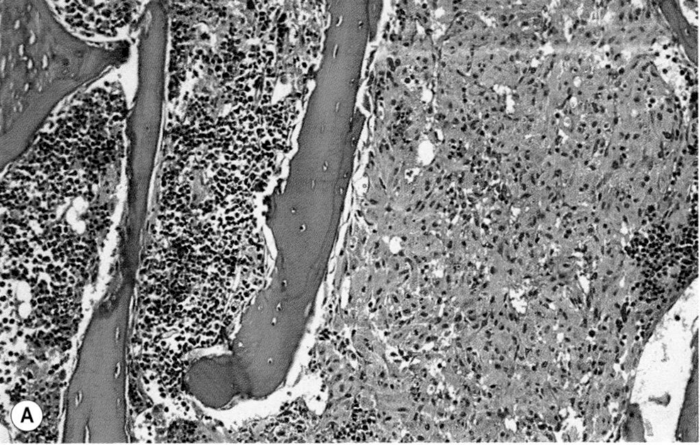
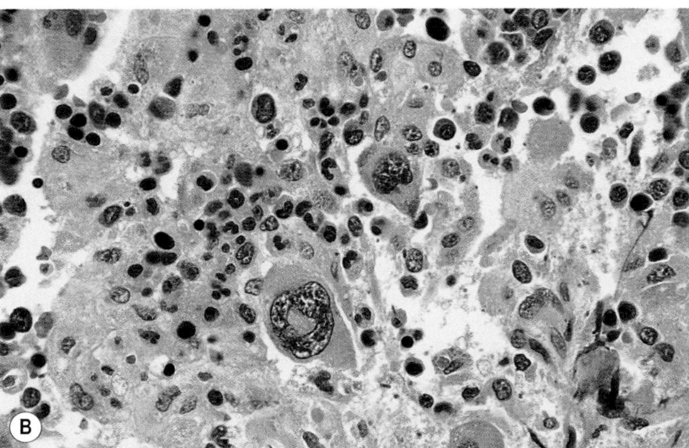
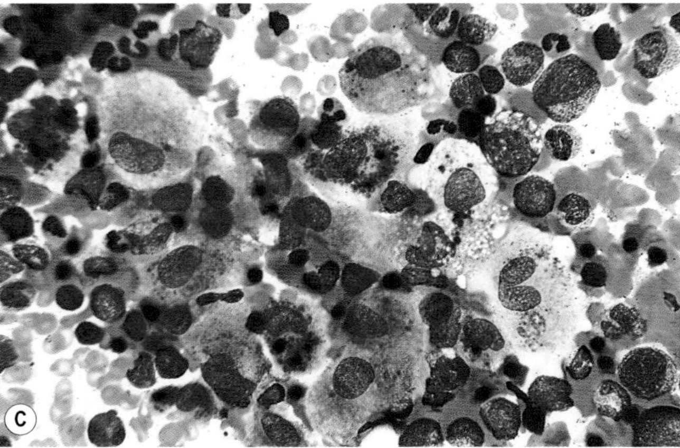

Fig. 23.105 **A**, Marrow biopsy from a child with Langerhans cell histiocytosis showing extensive replacement. **B**, High magnification of the lesion in **A** showing giant cells and several histiocytes. Some residual myeloid cells are present. **C**, Bone marrow smear from the case illustrated in **A** and **B**. The Langerhans cells are very large with abundant cytoplasm; several histiocytes contain nonspecific debris and occasionally red blood cells.

or lobulated with dispersed chromatin and inconspicuous nucleoli. Hemosiderin and lipofuscin-like granules may be present in the cytoplasm. Mitotic activity is variable The lesions may be relatively monocellular or polycellular with admixed phagocytic histiocytes, multinucleate giant cells, lymphocytes, plasma cells, eosinophils, and neutrophils. Stains for reticulin show an increased number of reticulin fibers. Immunohistochemical reactions for S-100 protein, langerin, and CD1a highlight the Langerhans cell infiltrate. However, with some fixatives and decalcifying agents, the reaction with antibody to CD1a may be suboptimal in bone marrow biopsies. The cells are variably reactive for CD68 (KP-1), HLA-DR, CD45, lysozyme, and nonspecific esterase.[612] In smear preparations and touch imprints, the Langerhans cell has abundant cytoplasm which frequently contains particulate green–blue debris (Fig. 23.105C). Characteristic Birbeck granules are observed on ultrastructural examination.

Box 23.9 Plasma cell neoplasms[a]

- Plasma cell myeloma
  - Variants:
    - Nonsecretory myeloma
    - Asymptomatic myeloma (smoldering myeloma)
    - Plasma cell leukemia
    - Osteosclerotic myeloma
- Plasmacytoma
  - Solitary plasmacytoma of bone
  - Extramedullary plasmacytoma
- Immunoglobulin deposition diseases
  - Primary amyloidosis
  - Systemic light and heavy chain deposition diseases

[a]Modified from WHO.[614] Monoclonal gammopathy of undetermined significance (MGUS) excluded.

Plasma cell dyscrasias

The plasma cell dyscrasias are proliferations of immunosecretory cells generally associated with perturbation of serum immunoglobulins. This group of diseases includes the plasma cell proliferations and lymphoplasmacytic lymphoma. A modification of the WHO classification of plasma cell neoplasms is shown in Box 23.9.[614] Monoclonal gammopathy of undetermined significance (MGUS), which is not strictly a neoplasm, is excluded from the present table.

The prototype disorder for this group of diseases is plasma cell myeloma, of which the clinical syndrome is multiple myeloma. Monoclonal gammopathy of undetermined significance is viewed as a precursor lesion.

The criteria for the diagnosis of symptomatic and asymptomatic plasma cell myeloma are listed in Box 23.10.[614]

Plasma cell myeloma

Plasma cell myeloma (PCM) is a neoplastic proliferation of plasma cells accompanied by the production of a monoclonal immunoglobulin detectable in the serum, urine, or both.[639,640] There are several clinical variants including asymptomatic or smoldering myeloma, nonsecretory myeloma, and plasma cell leukemia. The peak incidence is in the seventh decade; the disease is slightly more frequent in males than females. Osteolytic lesions in the skull, ribs, sternum, vertebrae, and pelvis are present in approximately 70% of cases; in rare cases, x-ray films reveal osteosclerotic lesions.

Marrow involvement in myeloma may be patchy, and the percentage of plasma cells may vary in aspirates and biopsies from different sites. In trephine sections, the distribution of plasma cells may be focal, interstitial, diffuse, or a combination of these patterns[616,618,621,651] (Fig. 23.106). There is variability in the appearance of the plasma cells in different cases from very immature plasma cells with a blastlike appearance to pleomorphic cells to

Box 23.10 2008 WHO diagnostic criteria for plasma cell myeloma[614]

Symptomatic plasma cell myeloma

M-protein in serum or urine[a]
Bone marrow clonal plasma cells or plasmacytoma[b]
Related end-organ damage (end-organ damage or bone lesions: hypercalcemia, renal impairment, anemia, bone lesions or myeloma-related symptoms)

Asymptomatic (smoldering) myeloma

M-protein in serum or urine (>30 g/L), and/or
10% or more clonal plasma cells in marrow
No related organ damage or tissue impairment

[a]No level of serum or urine protein is included. The M-protein in most cases is >30 g/L of IgG or >25 g/L of IgA or 1 g/24 hours of urine light chain; some patients with symptomatic myeloma have levels which are lower.
[b]Monoclonal plasma cells usually exceed 10% in the marrow but no minimum level is designated; about 5% of patients with symptomatic myeloma have <10% monoclonal plasma cells in the marrow.

mature-appearing plasma cells[619,627,631] (Fig. 23.107). Nucleoli may be very prominent in some of the more immature types, and binucleate cells resembling Reed–Sternberg cells may be found. Nuclear and cytoplasmic inclusions of varying types may be noted; these are usually related to immunoglobulin production (Fig. 23.108). The marrow in approximately 10–20% of cases shows an associated fibrosis[620,637] (Fig. 23.109).

Several approaches to the staging of myeloma have been introduced: these have included the correlation of myeloma cell mass with presenting laboratory findings, including hemoglobin, monoclonal immunoglobulin, and calcium levels, and the presence of osteolytic bone lesions.[622,623,628,633,648] The serum β_2-microglobulin level and the plasma cell labeling index have been found to be significant prognostic factors.[617,624,630,631] β_2-Microglobulin levels above 4 ng/μL and plasma cell labeling index greater than 0.4% are associated with a shorter survival than β_2-microglobulin levels less than 1 ng/μL and labeling index of 0.[624,629,630,632]

The occurrence of genetic abnormalities detected by interphase fluorescent in situ hybridization (FISH) has been reported in up to 90% of patients with PCM. The most frequent abnormalities are del(13q14), hyperdiploidy, t(11;14), t(4;14), *MYC* translocations, and del(17p13). del(13q14) is frequently associated with t(4;14) or del(17p13).[636,646] The most frequent translocations involve 14q32 and occur in 55–70% of cases. The five major translocations involving 14q32 are t(4;11), t(4;14), t(14;16), t(14;14), and t(14;20); combined these translocations occur in approximately 40% of cases.[636,640,641] t(4;14), t(14;16), and t(14;20) have been associated with poor response to conventional induction therapy and short overall median survival.[641] del(17p13) has also been associated with a poor prognosis. The prognosis of cases with monosomy 13 or del(13q14) with concurrent t(4;14) or del(17p13) appears to be dictated by the non 13 abnormality. In a large multi-institutional study, the most important predictive genetic factors for survival were t(4;14) and del(17p13) combined with the serum β_2-microglobulin level. The combination of one of these genetic abnormalities and an elevated β_2-microglobulin level was an adverse predictive factor.[615]

Similar to mantle cell lymphoma with t(11;14)(q13;q32), the nuclei of the myeloma cells in patients with this translocation are cyclin D1 positive.[626,634]

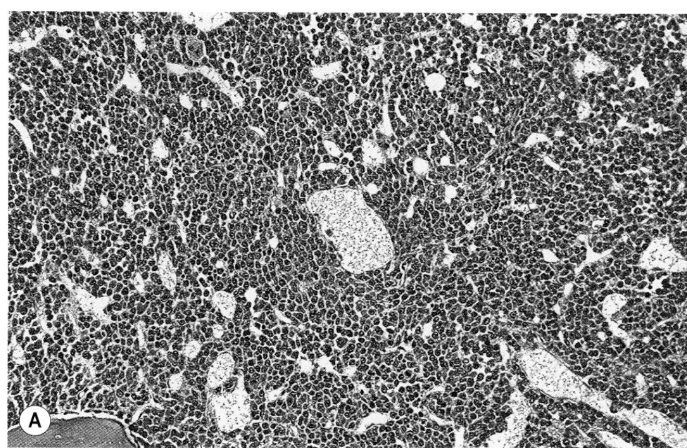

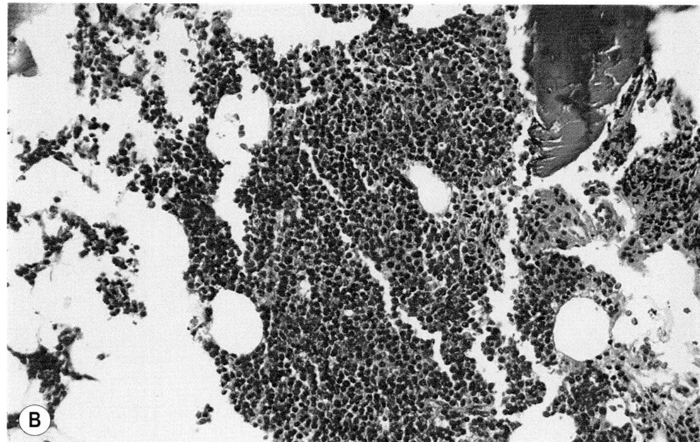

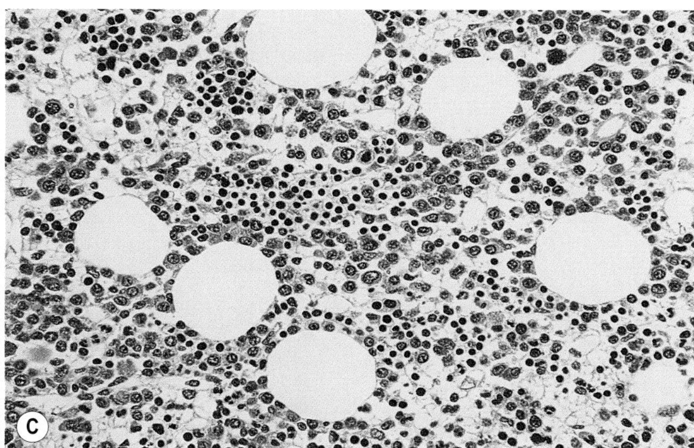

Fig. 23.106 **A**, Marrow biopsy from a patient with multiple myeloma with extensive diffuse replacement by myeloma cells. **B**, Marrow biopsy with a large focus of myeloma cells. **C**, Marrow biopsy showing essentially normal marrow architecture and interstitial infiltration by myeloma cells.

Histopathologic staging of myeloma in bone marrow biopsies based on cytologic features of the myeloma cells and the degree of plasma cell infiltration has been shown to have prognostic significance.[640] The more mature type of plasma cell myeloma, plasmacytic, and less than 20% marrow replacement are favorable prognostic factors. The more immature or poorly differentiated the myeloma cells, i.e., plasmablastic, and the more extensive the marrow involvement (>50% replacement), the more unfavorable

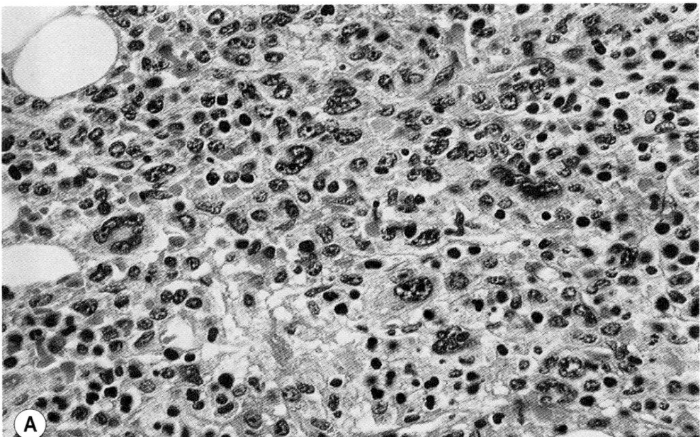

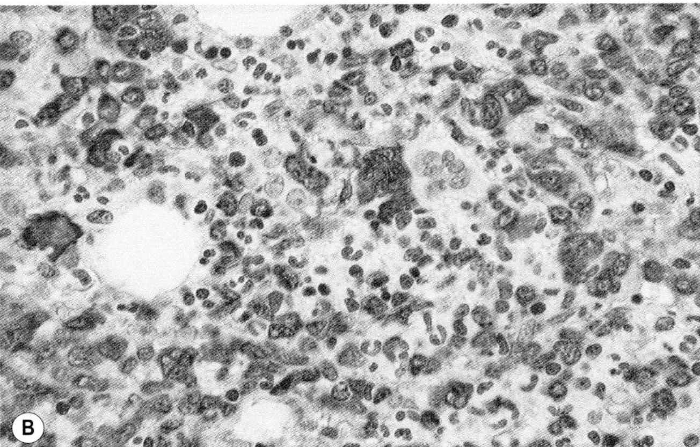

Fig. 23.107 **A**, Marrow from a patient with anaplastic myeloma; many of the plasma cells are large with lobulated nuclei. **B**, Specimen in **A** reacted with antibody to lambda light chains. The plasma cells show intense cytoplasmic reactivity. Numerous nonreactive residual myeloid cells are present. (**B**, Immunoperoxidase)

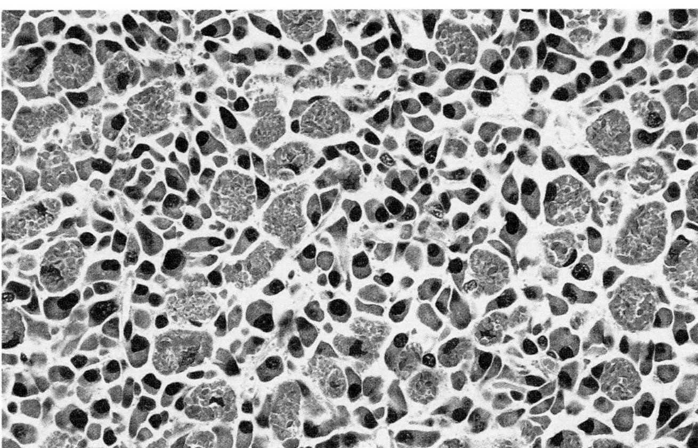

Fig. 23.108 Marrow biopsy from a 63-year-old patient with multiple myeloma with hypogammaglobulinemia and kappa light chain Bence Jones proteinuria. The cytoplasm of myeloma cells is distended by numerous, frequently confluent eosinophilic inclusions.

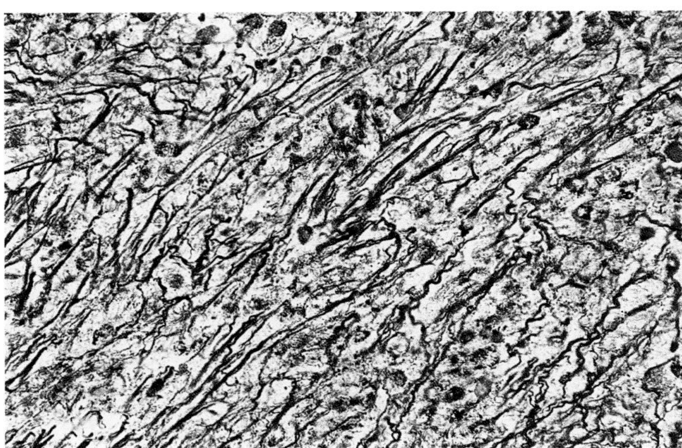

Fig. 23.109 Marrow biopsy from a patient with plasma cell myeloma and marked reticulin fibrosis.

the prognosis. An anaplastic evolution of myeloma may occur, and some of these cases have the histopathologic features of immunoblastic lymphoma.[625] Studies comparing anaplastic myeloma with B-immunoblastic lymphoma have demonstrated clinical and immunologic differences.[649,650] The plasma cells in anaplastic myeloma are usually of the IgG or IgA heavy chain class in contrast to B-immunoblastic lymphoma in which the cells are IgM. The cells in immunoblastic lymphoma usually express pan-B-cell antigens; the plasma cells in approximately 80% of cases of myeloma do not express pan-B-cell antigens. Exceptions to these generalizations occur. All clinical and laboratory findings should be considered. Histopathologic staging of myeloma in the marrow, using an approach similar to that used for CLL, has shown good correlation between pattern of marrow involvement and clinical stage; a diffuse pattern of involvement is usually associated with a more advanced clinical stage.[651] In some patients, the pattern of marrow involvement may be somewhat inconsistent from biopsy to biopsy, and focal involvement may be associated with an advanced clinical stage. Immunohistologic studies on paraffin-embedded biopsy specimens, utilizing antibodies to CD38 and CD138, are very useful in identifying myeloma cells and detecting extent of marrow involvement.[642–644,652] Anti-kappa and anti-lambda antibodies are used for detection and determining monoclonality. Immunohistochemistry is particularly helpful following chemotherapy and hematopoietic stem cell transplant for detecting residual disease.

As noted, the myeloma cells in patients with an associated t(11;14)(q13;q32) translocation are usually cyclin D1 positive; a substantial number of these cases are reported as having lymphoplasmacytoid morphology and extensive marrow infiltration.[626,634]

Nonsecretory myeloma

Approximately 3% of patients with PCM present with the clinical, radiographic, and histopathologic features of multiple myeloma but lack evidence of monoclonal immunoglobulin production in the serum or urine. These cases have been referred to as 'nonsecretory' myeloma.[645,647] Considerable caution should be exercised in the use of this term, since striking reactive plasmacytosis may be observed with nonmalignant conditions, including liver disease, connective tissue disorders, chronic granulomatous disorders, hypersensitivity states, and drug-related agranulocytosis.[635] When a nonsecretory myeloma is suspected, the monoclonal nature of the proliferating plasma cells should be confirmed by immunoperoxidase or immunofluorescent techniques that will demonstrate kappa or lambda light chain restriction.[633,642,652] An increase in reactive plasma cells will be characterized by a relatively balanced population of kappa- and lambda-containing cells.

Asymptomatic (smoldering) plasma cell myeloma

Asymptomatic or smoldering myeloma are the terms used for cases of plasma cell myeloma in which the criteria for myeloma are present but there is no related organ or tissue impairment, i.e., no symptomatology.[638,640] Approximately 8% of patients presenting with myeloma are of this type. The majority of these cases have between 10% and 20% plasma cells in the marrow. The cumulative probability of progression to symptomatic myeloma is 10% per year for the first 5 years following diagnosis and approximately 1% per year for the next 10 years.

Plasma cell leukemia

The term plasma cell leukemia is applied to those processes in which a patient presents with a plasma cell proliferation in the blood; the plasma cells exceed 20% of the blood leukocytes, or the absolute plasma cell count exceeds $20 \times 10^9/L$[654,655,657] (Fig. 23.110). The term should be reserved for cases with this finding at initial presentation. In contrast to cases of PCM presenting with detectable monoclonal immunoglobulin production, usually of IgG or IgA type, cases of plasma cell leukemia frequently present with a higher incidence of light chain disease, IgD or IgE paraprotein than the other forms of myeloma.[653,657] The marrow in plasma cell leukemia usually shows diffuse and extensive replacement of normal hematopoietic cells by the plasma cells. In some cases, the myeloma cells have a lymphoid appearance. Patients with plasma cell leukemia have a higher incidence of organomegaly than those with other forms of myeloma, and the disease is usually associated with an unfavorable prognosis with a higher incidence of unfavorable cytogenetic profiles than other patients with PCM. Osteolytic lesions and bone pain are less frequent than other forms of myeloma.

Multiple myeloma or amyloidosis may occur in patients with the adult Fanconi syndrome; the renal abnormalities may precede the overt manifestations of the plasma cell dyscrasia by several years. Bence Jones proteinuria of kappa light chain type is a common finding. A high percentage of the patients with this variant of myeloma manifest crystalline inclusions in the cytoplasm of the proliferating plasma cells and renal tubular cells.[656]

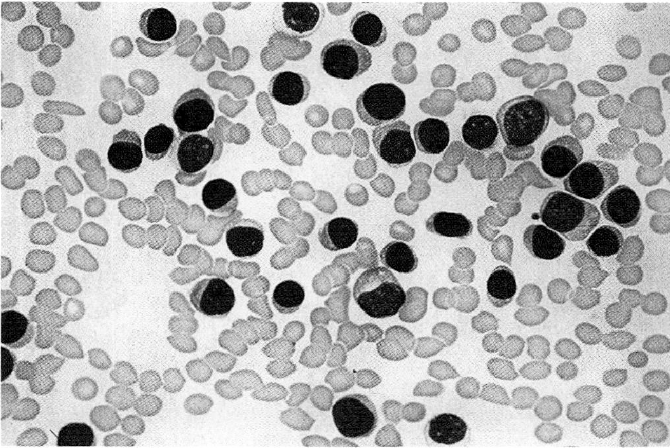

Fig. 23.110 Blood smear from a 47-year-old woman with leukocytosis of $24.0 \times 10^9/L$ and 90% plasma cells. Many of the plasma cells have 'lymphoid' features. There was a serum IgG kappa monoclonal protein. (Wright–Giemsa)

(Reproduced from Brunning RD, McKenna RW. Tumors of the hematopoietic system. Atlas of tumor pathology, series 3, fascicle 9. Washington DC, 1994, Armed Forces Institute of Pathology)

Osteosclerotic myeloma (POEMS syndrome)

Osteosclerotic myeloma is a form of plasma cell dyscrasia characterized by sclerotic bone lesions and progressive demyelinating polyneuropathy.[659–664] The bone marrow aspirate usually contains less than 10% plasma cells. The plasma cell proliferation is usually evident as a plasmacytoma in the sclerotic lesions or in lymph nodes (Fig. 23.111A,B). The marrow from areas uninvolved by the sclerotic process may show typical myeloma cell infiltration. The megakaryocytes in the noninvolved areas may be increased and large with hyperlobulated nuclei (Fig. 23.111C). The involved lymph nodes may show angiofollicular hyperplasia with a parafollicular infiltration of monoclonal plasma cells, the plasma cell variant of Castleman disease.[658] A high percentage of patients with osteosclerotic myeloma have multiorgan involvement, including polyneuropathy, organomegaly, endocrinopathy, and skin changes, the so-called 'POEMS' syndrome.[658–666] Approximately 75% of patients have a thrombocytosis. Polycythemia and leukocytosis are present in about one-third of cases. There is usually a low level of monoclonal protein of IgG or IgA class, with a predominance of lambda light chain type.

The median age of onset is 51 years compared with 64 years for typical myeloma; median survival is 14.7 years, in contrast to 3–4 years for typical myeloma. The disease appears to be more common in Japan than in the United States or Europe.

An association of giant lymph node hyperplasia with osteoblastic bone lesions and the POEMS syndrome has been reported.[658,659]

Plasmacytoma

A solitary plasmacytoma, in contrast to the disseminated proliferation of plasma cells in multiple myeloma, is a single focus of plasma cells occurring in either bone or soft tissue.[667–682] Solitary plasmacytomas are more frequent in males than females and have a peak incidence in the sixth decade, slightly earlier than multiple myeloma. Plasmacytomas are generally divided into two broad groups based on location: plasmacytoma of bone and extramedullary or soft tissue plasmacytoma. The recommended diagnostic criteria for solitary plasmacytoma of bone are shown in Box 23.11.[670]

Evidence for different biologic behavior of these two types has been reported: plasmacytoma of bone has been reported to have a greater predilection to progress to multiple myeloma than soft tissue plasmacytoma. Other studies have shown no significant difference between these two locations and the incidence of evolution to myeloma.[675] The solitary plasmacytoma of bone may occur in both flat and long bones; the most common site is the axial skeleton, particularly a vertebra.[668,669,671,673–675] The thoracic vertebrae are more frequently involved than the cervical or lumbar vertebrae. Soft tissue extension from bone lesions may occur. The majority of plasmacytomas of bone show osteolytic change on radiologic examination, although osteolytic/osteoblastic lesions may occur.[682] The most frequent sites of extramedullary or soft tissue plasmacytomas are the nasal fossa, maxillary sinus, and nasopharynx.[673,675]

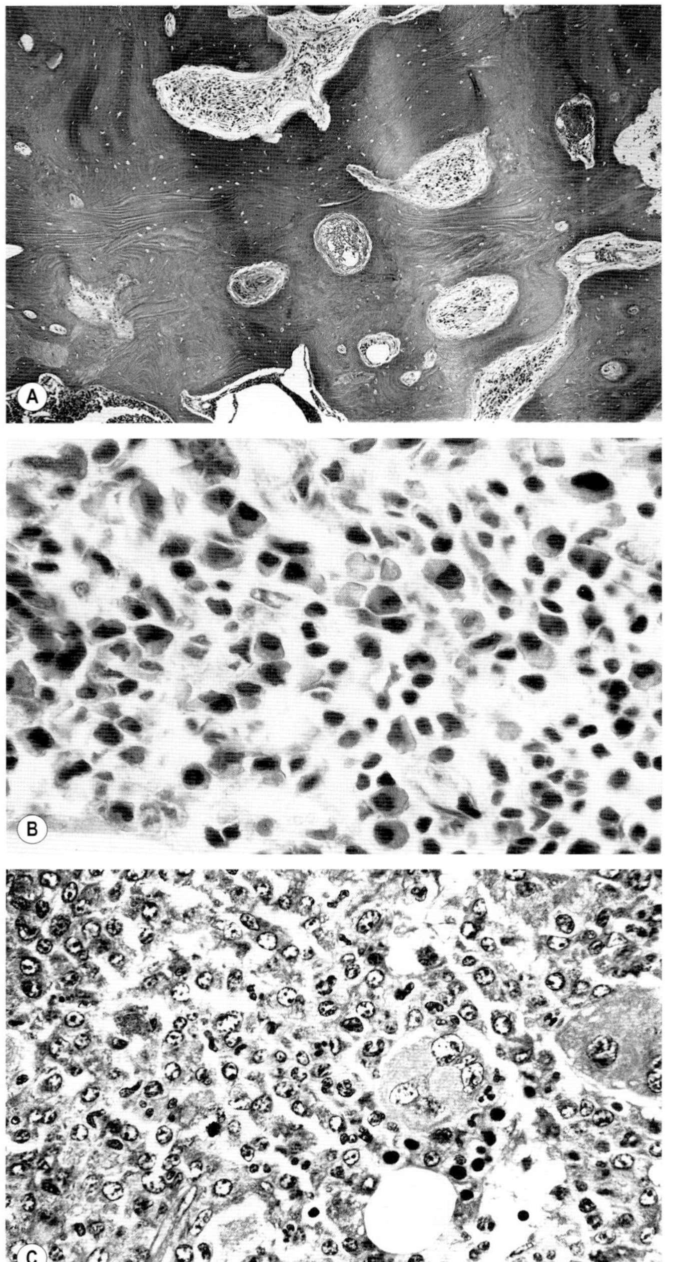

Fig. 23.111 **A**, An osteosclerotic bone lesion from a patient with osteosclerotic myeloma. **B**, High magnification of the marrow in the specimen in **A**. This area shows a large number of plasma cells that were lambda light chain restricted on immunohistochemical study. **C**, Marrow biopsy from a nonsclerotic area from a patient with osteosclerotic myeloma with POEMS syndrome. There was a thrombocytosis. The marrow in this area shows an infiltration by immature plasma cells. There was also an increase in large megakaryocytes, two of which are at right.

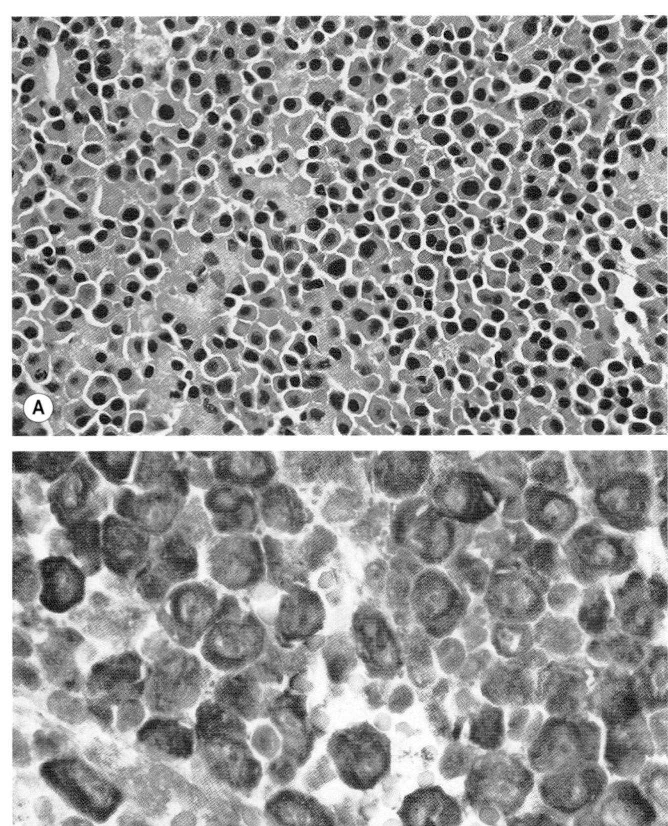

Fig. 23.112 **A**, Extramedullary plasmacytoma from the region of the nasopharynx. **B**, Plasmacytoma reacted with antibody to kappa light chains. The plasma cells show intense cytoplasmic reactivity. (**B**, Immunoperoxidase)

Box 23.11 Criteria for diagnosis of solitary plasmacytoma[670]

- Single area of bone destruction due to clonal plasma cells
- Normal marrow biopsy without clonal disease
- Normal results on a radiologic skeletal survey and MRI of the spine, pelvis, proximal femurs, and humeri
- No anemia, hypercalcemia or renal impairment attributable to myeloma
- No or low serum or urinary level of monoclonal protein and preserved levels of uninvolved immunoglobulins

The criteria for a soft tissue plasmacytoma are essentially similar.

Extension into adjacent bone tissue may occur, and multiple lesions may be present.

On microscopic examination the plasmacytoma is frequently very vascular with a minimal stromal component and consists of sheets of plasma cells of varying degrees of differentiation[668] (Fig. 23.112). The plasmacytic nature of the proliferating cells is readily recognized in the better-differentiated lesions. In plasmacytomas with a predominant population of more immature cells with a dispersed nuclear chromatin and single prominent nucleolus, there usually is a minor population of more differentiated plasma cells. Amyloid may be present and was noted in 25% of the lesions in one series.[675]

Immunocytochemical study with antibodies to kappa and lambda light chains is an important approach to the evaluation of a suspected plasmacytoma.[678] A kappa or lambda light chain-restricted population confirms a diagnosis of plasmacytoma (Fig. 23.112B). There is a predominance of IgG heavy chain type in solitary plasmacytoma of bone and IgA heavy chain type in plasmacytomas from the upper respiratory tract.

Patients with an apparent solitary plasmacytoma should be carefully evaluated for the presence of disseminated disease; studies should include bilateral iliac crest bone marrow biopsies, radiologic skeletal survey, MRI of the spine, pelvis, humeri, and femurs, immunoelectrophoretic examination of the serum and urine, and β_2-microglobulin assay. The patient with a solitary plasmacytoma usually has a normal hemoglobin level and no hypercalcemia. The diagnosis of a solitary plasmacytoma should be made only if all studies for disseminated disease are negative.

Approximately 50% of patients with a plasmacytoma have a monoclonal protein in the serum and/or urine; the level almost invariably is less than 20 g/L, and the nonmonoclonal immunoglobulins are normal in contrast to multiple myeloma, in which they are generally decreased. A marked reduction or disappearance of the monoclonal immunoglobulin will usually occur following tumoricidal radiation; the maximum reduction may not occur for several years.[675] Persistence of the monoclonal protein for more than 1 year after radiotherapy of the plasmacytoma has been identified as an adverse prognostic factor.[680]

Approximately 35% of patients with a solitary plasmacytoma who receive treatment, including radiation, chemotherapy, and surgical excision, will eventually develop multiple myeloma; this evolution may occur up to 12 years following initial diagnosis.[675,677] The presence of nuclear immaturity with prominent nucleoli appears to have some positive predictive value for the development of multiple myeloma. However, the presence of a monoclonal protein in serum, urine, or both does not predict the development of disseminated disease. Plasmacytomas of non-IgG class have been reported to have a higher predilection for systemic spread than IgG-producing tumors. Local recurrence of the lesion is uncommon.

The differential diagnosis of a plasmacytoma includes plasma cell granuloma, plasmacytoid lymphoma, and large cell lymphoma of immunoblastic type. The plasma cell granuloma shows a balanced proliferation of kappa- and lambda-reacting cells on immunocytochemical evaluation. The plasmacytoid lymphoma comprises a mixture of lymphocytes and plasma cells. Some of the large cell lymphomas, particularly the B-immunoblastic lymphoma, may be difficult to distinguish from a plasmacytoma. Immunoblastic lymphoma will usually involve lymph nodes in contrast to plasmacytoma. Immunophenotypic studies of plasmacytoma and immunoblastic lymphoma using a panel of monoclonal antibodies have shown significant immunophenotypic differences between these two processes.[679] The immunoblastic lymphomas have cytoplasmic IgM heavy chain and express pan-B-cell surface antigens such as CD19 and CD20. The plasmacytomas contain IgA or IgG heavy chain and are generally negative for pan-B-surface antigens; approximately 20% of plasmacytomas and myelomas are positive with pan-B-cell antibodies.

Monoclonal gammopathy of undetermined significance

Approximately 3–5% of individuals over the age of 50 and 2–3% of patients over age 65 have a serum monoclonal gammopathy without other evidence of a plasma cell dyscrasia; this constellation of findings is referred to as monoclonal gammopathy of undetermined significance (MGUS).[686,688,689] The monoclonal protein in these individuals is usually less than 30 g/L and there is usually no or minimal Bence Jones protein in the urine. There is no associated hypercalcemia, anemia, renal impairment, or radiologic evidence of bone lesions.[685] The bone marrow in these patients may be entirely normal or may manifest a slight increase in mature-appearing plasma cells; the increase is less than 10%. Some of these cases represent incipient myeloma or another type of plasma cell dyscrasia or lymphoproliferative disorder; others continue for several years without undergoing an obvious neoplastic evolution. In a study from the Mayo Clinic, MGUS constituted approximately 50% of the cases of monoclonal gammopathy.[688]

The incidence of MGUS varies in different studies. In one very large contemporary study of the population of Olmsted County in Minnesota in the USA using sensitive laboratory techniques, MGUS was identified in 3.2% of individuals 50 years of age or older and 5.3% of patients 70 years of age or older.[689] The concentration of monoclonal immunoglobulin was <10 g/L in 63.5% of individuals and >20 g/L in 4.5%. The incidence of MGUS is higher in black individuals than in whites.

Two important issues must be addressed when contemplating a diagnosis of MGUS: distinction from overt myeloma and probability of progression to an overt plasma cell dyscrasia if a diagnosis of MGUS is made. If the morphologic findings are suspicious for but not diagnostic of overt myeloma, the patient should be followed with marrow examination and repeat protein electrophoresis at 6-month intervals. An increase in the number of abnormal plasma cells or light chain-restricted plasma cells and an increase in the amount of monoclonal immunoglobulin suggest evolution to a neoplastic process.[683,685,690,691] A stable immunoglobulin level and plasma cell percentage are more reflective of MGUS. The plasma cell labeling index as described by Greipp and Kyle has been useful in distinguishing MGUS and smoldering myeloma from overt multiple myeloma.[685] The diagnostic accuracy of a plasma cell labeling index of greater than 0.4 was 83% in distinguishing myeloma from MGUS and smoldering myeloma. The accuracy is increased when combined with the percentage of marrow plasma cells. Approximately 8% of patients with MGUS eventually develop a neoplastic plasma cell dyscrasia or related process; the interval to occurrence ranges up to 29 years, and the rate of progression is approximately 1% per year.[687,690,691] Factors predicting transformation have varied in different studies: percentage of marrow plasma cells greater than or equal to 5% and paraprotein isotype at initial presentation have been found to have some value. Bone marrow angiogenesis is reported to increase progressively in those patients who manifest progression of MGUS to overt myeloma; median microvessel density correlated with the bone marrow plasma cell labeling index and the percentage of marrow plasma cells.[693] In a large series of patients with MGUS, the only independent risk factors for progression to an overt myeloma or related plasma cell dyscrasia was concentration of the serum monoclonal protein at diagnosis and the type of monoclonal protein. The risk for progression to myeloma or a related disorder at 10 years was 6% for an initial monoclonal protein of 5 g/L or less compared to 34% for an initial monoclonal protein of 30 g/L. Monoclonal proteins of IgM or IgA type had a higher risk of progression than an IgG paraprotein.[691] Patients with an abnormal serum light chain ratio have a significantly higher rate of progression to an overt plasma cell malignancy. Several cytogenetic abnormalities, including monosomy 13, t(4;14)(p16.3;q32), and t(14;16)(q32;q23), have been found in MGUS; no obvious clinical or biologic correlations have been established. Similar cytogenetic findings are present in overt myeloma.[684]

Immunocytochemistry on paraffin-embedded specimens using antibodies to kappa and lambda light chains can be a very important approach to the study of myeloma and related disorders.[692] The primary use of the technique in this group of diseases is to determine the relative proportion of kappa- or lambda-reacting cells; a predominant population of plasma cells reacting with a single light chain antibody is evidence for a monoclonal proliferation (see Fig. 23.2). A balanced proliferation of kappa- and lambda-reacting plasma cells usually indicates a benign process. A light chain ratio determined by dividing the number of positively reacting plasma cells for the predominant light chain by the number of positively reacting cells for the other light chain has been proposed as an aid in the distinction of myeloma from MGUS or a reactive increase in plasma cells.[692] Patients with overt myeloma generally have values above 16; patients with MGUS or a reactive process have values less than 16. These results should not be viewed in isolation but should be combined with the plasma cell labeling index.

Lymphoplasmacytic lymphoma

In 1944, Waldenström described a clinical syndrome characterized by hyperglobulinemia, increased serum viscosity, and a proliferation of lymphocytes in hematopoietic tissue as well as other organs.[707] The clinical syndrome is referred to as Waldenström macroglobulinemia in recognition of the original description and identification of the globulin as a macroglobulin in the majority of patients. The median age of onset is 60 years and there is a slight male predominance. Hepatosplenomegaly, lymphadenopathy, and neurologic abnormalities are frequent findings; anemia and hyperviscosity are commonly noted laboratory abnormalities.[701,704,707] The lymphoproliferative process associated with this syndrome usually involves the small B lymphocyte or the small B lymphocyte and plasmacytoid lymphocyte, i.e., lymphoplasmacytic lymphoma in the WHO classification.[700,702,704] Although commonly used to describe the histopathologic lesion occurring in patients with this syndrome, the term Waldenström macroglobulinemia should be reserved for those patients with IgM paraproteinemia and bone marrow involvement by lymphoplasmacytic lymphoma.[704] Cases of lymphoplasmacytic lymphoma may also be associated with paraprotein of IgG and IgA type.[706] Some cases of lymphoplasmacytic lymphoma have no associated serum gammopathy.[704] IgM gammopathy may occur with other hematopoietic tumors and has been reported in cases of multiple myeloma and marginal zone lymphoma.[695,699,705]

The peripheral blood shows a leukemic picture in approximately 30% of cases; the predominant cells are small lymphocytes or a mixture of small lymphocytes and plasmacytoid lymphocytes. A similar population of cells predominates in the bone marrow[698,702,703] (Fig. 23.113). Mature plasma cells, tissue mast cells, and histiocytes may also be increased. In some cases, plasma cells may predominate. In marrow sections, the infiltrate may be focal or diffuse; the focal lesions may be preferentially paratrabecular, interstitial or nonparatrabecular.[694] Marrow involvement may be very extensive with a marked decrease in normal hematopoietic cells. Intranuclear inclusions, frequently referred to as Dutcher bodies, may be observed in some of the lymphocytes and plasma cells;[698] these inclusions, which are variably PAS positive, may be observed in other lymphomas, multiple myeloma, and reactive proliferations, and are not diagnostic of lymphoplasmacytic lymphoma.[696] In some cases of plasmacytoid lymphoma, the plasma cells and plasmacytoid lymphocytes contain abundant cytoplasmic inclusions. These inclusions may be numerous, and some of these cells resemble histiocytes; the inclusions are usually intensely PAS positive (Fig. 23.114). Plasma cells with similar inclusions may occasionally predominate in multiple myeloma. Like other small lymphocytic lymphomas, the lymphoplasmacytic lymphoma associated with Waldenström macroglobulinemia may terminate with a clinicopathologic picture of Richter syndrome.[697]

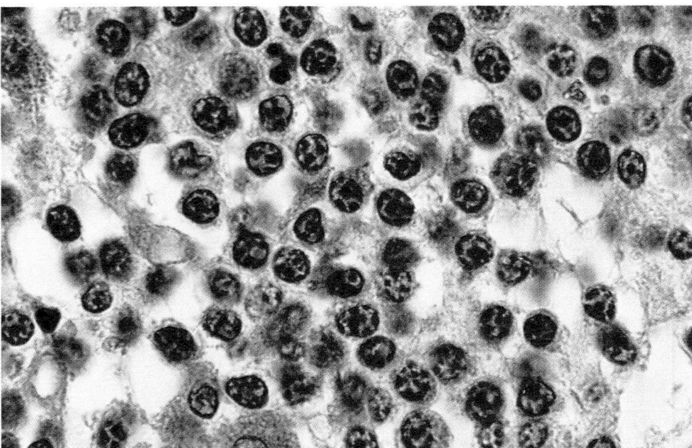

Fig. 23.113 Marrow from a patient with lymphoplasmacytic lymphoma and associated IgM gammopathy. The predominant lymphocytes have nuclei with very clumped chromatin and a slight to moderate amount of cytoplasm. Some lymphocytes contain small cytoplasmic and intranuclear inclusions. There is an increased number of tissue mast cells.

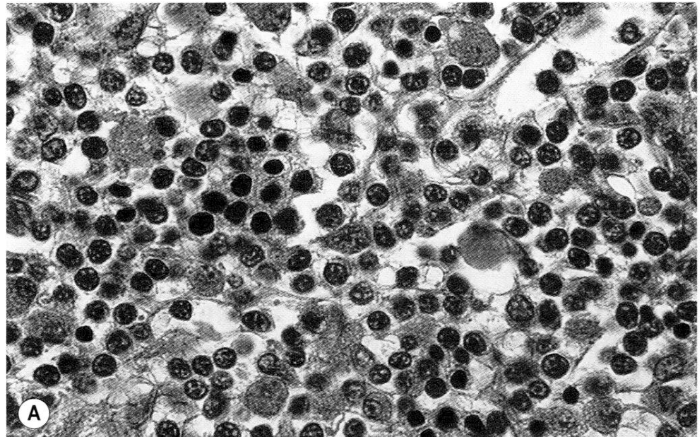

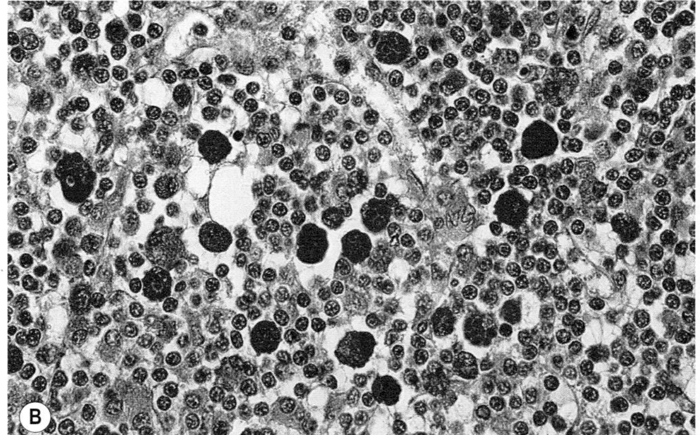

Fig. 23.114 **A**, Marrow section from a patient with lymphoplasmacytic lymphoma associated with serum IgM monoclonal gammopathy. Marrow is replaced by an infiltrate of lymphocytes and plasma cells; many of the plasma cells contain numerous cytoplasmic inclusions. Some lymphocytes contain prominent intranuclear inclusions (Dutcher bodies). **B**, Specimen illustrated in **A** reacted with PAS stain. Inclusions in plasma cells are strongly positive.

The differential diagnosis of lymphoplasmacytic lymphoma in the marrow includes multiple myeloma and marginal zone lymphoma. The presence of an IgM paraprotein, as well as lack of clinical features of multiple myeloma, would favor lymphoplasmacytic lymphoma. Correlation with clinical features and lymph node morphology is often necessary to exclude marginal zone lymphoma and this differential diagnosis cannot always be resolved on marrow biopsy tissue alone.[694,695]

Heavy chain disease

The heavy chain diseases are clinical syndromes that are associated with the production of heavy chain fragments of the immunoglobulin molecule.[708–713] Gamma-chain disease has more of the features of a malignant lymphoma, lymphoplasmacytic type, than of multiple myeloma. The median age for this disease is 61 years, but it has been reported in individuals younger than 20.[712] Weakness, fatigue, fever, and lymphadenopathy are common symptoms; hepatomegaly, splenomegaly, and peripheral lymphadenopathy are each present in slightly more than half of the cases. There are frequently anemia, leukopenia, and thrombocytopenia. Atypical lymphocytes and plasma cells may be found in the peripheral blood. The bone marrow is usually abnormal and shows an increase in lymphocytes, plasma cells, or both. Occasionally the marrow is normal. There may be an accompanying eosinophilia. Most of the reported cases of mu-chain disease have features similar to CLL, but the patients usually have hepatosplenomegaly rather than the typical lymphadenopathy of CLL.[709–711] The marrow in several of the reported cases contained vacuolated plasma cells. Alpha-chain disease, also known as immunoproliferative small intestinal disease or Mediterranean lymphoma, is considered a variant of extranodal marginal zone B-cell lymphoma (MALToma); the marrow is not usually involved. The occurrence of tumors composed of undifferentiated lymphoid cells in patients with heavy chain disease has been reported.[711,714]

Amyloidosis

Amyloidosis is the primary monoclonal immunoglobulin deposition disease to involve the bone marrow.[721,724] Bone marrow biopsies in patients with systemic amyloidosis are performed to detect evidence of the disease and to ascertain the number of plasma cells and whether there is a light chain predominant population of plasma cells. In a large single institution study of 474 patients with primary systemic amyloidosis, 56% of marrow biopsies were positive; abdominal fat aspirate was positive in 80%.[722] One or both sites were positive in 89% of patients. In rare cases, amyloid may be detected in marrow biopsies from patients without any clinical evidence of disease.

Primary systemic amyloidosis is associated with another form of plasma cell dyscrasia in approximately 35% of patients; the two most common disorders are multiple myeloma and monoclonal gammopathy of undetermined significance,[717,719,720,722,723] although amyloidosis may also occur with lymphoplasmacytic lymphoma. The distinction between primary amyloidosis with or without associated myeloma can be difficult and is usually based on a constellation of clinical and morphologic findings. The majority of patients with concurrent myeloma and primary systemic amyloidosis have more than 10% marrow plasma cells which show either lambda or kappa light chain predominance demonstrated by flow cytometric or immunohistochemical studies.

Marrow involvement may manifest either as small focal lesions or as extensive marrow replacement.[726] Early involvement is characterized by focal deposits of amyloid in the medullary vessels; these range from small deposits in the media to large accumulations that greatly expand the vessel walls, resulting in narrowing of the lumen. With more extensive involvement, the accumulation of amyloid is present in the perivascular tissue and marrow substance (Fig. 23.115). Congo red staining should be performed to confirm the diagnosis.

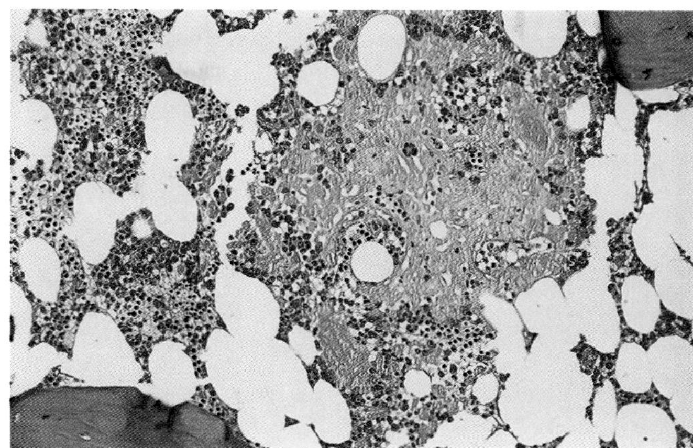

Fig. 23.115 Marrow with amyloid accumulation from a 50-year-old woman with primary amyloidosis.

Very rarely a proteinaceous deposition resembling amyloid but lacking the histochemical and electron microscopic characteristics of amyloid, similar to the findings in proteinaceous lymphadenopathy, may occur in the marrow in association with immune disorders (Fig. 23.116). The origin of the proteinaceous substance appears to be immunoglobulin or portions of the immunoglobulin molecule produced by cells of the immune system, and the findings have been referred to as monoclonal light and heavy chain deposition diseases.[715,716,718,724,725]

Systemic polyclonal B-immunoblastic proliferation

A florid polyclonal proliferation of B immunoblasts accompanied by a polyclonal hypergammaglobulinemia may occur in patients with a variety of immune disorders and involve blood, bone marrow, and lymph nodes.[727,728,730,731] The leukocyte count may be elevated with a high percentage of B immunoblasts, cells with intensely basophilic cytoplasm, relatively coarse nuclear chromatin, and distinct nucleoli. There frequently is some evidence of maturation of these cells to plasma cells. The bone marrow may show extensive infiltration and may resemble lymphoma or plasmablastic myeloma with immunoblasts, plasma cells, and intermediate forms (Fig. 23.117). Lymph nodes may show a similar infiltrate, with complete effacement of the normal architecture. Immunologic studies are critical in the evaluation of these lesions. The polyclonal nature of the infiltrate is demonstrated with immunocytochemical reactions that show essentially a balanced population of kappa- and lambda-reacting cells[729] (Fig. 23.117B,C).

The biology of this process is not completely clear; in some patients it appears to represent an acute immune reaction, and it has been observed in patients with laboratory findings of acute lupus erythematosus. It may in some instances be analogous to the polymorphous lymphoid lesions observed in transplant patients. There may be dramatic regression following steroid therapy.[730,731]

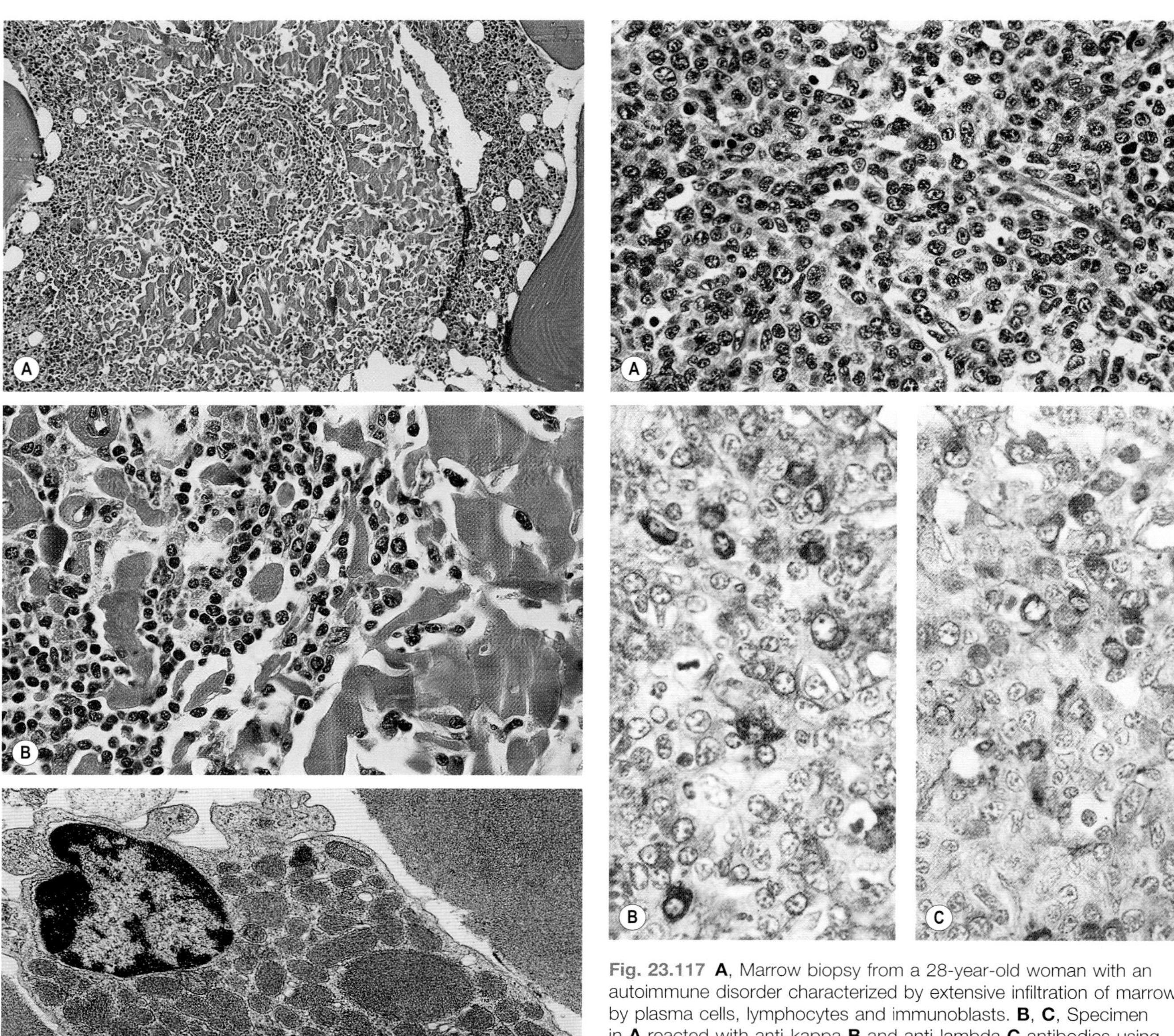

Fig. 23.116 Proteinaceous myelopathy. **A**, Marrow biopsy from a 25-year-old female with a 10-year history of lupus erythematosus. There is extensive intercellular accumulation of an amorphous eosinophilic substance resembling amyloid but lacking the histochemical and ultrastructural findings of amyloid. There is an associated proliferation of plasma cells and small lymphocytes. The plasma cells consisted of both kappa and lambda light chain positive populations. **B**, High magnification of the specimen in **A**. **C**, Ultrastructure of the intracellular and extracellular material. There was complete regression of the finding following high dose steroid and vinblastine therapy.

Fig. 23.117 **A**, Marrow biopsy from a 28-year-old woman with an autoimmune disorder characterized by extensive infiltration of marrow by plasma cells, lymphocytes and immunoblasts. **B**, **C**, Specimen in **A** reacted with anti-kappa **B** and anti-lambda **C** antibodies using peroxidase–antiperoxidase–immunoperoxidase technique. There is balanced reactivity for kappa- and lambda-reacting cells. (**B** and **C**, Immunoperoxidase)

Metastatic tumors

Bone marrow biopsies are used frequently for the staging of patients with histologically documented malignancies; they also may be performed on patients with suspected malignancy in an attempt to obtain material for a histologic diagnosis.[739,743,750,757,758,763,766,767] Due to the focal nature of marrow involvement by metastatic disease, the yield of marrow biopsies is increased by the amount of biopsy tissue obtained. For this reason, either bilateral iliac crest biopsies or two biopsies from a single site are recommended for adequate staging.[738,767] The tumors most frequently detected in bone marrow biopsies in adults are carcinoma of the breast, lung, prostate, stomach, colon, kidney, and thyroid gland. The bone marrow biopsy is widely used for staging small cell carcinoma of the lung.[732,734,741,746–749,752–757] Sarcomas have a relatively low incidence

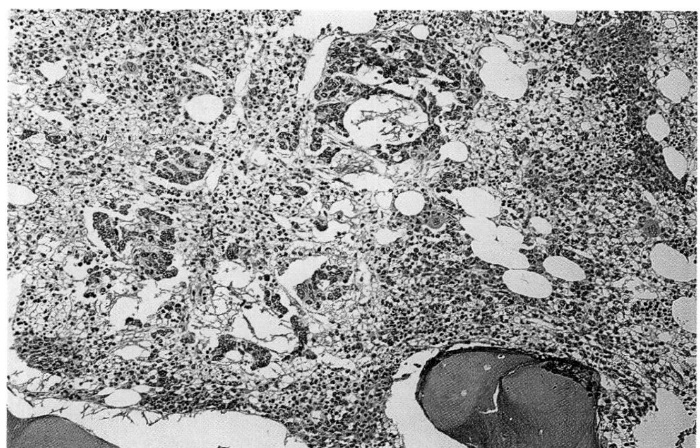

Fig. 23.118 Marrow biopsy from a child with metastatic neuroblastoma. Several foci of tumor are present.

of marrow metastasis in adults.[736] In the pediatric age group, neuroblastoma is the most common metastatic lesion, followed by rhabdomyosarcoma, Ewing sarcoma, and retinoblastoma.[745,750,760,764] Wilms tumor metastatic to marrow is extremely uncommon.

In smears, tumor cells frequently, but not invariably, occur in clusters. This may be an important diagnostic feature because tumors of hematopoietic origin generally do not occur in cohesive aggregates. In marrows with extensive involvement, both clusters and individual cells may be present. In some small cell tumors the individual cells may resemble malignant lymphoid cells. In trephine sections, metastatic tumor may occur as small focal lesions surrounded by normal hematopoietic cells, or it may replace virtually the entire specimen. In focal lesions or those occupying only a portion of the biopsy, the tumor foci may be sharply demarcated from the adjacent hematopoietic tissue or may be associated with an irregularly shaped area of fibrosis (Figs 23.118 and 23.119). Many tumors, most notably breast and prostate, may be associated with a marked desmoplastic reaction, and attempts at aspiration may be unsuccessful. These tumors also may be accompanied by marked osteosclerosis (Figs 23.120 and 23.121). In the unusual occurrence of a metastatic sarcoma in the marrow, the lesion may resemble primary myelofibrosis.

In the majority of cases of metastatic tumor in marrow smears and aspirates, the tumor cells have characteristics that clearly distinguish them from normal hematopoietic cells. This distinction is aided by the frequent desmoplastic reaction that accompanies some of the tumors that most commonly metastasize to the marrow. In some instances the metastatic tumor cells may have features suggesting a hematopoietic origin, particularly megakaryocytes. This may be a particular problem with some cases of rhabdomyosarcoma in which the tumor cells may react with antibodies to platelet glycoproteins (Fig. 23.122). Antibody studies for actin, desmin, and myogenin and cytogenetic studies may be useful in recognizing this tumor (Fig. 23.122B). Less commonly, individual tumor cells may involve the marrow and such cases may require immunohistochemical studies even in the absence of obvious marrow involvement on hematoxylin–eosin-stained slides. Metastatic lobular carcinoma and neuroblastoma are the two most common tumors to infiltrate the marrow as individual tumor cells, and routine immunohistochemical studies may be warranted if either of these diagnoses is suspected.[751,756]

The approach to determining the site of origin of a metastatic tumor in a patient without a known primary lesion should be the same as for determining metastatic lesions in other sites. Immunocytochemical techniques may be particularly useful both for determining the possible site of origin and for detecting small lesions.[750,756,758] Antibodies to the common leukocyte antigen are useful in distinguishing a malignant lymphoma from metastatic carcinoma or sarcoma. As with other tissue, it is important to use a panel of antibodies that has the capacity to recognize all reasonable possibilities. For metastatic carcinoma of unknown primary, a panel that includes cytokeratins 7 and 20 as well as synaptophysin, TTF-1, and estrogen receptor and BRST-1 in women and prostate specific antigen in men will suggest a primary tumor in most cases.[750] In instances in which small foci are identified with the immunocytochemical reaction, the tumor should be found in adjacent sections stained with hematoxylin and eosin.

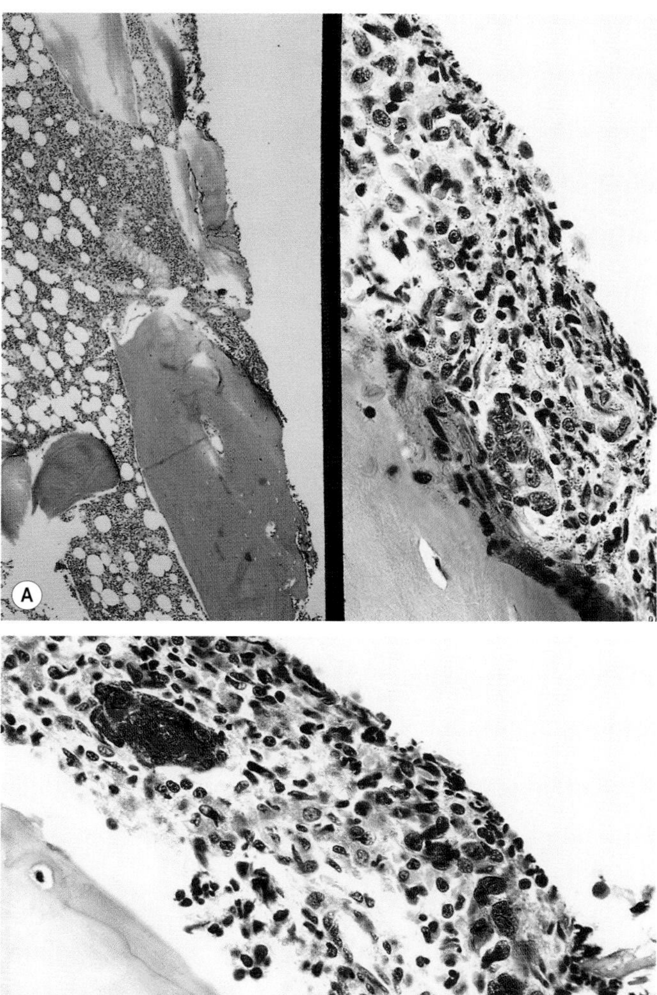

Fig. 23.119 **A**, Low (left) and high (right) magnification of a marrow biopsy from a child with metastatic neuroblastoma with small focal lesions. **B**, Specimen reacted with antibody to neuron-specific enolase. Small clusters of reactive cells are present. This was the only involved area in the biopsy. (**B**, Immunoperoxidase)

Detection of micrometastasis from lung and breast carcinoma in bone marrow is increased with the use of immunologic markers applied to smears prepared from Ficoll Hypaque-separated specimens of bone marrow aspirate.[742,744,759] Molecular techniques

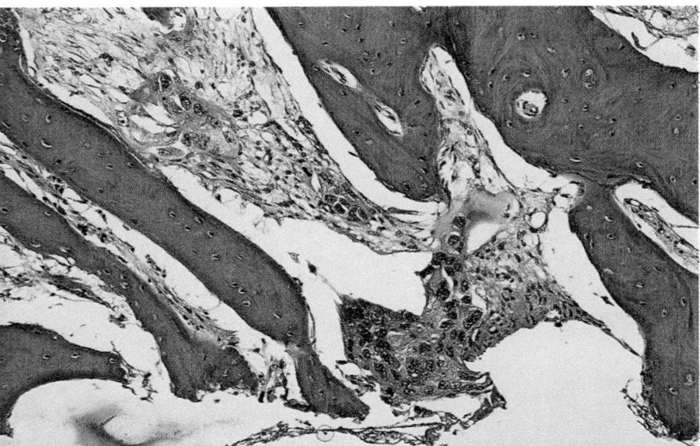

Fig. 23.120 Marrow from a patient with metastatic carcinoma of breast with osteosclerotic reaction and foci of tumor cells.

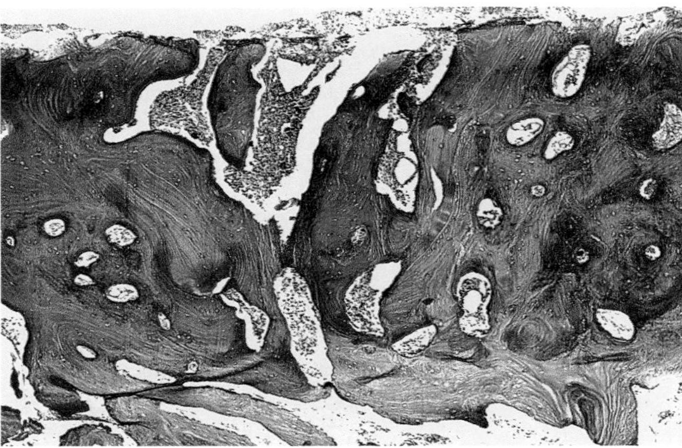

Fig. 23.121 Marrow biopsy from a patient with metastatic carcinoma of prostate with a marked osteoblastic lesion.

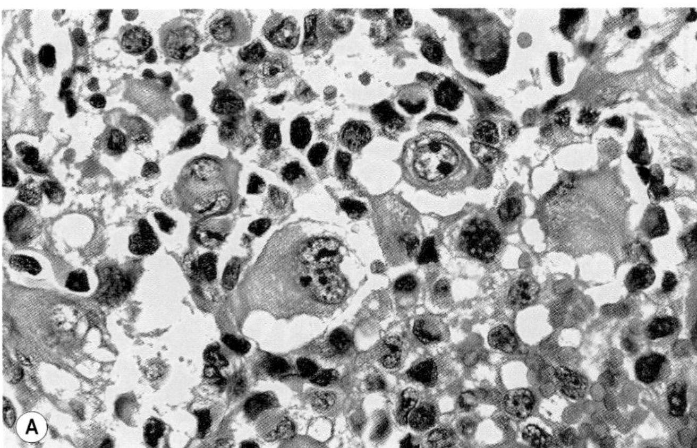

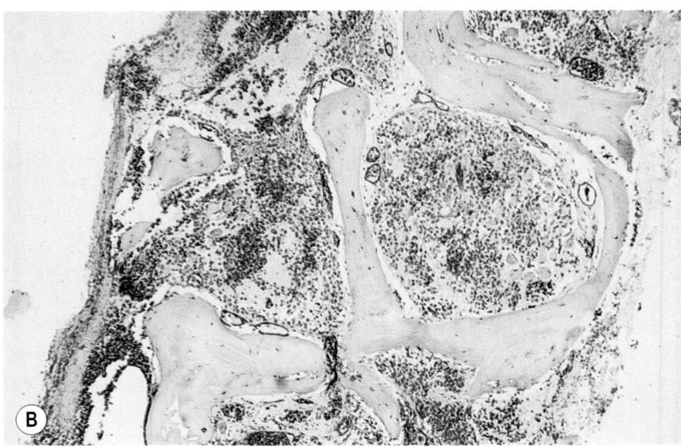

Fig. 23.122 **A**, Bone marrow biopsy from a 17-year-old male with partial replacement of marrow by a pleomorphic population of cells, some of which are large with very abundant cytoplasm. Larger cells have one or two nuclei with distinct and frequently prominent nucleoli. The majority of the cells reacted with antibodies to actin (**B**) and desmin; chromosome studies of the cells showed a t(2;13)(q35;q14) abnormality, a characteristic cytogenetic finding in alveolar rhabdomyosarcoma.

for the identification of markers increase the detection level of micrometastasis.[733]

Special note is made here of neuroblastoma because the bone marrow biopsy may serve as the primary diagnostic specimen in patients with neuroblastoma if the aspirate or trephine biopsy specimen contains unequivocal tumor cells and there is significantly increased serum or urinary catecholamines or metabolites.[735,737,762] Because the detection rate increases with multiple biopsies, two aspirates and one trephine biopsy specimen from each posterior iliac crest are recommended for assessment of marrow involvement. Patients with stage 4S disease have less than 10% involvement; if there is more than 10%, the disease is stage 4.[737]

Tumor cells may be detected in bone marrow smears, particle sections, trephine imprints, or trephine biopsies. The relative merits of these various techniques for detecting tumor have been the subject of considerable discussion. The yield of positive results has increased with the performance of multiple trephine biopsies. Metastatic neuroblastoma in marrow sections may show varying degrees of differentiation. Following therapy, the lesions may show marked differentiation to ganglion cells (Fig. 23.123).

Immunologic markers may be used for the identification of neuroblastoma cells; antibodies to neuron-specific enolase, synaptophysin, and chromogranin have been recommended by the Second International Neuroblastoma Staging System Conference.[737] Newer and more specific markers of neuroblastoma, including GD2 synthetase, also appear to be useful in the primary diagnosis of neuroblastoma.[740,751,761] Immunocytologic quantification of neuroblastoma cells in bone marrow and blood at diagnosis and in marrow during induction therapy can identify patients with very high risk disease.[765]

Lipid storage diseases

Gaucher disease

Gaucher disease is an autosomal recessive sphingolipid storage disorder resulting from the accumulation of glucosylceramide (glucocerebroside) in organs and tissues as a result of a deficiency in lysosomal β-glycosidase (glucocerebrosidase) which is encoded by a gene on chromosome 1q21.[768,770,773,777] It occurs in three forms: type I, chronic non-neuronopathic (adult) type; type II, acute neuronopathic type; and type III, subacute neuronopathic (juvenile) type. It is most frequent in Ashkenazi Jews.

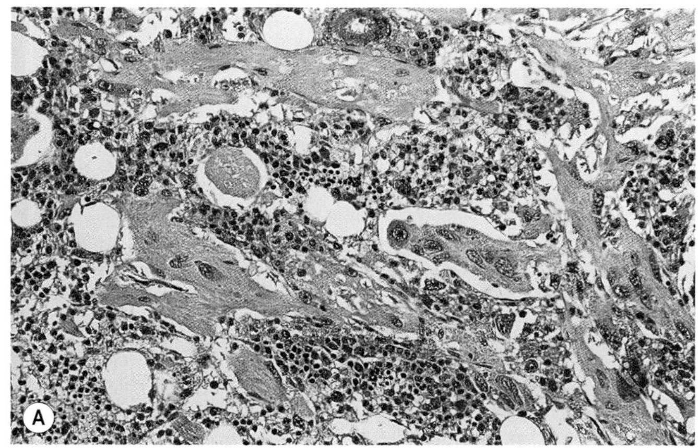

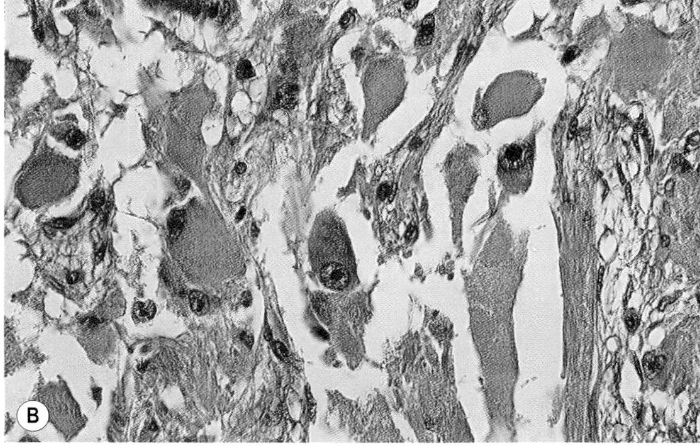

Fig. 23.123 **A**, Marrow biopsy from a child with metastatic neuroblastoma with ganglion differentiation. **B**, High magnification of the specimen in **A** showing marked variability in size of the tumor cells. In contrast to megakaryocytes, some tumor cells contain single, very prominent, nuclei. (See Fig. 23.10, which is the same specimen reacted with antibody to neuron-specific enolase.)

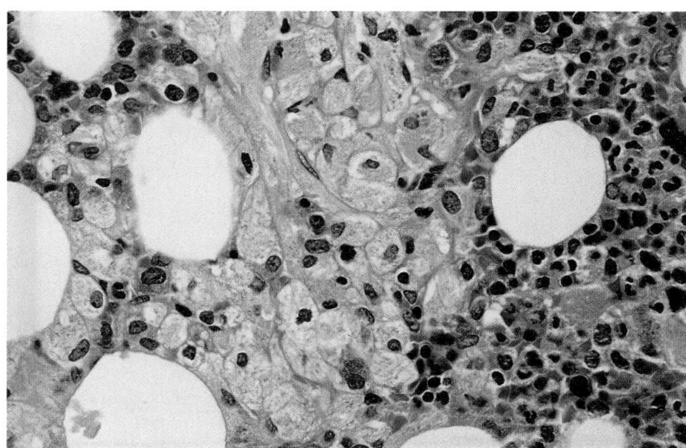

Fig. 23.124 Bone marrow section from an adult with type I chronic non-neuronopathic Gaucher disease. The cytoplasm of many Gaucher cells has a fibrillary or granular appearance. Nuclei are small and usually eccentric in location.

The characteristic diagnostic morphologic feature of the disorder is the presence of Gaucher cells in the bone marrow, spleen, liver, and lymph nodes and other organs.

In the bone marrow sections, Gaucher cells may be found in small focal accumulations or may replace large portions of a biopsy. There is an associated increase in reticulin fibers. In imprint and smear preparations, the Gaucher cell is large, 30–100 μm in diameter, and has one or more centrally or eccentrically located nuclei.[771,776] The cytoplasm has a characteristic fibrillary or striated pattern and is pale blue–gray in color. In sections stained with hematoxylin and eosin, the cytoplasm is slightly eosinophilic; a fibrillary pattern may be very prominent (Fig. 23.124). The Gaucher cells are variably and often intensely positive with the PAS reaction. The cells also stain positively for iron in older children and adults. Cells similar to Gaucher cells, pseudo-Gaucher cells, may be found in the marrow of some patients with chronic myelogenous leukemia,[769,772,774,775,778] type II congenital dyserythropoietic anemia, and thalassemia.[781]

A monoclonal gammopathy may be present in patients with chronic Gaucher disease and may be associated with a marrow plasmacytosis.[779] The coincidence of multiple myeloma, plasmacytoid lymphoma, and Gaucher disease has been reported.[780]

Treatment of patients with type I (adult type) Gaucher disease with recombinant β-glucocerebrosidase (imiglucerase) results in a decrease in the relative volume of bone replaced by Gaucher cells and an increase in hematopoietic and fat cells and a decreased cortical bone structure. The decrease in amount of marrow replaced by Gaucher cells is the result of a decrease in both the number and size of Gaucher cells.[769,772,778] An additional form of therapy is directed at substrate reduction which may be used in addition to enzyme replacement.

Niemann–Pick disease

Niemann–Pick (NP) disease comprises a group of autosomal recessive sphingomyelin–cholesterol lipidoses characterized by organomegaly and the accumulation of sphingomyelin and other lipids throughout the tissues of the body as a result of a deficiency of lysosomal acid sphingomyelinase.[784,785–787] The gene encoding acid sphingomyelinase in types NPA and NPB has mapped to chromosome 11 bands p15.1–15.4. Three major clinical types are recognized: an acute neuronopathic form (A); a chronic form without nervous system involvement (B); and chronic neuronopathic forms (C1 and C2).[784,785–787] The foam cell, as seen in the bone marrow in Niemann–Pick disease, does not have diagnostic specificity and may be found in other disorders of lipid metabolism such as hypercholesterolemia and Tangier disease; in Niemann–Pick disease type C1 the enzymatic defect results in cholesterol accumulation in the macrophages in the marrow and elsewhere.[782,783] In Romanowsky-stained smears, the cell measures 20–50 μm; the cytoplasm is filled with clear vacuoles of varying size.[782,783] In sections, the cells are randomly scattered singly and in aggregates; the cytoplasm of the Niemann–Pick cell is marked by confluent clear vacuoles of varying size. The cells may be difficult to appreciate because of the very light-staining cytoplasm. The nucleus is randomly located (Fig. 23.125). The vacuoles are PAS negative and positive with lipid stains.

Niemann–Pick disease types C1 and C2 are panethnic autosomal recessive lipidoses with linkage to chromosome 18.[784,785,787] The basic defect involves a unique error in cellular trafficking of exogenous cholesterol that is associated with a lysosomal accumulation of unesterified cholesterol; the disease is distinct from the sphingomyelin lipidoses, Niemann–Pick disease types A and B. Foam cells or sea-blue histiocytes may be present in the marrow; these, however, are not distinctive and may be observed in several different lipidoses.

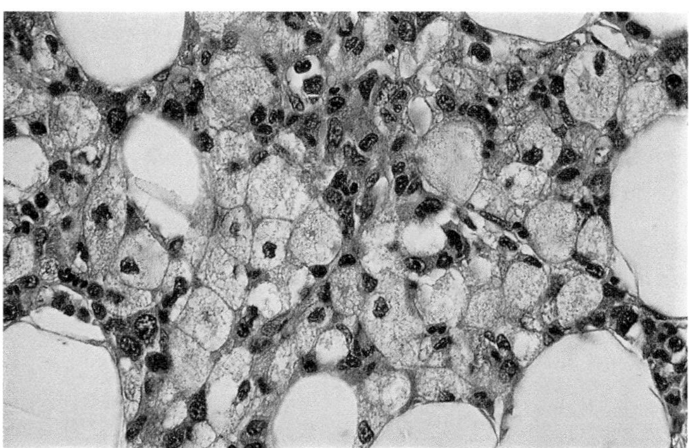

Fig. 23.125 Biopsy from a 14-month-old child with Niemann–Pick disease. Focal accumulations of foam cells are present. The cytoplasm of the foam cells is clear, with the suggestion of numerous confluent vacuoles.

Fabry disease

Fabry disease is an X-linked recessive inborn error of glycosphingolipid metabolism caused by deficient activity of α-galactosidase. It is characterized by multiorgan involvement with accumulation of globotriaosylceramide in cells throughout the body, including macrophages in the marrow. The characteristic storage cells in bone marrow specimens in this disease are filled with small globular inclusions that stain blue in Romanowsky-stained smears and are lightly eosinophilic in sections stained with hematoxylin and eosin.[788] The cytoplasmic substance reacts intensely with the PAS and Sudan black B stains.

Similar to Gaucher disease, therapy for Fabry disease consists of enzyme replacement, substrate reduction, and enzyme enhancement.[789]

Sea-blue histiocyte syndrome

The macrophages of the sea-blue histiocyte syndrome[790,792] contain a substance that stains blue in Romanowsky-stained smears and yellow to tan in sections stained with hematoxylin and eosin. Positive reactions occur with the PAS and Sudan black B stains. In some instances, the substance appears to be ceroid; in others the material has not been well characterized. Macrophages containing blue pigment may be observed in several unrelated disorders and lack diagnostic specificity. This cell type has also been reported in some cases of Niemann–Pick disease. The sea-blue histiocytes may resemble the macrophages in Whipple disease, which may rarely be detected in marrow specimens.[791]

Hematopoietic stem cell transplantation

Hematopoietic stem cell transplantation, using either bone marrow or peripheral blood stem cells, is being increasingly used as a therapeutic approach in patients with primary bone marrow disease.[794] Bone marrow examination is performed for a variety of reasons following hematopoietic stem cell transplantation. While evaluation for residual or recurrent disease in these specimens remains important, the marrow also provides clues to the success of engraftment and to possible infectious complications of the procedure.

The objective of hematopoietic stem cell transplantation is reconstitution of normal hematopoiesis in marrows that are aplastic; the aplasia may be the result of aplastic anemia or the marrow is rendered aplastic with chemotherapy and radiation in the preparative regimen employed prior to marrow transplantation for various neoplastic processes or, less commonly, inherited disorders.

The source of the graft may be the patient's own marrow or peripheral blood stem cells that have been harvested prior to the preparatory regimen (autologous) or from another individual (allogeneic). Autologous stem cells in some cases are 'purged' with chemotherapeutic agents and/or monoclonal antibodies to eradicate malignant cells. Umbilical cord blood stem cells are also being used.[795]

Hematopoietic stem cell transplant involves preparing the patient for transplant with a regimen utilizing chemotherapy with or without total body irradiation therapy. The preparative regimen has two purposes: to immunosuppress the patient and to eradicate malignant cells that may be present in the recipient. For patients with severe aplastic anemia, cyclophosphamide alone or cyclophosphamide plus antithymocyte globulin or cyclophosphamide plus total lymphoid irradiation has been utilized most commonly and now provides long-term success rates of over 80% in matched sibling donor patients. For patients with leukemia, regimens including chemotherapy and total body irradiation have most commonly been used; the combination of busulfan and cyclophosphamide has been successful in the preparation of patients with acute myeloid leukemia.

The major complications associated with hematopoietic stem cell transplantation involve infection in the severely immunosuppressed host, graft rejection, and graft-versus-host disease.[799] Recurrent disease is also a cause of failure in patients with malignant diseases. Infection continues to be a major cause of peritransplant morbidity and, in some cases, mortality. The use of better antibiotics and growth factors to accelerate white blood cell production has decreased but not eliminated infectious complications. Graft rejection is an infrequent complication of matched sibling donor transplant; however, it is a significant complication in patients undergoing unrelated donor transplant, especially for diseases such as aplastic anemia. Certain methods of graft-versus-host disease prophylaxis, specifically T-cell depletion, may be associated with an increased risk of graft rejection.

The rate of engraftment following hematopoietic stem cell transplantation is influenced by several factors, and although some generalizations can be made about reconstitution of hematopoiesis, there are frequent exceptions.[796–800] The amount of marrow damage incurred prior to the transplant from chemotherapy and radiation used for treatment of the disease for which the transplant is necessary may influence the success rate. Autologous marrow specimens that have been purged with antibodies or chemotherapeutic agents may reconstitute less quickly than allogeneic marrow grafts. The disease for which the transplant was performed may recur early in the transplant period.

Marrow biopsies are not usually performed in the first 7 days following transplantation. However, the marrow biopsies performed during this period show marked hypocellularity with hemorrhage and proteinaceous debris. Scattered fat cells and macrophages are present. The findings are similar to those in patients treated with myelotoxic agents for acute leukemia.[796–798,800] At 7–14 days, adipose tissue is reconstituted. The appearance of the marrow in the second to third week is variable; there may be evidence of hematopoiesis, or the marrow may be markedly hypocellular (Figs 23.126 and 23.127). The initial stages of engraftment are usually characterized by foci of hematopoietic cells scattered throughout the adipose tissue in what appears to be a random distribution. These foci initially are usually unilineage and

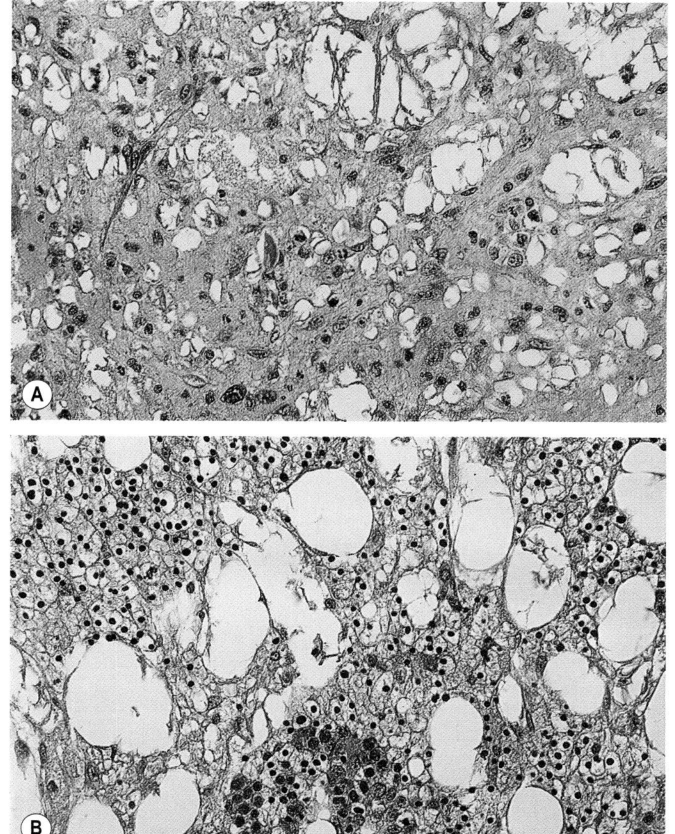

Fig. 23.126 **A**, Marrow biopsy 4 days post allogeneic marrow transplant for blast crisis of chronic myelogenous leukemia. The marrow is markedly hypocellular with scattered cells and abundant interstitial proteinaceous debris. **B**, Marrow biopsy from the patient illustrated in **A** 28 days post transplant. Evidence of engraftment is characterized principally by erythroid precursors at a late stage of maturation and foci of more immature forms. There was no evidence of a t(9;22) cytogenetic abnormality in either biopsy.

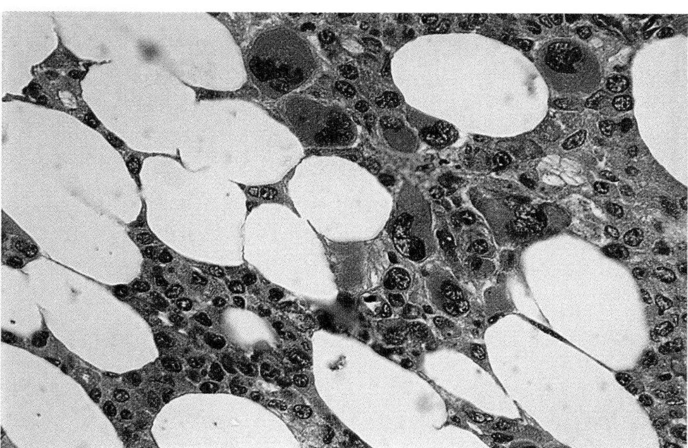

Fig. 23.128 Marrow from an adult male 18 days post unrelated marrow transplant for acute myeloid leukemia. The marrow is markedly hypocellular with scattered clusters of normal-appearing megakaryocytes; there is no evidence of leukemia.

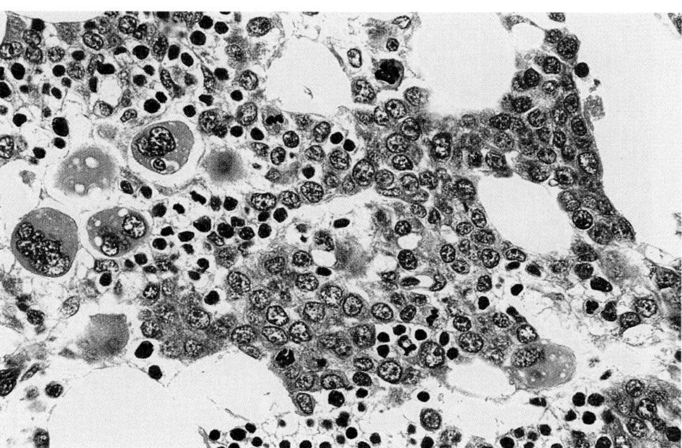

Fig. 23.129 Marrow from an adult female 21 days post autologous marrow transplant for chronic myelogenous leukemia illustrating a focus of erythroid precursors at an early stage of maturation in an overall hypocellular marrow. Erythroid precursors at a late stage of maturation are located in the surrounding interstitium; there are several normal-appearing megakaryocytes.

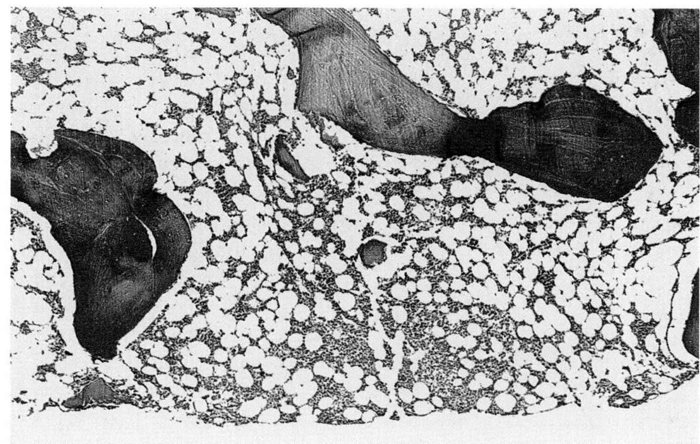

Fig. 23.127 Marrow biopsy from a 7-year-old child 14 days post allogeneic bone marrow transplant for aplastic anemia. The marrow is moderately to markedly hypocellular. Subsequent biopsies showed failure of engraftment.

composed of tight clusters of erythroid precursors followed by aggregates of promyelocytes and myelocytes (Fig. 23.126B). Blasts are not increased. There is no preferential paratrabecular distribution of the promyelocyte and myelocyte islands in this period. Megakaryocytes are usually sparse. Following this stage there is progressive spreading of the hematopoietic cells throughout the interstitium and gradual regression of adipose tissue; the foci of hematopoiesis at this stage of recovery are usually multilineage, although predominantly monolineage proliferation may persist (Figs 23.128 and 23.129). Megakaryocyte reconstitution may lag behind the granulocytic and erythroid cells for prolonged periods. In some patients, megakaryocytes appear early in the engraftment period and may form small aggregates. There may be considerable variability in the amount of hematopoietic tissue in different areas of a large biopsy specimen; clot sections, small specimens, or fragmented specimens may be misleading.

There may be a marked shift to promyelocytes and myelocytes early in the post-transplant period; this is accentuated by the administration of recombinant granulocyte growth factor

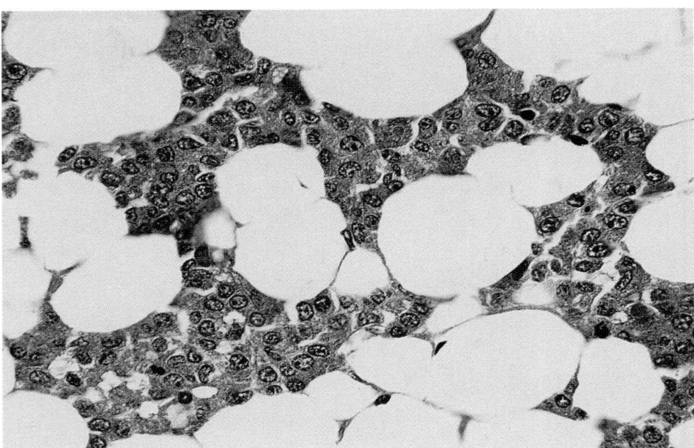

Fig. 23.130 Marrow biopsy 20 days post allogeneic sibling transplant for chronic myelogenous leukemia; 3 days prior to the biopsy the patient received granulocyte colony stimulating factor for marked neutropenia. The cells in the interstitium are neutrophil precursors at the promyelocyte–myelocyte stage of maturation, a characteristic early effect of growth factor stimulation.

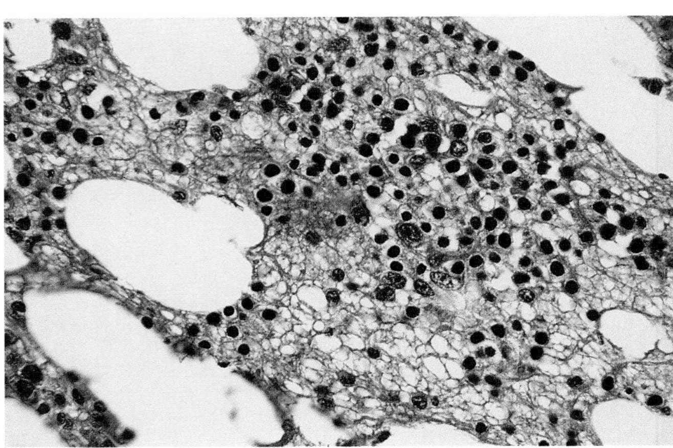

Fig. 23.132 Marrow biopsy from an adult 8 months following autologous marrow transplant for chronic myeloid leukemia. The marrow is markedly hypocellular with markedly decreased granulocytes and megakaryocytes. The interstitium is markedly depleted with principally late stage erythroid precursors.

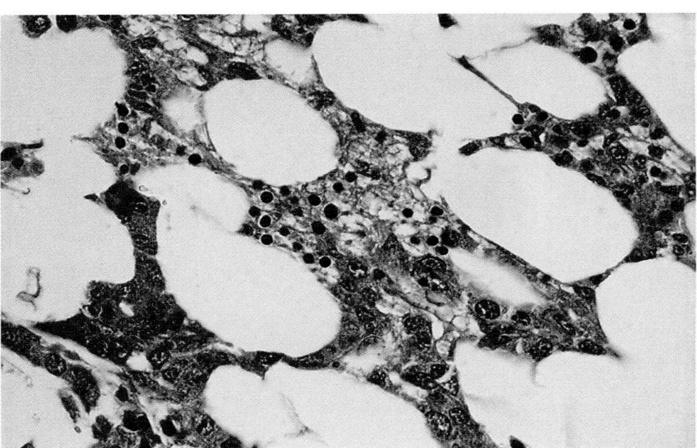

Fig. 23.131 Marrow biopsy from an 11-year-old child 100 days following unrelated donor marrow transplant for chronic myelogenous leukemia. The marrow is moderately to markedly hypocellular with erythroid and granulocyte precursors and only rare megakaryocytes.

(Fig. 23.130). This shift to immaturity is not usually accompanied by an increase in blasts. During this period, patients frequently receive a large number of drugs, some of which may be associated with agranulocytosis. This factor should be considered in patients who manifest prolonged neutropenia with a morphologic appearance of 'maturation arrest' of neutrophils in the marrow specimen.

Granulomas occur with greater frequency in post-transplant marrows than in marrows from other groups of patients; these granulomas usually consist of only a small collection of epithelioid histiocytes. In some cases, giant cells are present. Phagocytic histiocytes may be increased and diffusely scattered throughout the marrow. The histiocytes may manifest marked phagocytic activity; this finding warrants evaluation for an infectious process.

The rate of growth of the graft varies substantially in the first 3–4 weeks. In some cases the marrow may remain hypocellular for many months or years; in other cases one of the major myeloid cell lines remains depressed (Figs 23.131 and 23.132). Remission of myelofibrosis and osteosclerosis may occur (Fig. 23.133).

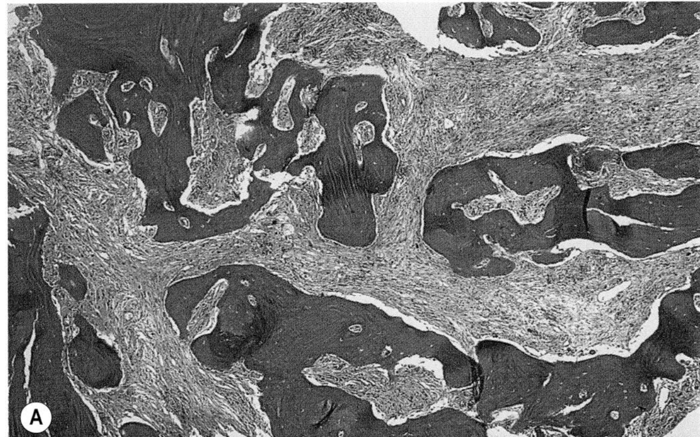

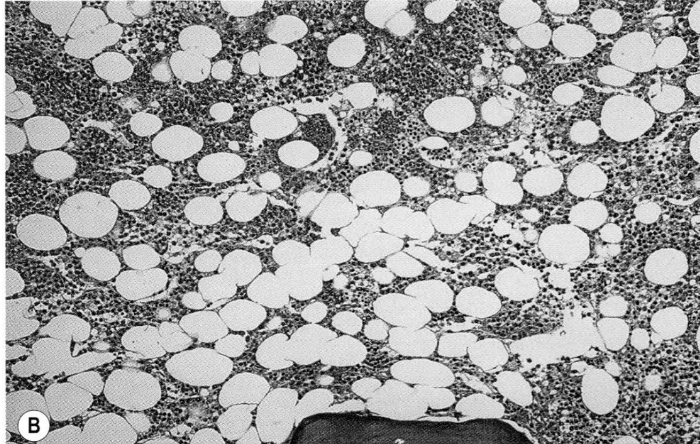

Fig. 23.133 **A**, Marrow biopsy with marked osteosclerosis from a 32-year-old patient with Philadelphia chromosome-positive chronic myelogenous leukemia immediately prior to marrow transplant. **B**, Marrow biopsy from the patient illustrated in **A** 5 months post allogeneic marrow transplant. There is complete resolution of the osteosclerosis. The cytogenetics from this specimen were normal.

Loss of graft is reflected by decreasing marrow cellularity and progressive cytopenias. This may occur gradually or abruptly. In some instances, there is a dissociation between the blood counts and marrow cellularity, with very hypocellular marrows and normal blood counts or normocellular marrows and blood cytopenias. Marrow sampling may be the basis of the discrepancy when normal blood counts occur with hypocellular marrow. There are no specific marrow findings reflecting graft-versus-host disease.

Marrow transplants in patients with leukemia present the additional problem of recognition of recurrent disease. Cytogenetics, membrane surface markers, and molecular studies are very important adjuncts to morphology in the evaluation of these patients. In addition, molecular genetic studies for engraftment now focus primarily on the ratio of donor to recipient histocompatibility markers.[793]

References

BIOPSY PROCEDURE AND PROCESSING OF SPECIMEN

1 Bain BJ. Bone marrow aspiration. J Clin Pathol 2001, **54**: 657–663.

2 Bain BJ. Bone marrow trephine biopsy. J Clin Pathol 2001, **54**: 737–742.

3 Brinn NT, Pickett JP. Glycol methacrylate for routine, special stains, histochemistry, enzyme histochemistry and immunohistochemistry. A simplified method for surgical biopsy tissue. J Histotechnol 1979, **2**: 125–130.

4 Brunning RD, Bloomfield CD, McKenna RW, Peterson L. Bilateral trephine bone marrow biopsies in lymphoma and other neoplastic diseases. Ann Intern Med 1975, **82**: 365–366.

5 Burkhardt R, Frisch B, Bartl R. Bone biopsy in haematological disorders. J Clin Pathol 1982, **35**: 257–284.

6 Contreras E, Ellis LD, Lee RE. Value of the bone marrow biopsy in the diagnosis of metastatic carcinoma. Cancer 1972, **29**: 778–783.

7 Dee JW, Valdivieso M, Drewinko B. Comparison of the efficacies of closed trephine needle biopsy, aspirated paraffin-embedded clot section, and smear preparation in the diagnosis of bone marrow involvement by lymphoma. Am J Clin Pathol 1976, **65**: 183–194.

8 Ellman L. Bone marrow biopsy in the evaluation of lymphoma, carcinoma, and granulomatous disorders. Am J Med 1976, **60**: 1–7.

9 Fend F, Bock O, Kremer M, Specht K, Quintanilla-Martinez L. Ancillary techniques in bone marrow pathology: molecular diagnostics on bone marrow trephine biopsies. Virchows Arch 2005, **447**: 909–919.

10 Garrett TJ, Gee TS, Leiberman PH, McKenzie S, Clarkson BD. The role of bone marrow aspiration and biopsy in detecting marrow involvement by non-hematologic malignancies. Cancer 1976, **38**: 2401–2403.

11 Gatter KC, Heryet A, Brown DC, Mason DY. Is it necessary to embed bone marrow biopsies in plastic for haematological diagnosis? Histopathology 1987, **11**: 1–7.

12 Gruppo RA, Lampkin BC, Granger S. Bone marrow cellularity determination. Comparison of the biopsy, aspirate and buffy coat. Blood 1977, **49**: 29–31.

13 Jamshidi K, Swaim WR. Bone marrow biopsy with unaltered architecture: a new biopsy device. J Lab Clin Med 1971, **77**: 335–342.

14 Liao KT. The superiority of histologic sections of aspirated bone marrow in malignant lymphomas. Cancer 1971, **27**: 618–628.

15 McCarthy DM. Annotation, fibrosis of the bone marrow: content and causes. Br J Haematol 1985, **59**: 1–7.

16 Peterson LC, Brunning RD. Bone marrow specimen processing. In Knowles DM (ed): Neoplastic hematopathology, ed. 2. Philadelphia, 2001, Lippincott Williams & Wilkins, pp. 1391–1406.

17 Torlakovic EE, Naresh KN, Brunning RD. Bone marrow immunohistochemistry. Chicago 2008, American Society for Clinical Pathology Press.

18 Wang J, Weiss LM, Chang KL, Slovak ML, Gaal K, Forman SJ, Arber DA. Diagnostic utility of bilateral bone marrow examination, significance of morphologic and ancillary technique study in malignancy. Cancer 2002, **94**: 1522–1531.

IMMUNOHISTOLOGY

19 Arber DA, Jenkins KA. Paraffin section immunophenotyping of acute leukemias in bone marrow specimens. Am J Clin Pathol 1996, **106**: 462–468.

20 Arber DA, Snyder DS, Fine M, Dagis A, Niland J, Slovok ML. Myeloperoxidase immunoreactivity in adult lymphoblastic leukemia. Am J Clin Pathol 2001, **116**: 25–33.

21 Bluth RF, Casey TT, McCurley TL. Differentiation of reactive from neoplastic small-cell lymphoid aggregates in paraffin-embedded marrow particle preparations using L-26 (CD20) and UCHL-1 (CD45RO) monoclonal antibodies. Am J Clin Pathol 1993, **99**: 150–156.

22 Brown DC, Gatter KC. Monoclonal antibody Ki-67: its use in histopathology. Histopathology 1990, **17**: 489–503.

23 Brown DC, Gatter KC. The bone marrow trephine biopsy: a review of normal histology. Histopathology 1993, **22**: 411–422.

24 Chuang SS, Li CY. Useful panel of antibodies for the classification of acute leukemia by immunohistochemical methods in bone marrow trephine biopsy specimens. Am J Clin Pathol 1997, **107**: 410–418.

25 Dhillon AP, Rode J, Leathem A. Neuron specific enolase. An aid to the diagnosis of melanoma and neuroblastoma. Histopathology 1982, **5**: 81–92.

26 Dunphy C, Polski JM, Evans HL, Gardner LJ. Evaluation of bone marrow specimens with acute myelogenous leukemia for CD34, CD15, CD117 and myeloperoxidase. Arch Pathol Lab Med 2001, **125**: 1063–1069.

27 Erber WN, Gibbs TA, Ivey JG. Antigen retrieval by microwave oven heating for immunohistochemical analysis of bone marrow trephine biopsies. Pathology 1996, **28**: 45–50.

28 Erber WN, Willis JI, Hoffman GJ. An enhanced immunocytochemical method for staining bone marrow trephine sections. J Clin Pathol 1997, **50**: 389–393.

29 Fend F, Bock O, Kremer M, Specht K, Quintanilla-Martinez L. Ancillary techniques in bone marrow pathology: molecular diagnostics on bone marrow trephine biopsies. Virchows Arch 2005, **447**: 909–919.

30 Fend F, Tzankov A, Bink K, Seidl S, Quintanilla-Martinez L, Kremer M, Dirnhofer S. Modern techniques for the diagnostic evaluation of the trephine bone marrow biopsy: methodological aspects and application. Prog Histochem Cytochem 2008, **42**: 203–252.

31 Horny HP, Wehrmann M, Grisser H, Tiemann M, Bultmann B, Kaiserling E. Investigation of bone marrow lymphocyte subsets in normal, reactive, and neoplastic states, using paraffin-embedded biopsy specimens. Am J Clin Pathol 1993, **99**: 142–149.

32 Kremer M, Dirnhofer S, Nickl A, Hoefler H, Quintanilla-Martinez L, Fend F. p27kip1 immunostaining for the differential diagnosis of small B-cell neoplasms in trephine bone marrow biopsies. Mod Pathol 2001, **14**: 1022–1029.

33 Kremer M, Quintanilla-Martinez L, Nährig J, Von Schilling C, Fend F. Immunohistochemistry in bone marrow pathology: a useful adjunct for morphologic diagnosis. Virchows Arch 2005, **447**: 920–937.

34 Kronland R, Grogan T, Spier C, Wirt D, Rangel C, Richter L, Durie B, Greenberg B, Miller T, Jones S. Immunotopographic assessment of lymphoid and plasma cell malignancies in the bone marrow. Hum Pathol 1985, **16**: 1247–1254.

35 Kubic VL, Brunning RD. Immunohistochemical evaluation of neoplasms in bone marrow biopsies using monoclonal antibodies reactive in paraffin embedded tissue. Mod Pathol 1989, **2**: 618–629.

36 Manion EM, Rosenthal NS. Bone marrow biopsies in patients 85 years or older. Am J Clin Pathol 2008, **130**: 832–835.

37 Mason DY, Comans-Bitter WM, Cordell JL, Verhoeven MAJ, von Dongen JJM. Antibody L26 recognizes an intracellular epitope on the B cell associated CD20 antigen. Am J Pathol 1990, **136**: 1215–1222.

38 Norton AJ, Isaacson PG. Monoclonal antibody L26: an antibody that is reactive with normal and neoplastic B lymphocytes in routinely fixed and paraffin wax embedded tissues. J Clin Pathol 1987, **40**: 1405–1412.

39 Peterson LC, Brown BA, Crosson JT, Mladenovic J. Application of the immunoperoxidase technic to bone marrow trephine biopsies in the classification of patients with monoclonal gammopathies. Am J Clin Pathol 1986, **85**: 688–693.

40 Pileri SA, Ascani S, Milani M, Visani G, Piccioli M, Orcioni GF, Poggi S, Sabattini E, Santini D, Falini B. Acute leukemia immunophenotyping in bone marrow routine sections. Br J Haematol 1999, **105**: 394–401.

41 Pinkus GS, Pinkus JL. Myeloperoxidase. A specific marker for myeloid cells in paraffin sections. Mod Pathol 1991, **4**: 733–741.

42 Poje EJ, Soori GS, Weisenburger DS. Systemic polyclonal immunoblastic proliferation with marked peripheral blood and bone marrow plasmacytosis. Am J Clin Pathol 1992, **98**: 222–226.

43 Seshi B, True L, Carter D, Rosai J. Immunohistochemical characterization of a set of monoclonal antibodies to human neuron-specific enolase. Am J Pathol 1988, **131**: 258–269.

44 Torlakovic E, Torlakovic G, Nguyen PI, Brunning RD, Delabie J. The value of anti-Pax-5 immunostaining in routinely fixed and paraffin embedded sections: a novel pan pre-B and B-cell marker. Am J Surg Pathol 2002, **26**: 1343–1350.

45 Torlakovic EE, Naresh KN, Brunning RD. Bone marrow immunohistochemistry. Chicago, 2008, America Society for Clinical Pathology Press.

46 Tsang WYW, Chan JKC, Ng CS, Pau MY. Utility of a paraffin section reactive CD56 antibody (123C3) for characterization and diagnosis of lymphoma. Am J Surg Pathol 1996, **20**: 202–210.

47 Walls AF, Jones DB, Williams JH, Church MK, Holgate ST. Immunohistochemical identification of mast cells in formaldehyde-fixed tissue using monoclonal antibodies specific for tryptase. J Clin Pathol 1990, **162**: 119–126.

48 Zutter M, Hockenbery D, Silverman GA, Korsmeyer SJ. Immunolocalization of the bcl-2 protein within hematopoietic neoplasms. Blood 1991, **78**: 1062–1068.

NORMOCELLULAR BONE MARROW

49 Hartsock RJ, Smith EB, Petty CS. Normal variations with aging of the amount of hematopoietic tissue in bone marrow from the anterior iliac crest. Am J Clin Pathol 1965, **43**: 326–331.

50 Ricci C, Cova M, Kang YS, Yang A, Rahmouni A, Scott WW, Zerhouni EA. Normal age-related patterns of cellular and fatty bone marrow distribution in the axial skeleton: MR imaging study. Radiology 1990, **177**: 83–88.

51 Wickramasinghe SN. Bone marrow. In Sternberg S (ed.): Histopathology for pathologists, ed. 2. Philadelphia, 1997, Lippincott-Raven, pp. 707–744.

ALTERATIONS IN CELLULARITY

APLASTIC ANEMIA

52 Ajlouni K, Doeblin T. The syndrome of hepatitis and aplastic anemia. Br J Haematol 1974, **27**: 345–355.

53 Alter BP, Potter NU, Li FP. Classification and aetiology of the aplastic anemias. Clin Haematol 1978, **7**: 431–465.

54 Crook TW, Rogers BB, McFarland RD, Kroft SH, Muretto P, Hernandez JA, Latimer MJ, McKenna RW. Unusual bone marrow manifestations of parvovirus B19 infection in immunocompromised patients. Human Pathol 2000, **31**: 161–168.

55 Dawson JP. Congenital pancytopenia associated with multiple congenital anomalies (Fanconi type). Review of the literature and report of a 20-year-old female with a 10-year follow-up and apparently good response to splenectomy. Pediatrics 1955, **15**: 325–333.

56 Dessypris EN. The biology of pure red cell aplasia. Semin Hematol 1991, **28**: 275–284.

57 Dokal I, Vulliamy T. Inherited aplastic anaemias/bone marrow failure syndromes. Blood Rev 2008, **22**: 141–153.

58 Dokal I, Ganly P, Riebero I, Marsh J, Steed A, Kendra J, Drysdale C, Hows J. Late onset bone marrow failure associated with proximal fusion of radius and ulna: a new syndrome. Br J Haematol 1989, **71**: 277–280.

59 Estren S, Dameshek W. Familial hypoplastic anemia of childhood. Am J Dis Child 1947, **73**: 671–687.

60 Evans DI. Congenital defects of the marrow stem cell. Bailliere's Clin Haematol 1989, **2**: 162–190.

61 Gordon-Smith EC, Rutherford TR. Fanconi anaemia – constitutional, familial aplastic anaemia. Bailliere's Clin Haematol 1989, **2**: 139–153.

62 Goswitz FA, Andrews GA, Kniseley RM. Effects of local irradiation (Co60 teletherapy) on the peripheral blood and bone marrow. Blood 1963, **21**: 605–619.

63 Haak HL, Hartgrink-Groeneveld CA, Eernisse JG, Speck B, Van Rood JJ. Acquired aplastic anemia in adults. Acta Haematol 1977, **58**: 257–277.

64 Kurtzman G, Young N. Viruses and bone marrow failure. Bailliere's Clin Haematol 1989, **2**: 51–67.

65 Maciejewski JP, Risitano A, Sloand EM, Nunez O, Young NS. Distinct clinical outcomes for cytogenetic abnormalities evolving from aplastic anemia. Blood 2002, **99**: 3129–3135.

66 Mark M, Rijli FM, Chambon P. Homeobox gene in embryogenesis and pathogenesis. Pediatr Res 1997, **42**: 421–429.

67 Naeim F, Smith GS, Gale RP. Morphologic aspects of bone marrow transplantation in patients with aplastic anemia. Hum Pathol 1978, **9**: 295–308.

68 Nissen C. The pathophysiology of aplastic anemia. Semin Hematol 1991, **28**: 313–318.

69 Orazi A, Albitar M, Heerema NA, Haskins NS, Neiman RS. Hypoplastic myelodysplastic syndrome can be distinguished from acquired aplastic anemia by CD34 and PCNA immunostaining of bone marrow biopsy specimens. Am J Clin Pathol 1997, **107**: 268–274.

70 Rosse WF. Paroxysmal nocturnal hemoglobinuria in aplastic anemia. Clin Haematol 1978, **7**: 541–553.

71 Saarinen UM, Chorba TL, Tattersall P, Young NS, Anderson LJ, Palmer E, Coccia PF. Human parvovirus B-19 induced epidemic acute red cell aplasia in patients with hereditary hemolytic anemia. Blood 1986, **67**: 1411–1417.

72 Sale GE, Marmont BS. Marrow mast cell counts do not predict bone marrow graft rejection. Hum Pathol 1980, **12**: 605–608.

73 Shwachman H, Diamond LK, Oski FA, Khaw KT. The syndrome of pancreatic insufficiency and bone marrow dysfunction. J Pediatr 1964, **65**: 645–663.

74 Shimamura A. Inherited bone marrow failure syndromes: molecular features. Hematology Am Soc Hematol Educ Program 2006, 63–71.

75 Smith GP, Perkins SL, Segal GH, Kjeldsberg CR. T-cell lymphocytosis associated with invasive thymomas. Am J Clin Pathol 1994, **102**: 447–453.

76 Thompson AA, Nguyen LT. Amegakaryocytic thrombocytopenia and radio-ulnar synostosis are associated with HOX A11 mutation. Nat Genet 2000, **26**: 397–398.

77 Young NS, Maciejewski J. The pathophysiology of aplastic anemia. N Engl J Med 1997, **336**: 1365–1372.

78 Young NS, Calado RT, Scheinberg P. Current concepts in the pathophysiology and treatment of aplastic anemia. Blood 2006, **108**: 2509–2519.

GELATINOUS TRANSFORMATION (SEROUS DEGENERATION)

79 Abella E, Feliu E, Granada I, Millá F, Oriol A, Ribera JM, Sánchez-Planell L, Berga LI, Reverter JC, Rozman C. Bone marrow changes in anorexia nervosa are correlated with the amount of weight loss and not with other clinical findings. Am J Clin Pathol 2002, **118**: 582–588.

80 Bohm J. Gelatinous transformation of the bone marrow; the spectrum of underlying disease. Am J Surg Pathol 2000, **24**: 56–65.

81 Jain R, Singh ZN, Khurana N, Singh T. Gelatinous transformation of bone marrow: a study of 43 cases. Indian J Pathol Microbiol 2005, **48**: 1–3.

82 Mehta K, Gascon P, Robboy S. The gelatinous bone marrow (serous atrophy) in patients with acquired immunodeficiency syndrome. Evidence of excess sulfated glycosaminoglycan. Arch Pathol Lab Med 1992, **116**: 504–508.

83 Seaman JP, Kjeldsberg CR, Linker A. Gelatinous transformation of the bone marrow. Hum Pathol 1978, **9**: 685–692.

84 Sen R, Singh S, Singh H, Gupta A, Sen J. Clinical profile in gelatinous bone marrow transformation. J Assoc Physicians India 2003, **51**: 585–588.

OSTEOPETROSIS

85 Asskmyr MK, Fasth A, Richter J. Toward a better understanding and new therapeutics of osteopetrosis. Br J Haematol 2008, **140**: 597–609.

86 Coccia PF, Krivit W, Cervenka J, Clawson C, Kersey JH, Kim TH, Nesbit ME, Ramsay NK, Warkentin PI, Teitelbaum SL, Kahn AJ, Brown DM. Successful bone marrow transplantation for infantile malignant osteopetrosis. N Engl J Med 1980, **302**: 701–708.

87 Del Fattore A, Cappariello A, Teti A. Genetics, pathogenesis and complications of osteopetrosis. Bone 2008, **42**: 19–29.

88 Gerritsen EJ, Vossen JM, van Loo IH, Hermans J, Helfrich MH, Griscelli C, Fischer A. Autosomal recessive osteopetrosis: variability of findings at diagnosis and during the natural course. Pediatrics 1994, **93**: 247–253.

89 Gerritsen JA, Vossen JM, Fasth A, Friedrich W, Morgan G, Padmos A, Vellodi A, Porras O, O'Meara A, Porta F, et al. Bone marrow transplantation for autosomal recessive osteopetrosis. A report from the Working Party on Inborn Errors of the European Bone Marrow Transplantation Group. J Pediatr 1994, **125**: 896–902.

90 Helfrich MH, Aronson DC, Everts V, Mieremet RH, Gerritsen EJ, Eckhardt PG, Groot CG, Scherft JP. Morphologic features of bone in human osteopetrosis. Bone 1991, **12**: 411–419.

91 Kilpatrick L. Osteopetrosis. In Damjanov I, Linder J (eds): Anderson's pathology, ed. 10. St Louis, 1996, Mosby, pp. 2585, 2586.

92 Tolar J, Teitelbaum SL, Orchard PJ. Osteopetrosis. N Engl J Med 2004, **351**: 2839–2849.

BONE MARROW NECROSIS

93 Brown CH. Bone marrow necrosis. A study of seventy cases. Johns Hopkins Med J 1972, **131**: 189–203.

94 Goodall HB. Atypical changes in the bone marrow in acute infections. In Clark WJ, Howard EB, Hachett PL (eds): Myeloproliferative disorder of animal and man. Oak Ridge, Tennessee, 1970, United States Energy Commission, pp. 314–339.

95 Kundel DW, Brecher G, Bodey GP, Brittin GM. Reticulin fibrosis and bone infarction in acute leukemia. Implications for prognosis. Blood 1964, **23**: 526–544.

96 Niebrugge DJ, Benjamin DR. Bone marrow necrosis preceding acute lymphoblastic leukemia in childhood. Cancer 1983, **52**: 2162–2164.

97 Pui CH, Stass S, Green A. Bone marrow necrosis in children with malignant disease. Cancer 1985, **56**: 1522–1525.

98 Smith RR, Spivak JL. Marrow cell necrosis in anorexia nervosa and in voluntary starvation. Br J Haematol 1985, **60**: 525–530.

INFLAMMATORY DISORDERS

GRANULOMATOUS INFLAMMATION

99 Browne PM, Sharma OP, Salkin D. Bone marrow sarcoidosis. JAMA 1978, **240**: 2654–2655.

100 Choe JK, Hyun BH, Salazar GH, Ashton JK, Sung C. Epithelioid granulomas of the bone marrow in non-Hodgkin's lymphoproliferative malignancies. Am J Clin Pathol 1983, **80**: 19–24.

101 Cruikshank B, Thomas MJ. Mineral oil (follicular) lipidosis. II. Histologic studies of spleen, liver, lymph nodes, and bone marrow. Hum Pathol 1984, **15**: 731–737.

102 Delsol G, Pellegrin M, Familiades J, Auvergnat JC. Bone marrow lesions in Q fever. Blood 1978, **52**: 637–638.

103 Diebold J, Molina T, Camilleri-Broet S, Le Tournea A, Audouin J. Bone marrow manifestations of infection and systemic diseases observed in bone marrow trephine biopsy review. Histopathology 2000, **37**: 199–211.

104 Farhi DC, Mason UG, Horsburgh CR Jr. The bone marrow in disseminated *Mycobacterium avium-intracellulare* infection. Am J Clin Pathol 1985, **83**: 463–468.

105 Hakawi AM, Airajhi AA. Tuberculosis of the bone marrow: clinico-pathological study of 22 cases from Saudi Arabia. Int J Tuberc Lung Dis 2006, **10**: 1041–1044.

106 Hussong J, Peterson LR, Warren JR, Peterson LC. Detecting disseminated *Mycobacterium avium* complex infections in HIV-positive patients, the usefulness of bone marrow trephine biopsy specimens, aspirate cultures, and blood cultures. Am J Clin Pathol 1998, **110**: 806–809.

107 Kadin ME, Donaldson SS, Dorfman RF. Isolated granulomas in Hodgkin's disease. N Engl J Med 1970, **283**: 859–861.

108 Ker CC, Hung CC, Huang SY, Chen MY, Hsieh SM, Lin CC, Chang SC, Luh KT. Comparison of bone marrow studies with blood culture for etiological diagnosis of disseminated mycobacterial and fungal infection in patients with acquired immunodeficiency syndrome. Microbiol Immunol Infect 2002, **35**: 89–93.

109 Kilby JM, Marques MB, Jaye DL, Tabereaux PB, Reddy VB, Waites KB. The yield of bone marrow biopsy and culture compared with blood culture in the evaluation of HIV-infected patients for mycobacterial and fungal infections. Am J Med 1998, **104**: 123–128.

110 Kvasnicka HM, Thiele J. Differentiation of granulomatous lesions in the bone marrow. Pathologie 2002, **23**: 465–471.

111 McKenna RW, Dehner LP. Oxalosis. An unusual cause of myelophthisis in childhood. Am J Clin Pathol 1976, **66**: 991–997.

112 Mohamed T, Sanjay R, Sycheva T, Aish L, Schneider D, Oo TH. Amiodarone-associated bone marrow granulomas: a report of 2 cases and review of the literature. Int J Hematol 2007, **85**: 101–104.

113 Mukhopadhyay S, Mukhopadhyay S, Abraham NZ Jr, Jones LA, Howard L, Gajra A. Unexplained bone marrow granulomas: is amiodarone the culprit? A report of 2 cases. Am J Hematol 2004, **75**: 110–112.

114 Park DY, Kim JY, Choi KU, Lee JS, Lee CH, Sol MY, Suh KS. Comparison of polymerase chain reaction with histopathologic feature for diagnosis of tuberculosis in formalin-fixed, paraffin-embedded histologic specimens. Arch Pathol Lab Med 2003, **127**: 326–330.

115 Riley UB, Crawford S, Barrett SP, Abdalla SH. Detection of mycobacteria in bone marrow biopsy specimens taken to investigate pyrexia of unknown origin. J Clin Pathol 1995, **48**: 706–709.

116 Rywlin AM, Ortega R. Lipid granulomas of the bone marrow. Am J Clin Pathol 1972, **57**: 457–462.

117 Rywlin AM. A pathologist's view of the bone marrow. J Fla Med Assoc 1980, **67**: 121–124.

118 Srigley JR, Vellend H, Palmer N, Phillips MJ, Geddie WR, Van Nostrand AW, Edwards VD. Q-fever. The liver and bone marrow pathology. Am J Surg Pathol 1985, **9**: 752–758.

119 Swerdlow SH, Collins RD. Marrow granulomas. In Ioachim HE (ed.): Pathology of granulomas. New York, 1983, Raven Press, pp. 125–150.

120 Vilalta-Castel E, Valdés-Sanchez MD, Guerra-Vales JM, Teno-Esteban C, Garzón A, López JI, Ricard MP, Abarca M, Garcia-Diaz JD. Significance of granulomas in bone marrow: a study of 40 cases. Eur J Haematol 1988, **41**: 12–16.

121 Volk EE, Miller ML, Kirkley BA, Washington JA. The diagnostic usefulness of bone marrow cultures in patients with fever of unknown origin. Am J Clin Pathol 1998, **110**: 150–153.

122 White RM, Johnston CL. Granulomatous bone marrow disease in Virginia. Study of 50 cases. Va Med 1985, **112**: 316–319.

123 Williams HE, Smith LH Jr. Primary hyperoxaluria. In Stanbury JB, Wyngaarden JB, Fredrickson DS, Goldstein JL, Brown MS (eds): The metabolic basis of inherited disease. New York, 1983, McGraw-Hill Book Co., pp. 204–228.

124 Young N. Hematologic and hematopoietic consequences of B19 parvovirus infection. Semin Hematol 1988, **25**: 159–172.

NONSPECIFIC INFLAMMATORY REACTIONS

125 Custer RP. An atlas of the blood and bone marrow. Philadelphia, 1974, W.B. Saunders.

126 Georgii A, Vykoupil KF. Unspecific mesenchymal reaction in bone marrow in patients with Hodgkin's disease. Recent Results Cancer Res 1974, **46**: 39–44.

HUMAN IMMUNODEFICIENCY VIRUS SYNDROME (HIV, AIDS)

127 Abrams DI, Kirpov DD, Goedert JJ, Sarngadharan MG, Gallo RC, Volberding PA. Antibodies to human T lymphotropic virus type III and development of the acquired immunodeficiency syndrome in homosexual men presenting with immune thrombocytopenia. Ann Intern Med 1986, **104**: 47–50.

128 Brynes RK, Ewing EP Jr, Joshi VV, Chan WC. The histopathology of HIV infection: an overview. Prog AIDS Pathol 1989, **1**: 1–28.

129 Castella A, Croxson TS, Mildvan D, Witt DH, Zalusky R. The bone marrow in AIDS. A histologic, hematologic, and microbiologic study. Am J Clin Pathol 1985, **84**: 425–432.

130 Crook TW, Rogers BB, McFarland RD, Kroft SH, Muretto P, Hernandez JA, Latimer MJ, McKenna RW. Unusual bone marrow manifestations of parvovirus B19 infection in immunocompromised patients. Hum Pathol 2000, **31**: 161–168.

131 Frickhofen N, Abkowitz JL, Safford M, Berry JM, Antunez-de-Mayolo J, Astrow A, Cohen R, Halperin I, King L, Mintzer D, et al. Persistent B19 parvovirus infection in patients infected with human immunodeficiency virus type 1 (HIV-1). A treatable cause of anemia in AIDS. Ann Intern Med 1990, **113**: 926–933.

132 Geller SA, Muller R, Greenberg ML, Siegal FP. Acquired immunodeficiency syndrome. Distinctive features of bone marrow biopsies. Arch Pathol Lab Med 1985, **109**: 138–141.

133 Hussong J, Peterson LR, Warren JR, Peterson LC. Detecting disseminated *Mycobacterium avium* complex infections in HIV-positive patients. The usefulness of bone marrow trephine biopsy specimens, aspirate cultures, and blood cultures. Am J Clin Pathol 1998, **110**: 806–809.

134 Ioachim HL, Dorsett B, Cronin W, Maya M, Wall S. Acquired immunodeficiency syndrome-associated lymphomas: clinical, pathologic, immunologic, and viral characteristics of 111 cases. Hum Pathol 1991, **22**: 659–673.

135 Karcher DS, Frost AR. The bone marrow in human immunodeficiency virus (HIV)-related disease. Morphology and clinical correlation. Am J Clin Pathol 1991, **95**: 63–71.

136 Luther JM, Lakey DL, Larson RS, Kallianpur AR, D'Agata E, Cousar JB, Haas DW. Utility of bone marrow biopsy for rapid diagnosis of febrile illnesses in patients with human immunodeficiency viral infection. South Med J 2000, **93**: 692–697.

137 Morris L, Distenfeld A, Amorosi E, Karpatkin S. Autoimmune thrombocytopenic purpura in homosexual men. Ann Intern Med 1982, **96**: 714–717.

138 Namiki TS, Boone DC, Meyer PR. A comparison of bone marrow findings in patients with acquired immunodeficiency syndrome (AIDS) and AIDS related conditions. Hematol Oncol 1987, **5**: 99–106.

139 Nasr SA, Brynes RK, Garrison CP, Chan WC. Peripheral T-cell lymphoma in a patient with acquired immunodeficiency syndrome. Cancer 1988, **61**: 947–951.

140 Nichols L, Florentine B, Lewis W, Sattler F, Rarrick MU, Byrnes RK. Bone marrow examination for the diagnosis of mycobacterial and fungal infections in the acquired immunodeficiency syndrome. Arch Pathol Lab Med 1991, **115**: 1125–1132.

141 Osborne BM, Guarda LA, Butler JJ. Bone marrow biopsies in patients with the acquired immunodeficiency syndrome. Hum Pathol 1984, **15**: 1048–1053.

142 Ponzoni M, Fumagalli L, Rossi G, Freschi M, Re A, Viganò MG, Guidoboni M, Dolcetti R, McKenna RW, Facchetti F. Isolated bone marrow manifestation of HIV-associated Hodgkin lymphoma. Mod Pathol 2002, **15**: 1273–1278.

143 Richman DD, Fischl MA, Grieco MH, Gottlieb MS, Volberding PA, Laskin OL, Leedom JM, Groopman JE, Mildvan D, Hirsch MS, Jackson GG, Durack DT, Nusinoff-Lehrman S, and the AZT Collaborative Working Group. The efficacy of azidothymidine (AZT) in the treatment of patients with AIDS and AIDS related complex. A double-blind, placebo-controlled trial. N Engl J Med 1987, **317**: 192–197.

144 Savona S, Nardi MA, Lennette ET, Karpatkin S. Thrombocytopenic purpura in narcotics addicts. Ann Intern Med 1985, **102**: 737–741.
145 Schneider DR, Picker LJ. Myelodysplasia in the acquired immune deficiency syndrome. Am J Clin Pathol 1985, **84**: 144–152.
146 Spivak JL, Bender BS, Quinn TC. Hematologic abnormalities in the acquired immune deficiency syndrome. Am J Med 1984, **77**: 224–228.
147 Treacy M, Lai L, Costello C, Clark A. Peripheral blood and bone marrow abnormalities in patients with HIV and related disease. Br J Haematol 1987, **65**: 289–294.
148 Zon LI, Arkin C, Groopman JE. Haematologic manifestations of the human immune deficiency virus (HIV). Br J Haematol 1987, **66**: 251–256.

LEUKEMIAS AND RELATED DISORDERS

ACUTE LEUKEMIA

149 Arber DA. Acute myeloid leukemia. In Hsi ED (ed.): Foundations in diagnostic pathology, hematopathology. Philadelphia, 2007, Churchill Livingstone, pp. 397–432.
150 Arber DA, Brunning RD, LeBeau MM, Falini B, Vardiman JW, Porwit A, et al. Acute myeloid leukaemia with recurrent genetic abnormalities. In Swerdlow SH, Campo E, Harris NL, Jaffe ES, Pileri SA, Stein H, Thiele J, Vardiman JW (eds): WHO classification of tumours of haematopoietic and lymphoid tissues. Lyon, 2008, IARC Press, pp. 110–123.
151 Arber DA, Brunning RD, Orazi A, Bain BJ, Porwit A, Vardiman JW, et al. Acute myeloid leukaemia with myelodysplasia-related changes. In Swerdlow SH, Campo E, Harris NL, Jaffe ES, Pileri SA, Stein H, Thiele J, Vardiman JW (eds): WHO classification of tumours of haematopoietic and lymphoid tissues. Lyon, 2008, IARC Press, pp. 124–126.
152 Arber DA, Brunning RD, Orazi A, Porwit A, Paterson L, Thiele J, Le Beau MM. Acute myeloid leukaemia, not otherwise specified. In Swerdlow SH, Campo E, Harris NL, Jaffe ES, Pileri SA, Stein H, Thiele J, Vardiman JW (eds): WHO classification of tumours of haematopoietic and lymphoid tissues. Lyon, 2008, IARC Press, pp. 130–139.
153 Arber DA, Cousar JB. Hematopoietic tumors: principles of pathologic diagnosis. In Greer JP, Foerster J, Rodgers GM, Paraskevas F, Glader B, Arber DA, Means RT Jr (eds): Wintrobe's clinical hematology, ed. 12. Philadelphia, 2009, Lippincott Williams & Wilkins, pp. 1663–1668.
154 Arber DA, Jenkins KA. Paraffin section immunophenotyping of acute leukemias in bone marrow specimens. Am J Clin Pathol 1996, **106**: 462–468.
155 Arber DA, Stein AS, Carter NH, Ikle D, Forman SJ, Slovak ML. Prognostic impact of acute myeloid leukaemia classification. Importance of detection of recurring cytogenetic abnormalities and multilineage dysplasia on survival. Am J Clin Pathol 2003, **119**: 672–680.
156 Barcos MP, Lukes RJ. Malignant lymphomas of convoluted lymphocytes. A new entity of possible T-cell type. In Sinks LR, Godden JO (eds): Conflicts in childhood cancer. An evaluation of current management, vol. 4. New York, 1975, Alan R. Liss, pp. 147–178.
157 Baumann I, Niemeyer CM, Brunning RD, Arber DA, Porwit A. Myeloid proliferations related to Down syndrome. In Swerdlow SH, Campo E, Harris NL, Jaffe ES, Pileri SA, Stein H, Thiele J, Vardiman JW (eds): WHO classification of tumours of haematopoietic and lymphoid tissues. Lyon, 2008, IARC Press, pp. 142–144.
158 Bennett JM, Catovsky D, Daniel MT, Sultan C, Flandrin G, Galton DAG, Gralnick HR. Proposals for the classification of the acute leukaemias. French–American–British (FAB) co-operative group. Br J Haematol 1976, **33**: 451–458.
159 Berdeaux DH, Glasser L, Serokmann R, Moon T, Durie BG. Hypoplastic acute leukemia. Review of 70 cases with multivariate regression analysis. Hematol Oncol 1986, **4**: 291–305.
160 Borowitz MJ, Béné M-C, Harris NL, Porwit A, Matutes E. Acute leukaemias of ambiguous lineage. In Swerdlow SH, Campo E, Harris NL, Jaffe ES, Pileri SA, Stein H, Thiele J, Vardiman JW (eds): WHO classification of tumours of haematopoietic and lymphoid tissues. Lyon, 2008, IARC Press, pp. 150–155.
161 Borowitz MJ, Chan JKC. B lymphoblastic leukaemia/lymphoma, not otherwise specified. In Swerdlow SH, Campo E, Harris NL, Jaffe ES, Pileri SA, Stein H, Thiele J, Vardiman JW (eds): WHO classification of tumours of haematopoietic and lymphoid tissues. Lyon, 2008, IARC Press, pp. 168–170.
162 Borowitz MJ, Chan JKC. B lymphoblastic leukaemia/lymphoma with recurrent genetic abnormalities. In Swerdlow SH, Campo E, Harris NL, Jaffe ES, Pileri SA, Stein H, Thiele J, Vardiman JW (eds): WHO classification of tumours of haematopoietic and lymphoid tissues. Lyon, 2008, IARC Press, pp. 171–175.
163 Borowitz MJ, Chan JKC. T lymphoblastic leukaemia/lymphoma. In Swerdlow SH, Campo E, Harris NL, Jaffe ES, Pileri SA, Stein H, Thiele J, Vardiman JW (eds): WHO classification of tumours of haematopoietic and lymphoid tissues. Lyon, 2008, IARC Press, pp. 176–178.
164 Breatnach F, Chessells JM, Greaves MF. The aplastic presentation of childhood leukaemia. A feature of common-ALL. Br J Haematol 1981, **49**: 387–393.
165 Brunning R. The effects of leukemia and lymphoma therapy on hematopoietic cells. Am J Med Technol 1973, **39**: 165–174.
166 Chuang SS, Li CY. Useful panel of antibodies for the classification of acute leukemia by immunohistochemical methods in bone marrow trephine biopsy specimens. Am J Clin Pathol 1997, **107**: 410–418.
167 Howe RB, Bloomfield CD, McKenna RW. Hypocellular acute leukemia. Am J Med 1982, **72**: 391–395.
168 Lin P, Jones O, Dorfman DM, Medeiros LJ. Precursor B-cell lymphoblastic lymphoma: a predominantly extranodal tumor with low propensity for leukemic involvement. Am J Surg Pathol 2000, **24**: 1480–1490.
169 Manoharan A, Horsley R, Pitney WR. The reticulin content of bone marrow in acute leukaemia in adults. Br J Haematol 1979, **43**: 185–190.
170 Murphy SB, Hustu HO. A randomized trial of combined modality theory of childhood non-Hodgkin's lymphoma. Cancer 1980, **45**: 630–637.
171 Pileri SA, Ascani S, Milani M, Visani G, Piccioli M, Orcioni GF, Poggi S, Sabattini E, Santini D, Falini B. Acute leukemia immunophenotyping in bone marrow routine sections. Br J Haematol 1999, **105**: 394–401.
172 Rimsza LM, Larson RS, Winter SS, Foucar K, Chong YY, Garner KW, Leith CP. Benign hematogone-rich lymphoid proliferations can be distinguished from B-lineage acute lymphoblastic leukemia by integration of morphology, immunophenotype, adhesion molecule expression, and architectural features. Am J Clin Pathol 2000, **114**: 66–75.
173 Vardiman JW, Arber DA, Brunning RD, Larson RA, Matutes E, Baumann I, Thiele J. Therapy-related myeloid neoplasms. In Swerdlow SH, Campo E, Harris NL, Jaffe ES, Pileri SA, Stein H, Thiele J, Vardiman JW (eds): WHO classification of tumours of haematopoietic and lymphoid tissues. Lyon, 2008, IARC Press, pp. 127–129.
174 Vardiman JW, Brunning RD, Arber DA, LeBeau M, Porwit A, Tefferi A, Bloomfield CD, Thiele J. Introduction and overview of the classification of the myeloid neoplasms. In Swerdlow SH, Campo E, Harris NL, Jaffe ES, Pileri SA, Stein H, Thiele J, Vardiman JW (eds): WHO classification of tumours of haematopoietic and lymphoid tissues. Lyon, 2008, IARC Press, pp. 18–30.
175 Vardiman JW, Thiele J, Arber DA, Brunning RD, Borowitz MJ, Porwit A, Harris NL, Le Beau MM, Hellstrom-Lindberg E, Tefferi A, Bloomfield CD. The 2008 revision of the WHO classification of myeloid neoplasms and acute leukemia: rationale and important changes. Blood 2009, **114**: 937–951.
176 Yunis JJ, Brunning RD. Prognostic significance of chromosomal abnormalities in acute leukaemias and myelodysplastic syndromes. Clin Haematol 1986, **15**: 597–620.

ACUTE PANMYELOSIS WITH MYELOFIBROSIS (ACUTE MYELOFIBROSIS)

177 Arber DA, Brunning RD, Orazi A, Porwit A, Paterson L, Thiele J, Le Beau MM. Acute myeloid leukaemia, not otherwise specified. In Swerdlow SH, Campo E, Harris NL, Jaffe ES, Pileri SA, Stein H, Thiele J, Vardiman JW (eds): WHO classification of tumours of haematopoietic and lymphoid tissues. Lyon, 2008, IARC Press, pp. 130–139.
178 Bain B, Catovsky D, O'Brien M, Prentice HG, Lawlor E, Kumaran TO, McCann SR, Matutes E, Galton DA. Megakaryoblastic leukemia presenting as acute myelofibrosis. A study of four cases with the platelet–peroxidase reaction. Blood 1981, **58**: 206–213.
179 Bearman RM, Pangalis GA, Rappaport H. Acute (malignant) myelosclerosis. Cancer 1979, **43**: 279–293.
180 Hruban RH, Kuhajda FP, Mann RB. Acute myelofibrosis. Immunohistochemical study of four cases and comparison with acute megakaryoblastic leukemia. Am J Clin Pathol 1987, **88**: 578–588.
181 Sultan C, Sigaux F, Imbert M, Reyes F. Acute myelodysplasia with myelofibrosis. A report of eight cases. Br J Haematol 1981, **49**: 11–16.
182 Suvajdzic N, Marisavljevic D, Kraguljac N, Pantic M, Djordjevic V, Jankovic G, Cemerikic-Martinovic V, Colovic M. Acute panmyelosis with myelofibrosis: clinical, immunophenotypic and cytogenetic study of twelve cases. Leuk Lymphoma 2004, **45**: 1873–1879.
183 Thiele J, Kvasnicka HM, Zerhusen G, Vardiman J, Diehl V, Luebbert M, Schmitt-Graeff A. Acute panmyelosis with myelofibrosis: a clinicopathological study on 46 patients including histochemistry of bone marrow biopsies and follow-up. Ann Hematol 2004, **83**: 513–521.

MYELOID SARCOMA

184 Beckman EN, Oehrle JS. Fibrous hematopoietic tumors arising in agnogenic myeloid metaplasia. Hum Pathol 1982, **13**: 804–810.
185 Brunning R, McKenna RW. Tumors of the hematopoietic system. Atlas of tumor pathology, series 3, fascicle 29. Washington DC, 1994, Armed Forces Institute of Pathology, pp. 93–100.

186 Cavdar AO, Arcasoy A, Babacan E, Gözdasoglu S, Topuz Ü, Fraumeni JF. Ocular granulocytic sarcoma (chloroma) with acute myelomonocytic leukemia in Turkish children. Cancer 1978, **41**: 1606–1609.

187 Garfinkel LS, Bennett DE. Extramedullary myeloblastic transformation in chronic myelocytic leukemia simulating a coexistent malignant lymphoma. Am J Clin Pathol 1969, **51**: 638–645.

188 Gralnick HR, Dittmar K. Development of myeloblastoma with massive breast and ovarian involvement during remission in acute leukemia. Cancer 1969, **24**: 746–749.

189 Leder LD. The selective enzymochemical demonstration of neutrophilic myeloid cells and tissue mast cells in paraffin sections. Klin Wochenschr 1964, **42**: 553.

190 McKenna RW, Bloomfield CD, Dick F, Nesbitt ME, Brunning RD. Acute monoblastic leukemia. Diagnosis and treatment of ten cases. Blood 1975, **46**: 481–494.

191 Mason TE, Damaree R, Margolis CI. Granulocytic sarcoma (chloroma) two years preceding myelogenous leukemia. Cancer 1973, **31**: 423–432.

192 Meis JM, Butler JJ, Osborne BM, Manning JT. Granulocytic sarcoma in non-leukemic patients. Cancer 1986, **58**: 2697–2709.

193 Muller S, Sangster G, Crocker J, Nar P, Burnett D, Brown G, Leyland MJ. An immunohistochemical and clinicopathological study of granulocytic sarcoma ('chloroma'). Hematol Oncol 1986, **4**: 101–112.

194 Neiman RS, Barcos M, Berard C, Bonner H, Mann R, Rydell RE, Bennett JM. Granulocytic sarcoma. A clinicopathologic study of 61 biopsied cases. Cancer 1981, **48**: 1426–1437.

195 Peterson LC, Dehner L, Brunning RD. Extramedullary masses as presenting features of acute monoblastic leukemia. Am J Clin Pathol 1980, **75**: 140–148.

196 Pileri AS, Ascani S, Cox MC, Campidelli C, Bacci F, Piccioli M, Piccaluga PP, Agostinelli C, Asioli S, Novero D, Bisceglia M, Ponzoni M, Gentile A, Rinaldi P, Franco V, Vincelli D, Pileri A Jr, Gasbarra R, Falini B, Zinzani PL, Baccarani M. Myeloid sarcoma: clinico-pathologic, phenotypic and cytogenetic analysis of 92 adult patients. Leukemia 2007, **21**: 340–350.

197 Pileri SA, Orazi A, Falini B. Myeloid sarcoma. In Swerdlow SH, Campo E, Harris NL, Jaffe ES, Pileri SA, Stein H, Thiele J, Vardiman JW (eds): WHO classification of tumours of haematopoietic and lymphoid tissues. Lyon, 2008, IARC Press, pp. 140–141.

198 Pinkus GS, Pinkus JL. Myeloperoxidase. A specific marker for myeloid cells in paraffin sections. Mod Pathol 1991, **4**: 733–741.

199 Tallman MS, Hakimian D, Shaw JM, Lissner GS, Russell EJ, Variakojis D. Granulocytic sarcoma is associated with the 8;21 translocation in acute myeloid leukemia. J Clin Oncol 1993, **11**: 690–697.

200 Traweek ST, Arber DA, Rappaport H, Brynes RK. Extramedullary myeloid cell tumors: an immunohistochemical and morphologic study of 28 cases. Am J Surg Pathol 1993, **17**: 1011–1019.

201 Wiernik PH, Serpick AA. Granulocytic sarcoma (chloroma). Blood 1970, **35**: 361–369.

MYELODYSPLASTIC SYNDROMES

202 Baumann I, Niemeyer CM, Bennett JM, Shannon K. Childhood myelodysplastic syndrome. In Swerdlow SH, Campo E, Harris NL, Jaffe ES, Pileri SA, Stein H, Thiele J, Vardiman JW (eds): WHO classification of tumours of haematopoietic and lymphoid tissues. Lyon, 2008, IARC Press, pp. 104–107.

203 Bennett JM, Catovsky D, Daniel MT, Flandrin G, Galton DA, Gralnick HR, Sultan C. Proposals for the classification of the myelodysplastic syndromes. Br J Haematol 1982, **51**: 189–199.

204 Brunning RD, Orazi A, Germing U, Le Beau MM, Porwit A,. Baumann I, Vardiman JW, Hellstrom-Lindberg E. Myelodysplastic syndromes/neoplasms. In Swerdlow SH, Campo E, Harris NL, Jaffe ES, Pileri SA, Stein H, Thiele J, Vardiman JW (eds): WHO classification of tumours of haematopoietic and lymphoid tissues. Lyon, 2008, IARC Press, pp. 89–93.

205 Delacretaz F, Schmidt PM, Piguet D, Bachmann F, Costa J. Histopathology of myelodysplastic syndromes. The FAB classification (proposals) applied to bone marrow biopsy. Am J Clin Pathol 1987, **87**: 180–186.

206 Hasserjian RP, LeBeau MM, List AF, Bennett JM, Thiele J. Myelodysplastic syndrome with isolated del(5q–). In Swerdlow SH, Campo E, Harris NL, Jaffe ES, Pileri SA, Stein H, Thiele J, Vardiman JW (eds): WHO classification of tumours of haematopoietic and lymphoid tissues. Lyon, 2008, IARC Press, pp. 102, 103.

207 Horny H-P, Sotlar K, Valent P. Diagnostic value of histology and immunohistochemistry in myelodysplastic syndromes. Leuk Res 2007, **31**: 1609–1616.

208 Lim ZY, Killick S, Germing U, Cavenagh J, Culligan D, Bacigalupo A, Marsh J, Mufti GJ. Low IPSS score and bone marrow hypocellularity in MDS patients predict hematological responses to antithymocyte globulin. Leukemia 2007, **21**: 1436–1441.

209 List AF, Garewal HS, Sandberg AA. The myelodysplastic syndromes, biology and implications for management. J Clin Oncol 1990, **8**: 1424–1441.

210 Liu Y-C, Ito Y, Hsiao H-H, Sashida G, Kodama A, Ohyashiki JH, Ohyashiki K. Risk factor analysis in myelodysplastic syndrome patients with del(20q): prognosis revisited. Cancer Genet Cytogenet 2006, **171**: 9–16.

211 Maschek H, Georgii A, Kaloutal V, Werner M, Bandecar K, Kressel MG, Choritz H, Freund M, Hufnagl D. Myelofibrosis in primary myelodysplastic syndromes. A retrospective study of 352 patients. Eur J Haematol 1992, **48**: 208–214.

212 Mathew P, Tefferi A, Dewald GW, Goldberg SL, Hoagland HC, Noel P. The 5q– syndrome. A single institution study of 43 consecutive cases. Blood 1993, **81**: 1040–1045.

213 Orazi A. Histopathology in the diagnosis and classification of acute myeloid leukemia, myelodysplastic syndromes, and myelodysplastic/myeloproliferative diseases. Pathobiology 2007, **74**: 97–114.

214 Orazi A, Albitar M, Heerema NA, Haskins NS, Neiman RS. Hypoplastic myelodysplastic syndrome can be distinguished from acquired aplastic anemia by CD34 and PCNA immunostaining of bone marrow biopsy specimens. Am J Clin Pathol 1997, **107**: 268–274.

215 Orazi A, Brunning RD, Hasserjian RO, Germing U, Thiele J. Refractory anaemia with excess blasts. In Swerdlow SH, Campo E, Harris NL, Jaffe ES, Pileri SA, Stein H, Thiele J, Vardiman JW (eds): WHO classification of tumours of haematopoietic and lymphoid tissues. Lyon, 2008, IARC Press, pp. 100, 101.

216 Orazi A, Bennett JM, Germing U, Brunning R, Bain BJ, Thiele J. Chronic myelomonocytic leukaemia. In Swerdlow SH, Campo E, Harris NL, Jaffe ES, Pileri SA, Stein H, Thiele J, Vardiman JW (eds): WHO classification of tumours of haematopoietic and lymphoid tissues. Lyon, 2008, IARC Press, pp. 76–79.

217 Tricot G, Vlietnick R, Boogaerts MA, Hendrickx B, De Wolf-Peeters C, Van den Berghe H, Verwilghen RL. Prognostic factors in the myelodysplastic syndromes. Importance of initial data on peripheral blood counts, bone marrow, cytology, trephine biopsy and chromosomal analysis. Br J Haematol 1985, **60**: 19–32.

218 Vardiman JW, Arber DA, Brunning RD, Larson RA, Matutes E, Baumann I, Thiele J. Therapy-related myeloid neoplasms. In Swerdlow SH, Campo E, Harris N, Jaffee ES, Pileri SA, Stein H, Thiele J, Vardiman JW (eds): WHO classification of tumours of the haematopoietic and lymphoid tissues. Lyon, 2008, IARC Press, pp. 127–129.

219 Vardiman JW, Brunning RD, Arber DA, Le Beau MM, Porwit A, Tefferi A, et al. Introduction and overview of the classification of the myeloid neoplasms. In Swerdlow SH, Campo E, Harris N, Jaffee ES, Pileri SA, Stein H, Thiele J, Vardiman JW (eds): WHO classification of tumours of the haematopoietic and lymphoid tissues. Lyon, 2008, IARC Press, pp. 18–30.

220 Verburgh E, Achten R, Maes B, Hagemeijer A, Boogaerts M, De Wolf-Peeters C, Verhoef G. Additional prognostic value of bone marrow histology in patients subclassified according to the International Prognostic Scoring System for Myelodysplastic Syndromes. J Clin Oncol 2003, **21**: 273–282.

MYELOPROLIFERATIVE NEOPLASMS

Chronic myelogenous leukemia

221 Braziel RM, Launder TM, Druker BJ, Olson SB, Magenis RE, Mauro MJ, Sawyers CL, Paquette RL, O'Dwyer ME. Hematopathologic and cytogenetic findings on imatinib mesylate-treated chronic myelogenous leukemia patients: 14 months' experience. Blood 2002, **100**: 435–441.

222 Clough V, Geary CG, Hashmi K, Davson J, Knowlson T. Myelofibrosis in chronic granulocytic leukaemia. Br J Haematol 1979, **42**: 515–526.

223 Dekmezian R, Kantarjian HM, Keating MJ, Talpaz M, McCredie KB, Freireich EJ. The relevance of reticulin stain-measured fibrosis at diagnosis in chronic myelogenous leukemia. Cancer 1987, **59**: 1739–1743.

224 Kantarjian HM, Cortes JE, O'Brien S, Giles F, Garcia-Manero G, Faderl S, Thomas D, Jeha S, Rios MB, Letvak L, Bochinski K, Arlinghaus R, Talpaz M. Imatinib mesylate therapy in newly diagnosed patients with Philadelphia chromosome-positive chronic myelogenous leukemia; high incidence of early complete and major cytogenetic responses. Blood 2002, **101**: 97–100.

225 Kantarjian HM, Deisseroth A, Kurzrock R, Estrov Z, Talpaz M. Chronic myelogenous leukemia. A concise update. Blood 1993, **82**: 691–703.

226 Kantarjian H, Sawyers C, Hochhaus A, Guilhot F, Schiffer C, Gambacorti-Passerini C, Niederwieser D, Resta D, Capdeville R, Zoellner U, Talpaz M, Druker B, Goldman J, O'Brien SG, Russell N, Fischer T, Ottmann O, Cony-Makhoul P, Facon T, Stone R, Miller C, Tallman M, Brown R, Schuster M, Loughran T, Gratwohl A, Mandelli F, Saglio G, Lazzarino M, Russo D, Baccarani M, Morra E; International STI571 CML Study Group. Hematologic and cytogenetic responses to imatinib mesylate in chronic myelogenous leukemia. N Engl J Med 2002, **346**: 645–652.

227 Kvasnicka HM, Thiele J, Staib P, Engels K, Kriener S, Schmitt-Graeff A. Therapy-related changes of angiogenesis in Philadelphia chromosome positive chronic myelogenous leukemia. Pathologe 2004, **25**: 127–134.

228 Kvasnicka HM, Thiele J. Bone marrow angiogenesis: methods of quantification and changes evolving in chronic myeloproliferative disorders. Histol Histopathol 2004, **19**: 1245–1260.

229 Lugli A, Ebnother M, Tichelli A, Gratwohl A, Zimpfer A, Cogliatti S, Linn M, Dirnhofer S. Bone marrow morphology in CML patients during treatment with STI571 (Glivec): evidence of complete morphological remission and correlation to hematologic and cytogenetic response. J Clin Pathol 2002, **55**: A6.

230 McGlave PB, Brunning RD, Hurd DD, Kim TH. Reversal of severe bone marrow fibrosis and osteosclerosis following allogeneic bone marrow transplantation for chronic granulocytic leukaemia. Br J Haematol 1982, **52**: 189–194.

231 Muehleck SD, McKenna RW, Arthur DC, Parkin JL, Brunning RD. Transformation of chronic myelogenous leukemia. Clinical, morphologic and cytogenetic features. Am J Clin Pathol 1984, **82**: 1–14.

232 Palandri F, Castagnetti F, Alimena G, Testoni N, Breccia M, Luatti S, Rege-Cambrin G, Stagno F, Specchia G, Martino B, Levato L, Merante S, Liberati AM, Pane F, Saglio G, Alberti D, Martinelli G, Baccarani M, Rosti G. The long-term durability of cytogenetic responses in patients with accelerated phase chronic myeloid leukemia treated with imatinib 600 mg: the GIMEMA CML Working Party experience after a 7-year follow-up. Haematologica 2009, **94**: 205–212.

233 Thiele J, Kvasnicka NM, Beelen DW, Flucke U, Spoer C, Paperno S, Leder LD, Schaefer UW. Megakaryopoiesis and myelofibrosis in chronic leukemia after allogeneic bone marrow transplantation: an immunohistochemical study of 127 patients. Mod Pathol 2000, **14**: 129–138.

234 Thiele J, Kvasnicka HM, Orazi A. Bone marrow histopathology in myeloproliferative disorders – current diagnostic approach. Semin Haematol 2005, **42**: 184–195.

235 Thiele J, Kvasnicka HM. Myelofibrosis – what's in a name? Consensus on definition and EUMNET grading. Pathobiology 2007, **74**: 89–96.

236 Thiele J, Kvasnicka HM, Schmitt-Graeff A, Bundschuh S, Biermann T, Roessler G, Wasmus M, Diehl V, Zankovich R, Schaefer HE. Effects of chemotherapy (busulfan-hydroxyurea) and interferon-alfa on bone marrow morphologic features in chronic myelogenous leukemia: histochemical and morphometric study on sequential bone marrow biopsy specimens with special emphasis on dynamic features. Am J Clin Pathol 2000, **114**: 57–65.

237 Vardiman JW, Bennett JM, Bain BJ, Baumann I, Thiele J, Orazi A. Atypical chronic myeloid leukaemia, BCR/ABL1 negative. In Swerdlow SH, Campo E, Harris NL, Jaffee ES, Pileri SA, Stein H, Thiele J, Vardiman JW (eds): WHO classification of tumours of haematopoietic and lymphoid tissues. Lyon, 2008, IARC Press, pp. 80, 81.

238 Vardiman JW, Brunning RD, Arber DA, Le Beau MM, Porwit A, Tefferi A, et al. Introduction and overview of the classification of the myeloid neoplasms. In Swerdlow SH, Campo E, Harris N, Jaffee ES, Pileri SA, Stein H, Thiele J, Vardiman JW (eds): WHO classification of tumours of the haematopoietic and lymphoid tissues. Lyon, 2008, IARC Press, pp. 18–30.

239 Vardiman JW, Melo JV, Baccarinii M, Thiele J. Chronic myelogenous leukaemia, BCR/ABL1 positive. In Swerdlow SH, Campo E, Harris N, Jaffee ES, Pileri SA, Stein H, Thiele J, Vardiman JW (eds): WHO classification of tumours of haematopoietic and lymphoid tissues. Lyon, 2008, IARC Press, pp. 32–37.

Polycythemia vera

240 Ellis JT, Peterson P, Geller SA, Rappaport H. Studies of the bone marrow in polycythemia vera and the evolution of myelofibrosis and second hematologic malignancies. Semin Hematol 1986, **12**: 144–155.

241 Ellis JT, Silver RT, Coleman M, Geller SA. The bone marrow in polycythaemia vera. Semin Hematol 1975, **12**: 433–444.

242 Gianelli U, Iurlo A, Vener C, Moro A, Fermo E, Bianchi P, Graziani D, Radaelli F, Coggi G, Bosari S, Deliliers GL, Zanella A. The significance of bone marrow biopsy and JAK2V617F mutation in the differential diagnosis between the 'early' prepolycythemic phase of polycythemia vera and essential thrombocytopenia. Am J Clin Pathol 2008, **130**: 336–342.

243 Klein H. Morphology of the hematopoietic tissues. In Klein H (ed.): Polycythemia, theory and management. Springfield, Ill., 1973, Charles Thomas, pp. 201–208.

244 Kralovics R, Passamonti F, Buser AS, Teo SS, Tiedt R, Passweg JR, Tichelli A, Cazzola M, Skoda RC. A gain-of-function mutation of JAK2 in myeloproliferative disorders. N Engl J Med 2005, **352**: 1779–1790.

245 Kvasnicka HM, Thiele J. The impact of clinicopathological studies on staging and survival in essential thrombocythemia, chronic idiopathic myelofibrosis, and polycythemia rubra vera. Semin Thromb Hemost 2006, **32**: 362–371.

246 Kvasnicka HM, Thiele J. Bone marrow angiogenesis: methods of quantification and changes evolving in chronic myeloproliferative disorders. Histol Histopathol 2004, **19**: 1245–1260.

247 Landaw SA. Acute leukemia in polycythemia vera. Semin Hematol 1986, **23**: 156–165.

248 Lawrence JH, Winchell HS, Donald WG. Leukemia in polycythemia vera. Relationship to splenic myeloid metaplasia and therapeutic radiation dose. Ann Intern Med 1969, **70**: 763–771.

249 Lazslo J. Myeloproliferative disorders (MPD). Myelofibrosis, myelosclerosis, extramedullary hematopoiesis, undifferentiated MPD and hemorrhagic thrombocythemia. Semin Hematol 1975, **12**: 409–432.

250 Levine RL, Gilliland DG. Myeloproliferative disorders. Blood 2008, **112**: 2190–2198.

251 Levine RL, Wadleigh M, Cools J, Ebert BL, Wernig G, Huntly BJ, Boggon TJ, Wlodarska I, Clark JJ, Moore S, Adelsperger J, Koo S, Lee JC, Gabriel S, Mercher T, D'Andrea A, Fröhling S, Döhner K, Marynen P, Vandenberghe P, Mesa RA, Tefferi A, Griffin JD, Eck MJ, Sellers WR, Meyerson M, Golub TR, Lee SJ, Gilliland DG. Activating mutation in the tyrosine kinase JAK2 in polycythemia vera, essential thrombocythemia, and myeloid metaplasia with myelofibrosis. Cancer Cell 2005, **7**: 387–397.

252 Lundberg LG, Lerner R, Sundelin P, Rogers R, Folkman J, Palmblad J. Bone marrow in polycythemia vera, chronic myelocytic leukemia, and myelofibrosis has an increased vascularity. Am J Pathol 2000, **157**: 15–19.

253 Mesa RA, Verstovsek S, Cervantes F, Barosi G, Reilly JT, Dupriez B, Levine R, Le Bousse-Kerdiles MC, Wadleigh M, Campbell PJ, Silver RT, Vannucchi AM, Deeg HJ, Gisslinger H, Thomas D, Odenike O, Solberg LA, Gotlib J, Hexner E, Nimer SD, Kantarjian H, Orazi A, Vardiman JW, Thiele J, Tefferi A; International Working Group for Myelofibrosis Research and Treatment (IWG-MRT). Primary myelofibrosis (PMF), post polycythemia vera myelofibrosis (post-PV MF), post essential thrombocythemia myelofibrosis (post-ET MF), blast phase PMF (PFM-BP): consensus on terminology by the international working group for myelofibrosis research and treatment (IWG-MRT). Leuk Res 2007, **31**: 737–740.

254 Modan B, Lilienfield AM. Polycythemia vera and leukemia. The role of radiation treatment. Medicine (Baltimore) 1965, **44**: 305–344.

255 Roberts BE, Miles DW, Woods CG. Polycythaemia vera and myelosclerosis. A bone marrow study. Br J Haematol 1969, **16**: 75–85.

256 Rossi D, Cortini F, Deambrogi C, Barbieri C, Cerri M, Franceschetti S, Conconi A, Capello D, Gaidano G. Usefulness of JAK2V617F mutation in distinguishing idiopathic erythrocytosis from polycythemia vera. Leuk Res 2007, **31**: 97–101.

257 Silverstein MN. The evolution into and the treatment of late stage polycythemia vera. Semin Hematol 1976, **13**: 79–84.

258 Spivak JL. Polycythemia vera: myths, mechanisms, and management. Blood 2002, **100**: 4272–4290.

259 Spivak JL. MPDs: it's all in the family. Blood 2008, **112**: 2173–2174.

260 Tefferi A, Theile J, Orazi A, Kvasnicka HM, Barbui T, Hanson CA, Barosi G, Verstovsek S, Birgegard G, Mesa R, Reilly JT, Gisslinger H, Vannucchi AM, Cervantes F, Finazzi G, Hoffman R, Gilliland DG, Bloomfield CD, Vardiman JW. Proposals and rationale for revision of the World Health Organization diagnostic criteria for polycythemia vera, essential thrombocythemia, and primary myelofibrosis: recommendations from an ad hoc international expert panel. Blood 2007, **110**: 1092–1097.

261 Tefferi A, Lasho TL, Gilliland G. JAK2 mutations in myeloproliferative disorders. N Engl J Med 2005, **353**: 1416–1417.

262 Thiele J, Kvasnicka HM. Diagnostic impact of bone marrow histopathology in polycythemia vera (PV). Histol Histopathol 2005, **20**: 317–328.

263 Thiele J, Kvasnicka HM, Diehl V. Initial (latent) polycythemia vera with thrombocytosis mimicking essential thrombocythemia. Acta Haematol 2005, **113**: 213–219.

264 Thiele J, Kvasnicka HM, Orazi A, Tefferi A, Birgegard G. Polycythemia vera. In Swerdlow SH, Campo E, Harris NL, Jaffe ES, Pileri SA, Stein H, Thiele J, Vardiman JW (eds): WHO classification of tumours of haematopoietic and lymphoid tissues. Lyon, 2008, IARC Press, pp. 40–43

265 Vykoupil KF, Thiele J, Stangel W, Krmpotic E, Georgii A. Polycythemia vera. II. Transgression towards leukemia with special emphasis on histological differential diagnosis, cytogenetics and survival. Virchows Arch [A] 1980, **389**: 325–341.

Essential thrombocythemia

266 Buss DH, O'Connor ML, Woodruff RD, Richards F II, Brockschmidt JK. Bone marrow and peripheral blood findings in patients with extreme thrombocytosis. A report of 63 cases. Arch Pathol Lab Med 1991, **115**: 475–480.

267 Gisslinger H. Update on diagnosis and management of essential thrombocythemia. Semin Thromb Hemost 2006, **32**(4 pt 2): 430–436.

268 Kralovics R, Passamonti F, Buser AS, Teo SS, Tiedt R, Passweg JR, Tichelli A, Cazzola M, Skoda RC. A gain-of-function mutation of JAK2 in myeloproliferative disorders. N Engl J Med 2005, **352**: 1779–1790.

269 Kvasnicka HM, Thiele J. The impact of clinicopathological studies on staging and survival in essential thrombocythemia, chronic idiopathic myelofibrosis, and polycythemia rubra vera. Semin Thromb Hemost 2006, **32**: 362–371.

270 Levine RL, Gilliland DG. Myeloproliferative disorders. Blood, 2008, **112**: 2190–2198.

271 Levine RL, Wadleigh M, Cools J, Ebert BL, Wernig G, Huntly BJ, Boggon TJ, Wlodarska I, Clark JJ, Moore S, Adelsperger J, Koo S, Lee JC, Gabriel S, Mercher T, D'Andrea A, Fröhling S, Döhner K, Marynen P, Vandenberghe P, Mesa RA, Tefferi A, Griffin JD, Eck MJ, Sellers WR, Meyerson M, Golub TR, Lee SJ, Gilliland DG. Activating mutation in the tyrosine kinase JAK2 in polycythemia vera, essential thrombocythemia, and myeloid metaplasia with myelofibrosis. Cancer Cell 2005, **7**: 387–397.

272 Mesa RA, Hanson CA, Li CY, Yoon S-Y, Rajkumar SV, Schroeder G, Tefferi A. Diagnostic and prognostic value of bone marrow angiogenesis and megakaryocyte c-mpl expression in essential thrombocythemia. Blood 2002, **99**: 4131–4137.

273 Murphy S, Iland H, Rosenthal D, Laszlo J. Essential thrombocythemia. An interim report from the Polycythemia Vera Study Group. Semin Hematol 1986, **23**: 177–182.

274 Thiele J, Kvasnicka HM, Orazi A, Tefferi A, Gisslikngher H. Essential thrombocythaemia. In Swerdlow SH, Campo E, Harris NL, Jaffe ES, Pileri SA, Stein H, Thiele J, Vardiman JW (eds): WHO classification of tumours of haematopoietic and lymphoid tissues. Lyon, 2008, IARC Press, pp. 48–50.

Primary myelofibrosis

275 Akikusa B, Komatsu T, Kondo Y, Yokota T, Uchino F, Yonemitsu H. Amyloidosis complicating idiopathic myelofibrosis. Arch Pathol Lab Med 1987, **111**: 525–529.

276 Bass RD, Pullarkat V, Feinstein DI, Kaul A, Winberg CD, Brynes RK. Pathology of autoimmune myelofibrosis. A report of three cases and a review of the literature. Am J Clin Pathol 2001, **116**: 211–216.

277 Bearman RM, Pangalis GA, Rappaport H. Acute ('malignant') myelosclerosis. Cancer 1979, **43**: 279–293.

278 Beckman EN, Oehrle JS. Fibrous hematopoietic tumors arising in agnogenic myeloid metaplasia. Hum Pathol 1982, **13**: 804–810.

279 Block M, Burkhardt R, Chelloul N, Demmler K, Duhamel G, Georgii A, Kirsten WH, Lennert K, Nezelof C, Te Velde J. Myelofibrosis–osteosclerosis syndrome. Pathology and morphology. Adv Biosci 1975, **16**: 219–240.

280 Bock O, Schlue J, Lehmann U, von Wasielewski R, Langer F, Kreipe H. Megakaryocytes from chronic myeloproliferative disorders show enhanced nuclear bFGB expression. Blood 2002, **100**: 2274–2275.

281 Burston J, Pinniger JL. The reticulin content of bone marrow in haematological disorders. Br J Haematol 1963, **9**: 172–184.

282 Georgii A, Buesche G, Kreft A. The histopathology of chronic myeloproliferative diseases. Bailliere's Clin Hematol 1998, **11**: 721–749.

283 Lubin J, Rozen S, Rwylin AM. Malignant myelosclerosis. Arch Intern Med 1976, **136**: 141–145.

284 Kralovics R, Passamonti F, Buser AS, Teo SS, Tiedt R, Passweg JR, Tichelli A, Cazzola M, Skoda RC. A gain-of-function mutation of JAK2 in myeloproliferative disorders. N Engl J Med 2005, **352**: 1779–1790.

285 Kvasnicka HM, Thiele J. Bone marrow angiogenesis: methods of quantification and changes evolving in chronic myeloproliferative disorders. Histol Histopathol 2004, **18**: 1245–1260.

286 Lebwaze BM, Le Tourneau A, Rio B, Perrot JY, Heuberger L, Kabongo JM, Kalengayi RM, Molina T, Diebold J, Audouin J. Histopathologic pattern of hyperplasia of bone marrow hematogones (medullar B lymphoid cell precursors) occurring after treatment of idiopathic myelofibrosis. Ann Pathol 2008, **28**: 27–31.

287 Levine RL, Gilliland DG. Myeloproliferative disorders. Blood 2008, **112**: 2190–2198.

288 Levine RL, Wadleigh M, Cools J, Ebert BL, Wernig G, Huntly BJ, Boggon TJ, Wlodarska I, Clark JJ, Moore S, Adelsperger J, Koo S, Lee JC, Gabriel S, Mercher T, D'Andrea A, Fröhling S, Döhner K, Marynen P, Vandenberghe P, Mesa RA, Tefferi A, Griffin JD, Eck MJ, Sellers WR, Meyerson M, Golub TR, Lee SJ, Gilliland DG. Activating mutation in the tyrosine kinase JAK2 in polycythemia vera, essential thrombocythemia, and myeloid metaplasia with myelofibrosis. Cancer Cell 2005, **7**: 387–397.

289 Lundberg LG, Lerner R, Sundelin P, Rogers R, Folkman J, Palmblad J. Bone marrow in polycythemia vera, chronic myelocytic leukemia, and myelofibrosis has an increased vascularity. Am J Pathol 2000, **157**: 15–19.

290 Mesa RA, Verstovsek S, Cervantes F, Barosi G, Reilly JT, Dupriez B, Levine R, Le Bousse-Kerdiles MC, Wadleigh M, Campbell PJ, Silver RT, Vannucchi AM, Deeg HJ, Gisslinger H, Thomas D, Odenike O, Solberg LA, Gotlib J, Hexner E, Nimer SD, Kantarjian H, Orazi A, Vardiman JW, Thiele J, Tefferi A; International Working Group for Myelofibrosis Research and Treatment (IWG-MRT). Primary myelofibrosis (PMF), post polycythemia vera myelofibrosis (post-PV MF), post essential thrombocythemia myelofibrosis (post-ET MF), blast phase PMF (PFM-BP): consensus on terminology by the international working group for myelofibrosis research and treatment (IWG-MRT). Leuk Res 2007, **31**: 737–740.

291 Mesa RA, Hanson CA, Rajkuman V, Schroeder G, Tefferi A. Evaluation and clinical correlations of bone marrow angiogenesis in myelofibrosis with myeloid metaplasia. Blood 2000, **96**: 3374–3380.

292 Ponzoni M, Shendrik U, Ferreri AJM, Pruneri G, Saruida P, Bertolini F, Urazi A. Endoglin (CD105)-positive vessels are increased in chronic idiopathic myelofibrosis. J Clin Pathol 2002, **55**(Suppl 1): A7.

293 Reilly JT. Cytogenetic and molecular genetic abnormalities in agnogenic myeloid metaplasia. Semin Oncol 2005, **32**: 359–364.

294 Rondeau E, Solal-Celigny P, Dhermy D, Vroclans M, Brousse N, Bernard JF, Boivin P. Immune disorders in agnogenic myeloid metaplasia. Relations to myelofibrosis. Br J Haematol 1983, **53**: 467–475.

295 Tefferi A. Myelofibrosis with myeloid metaplasia. N Engl J Med 2000, **342**: 1255–1265.

296 Thiele J, Kvasnicka HM. Diagnostic differentiation of essential thrombocythaemia from thrombocythaemias associated with chronic idiopathic myelofibrosis by discriminate analysis of bone marrow features – a clinicopathological study on 272 patients. Histol Histopathol 2003, **18**: 93–102.

297 Thiele J, Kvasnicka HM. Prefibrotic chronic idiopathic myelofibrosis – a diagnostic enigma? Acta Haematol 2004, **111**: 155–159.

298 Thiele J, Kvasnicka HM. Hematopathologic findings in chronic idiopathic myelofibrosis. Semin Oncol 2005, **32**: 380–394.

299 Thiele J, Kvasnicka HM, Facchetti F, Franco V, van der Walt J, Orazi A. European consensus on grading bone marrow fibrosis and assessment of cellularity. Haematologica 2005, **90**: 1128–1132.

300 Thiele J, Kvasnicka HM, Tefferi A, Barosi G, Orazi A, Vardiman JW. Primary myelofibrosis. In Swerdlow SH, Campo E, Harris NL, Jaffee ES, Pileri SA, Stein H, Thiele J, Vardiman JW (eds): WHO classification of tumours of haematopoietic and lymphoid tissues. Lyon, 2008, IARC Press, pp. 44–47.

301 Thiele J, Zankovich R, Steinberg T, Fischer R, Diehl V. Agnogenic myeloid metaplasia (AMM). Correlation of bone marrow lesions with laboratory data. A longitudinal clinicopathological study on 114 patients. Hematol Oncol 1989, **7**: 327–343.

302 Tobin MS, Tan C, Argano SAP. Myelofibrosis in pediatric age group. N Y State J Med 1969, **69**: 1080–1083.

303 Varki A, Lottenberg R, Griffith R, Reinhard E. The syndrome of idiopathic myelofibrosis. A clinicopathologic review with emphasis on the prognostic variables predicting survival. Medicine (Baltimore) 1983, **62**: 353–371.

304 Ward HP, Block MH. The natural history of agnogenic myeloid metaplasia (AMM) and a critical evaluation of its relationship with the myeloproliferative syndrome. Medicine (Baltimore) 1971, **50**: 357–420.

305 Weinstein IM. Idiopathic myelofibrosis. Historical review, diagnosis, and management. Blood Rev 1991, **5**: 98–104.

306 Wolf BC, Neiman RS. Myelofibrosis with myeloid metaplasia: pathophysiologic implications of the correlation between bone marrow changes and progression of splenomegaly. Blood 1985, **65**: 803–809.

Hematopoietic neoplasms associated with eosinophilia and abnormalities of *PDGFRA*, *PDGFRB* or *FGFR1*

307 Bain BJ, Gilliland DG, Horny HP, Vardiman JW. Myeloid and lymphoid neoplasms with eosinophilia and abnormalities of PDGFRA, PDGFRB or FGFR1. In Swerdlow SH, Campo E, Harris NL, Jaffee ES, Pileri SA, Stein H, Thiele J, Vardiman JW (eds): WHO classification of tumours of haematopoietic and lymphoid tissues. Lyon, 2008, IARC Press, pp. 68–73.

308 Cools J, DeAngelo DJ, Gotlib J, Stover EH, Legare RD, Cortes J, Kutok J, Clark J, Galinsky I, Griffin JD, Cross NC, Tefferi A, Malone J, Alam R, Schrier SL, Schmid J, Rose M, Vandenberghe P, Verhoef G, Boogaerts M, Wlodarska I, Kantarjian H, Marynen P, Coutre SE, Stone R, Gilliland DG. A tyrosine kinase created by fusion of the PDGFRA and FIP1L1 genes as a therapeutic target of imatinib in idiopathic hypereosinophilic syndrome. N Engl J Med 2003, **348**: 1201–1214.

309 Curtis CE, Grand FH, Waghorn K, Sahoo TP, Goergoe J, Cross NCP. A novel ETV6-PDGFRB fusion transcript missed by standard screening in a patient with an imatinib responsive

chronic myeloproliferative disease. Leukemia 2007, **21**: 1839–1841.

310 Fink SR, Belongie KJ, Paternoster SF, Smoley SA, Pardanani AD, Tefferi A, Van Dyke DL, Ketterling RP. Validation of a new three-color fluorescence in situ hybridization (FISH) method to detect CHIC2 deletion, FIP1L1/PDGFRA fusion and PDGFRA translocations. Leuk Res 2009, **33**: 843–846.

311 Gotlib J, Cools J. Five years since the discovery of FIP1L1–PDGFRA: what we have learned about the fusion and other molecularly defined eosinophilias? Leukemia 2008, **22**: 1999–2010.

312 Kilon AD, Noel P, Akin C, Law MA, Gilliland DG, Cools J, Metcalfe DD, Nutman TB. Elevated serum tryptase levels identify a subset of patients with a myeloproliferative variant of idiopathic hypereosinophilic syndrome associated with tissue fibrosis, poor prognosis and imatinib responsiveness. Blood 2003, **102**: 4060–4066.

313 Kilon AD, Akin C, Nutman TB. Hypereosinophilic syndrome with elevated serum tryptase is a syndrome that differs from systemic mast cell disease with eosinophilia. Blood 2003, **102**: 3074.

314 Maric I, Robyn J, Metcalfe DD, Fay MP, Carter M, Wilson T, Fu W, Stoddard J, Scott L, Hartsell M, Kirshenbaum A, Akin C, Nutman TB, Noel P, Klion AD. KIT D816V-associated systemic mastocytosis with eosinophilia and FIP1L1/PDGFRA-associated chronic eosinophilic leukemia are distinct entities. J Allergy Clin Immunol 2007, **120**: 680–687.

315 Pardanani A, Ketterling RP, Li CY, Patnaik MM, Wolanskyj AP, Elliott MA, Camoriano JK, Butterfield JH, Dewald GW, Tefferi A. FIP1L1–PDGFRA in eosinophilic disorders: prevalence in routine clinical practice, long-term experience with imatinib therapy, and a critical review of the literature. Leuk Res 2006, **30**: 965–970.

316 Pardanini AD, Ketterling RP, Brockman SR, Flynn HC, Paternoster SF, Shearer BM, Reeder TL, Li CY, Cross NC, Cools J, Gilliland DG, Dewald GW, Tefferi A. CHIC2 deletion, a surrogate for FIP1L1-PDGFRA fusion, occurs in systemic mastocytosis associated with eosinophilia and predicts response to imatinib mesylate therapy. Blood 2003, **102**: 3093–3096.

317 Tefferi A, Pardanani A, Li C-Y. Hypereosinophilic syndrome with elevated serum tryptase versus systemic mast cell disease associated with eosinophilia: two distinct entities? Blood 2003, **102**: 3073.

SYSTEMIC MASTOCYTOSIS

318 Brunning RD, McKenna RW, Rosai J, Parkin JL, Risdall R. Systemic mastocytosis. Am J Surg Pathol 1983, **7**: 425–438.

319 Czarnetzki BM, Kolde G, Schoemann A, Urbanitz S, Urbanitz D. Bone marrow findings in adult patients with urticaria pigmentosa. J Am Acad Dermatol 1980, **18**: 45–51.

320 Horny H-P, Metcalf DD, Bennett JM, Bain BJ, Akin C, Escribano L, Valent P. Systemic mastocytosis. In Swerdlow SH, Campo E, Harris NL, Jaffee ES, Pileri SA, Stein H, Thiele J, Vardiman JW (eds): WHO classification of tumours of the haematopoietic and lymphoid tissues. Lyon, 2008, IARC Press, pp. 54–63.

321 Horny HP, Parwaresch MR, Lennert K. Bone marrow findings in systemic mastocytosis. Hum Pathol 1985, **16**: 808–814.

322 Horny HP, Reimann O, Kaiserling E. Immunoreactivity of normal and neoplastic tissue mast cells. Am J Clin Pathol 1988, **89**: 335–340.

323 Horny HP, Ruck M, Wehrmann M, Kaiserling E. Blood findings in generalized mastocytosis. Evidence of frequent simultaneous occurrence of myeloproliferative disorders. Br J Haematol 1990, **76**: 186–193.

324 Lawrence JB, Friedman BS, Travis WD, Chinchilli VM, Metcalfe DD, Gralnick HR. Hematologic manifestations of systemic mast cell disease. A prospective study of laboratory and morphologic features and their relation to prognosis. Am J Med 1991, **91**: 612–624.

325 Natkunam Y, Rouse RV. Utility of paraffin section immunohistochemistry for c-kit (CD117) in the differential diagnosis of systemic mast cell disease involving the bone marrow. Am J Surg Pathol 2000, **24**: 81–99.

326 Rappaport H. Tumors of the hematopoietic system. In Atlas of tumor pathology, series 3, fascicle 8. Washington DC, 2001, Armed Forces Institute of Pathology, pp. 336–344.

327 Rywlin AM. Mastocytic eosinophilic fibrohistiocytic lesion of the bone marrow. Hematology 1982, **24**: 330.

328 Scully RE, Mark EJ, McNeely BU. Case records of the Massachusetts General Hospital. N Engl J Med 1986, **315**: 816.

329 Stevens EC, Rosenthal NS. Bone marrow mast cell morphologic features and hematopoietic dyspoiesis in systemic mast cell disease. Am J Clin Pathol 2001, **116**: 177–182.

330 Tefferi A, Li C-Y, Butterfield JH, Hoagland HC. Treatment of systemic mast cell disease with cladribine. N Engl J Med 2001, **344**: 307–308.

331 Travis W, Li C-Y, Bergstralh EJ, Yam LT, Swee RG. Systemic mast cell disease. Analysis of 58 cases and literature review. Medicine (Baltimore) 1988, **67**: 345–368.

332 Valent P, Akin C, Sperr WR, Horny HP, Arock M, Lechner K, Bennett JM, Metcalfe DD. Diagnosis and treatment of systemic mastocytosis: state of the art. Br J Haematol 2003, **122**: 695–717.

333 Valent P, Horny HO, Escribano L, Longley BJ, Li CY, Schwartz LB, Marone G, Nuñez R, Akin C, Sotlar K, Sperr WR, Wolff K, Brunning RD, Parwaresch RM, Austen KF, Lennert K, Metcalfe DD, Vardiman JW, Bennett JM. Diagnostic criteria and classification of mastocytosis: a consensus proposal. Leuk Res 2001, **25**: 603–625.

334 Walls AF, Jones DB, Williams JH, Church MK, Holgate ST. Immunohistochemical identification of mast cells in formalin-fixed tissue using monoclonal antibodies specific for tryptase. J Clin Pathol 1990, **162**: 119–126.

335 Webb TA, Li C-Y, Yam LT. Systemic mast cell disease. A clinical and hematopathologic study of 26 cases. Cancer 1982, **49**: 927–938.

336 Wilkins BS, Buchan SL, Webster J, Jones DB. Tryptase-positive mast cells accompany lymphocytic as well as lymphoplasmacytic lymphoma infiltrates in bone marrow biopsies. Histopathology 2001, **39**: 150–155.

337 Yang F, Tran TA, Carlson JA, Hsi ED, Ross CW, Arber DA. Paraffin section immunophenotype of cutaneous and extracutaneous mast cell disease. Comparison to other hematopoietic neoplasms. Am J Surg Pathol 2000, **24**: 703–709.

MATURE B-CELL NEOPLASMS

CHRONIC LYMPHOCYTIC LEUKEMIA

338 Bennett JM, Catovsky D, Daniel M-T, Flandrin G, Galton DAG, Gralnick JR, Sultan C. Proposals for the classification of chronic (mature) B and T lymphoid leukaemias. J Clin Pathol 1989, **42**: 567–584.

339 Binet L, Catovsky D, Chandra P, Dighiero G, Montserrat E, Rai KR, Sawitsky A. Chronic lymphocytic leukaemia. Proposals for a revised prognostic staging system. Br J Haematol 1981, **48**: 365–367.

340 Brouet JC, Fermand JP, Laurent G, Grange MJ, Chevalier A, Jacquillat C, Seligmann M. The association of chronic lymphocytic leukaemia and multiple myeloma. A study of eleven patients. Br J Haematol 1985, **59**: 55–66.

341 Brouet JC, Flandrin G, Sasportes M, Preud'Homme JL, Seligmann M. Chronic lymphocytic leukemia of T-cell origin. Lancet 1975, **2**: 890–893.

342 Crespo M, Bosch F, Villamor N, Bellosillo B, Colomer D, Rozman M, Marcé S, López-Guillermo A, Campo E, Montserrat E. ZAP-70 expression as a surrogate for immunoglobulin-variable-region mutations in chronic lymphocytic leukemia. N Engl J Med 2003, **348**: 1764–1775.

343 Damle RN, Wasil T, Fais F, Ghiotto F, Valetto A, Allen SL, Buchbinder A, Budman D, Dittmar K, Kolitz J, Lichtman SM, Schulman P, Vinciguerra VP, Rai KR, Ferrarini M, Chiorazzi N. Ig V mutation status and CD38 expression as novel prognostic indicators in chronic lymphocytic leukemia. Blood 1999, **94**: 1840–1847.

344 Döhner H, Stilgenbauer S, Benner A, Leupolt E, Kröber A, Bullinger L, Döhner K, Bentz M, Lichter P. Genomic aberrations and survival in chronic lymphocytic leukemia. N Engl J Med 2000, **343**: 1910–1916.

345 Enno A, Catovsky D, O'Brien M, Cherchi M, Kumaran TO, Galton DA. 'Prolymphocytoid' transformation of chronic lymphocytic leukaemia. Br J Haematol 1979, **41**: 9–18.

346 Hallek M, Cheson BD, Catovsky D, Caligaris-Cappio F, Dighiero G, Döhner H, Hillmen P, Keating MJ, Montserrat E, Rai KR, Kipps TJ; International Workshop on Chronic Lymphocytic Leukemia. Guidelines for the diagnosis and treatment of chronic lymphocytic leukemia: a report from the International Workshop on Chronic Lymphocytic Leukemia (IWCLL) updating the National Cancer Institute-Working Group (NCI-WG) 1996 guidelines. Blood 2008, **111**: 5446–5456.

347 Lens D, Dyer MJ, Garcia-Marco JM, De Schouwer PJ, Hamoudi RA, Jones D, Farahat N, Matutes E, Catovsky D. p53 abnormalities in CLL are associated with excess of prolymphocytes and poor prognosis. Br J Haematol 1997, **99**: 848–857.

348 Litz CE, Brunning RD. Chronic lymphoproliferative disorders. Classification and prognosis. Bailliere's Clin Haematol 1993, **6**: 767–783.

349 Montserrat E, Marques-Pereira JP, Gallart T, Rosman C. Bone marrow histopathologic patterns and immunologic findings in B chronic lymphocytic leukemia. Cancer 1984, **54**: 447–451.

350 Montserrat E, Rozman CR. Chronic lymphocytic leukemia. Prognostic factors and natural history. Bailliere's Clin Haematol 1993, **6**: 849–866.

351 Müller-Hermelink HK, Montserrat E, Catovsky D, Harris NL. Chronic lymphocytic leukaemia/small lymphocytic lymphoma. In Swerdlow SH, Campo E, Harris NL, Jaffee ES, Pileri SA, Stein H, Thiele J, Vardiman JW (eds): WHO classification of tumours of haematopoietic and lymphoid tissues. Lyon, 2008, IARC Press, pp. 180–182.

352 Pangalis GA, Roussou PA, Kittas C, Kokkinou S, Fessas P. B-chronic lymphocytic leukemia. Prognostic implication of bone marrow histology in 120 patients experience from a single hematology unit. Cancer 1987, **59**: 767–771.

353 Pangalis GA, Roussou PA, Kittas C, Mitsoulis-Mentzikoff C, Matsouka-Alexandridis P, Anagnostopoulos N, Rombos I, Fessas P. Patterns of bone marrow involvement in chronic lymphocytic leukemia and small lymphocytic (well-differentiated) non-Hodgkin's lymphoma. Its clinical significance in relation to their differential diagnosis and prognosis. Cancer 1984, **54**: 702–708.

354 Rai KR, Sawitsky A, Cronkite EP, Chanana AD, Levy RN, Pasternack BS. Clinical staging of chronic lymphocytic leukemia. Blood 1975, **46**: 219–234.

355 Rassenti LZ, Huynh L, Toy TL, Chen L, Keating MJ, Gribben JG, Neuberg DS, Flinn IW, Rai KR, Byrd JC, Kay NE, Greaves A, Weiss A, Kipps TJ. ZAP-70 compared with immunoglobulin heavy-chain gene mutation status as a predictor of disease progression in chronic lymphocytic leukemia. N Engl J Med 2004, **351**: 893–901.

356 Rausig A. Lymphocytic leukemia and malignant lymphoma in the adult. Acta Med Scand 1976, **595**(Suppl): 1–270.

357 Rozman C, Hernandez-Nieto L, Montserrat E, Brugues R. Prognostic significance of bone marrow patterns in chronic lymphocytic leukaemia. Br J Haematol 1981, **47**: 529–537.

RICHTER SYNDROME

358 Brecher M, Banks P. Hodgkin's disease variant of Richter's syndrome. Am J Clin Pathol 1990, **93**: 333–339.

359 Brousse N, Solal-Celigny P, Herrera A, Breil P, Molas G, Flejou JF, Boivin P, Potet F. Gastrointestinal Richter's syndrome. Hum Pathol 1985, **16**: 854–857.

360 Case record of the Massachusetts General Hospital (Case 6–1978). N Engl J Med 1978, **298**: 387–396.

361 Foucar K, Rydell RE. Richter's syndrome in chronic lymphocytic leukemia. Cancer 1980, **46**: 118–134.

362 Goldstein J, Baden J. Richter's syndrome. South Med J 1977, **70**: 1381–1382.

363 Kroft SH. Lymphoma transformation. Genetic relatedness, stealth lymphomas, and the final frontier. Am J Clin Pathol 2001, **116**: 811–814.

364 Litz CE, Arthur DC, Gajl-Peczalska KJ, Rausch D, Copenhaver C, Coad JE, Brunning RD. Transformation of chronic lymphocytic leukemia to small non-cleaved cell lymphoma. A cytogenetic, immunological, and molecular study. Leukemia 1991, **5**: 972–978.

365 Long JC, Aisenberg AC. Richter's syndrome. A terminal complication of chronic lymphocytic leukemia with distinct clinicopathologic features. Am J Clin Pathol 1975, **63**: 786–795.

366 Mao Z, Quintanilla-Martinez L, Raffeld M, Richter M, Krugmann J, Burek C, Hartmann E, Rudiger T, Jaffe ES, Müller-Hermelink HK, Ott G, Fend F, Rosenwald A. IgVH mutational status and clonality analysis of Richter's transformation: diffuse large B-cell lymphoma and Hodgkin lymphoma in association with B-cell chronic lymphocytic leukemia (B-CLL) represent 2 different pathways of disease evolution. Am J Surg Pathol 2007, **31**: 1605–1614.

367 Momose H, Jaffe ES, Shin SS, Chen YY, Weiss LM. Chronic lymphocytic leukemia/small lymphocytic lymphoma with Reed–Sternberg-like cells and possible transformation to Hodgkin's disease. Mediation by Epstein–Barr virus. Am J Surg Pathol 1992, **16**: 859–867.

368 Richter MN. Generalized reticular cell sarcoma of lymph nodes associated with lymphatic leukemia. Am J Pathol 1928, **4**: 285–292.

369 Seligmann M, Preud'Homme JL, Brouet JC. Membrane markers in human lymphoid malignancies. Clinicopathologic correlations and insights into the differentiation of normal and neoplastic cells. In Clarkson B, Marks P, Till JR (eds): Differentiation of normal and neoplastic cells. Cold Spring Harbor, NY, 1978, Cold Spring Harbor Laboratory, pp. 859–876.

370 Traweek ST, Liu J, Johnson RM, Winberg CD, Rappaport H. High-grade transformation of chronic lymphocytic leukemia and low-grade non-Hodgkin's lymphoma. Genotypic confirmation of clonal identity. Am J Clin Pathol 1993, **100**: 519–526.

371 Trump DL, Mann RB, Phelps R, Roberts H, Conley CL. Richter's syndrome: diffuse histiocytic lymphoma in patients with chronic lymphocytic leukemia. Am J Med 1980, **68**: 539–548.

PROLYMPHOCYTIC LEUKEMIA

372 Bearman RM, Pangalis GA, Rappaport H. Prolymphocytic leukemia: clinical, histological, and cytochemical observations. Cancer 1978, **42**: 2360–2372.

373 Brito-Babapulle V, Catovsky D. Inversions and tandem translocations involving chromosome 14q11 and 14q32 in T-prolymphocytic leukemia and T-cell leukemias in patients with ataxia telangiectasia. Cancer Genet Cytogenet 1991, **55**: 1–9.

374 Campo E, Catovsky D, Montserrat E, Müller-Hermelink HK, Harris NL, Stein H. B-cell prolymphocytic leukaemia. In Swerdlow SH, Campo E, Harris NL, Jaffee ES, Pileri SA, Stein H, Thiele J, Vardiman JW (eds): WHO classification of tumours of haematopoietic and lymphoid tissues. Lyon, 2008, IARC Press, pp. 183–184.

375 Catovsky D, Müller-Hermelink HK, Ralfkiaer E. T-cell prolymphocytic leukaemia. In Swerdlow SH, Campo E, Harris NL, Jaffee ES, Pileri SA, Stein H, Thiele J, Vardiman JW (eds): WHO classification of tumours of haematopoietic and lymphoid tissues. Lyon, 2008, IARC Press, pp. 270–271.

376 Galton DA, Goldman JM, Wiltshaw E, Catovsky D, Henry K, Goldenberg GJ. Prolymphocytic leukaemia. Br J Haematol 1974, **27**: 7–23.

377 Matutes E, Brito-Babapulle V, Swansbury J, Ellis J, Morilla R, Dearden C, Sempere A, Catovsky D. Clinical and laboratory features of 78 cases of T-prolymphocytic leukemia. Blood 1991, **78**: 3269–3274.

378 Melo JV, Catovsky D, Galton DAG. The relationship between chronic lymphocytic leukaemia and prolymphocytic leukaemia. I. Clinical and laboratory features of 300 patients and characterization of an intermediate group. Br J Haematol 1986, **63**: 377–387.

379 Melo JV, Catovsky D, Galton DAG. The relationship between chronic lymphocytic leukaemia and prolymphocytic leukaemia. II. Patterns of evolution of 'prolymphocytoid' transformation. Br J Haematol 1986, **64**: 77–86.

380 Onciu M, Schlette E, Bueso-Ramos C, Medeiros LJ. Leukemic mantle cell lymphoma with cells resembling prolymphocytes. Am J Clin Pathol 2002, **118**: 305–306.

381 Owens MR, Strauchen JA, Rowe JM, Bennett JM. Prolymphocytic leukemia: histologic features in atypical cases. Hematol Oncol 1984, **2**: 249–257.

382 Wong K-F, Chan JKC, So JCC, Yu PH. Mantle cell lymphoma in leukemic phase. Characterization of its broad cytologic spectrum with emphasis on the importance of distinction from other chronic lymphoproliferative disorders. Cancer 1999, **86**: 850–857.

HAIRY CELL LEUKEMIA, HAIRY CELL LEUKEMIA VARIANT

383 Bartl R, Frisch B, Hill W, Burkhardt R, Sommerfeld W, Sund M. Bone marrow histology in hairy cell leukemia. Identification of subtypes and their prognostic significance. Am J Clin Pathol 1983, **79**: 531–545.

384 Bennett JM, Catovsky D, Daniel MT, Flandrin G, Galton DA, Gralnick HR, Sultan C. Proposals for the classification of chronic (mature) B and T lymphoid leukemias. J Clin Pathol 1989, **42**: 567–584.

385 Burke JS. The value of the bone marrow biopsy in the diagnosis of hairy cell leukemia. Am J Clin Pathol 1978, **70**: 876–884.

386 Burke JS, Byrne GE Jr, Rappaport H. Hairy cell leukemia (leukemic reticuloendotheliosis). I. A clinical pathologic study of 21 patients. Cancer 1974, **33**: 1399–1410.

387 Catovsky D, O'Brien M, Melo JV, Wardle J, Brozovic M. Hairy cell leukemia (HCL) variant. An intermediate disease between HCL and B prolymphocytic leukemia. Semin Oncol 1984, **11**: 362–369.

388 Chen YH, Tallman MS, Goolsby C, Peterson L. Immunophenotypic variations in hairy cell leukemia. Am J Clin Pathol 2006, **125**: 251–259.

389 Demanes DJ, Lane N, Beckstead JH. Bone involvement in hairy cell leukemia. Cancer 1982, **49**: 1697–1701.

390 Falini B, Tiacci E, Liso A, Basso K, Sabattini E, Pacini R, Foa R, Pulsoni A, Dalla Favera R, Pileri S. Simple diagnostic assay for hairy cell leukaemia by immunocytochemical detection of annexin A1 (ANXA1). Lancet 2004, **363**: 1869–1870.

391 Foucar K, Falini B, Catovsky D, Stein H. Hairy cell leukaemia. In Swerdlow SH, Campo E, Harris NL, Jaffee ES, Pileri SA, Stein H, Thiele J, Vardiman JW (eds): WHO classification of tumours of haematopoietic and lymphoid tissues. Lyon, 2008, IARC Press, pp. 188–190.

392 Golomb HM, Catovsky D, Golde DW. Hairy cell leukemia: a clinical review based on 71 cases. Ann Intern Med 1978, **89**: 677–683.

393 Hakimian D, Tallman MS, Kiley C, Peterson L. Detection of minimal residual disease by immunostaining of bone marrow biopsies after 2-chlorodeoxyadenosine for hairy cell leukemia. Blood 1993, **82**: 1798–1802.

394 Hanson CA, Ward PC, Schnitzer B. A multilobular variant of hairy cell leukemia with morphologic similarities to T-cell lymphoma. Am J Surg Pathol 1989, **13**: 671–679.

395 Herold CJ, Wittlich GR, Schwarzinger I, Haller J, Chott A, Mostbeck G, Hajek PC. Skeletal involvement in hairy cell leukemia. Skeletal Radiol 1988, **17**: 171–175.

396 Hoyer JD, Li CY, Yam LT, Hanson CA, Kurtin PJ. Immunohistochemical demonstration of acid phosphatase isoenzyme 5(tartrate-resistant) in paraffin sections of hairy cell leukemia and other hematologic disorders. Am J Clin Pathol 1997, **108**: 308–315.

397 Johrens K, Stein H, Anagnostopoulos I. T-bet transcription factor detection facilitates the diagnosis of minimal hairy cell leukemia infiltrates in bone marrow trephines. Am J Surg Pathol 2007, **31**: 1181–1185.

398 Katayama I, Schneider GB. Further ultrastructural characterization of hairy cells of leukemic reticuloendotheliosis. Am J Pathol 1977, **86**: 163–182.

399 Lal A, Tallman MS, Soble MB, Golubovich I, Peterson L. Hairy cell leukemia presenting as localized skeletal involvement. Leuk Lymphoma 2003, **43**: 2207–2211.

400 Lee WMF, Beckstead JH. Hairy cell leukemia with bone marrow hypoplasia. Cancer 1982, **50**: 2207–2210.

401 Lembersky BC, Ratain MJ, Golomb H. Skeletal complications in hairy cell leukemia: diagnosis and therapy. J Clin Oncol 1988, **6**: 1280–1284.

402 Matutes E, Wotherspoon A, Brito-Babapulle V, Catovsky D. The natural history and clinico-pathological features of the variant form of hairy cell leukemia. Leukemia 2001, **15**: 184–186.

403 Mercieca J, Matutes E, Moskovic E, MacLennan K, Matthey F, Costello C, Behrens J, Basu S, Roath S, Fairhead S, et al. Massive abdominal lymphadenopathy in hairy cell leukaemia: a report of 12 cases. Br J Haematol 1992, **82**: 547–554.

404 Naeim F, Jacobs AD. Bone marrow changes in patients with hairy cell leukemia treated by recombinant alpha 2-interferon. Hum Pathol 1985, **16**: 1200–1205.

405 Paoletti M, Bitter MA, Vardiman JW. Hairy cell leukemia. Morphologic, cytochemical, and immunologic features. Clin Lab Med 1988, **8**: 179–195.

406 Piris M, Foucar K, Mollejo M, Campo E, Falini B. Splenic B-cell lymphoma/leukaemia, unclassifiable. In Swerdlow SH, Campo E, Harris NL, Jaffe ES, Pileri SA, Stein H, Thiele J, Vardiman JW (eds): WHO classification of tumours of haematopoietic and lymphoid tissues. Lyon, 2008, IARC Press, pp. 191–193.

407 Piro LD, Carrera CJ, Carson DA, Beutler E. Lasting remissions in hairy cell leukemia induced by a single infusion of 2-chlorodeoxyadenosine. N Engl J Med 1990, **322**: 1117–1121.

408 Pittaluga S, Tierans A, Dodoo YL, Delabie J, De Wolf-Peeters C. How reliable is histologic examination of bone marrow trephine biopsy specimens for the staging of non-Hodgkin lymphoma? A study of hairy cell leukemia and mantle cell lymphoma involvement of the bone marrow trephine specimen by histologic, immunohistochemical, and polymerase chain reaction techniques. Am J Clin Pathol 1999, **111**: 179–184.

409 Platanias LC, Golomb H. Hairy cell leukaemia. Bailliere's Clin Haematol 1993, **6**: 887–898.

410 Robak T. Current treatment options in hairy cell leukemia and hairy cell leukemia variant. Cancer Treat Rev 2006, **32**: 365–376.

411 Robbins BA, Ellison DJ, Spinosa JC, Carey CA, Lukes RJ, Poppema S, Saven A, Piro LD. Diagnostic application of two-color flow cytometry in 161 cases of hairy cell leukemia. Blood 1993, **82**: 1277–1287.

412 Sigal DS, Sharpe R, Burian C, Saven A. Very long-term eradication of minimal residual disease in patients with hairy cell leukemia after a single course of cladribine. Blood 2010, **115**: 1893–1896.

413 Spiers AD, Moore D, Cassileth PA, Harrington DP, Cummings FJ, Neiman RS, Bennett JM, O'Connell MJ. Remissions in hairy cell leukemia with pentostatin (2' deoxycoformycin). N Engl J Med 1987, **316**: 825–830.

414 Vykoupil KF, Thiele J, Georgii A. Hairy cell leukemia. Bone marrow findings in 24 patients. Virchows Arch [A] 1976, **370**: 273–289.

SPLENIC MARGINAL ZONE LYMPHOMA

415 Arber DA, George TI. Bone marrow biopsy involvement by non-Hodgkin's lymphoma: frequency of lymphoma types, patterns, blood involvement, and discordance with other sites in 450 specimens. Am J Surg Pathol 2005, **29**: 1549–1557.

416 Audouin J, Le Tourneau A, Molina T, Camilleri-Broët S, Adida C, Comperat E, Benattar L, Delmer A, Devidas A, Rio B, Diebold J. Patterns of bone marrow involvement in 58 patients presenting primary splenic marginal zone lymphoma with or without circulating villous lymphocytes. Br J Haematol 2003, **122**: 404–412.

417 Camacho FI, Mollejo M, Mateo MS, Algara P, Navas C, Hernández JM, Santoja C, Solé F, Sánchez-Beato M, Piris MA. Progression to large B-cell lymphoma in splenic marginal zone lymphoma – a description of a series of 12 cases. Am J Surg Pathol 2001, **25**: 1268–1276.

418 Catovsky D, Matutes E. Splenic lymphoma with villous lymphocytes/splenic marginal zone lymphoma. Semin Hematol 1999, **36**: 148–154.

419 Franco V, Florena AM, Campesi G. Intrasinusoidal bone marrow infiltration: a possible hallmark of splenic lymphoma. Histopathology 1996, **29**: 571–575.

420 Franco V, Florena A-M, Stella M, Rizzo A, Iannitto E, Quintini G, Campesi G. Splenectomy influences bone marrow infiltration in patients with splenic marginal zone cell lymphoma with or without villous lymphocytes. Cancer 2000, **91**: 294–301.

421 Hermine O, Lefrère F, Bronowicki JP, Mariette X, Jondeau K, Eclache-Saudreau V, Delmas B, Valensi F, Cacoub P, Brechot C, Varet B, Troussard X. Regression of splenic lymphoma with villous lymphocytes after treatment of hepatitis C infection. N Engl J Med 2002, **347**: 89–94.

422 Isaacson PG, Matutes E, Burke M, Catovsky D. The histopathology of splenic lymphoma with villous lymphocytes. Blood 1994, **84**: 3828–3834.

423 Isaacson PG, Piris MA, Berger F, Swerdlow SH, Thieblemont C, Pittaluga S, Harris NL. Splenic B-cell marginal zone lymphoma. In Swerdlow SH, Campo E, Harris NL, Jaffe ES, Pileri SA, Stein H, Thiele J, Vardiman JW (eds): WHO classification of tumours of haematopoietic and lymphoid tissues. Lyon, 2008, IARC Press, pp. 185–187.

424 Kent SA, Variakojis D, Peterson LC. Comparative study of marginal zone lymphoma involving bone marrow. Am J Clin Pathol 2002, **117**: 698–708.

425 Matutes E, Morilla R, Owusu-Ankomah K, Houlihan A, Catovsky D. The immunophenotype of splenic lymphoma with villous lymphocytes and its relevance to the differential diagnosis with other B-cell disorders. Blood 1993, **83**: 1558–1562.

426 Melo JV, Hegde U, Parreira A, Thompson I, Lampert IA, Catovsky D. Splenic B cell lymphoma with circulating villous lymphocytes. Differential diagnosis of B cell leukaemias with large spleens. J Clin Pathol 1987, **40**: 642–651.

427 Oscier D, Matutes E, Gardiner A, Glide S, Mould S, Brito-Babapulle V, Ellis J, Catovsky D. Cytogenetic studies in splenic lymphoma with villous lymphocytes. Br J Haematol 1993, **85**: 487–491.

BURKITT LYMPHOMA/LEUKEMIA

428 Banks PM, Arseneau JC, Gralnick HR, Canellos GP, DeVita VT Jr, Berard CW. American Burkitt's lymphoma. A clinicopathologic study of 30 cases II. Pathologic correlations. Am J Med 1975, **58**: 322–329.

429 Bennett JM, Catovsky D, Daniet MT, Flandrin G, Galton DA, Gralnick HR, Sultan C. Proposals for the classification of the acute leukaemias. Br J Haematol 1976, **33**: 451–458.

430 Brunning RD, McKenna RW, Bloomfield CD, Coccia P, Gajl-Peczalska KJ. Bone marrow involvement in Burkitt's lymphoma. Cancer 1977, **40**: 1771–1779.

431 Dayton VD, Arthur DC, Gajl-Peczalsak KJ, Brunning R. L3 acute lymphoblastic leukaemia. Comparison with small noncleaved cell lymphoma involving the bone marrow. Am J Clin Pathol 1994, **101**: 130–139.

432 Dorfman RF. Childhood lymphosarcoma in St. Louis, Missouri, clinically and histologically resembling Burkitt's tumor. Cancer 1965, **18**: 418–430.

433 Leoncini L, Raphaël M, Stein H, Harris NL, Jaffe ES, Kluin PM. Burkitt lymphoma. In Swerdlow SH, Campo E, Harris NL, Jaffe ES, Pileri SA, Stein H, Thiele J, Vardiman JW (eds): WHO classification of tumours of haematopoietic and lymphoid tissues. Lyon, 2008, IARC Press, pp. 185–187.

434 O'Connor GT, Rappaport H, Smith EB. Childhood lymphoma resembling 'Burkitt tumor' in the United States. Cancer 1978, **18**: 411–417.

NON-HODGKIN LYMPHOMA

B-CELL LYMPHOMA

435 Arber DA, George TI. Bone marrow biopsy involvement by non-Hodgkin's lymphoma: frequency of lymphoma types, patterns, blood involvement, and discordance with other sites in 450 specimens. Am J Surg Pathol 2005, **29**: 1549–1557.

436 Bain B, Matutes E, Robinson D, Lampert IA, Brito-Babapulle V, Morilla R, Catovsky D. Leukaemia as a manifestation of large cell lymphoma. Br J Haematol 1991, **77**: 301–310.

437 Bartl R, Frisch B, Burkhardt R, Kettner G, Mahl G, Fateh-Moghadam A, Sund M. Assessment of bone marrow histology in the malignant lymphoma (non-Hodgkin's): correlation with clinical factors for diagnosis, prognosis, classification and staging. Br J Haematol 1982, **51**: 511–530.

438 Bartl R, Hansmann ML, Frisch B, Burkhardt R. Comparative histology of malignant lymphomas in lymph node and bone marrow. Br J Haematol 1988, **69**: 229–237.

439 Choe JK, Hyun BH, Salazar GH, Ashton JK, Sung C. Epithelioid granulomas of the bone marrow in non-Hodgkin's lymphoproliferative malignancies. Am J Clin Pathol 1983, **80**: 19–24.

440 Cohen PL, Kurtin PJ, Donovan KA, Hanson CA. Bone marrow and peripheral blood involvement in mantle cell lymphoma. Br J Haematol 1998, **101**: 302–310.

441 Conlan MG, Bast M, Armitage JO, Weisenburger DD for the Nebraska Lymphoma Study Group. Bone marrow involvement by non-Hodgkin's lymphoma: the clinical significance of morphologic discordance between the lymph node and bone marrow. J Clin Oncol 1990, **8**: 1163–1172.

442 Crotty RPL, Smith BR, Tallini G. Morphologic, immunophenotypic, and molecular evaluation of bone marrow involvement in

non-Hodgkin's lymphoma. Diagn Mol Pathol 1998, **7**: 90–95.

443 De Oliveira MS, Jaffe ES, Catovsky D. Leukaemic phase of mantle zone (intermediate) lymphoma: its characterization in 11 cases. J Clin Pathol 1989, **42**: 962–972.

444 Delabie J, Vandenberghe E, Kennes C, Verhoef G, Foschini MP, Stul M, Cassiman JJ, De Wolf-Peeters C. Histiocyte rich B-cell lymphoma. A distinct clinicopathologic entity possibly related to lymphocyte predominant Hodgkin's disease, paragranuloma type. Am J Surg Pathol 1992, **16**: 37–48.

445 Dick F, Bloomfield CD, Brunning RD. Incidence, cytology, and histopathology of non-Hodgkin's lymphomas in the bone marrow. Cancer 1974, **33**: 1382–1398.

446 Diebold J, Jaffe ES, Raphael M, Warnke RA. Burkitt lymphoma. In Jaffe ES, Harris NL, Stein H, Vardiman JW (eds): World Health Organization classification of tumors. Pathology and genetics of tumours of haematopoietic and lymphoid tissues. Lyon, 2001, IARC Press, pp. 181–184.

447 Douglas VK, Gordon LI, Goolsby CL, White CA, Peterson LC. Lymphoid aggregates in bone marrow mimic residual lymphoma after rituximab therapy for non-Hodgkin lymphoma. Am J Clin Pathol 1999, **112**: 844–853.

448 Estabilla OC, Kou CH, Byrnes RK, Medeiros LJ. Intravascular large B-cell lymphoma. Am J Clin Pathol 1999, **112**: 248–255.

449 Fisher DE, Jacobson JO, Ault KA, Harris NL. Diffuse large cell lymphoma with discordant bone marrow histology. Clinical features and biologic implications. Cancer 1989, **64**: 1879–1887.

450 Foon KA, Todd RF. Immunologic classification of leukemia and lymphoma. Blood 1986, **68**: 1–31.

451 Foucar K, McKenna RW, Frizzera G, Brunning RD. Incidence and patterns of bone marrow and blood involvement by lymphoma in relationship to the Lukes–Collins classification. Blood 1979, **54**: 1417–1422.

452 Foucar K, McKenna RW, Frizzera G, Brunning RD. Bone marrow and blood involvement by lymphoma in relationship to the Lukes–Collins classification. Cancer 1982, **49**: 888–897.

453 Fraga M, Brousset P, Schlaifer D, Payen C, Robert A, Rubie H, Huguet-Rigal F, Delsol G. Bone marrow involvement in anaplastic large cell lymphoma. Immunohistochemical detection of minimal disease and its prognostic significance. Am J Clin Pathol 1995, **103**: 82–89.

454 Gaulard P, Kanavaros P, Farcet JP, Rocha FD, Haioun C, Divine M, Reyes F, Zafrani ES. Bone marrow histologic and immunohistochemical findings in peripheral T-cell lymphoma. A study of 38 cases. Hum Pathol 1991, **22**: 331–338.

455 Hanson CA, Brunning RD, Gajl-Peczalska KJ, Frizzera G, McKenna RW. Bone marrow manifestation of peripheral T-cell lymphoma. A study of 30 cases. Am J Clin Pathol 1986, **86**: 449–460.

456 Swerdlow SH, Webber SA, Chadburn A, Ferry JA. Post-transplant lymphoproliferative disorders. In Swerdlow SH, Campo E, Harris NL, Jaffe ES, Pileri SA, Stein H, Thiele J, Vardiman JW (eds): WHO classification of tumours of haematopoietic and lymphoid tissues. Lyon, 2008, IARC Press, pp. 343–349.

457 Kent SA, Variakojis D, Peterson LC. Comparative study of marginal zone lymphoma involving bone marrow. Am J Clin Pathol 2002, **117**: 698–708.

458 Kinney MC, Collins RD, Greer JP, Whitlock JA, Sioutes N, Kadin ME. A small-cell-predominant variant of primary Ki-1 (CD30)+ T-cell lymphoma. Am J Surg Pathol 1993, **17**: 859–968.

459 Koeppen H, Newell K, Baunoch DA, Vardiman JW. Morphologic bone marrow changes in patients with post-transplantation lymphoproliferative disorders. Am J Surg Pathol 1998, **22**: 208–214.

460 Kremer M, Dirnhofer S, Nickl A, Hoefler H, Quintanilla-Martinez L, Fend F. p27(kip1) immunostaining for the differential diagnosis of small B-cell neoplasms in trephine bone marrow biopsies. Mod Pathol 2001, **14**: 1022–1029.

461 Kremer M, Spitzer M, Mandl-Weber S, Stecker K, Quintanilla-Martinez L, Fend F. Discordant bone marrow involvement in diffuse large B-cell lymphoma; molecular analysis of microdissected bone marrow infiltrates reveals a heterogeneous group of disorders. J Clin Pathol 2002, **55**(Suppl 1): A5.

462 Litz CE, Brunning RD. Chronic lymphoproliferative disorders. Classification and diagnosis. Bailliere's Clin Haematol 1993, **6**: 767–789.

463 McKenna RW, Bloomfield CD, Brunning RD. Nodular lymphoma. Bone marrow and blood manifestations. Cancer 1975, **36**: 428–440.

464 McKenna RW, Brunning RD. Reed–Sternberg-like cells in nodular lymphoma involving the bone marrow. Am J Clin Pathol 1975, **63**: 779–785.

465 McKenna RW, Hernandez JA. Bone marrow in malignant lymphoma. Hematol Oncol Clin North Am 1988, **2**: 617–619.

466 Momose H, Jaffe ES, Shin SS, Chen YY, Weiss LM. Chronic lymphocytic leukemia/small lymphocytic lymphoma with Reed–Sternberg-like cells and possible transformation to Hodgkin's disease. Mediation by Epstein–Barr virus. Am J Surg Pathol 1992, **16**: 859–867.

467 Onciu M, Schlette E, Bueso-Ramos C, Medeiros LJ. Leukemic mantle cell lymphoma with cells resembling prolymphocytes. Am J Clin Pathol 2002, **118**: 305–306.

468 Perry DA, Bast MA, Armitage JO, Weisenburger DD. Diffuse intermediate lymphocyte lymphoma. A clinicopathologic study and comparison with small lymphocytic lymphoma and small cleaved cell lymphoma. Cancer 1990, **66**: 1995–2000.

469 Pittaluga S, Tierans A, Dodoo YL, Delabie J, De Wolf-Peeters C. How reliable is histologic examination of bone marrow trephine biopsy specimens for the staging of non-Hodgkin lymphoma? A study of hairy cell leukemia and mantle cell lymphoma involvement of the bone marrow trephine specimen by histologic, immunohistochemical, and polymerase chain reaction techniques. Am J Clin Pathol 1999, **111**: 179–184.

470 Pittaluga S, Verhoef G, Criel A, Maes A, Nuyts J, Boogaerts M, De Wolf Peeters C. Prognostic significance of bone marrow trephine and peripheral blood smears in 55 patients with mantle cell lymphoma. Leuk Lymphoma 1996, **21**: 115–125.

471 Robertson LE, Redman JR, Butler JJ, Osborne BM, Velasquez WS, McLaughlin P, Swan F, Rodriguez MA, Hagemeister FB, Fuller LM, et al. Discordant bone marrow involvement in diffuse large-cell lymphoma. A distinct clinical–pathologic entity associated with a continuous risk of relapse. J Clin Oncol 1991, **9**: 236–242.

472 Schlette E, Lai R, Onciu M, Doherty D, Bueso-Ramos C, Medieros LJ. Leukemic mantle cell lymphoma: clinical and pathologic spectrum of twenty-three cases. Mod Pathol 2001, **14**: 1133–1140.

473 Thieblemont C, Berger F, Dumontet C, Moullet I, Bouafia F, Felman P, Salles G, Coiffier B. Mucosa-associated lymphoid tissue lymphoma is a disseminated disease in one-third of 158 patients analyzed. Blood 2000, **95**: 802–806.

474 Torlakovic B, Torlakovic G, Brunning RD. Follicular pattern of bone marrow involvement by follicular lymphoma. Am J Clin Pathol 2002, **118**: 780–786.

475 Van Huyen JP, Molina T, Delmer A, Audouin J, Le Tourneau A, Zittoun R, Bernadou A, Diebold J. Splenic marginal zone lymphoma with or without plasmacytic differentiation. Am J Surg Pathol 2000, **24**: 1581–1592.

476 Vasef MA, Medeiros LJ, Koo C, McCourty A, Brynes RK. Cyclin D1 immunohistochemical staining is useful in distinguishing mantle cell lymphoma from other low-grade B-cell neoplasms. Am J Clin Pathol 2000, **108**: 302–307.

477 Wasman J, Rosenthal NS, Farhi DC. Mantle cell lymphoma. Morphologic findings in bone marrow involvement. Am J Clin Pathol 1996, **106**: 196–200.

478 Weinberg OK, Seo K, Arber DA. Prevalence of bone marrow involvement in systemic anaplastic large cell lymphoma: are immunohistochemical studies necessary? Hum Pathol 2008, **39**: 1331–1340.

479 Weir EG, Borowitz MJ, Racke FR. Germinal centers in bone marrow specimens are associated with marginal zone lymphoma. Mod Pathol 2001, **14**: 182A.

480 Zukerberg LR, Medeiros LJ, Ferry JA, Harris NL. Diffuse low-grade B-cell lymphomas. Four clinically distinct subtypes defined by a combination of morphologic and immunophenotypic features. Am J Clin Pathol 1993, **100**: 373–385.

T- AND NK-CELL LYMPHOMAS/ LEUKEMIAS

Peripheral T-cell lymphoma, not otherwise specified

481 Dogan A, Morice WG. Bone marrow histopathology in peripheral T-cell lymphomas. Br J Haematol 2004, **127**: 140–154.

482 Gaulard P, Kanavaros P, Farcet JP, Rocha FD, Haioun C, Divine M, Reyes F, Zafrani ES. Bone marrow histologic and immunohistochemical findings in peripheral T-cell lymphoma. A study of 38 cases. Hum Pathol 1991, **22**: 331–338.

483 Gebhard S, Benhatter J, Bricod C, Meuge-Moraw C, Delacratez F. Polymerase chain reaction in the diagnosis of T-cell lymphoma in paraffin embedded bone marrow biopsies: a comparative study. Histopathology 2001, **38**: 37–44.

484 Hanson CA, Brunning RD, Gajl-Peczalska KJ, Frizzera G, McKenna RW. Bone marrow manifestation of peripheral T cell lymphoma. Am J Clin Pathol 1986, **86**: 449–460.

485 Jaffe ES. Pathologic and clinical spectrum of post-thymic T-cell malignancies. Cancer Invest 1984, **2**: 413–426.

486 Pileri SA, Weisenburger DD, Sng I, Jaffe ES, Ralfkiaer E, Nakamura S, Müller-Hermelink HK. Peripheral T-cell lymphoma, not otherwise specified. In Swerdlow SH, Campo E, Harris NL, Jaffe ES, Pileri SA, Stein H, Thiele J, Vardiman JW (eds): WHO classification of tumours of haematopoietic and lymphoid tissues. Lyon, 2008, IARC Press, pp. 306–308.

487 Rizvi MA, Evens AM, Tallman MS, Nelson BP, Rosen ST. T-cell non-Hodgkin lymphoma. Blood 2006, **107**: 1255–1264.

488 Tan BT, Seo K, Warnke RA, Arber DA. The frequency of immunoglobulin heavy chain gene and T-cell receptor gamma-chain gene rearrangements and Epstein–Barr virus in ALK+ and ALK– anaplastic large cell lymphoma and other peripheral T-cell lymphomas. J Mol Diagn 2008, **10**: 502–512.

Adult T-cell leukemia/lymphoma

489 Kiyokawa T, Yamaguchi K, Takeya M, Takahashi K, Watanabe T, Matsumoto T, Lee SY, Takatsuki K. Hypercalcemia and osteoclast proliferation in adult T-cell leukemia. Cancer 1987, **59**: 1187–1191.

490 Ohshima K. Pathological features of diseases associated with human T cell leukemia virus type 1. Cancer Sci 2007, **98**: 772–778.

491 Ohshima K, Jaffe ES, Kikuchi M. Adult T-cell leukaemia/lymphoma. In Swerdlow SH, Campo E, Harris NL, Jaffe ES, Pileri SA, Stein H, Thiele J, Vardiman JW (eds): WHO classification of tumours of haematopoietic and lymphoid tissues. Lyon, 2008, IARC Press, pp. 281–284.

492 Yamaguchi K, Takatsuki K. Adult T cell leukaemia lymphoma. Bailliere's Clin Haematol 1993, **6**: 899–915.

Sézary syndrome

493 Flandrin G, Brouet J. The Sézary cell: cytologic, cytochemical and immunologic studies. Mayo Clin Proc 1974, **49**: 575–583.

494 Lutzner MA, Jordan HW. The ultrastructure of an abnormal cell in Sézary's syndrome. Blood 1968, **31**: 719–726.

495 Ralfkiaer E, Willemze R, Whittaker SJ. Sézary syndrome. In Swerdlow SH, Campo E, Harris NL, Jaffe ES, Pileri SA, Stein H, Thiele J, Vardiman JW (eds): WHO classification of tumours of haematopoietic and lymphoid tissues. Lyon, 2008, IARC Press, pp. 306–308.

496 Sibaud V, Beylot-Barry M, Thiébaut R, Parrens M, Vergier B, Delaunay M, Beylot C, Chêne G, Ferrer J, de Mascarel A, Dubus P, Merlio JP. Bone marrow histopathologic and molecular staging in epidermotropic T-cell lymphomas. Am J Clin Pathol 2003, **119**: 414–423.

497 Taswell HF, Winkelman RK. Sézary syndrome. A malignant reticulemic erythroderma. JAMA 1961, **177**: 465–472.

498 Variakojis D, Rosas-Uribe A, Rappaport H. Mycosis fungoides. Pathologic findings in staging laparotomies. Cancer 1974, **33**: 1589–1600.

499 Zucker-Franklin D, Melton JW, Quagliata F. Ultrastructural, immunologic and functional studies on Sézary cells: a neoplastic variant of thymus derived (T) lymphocytes. Proc Natl Acad Sci U S A 1974, **71**: 1877–1881.

Large granulated T-cell lymphocytic leukemia

500 Alekshun TJ, Sokol L. Diseases of large granular lymphocytes. Cancer Control 2007, **14**: 141–150.

501 Cady FM, Morice WG. Flow cytometric assessment of T-cell chronic lymphoproliferative disorders. Clin Lab Med 2007, **27**: 513–532, vi.

502 Chan WC, Foucar K, Morice WG, Catovsky D. T-cell large granular lymphocytic leukaemia. In Swerdlow SH, Campo E, Harris NL, Jaffe ES, Pileri SA, Stein H, Thiele J, Vardiman JW (eds): WHO classification of tumours of haematopoietic and lymphoid tissues. Lyon, 2008, IARC Press, pp. 272, 273.

503 Costes, V, Duchayne E, Taib J, Delfour C, Rousset T, Baldet P, Delsol G, Brousset P. Intrasinusoidal bone marrow infiltration: a common growth pattern for different lymphoma subtypes. Br J Haematol 2002, **119**: 916–922.

504 Evans HL, Burks E, Viswanatha D, Larson RS. Utility of immunohistochemistry I bone marrow evaluation of T-lineage large granular lymphocyte leukemia. Hum Pathol 2000, **31**: 1266–1273.

505 Lundell R, Hartung L, Hill S, Perkins SL, Bahler DW. T-cell large granular lymphocyte leukemias have multiple phenotypic abnormalities involving pan-T-cell antigens and receptors of MHC molecules. Am J Clin Pathol 2005, **124**: 937–946.

506 Morice WG. The immunophenotypic attributes of NK cells and NK-cell lineage lymphoproliferative disorders. Am J Clin Pathol 2007, **127**: 881–886.

507 Morice WG, Jevremovic D, Hanson CA. The expression of the novel cytotoxic protein granzyme M by large granular lymphocytic leukemias of both T-cell and NK-cell lineage: an unexpected finding with implications regarding the pathobiology of these disorders. Br J Haematol 2007, **137**: 237–239.

508 Morice WG, Kurtin PJ, Tefferi A, Hanson CA. Distinct bone marrow findings in T-cell granular lymphocytic leukemia revealed by paraffin section immunoperoxidase stains for CD8, TIA-1, granzyme B. Blood 2002, **99**: 268–274.

509 O'Malley DP. T-cell large granular leukemia and related proliferations. Am J Clin Pathol 2007, **127**: 850–859.

510 Osuji N, Matutes E, Catovsky D, Lampert I, Wotherspoon A. Histopathology of the spleen in T-cell large granular lymphocyte leukemia and T-cell prolymphocytic leukemia: a comparative review. Am J Surg Pathol 2005, **29**: 935–941.

511 Tefferi A, Li CY, Witzig TE, Dhodapkar MV, Okuno SH, Phyliky RL. Chronic natural killer cell lymphocytosis: a descriptive clinical study. Blood 1994, **84**: 2721–2725.

512 Wlodarski MW, Schade AE, Maciejewski JP. T-large granular lymphocyte leukemia: current molecular concepts. Hematology 2006, **11**: 245–256.

Angioimmunoblastic T-cell lymphoma

513 Frizzera G, Moran EM, Rappaport H. Angio-immunoblastic lymphadenopathy with dysproteinaemia. Lancet 1974, **1**: 1070–1073.

514 Frizzera G, Moran EM, Rappaport H. Angio-immunoblastic lymphadenopathy. Diagnosis and clinical course. Am J Med 1975, **59**: 803–818.

515 Ghani AM, Krause JR. Bone marrow biopsy findings in angioimmunoblastic lymphadenopathy. Br J Haematol 1985, **61**: 203–231.

516 Grogg KL, Morice WG, Macon WR. Spectrum of bone marrow findings in patients with angioimmunoblastic T-cell lymphoma. Br J Haematol 2007, **137**: 416–422.

517 Higgins JP, van de Rijn M, Jones CD, Zehnder JL, Warnke RA. Peripheral T-cell lymphoma complicated by a proliferation of large B cells. Am J Clin Pathol 2000, **114**: 236–247.

518 Lukes RJ, Tindle BH. Immunoblastic lymphadenopathy. A hyperimmune entity resembling Hodgkin's disease. N Engl J Med 1975, **292**: 1–8.

519 Pangalis GA, Moran EM, Rappaport H. Blood and bone marrow findings in angio-immunoblastic lymphadenopathy. Blood 1978, **51**: 71–83.

520 Schnaidt U, Vykoupil KF, Thiele J, Georgii A. Angioimmunoblastic lymphadenopathy. Histopathology of bone marrow involvement. Virchows Arch [A] 1980, **389**: 369–380.

521 Tan BT, Warnke RA, Arber DA. The frequency of B- and T-cell gene rearrangements and Epstein–Barr virus in T-cell lymphomas: a comparison between angioimmunoblastic T-cell lymphoma and peripheral T-cell lymphoma, unspecified with and without associated B-cell proliferations. J Mol Diagn 2006, **8**: 466–475.

Anaplastic large cell lymphoma

522 Bovio IM, Allan RW. The expression of myeloid antigens CD13 and/or CD33 is a marker of ALK+ anaplastic large cell lymphomas. Am J Clin Pathol 2008, **130**: 628–634.

523 Delsol G, Falini B, Müller-Hermelink HK, Campo E, Jaffe ES, Gascoyne RD, Stein H,. Kiney MC. Anaplastic large cell lymphoma (ALCL), ALK-positive. In Swerdlow SH, Campo E, Harris NL, Jaffe ES, Pileri SA, Stein H, Thiele J, Vardiman JW (eds): WHO classification of tumours of haematopoietic and lymphoid tissues. Lyon, 2008, IARC Press, pp. 312–316.

524 Fraga M, Brousset P, Schlaifer D, Payen C, Robert A, Rubie H, Huguet-Rigal F, Delsol G. Bone marrow involvement in anaplastic large cell lymphoma. Immunohistochemical detection of minimal disease and its prognostic significance. Am J Clin Pathol 1995, **103**: 82–89.

525 Grewal JS, Smith LB, Winegarden JD 3rd, Krauss JC, Tworek JA, Schnitzer B. Highly aggressive ALK-positive anaplastic large cell lymphoma with a leukemic phase and multi-organ involvement: a report of three cases and a review of the literature. Ann Hematol 2007, **86**: 499–508.

526 Juco J, Holden JT, Mann KP, Kelley LG, Li S. Immunophenotypic analysis of anaplastic large cell lymphoma by flow cytometry. Am J Clin Pathol 2003, **119**: 205–212.

527 Kinney MC, Collins RD, Greer JP, Whitlock JA, Sioutos N, Kadin ME. A small-cell-predominant variant of primary Ki-1 (CD30)+ T-cell lymphoma. Am J Surg Pathol 1993, **17**: 859–868.

528 Mason DY, Harris NL, Delsol G, Stein H. Anaplastic large cell lymphoma, ALK-negative. In Swerdlow SH, Campo E, Harris NL, Jaffe ES, Pileri SA, Stein H, Thiele J, Vardiman JW (eds): WHO classification of tumours of haematopoietic and lymphoid tissues. Lyon, 2008, IARC Press, pp. 317–319.

529 Weinberg OK, Seo K, Arber DA. Prevalence of bone marrow involvement in systemic anaplastic large cell lymphoma: are immunohistochemical studies necessary? Hum Pathol 2008, **39**: 1331–1340.

Hepatosplenic T-cell lymphoma, post-transplant T-cell lymphoma, and aggressive NK-cell lymphoma

530 Alonsozana ELC, Stamberg J, Kumar D, Jaffe ES, Medeiros LJ, Frantz C, Schiffer CA, O'Connell BA, Kerman S, Stass SA, Abruzzo LV. Isochromosome 7q: the primary cytogenetic abnormality in hepatosplenic gamma delta T cell lymphoma. Leukemia 1997, **11**: 1367–1372.

531 Chan J, Sin VC, Wong KF, Ng CS, Tsang WY, Chan CH, Cheung MM, Lau WH. Nonnasal lymphoma expressing the natural killer cell marker CD56: a clinicopathologic study of 49

cases of an uncommon aggressive neoplasm. Blood 1997, **89**: 4501–4513.

532 de Wolf-Peeters C, Achten R. Gamma/delta T-cell lymphomas: a homogeneous entity? Histopathology 2000, **36**: 294–305.

533 Gaulard P, Jaffe ES, Krenacs L, Macin WR. Hepatosplenic T-cell lymphoma. In Swerdlow SH, Campo E, Harris NL, Jaffe ES, Pileri SA, Stein H, Thiele J, Vardiman JW (eds): WHO classification of tumours of haematopoietic and lymphoid tissues. Lyon, 2008, IARC Press, pp. 292, 293.

534 Jaffe ES. Pathologic and clinical spectrum of post-thymic T-cell malignancies. Cancer Invest 1984, **2**: 413–426.

535 Jonveaux P, Daniel MT, Martel V, Maarek O, Berger R. Isochromosome 7q and trisomy 8 are consistent primary non-random chromosome abnormalities associated with hepatosplenic T gamma/delta lymphoma. Leukemia 1996, **10**: 1453–1455.

536 Macon WR, Levy NB, Kurtin PJ, Salhany KE, Elkhalifa MY, Casey TT, Craig FE, Vnencak-Jones CL, Gulley ML, Park JP, Cousar JB. Hepatosplenic αβ T-cell lymphomas: a report of 14 cases and comparison with hepatosplenic gamma delta T-cell lymphomas. Am J Surg Pathol 2001, **25**: 285–296.

537 Shaw PH, Cohn SL, Morgan ER, Kovarik P, Haut PR, Kletzel M, Murphy SB. Natural killer cell lymphoma: report of two pediatric cases, therapeutic options and review of the literature. Cancer 2001, **91**: 642–646.

538 Vega F, Medeiros LJ, Buesa-Ramos C, Jones D, Lai R, Luthra R, Abruzzo LV. Hepatosplenic gamma/delta T-cell lymphoma in bone marrow. A sinusoidal neoplasm with blastic cytologic features. Am J Clin Pathol 2001, **116**: 410–419.

539 Wong KF, Chan JK, Cheung MMC, So JC. Bone marrow involvement by nasal NK cell lymphoma at diagnosis is uncommon. Am J Clin Pathol 2001, **115**: 226–270.

BENIGN LYMPHOCYTIC AGGREGATES

540 Bluth RF, Casey TT, McCurley TL. Differentiation of reactive from neoplastic small-cell lymphoid aggregates in paraffin-embedded marrow particle preparations using L-26 (CD20) and UCHL-1 (CD45RO) monoclonal antibodies. Am J Clin Pathol 1993, **99**: 150–156.

541 Cheson BD, Horning SJ, Coiffier B, Shipp MA, Fisher RI, Connors JM, Lister TA, Vose J, Grillo-López A, Hagenbeek A, Cabanillas F, Klippensten D, Hiddemann W, Castellino R, Harris NL, Armitage JO, Carter W, Hoppe R, Canellos GP. Report of an international workshop to standardize response criteria for non-Hodgkin's lymphomas. J Clin Oncol 1999, **17**: 1244–1253.

542 Cheson BD, Pfistner B, Juweid ME, Gascoyne RD, Specht L, Horning SJ, Coiffier B, Fisher RI, Hagenbeek A, Zucca E, Rosen ST, Stroobants S, Lister TA, Hoppe RT, Dreyling M, Tobinai K, Vose JM, Connors JM, Federico M, Diehl V; International Harmonization Project on Lymphoma. Revised response criteria for malignant lymphoma. J Clin Oncol 2007, **25**: 579–586.

543 Chu PG, Chen Y-Y, Molina A, Arber DA, Weiss LM. Recurrent B-cell neoplasms after rituximab therapy: an immunophenotypic and genotypic study. Leuk Lymphoma 2002, **43**: 2335–2341.

544 Douglas VK, Gordon LI, Goolsby CL, White CA, Peterson LC. Lymphoid aggregates in bone marrow mimic residual lymphoma after rituximab therapy for non-Hodgkin lymphoma. Am J Clin Pathol 1999, **112**: 844–853.

545 Engels K, Oeschger S, Hansmann ML, Hillebrand M, Kriener S. Bone marrow trephines containing lymphoid aggregates from patients with rheumatoid and other autoimmune disorders frequently show clonal B-cell infiltrates. Hum Pathol 2007, **38**: 1402–1411.

546 Faulkner-Jones BE, Howie AJ, Boughton BJ, Franklin IM. Lymphoid aggregates in bone marrow: study of eventual outcome. J Clin Pathol 1988, **41**: 768.

547 Hashimoto H, Hashimoto N. The occurrence of lymph nodules in human bone marrow with particular reference to their number. Kyushu J Med Sci 1963, **14**: 343–354.

548 Hashimoto M, Higuchi M, Saito T. Lymph nodules in human bone marrow. Acta Pathol Jpn 1957, **7**: 33–52.

549 Horny HP, Wehrmann M, Grisser H, Tiemann M, Bultmann B, Kaiserling E. Investigation of bone marrow lymphocyte subsets in normal, reactive, and neoplastic states, using paraffin-embedded biopsy specimens. Am J Clin Pathol 1993, **99**: 142–149.

550 Maeda K, Hyun BH, Rebuck JW. Lymphoid follicles in bone marrow aspirates. Am J Clin Pathol 1977, **67**: 41–48.

551 Rywlin AM, Ortega RS, Dominguez CJ. Lymphoid nodules of bone marrow: normal and abnormal. Blood 1974, **43**: 389–400.

552 Thiele J, Zirbes TK, Kvasnicka HM, Fischer R. Focal lymphoid aggregates (nodules) in bone marrow biopsies: differentiation between hyperplasia and malignant lymphoma – a practical guideline. J Clin Pathol 1999, **52**: 294–300.

HODGKIN LYMPHOMA

553 Bartl R, Frisch B, Burkhardt R, Huhn D, Pappenberger R. Assessment of bone marrow histology in Hodgkin's disease: correlation with clinical factors. Br J Haematol 1982, **51**: 345–360.

554 Chang KL, Kamel OW, Arber DA, Horyd ID, Weiss LM. Pathologic features of nodular lymphocyte predominance Hodgkin's disease in extranodal sites. Am J Surg Pathol 1995, **19**: 1313–1324.

555 Diehl V, Sextro M, Franklin J, Hansmann ML, Harris N, Jaffe E, Poppema S, Harris M, Franssila K, van Krieken J, Marafioti T, Anagnostopoulos I, Stein H. Clinical presentation, course, and prognostic factors in lymphocyte-predominant Hodgkin's disease: report from the European Task Force on Lymphoma Project on Lymphocyte-Predominant Hodgkin's Disease. J Clin Oncol 1999, **17**: 776–783.

556 Dorfman RF. In discussion of Lukes RJ: Criteria for involvement of lymph node, bone marrow, spleen, and liver in Hodgkin's disease. Cancer Res 1971, **31**: 1768–1769.

557 Kinney MC, Greer JP, Stein RS, Collins RD, Cousar JB. Lymphocyte-depletion Hodgkin's disease. Histopathologic diagnosis of marrow involvement. Am J Surg Pathol 1986, **10**: 219–226.

558 Koene-Bogman J. Granulomas and the diagnosis of Hodgkin's disease. N Engl J Med 1978, **299**: 533.

559 Lukes RJ. Criteria for involvement of lymph node, bone marrow, spleen and liver in Hodgkin's disease. Cancer Res 1971, **31**: 1755–1767.

560 McKenna RW, Brunning RD. Reed–Sternberg-like cells in nodular lymphoma involving the bone marrow. Am J Clin Pathol 1975, **63**: 779–785.

561 Munker R, Hasenclever D, Brosteanu O, Hiller E, Diehl V. Bone marrow involvement in Hodgkin's disease: an analysis of 135 consecutive cases. J Clin Oncol 1995, **13**: 403–409.

562 Neiman RS, Rosen PJ, Lukes RJ. Lymphocyte-depletion Hodgkin's disease. A clinicopathologic entity. N Engl J Med 1973, **288**: 751–755.

563 O'Carroll DI, McKenna RW, Brunning RD. Bone marrow manifestations of Hodgkin's disease. Cancer 1976, **38**: 1717–1728.

564 Ponzoni M, Fumagalli L, Rossi G, Freschi M, Re A, Viganò MG, Guidoboni M, Dolcetti R, McKenna RW, Facchetti F. Isolated bone marrow involvement in human immunodeficiency virus-associated Hodgkin lymphoma. Mod Pathol 2002, **15**: 1273–1278.

565 Poppema S, Delsol G, Pileri SA, Stein H, Swerdlow SH, Warnke RA, et al. Nodular lymphocyte predominant Hodgkin lymphoma. In Swerdlow SH, Campo E, Harris NL, Jaffe ES, Pileri SA, Stein H, Thiele J, Vardiman JW (eds): WHO classification of tumours of haematopoietic and lymphoid tissues. Lyon, 2008, IARC Press, pp. 323–325.

566 Rappaport H, Berard CW, Butler JJ, Dorfman RF, Lukes RJ, Thomas LB. Report of the Committee of Histopathological Criteria contributing to staging of Hodgkin's disease. Cancer Res 1971, **31**: 1864–1865.

567 Siebert JD, Stuckey JH, Kurtin PJ, Banks PM. Extranodal lymphocyte predominance Hodgkin's disease. Clinical and pathologic features. Am J Clin Pathol 1995, **103**: 485–491.

568 Stein H, Delsol G, Pileri SA, Weiss LM, Poppema S, Jaffee ES. Classical Hodgkin lymphoma, introduction. In Swerdlow SH, Campo E, Harris NL, Jaffe ES, Pileri SA, Stein H, Thiele J, Vardiman JW (eds): WHO classification of tumours of haematopoietic and lymphoid tissues. Lyon, 2008, IARC Press, pp. 326–329.

569 Te Velde J, Den Ottolander GJ, Spaander PJ, Van den Berg C, Hartgrink-Groeneveld CA. The bone marrow in Hodgkin's disease: the non-involved marrow. Histopathology 1978, **2**: 31–46.

HISTIOCYTIC DISORDERS

MALIGNANT HISTIOCYTOSIS

570 Copie-Bergman C, Wotherspoon AC, Norton AJ, Diss TC, Isaacson PG. True histiocytic lymphoma: a morphologic, immunohistochemical, and molecular genetic study of 13 cases. Am J Surg Pathol 1998, **22**: 1386–1392.

571 Grogan TM, Pileri SA, Chan JKC, Weiss LM, Fletcher CDM. Histiocytic sarcoma. In Swerdlow SH, Campo E, Harris NL, Jaffe ES, Pileri SA, Stein H, Thiele J, Vardiman JW (eds): WHO classification of tumours of haematopoietic and lymphoid tissues. Lyon, 2008, IARC Press, pp. 356, 357.

572 Jaffe R, Pileri SA, Fachetti F, Jones DM, Jaffee ES. Histiocytic and dendritic cell neoplasms. Introduction. In Swerdlow SH, Campo E, Harris NL, Jaffe ES, Pileri SA, Stein H, Thiele J, Vardiman JW (eds): WHO classification of tumours of haematopoietic and lymphoid tissues. Lyon, 2008, IARC Press, pp. 354, 355.

573 Lampert IA, Catovsky D, Bergier N. Malignant histiocytosis: a clinico-pathological study of 12 cases. Br J Haematol 1978, **40**: 65–77.

574 Rappaport H. Tumors of the hematopoietic system. In Atlas of tumor pathology, series 3, fascicle 8. Washington DC, 2001, Armed Forces Institute of Pathology.

575 Rousseau-Merck MF, Jaubert E, Nezelof C. Malignant histiocytosis in childhood. Hum Pathol 1985, **16**: 321.

576 Van Heerde P, Feltkamp CA, Hart AA, Somers R. Malignant histiocytosis and related tumors. A clinicopathologic study of 42 cases using cytological, histochemical, and ultrastructural parameters. Hematol Oncol 1984, **2**: 13–32.

577 Warnke RA, Kim H, Dorfman RF. Malignant histiocytosis (histiocytic medullary reticulosis) I. Clinicopathologic study of 29 cases. Cancer 1975, **35**: 215–230.

578 Weiss LM, Azzi R, Dorfman RF, Warnke RA. Sinusoidal hematolymphoid malignancy ('malignant histiocytosis') presenting as atypical sinusoidal proliferation. A study of nine cases. Cancer 1986, **58**: 1681–1688.

579 Wilson MS, Weiss LM, Gatter KC, Mason DY, Dorfman RF, Warnke RA. Malignant histiocytosis. A reassessment of cases previously reported in 1975 based on paraffin section immunophenotyping studies. Cancer 1990, **66**: 530–536.

HEMOPHAGOCYTIC SYNDROMES

580 Allory Y, Challine D, Haioun C, Copie-Bergman C, Delfau-Larue MH, Boucher E, Charlotte F, Fabre M, Michel M, Gaulard P. Bone marrow involvement in lymphomas with hemophagocytic syndrome at presentation. A clinicopathologic study of 11 patients in a western institution. Am J Surg Pathol 2001, **25**: 865–874.

581 Ashby MA, Williams CJ, Buchanan RB, Bleehan NM, Arno J. Mediastinal germ cell tumor associated with malignant histiocytosis and high rubella titres. Hematol Oncol 1986, **4**: 183–194.

582 Chen R-L, Su I-J, Lin K-H, Lee SH, Lin DT, Chuu WM, Lin KS, Huang LM, Lee CY. Fulminant childhood hemophagocytic syndrome mimicking histiocytic medullary reticulosis. Am J Clin Pathol 1991, **96**: 171–176.

583 Chott A, Kaserer K, Augustin I, Vesely M, Heinz R, Oehlinger W, Hanak H, Radaszkiewicz T. Ki-1 positive large cell lymphoma. A clinicopathologic study of 41 cases. Am J Surg Pathol 1990, **14**: 439–448.

584 Daum GS, Sullivan JL, Ansell J, Mulder C, Woda BA. Virus-associated hemophagocytic syndrome. Identification of an immunoproliferative precursor lesion. Hum Pathol 1987, **18**: 1071–1074.

585 Falini B, Pileri S, De Solas I, Martelli MF, Mason DY, Delsol G, Gatter KC, Fagioli M. Peripheral T-cell lymphoma associated with hemophagocytic syndrome. Blood 1990, **75**: 434–444.

586 Filipovich AH. Hemophagocytic lymphohistiocytosis and other hemophagocytic disorders. Immunol Allergy Clin North Am 2008, **28**: 293–313.

587 Gaffey MJ, Frierson HF, Medeiros LJ, Weiss LM. The relationship of Epstein–Barr virus (sporadic) and familial hemophagocytic syndrome and secondary (lymphoma-related) hemophagocytosis. An in situ hybridization study. Hum Pathol 1993, **24**: 657–667.

588 Henter J-I, Aricò M, Elinder G, Imashuku S, Janka G. Familial hemophagocytic lymphohistiocytosis; primary hemophagocytic lymphohistiocytosis. Hematol Oncol Clin North Am 1998, **12**: 417–433.

589 Henter JI, Elinder G, Ost A. Diagnostic guidelines for hemophagocytic lymphohistiocytosis. Semin Oncol 1991, **18**: 29–33.

590 Imashuku S, Kuriyama K, Tearmura T, Ishii E, Kinugawa N, Kato M, Sako M, Hibi S. Requirement for etoposide in the treatment of Epstein–Barr virus-associated hemophagocytic lymphohistiocytosis. J Clin Oncol 2001, **19**: 2665–2673.

591 Jaffe ES, Costa J, Fauci AS, Cossman J, Tsosos M. Malignant lymphoma and erythrophagocytosis simulating malignant histiocytosis. Am J Med 1983, **75**: 741–749.

592 Janka G, Imashuku S, Elinder G, Schneider M, Henter JI. Infection- and malignancy-associated hemophagocytic syndromes. Secondary hemophagocytic lymphohistiocytosis. Hematol Oncol Clin North Am 1998, **12**: 435–444.

593 Kikuta H, Sakiyama Y, Matsumoto S, Oh-Ishi T, Nakano T, Nagashima T, Oka T, Hironaka T, Hirai K. Fatal Epstein–Barr virus-associated hemophagocytic syndrome. Blood 1993, **82**: 3259–3264.

594 Kimura H, Hoshino Y, Kanegane H, Tsuge I, Okamura T, Kawa K, Morishima T. Clinical and virologic characteristics of chronic active Epstein–Barr virus infections. Blood 2001, **98**: 280–286.

595 Kogawa K, Lee SM, Villaneuva J, Marmer D, Sumegi J, Filipovich AH. Perforin expression in cytotoxic lymphocytes from patients with hemophagocytic lymphohistiocytosis and their family members. Blood 2002, **99**: 61–66.

596 Lay J-D, Tsao C-J, Chen J-Y, Kadin M, Su I-J. Upregulation of tumor necrosis factor-α gene by Epstein–Barr virus and activation of macrophages in Epstein–Barr virus-infected T cells in the pathogenesis of hemophagocytic syndrome. J Clin Invest 1997, **100**: 1969–1979.

597 Mroczek EC, Weisenburger DD, Grierson HL, Markin R, Purtilo DT. Fatal infectious mononucleosis and virus-associated hemophagocytic syndrome. Arch Pathol Lab Med 1987, **111**: 530–535.

598 Ravelli A. Macrophage activation syndrome. Curr Opin Rheumatol 2002, **14**: 548–552.

599 Ravelli A, Magni-Manzoni S, Postorio A, Besana C, Foti T, Ruperto N, Viola S, Martini A. Preliminary diagnostic guidelines for macrophage activation syndrome complicating systemic juvenile idiopathic arthritis. J Pediatr 2005, **146**: 598–604.

600 Reiner AP, Spivak JL. Hematophagocytic histiocytosis. A report of 23 new patients and a review of the literature. Medicine (Baltimore) 1988, **67**: 349–368.

601 Reisman RP, Greco MA. Virus-associated hemophagocytic syndrome due to Epstein–Barr virus. Hum Pathol 1984, **15**: 290–293.

602 Risdall RJ, Brunning RD, Hernandez JI, Gordon DH. Bacteria-associated hemophagocytic syndrome. Cancer 1984, **54**: 2968–2972.

603 Risdall RJ, McKenna RW, Nesbit ME, Krivit W, Balfour HH, Simmons RL, Brunning RD. Virus associated hemophagocytic syndrome. Hum Pathol 1981, **12**: 395–398.

604 Shimazaki C, Inaba T, Shimura K, Okamoto A, Takahashi R, Hirai H, Sudo Y, Ashihara E, Adachi Y, Murakami S, Saigo K, Fujita N, Nakagawa M. B-cell lymphoma associated with hemophagocytic syndrome: a clinical, immunological and cytogenetic study. Br J Haematol 1999, **104**: 672–679.

605 Shirono K, Tsuda H. Parvovirus B19-associated hemophagocytic syndrome in healthy adults. Br J Haematol 1995, **89**: 923–926.

606 Stepp SE, Dufourcq-Lagelouse R, LeDeist F, Bhawan S, Certain S, Mathew PA, Henter JI, Bennett M, Fischer A, de Saint Basile G, Kumar V. Perforin gene defect in familial hemophagocytic lymphohistiocytosis. Science 1999, **286**: 1957–1959.

607 Su I-J, Wang C-H, Cheng A-L, Chen R-L. Hemophagocytic syndrome in Epstein–Barr virus associated T-lymphoproliferative disorders: disease spectrum, pathogenesis and management. Leuk Lymphoma 1995, **19**: 401–406.

608 Sullivan JL, Woda BA, Herrod HG, Koh G, Rivara FP, Mulder C. Epstein–Barr virus-associated hemophagocytic syndrome. Virological and immunopathological studies. Blood 1985, **65**: 1097–1104.

609 Teruya-Feldstein J, Setsuda J, Yao X, Kingma DW, Straus S, Tosato G, Jaffe ES. MIP-1 alpha expression in tissues from patients with hemophagocytic syndrome. Lab Invest 1999, **79**: 1583–1590.

610 Verbsky JW, Grossman WJ. Hemophagocytic lymphohistiocytosis: diagnosis, pathophysiology, treatment, and future perspectives. Ann Med 2006, **38**: 20–31.

611 Woda BA, Sullivan JL. Reactive histiocytic disorders. Am J Clin Pathol 1993, **99**: 459–463.

LANGERHANS CELL HISTIOCYTOSIS

612 Jaffee R, Weiss LM, Fachetti F. Tumours derived from Langerhans cells. In Swerdlow SH, Campo E, Harris NL, Jaffe ES, Pileri SA, Stein H, Thiele J, Vardiman JW (eds): WHO classification of tumours of haematopoietic and lymphoid tissues. Lyon, 2008, IARC Press, pp. 358–360.

613 McClain K, Ramsay NKC, Robison L, Sundberg RD, Nesbit M Jr. Bone marrow involvement in histiocytosis X. Med Pediatr Oncol 1983, **11**: 167–171.

PLASMA CELL DYSCRASIAS

614 McKenna RW, Kyle RA, Kuehl WM, Grogan TM, Harris NL, Coupland RW. Plasma cell neoplasms. In Swerdlow SH, Campo E, Harris NL, Jaffe ES, Pileri SA, Stein H, Thiele J, Vardiman JW (eds): WHO classification of tumours of haematopoietic and lymphoid tissues. Lyon, 2008, IARC Press, pp. 200–213.

PLASMA CELL MYELOMA, NONSECRETORY MYELOMA, ASYMPTOMATIC (SMOLDERING) PLASMA CELL MYELOMA

615 Avet-Loiseau H, Attal M, Moreau P, Charbonnel C, Garban F, Hulin C, Leyvraz S, Michallet M, Yakoub-Agha I, Garderet L, Marit G, Michaux L, Voillat L, Renaud M, Grosbois B, Guillerm G, Benboubker L, Monconduit M, Thieblemont C, Casassus P, Caillot D, Stoppa AM, Sotto JJ, Wetterwald M, Dumontet C, Fuzibet JG, Azais I, Dorvaux V, Zandecki M, Bataille R, Minvielle S, Harousseau JL, Facon T, Mathiot C. Genetic abnormalities and survival in multiple myeloma: the experience of the Intergroupe Francophone du Myélome. Blood 2007, **109**: 3489–3495.

616 Bartl R, Frisch B, Fateh-Moghadam A, Kettner G, Jaeger K, Sommerfeld W. Histologic classification and staging of multiple myeloma. A retrospective study of 674 cases. Am J Clin Pathol 1987, **87**: 342–355.

617 Bataille R, Durie BGM, Grenier J. Serum beta2 microglobulin and survival duration in multiple myeloma. A simple reliable marker for staging. Br J Haematol 1983, **55**: 439–447.

618 Carbone A, Volpe R, Manconi R, Poletti A, Tirelli U, Monfardini S. Bone marrow pattern and clinical staging in multiple myeloma. Br J Haematol 1987, **65**: 502.

619 Carter A, Hocherman I, Linn S, Cohen Y, Tatarsky I. Prognostic significance of plasma

cell morphology in multiple myeloma. Cancer 1987, **60**: 1060–1065.

620 Case record of the Massachusetts General Hospital; Case 4–1992. N Engl J Med 1992, **326**: 255–263.

621 Cavo M, Baccarani M, Gobbi M, Lipizer A, Tura S. Prognostic value of bone marrow plasma cell infiltration in stage I multiple myeloma. Br J Haematol 1983, **55**: 683–690.

622 Durie BG. Staging and kinetics of multiple myeloma. Semin Oncol 1986, **13**: 300–309.

623 Durie BGM, Salmon SE, Moon TE. Pretreatment tumor mass, cell kinetics, and prognosis in multiple myeloma. Blood 1980, **55**: 364–372.

624 Facon T, Avet-Loiseau H, Guillerm G, Moreau P, Geneviève F, Zandecki M, Laï JL, Leleu X, Jouet JP, Bauters F, Harousseau JL, Bataille R, Mary JY; Intergroupe Francophone du Myélome. Chromosome 13 abnormalities identified by FISH analysis and serum B2-microglobulin produce a powerful myeloma staging system for patients receiving high-dose therapy. Blood 2001, **97**: 1566–1571.

625 Falini B, DeSolas I, Levine AM, Parker JW, Lukes RJ, Taylor CR. Emergence of B-immunoblastic sarcoma in patients with multiple myeloma. A clinico-pathologic study of 10 cases. Blood 1982, **59**: 923–933.

626 Fonseca R, Blood EA, Oken MM, Kyle RA, Dewald GW, Bailey RJ, Van Wier SA, Henderson KJ, Hoyer JD, Harrington D, Kay NE, Van Ness B, Greipp PR. Myeloma and the t(11;14)(q13;q32); evidence for a biologically defined unique subset of patients. Blood 2002, **99**: 3735–3741.

627 Fritz E, Ludwig H, Kundi M. Prognostic relevance of cellular morphology in multiple myeloma. Blood 1984, **63**: 1072–1079.

628 Gassmann W, Pralle H, Haferlach T, Pandurevic S, Graubner M, Schmitz N, Löffler H. Staging systems for multiple myeloma. A comparison. Br J Haematol 1985, **59**: 703–711.

629 Gertz MA, Kyle RA, Greipp PR. The plasma cell labeling index; a valuable tool in primary systemic amyloidosis. Blood 1989, **74**: 1108–1111.

630 Greipp PR, Katzmann JA, O'Fallon WM, Kyle RA. Impact of pretreatment β2 microglobulin levels on survival in patients with multiple myeloma. Blood 1985, **66**: 188a.

631 Greipp PR, Raymond NM, Kyle RA, O'Fallon WM. Multiple myeloma. Significance of plasmablastic subtype in morphological classification. Blood 1985, **65**: 305–310.

632 Greipp PR, Witzig TE, Gonchoroff NJ, Habermann TM, Katzmann JA, O'Fallon WM, Kyle RA. Immunofluorescence labeling indices in myeloma and related monoclonal gammopathies. Mayo Clin Proc 1987, **62**: 969–977.

633 Greipp PR. Advances in the diagnosis and management of myeloma. Semin Hematol 1992, **29**: 24–45.

634 Hoyer JD, Hanson CA, Fonseca R, Greipp PR, Dewald G, Kurtin PJ. The (11;14)(q13;q32) translocation in multiple myeloma. Am J Clin Pathol 2000, **113**: 831–837.

635 Hyun BK, Kwa D, Gabaldon H, Ashton JK. Reactive plasmacytic lesions of the bone marrow. Am J Clin Pathol 1976, **65**: 921–928.

636 Konigsberg R, Zojer N, Ackermann J, Krömer E, Kittler H, Fritz E, Kaufmann H, Nösslinger T, Riedl L, Gisslinger H, Jäger U, Simonitsch I, Heinz R, Ludwig H, Huber H, Drach J. Predictive role of interphase cytogenetics for survival of patients with multiple myeloma. J Clin Oncol 2000, **18**: 804–812.

637 Krzyzaniak RL, Buss DH, Cooper R, Wells HB. Marrow fibrosis and multiple myeloma. Am J Clin Pathol 1988, **89**: 63–68.

638 Kyle RA, Remstein ED, Therneau TM, Dispenzieri A, Kurtin PJ, Hodnefield JM, Larson DR, Plevak MF, Jelinek DF, Fonseca R, Melton LJ 3rd, Rajkumar SV. Clinical course and prognosis of smoldering (asymptomatic) multiple myeloma. N Engl J Med 2007, **356**: 2582–2590.

639 Kyle RA, Gertz MA, Witzig TE, Lust JA, Lacy MQ, Dispenzieri A, Fonseca R, Rajkumar SV, Offord JR, Larson DR, Plevak ME, Therneau TM, Greipp PR. Review of 1027 patients with newly diagnosed multiple myeloma. Mayo Clinic Proc 2003, **78**: 21–33.

640 McKenna RW, Kyle RA, Kuehl WM, Grogan TM, Harris NL, Coupland RW. Plasma cell neoplasms. In Swerdlow SH, Campo E, Harris NL, Jaffe ES, Pileri SA, Stein H, Thiele J, Vardiman JW (eds): WHO classification of tumours of haematopoietic and lymphoid tissues. Lyon, 2008, IARC Press, pp. 200–213.

641 Moreau P, Facon T, Leleu X, Morineau N, Huyghe P, Harousseau JL, Bataille R, Avet-Loiseau H; Intergroupe Francophone du Myélome. Recurrent 14q32 translocations determine the prognosis of multiple myeloma, especially in patients receiving intensive chemotherapy. Blood 2002, **100**: 1579–1583.

642 Peterson LC, Brown BA, Crosson JT, Mladenovic J. Application of the immunoperoxidase technic to bone marrow trephine biopsies in the classification of patients with monoclonal gammopathies. Am J Clin Pathol 1986, **85**: 688–693.

643 Petruch UR, Horny HP, Kaiserling E. Frequent expression of haemopoietic and non-haemopoietic antigens by neoplastic plasma cells. An immunohistochemical study using formalin-fixed, paraffin-embedded tissue. Histopathology 1992, **20**: 35–40.

644 Pileri S, Poggi S, Baglioni P, Montanari M, Sabattini E, Galieni P, Tazzari PL, Gobbi M, Cavo M, Falini B, et al. Histology and immunohistology of bone marrow biopsy in multiple myeloma. Eur J Haematol 1989, **43**: 52–59.

645 Preud'Homme JL, Hurez D, Danon F, Brouet JC, Seligmann M. Intracytoplasmic and surface-bound immunoglobulins in 'nonsecretory' and Bence Jones myeloma. Clin Exp Immunol 1976, **25**: 428–436.

646 Smadja NV, Bastard C, Brigaudeau C, Leroux D, Fruchart C. Hypodiploidy is a major prognostic factor in multiple myeloma. Blood 2001, **98**: 2229–2238.

647 Smith DB, Harris M, Gowland E, Chaang J, Scargge JH. Non-secretory multiple myeloma. A report of 13 cases with a review of the literature. Hematol Oncol 1986, **4**: 307–313.

648 Stewart AK, Bergasagel PL, Greipp PR, Dispenzieri A, Gertz MA, Hayman SR, Kumar S, Lacy MQ, Lust JA, Russell SJ, Witzig TE, Zeldenrust SR, Dingli D, Reeder CB, Roy V, Kyle RA, Rajkumar SV, Fonseca R. A practical guide to defining high-risk myeloma for clinical trials, patient counseling and choice of therapy. Leukemia 2007, **21**: 529–534.

649 Strand WR, Banks PM, Kyle RA. Anaplastic plasma cell myeloma and immunoblastic lymphoma. Clinical, pathologic, and immunologic comparison. Am J Med 1984, **76**: 861–867.

650 Strickler JG, Audeh MW, Copenhaver CM, Warnke RA. Immunophenotypic differences between plasmacytoma/multiple myeloma and immunoblastic lymphoma. Cancer 1988, **61**: 1782–1786.

651 Supkanichnant S, Cousar JB, Leelasiri A, Graber SE, Greer JP, Collins RD. Diagnostic criteria and histologic grading in multiple myeloma. Histologic and immunohistologic analysis of 176 cases with clinical correlation. Hum Pathol 1994, **25**: 308–318.

652 Thiry A, Delvenne P, Fontaine MA, Bonvier J. Comparison of bone marrow sections, smears, and immunohistological staining for immunoglobulin light chains in the diagnosis of benign and malignant plasma cell proliferations. Histopathology 1993, **22**: 423–428.

Plasma cell leukemia

653 García-Sanz R, Orfão A, González M, Tabernero MD, Bladé J, Moro MJ, Fernández-Calvo J, Sanz MA, Pérez-Simón JA, Rasillo A, Miguel JF. Primary plasma cell leukemia: clinical, immunophenotypic, DNA ploidy, and cytogenetic characteristics. Blood 1999, **93**: 1032–1037.

654 Kosmo MA, Gale RP. Plasma cell leukemia. Semin Hematol 1987, **24**: 202–208.

655 Kyle RA, Maldonado JE, Baryd ED. Plasma cell leukemia. Report on 17 cases. Arch Intern Med 1974, **133**: 813–818.

656 Maldonado J, Velosa JA, Kyle RA, Wagoner RD, Holley KE, Salassa RM. Fanconi syndrome in adults. A manifestation of a latent form of myeloma. Am J Med 1974, **58**: 354–364.

657 McKenna RW, Kyle RA, Kuehl WM, Grogan TM, Harris NL, Coupland RW. Plasma cell neoplasms. In Swerdlow SH, Campo E, Harris NL, Jaffe ES, Pileri SA, Stein H, Thiele J, Vardiman JW (eds): WHO classification of tumours of haematopoietic and lymphoid tissues. Lyon, 2008, IARC Press, pp. 200–213.

OSTEOSCLEROTIC MYELOMA (POEMS SYNDROME)

658 Bitter MA, Komaiko W, Franklin WA. Giant lymph node hyperplasia with osteoblastic bone lesions and the POEMS (Takatsuki's) syndrome. Cancer 1985, **56**: 188–194.

659 Case record of the Massachusetts General Hospital; Case 39–1992. N Engl J Med 1992, **327**: 1014–1021.

660 Diego Miralles G, O'Fallon JR, Talley NJ. Plasma-cell dyscrasia with polyneuropathy. The spectrum of POEMS syndrome. N Engl J Med 1992, **327**: 1919–1923.

661 Dispenzieri A, Kyle RA, Lacy MQ, Rajkumar SV, Therneau TM, Larson DR, Greipp PR, Witzig TE, Basu R, Suarez GA, Fonseca R, Lust JA, Gertz MA. POEMS syndrome: definitions and long-term outcome. Blood 2002, **101**: 2496–2506.

662 Imawari M, Akatsuka N, Beppu H, Suzuki H, Ishibashi M. Syndrome of plasma cell dyscrasia, polyneuropathy, and endocrine disturbances. Ann Intern Med 1974, **81**: 490–493.

663 McKenna RW, Kyle RA, Kuehl WM, Grogan TM, Harris NL, Coupland RW. Plasma cell neoplasms. In Swerdlow SH, Campo E, Harris NL, Jaffe ES, Pileri SA, Stein H, Thiele J, Vardiman JW (eds): WHO classification of tumours of haematopoietic and lymphoid tissues. Lyon, 2008, IARC Press, pp. 200–213.

664 Miralles GD, O'Fallon JR, Talley NJ. Plasma-cell dyscrasia with polyneuropathy. The spectrum of POEMS syndrome. N Engl J Med 1992, **327**: 1919–1923.

665 Soubrier MJ, Dubost J-J, Sauvezie BJH. POEMS syndrome. A study of 25 cases and a review of the literature. Am J Med 1994, **97**: 543–553.

666 Takatsuki K, Sanada I. Plasma cell dyscrasia with polyneuropathy and endocrine disorder. Clinical and laboratory features of 109 reported cases. Jpn J Clin Oncol 1983, **13**: 543–556.

PLASMACYTOMA

667 Alexanian R. Localized and indolent myeloma. Blood 1980, **56**: 521–525.

668 Alexiou C, Kau RJ, Dietzfelbinger H, Kremer M, Spiess JC, Schratzenstaller B, Arnold W. Extramedullary plasmacytoma. Tumor occurrence and therapeutic concepts. Cancer 1999, **85**: 2305–2315.

669 Corwin J, Lindberg RD. Solitary plasmacytoma of bone vs. extramedullary plasmacytoma and their relationship to multiple myeloma. Cancer 1979, **43**: 1007–1013.

670 Dimopoulos MA, Moulopoulos LA, Maniatis A, Alexanian R. Solitary plasmacytoma of bone and asymptomatic multiple myeloma. Blood 2000, **96**: 2037–2044.

671 Galieni P, Cavo M, Avvisati G, Pulsoni A, Falbo R, Bonelli MA, Russo D, Petrucci MT, Bucalossi A, Tura S. Solitary plasmacytoma of bone and extramedullary plasmacytoma: two different entities? Ann Oncol 1995, **6**: 687–691.

672 Holland J, Trenkner DA, Wasserman TH, Fineberg B. Plasmacytoma. Treatment results and conversion to myeloma. Cancer 1992, **69**: 1513–1517.

673 Kotner LM, Wang CC. Plasmacytoma of the upper air and food passages. Cancer 1972, **30**: 414–418.

674 McKenna RW, Kyle RA, Kuehl WM, Grogan TM, Harris NL, Coupland RW. Plasma cell neoplasms. In Swerdlow SH, Campo E, Harris NL, Jaffe ES, Pileri SA, Stein H, Thiele J, Vardiman JW (eds): WHO classification of tumours of haematopoietic and lymphoid tissues. Lyon, 2008, IARC Press, pp. 200–213.

675 Meis JM, Butler JJ, Osborne BM, Ordonez MG. Solitary plasmacytomas of bone and extramedullary plasmacytomas. A clinicopathologic and immunohistochemical study. Cancer 1987, **59**: 1475–1485.

676 Meyer JE, Schulz MD. 'Solitary' myeloma of bone. A review of 12 cases. Cancer 1974, **34**: 438–440.

677 Mill WB, Griffith R. The role of radiation therapy in the management of plasma cell tumors. Cancer 1980, **45**: 647–652.

678 Peterson LC, Brown BA, Crosson JT, Mladenovic J. Application of the immunoperoxidase technic to bone marrow trephine biopsies in the classification of patients with monoclonal gammopathies. Am J Clin Pathol 1986, **85**: 688–693.

679 Strickler JG, Audeh MW, Copenhaver CM, Warnke A. Immunophenotypic differences between plasmacytoma/multiple myeloma and immunoblastic lymphoma. Cancer 1988, **61**: 1782–1786.

680 Wilder RB, Ha CS, Cox JD, Weber D, Delasalle K, Alexanian R. Persistence of myeloma protein for more than one year after radiotherapy is an adverse prognostic factor in solitary plasmacytoma of bone. Cancer 2002, **94**: 1532–1537.

681 Wiltshaw E. The natural history of extramedullary plasmacytoma and its relation to solitary myeloma of bone and myelomatosis. Medicine (Baltimore) 1976, **55**: 217–238.

682 Woodruff RK, Whittle JM, Malplas JS. Solitary plasmacytoma. Extramedullary soft tissue plasmacytoma. Cancer 1979, **43**: 2340–2343.

MONOCLONAL GAMMOPATHY OF UNDETERMINED SIGNIFICANCE

683 Cesana C, Klersy C, Barbarano L, Nosari AM, Crugnola M, Pungolino E, Gargantini L, Granata S, Valentini M, Morra E. Prognostic factors for malignant transformation in monoclonal gammopathy of undetermined significance and smoldering multiple myeloma. J Clin Oncol 2002, **20**: 1625–1634.

684 Fonseca R, Bailey RJ, Ahmann GJ, Rajkumar SV, Hoyer JD, Lust JA, Kyle RA, Gertz MA, Greipp PR, Dewald GW. Genomic abnormalities in monoclonal gammopathy of undetermined significance. Blood 2002, **100**: 1417–1424.

685 Greipp PR, Kyle RA. Clinical, morphological and cell kinetic differences among multiple myeloma, monoclonal gammopathy of undetermined significance, and smoldering multiple myeloma. Blood 1983, **62**: 166–171.

686 Kyle RA. 'Benign' monoclonal gammopathy. After 20–35 years of follow-up. Mayo Clin Proc 1993, **68**: 26–36.

687 Kyle RA, Rajkumar SV, Thermeau TM, Larson DR, Plevak MF, Melton LJ 3rd. Prognostic factors and predictors of outcome of immunoglobulin M monoclonal gammopathy of undetermined significance. Clin Lymphoma 2005, **5**: 257–260.

688 Kyle RA, Rajkumar SV. Monoclonal gammopathy of undetermined significance. Br J Haematol 2006, **134**: 573–589.

689 Kyle RA, Thermeau TM, Rajikumar SV, Larson DR, Plevak MF, Offord JR, Dispenzieri A, Katzmann JA, Melton LJ 3rd. Prevalence of monoclonal gammopathy of undetermined significance. N Engl J Med 2006, **354**: 1362–1369.

690 Kyle RA, Thermeau TM, Rajikumar SV, Remstein ED, Offord JR, Larson DR, Plevak MF, Melton LJ 3rd. Long-term follow-up of IgM monoclonal gammopathy of undetermined significance. Blood 2003, **102**: 3759–3764.

691 Kyle RA, Therneau TM, Rajkumar SV, Offord JR, Larson DR, Plevak MF, Melton LJ 3rd. A long-term study of prognosis in monoclonal gammopathy of undetermined significance. N Engl J Med 2002, **346**: 564–569.

692 Peterson LC, Brown BA, Crosson JT, Mladenovic J. Application of the immunoperoxidase technic to bone marrow trephine biopsies in the classification of patients with monoclonal gammopathies. Am J Clin Pathol 1986, **85**: 688–693.

693 Rajkumar SV, Mesa RA, Fonseca R, Schroeder G, Plevak MF, Dispenzieri A, Lacy MQ, Lust JA, Witzig TE, Gertz MA, Kyle RA, Russell SJ, Greipp PR. Bone marrow angiogenesis in 400 patients with monoclonal gammopathy of undetermined significance, multiple myeloma, and primary amyloidosis. Clin Cancer Res 2002, **8**: 2210–2216.

LYMPHOPLASMACYTIC LYMPHOMA

694 Arber DA, George TI. Bone marrow biopsy involvement by non-Hodgkin's lymphoma: frequency of lymphoma types, patterns, blood involvement, and discordance with other sites in 450 specimens. Am J Surg Pathol 2005, **29**: 1549–1557.

695 Berger F, Traverse-Glehen A, Felman P, Callet-Bauchu E, Baseggio L, Gazzo S, Thieblemont C, French M, Magaud JP, Salles G, Coiffer B. Clinicopathologic features of Waldenström's macroglobulinemia and marginal zone lymphoma: are they distinct or the same entity? Clin Lymphoma 2005, **5**: 220–224.

696 Brittin G, Tanaka Y, Brecher G. Intranuclear inclusions in multiple myeloma and macroglobulinemia. Blood 1963, **21**: 335–351.

697 Case records of the Massachusetts General Hospital (Case 6–1978). N Engl J Med 1978, **298**: 387–396.

698 Dutcher TF, Fahey JL. The histopathology of the macroglobulinemia of Waldenström. J Natl Cancer Inst 1959, **22**: 887–917.

699 Lin P, Bueso-Ramos C, Wilson CS, Mansoor A, Medeiros LJ. Waldenström macroglobulinemia involving extramedullary sites: morphologic and immunophenotypic findings in 44 patients. Am J Surg Pathol 2003, **27**: 1104–1113.

700 Non-Hodgkin's Lymphoma Classification Project. National Cancer Institute Sponsored Study of Classification of Non-Hodgkin's Lymphomas. Summary and description of a working formulation for clinical usage. Cancer 1982, **49**: 2112–2135.

701 Owen RG, Treon SP, Al-Katib A, Fonseca R, Greipp PR, McMaster ML, Morra E, Pangalis GA, San Miguel JF, Branagan AR, Dimopoulos MA. Clinicopathological definition of Waldenström's macroglobulinemia: consensus panel recommendations from the Second International Workshop on Waldenström's Macroglobulinemia. Semin Oncol 2003, **30**: 110–115.

702 Pangalis GA, Nathwani BN, Rappaport H. Malignant lymphoma, well differentiated lymphocytic. Its relationship with chronic lymphocytic leukemia and macroglobulinemia of Waldenström. Cancer 1977, **39**: 999–1010.

703 Rywlin AW, Civantos F, Ortega RS, Dominguez CJ. Bone marrow histology in monoclonal macroglobulinemia. Am J Clin Pathol 1975, **63**: 769–778.

704 Swerdlow SH, Berger F, Pileri SA, Harris NL, Jaffee ES, Stein H. Lymphoplasmacytic lymphoma. In Swerdlow SH, Campo E, Harris NL, Jaffe ES, Pileri SA, Stein H, Thiele J, Vardiman JW (eds): WHO classification of tumours of haematopoietic and lymphoid tissues. Lyon, 2008, IARC Press, pp. 194–195.

705 Tubbs RR, Hoffman GC, Deodhar SD, Hewlett JS. IgM monoclonal gammopathy. Histopathologic and clinical spectrum. Cleve Clin Q 1976, **43**: 217–235.

706 Tursz T, Brouet J, Flandrin G, Danon F, Clauvel JP, Seligmann M. Clinical and pathologic features of Waldenström's macroglobulinemia in seven patients with serum monoclonal IgG or IgA. Am J Med 1977, **63**: 499–502.

707 Waldenström J. Incipient myelomatosis or 'essential' hypergammaglobulinemia with fibrinogenopenia. A new syndrome. Acta Med Scand 1944, **117**: 216–247.

HEAVY CHAIN DISEASE

708 Frangione B, Franklin EC. Heavy chain diseases. Clinical features and molecular significance of the disordered immunoglobulin structure. Semin Hematol 1973, **10**: 53–64.

709 Franklin EC. Mu-chain disease. Arch Intern Med 1975, **135**: 71–72.

710 Harris NL, Isaacson PG, Grogan TM, Jaffee ES. Heavy chain diseases. In Swerdlow SH, Campo E, Harris NL, Jaffe ES, Pileri SA, Stein H, Thiele J, Vardiman JW (eds): WHO classification of tumours of haematopoietic and lymphoid tissues. Lyon, 2008, IARC Press, pp. 196–199.

711 Jonsson V, Videbaek A, Axelsen NH, Harboe M. Mu-chain disease in a case of chronic lymphocytic leukemia and malignant histiocytoma. I. Clinical aspects. Scand J Haematol 1976, **16**: 209–217.

712 Kyle RA, Greipp PR, Banks PM. The diverse picture of gamma heavy-chain disease. Report of seven cases and review of literature. Mayo Clin Proc 1981, **56**: 439–451.

713 Seligmann M, Preud'Homme JL, Brouet JC. Membrane markers in human lymphoid malignancies. Clinicopathological correlations

and insights into the differentiation of normal and neoplastic cells. In Clarkson B, Marks P, Till JR (eds): Differentiation of normal and neoplastic hematopoietic cells. Cold Spring Harbor, NY, 1978, Cold Spring Harbor Laboratory, pp. 859–876.

714 Seligmann M. Immunochemical, clinical, and pathologic features of alpha-chain disease. Arch Intern Med 1975, **135**: 78–82.

AMYLOIDOSIS

715 Banerjee D, Mills DM, Hearn SA, Meek M, Turner KL. Proteinaceous lymphadenopathy due to monoclonal nonamyloid immunoglobulin deposit disease. Arch Pathol Lab Med 1990, **114**: 34–39.

716 Buxbaum JN, Chuba JV, Hellman GC, Solomon A, Gallo GR. Monoclonal immunoglobulin deposition disease: light chain and light and heavy chain deposition diseases and their relation to light chain amyloidosis. Clinical features, immunopathology and molecular analysis. Ann Intern Med 1990, **112**: 455–464.

717 Falk RH, Comenzo RL, Skinner M. The systemic amyloidoses. N Engl J Med 1997, **337**: 898–909.

718 Feiner HD. Pathology of dysproteinemia: light chain amyloidosis, non-amyloid immunoglobulin deposition disease, cryoglobulinemia syndromes, and macroglobulinemia of Waldenström. Hum Pathol 1988, **19**: 1255–1272.

719 Gertz MA, Greipp PR, Kyle RA. Classification of amyloidosis by the detection of clonal excess of plasma cells in the bone marrow. J Lab Clin Med 1991, **118**: 33–39.

720 Gertz MA, Kyle RA. Primary systemic amyloidosis. A diagnostic primer. Mayo Clin Proc 1989, **64**: 1505–1519.

721 Jacobs P, Ruff P, Wood L, Moodley D, Mansvelt E. Amyloidosis: a changing clinical perspective. Hematology 2007, **12**: 163–167.

722 Kyle RA, Gertz M. Primary systemic amyloidosis. Clinical and laboratory features in 474 cases. Semin Hematol 1995, **32**: 45–59.

723 Kyle RA, Greipp PR. Amyloidosis (AL). Clinical and laboratory features in 229 cases. Mayo Clin Proc 1983, **58**: 665–683.

724 McKenna RW, Kyle RA, Kuehl WM, Grogan TM, Harris NL, Coupland RW. Plasma cell neoplasms. In Swerdlow SH, Campo E, Harris NL, Jaffe ES, Pileri SA, Stein H, Thiele J, Vardiman JW (eds): WHO classification of tumours of haematopoietic and lymphoid tissues. Lyon, 2008, IARC Press, pp. 200–213.

725 Osborne BM, Butler JJ, Mackay B. Proteinaceous lymphadenopathy with hypergammaglobulinemia. Am J Surg Pathol 1979, **3**: 137–145.

726 Wolf BC, Kumar A, Vera JC, Neiman RS. Bone marrow morphology and immunology in systemic amyloidosis. Am J Clin Pathol 1986, **86**: 84–88.

SYSTEMIC POLYCLONAL B-IMMUNOBLASTIC PROLIFERATION

727 Hanto DW, Frizzera G, Purtilo DT, Sakamoto K, Sullivan JL, Saemundsen AK, Klein G, Simmons RL, Najarian JS. Clinical spectrum of lymphoproliferative disorders in renal transplant recipients and evidence for the role of Epstein–Barr virus. Cancer Res 1981, **41**: 4253–4261.

728 Koo CH, Nathwani BN, Winberg CD, Hill LR, Rappaport H. Atypical lymphoplasmacytic and immunoblastic proliferation in lymph nodes of patients with autoimmune disease (autoimmune disease-associated lymphadenopathy). Medicine (Baltimore) 1984, **63**: 274–290.

729 Peterson LC, Brown BA, Crosson JT, Mladenovic J. Application of the immunoperoxidase technic to bone marrow trephine biopsies in the classification of patients with monoclonal gammopathies. Am J Clin Pathol 1986, **85**: 688–693.

730 Peterson LC, Kueck B, Arthur DC, Dedeker K, Brunning RD. Systemic polyclonal immunoblastic proliferations. Cancer 1988, **61**: 1350–1358.

731 Poje EJ, Soori GS, Weisenburger DD. Systemic polyclonal B-immunoblastic proliferation with marked peripheral blood and bone marrow plasmacytosis. Am J Clin Pathol 1992, **98**: 222–226.

METASTATIC TUMORS

732 Anner RM, Drewinko B. Frequency and significance of bone marrow involvement by metastatic solid tumors. Cancer 1977, **39**: 1337–1344.

733 Ballestrero A, Coviello DA, Garuti A, Nencioni A, Famà A, Rocco I, Bertorelli R, Ferrando F, Gonella R, Patrone F. Reverse-transcriptase polymerase chain reaction of the maspin gene in the detection of bone marrow breast carcinoma cell contamination. Cancer 1992, **92**: 2030–2035.

734 Bezwoda WR, Lewis D, Livini N. Bone marrow involvement in anaplastic small cell lung cancer. Cancer 1986, **58**: 1762–1765.

735 Bostrom BB, Nesbitt ME, Brunning RD. The value of bone marrow biopsy in the diagnosis of metastatic neuroblastoma. Am J Pediatr Hematol Oncol 1985, **7**: 301–305.

736 Bramwell VHC, Littley MB, Chang J, Crowther D. Bone marrow involvement in adult soft tissue sarcoma. Eur J Cancer Clin Oncol 1982, **18**: 1099–1106.

737 Brodeur GM, Pritchard J, Berthold F, Carlsen NL, Castel V, Castelberry RP, De Bernardi B, Evans AE, Favrot M, Hedborg F, et al. Revisions of the international criteria for neuroblastoma diagnosis, staging, and response to treatment. J Clin Oncol 1993, **11**: 1466–1477.

738 Brunning RD, Bloomfield CD, McKenna RW, Peterson LA. Bilateral trephine bone marrow biopsies in lymphoma and other neoplastic diseases. Ann Intern Med 1975, **82**: 365–366.

739 Ceci G, Franciosi V, Passalacqua R, Di Blasio B, Boni C, Lottici R, De Lisi V, Nizzoli R, Guazzi A, Cocconi G. The value of bone marrow biopsy in breast cancer at the time of first relapse. A prospective study. Cancer 1988, **61**: 1041–1045.

740 Cheung NK, Heller G, Kushner BH, Liu C, Cheung IY. Detection of metastatic neuroblastoma in bone marrow: when is routine histology insensitive? J Clin Oncol 1997, **15**: 2807–2817.

741 Clamon GH, Edwards WR, Hamous JE, Scupham RK. Patterns of bone marrow involvement with small cell lung cancer. Cancer 1984, **54**: 100–102.

742 Cote RJ, Rosen PP, Hakes TB, Sedira M, Bazinet M, Kinne DW, Old LJ, Osborne MP. Monoclonal antibodies detect occult breast carcinoma metastases in the bone marrow of patients with early stage disease. Am J Surg Pathol 1988, **12**: 333–340.

743 Cote RJ, Rosen PP, Lesser ML, Old LJ, Osborne MP. Prediction of early relapse in patients with operable breast cancer by detection of occult bone marrow micrometastases. J Clin Oncol 1991, **9**: 1749–1756.

744 Diel IJ, Kaufmann M, Goerner R, Costa SD, Kaul S, Bastert G. Detection of tumor cells in bone marrow of patients with primary breast cancer. A prognostic factor for distant metastasis. J Clin Oncol 1992, **10**: 1534–1539.

745 Finklestein JZ, Ekert H, Isaacs H, Higgins G. Bone marrow metastases in children with solid tumors. Am J Dis Child 1976, **119**: 49–52.

746 Hansen HH, Muggia FM, Selawry OS. Bone-marrow examination in 100 consecutive patients with bronchogenic carcinoma. Lancet 1971, **2**: 443–445.

747 Hirsch F, Hansen HH, Dombernowsky P, Hainau B. Bone-marrow examination in the staging of small-cell anaplastic carcinoma of the lung with special reference to subtyping. Cancer 1977, **39**: 2563–2567.

748 Ingle JN, Tormey DC, Tan HK. The bone marrow examination in breast cancer. Diagnostic considerations and clinical usefulness. Cancer 1978, **41**: 670–674.

749 Kelly BW, Morris JF, Harwood BP, Bruya TE. Methods and prognostic value of bone marrow examination in small cell carcinoma of the lung. Cancer 1984, **53**: 99–102.

750 Krishnan C, George TI, Arber DA. Bone marrow metastases: survey of non-hematologic metastases with immunohistochemical study of metastatic carcinomas. Appl Immunohistochem Mol Morphol 2007, **15**: 1–7.

751 Krishnan C, Twist CJ, Fu T, Arber DA. Detection of isolated tumor cells in neuroblastoma by immunohistochemical analysis in bone marrow biopsy specimens: improved detection with use of beta-catenin. Am J Clin Pathol 2009, **131**: 49–57.

752 Kristjansen PEG, Osterlind K, Hansen M. Detection of bone marrow relapse in patients with small cell carcinoma of the lung. Cancer 1986, **58**: 2538–2541.

753 Landys K. Prognostic value of bone marrow biopsy in breast cancer. Cancer 1982, **49**: 513–518.

754 Lawrence JB, Eleff M, Behm FG, Johnston CL Jr. Bone marrow examination in small cell carcinoma of the lung. Comparison of trephine biopsy with aspiration. Cancer 1984, **53**: 2188–2190.

755 Levitan N, Byrne RE, Bromer RH, Faling LJ, Caslowitz P, Pattern DH, Hong WK. The value of the bone scan and bone marrow biopsy in staging small cell lung cancer. Cancer 1985, **56**: 652–654.

756 Lyda MH, Tetef M, Carter N, Ikle D, Weiss L, Arber DA. Keratin immunohistochemistry detects clinically significant metastases in bone marrow biopsy specimens in women with lobular breast carcinoma. Am J Surg Pathol 2000, **24**: 1593–1599.

757 Mead GM, Williams CJ, Thompson J, Smith AG, Whitehouse JMA. Bone marrow examination in small cell carcinoma of the bronchus. An unnecessary procedure? Hematol Oncol 1985, **3**: 159–163.

758 Meinhausen J, Choritz H, Georgii A. Frequency of skeletal metastases as revealed by routinely taken bone marrow biopsies. Virchows Arch [A] 1980, **389**: 409–417.

759 Pantel K, Izbicki JR, Angstwurm M, Braun S, Passlick B, Karg O, Thetter O, Riethmüller G. Immunocytological detection of bone marrow micrometastasis in operable non-small cell lung cancer. Cancer Res 1993, **53**: 1027–1031.

760 Penchansky L. Bone marrow biopsy in the metastatic work-up of solid tumors in children. Cancer 1984, **54**: 1447–1448.

761 Lo Piccolo MSL, Cheung NK, Cheung IY. GD2 synthase: a new molecular marker for detecting neuroblastoma. Cancer 2001, **92**: 924–931.

762 Reid MM, Hamilton PJ. Histology of neuroblastoma involving bone marrow. The problem of detecting residual tumour after initiation of chemotherapy. Br J Haematol 1988, **69**: 487–490.

763 Ridell B, Landys K. Incidence and histopathology of metastases of mammary carcinoma in biopsies from the posterior iliac crest. Cancer 1979, **44**: 1782–1788.

764 Ruymann FB, Newton WA, Ragab AH, Donaldson MH, Foulkes M. Bone marrow metastases at diagnosis in children and adolescents with rhabdomyosarcoma. A report from the Intergroup Rhabdomyosarcoma Study. Cancer 1984, **53**: 368–373.

765 Seeger RC, Reynolds CP, Gallego R, Strum DO, Gerbing RB, Matthay KK. Quantitative tumor cell content of bone marrow and blood as a prediction of outcome in stage IV neuroblastoma: a children's cancer group study. J Clin Oncol 2000, **18**: 4067–4076.

766 Singh G, Krause JR, Breitfeld V. Bone marrow examination for metastatic tumor, aspiration and biopsy. Cancer 1977, **40**: 2317–2321.

767 Wang J, Weiss LM, Chang KL, Slovak ML, Gaal K, Forman SJ, Arber DA. Diagnostic utility of bilateral bone marrow examination: significance of morphologic and ancillary technique study in malignancy. Cancer 2002, **94**: 1522–1531.

LIPID STORAGE DISEASES

GAUCHER DISEASE

768 Barranger JA, Ginns BI. Glucosylceramide lipidoses: Gaucher disease. In Scriver CR, Beaudet AL, Sly WS, Valle E (eds): The metabolic basis of inherited disease, ed. 6. New York, 1989, McGraw-Hill Book Co., pp. 1655–1676.

769 Beck M. New therapeutic options for lysosomal storage disorders: enzyme replacement, small molecules and gene therapy. Hum Genet 2007, **121**: 1–22.

770 Brady RO, Barranger JA. Glucosyl ceramide lipidosis. Gaucher's disease. In Stanbury JB, Wyngaarden JB, Fredrickson DS, Goldstein JL, Brown MS (eds): The metabolic basis of inherited disease. New York, 1983, McGraw-Hill Book Co., pp. 842–856.

771 Brunning RD. Morphologic alterations in nucleated blood and marrow cells in genetic disorders. Hum Pathol 1970, **1**: 99–124.

772 Burrow TA, Hopkin RJ, Leslie ND, Tinkle BT, Grabowski GA. Enzyme reconstitution/replacement therapy for lysosomal storage diseases. Curr Opin Pediatr 2007, **19**: 628–635.

773 Chen M, Wang J. Gaucher disease: review of the literature. Arch Pathol Lab Med 2008, **132**: 851–853.

774 Dosik H, Rosner F, Sawitsky A. Acquired lipidosis. Gaucher-like cells and 'blue cells' in chronic granulocytic leukemia. Semin Hematol 1972, **9**: 309–316.

775 Grabowski A, Leslie N. Lysosomal storage diseases: perspectives and principles. In Hoffman R, Benz EJ, Shattil SJ, Furie B, Cohen HJ, Silberstein LE, McGlave P (eds): Hematology: basic principles and practice, ed. 4. Edinburgh, 2005, Churchill Livingstone, pp. 873–890.

776 Hansen HG, Graucob E. Hematologic cytology of storage disease. New York, 1985, Springer-Verlag.

777 Imcerti C. Gaucher disease: an overview. Semin Hematol 1995, **32**(Suppl): 3–9.

778 Jmoudiak M, Futerman AH. Gaucher disease: pathological mechanisms and modern management. Br J Haematol 2005, **129**: 178–188.

779 Pratt PW, Estren S, Kochwa S. Immunoglobulin abnormalities in Gaucher's disease. Report of 16 cases. Blood 1968, **31**: 633–640.

780 Ruestow PC, Levinson DJ, Catchatourian R, Sreekanth S, Cohen H, Rosenfeld S. Coexistence of IgA myeloma and Gaucher's disease. Arch Intern Med 1980, **140**: 1115–1116.

781 Zaino EC, Rossi MB, Pham TD, Azar H. Gaucher's cells in thalassemia. Blood 1971, **38**: 457–462.

NIEMANN–PICK DISEASE

782 Brunning RD. Morphologic alterations in nucleated blood and marrow cells in genetic disorders. Hum Pathol 1970, **1**: 99–124.

783 Burrow TA, Hopkin RJ, Leslie ND, Tinkle BT, Grabowski GA. Enzyme reconstitution/replacement therapy for lysosomal storage diseases. Curr Opin Pediatr 2007, **19**: 628–635.

784 Grabowski A, Leslie N. Lysosomal storage diseases: perspectives and principles. In Hoffman R, Benz EJ, Shattil SJ, Furie B, Cohen HJ, Silberstein LE, McGlave P (eds): Hematology: basic principles and practice, ed. 4. Edinburgh, 2005, Churchill Livingstone, pp. 873–890.

785 Hansen HG, Graucob E. Hematologic cytology of storage disease. New York, 1985, Springer-Verlag.

786 Patterson MC, Vanier MT, Suzuki K, Morris JA, Carsteu E, Neufeld EB, Blanchette-Mackie JE, Pentcheu DG. Niemann–Pick disease type C. A lipid trafficking disorder. In Scriver CR, Beaudet AL, Sly WS, Valle D (eds): The metabolic and molecular basis of inherited disease, ed. 8, vol. II. New York, 2001, Mulencer Hill, pp. 3611–3634.

787 Schuchman EH, Desnick RJ. Niemann–Pick disease types A and B. Acid sphingomyelinase deficiencies. In Scriver CR, Beaudet AL, Sly WS, Valle D (eds): The metabolic and molecular basis of inherited disease, ed. 8, vol. II. New York, 2001, Mulencer Hill, pp. 3589–3610.

FABRY DISEASE

788 Brunning RD. Morphologic alterations in nucleated blood and marrow cells in genetic disorders. Hum Pathol 1970, **1**: 99–124.

789 Burrow TA, Hopkin RJ, Leslie ND, Tinkle BT, Grabowski GA. Enzyme reconstitution/replacement therapy for lysosomal storage diseases. Curr Opin Pediatr 2007, **19**: 628–635.

SEA-BLUE HISTIOCYTE SYNDROME

790 Hansen HG, Graucob E. Hematologic cytology of storage disease. New York, 1985, Springer-Verlag.

791 Rausing A. Bone marrow biopsy in diagnosis of Whipple's disease. Acta Med Scand 1973, **193**: 5–8.

792 Silverstein MN, Ellefson RD, Ahern EF. The syndrome of the sea-blue histiocyte. N Engl J Med 1970, **282**: 1–4.

HEMATOPOIETIC STEM CELL TRANSPLANTATION

793 Baron F, Sandmaier BM. Chimerism and outcomes after allogeneic hematopoietic cell transplantation following nonmyeloablative conditioning. Leukemia 2006, **20**: 1690–1700.

794 Blume KG, Forman SJ, Appelbaum FR (eds): Hematopoietic cell transplantation, ed. 3. London, 2004, Blackwell Publishing Ltd.

795 Eapen M, Rubinstein P, Zhang MJ, Stevens C, Kurtzberg J, Scaradavou A, Loberiza FR, Champlin RE, Klein JP, Horowitz MM, Wagner JE. Outcomes of transplantation of unrelated donor umbilical cord blood and bone marrow in children with acute leukaemia: a comparison study. Lancet 2007, **369**: 1947–1954.

796 Hurwitz N. Bone marrow changes following chemotherapy and/or bone marrow transplantation. Curr Diagn Pathol 1997, **4**: 196–200.

797 Naeim F, Smith GS, Gale RP. Morphologic aspects of bone marrow transplantation in patients with aplastic anemia. Hum Pathol 1978, **9**: 295–308.

798 Sale GB, Buckner CD. Pathology of bone marrow in transplant recipients. Hematol Oncol Clin North Am 1988, **2**: 735–756.

799 Sloane JP, Norton J. The pathology of bone marrow transplantation. Histopathology 1993, **22**: 201–209.

800 Van Den Berg H, Kluin PhM, Zwaan FE, Vossen JM. Histopathology of bone marrow reconstitution after allogeneic bone marrow transplantation. Histopathology 1989, **15**: 363–373.

Bone and joints

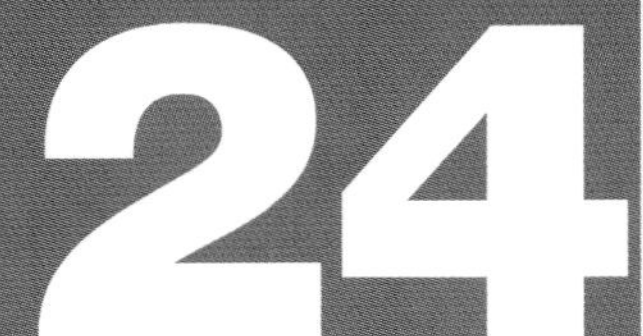

CHAPTER CONTENTS

Bone

Normal anatomy

Adult bones are classified according to their shape into long (such as femur), flat (such as pelvis), and short (such as bones of hand and feet). Long bones (and some short bones such as metacarpal bones) are divided topographically into three regions: diaphysis, epiphysis, and metaphysis. The diaphysis is the shaft. The epiphysis is at both ends of the bone and is partially covered by articular cartilage. The metaphysis is at the junction of the diaphysis and epiphysis. In the growing bone, it begins at the epiphyseal plate (epiphyseal disk, physis). This is the place where endochondral ossification takes place, a process by which longitudinal, regularly spaced columns of vascularized cartilage are replaced by bone.[19] When the bone has reached its adult length, this process ends, and the epiphysis 'closes' by becoming totally ossified. The time of closure of the epiphysis differs in various bones and in the sexes. The epiphyseal plate is very important in bone pathology because it is by far the most common site of occurrence of most primary bone tumors. In addition, whether the epiphysis is closed or open influences the extension of pathologic processes, in the sense that cartilage is often at least a partial barrier to spreading osteosarcoma. If the epiphysis is closed and cartilage is no longer present, this area is more easily invaded.[8]

Bones are also classified according to their embryologic development. The two main categories are *membranous* (such as the skull), if formed de novo from primitive connective tissue, and *endochondral* (such as long bones), if their formation is preceded by a cartilaginous anlage.[4,19]

On cross section, mature bones are seen formed by an outer *compact layer* (cortex, cortical bone, compact bone) and a central *spongy region* (spongiosa, medulla, cancellous bone). Compact bone contains vascular channels, which are divided into two types on the basis of their orientation and their relation to the lamellar structure of the surrounding bone: longitudinal (haversian canals) and transverse/oblique (Volkmann canals). Except for the region of the articular cartilage, the cortex is surrounded by the *periosteum*, which consists of an outer fibrous layer and an inner cellular (cambium) layer of osteoprogenitor cells (fibroblasts and osteoblasts). It contains nerve filaments that carry proprioceptive and sensory impulses; small nerve filaments also may pass with the nutrient vessels into the medullary canal. Coarse bundles of collagenous fibers penetrating the outer compact layer from the outer layer of the periosteum are called Sharpey fibers or perforating fibers.[19]

The periosteum may become detached and elevated from the bone in pathologic processes such as trauma, infection, and primary or secondary malignant tumors. Whenever this happens, new bone formation between the elevated periosteum and the bone will occur. This appears by radiographic examination as fine spicules placed perpendicular to the long axis of the bone. This finding is often considered a manifestation of a primary malignant neoplasm, particularly osteosarcoma and Ewing sarcoma. However, periosteal bone proliferation also can occur in syphilis, tuberculosis, metastatic carcinoma, and subperiosteal hematoma. In some lesions, such as plasma cell myeloma, the periosteum may be destroyed or encroached upon so that no radiographic changes occur.

An understanding of the blood supply of bone helps to explain the spread and limitation of infection, the healing of fractures, and the involvement of bone by primary or secondary neoplasms. The metaphysis is mainly supplied by end arteries that enter from the diaphysis and terminate at the level of the epiphyseal plate. The epiphyses receive their blood supply from a network of widely anastomosing vessels. The diaphyseal cortex is supplied by vessels that enter through Volkmann canals and communicate with the haversian system. A nutrient artery enters the medullary canal at about the center of the diaphysis, divides, and extends both distally and proximally. The metabolic exchange of calcium and phosphorus occurs primarily in the metaphysis. Lymph vessels exist in the connective tissue overlying the periosteum, but apparently not in the cortex or medulla.[7]

Osteoblasts are bone-producing cells derived from marrow-residing mesenchymal cells. They have a plump appearance and often exhibit a perinuclear halo resulting from a prominent Golgi zone that gives them a resemblance to plasma cells. They have a high cytoplasmic content of alkaline phosphatase. Ultrastructurally, they resemble fibroblasts by virtue of a well-developed rough endoplasmic reticulum and Golgi apparatus. Indeed, osteoblasts are regarded as a specialized ('sophisticated') form of fibroblast.[6] Once these are incorporated into the bone matrix and housed in lacunae, they are referred to as *osteocytes*.

Osteoclasts are multinucleated giant cells involved in bone resorption.[20] As such, they often are found in shallow concavities in the surface of bone called *Howship lacunae*. Osteoclasts arise from mononuclear monocyte–macrophage precursors.[21] Osteoclasts contain abundant tartrate-resistant acid phosphatase, respond to osteotropic hormones, and contract under the influence of calcitonin. They express osteoclast-specific antigens (detected by monoclonal antibodies 13c2 and 23c6) and various matrix metalloproteinases;[16] they are instead unreactive for T-cell antigens, most myeloid antigens, and mature macrophage antigens.[13]

Ultrastructurally, the cytoplasm of osteoclasts has a very large number of mitochondria and scanty lysosomes; a ruffled edge is present in the area of the cell membrane that is in the process of bone resorption.

Osteoid is the unmineralized organic precursor matrix of bone. It is composed of a mixture of collagen (mainly type I), acid mucopolysaccharides, and noncollagen proteins.[11] These include osteopontin,[15,18] osteocalcin,[17] and bone morphogenetic protein.[22] The latter is thought to play a critical role in initiating the process that begins with cartilage resorption and ends with bone formation.[23] Osteoid is not a homogeneous mass but rather shows a constant, patterned sequence of maturation and organization.[9] It has

acidophilic properties in hematoxylin–eosin-stained sections, and it may be difficult to distinguish from hyalinized collagen.

Bone is formed through mineralization of the organic matrix of the osteoid.[10] Extracellular matrix vesicles are present at or near the mineralization front and constitute the initial site of hydroxyapatite mineral deposition.[2] In *woven bone* (fiber bone), there is a haphazard arrangement of collagen fibers within the matrix, which is best appreciated with reticulum stains or under polarized light. Formation of woven bone is the key criterion for the diagnosis of fibrous dysplasia, but it also appears in any condition associated with accelerated bone turnover, such as the callus of a healing fracture or osteitis fibrosa cystica. The difference resides in the fact that in the latter group the woven bone eventually becomes lamellar bone, whereas in fibrous dysplasia it does not. *Lamellar bone* is characterized by concentric parallel lamellae, as seen with examination under polarizing lenses.

Normal skeletal growth results from a balance between the processes of bone matrix synthesis and resorption, these activities being regulated by systemic and local factors.[1,4,14] Of these, transforming growth factor (TGF)-β activity is particularly important for bone matrix production.[5] Vitamin D and parathyroid hormone (PTH) also play an important role.[12] Molecules thought to regulate the growth plate thickness and bone length through their action on chondrocytes during endochondral ossification are fibroblast growth factor receptor-3, PTH-related protein, and tartrate-resistant acid phosphatase.[4] Some proteins seem to act as negative regulators of bone cell function, e.g., osteoprotegerin in osteoclasts, and osteocalcin, bone sialoprotein, and 5-lipoxygenase in osteoblasts.[4]

Bone necrosis can be recognized by the staining quality of the dead bone, which is a deeper blue than normal bone. Lacunar cells are absent, and the margins of the bone are ragged (Fig. 24.1). The presence of osteoclasts on these margins indicates that the necrotic bone is already being reabsorbed.

Bone production can be recognized by the presence of well-stained small spicules of bone with cells in their lacunae and a prominent row of osteoblasts along their margins. New bone formation can be found in a variety of physiologic and pathologic processes, such as a healing fracture, Paget disease, metaplastic ossification, myositis ossificans, and osteitis fibrosa cystica.

Bone resorption (*destruction*) can be recognized by the presence of numerous osteoclasts in the bone margins and in Howship lacunae. It can involve necrotic bone, as indicated above, or viable bone, as in osteitis fibrosa cystica.

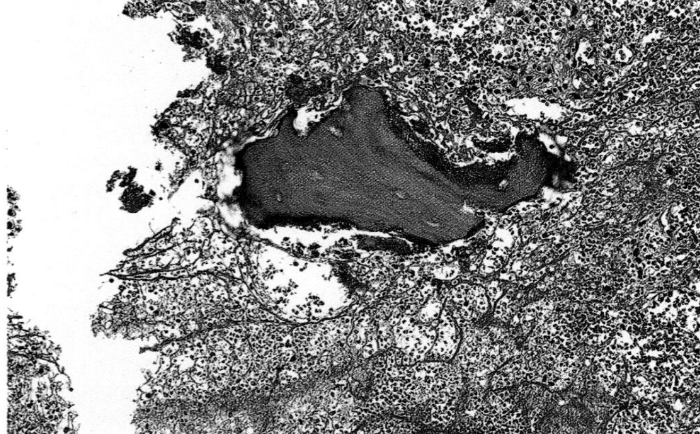

Fig. 24.1 The necrotic nature of this bone fragment is recognized because of the ragged basophilic edges and the empty lacunae.

Skeletal substitute material of an increasingly varying nature is being used by orthopedic surgeons to replace or 'extend' bone autographs, and these can be found by the pathologist in biopsy and resection specimens in which a previous operation had taken place. Bauer[3] has provided a useful list of these substitutes and the criteria for their recognition.

Metabolic bone diseases

A thorough discussion of metabolic bone diseases is outside the scope of this chapter. Some metabolic bone diseases will be mentioned briefly, but for a detailed discussion the reader is referred to the books, monographs, and excellent articles that have been written on the subject.[24,25,28,30,32,33,36–38,44–46]

Osteoporosis refers to a decreased mass of normally mineralized bone.[39,48] It develops when an individual is unable to repair and maintain the mass of bone tissue that has been acquired throughout growth and maturation.[41] Quantitative microradiographic studies have shown that the main difference between the bone in most forms of osteoporosis and normal bone is an increase in the amount of resorption, bone formation levels being generally normal.[34] Osteoporosis occurs frequently after menopause, presumably because of estrogen deficiency. The causes of osteoporosis are multiple.[40] Fluoride consumption has been shown to be important in its prevention.[27,42]

A good biopsy specimen from the iliac crest will show changes that correspond well with those in the spine.[26] Routine radiographic examination of the spine is not reliable, since the changes cannot be seen until they are advanced. Studies made at autopsy by Caldwell[29] have helped to clarify some issues. For instance, he showed that vertebral biconcavity is not a reliable index of osteoporosis, as commonly believed at the time.

The treatment of osteoporosis is based on medications that slow down bone resorption by inhibiting the formation or activity of osteoclasts, and on those that promote bone formation, such as growth factors and hormones.[43]

Osteomalacia (comparable to rickets in a young person in whom the epiphyses are not yet closed) refers to the accumulation of unmineralized bone matrix resulting from a diminished rate of mineralization. It may be secondary to a wide spectrum of congenital and acquired metabolic abnormalities that result in sufficient decrease in serum calcium, phosphorus, or both to impair mineralization of the skeleton and epiphyseal growth.[35] Some cases have been seen as a complication of bone and soft tissue neoplasms (see Chapter 25). Osteomalacia changes can be demonstrated in adequate biopsies from long bones and iliac crests with preparation of nondecalcified specimens and examination with bright-field and phase-contrast microscopes and with the use of fluorescent tetracycline markers.[31]

Sophisticated methods of investigating these metabolic bone processes have been devised, but many of them are difficult to implement in the routine pathology laboratory.[47]

Fractures

Fractures are breaks in the continuity of bone, usually with severance of periosteum, blood vessels, and sometimes muscles. The speed of return of bone to a normal state following fracture depends on factors such as the age and nutrition of the patient, severity of the fracture, vascularity of the area, and type of treatment. Fractures may fail to heal because of improper immobilization, complete devascularization of the fractured bone segments, persistent infection, and interposition of soft tissue between the ends of the bone.

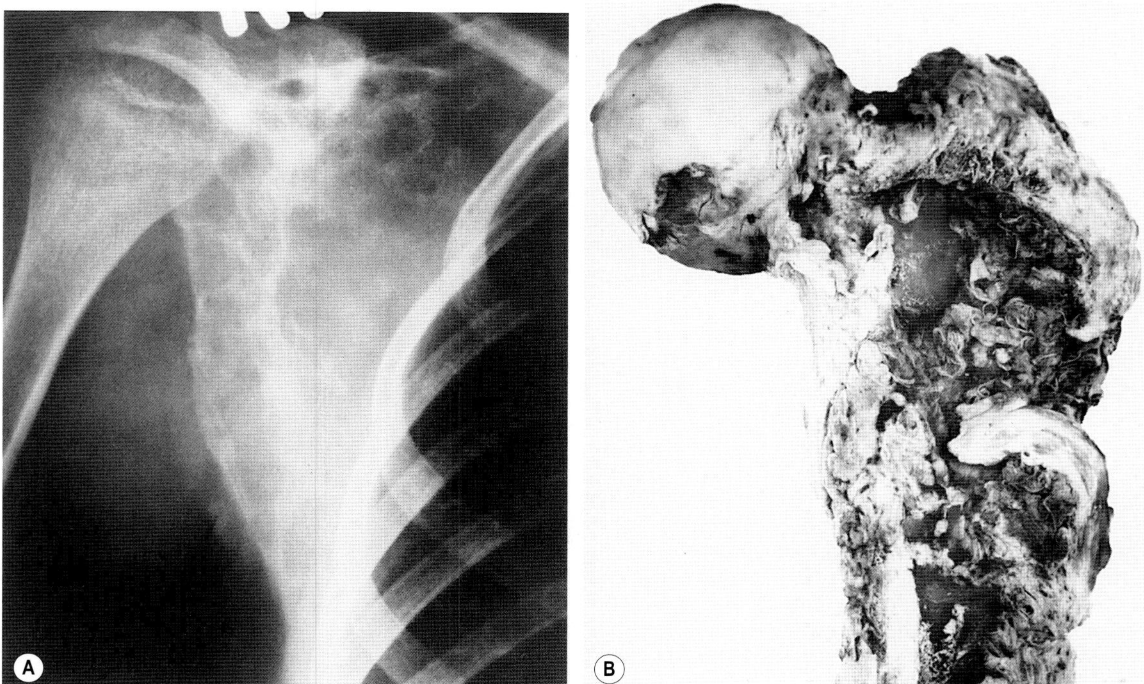

Fig. 24.2 **A**, Extensive involvement of scapula by osteomyelitis of staphylococcal origin in an 8-year-old child. This was apparently the only bone involved. **B**, Osteomyelitis of upper femur with massive bone destruction and reactive sclerosis.
*(**A**, Courtesy of Dr P Flynn, Redding, CA)*

Following a fracture, a hematoma forms between the two severed ends of bone. Organization of this hematoma begins with the ingrowth of young capillaries. After about 3 days, the devitalized bone fragments begin to be reabsorbed. Intramembranous bone growth makes its appearance from the inner layer of the periosteum, both proximal and distal to the fracture site. The newly formed trabeculae begin to calcify as the cartilage is replaced by bone. This process on each side of the fracture meets at the fracture site to form the primary callus. This is later reabsorbed and replaced by the secondary callus, which is made up of mature lamellar bone. The new bone is laid down predominantly along lines of stress. The formation and persistence of cartilage largely depend on mechanical factors.[51]

With early proper reduction of the fracture, adequate blood supply, no infection, and normal metabolism, the fracture heals rapidly with little visible callus. Exuberant callus usually means slow fracture healing. In children, even with prominent angulation or deformity, the bone remodels itself to an astonishing degree. For this reason, open reduction and internal fixation of fractures in children are seldom justified. Shortening of a long bone resulting from overriding of fragments will nearly always correct itself in children by overgrowth of bone.

The formation of exuberant cartilage and disorderly membranous bone in rapidly forming primary callus results in a bewildering microscopic pattern that may be confused with osteosarcoma. This phenomenon is particularly luxuriant in osteogenesis imperfecta.[52]

When a noncorrosive nail is driven into a bone to immobilize a fracture, it eventually becomes completely isolated from the bone substance.[49] The nail is separated from the medullary cavity by fibrous tissue that is continuous with the periosteum. Compact-type bone forms adjacent to the fibrous tissue. At a later stage, this becomes continuous with the original bone cortex. No foreign body giant cell reaction is observed.[50]

Osteomyelitis

Bacterial osteomyelitis may be caused by a large variety of microorganisms. About 70–90% of the cases are due to coagulase-positive staphylococci[68] (Fig. 24.2A). Other organisms involved are *Klebsiella, Aerobacter, Proteus, Pseudomonas, Streptococcus*, pneumococcus, gonococcus, meningococcus, *Brucella*, and *Salmonella*.[64,70] The latter organism is often involved in the osteomyelitis that affects individuals with abnormal hemoglobin, particularly sickle cell disease.[56]

Osteomyelitis may be due to local or exogenous causes (such as compound fractures)[54] or may develop through the hematogenous route. The latter occurs most often in patients under 20 years of age and involves the bones of the lower extremity in about 75% of cases. It can be acute, subacute, or chronic, these designations referring to the duration of the disease rather than the microscopic composition of the inflammatory infiltrate. A form of osteomyelitis characterized by recurrent multifocal involvement in children, sometimes associated with palmoplantar pustulosis, has been described; bacterial cultures are negative and the etiology is unknown.[61]

Subacute and chronic osteomyelitis can closely simulate clinically and radiographically a malignant bone tumor (particularly Ewing sarcoma, malignant lymphoma, and osteosarcoma) by virtue of the combination of destructive and regenerative bone changes[55] (Fig. 24.2B). Hematogenous pyogenic vertebral osteomyelitis is frequently underdiagnosed radiographically because of the subtle nature of the disease.[60] A variant of osteomyelitis characterized by very extensive regenerative bone changes is referred to as Garre

osteomyelitis, sclerosing osteomyelitis, or periostitis ossificans. This form is particularly common in the jawbone.[59]

The morphologic changes in osteomyelitis are conditioned by the age of the patient, bone involved (particularly in regard to its blood supply), virulence of the organism, and resistance of the host.[67] In the infant under 1 year of age, permanent epiphyseal damage and joint infection occur, but there is little damage to the metaphysis or diaphysis. In children over 1 year of age the reverse is true, in the sense that cortical metaphyseal involvement is extensive, whereas permanent damage to cartilage and joints is rare. From its center in the metaphysis, the infection permeates the cortex through the vessels of Volkmann canals and may spread along the medullary canal to the rest of the bone. If pus accumulates beneath the periosteum, perforation through it usually takes place. The dead bone (sequestrum) is later surrounded by new bone laid down by the cambium layer of the periosteum (involucrum), and this may eventually extend around the entire bone (Figs 24.3 and 24.4).

Chronic osteomyelitis persists as long as infected dead bone remains. The dead bone is surrounded by granulation tissue that attacks the sequestrum, making it pitted on the surface next to the marrow cavity. The cortical surface remains smooth. Surgical removal of the sequestrum at the proper time usually allows the osteomyelitis to heal. However, the osteomyelitis may recur many years later if bacteria remain within the scar.

In the adult, there is again a high incidence of joint infection, but this time in association with involvement of extensive portions of bone.

Microscopically, the changes of osteomyelitis are represented by an admixture of inflammatory cells (including neutrophils, lymphocytes, and plasma cells), fibrosis, bone necrosis, and new bone formation. When the plasma cell population is particularly prominent, the disease has been designated *plasma cell osteomyelitis*,[71] and when foamy macrophages are abundant, it has been called *xanthogranulomatous osteomyelitis*.[57] Chronic osteomyelitis may be accompanied by prominent periosteal bone proliferation (Fig. 24.5).

Osteomyelitic sinuses in the adult may become lined by squamous epithelium that extends deeply in the bone and becomes discontinuous with the cutaneous surface. Despite apparent healing

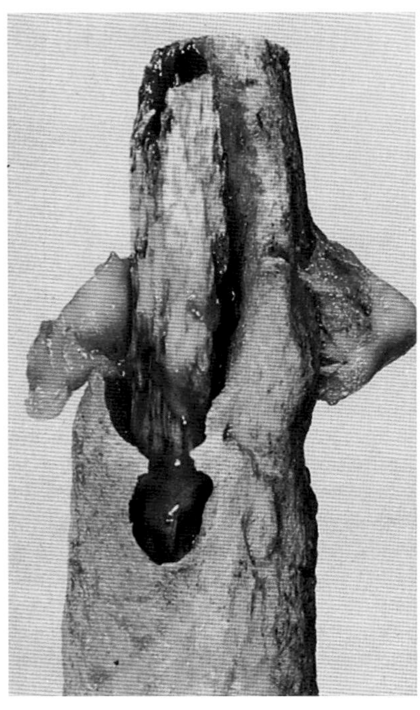

Fig. 24.4 Resected fibula showing dense outer involucrum surrounding loosened sequestrum with its pitted surface.

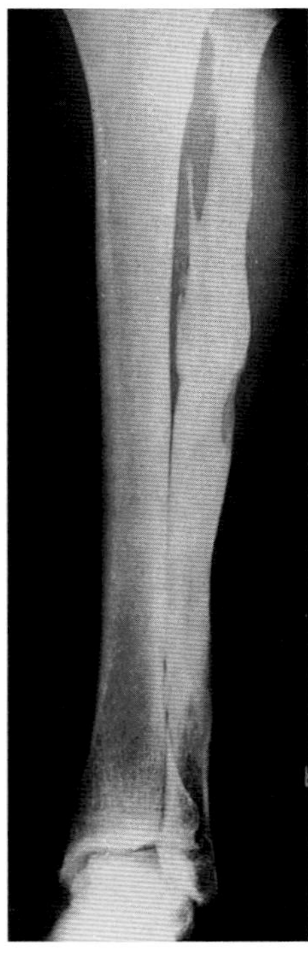

Fig. 24.3 Chronic osteomyelitis of fibula. Note dense, irregular bone.

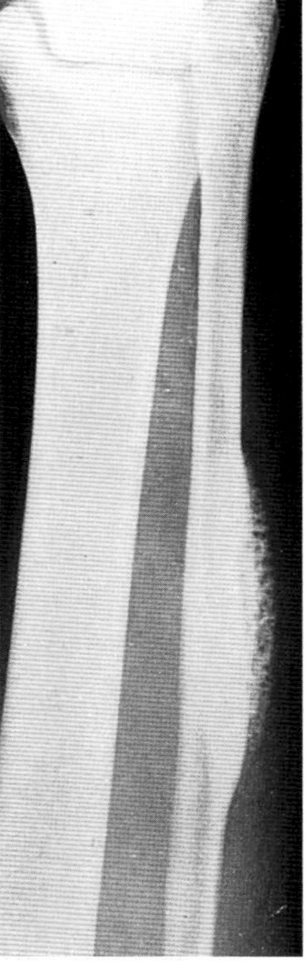

Fig. 24.5 Prominent periosteal bone proliferation in chronic osteomyelitis.

of the overlying skin, large epidermal inclusion cysts can slowly develop in the underlying bone. These are filled with keratin-containing debris similar to those present in epidermal inclusion cysts of the skin. Rarely, after a long period, squamous cell carcinoma develops within these sinuses. This complication is heralded by the appearance of pain and increasingly malodorous discharge.[58,63]

Tuberculous osteomyelitis as a hematogenous infection is usually seen in young adults or children. The bones most often infected are the vertebrae, pelvis, knee, ankle, elbow, and wrist. The areas usually involved are the metaphysis, epiphysis, and synovium.[53]

There has been considerable controversy as to which of these areas is the one first involved. Metaphyseal infection is more common in children, and epiphyseal infection is more common in adults; however, with progression of the disease, all zones become affected. Tuberculous granulation tissue forming in the synovia destroys the synovial attachments. The cartilage, no longer nourished from the synovia, undergoes progressive destruction, allowing the inflammation to extend into the epiphysis and finally into the metaphyseal area. If the process begins in the epiphysis, the tuberculous granulation tissue quickly extends into the adjacent joint. When the process begins in the metaphyseal area, extension into the joint may be heralded by the development of fluid in it.

Cutaneous sinuses may occur in advanced tuberculosis. These sinuses allow entry of secondary bacterial infection that modifies the pathologic changes. When the tuberculous process begins to heal, fusion of the joint may be associated with complete or partial denudation of cartilage and 'kissing sequestra'. Sequestra are cortical in pyogenic processes, but in tuberculous osteomyelitis they are cancellous.

Fungal infections of bone include blastomycosis, actinomycosis, histoplasmosis, and coccidioidomycosis.[65,66] Actinomycosis is particularly common following osteoradionecrosis.[62]

Tertiary syphilis may involve the bone and cause both osseous destruction and production, often in association with conspicuous periosteal bone proliferation (Fig. 24.6). The necrotic, well-defined defects are mainly cortical and periosteal, and are surrounded by sclerotic bone. They may occur in the vertebrae, flat bones of the hands and feet, and diaphysis of long tubular bones. The radiographic diagnosis is usually apparent if multiple x-ray studies of the bones are taken, but it may be difficult in single or isolated lesions, some of which closely resemble the appearance of osteosarcoma. Biopsy will show a granulomatous process associated with bone destruction and production.

Malakoplakia of bone has been described. As in the bladder and other sites, it probably represents an unusual host reaction to bacterial infection.[69]

Bone necrosis

Infarct

Bone infarct can be the result of a large number of etiologic factors. Radiographically, the changes depend on the age of the lesion and the degree of repair. During the first 1 or 2 weeks, no abnormalities are detected on a plain x-ray. Resorption of the dead bone results in areas of decreased density, whereas new bone formation growing in apposition to dead trabeculae ('creeping apposition') leads to an increase in bone density. The process of reossification is often irregular, and the combination of incomplete resorption of dead bone and focal deposition of new bone results in a mottled and irregular radiographic appearance (Fig. 24.7).

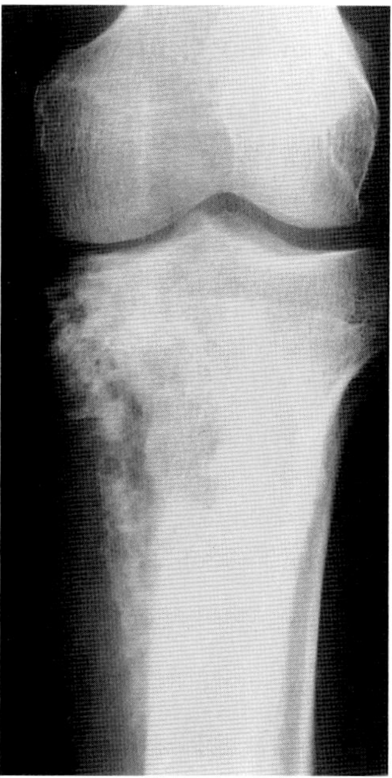

Fig. 24.6 Gummatous involvement of tibia in a 45-year-old woman. *(Courtesy of Dr RJ Reed, New Orleans)*

An increased incidence of primary malignant bone tumors has been seen in association with large infarcts of long bones. Most of the reported cases have occurred in the medulla of the femur or tibia of male adults and have been diagnosed as malignant fibrous histiocytoma, osteosarcoma, fibrosarcoma, or angiosarcoma.[72–76]

Aseptic (avascular) bone necrosis

Aseptic bone necrosis (avascular necrosis, osteonecrosis) is a common abnormality that has been reported in practically every secondary epiphysis and in many primary epiphyses[79] (Fig. 24.8). Many of these sites have been described separately and given eponymic designations such as Osgood–Schlatter disease (for necrosis of the tibial tuberosity) and Legg–Calvé–Perthes disease (for necrosis of the upper femoral epiphysis).

The pathogenetic mechanism is thought to be interruption of the blood supply induced in most cases by a mechanical disruption, such as fracture or dislocation,[77,81] but sometimes by thrombosis induced by sickle cell disease.[78] The responsible injury seems to be a single event, inasmuch as extension of the osteonecrosis once developed is extremely rare.[80]

The initial necrosis of epiphyseal bone is followed by hyperemia of the surrounding tissues. The epiphyseal cartilage may or may not remain viable. The dead bone gradually undergoes resorption by a mechanism of 'creeping substitution'. This is a slow process that may take months or even years and that results in a dense radiographic appearance, particularly well appreciated in lesions of the femoral neck.[77] Microscopically, it is typical to see osteoclastic activity on one side of the dead trabeculae and osteoblastic activity on the other. The newly formed bone, which is of soft consistency, may flatten because of pressure, resulting in degenerative joint disease.

Osteochondritis dissecans

Osteochondritis dissecans results from a small area of necrosis involving the articular cartilage and subchondral bone that totally

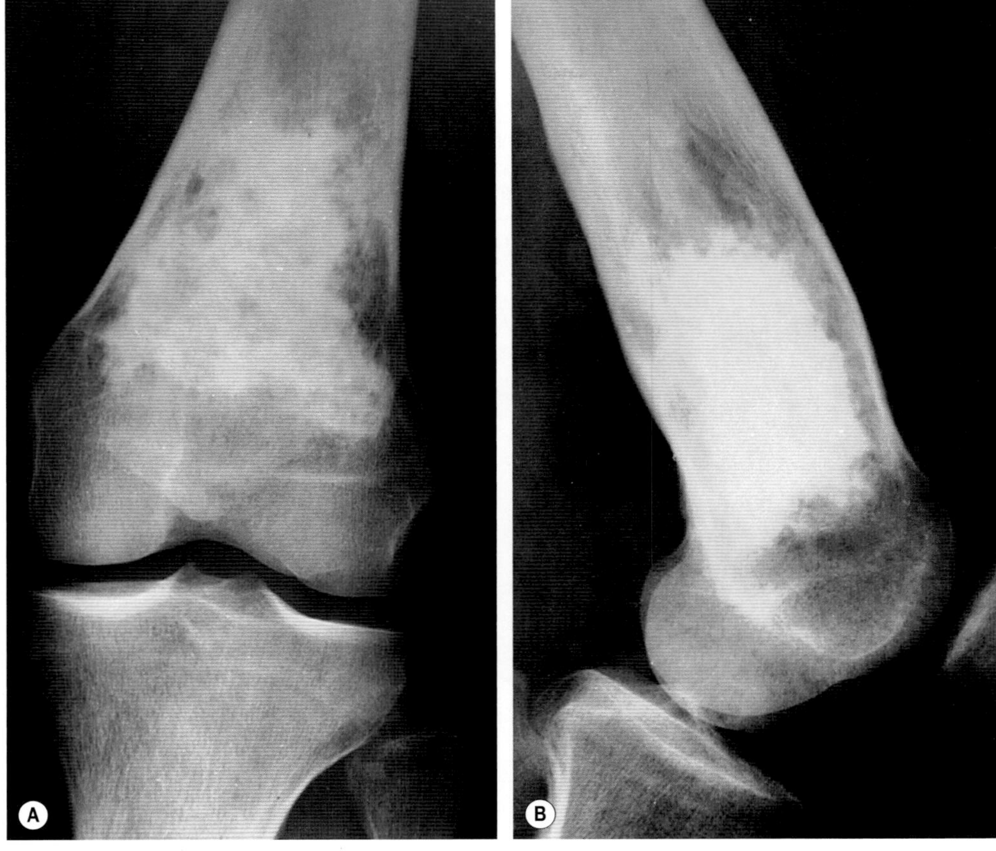

Fig. 24.7 Large diaphysometaphyseal bone infarct of femur. The irregular area of increased radiodensity is indicative of new bone production superimposed on necrosis. *(Courtesy of Dr H Danziger, Welland, Ontario, Canada)*

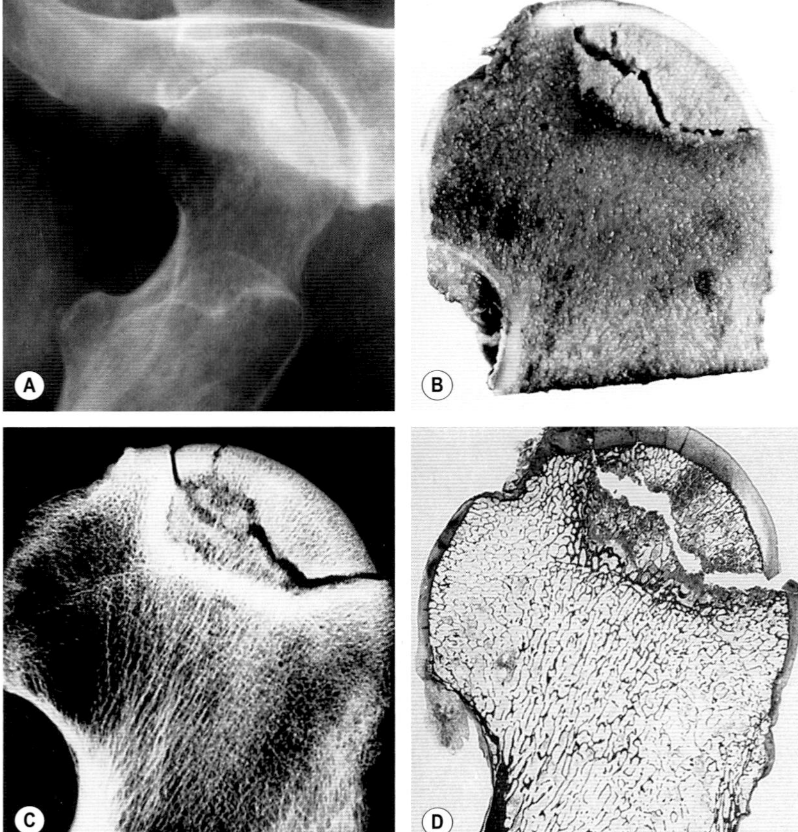

Fig. 24.8 A–D, Aseptic necrosis of femoral head with superimposed fracture. **A**, Radiograph. **B**, Cross section of excised specimen. **C**, Radiograph of a slice of the same specimen, emphasizing peripheral eburnation. **D**, The whole-mount specimen shows a well-delimited focus of necrosis.

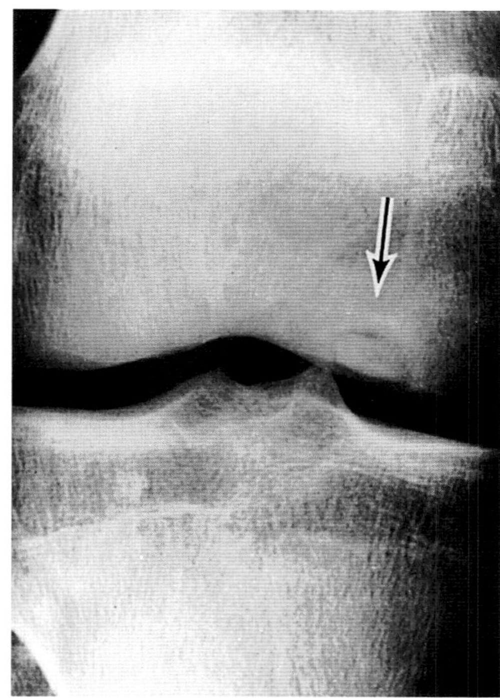

Fig. 24.9 Sharply delimited area of osteochondritis dissecans of medial condyle (arrow). This was easily enucleated.

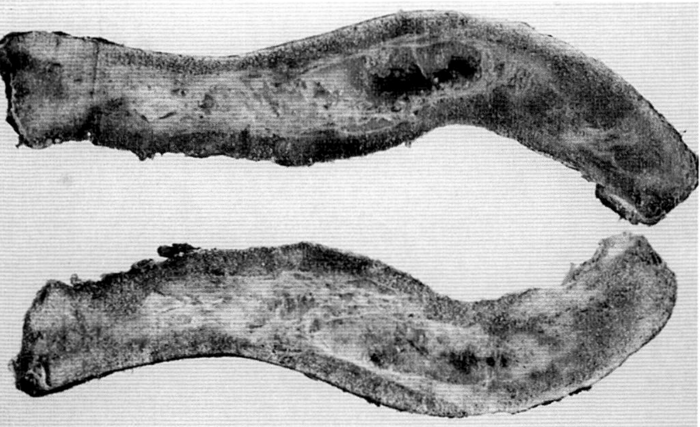

Fig. 24.10 Extensive Paget disease of clavicle in a 60-year-old man. Note distortion and changes in cortex.

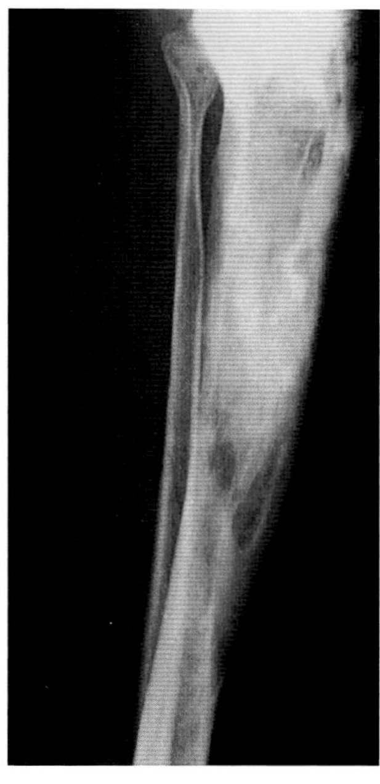

Fig. 24.11 Monostotic Paget disease of tibia with bone destruction and bone formation. The nature of the process was obscure until biopsy.

or partially separates from the adjacent structures. The etiology is uncertain but is probably related to trauma in most of the cases.[82,84] It occurs most frequently on the lateral aspect of the medial femoral condyle, near the intercondylar notch (Fig. 24.9). Microscopically, a portion of articular cartilage is always present, often exhibiting secondary calcification; in addition, a fragment of subchondral bone is found in approximately half of the cases.[83,84] If this osteochondromatous body remains attached to the joint surface or synovium, both components remain viable. If, instead, it becomes completely detached, its osseous portion dies, but the cartilage remains alive, apparently through nutrients obtained from the synovial fluid.

Patients with bilateral symmetric involvement and cases with familial incidence have been described.

Radiation necrosis

Damage to the underlying bone can be a major complication of radiation therapy, whether alone or combined with chemotherapy.[85] Radiation changes resulting in serious complications have been reported in the jaw, ribs, pelvis, spine, humerus, and several other bones.[87] The changes usually occur within 3 years of the therapy. Microscopically, these changes consist of necrotic bone, fibrosis of the bone marrow, and neovascularization. Irregular, heavily staining cement lines may develop and lead to confusion with Paget disease. Radiation necrosis of the jaw can be complicated by actinomycosis, an often underdiagnosed occurrence.[86]

Paget disease

About 90% of the patients with Paget disease are over 55 years of age. The disease is rare before the age of 40 years and uncommon between the ages of 40 and 55 years, although several cases of precocious onset are on record.[95] It affects men slightly more often than women (4:3). It has a very peculiar geographic distribution. The highest incidence is in England, Australia, and the Western European plain.[88,96] In an often quoted autopsy series from England, about one of 30 patients over 40 years of age had Paget disease.[89] The most common sites are the lumbosacral spine, pelvis, and skull. It may also occur in the femur, tibia, clavicle (Fig. 24.10), radius, ulna, fibula, and jaws,[105] but is extremely rare in the ribs.

The disease is usually polyostotic and accompanied by elevations of serum alkaline phosphatase levels. However, it can also appear as a monostotic process in a long bone, jaw, or vertebra (Fig. 24.11). In such cases, the alkaline phosphatase levels may be normal.

The basic abnormality of Paget disease is a focal acceleration of bone turnover, but its etiology remains obscure. Recent evidence

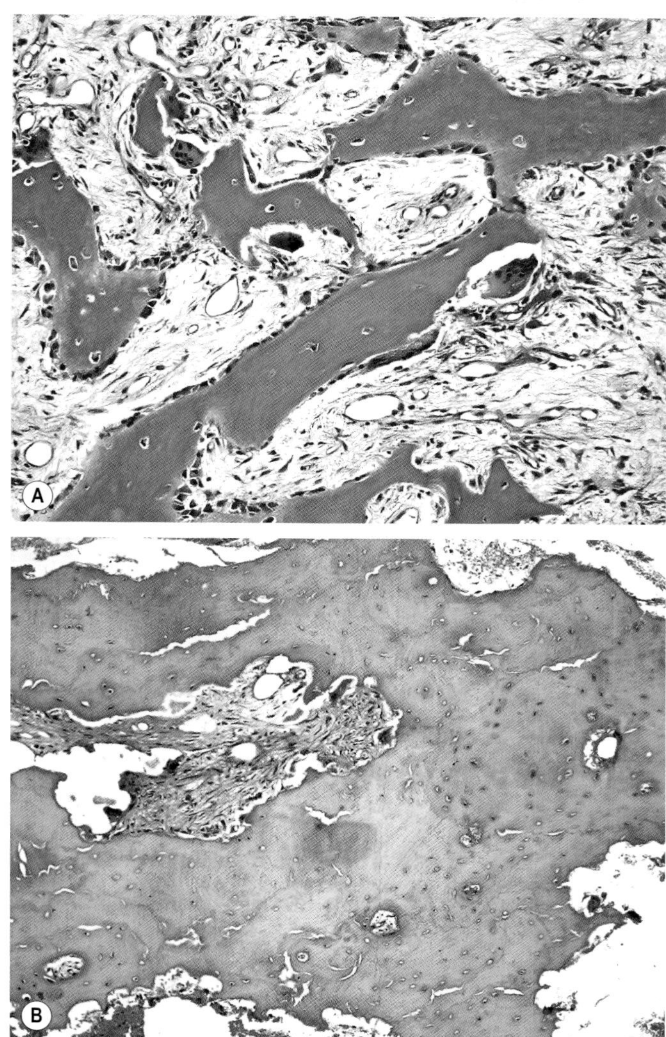

Fig. 24.12 **A** and **B**, Paget disease. **A**, Early changes. There is prominent osteoclastic activity, resulting in bone resorption. **B**, A well-established case, with thick, irregularly shaped bone trabeculae.

strongly implicates both genetic and environmental factors.[91,104] The suggestion that it might be of viral origin has been raised by the finding of nuclear inclusions resembling viral nucleocapsids of the measles type in the lesional osteoclasts,[94,101,102] but the evidence remains inconclusive.

The initial lesion is osteoclastic and therefore lytic ('osteoporosis circumscripta')[90,93] (Fig. 24.12A). Abnormal hyperplasia soon follows, as evidenced by the deposition of primitive coarse-fibered bone in discontinuous trabeculae, which in turn is replaced by thick trabeculae with a disjointed lamellar pattern (Figs 24.12B and 24.13). This evolution in the morphogenesis of the disease can be better appreciated with reticulin stains than with the use of polarized light. The disorganization in the structure of the lamellar bone leads to the formation of *cement lines*. These are caused by the abrupt interruptions and changes in direction of bone lamellae and fibers resulting from resorption and regeneration of masses of bone during the course of the disease and represent the key to the diagnosis of Paget disease. However, they are not specific for it; there are many pathologic processes that involve active reparative change accompanied by new bone formation with cement lines. These

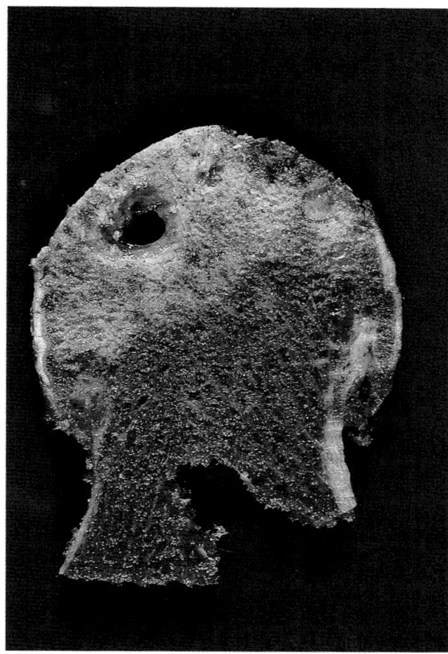

Fig. 24.13 Paget disease of femoral head, accompanied by degenerative joint disease.

include irradiation effect, chronic osteomyelitis, reactive bone surrounding metastatic cancer, and polyostotic fibrous dysplasia. In general, the cement lines seen in these conditions are more orderly and structurally better oriented than those of Paget disease. The marrow space is commonly replaced by richly vascularized loose connective tissue.

Two important complications of Paget disease are fractures and development of bone tumors. The fractures are usually of the transverse type.[98] Patients who are immobilized because of long bone fractures may undergo rapid dissolution of bone substance.[100]

The overall incidence of bone sarcoma in Paget disease (so-called Paget sarcoma) is relatively low if one considers the worldwide prevalence of the latter disorder.[89] Osteosarcoma is by far the most common type (about 80% of all cases), but chondrosarcoma, fibrosarcoma, and giant cell tumors have also been observed.[92,97,103] Instances of familial or geographic clustering of this complication have been seen. The most common locations of sarcomas arising in Paget disease are the femur, humerus, pelvis, tibia, and skull. Osteosarcoma should be distinguished from the periosteal (juxtacortical) bone masses that can be seen as an exaggerated expression of the basic pathologic process of Paget disease.[99] The prognosis of Paget sarcoma remains very poor.[92]

Osteopetrosis

Osteopetrosis (Albers–Schönberg disease, marble-bone disease) is a family of genetically determined disorders resulting from a defect in bone remodeling secondary to malfunction or, less commonly, failure of development of osteoclasts.[108,111] At least 10 genes have been identified as causative, such as those encoding molecules involved in acidification machinery (e.g., proton pump vacuolar ATPase, chloride channel and carbonic anhydrase II) and those affecting osteoclast differentiation which result in the osteoclast-poor form of the disease (e.g., *IKBKG, RANK, RANKL*).[111] Microscopically, the disorder is characterized by persistence in the marrow cavity of unresorbed osteocartilaginous matrix.[106,110] The disease has been reversed by bone marrow transplantation[107] and has been successfully treated with recombinant human interferon gamma.[109]

Tumors

Classification and distribution

The terminology and classification of bone tumors and tumorlike lesions we use are largely those recommended by the World Health Organization (WHO) Committee for the Histological Definition and Classification of Bone Tumours,[114] slightly modified to accommodate some new concepts and entities.

In the WHO classification, most neoplasms are classified as either benign or malignant. Although a sharp separation between these two categories is feasible in most of them, some neoplasms (such as giant cell tumors and some well-differentiated cartilaginous tumors) exhibit borderline or intermediate characteristics. Most malignant bone tumors arise de novo, but there is a small number of benign bone lesions that predispose the patient to the development of skeletal malignancies; these include Paget disease, chondromatosis, osteochondromatosis, fibrous dysplasia, osteofibrous dysplasia, and osteogenesis imperfecta.[112]

Tumors of the skeletal system are relatively constant in their pattern of presentation.[113] The five basic parameters of importance in this regard are the age of the patient, bone involved, specific area within the bone (epiphysis, metaphysis, or diaphysis; cortex, medulla, or periosteum), radiographic appearance, and microscopic appearance. The pathologist should be fully aware of the first four before trying to evaluate the fifth.[115] Otherwise, serious mistakes may occur. Table 24.1 should help in providing a quick orientation for the pathologist confronted with a bone neoplasm.

Bone-forming tumors

Osteoma

Osteoma is seen almost exclusively in the flat bones of the skull and face, where it has been divided into central and peripheral (periosteal). It may protrude inside a paranasal sinus (particularly the frontal and ethmoid) and block the normal drainage from these sinuses. Microscopically, it is composed of dense, mature, predominantly lamellar bone. This lesion is benign and probably not a true neoplasm. Some cases may represent end stages of fibrous dysplasia or related fibro-osseous lesions. Patients with Gardner syndrome (intestinal polyposis and soft tissue tumors) may have multiple osteomas and other abnormalities,[117] whereas cases of solitary osteoma are usually nonsyndromic.[118] Occasionally, osteomas involve bones other than skull and face. Most of these have a parosteal location and need to be distinguished from parosteal osteosarcoma.[116]

Osteoid osteoma and osteoblastoma

Osteoid osteoma is a benign bone neoplasm that is found more frequently in patients between 10 and 30 years of age, and that exhibits a 2 : 1 male–female ratio. Intense pain is the most prominent symptom; this is often sharply localized and unaccompanied by clinical or laboratory evidence of infection. Vertebral lesions may be associated with scoliosis.[140]

Osteoid osteoma has been reported in practically every bone but occurs most frequently in the femur, tibia, humerus, bones of the hands and feet, vertebrae, and fibula.[133,138] Lesions of long bones are usually metaphyseal, but they may be epiphyseal and even juxta- or intra-articular.[121,132] Most are centered in the cortex (85%), but they may also occur in the spongiosa (13%) or subperiosteal region (2%).[141] Vertebral lesions usually affect the pedicle or the arch.[135]

Radiographically, the typical finding is a radiolucent central nidus that is seldom larger than 1.5 cm and that may or may not contain a dense center (Fig. 24.14). This nidus is surrounded by a peripheral sclerotic reaction that may extend for several centimeters along both sides of the cortex and that may lead to a mistaken radiographic diagnosis of Garre osteomyelitis (Fig. 24.15).

Microscopically, the sharply delineated central nidus is composed of more or less calcified osteoid lined by plump osteoblasts and growing within highly vascularized connective tissue, without evidence of inflammation (Figs 24.16 and 24.17). The appearance is so characteristic that the lesion can still be diagnosed when removed

Table 24.1 Usual age and sex of patient and location and behavior of most common primary bone tumors and tumorlike lesions[a]

TUMOR OR TUMORLIKE LESION	AGE (YR)	SEX (M:F)	BONES MORE COMMONLY AFFECTED (IN ORDER OF FREQUENCY)	USUAL LOCATION WITHIN LONG BONE	BEHAVIOR
Osteoma	40–50	2:1	Skull and facial bones	–	Benign
Osteoid osteoma	10–30	2:1	Femur, tibia, humerus, hands and feet, vertebrae, fibula	Cortex of metaphysis	Benign
Osteoblastoma	10–30	2:1	Vertebrae, tibia, femur, humerus, pelvis, ribs	Medulla of metaphysis	Benign
Osteosarcoma	10–25	3:2	Femur, tibia, humerus, pelvis, jaw, fibula	Medulla of metaphysis	Malignant; 20% 5-yr survival rate
Juxtacortical (parosteal) osteosarcoma	30–60	1:1	Femur, tibia, humerus	Juxtacortical area of metaphysis	Malignant; 80% 5-yr survival rate
Chondroma	10–40	1:1	Hands and feet, ribs, femur, humerus	Medulla of diaphysis	Benign

Continued

Table 24.1 Usual age and sex of patient and location and behavior of most common primary bone tumors and tumorlike lesions[a]—cont'd.

TUMOR OR TUMORLIKE LESION	AGE (YR)	SEX (M:F)	BONES MORE COMMONLY AFFECTED (IN ORDER OF FREQUENCY)	USUAL LOCATION WITHIN LONG BONE	BEHAVIOR
Osteochondroma	10–30	1:1	Femur, tibia, humerus, pelvis	Cortex of metaphysis	Benign
Chondroblastoma	10–25	2:1	Femur, humerus, tibia, feet, pelvis, scapula	Epiphysis, adjacent to cartilage plate	Practically always benign
Chondromyxoid fibroma	10–25	1:1	Tibia, femur, feet, pelvis	Metaphysis	Benign
Chondrosarcoma	30–60	3:1	Pelvis, ribs, femur, humerus, vertebrae	Central: medulla of diaphysis; peripheral: cortex or periosteum of metaphysis	Malignant. 5-yr survival rate: low grade, 78%; moderate grade, 53%; high grade, 22%
Mesenchymal chondrosarcoma	20–60	1:1	Ribs, skull and jaw, vertebrae, pelvis	Medulla or cortex of diaphysis	Malignant; extremely poor prognosis
Giant cell tumor	20–40	4:5	Femur, tibia, radius	Epiphysis and metaphysis	Potentially malignant; 50% recur; 10% metastasize
Ewing sarcoma/PNET	5–20	1:2	Femur, pelvis, tibia, humerus, ribs, fibula	Medulla of diaphysis or metaphysis	Highly malignant; 20–30% 5-yr survival rate in recent series
Malignant lymphoma, large cell, and mixed cell types	30–60	1:1	Femur, pelvis, vertebrae, tibia, humerus, jaw, skull, ribs	Medulla of diaphysis or metaphysis	Malignant; 22–50% 5-yr survival rate
Plasma cell myeloma	40–60	2:1	Vertebrae, pelvis, ribs, sternum, skull	Medulla of diaphysis, metaphysis, or epiphysis	Malignant; diffuse form uniformly fatal, localized form often controlled with radiation therapy
Hemangioma	20–50	1:1	Skull, vertebrae, jaw	Medulla	Benign
Desmoplastic fibroma	20–30	1:1	Humerus, tibia, pelvis, jaw, femur, scapula	Metaphysis	Benign
Fibrosarcoma	20–60	1:1	Femur, tibia, jaw, humerus	Medulla of metaphysis	Malignant; 28% 5-yr survival rate
Chordoma	40–60	2:1	Sacrococcygeal, spheno-occipital, cervical vertebrae	–	Malignant; slow course; locally invasive; 48% distant metastases
Solitary bone cyst	10–20	3:1	Humerus, femur	Medulla of metaphysis	Benign
Aneurysmal bone cyst	10–20	1:1	Vertebrae, flat bones, femur, tibia	Metaphysis	Benign, sometimes secondary to another bone lesion
Metaphyseal fibrous defect	10–20	1:1	Tibia, femur, fibula	Metaphysis	Benign
Fibrous dysplasia	10–30	3:2	Ribs, femur, tibia, jaw, skull	Medulla of diaphysis or metaphysis	Locally aggressive; rarely complicated by sarcoma
Langerhans cell histiocytosis	5–15	3:2	Skull, jaw, humerus, rib, femur	Metaphysis or diaphysis	Benign

[a]It should be emphasized that these data correspond to the typical case and should not be taken in an absolute sense. Isolated exceptions to practically every one of these statements have occurred.

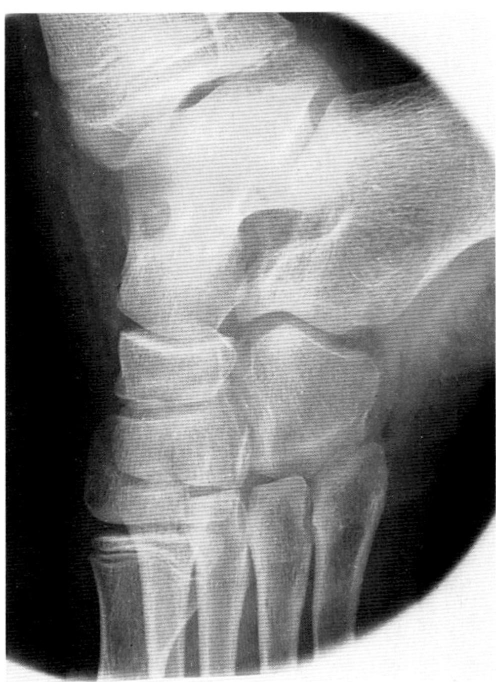

Fig. 24.14 Osteoid osteoma of talus. Note the small central osteolytic nidus surrounded by dense bone.

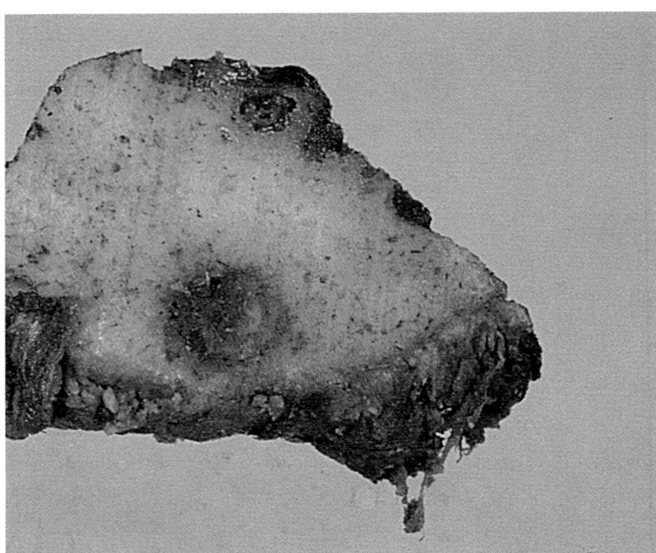

Fig. 24.15 Gross appearance of osteoid osteoma measuring 5 mm. The small, reddish central nidus is surrounded by a thick layer of sclerotic bone.

piecemeal. Surrounding the nidus, there is a variably thick layer of dense bone.

The pain associated with osteoid osteoma is characteristically more intense at night, relieved by nonsteroidal anti-inflammatory drugs such as aspirin, and eliminated by excision of the lesion. It has been attributed by some authors to the effect on nerves and vessels of osteoblast-produced prostaglandin E2, which is typically present in large amounts in these lesions.[131,144] Others believe that the pain is simply related to the presence of entrapped and proliferating nerves within and particularly around the nidus.[130,139]

Preoperative localization with CT scan and intraoperative monitoring of the location and resection with radioscintigraphy have markedly reduced the recurrence rate.[131,136] The nidus can also be demonstrated by administering tetracycline preoperatively and examining the lesion under ultraviolet light at operation.[120]

Osteoblastoma (benign osteoblastoma, giant osteoid osteoma) is a tumor closely related to osteoid osteoma both microscopically and ultrastructurally[126,143] (Fig. 24.18). It is distinguished from the latter by the larger size of the nidus, the absence or inconspicuousness of a surrounding area of reactive bone formation, and the lack of intense pain.[128] A cartilaginous matrix is present in some cases.[123] Most cases arise in the spongiosa of the bone, but cortical and subperiosteal forms also occur.[141] The majority of the cases are located in the spine or major bones of the lower extremity.[133,137] Osteomalacia can be seen as a complication.[145]

The differential diagnosis between osteoblastoma and osteosarcoma can be extremely difficult because the latter may be very well differentiated and the former is sometimes accompanied by the presence of scattered bizarre tumor cells probably of a degenerative nature,[124,127] or may be composed of large epithelioid cells accompanied by telangiectatic features.[119] As is the case in many other bone tumors, the radiographic pattern is of great assistance in this differential diagnosis. However, in some cases of osteoblastoma the radiographic picture suggests a malignant neoplasm.[134,137]

Aggressive osteoblastoma and related lesions. Some lesions with the radiographic and architectural features of osteoblastoma show atypical cytologic features that correlate with a tendency for local recurrence. These tumors have been designated aggressive osteoblastomas. According to Dorfman and Weiss,[129] they are distinguished microscopically from the ordinary osteoblastomas because of the presence of wider or more irregular trabeculae, by the focal lack of a trabecular pattern of the osteoid proliferation, and – most of all – by the fact that the osteoid trabeculae are bordered by epithelioid-appearing osteoblasts They are distinguished from conventional osteosarcomas because of a low mitotic rate and the absence of the following features: lace-like osteoid, permeation of surrounding intertrabecular spaces, and atypical mitoses. Some of these tumors grow in a multinodular fashion, as defined by the presence of multiple nidi in a single tumor.[146]

The entity of aggressive osteoblastoma merges with – and may indeed be identical to – tumors described as epithelioid osteoblastoma,[146] malignant osteoblastoma,[142] osteosarcoma resembling osteoblastoma,[124] and osteoblastoma-like osteosarcoma,[122] some of which have metastasized. To complicate the issue further, there are several reported cases of supposedly ordinary osteoblastomas that have undergone malignant transformation toward osteosarcomas.[125,129]

Osteosarcoma

Generalities. Osteosarcoma is the most frequent primary malignant bone tumor, exclusive of hematopoietic malignancy.[186] It usually occurs in patients between 10 and 25 years of age and is exceptionally rare in preschool children.[219] Another peak age incidence occurs after 40, in association with other disorders (see the following discussion). There is a slight male predominance (1.5 : 1).

Predisposing factors. Most osteosarcomas arise de novo, but others arise within the context of a preexisting condition:

1 *Paget disease*. A high number of osteosarcomas developing in patients over the age of 40 are located in bones affected by Paget disease[204] (see p. 2020).

2 *Radiation exposure*. One of the classic cases of human carcinogenesis occurred in a group of factory workers in Illinois who developed osteosarcomas from moistening brushes in their mouths when applying radium paint to create luminous numerals on watches.[231,251] Some cases of osteosarcoma have also been reported years after Thorotrast administration.[270] Many others have been seen, in both adults and children, as a complication of external radiation therapy.[235,293] The average latency period ranges from 10 to 15 years in the various reported series.[209,297] It could be noted here that the majority of post-radiation sarcomas of bone and soft tissues remain unclassified at the microscopic and immunohistochemical level.[235]

3 *Chemotherapy*. Children treated with alkylating agents for retinoblastoma and other malignancies have an increased risk of osteosarcoma.[286] The genetic factor probably plays an important contributory role.

4 *Preexisting benign bone lesions*. These include fibrous dysplasia, osteochondromatosis, chondromatosis, and osteogenesis imperfecta[271,283] (see respective sections).

5 *Foreign bodies*. A few but well-documented cases of osteosarcoma have been reported arising at the site of a total hip replacement or at sites of other orthopedic implants.[215,249]

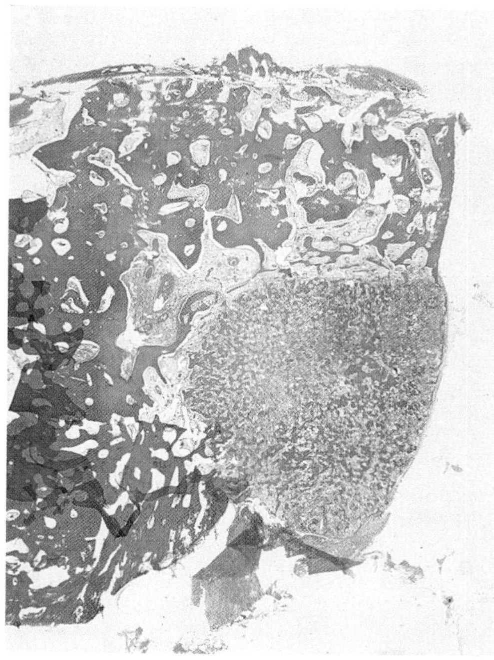

Fig. 24.16 Low-power microscopic view of osteoid osteoma showing a wedge-shaped nidus protruding slightly above the surface and surrounded by sclerotic bone.

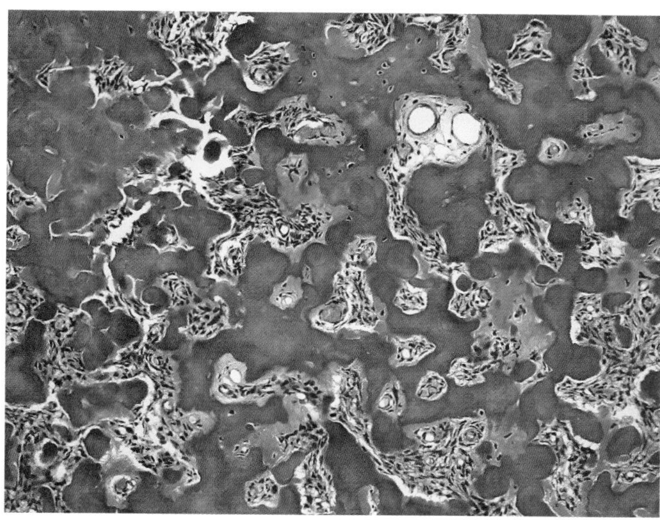

Fig. 24.18 Microscopic appearance of recurrent osteoblastoma. The appearance is similar to that of osteoid osteoma.

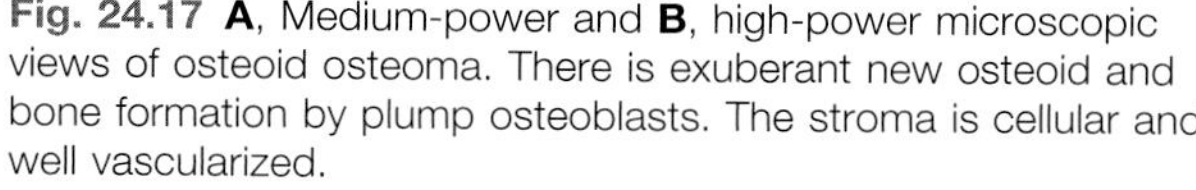

Fig. 24.17 **A**, Medium-power and **B**, high-power microscopic views of osteoid osteoma. There is exuberant new osteoid and bone formation by plump osteoblasts. The stroma is cellular and well vascularized.

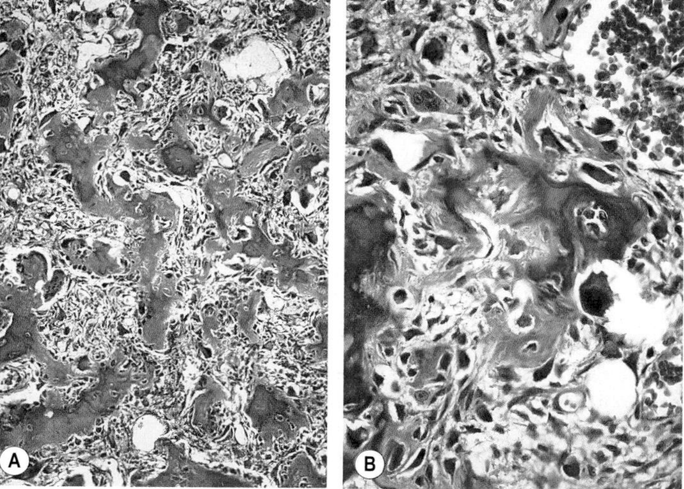

6 *Trauma*. Isolated trauma, no matter how intense, does not cause osteosarcoma or other bone tumors.[194] If it did, one would expect to find an increased incidence of bone tumors after fractures, various orthopedic procedures, or other severe injuries. Trauma usually only calls attention to an already present advanced bone tumor (so-called traumatic determinism).
7 *Genetic predisposition*. Patients with Li-Fraumeni syndrome (usually caused by germline mutation of the *TP53* gene), hereditary retinoblastoma (caused by germline mutation of the *RB1* gene), Rothmund–Thomson syndrome, Werner syndrome, and familial Paget disease have an increased risk of developing osteosarcoma.[232,246]

Location. Most osteosarcomas arising de novo are located in the metaphyseal area of the long bones, particularly the lower end of the femur, the upper end of the tibia, and the upper end of the humerus.[175] A few cases arise in the diaphyses and an even smaller number in the epiphyses. Less commonly, osteosarcomas are found in flat bones (such as craniofacial bones, pelvis, and scapula),[195,216] spine,[244] and short bones.[242] Occasionally, osteosarcomas are multicentric, in either a synchronous or a metachronous fashion: most of these multicentric cases occur in children and tend to be densely sclerotic radiographically and extremely aggressive.[247] Germline and somatic mutations of *TP53* have been found in some of these cases.[210]

The large majority of osteosarcomas arise within the medullary cavity, from which they extend into the cortex; only occasionally will they begin within the cortex itself[294] – when they do, they seem to have a predilection for the diaphysis.[222]

Gross appearance and spread. The gross appearance of the cut surface of an osteosarcoma varies a great deal, depending on the relative amounts of bone, cartilage, cellular stroma, and vessels (Figs 24.19 and 24.20). The range extends from bony hard to cystic, friable, and hemorrhagic. From its usual origin in the metaphysis of a long bone, the tumor may:

1 Spread along the marrow cavity.
2 Invade the adjacent cortex.
3 Elevate or perforate the periosteum. In the latter circumstance, a radiographic sign known as Codman triangle develops. The two long sides of this triangle are formed by the elevated periosteum and the underlying bone; the space within them is mainly occupied by reactive new bone, arranged perpendicular to the bone surface, but it may also contain malignant tumor. This radiographic sign, although useful, is not specific for osteosarcoma or even for a malignant tumor; it can be produced by any lesion that elevates the periosteum, including hematoma.
4 Extend into the soft tissues. It may even reach beneath the skin, although cutaneous ulceration is very rare.
5 Extend into the epiphysis. This happens frequently after the epiphysis is closed, but it may also be seen when the epiphyseal growth line is still present.[268]
6 Extend into the joint space. This invasion occurs when the tumor extends under the capsule insertion to involve the margin of the articular cartilage. In the knee, the tumor may extend across or around the osseous–tendinous junction of the cruciate ligaments into the joint space.[269]
7 Form satellite nodules independent from the main tumor mass proximal to the primary lesion, either in the same bone or transarticularly (Fig. 24.21). These have been called 'skip' metastases[187] and may be responsible for an increased incidence of local recurrences and subsequent metastases.[227]
8 Metastasize through the bloodstream to distant sites, particularly the lung. In an autopsy series of 54 cases, the four main sites of metastases were lung (98%), other bones (37%), pleura (33%), and heart (20%).[290] Conversely, metastases to regional lymph nodes are so rare that they should be disregarded for purposes of therapy. On occasion, the lung metastases present in the form of extensive intraluminal tumor growth in the pulmonary arteries.[296]

Microscopic features. Microscopically, osteosarcoma may destroy the preexisting bone trabeculae or grow around them in an appositional fashion (Fig. 24.22). The key feature for the diagnosis is the detection, somewhere in the tumor, of osteoid and/or bone

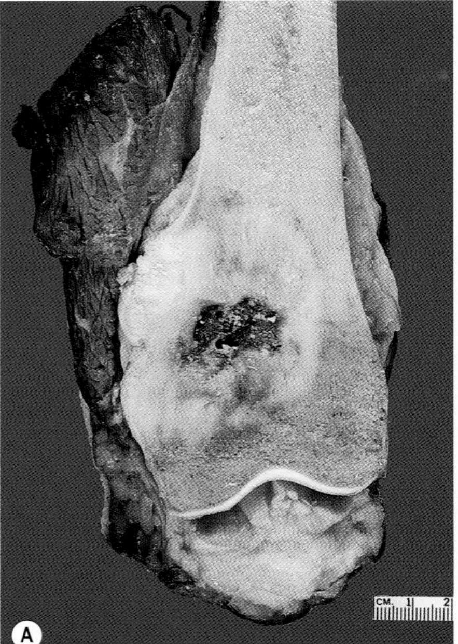

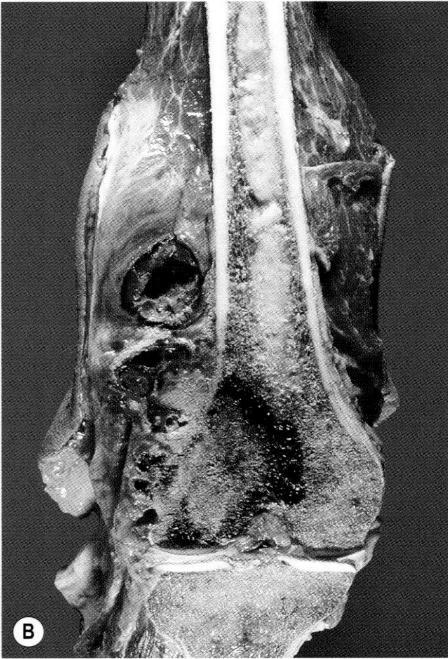

Fig. 24.19 A and **B**, Gross appearances of osteosarcoma of femur. In both instances the tumor is located at the typical metaphyseal site. The tumor shown in **A** is largely restricted to bone, whereas that illustrated in **B** is accompanied by massive soft tissue extension.

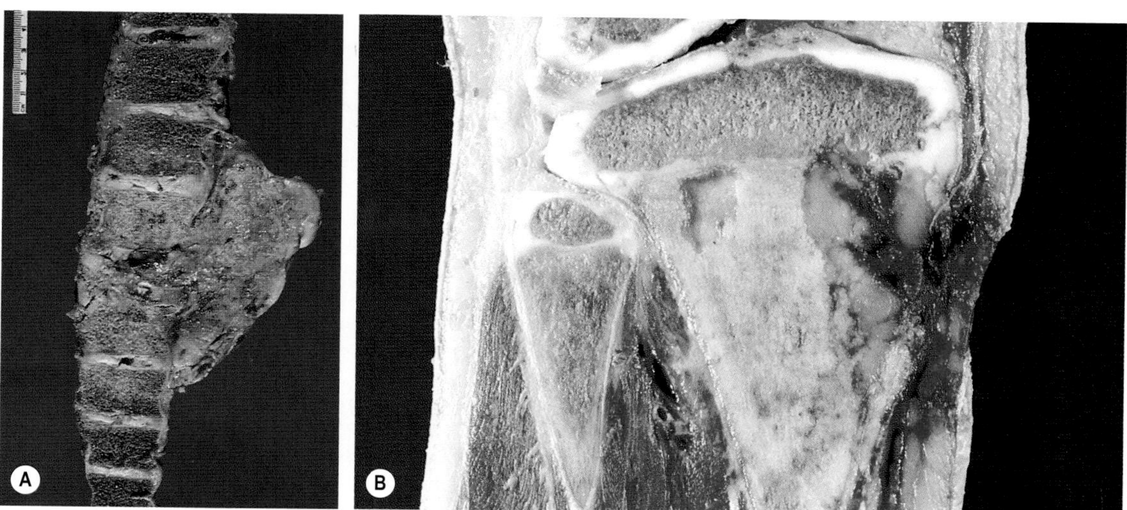

Fig. 24.20 **A** and **B**, Other gross appearances of osteosarcoma. **A**, Tumor extensively involving spine and producing a large soft tissue mass. **B**, This tumor of the upper tibial metaphysis is being temporarily restrained by the cartilage of the epiphyseal line. The hemorrhagic area represents the biopsy site.

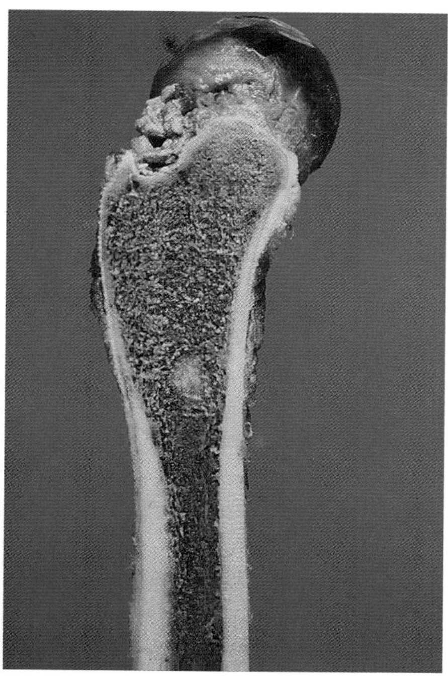

Fig. 24.21 So-called 'skip metastasis' located in the upper half of the femur. The primary tumor was located in the lower metaphysis of the same bone.

(calcified osteoid) produced directly by the tumor cells without interposition of cartilage (Fig. 24.23). Osteoid is recognized by its eosinophilic-staining quality, its glassy appearance, irregular contours, and the fact that it is surrounded by a rim of osteoblasts. It may be very difficult to distinguish osteoid from hyalinized collagen; a homogeneous rather than fibrillary appearance, beginning punctate calcification, and a plump appearance of the cells around it are more in keeping with osteoid. A different but highly characteristic type of bone tumor is characterized by thin tubular

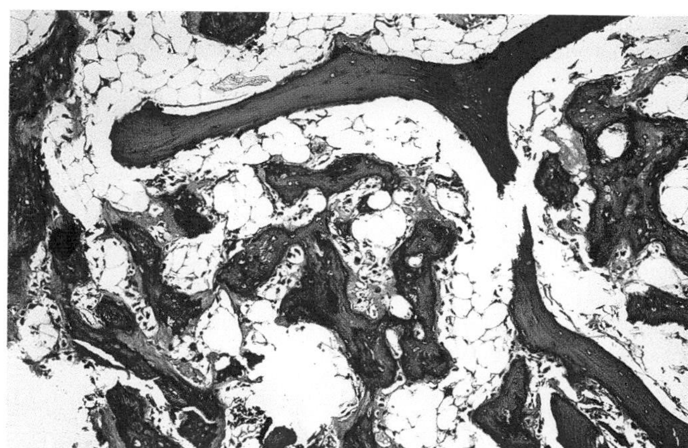

Fig. 24.22 Osteosarcoma. The malignant bone is more basophilic and has more irregular borders than the preexisting bone trabeculae.

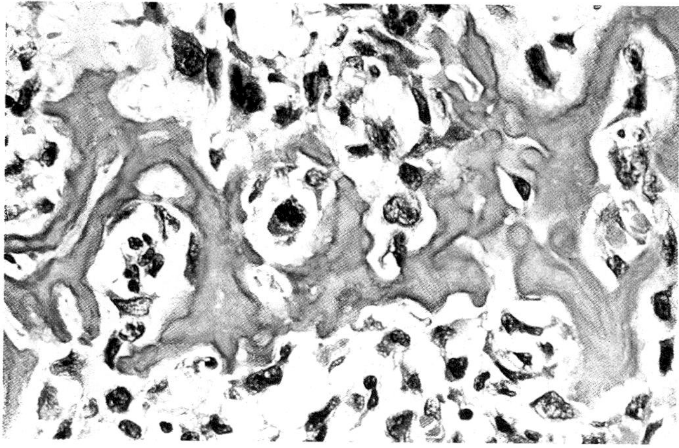

Fig. 24.23 Malignant bone formation by the tumor cells of osteosarcoma without interposition of cartilage.

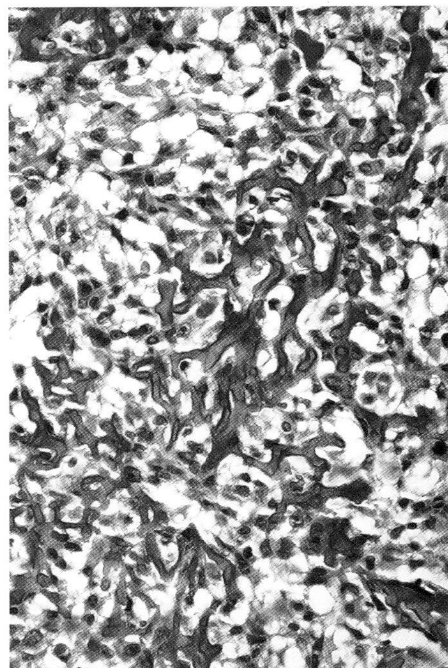

Fig. 24.24 Microscopic appearance of osteosarcoma showing characteristic basophilic thin trabeculae of neoplastic bone with an appearance that is reminiscent of fungal hyphae.

anastomosing 'microtrabeculae', which are very basophilic and vaguely reminiscent of the appearance of fungal hyphae (Fig. 24.24).

These osteoblastic areas are often mixed with fibroblastic and chondroblastic foci, the relative proportions among these three components varying a great deal from case to case. Depending on which component predominates, osteosarcomas have been divided into osteoblastic, fibroblastic, and chondroblastic, but there seems to be no prognostic significance to this division. The important fact to remember is that a malignant bone tumor should be designated as osteosarcoma whenever osteoid is seen unconnected with cartilage and being formed directly from the tumor cells, no matter how much neoplastic cartilage (with or without endochondral ossification) or fibrous tissue is present elsewhere.

Morphologic variations in osteosarcoma are plentiful.[176,263,310] The osteoid may be sparse or massive, surrounded by pleomorphic bizarre cells or relatively acellular, irregularly shaped, or with a rosettelike configuration (the latter allegedly being a more aggressive variant).[240] The tumor cells may grow in diffuse, nesting, or pseudopapillary arrangements. The vessels may be scanty or numerous, sometimes with a dilated or hemangiopericytomatous appearance. The tumor cells may be spindle, oval, or round, and their size may range from small to giant; exceptionally, they have a distinctly epithelial-like appearance.[177,201,220,306] Osteoclast-like multinucleated giant cells are present in one-fourth of the cases and may dominate the picture focally (so-called giant cell-rich osteosarcoma); the cartilage may be immature, mineralized, or highly myxoid. In the latter instance, the tumor may simulate a chondromyxoid fibroma.[173]

Depending on which one of the previously mentioned microscopic patterns happens to be present, the differential diagnosis of osteosarcoma may include a remarkably high number of benign and malignant lesions, such as fracture callus, myositis ossificans, fibrous dysplasia, osteoblastoma, fibrosarcoma, chondrosarcoma, giant cell tumor, malignant lymphoma, and metastatic carcinoma.[310] Exuberant fracture callus is particularly likely to be misdiagnosed as osteosarcoma by the unwary, with disastrous consequences for the patient. This callus may be secondary to a pathologic fracture in a benign lesion such as a metaphyseal fibrous defect or aneurysmal bone cyst, in a metastatic carcinoma, or in osteogenesis imperfecta (where it may be particularly exuberant).[156,213] Myositis ossificans is a reactive lesion pathogenetically closely related to fracture callus and may induce similar diagnostic problems (see p. 2066).

Other entities that need to be considered in the differential diagnosis are discussed in connection with the osteosarcoma variants described in the following section.

Histochemical, immunohistochemical, and electron microscopic features. Osteosarcoma cells usually exhibit strong alkaline phosphatase activity, regardless of their appearance (osteoblastic or fibroblastic), a feature of diagnostic value.[276,305] Ultrastructurally, the better differentiated tumor cells resemble normal osteoblasts in their abundance of dilated cisternae of granular endoplasmic reticulum and sparse mitochondria.[192,230,264,273,300] Other cells present are osteocytes, chondroblasts, undifferentiated cells, and myofibroblasts.[255,274,275] The matrix is formed of nonperiodic fibrils, scattered collagen fibers, and focal calcium deposits of hydroxyapatite crystals.[196]

Immunohistochemically, the cells of osteosarcoma consistently express vimentin. In some cases they are also positive for smooth muscle actin and desmin (suggesting myofibroblastic or myoid differentiation) and exceptionally for keratin and epithelial membrane antigen (EMA).[192,200,281] S-100 protein is always present in foci of chondroid differentiation, but it may also be seen in osteoblastic areas.[200]

Proteins specifically associated with bone metabolism – osteonectin, osteocalcin, osteopontin bone morphogenetic protein, and bone GLA protein – have been identified immunohistochemically in the cells of osteosarcoma and may be of utility in the differential diagnosis of this tumor.[166,188,211,261,280,307,308] Type I collagen is consistently found in the extracellular material; in addition, type II collagen is present in chondroid foci, and type IV collagen may also be encountered.[224]

Molecular genetic features. Osteosarcoma typically shows complex karyotypes, with structural alterations (including translocations) and numerical alterations (gain and loss) involving multiple chromosomes.[167,234,245,257] At the molecular level, alterations of both the *TP53* gene and retinoblastoma gene pathways are found in most cases, not unexpectedly since germline mutations in these genes are known to predispose to development of osteosarcoma.[295] The *TP53* pathway is altered through loss-of-function mutation in *TP53* (50%), *MDM2* amplification (14–27%), and deletion or hypermethylation of *P14/ARF* (10–34%). The retinoblastoma gene pathway is altered through loss of *RB1* and *CDKN2A*, and amplification of *CDK4* and *CCND1*.[160,181,214] Increased copies of *MYC* and *PRIM1* genes are also common (about 40% of cases).[278,309]

Microscopic variants and special types. In addition to the wide range in morphologic appearance already described in osteosarcoma, there are some cases in which the cytoarchitectural characteristics depart enough from the norm to justify recognition as a special category.[218] It should be realized that these variations may be present only focally and that they may occur in combination; their main importance rests on their ability to simulate other bone processes microscopically and also on the fact that some of them carry distinctive prognostic connotations:

1 *Telangiectatic*. Blood-filled cystic formations are prominent, resulting in an appearance similar to that of aneurysmal bone cyst radiographically and pathologically, although the arteriographic pattern is usually different (Fig. 24.25).

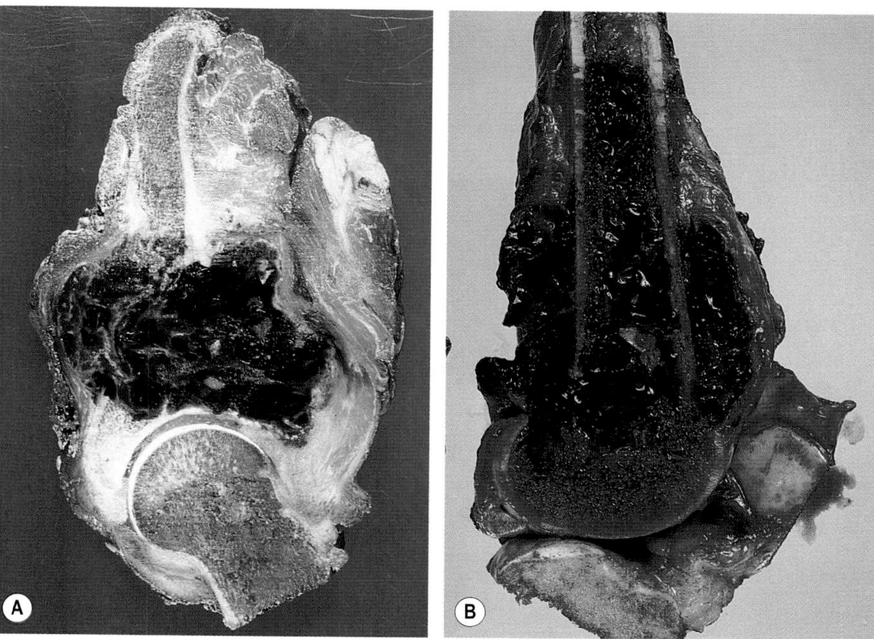

Fig. 24.25 **A** and **B**, Gross appearances of telangiectatic osteosarcoma.

Pathologic fractures are very frequent.[207] The lesion is identified as osteosarcoma through the detection of malignant stroma in the septa that separate the bloody cysts[162] (Fig. 24.26). Telangiectatic osteosarcoma has been found to be associated with a more aggressive course than the conventional variety in one large series[233] but not in two others.[162,207]

2 *Small cell.* The small size and uniformity of the tumor cells and their diffuse pattern of growth closely simulate the appearance of Ewing sarcoma/PNET and malignant lymphoma.[236,248] In some cases, these cells are spindle rather than round.[151] Focal production of osteoid (sometimes mixed with cartilage) by these small cells is the distinguishing feature.[163,267] Areas of cartilage formation can also be present.[151] In contrast to Ewing sarcoma/PNET, most cases of small cell osteosarcoma lack immunoreactivity for CD99,[182] although a recent study challenged this conclusion.[226] There are no pathognomonic ultrastructural features, and it is difficult to distinguish small cell osteosarcoma from Ewing sarcoma/PNET at this level when osteoid is not present in the sample.[183]

3 *Fibrohistiocytic.* The appearance in most areas is indistinguishable from that of so-called malignant fibrous histiocytoma, especially in the areas of soft tissue extension and in the distant metastases; however, tumor osteoid is focally present.

4 *Anaplastic.* The tumor is so bizarre and undifferentiated as to raise the possibility of any type of pleomorphic sarcoma or metastatic carcinoma. Once again, the key to the diagnosis is the identification of tumor osteoid.

5 *Well-differentiated (low-grade) intramedullary (intraosseous)* (Fig. 24.27). This tumor is microscopically so bland looking as to be often underdiagnosed as a benign lesion, particularly fibrous dysplasia.[289] Other cases resemble histologically parosteal osteosarcoma[161] or Paget disease.[193] These morphologic similarities are retained at the electron microscopic level.[277] Most patients are adults, the femur and

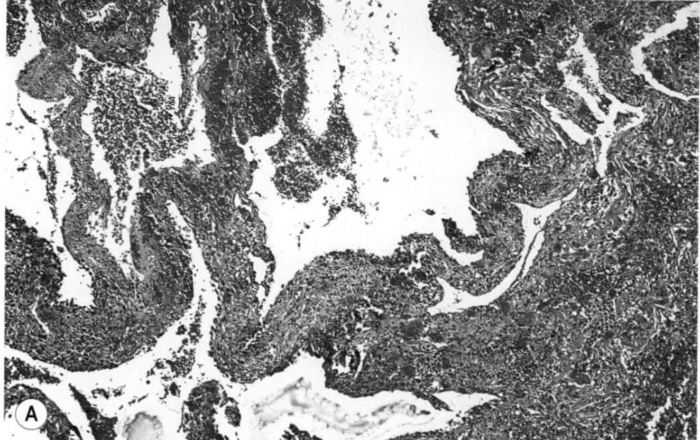

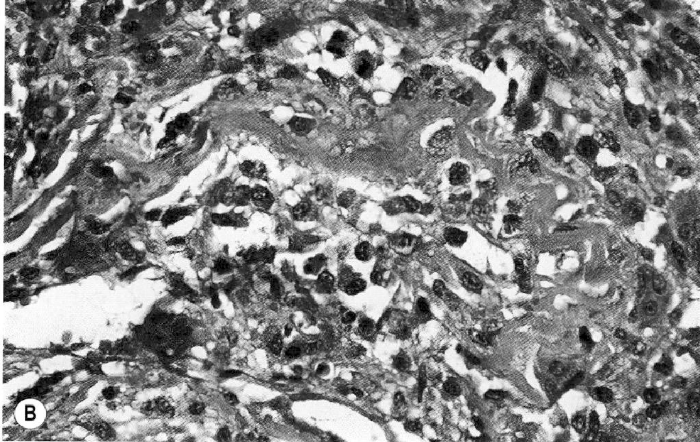

Fig. 24.26 **A** and **B**, Microscopic appearance of telangiectatic osteosarcoma. **A**, The low-power architecture closely simulates the appearance of an aneurysmal bone cyst. **B**, Malignant osteoid is present in the septa.

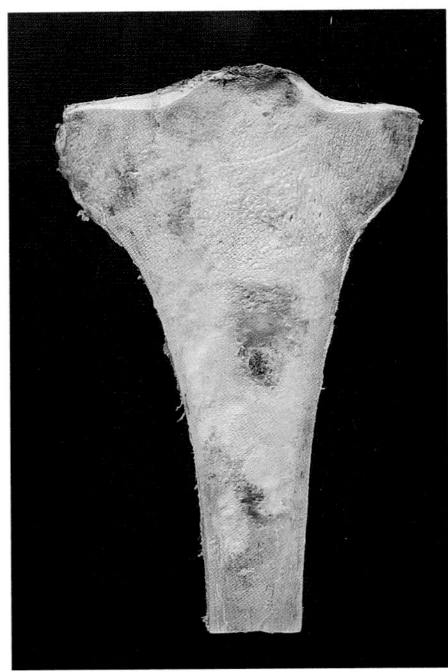

Fig. 24.27 Gross appearance of intraosseous well-differentiated osteosarcoma of tibia.
(Courtesy of Dr Juan José Segura, San José, Costa Rica)

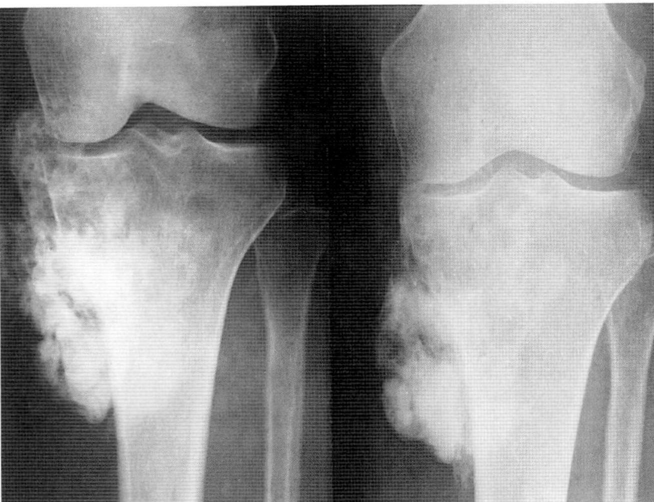

Fig. 24.28 Juxtacortical osteosarcoma occurring in a 40-year-old woman. Note the large extracortical component.

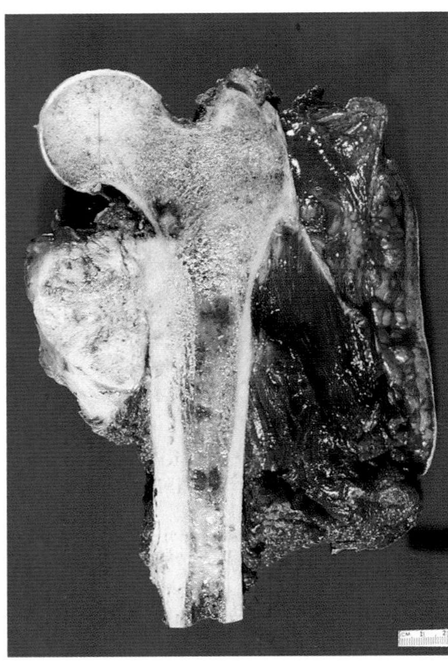

Fig. 24.29 Juxtacortical osteosarcoma of upper femur. There is only minimal involvement of the cortex.

tibia being the most commonly involved sites. Exceptionally, the small phalangeal bones are affected.[279] Spindle cells with minimal atypia and scanty mitoses are seen mixed with abundant osteoid. Recurrences are common, but metastases are very rare (unless the tumor converts in the recurrence into a conventional high-grade osteosarcoma), i.e., undergoes 'dedifferentiation'.[221,239] In contrast to fibrous dysplasia, this tumor shows radiographic evidence of cortical destruction.[221] Microscopically, atypia is minimal but still present. This feature and the invasive growth pattern are helpful in distinguishing this tumor from fibrous dysplasia.[221] The *GNAS1* gene mutation consistently found in fibrous dysplasia is generally absent in low-grade central osteosarcoma, pointing to a different pathogenesis for each of the two processes and providing a tool for their differential diagnosis.[252] Comparative genomic hybridization reveals a low number of chromosomal imbalances, which contrasts with the complex aberrations seen in conventional high-grade osteosarcoma.[284]

Other variants of osteosarcoma are defined on the basis of topographic, clinical, or radiographic features, or a combination of them:

1 *Juxtacortical (parosteal) osteosarcoma*. This infrequent variant occurs in a slightly older age group than the conventional variety.[287] It usually arises in a juxtacortical position in the metaphyses of long bones (usually the posterior aspect of the lower femoral shaft) and grows very slowly, some cases having a life history of up to 15 years. Eventually, it forms a large lobulated mass with a tendency to encircle the bone (Figs 24.28 and 24.29). Later in its evolution, it may penetrate into the medullary cavity, a feature associated with a higher microscopic grade and decreased survival.[172] Satellite nodules may be present. Rare cases have been described at other sites, such as the mandible and small bones of the hand.[292] The radiographic appearance is highly characteristic.[291] Microscopically, there is a disorderly pattern of well-formed bone, osteoid, occasional cartilage, and a highly fibrous spindle-cell stroma (Fig. 24.30). The cytologic signs of malignancy in the fibrous stroma are often subtle, thus accounting for the great frequency of misdiagnoses made in this tumor.[185] Exceptionally, the tumor is rich in osteoclast-like giant cells.[262] The most important differential diagnosis is with myositis ossificans, which is distinguished mainly on the basis of its orderly pattern of maturation (see p. 2066). The prognosis for juxtacortical osteosarcoma is very good, even

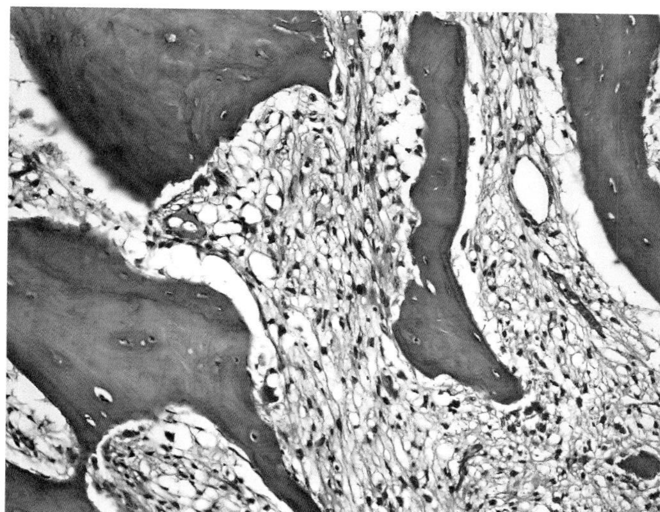

Fig. 24.30 Juxtacortical osteosarcoma. Moderately atypical spindle tumor cells grow between irregularly shaped bone trabeculae.

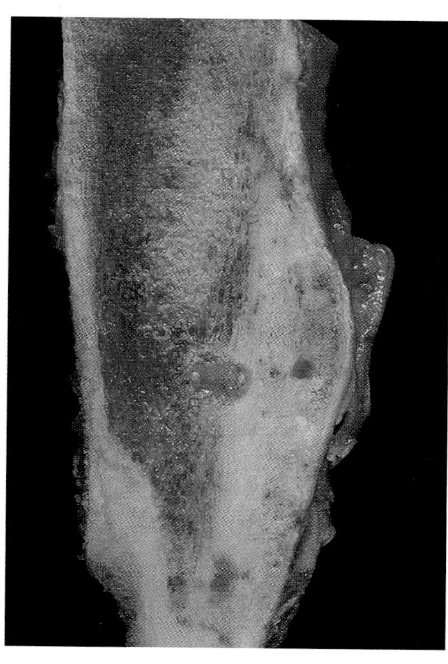

Fig. 24.31 Periosteal osteosarcoma. The white shining appearance is due to the high content of cartilage.

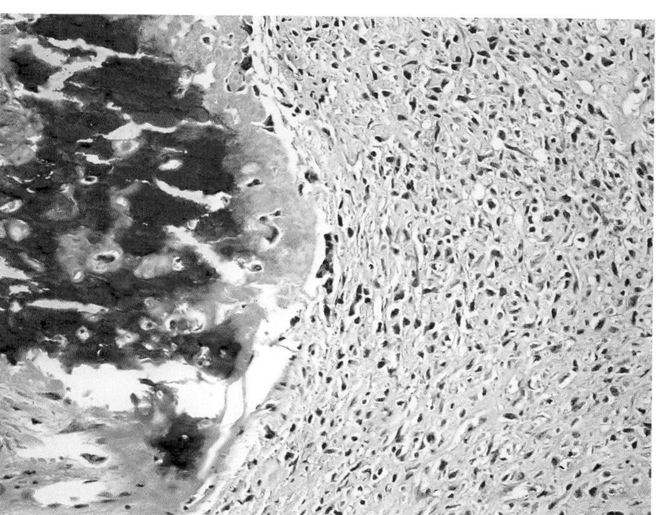

Fig. 24.32 Microscopic appearance of periosteal chondrosarcoma. There is a predominance of myxochondroid areas.

with segmental excision. It should be emphasized that not all osteosarcomas located juxtacortically belong to this variety. Those having morphologic features equivalent to those of the conventional intramedullary osteosarcoma are referred to as *high-grade surface osteosarcomas* and behave as aggressively as the former.[189,241,302] This is also true for the conventional intramedullary osteosarcoma with periosteal spread. Sometimes, features of high-grade osteosarcoma are seen focally in what is otherwise a typical juxtacortical osteosarcoma, either initially or – more commonly – following repeated tumor recurrences; this phenomenon, which is referred to as 'dedifferentiation', is associated with a markedly decreased survival rate.[147,265,287,303] The molecular genetic makeup of juxtacortical osteosarcoma is different from that of conventional osteosarcoma. It is characterized by a supernumerary ring chromosome as the sole aberration, effecting gain of 12q13–15, which results in coamplification of the *SAS*, *CDK4*, and *MDM2* genes.[202,282,304]

2 *Periosteal osteosarcoma.* This tumor type, which is very different from juxtacortical (parosteal) osteosarcoma despite the similarities in the misleading terminology chosen, grows on the surface of long bones.[288] Most of the reported cases have been located in the upper tibial shaft or femur and have presented as small lucent lesions on the bone surface, accompanied by bone spicules arranged perpendicular to the shaft. Exceptionally, they have been found in the small bones of digits.[184] The lesions are limited to the cortex and only rarely invade the medullary cavity[180,198] (Fig. 24.31). Microscopically, the tumors are relatively high-grade osteosarcomas, with a prominent cartilaginous component (Fig. 24.32). The prognosis is better than for conventional osteosarcoma.[288] This entity is closely related to the one discussed on page 2038 under the term juxtacortical (periosteal) chondrosarcoma, but some minor differences in location, microscopic grade, and behavior between the two have been described.

3 *Osteosarcoma of the jaw.* Gnathic osteosarcoma is distinctive enough to be treated separately from the rest.[174] Patients affected are slightly older (average age, 34 years), and most lesions show a prominent chondroblastic component. The most common sites of involvement are the body of the mandible and the alveolar ridge of the maxilla. The prognosis is relatively good.[174]

4 *Osteosarcoma in Paget disease.* Nearly all the cases of Paget disease complicated by osteosarcoma are of the polyostotic type. The tumors themselves are often multicentric. The most common locations are the pelvis, humerus, femur, tibia, and skull.[205,208,299] According to Schajowicz et al.,[259] these osteosarcomas are characterized microscopically by a large number of osteoclasts alternating with atypical osteoblasts. The prognosis is extremely poor.[205,299]

Diagnosis. Although most osteosarcomas have a very characteristic radiographic appearance, there is sufficient overlap with other malignant bone tumors and with benign conditions to make imperative a pathologic diagnosis before instituting definitive therapy. Depending on the size and location of the tumor and the skill and experience of the diagnostic team, the choice of procedure may be open biopsy, needle biopsy, fine needle aspiration, or frozen section.[191]

When performing an open biopsy, an attempt should be made to include tumor and adjacent non-neoplastic tissue; excessive trauma should be avoided, and the biopsy incision should be so placed that it will be entirely removed by the subsequent surgical excision.[229] There is no evidence that the performance of an incisional biopsy affects survival in these patients.[168]

Needle biopsy in experienced hands is extremely reliable and is of particular use in locations that are difficult to reach by open biopsy, such as the vertebral column.[150,179,258] Fine needle aspiration has also been used extensively with very good results.[165,298]

Laboratory tests are of no great value in the diagnosis of osteosarcoma. The only abnormality detected with some frequency is elevation of serum alkaline phosphatase, but this is merely an expression of bone production and, as such, is nonspecific. It can also be elevated in hyperparathyroidism, Paget disease, and metastatic carcinoma from the breast or prostate. Conversely, it is apt to be negative in a predominantly osteolytic osteosarcoma.

Therapy. Formerly, the therapy of osteosarcoma of the extremities has usually consisted of amputation or disarticulation, depending on the location of the tumor. At present, more limited forms of surgery (limb-sparing procedures) have been coupled with other therapeutic modalities, particularly preoperative and postoperative neoadjuvant chemotherapy.[154,169,170,253] The preoperative chemotherapy can be administered systemically or intra-arterially.[212,301]

Microscopic studies of the tumor successfully treated with chemotherapy show extensive areas of necrosis and hemorrhage;[149] sites where viable tumor is more likely to persist are the soft tissue, cortex and subcortex, ligaments, and areas in contact with cartilage.[250] These morphologic changes correlate well with functional bone imaging, which therefore provides an accurate presurgical assessment of tumor response.[272] The presence of extensive tumor necrosis following chemotherapy constitutes a good prognostic sign[254] (see next section).

Surgical removal of metastatic nodules of osteosarcoma in the lungs prolongs survival in selected patients.[153,159,260]

Prognosis. The overall prognosis for osteosarcoma has significantly improved. For many years, the 5-year survival rate fluctuated very little from the figure of 20% in most series. Lately, many reports listing 5-year disease-free rates of 70% or more have appeared;[197,223] it is not clear how much of this apparent improvement is due to change in treatment (particularly the administration of multidrug chemotherapy following surgery), as opposed to a better selection of surgical candidates through more detailed radiographic studies.[199,256] When making these calculations, it is important to exclude cases of chondrosarcoma or fibrosarcoma, both of which carry a better prognosis than osteosarcoma.

Factors to be considered in regard to prognosis of osteosarcoma are the following:

1 *Age, sex, and pregnancy*. No apparent prognostic differences have been related to any of these parameters.[171,175,206]
2 *Presence of Paget disease*. These tumors are usually highly malignant; most of the reported cases have proved fatal.[205,299]
3 *History of prior irradiation*. Radiation-induced osteosarcomas do not behave significantly differently from those arising de novo; in one large series, the 5-year survival rate was 28%.[148]
4 *Specific bone involved*. Osteosarcomas of the jaw and distal extremities (below the elbows and knees) have a better prognosis than the others.[175,238] With osteosarcoma of the jaw, survival figures of over 80% have been achieved with current surgical modalities. In contrast, osteosarcomas of other craniofacial bones and vertebrae (many of which arise within the context of Paget disease) have a very poor prognosis.[157,208,237,266]
5 *Multifocal osteosarcoma*. This form is almost uniformly fatal.[247]
6 *Osteoblastic, chondroblastic, and fibroblastic types*. Some authors have claimed a better prognosis for the fibroblastic type, but the difference is so small as to be of no statistical significance. The chondroblastic type of osteosarcoma is said to be less responsive to chemotherapy than the osteoblastic or fibroblastic types.[152]
7 *Microscopic grading*. There is no definite relationship with prognosis[175,238] once the osteosarcoma variants are excluded.
8 *Parosteal and periosteal osteosarcoma*. As already indicated, both of these variants are associated with an improved prognosis, particularly the former.
9 *Microscopic variants*. Telangiectatic osteosarcoma has a worse prognosis (at least in one series), and well-differentiated intramedullary osteosarcoma has a better prognosis than conventional osteosarcoma. Small cell osteosarcoma has a prognosis that is the same as or slightly worse than conventional osteosarcoma.[151,163]
10 *Serum elevation of alkaline phosphatase*. Tumors associated with serum elevations of this enzyme have been found to have an increased metastatic rate.[225]
11 *Postchemotherapy tumor necrosis*. It has been shown by several independent studies that the amount of tumor necrosis following chemotherapy is directly related to survival rate.[164,254] As a matter of fact, this feature has emerged as the single most important prognostic parameter in conventional osteosarcoma of extremities with no evidence of distant metastases at presentation.[178]
12 *Aneuploidy*. Alteration of DNA ploidy as measured by flow cytometry is correlated with the microscopic grade of the tumor and may prove of prognostic value.[203,228] The technique may also be of help in the differential diagnosis, since most osteosarcomas are hyperploid or aneuploid, whereas the vast majority of benign bone tumors are diploid; however, periosteal and well-differentiated osteosarcomas are also usually diploid.[158]
13 *Heat shock protein*. The claim has been advanced that expression of heat shock protein 72 correlates with good response to neoadjuvant chemotherapy in osteosarcomas.[285]
14 *RB gene*. Loss of heterozygosity of the *RB* gene is a poor prognostic factor.[190]
15 *HER2/neu expression*. The expression of this surface protein has been said to correlate with poor prognosis.[243] However, this claim has not been substantiated by other authors.[217]
16 *P-glycoprotein*. A widespread pattern of P-glycoprotein expression in tumor cells at the time of diagnosis is associated with an increased rate of systemic relapse.[155]

Cartilage-forming tumors

Chondroma

Chondroma is a common benign cartilaginous tumor that occurs most frequently in the small bones of the hands and feet, particularly the proximal phalanges. **Enchondromas** begin in the spongiosa of the diaphysis from which they expand and thin the cortex.

Chondromas of the thumb and terminal phalanges are distinctly uncommon. About 30% of chondromas are multiple.[324]

Multiple enchondromas having a predominantly unilateral distribution are referred to as *Ollier disease*. The association of multiple enchondromas with soft tissue hemangiomas (including spindle cell hemangioendotheliomas) is known as *Maffucci syndrome*[318] (Fig. 24.33). In both conditions, there is a significant risk of malignant transformation, usually in the form of chondrosarcoma,[312,316,319,323] sometimes developing in multiple bones.[315] Ollier disease is also associated with ovarian sex cord-stromal tumors.[325]

Enchondromas of the ribs and long bones are distinctly unusual. A variant of the latter, presenting in the metaphysis of long bones, is characterized by massive calcification within the neoplasm (*calcifying enchondroma*)[317] (Fig. 24.34).

Juxtacortical (periosteal) chondromas are much less common than enchondromas; they arise from the periosteal region of a long bone or a small bone of the hand or foot.[311] They characteristically erode and induce sclerosis of the contiguous cortex (Fig. 24.35). Radiographically, juxtacortical chondromas are smaller and better marginated than their malignant counterpart[321] (see p. 2038). Recurrence may follow incomplete excision.[322]

Microscopically, chondromas are composed of mature lobules of hyaline cartilage (Fig. 24.36). Foci of myxoid degeneration, calcification, and endochondral ossification are common. Juxtacortical chondroma tends to be more cellular than its medullary counterpart and may contain occasional plump or double nuclei.[311]

Although not strictly a chondroma, the peculiar chest wall lesion of infancy known as **cartilaginous and vascular hamartoma (mesenchymoma)** is discussed here because of its benign nature and predominant cartilaginous composition.[313,314,320] These chondroid areas, which often exhibit endochondral ossification, are mixed with spindle areas with an aneurysmal bone cyst-like appearance. Most of the cases are already present at birth, and the behavior is benign.

Osteochondroma and related lesions

Osteochondroma is the most frequent benign bone tumor. It is usually asymptomatic, but it may lead to deformity or interfere with the function of adjacent structures such as tendons and blood vessels.[338] It may also undergo spontaneous regression.[333] The most common locations are the metaphyses of the lower femur, upper tibia, upper humerus, and pelvis. The radiographic appearance of osteochondroma is very characteristic; one of the most typical features is the fact that the lesions, when located in metaphyses of long bones, grow out in a direction opposite to the adjacent joint.

The average age of the patient at onset is approximately 10 years; in the large majority of the cases, the tumor appears before the patient is 20 years old.

The average greatest diameter is approximately 4 cm, but the tumors may reach sizes of 10 cm or more. The smaller tumors are sessile, whereas the larger ones tend to be pedunculated. Characteristically, there is a cap of cartilage covered by a fibrous membrane, which is continuous with the periosteum of the adjacent bone. This cap is usually lobulated in the large lesions (Figs 24.37 and 24.38). Its average thickness is about 0.6 cm; it is rare for it to exceed 1 cm. Microscopically, the cells resemble those of normal hyaline cartilage. Eosinophilic, periodic acid–Schiff (PAS)-positive inclusions may be seen in the cytoplasm.[334,340] The bulk of the lesion is made up of mature bone trabeculae located beneath the cartilaginous cap and containing normal bone marrow. At the interphase between cartilage and bone, there is active endochondral ossification. In older lesions, the cap thins out and may disappear altogether.

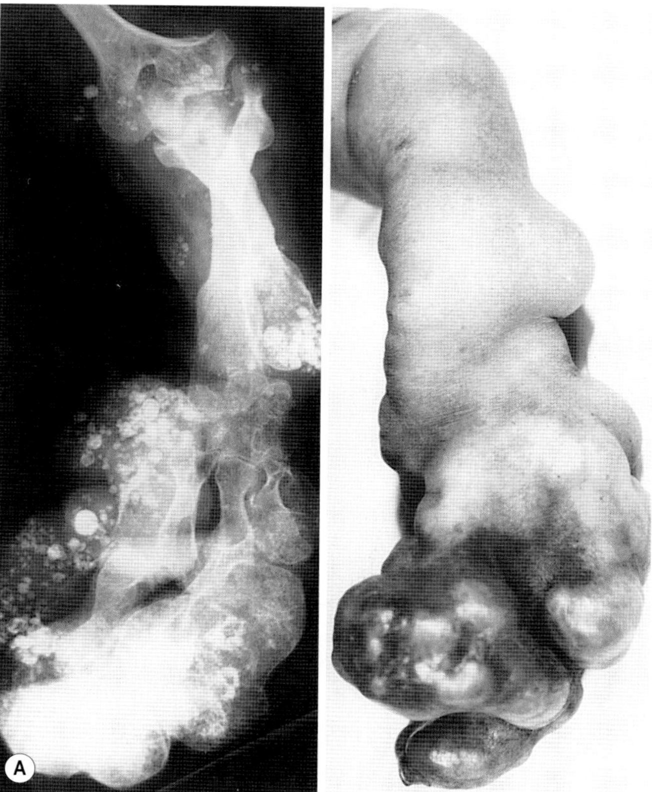

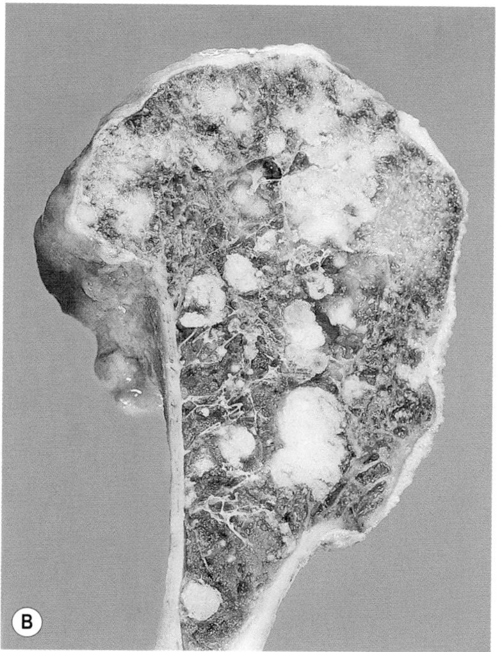

Fig. 24.33 **A**, Arm of a patient affected by Maffucci syndrome. Innumerable chondromas are seen concentrated in the distal aspect of the extremity. The patient developed chondrosarcoma in the innominate bone, with pulmonary metastases. **B**, Gross appearance of head of humerus affected by multiple chondromas in a patient with Ollier disease.

*(**A**, Courtesy of Dr O Urteaga, Lima, Perú; **B**, Courtesy of Dr RA Cooke, Brisbane, Australia; from Cooke RA, Stewart B. Colour Atlas of Anatomical Pathology. Edinburgh, 2004, Churchill Livingstone)*

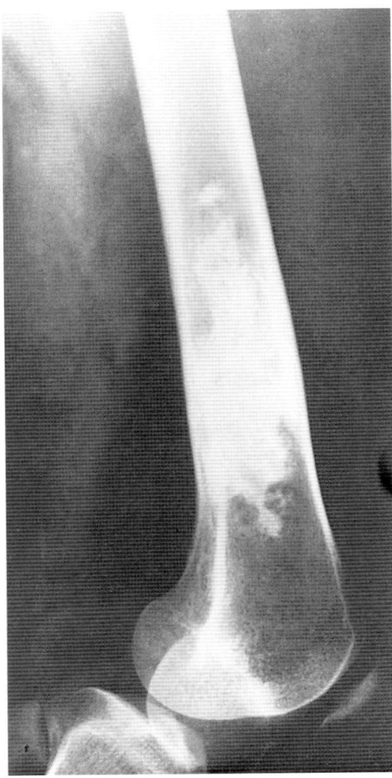

Fig. 24.34 Large asymptomatic enchondroma of femur in a 42-year-old woman. The tumor is extensively calcified.

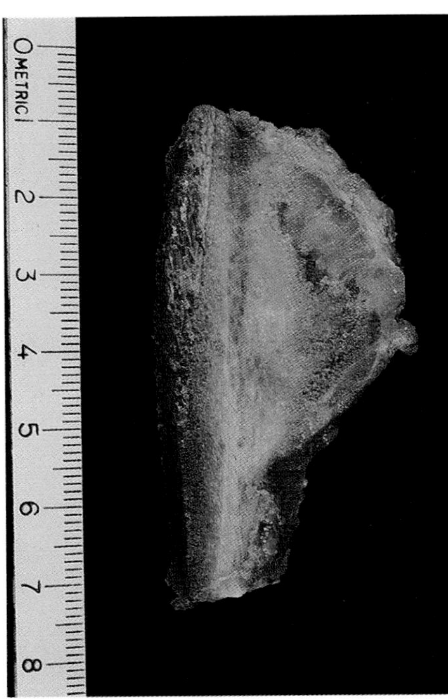

Fig. 24.35 Gross appearance of juxtacortical chondroma. The tumor produces a semispherical expansion of the involved bone.

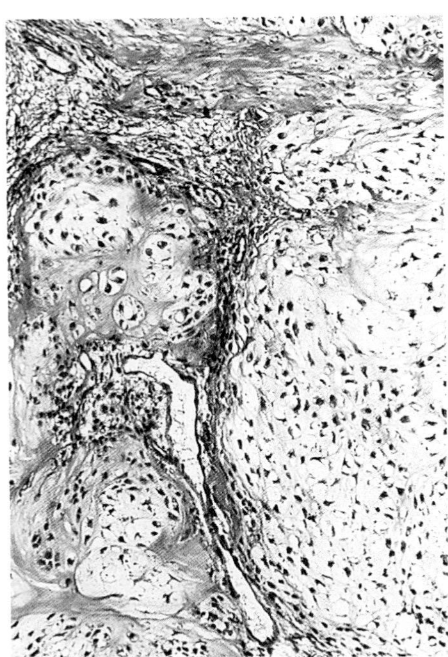

Fig. 24.36 Enchondroma of phalanx. The tumor has a typical lobulated appearance.

A bursa may develop around the head of a long-standing osteochondroma; in turn, this bursa may develop complications such as osteocartilaginous loose bodies, synovial chondrometaplasia, and – exceptionally – chondrosarcoma.[341]

The gross and microscopic appearance of a single lesion of the familial condition known as **osteochondromatosis** (multiple cartilaginous exostoses, Ehrenfried hereditary deforming chondrodysplasia, diaphyseal aclasis) cannot be distinguished from solitary osteochondroma.[347] Osteochondromatosis is caused by germline mutation in the *EXT1* (at 8q24) or *EXT2* (at 11p11–p12) gene.[328] These genes are implicated in the formation of both sporadic and hereditary osteochondromas, in that both alleles of the gene (more often *EXT1*) are inactivated through deletion or mutation (with one allele showing germline mutation for the hereditary form).[330,331,335]

A very small proportion of the solitary tumors evolve into chondrosarcomas, but the incidence reaches 10% in the cases with multiple lesions. The progression from osteochondroma to chondrosarcoma is associated with upregulation of PTHrP and BCL2 expression.[327] The supervening chondrosarcoma characteristically shows genetic instability, a high frequency of loss of heterozygosity, a broad range of DNA ploidy, and additional gene mutations (such as *TP53*).[329,337]

Osteochondroma should be distinguished from the **bizarre parosteal osteochondromatous proliferation (Nora lesion)**, which may occur in the bones of the hands and feet[339,346] and occasionally in long bones;[326] these lesions are radiographically distinctive but can simulate chondrosarcoma microscopically because of the presence of enlarged, bizarre, and binucleated chondrocytes.[343,346] Recurrent chromosomal alterations have been found, suggesting that this condition is of neoplastic nature.[345,348]

Subungual exostosis (Dupuytren exostosis) is usually located on the great toe. It is thought to represent a different entity from osteochondromas but is also composed of a proliferating cartilaginous

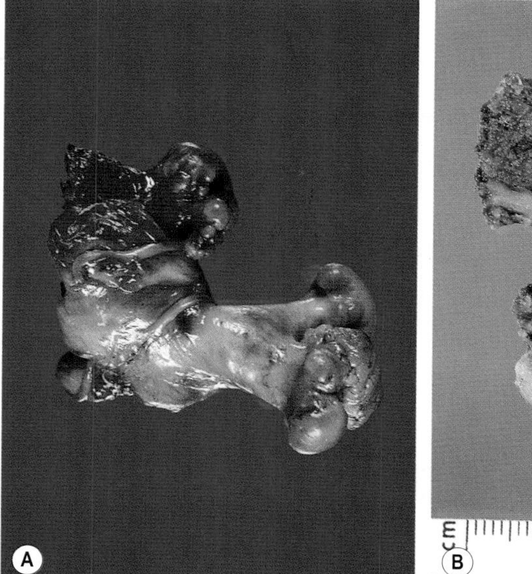
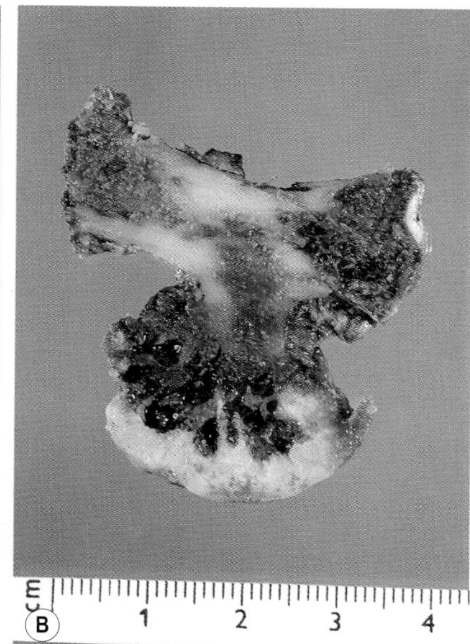

Fig. 24.37 **A**, Large osteochondroma of femur with a bilobed appearance. **B**, Cut surface of osteochondroma of rib. Note the thick cartilaginous cup.
(Courtesy of Dr RA Cooke, Brisbane, Australia; from Cooke RA, Stewart B. Colour Atlas of Anatomical Pathology. Edinburgh, 2004, Churchill Livingstone)

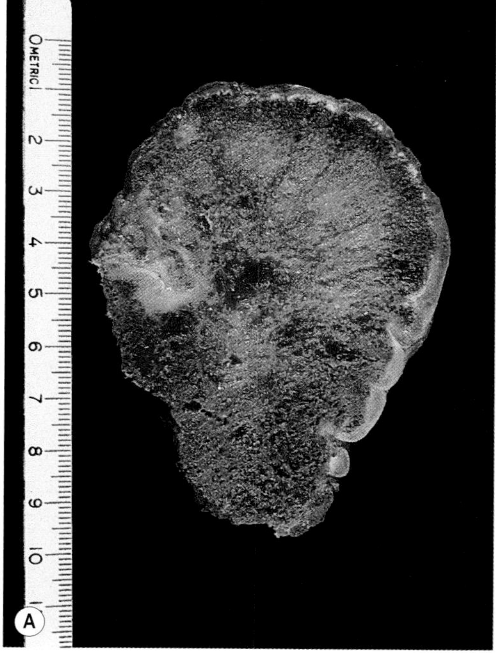
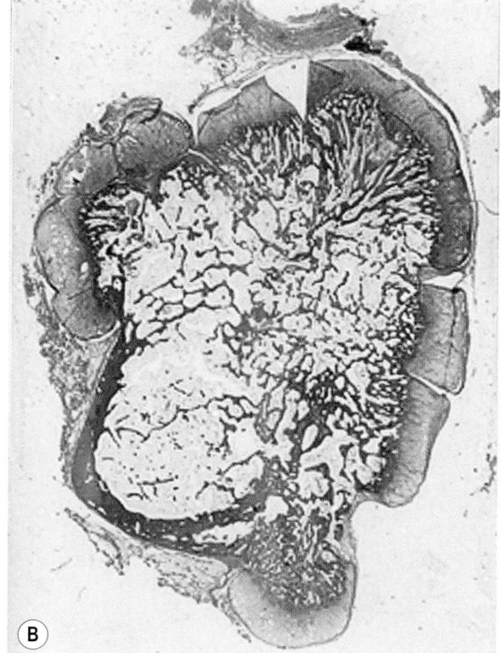

Fig. 24.38 **A** and **B**, Gross and whole-mount appearance of osteochondroma. Mature bone is covered by a well-differentiated cartilaginous cap.

cap that merges into mature trabecular bone at its base. These exostoses may recur but are invariably benign.[342,344] Like for Nora lesion, cytogenetic studies have demonstrated recurrent chromosomal rearrangements consistent with a neoplastic process.[348]

Dysplasia epiphysealis hemimelica (Trevor disease), a rare developmental disorder of childhood characterized by asymmetric enlargement of the epiphyseal cartilage of long bones, is yet another condition that can mimic osteochondroma.[336]

Osteochondromyxoma is a recently described congenital neoplasm associated with lentigines and other extraskeletal disorders; the syndrome seems to represent a variation of the Carney complex.[332]

Chondroblastoma

Chondroblastoma occurs predominantly in males under 20 years of age, and it can be quite painful.[371] It usually arises in the epiphyseal end of long bones before the epiphyseal cartilage has disappeared, particularly in the distal end of the femur, proximal end of the humerus, and proximal end of the tibia[371] (Fig. 24.39).

Radiographically, the tumor usually is fairly well delimited and contains areas of rarefaction (Fig. 24.40). From the epiphysis it may extend into the metaphyseal area or the articular cavity. Occasionally, it is found entirely in a metaphyseal location or in a small bone.[349,351]

Microscopically, this lesion may be confusing because of its extreme cellularity and variability.[354] The occasional scattered collections of giant cells may lead to an erroneous diagnosis of giant cell tumor (Fig. 24.41). The basic tumor cell is an embryonic chondroblast with only a limited capacity for the production of a cartilaginous matrix. The shape of this cell is usually polyhedral, although spindle elements can also be present. The cell membrane appears thick and sharply defined. The nuclei vary in shape from round to indented and lobulated; some resemble those of Langerhans cells[362] (Fig. 24.42). Mitoses are exceptional. Intracytoplasmic glycogen granules are present, sometimes in large numbers. Reticulin fibers surround each individual cell. Recurrent lesions may show some degree of atypia, a feature that should not be interpreted as a sign of malignant transformation. A distinctive microscopic change is the presence of small zones of focal calcification. These zones range from a network of thin lines ('chicken wire') to obvious deposits surrounded by giant cells.

In approximately one-fourth of the cases, areas resembling aneurysmal bone cyst are seen engrafted on the primary bone lesion[371] (Fig. 24.39). In patients with recurrent lesions, the incidence of this phenomenon rises to 50%.

By electron microscopy, the cells of chondroblastoma closely resemble normal epiphyseal cartilage cells grown in tissue culture.[372,374] They often have a prominent 'fibrous lamina' lying

Fig. 24.39 Gross appearance of chondroblastoma of upper end of the humerus, associated with aneurysmal bone cyst-like changes.

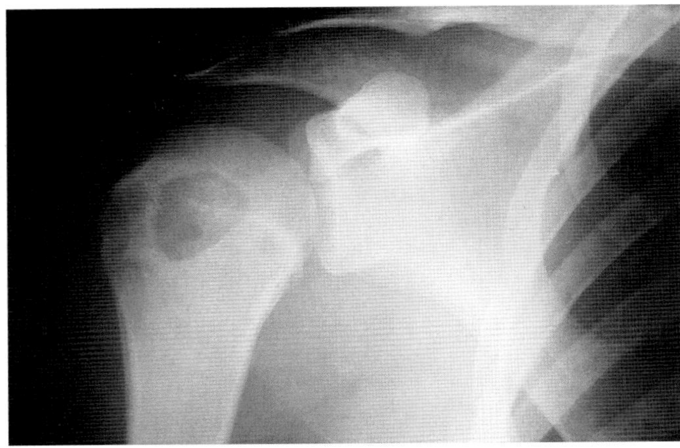

Fig. 24.40 Typical sharply delineated lytic appearance of chondroblastoma of humeral head.

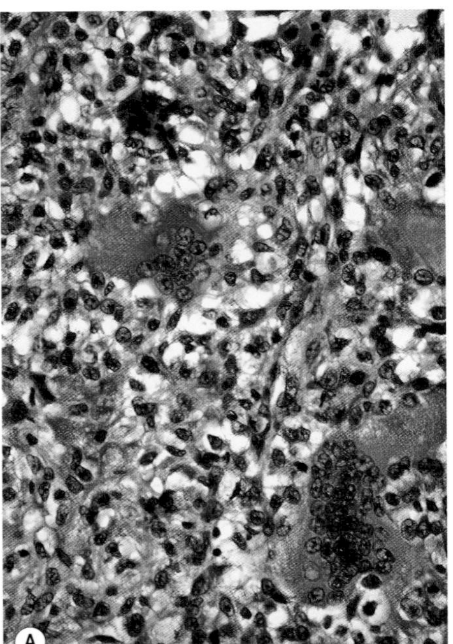

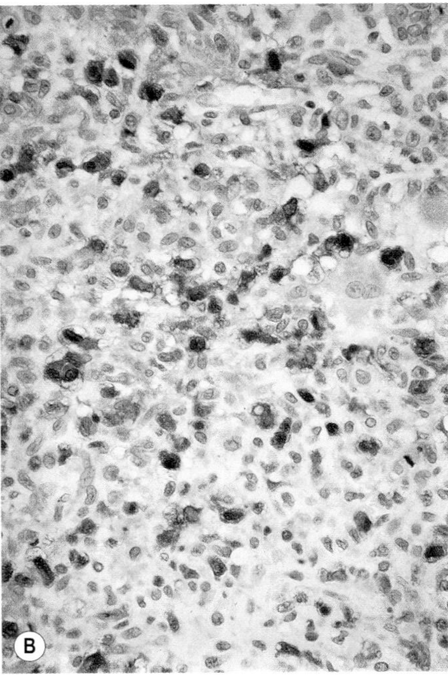

Fig. 24.41 **A** and **B**, Chondroblastoma. **A**, Small tumor cells of round shape are accompanied by scattered osteoclasts. **B**, Immunoreactivity for S-100 protein in the neoplastic component.

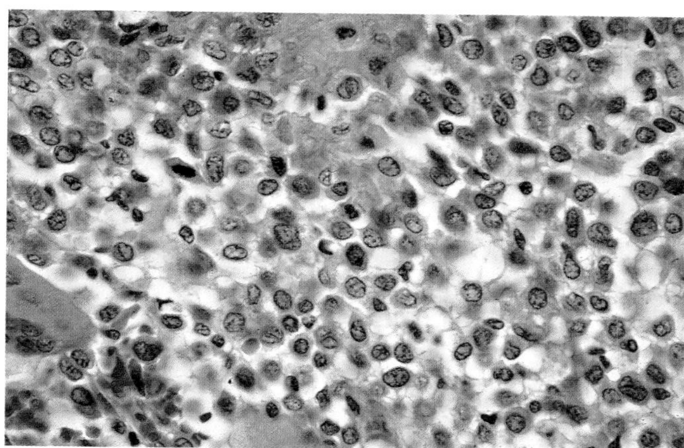

Fig. 24.42 Histiocyte-like appearance of the nuclei of chondroblastoma cells.

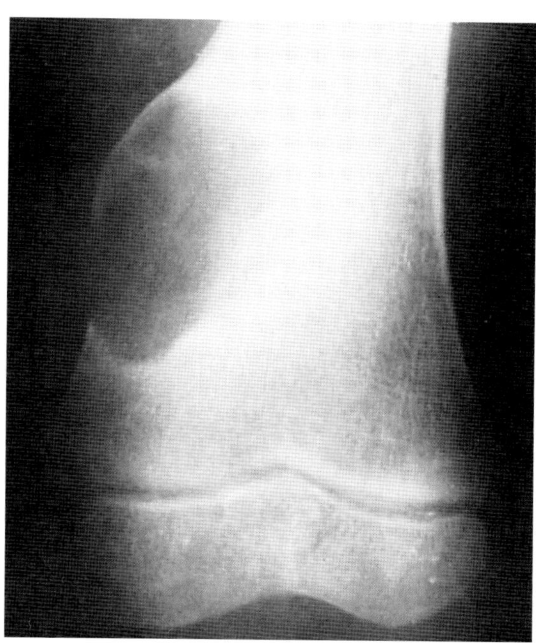

Fig. 24.43 Sharply delimited chondromyxoid fibroma of lower femoral metaphysis in a young boy.

against the inner aspect of the nuclear membrane, resulting in the membrane thickening seen by light microscopy.[357] Cytoplasmic glycogen is usually abundant. Proteoglycans and calcium have been demonstrated by ultrastructural cytochemistry in the extracellular matrix.[363] Immunohistochemically, the cells of osteoblastoma coexpress vimentin and S-100 protein (Fig. 24.41B). They may also be immunoreactive for neuron-specific enolase, muscle-specific actin, low molecular weight keratins, and Sox9.[351,359,367,370]

The histogenesis of chondroblastoma has been controversial. It has been variously regarded as a 'chondromatous' variant of giant cell tumor, as arising from histiocytic or 'reticuloendothelial cells', and as a truly cartilaginous neoplasm. The frequent areas of calcification, the occasional foci of well-developed cartilaginous stroma, the histochemical and ultrastructural profile, and the immunohistochemical positivity for S-100 protein and Sox9 all point toward a cartilaginous nature.[352,356,362–365]

The diagnosis is possible on the basis of fine needle aspiration material, which in a typical case will consist of neoplastic chondroblasts, multinucleated osteoclast-like giant cells, and chondroid matrix fragments.[355] Curetting with bone grafting, which is the preferred treatment, provides local control in over 80% of the cases.[353] Local recurrences can be treated similarly.[373]

Several cases of chondroblastoma, microscopically indistinguishable from the rest, have behaved locally in an aggressive fashion, invading the soft tissues and developing tumor thrombi in lymph channels. Most of these aggressive tumors were located in the pelvis.[368] A few others have given rise to distant metastases, usually to the lungs.[350,358,361,366] In nearly all of the reported cases of this phenomenon, the metastases have occurred after surgical manipulation of the primary tumor.[360,361,369]

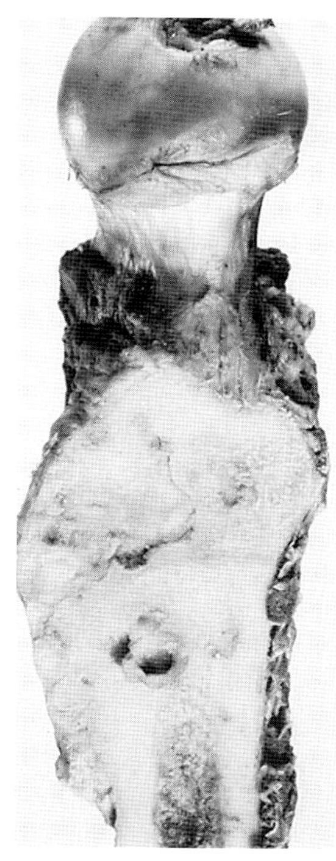

Fig. 24.44 Chondromyxoid fibroma of proximal femur extending into soft tissue. This rare event should not be regarded as evidence of malignancy.

Chondromyxoid fibroma and related tumors

Chondromyxoid fibroma of bone is an unusual benign tumor of cartilaginous nature.[385,394] It usually occurs in a long bone of a young adult, but it has also been reported in the small bones of the hands and feet, pelvis, ribs, vertebrae, and skull base; in the latter location there is a risk of it being misdiagnosed as chordoma or chondrosarcoma.[382]

Radiographically, it is sharply defined and may attain a large size (Fig. 24.43). It is usually located in the medullary portion of the bone, but a juxtacortical variant arising on the bone surface has been described.[376] Grossly, it is solid and yellowish white or tan, replaces bone, and thins the cortex (Fig. 24.44). Microscopically, it comprises hypocellular lobules with a myxochondroid appearance, separated by intersecting bands of highly cellular tissue composed of fibroblast-like spindle cells and osteoclasts[380] (Fig. 24.45). Calcification may occur, particularly in the juxtacortical variant.[376]

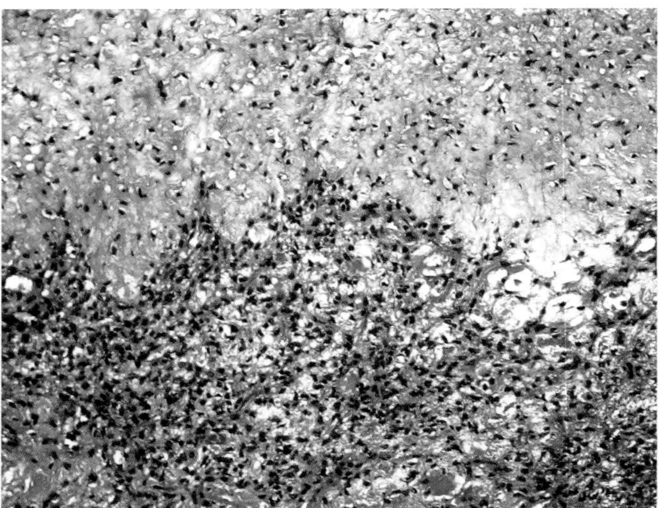

Fig. 24.45 Chondromyxoid fibroma. The tumor has a lobulated appearance, in which myxochondroid islands alternate with more cellular foci.

The occasional presence of large pleomorphic cells may result in an erroneous diagnosis of chondrosarcoma.[375,392,395] However, mitotic figures are exceptional. Some tumors show a combination of the features of chondroblastoma and chondromyxoid fibroma.[378]

Immunohistochemical reactivity for S-100 protein is the rule, in keeping with its presumed cartilaginous nature,[377] but there are also cells with myofibroblastic and myochondroblastic features.[379,390] Although the intercellular matrix is primarily of a cartilaginous nature, it exhibits significant differences from that present in any other cartilaginous neoplasm.[393] The basic cartilaginous nature of this tumor has been demonstrated through its immunoreactivity for Sox9 (an essential regulator of chondrogenesis) and further supported by the presence of type II collagen. In contrast to chondroblastoma, it is consistently negative for keratin.[384]

Cytogenetically, chondromyxoid fibroma is characterized by rearrangements of chromosome 6 at band q13 or q25.[381,391]

Local recurrence follows curettage of chondromyxoid fibroma in about 25% of the cases, sometimes after an interval as long as 30 years.[383] Because of this, en bloc excision is recommended whenever possible. Soft tissue extension or implantation may occur,[386,395] but distant metastases have not been reported.

Fibromyxoma is microscopically similar to chondromyxoid fibroma but lacks cartilaginous areas and tends to occur in older individuals.[387,388] Its existence as an entity distinct from chondromyxoma remains doubtful.

Myxoma of long bones is characterized by an expansile radiographic appearance, distal location, benign behavior, and microscopic appearance similar to soft tissue myxoma.[389]

Chondrosarcoma

Chondrosarcoma, a malignant tumor of cartilage-forming tissues, is divided into two major categories on the basis of microscopic criteria: conventional chondrosarcoma and chondrosarcoma variants. Each of these categories comprises several distinct types, some defined on microscopic grounds and others on the basis of location within the affected bone.

Conventional chondrosarcoma. The majority of the patients with conventional chondrosarcoma are between 30 and 60 years of age. Chondrosarcoma in childhood is distinctly uncommon[413,456] and tends more often to be located in the extremities than its adult counterpart;[421] most malignant bone tumors in this age group exhibiting cartilage formation are actually osteosarcomas with a predominant cartilaginous component.

Chondrosarcomas are divided according to location into central, peripheral, and juxtacortical (periosteal) forms.[405] **Central chondrosarcomas** are located in the medullary cavity, usually of a flat or long bone[401] (Fig. 24.46). Radiographically, they present a rather characteristic picture of an osteolytic lesion with splotchy calcification (Fig. 24.47). Ill-defined margins, fusiform thickening of the shaft, and perforation of the cortex are three important diagnostic signs.[398] In advanced stages, they may break through the cortex but only rarely grow beyond the periosteum. The pelvic bones, ribs (usually at the costochondral junction), and shoulder girdle are the most common locations. Chondrosarcomas of the small bones of the hands and feet are exceptional but have been described by several authors, particularly in the os calcis.[404,408,428,438,442] Chondrosarcoma can also involve the bones of the skull, especially the temporal bone and base of the skull, where the differential diagnosis includes chordoma, meningioma, and glomus jugulare tumor.[406,444]

Peripheral chondrosarcomas may arise de novo or from the cartilaginous cap of a preexisting osteochondroma (Fig. 24.48). Osteochondromatosis is particularly prone to this complication, as already indicated. In the 212 cases of chondrosarcoma reported by Dahlin and Henderson,[407] 19 apparently arose from osteochondroma. The risk of malignant transformation in a solitary osteochondroma is believed to be between 1% and 2%. The signs of malignancy in an osteochondroma include increased growth during adolescence, a diameter over 8 cm, and a cartilaginous cap that is irregular and thicker than 3 cm. Radiographically, peripheral chondrosarcomas present as large tumors, with a heavily calcified center surrounded by a lesser denser periphery with splotchy calcification (Fig. 24.49). Malignant change should be suspected radiographically in an osteochondroma if the cartilage cap has irregular margins or if there are lucent zones within the lesion.[414]

Juxtacortical (periosteal) chondrosarcoma involves the shaft of a long bone (most often the femur) and is characterized by a cartilaginous lobular pattern with areas of spotty calcification and endochondral ossification.[449] This tumor is closely related to the entity reported as periosteal osteosarcoma (see p. 2031); however, some minor differences in location, microscopic grade, and behavior between the two have been described that may justify their separation.[400]

Microscopically, conventional chondrosarcomas of central, peripheral, or juxtacortical types show a remarkably wide range of differentiation, the common denominator being the production of a cartilaginous matrix and the lack of direct bone formation by the tumor cells. This range in differentiation is the basis for the grading of these tumors into well, moderately, and poorly differentiated. The differential diagnosis between well-differentiated chondrosarcoma and chondroma rests on a combination of radiographic, architectural, and cytologic features[450] (Fig. 24.50). This differentiation can be very difficult and is subject to a distressingly high degree of interobserver variability.[410] In well-differentiated chondrosarcoma, the nuclei are plump and hyperchromatic; there may be two or more nuclei per cell and two or more cells per lacuna (Fig. 24.51). Mirra et al.[436] have emphasized permeation of the bone marrow with trapping of host lamellar bone on all sides in well-differentiated chondrosarcoma as an important sign in the differential diagnosis with chondroma. Both the nuclear and architectural abnormalities of chondrosarcoma are often better seen at the growing edge of the tumor. Correlation of the microscopic features

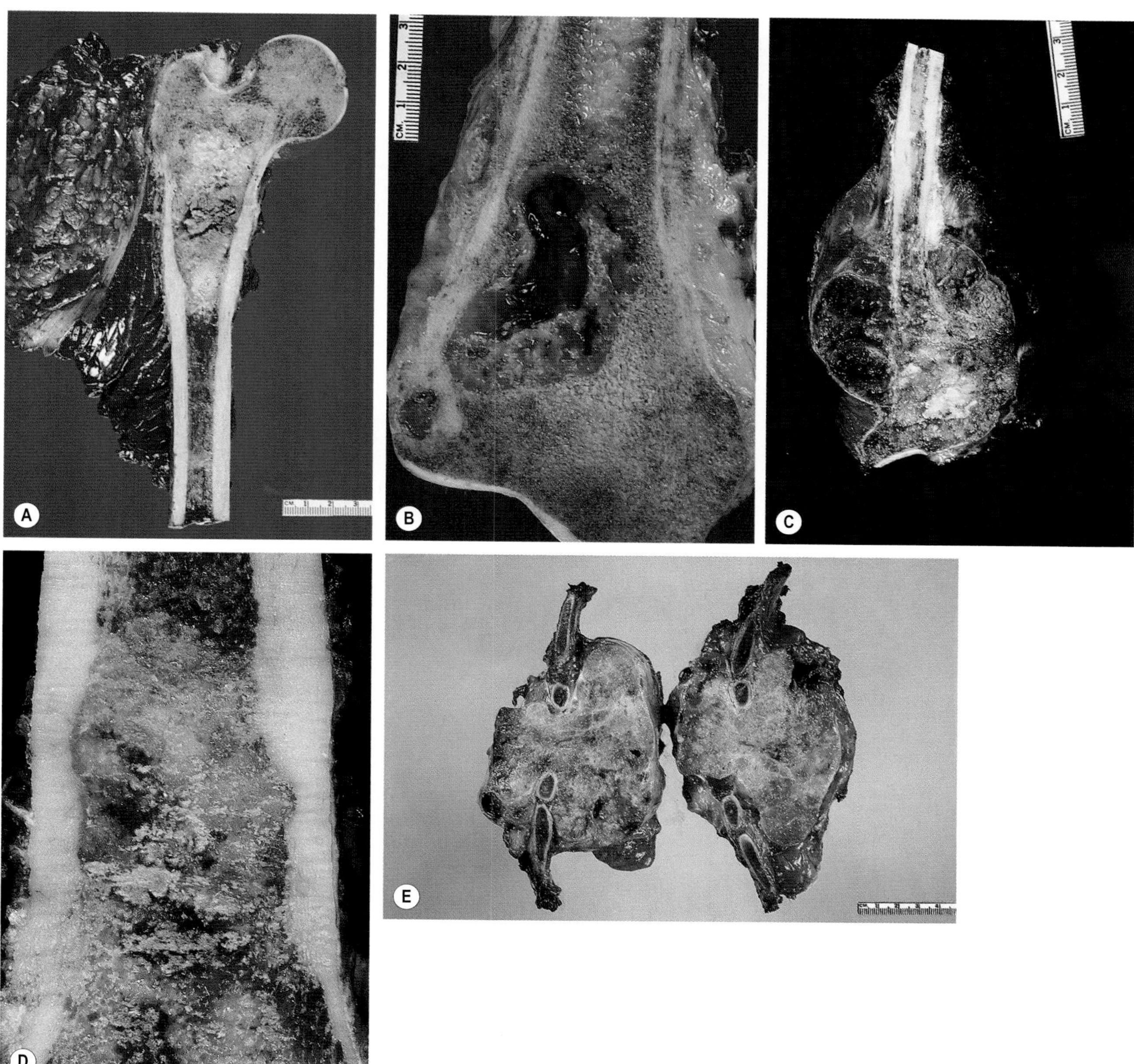

Fig. 24.46 Gross appearances of central chondrosarcoma: **A–D**, all of these tumors were located in the femur, the single most common site of occurrence; **E**, chondrosarcoma of rib, resulting in massive expansion of the bone.

with the clinical and especially the radiographic findings is essential. Large tumors of the long bones or ribs or those that begin to grow rapidly over adolescence and reach a size of 8 cm or more are almost invariably malignant.[433] Minor degrees of atypia in the cartilaginous cells under these circumstances justify a diagnosis of chondrosarcoma, whereas similar or even greater atypical changes in cartilaginous tumors of the hands and feet, osteochondromas, synovial osteochondromatosis, and soft tissue neoplasms are much less significant. It also should be noted that the minor atypical changes on which the diagnosis of malignancy are based are often focal, a point to remember when examining a small sample of a cartilaginous neoplasm.

Chondrosarcoma is distinguished from osteosarcoma by the lack of direct osteoid or bone formation by the tumor cells. Bone can be present in a bona fide chondrosarcoma, but this is non-neoplastic and probably originates from reabsorption of the tumor cartilage by a mechanism of endochondral ossification.

Histochemically, well-differentiated chondrosarcomas have a staining reaction similar to that of adult cartilage, whereas poorly differentiated tumors resemble fetal cartilage.[422] Biochemically, a marked variability in composition has been observed.[431,432] Ultrastructurally, the cells of well-differentiated tumors show cytoplasmic accumulation of glycogen, lipid droplets, and dilated cisternae of granular endoplasmic reticulum.[411] Immunohistochemically, there is reactivity for S-100 protein, estrogen receptors, and Sox9, the latter being an essential regulator of chondrogenesis[416,423,437,439] (Fig. 24.52). BCL2 is positive in over half of the cases, whereas it is negative in 95% of osteochondromas.[418]

Chondrosarcomas also show positivity for MCM6 (minichromosome maintenance protein) and CXCR4, the degree of staining being related in both instances to the tumor grade.[397,420] The surprising claim has been made that ezrin (a cytoskeletal linker protein) is consistently absent in chondrosarcoma while often present in osteosarcoma, including the chondroblastic subtype of this tumor.[445]

Cytogenetically, there is considerable heterogeneity among chondrosarcomas but also evidence that some of the karyotypic anomalies are not random.[429,430,446] In contrast to peripheral secondary chondrosarcoma (see above section on enchondroma), primary conventional chondrosarcoma is characterized by peridiploidy and a low frequency of loss of heterozygosity.[403] Inactivation of *CDKN2A* is a common occurrence.[417,454] Hemizygous deletion of *EXT1* or *EXT2* (genes implicated in osteochondroma and osteochondromatosis) occurs in 27% of cases.[417]

Overexpression of *TP53* is limited to the high-grade (poorly differentiated) types.[409,441,453] Use of gene expression profiling to identify a pre-chondrogenic and a chondrogenic phenotype for chondrosarcoma can help predict the clinical behavior.[402]

Soft tissue implantation following biopsy is a well-known complication of chondrosarcoma. Therefore, if a large cartilaginous tumor is so located that the biopsy site cannot be entirely excised, the initial excision should be complete. If an extremely large tumor involves the pelvic bone, wide block excision or even

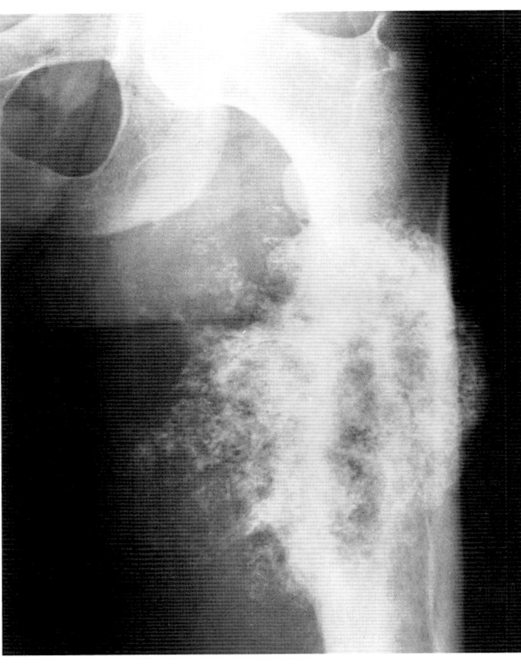

Fig. 24.47 Typical chondrosarcoma of femur showing splotchy calcification and extensive cortical destruction.

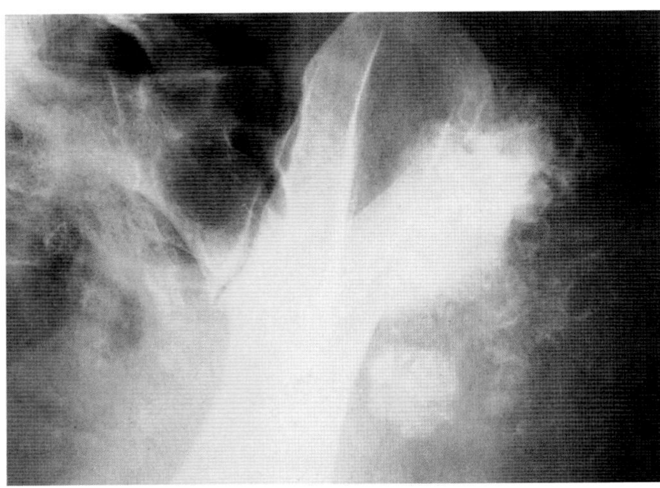

Fig. 24.49 Typical radiographic appearance of peripheral chondrosarcoma of innominate bone.
(Courtesy of Dr WT Hill, Houston)

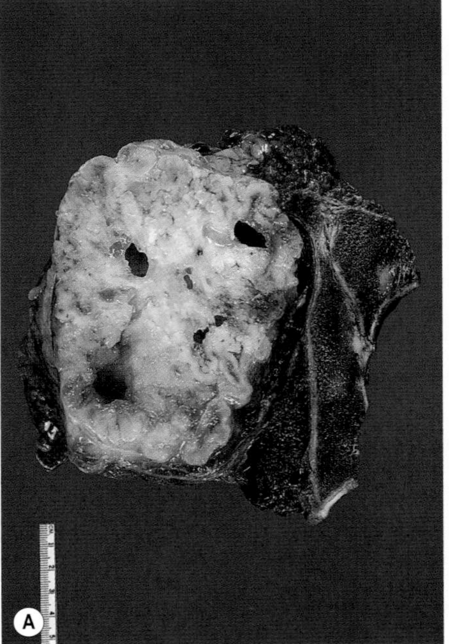

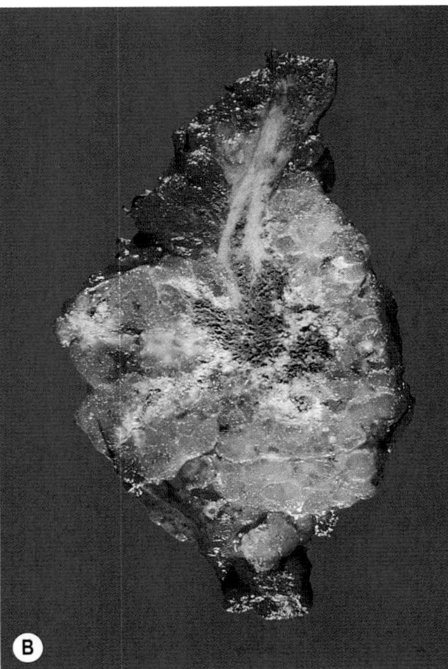

Fig. 24.48 **A** and **B**, Gross appearances of chondrosarcoma. **A**, Peripheral chondrosarcoma of femur resulting in a huge exophytic mass. **B**, Large expansile chondrosarcoma of sternum.
*(**A**, Courtesy of Dr Juan José Segura, San José, Costa Rica)*

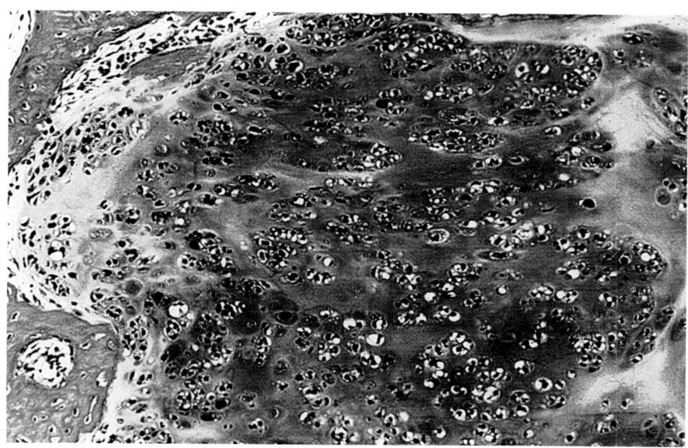

Fig. 24.50 Well-differentiated chondrosarcoma. The tumor has a distinctly lobulated quality.

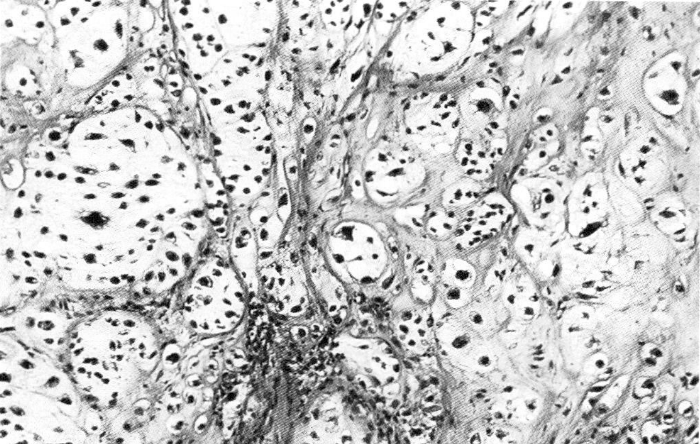

Fig. 24.51 Microscopic appearance of well-differentiated chondrosarcoma. The tumor retains a lobulated appearance, but nuclear atypicality is obvious.

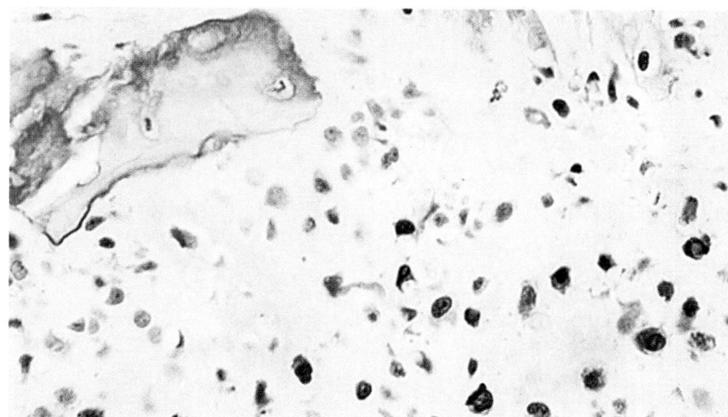

Fig. 24.52 Chondrosarcoma of bone. There is both cytoplasmic and nuclear staining for S-100 protein.

hemipelvectomy is justified without prior histologic diagnosis. Chondrosarcomas of the rib should be excised en bloc with the adjacent uninvolved ribs and pleura.[434,440] Well-differentiated chondrosarcomas of the extremities are amenable to conservative therapy in the form of segmental resection.[452] It should be noted, however, that skip metastases of the type more commonly seen in osteosarcoma also exceptionally occur in chondrosarcoma.[455]

In contrast to osteosarcoma, microscopic grading of chondrosarcomas, whether done by a combination of cytoarchitectural features[412] or by nuclear grade alone,[425] is of value in predicting the final outcome. In the series reported by McKenna et al.,[435] the 5-year survival rates were 78%, 53%, and 22% for low-, moderate-, and high-grade tumors, respectively. In three other series, the overall survival figures were generally better, but the differences between the three grades were still obvious.[412,415,419,443,447] Recurrences often are of a higher microscopic grade than the original tumor.[426] Equally important prognostically is the adequacy of initial therapy.[399,415,451] Preliminary results with flow cytometry suggest that determination of DNA ploidy may be an important prognostic determinator.[396,424,427] An association between 6q13–21 chromosome aberrations and locally aggressive behavior has been described.[448] High-grade chondrosarcomas metastasize early, particularly to the lungs. Lymph node metastases are practically nonexistent.

Chondrosarcoma variants

Clear cell chondrosarcoma

Clear cell chondrosarcoma is characterized by tumor cells with an abundant clear or ground glass cytoplasm and sharply defined borders, often interspersed with small trabeculae of woven bone.[462,463] It may be confused with chondroblastoma and may actually represent its malignant counterpart[464] (Fig. 24.53). Ultrastructurally, it shows chondroid cells in various stages of differentiation[460] and, immunohistochemically, exhibits immunoreactivity for S-100 protein and collagens types II and X (but not I).[457,463–466] Most patients are older than those affected by chondroblastoma.[458] Radiographically, the lesion is usually entirely lytic, slightly expansile, and sharply marginated.[458] Most of the cases have involved the proximal end of the femur or humerus, and the behavior has generally been that of a low-grade malignancy, with some outstanding exceptions.[459] In addition – and like conventional chondrosarcoma – it can undergo dedifferentiation.[461]

Myxoid chondrosarcoma (chordoid sarcoma)

This variant of chondrosarcoma can occur in bone but is much more common in the soft tissues (see Chapter 25).[467,469] It is morphologically reminiscent of chordoma because of the rows of cuboidal cells separated by a myxoid background.[470] It reacts immunohistochemically for S-100 protein and vimentin but, in contrast to chordoma, is negative for keratin.[471] Ultrastructurally, it is closer in appearance to conventional chondrosarcoma than to chordoma.[472] Whether the tumor reported by Dabska[468] as **parachordoma** is also histogenetically related to myxoid chondrosarcoma or a type of myoepithelioma remains to be determined.[473]

Dedifferentiated chondrosarcoma

The term dedifferentiated chondrosarcoma refers to the presence of a poorly differentiated sarcomatous component at the periphery of an otherwise typical low-grade chondrosarcoma.[479,484,489] The chondrosarcoma is usually of the central type, but it can also be peripheral[477,486] (Fig. 24.54). The dedifferentiation can be found in the initial lesion but occurs more often in specimens from recurrent tumor. The microscopic appearance of this component may be that of osteosarcoma, fibrosarcoma, pleomorphic sarcoma with MFH-like features or rhabdomyosarcoma (Fig. 24.55).[482,487] As such, it is phenotypically different from the preexisting chondrosarcoma. Accordingly, these areas may acquire immunohistochemical positivity for α_1-antichymotrypsin, actin, desmin, myoglobin,

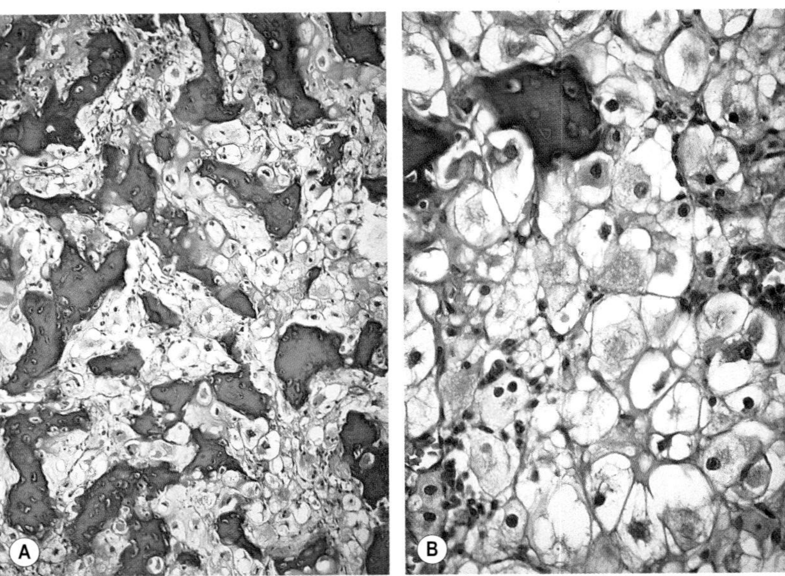

Fig. 24.53 **A** and **B**, Clear cell chondrosarcoma. **A**, Low-power appearance showing numerous bone trabeculae that may result in a mistaken diagnosis of osteosarcoma. **B**, High-power view showing plump and vacuolated appearance of the tumor cells. S-100 protein was strongly immunoreactive.

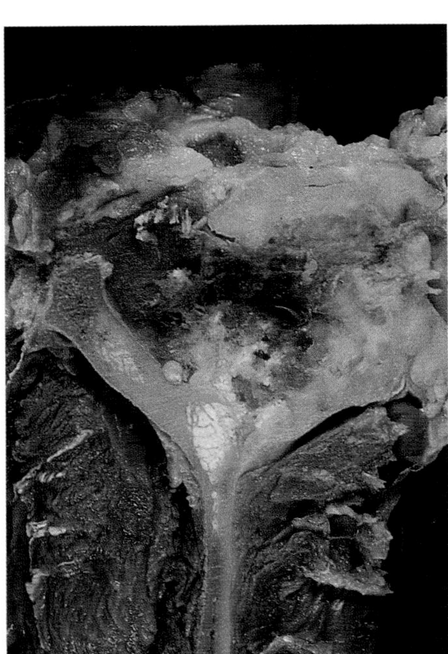

Fig. 24.54 Gross appearance of dedifferentiated chondrosarcoma of pelvic bone.

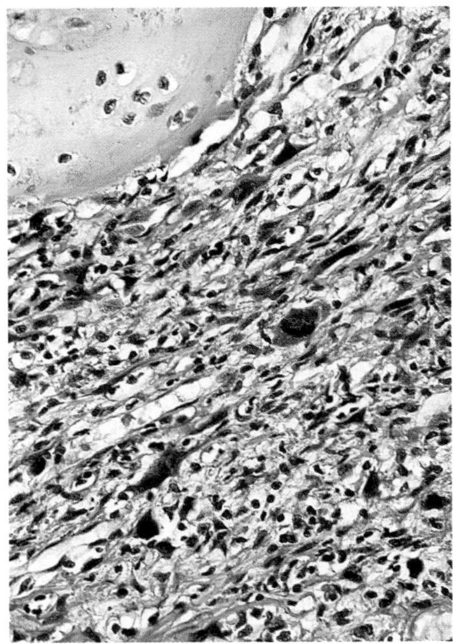

Fig. 24.55 Microscopic appearance of dedifferentiated chondrosarcoma. The edge of an island of well-differentiated cartilage (upper left) is surrounded by highly pleomorphic sarcoma containing tumor giant cells.

myogenin, and exceptionally even keratin.[480,490] In some cases, however, there is some ultrastructural and immunohistochemical (S-100 protein) preservation of the cartilaginous character of the tumor in the anaplastic portion.[474,481] Simultaneous cytogenetic and immunophenotyping studies indicate that both the differentiated and the 'dedifferentiated' components originate from a common primitive mesenchymal cell progenitor, and that the term 'dedifferentiated' may be an inaccurate designation.[475,478] At the molecular level, the process of anaplastic transformation is accompanied by overexpression of *TP53* and *HRAS* mutation.[488]

Regardless of terminology, the development of this component in chondrosarcoma is accompanied by a marked acceleration of the clinical course and a decidedly worsened prognosis.[483,485] The overall 5-year survival rate is quoted at 10% but in the pelvis it is in the neighborhood of 35%.[476]

Mesenchymal chondrosarcoma

Mesenchymal chondrosarcoma is a specific variant of chondrosarcoma characterized microscopically by a dimorphic pattern in which areas of well-differentiated cartilage alternate with undifferentiated stroma[491,502] (Fig. 24.56). The boundaries between the two components are usually abrupt. The undifferentiated element is

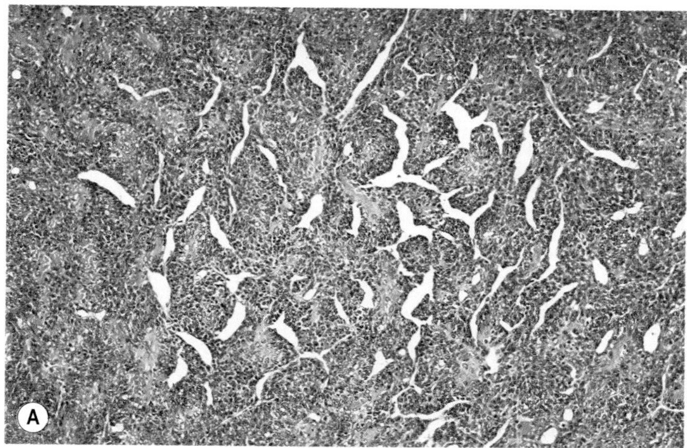

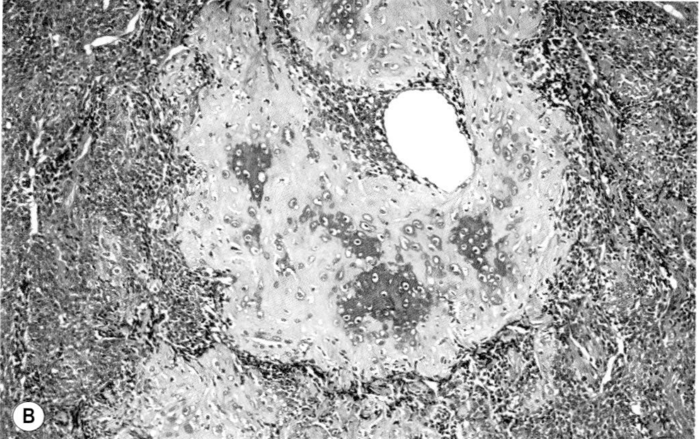

Fig. 24.56 Mesenchymal chondrosarcoma: **A** illustrates a cellular, hemangiopericytoma-like component; **B** shows an island of well-differentiated cartilage in the center.

composed of small cells and can be confused with malignant lymphoma, hemangiopericytoma, and Ewing sarcoma/PNET. It should be noted that despite the apparently undifferentiated nature of this component at both the light and electron microscopic level, pleomorphism and mitotic activity are inconspicuous.[503] Immunohistochemically, the small cell component is positive for vimentin, CD99, and Leu7 but not for S-100 protein;[497,504] the latter is found instead in the chondroid areas. There is also nuclear immunoreactivity for Sox9 (a master regulator of chondrogenesis) and for osteocalcin.[494,505] Surprisingly, immunoreactivity for desmin and myogenin has been found in exceptional instances.[496]

Most patients are females in the second or third decade of life. The radiographic appearance resembles that of conventional chondrosarcomas. The bones most commonly affected are the jaw, pelvis, femur, ribs, and spine.[502] A high percentage of these neoplasms involve extraosseous structures, such as the orbit, paraspinal region, meninges, or soft tissues of the extremities.[498] The prognosis is generally poor, although there is great variability in the clinical course.[499]

It has been proposed that mesenchymal chondrosarcoma represents a neoplastic caricature of embryonal endochondral osteogenesis.[493,494] Jacobson[500] postulated that mesenchymal chondrosarcoma is one morphologic type of the bone tumor that he proposes to call *polyhistioma*. He defines it as a malignant neoplasm whose basic cells are small and round, like those of Ewing sarcoma, but that differentiate into various mesenchymal structures, such as bone and cartilage, and sometimes even into epithelial tissues. Additional case reports have confirmed the existence of multipotential bone tumors composed of a mixture of mesenchymal (chondrosarcoma) and epithelial (squamous cell carcinoma) elements.[495,501]

Granular cell chondrosarcoma refers to a unique case we have recently seen of a tumor of the humerus which combined in a biphasic fashion the typical features of a well-differentiated chondrosarcoma with those of an equally typical granular cell tumor.[492] Interestingly, the latter component metastasized to the lung.

Giant cell tumor

Giant cell tumor (osteoclastoma) is usually seen in patients over 20 years of age.[519] It is more common in women than in men and seems to occur more frequently in Oriental than in Western countries.[570]

The classic location is the epiphysis of a long bone, from which it may spread into the metaphyseal area, break through the cortex, invade intermuscular septa, or even cross a joint space. The sites most commonly affected (in order of frequency) are the lower end of the femur, the upper end of the tibia, and the lower end of the radius.[519] It also occurs in the humerus, fibula, and skull, particularly the sphenoid bone.[513,523,576] Occasionally, a giant cell tumor will be seen in a child[554] and/or in a metaphyseal or diaphyseal location.[525] Involvement of the bones of the hands and feet, jaw, and vertebrae (other than sacrum) is distinctly unusual. Although giant cell tumor has been documented at all of these sites,[514,562,575] the occurrence of a giant cell-containing lesion in any of these locations should suggest an alternative diagnosis. Multicentricity has been reported, particularly in young patients and in the small bones of hands and feet[530] (see p. 2045).

Radiographically, the typical appearance of a giant cell tumor is that of an entirely lytic, expansile lesion in the epiphysis, usually without peripheral bone sclerosis or periosteal reaction (Fig. 24.57).

Grossly, the size of the tumor varies considerably; when large, it may be associated with a pathologic fracture. The cut surface is solid and tan or light brown, traversed by fibrous trabeculae, and often contains hemorrhagic areas (Figs 24.58 and 24.59). The cortex is thinned, but periosteal new bone formation is rare.

Microscopically, the two main components of giant cell tumor are the so-called stromal cells and giant cells (Fig. 24.60). The giant cells are usually large and have over 20 or 30 nuclei, most of them arranged toward the center. They resemble osteoclasts at all levels: morphologic, ultrastructural (ruffled border and abundant mitochondria),[529,548,568] enzyme histochemical (abundant tartrate-resistant acid phosphatase, cathepsin K, and other hydrolytic enzymes),[506,537,578] and immunohistochemical (positivity for microphthalmia-associated transcription factor (Mitf), lysozyme, α_1-antitrypsin, α_1-antichymotrypsin, and other histiocytic markers)[510,545,556,567] (Fig. 24.61). They have also been found to contain receptors for calcitonin (a phenotypic marker for osteoclasts), estrogen receptors, vitronectin, and matrix metalloproteinases (allegedly associated with vascular invasion).[528,534,552,565,573]

It is the prominence of these multinucleated giant cells that gives the tumor its name. Yet, all evidence indicates that these are not neoplastic elements but rather the result of fusion of circulating monocytes that have been recruited into the lesion. Possible mechanisms that have been proposed to account for this phenomenon include an autocrine or paracrine loop mediated by TGF-β,[579] production of osteoprotegerin ligand, a factor known to be essential for osteoclastogenesis,[531] and expression of the ligand for RANK (receptor activator of nuclear factor kappa B).[559]

By contrast, the mononuclear stromal cell is to be interpreted as neoplastic. It is the only proliferating element in the lesion (as confirmed by autoradiographic studies)[558] and the one exhibiting atypia in the rare cytologically malignant examples of this tumor[532,549] (see later section). Parenthetically, these changes may be focal, rendering imperative a thorough sampling.

The nature of the neoplastic stromal cell remains controversial. They are clearly mesenchymal rather than hematopoietic in nature, and they share many features with normal mesenchymal stromal cells.[577] At the ultrastructural level they resemble fibroblasts or osteoblasts.[507–509] That a close histogenetic relationship with osteoblasts exists is suggested by the fact that focal deposition of osteoid or bone (possibly induced by the secretion of transforming growth factors)[572] is seen in one-third of the cases. This stromal cell produces types I and III collagen and has receptors for parathyroid hormone.[528] It does not express macrophage surface antigen, but it

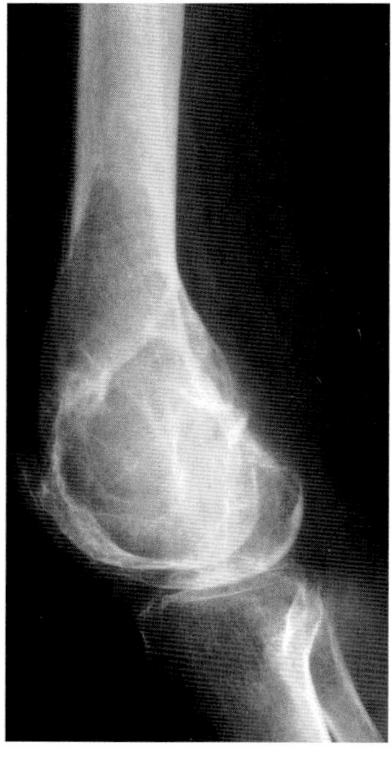

Fig. 24.57 Typical radiograph of giant cell tumor of distal end of femur involving epiphysis and metaphyseal area. The lesion was resected surgically.
(From Sissons HA. Malignant tumors of bone and cartilage. In Raven RW (ed.): Cancer, vol. 2. London, 1958, Butterworth)

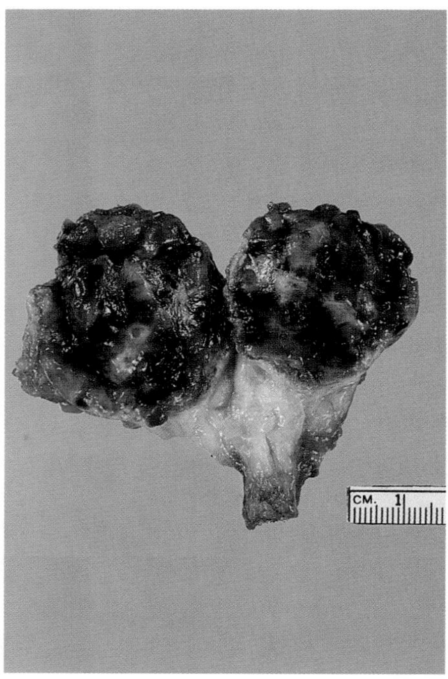

Fig. 24.59 Gross appearance of giant cell tumor of ulna. Note the well-circumscribed character, expansile quality, and brownish-red discoloration.

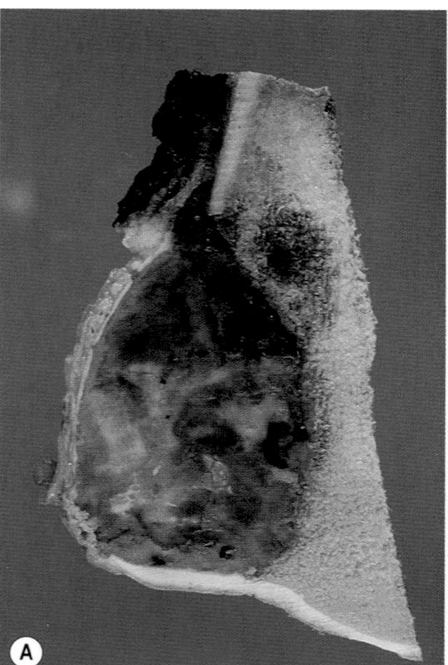

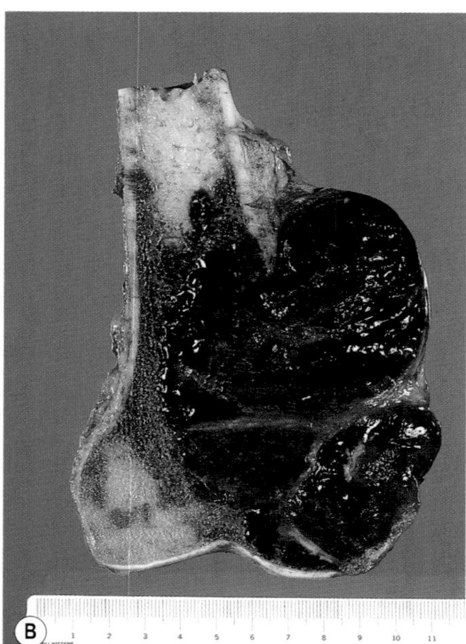

Fig. 24.58 **A**, Gross appearance of giant cell tumor of lower end of femur. The lesion is characteristically peripheral, expansile, well circumscribed, and hemorrhagic. **B**, Giant cell tumor of lower end of femur. The lesion, which has a very hemorrhagic quality, has destroyed the cortex and extended into the adjacent soft tissues.
(Courtesy of Dr RA Cooke, Brisbane, Australia; from Cooke RA, Stewart B. Colour Atlas of Anatomical Pathology. Edinburgh, 2004, Churchill Livingstone)

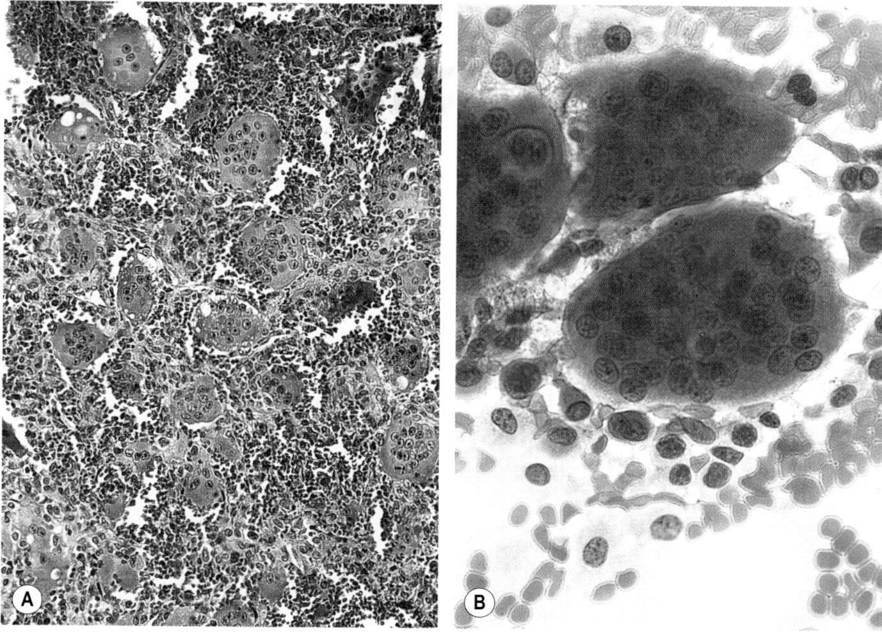

Fig. 24.60 Giant cell tumor of bone: **A**, microscopic appearance; **B**, cytologic preparation.

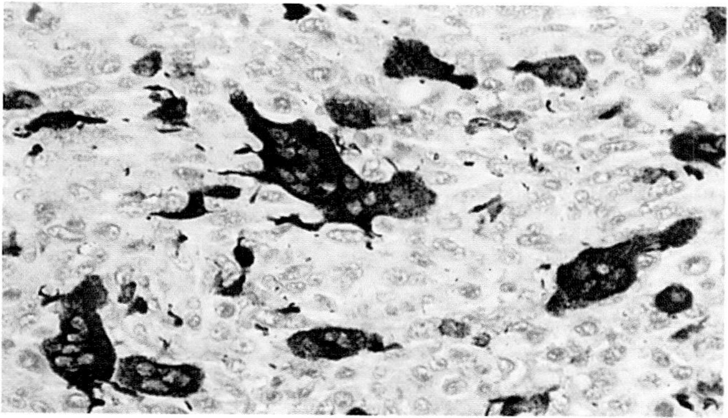

Fig. 24.61 Specimen from giant cell tumor of bone fixed in formalin and embedded in paraffin, stained for acid phosphatase.
(Courtesy of Dr Paul Duray, Bethesda, MD)

may contain lysozyme and α_1-antitrypsin.[515,524,541] Frequent positivity for actin and focal reactivity for S-100 protein have also been described.[539,574] Most true giant cell tumors express *TP63*, whereas this is true for only a small minority of the lesions that simulate it.[521,536,538] A provocative ultrastructural finding has been the presence of viral-like and other intranuclear inclusions in the cells of giant cell tumor, some of them being similar to those of Paget disease of bone.[526,550,564]

Many benign lesions with giant cells have been misdiagnosed as giant cell tumor in the past. These lesions include entities such as metaphyseal fibrous defect and nonossifying fibroma, chondromyxoid fibroma, chondroblastoma, Langerhans cell histiocytosis, solitary bone cyst, osteitis fibrosa cystica of hyperparathyroidism, giant cell reparative granuloma, aneurysmal bone cyst, osteoid osteoma, and osteoblastoma. So-called giant cell tumors of tendon sheath are also unrelated to giant cell tumors of bone. One of the main microscopic differences between true giant cell tumor and these so-called variants resides in the spatial relationship between the giant and stromal cells. The former tend to be distributed regularly and uniformly in giant cell tumor (except in areas showing secondary changes such as hemorrhage, fibrosis or fibrohistiocytic reaction), whereas in the lesions that simulate it, foci containing numerous, clumped giant cells alternate with large areas completely lacking this component. The giant cells themselves do not differ significantly in the two groups of diseases, morphologically, histochemically, or immunohistochemically.[547,556,563] Statistically, those of giant cell tumor may be larger and have more nuclei than those of the other lesions, but there is enough overlap to render this feature of no differential value. Although exceptions to all of the following statements have been recorded, a diagnosis of a lesion *other than* giant cell tumor should be favored if: (1) the patient is a child; (2) the lesion is located in the metaphysis or diaphysis of a long bone rather than the epiphysis; (3) the lesion is multiple (except if a patient has Goltz syndrome);[571] and (4) the lesion is located in the vertebrae (other than sacrum), jaw (except for patients with Paget disease), or bones of the hands or feet. The distinction is of clinical importance because of the better prognosis associated with most of the giant cell-containing lesions that simulate giant cell tumor.

The treatment of giant cell tumor should be surgical whenever technically feasible. It consists of curettage with bone grafting or en bloc excision with replacement with allograft or artificial material, depending on the location.[522,540,544,553] Special care should be taken to prevent implantation of the tumor into the adjoining soft tissues.

The use of radiation therapy should be reserved only for cases in which surgical removal is impossible, in view of the relatively high number of reported cases of malignant transformation following this therapeutic modality. As a matter of fact, review of series of postradiation sarcoma of bone shows that in a disproportionate number of cases the initial lesion was a giant cell tumor. Giant cell tumors of the spine have been traditionally treated with radiation therapy, but they are also amenable to surgical excision.[562]

The natural history of giant cell tumor is that of a low-grade malignancy. In most reported series, the incidence of clinical malignancy (expressed by uncontrollable local recurrence or metastases) has been in the range of 10%.[520] The type of initial surgical removal is the most significant factor in recurrence; in one large series, the recurrence rate was 34% following curettage and 7% following wide resection.[544] A good relation also exists between surgical stage and prognosis;[555] in one series all cases of metastasizing giant cell tumor were deemed to be stage III lesions, with interruption of the cortex and soft tissue extension.[512]

It is also of interest that nearly all cases of metastases of giant cell tumor have occurred after a surgical intervention to the primary tumor, suggesting the possibility of mechanical disruption with access to the bloodstream. However, no relationship has been found between the presence of giant cells in blood vessels and prognosis. Microscopic grading of giant cell tumors is not of great value except for the obviously sarcomatous (grade III) lesions.[518,560] Indeed, some of these metastases have occurred in tumors with an entirely benign microscopic appearance (1–2% of all cases), and the metastases themselves may have a very innocuous look;[557] those developing in the lung, which are by far the most common, are often surrounded by a rim of mature bone. It should be mentioned here that grade III lesions are those characterized by the combination of pleomorphism, marked nuclear atypia, and high mitotic activity in the neoplastic mononuclear component, often accompanied by necrosis; exceptionally, bizarre (symplastic) nuclear forms are seen in the absence of the other features, and these should not be labeled as malignant.[535]

Most cases of giant cell tumor exhibit chromosomal abnormalities, usually in the form of telomeric association that can involve a variety of chromosomes, such as 11p, 13p, 14p, 15p, 19q, 20q, and 21p.[517,566] Telomeric association is a rare form of cytogenetic abnormality characterized by end-to-end fusion of intact chromosomes. Clonal structural abnormalities may be present in addition.[543] Chromosomal aberrations seem to be more common in the clinically more aggressive neoplasms.[516]

DNA ploidy analysis of giant cell tumors has not yet been shown to have prognostic value above and beyond that provided by the more conventional parameters.[527,533,561]

Similarly, no statistically significant relationship seems to exist between prognosis and either proliferation index or vascular density.[569] Instead, it has been claimed that tumors overexpressing *TP53* have a higher potential for recurrence and metastases.[542] As a matter of fact, the suggestion has been made that molecular abnormalities of *TP53* and *HRAS* underlie the process of malignant transformation in these tumors.[551]

Malignant giant cell tumor

As already mentioned, all giant cell tumors of bone should be regarded as potentially low-grade malignancies because of their tendency to recur and their occasional capacity to metastasize regardless of histologic appearance. A contentious issue is the existence of a cytologically malignant giant cell tumor (i.e., a lesion that retains the clinical, topographic, and general microscopic features of giant cell tumor but that exhibits clearcut evidence of malignancy in the mononuclear stromal component). As such, it is equivalent to a grade III giant cell tumor. It represents a most unusual process, part of the reason being the conceptual and practical difficulties in separating it from other malignant tumors, particularly so-called giant cell-rich osteosarcoma (when osteoid production is present) and other pleomorphic sarcomas (when osteoid production is absent).

On occasion, a typical benign-appearing giant cell tumor is seen in combination with but sharply segregated from a high-grade sarcoma. This phenomenon has been referred to as dedifferentiation, in analogy to the situation occurring more commonly with chondrosarcoma and chordoma.[546] In other instances a high-grade sarcoma is seen developing at the site of a previously treated giant cell tumor[511] (Fig. 24.62).

Marrow tumors

Ewing sarcoma/primitive neuroectodermal tumor (PNET)

Ewing sarcoma, initially regarded as an undifferentiated type of bone sarcoma of children, is now linked with the neoplasm originally described in the soft tissues as primitive (or peripheral) neuroectodermal tumor (PNET), and the term Ewing sarcoma/PNET (ES/PNET) is currently favored for this tumor family.[589] The best evidence for the pathogenetic unity of these processes is provided by the nearly universal presence of the gene fusion to be described below, resulting from the 11;22 chromosomal translocation.[600,616,633,651,667] It has been commented that the bone tumors tend to be undifferentiated (and therefore more in keeping with the original definition of James Ewing), whereas their soft tissue counterparts tend to show better evidence of neuroectodermal differentiation.[664,676] However, the overlap is considerable, as reflected by terms such as extraskeletal Ewing sarcoma on one hand and PNET of bone on the other.[595,623,672,687,688] The link is also supported by the fact that neural differentiation can be induced in conventional Ewing sarcoma of bone by agents such as dibutyril cyclic AMP and retinoic acid,[654] and that it can become very evident in post-therapy specimens. This unitary concept has also embraced the malignant small round cell tumor of the thoracopulmonary region (so-called Askin tumor), which is now simply regarded as an example of ES/PNET located in the chest wall.[585]

It should be made clear that this unitary concept does not include neuroblastoma and related tumors of the sympathetic nervous system, which lack the molecular aberrations of ES/PNET.[584]

Clinical features. ES/PNET of bone is usually seen in patients between the ages of 5 and 20 years,[629,696] with only a minority of the cases presenting in infancy or adulthood.[609,635,644,690] Clinically the tumor may simulate osteomyelitis because of pain, fever, and leukocytosis. It occurs most often in long bones (femur, tibia, humerus, and fibula) and in bones of the pelvis, rib, vertebrae, mandible, and clavicle.[625,677,684] It generally arises in the medullary canal of the shaft (hence its traditional inclusion among the 'marrow tumors'), from which it permeates the cortex and invades the soft tissues (Fig. 24.63). Rarely, it is predominantly periosteal in location.[588] As already indicated, tumors with the appearance of ES/PNET can present clinically as a soft tissue neoplasm with a normal appearance of the underlying bone on plain x-ray films. However, CT scans, MRI, and microscopic examination of these cases may reveal that the tumor arose in the medullary canal and that it diffusely permeated the marrow spaces to extend outside the bone without destroying a significant amount of bone trabeculae, thus remaining undetectable by conventional radiography. This possibility should always be kept in mind before making a diagnosis of primary extraskeletal ES/PNET (see Chapter 25).[627]

Following the reassessment of ES/PNET on the basis of its distinct molecular alterations, it has become apparent that, in addition to bone and soft tissue, the lesion can occur in a wide variety of sites, including skin and viscera;[622,655] these are discussed in the respective chapters.

The typical radiographic changes in bone associated with ES/PNET are cortical thickening and widening of the medullary canal. With progression of the lesion, reactive periosteal bone may be deposited in layers parallel to the cortex (onion-skin appearance) or at right angles to it (sun-ray appearance) (Fig. 24.64).

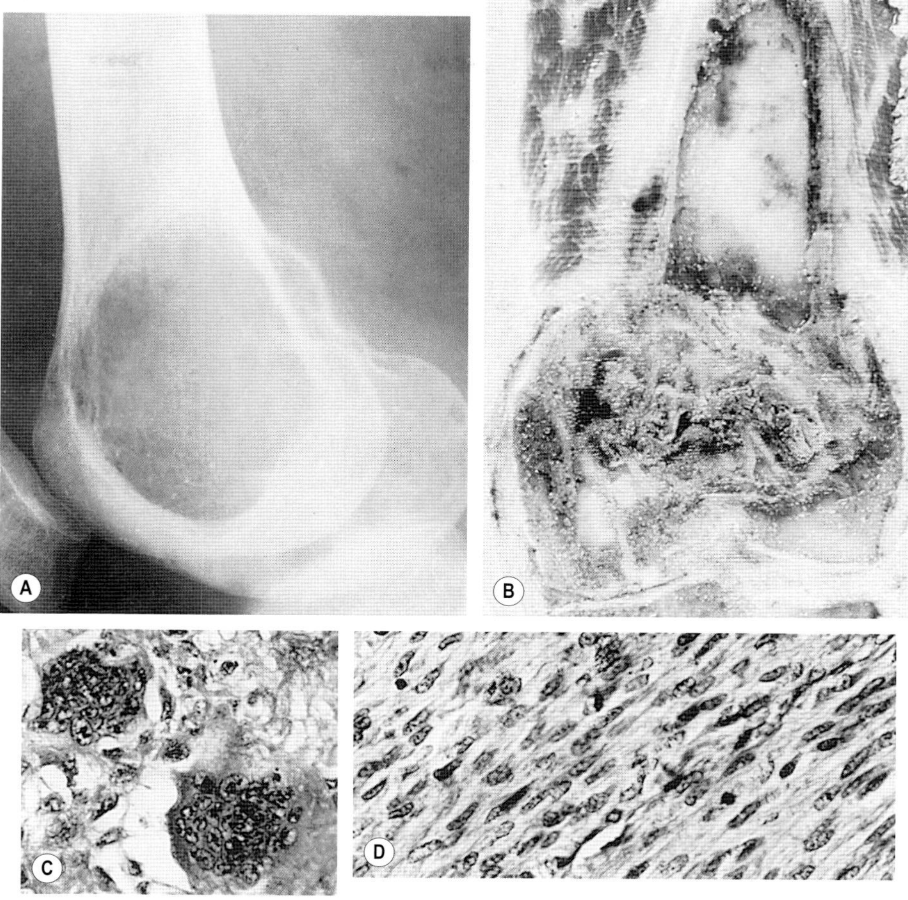

Fig. 24.62 **A**, Giant cell tumor of distal end of femur. The lesion was curetted and replaced with bone chips. **B**, The giant cell tumor shown in **A** recurred, necessitating amputation. Gross specimen demonstrates bone chips still in place with tumor replacing femur. Review of original sections showed benign giant cell tumor, but re-cuts of curetted material demonstrated malignant stroma. **C**, Original section of curettings referred to in **B** showing areas of rather innocuous-appearing stroma with typical multinucleated giant cells. These changes were called benign. **D**, Later tissue section of malignant giant cell tumor referred to in **B** and **C** that has the appearance of fibrosarcoma. There was no evidence of osteoid formation. The patient died of pulmonary metastases.

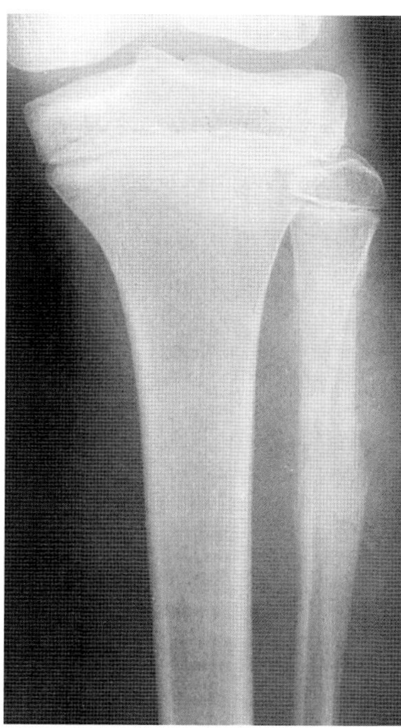

Fig. 24.63 Ewing sarcoma of fibula. Growth is ill defined and accompanied by a prominent periosteal reaction.

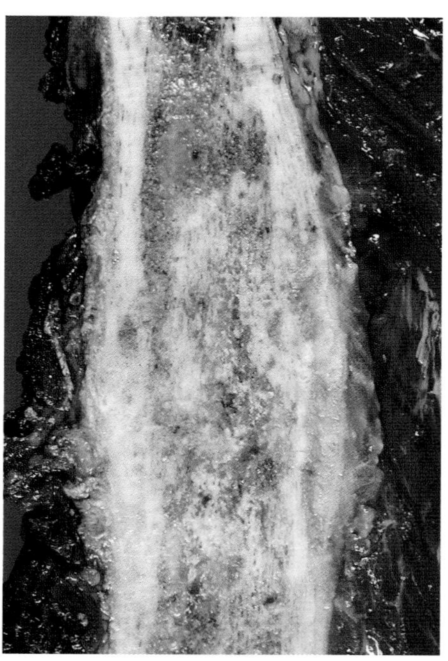

Fig. 24.64 Gross appearance of Ewing sarcoma. It has a typical ill-defined quality, with extensive involvement of medulla and cortex associated with elevation of periosteum.

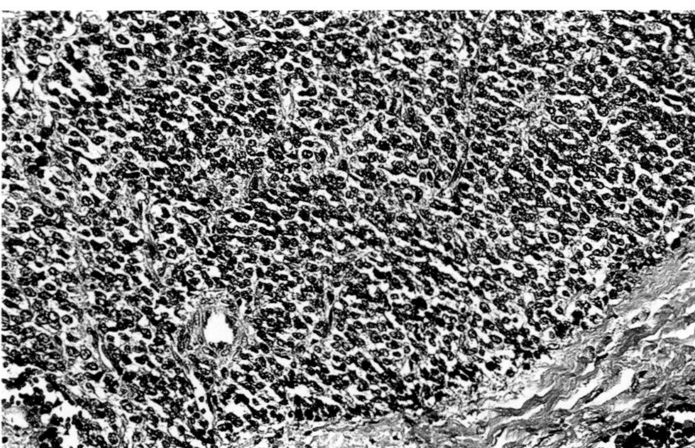

Fig. 24.65 Diffuse pattern of growth and monotonous cytologic appearance in Ewing sarcoma/PNET.

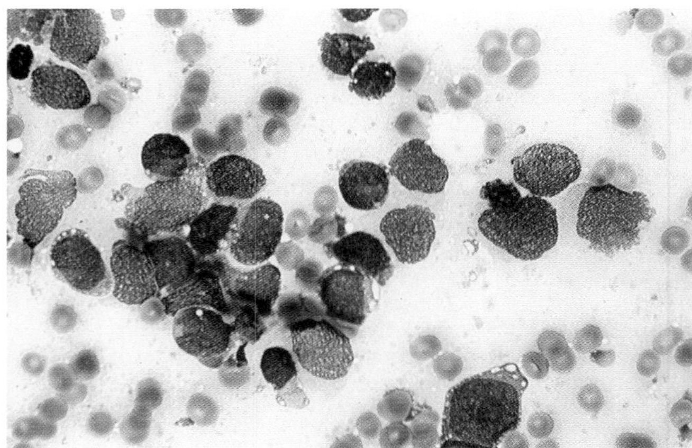

Fig. 24.67 Cytologic appearance of Ewing sarcoma/PNET as seen in a fine needle aspiration specimen.

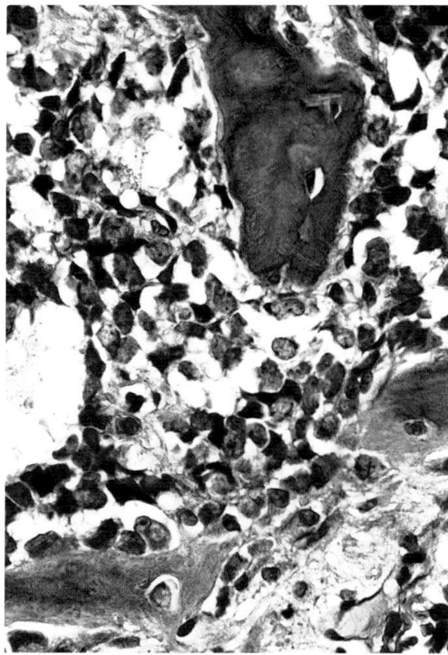

Fig. 24.66 Microscopic appearance of Ewing sarcoma/PNET. Uniform cells with darkly staining nuclei and very scanty cytoplasm infiltrate the marrow spaces around bone trabeculae.

Microscopic features. Microscopically, the typical ES/PNET consists of solid sheets of cells divided into irregular masses by fibrous strands (Fig. 24.65). Individual cells are small and uniform. The cell outlines are indistinct, resulting in a 'syncytial' appearance. The nuclei are round, with frequent indentations, small nucleoli, and variable but usually brisk mitotic activity (Fig. 24.66). There is a well-developed vascular network. Some of the tumor cells may arrange themselves around the vessels in a pseudorosette fashion. Exceptionally, a few true rosettes (without central lumen) are formed, these having provided some of the earlier evidence for a neuroepithelial differentiation in these neoplasms.[626] Necrosis is common and may dominate the microscopic picture. A fair degree of histologic heterogeneity exists.[638] Some tumors are composed of larger and more pleomorphic cells exhibiting conspicuous nucleoli (so-called large cell or atypical variant).[650] Other tumors display an organoid pattern characterized by bicellular strands of tissue separated by a 'filmy' vascular stroma, referred to as the 'filigree pattern'.[628]

The morphologic features of the ES/PNET tumor cells can be recognized on cytologic examination, which represents an important diagnostic tool, both in bone and in soft tissue lesions[619] (Fig. 24.67).

The differential diagnosis of ES/PNET includes practically all other 'small round cell tumors', particularly lymphoblastic lymphoma, desmoplastic small cell tumor, and embryonal/alveolar rhabdomyosarcoma.[620,645] The immunohistochemical and molecular genetic features (described below) are very useful and often indispensable to achieve this end.[611]

A most peculiar morphologic variation in the theme is the lesion combining features of ES/PNET and adamantinoma, and variously called adamantinoma-like Ewing sarcoma and Ewing sarcoma-like adamantinoma.[590,613] The fact that these cases display the 11;22 translocation would seem to indicate that they represent a subtype of ES/PNET resembling adamantinoma rather than the reverse.[612] Cases of ES/PNET exhibiting complex epithelial differentiation (including expression of high-molecular-weight keratin) are probably an expression of the same theme.[694]

Histochemical, electron microscopic, and immunohistochemical features. The cells of ES/PNET usually contain large amounts of cytoplasmic glycogen, as demonstrated by a PAS stain with diastase control or by electron microscopy (Figs 24.68 and 24.69). Traditionally, this has represented an important feature for the differential diagnosis with other small round cell tumors.[669] However, it is far from being specific. Some cases of this entity show little or no glycogen (at least in routine formalin-fixed and paraffin-embedded preparations), whereas sizable amounts of this substance can be found in metastatic neuroblastoma and malignant lymphoma occasionally, and in embryonal rhabdomyosarcoma commonly.[686,697]

Ultrastructurally, the cells of ES/PNET show a rather primitive appearance. Occasionally, a few dense core granules will be found, either in the cytoplasm or in cell prolongations.[639,643,682] Some cases (corresponding to those immunoreactive to keratin, see below) show signs of epithelial differentiation, such as desmosomes and tonofilaments.[679]

Immunohistochemically, there is the expected consistent positivity for vimentin. In addition, there is frequent reactivity for low-molecular-weight keratin and other epithelial markers, a fact not widely appreciated.[602,618,671,689] Furthermore, positivity has been

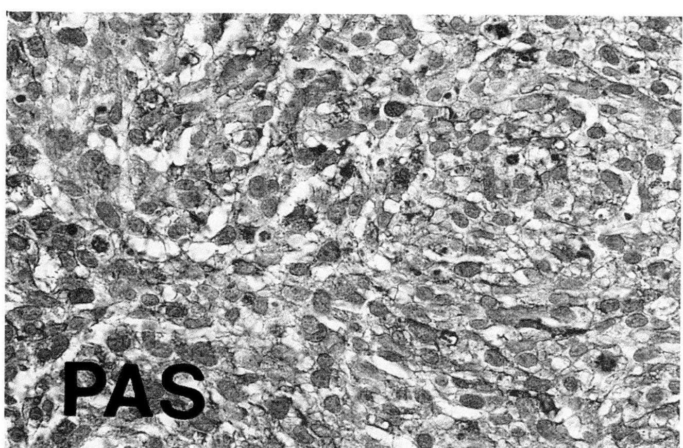

Fig. 24.68 PAS stain in Ewing sarcoma/PNET showing large amounts of cytoplasmic glycogen. The material was entirely removed by diastase digestion.

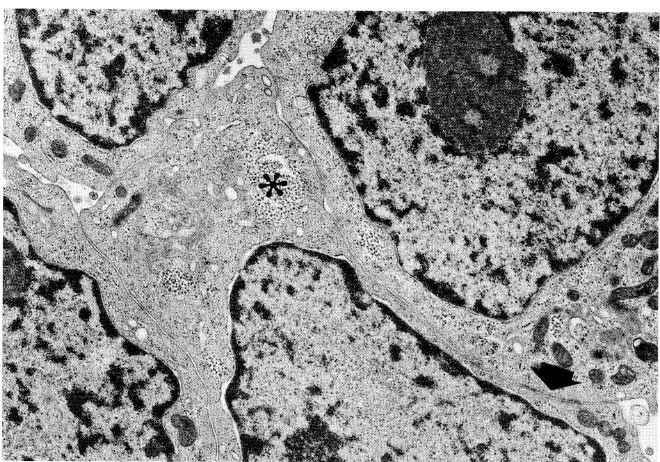

Fig. 24.69 Electron microscopic appearance of Ewing sarcoma/PNET. Undifferentiated tumor cells with multiple small foci of cytoplasmic glycogen (asterisk) are joined by two rudimentary cell junctions (arrow).
(×12 000; courtesy of Dr Robert A Erlandson, Memorial Sloan-Kettering Cancer Center)

described for neuron-specific enolase, protein gene product 9.5, Leu7 (CD57), secretogranin II, and neurofilaments, these reactions again providing evidence for neuroepithelial differentiation.[594,636,641,647,648,657,662,675] The latter has also been evidenced by the demonstration of chromogranin mRNA by reverse transcriptase polymerase chain reaction (RT-PCR).[658] The expression of some of these neural (including glial) markers seems to be related to the type of gene fusion described in the following section.[581]

CD99 (013; HBA71; p30/32; MIC2) is a cell membrane protein coded by a gene located on the short arms of the X and Y chromosomes that is consistently expressed by the cells of ES/PNET (Fig. 24.70).[582,673] It is, however, far from being pathognomonic for this family of tumors, inasmuch as expression of this marker has also been documented in embryonal rhabdomyosarcoma, other soft tissue sarcomas, and lymphoblastic lymphoma.[607,624,660,681,693] The *EWS–FLI1* fusion described in the following section results in the expression of the FLI1 protein, which can be detected at the immunohistochemical level; it should be noted, however, that there are several cell types – such as endothelial cells – that express this protein under normal conditions.[610,640]

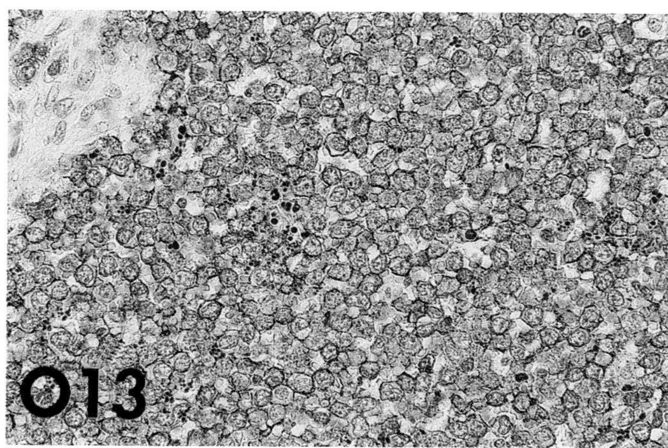

Fig. 24.70 CD99 (013) stain in Ewing sarcoma/PNET. All of the tumor cells show strong membrane immunoreactivity.

Desmosome-associated proteins are demonstrable immunohistochemically in the areas of cell junctions, but neural cell adhesion molecules are not.[614] Various types of collagen are found in the extracellular matrix.[668]

Molecular genetic features. About 95% of cases of ES/PNET show on cytogenetic examination the reciprocal translocation t(11;22)(q24;q12) or t(21;22)(q22;q12), which results in the fusion of the *EWS* (Ewing sarcoma) gene at 22q12 with the *FLI1* or *ERG* gene, respectively.[600,604,616,634] The most common fusion is the one that results in 'in frame linking' of *EWS* exon 7 with *FLI1* exon 6. In the remaining cases, *EWS* is fused with other genes, such as *FEV*, *ETV1*, and *E1AF*.[587,691] These translocations, which are detectable in frozen or paraffin-embedded material by RT-PCR, can be used for the primary diagnosis and for the detection of metastatic or residual disease in tissue or body fluids, including peripheral blood.[580,605,608,642,674,678,680,695] The *EWS* rearrangement can also be detected by the fluorescent in situ hybridization (FISH) technique in cytologic preparations, frozen sections, or paraffin sections.[591,632,637,649] Apparently there are no phenotypic differences among cases of ES/PNET associated with *EWS–FLI1* and those associated with *EWS–ERG*.[617]

It needs to be noted that therapy-induced neural differentiation in Ewing sarcoma may result in loss of expression of *EWS–FLI1*.[630]

The fact that there is a remarkable correlation between this gene fusion and ES/PNET is undeniable; whether it can be regarded as pathognomonic of the entity remains controversial. Suffice it to say that a few cases have been reported in which the ES/PNET transcript was found in tumors having phenotypic features of other tumor types.[685]

Additional genetic aberrations exist in ES/PNET, such as inactivation of *INK4A* (encoding CDKN2A) in up to one-third of cases.[631,692] Loss of this cell cycle inhibitor stabilizes the chimeric oncoprotein EWS/FLI1, and is associated with a worse prognosis.[601,692]

Another gene that has been found to be activated in ES/PNET is *TRK*, this phenomenon being supposedly associated with neural differentiation.[653]

Spread and metastases. The metastatic spread of ES/PNET is to the lungs and pleura, other bones (particularly the skull), central nervous system, and (rarely) regional lymph nodes. About 25% of the patients have multiple bone and/or visceral lesions at the time of presentation.[593,615]

Treatment. The treatment of ES/PNET represents one of the success stories of medical oncology. In the past, surgical excision (including amputation) and radiation therapy resulted in a 5-year survival rate of less than 10%, and the pathologist was warned to question a previous diagnosis of Ewing sarcoma in a long-term survivor.[652] The combination of high-dose irradiation and multi-drug chemotherapy – sometimes combined with limited surgery – has dramatically changed the picture.[586,663,665] Local control is achieved in over 85% of the cases, and the actuarial 5-year disease-free survival is 75%. Parenthetically, it should be noted that therapy may result in increased pleomorphism, appearance of bizarre giant cells, or increased neural differentiation.[596,683] Radiographic evidence of effective treatment consists of reconstitution of the cortical pattern, 'periostitis', and regression of the extraosseous soft tissue mass if one was present; any localized lysis at the primary site should be regarded as suspicious for recurrence.[606]

Prognosis. Prognostic factors related to ES/PNET are listed below.

1. *Osseous versus extraosseous location*. The claim has been made that classical Ewing sarcoma of bone has a better prognosis than PNET of soft tissue.[592,621]
2. *Soft tissue extension*. Direct extension of an osseous Ewing sarcoma into soft tissues is a bad prognostic sign.[646]
3. *Metastases*. Not surprisingly, presence of metastases at presentation is a poor prognostic sign, particularly if these metastases are in the skeletal system rather than the lung.[597]
4. *Surgical margins*. Although surgery plays a role in the treatment of ES/PNET, the prognostic importance of the status of the surgical margins has diminished considerably with current chemotherapeutic regimes.[656]
5. *Therapy-induced necrosis*. As for osteosarcoma, there is a close relationship between presence and amount of tumor necrosis following chemotherapy and outcome. It has been recommended that the changes be graded as follows: I, gross viable tumor; II, microscopic viable tumor; III, no viable tumor cells.[661,666]
6. *Microscopic features*. A filigree microscopic pattern is said to represent an unfavorable prognostic indicator, at least with the therapy used at the time that the observation was made.[621,628]
7. *Neural differentiation*. The claim was originally made that presence of neural (neuroepithelial, neuroectodermal) differentiation in ES/PNET was associated with a poor outcome, but more recent series have failed to find a statistically significant difference.[659]
8. *Type of gene fusion transcript*. The claim has been made that patients with the most common type of gene fusion (*EWS* exon 7 linked in frame with exon 6 of *FLI1*) are less likely to metastasize and have a better prognosis than patients having any other type of fusion.[600,698] This may be related to the fact that tumors with *EWS–FLI1*-type fusion seem to have a lower proliferation rate.[599]
9. *TP53*. Overexpression of *TP53* seems to define a small subset of cases with a markedly unfavorable outcome.[583,598]
10. *MYC*. In one study, *MYC* amplification has been found to be a marker of poor prognosis.[670]
11. *INK4A*. The suggestion has been advanced that deletion of this gene may identify a subgroup of patients with poor prognosis.[692]
12. *DNA content*. DNA content, as determined by flow cytometry or cytophotometry, seems to correlate with prognosis, in that patients with diploid tumors do better than those with aneuploid ones.[603]

Malignant lymphoma and related lesions

Malignant lymphomas can involve the skeletal system primarily or as a manifestation of systemic disease.[702,716]

Large B-cell lymphoma is the most common type of primary bone lymphoma in adults, 60% of the cases occurring in patients over the age of 30 years.[706] However, they can also affect children.[737] There is no sex predilection. Most cases are solitary, but there are also polyostotic examples limited to the skeletal system, without visceral or lymph node involvement.[700]

Grossly, most cases involve the diaphysis or metaphysis of a long bone or the vertebrae, producing patchy cortical and medullary destruction.[736] This is associated with minimal to moderate periosteal reaction, usually of the lamellated type. The tumor, which is pinkish gray and granular, frequently extends into the soft tissues and invades the muscle.

Radiographically, a combination of bone production and bone destruction often involves a wide area of a long bone[711] (Fig. 24.71). This pattern is very suggestive of the diagnosis, but osteosarcoma and chronic osteomyelitis may closely simulate it.

Microscopically, the appearance is similar to that of large cell lymphomas in nodal and other extranodal sites.[707,711,730,735] Some cases are accompanied by prominent fibrosis, which may result in compression and spindling of the tumor cells, thus simulating a sarcoma. Traditionally, the main source of diagnostic difficulty has resided in their distinction from Ewing sarcoma.[718,721,734] The cells of large cell malignant lymphoma are larger, and their nuclei are somewhat pleomorphic, with many indented, multilobulated, or horseshoe-shaped forms. They usually have prominent nucleoli, unlike the fine nucleoli of Ewing sarcoma (Fig. 24.72). Cytoplasmic outlines of large cell lymphoma are well defined, whereas those of Ewing tumor are indistinct. The cytoplasm is more abundant and often amphophilic. Reticulin fibers occur between individual cells

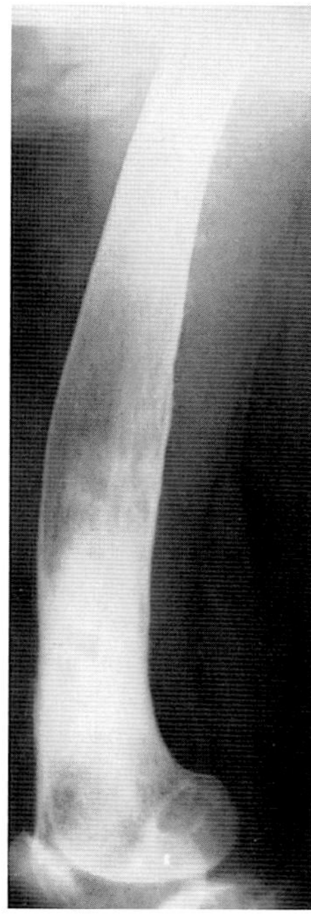

Fig. 24.71 Malignant lymphoma involving lower end of femur associated with bone destruction and bone production. These lesions are often erroneously diagnosed as chronic osteomyelitis.

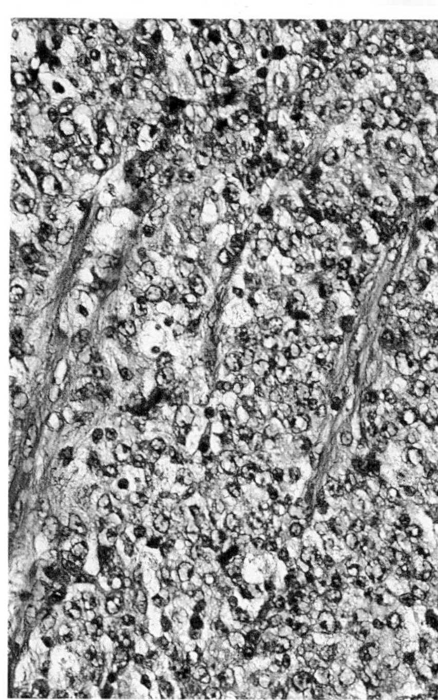

Fig. 24.72 Malignant lymphoma of bone. The tumor is of large cell type and is associated with some fibrosis.

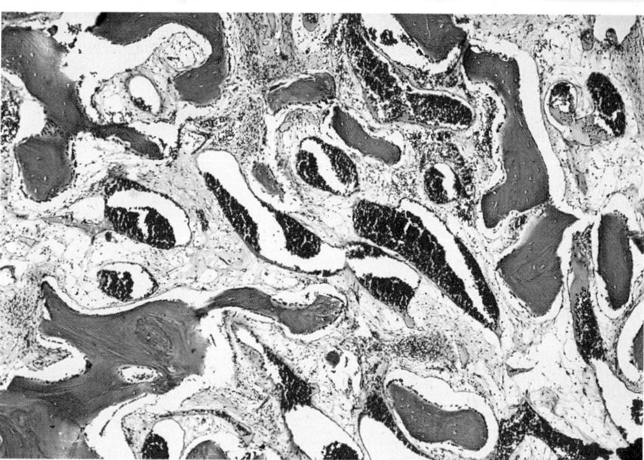

Fig. 24.73 Cavernous hemangioma of bone. Large dilated vessels with thin walls expand marrow spaces and elicit some new bone formation in surrounding trabeculae.

and groups of cells, whereas in Ewing sarcoma they are mainly restricted to perivascular areas. Ultrastructurally, the features are analogous to those of nodal and other extranodal lymphomas. Immunohistochemically, there is positivity for CD45 and – in the large majority of cases – for B-cell markers.[714,719,728,729] BCL2 is expressed in approximately 70% of the cases.[712]

The 5-year survival rate for localized large B-cell lymphomas of bone, which for many years has ranged from 30% to 60%,[703] has now reached a figure of 95%.[705] Although the stage of the disease is the single most important prognostic determinator,[725] there is also a definite relation with cell type.[713] Tumors expressing antigens associated with germinal centers are said to behave better than the others.[712] The workup of these patients should include skeletal survey and bone marrow examination. The treatment usually consists of a combination of radiation therapy and chemotherapy.[701]

Hodgkin lymphoma produces radiographically detectable bone lesions in approximately 15% of the patients. The involvement is multifocal in about 60% of the cases, the most frequent sites being vertebrae, pelvis, ribs, sternum, and femur.[717] The osseous lesions of Hodgkin lymphoma are often asymptomatic and in half of the cases are not demonstrable radiographically. When they become apparent in the x-ray film, the foci may be osteolytic, mixed, or purely osteoblastic. The latter appearance is particularly common in vertebrae. Exceptionally, Hodgkin lymphoma will present initially as a bone mass,[710] with or without associated involvement of the adjacent soft tissues.[699,710,724,726] Osteonecrosis of the femoral or humeral head can occur as a complication of therapy for Hodgkin lymphoma or non-Hodgkin lymphoma.[731]

Anaplastic large cell lymphoma exhibiting CD30, EMA, and variably anaplastic lymphoma kinase (ALK) immunoreactivity and either a null or a T-cell phenotype occurs as a primary bone lesion and needs to be distinguished mainly from Hodgkin lymphoma.[709,723] Most patients are adults, but children can also be affected.[704] The outcome is poor.

Burkitt lymphoma, as originally reported from Africa, typically presents with massive jawbone involvement. It can also result in tumor masses in the long bones and pelvis.[715]

Lymphoblastic lymphoma of precursor B-cell type can present as a solitary bone tumor and simulate Ewing sarcoma.[720] Immunohistochemically, the tumor cells are positive for terminal deoxynucleotidyl transferase (TdT), PAX5, CD43, CD99, CD79a, and inconstantly for CD20.[720]

Acute leukemia of childhood is associated with radiographic abnormalities in the skeletal system in 70–90% of the cases.[722,733] In the large majority of instances, the changes are widespread and therefore unlikely to be confused with a primary bone neoplasm.[732] In contrast, destructive bone lesions are extremely rare in the chronic leukemias. Chabner et al.[708] reported six cases in a series of 205 patients with chronic granulocytic leukemia. In three of the patients, the bone lesion appeared at the time of blastic transformation.

Plasma cell myeloma and **plasmacytoma** are discussed in Chapter 23. *Amyloidoma* of bone is regarded as a manifestation of plasma cell neoplasm and is also addressed in the chapter dealing with bone marrow.[727]

Vascular tumors

Hemangiomas of bone are often seen in the vertebrae as an incidental post mortem finding. In a classic autopsy study by Töpfer,[768] hemangiomas were detected in 11.9% of 2154 cases. They were multiple in 34% of the cases. These lesions should probably be regarded as vascular malformations rather than true neoplasms.

The most common locations of clinically significant osseous hemangiomas are skull, vertebrae, and jawbones.[770,774] Hemangiomas in the long bones are extremely rare. When a lesion involves the flat bones (particularly the skull), sunburst trabeculation occurs because of elevation of the periosteum. Grossly, the cut section of these tumors often has a currant jelly appearance. Microscopically, there is a thick-walled lattice-like pattern of endothelial-lined cavernous spaces filled with blood (Fig. 24.73).

Multiple hemangiomas are mainly seen in children and are associated in about half of the cases with cutaneous, soft tissue, or visceral hemangiomas ('angiomatosis').[739,766] Hemangiomas of the sacrum in infants are often accompanied by a variety of congenital abnormalities.[746]

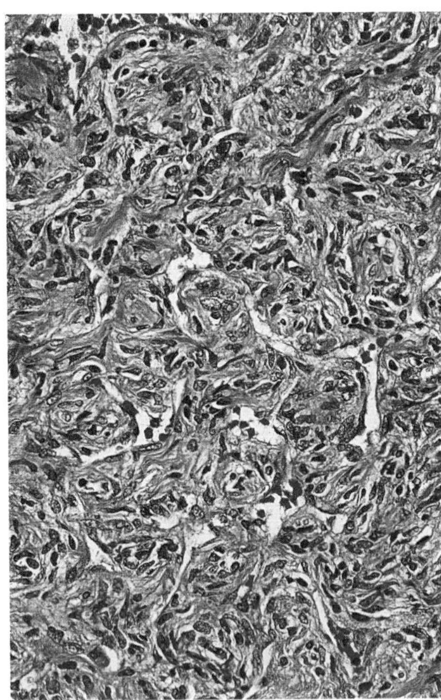

Fig. 24.74 Primary hemangiopericytoma of bone. The appearance is similar to that of its more common counterpart in the soft tissues.

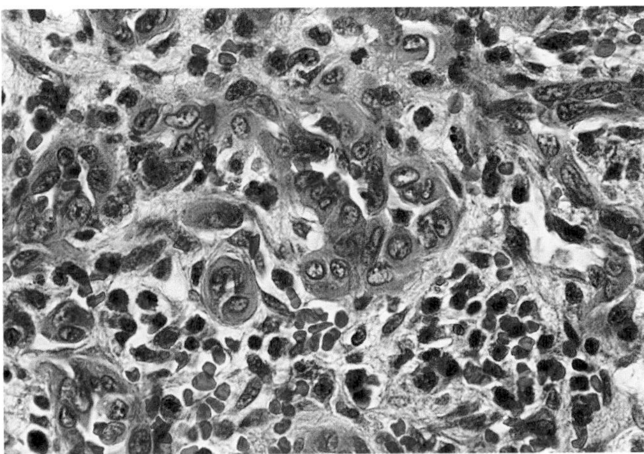

Fig. 24.75 Epithelioid hemangioendothelioma. The tumor cells have a plump appearance and acidophilic cytoplasm. The stroma contains an inflammatory infiltrate rich in eosinophils.

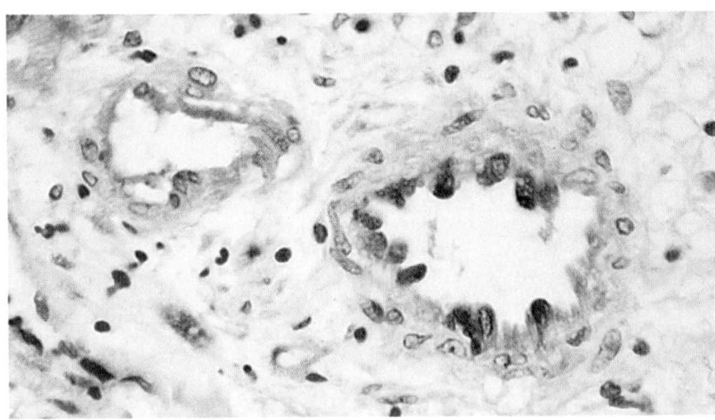

Fig. 24.76 Epithelioid hemangioendothelioma of bone (immunostained with factor VIII-related antigen).

Massive osteolysis (Gorham disease) is probably not a vascular neoplasm but is included in this discussion because of its microscopic similarities with skeletal angiomatosis. It has a destructive character that the latter lacks. It results in reabsorption of a whole bone or several bones and the filling of the residual spaces by a heavily vascularized fibrous tissue.[747,748]

Lymphangiomas of bone are exceptional.[750] Most cases are multiple and associated with soft tissue tumors of similar appearance; variations on the theme have been termed *cystic angiomatosis* and *hamartomatous hemolymphangiomatosis*.[764]

Glomus tumor of the subungual soft tissues may erode the underlying bone. Much rarer is the occurrence of a purely intraosseous glomus tumor involving the terminal phalanx.[755]

Hemangiopericytoma has been reported as a primary bone lesion, most commonly in the pelvis[765,776] (Fig. 24.74). Both benign and malignant forms have been described. The differential diagnosis includes metastatic hemangiopericytoma of meninges, which is actually more common than primary hemangiopericytoma of bone. As a matter of fact, it is likely that most if not all cases of reported primary hemangiocytomas of bone are in reality examples of nonvascular tumors sharing the so-called hemangiopericytomatous pattern of growth, including solitary fibrous tumor and synovial sarcoma.[773]

Epithelioid hemangioendothelioma of bone is the most common and distinctive member of the family of epithelioid (histiocytoid) vascular neoplasms, originally embraced in the histiocytoid hemangioma concept.[742,752,763] It is a borderline type of vascular neoplasm characterized microscopically by the presence of epithelial- or histiocyte-like endothelial cells with abundant acidophilic and often vacuolated cytoplasm, large vesicular nucleus (sometimes with prominent grooves), modest atypia, scanty mitotic activity, inconspicuous or absent anastomosing channels, recent and old hemorrhage, and an inconstant but sometimes prominent inflammatory component rich in eosinophils (Figs 24.75 and 24.76).[772] A myxoid stroma is prominent in some cases and may produce confusion with a cartilaginous neoplasm.[756] Many of the tumors classified as grade I (and perhaps grade II) hemangioendotheliomas of bone in some series[740,762] belong in this category.

In this regard, it should be emphasized that a range of cytologic atypia exists among epithelioid vascular tumors of bone. Those showing only a modest degree of atypia fit better the category of epithelioid hemangioendothelioma described above and are the most numerous. Those showing little or no atypia could be termed epithelioid hemangiomas (although controversy persists about the use of this term),[744,745,753,758–760] whereas those exhibiting marked atypia (often accompanied by mitotic activity and necrosis) are better designated as epithelioid angiosarcomas (see later discussion). It should also be noted that the epithelioid features may be admixed with spindle cell forms in all three subtypes, whether one regards these combined forms as distinct tumor entities[751] or simply as morphologic variations of a continuous spectrum, as we prefer to.

Immunohistochemically, the cells of epithelioid vascular neoplasms display endothelial cell markers, such as factor VIII, CD31, CD34, and FLI1. However, these antigens can be poorly expressed and/or coexist with epithelial markers such as keratin.[771]

Epithelioid hemangioendothelioma of bone is often multiple[738] and may be associated with similar lesions in the skin or soft tissue, which are characteristically located in close proximity to the osseous

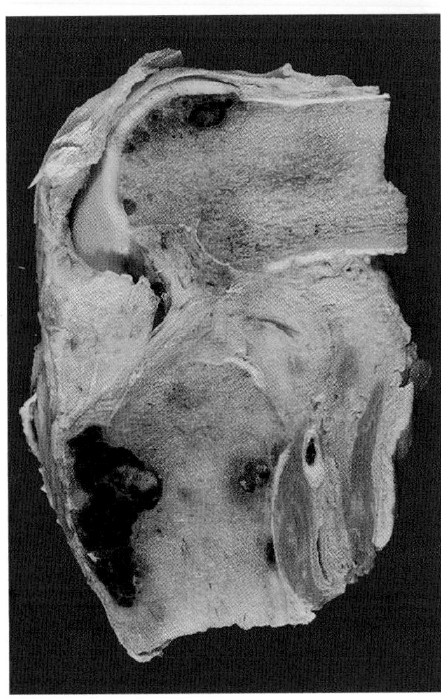

Fig. 24.77 Gross appearance of multicentric epithelioid hemangioendothelioma involving femur and tibia.

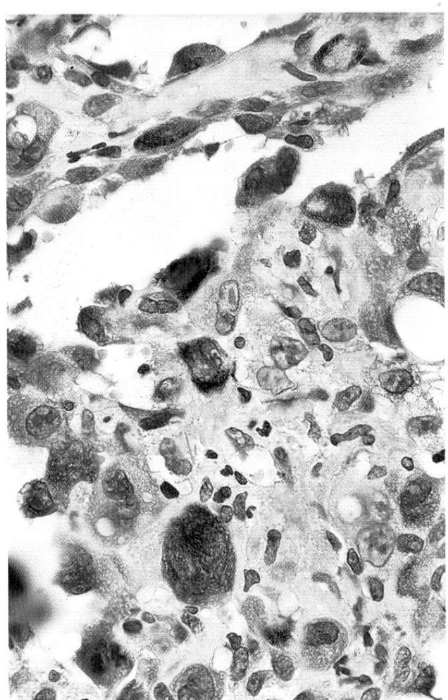

Fig. 24.79 Immunoreactivity for factor VIII in the highly atypical cells of angiosarcoma of bone.

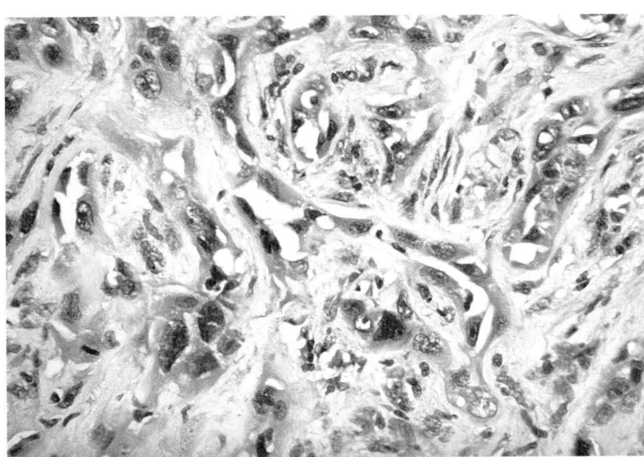

Fig. 24.78 Angiosarcoma of bone. Anastomosing vascular channels lined by highly atypical endothelial cells are seen.

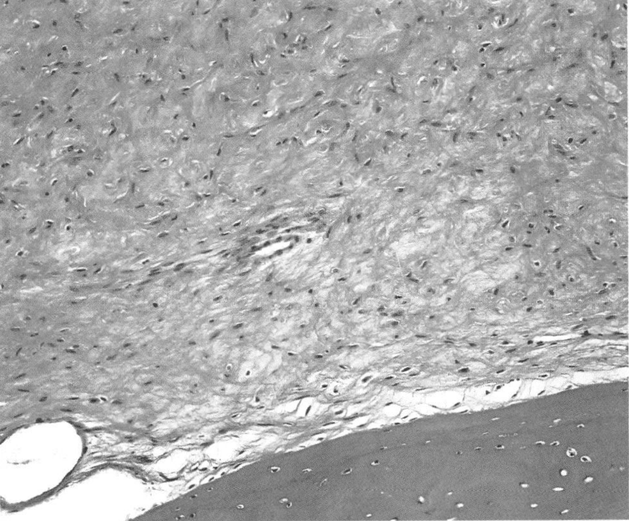

Fig. 24.80 Hypocellular quality and heavy collagen deposition in desmoplastic fibroma.

foci[761] (Fig. 24.77). The clinical course is protracted, especially for the multicentric tumors; distant metastases are exceptional.[769]

Angiosarcoma (malignant hemangioendothelioma, hemangioendothelial sarcoma) exhibits obvious atypia of the tumor cells, formation of solid areas alternating with others with anastomosing vascular channels, and foci of necrosis and hemorrhage[743,754] (Fig. 24.78). A wide range of differentiation exists from tumor to tumor and sometimes within the same case.[775] As already mentioned, in some cases the cells have an epithelioid or histiocytoid appearance.[741,749] Ultrastructurally and immunohistochemically, the large majority of tumor elements have the phenotype of endothelial cells, with only an occasional admixture of pericytes[767] (Fig. 24.79). Multicentric examples occur.[757] Distant metastases are common, particularly to the lungs. Before a diagnosis of angiosarcoma in a bone lesion is made, the more common possibilities of well-vascularized osteosarcoma and metastatic carcinoma (particularly of renal origin) should be ruled out.[770]

Other mesenchymal tumors

Fibrous and related tumors

Desmoplastic fibroma is a rare neoplasm formed by mature fibroblasts separated by abundant collagen.[782,784] Pleomorphism, necrosis, and mitotic activity are lacking (Fig. 24.80). Ultrastructurally and immunohistochemically, the predominant cells are myofibroblasts, with a lesser component of fibroblasts and primitive mesenchymal cells.[793,801] This lesion has been regarded by some authors as the osseous counterpart of soft tissue fibromatosis, but immunohistochemical and molecular genetic studies have not shown the type of β-catenin pathway alteration that is typical of the latter.[793]

Desmoplastic fibroma occurs most often in the long bones and jaw.[799] There is a male predominance, and three-fourths of the patients are below the age of 30 years.[799] Radiographically, it has a purely lytic, honeycombed appearance. It is destructive locally and often recurs following incomplete excision, but metastases do not occur.[791,808]

Infantile myofibromatosis can present as a solitary lesion in bone. Most of the cases occur in patients 2 years old or younger, and they involve almost always the craniofacial bones.[792,798] The microscopic appearance is the same as for its more common soft tissue counterpart.

Solitary fibrous tumor has been described as a pedunculated periosteal mass,[807] as well as an intraosseous lesion.[813]

Fibrosarcoma of bone often arises in the metaphyseal area of the long bones.[786,796] Approximately 50% of these occur in the distal segment of the femur or proximal portion of the tibia. The majority arise in the medullary portion, from where they destroy the cortex and often extend into the soft tissues. A less common location is the periosteum.

Radiographically, these tumors are osteolytic, with a 'soap-bubble' appearance. Well-differentiated lesions have well-defined margins, whereas high-grade tumors appear more invasive[783] (Fig. 24.81).

Microscopically, this tumor is similar to its soft tissue counterpart (Fig. 24.82). By definition, it should not contain any areas of tumor osteoid. It has also, somewhat arbitrarily, been agreed that the presence of prominent pleomorphism in a lesion of this type removes it from the fibrosarcoma category and places it into the malignant fibrous histiocytoma group.[811] The alternative possibility, which is being increasingly favored, is that these tumors represent pleomorphic fibrosarcomas;[779] after all, there is no reason why among the major types of bone and soft tissue sarcomas, only fibrosarcomas should be lacking the potential to undergo this type of change.

Other morphologic variations on the theme of fibrosarcoma of bone are the sclerosing epithelioid variety,[777] and a type characterized by myoid or myofibroblastic features, i.e., *myofibroblastic sarcoma* (*myofibrosarcoma*),[814] including the subtype accompanied by a heavy inflammatory infiltrate (*inflammatory myofibroblastic tumor*).[809]

Extremely well-differentiated fibrosarcomas may be misdiagnosed as benign lesions of fibrous tissue, but the radiographic appearance usually suggests their malignant nature. Microscopically, the presence of cellular areas, mitotic figures, and hyperchromasia are all features that favor a diagnosis of fibrosarcoma over one of desmoplastic fibroma. Fibrosarcoma also should be distinguished from the variety of osteosarcoma mainly composed of fibroblastic elements.[787] Wide local excision and amputation are the two choices of therapy, depending on the location, size, and microscopic grade of the tumor.

A good correlation exists between microscopic grade and prognosis.[783,811] In one series, the 10-year survival rate was 83% for low-grade lesions and 34% for high-grade tumors.[783]

Occasionally, fibrosarcoma can present as a multicentric process involving numerous bones.[793a] Before this diagnosis is made, the possibility of metastatic sarcomatoid carcinoma (particularly from the kidney) should be ruled out.

Malignant fibrous histiocytoma having a morphologic appearance analogous to that of the more common soft tissue sarcoma bearing that name occurs in bone[795,800,804,806,810] (Fig. 24.83). Many of the reported cases have been located in long bones or the jaw.[778,795] Close to 30% of these tumors arise in bone infarcts (often secondary to sickle cell disease),[789,790,794] around foreign bodies,[780,802] following irradiation,[797] in Paget disease, or as expression of 'dedifferentiation' or anaplastic transformation in chondrosarcoma, chordoma, or giant cell tumor.[781,805] The mean age at the time of presentation is 40 years.[795] The morphologic, ultrastructural, and immunohistochemical features of most tumor cells correspond to those of fibroblasts and myofibroblasts.[803,812]

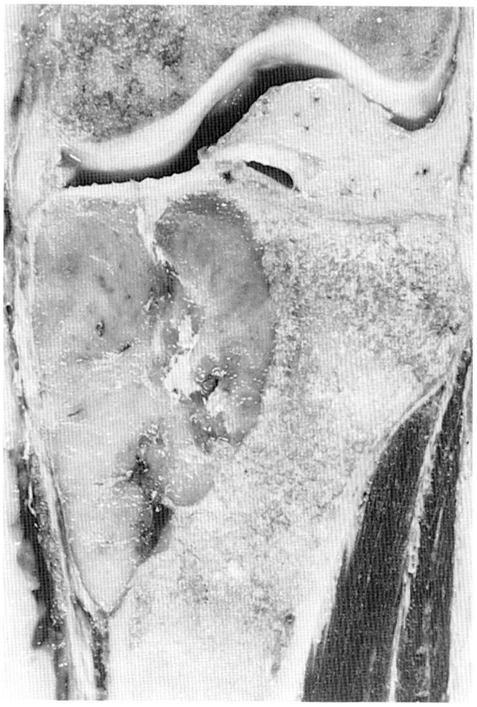

Fig. 24.81 Fibrosarcoma of tibia. The lesion produced an osteolytic defect and was confused radiographically with giant cell tumor.

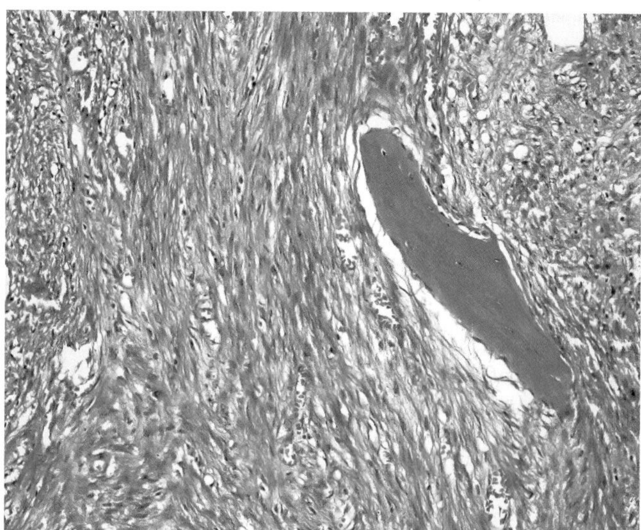

Fig. 24.82 Fibrosarcoma of bone. The tumor is more cellular than desmoplastic fibroma, but pleomorphism remains minimal.

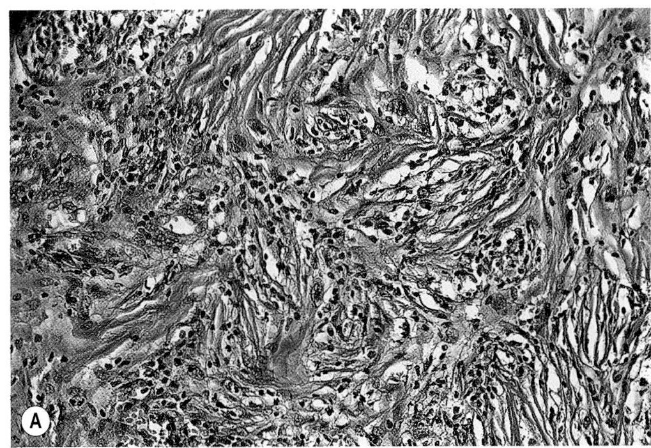

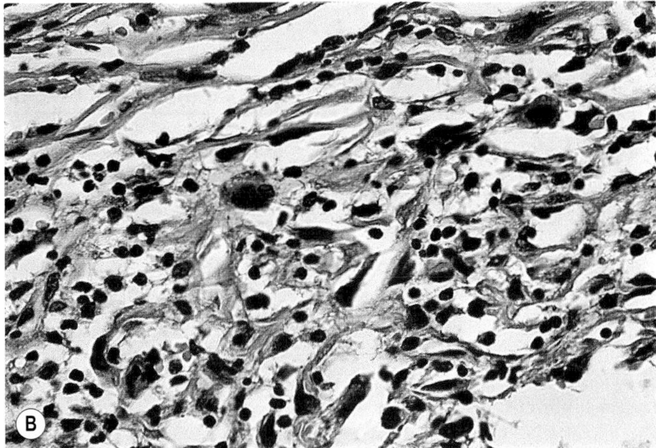

Fig. 24.83 So-called malignant fibrous histiocytoma of bone: **A**, storiform area; **B**, pleomorphic area.

The histogenesis and differential diagnosis of this tumor when involving bone are just as controversial as for its more common soft tissue counterpart, if not more so. As Dahlin et al.[788] have pointed out, areas indistinguishable from those of malignant fibrous histiocytoma can be found in otherwise typical examples of osteosarcoma or chondrosarcoma. Only when thorough sampling of the tumor reveals no areas suggestive of any of these lesions can a diagnosis of malignant fibrous histiocytoma of bone be justified. Even under these circumstances, it is doubtful whether this is a real entity as opposed to a pleomorphic, poorly differentiated sarcoma. The latter interpretation would explain why the overall prognosis is so poor, at least in some series.[785,810] In one group of cases, tumors with marked desmoplasia had a worse prognosis (5-year survival rate of 20%) than those with a prominent chronic inflammatory infiltrate (5-year survival rate of 78%).[815]

Muscle tumors

Leiomyomas of bone are practically nonexistent. **Leiomyosarcomas** are very rare, most of the reported cases being located in the jaw and in long bones, particularly the femur.[817–819,822,829] The morphologic, ultrastructural, and immunohistochemical features are analogous to those of its soft tissue counterpart.[819,821] Specifically, the tumor cells are immunoreactive for common and smooth muscle actin, desmin, and h-caldesmon, and they are enveloped by type IV collagen.[830] They may also be positive for keratin and S-100 protein.[820,831] Ultrastructurally, cytoplasmic microfilaments with focal densities are found.[826] Exceptional cases have been seen of the epithelioid variety (leiomyoblastoma).[824] About half of the patients present with metastatic disease or develop metastases within 1 year of diagnosis.[816]

Isolated examples of primary **rhabdomyosarcomas** of bone are on record.[823,827] Some have been of the pleomorphic type and others had embryonal features.[825,828]

Adipose tissue tumors

Lipoma of bone is a very rare tumor. The few reported cases have occurred in the long bones of adults and have presented radiographically as sharply outlined lytic lesions with sclerotic margins.[834,837] Microscopically, they are composed of mature adipose tissue devoid of hematopoietic elements; dystrophic calcification, fat necrosis, and hemorrhage may be present.[832,833]

Liposarcoma of bone is even more exceptional.[835,836] It is likely that many of the cases reported as such in the past would be reclassified today in other categories.

Chordoma and other notochordal lesions

The notochord is a phylogenetic structure representing a primitive spine which in higher organisms is replaced by the vertebrae and sacrum. **Notochordal remnants** are found in humans within the vertebral bodies and intervertebral disks.[867,878,891,909] *Ecchordosis physaliphora* is the name given to a grossly visible notochordal remnant found incidentally at autopsy as a discrete gelatinous nodule attached to the clivus or overlying the anterior surface of the pons.[897] Other sites where ectopic notochordal tissues can be found are the odontoid process of the axis, the nasopharynx, and the coccyx and adjacent presacral soft tissues.[862]

Giant notochordal hamartoma (benign notochordal cell tumor) is thought to be an exaggerated form of the same process located within the vertebral bodies, usually solitary but sometimes multifocal.[899] This lesion can be easily overdiagnosed as chordoma, from which it is distinguished by a combination of clinical, radiographic, and microscopic features.[870,879] The nuclei are round and bland, there are cytoplasmic hyaline globules, and there is no myxoid matrix or necrosis.[913] Although benign, they are regarded by some authors as precursors of chordomas.[851,914]

Chordoma is more frequent in the fifth and sixth decades but occurs in all ages and in both sexes. Chordomas grow slowly, the duration of the symptoms before diagnosis usually being over 5 years. About 50% arise in the sacrococcygeal area, 35% in the spheno-occipital area, and the remainder along the cervico-thoraco-lumbar ('mobile') spine.[842,858] The sacrococcygeal tumors are more common in the fifth and sixth decades of life, whereas many of the spheno-occipital neoplasms occur in children and adolescents.[850,860,861,912] In the former, a portion of the sacrum is seen destroyed by an osteolytic or rarely an osteoblastic process (Fig. 24.84). If the tumor encroaches on the spine, symptoms of spinal cord compression arise. The retroperitoneal space is often involved by direct extension. The tumor may grow large enough to narrow the lumen of the large bowel, impinge on the bladder, or invade the skin by direct extension.[855] It can be felt as a firm extrarectal mass. Spheno-occipital chordomas may present with a nasal, paranasal, or nasopharyngeal mass; multiple cranial nerve involvement; and destruction of bone.[844,892] Exceptionally, they may lead to fatal acute pontocerebellar hemorrhage.[854]

Grossly, chordoma is gelatinous and soft and contains areas of hemorrhage (Fig. 24.85). Microscopically, it closely resembles normal notochord tissue in its different stages of development.[857] It grows in cell cords and lobules separated by a variable but usually

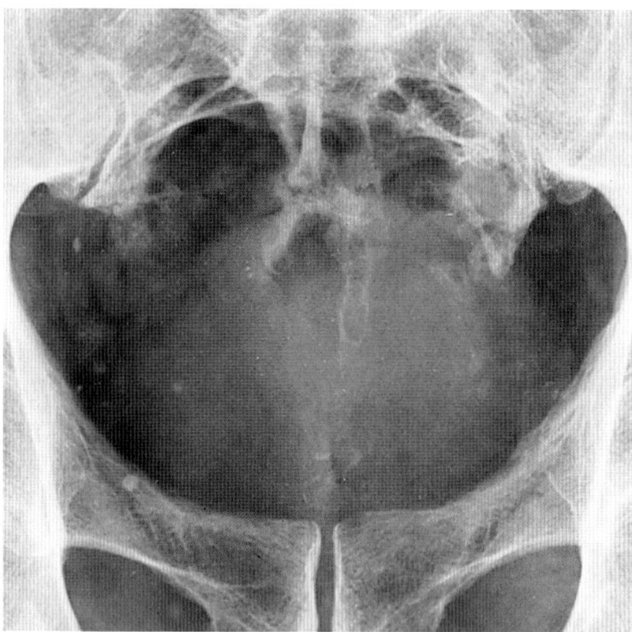

Fig. 24.84 Osteolytic destruction of sacrum by chordoma.

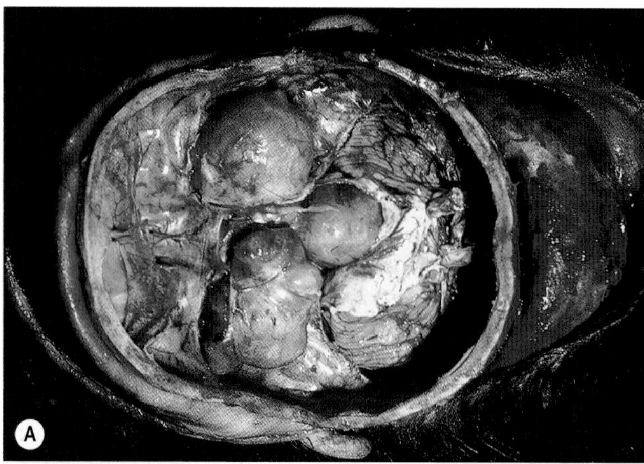

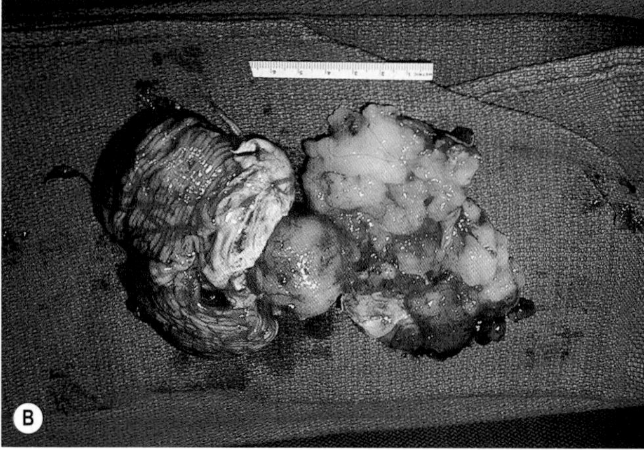

Fig. 24.85 **A** and **B**, Chordoma of spheno-occipital region as seen at autopsy. The gelatinous appearance of the tumor is well appreciated in **B**.

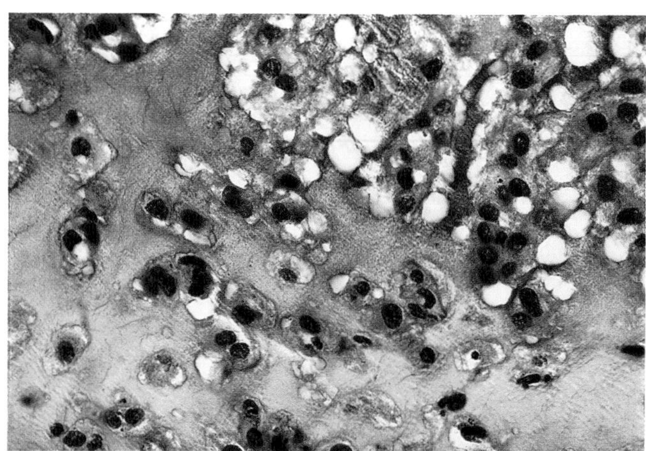

Fig. 24.86 Microscopic appearance of chordoma. The bubbly appearance of the myxoid stroma is characteristic.

extensive amount of mucoid intercellular tissue and by fibrous septa[884] (Fig. 24.86). Some of the tumor cells (known as physaliferous) are extremely large, with vacuolated cytoplasm and prominent vesicular nucleus; some of the cytoplasmic vacuoles contain glycogen, presumably in the process of being broken down.[872] Other tumor cells are small, with inconspicuous nuclei and no visible nucleoli. Mitotic figures are generally scanty or absent. Areas of cartilage and bone may be present. In some areas, the tumor may simulate carcinoma, particularly of renal cell origin.[853] The microscopic differential diagnosis also includes chondrosarcoma, signet cell adenocarcinoma of the rectum, myxopapillary ependymoma, and chordoid meningioma.[847]

Ultrastructurally, chordoma cells may contain peculiar mitochondrial–endoplasmic reticulum complexes, as well as parallel bundles of crisscrossing microtubules within the granular endoplasmic reticulum, two interesting albeit nonspecific features[852,866,903] (Fig. 24.87). They also have desmosomes, in keeping with their epithelial nature.[895] Immunohistochemically, chordoma shows reactivity for S-100 protein, keratin, epithelial membrane antigen (EMA), HBME-1, SOX9, sonic hedgehog (SHH; a morphogen secreted by the notochord), cathepsin K, and cadherin,[838,845,849,856,874,877,881,885,886,888,896] but only rarely for carcinoembryonic antigen (CEA)[838] (Fig. 24.88). Decreased expression of E-cadherin and increased expression of N-cadherin are said to indicate a more aggressive tumor phenotype.[902] Among the keratins, those regularly expressed are CK8, CK19, and (less consistently) CK5; they are instead usually negative for CK7 and CK20.[883,888] Microtubule-associated (Tau) proteins are also commonly expressed.[864] Glial fibrillary acidic protein (GFAP) reactivity is commonly encountered with the use of polyclonal antibodies, less so with their monoclonal counterparts.[910] Strong 5-nucleotidase positivity has been found in the cell membrane of the tumor cells, another feature of potential diagnostic utility.[843] Yet another potentially useful marker of chordoma is brachyury, a transcription factor involved in mesodermal differentiation, including notochord development.[886,901] The lectin-binding pattern of chordoma closely recapitulates that of the human fetal notochord.[868] The extracellular material contains collagen of nearly all types (I, II, III, IV, V, and VI); laminin is also present, as evidence of basement membrane deposition.[904]

The characteristic physaliferous cells of chordoma can be identified in material from fine needle aspiration, which is also amenable to histochemical and immunohistochemical evaluation.[907]

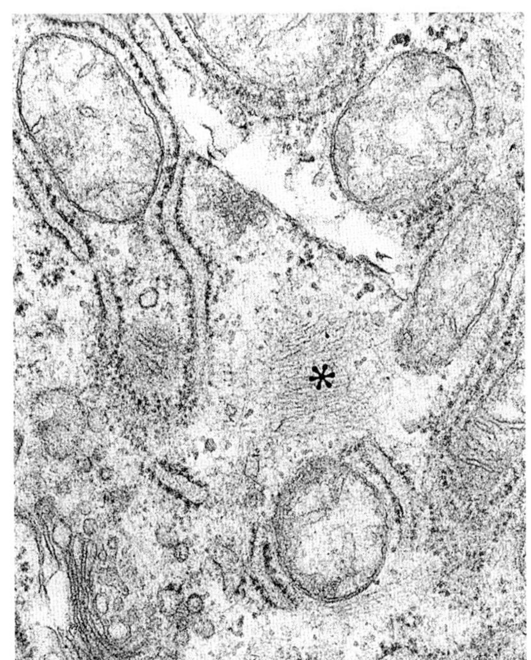

Fig. 24.87 Electron microscopic appearance of chordoma of sacrum. Mitochondria surrounded by cisternae of rough endoplasmic reticulum and aggregates of cytokeratin filaments (asterisk) are illustrated. *(Courtesy of Dr Robert A Erlandson, Memorial Sloan-Kettering Cancer Center)*

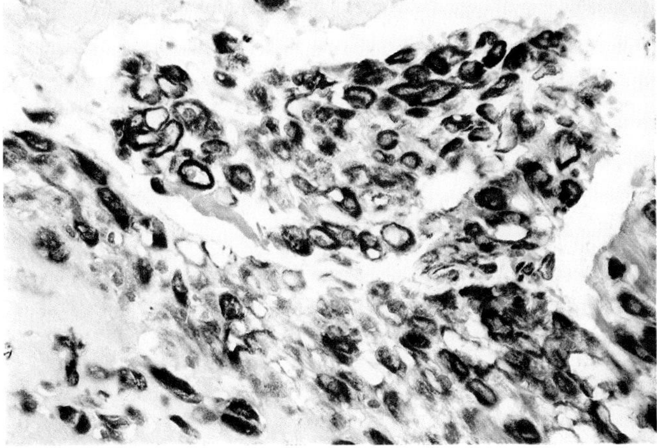

Fig. 24.88 Strong immunoreactivity of chordoma for keratin. This tumor was also positive for S-100 protein.

Chordomas commonly show hypodiploid karyotype, frequently with loss of chromosomes 3 (especially 3p), 4, 10, and 13.[871,876,900] Comparative genomic hybridization shows that the most frequent changes are: −1p, −3p, +5q, +7q, +12q, and +20.[898] The candidate region for sporadic and inherited chordoma development has been mapped to 1p36.13.[893]

The natural history of chordoma is characterized by repeated episodes of local recurrence and an often fatal outcome. Recurrences may develop 10 years or longer after the initial therapy.[839] Distant metastases are also late in the evolution of the disease.[846] In one series, the frequency of metastatic disease was 43%.[859] The most common sites are the skin (where they can simulate a sweat gland tumor) and bone, but they can occur in many other places, including the ovary.[855,916]

Treatment is in the form of surgical excision, radiation therapy, or a combination of both modalities.[887,889,891,915] The recurrence rate is very high following surgery, particularly when the tumor is entered during the procedure.[867] Adverse prognostic factors are represented by large tumor size, positive surgical margins, tumor necrosis, and high proliferative activity.[840,869,873,882]

Foci of high-grade spindle cell and/or pleomorphic sarcoma can be present in conjunction with areas of typical chordoma, either in the primary tumor or in the recurrences.[863] This phenomenon is analogous to that of 'dedifferentiated' chondrosarcoma and carries an equally ominous prognostic significance.[875,906] Like in the latter, these foci may exhibit 'divergent differentiation' in the form of rhabdomyoblasts or other cell types.[841] The high-grade foci exhibit a high proliferative index and have an aneuploid–hyperploid pattern on flow cytometry, in stark contrast to that of the conventional chordomatous component.[863] Indeed, some of the prognostic factors noted above relate to the presence of these high-grade foci.

Chondroid chordoma is a controversial tumor entity, originally defined as a chordoma with prominent cartilaginous foci.[858] It occurs most often in the spheno-occipital region, but it may also be seen in the sacro-coccygeal area.[848] The overall prognosis is better than that of conventional chordoma, although the differences in recent series are not as pronounced as in previous work.[880]

Ultrastructurally and immunohistochemically, the tumor seems to share features of chordoma and chondrosarcoma.[905] Immunohistochemically, most authors have found reactivity for S-100 protein, keratin, and – less commonly – EMA and CEA.[865,880,890,894,908,911] Although the two extreme suggestions have been made that this tumor is a chondrosarcoma with no relation to chondroma[908] or a chordoma with no cartilaginous features,[865] most evidence suggests that both components are present.

Adamantinoma of long bones

Adamantinoma of long bones characteristically involves the tibia but has been reported in other long bones, such as the femur, ulna, and fibula.[927,930] Occasionally, adamantinoma of the tibia is seen also involving the adjacent fibula.[935] It may be located in the shaft or in the metaphyseal area of the bone.[918]

Radiographically, it presents as single or multiple lytic areas in the cortex or medulla, surrounded by marked sclerosis. Grossly, it is poorly defined and may extend into the overlying soft tissues.

Microscopically, several patterns of growth have been described. The most common consists of solid nests of basaloid cells with palisading at the periphery and sometimes a stellate configuration in the center. Less frequent forms have been described as spindle, squamoid, and tubular; the latter simulates closely the appearance of a vascular neoplasm[918] (Fig. 24.89). Electron microscopic and immunohistochemical studies have confirmed the epithelial nature of the tumor cells[925,931–933,937] (Figs 24.90 and 24.91). The keratins expressed by adamantinoma are mainly 14 and 19, with lesser representation of keratins 5, 17, 7, and 13.[921] In contrast to other bone and soft tissue tumors with epithelial phenotypes – such as synovial sarcoma, chordoma, and epithelioid sarcoma – it lacks immunoreactivity for keratins 8 and 18.[921] Adamantinomas commonly show recurrent numerical chromosomal abnormalities, mainly gain of chromosomes 7, 8, 12, 19, and 21.[926]

On occasion adamantinoma is accompanied by osteofibrous dysplasia (see p. 2066), the relative proportions of the two lesions varying greatly from case to case.[919,934,936] Of great interest is the fact

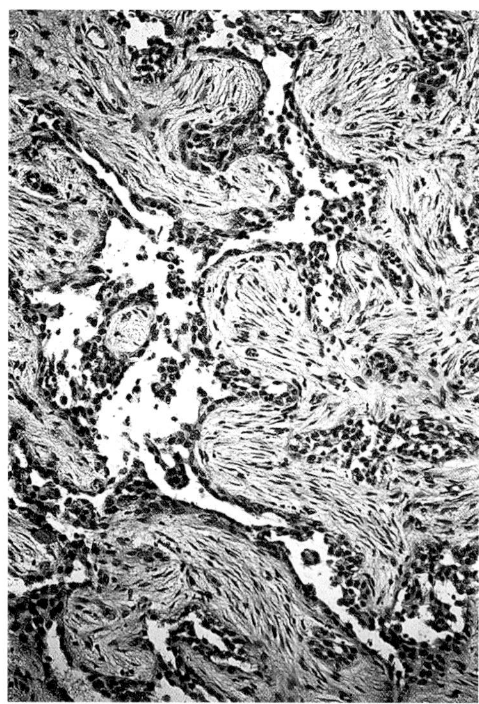

Fig. 24.89 Adamantinoma of tibia. Lack of cohesiveness of tumor cells in some of the islands results in a pseudovascular appearance.

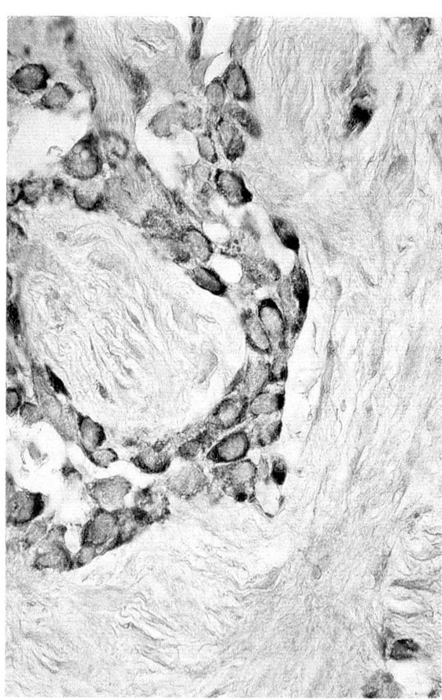

Fig. 24.91 Immunoreactivity for keratin in the tumor cells of adamantinoma of tibia.

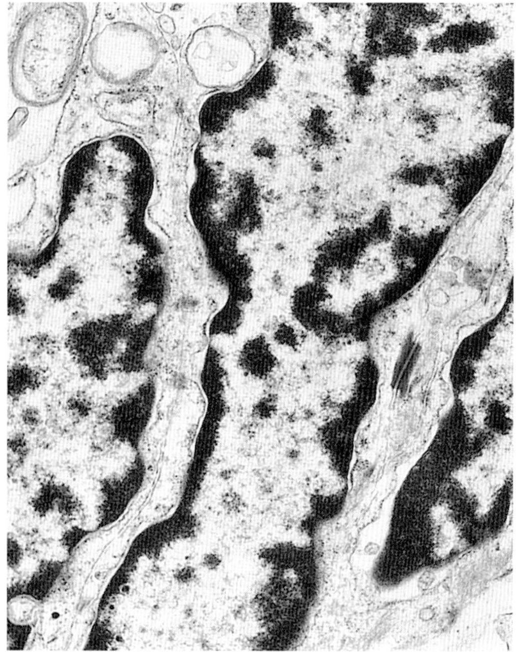

Fig. 24.90 Electron microscopic appearance of adamantinoma of tibia showing spindle-shaped epithelial tumor cells joined by desmosomes. *(×15 600; courtesy of Dr Robert A Erlandson, Memorial Sloan-Kettering Cancer Center)*

that the spindle cells of the latter component are also immunoreactive for keratin, suggesting a common histogenesis.[917,928]

The histogenesis of this tumor remains controversial. Now that the presence of epithelial differentiation has been proved beyond doubt, the two favored possibilities are origin from intraosseous epithelial rests, possibly of skin adnexal type,[920] or epithelial metaplasia in a primary mesenchymal process, the latter being suggested by the above-mentioned immunoreactivity for keratin, the distribution pattern of the extracellular matrix components, and the type of cytogenetic abnormalities present.[922,923,928] It is of interest that morphologically identical tumors can occur in the soft tissues of the pretibial area in the absence of bone involvement.[929] The odd tumor type combining features of adamantinoma and Ewing sarcoma (variously called adamantinoma-like Ewing sarcoma and Ewing-like adamantinoma) is discussed on page 2048.

Adamantinoma of bone is a low-grade malignant tumor characterized by a tendency for local recurrence and the occasional development of lymph node and distant metastases, particularly to lung.[927] En bloc excision and amputation are the therapeutic choices, depending on the circumstances of the case.[927] A unique case has been described with complete sarcomatoid dedifferentiation.[924]

Peripheral nerve tumors

Schwannoma rarely presents as an intraosseous mass.[939,941] A strong predilection for the mandible has been noted, and origin from the mandibular nerve sometimes has been demonstrated.[945] Schwannomas of the sacrum can reach huge dimensions and present as retrorectal masses; they may simulate a malignant tumor on radiographic grounds (particularly chordoma) and present great technical difficulties for their surgical removal.[944] A few of the reported cases of intraosseous schwannoma have been of the *melanotic* variety.[943]

Recklinghausen disease often results in several types of skeletal abnormalities (such as scoliosis, bowing, pseudoarthrosis, and other disorders of growth)[942] and may be accompanied by malignant bone tumors such as fibrosarcoma or so-called malignant fibrous histiocytoma;[940] however, intraosseous neurofibromas are extremely rare.

Malignant peripheral nerve sheath tumor has been rarely seen in bone in patients with or without Recklinghausen disease; several of the cases have involved jawbones.[938]

Xanthoma

Xanthoma of bone presents in patients over the age of 20 years and has a male : female ratio of 2 : 1. It is almost always solitary, and the flat bones (pelvis, ribs, skull) are the most frequent sites. Radiographically, it presents as a well-defined, sometimes expansile lytic lesion, often with a sclerotic margin. Microscopically, an admixture of foamy cells, multinucleated giant cells, cholesterol clefts, and fibrosis is seen. The differential diagnosis includes Rosai–Dorfman disease and secondary xanthomatous changes in other bone lesions, such as Langerhans cell histiocytosis and fibrous/post-traumatic dysplasia.[946]

Fibrocartilaginous mesenchymoma

Fibrocartilaginous mesenchymoma is a term that has been applied to a rare benign condition affecting the metaphysis of long bones (particularly the fibula) and characterized microscopically by an admixture of spindle cells, bone trabeculae, and islands of cartilage. Some of the cartilage is in the form of structures resembling epiphyseal plates. The condition is also known as subperiosteal fibrocartilaginous pseudotumor of long bones and focal fibrocartilaginous dysplasia.[948] Recurrences may supervene, but metastases have not been reported.[947]

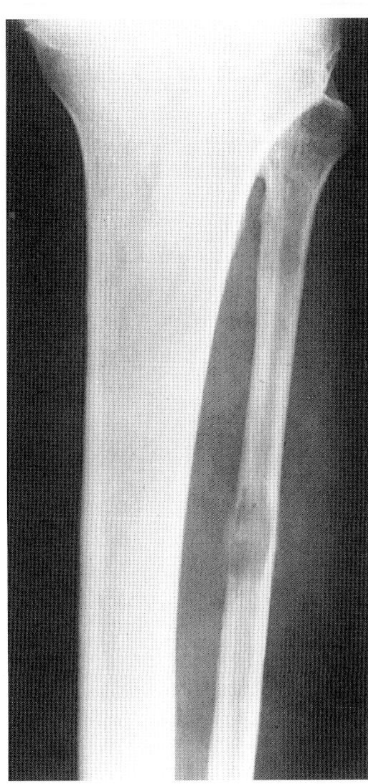

Fig. 24.92 Ill-defined lytic lesion in midshaft of fibula produced by metastasis of lung carcinoma.

Phosphaturic mesenchymal tumor

Phosphaturic mesenchymal tumor (also known as osteomalacia-associated mesenchymal tumor) is responsible for oncogenic osteomalacia, a rare paraneoplastic syndrome due to phosphate wasting. Microscopically, areas with a hemangiopericytoma-like appearance are seen combined with foci of giant cells.[952] There is also osteoid production and poorly developed cartilaginous areas. A distinctive type of calcified matrix (imaginatively described as 'grungy') is often present. These peculiar tumors of bone or soft tissue cause osteomalacia or rickets through the production of a renal phosphaturic substance that depletes total body phosphates by reducing tubular reabsorption of phosphate.[949] This substance has been identified as fibroblastic growth factor 23.[951] Their behavior is usually benign, but malignant cases associated with lung metastases are also on record.[950,953]

Others

Other types of mesenchymal neoplasms that have exceptionally presented as primary bone lesions include clear cell sarcoma (malignant melanoma of soft part type),[962] alveolar soft part sarcoma,[958] dendritic reticulum cell tumor,[956] desmoplastic small cell tumor,[954] malignant mesenchymoma,[959,961] and monotypic epithelioid angiomyolipoma (PEComa).[955,957,960]

Metastatic tumors

Metastatic tumors are the most frequent malignant neoplasms of bone[980] (Fig. 24.92). Since in most cases the lesions are multiple and the presence of a tumor elsewhere is known, the diagnosis is obvious. However, solitary metastases from occult primaries can be confused with primary bone tumors. More than 80% of all bone metastases originate in the breast, lung, prostate, thyroid, or kidney. These metastases can be accompanied by visceral deposits or represent the only apparent site of dissemination.[964,983] Soft tissue sarcomas rarely metastasize to the skeletal system,[974] the outstanding exception being embryonal rhabdomyosarcoma of the soft tissues in children.[965]

About 70% of bone metastases affect the axial skeleton (cranium, ribs, spine, sacrum), and the remaining involve the appendicular skeleton (long bones) or both compartments. In all bones, metastases are preferentially situated in the red bone marrow.[963] When located in long bones, the area usually involved is the metaphysis.

Metastatic bone lesions are usually osteolytic but may be osteoblastic or mixed. Tumors with a tendency to produce pure osteoblastic metastases are prostatic carcinoma, carcinoid tumor, and other neuroendocrine neoplasms, and – less commonly – breast carcinoma.[966,981] The mechanism is thought to be the production of bone growth factors by the tumor cells, such as transforming growth factor (TGF)-β, fibroblast growth factor, and bone morphogenetic proteins.[969,976] If the osteoblastic bone metastases of prostatic carcinoma are extensive, they can be accompanied by osteomalacia, possibly because the organism cannot satisfy the high calcium demand for new bone formation.[967]

The bone(s) involved and the character of the changes seen radiographically are helpful in predicting the site of the primary neoplasm. Thyroid carcinoma usually metastasizes to the bones of the shoulder girdle, skull, ribs, and sternum. Carcinoma of the kidney tends to involve the skull, sternum, flat bones of the pelvis, femur, and scapula[971] (Fig. 24.93). Bone metastases peripheral to the knees or elbows are rare, but they certainly occur, as distally as the terminal phalanges.[972,975,982]

Periosteal bone proliferation may rarely accompany a metastatic lesion.[977] This is more likely to occur in certain sclerosing lesions such as those of the prostate. Exuberant new bone formation can also occur because of a pathologic fracture associated with metastatic carcinoma and lead to diagnostic confusion with osteosarcoma[973] (Fig. 24.94). Metastatic malignant tumors – including

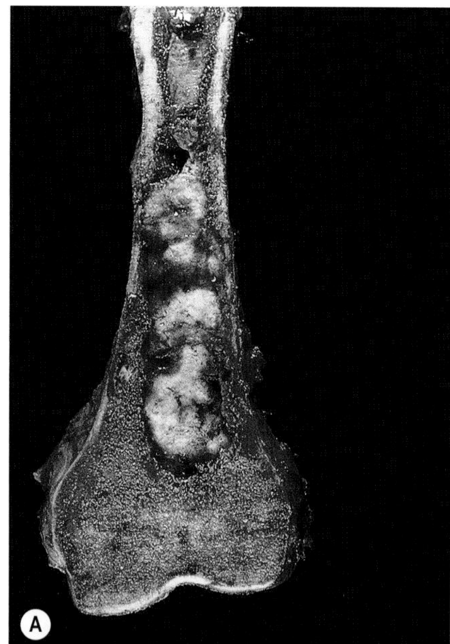

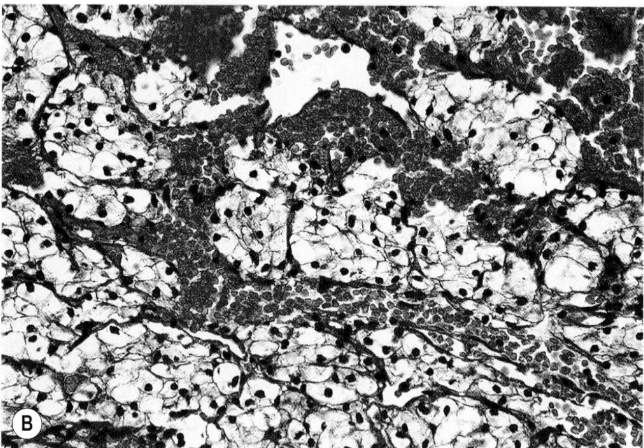

Fig. 24.93 **A**, Gross appearance of femur with medullary involvement by metastatic renal cell carcinoma. **B**, Microscopic appearance. The optically clear appearance of the cytoplasm and the extensive hemorrhage are characteristic features.

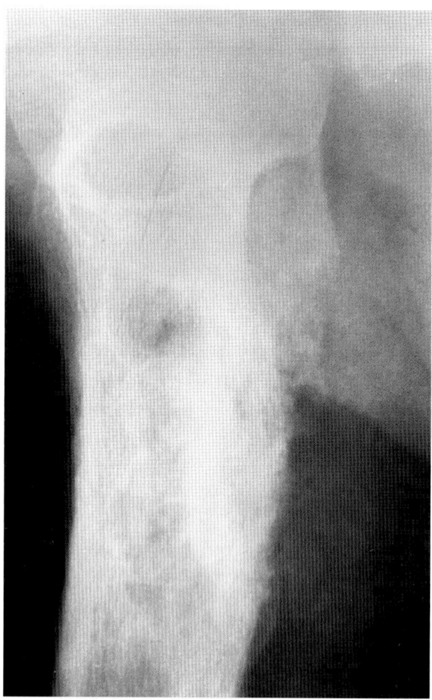

Fig. 24.94 Metastatic carcinoma in femur, with extensive callus formation, which simulated osteosarcoma both radiographically and microscopically. The primary tumor was probably in lung.

carcinoma and melanoma – can be accompanied by a prominent population of osteoclasts and simulate a giant cell tumor.[968] A soft tissue component may be present, particularly in bone metastases from the sternum or spine; sometimes, a pulsating mass will form as a result. Any tumor metastatic to bone, if extensive enough, may lead to hypercalcemia and elevation of serum acid phosphatase.

The mechanism of bone resorption is thought to be related to the transformation of tumor-infiltrating macrophages into osteoclasts.[979] Tumor-produced PTH-related protein is thought to be a mediator of the osteolytic process. In turn, the production of this protein is said to be stimulated by the secretion of TGF-β by the tumor cells.[970]

Most metastatic bone lesions cause pain. Treatment is for its relief and to prevent fracture of weight-bearing bones. Localized radiation therapy is highly effective, inducing partial or complete relief of pain in over 80% of the cases. When a pathologic fracture supervenes, internal fixation and radiation therapy provide the best results.[978] Palliative measures such as estrogen therapy and/or orchiectomy may afford relief in patients with disseminated metastases from carcinoma of the prostate. Hormonal therapy with estrogens or tamoxifen, or ovarian ablation provides pain relief in 25–50% of patients with metastatic breast cancer. Strontium-89 and hormonal manipulation have proved equally successful for pain relief in prostatic carcinoma. In a few instances, a single metastatic focus, particularly from the thyroid or kidney, may be excised with benefit.

Tumorlike lesions

Solitary bone cyst

Solitary (unicameral) bone cysts usually occur in long bones, most often in the upper portion of the shaft of the humerus and femur (Fig. 24.95). They also may be seen in short bones, particularly the calcaneus.[987] Most cases are seen in males, and almost all occur in patients under 20 years of age.

These lesions usually are advanced when first seen. Most are centered in the metaphysis and their natural evolution is to migrate away from the epiphyseal line. The cortex is thinned, but periosteal bone proliferation does not take place except in areas of fracture. Bones affected by these lesions often fracture, usually in the proximal portion of the cystic area.

The cyst contains a clear or yellow fluid and is lined by a smooth fibrous membrane that may be brown (Fig. 24.96). The fluid may be hemorrhagic if a previous fracture has occurred. Microscopically, well-vascularized connective tissue, hemosiderin (often within macrophages), and cholesterol clefts are frequent. The bone surrounding the cyst may have a dense quality, with irregular cement lines.[984–986]

The diagnosis may be difficult in the presence of reparative changes following fracture, in recurrent lesions after bone grafting,

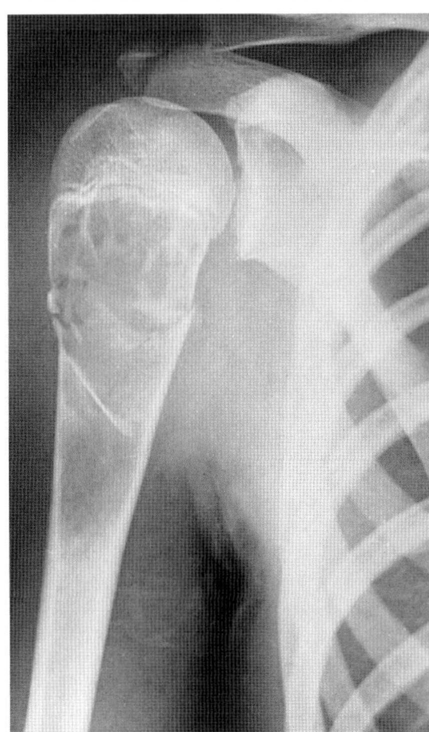

Fig. 24.95 Typical solitary bone cyst of upper end of humerus abutting against epiphyseal plate in a 13-year-old boy.

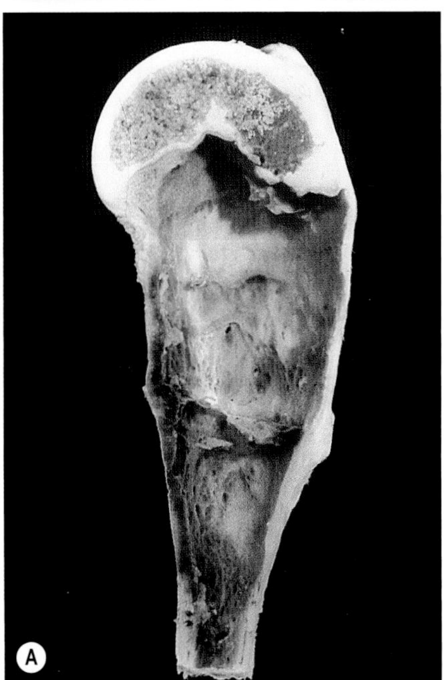

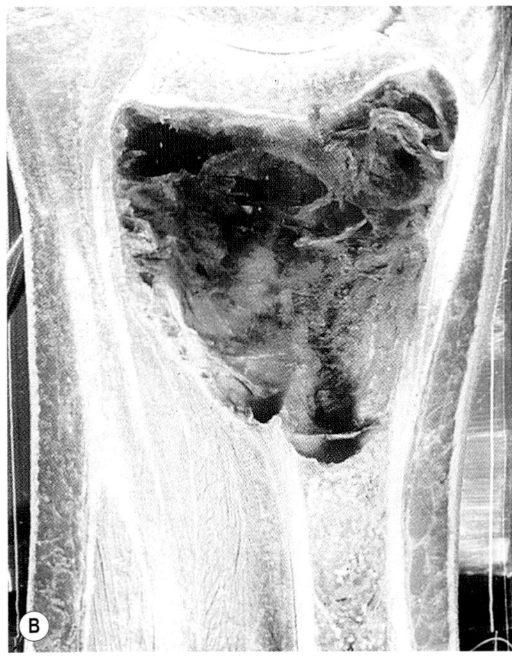

Fig. 24.96 **A** and **B**, Gross appearances of solitary bone cyst. **A**, A large lesion located in the upper metaphysis of the humerus. **B**, A triangular lesion located in the upper end of the tibia. There has been secondary hemorrhage, leading to an appearance not too dissimilar to that of an aneurysmal bone cyst.

and when articular cartilage is included in the curettings, but it becomes clear if the history and the x-ray films are available.

It is believed that this lesion arises on the basis of a local disorder of development and bone growth. A synovial origin has been suggested as an alternative pathogenesis.[986]

The treatment of choice is curettement and replacement of the cyst with bone chips. The results of therapy correlate well with the cyst 'activity' as determined by its location. Good results are obtained when the cyst has migrated away from the epiphyseal line, but recurrences often develop when it has not.[987]

Aneurysmal bone cyst

Aneurysmal bone cyst is seen usually in patients between 10 and 20 years of age[996,1018] and is slightly more common in females.[1004] It occurs mainly in the vertebrae and flat bones but can also arise in the shaft of long bones.[993] Multiple involvement is frequent in the vertebral lesions. Exceptionally, a lesion with the features of an osseous aneurysmal bone cyst is seen in a soft tissue location and even within the wall of a major artery.[1011,1012,1016]

Radiographically, aneurysmal bone cyst shows eccentric expansion of the bone, with erosion and destruction of the cortex and a small peripheral area of periosteal new bone formation (Fig. 24.97). Grossly, it forms a spongy hemorrhagic mass covered by a thin shell of reactive bone, which may extend into the soft tissue. Microscopically, large spaces filled with blood are seen. They do not have an endothelial lining but are rather delimited by cells with the morphologic, ultrastructural, and immunohistochemical features of fibroblasts, myofibroblasts, and histiocytes.[988,989] These cells also occupy the septa that separate the cysts.[989] A row of osteoclasts is often seen immediately beneath the surface (Figs 24.98 and 24.99). The septa also contain blood vessels and foci of osteoid and bone. An additional feature of great diagnostic significance is the deposition of a peculiar degenerated calcifying fibromyxoid tissue.[1017]

The differential diagnosis includes solitary bone cyst, giant cell tumor, hemangioma, telangiectatic osteosarcoma, and – especially for the lesions located in the jaw – giant cell reparative granuloma.

The pathogenesis of aneurysmal bone cyst remains elusive. In a few cases, the lesion is preceded by trauma with fracture or subperiosteal hematoma.[995] In others, it seems to arise in some preexisting

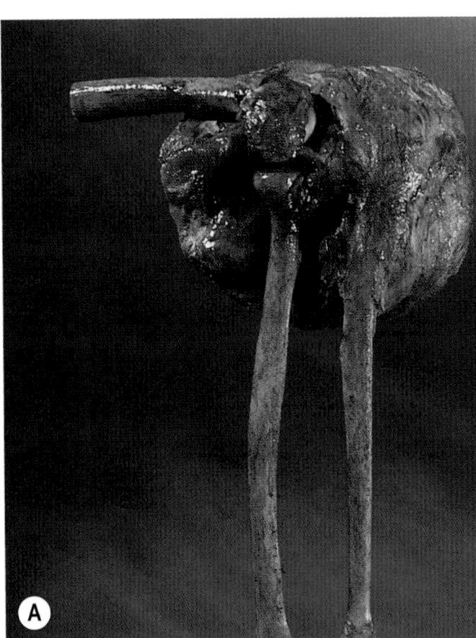

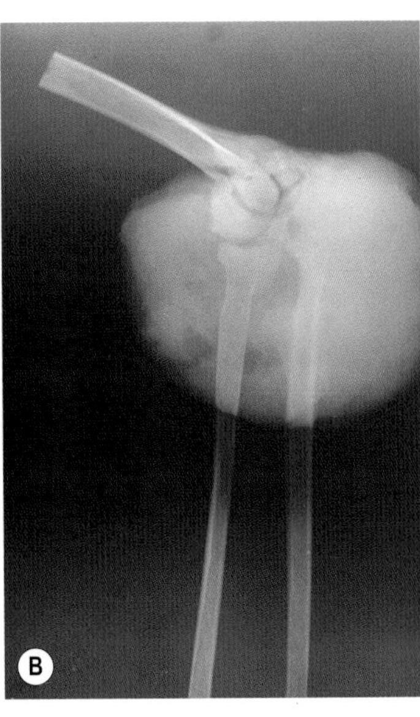

Fig. 24.97 **A**, Gross and **B**, radiographic appearances of large aneurysmal bone cyst of ulna.
(Courtesy of Dr Juan José Segura, San José, Costa Rica)

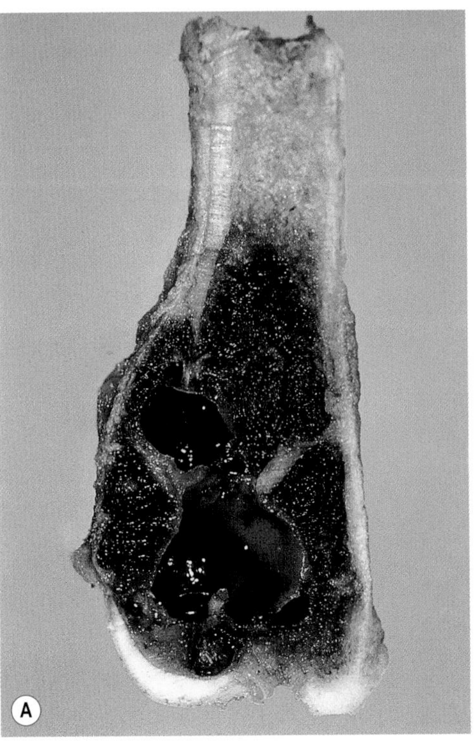

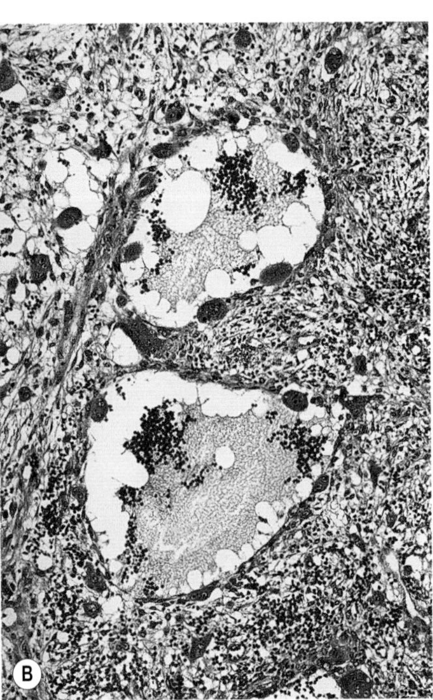

Fig. 24.98 **A** and **B**, Aneurysmal bone cyst of lower end of ulna. **A**, The large blood-filled cavities expand the metaphysis. **B**, Microscopic appearance, showing two cavities lined by osteoclast-like multinucleated giant cells. The intervening stroma is cellular but contains no neoplastic osteoid.
*(**A**, Courtesy of Dr RA Cooke, Brisbane, Australia; from Cooke RA, Stewart B. Colour Atlas of Anatomical Pathology. Edinburgh, 2004, Churchill Livingstone)*

bone lesion as a result of changed hemodynamics.[992,1000,1005] Areas grossly and microscopically indistinguishable from aneurysmal bone cyst can occur in chondroblastoma, giant cell tumor, fibrous dysplasia, nonossifying fibroma, osteoblastoma, chondrosarcoma, and in the vascular and cartilaginous hamartoma of the chest wall in infants (so-called secondary aneurysmal bone cysts).[1006] However, in most aneurysmal bone cysts, an underlying lesion is not encountered.[994,1017] Naturally, this might be the result of sampling or the fact that the aneurysmal bone cyst destroyed all evidence of the preexisting lesion. It has been suggested that insulin-like growth factor-1, which has been consistently found in this lesion, may play a role in its pathogenesis.[1003] The fact that nonrandom cytogenetic aberrations are found in primary aneurysmal bone cysts suggests that they are true neoplasms.[990,1015] Through chromosomal translocation, the *USP6* (ubiquitin-specific protease) gene on chromosome 17p13 can be fused with a number of partner genes, such as *CDH11* (osteoblast cadherin 11 gene) on 16q22 which is most common, *ZNF9* (zinc finger 9), *COL1A1* (collagen 1A1), *TRAP150* (thyroid receptor-associated protein 150), and *OMD* (osteomodulin).[1008,1009] Interestingly, these genetic alterations are not found in the secondary type of aneurysmal bone cyst.[1008]

Recurrence supervenes in approximately one-fourth of the cases treated by curettage alone because of incompleteness of surgical excision.[1013,1018] En bloc resection or curettage with bone grafting affords better results.[1001] It has been claimed that lesions containing fibromyxoid areas and immature osteoid are more likely to recur.[999]

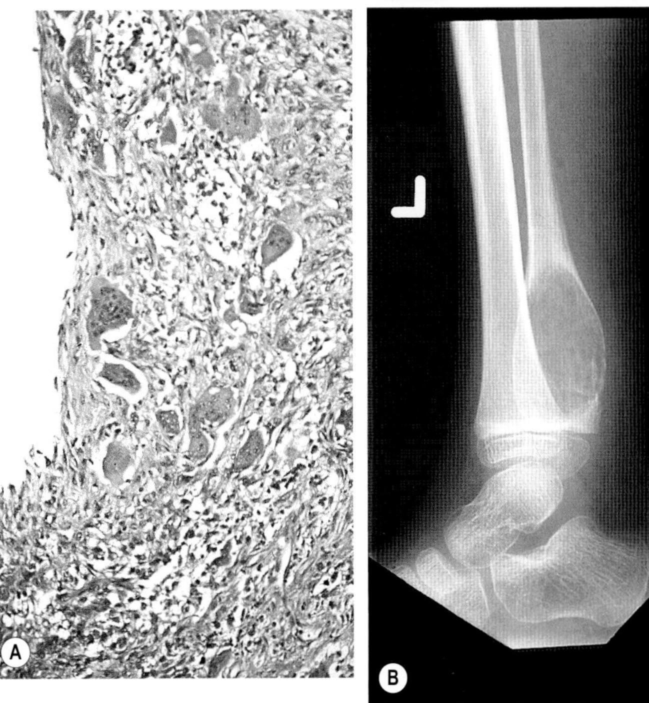

Fig. 24.99 **A**, Microscopic and **B**, radiographic appearances of aneurysmal bone cyst of lower end of fibula.

A few cases of reasonably convincing malignant transformation of aneurysmal bone cyst into osteosarcoma have been described; this exceptionally rare phenomenon should be distinguished from telangiectatic osteosarcoma and osteosarcoma with aneurysmal cyst-like areas.[1002]

Sometimes lesions with the features of aneurysmal bone cysts are seen in association with solid areas composed of an admixture of fibrous tissue, new bone formation, and osteoclasts. In other instances, solid areas with this mixed appearance are seen in the absence of typical aneurysmal bone cyst features. Depending on the location of the lesion, variation in microscopic appearance, and the pathologist's bias, these lesions have been variously referred to as *giant cell reaction*, *(extragnathic) giant cell reparative granuloma*, *giant cell-containing fibrous lesion*, and *solid variant of aneurysmal bone cyst*.[997,998,1007,1010,1014,1019,1020] Locations include the small bones of the hand and feet, vertebrae, sacrum, and – less commonly – long bones. In the latter locations, they tend to have a metaphyseal location[991] (Fig. 24.100). Determining whether these lesions are reactive or neoplastic and establishing their exact place in the classification of bone diseases remain to be accomplished.

Other cysts

Ganglion cysts morphologically indistinguishable from those commonly seen in the periarticular soft tissue are occasionally found in an intraosseous location, always close to a joint space[1022,1023] (Fig. 24.101).

The cyst is surrounded by a zone of condensed bone, is often multiloculated, and has a gelatinous content and a wall of attenuated fibrous tissue. The bones of the ankle, particularly the tibia, are those most commonly affected.[1024] Intraosseous ganglia need to be distinguished from solitary bone cysts and the periarticular cysts seen in association with degenerative joint diseases.

Subpubic cartilaginous cyst is the name given to a fibrocartilaginous mass with extensive degenerative cystic changes that has been observed in the proximity of the symphysis pubis.[1021]

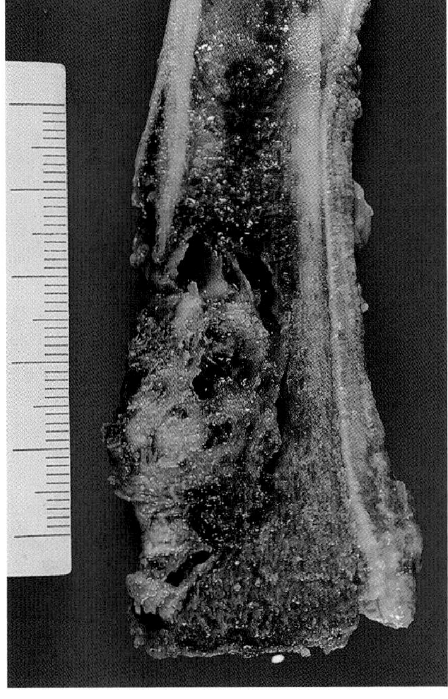

Fig. 24.100 Gross appearance of so-called 'solid variant' of aneurysmal bone cyst. A few hemorrhagic cystic areas are present at the periphery.

Metaphyseal fibrous defect (nonossifying fibroma)

Metaphyseal fibrous defects are distinctive lesions of bone that occur in adolescents, most often in long tubular bones, particularly the upper or lower tibia or the lower femur.[1028] They are eccentric, sharply delimited lesions not too distant from the epiphysis and sometimes accompanied by epiphyseal disorders (Fig. 24.102).

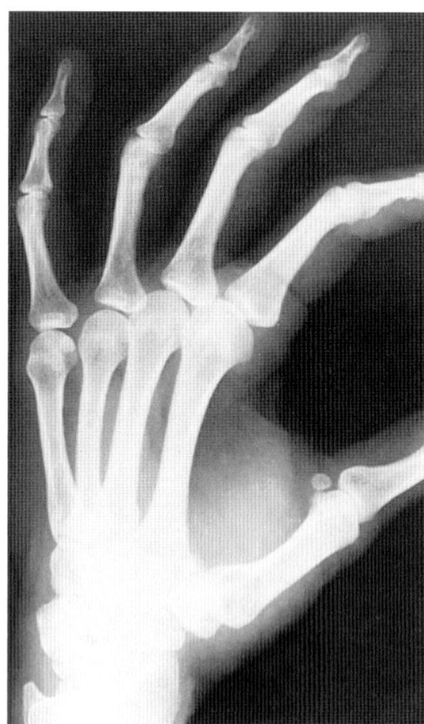

Fig. 24.101 Intraosseous ganglion cyst involving base of first metacarpal. It was associated with a larger ganglion of adjacent soft tissue, which is also apparent in the radiograph.
(Courtesy of Dr G Davis, St Louis)

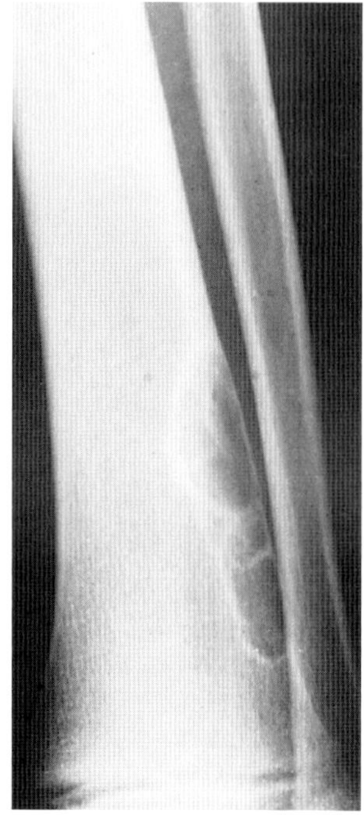

Fig. 24.102 Metaphyseal fibrous defect of lower end of tibia. Note its sharp delineation and sclerotic margins.

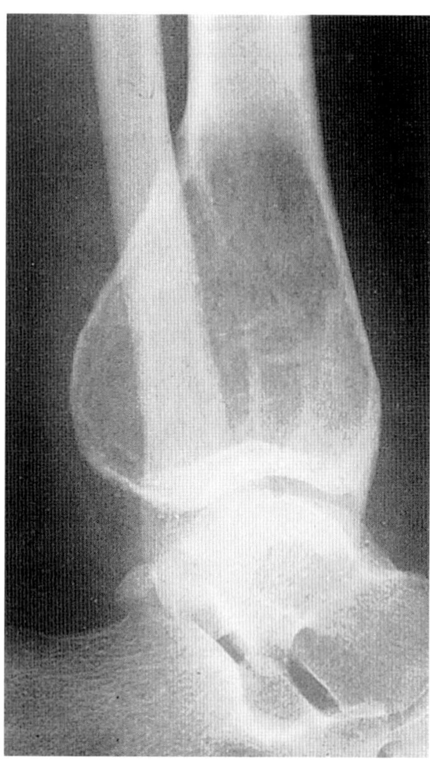

Fig. 24.103 Large metaphyseal fibrous defect expanding lower tibial metaphysis. Lesions of this size are sometimes called nonossifying fibroma.

When loose and associated with an intramedullary component, they have been designated as nonossifying or nonosteogenic fibromas (Fig. 24.103). There has been a long-standing and still unresolved controversy regarding whether these lesions are neoplastic or whether they represent developmental aberrations of the epiphyseal plate.

Grossly, the lesion is granular and brown or dark red. Microscopically, it consists of cellular masses of fibrous tissue, often arranged in a storiform pattern (Figs 24.104 and 24.105). Scattered osteoclasts and collections of foamy and hemosiderin-laden macrophages are frequent. The microscopic appearance is very reminiscent of a benign fibrous histiocytoma and is designated as such by some authors, especially when it occurs in adult patients in places other than metaphyses of long bones.[1026] Exceptionally, bizarre nuclear features are present, which are not necessarily indicative of a malignant nature.[1027]

Clinically, there are few or no symptoms except pain. The lesion is usually found incidentally on x-ray examination. Fractures can occur through the thinned cortex.[1025]

Fibrous dysplasia and related lesions

Fibrous dysplasia can present in two forms: monostotic and polyostotic. The monostotic variety is usually seen in older children and young adults, and most commonly affects the rib, femur, and tibia.[1039] The less common polyostotic type is characterized by a unilateral distribution and is usually associated with endocrine dysfunction, precocious puberty in female individuals, and areas of cutaneous hyperpigmentation (McCune–Albright syndrome). Monostotic fibrous dysplasia, polyostotic fibrous dysplasia, and McCune–Albright syndrome all occur sporadically, and are caused by activating mutations in the *GNAS1* gene (located in 20q13, encoding the α-stimulatory subunit of heterotrimeric G proteins) that occur postzygotically in a somatic cell.[1033,1034,1047] The differences in clinical manifestations relate to the time in which the mutation takes place, with mutation occurring during embryonic life being more likely to result in McCune–Albright syndrome, and mutation occurring in postnatal life more likely to cause monostotic disease. The gene mutation can be detected in paraffin-embedded material.[1058] The bone lesions of fibrous dysplasia have been found to be clonal, in keeping with a neoplastic process.[1049]

Radiographs of these lesions in the rib show a fusiform, expanded mass with thinning of the cortex. In the tibia, a lobulated, sharply delimited lesion of the shaft is formed (Fig. 24.106). This lesion may have a multilocular appearance because of endosteal cortical scalloping. Comparable lesions in membranous bone, particularly in the maxilla or the mandible, may show an overgrowth of dense bone. Occasionally the lesion protrudes far beyond the normal bone contour ('fibrous dysplasia protuberans').[1035]

Grossly, the tissue cuts with a gritty consistency and is grayish white (Fig. 24.107). The cortical bone often is thinned and expanded.

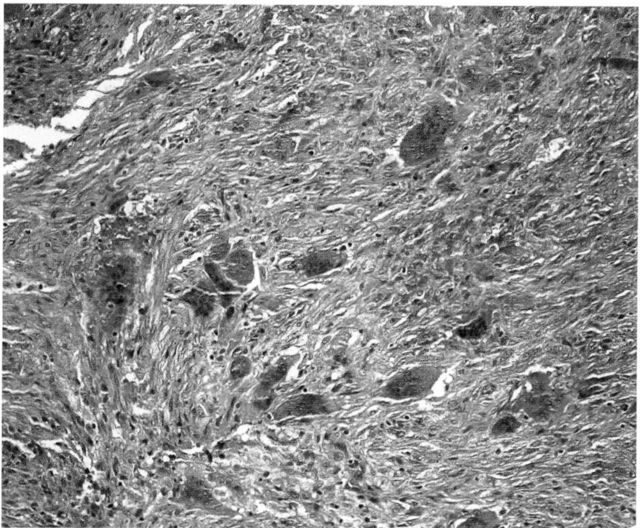

Fig. 24.104 Metaphyseal fibrous defect. The predominant element is a spindle cell of fibroblastic appearance. There are also irregularly scattered osteoclasts.

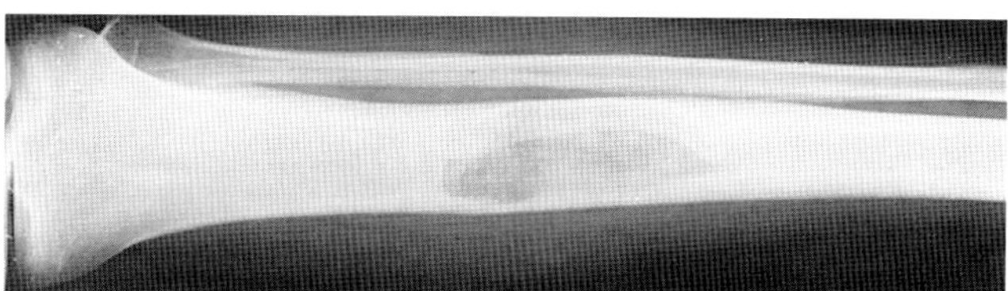

Fig. 24.106 Fibrous dysplasia of tibia forming a sharply delimited lesion.

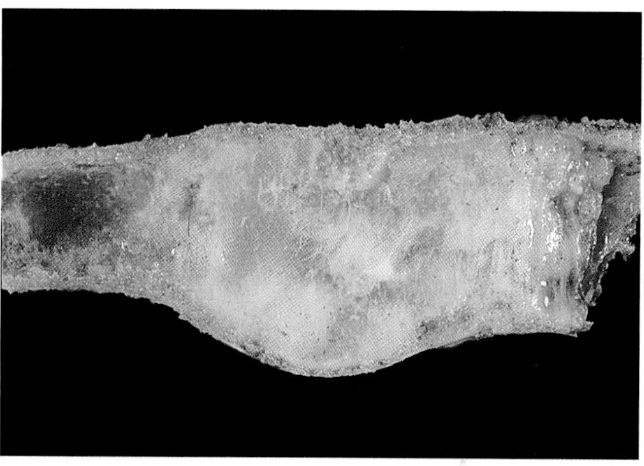

Fig. 24.107 Gross appearance of fibrous dysplasia of the rib. The lesion forms a fusiform, expanded mass that is grayish white.

Fig. 24.105 **A**, Radiographic and **B**, microscopic appearances of metaphyseal fibrous defect involving the upper metaphysis of the tibia.

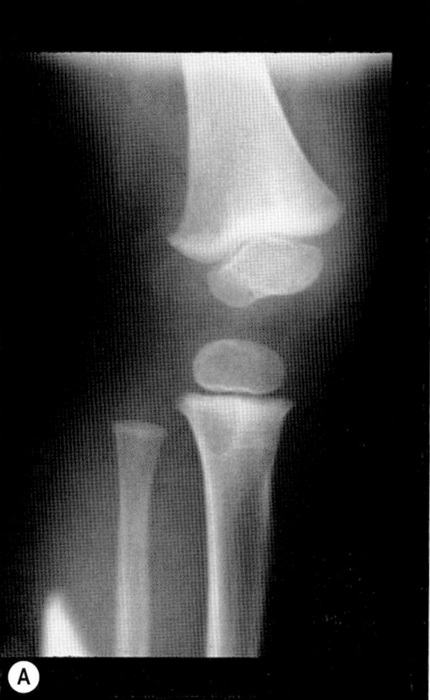

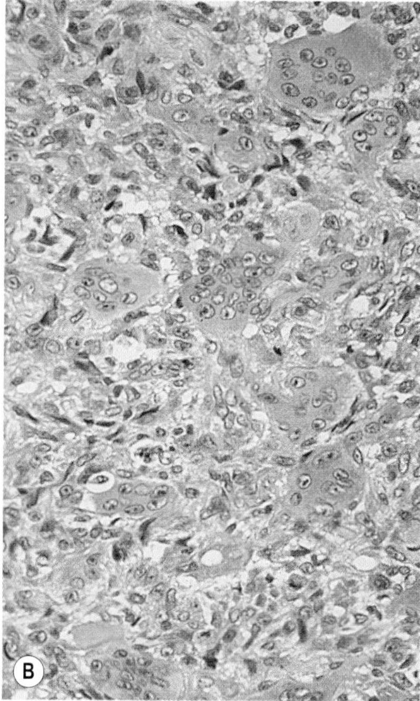

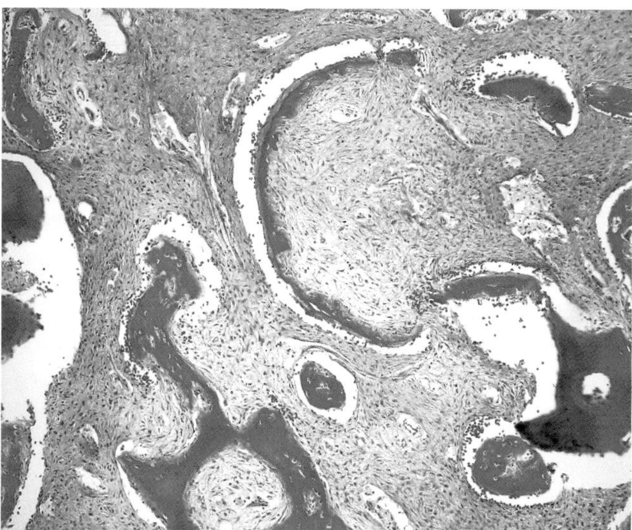

Fig. 24.108 Typical low-power appearance of fibrous dysplasia.

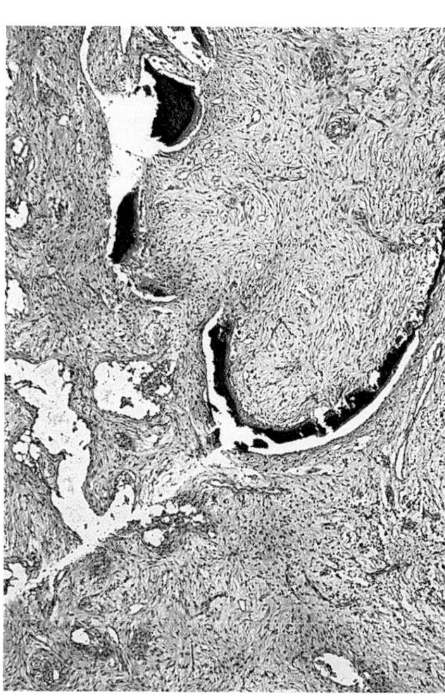

Fig. 24.109 Osteofibrous dysplasia. The low-power view is similar to that of fibrous dysplasia, but on high power there was osteoblastic rimming of the bone trabeculae.

Microscopically, narrow, curved, and misshaped bone trabeculae, often having a characteristic fishhook configuration, are interspersed with fibrous tissue of variable cellularity[1055] (Fig. 24.108). The coarse fiber ('woven') bone present in this condition does not transform into lamellar bone, suggesting that fibrous dysplasia represents a maturation defect so that the process of bone formation is arrested at an early stage resembling membranous ossification. Rows of cuboidal appositional osteoblasts do not appear on the surface of the trabeculae except as a pattern of reaction following local trauma. Silver stains are helpful in showing this failure of maturation. Ultrastructurally, the immature woven bone trabeculae are lined by abnormal osteoblasts with a fibroblast-like appearance.[1038] Immunohistochemically, they have been found to express periostin, a marker of intramembranous ossification.[1044]

If a lesion of fibrous dysplasia is biopsied over a period of years, maturation is still absent. This fundamental histologic abnormality makes it possible to distinguish fibrous dysplasia from other lesions. In some instances, however, particularly in femoral lesions, the differential diagnosis becomes nearly impossible.[1054]

Occasionally, lesions of fibrous dysplasia show calcified spherules similar to those seen in cementifying fibromas.[1053,1060,1062] Other cases show highly cellular areas that may be diagnosed incorrectly as sarcoma. Focal areas of hyaline cartilage and cystic areas may also be present. The former are more common in the polyostotic variety and can dominate the microscopic picture to such a degree that a mistaken diagnosis of a cartilaginous tumor can be made (fibrochondrodysplasia).[1052] The transition of normal to abnormal bone is often abrupt. This is helpful in distinguishing it radiographically from osteitis fibrosa cystica resulting from hyperparathyroidism.

It has been suggested that some rib lesions resembling fibrous dysplasia but showing progressive maturation of the bone toward the periphery are secondary to trauma ('post-traumatic dysplasia or lesion').[1043,1048] Some of these lesions are bilateral and strikingly symmetrical.[1037] A conceptually related issue is the so-called *liposclerosing myxofibrous tumor*, which some authors have hypothesized represents a form of fibrous dysplasia with secondary trauma-induced changes.[1040]

Fibrous dysplasia may be accompanied by intramuscular myxoma of the same extremity.[1029] In addition, fibrous dysplasia of either monostotic or polyostotic type can be complicated not only by the development of a primary bone sarcoma, particularly osteosarcoma,[1041] but also chondrosarcoma and so-called malignant fibrous histiocytoma.[1042,1056]

Resection cures fibrous dysplasia in bones such as the rib. Curettement is adequate in long bones such as the tibia. In the maxilla, where some deformity may exist, partial removal of the lesion is all that is necessary.

Osteofibrous dysplasia (fibro-osseous dysplasia, ossifying fibroma; Campanacci lesion) is distinguished microscopically from fibrous dysplasia by the osteoblastic rimming of the bone trabeculae and the presence of lamellar bone and radiographically by its cortical rather than medullary location and its greater tendency to recur[1031,1032,1045] (Fig. 24.109). The tibia and fibula are the bones usually affected, the lesions usually being eccentrically located.[1031,1050]

Clonal chromosomal abnormalities have been identified in this lesion, suggesting a neoplastic nature.[1030,1036] Immunohistochemically, reactivity for keratin, neurofibromin, S-100 protein, and Leu7 are commonly found in osteofibrous dysplasia, in contrast to fibrous dysplasia[1051,1059,1061] (Fig. 24.110). A peculiar and as yet unexplained relationship exists between osteofibrous dysplasia and adamantinoma of long bones[1036,1046] (see p. 2057). In contrast to fibrous dysplasia, there are no activating mutations of *GNAS1*, suggesting that the two disorders are not pathogenetically related, despite their morphologic and some phenotypic similarities.[1057,1058]

Myositis ossificans

Localized myositis ossificans is a reactive condition that is sometimes mistaken microscopically for osteosarcoma.[1063,1065,1072] The term is inaccurate because the muscle may not be involved, and inflammation is virtually absent. A history of trauma is obtained in only half of the patients. The most common locations are the flexor muscles of the upper arm (especially the brachialis anticus), the quadriceps femoris, the adductor muscles of the thigh, the gluteal muscles, and the soft tissues of the hand. Radiographic studies show periosteal reaction and faint soft tissue calcification within 3–6

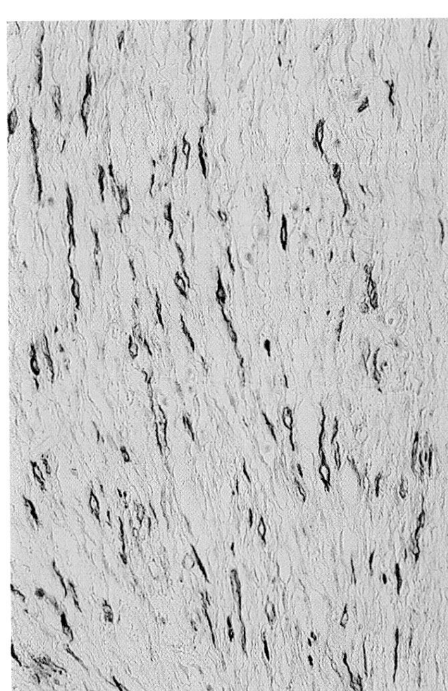

Fig. 24.110 Immunoreactivity of spindle cells of osteofibrous dysplasia for keratin. This does not occur in fibrous dysplasia.

weeks of the injury; these are gradually replaced by mature heterotopic bone by 10–12 weeks (Fig. 24.111). Arteriography done during the active stage of the disease shows numerous fine vessels followed by a dense, poorly defined stain in the mass.[1073]

Microscopically, there is a highly cellular stroma associated with new bone and, less commonly, cartilage formation. In an early lesion, the centrally placed areas may be very difficult to distinguish from osteosarcoma because of their extreme cellularity. As the process evolves, osteoid appears in an orderly pattern at the periphery of this mass and subsequently matures into well-developed bone. Several microscopic subtypes have been described, which correspond to different stages of the process.[1072] The most important diagnostic feature is provided by the maturation pattern ('zonal phenomenon'), characterized by a central cellular area, an intermediate zone of osteoid formation, and a peripheral shell of highly organized bone[1063] (Figs 24.112 and 24.113). Ultrastructurally, cells with features of myofibroblasts are prominent, as is also the case with other reactive conditions of mesenchymal tissues.[1068] The demonstration of *USP6* gene rearrangement in two of 12 cases of myositis ossificans in a recent study argues for a relationship of a subset of cases with aneurysmal bone cyst.[1071]

The most important differential diagnosis is with extraosseous and juxtacortical osteosarcoma. In the former condition, there should be greater cytologic atypia, and the zonal phenomenon does not occur (see Chapter 25). It is doubtful whether myositis ossificans ever develops into osteosarcoma. It is likely that many of the reported cases of this complication actually represent misdiagnosed instances of juxtacortical or extraosseous osteosarcoma.

A reactive lesion histologically and pathogenetically probably related to myositis ossificans has been reported in the small bones of the hand as *florid reactive periostitis, parosteal fasciitis, fibro-osseous tumor of the digits,* and other descriptive terms.[1064–1066,1070] Localized myositis ossificans also needs to be distinguished from multicentric myositis ossificans, also known as *progressive osseous heteroplasia,* which results from mutations of the *GNAS1* gene.[1067,1069]

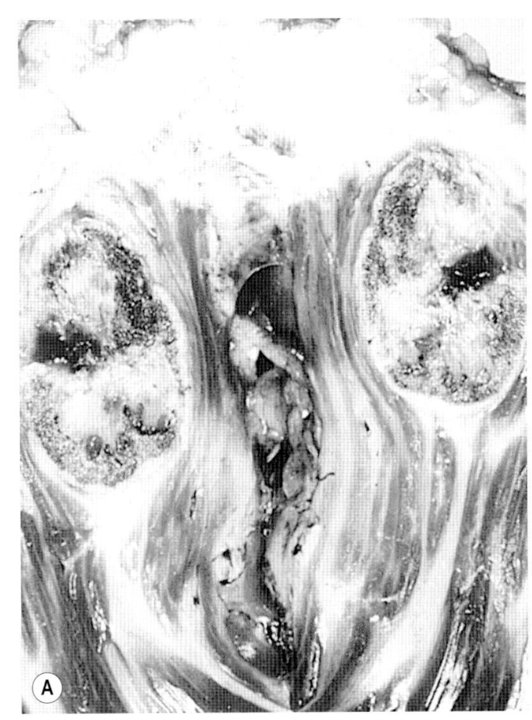

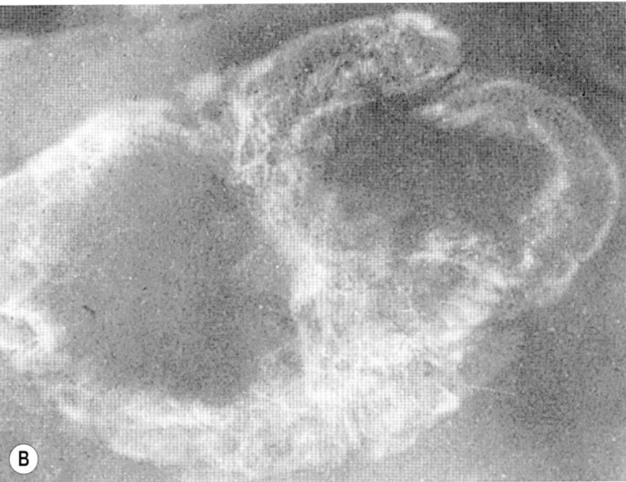

Fig. 24.111 **A**, Well-defined myositis ossificans occurring in muscle. **B**, Same lesion, illustrating bone formation in periphery.
(From Ackerman LV. Extraosseous localized nonneoplastic bone and cartilage formation [so-called myositis ossificans]. J Bone Joint Surg 1958, ***40A:*** *279–298)*

Langerhans cell histiocytosis

The unifying feature of the group of conditions designated as Langerhans cell histiocytosis (histiocytosis X, eosinophilic granuloma) is an infiltration by a cell of the accessory immune system known as Langerhans cell. This is accompanied by a variable admixture of eosinophils, giant cells, neutrophils, foamy cells, and areas of fibrosis (Fig. 24.114). Langerhans cells have a characteristic morphologic appearance (Fig. 24.115). Their nuclei often are lobulated or indented, sometimes with a longitudinal groove; their cytoplasm is, for the most part, distinctly acidophilic. A specific intracytoplasmic organelle, known as Langerhans or Birbeck granule, is regularly present on electron microscopic examination (Fig. 24.116).

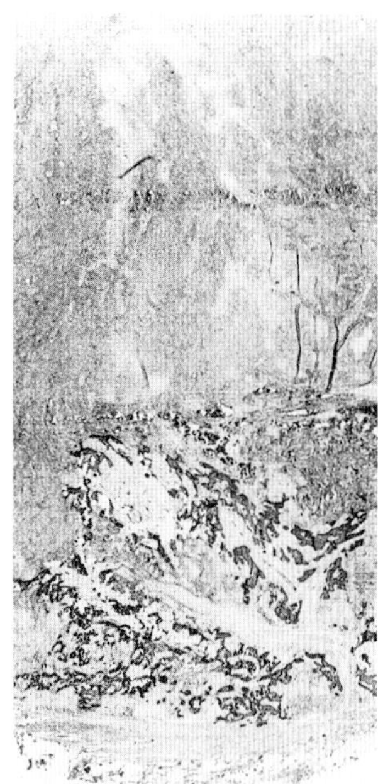

Fig. 24.112 Schematic representation of zonal phenomenon in myositis ossificans.
(From Ackerman LV. Extraosseous localized nonneoplastic bone and cartilage formation [so-called myositis ossificans]. J Bone Joint Surg 1958, ***40A:*** *279–298)*

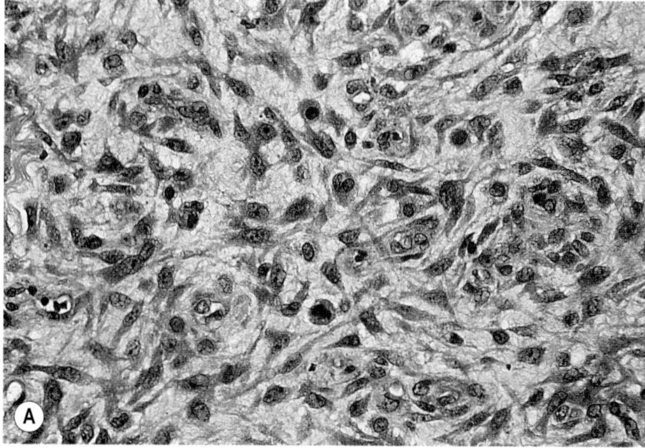

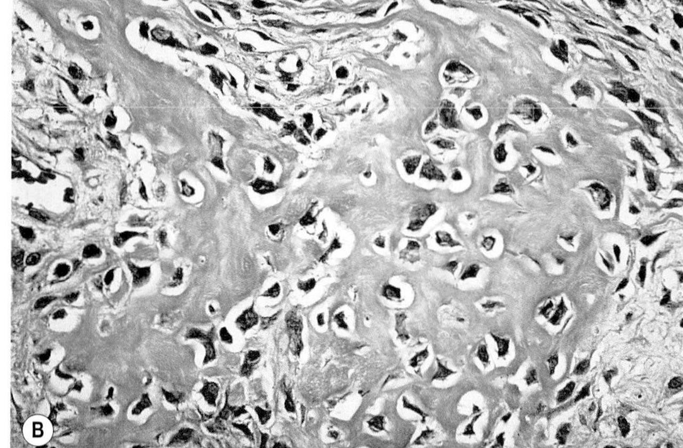

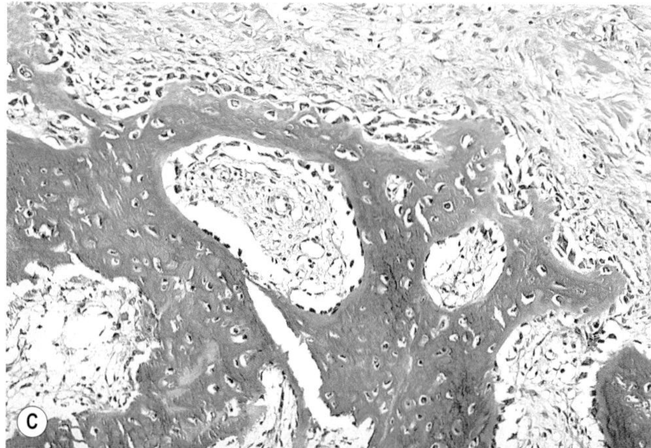

Fig. 24.113 A–C, Various appearances of myositis ossificans. **A**, Deep region showing a highly cellular appearance that can simulate a soft tissue sarcoma. **B**, Midportion showing osteoid formation by plump osteoblasts. **C**, Peripheral portion showing a shell of well-formed bone.

Diagnostic immunohistochemical markers include S100 protein, CD1a and langerin (CD207).[1076]

Langerhans cell histiocytosis of bone can be divided into three major categories on the basis of type and extent of the organ involvement:

1 Solitary bone involvement
2 Multiple bone involvement (with or without skin involvement)
3 Multiple organ involvement (bone, liver, spleen, and others).

The cases with solitary bone involvement, which represent the most common variety, have been traditionally referred to as eosinophilic granuloma.[1078] Young adults are most commonly affected.[1079] Any bone can be involved, with the possible exception of the hands and feet. The most common sites are the cranial vault, jaw, humerus, rib, and femur[1074] (Fig. 24.117). Radiographically, they present as an osteolytic lesion often in the metaphyseal area of long bones, sometimes associated with periosteal bone proliferation. They can be confused radiographically with metastatic carcinoma (Fig. 24.118) or Ewing sarcoma (Fig. 24.119). After fracture, this process may extend into adjacent soft tissues. Recurrences may develop in soft tissue after surgery. These lesions may spontaneously regress. They are extremely radiosensitive and can be cured with small amounts of radiation. The long-term prognosis is excellent.[1075] It is exceptional for these patients to develop other bone lesions or involvement of other organs.

Cases of multiple bone involvement have been traditionally designated as multiple or polyostotic eosinophilic granulomas.[1077] Depending on the location, the bony infiltration may result in proptosis, diabetes insipidus, chronic otitis media, or a combination of these conditions. The eponym of Hand–Schüller–Christian disease has been applied to this variety. Since the circumstances on which this designation is based are fortuitous and erratic, it would probably be better to drop the term entirely. This form is characterized by a prolonged clinical course, often marked by alternating episodes of regressions and recrudescences. The eventual outcome is favorable in most cases.

This type of Langerhans cell histiocytosis blends imperceptibly with the form having multiple organ involvement. Following the skeletal system, the skin and the lungs are the two most common sites affected. It is difficult to predict the outcome of the disease in a particular case, but there are several parameters that can be used

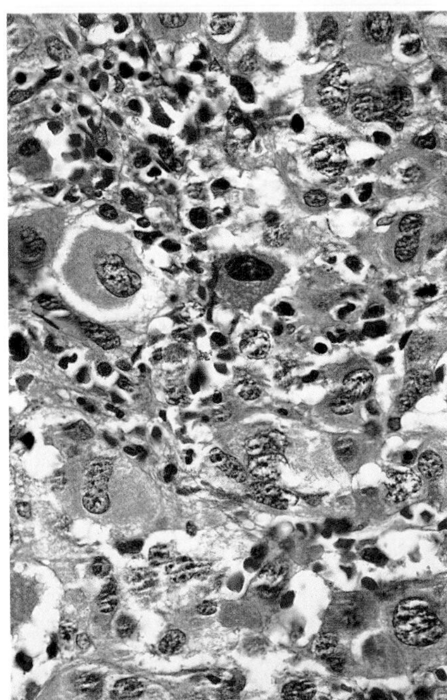

Fig. 24.114 Langerhans cell histiocytosis. Polymorphic appearance resulting from an admixture of Langerhans cells, nonspecific histiocytes, lymphocytes, and eosinophils. There is a mild atypia in the Langerhans cells that can simulate a malignant process.

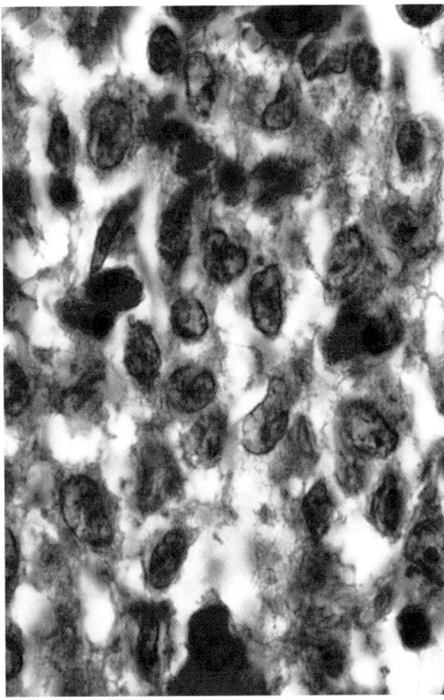

Fig. 24.115 High-power view showing elongated nuclei with occasional longitudinal grooves in the Langerhans cells.

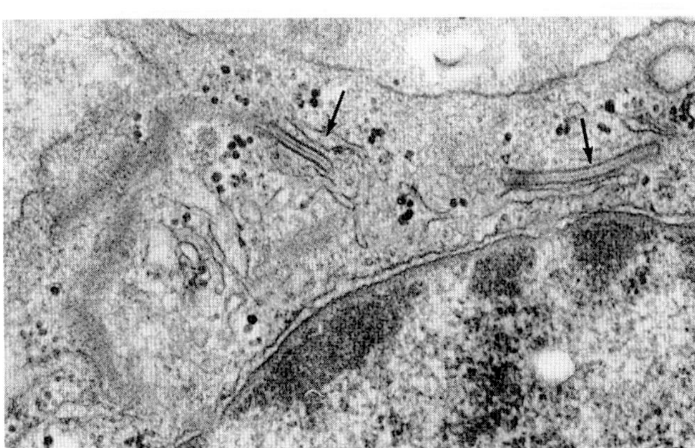

Fig. 24.116 At the ultrastructural level, this cell from Langerhans cell histiocytosis of bone contains several Birbeck granules (arrows). This is a constant feature of Langerhans cells.

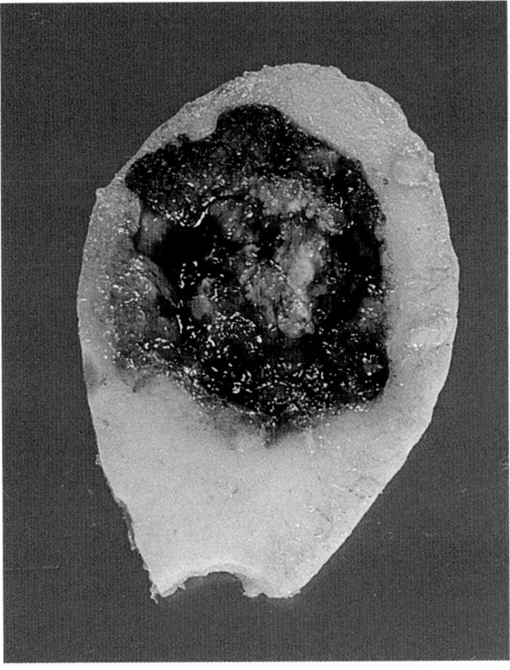

Fig. 24.117 Gross appearance of Langerhans cell histiocytosis of skull. A sharply circumscribed, dark brown lesion is seen.
(Courtesy of Dr Juan José Segura, San José, Costa Rica)

as guidelines. Poor prognostic factors are young age (under 18 months) at the time of diagnosis, hepatomegaly, anemia and/or thrombocytopenia, bone marrow involvement, and hemorrhagic skin lesions. Features not associated with a poor prognosis are seborrhea-like skin lesions, diabetes insipidus, and pulmonary lesions.[1081] Microscopically, it is very difficult to separate the aggressive from the more indolent forms. In a typical case of the former, the infiltrate is more monomorphic, with more mitoses and necrosis and fewer giant cells and eosinophils than in a typical case of the latter,[1080] but in our experience the overlap has been too great to rely on these features alone.

The differential diagnosis of Langerhans cell histiocytosis of bone at the microscopic level includes osteomyelitis and the osseous manifestations of Rosai–Dorfman disease.[1082]

Other histiocytic lesions

Rosai–Dorfman disease (sinus histiocytosis with massive lymphadenopathy) can involve the skeletal system either as a manifestation of multisystem disease or – less commonly – as a mass limited to this site.[1085] The morphologic features are similar to those

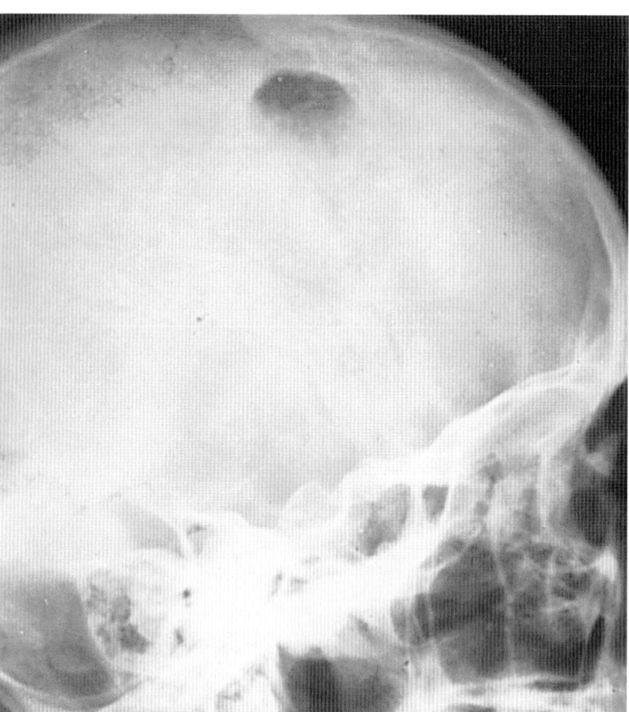

Fig. 24.118 Osteolytic lesion of skull in a 25-year-old woman. Radiographically, the lesion was thought to be metastatic carcinoma but proved to be a solitary lesion of Langerhans cell histiocytosis.

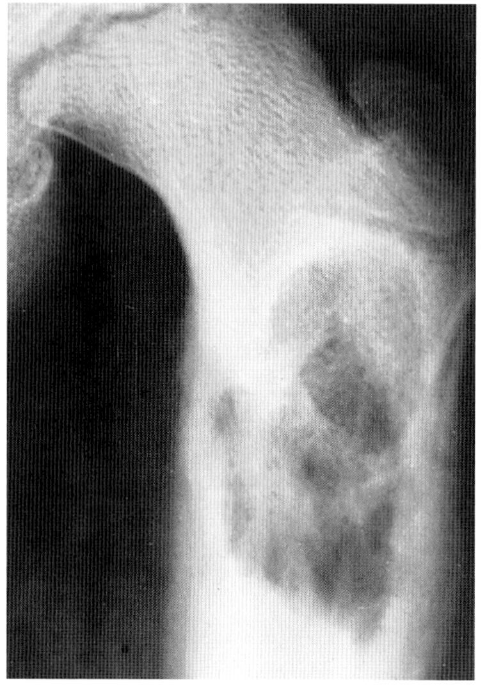

Fig. 24.119 Osteolytic lesion of femur in a 12-year-old boy. This was thought to be Ewing sarcoma but proved microscopically to be Langerhans cell histiocytosis.

seen at other extranodal sites, in the sense that secondary xanthomatous changes and fibrosis are common. These features, plus the paucity of emperipolesis, can render its recognition difficult.[1088]

Erdheim–Chester disease is a lipid-storing histiocytosis of non-Langerhans cell type which may be restricted to the bones or involve multiple organ systems, including lung and central nervous system. The foamy histiocytes that accumulate in this disease are CD68+ and CD1*a*–. The disease may be accompanied by extensive necrosis.[1087] In the lung the involvement is primarily septal, a fact of diagnostic significance both radiographically and morphologically. As in the case of Langerhans cell histiocytosis, there is controversy as to whether the disease is reactive or neoplastic.[1083,1084,1086]

Joints and related structures

Normal anatomy

Joints that permit free movements of the bone, referred to as *diarthroses*, are covered by hyaline cartilage and enclosed in a capsule. This capsule is composed of an outer fibrous layer of dense connective tissues, which is continuous with the periosteum of the bones, and an inner synovial layer.[1090] The latter, also referred to as *synovial membrane*, contains fibroblast-like cells (synoviocytes, type B cells)[1093] and macrophages of presumed bone marrow derivation (type A cells).[1090] Synoviocytes secrete collagen and proteoglycan and have a highly characteristic phenotype that includes the strong expression of vascular cell adhesion molecule-1 (VCAM-1),[1092] the antigen detected by Mab67,[1091] and clusterin (a follicular dendritic cell-associated apolipoprotein).[1089] They also exhibit high activity of the enzyme uridine diphosphoglucose dehydrogenase. Synoviocytes are immunoreactive for vimentin but not for keratin or other epithelial markers.

A layer of loose connective tissue or adipose tissue is present in some regions of the joint between the synovial and the fibrous layers, resulting in the formation of folds or 'villi', which protrude into the joint cavity. In old age, these villi may contain islands of cartilage.

Tendons are composed of closely packed parallel type I collagen fibers. They are surrounded by a layer of connective tissue known as the *tendon sheath*. In long tendons, this sheath is composed of an inner layer adjacent to the collagen and an outer layer that is loosely bound to the tissues surrounding the tendon. The space between these two layers is somewhat reminiscent of a joint cavity.

Non-neoplastic diseases

Ganglia and cystic meniscus

Ganglia (ganglion cysts) occur around joints and – less commonly – around tendon sheaths. They are annoying deformities that may cause pain, weakness, partial disability of the joint, and bone changes. Ganglia located in the popliteal space can result in pain or foot drop because of compression of the common peroneal nerve.[1096] Individuals overusing the wrist and fingers (pianists, computer operators) are prone to this condition. A history of injury preceding ganglion formation may exist.

Ganglia develop by myxoid degeneration and cystic softening of the connective tissue of the joint capsule or tendon sheath. The theory of a rent in the synovial membrane of a joint leading to the collection of synovial fluid and the formation of a false capsule can seldom be substantiated.

The most common location of ganglia is on the dorsal carpal area of the hand, where the cystic lesion pushes its way toward the surface between the tendons of the extensor indicis proprius and the extensor carpi radialis (Figs 24.120 and 24.121). The second most frequent location is the volar surface of the wrist, superficial and medial to the radial artery. Ganglia also arise on the volar surfaces of the fingers just distal to the metacarpophalangeal joints, in the dorsum of the foot, around the ankle and knee, and in the various articular and ligamentous areas of the spine. Intraosseous ganglia are discussed on page 2063. Ganglia are not lined by synovia and do not communicate with the joint cavity, two features distinguishing them from Baker cysts (see next section) (Fig. 24.122).

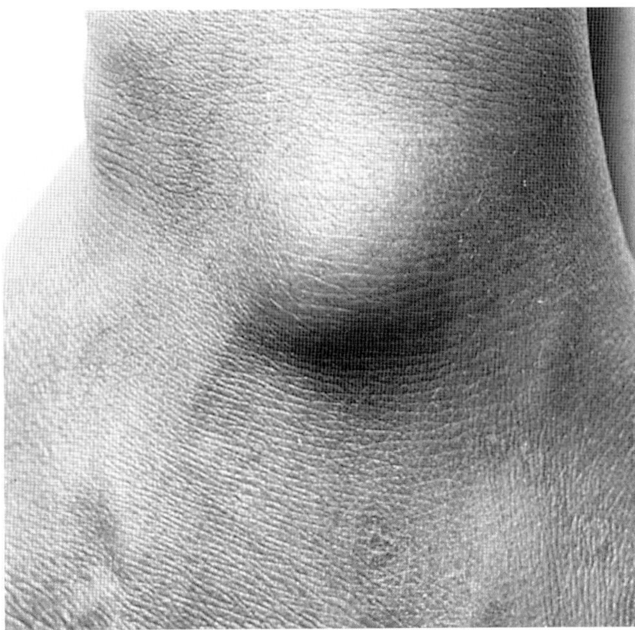

Fig. 24.120 Typical location and appearance of ganglion.

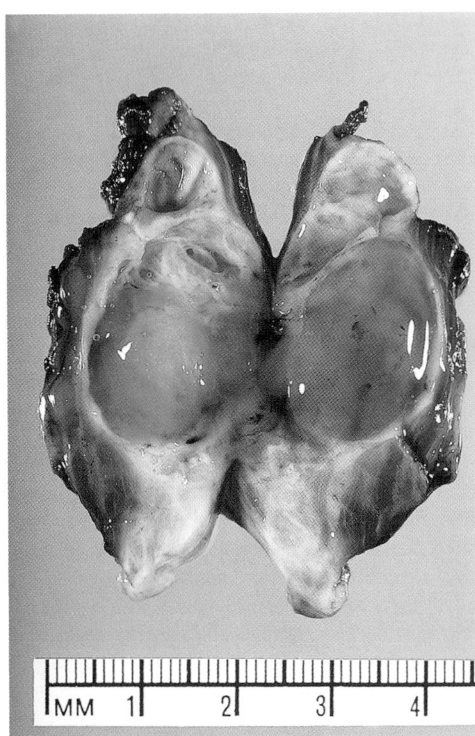

Fig. 24.121 Gross appearance of ganglion cyst.
(Courtesy of Dr RA Cooke, Brisbane, Australia; from Cooke RA, Stewart B. Colour Atlas of Anatomical Pathology. Edinburgh, 2004, Churchill Livingstone)

A lesion microscopically similar to soft tissue ganglion may occur in the menisci of the knee and is referred to simply as *cystic meniscus*. The most common site is the peripheral portion of the middle third of the lateral meniscus.[1094,1095] It may remain confined to the meniscus or extend extracapsularly. A traumatic etiology is favored.

Bursae and Baker cyst

Bursae are found where muscles, tendons, and skin glide over bony prominences. They are composed of a fibrohyaline wall with no inner lining. Bursae are subject to all the diseases that occur in large joint spaces. Inflammation may be associated with the formation of cysts, fluid, and loose bodies (Fig. 24.123). The incomplete removal of loose bodies may be followed by the disappearance of the remaining ones from the bursa.

A related lesion is *subdeltoid bursitis* associated with *calcareous tendonitis*. This entity is primarily a degeneration of a tendon or muscle in the rotator cuff of the shoulder followed by deposition of calcium in necrotic collagenous tissue. This calcific material stimulates a secondary inflammatory reaction.[1097] Psammomatous-type formations can be present.[1098]

Baker cyst occurs in the popliteal space from herniation of the synovial membrane through the posterior part of the capsule or from escape of joint fluid through normal anatomic connections of the knee joint with the semimembranous bursa (Fig. 24.124). The cyst is lined by true synovium and may have cartilage in its wall. Any joint disease leading to increased intra-articular pressure, such as degenerative joint disease, neuropathic arthropathy, and rheumatoid arthritis, may result in the formation of Baker cysts.[1099]

Carpal tunnel syndrome

The carpal tunnel is the space between the flexor retinaculum or transverse carpal ligament and the carpal bones. The medial nerve courses through this tunnel and its compression in this location by a variety of causes produces the symptoms of carpal tunnel

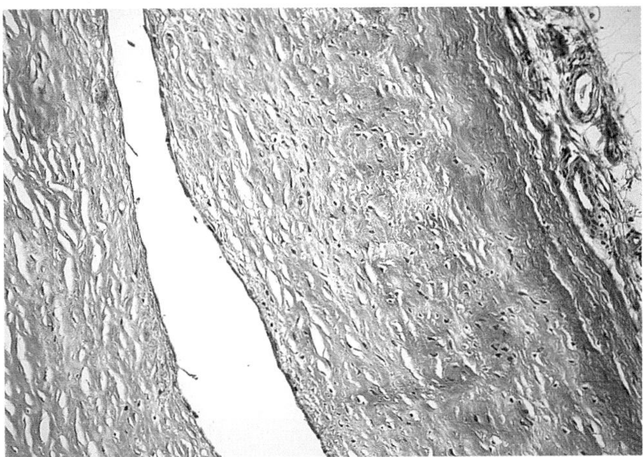

Fig. 24.122 Microscopic appearance of ganglion cyst. The wall is composed of dense fibrous tissue, and there is no synovial lining.

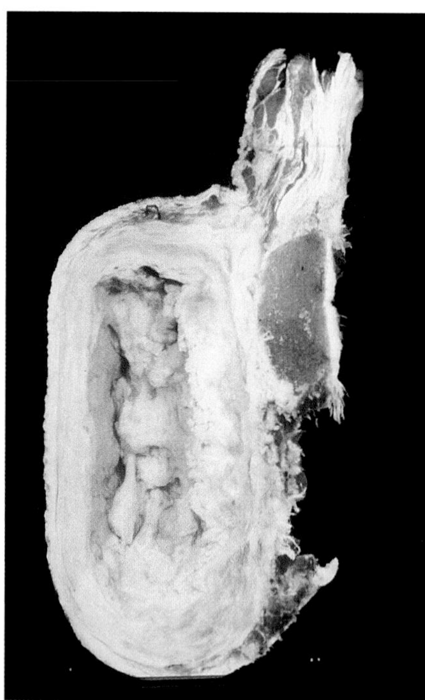

Fig. 24.123 Gross appearance of prepatellar bursa with chronic inflammation.

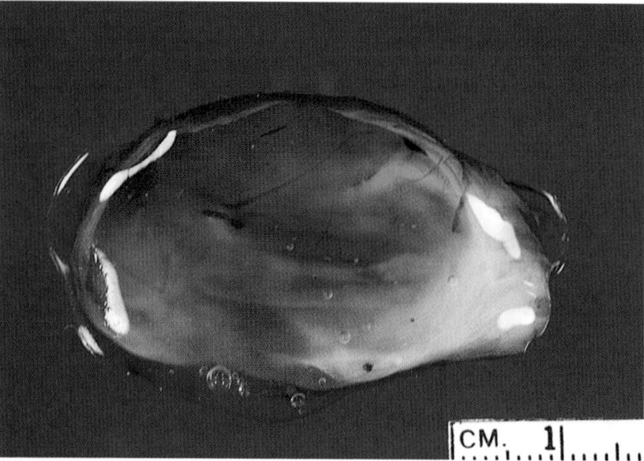

Fig. 24.124 Gross appearance of Baker cyst.

syndrome.[1101–1103] These include bony deformity following trauma, masses within the canal (i.e., hemangiomas, lipomas, ganglia), rheumatoid arthritis, and amyloidosis.[1100] Often, no specific etiology can be demonstrated.[1104]

Arthritis

Synovial biopsy

Needle biopsy of the synovium, particularly of the knee joint, is of aid in the assessment of synovial inflammatory conditions[1107,1108,1112] (Fig. 24.125). The specimen can be obtained either by blind needle biopsy or minimally invasive arthroscopy.[1113] The procedure is safe, simple, and easily repeated. It is indicated for inflammatory joint diseases when the etiology remains in doubt, particularly when only one joint is affected. Examination of the synovial fluid should always be performed before biopsy. It is possible to diagnose tuberculosis and other specific granulomatous lesions by this method.[1105,1107–1112] Other diagnosable diseases are pigmented villonodular synovitis, amyloidosis, Whipple disease, hemochromatosis, gout, and metastatic tumor. A heavy neutrophilic infiltrate is highly characteristic of infectious arthritis, although it also may be seen in Behçet disease and familial Mediterranean fever. Unfortunately, the histologic findings in the most common rheumatic diseases are often nonspecific;[1105] however, the combination of prominent lymphoid follicles and marked hyperplasia of synovial cells is highly suggestive of rheumatoid arthritis. By the use of a small-caliber synovial biopsy needle (Parker–Pearson technique), Schumacher and Kulka[1110] were able to obtain sufficient synovial tissue for diagnosis in 92% of the 109 joint biopsies they performed. Histologic examination proved to be of direct diagnostic value in 38 cases. In cases of synovitis, the process can be graded into low and high grade by using a score system based on hyperplasia of the lining cell layer, cellularity of the underlying stroma, and number of inflammatory cells.[1106]

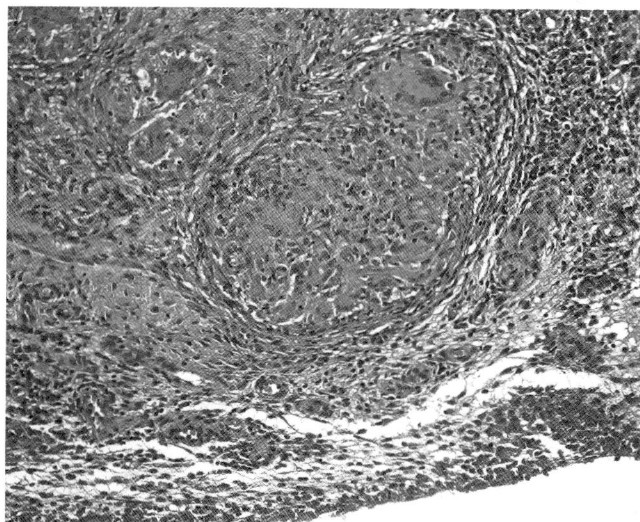

Fig. 24.125 Synovitis with non-necrotizing granulomas consistent with sarcoidosis.

Degenerative joint disease (osteoarthrosis)

The term *osteoarthritis* used in the past for this disease is inaccurate because this type of joint disease is degenerative and not inflammatory.[1118] The pathologic changes are related directly to age and are conditioned by use and occupation of the patient. These morphologic changes have been beautifully described in the classical works of Bennett et al.,[1115] Collins,[1116] and Hirsch et al.[1122]

The earliest change is an even degeneration of the hyaline cartilage of the articular surface, first detected as a fibrillation of the cartilaginous matrix at a right angle to the surface, and eventually resulting in a papillary appearance and sometimes in the freeing of fragments of cartilage. This leads to thinning of cartilage and compensatory overgrowth of the apposite joint surface. Once the articular cartilage disappears, the two bony surfaces are brought into contact, with progressive thickening of the trabeculae ('eburnation') (Figs 24.126 and 24.127). There is also increased activity of the perichondrium at the periphery of the joint, with formation of so-called *Heberden nodes*. The synovial membrane may remain

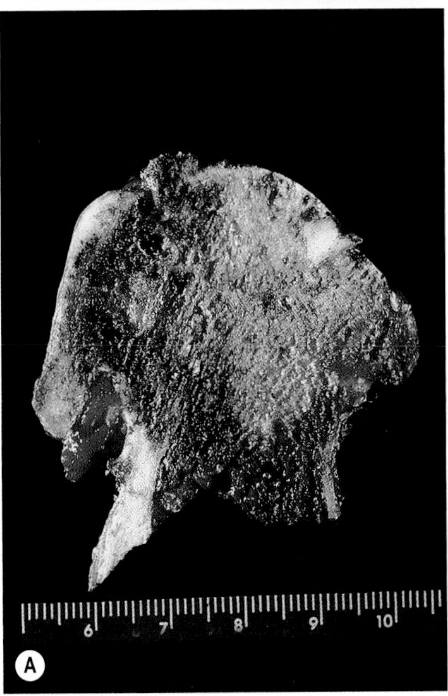

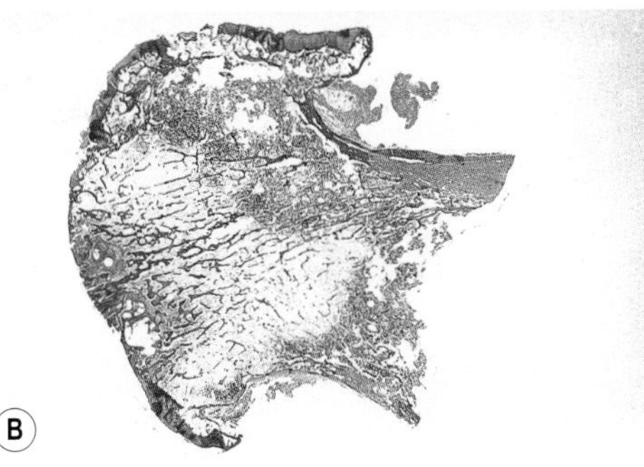

Fig. 24.126 Advanced osteoarthritis of femoral head: **A**, gross appearance, showing near-total disappearance of articular cartilage; **B**, whole mount of the same case.

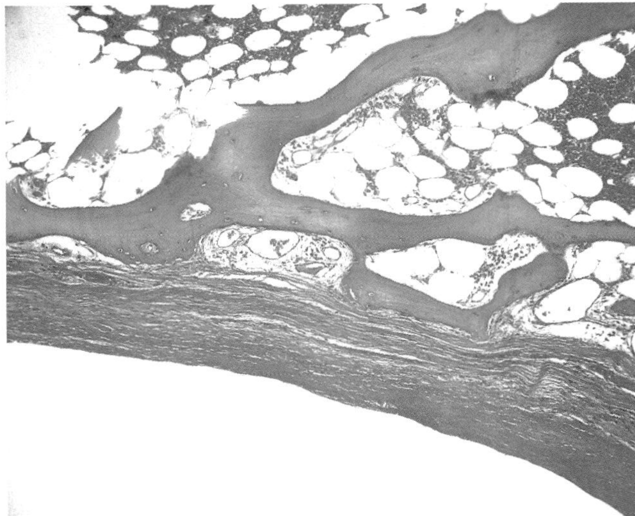

Fig. 24.127 Osteoarthritis. The articular cartilage has been replaced by a thin layer of fibrous tissue.

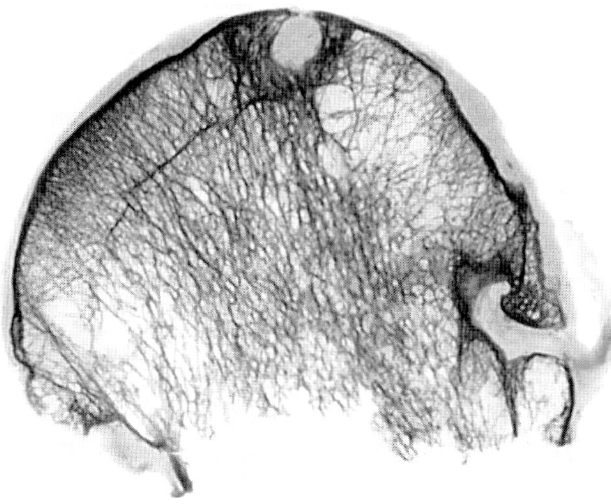

Fig. 24.128 Specimen radiograph of femoral head with osteoarthrosis. Note irregular thinning of articular cartilage and formation of a subchondral cyst surrounded by sclerotized bone.

normal or undergo thickening, with formation of papillary metaplastic masses of cartilage, bone, or adipose tissue. Detachment of these masses gives rise to intra-articular loose bodies known as *rice bodies*.

In some cases of severe osteoarthrosis there are foci of subchondral acute inflammation resembling osteomyelitis, but these are probably of a noninfectious nature.[1127]

It should be emphasized that the changes of degenerative joint disease are centered in the cartilage, a type of tissue notorious for its poor capacity for repair.[1120,1132] These changes are more prominent on the joint surface exposed to friction, weight bearing, or movement, but they also occur in areas of the joint not subject to these mechanical forces.[1121] The mechanical attrition of the cartilage is preceded by a loss of chondroitin sulfate matrix. Loss of cartilage thickness leads to narrowing of the joint space and loss of stability of the chondro-osseous junction. The osteophytes seen at the margins of osteoarthritic joints progress through discrete stages of cartilage differentiation that can be followed with collagen type-specific probes.[1114] The cartilage degradation in osteoarthritis is believed to be mediated by cytokines, in particular interleukin 1 (IL-1).[1131]

Some degree of synovial hyperplasia with hyperemia and lymphocytic infiltration can be seen in advanced stages of the disease, especially in the hip; these changes should not be confused with rheumatoid arthritis.

A secondary change sometimes seen in the osteoarthrotic head of a femur is the presence of cysts located close to the surface. These are surrounded by dense bone and contain fluid or loose connective tissue[1121,1124,1125,1130] (Fig. 24.128). Other secondary features of the disease are represented by changes in the capsular and synovial nerves.[1117,1129]

Neuropathic arthropathy (Charcot joint) is a particularly destructive variant of degenerative joint disease (Fig. 24.129). The process is usually slowly progressive, although on rare occasions it may have an extremely rapid evolution.[1126] Particles of dead bone and cartilage often are seen in large amounts embedded in the synovial membrane.[1123] However, they are not specific for this condition.

Chondromalacia patellae is the name given to a condition of obscure etiology characterized by softening, fibrillation, fissuring,

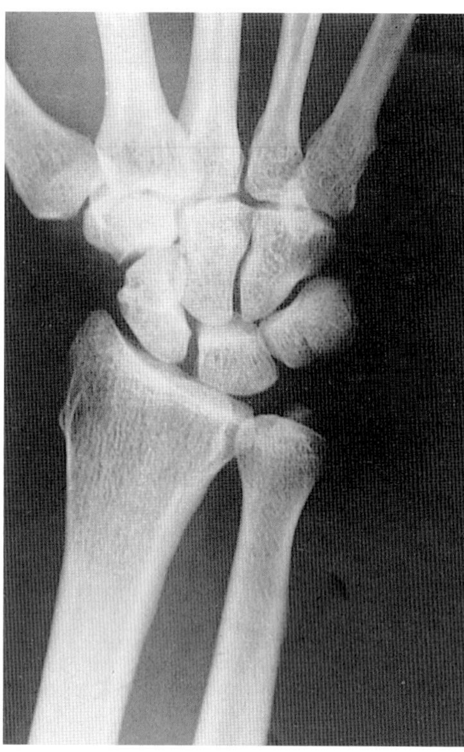

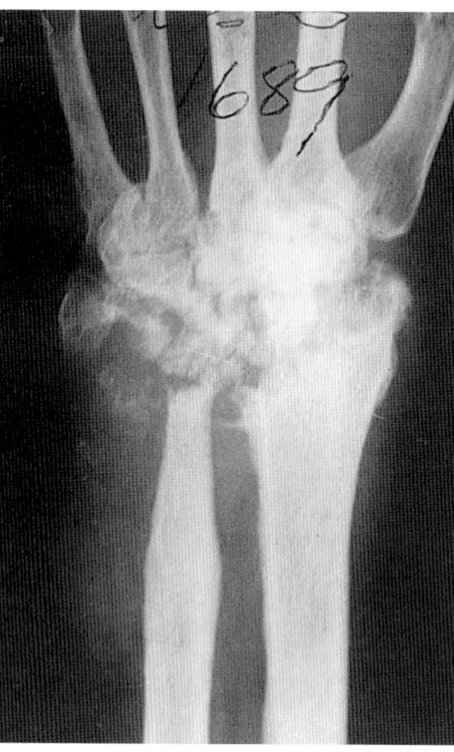

Fig. 24.129 Neuropathic changes in wrist secondary to syringomyelia.

and erosion of the articular cartilage of the patella.[1128] Microscopically, the changes are indistinguishable from those of degenerative joint disease.[1119]

Rheumatoid arthritis

Rheumatoid arthritis is an immune-complex disease that manifests as a chronic polyarticular arthritis. It is mostly seen in women during the second and third decades of life.[1157] The joints of the feet and hands are nearly always involved. Other joints frequently affected are the elbows, knees, wrists, ankles, hips, spine, and temporomandibular articulations.

Lysosomes and interleukins are mediators of the inflammatory reaction seen in this disease and in other joint diseases.[1133,1141,1162] Basic fibroblastic growth factor may play a role in synovial hyperplasia and joint destruction.[1154] The etiology of rheumatoid arthritis is unknown, but a viral participation has long been suspected on the basis of epidemiologic, morphologic, and immunohistologic findings.[1161] The human leukocyte antigen (HLA) linkage and the autoantibody production observed in most patients support an autoimmune element in this disease.[1160]

The earliest morphologic changes occur in the synovial membrane. Hyperemia of the synovium is followed by proliferation of the synovial lining cells and infiltration by plasma cells and lymphocytes[1148] (Fig. 24.130). Lymphoid follicles are often present.[1145] The small synovial blood vessels are lined by plump endothelial cells, and fibrin deposits often are seen close to the synovial lining or within the stroma. Two additional microscopic features, which are also nonspecific, include the presence of synovial giant cells and bone and cartilage fragments within the actual synovial membrane.[1152] They need to be distinguished from multinucleated plasma cells, foreign body cells, and Touton giant cells that can also occur in joints with rheumatoid arthritis. These synovial giant cells tend to be present in patients with active, seropositive disease, but there is no correlation with the serologic titer.[1139] Bhan and Roy[1136] found them in seropositive and seronegative cases, as well as in tuberculosis, traumatic arthritis, and villonodular synovitis. The cartilage and bone fragments tend to occur in joints with advanced disease. They appear to arise as a result of the erosive destructive process of the articular surface, and can be distinguished by virtue of their position and clear demarcation from the metaplastic cartilage and bone that sometimes arises from synovial cells. They also have been seen in synovial membranes of osteoarthritis, osteochondritis dissecans, chondromalacia patellae, and particularly in neuropathic joints.[1144,1152]

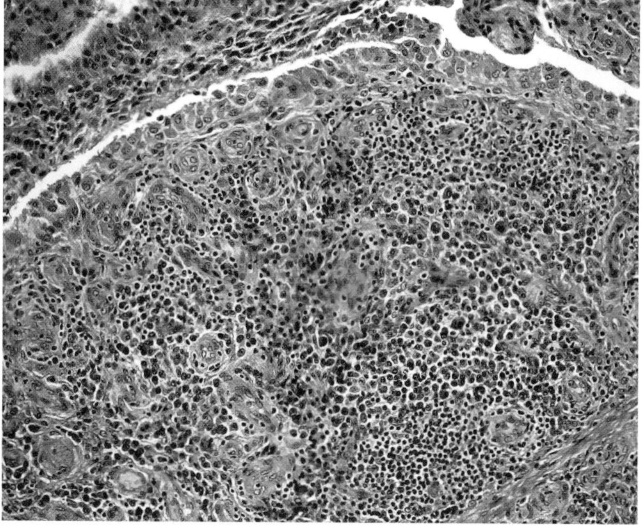

Fig. 24.130 Synovial hyperplasia and heavy lymphoplasmacytic infiltrate in rheumatoid arthritis.

In the second phase, granulation tissue grows into the subchondral marrow of the bone. Osteoporosis occurs early and may result

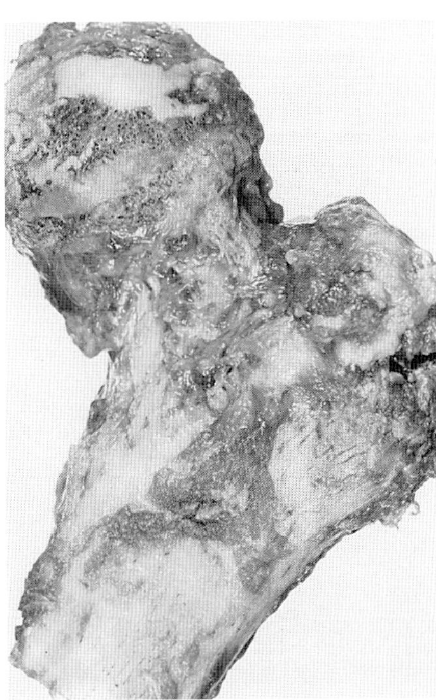

Fig. 24.131 Advanced rheumatoid arthritis involving femur. There is prominent proliferation of synovium and almost complete destruction of overlying articular cartilage.

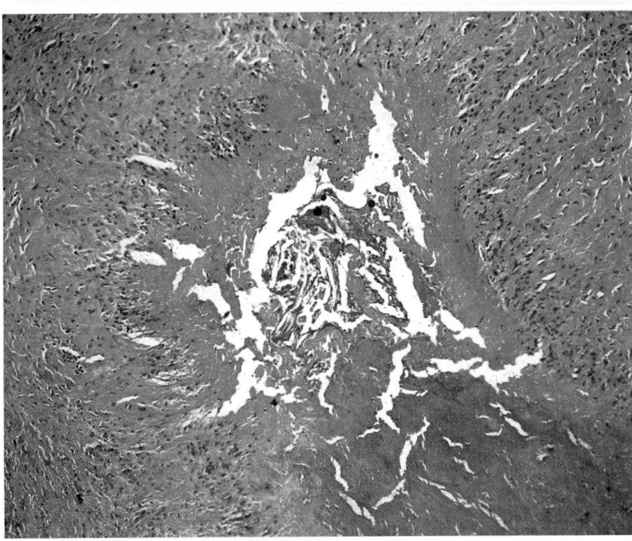

Fig. 24.132 Rheumatoid nodule with early cystic change of the 'necrobiotic' center. Note the peripheral palisading of histiocytes.

in spontaneous fractures of long bones (particularly the femoral neck) and the pelvis.[1159] Prominent pannus is formed over the articular cartilage (Fig. 24.131). Cartilage and even bone form in this pannus. The granulation tissue of the subchondral area and the pannus within the joint attack the cartilage.[1137] Its destruction may be followed by fibrous ankylosis and eventually bony ankylosis. Increased articular pressure may lead to bursting of the joint capsule and acute joint rupture,[1138] bone cysts ('rheumatoid geodes'),[1153] or herniation of the capsule into the soft tissues.[1146] The bone cysts are radiographically similar to those seen in association with degenerative joint disease, but in rheumatoid arthritis they contain granulation tissue instead of fluid or myxoid material. The microscopic changes of rheumatoid arthritis correlate well with the radiographic findings, but not too closely with the clinical findings.[1150]

Tenosynovitis and 'rheumatoid nodules' are the two most common extra-articular manifestations of rheumatoid arthritis.[1142,1143] The changes seen in the former are indistinguishable from those seen in the joint membrane.[1147] Rheumatoid nodules, which are seen in approximately 20% of the patients, occur most often in tendons and tendon sheaths and periarticular subcutaneous tissue but also have been seen in the heart and large vessels, lung and pleura, kidney, meninges, and synovial membrane itself.[1155] Microscopically, they are composed of a necrotic center impregnated with fibrin, surrounded by a predominantly histiocytic inflammatory reaction, often arranged in a palisading fashion (Fig. 24.132). They are not specific to rheumatoid arthritis. Nodules morphologically indistinguishable can occur in rheumatic fever, in systemic lupus erythematosus, and in children in the absence of any apparent disease.[1134,1140] Berardinelli et al.[1135] followed 10 cases of the latter and found rheumatoid factor 2–16 years after the appearance of the nodules. Rheumatoid nodules also need to be distinguished from suture granulomas from previous surgical procedures.[1149]

Sokoloff et al.[1158] found non-necrotizing arteritis in 10% of patients with rheumatoid arthritis. Necrotizing arteritis has also been described.[1151,1156] Polyneuritis can be observed.

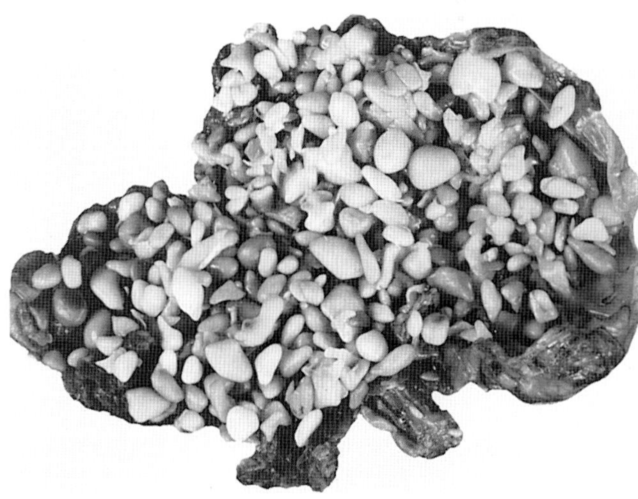

Fig. 24.133 Tuberculous bursitis with innumerable 'rice bodies'. The latter are mainly composed of fibrin and have no diagnostic significance.
(Courtesy of Dr EF Lascano, Buenos Aires)

The pulmonary manifestations of rheumatoid arthritis have been discussed in Chapter 7 and the lymph node changes in Chapter 21.

Amyloidosis is a significant complication of the disease. As a matter of fact, in the United States, rheumatoid arthritis has displaced tuberculosis as the most common underlying disorder associated with amyloid deposition.

Infectious arthritis

Bacterial, fungal, and parasitic infections can reach the joints either by hematogenous spread or by contiguous extension from a neighboring osteomyelitis (Fig. 24.133). A form of infectious arthritis that has risen dramatically in recognition and frequency in recent years is *Lyme disease*, an arthropod-transmitted spirochetosis that also involves skin, heart, and nervous system.[1163,1165,1166,1168] The microscopic changes in the synovium are those of a nonspecific chronic synovitis, but the spirochete can occasionally be detected with the Liederle stain.[1164] Spirochetal antigens have also been demonstrated ultrastructurally in cases of chronic Lyme disease.[1167]

Gout and pseudogout

About 2–5% of chronic joint disease is caused by gout. The metatarsophalangeal joints are often the first to be involved, but other joints of the hands and feet are also frequently involved. The disease may also involve the joints of the long bones (Fig. 24.134A).

Calcification and even ossification of tophi occur frequently.[1172] The urate deposits progressively destroy the cartilage and may cause osteolytic, irregular destruction of subchondral bone. These deposits may extend out from a joint into the soft tissue and cause destruction of the ligaments. This destruction eventually leads to subcutaneous deposits that may erode through the skin. The microscopic pattern of gout is unmistakable. Fixation in alcohol is important for the preservation of sodium urate monohydrate deposits that appear as needle-shaped, doubly refractile crystals. The deGalantha stain is particularly suited for their demonstration. Even if alcohol fixation is not done, the appearance of tophi is usually diagnostic because of the typical granulomatous response that they elicit (Fig. 24.134B). Furthermore, the negative birefringence of these crystals can still be demonstrated after staining with nonaqueous alcoholic eosin.[1170,1174] Histiocytes and foreign body giant cells predominate in the infiltrate. Palisading of the histiocytes sometimes occurs and may be a source of confusion with rheumatoid nodules.

Gout should also be distinguished from *chondrocalcinosis* (pseudogout, calcium pyrophosphate dihydrate crystal deposition disease), a rare condition in which the symptoms result from diffuse deposition of calcium pyrophosphate crystals in the articular cartilage.[1169,1171,1173] Many of these cases involve the temporomandibular joint and are discussed further in Chapter 6. Others are centered in the spinal yellow ligaments, from which they may protrude into the vertebral canal.

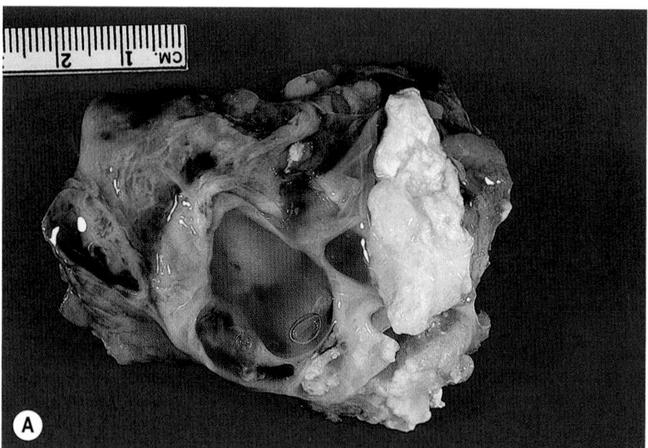

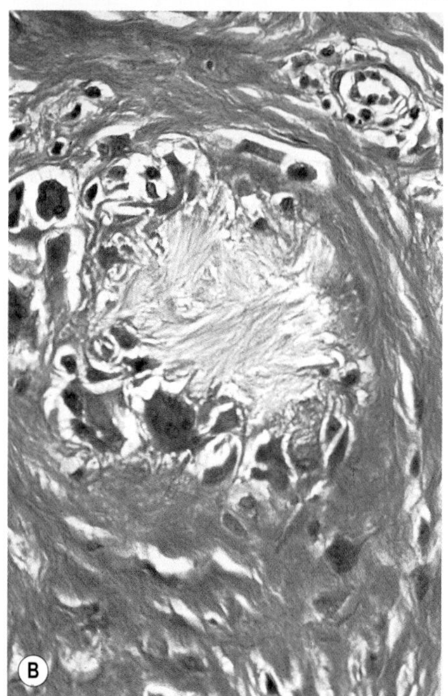

Fig. 24.134 A and **B**, Gout. **A**, Gross appearance of large gouty deposit in the posterior knee. **B**, A lesion of periarticular gout showing a foreign body-type giant cell reaction to the deposited crystals. The crystalline nature of this material is not obvious in this formalin-fixed specimen.

Intervertebral disk prolapse

Prolapse of intervertebral disks is a complication of mechanical overload-induced degeneration of the disk. This process seems to be mediated through the mitochondrial apoptotic pathway.[1176] Material curetted from an intervertebral disk because of prolapse is a very common surgical specimen. Features such as fibrillation, clustering of chondrocytes, and granular change are generally regarded as indicators of degeneration related to prolapse.[1175] Weidner and Rice[1177] found instead that the feature that better correlated with prolapse was neovascularization occurring at the edges of the fibrocartilaginous fragments.

Other articular and periarticular diseases

Hemophilia is characterized by the accumulation of hemosiderin-laden macrophages in the synovium. In contrast to pigmented villonodular synovitis (PVNS), there are few if any foamy macrophages or spindle cells. The morphologic features of hemophilic arthropathy are those of a degenerative rather than an inflammatory process.[1188]

Scleroderma (progressive systemic sclerosis) is often accompanied by arthralgia or arthritis, and sometimes these dominate the clinical picture. The main microscopic changes in the synovial membrane are superficial deposition of fibrin, mild mononuclear infiltrate, minimal hyperplasia of synovial lining cells, proliferation of collagen fibers, and focal obliteration of small vessels.[1187]

Lupus erythematosus may be accompanied by microscopic changes in the synovium which are indistinguishable from those of rheumatoid arthritis. As a rule, however, there is a more intense surface fibrin deposition and a lesser degree of proliferation of synovial cells.[1180]

Amyloid can deposit in the synovium, articular cartilage, menisci, periarticular tissue, and intervertebral disk in old age, apparently unrelated to osteoarthritis and in the absence of systemic amyloidosis.[1178,1179,1183,1184,1189] Heavier amounts can be seen as an expression of primary amyloidosis or multiple myeloma.[1185] Amyloidosis is one of the causes of the carpal tunnel syndrome[1181,1182] (see p. 2071). The amyloid material usually consists of transthyretin (AF/ASCI, prealbumin).[1184]

SAPHO is a peculiar syndrome of unknown etiology in which synovitis is seen in combination with acne, pustulosis, hyperostosis, and osteitis.[1186]

Tumors and tumorlike conditions

Tenosynovial giant cell tumor

Tenosynovial giant cell tumor (TSGCT, nodular tenosynovitis, fibrous histiocytoma of tendon sheath, xanthogranuloma, benign synovioma) is a common lesion that occurs more frequently in women than men, usually appearing in young and middle-aged persons. Most cases are distributed between the wrist and fingertips and between the ankle and toe tips. It is more often proximal than distal on both the hands and feet and occurs most frequently on their flexor surfaces. Other sites can be affected, including the vertebral column.[1197]

Grossly, it presents as a single mass usually measuring 1–3 cm in diameter. It has a fairly well-defined capsule, may be somewhat lobulated, and varies in color from whitish gray to yellowish brown (Fig. 24.135). The so-called diffuse form tends to have a larger size and infiltrative margins.[1196,1203]

Microscopically, this lesion contains closely packed medium-sized polyhedral cells with a variable admixture of giant cells containing fat and hemosiderin (Fig. 24.136). Cells in zones of active proliferation may show mitotic figures. Focal zones of hyalinization constitute the more quiescent areas. Sometimes, the whole lesion adopts a hypocellular fibrohyalinized appearance. We suspect that the cases reported as *tendon sheath fibromas* are histogenetically related to TSGCT.[1193,1200] Their location, clinical presentation, and recurrence rate are certainly comparable. Ultrastructural and immunohistochemical studies of TSGCT have shown cells with the features of synovial cells admixed with fibroblastic elements, histiocytes, and lymphocytes.[1190,1201,1204] This includes the expression of clusterin, an apoprotein expressed by normal synoviocytes and follicular dendritic cells.[1192] The multinucleated giant cells have the phenotypic features of osteoclasts.[1195]

The great cellularity of this tumor, its variable pattern, and the presence of mitotic figures may lead to an erroneous diagnosis of sarcoma. However, these tumors are nearly always benign. They may erode contiguous bone by pressure. If incompletely removed, they may recur locally.

The nature of this lesion is still controversial: Jaffe et al.[1198] considered it a reactive process – hence the name of nodular tenosynovitis. Most authors currently regard it as neoplastic, a hypothesis supported by the presence in this lesion of clonal chromosomal aberrations.[1202] Chromosomal translocation involving the *CSF1* gene (located at 1p13 and encoding ligand of the tyrosine kinase receptor) is often present.[1194] Interestingly, the translocation is present in only 2–16% of the lesional cells.[1206] There is high expression of *CSF1* mRNA and protein, even in tumors lacking demonstrable *CSF1* translocation.[1194]

A very rare malignant counterpart of this lesion has been described in both the localized and diffuse forms.[1199] Features that should suggest malignancy are a high number of mitotic figures, marked nuclear hyperchromasia, and lack or paucity of multinucleated giant cells.[1191,1205] The main differential diagnosis of TSGCT is epithelioid sarcoma. The presence of granuloma-like formations, necrosis, invasiveness, epithelioid features, and keratin immunoreactivity favors the latter.

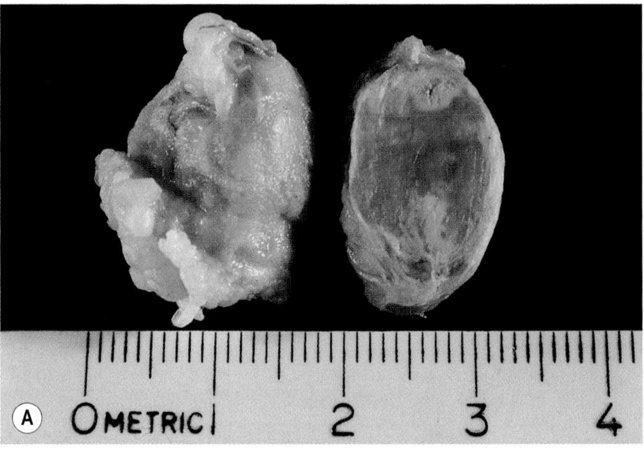

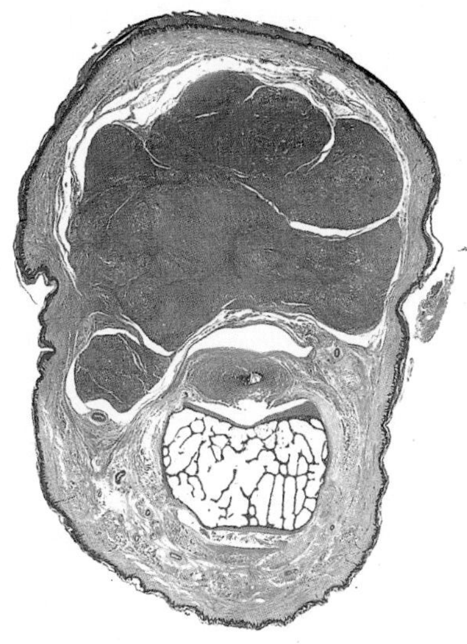

Fig. 24.135 A, Gross appearance of tenosynovial giant cell tumor. The lesion is small, well circumscribed, solid, and with a brownish cast. **B**, Whole-mount appearance of the cross section of a lesion located in the finger. Note the lobulated quality.

Pigmented villonodular synovitis and bursitis

PVNS is believed to be closely related to TSGCT, to the point that the diffuse type of the latter is also known as extra-articular PVNS.[1220]

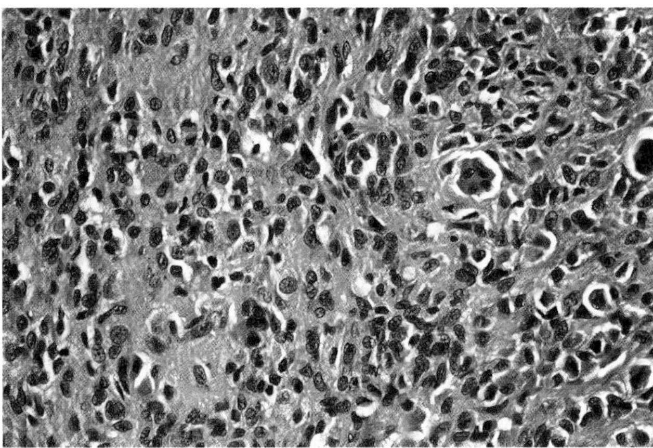

Fig. 24.136 Microscopic appearance of tenosynovial giant cell tumor. A polymorphic infiltrate of small histiocytes and multinucleated giant cells is embedded in dense fibrous tissue.

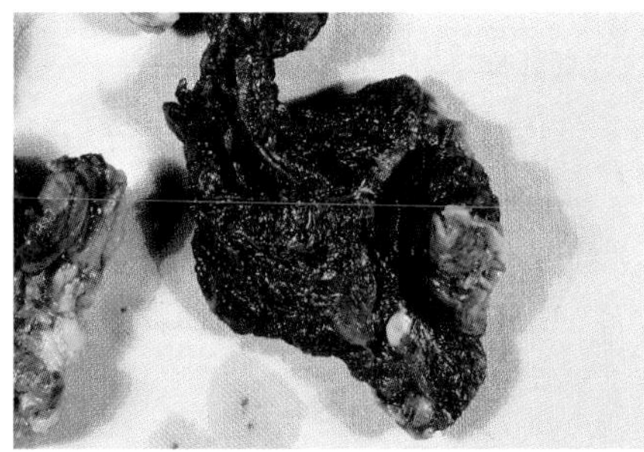

Fig. 24.137 Gross appearance of pigmented villonodular synovitis of knee joint. The lesion has a characteristic dark brown color resulting from extensive hemosiderin deposition.
(Courtesy of Dr Jack Uecker, St Paul, MN)

PVNS tends to occur in young adults.[1213,1214] Although the knee joint is the usual site, the process may also involve the ankle, hip, shoulder, or even the elbow joint.[1216] Usually only one articulation is affected, instances of bilateral disease being exceptional. Occasionally, the lesion may penetrate within the underlying bone.[1219]

The process may be focal or diffuse. When diffuse, it is made up of brownish yellow spongy tissue. Its appearance depends on the content of hemosiderin pigment. Large amounts of tissue often are present, and complete removal may be impossible (Fig. 24.137). Microscopically, the cellular component is similar to that of TSGCT, but in addition there are papillary projections made up of foamy cells and hemosiderin-containing phagocytes (Fig. 24.138). Large clefts and pseudoglandular or alveolar spaces lined by synovial cells are also present.[1221] Occasionally, foci of chondroid metaplasia resembling osseous chondroblastoma are found.[1215] Immunohistochemically, there is expression of both histiocytic and synoviocyte-associated markers, the latter including clusterin.[1208,1222]

The capacity of this lesion to result in bone cyst formation and late cartilage and bone loss has been attributed to the production of metalloproteinases such as collagenase and stromelysin.[1211] Clonal chromosomal aberrations similar to those of TSGCT have been found in PVNS, supporting a pathogenetic link between the two conditions and the neoplastic nature of both.[1207,1217,1218]

This disease can be treated by excision. It may recur locally because complete removal is often impossible.[1209] If it recurs locally, radiation therapy may be helpful. As for TSGCT, isolated examples of malignant PVNS have been described.[1210,1212,1220]

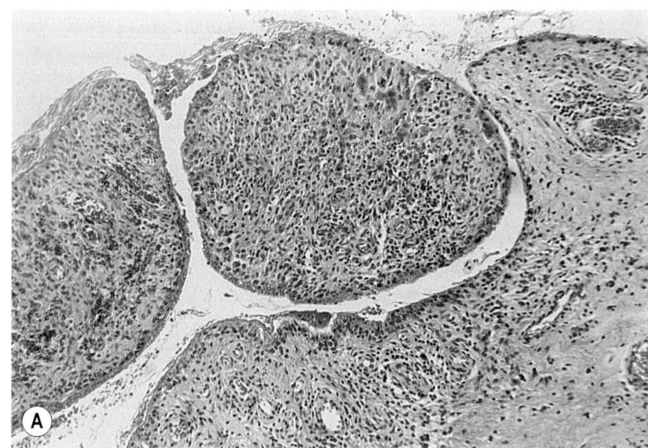

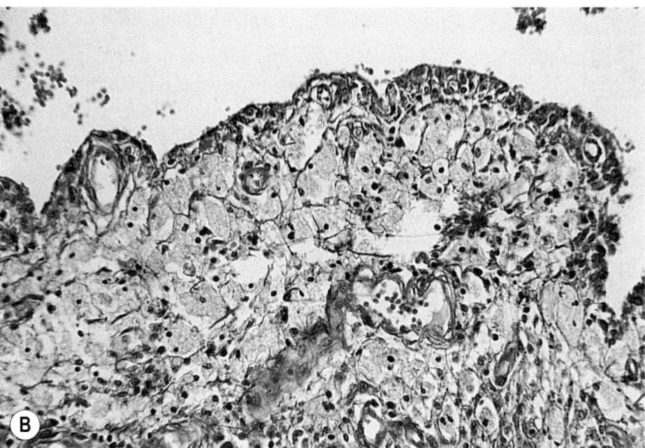

Fig. 24.138 **A** and **B**, Microscopic appearance of pigmented villonodular synovitis. **A**, Low-power view showing the villous appearance of the proliferation and hyperplastic synovium. **B**, High-power view. In this area, foamy cells predominate. In others, there were large collections of hemosiderin-laden macrophages.

Synovial osteochondromatosis and chondrosarcoma

Synovial osteochondromatosis (synovial chondrometaplasia) is characterized by the formation of osteocartilaginous bodies in the synovial membrane.[1223] This condition most often is monoarticular, affecting the knee or hip and communicating bursae. It is aggravated by infection and trauma. Sometimes a similar condition is seen in the soft tissue adjacent to but not communicating with the joint.[1232] This is referred to as tenosynovial or extra-articular chondromatosis.[1226] The etiology is unknown, but the presence of clonal chromosomal aberrations suggests that it represents a neoplastic condition.[1231]

Grossly, the osteocartilaginous bodies may remain confined to the synovium or be extruded within the joint cavity. They usually are partially calcified (Fig. 24.139). Innumerable small bodies can

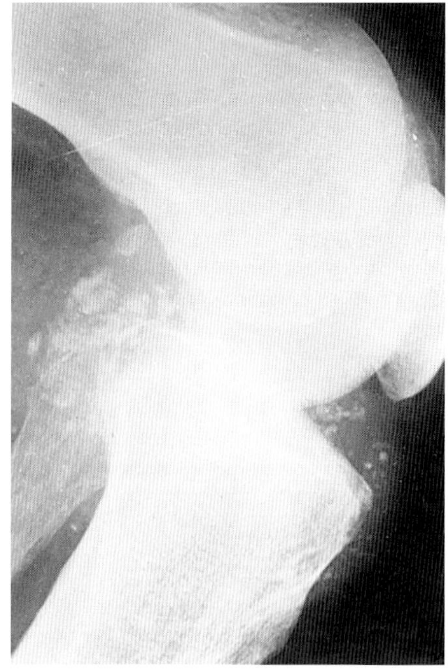

Fig. 24.139 Synovial osteochondromatosis. Nodules can be seen clearly in the joint space.

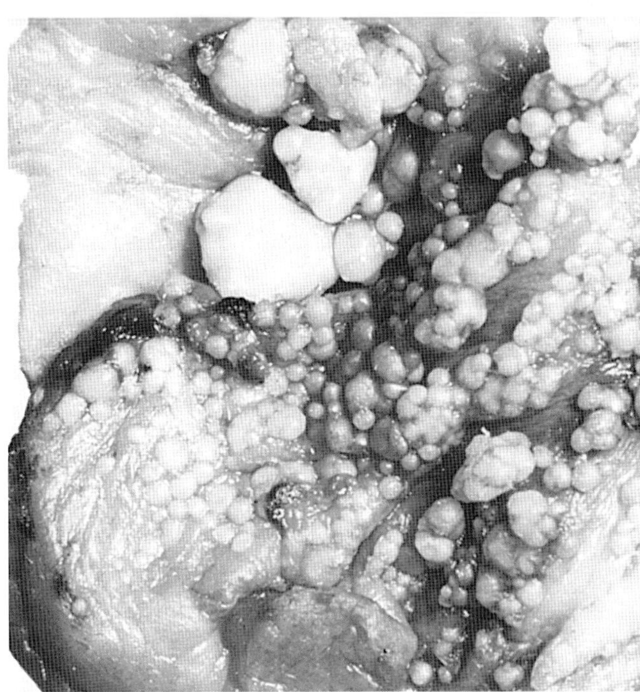

Fig. 24.140 Extensive involvement of synovium of knee joint by osteochondromatosis.

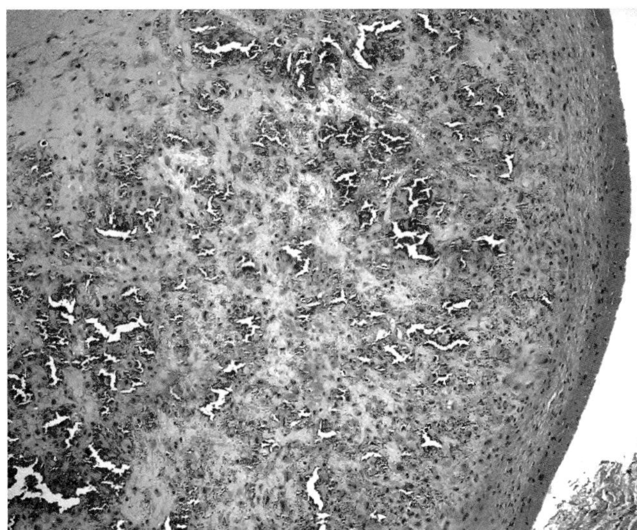

Fig. 24.141 Microscopic appearance of one of the nodules of synovial osteochondromatosis. The lesion has undergone focal calcification, as is usually the case.

be seen grossly in the resected lesion (Figs 24.140 and 24.141). The disease seems to follow this sequence:

1 active intrasynovial disease with no loose bodies,
2 intrasynovial proliferation and free loose bodies, and
3 multiple free osteochondral bodies with no demonstrable intrasynovial disease.[1229]

To make a diagnosis of synovial osteochondromatosis, one should find cartilaginous or osteocartilaginous bodies attached to the synovial membrane in addition to those free in the joint spaces. The latter also can occur in degenerative joint disease, neuropathic arthropathy, and osteochondritis dissecans, in which case the process is referred to as *secondary synovial chondrometaplasia*.[1233] Microscopically, the chondrocytes of primary synovial osteochondromatosis may show some degree of atypia and even binucleated forms, but this does not necessarily indicate malignancy.[1230] Local recrudescence after treatment may supervene. Rare cases of malignant transformation have been reported that should be distinguished from the condition described below.[1225]

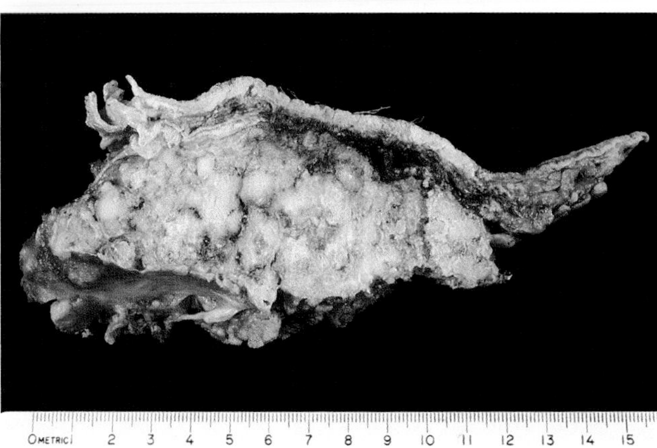

Fig. 24.142 Gross appearance of synovial chondrosarcoma. The lesion has a more expansile quality than the usual synovial osteochondromatosis.

Synovial chondrosarcoma is an exceptionally rare entity that closely resembles synovial chondromatosis radiographically and grossly[1224,1227,1228] (Fig. 24.142). The distinction, which may be quite difficult, is based on the presence in the chondrosarcoma of obvious cytologic features of malignancy in the chondrocytes.[1228]

Other tumors and tumorlike conditions

Most tumors involving the joint space represent direct extension from neoplasms initially located in the adjacent bones.

The only primary tumor of the joints that is seen with any frequency in addition to those already mentioned is **synovial hemangioma**. Most patients are young adults, and there is a predominance for the male sex. The knee is the most common site, followed by the elbow and finger. In most cases the tumor is confined to the intra-articular synovium, but sometimes it is located in a bursa adjacent to a joint. The most common microscopic pattern is cavernous hemangioma, followed by lobular capillary hemangioma, arteriovenous hemangioma, and venous hemangioma.[1234]

Isolated cases of *intra-articular hemangiopericytoma*, *intracapsular chondroma*, *synovial sarcoma*, *epithelioid sarcoma*, arthroplasty-associated *malignant fibrous histiocytoma*, and *malignant lymphoma* around joints involved by rheumatoid arthritis have been reported.[1235,1237–1239]

Nodular fasciitis can be seen in an intra-articular location. It is microscopically similar to its more common soft tissue counterpart, except for a greater tendency to stromal hyalinization and adjacent hemosiderin deposition.[1236]

References

BONE

NORMAL ANATOMY

1 Alliston T, Derynck D. Interfering with bone remodelling. Nature 2002, **416**: 686–687.

2 Anderson HC. Mechanism of mineral formation in bone. Lab Invest 1989, **60**: 320–330.

3 Bauer TW. An overview of the histology of skeletal substitute materials. Arch Pathol Lab Med 2007, **131**: 217–224.

4 Boyce BF, Hughes DE, Wright KR, Xing L, Dai A. Recent advances in bone biology provide insight into the pathogenesis of bone disease. Lab Invest 1999, **79**: 83–94.

5 Centrella M, McCarthy TL, Canalis E. Skeletal tissue and transforming growth factor beta. FASEB J 1988, **2**: 3066–3073.

6 Ducy P, Schinke T, Karsenty G. The osteoblast: a sophisticated fibroblast under central surveillance. Science 2000, **289**: 1501–1504.

7 Edwards JR, Williams K, Kindblom LG, Meis-Kindblom JM, Hogendoorn PC, Hughes D, Forsyth RG, Jackson D, Athanasou NA. Lymphatics and bone. Hum Pathol 2008, **39**: 49–55.

8 Enneking WF, Kagan A. Transepiphyseal extension of osteosarcoma. Incidence, mechanism, and implications. Cancer 1978, **41**: 1526–1537.

9 Fornasier VL. Osteoid. An ultrastructural study. Hum Pathol 1977, **8**: 243–254.

10 Glimcher MJ. Mechanism of calcification. Role of collagen fibrils and collagen-phosphoprotein complexes *in vitro* and *in vivo*. Anat Rec 1989, **224**: 139–153.

11 Heinegard D, Oldberg A. Structure and biology of cartilage and bone matrix non-collagenous macromolecules. FASEB J 1989, **3**: 2042–2051.

12 Huffer WE. Morphology and biochemistry of bone remodeling. Possible control by vitamin D, parathyroid hormone, and other substances. Lab Invest 1988, **59**: 418–442.

13 Kukita T, McManus LM, Miller M, Civin C, Roodman GD. Osteoclast-like cells formed in long-term human bone marrow cultures express a similar surface phenotype as authentic osteoclasts. Lab Invest 1989, **60**: 532–538.

14 Marks SJ Jr, Popoff SN. Bone cell biology. The regulation of development, structure, and function in the skeleton. Am J Anat 1988, **83**: 1–44.

15 Noda M, Vogel RL, Craig AM, Prahl J, DeLuca HF, Denhardt DT. Identification of a DNA sequence responsible for binding of the 1,25-dihydroxyvitamin D3 receptor and 1,25-dihydroxyvitamin D3 enhancement of mouse secreted phosphoprotein 1 (SPP-1 or osteopontin) gene expression. Proc Natl Acad Sci U S A 1990, **87**: 9995–9999.

16 Okada Y, Naka K, Kawamura K, Matsumoto T, Nakanishi I, Fujimoto N, Sato H, Seiki M. Localization of matrix metalloproteinase 9 (92-Kilodalton gelatinase/type IV collagenase = gelatinase B) in osteoclasts. Implications for bone resorption. Lab Invest 1995, **72**: 311–322.

17 Owen TA, Bortell R, Yocum SA, Smock SL, Zhang M, Abate C, Shalhoub V, Aronin N, Wright KL, van Wijnen AJ, et al. Coordinate occupancy of AP-1 sites in the vitamin D-responsive and CCAAT box elements by Fos–Jun in the osteocalcin gene: model for phenotype suppression of transcription. Proc Natl Acad Sci U S A 1990, **87**: 9990–9994.

18 Reinholt FP, Hultenby K, Oldberg A, Heinegard D. Osteopontin. A possible anchor of osteoclasts to bone. Proc Natl Acad Sci U S A 1990, **87**: 4473–4475.

19 Rosenberg AE, Sanford IR. Bone. In Mills SE (ed.): Histology for pathologists, ed. 3. Philadelphia, 2007, Lippincott Williams & Wilkins.

20 Teitelbaum SL. Bone resorption by osteoclasts. Science 2000, **289**: 1504–1508.

21 Udagawa N, Takahashi N, Akatsu T, Tanaka H, Sasaki T, Nishihara T, Koga T, Martin TJ, Suda T. Origin of osteoclasts. Mature monocytes and macrophages are capable of differentiating into osteoclasts under a suitable microenvironment prepared by bone marrow-derived stromal cells. Proc Natl Acad Sci U S A 1990, **87**: 7260–7264.

22 Wozney JM, Rosen V, Celeste AJ, Mitsock LM, Whitters MJ, Kriz RW, Hewick RM, Wang EA. Novel regulators of bone formation. Molecular clones and activities. Science 1988, **242**: 1528–1534.

23 Zheng MH, Wood DJ, Papadimitriou JM. What's new in the role of cytokines on osteoblast proliferation and differentiation? Pathol Res Pract 1992, **188**: 1104–1121.

METABOLIC BONE DISEASES

24 Avioli LV, Krane SM (eds). Metabolic bone disease, vol. I. New York, 1977, Academic Press.

25 Avioli LV, Teitelbaum SL. The renal osteodystrophies. In Brenner BM, Rector FC (eds): The kidney. Philadelphia, 1976, W.B. Saunders, pp. 1542–1591.

26 Becks JS, Nordin BEC. Histological assessment of osteoporosis by iliac crest biopsy. J Pathol Bacteriol 1960, **80**: 391–397.

27 Bernstein DS, Sadowsky N, Hegsted DM, Guri CD, Stare FJ. Prevalence of osteoporosis in high- and low-fluoride areas in North Dakota. JAMA 1966, **198**: 499–504.

28 Bullough PG. Atlas of orthopedic pathology, ed. 2. St Louis, 1992, Mosby.

29 Caldwell RA. Observations on the incidence, aetiology and pathology of senile osteoporosis. J Clin Pathol 1962, **15**: 421–431.

30 Coe FL, Favus MJ (eds). Disorders of bone and mineral metabolism. New York, 1992, Raven Press.

31 Fallon MD, Teitelbaum SL. The interpretation of fluorescent tetracycline markers in the diagnosis of metabolic bone diseases. Hum Pathol 1982, **13**: 416–417.

32 Falvo KA, Bullough PG. Osteogenesis imperfecta. A histometric analysis. J Bone Joint Surg (Am) 1973, **55**: 275–286.

33 Gueldner SH (ed.). Osteoporosis: clinical guidelines for prevention, diagnosis, and management. New York, 2008, Springer.

34 Jowsey J, Kelly PJ, Riggs BL, Bianco AJ Jr, Scholz DA, Gershon-Cohen J. Quantitative microradiographic studies of normal and osteoporotic bone. J Bone Joint Surg (Am) 1965, **47**: 785–806.

35 Mankin HJ. Rickets, osteomalacia, and renal osteodystrophy. Part II. J Bone Joint Surg (Am) 1974, **56**: 352–386.

36 Mankin HJ (ed.). Pathophysiology of orthopaedic diseases. Rosemont, IL, 2006, American Academy of Orthopaedic Surgeons.

37 Marcus R (ed.). Osteoporosis, ed. 3. Amsterdam, 2008, Elsevier Academic Press.

38 Mattingly BE, Pillare AC (eds). Osteoporosis: etiology, diagnosis, and treatment. Hauppauge, NY, 2009, Nova Science Publishers.

39 Orwoll ES, Bliziotes M. Osteoporosis: pathophysiology and clinical management. N Engl J Med 2003, **348**: 2269–2270.

40 Raisz LG. Local and systemic factors in the pathogenesis of osteoporosis. N Engl J Med 1988, **318**: 818–828.

41 Riggs BL, Melton LJ III. Involutional osteoporosis. N Engl J Med 1986, **314**: 1676–1686.

42 Riggs BL, Melton LJ. The prevention and treatment of osteoporosis. N Engl J Med 1992, **327**: 620–627.

43 Rodan GA, Martin TJ. Therapeutic approaches to bone disease. Science 2000, **289**: 1508–1514.

44 Sillence DO, Horton WA, Rimoin DL. Morphologic studies in the skeletal dysplasias. A review. Am J Pathol 1979, **96**: 811–870.

45 Stevenson JC (ed.). New techniques in metabolic bone diseases. London, 1990, Wright.

46 Teitelbaum SL, Bullough PG. The pathophysiology of bone and joint disease. Am J Pathol 1979, **96**: 283–354.

47 Vigorita VJ. The bone biopsy protocol for evaluating osteoporosis and osteomalacia. Am J Surg Pathol 1984, **8**: 925–930.

48 Vigorita VJ. Osteoporosis. A diagnosable disorder? Pathol Annu 1988, **23**(Pt 2): 185–212.

FRACTURES

49 Collins DH. Structural changes around nails and screws in human bones. J Pathol Bacteriol 1953, **65**: 109–121.

50 Collins DH. Tissue changes in human femurs containing plastic appliances. J Bone Joint Surg (Br) 1954, **36**: 458–563.

51 Mindell ER, Rodbard S, Kwasman BG. Chrondrogenesis in bone repair. A study of the healing fracture callus in the rat. Clin Orthop 1971, **79**: 187–196.

52 Schwarz E. Hypercallosis in osteogenesis imperfecta. Am J Roentgenol Radium Ther Nucl Med 1961, **85**: 645–648.

OSTEOMYELITIS

53 Berney S, Goldstein M, Bishko F. Clinical and diagnostic features of tuberculous arthritis. Am J Med 1972, **53**: 36–42.

54 Bohm E, Josten C. What's new in exogenous osteomyelitis? Pathol Res Pract 1992, **188**: 254–258.

55 Cabanela ME, Sim FH, Beabout JW, Dahlin DC. Osteomyelitis appearing as neoplasms. A diagnostic problem. Arch Surg 1974, **109**: 68–72.

56 Chambers JB, Forsythe DA, Bertrand SL, Iwinski HJ, Steflik DE. Retrospective review of osteoarticular infections in a pediatric sickle cell age group. J Pediatr Orthop 2000, **20**: 682–685.

57 Cozzutto C. Xanthogranulomatous osteomyelitis. Arch Pathol Lab Med 1984, **108**: 973–976.

58 Farrow R, Cureton RJR. Carcinomatous invasion of bone in osteomyelitis. Br J Surg 1962, **50**: 107–109.

59 Felsberg GJ, Gore RL, Schweitzer ME, Jui V. Sclerosing osteomyelitis of Garrè (periostitis ossificans). Oral Surg Oral Med Oral Pathol 1990, **70**: 117–120.

60 Garcia A Jr, Grantham SA. Hematogenous pyogenic vertebral osteomyelitis. J Bone Joint Surg (Am) 1960, **42**: 429–436.

61 Girschick HJ, Huppertz HI, Harmsen D, Krauspe R, Muller-Hermelink HK, Papadopoulos T. Chronic recurrent multifocal osteomyelitis in children: diagnostic value of histopathology and microbial testing. Hum Pathol 1999, **30**: 59–65.

62 Hansen T, Kunkel M, Kirkpatrick CJ, Weber A. Actinomyces in infected osteoradionecrosis – underestimated? Hum Pathol 2006, **37**: 61–67.

63 Johnson LL, Kempson RL. Epidermoid carcinoma in chronic osteomyelitis. Diagnostic problems and management. J Bone Joint Surg (Am) 1965, **47**: 133–145.

64 Lewis P, Sutter VL, Finegold M. Bone infections involving anaerobic bacteria. Medicine (Baltimore) 1978, **57**: 279–305.

65 Moore RM, Green NE. Blastomycosis of bone. A report of six cases. J Bone Joint Surg (Am) 1982, **64**: 1097–1101.

66 Schwarz J. What's new in mycotic bone and joint diseases? Pathol Res Pract 1984, **178**: 617–634.

67 Trueta J. The three types of acute haematogenous osteomyelitis. J Bone Joint Surg (Br) 1959, **41**: 671–680.

68 Waldvogel FA, Vasey H. Osteomyelitis. The past decade. N Engl J Med 1980, **300**: 360–370.

69 Weisenburger DD, Vinh TN, Levinson B. Malakoplakia of bone. An unusual cause of pathologic fracture in an immunosuppressed patient. Clin Orthop 1985, **201**: 106–110.

70 Wu P-C, Khin N-M, Pang S-W. Salmonella osteomyelitis. An important differential diagnosis of granulomatous osteomyelitis. Am J Surg Pathol 1985, **9**: 531–537.

71 Yasuma T, Nakajima Y. Clinicopathological study on plasma cell osteomyelitis. Acta Pathol Jpn 1981, **31**: 835–844.

BONE NECROSIS

INFARCT

72 Cerilli LA, Fechner RE. Angiosarcoma arising in a bone infarct. Ann Diagn Pathol 1999, **3**: 370–373.

73 Desai P, Perino G, Present D, Steiner GC. Sarcoma in association with bone infarcts: report of five cases. Arch Pathol Lab Med 1996, **120**: 482–489.

74 Galli SJ, Weintraub HP, Proppe KH. Malignant fibrous histiocytoma and pleomorphic sarcoma in association with medullary bone infarcts. Cancer 1978, **41**: 607–619.

75 Mirra JM, Bullough PG, Marcove RC, Jacobs B, Huvos AG. Malignant fibrous histiocytoma and osteosarcoma in association with bone infarcts. Report of four cases, two in caisson workers. J Bone Joint Surg (Am) 1974, **56**: 932–940.

76 Torres FX, Kyriakos M. Bone infarct-associated osteosarcoma. Cancer 1992, **70**: 2418–2430.

ASEPTIC (AVASCULAR) BONE NECROSIS

77 Bohr H, Larsen EJ. On necrosis of the femoral head after fracture of the neck of the femur. J Bone Joint Surg (Br) 1965, **47**: 330–338.

78 Golding JSR, Maciver JF, Went LN. The bone changes in sickle-cell anaemia and its genetic variants. J Bone Joint Surg (Br) 1959, **41**: 711–718.

79 Mankin HJ. Nontraumatic necrosis of bone (osteonecrosis). N Engl J Med 1992, **326**: 1473–1479.

80 Yamamoto T, DiCarlo EF, Bullough PG. The prevalence and clinicopathological appearance of extension of osteonecrosis in the femoral head. J Bone Joint Surg (Br) 1999, **81**: 328–332.

81 Yamamoto T, Yamaguchi T, Lee KB, Bullough PG. A clinicopathologic study of osteonecrosis in the osteoarthritic hip. Osteoarthritis Cartilage 2000, **8**: 303–308.

OSTEOCHONDRITIS DISSECANS

82 Franceschi L, Grigolo B, Roseti L, Marconi E, Facchini A, Buda R, Vannini F, Giannini S. Osteochondritis dissecans. Histopathology 2007, **51**: 133–135.

83 Kusumi T, Ishibashi Y, Tsuda E, Kusumi A, Tanaka M, Sato F, Toh S, Kijima H. Osteochondritis dissecans of the elbow: histopathological assessment of the articular cartilage and subchondral bone with emphasis on their damage and repair. Pathol Int 2006, **56**: 604–612.

84 Milgram JW. Radiological and pathological manifestations of osteochondritis of the distal femur. A study of 50 cases. Radiology 1978, **126**: 305–311.

RADIATION NECROSIS

85 Dzik-Jurasz AS, Brooker S, Husband JE, Tait D. What is the prevalence of symptomatic or asymptomatic femoral head osteonecrosis in patients previously treated with chemoradiation? A magnetic resonance study of anal cancer patients. Clin Oncol 2001, **13**: 130–134.

86 Hansen T, Kunkel M, Kirkpatrick CJ, Weber A. Actinomyces in infected osteoradionecrosis – underestimated? Hum Pathol 2006, **37**: 61–67.

87 Sengupta S, Prathap K. Radiation necrosis of the humerus. A report of three cases. Acta Radiol 1973, **12**: 313–320.

PAGET DISEASE

88 Barry HC. Paget's disease of bone. Edinburgh, 1969, E & S Livingstone, Ltd.

89 Collins DH. Paget's disease of bone. Incidence and subclinical forms. Lancet 1956, **2**: 51–57.

90 Collins DH, Winn JM. Focal Paget's disease of the skull (osteoporosis circumscripta). J Pathol Bacteriol 1955, **69**: 1–9.

91 Cundy T, Bolland M. Paget disease of bone. Trends Endocrinol Metab 2008, **19**: 246–253.

92 Deyrup AT, Montag AG, Inwards CY, Xu Z, Swee RG, Krishnan Unni K. Sarcomas arising in Paget disease of bone: a clinicopathologic analysis of 70 cases. Arch Pathol Lab Med 2007, **131**: 942–946.

93 Eisman JA, Martin TJ. Osteolytic Paget's disease. Recognition and risks of biopsy. J Bone Joint Surg (Am) 1986, **68**: 112–117.

94 Fallon MD, Schwamm HA. Paget's disease of bone. An update on the pathogenesis, pathophysiology, and treatment of osteitis deformans. Pathol Annu 1989, **24**(Pt 1): 115–159.

95 Greenspan A, Norman A, Sterling AP. Precocious onset of Paget's disease – a report of three cases and review of the literature. J Can Assoc Radiol 1977, **28**: 69–72.

96 Hadjipavlou AG, Gaitanis IN, Kontakis GM. Paget's disease of the bone and its management. J Bone Joint Surg (Br) 2002, **84**: 160–169.

97 Hadjipavlou A, Lander P, Srolovitz H, Enker IP. Malignant transformation in Paget disease of bone. Cancer 1992, **70**: 2802–2808.

98 Lake ME. The pathology of fracture in Paget's disease. Aust NZ J Surg 1958, **27**: 307–312.

99 Lamovec J, Rener M, Spiler M. Pseudosarcoma in Paget's disease of bone. Ann Diagn Pathol 1999, **3**: 99–103.

100 Melton LJ 3rd, Tiegs RD, Atkinson EJ, O'Fallon WM. Fracture risk among patients with Paget's disease: a population-based cohort study. J Bone Miner Res 2000, **15**: 2123–2128.

101 Mii Y, Miyauchi Y, Honoki K, Morishita T, Miura S, Aoki M, Tamai S, Tsunoda S, Nishitani M, Sakaki T. Electron microscopic evidence of a viral nature for osteoclast inclusions in Paget's disease of bone. Virchows Arch Pathol 1994, **424**: 99–104.

102 Mills BG, Singer FR. Nuclear inclusions in Paget's disease of bone. Science 1976, **194**: 201–202.

103 Price CHG, Goldie W. Paget's sarcoma of bone. A study of 80 cases from the Bristol and the Leeds bone tumour registries. J Bone Joint Surg (Br) 1969, **51**: 205–224.

104 Ralston SH. Pathogenesis of Paget's disease of bone. Bone 2008, **43**: 819–825.

105 Smith BJ, Eveson JW. Paget's disease of bone with particular reference to dentistry. J Oral Pathol 1981, **10**: 233–247.

OSTEOPETROSIS

106 Boyce BF, Hughes DE, Wright KR, Xing L, Dai A. Recent advances in bone biology provide insight into the pathogenesis of bone disease. Lab Invest 1999, **79**: 83–94.

107 Coccia PF, Krivit W, Cervenka J, Clawson C, Kersey JH, Kim TH, Nesbit ME, Ramsay MKC, Warkentin PI, Teitelbaum SL, Kahn AJ, Brown DM. Successful bone marrow transplantation for infantile malignant osteopetrosis. N Engl J Med 1980, **302**: 701–708.

108 Del Fattore A, Cappariello A, Teti A. Genetics, pathogenesis and complications of osteopetrosis. Bone 2008, **42**: 19–29.

109 Key LL Jr, Rodriguiz RM, Willi SM, Wright NM, Hatcher HC, Eyre DR, Cure JK, Griffin PP, Ries WL. Long-term treatment of osteopetrosis with recombinant human interferon gamma. N Engl J Med 1995, **332**: 1594–1599.

110 Milgram JW, Murali J. Osteopetrosis. A morphological study of twenty-one cases. J Bone Joint Surg (Am) 1982, **64**: 912–919.

111 Stark Z, Savarirayan R. Osteopetrosis. Orphanet J Rare Dis 2009, **4**: 5.

TUMORS

CLASSIFICATION AND DISTRIBUTION

112 Dorfman HD. Malignant transformation of benign bone lesions. In Proceedings of the Seventh National Cancer Conference, vol. 7. Philadelphia, 1973, JB Lippincott Co., pp. 901–913.

113 Dorfman HD, Czerniak B. Bone cancers. Cancer 1995, **75**: 203–210.

114 Fletcher CDM, Unni KK, Mertens F (eds). Tumors of soft tissue and bone, pathology and genetics. World Health Organization classification of tumours. Lyon, 2002, IARC Press.

115 Hudson TM. Radiologic–pathologic correlation of musculoskeletal lesions. Baltimore, 1987, Williams & Wilkins.

BONE-FORMING TUMORS

Osteoma

116 Bertoni F, Unni KK, Beabout JW, Sim FH. Parosteal osteoma of bones other than of the skull and face. Cancer 1995, **75**: 2466–2473.

117 Chang CHJ, Piatt ED, Thomas KE, Watne AL. Bone abnormalities in Gardner's syndrome. Am J Roentgenol Radium Ther Nucl Med 1968, **103**: 645–652.

118 Kaplan I, Nicolaou Z, Hatuel D, Calderon S. Solitary central osteoma of the jaws: a diagnostic dilemma. Oral Surg Oral Med Oral Pathol Oral Radiol Endod 2008, **106**: e22–e29.

Osteoid osteoma and osteoblastoma

119 Angervall L, Persson S, Stenman G, Kindblom LG. Large cell, epithelioid, telangiectatic osteoblastoma: a unique pseudosarcomatous variant of osteoblastoma. Hum Pathol 1999, **30**: 1254–1259.

120 Ayala AG, Murray JA, Erling MA, Raymond AK. Osteoid-osteoma. Intraoperative tetracycline-fluorescence demonstration of the nidus. J Bone Joint Surg (Am) 1986, **68**: 747–751.

121 Bauer TW, Zehr RJ, Belhobek GH, Marks KE. Juxta-articular osteoid osteoma. Am J Surg Pathol 1991, **15**: 381–387.

122 Bertoni F, Bacchini P, Donati D, Martini A, Picci P, Campanacci M. Osteoblastoma-like osteosarcoma. The Rizzoli Institute experience. Mod Pathol 1993, **6**: 707–716.

123 Bertoni F, Unni KK, Lucas DR, McLeod RA. Osteoblastoma with cartilaginous matrix. An unusual morphologic presentation in 18 cases. Am J Surg Pathol 1993, **17**: 69–74.

124 Bertoni F, Unni KK, McLeod RA, Dahlin DC. Osteosarcoma resembling osteoblastoma. Cancer 1985, **55**: 416–426.

125 Beyer WF, Kühn H. Can an osteoblastoma become malignant? Virchows Arch [A] 1985, **408**: 297–305.

126 Byers PD. Solitary benign osteoblastic lesions of bone – osteoid osteoma and benign osteoblastoma. Cancer 1968, **22**: 43–57.

127 Cheung FMF, Wu WC, Lam CK, Fu YK. Diagnostic criteria for pseudomalignant osteoblastoma. Histopathology 1997, **31**: 196–200.

128 Della Rocca C, Huvos AG. Osteoblastoma: varied histological presentations with a benign clinical course: an analysis of 55 cases. Am J Surg Pathol 1996, **20**: 841–850.

129 Dorfman HD, Weiss SW. Borderline osteoblastic tumors. Problems in the differential diagnosis of aggressive osteoblastoma and low-grade osteosarcoma. Semin Diagn Pathol 1984, **1**: 215–234.

130 Hasegawa T, Hirose T, Sakamoto R, Seki K, Ikata T, Hizawa K. Mechanism of pain in osteoid osteomas. An immunohistochemical study. Histopathology 1993, **22**: 487–491.

131 Healey JH, Ghalman B. Osteoid osteoma and osteoblastoma. Current concepts and recent advances. Clin Orthop 1986, **204**: 76–85.

132 Kawaguchi Y, Sato C, Hasegawa T, Oka S, Kuwahara H, Norimatsu H. Intraarticular osteoid osteoma associated with synovitis: a possible role of cyclooxygenase-2 expression by osteoblasts in the nidus. Mod Pathol 2000, **13**: 1086–1091.

133 Loizaga JM, Calvo M, Lopez Barea F, Martinez Tello FJ, Perez Villanueva J. Osteoblastoma and osteoid osteoma. Clinical and morphological features of 162 cases. Pathol Res Pract 1993, **189**: 33–41.

134 Lucas DR, Unni KK, McLeod RA, O'Connor MI, Sim FH. Osteoblastoma. Clinicopathologic study of 306 cases. Hum Pathol 1994, **25**: 117–134.

135 MacLennan DI, Wilson FC Jr. Osteoid osteoma of the spine. A review of the literature and report of six new cases. J Bone Joint Surg (Am) 1967, **49**: 111–121.

136 Marcove RC, Heelan RT, Huvos AG, Healey J, Lindeque BG. Osteoid osteoma. Diagnosis, localization, and treatment. Clin Orthop 1991, **267**: 197–201.

137 Marsh BW, Bonfiglio M, Brady LP, Enneking WF. Benign osteoblastoma. Range of manifestations. J Bone Joint Surg (Am) 1975, **57**: 1–9.

138 McLeod RA, Dahlin DC, Beabout JW. The spectrum of osteoblastoma. Am J Roentgenol 1976, **126**: 321–335.

139 O'Connell JX, Nanthakumar SS, Nielsen GP, Rosenberg AE. Osteoid osteoma: the uniquely innervated bone tumor. Mod Pathol 1998, **11**: 175–180.

140 Pettine KA, Klassen RA. Osteoid-osteoma and osteoblastoma of the spine. J Bone Joint Surg (Am) 1986, **68**: 354–361.

141 Schajowicz F, Lemos C. Osteoid osteoma and osteoblastoma. Acta Orthop Scand 1970, **41**: 272–291.

142 Schajowicz F, Lemos C. Malignant osteoblastoma. J Bone Joint Surg 1976, **58**: 202–211.

143 Steiner GC. Ultrastructure of osteoid osteoma. Hum Pathol 1976, **7**: 309–325.

144 Wold LE, Pritchard DJ, Bergert J, Wilson DM. Prostaglandin synthesis by osteoid osteoma and osteoblastoma. Mod Pathol 1988, **1**: 129–131.

145 Yoshikawa S, Nakamura T, Takagi M, Imamura T, Okano K, Sasaki S. Benign osteoblastoma as a cause of osteomalacia. A report of two cases. J Bone Joint Surg (Br) 1977, **59**: 279–286.

146 Zon Filippi R, Swee RG, Krishnan Unni K. Epithelioid multinodular osteoblastoma: a clinicopathologic analysis of 26 cases. Am J Surg Pathol 2007, **31**: 1265–1268.

Osteosarcoma

147 Ahuja SC, Villacin AB, Smith J, Bullough PG, Huvos AG, Marcove RC. Juxtacortical (parosteal) osteogenic sarcoma. Histologic grading and prognosis. J Bone Joint Surg (Am) 1977, **59**: 632–647.

148 Arlen M, Higinbotham NL, Huvos AG, Marcove RC, Miller T, Shah IC. Radiation-induced sarcoma of bone. Cancer 1971, **28**: 1087–1099.

149 Ayala AG, Raymond AK, Jaffe N. The pathologist's role in the diagnosis and treatment of osteosarcoma in children. Hum Pathol 1984, **15**: 258–266.

150 Ayala AG, Raymond AK, Ro JY, Carrasco CH, Fanning CV, Murray JA. Needle biopsy of primary bone lesions. M.D. Anderson experience. Pathol Annu 1989, **24**(Pt 1): 219–251.

151 Ayala AG, Ro JY, Raymond AK, Jaffe N, Chawla S, Carrasco H, Link M, Jimenez J, Edeiken J, Wallace S, et al. Small cell osteosarcoma. A clinicopathologic study of 27 cases. Cancer 1989, **64**: 2162–2173.

152 Bacci G, Ferrari S, Delepine N, Bertoni F, Picci P, Mercuri M, Bacchini P, Brach Del Prever A, Tienghi A, Comandone A, Campanacci M. Predictive factors of histologic response to primary chemotherapy in osteosarcoma of the extremity: study of 272 patients preoperatively treated with high-dose methotrexate, doxorubicin, and cisplatin. J Clin Oncol 1998, **16**: 658–663.

153 Bacci G, Mercuri M, Briccoli A, Ferrari S, Bertoni F, Donati D, Monti C, Zanoni A, Forni C, Manfrini M. Osteogenic sarcoma of the extremity with detectable lung metastases at presentation: results of treatment of 23 patients with chemotherapy followed by simultaneous resection and metastatic lesions. Cancer 1997, **79**: 245–254.

154 Bacci G, Picci P, Ruggieri P, Mercuri M, Avella M, Capanna R, Brach Del Prever A, Mancini A, Gherlinzoni F, Padovani G, et al. Primary chemotherapy and delayed surgery (neoadjuvant chemotherapy) for osteosarcoma of the extremities. The Istituto Rizzoli Experience in 127 patients treated preoperatively with intravenous methotrexate (high versus moderate doses) and intraarterial cisplatin. Cancer 1990, **65**: 2539–2553.

155 Baldini N, Scotlandi K, Serra M, Picci P, Bacci G, Sottili S, Campanacci M. P-glycoprotein expression in osteosarcoma: a basis for risk-adapted adjuvant chemotherapy. J Orthop Res 1999, **17**: 629–632.

156 Banta JV, Schreiber RR, Kulik WJ. Hyperplastic callus formation in osteogenesis imperfecta simulating osteosarcoma. J Bone Joint Surg (Am) 1971, **53**: 115–122.

157 Barwick KW, Huvos AG, Smith J. Primary osteogenic sarcoma of the vertebral column. A clinicopathologic correlation of ten patients. Cancer 1980, **46**: 595–604.

158 Bauer HC, Kreicbergs A, Silversward C, Tribukait B. DNA analysis in the differential diagnosis of osteosarcoma. Cancer 1988, **61**: 2532–2540.

159 Belli L, Scholl S, Livartowski A, Ashby M, Palangie T, Levasseur P, Pouillart P. Resection of pulmonary metastases in osteosarcoma. A retrospective analysis of 44 patients. Cancer 1989, **63**: 2546–2550.

160 Benassi MS, Molendini L, Gamberi G, Magagnoli G, Ragazzini P, Gobbi GA, Sangiorgi L, Pazzaglia L, Asp J, Bransting C, Picci P. Involvement of INK4A gene products in the pathogenesis and development of human osteosarcoma. Cancer 2001, **92**: 3062–3067.

161 Bertoni F, Bacchii P, Fabbri N, Mercuri M, Picci P, Ruggieri P, Campanacci M. Osteosarcoma. Low-grade intraosseous-type osteosarcoma, histologically resembling parosteal osteosarcoma, fibrous dysplasia, and desmoplastic fibroma. Cancer 1993, **71**: 338–345.

162 Bertoni F, Pignatti G, Bachini P, Picci P, Bacci G, Campanacci M. Telangiectatic or hemorrhagic osteosarcoma of bone. A clinicopathologic study of 41 patients at the Rizzoli Institute. Progr Surg Pathol 1989, **10**: 63–82.

163 Bertoni F, Present D, Bacchini P, Pignatti G, Picci P, Campanacci M. The Istituto Rizzoli experience with small cell osteosarcoma. Cancer 1989, **64**: 2591–2599.

164 Björnsson J, Inwards CY, Wold LE, Sim FH, Taylor WF. Prognostic significance of spontaneous tumour necrosis in osteosarcoma. Virchows Arch [A] 1993, **423**: 195–199.

165 Bommer KK, Ramzy I, Mody D. Fine-needle aspiration biopsy in the diagnosis and management of bone lesions: a study of 450 cases. Cancer 1997, **81**: 148–156.

166 Bosse A, Vollmer E, Bocker W, Roessner A, Wuisman P, Jones D, Fisher LW. The impact of osteonectin for differential diagnosis of bone tumors. An immunohistochemical approach. Pathol Res Pract 1990, **186**: 651–657.

167 Bridge JA, Nelson M, McComb E, McGuire MH, Rosenthal H, Vergara G, Maale GE, Spanier S, Neff JR. Cytogenetic findings in 73 osteosarcoma specimens and a review of the literature. Cancer Genet Cytogenet 1997, **95**: 74–87.

168 Broström L-A, Harris MA, Simon MA, Cooperman DR, Nilsonne U. The effect of biopsy on survival of patients with osteosarcoma. J Bone Joint Surg (Br) 1979, **61**: 209–212.

169 Burgers JM, van Glabbeke M, Busson A, Cohen P, Mazabraud AR, Abbatucci JS, Kalifa C, Tubiana M, Lemerle JS, Voute PA, et al. Osteosarcoma of the limbs. Report of the EORTC-SIOP 03 trial 20781 investigating the value of adjuvant treatment with chemotherapy and/or prophylactic lung irradiation. Cancer 1988, **61**: 1024–1031.

170 Campanacci M, Bacci G, Gertoni F, Picci P, Minutillo A, Franceschi C. The treatment of osteosacoma of the extremities. Twenty years' experience at the Istituto Ortopedico Rizzoli. Cancer 1981, **48**: 1569–1581.

171 Campanacci M, Cervellati G. Osteosarcoma. A review of 345 cases. Ital J Orthop Traumatol 1975, **1**: 5–22.

172 Campanacci M, Picci P, Gherlinzoni F, Guerra A, Bertoni F, Neff JR. Parosteal osteosarcoma. J Bone Joint Surg (Br) 1984, **66**: 313–321.

173 Chow LT, Lin J, Yip KM, Kumta SM, Ahuja AT, King WW, Lee JC. Chondromyxoid fibroma-like osteosarcoma: a distinct variant of low-grade osteosarcoma. Histopathology 1996, **29**: 429–436.

174 Clark JL, Unni KK, Dahlin DC, Devine KD. Osteosarcoma of the jaw. Cancer 1983, **51**: 2311–2316.

175 Dahlin DC, Coventry MB. Osteogenic sarcoma. A study of 600 cases. J Bone Joint Surg (Am) 1967, **49**: 101–110.

176 Dahlin DC, Unni KK. Osteosarcoma of bone and its important recognizable varieties. Am J Surg Pathol 1977, **1**: 61–72.

177 Dardick I, Schatz J, Colgan T. Osteogenic sarcoma with epithelial differentiation. Ultrastruct Pathol 1992, **16**: 463–474.

178 Davis AM, Bell RS, Goodwin PJ. Prognosic factors in osteosarcoma. A critical review. J Clin Oncol 1994, **12**: 423–431.

179 deSantos LA, Murray JA, Ayala AG. The value of percutaneous needle biopsy in the management of primary bone tumors. Cancer 1979, **43**: 735–744.

180 deSantos LA, Murray JA, Finklestein JB, Spjut HJ, Ayala AG. The radiographic spectrum of periosteal osteosarcoma. Radiology 1978, **127**: 123–129.

181 Deshpande A, Hinds PW. The retinoblastoma protein in osteoblast differentiation and osteosarcoma. Curr Mol Med 2006, **6**: 809–817.

182 Devaney K, Vinh TN, Sweet DE. Small cell osteosarcoma of bone. An immunohistochemical study with differential diagnostic considerations. Hum Pathol 1993, **24**: 1211–1225.

183 Dickersin GR, Rosenberg AE. The ultrastructure of small-cell osteosarcoma, with a review of the light microscopy and differential diagnosis. Hum Pathol 1991, **22**: 267–275.

184 Dominguez-Malagon H, Ro JY, Ayala AG. Periosteal osteosarcoma of the digits: a case report. Int J Surg Pathol 1996, **4**: 55–59.

185 Edeiken J, Farrell C, Ackerman LV, Spjut HJ. Parosteal sarcoma. Am J Roentgenol Radium Ther Nucl Med 1971, **111**: 579–583.

186 Enneking WF (ed). Osteosarcoma. Symposium. Clin Orthop 1975, **111**: 1–104.

187 Enneking WF, Kagan A. 'Skip' metastases in osteosarcoma. Cancer 1975, **36**: 2192–2205.

188 Fanburg JC, Rosenberg AE, Weaver DL, Leslie KO, Mann KG, Taatjes DJ, Tracy RP. Osteocalcin and osteonectin immunoreactivity in the diagnosis of osteosarcoma. Am J Clin Pathol 1997, **108**: 464–473.

189 Farr GH, Huvos AG. Juxtacortical osteogenic sarcoma. J Bone Joint Surg (Am) 1972, **51**: 1205–1216.

190 Feugeas O, Guriec N, Babin-Boilletot A, Marcellin L, Simon P, Babin S, Thyss A, Hofman P, Terrier P, Kalifa C, Brunat-Mentigny M, Patricot LM, Oberling F. Loss of heterozygosity of the RB gene is a poor prognostic factor in patients with osteosarcoma. J Clin Oncol 1996, **14**: 467–472.

191 Fechner RE, Huvos AG, Mirra JM, Spjut HJ, Unni KK. A symposium on the pathology of bone tumors. Pathol Annu 1984, **9**(Pt 1): 125–194.

192 Franchi A, Comin CE, Santucci M. Submicroscopic and immunohistochemical profile of surface osteosarcomas. Ultrastruct Pathol 1999, **23**: 233–240.

193 Franchi A, Bacchini P, Della Rocca C, Bertoni F. Central low-grade osteosarcoma with pagetoid bone formation: a potential diagnostic pitfall. Mod Pathol 2004, **17**: 288–291.

194 Frentzel-Beyme R, Wagner G. Malignant bone tumours. Status of aetiological knowledge and needs of epidemiological research. Arch Orthop Trauma Surg 1979, **94**: 81–89.

195 Gadwal SR, Gannon FH, Fanburg-Smith JC, Becoskie EM, Thompson LD. Primary osteosarcoma of the head and neck in pediatric patients: a clinicopathologic study of 22 cases with review of the literature. Cancer 2001, **91**: 598–605.

196 Garbe LR, Monges GM, Pellegrin EM, Payan HL. Ultrastructural study of osteosarcomas. Hum Pathol 1981, **12**: 891–896.

197 Glasser DB, Lane JM, Huvos AG, Marcove RC, Rosen G. Survival, prognosis, and therapeutic response in osteogenic sarcoma. The Memorial Hospital experience. Cancer 1992, **69**: 698–708.

198 Hall RB, Robinson LH, Malawar MM, Dunham WK. Periosteal osteosarcoma. Cancer 1985, **55**: 165–171.

199 Harvei S, Solheim O. The prognosis in osteosarcoma. Norwegian national data. Cancer 1981, **48**: 1719–1723.

200 Hasegawa T, Hirose T, Kudo E, Hizawa K, Usui M, Ishii S. Immunophenotypic heterogeneity in osteosarcomas. Hum Pathol 1991, **22**: 583–590.

201 Hasegawa T, Shibata T, Hirose T, Seki K, Hizawa K. Osteosarcoma with epithelioid features. An immunohistochemical study. Arch Pathol Lab Med 1993, **117**: 295–298.

202 Heidenblad M, Hallor KH, Staaf J, Jönsson G, Borg A, Höglund M, Mertens F, Mandahl N. Genomic profiling of bone and soft tissue tumors with supernumerary ring chromosomes using tiling resolution bacterial artificial chromosome microarrays. Oncogene 2006, **25**: 7106–7116.

203 Hiddemann W, Roessner A, Wörmann B, Mellin W, Klockenkemper B, Bösing T, Büchner T, Grundmann E. Tumor heterogeneity in osteosarcoma as identified by flow cytometry. Cancer 1987, **59**: 324–328.

204 Huvos AG. Osteogenic sarcoma of bones and soft tissues in older persons. A clinicopathologic analysis of 117 patients older than 60 years. Cancer 1986, **57**: 1442–1449.

205 Huvos AG, Butler A, Bretsky SS. Osteogenic sarcoma associated with Paget's disease of bone. A clinicopathologic study of 65 patients. Cancer 1983, **52**: 1489–1495.

206 Huvos AG, Butler A, Bretsky SS. Osteogenic sarcoma in pregnant women. Prognosis, therapeutic implications, and literature review. Cancer 1985, **56**: 2326–2331.

207 Huvos AG, Rosen G, Bretsky SS, Butler A. Telangiectatic osteogenic sarcoma. A clinicopathologic study of 124 patients. Cancer 1982, **49**: 1679–1689.

208 Huvos AG, Sundaresan N, Bretsky SS, Butler A. Osteogenic sarcoma of the skull. A clinicopathologic study of 19 patients. Cancer 1985, **56**: 1214–1221.

209 Huvos AG, Woodard HQ, Cahan WG, Higinbotham NL, Stewart FW, Butler A, Bretsky SS. Postradiation osteogenic sarcoma of bone and soft tissues. A clinicopathologic study of 66 patients. Cancer 1985, **55**: 1244–1255.

210 Iavarone A, Matthay KK, Steinkirchner TM, Israel MA. Germ-line and somatic p53 gene mutations in multifocal osteogenic sarcoma. Proc Natl Acad Sci U S A 1992, **89**: 4207–4209.

211 Iwasaki R, Yamamuro T, Kotoura Y, Okumura H, Kasai R, Nakashima Y. Immunohistochemical study of bone GLA protein in primary bone tumors. Cancer 1992, **70**: 619–624.

212 Jaffe N, Raymond AK, Ayala A, Carrasco CH, Wallace S, Robertson R, Griffiths M, Wang YM. Effect of cumulative courses of intraarterial cisdiamminedichloroplatin-II on the primary tumor in osteosarcoma. Cancer 1989, **63**: 63–67.

213 Kahn LB, Wood FW, Ackerman LV. Fracture callus associated with benign and malignant bone lesions and mimicking osteosarcoma. Am J Clin Pathol 1969, **52**: 14–24.

214 Kansara M, Thomas DM. Molecular pathogenesis of osteosarcoma. DNA Cell Biol 2007, **26**: 1–18.

215 Keel SB, Jaffe KA, Petur Nielsen G, Rosenberg AE. Orthopaedic implant-related sarcoma: a study of twelve cases. Mod Pathol 2001, **14**: 969–977.

216 Kellie SJ, Pratt CB, Parham DM, Fleming ID, Meyer WH, Rao BN. Sarcomas (other than Ewing's) of flat bones in children and adolescents. A clinicopathologic study. Cancer 1990, **65**: 1011–1016.

217 Kilpatrick SE, Geisinger KE, King TS, Sciarrotta J, Ward WG, Gold SH, Bos GD. Clinicopathologic analysis of HER-2neu immunoexpression among various histologic subtypes and grades of osteosarcoma. Mod Pathol 2001, **14**: 1277–1283.

218 Klein MJ, Siegal GP. Osteosarcoma: anatomic and histologic variants. Am J Clin Pathol 2006, **125**: 555–581.

219 Kozakewich H, Perez-Atayde AR, Goorin AM, Wilkinson RH, Gebhardt MC, Vawter GF. Osteosarcoma in young children. Cancer 1991, **67**: 638–642.

220 Kramer K, Hicks DG, Palis J, Rosier RN, Oppenheimer J, Fallon MD, Cohen HJ. Epithelioid osteosarcoma of bone. Immunocytochemical evidence suggesting divergent epithelial and mesenchymal differentiation in a primary osseous neoplasm. Cancer 1993, **71**: 2977–2982.

221 Kurt AM, Unni KK, McLeod RA, Pritchard DJ. Low-grade intraosseous osteosarcoma. Cancer 1990, **65**: 1418–1428.

222 Kyriakos M. Intracortical osteosarcoma. Cancer 1980, **56**: 2525–2533.

223 Lane JM, Hurson B, Boland PJ, Glasser DB. Osteogenic sarcoma. Clin Orthop 1986, **204**: 93–110.

224 Lanzer WL, Liotta LA, Yee C, Azar HA, Costa J. Synthesis of pro-collagen type II by a xenotransplanted human chondroblastic osteosarcoma. Am J Pathol 1981, **104**: 217–226.

225 Levine AM, Resenberg SA. Alkaline phosphatase levels in osteosarcoma tissue are related to prognosis. Cancer 1979, **44**: 2291–2293.

226 Machado I, Alberghini M, Giner F, Corrigan M, O'Sullivan M, Noguera R, Pellin A, Bertoni F, Llombart-Bosch A. Histopathological characterization of small cell osteosarcoma with immunohistochemistry and molecular genetic support. A study of 10 cases. Histopathology 2010, **57**: 147–167/

227 Malawer MM, Dunham WK. Skip metastases in osteosarcoma. Recent experience. J Surg Oncol 1983, **22**: 236–245.

228 Mankin HJ, Conner JF, Schiller AL, Perlmutter N, Alho A, McGuire M. Grading of bone tumors by analysis of nuclear DNA content using flow cytometry. J Bone Joint Surg (Am) 1985, **67**: 404–413.

229 Mankin HJ, Lange TA, Spanier SS. The hazards of biopsy in patients with malignant primary bone and soft-tissue tumors. J Bone Joint Surg (Am) 1982, **64**: 1121–1127.

230 Martínez-Tello FJ, Navas-Palacios JJ. The ultrastructure of conventional, parosteal, and periosteal osteosarcomas. Cancer 1982, **50**: 949–961.

231 Martland HS, Humphries RE. Osteogenic sarcoma in dial painters using luminous paint. Arch Pathol 1929, **7**: 406–417.

232 Matsunaga E. Hereditary retinoblastoma: host resistance and second primary tumors. J Natl Cancer Inst 1980, **65**: 47–51.

233 Matsuno T, Unni KK, McLeod RA, Dahlin DC. Telangiectatic osteogenic sarcoma. Cancer 1976, **38**: 2538–2547.

234 Mitelman F. Recurrent chromosome aberrations in cancer. Mutat Res 2000, **462**: 247–253.

235 Morgan EA, Kozono DE, Butrynski JE, Baldini EH, Raut CP, Nascimento AF. Radiation-associated sarcoma of soft tissue and bone: a clinicopathologic study of 70 cases in a single institution. Lab Invest 2009, **89**(Suppl 1): 19A.

236 Nakajima H, Sim FH, Bond JR, Unni KK. Small cell osteosarcoma of bone: review of 72 cases. Cancer 1997, **79**: 2095–2106.

237 Nora FE, Unni KK, Pritchard DJ, Dahlin DC. Osteosarcoma of extragnathic craniofacial bones. Mayo Clin Proc 1983, **58**: 268–272.

238 O'Hara JM, Hutter RVP, Foote FW Jr, Miller T, Woodward HQ. An analysis of 30 patients surviving longer than ten years after treatment for osteogenic sarcoma. J Bone Joint Surg (Am) 1968, **50**: 335–354.

239 Ogose A, Hotta T, Emura I, Imaizumi S, Takeda M, Yamamura S. Repeated dedifferentiation of low-grade intraosseous osteosarcoma. Hum Pathol 2000, **31**: 615–618.

240 Okada K, Hasegawa T, Yokoyama R. Rossette-forming epithelioid osteosarcoma: a histologic subtype with highly aggressive clinical behaviour. Hum Pathol 2001, **32**: 726–733.

241 Okada K, Unni KK, Swee RG, Sim FH. High grade surface osteosarcoma: a clinicopathologic study of 46 cases. Cancer 1999, **85**: 1044–1054.

242 Okada K, Wold LE, Beabout JW, Shives TC. Osteosarcoma of the hand. A clinicopathologic study of 12 cases. Cancer 1993, **72**: 719–725.

243 Onda M, Matsuda S, Higaki S, Lijima T, Fukushima J, Yokokura A, Kojima T, Horiuchi H, Kurokawa T, Yamamoto T. ErB-2 expression is correlated with poor prognosis for patients with osteosarcoma. Cancer 1996, **77**: 71–78.

244 Ozaki T, Flege S, Liljenqvist U, Hillman A, Delling G, Salzer-Kuntschik M, Jurgens H, Kotz R, Winkelmann W, Bielack SS. Osteosarcoma of the spine: experience of the cooperative osteosarcoma study group. Cancer 2002, **94**: 1069–1077.

245 Ozisik YY, Meloni AM, Peier A, Altungoz O, Spanier SS, Zalupski MM, Leong SP, Sandberg AA. Cytogenetic findings in 19 malignant bone tumors. Cancer 1994, **74**: 2268–2275.

246 Palmero EI, Achatz MI, Ashton-Prolla P, Olivier M, Hainaut P. Tumor protein 53 mutations and inherited cancer: beyond Li-Fraumeni syndrome. Curr Opin Oncol 2010, **22**: 64–69.

247 Parham DM, Prat CB, Parvey LS, Webber BL, Champion J. Childhood multifocal osteosarcoma. Clinicopathologic and radiologic correlates. Cancer 1985, **55**: 2653–2658.

248 Park S-H, Kim I. Small cell osteogenic sarcoma of the ribs: cytological, immunohistochemical and ultrastructural study with literature review. Ultrastruct Pathol 1999, **23**: 133–140.

249 Penman HG, Ring PA. Osteosarcoma in association with total hip replacement. J Bone Joint Surg (Br) 1984, **66**: 632–634.

250 Picci P, Bacci G, Campanacci M, Gasparini M, Pilotti S, Cerasoli S, Bertoni F, Guerra A, Capanna R, Albisinni U, Galletti S, Gherlinzoni F, Calderoni P, Sudanese A, Baldini N, Bernini M, Jaffe N. Histologic evaluation of necrosis in osteosarcoma induced by chemotherapy. Regional mapping of viable and nonviable tumor. Cancer 1985, **56**: 1515–1521.

251 Polednak AP. Bone cancer among female radium dial workers. Latency periods and incidence rates by time after exposure. Brief communication. J Natl Cancer Inst 1978, **60**: 77–82.

252 Pollandt K, Engels C, Kaiser E, Werner M, Delling G. Gsalpha gene mutations in monostotic fibrous dysplasia of bone and fibrous dysplasia-like-low-grade central osteosarcoma. Virchows Arch 2001, **439**: 170–175.

253 Rao BN, Champion JE, Pratt CB, Carnesale P, Dilawari R, Fleming I, Green A, Austin B, Wrenn E, Kumar M. Limb salvage procedures for children with osteosarcoma. An alternative to amputation. J Pediatr Surg 1983, **18**: 901–908.

254 Raymond AK, Chawla SP, Carrasco CH, Ayala AG, Fanning CV, Grice B, Armen T, Plager C, Papadopoulos NEJ, Edeiken J, Wallace S, Jaffe N, Murray JA, Benjamin RS. Osteosarcoma chemotherapy effect. A prognostic factor. Semin Diagn Pathol 1987, **4**: 212–236.

255 Reddick RL, Michelitch HJ, Levine AM, Triche TJ. Osteogenic sarcoma. A study of the ultrastructure. Cancer 1980, **45**: 64–71.

256 Rosen G, Marcove RC, Caparros B, Nirenberg A, Kosloff C, Huvos AG. Primary osteogenic sarcoma. The rationale for preoperative chemotherapy and delayed surgery. Cancer 1979, **43**: 2163–2177.

257 Sandberg AA. Cytogenetics and molecular genetics of bone and soft-tissue tumors. Am J Med Genet 2002, **115**: 189–193.

258 Schajowicz F, Derqui JC. Puncture biopsy in lesions of the locomotor system. Review of results in 4,050 cases, including 941 vertebral punctures. Cancer 1968, **21**: 531–548.

259 Schajowicz F, Santini Araujo E, Berenstein M. Sarcoma complicating Paget's disease of bone. A clinicopathological study of 62 cases. J Bone Joint Surg (Br) 1983, **65**: 299–307.

260 Schaller RT Jr, Haas J, Schaller J, Morgan A, Bleyer A. Improved survival in children with osteosarcoma following resection of pulmonary metastases. J Pediatr Surg 1982, **17**: 546–550.

261 Schulz A, Jundt G, Berghäuser K-H, Gehron-Robey P, Termine JD. Immunohistochemical study of osteonectin in various types of osteosarcoma. Am J Pathol 1988, **132**: 233–238.

262 Sciot R, Samson I, Dal Cin P, Lateur L, Van Damme B, Van Den Berghe H, Desmet V. Giant cell rich parosteal osteosarcoma. Histopathology 1995, **27**: 51–55.

263 Scranton PE, DeCicco FA, Totten RS, Yunis EJ. Prognostic factors in osteosarcoma. A review of 20 years' experience at the University of Pittsburgh Health Center Hospitals. Cancer 1975, **36**: 2179–2191.

264 Shapiro F. Ultrastructural observations on osteosarcoma tissue. A study of 10 cases. Ultrastruct Pathol 1983, **4**: 151–161.

265 Sheth DS, Yasko AW, Raymond AK, Ayala AG, Carrasco CH, Benjamin RS, Jaffe N, Murray JA. Conventional and dedifferentiated parosteal osteosarcoma: diagnosis, treatment, and outcome. Cancer 1996, **78**: 2136–2145.

266 Shives TC, Dahlin DC, Sim FH, Pritchard DJ, Earle JD. Osteosarcoma of the spine. J Bone Joint Surg (Am) 1986, **68**: 660–668.

267 Sim FH, Unni KK, Beabout JW, Dahlin DC. Osteosarcoma with small cells simulating Ewing's tumor. J Bone Joint Surg (Am) 1979, **62**: 207–215.

268 Simon MA, Bos GD. Epiphyseal extension of metaphyseal osteosarcoma in skeletally immature individuals. J Bone Joint Surg (Am) 1980, **62**: 195–204.

269 Simon MA, Hecht JD. Invasion of joints by primary bone sarcomas in adults. Cancer 1982, **50**: 1649–1655.

270 Sindelar WF, Costa J, Ketcham AS. Osteosarcoma associated with Thorotrast administration. Cancer 1978, **42**: 2604–2609.

271 Smith GD, Chalmers J, McQueen MM. Osteosarcoma arising in relation to an enchondroma. A report of three cases. J Bone Joint Surg (Br) 1986, **68**: 315–319.

272 Sommer H-J, Knop J, Heise U, Winkler K, Delling G. Histomorphometric changes of osteosarcoma after chemotherapy. Correlation with 99^{m}TC methylene diphosphonate functional imaging. Cancer 1987, **59**: 252–258.

273 Stark A, Aparisi T, Ericsson JLE. Human osteogenic sarcoma. Fine structure of the osteoblastic type. Ultrastruct Pathol 1983, **4**: 311–329.

274 Stark A, Aparisi T, Ericsson JLE. Human osteogenic sarcoma. Fine structure of the chondroblastic type. Ultrastruct Pathol 1984, **6**: 51–67.

275 Stark A, Aparisi T, Ericsson JLE. Human osteogenic sarcoma. Fine structure of the fibroblastic type. Ultrastruct Pathol 1984, **7**: 301–319.

276 Stark A, Aparisi T, Ericsson JLE. Human osteogenic sarcoma. Fine structural localization of alkaline phosphatase. Ultrastruct Pathol 1985, **8**: 143–154.

277 Steiner GC, Forest M, Vacher-Lavenu MC. Ultrastructure of low-grade intraosseous osteosarcoma of bone: a comparative study with fibrous dysplasia and parosteal osteosarcoma. Ultrastruct Pathol 2006, **30**: 293–299.

278 Stock C, Kager L, Fink FM, Gadner H, Ambros PF. Chromosomal regions involved in the pathogenesis of osteosarcomas. Genes Chromosomes Cancer 2000, **28**: 329–336.

279 Sugano I, Tajima Y, Ishida Y, Nagao K, Saga N, Ohno T, Miyakawa E. Phalangeal intraosseous well-differentiated osteosarcoma of the hand. Virchows Arch 1997, **430**: 185–189.

280 Sulzbacher I, Birner P, Trieb K, Lang S, Chott A. Expression of osteopontin and vascular endothelial growth factor in benign and malignant bone tumors. Virchows Arch 2002, **441**: 345–349.

281 Swanson PE, Dehner LP, Sirgi KE, Wick MR. Cytokeratin immunoreactivity in malignant tumors of bone and soft tissue. A reappraisal of cytokeratin as a reliable marker in diagnostic immunohistochemistry. Appl Immunohistochem 1994, **2**: 103–112.

282 Szymanska J, Mandahl N, Mertens F, Tarkkanen M, Karaharju E, Knuutila S. Ring chromosomes in parosteal osteosarcoma contain sequences from 12q13–15: a combined cytogenetic and comparative genomic hybridization study. Genes Chromosomes Cancer 1996, **16**: 31–34.

283 Takahashi S, Okada K, Nagasawa H, Shimada Y, Sakamoto H, Itoi E. Osteosarcoma occurring in osteogenesis imperfecta. Virchows Arch 2004, **444**: 454–458.

284 Tarkkanen M, Böhling T, Gamberi G, Ragazzini P, Benassi MS, Kivioja A, Kallio P, Elomaa I, Picci P, Knuutila S. Comparative genomic hybridization of low-grade central osteosarcoma. Mod Pathol 1998, **11**: 421–426.

285 Trieb K, Lechleitner T, Lang S, Windhager R, Kotz R, Dirnhofer S. Heat shock protein 72 expression in osteosarcomas correlates with good response to neoadjuvant chemotherapy. Hum Pathol 1998, **29**: 1050–1055.

286 Tucker MA, Dángio GJ, Boice JD Jr, Strong LC, Li FP, Stovall M, Stone BJ, Green DM, Lombardi F, Newton W, Hoover RN, Fraumeni JF Jr. Bone sarcomas linked to radiotherapy and chemotherapy in children. N Engl J Med 1987, **317**: 588–593.

287 Unni KK, Dahlin DC, Beabout JW, Ivins JC. Parosteal osteogenic sarcoma. Cancer 1976, **37**: 2466–2475.

288 Unni KK, Dahlin DC, Beabout JW. Periosteal osteogenic sarcoma. Cancer 1976, **37**: 2476–2485.

289 Unni KK, Dahlin DC, McLeod RA, Pritchard DJ. Intraosseous well-differentiated osteosarcoma. Cancer 1977, **40**: 1337–1347.

290 Uribe-Botero G, Russell WO, Sutow WW, Martin RG. Primary osteosarcoma of bone. A clinicopathologic investigation of 243 cases, with necropsy studies in 54. Am J Clin Pathol 1977, **67**: 427–435.

291 Van der Heul RO, Von Ronnen JR. Juxtacortical osteosarcoma. Diagnosis, differential diagnosis, treatment, and an analysis of eighty cases. J Bone Joint Surg (Am) 1967, **49**: 415–439.

292 van der Walt JD, Ryan JF. Parosteal osteogenic sarcoma of the hand. Histopathology 1990, **16**: 75–78.

293 Varela-Duran J, Dehner LP. Postirradiation osteosarcoma in childhood. A clinicopathologic study of three cases and review of the literature. Am J Pediatr Hematol Oncol 1980, **2**: 263–271.

294 Vigorita VJ, Jones JK, Ghelman B, Marcove RC. Intracortical osteosarcoma. Am J Surg Pathol 1984, **8**: 65–71.

295 Wang LL. Biology of osteogenic sarcoma. Cancer J 2005, **11**: 294–305.

296 Wakasa K, Sakurai M, Uchida A, Yoshikawa H, Maeda A. Massive pulmonary tumor emboli in osteosarcoma. Occult and fatal complication. Cancer 1990, **66**: 583–586.

297 Weatherby RP, Dahlin DC, Ivins JC. Postradiation sarcoma of bone. Review of 78 Mayo Clinic cases. Mayo Clin Proc 1981, **56**: 294–306.

298 White VA, Fanning CV, Ayala AG, Raymond AK, Carrasco CH, Murray JA. Osteosarcoma and the role of fine-needle aspiration. A study of 51 cases. Cancer 1988, **62**: 1238–1246.

299 Wick MR, Siegal GP, Unni KK, McLeod RA, Greditzer HG III. Sarcomas of bone complicating osteitis deformans (Paget's disease). Fifty years' experience. Am J Surg Pathol 1981, **5**: 47–59.

300 Williams AH, Schwinn CP, Parker JW. The ultrastructure of osteosarcoma. A review of twenty cases. Cancer 1976, **37**: 1293–1301.

301 Winkler K, Bielack S, Delling G, Salzer-Kuntschik M, Kotz R, Greenshaw C, Jurgens H, Ritter J, Kusnierz-Glaz C, Erttmann R, et al. Effect of intraarterial versus intravenous cisplatin in addition to systemic doxorubicin, high-dose methotrexate, and ifosfamide on histologic tumor response in osteosarcoma (study COSS-86). Cancer 1990, **66**: 1703–1710.

302 Wold LE, Unni KK, Beabout JW, Pritchard DJ. High-grade surface osteosarcomas. Am J Surg Pathol 1984, **8**: 181–186.

303 Wold LE, Unni KK, Beabout JW, Sim FH, Dahlin DC. Dedifferentiated parosteal osteosarcoma. J Bone Joint Surg (Am) 1984, **66**: 53–59.

304 Wunder JS, Eppert K, Burrow SR, Gokgoz N, Bell RS, Andrulis IL. Co-amplification and overexpression of CDK4, SAS and MDM2 occurs frequently in human parosteal osteosarcomas. Oncogene 1999, **18**: 783–788.

305 Yoshida H, Adachi H, Hamada Y, Aki T, Yumoto T, Morimoto K, Orido T. Osteosarcoma. Ultrastructural and immunohistochemical studies on alkaline phosphatase-positive tumor cells constituting a variety of histologic types. Acta Pathol Jpn 1988, **38**: 325–338.

306 Yoshida H, Yumoto T, Adachi H, Minamizaki T, Maeda N, Furuse K. Osteosarcoma with prominent epithelioid features. Acta Pathol Jpn 1989, **39**: 439–445.

307 Yoshikawa H, Rettig WJ, Takaoka K, Alderman E, Rup B, Rosen V, Wozney JM, Lane JM, Huvos AG, Garin-Chesa P. Expression of bone morphogenetic proteins in human osteosarcoma. Immunohistochemical detection with monoclonal antibody. Cancer 1994, **73**: 85–91.

308 Yoshikawa H, Rettig WJ, Lane JM, Takaoka K, Alderman E, Rup B, Rosen V, Healey JH, Huvos AG, Garin-Chesa P. Immunohistochemical detection of bone morphogenetic proteins in bone and soft-tissue sarcomas. Cancer 1994, **74**: 842–847.

309 Yotov WV, Hamel H, Rivard GE, Champagne MA, Russo PA, Leclerc JM, Bernstein ML, Levy E. Amplifications of DNA primase 1 (PRIM1) in human osteosarcoma. Genes Chromosomes Cancer 1999, **26**: 62–69.

310 Yunis EJ, Barnes L. The histologic diversity of osteosarcoma. Pathol Annu 1986, **21**(Pt 1): 121–141.

CARTILAGE-FORMING TUMORS

Chondroma

311 Boriani S, Bacchini P, Bertoni F, Campanacci M. Periosteal chondroma. A review of twenty cases. J Bone Joint Surg (Am) 1983, **65**: 205–212.

312 Bovée JV, van Roggen JF, Cleton-Jansen AM, Taminiau AH, van der Woude HJ, Hogendoom PCW. Malignant progression in multiple enchondromatosis (Ollier's disease): an autopsy-based molecular genetic study. Hum Pathol 2000, **31**: 1299–1303.

313 Brand T, Hatch EI, Schaller RT, Stevenson JK, Arensman RM, Schwartz MC. Surgical management of the infant with mesenchymal hamartoma of the chest wall. J Pediatr Surg 1986, **21**: 556–558.

314 Campbell AN, Wagget J, Mott MG. Benign mesenchymoma of the chest wall in infancy. J Surg Oncol 1982, **21**: 267–270.

315 Cannon SR, Sweetnam DR. Multiple chondrosarcomas in dyschondroplasia (Ollier's disease). Cancer 1985, **55**: 836–840.

316 Cowan WK. Malignant change and multiple metastases in Ollier's disease. J Clin Pathol 1965, **18**: 650–653.

317 Laurence W, Franklin EL. Calcifying enchondroma of long bones. J Bone Joint Surg (Br) 1953, **35**: 224–228.

318 Lewis RJ, Ketcham AS. Maffucci's syndrome. Functional and neoplastic significance. Case report and review of the literature. J Bone Joint Surg (Am) 1973, **55**: 1465–1479.

319 Liu J, Hudkins PG, Swee RG, Unni KK. Bone sarcomas associated with Ollier's disease. Cancer 1987, **59**: 1376–1385.

320 McCarthy EF, Dorfman HD. Vascular and cartilaginous hamartoma of the ribs in infancy with secondary aneurysmal bone cyst formation. Am J Surg Pathol 1980, **4**: 247–253.

321 Nojima T, Unni KK, McLeod RA, Pritchard DJ. Periosteal chondroma and periosteal chondrosarcoma. Am J Surg Pathol 1985, **9**: 666–677.

322 Nosanchuk JS, Kaufer H. Recurrent periosteal chondroma. Report of two cases and a review of the literature. J Bone Joint Surg (Am) 1969, **51**: 375–380.

323 Sun T-C, Swee RG, Shives TC, Unni KK. Chondrosarcoma in Maffucci's syndrome. J Bone Joint Surg (Am) 1985, **67**: 1214–1215.

324 Takigawa K. Chondroma of the bones of the hand. J Bone Joint Surg (Am) 1971, **53**: 1591–1600.

325 Tamimi HK, Bolen JW. Enchondromatosis (Ollier's disease) and ovarian juvenile granulosa cell tumor. A case report and review of the literature. Cancer 1984, **53**: 1605–1608.

Osteochondroma and related lesions

326 Abramovici L, Steiner GC. Bizarre parosteal osteochondromatous proliferation (Nora's lesion): a retrospective study of 12 cases, 2 arising in long bones. Hum Pathol 2002, **33**: 1205–1210.

327 Bovée JV, van den Broek LJ, Cleton-Jansen AM, Hogendoorn PC. Up-regulation of PTHrP and Bcl-2 expression characterizes the progression of osteochondroma towards peripheral chondrosarcoma and is a late event in central chondrosarcoma. Lab Invest 2000, **80**: 1925–1934.

328 Bovée JV. Multiple osteochondromas. Orphanet J Rare Dis 2008, **3**: 3.

329 Bovée JV, Cleton-Jansen AM, Kuipers-Dijkshoorn NJ, van den Broek LJ, Taminiau AH, Cornelisse CJ, Hogendoorn PC. Loss of heterozygosity and DNA ploidy point to a diverging genetic mechanism in the origin of peripheral and central chondrosarcoma. Genes Chromosomes Cancer 1999, **26**: 237–246.

330 Bovée JV, Cleton-Jansen AM, Wuyts W, Caethoven G, Taminiau AH, Bakker E, Van Hul W, Cornelisse CJ, Hogendoorn PC. EXT-mutation analysis and loss of heterozygosity in sporadic and hereditary osteochondromas and secondary chondrosarcomas. Am J Hum Genet 1999, **65**: 689–698.

331 Bridge AJ, Nelson M, Orndal C, Bhatia P, Neff JR. Clonal karyotypic abnormalities of the hereditary multiple exostoses chromosomal loci 8q24.1(EX1) and 11p11-12(EXT2) in patients with sporadic and hereditary osteochondromas. Cancer 1998, **82**: 1657–1663.

332 Carney JA, Boccon-Gibod L, Jarka DE, Tanaka Y, Swee RG, Unni KK, Stratakis CA. Osteochondromyxoma of bone: a congenital tumor associated with lentigines and other unusual disorders. Am J Surg Pathol 2001, **25**: 164–176.

333 Copeland RL, Meehan PL, Morrissy RT. Spontaneous regression of osteochondromas. Two case reports. J Bone Joint Surg (Am) 1985, **67**: 971–973.

334 del Rosario AD, Bui HX, Singh J, Ginsburg R, Ross JS. Intracytoplasmic eosinophilic hyaline globules in cartilaginous neoplasms. A surgical, pathological, ultrastructural, and electron probe x-ray microanalytic study. Hum Pathol 1994, **25**: 1283–1289.

335 Feely MG, Boehm AK, Bridge RS, Krallman PA, Neff JR, Nelson M, Bridge JA. Cytogenetic and molecular cytogenetic evidence of recurrent 8q24.1 loss in osteochondroma. Cancer Genet Cytogenet 2002, **137**: 102–107.

336 Glick R, Khaldi L, Ptaszynski K, Steiner GC. Dysplasia epiphysealis hemimelica (Trevor disease): a rare developmental disorder of bone mimicking osteochondroma of long bones. Hum Pathol 2007, **38**: 1265–1272.

337 Hallor KH, Staaf J, Bovée JV, Hogendoorn PC, Cleton-Jansen AM, Knuutila S, Savola S, Niini T, Brosjö O, Bauer HC, Vult von Steyern F, Jonsson K, Skorpil M, Mandahl N, Mertens F. Genomic profiling of chondrosarcoma: chromosomal patterns in central and peripheral tumors. Clin Cancer Res 2009, **15**: 2685–2694.

338 Han SK, Henein HG, Novin N, Giargiana FA Jr. An unusual arterial complication seen with a solitary osteochondroma. Am Surg 1977, **43**: 471–472.

339 Horiguchi H, Sakane M, Matsui M, Wadano Y. Bizarre parosteal osteochondromatous proliferation (Nora's lesion) of the foot. Pathol Int 2001, **51**: 816–823.

340 Hwang W-S, McQueen D, Monson RC, Reed MH. The significance of cytoplasmic chondrocyte inclusions in multiple osteochondromatosis, solitary osteochondromas, and chondrodysplasias. Am J Clin Pathol 1982, **78**: 89–91.

341 Josefczyk MA, Huvos AG, Smith J, Urmacher C. Bursa formation in secondary chondrosarcoma with intrabursal chondrosarcomatosis. Am J Surg Pathol 1985, **9**: 309–314.

342 Landon GC, Johnson KA, Dahlin DC. Subungual exostoses. J Bone Joint Surg (Am) 1979, **61**: 256–259.

343 Meneses MF, Unni KK, Swee RG. Bizarre parosteal osteochondromatous proliferation of bone (Nora's lesion). Am J Surg Pathol 1993, **17**: 691–697.

344 Miller-Breslow A, Dorfman HD. Dupuytren's (subungual) exostosis. Am J Surg Pathol 1988, **12**: 368–378.

345 Nilsson M, Domanski HA, Mertens F, Mandahl N. Molecular cytogenetic characterization of recurrent translocation breakpoints in bizarre parosteal osteochondromatous proliferation (Nora's lesion). Hum Pathol 2004, **35**: 1063–1069.

346 Nora FE, Dahlin DC, Beabout JW. Bizarre parosteal osteochondromatous proliferations of the hands and feet. Am J Surg Pathol 1983, **7**: 245–250.

347 Unni KK, Dahlin DC. Premalignant tumors and conditions of bone. Am J Surg Pathol 1979, **3**: 47–60.

348 Zambrano E, Nosé V, Perez-Atayde AR, Gebhardt M, Hresko MT, Kleinman P, Richkind KE, Kozakewich HP. Distinct chromosomal rearrangements in subungual (Dupuytren) exostosis and bizarre parosteal osteochondromatous proliferation (Nora lesion). Am J Surg Pathol 2004, **28**: 1033–1039.

Chondroblastoma

349 Aronsohn RS, Hart WR, Martel W. Metaphyseal chondroblastoma of bone. Am J Roentgenol 1976, **127**: 686–688.

350 Birch PJ, Buchanan R, Golding P, Pringle JAS. Chondroblastoma of the rib with widespread bone metastases. Histopathology 1994, **25**: 583–585.

351 Bousdras K, O'Donnell P, Vujovic S, Henderson S, Boshoff C, Flanagan AM. Chondroblastomas but not chondromyxoid fibromas express cytokeratins: an unusual presentation of a chondroblastoma in the metaphyseal cortex of the tibia. Histopathology 2007, **51**: 414–416.

352 Brecher ME, Simon MA. Chondroblastoma. An immunohistochemical study. Hum Pathol 1988, **19**: 1043–1047.

353 Coleman SS. Benign chondroblastoma with recurrent soft-tissue and intra-articular lesions. J Bone Joint Surg (Am) 1966, **48**: 1554–1560.

354 De Silva MV, Reid R. Chondroblastoma: varied histologic appearance, potential diagnostic pitfalls, and clinicopathologic features associated with local recurrence. Ann Diagn Pathol 2003, **7**: 205–213.

355 Fanning CV, Sneige NS, Carrasco CH, Ayala AG, Murray JA, Raymond AK. Fine needle aspiration cytology of chondroblastoma of bone. Cancer 1990, **65**: 1847–1863.

356 Hicks DG, Krasinskas AM, Sickel JZ, Hughes SS, Puzas JE, Moynas R, Rosier RN. Chondroblastoma. In situ hybridization and immunohistochemical evidence supporting a cartilaginous origin. Int J Surg Pathol 1994, **1**: 155–162.

357 Huvos AG, Marcove RC, Erlandson RA, Mike V. Chondroblastoma of bone. A clinicopathologic and electron microscopic study. Cancer 1972, **29**: 760–771.

358 Kahn LB, Wood FM, Ackerman LV. Malignant chondroblastoma. Report of two cases and review of the literature. Arch Pathol 1969, **88**: 371–376.

359 Konishi E, Nakashima Y, Iwasa Y, Nakao R, Yanagisawa A. Immunohistochemical analysis for Sox9 reveals the cartilaginous character of chondroblastoma and chondromyxoid fibroma of the bone. Hum Pathol 2010, **41**: 208–213.

360 Kunze E, Graewe TH, Peitsch E. Histology and biology of metastatic chondroblastoma. Report of a case with a review of the literature. Pathol Res Pract 1987, **182**: 113–120.

361 Kyriakos M, Land VJ, Penning HL, Parker SG. Metastatic chondroblastoma. Report of a fatal case with a review of the literature on atypical, aggressive, and malignant chondroblastoma. Cancer 1985, **55**: 1770–1789.

362 Levine GD, Bensch KG. Chondroblastoma – the nature of the basic cell. A study by means of histochemistry, tissue culture, electron microscopy, and autoradiography. Cancer 1972, **29**: 1546–1562.

363 Mii Y, Miyauchi Y, Honoki K, Morishita T, Miura S, Aoki M, Tamai S. Ultrastructural cytochemical demonstration of proteoglycans and calcium in the extracellular matrix of chondroblastomas. Hum Pathol 1994, **25**: 1290–1294.

364 Monda L, Wick MR. S-100 protein immunostaining in the differential diagnosis of chondroblastoma. Hum Pathol 1985, **16**: 287–293.

365 Nakamura Y, Becker LE, Marks A. S-100 protein in tumors of cartilage and bone. An immunohistochemical study. Cancer 1983, **58**: 1820–1824.

366 Posl M, Werner M, Amling M, Ritzel H, Delling G. Malignant transformation of chondroblastoma. Histopathology 1996, **29**: 477–480.

367 Povysil C, Tomanova R, Matejovsky Z. Muscle-specific actin expression in chondroblastomas. Hum Pathol 1997, **28**: 316–320.

368 Reyes CV, Kathuria S. Recurrent and aggressive chondroblastoma of the pelvis with late malignant neoplastic changes. Am J Surg Pathol 1979, **3**: 449–455.

369 Schajowicz F, Gallardo H. Epiphysial chondroblastoma of bone. A clinicopathological study of sixty-nine cases. J Bone Joint Surg (Br) 1970, **52**: 205–226.

370 Semmelink HJ, Pruszczynski M, Wiersma-van Tilburg A, Smedts F, Ramaekers FC. Cytokeratin expression in chondroblastomas. Histopathology 1990, **16**: 257–263.

371 Springfield DS, Capanna R, Gherlinzoni F, Picci P, Campanacci M. Chondroblastoma. A review of seventy cases. J Bone Joint Surg (Am) 1985, **67**: 748–754.

372 Steiner GC. Ultrastructure of benign cartilaginous tumors of intraosseous origin. Hum Pathol 1979, **10**: 71–86.

373 Turcotte RE, Kurt AM, Sim FH, Unni KK, McLeod RA. Chondroblastoma. Hum Pathol 1993, **24**: 944–949.

374 Welsh RA, Meyer AT. A histogenetic study of chondroblastoma. Cancer 1964, **17**: 578–589.

Chondromyxoid fibroma and related tumors

375 Bahk WJ, Mirra JM, Sohn KR, Shin DS. Pseudoanaplastic chondromyxoid fibroma. Ann Diagn Pathol 1998, **2**: 241–246.

376 Baker AC, Rezeanu L, O'Laughlin S, Unni K, Klein MJ, Siegal GP. Juxtacortical chondromyxoid fibroma of bone: a unique variant: a case study of 20 patients. Am J Surg Pathol 2007, **31**: 1662–1668.

377 Bleiweiss IJ, Klein MJ. Chondromyxoid fibroma. Report of six cases with immunohistochemical studies. Mod Pathol 1990, **3**: 664–666.

378 Dahlin DC. Chondromyxoid fibroma of bone, with emphasis on its morphological relationship to benign chondroblastoma. Cancer 1956, **9**: 195–203.

379 Fanburg-Smith JC, Auerbach A, Marwaha JS, Wang Z, Santi M, Judkins AR, Rushing EJ. Immunoprofile of mesenchymal chondrosarcoma: aberrant desmin and EMA expression, retention of INI1, and negative estrogen receptor in 22 female-predominant central nervous system and musculoskeletal cases. Ann Diagn Pathol 2010, **14**: 8–14.

380 Gherlinzoni F, Rock M, Picci P. Chondromyxoid fibroma. The experience at the Istituto Ortopedico Rizzoli. J Bone Joint Surg (Am) 1983, **65**: 198–204.

381 Granter SR, Renshaw AA, Kozakewich HP, Fletcher JA. The pericentromeric inversion, inv (6)(p25q13), is a novel diagnostic marker in chondromyxoid fibroma. Mod Pathol 1998, **11**: 1071–1074.

382 Keel SB, Bhan AK, Liebsch NJ, Rosenberg AE. Chondromyxoid fibroma of the skull base: a tumor which may be confused with chordoma and chondrosarcoma: a report of three cases and review of the literature. Am J Surg Pathol 1997, **21**: 577–582.

383 Kikuchi F, Dorfman HD, Kane PB. Recurrent chondromyxoid fibroma of the thoracic spine 30 years after primary excision: case report and review of the literature. Int J Surg Pathol 2001, **9**: 323–330.

384 Konishi E, Nakashima Y, Iwasa Y, Yanagisawa A. Immunohistochemical comparative study of chondromyxoid fibroma, chondroblastoma and chondrosarcoma, using Sox9, p63 and CAM 5.2. Lab Invest 2009, **89**(Suppl 1): 16A.

385 Kreicbergs A, Lönnquist PA, Willems J. Chondromyxoid fibroma. A review of the literature and a report on our own experience. Acta Pathol Microbiol Immunol Scand (A) 1985, **93**: 189–197.

386 Kyriakos M. Soft tissue implantation of chondromyxoid fibroma. Am J Surg Pathol 1979, **3**: 363–372.

387 Marcove RC, Kambolis C, Bullough PG, Jaffe HL. Fibromyxoma of bone. Cancer 1964, **17**: 1209–1213.

388 Marcove RC, Lindeque BG, Huvos AG. Fibromyxoma of the bone. Surg Gynecol Obstet 1989, **169**: 115–118.

389 McClure DK, Dahlin DC. Myxoma of bone. Report of three cases. Mayo Clin Proc 1977, **52**: 249–253.

390 Nielsen GP, Keel SB, Dickersin GR, Selig MK, Bhan AK, Rosenberg AE. Chondromyxoid fibroma: a tumor showing myofibroblastic, myochondroblastic, and chondrocytic differentiation. Mod Pathol 1999, **12**: 514–517.

391 Safar A, Nelson M, Neff JR, Maale GE, Bayani J, Squire J, Bridge JA. Recurrent anomalies of 6q25 in chondromyxoid fibroma. Hum Pathol 2000, **31**: 306–311.

392 Schajowicz F, Gallardo H. Chondromyxoid fibroma (fibromyxoid chondroma) of bone. A clinico-pathological study of thirty-two cases. J Bone Joint Surg (Br) 1971, **53**: 198–216.

393 Soder S, Inwards C, Muller S, Kirchner T, Aigner T. Cell biology and matrix biochemistry of chondromyxoid fibroma. Am J Clin Pathol 2001, **116**: 271–277.

394 Wu CT, Inwards CY, O'Laughlin S, Rock MG, Beabout JW, Unni KK. Chondromyxoid fibroma of bone: a clinicopathologic review of 27 cases. Hum Pathol 1998, **29**: 438–446.

395 Zillmer DA, Dorfman HD. Chondromyxoid fibroma of bone. Thirty-six cases with clinicopathologic correlation. Hum Pathol 1989, **20**: 952–964.

Chondrosarcoma

396 Alho A, Connor JF, Mankin HJ, Schiller AL, Campbell CJ. Assessment of malignancy of cartilage tumors using flow cytometry. A preliminary report. J Bone Joint Surg (Am) 1983, **65**: 779–785.

397 Bai S, Wang D, Klein MJ, Siegal GB. Characterization of CXCR4 expression in chondrosarcoma of bone. Lab Invest 2009, **89**(Suppl 1): 12A.

398 Barnes R, Catto M. Chondrosarcoma of bone. J Bone Joint Surg (Br) 1966, **48**: 729–764.

399 Bergh P, Gunterberg B, Meis-Kindblom JM, Kindblom LG. Prognostic factors and outcome of pelvic, sacral, and spinal chondrosarcomas: a center-based study of 69 cases. Cancer 2001, **91**: 1201–1212.

400 Bertoni F, Boriani S, Laus M, Campanacci M. Periosteal chondrosarcoma and periosteal osteosarcoma. Two distinct entities. J Bone Joint Surg (Br) 1982, **64**: 370–376.

401 Björnsson J, McLeod RA, Unni KK, Ilstrup DM, Pritchard DJ. Primary chondrosarcoma of long bones and limb girdles. Cancer 1998, **83**: 2105–2119.

402 Boeuf S, Kunz P, Hennig T, Lehner B, Hogendoorn P, Bovée J, Richter W. A chondrogenic gene expression signature in mesenchymal stem cells is a classifier of conventional central chondrosarcoma. J Pathol 2008, **216**: 158–166.

403 Bovée JV, Cleton-Jansen AM, Kuipers-Dijkshoorn NJ, van den Broek LJ, Taminiau AH, Cornelisse CJ, Hogendoorn PC. Loss of heterozygosity and DNA ploidy point to a diverging genetic mechanism in the origin of peripheral and central chondrosarcoma. Genes Chromosomes Cancer 1999, **26**: 237–246.

404 Bovée JV, van Der Heul RO, Taminiau AH, Hogendoom PC. Chondrosarcoma of the phalanx: a locally aggressive lesion with minimal metastatic potential: a report of 35 cases and a review of the literature. Cancer 1999, **86**: 1724–1732.

405 Campanacci M, Guernelli N, Leonessa C, Boni A. Chondrosarcoma. A study of 133 cases, 80 with long term follow up. Ital J Orthop Traumatol 1975, **1**: 387–414.

406 Coltrera MD, Googe PB, Harrist TJ, Hyams VJ, Schiller AL, Goodman ML. Chondrosarcoma of the temporal bone. Diagnosis and treatment of 13 cases and review of the literature. Cancer 1986, **58**: 2689–2696.

407 Dahlin DC, Henderson ED. Chondrosarcoma, a surgical and pathological problem. J Bone Joint Surg (Am) 1956, **38**: 1025–1038.

408 Dahlin DC, Salvador AH. Chondrosarcomas of bones of the hands and feet. A study of 30 cases. Cancer 1974, **34**: 755–760.

409 Dobashi Y, Sugimura H, Sato A, Hirabayashi T, Kanda H, Kitagawa T, Kawaguchi N, Imamura T, Machinami R. Possible association of p53 overexpression and mutation with high-grade chondrosarcoma. Diagn Mol Pathol 1993, **2**: 257–263.

410 Eefting D, Schrage YM, Geirnaerdt MJ, Le Cessie S, Taminiau AH, Bovée JV, Hogendoorn PC; EuroBoNeT consortium. Assessment of interobserver variability and histologic parameters to improve reliability in classification and grading of central cartilaginous tumors. Am J Surg Pathol 2009, **33**: 50–57.

411 Erlandson RA, Huvos AG. Chondrosarcoma. A light and electron microscopic study. Cancer 1974, **34**: 1642–1652.

412 Evans HL, Ayala AG, Romsdahl MM. Prognostic factors in chondrosarcoma of bone. A clinicopathologic analysis with emphasis on histologic grading. Cancer 1977, **40**: 818–831.

413 Gadwal SR, Fanburg-Smith JC, Gannon FH, Thompson LD. Primary chondrosarcoma of the head and neck in pediatric patients: a clinicopathologic study of 14 cases and review of the literature. Cancer 2000, **88**: 2181–2188.

414 Garrison RC, Unni KK, McLeod RA, Pritchard DJ, Dahlin DC. Chondrosarcoma arising in osteochondroma. Cancer 1982, **49**: 1890–1897.

415 Gitelis S, Bertoni F, Picci P, Campanacci M. Chondrosarcoma of bone. The experience at the Istituto Ortopedico Rizzoli. J Bone Joint Surg (Am) 1981, **63**: 1248–1257.

416 Grifone TJ, Haupt HM, Podolski V, Brooks JJ. Immunohistochemical expression of estrogen receptors in chondrosarcomas and enchondromas. Int J Surg Pathol 2008, **16**: 31–37.

417 Hallor KH, Staaf J, Bovée JV, Hogendoorn PC, Cleton-Jansen AM, Knuutila S, Savola S, Niini T, Brosjö O, Bauer HC, Vult von Steyern F, Jonsson K, Skorpil M, Mandahl N, Mertens F. Genomic profiling of chondrosarcoma: chromosomal patterns in central and peripheral tumors. Clin Cancer Res 2009, **15**: 2685–2694.

418 Hameetman L, Kok P, Eilers PH, Cleton-Jansen AM, Hogendoorn PC, Bovée JV. The use of Bcl-2 and PTHLH immunohistochemistry in the diagnosis of peripheral chondrosarcoma in a clinicopathological setting. Virchows Arch 2005, **446**: 430–437.

419 Healey JH, Lane JM. Chondrosarcoma. Clin Orthop 1986, **204**: 119–129.

420 Helfenstein A, Frahm SO, Krams M, Drescher W, Parwaresch R, Hassenpflug J. Minichromosome maintenance protein (MCM6) in low-grade chondrosarcoma: distinction from enchondroma and identification of progressive tumors. Am J Clin Pathol 2004, **122**: 912–918.

421 Huvos AG, Marcove RC. Chondrosarcoma in the young. A clinicopathologic analysis of 790 patients younger than 21 years of age. Am J Surg Pathhol 1987, **11**: 930–942.

422 Kindblom L, Angervall L. Histochemical characterization of mucosubstances in bone and soft tissue tumors. Cancer 1975, **36**: 985–994.

423 Konishi E, Nakashima Y, Iwasa Y, Yanagisawa A. Immunohistochemical comparative study of chondromyxoid fibroma, chondroblastoma and chondrosarcoma, using Sox9, p63 and CAM 5.2. Lab Invest 2009, **89**(Suppl 1): 16A.

424 Kreicbergs A, Boquist L, Borssén B, Larsson S-E. Prognostic factors in chondrosarcoma. A comparative study of cellular DNA content and clinicopathologic features. Cancer 1982, **50**: 577–583.

425 Kreicbergs A, Slezak E, Söderberg G. The prognostic significance of different histomorphologic features in chondrosarcoma. Virchows Arch [A] 1981, **390**: 1–10.

426 Kristensen IB, Sunde LM, Jensen OM. Chondrosarcoma. Increasing grade of malignancy in local recurrence. Acta Pathol Microbiol Immunol Scand (A) 1986, **94**: 73–77.

427 Kusuzaki K, Murata H, Takeshita H, Hirata M, Hashiguchi S, Tsuji Y, Nakamura S, Ashihara T, Hirasawa Y. Usefulness of cytofluorometric DNA ploidy analysis in distinguishing benign cartilaginous tumors from chondrosarcomas. Mod Pathol 1999, **12**: 863–872.

428 Lansche WE, Spjut HJ. Chondrosarcoma of the small bones of the hand. J Bone Joint Surg (Am) 1958, **40**: 1139–1149.

429 Larramendy ML, Mandahl N, Mertens F, Blomqvist C, Kivioja AH, Karaharju E, Valle J, Böhling T, Tarkkanen M, Rydholm A, Akerman M, Bauer HC, Anttila JP, Elomaa I, Knuutila S. Clinical significance of genetic imbalances revealed by comparative genomic hybridization in chondrosarcomas. Hum Pathol 1999, **30**: 1247–1253.

430 Mandahl N, Heim S, Arheden K, Rydholm A, Willen H, Mitelman F. Chromosomal rearrangements in chondromatous tumors. Cancer 1990, **65**: 242–248.

431 Mankin HJ, Cantley KP, Lippiello L, Schiller AL, Campbell CJ. The biology of human chondrosarcoma. I. Description of the cases, grading, and biochemical analyses. J Bone Joint Surg (Am) 1980, **62**: 160–176.

432 Mankin HJ, Cantley KP, Schiller AL, Lippiello L. The biology of human chondrosarcoma. II. Variation in chemical composition among types and subtypes of benign and malignant cartilage tumors. J Bone Joint Surg (Am) 1980, **62**: 176–188.

433 Marcove RC, Huvos AG. Cartilaginous tumors of the ribs. Cancer 1971, **27**: 794–801.

434 McAfee MK, Pairolero PC, Bergstralh EJ, Piehler JM, Unni KK, McLeod RA, Bernatz PE, Payne WS. Chondrosarcoma of the chest wall. Factors affecting survival. Ann Thorac Surg 1985, **40**: 535–541.

435 McKenna RJ, Schwinn CP, Soong KY, Higinbotham NL. Sarcomata of the osteogenic series (osteosarcoma, fibrosarcoma, chondrosarcoma, parosteal osteogenic sarcoma, and sarcomata arising in abnormal bone). J Bone Joint Surg (Am) 1966, **48**: 1–26.

436 Mirra JM, Gold R, Downs J, Eckardt JJ. A new histologic approach to the differentiation of enchondroma and chondrosarcoma of the bones. A clinicopathologic analysis of 51 cases. Clin Orthop 1985, **201**: 214–237.

437 Nakamura Y, Becker LE, Marks A. S-100 protein in tumors of cartilage and bone. An immunohistochemical study. Cancer 1983, **58**: 1820–1824.

438 Ogose A, Unni KK, Swee RG, May GK, Rowland CM, Sim FH. Chondrosarcoma of small bones of the hands and feet. Cancer 1997, **80**: 50–59.

439 Okajima K, Honda I, Kitagawa T. Imunohistochemical distribution of S-100 protein in tumors and tumorlike lesions of bone and cartilage. Cancer 1988, **61**: 792–799.

440 O'Neal LW, Ackerman LV. Cartilaginous tumors of ribs and sternum. J Thorac Surg 1951, **21**: 71–108.

441 Oshiro Y, Chaturvedi V, Hayden D, Nazeer T, Johnson M, Johnston DA, Ordóñez NG, Ayala AG, Czerniak B. Altered p53 is associated with aggressive behavior of chondrosarcoma: a long term follow-up study. Cancer 1998, **83**: 2324–2334.

442 Ostrowski ML, Spjut HJ. Lesions of the bones of the hands and feet. Am J Surg Pathol 1997, **21**: 676–690.

443 Pritchard DJ, Lunke RJ, Taylor WF, Dahlin DC, Medley BE. Chondrosarcoma. A clinicopathologic and statistical analysis. Cancer 1980, **45**: 149–157.

444 Rosenberg AE, Neilsen GP, Keel SB, Renard LG, Fitzek MM, Munzenrider JE, Liebsch NJ. Chondrosarcoma of the base of the skull: a clinicopathologic study of 200 cases with emphasis on its distinction from chordoma. Am J Surg Pathol 1999, **23**: 1370–1378.

445 Salas S, de Pinieux G, Gomez-Brouchet A, Larrousserie F, Leroy X, Aubert S, Decouvelaere AV, Giorgi R, Fernandez C, Bouvier C. Ezrin immunohistochemical expression in cartilaginous tumours: a useful tool for differential diagnosis between chondroblastic osteosarcoma and chondrosarcoma. Virchows Arch 2009, **454**: 81–87.

446 Sandberg AA, Bridge JA. Updates on the cytogenetics and molecular genetics of bone soft tissue tumors: chondrosarcoma and other cartilaginous neoplasms. Cancer Genet Cytogenet 2003, **143**: 1–31.

447 Sanerkin NG, Gallagher P. A review of the behaviour of chondrosarcoma of bone. J Bone Joint Surg (Br) 1979, **61**: 395–400.

448 Sawyer JR, Swanson CM, Lukacs JL, Nicholas RW, North PE, Thomas JR. Evidence of an association between 6q13–21 chromosome aberrations and locally aggressive behavior in patients with cartilage tumors. Cancer 1998, **82**: 474–483.

449 Schajowicz F. Juxtacortical chondrosarcoma. J Bone Joint Surg (Br) 1977, **59**: 473–480.

450 Schiller AL. Diagnosis of borderline cartilage lesions of bone. Semin Diagn Pathol 1985, **2**: 42–62.

451 Sheth DS, Yasko AW, Johnson ME, Ayala AG, Murray JA, Romsdahl MM. Chondrosarcoma of the pelvis: prognostic factors for 67 patients treated with definitive surgery. Cancer 1996, **78**: 745–750.

452 Smith WS, Simon MA. Segmental resection for chondrosarcoma. J Bone Joint Surg (Am) 1975, **57**: 1097–1103.

453 Terek RM, Healey JH, Garin-Chesa P, Mak S, Huvos A, Albino AP. p53 mutations in chondrosarcoma. Diagn Mol Pathol 1998, **7**: 51–56.

454 van Beerendonk HM, Rozeman LB, Taminiau AH, Sciot R, Bovée JV, Cleton-Jansen AM, Hogendoorn PC. Molecular analysis of the INK4A/INK4A-ARF gene locus in conventional (central) chondrosarcomas and enchondromas: indication of an important gene for tumour progression. J Pathol 2004, **202**: 359–366.

455 Wang W-L, Hilliard NJ, Deavers MT, Lewis VO, Raymond AK. Chondrosarcomas: skip metastasis. Lab Invest 2009, 89(Suppl 1): 25A.

456 Young CL, Sim FH, Unni KK, McLeod RA. Chondrosarcoma of bone in children. Cancer 1990, **66**: 1641–1648.

Chondrosarcoma variants

Clear cell chondrosarcoma

457 Aigner T, Dertinger S, Belke J, Kirchner T. Chondrocytic cell differentiation in clear cell chondrosarcoma. Hum Pathol 1996, **27**: 1301–1305.

458 Bjornsson J, Unni KK, Dahlin DC, Beabout JW, Sim FH. Clear cell chondrosarcoma of bone. Observations in 47 cases. Am J Surg Pathol 1984, **8**: 223–230.

459 Corradi D, Bacchini P, Campanini N, Bertoni F. Aggressive clear cell chondrosarcomas: do distinctive characteristics exist? A report of four cases. Arch Pathol Lab Med 2006, **130**: 1673–1679.

460 Faraggiana T, Sender B, Glicksman P. Light- and electron-microscopic study of clear cell chondrosarcoma. Am J Clin Pathol 1981, **75**: 117–121.

461 Kalil RK, Inwards CY, Unni KK, Bertoni F, Bacchini P, Wenger DE, Sim FH. Dedifferentiated clear cell chondrosarcoma. Am J Surg Pathol 2000, **24**: 1079–1086.

462 Masui F, Ushigome S, Fujii K. Clear cell chondrosarcoma: a pathological and immunohistochemical study. Histopathology 1999, **34**: 447–452.

463 Swanson PE. Clear cell tumors of bone. Semin Diagn Pathol 1998, **14**: 281–291.

464 Unni KK, Dahlin DC, Beabout JW, Sim FH. Chondrosarcoma. Clear-cell variant. A report of sixteen cases. J Bone Joint Surg (Am) 1976, **58**: 676–683.

465 Wang LT, Liu TC. Clear cell chondrosarcoma of bone. A report of three cases with immunohistochemical and affinity histochemical observations. Pathol Res Pract 1993, **189**: 411–415.

466 Weiss A-PC, Dorfman HD. S-100 protein in human cartilage lesions. J Bone Joint Surg (Am) 1986, **68**: 521–526.

Myxoid chondrosarcoma (chordoid sarcoma)

467 Antonescu CR, Argani P, Erlandson RA, Healey JH, Ladanyi M, Huvos AG. Skeletal and extraskeletal myxoid chondrosarcoma: a comparative clinicopathologic, ultrastructural, and molecular study. Cancer 1998, **83**: 1504–1521.

468 Dabska M. Parachordoma. A new clinicopathologic entity. Cancer 1977, **40**: 1586–1592.

469 Kilpatrick SE, Inwards CY, Fletcher CD, Smith MA, Gitelis S. Myxoid chondrosarcoma (chordoid sarcoma) of bone: a report of two cases and review of the literature. Cancer 1997, **79**: 1903–1910.

470 Martin RF, Melnick PJ, Warner NE, Terry R, Bullock WK, Schwinn CP. Chordoid sarcoma. Am J Clin Pathol 1972, **59**: 623–635.

471 Miettinen M, Lehto V-P, Dahl D, Virtanen I. Differential diagnosis of chordoma, chondroid, and ependymal tumors as aided by anti-intermediate filament antibodies. Am J Pathol 1983, **112**: 160–169.

472 Pardo-Mindan FJ, Guillen FJ, Villas C, Vazquez JJ. A comparative ultrastructural study of chondrosarcoma, chordoid sarcoma, and chordoma. Cancer 1981, **47**: 2611–2619.

473 Shin HJ, Mackay B, Ichinose H, Ayala AG, Romsdahl MM. Parachordoma. Ultrastruct Pathol 1994, **18**: 249–256.

Dedifferentiated chondrosarcoma

474 Abenoza P, Neumann MP, Manivel JC, Wick MR. Dedifferentiated chondrosarcoma. An ultrastructural study of two cases, with immunocytochemical correlations. Ultrastruct Pathol 1986, **10**: 529–538.

475 Aigner T, Dertinger S, Neureiter D, Kirchner T. De-differentiated chondrosarcoma is not a 'de-differentiated' chondrosarcoma. Histopathology 1998, **33**: 11–19.

476 Bertoni F, El Ghoneimy A, Bacchini P, Inwards CY, Donati D. Dedifferentiated chondrosarcoma of the pelvis. A report of the

clinicopathologic features of fourteen cases treated at the Istituto Rizzoli [abstract]. Mod Pathol 2003, **16**: 9a.

477 Bertoni F, Present D, Bacchini P, Picci P, Pignatti G, Gherlinzoni F, Campanacci M. Dedifferentiated peripheral chondrosarcomas. A report of seven cases. Cancer 1989, **63**: 2054–2059.

478 Bridge JA, De Boer J, Travis J, Johansson SL, Elmberger G, Noel SM, Neff JR. Simultaneous interphase cytogenetic analysis and fluorescence immunophenotyping of dedifferentiated chondrosarcoma. Implications for histopathogenesis. Am J Pathol 1994, **144**: 215–220.

479 Dahlin DC, Beabout JW. Dedifferentiation of low-grade chondrosarcomas. Cancer 1971, **28**: 461–466.

480 Dervan PA, O'Loughlin J, Hurson BJ. Dedifferentiated chondrosarcoma with muscle and cytokeratin differentiation in the anaplastic component. Histopathology 1988, **12**: 517–526.

481 Jaworski RC. Dedifferentiated chondrosarcoma. An ultrastructural study. Cancer 1984, **53**: 2674–2678.

482 Johnson S, Tetu B, Ayala AG, Chawla SP. Chondrosarcoma with additional mesenchymal component (dedifferentiated chondrosarcoma). I. A clinicopathologic study of 26 cases. Cancer 1986, **58**: 278–286.

483 McCarthy EF, Dorfman HD. Chondrosarcoma of bone with dedifferentiation. A study of eighteen cases. Hum Pathol 1982, **13**: 36–40.

484 McFarland GB, McKinley LM, Reed RJ. Dedifferentiation of low-grade chondrosarcomas. Clin Orthop 1977, **122**: 157–164.

485 Meis JM. 'Dedifferentiation' in bone and soft-tissue tumors. A histological indicator of tumor progression. Pathol Annu 1991, **26**(Pt 1): 37–62.

486 Mitchel A, Rudan JR, Fenton PV. Juxtacortical dedifferentiated chondrosarcoma from a primary periosteal chondrosarcoma. Mod Pathol 1996, **9**: 279–283.

487 Reith JD, Bauer TW, Fischler DF, Joyce MJ, Marks KE. Dedifferentiated chondrosarcoma with rhabdomyosarcomatous differentiation. Am J Surg Pathol 1996, **20**: 293–298.

488 Sakamoto A, Oda Y, Adachi T, Oshiro Y, Tamiya S, Tanaka K, Matsuda S, Iwamoto Y, Tsuneyoshi M. H-ras oncogene mutation in dedifferentiated chondrosarcoma: polymerase chain reaction-restriction fragment length polymorphism analysis. Mod Pathol 2001, **14**: 343–349.

489 Staals EL, Bacchini P, Bertoni F. Dedifferentiated central chondrosarcoma. Cancer 2006, **106**: 2682–2691.

490 Tetu B, Ordóñez NG, Ayala AG, Mackay B: Chondrosarcoma with additional mesenchymal component (dedifferentiated chondrosarcoma). II. An immunohistochemical and electron microscopic study. Cancer 1986, **58**: 287–298.

Mesenchymal chondrosarcoma

491 Bertoni F, Picci P, Bacchini P, Capanna R, Innao V, Bacci G, Campanacci M. Mesenchymal chondrosarcoma of bone and soft tissues. Cancer 1983, **52**: 533–541.

492 Cremonini A, Kuhn E, De Biase P, Franchi A. Well-differentiated chondrosarcoma of the humerus with prominent granular cell component: a hitherto unreported occurrence. Int J Surg Pathol 2006, **14**: 147–154.

493 Dabska M, Huvos AG. Mesenchymal chondrosarcoma in the young. A clinicopathologic study of 19 patients with explanation of histogenesis. Virchows Arch [A] 1983, **399**: 89–104.

494 Fanburg-Smith JC, Auerbach A, Marwaha JS, Wang Z, Rushing EJ. Reappraisal of mesenchymal chondrosarcoma: novel morphologic observations of the hyaline cartilage and endochondral ossification and beta-catenin, Sox9, and osteocalcin immunostaining of 22 cases. Hum Pathol 2010, **41**: 653–662.

495 Frydman CP, Klein MJ, Abdelwahab IF, Zwass A. Primitive multipotential primary sarcoma of bone. A case report and immunohistochemical study. Mod Pathol 1991, **4**: 768–772.

496 Gengler C, Letovanec I, Taminelli L, Egger JF, Guillou L. Desmin and myogenin reactivity in mesenchymal chondrosarcoma: a potential diagnostic pitfall. Histopathology 2005, **48**: 200–219.

497 Granter SR, Renshaw AA, Fletcher CD, Bhan AK, Rosenberg AE. CD99 reactivity in mesenchymal chondrosarcoma. Hum Pathol 1996, **27**: 1273–1276.

498 Guccion JG, Font RL, Enzinger FM, Zimmerman LE. Extraskeletal mesenchymal chondrosarcoma. Arch Pathol 1973, **95**: 336–340.

499 Huvos AG, Rosen G, Dabska M, Marcove RC. Mesenchymal chondrosarcoma. A clinicopathologic analysis of 35 patients with emphasis on treatment. Cancer 1983, **51**: 1230–1237.

500 Jacobson SA. Polyhistioma. A malignant tumor of bone and extraskeletal tissues. Cancer 1977, **40**: 2116–2130.

501 Ling LL-L, Steiner GC. Primary multipotential malignant neoplasm of bone. Chondrosarcoma associated with squamous cell carcinoma. Hum Pathol 1986, **17**: 317–320.

502 Nakashima Y, Unni KK, Shives TC, Swee RG, Dahlin DC. Mesenchymal chondrosarcoma of bone and soft tissue. A review of 111 cases. Cancer 1986, **57**: 2444–2453.

503 Steiner GC, Mirra JM, Bullough PG. Mesenchymal chondrosarcoma. A study of the ultrastructure. Cancer 1973, **32**: 926–939.

504 Swanson PE, Lillemoe TJ, Manivel JC, Wick MR. Mesenchymal chondrosarcoma. An immunohistochemical study. Arch Pathol Lab Med 1990, **114**: 943–948.

505 Wehrli BM, Huang W, De Cromrugghe B, Ayala AG, Czerniak B. Sox9, a master regulator of chondrogenesis, distinguishes mesenchymal chondrosarcoma from other small blue round cell tumors. Hum Pathol 2003, **34**: 263–269.

GIANT CELL TUMOR

506 Anazawa U, Hanaoka H, Shiraishi T, Morioka H, Morii T, Toyama Y. Similarities between giant cell tumor of bone, giant cell tumor of tendon sheath, and pigmented villonodular synovitis concerning ultrastructural cytochemical features of multinucleated giant cells and mononuclear stromal cells. Ultrastruct Pathol 2006, **30**: 151–158.

507 Aparisi T. Giant cell tumor of bone. Acta Orthop Scand 1978, **173**(Suppl): 1–38.

508 Aparisi T, Arborgh B, Ericsson JLE. Giant cell tumor of bone. Virchows Arch [A] 1979, **381**: 159–178.

509 Aqel NM, Pringle JA, Horton MA. Cellular heterogeneity in giant cell tumour of bone (osteoclastoma). An immunohistological study of 16 cases. Histopathology 1988, **13**: 675–685.

510 Athanasou NA, Bliss E, Gatter KC, Heryet A, Woods CG, McGee JO. An immunohistological study of giant-cell tumour of bone. Evidence for an osteoclast origin of the giant cells. J Pathol 1985, **147**: 153–158.

511 Bertoni F, Bacchini P, Staals EL. Malignancy in giant cell tumor of bone. Cancer 2003, **97**: 2520–2590.

512 Bertoni F, Present D, Enneking WF. Giant-cell tumor of bone with pulmonary metastases. J Bone Joint Surg (Am) 1985, **67**: 890–900.

513 Bertoni F, Unni KK, Beabout JW, Ebersold MJ. Giant cell tumor of the skull. Cancer 1992, **70**: 1124–1132.

514 Biscaglia R, Bacchini P, Bertoni F. Giant cell tumor of the bones of the hand and foot. Cancer 2000, **88**: 2022–2032.

515 Bouropoulou V, Kontogeorgos G, Manika Z. A histological and immunoenzymatic study on the histogenesis of 'giant cell tumor of bones'. Pathol Res Pract 1985, **180**: 61–67.

516 Bridge JA, Neff JR, Bhatia PS, Sanger WG, Murphey MD. Cytogenetic findings and biologic behavior of giant cell tumors of bone. Cancer 1990, **65**: 2697–2703.

517 Bridge JA, Neff JR, Mouron BJ. Giant cell tumor of bone. Chromosomal analysis of 48 specimens and review of the literature. Cancer Genet Cytogenet 1992, **58**: 2–13.

518 Brimo F, Aziz M, Rosen G, Turcotte R, Nahal A. Malignancy in giant cell tumour of bone: is there a reproducible histological threshold? A study of three giant cell tumours with worrisome features. Histopathology 2007, **51**: 864–866.

519 Campanacci M, Giunti A, Olmi R. Giant-cell tumours of bone. A study of 209 cases with long-term follow-up in 130. Ital J Orthop Traumatol 1975, **1**: 249–277.

520 Dahlin DC, Cupps RE, Johnson EW Jr. Giant-cell tumor. A study of 195 cases. Cancer 1970, **25**: 1061–1070.

521 Dickson BC, Li SQ, Wunder JS, Ferguson PC, Eslami B, Werier JA, Turcotte RE, Kandel RA. Giant cell tumor of bone express p63. Mod Pathol 2008, **21**: 369–375.

522 Eckardt JJ, Grogan TJ. Giant cell tumor of bone. Clin Orthop 1986, **204**: 45–58.

523 Emley WE. Giant cell tumor of the sphenoid bone. A case report and review of literature. Arch Otolaryngol 1971, **94**: 369–374.

524 Emura I, Inoue Y, Ohnishi Y, Morita T, Saito H, Tajima T. Histochemical, immunohistochemical and ultrastructural investigations of giant cell tumors of bone. Acta Pathol Jpn 1986, **36**: 691–702.

525 Fain JS, Unni KK, Beabout JW, Rock MG. Nonepiphyseal giant cell tumor of the long bones. Clinical, radiologic, and pathologic study. Cancer 1993, **71**: 3514–3519.

526 Fornasier VL, Flores L, Hastings D, Sharp T. Virus-like filamentous intranuclear inclusions in a giant-cell tumor, not associated with Paget's disease of bone. A case report. J Bone Joint Surg (Am) 1985, **67**: 333–336.

527 Fukunaga M, Nikaido T, Shimoda T, Ushigoma S, Nakamori K. A flow cytometric DNA analysis of giant cell tumors of bone including two cases with malignant transformation. Cancer 1992, **70**: 1886–1894.

528 Goldring SR, Schiller AL, Mankin HJ, Dayer J-M, Krane SM. Characterization of cells from human giant cell tumors of bone. Clin Orthop 1986, **204**: 59–75.

529 Hanaoka H, Friedman B, Mack RP. Ultrastructure and histogenesis of giant-cell tumor of bone. Cancer 1970, **25**: 1408–1423.

530 Hoch BL, Inwards C, Rosenberg AE. Multicentric giant cell tumor of bone: a clinicopathologic analysis of thirty cases [abstract]. Mod Pathol 2003, **16**: 13a–14a.

531 Huang L, Xu J, Wood DJ, Zheng MH. Gene expression of osteoprotegerin ligand, osteoprotegerin, and receptor activator of NF-κB in giant cell tumor of bone: possible involvement in tumor cell-induced osteoclast-like cell formation. Am J Pathol 2000, **156**: 761–767.

532 Kasahara K, Yamamuro T, Kasahara A. Giant-cell tumour of bone. Cytological studies. Br J Cancer 1979, **40**: 201–209.

533 Ladanyi M, Traganos F, Huvos AG. Benign metastasizing giant cell tumors of bone. A DNA flow cytometric study. Cancer 1989, **64**: 1521–1526.

534 Lau YS, Sabokbar A, Gibbons CL, Giele H, Athanasou N. Phenotypic and molecular studies of giant-cell tumors of bone and soft tissue. Hum Pathol 2005, **36**: 945–954.

535 Layfield LJ, Bentley RC, Mirra JM. Pseudoanaplastic giant cell tumor of bone. Arch Pathol Lab Med 1999, **123**: 163–166.

536 Lee CH, Espinosa I, Jensen KC, Subramanian S, Zhu SX, Varma S, Montgomery KD, Nielsen TO, van de Rijn M, West RB. Gene expression profiling identifies p63 as a diagnostic marker for giant cell tumor of the bone. Mod Pathol 2008, **21**: 531–539.

537 Lindeman JH, Hanemaaijer R, Mulder A, Dijkstra PD, Szuhai K, Bromme D, Verheijen JH, Hogendoorn PC. Cathepsin K is the principal protease in giant cell tumor of bone. Am J Pathol 2004, **165**: 593–600.

538 Linden MD. Giant cell lesions of bone and soft tissues: diagnostic value of immunohistochemistry. Lab Invest 2009, **89**(Suppl 1): 18A.

539 Liu TC, Ji ZM, Wang LT. Giant cell tumors of bone. An immunohistochemical study. Pathol Res Pract 1989, **185**: 448–453.

540 Mankin HJ, Fogelson FS, Thrasher AZ, Jaffer F. Massive resection and allograft transplantation in the treatment of malignant bone tumors. N Engl J Med 1976, **294**: 1247–1255.

541 Masui F, Ushigome S, Fujii K. Giant cell tumor of bone: an immunohistochemical comparative study. Pathol Int 1998, **48**: 355–361.

542 Masui F, Ushigome S, Fujii K. Giant cell tumor of bone: a clinicopathologic study of prognostic factors. Pathol Int 1998, **48**: 723–729.

543 McComb EN, Johansson SL, Neff JR, Nelson M, Bridge JA. Chromosomal anomalies exclusive of telomeric associations in giant cell tumor of bone. Cancer Genet Cytogenet 1996, **88**: 163–166.

544 McDonald DJ, Sim FH, McLeod RA, Dahlin DC. Giant-cell tumor of bone. J Bone Joint Surg (Am) 1986, **68**: 235–242.

545 Medeiros J, Beckstead J, Rosenberg A, Warnke R, Wood G. Giant cells and mononuclear cells of giant cell tumor of bone resemble histiocytes. Appl Immunohistochem 1993, **1**: 115–122.

546 Meis JM, Dorfman HD, Nathanson SD, Haggar AM, Wu KK. Primary malignant giant cell tumor of bone. 'Dedifferentiated' giant cell tumor. Mod Pathol 1989, **2**: 541–546.

547 Metze K, Ciplea AG, Hettwer H, Barckhaus RH. Size dependent enzyme activities of multinucleated (osteoclastic) giant cells in bone tumors. Pathol Res Pract 1987, **182**: 214–221.

548 Mii Y, Miyauchi Y, Morishita T, Miura S, Honoki K, Aoki M, Tamai S. Osteoclast origin of giant cells in giant cell tumors of bone. Ultrastructural and cytochemical study of six cases. Ultrastruct Pathol 1991, **15**: 623–629.

549 Nascimento AG, Huvos AG, Marcove RC. Primary malignant giant cell tumor of bone. A study of eight cases and review of the literature. Cancer 1979, **44**: 1393–1402.

550 Negoescu A, Mandache E. The ultrastructure of nuclear inclusions in the giant-cell tumor of bone. Pathol Res Pract 1989, **184**: 410–417.

551 Oda Y, Sakamoto A, Saito T, Matsuda S, Tanaka K, Iwamoto Y, Tsuneyoshi M. Secondary malignant giant-cell tumour of bone: molecular abnormalities of p53 and H-ras gene correlated with malignant transformation. Histopathology 2001, **39**: 629–637.

552 Oliveira P, Perez E, Ortega A, Terual R, Gomes C, Moreno LF, Duenas A, De La Garza J, Melendez-Zajgla J, Maldonado V. Estrogen receptor expression in giant cell tumors of the bone. Hum Pathol 2002, **33**: 165–169.

553 Parrish FF. Allograft replacement of all or part of the end of a long bone following excision of a tumor. Report of twenty-one cases. J Bone Joint Surg (Am) 1973, **55**: 1–22.

554 Picci P, Manfrini M, Zucchi V, Gherlinzoni F, Rock M, Bertoni F, Neff JR. Giant-cell tumor of bone in skeletally immature patients. J Bone Joint Surg (Am) 1983, **65**: 486–490.

555 Present D, Bertoni F, Hudson T, Enneking WF. The correlation between the radiologic staging studies and histopathologic findings in aggressive stage 3 giant cell tumor of bone. Cancer 1986, **57**: 237–244.

556 Regezi JA, Zarbo RJ, Lloyd RV. Muramidase, α-1 antitrypsin, α-1 antichymotrypsin, and S-100 protein immunoreactivity in giant cell lesions. Cancer 1987, **59**: 64–68.

557 Rock MG, Pritchard DJ, Unni KK. Metastases from histologically benign giant-cell tumor of bone. J Bone Joint Surg (Am) 1984, **66**: 269–274.

558 Roessner A, Bassewitz DBv, Schlake W, Thorwesten G, Grundmann E. Biologic characterization of human bone tumors. III. Giant cell tumor of bone. A combined electron microscopical, histochemical, and autoradiographical study. Pathol Res Pract 1984, **178**: 431–440.

559 Roux S, Amazit L, Meduri G, Guiochon-Mantel A, Milgrom E, Mariette X. RANK (receptor activator of nuclear factor kappa B) and RANK ligand are expressed in giant cell tumors of bone. Am J Clin Pathol 2002, **117**: 210–216.

560 Sanerkin NG. Malignancy, aggressiveness, and recurrence in giant cell tumor of bone. Cancer 1980, **46**: 1641–1649.

561 Sara AS, Ayala AG, el-Naggar A, Ro JY, Raymond AK, Murray JA. Giant cell tumor of bone. A clinicopathologic and DNA flow cytometric analysis. Cancer 1990, **66**: 2186–2190.

562 Savini R, Gherlinzoni F, Morandi M, Neff JR, Picci P. Surgical treatment of giant-cell tumor of the spine. Istituto Ortopedico Rizzoli. J Bone Joint Surg (Am) 1983, **65**: 1283–1290.

563 Schajowicz F. Giant-cell tumors of bone (osteoclastoma). A pathological and histochemical study. J Bone Joint Surg (Am) 1961, **43**: 1–29.

564 Schajowicz F, Ubios AM, Santini Araujo E, Cabrini RL. Virus-like intranuclear inclusions in giant cell tumor of bone. Clin Orthop 1985, **201**: 247–250.

565 Schoedel KE, Greco MA, Stetler-Stevenson WG, Ohori NP, Goswami S, Present D, Steinger GC. Expression of metalloproteinases and tissue inhibitors of metalloproteinases in giant cell tumor of bone: an immunohistochemical study with clinical correlation. Hum Pathol 1996, **27**: 1144–1148.

566 Sciot R, Dorfman H, Brys P, Dal Cin P, De Wever I, Fletcher CD, Jonson K, Mandahl N, Mertens F, Mitelman F, Rosai J, Rydholm A, Samson I, Tallini G, Van den Berghe H, Vanni R, Willén H. Cytogenetic–morphologic correlations in aneurysmal bone cyst, giant cell tumor of bone and combined lesions. A report from the CHAMP study group. Mod Pathol 2000, **13**: 1206–1210.

567 Seethala RR, Goldblum JR, Hicks DG, Lehman M, Khurana JS, Pasha TL, Zhang PJ. Immunohistochemical evaluation of microphthalmia-associated transcription factor expression in giant cell lesions. Mod Pathol 2004, **17**: 1491–1496.

568 Steiner GC, Ghosh L, Dorfman HD. Ultrastructure of giant cell tumors of bone. Hum Pathol 1972, **3**: 569–586.

569 Sulh MA, Greco MA, Jiang T, Goswami SB, Present D, Steiner G. Proliferation index and vascular density of giant cell tumors of bone: are they prognostic markers? Cancer 1996, **77**: 2044–2051.

570 Sung HW, Kuo DP, Shu WP, Chai YB, Liu CC, Li SM. Giant-cell tumor of bone. Analysis of two hundred and eight cases in Chinese patients. J Bone Joint Surg (Am) 1982, **64**: 755–761.

571 Sybrandy S, de la Fuente AA. Multiple giant tumour of bone. Report of a case. J Bone Joint Surg (Br) 1973, **55**: 350–356.

572 Teot LA, O'Keefe RJ, Rosier RN, O'Connell JX, Fox EJ, Hicks DG. Extraosseous primary and recurrent giant cell tumors: transforming growth factor-beta1 and -beta2 expression may explain metaplastic bone formation. Hum Pathol 1996, **27**: 625–632.

573 Ueda Y, Imai K, Tsuchiya H, Fujimoto N, Nakanishi I, Katsuda S, Seiki M, Okada Y. Matrix metalloproteinase 9 (gelatinise B) is expressed in multinucleated giant cells of human giant cell tumor of bone and is associated with vascular invasion. Am J Pathol 1996, **148**: 611–622.

574 Watanabe K, Tajino T, Kusakabe T, Saitoh A, Suzuki T. Giant cell tumor of bone: frequent actin immunoreactivity in stromal tumor cells. Pathol Int 1997, **47**: 680–684.

575 Wold LE, Swee RG. Giant cell tumor of the small bones of the hands and feet. Semin Diagn Pathol 1984, **1**: 173–184.

576 Wolfe JT III, Scheithauer BW, Dahlin DC. Giant-cell tumor of the sphenoid bone. Review of 10 cases. J Neurosurg 1983, **59**: 322–327.

577 Wülling M, Delling G, Kaiser E. The origin of the neoplastic stromal cell in giant cell tumor of bone. Hum Pathol 2003, **34**: 983–993.

578 Yoshida H, Akeho M, Yumoto T. Giant cell tumor of bone. Enzyme histochemical, biochemical and tissue culture studies. Virchows Arch [A] 1982, **395**: 319–330.

579 Zheng MH, Fan Y, Wysocki SJ, Lau AT, Robertson T, Beilharz M, Wood DJ, Papadimitriou JM. Gene expression of transforming growth factor-beta 1 and its type II receptor in giant cell tumors of bone. Possible involvement in osteoclast-like cell migration. Am J Pathol 1994, **145**: 1095–1104.

MARROW TUMORS

Ewing sarcoma/primitive neuroectodermal tumor (PNET)

580 Adams V, Hany MA, Schmid M, Hassam S, Briner J, Niggli FK. Detection of t(11;22)(q24;q12) translocation breakpoint in paraffin-embedded tissue of the Ewing's sarcoma family by nested reverse transcription-polymerase chain reaction. Diagn Mol Pathol 1996, **5**: 107–113.

581 Amann G, Zoubek A, Salzer-Kuntschik M, Windhager R, Kovar H. Relation of neuroglial marker expression and EWS gene fusion types in MIC2/CD99-positive tumors of the Ewing family. Hum Pathol 1999, **30**: 1058–1064.

582 Ambros IM, Ambros PF, Strehl S, Kovar H, Gadner H, Salzer-Kuntschik M. MIC2 is a specific marker for Ewing's sarcoma and peripheral primitive neuroectodermal tumors. Evidence for a common histogenesis of Ewing's sarcoma and peripheral primitive neuroectodermal tumors from MIC2 expression and specific chromosome aberration. Cancer 1991, **67**: 1886–1893.

583 Amir G, Issakov J, Meller I, Sucher E, Peyser A, Cohen IJ, Yaniv I, Arush MWB, Tavori U, Kollender Y, Ron N, Peylan-Ramu N. Expression of p53 gene product and cell proliferation marker Ki-67 in Ewing's sarcoma: correlation with clinical outcome. Hum Pathol 2002, **33**: 170–174.

584 Askin FB, Perlman EJ. Neuroblastoma and peripheral neuroectodermal tumors. Am J Clin Pathol 1998, **109**: S23–S30.

585 Askin FB, Rosai J, Sibley RK, Dehner LP, McAlister WH. Malignant small cell tumor of the thoracopulmonary region in childhood; a distinctive clinicopathologic entity of uncertain histogenesis. Cancer 1979, **43**: 2438–2451.

586 Bacci G, Toni A, Avella M, Manfrini M, Sudanese A, Ciaroni D, Boriani S, Emiliani E, Campanacci M. Long-term results in 144 localized Ewing's sarcoma patients treated with combined therapy. Cancer 1989, **63**: 1477–1486.

587 Barr FG, Womer RB. Molecular diagnosis of Ewing family tumors: too many fusions … ? J Mol Diagn 2007, **9**: 437–440.

588 Bator SM, Bauer TW, Marks KE, Norris DG. Periosteal Ewing's sarcoma. Cancer 1986, **58**: 1781–1784.

589 Batsakis JG, El-Naggar AK. Ewing's sarcoma and primitive neuroectodermal tumors; cytogenetic cynosures seeking a common histogenesis. Adv Anat Pathol 1997, **4**: 207–220.

590 Bridge JA, Fidler ME, Neff JR, Degenhardt J, Wang M, Walker C, Dorfman HD, Baker KS, Seemayer TA. Adamantinoma-like Ewing's sarcoma: genomic confirmation, phenotypic drift. Am J Surg Pathol 1999, **23**: 159–165.

591 Bridge RS, Rajaram V, Dehner LP, Pfeifer JD, Perry A. Molecular diagnosis of Ewing sarcoma/primitive neuroectodermal tumor in routinely processed tissue: a comparison of two FISH strategies and RT-PCR in malignant round cell tumors. Mod Pathol 2006 **19**: 1–8.

592 Brinkhuis M, Winjnaendts LC, van der Linden JC, van Unnik AJ, Voute PA, Baak JP, Meijer CJ. Peripheral primitive neuroectodermal tumour and extraosseous Ewing's sarcoma; a histological, immunohistochemical and DNA flow cytometric study. Virchows Arch 1995, **425**: 611–616.

593 Cangir A, Vietti TJ, Gehan EA, Burgert EO Jr, Thomas P, Tefft M, Nesbit ME, Kissane J, Pritchard D. Ewing's sarcoma metastatic at diagnosis. Results and comparisons of two intergroup Ewing's sarcoma studies. Cancer 1990, **66**: 887–893.

594 Carter RL, al-Sams SZ, Corbett RP, Clinton S. A comparative study of immunohistochemical staining for neuron-specific enolase, protein gene product 9.5 and S-100 protein in neuroblastoma, Ewing's sarcoma and other round cell tumours in children. Histopathology 1990, **16**: 461–467.

595 Cavazzana AO, Miser JS, Jefferson J, Triche TJ. Experimental evidence for a neural origin of Ewing's sarcoma of bone. Am J Pathol 1987, **127**: 507–518.

596 Coffin CM, Lowichik A, Zhou H. Treatment effects in pediatric soft tissue and bone tumors: practical considerations for the pathologist. Am J Clin Pathol 2005, **123**: 75–90.

597 Cotterill SJ, Ahrens S, Paulussen M, Jurgens HF, Voute PA, Gadner H, Craft AW. Prognostic factors in Ewing's tumor of bone: analysis of 975 patients from the European intergroup cooperative Ewing's sarcoma study group. J Clin Oncol 2000, **18**: 3108–3114.

598 de Alava E, Antonescu CR, Panizo A, Leung D, Meyers PA, Huvos AG, Pardo-Mindan FJ, Healey JH, Ladanyi M. Prognostic impact of p53 status in Ewing sarcoma. Cancer 2000, **89**: 783–792.

599 de Alava E, Panizo A, Antonescu CR, Huvos AG, Pardo-Mindan FJ, Barr FG, Ladanyi M. Associaton of EWS-FLI1 type 1 fusion with lower proliferative rate in Ewing's sarcoma. Am J Pathol 2000, **156**: 849–855.

600 de Alava E, Pardo J. Ewing tumor: tumor biology and clinical applications. Int J Surg Pathol 2001, **9**: 7–17.

601 Deneen B, Denny CT. Loss of p16 pathways stabilizes EWS/FLI1 expression and complements EWS/FLI1 mediated transformation. Oncogene 2001, **20**: 6731–6741.

602 Devoe K, Weidner N. Immunohistochemistry of small round-cell tumors. Semin Diagn Pathol 2000, **17**: 216–224.

603 Dierick AM, Langlois M, Van Oostveldt P, Roels H. The prognostic significance of the DNA content in Ewing's sarcoma. A retrospective cytophotometric and flow cytometric study. Histopathology 1993, **23**: 333–339.

604 Dockhorn-Dworniczak B, Schafer KL, Dantcheva R, Blasius S, Winkelmann W, Strehl S, Burdach S, van Valen F, Jurgens H, Bocker W. Diagnostic value of the molecular genetic detection of the t(11;22) translocation in Ewing's tumours. Virchows Arch 1994, **425**: 107–112.

605 Downing JR, Head DR, Parham DM, Douglass EC, Hulshof MG, Link MP, Motroni TA, Grier HE, Curcio-Brint AM, Shapiro DN. Detection of the (11;22)(q24;q12) translocation of Ewing's sarcoma and peripheral neuroectodermal tumor by reverse transcription polymerase chain reaction. Am J Pathol 1993, **143**: 1294–1300.

606 Ehara S, Kattapuram SV, Egglin TK. Ewing's sarcoma. Radiographic pattern of healing and bony complications in patients with long-term survival. Cancer 1991, **68**: 1531–1535.

607 Fellinger EJ, Garin-Chesa P, Glasser DB, Huvos AG, Rettig WJ. Comparison of cell surface antigen HBA71 (p30/32MIC2), neuron-specific enolase, and vimentin in the immunohistochemical analysis of Ewing's sarcoma of bone. Am J Surg Pathol 1992, **16**: 746–755.

608 Fidelia-Lambert MN, Zhuang Z, Tsokos M. Sensitive detection of rare Ewing's sarcoma cells in peripheral blood by reverse transcriptase polymerase chain reaction. Hum Pathol 1999, **30**: 78–80.

609 Fizazi K, Dohollou N, Blay J-Y, Guérin S, Le Cesne AL, André F, Pouillart P, Tursz T, Nguyen BB. Ewing's family of tumors in adults: multivariate analysis of survival and long-term results of multimodality therapy in 182 patients. J Clin Oncol 1998, **16**: 3736–3743.

610 Folpe AL, Hill CE, Parham DM, O'Shea PA, Weiss SW. Immunohistochemical detection of FLI-1 protein expression: a study of 132 round cell tumors with emphasis on CD99-positive mimics of Ewing's sarcoma/primitive neuroectodermal tumor. Am J Surg Pathol 2000, **24**: 1657–1662.

611 Folpe AL, Goldblum JR, Rubin BP, Shehata BM, Liu W, Dei Tos AP, Weiss SW. Morphologic and immunophenotypic diversity in Ewing family tumors: a study of 66 genetically confirmed cases. Am J Surg Pathol 2005, **29**: 1025–1033.

612 Fujii H, Honoki K, Enomoto Y, Kasai T, Kido A, Amano I, Kumamoto M, Morishita T, Mii Y, Nonomura A, Takakura Y. Adamantinoma-like Ewing's sarcoma with EWS-FLI1 fusion gene: a case report. Virchows Arch 2006, **449**: 579–584.

613 Fukunaga M, Ushigome S. Periosteal Ewing-like adamantinoma. Virchows Arch 1998, **433**: 385–389.

614 Garin-Chesa P, Fellinger EJ, Huvos AG, Beresford HR, Melamed MR, Triche TJ, Rettig WJ. Immunohistochemical analysis of neural cell adhesion molecules. Differential expression in small round cell tumors of childhood and adolescence. Am J Pathol 1991, **139**: 275–286.

615 Gasparini M, Barni S, Lattuada A, Musumeci R, Bonadonna G, Fossati-Bellani F. Ten years experience with Ewing's sarcoma. Tumori 1977, **63**: 77–90.

616 Gerald WL. A practical approach to the differential diagnosis of small round cell tumors of infancy using recent scientific and technical advances. Int J Surg Pathol 2000, **8**: 87–97.

617 Ginsberg JP, de Alava E, Ladanyi M, Wexler LH, Kovar H, Paulussen M, Zoubek A, Dockhorn-Dworniczak B, Juergens H, Wunder JS, Andrulis IL, Malik R, Sorensen PH, Womer RB, Barr FG. EWS-FLI1 and EWS-ERG gene fusions are associated with similar clinical phenotypes in Ewing's sarcoma. J Clin Oncol 1999, **17**: 1809–1814.

618 Gu M, Antonescu CR, Guiter G, Huvos AG, Ladanyi M, Zakowski MF. Cytokeratin immunoreactivity in Ewing's sarcoma: prevalence in 50 cases confirmed by molecular studies. Am J Surg Pathol 2000, **24**: 410–416.

619 Guiter GE, Gamboni MM, Zakowski MF. The cytology of extraskeletal Ewing sarcoma. Cancer 1999, **87**: 141–148.

620 Hameed M. Small round cell tumors of bone. Arch Pathol Lab Med 2007, **131**: 192–204.

621 Hartman KR, Triche TJ, Kinsella TJ, Miser JS. Prognostic value of histopathology in Ewing's sarcoma. Long-term follow-up of distal extremity primary tumors. Cancer 1991, **67**: 163–171.

622 Hasegawa SL, Davison JM, Rutten A, Fletcher JA, Fletcher CD. Primary cutaneous Ewing's sarcoma: immunophenotypic and molecular cytogenetic evaluation of five cases. Am J Surg Pathol 1998, **22**: 310–318.

623 Hasegawa T, Hirose T, Kudo E, Hizawa K, Yamawaki S, Ishii S. Atypical primitive neuroectodermal tumors. Comparative light and electron microscopic and immunohistochemical studies on peripheral neuroepitheliomas and Ewing's sarcomas. Acta Pathol Jpn 1991, **41**: 444–454.

624 Hess E, Cohen C, DeRose PB, Yost BA, Costa MJ. Nonspecificity of p30/32[MIC2] immunolocalization with the 013 monoclonal antibody in the diagnosis of Ewing's sarcoma: application of an algorithmic immunohistochemical analysis. Appl Immunohistochem 1997, **5**: 94–103.

625 Hoffmann C, Ahrens S, Dunst J, Hillmann A, Winkelmann W, Craft A, Gobel U, Rube C, Voute PA, Harms D, Jurgens H. Pelvic Ewing sarcoma: a retrospective analysis of 241 cases. Cancer 1999, **85**: 869–877.

626 Jaffe R, Santamaria M, Yunis EJ, Tannery NH, Agostini RM Jr, Medina J, Goodman M. The neuroectodermal tumor of bone. Am J Surg Pathol 1984, **8**: 885–898.

627 Kaspers GJ, Kamphorst W, van de Graaff M, van Alphen HA, Veerman AJ. Primary spinal epidural extraosseous Ewing's sarcoma. Cancer 1991, **68**: 648–654.

628 Kissane JM, Askin FB, Foulkes M, Stratton LB, Shirley SF. Ewing's sarcoma of bone. Clinicopathologic aspects of 303 cases from the Intergroup Ewing's Sarcoma Study. Hum Pathol 1983, **14**: 773–779.

629 Kissane JM, Askin FB, Nesbit M, Vietti T, Burgert EO Jr, Cangir A, Gehan EA, Perez CA, Pritchard DJ, Tefft M. Sarcomas of bone in childhood. Pathologic aspects. In Glicksmann A, Tefft M (eds): Bone and soft tissue sarcomas. J Natl Cancer Inst Monograph 1981, **56**: 29–41.

630 Knezevich SR, Hendson G, Mathers JA, Carpenter B, Lopez-Terrada D, Brown KL, Sorensen PH. Absence of detectable EWS/FLI1 expression after therapy-induced neural differentiation in Ewing sarcoma. Hum Pathol 1998, **29**: 289–294.

631 Kovar H, Jug G, Aryee DN, Zoubek A, Ambros P, Gruber B, Windhager R, Gadner H. Among genes involved in the RB dependent cell cycle regulatory cascade, the p16 tumor suppressor gene is frequently lost in the Ewing family of tumors. Oncogene 1997, **15**: 2225–2232.

632 Kumar S, Pack S, Kumar D, Walker R, Quezado M, Zhuang Z, Meltzer P, Tsokos M. Detection of EWS-FLI-1 fusion in Ewing's sarcoma/peripheral primitive neuroectodermal tumor by fluorescence in situ hybridisation using formalin-fixed paraffin-embedded tissue. Hum Pathol 1999, **30**: 324–330.

633 Ladanyi M, Heinemann FS, Huvos AG, Rao PH, Chen QG, Jhanwar SC. Neural differentiation in small round cell tumors of bone and soft tissue with the translocation t(11;22)(q24;q12). An immunohistochemical study of 11 cases. Hum Pathol 1990, **21**: 1245–1251.

634 Ladanyi M, Lewis R, Garin-Chesa P, Rettig WJ, Huvos AG, Healey JH, Jhanwar SC. EWS rearrangement in Ewing's sarcoma and peripheral neuroectodermal tumor. Molecular detection and correlation with cytogenetic analysis and MIC2 expression. Diagn Mol Pathol 1993, **2**: 141–146.

635 Lawlor ER, Mathers JA, Bainbridge T, Horsman DE, Kawai A, Healey JH, Huvos AG, Bridge JA, Ladanyi M, Sorensen PH. Peripheral primitive neuroectodermal tumors in adults: documentation by molecular analysis. J Clin Oncol 1998, **16**: 1150–1157.

636 Leong A S-Y, Milios J. Small round cell tumors in childhood. Immunohistochemical studies in rhabdomyosarcoma, neuroblastoma, Ewing's sarcoma, and lymphoblastic lymphoma. Surg Pathol 1989, **2**: 5–18.

637 Lewis TB, Coffin CM, Bernard PS. Differentiating Ewing's sarcoma from other round blue cell tumors using a RT-PCR translocation panel on formalin-fixed paraffin-embedded tissues. Mod Pathol 2007, **20**: 397–404.

638 Llombart-Bosch A, Machado I, Navarro S, Bertoni F, Bacchini P, Alberghini M, Karzeladze A, Savelov N, Petrov S, Alvarado-Cabrero I, Mihaila D, Terrier P, Lopez-Guerrero JA, Picci P. Histological heterogeneity of Ewing's sarcoma/PNET: an immunohistochemical analysis of 415 genetically confirmed cases with clinical support. Virchows Arch 2009, **455**: 397–411.

639 Llombart-Bosch A, Contesso G, Reydro-Olaya A. Histology, immunohistochemistry, and electron microscopy of small round cell tumors of bone. Semin Diagn Pathol 1996, **13**: 153–170.

640 Llombart-Bosch A, Navarro S. Immunohistochemical detection of EWS and FLI-1 proteins in Ewing sarcoma and primitive neuroectodermal tumors: comparative analysis with CD99(MIC-2) expression. Appl Immunohistochem Molecul Morphol 2001, **9**: 255–260.

641 Löning TH, Liebsch J, Delling G. Osteosarcomas and Ewing's sarcomas. Comparative immunocytochemical investigation of filamentous proteins and cell membrane determinants. Virchows Arch [A] 1985, **407**: 323–336.

642 Mangham DC, Williams A, McMullan DJ, McClure J, Sumathi VP, Grimer RJ, Davies AM. Ewing's sarcoma of bone: the detection of specific transcripts in a large, consecutive series of formalin-fixed, decalcified, paraffin-embedded tissue samples using the reverse transcriptase-polymerase chain reaction. Histopathology 2006, **48**: 363–376.

643 Mawad JK, Mackay B, Raymond AK, Ayala AG. Electron microscopy in the diagnosis of small round cell tumors of bone. Ultrastruct Pathol 1994, **18**: 263–268.

644 Maygarden SJ, Askin FB, Siegal GP, Gilula LA, Schoppe J, Foulkes M, Kissane JM, Nesbit M. Ewing sarcoma of bone in infants and toddlers. A clinicopathologic report from the Intergroup Ewing's Study. Cancer 1993, **71**: 2109–2118.

645 Meis-Kindblom JM, Stenman G, Kindblom LG. Differential diagnosis of small round cell tumors. Semin Diagn Pathol 1996, **13**: 213–241.

646 Mendenhall CM, Marcus RB Jr, Enneking WF, Springfield DS, Thar TL, Million RR. The prognostic significance of soft tissue extension in Ewing's sarcoma. Cancer 1983, **51**: 913–917.

647 Miettinen M, Lehto V-P, Virtanen I. Histogenesis of Ewing's sarcoma. An evaluation of intermediate filaments and endothelial cell markers. Virchows Arch [Cell Pathol] 1982, **41**: 277–284.

648 Moll R, Lee I, Gould VE, Berndt R, Roessner A, Franke WW. Immunocytochemical analysis of Ewing's tumors. Patterns of expression of intermediate filaments and desmosomal proteins indicate cell type heterogeneity and pluripotential differentiation. Am J Pathol 1987, **127**: 288–304.

649 Montforte-Muñoz H, Lopez-Terrada D, Affendie H, Rowland JM, Triche TJ. Documentation of EWS gene rearrangements by fluorescence in-situ hybridization (FISH) in frozen sections of Ewing's sarcoma-peripheral primitive neuroectodermal tumor. Am J Surg Pathol 1999, **23**: 309–315.

650 Nascimento AG, Unni KK, Pritchard DJ, Cooper KL, Dahlin DC. A clinicopathologic study of 20 cases of large-cell (atypical) Ewing's sarcoma of bone. Am J Surg Pathol 1980, **4**: 29–36.

651 Navarro S, Cavazzana AO, Llombart-Bosch A, Triche TJ. Comparison of Ewing's sarcoma of bone and peripheral neuroepithelioma. An immunocytochemical and ultrastructural analysis of two primitive neuroectodermal neoplasms. Arch Pathol Lab Med 1994, **118**: 608–615.

652 Neff JR. Nonmetastatic Ewing's sarcoma of bone. The role of surgical therapy. Clin Orthop 1980, **204**: 111–118.

653 Nogueira E, Navarro S, Pellín A, Llombart-Bosch A. Activation of TRK genes in Ewing's sarcoma. Trk A receptor expression linked to neural differentiation. Diagn Mol Pathol 1997, **6**: 10–16.

654 Noguera R, Triche TJ, Navarro S, Tsokos M, Llombart-Bosch A. Dynamic model of differentiation in Ewing's sarcoma cells. Comparative analysis of morphologic, immunocytochemical, and oncogene expression parameters. Lab Invest 1992, **66**: 143–151.

655 O'Sullivan MJ, Perlman EJ, Furman J, Humphrey PA, Dehner LP, Pfeifer JD. Visceral primitive peripheral neuroectodermal tumors: a clinicopathologic and molecular study. Hum Pathol 2001, **32**: 1109–1115.

656 Ozaki T, Hillmann A, Hoffmann C, Rube C, Blasius S, Dunst J, Jurgens H, Winkelmann W. Significance of surgical margin on the prognosis of patients with Ewing's sarcoma: a report from the Cooperative Ewing's Sarcoma Study. Cancer 1996, **78**: 892–900.

657 Pagani A, Fischer-Colbrie R, Sanfilippo B, Winkler H, Cerrato M, Bussolati G. Secretogranin II expression in Ewing's sarcomas and primitive neuroectodermal tumors. Diagn Mol Pathol 1992, **1**: 165–172.

658 Pagani A, Macri L, Rosolen A, Toffolatti L, Stella A, Bussolati G. Neuroendocrine differentiation in Ewing's sarcoma and primitive neuroectodermal tumors revealed by reverse transcriptase-polymerase chain reaction of chromogranin mRNA. Diagn Mol Pathol 1998, **7**: 36–43.

659 Parham DM, Hijazi Y, Steinberg SM, Meyer WH, Horowitz M, Tzen CY, Wexler LH, Tsokos M. Neuroectodermal differentiation in Ewing's sarcoma family of tumors does not predict tumor behavior. Hum Pathol 1999, **30**: 911–918.

660 Perlman EJ, Dickman PS, Askin FB, Grier HE, Miser JS, Link MP. Ewing's sarcoma – routine diagnostic utilization of MIC2 analysis. A Pediatric Oncology Group/Children's Cancer Group Intergroup Study. Hum Pathol 1994, **25**: 304–307.

661 Picci P, Bohling T, Bacci G, Ferrari S, Sangiorgi L, Mercuri M, Ruggieri P, Manfrini M, Ferraro A, Casadei R, Benassi MS, Mancini AF, Rosito P, Cazzola A, Barbieri E, Tienghi A, Brach del Prever A, Comandone A, Bacchini P, Bertoni F. Chemotherapy-induced tumor necrosis as a prognostic factor in localized Ewing's sarcoma of the extremities. J Clin Oncol 1997, **15**: 1553–1559.

662 Pinto A, Grant LH, Hayes FA, Schell MJ, Parham DM. Immunohistochemical expression of neuron-specific enolase and Leu 7 in Ewing's sarcoma of bone. Cancer 1989, **64**: 1266–1273.

663 Razek A, Perez CA, Tefft M, Nesbit M, Vietti T, Burgert EO Jr, Kissane J, Pritchard DJ, Gehan EA. Intergroup Ewing's sarcoma study. Local

control related to radiation dose, volume, and site of primary lesion in Ewing's sarcoma. Cancer 1980, **46**: 516–521.

664 Roessner A, Jurgens H. Round cell tumours of bone. Pathol Res Pract 1993, **189**: 111–136.

665 Rosen G, Caparros B, Nirenberg A, Marcove RC, Huvos AG, Kosloff C, Lane J, Murphy ML. Ewing's sarcoma. Ten-year experience with adjuvant chemotherapy. Cancer 1981, **47**: 2204–2213.

666 Rosito P, Mancini AF, Rondelli R, Abate ME, Pession A, Bedei L, Bacci G, Picci P, Mercuri M, Ruggieri P, Frezza G, Campanacci M, Paolucci G. Italian cooperative study for the treatment of children and young adults with localized Ewing sarcoma of bone: a preliminary report of 6 years of experience. Cancer 1999, **86**: 421–428.

667 Sandberg AA, Bridge JA. Updates of cytogenetics and molecular genetics of bone and tissue tumors: Ewing sarcoma and peripheral primitive neuroectodermal tumors. Cancer Genet Cytogenet 2000, **123**: 1–26.

668 Scarpa S, Modesti A, Triche TJ. Extracellular matrix synthesis by undifferentiated childhood tumor cell lines. Am J Pathol 1987, **129**: 74–85.

669 Schajowicz F. Ewing's sarcoma and reticulum-cell sarcoma of bone. With special reference to the histochemical demonstration of glycogen as an aid to differential diagnosis. J Bone Joint Surg (Am) 1959, **41**: 349–356.

670 Scheurlen WG, Schwabe GC, Joos S, Mollenhauer J, Sorensen N, Kuhl J. Molecular analysis of childhood primitive neuroectodermal tumors defines markers associated with poor outcome. J Clin Oncol 1998, **16**: 2478–2485.

671 Schuetz AN, Rubin BP, Goldblum JR, Shehata B, Weiss SW, Liu W, Wick MR, Folpe AL. Intercellular junctions in Ewing sarcoma/primitive neuroectodermal tumor: additional evidence of epithelial differentiation. Mod Pathol 2005, **18**: 1403–1410.

672 Schmidt D, Mackay B, Ayala AG. Ewing's sarcoma with neuroblastoma-like features. Ultrastruct Pathol 1982, **3**: 143–151.

673 Scotlandi K, Serra M, Manara MC, Benini S, Sarti M, Maurici D, Lollini PL, Picci P, Bertoni F, Baldini N. Immunostaining of the p30/32^{MIC2} antigen and molecular detection of EWS rearrangements for the diagnosis of Ewing's sarcoma and peripheral neuroectodermal tumor. Hum Pathol 1996, **27**: 408–416.

674 Selleri L, Hermanson GG, Eubanks JH, Lewis KA, Evans GA. Molecular localization of the t(11;22)(q24;q12) translocation of Ewing sarcoma by chromosomal in situ suppression hybridization. Proc Natl Acad Sci U S A 1991, **88**: 887–891.

675 Shanfeld RL, Edelman J, Willis JE, Tuason L, Goldblum JR. Immunohistochemical analysis of neural markers in peripheral primitive neuroectodermal tumors (pNET) without light microscopic evidence of neural differentiation. Appl Immunohistochem 1997, **5**: 78–86.

676 Shishikura A, Ushigome S, Shimoda T. Primitive neuroectodermal tumors of bone and soft tissue. Histological subclassification and clinicopathologic correlations. Acta Pathol Jpn 1993, **43**: 176–186.

677 Siegal GP, Oliver WR, Reinus WR, Gilula LA, Foulkes MA, Kissane JM, Askin FB. Primary Ewing's sarcoma involving the bones of the head and neck. Cancer 1987, **60**: 2829–2840.

678 Sorensen P, Liu X, Delattre O, Rowland J, Biggs C, Thomas G, Triche T. Reverse transcriptase PCR amplification of EWS/FLI-1 fusion transcripts as a diagnostic test for peripheral primitive neuroectodermal tumors of childhood. Diagn Mol Pathol 1993, **2**: 147–157.

679 Srivastava A, Rosenberg AE, Selig M, Rubin BP, Nielsen GP. Keratin-positive Ewing's sarcoma: an ultrastructural study of 12 cases. Int J Surg Pathol 2005, **13**: 43–50.

680 Stephenson CF, Bridge JA, Sandberg AA. Cytogenetic and pathologic aspects of Ewing's sarcoma and neuroectodermal tumors. Hum Pathol 1992, **23**: 1270–1277.

681 Stevenson AJ, Chatten J, Bertoni P, Miettinen M. CD99 (p30/32MIC) neuroectodermal/Ewing's sarcoma antigen as an immunohistochemical marker. Review of more than 600 tumors and the literature experience. Appl Immunohistochem 1994, **2**: 231–240.

682 Suh CH, Ordóñez NG, Hicks J, Mackay B. Ultrastructure of the Ewing's sarcoma family of tumors. Ultrastruct Pathol 2002, **26**: 67–76.

683 Telles NC, Rabson AS, Pomeroy TC. Ewing's sarcoma. An autopsy study. Cancer 1978, **41**: 2321–2329.

684 Thomas PRM, Foulkes MA, Gilula LA, Burgert EO, Evans RG, Kissane J, Nesbit ME, Pritchard DJ, Tefft M, Vietti TJ. Primary Ewing's sarcoma of the ribs. A report from the Intergroup Ewing's Sarcoma Study. Cancer 1983, **51**: 1021–1027.

685 Thorner P, Squire J, Chilton-MacNeill S, Marrano P, Bayani J, Malkin D, Greenberg M, Lorenzana A, Zielenska M. Is the EWS/FLI-1 fusion transcript specific for Ewing sarcoma and peripheral primitive neuroectodermal tumor? A report of four cases showing this transcript in a wider range of tumor types. Am J Pathol 1996, **148**: 1125–1138.

686 Triche TJ, Ross WE. Glycogen-containing neuroblastoma with clinical and histopathologic features of Ewing's sarcoma. Cancer 1978, **41**: 1425–1432.

687 Tsuneyoshi M, Yokoyama R, Hashimoto H, Enjoji M. Comparative study of neuroectodermal tumor and Ewing's sarcoma of the bone. Histopathologic, immunohistochemical and ultrastructural features. Acta Pathol Jpn 1989, **39**: 573–581.

688 Ushigome S, Shimoda T, Takaki K, Nikaido T, Takakuwa T, Ishikawa E, Spjut HJ. Immunocytochemical and ultrastructural studies of the histogenesis of Ewing's sarcoma and putatively related tumors. Cancer 1989, **64**: 52–62.

689 Vakar-López F, Ayala AG, Raymond AK, Czerniak B. Epithelial phenotype in Ewing's sarcoma/primitive neuroectodermal tumor. Int J Surg Pathol 2001, **8**: 59–65.

690 Verrill MW, Judson IR, Harmer CL, Fisher C, Thomas JM, Wiltshaw E. Ewing's sarcoma and primitive neuroectodermal tumor in adults: are they different from Ewing's sarcoma and primitive neuroectodermal tumor in children? J Clin Oncol 1997, **15**: 2611–2621.

691 Wang L, Bhargava R, Zheng T, Wexler L, Collins MH, Roulston D, Ladanyi M. Undifferentiated small round cell sarcomas with rare EWS gene fusions: identification of a novel EWS-SP3 fusion and of additional cases with the EWS-ETV1 and EWS-FEV fusions. J Mol Diagn 2007, **9**: 498–509.

692 Wei G, Antonescu CR, de Alava E, Leung D, Huvos AG, Meyers PA, Healey JH, Ladanyi M. Prognostic impact of INK4A deletion in Ewing sarcoma. Cancer 2000, **89**: 793–799.

693 Weidner N, Tjoe J. Immunohistochemical profile of monoclonal antibody O13. Antibody that recognizes glycoprotein p30/32MIC2 and is useful in diagnosing Ewing's sarcoma and peripheral neuroepithelioma. Am J Surg Pathol 1994, **18**: 486–494.

694 Weinreb I, Goldstein D, Perez-Ordoñez B. Primary extraskeletal Ewing family tumor with complex epithelial differentiation: a unique case arising in the lateral neck presenting with Horner syndrome. Am J Surg Pathol 2008, **32**: 1742–1748.

695 West DC, Grier HE, Swallow MM, Demetri GD, Granowetter L, Sklar J. Detection of circulating tumor cells in patients with Ewing's sarcoma and peripheral primitive neuroectodermal tumor. J Clin Oncol 1997, **15**: 583–588.

696 Wilkins RM, Pritchard DJ, Burgert EO Jr, Unni KK. Ewing's sarcoma of bone. Experience with 140 patients. Cancer 1986, **58**: 2551–2555.

697 Yunis EJ, Agostini RM Jr, Walpusk JA, Hubbard JD. Glycogen in neuroblastomas. A light- and electron-microscopic study of 40 cases. Am J Surg Pathol 1979, **3**: 313–323.

698 Zoubek A, Dockhorn-Dworniczak B, Delattre O, Christiansen H, Niggli F, Gatterer-Menz I, Smith TL, Jurgens H, Gadner H, Kovar H. Does expression of different EWS chimeric transcripts define clinically distinct risk groups of Ewing tumor patients? J Clin Oncol 1996, **14**: 1245–1251.

Malignant lymphoma and related lesions

699 Abbondanzo SL, Devaney K. Hodgkin's disease involving bone and adjacent soft tissue in adults: a clinicopathologic and immunophenotypic study of seven cases. Int J Surg Pathol 1996, **3**: 147–154.

700 Adams H, Tzankov A, d'Hondt S, Jundt G, Dirnhofer S, Went P. Primary diffuse large B-cell lymphomas of the bone: prognostic relevance of protein expression and clinical factors. Hum Pathol 2008, **39**: 1323–1330.

701 Baar J, Burkes RL, Bell R, Blackstein ME, Fernandes B, Langer F. Primary non-Hodgkin's lymphoma of bone. A clinicopathologic study. Cancer 1994, **73**: 1194–1199.

702 Baar J, Burkes RL, Gospodarowicz M. Primary non-Hodgkin's lymphoma of bone. Semin Oncol 1999, **26**: 270–275.

703 Bacci G, Jaffe N, Emiliani E, Van Horn J, Manfrini M, Picci P, Bertoni F, Gherlinzoni F, Campanacci M. Therapy for primary non-Hodgkin's lymphoma of bone and a comparison of results with Ewing's sarcoma. Ten years' experience at the Istituto Ortopedico Rizzoli. Cancer 1986, **57**: 1468–1472.

704 Bakshi NA, Ross CW, Finn WG, Valdez R, Ruiz R, Koujok K, Schnitzer B. ALK-positive anaplastic large cell lymphoma with primary bone involvement in children. Am J Clin Pathol 2006, **125**: 57–63.

705 Beal K, Allen L, Yahalom J. Primary bone lymphoma: treatment results and prognostic factors with long-term follow-up of 82 patients. Cancer 2006, **106**: 2652–2656.

706 Bhagavathi S, Micale MA, Les K, Wilson JD, Wiggins ML, Fu K. Primary bone diffuse large B-cell lymphoma: clinicopathologic study of 21 cases and review of literature. Am J Surg Pathol 2009, **33**: 1463–1469.

707 Boston HC, Dahlin DC, Ivins JC, Cupps RE. Malignant lymphoma (so-called reticulum cell sarcoma) of bone. Cancer 1974, **34**: 1131–1137.

708 Chabner BA, Haskell CM, Canellos GP. Destructive bone lesions in chronic granulocytic leukemia. Medicine (Baltimore) 1969, **48**: 401–410.

709 Chan JK, Ng CS, Hui PK, Leung WT, Sin VC, Lam TK, Chick KW, Lam WY. Anaplastic large cell Ki-1 lymphoma of bone. Cancer 1991, **68**: 2186–2191.

710 Chan K-W, Rosen G, Miller DR, Tan CTC. Hodgkin's disease in adolescents presenting as a primary bone lesion. A report of four cases and review of literature. Am J Pediatr Hematol Oncol 1982, **4**: 11–17.

711 Clayton F, Butler JJ, Ayala AG, Ro JY, Zornoza J. Non-Hodgkin's lymphoma in bone. Pathologic and radiologic features with clinical correlates. Cancer 1987, **60**: 2494–2501.

712 De Leval L, Braaten KM, Ancukiewicz M, Kiggundu E, Delaney T, Mankin HJ, Harris NL. Diffuse large B-cell lymphoma of bone. An analysis of differentiation-associated antigens with clinical correlation. Am J Surg Pathol 2003, **27**: 1269–1277.

713 Dosoretz DE, Raymond AK, Murphy GF, Doppke KP, Schiller AL, Wang CC, Suit HD. Primary lymphoma of bone. The relationship of morphologic diversity to clinical behavior. Cancer 1982, **50**: 1009–1014.

714 Falini B, Binazzi R, Pileri S, Mori A, Bertoni F, Canino S, Fagioli M, Minelli O, Ciani C, Pellicioli P. Large cell lymphoma of bone. A report of three cases of B-cell origin. Histopathology 1988, **12**: 177–190.

715 Fowles JV, Olweny CLM, Katongole-Mbidde E, Lukanga-Ndawula A, Owor R. Burkitt's lymphoma in the appendicular skeleton. J Bone Joint Surg (Br) 1983, **65**: 464–471.

716 Gianelli U, Patriarca C, Moro A, Ponzoni M, Giardini R, Massimino M, Alfano RM, Armiraglio E, Nuciforo P, Bosari S, Coggi G, Parafioriti A. Lymphomas of the bone: a pathological and clinical study of 54 cases. Int J Surg Pathol 2002, **10**: 257–266.

717 Horan FT. Bone involvement in Hodgkin's disease. Br J Surg 1969, **56**: 277–281.

718 Howat AJ, Thomas HUW, Waters KD, Campbell PE. Malignant lymphoma of bone in children. Cancer 1987, **59**: 335–339.

719 Huebner-Chan D, Fernandes B, Yang G, Lim MS. An immunophenotypic and molecular study of primary large B-cell lymphoma of the bone. Mod Pathol 2001, **14**: 1000–1007.

720 Iravani S, Singleton TP, Ross CW, Schnitzer B. Precursor B lymphoblastic lymphoma presenting as lytic bone lesions. Am J Clin Pathol 1999, **112**: 836–843.

721 Llombart-Bosch A, Blache R, Peydro-Olaya A. Round-cell sarcomas of bone and their differential diagnosis (with particular emphasis on Ewing's sarcoma and reticulosarcoma). A study of 233 tumors with optical and electron microscopic techniques. Pathol Annu 1982, **17**(Pt 2): 113–145.

722 Marsh WL Jr, Bylund DJ, Heath VC, Anderson MJ. Osteoarticular and pulmonary manifestations of acute leukemia. Case report and review of the literature. Cancer 1986, **57**: 385–390.

723 Nagasaka T, Nakamura S, Medeiros LJ, Juco J, Lai R. Anaplastic large cell lymphomas presented as bone lesions: a clinicopathologic study of six cases and review of the literature. Mod Pathol 2000, **13**: 1143–1149.

724 Ostrowski ML, Inwards CY, Strickler JG, Witzig TE, Wenger DE, Unni KK. Osseous Hodgkin disease. Cancer 1999, **85**: 1166–1178.

725 Ostrowski ML, Unni KK, Banks PM, Shives TC, Evans RG, O'Connell MJ, Taylor WF. Malignant lymphoma of bone. Cancer 1986, **58**: 2646–2655.

726 Ozdemirli M, Mankin HJ, Aisenberg AC, Harris NL. Hodgkin's disease presenting as a solitary bone tumor: a report of four cases and a review of the literature. Cancer 1996, **77**: 79–88.

727 Pambuccian SE, Horyd ID, Cawte T, Huvos AG. Amyloidoma of bone, a plasma cell/plasmacytoid neoplasm: report of three cases and review of the literature. Am J Surg Pathol 1997, **21**: 179–186.

728 Pettit CK, Zukerberg LR, Gray MH, Ferry JA, Rosenberg AE, Harmon DC, Harris NL. Primary lymphoma of bone. A B-cell neoplasm with a high frequency of multilobated cells. Am J Surg Pathol 1990, **14**: 329–334.

729 Radaszkiewicz T, Hansmann ML. Primary high-grade malignant lymphomas of bone. Virchows Arch [A] 1988, **413**: 269–274.

730 Reimer RR, Chabner BA, Young RC, Reddick R, Johnson RE. Lymphoma presenting in bone. Results of histopathology, staging, and therapy. Ann Intern Med 1977, **87**: 50–55.

731 Rossleigh MA, Smith J, Straus DJ, Engel IA. Osteonecrosis in patients with malignant lymphoma. A review of 31 cases. Cancer 1986, **58**: 1112–1116.

732 Simmons CR, Harle TS, Singleton EB. The osseous manifestations of leukemia in children. Radiol Clin North Am 1968, **6**: 115–129.

733 Thomas LB, Forkner CE, Frei E, Besse BE, Stabenau JR. The skeletal lesions of acute leukemia. Cancer 1961, **14**: 608–621.

734 Triche TJ, Askin FB, Kissane JM. Neuroblastoma, Ewing's sarcoma, and the differential diagnosis of small-, round-, blue-cell tumors. In Finegold M (ed.): Pathology of neoplasia in children and adolescents, vol. 18. Major Series in Pathology. Philadelphia, 1986, W.B. Saunders.

735 Vassallo J, Roessner A, Vollmer E, Grundmann E. Malignant lymphomas with primary bone manifestation. Pathol Res Pract 1987, **182**: 381–389.

736 Wu SL, McGregor DK, Medeiros LJ, Raymond AK, Deavers MT. Primary lymphoma of bone: a clinicopathologic study of 15 cases [abstract]. Mod Pathol 2003, **16**: 20a.

737 Zhao XF, Young KH, Frank D, Goradia A, Glotzbecker MP, Pan W, Kersun LS, Leahey A, Dormans JP, Choi JK. Pediatric primary bone lymphoma–diffuse large B-cell lymphoma: morphologic and immunohistochemical characteristics of 10 cases. Am J Clin Pathol 2007, **127**: 47–54.

VASCULAR TUMORS

738 Bollinger BK, Laskin WB, Knight CB. Epithelioid hemangioendothelioma with multiple site involvement. Literature review and observations. Cancer 1994, **73**: 610–615.

739 Bruder E, Perez-Atayde AR, Jundt G, Alomari AI, Rischewski J, Fishman SJ, Mulliken JB, Kozakewich HPW. Vascular lesions of bone in children, adolescents, and young adults. A clinicopathologic reappraisal and application of the ISSVA classification. Virchows Arch 2009, **454**: 161–179.

740 Campanacci M, Boriani S, Giunti A. Hemangioendothelioma of bone. A study of 29 cases. Cancer 1980, **46**: 804–814.

741 Deshpande V, Rosenberg AE, O'Connell JX, Nielsen GP. Epithelioid angiosarcoma of the bone. A series of 10 cases. Am J Surg Pathol 2003, **27**: 709–716.

742 Deyrup AT, Montag AG. Epithelioid and epithelial neoplasms of bone. Arch Pathol Lab Med 2007, **131**: 205–216.

743 Dorfman HD, Steiner GC, Jaffe HL. Vascular tumors of bone. Hum Pathol 1971, **2**: 349–376.

744 Evans HL, Raymond K, Ayala AG. Vascular tumors of bone: a study of 17 cases other than ordinary hemangioma, with an evaluation of the relationship of hemangioendothelioma of bone to epithelioid hemangioma, epithelioid hemangioendothelioma, and high-grade angiosarcoma. Hum Pathol 2003, **34**: 680–689.

745 Floris G, Deraedt K, Samson I, Brys P, Sciot R. Epithelioid hemangioma of bone: a potentially metastasizing tumor? Int J Surg Pathol 2006, **14**: 9–15; discussion 16–20.

746 Goldberg NS, Hebert AA, Esterly NB. Sacral hemangiomas and multiple congenital abnormalities. Arch Dermatol 1986, **122**: 684–687.

747 Gorham LW, Stout AP. Massive osteolysis (acute spontaneous absorption of bone, phantom bone, disappearing bone). Its relation to hemangiomatosis. J Bone Joint Surg (Am) 1955, **37**: 985–1004.

748 Halliday DR, Dahlin DC, Pugh DG, Young HH. Massive osteolysis and angiomatosis. Radiology 1964, **82**: 627–644.

749 Hasegawa T, Fujii Y, Seki K, Yang P, Hirose T, Matsuzaki K, Sano T. Epithelioid angiosarcoma of the bone. Hum Pathol 1997, **28**: 985–989.

750 Jumbelic M, Feuerstein IM, Dorfman HD. Solitary intraosseous lymphangioma. A case report. J Bone Joint Surg (Am) 1984, **66**: 1479–1480.

751 Keel SB, Rosenberg AE. Hemorrhagic epithelioid and spindle cell hemangioma: a newly recognized, unique vascular tumor of bone. Cancer 1999, **85**: 1966–1972.

752 Kleer CG, Unni KK, McLeod RA. Epithelioid hemangioendothelioma of bone. Am J Surg Pathol 1996, **20**: 1301–1311.

753 Lamovec J, Bracko M. Epithelioid hemangioma of small tubular bones: a report of three cases, two of them associated with pregnancy. Mod Pathol 1996, **9**: 821–827.

754 Larsson S-E, Lorentzon R, Boquist L. Malignant hemangioendothelioma of bone. J Bone Joint Surg (Am) 1975, **57**: 84–89.

755 Mackenzie DH. Intraosseous glomus tumors. Report of two cases. J Bone Joint Surg (Br) 1962, **44**: 648–651.

756 Mirra JM, Kameda N. Myxoid angioblastomatosis of bones. A case report of a rare, multifocal entity with light, ultramicroscopic, and immunopathologic correlation. Am J Surg Pathol 1985, **9**: 450–458.

757 Mitsuhashi T, Shimizu Y, Ban S, Ogawa F, Hirose T, Tanaka J, Shimizu M. Multicentric contiguous variant of epithelioid angiosarcoma of the bone. A rare variant showing angiotropic spread. Ann Diagn Pathol 2005, **9**: 33–37.

758 Nielsen GP, Srivastava A, Kattapuram S, Deshpande V, O'Connell JX, Mangham CD, Rosenberg AE. Epithelioid hemangioma of bone revisited: a study of 50 cases. Am J Surg Pathol 2009, **33**: 270–277.

759 O'Connell JX, Kattapuram SV, Mankin HJ, Bhan AK, Rosenberg AE. Epithelioid hemangioma of bone. A tumor often mistaken for low-grade angiosarcoma or malignant hemangioendothelioma. Am J Surg Pathol 1993, **17**: 610–617.

760 O'Connell JX, Nielsen GP, Rosenberg AE. Epithelioid vascular tumors of bone: a review and proposal of a classification scheme. Adv Anat Pathol 2001, **8**: 74–82.

761 Ose D, Vollmer R, Shelburne J, McComb R, Harrelson J. Histiocytoid hemangioma of the

skin and scapula. A case report with electron microscopy and immunohistochemistry. Cancer 1983, **51**: 1656–1662.

762 Otis J, Hutter RVP, Foote FW Jr, Marcove RC, Stewart FW. Hemangioendothelioma of bone. Surg Gynecol Obstet 1968, **127**: 295–305.

763 Rosai J, Gold J, Landy R. The histiocytoid hemangiomas. A unifying concept embracing several previously described entities of skin, soft tissue, large vessels, bone, and heart. Hum Pathol 1979, **10**: 707–730.

764 Schajowicz F, Aiello CL, Francone MV, Giannini RE. Cystic angiomatosis (hamartomatous haemolymphangiomatosis) of bone. A clinicopathological study of three cases. J Bone Joint Surg (Br) 1978, **60**: 100–106.

765 Sellke FW, Laszewski MJ, Robinson RA, Davis R, Rossi NP. Hemangiopericytoma of the sternum. Arch Pathol Lab Med 1991, **115**: 242–244.

766 Spjut HJ, Lindbom A. Skeletal angiomatosis. Report of two cases. Acta Pathol Microbiol Scand 1962, **55**: 49–58.

767 Steiner GC, Dorfman HD. Ultrastructure of hemangioendothelial sarcoma of bone. Cancer 1972, **29**: 122–135.

768 Töpfer DI. Ueber ein infiltrierend wachsendes Hämangiom der Haut und multiple Kapillarektasien der Haut und innergen Organe. II. Zur Kenntnis der Wirbelangiome. Frankfurt Z Pathol 1928, **36**: 337–345.

769 Tsuneyoshi M, Dorfman HD, Bauer TW. Epithelioid hemangioendothelioma of bone. A clinicopathologic, ultrastructural, and immunohistochemical study. Am J Surg Pathol 1986, **10**: 754–764.

770 Unni KK, Ivins JC, Beabout JW, Dahlin DC. Hemangioma, hemangiopericytoma, and hemangioendothelioma (angiosarcoma) of bone. Cancer 1971, **27**: 1403–1414.

771 van Haelst UJ, Pruszczynski M, ten Cate LN, Mravunac M. Ultrastructural and immunohistochemical study of epithelioid hemangioendothelioma of bone. Coexpression of epithelial and endothelial markers. Ultrastruct Pathol 1990, **14**: 141–149.

772 Verbeke SL, Bertoni F, Bacchini P, Sciot R, Mertens BJ, Kroon HM, Hogendoorn PC, Bovée JV. Hemangioendothelioma and angiosarcoma of bone: distinct histological criteria predicting clinical behavior. Lab Invest 2009, **89**(Suppl 1): 24A.

773 Verbeke SL, Fletcher CD, Alberghini M, Daugaard S, Flanagan AM, Parratt T, Kroon HM, Hogendoorn PC, Bovée JV. A reappraisal of hemangiopericytoma of bone; analysis of cases reclassified as synovial sarcoma and solitary fibrous tumor of bone. Am J Surg Pathol 2010, **34**: 777–783.

774 Wold LE, Swee RG, Sim FH. Vascular lesions of bone. Pathol Annu 1985, **20**(Pt 2): 101–137.

775 Wold LE, Unni KK, Beabout JW, Ivins JC, Bruckman JE, Dahlin DC. Hemangioendothelial sarcoma of bone. Am J Surg Pathol 1982, **6**: 59–70.

776 Wold LE, Unni KK, Cooper KL, Sim FH, Dahlin DC. Hemangiopericytoma of bone. Am J Surg Pathol 1982, **6**: 53–58.

OTHER MESENCHYMAL TUMORS

Fibrous and related tumors

777 Abdulkader I, Cameselle-Teijeiro J, Fraga M, Caparrini A, Forteza J. Sclerosing epithelioid fibrosarcoma primary of the bone. Int J Surg Pathol 2002, **10**: 227–230.

778 Abdul-Karim FW, Ayala AG, Chawla SP, Jing B-S, Goepfert H. Malignant fibrous histiocytoma of jaws. A clinicopathologic study of 11 cases. Cancer 1985, **56**: 1590–1596.

779 Antonescu CR, Erlandson RA, Huvos AG. Primary fibrosarcoma and malignant fibrous histiocytoma of bone – a comparative ultrastructural study: evidence of a spectrum of fibroblastic differentiation. Ultrastruct Pathol 2000, **24**: 83–91.

780 Bagó-Granell J, Aguirre-Canyadell M, Nardi J, Tallada N. Malignant fibrous histiocytoma of bone at the site of a total hip arthroplasty. A case report. J Bone Joint Surg (Br) 1984, **66**: 38–40.

781 Belza MG, Urich H. Chordoma and malignant fibrous histiocytoma. Evidence for transformation. Cancer 1986, **58**: 1082–1087.

782 Bertoni F, Calderoni P, Bacchini P, Campanacci M. Desmoplastic fibroma of bone. A report of six cases. J Bone Joint Surg (Br) 1984, **66**: 265–268.

783 Bertoni F, Capanna R, Calderoni P, Bacchini P, Campanacci M. Primary central (medullary) fibrosarcoma of bone. Semin Diagn Pathol 1984, **1**: 185–198.

784 Bohm P, Krober S, Greschniok A, Laniado M, Kaiserling E. Desmoplastic fibroma of the bone: a report of two patients, review of the literature, and therapeutic implications. Cancer 1996, **78**: 1011–1023.

785 Boland PJ, Huvos AG. Malignant fibrous histiocytoma of bone. Clin Orthop 1986, **204**: 130–134.

786 Cunningham MP, Arlen M. Medullary fibrosarcoma of bone. Cancer 1968, **21**: 31–37.

787 Dahlin DC, Ivins JC. Fibrosarcoma of bone. A study of 114 cases. Cancer 1969, **23**: 35–41.

788 Dahlin DC, Unni KK, Matsuno T. Malignant (fibrous) histiocytoma of bone – fact or fancy? Cancer 1977, **39**: 1508–1516.

789 Duong S, Sallis JG, Zee SY. Malignant fibrous histiocytoma arising within a bone infarct in a patient with sickle cell trait. Int J Surg Pathol 2004, **12**: 67–73.

790 Frierson HF Jr, Fechner RE, Stallings RG, Wang G-J. Malignant fibrous histiocytoma in bone infarct. Association with sickle cell trait and alcohol abuse. Cancer 1987, **59**: 496–500.

791 Gebhardt MC, Campbell CJ, Schiller AL, Mankin HJ. Desmoplastic fibroma of bone. A report of eight cases and review of the literature. J Bone Joint Surg (Am) 1985, **67**: 732–747.

792 Hasegawa T, Hirose T, Seki K, Hizawa K, Okada J, Nakanishi H. Solitary infantile myofibromatosis of bone. An immunohistochemical and ultrastructural study. Am J Surg Pathol 1993, **17**: 308–313.

793 Hauben EI, Jundt G, Cleton-Jansen AM, Yavas A, Kroon HM, Van Marck E, Hogendoorn PC. Desmoplastic fibroma of bone: an immunohistochemical study including beta-catenin expression and mutational analysis for beta-catenin. Hum Pathol 2005, **36**: 1025–1030.

793a Hernandez FJ, Fernandez BB. Multiple diffuse fibrosarcoma of bone. Cancer 1976, **37**: 939–945.

794 Heselson NG, Price SK, Mills EED, Conway SSM, Marks RK. Two malignant fibrous histiocytomas in bone infarcts (case report). J Bone Joint Surg (Am) 1983, **65**: 1166–1171.

795 Huvos AG, Heilweil M, Bretsky SS. The pathology of malignant fibrous histiocytoma of bone. A study of 130 patients. Am J Surg Pathol 1985, **9**: 853–871.

796 Huvos AG, Higinbotham NL. Primary fibrosarcoma of bone. A clinicopathologic study of 130 patients. Cancer 1975, **35**: 837–847.

797 Huvos AG, Woodard HQ, Heilweil M. Postradiation malignant fibrous histiocytoma of bone. A clinicopathologic study of 20 patients. Am J Surg Pathol 1986, **10**: 9–18.

798 Inwards CY, Unni KK, Beabout JW, Shives TC. Solitary congenital fibromatosis (infantile myofibromatosis) of bone. Am J Surg Pathol 1991, **15**: 935–941.

799 Inwards CY, Unni KK, Beabout JW, Sim FH. Desmoplastic fibroma of bone. Cancer 1991, **68**: 1978–1983.

800 Kahn LB, Webber B, Mills E, Antsey L, Heleson NG. Malignant fibrous histiocytoma (malignant fibrous xanthoma: xanthosarcoma) of bone. Cancer 1978, **42**: 640–651.

801 Lagacé R, Bouchard HL, Delage C, Seemayer TA. Desmoplastic fibroma of bone. An ultrastructural study. Am J Surg Pathol 1979, **3**: 423–430.

802 Lee Y-S, Pho RWH, Nather A. Malignant fibrous histiocytoma at site of metal implant. Cancer 1984, **54**: 2286–2289.

803 Martorell M, Calabuig C, Peydro-Olaya A, Llombart-Bosch A, Terrier-Lacombe MJ, Contesso G. Fibroblast and myofibroblast participation in malignant fibrous histiocytoma (MFH) of bone. Ultrastructural study of eight cases with immunohistochemical support. Pathol Res Pract 1989, **184**: 582–590.

804 McCarthy EF, Matsuno T, Dorfman HD. Malignant fibrous histiocytoma of bone. A study of 35 cases. Hum Pathol 1979, **10**: 57–70.

805 Miettinen M, Lehto V-P, Virtanen I. Malignant fibrous histiocytoma within a recurrent chordoma. A light microscopic, electron microscopic, and immunohistochemical study. Am J Clin Pathol 1984, **82**: 738–743.

806 Nishida J, Sim FH, Wenger DE, Unni KK. Malignant fibrous histiocytoma of bone: a clinicopathologic study of 81 patients. Cancer 1997, **79**: 482–493.

807 O'Connell JX, Logan PM, Beauchamp CP. Solitary fibrous tumor of the periosteum. Hum Pathol 1995, **26**: 460–462.

808 Rabham WN, Rosai J. Desmoplastic fibroma. Report of ten cases and review of the literature. J Bone Joint Surg (Am) 1968, **50**: 487–502.

809 Sciot R, Dal Cin P, Fletcher CD, Hernandez JM, Garcia JL, Samson I, Ramos L, Brys P, Van Damme B, Van Den Berghe H. Inflammatory myofibroblastic tumor of bone: report of two cases with evidence of clonal chromosomal changes. Am J Surg Pathol 1997, **21**: 1166–1172.

810 Spanier SS, Enneking WF, Enriquez P. Primary malignant fibrous histiocytoma of bone. Cancer 1975, **36**: 2084–2098.

811 Taconis WK, Van Rijssel ThG. Fibrosarcoma of long bones. A study of the significance of areas of malignant fibrous histiocytoma. J Bone Joint Surg (Br) 1985, **67**: 111–116.

812 Ushigome S, Shimoda T, Fukunaga M, Takakuwa T, Nakajima H. Immunohistochemical aspects of the differential diagnosis of osteosarcoma and malignant fibrous histiocytoma. Surg Pathol 1988, **1**: 347–358.

813 Verbeke SL, Fletcher CD, Picci P, Daugaard S, Kroon HM, Hogendoorn PC, Bovée JV. Haemangiopericytoma of bone: real or imagined? Lab Invest 2009, **89**(Suppl 1): 24A.

814 Watanabe K, Ogura G, Tajino T, Hoshi N, Suzuki T. Myofibrosarcoma of the bone: a clinicopathologic study. Am J Surg Pathol 2001, **25**: 1501–1507.

815 Yokoyama R, Tsuneyoshi M, Enjoji M, Shinohara N, Masuda S. Prognostic factors of malignant fibrous histiocytoma of bone. A clinical and histopathologic analysis of 34 cases. Cancer 1993, **72**: 1902–1908.

Muscle tumors

816 Adelani MA, Schultenover SJ, Holt GE, Cates JMM. Primary leiomyosarcoma of extragnathic bone: clinicopathologic features and reevaluation of prognosis. Arch Pathol Lab Med 2009, **133**: 1448–1456.

817 Amstalden EM, Barbosa CS, Gamba R. Primary leiomyosarcoma of bone: report of two cases in extragnathic bones. Ann Diagn Pathol 1998, **2**: 103–110.

818 Angervall L, Berlin Ö, Kindblom L-G, Stener B. Primary leiomyosarcoma of bone. A study of five cases. Cancer 1980, **46**: 1270–1279.

819 Antonescu CR, Erlandson RA, Huvos AG. Primary leiomyosarcoma of bone: a clinicopathologic, immunohistochemical, and ultrastructural study of 33 patients and a literature review. Am J Surg Pathol 1997, **21**: 1281–1294.

820 Jundt G, Moll C, Nidecker A, Schilt R, Remagen W. Primary leiomyosarcoma of bone. Report of eight cases. Hum Pathol 1994, **25**: 1205–1212.

821 Kawai T, Suzuki M, Mukai M, Hiroshima K, Shinmei M. Primary leiomyosarcoma of bone. An immunohistochemical and ultrastructural study. Arch Pathol Lab Med 1983, **107**: 433–437.

822 Khoddami M, Bedard YC, Bell RS, Kandel RA. Primary leiomyosarcoma of bone: report of seven cases and review of the literature. Arch Pathol Lab Med 1996, **120**: 671–675.

823 Lamovec J, Zidar A, Bracko M, Golouh R. Primary bone sarcoma with rhabdomyosarcomatous component. Pathol Res Pract 1994, **190**: 51–60.

824 Lopez-Barea F, Rodriguez-Peralto JL, Sancez-Herrera S, Gonzalez-Lopez J, Burgos-Lizaldez E. Primary epithelioid leiomyosarcoma of bone. Case report and literature review. Virchows Arch 1999, **434**: 367–371.

825 Lucas DR, Ryan JR, Zalupski MM, Gross ML, Ravindranth Y, Ortman B. Primary embryonal rhabdomyosarcoma of long bone: case report and review of the literature. Am J Surg Pathol 1996, **20**: 239–244.

826 Myers JL, Arocho J, Bernreuter W, Dunham W, Mazur MT. Leiomyosarcoma of bone. A clinicopathologic, immunohistochemical, and ultrastructural study of five cases. Cancer 1991, **67**: 1051–1056.

827 Oda Y, Tsuneyoshi M, Hashimoto H, Iwashita T, Ushijima M, Masuda S, Iwamoto Y, Sugioka Y. Primary rhabdomyosarcoma of the iliac bone in an adult. A case mimicking fibrosarcoma. Virchows Arch [A] 1993, **423**: 65–69.

828 Rashid A, Dickersin GR, Rosenthal DI, Mankin H, Rosenberg AE. Rhabdomyo-sarcoma of the long bone in an adult. A case report and literature review. Int J Surg Pathol 1994, **1**: 253–260.

829 von Hochstetter AR, Eberle H, Rüttner JR. Primary leiomyosarcoma of extragnathic bones. Case report and review of literature. Cancer 1984, **53**: 2194–2200.

830 Watanabe K, Tajino T, Sekiguchi M, Suzuki T. H-caldesmon as a specific marker for smooth muscle tumors. Comparison with other smooth muscle markers in bone tumors. Am J Clin Pathol 2000, **113**: 663–668.

831 Young MP, Freemont AJ. Primary leiomyosarcoma of bone. Histopathology 1991, **19**: 257–262.

Adipose tissue tumors

832 Barcelo M, Pathria MN, Abdul-Karim FW. Intraosseous lipoma. A clinicopathologic study of four cases. Arch Pathol Lab Med 1992, **116**: 947–950.

833 Chow LT, Lee KC. Intraosseous lipoma. A clinicopathologic study of nine cases. Am J Surg Pathol 1992, **16**: 401–410.

834 Eyzaguirre E, Liqiang W, Karla GM, Rajendra K, Alberto A, Gatalica Z. Intraosseous lipoma. A clinical, radiologic, and pathologic study of 5 cases. Ann Diagn Pathol 2007, **11**: 320–325.

835 Mandard JC, Mandard AM, Le Gal Y. Les liposarcomes primitifs de l'os. A propos de 5 cas revue de la littérature. Ann Anat Pathol (Paris) 1973, **18**: 329–346.

836 Pardo-Mindan FJ, Ayala H, Joly M, Gimeno E, Vazquez JJ. Primary liposarcoma of bone. Light and electron microscopic study. Cancer 1981, **48**: 274–280.

837 Yamamoto T, Marui T, Akisue T, Hitora T, Nagira K, Ohta R, Yoshiya S, Kurosaka M. Intracortical lipoma of the femur. Am J Surg Pathol 2002, **26**: 804–808.

CHORDOMA AND OTHER NOTOCHORDAL LESIONS

838 Abenoza P, Sibley RK. Chordoma. An immunohistologic study. Hum Pathol 1986, **17**: 744–747.

839 Ariel IM, Verdu C. Chordoma. An analysis of twenty cases treated over a twenty-year span. J Surg Oncol 1975, **7**: 27–44.

840 Bergh P, Kindblom LG, Gunterberg B, Remotti F, Ryd W, Meis-Kindblom JM. Prognostic factors in chordoma of the sacrum and mobile spine: a study of 39 patients. Cancer 2000, **88**: 2122–2134.

841 Bisceglia M, D'Angelo VA, Guglielmi G, Dor DB, Pasquinelli G. Dedifferentiated chordoma of the thoracic spine with rhabdomyosarcomatous differentiation. Report of a case and review of the literature. Ann Diagn Pathol 2007, **11**: 262–273.

842 Bjornsson J, Wold LE, Ebersold MJ, Laws ER. Chordoma of the mobile spine. A clinicopathologic analysis of 40 patients. Cancer 1993, **71**: 735–740.

843 Bottles K, Beckstead JH. Enzyme histochemical characterization of chordomas. Am J Surg Pathol 1984, **8**: 443–447.

844 Campbell WM, McDonald TJ, Unni KK, Laws ER Jr. Nasal and paranasal presentations of chordomas. Laryngoscope 1980, **90**: 612–618.

845 Cates JM, Itani DM, Homlar KC, Olson SJ, Holt GE, Schwartz HS, Coffin CM, Harfe BD. The sonic hedgehog pathway in chordoma. Lab Invest 2009, **89**(Suppl 1): 12A.

846 Chambers PW, Schwinn CP. Chordoma. A clinicopathologic study of metastasis. Am J Clin Pathol 1979, **72**: 765–776.

847 Cho HY, Lee M, Takei H, Dancer J, Ro JY, Zhai QJ. Immunohistochemical comparison of chordoma with chondrosarcoma, myxopapillary ependymoma, and chordoid meningioma. Appl Immunohistochem Mol Morphol 2009, **17**: 131–138.

848 Chu TA. Chondroid chordoma of the sacrococcygeal region. Arch Pathol Lab Med 1987, **111**: 861–864.

849 Coffin CM, Swanson PE, Wick MR, Dehner LP. An immunohistochemical comparison of chordoma with renal cell carcinoma, colorectal adenocarcinoma, and myxopapillary ependymoma. A potential diagnostic dilemma in the diminutive biopsy. Mod Pathol 1993, **6**: 531–538.

850 Coffin CM, Swanson PE, Wick MR, Dehner LP. Chordoma in childhood and adolescence. A clinicopathologic analysis of 12 cases. Arch Pathol Lab Med 1993, **117**: 927–933.

851 Deshpande V, Nielsen GP, Rosenthal DI, Rosenberg AE. Intraosseous benign notochord cell tumors (BNCT): further evidence supporting a relationship to chordoma. Am J Surg Pathol 2007, **31**: 1573–1577.

852 Erlandson RA, Tandler B, Lieberman PH, Higinbotham NL. Ultrastructure of human chordoma. Cancer Res 1968, **28**: 2115–2125.

853 Fan F, Templeton K, Damjanov I. Epithelioid cellular chordoma of the sacrum: a potential diagnostic problem. Ann Diagn Pathol 2005, **9**: 139–142.

854 Franquemont DW, Katsetos CD, Ross GW. Fatal acute pontocerebellar hemorrhage due to an unsuspected spheno-occipital chordoma. Arch Pathol Lab Med 1989, **113**: 1075–1078.

855 Gagne EJ, Su WP. Chordoma involving the skin. An immunohistochemical study of 11 cases. J Cutan Pathol 1992, **19**: 469–475.

856 Haeckel C, Kruger S, Kuester D, Ostertag H, Samil M, Buehling F, Broemme D, Czerniak B, Roessner A. Expression of cathepsin K in chordoma. Hum Pathol 2000, **31**: 834–840.

857 Heaton JM, Turner DR. Reflections on notochordal differentiation arising from a study of chordomas. Histopathology 1985, **9**: 543–550.

858 Heffelfinger MJ, Dahlin DC, MacCarty CS, Beabout JW. Chordomas and cartilaginous tumors at the skull base. Cancer 1973, **32**: 410–420.

859 Higinbotham NL, Phillips RF, Farr HW, Hustu O. Chordoma. Thirty-five-year study at Memorial Hospital. Cancer 1967, **20**: 1841–1850.

860 Hoch BL, Neilsen GP, Leibsch NJ, Rosenberg AE. Base of skull chordomas in children and adolescents: a clinicopathologic analysis of 72 cases [abstract]. Mod Pathol 2003, **16**: 13a.

861 Hoch BL, Nielsen GP, Liebsch NJ, Rosenberg AE. Base of skull chordomas in children and adolescents: a clinicopathologic study of 73 cases. Am J Surg Pathol 2006, **30**: 811–818.

862 Houghton J, Korda M, Quick C, McClure M. Diagnostic dilemma of ectopic notochord tissue in the nasopharynx. Histopathology 2008, **52**: 518–519.

863 Hruban RH, May M, Marcove RC, Huvos AG. Lumbo-sacral chordoma with high-grade malignant cartilaginous and spindle cell components. Am J Surg Pathol 1990, **14**: 384–389.

864 Hu B, McPhaul L, Cornford M, Gaal K, Mirra J, French SW. Expression of Tau proteins and tubulin in extraskeletal myxoid chondrosarcoma, chordoma, and other chondroid tumors. Am J Clin Pathol 1999, **112**: 189–193.

865 Jeffrey PB, Biava CG, Davis RL. Chondroid chordoma. A hyalinized chordoma without cartilaginous differentiation. Am J Clin Pathol 1995, **103**: 271–279.

866 Jeffrey PB, Davis RL, Biava C, Rosenblum M. Microtubule aggregates in a clival chordoma. Arch Pathol Lab Med 1993, **117**: 1055–1057.

867 Kaiser TE, Pritchard DJ, Unni KK. Clinicopathologic study of sacrococcygeal chordoma. Cancer 1984, **54**: 2574–2578.

868 Kaneko Y, Iwaki T, Fukui M. Lectin histochemistry of human fetal notochord,

ecchordosis physaliphora, and chordomas. Arch Pathol Lab Med 1992, **116**: 60–64.

869 Kilgore S, Prayson RA. Apoptotic and proliferative markers in chordomas: a study of 26 tumors. Ann Diagn Pathol 2002, **6**: 222–228.

870 Knapik JA, Vlasak R, Reith JD. Notochordal hamartoma and its necessary distinction from chordoma. Mod Pathol 2003, **16**: 15a.

871 Kuzniacka A, Mertens F, Strombeck B, Wiegant J, Mandahl N. Combined binary ratio labeling fluorescence in situ hybridization analysis of chordoma. Cancer Genet Cytogenet 2004, **151**: 178–181.

872 Lam R. The nature of cytoplasmic vacuoles in chordoma cells. A correlative enzyme and electron microscopic histochemical study. Pathol Res Pract 1990, **186**: 642–650.

873 Matsuno A, Sasaki T, Nagashima T, Matsuura R, Tanaka H, Hirakawa M, Murakami M, Kirini T. Immunohistochemical examination of proliferative potentials and the expression of cell cycle-related proteins of intracranial chordomas. Hum Pathol 1997, **28**: 714–719.

874 Meis JM, Giraldo AA. Chordoma. An immunohistochemical study of 20 cases. Arch Pathol Lab Med 1988, **112**: 553–556.

875 Meis JM, Raymond AK, Evans HL, Charles RE, Giraldo AA. 'Dedifferentiated' chordoma. A clinicopathologic and immunohistochemical study of three cases. Am J Surg Pathol 1987, **11**: 516–525.

876 Mertens F, Kreicbergs A, Rydholm A, Willén H, Carlén B, Mitelman F, Mandahl N. Clonal chromosome aberrations in three sacral chordomas. Cancer Genet Cytogenet 1994, **73**: 147–151.

877 Miettinen M. Chordoma. Antibodies to epithelial membrane antigen and carcinoembryonic antigen in differential diagnosis. Arch Pathol Lab Med 1984, **108**: 891–892.

878 Mindell ER. Current concepts review. Chordoma. J Bone Joint Surg (Am) 1981, **63**: 501–505.

879 Mirra JM, Brien EW. Giant notochordal hamartoma of intraosseous origin: a newly reported benign entity to be distinguished from chordoma. Report of two cases. Skeletal Radiol 2001, **30**: 698–709.

880 Mitchell A, Scheithauer BW, Unni KK, Forsyth PJ, Wold LE, McGivney DJ. Chordoma and chondroid neoplasms of the spheno-occiput. An immunohistochemical study of 41 cases with prognostic and nosologic implications. Cancer 1993, **72**: 2943–2949.

881 Mori K, Chano T, Kushima R, Huduka S, Okabe H. Expression of E-cadherin in chordomas: diagnostic marker and possible role of tumor cell affinity. Virchows Arch 2002, **440**: 123–127.

882 Naka T, Fukuda T, Chuman H, Iwamoto Y, Sugioka Y, Fukui M, Tsuneyoshi M. Proliferative activities in conventional chordoma: a clinicopathologic, DNA flow cytometric, and immunohistochemical analysis of 17 specimens with special reference to anaplastic chordoma showing a diffuse proliferation and nuclear atypia. Hum Pathol 1996, **27**: 381–388.

883 Naka T, Iwamoto Y, Shinohara N, Chuman H, Fukui M, Tsuneyoshi M. Cytokeratin subtyping in chordomas and the fetal notochord: an immunohistochemical analysis of aberrant expression. Mod Pathol 1997, **10**: 545–551.

884 Naka T, Boltze C, Kuester D, Samii A, Herold C, Ostertag H, Iwamoto Y, Oda Y, Tsuneyoshi M, Roessner A. Intralesional fibrous septum in chordoma: a clinicopathologic and immunohistochemical study of 122 lesions. Am J Clin Pathol 2005, **124**: 288–294.

885 Nakamura Y, Becker LE, Marks A. S 100 protein in human chordoma and human and rabbit notochord. Arch Pathol Lab Med 1983, **107**: 118–120.

886 Oakley GJ, Fuhrer K, Seethala RR. Brachyury, SOX-9, and podoplanin, new markers in the skull base chordoma vs chondrosarcoma differential: a tissue microarray-based comparative analysis. Mod Pathol 2008, **21**: 1461–1469.

887 O'Connell JX, Renard LG, Liebsch NJ, Efird JT, Munzenrider JE, Rosenberg AE. Base of skull chordoma. A correlative study of histologic and clinical features of 62 cases. Cancer 1994, **74**: 2261–2267.

888 O'Hara BJ, Paetau A, Miettinen M. Keratin subsets and monoclonal antibody HBME-1 in chordoma: immunohistochemical differential diagnosis between tumors simulating chordoma. Hum Pathol 1998, **29**: 119–126.

889 Pearlman AW, Friedman M. Radical radiation therapy of chordoma. Am J Roentgenol Radium Ther Nucl Med 1970, **108**: 333–341.

890 Persson S, Kindblom LG, Angervall L. Classical and chondroid chordoma. A light-microscopic, histochemical, ultrastructural and immunohistochemical analysis of the various cell types. Pathol Res Pract 1991, **187**: 828–838.

891 Rich TA, Schiller A, Suit HD, Mankin HJ. Clinical and pathologic review of 48 cases of chordoma. Cancer 1985, **56**: 182–187.

892 Richter HJ, Batsakis JG, Boles R. Chordomas. Nasopharyngeal presentation and atypical long survival. Ann Otol Rhinol Laryngol 1975, **84**: 327–332.

893 Riva P, Crosti F, Orzan F, Dalprà L, Mortini P, Parafioriti A, Pollo B, Fuhrman Conti AM, Miozzo M, Larizza L. Mapping of candidate region for chordoma development to 1p36.13 by LOH analysis. Int J Cancer 2003, **107**: 493–497.

894 Rosenberg AE, Brown GA, Bhan AK, Lee JM. Chondroid chordoma – a variant of chordoma. A morphologic and immunohistochemical study. Am J Clin Pathol 1994, **101**: 36–41.

895 Rutherfoord GS, Davies AG. Chordomas – ultrastructure and immunohistochemistry. A report based on the examination of six cases. Histopathology 1987, **11**: 775–787.

896 Salisbury JR, Isaacson PG. Demonstration of cytokeratins and an epithelial membrane antigen in chordomas and human fetal notochord. Am J Surg Pathol 1985, **9**: 791–797.

897 Sarasa JL, Fortes J. Ecchordosis physaliphora. An immunohistochemical study of two cases. Histopathology 1991, **18**: 273–275.

898 Scheil S, Brüderlein S, Liehr T, Starke H, Herms J, Schulte M, Möller P. Genome-wide analysis of sixteen chordomas by comparative genomic hybridization and cytogenetics of the first human chordoma cell line, U-CH1. Genes Chromosomes Cancer 2001, **32**: 203–211.

899 Smith DS, French G, Miller M. Multifocal benign notochordal cell tumours. Histopathology 2007, **51**: 412–414.

900 Tallini G, Dorfman H, Brys P, Dal Cin P, De Wever I, Fletcher CD, Jonson K, Mandahl N, Mertens F, Mitelman F, Rosai J, Rydholm A, Samson I, Sciot R, Van den Berghe H, Vanni R, Willén H. Correlation between clinicopathological features and karyotype in 100 cartilaginous and chordoid tumours. A report from the Chromosomes and Morphology (CHAMP) Collaborative Study Group. J Pathol 2002, **196**: 194–203.

901 Tirabosco R, Mangham DC, Rosenberg AE, Vujovic S, Bousdras K, Pizzolitto S, De Maglio G, den Bakker MA, Di Francesco L, Kalil RK, Athanasou NA, O'Donnell P, McCarthy EF, Flanagan AM. Brachyury expression in extra-axial skeletal and soft tissue chordomas: a marker that distinguishes chordoma from mixed tumor/myoepithelioma/parachordoma in soft tissue. Am J Surg Pathol 2008, **32**: 572–580.

902 Triana A, Sen C, Wolfe D, Hazan R. Cadherins and catenins in clival chordomas: correlation of expression with tumor aggressiveness. Am J Surg Pathol 2005, **29**: 1422–1434.

903 Ueda Y, Nakanishi I, Tsuchiya H, Tomita K. Microtubular aggregates in the rough endoplasmic reticulum of sacrococcygeal chordoma. Ultrastruct Pathol 1991, **15**: 77–82.

904 Ueda Y, Oda Y, Kawashima A, Tsuchiya H, Tomita K, Nakanishi I. Collagenous and basement membrane proteins of chordoma. Immunohistochemical analysis. Histopathology 1992, **21**: 345–352.

905 Valderrama E, Kahn LB, Lipper S, Marc J. Chondroid chordoma. Electron-microscopic study of two cases. Am J Surg Pathol 1983, **7**: 625–632.

906 Volpe R, Mazabraud A. A clinicopathologic review of 25 cases of chordoma (a pleomorphic and metastasizing neoplasm). Am J Surg Pathol 1983, **7**: 161–170.

907 Walaas L, Kindblom LG. Fine-needle aspiration biopsy in the preoperative diagnosis of chordoma. A study of 17 cases with application of electron microscopic, histochemical, and immunocytochemical examination. Hum Pathol 1991, **22**: 22–28.

908 Walker WP, Landas SK, Bromley CM, Sturm MT. Immunohistochemical distinction of classic and chondroid chordomas. Mod Pathol 1991, **4**: 661–666.

909 Wang WL, Abramson JH, Ganguly A, Rosenberg AE. The surgical pathology of notochordal remnants in adult intervertebral disks: a report of 3 cases. Am J Surg Pathol 2008, **32**: 1123–1129.

910 Wittchow R, Landas SK. Glial fibrillary acidic protein expression in pleomorphic adenoma, chordoma, and astrocytoma. A comparison of three antibodies. Arch Pathol Lab Med 1991, **115**: 1030–1033.

911 Wojno KJ, Hruban RH, Garin-Chesa P, Huvos AG. Chondroid chordomas and low-grade chondrosarcomas of the craniospinal axis. An immunohistochemical analysis of 17 cases. Am J Surg Pathol 1992, **16**: 1144–1152.

912 Wold LE, Laws ER Jr. Cranial chordomas in children and young adults. J Neurosurg 1983, **59**: 1043–1047.

913 Yamaguchi T, Suzuki S, Ishiiwa H, Shimizu K, Ueda Y. Benign notochordal cell tumors: a comparative histological study of benign notochordal cell tumors, classic chordomas, and notochordal vestiges of fetal intervertebral discs. Am J Surg Pathol 2004, **28**: 756–761.

914 Yamaguchi T, Suzuki S, Ishiiwa H, Ueda Y. Intraosseous benign notochordal cell tumours: overlooked precursors of classic chordomas? Histopathology 2004, **44**: 597–602.

915 Yonemoto T, Tatezaki SI, Takenouchi T, Ishii T, Satoh T, Moriya H. The surgical management of sacrococcygeal chordoma. Cancer 1999, **85**: 878–883.

916 Zukerberg LR, Young RH. Chordoma metastatic to the ovary. Arch Pathol Lab Med 1990, **114**: 208–210.

Adamantinoma of long bones

917 Benassi MS, Campanacci L, Gamberi G, Ferrari C, Picci P, Sangiorgi L, Campanacci M. Cytokeratin expression and distribution in adamantinoma of the long bones and osteofibrous dysplasia of tibia and fibula. An immunohistochemical study correlated to histogenesis. Histopathology 1994, **25**: 71–76.

918 Campanacci M, Giunti A, Bertoni F, Laus M, Gitelis S. Adamantinoma of the long bones. The experience at the Istituto Ortopedico Rizzoli. Am J Surg Pathol 1981, **5**: 533–542.

919 Czerniak B, Rojas-Corona RR, Dorfman HD. Morphologic diversity of long bone adamantinoma. The concept of differentiated (regressing) adamantinoma and its relationship to osteofibrous dysplasia. Cancer 1989, **64**: 2319–2334.

920 Eisenstein W, Pitcock JA. Adamantinoma of the tibia. An eccrine carcinoma. Arch Pathol Lab Med 1984, **108**: 246–250.

921 Hazelbag HM, Fleuren GJ, vd Broek LJ, Taminiau AH, Hogendoorn PC. Adamantinoma of the long bones. Keratin subclass immunoreactivity pattern with reference to its histogenesis. Am J Surg Pathol 1993, **17**: 1225–1233.

922 Hazelbag HM, Van den Broek LJ, Fleuren GJ, Taminiau AH, Hogendoorn PC. Distribution of extracellular matrix components in adamantinoma of long bones suggests fibrous-to-epithelial transformation. Hum Pathol 1997, **28**: 183–188.

923 Hazelbag HM, Wessels JW, Mollevangers P, van den Berg E, Molenaar WH, Hogendoorn PC. Cytogenetic analysis of adamantinoma of long bones: further indications for a common histogenesis with osteofibrous dysplasia. Cancer Genet Cytogenet 1997, **97**: 5–11.

924 Izquierdo FM, Ramos LR, Sánchez-Herráez S, Hernández T, de Alava E, Hazelbag HM. Dedifferentiated classic adamantinoma of the tibia: a report of a case with eventual complete revertant mesenchymal phenotype. Am J Surg Pathol 2010, **34**: 1388–1392.

925 Jundt G, Remberger K, Roessner A, Schulz A, Bohndorf K. Adamantinoma of long bones. A histopathological and immunohistochemical study of 23 cases. Pathol Res Pract 1995, **191**: 112–120.

926 Kanamori M, Antonescu CR, Scott M, Bridge RS Jr, Neff JR, Spanier SS, Scarborough MT, Vergara G, Rosenthal HG, Bridge JA. Extra copies of chromosomes 7, 8, 12, 19, and 21 are recurrent in adamantinoma. J Mol Diagn 2001, **3**: 16–21.

927 Keeney GL, Unni KK, Beabout JW, Pritchard DJ. Adamantinoma of long bones. A clinicopathologic study of 85 cases. Cancer 1989, **64**: 730–737.

928 Kuruvilla G, Steiner GC. Osteofibrous dysplasia-like adamantinoma of bone: a report of five cases with immunohistochemical and ultrastructural studies. Hum Pathol 1998, **29**: 809–814.

929 Mills SE, Rosai J. Adamantinoma of the pretibial soft tissue. Clinicopathologic features, differential diagnosis, and possible relationship to intraosseous disease. J Clin Pathol 1985, **83**: 108–114.

930 Moon NF, Mori H. Adamantinoma of the appendicular skeleton – updated. Clin Orthop 1986, **204**: 215–237.

931 Perez-Atayde AR, Kozakewich HPW, Vawter GF. Adamantinoma of the tibia. An ultrastructural and immunohistochemical study. Cancer 1985, **55**: 1015–1023.

932 Rosai J. Adamantinoma of the tibia. Electron microscopic evidence of its epithelial origin. Am J Clin Pathol 1969, **51**: 786–792.

933 Rosai J, Pinkus GS. Immunohistochemical demonstration of epithelial differentiation in adamantinoma of the tibia. Am J Surg Pathol 1982, **6**: 427–434.

934 Ueda Y, Roessner A, Boose A, Edel G, Bocker W, Wuisman P. Juvenile intracortical adamantinoma of the tibia with predominant osteofibrous dysplasia-like features. Pathol Res Pract 1991, **187**: 1039–1043.

935 Unni KK, Dahlin DC, Beabout JW, Ivins JC. Adamantinomas of long bones. Cancer 1974, **34**: 1796–1805.

936 Weiss SW, Dorfman HD. Adamantinoma of long bone. An analysis of nine new cases with emphasis on metastasizing lesions and fibrous dysplasia-like changes. Hum Pathol 1977, **8**: 141–153.

937 Yoneyama T, Winter WG, Milsow L. Tibial adamantinoma. Its histogenesis from ultrastructural studies. Cancer 1977, **40**: 1138–1142.

Peripheral nerve tumors

938 Bullock MJ, Bedard YC, Bell RS, Kandel R. Intraosseous malignant peripheral nerve sheath tumor. Report of a case and review of the literature. Arch Pathol Lab Med 1995, **119**: 367–370.

939 De La Monte SM, Dorfman HD, Chandra R, Malawer M. Intraosseous schwannoma. Histologic features, ultrastructure, and review of the literature. Hum Pathol 1984, **15**: 551–558.

940 Ducatman BS, Scheithauer BW, Dahlin DC. Malignant bone tumors associated with neurofibromatosis. Mayo Clin Proc 1983, **58**: 578–582.

941 Fawcett KJ, Dahlin DC. Neurilemoma of bone. Am J Clin Pathol 1967, **47**: 759–766.

942 Hunt JC, Pugh DG. Skeletal lesions in neurofibromatosis. Radiology 1961, **76**: 1–19.

943 Myers JL, Bernreuter W, Dunham W. Melanotic schwannoma. Clinicopathologic, immunohistochemical, and ultrastructural features of a rare primary bone tumor. Am J Clin Pathol 1990, **93**: 424–429.

944 Turk PS, Peters N, Libbey NP, Wanebo HJ. Diagnosis and management of giant intrasacral schwannoma. Cancer 1992, **70**: 2650–2657.

945 Wirth WA, Bray CB. Intra-osseous neurilemoma. Case report and review of thirty-one cases from the literature. J Bone Joint Surg (Am) 1977, **59**: 252–255.

Xanthoma

946 Bertoni F, Unni KK, McLeod RA, Sim FH. Xanthoma of bone. Am J Clin Pathol 1988, **90**: 377–384.

Fibrocartilaginous mesenchymoma

947 Bulychova IV, Unni KK, Bertoni F, Beabout JW. Fibrocartilaginous mesenchymoma of bone. Am J Surg Pathol 1993, **17**: 830–836.

948 Kim CJ, Choi IH, Cho TJ, Chung CY, Chi JG. The histological spectrum of subperiosteal fibrocartilaginous pseudotumor of long bone (focal fibrocartilaginous dysplasia). Pathol Int 1999, **49**: 1000–1006.

Phosphaturic mesenchymal tumor

949 Cai Q, Hodgson SF, Kao PC, Lennon VA, Klee GG, Zinsmiester AR, Kumar R. Brief report. Inhibition of renal phosphate transport by a tumor product in a patient with oncogenic osteomalacia. N Engl J Med 1994, **330**: 1645–1649

950 Folpe AL, Fanburg-Smith JC, Billings SD, Bisceglia M, Bertoni F, Cho JY, Econs MJ, Inwards CY, Jan de Beur SM, Mentzel T, Montgomery E, Michal M, Miettinen M, Mills SE, Reith JD, O'Connell JX, Rosenberg AE, Rubin BP, Sweet DE, Vinh TN, Wold LE, Wehrli BM, White KE, Zaino RJ, Weiss SW. Most osteomalacia-associated mesenchymal tumors are a single histopathologic entity: an analysis of 32 cases and a comprehensive review of the literature. Am J Surg Pathol 2004, **28**: 1–30.

951 Jonsson KB, Zahradnik R, Larsson T, White KE, Sugimoto T, Imanishi Y, Yamamoto T, Hampson G, Koshiyama H, Ljunggren O, Oba K, Yang IM, Miyauchi A, Econs MJ, Lavigne J, Juppner H. Fibroblast growth factor 23 in oncogenic osteomalacia and X-linked hypophosphatemia. N Engl J Med 2003, **348**: 1656–1663

952 Nuovo MA, Dorfman HD, Sun CC, Chalew SA. Tumor-induced osteomalacia and rickets. Am J Surg Pathol 1989, **13**: 588–599.

953 Weidner N, Santa Cruz D. Phosphaturic mesenchymal tumors. A polymorphous group causing osteomalacia or rickets. Cancer 1987, **59**: 1442–1454.

Others

954 Adsay V, Cheng J, Athanasian E, Gerald W, Rosai J. Primary desmoplastic small cell tumor of soft tissues and bone of the hand. Am J Surg Pathol 1999, **23**: 1408–1413.

955 Insabato L, De Rosa G, Terracciano LM, Fazioli F, Di Santo F, Rosai J. Primary monotypic epithelioid angiomyolipoma of bone. Histopathology 2002, **40**: 286–290.

956 Jones D, Amin M, Ordonez NG, Glassman AB, Hayes KJ, Medeiros LJ. Reticulum cell sarcoma of lymph node with mixed dendritic and fibroblastic features. Mod Pathol 2001, **14**: 1059–1067.

957 Lehman NL. Malignant PEComa of the skull base. Am J Surg Pathol 2004, **28**: 1230–1232.

958 Park YK, Unni KK, Kim YW, Han CS, Yang MH, Wenger DE, Sim FH, Lucas DR, Ryan JR, Nadim YA, Nojima T, Fletcher CD. Primary alveolar soft part sarcoma of bone. Histopathology 1999, **35**: 411–417.

959 Scheele PM Jr, Von Kuster LC, Krivchenia G. Primary malignant mesenchymoma of bone. Arch Pathol Lab Med 1990, **114**: 614–617.

960 Torii I, Kondo N, Takuwa T, Matsumoto S, Okumura Y, Sato A, Tanaka F, Nishigami T, Hasegawa S, Tsujimura T. Perivascular epithelioid cell tumor of the rib. Virchows Arch 2008, **452**: 697–702.

961 Van Dorpe J, Sciot R, Samson I, De Vos R, Brys P, Van Damme B. Primary osteorhabdomyosarcoma (malignant mesenchymoma) of bone: a case report and review of the literature. Mod Pathol 1997, **10**: 1047–1053.

962 Yokoyama R, Mukai K, Hirota T, Beppu Y, Fukuma H. Primary malignant melanoma (clear cell sarcoma) of bone: report of a case arising in the ulna. Cancer 1996, **77**: 2471–2475.

METASTATIC TUMORS

963 Berrettoni BA, Carter JR. Mechanisms of cancer metastasis to bone. J Bone Joint Surg (Am) 1986, **68**: 308–312.

964 Briasoulis E, Karavasilis V, Kostadima L, Ignatiadis M, Fountzilas G, Pavlidis N. Metastatic breast carcinoma confined to bone: portrait of a clinical entity. Cancer 2004, **101**: 1524–1528.

965 Caffey J, Andersen DH. Metastatic embryonal rhabdomyosarcoma in the growing skeleton. Clinical, radiographic, and microscopic features. Am J Dis Child 1958, **95**: 581–600.

966 Carlin BI, Andriole GL. The natural history, skeletal complications, and management of bone metastases in patients with prostate carcinoma. Cancer 2000, **88**: 2989–2994.

967 Charhon SA, Chapuy MC, Delvin EE, Valentin-Opran A, Edouard CM, Meunier PJ. Histomorphometric analysis of sclerotic bone metastases from prostatic carcinoma with special reference to osteomalacia. Cancer 1983, **51**: 918–924.

968 Daroca PJ Jr, Reed RJ, Martin PC. Metastatic amelanotic melanoma simulating giant-cell tumor of bone. Hum Pathol 1990, **21**: 978–980.

969 Goltzman D. Mechanisms of the development of osteoblastic metastases. Cancer 1997, **80**: 1581–1587.

970 Guise TA. Molecular mechanisms of ostelytic bone metastases. Cancer 2000, **88**: 2892–2898.

971 Gurney H, Larcos G, McKay M, Kefford R, Langlands A. Bone metastases in hypernephroma. Frequency of scapular involvement. Cancer 1989, **64**: 1429–1431.

972 Healey JH, Turnbull ADM, Miedema B, Lane JM. Acrometastases. A study of twenty-nine patients with osseous involvement of the hands and feet. J Bone Joint Surg (Am) 1986, **68**: 743–746.

973 Kahn LB, Wood FW, Ackerman LV. Fracture callus associated with benign and malignant bone lesions and mimicking osteosarcoma. Am J Clin Pathol 1969, **52**: 14–24.

974 Lucas DR, Kolodziej P, Gross ML, Mott MP, Budev H, Zalupski MM, Ryan JR. Metastatic uterine leiomyosarcoma to bone: a clinicopathologic study. Int J Surg Pathol 1996–1997, **4**: 159–168.

975 Morris DM, House HC. The significance of metastasis to the bones and soft tissues of the hand. J Surg Oncol 1985, **28**: 146–150.

976 Mundy GR. Mechanisms of bone metastasis. Cancer 1997, **80**: 1546–1556.

977 Norman A, Ulin R. A comparative study of periosteal new-bone response in metastatic bone tumors (solitary) and primary bone sarcomas. Radiology 1969, **92**: 705–708.

978 Perez CA, Bradfield JS, Morgan HC. Management of pathologic fractures. Cancer 1972, **29**: 1027–1037.

979 Quinn JM, Matsumura Y, Tarin D, McGee JO, Athanasou NA. Cellular and hormonal mechanisms associated with malignant bone resorption. Lab Invest 1994, **71**: 465–471.

980 Simon MA, Bartucci EJ. The search for the primary tumor in patients with skeletal metastases of unknown origin. Cancer 1986, **58**: 1088–1095.

981 Thomas BM. Three unusual carcinoid tumours, with particular reference to osteoblastic bone metastases. Clin Radiol 1968, **19**: 221–225.

982 Troncoso A, Ro JY, Grignon DJ, Han WS, Wexler H, von Eschenbach A, Ayala AG. Renal cell carcinoma with acrometastasis. Report of two cases and review of the literature. Mod Pathol 1991, **4**: 66–69.

983 Yamashita K, Ueda T, Komatsubara Y, Koyama H, Inaji H, Yonenobu K, Ono K. Breast cancer with bone-only metastases. Visceral metastases-free rate in relation to anatomic distribution of bone metastases. Cancer 1991, **68**: 634–637.

TUMORLIKE LESIONS

SOLITARY BONE CYST

984 Amling M, Werner M, Posl M, Maas R, Korn U, Delling G. Calcifying solitary bone cyst. Morphologic aspects and differential diagnosis of sclerotic bone tumours. Virchows Arch 1995, **426**: 235–242.

985 Campanacci M, Capanna R, Picci P. Unicameral and aneurysmal bone cysts. Clin Orthop 1986, **204**: 25–36.

986 Mirra JM, Bernard GW, Bullough PG, Johnston W, Mink G. Cementum-like bone production in solitary bone cysts (so-called 'cementoma' of long bones). Report of three cases. Electron microscopic observations supporting a synovial origin to the simple bone cyst. Clin Orthop 1978, **135**: 295–307.

987 Smith RW, Smith CF. Solitary unicameral bone cyst of the calcaneus. A review of twenty cases. J Bone Joint Surg (Am) 1974, **56**: 49–56.

ANEURYSMAL BONE CYST

988 Aho HJ, Aho AJ, Einola S. Aneurysmal bone cyst. A study of ultrastructure and malignant transformation. Virchows Arch [A] 1982, **395**: 169–179.

989 Alles JU, Schulz A. Immunocytochemical markers (endothelial and histiocytic) and ultrastructure of primary aneurysmal bone cysts. Hum Pathol 1986, **17**: 39–45.

990 Althof PA, Ohmori K, Zhou M, Bailey JM, Bridge RS, Nelson M, Neff JR, Bridge JA. Cytogenetic and molecular cytogenetic findings in 43 aneurysmal bone cysts: aberrations of 17p mapped to 17p13.2 by fluorescence in situ hybridization. Mod Pathol 2004, **17**: 518–525.

991 Bertoni F, Bacchini P, Capanna R, Ruggieri P, Biagini R, Ferruzzi A, Bettelli G, Picci P, Campanacci M. Solid variant of aneurysmal bone cyst. Cancer 1993, **71**: 729–734.

992 Buraczewski J, Dabska M. Pathogenesis of aneurysmal bone cyst. Relationship between the aneurysmal bone cyst and fibrous dysplasia of bone. Cancer 1971, **28**: 597–604.

993 Capanna R, Albisinni U, Picci P, Calderoni P, Campanacci M, Springfield DS. Aneurysmal bone cyst of the spine. J Bone Joint Surg (Am) 1985, **67**: 527–531.

994 Clough JR, Price CHG. Aneurysmal bone cyst. Pathogenesis and long term results of treatment. Clin Orthop 1973, **97**: 52–63.

995 Dabezies EJ, D'Ambrosia RD, Chuinard RG, Ferguson AB. Aneurysmal bone cyst after fracture. A report of three cases. J Bone Joint Surg (Am) 1982, **64**: 617–621.

996 Dabska M, Buraczewski J. Aneurysmal bone cyst. Pathology, clinical course and radiologic appearances. Cancer 1969, **23**: 371–389.

997 D'Alonzo RT, Pitcock JA, Milford LW. Giant cell reaction of bone. Report of two cases. J Bone Joint Surg (Am) 1972, **54**: 1267–1271.

998 Dehner LP, Risdall RJ, L'Heureux P. Giant cell-containing 'fibrous' lesion of the sacrum. Am J Surg Pathol 1978, **2**: 55–70.

999 de Silva MV, Raby N, Reid R. Fibromyxoid areas and immature osteoid are associated with recurrence of primary aneurysmal bone cysts. Histopathology 2003, **43**: 180–188.

1000 Edling NPG. Is the aneurysmal bone cyst a true entity? Cancer 1965, **18**: 1127–1130.

1001 Koskinen EVS, Visuri TI, Holmström T, Roukkula MA. Aneurysmal bone cyst. Evaluation of resection and of curettage in 20 cases. Clin Orthop 1976, **118**: 136–146.

1002 Kyriakos M, Hardy D. Malignant transformation of aneurysmal bone cyst, with an analysis of the literature. Cancer 1991, **68**: 1770–1780.

1003 Leithner A, Lang S, Windhager R, Leithner K, Karlic H, Kotz R, Haas OA. Expression of insulin-like growth factor-1 (IGF-1) in aneurysmal bone cyst. Mod Pathol 2001, **14**: 1100–1104.

1004 Leithner A, Windhager R, Lang S, Haas OA, Kainberger F, Kotz R. Aneurysmal bone cyst. A population based epidemiologic study and literature review. Clin Orthop 1999, **363**: 176–179.

1005 Levy WM, Miller AS, Bonakdarpour A, Aegerter E. Aneurysmal bone cyst secondary to other osseous lesions. Report of 57 cases. Am J Clin Pathol 1975, **63**: 1–8.

1006 McCarthy EF, Dortman HD. Vascular and cartilaginous hamartoma of the ribs in infancy with secondary aneurysmal bone cyst formation. Am J Surg Pathol 1980, **4**: 247–253.

1007 Oda Y, Tsuneyoshi M, Shinohara N. 'Solid' variant of aneurysmal bone cyst (extragnathic giant cell reparative granuloma) in the axial skeleton and long bones. A study of its morphologic spectrum and distinction from allied giant cell lesions. Cancer 1992, **70**: 2642–2649.

1008 Oliveira AM, Perez-Atayde AR, Inwards CY, Medeiros F, Derr V, Hsi BL, Gebhardt MC, Rosenberg AE, Fletcher JA. USP6 and CDH11 oncogenes identify the neoplastic cell in primary aneurysmal bone cysts and are absent in so-called secondary aneurysmal bone cysts. Am J Pathol 2004, **165**: 1773–1780.

1009 Oliveira AM, Perez-Atayde AR, Dal Cin P, Gebhardt MC, Chen CJ, Neff JR, Demetri GD, Rosenberg AE, Bridge JA, Fletcher JA. Aneurysmal bone cyst variant translocations upregulate USP6 transcription by promoter swapping with the ZNF9, COL1A1, TRAP150, and OMD genes. Oncogene 2005, **24**: 3419–3426.

1010 Panico L, Passeretti U, De Rosa N, D'Antonio A, De Rosa G. Giant cell reparative granuloma of the distal skeletal bones. A report of five cases with immunohistochemical findings. Virchows Arch 1994, **425**: 315–320.

1011 Petrik PK, Findlay JM, Sherlock RA. Aneurysmal cyst, bone type, primary in an artery. Am J Surg Pathol 1993, **17**: 1062–1066.

1012 Rodriguez-Peralto JL, Lopez-Barea F, Sanchez-Herrera S, Atienza M. Primary aneurysmal cyst of soft tissues (extraosseous aneurysmal cyst). Am J Surg Pathol 1994, **18**: 632–636.

1013 Ruiter DJ, van Rijssel ThG, van der Velde EA. Aneurysmal bone cysts. A clinicopathological study of 105 cases. Cancer 1977, **39**: 2231–2239.

1014 Sanerkin NG, Mott MG, Roylance J. An unusual intraosseous lesion with fibroblastic, osteoclastic, osteoblastic, aneurysmal and fibromyxoid elements. 'Solid' variant of aneurysmal bone cyst. Cancer 1983, **51**: 2278–2286.

1015 Sciot R, Dorfman H, Brys P, Dal Cin P, De Wever I, Fletcher CD, Jonson K, Mandahl N, Mertens F, Mitelman F, Rosai J, Rydholm A, Samson I, Tallini G, Van den Berghe H, Vanni R, Willen H. Cytogenetic–morphologic correlations in aneurysmal bone cyst, giant cell tumor of bone and combined lesions. A report from the CHAMP study group. Mod Pathol 2000, **13**: 1206–1210.

1016 Shannon P, Bedard Y, Bell R, Kandel R. Aneurysmal cyst of soft tissue: report of a case with serial magnetic resonance imaging and biopsy. Hum Pathol 1997, **28**: 255–257.

1017 Tillman BP, Dahlin DC, Lipscomb PR, Stewart JR. Aneurysmal bone cyst. An analysis of 95 cases. Mayo Clin Proc 1968, **43**: 478–495.

1018 Vergel De Dios AM, Bond JR, Shives TC, McLeod RA, Unni KK. Aneurysmal bone cyst. A clinicopathologic study of 238 cases. Cancer 1992, **69**: 2921–2931.

1019 Wold LE, Dobyns JH, Swee RG, Dahlin DC. Giant cell reaction (giant cell reparative granuloma) of the small bones of the hands and feet. Am J Surg Pathol 1986, **10**: 491–496.

1020 Yamaguchi T, Dorfman HD. Giant cell reparative granuloma. A comparative clinicopathologic study of lesions in gnathic and extragnathic sites. Int J Surg Pathol 2001, **9**: 189–200.

OTHER CYSTS

1021 Alguacil-Garcia A, Littman CD. Subpubic cartilaginous cyst: report of two cases. Am J Surg Pathol 1996, **20**: 975–979.

1022 Bauer TW, Dorfman, HD. Intraosseous ganglion. A clinicopathologic study of 11 cases. Am J Surg Pathol 1982, **6**: 207–213.

1023 Schajowicz F, Sainz MC, Slullitel JA. Juxta-articular bone cysts (intra-osseous ganglia). J Bone Joint Surg (Br) 1979, **61**: 107–116.

1024 Sim FH, Dahlin DC. Ganglion cysts of bone. Mayo Clin Proc 1971, **46**: 484–488.

METAPHYSEAL FIBROUS DEFECT (NONOSSIFYING FIBROMA)

1025 Arata MA, Peterson HA, Dahlin DC. Pathological fractures through non-ossifying fibromas. Review of the Mayo Clinic experience. J Bone Joint Surg (Am) 1981, **63**: 980–988.

1026 Clarke BE, Xipell JM, Thomas DP. Benign fibrous histiocytoma of bone. Am J Surg Pathol 1985, **9**: 806–815.

1027 Craver RD, Heinrich S, Mirra J. Fibrous cortical defect with bizarre nuclear features. Ann Diagn Pathol 1997, **1**: 26–30.

1028 Cunningham JB, Ackerman LV. Metaphyseal fibrous defects. J Bone Joint Surg (Am) 1956, **38**: 797–808.

FIBROUS DYSPLASIA AND RELATED LESIONS

1029 Aoki T, Kouho H, Hisaoka M, Hashimoto H, Nakata H, Sakai A. Intramuscular myxoma with fibrous dysplasia. A report of two cases with a review of the literature. Pathol Int 1995, **45**: 165–171.

1030 Bridge JA, Dembinski A, De Boer J, Travis J, Neff JR. Clonal chromosomal abnormalities in osteofibrous dysplasia. Implications for histopathogenesis and its relationship with adamantinoma. Cancer 1994, **73**: 1746–1752.

1031 Campanacci M, Laus M. Osteofibrous dysplasia of the tibia and fibula. J Bone Joint Surg (Am) 1981, **63**: 367–375.

1032 Campbell CJ, Hawk T. A variant of fibrous dysplasia (osteofibrous dysplasia). J Bone Joint Surg (Am) 1982, **64**: 231–236.

1033 Cohen MM Jr. The new bone biology: pathologic, molecular, and clinical correlates. Am J Med Genet A 2006, **140**: 2646–2706.

1034 de Sanctis L, Delmastro L, Russo MC, Matarazzo P, Lala R, de Sanctis C. Genetics of McCune–Albright syndrome. J Pediatr Endocrinol Metab 2006, **19**(Suppl 2): 577–582.

1035 Dorfman HD, Ishida T, Tsuneyoshi M. Exophytic variant of fibrous dysplasia (fibrous dysplasia protuberans). Hum Pathol 1994, **25**: 1234–1237.

1036 Gleason BC, Liegl-Atzwanger B, Kozakewich HP, Connolly S, Gebhardt MC, Fletcher JA, Perez-Atayde AR. Osteofibrous dysplasia and adamantinoma in children and adolescents: a clinicopathologic reappraisal. Am J Surg Pathol 2008, **32**: 363–376.

1037 Gouldesbrough DR. Symmetrical fibro-osseous dysplasia of rib – evidence for a traumatic aetiology. Histopathology 1990, **17**: 267–270.

1038 Greco MA, Steiner GC. Ultrastructure of fibrous dysplasia of bone. A study of its fibrous, osseous, and cartilaginous components. Ultrastruct Pathol 1986, **10**: 55–66.

1039 Harris WH, Dudley HR, Barry RJ. The natural history of fibrous dysplasia. J Bone Joint Surg (Am) 1962, **44**: 207–233.

1040 Heim-Hall JM, Williams RP. Liposclerosing myxofibrous tumour: a traumatized variant of fibrous dysplasia? Report of four cases and review of the literature. Histopathology 2004, **45**: 369–376.

1041 Huvos AG, Higinbotham NL, Miller TR. Bone sarcomas arising in fibrous dysplasia. J Bone Joint Surg (Am) 1972, **54**: 1047–1056.

1042 Ishida T, Machinami R, Kojima T, Kikuchi F. Malignant fibrous histiocytoma and osteosarcoma in association with fibrous dysplasia of bone. Report of three cases. Pathol Res Pract 1992, **188**: 757–763.

1043 Kandel RA, Pritzker KPH, Bedard YC. Symmetrical fibro-osseous dysplasia of rib – post-traumatic dysplasia? Histopathology 1981, **5**: 651–658.

1044 Kashima TG, Nishiyama T, Shimazu K, Shimazaki M, Kii I, Grigoriadis AE, Fukayama M, Kudo A. Periostin, a novel marker of intramembranous ossification, is expressed in fibrous dysplasia and in c-Fos-overexpressing bone lesions. Hum Pathol 2009, **40**: 226–237.

1045 Kempson RL. Ossifying fibroma of the long bones. Arch Pathol 1966, **82**: 218–233.

1046 Maki M, Athanasou N. Osteofibrous dysplasia and adamantinoma: correlation of proto-oncogene product and matrix protein expression. Hum Pathol 2004, **35**: 69–74.

1047 Marie PJ, De Pollak C, Chanson P, Lomri A. Increased proliferation of osteoblastic cells expressing the activating GS alpha mutation in monostotic and polyostotic fibrous dysplasia. Am J Pathol 1997, **150**: 1059–1069.

1048 McDermott MB, Kyriakos M, Flanagan FL. Posttraumatic fibro-osseous lesion of rib. Hum Pathol 1999, **30**: 770–780.

1049 Mikami M, Koizumi H, Ishii M, Nakajima H. The identification of monoclonality in fibrous dysplasia by methylation-specific polymerase chain reaction for the human androgen receptor gene. Virchows Arch 2004, **444**: 56–60.

1050 Nakashima Y, Yamamuro T, Fujiwara Y, Kotoura Y, Mori E, Hamashima Y. Osteofibrous dysplasia (ossifying fibroma of long bones). A study of 12 cases. Cancer 1983, **52**: 909–914.

1051 Park YK, Unni KK, McLeod RA, Pritchard DJ. Osteofibrous dysplasia. Clinico-pathologic study of 80 cases. Hum Pathol 1993, **24**: 1339–1347.

1052 Pelzmann KS, Nagel DZ, Salyer WR. Polyostotic fibrous dysplasia and fibrochondrodysplasia. Skeletal Radiol 1980, **5**: 116–118.

1053 Povysil C, Matejovsky Z. Fibro-osseous lesion with calcified spherules (cementifying fibromalike lesion) of the tibia. Ultrastruct Pathol 1993, **17**: 25–34.

1054 Ragsdale BD. Polymorphic fibro-osseous lesions of bone. An almost site-specific diagnostic problem of the proximal femur. Hum Pathol 1993, **24**: 505–512.

1055 Reed RJ. Fibrous dysplasia of bone. A review of 25 cases. Arch Pathol 1963, **75**: 480–495.

1056 Ruggieri P, Sim FH, Bond JR, Unni KK. Malignancies in fibrous dysplasia. Cancer 1994, **73**: 1411–1424.

1057 Sakamoto A, Oda Y, Iwamoto Y, Tsuneyoshi M. A comparative study of fibrous dysplasia and osteofibrous dysplasia with regard to expression of c-fos and c-jun products and bone matrix proteins: a clinicopathologic review and immunohistochemical study of c-fos, c-jun type I collagen, osteonectin, osteopontin, and osteocalcin. Hum Pathol 1999, **30**: 1418–1426.

1058 Sakamoto A, Oda Y, Iwamoto Y, Tsuneyoshi M. A comparative study of fibrous dysplasia and osteofibrous dysplasia with regard to Gsalfa mutation at the Arg 201 codon: polymerase chain reaction-restriction fragment length polymorphism analysis of paraffin-embedded tissue. J Mol Diagn 2000, **2**: 67–72.

1059 Sakamoto A, Oda Y, Oshiro Y, Tamiya S, Iwamoto Y, Tsuneyoshi M. Immunoexpression of neurofibromin, S-100 protein, and leu-7 and mutation analysis of the NF1 gene at codon 1423 in osteofibrous dysplasia. Hum Pathol 2001, **32**: 1245–1251.

1060 Sissons HA, Steiner GC, Dorfman HD. Calcified spherules in fibro-osseous lesions of bone. Arch Pathol Lab Med 1993, **117**: 284–290.

1061 Sweet DE, Vinh TN, Devaney K. Cortical osteofibrous dysplasia of long bone and its relationship to adamantinoma. A clinicopathologic study of 30 cases. Am J Surg Pathol 1992, **16**: 282–290.

1062 Voytek TM, Ro JY, Edeiken J, Ayala AG. Fibrous dysplasia and cemento-ossifying fibroma. A histologic spectrum. Am J Surg Pathol 1995, **19**: 775–781.

MYOSITIS OSSIFICANS

1063 Ackerman LV. Extraosseous localized nonneoplastic bone and cartilage formation (so-called myositis ossificans). J Bone Joint Surg (Am) 1958, **40**: 279–298.

1064 Craver RD, Correa-Gracian H, Heinrich S. Florid reactive periostitis. Hum Pathol 1997, **28**: 745–747.

1065 de Silva MV, Reid R. Myositis ossificans and fibroosseous pseudotumor of digits: a clinicopathological review of 64 cases with emphasis on diagnostic pitfalls. Int J Surg Pathol 2003, **11**: 187–195.

1066 Dupree WB, Enzinger FM. Fibro-osseous pseudotumor of the digits. Cancer 1986, **58**: 2103–2109.

1067 Jüppner H. The genetic basis of progressive osseous heteroplasia. N Engl J Med 2002, **346**: 128–130.

1068 Povysil C, Matejovsky Z. Ultrastructural evidence of myofibroblasts in pseudo-malignant myositis ossificans. Virchows Arch [A] 1979, **381**: 189–203.

1069 Shore EM, Ahn J, Jan de Beur S. Paternally inherited inactivating mutations of the *GNAS1* gene in progressive osseous heteroplasia. N Engl J Med 2002, **346**: 99–106.

1070 Spjut HJ, Dorfman HD. Florid reactive periostitis of the tubular bones of the hands and feet. Am J Surg Pathol 1981, **5**: 423–433.

1071 Sukov WR, Franco MF, Erickson-Johnson M, Chou MM, Unni KK, Wenger DE, Wang X, Oliveira AM. Frequency of USP6 rearrangements in myositis ossificans, brown tumor, and cherubism: molecular cytogenetic evidence that a subset of 'myositis ossificans-like lesions' are the early phases in the formation of soft-tissue aneurysmal bone cyst. Skeletal Radiol 2008, **37**: 321–327.

1072 Sumiyoshi K, Tsuneyoshi M, Enjoji M. Myositis ossificans. A clinicopathologic study of 21 cases. Acta Pathol Jpn 1985, **35**: 1109–1122.

1073 Yaghmai I. Myositis ossificans. Diagnostic value of arteriography. AJR 1977, **128**: 811–816.

LANGERHANS CELL HISTIOCYTOSIS

1074 Gibson SE, Prayson RA. Primary skull lesions in the pediatric population: a 25-year experience. Arch Pathol Lab Med 2007, **131**: 761–766.

1075 Howarth DM, Gilchrist GS, Mullan BP, Wiseman GA, Edmonson JH, Schomberg PJ. Langerhans cell histiocytosis: diagnosis, natural history, management and outcome. Cancer 1999, **85**: 2278–2290.

1076 Lau SK, Chu PG, Weiss LM. Immunohistochemical expression of Langerin in Langerhans cell histiocytosis and non-Langerhans cell histiocytic disorders. Am J Surg Pathol 2008, **32**: 615–619.

1077 Lieberman PH, Jones CR, Dargeon HWK, Begg CF. A reappraisal of eosinophilic granuloma of bone. Hand–Schüller–Christian syndrome and Letterer–Siwe syndrome. Medicine (Baltimore) 1969, **48**: 375–400.

1078 Makley JT, Carter JR. Eosinophilic granuloma of bone. Clin Orthop 1986, **204**: 37–44.

1079 McGavran MH, Spady HA. Eosinophilic granuloma of bone. A study of 28 cases. J Bone Joint Surg (Am) 1960, **42**: 979–992.

1080 Newton WA, Hamoudi AB. Histiocytosis. A histologic classification with clinical correlation. Perspect Pediatr Pathol 1973, **1**: 251–283.

1081 Nezelof C, Frileux-Herbet F, Cronier-Sachot J. Disseminated histiocytosis X. Analysis of prognostic factors based on a retrospective study of 50 cases. Cancer 1979, **44**: 1824–1838.

1082 Walker PD, Rosai J, Dorfman RF. The osseous manifestations of sinus histiocytosis with massive lymphadenopathy. Am J Clin Pathol 1981, **75**: 131–139.

OTHER HISTIOCYTIC LESIONS

1083 Al-Quran S, Rieth J, Bradley J, Rimsza L. Erdheim–Chester disease: case report, PCR-based analysis of clonality, and review of literature. Mod Pathol 2002, **15**: 666–672.

1084 Chetritt J, Paradis V, Dargere D, Adle-Biassette H, Maurage CA, Mussini JM, Vital A, Wechsler J, Bedossa P. Chester-Erdheim disease: a neoplastic disorder. Hum Pathol 1999, **30**: 1093–1096.

1085 Demicco EG, Rosenberg AE, Björnsson J, Rybak LD, Unni KK, Nielsen GP. Primary Rosai–Dorfman disease of bone: a clinicopathologic study of 15 cases. Am J Surg Pathol 2010, **34**: 1324–1333.

1086 Kenn W, Eck M, Allolio B, Jacob F, Illg A, Marx A, Mueller-Hermelink HK, Hahn D. Erdheim–Chester disease: evidence for a disease entity different from Langerhans cell histiocytosis? Three cases with detailed radiological and immunohistochemical analysis. Hum Pathol 2000, **31**: 734–739.

1087 Kim N-R, Ko Y-H, Choe YH, Lee H-G, Huh B, Ahn G-H. Erdheim–Chester disease with extensive marrow necrosis. A case report and literature review. Int J Surg Pathol 2001, **9**: 73–79.

1088 Walker PD, Rosai J, Dorfman RF. The osseous manifestations of sinus histiocytosis with massive lymphadenopathy. Am J Clin Pathol 1981, **75**: 131–139.

JOINTS AND RELATED STRUCTURES

NORMAL ANATOMY

1089 Boland JM, Folpe AL, Hornick JL, Grogg KL. Clusterin, a follicular dendritic cell-associated apolipoprotein, is expressed in normal synoviocytes and in tenosynovial giant cell tumors of localized and diffuse types: Diagnostic and histogenetic implications. Lab Invest 2009, **89**(Suppl 1): 12A.

1090 Bullough PG. Joints. In Mills SE (ed.): Histology for pathologists, ed. 3. Philadelphia, 2007, Lippincott Williams & Wilkins, pp. 97–122.

1091 Stevens CR, Map PI, Revell PA. A monoclonal antibody (Mab 67) marks type B synoviocytes. Rheumatol Int 1990, **10**: 103–106.

1092 Wilkinson LS, Edwards JCW, Poston RN, Haskard DO. Expression of vascular cell adhesion molecule-1 in normal and inflamed synovium. Lab Invest 1993, **68**: 82–88.

1093 Wilkinson LS, Pitsillides AA, Worrall JG, Edwards JCW. Light microscopic characterization of the fibroblast-like synovial intimal cell (synoviocyte). Arthritis Rheum 1992, **35**: 1179–1184.

NON-NEOPLASTIC DISEASES

GANGLIA AND CYSTIC MENISCUS

1094 Glasgow MM, Allen PW, Blakeway C. Arthroscopic treatment of cysts of the lateral meniscus. J Bone Joint Surg Br 1993, **75**: 299–302.

1095 Romanini L, Calvisi V, Collodel M, Masciocchi C. Cystic degeneration of the lateral meniscus. Pathogenesis and diagnostic approach. Ital J Orthop Traumatol 1988, **14**: 493–500.

1096 Stack RE, Bianco AH Jr, MacCarthy CS. Compression of the common peroneal nerve by ganglion cyst. Report of nine cases. J Bone Joint Surg (Am) 1965, **47**: 773–778.

BURSAE AND BAKER CYST

1097 Pederson HE, Key JA. Pathology of calcareous tendinitis and subdeltoid bursitis. Arch Surg 1951, **62**: 50–63.

1098 Shon W, Folpe AL. Tenosynovitis with psammomatous calcification: a poorly recognized pseudotumor related to repetitive tendinous injury. Am J Surg Pathol 2010, **34**: 892–895.

1099 Wagner T, Abgarowicz T. Microscopic appearance of Baker's cyst in cases of rheumatoid arthritis. Rheumatologia 1970, **8**: 21–26.

CARPAL TUNNEL SYNDROME

1100 Bastian FO. Amyloidosis and the carpal tunnel syndrome. Am J Clin Pathol 1974, **61**: 711–717.

1101 Entin MA. Carpal tunnel syndrome and its variants. Surg Clin North Am 1968, **48**: 1097–1112.

1102 Phalen GS. The carpal-tunnel syndrome. Seventeen years' experience in diagnosis and treatment of six hundred and fifty-four hands. J Bone Joint Surg (Am) 1966, **48**: 211–228.

1103 Spinner RJ, Bachman JW, Amadio PC. The many faces of carpal tunnel syndrome. Mayo Clin Proc 1989, **64**: 829–836.

1104 Uchiyama S, Itsubo T, Nakamura K, Kato H, Yasutomi T, Momose T. Current concepts of carpal tunnel syndrome: pathophysiology, treatment, and evaluation. J Orthop Sci 2010, **15**: 1–13.

ARTHRITIS

Synovial biopsy

1105 Goldenberg DL, Cohen AS. Synovial membrane histopathology in the differential diagnosis of rheumatoid arthritis, gout, pseudogout, systemic lupus erythematosus, infectious arthritis and degenerative joint disease. Medicine 1978, **57**: 239–252.

1106 Krenn V, Morawietz L, Burmester GR, Kinne RW, Mueller-Ladner U, Muller B, Haupl T. Synovitis score: discrimination between chronic low-grade and high-grade synovitis. Histopathology 2006, **49**: 358–364.

1107 O'Connell JX. Pathology of the synovium. Am J Clin Pathol 2000, **114**: 773–784.

1108 Revell PA. The synovial biopsy. In Anthony PP, MacSween RNM (eds): Recent advances in histopathology, vol. 13. Edinburgh, 1987, Churchill Livingstone.

1109 Rodnan GP, Yunis EJ, Totten RS. Experience with punch biopsy of synovium in the study of joint disease. Ann Intern Med 1960, **53**: 319–331.

1110 Schumacher HR, Kulka JP. Needle biopsy of the synovial membrane. Experience with the Parker–Pearson technic. N Engl J Med 1972, **286**: 416–419.

1111 Schwartz S, Cooper N. Synovial membrane punch biopsy. Arch Intern Med 1961, **108**: 400–406.

1112 Soren A. Histodiagnosis and clinical correlation of rheumatoid and other synovitis. Philadelphia, 1978, JB Lippincott Co.

1113 Vordenbäumen S, Joosten LA, Friemann J, Schneider M, Ostendorf B. Utility of synovial biopsy. Arthritis Res Ther 2009, **11**: 256.

Degenerative joint disease (osteoarthrosis)

1114 Aigner T, Dietz U, Stöss H, Von der Mark K. Differential expression of collagen types I, II, III, and X in human osteophytes. Lab Invest 1995, **73**: 236–243.

1115 Bennett GA, Waine H, Bauer W. Changes in the knee joint at various ages. New York, 1942, Commonwealth Fund.

1116 Collins DH. The pathology of articular and spinal diseases. London, 1949, Edward Arnold & Co.

1117 Di Francesco L, Sokoloff L. Lipochondral degeneration of capsular tissue in osteoarthritic hips. Am J Surg Pathol 1995, **19**: 278–283.

1118 Gardner DL, Salter DM, Oates K. Advances in the microscopy of osteoarthritis. Microsc Res Tech 1997, **37**: 245–270.

1119 Haliburton RA, Sullivan CR. The patella in degenerative joint disease. A clinicopathologic study. Arch Surg 1958, **77**: 677–683.

1120 Hamerman D. The biology of osteoarthritis. N Engl J Med 1989, **320**: 1322–1330.

1121 Harrison MHM, Schajowicz F, Tureta J. Osteoarthritis of the hip. A study of the nature and evolution of the disease. J Bone Joint Surg (Br) 1953, **35**: 598–626.

1122 Hirsch C, Schajowicz F, Galante J. Structural changes in the cervical spine. A study on autopsy specimens in different age groups. Acta Orthop Scand (Suppl) 1967, **109**: 7–77.

1123 Horwitz T. Bone and cartilage debris in the synovial membrane. Its significance in the early diagnosis of neuro-arthropathy. J Bone Joint Surg (Am) 1948, **30**: 579–588.

1124 Jayson MI, Rubenstein D, Dixon AS. Intra-articular pressure and rheumatoid geodes (bone 'cysts'). Ann Rheum Dis 1970, **29**: 496–502.

1125 Mankin HJ. The reaction of articular cartilage to injury and osteoarthritis. N Engl J Med 1974, **291**: 1285–1292, 1335–1340.

1126 Norman A, Robbins H, Milgram JE. The acute neuropathic arthropathy. A rapid, severely disorganizing form of arthritis. Radiology 1968, **90**: 1159–1164.

1127 O'Connell JX, Nielsen GP, Rosenberg AE. Subchondral acute inflammation in severe arthritis: a sterile osteomyelitis? Am J Surg Pathol 1999, **23**: 192–197.

1128 Outerbridge RE. The etiology of chrondromalacia patellae. J Bone Joint Surg (Br) 1961, **43**: 752–757.

1129 Rabinowicz T, Jacqueline F. Pathology of the capsular and synovial hip nerves in chronic hip diseases. Pathol Res Pract 1990, **186**: 283–292.

1130 Rhaney K, Lamb DW. The cysts of osteoarthritis of the hip. A radiological and pathological study. J Bone Joint Surg (Br) 1955, **37**: 663–675.

1131 Sadouk M, Pelletier J-P, Tardif G, Klansa D, Cloutier J-M, Martel-Pelletier J. Human synovial fibroblasts coexpress IL-1 receptor Type I and Type II mRNA. The increased level of the IL-I receptor in osteoarthritic cells is related to an increased level of the Type I receptor. Lab Invest 1995, **74**: 347–355.

1132 Sokoloff L. Pathology and pathogenesis of osteoarthritis. In McCarty DJ (ed.): Arthritis and applied conditions, ed. 9. Philadelphia, 1979, Lea & Febiger, pp. 1135–1153.

Rheumatoid arthritis

1133 Baumann H, Kushner I. Production of interleukin-6 by synovial fibroblasts in rheumatoid arthritis. Am J Pathol 1998, **152**: 641–644.

1134 Beatty EC Jr. Rheumatic-like nodules occurring in nonrheumatic children. Arch Pathol 1959, **68**: 154–159.

1135 Berardinelli JL, Hyman CJ, Campbell EE, Fireman P. Presence of rheumatoid factor in ten children with isolated rheumatoid-like nodules. J Pediatr 1972, **81**: 751–757.

1136 Bhan AK, Roy S. Synovial giant cells in rheumatoid arthritis and other joint diseases. Ann Rheum Dis 1971, **30**: 294–298.

1137 Cooper NS. Pathology of rheumatoid arthritis. Med Clin North Am 1968, **52**: 607–621.

1138 Dixon AStJ, Grant C. Acute synovial rupture in rheumatoid arthritis. Clinical and experimental observations. Lancet 1964, **1**: 742–745.

1139 Grimley PM, Sokoloff L. Synovial giant cells in rheumatoid arthritis. Am J Pathol 1966, **49**: 931–954.

1140 Hahn BH, Yardley JH, Stevens MB. 'Rheumatoid' nodules in systemic lupus erythematosus. Ann Intern Med 1970, **72**: 49–58.

1141 Harris ED Jr. Rheumatoid arthritis. Pathophysiology and implications for therapy. N Engl J Med 1990, **322**: 1277–1289.

1142 Hart FD. Rheumatoid arthritis. Extra-articular manifestations. Br Med J 1969, **3**: 131–136.

1143 Hart FD. Rheumatoid arthritis. Extra-articular manifestations. Part II. Br Med J 1970, **2**: 747–752.

1144 Horwitz T. Bone and cartilage debris in the synovial membrane. Its significance in the early diagnosis of neuro-arthropathy. J Bone Joint Surg (Am) 1948, **30**: 579–588.

1145 Imai Y, Sato T, Yamakava M, Kasajima T, Suda A, Watanabe Y. A morphological and immunohistochemical study of lymphoid germinal centers in synovial and lymph node tissues from rheumatoid arthritis patients with special reference to complement components and their receptors. Acta Pathol Jpn 1989, **39**: 127–134.

1146 Jayson MI, Dixon AS, Kates A, Pinder I, Coomes EN. Popliteal and calf cysts in rheumatoid arthritis. Treatment by anterior synovectomy. Ann Rheum Dis 1972, **31**: 9–15.

1147 Kaibara N, Yamada H, Shuto T, Nakashima Y, Okazaki K, Miyahara H, Esaki Y, Hirata G, Iwamoto Y. Comparative histopathological analysis between tenosynovitis and joint synovitis in rheumatoid arthritis. Histopathology 2008, **52**: 856–864.

1148 Koizumi F, Matsuno H, Wakaki K, Ishii Y, Kurashige Y, Nasamura H. Synovitis in rheumatoid arthritis: scoring of characteristic histopathological features. Pathol Int 1999, **49**: 298–304.

1149 Marcus VA, Roy I, Sullivan JD, Sutton JR. Necrobiotic palisading suture granulomas involving bone and joint: report of two cases. Am J Surg Pathol 1997, **21**: 563–565.

1150 Matsuno H, Yodoh K, Nakazawa F, Koizumi F. Relationship between histological findings and clinical findings in rheumatoid arthritis. Pathol Int 2002, **52**: 527–533.

1151 Mongan ES, Cass FM, Jacox RF, Vaughan JH. A study of the relation of seronegative and seropositive rheumatoid arthritis to each other and to necrotizing vasculitis. Am J Med 1969, **47**: 23–25.

1152 Muirden KD. Giant cells, cartilage and bone fragments within rheumatoid synovial membrane. Clinicopathological correlations. Aust Ann Med 1970, **2**: 105–110.

1153 Palmer DG. Synovial cysts in rheumatoid disease. Ann Intern Med 1969, **70**: 61–68.

1154 Qu Z, Huang X-N, Almadi P, Andresevic J, Planck SR, Hart CE, Rosenbaum JT. Expression of basic fibroblast growth factor in synovial tissue from patients with rheumatoid arthritis and degenerative joint disease. Lab Invest 1995, **73**: 339–346.

1155 Roberts WC, Kehol JA, Carpenter DF, Golden A. Cardiac valvular lesions in rheumatoid arthritis. Arch Intern Med 1968, **122**: 141–146.

1156 Schmid FR, Cooper NS, Ziff M, McEwen C. Arteritis in rheumatoid arthritis. Am J Med 1961, **30**: 56–83.

1157 Sokoloff L. Pathology of rheumatoid arthritis and allied disorders. In McCarty DJ (ed.): Arthritis and applied conditions, ed 9. Philadelphia, 1979, Lea & Febiger, pp. 429–447.

1158 Sokoloff L, Wilen SL, Bunim JJ. Arteritis of striated muscle in rheumatoid arthritis. Am J Pathol 1951, **27**: 157–173.

1159 Taylor RT, Huskisson EC, Whitehouse GH, Hart FD. Spontaneous fractures of pelvis in rheumatoid arthritis. Br Med J 1971, **4**: 663–664.

1160 Winchester R. The molecular basis of susceptibility to rheumatoid arthritis. Adv Immunol 1994, **56**: 389–466.

1161 Ziegler B, Gay RE, Huang GQ, Fassbender HG, Gay S. Immunohistochemical localization of HTLV-I p19- and p24-related antigens in synovial joints of patients with rheumatoid arthritis. Am J Pathol 1989, **135**: 1–5.

1162 Zvaifer NJ. Rheumatoid arthritis. The multiple pathways to chronic synovitis (editorial). Lab Invest 1995, **73**: 307–310.

Infectious arthritis

1163 Baumgarten JM, Montiel NJ, Sinha AA. Lyme disease-part 1: epidemiology and etiology. Cutis 2002, **69**: 349–352.

1164 Johnston YE, Duray PH, Steere AC, Kashgarian M, Buza J, Malawista SE, Askenase PW. Lyme arthritis. Spirochetes found in synovial microangiopathic lesions. Am J Pathol 1985, **118**: 26–34.

1165 Meyerhoff J. Lyme disease. Am J Med 1983, **75**: 663–670.

1166 Montiel NJ, Baumgarten JM, Sinha AA. Lyme disease – part II: clinical features and treatment. Cutis 2002, **69**: 443–448.

1167 Nanagara R, Duray PH, Schumacher HR Jr. Ultrastructural demonstration of spirochetal antigens in synovial fluid and synovial membrane in chronic Lyme disease. Possible factors contributing to persistence of organisms. Hum Pathol 1996, **27**: 1025–1034.

1168 Steere AC. Lyme disease. N Engl J Med 1989, **321**: 586–596.

Gout and pseudogout

1169 Chaplin AJ. Calcium pyrophosphate. Histological characterization of crystals in pseudogout. Arch Pathol Lab Med 1976, **100**: 12–15.

1170 Darby AJ, Harness NF, Pritchard MS. Demonstration of urate crystals after formalin fixation. Histopathology 1998, **32**: 382–383.

1171 Ishida T, Dorfman HD, Bullough PG. Tophaceous pseudogout (tumoral calcium pyrophosphate dihydrate crystal deposition disease). Hum Pathol 1995, **26**: 587–593.

1172 Lichtenstein L, Scott HW, Levin MH. Pathologic changes in gout – survey of eleven necropsied cases. Am J Pathol 1956, **32**: 871–895.

1173 Moskowitz RW, Katz D. Chondrocalcinosis and chondrocalsynovitis (pseudogout syndrome). Analysis of 24 cases. Am J Med 1967, **43**: 322–334.

1174 Shidham V, Chivukula M, Basir Z, Shidham G. Evaluation of crystals in formalin fixed, paraffin-embedded tissue sections for the differential diagnosis of pseudogout, gout, and tumoral calcinosis. Mod Pathol 2001, **14**: 806–810.

INTERVERTEBRAL DISK PROLAPSE

1175 Ford JL, Downes S. Cellularity of human annulus tissue: an investigation into the cellularity of tissue of different pathologies. Histopathology 2002, **41**: 531–537.

1176 Rannou F, Lee TS, Zhou RH, Chin J, Lotz JC, Mayoux-Benhamou MA, Barbet JP, Chevrot A, Shyy JY. Intervertebral disc degeneration: the role of the mitochondrial pathway in annulus fibrosus cell apoptosis induced by overload. Am J Pathol 2004, **164**: 915–924.

1177 Weidner N, Rice DT. Intervertebral disk material. Criteria for determining probable prolapse. Hum Pathol 1988, **19**: 406–410.

OTHER ARTICULAR AND PERIARTICULAR DISEASES

1178 Athanasou NA, Sallie B. Localized deposition of amyloid in articular cartilage. Histopathology 1992, **20**: 41–46.

1179 Cary NRB. Clinicopathological importance of deposits of amyloid in the femoral head. J Clin Pathol 1985, **38**: 868–872.

1180 Goldenberg DL, Cohen AS. Synovial membrane histopathology in the differential diagnosis of rheumatoid arthritis, gout, pseudogout, systemic lupus erythematosus, infectious arthritis and degenerative joint disease. Medicine (Baltimore) 1978, **57**: 239–252.

1181 Kyle RA, Eilers SG, Linscheid RL, Gaffey TA. Amyloid localized to tenosynovium at carpal tunnel release. Natural history of 124 cases. Am J Clin Pathol 1989, **91**: 393–397.

1182 Kyle RA, Gertz MA, Linke RP. Amyloid localized to tenosynovium at carpal tunnel release. Immunohistochemical identification of amyloid type. Am J Clin Pathol 1992, **97**: 250–253.

1183 Ladefoged C, Merrild U, Jorgensen B. Amyloid deposits in surgically removed articular and periarticular tissue. Histopathology 1989, **15**: 289–296.

1184 Mihara S, Kawai S, Gondo T, Ishihara T. Intervertebral disc amyloidosis. Histochemical, immunohistochemical and ultrastructural observations. Histopathology 1994, **25**: 415–420.

1185 Pambuccian SE, Horyd ID, Cawte T, Huvos AG. Amyloidoma of bone, a plasma cell/plasmacytoid neoplasm: report of three cases and review of the literature. Am J Surg Pathol 1997, **21**: 179–186.

1186 Reith JD, Bauer TW, Schils JP. Osseous manifestations of SAPHO (synovitis, acne, pustolsis, hyperostosis, osteitis) syndrome. Am J Surg Pathol 1996, **20**: 1368–1377.

1187 Rodnan GP, Medsger TA. The rheumatic manifestations of progressive systemic sclerosis (scleroderma). Clin Orthop 1968, **57**: 81–93.

1188 Roosendaal G, van Rinsum AC, Vianen ME, van den Berg HM, Lafeber FPJG, Bijlsma JW. Haemophilic arthropathy resembles degenerative rather than inflammatory joint disease. Histopathology 1999, **34**: 144–153.

1189 Rumpelt HJ, Braun A, Spier R, Suren EG, Thies E. Localized amyloid in the menisci of the knee joint. Pathol Res Pract 1996, **192**: 547–551.

TUMORS AND TUMORLIKE CONDITIONS

TENOSYNOVIAL GIANT CELL TUMOR

1190 Alguacil-Garcia A, Unni KK, Goellner JR. Giant cell tumor of tendon sheath and pigmented villonodular synovitis. An ultrastructural study. Am J Clin Pathol 1978, **69**: 6–17.

1191 Bertoni F, Unni KK, Beabout JW, Sim FH. Malignant giant cell tumor of the tendon sheaths and joints (malignant pigmented villonodular synovitis). Am J Surg Pathol 1997, **21**: 153–163.

1192 Boland JM, Folpe AL, Hornick JL, Grogg KL. Clusterin is expressed in normal synoviocytes and in tenosynovial giant cell tumors of localized and diffuse types: diagnostic and histogenetic implications. Am J Surg Pathol 2009, **33**: 1225–1229.

1193 Chung EB, Enzinger FM. Fibroma of tendon sheath. Cancer 1979, **44**: 1945–1954.

1194 Cupp JS, Miller MA, Montgomery KD, Nielsen TO, O'Connell JX, Huntsman D, van de Rijn M, Gilks CB, West RB. Translocation and expression of CSF1 in pigmented villonodular synovitis, tenosynovial giant cell tumor, rheumatoid arthritis and other reactive synovitides. Am J Surg Pathol 2007, **31**: 970–976.

1195 Darling JM, Goldring SR, Harada Y, Handel ML, Glowacki J, Gravallese EM. Multinucleated cells in pigmented villondular synovitis and giant cell tumor of tendon sheath express features of osteoclasts. Am J Pathol 1997, **150**: 1383–1393.

1196 Ferrer J, Namiq A, Carda C, Lopez-Gines C, Tawfik O, Llombart-Bosch A. Diffuse type of giant-cell tumor of tendon sheath: an ultrastructural study of two cases with cytogenetic support. Ultrastruct Pathol 2002, **26**: 15–22.

1197 Furlong MA, Motamedi K, Laskin WB, Vinh TN, Murphey M, Sweet DE, Fetsch JF. Synovial-type giant cell tumors of the vertebral column: a clinicopathologic study of 15 cases, with a review of the literature and discussion of the differential diagnosis. Hum Pathol 2003, **34**: 670–679.

1198 Jaffe HL, Lichtenstein L, Sutro CJ. Pigmented villonodular synovitis, bursitis, and tenosynovitis. Arch Pathol 1941, **31**: 731–765.

1199 Li CF, Wang JW, Huang WW, Hou CC, Chou SC, Eng HL, Lin CN, Yu SC, Huang HY. Malignant diffuse-type tenosynovial giant cell tumors: a series of 7 cases comparing with 24 benign lesions with review of the literature. Am J Surg Pathol 2008, **32**: 587–599.

1200 Maluf HM, DeYoung BR, Swanson PE, Wick MR. Fibroma and giant cell tumor of tendon sheath. A comparative histological and immunohistological study. Mod Pathol 1995, **8**: 155–159.

1201 O'Connel JX, Fanburg JC, Rosenberg AE. Giant cell tumor of tendon sheath and pigmented villonodular synovitis. Immunophenotype suggests a synovial cell origin. Hum Pathol 1995, **26**: 771–775.

1202 Sciot R, Rosai J, Dal Cin P, De Wever I, Fletcher CD, Mandahl N, Mertens F, Mitelman F, Rydholm A, Tallini G, van den Berghe H, Vanni R, Willen H. Analysis of 35 cases of localized and diffuse tenosynovial giant cell tumor: a report from the Chromosomes and Morphology (CHAMP) Study Group. Mod Pathol 1999, **12**: 576–579.

1203 Somerhausen NS, Fletcher CD. Diffuse-type giant cell tumor: clinicopathologic and immunohistochemical analysis of 50 cases with extraarticular disease. Am J Surg Pathol 2000, **24**: 479–492.

1204 Tashiro H, Iwasaki H, Kikuchi M, Ogata K, Okazaki M. Giant cell tumors of tendon sheath. A single and multiple immunostaining analysis. Pathol Int 1995, **45**: 147–155.

1205 Ushijima M, Hashimoto H, Tsuneyoshi M, Enjoji M, Miyamoto Y, Okue A. Malignant giant cell tumor of tendon sheath. Report of a case. Acta Pathol Jpn 1985, **35**: 699–709.

1206 West RB, Rubin BP, Miller MA, Subramanian S, Kaygusuz G, Montgomery K, Zhu S, Marinelli RJ, De Luca A, Downs-Kelly E, Goldblum JR, Corless CL, Brown PO, Gilks CB, Nielsen TO, Huntsman D, van de Rijn M. A landscape effect in tenosynovial giant-cell tumor from activation of CSF1 expression by a translocation in a minority of tumor cells. Proc Natl Acad Sci U S A 2006, **103**: 690–695.

PIGMENTED VILLONODULAR SYNOVITIS AND BURSITIS

1207 Berger I, Weckauf H, Helmchen B, Ehemann V, Penzel R, Fink B, Bernd L, Autschbach F. Rheumatoid arthritis and pigmented villonodular synovitis: comparative analysis of cell polyploidy, cell cycle phases and expression of macrophage and fibroblast markers in proliferating synovial cells. Histopathology 2005, **46**: 490–497.

1208 Boland JM, Folpe AL, Hornick JL, Grogg KL. Clusterin is expressed in normal synoviocytes and in tenosynovial giant cell tumors of localized and diffuse types: diagnostic and histogenetic implications. Am J Surg Pathol 2009, **33**: 1225–1229.

1209 Byers PD, Cotton RE, Deacon OW, Lowy M, Newman PH, Sissons HA, Thomson AD. The diagnosis and treatment of pigmented villonodular synovitis. J Bone Joint Surg (Br) 1968, **50**: 290–305.

1210 Choong PF, Willen H, Nilbert M, Mertens F, Mandahl N, Carlen B, Rydholm A. Pigmented villonodular synovitis. Monoclonality and metastasis – a case for neoplastic origin? Acta Orthop Scand 1998, **66**: 64–68.

1211 Darling JM, Glimcher LH, Shortkroff S, Albano B, Gravallese EM. Expression of metalloproteinases in pigmented villonodular synovitis. Hum Pathol 1994, **25**: 825–830.

1212 Layfield LJ, Meloni-Ehrig A, Liu K, Shepard R, Harrelson M. Malignant giant cell tumor of synovium (malignant pigmented villonodular synovitis). Arch Pathol Lab Med 2000, **124**: 1636–1641.

1213 Myers BW, Masi AT. Pigmented villonodular synovitis and tenosynovitis. A clinical epidemiologic study of 166 cases and literature review. Medicine 1980, **59**: 223–238.

1214 Nilsonne U, Moberger G. Pigmented villonodular synovitis of joints. Histological and clinical problems in diagnosis. Acta Orthop Scand 1969, **40**: 448–460.

1215 Oda Y, Izumi T, Harimaya K, Segawa Y, Ishihara S, Komune S, Iwamoto Y, Tsuneyoshi M. Pigmented villonodular synovitis with chondroid metaplasia, resembling chondroblastoma of the bone: a report of three cases. Mod Pathol 2007, **20**: 545–551.

1216 Rao AS, Vigorita VJ. Pigmented villonodular synovitis (giant-cell tumor of the tendon sheath and synovial membrane). A review of eighty-one cases. J Bone Joint Surg (Am) 1984, **66**: 76–94.

1217 Ray RA, Morton CC, Lipinski KK, Corson JM, Fletcher JA. Cytogenetic evidence of clonality in a case of pigmented villonodular synovitis. Cancer 1991, **67**: 121–125.

1218 Sciot R, Rosai J, Dal Cin P, De Wever I, Fletcher CD, Mandahl N, Mertens F, Mitelman F, Rydholm A, Tallini G, van den Berghe H, Vanni R, Willen H. Analysis of 35 cases of localized and diffuse tenosynovial giant cell tumor: a report from the Chromosomes and Morphology (CHAMP) Study Group. Mod Pathol 1999, **12**: 576–579.

1219 Scott FM. Bone lesions in pigmented villonodular synovitis. J Bone Joint Surg (Br) 1968, **50**: 306–311.

1220 Somerhausen NS, Fletcher CD. Diffuse-type giant cell tumor: clinicopathologic and immunohistochemical analysis of 50 cases with extraarticular disease. Am J Surg Pathol 2000, **24**: 479–492.

1221 Ushijima M, Hashimoto H, Tsuneyoshi M, Enjoji M. Pigmented villonodular synovitis. A clinicopathologic study of 52 cases. Acta Pathol Jpn 1986, **36**: 317–326.

1222 Yoshida W, Uzuki M, Kurose A, Yoshida M, Nishida J, Shimamura T, Sawai T. Cell characterization of mononuclear and giant cells constituting pigmented villonodular synovitis. Hum Pathol 2003, **34**: 65–73.

SYNOVIAL OSTEOCHONDROMATOSIS AND CHONDROSARCOMA

1223 Baunsgaard P, Nielsen BB. Primary synovial chondrometaplasia. Histologic variations in the structure of metaplastic nodules. Acta Pathol Microbiol Immunol Scand (A) 1984, **92**: 455–460.

1224 Bertoni F, Unni KK, Beabout JW, Sim FH. Chondrosarcomas of the synovium. Cancer 1991, **67**: 155–162.

1225 Davis RI, Hamilton A, Biggart JD. Primary synovial chondromatosis: a clinicopathologic review and assessment of malignant potential. Hum Pathol 1998, **29**: 683–688.

1226 Fetsch JF, Vinh TN, Remotti F, Walker EA, Murphey MD, Sweet DE. Tenosynovial (extraarticular) chondromatosis. An analysis of 37 cases of an underrecognized clinicopathologic entity with a strong predilection for the hands and feet and a high local recurrence rate. Am J Surg Pathol 2003, **27**: 1260–1268.

1227 Goldman RL, Lichtenstein L. Synovial chondrosarcoma. Cancer 1964, **12**: 1233–1240.

1228 King JW, Spjut HJ, Fechner RE, Vanderpool DW. Synovial chondrosarcoma of the knee joint. J Bone Joint Surg (Am) 1967, **49**: 1389–1396.

1229 Milgram JW. Synovial osteochondromatosis. A histopathological study of thirty cases. J Bone Joint Surg (Am) 1977, **59**: 792–801.

1230 Murphy FP, Dahlin DC, Sullivan CR. Articular synovial chondromatosis. J Bone Joint Surg (Am) 1962, **44**: 77–86.

1231 Sciot R, Dal Cin P, Bellemans J, Samson I, Van den Berghe H, Van Damme B. Synovial chondromatosis: clonal chromosome changes provide further evidence for a neoplastic disorder. Virchows Arch 1998, **433**: 189–191.

1232 Sviland L, Malcolm AJ. Synovial chondromatosis presenting as painless soft tissue mass. A report of 19 cases. Histopathology 1995, **27**: 275–279.

1233 Villacin AB, Brigham LN, Bullough PG. Primary and secondary synovial chondrometaplasia. Histopathologic and clinicoradiologic differences. Hum Pathol 1979, **10**: 439–451.

OTHER TUMORS AND TUMORLIKE CONDITIONS

1234 Devaney K, Vinh TN, Sweet DE. Synovial hemangioma. A report of 20 cases with differential diagnostic considerations. Hum Pathol 1993, **24**: 737–745.

1235 Goodlad JR, Hollowood K, Smith MA, Chan JK, Fletcher CD. Primary juxtaarticular soft tissue lymphoma arising in the vicinity of inflamed joints in patients with rheumatoid arthritis. Histopathology 1999, **34**: 199–204.

1236 Hornick JL, Fletcher CD. Intraarticular nodular fasciitis – a rare lesion: clinicopathologic analysis of a series. Am J Surg Pathol 2006, **30**: 237–241.

1237 Ladefoged C, Jensen NK. Synovial haemangiopericytoma of the knee joint. Histopathology 1989, **15**: 635–637.

1238 Lucas DR, Miller PR, Mott MP, Kronick JL, Unni KK. Arthroplasty-associated malignant fibrous histiocytoma: two case reports. Histopathology 2001, **39**: 620–628.

1239 Rodriguez-Peralto JL, Lopez-Barea F, Gonzalez-Lopez J. Intracapsular chondroma of the knee: an unusual neoplasm. Int J Surg Pathol 1997, **5**: 49–54.

Soft tissues

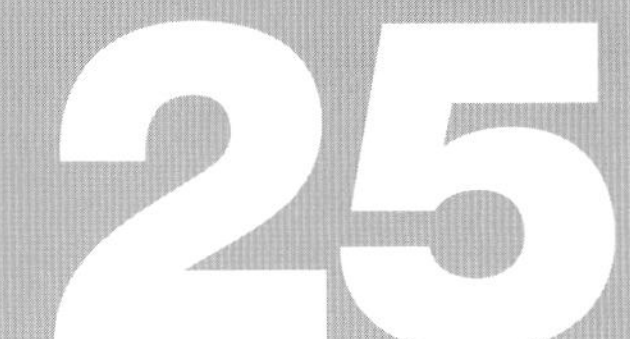

CHAPTER CONTENTS

Normal anatomy

Soft tissue is loosely defined as the complex of nonepithelial extraskeletal structures of the body exclusive of the supportive tissue of the various organs and the hematopoietic/lymphoid tissue. It is composed of fibrous (connective) tissue, adipose tissue, skeletal muscle, blood and lymph vessels, and peripheral nervous system. Most of the soft tissue is derived embryologically from mesoderm, with a neuroectodermal contribution corresponding to the peripheral nerves, and presumably to some of the soft tissues of the head and neck region.[9]

Fibrous tissue consists primarily of fibroblasts and an extracellular matrix that contains fibrillary structures (collagen and elastin) and nonfibrillary extracellular matrix ('ground substance'). Fibrous tissue is classified according to its texture into loose (most locations) and dense (tendons, aponeuroses, and ligaments). *Fibroblasts* are responsible for the production of the various extracellular materials, including the many types of collagen. Their shape varies from spindle (especially when stretched along bundles of collagen fibers) to stellate (in myxoid areas). Immunohistochemically, they are reactive for vimentin and focally for actin. *Fibrocytes* represent the quiescent stage of fibroblasts. *Myofibroblasts* are modified fibroblasts that show features intermediate between fibroblasts and smooth muscle cells.[25-27]

Adipose tissue is divided into two major types: *white fat*, mainly located in the subcutaneous tissue, mediastinum, abdomen, and retroperitoneum; and *brown fat*, which is concentrated in the interscapular region, neck, mediastinum, axillae, and retroperitoneum (especially perirenal region).[3] Brown fat, whose main function is heat production, is much more conspicuous in infants and children. White fat consists of *lipocytes*. These are round or oval cells having most of the cytoplasm occupied by a single large lipid droplet that pushes the crescent-shaped nucleus to the periphery. *Brown fat cells* are smaller, with an acidophilic multivacuolated cytoplasm and a centrally located nucleus showing fine indentations; mitochondria are numerous at the ultrastructural level.

Skeletal muscle is mainly derived from within myotomes (but also from mesectoderm in the head and neck region) through the formation of myoblasts and eventually of myotubes (muscle fibers).[14] The most distinguishing feature of these fibers is the presence of myofibrils, which are composed of two types of microfilament: thin (made of actin) and thick (made of myosin). The periodic arrangement and interdigitation of thin and thick filaments results in the cross-banding seen at a light microscopic level. The I (isotropic) band is made only of thin filaments, the adjacent A (anisotropic) band is a zone of overlapping thin and thick filaments, and the H band is made up only of thick myofilaments. The I band is divided in its center by the Z line or disc, which is thought to serve as an attachment site for the *sarcomere* (that is, the repeating individual unit of the muscle fiber).

Vessels are divided into blood vessels and lymph vessels. *Blood vessels* are further subdivided into arterial and venous compartments joined by a network of capillaries. The several types of cell present in blood vessels are divided into two major types: endothelial cells (located toward the lumen) and a closely related group composed of pericytes, smooth muscle cells, and glomus cells (located toward the outside).[12] Endothelial cells are usually recognized with ease by their shape and location, but both of these can be greatly altered in neoplastic conditions; therefore one has to rely on the presence of other features to identify them. Ultrastructurally, endothelial cells exhibit numerous pinocytotic vesicles, cytoplasmic microfilaments, specialized cell junctions, microvilli, continuous basal lamina, and – most important – the Weibel–Palade body, a membrane-bound organelle thought to be specific to this cell type[6] and shown to contain the von Willebrand factor (factor VIII-related antigen).[34]

Immunohistochemically, endothelial cells exhibit reactivity for vimentin, factor VIII-related antigen (FVIII-RA), *Ulex europaeus* I lectin, CD31, CD34, endothelin, FLI-1, thrombomodulin, FKBP12 (a cytosolic binding protein that interacts with calcineurin), and basal lamina components.[1,5,7,8,11,13,15,19-21,24,28-31,33] Of these, CD31 appears the most useful by virtue of its sensitivity and specificity, although histiocytes and plasma cells are also positive. FVIII-RA is also very specific (the only other positive cell type being the megakaryocyte), but the labile nature of this antigen and its tendency to diffuse out in the tissues limit its utility. FLI-1 (a nuclear transcription factor involved in the pathogenesis of Ewing sarcoma/primitive neuroectodermal tumor [PNET]) seems also extremely promising.[11] Use of monoclonal antibodies for other endothelial markers indicates that phenotypic diversity exists among these cells, a fact of potential diagnostic utility.[10,23,32]

The cells of the pericyte–smooth muscle–glomus family are characterized ultrastructurally by cytoplasmic microfilaments exhibiting focal condensations, numerous pinocytotic vesicles, and a thick continuous basal lamina. Immunohistochemically, they show reactivity for actin, vimentin, and myosin; positivity for desmin is largely restricted to smooth muscle cells, and is not as strong as that exhibited by the 'parenchymal' (non-blood vessel-related) cells. An additional marker of pericytes known as RGS5 has been identified through microarray analysis.[2]

Lymph vessels are lined by endothelial cells exhibiting a much weaker staining for FVIII-RA than endothelial cells from blood vessels, but a similar degree of reactivity for *Ulex*,[5,17] and thrombomodulin.[1] They also stain for Lyve-1 and podoplanin (D2-40).[18] The provocative proposal has been made that the majority of soft tissue sarcomas (with the outstanding exception of epithelioid sarcoma) and benign soft tissue tumors lack intratumoral lymph vessels, in contrast with reactive and proliferative conditions, including nodular fasciitis and related pseudosarcomatous processes.

Peripheral nerves are formed by axons, Schwann cells, perineurial cells, and fibroblasts.[22] Most of the fibroblasts are located in the *epineurium*, which is the outer sheath of fully developed nerves. They are immunoreactive for CD34.[16] Each nerve fascicle is surrounded by the *perineurium*, a structure continuous with the pia arachnoid of the central nervous system; *perineurial cells* are immunoreactive for epithelial membrane antigen (EMA) and Glut-1 and negative for S-100 protein.[16] *Schwann cells* look somewhat similar to fibroblasts at the light microscopic level but are easily distinguished from them immunohistochemically because of their strong immunoreactivity for S-100 protein and ultrastructurally by an intimate relationship to axons (with the formation of mesoaxons) and the presence of a continuous basal lamina that coats the surface of the cell facing the endoneurium. Schwann cells are of neuroectodermal derivation, whereas perineurial cells apparently originate from fibroblasts.[4]

Infections and hematomas

Soft tissue involvement by infectious processes usually is the result of direct extension from cutaneous, visceral, or osseous foci or the complication of trauma or surgery. Rarely, the process has a hematogenous source.

The severity of the inflammatory reaction and the type of tissue response observed pathologically depend on the type, dose, and virulence of the infecting organism; the resistance of the host tissues; the presence or absence of necrotic tissue, hematoma, or foreign body; and the anatomic features of the infected area.

Clinical types of infectious processes, such as hemolytic streptococcal gangrene, necrotizing fasciitis, and Meleney synergistic gangrene, must be diagnosed by clinical appearance and bacteriologic study. In **necrotizing fasciitis** the process is accompanied by severe systemic toxicity; it is usually caused by group A streptococci, but other bacteria and fungi may be involved, including zygomycosis.[36,40] All of the pyogenic and necrotizing infections result in acute inflammatory tissue reactions indistinguishable microscopically. **Granulomatous inflammations** of soft tissue include *tuberculosis, atypical mycobacteriosis, actinomycosis, blastomycosis, coccidioidomycosis, sporotrichosis, cryptococcosis,* and *dirofilariasis*.[35,38,39] A proper search for microorganisms should be made with special stains and cultures.

Hematoma, if deep and encysted, can simulate clinically and radiographically a malignant soft tissue tumor. They occur most commonly in and around the tensor fasciae latae and have been variously referred to as ancient hematoma, calcifying myonecrosis, chronic expanding hematoma, and post-traumatic cyst of soft tissues.[37]

Tumors

Classification

Soft tissue tumors constitute a large and heterogeneous group of neoplasms. This chapter deals primarily with tumors located in the somatic soft tissues; it excludes those arising from the soft tissues of the mediastinum, retroperitoneum, and visceral organs and those primarily involving the dermis, such as Kaposi sarcoma and dermatofibrosarcoma protuberans.

Traditionally, soft tissue sarcomas have been classified according to a histogenetic concept (e.g., fibrosarcoma as a tumor arising from fibroblasts, osteosarcoma as a tumor arising from osteoblasts, and so on). However, morphologic, immunohistochemical, and data from experimental animals suggest that most if not all sarcomas arise from primitive multipotential mesenchymal cells, which in the course of neoplastic transformation undergo differentiation along one or more lines.[42] The acceptance of this alternative scheme does not require a change in terminology: a liposarcoma remains as such but is now viewed not as a tumor arising from a lipoblast but as a tumor exhibiting lipoblastic differentiation. At a practical level, the importance of this classification based on histogenesis and/or differentiation is that it correlates with a variety of clinical parameters, such as location, pattern of growth, multiplicity, likelihood of recurrence, incidence and distribution of metastases, therapeutic response (such as the good response to ifosfamide-based regimens in synovial sarcoma and the greater resistance to chemotherapeutic agents in leiomyosarcoma), prognosis, and patient's age.[41,43]

Clinical features

A definite relationship exists between soft tissue tumor type and the age of presentation.[46,47] For instance, embryonal rhabdomyosarcoma is typically a tumor of infants and children, synovial sarcoma mainly affects adolescents and young adults, and liposarcomas and so-called malignant fibrous histiocytomas are usually seen in middle-aged and elderly patients. Some of the pediatric cases are congenital. It is interesting that congenital soft tissue tumors rarely behave in a malignant fashion, even if an aggressive behavior might have been expected from their microscopic appearance.[45]

Most soft tissue sarcomas are solitary. Synchronous or metachronous multiple sarcomas represent only 0.2% of all cases.[44] Liposarcomas account for a high percentage of these cases.

Diagnosis and special techniques

For any large soft tissue tumor in which the possibility of malignancy exists, the proper initial diagnostic procedure is to obtain material through incisional biopsy or fine needle aspiration. The latter technique is being used with increasing frequency in the United States, with rates of accuracy equivalent to those obtainable with frozen section.[62] After the tumor has been accurately classified, it can be treated properly. Incisional biopsy has not been shown to result in an increase of recurrence or metastases; on the contrary, when followed by adequate treatment, it is associated with a lower incidence of local recurrence than is primary excision of the sarcoma performed without prior biopsy. At the time of the definitive surgery the area of the biopsy or aspiration should be excised in continuity with the tumor.

Performance of frozen sections is useful in determining the type of neoplasm, the degree of malignancy, and the adequacy of surgical margins.

Light microscopic evaluation of hematoxylin–eosin-stained sections remains the standard technique for the initial diagnostic approach to these tumors and is sufficient in the majority of the cases.[54] However, there are special techniques that have been successfully applied to increase diagnostic accuracy and which sometimes are indispensable, this development applying both to adult and pediatric tumors.[59,60] These techniques include conventional special stains, electron microscopy, immunohistochemistry, and molecular genetic methods. Examples of the first category are reticulin stain for vascular tumors and synovial sarcomas, periodic acid–Schiff (PAS) for alveolar soft part sarcomas (for the demonstration of intracytoplasmic crystals), phosphotungstic acid–hematoxylin or Masson trichrome for tumors of striated muscle, and mucin stains for synovial sarcomas and myxoid tumors in general.

Electron microscopy also can be very helpful, the currently dismissive attitude toward its use notwithstanding.[55,72] Smooth and striated muscle cells, Schwann cells, endothelial cells, glomus cells, and the cells of granular cell tumor and alveolar soft part sarcoma have distinctive ultrastructural features that often lead to a specific diagnosis.[53,66] These ultrastructural studies can also be performed on material obtained from fine needle aspiration.[61]

Enzyme histochemical determinations are of limited use. Alkaline phosphatase is particularly strong in osteosarcoma and vascular endothelial tumors, whereas acid phosphatase and nonspecific esterase are demonstrable in giant cell tumors and histiocytic tumors in general.[49]

Immunohistochemistry for tissue-related markers (such as smooth muscle actin or FVIII-RA) has proved to be of great value and is now extensively used to accurately classify these neoplasms: the specificity, sensitivity, and applicability of this technique to routinely processed material clearly render it the method of choice in most circumstances.[52,58,63,68] The number of available markers is very large and continues to grow.[67] An area of particular expansion is that of the transcription factors, as exemplified by myogenin, WT1, and FLI-1. These nuclear-based markers have a degree of sensitivity and specificity that in many cases surpasses those of the conventional markers located in the cytoplasm, cell membrane, or extracellular space. It should be noted, however, that the immunophenotype of a soft tissue sarcoma may undergo changes following radiation/chemotherapy.[51,64]

The systematic use of cytogenetics has shown the existence of nonrandom chromosomal alterations (mainly translocations) in association with many types of soft tissue tumor.[56,57,65,69,71] The findings have validated the morphologic approach to classification of soft tissue tumors, helped to refine the boundaries of some entities (such as broadening morphology and location of desmoplastic small cell tumor, merging of spindle cell lipoma with pleomorphic lipoma, and merging of round cell liposarcoma into myxoid liposarcoma), and offered insight into the genesis of the tumors. Furthermore, the molecular alterations (gene fusions) that result from the chromosomal translocations can now be readily demonstrated in routine paraffin-embedded tissues by reverse transcriptase-polymerase chain reaction (RT-PCR) or fluorescent in situ hybridization (FISH), and such studies can be extremely helpful in the diagnosis of these tumors, especially in small biopsies, tumors with unusual morphology, or tumors in unusual sites[48,50] (see Table 3.1, Chapter 3). A breakapart FISH probe against the *EWS* (also known as *EWSR1*) gene is particularly helpful since this gene is implicated in many different soft tissue tumor types, including Ewing sarcoma/PNET, angiomatoid fibrous histiocytoma, extraskeletal myxoid chondrosarcoma, myxoid liposarcoma, clear cell sarcoma of tendons and aponeurosis, and desmoplastic small cell tumor. Similarly, a breakapart FISH probe against the *FUS* (also known as *TLS*) gene can aid in the diagnosis of low-grade fibromyxoid sarcoma, myxoid liposarcoma, and angiomatoid fibrous histiocytoma. Such probes can serve as good screening tools, but fail to provide information on the identity of partner fusion genes.

As in other fields of oncology, attempts are being made to classify soft tissue tumors on the basis of their gene expression profile.[70]

The specific applications of these various methods are described under the respective tumor types.

Grading and staging

Some degree of microscopic grading of soft tissue is already built into the conventional microscopic classification of these tumors. Thus dermatofibrosarcoma protuberans is by definition a low-grade neoplasm, whereas all alveolar rhabdomyosarcomas are high-grade tumors. In addition, several attempts have been made to establish some general guidelines for the grading of soft tissue sarcomas independent of their microscopic type.[73,76,87–90] The number of grades has varied in the different systems: two (low-grade and high-grade), three (I, II, and III, or low-grade, intermediate-grade, and high-grade), and four (I, II, III, and IV) grades have been recognized.

In a two-grade system, tumors are assigned to the low-grade category when their metastasizing potential is nil to low (15% or less).[79,82] Understandably, many clinicians prefer such a system because it makes their therapeutic decision easier. Yet we believe that a three-grade system reflects better the morphologic and behavioral span of these neoplasms.

The criteria used have included degree of cellularity, pleomorphism, mitotic activity, and necrosis, and have been found to be of definite prognostic value for both adult and pediatric soft tissue tumors;[76,86,87] however, it is misleading to overemphasize grading that is independent of the specific microscopic type of the sarcoma and the circumstances in which it occurs, such as the patient's age or the depth and size of the tumor.[81,85] For instance, a congenital fibrosarcoma and a superficially located leiomyosarcoma may both be regarded as grade III tumors, yet their incidence of metastatic spread is extremely low; conversely, a deeply seated malignant peripheral nerve sheath tumor (MPNST) in a patient with Recklinghausen disease may appear as a grade I tumor because of uniformity of proliferation and low mitotic count, yet it will usually behave in a very aggressive fashion. Additional difficulties relate to the inherently subjective nature of the evaluation, the sampling issue in biopsy material, and the confounding effect of preoperative therapy.[75,78] It is remarkable that, despite these severe limitations, microscopic grading (within the various histotypes and whenever applicable) remains one of the best prognostic indicators. The two grading schemes that have been most widely applied are those of the French Federation of Cancer Centers Sarcoma Groups and the National Cancer Institute.[77,80] The results that have been obtained with these two methods are roughly equivalent, but the French system seems to have a slight edge.[84] It is based on the evaluation of three separate parameters: tumor differentiation, mitotic rate, and amount of tumor necrosis, according to the scheme outlined in Box 25.1.[77]

Two main staging systems for soft tissue sarcoma have been proposed. The one espoused by the American Joint Committee (AJC) is largely based on the TNM system, in that it uses the size of the primary tumor (T), the status of lymph nodes (N), the presence of distant metastases (M), and the tumor's histologic grade (G)[74] (see Appendix C).

In the Enneking system,[83] which is also applied to tumors of bone and which is better suited to lesions in the extremities, soft tissue sarcomas are grouped according to anatomic settings (T1, intracompartmental, or T2, extracompartmental); grades (G1, low, and G2, high) and presence or absence of metastases, giving the scheme shown in Box 25.1.

Prognosis

The prognosis of soft tissue tumors depends on a variety of parameters, many of which are interrelated.

Box 25.1 French Federation of Cancer Centers Sarcoma Group grading system

Tumor differentiation

Score 1: Sarcomas closely resembling normal adult mesenchymal tissue. Examples: well-differentiated liposarcomas and well-differentiated fibrosarcoma.
Score 2: Sarcomas for which the histologic typing is certain. Examples: biphasic synovial sarcoma, alveolar soft-part sarcoma, myxoid liposarcoma.
Score 3: Embryonal sarcomas, undifferentiated sarcomas, and sarcomas of doubtful tumor type.

Mitosis count

The count is made at g × 400 in 10 successive fields. This count is taken to establish the score:
Score 1: 0–9 mitoses per 10 fields
Score 2: 10–19 mitoses per 10 fields
Score 3: More than 20 mitoses per 10 fields

Tumor necrosis

Score 0: No necrosis on any examined slides
Score 1: Less than 50% tumor necrosis for all the examined tumor surface
Score 2: Tumor necrosis on more than half of the examined tumor surface

The three-grade system is set up as follows: Grade I is defined as a total of 2 or 3 when summing the scores obtained for each of the three histologic criteria; Grade II represents a total of 4 or 5; Grade III represents a total of 6, 7, or 8.

Enneking staging system for soft tissue sarcoma

Stage I:

G1	Without metastases	T1
G1	Without metastases	T2

Stage II:

G2	Without metastases	T1
G2	Without metastases	T2

Stage III:

G1 or G2	With metastases	T1
G1 or G2	With metastases	T2

1 **Tumor size.** There is a definite relationship between tumor size and outcome. This is true for practically all tumor types in which this parameter has been analyzed.[108,111]
2 **Depth.** Superficially located tumors (dermis and subcutaneous tissue) have a much better prognosis than deep-seated ones (intermuscular or intramuscular, retroperitoneal) of similar microscopic type.[100,107] The difference is largely due to the fact that superficial lesions tend to be considerably smaller at the time of excision. Along similar lines, soft tissue sarcomas featuring histologic evidence of bone invasion have a poorer prognosis.[99]
3 **Location.** Tumors of the retroperitoneum do much worse than microscopically similar lesions located in the extremities. Among the latter, local recurrence has been found to be more frequent with those of the upper extremity than those of the lower extremity.[100]
4 **Microscopic type.** Some soft tissue neoplasms (such as atypical lipomatous tumors) are low-grade lesions with no capacity to metastasize, whereas other neoplasms of similar cell type (such as pleomorphic liposarcoma) are highly aggressive and prone to spread distantly.
5 **Vascular invasion.** This has been shown to be the strongest predictor of distant metastases in several series.[96]
6 **Surgical margins.** Not surprisingly, adequacy of surgical margins is statistically associated with local relapse.[92,98,103,104,110,115] Parenthetically, local recurrence is of relatively minor importance in the development of distant metastases.[101,113]
7 **Microscopic grade.** As already indicated, a relationship has been found between various microscopic grading systems and outcome, which in some cases is directly related to the histotype but in others it is applied within a given histotype.
8 **Clinical stage.** As for most other tumors, this determination – which incorporates several of the previously mentioned parameters, as well as the presence or absence of metastases – is the most powerful prognostic determinator.
9 **DNA ploidy.** Several flow cytometric studies performed in soft tissue sarcomas of various microscopic types have shown – as expected – that DNA aneuploidy correlates with a higher microscopic grade, a higher rate of cell proliferation, and decreased survival rates.[91,106] However, it is doubtful whether ploidy analysis is an independent prognostic factor when applied to soft tissue sarcomas that have been segregated by microscopic type, anatomic site, stage, grade, margin status, and type of therapy.[94]
10 **Cell proliferation.** As already indicated, mitotic activity is incorporated into most grading schemes. Evaluation of proliferation markers such as MIB-1 and p105 has been shown to correlate with prognosis but – as for ploidy values – it remains to be seen whether it qualifies as an independent variable.[97,102,112,114]
11 **Genetic alterations.** It has been shown that soft tissue tumors exhibiting mutations of *TP53* or altered expression of the retinoblastoma gene behave more aggressively than those lacking these changes,[93,95,105] but similar provisos apply. Along similar lines, claims have been made of a relationship between the type of gene fusion in the sarcomas associated with chromosomal translocations and prognosis (as in alveolar rhabdomyosarcoma and synovial sarcoma; these are discussed in the respective sections). Expression of epidermal growth factor receptor is said to be associated with a higher microscopic grade and a poorer prognosis.[109]

Therapy

Soft tissue tumors that are relatively small and/or clearly benign on clinical grounds (such as superficially located lipomas, schwannomas, hemangiomas, and tenosynovial giant cell tumors) can be removed directly, but in most others the excision should be preceded by an incisional or core needle biopsy, or at least a fine needle aspiration. A few tumors (such as schwannomas) can be safely enucleated, but for most others – even if benign – a rim of uninvolved normal tissue should be excised in continuity with the neoplasm to prevent recurrence. Many soft tissue sarcomas, such as fibrosarcoma, myxoid liposarcoma, and leiomyosarcoma, may appear grossly encapsulated, but microscopic examination will often show tumor cells beyond the apparent capsule; therefore enucleation will usually fail. A wide local excision is particularly important for infiltrative lesions such as fibromatosis and dermatofibrosarcoma protuberans.

Full-fledged soft tissue sarcomas in children are currently treated, for the most part, by a combination of surgery, radiation therapy, and multidrug chemotherapy, with results that are vastly superior to those obtained in the prechemotherapy era.[122]

The treatment of high-grade soft tissue sarcomas in adults has undergone radical changes.[124] It has been thought for many years that amputation or disarticulation offered the best chances of cure for sarcomas involving an extremity. Contrariwise, many studies done during the past 40 years have shown that for several types of soft tissue sarcoma, a wide local excision offers as good a chance of survival as an amputation, especially if supplemented by other types of therapy.[120,130] Very good results along this line have been obtained by combining limited (even incomplete) surgery with radical-dose radiation therapy (6300–7000 rad over 6½ to 7½ weeks).[125,126] Tumor histologic grade correlates well with the incidence of local recurrence and disease-free survival following this therapeutic modality.[125,126,129]

A controversial issue is the usefulness of adjuvant preoperative or postoperative chemotherapy for sarcomas of adult patients.[117,121,127] Results from a randomized study conducted at the National Cancer Institute strongly suggest that chemotherapy diminishes the likelihood of tumor recurrence, at least on a short-term basis, whether the sarcoma is located in the extremities, head and neck region, or trunk.[119,123] Inspired by the success story of Gleevec therapy in patients with gastrointestinal stromal tumors, targeted therapy is increasingly used and tried for patients with recurrent or metastatic soft tissue sarcoma.[116,128]

Finally, surgical resection of pulmonary metastases has proved of value in 20–25% of the patients who develop this complication.[118]

Pathogenesis

Much has been written in the medical and legal literature on the possible relationship between trauma and soft tissue sarcoma, but no convincing evidence has been provided for a definite cause–effect relationship between the two.[143] Individuals subjected to repeated serious trauma (such as football players) do not have an increased incidence of soft tissue tumors. In the overwhelming majority of the cases in which a relation between tumor and trauma seems to exist, careful review of the evidence and doubling rates studies will show that the tumor antedated the trauma and that the latter simply called the attention of the patient to its presence (so-called 'traumatic determinism').

The large majority of soft tissue sarcomas arise de novo rather than from malignant degeneration of preexisting benign tumors. Although the latter phenomenon may occur (as in neurofibromas), in most cases in which a given benign tumor is said to have become malignant, review of the original material will show that it was malignant from its inception. Conclusive evidence has accumulated that a variety of soft tissue sarcomas can arise as a complication of radiation therapy.[139,142] So-called malignant fibrous histiocytomas and soft tissue (extraskeletal) osteosarcomas are the most common types. The average latent period is approximately 10 years, and the prognosis is poor. Soft tissue sarcomas have also developed around foreign bodies, such as bullets, shrapnel, and surgically implanted material.[138] The latency period has varied from 2 years to over 50 years, and the most common microscopic types have been so-called malignant fibrous histiocytoma and angiosarcoma.[136]

A possible association between exposure to phenoxy herbicides and development of soft tissue sarcoma has been suggested.[135,141,145] However, several case control studies have failed to show any significant association among the United States soldiers stationed in Vietnam and exposed to Agent Orange, a defoliant that contained dioxin as a contaminant.[134,137]

Viruses play a role in the development of certain soft tissue tumors, such as human herpes virus 8 (HHV8) in Kaposi sarcoma, and Epstein–Barr virus (EBV) in smooth muscle tumors and myopericytomas arising in patients with immunodeficiency.[131,133,140]

Some hereditary diseases predispose to the development of soft tissue tumors. Examples include: neurofibromatosis (benign and malignant peripheral nerve sheath tumors); Gardner syndrome (fibromatosis and Gardner fibroma); Li–Fraumeni syndrome caused by germline mutation of the *TP53* gene (various sarcomas), Carney complex (psammomatous melanotic schwannoma, cutaneous myxoma), and tuberous sclerosis (PEComas).[132,144]

Tumors and tumorlike conditions of fibroblasts and myofibroblasts

Calcifying aponeurotic fibroma

Calcifying aponeurotic fibroma is a distinctive lesion originally described as juvenile aponeurotic fibroma, typically presenting as a soft tissue mass in the hand or wrist of a child or adolescent,[151] but sometimes also occurring in the proximal extremities or trunk.[148] At surgery, it may appear as a nodule or as an ill-defined infiltrating mass in the subcutaneous tissue or attached to a tendon (Fig. 25.1). Sometimes, foci of calcification may be detected on gross inspection.[147]

Microscopically, the lesion is characterized by a diffuse fibroblastic growth in which spotty calcification occurs (Fig. 25.2). Infiltration of fat and striated muscle is often seen at the periphery. Mitoses are scarce, and atypical cytologic features are absent. Scattered osteoclast-like giant cells are frequently seen. The cells inside and surrounding the calcified foci have a strong resemblance to chondrocytes. It is this feature that led some authors to postulate that this lesion is basically of cartilaginous origin and that it represents the cartilaginous analog of fibromatosis.[149,150,152] Immunohistochemically, the proliferating cells are reactive for vimentin, common and

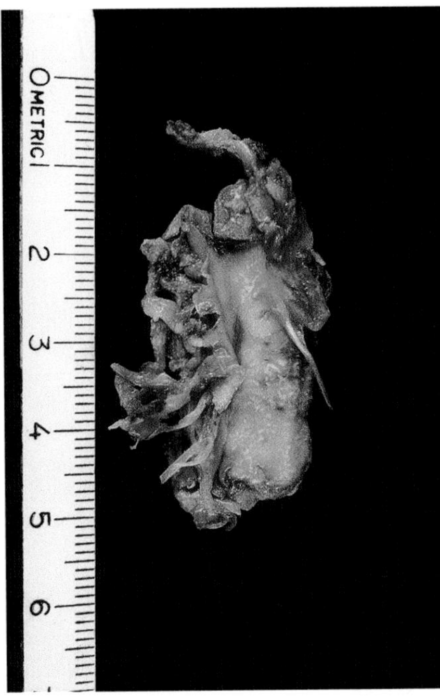

Fig. 25.1 Gross appearance of calcifying aponeurotic fibroma. The mass is unencapsulated and ill defined.

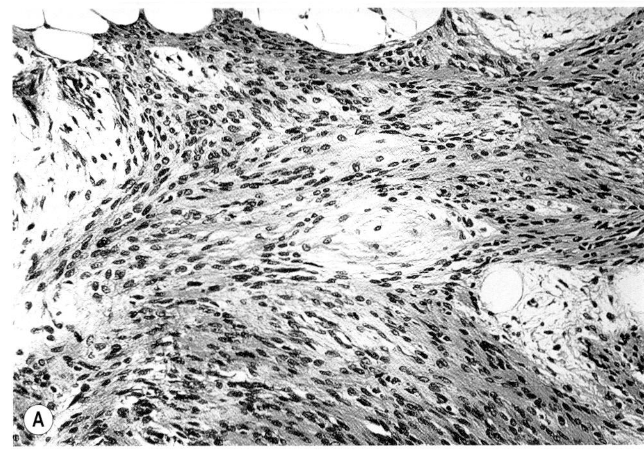

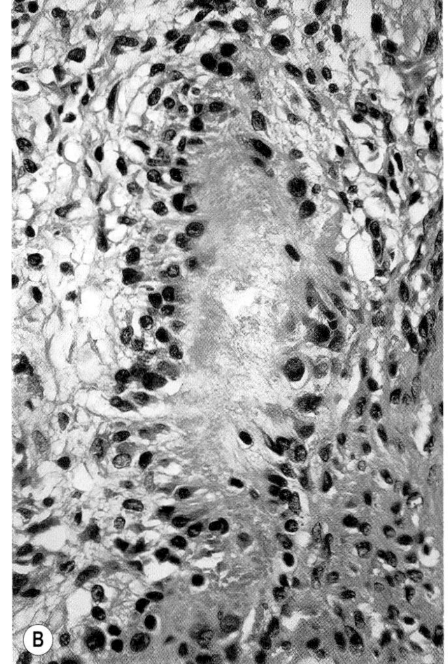

Fig. 25.2 **A** and **B**, Low- and high-power appearance of calcifying aponeurotic fibroma. The tumor cells arrange themselves in a palisading fashion around finely calcified material.

smooth muscle actin (sometimes), CD99, S-100 protein, and CD68.[148]

Calcifying aponeurotic fibroma can be confused with rheumatoid nodule, schwannoma, and fibromatosis. Local recurrence is common, especially in young children. However, distant metastases do not occur.[146]

Fibroma of tendon sheath

Fibroma of tendon sheath is a well-circumscribed, often lobulated tumor found attached to tendon or tendon sheath.[156] Microscopically, it is composed of dense fibrous tissue containing spindle and sometimes stellate mesenchymal cells (Fig. 25.3). Frequently, there are dilated or slit-like channels, some of them resembling tenosynovial spaces.[153,155,161] Occasionally, a component of bizarre tumor cells unaccompanied by mitoses is seen.[157] Ultrastructurally, most of the cells have features of myofibroblasts.[155] The behavior is benign. It is not clear whether this is a distinct entity or a heterogeneous process representing the end stage of a variety of lesions, particularly tenosynovial giant cell tumor or nodular fasciitis.[158–160] We favor the latter interpretation. The translocation t(2;11)(q31–32;q12) has been found in one case, suggesting that at least some examples are of neoplastic nature.[154]

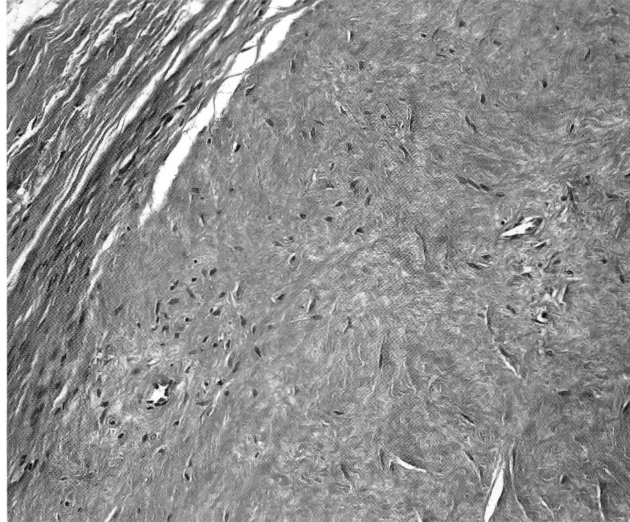

Fig. 25.3 Tendon sheath fibroma. The lesion is hypocellular and contains abundant collagen.

Other types of fibroma

Collagenous fibroma (desmoplastic fibroblastoma) is a benign lesion usually centered in the subcutaneous tissue and with a wide anatomic distribution. The most distinctive microscopic feature is the presence of stellate fibroblasts (together with ordinary spindle-shaped fibroblasts) separated by a collagenous matrix with or without myxoid features.[163,168,169] Ultrastructurally, some of the cells show myofibroblastic features.[162] This lesion, which is cured by a conservative excision, could be viewed as the skin and soft tissue equivalent of the generally polypoid lesions containing similar stellate cells that occur in various mucosa-lined sites, such as oral cavity, anus, and vulvovaginal region. On the other hand, the presence of a clonal chromosomal translocation involving 11q12 suggests a neoplastic process, as well as a possible link with fibroma of tendon sheath.[166,170,171]

Nuchal-type fibroma is a benign lesion found in the posterior aspect of the neck and characterized microscopically by hypocellular bundles of thick collagen fibers, with entrapped adipose tissue and traumatic neuroma-like structures. A high percentage of the patients are diabetic.[167] This process is probably closely related to **nuchal fibrocartilaginous pseudotumor**, which is characteristically located in the deep soft tissue overlying the posterior aspect of the lower cervical vertebrae and thought to be due to fibrocartilaginous metaplasia of the nuchal ligament, probably trauma-induced.[165]

Superficial acral fibromyxoma is the name given to a soft tissue tumor with a predilection for the fingers and toes and composed of spindle and stellate bland-looking tumor cells with a nondescript, storiform, or fascicular pattern of growth, embedded in a myxoid or collagenous stroma.[164]

Giant cell fibroblastoma

Giant cell fibroblastoma is a mesenchymal neoplasm occurring almost exclusively in children younger than 10 years of age,[174,182]

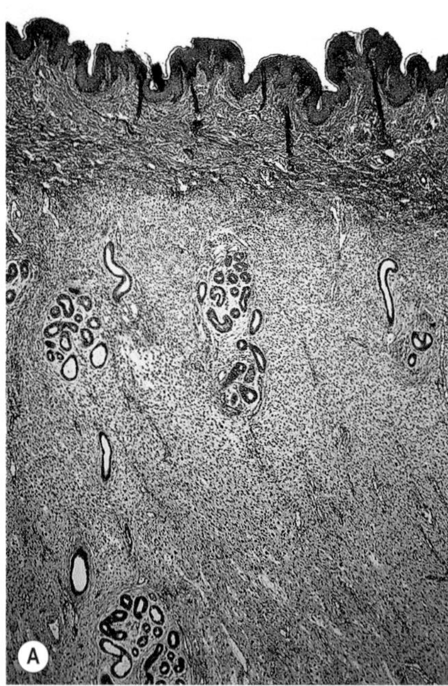

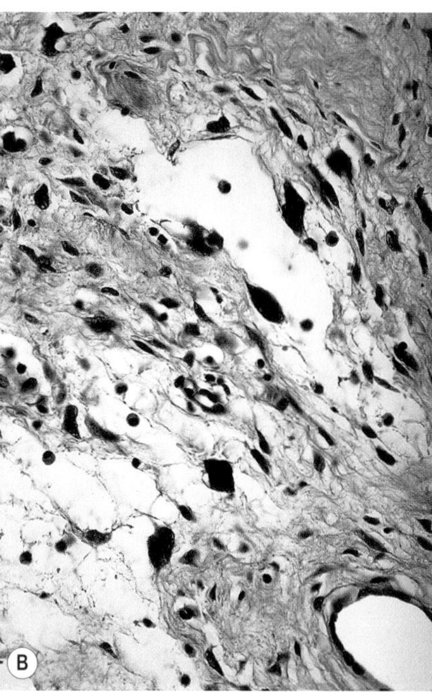

Fig. 25.4 A and **B**, Low- and high-power appearance of giant cell fibroblastoma. Some of the tumor cells line empty spaces that simulate vascular structures.

but which is exceptionally also seen in adults. Most of these lesions are located in the superficial soft tissues of back or thigh. Microscopically, an ill-defined proliferation of fibroblasts is seen in a heavily collagenized and focally myxoid stroma. Typical features include the presence of multinucleated cells with a floret-like appearance, other types of atypical tumor cells, and the formation of cystic and sinusoidal structures lined by spindle and floret cells[176,183] (Fig. 25.4). Another typical feature is the presence of perivascular lymphocytes arranged in an onion-skin pattern.[179] Ultrastructurally and immunohistochemically, the cells have the features of primitive mesenchymal cells.[172] At the molecular level they are characterized by the gene fusion transcripts resulting from the balanced translocation t(17;22)(q22;q13).[182,184] Local recurrence is frequent, but distant metastases do not occur.[175,177]

The suggestion that giant cell fibroblastoma is related to dermatofibrosarcoma protuberans and that it may represent its infantile counterpart[183] has received strong support from the similarities of the ultrastructural, immunohistochemical, and molecular profiles of these two lesions,[177,181] the fact that both lesions can undergo so-called fibrosarcomatous transformation,[179] and the description of hybrid and combined cases, whether in the original lesion or in the recurrence.[173,178,180] In one such case the dermatofibrosarcoma component had pigmented features (Bednar tumor, see below).[185]

Nodular fasciitis and related lesions

Nodular fasciitis is the preferred designation for the condition originally designated as subcutaneous pseudosarcomatous fibromatosis.[205] It is a distinctive lesion and a very important one because of its ability to simulate a malignant process.[186,188,204,215,219] It can affect patients of all ages but is most prevalent in young adults, the peak age being 40 years.[202,217,219]

The most common locations are the upper extremities (particularly the flexor aspect of the forearms), trunk, and neck, but they have been described almost anywhere. Two important clinical features of nodular fasciitis are a history of rapid growth (usually a few weeks) and its small size. It usually extends above the fascia into the subcutis, but it may grow beneath it into skeletal muscle, remain within the fascia as a fusiform expansion of this structure, or be centered in the dermis[193,206,210,216] (Fig. 25.5). Exceptionally, it may be found within a joint cavity.[201] Like other soft tissue reactive conditions of fibrous tissue nature, nodular fasciitis has infiltrative margins.

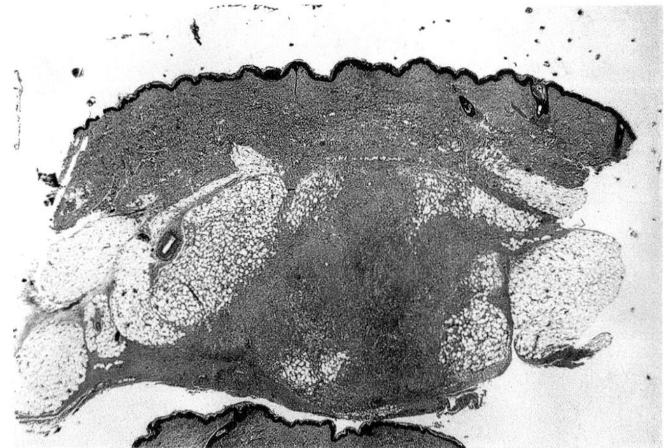

Fig. 25.5 Panoramic view of nodular fasciitis. The lesion is small, ill defined, and centered in the subcutaneous tissue.

Microscopically, the lesion is characterized by a cellular spindle cell growth set in a loosely textured myxoid matrix (Figs 25.6 and 25.7). Vascular proliferation, lymphocytic infiltration, and extravasated red blood cells are also present. A feature of diagnostic significance is the presence of undulating wide bands of collagen lined on the sides by spindle cells, similar to those seen in keloid scars (Fig. 25.8). Storiform areas may be seen focally. Focal metaplastic bone formation may be present, establishing a link between nodular fasciitis and myositis ossificans.[191,192] The high cellularity of the lesion and the presence of mitotic figures are responsible for the frequent confusion of this lesion with a sarcoma. Small size, short

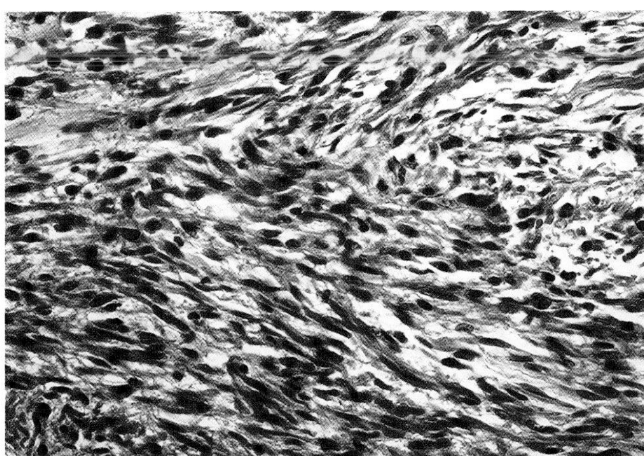

Fig. 25.6 A highly cellular example of nodular fasciitis.

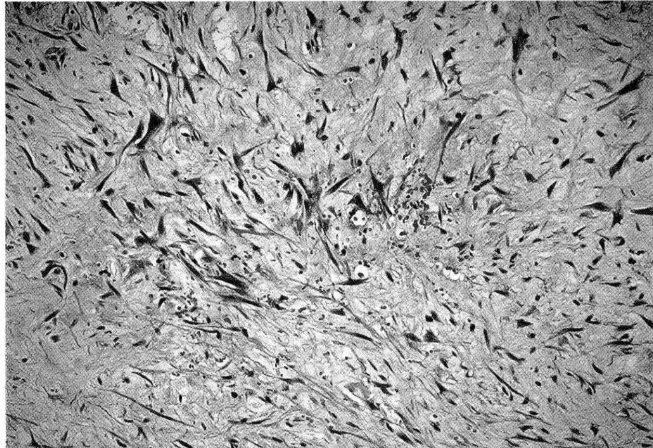

Fig. 25.7 Nodular fasciitis with marked myxoid features.

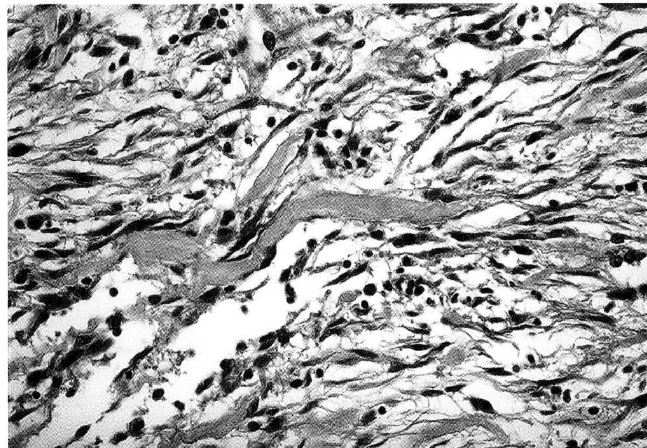

Fig. 25.8 Keloid-like collagen deposition in nodular fasciitis.

duration, red blood cell extravasation, keloid-type collagen, and lack of markedly atypical cells are the main features favoring a diagnosis of nodular fasciitis. In other words, it is acceptable for nodular fasciitis to be hypercellular, infiltrative, and mitotically active, but not to have cells with large atypical hyperchromatic nuclei.

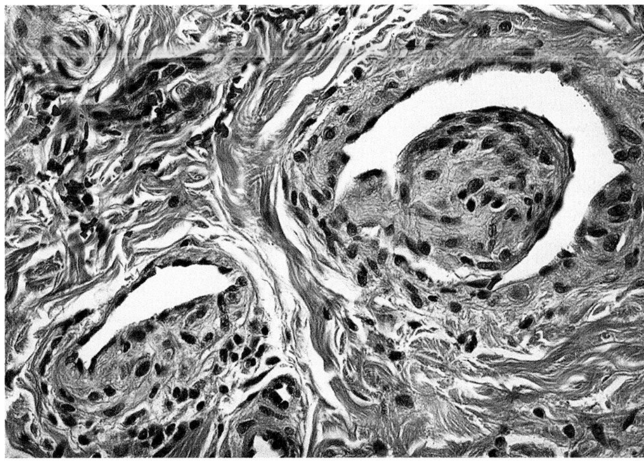

Fig. 25.9 Involvement of wall and lumen of blood vessels in nodular fasciitis.

Ultrastructurally and immunohistochemically, many of the proliferating spindle cells have features of myofibroblasts.[211,223] The DNA pattern is always diploid.[196] Follow-up studies of this entity have conclusively shown that it is perfectly benign, and often resolves spontaneously.[202,204,215,224] Traditionally, it has been regarded as the prototypical pattern of mesenchymal reaction to injury, but the recent finding of clonal chromosomal rearrangements has led some authors to favor the interpretation that it is a neoplastic process.[194] Perhaps it is, depending on how one defines a neoplasm, but benign it remains.

In addition to sarcoma, the differential diagnosis of nodular fasciitis includes the exuberant mesenchymal reactions that can accompany malignant tumors, particularly papillary thyroid carcinoma.[222]

Cranial fasciitis is a distinct variant of nodular fasciitis seen generally in children and sometimes in adults and characterized by involvement of the skull with erosion of the underlying cranium.[207]

Intravascular fasciitis is another morphologic variant of fasciitis in which involvement of the wall and lumen of the medium-sized veins and arteries occurs.[213,216] This is an exaggerated expression of a phenomenon seen frequently in ordinary nodular fasciitis and which constitutes a useful diagnostic sign, i.e., the fact that, at the periphery of the lesion, the walls of small to medium-sized vessels are involved by the reactive mesenchymal process (Fig. 25.9).

In *proliferative fasciitis* the location of the lesion, rapidity of growth, and self-limited nature are the same as those of nodular fasciitis, but the presence of large basophilic cells resembling ganglion cells indicates a link with proliferative myositis (see subsequent discussion) (Fig. 25.10). It usually affects adults, although it can also be seen in children.[209] It follows a benign clinical course.[189,218] As in the other conditions described in this section, myofibroblasts are the cells that predominate ultrastructurally.[190] It should be mentioned here that the presence in a soft tissue lesion of the ganglion-like cells mentioned above does not guarantee that the condition is of a reactive nature. Indeed, we have seen several cases of soft tissue sarcoma containing these cells that could be regarded as the malignant counterpart of proliferative fasciitis/myositis.

Nodular fasciitis and the variants described previously are characteristically located in the somatic soft tissues, but fasciitis-like lesions with a somewhat different morphologic appearance (even more sarcomatoid) can develop from the stromal tissue of a variety

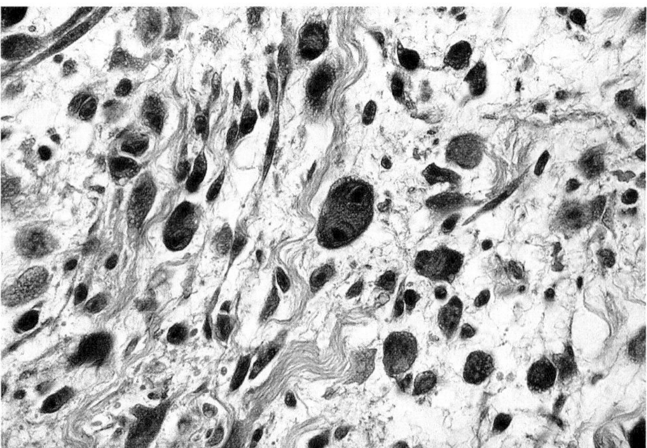

Fig. 25.10 Ganglion-like cells in proliferative fasciitis.

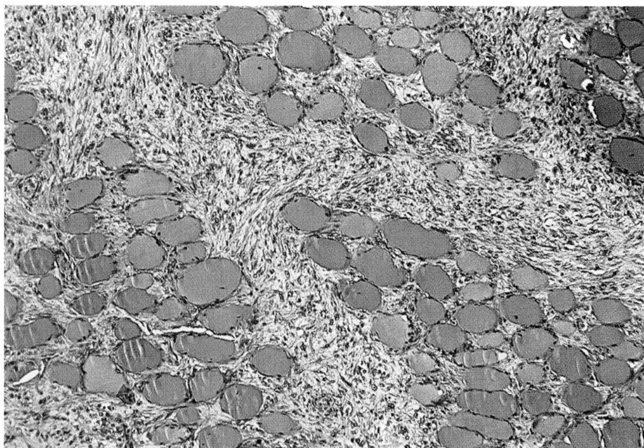

Fig. 25.12 Low-power appearance of proliferative myositis.

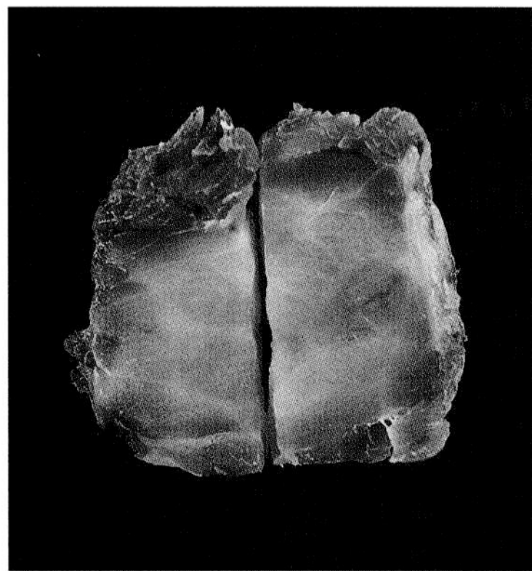

Fig. 25.11 Gross appearance of proliferative myositis. There is an ill-defined whitish material in between the skeletal muscle fibers.

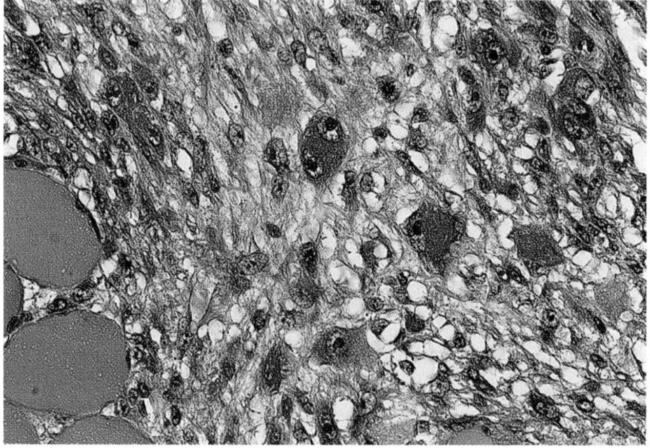

Fig. 25.13 On high power, the ganglion-like cells of proliferative myositis look similar to those of proliferative fasciitis (compare with Figure 25.10).

of organs, such as the bladder, prostate, vulva, vagina, and cervix (see respective chapters).

Proliferative myositis can be confused with sarcoma not only clinically and at surgery but also microscopically.[203] The skeletal muscles of the shoulder, thorax, and thigh are those most commonly affected. Most patients are over the age of 45 years, but it can also present in children.[209] Grossly, the lesion does not look like a sarcoma but rather like an ill-defined scar-like induration of the muscle (Fig. 25.11). Microscopically, a cellular proliferation rich in fibroblasts is seen surrounding individual fibers (Fig. 25.12). The hallmark of the lesion is the presence of very large basophilic cells with vesicular nuclei and very prominent nucleoli, resembling ganglion cells or rhabdomyoblasts (Fig. 25.13). Their appearance and immunohistochemical profile suggest a myofibroblastic nature.[195] Conservative surgery is curative.[197]

Focal myositis is an altogether different inflammatory condition that affects children and adults. It typically evolves over a period of a few weeks as a localized, painful swelling of the soft tissues.[187,198,220] Most cases occur in the lower extremities. Both clinically and at surgery, the impression given is often of a neoplasm. Grossly, the lesion is pale and ill defined. Microscopically, degeneration and regeneration of muscle fibers are seen in association with interstitial inflammation and fibrosis. The inflammatory infiltrate is mainly composed of T lymphocytes, with few accompanying CD4+ cells.[221] The lesion is solitary and self-limited and should be distinguished from polymyositis. Enzyme histochemical and electron microscopic studies suggest that the disease may be the result of a denervation process.[199] Search for a viral agent has so far proved elusive.[221]

Other pseudoneoplastic myofibroblastic processes pathogenetically related to nodular fasciitis and representing an exaggerated reaction to injury include *proliferative funiculitis* (involving the spermatic cord and probably secondary to ischemia or torsion)[200] and *atypical decubital fibroplasia* (occurring primarily but not exclusively in physically debilitated or immobilized patients).[212] The latter condition merges with *ischemic fasciitis*, in which a central area of necrosis is seen surrounded by a ring of neoformed vessels and proliferating fibroblasts/myofibroblasts.[208,214]

Myositis ossificans

Although myositis ossificans and related conditions such as *fibro-osseous pseudotumor of the digits*[225] are located in the soft tissue and are pathogenetically and histologically linked to the previous

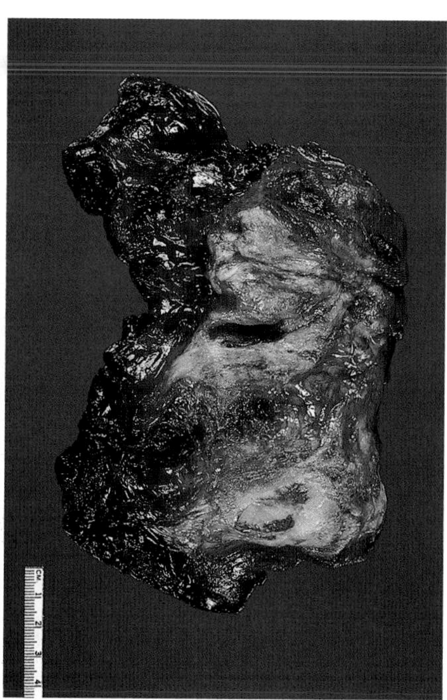

Fig. 25.14 Gross appearance of elastofibroma.

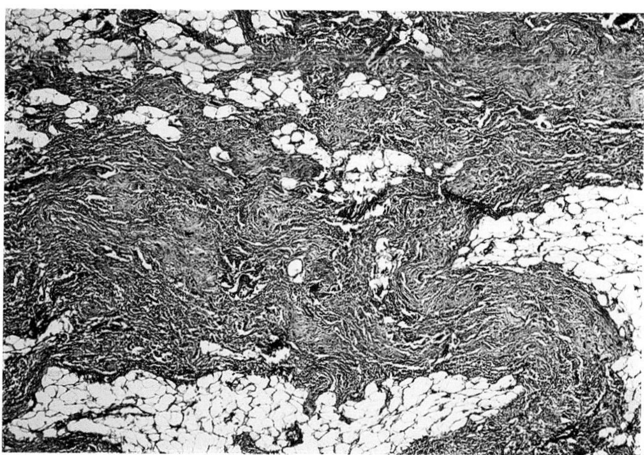

Fig. 25.15 On low power, elastofibroma appears as an irregularly shaped fibrohyaline mass within adipose tissue.

entities, they are discussed in Chapter 24 because of their intimate relation to bone and periosteum.

Elastofibroma

Elastofibroma is a benign, poorly circumscribed process involving almost exclusively the subscapular region of elderly individuals, although isolated cases have been seen in the deltoid muscle, infraolecranon area, hip, thigh, and stomach.[227] Multicentric and familial cases have been described, suggesting the existence of a constitutional background.[237] There is often a history of strenuous manual labor. At surgery, the lesions usually are found at the apex of the scapula, beneath the rhomboid and latissimus dorsi muscles (Fig. 25.14). The right side is affected more commonly than the left but bilaterality is frequent. A periosteal origin has been suggested.[235]

Microscopically, collagen bundles alternate with numerous acidophilic, refractive cylinders often containing a central dense core, both of which stain strongly with elastic stains (Figs 25.15 and 25.16). Ultrastructurally, the cylinders are made up of immature amorphous elastic tissue, whereas the central core contains mature fibers.[226,230,239] Elastase digestion fully removes this material.[238] Immunohistochemically, the cells present in the lesion are positive for CD34, MEF-2, prominin 2 (CD133), and factor XIIIa.[240]

Occasionally, adipose tissue is found intermingled with the collagen and elastic fibers, a variation in the theme that has been dignified with the name *elastofibrolipoma*.[228]

The biochemical composition of the fibers is that of elastin but with an amino acid composition slightly different from that of normal elastic tissue.[233,238] The collagen deposited in the lesion is a mixture of types I, II, and III; the presence of type II collagen is perplexing because this is normally present only in articular cartilage and some ocular structures.[236] It would seem that the new material synthesized by the spindle cells is laid down around preexisting elastic fibers.[234] Traditionally, this lesion has not been regarded as a true neoplasm but rather a reactive hyperplasia

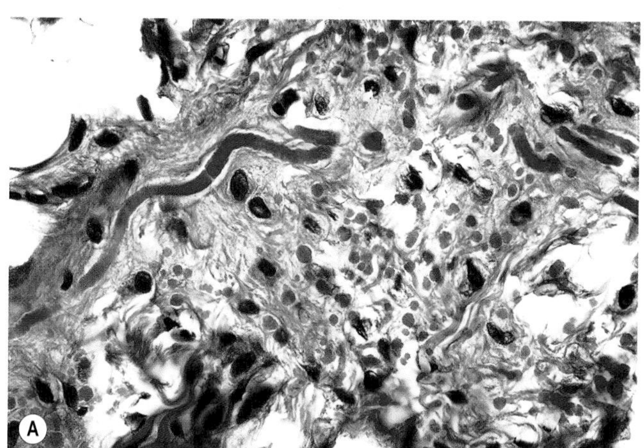

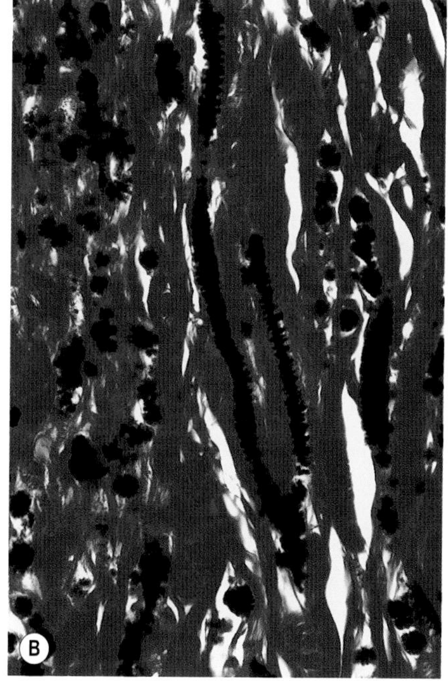

Fig. 25.16 **A** and **B**, High-power view of elastofibroma showing diagnostic rods of elastic tissue. (**B**, Elastic tissue stain.)

involving abnormal elastogenesis;[229,232] however, a recent study has shown that the lesion is a clonal proliferation.[231]

Solitary fibrous tumor

This soft tissue neoplasm, formerly thought to be of mesothelial nature and limited to mesothelium-covered surfaces, is now known to be composed of a subset of fibroblast-like cells and to be quite ubiquitous. Curiously, the soft tissues of the extremities are among the rarest sites of occurrence of this entity; however, well-documented examples are on record.[241,249] As in other sites, both benign and malignant varieties exist. Microscopically, the alternation of hyper- and hypocellular areas, the deposition of dense keloid-type collagen, and the occurrence of hemangiopericytoma-like areas are the most distinguishing features. Occasionally the stroma is very myxoid.[242] In rare instances there is an associated component of mature adipose tissue, in which case the term *lipomatous hemangiopericytoma* has been used.[244,245] It seems likely that the tumor originally described as *giant cell angiofibroma*[243] is a giant cell-rich variant of solitary fibrous tumor.[246] Solitary fibrous tumor can undergo dedifferentiation in a fashion similar to that seen in atypical lipomatous tumor and chondrosarcoma.[247,248]

Fibromatosis

The generic term **fibromatosis** was originally proposed by Stout[325] for a group of related conditions having in common the following features:

1. Proliferation of well-differentiated fibroblasts (later shown to be mainly myofibroblasts)
2. Infiltrative pattern of growth
3. Presence of a variable (but usually abundant) amount of collagen between the proliferating cells
4. Lack of cytologic features of malignancy
5. Scanty or absent mitotic activity
6. Aggressive clinical behavior characterized by repeated local recurrences but lack of capacity to metastasize distantly.

Grossly, these lesions are often large, firm, and whitish, with ill-defined outlines and an irregularly whorled cut surface[251] (Figs 25.17 and 25.18). They often arise in a muscular fascia. Microscopically, most of the proliferating cells have features intermediate between those of fibroblasts and smooth muscle cells (i.e., of myofibroblasts) (Figs 25.19 and 25.20). This was first described in a classic ultrastructural study of palmar fibromatosis by Gabbiani and Majno.[284] The authors noted nuclear deformations of the type found in contracted cells (retrospectively identified by light microscopy as cross-banded nuclei) and a cytoplasmic fibrillary system similar to that seen in smooth muscle cells. They suggested that the

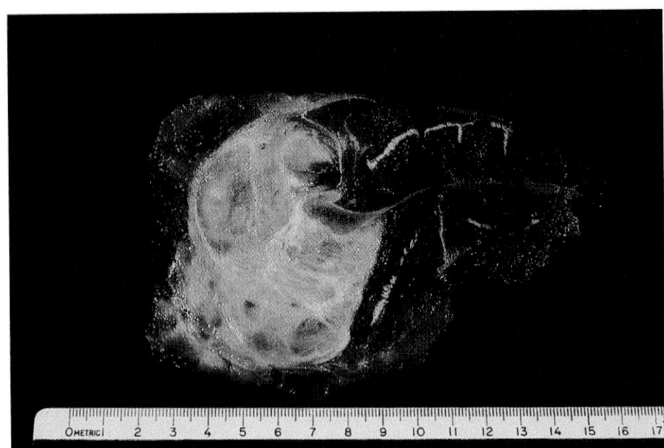

Fig. 25.18 Deep-seated fibromatosis embedded within major skeletal muscle.

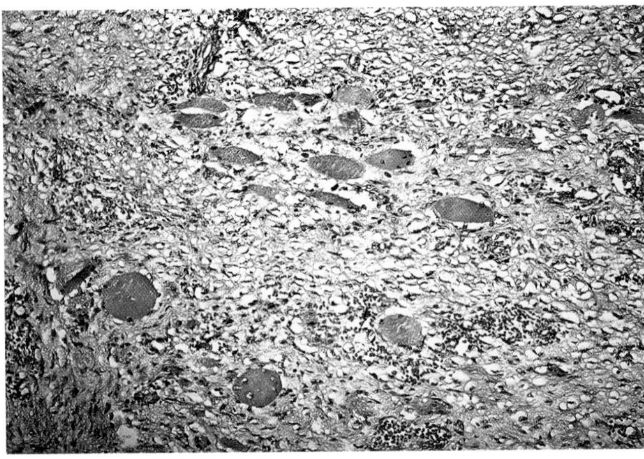

Fig. 25.19 The spindle cells of fibromatosis grow diffusely between skeletal muscle fibers.

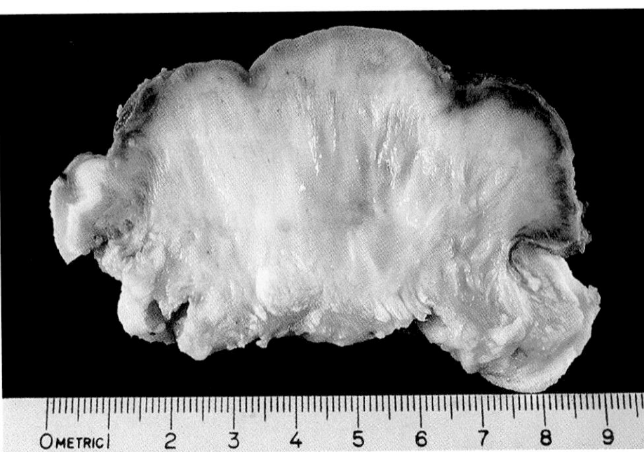

Fig. 25.17 Plantar fibromatosis. The tissue is whitish and unencapsulated, with an elastic consistency.

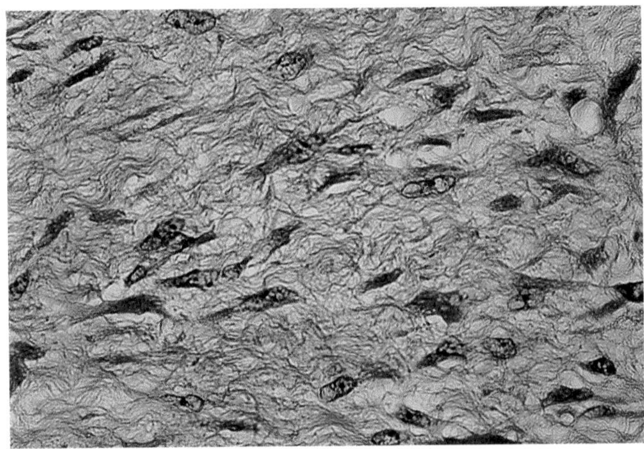

Fig. 25.20 On high power, the cells of fibromatosis have features consistent with myofibroblasts.

proliferating fibroblasts had modulated toward a contractile cell – which they proposed to designate the myofibroblast – and that this was responsible for the contracture evident clinically. The myofibroblastic appearance of the cells of fibromatosis has been confirmed by many,[286,302] as has the fact that this cell type is implicated in a large number of reactive conditions as well as neoplasms of soft tissue.[271] In an ultrastructural study of fibromatosis, Welsh[329] described intracytoplasmic collagen formation, probably representing a disruption of collagen synthesis. This alteration is, however, nonspecific; it has also been detected in a variety of collagen-producing soft tissue sarcomas.[305] Clonal chromosomal aberrations are present in approximately half of the deep-seated fibromatoses but only in 10% of those located superficially. Trisomies 8 and 20 and loss of 5q material represent the recurring cytogenetic changes.[268] At the molecular level, there are activating mutations of *CTNNB1* (encoding β-catenin), leading to frequent nuclear expression of β-catenin.[256,303,308,310] For cases associated with Gardner syndrome, there is germline mutation of the *APC* gene (5q22–22), together with loss of heterozygosity at the locus.[290] The end result is similar, since both APC and β-catenin are components of the Wnt signaling pathway. The cells of fibromatosis are also immunoreactive for alpha-smooth muscle actin, desmin (focally and erratically), calponin, and estrogen receptor-beta (but not estrogen receptor-alpha or CD34).[269]

Other light microscopic features commonly encountered in fibromatosis are a perivascular lymphocytic infiltrate located at the advancing edge of the lesion, and thick-walled vessels sharply outlined from the surrounding tissue. Dystrophic calcification and metaplastic ossification have also been described.[282]

Some pathologists add the adjective *aggressive* to some forms of fibromatosis to emphasize its potential behavior. We do not use the term, since we regard it as redundant, being that all deep-seated fibromatoses are potentially aggressive. Besides, there is little correlation between the cellularity or other microscopic features of these lesions and their biologic behavior.[332] Other authors have gone even further and have used *well-differentiated fibrosarcoma* as a synonym for the histologically more cellular or clinically more aggressive types of fibromatosis. We are opposed to this terminology because the designation of sarcoma endows this lesion in the mind of many surgeons with a metastasizing potential that it does not possess. Although we recognize the difficulties involved, we always attempt to make a distinction between fibromatosis and well-differentiated fibrosarcoma, reserving the latter term for tumors showing atypical cytologic features and/or a significant number of mitotic figures (more than one per high-power field). As Enzinger[275] remarked, it is usually not possible on the basis of the histologic examination to predict whether or not a fibromatosis will recur, but it is possible to predict whether a fibrous tumor is or is not capable of metastasizing.

Most soft tissue fibromatoses are in intimate contact with skeletal muscles and their aponeuroses – hence their designation as *musculoaponeurotic fibromatosis*.[276] This is preferable to the obsolete term *desmoid tumor*, traditionally used for a neoplasm of the abdominal wall appearing in women during or following pregnancy. In our experience, this lesion is almost as common in men and in other locations, such as the shoulder girdle, head and neck area, and thigh.[307,314] It can also occur in the mediastinum, pleural cavity (with lung invasion), retroperitoneum, abdominal cavity (see subsequent discussion), and breast.[252,260,261,319]

The treatment of choice is a prompt radical excision, including a wide margin of involved tissue. Sometimes this requires the removal of the entire muscle involved. The incidence of local recurrence is lower in fibromatoses of the abdominal wall than in those located elsewhere. Some of the latter have recurred as many as five times or more. Only rarely, however, has local aggressiveness forced amputation. Actually, cessation of attempts to excise persistent tissue locally may be followed by failure of the lesion to enlarge further. Because of this observation, some authors have advised against the reexcision of a recurrent lesion that does not appear to be growing.[316] Enzinger and Shiraki[276] analyzed 30 cases located in the shoulder girdle that had been followed for a minimum of 10 years. In 57% of the patients the tumor recurred one or more times. However, at the end of the follow-up period, *all patients* were living without any evidence of continuing tumor growth. A higher incidence of recurrence was seen in young individuals and in those patients with tumors of large size. It has been claimed that cases of fibromatosis expressing nuclear β-catenin and p53 have a greater tendency for recurrence.[285]

Radiation therapy may be effective in achieving local control. It has been used in the form of external radiation following conservative (and sometimes inadequate) surgery[300] and in the form of iridium implantation coupled with surgery for the treatment of recurrences.[334] Some cases of fibromatosis have also been successfully managed with endocrine therapy, such as tamoxifen.[323,330]

Juvenile fibromatosis is a term that has often been applied to examples of fibromatosis occurring in children and adolescents.[253,287,320] Except for their greater frequency in this age group and, in some specific instances, their greater propensity for local recurrence, there is very little either on clinical or microscopic grounds that differentiates fibromatosis in children from that occurring in other age groups.[265] There are, however, three variants of fibromatosis apparently restricted to childhood that present a distinctive clinicopathologic picture: fibromatosis colli (congenital torticollis), infantile digital fibromatosis, and infantile myofibromatosis.

Fibromatosis colli (congenital torticollis) is a type of fibromatosis affecting the lower third of the sternomastoid muscle and appearing at birth or shortly thereafter, sometimes bilaterally.[266] Fibromatosis colli is frequently associated with various congenital anomalies. Thus, Iwahara and Ikeda[296] found congenital (usually ipsilateral) dislocations of the hip in 14% of their patients. An association between complicated deliveries (particularly breech deliveries) and fibromatosis colli has been established. Although some instances of spontaneous disappearance have been recorded, this condition usually necessitates resection of the muscle. Microscopically, the cellularity of the fibrous tissue depends on the age of the process. This condition has been considered to be caused by birth injury, but there is rarely evidence of previous hemorrhage.

Infantile digital fibromatosis (inclusion body fibromatosis) is a form of fibromatosis usually restricted to childhood.[315] The typical location is on the exterior surface of the end phalanges of the fingers and toes, but it may also occur outside the digits and at sites such as the oral cavity and breast[311,313] (Fig. 25.21). The lesions can be solitary or multiple and either present at birth or appear during the first 2 years of life. However, morphologically identical lesions in adults are on record.[326] The component cells show immunoreactivity for calponin, desmin, alpha-smooth muscle actin, CD99, and CD117.[257,304] A distinctive microscopic feature, generally not observed in other forms of fibromatosis, is the presence of peculiar eosinophilic cytoplasmic inclusions (Fig. 25.22). These have been examined ultrastructurally and found to be composed of compact masses of granules and filaments without a limiting membrane.[254,262] Their significance is obscure; their similarity with the 'virus factories' seen in cells with certain viruses has been commented on, but they are currently thought to derive from cytoplasmic contractile proteins, probably actin.[277,293,297,309,333] Other ultrastructural features include the presence of intracellular collagen and fibronexus, the latter being regarded as one of the most distinguishing features of

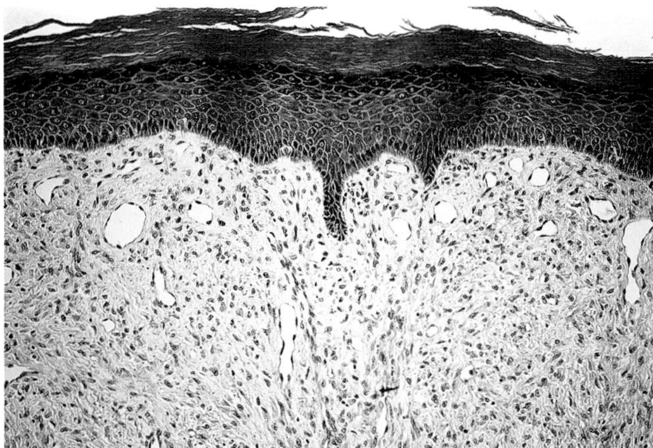

Fig. 25.21 Low-power view of infantile digital fibromatosis growing beneath a flattened epidermis.

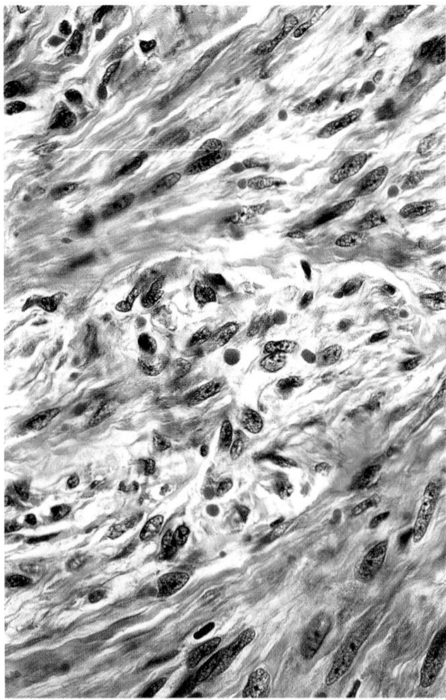

Fig. 25.22 On high power, the cells of infantile digital fibromatosis are seen to contain cytoplasmic hyaline globules.

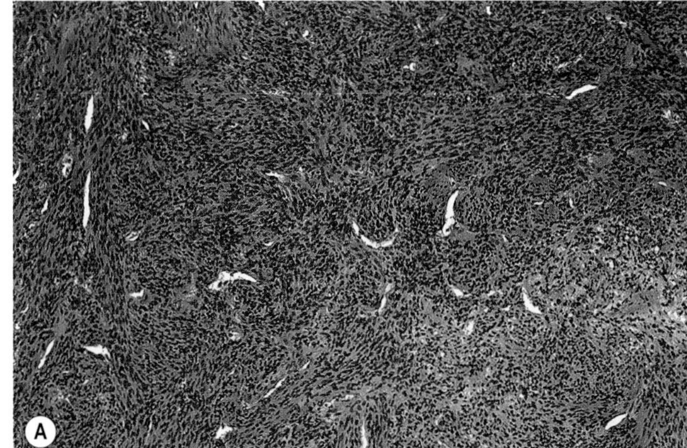

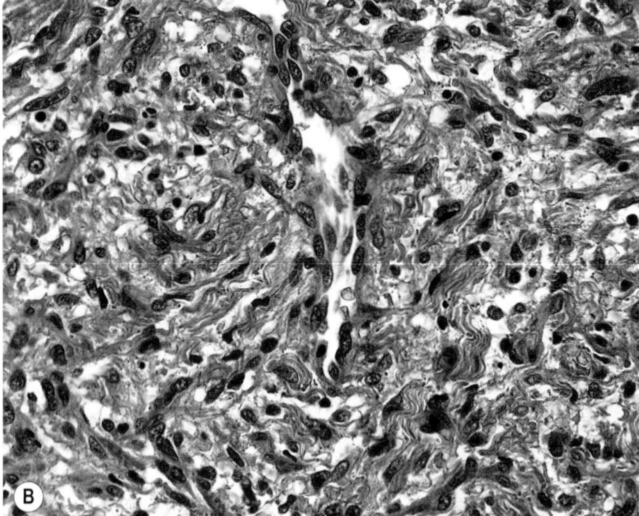

Fig. 25.23 **A** and **B**, Infantile myofibromatosis. The field shown in **A** contains hemangiopericytoma-like features. The higher power shown in **B** emphasizes the hypercellularity of the lesion.

myofibroblasts.[272] Infantile digital fibromatosis has a high tendency for local recurrence.[321]

Cases of infantile digital fibromatosis lacking inclusion bodies may be a component (and sometimes the first clinical manifestation) of the syndrome known as *terminal osseous dysplasia with pigmentary defects*.[274]

Infantile myofibromatosis presents as solitary (myofibroma)[327] or multiple (myofibromatosis)[259,270,281] nodules in the skin, soft tissues, or bone, either limited to these sites or associated with internal organ involvement.[292,327] A large majority of the cases occur before the age of 2 years, and approximately 60% are congenital.[263] However, this lesion can also occur in adults.[255,267,294] Solitary forms are more common in males, and multicentric forms are more common in females.[236] A familial incidence has been detected, and evidence for an autosomal dominant pattern of transmission has been obtained.[299] Microscopically, peripheral areas that resemble smooth muscle alternate with hemangiopericytoma-like areas and foci having a more typical fibroblastic configuration (Fig. 25.23). Central necrosis and intravascular growth may be present.[263] Ultrastructurally, the lesion is largely composed of myofibroblasts, hence its name; however, a whole range of differentiation exists between fibroblasts and fully developed, desmin-positive smooth muscle cells.[280] Indeed, myofibromatosis seems to be a member of a family of tumors showing vessel-related myoid differentiation, which also includes glomangiopericytoma, myopericytoma, and hemangiopericytoma, particularly the infantile form of the latter (see p. 2155).[288] This impression is supported by the existence of combined and hybrid forms.[250] Infantile myofibromatosis can undergo spontaneous regression, allegedly through the mechanism of apoptosis.[283]

Lipofibromatosis is a minor variation on the theme of infantile fibromatosis, in which a spindle cell component of fibroblastic appearance (mainly located in septa and skeletal muscle) is admixed with mature adipose tissue.[278] It resembles fibrous hamartoma of infancy (see p. 2179) but for the lack of a primitive nodular fibromyxoid component; local recurrence is very common.[278]

Fibromatosis hyalinica multiplex (multiple juvenile hyaline fibromatosis, systemic hyalinosis) is a morphologically distinctive type of familial multiple fibromatosis affecting children but not present at birth,[295] characterized microscopically by a conspicuous hyalinization of the connective tissue of the skin, oral cavity, articular capsule, and bone.[273] Multinucleated histiocytic giant cells can be present.[289] Ultrastructurally, the cells have the features of fibroblasts; numerous cisternae of endoplasmic reticulum are seen, many of which are dilated ('fibril-filled balls'). Entangled cytoplasmic tubules may also be present.[328,331] It has been claimed that the disease is the result of mutations in the gene encoding capillary morphogenesis protein 2.[291]

Some forms of fibromatosis derive their names from their particular location.[251] **Penile fibromatosis** (Peyronie disease) is discussed in Chapter 18. **Palmar fibromatosis** is also known as Dupuytren contracture, and **plantar fibromatosis** as Ledderhose disease.[298,312,322] These conditions occur predominantly in adults but can also be seen in children and adolescents.[279] Contracture of the fingers or toes is the leading clinical manifestation. The lesions can be multiple and bilateral, and may coexist in the upper and lower extremities. The plantar form tends to be more localized than its palmar counterpart. Microscopically, they have been classified into three phases: proliferative, involutive, and residual.[326] During the proliferative phase, cellularity may be marked (especially for the plantar lesions), and this may lead to a mistaken diagnosis of fibrosarcoma. It is well to remember that fibrosarcoma of the palmar and plantar areas is exceptional and that the differential diagnosis of a cellular spindle cell tumor of the sole is usually between fibromatosis, synovial sarcoma, malignant melanoma, and Kaposi sarcoma.

Fibromatoses also have been named according to the presumed inciting cause, such as **cicatricial fibromatosis** and **postirradiation fibromatosis**. The cicatricial form may follow accidental trauma or arise in the scar of surgical procedures. Postirradiation fibromatosis differs from the other forms by virtue of the common occurrence of bizarre cells with large hyperchromatic nuclei. This feature, which in the absence of radiation exposure would be strong evidence of malignancy, should be interpreted more conservatively under these circumstances.

The association of soft tissue tumors, usually of the fibromatosis type, with multiple colonic polyposis and occasionally multiple osteomas is known as **Gardner syndrome**.[258,318,324] In this condition, the fibromatosis has a particular tendency to involve intra-abdominal structures, such as the omentum and mesentery,[260,261,301] and to manifest itself following a surgical procedure in the area. It is important not to misdiagnose intra-abdominal fibromatosis involving the intestinal wall (a not uncommon occurrence) as a gastrointestinal stromal tumor (GIST).[317] Along these lines, it should be mentioned that – despite early statements to the contrary – fibromatosis seems to be a CD117-negative tumor, as opposed to bona fide GIST.[306] Patients with Gardner syndrome can also develop so-called *Gardner fibroma*, a soft tissue tumor most often located in the back or paraspinal region and characterized microscopically by a bland hypocellular proliferation of spindle cells embedded in a background of haphazardly oriented coarse collagen fibers, similar to nuchal-type fibroma.[264]

Fibrosarcoma

Fibrosarcomas are commonly tumors of adults, although they can occur in any age group and even be present as congenital neoplasms.[338,342,346,353,358] The latter are to be regarded as a special category (see below). Fibrosarcomas can arise from superficial and deep connective tissues such as fascia, tendon, periosteum, and scar; grow slowly or rapidly; and often appear well circumscribed[355] (Fig. 25.24). They usually are soft and cellular and may contain areas of necrosis and hemorrhage.

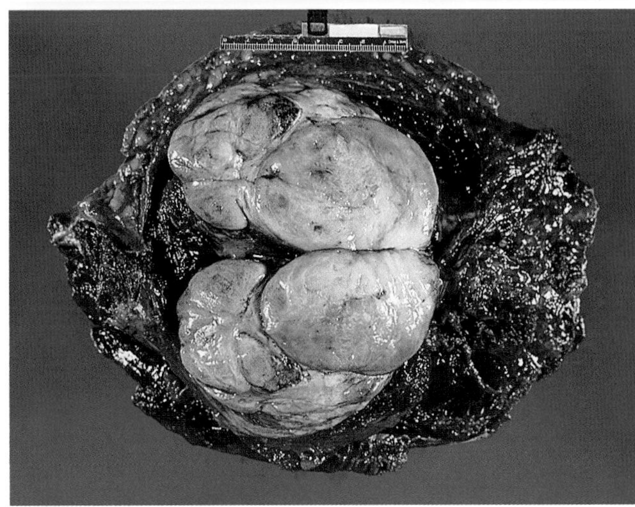

Fig. 25.24 Well-circumscribed fibrosarcoma growing within skeletal muscle.

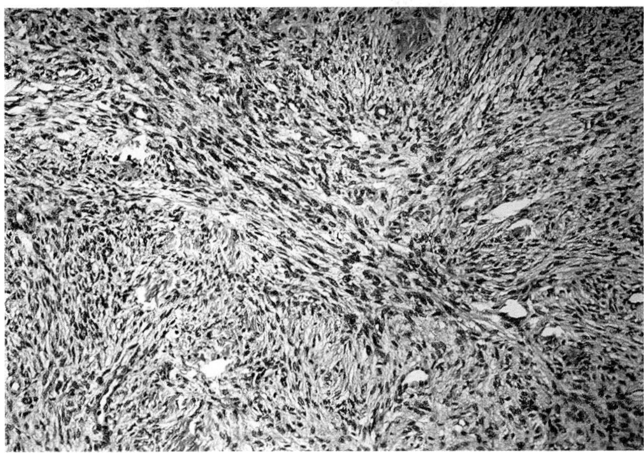

Fig. 25.25 Low-power appearance of well-differentiated fibrosarcoma. The tumor has a monotonous hypercellular look.

Microscopically, the well-differentiated tumors are easily recognized as fibroblastic (Fig. 25.25). The cells are arranged in fascicles that intersect each other at acute angles, resulting in a herringbone appearance. The individual cells resemble normal fibroblasts, and a reticulin stain demonstrates abundant fibers *wrapped around each cell*.[357] The fibroblastic nature is more difficult to recognize in the undifferentiated tumors (Fig. 25.26). It should be remembered that many other soft tissue tumors, particularly synovial sarcoma, liposarcoma, so-called malignant fibrous histiocytoma, and MPNST, often contain areas closely resembling fibrosarcoma. Only careful examination of different blocks of the tumor will provide the correct diagnosis in these instances. Although a pleomorphic type of fibrosarcoma probably exists (see under 'Malignant fibrous histiocytoma'), one should question the diagnosis of fibrosarcoma in the presence of a soft tissue sarcoma with numerous tumor giant cells. As a matter of fact, the diagnosis of fibrosarcoma (especially the low-grade type) should be viewed as a diagnosis of exclusion.[345] Ultrastructurally, most of the tumor cells of fibrosarcoma recapitulate the morphology of normal fibroblasts, whereas others have

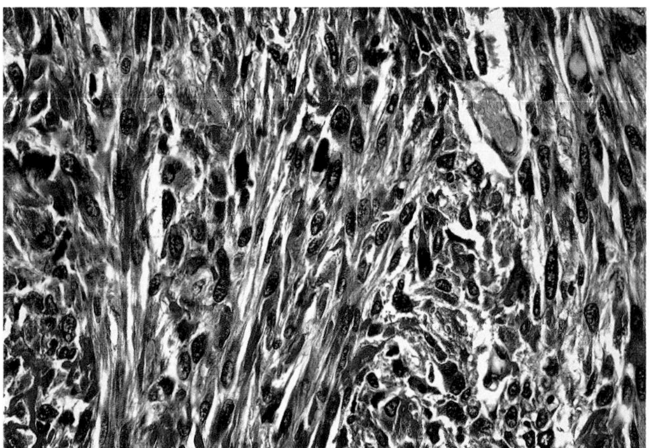

Fig. 25.26 Fibrosarcoma showing a moderate degree of nuclear pleomorphism.

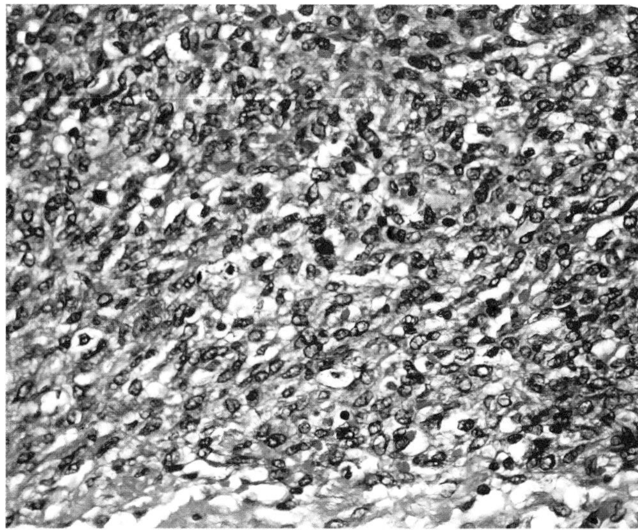

Fig. 25.27 Congenital fibrosarcoma. The tumor is extremely cellular and mitotically active.

features of myofibroblasts[339] or other features that reflect the remarkable phenotypic plasticity of this cell type.[341] Immunohistochemically, the prototypical fibrosarcoma should have reactivity for vimentin and type I collagen but not for smooth muscle markers, histiocytic markers, or basal lamina components.[344] The presence of focal immunoreactivity for smooth muscle actin, laminin, or collagen (not an unusual occurrence) should be taken to indicate incipient differentiation along myoid or possibly myofibroblastic lines.

As already indicated, another important differential diagnosis is with fibromatosis. The main light microscopic differences are discussed on page 2117. With special techniques and allowing for some degree of overlap, fibrosarcoma is more likely than fibromatosis to have a high proliferative index, an aneuploid DNA pattern, and p53 positivity.[349] In contrast to the fibromatoses, fibrosarcomas are capable of distant metastases. The survival rate in a recent large series was 41% at 5 years and 29% at 10 years.[360] Generally, the more superficial and differentiated the tumor, the better the prognosis. Increased mitotic activity and marked cellularity (as expressed by a grading system) are associated with an increased incidence of metastases.[360] In two large series,[350,359] fibrosarcomas in children under 5 years of age at the time of diagnosis were shown to have a high recurrence rate but an incidence of distant metastases of only 7–8%. Many of these belong to the category of congenital fibrosarcoma discussed below. Instead, fibrosarcomas occurring in children 10 years old or older have a metastatic rate close to that of adult patients (i.e., 50%).[356] The treatment of choice is radical excision. Postoperative radiation therapy should be considered if microscopic residual or positive margins are encountered. Since subclinical microscopic metastases are presumed to exist in many patients at the time of surgery, adjuvant chemotherapy has been recommended following the surgical excision of the tumor in high-grade lesions.[360]

Congenital fibrosarcoma (infantile fibrosarcoma) is an extremely cellular tumor characterized by very rapid growth and the capability for extensive local invasion, but its metastatic rate is negligible[340] (Fig. 25.27). At the molecular level, it is characterized by the *ETV6–NTRK3* gene fusion, which results from the chromosomal translocation t(12;15)(p13;q25).[337,352] This gene fusion is not present in the conditions that enter in the differential diagnosis with congenital fibrosarcoma, namely adult-type fibrosarcoma, infantile fibromatosis, infantile myofibromatosis, and the newly described *congenital/infantile myxoid mesenchymal tumor* which has not yet been well characterized.[335] In addition, trisomies of chromosomes 8, 11, 17, and 20 are common.[354] Of interest, congenital mesoblastic nephroma of the kidney shows identical genetic alterations, suggesting that these two entities are closely related.[347]

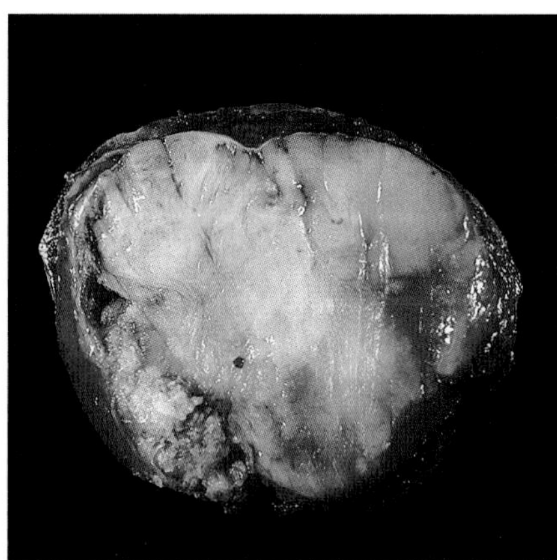

Fig. 25.28 Gross appearance of sclerosing epithelioid fibrosarcoma.

Sclerosing epithelioid fibrosarcoma is a variant of fibrosarcoma that simulates the appearance of infiltrating carcinoma[348,351] (Fig. 25.28). It is composed of small, round to ovoid tumor cells embedded in a dense fibrohyaline stroma. The scanty cytoplasm often has a clear appearance, and there may be an Indian file pattern of growth (Fig. 25.29). Necrosis and bone invasion may be found.[336] There is consistent positivity for vimentin, and occasional positivity for EMA and even for keratin.[348] The tumor is associated with a high incidence of local recurrence and distant metastases. Some cases exhibit the same distinctive chromosomal translocation of low-grade fibromyxoid sarcoma, raising the possibility of a close relationship between these two tumor types.[343]

Myofibroblastic tumors

A particularly difficult issue in the classification of soft tissue tumors is the role played by myofibroblasts. Some authors have taken a very restrictive view of the definition of a myofibroblast (including the requirement of ultrastructural confirmation), whereas others use

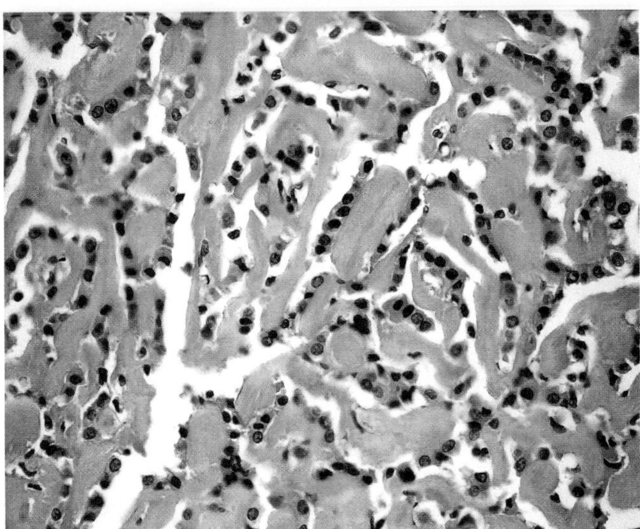

Fig. 25.29 Sclerosing epithelioid fibrosarcoma. The Indian file disposition simulates carcinoma.

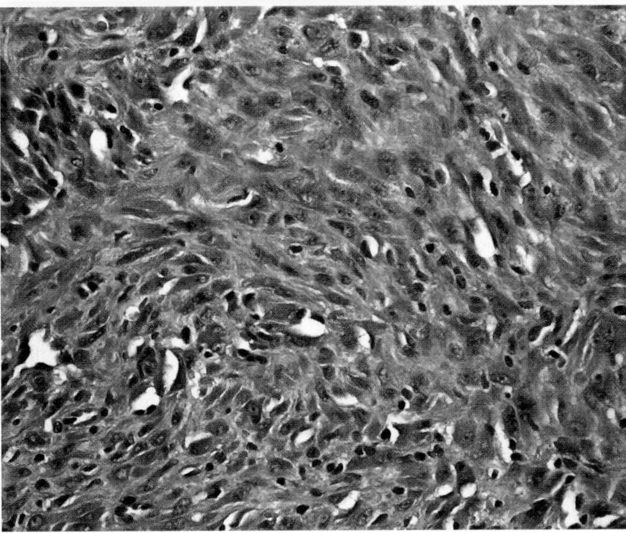

Fig. 25.30 So-called 'myofibrosarcoma'. Some of the tumor cells have a polygonal shape and a basophilic cytoplasm.

the term rather liberally for any cells having features intermediate between those of a fibroblast and a smooth muscle cell.[375,381] This being the case, it is not surprising that this hybrid cell is undergoing the same swings in popularity that have previously affected the pericyte. Part of the problem is the fact that there are no specific immunohistochemical markers for myofibroblasts, although endosialin (Tem1) has been recently proposed as a candidate.[362] Perhaps it would be better to use the alternative and less committal term *myoid cell* to avoid unwarranted histogenetic and functional assumptions.

The other problem concerns the fact that cells with myofibroblastic (myoid) features can be found in a large number of benign and malignant soft tissue lesions, which means that we are in danger of creating a waste-basket category, just as large as if not larger than that of malignant fibrous histiocytoma. Therefore, if there is to be a category of myofibroblastic tumors, it would be wise to reserve it for lesions that are composed almost entirely of cells having the hybrid features above described, and which do not fit the criteria of already established entities, such as nodular fasciitis, fibromatosis, or, for that matter, myofibromatosis. Tumors that have been placed into this category include *myofibroblastoma*, including its *desmoplastic variant*, and *myofibrosarcoma* (*myofibroblastic sarcoma*), including its *low-grade variant*.[366,368,369,372,375,376,378] The claim has been made that myofibrosarcomas express calponin but not caldesmon, whereas leiomyosarcomas are said to exhibit both markers[367] (Fig. 25.30).

Inflammatory myofibroblastic tumor is a distinctive entity, which blends imperceptibly with cases that have been reported as inflammatory pseudotumor on one hand and inflammatory fibrosarcoma on the other.[363,374,379,382] Many of the cases have occurred in the mesentery or retroperitoneum of children or adolescents, and have often been accompanied by anemia and fever.[364] Whether the proliferating spindle cells are truly myofibroblastic or members of the accessory immune system (reticulum fibroblastic cells) remains to be determined.[377] ALK is often expressed at the immunohistochemical level.[361,370] This results from a rearrangement of the *ALK* gene on chromosome 2p23, and is more commonly seen in pediatric than in adult cases, suggesting a different molecular pathogenetic mechanism among the two groups.[380,383] Many partner genes can be fused with *ALK*, including *TPM3, TPM4, CLTC, CARS, ATIC, SEC31L1*, and *RANBP2*, and some of these genes are the same partner genes involved in ALK+ anaplastic large cell lymphoma (*TPM3, TPM4, CLTC, ATIC*) and ALK+ large B-cell lymphoma (*CLTC*).[365,371] *TP53* mutation and MDM2 amplification are rare.[383] The behavior is generally indolent but sometimes aggressive.[373]

So-called fibrohistiocytic tumors

This large, complex, and controversial family of tumors was originally defined by the presence of a dual cellular composition: cells with a fibroblastic appearance intimately mixed with others having some of the morphologic and functional attributes of histiocytes.[441,512] Stout and his colleagues at Columbia Presbyterian Hospital in New York City[474,505,513] first proposed that these tumors originate from tissue histiocytes, some of which were said to acquire fibroblastic features; that is, they became 'facultative fibroblasts', a property supposedly shared by Schwann cells, smooth muscle cells, and other mesenchymal cells. Another proposed interpretation of these lesions is that they arise from primitive mesenchymal cells with the capacity for dual differentiation into histiocytes and fibroblasts.[386,433] Both theories assume the existence in these lesions of a true neoplastic histiocytic component, in addition to the population of reactive histiocytes that is undoubtedly present. To be sure, some of the cells in these tumors do show phagocytic properties, accumulate fat and hemosiderin, exhibit lysosomes ultrastructurally, and manifest immunocytochemical reactivity for hydrolytic enzymes;[456,522] however, the specific cell markers of 'true histiocytes' derived from bone marrow have been found to be absent in the tumor cells and present only in the osteoclast-like giant cells occasionally seen in these lesions.[402,418,528,558] In these and other studies, the tumor cells had a phenotypic appearance resembling that of fibroblasts or myofibroblasts.[455] Furthermore, the existence of a cell of hematopoietic lineage in a mesenchymal neoplasm would seem highly unlikely on conceptual grounds. There is also the fact that patterns indistinguishable from those of malignant fibrous histiocytoma (MFH) can be seen in otherwise typical mesenchymal tumors of various well-defined types, particularly liposarcoma and MPNST.[418,444] It seems increasingly evident that the tumors in the fibrous histiocytoma group (particularly the malignant ones) do not represent a specific type but rather a common pathway for a variety of other soft tissue tumors, including fibrosarcoma, leiomyosarcoma, liposarcoma, and MPNST.[426,455] In any event, these lesions have enough features in common to justify discussing them as a group.

Histiocytoma. Pure histiocytoma of skin and soft tissue is probably the only tumor composed of true histiocytes listed in this section. As such, it may be totally unrelated to all the other types of described 'fibrohistiocytic' tumors, in the sense of being composed not of fibroblasts or other cells of conventional mesenchymal lineage but rather of one of the cells belonging to the accessory immune system, which includes histiocytes (macrophages) and the various subtypes of reticulum/dendritic cells.

Most cases of histiocytoma occur in children. Microscopically, the typical case is made up of closely packed polygonal cells with little or no intervening stroma.[461] The cytoplasm is eosinophilic and may contain lipid droplets. Inflammatory cells are frequently present. Fibrosis, which may be present in the older lesions, should be distinguished from the active fibroblastic proliferation of fibrous histiocytomas. The benign tumors greatly predominate over those exhibiting a malignant behavior, and the differential diagnosis between them may be difficult. Histiocytomas with clinical and/or pathologic features that single them out from the rest are **juvenile xanthogranuloma**,[459] **reticulohistiocytoma**, and **generalized eruptive histiocytoma**, all of which are benign. Most of these varieties are discussed in Chapter 4. Although most of these lesions are cutaneous, deep soft tissue examples exist.[423,458] We have seen several such cases that have been overinterpreted as embryonal rhabdomyosarcoma or other malignant neoplasms.

Benign fibrous histiocytoma. Well-defined examples of lesions regarded at the time as examples of benign forms of fibrous histiocytoma include **dermatofibroma**, **tenosynovial giant cell tumor**,[547] and the closely related **pigmented villonodular synovitis**, including its diffuse variant (see Chapter 24). The microscopic diagnosis is usually simple. A variable mixture of histiocyte-like cells (some foamy, others multinucleated, still others containing hemosiderin) and fibroblast-like cells is always present.[401,504] Some lesions can be extremely cellular (cellular variant), and some may have large atypical nuclei (atypical variant),[538] and a variable degree of mitotic activity. The classic benign fibrous histiocytoma is superficially located in the skin, but deeply seated examples occur.[427] These have a better developed storiform pattern, are more circumscribed, and may exhibit prominent hemangiopericytoma-like vessels. They have a 20% incidence of local recurrence. More disturbingly, exceptionally they metastasize to distant sites.[434]

The recently described *hemosiderotic fibrohistiocytic lipomatous lesion* (*hemosiderotic fibrolipomatous tumor*), characteristically occurring almost exclusively in the ankle region of elderly patients (usually females), should be mentioned in this section despite the fact that its pathogenesis is thought to be reactive (secondary to repeated minor trauma) rather than neoplastic.[482] Local recurrence is common.[403] Of interest, a recent study identifies chromosomal translocation identical to that of myxoinflammatory fibroblastic sarcoma, raising the possibility that it may represent a possible precursor of the latter tumor.[440]

Pure **xanthomas** are regarded as the tissue expression of an abnormality of lipid metabolism and not as members of the fibrous histiocytoma group. It is probable that the cases reported as *plexiform xanthomatous tumor*[495] represent a morphologic variant on the theme of xanthoma, as suggested by their usual periarticular location and not infrequent multiplicity.

Intermediate (borderline) fibrous histiocytoma. This vaguely defined group of tumors is characterized by local aggressiveness (manifested by a high tendency for local occurrence) but an extremely low rate of distant metastases.[398,490] Furthermore, the few metastases that develop generally do so only after repeated failures at local control.[424,539,549] The best example in this category is the tumor traditionally known as **dermatofibrosarcoma protuberans (DFSP)** and also discussed in Chapter 4.[392,404,428,436] It is typically centered in the dermis, but it can also occur in deeper soft tissues.[391] This lesion is characterized microscopically by lack of circumscription; high cellularity; a relatively monomorphic appearance; nuclear hyperchromasia; moderate to high mitotic activity; lack or inconspicuousness of giant, foamy, or hemosiderin-laden cells; and the presence of what has been called a *storiform* pattern of growth (Fig. 25.31). This refers to a peculiar arrangement of the tumor cells

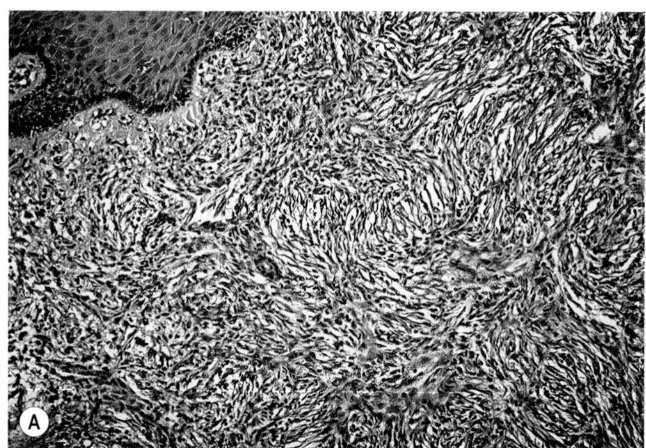

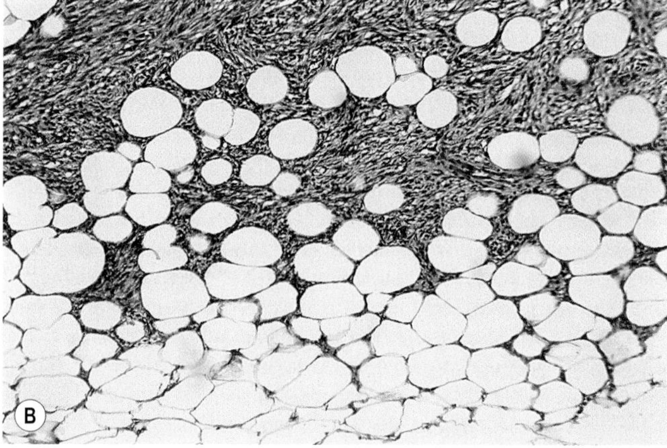

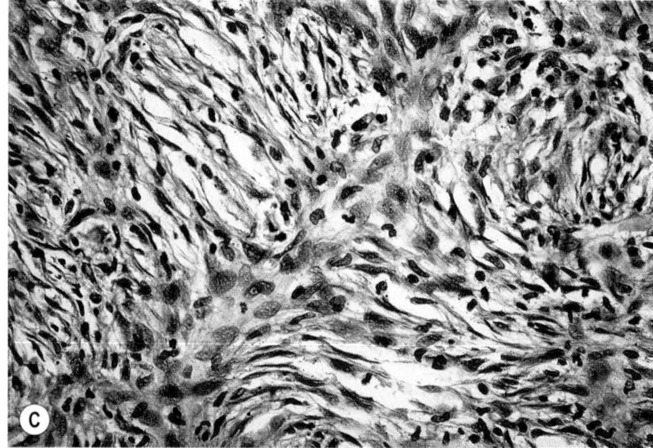

Fig. 25.31 Dermatofibrosarcoma protuberans: **A**, diffuse hypercellular growth in the dermis; **B**, typical pattern of infiltration of the subcutaneous fat; **C**, storiform pattern of growth.

around a central point, producing radiating 'spokes' grouped at right angles to each other. Tridimensional reconstruction studies suggest that this structure develops at the periphery of adjacent proliferating cell groups.[486] This pattern can also be seen in benign fibrous histiocytomas as well as in tumors of totally unrelated types, such as thymoma. The collagen deposited in dermatofibrosarcoma appears as nonpolarizable thin strands, in contrast to that present in most dermatofibromas.[393] Sometimes the tumor has prominent myxoid features.[493,525]

The histogenesis of dermatofibrosarcoma protuberans remains controversial; the immunohistochemical profile is more in keeping with a fibroblastic than a fibrohistiocytic or neural derivation,[413,475] although the existence of a pigmented variant (Bednar tumor, see below) suggests otherwise.

Virtually all cases of dermatofibrosarcoma protuberans have a translocation that involves chromosomes 17 and 22, resulting in fusion of the collagen type I α I (*COL1A1*) and platelet-derived growth factor β (*PDGFβ*) genes, which can be detected by RT-PCR or FISH.[516] They have also been shown to have a distinctive gene expression profile.[479]

The main differential diagnosis is with deep-seated benign fibrous histiocytoma;[460] stains for CD34 and apolipoprotein A (positive in dermatofibrosarcoma protuberans), as well as factor XIIIa and HMGA1/HMGA2 (positive in benign fibrous histiocytoma of skin), are helpful in this regard.[478,554]

As previously noted, a close link exists between dermatofibrosarcoma protuberans and giant cell fibroblastoma, which also applies to the genetic molecular alterations.[533,541] Indeed, the latter is regarded by most as the juvenile variant of the former.[394] It should be noted, however, that classic forms of dermatofibrosarcoma can also be seen in the pediatric age group.[484]

Sometimes tumors with the typical appearance of dermatofibrosarcoma protuberans develop foci indistinguishable from conventional fibrosarcoma, myofibrosarcoma, or pleomorphic (MFH-like) sarcoma.[435,491,507,510,559] Significantly, there is usually a loss of CD34 immunoreactivity in these foci.[435] There is disagreement among the various series as to whether this development is accompanied by a more aggressive clinical course,[407,411] but most evidence suggests that this is indeed the case.[384,491]

Pigmented dermatofibrosarcoma (Bednar tumor) looks like the usual dermatofibrosarcoma protuberans except for the presence of a population of dendritic cells heavily loaded with melanin (Fig. 25.32); the occurrence of this variant is of interest because it raises the possibility of a peripheral nerve sheath origin,[416,499] a possibility that others have also raised for the usual type of dermatofibrosarcoma protuberans.[442] An alternative possibility, i.e., that the melanin-containing dendritic cells are not neoplastic but rather represent secondary melanocyte colonization, has been suggested.[412,429] A case with the Bednar tumor pattern has been seen in the recurrence of a giant cell fibroblastoma, further supporting the relationship between these various neoplasms.[409]

Atypical fibroxanthoma is another tumor that can be placed in an intermediate or borderline category. It typically presents as a small nodule in the sun-exposed skin of elderly individuals.[464,468] Less commonly, it appears as a large mass in the trunk and limbs of younger patients.[432] Some cases develop in parts of the body previously subjected to radiation therapy.[520] The main differential diagnosis is with spindle cell squamous cell carcinoma and spindle cell (desmoplastic) malignant melanoma. Immunohistochemical stains for S-100 protein and keratin are useful in this regard.[469] The large majority of atypical fibroxanthomas are cured by local excision,[432,451] but a few cases accompanied by metastases are on record.[443] This tumor type is discussed in more detail in Chapter 4.

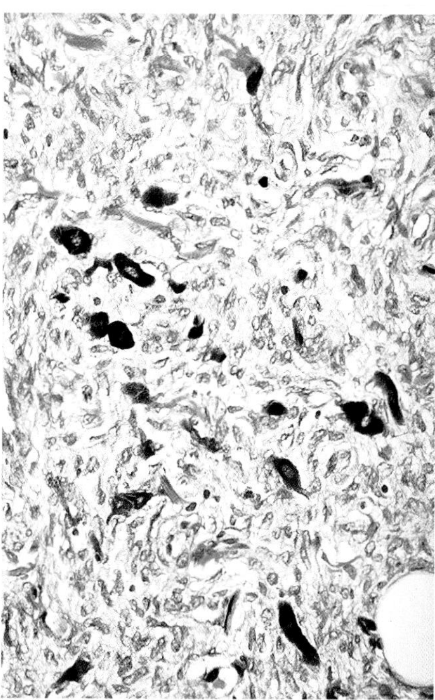

Fig. 25.32 Pigmented dermatofibrosarcoma protuberans (Bednar tumor). Scattered, heavily pigmented cells are seen among the spindle neoplastic elements.

Malignant fibrous histiocytoma (MFH) and related tumors. This tumor, also known as fibroxanthosarcoma and fibrohistiocytic sarcoma, was regarded in the seventies and eighties as the most common type of soft tissue sarcoma. Many tumors formerly designated pleomorphic rhabdomyosarcoma or pleomorphic liposarcoma were renamed MFH during that period. However, as already mentioned, serious doubts have been raised about the existence of MFH as a specific entity.[426] It may well be that this designation embraces sarcomas of various types (such as fibrosarcomas and leiomyosarcomas[420]) having some common morphologic features, such as pleomorphism and a storiform pattern of growth, a hypothesis well supported by gene expression profiling studies which show that MFH cases fail to form discrete clusters.[477,501] In retrospect, the somewhat arbitrary assumption that fibrosarcomas are almost never pleomorphic is at least partially responsible for the almost epidemic proportions that MFH reached at one point. Although the term MFH is retained in this book for the purposes of discussion, a more accurate term to use for cases with this appearance would be that of *undifferentiated pleomorphic sarcoma, NOS (so-called MFH)*.[385,410]

Several morphologic variants of MFH have been described. **Storiform-pleomorphic MFH** is the prototypic and most common member of this group.[488,489,536,550] Most cases occur in the deep soft tissues of extremities in adults, with a peak in the seventh decade, but cases have also been recorded in children[521,529,543] (Fig. 25.33). Some develop at the site of previous radiation therapy.[519] Still others have appeared around an infarct or a foreign body or at the site of a surgical scar.[452] Nearly half of them involve the deep fascia or the substance of a skeletal muscle.[463,551] Often they are quite large at the time of excision. As the name indicates, the presence of highly pleomorphic tumor cells and a storiform pattern of growth are the two most important microscopic features, even if the latter is not essential for the diagnosis[487,488] (Fig. 25.34). Sometimes the cytoplasm of the giant tumor cells is seen to contain numerous variably sized hyaline globules, thought to be related to apoptosis and

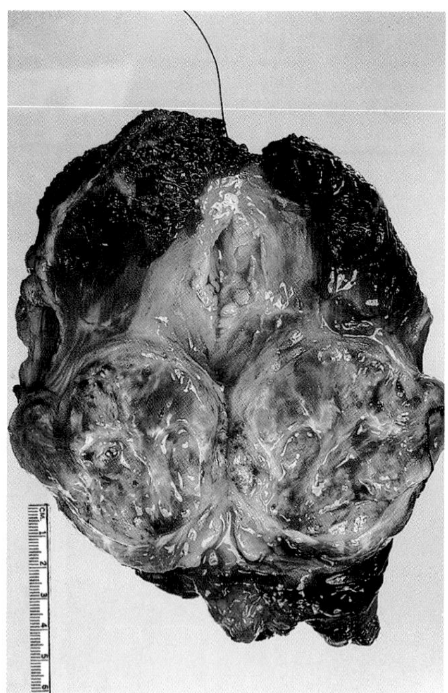

Fig. 25.33 Large so-called malignant fibrous histiocytoma with areas of cystic change and necrosis.

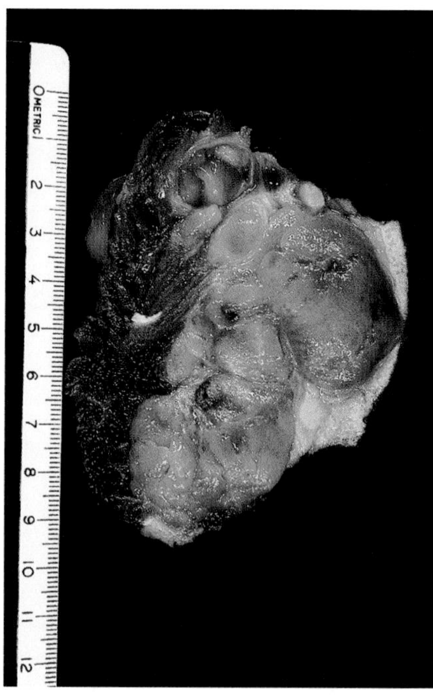

Fig. 25.35 Gross appearance of myxofibrosarcoma (myxoid MFH).

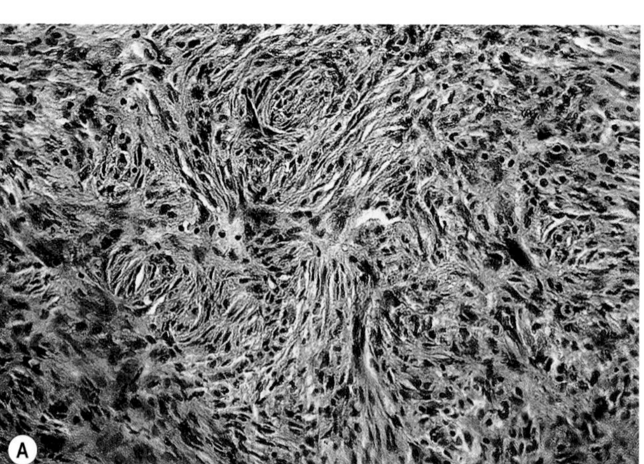

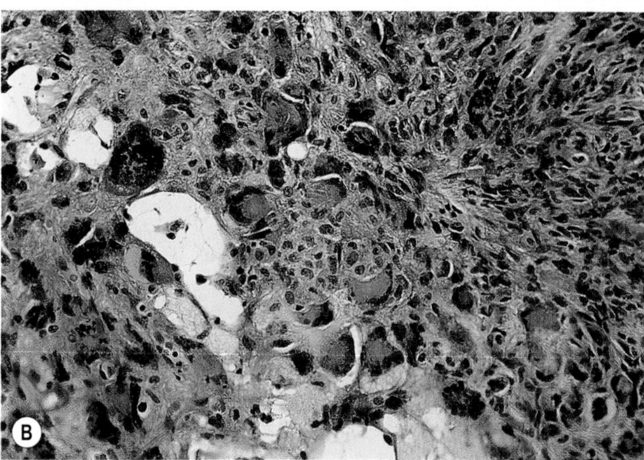

Fig. 25.34 So-called malignant fibrous histiocytoma of storiform–pleomorphic type: **A**, storiform pattern of growth; **B**, marked pleomorphism, with numerous multinucleated giant cells.

lugubriously called *thanatosomes*.[515] Inflammatory elements, such as lymphocytes, plasma cells, and eosinophils, are usually mixed with the neoplastic cells. Metaplastic bone and cartilage formation may be present focally.[397] Ultrastructurally, MFH consists of a mixture of cells resembling fibroblasts, myofibroblasts, histiocytes, and primitive mesenchymal cells.[447,471,540,545] Peculiar intranuclear inclusions consisting of closely packed undulating fibrils have been found in some cases.[544] Immunohistochemically, there is usually reactivity for vimentin, α_1-antitrypsin, α_1-antichymotrypsin, KP-1 (CD68), factor XIIIa, ferritin, and the plasma proenzyme factor XIII, and sometimes also for actin, desmin, and lysozyme.[400,414,445,453,454,466,476,496,503,523,558] A variety of lysosomal enzymes have also been detected using standard enzyme histochemical techniques.[395,500] It should be remarked that none of these antigens is specific for histiocytes.[535] Some cases of MFH have also shown immunoreactivity for keratin.[446,480,530]

This tumor is prone to local recurrence and has the capacity to metastasize to distant sites, especially the lungs and regional lymph nodes.[536] The most important prognostic factors are size and depth of its location, two parameters that are closely related.[396,462,518,529,531] In the classic series of 200 cases reported by Weiss and Enzinger,[552] tumors that were small, were superficially located, or had a prominent inflammatory component (other than neutrophilic) metastasized only rarely.

Myxofibrosarcoma is the term currently preferred for the tumor also known as myxoid MFH.[387,467] Most of these tumors arise in the extremities of adults. They are usually attached to the fascia or within a major muscle, but they can also be very superficial.[481] Grossly, they are mucoid and resemble myxoid liposarcomas (Fig. 25.35). Microscopically, the low-grade forms exhibit an abundant matrix of acid mucopolysaccharides, high vascularity, and the presence of cells resembling lipoblasts[438,492] (Fig. 25.36). They are distinguished from myxoid liposarcomas by the presence elsewhere in the tumor of typical areas with the storiform–pleomorphic MFH pattern and the absence of true lipoblasts, which should contain neutral fat in the cytoplasmic vacuoles rather than acid

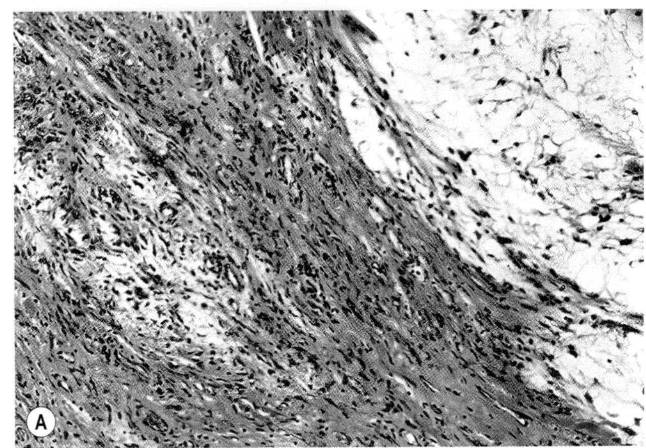

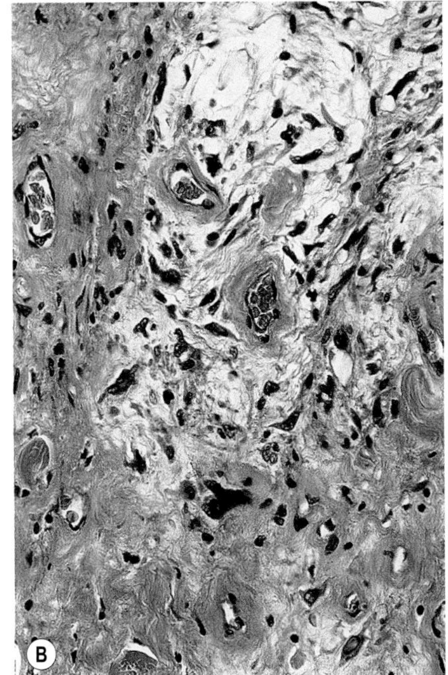

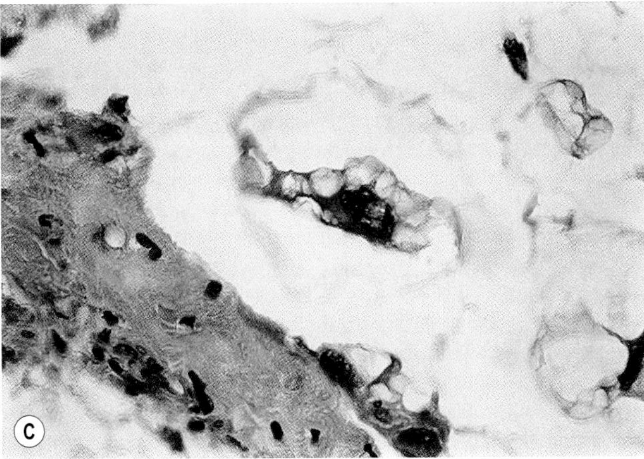

Fig. 25.36 Myxofibrosarcoma (myxoid MFH): **A**, alternation of cellular and myxoid areas; **B**, moderate pleomorphism of tumor cells; **C**, lipoblast-like tumor cells floating in myxoid material.

mucopolysaccharides. Generally speaking, however, the histochemical evaluation of the myxoid extracellular matrix is of little utility in the differential diagnosis of myxoid soft tissue tumors, largely composed of glycosaminoglycans and albumin but rather heterogeneous in the relative proportions and specific nature of these substances.[556]

Other features of differential value include the presence in myxoid MFH of a greater degree of pleomorphism in the myxoid areas and the fact that the vessels have a coarser quality and an elongated curvilinear disposition.[509] Some electron microscopic differences between the two tumors have also been found.[472,546]

A variant of myxofibrosarcoma with a predominantly epithelioid morphology has been recently described.[502] The overall prognosis of myxoid MFH is better than for the conventional storiform–pleomorphic MFH.[552] Altered expression of cell cycle regulators (such as reduced expression of p21) is said to be a poor prognostic factor.[508] There is a relationship between microscopic grade and prognosis, but even the lower-grade tumors have a potential for recurrence.[449,450] Recurrent tumors tend to exhibit a higher histologic grade.[555]

Low-grade fibromyxoid sarcoma (Evans tumor) is a soft tissue neoplasm (usually deep but sometimes superficial, especially in children[399]) characterized by alternating fibrous and myxoid areas, a focally whorled pattern of growth, low cellularity, and a bland appearance of the fibroblastic spindle cells[421] (Fig. 25.37). Curvilinear capillaries and pseudolipoblasts are not seen. Areas of

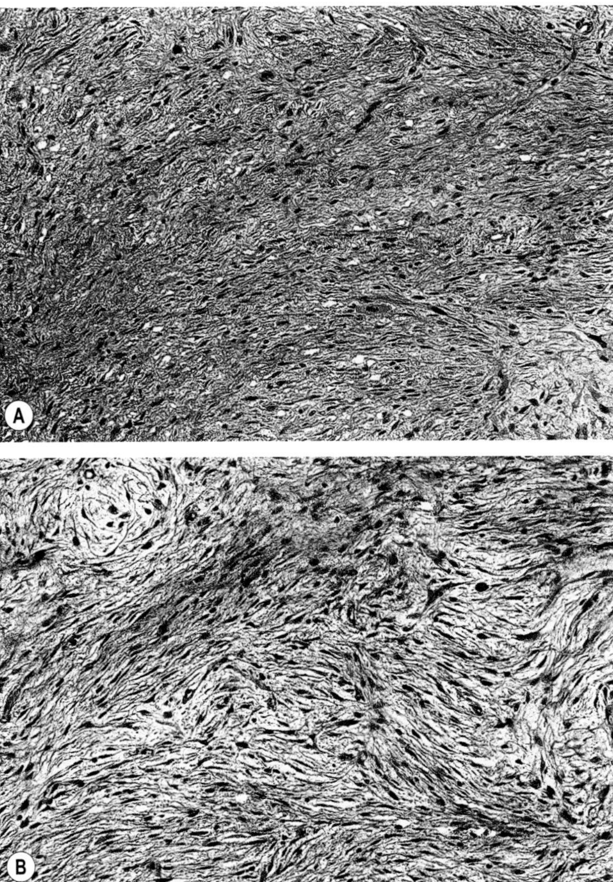

Fig. 25.37 A and **B**, Low- and high-power views of low-grade fibromyxoid sarcoma. There is very little pleomorphism. The fibrosis predominates over the myxoid change.

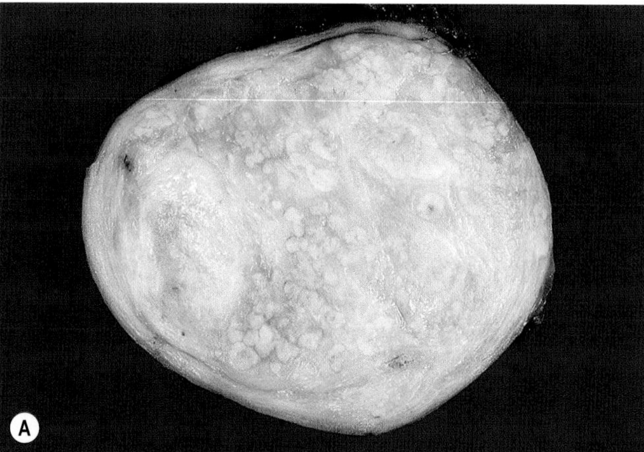

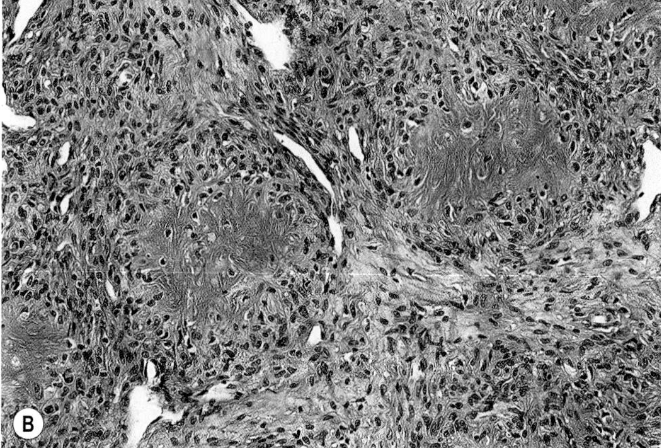

Fig. 25.38 Hyalinizing spindle cell tumor with giant rosettes: **A**, gross appearance of tumor located in anterior abdominal wall; **B**, giant rosettelike structures surrounded by tumor cells.

hypercellularity and necrosis may be seen.[430] Both local recurrences and distant metastases have been common in the cases reported from a single institution.[421,437] The main differential diagnosis is with myxofibrosarcoma. Low-grade fibromyxoid sarcoma has a biphasic fibrous and myxoid appearance, and the vascular network is less well developed. Ultrastructurally, low-grade fibromyxoid sarcoma is composed of cells with primarily fibroblastic features, including well-developed cisternae of rough endoplasmic reticulum which are often distended.[388]

It is now accepted that the neoplasm originally described as *hyalinizing spindle cell tumor with giant rosettes* is a morphologic variant of low-grade fibromyxoid sarcoma characterized by the presence of huge rosettelike formations made up of hyalinized collagen[473] (Fig. 25.38). The similarities also apply to the clinical behavior, including the capability for distant metastases.[430,511] These two tumor types also share the t(7;16)(q33;p11) translocation which results in *FUS–CREB3L2* gene fusion or, rarely, t(11;16)(p11;p11) with *FUS–CREB3L1* fusion,[494,514,524] and a variety of ultrastructural features.[431] Molecular study is particularly helpful for the diagnosis of this malignant neoplasm which has a deceptively bland morphology.[483] Although both low-grade fibromyxoid sarcoma and its alleged variant, hyalinizing spindle cell tumor with giant rosettes, are generally located in the soft tissues, they have also been described in the lung, ovary, and other internal sites.[465,557] Another tumor type for which a relationship with low-grade fibromyxoid sarcoma has been suggested (based on

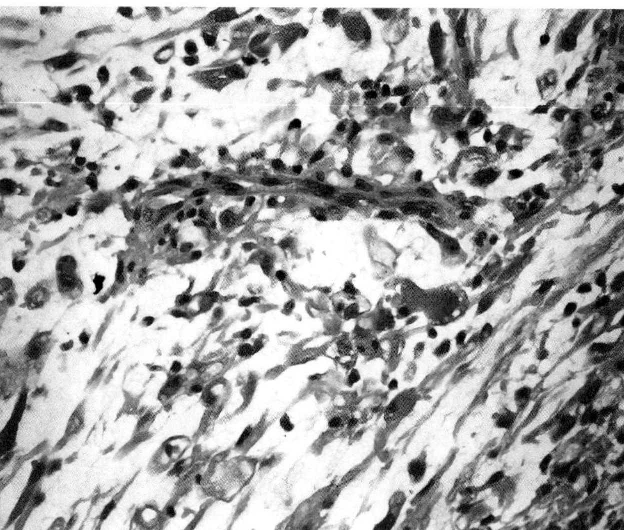

Fig. 25.39 Inflammatory myxohyaline tumor. Note the atypical cells with large nucleoli.

morphologic and molecular similarities) is sclerosing epithelioid fibrosarcoma (see above).

Inflammatory myxohyaline tumor (acral myxoinflammatory fibroblastic sarcoma) is a low-grade malignant tumor usually found in the distal extremities that can simulate an inflammatory condition, Hodgkin lymphoma, and various types of soft tissue sarcoma. Microscopically, it has an infiltrative multinodular quality and a polymorphic cellular composition in a hyaline or myxoid background (Fig. 25.39). There is a dense mononuclear inflammatory infiltrate containing scattered stromal cells of either epithelioid or spindle shape. Some of the latter are very large, with bizarre nuclei and prominent nucleoli, resulting in a resemblance to Reed–Sternberg cells or virus-infected cells.[485,497] The immunohistochemical profile, which is nonspecific, includes occasional focal reactivity for keratin. Local recurrence is common, but distant metastases are exceptional.[532] Recently, this neoplasm is shown to exhibit a recurrent genetic aberration t(1;10)(p22;q24), with the involved gene on 1p22 being identified as *TGFBR3*.[440]

Plexiform fibrohistiocytic tumor occurs chiefly in children and young adults.[526] It usually presents as a small, slow-growing dermal or subcutaneous mass, often in an upper extremity. Microscopically, there is a multinodular or plexiform proliferation of fibroblast-like and histiocyte-like cells admixed with osteoclast-like giant cells[419] (Fig. 25.40). They have been divided morphologically into three subtypes: fibroblastic, histiocytic (often with osteoclast-type giant cells), and mixed.[498] The immunohistochemical and ultrastructural features have been rather erratic, but have been generally interpreted as being consistent with a myofibroblastic derivation.[448] Local recurrence is very common, and a few cases have resulted in regional lymph node metastases.[419] We have seen several cases in which the typical appearance of this tumor type merged with a pattern highly reminiscent of neurothekeoma, suggesting a histogenetic link between the two entities.[457]

Inflammatory MFH is a tumor in which the neoplastic cells (some with a bland appearance and others that are bizarre and anaplastic) are mixed with, and even obscured by, an intense inflammatory infiltrate rich in neutrophils[470] (Fig. 25.41). Some of the tumor cells contain phagocytosed neutrophils in their cytoplasm. Storiform pattern, collections of foamy cells, and areas of

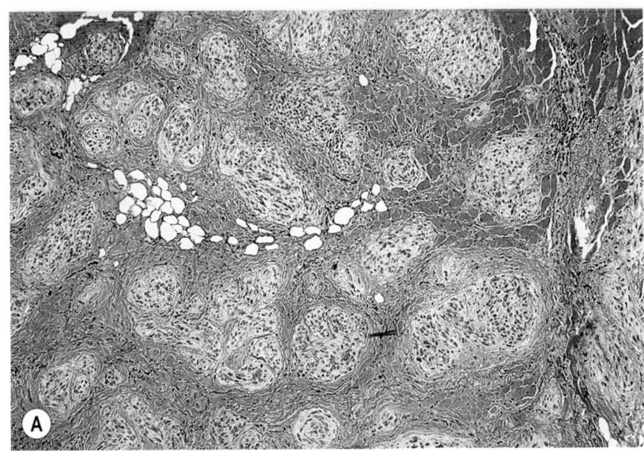

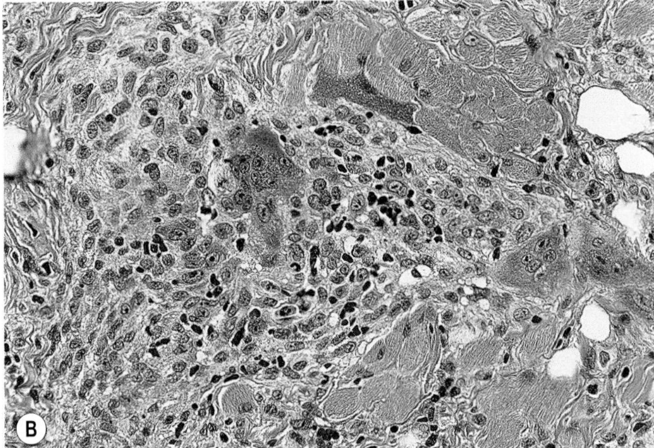

Fig. 25.40 **A** and **B**, Plexiform fibrohistiocytic tumor. **A**, Low-power view, showing nodular and plexiform pattern of growth. **B**, High-power view of one of the nodules, showing mononuclear tumor cells and scattered osteoclast-like giant cells.

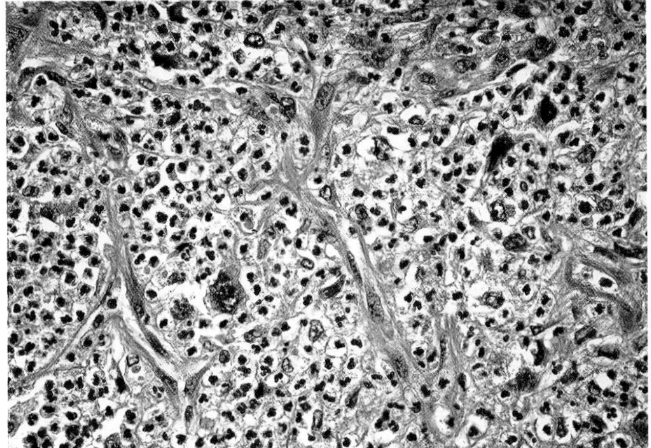

Fig. 25.41 So-called 'inflammatory MFH'. In this case the infiltrate is largely of neutrophilic nature.

tissue necrosis are also consistently present. In all likelihood this is a pattern of growth rather than a specific tumor type, in the sense that the same microscopic appearance (i.e., intense neutrophilic infiltration in a pleomorphic tumor associated with phagocytosis of neutrophils by the tumor cells) can be seen in otherwise typical liposarcomas, irradiated osteosarcomas, and metastatic

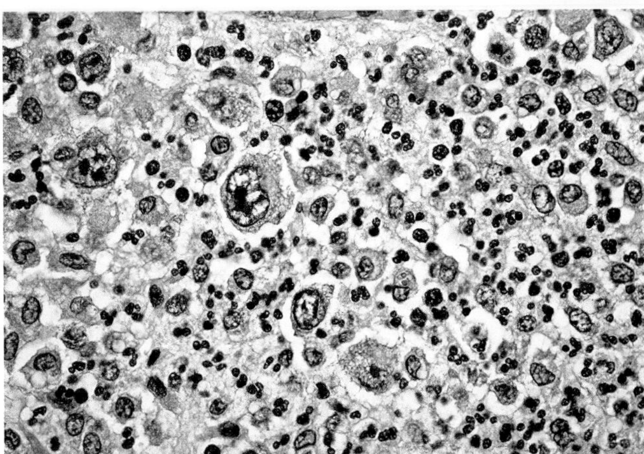

Fig. 25.42 Inflammatory MFH pattern in a case of lung carcinoma.

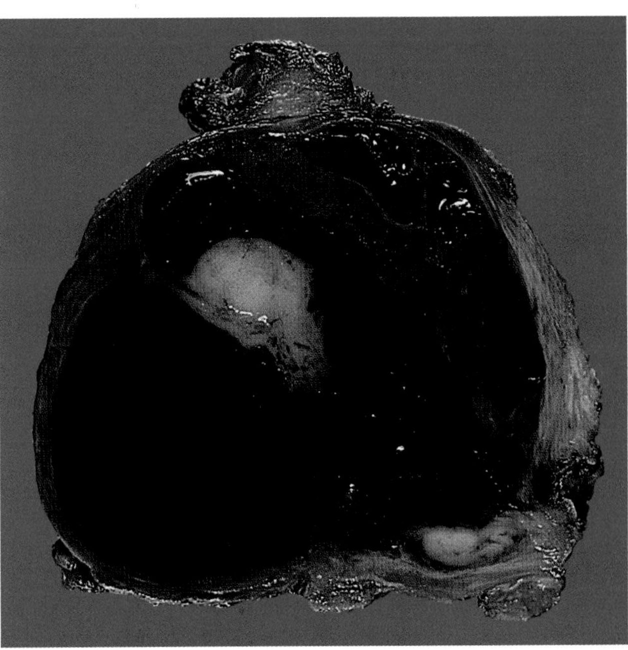

Fig. 25.43 Angiomatoid MFH. A small solid focus of white tumor is seen within a large hemorrhagic cyst.
(Courtesy of Dr Hector Rodriguez-Martinez, Mexico City)

carcinomas from various sites, such as lung, adrenal cortex, and kidney (Fig. 25.42). As a matter of fact, it would appear that most tumors with the inflammatory MFH pattern are dedifferentiated liposarcomas.[405] Sometimes this intratumoral inflammatory reaction is accompanied by a peripheral leukemoid reaction and eosinophilia.[548] In other instances the inflammatory infiltrate is predominantly composed of lymphocytes and plasma cells rather than neutrophils; in the case of liposarcomas, these tumors are referred to as *lymphocyte rich* or *inflammatory* (see p. 2148).

Angiomatoid MFH (angiomatoid fibrous histiocytoma) usually appears in the extremities of children and young adults as a circumscribed, multinodular, or multicystic hemorrhagic mass[408,417,517] (Fig. 25.43). Occasional congenital examples have been described.[389] Exceptional examples occurring outside somatic soft tissues, such as mediastinum, brain, and lung, have been reported.[390,415,527]

Microscopically, highly cellular foci are mixed with focal areas of hemorrhagic cyst-like spaces and large aggregates of chronic inflammatory cells. The latter are often arranged at the periphery of the tumor in the form of lymphoid follicles and may simulate the appearance of a lymph node (Fig. 25.44A,B).

Although this tumor was originally placed under the MFH umbrella on the basis of morphologic, immunohistochemical, and ultrastructural features, several studies have provided evidence to suggest a vascular or myoid nature.[422,425,537] Also, immunoreactivity for desmin has been found in over half of the cases[425] (Fig. 25.44C). We favor the interpretation that angiomatoid MFH is a tumor of vessel-related myoid cells with associated inflammatory features. Indeed, we have seen several cases in which the typical features of this entity merged with those of an inflammation-free component having hemangiopericytoid/glomoid features (Fig. 25.45). We have also seen cases lacking the central hemorrhagic cavity (a 'solid variant', so to speak) (Fig. 25.46). Recurrent chromosomal aberrations have been detected in angiomatoid MFH, mostly commonly t(2;22)(q33;q12) with *EWS–CRBE1* fusion, and less commonly t(12;16)(q13;p11) with *FUS–ATF1* fusion and t(12;22)(q13;q12) with *EWS–ATF1* fusion.[388,415,439,542] Of interest, the latter chromosomal translocation is also found in clear cell sarcoma of tendon sheaths and aponeurosis.

Angiomatoid MFH is a low-grade malignant tumor that has a tendency for local recurrence and that can also metastasize distantly.[408,417] It is important to recognize that perfectly benign dermal fibrous histiocytomas (so-called 'dermatofibromas') also can be accompanied by hemorrhagic foci and that this does not endow them with any particular aggressive behavior[534] (see Chapter 4).

Most of the retroperitoneal and mediastinal lesions formerly called **xanthogranuloma**[506] are examples of liposarcoma or fibrous histiocytoma (usually malignant), whereas others probably represent idiopathic mediastinal or retroperitoneal inflammatory fibrosclerosis, malakoplakia, or Rosai–Dorfman disease[406] (see Chapter 21). We think therefore that the term xanthogranuloma should not be used as a specific diagnosis.

It has been suggested that epithelioid sarcoma and malignant giant cell tumor of soft parts also represent malignant tumors of histiocytes; however, until more definite evidence for this is obtained, it is preferable to categorize them as tumors of uncertain cell type (a designation which, to be candid, would also fit many of the tumors described in this section) (see pp. 2185 and 2186, respectively).

The microscopic appearance of benign and malignant fibrous histiocytoma can be closely simulated by a number of benign and malignant conditions, including malakoplakia,[406] silica reaction,[553] histoid leprosy, and metastatic carcinoma (particularly from the kidney).

Tumors and tumorlike conditions of peripheral nerves

Proliferative lesions of peripheral nerves are divided into non-neoplastic (such as traumatic neuroma), benign tumors (such as schwannomas, neurofibromas, and perineuriomas), and malignant tumors, collectively designated as malignant peripheral nerve sheath tumors (MPNSTs). Despite the fact that these lesions may overlap and coexist with each other, it is important to make a distinction among them in view of their markedly different natural history. For a discussion on the features of schwannoma and neurofibroma in the mediastinum and retroperitoneal areas, see Chapters 8 and 26, respectively.

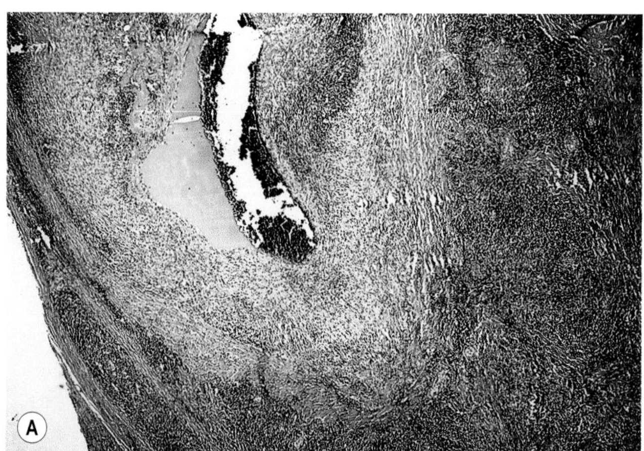

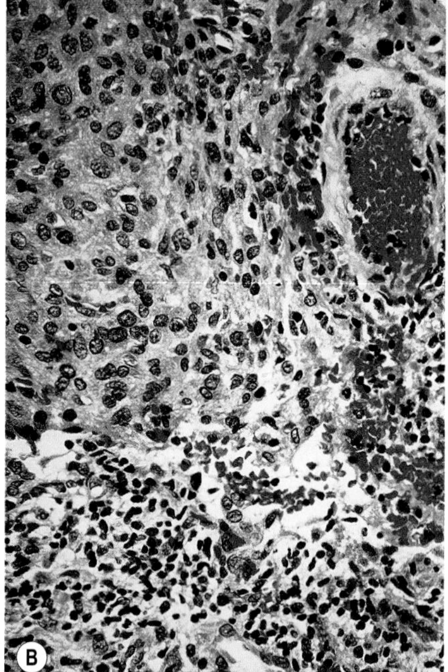

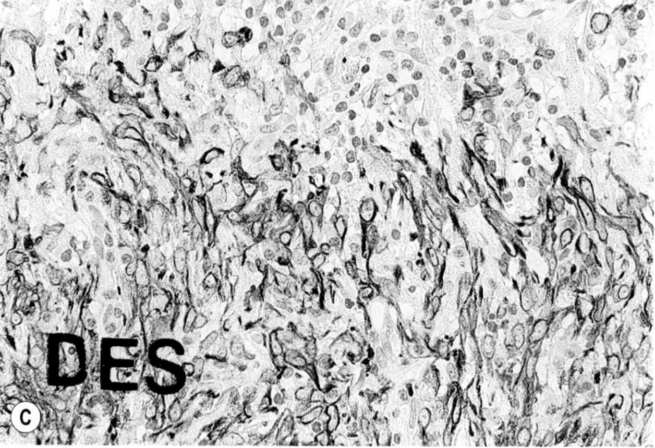

Fig. 25.44 A–C, Angiomatoid MFH. **A**, Low-power view showing a blood-filled space surrounded by a wall of tumor cells and a peripheral rim of lymphocytes. **B**, High-power view of the tumor cell component. **C**, Strong immunoreactivity for desmin.

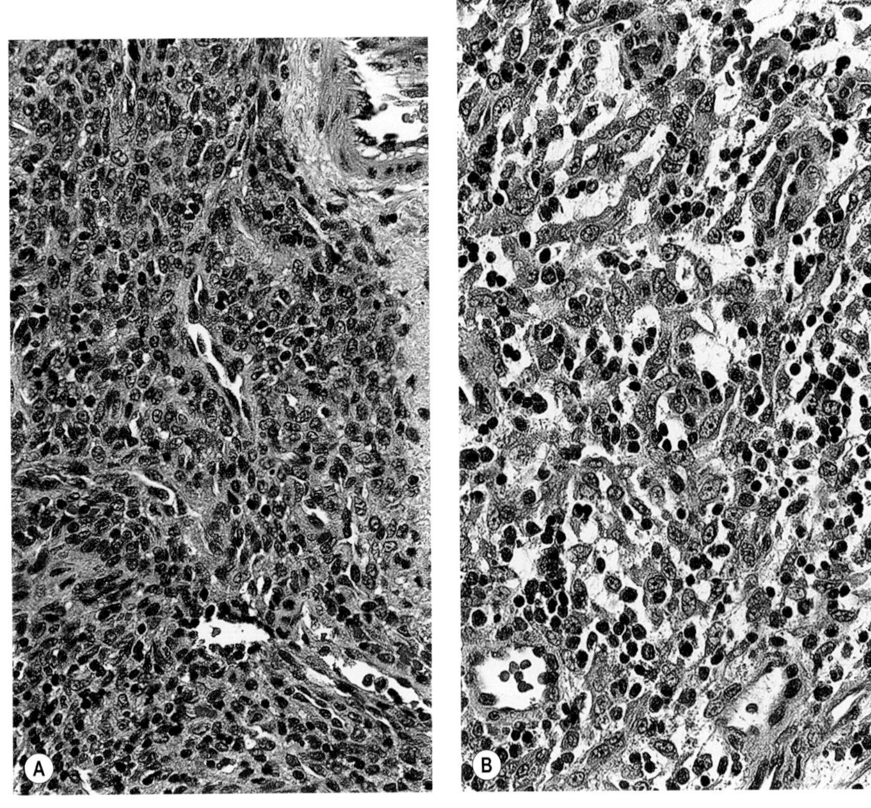

Fig. 25.45 Angiomatoid MFH (**A**) blending with tumor tissue having a glomangiopericytoid appearance (**B**).

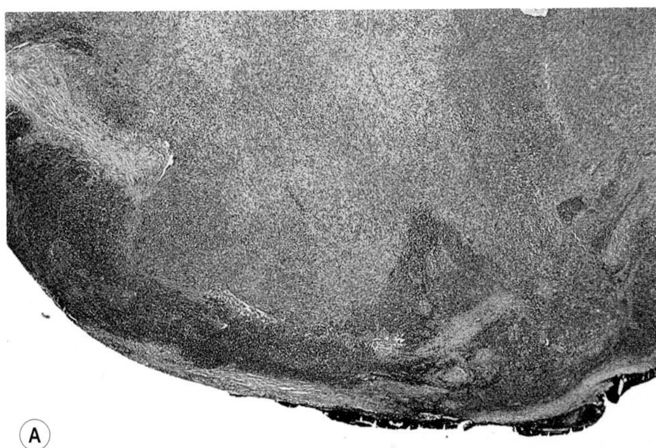

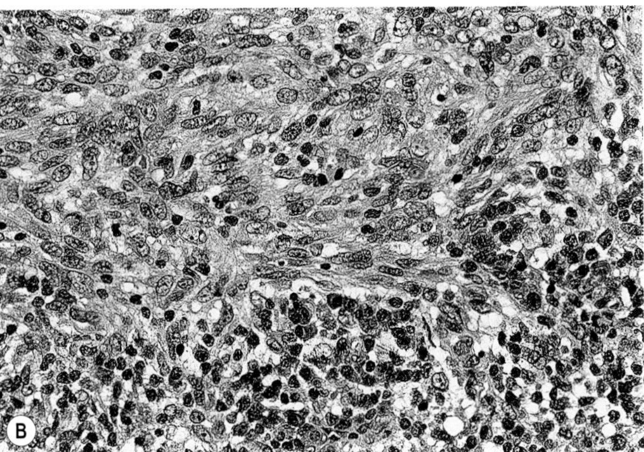

Fig. 25.46 A and **B**, Soft tissue tumor with an angiomatoid MFH pattern but lacking the central hemorrhagic area.

Neuroma

The large majority of neuromas follow trauma – hence their designation as **traumatic neuromas**. When a peripheral nerve is severed or crushed, the distal end undergoes wallerian degeneration, whereas the proximal end regenerates. If it fails to meet the distal end, a tangled mass of nerve fibers results. Microscopically, all the elements of a nerve can be recognized: axons, Schwann cells, perineurial cells, and fibroblasts (Fig. 25.47). In addition, scar tissue is often present. Not surprisingly, this lesion may be exquisitely painful. Immunohistochemically, the Schwann cells of traumatic neuroma show aberrant expression of the macrophage-associated antigens CD68 and Ki-M1-P, in keeping with the macrophagic properties that they are known to acquire under these circumstances.[564] **Amputation neuroma**, a term made popular during the First World War, is a type of traumatic neuroma in which the original trauma involves the loss of part or all of an extremity.

Morton neuroma (Morton metatarsalgia) can be regarded as a subtype of traumatic neuroma caused by repeated mild trauma to the region.[563] Its typical location is the interdigital plantar nerve between the third and fourth toes. The lesion is more common in female adults. Microscopically, the affected nerve is markedly distorted. There is extensive perineurial fibrosis, often arranged in a concentric fashion. The arterioles are thickened and sometimes occluded by thrombi.[565]

Palisaded encapsulated neuroma (solitary circumscribed neuroma) presents as a small, solitary, asymptomatic papule in the skin (see Chapter 4). Its most common location is the face of middle-aged individuals. Microscopically, the lesion is centered in the dermis (in contrast to schwannoma, which is rarely seen in this location) and is characterized by a proliferation of Schwann cells and numerous axons located within a capsule derived from perineurium.[562] Immunohistochemically, the Schwann cells are reactive for S-100 protein, the axons for neurofilaments, and the capsule for EMA, the latter indicating the presence of perineurial cells.[560,561]

Schwannoma (neurilemoma)

Schwannoma (neurilemoma) is one of the few *truly encapsulated* neoplasms of the human body and is almost always solitary (unless seen as a component of Recklinghausen disease type 2). Its most common locations are the flexor surfaces of the extremities, neck, mediastinum, retroperitoneum, posterior spinal roots, and cerebellopontine angle.[612] The nerve of origin often can be demonstrated in the periphery, flattened along the capsule but not penetrating the substance of the tumor (Fig. 25.48). Since this is a benign neoplasm that only rarely recurs locally, every attempt should be made to preserve the nerve, if this is of any clinical significance (e.g., facial nerve or vagus nerve). The great majority of cases occur sporadically, while a small percentage of cases are associated with neurofibromatosis type 2 (caused by a germline mutation in the *NF2* gene located on 22q12, which encodes merlin, also known as schwannomin).

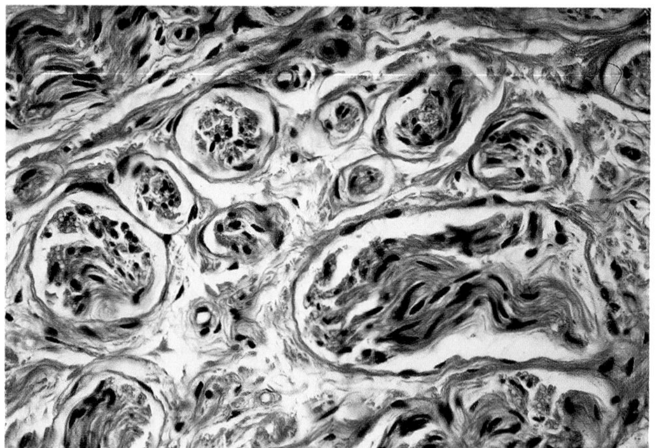

Fig. 25.47 Traumatic neuroma. The haphazardly distributed nerve trunks are surrounded by fibrous tissue.

Grossly, the larger schwannomas often contain cystic areas (Fig. 25.49). The microscopic appearance is distinctive. Two different patterns usually can be recognized, designated by Antoni as A and B. The type A areas, which in small tumors comprise almost their entirety, are quite cellular, composed of spindle cells often arranged in a palisading fashion or in an organoid arrangement (Verocay bodies) (Fig. 25.50).

In type B areas the tumor cells are separated by abundant edematous fluid that may form cystic spaces. Occasionally, isolated cells with bizarre hyperchromatic nuclei are observed;[606] they are particularly common in so-called *ancient schwannomas* and are of no particular significance[575] (Fig. 25.51). Mitoses are usually absent or extremely scanty. Blood vessels can be of such prominence as to simulate a vascular neoplasm (Fig. 25.52). By electron microscopy, they have been found to be of the fenestrated type, a rather surprising feature.[594] Thrombosis and hyaline thickening of the adventitia are common. Sometimes, large nodular masses of collagen with radiating edges are seen, a feature sometimes descriptively designated as ‘amianthoid’ fibers or collagenous spherules. The majority of soft tissue tumors exhibiting these formations are of peripheral nerve sheath derivation,[574,615,618] but this does not apply to lesions of lymph nodes containing similar structures (see Chapter 21).

Palisading of nuclei is not unique to schwannoma. It can also occur in leiomyoma, leiomyosarcoma, GIST, calcifying aponeurotic fibroma, and even in non-neoplastic smooth muscle (most commonly in the appendiceal wall). The traditional wisdom is that (in contrast to neurofibromas, see below) axons are not present in schwannoma, except in the portion of the capsule where the nerve is attached; however, recent studies employing an antibody against neurofilament have challenged that assumption.[611] Collections of foamy macrophages are sometimes seen, especially in the larger neoplasms. More unusual is the presence of clusters of granular cells similar to those seen in granular cell tumors.[570] The rare occurrence of plexiform areas in schwannoma may cause them to be mistaken for neurofibroma.[584,600] Most of these *plexiform schwannomas* are

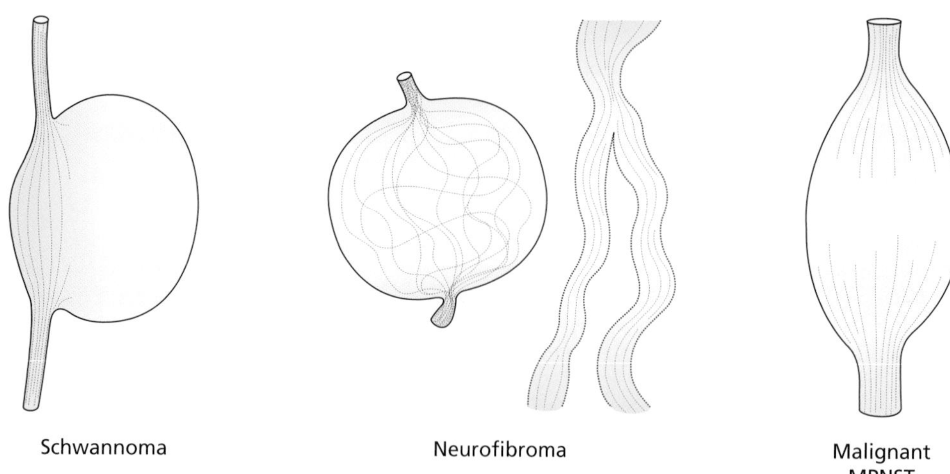

Fig. 25.48 Schematic drawing emphasizing the main differences between the three major types of peripheral nerve tumors. Note diameter of nerve involved and behavior of neurites (thin black lines) in relation to neoplasm.

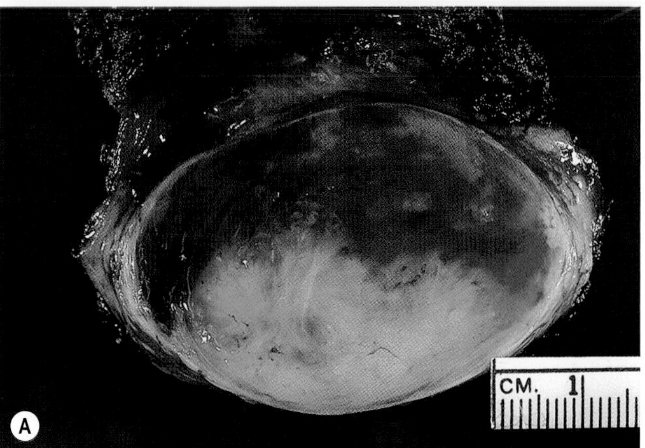

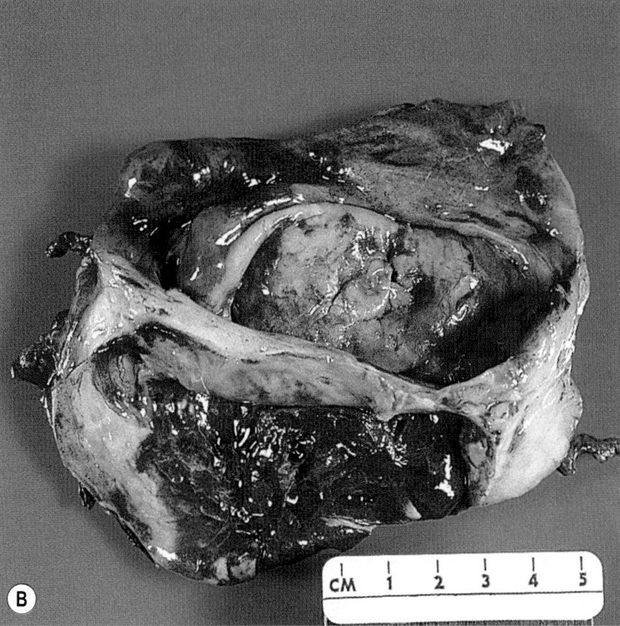

Fig. 25.49 **A** and **B**, Gross appearances of schwannoma. The tumor shown in **B** has undergone marked secondary cystic changes.

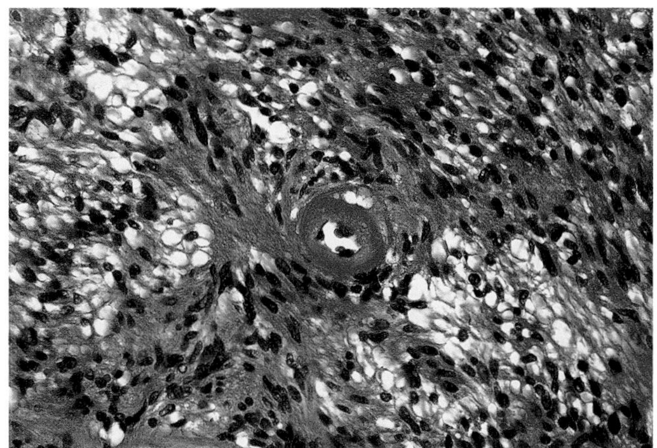

Fig. 25.50 Schwannoma with a suggestion of nuclear palisading and hyaline thickening of vessel walls.

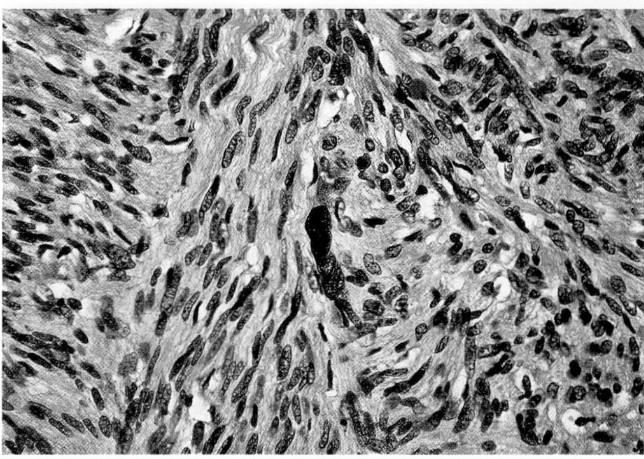

Fig. 25.51 Large hyperchromatic nuclei in schwannoma. This is not necessarily an indication of malignant change.

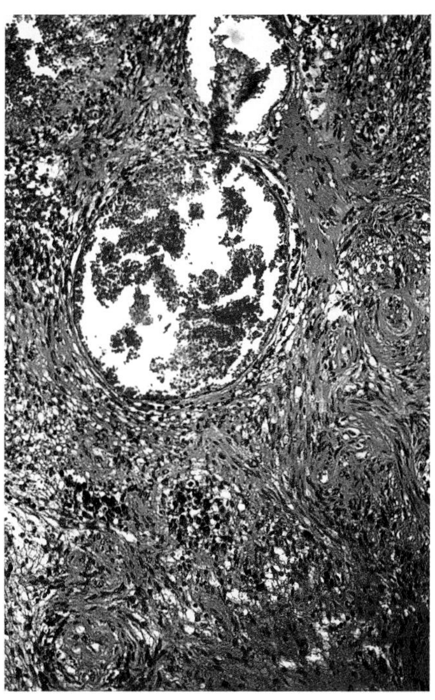

Fig. 25.52 Schwannoma showing large vascular spaces that may lead to confusion with a vascular neoplasm. Hemosiderin-laden macrophages are also present as evidence of previous hemorrhage.

found superficially in the dermis or subcutaneous tissue, but they can also be deep-seated.[566,567] Epithelioid areas can also be present, although much less commonly than in neurofibroma and MPNST.[587,603,620] When these areas predominate, the tumor has been referred to as *benign epithelioid schwannoma*.[602] A few cases containing a glandular component have been described (*benign glandular schwannomas*).[568,572,613] These should be distinguished from the pseudoglandular formations lined by low columnar or cuboidal Schwann cells having an epithelial-like appearance[617] as well as from entrapped sweat glands.

Rare schwannomas are found to contain melanin pigment.[619] When this feature is prominent and accompanied by psammoma body formation, the possibility of the tumor representing a psammomatous melanotic schwannoma should be considered[569] (see

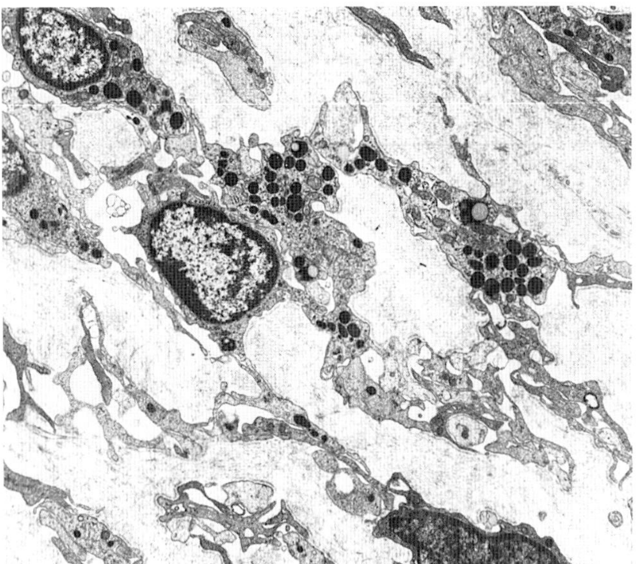

Fig. 25.53 Electron microscopic appearance of schwannoma of retroperitoneum. Elongated cells with processes are partially covered by basal lamina. Cells contain lipid of varied density.

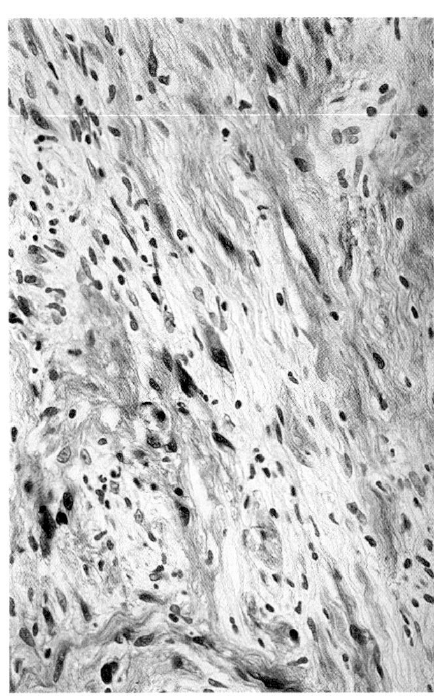

Fig. 25.54 S-100 protein immunoreactivity in schwannoma.

subsequent sections). Rarely, schwannomas (and neurofibromas) can exhibit a lipoblastic component, accompanied by cells with signet ring-like features.[616] Other schwannomas have a predominant *microcystic/reticular* appearance; these manifest a predilection for visceral locations, particularly the gastrointestinal tract.[605]

Exceptionally, otherwise typical schwannomas or those with epithelioid features have been found to contain foci of small, round hyperchromatic Schwann cells with scanty cytoplasm, sometimes forming rosettes and simulating neuroblastoma.[581,589]

It is generally agreed that the neoplasm described in this section originates from Schwann cells, hence the current preference for the term schwannoma.[583] By electron microscopy, the tumor cells have a continuous and often reduplicated basal lamina; numerous, extremely thin cytoplasmic processes; aggregates of intracytoplasmic microfibrils; peculiar intracytoplasmic lamellar bodies; and extracellular long-spacing collagen[577,588,595,596,621] (Fig. 25.53). Parenthetically, the latter feature is not specific for peripheral nerve cell tumors.[582] Immunohistochemically, the tumor cells show immunoreactivity for S-100 protein, calretinin (in contrast to neurofibromas), calcineurin, basal lamina components (such as laminin, type IV collagen, and merosin), vimentin, nerve growth factor receptor, lipocortin-1, and sometimes glial fibrillary acidic protein and KP-l (CD68)[576,580,588,590–592,598,599,601,604,607,608,610,614] (Fig. 25.54). Whether they also exhibit positivity for myelin markers – such as myelin basic protein and P2 protein – remains a disputed issue.[573] Curiously, keratin is often expressed in retroperitoneal schwannomas but virtually never in peripheral schwannomas.[579] Desmoplakin and desmin are consistently negative[591] but smooth muscle can be present.[578] Genetically, schwannoma, whether sporadic or associated with neurofibromatosis type 2, is characterized by somatic mutation (sporadic form) or germline mutation (neurofibromatosis type 2) of the *NF2* gene in one allele, and loss of *NF2* in the remaining allele through deletion or monosomy 22.[597,609]

Malignant transformation of schwannoma is – in contrast to neurofibroma – an exceptionally rare event. However, several indubitable cases are on record.[593,624] Interestingly, in most of them the malignant component has exhibited an epithelioid morphology.

Cellular schwannoma is the term used for highly cellular schwannomas that are exclusively composed of Antoni A areas but lack Verocay bodies[585,623] (Fig. 25.55). These changes can be accompanied by nuclear atypia, mitotic activity, and focal necrosis. Most reported cases have been in the retroperitoneum, pelvis, and mediastinum.[571,622] The differential diagnosis with a low-grade MPNST remains a difficult and controversial subject.

Psammomatous melanotic schwannoma is a distinctive type of peripheral nerve sheath tumor that occurs as a component of the Carney complex.[569] Most arise from the spinal nerve roots.[586] As the name indicates, the tumor is characterized microscopically by the presence of melanin pigmentation and the deposition of psammoma bodies (Fig. 25.56). In contrast to all other types of schwannoma described in this section, the psammomatous melanotic variety is regarded as a low-grade malignancy because of its tendency for local recurrence and the fact that a few of the reported cases have metastasized.[569]

Neurofibroma

The gross, microscopic, and ultrastructural features of neurofibroma, as well as its natural history, are distinct from those of schwannoma. The fact that in some instances the differential diagnosis may be difficult or that in isolated cases features of both lesions may coexist does not justify lumping them together.

The gross appearance of neurofibroma varies a great deal from lesion to lesion. As a rule, the tumors are not encapsulated and have a softer consistency than schwannoma (Fig. 25.57). The more superficial tumors appear as small, soft, pedunculated nodules protruding from the skin ('molluscum pendulum'). Deeper tumors grow larger. Tumors resulting in diffuse tortuous enlargement of peripheral nerves are designated as *plexiform neurofibromas* and are usually seen in the context of type 1 neurofibromatosis (caused by a germline mutation in the *NF1* gene located on 17q11.2, which encodes neurofibromin)[659] (Fig. 25.58). The diffuse involvement

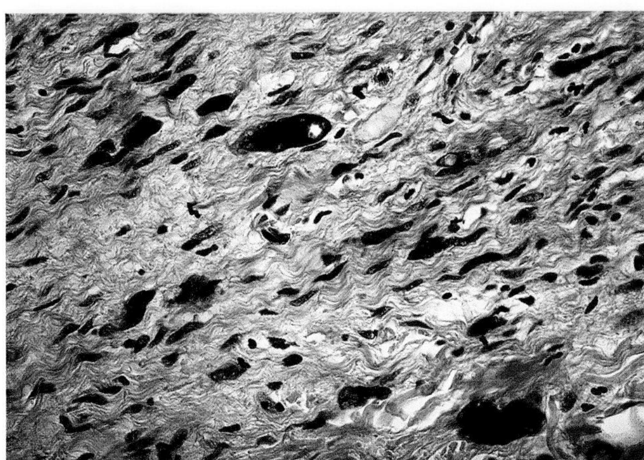
Fig. 25.62 Neurofibroma with large bizarre hyperchromatic nuclei.

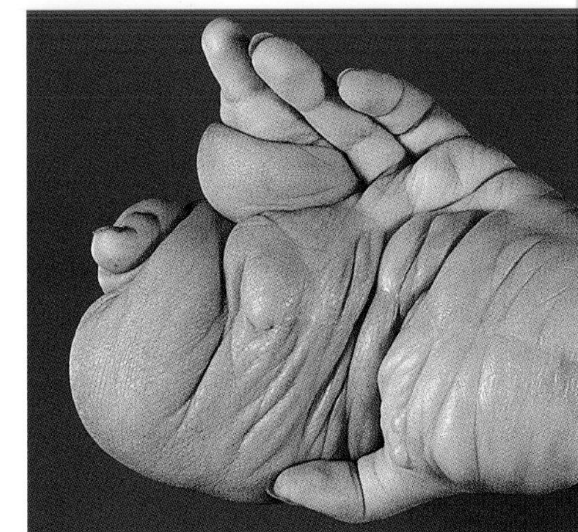
Fig. 25.63 Marked deformation of distal upper extre
neurofibromatosis. This patient developed a maligna
sheath tumor.

to whether the latter lesions are of neoplastic or hyperplastic nature.[639]

In contrast to schwannomas, Verocay bodies, palisading of nuclei, and hyaline thickening of the vessel wall are almost always absent in neurofibromas. Sometimes, otherwise typical neurofibromas are seen to contain melanin, a feature not unexpected in view of the embryologic relationship between Schwann cells and melanocytes.[628,630] These *pigmented neurofibromas* should be differentiated from blue nevi and malignant melanomas.[637,663] Occasionally, an otherwise typical neurofibroma will show foci of skeletal muscle differentiation (*neuromuscular hamartoma; benign triton tumor*).[625,657] Some neurofibromas (as well as other types of benign and malignant peripheral nerve tumors) may be partially composed of granular cells, similar in all respects to those of granular cell tumor.[638] Other have prominent epithelioid features, similar to those also seen in schwannoma and MPNST.[653] Still others – of somewhat disputed histogenesis – have a dendritic cell morphology and contain pseudorosettes.[661]

Neurofibromas that occur in the setting of type 1 neurofibromatosis typically show germline mutation of *NF1* in one allele and loss or mutation of *NF1* in the other allele, conforming to the 'two-hit hypothesis' in tumorigenesis.[636,671,674,675] The genetic alterations are less clear in sporadic neurofibromas, but *NF1* alterations are present in at least some cases.[675,678]

Malignant transformation of neurofibroma should be suspected in the presence of frequent mitoses, overly expressed cell proliferation markers, and the presence of p53 in many tumor cells.[652]

Neurofibromatosis (Recklinghausen disease). Multiple neurofibromas represent the most important component of the genetically determined disorder known as neurofibromatosis or Recklinghausen disease type 1.[666] This is one of the most common autosomal dominant diseases in humans, the prevalence being 1 in 2500 to 3300. The responsible gene (*NF1*) is located on chromosome 17q11.2[626,640,688] and encodes a ubiquitous protein known as neurofibromin, which is necessary for the correct negative regulation of RAS proteins.[627,635,643,644] It has been shown that the tumors developing in this syndrome require a loss of *NF1* in the cells destined to become neoplastic, as well as heterozygosity in the non-neoplastic cells.[689] In neurofibromatosis type 1, neurofibromas may occur in every conceivable site: axilla, thigh, buttock, deep-lying soft tissue, orbit, mediastinum, retroperitoneum, tongue, gastrointestinal tract, and many others.[668] Plexiform neurofibromas may result in massive enlargement of a limb or some other part of the body

('elephantiasis neuromatosa') (Fig. 25.63). In ad
bromas, patients with type 1 Recklinghausen d
many other associated lesions, the most common
lait spot. This consists microscopically of an increa
of melanin in the epidermal basal layer and is
overlying a neurofibroma. It can be distinguish
mented spots associated with Albright syndrom
distribution and smooth, delicate margins.[629] So
spots are common in normal individuals. Onl
present in a number of five or more can a signi
with neurofibromatosis be detected.[686] Other le
seen in patients with Recklinghausen disease in
malformations of various types,[646] megacolon, var
cular lesions,[656,670] fibrosing alveolitis,[683] schwa
pheochromocytoma, neuroblastoma,[632,687] ganglic
cinoid tumor,[647] gastrointestinal stromal tumor
Wilms tumor.[631,677] Increased serum levels of ner
have been detected in these patients.[673]

Type 2 (central) Recklinghausen disease is gen
from type 1, resulting from an alteration of the N
in chromosome 22q12 encoding merlin.[669,685] It is
the presence of a variety of neoplasms in the centra
the most distinctive of which are bilateral acoust
(see Chapter 28). Meningiomas, astrocytomas, and
types also occur.[648]

A small proportion of patients with type 1 n
develop MPNST. The incidence quoted ranges b
13%.[676] The malignant tumors arise almost alwa
trunks of the neck or extremities. For practical pur
superficial neurofibromas never become maligna
reasons for surgical removal are size and unsightlin
incidence of nonlymphatic leukemia seems to exist
type 1 Recklinghausen disease.[642]

Perineurioma

Benign tumors of the peripheral nerve composed
or exclusively of perineurial cells are being inc
nized.[708,717] Microscopically, they are composed of
gated cells arranged in parallel bundles, the appea
too dissimilar from that of neurofibroma or p
broma[702] (Fig. 25.64). Some cases have a storif

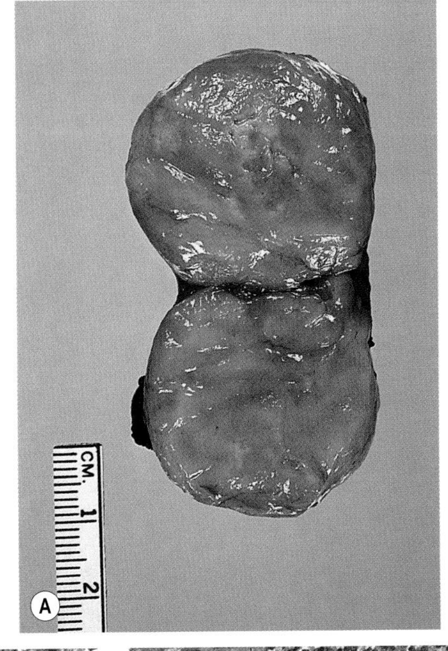

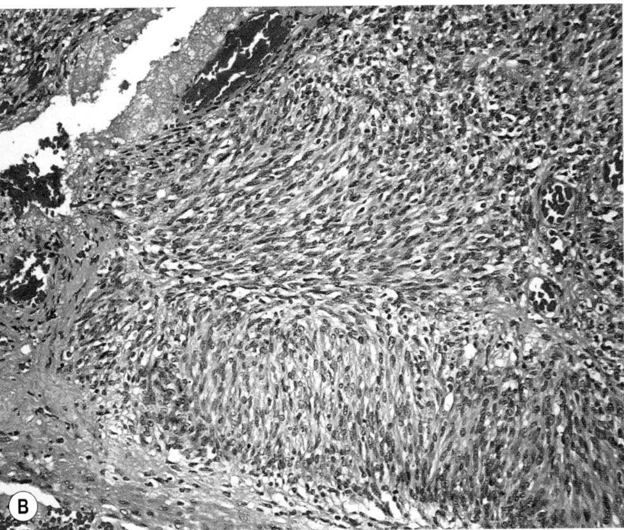

Fig. 25.55 Cellular schwannoma: **A**, gross appearance; **B**, microscopic appearance. The tumor has a homogeneous hypercellular quality.

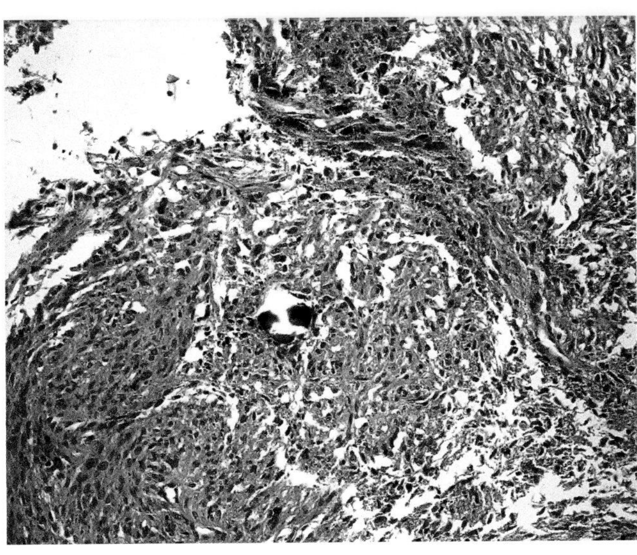
Fig. 25.56 Melanocytic psammomatous schwannoma in a patient with Carney syndrome.

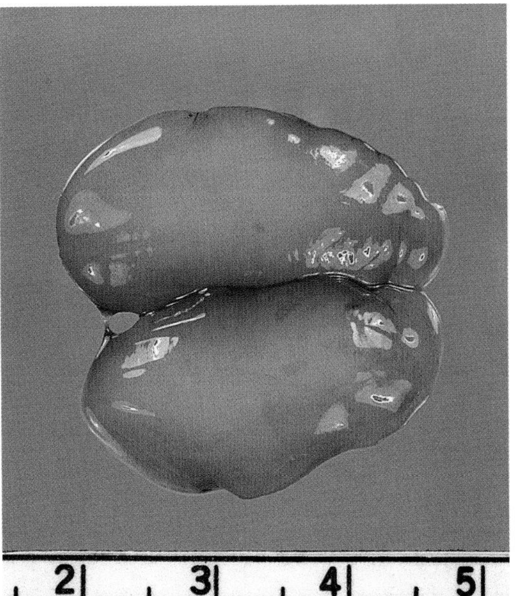

Fig. 25.57 Well-circumscribed neurofibroma of soft tissue. The tumor has a gelatinous appearance.

of the nerves may make a complete resection impossible. This particular form of neurofibroma is more commonly seen in the orbit, neck, back, and inguinal region.

Microscopically, neurofibromas are formed by a combined proliferation of all the elements of a peripheral nerve: axons, Schwann cells, fibroblasts, and (in the plexiform type) perineurial cells (Fig. 25.59). Axons can be demonstrated by silver or acetylcholinesterase stains or by immunostaining for neuron-specific enolase (NSE), neurofilaments, or various neuropeptides.[651,681] Schwann cells usually represent the predominant cellular element. Most have markedly elongated nuclei, with a wavy, serpentine configuration and pointed ends (Fig. 25.60). Ultrastructurally, they are seen to enclose axons in plasmalemmal invaginations (mesaxons)[682] (Fig. 25.61). They are immunoreactive for S-100 protein and surrounded by basement membrane components.[634] A population of factor XIIIa-positive and CD34-positive cells is also present; the nature of these cells and their histogenetic relationship with normal nerve constituents is not clear.[679,684] EMA-positive perineurial cells are common in plexiform but not in ordinary neurofibromas.[680] Immunoreactivity for protein gene product (PGP) 9.5 is the rule, but its degree of specificity in relation to other nerve sheath tumors and other mesenchymal neoplasm is very low.[633] The stroma contains a rich network of collagen fibers, among which almost all major types are represented (I, III, IV, V, and VI).[634,664,665] Mucinous changes in the stroma may be prominent and result in a mistaken diagnosis of myxoma or myxoid liposarcoma.[660] As with schwannomas, neurofibromas may exhibit scattered large hyperchromatic nuclei; these

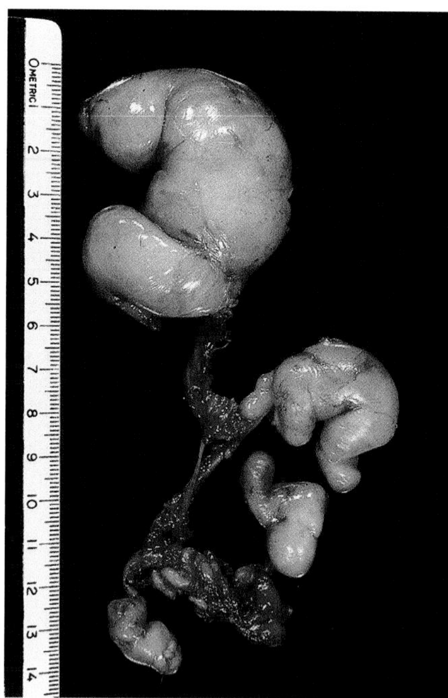

Fig. 25.58 Typical gross appearance of plexiform neurofibroma. This tumor variety is indicative of Recklinghausen disease.

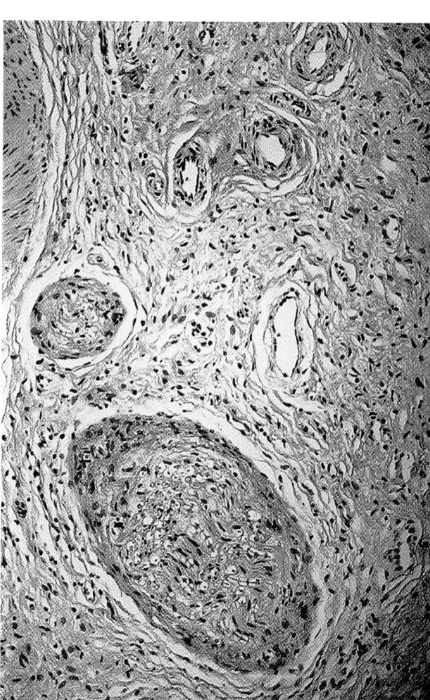

Fig. 25.59 Neurofibroma with plexiform features.

neurofibromas with atypia may also have increased cellularity but mitotic activity is scanty or absent, and the MIB-1 index is very low[654] (Fig. 25.62).

The stroma of neurofibromas often contains numerous mast cells.[649,667] Distorted organoid structures resembling Wagner–Meissner or Pacini corpuscles are sometimes seen. Tumors in which these formations are particularly prominent have sometimes been designated as *tumors of tactile end organs*, and *pacinian neurofibromas*, respectively.[645,650,655,672] There is some question, however, as

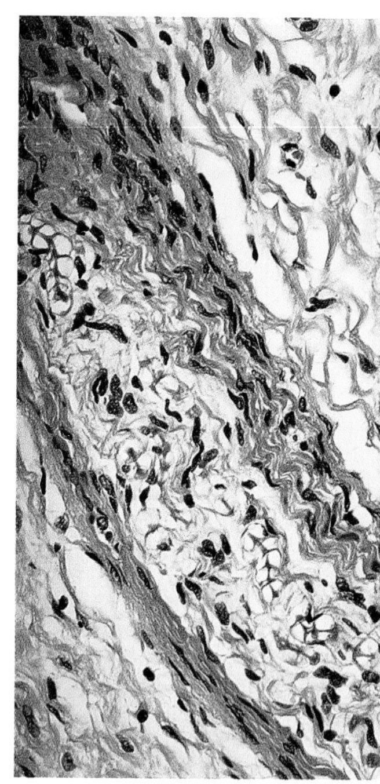

Fig. 25.60 The nuclei of the tumor cells of neur typical fascicular pattern of growth and serpentir

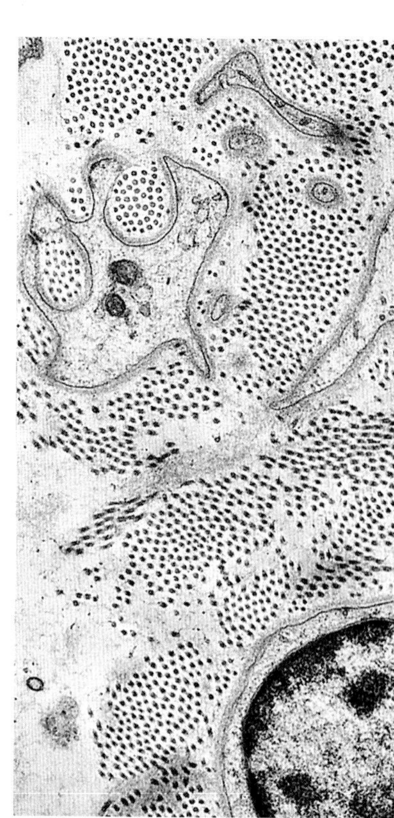

Fig. 25.61 Electron microscopic appearance of p neurofibroma in a patient with Recklinghausen dis shows Schwann cell processes, one of which (up collagen fibrils. Note the continuous basal lamina. *(×14 900; courtesy of Dr Robert A Erlandson, Memorial S Center)*

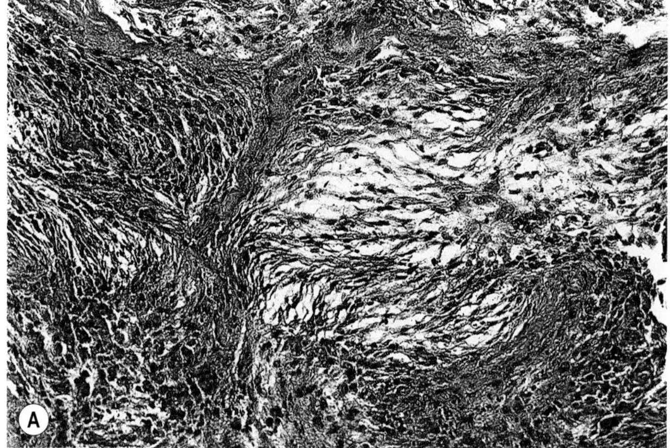

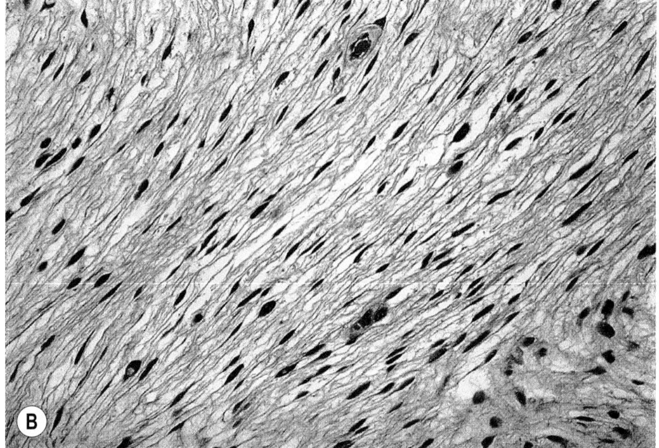

Fig. 25.64 **A** and **B**, Two morphologic aspects of perineurioma. The tumor shown in **A** can simulate myxofibrosarcoma.

growth and may correspond to the former *storiform perineurial fibromas*.[709] The diagnosis of perineurioma should be suspected in myxoid lesions of soft tissue in which a storiform or fascicular pattern of growth is evident.[713,718] There is an *intraneural* variant of perineurioma, associated with nonrandom chromosomal abnormalities and therefore presumably neoplastic.[694,699] It seems likely that at least some of the cases reported in the past as *localized hypertrophic neuropathy*[693,716] belong to the same category.[699] Other recently recognized variants of this tumor include *sclerosing perineurioma*, which has a predilection for the fingers and palms of young adults;[697] *reticular* (*retiform*) *perineurioma*, with a predominant lace-like or reticular growth pattern composed of anastomosing cords of spindle cells;[700,710] *plexiform perineurioma*;[710] and the exceptionally rare *granular cell perineurioma*.[691,719] *Hybrid forms* of schwannoma and perineurioma have also been described,[703–705,711] as well as **malignant** forms of perineurioma, the latter representing a subtype of MPNST (see below).

Ultrastructurally, perineurioma is characterized by nonbranching, thin cytoplasmic processes coated by an external lamina and joined at their ends by a tight junction, few organelles, actin and vimentin filaments, and numerous pinocytotic vesicles[696,707,713] (Fig. 25.65). Immunohistochemically, the tumor cells are positive for EMA, Glut-1, and CD34, and negative for S-100 protein, recapitulating the profile of normal perineurial cells[690,692,701,714,715] (Fig. 25.66). There is also frequent expression of claudin-1, a recently described tight junction-associated protein.[698] At the cytogenetic level, many cases show deletion of part or all of chromosome 22.[695,699] In

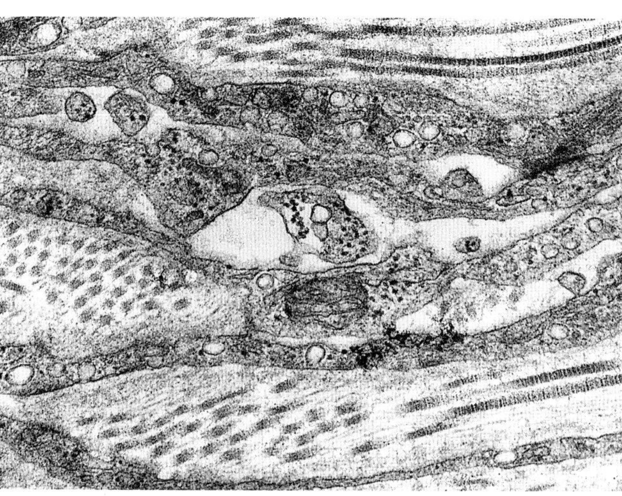

Fig. 25.65 Electron microscopic appearance of perineurioma. Thin perineurial cell cytoplasmic processes with prominent pinocytotic vesicles. The processes are coated by a continuous basal lamina. *(×42 000; courtesy of Dr Robert A Erlandson, Memorial Sloan-Kettering Cancer Center)*

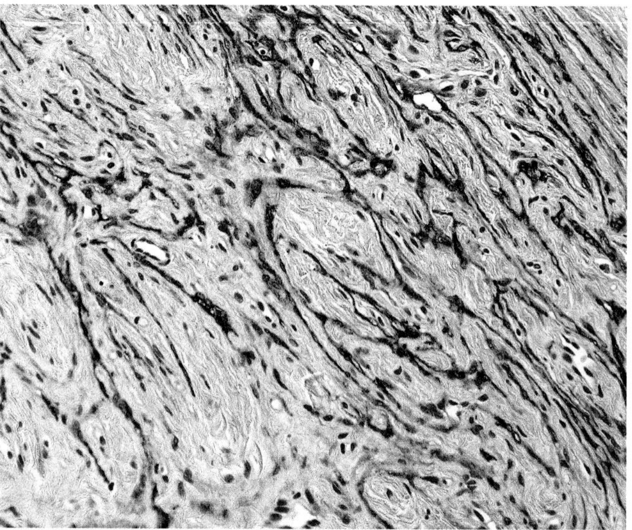

Fig. 25.66 EMA immunoreactivity in perineurioma.

addition, mutations of the *NF2* gene and loss of chromosome 13 have also been documented.[706,712]

Nerve sheath myxoma

This controversial benign tumor of peripheral nerves can occur in the skin, soft tissues, or an intraspinal location.[726] In most instances, it involves the distal extremities.[722] It has a gross and microscopic appearance reminiscent of myxoma, except for the prominent multinodularity with a fibrous border and the presence of plumper, epithelial-like cells and a distinct fascicular or plexiform arrangement; the latter feature is sometimes so pronounced that some authors have suggested the less committal designation of *plexiform myxoma*.[720,727] It seems likely that nerve sheath myxoma and the cutaneous tumor described as *neurothekeoma*[724] are closely related, if not identical (see Chapter 4) (Fig. 25.67). As mentioned in the

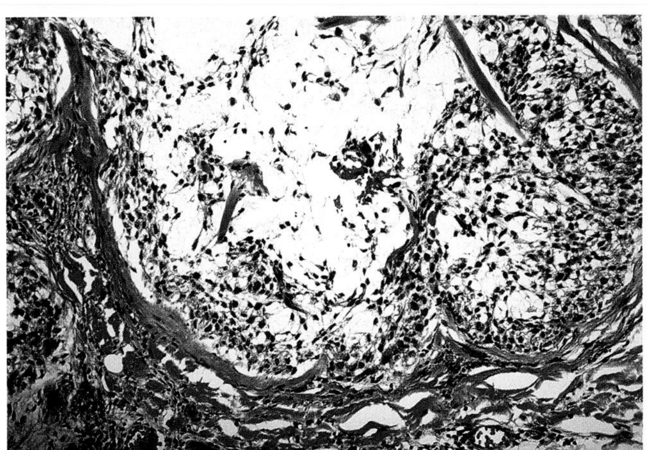

Fig. 25.67 Lobulated appearance of neurothekeoma. There is focal hypercellularity.

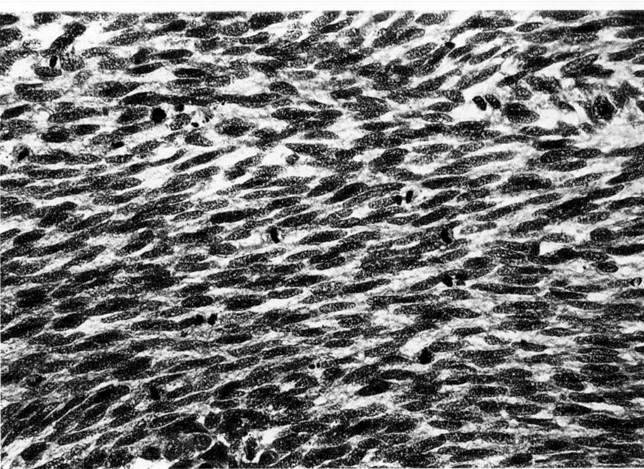

Fig. 25.68 Malignant peripheral nerve sheath tumor. The marked hypercellularity and the high mitotic activity in the absence of significant pleomorphism are commonly seen in this tumor type.

previous section, the differential diagnosis includes perineurioma (which can show prominent myxoid features and a fascicular or storiform pattern of growth) and myxoid neurofibroma.[721,723,725] Immunohistochemically, some of the cells of nerve sheath myxoma stain for S-100 protein, others (very few) for EMA, and still others for CD34.[722]

Malignant peripheral nerve sheath tumor

Malignant peripheral nerve sheath tumor (MPNST) is the currently preferred term for the neoplasm also known over the years as *malignant schwannoma, neurogenic sarcoma,* and *neurofibrosarcoma.*[759] Approximately half of these tumors arise de novo, and the other half from nerves involved by neurofibromas as part of type 1 Recklinghausen disease. Some have occurred in areas of previous irradiation,[752,786] and a few have originated from the Schwann cell-like (satellite cell) component of ganglioneuroma.[731,756,758,792] The development of MPNST in Recklinghausen disease has been found to be associated with chromosome 17p deletions and *TP53* gene mutations.[781]

Because of its difficult microscopic recognition, errors are often made, more often than not by diagnosing MPNST as some other type of soft tissue sarcoma. There are two circumstances in which the diagnosis of MPNST should be the primary consideration in the presence of a malignant tumor of soft tissues composed of spindle cells: (1) when the tumor develops in a patient with type 1 Recklinghausen disease; or (2) when the tumor is obviously arising within the anatomic compartment of a major nerve or in continuity with a neurofibroma.[745] In the absence of these circumstances the light microscopic diagnosis of MPNST is often only presumptive and dependent on a combination of features, none of which is diagnostic by itself. They include: serpentine shape of the tumor cells; arrangement in palisades or whorls; marked contrast between the deeply hyperchromatic nuclei and the pale cytoplasm ('punched-out nuclei'); perivascular concentration of tumor cells, with a plumper shape; epithelioid appearance of the endothelial cells of these vessels; presence of large gaping vascular spaces, resulting in a hemangiopericytoma-like appearance; and geographic areas of necrosis, with tumor palisading at the edges[761] (Figs 25.68–25.70). In most areas the appearance is that of an extremely cellular spindle cell neoplasm. Mitoses are usually abundant. Although most tumors are quite monomorphic (a feature they share with fibrosarcoma and monophasic synovial sarcoma), some can be extremely bizarre. At the light microscopic level the latter can simulate the appearance of a pleomorphic liposarcoma or so-called malignant fibrous histiocytoma very closely and may be identified as neural only on ultrastructural examination.[763] Metaplastic tissues such as cartilage, bone, muscle, or blood vessels are present in approximately 15% of the cases[753,754,785] (Fig. 25.71). The most spectacular variant is characterized by the presence of well-developed skeletal muscle and has been dignified by the picturesque term *malignant triton tumor*[737,749,791,813] (Fig. 25.72). Areas of recognizable MPNST should

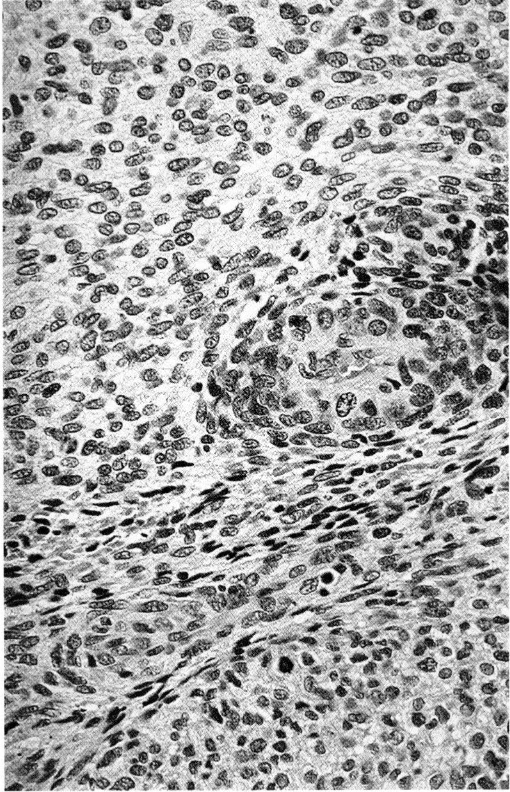

Fig. 25.69 Malignant peripheral nerve sheath tumor. The plump and almost epithelioid appearance of the cells surrounding the vessels is a common feature in this tumor type.

be present to make such a diagnosis in these metaplastic tumors; otherwise a diagnosis corresponding to the morphologic appearance of the tumor is appropriate, even if the patient has Recklinghausen disease.[738,784] This applies, for instance, to *angiosarcoma* of peripheral nerves, of which several examples have been reported, including the *epithelioid* variety.[778]

In some MPNSTs, part or most of the tumor is composed of plump cells with polygonal acidophilic cytoplasm and an epithelioid-like appearance; these are designated as *epithelioid malignant MPNST* [729,750,772] (Figs 25.73 and 25.74). One such case exhibited squamous differentiation.[730] Epithelioid MPNST of the skin may be associated with HMB-45 immunoreactivity and be indistinguishable from some neurotropic/spindle cell/desmoplastic forms of malignant melanoma.[797,801] Interestingly, and as already mentioned, most of the MPNSTs that have arisen from malignant transformation of benign schwannomas have been of the epithelioid type.[790,793,815] Occasionally, MPNST show foci of *glandular differentiation*, with or without mucin production and with positivity for keratin, EMA, carcinoembryonic antigen (CEA), chromogranin, somatostatin, serotonin, and some peptide hormones;[742,747,812,814] it has been suggested that these formations represent foci of ependymal or neuroendocrine differentiation, but this view has been contested.[748,807] Glands, skeletal muscle, and other tissues can coexist in the same tumor[794] (Fig. 25.71). In general, any peripheral nerve

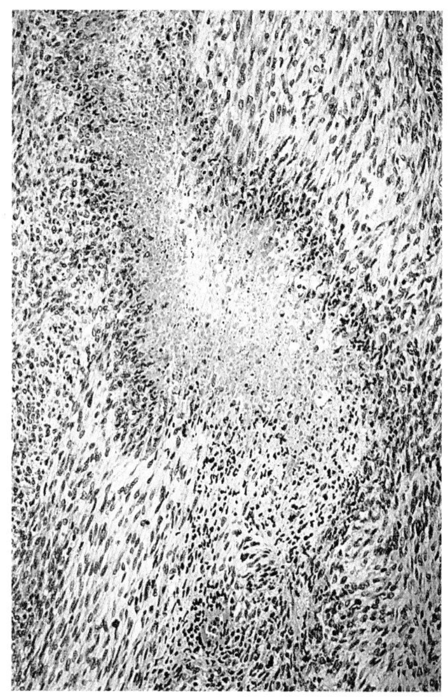

Fig. 25.70 MPNST. The area of necrosis with irregular borders and palisading at the edges is similar to that seen in glioblastoma multiforme of the central nervous system.

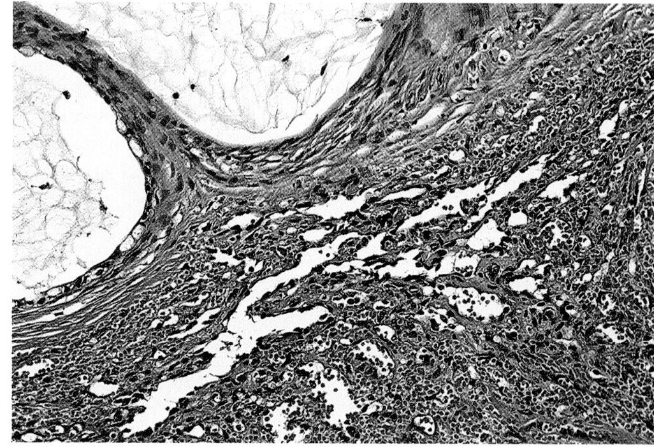

Fig. 25.71 Malignant peripheral nerve sheath tumor with divergent differentiation into blood vessels and mucin-producing glands.

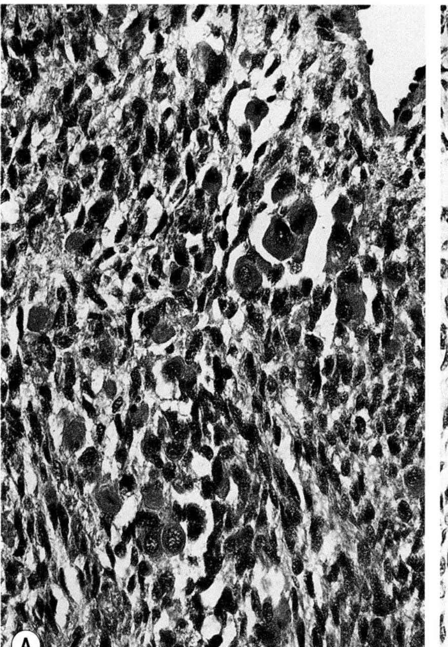

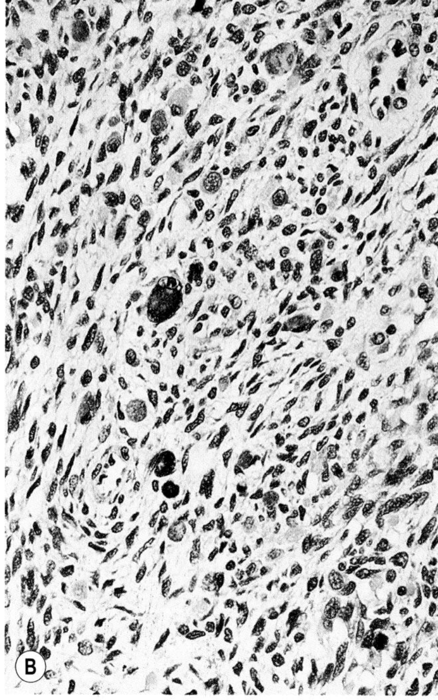

Fig. 25.72 **A** and **B**, Malignant peripheral nerve sheath tumor with skeletal muscle differentiation (so-called 'triton tumor'). **B**, Positive immunostain for myoglobin.

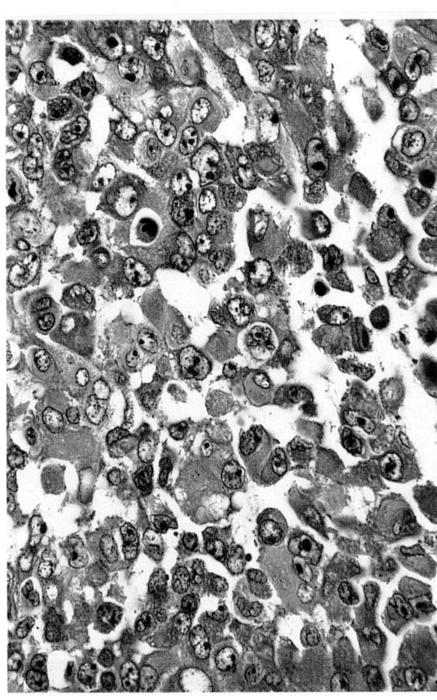

Fig. 25.73 Malignant peripheral nerve sheath tumor of epithelioid type.

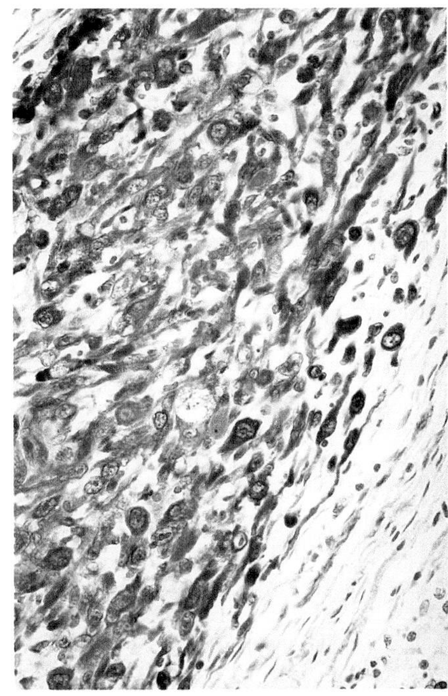

Fig. 25.74 Same case as Figure 25.73 showing strong immunoreactivity for S-100 protein.

tumor should be suspected of being malignant if it contains epithelial glandular structures, no matter how well differentiated they are. Melanin can be present in the tumor cells, particularly if the tumor arises from spinal nerve roots; the distinction between melanocytic MPNST and primary malignant melanoma of nerves has little practical significance and may not be warranted from a conceptual standpoint.[771]

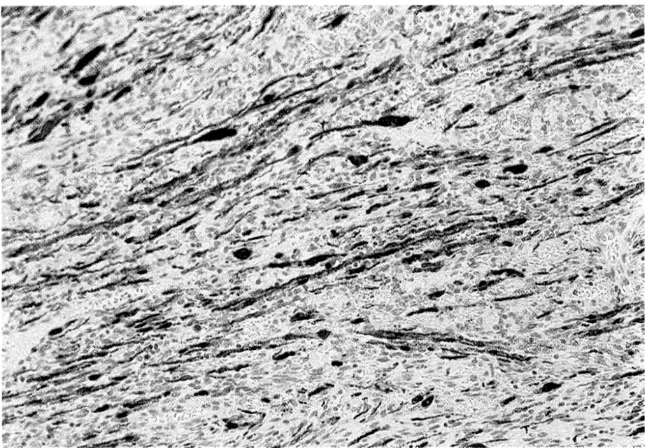

Fig. 25.75 Patchy immunoreactivity for S-100 protein in malignant peripheral nerve sheath tumor.

The belief that these MPNSTs generally originate in Schwann cells is largely based on circumstantial evidence, the reasoning being that if these tumors represent the malignant counterpart of neurofibromas and the latter arise primarily from Schwann cells, then the former also must have that origin. Some of the microscopic features just mentioned and tissue culture studies favor this hypothesis, which is also supported by the electron microscope description of infoldings of the cell membrane with lamellar configuration, presence of discontinuous basal lamina material, conspicuous intercellular junctions, and occasional dense-core granules.[740,741,751,762,803,806] Further support comes from the fact that immunohistochemically the tumor cells show reactivity for Schwann cell markers, such as S-100 protein and Leu7, in approximately half of the cases,[760,769,809,811] the former being particularly prominent in neurofibroma-like areas and in foci of melanocytic differentiation.[777] However, some MPNSTs show no discernible schwannian features at any level and may actually exhibit features suggestive of perineurial or fibroblastic nature.[755,764,765] Indeed, the existence of a *perineurial MPNST* (*malignant perineurioma*) has been supported on morphologic, immunohistochemical, and ultrastructural grounds.[766,802] Because of this fact, a histogenetically noncommittal term, such as MPNST, seems preferable to the time-honored malignant schwannoma. Regarding immunoreactivity to S-100 protein, it tends to be focal and not particularly strong, except in the epithelioid variant of this tumor;[817] therefore, the presence of *strong and diffuse* immunoreactivity for S-100 protein in a malignant spindle cell tumor with morphologic features suggestive of MPNST should raise the possibility of the alternative diagnosis of malignant melanoma, particularly if the lesion is located in the skin or a lymph node[770] (Figs 25.75 and 25.76). Other immunohistochemical markers for MPNST are nestin (an intermediate filament protein normally expressed by neuroectodermal stem cells[796]), HMGA2 protein,[768] and Sox10 (a neural crest transcription factor crucial for specification, maturation, and maintenance of Schwann cells and melanocytes).[787] Alas, most of these markers are also present in many benign schwannomas. Some cases express p53 protein, and this feature is a strong predictor for poor survival.[736]

The large majority of MPNSTs arise in adults, but they have also been recorded in children.[779,780,789] The most common locations are the neck, forearm, lower leg, and buttock.[739,767] They can also arise from cranial nerves or their branches.[795] Grossly, the finding of a large mass producing fusiform enlargement of a major nerve, such as the sciatic nerve, is characteristic[804] (Fig. 25.77). Most MPNSTs

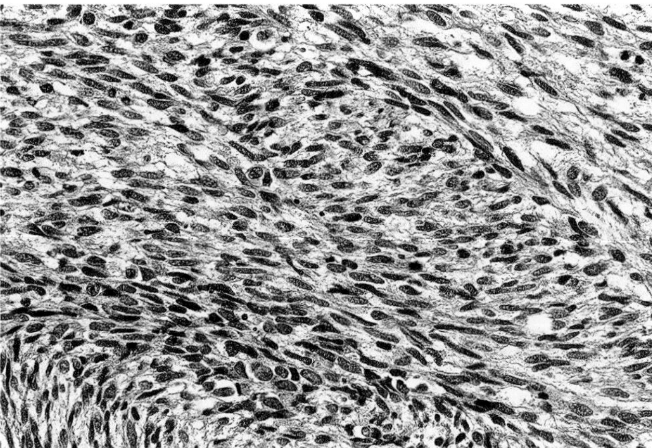

Fig. 25.76 The contrast between the dark hyperchromatic nuclei and the light cytoplasm is typical of malignant peripheral nerve sheath tumor.

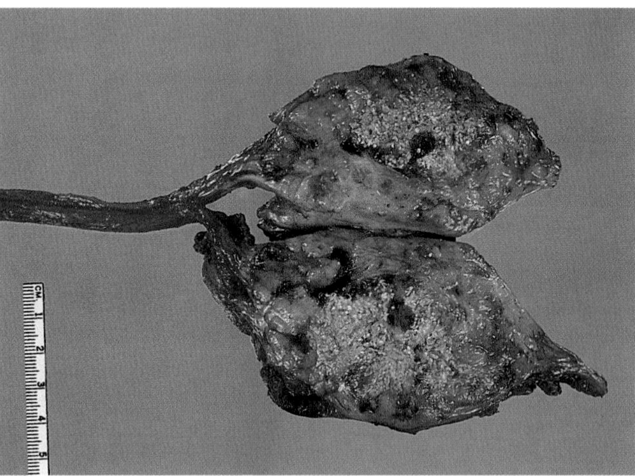

Fig. 25.77 Malignant peripheral nerve sheath tumor producing a characteristic fusiform expansion of the sciatic nerve. Foci of necrosis and hemorrhage are present.

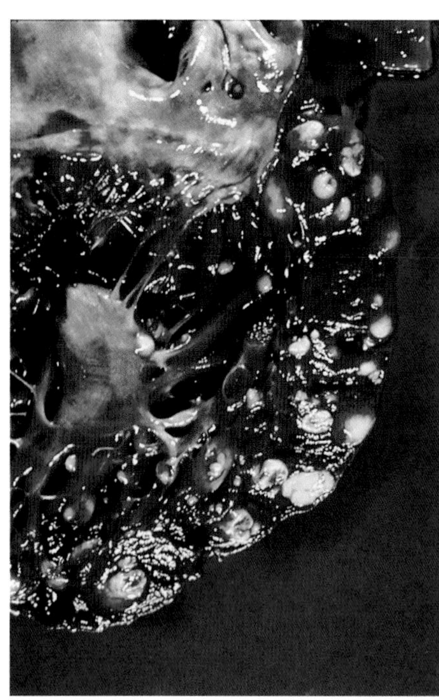

Fig. 25.78 Multiple tumor nodules in the heart in a case of widely metastatic malignant peripheral nerve sheath tumor.

are deep-seated, but they can occur in the subcutis or even in the skin.[728,744,757]

The clinical evolution is generally that of a highly malignant neoplasm, despite the relatively slow growth rate of some cases.[734,746,800,808] Local recurrence (often in the cut nerve ends) and distant metastases are frequent[746,810] (Fig. 25.78). In general, there is little correlation between microscopic grading and prognosis.[754,805] However, the *plexiform variant* of MPNST occurring in a superficial location in children has been associated with a better prognosis.[780] As a matter of fact, the lack of well-documented metastasizing examples of this entity has led some authors to question their placement into a malignant category.[816] Semantics aside, the fact remains that these tumors have a high tendency for recurrence and may be very troublesome to treat, as we have had the opportunity to observe on several occasions.

Occasionally, malignant tumors are found in major peripheral nerves or elsewhere in the soft tissue, having a light and electron microscopic appearance suggestive of primitive neuroectodermal origin. Sometimes these features are seen together with areas of typical MPNST and sometimes in a pure form.[773,776] The latter form, known as peripheral neuroepithelioma, peripheral or adult neuroblastoma, or primitive neuroectodermal tumor (PNET), is discussed on page 2188. The rare occurrence of neuroblastoma-like areas in benign schwannoma has already been mentioned (see p. 2131).

MPNSTs usually show a complex karyotype with numerical and structural abnormalities.[782,783] A claim that a high proportion of these tumors are associated with the t(X;18) translocation that is typical of synovial sarcoma has not been substantiated by subsequent studies.[743] Whether occurring sporadically or in the setting of type 1 neurofibromatosis, both alleles of the *NF1* gene are often inactivated in MPNST.[735,775,798] In addition, there are commonly mutations in the *TP53* gene, deletion of *CDKN2A* (9p21), and gain or amplification of 17q25, probably involving *BIRC5/SURVIVIN*.[732,733,774,788,799]

Other tumors of peripheral nerves

In addition to benign and malignant tumors composed of the constitutive cells of peripheral nerves, these structures are occasionally involved in a selective fashion by mesenchymal or other neoplasms. Thus, isolated cases of *hemangioma, fibrolipomatous hamartoma* (Fig. 25.79), *angiosarcoma,* and *malignant lymphoma* have been described.[818,819,822,823] Some of these tumors have occurred in nerves affected by neurofibroma and/or in patients with type 1 Recklinghausen disease.[821] Most of the lymphomas have been of B-cell type.[820]

Tumors of adipose tissue

Lipoma

Benign fatty tumors can arise in any location in which fat is normally present. The majority occur in the upper half of the body, particularly the trunk and neck, but they can develop in any other site, including hands and feet.[852] Most lipomas are subcutaneous,

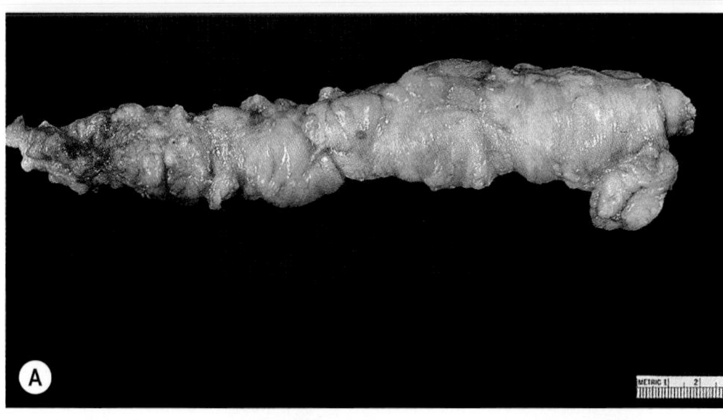

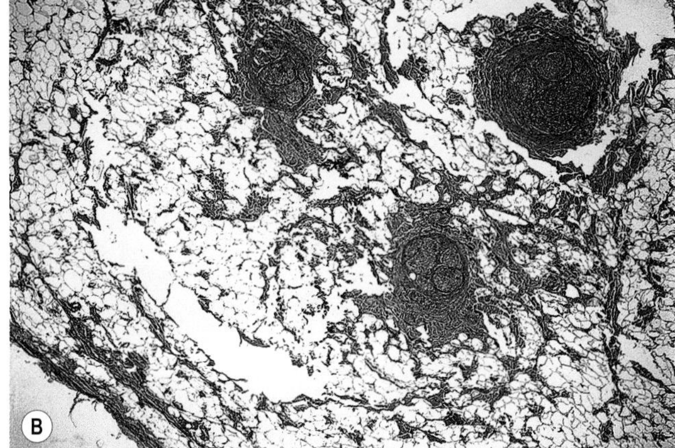

Fig. 25.79 **A** and **B**, Gross and microscopic appearance of fibrolipomatous hamartoma of nerve.

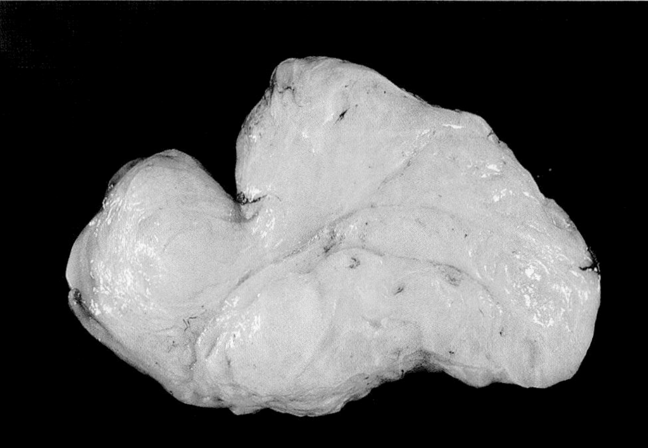

Fig. 25.80 Gross appearance of lipoma. Except for the circumscription, the appearance is indistinguishable from that of normal fat.

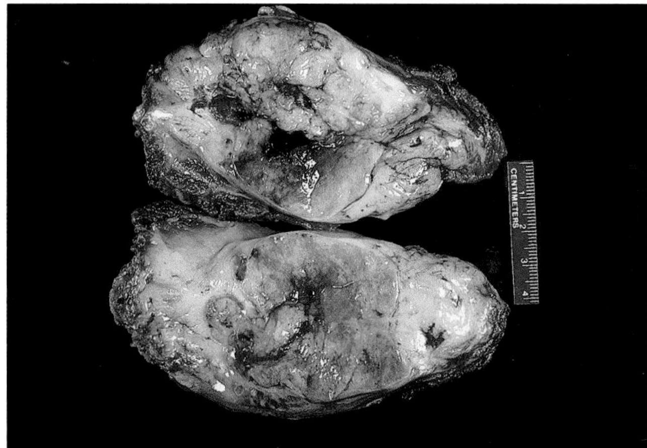

Fig. 25.81 Gross appearance of chondroid lipoma.

an important point in the differential diagnosis with liposarcomas, which are almost always deep-seated. However, lipomas can also occur in the deep soft tissues; these are subclassified into *intramuscular* (most common in the trunk) and *intermuscular* (most common in the anterior abdominal wall).[835] Most patients are in the fifth or sixth decade of life. Only rarely are children affected. Lipomas may be single or multiple. Multiple lipomas are more common in women; many are seen in a familial setting, and some occur in patients with neurofibromatosis or multiple endocrine neoplasia. In **diffuse lipomatosis**, massive enlargement of a limb may be seen as a result of diffuse proliferation of mature adipose tissue. In the familial variant of this process, lipomatosis has a symmetric distribution.[831]

Lipomas can grow to a large size; they are usually encapsulated when located in the superficial soft tissues but tend to be poorly circumscribed when arising in deeper structures.[838,845] Grossly, lipomas consist of bright yellow fat separated by fine fibrous trabeculae (Fig. 25.80). Microscopically, they are composed of mature adipose tissue with no cellular atypia. They are cytologically and immunohistochemically indistinguishable from normal fat, including positivity for S-100 protein and calretinin.[828]

Areas of fat necrosis, infarct, and calcification may be present. It is important not to confuse the histiocytes associated with fat necrosis with lipoblasts. The fact that they are often seen arranged in a circumferential fashion around a large lipid droplet (as is also the case in fat necrosis at other sites) is a helpful diagnostic sign. Rarely, lipomas are seen to contain foci of mature metaplastic cartilage and bone.[843]

Ultrastructurally, only univacuolar mature adipocytes are present in typical lipomas.[844] Although the light microscopic and electron microscopic appearance of a lipoma does not differ significantly from that of normal adult fat, its lipid content as determined by biochemical extraction and the activity of lipoprotein lipase is different.[853,861]

Morphologic variations that lipomas may exhibit include the following:

1 **Fibrolipoma** (sclerotic lipoma; fibroma-like lipoma). This is characterized by the presence of prominent bundles of *mature* collagenous or myxocollagenous stroma intermixed with mature adipocytes.[847] It affects mainly the distal extremities and should not be equated with spindle cell lipoma (see later section).

2 **Myxolipoma.** This tumor features focally well-developed myxoid changes. It should not be overdiagnosed as myxoid liposarcoma.

3 **Chondroid lipoma.** This variant is usually deep-seated (Fig. 25.81). It is characterized by a component of eosinophilic and vacuolated cells containing glycogen and lipid that resembles brown fat cells, lipoblasts, and chondroblasts[851] (Fig. 25.82). These cells are immunoreactive for vimentin, S-100 protein, and CD68; curiously, some are also positive for keratin.[846,851]

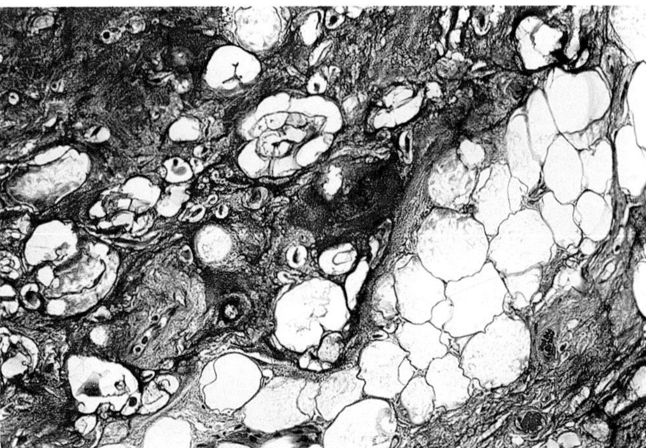

Fig. 25.82 Microscopic appearance of chondroid lipoma, showing admixture of mature fat and chondroid tissue.

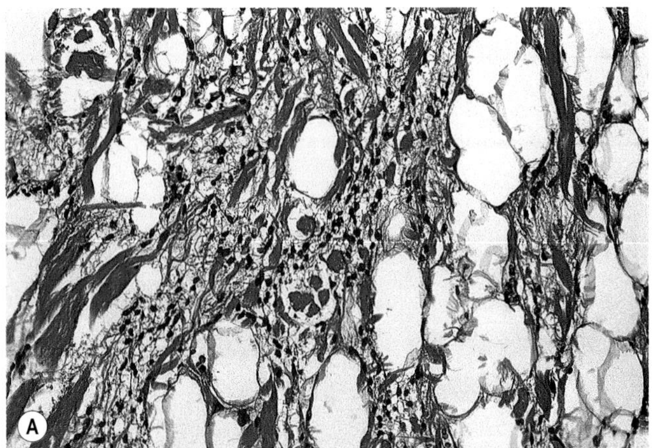

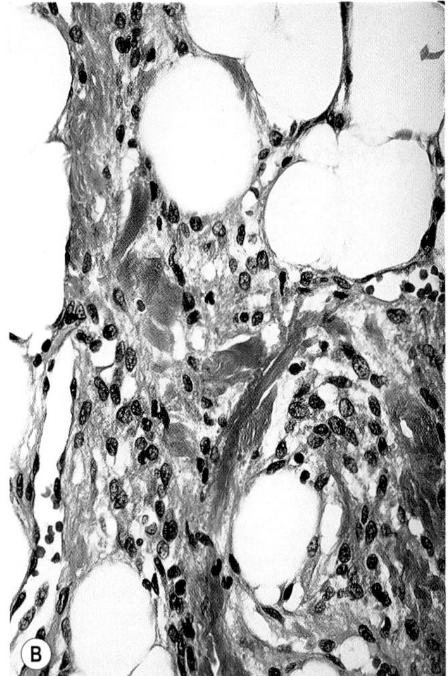

Fig. 25.83 **A** and **B**, Low- and high-power views of spindle cell lipoma. The oval to spindle cells are concentrated in the fibrous bands within lobules of mature adipose tissue.

4 **Myolipoma.** This tumor is characterized by an admixture in variable proportions of mature adipose tissue and bundles of well-differentiated smooth muscle.[850]

5 **Spindle cell lipoma.** This is a benign fatty tumor characteristically located in the regions of the shoulder and posterior neck of adults, but also found in many other locations, including the limbs, face, oral cavity, trunk, and anus.[837,854] It is composed of an admixture of mature lipocytes and uniform spindle cells set in a mucinous and fibrous background[833] (Fig. 25.83). Features that assist in distinguishing it from myxoid liposarcoma include the absence of lipoblasts and of a prominent plexiform vascular pattern, the presence of thick ('ropy') collagen bundles, and the great uniformity of the proliferating small spindle cells. In some instances the presence of irregular branching spaces with villiform projections results in an angiomatoid appearance.[839] Although the spaces were originally thought to be nonvascular ('pseudoangiomatous'), they have been found to be lined by cells with the immunohistochemical features of endothelial cells[863] (Fig. 25.84).

Cases of spindle cell lipoma in which mature fat is scanty or absent can be misdiagnosed as neurofibromas or low-grade sarcomas.[826] Immunohistochemically, there may be expression of desmin, an unexpected and potentially misleading finding.[862] Ultrastructurally, spindle cell lipomas are composed of a mixture of spindle mesenchymal cells and mature lipocytes.[827]

6 **Pleomorphic lipoma.** This is a lipoma containing hyperchromatic multinucleated ('floret-like') tumor cells within the fibrous septa traversing the neoplasm (Fig. 25.85). As for spindle cell lipoma, its most common location is the shoulder and posterior neck region.[860] We have also seen them in the dermis and beneath mucosal membranes. The most difficult differential diagnosis is with the sclerosing form of well-differentiated liposarcoma (atypical lipomatous tumor). The location of the lesion is an important clue, and the proportion of floret-type giant cells and lipoblasts is the most important distinguishing feature at the microscopic level.[824]Pleomorphic lipoma with little or no fat may be a diagnostic challenge.[856] Pleomorphic lipoma (and atypical lipomatous tumor, see below) can be simulated microscopically by *subconjunctival herniated orbital fat*, a non-neoplastic process due to prolapse of the subconjunctival intraconal orbital fat.[858]

7 **Angiolipoma.** These well-circumscribed small tumors occur shortly after puberty. They are often painful and characteristically multiple. They are located in the subcutis, most commonly on the trunk or extremities. Vascularity often is limited to a band of tissue on the periphery of the neoplasm (Fig. 25.86). Hyaline thrombi are common and constitute an important diagnostic sign[830] (Fig. 25.87). Angiolipomas in which the vascular component predominates (*cellular angiolipomas*) can be confused with Kaposi sarcoma or angiosarcoma[842] (Fig. 25.88). The pain correlates well with the degree of vascularity.[841] The fact that angiolipomas lack chromosomal aberrations (like hemangiomas and unlike lipomas) suggests that they are hemangiomas with fat rather than true mixed tumors.[859]

So-called *infiltrating angiolipomas* are unrelated to the lesion just described. They are probably not true mixed tumors but

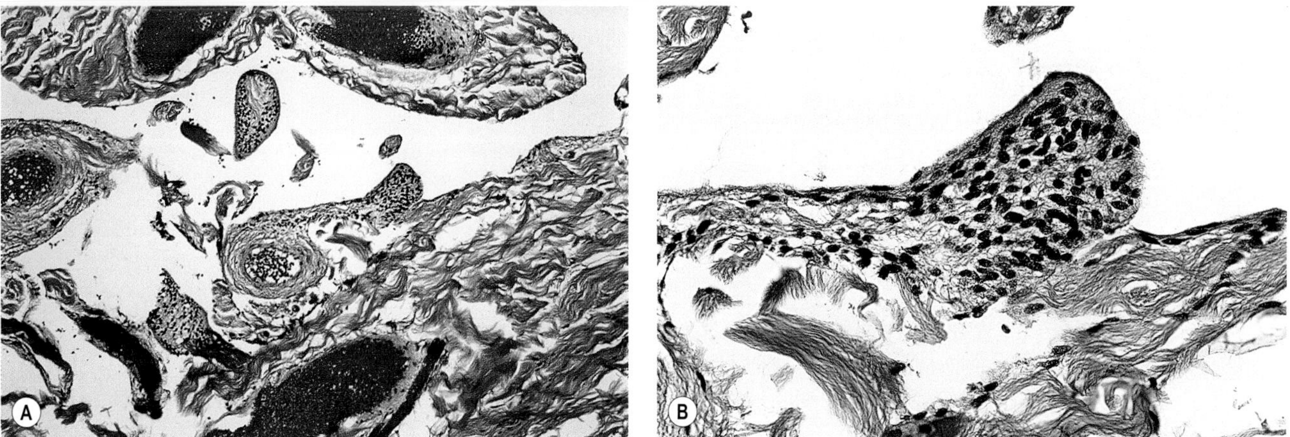

Fig. 25.84 **A** and **B**, Spindle cell lipoma with pseudoangiomatous appearance resulting from accumulation of tumor cells beneath artifactual tissue spaces.

Fig. 25.85 **A** and **B**, Pleomorphic lipoma. The high-power view (**B**) highlights the floret cells.

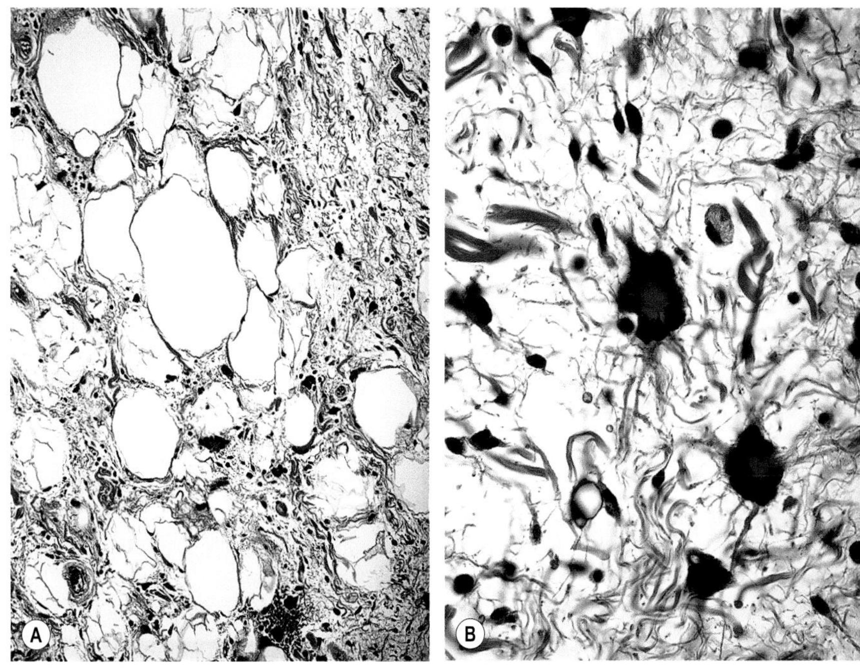

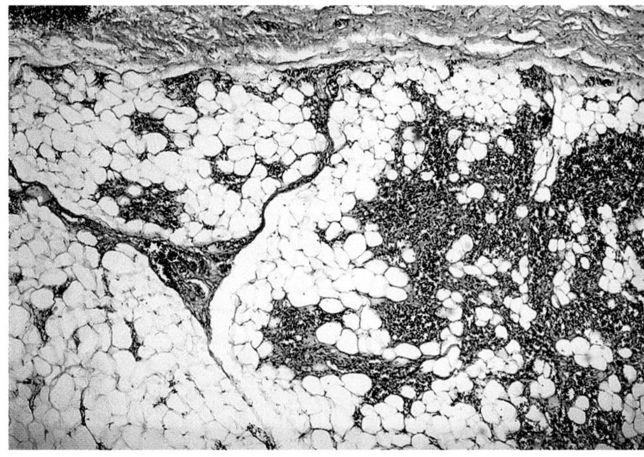

Fig. 25.86 Angiolipoma showing intimate admixture of blood vessels and mature adipose tissue.

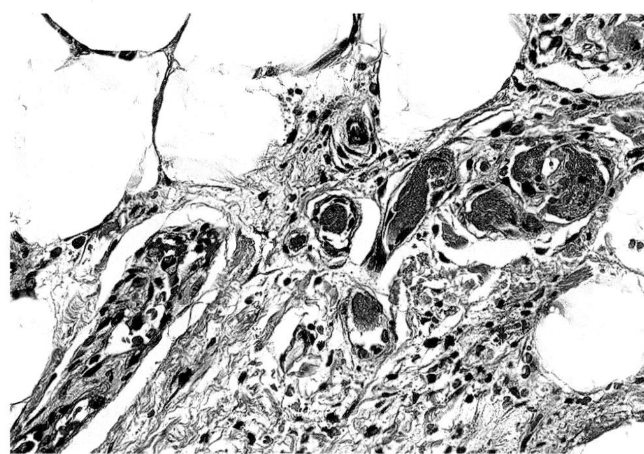

Fig. 25.87 Numerous hyaline thrombi in angiolipoma.

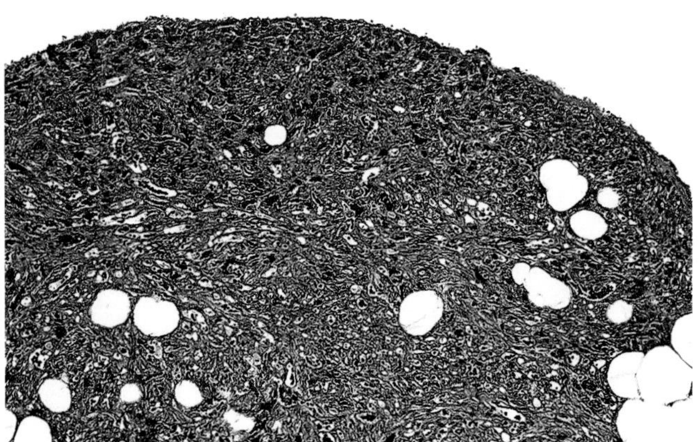

Fig. 25.88 Cellular angiolipoma. This benign tumor should not be confused with Kaposi sarcoma.

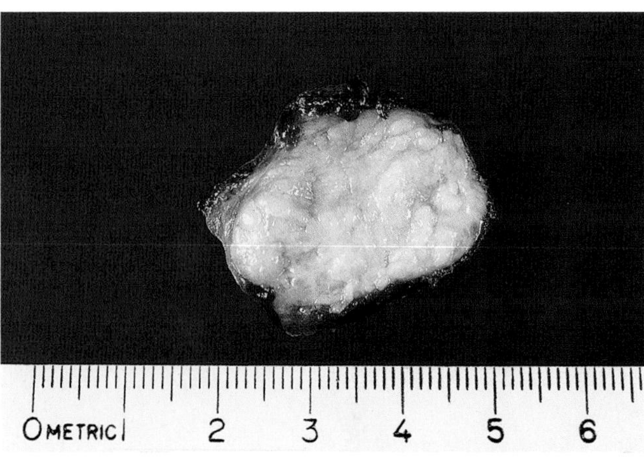

Fig. 25.89 Gross appearance of lipoblastoma. The tumor has a mucoid cut surface.

rather intramuscular large-vessel hemangiomas in which portions of the affected muscle tissue have been replaced by fat.[832]

Cytogenetically, 80% of solitary lipomas exhibit chromosomal aberrations, such as rearrangements of 12q14–15, rearrangements of 6p21–22, or deletions of 13q12–14 and 13q22.[825,834,855,857] The gene involved in 12q14–15 is *HMGA2* (also known as *HMGIC*, which encodes a high mobility group protein), and the gene involved in 6p21–22 is *HMGA1*.[848] In contrast with atypical lipomatous tumors, marker ring or giant chromosomes are extremely rare. Multiple lipomas usually exhibit a normal karyotype.

Nearly all spindle cell and pleomorphic lipomas show deletions or unbalanced rearrangements of chromosome 13q and/or 16q. This finding supports the close link between these two tumor types and the fact that they are distinct from atypical lipomatous tumors.[829,836,840,849]

Lipoblastoma/lipoblastomatosis

Lipoblastoma/lipoblastomatosis affects almost exclusively infants and young children (below the age of 5 years),[867,871,873,875,876] but occasional cases in adolescents and young adults are on record.[866a,868] It commonly involves the proximal portion of the lower and upper extremities. Grossly, the lesion is soft and lobulated (Fig. 25.89). It is subdivided into (benign) lipoblastoma (sometimes also designated as embryonal or fetal lipoma) when well circumscribed and lipoblastomatosis when deep-seated and ill defined. Microscopically, it closely resembles fetal fat.[866] It may be confused with myxoid liposarcoma because of the presence of lipoblasts, a plexiform vascular pattern, and an abundant myxoid stroma (Fig. 25.90). Its ultrastructural appearance is also very similar to that of myxoid liposarcoma.[864] It is distinguished from the latter by virtue of the young age of the patient, distinct lobulation, and absence of giant cells or pleomorphic nuclei.[865,873] Cytogenetically, lipoblastoma/lipoblastomatosis is often associated with rearrangements of 8q11–13, with the implicated gene being *PLAG1* (pleomorphic adenoma gene).[866a,869,870,872,875] A number of partner genes have been identified, such as *HAS2* in 8q24 and *COL1A2* in 7q22. Some cases show gain of chromosome 8, with or without simultaneous 8q11–13 rearrangement. The clinical course is benign. In the series of Chung and Enzinger,[865] the recurrence rate was 14% and was attributed to incomplete removal of the tumor.

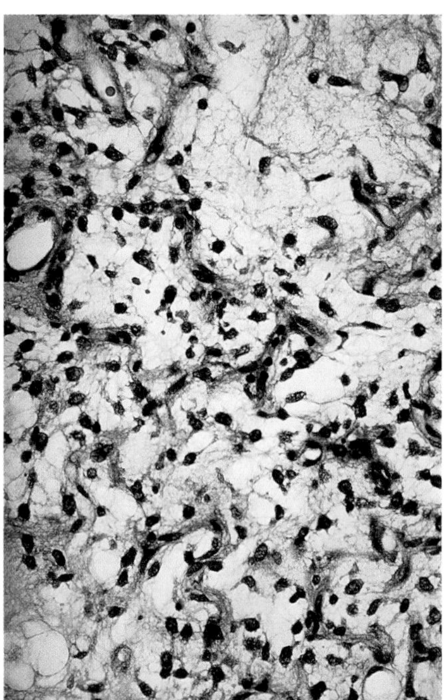

Fig. 25.90 Lipoblastoma. On high power, the appearance is reminiscent of myxoid liposarcoma.

Lipoblastomas that are not removed in infancy mature into lipomas, a clue to their primeval nature being the prominent fibrous septa that still divide them into distinct lobules[874] (Fig. 25.91).

Hibernoma

Hibernoma is a rare benign neoplasm occurring usually in the interscapular region, axilla, and thigh, but also in the mediastinum and retroperitoneum.[880] Its cut surface has a typical brown color, and its microscopic pattern is characteristic – an organoid arrangement of large cells with centrally located nucleus and a cytoplasm filled with many small vacuoles that stain for neutral fat (Figs 25.92 and 25.93). Cytogenetically, it is often associated with rearrangements involving 11q13.[879,884]

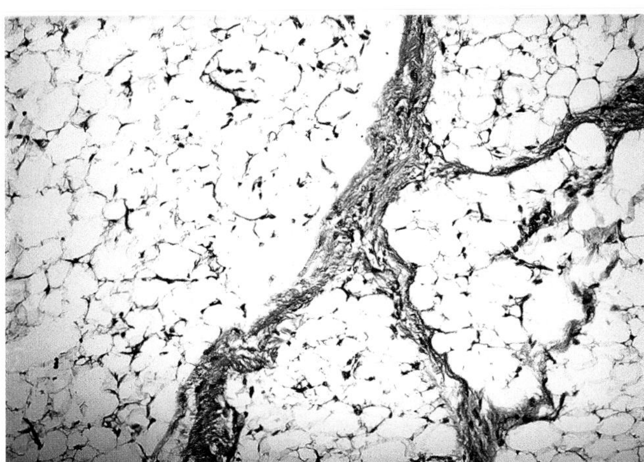

Fig. 25.91 'Mature' lipoblastoma. The lesion retains the lobulation that is characteristic of this tumor type.

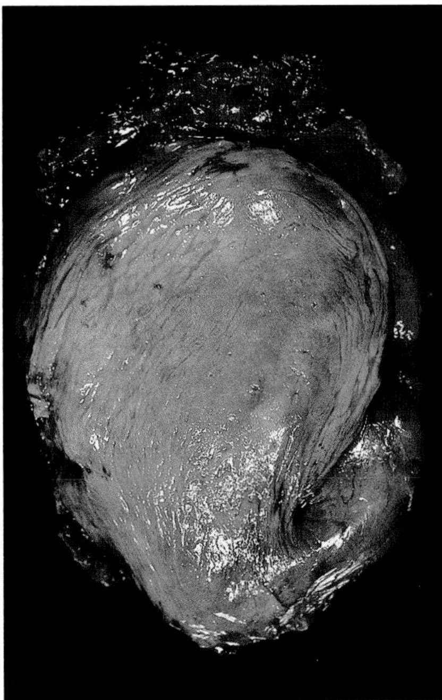

Fig. 25.92 Gross appearance of hibernoma exhibiting the typical light brown cut surface.

This tumor has received its name because it resembles the brown fat of the hibernating glands of animals, a similarity that is maintained at the electron microscopic level.[881,882,885] Interestingly, endocrine-like activity resembling that of adrenal cortical tissue has been detected in one case.[877] Sometimes the features of hibernoma are seen mixed with those of ordinary lipoma or of spindle cell lipoma (hybrid tumors) (Fig. 25.94). Other hibernomas are accompanied by a myxoid matrix.[878,880] Malignant soft tissue tumors in which many of the tumor cells have features of brown fat occur and are regarded as a morphologic variant of liposarcoma. Interestingly, hibernomas of the interscapular region develop regularly in transgenic mice containing the adipocyte-specific regulatory region from the adipocyte *P2* gene linked to the simian virus 40 transforming genes.[883]

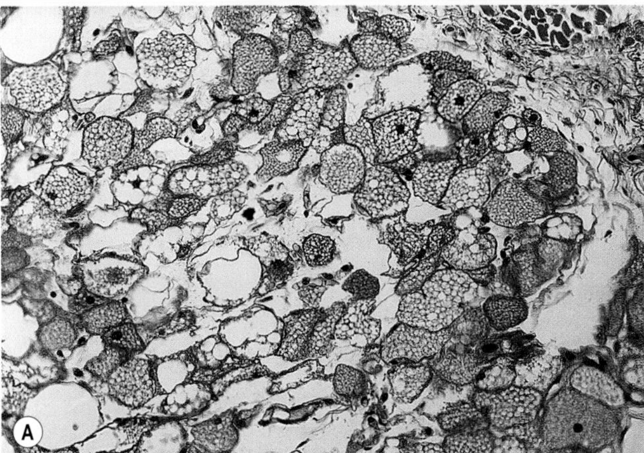

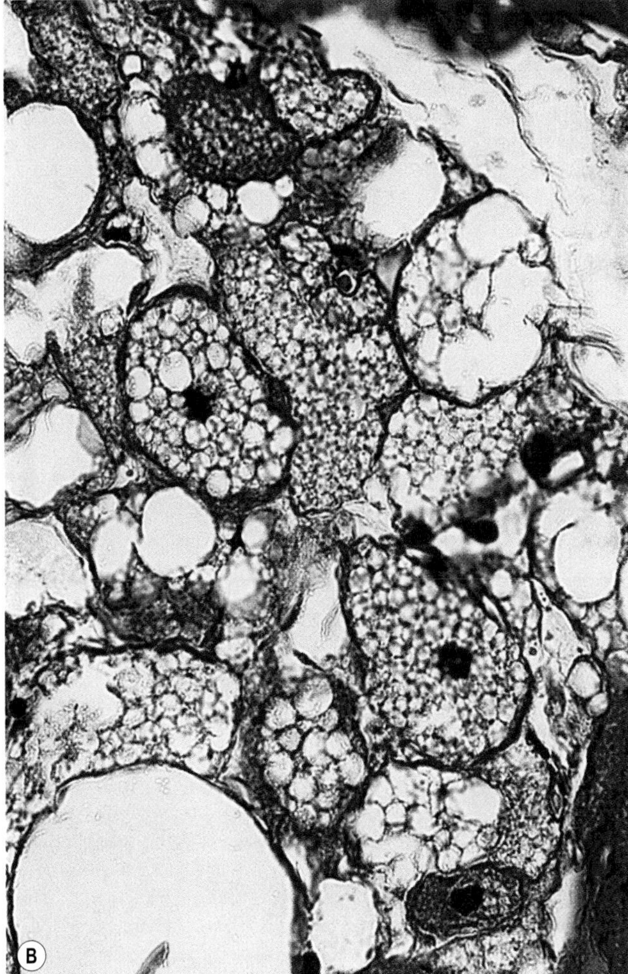

Fig. 25.93 **A** and **B**, Low- and high-power appearance of hibernoma. Note the central location of the indented nuclei.

Liposarcoma (including atypical lipomatous tumor)

Liposarcoma is the most frequent soft tissue sarcoma in adults.[914] Indubitable cases of liposarcoma have also been observed in adolescents and children.[889,903,939,945,968,971] However, most cases so diagnosed in this age group (particularly in the past) were in reality examples of lipoblastomatosis or giant cell fibroblastoma.[905]

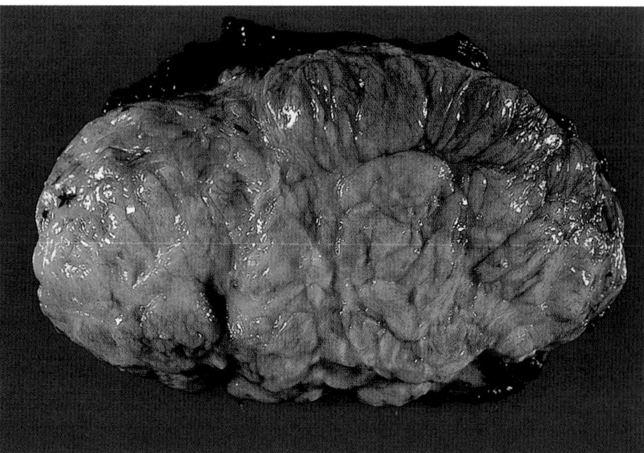

Fig. 25.94 Gross appearance of benign adipose tissue tumor that combines features of hibernoma and lipoma.

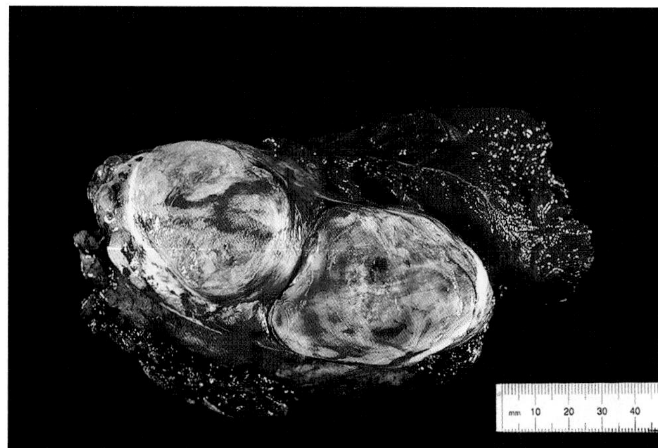

Fig. 25.96 Gross appearance of myxoid liposarcoma of thigh, characteristically located in the intermuscular spaces.

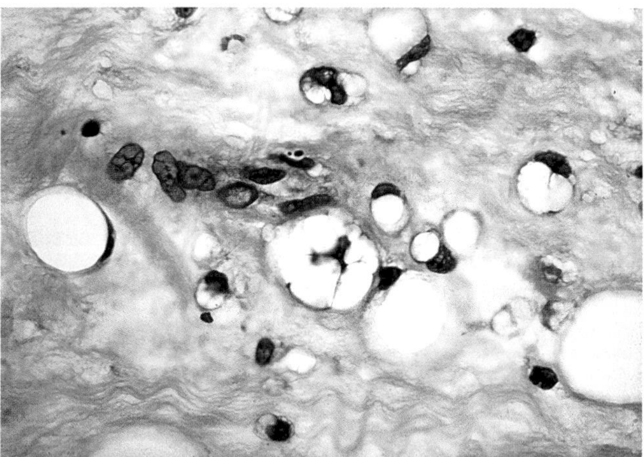

Fig. 25.95 Typical lipoblast from a case of metastatic liposarcoma, showing nuclear indentation by lipid-containing cytoplasmic vacuoles.

Liposarcomas are usually large and occur most frequently in the lower extremities (popliteal fossa and medial thigh); retroperitoneal, perirenal, and mesenteric region; and shoulder area.[964] Their relative frequency at these various sites is greatly dependent on the tumor subtype (see below). Although liposarcomas of the posterior neck, upper back, and shoulder certainly occur, it should be remembered that this is the classic site for benign adipose tissue tumors that can simulate liposarcoma, including spindle cell lipoma, pleomorphic lipoma, lipoblastoma/lipoblastomatosis, and hibernoma. Grossly, liposarcomas are well circumscribed but not encapsulated.[974] Depending on the subtype, they may have a mucoid, slimy surface suggestive of myxoma, a bright yellow appearance mimicking lipoma, or a surface resembling cerebral convolutions. Rarely, liposarcomas present as multicentric tumors[886,927] and/or are associated with independent benign multiple lipomas in the same patient.

The common morphologic denominator of liposarcoma is the *lipoblast*. This appears as a mononuclear or multinucleated cell with one or more cytoplasmic vacuoles that contain fat. The nucleus may be pushed aside by a single large vacuole, resulting in a signet ring configuration, or it may remain centrally located but exhibit small indentations by multiple small vacuoles, the appearance being similar to that of mature sebaceous cells or spongiocytes of adrenal cortex (Fig. 25.95). This highly characteristic scalloped nuclear appearance can also be appreciated in specimens obtained from fine needle aspiration.[979] It has been shown that both lipoblasts and mature adipocytes stain for topoisomerase-II alpha (a cycle-related intranuclear marker), a finding of potential diagnostic significance.[912]

In their classic article on liposarcoma, Enzinger and Winslow[915] divided liposarcomas into four types: myxoid, round cell, well differentiated, and pleomorphic, acknowledging the existence of mixed forms. Several modifications have been incorporated into this classification in subsequent years, but the basic scheme remains essentially intact, a tribute to the prescience of Dr Franz Enzinger. It has been suggested that the various liposarcoma types relate to various stages of differentiation of stem cells, in a fashion similar to that believed to be operating in hematologic malignancies.[900,949]

Myxoid liposarcoma, which is the most common type of liposarcoma, shows a marked predilection for the lower extremities, particularly the thigh (Fig. 25.96). It practically never occurs in the retroperitoneum, most cases so diagnosed being in reality examples of atypical lipomatous tumor with prominent myxoid change (see below).[910] Microscopically, myxoid liposarcoma has few or no mitotic figures and is characterized by proliferating lipoblasts in different stages of differentiation, a prominent anastomosing capillary network, and a mucoid matrix rich in hyaluronidase-sensitive acid mucopolysaccharides[983] (Fig. 25.97). The presence of a delicate network of thin-walled vessels is an important feature in the differential diagnosis with myxoma and other myxoid tumors. The mucoid extracellular material may accumulate in large pools, thus simulating a tumor of lymph vessel origin. Metaplastic cartilage is found in rare instances.[969,981] Ultrastructurally, cells varying in appearance from primitive mesenchymal cells to typical multivacuolated and univacuolated lipoblasts are seen.[895,966] The abundant capillaries are intimately related to all of these various cell types in a manner analogous to that of developing fetal adipose tissue.[895,942,944]

Cytogenetically, myxoid liposarcoma is characterized by the reciprocal translocation t(12;16)(q13;p11), which results in the *FUS–DDIT3* (formerly known as *TLS–CHOP*) fusion, and less commonly, t(12;22)(q13;q12) with *EWS–DDIT3* fusion.[891,913,959] *DDIT3* is a gene involved in adipocyte differentiation.[890,908,924,928,973] The chimeric protein encoded by *FUS–DDIT3* can be detected immunohistochemically.[956]

In the **round cell type** the tumor cells are small and have a distinctly acidophilic cytoplasm (Fig. 25.98). The presence among

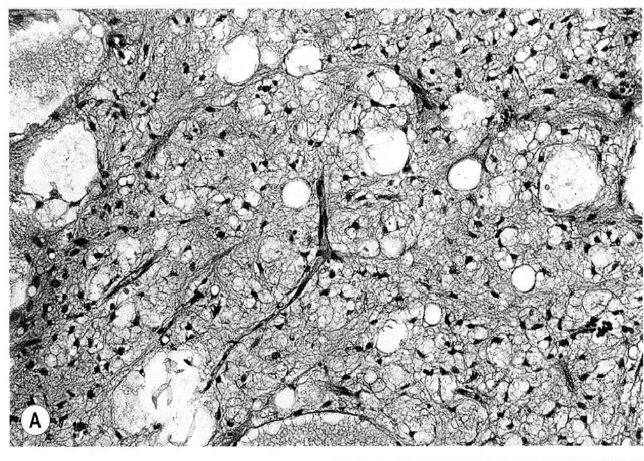

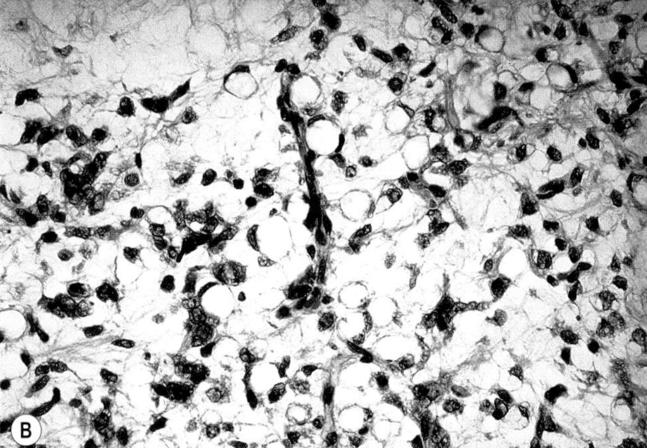

Fig. 25.97 **A** and **B**, Low- and high-power appearance of myxoid liposarcoma.

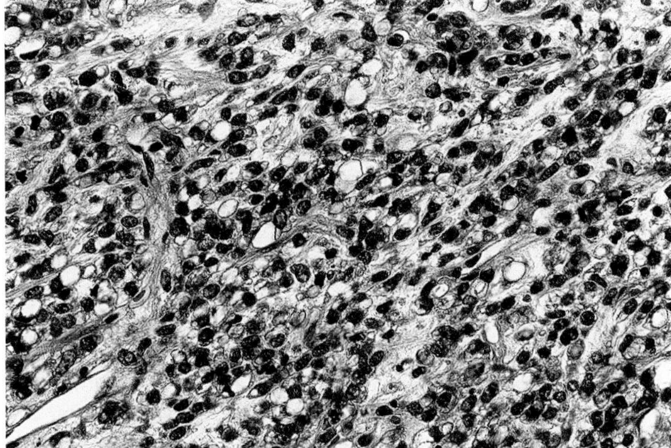

Fig. 25.98 Round cell liposarcoma. This tumor is to be viewed as a poorly differentiated form of myxoid liposarcoma.

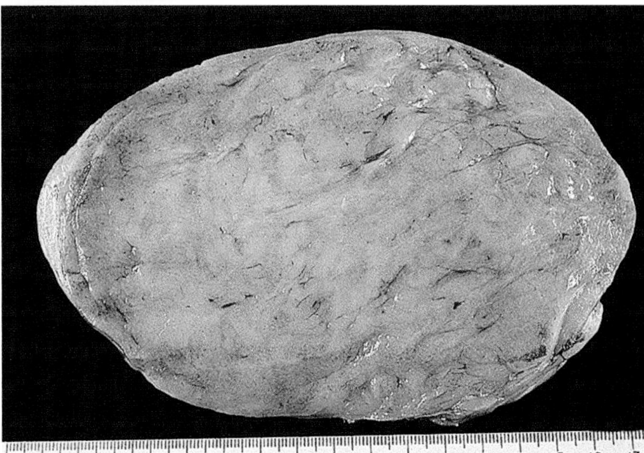

Fig. 25.99 Atypical lipomatous tumor. The neoplasm is well circumscribed and not very different from an ordinary lipoma.

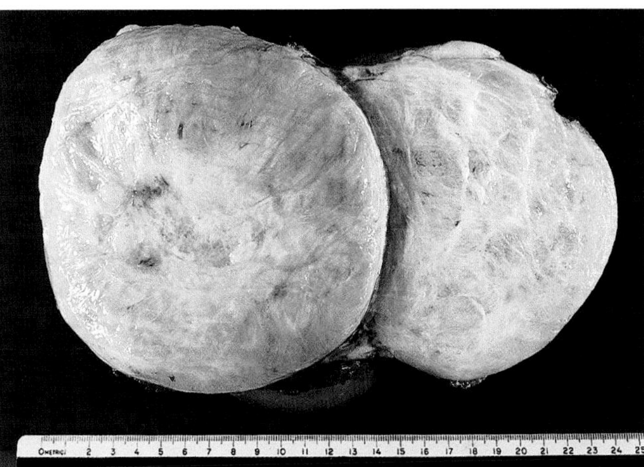

Fig. 25.100 Gross appearance of a retroperitoneal atypical lipomatous tumor that microscopically combined features of the sclerosing and lipoma-like subtypes.

them of scattered lipoblasts establishes the diagnosis. Mitoses are more common than in the myxoid form, whereas the vascular network is less prominent. Pseudoglandular arrangement of the tumor cells is frequent. Immunoreactivity for S-100 protein is a constant and diagnostically useful feature.

It has been established that round cell liposarcoma is not a specific subtype but rather a poorly differentiated form of myxoid liposarcoma, as supported by the presence of a common chromosomal translocation and gene fusion.[977] Actually, a whole range exists in the prevalence of round cells in myxoid liposarcoma, an increasing number of these cells indicating a greater degree of tumor aggressiveness, with the pure round cell liposarcoma representing the end of the spectrum.[940,971] Notably, even a round cell component of 1–5% is associated with an increased risk of local recurrence and poorer disease-specific survival.[975] Along these lines, a very rare form of myxoid liposarcoma exists in which the poorly differentiated nature is manifested not through the presence of round cells but of spindle or pleomorphic elements.[977]

Atypical lipomatous tumor resembles ordinary lipoma grossly (Figs 25.99 and 25.100). It also resembles it on low-power examination, but closer inspection shows scattered tumor cells with large, deep-staining nuclei. These atypical cells may concentrate on the fibrous strands that traverse the adipose tissue lobules (*sclerosing subtype*) (Fig. 25.101) or be scattered among the mature adipocytes (*lipoma-like subtype*) (Fig. 25.102). Some of the atypical cells have features of lipoblasts by virtue of the cytoplasmic vacuoles producing nuclear indentations, but most do not. Some of the nuclei have sharply outlined vacuoles ('Lochkern'), which at the ultrastructural

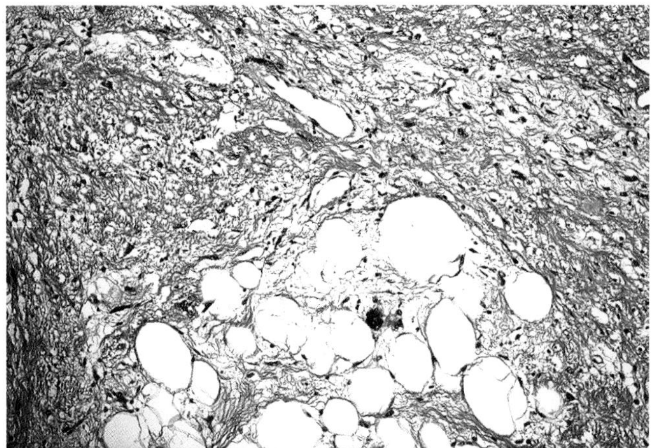

Fig. 25.101 Low-power microscopic view of an atypical lipomatous tumor with prominent sclerosing pattern. This corresponds to the well-differentiated liposarcoma, sclerosing type, of other classification schemes.

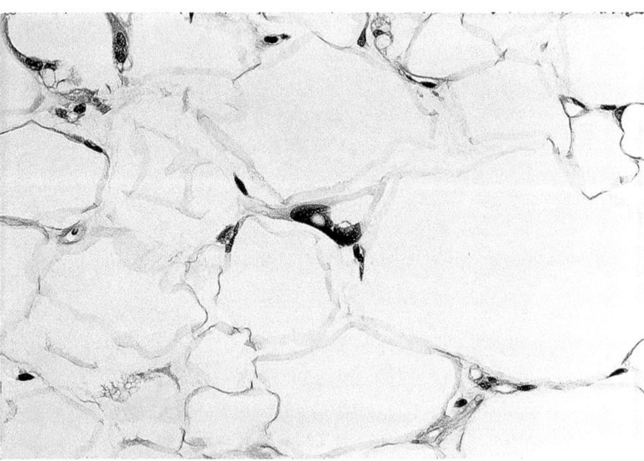

Fig. 25.102 Lipoma-like subtype of atypical lipomatous tumor. A single atypical cell with a nuclear vacuole ('Lochkern') is seen in the center of the field.

level are seen to correspond to invaginations of the nuclear membrane, i.e., pseudoinclusions. It should be pointed out that occasional adipocytes with hyperchromatic and slightly enlarged nuclei containing pseudoinclusions can be seen in the non-neoplastic fat of somatic soft tissues and other sites, such as breast.

Atypical lipomatous tumor was included in the category of *well-differentiated liposarcoma* in the Enzinger–Winslow classification,[915] but the proposed switch in terminology is justified by the fact that this is a nonmetastasizing neoplasm (unless it were to undergo differentiation, see below).[893,902,917,920,941] The term *atypical lipoma* has been used by some authors as a synonym for atypical lipomatous tumor and by others for the tumors in this category showing only a minimal degree of atypia; it is probably better to avoid it. The behavior of atypical lipomatous tumors is substantially different depending on their location.[946] Those situated in the somatic soft tissues may recur, but these recurrences are controllable so that tumor-related deaths are practically nonexistent; instead, those originating in the retroperitoneum have a very high incidence of recurrence (some of these recurrences having a 'dedifferentiated' appearance, see subsequent discussion), and some of the patients die as a result. In view of these findings and based on pragmatic criteria, the proposal has been made to use the term *atypical lipoma* for the former and *well-differentiated liposarcoma* for the latter.[893] We prefer to designate the entire group as *atypical lipomatous tumor*, followed by a statement as to the predicted natural history based on the size and location of the mass.

It is not unusual for atypical lipomatous tumors to exhibit secondary myxoid changes; when prominent, these tumors may be confused with myxoid liposarcoma. True mixed myxoid/well-differentiated liposarcomas exist, but they are vanishingly rare.[952]

Occasionally, smooth muscle bundles are seen in these neoplasms, a phenomenon akin to that already mentioned in connection with lipomas.[918] These tumors, which have been referred to as *lipoleiomyosarcomas*, should not be overinterpreted as dedifferentiated liposarcomas.[925] In other instances a heavy inflammatory infiltrate of either neutrophilic or lymphoplasmacytic nature is present, with some of the inflammatory cells being located within the cytoplasm of the giant tumor cells. Tumors with this appearance have been called *inflammatory liposarcoma* and *lymphocyte-rich liposarcoma*[892,943] (Fig. 25.103). This inflammatory pattern can be seen in association with or independently from dedifferentiation.

Spindle cell liposarcoma is an unusual and controversial variant of atypical lipomatous tumor characterized by a population of relatively bland spindle cells arrayed in fascicles and whorls, set in a variably myxoid stroma (Fig. 25.104). Most of the reported cases were located in the subcutaneous tissue of the shoulder girdle or upper limbs and therefore appeared different from the tumors that were described as fibroblastic or spindle cell liposarcomas in previous works.

The recently described *sclerosing poorly differentiated liposarcoma*[976] seems also to be a variation in the theme of the sclerosing subtype of atypical lipomatous tumor.

Cytogenetically, close to 80% of the atypical lipomatous tumors (including the dedifferentiated examples) show supernumerary ring or giant marker chromosomes, in stark contrast to lipomas of either ordinary or spindle/pleomorphic type.[924,965] At the molecular level, these chromosomal changes result in amplification of the 12q13–15 region, which includes *MDM2*, *SAS*, *HMGA2*, and *CDK4* genes.[887,970] Demonstration of *MDM2* or *CDK4* amplification in tissue sections with the FISH technique,[907,980] or overexpression of the proteins by immunohistochemistry, even in Tru-cut biopsies, may be of help in distinguishing well-differentiated liposarcoma from lipoma.[897,901] Recently, it has been shown that p16 (an important cell cycle regulator) is expressed in the majority of atypical lipomatous tumors but apparently not in lipomas.[933]

Pleomorphic liposarcoma is a highly cellular, poorly differentiated neoplasm containing numerous tumor giant cells, some of them having the features of lipoblasts[911,935,957] (Fig. 25.105). Mitoses and foci of necrosis are frequent. The differential diagnosis includes so-called malignant fibrous histiocytoma and pleomorphic rhabdomyosarcoma. In addition to the expected positivity for S-100 protein (which is actually seen in only one-third of the cases), there may be reactivity for smooth muscle actin and desmin.[935] In addition, an *epithelioid variant* of pleomorphic liposarcoma has been described that simulates undifferentiated carcinoma at the morphologic and immunohistochemical level (focal reactivity for keratin)[938,953] (Fig. 25.106).

Dedifferentiated liposarcoma is the term used for the emergence of a generally nonlipogenic component within an atypical lipomatous tumor or, much more rarely, in myxoid liposarcoma.[951,961] The dedifferentiated component may already be present at the time of the original excision but is much more commonly seen in recurrent or metastatic foci. It is much more common in retroperitoneal neoplasms, but it has also been documented in tumors of the

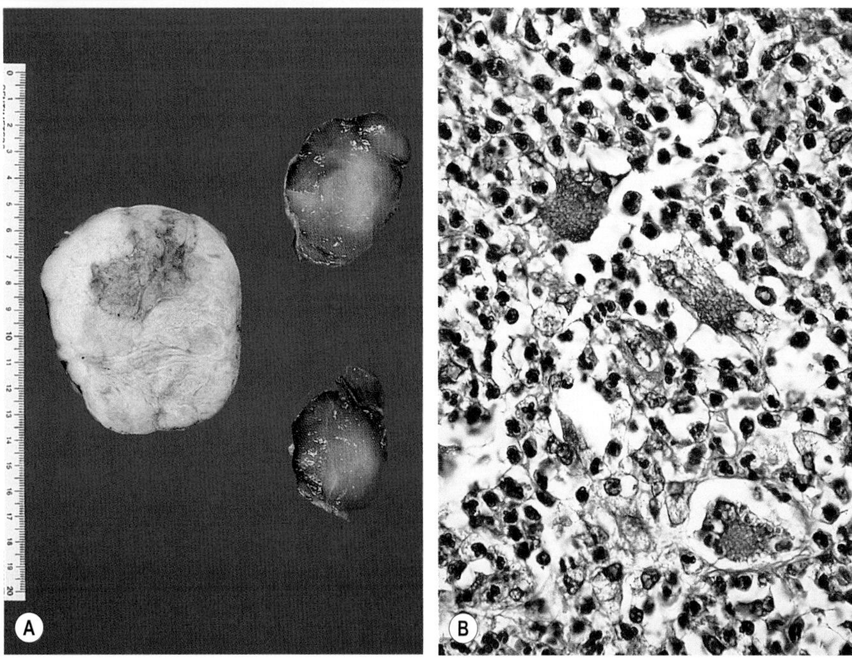

Fig. 25.103 A and B, Inflammatory liposarcoma. A, Gross appearance. The inflammatory liposarcoma is represented by the larger mass, whereas the others were atypical lipomatous tumors. All three masses were located in the retroperitoneum. B, Microscopic appearance showing highly pleomorphic tumor cells surrounded by numerous neutrophils. The appearance is that of so-called 'inflammatory MFH'. (Compare with Figures 25.41 and 25.42.)

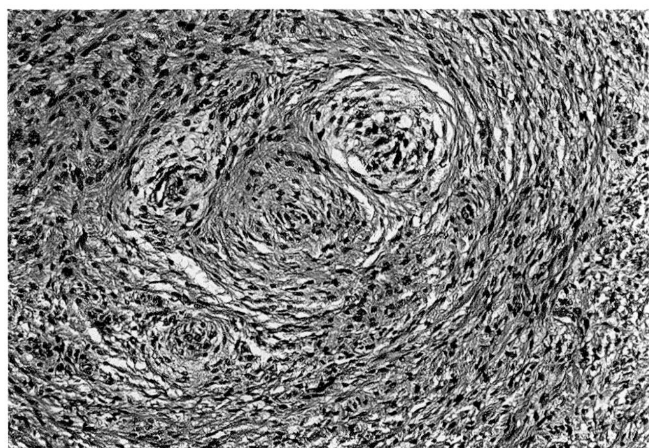

Fig. 25.104 So-called 'spindle cell liposarcoma' exhibiting a whorling pattern of growth.

extremities[894,950] (Fig. 25.107). Microscopically, the dedifferentiated component is usually high grade, with an appearance reminiscent of fibrosarcoma or so-called malignant fibrous histiocytoma, with or without myxoid features[916,932,972,982] (Fig. 25.108). Heterologous elements, such as skeletal muscle (particularly frequent[898,978]), cartilage or blood vessels, may be present;[919] these foci, which are viewed as evidence of divergent differentiation, are accompanied by their respective immunohistochemical markers[931,960] (Fig. 25.109). Recently, the existence of a 'homologous' form of dedifferentiation (with the appearance of a pleomorphic liposarcoma) has been proposed.[948] Occasionally, the dedifferentiated component appears in the form of a discontinuous micronodular pattern throughout the tumor.[950] In other cases, it exhibits a whorling pattern with a neural-like or meningothelial-like appearance associated with metaplastic bone formation.[922,954] A high percentage of dedifferentiated liposarcomas stain for PPAR-gamma, whereas this is true for only one-fourth of other sarcoma types.[936]

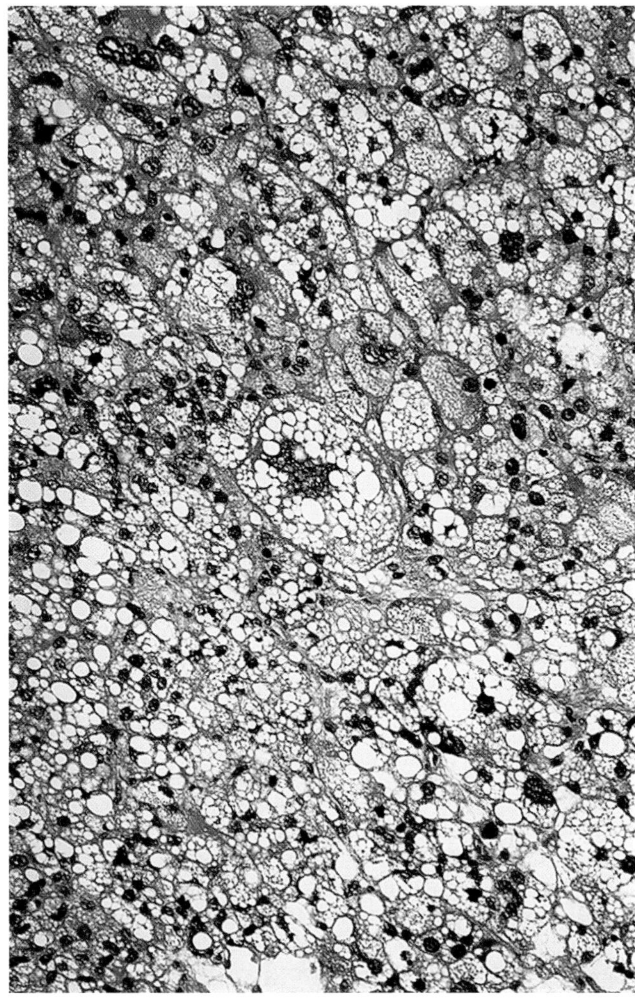

Fig. 25.105 Pleomorphic liposarcoma with numerous giant lipoblasts.

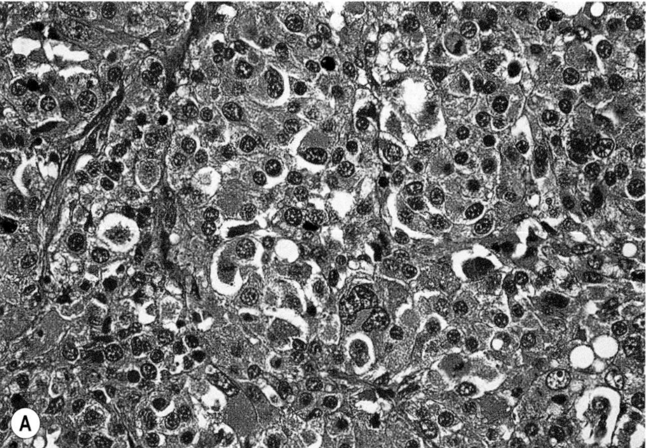

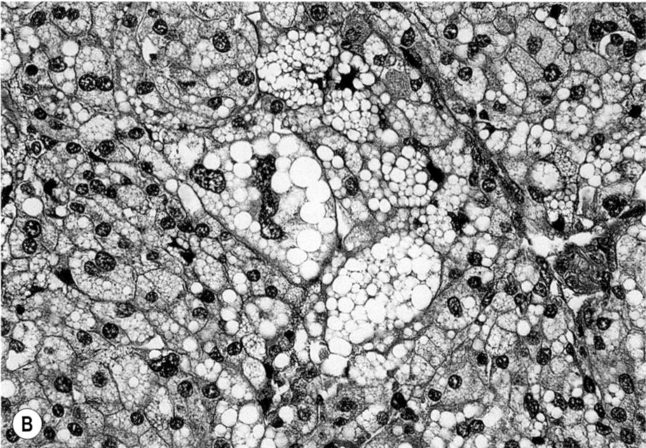

Fig. 25.106 **A** and **B**, Epithelioid variant of pleomorphic liposarcoma. The epithelioid features are better demonstrated in **A**, whereas the liposarcomatous nature of the tumor is better shown in **B**.

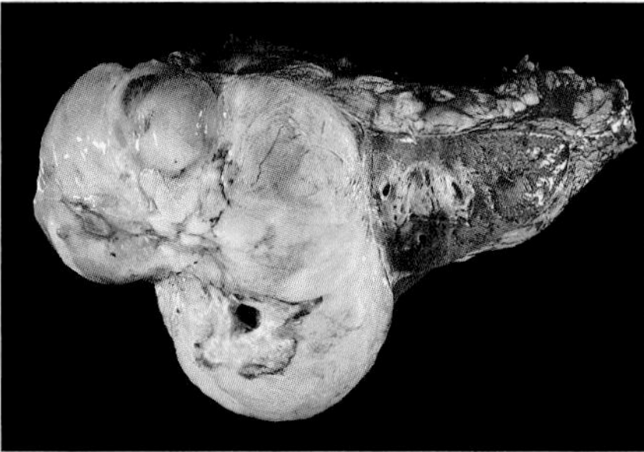

Fig. 25.107 Dedifferentiated liposarcoma of retroperitoneum abutting on the kidney, a common occurrence.

Dedifferentiated liposarcoma shows the same genetic changes as the preexisting well-differentiated liposarcoma, but often shows additional genetic changes, such as amplifications (e.g., gain of 1q21–24, 6q22–24, 20q13, or 12q24), deletions (e.g., loss of 13q14–21 or 11q22–23), and *TP53* mutation.[937,962]

It should be noted that the dedifferentiated component can also be low grade, with a resemblance to fibromatosis, well-differentiated fibrosarcoma,[934] or osteosarcoma.[984] Along these lines, Evans has proposed the existence of a *cellular atypical lipomatous tumor*, as defined by atypical lipomatous tumors with increased cellularity but fewer than five mitoses per 10 high-power fields in the nonlipogenic component. Regardless of terminology, these cellular tumors are not to be equated with conventional high-grade dedifferentiated tumors in view of their significantly different behavior.[921] Parenthetically, dedifferentiation is accompanied by overexpression of p53.[929]

Histochemical and immunohistochemical features. Fat stains are of little help in the diagnosis of liposarcoma, since they can be almost absent in the pure round cell and pleomorphic forms, whereas they may be present in a host of nonlipogenic soft tissue neoplasms. S-100 protein is focally but consistently found immunohistochemically in the cells of both benign and malignant adipose tissue tumors.[906,930] Other markers usually found in this family of neoplasms are caveolin (also present in smooth muscle neoplasms)[896] and leptin (a cytokine-like peptide).[958]

Differential diagnosis. The benign lesions most commonly confused with liposarcoma are lipoblastoma/lipoblastomatosis; spindle cell and pleomorphic lipoma; myxoid, inflamed, or necrotic lipoma; lipogranuloma (such as that resulting from injection of liquid silicone); *localized lipoatrophy* (such as that seen at sites of insulin or steroid injections); *subconjunctival herniated orbital fat* (prolapse of subconjunctival intraconal orbital fat); and *massive localized lymphedema* (a non-neoplastic disease most often occurring in the lower extremities of morbidly obese patients).[888,899,909,923,947,967] We have also been impressed by the similarity to myxoid liposarcoma that lipomas present in individuals who have subjected themselves to a drastic diet program can have. As a general rule, the diagnosis of liposarcoma should be questioned for any tumor seen in the pediatric age group or any tumor that is small, superficial, embedded within a major muscle, or located in the neck region. Although bona fide liposarcomas have been documented in all of these situations, the features of malignancy need to be assessed in a particularly critical fashion because of the high frequency with which benign lesions that simulate liposarcoma occur in these settings.

Treatment and prognosis. The primary treatment of all types of liposarcoma is surgical, inasmuch as radiation therapy and chemotherapy are generally of only dubious value.

Tumor location, size, and histologic subtype are the most important prognostic indicators.[963] Both the pure myxoid liposarcomas and the atypical lipomatous tumors (particularly the latter) tend to recur locally rather than to metastasize.[904] By contrast, the pure round cell, pleomorphic, and dedifferentiated types often give rise to metastases, most often to the lungs and sometimes widespread.[911,926,955] In the classic series of Enzinger and Winslow,[915] the 5-year survival rate of patients with myxoid and well-differentiated forms (atypical lipomatous tumors) exceeded 70%, whereas for the round cell pleomorphic varieties it was only 18%.

Tumors and tumorlike conditions of blood and lymph vessels

Hemangioma

Hemangiomas occupy a gray zone between hamartomatous malformations and true neoplasms.[1028] They are frequently designated and regarded as tumors because of their usually localized nature and mass effect. However, the fact that they consistently lack chromosomal alterations speaks against a true neoplastic nature. The presence or absence of nerve bundles intimately admixed with the vascular proliferation has been used to place them into a malformative or a neoplastic category, respectively.[985,1015] Although clearly benign, they can become very large and unsightly, and can even be fatal if they affect vital structures. They almost never

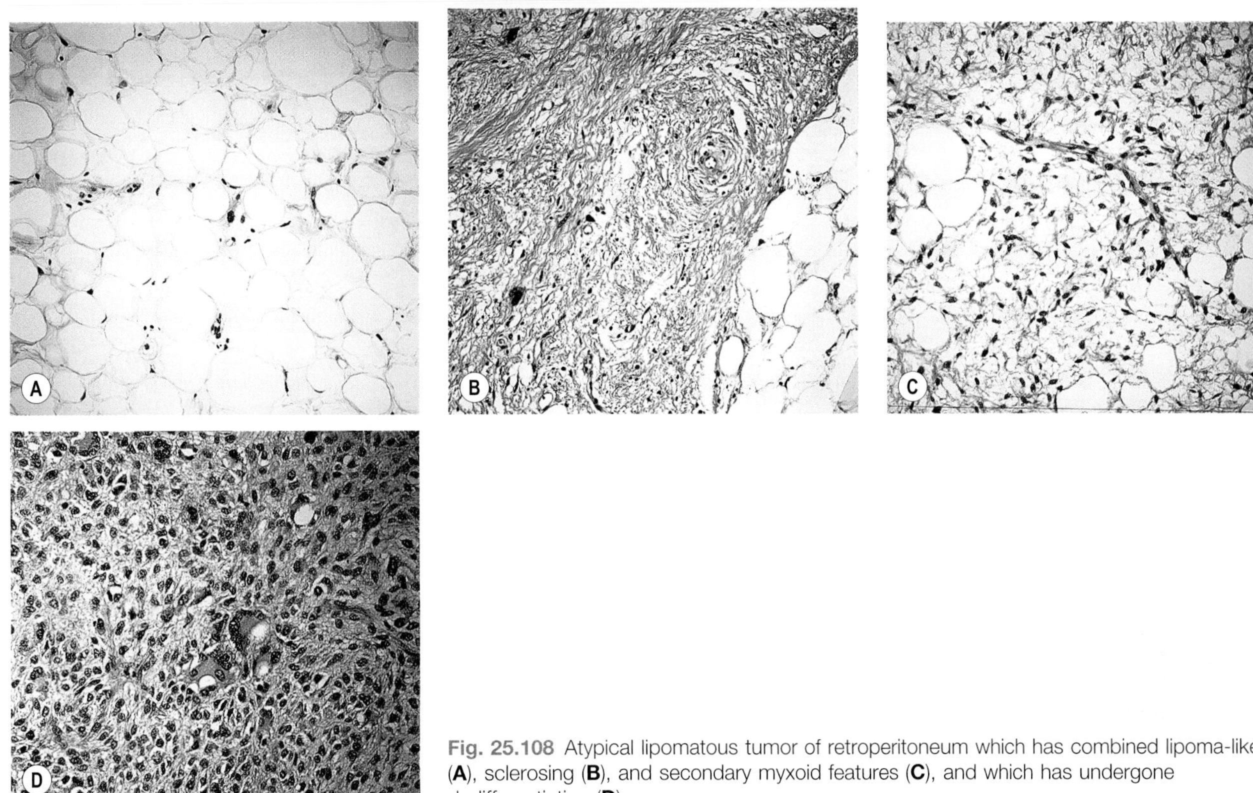

Fig. 25.108 Atypical lipomatous tumor of retroperitoneum which has combined lipoma-like (**A**), sclerosing (**B**), and secondary myxoid features (**C**), and which has undergone dedifferentiation (**D**).

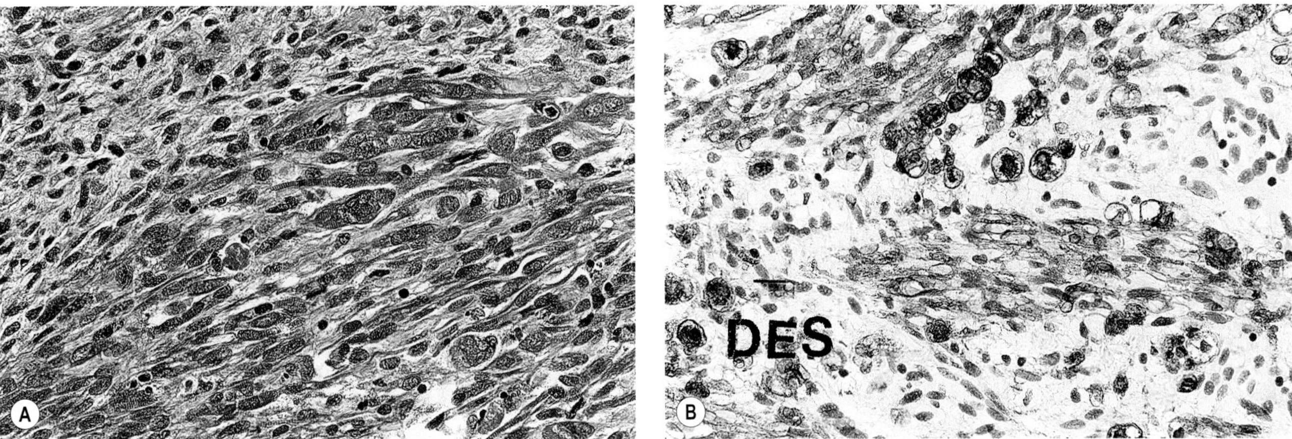

Fig. 25.109 **A** and **B**, Dedifferentiated retroperitoneal liposarcoma with divergent differentiation toward skeletal muscle. **B**, Desmin immunostain.

become malignant, although a few well-documented examples of this complication are on record. A high percentage occurs in children, and many are already present at birth.[992,1018] Over half of the cases are in the head and neck area; they can also occur in the trunk or extremities. Most hemangiomas are solitary; when multiple (with or without associated lesions in internal organs) or affecting a large segment of the body, the condition is known as (*multifocal*) *angiomatosis*.[1008,1024]

Hemangiomas have been classified according to their clinical appearance and the caliber of vessel involved. A close correlation exists between these two parameters.

Capillary hemangiomas are made up of small vessels of capillary caliber and can occur in any organ. The most distinctive and common variant of this type is known as *benign hemangioendothelioma* or *juvenile* or *hyperplastic hemangioma*. Its most common location is the skin, where it appears as an elevated nodule with an intense crimson color. Such a hemangioma is traditionally known to dermatologists as a *strawberry hemangioma* because of its clinical appearance. It is usually present at birth or appears during the first month of life and enlarges rapidly during the first few months, only to stop growing when the child is approximately 6 months old. Subsequently, it becomes flaccid, pale blue,

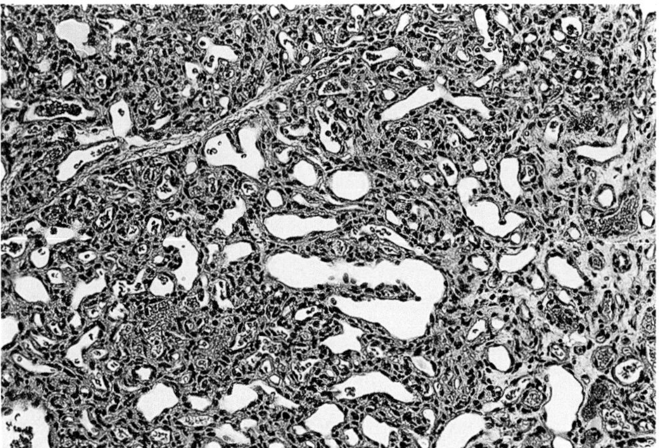

Fig. 25.110 Infantile hemangioendothelioma showing vaguely lobulated architecture.

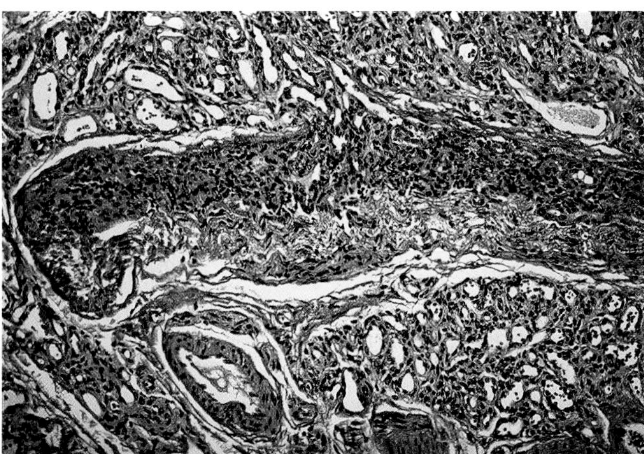

Fig. 25.112 Perineurial spread in juvenile hemangioendothelioma.

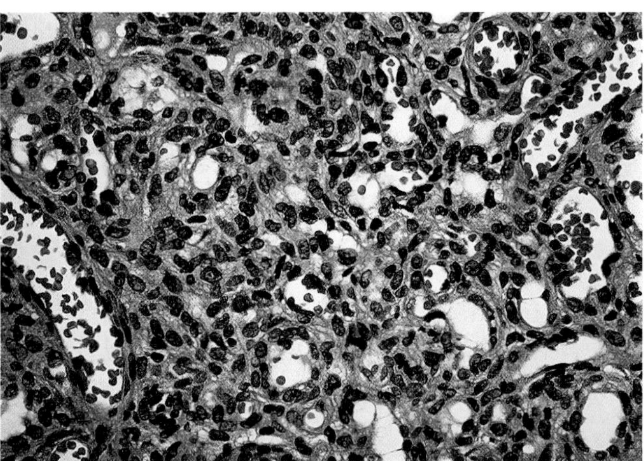

Fig. 25.111 The high cellularity and mitotic activity of juvenile hemangioendothelioma should not lead to an overdiagnosis of malignancy.

and covered with tiny wrinkles, and it eventually disappears completely.[999,1017]

Other locations for this lesion include the salivary gland and breast. Microscopically, the lesion exhibits a vaguely lobular configuration on low-power examination (Fig. 25.110). Masses of closely packed spindle cells are seen with neoformed spaces that contain little blood (Fig. 25.111). Mitotic figures are usually present and can be numerous. At the periphery, the tumor may be seen to invade subcutaneous tissue or skeletal muscle. Perineurial involvement has also been observed[990,1022] (Fig. 25.112). Mast cells may be numerous.[996]

Ultrastructurally and immunohistochemically, most of the cells have the features of endothelial cells, including positivity for FVIII-RA, CD31, CD34, FLI-1, estrogen receptor beta, annexin II (ANX2, a cell surface receptor for angiostatin), and LMO2 (a transcription factor involved in vascular and hematopoietic development).[997,1004,1030,1037] Interestingly, these cells also exhibit myeloid markers, such as CD83, CD32, CD14, and CD15.[1025] The issue whether they also express lymph vessel-type markers, such as LYVE-1, remains controversial.[994,1019] Hemangiomas also have a component of pericytes/smooth muscle cells and fibroblasts.[1003,1009,1029,1031]

Kaposi-like or kaposiform hemangioendothelioma is a distinct type of benign hemangioendothelioma with an appearance that closely simulates Kaposi sarcoma, as indicated by its name.[1014] It is usually located in the retroperitoneum or deep soft tissue of the extremities and is often associated with thrombocytopenia and hemorrhage (Kasabach–Merritt syndrome).[993,1001,1032,1038] It is seen mainly in infants and children, but it can also occur in adults.[1016] Microscopically, highly cellular nodules of compressed vessels resembling those seen in conventional benign hemangioendothelioma and Kaposi sarcoma are seen admixed with variously sized lymph vessels.[1014] Immunohistochemically, the endothelial cells are reactive for CD31, CD34, and FLI-1.[1014] In contrast to Kaposi sarcoma, kaposiform hemangioendothelioma is not associated with HHV8.[1014] In contrast to the usual type of benign (juvenile) hemangioendothelioma, it is negative for Glut-1 and Lewis Y antigen,[1014] but positive for D2-40.[995] Involvement of regional nodes has been documented, but not distant metastases.[1014]

Cavernous hemangiomas are composed of larger vessels with cystically dilated lumina and thin walls. Those occurring in the skin are traditionally known as *port-wine nevus* or *nevus flammeus*. This lesion, which is present at birth, grows very slowly and in proportion to the growth of the patient; in time, it becomes nodular and soft. In contrast to the strawberry nevus, it does not regress spontaneously.[999] Large, deep cavernous hemangiomas may undergo thrombosis, ulceration, and infection (Fig. 25.113). The thrombi may be seen in various stages of organization and recanalization, the latter including papillary endothelial hyperplasia (Masson lesion). They can also be associated with thrombocytopenia and with intravascular coagulation, which are corrected by removal of the tumor.[1034] Cavernous hemangiomas containing dilated, interconnecting thin-walled channels with occasional pseudopapillary projections have been designated as *sinusoidal hemangiomas*[989] (Fig. 25.114).

Large-vessel hemangiomas may be composed of vessels with the structure of veins (*venous hemangiomas*) or a combination of veins and arteries (*racemose, cirsoid,* or *arteriovenous hemangiomas*).[1010] The structure of the vessel wall is often abnormal and not easily identifiable as arterial or venous. They occur in the back, gluteal region, thigh, and other sites; sometimes an entire extremity is involved. The association of varicose veins, (dysplastic) cutaneous hemangiomas, and soft tissue and bone hypertrophy is known as *Klippel–Trenaunay syndrome*.[1012,1013] Venous hemangiomas of the feet have been seen in patients with Turner syndrome.[1035] Thrombosis and

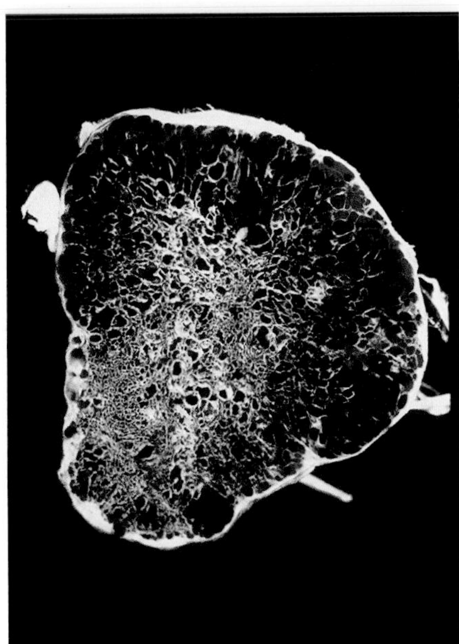

Fig. 25.113 Cavernous hemangioma of soft tissues of orbit.

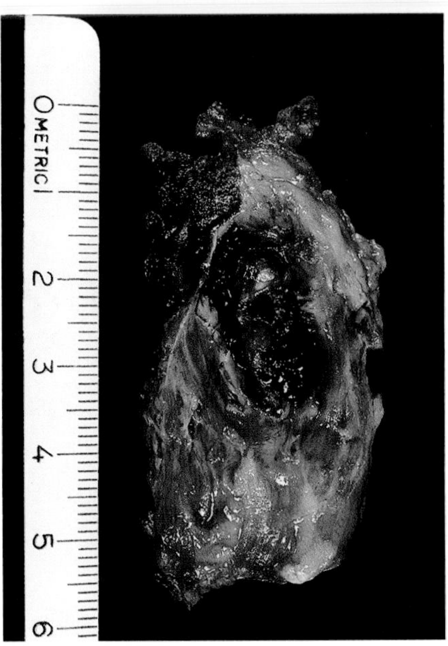

Fig. 25.115 Gross appearance of skeletal hemangioma.

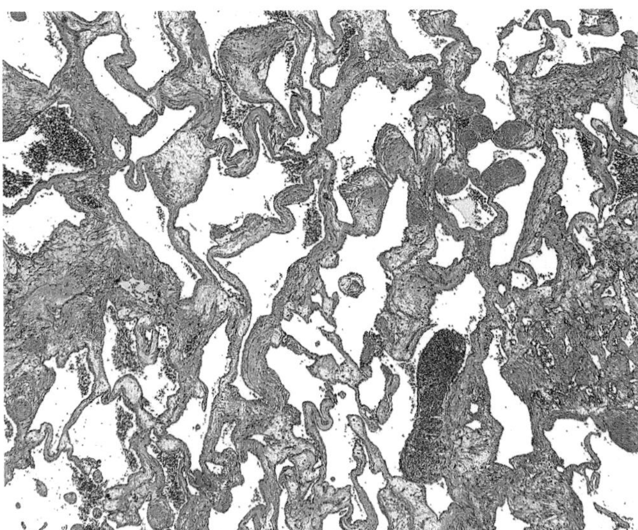

Fig. 25.114 Sinusoidal hemangioma. The vascular spaces are widely dilated.

calcification are common in large-vessel hemangiomas; the latter can be large enough to be detectable radiographically.

Skeletal muscle (intramuscular) hemangiomas usually have a venous or cavernous microscopic appearance[988] (Fig. 25.115). In other cases, they are very cellular, with plump nuclei, mitotic figures, intraluminal papillary projections, and even infiltration of perineurial spaces.[987] It should be remembered that bona fide angiosarcomas of skeletal muscle are exceptionally rare.

Intravascular papillary endothelial hyperplasia (Masson hemangioma or Masson lesion) is probably not a true neoplasm but is discussed here because of its capacity to simulate microscopically benign and malignant vascular tumors.[991,1011] First described by Masson in hemorrhoidal vessels as 'vegetant intravascular hemangioendothelioma', it is currently thought to represent an exuberant organization and recanalization of a thrombus, an interpretation supported by immunohistochemical studies.[986] It can occur in previously normal vessels or in varices, hemorrhoids, hematomas, pyogenic granulomas, hemangiomas, and angiosarcomas.[1011,1020,1023,1026] The de novo ('pure') form is usually found in the extremities (particularly the fingers) and the head and neck region, whereas the type engrafted on a preexisting vascular disorder ('mixed') tends to be in the trunk.[1006] It simulates angiosarcoma because of the presence of papillary formations, anastomosing vascular channels, and plump endothelial cells. It is identified because of the exclusively intravascular nature of the process; the lack of necrosis, bizarre cells, and atypical mitoses; the characteristically fibrinous and/or hyaline (deeply eosinophilic) appearance of the papillary stalks; and the frequent finding of residual organizing thrombi (Fig. 25.116).

Spindle cell hemangioma, a vascular tumor originally described as spindle cell hemangioendothelioma,[1036] may present at any age, has a male predominance, occurs preferentially in the dermis and subcutaneous tissue of the distal extremities, and combines histologically the features of cavernous hemangioma and Kaposi sarcoma[1021,1027,1033] (Fig. 25.117). The latter areas often have a component of epithelioid (histiocytoid) endothelial cells. The immunohistochemical features are those of endothelial cells.[1002] Development of recurrences or new lesions is common, but metastases have been documented in only one case, following repeated recurrences and radiation therapy.[1036] Some cases have occurred in patients with Maffucci or Klippel–Trenaunay syndrome.[998,1000] Variously described as a low-grade angiosarcoma[1036] and a non-neoplastic lesion related to a vascular malformation,[1000,1007] it is currently classified as a benign endothelial neoplasm.

Hobnail hemangioma[1005] is discussed in Chapter 4.

Glomus tumor

Glomus tumor, also known as *glomangioma,* originates in the neuromyoarterial glomus, a normal arteriovenous shunt abundantly supplied with nerve fibers and fulfilling a temperature-regulating function.[1057] The classic location of the glomus tumor is the subungual region, but it can occur elsewhere in the skin, soft tissues

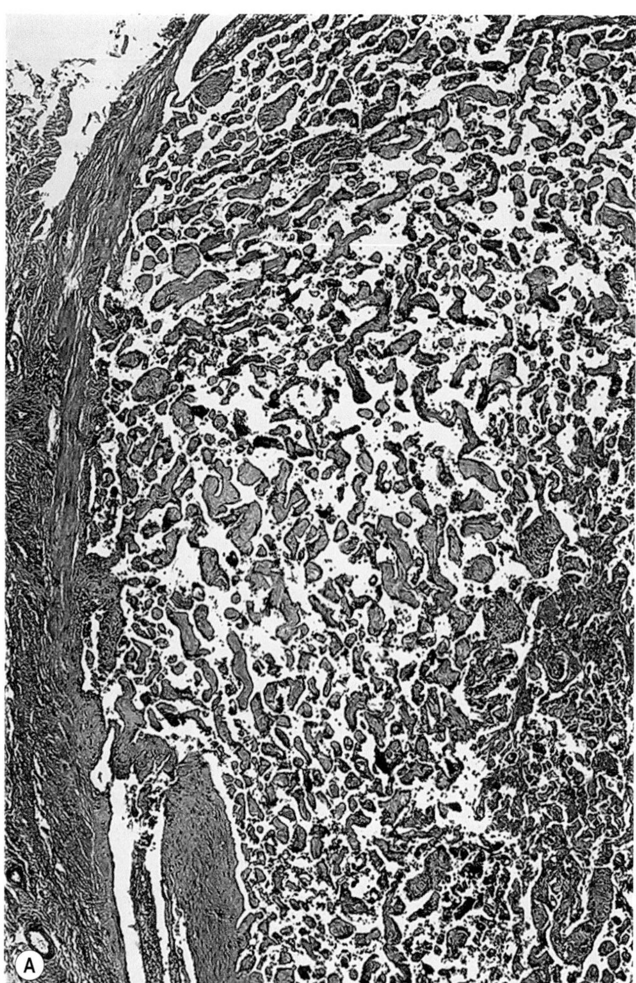

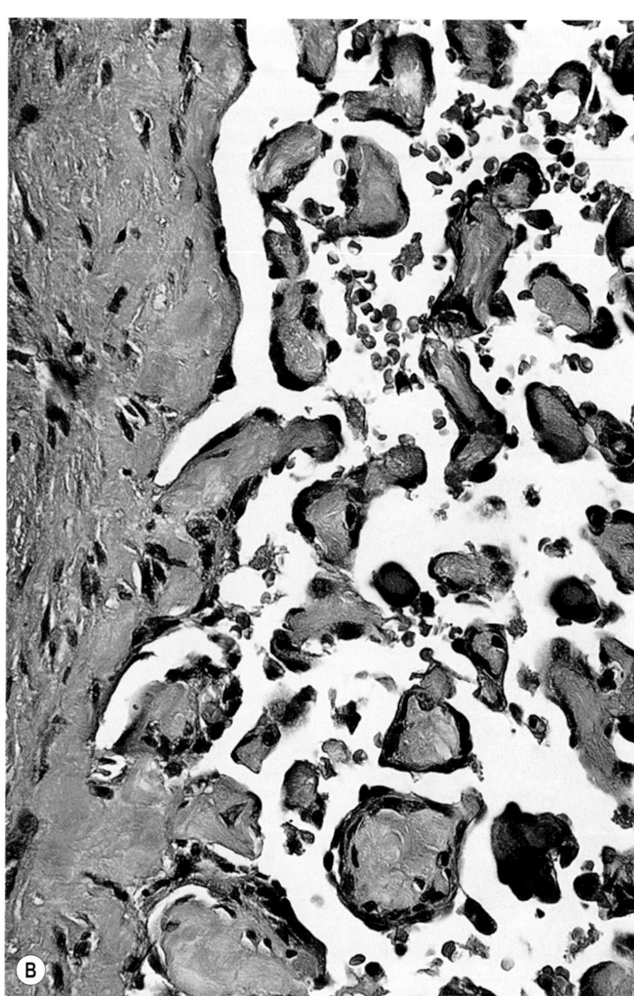

Fig. 25.116 **A** and **B**, Intravascular papillary endothelial hyperplasia. The confinement of the lesion to the vascular lumen and the hyaline core of the papillae are characteristic features.

(particularly in the flexor surface of the arms and about the knee), nerves, stomach (see Chapter 11), nasal cavity, and trachea.[1042,1043,1049,1057,1063] It has also been reported in the sacrococcygeal region, arising from the coccygeal body (glomus coccygeum) and associated with coccydynia,[1046] but there is some question as to whether this is a true neoplasm or simply a normal structure of this region.[1040,1041,1060]

Subungual lesions are always supplied by numerous nerve fibers and are exquisitely painful, two features often absent in glomus tumors arising elsewhere. The tumor may erode the terminal phalanx or even present as an intraosseous lesion in this location.[1054] Superficial lesions are well circumscribed. Glomus tumors in children tend to be multiple and of an infiltrative nature.[1053] They may present clinically as varicosities of the lower extremities.

Microscopically, glomus tumors consist of blood vessels lined by normal endothelial cells and surrounded by a solid proliferation of round or cuboidal 'epithelioid' cells with perfectly round nuclei and acidophilic cytoplasm (Fig. 25.118). As seen under an electron microscope, the tumor cells have features of smooth muscle rather than of pericytes.[1065] Immunohistochemically, they manifest reactivity for myosin, vimentin, actin, and basal lamina components but usually not for desmin[1044,1045,1056,1059] (Fig. 25.119). Numerous substance P-containing nerve fibers have been detected among the glomus cells.[1052]

Three microscopic types of glomus tumor have been recognized: *solid*, *angiomatous*, and *myxoid* [1055,1064] (Fig. 25.120). The solid type can be confused with sweat gland tumor, melanocytic nevus, or metastatic carcinoma.[1050] This is particularly the case when the tumor cells are very epithelioid and/or grow in an Indian-file fashion.[1061] The angiomatous type can have a diffuse quality, in the sense of looking like an angiomatosis with an increased number of glomus cells in the vessel wall[1047] (Fig. 25.121). An *oncocytic variant* of glomus tumor, in which the cytoplasm of the glomus cells is packed with mitochondria, has also been described.[1062] Often the tell-tale relationship between tumor cells and blood vessels can be clearly seen only at the very periphery of the neoplasm. Mast cells are common (Fig. 25.122).

On rare occasions, glomus tumors behave in an aggressive fashion, with local recurrences, invasion of adjacent structures and exceptionally even distant metastases.[1047,1048,1051] In other instances, lesions with the typical cytoarchitectural features of glomus tumor merge with a cytologically malignant tumor; these have been designated *glomangiosarcomas*.[1039,1048,1058]

There are also examples of cytologically atypical glomus tumors. A proposal has recently been made to subclassify these as symplastic, of uncertain malignant potential, and malignant.[1047] Those called malignant (the only ones to metastasize) were defined as glomus tumors with a deep location and a size of more than 2 cm,

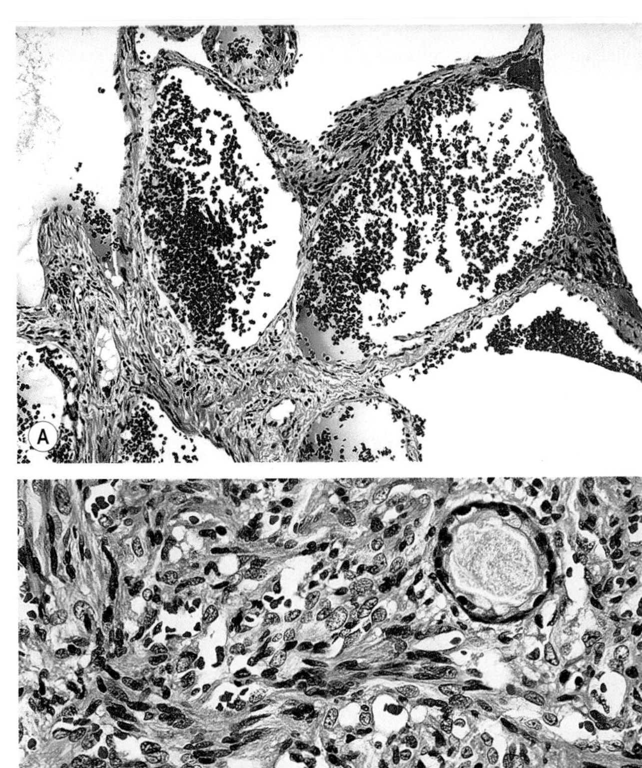

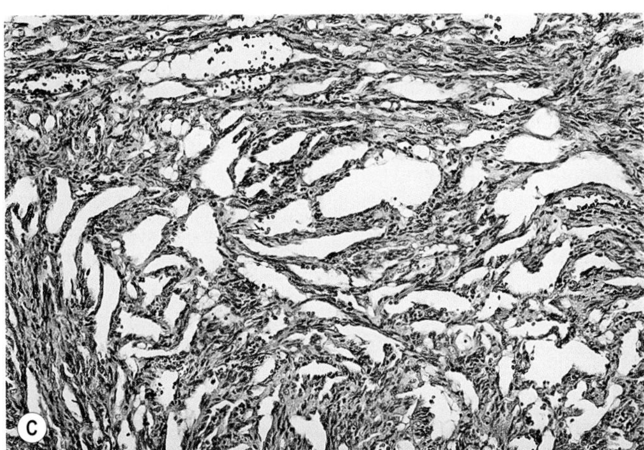

Fig. 25.117 Spindle cell hemangioendothelioma: **A**, cavernous hemangioma-like area; **B**, Kaposi sarcoma-like area; **C**, characteristic 'spongy' low-power appearance.

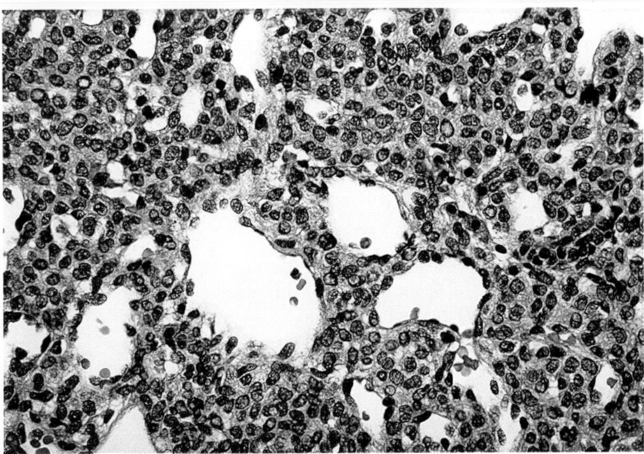

Fig. 25.118 Glomus tumor. The distribution of round glomus cells around the open vascular lumen is a key to the diagnosis.

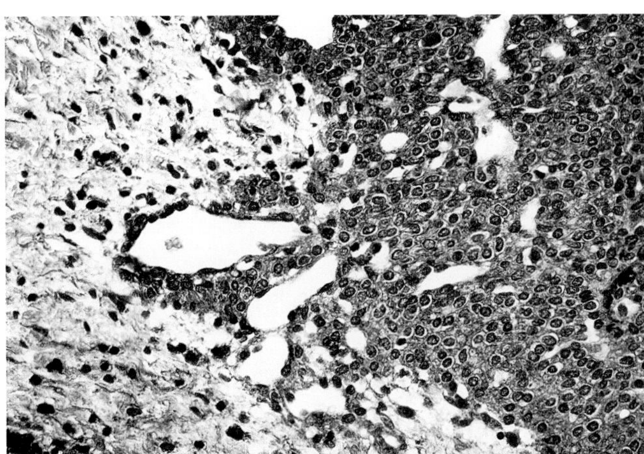

Fig. 25.119 Immunoreactivity for smooth muscle actin in glomus tumor.

or atypical mitotic figures, or moderate to high nuclear grade and five or more mitoses per 50 high-power fields.[1047] These malignant glomus tumors overlap considerably with the malignant myopericytomas mentioned in the next section.

Hemangiopericytoma

Stout originally defined hemangiopericytoma as a tumor of Zimmerman pericytes.[1076] The concept proved controversial from its inception and has been under heavy attack in recent times.[1067] There is no question that the term has been abused and that a large variety of tumor types have been inappropriately placed under this rubric, as Stout himself decried.[1077] At the same time, we believe that the concept is theoretically sound and that it could be rescued if the following considerations were accepted:

1 There is a family of tumor types composed of cells with pericytic features, which blend on one side with vascular smooth muscle cells and on the other with vascular glomus cells. Parenthetically, this was Stout's original contention, in that he considered hemangiopericytoma a less organoid type of glomus tumor. This tumor is usually found in the soft tissues of the extremities (usually distal), tends to have a multinodular pattern of growth, and can be multiple (Fig. 25.123). The most typical cases we have seen have presented as multinodular growths around the ankle of young adults.[1071] Depending on some variations of their microscopic appearance along the pericytic/smooth muscle/glomus cell lines, and in order to avoid the persisting confusion surrounding the generic term hemangiopericytoma, it has been proposed that this tumor be subdivided into (and renamed) glomangiopericytoma, myopericytoma, and adult myofibromatosis.[1070,1074] This is fine, as long as one realizes

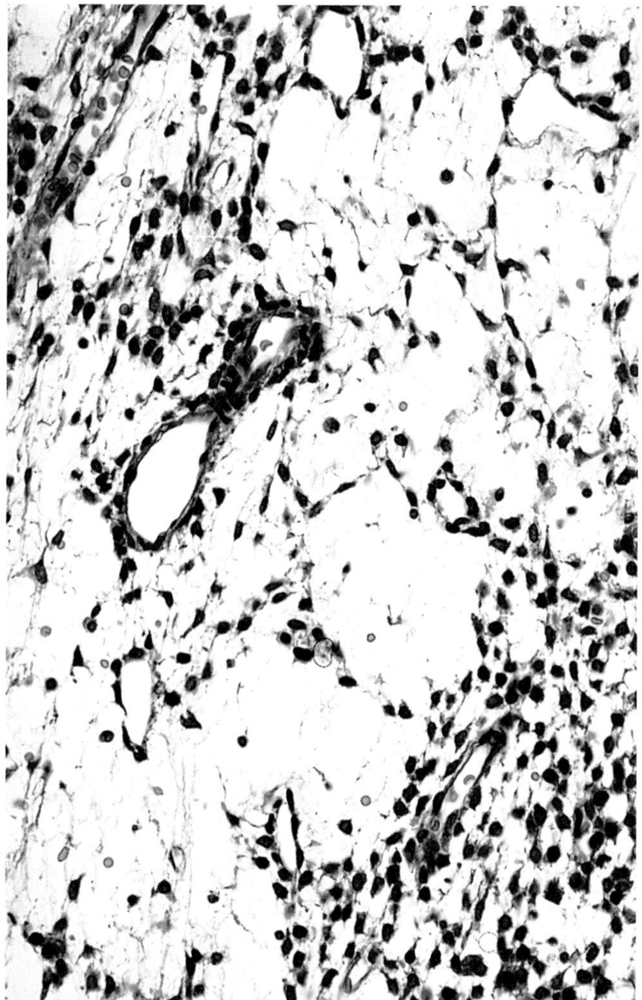

Fig. 25.120 Glomus tumor showing prominent secondary edematous changes.

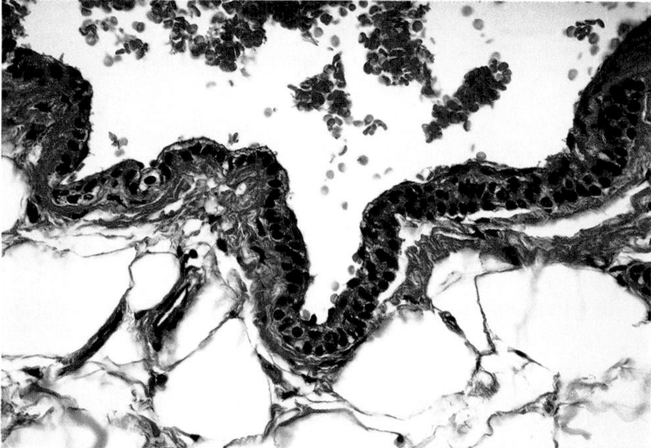

Fig. 25.121 Angiomatous type of glomus tumor. The appearance is somewhat similar to that of a cavernous hemangioma, but the dilated vessel contains a continuous layer of glomus cells.

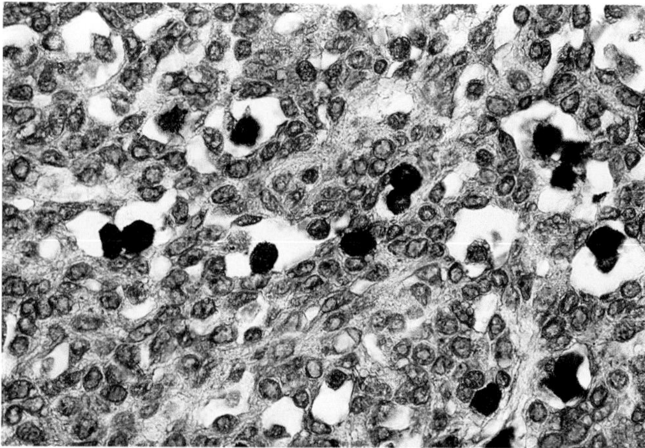

Fig. 25.122 Numerous mast cells in glomus tumor demonstrated with a metachromatic stain (toluidine blue).

that this tumor complex comes very close to Stout's original concept of hemangiopericytoma. The natural history of these lesions is characterized by a tendency to local recurrence, not surprising in view of their multinodular pattern of growth. Metastasizing examples are also on record.[1073] Myopericytomas that occur in the setting of immunodeficiency are associated with EBV.[1072]

2 The other large major category that Stout, in later papers and perhaps inappropriately, included in the category of hemangiopericytoma is that currently designated as solitary fibrous tumor, the main reason being the presence of branching vessels with a staghorn appearance[1068,1069] (Fig. 25.124). Most of these tumors are found in the pleural space, peritoneal cavity (particularly pelvis), and orbit, but can occur in many other sites and can be benign or malignant. There is no evidence that the cells of this tumor are related to pericytes. These considerations also apply to myxoid hemangiopericytoma (Fig. 25.125) and to the tumor recently described as lipomatous hemangiopericytoma (which for all practical purposes can be considered a fat-containing solitary fibrous tumor),[1075] and to most cases of so-called 'angioblastic meningioma' (to be regarded as solitary fibrous tumor of the meninges, see Chapter 28).[1066]

3 There are many other tumor types that can have a hemangiopericytoma-like pattern of growth similar to that described in the preceding paragraph, most but not all of them of malignant mesenchymal nature.[1078] They include: synovial sarcoma (particularly the monophasic variant); MPNST; mesenchymal chondrosarcoma (which also contains areas of relatively mature cartilage); so-called 'phosphaturic mesenchymal tumor' (in which the hemangiopericytoma-like areas are associated with osteoclast-like cells, cartilage, and other patterns, see p. 2189); infantile fibrosarcoma; and even thymoma (which will exhibit epithelial markers at the immunohistochemical and ultrastructural level) (Fig. 25.126).

Hemangioendothelioma

The term *hemangioendothelioma* has been used over the years for both benign and malignant vascular tumors composed of endothelial cells, and therefore lacks specificity. Currently, its preferred use is for vascular tumors of an endothelial nature that occupy

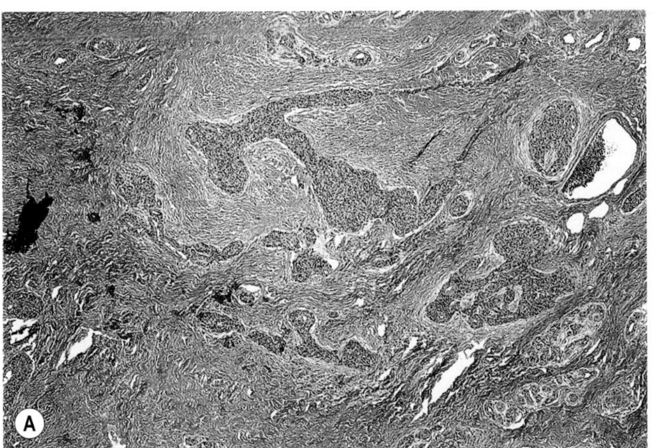

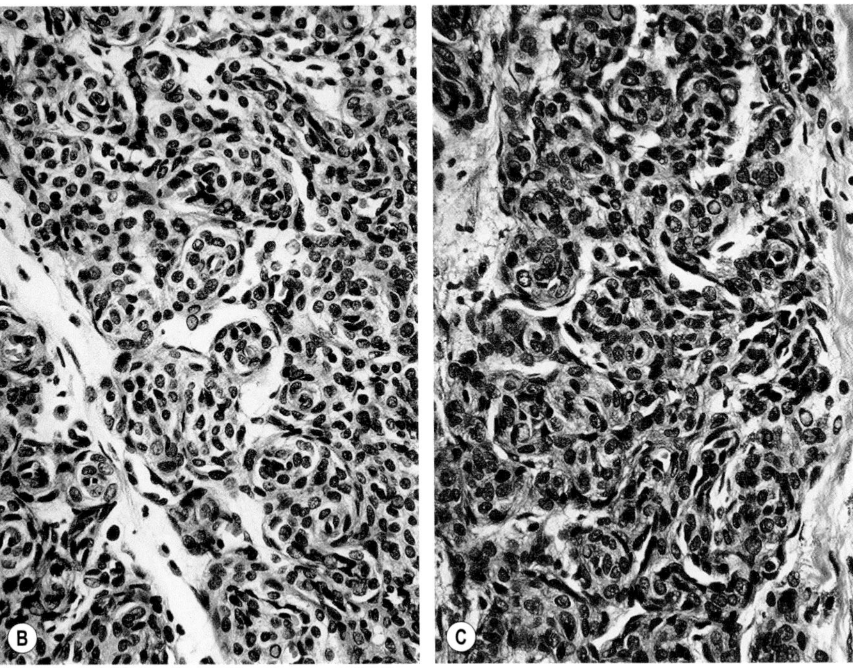

Fig. 25.123 A–C, Tumor of soft tissues of the ankle showing hybrid features between glomus tumor and hemangiopericytoma. **A**, Characteristic multinodular quality as seen on low power. **B** and **C**, High-power view showing a cytologic appearance intermediate between that of glomus cells and pericytes.

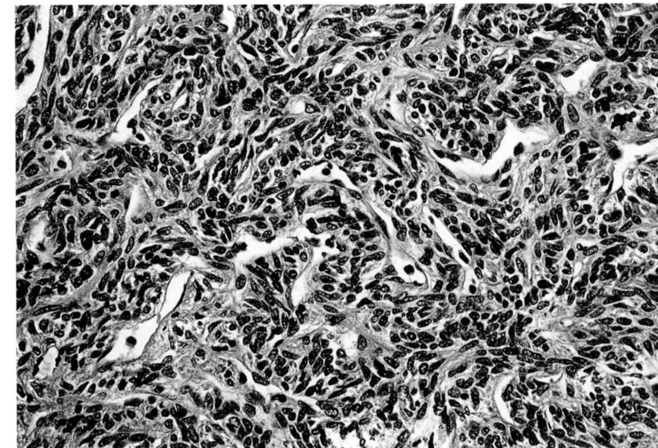

Fig. 25.124 This lesion, traditionally included among the hemangiopericytomas, is now regarded as a solitary fibrous tumor.

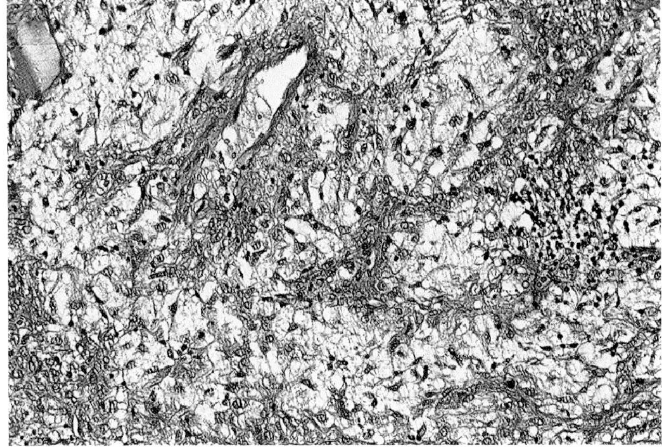

Fig. 25.125 So-called 'myxoid hemangiopericytoma'. This neoplasm should probably be viewed as a myxoid variant of solitary fibrous tumor.

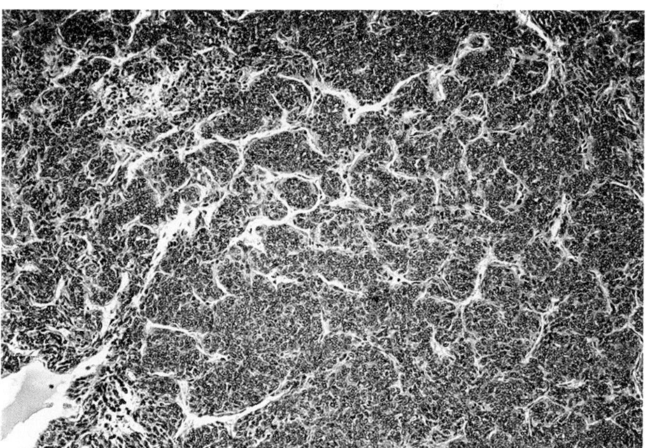

Fig. 25.126 Hemangiopericytoma-like pattern in thymoma.

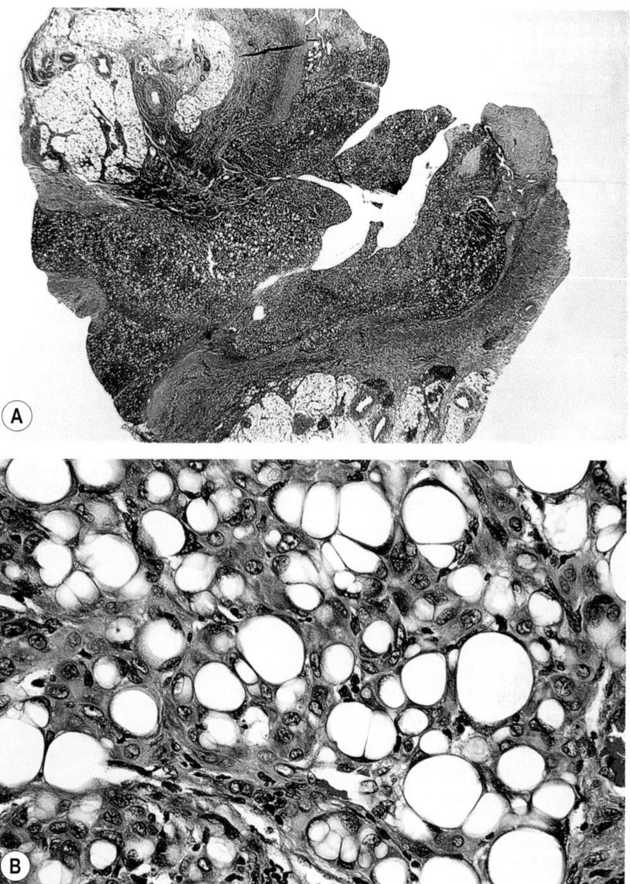

Fig. 25.127 **A** and **B**, Epithelioid hemangioendothelioma. **A**, The tumor partially fills the lumen of the femoral vein. **B**, Prominent cytoplasmic vacuolization is apparent on high-power examination of the same case.

(Courtesy of Dr Antonio Cubilla, Asunción, Paraguay)

an *intermediate* position between the benign hemangioma and the full-blown angiosarcoma.[1080,1084] Because of the possibility of misunderstanding, it is better to always use the term with one of the qualifiers that follow.

Epithelioid hemangioendothelioma is composed of a distinctive type of endothelial cells having an epithelial-like or histiocyte-like appearance. The cytoplasm is abundant and eosinophilic, often vacuolated. The nucleus is round, vesicular, and occasionally indented. Vascular lumina are present, most of them small; some are located intracellularly and are responsible for the cytoplasmic vacuolation (Fig. 25.127). Mitoses, pleomorphism, and necrosis are variable but usually scanty or absent. An inflammatory infiltrate is often present at the periphery; this may contain well-formed germinal centers and/or a large number of eosinophils. The stroma may be scanty or have a prominent myxoid appearance. Osteoclast-like multinucleated giant cells may be present.[1103] The endothelial nature of the tumor cells has been confirmed ultrastructurally and immunohistochemically. The acidophilic staining quality of the cytoplasm is due to the presence of packed intermediate filaments of vimentin type.

Tumors with this set of morphologic features have been described in a large number of sites, including skin, bone, lung, pleura, liver, peritoneum, and lymph nodes.[1104] Those located in the soft tissue are seen in adults and often arise from the wall of a vein in an extremity.[1080,1101,1102] They also occur in the head and neck area.[1085] Local recurrences and distant metastases can develop, but the prognosis remains better than for angiosarcoma of either the conventional or epithelioid type (see below).[1093] Mitotic activity and tumor size are associated with increased clinical aggressivity.[1084]

Epithelioid hemangioendothelioma is one of several related proliferative lesions of endothelial cells having as a common denominator an epithelioid or histiocytoid morphology, often accompanied by immunoreactivity for keratin.[1090] These were originally embraced under the generic category of *histiocytoid hemangioma*,[1079,1082,1097] but it has become clear that lesions composed of epithelioid (histiocytoid) cells can be present in infectious processes (such as Peruvian verruca and bacillary angiomatosis), in the skin disorder of unknown pathogenesis traditionally known as angiolymphoid hyperplasia with eosinophilia (also designated as epithelioid hemangioma), in the low-grade neoplasm described here, and in the fully malignant epithelioid angiosarcoma (see next section).[1087,1098] Despite early statements to the contrary, Kimura disease as seen more commonly in the Orient does not seem to belong to this group.[1100]

A morphologically distinct subtype of epithelioid hemangioendothelioma is characterized by a marked histologic resemblance to epithelioid sarcoma, to the point of having been named *epithelioid sarcoma-like hemangioendothelioma*.[1081] One of the clues to the diagnosis is the presence of cytoplasmic vacuoles consistent with intracytoplasmic vascular lumen formation. Immunohistochemically, the tumor cells are reactive for keratin, vimentin, CD31, and FLI-1, but not CD34.[1081] The existence of this tumor makes one wonder about the nature of classic epithelioid sarcoma, which could conceivably represent the extreme form of epithelioid transformation of an endothelial vascular neoplasm. A recurrent chromosomal aberration t(1;3)(p36.3;q25) is recognized, but other chromosomal translocations and aberrations have also been reported.[1091,1092,1099]

Malignant endovascular papillary angioendothelioma (Dabska tumor; papillary intralymphatic angioendothelioma) is an extremely rare but distinctive tumor usually seen in children but also reported in adults, located in the skin or soft tissues and characterized by papillary tufts that are lined by plump endothelial cells located within dilated vascular lumina, some of which have a glomeruloid configuration (Fig. 25.128). Many of the tumor cells have epithelioid or histiocytoid features, including cytoplasmic eosinophilia and vacuolation. There may be an associated lymphedema.[1089] The lesion has a uniformly good prognosis, although nodal metastases have occurred in a few instances.[1083,1086,1094,1096]

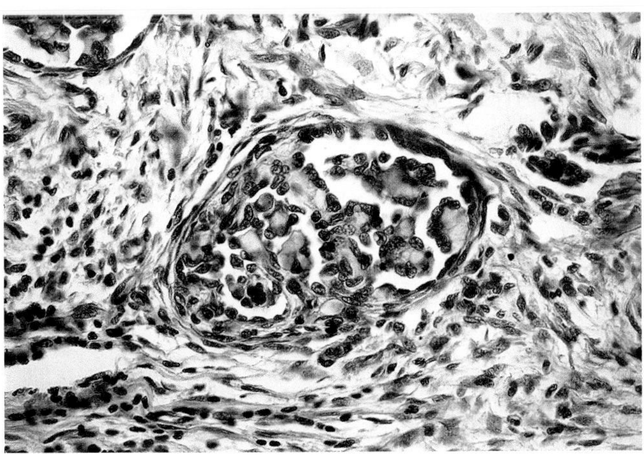

Fig. 25.128 Malignant endovascular papillary angioendothelioma (Dabska tumor). The papillary configuration of the endothelial fronds can be appreciated.

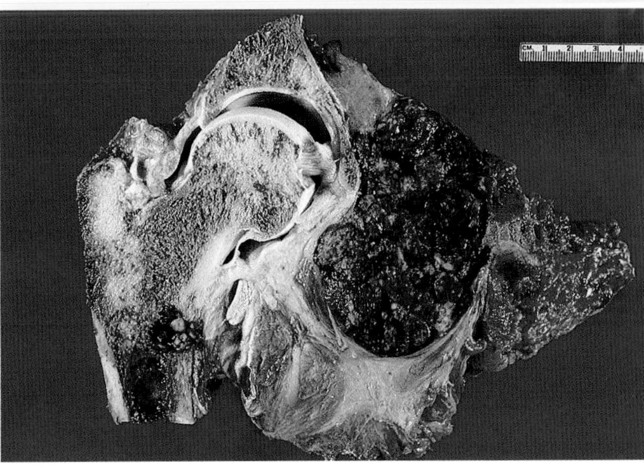

Fig. 25.129 Gross hemorrhagic appearance of angiosarcoma in the region of the hip.

Retiform hemangioendothelioma. See Chapter 4.

Composite hemangioendothelioma is the name that has been proposed for a vascular neoplasm showing various combinations of benign, low-grade malignant, and malignant components.[1088,1095] The two most common patterns are those of epithelioid and retiform hemangioendothelioma. This probably does not represent a specific entity but rather the manifestation of the fact that there is a great deal of overlap between the seemingly endless number of types and subtypes of vascular tumors that are being described.

Angiosarcoma

The term *angiosarcoma,* if used without adjectives or prefixes, refers to a malignant neoplasm arising from the *endothelial cells of blood vessels,* and is therefore synonymous with malignant hemangioendothelioma.[1129,1133] It is usually seen in adults and the elderly, but it can also occur in children.[1112] The most common locations are the skin, soft tissue, breast, bone, liver, and spleen. Some soft tissue angiosarcomas arise from major vessels, such as the inferior vena cava, pulmonary artery, or aorta.[1105,1121] These tend to have a very undifferentiated appearance and a solid pattern of growth,[1134] to such an extent that they may not be identifiable as being of endothelial nature.[1107,1108] Accordingly, topographic terms such as intimal sarcoma, luminal sarcoma, and arterial/venous trunk sarcoma have been used for them.[1113,1121]

Angiosarcomas have been reported in previously irradiated fields,[1111,1125] around long-standing foreign bodies,[1116,1118] in arteriovenous fistulas[1109] (including surgically constructed ones),[1132] as a secondary somatic-type development in mediastinal or retroperitoneal germ cell tumors,[1130] or arising within preexisting benign tumors, such as hemangioma/vascular malformation, neurofibroma, intramuscular lipoma, or leiomyoma.[1110,1124,1128,1135]

Grossly, angiosarcomas tend to be highly hemorrhagic and deeply invasive (Fig. 25.129). Their microscopic appearance ranges from a pattern so well differentiated as to simulate a benign hemangioma to one so undifferentiated and solid as to simulate carcinoma, malignant melanoma, or other types of sarcoma.[1123] The diagnostic areas of angiosarcoma are represented by the freely anastomosing vascular channels lined by atypical endothelial cells (Fig. 25.130), a pattern that is accentuated by silver reticulin stains or immunostains for basement membrane components.[1127] Clusters of reactive lymphocytes and clumps of hemosiderin are common.

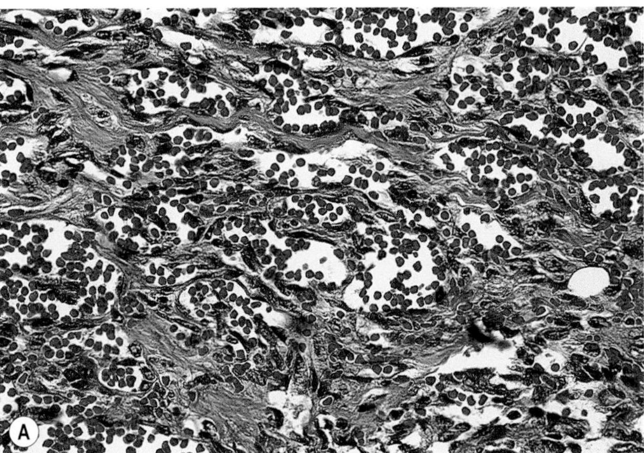

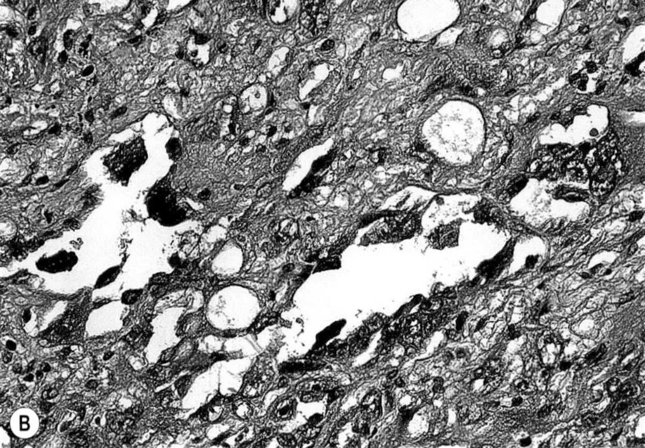

Fig. 25.130 **A** and **B**, Angiosarcoma of mediastinal soft tissues. **A**, Anastomosing vascular channels. **B**, On high power, the channels are seen to be lined by highly atypical endothelial cells.

Variations in the appearance of the neoplastic endothelial cells are great. Their shape ranges from very elongated to plump and epithelioid, and their size from small to giant, with occasional development of multinucleated forms[1114] (Fig. 25.131). The latter are sometimes seen to display prominent hyaline globules containing α_1-antitrypsin and α_1-antichymotrypsin.[1131] In rare cases, foci of

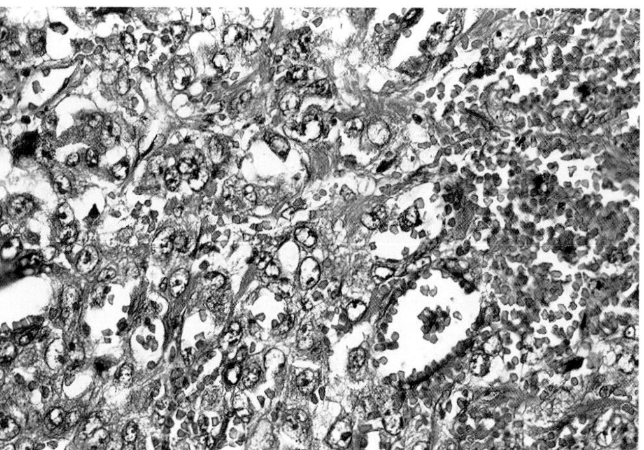

Fig. 25.131 Epithelioid angiosarcoma arising from the region of the seminal vesicle.

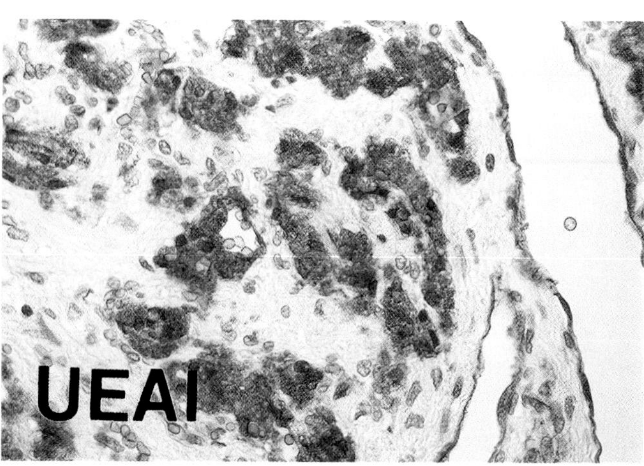

Fig. 25.132 *Ulex europaeus* lectin I reactivity in angiosarcoma.

granular cells similar to those seen in granular cell tumors are present.[1122] The predominantly epithelioid appearance of the neoplastic endothelial cells can also be seen in the primarily intraluminal ('intimal') tumors of large vessels.[1117]

The differential diagnosis of angiosarcoma includes hemangioma for the better differentiated lesions, Kaposi sarcoma for those with a predominantly spindle component, and carcinoma or amelanotic melanoma for the poorly differentiated types. Metastatic renal cell carcinoma, because of its high degree of vascularity, is particularly notorious for its ability to simulate angiosarcoma; in this regard, it should be kept in mind that clear tumor cells are not a feature of angiosarcoma.

Immunohistochemically and ultrastructurally, various endothelial markers can be demonstrated depending on the degree of differentiation[1119] (Fig. 25.132); of these, CD31 and FLI-1 are the most reliable. In some cases (particularly the epithelioid variant) there is coexpression of keratin.[1106,1114] In other cases there is expression of D2-40, suggesting differentiation toward lymph vessel endothelial cells.[1126]

A well-defined clinicopathologic form of angiosarcoma involves the head and neck region (particularly the scalp) of elderly individuals. It begins in the skin but often extends into the subcutis. The clinical course includes repeated local occurrences over a long period of time, followed in some cases by lymph node and pulmonary metastases.[1115,1120,1127]

Neoplastic angioendotheliomatosis, once regarded as a form of multicentric angiosarcoma, is now viewed as a type of malignant lymphoma with a particular tropism for vascular lumina; this entity is discussed in Chapter 4.

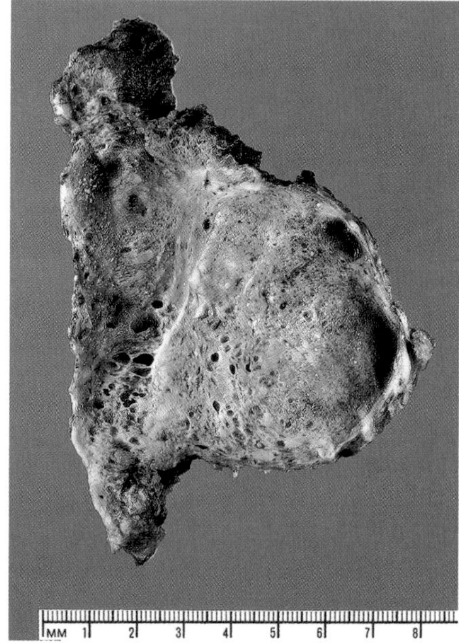

Fig. 25.133 Cavernous lymphangioma.
(Courtesy of Dr RA Cooke, Brisbane, Australia; from Cooke RA, Stewart B. Colour atlas of anatomical pathology. Edinburgh, 2004, Churchill Livingstone)

Lymphangioma and lymphangiomyoma

Most **lymphangiomas** represent malformations rather than true neoplasms and are thought to result from failure of the lymphatic system to communicate with the venous system.[1140,1162] Three forms exist: *capillary*, *cavernous*, and *cystic* (Fig. 25.133). The capillary form occurs in the skin, whereas the cavernous variety prefers deep soft tissues. Cystic lymphangioma has been traditionally known as *hygroma*. Its most common presentation is in the form of a poorly defined soft tissue mass in the neck of children, usually situated posterior to the sternocleidomastoid muscle and sometimes extending into the mediastinum (Figs 25.134 and 25.135). Those developing in utero often progress to hydrops and cause fetal death. Many of the fetuses have karyotypes consistent with Turner syndrome[1137,1140] or other chromosomal abnormalities. Some lymphangiomas are diffuse and/or multicentric, the condition being designated as *lymphangiomatosis*. These cases may be limited to the soft tissues or be accompanied by osseous and/or visceral manifestations.[1160] A preferred location is the thoracic cavity, with resulting chylous pleural effusion and/or chylopericardium.[1138] Other cases affect diffusely the extremities.[1148]

Microscopically, lymphangioma consists of large lymphatic channels growing in loose connective tissue (Fig. 25.136). A few disorganized bundles of smooth muscle can be present in the wall of the larger channels. Focal areas of papillary endothelial proliferation similar to those described by Masson in blood vessels are sometimes found.[1156] Large collections of lymphocytes may be present in the stroma and cause mistakes in interpretation. Lymphangioma practically never becomes malignant and is curable by excision.[1150]

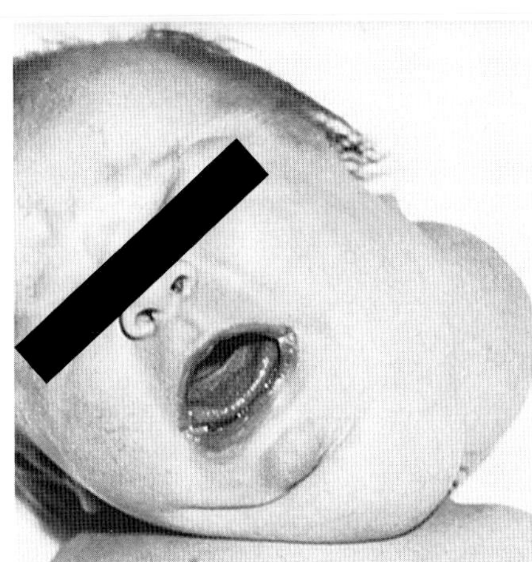

Fig. 25.134 Large cystic hygroma in an infant.
*(From Maxwell JH. Tumors of the face and neck in infancy and childhood. South Med J 1952, **45:** 292–299)*

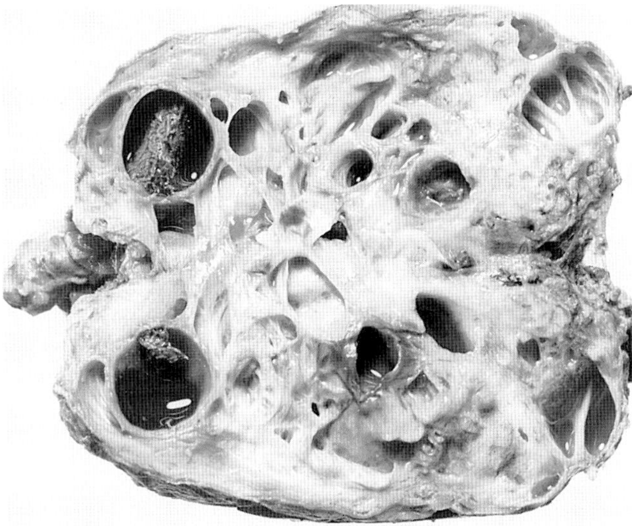

Fig. 25.135 Large cystic hygroma in the neck of an 18-month-old infant. The tumor extended into the superior portion of the mediastinum.

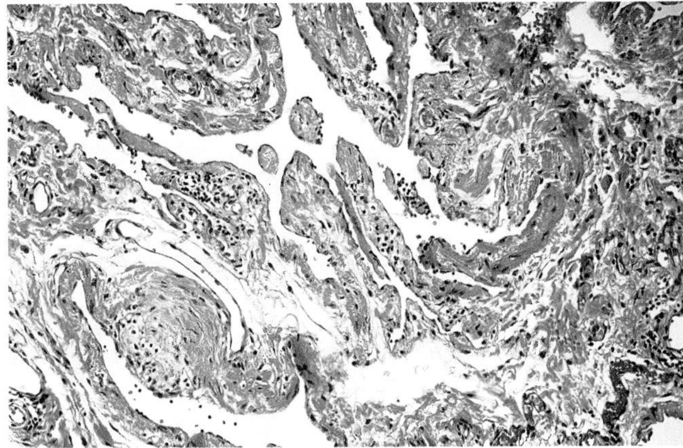

Fig. 25.136 Lymphangioma of soft tissue showing dilated spaces lined by flattened endothelium. A scattering of lymphocytes is present in the stroma.

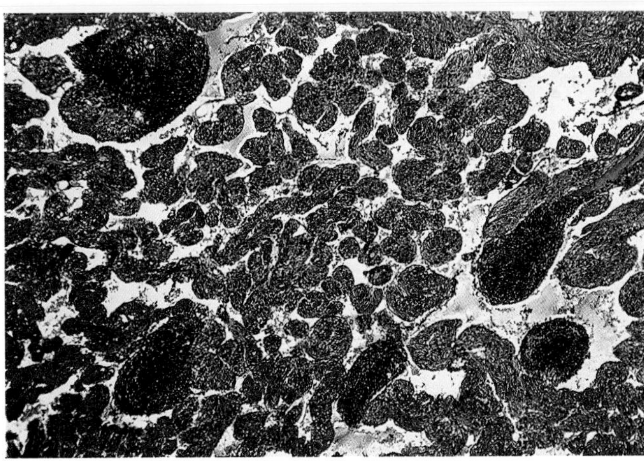

Fig. 25.137 Microscopic appearance of lymphangioma.

The variant of cutaneous lymphangioma originally named acquired progressive lymphangioma and recently redesignated benign lymphangioendothelioma[1151] is discussed in Chapter 4.

Lymphangiomyoma is the preferred term for a benign neoplasm seen exclusively in females and originally described as lymphangiopericytoma.[1143,1164] The localized form is restricted to the mediastinum and retroperitoneum. It is often seen in close association with the thoracic duct and its tributaries, and often results in chylothorax.[1141] Chylous ascites and chyluria (secondary to ureteral wall involvement) may also be present. The diffuse form of the disease, known as *lymphangio(leio)myomatosis*, typically involves the lung[1161] (see Chapter 7).

Microscopically, there is a proliferation of intimately mingled lymph vessels and smooth muscle elements (Fig. 25.137). Immunohistochemically, the lining cells show lymph vessel markers such as D2-40,[1152] whereas the tumor cells (which are plumper and paler than those of ordinary leiomyomas) are reactive for actin, desmin, HMB-45, and other melanocytic markers, such as MiTF, tyrosinase, and melan-A.[1139] This profile (particularly the HMB-45 immunoreactivity), plus their occurrence in patients with the tuberous sclerosis complex,[1155] links these tumors with renal and extrarenal angiomyolipomas (including their epithelioid and monotypic variants), pulmonary clear cell ('sugar') tumor, clear cell myomelanocytic tumor,[1144,1145] and other neoplasms into the continuously enlarging **PEComa** concept.[1154] Indeed, cases are increasingly being reported of primary **angiomyolipomas** and **PEComas** of soft tissue of both benign and malignant nature.[1146,1153,1157,1163] Their histogenesis (whether mesenchymal or neural) remains controversial. The consistent lack of reactivity for Sox10 (a neuroectodermal stem cell marker) speaks against a neural derivation,[1147] whereas the common expression of TFE3 (a DNA-binding factor closely linked to MiTF) suggests a perplexing partnership with alveolar soft part sarcoma and some types of renal cell carcinoma.[1142]

Although immunohistochemical evaluation of hormone receptors in lymphangiomyoma/lymphangiomyomatosis has resulted in conflicting findings,[1149,1159] good therapeutic results have been reported with progesterone therapy[1158] or oophorectomy.[1136]

Lymphangiosarcoma and related lesions

Lymphangiosarcoma is regarded as the lymph vessel counterpart of angiosarcoma, the latter term implying – when used without a qualifier – an origin from blood vessels.[1173] The cutaneous examples of lymphangiosarcoma, which are the most common, present

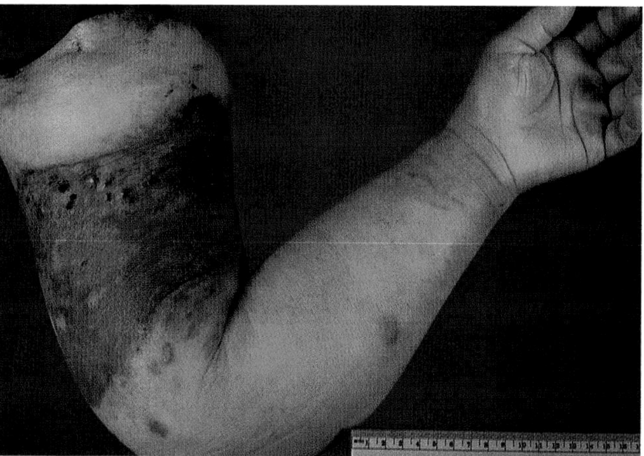

Fig. 25.138 Amputated upper extremity in a case of post-mastectomy lymphangiosarcoma.

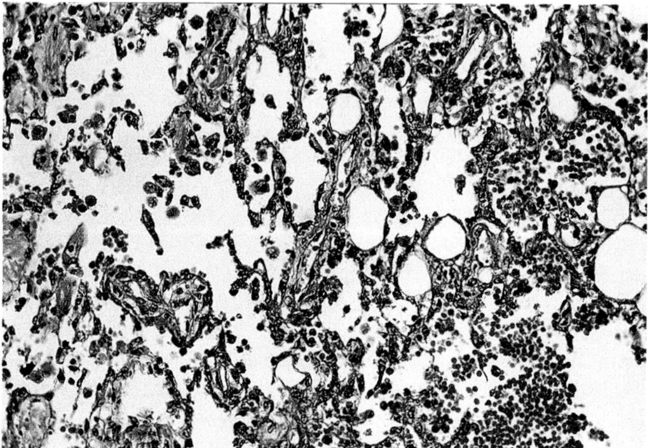

Fig. 25.139 Post-mastectomy lymphangiosarcoma showing an intricate network of neoplastic vessels.

clinically as bluish or purple elevations. They are often multiple, although in late stages they coalesce to form a large hemorrhagic mass (Fig. 25.138). Microscopically, they show a wide variation of patterns, ranging from solid undifferentiated areas that can simulate carcinoma[1170] to others so well differentiated as to be indistinguishable from lymphangioma or lymphangiectasia (Fig. 25.139). As in the case of (hem)angiosarcoma, the most typical areas are represented by freely anastomosing channels lined by atypical endothelial cells. Ultrastructural and immunohistochemical studies have not only documented the presence of endothelial markers such as D2-40,[1169] but have also shown that some of these tumors differentiate in the direction of blood vessels rather than lymph vessels.[1165,1172,1174]

The behavior of full-blown lymphangiosarcoma is extremely malignant. In an often-quoted series of 129 patients, only 11 survived over 5 years.[1181]

Generally, the diagnosis of lymphangiosarcoma has been made in the presence of malignant vascular tumors superimposed on areas of chronic lymphedema, the prototypical example being the lymphangiosarcoma developing in patients who have had long-standing massive lymphedema after radical mastectomy for breast carcinoma (Stewart–Treves syndrome).[1175,1179,1180] The average interval is approximately 10 years. A pathogenetically analogous situation is the lymphangiosarcoma developing secondarily to chronic lymphedema of the lower leg.[1171,1176] In these instances, it is extremely difficult to detect the early neoplastic changes in the lymphangiectatic vessels, and all the pathologist can do is to indicate the presence of 'atypical vascular hyperplasia', which may be an indicator of early neoplasia or a preneoplastic process.

With the decrease in the number of radical mastectomies performed during the last few decades, and the corresponding increase in the number of conservative breast operations followed by radiation, the pattern of breast carcinoma-associated vascular proliferative processes has changed. The malignant tumors developing under these circumstances have similar morphologic features, but the interval from the time of therapy is generally shorter, the tumor is in the skin overlying the breast rather than in the arm, and there is no accompanying lymphedema.[1178] The matter is complicated by the fact that radiation therapy may also induce lymph vessel proliferations with the appearance of lymphangioma circumscriptum[1167] or progressive acquired lymphangioma.[1177] Furthermore, an increasingly large number of cases are being described of *atypical vascular lesions* in the skin of radiated breast.[1168] These lesions are characterized by dermal vascular proliferation and associated inflammation, but not enough architectural or cytologic atypia to justify a diagnosis of malignancy. Time will tell whether these are entirely benign lesions of reactive nature or whether they are the forerunners of angiosarcoma. Our own experience suggests that in some cases the latter is true, particularly when the lesions exhibit scattered hypercellular vascular lobules.[1166]

Hemangioblastoma

So-called hemangioblastoma, a tumor characteristically located in the central nervous system and linked with the von Hippel–Lindau syndrome, can occasionally involve other sites, including soft tissues.[1182,1183] Some of the reported cases have been anatomically associated with a peripheral nerve.[1184] As in the case for its more common CNS counterpart, the nature of the 'stromal cells' located in between the numerous vessels remains controversial. It is our impression that these 'stromal cells' can demonstrate a variety of phenotypes depending on the location.[1183]

Tumors of smooth muscle

Leiomyoma

Several types of leiomyoma exist. **Cutaneous leiomyomas** located in the dermis (also discussed in Chapter 4) arise from arrectores pilorum muscles; they are characteristically superficial, small, multiple, and grouped.

Genital leiomyomas are solitary tumors that arise from smooth muscle bundles located in the superficial subcutaneous tissue of genital areas and structures that are topographically and functionally related to them, such as the nipple, areola, axilla, scrotum, penis, vulvar labia, and anal skin.

Vascular leiomyomas (angioleiomyomas) arise from the smooth muscle of blood vessels. They occur more frequently in females and are usually located in the soft tissues of the lower limbs.[1189,1193,1195] They constitute, together with traumatic neuroma, glomus tumor, eccrine spiradenoma, and angiolipoma, the classic five spontaneously painful nodules of skin and soft tissues.

Grossly, vascular leiomyomas are yellow or yellowish pink, sharply circumscribed, and fairly firm (Fig. 25.140). Microscopically, they are made up of intersecting fascicles of smooth muscle cells encircling vascular lumina lined by normal endothelial cells

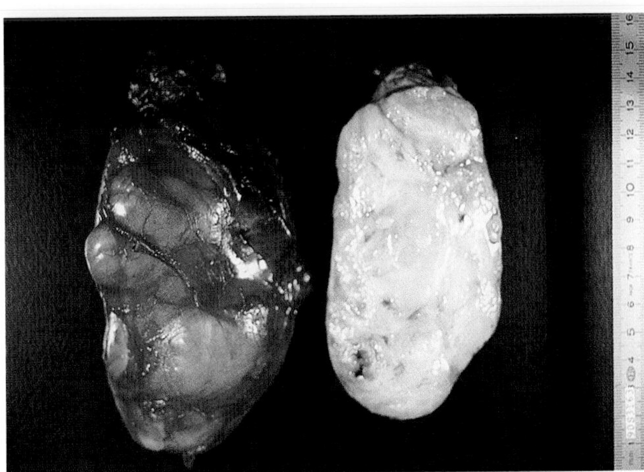

Fig. 25.140 Gross appearance of a soft tissue leiomyoma located in the leg of a child.

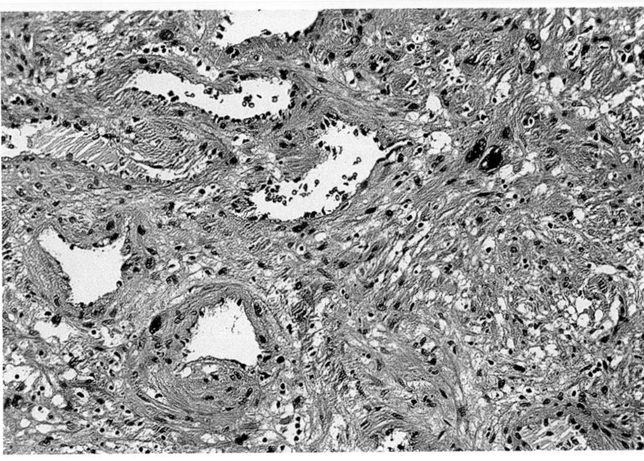

Fig. 25.142 Vascular leiomyoma with scattered bizarre tumor cells, a feature of no prognostic significance.

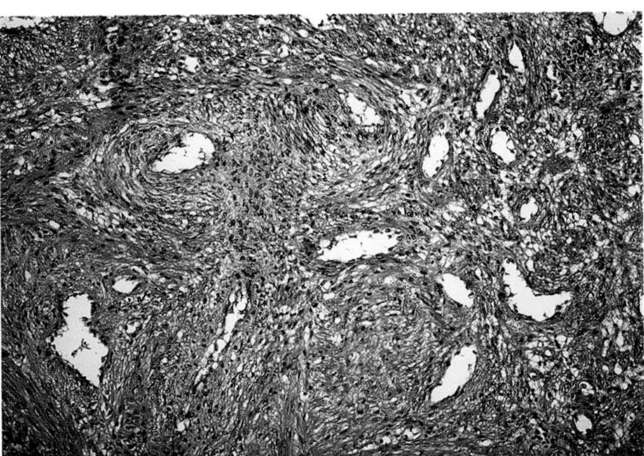

Fig. 25.141 Vascular leiomyoma. The neoplastic smooth muscle cells are clearly related to vessel walls.

(Fig. 25.141). The vascular organoid appearance resulting from this feature is marked, but the vascular elastic lamina is absent. Mitotic activity is absent, and there is no necrosis or hemorrhage. Foci of cartilaginous metaplasia may be present.[1191] Islands of mature fat may be present in between the smooth muscle fibers. Tumors composed of smooth muscle and adipose tissue (*myolipoma*) are discussed on page 2142. Occasionally, bizarre nuclear forms similar to those seen in uterine symplastic leiomyoma are encountered[1186] (Fig. 25.142). Vascular leiomyomas have been subdivided into capillary (solid), cavernous, and venous types;[1189] as already indicated, transitional forms with glomus tumor and hemangiopericytoma also occur, the latter known as myopericytomas.[1194]

The pain often associated with vascular leiomyomas is thought to be mediated by the nerves present within the tumor and in the capsule, whether by mechanical stretching or through mast cell mediation.[1187,1188,1190] The behavior of these tumors is benign. Their ultrastructure, immunohistochemistry, and differential diagnosis with leiomyosarcoma are discussed in connection with the latter.

Deep-seated leiomyomas of nonvascular type occur most commonly in the extremities;[1192] they can also be seen in the pelvic region of females (see Chapter 26).[1185]

Leiomyosarcoma

Leiomyosarcoma of soft tissue is relatively rare.[1202,1203,1205,1209] It is typically a tumor of adults and the elderly, although cases in children are on record.[1205,1243,1249] The leiomyosarcomas seen with increasing frequency in immunosuppressed patients (HIV-infected individuals and organ transplant recipients) have been found to be associated with the Epstein–Barr virus[1221,1225] (Fig. 25.143).

Most soft tissue leiomyosarcomas are located in the extremities, but they can occur anywhere, including the head and neck region.[1230] Many arise from the walls of arteries and veins of widely differing caliber, ranging from large ones (inferior vena cava, saphenous vein, femoral vein, pulmonary artery, femoral artery, and aorta, in that order of frequency) to venules and arterioles.[1213,1219,1220,1236] Those located in the inferior vena cava can result in Budd–Chiari syndrome.[1215]

Grossly, leiomyosarcomas can be as well circumscribed as the leiomyomas but are larger and softer and have a tendency for fresh tumor necrosis, hemorrhage, and cystic degeneration (Fig. 25.144). Those arising from major vessels can protrude in a polypoid fashion within the lumen[1198] or be predominantly intramural[1222] (Figs 25.145 and 25.146). The intraluminal growth can be demonstrated by phlebography or CT scanning.[1198]

Microscopically, the pattern of growth is predominantly fascicular, with the tumor bundles intersecting each other at wide angles. Merging of tumor cells with blood vessel walls is an important diagnostic clue (Fig. 25.147). In some cases the vascular pattern is particularly prominent, resulting in a hemangiopericytoma-like appearance. We regard these tumors as the malignant counterpart of vascular leiomyoma and have designated them *vascular leiomyosarcomas*[1245] (Fig. 25.148). The individual cells have elongated, blunt-ended nuclei and acidophilic fibrillary cytoplasm, features that are also apparent in cytologic preparations.[1203] Palisading of nuclei may occur, a feature that may cause confusion with peripheral nerve sheath tumors. The degree of nuclear atypia is highly variable; in extreme cases, it may result in an MFH-like picture.[1231] As a matter of fact, the most commonly demonstrable pattern of differentiation of soft tissue sarcomas with the morphologic appearance of MFH is toward smooth muscle lines.[1210,1212] Cytoplasmic vacuoles located at both ends of the nucleus, sometimes indenting them, represent another diagnostic clue. Focal granular changes can be present in the cytoplasm, approaching those seen in granular cell tumor.[1227,1232] Myxoid changes,[1238,1240] inflammatory changes ('inflammatory leiomyosarcoma'),[1201] and osteoclast-like

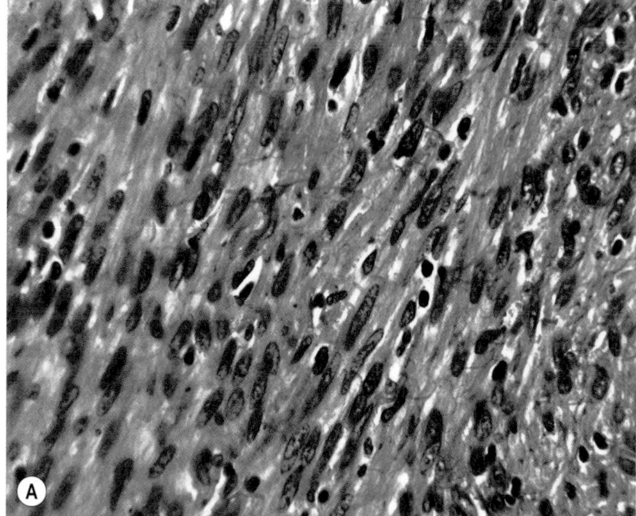

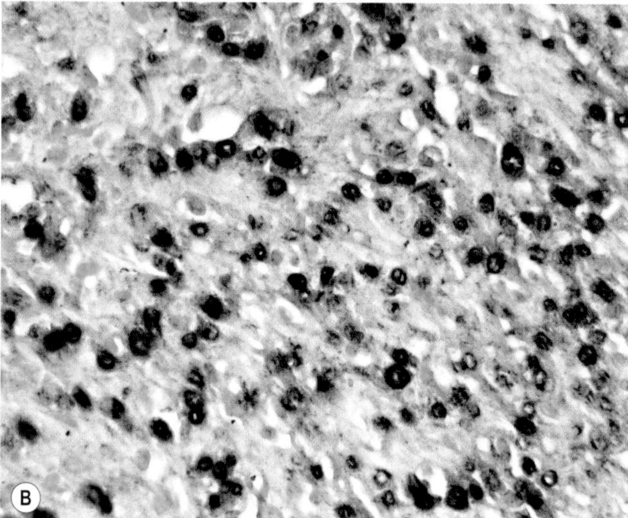

Fig. 25.143 **A** and **B**, Leiomyosarcoma in an immunosuppressed patient. **B**, EBER demonstration by in situ hybridization.

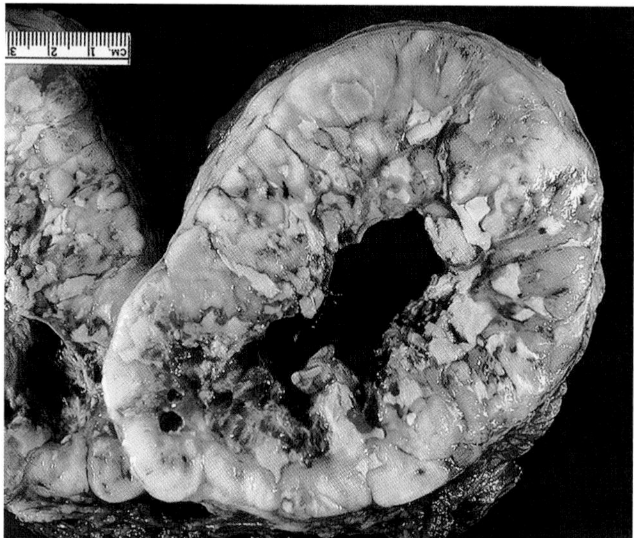

Fig. 25.144 Gross appearance of recurrent leiomyosarcoma. The central cystic cavity is a common feature of this tumor type.

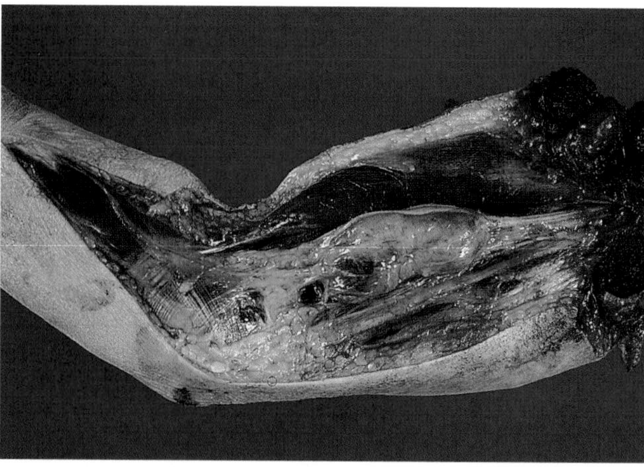

Fig. 25.145 Leiomyosarcoma of soft tissues of arm. The fusiform shape of the tumor is due to the fact that the tumor is following the course of the large blood vessels from which it arose.

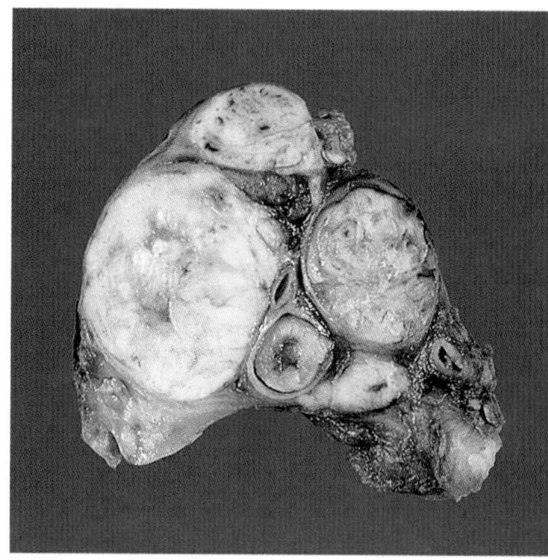

Fig. 25.146 Leiomyosarcoma filling the lumen of the popliteal vein and its branches, as seen on cross section. The popliteal artery is uninvolved.

multinucleated giant cells[1226,1248] may be prominent. Rhabdoid features can be present; as for other tumor types, this feature is an indicator of aggressive behavior.[1235] The EBV-related tumors lack significant pleomorphism and often have a component of primitive round cells and numerous intratumoral T cells.[1207]

Ultrastructurally, the tumor cells exhibit numerous cytoplasmic filaments with focal densities, pinocytotic vesicles, and a thick basal lamina.[1223] Myofibrils can be demonstrated in well-differentiated tumors with PTAH. Reticulin stain shows wavy, undulating fibers between long lines of tumor cells, without individual cells being wrapped within. Immunohistochemically, both leiomyomas and well-differentiated leiomyosarcomas show reactivity for vimentin (particularly in those of vascular origin), actin, smooth muscle myosin, desmin, H-caldesmon, and basal lamina components, including laminin and type IV collagen[1208,1214,1228,1234,1239,1241] (Fig. 25.147B). Surprisingly, normal and neoplastic smooth muscle cells have been found also to react for keratin and EMA; this feature seems to be particularly prominent in tumors of the female genital tract and large vessels[1199,1216,1233,1244] (Fig. 25.149). Other markers that have been detected in smooth muscle tumors of soft tissues

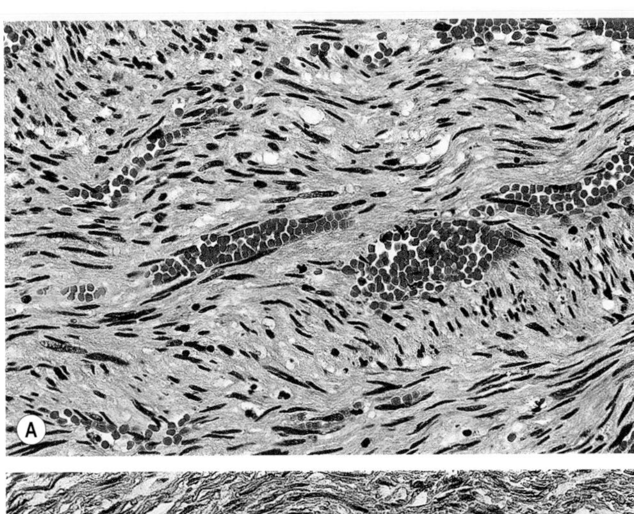

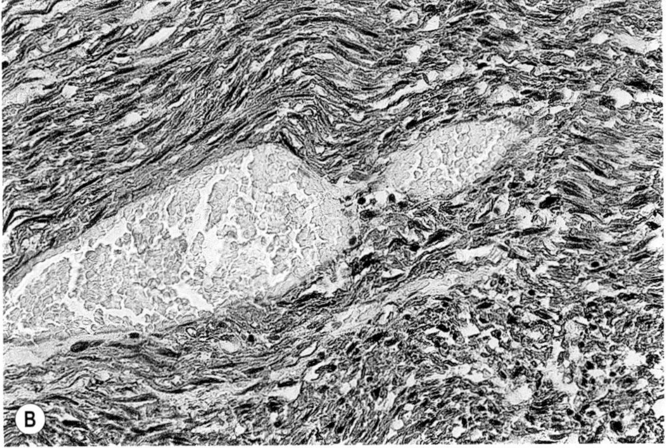

Fig. 25.147 **A** and **B**, The intimate relationship of the tumor cells with the vessel walls is a clue to the diagnosis of leiomyosarcoma. **B**, Smooth muscle actin immunostain.

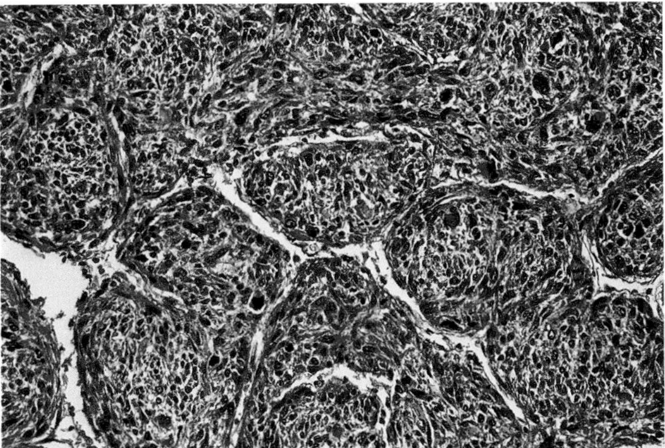

Fig. 25.148 Leiomyosarcoma of soft tissues with a vascular (hemangiopericytoma-like) pattern of growth.

are estrogen receptors,[1246] caveolin (a member of the membrane-scaffolding proteins, also present in adipose tissue tumors),[1196] and placental alkaline phosphatase (although not as frequently as in rhabdomyosarcomas).[1211] Estrogen receptor protein has also been detected in some of these tumors, raising the possibility of hormonal responsiveness.[1218,1246]

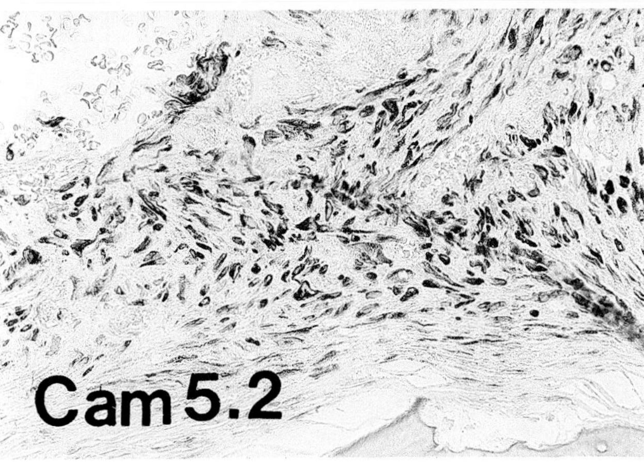

Fig. 25.149 Immunoreactivity for low molecular weight keratin (CAM 5.2) in leiomyosarcoma.

Cytogenetic analysis has shown a variety of chromosomal aberrations but no specific karyotypic marker; curiously, a relatively high number of these tumors show no detectable karyotypic abnormalities.[1224,1229,1242] Common genetic alterations include *RB1, CDKN2A, CCND1,* and *CCND3*.[1204] The gene expression profiles of leiomyosarcomas greatly overlap with those of undifferentiated pleomorphic sarcomas, and a recent study utilizes such data to identify distinctive molecular subtypes of leiomyosarcoma.[1197,1200,1237]

The differential diagnosis between leiomyoma and leiomyosarcoma of the soft tissues depends on a combination of gross and microscopic features. High mitotic activity is virtually diagnostic of malignancy. A diagnosis of leiomyosarcoma should also be strongly suspected for tumors that are overly large, necrotic, or hemorrhagic, even if their mitotic count is low. Prognosis in leiomyosarcoma correlates primarily with tumor size and depth, two parameters that are closely related.[1209,1217] In one large series, 40% of the cutaneous leiomyosarcomas recurred, but none metastasized; among the subcutaneous tumors, one-half recurred, and one-third resulted in metastases or tumor-related deaths.[1209] Prognosis is even worse for the tumors located intramuscularly. Mitotic activity also correlates with prognosis;[1247] however, the fact remains that in many metastasizing leiomyosarcomas of soft tissue, there are fewer than 10 mitoses per high-power field. It has been shown recently that the very presence of smooth muscle differentiation in pleomorphic spindle cell sarcomas of the extremities is an independent indicator of poor prognosis.[1206] Simple enucleation of the tumor virtually guarantees local recurrence. The majority of these tumors eventually give rise to distant metastases, sometimes 15 years or more after the original excision.

It should be noted that all the comments made above are intended for the smooth muscle tumors located in soft tissues and do not necessarily apply to those in the uterus or gastrointestinal tract.

Clear cell (epithelioid) smooth muscle tumors

Smooth muscle tumors of soft tissues may have a round cell (clear cell, epithelioid) configuration, in whole or in part, similar to that seen more often in mesenchymal tumors of the stomach and other intra-abdominal sites[1252] (Fig. 25.150). The term *bizarre leiomyoblastoma* has been used for this tumor type, which has benign and malignant forms. An intravascular variant has also been described.[1250] We prefer to designate these tumors as *leiomyomas* or *leiomyosarcomas, clear cell (epithelioid) variant,* and classify them as benign or

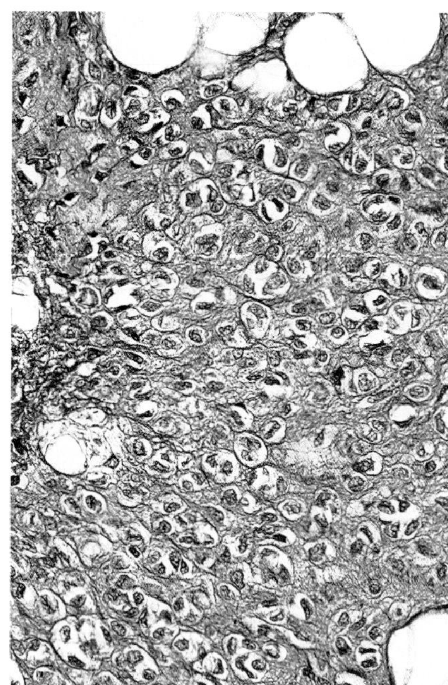

Fig. 25.150 Epithelioid smooth muscle tumor. The PAS stain highlights the thick basement membrane that surrounds individual tumor cells.

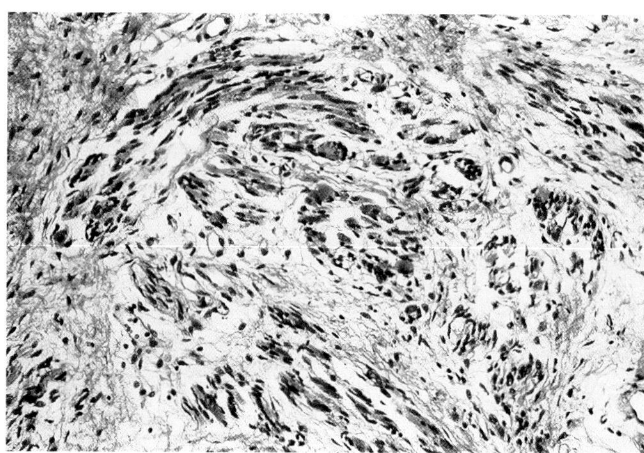

Fig. 25.151 Fetal rhabdomyoma.
(Courtesy of Dr Louis Dehner, St Louis, MO)

malignant by using similar criteria to those we apply for smooth muscle tumors in general, although acknowledging the fact that this distinction can be extremely difficult to make in the individual case. Immunohistochemical or ultrastructural markers of smooth muscle differentiation tend to be expressed only focally and imperfectly in these tumors.[1251,1252]

The morphologic similarities that these tumors exhibit with the gastrointestinal stromal neoplasms currently known as GISTs suggests a possible histogenetic relationship and the need for an immunohistochemical and molecular study of these tumors when encountered in the soft tissues.

Tumors of striated muscle

Rhabdomyoma

Bona fide soft tissue benign tumors of skeletal muscle origin are exceedingly rare.[1253] They can be divided into distinct subtypes, although some overlap exists.[1254,1263,1267,1268] Those known as the *adult* type are found almost exclusively in the oral cavity and its vicinity in adult patients.[1258] Sometimes they represent an incidental microscopic finding.[1265] They can be multifocal and may recur locally.[1257,1266] Microscopically, the cells are well differentiated, large, rounded or polygonal, with abundant acidophilic cytoplasm containing variable amounts of lipid and glycogen. Some cells have features of 'spider cells'. Cross striations and intracytoplasmic rod-like ('jack straw') inclusions are frequent, and intranuclear inclusions may be seen. There is no mitotic activity or nuclear atypia. The differential diagnosis includes granular cell tumor, hibernoma, and the peculiar condition known as crystal-storing histiocytosis.[1259]

The *fetal* form of rhabdomyoma is seen almost exclusively in two locations: the head and neck area (particularly the retroauricular area) in children under 3 years of age and the vulvovaginal region of middle-aged women.[1255,1256,1260] The latter, also referred to as *genital rhabdomyoma*, is separated by some authors from the other fetal types. Microscopically, both forms are very cellular, formed by immature skeletal muscle fibers (some containing cross striations) and primitive mesenchymal cells (Fig. 25.151). Their development is equivalent to that of fetal skeletal muscle of 7–12 weeks' gestation. Nuclear aberrations are absent, and mitoses are generally rare. The vulvovaginal cases tend to have a myxoid quality. Kapadia et al.[1260] have divided their cases of fetal rhabdomyoma into 'classic' (having the above described features) and 'intermediate'. The latter were characterized by the presence of large, ganglion cell-like rhabdomyoblasts with vesicular nuclei and prominent nucleoli, interlacing ribbon- or strap-like rhabdomyoblasts with deeply acidophilic cytoplasm, fascicles simulating smooth muscle, plexiform patterns with infiltration of fat, and intimate relationship with peripheral nerves.

The main differential diagnosis of fetal rhabdomyoma is with well-differentiated rhabdomyosarcoma. The distinction can be very difficult because of the overlap of many histologic features; nuclear atypia is said to be the most important distinguishing feature.[1260,1262]

The immunohistochemical features of rhabdomyoma (especially the adult type) recapitulate those of normal skeletal muscle cells;[1261,1264] the markers that these cells can exhibit are listed in the section on rhabdomyosarcoma. Ultrastructurally, hypertrophied Z-band material, thick and thin filaments, numerous mitochondria (some with abnormal configuration or with inclusions), intranuclear bodies, and cytoplasmic bodies have been observed.

It is likely that so-called 'cardiac rhabdomyoma', seen in association with the tuberous sclerosis syndrome, is not a true neoplasm (see Chapter 27).

Rhabdomyosarcoma

There are three major categories of rhabdomyosarcoma: pleomorphic, embryonal, and alveolar,[1269,1321] as well as several subtypes and possibly minor categories.[1367,1370]

Pleomorphic rhabdomyosarcoma. This tumor, which constituted practically all the cases of rhabdomyosarcoma in the older literature, is actually the least common of the three categories. It arises in areas where myotome-derived skeletal muscle occurs and is therefore usually located in an extremity, especially the thigh.[1338,1391] It occurs almost exclusively in adults, but isolated cases in children have been reported.[1309,1310,1390] Grossly, it may be

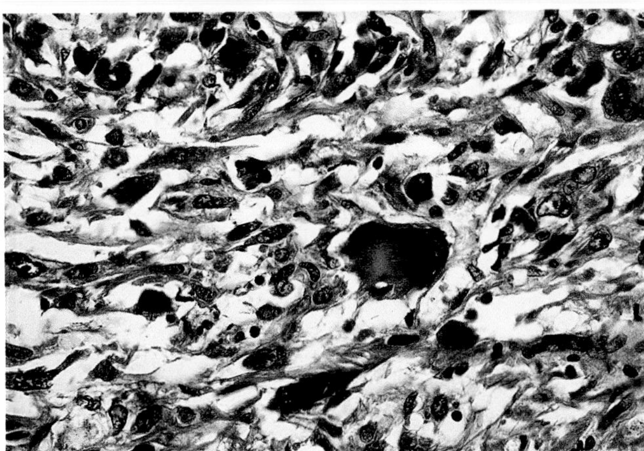

Fig. 25.152 Pleomorphic rhabdomyosarcoma. The tumor was immunoreactive for desmin and skeletal muscle actin.

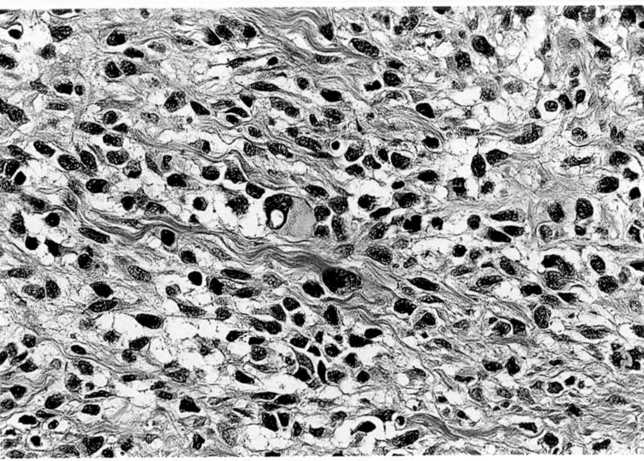

Fig. 25.153 Embryonal rhabdomyosarcoma. Most of the nuclei are oval; the cytoplasm is scanty and acidophilic.

confined within fascial compartments and have the shape of the muscle from which it arises. Microscopically, the tumor is very pleomorphic, with numerous tumor giant cells[1383] (Fig. 25.152). Making a differential diagnosis with pleomorphic liposarcoma and other types of pleomorphic sarcoma is so difficult that a diagnosis of pleomorphic rhabdomyosarcoma should not be made unless there is incontrovertible evidence of skeletal muscle differentiation in the form of cross striations (good luck!) or through the demonstration of specific ultrastructural or immunohistochemical markers (see subsequent discussion). One should be very careful to avoid the following pitfalls: (1) entrapped non-neoplastic skeletal muscle fibers; (2) release of myoglobin from necrotic muscle with subsequent nonspecific absorption by tumor cells, which thus become immunoreactive;[1301] and (3) presence of skeletal muscle differentiation in other malignant tumors.[1303] In regard to the latter event, it is somewhat ironic that the best evidence of skeletal muscle differentiation in malignant tumors is often found not in rhabdomyosarcoma per se but rather in tumors such as MPNST (see p. 2169), malignant thymoma (see Chapter 8), mixed müllerian tumor of the female genital tract (see Chapter 19), malignant germ cell tumors (particularly extragonadal ones), medulloblastoma (see Chapter 28), and Wilms tumor (see Chapter 17).

When defined by the restrictive criteria listed previously, pleomorphic rhabdomyosarcoma becomes a very rare neoplasm;[1351] however, well-documented cases exist,[1288,1311] some of them following radiation therapy of other types of malignant tumor.[1374] The behavior of pleomorphic rhabdomyosarcoma seems not to be substantially different from that of other pleomorphic sarcomas of soft tissue.

The other two major types of rhabdomyosarcomas occur primarily in children and adolescents and actually constitute the most common form of soft tissue sarcoma in this age group.[1312,1394,1396] Sometimes these two types are grouped under the term 'juvenile',[1360] a potentially misleading practice considering the vast clinical, morphologic, molecular, and behavioral differences that exist between the two.

Embryonal rhabdomyosarcoma. This tumor type arises from unsegmented and undifferentiated mesoderm and is common in the head and neck region (particularly the orbit, nasopharynx, middle ear, and oral cavity), retroperitoneum, bile ducts, and urogenital tract.[1324,1342,1372] A smaller percentage occur in the extremities, and these are associated with a higher relapse rate and a lower survival rate.[1317,1389] A few grow predominantly within the thoracic cavity.[1285] Cases with primary presentation in the skin are also on record.[1381] The large majority occur in children between the ages of 3 and 12 years, but they can also be seen in younger patients[1373] and adults.[1291,1305,1320,1339] Some cases have been associated with hypercalcemia or with elevated parathormone levels.[1297] Grossly, the tumor is poorly circumscribed, white, and soft.

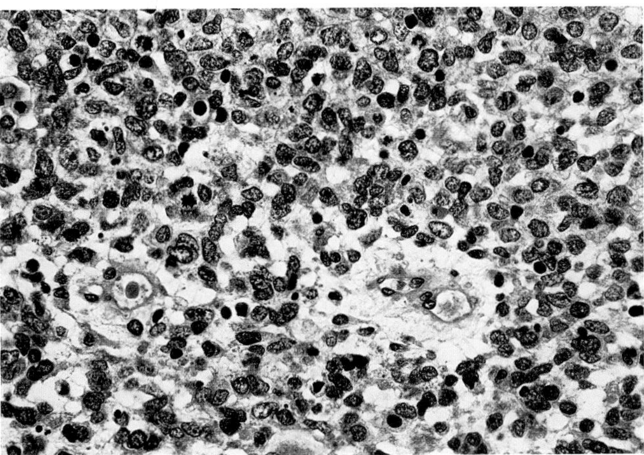

Fig. 25.154 Embryonal rhabdomyosarcoma composed predominantly of round cells. There is a perivascular pseudorosette around a blood vessel.

Microscopically, the tumor cells are small and spindle shaped. Some have a deeply acidophilic cytoplasm (Fig. 25.153). A feature of diagnostic value is the presence of highly cellular areas usually surrounding blood vessels, alternating with paucicellular regions that have abundant myxoid intercellular material (Fig. 25.154). Cross striations may or may not be present; in contrast to pleomorphic rhabdomyosarcoma in adults, their presence is not indispensable for the light microscopic diagnosis, as long as all the other features are present. Confirmation of the diagnosis, always desirable, can be obtained with ultrastructural and particularly the numerous immunohistochemical markers that are available (see the subsequent discussion).

The most common sites of metastatic involvement are the soft tissues, serosal surfaces, lung, bone marrow, and lymph nodes.[1281,1375,1379] Cases associated with diffuse bone marrow

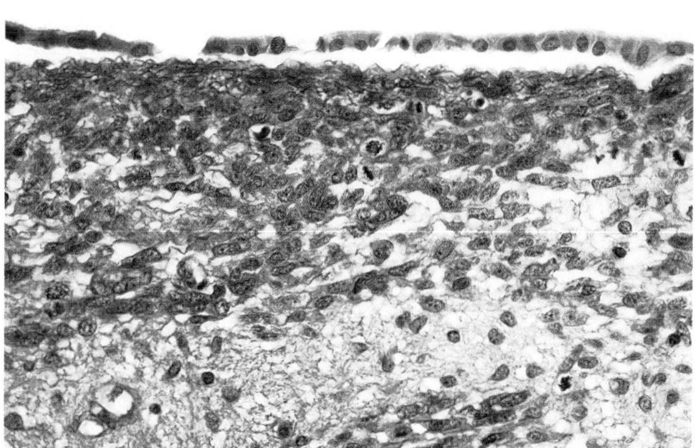

Fig. 25.155 Botryoid rhabdomyosarcoma of common bile duct showing a concentration of tumor cells immediately beneath the epithelium ('cambium layer').

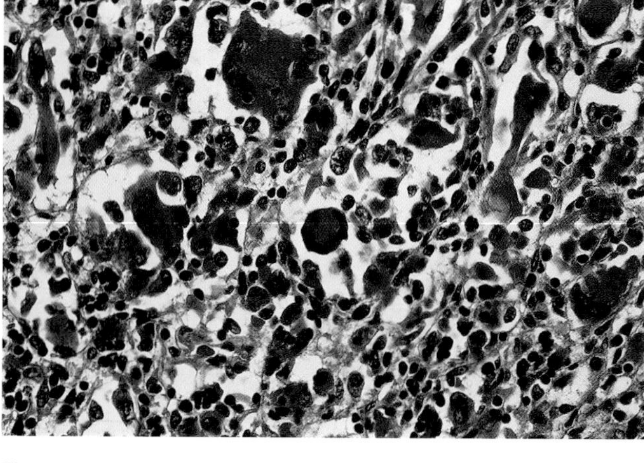

Fig. 25.156 Embryonal rhabdomyosarcoma with pleomorphic features in a child.

involvement may simulate acute leukemia.[1315] Rhabdomyosarcomas arising from genitourinary sites or extremities are particularly prone to metastasize to lymph nodes,[1335] whereas tumors originating in head and neck structures adjacent to meningeal surfaces have a high incidence of direct meningeal extension.

The prognosis of embryonal rhabdomyosarcoma has markedly improved following multimodality treatment with excision, radiation therapy, and multidrug chemotherapy.[1273,1306] Over 80% of children now survive when the disease is localized to the region of origin.[1343,1344] Age at diagnosis is an independent predictor of outcome.[1334]

Embryonal rhabdomyosarcoma: variants and related tumors. When growing beneath a mucosal membrane, such as the vagina, urinary bladder, or nasal cavity, it frequently forms large polypoid masses resembling a bunch of grapes – hence the name *sarcoma botryoides*. This is regarded as a variation in the pattern of growth of embryonal rhabdomyosarcoma and is referred to as the *botryoid subtype*. The appearance is reminiscent of an allergic nasal polyp, and, as such, is deceptively benign. A highly characteristic feature of these polypoid ('botryoid') tumors is the presence of a dense zone of undifferentiated tumor cells immediately beneath the epithelium, a formation known as *Nicholson cambium layer* (Fig. 25.155).

Occasional tumors within the embryonal category have focally anaplastic features, with bizarre nuclear forms; these should not be classified as pleomorphic rhabdomyosarcomas but rather as *pleomorphic subtypes of embryonal (and rarely alveolar) rhabdomyosarcoma*[1330] (Fig. 25.156). It has been suggested that they are associated with a more aggressive clinical course, especially when the pleomorphic features are extensive;[1314,1330] conversely, well-differentiated tumors (with over 50% rhabdomyoblasts) are associated with an excellent response to chemotherapy.[1382]

Tumors examined following multidrug chemotherapy tend to show a greater degree of differentiation than the pretherapy specimen, suggesting that the drugs have either induced maturation or resulted in a selection of the better differentiated components.[1286,1352]

Very rarely, accumulation of cytoplasmic glycogen or lipids in embryonal rhabdomyosarcoma results in a *clear cell appearance* that can simulate clear cell carcinoma.[1280,1406]

Another morphologic variation is represented by tumor cells containing cytoplasmic globular inclusions composed of intermediate filaments and resulting in a *rhabdoid appearance*.[1329]

Occasionally, in infants and children, tumors with a location and appearance otherwise characteristic of embryonal rhabdomyosarcoma are seen to contain collections of cells exhibiting neuronal, melanocytic, and/or schwannian differentiation; these have been interpreted by some as originating from the migratory neural crest (ectomesenchyme) and designated as *ectomesenchymomas*.[1325,1326] Most of these tumors have been located in the head and neck region, but cases have also been reported involving the distal extremities.[1364] Tumors with similar appearance have been given the histogenetically less committal name of *gangliorhabdomyosarcoma*.[1328] Little is known about their natural history, which does not seem to differ much from that of the ordinary embryonal rhabdomyosarcoma.

A distinct variant of embryonal rhabdomyosarcoma is represented by the *spindle cell* type, which is composed of elongated spindle cells arranged in a fasciculated or storiform pattern.[1278] Most of the initially published cases were in male children. The most common locations were the paratesticular area and the head and neck region, and their prognosis was favorable.[1336] Conversely, spindle cell rhabdomyosarcomas occurring in adults predilect the head and neck region and seem to be more aggressive than their pediatric counterparts.[1345,1361] Spindle cell rhabdomyosarcoma bears some resemblance to the tumors described by Lundgren et al.[1341] as *infantile rhabdomyofibrosarcomas*, but it is not clear whether the two are identical. The latter tumors microscopically simulated fibrosarcoma and were characterized by an aggressive clinical course.

Sclerosing (pseudovascular) rhabdomyosarcoma refers to a type of rhabdomyosarcoma accompanied by such a prominent deposition of matrix material as to simulate an osteosarcoma or a chondrosarcoma.[1307,1332] It may also feature a pseudovascular growth pattern, mimicking angiosarcoma. The initial reported cases were in adults, but lately they have also been identified in children.[1398,1405] It is not clear whether this tumor is a variety of either alveolar or embryonal rhabdomyosarcoma or a distinct subtype.

Alveolar rhabdomyosarcoma may be related to the embryonal form and is said to occasionally coexist with it; however, it should be regarded as a separate entity because it differs from the latter in several ways. For instance, it predominates in an older age group (10–25 years) and occurs more frequently in the extremities, the most common locations being forearms, arms, and perirectal and perineal regions (Fig. 25.157). It also occurs in the head and neck region, including the parameningeal region.[1354,1402]

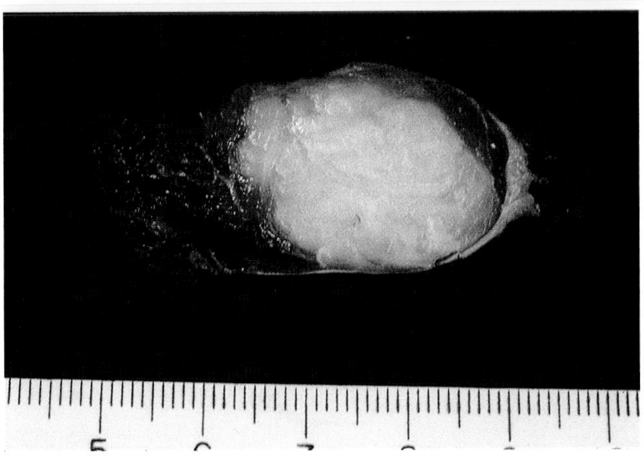

Fig. 25.157 Gross appearance of alveolar rhabdomyosarcoma. The tumor is embedded within skeletal muscle.

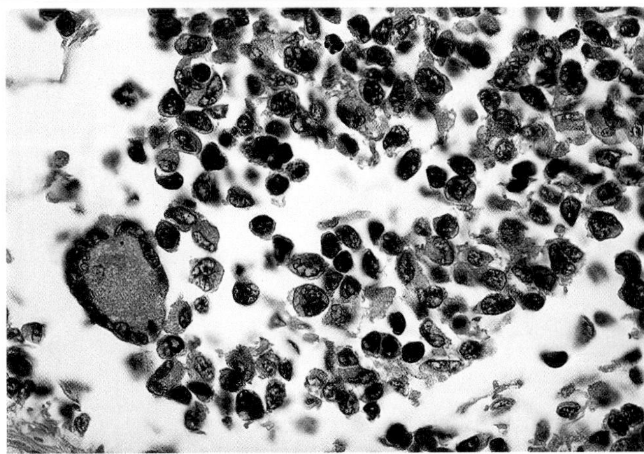

Fig. 25.159 On high power, this rhabdomyosarcoma shows a single multinucleated tumor giant cell among the mononuclear small cells, an important diagnostic clue.

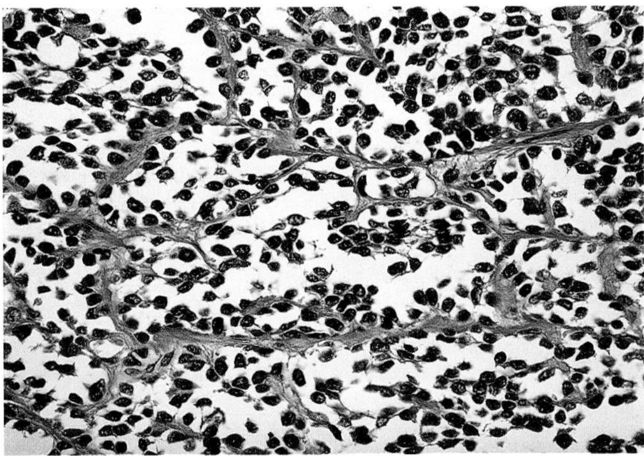

Fig. 25.158 Typical low-power appearance of alveolar rhabdomyosarcoma. Note the small size of the tumor cells.

Microscopically, small, round, or oval tumor cells are seen separated in nests by connective tissue septa (Fig. 25.158). The tumor cells in contact with these fibrous strands remain firmly attached to them, but the others tend to detach because of a lack of cohesiveness, which results in a typical alveolar or pseudoglandular appearance. The deep acidophilia of the cytoplasm and the presence of occasional multinucleated giant cells are important diagnostic features[1385] (Fig. 25.159). Cases in which the alveolar pattern is poorly developed are referred to as the 'solid' variant of alveolar rhabdomyosarcoma and are particularly difficult to diagnose.[1318] Before identification of this entity,[1298,1377] many of these tumors were misdiagnosed as primary malignant lymphoma ('reticulum cell sarcoma') of the soft tissues. The comments made regarding cross striations and special studies for the diagnosis of embryonal rhabdomyosarcomas also apply for the alveolar type.

The prognosis of alveolar rhabdomyosarcoma is distinctly worse than for the embryonal variety, even with the current multimodality therapies.[1316,1376,1386,1401] In the classic series reported by Enzinger[1299] (which antedates current therapeutic regimens), 92% of the patients had died from widespread metastasis within the first 4 years after diagnosis. The lung and regional lymph nodes are the most common metastatic sites. The ovary can also be involved.[1403] Peripheral lymph node involvement, sometimes in a multiple fashion, may be the first manifestation of the disease ('lymphadenopathic form'). A common site for occult primary alveolar rhabdomyosarcoma is the perirectal–perineal region.

Special techniques in rhabdomyosarcoma

Electron microscopic features. Ultrastructural examination may confirm a diagnosis of rhabdomyosarcoma through the identification of sarcomere-related structures, such as Z bands, thick and thin filaments in a hexagonal array, an A band containing thick filaments, and H and M bands, or leptomeric structures[1275,1300,1347,1355] (Fig. 25.160). There is a good correlation between the light and electron microscopic features of these tumors.[1384] Drawbacks of this technique are those related to sampling and the absence of these features in the poorly differentiated cells.[1283] These facts, plus the availability of a large panel of relatively specific immunohistochemical (and, in the case of alveolar rhabdomyosarcoma, molecular) markers, has greatly diminished the diagnostic utility of electron microscopy in this field. However, the two techniques should be viewed as complementary rather than mutually exclusive.[1308]

Histochemical and immunohistochemical features. Conventional special stains such as PTAH, Masson trichrome, and silver impregnation technique are of only relative use in the diagnosis of rhabdomyosarcoma.[1380] They highlight the cross striations when these are already appreciated in a good H&E preparation, but they only rarely detect them if they are not already apparent in the routine preparations.

Immunohistochemistry, on the other hand, has proved of great value. Hardly any other tumor type has been described for which the array of markers is as varied as for rhabdomyosarcoma, and the list continues to grow.[1270,1302,1393,1395] There is a range of specificity and sensitivity among these markers and this translates into their relative practical utility. Algorithms have been proposed to guide the uninitiated in the search for striated muscle differentiation in a soft tissue tumor.[1356] The most important markers are as follows.

1 **Myogenin.** The myogenin gene codes for a phosphoprotein that induces skeletal muscle differentiation in mesenchymal cells. The protein, which has a high degree of specificity,[1279,1333] can be demonstrated in the nuclei of the tumor cells in all types and virtually all cases of rhabdomyosarcoma, but it is expressed in a particularly strong and widespread fashion in the alveolar type[1292] (Fig. 25.161). Probably because of this

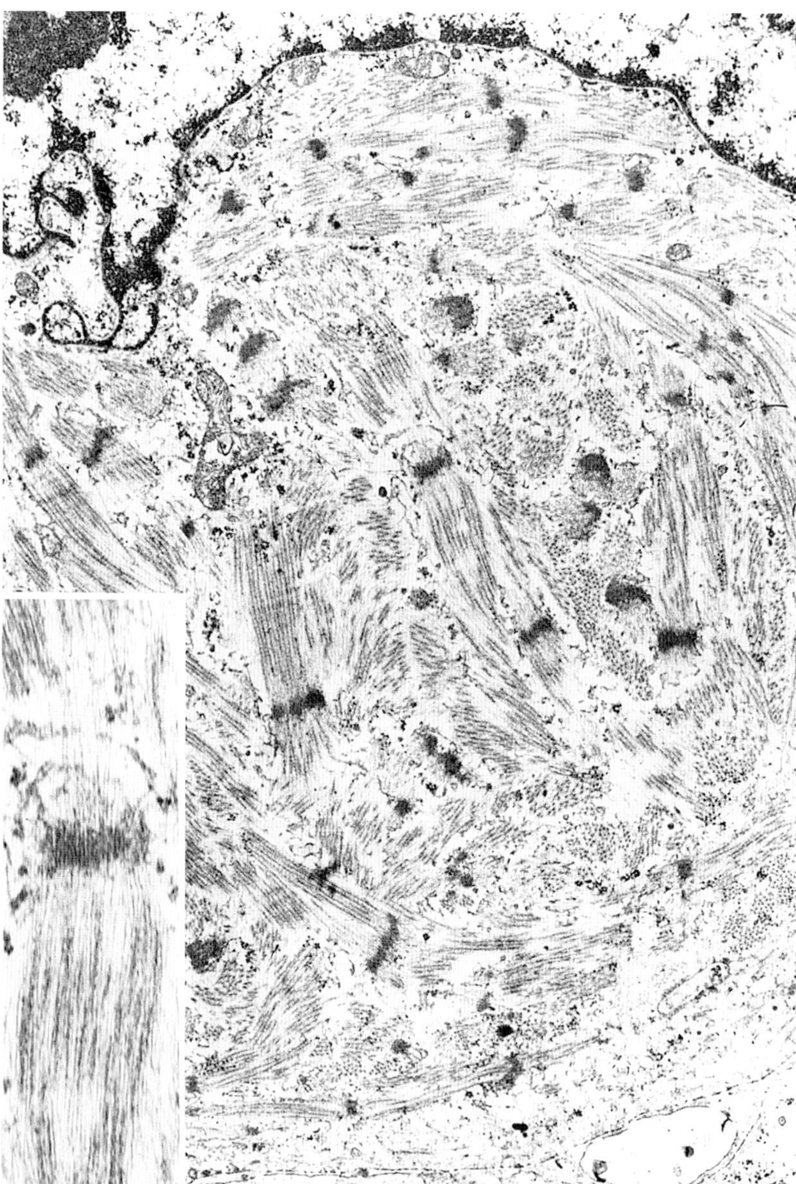

Fig. 25.160 Electron micrograph of embryonal rhabdomyosarcoma. The cytoplasm of tumor cells contains abortive cross striations, too small and haphazardly oriented to be visible with the light microscope. Inset shows a Z band and clearly visible double set of filaments.
(×18 000; inset ×45 000; courtesy of Dr B Lane, New York)

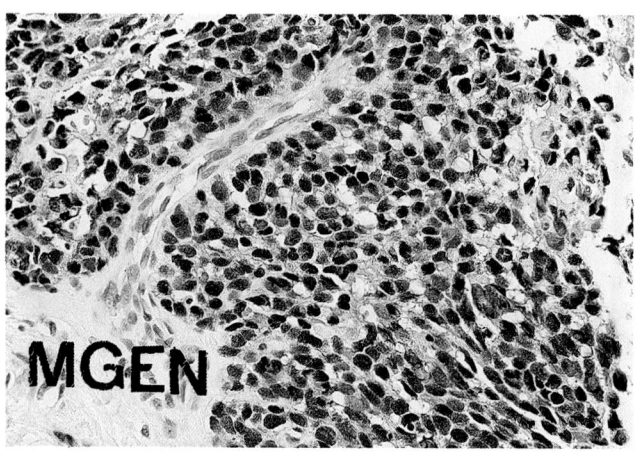

Fig. 25.161 Widespread nuclear immunoreactivity for myogenin in alveolar rhabdomyosarcoma.

very fact, diffuse expression of myogenin is a marker of poor prognosis.[1319]

MyoD1 is a related nuclear protein with a similar degree of specificity, but – in contrast to myogenin – not well demonstrated in formalin-fixed paraffin-embedded material, and therefore of lesser diagnostic utility.[1282,1293,1294,1399] The MyoD1 protein present in these tumors binds DNA but it is relatively nonfunctional as a transcriptional activator, suggesting the lack of a factor needed for its activity.

2 **Desmin.** This intermediate filament is a specific indicator for muscle differentiation, but it is present in both smooth and striated muscle. In general, only tumors with round rhabdomyoblasts or strap cells show positivity for this marker.[1353]
3 **Sarcomeric actin.** Rhabdomyosarcomas consistently express sarcomeric actin, which represents one of the best markers for this tumor.[1289,1348,1358,1387] The interesting and surprising observation has been made that the specific sarcomeric actin

expressed by these tumors is not of the alpha-skeletal muscle but the alpha-cardiac type.[1284] Rhabdomyosarcoma cells also express common muscle actin, but little or no smooth muscle actin.

4 **Myosin.** This marker has proved very effective for the identification of skeletal muscle differentiation.[1331,1393] Adult sarcomeric and fetal forms of myosin exist; expression of fetal heavy chain skeletal myosin, viewed as the expression of an oncofetal antigen, was found in one series in 81% of rhabdomyosarcomas.[1287,1288,1304]
5 **Myoglobin.** This protein appears to be specific for striated muscle differentiation, and it would therefore seem well suited for this purpose.[1274,1327,1357] Unfortunately, it is expressed only when the tumor cell has acquired a high degree of differentiation. It is therefore often negative in poorly differentiated tumors.[1277] One should also be careful of diffusion from neighboring injured skeletal muscle fibers.[1301]
6 **Tropomyosin α-actinin, titin, and Z protein.** These are constituent proteins of sarcomeric muscle and show a high degree of specificity. Unfortunately, most of them stain only well-differentiated cells in a minority of the tumors, a fact that greatly limits their diagnostic application.[1359,1365]
7 **Vimentin.** This antigen is consistently positive, particularly in the lesser differentiated tumors, but of course it lacks specificity as a skeletal muscle marker.[1353] It is the first marker to appear in the tumor cells, followed sequentially by actin, desmin, fast myosin, and myoglobin.[1276,1400]
8 **Enzymes.** These can be demonstrated immunohistochemically or through standard enzymatic histochemical techniques; most of the latter require fresh frozen tissue. They include *creatine kinase subunit M* (*muscle type*[1290]), myophosphorylase, acetylcholinesterase, adenosine triphosphatase,[1397] and *β-enolase*.[1369,1378]
9 **CARP.** This cardiac ankyrin-related protein and its homolog *arpp* are expressed in all types of rhabdomyosarcoma, the expression patterns being different from those of muscle actin or desmin.[1322,1323]
10 **Basal lamina components (type IV collagen, laminin).** No specificity can be ascribed to these markers, since they are also present in other types of mesenchymal cells and in epithelial cells.[1271]
11 **Antiskeletal muscle antibody from myasthenic patients.** The specific antigen against which this antibody is directed is not known, but it is clearly associated with the skeletal muscle fiber.[1363]
12 **Insulin-like growth factor II.** This has been found to be consistently expressed in rhabdomyosarcomas, in contrast to most other types of childhood malignancy.[1404]
13 **Other markers.** Rhabdomyosarcomas (especially the alveolar type) have been found to show focal immunoreactivity for keratin, neurofilaments and other neural/neuroendocrine markers, PAX, and S-100 protein.[1272,1349,1392]

This is a wide and somewhat confusing choice of options. In our institution, we have chosen the battery of myogenin, sarcomeric actin, and desmin for the routine investigation of these neoplasms.

Molecular genetic features. Alveolar rhabdomyosarcomas are consistently associated with the translocation t(2;13) or t(1;13), which results in the gene fusions *PAX3–FOXO1A* and *PAX7–FOXO1A*, respectively (*FOXO1A* being previously known as *FKHR*).[1295,1346,1368,1388] The translocations can be detected in paraffin-embedded tissue with the FISH technique.[1362] There is limited correlation between the morphologic appearance and the presence or absence of *PAX/FOXO1A* fusion or type of fusion.[1371] In a recent study, it was concluded that alveolar rhabdomyosarcomas with *PAX3–FOXO1A* are associated with a more aggressive clinical course than those having *PAX7–FOXO1A*.[1388] *MYCN* amplification has been detected in close to half of the alveolar rhabdomyosarcomas but not in the embryonal types.[1296]

Embryonal rhabdomyosarcomas do not exhibit the distinctive genetic alterations of alveolar rhabdomyosarcomas. They often show complex karyotypes, commonly with gains of chromosomes 2, 8, and 13.[1313] Most cases show allelic loss of 11p15, the same genetic region altered in Beckwith–Wiedemann syndrome (an imprinting disorder resulting from mutations or epigenetic events affecting imprinted genes at 11p15.5).[1337,1340]

Most rhabdomyosarcomas have been shown to be aneuploid, in contrast to other types of childhood sarcomas.[1350] It has been suggested that DNA content is a predictor of outcome in some subsets of embryonal rhabdomyosarcoma.[1366]

Tumors of pluripotential mesenchyme

Mesenchymoma was the term coined by Stout[1414] for tumors consisting of two or more mesenchymal elements in addition to fibrous tissue. Benign and malignant forms exist. The prototypical benign variant is composed of smooth muscle, fat, and blood vessels (angiomyolipoma). Cartilage may also be present in benign mesenchymoma, establishing a histogenetic link with the tumors described in the following section.[1409–1411] It is debatable whether benign mesenchymoma is of a neoplastic or hamartomatous nature.[1408] The malignant variant contains in the same neoplasm multiple varieties of soft tissue sarcomas, such as chondrosarcoma, liposarcoma, and leiomyosarcoma. The retroperitoneum and thigh are the most common sites.[1407] Nash and Stout[1412] reviewed 42 cases occurring in children, in nine of which the tumor was present at birth. Most malignant mesenchymomas are high-grade neoplasms,[1407] but some cases have been characterized by a low-grade histology and an indolent clinical course.[1413]

Tumors of metaplastic mesenchyme

Soft tissue (extraskeletal) chondromas are seen most frequently in the soft tissues of the hands and feet of adults.[1444,1450] Grossly, they are lobulated, have a typical hyaline appearance, and are often calcified (Fig. 25.162). Some nuclear hyperchromasia may be present and should not be interpreted as evidence of malignancy.[1465] Chondrosarcomas of the hands and feet exist, but they are exceptionally rare.[1428] The occasional presence of a cellular fibroblastic growth around the lobules may prompt confusion with calcifying

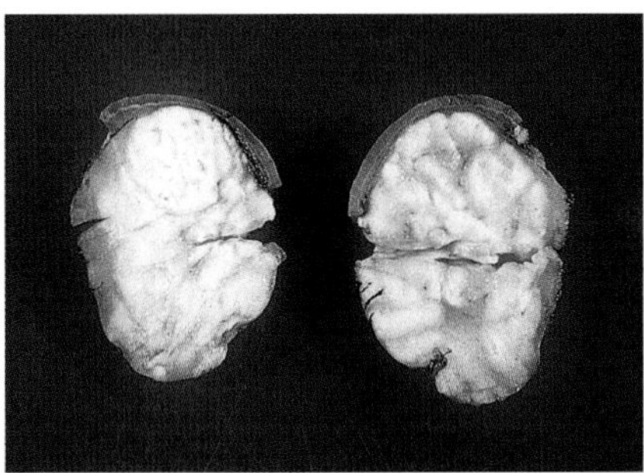

Fig. 25.162 Gross appearance of chondroma of soft tissues of hand. The tumor was partially calcified.

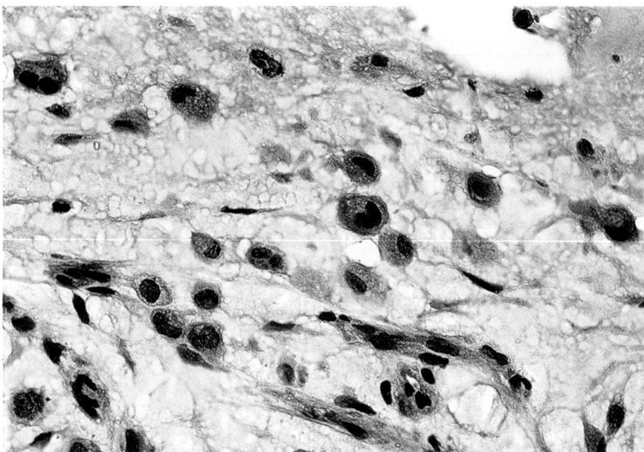

Fig. 25.163 The tumor cells of this soft tissue chondroma have a histiocyte-like quality, similar to that seen in chondroblastoma of bone.

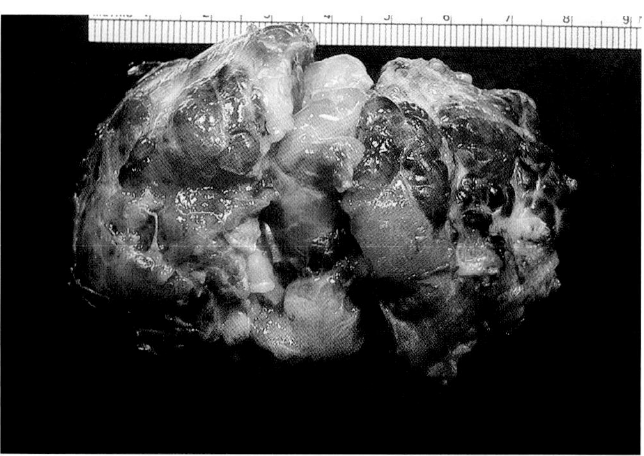

Fig. 25.165 Lobulated outer appearance of myxoid chondrosarcoma.

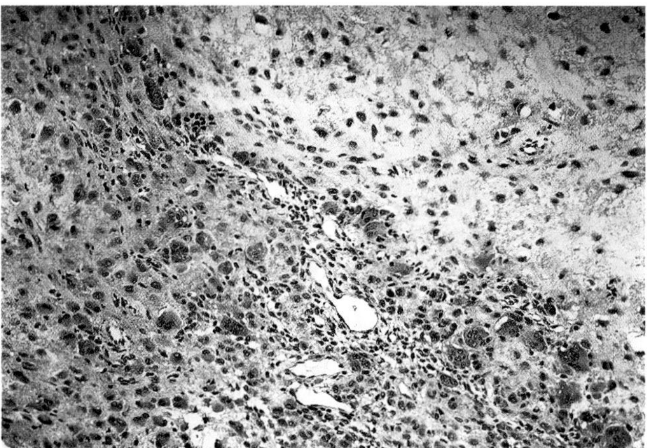

Fig. 25.164 Soft tissue chondroma with a hypercellular component having osteoclast-like giant cells and resembling chondromyxoid fibroma of bone.

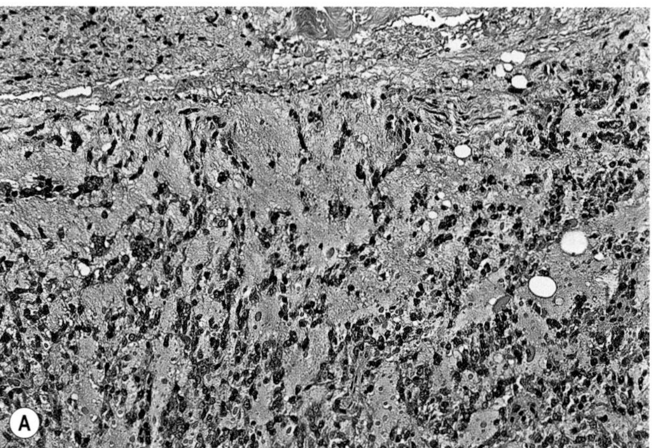

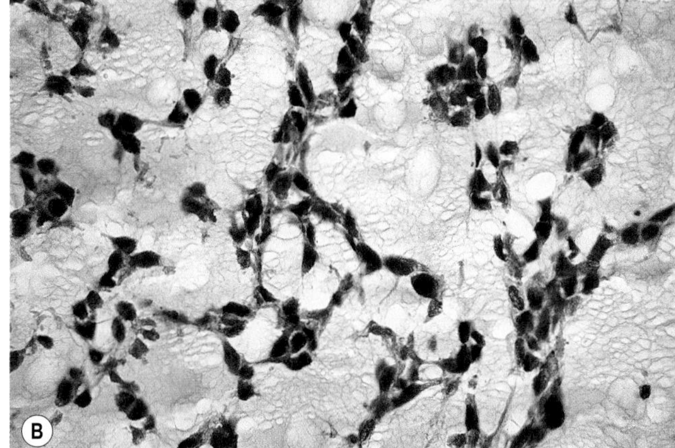

Fig. 25.166 **A** and **B**, Low- and high-power views of myxoid chondrosarcoma. Note the thin anastomosing strands of tumor cells surrounded by an abundant myxoid matrix. In contrast to myxoid liposarcoma, vascularity is scanty.

aponeurotic fibroma. Also confusing is the fact that sometimes the cartilaginous cells have an acidophilic cytoplasm simulating that of a histiocyte and sometimes a vacuolated appearance reminiscent of a lipoblast (Fig. 25.163). A histologic variant with proliferation of osteoclast-like giant cells and a chondroblastoma-like appearance has been described[1423,1425] (Fig. 25.164). Local recurrence is not infrequent.

Soft tissue (extraskeletal) chondrosarcoma, when used without a qualifier, refers to a soft tissue neoplasm composed of lobules of well-differentiated cartilage. In general, these tumors exhibit a less aggressive behavior than their skeletal counterparts.[1471,1476]

(Extraskeletal) myxoid chondrosarcoma is a specific type of soft tissue tumor which may have been incorrectly named, evidence accumulating to the effect that it is unrelated to cartilage.[1416,1441] This tumor type rarely if ever occurs within bone.[1418,1466] Most of the reported cases have been in the extremities of adult patients,[1433,1456,1460] but they have also been reported in the trunk and/or in children[1440] (Fig. 25.165). Microscopically, there are strands and cords of relatively small cells with acidophilic cytoplasm that are occasionally vacuolated, embedded in an abundant myxoid matrix[1439,1472] (Fig. 25.166). Well-differentiated chondrocytes are absent. Glycogen is present in many of the tumor cells. Acid mucopolysaccharides are abundant in the stroma. In contrast with those present in myxoma and myxoid liposarcoma, they are partially resistant to testicular hyaluronidase treatment because they are largely composed of chondroitin-4-sulfate, chondroitin-6-sulfate, and keratan sulfate. In some tumors, this myxochondroid stroma is scanty, and the diagnosis may consequently be missed.[1452,1464] Rhabdoid features may

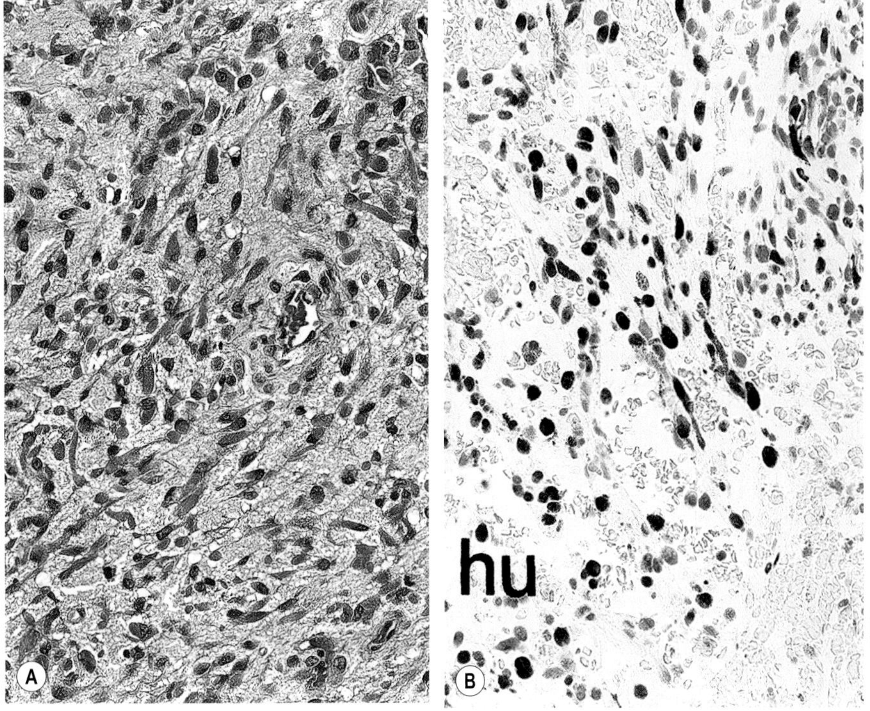

Fig. 25.167 **A** and **B**, Myxoid chondrosarcoma with immunohistochemical evidence of neuroendocrine differentiation. **B**, Hu immunostain showing nuclear reactivity.

be present; as usual, they portend an aggressive behavior.[1461] A high-grade form of myxoid chondrosarcoma has been described, characterized by the presence of numerous large epithelioid cells and a very aggressive behavior.[1451]

Ultrastructurally, the most conspicuous features of the cells of myxoid chondrosarcoma are a well-developed granular endoplasmic reticulum (sometimes containing peculiar parallel microtubules, a very distinctive feature of this entity), abundant cytoplasmic filaments, and cytoplasmic glycogen.[1430,1455,1463,1472,1475] In addition, some tumor cells have been shown to contain microtubules and neuroendocrine-type granules.[1424,1438] Immunohistochemically, myxoid chondrosarcomas are only focally and erratically positive for S-100 protein, much less so than one would expect in a true cartilaginous neoplasm. We and others have found that a high proportion of the cases show focal immunoreactivity for neural/neuroendocrine markers, such as NSE, Leu7, synaptophysin, Hu (a marker of primitive neural/neuroendocrine cells) and Tau proteins (microtubule-associated proteins required for polymerization of tubulin), but not for keratin[1424,1432,1436,1443] (Fig. 25.167). These surprising results, which are supported by microarray analyses,[1469] suggest that this peculiar lesion may represent a primary myxoid neuroendocrine tumor of soft tissue.[1424]

Cytogenetically, myxoid chondrosarcoma is characterized by a specific chromosomal translocation t(9;22)(q22–31;q11–12),[1468] or t(9;17)(q22;q11) which results in the gene fusions *EWS–NR4A3* (formerly *EWS–CHN*) or *RBP56–NR4A3* (formerly *RBP56–CHN*), respectively.[1462] These alterations are detectable in paraffin-embedded material with the FISH technique.[1473]

Myxoid chondrosarcoma is an aggressive neoplasm that recurs locally and metastasizes distantly, particularly to the lungs;[1449,1467] in some instances, the lung metastasis is the first manifestation of the tumor.[1429]

It seems likely that cases reported as *chordoid sarcoma* or *chordoid tumor*[1422,1454,1474] belong to the same category as myxoid chondrosarcoma, whereas the cases published as *parachordomas*[1427] may be related to myoepitheliomas of soft tissue (see p. 2191).

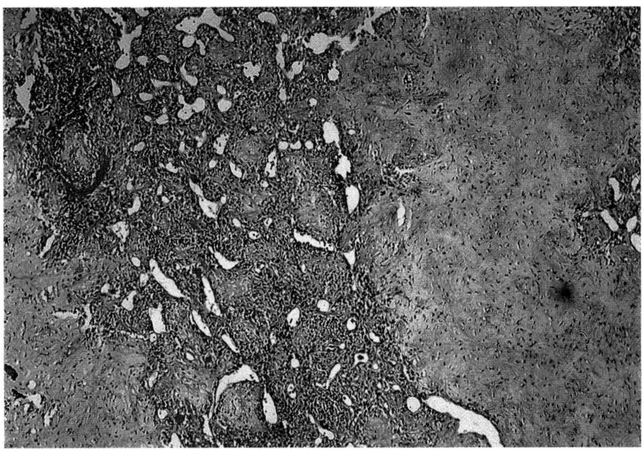

Fig. 25.168 Mesenchymal chondrosarcoma. Hypercellular areas with hemangiopericytoma-like features are admixed with islands of well-differentiated cartilage.

Mesenchymal chondrosarcoma has been described in the orbit, dura, trunk, retroperitoneum, extremities, and kidney.[1420,1439,1453,1459,1477] Like its counterpart in bone, it is characterized microscopically by an alternating pattern of highly cellular undifferentiated small cells (often growing in a hemangiopericytomatous fashion) and islands of well-differentiated cartilage (Fig. 25.168) (see Chapter 24). Immunohistochemically, it may show a polyphenotypic profile, including expression of CD99 (in the small cell component), S-100 protein (in the cartilaginous component), and focal positivity for actin, desmin, myogenin, and NSE.[1437,1442] The extracellular matrix contains type II collagen, a feature of diagnostic significance.[1458] Despite the morphologic resemblance of the small cell component of mesenchymal chondrosarcoma to Ewing sarcoma/PNET, the chromosomal

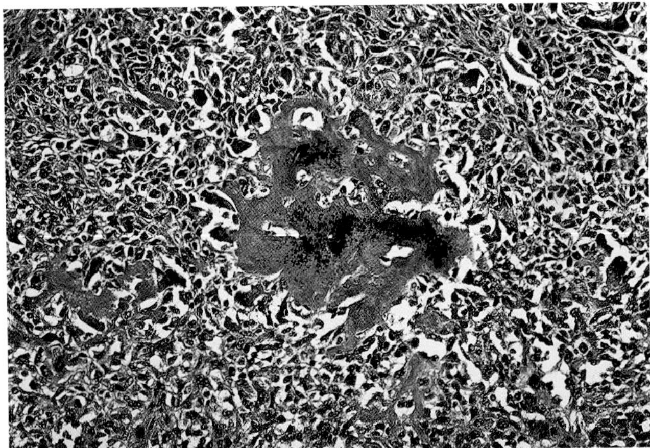

Fig. 25.169 Extraskeletal osteosarcoma with a central nidus of neoplastic bone.

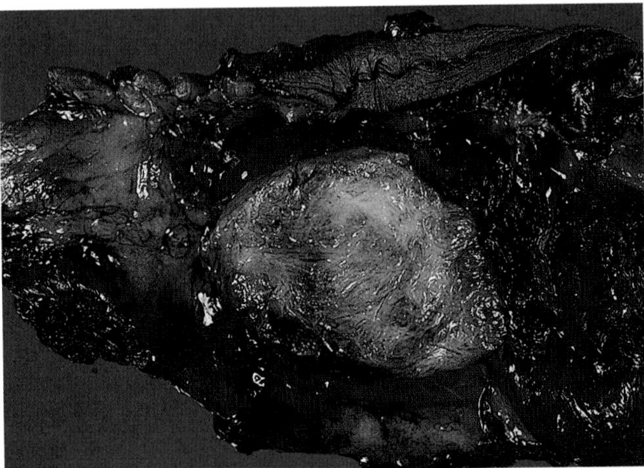

Fig. 25.170 Extraskeletal osteosarcoma. The neoplasm is embedded within skeletal muscle and is relatively well circumscribed.

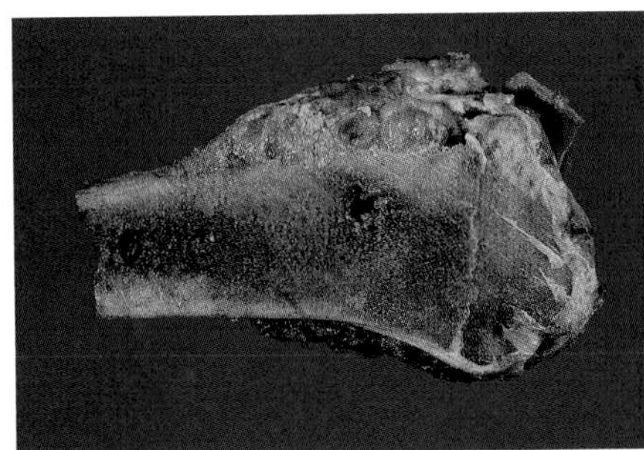

Fig. 25.171 Gross appearance of deep-seated synovial sarcoma involving periosteum of femur in an adolescent boy.

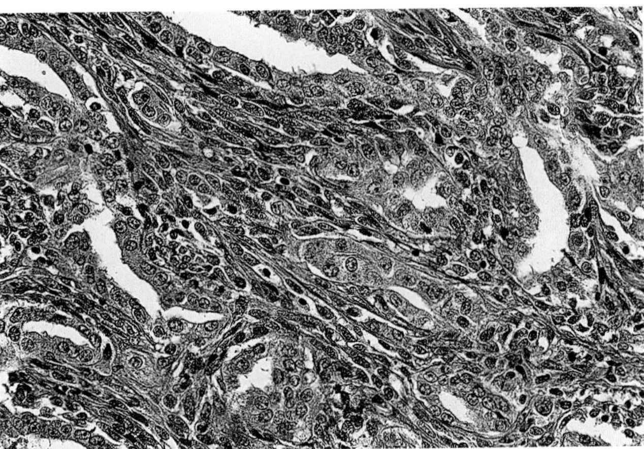

Fig. 25.172 Typical biphasic appearance of synovial sarcoma.

translocation associated with the latter is uniformly absent.[1447] The prognosis is poor.[1459]

Soft tissue (extraskeletal) osteosarcoma is distinguished from chondrosarcoma by applying the same criteria used for skeletal tumors (i.e., the occurrence of osteoid and bone formation directly produced by the tumor cells, without interposition of cartilage)[1448] (Fig. 25.169). It usually occurs in the extremities of adults[1417,1435,1445,1470] (Fig. 25.170). A small proportion of these tumors arise following exposure to x-rays.[1446] As for their most common counterpart in the skeletal system, the predominant histologic pattern may be osteoblastic, chondroblastic, fibroblastic, MFH-like, telangiectatic, or well differentiated (the latter being analogous to parosteal osteosarcoma).[1419,1457,1478] The immunohistochemical profile is also analogous to that of skeletal osteosarcoma, including expression of osteocalcin and osteonectin.[1434] In general, the prognosis is much worse than for chondrosarcoma, the overall mortality rate being over 60%.[1426] However, well-differentiated variants associated with an indolent clinical course and isolated cases of aggressive (epithelioid) osteoblastomas have been described.[1415,1431] The most important differential diagnosis of extraskeletal osteosarcoma is with myositis ossificans (see Chapter 24).[1465] The presence of marked nuclear atypia and lack of differentiation ('zone phenomenon') are the most important identifying features. It should also be distinguished from other soft tissue tumors in which metaplastic bone is formed, such as fibrosarcoma, synovial sarcoma, and so-called MFH.[1421]

Tumors resembling synovial tissue

Synovial sarcoma typically arises about the knee and ankle joints of children and young adults,[1500,1519,1538,1545,1567] but it can also occur in older patients[1488] (Fig. 25.171). It also occurs around other joints, such as shoulder and hip.[1497] It often grows close to the joints, tendon sheaths, and bursae, but it is extremely rare for it to invade the joint space and synovial membrane, with which it is probably unrelated. It can also be seen in many other soft tissue locations, including neck (particularly the retropharyngeal area),[1485,1549,1558] anterior abdominal wall,[1498] abdominal cavity,[1503] retroperitoneum,[1557] mediastinum,[1562,1572] blood vessels,[1534,1554] and nerves.[1541] Lately, it has become evident that the distribution of this tumor is even wider, with cases reported in the oral cavity,[1274] salivary glands,[1480] lung,[1510,1574] gastrointestinal tract,[1529,1553] kidney, prostate,[1505] and vulva.[1571]

Grossly, it tends to be well-circumscribed, firm, and grayish pink. Focal calcification is frequent and may be detected radiographically.[1570] When located in the hands or feet, it may have extremely small dimensions.[1530]

Microscopically, the classic form of synovial sarcoma is that of a *biphasic* tumor composed of sharply segregated epithelial and sarcomatous components (the terms being used descriptively and not histogenetically) (Figs 25.172 and 25.173). The epithelial areas usually appear in the form of gland-like spaces lined by cuboidal (synovial-like) or columnar cells, but can also present as solid nests of large pale cells. It is exceptional for this component to exhibit squamous features.[1537]

The sarcomatous component is made up of spindle cells with a fibroblast-like appearance. It tends to be hypercellular but with a relatively monotonous appearance, plump nuclei, a focally whorled pattern, distinct lobulation or fasciculation, hemangiopericytoma-like areas, and a large number of mast cells (Fig. 25.174). Hyalinization, calcification, and osseous metaplasia can be present. When the calcification is particularly heavy, the term *calcifying synovial sarcoma* has been used[1570] (Fig. 25.175). The osteoid and bone formation can be extensive enough to obscure the true nature of the tumor.[1536] In other instances, the stroma may have a prominent myxoid quality.[1518]

Monophasic synovial sarcoma is composed of only one of the two components. In the large majority of cases, this applies to the spindle cell sarcomatous component, which is easily misdiagnosed as fibrosarcoma, hemangiopericytoma, or some other spindle cell neoplasm by the unwary[1527,1532] (Fig. 25.176). A search for epithelial-looking foci should be carried out in these situations, as well as a thorough immunohistochemical (and possibly molecular) evaluation (see below).

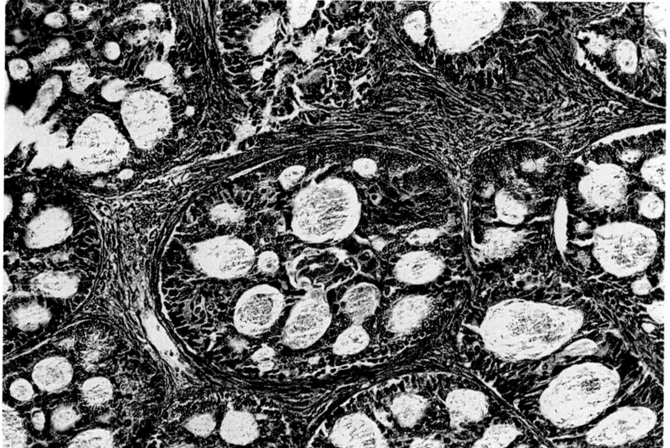

Fig. 25.173 Synovial sarcoma with an adenocarcinoma-like appearance of the epithelial component.

Theoretically, a monophasic form of synovial sarcoma composed only of the epithelial elements of the tumor should also exist. The fact that in some neoplasms the glandular elements are so prominent as to simulate a metastatic adenocarcinoma cannot be denied.[1512,1528] It has also been suggested that some of the reported cases of carcinoma of soft tissue and of epithelioid sarcoma are epithelial-rich forms of synovial sarcoma, the latter supposition being based on the occasional coexistence of the two tumors[1552] and their ultrastructural similarities.[1517,1522] However, the existence of a pure form of monophasic epithelial synovial sarcoma has yet to be convincingly demonstrated at the cytogenetic/molecular level.

A *poorly differentiated* form of synovial sarcoma is being increasingly recognized, characterized by a greater degree of cellularity, atypia, and mitotic activity.[1493,1504,1546] The tumor cells may be spindle, small, or large and clear.[1569] Here too, immunohistochemical and particularly cytogenetic/molecular confirmation (see below) becomes crucial.

In terms of special stains, the biphasic quality of the classic synovial sarcoma is highlighted by the reticulin preparations. Mucin stains reveal the presence of acid mucopolysaccharides (hyaluronic acid, chondroitin sulfate, heparitin sulfate) in the spindle cell areas and of PAS-positive, sialic acid-containing glycoproteins in the epithelial foci.[1540]

Ultrastructurally, the epithelial areas have features of true glandular epithelium; subtle features of epithelial differentiation are sometimes also found in the spindle cell component, such as intercellular spaces within processes and specialized cell junctions[1491,1492,1494,1495,1499,1517,1524,1567] (Figs 25.177 and 25.178).

Immunohistochemically, there is strong reactivity for keratin in the epithelial areas and often in the spindle cells as well.[1479,1489,1523,1550] Since normal or reactive synovial cells do not express keratin, the possibility has been raised that synovial sarcoma is not

Fig. 25.174 **A** and **B**, Mast cells in monophasic synovial sarcoma, a useful diagnostic clue. **B**, Toluidine blue metachromatic stain.

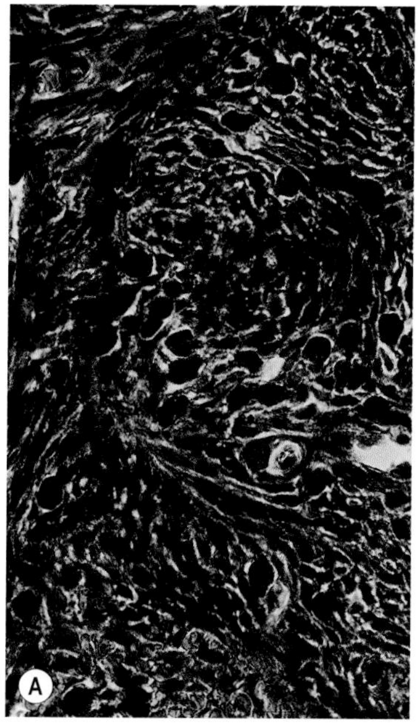

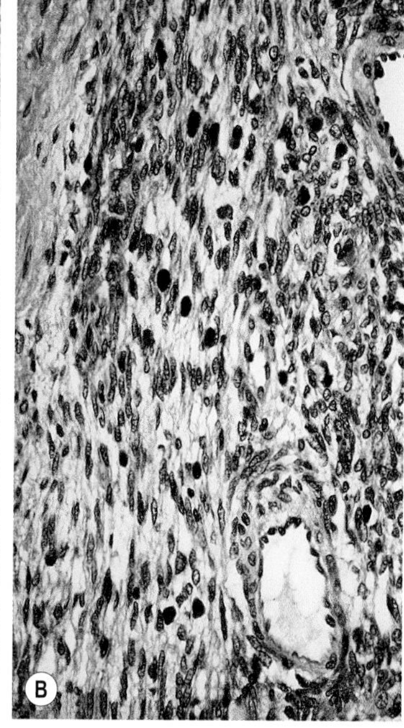

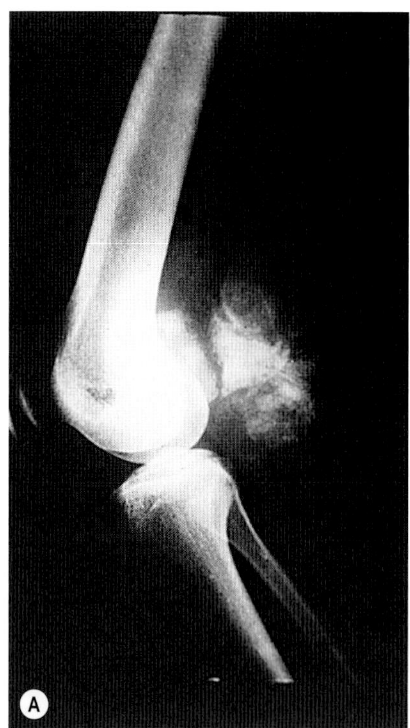

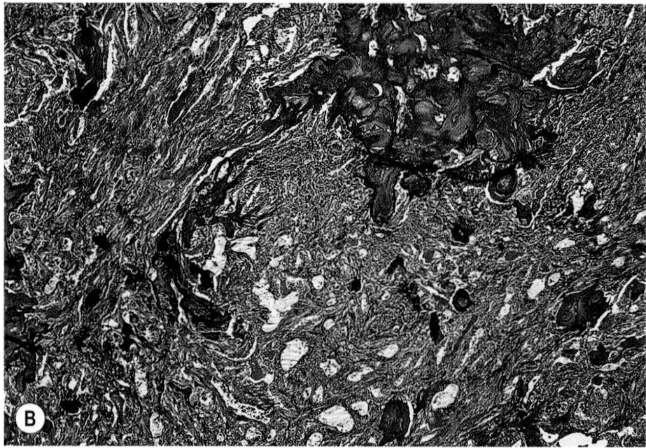

Fig. 25.175 **A** and **B**, Calcifying synovial sarcoma. **A**, Radiographic appearance of tumor located in popliteal space. **B**, Microscopic appearance.
(*A From Varela-Durán J, Enzinger FM. Calcifying synovial sarcoma. A clinicopathologic study of 32 cases. Cancer 1982, **50:** 345–352*)

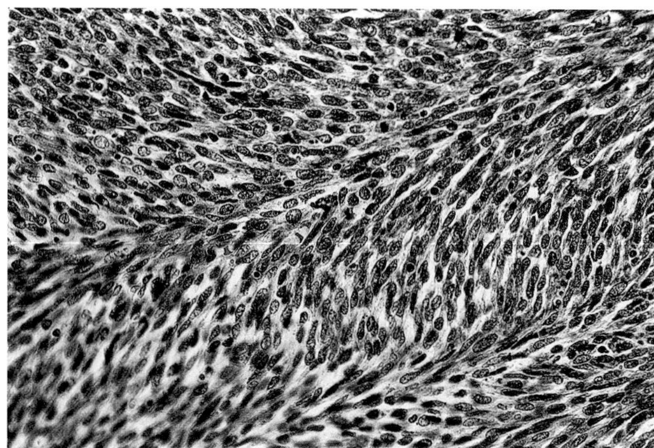

Fig. 25.176 Monophasic synovial sarcoma. The tumor is hypercellular but remarkably monomorphic.

differentiating toward synovial structures, as traditionally believed, but toward true epithelium. The corollary of this theory is that the tumor should be viewed as a primary carcinoma (or carcinosarcoma) of soft tissue,[1506,1520,1535] whether arising from epithelial rests or – more likely – from mesenchymal tissues that have undergone epithelial metaplasia. Of importance in this regard is the fact that, whereas many types of soft tissue sarcoma (including epithelioid sarcoma) exhibit immunoreactivity for keratins 8 and 18, only synovial sarcoma shows positivity for keratins 7, 14, and 19, as well as for the specialized cell junction-associated protein desmoplakin ZO-1, claudin-1, and occludin.[1486,1531] Vimentin, EMA, CEA, calponin, HBME-1, and occasionally S-100 protein are also expressed by this tumor.[1479,1489,1501,1502,1509,1520,1533,1544,1547] As a matter of fact, it is not rare to find monophasic synovial sarcomas that are focally reactive for EMA but not keratin. It has also been found that a significant number of cases of synovial sarcoma are immunoreactive for CD99, the marker characteristically associated with Ewing sarcoma/PNET (see p. 2188),[1492] BCL2,[1525] HER2/NEU,[1542] MAGE-CT (a cancer testis antigen),[1482] the oncogene *MYCN*,[1555] and TLE1 (a transcriptional corepressor that inhibits Wnt signaling, the specificity of which has been questioned)[1515,1516,1565] (Fig. 25.179). Finally, it has been observed that synovial sarcomas may exhibit focal reactivity for calretinin (but not for WT1), a point of importance in the differential diagnosis with mesothelioma, a tumor which they may closely resemble.[1533]

Synovial sarcoma exhibits in over 90% of the cases the chromosomal translocation t(X;18)(p11.2;q11.2), which results in the fusion of the *SS18* (formerly known as *SYT*) gene on chromosome 18 with either *SSX1* (in two-thirds of the cases) or *SSX2* (the other third) on chromosome X.[1551] Other molecular variants exist. This highly specific genetic alteration can be detected with RT-PCR in fresh or paraffin-embedded material,[1484,1508] conventional cytogenetics or FISH,[1539,1556,1564] and the hybrid protein SS18/SSX can be visualized immunohistochemically.[1481,1511] Notably, a high degree of correlation exists between the type of gene fusion and the tumor subtype, in the sense that nearly all biphasic tumors carry the *SS18–SSX1* fusion, whereas most of those with *SS18–SSX2* are monophasic. There is instead no association between the fusion type and the immunohistochemical expression of epithelial markers.[1483]

Synovial sarcoma can recur locally and metastasize distantly, particularly to the lung and lymph nodes. The incidence of nodal metastases is in the range of 10–15% (i.e., much higher than that of most soft tissue sarcomas of adults). The preferred treatment is local excision, with wide margins of normal tissue, supplemented by a high dose of radiation therapy.[1561] Synovial sarcoma has been traditionally regarded as a tumor of ominous prognosis; in several series, however, the 5-year survival rate has approached 50%.[1490,1526,1568] The prognosis is even better for the synovial sarcomas associated with heavy calcification (calcifying synovial sarcoma), where the survival rate reaches the figure of 80%.[1570] The prognosis is also related to age (better in young patients), site (better for distal lesions),[1521,1566] size (better for tumors less than 5 cm in diameter),[1559,1560,1573] status of the surgical margins,[1559] mitotic activity (better for tumors having fewer than 15 mitoses per 10 high-power fields),[1487] necrosis (worse for tumors having tumor necrosis of more than 50%), rhabdoid cells (worse when present), microscopic grade (which takes into account some of parameters just listed), dysadherin expression (worse when present, indicating

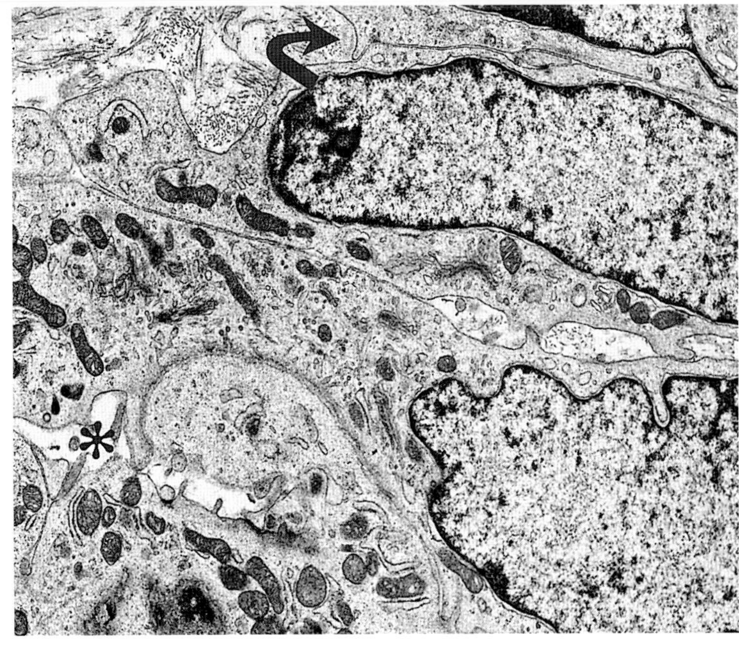

Fig. 25.177 Electron microscopic appearance of monophasic synovial sarcoma with spindle-shaped tumor cells. Note the rudimentary lumen with microvilli (asterisk) and the remnants of basal lamina (arrow).
(×7700; courtesy of Dr Robert A Erlandson, Memorial Sloan-Kettering Cancer Center)

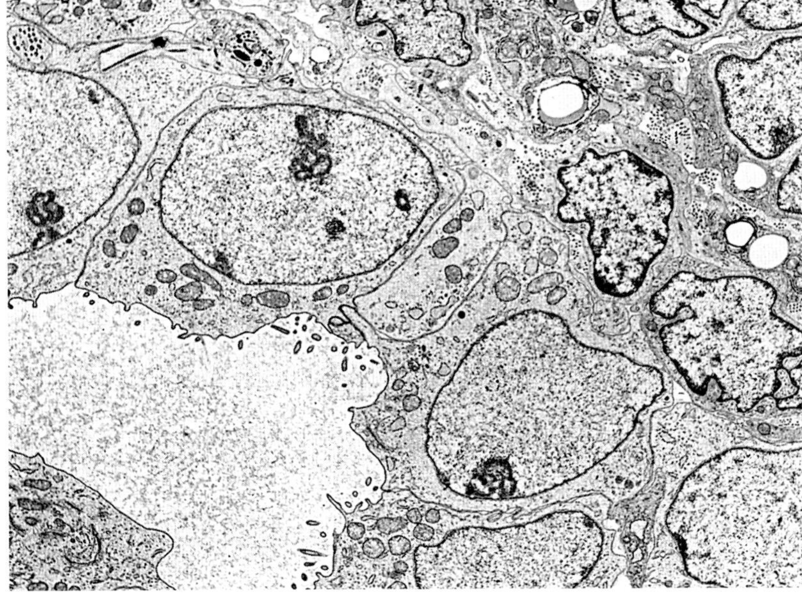

Fig. 25.178 Electron microscopic appearance of biphasic synovial sarcoma. There is a glandular formation of epithelioid tumor cells with sparse luminal microvilli (lower left).
(×4300; courtesy of Dr Robert A Erlandson, Memorial Sloan-Kettering Cancer Center)

E-cadherin dysfunction),[1513] and DNA ploidy pattern (worse for aneuploid tumors).[1496,1543,1548] Early reports that the type of gene fusion showed a significant association with prognosis[1514] have not been confirmed in other series.[1507,1563]

Tumors of extragonadal germ cells

Soft tissue teratomas are more frequent in females and present either at birth or in early childhood.[1575,1582] In some cases, there is an association with twinning or malformations. The most common locations, in descending order of frequency, are the sacrococcygeal area, head and neck, retroperitoneum, mediastinum, and central nervous system.[1576,1580,1584,1585] Taken as a whole, approximately three-fourths are benign. However, there are important variations in the incidence of malignancy according to location, completeness of resection, age, and sex.[1578,1579,1582] Nearly all the teratomas presenting in the neck during infancy are benign, usually asymmetric, and massive; the rare teratomas of the neck presenting in adults have a high incidence of malignancy.[1577,1583]

The terminology and diagnostic criteria used in the evaluation of these lesions are the same as for those of gonadal origin (see Chapters 18 and 19). The benign form is often multicystic and contains a variety of well-differentiated tissues. The malignant types may have the appearance of teratocarcinoma, embryonal carcinoma, or yolk sac tumor. Immature neuroectodermal components are common in otherwise mature teratomas; although they occasionally exhibit metastasizing capacity, their natural tendency is toward spontaneous maturation.[1581]

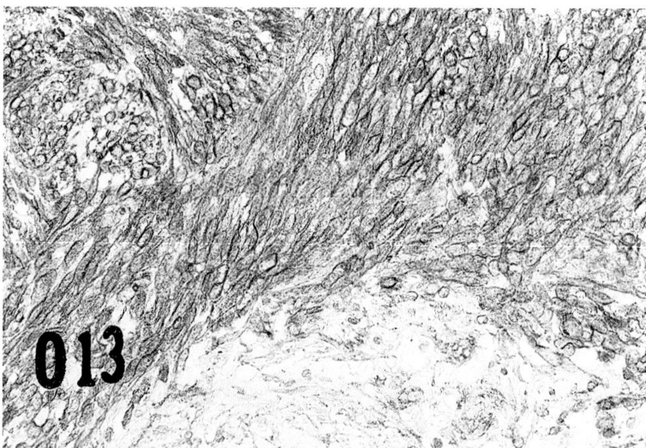

Fig. 25.179 Strong CD99 (O13) immunoreactivity in monophasic synovial sarcoma.

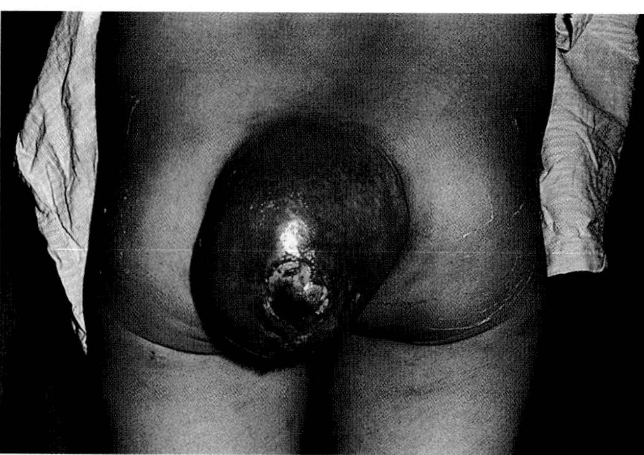

Fig. 25.181 Myxopapillary ependymoma of the sacrococcygeal region resulting in a huge protruding mass that is focally ulcerated.
(Courtesy of Dr Juan José Segura, San José, Costa Rica)

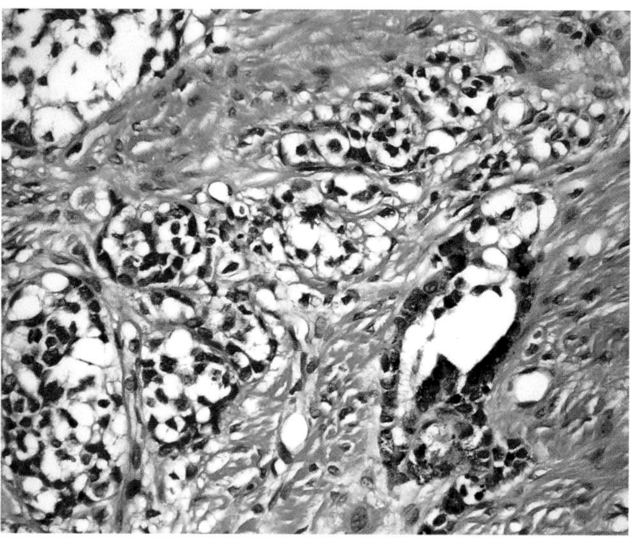

Fig. 25.180 Pigmented neuroectodermal tumor of infancy. Nests of neuroblast-like cells are adjacent to gland-like spaces lined by larger cells containing neural-type melanin.

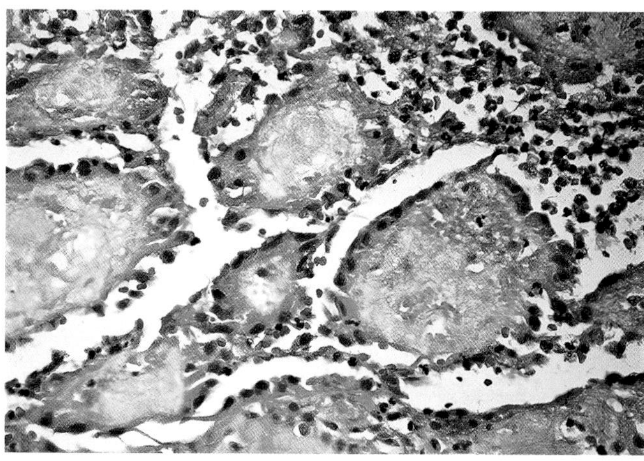

Fig. 25.182 Myxopapillary ependymoma involving soft tissues of buttock. The tumor papillae have an abundant hyalinized core.

Tumors of neural tissue (other than peripheral nerves)

Pigmented neuroectodermal tumor of infancy

Pigmented neuroectodermal tumor of infancy, also known as melanotic progonoma and retinal anlage tumor, is a neurally derived neoplasm.[1587,1590,1591] The classic location is the maxilla, but it also has been reported in the mandible, skull, and other bones, mediastinum, soft tissues (thigh, forearm, cheek), and epididymis.[1589,1591,1594,1596] Microscopically, most tumor cells are small and round, with the appearance of neuroblasts. As a result, this tumor may be misdiagnosed as neuroblastoma. The diagnostic feature is the presence of pseudoglandular or alveolar formations lined by a wall of larger cells containing abundant CNS-type (spiculated) melanin in their cytoplasm (Fig. 25.180). Rarely, a skeletal muscle component is present.[1592] Immunohistochemically, the large cells are strongly reactive for keratin and HMB-45 and less so for vimentin and NSE, whereas the small cells show only positivity for NSE. Both cell components are negative for S-100 protein.[1586,1592,1593,1595] Ultrastructurally, there are melanosomes at various stages of maturation in the large cells, and neurosecretory granules and cytoplasmic processes in the small cells.[1592]

The clinical course is usually benign. Most supposedly malignant varieties probably represent malignant teratomas with a pigmented neuroectodermal component. However, unquestionable recurrent and metastatic cases of pigmented neuroectodermal tumor of infancy have been seen.[1588,1589,1592]

Other neural tumors

Meningiomas can present as a soft tissue mass at the base of the nose or scalp[1598,1601] (see Chapters 4 and 7).

Myxopapillary ependymomas can appear as soft tissue masses over the sacrococcygeal area, unconnected with the spine or spinal cord structures[1597,1600] (Fig. 25.181). The clinical diagnosis is usually that of pilonidal cyst. Grossly, they are well circumscribed and can be shelled out easily. Their microscopic appearance is homologous to that of their more common counterpart in the filum terminale and cauda equina (see Chapter 28) (Fig. 25.182). Metastases have occurred in approximately one-fifth of the cases.[1599]

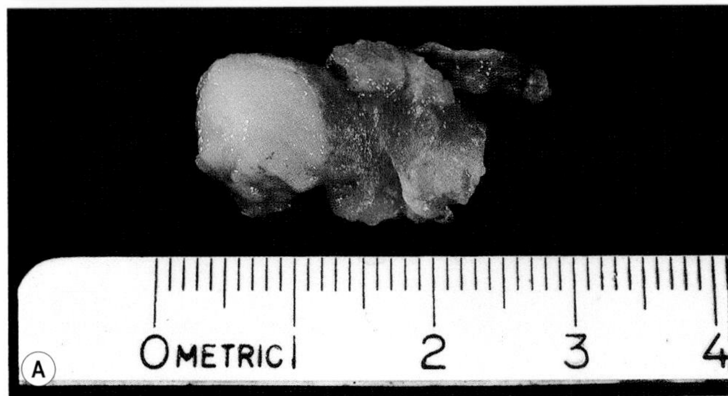

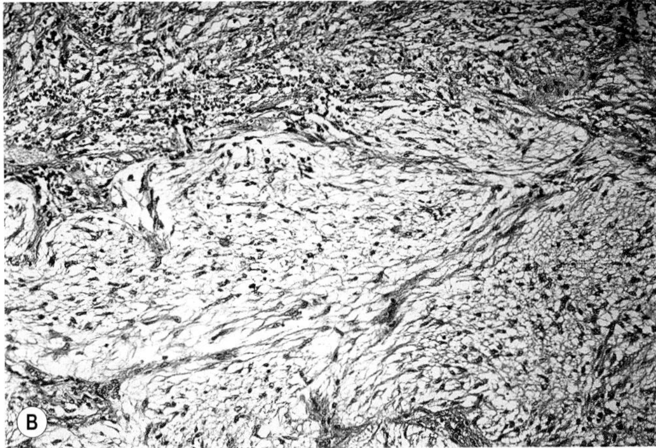
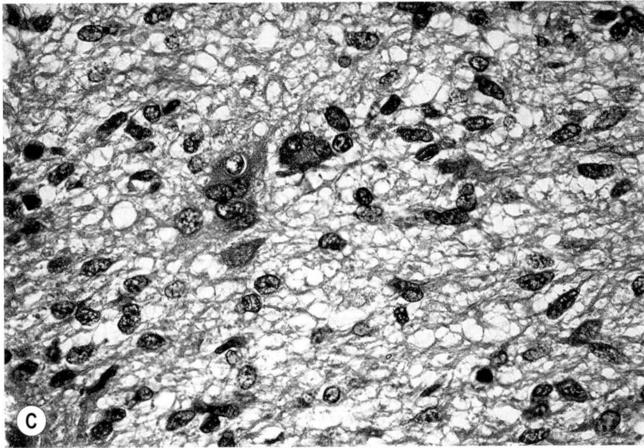

Fig. 25.183 Soft tissue 'glioma' involving the orbit: **A**, gross appearance; **B**, low-power view; **C**, high-power view showing the glial fibrillary background and scattered multinucleated cells. This lesion is probably of malformative rather than neoplastic nature.

Myxopapillary ependymomas should be distinguished from sacrococcygeal ependymal rests, which probably represent their precursors. These are small (less than 0.5 cm) nodules that are usually found incidentally in tissue from pilonidal sinuses and that consist of clusters of ependymal cells near the junction of dermis and subcutis.[1603]

Gliomas of soft tissue have been generally located at the root of the nose in infants, but they can occur in other sites such as orbit, scalp, chest wall, and gluteal region;[1602] they are probably not neoplasms but examples of heterotopic glial tissue[1604] (Fig. 25.183).

Primitive neuroectodermal tumors (PNET) are discussed on page 2188.

Tumors of hematopoietic tissue

Malignant lymphomas may exceptionally manifest themselves initially as soft tissue masses, usually located in an extremity.[1614] This occurrence is more common with non-Hodgkin lymphomas than with Hodgkin lymphoma, but both of these major types occur.[1605,1613] Most cases are of B-cell derivation, but examples of peripheral T-cell lymphoma (including NK and NK-like T-cell lymphomas) with primary involvement of soft tissues are on record.[1607,1611,1612] Exceptionally, these lymphomas develop in areas of post-mastectomy lymphedema and are confused clinically with angiosarcoma.[1609]

True histiocytic sarcomas have been described outside lymphoid structures, including soft tissues.[1610] Microscopically, they are composed of sheets of large epithelioid cells with abundant eosinophilic cytoplasm, round to oval (sometimes indented) nuclei, and large nucleoli. Some of the tumor cells are bi- or multinucleated. Immunohistochemically, they are reactive to CD45, CD45RO, CD68, and CD163. They also often express CD4, lysozyme, and CD31.[1610]

Plasmacytomas of soft tissue represent, for the most part, direct extension from underlying osseous foci.[1606] However, isolated soft tissue masses also can occur in the absence of bone involvement. They have a tendency to become disseminated.

Extramedullary hematopoiesis may present in the form of nodules in the mediastinum, retroperitoneum, or other soft tissue areas; they have been described in agnogenic myeloid metaplasia and congenital spherocytosis and in other types of anemia,[1608] and should be distinguished from myelolipoma (see Chapter 16).

Tumors of uncertain cell type

Fibrous hamartoma of infancy

Fibrous hamartoma of infancy is a tumorlike condition seen almost exclusively during the first 2 years of life and sometimes present at birth.[1615,1618] It predominates in boys, and the most common locations are the region of the shoulder, axilla, and upper arm. It is almost always solitary. Grossly, it is poorly circumscribed and composed of whitish tissue of fibrous appearance intermixed with islands of fat.

Microscopically, the distinctive feature of this lesion is an organoid pattern, three distinct types of tissue being present: (1) well-differentiated spindle cells of fibroblastic/myofibroblastic appearance accompanied by deposition of collagen; (2) mature adipose tissue; and (3) immature cellular areas arranged in a whorl-like pattern and resembling primitive mesenchyme (Fig. 25.184). Positivity for vimentin occurs in both fibrous and immature areas, whereas reactivity for actin (and sometimes desmin) is found mainly in the spindle cell areas, suggesting the existence of a myofibroblastic component.[1616,1617,1619] Although there may be local recurrence, the clinical course is basically that of a benign disease.[1615]

Myxoma and related tumors

Myxomas are rare neoplasms that have a mucoid, slimy gross appearance (Fig. 25.185). They almost always occur in adults and are more common in females.[1624] The diagnosis of myxoma in a child should be seriously questioned. A high proportion of myxomas arise within skeletal muscle (intramuscular myxoma), especially in the thigh region. The prognosis is excellent. In most of the reported series, there was not a single case of local recurrence.[1624,1626] Multiple intramuscular myxomas are nearly always seen in association with fibrous dysplasia of the bones of the same extremity.[1621,1627,1637] The presence of multiple myxomas in the skin, breast, or other locations should raise the possibility of Carney complex, which also includes

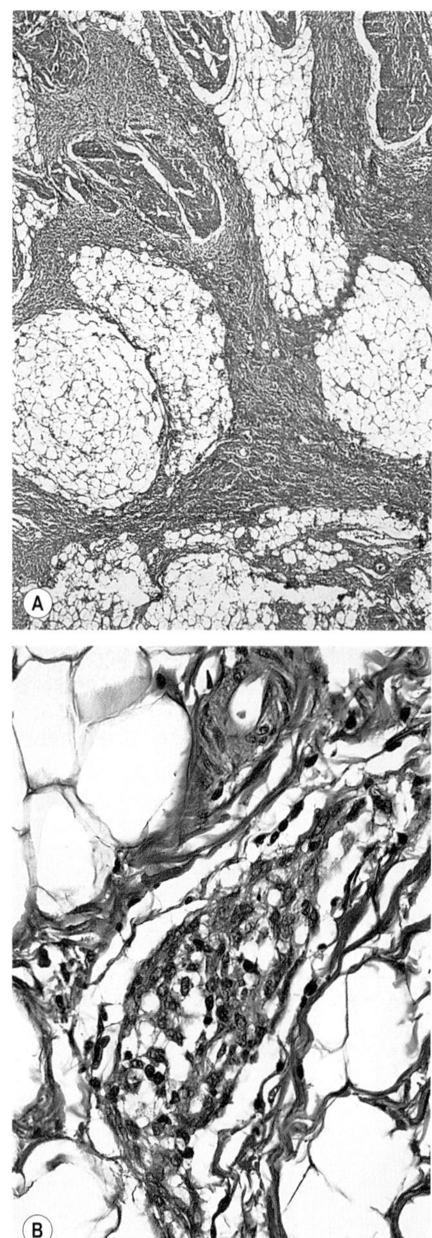

Fig. 25.184 **A** and **B**, Fibrous hamartoma of infancy. **A**, Low-power microscopic view showing an admixture of islands of mature adipose tissue and cellular fibrous foci. **B**, High-power view showing an oval cluster of plump mesenchymal cells.

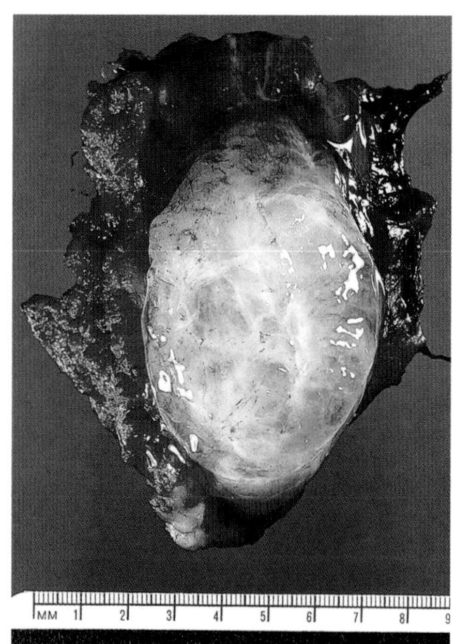

Fig. 25.185 Typical gross appearance of intramuscular myxoma. *(Courtesy of Dr RA Cooke, Brisbane, Australia; from Cooke RA, Stewart B. Colour atlas of anatomical pathology. Edinburgh, 2004, Churchill Livingstone)*

spotty cutaneous pigmentation, nodular pigmented adrenal disease, and other endocrine abnormalities.[1623] Another important location of myxoma is the juxta-articular region (*juxta-articular myxoma*), particularly in the knee.[1631]

Microscopically, a typical myxoma has a bland and hypocellular appearance throughout, mitotic activity is practically absent, and blood vessels are extremely scanty (Fig. 25.186), the latter feature having been well documented with angiographic and microangiographic studies. Focal aggregates of foamy histiocytes may be present; these contain neutral fat with the oil red O stain and should not be confused with the lipoblasts of myxoid liposarcoma.[1626]

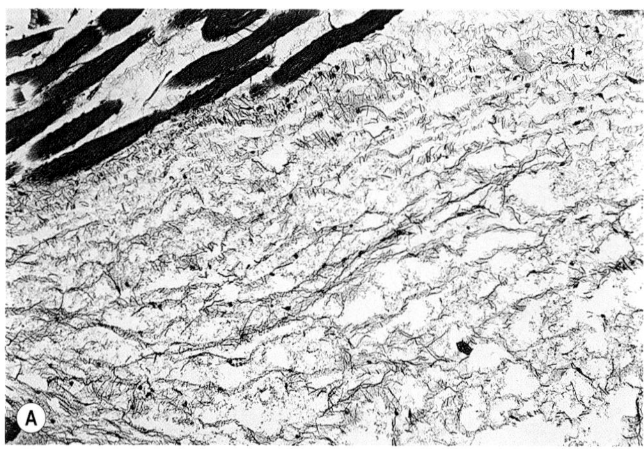

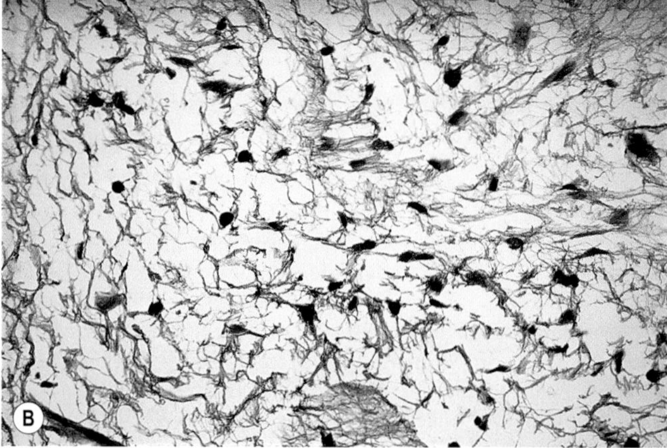

Fig. 25.186 **A** and **B**, Intramuscular myxoma. **A**, Note the hypocellular quality, lack of encapsulation, and intramuscular location. **B**, The high-power view highlights the lack of atypia and paucity of vessels.

Ultrastructurally, the principal cell of intramuscular myxoma resembles a fibroblast, with prominent granular endoplasmic reticulum, well-developed Golgi apparatus, and cytoplasmic filaments.[1625] Immunohistochemically, myxoma shows no reactivity for S-100 protein, this being another difference with myxoid liposarcoma.[1626] Desmin is also absent, but vimentin is expressed.[1632] The myxoid material is entirely digestible by hyaluronidase.

Genetically, intramuscular myxoma commonly exhibits activating mutations in the *GNAS1* gene, the same gene involved in the genesis of fibrous dysplasia of bone.[1634,1636] The result of the mutation is downstream activation of cellular oncogene protein c-Fos.[1636] Mutations of *GNAS1*, on the other hand, are not seen in juxta-articular myxomas.[1634]

The differential diagnosis of myxoma comprises two types of disease. The first is a group of neoplasms in which myxoid change can be a prominent secondary feature, such as liposarcoma, myxofibrosarcoma, chondrosarcoma, leiomyosarcoma, embryonal rhabdomyosarcoma, neurofibroma, nerve sheath myxoma/neurothekeoma, and aggressive angiomyxoma.[1630] The latter occurs preferentially in the soft tissues of the female genital tract (see Chapter 19), but a counterpart located in the superficial soft tissue has been described.[1621,1622] If a myxoid tumor is hypercellular and hypervascular, the alternative possibility of low-grade myxofibrosarcoma should be considered. However, a *cellular variant* of myxoma has been described which is more cellular and more vascular than the ordinary type;[1633,1635] this tumor lacks the pleomorphism, nuclear atypia, and curvilinear vascular pattern of low-grade myxofibrosarcoma.[1635]

The second group of diseases from which myxoma should be distinguished is a variety of non-neoplastic disorders resulting in focal mucinous degeneration of the skin or soft tissues, such as nodular fasciitis, localized myxedema, mucous (myxoid) cyst, ganglion, follicular mucinosis (alopecia mucinosa), papular mucinosis, and cutaneous focal mucinosis.[1628]

Superficial acral fibromyxoma presents as a solitary mass or nodule in the distal extremities (usually digits but also heels).[1620] Microscopically, it is composed of spindle cells with vaguely storiform and fascicular patterns, embedded in a myxoid, fibromyxoid, or collagenous stroma. Immunohistochemically, they are CD34 positive and sometimes also stain for CD99 and/or EMA. A *cellular variant* of this tumor has been described.[1629]

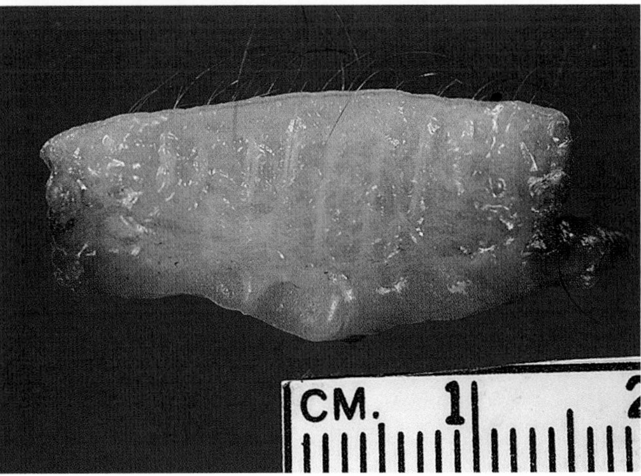

Fig. 25.187 Granular cell tumor of skin. There is an ill-defined permeation of the dermis by whitish tissue.

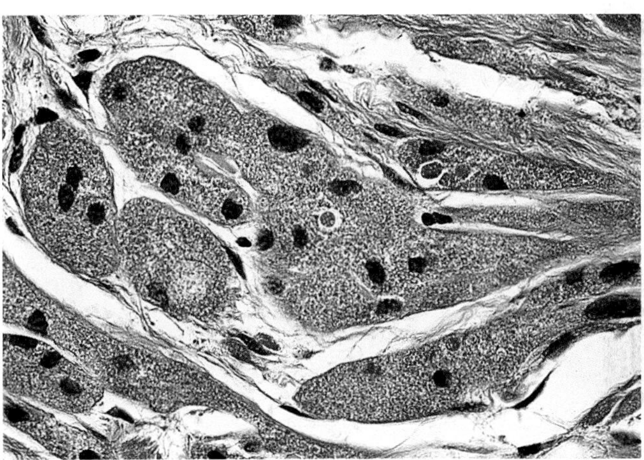

Fig. 25.188 Granular cell tumor. The cells contain innumerable fine cytoplasmic granules as well as scattered larger eosinophilic globules.

Granular cell tumor

The classic location of granular cell tumor, classically known as granular cell myoblastoma, is the tongue. It has been seen, however, in innumerable other locations, such as skin, vulva, breast, larynx, bronchus, esophagus, stomach, appendix, rectum, anus, salivary glands, bile ducts, pancreas, urinary bladder, uterus, brain, pituitary gland, and soft tissue.[1642,1646,1649,1650,1655,1658,1659,1671,1684,1692] Multiplicity of lesions can be observed, particularly in black patients.[1669,1671,1685] Congenital examples have been reported, most of them located in the gingiva,[1648,1660,1663] but some exhibiting systemic involvement.[1680]

These tumors are usually small, although we have seen cases measuring up to 5 cm in diameter. They have a hard consistency and ill-defined margins (Fig. 25.187). This, together with the ulceration sometimes complicating the larger cutaneous tumors, explains why they are sometimes confused clinically and on gross inspection with a malignant neoplasm. Rarely, they have a polypoid shape,[1643,1656,1662] these being usually negative for S-100 protein (see below). The individual cells are large and their cytoplasm is highly granular (Fig. 25.188). Most granules are small and regular. They alternate with larger round droplets having a homogeneous eosinophilic appearance and a stronger PAS positivity. The pattern of growth is ill-defined and pseudoinvasive. Some of the granular cells can be found in the wall or lumen of blood vessels, not to be taken as a sign of malignancy.[1647] If the tumor grows near an epithelial surface, in sites such as skin, vulva, or larynx, secondary epithelial hyperplasia occurs that may be incorrectly diagnosed as carcinoma[1688] (Fig. 25.189). Elastosis is often present in the stroma.[1666]

Histochemically, the cytoplasmic granules contain large amounts of hydrolytic enzymes (such as acid phosphatase), and they are consistently positive for Luxol fast blue.[1670] Ultrastructurally, they have the appearance of lysosomes. Other interesting electron microscopic findings are the presence of a second cell population with 'angulated bodies' resulting in a Gaucher cell-like appearance[1640,1654] and of replicated basal lamina material around the granular cells, the latter suggesting repeated cycles of cellular injury and repair. Immunohistochemically, positivity has been described (in at least some of the lesions) for S-100 protein, laminin, calretinin, the alpha subunit of inhibin HLA-DR, PGP 9.5, CD68, osteopontin, myelin basic protein, and CEA.[1652,1657,1661,1665,1672–1674,1677,1681] The presence of the latter two markers remains controversial;[1645] the apparent CEA

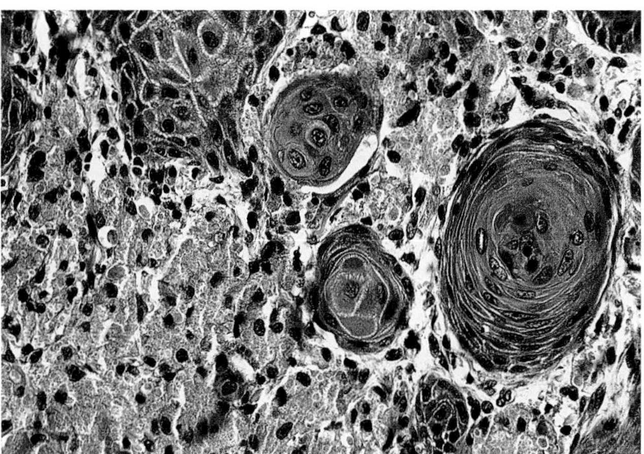

Fig. 25.189 Pseudoepitheliomatous hyperplasia in squamous epithelium overlying granular cell tumor.

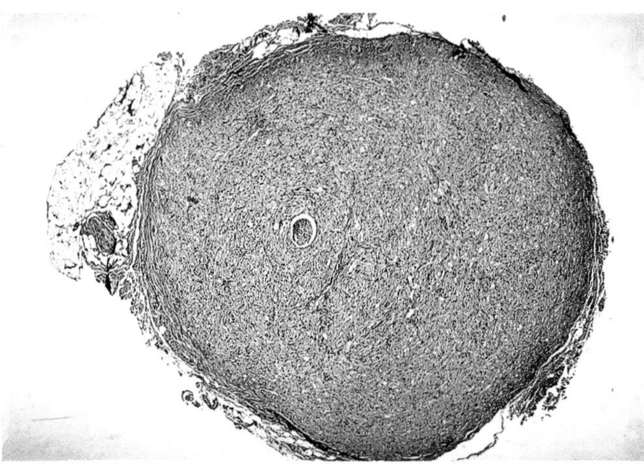

Fig. 25.190 Granular cell tumor growing concentrically within and around a nerve cut transversally.

reactivity may be caused by the presence of a cross-reacting antigen.[1664,1676] The expression of HLA-DR is thought to be related not to the cell of origin but rather to some common immunologic pathogenesis.[1682] Granular cell tumors of the gastrointestinal tract also express the intermediate filament protein nestin.[1679]

The large majority of the granular cell tumors pursue a benign clinical course. Most cases reported in the old literature as malignant granular cell myoblastomas are in reality examples of alveolar soft part sarcoma. However, there have been several well-documented cases of tumors with a light and electron microscopic appearance entirely consistent with that of granular cell tumor that have resulted in distant metastases.[1638,1683,1689–1691] Features favoring malignancy in granular cell tumor (especially when seen in combination) are necrosis, high mitotic activity, spindling of tumor cells, vesicular nuclei with large nucleoli, and high MIB-1 values.[1651]

The histogenesis of this lesion is still being argued.[1678] Most writers on the subject favor a Schwann cell origin, based on histochemical, immunohistochemical, and ultrastructural findings and on the occurrence of typical lesions, within nerves[1639,1641,1654,1686] (Fig. 25.190). However, in some lesions, there is no evidence of Schwann cell participation.[1662] Furthermore, changes histochemically and ultrastructurally indistinguishable from those previously discussed have been documented in neoplastic and non-neoplastic smooth muscle cells and in tumoral ameloblasts.[1644,1675,1687] We therefore favor the view that granular cell tumor is not a specific entity but rather the expression of a degenerative change resulting in a cytoplasmic accumulation of lysosomes that occur primarily in Schwann cells as well as in a variety of other cell types, whether previously normal or forming part of a benign or a malignant neoplasm, such as MPNST, leiomyosarcoma, or angiosarcoma.[1653,1667,1668,1677] We favor making the diagnosis of granular cell tumor only when the entire lesion is granular and to designate the other cases according to their basic component, noting that focal granular changes are present.

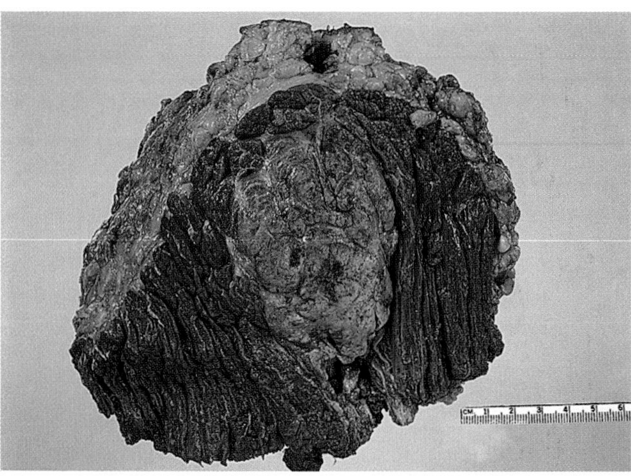

Fig. 25.191 Alveolar soft part sarcoma. The tumor is multinodular, relatively well circumscribed, and embedded within skeletal muscle.

Alveolar soft part sarcoma

Alveolar soft part sarcoma, a malignant soft tissue tumor designated in the past as malignant organoid granular cell myoblastoma and malignant nonchromaffin paraganglioma, involves most often the deep soft tissues of the thigh and leg.[1709] It has also been seen in the oral cavity and pharynx (including tongue), mediastinum (sometimes arising from the pulmonary vein), stomach, retroperitoneum, orbit, bladder, uterus, and vagina.[1693,1700,1702,1705,1722,1727,1729] We have also seen it inside the patella. Most patients are young females. Grossly, the tumors are well circumscribed, usually large, moderately firm, and gray or yellowish (Fig. 25.191). Areas of necrosis or hemorrhage are common in the larger neoplasms.[1730]

Microscopically, the tumor cells are separated by fibrous tissue into well-defined nests. Detachment of the central cells results in a typical alveolar pattern (Fig. 25.192). The individual cells are large and have vesicular nuclei, prominent nucleoli, and a granular cytoplasm. Mitoses are exceptional. PAS stain sometimes demonstrates the presence of diastase-resistant intracytoplasmic needle-like structures (Fig. 25.193). These are seen by electron microscopy as membrane-bound crystals with a periodicity of 58–100 nm, sometimes arranged in a cross-grid pattern[1701] (Fig. 25.194). This feature is of great diagnostic value in lesions of controversial nature.[1726] Other ultrastructural features include numerous vesicles with an electron-dense content in the Golgi region (possibly representing the precursors of the crystals) and smooth tubular aggregates associated with plasmalemmal invaginations.[1718]

Alveolar soft part sarcomas occurring in children are often associated with a more solid pattern of growth, and therefore tend to be misdiagnosed (Fig. 25.195). Conversely, the alveolar appearance

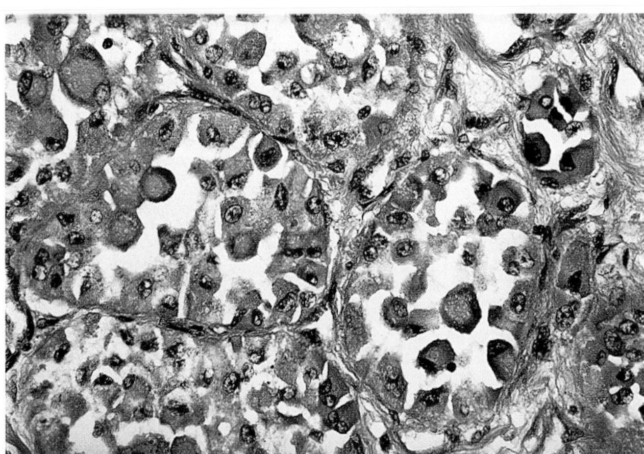

Fig. 25.192 Typical microscopic appearance of alveolar soft part sarcoma. Note the lack of mitoses.

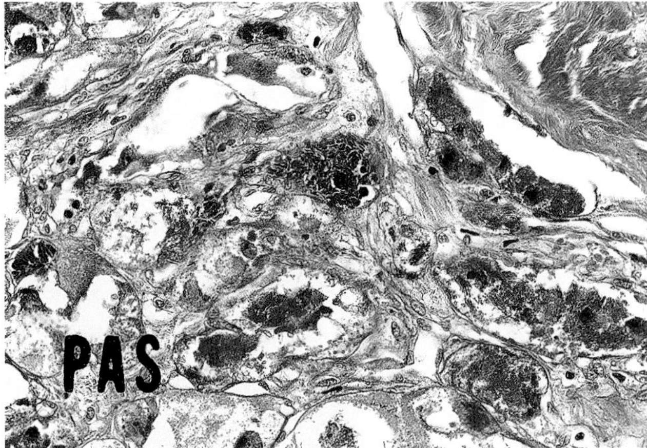

Fig. 25.193 PAS-positive cytoplasmic granules in alveolar soft part sarcoma, some having a crystalline appearance.

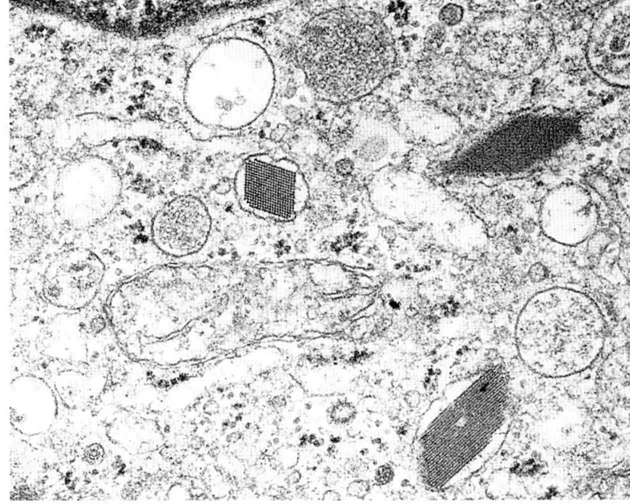

Fig. 25.194 Electron microscopic appearance of alveolar soft part sarcoma. Detailed view of characteristic crystalloid inclusions that demonstrate orderly 70 Å periodicity. Both linear and cross-hatched crystalloid patterns may be noted.
(×70 000; courtesy of Dr J Sciubba, New Hyde Park, NY)

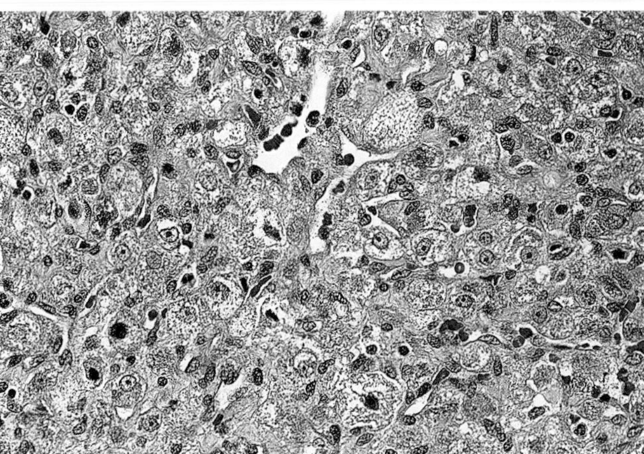

Fig. 25.195 Alveolar soft part sarcoma with a nesting pattern of growth and lack of alveolar formations. This variant, which is particularly common in children, is likely to be misdiagnosed.

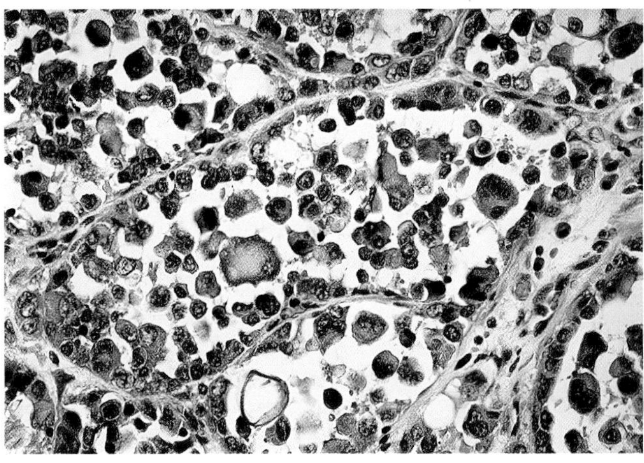

Fig. 25.196 Metastatic malignant melanoma closely simulating the appearance of alveolar soft part sarcoma.

of this entity can be closely simulated by other malignant neoplasms, notably malignant melanoma and renal cell carcinoma (Fig. 25.196).

Alveolar soft part sarcoma is highly malignant, despite its deceptively slow and indolent clinical course. Vein invasion is common. Blood-borne metastases appear in the lungs and other organs as long as 30 years or more following excision of the primary tumor.[1710,1711] Not infrequently, a metastasis in the lung or in another organ is the first manifestation of the disease. There is a good correlation between tumor size and survival.[1699]

The histogenesis of this strange neoplasm has not yet been definitely established.[1696,1715] We believe there is no convincing evidence to support the theory that this tumor represents a malignant counterpart of granular cell tumor, that it arises from nonchromaffin paraganglia, or that it is related to renin-producing cells of blood vessel walls.[1698] Instead, a wealth of data has accumulated in recent years supporting the interpretation that alveolar soft part sarcoma is of myogenous derivation and that it represents a distinct variant of rhabdomyosarcoma.[1704] This includes the (admittedly inconsistent) immunohistochemical demonstration of smooth muscle and sarcomeric actin, desmin, Z-protein, fast myosin, β-enolase, and the MM isozyme of creatine kinase[1703,1706,1713,1714,1716,1717,1719,1720,1723]

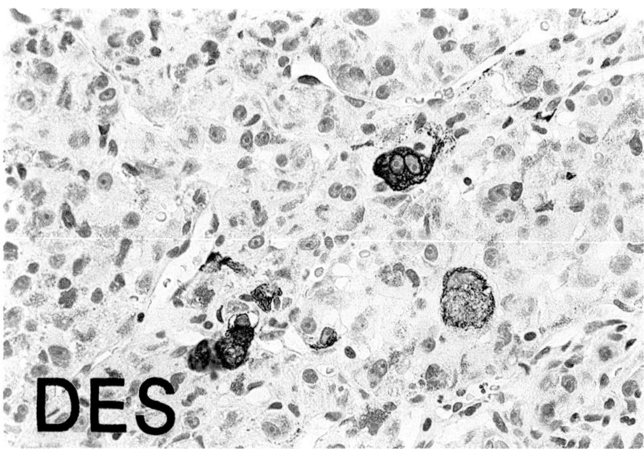

Fig. 25.197 Desmin immunoreactivity in scattered tumor cells of alveolar soft part sarcoma.

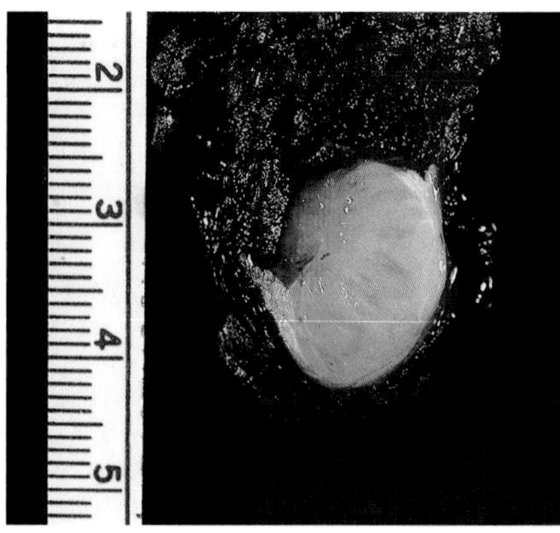

Fig. 25.198 Gross appearance of clear cell sarcoma (malignant melanoma of soft parts) located in the posterior thigh.

(Fig. 25.197); the demonstration of ATPase activity in the crystalline inclusions;[1712] the detection of similar membrane-bound cytoplasmic crystals in a normal human muscle spindle;[1697] the presence of T-tubule-like structures at the ultrastructural level;[1718] and the (not independently confirmed) demonstration of MyoD1 protein, a nuclear phosphoprotein that is the product of a regulatory gene that controls the commitment of a cell to a myogenic lineage.[1724] However, we freely admit that the matter is far from settled.[1721,1728] Along these lines, the demonstration that the precrystalline cytoplasmic granules of this tumor contain monocarboxylate transporter 1 and CD147[1707] is of interest but does not particularly contribute to the solution of the histogenetic riddle that surrounds this tumor.

At the cytogenetic level, alveolar soft part sarcoma has been found to be associated with the chromosomal unbalanced translocation der(17)t(X;17)(p11.2;q25), which results in the fusion of the *TFE3* transcription factor gene to the *ASPSCR1* (formerly known as *ASPL*) gene.[1708,1715,1725] Interestingly, a similar but balanced translocation has been detected in a type of renal neoplasm which is probably epithelial but which bears some morphologic resemblance to alveolar soft part sarcoma (see also Chapter 17).[1694] The presence of aberrant nuclear expression of TFE3 can be demonstrated in these tumors by immunohistochemistry.[1695]

Clear cell sarcoma of tendons and aponeuroses (malignant melanoma of soft parts)

This malignant tumor arises chiefly from large tendons and aponeuroses of the extremities.[1738,1739,1741,1751] The feet are the most common site, but it has been described in several other sites, including penis and gastrointestinal tract (see below).[1754,1757] Most of the patients are young adults, and there is a male predominance.[1743]

Grossly, the tumors are firm, well circumscribed, and gray or white, and are cut with a gritty sensation (Fig. 25.198). Microscopically, solid nests and fascicles of pale fusiform or cuboidal cells are present (Fig. 25.199). The nucleoli are large and deeply basophilic. Multinucleated giant cells are often seen. Abundant extracellular and intracellular iron is present. In many of the cases the tumor cells also contain cytoplasmic melanin,[1733,1736,1756] strongly suggesting that this neoplasm is of neuroectodermal derivation and that it represents a peculiar type of malignant melanoma of soft parts.[1732,1736,1749] In keeping with this interpretation is the fact that the tumor cells consistently exhibit immunoreactivity for S-100

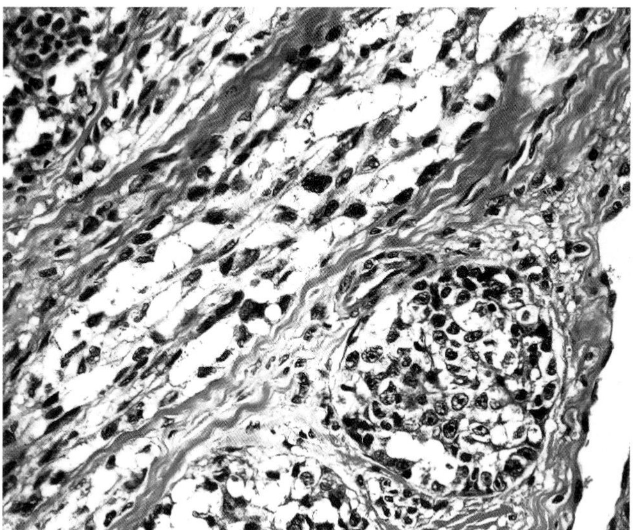

Fig. 25.199 Clear cell sarcoma of soft parts. Note the fascicular pattern of growth and the prominent nucleoli.

protein, HMB-45, Leu7, NSE, and vimentin,[1736,1742,1744,1755] and that ultrastructurally there are melanosomes plus features consistent with a neural derivation.[1734,1750] When compared with conventional melanoma of skin metastatic to soft tissue by DNA ploidy analysis, clear cell sarcoma is more likely to be diploid or to show a lesser degree of aneuploidy.[1740] Like conventional melanoma, clear cell sarcoma may exhibit immunoreactivity for keratin.[1748]

Clear cell sarcoma is associated with the chromosomal translocation t(12;22)(q13;q12),[1735,1752] which results in the *EWS–ATF1* gene fusion and the expression of the melanocyte-specific splice form of the MIFT transcript.[1731] Interestingly, this molecular genetic aberration, which is not present in cutaneous melanomas, has also been found in some morphologically conventional melanomas located in the gastrointestinal tract,[1746] as well as in a peculiar osteoclast-rich tumor of the upper gastrointestinal tract which is positive for S-100 protein but negative for melanin stains and melanoma-associated immunostains, such as HMB-45.[1758]

The clinical course of clear cell sarcoma is characterized by slow but relentless progression with frequent local recurrences and eventual nodal and distant metastases.[1737,1741] Large tumor size and necrosis are statistically significant predictors of poor prognosis.[1745,1747,1753]

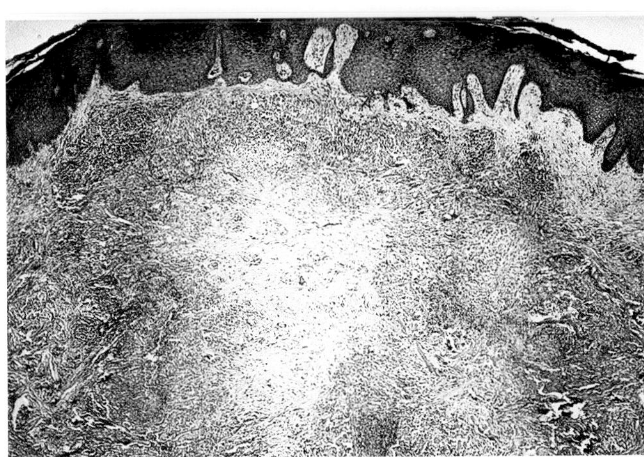

Fig. 25.200 The low-power appearance of this dermally located epithelioid sarcoma simulates a granuloma annulare or rheumatoid nodule.

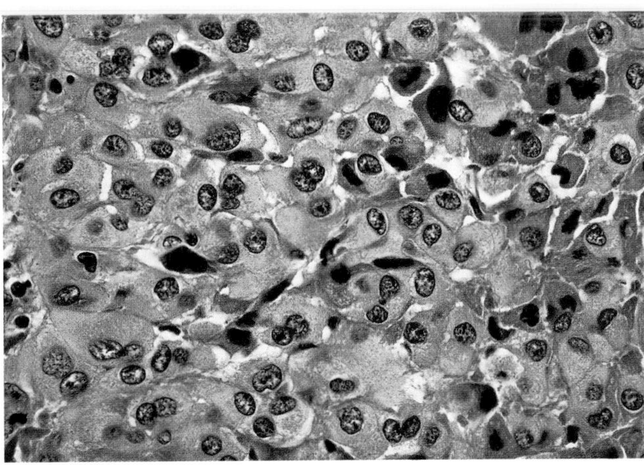

Fig. 25.202 Remarkable epithelioid quality of tumor cells in epithelioid sarcoma. Note the diffuse tissue eosinophilia.

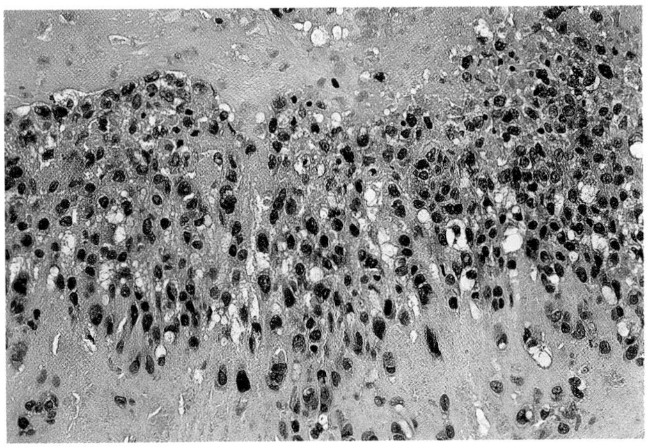

Fig. 25.201 Tightly clustered epithelioid tumor cells around the necrotic center in epithelioid sarcoma.

Epithelioid sarcoma

Epithelioid sarcoma usually affects adolescents and young adults.[1768,1773] A few cases have been reported in patients with neurofibromatosis.[1791] The extremities are the most common location, particularly the hands and fingers. Several instances of vulvar involvement have also been recorded.[1797] The tumors tend to be superficially located and are sometimes centered in the reticular dermis. Others are found in the subcutis or deeper soft tissues, particularly fascial planes, aponeuroses, and tendon sheaths.[1792] The necrosis often seen in the center of the nodules and the epithelioid appearance of the tumor cells may result in a mistaken diagnosis of infectious granuloma or, more frequently, necrobiotic collagen granuloma[1792] (Fig. 25.200).

One of the most characteristic features of this lesion is the striking acidophilia of the tumor tissue, which is due to the combined effect of the staining characteristics of the cytoplasm and the extensive desmoplasia (Figs 25.201 and 25.202). Metaplastic elements such as bone and cartilage may be present.[1765,1778] Sometimes, most of the tumor cells have a spindle shape and simulate a fibroma or a dermatofibrosarcoma protuberans.[1785] In other cases the tumor cells are unusually large (*large cell subtype*).[1764] Some epithelioid sarcomas of the soft tissue or vulva exhibit rhabdoid features; this is particularly common in the so-called 'proximal type' (see below).[1786,1789]

Ultrastructurally, the tumor cells exhibit abundant intermediate filaments, desmosome-like cell junctions, and small intercellular spaces surrounded by filopodia or microvilli[1771,1783,1787] (Fig. 25.203). Immunohistochemically, there is positivity for keratin, EMA, vimentin, CD34, tissue polypeptide antigen, and occasionally CEA[1762,1763,1766,1770,1781,1782,1787] (Fig. 25.204). The coexpression of vimentin and keratin is thought to be characteristic of this tumor; however, vimentin-negative cases that still retain positivity for keratin and CD34 have been reported.[1759] Similar to rhabdoid tumor, INI1 expression is commonly lost.[1775,1777] Regarding keratin subtypes, Miettinen et al.[1783] found positivity for CK8 in 94% of the cases, CK19 in 72%, 34βEH12 in 48%, and CK7 in 22%. Keratin 5/6 is usually negative or expressed only focally, in contrast to squamous cell carcinoma.[1779]

Genetically, translocations involving chromosomes 7, 8, 14, 18, 20, and 22 have been described.[1780] Deletions of the *INI1* gene on chromosome 22q11.2 are recognized in a subset of cases.[1777]

The histogenesis of this tumor remains obscure. It clearly exhibits features of epithelial differentiation and therefore could be regarded as a form of carcinoma of soft tissue, together with synovial sarcoma and the exceptionally rare adamantinoma of soft tissues.[1784] Whether the epithelial features present in these tumors derive from metaplasia of mesenchymal elements remains to be determined. Another possibility, already mentioned in this chapter, is that epithelioid sarcoma may represent a peculiar form of epithelioid hemangioendothelioma.[1767] Yet another is that of epithelioid sarcoma possibly representing a form of malignant perineurioma.[1795]

The tumor spreads to noncontiguous areas of skin, soft tissue, fascia, and bone, as well as by direct extension along fascial planes.[1760,1788] Local recurrence is the rule, although it may take years for this to develop. Lymph node metastases are relatively common and constitute an ominous prognostic sign.[1790] Metastases also occur in the lungs, other organs, and skin; for some peculiar reason, the scalp is a preferred site.[1797] Sometimes a lymph node metastasis is the first clinical manifestation of the disease.[1796] Excision plus radiation therapy achieves a low rate of local recurrence.[1793] A more aggressive clinical course is associated with a proximal or axial tumor location, increased size and depth, hemorrhage, mitotic figures, necrosis, rhabdoid features, and vascular invasion.[1761,1769] Some of these features may be seen in combination. Indeed, the proposal has been made for the existence of a *proximal type* of

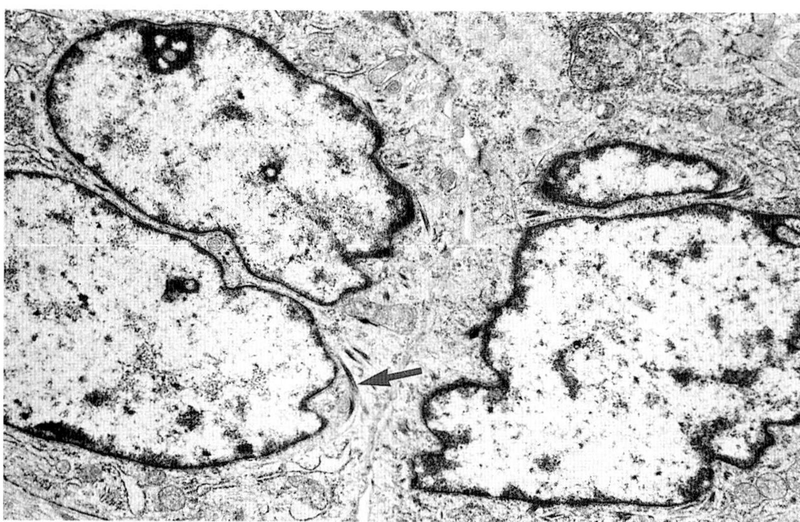

Fig. 25.203 Electron microscopic appearance of epithelioid sarcoma. Small tonofibrils (arrow) are present in the epithelioid tumor cells.
(×11 100; courtesy of Dr Robert A Erlandson, Memorial Sloan-Kettering Cancer Center)

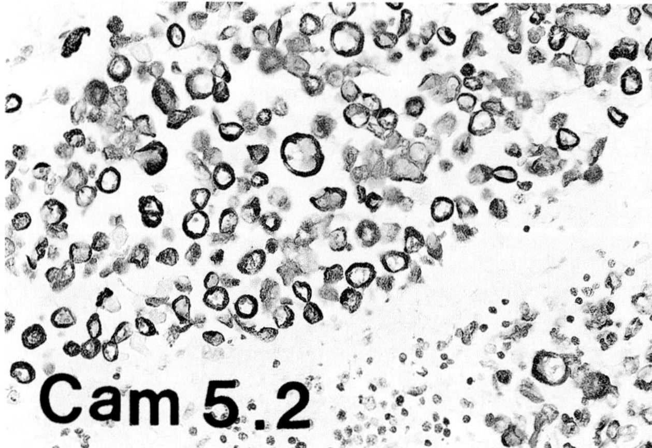

Fig. 25.204 Strong keratin immunoreactivity (CAM 5.2) in epithelioid sarcoma.

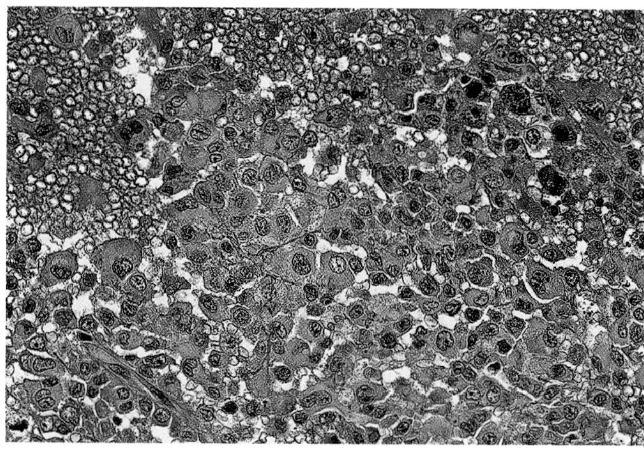

Fig. 25.205 So-called 'proximal variant' of epithelioid sarcoma. Many of the tumor cells have a rhabdoid quality.

epithelioid sarcoma characterized by a proximal location (pelvis, perineal and pubic region, vulva, buttock), deep invasion, necrosis, and sometimes prominent rhabdoid features[1772,1774] (Fig. 25.205). The keratin profile of this variant is more restricted than that of conventional epithelioid sarcoma and more in keeping with rhabdoid tumors of other types.[1794] Dysadherin (a cell membrane glycoprotein which downregulates E-cadherin) is expressed more commonly in proximal-type epithelioid sarcoma than in the conventional distal type.[1776] We believe this is a valid concept, but warn the pathologist always to consider the alternative possibility of undifferentiated carcinoma before making a diagnosis of proximal type epithelioid sarcoma, especially if the patient is old and the tumor is 'too central' (pelvic, retroperitoneal).

Giant cell tumor of soft parts

Giant cell tumor of soft parts is a rare neoplasm that mainly affects adults and the elderly and is usually located in the extremities. Most cases are located deeply, but a superficial variety in the subcutaneous tissue and fascia has also been described[1801] (Fig. 25.206). The tumor is composed of an admixture of osteoclast-like multinucleated giant cells and stromal cells[1798,1802,1807] (Fig. 25.207).

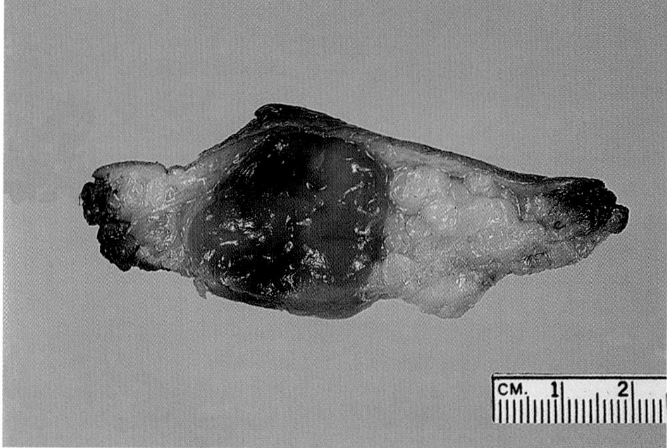

Fig. 25.206 Malignant giant cell tumor of soft parts. The tumor is relatively well circumscribed, bulges on the cut surface, and is focally hemorrhagic.

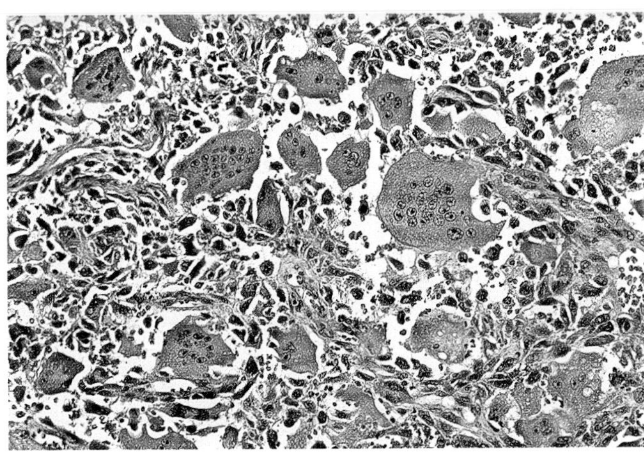

Fig. 25.207 Giant cell tumor of soft parts. The appearance is remarkably similar to that of giant cell tumor of bone.

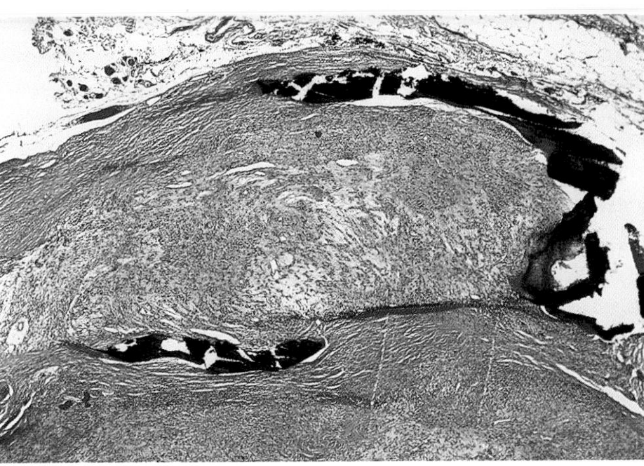

Fig. 25.209 Low-power view of ossifying fibromyxoid tumor. A shell of metaplastic bone partially surrounds the tumor periphery.

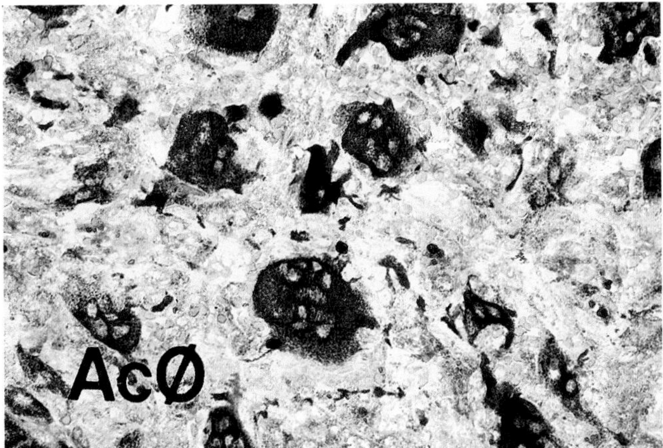

Fig. 25.208 Intense positivity for acid phosphatase in the multinucleated cells of giant cell tumor of soft tissues.

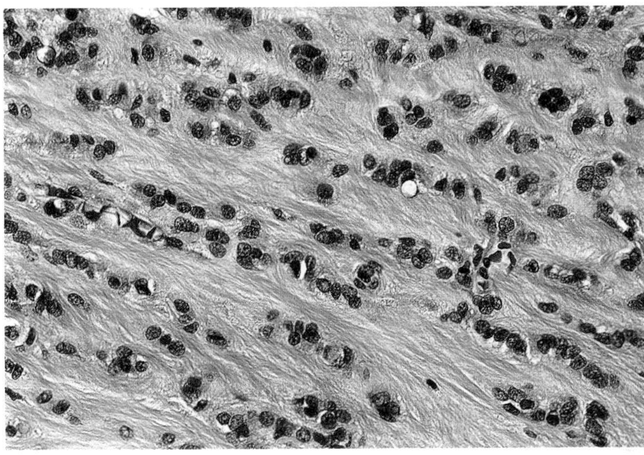

Fig. 25.210 On high power, the cells of ossifying fibromyxoid tumor are medium-sized, only moderately atypical, and embedded in a hyaline matrix.

The stromal cells are probably the only neoplastic component; some are elongated and fibroblast-like, whereas others are plump, resembling histiocytes. Some of the latter may be multinucleated but different from the osteoclast-like elements. Their phenotype is similar to that of osteoblasts, including the expression of alkaline phosphatase and osteoprotegerin.[1804] The giant cells resemble osteoclasts not only light microscopically, but also ultrastructurally and in their content of hydrolytic enzymes, such as acid phosphatase[1804] (Fig. 25.208). Metaplastic bone may be present, usually in the form of peripheral shell, perhaps induced by secretion of transforming growth factor (TGF) β1 and β2 by the tumor cells.[1808] The tumor has a characteristic multinodular configuration on low-power examination. Vascularity is pronounced, a fact also evident in angiographic studies.[1799] The overall appearance of the tumor is highly reminiscent of giant cell tumor of bones. The histogenesis is unclear.[1798,1802] In earlier schemes this tumor had been included as one of the histologic types of MFH,[1803] but this is no longer favored.

The behavior is dependent upon the location, size, and microscopic appearance. Low-grade (benign; of low malignant potential) and high-grade (malignant) forms have been separated from each other on the basis of the atypia, pleomorphism, and mitotic activity of the mononuclear neoplastic component.[1800,1805,1806]

Ossifying fibromyxoid tumor

Ossifying fibromyxoid tumor is a soft tissue neoplasm which usually presents in adult patients as a small, painless, well-circumscribed mass in the subcutaneous tissue or muscle of the extremities.[1810,1815] Microscopically, the tumor cells are typically arranged in a cord- or nest-like pattern within a myxoid matrix that blends with foci of fibrosis and osteoid formation. The low-power appearance is distinctive by virtue of lobulation and an incomplete shell of mature bone in the region corresponding to the tumor capsule[1810] (Fig. 25.209). The tumor cells are small and round, with scanty atypia and few mitoses (Fig. 25.210).

Immunohistochemically, there is widespread immunoreactivity for S-100 protein and vimentin, associated with focal reactivity for Leu7 and glial fibrillary acidic protein, and negativity for type II collagen. Ultrastructurally, there are complex cell processes and basement membrane deposition. This combination of features is more in keeping with a schwannian than a cartilaginous or some other type of mesenchymal derivation.[1809,1814] However, the detection of desmin, smooth muscle actin, and keratin, plus some ultrastructural features, suggests that – once again – a differentiation toward a smooth muscle or myoepithelial phenotype may be taking place in these tumors.[1812,1816–1818]

The behavior of this tumor is indolent, but local recurrences developed in one-fourth of the cases reported by Enzinger et al.[1810] and in an updated series from the same institution.[1815] However, distant metastases are practically nonexistent. Rare atypical and malignant cases have been reported by other authors.[1811,1813]

Extraskeletal Ewing sarcoma/PNET

Tumors morphologically indistinguishable from **Ewing sarcoma** of the skeletal system can present as soft tissue masses. In some cases, they simply represent soft tissue extensions of tumor originating in the underlying bone. In others, bone involvement is absent, and these are regarded as primary Ewing sarcomas of soft tissues.[1848,1853,1856] Most of the patients are adolescents or young adults, and the usual sites of involvement are the deep soft tissues of the lower extremity and paravertebral region.[1820] They have been described in many other sites, including digits and craniospinal vault.[1844] Occasionally, the tumors are superficial, with primary involvement of subcutis or skin.[1828,1860] Microscopically, like their skeletal counterpart, they are composed of uniform small, round, or oval cells containing cytoplasmic glycogen and sometimes arranged in a 'peritheliomatous' pattern (Figs 25.211 and 25.212). Ultrastructurally, the cells are rather primitive, with abundant cytoplasmic glycogen, poorly developed cell junctions (more complex in keratin-positive cases, see below[1857]), and no overt evidence of neural differentiation.[1833,1836,1859,1867] The course is aggressive and distant metastases are common, particularly to lung and skeleton.

As already discussed in Chapter 24, Ewing sarcoma of both osseous and extraosseous sites is currently regarded as merging imperceptibly with **primitive neuroectodermal tumor** (PNET)[1837,1849,1865] and subsuming the clinicopathologic entity originally described as malignant small cell tumor of the thoracopulmonary region[1821,1823,1834,1843] (Fig. 25.213). This group of lesions is colloquially referred to as the 'Ewing family' of tumors. The nosologic unity of Ewing sarcoma/PNET is strongly supported by the existence of numerous intermediate forms,[1838,1853,1854,1868] the strong immunoreactivity for CD99 (O13, HBA71, 12E7, RFB-1),[1847] and – most important – the presence of a consistent chromosomal translocation (11;22)(q24;q12),[1863] which leads to the fusion of the Ewing sarcoma gene (*EWS*) in chromosome 22 to the *FLI-1* gene or other partners in chromosome 11 and the production of a chimeric transcript, or variant forms of chromosomal translocation.[1824,1825] This genetic alteration can be detected with RT-PCR or FISH in fresh or paraffin-embedded material.[1827,1839,1841,1852,1855]

CD99 recognizes a cell membrane protein of yet unknown function (p30/32 MIC2; O13), which is the product of *MIC2*, a pseudoautosomal gene located on the short arm of the X and Y chromosomes.[1819,1829,1858,1866] It is not specific for Ewing sarcoma/PNET. Other markers that have been detected immunohistochemically in this family of tumors – some of them pointing toward a neuroectodermal line of differentiation – include NSE, synaptophysin, S-100 protein, PGP 9.5, secretogranin II, vimentin, and

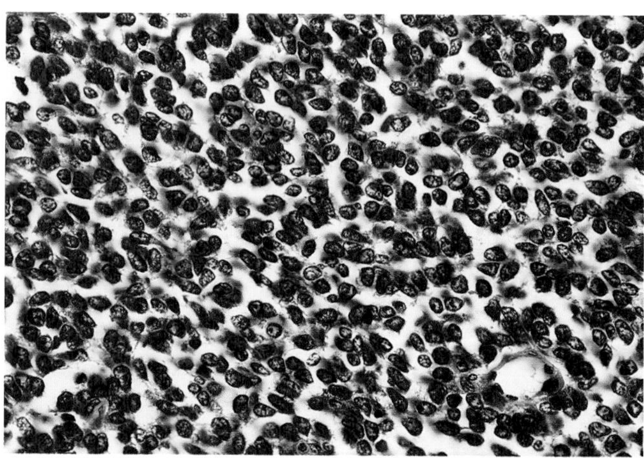

Fig. 25.211 Extraskeletal Ewing sarcoma/PNET. The tumor is extremely cellular, with hardly any intervening stroma. Some tumor cells are attached to a vessel wall in a pseudorosette arrangement.

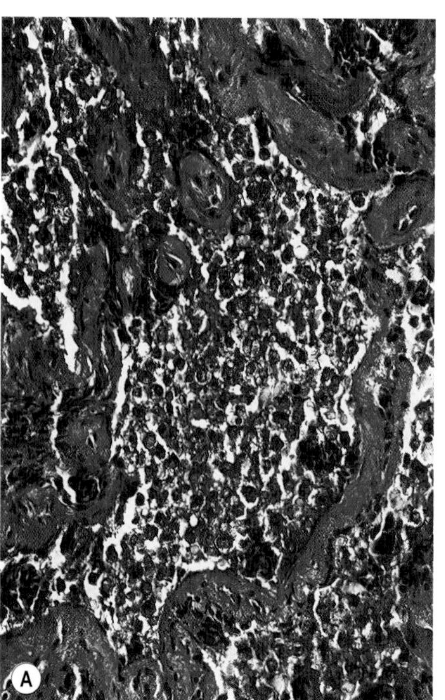

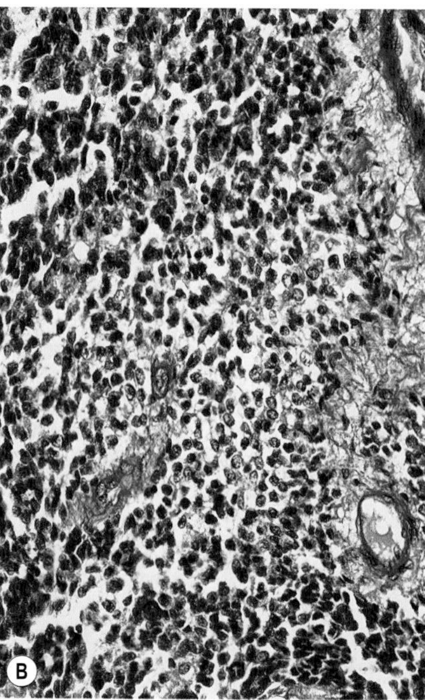

Fig. 25.212 Abundant cytoplasmic glycogen in the cells of Ewing sarcoma/PNET, as shown with PAS stain (**A**) with diastase control (**B**).

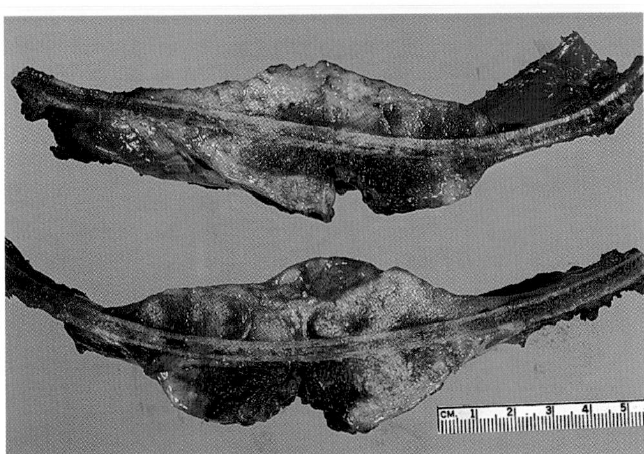

Fig. 25.213 Ewing sarcoma/PNET of thoracopulmonary region. The tumor is present on both sides of the rib, but the bone was only minimally involved.

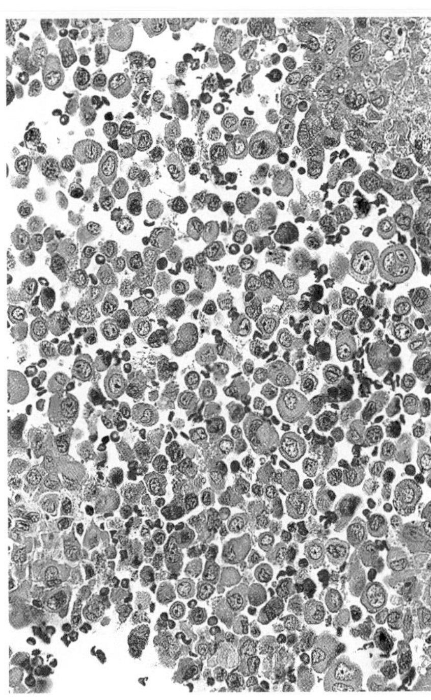

Fig. 25.214 Soft tissue tumor of the vulvar region with rhabdoid features. The tumor cells are small and round to oval, and their nuclei are displaced laterally.

keratin.[1822,1835,1840,1846] The keratin reactivity has been detected in close to a fifth of the cases, and it may be quite extensive.[1864] Cell junction-related proteins, such as claudin-1 and occludin, are sometimes expressed.[1850] The protein transcript of t(11;22) can be identified with the anti-FLI-1 antibody.[1830]

The claim that tumors having easily detectable neuroectodermal markers run a more aggressive clinical course than the others[1837] has not been substantiated.[1847] Furthermore, most attempts to subdivide them on phenotypic grounds have been unsuccessful.[1845,1855] The fact remains that – statistically speaking – tumors located in bone are more likely to exhibit a more undifferentiated phenotype (in keeping with the original Ewing sarcoma concept), whereas those located in soft tissues – including most thoracopulmonary examples – tend to display various degrees of neuroectodermal differentiation.[1843]

The differential diagnosis of Ewing sarcoma/PNET of soft tissues includes embryonal and alveolar rhabdomyosarcoma (especially the solid variant of the latter), malignant lymphoma, desmoplastic small cell tumor, and so-called 'rhabdoid tumor'.[1826,1862] A combined morphologic, immunohistochemical, and molecular approach will place most tumors into one or another of these categories, allowing for the existence of hybrid forms and of a sometimes bewildering phenotypic diversity.[1831,1832,1842,1851,1861]

Desmoplastic small cell tumor

Desmoplastic small cell tumor is typically located within the abdominal cavity (see Chapter 24), but has also been seen in the pleural cavity, CNS, orbit, and – more pertinently for the purposes of this chapter – in the soft tissues and bones of the hand.[1869,1870]

Rhabdoid tumor

Rhabdoid tumor was originally described as a primary renal neoplasm (see Chapter 17), but examples of a morphologically similar neoplasm have been subsequently identified in many other sites, particularly soft tissues.[1876,1879,1885] Some of the cases have involved major nerves. Most patients are infants or children, but it can also occur in adults. Microscopically, solid sheets of cells are present with areas of compartmentalization. The most striking morphologic feature is the deeply and homogeneously acidophilic cytoplasm of the tumor cells (the result of packing by intermediate filaments), with lateral displacement of the nucleus[1873] (Figs 25.214 and 25.215). Myxoid, pseudoalveolar, and hyalinized areas may be present.[1882] Immunohistochemically, there is positivity for vimentin and often for keratin and EMA but generally not for skeletal muscle markers or S-100 protein[1877] (Fig. 25.216). However, a great deal of phenotypic diversity has been recorded in these lesions,[1880,1884] including the common expression of neural/neuroendocrine markers.[1872] 'De novo' rhabdoid tumors (those that do not represent other specific tumor types showing rhabdoid morphology), like their renal and CNS counterparts, show alterations of chromosome 22, in the form of deletions or translocations involving 22q11.2 (harboring the *hSNF5/INI1* gene), which can be demonstrated by FISH or loss of heterozygosity studies.[1871,1878,1881] Alternatively, loss of expression of INI1 can be revealed by immunohistochemistry.[1875]

Metastases occur early (to the lungs, liver, and lymph nodes), response to therapy is poor, and the clinical course is extremely aggressive.[1883,1885] Most evidence suggests that rhabdoid tumor of soft tissues is not a specific tumor entity but rather the expression of a particular phenotype that can develop in a wide variety of tumor types, including epithelioid sarcoma, synovial sarcoma, intra-abdominal desmoplastic small cell tumor, rhabdomyosarcoma, malignant melanoma, and various types of carcinoma.[1880,1886,1887] Of practical importance is the fact that the emergence of the rhabdoid phenotype is invariably associated with an aggressive and often lethal clinical course.[1872,1874]

Phosphaturic mesenchymal tumor

An interesting association has been reported between some tumors of soft tissue or bone and osteomalacia or rickets.[1893] The syndrome results from tumor production of a renal phosphaturic substance that depletes total-body phosphates by inhibiting tubular

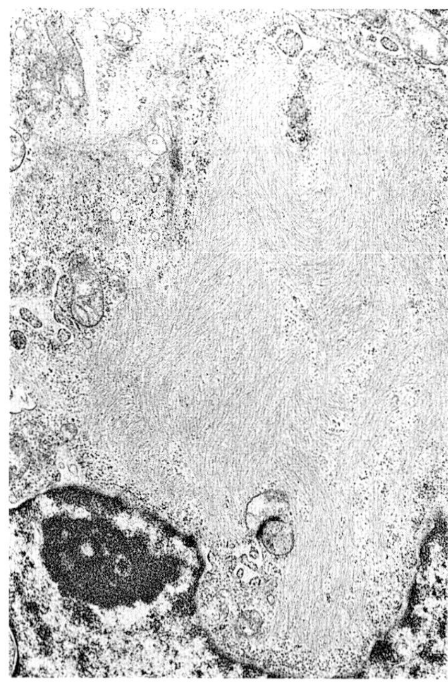

Fig. 25.215 Electron microscopic appearance of rhabdoid tumor of soft tissue. The cytoplasmic organelles of this rhabdoid cell are displaced by a large aggregate of intermediate filaments, immunohistochemically shown to be of vimentin type.
(×15 000; courtesy of Dr Robert A Erlandson, Memorial Sloan-Kettering Cancer Center)

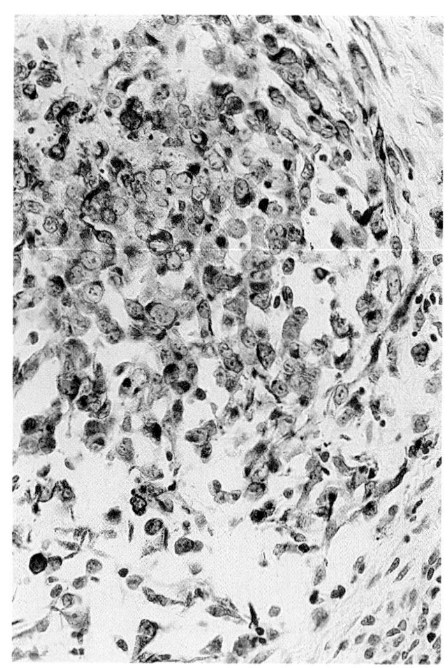

Fig. 25.216 Rhabdoid tumor immunostained for keratin. The reaction has a characteristic punctate quality.

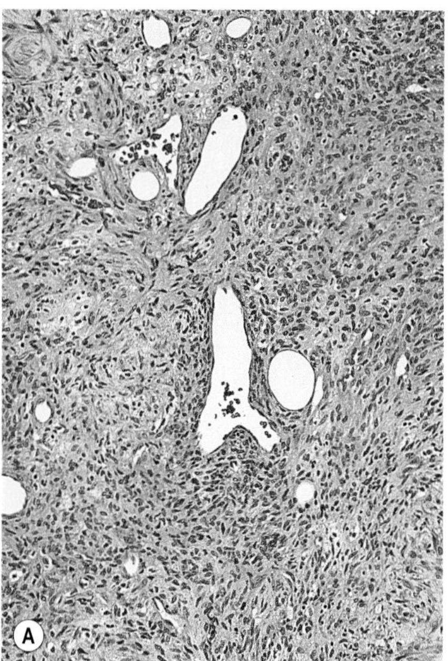

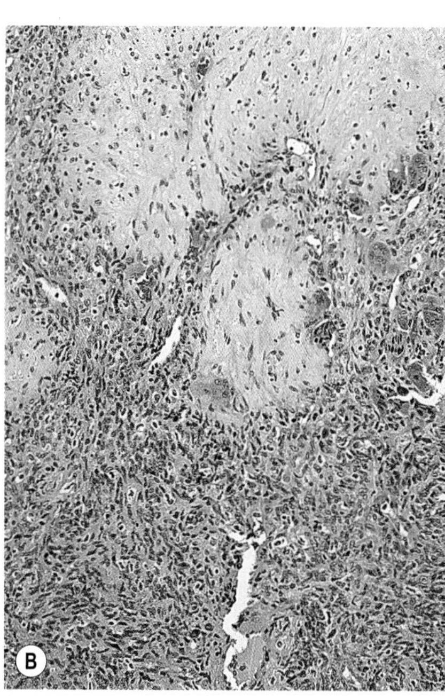

Fig. 25.217 A and **B**, Phosphaturic mesenchymal tumor. **A**, This area has a hemangiopericytoma-like quality. **B**, In this area from the same tumor, there is chondroid differentiation and a scattering of osteoclast-like giant cells.

reabsorption of phosphate.[1888,1892] It is characterized biochemically by hypophosphatemia, renal phosphate wasting, and decreased serum 1,25-dihydroxyvitamin D3 levels.[1891] The soft tissue tumors associated with this complication have shown an admixture of microscopic features.[1893] In our experience the most characteristic feature has been the association of hemangiopericytoma-like areas and osteoclast-like giant cells, with or without foci of osseous and cartilaginous metaplasia. A 'grungy' calcified matrix is said to be particularly distinctive[1888] (Fig. 25.217). Immunohistochemically, they usually express fibroblastic growth factor-23 (FGF-23), a protein implicated in renal tubular phosphate loss.[1890] It should be pointed out that not all cases with this morphology are associated with phosphaturia. The behavior has been generally benign,[1891,1893] but malignant examples are on record.[1889]

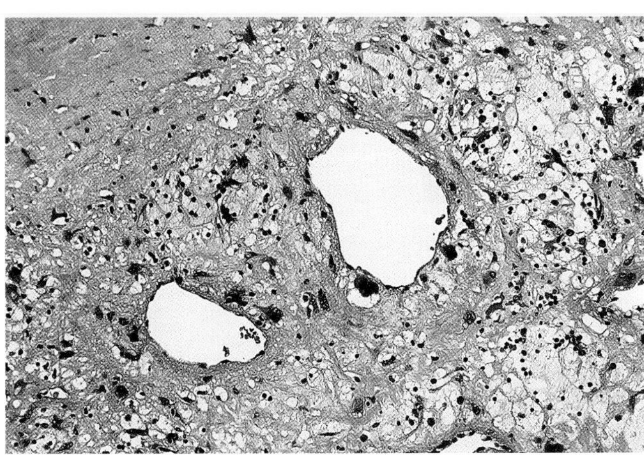

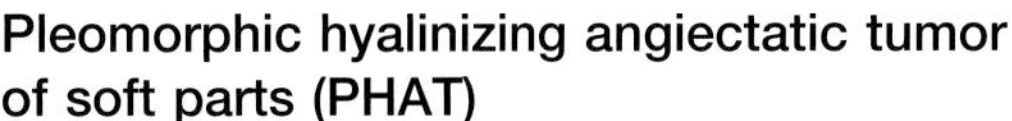

Fig. 25.218 Pleomorphic hyalinizing angiectatic tumor of soft parts. The pleomorphic tumor cells surround dilated vessels.

Pleomorphic hyalinizing angiectatic tumor of soft parts (PHAT)

This tumor type can simulate schwannoma by virtue of the angiectatic vasculature, the presence of hemosiderin-laden macrophages, and the occurrence of a spindle cell component with scattered bizarre nuclear forms but practically no mitotic activity (Fig. 25.218). Two diagnostic clues are represented by the nuclear pseudoinclusions and the fact that many of the bizarre cells are embedded within a fibrinous material surrounding the angiectatic vessels. CD34 is focally positive and S-100 protein is negative. Folpe et al.[1895] have identified in some of the cases a monomorphic, partially myxoid spindle cell component (sometimes present by itself) which they believe may be an early stage or precursor of the full-blown PHAT.

Cytogenetically, supernumerary ring chromosomes have been found, linking PHAT with other low-grade mesenchymal malignancies, such as dermatofibrosarcoma protuberans, parosteal osteosarcoma, and well-differentiated liposarcoma.[1894] Local recurrences have been described but not distant metastases.[1897] Some of the recurrences have exhibited a sarcomatous appearance, such as high-grade myxofibrosarcoma.[1896]

Myoepithelioma of soft tissue

The proposal has been made that there exists in the soft tissue a group of tumors showing differentiation toward myoepithelial cells (presumably related to skin adnexa), which can occur either in a pure form (myoepitheliomas) or in association with glandular structures (mixed tumors).[1901,1903] Microscopically, the myoepithelial component is present in the form of nests, cords, and ductules of epithelioid cells, and/or nests of spindle cells within a hyalinized or chondromyxoid stroma (Fig. 25.219A). Osteoid production and chondroid differentiation may be present. Immunohistochemically, there may be reactivity for keratin, S-100 protein, smooth muscle actin, desmin, glial fibrillary acidic protein (GFAP), and EMA[1901] (Fig. 25.219B,C). These tumors have the capability for local recurrence and distant metastases. The malignant forms of these tumors have been referred to as *myoepithelial carcinomas*, a relatively high percentage of them occurring in children.[1900]

It has further been suggested that the mysterious neoplasm originally reported by Dabska as *parachordoma*[1898,1902,1904,1905] may be part of this spectrum. Parachordoma has been typically described adjacent to tendons, synovium, and osseous structures within extremities. Microscopically, well-circumscribed lobules composed of small cellular aggregates embedded within a hyalinized and chondroid matrix are present.[1898,1899] Some of the tumor cells are reminiscent of physaliphorous cells, hence the name.

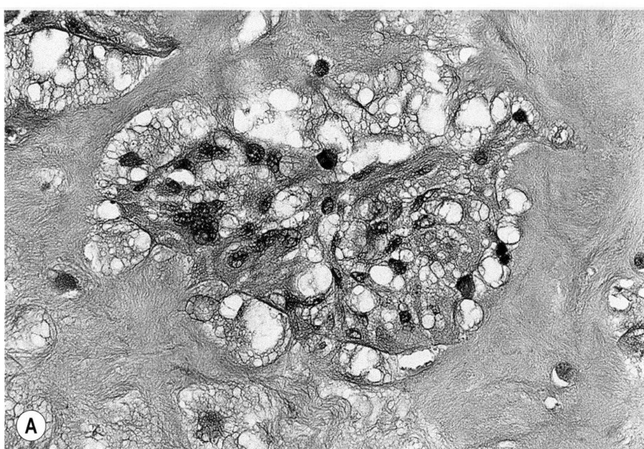

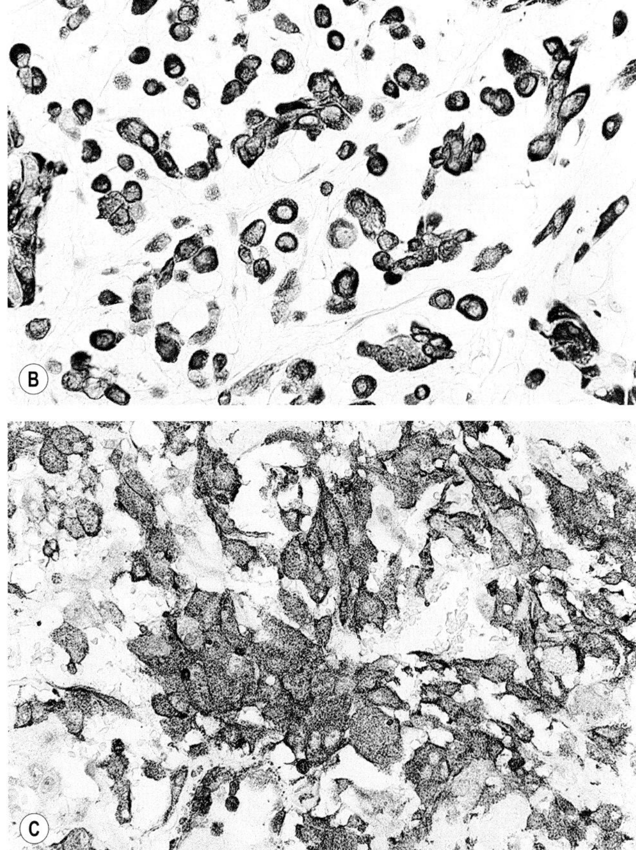

Fig. 25.219 **A–C**, Myoepithelioma of soft parts. The appearance is highly reminiscent of so-called 'parachordoma'. **B**, Keratin (CAM 5.2). **C**, Smooth muscle actin.

Other tumors

Oncocytoma has been reported as a primary tumor of soft tissues, and we have seen a similar example.[1906] The appearance does not

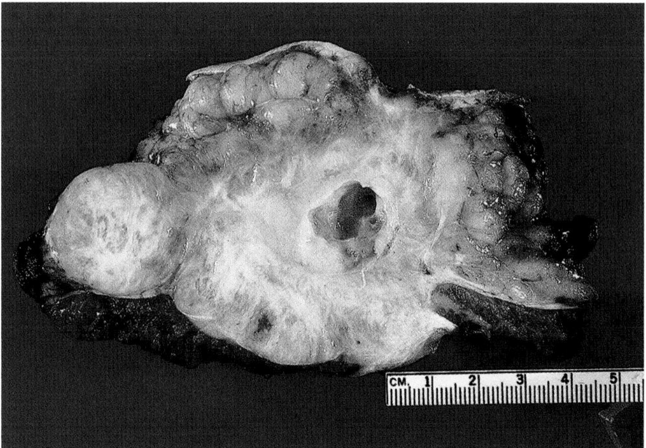

Fig. 25.220 Carcinoma of large bowel metastatic to soft tissues and skin.

differ from that of oncocytomas at other sites. Its origin may be related to deeply seated skin adnexa.

Metastatic tumors

Skeletal muscle or other deep soft tissue metastases of carcinoma or melanoma occur, but only rarely do they represent the first clinical manifestation of the disease. Reported cases include metastases from carcinoma of the kidney, lung, breast, stomach, and large bowel[1907,1908] (Fig. 25.220).

Other tumorlike conditions

Bronchogenic cysts of skin and soft tissue are usually discovered at or seen after birth in male infants. The most common location is the suprasternal notch and manubrium sterni;[1916] despite their name, they are probably of branchial arch derivation (i.e., *branchiogenic*)[1914,1929] (see Chapter 4).

Tumoral calcinosis is characterized by the formation of large, painless, calcified masses in the periarticular soft tissues, especially along extensor surfaces (Figs 25.221 and 25.222). The elbows and hips are the most common sites. Curiously, the knee is always spared. It is not clear whether the *calcareous lesions* encountered in the distal extremities, sometimes in patients with scleroderma, are the distal counterpart of tumoral calcinosis or a different process.[1922]

The disease can be inherited as an autosomal dominant trait with variable clinical expressivity. Germline mutations in the *FGF23* (encoding a potent phosphaturic protein), *GALNT3* (encoding a glycosyltransferase for initiating O-glycosylation) or *SAMD9* (encoding tumor necrosis factor-α responsive protein) gene have been described.[1911,1912,1931] The largest series have been reported from African countries.[1927] The serum calcium is usually normal, but there is hyperphosphatemia and elevated serum dihydroxyvitamin D levels.[1923] The disease may recur after excision.[1917]

Calcifying fibrous pseudotumor is a benign and probably nonneoplastic fibrous lesion characterized by the presence of abundant hyalinized collagen with psammomatous or dystrophic calcifications and a lymphoplasmacytic infiltrate (Fig. 25.223). Most patients are adolescents and young adults, and the behavior is benign.[1915]

There is immunoreactivity for CD34 in most cases, but not for ALK-1. The latter finding does not lend support to the suggestion that calcifying fibrous pseudotumor may represent a late stage of inflammatory myofibroblastic tumor.[1925]

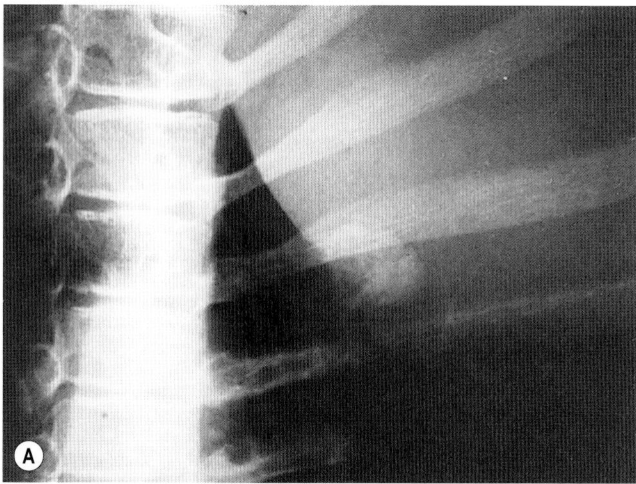

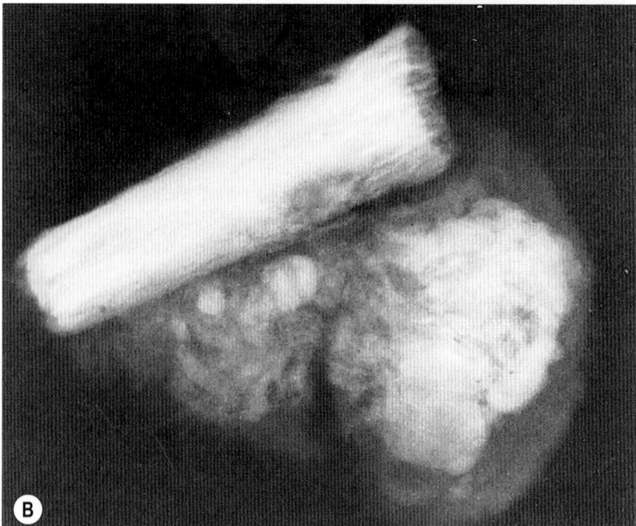

Fig. 25.221 **A** and **B**, Radiograph showing an area of tumoral calcinosis adjacent to a posterior rib in a 9-year-old child. **B**, Radiograph of excised specimen. Calcification is lobulated, splotchy, and independent of the eighth rib.

Amyloid tumor (amyloidoma) can present as a localized mass in the soft tissues. The mediastinum and retroperitoneum are the most common locations. The amyloid may be of AL (more frequently) or AA type.[1920]

Pseudorheumatoid nodules are characterized by a palisaded array of histiocytes surrounding an eosinophilic amorphous material ('necrobiotic collagen'). They occur most commonly in the lower legs and scalp of children and are thought to represent a deep form of granuloma annulare (see Chapter 4).[1909]

Aneurysmal (bone) cyst morphologically similar to that more commonly seen in the skeletal system can develop in the soft tissues.[1926,1928]

Rosai–Dorfman disease (sinus histiocytosis with massive lymphadenopathy) may present as a mass in the soft tissue, with or without associated lymph node involvement (Fig. 25.224). It is most commonly located in the extremities, but it can also occur in the trunk and head and neck region. As is also the case in other extranodal sites, emperipolesis is usually inconspicuous, and secondary collagen deposition is prominent.[1924]

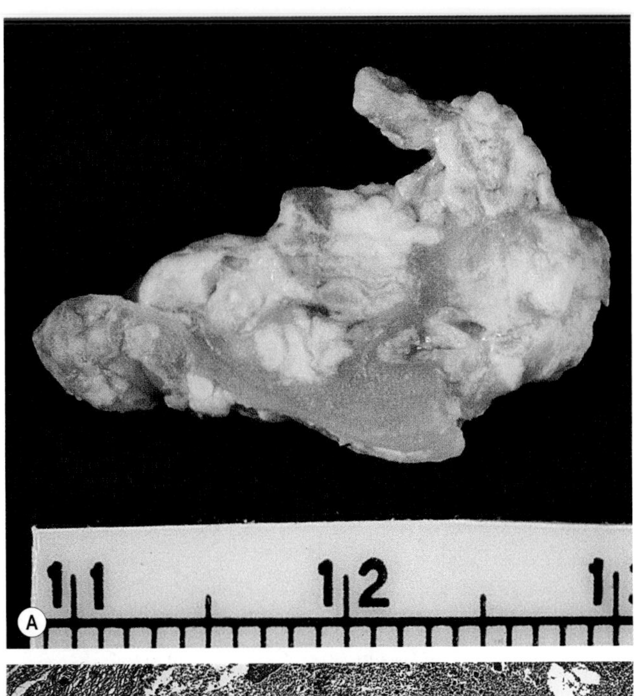

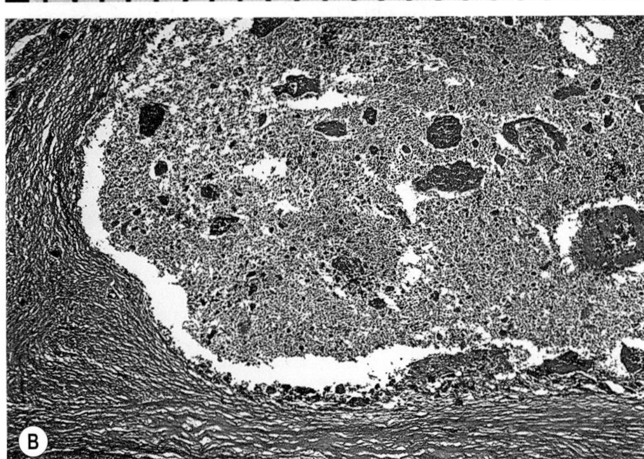

Fig. 25.222 Tumoral calcinosis. **A**, Gross appearance. The lesion is characteristically multinodular, and the material has a chalky quality. **B**, Microscopic appearance. Note the absence of cartilaginous features.

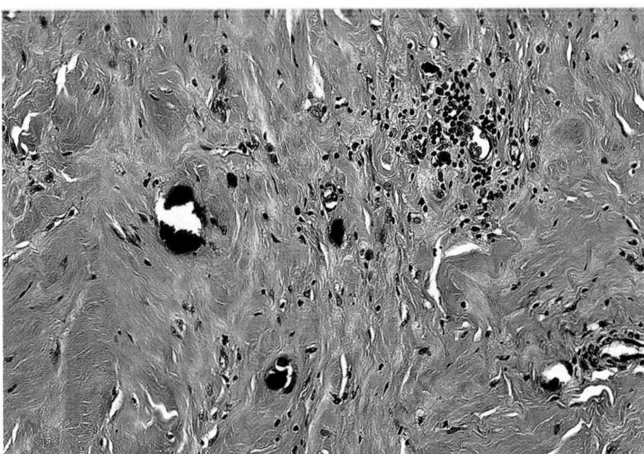

Fig. 25.223 Inflammatory calcifying pseudotumor. Round calcific concretions are seen against a fibrohyaline background containing scattered lymphocytes.

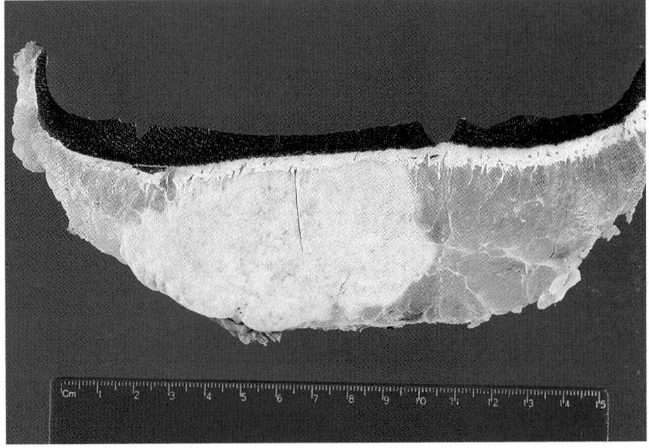

Fig. 25.224 Gross appearance of Rosai–Dorfman disease (sinus histiocytosis with massive lymphadenopathy) involving skin and soft tissues in the buttock region.

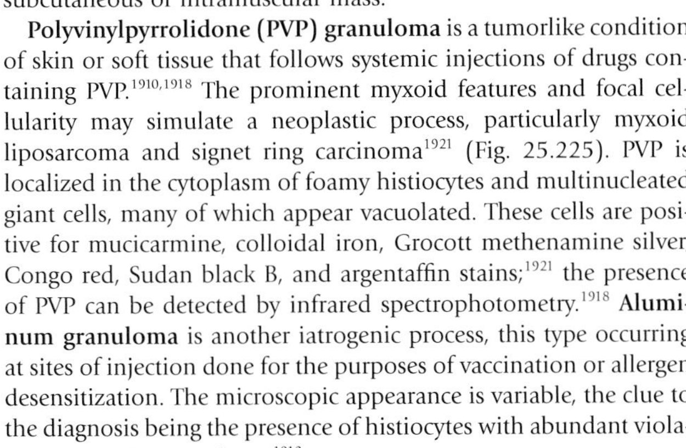

Castleman disease of the hyaline-vascular type can present as a subcutaneous or intramuscular mass.[1919,1930]

Polyvinylpyrrolidone (PVP) granuloma is a tumorlike condition of skin or soft tissue that follows systemic injections of drugs containing PVP.[1910,1918] The prominent myxoid features and focal cellularity may simulate a neoplastic process, particularly myxoid liposarcoma and signet ring carcinoma[1921] (Fig. 25.225). PVP is localized in the cytoplasm of foamy histiocytes and multinucleated giant cells, many of which appear vacuolated. These cells are positive for mucicarmine, colloidal iron, Grocott methenamine silver, Congo red, Sudan black B, and argentaffin stains;[1921] the presence of PVP can be detected by infrared spectrophotometry.[1918] **Aluminum granuloma** is another iatrogenic process, this type occurring at sites of injection done for the purposes of vaccination or allergen desensitization. The microscopic appearance is variable, the clue to the diagnosis being the presence of histiocytes with abundant violaceous granular cytoplasm.[1913]

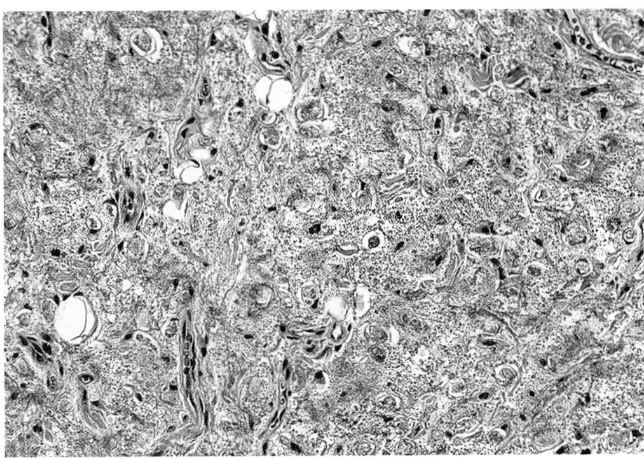

Fig. 25.225 So-called 'mucicarminophilic histiocytosis'. The highly myxoid quality of this lesion may induce confusion with a myxoid neoplasm.

References

NORMAL ANATOMY

1 Appleton MA, Attanoos RL, Jasani B. Thrombomodulin as a marker of vascular and lymphatic tumours. Histopathology 1997, **29**: 153–157.

2 Bondjers C, Kalén M, Hellström M, Scheidl SJ, Abramsson A, Renner O, Lindahl P, Cho H, Kehrl J, Betsholtz C. Transcription profiling of platelet-derived growth factor-B-deficient mouse embryos identifies RGS5 as a novel marker for pericytes and vascular smooth muscle cells. Am J Pathol 2003, **162**: 721–729.

3 Brooks JSJ, Perosio PM. Adipose tissue. In Mills SE (ed.): Histology for pathologists, ed. 3. Philadelphia, 2007, Lippincott Williams & Wilkins, pp. 165–194.

4 Bunge MB, Wood PM, Tynan LB, Bates ML, Sanes JR. Perineurium originates from fibroblasts. Demonstration in vitro with a retroviral marker. Science 1989, **243**: 229–231.

5 Burgdorf W, Mukai K, Rosai J. Immunohistochemical identification of factor VIII-related antigen in endothelial cells of cutaneous lesions of alleged vascular nature. Am J Clin Pathol 1981, **75**: 167–171.

6 Carstens PH. The Weibel–Palade body in the diagnosis of endothelial tumors. Ultrastruct Pathol 1981, **2**: 315–325.

7 Cohen PR, Rapini RP, Farhood AL. Expression of the human hematopoietic progenitor cell antigen CD34 in vascular and spindle cell tumors. J Cutan Pathol 1993, **20**: 15–20.

8 DeYoung BR, Swanson PE, Argenyi ZB, Ritter JH, Fitsgibbon JF, Stahl DJ, Hoover W, Wick MR. CD31 immunoreactivity in mesenchymal neoplasms of the skin and subcutis. Report of 145 cases and review of putative immunohistologic markers of endothelial differentiation. J Cutan Pathol 1995, **22**: 215–222.

9 Etchevers HC, Vincent C, Le Douarin NM, Couly GF. The cephalic neural crest provides pericytes and smooth muscle cells to all blood vessels of the face and forebrain. Development 2001, **128**: 1059–1068.

10 Fajardo LF. The complexity of endothelial cells. A review. Am J Clin Pathol 1989, **92**: 241–250.

11 Folpe AL, Chand EM, Goldblum JR, Weiss SW. Expression of Fli-1, a nuclear transcription factor, distinguishes vascular neoplasms from potential mimics. Am J Surg Pathol 2001, **25**: 1061–1066.

12 Gallagher PJ, van der Wal AC. Blood vessels. In Mills SE (ed.): Histology for pathologists, ed. 3. Philadelphia, 2007, Lippincott Williams & Wilkins, pp. 217–238.

13 Gottlieb AI, Langille BL, Wong MK, Kim DW. Structure and function of the endothelial cytoskeleton. Lab Invest 1991, **65**: 123–137.

14 Heffner RR Jr, Balos LL. Skeletal muscle. In Mills SE (ed.): Histology for pathologists, ed. 3. Philadelphia, 2007, Lippincott Williams & Wilkins, pp. 195–216.

15 Higgins JPT, Montgomary K, Wang L, Domanay E, Warnke RA, Brooks JD, van de Rijn M. Expression of FKBP12 in benign and malignant vascular endothelium: an immunohistochemical study on conventional sections and tissue microarrays. Am J Surg Pathol 2002, **27**: 58–64.

16 Hirose T, Tani T, Shimada T, Ishizawa K, Shimada S, Sano T. Immunohistochemical demonstration of EMA/Glut1-positive perineurial cells and CD34-positive firoblastic cells in peripheral nerve sheath tumors. Mod Pathol 2003, **16**: 293–298.

17 Hultberg BM, Svanholm H. Immunohistochemical differentiation between lymphangiographically verified lymphatic vessels and blood vessels. Virchows Arch [A] 1989, **414**: 209–215.

18 Mahendra G, Kliskey K, Williams K, Hollowood K, Jackson D, Athanasou NA. Intratumoural lymphatics in benign and malignant soft tissue tumours. Virchows Arch 2008, **453**: 457–464.

19 Miettinen M, Holthofer H, Lehto V-P, Miettinen A, Virtanen I. *Ulex europaeus* I lectin as a marker for tumors derived from endothelial cells. Am J Clin Pathol 1983, **79**: 32–36.

20 Miettinen M, Lindenmayer AE, Chaubal A. Endothelial cell markers CD31, CD34, and BNH9 antibody to H- and Y-antigens. Evaluation of their specificity and sensitivity in the diagnosis of vascular tumors and comparison with von Willebrand factor. Mod Pathol 1994, **7**: 82–90.

21 Mukai K, Rosai J, Burgdorf W. Localization of factor VIII-related antigen in vascular endothelial cells using an immunoperoxidase method. Am J Surg Pathol 1980, **4**: 273–276.

22 Ortiz-Hidalgo C, Weller RO. Peripheral nervous system. In Mills SE (ed.): Histology for pathologists, ed. 3. Philadelphia, 2007, Lippincott Williams & Wilkins, pp. 241–272.

23 Page C, Rose M, Yacoub M, Pigott R. Antigenic heterogeneity of vascular endothelium. Am J Pathol 1992, **141**: 673–683.

24 Rubanyi GM, Botelho LH. Endothelins. FASEB J 1991, **5**: 2713–2720.

25 Schmitt-Gräff A, Desmoulière A, Gabbiani G. Heterogeneity of myofibroblast phenotypic features. An example of fibroblastic cell plasticity. Virchows Arch 1994, **425**: 3–24.

26 Schurch W, Seemayer TA, Gabbiani G. The myofibroblast: a quarter century after its discovery. Am J Surg Pathol 1998, **22**: 141–147.

27 Schürch W, Seemayer TA, Hinz B, Gabbiani G. Myofibroblast. In Mills SE (ed.): Histology for pathologists, ed. 3. Philadelphia, 2007, Lippincott Williams & Wilkins, pp. 123–164.

28 Stephenson TJ, Mills PM. Monoclonal antibodies to blood group isoantigens. An alternative marker to factor VIII-related antigen for benign and malignant vascular endothelial cells. J Pathol 1985, **147**: 139–148.

29 Suzuki Y, Hashimoto K, Crissman J, Kanzaki T, Nishiyama S. The value of blood group-specific lectin and endothelial associated antibodies in the diagnosis of vascular proliferations. J Cutan Pathol 1986, **13**: 408–419.

30 Tokunaga O, Fan J, Watanabe T, Kobayashi M, Kumazaki T, Mitsui Y. Endothelin. Immunohistologic localization in aorta and biosynthesis by cultured human aortic endothelial cells. Lab Invest 1992, **67**: 210–217.

31 Traweek ST, Kandalaft PL, Mehta P, Battifora H. The human hematopoietic progenitor cell antigen (CD34) in vascular neoplasia. Am J Clin Pathol 1991, **96**: 25–31.

32 Turner RR, Beckstead JH, Warnke RA, Wood GS. Endothelial cell phenotypic diversity. In situ demonstration of immunologic and enzymatic heterogeneity that correlates with specific morphologic subtypes. Am J Clin Pathol 1987, **87**: 569–575.

33 Voigt J, Gorguet B, Szekeres G, Saati T, Delsol G. Comparison of the reactivities of monoclonal antibodies QBEND10 (CD34) and BNH9 in vascular tumors. Appl Immunohistochem 1993, **1**: 51–57.

34 Warhol MJ, Sweet JM. The ultrastructural localization of von Willebrand factor in endothelial cells. Am J Pathol 1984, **117**: 310–315.

INFECTIONS AND HEMATOMAS

35 Herzberg AJ, Boyd PR, Gutierrez Y. Subcutaneous dirofilariasis in Collier County, Florida, USA. Am J Surg Pathol 1995, **19**: 934–939.

36 Jain D, Kumar Y, Vasishta RK, Rajesh L, Pattari SK, Chakrabarti A. Zygomycotic necrotizing fasciitis in immunocompetent patients: a series of 18 cases. Mod Pathol 2006, **19**: 1221–1226.

37 Mentzel T, Goodlad JR, Smith MA, Fletcher CD. Ancient hematoma: an unifying concept for a post-traumatic lesion mimicking an aggressive soft tissue neoplasm. Mod Pathol 1997, **10**: 334–340.

38 Sing Y, Ramdial PK. Cryptococcal inflammatory pseudotumors. Am J Surg Pathol 2007, **31**: 1521–1527.

39 Taxy JB, Kodros S. Musculoskeletal coccidioidomycosis: unusual sites of disease in a nonendemic area. Am J Clin Pathol 2005, **124**: 693–696.

40 Woo ML, Patrick WGD, Simon MTP, French GL. Necrotising fasciitis caused by *Vibrio vulnificus*. J Clin Pathol 1984, **37**: 1301–1304.

TUMORS

CLASSIFICATION

41 Fletcher CD. The evolving classification of soft tissue tumours: an update based on the new WHO classification. Histopathology 2006, **48**: 3–12.

42 Mills SE. Sometimes we don't look like our parents [editorial]. Mod Pathol 1995, **8**: 347.

43 Ross J, Hendrickson MR, Kempson RL. The problem of the poorly differentiated sarcoma. Semin Oncol 1982, **9**: 467–483.

CLINICAL FEATURES

44 Grobmyer SR, Luther N, Antonescu CR, Singer S, Brennan MF. Multiple primary soft tissue sarcomas. Cancer 2004, **101**: 2633–2635.

45 Kauffman SL, Stout AP. Congenital mesenchymal tumors. Cancer 1965, **18**: 460–476.

46 Rydholm A, Berg NO, Gullberg B, Thorngren K-G, Persson BM. Epidemiology of soft-tissue sarcoma in the locomotor system. A retrospective population-based study of the inter-relationships between clinical and morphologic variables. Acta Pathol Microbiol Immunol Scand (A) 1984, **92**: 363–374.

47 Soule EH, Mahour GH, Mills SD, Lynn HB. Soft-tissue sarcomas of infants and children. A clinicopathologic study of 135 cases. Mayo Clin Proc 1968, **43**: 313–326.

DIAGNOSIS AND SPECIAL TECHNIQUES

48 Antonescu CR. The role of genetic testing in soft tissue sarcoma. Histopathology 2006, **48**: 13–21.

49 Bendix-Hansen K, Myhre-Jensen O. Enzyme histochemical investigations on bone and soft tissue tumours. Acta Pathol Microbiol Immunol Scand (A) 1985, **93**: 73–80.

50 Chang C-C, Shidham VB. Review. Molecular genetics of pediatric soft tissue tumors. Clinical application. J Mol Diagn 2003, **5**: 143–154.

51 Coffin CM, Lowichik A, Zhou H. Treatment effects in pediatric soft tissue and bone tumors: practical considerations for the pathologist. Am J Clin Pathol 2005, **123**: 75–90.

52 Coindre JM. Review. Immunohistochemistry in the diagnosis of soft tissue tumours. Histopathology 2003, **43**: 1–16.

53 Dickersin GR. Embryonic ultrastructure as a guide in the diagnosis of tumors. Ultrastruct Pathol 1987, **11**: 609–652.

54 Enjoji M, Hashimoto H. Diagnosis of soft tissue sarcomas. Pathol Res Pract 1984, **178**: 215–226.

55 Fisher C. The comparative roles of electron microscopy and immunohistochemistry in the diagnosis of soft tissue tumours. Histopathology 2006, **48**: 32–41.

56 Fletcher JA, Kozakewich HP, Hoffer FA, Lage JM, Weidner N, Tepper R, Pinkus GS, Morton CC, Corson JM. Diagnostic relevance of clonal cytogenetic aberrations in malignant soft-tissue tumors. N Engl J Med 1991, **324**: 436–442.

57 Goodlad JR, Fletcher CDM. Recent developments in soft tissue tumours. Histopathology 1995, **27**: 103–120.

58 Heim-Hall J, Yohe SL. Application of immunohistochemistry to soft tissue neoplasms. Arch Pathol Lab Med 2008, **132**: 476–489.

59 Hicks J, Mierau GW. The spectrum of pediatric tumors in infancy, childhood, and adolescence: a comprehensive review with emphasis on special techniques in diagnosis. Ultrastruct Pathol 2005, **29**: 175–202.

60 Iwasaki H, Nabeshima K, Nishio J, Jimi S, Aoki M, Koga K, Hamasaki M, Hayashi H, Mogi A. Pathology of soft-tissue tumors: daily diagnosis, molecular cytogenetics and experimental approach. Pathol Int 2009, **59**: 501–521.

61 Kindblom L-G, Walaas L, Widehn S. Ultrastructural studies in the preoperative cytologic diagnosis of soft tissue tumors. Semin Diagn Pathol 1986, **3**: 317–344.

62 Layfield LJ, Anders KH, Glasgow BJ, Mirra JM. Fine-needle aspiration of primary soft-tissue lesions. Arch Pathol Lab Med 1986, **110**: 420–424.

63 Miettinen M. Immunohistochemistry of soft-tissue tumors. Possibilities and limitations in surgical pathology. Pathol Annu 1990, **25**(Pt 1): 1–36.

64 Miller EC, Stevenson MA, Gebhardt MC, Anderson ME, Goldsmith JD. The effect of radiation/chemotherapy on the immunophenotype of soft tissue sarcomas. Lab Invest 2009, **89**(Suppl 1): 19A.

65 Molenaar WM, De Jong B, Buist J, Idenburg VJ, Seruca R, Vos AM, Hoekstra HJ. Chromosomal analysis and the classification of soft tissue sarcomas. Lab Invest 1989, **60**: 266–274.

66 Nakanishi I, Katsuda S, Ooi A, Kajikawa K, Matsubara F. Diagnostic aspect of spindle cell sarcomas by electron microscopy. Acta Pathol Jpn 1983, **33**: 425–437.

67 Ordóñez NG. Application of immunocytochemistry in the diagnosis of soft tissue sarcomas: a review and update. Adv Anat Pathol 1999, **5**: 67–85.

68 Parham DM. Immunohistochemistry of childhood sarcomas. Old and new markers. Mod Pathol 1993, **6**: 133–138.

69 Sandberg AA. Cytogenetics and molecular genetics of bone and soft-tissue tumors. Am J Med Genet 2002, **115**: 189–193.

70 Segal NH, Pavlidis P, Antonescu CR, Maki RG, Noble WS, DeSantis D, Woodruff JM, Lewis JJ, Brennan MF, Houghton AN, Cordon-Cardo C. Classification and subtype prediction of adult soft tissue sarcoma by functional genomics. Am J Pathol 2003, **163**: 691–700.

71 Sreekantaiah C, Ladanyi M, Rodriguez E, Chaganti RS. Chromosomal aberrations in soft tissue tumors. Relevance to diagnosis, classification, and molecular mechanisms. Am J Pathol 1994, **144**: 1121–1134.

72 van Haelst UJGM. General considerations on electron microscopy of tumors of soft tissues. Progr Surg Pathol 1980, **2**: 225–257.

GRADING AND STAGING

73 Angervall L, Kindblom L-G, Rydholm A, Stener B. The diagnosis and prognosis of soft tissue tumors. Semin Diagn Pathol 1986, **3**: 240–258.

74 Beahrs OH, Henson DE, Hutter RVP, Kennedy BJ. Manual for staging of cancer, ed. 4. Philadelphia, 1992, JB Lippincott Co.

75 Brown FM, Fletcher CD. Problems in grading soft tissue sarcomas. Am J Clin Pathol 2000, **114**: S82–S89.

76 Coindre JM, Nguyen BB, Bonichon F, de Mascarel I, Trojani M. Histopathologic grading in spindle cell soft tissue sarcomas. Cancer 1988, **61**: 2305–2309.

77 Coindre JM, Terrier P, Guillou L, Le Doussal V, Collin F, Ranchare D, Sastre X, Vilain MO, Bonichon F, N'Guyen Bui B. Predictive value of grade for metastasis development in the main histologic types of adult soft tissue sarcomas: a study of 1240 patients from the French Federation of Cancer Centers Sarcoma Group. Cancer 2001, **91**: 1914–1926.

78 Coindre JM, Trojani M, Contesso G, David M, Rouesse J, Bui NB, Bodaert A, De Mascarel I, De Mascarel A, Goussot J-F. Reproducibility of a histopathologic grading system for adult soft tissue sarcoma. Cancer 1986, **58**: 306–309.

79 Cooper JE, Allen PW. Low-grade sarcomas. Pathol Annu 1990, **25**(Pt 2): 1–18.

80 Costa J, Wesley RA, Glatstein E, Rosenberg SA. The grading of soft tissue sarcomas. Results of a clinicohistopathologic correlation in a series of 163 cases. Cancer 1984, **53**: 530–541.

81 Deyrup AT, Weiss SW. Grading of soft tissue sarcomas: the challenge of providing precise information in an imprecise world. Histopathology 2006, **48**: 42–50.

82 Donohue JH, Collin C, Friedrich C, Godbold J, Hajdu SI, Brennan MF. Lowgrade soft tissue sarcomas of the extremities. Analysis of risk factors for metastasis. Cancer 1988, **62**: 184–193.

83 Enneking WF. Musculoskeletal tumor staging. 1988 update. Cancer Treat Res 1989, **44**: 39–49.

84 Guillou L, Coindre JM, Bonichon F, N'Guyen BB, Terrier P, Collin F, Vilain MO, Mandard AM, Le Doussal V, Leroux A, Jacquemier J, Duplay H, Sastre-Garau X, Costa J. Comparative study of the National Cancer Institute and French Federation of Cancer Centres Sarcoma Group grading systems in a population of 410 adult patients with soft tissue sarcoma. J Clin Oncol 1997, **15**: 350–362.

85 Hashimoto H, Daimaru Y, Takeshita S, Tsuneyoshi M, Enjoji M. Prognostic significance of histologic parameters of soft tissue sarcomas. Cancer 1992, **70**: 2816–2822.

86 Heise HW, Myers MH, Russell WO, Suit HD, Enzinger FM, Edmonson JH, Cohen J, Martin RG, Miller WT, Hajdu SI. Recurrence-free survival time for surgically treated soft tissue sarcoma patients. Multivariate analysis of five prognostic factors. Cancer 1986, **57**: 172–177.

87 Myhre-Jensen O, Kaae S, Madsen EH, Sneppen O. Histopathological grading in soft-tissue tumours. Relation to survival in 261 surgically treated patients. Acta Pathol Microbiol Immunol Scand (A) 1983, **91**: 145–150.

88 Parham DM, Webber BL, Jenkins JJ III, Cantor AB, Maurer HM. Nonrhabdomyosarcomatous soft tissue sarcomas of childhood. Formulation of a simplified system for grading. Mod Pathol 1995, **8**: 705–710.

89 Russell WO, Cohen J, Enzinger F, Hajdu SI, Heise H, Martin RG, Meissner W, Miller WT, Schmidtz RL, Suit HD. A clinical and pathological staging system for soft tissue sarcomas. Cancer 1977, **40**: 1562–1570.

90 Trojani M, Contesso G, Coindre JM, Rouesse J, Bui NB, De Mascarel A, Goussot JF, David M, Bonichon F, Lagarde C. Soft-tissue sarcomas of adults. Study of pathological prognostic variables and definition of a histopathological grading system. Int J Cancer 1984, **33**: 37–42.

PROGNOSIS

91 Agarwal V, Greenebaum E, Wersto R, Koss LG. DNA ploidy of spindle cell soft-tissue tumors and its relationship to histology and clinical outcome. Arch Pathol Lab Med 1991, **115**: 558–562.

92 Bell RS, O'Sullivan B, Liu FF, Powell J, Langer F, Fornasier VL, Cummings B, Miceli PN, Hawkins N, Quirt I, et al. The surgical margin in soft-tissue sarcoma. J Bone Joint Surg (Am) 1989, **71**: 370–375.

93 Cance WG, Brennan MF, Dudas ME, Huang CM, Cordon-Cardo C. Altered expression of the retinoblastoma gene product in human sarcomas. N Engl J Med 1990, **323**: 1457–1462.

94 Dreinhofer KE, Baldetorp B, Akerman M, Ferno M, Rydholm A, Gustafson P. DNA ploidy in soft tissue sarcoma: comparison of flow and image cytometry with clinical follow-up in 93 patients. Cytometry 2002, **50**: 19–24.

95 Drobnjak M, Latres E, Pollack D, Karpeh M, Dudas M, Woodruff JM, Brennan MF, Cordon-Cardo C. Prognostic implications of p53 nuclear overexpression and high proliferation index of Ki-67 in adult soft-tissue sarcomas. J Natl Cancer Inst 1994, **86**: 549–554.

96 Engellau J, Bendahl PO, Persson A, Domanski HA, Akerman M, Gustafson P, Alvegård TA, Nilbert M, Rydholm A. Improved prognostication in soft tissue sarcoma: independent information from vascular invasion, necrosis, growth pattern, and immunostaining using whole-tumor sections and tissue microarrays. Hum Pathol 2005, **36**: 994–1002.

97 Engellau J, Persson A, Bendahl PO, Akerman M, Domanski HA, Bjerkehagen B, Lilleng P, Weide J, Rydholm A, Alvegård TA, Nilbert M. Expression profiling using tissue microarray in 211 malignant fibrous histiocytomas confirms the prognostic value of Ki-67. Virchows Arch 2004, **445**: 224–230.

98 Enneking WF, Maale GE. The effect of inadvertent tumor contamination of wounds during the surgical resection of musculoskeletal neoplasms. Cancer 1988, **62**: 1251–1256.

99 Ferguson PC, Griffin AM, O'Sullivan B, Catton CN, Davis AM, Murji A, Bell RS, Wunder JS. Bone invasion in extremity soft-tissue sarcoma: impact on disease outcomes. Cancer 2006, **106**: 2692–2700.

100 Gerrand CH, Bell RS, Wunder JS, Kandel RA, O'Sullivan B, Catton CN, Griffin AM, Davis AM. The influence of anatomic location on outcome in patients with soft tissue sarcoma of the extremity. Cancer 2003, **97**: 485–492.

101 Gustafson P, Rooser B, Rydholm A. Is local recurrence of minor importance for metastases in soft tissue sarcoma? Cancer 1991, **67**: 2083–2086.

102 Hasegawa T. Histological grading and MIB-1 labeling index of soft-tissue sarcomas. Pathol Int 2007, **57**: 121–125.

103 Herbert SH, Corn BW, Solin LJ, Lanciano RM, Schultz DJ, McKenna WG, Coia LR. Limb-preserving treatment for soft tissue sarcomas of the extremities. The significance of surgical margins. Cancer 1993, **72**: 1230–1238.

104 Heslin MJ, Woodruff J, Brennan MF. Prognostic significance of a positive microscopic margin in high-risk extremity soft tissue sarcoma: implications for management. J Clin Oncol 1996, **14**: 473–478.

105 Kawai A, Noguchi M, Beppu Y, Yokoyama R, Mukai K, Hirohashi S, Inoue H, Fukuma H. Nuclear immunoreaction of p53 protein in soft tissue sarcomas. A possible prognostic factor. Cancer 1994, **73**: 2499–2505.

106 Kroese MC, Rutgers DH, Wils IS, van Unnik JA, Roholl PJ. The relevance of the DNA index and proliferation rate in the grading of benign and malignant soft tissue tumors. Cancer 1990, **65**: 1782–1788.

107 Le Doussal V, Coindre JM, Leroux A, Hacene K, Terrier P, Bui NB, Bonichon F, Collin F, Mandard AM, Contesso G. Prognostic factors for patients with localized primary malignant fibrous histioctyoma: a multicenter study of 216 patients with multivariate analysis. Cancer 1996, **77**: 1823–1830.

108 Rooser B, Attewell R, Berg NO, Rydholm A. Prognostication in soft tissue sarcoma. A model with four risk factors. Cancer 1988, **61**: 817–823.

109 Sato O, Wada T, Kawai A, Yamaguchi U, Makimoto A, Kokai Y, Yamashita T, Chuman H, Beppu Y, Tani Y, Hasegawa T. Expression of epidermal growth factor receptor, ERBB2 and KIT in adult soft tissue sarcomas: a clinicopathologic study of 281 cases. Cancer 2005, **103**: 1881–1890.

110 Stojadinovic A, Leung DH, Hoos A, Jaques DP, Lewis JJ, Brennan M. Analysis of the prognostic significance of microscopic margin in 2084 localized primary adult soft tissue sarcomas. Ann Surg 2002, **235**: 424–434.

111 Stotter AT, A'Hern RP, Fisher C, Mott AF, Fallowfield ME, Westbury G. The influence of local recurrence of extremity soft tissue sarcoma on metastasis and survival. Cancer 1990, **65**: 1119–1129.

112 Swanson SA, Brooks JJ. Proliferation markers Ki-67 and p105 in soft-tissue lesions. Correlation with DNA flow cytometric characteristics. Am J Pathol 1990, **137**: 1491–1500.

113 Tanabe KK, Pollock RE, Ellis LM, Murphy A, Sherman N, Romsdahl MM. Influence of surgical margins on outcome in patients with preoperatively irradiated extremity soft tissue sarcomas. Cancer 1994, **73**: 1652–1659.

114 Ueda T, Aozasa K, Tsujimoto M, Ohsawa M, Uchida A, Aoki Y, Ono K, Matsumoto K. Prognostic significance of Ki-67 reactivity in soft tissue sarcomas. Cancer 1989, **63**: 1607–1611.

115 Zagars GK, Ballo MT, Pisters PWT, Pollock RE, Patel SR, Benjamin RS, Evans HL. Prognostic factors for patients with localized soft-tissue sarcoma treated with conservation surgery and radiation therapy. Cancer 2003, **97**: 2530–2543.

THERAPY

116 Aranha O, Agulnik M. Molecularly targeted therapies in adult soft tissue sarcomas: present approach and future directions. Expert Opin Ther Targets 2008, **12**: 197–207.

117 Casper ES, Gaynor JJ, Harrison LB, Panicek DM, Hajdu SI, Brennan MF. Preoperative and postoperative adjuvant combination chemotherapy for adults with high grade soft tissue sarcoma. Cancer 1994, **73**: 1644–1651.

118 Eilber FR, Huth JF, Mirra J, Rosen G. Progress in the recognition and treatment of soft tissue sarcomas. Cancer 1990, **65**: 660–666.

119 Glenn J, Kinsella T, Glatstein E, Tepper J, Baker A, Sugarbaker P, Sindelar W, Roth J, Brennan M, Costa J, Seipp C, Wesley R, Young RC, Rosenberg SA. A randomized, prospective trial of adjuvant chemotherapy in adults with soft tissue sarcomas of the head and neck, breast and trunk. Cancer 1985, **55**: 1206–1214.

120 Karakousis CP, Emrich LJ, Rao U, Krishnamsetty RM. Feasibility of limb salvage and survival in soft tissue sarcomas. Cancer 1986, **57**: 484–491.

121 Mazanet R, Antman KH. Adjuvant therapy for sarcomas. Semin Oncol 1991, **18**: 603–612.

122 Nesbit ME Jr. Advances and management of solid tumors in children. Cancer 1990, **65**: 696–702.

123 Potter DA, Kinsella T, Glatstein E, Wesley R, White DE, Seipp CA, Chang AE, Lack EE, Costa J, Rosenberg SA. High-grade soft tissue sarcomas of the extremities. Cancer 1986, **58**: 190–205.

124 Singer S, Demetri GD, Baldini EH, Fletcher CD. Management of soft-tissue sarcomas: an overview and update. Lancet Oncol 2002, **1**: 75–85.

125 Suit HD, Russell WO, Martin RG. Sarcoma of soft tissue. Clinical and histopathologic parameters and response to treatment. Cancer 1975, **35**: 1478–1483.

126 Tepper JE. Role of radiation therapy in the management of patients with bone and soft tissue sarcomas. Semin Oncol 1989, **16**: 281–288.

127 Ueda T, Aozasa K, Tsujimoto M, Hamada H, Hayashi H, Ono K, Matsumoto K. Multivariate analysis for clinical prognostic factors in 163 patients with soft tissue sarcoma. Cancer 1988, **62**: 1444–1450.

128 Wagner AJ, Malinowska-Kolodziej I, Morgan JA, Qin W, Fletcher CD, Vena N, Ligon AH, Antonescu CR, Ramaiya NH, Demetri GD, Kwiatkowski DJ, Maki RG. Clinical activity of mTOR inhibition with sirolimus in malignant perivascular epithelioid cell tumors: targeting the pathogenic activation of mTORC1 in tumors. J Clin Oncol 2010, **28**: 835–840.

129 Willett CG, Schiller AL, Suit HD, Mankin HJ, Rosenberg A. The histologic response of soft tissue sarcoma to radiation therapy. Cancer 1987, **60**: 1500–1504.

130 Yang JC, Rosenberg SA. Surgery for adult patients with soft tissue sarcomas. Semin Oncol 1989, **16**: 289–296.

PATHOGENESIS

131 Boshoff C, Chang Y. Kaposi's sarcoma-associated herpesvirus: a new DNA tumor virus. Annu Rev Med 2001, **52**: 453–470.

132 Carnevale A, Lieberman E, Cardenas R. Li-Fraumeni syndrome in pediatric patients with soft tissue sarcoma or osteosarcoma. Arch Med Res 1997, **28**: 383–386.

133 Deyrup AT. Epstein-Barr virus-associated epithelial and mesenchymal neoplasms. Hum Pathol 2008, **39**: 473–483.

134 Greenwald P, Kovasznay B, Collins DN, Therriault G. Sarcoma of soft tissues after Vietnam service. J Natl Cancer Inst 1984, **73**: 1107–1109.

135 Hardell L, Eriksson M. The association between soft tissue sarcomas and exposure to phenoxyacetic acids. A new case-referent study. Cancer 1988, **62**: 652–656.

136 Jennings TA, Peterson L, Axiotis CA, Friedlaender GE, Cooke RA, Rosai J. Angiosarcoma associated with foreign body material. A report of three cases. Cancer 1988, **62**: 2436–2444.

137 Kang H, Enzinger FM, Breslin P, Feil M, Lee Y, Shepard B. Soft tissue sarcoma and military service in Vietnam. A case control study. J Natl Cancer Inst 1987, **79**: 693–699.

138 Keel SB, Jaffe KA, Nielsen G, Rosenberg AE. Orthopaedic implant-related sarcoma: a study of twelve cases. Mod Pathol 2001, **14**: 969–977.

139 Laskin WB, Silverman TA, Enzinger FM. Postradiation soft tissue sarcomas. An analysis of 53 cases. Cancer 1988, **62**: 2330–2340.

140 Lau PP, Wong OK, Lui PC, Cheung OY, Ho LC, Wong WC, To KF, Chan JK. Myopericytoma in patients with AIDS: a new class of Epstein–Barr virus-associated tumor. Am J Surg Pathol 2009, **33**: 1666–1672.

141 Lynge E, Storm HH, Jensen OM. The evaluation of trends in soft tissue sarcoma according to diagnostic criteria and consumption of phenoxyherbicides. Cancer 1987, **60**: 1896–1901.

142 Mark RJ, Bailet JW, Poen J, Tran LM, Calcaterra TC, Abemayor E, Fu YS, Parker RG. Postirradiation sarcoma of the head and neck. Cancer 1993, **72**: 887–893.

143 Monkman GR, Orwoll G, Ivins JC. Trauma and oncogenesis. Mayo Clin Proc 1974, **49**: 157–163.

144 Wilkes D, McDermott DA, Basson CT. Clinical phenotypes and molecular genetic mechanisms of Carney complex. Lancet Oncol 2005, **6**: 501–508.

145 Wingren G, Fredrikson M, Brage HN, Nordenskjold B, Axelson O. Soft tissue sarcoma and occupational exposures. Cancer 1990, **66**: 806–811.

TUMORS AND TUMORLIKE CONDITIONS OF FIBROBLASTS AND MYOFIBROBLASTS

Calcifying aponeurotic fibroma

146 Allen PM, Enzinger FM. Juvenile aponeurotic fibroma. Cancer 1970, **26**: 857–867.

147 Chung EB. Pitfalls in diagnosing benign soft tissue tumors in infancy and childhood. Pathol Annu 1985, **20**(Pt 2): 323–386.

148 Fetsch JF, Miettinen M. Calcifying aponeurotic fibroma: a clinicopathologic study of 22 cases arising in uncommon sites. Hum Pathol 1998, **29**: 1504–1510.

149 Goldman RL. The cartilage analogue of fibromatosis (aponeurotic fibroma). Further observations based on 7 new cases. Cancer 1970, **26**: 1325–1331.

150 Iwasaki H, Kikuchi M, Eimoto T, Enjoji M, Yoh S, Sakurai H. Juvenile aponeurotic fibroma. An ultrastructural study. Ultrastruct Pathol 1983, **4**: 75–83.

151 Keasbey LE. Juvenile aponeurotic fibroma (calcifying fibroma). Cancer 1953, **6**: 338–346.

152 Lichtenstein L, Goldman RL. The cartilage analogue of fibromatosis. Cancer 1964, **17**: 810–816.

Fibroma of tendon sheath

153 Chung EB, Enzinger FM. Fibroma of tendon sheath. Cancer 1979, **44**: 1945–1954.

154 Dal Cin P, Sciot R, De Smet L, Van den Berghe H. Translocation 2;11 in a fibroma of tendon sheath. Histopathology 1998, **32**: 433–435.

155 Hashimoto H, Tsuneyoshi M, Daimaru Y, Ushijima M, Enjoji M. Fibroma of tendon sheath. A tumor of myofibroblasts. A clinicopathologic study of 18 cases. Acta Pathol Jpn 1985, **35**: 1099–1107.

156 Humphreys S, McKee PH, Fletcher CDM. Fibroma of tendon sheath. A clinicopathologic study. J Cutan Pathol 1986, **13**: 331–338.

157 Lamovec J, Bracko M, Voncina D. Pleomorphic fibroma of tendon sheath. Am J Surg Pathol 1991, **15**: 1202–1205.

158 Maluf HM, De Young BR, Swanson PE, Wick MR. Fibroma and giant cell tumor of tendon sheath. A comparative histological and immunohistological study. Mod Pathol 1995, **8**: 155–159.

159 Pulitzer DR, Martin PC, Reed RJ. Fibroma of tendon sheath. A clinicopathologic study of 32 cases. Am J Surg Pathol 1989, **13**: 472–479.

160 Satti MB. Tendon sheath tumours. A pathological study of the relationship between giant cell tumour and fibroma of tendon sheath. Histopathology 1992, **20**: 213–220.

161 Smith PS, Pieterse AS, McClure J. Fibroma of tendon sheath. J Clin Pathol 1982, **35**: 842–848.

Other types of fibroma

162 Alberghini M, Pasquinelli G, Zanella L, Bacchini P, Bertoni F. Desmoplastic fibroblastoma: a light and ultrastructural description of two cases. Ultrastruct Pathol 2004, **28**: 149–157.

163 Evans HL. Desmoplastic fibroblastoma. A report of seven cases. Am J Surg Pathol 1995, **19**: 1077–1081.

164 Fetsch JF, Laskin WB, Miettinen M. Superficial acral fibromyxoma: a clinicopathologic and immunohistochemical analysis of 37 cases of a distinctive soft tissue tumor with a predilection for the finger and toes. Hum Pathol 2001, **32**: 704–714.

165 Laskin WB, Fetsch JF, Miettinen M. Nuchal fibrocartilaginous pseudotumor: a clinicopathologic study of five cases and review of the literature. Mod Pathol 1999, **12**: 663–668.

166 Maghari A, Ma N, Aisner S, Benevenia J, Hameed M. Collagenous fibroma (desmoplastic fibroblastoma) with a new translocation involving 11q12: a case report. Cancer Genet Cytogenet 2009, **192**: 73–75.

167 Michal M, Fetsch JF, Hes O, Miettinen M. Nuchal-type fibroma. A clinicopathologic study of 52 cases. Cancer 1999, **85**: 156–163.

168 Miettinen M, Fetsch JF. Collagenous fibroma (desmoplastic fibroblastoma): a clinicopathologic analysis of 63 cases of a distinctive soft tissue lesion with stellate-shaped fibroblasts. Hum Pathol 1998, **29**: 676–682.

169 Nielsen GP, O'Connell JX, Dickersin GR, Rosenberg AE. Collagenous fibroma (desmoplastic fibroblastoma): a report of seven cases. Mod Pathol 1997, **9**: 781–785.

170 Sakamoto A, Yamamoto H, Yoshida T, Tanaka K, Matsuda S, Oda Y, Tsuneyoshi M, Iwamoto Y. Desmoplastic fibroblastoma (collagenous fibroma) with a specific breakpoint of 11q12. Histopathology 2007, **51**: 859–860.

171 Sciot R, Samson I, van den Berghe H, Van Damme B, Dal Cin P. Collagenous fibroma (desmoplastic fibroblastoma): genetic link with fibroma of tendon sheath? Mod Pathol 1999, **12**: 565–568.

Giant cell fibroblastoma

172 Abdul-Karim FW, Evans HL, Silva EG. Giant cell fibroblastoma. A report of three cases. Am J Clin Pathol 1985, **83**: 165–170.

173 Alguacil-García A. Giant cell fibroblastoma recurring as dermatofibrosarcoma protuberans. Am J Surg Pathol 1991, **15**: 798–801.

174 Chou P, Gonzalez-Crussi F, Mangkornkanok M. Giant cell fibroblastoma. Cancer 1989, **63**: 756–762.

175 Chung EB. Pitfalls in diagnosing benign soft tissue tumors in infancy and childhood. Pathol Annu 1985, **20**(Pt 2): 323–386.

176 Dymock RB, Allen PW, Stirling JW, Gilbert EF, Thornbery JM. Giant cell fibroblastoma. A distinctive, recurrent tumor of childhood. Am J Surg Pathol 1987, **11**: 263–271.

177 Fletcher CD. Giant cell fibroblastoma of soft tissue: a clinicopathological and immunohistochemical study. Histopathology 1988, **13**: 499–508.

178 Goldblum JR. Giant cell fibroblastoma: a report of three cases with histologic and immunohistochemical evidence of a relationship to dermatofibrosarcoma protuberans. Arch Pathol Lab Med 2002, **120**: 1052–1055.

179 Jha P, Moosavi C, Fanburg-Smith JC. Giant cell fibroblastoma: an update and addition of 86 new cases from the Armed Forces Institute of Pathology, in honor of Dr. Franz M. Enzinger. Ann Diagn Pathol 2007, **11**: 81–88.

180 Michal M, Zamecnik M. Giant cell fibroblastoma with a dermatofibrosarcoma protuberans component. Am J Dermatopathol 1992, **14**: 549–552.

181 Pinto A, Hwang W, Wong A, Seagram C. Giant cell fibroblastoma in childhood. Immunohistochemical and ultrastructural study. Mod Pathol 1992, **5**: 639–642.

182 Rubin BP, Fletcher JA, Fletcher CD. The histologic, genetic, and biological relationships between dermatofibrosarcoma protuberans and giant cell fibroblastoma: an unexpected story. Adv Anat Pathol 1997, **4**: 336–341.

183 Shmookler BM, Enzinger FM, Weiss SW. Giant cell fibroblastoma. A juvenile form of dermatofibrosarcoma protuberans. Cancer 1989, **64**: 2154–2161.

184 Terrier-Lacombe MJ, Guillou L, Maire G, Terrier P, Vince DR, de Saint Aubain Somerhausen N, Collin F, Pedeutour F, Coindre JM. Dermatofibrosarcoma protuberans, giant cell fibroblastoma, and hybrid lesions in children: clinicopathologic comparative analysis of 28 cases with molecular data – a study from the French Federation of Cancer Centers Sarcoma Group. Am J Surg Pathol 2003, **27**: 27–39.

185 Zámecník M, Michal M. Giant-cell fibroblastoma with pigmented dermatofibrosarcoma protuberans component. Am J Surg Pathol 1994, **18**: 736–740.

Nodular fasciitis and related lesions

186 Allen PW. Nodular fasciitis. Pathology 1972, **4**: 9–26.

187 Auerbach A, Fanburg-Smith JC, Wang G, Rushing EJ. Focal myositis: a clinicopathologic study of 115 cases of an intramuscular mass-like reactive process. Am J Surg Pathol 2009, **33**: 1016–1024.

188 Bernstein KE, Lattes R. Nodular (pseudosarcomatous) fasciitis, a nonrecurrent lesion. Cancer 1982, **49**: 1668–1678.

189 Chung EB, Enzinger FM. Proliferative fasciitis. Cancer 1975, **36**: 1450–1458.

190 Craver JL, McDivitt RW. Proliferative fasciitis. Ultrastructural study of two cases. Arch Pathol Lab Med 1981, **105**: 542–545.

191 Dahl I, Angervall L. Pseudosarcomatous proliferative lesions of soft tissue with or without bone formation. Acta Pathol Microbiol Scand (A) 1977, **85**: 577–589.

192 Daroca PJ Jr, Pulitzer DR, LoCicero J III. Ossifying fasciitis. Arch Pathol Lab Med 1982, **106**: 682–685.

193 de Feraudy S, Fletcher CDM. Intradermal nodular fasciitis: a rare lesion analyzed in a series of 24 cases. Am J Surg Pathol 2010, **34**: 1377–1381.

194 Donner LR, Silva T, Dobin SM. Clonal rearrangement of 15p11.2, 16p11.2, and 16p13.3 in a case of nodular fasciitis: additional evidence favoring nodular fasciitis as a benign neoplasm and not a reactive tumefaction. Cancer Genet Cytogenet 2002, **139**: 138–140.

195 el-Jabbour JN, Bennett MH, Burke MM, Lessells A, O'Halloran A. Proliferative myositis. An immunohistochemical and ultrastructural study. Am J Surg Pathol 1991, **15**: 654–659.

196 el-Jabbour JN, Wilson GD, Bennett MH, Burke MM, Davey AT, Eames K. Flow cytometric study of nodular fasciitis, proliferative fasciitis, and proliferative myositis. Hum Pathol 1991, **22**: 1146–1149.

197 Enzinger FM, Dulcey F. Proliferative myositis. Report of 33 cases. Cancer 1967, **20**: 2213–2223.

198 Heffner RR Jr, Armbrustmacher VW, Earle KM. Focal myositis. Cancer 1977, **40**: 301–306.

199 Heffner RR Jr, Barron SA. Denervating changes in focal myositis, a benign inflammatory pseudotumor. Arch Pathol Lab Med 1980, **104**: 261–264.

200 Hollowood K, Fletcher CD. Pseudosarcomatous myofibroblastic proliferations of the spermatic cord ('proliferative funiculitis'). Histologic and immunohistochemical analysis of a distinctive entity. Am J Surg Pathol 1992, **16**: 448–454.

201 Hornick JL, Fletcher CD. Intraarticular nodular fasciitis – a rare lesion: clinicopathologic analysis of a series. Am J Surg Pathol 2006, **30**: 237–241.

202 Hutter RVP, Stewart FW, Foote FW Jr. Fasciitis. A report of 70 cases with follow-up proving the benignity of the lesion. Cancer 1962, **15**: 992–1003.

203 Kern WH. Proliferative myositis. A pseudosarcomatous reaction to injury. Arch Pathol 1960, **69**: 209–216.

204 Kleinstiver BJ, Rodriguez HA. Nodular fasciitis. A study of 45 cases and review of the literature. J Bone Joint Surg (Am) 1968, **50**: 1204–1212.

205 Konwaler BE, Keasbey L, Kaplan L. Subcutaneous pseudosarcomatous fibromatosis (fasciitis). Report of 8 cases. Am J Clin Pathol 1955, **25**: 241–252.

206 Lai FM, Lam WY. Nodular fasciitis of the dermis. J Cutan Pathol 1993, **20**: 66–69.

207 Lauer DH, Enzinger FM. Cranial fasciitis of childhood. Cancer 1980, **45**: 401–406.

208 Liegl B, Fletcher CD. Ischemic fasciitis: analysis of 44 cases indicating an inconsistent association with immobility or debilitation. Am J Surg Pathol 2008, **32**: 1546–1552.

209 Meis JM, Enzinger FM. Proliferative fasciitis and myositis of childhood. Am J Surg Pathol 1992, **16**: 364–372.

210 Meister P, Bückmann FW, Konrad E. Extent and level of fascial involvement in 100 cases with nodular fasciitis. Virchows Arch [A] 1978, **380**: 177–185.

211 Montgomery EA, Meis JM. Nodular fasciitis. Its morphologic spectrum and immunohistochemical profile. Am J Surg Pathol 1991, **15**: 942–948.

212 Montgomery EA, Meis JM, Mitchell MS, Enzinger FM. Atypical decubital fibroplasia. A distinctive fibroblastic pseudotumor occurring in debilitated patients. Am J Surg Pathol 1992, **16**: 708–715.

213 Patchefsky AS, Enzinger FM. Intravascular fasciitis. A report of 17 cases. Am J Surg Pathol 1981, **5**: 29–36.

214 Perosio PM, Weiss SW. Ischemic fasciitis. A juxta-skeletal fibroblastic proliferation with a predilection for elderly patients. Mod Pathol 1993, **6**: 69–72.

215 Price EB Jr, Silliphant WM, Shuman R. Nodular fasciitis. A clinicopathologic analysis of 65 cases. Am J Clin Pathol 1961, **35**: 122–136.

216 Price SK, Kahn LB, Saxe N. Dermal and intravascular fasciitis. Unusual variants of nodular fasciitis. Am J Dermatopathol 1993, **15**: 539–543.

217 Rosenberg AE. Pseudosarcomas of soft tissue. Arch Pathol Lab Med 2008, **132**: 579–586.

218 Sasano H, Yamaki H, Ohashi Y, Ohtsuki S, Nagura H. Proliferative fasciitis of the forearm: case report with immunohistochemical, ultrastructural and DNA ploidy study and review of the literature. Pathol Int 1998, **48**: 486–490.

219 Shimuzu S, Hashimoto H, Enjoji M. Nodular fasciitis. An analysis of 250 patients. Pathology 1984, **16**: 161–166.

220 Toti P, Catella AM, Benvenuti A. Focal myositis. A pseudotumoral lesion. Histopathology 1994, **24**: 171–173.

221 Toti P, Ramano L, Villanova M, Zazzi M, Luzi P. Focal myositis: a polymerase chain reaction analysis for a viral etiology. Hum Pathol 1997, **28**: 111–113.

222 Toti P, Tanganelli P, Schurfeld K, Stumpo M, Barbagli L, Vatti R, Luzi P. Scarring in papillary carcinoma of the thyroid: report of two cases with exuberant nodular fasciitis-like stroma. Histopathology 1999, **35**: 418–422.

223 Wirman JA. Nodular fasciitis, a lesion of myofibroblasts. An ultrastructural study. Cancer 1976, **38**: 2378–2389.

224 Wong NL, Di F. Pseudosarcomatous fasciitis and myositis: diagnosis by fine-needle aspiration cytology. Am J Clin Pathol 2009, **132**: 857–865.

Myositis ossificans

225 Moosavi CA, Al-Nahar LA, Murphey MD, Fanburg-Smith JC. Fibroosseous pseudotumor of the digit: a clinicopathologic study of 43 new cases. Ann Diagn Pathol 2008, **12**: 21–28.

Elastofibroma

226 Dixon AY, Lee SH. An ultrastructural study of elastofibromas. Hum Pathol 1980, **11**: 257–262.

227 Enjoji M, Sumiyoshi K, Sueyuski K. Elastofibromatous lesion of the stomach in a patient with elastofibroma dorsi. Am J Surg Pathol 1985, **9**: 233–237.

228 Erkiliç S, Koçer NE, Sivrikoz C. Subscapular elastofibroma intermingled with adipose tissue: variant type of elastofibroma or lipoma? Ann Diagn Pathol 2005, **9**: 327–329.

229 Fukuda Y, Miyake H, Masuda Y, Masugi Y. Histogenesis of unique elastinophilic fibers of elastofibroma. Ultrastructural and immunohistochemical studies. Hum Pathol 1987, **18**: 424–429.

230 Govoni E, Severi B, Laschi R, Lorenzini P, Ronchetti IP, Baccarani M. Elastofibroma. An in vivo model of abnormal neoelastogenesis. Ultrastruct Pathol 1988, **12**: 327–339.

231 Hisaoka M, Hashimoto H. Elastofibroma: clonal fibrous proliferation with predominant CD34-positive cells. Virchows Arch 2006, **448**: 195–199.

232 Järvi OH, Saxén AE, Hopsu-Havu VK, Wartiovaara JJ, Vaissalo VT. Elastofibroma. A degenerative pseudotumor. Cancer 1969, **23**: 42–63.

233 Kahn HJ, Hanna WM. 'Abberrant elastic' in elastofibroma. An immunohistochemical and ultrastructural study. Ultrastruct Pathol 1995, **19**: 45–50.

234 Kindblom L-G, Spicer SS. Elastofibroma. A correlated light and electron microscopic study. Virchows Arch [A] 1982, **396**: 127–140.

235 Kumaratilake JS, Krishnan R, Lomax-Smith J, Cleary EG. Elastofibroma. Disturbed elastic fibrillogenesis by periosteal-derived cells? An immunoelectron microscopic and in situ hybridization study. Hum Pathol 1991, **22**: 1017–1029.

236 Madri JA, Dise CA, LiVolsi VA, Merino MJ, Bibro MC. Elastofibroma dorsi. An immunochemical study of collagen content. Hum Pathol 1981, **12**: 186–190.

237 Nagamine N, Nohara Y, Ito E. Elastofibroma in Okinawa. A clinicopathologic study of 170 cases. Cancer 1982, **50**: 1794–1805.

238 Nakamura Y, Okamoto K, Tanimura A, Kato M, Morimatsu M. Elastase digestion and biochemical analysis of the elastin from an elastofibroma. Cancer 1986, **58**: 1070–1075.

239 Stemmermann GN, Stout AP. Elastofibroma dorsi. Am J Clin Pathol 1962, **37**: 490–506.

240 Yamazaki K. An ultrastructural and immunohistochemical study of elastofibroma: CD34, MEF-2, prominin 2 (CD133), and factor XIIIa-positive proliferating fibroblastic stromal cells connected by Cx43-type gap junctions. Ultrastruct Pathol 2007, **31**: 209–219.

Solitary fibrous tumor

241 Brunnemann RB, Ro JY, Ordóñez NG, Mooney J, El-Naggar AK, Ayala AG. Extrapleural solitary fibrous tumor: a clinicopathologic study of 24 cases. Mod Pathol 1999, **12**: 1034–1042.

242 de Saint Aubain Somerhausen N, Rubin BP, Fletcher CD. Myxoid solitary fibrous tumor: a study of seven cases with emphasis on differential diagnosis. Mod Pathol 1999, **12**: 463–471.

243 Dei Tos AP, Seregard S, Calonje E, Chan JK, Fletcher CD. Giant cell angiofibroma. A distinctive orbital tumor in adults. Am J Surg Pathol 1995, **19**: 1286–1293.

244 Folpe AL, Devaney K, Weiss SW. Lipomatous hemangiopericytoma: a rare variant of hemangiopericytoma that may be confused with liposarcoma. Am J Surg Pathol 1999, **23**: 1201–1207.

245 Guillou L, Gebhard S, Coindre JM. Lipomatous hemangiopericytoma: a fat containing variant of solitary fibrous tumor? Clinicopathologic, immunohistochemical, and ultrastructural analysis of a series in favour of a unifying concept. Hum Pathol 2000, **31**: 1108–1115.

246 Guillou L, Gebhard S, Coindre JM. Orbital and extraorbital giant cell angiofibroma: a giant cell-rich variant of solitary fibrous tumor? Clinicopathologic and immunohistochemical analysis of a series in favour of a unifying concept. Am J Surg Pathol 2000, **24**: 971–979.

247 Macarenco RS, Erickson-Johnson MR, Wang X, Nascimento AG, Folpe AL, Oliveira AM. Dedifferentiated solitary fibrous tumors: a clinicopathologic study of 7 cases. Lab Invest 2009, **89**(Suppl 1): 18A.

248 Mosquera JM, Fletcher CDM. Expanding the spectrum of malignant progression in solitary fibrous tumors: a study of 8 cases with a discrete anaplastic component – is this dedifferentiated SFT? Am J Surg Pathol 2009, **33**: 1314–1321.

249 Nielsen GP, O'Connell JX, Dickersin GR, Rosenberg AE. Solitary fibrous tumor of soft tissue: a report of 15 cases, including 5 malignant examples with light microscopic, immunohistochemical, and ultrastructural data. Mod Pathol 1997, **10**: 1028–1037.

Fibromatosis

250 Alaggio R, Barisani D, Ninfo V, Rosolen A, Coffin CM. Morphologic overlap between infantile myofibromatosis and infantile fibrosarcoma: a pitfall in diagnosis. Pediatr Dev Pathol 2008, **11**: 355–362.

251 Allen PW. The fibromatoses. A clinicopathologic classification based on 140 cases. Am J Surg Pathol 1977, **1**: 255–270, 305–321.

252 Andino L, Cagle PT, Murer B, Lu L, Popper HH, Galateau-Salle F, Sienko AE, Barrios R, Zander DS. Pleuropulmonary desmoid tumors: immunohistochemical comparison with solitary fibrous tumors and assessment of beta-catenin and cyclin D1 expression. Arch Pathol Lab Med 2006, **130**: 1503–1509.

253 Ayala AG, Ro JY, Goepfert H, Cangir A, Khorsand J, Flake G. Desmoid fibromatosis. A clinicopathologic study of 25 children. Semin Diagn Pathol 1986, **3**: 138–150.

254 Battifora H, Hines JR. Recurrent digital fibromas of childhood. An electron microscope study. Cancer 1971, **27**: 1530–1536.

255 Beham A, Badve S, Suster S, Fletcher CD. Solitary myofibroma in adults.

Clinicopathological analysis of a series. Histopathology 1993, **22**: 335–341.

256 Bhattacharya B, Dilworth HP, Iacobuzio-Donahue C, Ricci F, Weber K, Furlong MA, Fisher C, Montgomery E. Nuclear beta-catenin expression distinguishes deep fibromatosis from other benign and malignant fibroblastic and myofibroblastic lesions. Am J Surg Pathol 2005, **29**: 653–659.

257 Bhawan J, Bacchetta C, Joris I, Majno G. A myofibroblastic tumor. Infantile digital fibroma (recurrent digital fibrous tumor of childhood). Am J Pathol 1979, **94**: 19–28.

258 Bochetto JF, Raycroft JE, Deinnocentes LW. Multiple polyposis, exostosis, and soft tissue tumors. Surg Gynecol Obstet 1963, **117**: 489–494.

259 Briselli MF, Soule EH, Gilchrist GS. Congenital fibromatosis. Report of 18 cases of solitary and 4 cases of multiple tumors. Mayo Clin Proc 1980, **55**: 554–562.

260 Burke AP, Sobin LH, Shekitka KM. Mesenteric fibromatosis. A follow-up study. Arch Pathol Lab Med 1990, **114**: 832–835.

261 Burke AP, Sobin LH, Shekitka KM, Federspiel BH, Helwig EB. Intraabdominal fibromatosis. A pathologic analysis of 130 tumors with comparison of clinical subgroups. Am J Surg Pathol 1990, **14**: 335–341.

262 Burry AF, Kerr JFR, Pope JH. Recurring digital fibrous tumour of childhood. An electron microscopic and virological study. Pathology 1970, **2**: 287–291.

263 Chung EB, Enzinger FM. Infantile myofibromatosis. Cancer 1981, **48**: 1807–1818.

264 Coffin CM, Hornick JL, Zhou H, Fletcher CD. Gardner fibroma: a clinicopathologic and immunohistochemical analysis of 45 patients with 57 fibromas. Am J Surg Pathol 2007, **31**: 410–416.

265 Cooper PH. Fibrous proliferations of infancy and childhood. J Cutan Pathol 1992, **19**: 257–267.

266 Coventry MB, Harris LE, Bianco AJ, Bulbulian AH. Congenital muscular torticollis (wry neck). Postgrad Med 1960, **28**: 383–392.

267 Daimaru Y, Hashimoto H, Enjoji M. Myofibromatosis in adults (adult counterpart of infantile myofibromatosis). Am J Surg Pathol 1989, **13**: 859–865.

268 De Wever I, Dal Cin P, Fletcher CD, Mandahl N, Mertens F, Mitelman F, Rosai J, Rydholm A, Sciot R, Tallini G, Van Den Berghe H, Vanni R, Willén H. Cytogenetic, clinical and morphologic correlations in 78 cases of fibromatosis: a report from the CHAMP study group, chromosomes and morphology. Mod Pathol 2000, **13**: 1080–1085.

269 Deyrup AT, Tretiakova M, Montag AG. Estrogen receptor-beta expression in extraabdominal fibromatoses: an analysis of 40 cases. Cancer 2006, **106**: 208–213.

270 Dimmick JE, Wood WS. Congenital multiple fibromatosis. Am J Dermatopathol 1983, **5**: 289–295.

271 Domínguez-Malagón H. Proliferative disorders of myofibroblasts. Ultrastruct Pathol 1993, **17**: 211–220.

272 Domínguez-Malagón H. Intracellular collagen and fibronexus in fibromatosis and other fibroblastic tumors. Ultrastruct Pathol 2004, **28**: 67–73.

273 Drescher E, Woyke S, Markiewicz C, Tegi S. Juvenile fibromatosis in siblings (fibromatosis hyalinica multiplex juvenilis). J Pediatr Surg 1967, **2**: 427–430.

274 Drut R, Pedemonte L, Rositto A. Noninclusion-body infantile digital fibromatosis: a lesion heralding terminal osseous dysplasia and pigmentary defects syndrome. Int J Surg Pathol 2005, **13**: 181–184.

275 Enzinger FM. Histological typing of soft tissue tumours. International histological classification of tumours. No 3. Geneva, 1969, World Health Organization.

276 Enzinger FM, Shiraki M. Musculo-aponeurotic fibromatosis of the shoulder girdle (extra-abdominal desmoid). Analysis of 30 cases followed up for ten or more years. Cancer 1967, **20**: 1131–1140.

277 Faraggiana T, Churg J, Strauss L. Ultrastructural histochemistry of infantile digital fibromatosis. Ultrastruct Pathol 1981, **2**: 241–247.

278 Fetsch JF, Miettinen M, Laskin WB, Michal M, Enzinger FM. A clinicopathologic study of 45 pediatric soft tissue tumors with an admixture of adipose tissue and fibroblastic elements, and a proposal for classification as lipofibromatosis. Am J Surg Pathol 2000, **24**: 1491–1500.

279 Fetsch JF, Laskin WB, Miettinen M. Palmar-plantar fibromatosis in children and preadolescents: a clinicopathologic study of 56 cases with newly recognized demographics and extended follow-up information. Am J Surg Pathol 2005, **29**: 1095–1105.

280 Fletcher CDM, Achu P, Van Noorden S, McKee PH. Infantile myofibromatosis. A light microscopic, histochemical and immunohistochemical study suggesting true smooth muscle differentiation. Histopathology 1987, **11**: 245–258.

281 Fletcher CDM, Stirling RW, Smith MA, Pambakian H, McKee PH. Multicentric extra-abdominal 'myofibromatosis'. Report of a case with ultrastructural findings. Histopathology 1986, **10**: 713–724.

282 Fromowitz FB, Hurst LC, Nathan J, Badalamente M. Infantile (desmoid type) fibromatosis with extensive ossification. Am J Surg Pathol 1987, **11**: 66–75.

283 Fukasawa Y, Ishikura H, Takada A, Yokoyama S, Imamura M, Yoshiki T, Sato H. Massive apoptosis in infantile myofibromatosis. A putative mechanism of tumor regression. Am J Pathol 1994, **144**: 480–485.

284 Gabbiani G, Majno G. Dupuytren's contracture. Fibroblast contraction? An ultrastructural study. Am J Pathol 1972, **66**: 131–138.

285 Gebert C, Hardes J, Kersting C, August C, Supper H, Winkelmann W, Buerger H, Gosheger G. Expression of beta-catenin and p53 are prognostic factors in deep aggressive fibromatosis. Histopathology 2007, **50**: 491–497.

286 Goellner JR, Soule EH. Desmoid tumors. An ultrastructural study of eight cases. Hum Pathol 1980, **11**: 43–50.

287 Goslee L, Clermont V, Bernstein J, Woolley PW Jr. Superficial connective tissue tumors in early infancy. J Pediatr 1964, **65**: 377–387.

288 Granter SR, Badizadegan K, Fletcher CD. Myofibromatosis in adults, glomangiopericytoma, and myopericytoma: a spectrum of tumors showing perivascular myoid differentiation. Am J Surg Pathol 1998, **22**: 513–525.

289 Haleem A, Al-Hindi HN, Al-Juboury M, Al Husseini H, Al Ajlan A. Juvenile hyaline fibromatosis: morphologic, immunohistochemical, and ultrastructural study of three siblings. Am J Dermatopathol 2002, **24**: 218–224.

290 Half E, Bercovich D, Rozen P. Familial adenomatous polyposis. Orphanet J Rare Dis 2009, **4**: 22.

291 Hanks S, Adams S, Douglas J, Arbour L, Atherton DJ, Balci S, Bode H, Campbell ME, Feingold M, Keser G, Kleijer W, Mancini G, McGrath JA, Muntoni F, Nanda A, Teare MD, Warman M, Pope FM, Superti-Furga A, Futreal PA, Rahman N. Mutations in the gene encoding capillary morphogenesis protein 2 cause juvenile hyaline fibromatosis and infantile systemic hyalinosis. Am J Hum Genet 2003, **73**: 791–800.

292 Hasegawa T, Hirose T, Seki K, Hizawa K, Okada J, Nakanishi H. Solitary infantile myofibromatosis of bone. An immunohistochemical and ultrastructural study. Am J Surg Pathol 1993, **17**: 308–313.

293 Hayashi T, Tsuda N, Chowdhury PR, Anami M, Kishikawa M, Iseki M, Kobayashi K. Infantile digital fibromatosis. A study of the development and regression of cytoplasmic inclusion bodies. Mod Pathol 1995, **8**: 548–552.

294 Hogan SF, Salassa JR. Recurrent adult myofibromatosis. A case report. Am J Clin Pathol 1992, **97**: 810–814.

295 Ishikawa H, Mori S. Systemic hyalinosis or fibromatosis hyalinica multiplex juvenilis as a congenital syndrome. A new entity based on the inborn error of the acid mucopolysaccharide metabolism in connective tissue cells? Acta Derm Venereol 1973, **53**: 185–191.

296 Iwahara T, Ikeda A. On the ipsilateral involvement of congenital muscular torticollis and congenital dislocation of the hip. J Jpn Orthop Assoc 1962, **35**: 1221–1226.

297 Iwasaki H, Kikuchi M, Ohtsuki I, Enjoji M, Suenaga N, Mori R. Infantile digital fibromatosis. Identification of actin filaments in cytoplasmic inclusions by heavy meromyosin binding. Cancer 1983, **52**: 1653–1661.

298 Iwasaki H, Müller H, Stutte HJ, Brennscheidt U. Palmar fibromatosis (Dupuytren's contracture). Ultrastructural and enzyme histochemical studies of 43 cases. Virchows Arch [A] 1984, **405**: 41–53.

299 Jennings TA, Duray PH, Collins FS, Sabetta J, Enzinger FM. Infantile myofibromatosis. Evidence for an autosomal-dominant disorder. Am J Surg Pathol 1984, **8**: 529–538.

300 Kiel KD, Suit HD. Radiation therapy in the treatment of aggressive fibromatoses (desmoid tumors). Cancer 1984, **54**: 2051–2055.

301 Kim D-H, Goldsmith HS, Quan SH, Huvos AG. Intraabdominal desmoid tumor. Cancer 1971, **27**: 1041–1043.

302 Kiryu H, Tsuneyoshi M, Enjoji M. Myofibroblasts in fibromatoses. An electron microscopic study. Acta Pathol Jpn 1985, **35**: 533–547.

303 Lazar AJ, Tuvin D, Hajibashi S, Habeeb S, Bolshakov S, Mayordomo-Aranda E, Warneke CL, Lopez-Terrada D, Pollock RE, Lev D. Specific mutations in the beta-catenin gene (CTNNB1) correlate with local recurrence in sporadic desmoid tumors. Am J Pathol 2008, **173**: 1518–1527.

304 Laskin WB, Miettinen M, Fetsch JF. Infantile digital fibroma/fibromatosis: a clinicopathologic and immunohistochemical study of 69 tumors from 57 patients with long-term follow-up. Am J Surg Pathol 2009, **33**: 1–13.

305 Levine AM, Reddick R, Triche T. Intracellular collagen fibrils in human sarcomas. Lab Invest 1978, **39**: 531–540.

306 Lucas DR, Al-Abbadi M, Tabaczka P, Hamre MR, Weaver DW, Mott MP. c-kit expression in desmoid fibromatosis: comparative immunohistochemical of two commercial antibodies [abstract]. Mod Pathol 2003, **16**: 16A.

307 Masson JK, Soule EH. Desmoid tumors of head and neck. Am J Surg 1966, **112**: 615–622.

308 Montgomery E, Lee JH, Abraham SC, Wu TT. Superficial fibromatoses are genetically distinct from deep fibromatoses. Mod Pathol 2001, **14**: 695–701.

309 Mukai M, Torikata C, Iri H, Hata J, Naito M, Shimoda T. Immunohistochemical identification of aggregated actin filaments in formalin-fixed, paraffin-embedded sections. I. A study of infantile digital fibromatosis by a new pretreatment. Am J Surg Pathol 1992, **16**: 110–115.

310 Ng TL, Gown AM, Barry TS, Cheang MC, Chan AK, Turbin DA, Hsu FD, West RB, Nielsen TO. Nuclear beta-catenin in mesenchymal tumors. Mod Pathol 2005, **18**: 68–74.

311 Pettinato G, Manivel JC, Gould EW, Albores-Saavedra J. Inclusion body fibromatosis of the breast. Two cases with immunohistochemical and ultrastructural findings. Am J Clin Pathol 1994, **101**: 714–718.

312 Pickren JW, Smith AG, Stevenson TW Jr, Stout AP. Fibromatosis of the plantar fascia. Cancer 1951, **4**: 846–856.

313 Purdy LJ, Colby TV. Infantile digital fibromatosis occurring outside the digit. Am J Surg Pathol 1984, **8**: 787–790.

314 Reitamo JJ, Hayry P, Nykyri E, Saxén AE. The desmoid tumor. Incidence, sex, age, and anatomical distribution in the Finnish population. Am J Clin Pathol 1982, **77**: 665–684.

315 Reye RDK. Recurring digital fibrous tumors of childhood. Arch Pathol 1965, **80**: 228–231.

316 Rock MG, Pritchard DJ, Reiman HM, Soule EH, Brewster RC. Extra-abdominal desmoid tumors. J Bone Joint Surg (Am) 1984, **66**: 1369–1374.

317 Rodriguez JA, Guarda LA, Rosai J. Mesenteric fibromatosis with involvement of the gastrointestinal tract. A GIST simulator: a study of 25 cases. Am J Clin Pathol 2004, **121**: 93–98.

318 Rodriguez-Bigas MA, Mahoney MC, Karakousis CP, Petrelli NJ. Desmoid tumors in patients with familial adenomatous polyposis. Cancer 1994, **74**: 1270–1274.

319 Rosen PP, Ernsberger D. Mammary fibromatosis. A benign spindle cell tumor with significant risk for local recurrence. Cancer 1989, **63**: 1363–1369.

320 Rosenberg HS, Stenback WA, Spjut HJ. The fibromatoses of infancy and childhood. Perspect Pediatr Pathol 1978, **4**: 269–348.

321 Santa Cruz DJ, Reiner CB. Recurrent digital fibroma of childhood. J Cutan Pathol 1978, **5**: 339–346.

322 Skoog T. Dupuytren's contracture. Pathogenesis and surgical treatment. Surg Clin North Am 1967, **47**: 433–444.

323 Sportiello DJ, Hoogerland DL. A recurrent pelvic desmoid tumor successfully treated with tamoxifen. Cancer 1991, **67**: 1443–1446.

324 Staley CJ. Gardner's syndrome. Simultaneous occurrence of polyposis coli, osteomatosis and soft tissue tumors. Arch Surg 1961, **82**: 420–422.

325 Stout AP. Juvenile fibromatosis. Cancer 1954, **7**: 953–978.

326 Viale G, Doglioni C, Iuzzolino P, Bontempini L, Colombi R, Coggi G, Dell'Orto P. Infantile digital fibromatosis-like tumour (inclusion body fibromatosis) of adulthood. Report of two cases with ultrastructural and immunocytochemical findings. Histopathology 1988, **12**: 415–424.

327 Walts AE, Asch M, Raj C. Solitary lesion of congenital fibromatosis. Am J Surg Pathol 1982, **6**: 255–260.

328 Wang N-S, Knaack J. Fibromatosis hyalinica multiplex juvenilis. Ultrastruct Pathol 1982, **3**: 153–160.

329 Welsh RA. Intracytoplasmic collagen formations in desmoid fibromatosis. Am J Pathol 1966, **49**: 515–535.

330 Wilcken N, Tattersall MH. Endocrine therapy for desmoid tumors. Cancer 1991, **68**: 1384–1388.

331 Woyke S, Domagala W, Olszewski W. Ultrastructure of a fibromatosis hyalinica multiplex juvenilis. Cancer 1970, **26**: 1157–1168.

332 Yokoyama R, Tsuneyoshi M, Enjoji M, Shinohara N, Masuda S. Extra-abdominal desmoid tumors. Correlations between histologic features and biologic behavior. Surg Pathol 1989, **2**: 29–42.

333 Yun K. Infantile digital fibromatosis. Immunohistochemical and ultrastructural observations of cytoplasmic inclusions. Cancer 1988, **61**: 500–507.

334 Zelefsky MJ, Harrison LB, Shiu MH, Armstrong JG, Hajdu SI, Brennan MF. Combined surgical resection and iridium 192 implantation for locally advanced and recurrent desmoid tumors. Cancer 1991, **67**: 380–384.

Fibrosarcoma

335 Alaggio R, Ninfo V, Rosolen A, Coffin CM. Primitive myxoid mesenchymal tumor of infancy: a clinicopathologic report of 6 cases. Am J Surg Pathol 2006, **30**: 388–394.

336 Antonescu CR, Rosenblum MK, Pereira P, Nascimento AG, Woodruff JM. Sclerosing epithelioid fibrosarcoma: a study of 16 cases and confirmation of a clinicopathologically distinct tumor. Am J Surg Pathol 2001, **25**: 699–709.

337 Bourgeois J, Knezevich SR, Mathers JA, Sorensen PH. Molecular detection of the ETV6–NTRK3 gene fusion differentiates congenital fibrosarcoma from other childhood spindle cell tumors. Am J Surg Pathol 2000, **24**: 937–946.

338 Chung EB, Enzinger FM. Infantile fibrosarcoma. Cancer 1976, **38**: 729–739.

339 Chung AM, Kahn LB. Myofibroblasts and related cells in malignant fibrous and fibrohistiocytic tumors. Hum Pathol 1977, **8**: 205–218.

340 Dehner LP, Askin FB. Tumors of fibrous tissue origin in childhood. A clinico-pathologic study of cutaneous and soft tissue neoplasms in 66 children. Cancer 1976, **38**: 888–900.

341 Eyden B. Fibroblast phenotype plasticity: relevance for understanding heterogeneity in 'fibroblastic' tumors. Ultrastruct Pathol 2004, **28**: 307–319.

342 Gonzalez-Crussi F, Wiederhold MD, Sotelo-Avila C. Congenital fibrosarcoma. Presence of a histiocytic component. Cancer 1980, **46**: 77–86.

343 Guillou L, Benhattar J, Gengler C, Gallagher G, Ranchère-Vince D, Collin F, Terrier P, Terrier-Lacombe MJ, Leroux A, Marquès B, Aubain Somerhausen Nde S, Keslair F, Pedeutour F, Coindre JM. Translocation-positive low-grade fibromyxoid sarcoma: clinicopathologic and molecular analysis of a series expanding the morphologic spectrum and suggesting potential relationship to sclerosing epithelioid fibrosarcoma: a study from the French Sarcoma Group. Am J Surg Pathol 2007, **31**: 1387–1402.

344 Hall J, Tseng SCG, Timpl R, Hendrix MJC, Stern R. Collagen types in fibrosarcoma. Absence of type III collagen in reticulin. Hum Pathol 1985, **16**: 439–446.

345 Hansen T, Katenkamp K, Brodhun M, Katenkamp D. Low-grade fibrosarcoma – report on 39 not otherwise specified cases and comparison with defined low-grade fibrosarcoma types. Histopathology 2006, **49**: 152–160.

346 Iwasaki H, Enjoji M. Infantile and adult fibrosarcomas of the soft tissues. Acta Pathol Jpn 1979, **29**: 377–388.

347 Knezevich SR, Garnett MJ, Pysher TJ, Beckwith JB, Grundy PE, Sorensen PH. ETV6-NTRK3 gene fusions and trisomy 11 establish a histogenetic link between mesoblastic nephroma and congenital fibrosarcoma. Cancer Res 1998, **58**: 5046–5048.

348 Meis-Kindblom JM, Kindblom L-G, Enzinger FM. Sclerosing epithelioid fibrosarcoma. A variant of fibrosarcoma simulating carcinoma. Am J Surg Pathol 1995, **19**: 979–993.

349 Oshiro Y, Fukuda T, Tsuneyoshi M. Fibrosarcoma versus fibromatoses and cellular nodular fasciitis. A comparative study of their proliferative activity using proliferating cell nuclear antigen, DNA flow cytometry, and p53. Am J Surg Pathol 1994, **18**: 712–719.

350 Pritchard DJ, Soule EH, Taylor WF, Ivins JC. Fibrosarcoma. A clinicopathologic and statistical study of 199 tumors of the soft tissues of the extremities and trunk. Cancer 1974, **33**: 888–897.

351 Reid R, Barrett A, Hamblen DL. Sclerosing epithelioid fibrosarcoma. Histopathology 1997, **28**: 451–455.

352 Sandberg AA, Bridge JA. Updates on the cytogenetics and molecular genetics of bone soft tissue tumors: congenital (infantile) fibrosarcoma and mesoblastic nephroma. Cancer Genet Cytogenet 2002, **132**: 1–13.

353 Schofield DE, Fletcher JA, Grier HE, Yunis EJ. Fibrosarcoma in infants and children. Application of new techniques. Am J Surg Pathol 1994, **18**: 14–24.

354 Schofield DE, Fletcher JA, Grier HE, Yunis EJ. Fibrosarcoma in infants and children. Application of new techniques. Am J Surg Pathol 1994, **18**: 14–24.

355 Scott SM, Reiman HM, Pritchard DJ, Ilstrup DM. Soft tissue fibrosarcoma. A clinicopathologic study of 132 cases. Cancer 1989, **64**: 925–931.

356 Soule EH, Pritchard DJ. Fibrosarcoma in infants and children. A review of 110 cases. Cancer 1977, **40**: 1711–1721.

357 Stout AP. Fibrosarcoma. The malignant tumor of fibroblasts. Cancer 1948, **1**: 30–63.

358 Stout AP. Fibrosarcoma in infants and children. Cancer 1962, **15**: 1028–1040.

359 van der Werf-Messing B, van Unnik JAM. Fibrosarcoma of the soft tissue. A clinicopathologic study. Cancer 1965, **18**: 1113–1123.

360 Weiss SW. Proliferative fibroblastic lesions. From hyperplasia to neoplasia. Am J Surg Pathol 1986, **10**(Suppl 1): 14–25.

Myofibroblastic tumors

361 Cessna MH, Zhou H, Sanger WG, Perkins SL, Tripp S, Pickering D, Daines C, Coffin CM. Expression of ALK1 and p80 in inflammatory

759 Ghosh BC, Ghosh L, Huvos AG, Fortner JG. Malignant schwannoma. A clinicopathologic study. Cancer 1973, **31**: 184–190.

760 Gray MH, Rosenberg AE, Dickersin GR, Bhan AK. Glial fibrillary acidic protein and keratin expression by benign and malignant nerve sheath tumors. Hum Pathol 1989, **20**: 1089–1096.

761 Guccion JG, Enzinger FM. Malignant schwannoma associated with von Recklinghausen's neurofibromatosis. Virchows Arch [A] 1979, **383**: 43–57.

762 Herrera GA, Pinto de Moraes H. Neurogenic sarcomas in patients with neurofibromatosis (von Recklinghausen's disease). Light, electron microscopy and immunohistochemistry study. Virchows Arch [A] 1984, **403**: 361–376.

763 Herrera GA, Reimann BE, Salinas JA. Malignant schwannomas presenting as malignant fibrous histiocytomas. Ultrastruct Pathol 1982, **3**: 253–261.

764 Hirose T, Hasegawa T, Kudo E, Seki K, Sano T, Hizawa K. Malignant peripheral nerve sheath tumors. An immunohistochemical study in relation to ultrastructural features. Hum Pathol 1992, **23**: 865–870.

765 Hirose T, Sano T, Hizawa K. Heterogeneity of malignant schwannomas. Ultrastruct Pathol 1988, **12**: 107–116.

766 Hirose T, Scheithauer BW, Sano T. Perineurial malignant peripheral nerve sheath tumor (MPNST): a clinicopathologic, immunohistochemical, and ultrastructural study of seven cases. Am J Surg Pathol 1998, **22**: 1368–1378.

767 Hruban RH, Shiu MH, Senie RT, Woodruff JM. Malignant peripheral nerve sheath tumors of the buttock and lower extremity. A study of 43 cases. Cancer 1990, **66**: 1253–1265.

768 Hui P, Li N, Johnson C, De Wever I, Sciot R, Manfioletti G, Tallini G. HMGA proteins in malignant peripheral nerve sheath tumor and synovial sarcoma: preferential expression of HMGA2 in malignant peripheral nerve sheath tumor. Mod Pathol 2005, **18**: 1519–1526.

769 Johnson TL, Lee MW, Meis JM, Zarbo RJ, Crissman JD. Immunohistochemical characterization of malignant peripheral nerve sheath tumors. Surg Pathol 1994, **4**: 121–135.

770 King R, Busam K, Rosai J. Metastatic malignant melanoma resembling malignant peripheral nerve sheath tumor: report of 16 cases. Am J Surg Pathol 1999, **23**: 1499–1505.

771 Krausz T, Azzopardi JG, Pearse E. Malignant melanoma of the sympathetic chain. With a consideration of pigmented nerve sheath tumours. Histopathology 1984, **8**: 881–894.

772 Laskin WB, Weiss SW, Bratthauer GL. Epithelioid variant of malignant peripheral nerve sheath tumor (malignant epithelioid schwannoma). Am J Surg Pathol 1991, **15**: 1136–1145.

773 Lattes R. Peripheral neuroepithelioma. Proceedings of the 39th Annual Anatomic Pathology Slide Seminar of the American Society of Clinical Pathologists. Chicago, 1975, American Society of Clinical Pathology, pp. 49–52.

774 Legius E, Dierick H, Wu R, Hall BK, Marynen P, Cassiman JJ, Glover TW. TP53 mutations are frequent in malignant NF1 tumors. Genes Chromosomes Cancer 1994, **10**: 250–255.

775 Legius E, Marchuk DA, Collins FS, Glover TW. Somatic deletion of the neurofibromatosis type 1 gene in a neurofibrosarcoma supports a tumour suppressor gene hypothesis. Nat Genet 1993, **3**: 122–126.

776 Mackay B, Luna MA, Butler JJ. Adult neuroblastoma. Electron microscopic observations in nine cases. Cancer 1976, **37**: 1334–1351.

777 Matsunou H, Shimoda T, Kakimoto S, Yamashita H, Ishikawa E, Mukai M. Histopathologic and immunohistochemical study of malignant tumors of peripheral nerve sheath (malignant schwannoma). Cancer 1985, **56**: 2269–2279.

778 McMenamin ME, Fletcher CD. Expanding the spectrum of malignant change in schwannomas: epithelioid malignant change, epithelioid malignant peripheral nerve sheath tumor, and epithelioid angiosarcoma: a study of 17 cases. Am J Surg Pathol 2000, **25**: 13–25.

779 Meis JM, Enzinger FM, Martz KL, Neal JA. Malignant peripheral nerve sheath tumors (malignant schwannomas) in children. Am J Surg Pathol 1992, **16**: 694–707.

780 Meis-Kindblom JM, Enzinger FM. Plexiform malignant peripheral nerve sheath tumor of infancy and childhood. Am J Surg Pathol 1994, **18**: 479–485.

781 Menon AG, Anderson KM, Riccardi VM, Chung RY, Whaley JM, Yandell DW, Farmer GE, Freiman RN, Lee JK, Li FP, et al. Chromosome 17p deletions and p53 gene mutations associated with the formation of malignant neurofibrosarcomas in von Recklinghausen neurofibromatosis. Proc Natl Acad Sci USA 1990, **87**: 5435–5439.

782 Mertens F, Rydholm A, Bauer HF, Limon J, Nedoszytko B, Szadowska A, Willén H, Heim S, Mitelman F, Mandahl N. Cytogenetic findings in malignant peripheral nerve sheath tumors. Int J Cancer 1995, **61**: 793–798.

783 Mertens F, Dal Cin P, De Wever I, Fletcher CD, Mandahl N, Mitelman F, Rosai J, Rydholm A, Sciot R, Tallini G, van Den Berghe H, Vanni R, Willén H. Cytogenetic characterization of peripheral nerve sheath tumours: a report of the CHAMP study group. J Pathol 2000, **190**: 31–38.

784 Millstein DI, Tang C-K, Campbell EW Jr. Angiosarcoma developing in a patient with neurofibromatosis (von Recklinghausen's disease). Cancer 1981, **47**: 950–954.

785 Morphopoulos GD, Banrjee SS, Ali HH, Stewart M, Vasudev KS, Eyden BTP, Harris M. Malignant peripheral nerve sheath tumour with vascular differentiation: a report of four cases. Histopathology 1997, **28**: 401–410.

786 Newbould MJ, Wilkinson N, Mene A. Post-radiation malignant peripheral nerve sheath tumour. A report of two cases. Histopathology 1990, **17**: 263–265.

787 Nonaka D, Chiriboga L, Rubin BP. Sox10: a pan-schwannian and melanocytic marker. Am J Surg Pathol 2008, **32**: 1291–1298.

788 Perrone F, Tabano S, Colombo F, Dagrada G, Birindelli S, Gronchi A, Colecchia M, Pierotti MA, Pilotti S. p15INK4b, p14ARF, and p16INK4a inactivation in sporadic and neurofibromatosis type 1-related malignant peripheral nerve sheath tumors. Clin Cancer Res 2003, **9**: 4132–4138.

789 Raney B, Schnaufer L, Ziegler M, Chatten J, Littman P, Jarrett P. Treatment of children with neurogenic sarcoma. Experience at the Children's Hospital of Philadelphia, 1958–1984. Cancer 1987, **59**: 1–5.

790 Rasbridge SA, Browse NL, Tighe JR, Fletcher CD. Malignant nerve sheath tumour arising in a benign ancient schwannoma. Histopathology 1989, **14**: 525–528.

791 Rekhi B, Jambhekar NA, Puri A, Agrawal M, Chinoy RF. Clinicomorphologic features of a series of 10 cases of malignant triton tumors diagnosed over 10 years at a tertiary cancer hospital in Mumbai, India. Ann Diagn Pathol 2008, **12**: 90–97.

792 Ricci A Jr, Parham DM, Woodruff JM, Callihan T, Green A, Erlandson RA. Malignant peripheral nerve sheath tumors arising from ganglioneuromas. Am J Surg Pathol 1984, **8**: 19–29.

793 Robson DK, Ironside JW. Malignant peripheral nerve sheath tumour arising in a schwannoma. Histopathology 1990, **16**: 295–297.

794 Rose DS, Wilkins MJ, Birch R, Evans DJ. Malignant peripheral nerve sheath tumour with rhabdomyoblastic and glandular differentiation. Immunohistochemical features. Histopathology 1992, **21**: 287–290.

795 Scheithauer BW, Erdogan S, Rodriguez FJ, Burger PC, Woodruff JM, Kros JM, Gokden M, Spinner RJ. Malignant peripheral nerve sheath tumors of cranial nerves and intracranial contents: a clinicopathologic study of 17 cases. Am J Surg Pathol 2009, **33**: 325–338.

796 Shimada S, Tsuzuki T, Kuroda M, Nagasaka T, Hara K, Takahashi E, Hayakawa S, Ono K, Maeda N, Mori N, Illei PB. Nestin expression as a new marker in malignant peripheral nerve sheath tumors. Pathol Int 2007, **57**: 60–67.

797 Shimizu S, Teraki Y, Ishiko A, Shimizu H, Harada T, Mukai M, Nishikawa T. Malignant epithelioid schwannoma of the skin showing partial HMB-45 positivity. Am J Dermatopathol 1993, **15**: 378–384.

798 Skuse GR, Kosciolek BA, Rowley PT. Molecular genetic analysis of tumors in von Recklinghausen neurofibromatosis: loss of heterozygosity for chromosome 17. Genes Chromosomes Cancer 1989, **1**: 36–41.

799 Storlazzi CT, Brekke HR, Mandahl N, Brosjö O, Smeland S, Lothe RA, Mertens F. Identification of a novel amplicon at distal 17q containing the BIRC5/SURVIVIN gene in malignant peripheral nerve sheath tumours. J Pathol 2006, **209**: 492–500.

800 Storm FK, Eilber FR, Mirra J, Morton DL. Neurofibrosarcoma. Cancer 1980, **45**: 126–129.

801 Suster S, Amazon K, Rosen LB, Ollague JM. Malignant epithelioid schwannoma of the skin. A low-grade neurotropic malignant melanoma? Am J Dermatopathol 1989, **11**: 338–344.

802 Suster D, Plaza JA, Shen R. Low-grade malignant perineurioma (perineurial sarcoma) of soft tissue: a potential diagnostic pitfall on fine needle aspiration. Ann Diagn Pathol 2005, **9**: 197–201.

803 Taxy JB, Battifora H, Trujillo Y, Dorfman HD. Electron microscopy in the diagnosis of malignant schwannoma. Cancer 1981, **48**: 1381–1391.

804 Thomas JE, Piepgras DG, Scheithauer B, Onofrio BM, Shives TC. Neurogenic tumors of the sciatic nerve. Mayo Clin Proc 1983, **58**: 640–647.

805 Trojanowski JQ, Kleinman GM, Proppe KH. Malignant tumors of nerve sheath origin. Cancer 1980, **46**: 1202–1212.

806 Tsuneyoshi M, Enjoji M. Primary malignant peripheral nerve tumors (malignant schwannomas). A clinicopathologic and electron microscopic study. Acta Pathol Jpn 1979, **29**: 363–375.

807 Uri AK, Witzelben CL, Raney RB. Electron microscopy of glandular schwannoma. Cancer 1984, **53**: 493–497.

808 Wanebo JE, Malik JM, Vanden Berg SR, Wanebo HJ, Driesen N, Persing JA. Malignant peripheral nerve sheath tumors. A clinicopathologic study of 28 cases. Cancer 1993, **71**: 1247–1253.

809 Weiss SW, Langloss JM, Enzinger FM. Value of S-100 protein in the diagnosis of soft tissue tumors with particular reference to benign and malignant Schwann cell tumors. Lab Invest 1983, **49**: 299–308.

810 White HR Jr. Survival in malignant schwannoma. An 18-year study. Cancer 1971, **27**: 720–729.

811 Wick MR, Swanson PE, Scheithauer BW, Manivel JC. Malignant peripheral nerve sheath tumor. An immunohistochemical study of 62 cases. Am J Clin Pathol 1987, **87**: 425–433.

812 Woodruff JM. Peripheral nerve tumors showing glandular differentiation (glandular schwannomas). Cancer 1976, **37**: 2399–2413.

813 Woodruff JM, Chevnik NL, Smith MC, Millett WB, Foote FW. Peripheral nerve tumors with rhabdomyosarcomatous differentiation (malignant 'triton' tumors). Cancer 1973, **32**: 426–439.

814 Woodruff JM, Christensen WN. Glandular peripheral nerve sheath tumors. Cancer 1993, **72**: 3618–3628.

815 Woodruff JM, Selig AM, Crowley K, Allen PW. Schwannoma (neurilemoma) with malignant transformation. A rare, distinctive peripheral nerve tumor. Am J Surg Pathol 1994, **18**: 882–895.

816 Woodruff JM, Scheithauer BW, Kurtkaya-Yapicier Ö, Raffel C, Amr SS, LaQuaglia MP, Antonescu CR. Congenital and childhood plexiform (multinodular) cellular schwannoma. A troublesome mimic of malignant peripheral nerve sheath tumor. Am J Surg Pathol 2003, **27**: 1321–1329.

817 Zhou H, Coffin CM, Perkins SL, Tripp SR, Liew M, Viskochil DH. Malignant peripheral nerve sheath tumor. A comparison of grade, immunophenotype, and cell cycle/growth. Activation marker expression in sporadic and neurofibromatosis 1-related lesions. Am J Surg Pathol 2003, **27**: 1337–1345.

Other tumors of peripheral nerves

818 Bisceglia M, Vigilante E, Ben-Dor D. Neural lipofibromatous hamartoma: a report of two cases and review of the literature. Adv Anat Pathol 2007, **14**: 46–52.

819 Eusebi V, Bondi A, Cancellieri A, Canedi L, Frizzera G. Primary malignant lymphoma of sciatic nerve. Report of a case. Am J Surg Pathol 1990, **14**: 881–885.

820 Misdraji J, Ino Y, Louis DN, Rosenberg AE, Chiocca EA, Harris NL. Primary lymphoma of peripheral nerve: report of four cases. Am J Surg Pathol 2000, **24**: 1257–1265.

821 Radi MJ, Foucar E, Palmer CH, Gooding RA. Malignant lymphoma arising in a large congenital neurofibroma of the head and neck. Report of a case. Cancer 1988, **61**: 1667–1673.

822 Silverman TA, Enzinger FM. Fibrolipomatous hamartoma of nerve: a clinicopathologic analysis of 26 cases. Am J Surg Pathol 1985, **9**: 7–14.

823 Vigna PA, Kusior MF, Collins MB, Ross JS. Peripheral nerve hemangioma. Potential for clinical aggressiveness. Arch Pathol Lab Med 1994, **118**: 1038–1041.

TUMORS OF ADIPOSE TISSUE

Lipoma

824 Azzopardi JG, Iocco J, Salm R. Pleomorphic lipoma. A tumour simulating liposarcoma. Histopathology 1983, **7**: 511–523.

825 Bartuma H, Hallor KH, Panagopoulos I, Collin A, Rydholm A, Gustafson P, Bauer HC, Brosjö O, Domanski HA, Mandahl N, Mertens F. Assessment of the clinical and molecular impact of different cytogenetic subgroups in a series of 272 lipomas with abnormal karyotype. Genes Chromosomes Cancer 2007, **46**: 594–606.

826 Billings SD, Folpe AL. Diagnostically challenging spindle cell lipomas: a report of 34 'low-fat' and 'fat-free' variants. Am J Dermatopathol 2007, **29**: 437–442.

827 Bolen JW, Thorning D. Spindle cell lipoma. A clinical, light- and electron-microscopic study. Am J Surg Pathol 1981, **5**: 435–441.

828 Cates JM, Coffing BN, Harris BT, Black CC. Calretinin expression in tumors of adipose tissue. Hum Pathol 2006, **37**: 312–321.

829 Dal Cin P, Sciot R, Polito P, Stas M, de Wever I, Cornelis A, Van den Berghe H. Lesions of 13q may occur independently of deletion of 16q in spindle cell/pleomorphic lipomas. Histopathology 1997, **31**: 222–225.

830 Dixon AY, McGregor DH, Lee SH. Angiolipomas. An ultrastructural and clinicopathological study. Hum Pathol 1981, **12**: 739–747.

831 Enzi G. Multiple symmetric lipomatosis. An updated clinical report. Medicine (Baltimore) 1984, **63**: 56–64.

832 Enzinger FM. Benign lipomatous tumors simulating a sarcoma. In M.D. Anderson Tumor Institute. Management of primary bone and soft tissue tumors. Chicago, 1977, Year Book Medical Publishers, pp. 11–24.

833 Enzinger FM, Harvey DA. Spindle cell lipoma. Cancer 1975, **36**: 1852–1859.

834 Fletcher CD, Akerman M, Dal Cin P, De Wever I, Mandahl N, Mertens F, Mitelman F, Rosai J, Rydholm A, Sciot R, Tallini G, Van Der Berghe H, Van de Ven W, Vanni R, Willén H. Correlation between clinicopathologic features and karyotype in lipomatous tumors. A report of 178 cases from the Chromosomes and Morphology (CHAMP) Collaborative Study Group. Am J Pathol 1996, **148**: 623–630.

835 Fletcher CD, Martin-Bates E. Intramuscular and intermuscular lipoma: neglected diagnoses. Histopathology 1988, **12**: 275–287.

836 Fletcher CD, Akerman M, Dal Cin P, De Wever I, Mandahl N, Mertens F, Mitelman F, Rosai J, Rydholm A, Sciot R, Tallini G, Van den Berghe H, Van de Ven W, Vanni R, Willen H. Correlation between clinicopathologic features and karyotype in lipomatous tumors. A report of 178 cases from the Chromosomes and Morphology (CHAMP) Collaborative Study Group. Am J Pathol 1996, **148**: 623–630.

837 Fletcher CDM, Martin-Bates E. Spindle cell lipoma. A clinicopathological study with some original observations. Histopathology 1987, **11**: 803–817.

838 Greenberg SD, Isensee C, Gonzalez-Angulo A, Wallace SA. Infiltrating lipomas of the thigh. Am J Clin Pathol 1963, **39**: 66–72.

839 Hawley IC, Krausz T, Evans DJ, Fletcher CD. Spindle cell lipoma – a pseudoangiomatous variant. Histopathology 1994, **24**: 565–569.

840 Heim S, Mandahl N, Rydholm A, Willén H, Mitelman F. Different karyotypic features characterize different clinico-pathologic subgroups of benign lipogenic tumors. Int J Cancer 1988, **42**: 863–867.

841 Howard WR, Helwig EB. Angiolipoma. Arch Dermatol 1960, **82**: 924–931.

842 Hunt SJ, Santa Cruz DJ, Barr RJ. Cellular angiolipoma. Am J Surg Pathol 1990, **14**: 75–81.

843 Katzer B. Histopathology of rare chondroosteoblastic metaplasias in benign lipomas. Pathol Res Pract 1989, **184**: 437–445.

844 Kin YH, Reiner L. Ultrastructure of lipoma. Cancer 1982, **50**: 102–106.

845 Kindblom L-G, Angervall L, Stener B, Wickbom I. Intermuscular and intramuscular lipomas and hibernomas. A clinical, roentgenologic, histologic, and prognostic study of 46 cases. Cancer 1974, **33**: 754–762.

846 Kindblom L-G, Meis-Kindblom JM. Chondroid lipoma. An ultrastructural and immunohistochemical analysis with further observations regarding its differentiation. Hum Pathol 1995, **26**: 706–715.

847 Laskin WB, Fetsch JF, Michal M, Miettinen M. Sclerotic (fibroma-like) lipoma: a distinctive lipoma variant with a predilection for the distal extremities. Am J Dermatopathol 2006, **28**: 308–316.

848 Lovell-Badge R. Developmental genetics. Living with bad architecture. Nature 1995, **376**: 725–726.

849 Mandahl N, Heim S, Arheden K, Rydholm A, Willén H, Mitelman F. Three major cytogenetic subgroups can be identified among chromosomally abnormal solitary lipomas. Hum Genet 1988, **79**: 203–208.

850 Meis JM, Enzinger FM. Myolipoma of soft tissue. Am J Surg Pathol 1991, **15**: 121–125.

851 Meis JM, Enzinger FM. Chondroid lipoma. A unique tumor simulating liposarcoma and myxoid chondrosarcoma. Am J Surg Pathol 1993, **17**: 1103–1112.

852 Paarlberg D, Linscheid RL, Soule EH. Lipomas of the hand. Including a case of lipoblastomatosis in a child. Mayo Clin Proc 1972, **47**: 121–124.

853 Popper H, Knipping G. A histochemical and biochemical study of a liposarcoma with several aspects on the development of fat synthesis. Pathol Res Pract 1981, **171**: 373–380.

854 Robb JA, Jones RA. Spindle cell lipoma in a perianal location. Hum Pathol 1982, **13**: 1052.

855 Rubin BP, Dal Cin P. The genetics of lipomatous tumors. Semin Diagn Pathol 2001, **18**: 286–293.

856 Sachdeva MP, Goldblum JR, Rubin BP, Billings SD. Low-fat and fat-free pleomorphic lipomas: a diagnostic challenge. Am J Dermatopathol 2009, **31**: 423–426.

857 Sandberg AA. Updates on the cytogenetics and molecular genetics of bone and soft tissue tumors: lipoma. Cancer Genet Cytogenet 2004, **150**: 93–115.

858 Schmack I, Patel RM, Folpe AL, Wojno T, Zaldivar RA, Balzer B, Kang SJ, Weiss SW, Grossniklaus HE. Subconjunctival herniated orbital fat: a benign adipocytic lesion that may mimic pleomorphic lipoma and atypical lipomatous tumor. Am J Surg Pathol 2007, **31**: 193–198.

859 Sciot R, Akerman M, Dal Cin P, De Wever I, Fletcher CD, Mandahl N, Mertens F, Mitelman F, Rosai J, Rydholm A, Tallini F, Van den Berghe H, Vanni R, Willén H. Cytogenetic analysis of subcutaneous angiolipoma: further evidence supporting its difference from ordinary pure lipomas: a report of the CHAMP Study Group. Am J Surg Pathol 1997, **21**: 441–444.

860 Shmookler BM, Enzinger FM. Pleomorphic lipoma. A benign tumor simulating liposarcoma. A clinicopathologic analysis of 48 cases. Cancer 1981, **47**: 126–133.

861 Solvonuk PF, Taylor GP, Hancock R, Wood WS, Frohlich J. Correlation of morphologic and biochemical observations in human lipomas. Lab Invest 1984, **51**: 469–474.

862 Tardío JC, Aramburu JA, Santonja C. Desmin expression in spindle cell lipomas: a potential diagnostic pitfall. Virchows Arch 2004, **445**: 354–358.

863 Zamecnik M, Michal M. Angiomatous spindle cell lipoma: report of three cases with immunohistochemical and ultrastructural study and reappraisal of former 'pseudoangiomatous' variant. Pathol Int 2007, **57**: 26–31.

Lipoblastoma/lipoblastomatosis

864 Bolen JW, Thorning D. Benign lipoblastoma and myxoid liposarcoma. A comparative light- and electron-microscopic study. Am J Surg Pathol 1980, **4**: 163–174.

865 Chung EB, Enzinger FM. Benign lipoblastomatosis. An analysis of 35 cases. Cancer 1973, **32**: 482–492.

866 Coffin CM. Lipoblastoma. An embryonal tumor of soft tissue related to organogenesis. Semin Diagn Pathol 1994, **11**: 98–103.

866a Coffin CM, Lowichik A, Putnam A. Lipoblastoma (LPB): a clinicopathologic and immunohistochemical analysis of 59 cases. Am J Surg Pathol 2009, **33**: 1705–1712.

867 Collins MH, Chatten J. Lipoblastoma/lipoblastomatosis: a clinicopathologic study of 25 tumors. Am J Surg Pathol 1997, **21**: 1131–1137.

868 de Saint Aubain Somerhausen N, Coindre JM, Debiec-Rychter M, Delplace J, Sciot R. Lipoblastoma in adolescents and young adults: report of six cases with FISH analysis. Histopathology 2008, **52**: 294–298.

869 Fletcher CD, Akerman M, Dal Cin P, De Wever I, Mandahl N, Mertens F, Mitelman F, Rosai J, Rydholm A, Sciot R, Tallini G, Van Der Berghe H, Van de Ven W, Vanni R, Willén H. Correlation between clinicopathologic features and karyotype in lipomatous tumors. A report of 178 cases from the Chromosomes and Morphology (CHAMP) Collaborative Study Group. Am J Pathol 1996, **148**: 623–630.

870 Gisselsson D, Hibbard MK, Dal Cin P, Sciot R, Hsi BL, Kozakewich HP, Fletcher JA. PLAG1 alterations in lipoblastoma: involvement in varied mesenchymal cell types and evidence for alternative oncogenic mechanisms. Am J Pathol 2001, **159**: 955–962.

871 Greco AMA, Garcia RL, Vuletin JC. Benign lipoblastomatosis. Ultrastructure and histogenesis. Cancer 1980, **45**: 511–515.

872 Hibbard MK, Kozakewich HP, Dal Cin P, Sciot R, Tan X, Xiao S, Fletcher JA. PLAG1 fusion oncogenes in lipoblastoma. Cancer Res 2000, **60**: 4869–4872.

873 Mentzel T, Calonje E, Fletcher CD. Lipoblastoma and lipoblastomatosis. A clinicopathological study of 14 cases. Histopathology 1993, **23**: 527–533.

874 Rosai J, Akerman M, Dal Cin P, DeWever I, Fletcher CDM, Mandahl M, Mertens F, Mitelman F, Rydholm A, Sciot R, Tallini G, Van Den Berghe H, Van DeVen W, Vanni R, Willén H. Combined morphologic and karyotypic study of 59 atypical lipomatous tumors: evaluation of their relationship and differential diagnosis with other adipose tissue tumors. Am J Surg Pathol 1996, **20**: 1182–1189.

875 Rubin BP, Dal Cin P. The genetics of lipomatous tumors. Semin Diagn Pathol 2001, **18**: 286–293.

876 Vellios F, Baez MF, Schumacher HB. Lipoblastomatosis. A tumor of fetal fat different from hibernoma. Am J Pathol 1958, **34**: 1149–1155.

Hibernoma

877 Allegra SR, Gmuer C, O'Leary GP Jr. Endocrine activity in a large hibernoma. Hum Pathol 1983, **14**: 1044–1052.

878 Chirieac LR, Dekmezian RH, Ayala AG. Characterization of the myxoid variant of hibernoma. Ann Diagn Pathol 2006, **10**: 104–106.

879 Fletcher CD, Akerman M, Dal Cin P, De Wever I, Mandahl N, Mertens F, Mitelman F, Rosai J, Rydholm A, Sciot R, Tallini G, Van Der Berghe H, Van de Ven W, Vanni R, Willén H. Correlation between clinicopathologic features and karyotype in lipomatous tumors. A report of 178 cases from the Chromosomes and Morphology (CHAMP) Collaborative Study Group. Am J Pathol 1996, **148**: 623–630.

880 Furlong MA, Fanburg-Smith JC, Miettinen M. The morphologic spectrum of hibernoma: a clinicopathologic study of 170 cases. Am J Surg Pathol 2001, **25**: 809–814.

881 Gaffney EF, Hargreaves HK, Semple E, Vellios F. Hibernoma. Distinctive light and electron microscopic features and relationship to brown adipose tissue. Hum Pathol 1983, **14**: 677–687.

882 Levine GD. Hibernoma. An electron microscopic study. Hum Pathol 1972, **3**: 351–359.

883 Ross SR, Choy L, Graves RA, Fox N, Solevjeva V, Klaus S, Ricquier D, Spiegelman BM. Hibernoma formation in transgenic mice and isolation of a brown adipocyte cell line expressing the uncoupling protein gene. Proc Natl Acad Sci USA 1992, **89**: 7561–7565.

884 Rubin BP, Dal Cin P. The genetics of lipomatous tumors. Semin Diagn Pathol 2001, **18**: 286–293.

885 Seemayer TA, Knaack J, Wang N, Ahmed MN. On the ultrastructure of hibernoma. Cancer 1975, **36**: 1785–1793.

Liposarcoma (including atypical lipomatous tumor)

886 Ackerman LV. Multiple primary liposarcomas. Am J Pathol 1944, **20**: 789–798.

887 Adachi T, Oda Y, Sakamoto A, Saito T, Tamiya S, Masuda K, Tsuneyoshi M. Immunoreactivity of p53, mdm2, and p21[WAF1] in dedifferentiated liposarcoma: special emphasis on the distinct immunophenotype of the well-differentiated component. Int J Surg Pathol 2001, **9**: 99–109.

888 Ahmed I. Post-injection involutional lipoatrophy: ultrastructural evidence for an activated macrophage phenotype and macrophage related involution of adipocytes. Am J Dermatopathol 2006, **28**: 334–337.

889 Alaggio R, Coffin CM, Weiss SW, Bridge JA, Issakov J, Oliveira AM, Folpe AL. Liposarcomas in young patients: a study of 82 cases occurring in patients younger than 22 years of age. Am J Surg Pathol 2009, **33**: 645–658.

890 Aman P, Ron D, Mandahl N, Fioretos T, Heim S, Arheden K, Willén H, Rydholm A, Mitelman F. Rearrangement of the transcription factor gene CHOP in myxoid liposarcomas with t(12;16)(q13;p11). Genes Chromosom Cancer 1992, **5**: 278–285.

891 Antonescu CR, Elahi A, Humphrey M, Lui MY, Healey JH, Brennan MF, Woodruff JM, Jhanwar SC, Ladanyi M. Specificity of TLS-CHOP rearrangement for classic myxoid/round cell liposarcoma: absence in predominantly myxoid well-differentiated liposarcomas. J Mol Diagn 2001, **2**: 132–138.

892 Argani P, Facchetti F, Inghirami G, Rosai J. Lymphocyte-rich well-differentiated liposarcoma: report of nine cases. Am J Surg Pathol 1997, **21**: 884–895.

893 Azumi N, Curtis J, Kempson RL, Hendrickson MR. Atypical and malignant neoplasms showing lipomatous differentiation. A study of 111 cases. Am J Surg Pathol 1987, **11**: 161–183.

894 Barbashina V, Singer S, Antonescu CR. Dedifferentiated liposarcoma of the extremities [abstract]. Mod Pathol 2003, **16**: 9A.

895 Battifora H, Núñez-Alonso C. Myxoid liposarcoma. Study of ten cases. Ultrastruct Pathol 1980, **1**: 157–169.

896 Bayer-Garner I, Morgan M, Smoller BR. Caveolin expression is common among benign and malignant smooth muscle and adipocyte neoplasms. Mod Pathol 2002, **15**: 1–5.

897 Binh MB, Sastre-Garau X, Guillou L, de Pinieux G, Terrier P, Lagacé R, Aurias A, Hostein I, Coindre JM. MDM2 and CDK4 immunostainings are useful adjuncts in diagnosing well-differentiated and dedifferentiated liposarcoma subtypes: a comparative analysis of 559 soft tissue neoplasms with genetic data. Am J Surg Pathol 2005, **29**: 1340–1347.

898 Binh MB, Guillou L, Hostein I, Château MC, Collin F, Aurias A, Binh BN, Stoeckle E, Coindre JM. Dedifferentiated liposarcomas with divergent myosarcomatous differentiation developed in the internal trunk: a study of 27 cases and comparison to conventional dedifferentiated liposarcomas and leiomyosarcomas. Am J Surg Pathol 2007, **31**: 1557–1566.

899 Bogusz AM, Hussey SM, Kapur P, et al. Massive localized lymphedema with unusual presentations: report of two cases and review of the literature. Int J Surg Pathol 2008, Jul 8. [Epub ahead of print]

900 Bolen JW, Thorning D. Liposarcomas. A histogenetic approach to the classification of adipose tissue neoplasms. Am J Surg Pathol 1984, **8**: 3–17.

901 Brimo F, Dion D, Huwait H, Turcotte R, Nahal A. The utility of MDM2 and CDK4 immunohistochemistry in needle biopsy interpretation of lipomatous tumours: a study of 21 Tru-Cut biopsy cases.Histopathology 2008, **52**: 889–904.

902 Brooks JJ, Connor AM. Atypical lipoma of the extremities and peripheral soft tissues with dedifferentiation. Implications for management. Surg Pathol 1990, **3**: 169–178.

903 Castleberry RP, Kelly DR, Wilson ER, Cain WS, Salter MR. Childhood liposarcoma. Report of a case and review of the literature. Cancer 1984, **54**: 579–584.

904 Chang HR, Hajdu SI, Collin C, Brennan MF. The prognostic value of histologic subtypes in primary extremity liposarcoma. Cancer 1989, **64**: 1514–1520.

905 Chung EB. Pitfalls in diagnosing benign soft tissue tumors in infancy and childhood. Pathol Annu 1985, **20**(Pt 2): 323–386.

906 Cocchia D, Lauriola L, Stolfi VM, Tallini G, Michetti F. S-100 antigen labels neoplastic cells in liposarcoma and cartilaginous tumours. Virchows Arch [A] 1983, **402**: 139–145.

907 Coindre JM, Pelmus M, Chibon F, Mariani O, Hostein I, Aurias A. Immunohistochemistry for Mdm2 and cdk4 in soft tissue sarcomas: analysis of a series of 322 cases and comparison to comparative genomic hybridization analysis [abstract]. Mod Pathol 2003, **16**: 10A.

908 Crozat A, Aman P, Mandahl N, Ron D. Fusion of CHOP to a novel RNA-binding protein in human myxoid liposarcoma. Nature 1993, **363**: 640–644.

909 Dahl PR, Zalla MJ, Winkelmann RK. Localized involutional lipoatrophy: a clinicopathologic study of 16 patients. J Am Acad Dermatol 1996, 35: 523–528.

910 de Vreeze RS, de Jong D, Tielen IH, Ruijter HJ, Nederlof PM, Haas RL, van Coevorden F. Primary retroperitoneal myxoid/round cell liposarcoma is a nonexisting disease: an immunohistochemical and molecular biological analysis. Mod Pathol 2009, **22**: 223–231.

911 Downes KA, Goldblum JR, Montgomery EA, Fisher C. Pleomorphic liposarcoma: a clinicopathologic analysis of 19 cases. Mod Pathol 2001, **14**: 179–184.

912 Endo H, Hirokawa M, Ishimaru N, Tanaka Y, Yamashita M, Sakaki M, Hayashi Y, Sano T. Unique cell membrane expression of topoisomerase-II alpha as a useful diagnostic marker of liposarcoma. Pathol Int 2004, **54**: 145–150.

913 Engström K, Willén H, Kåbjörn-Gustafsson C, Andersson C, Olsson M, Göransson M, Järnum S, Olofsson A, Warnhammar E, Aman P. The myxoid/round cell liposarcoma fusion oncogene FUS-DDIT3 and the normal DDIT3 induce a liposarcoma phenotype in transfected human fibrosarcoma cells. Am J Pathol 2006, **168**: 1642–1653.

914 Enterline HT, Culberson JD, Rochlin DB, Brady LW. Liposarcoma. A clinical and pathological study of 53 cases. Cancer 1960, **13**: 932–950.

915 Enzinger FM, Winslow DJ. Liposarcoma. A study of 103 cases. Virchows Arch [A] 1962, **335**: 367–388.

916 Evans HL. Liposarcoma. A study of 55 cases with a reassessment of its classification. Am J Surg Pathol 1979, **3**: 507–523.

917 Evans HL. Liposarcomas and atypical lipomatous tumors. A study of 66 cases followed for a minimum of 10 years. Surg Pathol 1988, **1**: 41–54.

918 Evans HL. Smooth muscle in atypical lipomatous tumors. A report of three cases. Am J Surg Pathol 1990, **14**: 714–718.

919 Evans HL, Khurana KK, Kemp BL, Ayala AG. Heterologous elements in the dedifferentiated component of dedifferentiated liposarcoma. Am J Surg Pathol 1994, **18**: 1150–1157.

920 Evans HL, Soule EH, Winkelmann RK. Atypical lipoma, atypical intramuscular lipoma, and well-differentiated retroperitoneal liposarcoma. A reappraisal of 30 cases formerly classified as well differentiated liposarcoma. Cancer 1979, **43**: 574–584.

921 Evans HL. Atypical lipomatous tumor, its variants, and its combined forms: a study of 61 cases, with a minimum follow-up of 10 years. Am J Surg Pathol 2007, **31**: 1–14.

922 Fanburg-Smith JC, Miettinen M. Liposarcoma with meningothelial-like whorls: a study of 17 cases of a distinctive histological pattern associated with dedifferentiated liposarcoma. Histopathology 1999, **33**: 414–424.

923 Farshid G, Weiss SW. Massive localized lymphedema in the morbidly obese: a histologically distinct reactive lesion simulating liposarcoma. Am J Surg Pathol 1998, **22**: 1277–1283.

924 Fletcher CDM, Akerman M, Dal Cin P, De Wever I, Mandahl N, Mertens F, Mitelman F, Rosai J, Rydholm A, Sciot R, Tallini G, Van den Berghe H, Van de Ven W, Vanni R, Willén H. Correlation between clinicopathologic features and karyotype in lipomatous tumors. A report of 178 cases from the Chromosomes and Morphology (CHAMP) Collaborative Study Group. Am J Pathol 1996, **148**: 623–630.

925 Folpe AL, Weiss SW. Lipoleiomyosarcoma (well-differentiated liposarcoma with leiomyosarcomatous differentiation): a clinicopathologic study of nine cases including one with dedifferentiation. Am J Surg Pathol 2002, **26**: 742–749.

926 Gebhard S, Coindre JM, Michels JM, Terrier P, Bertrand F, Trassard M, Taylor S, Château MC, Marquès B, Picot V, Guillou L. Pleomorphic liposarcoma: clinicopathologic, immunohistochemical, and follow-up analysis of 63 cases: a study from the French Federation of Cancer Centers Sarcoma Group. Am J Surg Pathol 2002, **26**: 601–616.

927 Georgiades DE, Alcalais CB, Karabela VG. Multicentric well-differentiated liposarcomas. A case report and a brief review of the literature. Cancer 1969, **24**: 1091–1097.

928 Gibas Z, Miettinen M, Limon J, Nedoszytko B, Mrozek K, Roszkiewicz A, Rys J, Niezabitowski A, Debiec-Rychter M. Cytogenetic and immunohistochemical profile of myxoid liposarcoma. Am J Clin Pathol 1995, **103**: 20–26.

929 Goldblum JR, Frank TS, Poy EL, Weiss SW. p53 mutations and tumor progression in well-differentiated liposarcoma and dermatofibrosarcoma protuberans. Int J Surg Pathol 1995, **3**: 35–42.

930 Hashimoto H, Daimaru Y, Enjoji M. S-100 protein distribution in liposarcoma. An immunoperoxidase study with special reference to the distinction of liposarcoma from myxoid malignant fibrous histiocytoma. Virchows Arch [A] 1984, **405**: 1–10.

931 Hashimoto H, Daimaru Y, Tsuneyoshi M, Enjoji M. Soft tissue sarcoma with additional anaplastic components. A clinicopathologic and immunohistochemical study of 27 cases. Cancer 1990, **66**: 1578–1589.

932 Hashimoto H, Enjoji M. Liposarcoma. A clinicopathologic subtyping of 52 cases. Acta Pathol Jpn 1990, **32**: 933–948.

933 He M, Das K, Blacksin M, Benevenia J, Hameed M. A translocation involving the placental growth factor gene is identified in an epithelioid hemangioendothelioma. Cancer Genet Cytogenet 2006, **168**: 150–154.

934 Henricks WH, Chu YC, Goldblum JR, Weiss SW. Dedifferentiated liposarcoma: a clinicopathological analysis of 155 cases with a proposal for an expanded definition of dedifferentiation. Am J Surg Pathol 1997, **21**: 271–281.

935 Hornick JL, Bosenberg MW, Mentzel T, McMenamin ME, Oliveira AM, Fletcher CD. Pleomorphic liposarcoma: clinicopathologic analysis of 57 cases. Am J Surg Pathol 2004, **28**: 1257–1267.

936 Horvai AE, Schaefer JT, Nakakura EK, O'Donnell RJ. Immunostaining for peroxisome proliferator gamma distinguishes dedifferentiated liposarcoma from other retroperitoneal sarcomas. Mod Pathol 2008, **21**: 517–524.

937 Horvai AE, DeVries S, Roy R, O'Donnell RJ, Waldman F. Similarity in genetic alterations between paired well-differentiated and dedifferentiated components of dedifferentiated liposarcoma. Mod Pathol 2009, **22**: 1477–1488.

938 Huang HY, Antonescu CR. Epithelioid variant of pleomorphic liposarcoma: a comparative immunohistochemical and ultrastructural analysis of six cases with emphasis on overlapping features with epithelial malignancies. Ultrastruct Pathol 2002, **26**: 299–308.

939 Kauffman SL, Stout AP. Lipoblastic tumors of children. Cancer 1959, **12**: 912–923.

940 Kilpatrick SE, Doyon J, Choong PF, Sim FH, Nascimento AG. The clinicopathologic spectrum of myxoid and round cell liposarcoma: a study of 95 cases. Cancer 1996, **77**: 1450–1458.

941 Kindblom L-G, Angervall L, Fassina AS. Atypical lipoma. Acta Pathol Microbiol Immunol Scand (A) 1982, **90**: 27–36.

942 Kindblom L-G, Säve-Söderbergh J. The ultrastructure of liposarcoma. A study of 10 cases. Acta Pathol Microbiol Scand (A) 1979, **87**: 109–121.

943 Kraus MD, Guillou L, Fletcher CD. Well-differentiated inflammatory liposarcoma: an uncommon and easily overlooked variant of a common sarcoma. Am J Surg Pathol 1997, **21**: 518–527.

944 Lagacé R, Jacob S, Seemayer TA. Myxoid liposarcoma. An electron microscopic study. Biological and histogenetic considerations. Virchows Arch [A] 1979, **384**: 159–172.

945 La Quaglia MP, Spiro SA, Ghavimi F, Hajdu SI, Meyers P, Exelby PR. Liposarcoma in patients younger than or equal to 22 years of age. Cancer 1993, **72**: 3114–3119.

946 Lucas DR, Nascimento AG, Sanjay BK, Rock MG. Well-differentiated liposarcoma. The Mayo Clinic experience with 58 cases. Am J Clin Pathol 1994, **102**: 677–683.

947 Manduch M, Oliveira AM, Nascimento AG, Folpe AL. Massive localized lymphedema: a clinicopathological study of 21 cases of still poorly recognized pseudosarcoma occurring in morbidly obese patients. Lab Invest 2009, **89**(Suppl 1): 18A.

948 Mariño-Enríquez A, Fletcher CD, Dal Cin P, Hornick JL. Dedifferentiated liposarcoma with 'homologous' lipoblastic (pleomorphic liposarcoma-like) differentiation: clinicopathologic and molecular analysis of a series suggesting revised diagnostic criteria. Am J Surg Pathol 2010, **34**: 1122–1131.

949 Matushansky I, Hernando E, Socci ND, Matos T, Mills J, Edgar MA, Schwartz GK, Singer S, Cordon-Cardo C, Maki RG. A developmental model of sarcomagenesis defines a differentiation-based classification for liposarcomas. Am J Pathol 2008, **172**: 1069–1080.

950 McCormick D, Mentzel T, Beham A, Fletcher CD. Dedifferentiated liposarcoma. Clinicopathologic analysis of 32 cases suggesting a better prognostic subgroup among pleomorphic sarcomas. Am J Surg Pathol 1994, **18**: 1213–1223.

951 Mentzel T, Fletcher CD. Dedifferentiated myxoid liposarcoma: a clinicopathological study suggesting a closer relationship between myxoid and well-differentiated liposarcoma. Histopathology 1997, **30**: 457–463.

952 Mentzel T, Palmedo G, Hantschke M, Woziwodzki J, Beck C. Mixed-type liposarcoma: clinicopathological, immunohistochemical, and molecular analysis of a case arising in deep soft tissues of the lower extremity. Virchows Arch 2008, **453**: 197–201.

953 Miettinen M, Enzinger FM. Epithelioid variant of pleomorphic liposarcoma: a study of 12 cases of a distinctive variant of high-grade liposarcoma. Mod Pathol 1999, **12**: 722–728.

954 Nascimento AG, Kurtin PJ, Guillou L, Fletcher CD. Dedifferentiated liposarcoma: a report of nine cases with a peculiar neuralike whorling pattern associated with metaplastic bone formation. Am J Surg Pathol 1998, **22**: 945–955.

955 Nicolas M, Moran CA, Suster S. Pulmonary metastasis from liposarcoma: a clinicopathologic and immunohistochemical study of 24 cases. Am J Clin Pathol 2005, **123**: 265–275.

956 Oikawa K, Ishida T, Imamura T, Yoshida K, Takanashi M, Hattori H, Ishikawa A, Fujita K, Yamamoto K, Matsubayashi J, Kuroda M, Mukai K. Generation of the novel monoclonal antibody against TLS/EWS-CHOP chimeric oncoproteins that is applicable to one of the most sensitive assays for myxoid and round cell liposarcomas. Am J Surg Pathol 2006, **30**: 351–356.

957 Oliveira AM, Nascimento AG. Pleomorphic liposarcoma. Semin Diagn Pathol 2001, **18**: 274–285.

958 Oliveira AM, Nascimento AG, Lloyd RV. Leptin and leptin receptor mRNA are widely expressed in tumors of adipocytic differentiation. Mod Pathol 2001, **14**: 549–555.

959 Panagopoulos I, Hoglund M, Mertens F, Mandahl N, Mitelman F, Aman P. Fusion of the EWS and CHOP genes in myxoid liposarcoma. Oncogene 1996, **12**: 489–494.

960 Panoussopoulos D, Theodoropoulos G, Lazaris AC, Papadimitriou K. Focal divergent chondrosarcomatous differentiation in a primary pleomorphic liposarcoma and expression of transforming growth factor β. Report of a case and review of the literature. Int J Surg Pathol 2004, **12**: 79–85.

961 Pytel P, Taxy JB, Krausz T. Divergent differentiation in malignant soft tissue neoplasms: the paradigm of liposarcoma and malignant peripheral nerve sheath tumor. Int J Surg Pathol 2005, **13**: 19–28.

962 Rieker RJ, Weitz J, Lehner B, Egerer G, Mueller A, Kasper B, Schirmacher P, Joos S, Mechtersheimer G. Genomic profiling reveals subsets of dedifferentiated liposarcoma to follow separate molecular pathways. Virchows Arch 2010, **456**: 277–285.

963 Reitan JB, Kaalhus O, Brennhovd IO, Sager EM, Stenwig AE, Talle K. Prognostic factors in liposarcoma. Cancer 1985, **55**: 2482–2490.

964 Reszel PA, Soule EH, Coventry MB. Liposarcoma of extremities and limb girdles. Study of 222 cases. J Bone Joint Surg (Am) 1966, **48**: 229–244.

965 Rosai J, Akerman M, Dal Cin P, DeWever I, Fletcher CDM, Mandahl M, Mertens F, Mitelman F, Rydholm A, Sciot R, Tallini G, Van Den Berghe H, Van DeVen W, Vanni R, Willén H. Combined morphologic and karyotypic study of 59 atypical lipomatous tumors: evaluation of their relationship and differential diagnosis with other adipose tissue tumors. Am J Surg Pathol 1996, **20**: 1182–1189.

966 Rossouw DJ, Cinti S, Dickersin GR. Liposarcoma. An ultrastructural study of 15 cases. Am J Clin Pathol 1986, **85**: 649–667.

967 Schmack I, Patel RM, Folpe AL, Wojno T, Zaldivar RA, Balzer B, Kang SJ, Weiss SW, Grossniklaus HE. Subconjunctival herniated orbital fat: a benign adipocytic lesion that may mimic pleomorphic lipoma and atypical lipomatous tumor. Am J Surg Pathol 2007, **31**: 193–198.

968 Schmookler BM, Enzinger FM. Liposarcoma occurring in children. An analysis of 17 cases and review of the literature. Cancer 1983, **52**: 567–574.

969 Siebert JD, Williams RP, Pulitzer DR. Myxoid liposarcoma with cartilaginous differentiation. Mod Pathol 1996, **9**: 249–252.

970 Sirvent N, Coindre JM, Maire G, Hostein I, Keslair F, Guillou L, Ranchere-Vince D, Terrier P, Pedeutour F. Detection of MDM2-CDK4 amplification by fluorescence in situ hybridization in 200 paraffin-embedded tumor samples: utility in diagnosing adipocytic lesions and comparison with immunohistochemistry and real-time PCR. Am J Surg Pathol 2007, **31**: 1476–1489.

971 Smith TA, Easley KA, Goldblum JR. Myxoid/round cell liposarcoma of the extremities: a clinicopathologic study of 29 cases with particular attention to extent of round cell liposarcoma. Am J Surg Pathol 1996, **20**: 171–180.

972 Snover DC, Sumner HW, Dehner LP. Variability of histologic pattern in recurrent soft tissue sarcomas originally diagnosed as liposarcoma. Cancer 1982, **49**: 1005–1015.

973 Sreekantaiah C, Karakousis CP, Leong SP, Sandberg AA. Cytogenetic findings in liposarcoma correlate with histopathologic subtypes. Cancer 1992, **69**: 2484–2495.

974 Stout AP. Liposarcoma. The malignant tumor of lipoblasts. Ann Surg 1944, **119**: 86–107.

975 Sumathi VP, Grimer RJ, Peake D, Kindblom L-G. Prognostic factors in a single-centre series of 160 cases of myxoid/round cell liposarcomas (MRLS). Lab Invest 2009, **89**(Suppl 1): 22A.

976 Suster S, Morrison C. Sclerosing poorly differentiated liposarcoma: clinicopathological, immunohistochemical and molecular analysis of a distinct morphological subtype of lipomatous tumour of soft tissue. Histopathology 2008, **52**: 283–293.

977 Tallini G, Akerman M, Dal Cin P, De Wever I, Fletcher CD, Mandahl N, Mertens F, Mitelman F, Rosai J, Rydholm A, Sciot R, Van Den Berghe H, Van Den Ven W, Vanni R, Willén H. Combined morphologic and karyotypic study of 28 myxoid liposarcomas: implications for a revised morphologic typing. A report of the CHAMP study group. Am J Surg Pathol 1996, **20**: 1047–1055.

978 Tallini G, Erlandson RA, Brennan MF, Woodruff JM. Divergent myosarcomatous differentiation in retroperitoneal liposarcoma. Am J Surg Pathol 1993, **17**: 546–556.

979 Walaas L, Kindblom L-G. Lipomatous tumors. A correlative cytologic and histologic study of 27 tumors examined by fine needle aspiration cytology. Hum Pathol 1985, **16**: 6–18.

980 Weaver J, Downs-Kelly E, Goldblum JR, Turner S, Kulkarni S, Tubbs RR, Rubin BP, Skacel M. Fluorescence in situ hybridization for MDM2 gene amplification as a diagnostic tool in lipomatous neoplasms. Mod Pathol 2008, **21**: 943–949.

981 Wei YC, Li CF, Eng HL, Yeh MC, Lin CN, Huang HY. Myxoid liposarcoma with cartilaginous differentiation: identification of the same type II TLS-CHOP fusion gene transcript in both lipogenic and chondroid components. Appl Immunohistochem Mol Morphol 2007, **15**: 477–480.

982 Weiss SW, Rao VK. Well-differentiated liposarcoma (atypical lipoma) of deep soft tissue of the extremities, retroperitoneum, and miscellaneous sites. A follow-up study of 92 cases with analysis of the incidence of 'dedifferentiation'. Am J Surg Pathol 1992, **16**: 1051–1058.

983 Winslow DJ, Enzinger FM. Hyaluronidase-sensitive acid mucopolysaccharides in liposarcomas. Am J Pathol 1960, **37**: 497–505.

984 Yoshida A, Ushiku T, Motoi T, Shibata T, Fukayama M, Tsuda H. Well-differentiated liposarcoma with low-grade osteosarcomatous component: an underrecognized variant. Am J Surg Pathol 2010, **34**: 1361–1366.

TUMORS AND TUMORLIKE CONDITIONS OF BLOOD AND LYMPH VESSELS

Hemangioma

985 Adegboyega PA, Qiu S. Hemangioma versus vascular malformation: presence of nerve bundle is a diagnostic clue for vascular malformation. Arch Pathol Lab Med 2005, **129**: 772–775.

986 Albrecht S, Kahn HJ. Immunohistochemistry of intravascular papillary endothelial hyperplasia. J Cutan Pathol 1990, **17**: 16–21.

987 Allen PW, Enzinger FM. Hemangioma of skeletal muscle. An analysis of 89 cases. Cancer 1972, **29**: 8–22.

988 Beham A, Fletcher CD. Intramuscular angioma. A clinicopathological analysis of 74 cases. Histopathology 1991, **18**: 53–59.

989 Calonje E, Fletcher CD. Sinusoidal hemangioma. A distinctive benign vascular neoplasm within the group of cavernous hemangiomas. Am J Surg Pathol 1991, **15**: 1130–1135.

990 Calonje E, Mentzel T, Fletcher CD. Pseudomalignant perineurial invasion in cellular ('infantile') capillary haemangiomas. Histopathology 1995, **26**: 159–164.

991 Clearkin KP, Enzinger FM. Intravascular papillary endothelial hyperplasia. Arch Pathol Lab Med 1976, **100**: 441–444.

992 Coffin CM, Dehner LP. Vascular tumors in children and adolescents. A clinicopathologic study of 228 tumors in 222 patients. Pathol Annu 1993, **28**(Pt 1): 97–120.

993 Dabashi Y, Eisen RN. Infantile hemangioendothelioma of the pelvis associated with Kasabach–Merritt syndrome. Pediatr Pathol 1990, **10**: 407–415.

994 Dadras SS, North PE, Bertoncini J, Mihm MC, Detmar M. Infantile hemangiomas are arrested in an early developmental vascular differentiation state. Mod Pathol 2004, **17**: 1068–1079.

995 Debelenko LV, Perez-Atayde AR, Mulliken JB, Liang MG, Archibald TH, Kozakewich HP. D2-40 immunohistochemical analysis of pediatric vascular tumors reveals positivity in kaposiform hemangioendothelioma. Mod Pathol 2005, **18**: 1454–1460.

996 Dethlefsen SM, Mulliken JB, Glowacki J. An ultrastructural study of mast cell interactions in hemangiomas. Ultrastruct Pathol 1986, **10**: 175–183.

997 Deyrup AT, Tretiakova M, Khramtsov A, Montag AG. Estrogen receptor beta expression in vascular neoplasia: an analysis of 53 benign and malignant cases. Mod Pathol 2004, **17**: 1372–1377.

998 Fanburg JC, Meis-Kindblom JM, Rosenberg AE. Multiple enchondromas associated with spindle cell hemangioendotheliomas. An overlooked variant of Maffucci's syndrome. Am J Surg Pathol 1995, **19**: 1029–1038.

999 Finn MC, Glowacki J, Mulliken JB. Congenital vascular lesions. Clinical application of a new classification. J Pediatr Surg 1983, **18**: 894–900.

1000 Fletcher CD, Beham A, Schmid C. Spindle cell haemangioendothelioma. A clinicopathological and immunohistochemical study indicative of a non-neoplastic lesion. Histopathology 1991, **18**: 291–301.

1001 Fukunaga M, Ushigome S, Ishikawa E. Kaposiform haemangioendothelioma associated with Kasabach–Merritt syndrome. Histopathology 1997, **28**: 281–284.

1002 Fukunaga M, Ushigome S, Nikaido T, Ishikawa E, Nakamori K. Spindle cell hemangioendothelioma. An immunohistochemical and flow cytometric study of six cases. Pathol Int 1995, **45**: 589–595.

1003 Gonzalez-Crussi F, Reyes-Mugica M. Cellular hemangiomas ('hemangioendotheliomas') in infants. Light microscopic, immunohistochemical, and ultrastructural observations. Am J Surg Pathol 1991, **15**: 769–778.

1004 Gratzinger D, Zhao S, West R, Rouse RV, Vogel H, Gil EC, Levy R, Lossos IS, Natkunam Y. The transcription factor LMO2 is a robust marker of vascular endothelium and vascular neoplasms and selected other entities. Am J Clin Pathol 2009, **131**: 264–278.

1005 Guillou L, Calonje E, Speight P, Rosai J, Fletcher CD. Hobnail hemangioma: a pseudomalignant vascular lesion with a reappraisal of targetoid hemosiderotic hemangioma. Am J Surg Pathol 1999, **23**: 97–105.

1006 Hashimoto H, Daimaru Y, Enjoji M. Intravascular papillary endothelial hyperplasia. A clinicopathologic study of 91 cases. Am J Dermatopathol 1983, **5**: 539–546.

1007 Imayama S, Murakamai Y, Hashimoto H, Hori Y. Spindle cell hemangioendothelioma exhibits the ultrastructural features of reactive vascular proliferation rather than of angiosarcoma. Am J Clin Pathol 1992, **97**: 279–287.

1008 Koblenzer PJ, Bukowski MJ. Angiomatosis (hamartomatous hem-lymphangiomatosis). Report of a case with diffuse involvement. Pediatrics 1961, **28**: 65–76.

1009 Kojimahara M, Baba Y, Nakajima T. Ultrastructural study of hemangiomas. Acta Pathol Jpn 1987, **37**: 605–609.

1010 Koutlas IG, Jessurun J. Arteriovenous hemangioma. A clinicopathological and immunohistochemical study. J Cutan Pathol 1994, **21**: 343–349.

1011 Kuo T-T, Sayers CP, Rosai J. Masson's 'vegetant intravascular hemangioen-dothelioma'. A lesion often mistaken for angiosarcoma. Study of seventeen cases located in the skin and soft tissues. Cancer 1976, **38**: 1227–1236.

1012 Lie JT. Pathology of angiodysplasia in Klippel–Trenaunay syndrome. Pathol Res Pract 1988, **183**: 747–755.

1013 Lindenauer SM. The Klippel–Trenaunay syndrome. Varicosity, hypertrophy and hemangioma with no arteriovenous fistula. Ann Surg 1965, **162**: 303–314.

1014 Lyons LL, North PE, Mac-Moune Lai F, Stoler MH, Folpe AL, Weiss SW. Kaposiform hemangioendothelioma: a study of 33 cases emphasizing its pathologic, immunophenotypic, and biologic uniqueness from juvenile hemangioma. Am J Surg Pathol 2004, **28**: 559–568.

1015 Meijer-Jorna LB, Breugem CC, de Boer OJ, Ploegmakers JP, van der Horst CM, van der Wal AC. Presence of a distinct neural component in congenital vascular malformations relates to the histological type and location of the lesion. Hum Pathol 2009, **40**: 1467–1473.

1016 Mentzel T, Massoleni G, Dei Tos AP, Fletcher CD. Kaposiform hemangioendothelioma in adults. Clinicopathologic and immunohistochemical analysis of three cases. Am J Clin Pathol 1997, **108**: 450–455.

1017 Modlin JJ. Capillary hemangiomas of the skin. Surgery 1955, **38**: 169–180.

1018 Mulliken JB, Young AE. Vascular birthmarks. Hemangiomas and malformations. Philadelphia, 1988, W.B. Saunders.

1019 Nguyen VA, Kutzner H, Fürhapter C, Tzankov A, Sepp N. Infantile hemangioma is a proliferation of LYVE-1-negative blood endothelial cells without lymphatic competence. Mod Pathol 2006, **19**: 291–298.

1020 Palomba A, Beltrami G, Campanacci D, Capanna R, Franchi A. Atypical organizing haematoma/seroma following treatment for soft tissue sarcoma. Histopathology 2009, **54**: 505–507.

1021 Perkins P, Weiss SW. Spindle cell hemangioendothelioma: an analysis of 78 cases with reassessment of its pathogenesis and biologic behavior. Am J Surg Pathol 1996, **20**: 1196–1204.

1022 Perrone T. Vessel-nerve intermingling in benign infantile hemangioendothelioma. Hum Pathol 1985, **16**: 198–200.

1023 Pins MR, Rosenthal DI, Springfield DS, Rosenberg AE. Florid extravascular papillary endothelial hyperplasia (Masson's pseudoangiosarcoma) presenting as a soft-tissue sarcoma. Arch Pathol Lab Med 1993, **117**: 259–263.

1024 Rao VK, Weiss SW. Angiomatosis of soft tissue. An analysis of the histologic features and clinical outcome in 51 cases. Am J Surg Pathol 1992, **16**: 764–771.

1025 Ritter MR, Reinisch J, Friedlander SF, Friedlander M. Myeloid cells in infantile hemangioma. Am J Pathol 2006, **168**: 621–628.

1026 Salyer WR, Salyer DC. Intravascular angiomatosis. Development and distinction from angiosarcoma. Cancer 1975, **36**: 995–1004.

1027 Scott GA, Rosai J. Spindle cell hemangioendothelioma. Report of seven additional cases of a recently described vascular neoplasm. Am J Dermatopathol 1988, **10**: 281–288.

1028 Sheth S, Lai CK, Dry S, Binder S, Fishbein MC. Benign vascular tumors and tumor-like proliferations. Semin Diagn Pathol 2008, **25**: 1–16.

1029 Smoller BR, Apfelberg DB. Infantile (juvenile) capillary hemangioma. A tumor of heterogeneous cellular elements. J Cutan Pathol 1993, **20**: 330–336.

1030 Syed SP, Martin AM, Haupt HM, Arenas-Elliot CP, Brooks JJ. Angiostatin receptor annexin II in vascular tumors including angiosarcoma. Hum Pathol 2007, **38**: 508–513.

1031 Taxy JB, Gray SR. Cellular angiomas of infancy. An ultrastructural study of two cases. Cancer 1979, **43**: 2322–2331.

1032 Tsang WY, Chan JK. Kaposi-like infantile hemangioendothelioma. A distinctive vascular neoplasm of the retroperitoneum. Am J Surg Pathol 1991, **15**: 982–989.

1033 Tsang WY, Chan JK, Fletcher CD. Recently characterized vascular tumours of skin and soft tissues. Histopathology 1991, **19**: 489–501.

1034 Weinblatt ME, Kahn E, Kochen JA. Hemangioendothelioma with intravascular coagulation and ischemic colitis. Cancer 1984, **54**: 2300–2304.

1035 Weiss SW. Pedal hemangioma (venous malformation) occurring in Turner's syndrome. An additional manifestation of the syndrome. Hum Pathol 1988, **19**: 1015–1018.

1036 Weiss SW, Enzinger FM. Spindle cell hemangioendothelioma. A low-grade angiosarcoma resembling a cavernous hemangioma and Kaposi's sarcoma. Am J Surg Pathol 1986, **10**: 521–530.

1037 Yasunga C, Sueishi K, Ohgami H, Suita S, Kawanami T. Heterogenous expression of endothelial cell markers in infantile hemangioendothelioma. Immunohisto-chemical study of two solitary cases and one multiple one. Am J Clin Pathol 1989, **91**: 673–681.

1038 Zukerberg LR, Nickoloff BJ, Weiss SW. Kaposiform hemangioendothelioma of infancy and childhood. An aggressive neoplasm associated with Kasabach–Merritt syndrome and lymphangiomatosis. Am J Surg Pathol 1993, **17**: 321–328.

Glomus tumor

1039 Aiba M, Hirayama A, Kuramochi S. Glomangiosarcoma in a glomus tumor. An immunohistochemical and ultrastructural study. Cancer 1988, **61**: 1467–1471.

1040 Albrecht S, Zbieranowski I. Incidental glomus coccygeum. When a normal structure looks like a tumor. Am J Surg Pathol 1990, **14**: 922–924.

1041 Bell RS, Goodman SB, Fornasier VL. Coccygeal glomus tumors. A case of mistaken identity? J Bone Joint Surg (Am) 1982, **64**: 595–597.

1042 Calonje E, Fletcher CDM. Cutaneous intraneural glomus tumor. Am J Dermatopathol 1995, **17**: 395–398.

1043 Carroll RE, Berman AT. Glomus tumors of the hand. Review of the literature and report of 28 cases. J Bone Joint Surg (Am) 1972, **54**: 691–703.

1044 Dervan PA, Tobbia IN, Casey M, O'Loughlin J, O'Brien M. Glomus tumours. An immunohistochemical profile of 11 cases. Histopathology 1989, **14**: 483–491.

1045 Di Sant'Agnese PA, De Mesy Jensen KL. Thick (myosin) filaments in a glomus tumor. Am J Clin Pathol 1983, **79**: 130–134.

1046 Duncan L, Halverson J, De Schryver-Kecskemeti K. Glomus tumor of the coccyx. A curable cause of coccygodynia. Arch Pathol Lab Med 1991, **115**: 78–80.

1047 Folpe AL, Fanburg-Smith JC, Miettinen M, Weiss SW. Atypical and malignant glomus tumor: analysis of 52 cases, with a proposal for the reclassification of glomus tumor. Am J Surg Pathol 2000, **25**: 1–12.

1048 Gould EW, Manivel JC, Albores-Saavedra J, Monforte H. Locally infiltrative glomus tumors and glomangiosarcomas. A clinical, ultrastructural, and immunohistochemical study. Cancer 1990, **65**: 310–318.

1049 Ito H, Motohiro K, Nomura S, Tahara E. Glomus tumor of the trachea. Immunohistochemical and electron microscopic studies. Pathol Res Pract 1988, **183**: 778–784.

1050 Kaye VM, Dehner LP. Cutaneous glomus tumor. A comparative immunohistochemical study with pseudoangiomatous intradermal melanocytic nevi. Am J Dermatopathol 1991, **13**: 2–6.

1051 Khoury T, Balos L, McGrath B, Wong MK, Cheney RT, Tan D. Malignant glomus tumor: a case report and review of literature, focusing on its clinicopathologic features and immunohistochemical profile. Am J Dermatopathol 2005, **27**: 428–431.

1052 Kishimoto S, Nagatani H, Miyashita A, Kobayashi K. Immunohistochemical demonstration of substance P-containing nerve fibers in glomus tumors. Br J Dermatol 1985, **113**: 213–218.

1053 Kohout E, Stout AR. The glomus tumor in children. Cancer 1961, **14**: 555–556.

1054 Lattes R, Bull DC. A case of glomus tumor with primary involvement of bone. Ann Surg 1948, **127**: 187–191.

1055 Masson P. Le glomus neuromyo-artérial des régions tactiles et ses tumeurs. Lyon Chir 1924, **21**: 259–280.

1056 Miettinen M, Lehto V-P, Virtanen I. Glomus tumor cells. Evaluation of smooth muscle and endothelial cell properties. Virchows Arch [Cell Pathol] 1983, **43**: 139–149.

1057 Murray MR, Stout AP. The glomus tumor. Investigations of its distribution and behavior, and the identity of its 'epithelioid' cell. Am J Pathol 1942, **18**: 183–203.

1058 Noer H, Krogdahl A. Glomangiosarcoma of the lower extremity. Histopathology 1991, **18**: 365–366.

1059 Nuovo MA, Grimes MM, Knowles DM. Glomus tumors. A clinicopathologic and immunohistochemical analysis of forty cases. Surg Pathol 1990, **3**: 31–46.

1060 Pambakian H, Smith MA. Glomus tumours of the coccygeal body associated with coccydynia. A preliminary report. J Bone Joint Surg (Br) 1981, **633**: 424–426.

1061 Pulitzer DR, Martin PC, Reed RJ. Epithelioid glomus tumor. Hum Pathol 1995, **26**: 1022–1027.

1062 Slater DN, Cotton DWK, Azzopardi JG. Oncocytic glomus tumour. A new variant. Histopathology 1987, **11**: 523–531.

1063 Stout AP. Tumors of the neuromyoarterial glomus. Am J Cancer 1935, **24**: 255–272.

1064 Tsuneyoshi M, Enjoji M. Glomus tumor. A clinicopathologic and electron microscopic study. Cancer 1982, **50**: 1601–1607.

1065 Venkatachalam MA, Greally JG. Fine structure of glomus tumor. Similarity of glomus cells to smooth muscle. Cancer 1969, **23**: 1176–1184.

Hemangiopericytoma

1066 D'Amore ES, Manivel JC, Sung JH. Soft-tissue and meningeal hemangiopericytomas. An immunohistochemical and ultrastructural study. Hum Pathol 1990, **21**: 414–423.

1067 Fletcher CDM. Haemangiopericytoma – a dying breed? Reappraisal of an 'entity' and its variants. A hypothesis. Curr Diagn Pathol 1994, **1**: 19–23.

1068 Folpe AL, Weiss SW. Hemangiopericytomas and solitary fibrous tumors of soft tissue: a study of 69 cases [abstract]. Mod Pathol 2003, **16**: 12A.

1069 Gengler C, Guillou L. Solitary fibrous tumour and haemangiopericytoma: evolution of a concept. Histopathology 2006, **48**: 63–74.

1070 Granter SR, Badizadegan K, Fletcher CD. Myofibromatosis in adults, glomangiopericytoma, and myopericytoma: a spectrum of tumors showing perivascular myoid differentiation. Am J Surg Pathol 1998, **22**: 513–525.

1071 Kuhn C III, Rosai J. Tumors arising from pericytes. Ultrastructure and organ culture of a case. Arch Pathol 1969, **88**: 653–663.

1072 Lau PP, Wong OK, Lui PC, Cheung OY, Ho LC, Wong WC, To KF, Chan JK. Myopericytoma in patients with AIDS: a new class of Epstein–Barr virus-associated tumor. Am J Surg Pathol 2009, **33**: 1666–1672.

1073 McMenamin ME, Fletcher CD. Malignant myopericytoma: expanding the spectrum of tumours with myopericytic differentiation. Histopathology 2002, **41**: 450–460.

1074 Mentzel T, Dei Tos AP, Sapi Z, Kutzner H. Myopericytoma of skin and soft tissues: clinicopathologic and immunohistochemical study of 54 cases. Am J Surg Pathol 2006, **30**: 104–113.

1075 Nielsen GP, Dickersin GR, Provenzal JM, Rosenberg AE. Lipomatous hemangiopericytoma. A histologic, ultrastructural and immunohistochemical study of a unique variant of hemangiopericytoma. Am J Surg Pathol 1995, **19**: 748–756.

1076 Stout AP. Hemangiopericytoma (a study of 25 new cases). Cancer 1949, **2**: 1027–1054.

1077 Stout AP. Tumors featuring pericytes. Glomus tumor and hemangiopericytoma. Lab Invest 1965, **5**: 217–223.

1078 Tsuneyoshi M, Daimaru Y, Enjoji M. Malignant hemangiopericytoma and other sarcomas with hemangiopericytoma-like pattern. Pathol Res Pract 1984, **178**: 446–453.

Hemangioendothelioma

1079 Allen PW, Ramakrishna B, MacCormac LB. The histiocytoid hemangiomas and other controversies. Pathol Annu 1992, **27**(Pt 2): 51–87.

1080 Angervall L, Kindblom L-G, Karlsson K, Stener B. Atypical hemangioendothelioma of venous origin. A clinicopathologic, angiographic, immunohistochemical, and ultrastructural study of two endothelial tumors within the concept of histiocytoid hemangioma. Am J Surg Pathol 1985, **9**: 504–516.

1081 Billings SD, Folpe AL, Weiss SW. Epithelioid sarcoma-like hemangioendothelioma. Am J Surg Pathol 2002, **27**: 48–57.

1082 Cooper PH. Is histiocytoid hemangioma a specific pathologic entity? Am J Surg Pathol 1988, **12**: 815–817.

1083 Dabska M. Malignant endovascular papillary angioendothelioma of the skin in childhood. Clinicopathologic study of six cases. Cancer 1969, **24**: 503–510.

1084 Deyrup AT, Tighiouart M, Montag AG, Weiss SW. Epithelioid hemangioendothelioma of soft tissue: a proposal for risk stratification based on 49 cases. Am J Surg Pathol 2008, **32**: 924–927.

1085 Ellis GL, Kratochvil FJ III. Epithelioid hemangioendothelioma of the head and neck. A clinicopathologic report of twelve cases. Oral Surg Oral Med Oral Pathol 1986, **61**: 61–68.

1086 Fanburg-Smith JC, Michal M, Partanen TA, Alitalo K, Miettinen M. Papillary intralymphatic angioendothelioma (PILA): a report of twelve cases of a distinctive vascular tumor with phenotypic features of lymphatic vessels. Am J Surg Pathol 1999, **23**: 1004–1010.

1087 Fetsch JF, Weiss SW. Observations concerning the pathogenesis of epithelioid hemangioma (angiolymphoid hyperplasia). Mod Pathol 1991, **4**: 449–455.

1088 Fukunaga M, Suzuki K, Saegusa N, Folpe AL. Composite hemangioendothelioma: report of 5 cases including one with associated Maffucci syndrome. Am J Surg Pathol 2007, **31**: 1567–1572.

1089 Fukunaga M, Ushigome S, Shishikura Y, Yokoi K, Ishikawa E. Endovascular papillary angioendothelioma-like tumour associated with lymphoedema. Histopathology 1995, **27**: 243–249.

1090 Gray MH, Rosenberg AE, Dickersin GR, Bhan AK. Cytokeratin expression in epithelioid vascular neoplasms. Hum Pathol 1990, **21**: 212–217.

1091 He M, Das K, Blacksin M, Benevenia J, Hameed M. A translocation involving the placental growth factor gene is identified in an epithelioid hemangioendothelioma. Cancer Genet Cytogenet 2006, **168**: 150–154.

1092 Mendlick MR, Nelson M, Pickering D, Johansson SL, Seemayer TA, Neff JR, Vergara G, Rosenthal H, Bridge JA. Translocation t(1;3)(p36.3;q25) is a nonrandom aberration in epithelioid hemangioendothelioma. Am J Surg Pathol 2001, **25**: 684–687.

1093 Mentzel T, Beham A, Calonje E, Katenkamp D, Fletcher CD. Epithelioid hemangioendothelioma of skin and soft tissues: clinicopathologic and immunohistochemical study of 30 cases. Am J Surg Pathol 1997, **21**: 363–374.

1094 Morgan J, Robinson MJ, Rosen LB, Unger H, Niven J. Malignant endovascular papillary angioendothelioma (Dabska tumor). A case report and review of the literature. Am J Dermatopathol 1989, **11**: 64–68.

1095 Nayler SJ, Rubin BP, Calonje E, Chan JK. Composite hemangioendothelioma: a complex, low grade vascular lesion mimicking angiosarcoma. Am J Surg Pathol 2000, **24**: 352–361.

1096 Patterson K, Chandra RS. Malignant endovascular papillary angioendothelioma. Cutaneous borderline tumor. Arch Pathol Lab Med 1985, **109**: 671–673.

1097 Rosai J, Gold J, Landy R. The histiocytoid hemangiomas. A unifying concept embracing several previously described entities of skin, soft tissue, large vessels, bone and heart. Hum Pathol 1979, **10**: 707–730.

1098 Tsang WY, Chan JK. The family of epithelioid vascular tumors. Histopathology 1993, **8**: 187–212.

1099 Tsarouha H, Kyriazoglou AI, Ribeiro FR, Teixeira MR, Agnantis N, Pandis N. Chromosome analysis and molecular cytogenetic investigations of an epithelioid hemangioendothelioma. Cancer Genet Cytogenet 2006, **169**: 164–168.

1100 Urabe A, Tsuneyoshi M, Enjoji M. Epithelioid hemangioma versus Kimura's disease. A comparative clinicopathologic study. Am J Surg Pathol 1987, **11**: 758–766.

1101 Weiss SW, Enzinger FM. Epithelioid hemangioendothelioma. A vascular tumor often mistaken for a carcinoma. Cancer 1982, **50**: 970–981.

1102 Weiss SW, Ishak KG, Dail DH, Sweet DE, Enzinger FM. Epithelioid hemangioendothelioma and related lesions. Semin Diagn Pathol 1986, **3**: 259–287.

1103 Williams SB, Butler BC, Gilkey FW, Kapadia SB, Burton DM. Epithelioid hemangioendothelioma with osteoclastlike giant cells. Arch Pathol Lab Med 1993, **117**: 315–318.

1104 Yousem SA, Hochholzer L. Unusual thoracic manifestations of epithelioid hemangioendothelioma. Arch Pathol Lab Med 1987, **111**: 459–463.

Angiosarcoma

1105 Abratt RP, Williams M, Dodd NF, Uys CJ. Angiosarcoma of the superior vena cava. Cancer 1983, **52**: 740–743.

1106 Al-Abbadi MA, Almasri NM, Al-Quran S, Wilkinson EJ. Cytokeratin and epithelial membrane antigen expression in angiosarcomas: an immunohistochemical study of 33 cases. Arch Pathol Lab Med 2007, **131**: 288–292.

1107 Baker PB, Goodwin RA. Pulmonary artery sarcomas. A review and report of a case. Arch Pathol Lab Med 1985, **109**: 35–39.

1108 Burke AP, Virmani R. Sarcomas of the great vessels. A clinicopathologic study. Cancer 1993, **71**: 1761–1773.

1109 Byers RJ, McMahon RF, Freemont AJ, Parrott NR, Newstead CG. Epithelioid angiosarcoma arising in an arteriovenous fistula. Histopathology 1992, **21**: 87–89.

1110 Chaudhuri B, Ronan SG, Manaligod JR. Angiosarcoma arising in a plexiform neurofibroma. A case report. Cancer 1980, **46**: 605–610.

1111 Davies JD, Rees GJG, Mera SL. Angiosarcoma in irradiated post-mastectomy chest wall. Histopathology 1983, **7**: 947–956.

1112 Deyrup AT, Miettinen M, North PE, Khoury JD, Tighiouart M, Spunt SL, Parham D, Weiss SW, Shehata BM. Angiosarcomas arising in the viscera and soft tissue of children and young adults: a clinicopathologic study of 15 cases. Am J Surg Pathol 2009, **33**: 264–269.

1113 Fitzmaurice RJ, McClure J. Aortic intimal sarcoma. An unusual case with pulmonary vasculature involvement. Histopathology 1990, **17**: 457–462.

1114 Fletcher CD, Beham A, Bekir S, Clarke AM, Marley NJ. Epithelioid angiosarcoma of deep soft tissue. A distinctive tumor readily mistaken for an epithelial neoplasm. Am J Surg Pathol 1991, **15**: 915–924.

1115 Girard C, Johnson WC, Graham JH. Cutaneous angiosarcoma. Cancer 1970, **26**: 868–883.

1116 Hayman J, Huygens H. Angiosarcoma developing around a foreign body. J Clin Pathol 1986, **36**: 515–518.

1117 Hottenrott G, Mentzel T, Peters A, Schrader A, Katenkamp D. Intravascular ('intimal') epithelioid angiosarcoma: clinicopathological and immunohistochemical analysis of three cases. Virchows Arch 2000, **435**: 473–478.

1118 Jennings TA, Peterson L, Friedlaender GE, Cooke RA, Axiotis A, Hayman JA, Rosai J. Angiosarcoma associated with foreign bodies. Report of three cases. Cancer 1988, **62**: 2436–2444.

1119 Mackay B, Ordóñez NG, Huang WL. Ultrastructural and immunocytochemical observations on angiosarcomas. Ultrastruct Pathol 1989, **13**: 97–110.

1120 Maddox JC, Evans HL. Angiosarcoma of skin and soft tissue. A study of 44 cases. Cancer 1981, **48**: 1907–1921.

1121 McGlennen RC, Manivel JC, Stanley SJ, Slater DL, Wick MR, Dehner LP. Pulmonary artery trunk sarcoma. A clinicopathologic, ultrastructural, and immunohistochemical study of four cases. Mod Pathol 1989, **2**: 486–494.

1122 McWilliam LJ, Harris M. Granular cell angiosarcoma of the skin. Histology, electron microscopy and immunohistochemistry of a newly recognized tumor. Histopathology 1985, **9**: 1205–1216.

1123 Meis-Kindblom JM, Kindblom LG. Angiosarcoma of soft tissue: a study of 80 cases. Am J Surg Pathol 1998, **22**: 683–697.

1124 Millstein DI, Tang C-K, Campbell EW Jr. Angiosarcoma developing in a patient with neurofibromatosis (von Recklinghausen's disease). Cancer 1981, **47**: 950–954.

1125 Nanus DM, Kelsen D, Clark DGC. Radiation-induced angiosarcoma. Cancer 1987, **60**: 777–779.

1126 Rao P, Lahat G, Dukah A, Halevi H, Xiao L, Changye Z, Smith KD, Pollock RE, Lev D, Lazar AJF. Angiosarcoma: clinical, pathological, and molecular predictors of disease-specific survival in 222 patients. Lab Invest 2009, **89**(Suppl 1): 20A.

1127 Rosai J, Sumner HW, Kostianovsky M, Perez-Mesa C. Angiosarcoma of the skin. A clinicopathologic and fine structural study. Hum Pathol 1976, **7**: 83–109.

1128 Rossi S, Fletcher CD. Angiosarcoma arising in hemangioma/vascular malformation: report of four cases and review of the literature. Am J Surg Pathol 2002, **26**: 1319–1329.

1129 Stout AP. Hemangio-endothelioma. A tumor of blood vessels featuring vascular endothelial cells. Ann Surg 1943, **118**: 445–464.

1130 Ulbright TM, Clark SA, Einhorn LH. Angiosarcoma associated with germ cell tumors. Hum Pathol 1985, **16**: 268–272.

1131 Vuletin JC, Wajsbort RR, Ghali V. Primary retroperitoneal angiosarcoma with eosinophilic globules. A combined light-microscopic, immunohistochemical, and ultrastructural study. Arch Pathol Lab Med 1990, **114**: 618–622.

1132 Wehrli BM, Janzen DL, Shokeir O, Masri BA, Bryne SK, O'Connel JX. Epithelioid angiosarcoma arising in a surgically constructed arteriovenous fistula: a rare complication of chronic immunosuppression in the setting of renal transplantation. Am J Surg Pathol 1998, **22**: 1154–1159.

1133 Wilson-Jones E. Malignant vascular tumours. Clin Exp Dermatol 1976, **1**: 287–312.

1134 Wright EP, Virmani R, Glick AD, Page DL. Aortic intimal sarcoma with embolic metastases. Am J Surg Pathol 1985, **9**: 890–897.

1135 Zagzag D, Yang G, Seidman I, Lusskin R. Malignant epithelioid hemangioendothelioma arising in an intramuscular lipoma. Cancer 1993, **71**: 764–768.

Lymphangioma and lymphangiomyoma

1136 Banner A, Carrington C, Emory W, Kittle F, Leonard G, Ringus J, Taylor P, Addington W. Efficacy of oophorectomy in lymphangioleiomyomatosis and benign metastasizing leiomyoma. N Engl J Med 1981, **305**: 204–210.

1137 Byrne J, Blanc WA, Warburton D, Wigger J. The significance of cystic hygroma in fetuses. Hum Pathol 1984, **15**: 61–67.

1138 Carlson KC, Parnassus WN, Klatt EC. Thoracic lymphangiomatosis. Arch Pathol Lab Med 1987, **111**: 475–477.

1139 Chan JK, Tsang WY, Pau MY, Tang MC, Pang SW, Fletcher CD. Lymphangiomyomatosis and angiomyolipoma. Closely related entities characterized by hamartomatous proliferation of HMB-45-positive smooth muscle. Histopathology 1993, **22**: 445–455.

1140 Chervenak FA, Isaacson G, Blakemore KJ, Breg WR, Hobbins JC, Berkowitz RL, Tortora M, Mayden K, Mahoney MJ. Fetal cystic hygroma. N Engl J Med 1983, **309**: 822–825.

1141 Cornog JL Jr, Enterline HT. Lymphangiomyoma, a benign lesion of chyliferous lymphatics synonymous with lymphangiopericytoma. Cancer 1966, **19**: 1909–1930.

1142 Dickson BC, Brooks JS, Pasha TL, Zhang PJ. Evaluation of TFE3 expression in tumors of microphthalmia-associated transcription factor (MiTF) family and its potential diagnostic significance. Lab Invest 2009, **89**(Suppl 1): 13A.

1143 Enterline HT, Roberts D. Lymphangiopericytoma. Case report of a previously undescribed tumor type. Cancer 1955, **8**: 582–587.

1144 Folpe AL, McKenney JK, Li Z, Smith SJ, Weiss SW. Clear cell myomelanocytic tumor of the thigh: report of a unique case. Am J Surg Pathol 2002, **26**: 809–812.

1145 Folpe AL, Goodman ZD, Ishak KG, Paulino AF, Taboada EM, Meehan SA, Weiss SW. Clear cell myomelanocytic tumor of the falciform ligament/ligamentum teres: a novel member of the perivascular epithelioid clear cell family of tumors with a predilection for children and young adults. Am J Surg Pathol 2000, **24**: 1239–1246.

1146 Folpe AL, Mentzel T, Lehr HA, Fisher C, Balzer BL, Weiss SW. Perivascular epithelioid cell neoplasms of soft tissue and gynecologic origin: a clinicopathologic study of 26 cases and review of the literature. Am J Surg Pathol 2005, **29**: 1558–1575.

1147 Francis F, Nonaka D. A study of MITF/TFE transcription factors and melanocytic differentiation markers in angiomyolipomas. Lab Invest 2009, **89**(Suppl 1): 13A.

1148 Gomez CS, Calonje E, Ferrar DW, Browse NL, Fletcher CDM. Lymphangiomatosis of the limbs: clinicopathologic analysis of a series with a good prognosis. Am J Surg Pathol 1995, **19**: 125–133.

1149 Graham ML II. Spelsberg TC, Dines DE, Payne WS, Bjornsson J, Lie JT. Pulmonary lymphangiomyomatosis. With particular reference to steroid-receptor assay studies and pathologic correlation. Mayo Clin Proc 1984, **59**: 3–11.

1150 Gross RE, Hurwitt ES. Cervicomediastinal and mediastinal cystic hygromas. Surg Gynecol Obstet 1948, **87**: 599–610.

1151 Guillou L, Fletcher CD. Benign lymphangioendothelioma (acquired progressive lymphangioma): a lesion not to be confused with well-differentiated angiosarcoma and patch stage Kaposi's sarcoma: clinicopathologic analysis of a series. Am J Surg Pathol 2000, **24**: 1047–1057.

1152 Hansen T, Katenkamp K, Bittinger F, Kirkpatrick CJ, Katenkamp D. D2-40 labeling in lymphangiomyoma/ lymphangiomyomatosis of the soft tissue: further evidence of lymphangiogenic tumor histogenesis. Virchows Arch 2007, **450**: 449–453.

1153 Harris GC, McCulloch TA, Perks G, Fisher C. Malignant perivascular epithelioid cell tumour ('PEComa') of soft tissue: a unique case. Am J Surg Pathol 2004, **28**: 1655–1658.

1154 Hornick JL, Fletcher CD. PEComa: what do we know so far? Histopathology 2006, **48**: 75–82.

1155 Jao J, Gilbert S, Messer R. Lymphangiomyoma and tuberous sclerosis. Cancer 1972, **29**: 1188–1192.

1156 Kuo T-T, Gomez LG. Papillary endothelial proliferation in cystic lymphangiomas. Arch Pathol Lab Med 1979, **103**: 306–308.

1157 Magro G, Lanzafame S. Sporadic subcutaneous angiomyolipoma with expression of estrogen and progesterone receptors. Virchows Arch 2007, **450**: 123–125.

1158 McCarty KS Jr, Mossler JA, McLelland R, Sieker HO. Pulmonary lymphangiomyomatosis responsive to progesterone. N Engl J Med 1980, **303**: 1461–1465.

1159 Ohori NP, Yousem SA, Sonmez-Alpan E, Colby TV. Estrogen and progesterone receptors in lymphangioleiomyomatosis, epithelioid hemangioendothelioma, and sclerosing hemangioma of the lung. Am J Clin Pathol 1991, **96**: 529–535.

1160 Ramani P, Shah A. Lymphangiomatosis. Histologic and immunohistochemical analysis of four cases. Am J Surg Pathol 1993, **17**: 329–335.

1161 Taylor JR, Ryu J, Colby TV, Raffin TA. Lymphangioleiomyomatosis. Clinical course in 32 patients. N Engl J Med 1990, **323**: 1254–1260.

1162 Wiegand S, Eivazi B, Barth PJ, von Rautenfeld DB, Folz BJ, Mandic R, Werner JA. Pathogenesis of lymphangiomas. Virchows Arch 2008, **453**: 1–8.

1163 Weinreb I, Howarth D, Latta E, Ghazarian D, Chetty R. Perivascular epithelioid cell neoplasms (PEComas): four malignant cases expanding the histopathological spectrum and a description of a unique finding. Virchows Arch 2007, **450**: 463–470.

1164 Wolff M. Lymphangiomyoma. Clinicopathologic study and ultrastructural confirmation of its histogenesis. Cancer 1973, **31**: 988–1007.

Lymphangiosarcoma and related lesions

1165 Capo V, Ozzello L, Fenoglio CM, Lombardi L, Rilke F. Angiosarcomas arising in edematous extremities. Immunostaining for factor VIII-related antigen and ultrastructural features. Hum Pathol 1985, **16**: 144–150.

1166 Di Tommaso L, Rosai J. The capillary lobule: a deceptively benign feature of post-radiation angiosarcoma of the skin: report of three cases. Am J Dermatopathol 2005, **27**: 301–305.

1167 Drachman D, Rosen L, Sharaf D, Weissmann A. Postmastectomy low-grade angiosarcoma. An unusual case clinically resembling a lymphangioma circumscriptum. Am J Dermatopathol 1988, **10**: 247–251.

1168 Fineberg S, Rosen PP. Cutaneous angiosarcoma and atypical vascular lesions of the skin and breast after radiation therapy for breast carcinoma. Am J Clin Pathol 1995, **102**: 757–763.

1169 Fukunaga M. Expression of D2-40 in lymphatic endothelium of normal tissues and in vascular tumours. Histopathology 2005, **46**: 396–402.

1170 Hashimoto K, Matsumoto M, Eto H, Lipinski J, LaFond AA. Differentiation of metastatic breast carcinoma from Stewart–Treves angiosarcoma. Use of anti-keratin and anti-desmosome monoclonal antibodies and factor VIII-related antibodies. Arch Dermatol 1985, **121**: 742–746.

1171 Herman JB. Lymphangiosarcoma of the chronically edematous extremity. Surg Gynecol Obstet 1965, **121**: 1107–1115.

1172 Lagacé R, Leroy J-P. Comparative electron microscopic study of cutaneous and soft tissue angiosarcomas, post-mastectomy angiosarcoma (Stewart–Treves syndrome) and Kaposi's sarcoma. Ultrastruct Pathol 1987, **11**: 161–173.

1173 Mankey CC, McHugh JB, Thomas DG, Lucas DR. Can lymphangiosarcoma be resurrected? A clinicopathological and immunohistochemical study of lymphatic differentiation in 49 angiosarcomas. Histopathology 2010, **56**: 364–371.

1174 McWilliam LJ, Harris M. Histogenesis of post-mastectomy angiosarcoma. An ultrastructural study. Histopathology 1985, **9**: 331–343.

1175 Miettinen M, Lehto V-P, Virtanen I. Postmastectomy angiosarcoma (Stewart–Treves syndrome). Light-microscopic, immunohistological, and ultrastructural characteristic of two cases. Am J Surg Pathol 1983, **7**: 329–339.

1176 Muller R, Hajdu SI, Brennan MF. Lymphangiosarcoma associated with chronic filarial lymphedema. Cancer 1987, **59**: 179–183.

1177 Rosso R, Gianelli U, Carnevali L. Acquired progressive lymphangioma of the skin following radiotherapy for breast carcinoma. J Cutan Pathol 1995, **22**: 164–167.

1178 Sener SF, Milos S, Feldman JL, Martz CH, Winchester DJ, Dieterich M, Locker GY, Khandekar JD, Brockstein B, Haid M, Michel A. The spectrum of vascular lesions in the mammary skin, including angiosarcoma, after breast conservation treatment for breast cancer. J Am Coll Surg 2001, **193**: 22–28.

1179 Sordillo PP, Chapman R, Hajdu SI, Magill GB, Golbey RB. Lymphangiosarcoma. Cancer 1981, **48**: 1674–1679.

1180 Stewart FW, Treves N. Lymphangiosarcoma in post-mastectomy lymphedema. A report of six cases in elephantiasis chirurgica. Cancer 1948, **1**: 64–81.

1181 Woodward AH, Ivins JC, Soule EH. Lymphangiosarcoma arising in chronic lymphedematous extremities. Cancer 1972, **30**: 562–572.

Hemangioblastoma

1182 Michal M, Vanecek T, Sima R, Mukensnabl P, Boudova L, Brouckova M, Koudepa K. Primary capillary hemangioblastoma of peripheral soft tissues. Am J Surg Pathol 2004, **28**: 962–966.

1183 Nonaka D, Rodriguez J, Rosai J. Extraneural hemangioblastoma: a report of 5 cases. Am J Surg Pathol 2007, **31**: 1545–1551.

1184 Patton KT, Satcher RL Jr, Laskin WB. Capillary hemangioblastoma of soft tissue: report of a case and review of the literature. Hum Pathol 2005, **36**: 1135–1139.

TUMORS OF SMOOTH MUSCLE

Leiomyoma

1185 Billings SD, Folpe AL, Weiss SW. Do leiomyomas of deep soft tissue exist? An analysis of highly differentiated smooth muscle tumors of deep soft tissue supporting two distinct subtypes. Am J Surg Pathol 2001, **25**: 1134–1142.

1186 Carla TG, Filotico R, Filotico M. Bizarre angiomyomas of superficial soft tissues. Pathologica 1991, **83**: 237–242.

1187 Fox SB, Heryet A, Khong TY. Angioleiomyomas. An immunohistological study. Histopathology 1990, **16**: 495–496.

1188 Geddy PM, Gray S, Reid WA. Mast cell density and PGP 9.5-immunostained nerves in angioleiomyoma. Their relationship to painful symptoms. Histopathology 1993, **22**: 387–390.

1189 Hachisuga T, Hashimoto H, Enjoji M. Angioleiomyoma. A clinicopathologic reappraisal of 562 cases. Cancer 1984, **54**: 126–130.

1190 Hasegawa T, Seki K, Yang P, Hirose T, Hizawa K. Mechanism of pain and cytoskeletal properties in angioleiomyomas. An immunohistochemical study. Pathol Int 1994, **44**: 66–72.

1191 Khalluf E, DeYoung BR, Swanson PE. Soft tissue leiomyoma with cartilaginous metaplasia. Report of an unusual phenomenon. Int J Surg Pathol 1994, **1**: 235–238.

1192 Kilpatrick SE, Mentzel T, Fletcher CD. Leiomyoma of deep soft tissue. Clinicopathologic analysis of a series. Am J Surg Pathol 1994, **18**: 576–582.

1193 MacDonald DM, Sanderson KV. Angioleiomyoma of the skin. Br J Dermatol 1974, **91**: 161–168.

1194 Matsuyama A, Hisaoka M, Hashimoto H. Angioleiomyoma: a clinicopathologic and immunohistochemical reappraisal with special reference to the correlation with myopericytoma. Hum Pathol 2007, **38**: 645–651.

1195 Yokoyama R, Hashimoto H, Daimaru Y, Enjoji M. Superficial leiomyomas. A clinicopathologic study of 34 cases. Acta Pathol Jpn 1987, **37**: 1415–1422.

Leiomyosarcoma

1196 Bayer-Garner I, Morgan M, Smoller BR. Caveolin expression is common among benign and malignant smooth muscle and adipocyte neoplasms. Mod Pathol 2002, **15**: 1–5.

1197 Beck AH, Lee CH, Witten DM, Gleason BC, Edris B, Espinosa I, Zhu S, Li R, Montgomery KD, Marinelli RJ, Tibshirani R, Hastie T, Jablons DM, Rubin BP, Fletcher CD, West RB, van de Rijn M. Discovery of molecular subtypes in leiomyosarcoma through integrative molecular profiling. Oncogene 2010, **29**: 845–854.

1198 Berlin O, Stener B, Kindblom L-G, Angervall L. Leiomyosarcomas of venous origin in the extremities. A correlated clinical, roentgenologic, and morphologic study with diagnostic and surgical implications. Cancer 1984, **54**: 2147–2159.

1199 Brown DC, Theaker JM, Banks PM, Gatter KC, Mason DY. Cytokeratin expression in smooth muscle and smooth muscle tumours. Histopathology 1987, **11**: 477–486.

1200 Carneiro A, Francis P, Bendahl PO, Fernebro J, Akerman M, Fletcher C, Rydholm A, Borg A, Nilbert M. Indistinguishable genomic profiles and shared prognostic markers in undifferentiated pleomorphic sarcoma and leiomyosarcoma: different sides of a single coin? Lab Invest 2009, **89**: 668–675.

1201 Chang A, Schuetze SM, Conrad EU 3rd, Swisshelm KL, Norwood TH, Rubin BP. So-called 'inflammatory leiomyosarcoma': a series of 3 cases providing additional insights into a rare entity. Int J Surg Pathol 2005, **13**: 185–195.

1202 Dahl I, Angervall L. Cutaneous and subcutaneous leiomyosarcoma. A clinicopathologic study of 47 patients. Pathol Europ 1974, **9**: 307–315.

1203 Dahl I, Hagmar B, Angervall L. Leiomyosarcoma of the soft tissue. A correlative cytological and histological study of 11 cases. Acta Pathol Microbiol Immunol Scand (A) 1981, **89**: 285–291.

1204 Dei Tos AP, Maestro R, Doglioni C, Piccinin S, Libera DD, Boiocchi M, Fletcher CD. Tumor suppressor genes and related molecules in leiomyosarcoma. Am J Pathol 1996, **148**: 1037–1045.

1205 de Saint Aubain Somerhausen N, Fletcher CD. Leiomyosarcoma of soft tissue in children: clinicopathologic analysis of 20 cases. Am J Surg Pathol 1999, **23**: 755–763.

1206 Deyrup AT, Haydon RC, Huo D, Ishikawa A, Peabody TD, He T-C, Montag AG. Myoid differentiation and prognosis in adult pleomorphic sarcomas of the extremity. An analysis of 92 cases. Cancer 2003, **98**: 805–813.

1207 Deyrup AT, Lee VK, Hill CE, Cheuk W, Toh HC, Kesavan S, Chan EW, Weiss SW. Epstein-Barr virus-associated smooth muscle tumors are distinctive mesenchymal tumors reflecting multiple infection events: a clinicopathologic and molecular analysis of 29 tumors from 19 patients. Am J Surg Pathol 2006, **30**: 75–82.

1208 Donner L, DeLanerolle P, Costa J. Immunoreactivity of paraffin-embedded normal tissues and mesenchymal tumors for smooth muscle myosin. Am J Clin Pathol 1983, **80**: 677–681.

1209 Fields JP, Helwig EB. Leiomyosarcoma of the skin and subcutaneous tissue. Cancer 1981, **47**: 156–169.

1210 Fletcher CD. Pleomorphic malignant fibrous histiocytoma: fact or fiction?: a critical reappraisal based on 159 tumors diagnosed as pleomorphic sarcoma. Am J Surg Pathol 1992, **16**: 213–228.

1211 Goldsmith JD, Pawel B, Goldblum JR, Pasha TL, Roberts S, Nelson P, Khurana JS, Barr FG, Zhang PJ. Detection and diagnostic utilization of placental alkaline phosphatase in muscular tissue and tumors with myogenic differentiation. Am J Surg Pathol 2002, **26**: 1627–1633.

1212 Hashimoto H, Daimaru Y, Tsuneyoshi M, Enjoji M. Leiomyosarcoma of the external soft tissues. A clinicopathologic, immunohistochemical, and electron microscopic study. Cancer 1986, **57**: 2077–2088.

1213 Hilliard NJ, Heslin MJ, Castro CY. Leiomyosarcoma of the inferior vena cava: three case reports and review of the literature. Ann Diagn Pathol 2005, **9**: 259–266.

1214 Hisaoka M, Wei-Qi S, Jian W, Morio T, Hashimoto H. Specific but variable expression of H-caldesmon in leiomyosarcomas: an immunohistochemical reassessment of a novel myogenic marker. Appl Immunohistochem Mol Morphol 2001, **9**: 302–308.

1215 Imakita M, Yutani C, Ishibashi-Ueda H, Hiraoka H, Naito H. Primary leiomyosarcoma of the inferior vena cava with Budd–Chiari syndrome. Acta Pathol Jpn 1989, **39**: 73–77.

1216 Iwata J, Fletcher CD. Immunohistochemical detection of cytokeratin and epithelial membrane antigen in leiomyosarcoma: a systemic study of 100 cases. Pathol Int 2000, **50**: 7–14.

1217 Jensen ML, Jensen OM, Michalski W, Nielsen OS, Keller J. Intradermal and subcutaneous leiomyosarcoma: a clinicopathological and immunohistochemical study of 41 cases. J Cutan Pathol 1997, **23**: 458–463.

1218 Kelley TW, Borden E, Patel R, Prok A, Goldblum JR. Estrogen and progesterone receptor expression in uterine and extra-uterine leiomyosarcomas (LMS): an immunohistochemical study [abstract]. Mod Pathol 2003, **16**: 15A.

1219 Kevoskian J, Cento DP. Leiomyosarcoma of large arteries and veins. Surgery 1973, **73**: 390–400.

1220 Laskin WB, Fanburg-Smith JC, Burke AP, Kraszewska E, Fetsch JF, Miettinen M. Leiomyosarcoma of the inferior vena cava: clinicopathologic study of 40 cases. Am J Surg Pathol 2010, **34**: 873–881.

1221 Lee ES, Locker J, Nalesnik M, Reyes J, Jaffe R, Alashari M, Nour B, Tzakis A, Dickman PS. The association of Epstein–Barr virus with smooth-muscle tumors occurring after organ transplantation. N Engl J Med 1995, **332**: 19–25.

1222 Leu HJ, Makek M. Intramural venous leiomyosarcomas. Cancer 1986, **57**: 1395–1400.

1223 Mackay B, Ro J, Floyd C, Ordóñez NG. Ultrastructural observations on smooth muscle tumors. Ultrastruct Pathol 1987, **11**: 593–607.

1224 Mandhal N, Fletcher CDM, Dal Cin P, deWever I, Mertens F, Mitelman F, Rosai J, Rydholm A, Sciot R, Tallini G, van den Berghe H, Vanni R, Willén H. Comparative cytogenetic study of spindle cell and pleomorphic leiomyosarcomas of soft tissue. A report from the CHAMP study group. Cancer Genet Cytogenet 2000, **116**: 66–73.

1225 McClain KL, Leach CT, Jenson HB, Joshi VV, Pollock BH, Parmley RT, Di Carlo FJ, Chadwick EG, Murphy SB. Association of Epstein–Barr virus with leiomyosarcomas in children with AIDS. N Engl J Med 1995, **332**: 12–18.

1226 Mentzel T, Calonje E, Fletcher CD. Leiomyosarcoma with prominent osteoclastlike giant cells. Analysis of eight cases closely mimicking the so-called giant cell variant of malignant fibrous histiocytoma. Am J Surg Pathol 1994, **18**: 258–265.

1227 Mentzel T, Wadden C, Fletcher CD. Granular cell change in smooth muscle tumours of skin and soft tissue. Histopathology 1994, **24**: 223–231.

1228 Miettinen M, Lehto V-P, Badley RA, Virtanen I. Expression of intermediate filaments in soft-tissue sarcomas. Int J Cancer 1982, **30**: 541–546.

1229 Miyajima K, Oda Y, Tamiya S, Shimizu K, Hachitanda Y, Tsuneyosi M. Cytogenetic and clinicopathological analysis of soft-tissue leiomyosarcomas. Pathol Int 2003, **53**: 163–168.

1230 Montgomery E, Goldblum JR, Fisher C. Leiomyosarcoma of the head and neck: a clinicopathological study. Histopathology 2002, **40**: 518–525.

1231 Nicolas MM, Tamboli P, Gomez JA, Czerniak BA. Pleomorphic and dedifferentiated leiomyosarcoma: clinicopathologic and immunohistochemical study of 41 cases. Hum Pathol 2010, **41**: 663 671.

1232 Nistal M, Paniagua R, Picazo ML, Cermeño deGiles F, Ramos Guerreira JL. Granular changes in vascular leiomyosarcoma. Virchows Arch [A] 1980, **386**: 239–248.

1233 Norton AJ, Thomas JA, Isaacson PG. Cytokeratin-specific monoclonal antibodies are reactive with tumours of smooth muscle derivation. An immunocytochemical and biochemical study using antibodies to intermediate filament cytoskeletal proteins. Histopathology 1987, **11**: 487–499.

1234 Ogawa K, Oguchi M, Yamabe H, Nakashima Y, Hamashima Y. Distribution of collagen type IV in soft tissue tumors. An immunohistochemical study. Cancer 1986, **58**: 269–277.

1235 Oshiro Y, Shiratsuchi H, Oda Y, Toyoshima S, Tsuneyoshi M. Rhabdoid features in leiomyosarcoma of soft tissue: with special reference to aggressive behaviour. Mod Pathol 2001, **13**: 1211–1218.

1236 Phelan JT, Sherer W, Perez-Mesa C. Malignant smooth-muscle tumors (leiomyosarcomas) of soft-tissue origin. N Engl J Med 1962, **266**: 1027–1030.

1237 Ren B, Yu YP, Jing L, Liu L, Michalopoulos GK, Luo J-H, Rao UNM. Gene expression analysis of human soft tissue leiomyosarcomas. Hum Pathol 2003, **34**: 549–558.

1238 Rubin BP, Fletcher CD. Myxoid leiomyosarcoma of soft tissue, an underrecognized variant. Am J Surg Pathol 2000, **24**: 927–936.

1239 Saku T, Tsuda N, Anami M, Okabe H. Smooth and skeletal muscle myosins in spindle cell tumors of soft tissue. An immunohistochemical study. Acta Pathol Jpn 1985, **35**: 125–136.

1240 Salm R, Evans DJ. Myxoid leiomyosarcoma. Histopathology 1985, **9**: 159–169.

1241 Schürch W, Skalli O, Seemayer TA, Gabbiani G. Intermediate filament proteins and actin isoforms as markers for soft tissue tumor differentiation and origin. I. Smooth muscle tumors. Am J Pathol 1987, **128**: 91–103.

1242 Sreekantaiah C, Davis JR, Sandberg AA. Chromosomal abnormalities in leiomyosarcomas. Am J Pathol 1993, **142**: 293–305.

1243 Swanson PE, Wick MR, Dehner LP. Leiomyosarcoma of somatic soft tissues in childhood. An immunohistochemical analysis of six cases with ultrastructural correlation. Hum Pathol 1991, **22**: 569–577.

1244 Tauchi K, Tsutsumi Y, Yoshimura S, Watanabe K. Immunohistochemical and immunoblotting detection of cytokeratin in smooth muscle tumors. Acta Pathol Jpn 1990, **40**: 574–580.

1245 Varela-Duran J, Oliva H, Rosai J. Vascular leiomyosarcoma. The malignant counterpart of vascular leiomyoma. Cancer 1979, **44**: 1684–1691.

1246 Weiss SW, Langloss JM, Shmookler BM, Malawer MM, D'Avis J, Enzinger FM, Stanton R. Estrogen receptor protein in bone and soft tissue tumors. Lab Invest 1986, **54**: 689–694.

1247 Wile AG, Evans HL, Romsdahl MM. Leiomyosarcoma of soft tissue. A clinicopathologic study. Cancer 1981, **48**: 1022–1032.

1248 Wilkinson N, Fitzmaurice RJ, Turner PG, Freemont AJ. Leiomyosarcoma with osteoclast-like giant cells. Histopathology 1992, **20**: 446–449.

1249 Yannopoulos K, Stout AP. Smooth muscle tumors in children. Cancer 1962, **15**: 958–971.

Clear cell (epithelioid) smooth muscle tumors

1250 Chen KTK, Ma CK. Intravenous leiomyoblastoma. Am J Surg Pathol 1983, **7**: 591–596.

1251 Evans DJ, Lampert IA, Jacobs M. Intermediate filaments in smooth muscle tumors. J Clin Pathol 1983, **36**: 57–61.

1252 Suster S. Epithelioid leiomyosarcoma of the skin and subcutaneous tissue. Clinicopathologic, immunohistochemical, and ultrastructural study of five cases. Am J Surg Pathol 1994, **18**: 232–240.

TUMORS OF STRIATED MUSCLE

Rhabdomyoma

1253 Agamanolis DP, Dasu S, Krill CE. Tumors of skeletal muscle. Hum Pathol 1986, **17**: 778–795.

1254 Crotty PL, Nakhleh RE, Dehner LP. Juvenile rhabdomyoma. An intermediate form of skeletal muscle tumor in children. Arch Pathol Lab Med 1993, **117**: 43–47.

1255 Dehner LP, Enzinger FM. Fetal rhabdomyoma. An analysis of nine cases. Cancer 1972, **30**: 160–166.

1256 di Sant'Agnese PA, Knowles DM II. Extracardiac rhabdomyoma. A clinicopathologic study and review of the literature. Cancer 1980, **46**: 780–789.

1257 Golz R. Multifocal adult rhabdomyoma. Case report and literature review. Pathol Res Pract 1988, **183**: 512–518.

1258 Hansen T, Katenkamp D. Rhabdomyoma of the head and neck: morphology and differential diagnosis. Virchows Arch 2005, **447**: 849–854.

1259 Kapadia SB, Enzinger FM, Heffner DK, Hyams VJ, Frizzera G. Crystal-storing histiocytosis associated with lymphoplasmacytic neoplasms: report of three cases mimicking adult rhabdomyoma. Am J Surg Pathol 1993, **17**: 461–467.

1260 Kapadia SB, Meis JM, Frisman DM, Ellis GL, Heffner DK. Fetal rhabdomyoma of the head and neck. A clinicopathologic and immunophenotypic study of 24 cases. Hum Pathol 1993, **24**: 754–765.

1261 Kapadia SB, Meis JM, Frisman DM, Ellis GL, Heffner DK, Hyams VJ. Adult rhabdomyoma of the head and neck. A clinicopathologic and immunophenotypic study. Hum Pathol 1993, **24**: 608–617.

1262 Kodet R, Fajstavr J, Kabelka Z, Koutecky J, Eckschlager T, Newton WA Jr. Is fetal cellular rhabdomyoma an entity or a differentiated rhabdomyosarcoma? A study of patients with rhabdomyoma of the tongue and sarcoma of the tongue enrolled in the intergroup rhabdomyosarcoma studies I, II, and III. Cancer 1991, **67**: 2907–2913.

1263 Konrad EA, Meister P, Hübner G. Extracardiac rhabdomyoma. Report of different types with light microscopic and ultrastructural studies. Cancer 1982, **49**: 898–907.

1264 Lehtonen E, Asikainen U, Badley RA. Rhabdomyoma. Ultrastructural features and distribution of desmin, muscle type of intermediate filament protein. Acta Pathol Microbiol Immunol Scand (A) 1982, **90**: 125–129.

1265 Rodriguez J, Andreola S. The world's smallest adult rhabdomyoma. Int J Surg Pathol 2004, **12**: 401.

1266 Scrivner D, Meyer JS. Multifocal recurrent adult rhabdomyoma. Cancer 1980, **46**: 790–795.

1267 Whitten RO, Benjamin DR. Rhabdomyoma of the retroperitoneum. A report of a tumor with both adult and fetal characteristics. A study by light and electron microscopy, histochemistry, and immunochemistry. Cancer 1987, **59**: 818–824.

1268 Willis J, Abdul-Karim FW, di Sant'Agnese PA. Extracardiac rhabdomyomas. Semin Diagn Pathol 1994, **11**: 15–25.

Rhabdomyosarcoma

1269 Agamanolis DP, Dasu S, Krill CE. Tumors of skeletal muscle. Hum Pathol 1986, **17**: 778–795.

1270 Altmannsberger M, Dirk T, Osborn M, Weber K. Immunohistochemistry of cytoskeletal filaments in the diagnosis of soft tissue tumors. Semin Diagn Pathol 1986, **3**: 306–316.

1271 Autio-Harmainen H, Apaja-Sarkkinen M, Martikainen J, Taipale A, Rapola J. Production of basement membrane laminin and type IV collagen by tumors of striated muscle. An immunohistochemical study of rhabdomyosarcomas of different histologic types and a benign vaginal rhabdomyoma. Hum Pathol 1986, **17**: 1218–1224.

1272 Bahrami A, Gown AM, Baird GS, Hicks MJ, Folpe AL. Aberrant expression of epithelial and neuroendocrine markers in alveolar rhabdomyosarcoma: a potentially serious diagnostic pitfall. Mod Pathol 2008, **21**: 795–806.

1273 Bale PM, Parsons RE, Stevens MM. Diagnosis and behavior of juvenile rhabdomyosarcoma. Hum Pathol 1983, **14**: 596–611.

1274 Brooks JJ. Immunohistochemistry of soft tissue tumors. Myoglobin as a tumor marker for rhabdomyosarcoma. Cancer 1982, **50**: 1757–1763.

1275 Carstens PHB. Soft tissue tumor with prominent leptomeric fibrils and complexes (rhabdomyosarcoma). Ultrastruct Pathol 1986, **10**: 137–144.

1276 Carter RL, Jameson CF, Philp ER, Pinkerton CR. Comparative phenotypes in rhabdomyosarcomas and developing skeletal muscle. Histopathology 1990, **17**: 301–309.

1277 Carter RL, McCarthy KP, Machin LG, Jameson CF, Philp ER, Pinkerton CR. Expression of desmin and myoglobin in rhabdomyosarcomas and in developing skeletal muscle. Histopathology 1989, **15**: 585–595.

1278 Cavazzana AO, Schmidt D, Ninfo V, Harms D, Tollot M, Carli M, Treuner J, Betto R, Salviati G. Spindle cell rhabdomyosarcoma. A prognostically favorable variant of rhabdomyosarcoma. Am J Surg Pathol 1992, **16**: 229–235.

1279 Cessna MH, Zhou H, Perkins SL, Tripp SR, Layfield L, Daines C, Coffin CM. Are myogenin and MyoD1 expression specific for rhabdomyosarcoma? A study of 150 cases, with emphasis on spindle cell mimics. Am J Surg Pathol 2001, **25**: 1150–1157.

1280 Chan JK, Ng HK, Wan KY, Tsao SY, Leung TW, Tse KC. Clear cell rhabdomyosarcoma of the nasal cavity and paranasal sinuses. Histopathology 1989, **14**: 391–399.

1281 Cho KR, Olson JL, Epstein JI. Primitive rhabdomyosarcoma presenting with diffuse bone marrow involvement. An immunohistochemical and ultrastructural study. Modern Pathol 1988, **1**: 23–28.

1282 Choi J, Costa ML, Mermelstein CS, Chagas C, Holtzer S, Holtzer H. MyoD converts primary dermal fibroblasts, chondroblasts, smooth muscle, and retinal pigmented epithelial cells into striated mononucleated myoblasts and multinucleated myotubes. Proc Natl Acad Sci USA 1990, **87**: 7988–7992.

1283 Churg A, Ringus J. Ultrastructural observations on the histogenesis of alveolar rhabdomyosarcoma. Cancer 1978, **41**: 1355–1361.

1284 Clement S, Orlandi A, Bocchi L, Pizzolato G, Foschini MP, Eusebi V, Gabbiani G. Actin isoform pattern expression: a tool for the diagnosis and biological characterization of human rhabdomyosarcoma. Virchows Arch 2003, **442**: 31–38.

1285 Crist WM, Raney RB Jr, Newton W, Lawrence W Jr, Tefft M, Foulkes MA. Intrathoracic soft tissue sarcomas in children. Cancer 1982, **50**: 598–604.

1286 D'Amore ES, Tollot M, Stracca-Pansa V, Menegon A, Meli S, Carli M, Ninfo V. Therapy associated differentiation in rhabdomyosarcomas. Mod Pathol 1994, **7**: 69–75.

1287 De Jong ASH, Albus-Lutter ChE, van Raamsdonk W, Voûte PA. Myosin and myoglobin as tumor markers in the diagnosis of rhabdomyosarcoma. Am J Surg Pathol 1984, **8**: 521–528.

1288 De Jong ASH, van Kessel-van Vark M, Albus-Lutter ChE. Pleomorphic rhabdomyosarcoma in adults. Immunohistochemistry as a tool for its diagnosis. Hum Pathol 1987, **18**: 298–303.

1289 De Jong ASH, van Kessel-van Vark M, Albus-Lutter ChE, van Raamsdonk W, Voûte PA. Skeletal muscle actin as tumor marker in the diagnosis of rhabdomyosarcoma in childhood. Am J Surg Pathol 1985, **9**: 467–474.

1290 De Jong ASH, van Kessel-van Vark M, Albus-Lutter ChE, Voûte PA. Creatine kinase subunits M and B as markers in the diagnosis of poorly differentiated rhabdomyosarcomas in children. Hum Pathol 1985, **16**: 924–928.

1291 Deyrup AT, Thway K, Fisher C, Wang W-L, Lazar AJ, Jones RL, Tighiouart M, Weiss SW. Clincopathologic analysis of adult alveolar and embryonal rhabdomyosarcoma: a study of 62 cases. Lab Invest 2009, **89**(Suppl 1): 13A.

1292 Dias P, Chen B, Dilday B, Palmer H, Hosoi H, Singh S, Wu C, Li X, Thompson J, Parham D, Qualman S, Houghton P. Strong immunostaining for myogenin in rhabdomyosarcoma is significantly associated with tumors of the alveolar subclass. Am J Pathol 2000, **156**: 399–408.

1293 Dias P, Dilling M, Houghton P. The molecular basis of skeletal muscle differentiation. Semin Diagn Pathol 1994, **11**: 3–14.

1294 Dias P, Parham DM, Shapiro DN, Webber BL, Houghton PJ. Myogenic regulatory protein (MyoD1) expression in childhood solid tumors. Diagnostic utility in rhabdomyosarcoma. Am J Pathol 1990, **137**: 1283–1291.

1295 Downing JR, Khandekar A, Shurtleff SA, Head DR, Parham DM, Webber BL, Pappo AS, Hulshof MG, Conn WP, Shapiro DN. Multiplex RT-PCR assay for the differential diagnosis of alveolar rhabdomyosarcoma and Ewing's sarcoma. Am J Pathol 1995, **146**: 626–634.

1296 Driman D, Thorner PS, Greenberg ML, Chilton-MacNeill S, Squire J. MYCN gene amplification in rhabdomyosarcoma. Cancer 1994, **73**: 2231–2237.

1297 Elomaa I, Lehto V-P, Selander R-K. Hypercalcemia and elevated serum parathyroid hormone level in association with rhabdomyosarcoma. Arch Pathol Lab Med 1984, **108**: 701–703.

1298 Enterline HT, Horn RC. Alveolar rhabdomyosarcoma. A distinctive tumor type. Am J Clin Pathol 1958, **20**: 356–366.

1299 Enzinger FM. Alveolar rhabdomyosarcoma. An analysis of 110 cases. Cancer 1969, **24**: 18–31.

1300 Erlandson RA. The ultrastructural distinction between rhabdomyosarcoma and other undifferentiated 'sarcomas'. Ultrastruct Pathol 1937, **11**: 83–101.

1301 Eusebi V, Bondi A, Rosai J. Immunohistochemical localization of myoglobin in nonmuscular cells. Am J Surg Pathol 1984, **8**: 51–55.

1302 Eusebi V, Ceccarelli C, Gorza L, Schiaffino S, Bussolati G. Immunocytochemistry of rhabdomyosarcoma. The use of four different markers. Am J Surg Pathol 1986, **10**: 293–299.

1303 Eusebi V, Damiani S, Pasquinelli G, Lorenzini P, Reuter VE, Rosai J. Small cell neuroendocrine carcinoma with skeletal muscle differentiation: report of three cases. Am J Surg Pathol 2000, **24**: 223–230.

1304 Eusebi V, Rilke F, Ceccarelli C, Fedeli F, Schiaffino S, Bussolati G. Fetal heavy chain skeletal myosin. An oncofetal antigen expressed by rhabdomyosarcoma. Am J Surg Pathol 1986, **10**: 680–686.

1305 Ferrari A, Dileo P, Casanova M, Bertulli R, Meazza C, Gandola L, Navarria P, Collini P, Gronchi A, Olmi P, Fossati-Bellani F, Casali PG. Rhabdomyosarcoma in adults. A retrospective analysis of 171 patients treated at a single institution. Cancer 2003, **98**: 571–580.

1306 Flamant F, Hill C. The improvement in survival associated with combined chemotherapy in childhood rhabdomyosarcoma. Cancer 1984, **53**: 2417–2421.

1307 Folpe AL, McKenney JK, Bridge JA, Weiss SW. Sclerosing rhabdomyosarcoma in adults: report of four cases of a hyalinzing matrix-rich variant of rhabdomyosarcoma that may be confused with osteosarcoma, chondrosarcoma, or angiosarcoma. Am J Surg Pathol 2002, **26**: 1175–1183.

1308 Franchi A, Massi D, Santucci M. The comparative role of immunohistochemistry and electron microscopy in the identification of myogenic differentiation in soft tissue pleomorphic sarcomas. Ultrastruct Pathol 2005, **29**: 295–304.

1309 Furlong MA, Fanburg-Smith JC. Pleomorphic rhabdomyosarcoma in children: four cases in the pediatric age group. Ann Diagn Pathol 2001, **5**: 199–206.

1310 Furlong MA, Fentzel T, Fanburg-Smith JC. Pleomorphic rhabdomyosarcoma in adults: a clinicopathologic study of 38 cases with emphasis on morphologic variants and recent skeletal muscle-specific markers. Mod Pathol 2001, **14**: 595–603.

1311 Gaffney EF, Dervan PA, Fletcher CD. Pleomorphic rhabdomyosarcoma in adulthood. Analysis of 11 cases with definition of diagnostic criteria. Am J Surg Pathol 1993, **17**: 601–609.

1312 Gonzalez-Crussi F, Black-Schaffer S. Rhabdomyosarcoma of infancy and childhood. Problems of morphologic classification. Am J Surg Pathol 1979, **3**: 157–171.

1313 Gordon T, McManus A, Anderson J, Min T, Swansbury J, Pritchard-Jones K, Shipley J; United Kingdom Children's Cancer Study Group; United Kingdom Cancer Cytogenetics Group. Cytogenetic abnormalities in 42 rhabdomyosarcoma: a United Kingdom Cancer Cytogenetics Group Study. Med Pediatr Oncol 2001, **36**: 259–267.

1314 Hawkins HK, Camacho-Velasquez JV. Rhabdomyosarcoma in children. A correlation of form and prognosis in one institution's experience. Am J Surg Pathol 1987, **11**: 531–542.

1315 Hayashi Y, Kikuchi F, Oka T, Itoyama S, Mohri N, Usuki K, Takaku F, Murakami T, Saitoh Y, Urano Y. Rhabdomyosarcoma with bone marrow metastasis simulating acute leukemia. Report of two cases. Acta Pathol Jpn 1988, **38**: 789–798.

1316 Hays DM, Newton W Jr, Soule EH, Foulkes MA, Raney RB, Tefft M, Ragab A, Maurer HM. Mortality among children with rhabdomyosarcomas of the alveolar histologic subtype. J Pediatr Surg 1983, **18**: 412–417.

1317 Hays DM, Soule EH, Lawrence W Jr, Gehan EA, Maurer HM, Donaldson M, Raney RB, Tefft M. Extremity lesions in the Intergroup Rhabdomyosarcoma Study (IRS-I). A preliminary report. Cancer 1982, **49**: 1–8.

1318 Heffner DK. The truth about alveolar rhadomyosarcoma. Ann Diagn Pathol 2003, **7**: 259–263.

1319 Heerema-McKenney A, Wijnaendts LC, Pulliam JF, Lopez-Terrada D, McKenney JK, Zhu S, Montgomery K, Mitchell J, Marinelli RJ, Hart AA, van de Rijn M, Linn SC. Diffuse myogenin expression by immunohistochemistry is an independent marker of poor survival in pediatric rhabdomyosarcoma: a tissue microarray study of 71 primary tumors including correlation with molecular phenotype. Am J Surg Pathol 2008, **32**: 1513–1522.

1320 Hollowood K, Fletcher CD. Rhabdomyosarcoma in adults. Semin Diagn Pathol 1994, **11**: 47–57.

1321 Horn RC Jr, Enterline HT. Rhabdomyosarcoma. A clinicopathological study and classification of 39 cases. Cancer 1958, **11**: 181–199.

1322 Ishiguro N, Baba T, Ishida T, Takeuchi K, Osaki M, Araki N, Okada E, Takahashi S, Saito M, Watanabe M, Nakaba C, Tsukamoto Y, Sato K, Ito K, Fukayama M, Mori S, Ito H, Moriyama M. Carp, a cardiac ankyrin-repeated protein, and its new homologue, Arpp, are differentially expressed in heart, skeletal muscle, and rhabdomyosarcomas. Am J Pathol 2002, **160**: 1767–1778.

1323 Ishiguro N, Motoi T, Osaki M, Araki N, Minamizaki T, Moriyama M, Ito H, Yoshida H. Immunohistochemical analysis of a muscle ankyrin-repeat protein, Arpp, in paraffin-embedded tumors: evaluation of Arpp as a tumor marker for rhabdomyosarcoma. Hum Pathol 2005, **36**: 620–625.

1324 Jaffe BF, Fox JE, Batsakis JG. Rhabdomyosarcoma of the middle ear and mastoid. Cancer 1971, **27**: 29–37.

1325 Karcioglu Z, Someren A, Mathes SJ. Ectomesenchymoma. A malignant tumor of migratory neural crest (ectomesenchyme) remnants showing ganglionic, schwannian, melanocytic and rhabdomyoblastic differentiation. Cancer 1977, **39**: 2486–2496.

1326 Kawamoto EH, Weidner N, Agostini RM Jr, Jaffe R. Malignant ectomesenchymoma of soft tissue. Report of two cases and review of the literature. Cancer 1987, **59**: 1791–1802.

1327 Kindblom L-G, Seidal T, Karlsson K. Immunohistochemical localization of myoglobin in human muscle tissue and embryonal and alveolar rhabdomyosarcoma. Acta Pathol Microbiol Immunol Scand [A] 1982, **90**: 167–174.

1328 Kodet R, Kasthuri N, Marsden HB, Coad NAG, Raafat F. Gangliorhabdomyosarcoma. A histopathological and immunohistochemical study of three cases. Histopathology 1986, **10**: 181–193.

1329 Kodet R, Newton WA Jr, Hamoudi AB, Asmar L. Rhabdomyosarcomas with intermediate-filament inclusions and features of rhabdoid tumors. Light microscopic and immunohistochemical study. Am J Surg Pathol 1991, **15**: 257–267.

1330 Kodet R, Newton WA Jr, Hamoudi AB, Asmar L, Jacobs DL, Maurer HM. Childhood rhabdomyosarcoma with anaplastic (pleomorphic) features. A report of the Intergroup Rhabdomyosarcoma Study. Am J Surg Pathol 1993, **17**: 443–453.

1331 Koh S-J, Johnson WW. Antimyosin and antirhabdomyoblast sera. Their use for the diagnosis of childhood rhabdomyosarcoma. Arch Pathol Lab Med 1980, **104**: 118–122.

1332 Kuhnen C, Herter P, Leuschner I, Mentzel T, Druecke D, Jaworska M, Johnen G. Sclerosing pseudovascular rhabdomyosarcoma – immunohistochemical, ultrastructural, and genetic findings indicating a distinct subtype of rhabdomyosarcoma. Virchows Arch 2006, **449**: 572–578.

1333 Kumar S, Pelman E, Haris CA, Raffeld M, Tsokos M. Myogenin is a specific marker for rhabdomyosarcomas: an immunohistochemical study of paraffin-embedded tissues. Mod Pathol 2001, **13**: 988–993.

1334 La Quaglia MP, Heller G, Ghavimi F, Casper ES, Vlamis V, Hajdu S, Brennan MF. The effect of age at diagnosis on outcome in rhabdomyosarcoma. Cancer 1994, **73**: 109–117.

1335 Lawrence W, Hays DM, Heyn R, Tefft M, Crist W, Beltangady M, Newton W Jr, Wharam M. Lymphatic metastases with childhood rhabdomyosarcoma. A report from the Intergroup Rhabdomyosarcoma Study. Cancer 1987, **60**: 910–915.

1336 Leuschner I, Newton WA Jr, Schmidt D, Sachs N, Asmar L, Hamoudi A, Harms D, Maurer HM. Spindle cell variants of embryonal rhabdomyosarcoma in the paratesticular region. A report of the Intergroup Rhabdomyosarcoma Study. Am J Surg Pathol 1993, **17**: 221–230.

1337 Lim D, Bowdin SC, Tee L, Kirby GA, Blair E, Fryer A, Lam W, Oley C, Cole T, Brueton LA, Reik W, Macdonald F, Maher ER. Clinical and molecular genetic features of Beckwith–Wiedemann syndrome associated with assisted reproductive technologies. Hum Reprod 2009, **24**: 741–747.

1338 Linscheid RL, Soule EH, Henderson ED. Pleomorphic rhabdomyosarcomata of the extremities and limb girdles. J Bone Joint Surg (Am) 1965, **47**: 715–726.

1339 Lloyd RV, Hajdu SI, Knapper WH. Embryonal rhabdomyosarcoma in adults. Cancer 1983, **51**: 557–565.

1340 Loh WE Jr, Scrable HJ, Livanos E, Arboleda MJ, Cavenee WK, Oshimura M, et al. Human chromosome 11 contains two different growth suppressor genes for embryonal rhabdomyosarcoma. Proc Natl Acad Sci USA 1992, **89**: 1755–1759.

1341 Lundgren L, Angervall L, Stenman G, Kindblom LG. Infantile rhabdomyofibrosarcoma. A high-grade sarcoma distinguishable from infantile fibrosarcoma and rhabdomyosarcoma. Hum Pathol 1993, **24**: 785–795.

1342 Masson JK, Soule EH. Embryonal rhabdomyosarcoma of head and neck. Report of 88 cases. Am J Surg 1965, **110**: 585–591.

1343 Maurer HM, Beltangady M, Gehan EA, Crist W, Hammond D, Hays DM, Heyn R, Lawrence W, Newton W, Ortega J, Ragab AH, Raney RB, Ruymann FB, Soule E, Tefft M, Webber B, Wharam M, Vietti TJ. The Intergroup Rhabdomyosarcoma Study. I. A final report. Cancer 1988, **61**: 209–220.

1344 Maurer HM, Gehan EA, Beltangady M, Crist W, Dickman PS, Donaldson SS, Fryer C, Hammond D, Hays DM, Herrmann J, et al. The Intergroup Rhabdomyosarcoma Study-II. Cancer 1993, **71**: 1904–1922.

1345 Mentzel T, Kuhnen C. Spindle cell rhabdomyosarcoma in adults: clinicopathological and immunohistochemical analysis of seven new cases. Virchows Arch 2006, **449**: 554–560.

1346 Mercado GE, Barr FG. Fusions involving PAX and FOX genes in the molecular pathogenesis of alveolar rhabdomyosarcoma: recent advances. Curr Mol Med 2007, **7**: 47–61.

1347 Mierau GW, Favara BE. Rhabdomyosarcoma in children. Ultrastructural study of 31 cases. Cancer 1980, **46**: 2035–2040.

1348 Miettinen M. Antibody specific to muscle actins in the diagnosis and classification of soft tissue tumors. Am J Pathol 1988, **130**: 205–215.

1349 Miettinen M, Rapola J. Immunohistochemical spectrum of rhabdomyosarcoma and rhabdomyosarcoma-like tumors. Expression of cytokeratin and the 68-kD neurofilament protein. Am J Surg Pathol 1989, **13**: 120–132.

1350 Molenaar WM, Dam-Meiring A, Kamps WA, Cornelisse CJ. DNA-aneuploidy in rhabdomyosarcomas as compared with other sarcomas of childhood and adolescence. Hum Pathol 1988, **19**: 573–579.

1351 Molenaar WM, Oosterhuis AM, Ramaekers FCS. The rarity of rhabdomyosarcomas in the adult. A morphologic and immunohistochemical study. Pathol Res Pract 1985, **180**: 400–404.

1352 Molenaar WM, Oosterhuis JW, Kamps WA. Cytologic 'differentiation' in childhood rhabdomyosarcomas following polychemotherapy. Hum Pathol 1984, **15**: 973–979.

1353 Molenaar WM, Oosterhuis JW, Oosterhuis AM, Ramaekers FCS. Mesenchymal and muscle-specific intermediate filaments (vimentin and desmin) in relation to differentiation in childhood rhabdomyosarcoma. Hum Pathol 1985, **16**: 838–843.

1354 Montone KT, Barr FG, Zhang PJ, Feldman MD, LiVolsi VA. Embryonal and alveolar rhabdomyosarcoma of parameningeal sites in adults: a report of 13 cases. Int J Surg Pathol 2009, **17**: 22–30.

1355 Morales AR, Fine G, Horn RC Jr. Rhabdomyosarcoma. An ultrastructural appraisal. Pathol Annu 1972, **7**: 81–106.

1356 Morotti RA, Nicol KK, Parham DM, Teot LA, Moore J, Hayes J, Meyer W, Qualman SJ; Children's Oncology Group. An immunohistochemical algorithm to facilitate diagnosis and subtyping of rhabdomyosarcoma: the Children's Oncology Group experience. Am J Surg Pathol 2006, **30**: 962–968.

1357 Mukai K, Rosai J, Hallaway BE. Localization of myoglobin in normal and neoplastic human skeletal muscle cells using an immunoperoxidase method. Am J Surg Pathol 1979, **3**: 373–376.

1358 Mukai K, Schollmeyer JV, Rosai J. Immunohistochemical localization of actin. Its applications in surgical pathology. Am J Surg Pathol 1981, **5**: 91–97.

1359 Mukai M, Iri H, Torikata C, Kageyama K, Morikawa Y, Shimizu K. Immunoperoxidase demonstration of a new muscle protein (Z-protein) in myogenic tumors as a diagnostic aid. Am J Pathol 1984, **114**: 164–170.

1360 Nakhleh RE, Swanson PE, Dehner LP. Juvenile (embryonal and alveolar) rhabdomyosarcoma of the head and neck in adults. A clinical, pathologic, and immunohistochemical study of 12 cases. Cancer 1991, **67**: 1019–1024.

1361 Nascimento AF, Fletcher CD. Spindle cell rhabdomyosarcoma in adults. Am J Surg Pathol 2005, **29**: 1106–1113.

1362 Nishio J, Althof PA, Bailey JM, Zhou M, Neff JR, Barr FG, Parham DM, Teot L, Qualman SJ, Bridge JA. Use of a novel FISH assay on paraffin-embedded tissues as an adjunct to diagnosis of alveolar rhabdomyosarcoma. Lab Invest 2006, **86**: 547–556.

1363 Om A, Ghose T. Use of anti-skeletal muscle antibody from myasthenic patients in the diagnosis of childhood rhabdomyosarcomas. Am J Surg Pathol 1987, **11**: 272–276.

1364 Oppenheimer O, Athanasian E, Meyers P, Antonescu CR, Gorlick R. Malignant ectomesenchymoma in the wrist of a child: case report and review of the literature. Int J Surg Pathol 2005, **13**: 113–116.

1365 Osborn M, Hill C, Altmannsberger M, Weber K. Monoclonal antibodies to titin in conjunction with antibodies to desmin separate rhabdomyosarcomas from other tumor types. Lab Invest 1986, **55**: 101–108.

1366 Pappo AS, Crist WM, Kuttesch J, Rowe S, Ashmun RA, Maurer HM, Newton WA, Asmar L, Luo X, Shapiro DN. Tumor-cell DNA content predicts outcome in children and adolescents with clinical group III embryonal rhabdomyosarcoma. The Intergroup Rhabdomyosarcoma Study Committee of the Children's Cancer Group and the Pediatric Oncology Group. J Clin Oncol 1993, **11**: 1901–1905.

1367 Parham DM. Pathologic classification of rhabdomyosarcomas and correlations with molecular studies. Mod Pathol 2001, **14**: 506–514.

1368 Parham DM, Shapiro DN, Downing JR, Webber BL, Douglass EC. Solid alveolar rhabdomyosarcomas with the t(2;13). Report of two cases with diagnostic implications. Am J Surg Pathol 1994, **18**: 474–478.

1369 Parham DM, Webber B, Holt H, Williams WK, Maurer H. Immunohistochemical study of childhood rhabdomyosarcomas and related neoplasms. Results of an Intergroup Rhabdomyosarcoma Study project. Cancer 1991, **67**: 3072–3080.

1370 Parham DM, Ellison DA. Rhabdomyosarcomas in adults and children: an update. Arch Pathol Lab Med 2006, **130**: 1454–1465.

1371 Parham DM, Qualman SJ, Teot L, Barr FG, Morotti R, Sorensen PH, Triche TJ, Meyer WH; Soft Tissue Sarcoma Committee of the Children's Oncology Group. Correlation between histology and PAX/FKHR fusion status in alveolar rhabdomyosarcoma: a report from the Children's Oncology Group. Am J Surg Pathol 2007, **31**: 895–901.

1372 Peters E, Cohen M, Altini M, Murray J. Rhabdomyosarcoma of the oral and paraoral region. Cancer 1989, **63**: 963–966.

1373 Ragab AH, Heyn R, Tefft M, Hays DN, Newton WA Jr, Beltangady M. Infants younger than 1 year of age with rhabdomyosarcoma. Cancer 1986, **58**: 2606–2610.

1374 Rajaram V, Hill DA, Doherty GM, Liapis H, Dehner LP. Pleomorphic rhabdomyosarcoma of the anterior abdominal wall following multimodality treatment for carcinoma of the rectum. Int J Surg Pathol 2004, **12**: 161–165.

1375 Raney RB Jr, Tefft M, Maurer HM, Ragab AH, Hays DM, Soule EH, Foulkes MA, Gehan EA. Disease patterns and survival rate in children with metastatic soft-tissue sarcoma. A report from the Intergroup Rhabdomyosarcoma Study (IRS)-I. Cancer 1988, **62**: 1257–1266.

1376 Reboul-Marty J, Quintana E, Mosseri V, Flamant F, Asselain B, Rodary C, Zucker JM. Prognostic factors of alveolar rhabdomyosarcoma in childhood. An International Society of Pediatric Oncology study. Cancer 1991, **68**: 493–498.

1377 Riopelle JL, Thériault JP. Sur une forme méconnue de sarcome des parties molles; le rhabdomyosarcome alvéolaire. Ann Anat Pathol (Paris) 1956, **1**: 88–111.

1378 Royds JA, Variend S, Timperley WR, Taylor CB. Comparison of β-enolase and myoglobin as histological markers of rhabdomyosarcoma. J Clin Pathol 1985, **38**: 1258–1260.

1379 Ruymann FB, Newton WA Jr, Ragab AH, Donaldson MH, Foulkes M. Bone marrow metastases at diagnosis in children and adolescents with rhabdomyosarcoma. A report from the Intergroup Rhabdomyosarcoma Study. Cancer 1984, **53**: 368–373.

1380 Sarnat HB, de Mello DE, Siddiqui SY. Diagnostic value of histochemistry in embryonal rhabdomyosarcoma. Am J Surg Pathol 1979, **3**: 177–183.

1381 Schmidt D, Fletcher CD, Harms D. Rhabdomyosarcoma with primary presentation in the skin. Pathol Res Pract 1993, **189**: 422–427.

1382 Schmidt D, Reimann O, Treuner J, Harms D. Cellular differentiation and prognosis in embryonal rhabdomyosarcoma. A report from the Cooperative Soft Tissue Sarcoma Study 1981 (CWS 81). Virchows Arch [A] 1986, **409**: 183–194.

1383 Schurch W, Begin LR, Seemayer TA, Lagace R, Boivin JC, Lamoureux C, Bluteau P, Piche J, Gabbiani G. Pleomorphic soft tissue myogenic sarcomas of adulthood: a reappraisal in the mid-1990s. Am J Surg Pathol 1996, **20**: 131–147.

1384 Seidal T, Kindblom L-G. The ultrastructure of alveolar and embryonal rhabdomyosarcoma. A correlative light and electron microscopic study of 17 cases. Acta Pathol Microbiol Immunol Scand (A) 1984, **92**: 231–248.

1385 Seidal T, Mark J, Hagmar B, Angervall L. Alveolar rhabdomyosarcoma. A cytogenetic and correlated cytological and histological study. Acta Pathol Microbiol Immunol Scand (A) 1982, **90**: 345–354.

1386 Shimada H, Newton WA Jr, Soule EH, Beltangady MS, Maurer HM. Pathology of fatal rhabdomyosarcoma. Report from Intergroup Rhabdomyosarcoma Study (IRS-I and IRS-II). Cancer 1987, **59**: 459–465.

1387 Skalli O, Gabbiani G, Babaï F, Seemayer TA, Pizzolato G, Schürch W. Intermediate filament proteins and actin isoforms as markers for soft tissue tumor differentiation and origin II. Rhabdomyosarcomas. Am J Pathol 1988, **130**: 515–531.

1388 Sorensen PH, Lynch JC, Qualman SJ, Tirabosco R, Lim JF, Maurer HM, Bridge JA, Crist WM, Triche TJ, Barr FG. PAX3-FKHR and PAX7-FKHR gene fusions are prognostic indicators in alveolar rhabdomyosarcoma: a report from the children's oncology group. J Clin Oncol 2002, **20**: 2672–2679.

1389 Soule EH, Geitz M, Henderson ED. Embryonal rhabdomyosarcoma of the limbs and limb-girdles. A clinicopathologic study of 61 cases. Cancer 1969, **23**: 1336–1346.

1390 Stock N, Chibon F, Binh MB, Terrier P, Michels JJ, Valo I, Robin YM, Guillou L, Ranchère-Vince D, Decouvelaere AV, Collin F, Birtwisle-Peyrottes I, Gregoire F, Aurias A, Coindre JM. Adult-type rhabdomyosarcoma: analysis of 57 cases with clinicopathologic description, identification of 3 morphologic patterns and prognosis. Am J Surg Pathol 2009, **33**: 1850–1859.

1391 Stout AP. Rhabdomyosarcoma of the skeletal muscles. Ann Surg 1946, **123**: 447–472.

1392 Sullivan LM, Atkins KA, LeGallo RD. PAX immunoreactivity identifies alveolar rhabdomyosarcoma. Am J Surg Pathol 2009, **33**: 775–780.

1393 Tsokos M. The role of immunocytochemistry in the diagnosis of rhabdomyosarcoma. Arch Pathol Lab Med 1986, **110**: 776–778.

1394 Tsokos M. The diagnosis and classification of childhood rhabdomyosarcoma. Semin Diagn Pathol 1994, **11**: 26–38.

1395 Tsokos M, Howard R, Costa J. Immunohistochemical study of alveolar and embryonal rhabdomyosarcoma. Lab Invest 1983, **48**: 148–155.

1396 Tsokos M, Webber BL, Parham DM, Wesley RA, Miser A, Miser JS, Etcubanas E, Kinsella T, Grayson J, Glatstein E, et al. Rhabdomyosarcoma. A new classification scheme related to prognosis. Arch Pathol Lab Med 1992, **116**: 847–855.

1397 Variend S, Loughlin MA. An evaluation of enzyme histochemistry in the diagnosis of childhood rhabdomyosarcoma. Histopathology 1985, **9**: 389–400.

1398 Wang J, Tu X, Sheng W. Sclerosing rhabdomyosarcoma: a clinicopathologic and immunohistochemical study of five cases. Am J Clin Pathol 2008, **129**: 410–415.

1399 Wesche WA, Fletcher CD, Dias P, Houghton PJ, Parham DM. Immunohistochemistry of MyoDI in adult pleomorphic soft tissue sarcomas. Am J Surg Pathol 1995, **19**: 261–269.

1400 Wijnaendts LC, van der Linden JC, van Unnik AJ, Delemarre JF, Barbet JP, Butler-Browne GS, Meijer CJ. Expression of developmentally regulated muscle proteins in rhabdomyosarcomas. Am J Pathol 1994, **145**: 895–901.

1401 Wijnaendts LC, van der Linden JC, van Unnik AJ, Delemarre JF, Voute PA, Meijer CJ. Histopathological classification of childhood rhabdomyosarcomas. Relationship with clinical parameters and prognosis. Hum Pathol 1994, **25**: 900–907.

1402 Yasuda T, Perry KD, Nelson M, Bui MM, Nasir A, Goldschmidt R, Gnepp DR, Bridge JA. Alveolar rhabdomyosarcoma of the head and neck region in older adults: genetic characterization and a review of the literature. Hum Pathol 2009, **40**: 341–348.

1403 Young RH, Scully RE. Alveolar rhabdomyosarcoma metastatic to the ovary. A report of two cases and a discussion of the differential diagnosis of small cell malignant tumors of the ovary. Cancer 1989, **64**: 899–904.

1404 Yun K. A new marker for rhabdomyosarcoma. Insulin-like growth factor II. Lab Invest 1992, **67**: 653–664.

1405 Zambrano E, Pérez-Atayde AR, Ahrens W, Reyes-Múgica M. Pediatric sclerosing rhabdomyosarcoma. Int J Surg Pathol 2006, **14**: 193–199.

1406 Zuppan CW, Mierau GW, Weeks DA. Lipid-rich rhabdomyosarcoma – a potential source of diagnostic confusion. Ultrastruct Pathol 1991, **15**: 353–359.

TUMORS OF PLURIPOTENTIAL MESENCHYME

1407 Brady MS, Perino GK, Tallini G, Russo P, Woodruff JM. Malignant mesenchymoma. Cancer 1996, **77**: 467–473.

1408 Bures C, Barnes L. Benign mesenchymomas of the head and neck. Arch Pathol Lab Med 1978, **102**: 237–241.

1409 Dorfman HD, Levin S, Robbins H. Cartilage-containing benign mesenchymomas of soft tissue. Report of two cases. J Bone Joint Surg (Am) 1980, **62**: 472–475.

1410 Hollingsworth H, Pogrebniak H, Baker A, Merino M. Unusual mesenchymoma with prominent chondro-osseous elements. Int J Surg Pathol 1993, **1**: 129–134.

1411 Milchgrub S, McMurry NK, Vuitch F, Dorfman HD. Chondrolipoangioma. A cartilage-containing benign mesenchymoma of soft tissue. Cancer 1990, **66**: 2636–2641.

1412 Nash A, Stout AP. Malignant mesenchymomas in children. Cancer 1961, **14**: 524–533.

1413 Newman PL, Fletcher CD. Malignant mesenchymoma. Clinicopathologic analysis of a series with evidence of low-grade behaviour. Am J Surg Pathol 1991, **15**: 607–614.

1414 Stout AP. Mesenchymoma, the mixed tumor of mesenchymal derivatives. Ann Surg 1948, **127**: 278–290.

TUMORS OF METAPLASTIC MESENCHYME

1415 Abramovici LC, Hytiroglou P, Klein RM, Karkavelas G, Drevelegas A, Panousi E, Steiner GC. Well-differentiated extraskeletal osteosarcoma: report of 2 cases, 1 with dedifferentiation. Hum Pathol 2005, **36**: 439–443.

1416 Aigner T, Oliveira AM, Nascimento AG. Extraskeletal myxoid chondrosarcomas do not show a chondrocytic phenotype. Mod Pathol 2004, **17**: 214–221.

1417 Allan CJ, Soule EH. Osteogenic sarcoma of the somatic soft tissues. Clinicopathologic study of 26 cases and review of literature. Cancer 1971, **27**: 1121–1133.

1418 Antonescu CR, Argani P, Erlandson RA, Healey JH, Ladanyi M, Huvos AG. Skeletal and extraskeletal myxoid chondrosarcoma: a comparative clinicopathologic, ultrastructural, and molecular study. Cancer 1998, **83**: 1504–1521.

1419 Bane BL, Evans HL, Ro JY, Carrasco CH, Grignon DJ, Benjamin RS, Ayala AG. Extraskeletal osteosarcoma. A clinicopathologic review of 26 cases. Cancer 1990, **65**: 2762–2770.

1420 Bertoni F, Picci P, Bacchini P, Capanna R, Innao V, Bacci G, Campanacci M. Mesenchymal chondrosarcoma of bone and soft tissues. Cancer 1983, **52**: 533–541.

1421 Bhagavan BS, Dorfman HD. The significance of bone and cartilage formation in malignant fibrous histiocytoma of soft tissue. Cancer 1982, **49**: 480–488.

1422 Carstens PHB. Chordoid tumor. A light, electron microscopic, and immunohistochemical study. Ultrastruct Pathol 1995, **19**: 291–296.

1423 Cates JM, Rosenberg AE, O'Connel JX, Neilsen GP. Chondroblastoma-like chondroma of soft tissue: an underrecognized variant and its differential diagnosis. Am J Surg Pathol 2001, **25**: 661–666.

1424 Chhieng DC, Erlandson RA, Antonescu C, Ladanyi M, Rosai J. Neuroendocrine differentiation in adult soft tissue sarcomas with features of extraskeletal myxoid chondrosarcoma: report of seven cases [abstract]. Mod Pathol 1998, **10**: 8A.

1425 Chung EB, Enzinger FM. Chondroma of soft parts. Cancer 1978, **41**: 1414–1424.

1426 Chung EB, Enzinger FM. Extraskeletal osteosarcoma. Cancer 1987, **60**: 1132–1142.

1427 Dabska M. Parachordoma. A new clinicopathologic entity. Cancer 1977, **40**: 1586–1592.

1428 Dahlin DC, Salvador AH. Cartilaginous tumors of the soft tissues of the hands and feet. Mayo Clin Proc 1974, **49**: 721–726.

1429 D'Ambrosio RG, Shiu MH, Brennan MF. Intrapulmonary presentation of extraskeletal myxoid chondrosarcoma of the extremity. Report of two cases. Cancer 1986, **58**: 1144–1148.

1430 De Blois G, Wang S, Kay S. Microtubular aggregates within rough endoplasmic reticulum. An unusual ultrastructural feature of extraskeletal myxoid chondrosarcoma. Hum Pathol 1986, **17**: 469–475.

1431 Deyrup AT, Monson DK, Dorfman HD. Aggressive (epithelioid) osteoblastoma arising in soft tissue. Int J Surg Pathol 2008, **16**: 308–310.

1432 Domanski HA, Carlén B, Mertens F, Åkerman M. Extraskeletal myxoid chondrosarcoma with neuroendocrine differentiation: a case report with fine-needle aspiration biopsy, histopathology, electron microscopy, and cytogenetics. Ultrastruct Pathol 2003, **27**: 363–368.

1433 Enzinger FM, Shiraki M. Extra-skeletal myxoid chondrosarcoma. An analysis of 34 cases. Hum Pathol 1972, **3**: 421–435.

1434 Fanburg-Smith JC, Bratthauer GL, Miettinen M. Osteocalcin and osteonectin immunoreactivity in extraskeletal osteosarcoma: a study of 28 cases. Hum Pathol 1999, **30**: 32–38.

1435 Fine G, Stout AP. Osteogenic sarcoma of the extraskeletal soft tissues. Cancer 1956, **9**: 1027–1043.

1436 Fletcher CDM, Powell G, McKee PH. Extraskeletal myxoid chondrosarcoma. A histochemical and immunohistochemical study. Histopathology 1986, **10**: 489–499.

1437 Gengler C, Letovanec I, Taminelli L, Egger JF, Guillou L. Desmin and myogenin reactivity in mesenchymal chondrosarcoma: a potential diagnostic pitfall. Histopathology 2005, **48**: 200–219.

1438 Goh Y-W, Spagnolo DV, Platten M, Caterina P, Fisher C, Oliveira AM, Nascimento AG. Extraskeletal myxoid chondrosarcoma: a light microscopic, immunohistochemical, ultrastructural and immuno-ultrastructural study indicating neuroendocrine differentiation. Histopathology 2001, **39**: 514–524.

1439 Guccion JG, Font RL, Enzinger FM, Zimmerman LE. Extraskeletal mesenchymal chondrosarcoma. Arch Pathol 1973, **95**: 336–340.

1440 Hachitanda Y, Tsuneyoshi M, Daimaru Y, Enjoji M, Nakagawara A, Ikeda K, Sueishi K. Extraskeletal myxoid chondrosarcoma in young children. Cancer 1988, **61**: 2521–2526.

1441 Hisaoka M, Hashimoto H. Extraskeletal myxoid chondrosarcoma: updated clinicopathological and molecular genetic characteristics. Pathol Int 2005, **55**: 453–463.

1442 Hoang MP, Suarez PA, Donner LR, Ro J, Ordóñez NG, Ayala AG, Czerniak B. Mesenchymal chondrosarcoma: a small cell neoplasm with polyphenotypic differentiation. Int J Surg Pathol 2000, **8**: 291–301.

1443 Hu B, McPhaul L, Cornford M, Gaal K, Mirra J, French SW. Expression of tau proteins and tubulin in extraskeletal myxoid chondrosarcoma, chordoma, and other chondroid tumors. Am J Clin Pathol 1999, **112**: 189–193.

1444 Humphreys S, Pambakian H, McKee PH, Fletcher CDM. Soft tissue chondroma. A study of 15 tumours. Histopathology 1986, **10**: 147–159.

1445 Huvos AG. Osteogenic sarcoma of bones and soft tissues in older persons. A clinicopathologic analysis of 117 patients older than 60 years. Cancer 1986, **57**: 1442–1449.

1446 Huvos AG, Woodard HQ, Cahan WG, Higinbotham NL, Stewart FW, Butler A, Bretsky SS. Postradiation osteogenic sarcoma of bone and soft tissues. A clinicopathologic study of 66 patients. Cancer 1985, **55**: 1244–1255.

1447 Isotalo Pa, Lae ME, Luzzato F, Rua AM, Lloyd RV, Sebo TJ, Riehle DL, Unni KK, Nascimento AG. Extraskeletal mesenchymal chondrosarcoma: a clinicopathologic and molecular study of 16 cases [abstract]. Mod Pathol 2003, **16**: 15A.

1448 Jensen ML, Schumacher B, Jensen OM, Neilsen OS, Keller J. Extraskeletal osteosarcomas: a clinicopathologic study of 25 cases. Am J Surg Pathol 1998, **22**: 588–594.

1449 Kawaguchi S, Wada T, Nagoya S, Ikeda T, Isu K, Yamashiro K, Kawai A, Ishii T, Araki N, Myoui A, Matsumoto S, Umeda T, Yoshikawa H, Hasegawa T. Extraskeletal myxoid chondrosarcoma. A multi-institutional study of 42 cases in Japan. Cancer 2003, **97**: 1285–1292.

1450 Lichtenstein L, Goldman RL. Cartilage tumors in soft tissues, particularly in the hand and foot. Cancer 1964, **17**: 1203–1208.

1451 Lucas DR, Fletcher CD, Adsay NV, Zalupski MM. High-grade extraskeletal myxoid chondrosarcoma: a high-grade epithelioid malignancy. Histopathology 1999, **35**: 201–208.

1452 Mackenzie DH. The unsuspected soft tissue chondrosarcoma. Histopathology 1983, **7**: 759–766.

1453 Malhotra CM, Doolittle CH, Rodil JV, Vezeridis MP. Mesenchymal chondrosarcoma of the kidney. Cancer 1984, **54**: 2495–2499.

1454 Martin RF, Melnick PJ, Warner NE, Terry R, Bullock WK, Schwinn CP. Chordoid sarcoma. Am J Clin Pathol 1973, **59**: 623–635.

1455 Martinez-Tello FJ, Navas-Palacios JJ. Ultrastructural study of conventional chondrosarcomas and myxoid- and mesenchymal-chondrosarcoma. Virchows Arch [A] 1982, **396**: 197–211.

1456 Meis-Kindblom JM, Bergh P, Gunterberg B, Kindblom LG. Extraskeletal myxoid chondrosarcoma: a reappraisal of its morphologic spectrum and prognostic factors based on 117 cases. Am J Surg Pathol 1999, **23**: 636–650.

1457 Mirra JM, Fain JS, Ward WG, Eckardt JJ, Eilber F, Rosen G. Extraskeletal telangiectatic osteosarcoma. Cancer 1993, **71**: 3014–3019.

1458 Müller S, Söder S, Oliveira AM, Inwards CY, Aigner T. Type II collagen as specific marker for mesenchymal chondrosarcomas compared to other small cell sarcomas of the skeleton. Mod Pathol 2005, **18**: 1088–1094.

1459 Nakashima Y, Unni KK, Shives TC, Swee RG, Dahlin DC. Mesenchymal chondrosarcoma of bone and soft tissue. A review of 111 cases. Cancer 1986, **57**: 2444–2453.

1460 Oliveira AM, Sebo TJ, McGrory JE, Gaffey TA, Rock MG, Nascimento AG. Extraskeletal myxoid chondrosarcoma: a clinicopathologic, immunohistochemical, and ploidy analysis of 23 cases. Mod Pathol 2000, **13**: 900–908.

1461 Oshiro Y, Shiratsuchi H, Tamiy S, Oda Y, Toyoshima S, Tsuneyoshi M. Extraskeletal myxoid chondrosarcoma with rhabdoid features, with special reference to its aggressive behaviour. Int J Surg Pathol 2001, **8**: 145–152.

1462 Panagopoulos I, Mertens F, Isaksson M, Domanski HA, Brosjo O, Heim S, Bjerkehagen B, Sciot R, Dal Cin P, Fletcher JA, Fletcher CD, Mandahl N. Molecular genetic characterization of the EWS/CHN and RBP56/CHN fusion genes in extraskeletal myxoid chondrosarcoma. Genes Chromosomes Cancer 2002, **35**: 340–352.

1463 Payne C, Dardick I, Mackay B. Extraskeletal myxoid chondrosarcoma with intracisternal microtubules. Ultrastruct Pathol 1994, **18**: 257–261.

1464 Reid R, de Silva VC, Paterson L. Poorly differentiated extraskeletal myxoid chondrosarcoma with t(9;22)(q22;q11) translocation presenting initially as a solid variant devoid of myxoid areas. Int J Surg Pathol 2003, **11**: 137–141.

1465 Reiman HM, Dahlin DC. Cartilage- and bone-forming tumors of the soft tissues. Semin Diagn Pathol 1986, **3**: 288–305.

1466 Rubin BP, Fletcher JA. Skeletal and extraskeletal myxoid chondrosarcoma: related or distinct tumors? Adv Anat Pathol 1999, **6**: 204–212.

1467 Saleh G, Evans HL, Ro JY, Ayala AG. Extraskeletal myxoid chondrosarcoma. A clinicopathologic study of ten patients with long-term follow-up. Cancer 1992, **70**: 2827–2830.

1468 Sciot R, Dal Cin P, Fletcher C, Samson I, Smith M, De Vos R, Van Damme B, Van den Berghe H. t(9;22)(q22–31;q11–12) is a consistent marker of extraskeletal myxoid chondrosarcoma. Evaluation of three cases. Mod Pathol 1995, **8**: 765–768.

1469 Sjögren H, Meis-Kindblom JM, Örndal C, Bergh P, Ptaszynski K, Åman P, Kindblom L-G, Stenman G. Studies on the molecular pathogenesis of extraskeletal myxoid chondrosarcoma – cytogenetic, molecular genetic, and cDNA microarray analyses. Am J Pathol 2003, **162**: 781–792.

1470 Sordillo PP, Hajdu SI, Magill GB, Golbey RB. Extraosseous osteogenic sarcoma. A review of 48 patients. Cancer 1983, **51**: 727–734.

1471 Stout AP, Verner EW. Chondrosarcoma of the extraskeletal soft tissue. Cancer 1953, **6**: 581–590.

1472 Tsuneyoshi M, Enjoji M, Iwasaki H, Shinohara N. Extraskeletal myxoid chondrosarcoma. A clinicopathologic and electron microscopic study. Acta Pathol Jpn 1981, **31**: 439–447.

1473 Wang WL, Mayordomo E, Czerniak BA, Abruzzo LV, Dal Cin P, Araujo DM, Lev DC, López-Terrada D, Lazar AJ. Fluorescence in situ hybridization is a useful ancillary diagnostic tool for extraskeletal myxoid chondrosarcoma. Mod Pathol 2008, **21**: 1303–1310.

1474 Weiss SW. Ultrastructure of the so-called 'chordoid sarcoma'. Evidence supporting cartilaginous differentiation. Cancer 1976, **37**: 300–306.

1475 Wolford JF, Bedetti CI. Skeletal myxoid chondrosarcoma with microtubular aggregates within rough endoplasmic reticulin. Arch Pathol Lab Med 1988, **112**: 77–81.

1476 Wu KK, Collon DJ, Guise ER. Extra-osseous chondrosarcoma. Report of five cases and review of the literature. J Bone Joint Surg (Am) 1980, **62**: 189–194.

1477 Wu WQ, Lapi A. Primary non-skeletal intracranial cartilaginous neoplasm. Report of a chondroma and a mesenchymal chondrosarcoma. J Neurol Neurosurg Psychiatry 1970, **33**: 469–475.

1478 Yi ES, Shmookler BM, Malawer MM, Sweet DE. Well-differentiated extraskeletal osteosarcoma. A soft-tissue homologue of parosteal osteosarcoma. Arch Pathol Lab Med 1991, **115**: 906–909.

TUMORS RESEMBLING SYNOVIAL TISSUE

1479 Abenoza P, Manivel JC, Swanson PE, Wick MR. Synovial sarcoma. Ultrastructural study and immunohistochemical analysis by a combined peroxidase-antiperoxidase/avidin-biotin-peroxidase complex procedure. Hum Pathol 1986, **17**: 1107–1115.

1480 Al-Daraji W, Lasota J, Foss R, Miettinen M. Synovial sarcoma involving the head: analysis of 36 cases with predilection to the parotid and temporal regions. Am J Surg Pathol 2009, **33**: 1494–1503.

1481 Amary MF, Berisha F, Bernardi Fdel C, Herbert A, James M, Reis-Filho JS, Fisher C, Nicholson AG, Tirabosco R, Diss TC, Flanagan AM. Detection of SS18–SSX fusion transcripts in formalin-fixed paraffin-embedded neoplasms: analysis of conventional RT-PCR, qRT-PCR and dual color FISH as diagnostic tools for synovial sarcoma. Mod Pathol 2007, **20**: 482–496.

1482 Antonescu CR, Busam KJ, Iversen K, Kolb D, Coplan K, Spagnoli GC, Ladanyi M, Old LJ, Jungbluth AA. MAGE antigen expression in monophasic and biphasic synovial sarcoma. Hum Pathol 2002, **33**: 225–229.

1483 Antonescu CR, Kawai A, Leung DH, Lonardo F, Woodruff JM, Healey JH, Landanyi M. Strong association of SYT–SSX fusion type and morphologic epithelial differentiation in synovial sarcoma. Diagn Mol Pathol 2000, **9**: 1–8.

1484 Argani P, Zakowski MF, Klimstra DS, Rosai J, Ladanyi M. Detection of the SYT–SSX chimeric RNA of synovial sarcoma in paraffin-embedded tissue and its application in problematic cases. Mod Pathol 1998, **11**: 65–71.

1485 Batsakis JG, Nishiyama RH, Sullinger GD. Synovial sarcomas of the neck. Arch Otolaryngol 1967, **85**: 327–331.

1486 Billings SD, Walsh SV, Fisher C, Nusrat A, Weiss SW, Folpe AL. Aberrant expression of tight junction-related proteins ZO-1, claudin-1 and occludin in synovial sarcoma: an immunohistochemical study with ultrastructural correlation. Mod Pathol 2004, **17**: 141–149.

1487 Cagle LA, Mirra JM, Storm FK, Roe DJ, Eilber FR. Histologic features relating to prognosis in synovial sarcoma. Cancer 1987, **59**: 1810–1814.

1488 Chan JA, McMenamin ME, Fletcher CDM. Synovial sarcoma in older patients: clinicopathological analysis of 32 cases with emphasis on unusual histological features. Histopathology 2003, **43**: 72–83.

1489 Corson JM, Weiss LM, Banks-Schlegel SP, Pinkus GS. Keratin proteins and carcinoembryonic antigen in synovial sarcomas. An immunohistochemical study of 24 cases. Hum Pathol 1984, **15**: 615–621.

1490 Crocker EW, Stout AP. Synovial sarcoma in children. Cancer 1959, **12**: 1123–1133.

1491 Dardick I, Ramjohn S, Thomas MJ, Jeans D, Hammar SP. Synovial sarcoma. Pathol Res Pract 1991, **187**: 871–885.

1492 Dei Tos AP, Wadden C, Calonje E, Sciot R, Pauwels P, Knight JC, Dal Cin P, Fletcher CDM. Immunohistochemical demonstration of glycoprotein p30/32^{MIC2} (CD99) in synovial sarcoma. A potential cause of diagnostic confusion. Appl Immunohistochem 1995, **3**: 168–173.

1493 de Silva MVC, McMahon AD, Paterson L, Reid R. Identification of poorly differentiated synovial sarcoma: a comparison of clinicopathological and cytogenetic features with those of typical synovial sarcoma. Histopathology 2003, **443**: 220–230.

1494 Dickersin GR. Synovial sarcoma. A review and update, with emphasis on the ultrastructural characterization of the nonglandular component. Ultrastruct Pathol 1991, **15**: 379–402.

1495 Dische FE, Darby AJ, Howard ER. Malignant synovioma. Electron microscopical findings in three patients and review of the literature. J Pathol 1978, **124**: 149–155.

1496 el-Naggar AK, Ayala AG, Abdul-Karim FW, McLemore D, Ballance WW, Garnsey L, Ro JY, Batsakis JG. Synovial sarcoma. A DNA flow cytometric study. Cancer 1990, **65**: 2295–2300.

1497 Ferrari A, Gronchi A, Casanova M, Meazza C, Gandola L, Collini P, Lozza L, Bertulli R, Olmi P, Casali PG. Synovial sarcoma: a retrospective analysis of 271 patients of all ages treated at a single institution. Cancer 2004, **101**: 627–634.

1498 Fetsch JF, Meis JM. Synovial sarcoma of the abdominal wall. Cancer 1993, **72**: 469–477.

1499 Fisher C. Synovial sarcoma. Ultrastructural and immunohistochemical features of epithelial differentiation in monophasic and biphasic tumors. Hum Pathol 1986, **17**: 996–1008.

1500 Fisher C. Synovial sarcoma. Ann Diagn Pathol 1999, **2**: 401–421.

1501 Fisher C, Montgomery E, Healy V. Calponin and h-caldesmon expression in synovial sarcoma; the use of calponin in diagnosis. Histopathology 2003, **42**: 588–593.

1502 Fisher C, Schofield JB. S-100 protein positive synovial sarcoma. Histopathology 1991, **19**: 375–377.

1503 Fisher C, Folpe AL, Hashimoto H, Weiss SW. Intra-abdominal synovial sarcoma: a clinicopathological study. Histopathology 2004, **45**: 245–253.

1504 Folpe AL, Schmidt RA, Chapman D, Gown AM. Poorly differentiated synovial sarcoma: immunohistochemical distinction from primitive peripheral nerve sheath tumors. Am J Surg Pathol 1998, **22**: 673–682.

1505 Fritsch M, Epstein JI, Perlman EJ, Watts JC, Argani P. Molecularly confirmed primary prostatic synovial sarcoma. Hum Pathol 2000, **31**: 246–250.

1506 Ghadially FN. Is synovial sarcoma a carcinosarcoma of connective tissue? Ultrastruct Pathol 1987, **11**: 147–151.

1507 Guillou L, Benhattar J, Terrier P, Gallagher G, Jundt G, Stauffer E, de St Aubain N, Michels JJ, Ranchere VD, Bertrand G, Trassard M, Collin F, Coindre JM. SYT–SSX fusion type is not a prognostic factor in synovial sarcoma patients. A multi-institutional study of 182 cases [abstract]. Mod Pathol 2003, **16**: 13A.

1508 Guillou L, Coindre JM, Gallagher G, Terrier P, Gebhard S, de Saint Aubain Somerhausen NA, Michels J, Jundt G, Vince DR, Collin F, Trassard M, Le Doussai V, Benhattar J. Detection of the synovial sarcoma translocation t(X;18)(SYT;SSX) in paraffin-embedded tissues using transcriptase-polymerase chain reaction: a reliable and powerful diagnostic tool for pathologists: a molecular analysis of 221 mesenchymal tumors fixed in different fixatives. Hum Pathol 2001, **32**: 105–112.

1509 Guillou L, Wadden C, Kraus MD, Dei Tos AP, Fletcher CD. S-100 protein reactivity in synovial sarcomas – a potentially frequent diagnostic pitfall: immunohistochemical analysis of 100 cases. Appl Immunohistochem 1996, **4**: 167–175.

1510 Hartel PH, Fanburg-Smith JC, Frazier AA, Galvin JR, Lichy JH, Shilo K, Franks TJ. Primary pulmonary and mediastinal synovial sarcoma: a clinicopathologic study of 60 cases and comparison with five prior series. Mod Pathol 2007, **20**: 760–769.

1511 He R, Patel RM, Alkan S, Hammadeh R, Weiss SW, Goldblum JR, Venkataraman G, Baila H. Immunostaining for SYT protein discriminates synovial sarcoma from other soft tissue tumors: analysis of 146 cases. Mod Pathol 2007, **20**: 522–528.

1512 Ishida T, Kojima T, Iijima T, Oka T, Kuroda M, Horiuchi H, Imamura T, Machinami R. Synovial sarcoma with a predominant epithelial component. Int J Surg Pathol 1994, **1**: 261–268.

1513 Izumi T, Oda Y, Hasegawa T, Nakanishi Y, Kawai A, Sonobe H, Takahira T, Kobayashi C, Yamamoto H, Tamiya S, Hirohashi S, Iwamoto Y, Tsuneyoshi M. Dysadherin expression as a significant prognostic factor and as a determinant of histologic features in synovial sarcoma: special reference to its inverse relationship with E-cadherin expression. Am J Surg Pathol 2007, **31**: 85–94.

1514 Kawai A, Woodruff J, Healey JH, Brennan MF, Antonescu CR, Ladanyi M. SYT–SSX gene fusion as a determinant of morphology and prognosis in synovial sarcoma. N Engl J Med 1998, **338**: 153–160.

1515 Knosel Th, Heretsch S, Altendorf-Hofmann A, Richter P, Katenkamp K, Katenkamp D, Berndt A, Petersen I. Overexpression of TLE1 is a robust biomarker for synovial sarcomas and correlates with t(X;18): analysis of 373 cases. Lab Invest 2009, **89**(Suppl 1): 15A.

1516 Kosemehmetoglu K, Vrana JA, Folpe AL. TLE1 expression is not specific for synovial sarcoma: a standard section study of 155 soft tissue and bone neoplasms. Lab Invest 2009, **89**(Suppl 1): 16A.

1517 Krall RA, Kostianovsky M, Patchefsky AS. Synovial sarcoma. A clinical, pathological, ultrastructural study of 26 cases supporting the recognition of a monophasic variant. Am J Surg Pathol 1981, **5**: 137–151.

1518 Krane JF, Bertoni F, Fletcher CD. Myxoid synovial sarcoma: an underappreciated morphologic subset. Mod Pathol 1999, **12**: 456–462.

1519 Ladenstein R, Treuner J, Koscielniak E, d'Oleire F, Keim M, Gadner H, Jurgens H, Niethammer D, Ritter J, Schmidt D. Synovial sarcoma of childhood and adolescence. Report of the German CWS-81 study. Cancer 1993, **71**: 3647–3655.

1520 Leader M, Patel J, Collins M, Kristin H. Synovial sarcomas. True carcinosarcomas? Cancer 1987, **59**: 2096–2098.

1521 Lewis JJ, Antonescu CR, Leung DH, Blumberg D, Healey JH, Woodruff JM, Brennan MF. Synovial sarcoma: a multivariate analysis of prognostic factors in 112 patients with primary localized tumors of the extremity. J Clin Oncol 2000, **18**: 2087–2094.

1522 Lombardi L, Rilke F. Ultrastructural similarities and differences of synovial sarcoma, epithelioid sarcoma, and clear cell sarcoma of the tendons and aponeuroses. Ultrastruct Pathol 1984, **6**: 209–219.

1523 Lopes JM, Bjerkehagen B, Holm R, Bruland O, Sobrinho-Simoes M, Nesland JM. Immunohistochemical profile of synovial sarcoma with emphasis on the epithelial-type differentiation. A study of 49 primary tumours, recurrences and metastases. Pathol Res Pract 1994, **190**: 168–177.

1524 Lopes JM, Bjerkehagen B, Sobrinho-Simoes M, Nesland JM. The ultrastructural spectrum of synovial sarcomas. A study of the epithelial type differentiation of primary tumors, recurrences, and metastases. Ultrastruct Pathol 1993, **17**: 137–151.

1525 Lopes JM, Nesland JM, Reis-Filho JS, Holm R. Differential Ki67 and bcl-2 immunoexpression in solid-glandular and spindle cell components of biphasic synovial sarcoma: a double immunostaining assessment with cytokeratin and vimentin. Histopathology 2002, **40**: 464–471.

1526 Mackenzie DH. Synovial sarcoma. A review of 58 cases. Cancer 1966, **19**: 169–180.

1527 Mackenzie DH. Monophasic synovial sarcoma – a histological entity? Histopathology 1977, **1**: 151–157.

1528 Majeste RM, Beckman EN. Synovial sarcoma with an overwhelming epithelial component. Cancer 1988, **61**: 2527–2531.

1529 Makhlouf HR, Ahrens W, Agarwal B, Dow N, Marshalleck JJ, Lee EL, Dotto JE, Hui P, Sobin LH, Oliveira A, Miettinen M. Synovial sarcoma of the stomach: a clinicopathologic, immunohistochemical, and molecular genetic study of 10 cases. Am J Surg Pathol 2008, **32**: 275–281.

1530 Michal M, Fanburg-Smith JC, Lasota J, Fetsch JF, Lichy J, Miettinen M. Minute synovial sarcomas of the hands and feet: a clinicopathologic study of 21 tumors less than 1 cm. Am J Surg Pathol 2006, **30**: 721–726.

1531 Miettinen M. Keratin subsets in spindle cell sarcomas. Keratins are widespread but synovial sarcoma contains a distinctive keratin polypeptide pattern and desmoplakins. Am J Pathol 1991, **138**: 505–513.

1532 Miettinen M, Lehto V-P, Virtanen I. Monophasic synovial sarcoma of spindle cell type. Virchows Arch [A] 1983, **44**: 187–199.

1533 Miettinen M, Limom J, Niezabitowski A, Lasota J. Calretinin and other mesothelioma markers in synovial sarcoma: analysis of antigenic similarities and differences with malignant mesothelioma. Am J Surg Pathol 2001, **25**: 610–617.

1534 Miettinen M, Santavirta S, Släts P. Intravascular synovial sarcoma. Hum Pathol 1987, **18**: 1075–1077.

1535 Miettinen M, Virtanen I. Synovial sarcoma – a misnomer. Am J Pathol 1984, **117**: 18–25.

1536 Milchgrub S, Ghandur-Mnaymneh L, Dorfman HD, Albores-Saavedra J. Synovial sarcoma with extensive osteoid and bone formation. Am J Surg Pathol 1993, **17**: 357–363.

1537 Mirra JM, Wang S, Bhuta S. Synovial sarcoma with squamous differentiation of its mesenchymal glandular elements. A case report with light-microscopic, ultramicroscopic, and immunologic correlation. Am J Surg Pathol 1984, **8**: 791–796.

1538 Moberger G, Nilsonne U, Friberg S Jr. Synovial sarcoma. Histologic features and prognosis. Acta Orthop Scand (Suppl) 1968, **3**: 1–38.

1539 Nagao K, Ito H, Yoshida H. Chromosomal translocation t(X;18) in human synovial sarcomas analysed by fluorescence in situ hybridisation using paraffin-embedded tissue. Am J Pathol 1996, **148**: 601–609.

1540 Nakamura T, Nakata K, Hata S, Ono K, Katsuyama T. Histochemical characterization of mucosubstances in synovial sarcoma. Am J Surg Pathol 1984, **8**: 429–434.

1541 O'Connell JX, Browne WL, Groppr PT, Berean KW. Intraneural biphasic synovial sarcoma: an alternative 'glandular' tumor of peripheral nerve. Mod Pathol 1997, **9**: 738–741.

1542 Nuciforo PG, Pellegrini C, Fasani R, Maggioni M, Coggi G, Parafioriti A, Bosari S. Molecular and immunohistochemical analysis of HER2/neu oncogene in synovial sarcoma. Hum Pathol 2003, **34**: 639–645.

1543 Oda Y, Hashimoto H, Tsuneyoshi M, Takeshita S. Survival in synovial sarcoma. A multivariate study of prognostic factors with special emphasis on the comparison between early death and long-term survival. Am J Surg Pathol 1993, **17**: 35–44.

1544 Ordóñez NG, Mahfouz SM, Mackay B. Synovial sarcoma. An immunohistochemical and ultrastructural study. Hum Pathol 1990, **21**: 733–749.

1545 Pappo AS, Fontanesi J, Luo X, Rao BN, Parham DM, Hurwitz C, Avery L, Pratt CB. Synovial sarcoma in children and adolescents. The St Jude Children's Research Hospital experience. J Clin Oncol 1994, **12**: 2360–2366.

1546 Pelmus M, Guillou L, Hostein I, Sierankowski G, Lussan C, Coindre JM. Monophasic fibrous and poorly differentiated synovial sarcoma: immunohistochemical reassessment of 60 t(X;18)(SYT-SSX)-positive cases. Am J Surg Pathol 2002, **26**: 1434–1440.

1547 Pinkus GS, Kurtin PJ. Epithelial membrane antigen – a diagnostic discriminant in surgical pathology. Immunohistochemical profile in epithelial, mesenchymal, and hematopoietic neoplasms using paraffin sections and monoclonal antibodies. Hum Pathol 1985, **16**: 929–940.

1548 Rooser B, Willén H, Hugoson A, Rydholm A. Prognostic factors in synovial sarcoma. Cancer 1989, **63**: 2182–2185.

1549 Roth JA, Enzinger FM, Tannenbaum M. Synovial sarcoma of the neck. A follow-up study of 24 cases. Cancer 1975, **35**: 1243–1253.

1550 Salisbury JR, Isaacson PG. Synovial sarcoma. An immunohistochemical study. J Pathol 1985, **147**: 49–57.

1551 Sandberg AA, Bridge JA. Updates on the cytogenetics and molecular genetics of bone soft tissue tumors. Synovial sarcoma. Cancer Genet Cytogenet 2002, **133**: 1–23.

1552 Schiffman R. Epithelioid sarcoma and synovial sarcoma in the same knee. Cancer 1980, **45**: 158–166.

1553 Schreiber-Facklam H, Bode-Lesniewska B, Frigerio S, Flury R. Primary monophasic synovial sarcoma of the duodenum with SYT/SSX2 type of translocation. Hum Pathol 2007, **38**: 946–949.

1554 Shaw GR, Lais CJ. Fatal intravascular synovial sarcoma in a 31-year-old woman. Hum Pathol 1993, **24**: 809–810.

1555 Somers GR, Zielenska M, Abdullah S, Sherman C, Chan S, Thorner PS. Expression of MYCN in pediatric synovial sarcoma. Mod Pathol 2007, **20**: 734–741.

1556 Shipley J, Crew J, Birdsall S, Gill S, Clark J, Fisher C, Kelsey A, Nojima T, Sonobe H, Cooper C, Gusterson B. Interphase fluorescence in situ hybridization and reverse transcription polymerase chain reaction as a diagnostic aid for synovial sarcoma. Am J Pathol 1996, **148**: 559–567.

1557 Shmookler BM. Retroperitoneal synovial sarcoma. Am J Clin Pathol 1982, **77**: 686–691.

1558 Shmookler BM, Enzinger FM, Brannon RB. Orofacial synovial sarcoma: a clinicopathologic study of 11 new cases and review of the literature. Cancer 1982, **50**: 269–272.

1559 Singer S, Baldini EH, Demetri GD, Fletcher JA, Corson JM. Synovial sarcoma: prognostic significance of tumor size, margin of resection, and mitotic activity for survival. J Clin Oncol 1996, **14**: 1201–1208.

1560 Soule EH. Synovial sarcoma. Am J Surg Pathol 1986, **10**(Suppl 1): 78–82.

1561 Suit HD, Russell WO, Martin RG. Management of patients with sarcoma of soft tissue in an extremity. Cancer 1973, **31**: 1247–1255.

1562 Suster S, Moran CA. Primary synovial sarcomas of the mediastinum: a clinicopathologic, immunohistochemical, and ultrastructural study of 15 cases. Am J Surg Pathol 2005, **29**: 569–578.

1563 ten Heuvel SE, Hoekstra HJ, Suurmeijer AJ. Diagnostic accuracy of FISH and RT-PCR in 50 routinely processed synovial sarcomas. Appl Immunohistochem Mol Morphol 2008, **16**: 246–250.

1564 ten Heuvel SE, Hoekstra HJ, Bastiaannet E, Suurmeijer AJ. The classic prognostic factors tumor stage, tumor size, and tumor grade are the strongest predictors of outcome in synovial sarcoma: no role for SSX fusion type or ezrin expression. Appl Immunohistochem Mol Morphol 2009, **17**: 189–195.

1565 Terry J, Saito T, Subramanian S, Ruttan C, Antonescu CR, Goldblum JR, Downs-Kelly E, Corless CL, Rubin BP, van de Rijn M, Ladanyi M, Nielsen TO. TLE1 as a diagnostic immunohistochemical marker for synovial sarcoma emerging from gene expression profiling studies. Am J Surg Pathol 2007, **31**: 240–246.

1566 Trassard M, Le Doussal V, Hacène K, Terrier P, Ranchère D, Guillou L, Fiche M, Collin F, Vilain MO, Bertrand G, Jacquemier J, Sastre-Garau X, Bui NB, Bonichon F, Coindre JM. Prognostic factors in localized primary synovial sarcoma: a multicenter study of 128 adult patients. J Clin Oncol 2001, **19**: 525–534.

1567 Tsuneyoshi M, Yokoyama K, Enjoji M. Synovial sarcoma. A clinicopathologic and ultrastructural study of 42 cases. Acta Pathol Jpn 1983, **33**: 23–36.

1568 van Andel JG. Synovial sarcoma. A review and analysis of treated cases. Radiol Clin Biol 1972, **41**: 145–159.

1569 van de Rijn M, Barr FG, Xiong QB, Hedges M, Shipley J, Fisher C. Poorly differentiated synovial sarcoma: an analysis of clinical, pathologic, and molecular genetic features. Am J Surg Pathol 1999, **23**: 106–112.

1570 Varela-Duran J, Enzinger FM. Calcifying synovial sarcoma. A clinicopathologic study of 32 cases. Cancer 1982, **50**: 345–352.

1571 White BE, Kaplan A, Lopez-Terrada DH, Ro JY, Benjamin RS, Ayala AG. Monophasic synovial sarcoma arising in the vulva: a case report and review of the literature. Arch Pathol Lab Med 2008, **132**: 698–702.

1572 Witkin GB, Rosai J. A biphasic tumor of the mediastinum with features of synovial sarcoma. A report of 4 cases [abstract]. Lab Invest 1988, **58**: 104A.

1573 Wright PH, Sim EH, Soule EH, Taylor WF. Synovial sarcoma. J Bone Joint Surg (Am) 1982, **64**: 112–122.

1574 Zeren H, Moran CA, Suster S, Fishback NF, Koss MN. Primary pulmonary sarcomas with features of monophasic synovial sarcoma: a clinicopathological, immunohistochemical, and ultrastructural study of 25 cases. Hum Pathol 1995, **26**: 474–480.

TUMORS OF EXTRAGONADAL GERM CELLS

1575 Berry CL, Keelnig J, Hilton C. Teratoma in infancy and childhood. A review of 91 cases. J Pathol 1969, **98**: 241–252.

1576 Billmire DF, Grosfeld JL. Teratomas in childhood. Analysis of 142 cases. J Pediatr Surg 1986, **21**: 548–551.

1577 Colton JJ, Batsakis JG, Work WP. Teratomas of the neck in adults. Arch Otolaryngol 1978, **104**: 271–272.

1578 Conklin J, Abell MR. Germ cell neoplasms of sacrococcygeal region. Cancer 1967, **20**: 2105–2117.

1579 Dehner LP. Intrarenal teratoma occurring in infancy. Report of a case with discussion of extragonadal germ cell tumors in infancy. J Pediatr Surg 1973, **8**: 369–378.

1580 Dehner LP, Mills A, Talerman A, Billman GF, Krous HF, Platz CE. Germ cell neoplasms of head and neck soft tissues. A pathologic spectrum of teratomatous and endodermal sinus tumors. Hum Pathol 1990, **21**: 309–318.

1581 Gonzalez-Crussi F, Winkler RF, Mirkin DL. Sacrococcygeal teratomas in infants and children. Relationship of histology and prognosis in 40 cases. Arch Pathol Lab Med 1978, **102**: 420–425.

1582 Heerema-McKenney A, Harrison MR, Bratton B, Farrell J, Zaloudek C. Congenital teratoma: a clinicopathologic study of 22 fetal and neonatal tumors. Am J Surg Pathol 2005, **29**: 29–38.

1583 Mochizuki Y, Noguchi S, Yokoyama S, Murakami N, Moriuchi A, Aisaka K, Yamashita H, Nakayama I. Cervical teratoma in a fetus and an adult. Two case reports and review of literature. Acta Pathol Jpn 1986, **36**: 935–943.

1584 Tapper D, Lack EE. Teratomas in infancy and childhood. A 54-year experience at the Children's Hospital Medical Center. Ann Surg 1983, **198**: 398–410.

1585 Willis RA. Pathology of tumors, ed. 4. London, 1968, Butterworth.

TUMORS OF NEURAL TISSUE (OTHER THAN PERIPHERAL NERVES)

Pigmented neuroectodermal tumor of infancy

1586 Argenyi ZB, Schelper RL, Balogh K. Pigmented neuroectodermal tumor of infancy. A light microscopic and immunohistochemical study. J Cutan Pathol 1991, **18**: 40–45.

1587 Borello ED, Gorlin RH. Melanotic neuroectodermal tumor of infancy – a neoplasm of neural crest origin. Report of a case associated with high urinary excretion of vanilmandelic acid. Cancer 1966, **19**: 196–206.

1588 Dehner LP, Sibley RK, Sauk JJ Jr, Vickers RA, Nesbit ME, Leonard AS, Waite DE, Neeley JE, Ophoven J. Malignant melanotic neuroectodermal tumor of infancy. A clinical, pathologic, ultrastructural and tissue culture study. Cancer 1979, **43**: 1389–1410.

1589 Johnson RE, Scheithauer BW, Dahlin DC. Melanotic neuroectodermal tumor of infancy. A review of seven cases. Cancer 1983, **52**: 661–666.

1590 Koudstaal J, Oldhoff J, Panders AK, Hardonk MJ. Melanotic neuroectodermal tumor of infancy. Cancer 1968, **22**: 151–161.

1591 Neustein HB. Fine structure of a melanotic progonoma or retinal anlage tumor of the anterior fontanel. Exp Mol Pathol 1967, **6**: 131–142.

1592 Pettinato G, Manivel JC, d'Amore ES, Jaszez W, Gorlin RJ. Melanotic neuroectodermal tumor of infancy. A reexamination of a histogenetic problem based on immunohistochemical, flow cytometric, and ultrastructural study of 10 cases. Am J Surg Pathol 1991, **15**: 233–245.

1593 Raju U, Zarbo R, Regezi J, Krutchkoff D, Perrin E. Melanotic, neuroectodermal tumors of infancy. Intermediate filament-, neuroendocrine-, and melanoma-associated antigen profiles. Appl Immunohistochem 1993, **1**: 69–76.

1594 Scheck O, Ruck P, Harms D, Kaiserling E. Melanotic neuroectodermal tumor of infancy occurring in the left thigh of a 6-month-old female infant. Ultrastruct Pathol 1989, **13**: 23–33.

1595 Stirling RW, Powell G, Fletcher CD. Pigmented neuroectodermal tumour of infancy. An immunohistochemical study. Histopathology 1988, **12**: 425–435.

1596 Young S, Gonzalez-Crussi F. Melanocytic neuroectodermal tumor of the foot. Report of a case with multicentric origin. Am J Clin Pathol 1985, **84**: 371–378.

Other neural tumors

1597 Anderson MS. Myxopapillary ependymomas presenting in the soft tissue over the sacrococcygeal region. Cancer 1966, **19**: 585–590.

1598 Bain GO, Shnitka TK. Cutaneous meningioma (psammoma). Arch Dermatol 1956, **74**: 590–594.

1599 Helwig EB, Stern JB. Subcutaneous sacrococcygeal myxopapillary ependymoma. A clinicopathologic study of 32 cases. Am J Clin Pathol 1984, **81**: 156–161.

1600 King P, Cooper PN, Malcolm AJ. Soft tissue ependymoma. A report of three cases. Histopathology 1993, **22**: 394–396.

1601 Lopez DA, Silvers DN, Helwig EB. Cutaneous meningiomas – a clinicopathologic study. Cancer 1974, **34**: 728–744.

1602 McDermott MB, Glasner SD, Nielsen PL, Dehner LP. Soft tissue gliomatosis: morphologic unity and histogenetic diversity. Am J Surg Pathol 1996, **20**: 148–155.

1603 Pulitzer DR, Martin PC, Collins PC, Ralph DR. Subcutaneous sacrococcygeal ('myxopapillary') ependymal rests. Am J Surg Pathol 1988, **12**: 672–677.

1604 Shepherd NA, Coates PJ, Brown AA. Soft tissue gliomatosis – heterotopic glial tissue in the subcutis. A case report. Histopathology 1987, **11**: 655–660.

TUMORS OF HEMATOPOIETIC TISSUE

1605 Abbondanzo SL, Devaney K. Hodgkin's disease involving bone and adjacent soft tissue in adults: a clinicopathologic and immunophenotypic study of seven cases. Int J Surg Pathol 1996, **3**: 147–154.

1606 Akosa AB, Ali MH. Extramedullary plasmacytoma of skeletal muscle. A case report with immunocytochemistry and ultrastructural study. Cancer 1989, **64**: 1504–1507.

1607 Axiotis CA, Fuks J, Jennings TA, Kadish AS. Peripheral T-cell lymphoma presenting as a soft-tissue mass of the extremity. Arch Pathol Lab Med 1988, **112**: 850–851.

1608 Condon WB, Safarik LR, Elzi EP. Extramedullary hematopoiesis simulating intrathoracic tumor. Arch Surg 1965, **90**: 643–648.

1609 d'Amore ES, Wick MR, Geisinger KR, Frizzera G. Primary malignant lymphoma arising in postmastectomy lymphedema. Another facet of the Stewart–Treves syndrome. Am J Surg Pathol 1990, **14**: 456–463.

1610 Hornick JL, Jaffe ES, Fletcher CD. Extranodal histiocytic sarcoma: clinicopathologic analysis of 14 cases of a rare epithelioid malignancy. Am J Surg Pathol 2004, **28**: 1133–1144.

1611 Ko YH, Cho E-Y, Kim J-E, Lee S-S, Huh J-R, Chang H-K, Yang W-I, Kim C-W, Kim S-W, Ree HJ. NK and NK-like T-cell lymphoma in extranasal sites: a comparative clinicopathological study according to site and EBV status. Histopathology 2004, **44**: 480–489.

1612 Lanham GR, Weiss SW, Enzinger FM. Malignant lymphoma. A study of 75 cases presenting in soft tissue. Am J Surg Pathol 1989, **13**: 1–10.

1613 Salamao DR, Nascimento AG, Lloyd RV, Chen MG, Habermann TM, Strickler JG. Lymphoma in soft tissue: a clinicopathologic study of 19 cases. Hum Pathol 1996, **27**: 253–257.

1614 Travis WD, Banks FM, Reiman HM. Primary extranodal soft tissue lymphoma of the extremities. Am J Surg Pathol 1987, **11**: 359–366.

TUMORS OF UNCERTAIN CELL TYPE

Fibrous hamartoma of infancy

1615 Enzinger FM. Fibrous hamartoma of infancy. Cancer 1965, **18**: 241–248.

1616 Fletcher CDM, Powell G, Van Noorden S, McKee PH. Fibrous hamartoma of infancy. A histochemical and immunohistochemical study. Histopathology 1988, **12**: 65–74.

1617 Groisman G, Lichtig C. Fibrous hamartoma of infancy. Am immunohistochemical and ultrastructural study. Hum Pathol 1991, **22**: 914–918.

1618 Maung R, Lindsay R, Trevenen C, Hwang WS. Fibrous hamartoma of infancy. Hum Pathol 1987, **18**: 652–653.

1619 Michal M, Mukensnabl P, Chlumska A, Kodet R. Fibrous hamartoma of infancy. A study of eight cases with immunohistochemical and electron microscopical findings. Pathol Res Pract 1992, **188**: 1049–1053.

Myxoma and related tumors

1620 Al-Daraji WI, Miettinen M. Superficial acral fibromyxoma: a clinicopathological analysis of 32 tumors including 4 in the heel. J Cutan Pathol 2008, **35**: 1020–1026.

1621 Allen PW, Dymock RB, MacCormac LB. Superficial angiomyxomas with and without epithelial components. Report of 30 tumors in 28 patients. Am J Surg Pathol 1988, **12**: 519–530.

1622 Calonje E, Guerin D, McCormick D, Fletcher CD. Superficial angiomyxoma: clinicopathologic analysis of a series of distinctive but poorly recognized cutaneous tumors with tendency for recurrence. Am J Surg Pathol 1999, **23**: 910–917.

1623 Carney JA, Gordon H, Carpenter PC, Shenoy BV, Go VLW. The complex of myxomas, spotty pigmentation, and endocrine overactivity. Medicine 1985, **64**: 270–283.

1624 Enzinger FM. Intramuscular myxoma. A review and follow-up study of 34 cases. Am J Clin Pathol 1965, **43**: 104–113.

1625 Feldman PS. A comparative study including ultrastructure of intramuscular myxoma and myxoid liposarcoma. Cancer 1979, **43**: 512–525.

1626 Hashimoto H, Tsuneyoshi M, Daimaru Y, Enjoji M, Shinohara N. Intramuscular myxoma. A clinicopathologic, immunohistochemical, and electron microscopic study. Cancer 1986, **58**: 740–747.

1627 Ireland DCR, Soule EH, Ivins JC. Myxoma of somatic soft tissues. A report of 58 patients, 3 with multiple tumors and fibrous dysplasia of bone. Mayo Clin Proc 1973, **48**: 401–410.

1628 Johnson WC, Helwig EB. Cutaneous focal mucinosis. A clinicopathological and histochemical study. Arch Dermatol 1966, **93**: 13–20.

1629 Luzar B, Calonje E. Superficial acral fibromyxoma: clinicopathological study of 14 cases with emphasis on a cellular variant. Histopathology 2009, **54**: 375–377.

1630 Mackenzie DH. The myxoid tumors of somatic soft tissues. Am J Surg Pathol 1981, **5**: 443–458.

1631 Meis JM, Enzinger FM. Juxta-articular myxoma. A clinical and pathologic study of 65 cases. Hum Pathol 1992, **23**: 639–646.

1632 Miettinen M, Hockerstedt K, Reitamo J, Totterman S. Intramuscular myxoma. A clinicopathological study of twenty-three cases. Am J Clin Pathol 1985, **84**: 265–272.

1633 Nielsen GP, O'Connell JX, Rosenberg AE. Intramuscular myxoma: a clinicopathologic study of 51 cases with emphasis on hypercellular and hypervascular variants. Am J Surg Pathol 1998, **22**: 1222–1227.

1634 Okamoto S, Hisaoka M, Ushijima M, Nakahara S, Toyoshima S, Hashimoto H. Activating Gs(alpha) mutation in intramuscular myxomas with and without fibrous dysplasia of bone. Virchows Arch 2000, **437**: 133–137.

1635 van Roggen JFG, McMenamin ME, Fletcher CD. Cellular myxoma of soft tissue: a clinicopathological study of 38 cases confirming indolent clinical behaviour. Histopathology 2001, **39**: 287–297.

1636 Willems SM, Mohseny AB, Balog C, Sewrajsing R, Briaire-de Bruijn IH, Knijnenburg J, Cleton-Jansen AM, Sciot R, Fletcher CD, Deelder AM, Szuhai K, Hensbergen PJ, Hogendoorn PC. Cellular/intramuscular myxoma and grade I myxofibrosarcoma are characterized by distinct genetic alterations and specific composition of their extracellular matrix. J Cell Mol Med 2009, **13**: 1291–1301.

1637 Wirth WA, Leavitt D, Enzinger FM. Multiple intramuscular myxomas. Another extraskeletal manifestation of fibrous dysplasia. Cancer 1971, **27**: 1167–1173.

Granular cell tumor

1638 Al-Sarraf M, Loud AV, Vaitkevicius VK. Malignant granular cell tumor. Histochemical and electron microscopic study. Arch Pathol 1971, **91**: 550–558.

1639 Bedetti CD, Martinez AJ, Beckford NS, May M. Granular cell tumor arising in myelinated peripheral nerves. Light and electron microscopy and immunoperoxidase study. Virchows Arch [A] 1983, **402**: 175–183.

1640 Bhawan J, Malhotra R, Naik DR. Gaucher-like cells in a granular cell tumor. Hum Pathol 1983, **14**: 730–733.

1641 Budzilovich GN. Granular cell 'myoblastoma' of vagus nerve. Acta Neuropathol 1968, **10**: 162–169.

1642 Chandrasoma P, Fitzgibbons P. Granular cell tumor of the intrapancreatic common bile duct. Cancer 1984, **53**: 2178–2182.

1643 Chaudhry IH, Calonje E. Dermal non-neural granular cell tumour (so-called primitive polypoid granular cell tumour): a distinctive entity further delineated in a clinicopathological study of 11 cases. Histopathology 2005, **47**: 179–185.

1644 Christ ML, Ozzello L. Myogenous origin of a granular cell tumor of the urinary bladder. Am J Clin Pathol 1971, **56**: 736–749.

1645 Clark HB, Minesky JJ, Agrawal D, Agrawal HC. Myelin basic protein and P2 protein are not immunohistochemical markers for Schwann cell neoplasms. A comparative study using antisera to S-100, P2, and myelin basic proteins. Am J Pathol 1985, **121**: 96–101.

1646 Copas P, Dyer M, Hall DJ, Diddle AW. Granular cell myoblastoma of the uterine cervix. Diagn Gynecol Obstet 1981, **3**: 251–254.

1647 Cserni G, Bori R, Sejben I. Vascular invasion demonstrated by elastic stain – a common phenomenon in benign granular cell tumors. Virchows Arch 2009, **454**: 211–215.

1648 de la Monte SM, Radowsky M, Hood AF. Congenital granular-cell neoplasms. An unusual case report with ultrastructural

1750 Ohno T, Park P, Utsunomiya Y, Hirahata H Inoue K. Ultrastructural study of a clear cell sarcoma suggesting Schwannian differentiation. Ultrastruct Pathol 1986, **10** 39–48.

1751 Pavlidis NA, Fisher C, Wiltshaw E. Clear-ce sarcoma of tendons and aponeuroses. A clinicopathologic study. Presentation of six additional cases with review of the literatu Cancer 1984, **54**: 1412–1417.

1752 Sandberg AA, Bridge JA. Updates on the cytogenetics and molecular genetics of bon soft tissue tumors: clear cell sarcoma (malignant melanoma soft parts). Cancer Genet Cytogenet 2001, **130**: 1–7.

1753 Sara AS, Evans HL, Benjamin RS. Malignan melanoma of soft parts (clear cell sarcoma A study of 17 cases, with emphasis on prognostic factors. Cancer 1990, **65**: 367–374.

1754 Saw D, Tse CH, Chan J, Watt CY, Ng CS, Poon YF. Clear cell sarcoma of the penis. Hum Pathol 1986, **17**: 423–425.

1755 Swanson PE, Wick MR. Clear cell sarcoma. An immunohistochemical analysis of six cases and comparison with other epithelioi neoplasms of soft tissue. Arch Pathol Lab Med 1989, **113**: 55–60.

1756 Tsuneyoshi M, Enjoji M, Kubo T. Clear cell sarcoma of tendons and aponeuroses. A comparative study of 13 cases with a provisional subgrouping into the melanoti and synovial types. Cancer 1978, **42**: 243–252.

1757 Zambrano E, Reyes-Mugica M, Franchi A, Rosai J. An osteoclast-rich tumor of the gastrointestinal tract with features resembli clear cell sarcoma of parts: reports of six ca of a GIST simulator. Int J Surg Pathol 2003, **11**: 75–81.

1758 Zambrano E, Reyes-Mugica M, Franchi A, Rosai J. An osteoclast-rich tumor of the gastrointestinal tract with features resembli clear cell sarcoma of soft parts: reports of 6 cases of a GIST simulator. Int J Surg Pathol 2003, **11**: 75–81.

Epithelioid sarcoma

1759 Arber DA, Kandalaft PL, Mehta P, Battifora Vimentin-negative epithelioid sarcoma. The value of an immunohistochemical panel th includes CD34. Am J Surg Pathol 1993, **17**: 302–307.

1760 Bryan RS, Soule EH, Dobyns JH, Pritchard I Linscheid RL. Primary epithelioid sarcoma the hand and forearm. J Bone Joint Surg (Am) 1974, **56**: 458–465.

1761 Chase DR, Enzinger FM. Epithelioid sarcom Diagnosis, prognostic indicators, and treatment. Am J Surg Pathol 1985, **9**: 241–263.

1762 Chase DR, Enzinger FM, Weiss SW, Langlos JM. Keratin in epithelioid sarcoma. An immunohistochemical study. Am J Surg Pathol 1984, **8**: 435–441.

1763 Chase DR, Enzinger FM, Weiss SW, Langlos JM. Coexpression of keratin and vimentin i epithelioid sarcoma. Am J Surg Pathol 1985 **9**: 460–463.

1764 Chbani L, Guillou L, Terrier P, Decouvelaere AV, Grégoire F, Terrier-Lacombe MJ, Ranchère D, Robin YM, Collin F, Fréneaux I Coindre JM. Epithelioid sarcoma: a clinicopathologic and immunohistochemica analysis of 106 cases from the French sarcoma group. Am J Clin Pathol 2009, **131** 222–227.

1765 Chetty R, Slavin JL. Epithelioid sarcoma wit extensive chondroid differentiation. Histopathology 1994, **24**: 400–401.

findings and a review of the literature. Am J Dermatopathol 1986, **8**: 57–63.

1649 Demay RM, Kay S. Granular cell tumor of the breast. Pathol Annu 1984, **19**(Pt 2): 121–148.

1650 Dimosthenous K, Righi A. Granular cell tumor of the parotid gland: an exceptionally rare occurrence. Int J Surg Pathol 2008, **16**: 213–214.

1651 Fanburg-Smith JC, Meis-Kindblom JM, Fante R, Kindblom LG. Malignant granular cell tumor of soft tissue: diagnostic criteria and clinicopathologic correlation. Am J Surg Pathol 1998, **22**: 779–794.

1652 Fine SW, Li M. Expression of calretinin and the alpha-subunit of inhibin in granular cell tumors. Am J Clin Pathol 2003, **119**: 259–264.

1653 Finkel G, Lane B. Granular cell variant of neurofibromatosis. Ultrastructure of benign and malignant tumors. Hum Pathol 1982, **13**: 959–963.

1654 Fisher ER, Wechsler H. Granular cell myoblastoma – a misnomer. Electron microscopic and histochemical evidence concerning its Schwann cell derivation and nature (granular cell schwannoma). Cancer 1962, **15**: 936–957.

1655 Garancis JC, Komorowski RA, Kuzma JF. Granular cell myoblastoma. Cancer 1970, **25**: 542–550.

1656 Habeeb AA, Salama S. Primitive nonneural granular cell tumor (so-called atypical polypoid granular cell tumor). Report of 2 cases with immunohistochemical and ultrastructural correlation. Am J Dermatopathol 2008, **30**: 156–159.

1657 Hoshi N, Sugino T, Suzuki T. Regular expression of osteopontin in granular cell tumor: distinctive feature among Schwannian cell tumors. Pathol Int 2005, **55**: 484–490.

1658 Johnston J, Helwig EB. Granular cell tumours of the gastrointestinal tract and perianal region. A study of 74 cases. Dig Dis Sci 1981, **26**: 807–816.

1659 Lack EE, Worsham GF, Callihan MD, Crawford BE, Klappenbach S, Rowden G, Chun B. Granular cell tumor. A clinicopathologic study of 110 patients. J Surg Oncol 1980, **13**: 301–316.

1660 Lack EE, Worsham GF, Callihan MD, Crawford BE, Vawter GF. Gingival granular cell tumors of the newborn (congenital 'epulis'). A clinical and pathologic study of 21 patients. Am J Surg Pathol 1981, **5**: 37–46.

1661 Le BH, Boyer PJ, Lewis JE, Kapadia SB. Granular cell tumor: immunohistochemical assessment of inhibin-alpha, protein gene product 9.5, S100 protein, CD68, and Ki-67 proliferative index with clinical correlation. Arch Pathol Lab Med 2004, **128**: 771–775.

1662 Le Boit PE, Barr RJ, Burall S, Metcalf JS, Yen TS, Wick MR. Primitive polypoid granular-cell tumor and other cutaneous granular-cell neoplasms of apparent nonneural origin. Am J Surg Pathol 1991, **15**: 48–58.

1663 Lifshitz MS, Flotte TJ, Greco MA. Congenital granular cell epulis. Immunohistochemical and ultrastructural observations. Cancer 1984, **53**: 1845–1848.

1664 Matthews JB, Mason GI. Granular cell myoblastoma. An immunoperoxidase study using a variety of antisera to human carcinoembryonic antigen. Histopathology 1983, **7**: 77–82.

1665 Mazur MT, Shultz JJ, Myers JL. Granular cell tumor. Immunohistochemical analysis of 21 benign tumors and one malignant tumor. Arch Pathol Lab Med 1990, **114**: 692–696.

1666 McMahon JN, Rigby HS, Davies JD. Elastosis in granular cell tumours. Prevalence and distribution. Histopathology 1990, **16**: 37–41.

1667 McWilliam LJ, Harris M. Granular cell angiosarcoma of the skin. Histology, electron microscopy and immunohistochemistry of a newly recognized tumor. Histopathology 1985, **9**: 1205–1216.

1668 Miettinen M, Lehtonen E, Lehtola H, Ekblom P, Lehto V, Virtanen I. Histogenesis of granular cell tumor. An immunohistochemical and ultrastructural study. J Pathol 1984, **142**: 221–229.

1669 Mitomi H, Matsumoto Y, Mori A, Arai N, Ishii K, Tanabe S, Kobayashi K, Sada M, Mieno H. Multifocal granular cell tumors of the gastrointestinal tract: immunohistochemical findings compared with those of solitary tumors. Pathol Int 2004, **54**: 47–51.

1670 Mittal KR, True LD. Origin of granules in granular cell tumor. Intracellular myelin formation with autodigestion. Arch Pathol Lab Med 1988, **112**: 302–303.

1671 Moscovic EA, Azar HA. Multiple granular cell tumors ('myoblastomas'). Case report with electron microscopic observations and review of the literature. Cancer 1967, **20**: 2032–2047.

1672 Mukai M. Immunohistochemical localization of S-100 protein and peripheral nerve myelin proteins (P2 protein, PO protein) in granular cell tumors. Am J Pathol 1983, **112**: 139–146.

1673 Nakazato Y, Ishizeki J, Takahashi K, Yamaguchi H. Immunohistochemical localization of S-100 protein in granular cell myoblastoma. Cancer 1982, **49**: 1624–1628.

1674 Nathrath WBJ, Remberger K. Immunohistochemical study of granular cell tumours. Demonstration of neurone specific enolase, S 100 protein, laminin and alpha-1-antichymotrypsin. Virchows Arch [A] 1986, **408**: 421–434.

1675 Navarrette AR, Smith M. Ultrastructure of granular cell ameloblastoma. Cancer 1971, **27**: 948–955.

1676 Nielsen K, Paulsen SM, Johansen P. Carcinoembryonic antigen like antigen in granular cell myoblastomas. An immunohistochemical study. Virchows Arch [A] 1983, **401**: 159–162.

1677 Nistal M, Paniagua R, Picazo ML, Cermeño de Giles F, Ramos Guerreira JL. Granular changes in vascular leiomyosarcoma. Virchows Arch [A] 1980, **386**: 239–248.

1678 Ordóñez NG, Mackay B. Granular cell tumor: a review of the pathology and histogenesis. Ultrastruct Pathol 1999, **23**: 207–222.

1679 Parfitt JR, McLean CA, Joseph MG, Streutker CJ, Al-Haddad S, Driman DK. Granular cell tumours of the gastrointestinal tract: expression of nestin and clinicopathological evaluation of 11 patients. Histopathology 2006, **48**: 424–430.

1680 Park SH, Kim TJ, Chi JG. Congenital granular cell tumor with systemic involvement. Immunohistochemical and ultrastructural study. Arch Pathol Lab Med 1991, **115**: 934–938.

1681 Penneys NS, Adachi K, Ziegels-Weissman J, Nadji M. Granular cell tumors of the skin contain myelin basic protein. Arch Pathol Lab Med 1983, **107**: 302–303.

1682 Regezi JA, Zarbo RJ, Courtney RM, Crissman JD. Immunoreactivity of granular cell lesions of skin, mucosa, and jaw. Cancer 1989, **64**: 1455–1460.

1683 Robertson AJ, McIntosh W, Lamont P, Guthrie W. Malignant granular cell tumour (myoblastoma) of the vulva. Report of a case and review of the literature. Histopathology 1981, **5**: 69–79.

1684 Sakurama N, Matsukado Y, Marubayashi T, Kodama T. Granular cell tumour of the brain and its cellular identity. Acta Neurochir (Wien) 1981, **56**: 81–94.

1685 Seo IS, Azzarelli B, Warner TF, Goheen MP, Senteney GE. Multiple visceral and cutaneous granular cell tumors. Ultrastructural and immunocytochemical evidence of Schwann cell origin. Cancer 1984, **53**: 2104–2110.

1686 Shimamura K, Osamura RY, Ueyama Y, Hata J-I, Tamaoki N, Machida N, Fukuda H, Uemura K. Malignant granular cell tumor of the right sciatic nerve. Report of an autopsy case with electron microscopic, immunohistochemical, and enzyme histochemical studies. Cancer 1984, **53**: 524–529.

1687 Sobel JH, Marquet E, Schwarz R. Granular degeneration of appendiceal smooth muscle. Arch Pathol 1971, **92**: 427–432.

1688 Strong EW, McDivitt RW, Brasfield RD. Granular cell myoblastoma. Cancer 1970, **25**: 415–422.

1689 Troncoso P, Ordóñez NG, Raymond AK, Mackay B. Malignant granular cell tumor. Immunocytochemical and ultrastructural observations. Ultrastruct Pathol 1988, **12**: 137–144.

1690 Usui M, Ishii S, Yamawaki S, Sasaki T, Minami A, Hizawa K. Malignant granular cell tumor of the radial nerve. Cancer 1977, **39**: 1547–1555.

1691 Uzoaru I, Firfer B, Ray V, Hubbard-Shepard M, Rhee H. Malignant granular cell tumor. Arch Pathol Lab Med 1992, **116**: 206–208.

1692 Vance SF III, Hudson RP. Granular cell myoblastoma. Clinicopathologic study of 42 patients. Am J Clin Pathol 1969, **52**: 208–211.

Alveolar soft part sarcoma

1693 Amin MB, Patel RM, Oliveira P, Cabrera R, Carneiro V, Preto M, Balzer B, Folpe AL. Alveolar soft-part sarcoma of the urinary bladder with urethral recurrence: a unique case with emphasis on differential diagnoses and diagnostic utility of an immunohistochemical panel including TFE3. Am J Surg Pathol 2006, **30**: 1322–1325.

1694 Argani P, Antonescu CR, Illei PB, Lui MY, Timmons CF, Newbury I, Reuter VE, Garvin AJ, Perez-Atayde AR, Fletcher JA, Beckwith JB, Bridge JA, Ladanyi M. Primary renal neoplasms with the ASPL–TFE3 gene fusion of alveolar soft part sarcoma: a distinctive tumor entity previously included among renal cell carcinomas of children and adolescents. Am J Pathol 2001, **159**: 179–192.

1695 Argani P, Lal P, Hutchinson B, Lui MY, Reuter VE, Ladanyi M. Aberrant nuclear immunoreactivity for TFE3 in neoplasms with TFE3 gene fusions. Am J Surg Pathol 2003, **27**: 750–761.

1696 Auerbach HE, Brooks JJ. Alveolar soft part sarcoma. A clinicopathologic and immunohistochemical study. Cancer 1987, **60**: 66–73.

1697 Carstens HB. Membrane-bound cytoplasmic crystals, similar to those in alveolar soft part sarcoma, in a human muscle spindle. Ultrastruct Pathol 1990, **14**: 423–428.

1698 DeSchryver-Kecskemeti K, Kraus FT, Engleman W, Lacy PE. Alveolar soft-part sarcoma – a malignant angioreninoma. Histochemical, immunocytochemical, and electron-microscopic study of four cases. Am J Surg Pathol 1982, **6**: 5–18.

1699 Evans HL. Alveolar soft-part sarcoma. of 13 typical examples and one with histologically atypical component. Ca 1985, **55**: 912–917.
1700 Fanburg-Smith JC, Miettinen M, Folp Weiss SW, Childers ELB. Alveolar soft sarcoma of the tongue: 14 cases [abst Mod Pathol 2003, **16**: 11A.
1701 Fisher ER, Reidford H. Electron micro evidence suggesting the myogenous derivation of the so-called alveolar so sarcoma. Cancer 1971, **27**: 150–159.
1702 Font RL, Jurco S III, Zimmerman LE. soft-part sarcoma of the orbit. A clinicopathologic analysis of 17 cases review of the literature. Hum Pathol 1 **13**: 569–579.
1703 Foschini MP, Ceccarelli C, Eusebi V, S Gabbiani G. Alveolar soft part sarcom Immunological evidence of rhabdom differentiation. Histopathology 1988, 101–108.
1704 Foschini MP, Eusebi V. Alveolar soft-p sarcoma. A new type of rhabdomyosa Semin Diagn Pathol 1994, **11**: 58–68.
1705 Gray GF Jr, Glick AD, Kurtin PJ, Jones Alveolar soft part sarcoma of the uter Pathol 1986, **17**: 297–300.
1706 Hirose T, Kudo E, Hasegawa T, Abe J, Hizawa K. Cytoskeletal properties of a soft part sarcoma. Hum Pathol 1990, 204–211.
1707 Ladanyi M, Antonescu CR, Drobnjak Baren A, Lui MY, Golde DW, Cordon- C. The precrystalline cytoplasmic gran alveolar soft part sarcoma contain monocarboxylate transporter 1 and C Am J Pathol 2002, **160**: 1215–1221.
1708 Ladanyi M, Lui MY, Antonescu CR, Krause-Boehm A, Meindl A, Argani P, JH, Ueda T, Yoshikawa H, Meloni-Ehr Sorens PH, Mertens F, Mandahl N, va Berghe H, Sciot R, Cin PD, Bride J. Th der(17)t(X;17)(p11;q25) of human al soft part sarcoma fuses the TFE3 trans factor gene to ASPL, a novel gene at 1 Oncogene 2001, **20**: 48–57.
1709 Lieberman PH, Brennan MF, Kimmel Erlandson RA, Garin-Chesa P, Fleking Alveolar soft-part sarcoma. A clinico- pathologic study of half a century. Ca 1989, **63**: 1–13.
1710 Lieberman PH, Foote FW, Stewart FW, JW. Alveolar soft-part sarcoma. JAMA **198**: 1047–1051.
1711 Lillehei KO, Kleinschmidt-De Masters Mitchell DH, Spector E, Kruse CA. Alv soft part sarcoma. An unusually long between presentation and brain meta Hum Pathol 1993, **24**: 1030–1034.
1712 Machinami R, Kikuchi F. Adenosine triphosphatase activity of crystalline inclusions in alveolar soft part sarcom ultrahistochemical study of a case. Pat Pract 1986, **181**: 357–361.
1713 Matsuno Y, Mukai K, Itabashi M, Yam Hirota T, Nakajima T, Shimosato Y. Al soft part sarcoma. A clinicopathologic immunohistochemical study of 12 cas Pathol Jpn 1990, **40**: 199–205.
1714 Miettinen M, Ekfors T. Alveolar soft p sarcoma. Immunohistochemical evide muscle cell differentiation. Am J Clin 1990, **93**: 32–38.
1715 Mukai M, Iri H, Nakajima T, Hirose S, Torikata C, Kageyama K, Ueno N, Mu K. Alveolar soft-part sarcoma. A review histogenesis and further studies based electron microscopy, immunohistoche and biochemistry. Am J Surg Pathol 1 679–689.

hormones and are probably the progenitors of lesions such as endometriosis, endosalpingiosis, ectopic decidual reaction, leiomyomatosis peritonealis disseminata, and tumors of ovarian or uterine type (see p. 2244). The large group of peritoneal disorders related to the female genital tract is also discussed in Chapter 19, Ovary and Uterus corpus.

Structures or regions topographically related to the peritoneum and retroperitoneum are the omentum, mesentery, hernia sacs, umbilicus, and sacrococcygeal region. Since an overlapping of pathologic processes exists among all of them, they are discussed in this chapter, with appropriate references to other sections of the text when indicated.

Inflammation

Chemical peritonitis can be caused by bile, pancreatic juice, gastric juice, meconium, and radiographic contrast media. Barium peritonitis was seen in the past following perforation of large bowel occurring during the course of radiographic examinations performed because of obstruction.[14]

Extravasation of *bile* as a result of trauma or disease of the gallbladder, bile ducts, or duodenum causes an acute or subacute peritonitis that is initially limited to the upper quadrant of the abdomen.[7] *Gastric juice* produces a severe peritoneal reaction because of its hydrochloric acid content, although it may be bacteriologically sterile. The release of *pancreatic juice* causes fat necrosis. The formation of calcium salts in large areas of fat necrosis may cause hypocalcemia.

Bacterial peritonitis may be either primary or secondary. The *primary* form usually is caused by streptococci and is seen more commonly in children (particularly in those affected by the nephrotic syndrome). Adult patients with ascites secondary to liver disease are also susceptible. This form of peritonitis tends to produce marked constitutional symptoms with minimal localizing findings. Aspiration of intra-abdominal fluid discloses an inflammatory exudate containing only a single type of organism. Large amounts of extracellular fluid are lost into the exudate, equivalent to those of a burn covering one-half to three-fourths of the cutaneous surface.

Perforation of a viscus such as the colon produces *secondary* peritonitis. If the fluid is aspirated, a mixture of bacterial flora rather than a single organism is usually found. *Tuberculous peritonitis* may occur with few constitutional symptoms, despite extensive involvement of the peritoneum.[5,10,11,17] In a review of 47 cases, Singh et al.[16] found radiographic evidence of pulmonary parenchymal lesions in only 6% of the cases. The search for acid-fast organisms on a direct smear of ascitic fluid is often unrewarding. The best diagnostic methods are culture of the fluid and percutaneous biopsy of the peritoneum.[12,13] Singh et al.[16] found the latter to be useful in 64% of their cases. Chemotherapy is the treatment of choice; surgery is reserved for those cases associated with enteritis leading to bowel obstruction, perforation, fistula, or a mass that does not resolve with drug therapy.[15] Other specific forms of peritonitis are *coccidioidomycosis* and *actinomycosis*.[6] Exceptionally, *Oxyuris vermicularis* may escape from the appendix or other portions of the gastrointestinal tract into the peritoneal cavity and elicit the formation of granulomas.[19]

Meconium peritonitis is the result of perforation of the small bowel during intrauterine life. It may present in infants as intestinal obstruction requiring surgical intervention. With healing, only scattered calcific foci remain. These can be located in the main peritoneal cavity, inguinal region, or scrotum; the latter can simulate clinically a testicular tumor.[8,18]

Vernix caseosa peritonitis represents a rare complication of cesarean section, and it has distinctive microscopic features.[9]

Adhesions

Adhesions, with the potential for intestinal obstruction, follow all intra-abdominal operations. They can be minimized by careful handling of tissues, re-peritonealization where feasible, and removal of intraperitoneal blood clots. Ryan et al.[26] showed in an experimental model that drying of the serosa plus bleeding consistently resulted in the formation of adhesions. There is good experimental evidence to suggest that the formation of peritoneal adhesions is related to a local depression of peritoneal plasminogen activator, which is the principal peritoneal fibrin-clearing system known.[20]

Innumerable agents, including sodium citrate, heparin, olive oil, liquid paraffin, adrenocorticotropic hormone (ACTH), cortisone, pepsin, fibrinolysin, and amniotic fluid, have been used over the years to prevent adhesions, but none has accomplished this goal in an entirely successful fashion. Adhesions become collagenous and strong as the cellularity of their fibrous tissue decreases with maturation. Postoperative adhesions are the most frequent cause of intestinal obstruction today.

Extensive peritoneal fibrosis (so-called *sclerosing* or *fibrosing peritonitis*) also has been described as a reaction to asbestos, to silica in drug abusers,[22] in patients with the carcinoid syndrome, in patients with lupus,[25] in women with luteinized thecomas/thecomatosis and related proliferative stromal lesions of the ovary,[23,27] and as a complication of the administration of beta-adrenergic-blocking drugs,[21] or of compounds containing fluoropyrimidines.[24] In many instances, the etiologic agent cannot be identified; some of these 'idiopathic' cases are probably pathogenetically related to mesenteric panniculitis and – as such – are part of the spectrum of the inflammatory fibrosclerosis group of diseases (see p. 2247). A few of the cases associated with ovarian tumors have proved fatal.[27]

Reaction to foreign materials

The peritoneum reacts briskly to foreign substances. The most spectacular (and easiest to recognize) are those accompanying retained sponges and instruments after surgery, an event still haunting the laparotomy procedure and more likely to occur in emergency situations and/or in obese patients.[36] Classically, one of the better known peritoneal reactions to foreign material is *talc powder granuloma*, which is secondary to the talc (hydrated magnesium silicate) used in the past on surgical gloves. Spillage of this material into the peritoneal cavity at surgery results in nodules that can be mistaken grossly for tuberculosis or metastatic carcinoma. Microscopically, they are formed by foreign body granulomas containing birefringent crystals. The latter are made apparent with polarizing lenses or simply by lowering the condenser of the microscope.

Talc used for surgical gloves has long been recognized as a hazard and has been replaced by other substances, such as modified starch. Although these materials elicit a lesser degree of reaction, intraperitoneal granulomas may still develop,[43] on average between 10 days and 4 weeks after a laparotomy. These usually have the appearance of foreign body granulomas but sometimes exhibit tuberculoid features with caseum-like necrosis.[42] At reoperation, the findings are ascites, miliary peritoneal nodules, serosal inflammation, and adhesions. The gross appearance can closely simulate metastatic carcinoma, tuberculosis, or Crohn disease. The nature of the granulomas can be identified by the presence of granules that are periodic acid–Schiff (PAS) positive and birefringent (with a Maltese cross pattern) within the cytoplasm of histiocytes and foreign body giant cells.[33,35]

1750 Ohno T, Park P, Utsunomiya Y, Hirahata H, Inoue K. Ultrastructural study of a clear cell sarcoma suggesting Schwannian differentiation. Ultrastruct Pathol 1986, **10**: 39–48.

1751 Pavlidis NA, Fisher C, Wiltshaw E. Clear-cell sarcoma of tendons and aponeuroses. A clinicopathologic study. Presentation of six additional cases with review of the literature. Cancer 1984, **54**: 1412–1417.

1752 Sandberg AA, Bridge JA. Updates on the cytogenetics and molecular genetics of bone soft tissue tumors: clear cell sarcoma (malignant melanoma soft parts). Cancer Genet Cytogenet 2001, **130**: 1–7.

1753 Sara AS, Evans HL, Benjamin RS. Malignant melanoma of soft parts (clear cell sarcoma). A study of 17 cases, with emphasis on prognostic factors. Cancer 1990, **65**: 367–374.

1754 Saw D, Tse CH, Chan J, Watt CY, Ng CS, Poon YF. Clear cell sarcoma of the penis. Hum Pathol 1986, **17**: 423–425.

1755 Swanson PE, Wick MR. Clear cell sarcoma. An immunohistochemical analysis of six cases and comparison with other epithelioid neoplasms of soft tissue. Arch Pathol Lab Med 1989, **113**: 55–60.

1756 Tsuneyoshi M, Enjoji M, Kubo T. Clear cell sarcoma of tendons and aponeuroses. A comparative study of 13 cases with a provisional subgrouping into the melanotic and synovial types. Cancer 1978, **42**: 243–252.

1757 Zambrano E, Reyes-Mugica M, Franchi A, Rosai J. An osteoclast-rich tumor of the gastrointestinal tract with features resembling clear cell sarcoma of parts: reports of six cases of a GIST simulator. Int J Surg Pathol 2003, **11**: 75–81.

1758 Zambrano E, Reyes-Mugica M, Franchi A, Rosai J. An osteoclast-rich tumor of the gastrointestinal tract with features resembling clear cell sarcoma of soft parts: reports of 6 cases of a GIST simulator. Int J Surg Pathol 2003, **11**: 75–81.

Epithelioid sarcoma

1759 Arber DA, Kandalaft PL, Mehta P, Battifora H. Vimentin-negative epithelioid sarcoma. The value of an immunohistochemical panel that includes CD34. Am J Surg Pathol 1993, **17**: 302–307.

1760 Bryan RS, Soule EH, Dobyns JH, Pritchard DJ, Linscheid RL. Primary epithelioid sarcoma of the hand and forearm. J Bone Joint Surg (Am) 1974, **56**: 458–465.

1761 Chase DR, Enzinger FM. Epithelioid sarcoma. Diagnosis, prognostic indicators, and treatment. Am J Surg Pathol 1985, **9**: 241–263.

1762 Chase DR, Enzinger FM, Weiss SW, Langloss JM. Keratin in epithelioid sarcoma. An immunohistochemical study. Am J Surg Pathol 1984, **8**: 435–441.

1763 Chase DR, Enzinger FM, Weiss SW, Langloss JM. Coexpression of keratin and vimentin in epithelioid sarcoma. Am J Surg Pathol 1985, **9**: 460–463.

1764 Chbani L, Guillou L, Terrier P, Decouvelaere AV, Grégoire F, Terrier-Lacombe MJ, Ranchère D, Robin YM, Collin F, Fréneaux P, Coindre JM. Epithelioid sarcoma: a clinicopathologic and immunohistochemical analysis of 106 cases from the French sarcoma group. Am J Clin Pathol 2009, **131**: 222–227.

1765 Chetty R, Slavin JL. Epithelioid sarcoma with extensive chondroid differentiation. Histopathology 1994, **24**: 400–401.

1766 Daimaru Y, Hashimoto H, Tsuneyoshi M, Enjoji M. Epithelial profile of epithelioid sarcoma. An immunohistochemical analysis of eight cases. Cancer 1987, **59**: 134–141.

1767 den Bakker MA, Flood SJ, Kliffen M. CD31 staining in epithelioid sarcoma. Virchows Arch 2003, **443**: 93–97.

1768 Enzinger FM. Epithelioid sarcoma. A sarcoma simulating a granuloma or a carcinoma. Cancer 1970, **25**: 1029–1041.

1769 Evans HL, Baer SC. Epithelioid sarcoma. A clinicopathologic and prognostic study of 26 cases. Semin Diagn Pathol 1993, **10**: 286–291.

1770 Fisher C. Epithelioid sarcoma. The spectrum of ultrastructural differentiation in seven immunohistochemically defined cases. Hum Pathol 1988, **19**: 265–275.

1771 Gabbiani G, Fu Y-S, Kaye GI, Lattes R, Majno G. Epithelioid sarcoma. A light and electron microscopic study suggesting a synovial origin. Cancer 1972, **30**: 486–499.

1772 Guillou L, Wadden C, Coindre JM, Krausz T, Fletcher CD. 'Proximal-type' epithelioid sarcoma, a distinctive aggressive neoplasm showing rhabdoid features: clinicopathologic, immunohistochemical, and ultrastructural study of a series. Am J Surg Pathol 1997, **21**: 130–146.

1773 Halling AC, Wollan PC, Pritchard DJ, Vlasak R, Nascimento AG. Epithelioid sarcoma: a clinicopathologic review of 55 cases. Mayo Clin Proc 1996, **71**: 636–642.

1774 Hasegawa T, Matsuno Y, Shimoda T, Umeda T, Yokoyama R, Hirohashi S. Proximal-type epithelioid sarcoma: a clinicopathologic study of 20 cases. Mod Pathol 2001, **14**: 655–663.

1775 Hornick JL, Dal Cin P, Fletcher CD. Loss of INI1 expression is characteristic of both conventional and proximal-type epithelioid sarcoma. Am J Surg Pathol 2009, **33**: 542–550.

1776 Izumi T, Oda Y, Hasegawa T, Nakanishi Y, Iwasaki H, Sonobe H, Goto H, Kusakabe H, Takahira T, Kobayashi C, Kawaguchi K, Saito T, Yamamoto H, Tamiya S, Iwamoto Y, Tsuneyoshi M. Prognostic significance of dysadherin expression in epithelioid sarcoma and its diagnostic utility in distinguishing epithelioid sarcoma from malignant rhabdoid tumor. Mod Pathol 2006, **19**: 820–831.

1777 Kohashi K, Izumi T, Oda Y, Yamamoto H, Tamiya S, Taguchi T, Iwamoto Y, Hasegawa T, Tsuneyoshi M. Infrequent SMARCB1/INI1 gene alteration in epithelioid sarcoma: a useful tool in distinguishing epithelioid sarcoma from malignant rhabdoid tumor. Hum Pathol 2009, **40**: 349–355.

1778 Koplin SA, Nielsen GP, Rosenberg AE. Heterotopic bone in epithelioid sarcomas: a histopathological review of 4 cases. Lab Invest 2009, **89**(Suppl 1): 16A.

1779 Laskin WB, Miettinen M. Epithelioid sarcoma. New insights based on an extended immunohistochemical analysis. Arch Pathol Lab Med 2003, **127**: 1161–1168.

1780 Lualdi E, Modena P, Debiec-Rychter M, Pedeutour F, Teixeira MR, Facchinetti F, Dagrada GP, Pilotti S, Sozzi G. Molecular cytogenetic characterization of proximal-type epithelioid sarcoma. Genes Chromosomes Cancer 2004, **41**: 283–290.

1781 Manivel JC, Wick MR, Dehner LP, Sibley RK. Epithelioid sarcoma. An immunohistochemical study. Am J Clin Pathol 1987, **87**: 319–326.

1782 Miettinen M, Fanburg-Smith JC, Virolainen M, Shmookler BM, Fetsch JF. Epithelioid sarcoma: an immunohistochemical analysis of 112 classical and variant cases and discussion of the differential diagnosis. Hum Pathol 1999, **30**: 934–942.

1783 Miettinen M, Lehto V-P, Vartio T, Virtanen I. Epithelioid sarcoma. Ultrastructural and immunohistologic features suggesting a synovial origin. Arch Pathol Lab Med 1982, **106**: 620–623.

1784 Mills SE, Rosai J. Adamantinoma of the pretibial soft tissue. Clinicopathologic features, differential diagnosis, and possible relationship to intraosseous disease. Am J Clin Pathol 1985, **83**: 108–114.

1785 Mirra JM, Kessler S, Bhuta S, Eckardt J. The fibroma-like variant of epithelioid sarcoma. A fibrohistiocytic/myoid cell lesion often confused with benign and malignant spindle cell tumours. Cancer 1992, **69**: 1382–1395.

1786 Molenaar WM, De Jong B, Dam-Meiring A, Postma A, De Vries J, Hoekstra HJ. Epithelioid sarcoma or malignant rhabdoid tumor of soft tissue? Epithelioid immunophenotype and rhabdoid karyotype. Hum Pathol 1989, **20**: 347–351.

1787 Mukai M, Torikata C, Iri H, Hanaoka H, Kawai T, Yakumaru K, Shimoda T, Mikata A, Kageyama K. Cellular differentiation of epithelioid sarcoma – electron-microscopic, enzyme-histochemical, and immunohistochemical study. Am J Pathol 1985, **119**: 44–56.

1788 Peimer CA, Smith RJ, Sirota RL, Cohen BE. Epithelioid sarcoma of the hand and wrist. Patterns of extension. J Hand Surg 1977, **2**: 275–282.

1789 Perrone T, Swanson PE, Twiggs L, Ulbright TM, Dehner LP. Malignant rhabdoid tumor of the vulva. Is distinction from epithelioid sarcoma possible? A pathologic and immunohistochemical study. Am J Surg Pathol 1989, **13**: 848–858.

1790 Prat J, Woodruff JM, Marcove RC. Epithelioid sarcoma. An analysis of 22 cases indicating the prognostic significance of vascular invasion and regional lymph node metastasis. Cancer 1978, **41**: 1472–1487.

1791 Rose DSC, Fisher C, Smith MEF. Epithelioid sarcoma arising in a patient with neurofibromatosis type 2. Histopathology 1994, **25**: 379–380.

1792 Santiago H, Feinerman LK, Lattes R. Epithelioid sarcoma. A clinical and pathologic study of nine cases. Hum Pathol 1972, **3**: 133–147.

1793 Shimm DS, Suit HD. Radiation therapy of epithelioid sarcoma. Cancer 1983, **52**: 1022–1025.

1794 Shiratsuchi H, Oshiro Y, Saito T, Itakura E, Kinoshita Y, Tamiya S, Oda Y, Komiyama S, Tsuneyoshi M. Cytokeratin subunits of inclusion bodies in rhabdoid cells: immunohistochemical and clinicopathological study of malignant rhabdoid tumor and epithelioid sarcoma. Int J Surg Pathol 2001, **9**: 37–48.

1795 Smith ME, Awasthi R, O'Shaughnessy S, Fisher C. Evaluation of perineurial differentiation in epithelioid sarcoma. Histopathology 2005, **47**: 575–581.

1796 Sugarbaker PH, Auda S, Webber BL, Triche TJ, Shapiro E, Cook WJ. Early distant metastases from epithelioid sarcoma of the hand. Cancer 1981, **48**: 852–855.

1797 Weissmann D, Amenta PS, Kantor GR. Vulvar epithelioid sarcoma metastatic to the scalp. A case report and review of the literature. Am J Dermatopathol 1990, **12**: 462–468.

Giant cell tumor of soft parts

1798 Alguacil-Garcia A, Unni KK, Goellner JR. Malignant giant cell tumor of soft parts. An ultrastructural study of four cases. Cancer 1977, **40**: 244–253.

1799 Angervall L, Hagmar B, Kindblom L-G, Merck C. Malignant giant cell tumor of soft tissues. A clinicopathologic, cytologic, ultrastructural, angiographic, and microangiographic study. Cancer 1981, **47**: 736–747.

1800 Folpe AL, Morris RJ, Weiss SW. Soft tissue giant cell tumor of low malignant potential: a proposal for the reclassification of malignant giant cell tumor of soft parts. Mod Pathol 1999, **12**: 894–902.

1801 Gould E, Albores-Saavedra J, Rothe M, Mnaymneh W, Menedez-Aponte S. Malignant giant cell tumor of soft parts presenting as a skin tumor. Am J Dermatopathol 1989, **11**: 197–201.

1802 Guccion JG, Enzinger FM. Malignant giant cell tumor of soft parts. An analysis of 32 cases. Cancer 1972, **29**: 1518–1529.

1803 Kearney MM, Soule EH, Ivins JC. Malignant fibrous histiocytoma. A retrospective study of 167 cases. Cancer 1980, **45**: 167–178.

1804 Lau YS, Sabokbar A, Gibbons CL, Giele H, Athanasou N. Phenotypic and molecular studies of giant-cell tumors of bone and soft tissue. Hum Pathol 2005, **36**: 945–954.

1805 O'Connell JX, Wehrli BM, Neilsen GP, Rosenberg AE. Giant cell tumors of soft tissue: a clinicopathologic study of 18 benign and malignant tumors. Am J Surg Pathol 2000, **24**: 386–395.

1806 Oliveira AM, Dei Tos AP, Fletcher CD, Nascimento AG. Primary giant cell tumor of soft tissues: a study of 22 cases. Am J Surg Pathol 2000, **24**: 248–256.

1807 Salm R, Sissons HA. Giant-cell tumours of soft tissues. J Pathol 1972, **107**: 27–39.

1808 Teot LA, O'Keefe RJ, Rosier RN, O'Connell JX, Fox EJ, Hicks DG. Extraosseous primary and recurrent giant cell tumors: transforming growth factor beta-1 and beta-2 expression may explain metaplastic bone formation. Hum Pathol 1996, **27**: 625–632.

Ossifying fibromyxoid tumor

1809 Donner LR. Ossifying fibromyxoid tumor of soft parts. Evidence supporting Schwann cell origin. Hum Pathol 1992, **23**: 200–202.

1810 Enzinger FM, Weiss SW, Liang CY. Ossifying fibromyxoid tumor of soft parts. A clinicopathological analysis of 59 cases. Am J Surg Pathol 1989, **13**: 817–827.

1811 Folpe AL, Weiss SW. Ossifying fibromyxoid tumor of soft parts. A clinicopathological study of 70 cases with emphasis on atypical malignant variants. Am J Surg Pathol 2003, **27**: 421–431.

1812 Hirose T, Shimada S, Tani T, Hasegawa T. Ossifying fibromyxoid tumor: invariable ultrastructural features and diverse immunophenotypic expression. Ultrastruct Pathol 2007, **31**: 233–239.

1813 Kilpatrick SE, Ward WG, Mozes M, Miettinen M, Fukunaga M, Fletcher CDM. Atypical and malignant variants of ossifying fibromyxoid tumor. Clinicopathologic analysis of six cases. Am J Surg Pathol 1995, **19**: 1039–1046.

1814 Miettinen M. Ossifying fibromyxoid tumor of soft parts. Additional observations of a distinctive soft tissue tumor. Am J Clin Pathol 1991, **95**: 142–149.

1815 Miettinen M, Finnell V, Fetsch JF. Ossifying fibromyxoid tumor of soft parts – a clinicopathologic and immunohistochemical study of 104 cases with long-term follow-up and a critical review of the literature. Am J Surg Pathol 2008, **32**: 996–1005.

1816 Min KW, Seo IS, Pitha J. Ossifying fibromyxoid tumor: modified myoepithelial cell tumor? Report of three cases with immunohistochemical and electron microscopic studies. Ultrastruct Pathol 2005, **29**: 535–548.

1817 Schofield JB, Krausz T, Stamp GW, Fletcher CD, Fisher C, Azzopardi JG. Ossifying fibromyxoid tumour of soft parts. Immunohistochemical and ultrastructural analysis. Histopathology 1993, **22**: 101–112.

1818 Yang P, Hirose T, Hasegawa T, Gao Z, Hizawa K. Ossifying fibromyxoid tumor of soft parts. A morphological and immunohistochemical study. Pathol Int 1994, **44**: 448–453.

Extraskeletal Ewing sarcoma/PNET

1819 Ambros IM, Ambros PF, Strehl S, Kovar H, Gadner H, Salzer-Kuntschik M. MIC2 is a specific marker for Ewing's sarcoma and peripheral primitive neuroectodermal tumors. Evidence for a common histogenesis of Ewing's sarcoma and peripheral primitive neuroectodermal tumors from MIC2 expression and specific chromosome aberration. Cancer 1991, **67**: 1886–1893.

1820 Angervall L, Enzinger FM. Extraskeletal neoplasm resembling Ewing's sarcoma. Cancer 1975, **36**: 240–251.

1821 Askin FB, Rosai J, Sibley RK, Dehner LP, McAlister WH. Malignant small cell tumor of the thoracopulmonary region in childhood. A distinctive clinicopathologic entity of uncertain histogenesis. Cancer 1979, **43**: 2438–2451.

1822 Cavazzana AO, Ninfo V, Roberts J, Triche TJ. Peripheral neuroepithelioma. A light microscopic, immunocytochemical, and ultrastructural study. Mod Pathol 1992, **5**: 71–78.

1823 Contesso G, Llombart-Bosch A, Terrier P, Peydro-Olaya A, Henry-Amar M, Oberlin O, Habrand JL, Dubousset J, Tursz T, Spielmann M, et al. Does malignant small round cell tumor of the thoracopulmonary region (Askin tumor) constitute a clinicopathologic entity? An analysis of 30 cases with immunohistochemical and electron-microscopic support treated at the Institute Gustave Roussy. Cancer 1992, **69**: 1012–1020.

1824 De Alava E, Pardo J. Ewing tumor: tumor biology and clinical applications. Int J Surg Pathol 2001, **9**: 7–17.

1825 Delattre O, Zucman J, Melot T, Garau XS, Zucker JM, Lenoir GM, Ambros PF, Sheer D, Turc-Carel C, Triche TJ, et al. The Ewing family of tumors – a sub group of small-round-cell tumors defined by specific chimeric transcripts. N Engl J Med 1994, **331**: 294–299.

1826 Dickman PS, Triche TJ. Extraosseous Ewing's sarcoma versus primitive rhabdomyosarcoma. Diagnostic criteria and clinical correlation. Hum Pathol 1986, **17**: 881–893.

1827 Downing JR, Head DR, Parham DM, Douglass EC, Hulshof MG, Link MP, Motroni TA, Grier HE, Curcio-Brint AM, Shapiro DN. Detection of the (11;22)(q24;q12) translocation of Ewing's sarcoma and peripheral neuroectodermal tumor by reverse transcription polymerase chain reaction. Am J Pathol 1993, **143**: 1294–1300.

1828 Ehrig T, Billings SD, Fanburg-Smith JC. Superficial primitive neuroectodermal tumor/Ewing sarcoma (PN/ES): same tumor as deep PN/ES or new entity? Ann Diagn Pathol 2007, **11**: 153–159.

1829 Fellinger EJ, Garin-Chesa P, Triche TJ, Huvos AG, Retting WJ. Immunohistochemical analysis of Ewing's sarcoma cell surface antigen p30/32MIC2. Am J Pathol 1991, **139**: 317–325.

1830 Folpe AL, Hill CE, Parham DM, O'Shea PA, Weiss SW. Immunohistochemical detection of FLI-1 protein expression: a study of 132 round cell tumors with emphasis on CD99-positive mimics of Ewing's sarcoma/primitive neuroectodermal tumor. Am J Surg Pathol 2000, **24**: 1657–1662.

1831 Folpe AL, Goldblum JR, Rubin BP, Shehata BM, Liu W, Dei Tos AP, Weiss SW. Morphologic and immunophenotypic diversity in Ewing family tumors: a study of 66 genetically confirmed cases. Am J Surg Pathol 2005, **29**: 1025–1033.

1832 Gerald WL. A practical approach to the differential diagnosis of small round cell tumors of infancy using recent scientific and technical advances. Int J Surg Pathol 2000, **8**: 87–97.

1833 Gillespie JJ, Roth LM, Wills ER, Einborn LH, Willman J. Extraskeletal Ewing's sarcoma. Histologic and ultrastructural observations in three cases. Am J Surg Pathol 1979, **3**: 99–108.

1834 Gonzalez-Crussi F, Wolfson SL, Misugi K, Nakajima T. Peripheral neuroectodermal tumors of the chest wall in childhood. Cancer 1984, **54**: 2519–2527.

1835 Harris MD, Moore IE, Steart PV, Weller RO. Protein gene product (PGP) 9.5 as a reliable marker in primitive neuroectodermal tumors – an immunohistochemical study of 21 childhood cases. Histopathology 1990, **16**: 271–277.

1836 Hashimoto H, Tsuneyoshi M, Daimaru Y, Enjoji M. Extraskeletal Ewing's sarcoma. A clinicopathologic and electron microscopic analysis of 8 cases. Acta Pathol Jpn 1985, **35**: 1087–1098.

1837 Jürgens H, Bier V, Harms D, Beck J, Brandeis W, Etspüler G, Gadner H, Schmidt D, Treuner J, Winkler K, Göbel U. Malignant peripheral neuroectodermal tumors. A retrospective analysis of 42 patients. Cancer 1988, **61**: 349–357.

1838 Kawaguchi K, Koike M. Neuron-specific enolase and leu-7 immunoreactive small round-cell neoplasm. The relationship to Ewing's sarcoma in bone and soft tissue. Am J Clin Pathol 1986, **86**: 79–83.

1839 Kumar S, Pack S, Kumar D, Walker R, Quezado M, Zhuang Z, Meltzer P, Tsokos M. Detection of EWS-FLI-1 fusion in Ewing's sarcoma/peripheral primitive neuroectodermal tumor by fluorescence in situ hybridization using formalin-fixed paraffin-embedded tissue. Hum Pathol 1999, **30**: 324–330.

1840 Ladanyi M, Heinemann FS, Huvos AG, Rao PH, Chen QG, Jhanwar SC. Neural differentiation in small round cell tumors of bone and soft tissue with the translocation t(11;22)(q24;q12). An immunohistochemical study of 11 cases. Hum Pathol 1990, **21**: 1245–1251.

1841 Ladanyi M, Lewis R, Garin-Chesa P, Rettig WJ, Huvos AG, Healey JH, Jhanwar SC. EWS rearrangement in Ewing's sarcoma and peripheral neuroectodermal tumor. Molecular detection and correlation with cytogenetic analysis and MIC2 expression. Diagn Mol Pathol 1993, **2**: 141–146.

1842 Lewis TB, Coffin CM, Bernard PS. Differentiating Ewing's sarcoma from other round blue cell tumors using a RT-PCR translocation panel on formalin-fixed paraffin-embedded tissues. Mod Pathol 2007, **20**: 397–404.

1843 Linnoila RI, Tsokos M, Triche TJ, Marangos PJ, Chandra RS. Evidence for neural origin and PAS-positive variants of the malignant small cell tumor of thoracopulmonary region ('Askin tumor'). Am J Surg Pathol 1986, **10**: 124–133.

1844 Mobley BC, Roulston D, Shah GV, Bijwaard KE, McKeever PE. Peripheral primitive neuroectodermal tumor/Ewing's sarcoma of the craniospinal vault: case reports and review. Hum Pathol 2006, **37**: 845–853.

1845 Navarro S, Cavazzana AO, Llombart-Bosch A, Triche TJ. Comparison of Ewing's sarcoma of bone and peripheral neuroepithelioma. An immunocytochemical and ultrastructural analysis of two primitive neuroectodermal neoplasms. Arch Pathol Lab Med 1994, **118**: 608–615.

1846 Pagani A, Fischer-Colbrie R, Sanfilippo B, Winkler H, Cerrato M, Bussolati G. Secretogranin II expression in Ewing's sarcomas and primitive neuroectodermal tumors. Diagn Mol Pathol 1992, **1**: 165–172.

1847 Parham DM, Hijazi Y, Steinberg SM, Meyer WH, Horowitz M, Tzen CY, Wexler LH, Tsokos M. Neuroectodermal differentiation in Ewing's sarcoma family of tumors does not predict tumor behavior. Hum Pathol 1999, **30**: 911–918.

1848 Rud NP, Reiman HM, Pritchard DJ, Frassica FJ, Smithson WA. Extraosseous Ewing's sarcoma. A study of 42 cases. Cancer 1989, **64**: 1548–1553.

1849 Schmidt D, Harms D, Burdach S. Malignant peripheral neuroectodermal tumours of childhood and adolescence. Virchows Arch [A] 1985, **406**: 351–365.

1850 Schuetz AN, Rubin BP, Goldblum JR, Shehata B, Weiss SW, Liu W, Wick MR, Folpe AL. Intercellular junctions in Ewing sarcoma/primitive neuroectodermal tumor: additional evidence of epithelial differentiation. Mod Pathol 2005, **18**: 1403–1410.

1851 Sebire NJ, Gibson S, Rampling D, Williams S, Malone M, Ramsay AD. Immunohistochemical findings in embryonal small round cell tumors with molecular diagnostic confirmation. Appl Immunohistochem Mol Morphol 2005, **13**: 1–5.

1852 Selleri L, Hermanson GG, Eubanks JH, Lewis KA, Evans GA. Molecular localization of the t(11; 22)(q24; q12) translocation of Ewing sarcoma by chromosomal in situ suppression hybridization. Proc Natl Acad Sci USA 1991, **88**: 887–891.

1853 Shimada H, Newton WA Jr, Soule EH, Qualman SJ, Aoyama C, Maurer HM. Pathologic features of extraosseous Ewing's sarcoma. A report from the Intergroup Rhabdomyosarcoma Study. Hum Pathol 1988, **19**: 442–453.

1854 Shishikura A, Ushigome S, Shimoda T. Primitive neuroectodermal tumors of bone and soft tissue. Histological subclassification and clinicopathologic correlations. Acta Pathol Jpn 1993, **43**: 176–186.

1855 Sorensen P, Liu X, Delattre O, Rowland J, Biggs C, Thomas G, Triche T. Reverse transcriptase PCR amplification of EWS/FLI-1 fusion transcripts as a diagnostic test for peripheral primitive neuroectodermal tumors of childhood. Diagn Mol Pathol 1993, **2**: 147–157.

1856 Soule EH, Newton W Jr, Moon TE, Tefft M. Extraskeletal Ewing's sarcoma – a preliminary review of 26 cases encountered in the Intergroup Rhabdomyosarcoma Study. Cancer 1978, **42**: 259–264.

1857 Srivastava A, Rosenberg AE, Selig M, Rubin BP, Nielsen GP. Keratin-positive Ewing's sarcoma: an ultrastructural study of 12 cases. Int J Surg Pathol 2005, **13**: 43–50.

1858 Stevenson AJ, Chatten J, Bertoni F, Miettinen M. CD99 (p30/32MIC2) neuroectodermal/Ewing's sarcoma antigen as an immunohistochemical marker. Review of more than 600 tumors and the literature experience. Appl Immunohistochem 1994, **2**: 231–240.

1859 Suh CH, Ordóñez NG, Hicks J, Mackay B. Ultrastructure of the Ewing's sarcoma family of tumors. Ultrastruct Pathol 2002, **26**: 67–76.

1860 Terrier-Lacombe MJ, Guillou L, Chibon F, Gallagher G, Benhattar J, Terrier P, Ranchère D, Coindre JM. Superficial primitive Ewing's sarcoma: a clinicopathologic and molecular cytogenetic analysis of 14 cases. Mod Pathol 2009, **22**: 87–94.

1861 Thorner P, Squire J, Chilton-MacNeill S, Marrano P, Bayani J, Malkin D, Greenberg M, Lorenzana A, Zielenska M. Is the EWS/FLI-1 fusion transcript specific for Ewing sarcoma and peripheral primitive neuroectodermal tumor? A report of four cases showing the transcript in a wider range of tumor types. Am J Pathol 1996, **148**: 1125–1138.

1862 Triche TJ, Askin FB, Kissane JM. Neuroblastoma. Ewing's sarcoma, and the differential diagnosis of small-, round-, blue-cell tumors. In Finegold M (ed.): Pathology of neoplasia in children and adolescents, vol 18. Philadelphia, 1986, WB Saunders, p. 145.

1863 Turc-Carel C, Philip I, Berger MP, Philip T, Lenoir GM. Chromosome study of Ewing's sarcoma (ES) cell lines. Consistency of a reciprocal translocation t(11;22)(q24;q12). Cancer Genet Cytogenet 1984, **12**: 1–12.

1864 Vakar-Lopez F, Ayala AG, Raymond AK, Czerniak B. Epithelial phenotype in Ewing's sarcoma/primitive neuroectodermal tumor. Int J Surg Pathol 2000, **8**: 59–65.

1865 Variend S. Small cell tumors in childhood. A review. J Pathol 1985, **145**: 1–25.

1866 Weidner N, Tjoe J. Immunohistochemical profile of monoclonal antibody O13. Antibody that recognizes glycoprotein p30/32MIC2 and is useful in diagnosing Ewing's sarcoma and peripheral neuroepithelioma. Am J Surg Pathol 1994, **18**: 486–494.

1867 Wigger HJ, Salazar GH, Blane WA. Extraskeletal Ewing sarcoma. An ultrastructural study. Arch Pathol Lab Med 1977, **101**: 446–449.

1868 Yunis EJ. Ewing's sarcoma and related small round cell neoplasms in children. Am J Surg Pathol 1986, **10**(Suppl 1): 54–62.

Desmoplastic small cell tumor

1869 Adsay V, Cheng J, Athanasian E, Gerald W, Rosai J. Primary desmoplastic small cell tumor of soft tissues and bone of the hand. Am J Surg Pathol 1999, **23**: 1408–1413.

1870 Hamazaki M, Okita H, Hata J, Shimizu S, Kobayashi H, Aoki K, Nara T. Desmoplastic small cell tumor of soft tissue: molecular variant of EWS-WT1 chimeric fusion. Pathol Int 2006, **56**: 543–548.

Rhabdoid tumor

1871 Biegel JA. Molecular genetics of atypical teratoid/rhabdoid tumor. Neurosurg Focus 2006, **20**: E11.

1872 Fanburg-Smith JC, Hengge M, Hengge UR, Smith JS, Miettinen M. Extrarenal rhabdoid tumors of soft tissue: a clinicopathologic and immunohistochemical study of 18 cases. Ann Diagn Pathol 1999, **2**: 351–362.

1873 Frierson HF, Mills SE, Innes DJ Jr. Malignant rhabdoid tumor of the pelvis. Cancer 1985, **55**: 1963–1967.

1874 Gururangan S, Bowman LC, Parham DM, Wilimas JA, Rao B, Pratt CB, Douglass EC. Primary extracranial rhabdoid tumors. Clinicopathologic features and response to ifosfamide. Cancer 1993, **71**: 2653–2659.

1875 Hoot AC, Russo P, Judkins AR, Perlman EJ, Biegel JA. Immunohistochemical analysis of hSNF5/INI1 distinguishes renal and extra-renal malignant rhabdoid tumors from other pediatric soft tissue tumors. Am J Surg Pathol 2004, **28**: 1485–1491.

1876 Kent AL, Mahoney DH Jr, Gresik MV, Steuber CP, Fernbach DJ. Malignant rhabdoid tumor of the extremity. Cancer 1987, **60**: 1056–1059.

1877 Kodet R, Newton WA Jr, Sachs N, Hamoudi AB, Raney RB, Asmar L, Gehan EA. Rhabdoid tumors of soft tissues. A clinicopathologic study of 26 cases enrolled on the Intergroup Rhabdomyosarcoma Study. Hum Pathol 1991, **22**: 674–684.

1878 Kohashi K, Izumi T, Oda Y, Yamamoto H, Tamiya S, Taguchi T, Iwamoto Y, Hasegawa T, Tsuneyoshi M. Infrequent SMARCB1/INI1 gene alteration in epithelioid sarcoma: a useful tool in distinguishing epithelioid sarcoma from malignant rhabdoid tumor. Hum Pathol 2009, **40**: 349–355.

1879 Oda Y, Tsuneyoshi M. Extrarenal rhabdoid tumors of soft tissue: clinicopathological and molecular genetic review and distinction from other soft-tissue sarcomas with rhabdoid features. Pathol Int 2006, **56**: 287–295.

1880 Parham DM, Weeks DA, Beckwith JB. The clinicopathologic spectrum of putative extrarenal rhabdoid tumors. An analysis of 42 cases studied with immunohistochemistry or electron microscopy. Am J Surg Pathol 1994, **18**: 1010–1029.

1881 Roberts CW, Biegel JA. The role of SMARCB1/INI1 in development of rhabdoid tumor. Cancer Biol Ther 2009, **8**: 412–416.

1882 Schmidt D, Leuschner I, Harms D, Sprenger E, Schafer HJ. Malignant rhabdoid tumor. A morphological and flow cytometric study. Pathol Res Pract 1989, **184**: 202–210.

1883 Sotelo-Avila C, Gonzalez-Crussi F, De Mello D, Vogler C, Gooch WM, Gale G, Pena R. Renal and extrarenal rhabdoid tumors in children. A clinicopathologic study of 14 patients. Semin Diagn Pathol 1986, **3**: 151–163.

1884 Tsokos M, Kouraklis G, Chandra RS, Bhagavan BS, Triche TJ. Malignant rhabdoid tumor of the kidney and soft tissues. Evidence for a diverse morphological and immunocytochemical phenotype. Arch Pathol Lab Med 1989, **113**: 115–120.

1885 Tsuneyoshi M, Daimaru Y, Hashimoto H, Enjoji M. Malignant soft tissue neoplasms with the histologic features of renal rhabdoid tumors. An ultrastructural and immunohistochemical study. Hum Pathol 1985, **16**: 1235–1242.

1886 Weeks DA, Beckwith JB, Mierau GW. Rhabdoid tumor. An entity or a phenotype? Arch Pathol Lab Med 1989, **113**: 113–114.

1887 Wick MR, Ritter JH, Dehner LP. Malignant rhabdoid tumors. A clinicopathologic review and conceptual discussion. Semin Diagn Pathol 1995, **12**: 233–248.

Phosphaturic mesenchymal tumor

1888 Cai Q, Hodgson SF, Kao PC, Lennon VA, Klee GG, Zinsmiester AR, Kumar R. Brief report. Inhibition of renal phosphate transport by a tumor product in a patient with oncogenic osteomalacia. N Engl J Med 1994, **330**: 1645–1649.

1889 Folpe AL, Fanburg-Smith JC, Wiess SW. Most phosphaturic mesenchymal tumors are a single entity: an analysis of 31 cases. Mod Pathol 2003, **16**: 12A.

1890 Folpe AL, Fanburg-Smith JC, Billings SD, Bisceglia M, Bertoni F, Cho JY, Econs MJ, Inwards CY, Jan de Beur SM, Mentzel T, Montgomery E, Michal M, Miettinen M, Mills SE, Reith JD, O'Connell JX, Rosenberg AE, Rubin BP, Sweet DE, Vinh TN, Wold LE, Wehrli BM, White KE, Zaino RJ, Weiss SW. Most osteomalacia-associated mesenchymal tumors are a single histopathologic entity: an analysis of 32 cases and a comprehensive review of the literature. Am J Surg Pathol 2004, **28**: 1–30.

1891 Weidner N. Review and update. Oncogenic osteomalacia-rickets. Ultrastruct Pathol 1991, **15**: 317–333.

1892 Weidner N, Bar RS, Weiss D, Strottmann MP. Neoplastic pathology of oncogenic osteomalacia/rickets. Cancer 1985, **55**: 1691–1705.

1893 Weidner N, Santa Cruz D. Phosphaturic mesenchymal tumors. A polymorphous group causing osteomalacia or rickets. Cancer 1987, **59**: 1442–1454.

Pleomorphic hyalinizing angiectatic tumor of soft parts

1894 Bridge JA, Gentry JD, Swarts SJ, Billings SD, Bridge RS Jr, Althof PA, Pickering D, Neff JR, Wiess SW. Supernumerary ring chromosomes in pleomorphic hyalinizing angiectatic tumor: a feature of potential diagnostic utility [abstract]. Mod Pathol 2003, **16**: 9A.

1895 Folpe AL, Weiss SW. Pleomorphic hyalinizing angiectatic tumor: analysis of 41 cases supporting evolution from a distinctive precursor lesion. Am J Surg Pathol 2004, **28**: 1417–1425.

1896 Kazakov DV, Pavlovsky M, Mukensnabl P, Michal M. Pleomorphic hyalinizing angiectatic tumor with a sarcomatous component recurring as high-grade myxofibrosarcoma. Pathol Int 2007, **57**: 281–284.

1897 Smith ME, Fisher C, Weiss SW. Pleomorphic hyalinizing angiectatic tumor of soft parts: a low-grade neoplasm resembling neurilemoma. Am J Surg Pathol 1996, **20**: 21–29.

Myoepithelioma of soft tissue

1898 Dabska M. Parachordoma. A new clinicopathologic entity. Cancer 1977, **40**: 1586–1592.

1899 Fisher C, Miettinen M. Parachordoma: a clinicopathologic and immunohistochemical study of four cases of an unusual soft tissue neoplasm. Ann Diagn Pathol 1999, **1**: 3–10.

1900 Gleason BC, Fletcher CD. Myoepithelial carcinoma of soft tissue in children: an aggressive neoplasm analyzed in a series of 29 cases. Am J Surg Pathol 2007, **31**: 1813–1824.

1901 Hornick JL, Fletcher CDM. Myoepithelial tumors of soft tissue. A clinicopathologic and immunohistochemical study of 101 cases with evaluation of prognostic parameters. Am J Surg Pathol 2003, **27**: 1183–1196.

1902 Ishida T, Oda H, Oka T, Imamura T, Machinami R. Parachordoma. An ultrastructural and immunohistochemical study. Virchows Arch [A] 1993, **422**: 239–246.

1903 Michal M, Miettinen M. Myoepitheliomas of the skin and soft tissues. Report of 12 cases. Virchows Arch 1999, **434**: 393–400.

1904 Sangueza OP, White CR Jr. Parachordoma. Am J Dermatopathol 1994, **16**: 185–188.

1905 Shin HJ, Mackay B, Ichinose H, Ayala AG, Romsdahl MM. Parachordoma. Ultrastruct Pathol 1994, **18**: 249–256.

Other tumors

1906 Polk P, Parker KM, Biggs PJ. Soft tissue oncocytoma. Hum Pathol 1996, **27**: 206–208.

METASTATIC TUMORS

1907 Alexiou G, Papadopoulou-Alexiou M, Karakousis CP. Renal cell carcinoma presenting as skeletal muscle mass. J Surg Oncol 1984, **27**: 23–25.

1908 Perez-Montiel DM, Plaza JA, Wakely P, Suster S. Metastases to soft tissue sites: review of 86 cases over a 30 year period [abstract]. Mod Pathol 2003, **16**: 19A.

OTHER TUMORLIKE CONDITIONS

1909 Barzilai A, Huszar M, Shpiro D, Nass D, Trau H. Pseudorheumatoid nodules in adults: a juxta-articular form of nodular granuloma annulare. Am J Dermatopathol 2005, **27**: 1–5.

1910 Cabanne F, Chapuis JL, Duperrat B, Putelat R. L'infiltration cutanée par la polyvinylpyrrolidone. Ann Anat Pathol 1966, **11**: 385–396.

1911 Chefetz I, Ben Amitai D, Browning S, Skorecki K, Adir N, Thomas MG, Kogleck L, Topaz O, Indelman M, Uitto J, Richard G, Bradman N, Sprecher E. Normophosphatemic familial tumoral calcinosis is caused by deleterious mutations in SAMD9, encoding a TNF-alpha responsive protein. J Invest Dermatol 2008, **128**: 1423–1429.

1912 Chefetz I, Heller R, Galli-Tsinopoulou A, Richard G, Wollnik B, Indelman M, Koerber F, Topaz O, Bergman R, Sprecher E, Schoenau E. A novel homozygous missense mutation in FGF23 causes familial tumoral calcinosis associated with disseminated visceral calcification. Hum Genet 2005, **118**: 261–266.

1913 Chong H, Brady K, Metze D, Calonje E. Persistent nodules at injection sites (aluminium granuloma) – clinicopathological study of 14 cases with a diverse range of histological reaction patterns. Histopathology 2006, **48**: 182–188.

1914 Coleman WR, Homer RS, Kaplan RP. Branchial cleft heterotopia of the lower neck. J Cutan Pathol 1989, **16**: 353–358.

1915 Fetsch JF, Montgomery EA, Meis JM. Calcifying fibrous pseudotumor. Am J Surg Pathol 1993, **17**: 502–508.

1916 Fraga S, Helwig EB, Rosen SM. Bronchogenic cysts in the skin and subcutaneous tissue. Am J Clin Pathol 1971, **56**: 230–238.

1917 Harkness JW, Peters HJ. Tumoral calcinosis, a report of six cases. J Bone Joint Surg (Am) 1967, **49**: 721–731.

1918 Hizawa K, Inaba H, Nakanishi S, Otsuka H, Izumi K. Subcutaneous pseudosarcomatous polyvinylpyrrolidone granuloma. Am J Surg Pathol 1984, **8**: 393–398.

1919 Kazakov DV, Fanburg-Smith JC, Suster S, Neuhauser TS, Palmedo G, Zamecnik M, Kempf W, Michal M. Castleman disease of the subcutis and underlying skeletal muscle: report of 6 cases. Am J Surg Pathol 2004, **28**: 569–577.

1920 Krishnan J, Chu WS, Elrod JP, Frizzera G. Tumoral presentation of amyloidosis (amyloidomas) in soft tissues. A report of 14 cases. Am J Clin Pathol 1993, **100**: 135–144.

1921 Kuo T-T, Hsueh S. Mucicarminophilic histiocytosis. A polyvinylpyrrolidone (PVP) storage disease simulating signet-ring cell carcinoma. Am J Surg Pathol 1984, **8**: 419–428.

1922 Laskin WB, Miettinen M, Fetsch JF. Calcareous lesions of the distal extremities resembling tumoral calcinosis (tumoral calcinosislike lesions): clinicopathologic study of 43 cases emphasizing a pathogenesis-based approach to classification. Am J Surg Pathol 2007, **31**: 15–25.

1923 Lyles KW, Burkes EJ, Ellis GJ, Lucas EJ, Dolan EA, Drezner MK. Genetic transmission of tumoral calcinosis. Autosomal dominant with variable clinical expressivity. J Clin Endocrinol Metab 1985, **60**: 1093–1096.

1924 Montgomery EA, Meis JM, Frizzera G. Rosai–Dorfman disease of soft tissue. Am J Surg Pathol 1992, **16**: 122–129.

1925 Nascimento AF, Ruiz R, Hornick JL, Fletcher CD. Calcifying fibrous 'pseudotumor'. Clinicopathologic study of 15 cases and analysis of its relationship to inflammatory myofibroblastic tumor. Int J Surg 2002, **10**: 189–196.

1926 Nielsen GP, Fletcher CD, Smith MA, Rybak L, Rosenberg AE. Soft tissue aneurysmal bone cyst: a clinicopathologic study of five cases. Am J Surg Pathol 2001, **26**: 64–69.

1927 Pakasa NM, Kalengayi RM. Tumoral calcinosis: a clinicopathological study of 111 cases with emphasis on the earliest changes. Histopathology 1997, **31**: 18–24.

1928 Rodriguez-Peralto JL, Lopez-Barea F, Sanchez-Herrera S, Atienza M. Primary aneurysmal cyst of soft tissues (extraosseous aneurysmal cyst). Am J Surg Pathol 1994, **18**: 632–636.

1929 Shareef DS, Salm R. Ectopic vestigial lesions of the neck and shoulders. J Clin Pathol 1981, **34**: 1155–1162.

1930 Sleater J, Mullins D. Subcutaneous Castleman's disease of the wrist. Am J Dermatopathol 1995, **17**: 174–178.

1931 Specktor P, Cooper JG, Indelman M, Sprecher E. Hyperphosphatemic familial tumoral calcinosis caused by a mutation in GALNT3 in a European kindred. J Hum Genet 2006, **51**: 487–490.

Peritoneum, retroperitoneum, and related structures

26

CHAPTER CONTENTS

Peritoneum

Normal anatomy

The peritoneal cavity is lined by mesodermally derived tissues consisting of a layer of surface mesothelium resting on vascularized subserosal tissue and separated from it by a continuous basal lamina.[2] It is characterized ultrastructurally by the presence of apical tight junctions, desmosomes, surface microvilli, and tonofilaments. Immunohistochemically, it exhibits strong reactivity to cytokeratin (including keratin 5/6), epithelial membrane antigen (EMA), calretinin, mesothelin, podoplanin (D2-40), thrombomodulin, and basal lamina components. It is negative for carcinoembryonic antigen (CEA), Leu-M1, Ber-EP4 and B72:3. The surprising fact that normal mesothelium expresses parathyroid hormone-like peptide activity has been noted.[4] More significant from a diagnostic standpoint is the fact that developing mesothelium in the embryo exhibits transient immunoreactivity for desmin before switching to its adult keratin-based intermediate filament profile, and that this capacity for desmin expression reappears under reactive and (less commonly) neoplastic conditions.[3]

The resting subserosal cells have the overall structure of fibroblasts, are negative for keratin, and express vimentin.[1] These cells are sometimes referred to as *multipotential subserosal cells* because they are thought to have the capacity to serve as replicative cells that can differentiate into surface mesothelium. In females, these subserosal cells can be conspicuous, especially in the pelvic parietal peritoneum and on the bladder dome. They are sensitive to sex hormones and are probably the progenitors of lesions such as endometriosis, endosalpingiosis, ectopic decidual reaction, leiomyomatosis peritonealis disseminata, and tumors of ovarian or uterine type (see p. 2244). The large group of peritoneal disorders related to the female genital tract is also discussed in Chapter 19, Ovary and Uterus corpus.

Structures or regions topographically related to the peritoneum and retroperitoneum are the omentum, mesentery, hernia sacs, umbilicus, and sacrococcygeal region. Since an overlapping of pathologic processes exists among all of them, they are discussed in this chapter, with appropriate references to other sections of the text when indicated.

Inflammation

Chemical peritonitis can be caused by bile, pancreatic juice, gastric juice, meconium, and radiographic contrast media. Barium peritonitis was seen in the past following perforation of large bowel occurring during the course of radiographic examinations performed because of obstruction.[14]

Extravasation of *bile* as a result of trauma or disease of the gallbladder, bile ducts, or duodenum causes an acute or subacute peritonitis that is initially limited to the upper quadrant of the abdomen.[7] *Gastric juice* produces a severe peritoneal reaction because of its hydrochloric acid content, although it may be bacteriologically sterile. The release of *pancreatic juice* causes fat necrosis. The formation of calcium salts in large areas of fat necrosis may cause hypocalcemia.

Bacterial peritonitis may be either primary or secondary. The *primary* form usually is caused by streptococci and is seen more commonly in children (particularly in those affected by the nephrotic syndrome). Adult patients with ascites secondary to liver disease are also susceptible. This form of peritonitis tends to produce marked constitutional symptoms with minimal localizing findings. Aspiration of intra-abdominal fluid discloses an inflammatory exudate containing only a single type of organism. Large amounts of extracellular fluid are lost into the exudate, equivalent to those of a burn covering one-half to three-fourths of the cutaneous surface.

Perforation of a viscus such as the colon produces *secondary* peritonitis. If the fluid is aspirated, a mixture of bacterial flora rather than a single organism is usually found. *Tuberculous peritonitis* may occur with few constitutional symptoms, despite extensive involvement of the peritoneum.[5,10,11,17] In a review of 47 cases, Singh et al.[16] found radiographic evidence of pulmonary parenchymal lesions in only 6% of the cases. The search for acid-fast organisms on a direct smear of ascitic fluid is often unrewarding. The best diagnostic methods are culture of the fluid and percutaneous biopsy of the peritoneum.[12,13] Singh et al.[16] found the latter to be useful in 64% of their cases. Chemotherapy is the treatment of choice; surgery is reserved for those cases associated with enteritis leading to bowel obstruction, perforation, fistula, or a mass that does not resolve with drug therapy.[15] Other specific forms of peritonitis are *coccidioidomycosis* and *actinomycosis*.[6] Exceptionally, *Oxyuris vermicularis* may escape from the appendix or other portions of the gastrointestinal tract into the peritoneal cavity and elicit the formation of granulomas.[19]

Meconium peritonitis is the result of perforation of the small bowel during intrauterine life. It may present in infants as intestinal obstruction requiring surgical intervention. With healing, only scattered calcific foci remain. These can be located in the main peritoneal cavity, inguinal region, or scrotum; the latter can simulate clinically a testicular tumor.[8,18]

Vernix caseosa peritonitis represents a rare complication of cesarean section, and it has distinctive microscopic features.[9]

Adhesions

Adhesions, with the potential for intestinal obstruction, follow all intra-abdominal operations. They can be minimized by careful handling of tissues, re-peritonealization where feasible, and removal of intraperitoneal blood clots. Ryan et al.[26] showed in an experimental model that drying of the serosa plus bleeding consistently resulted in the formation of adhesions. There is good experimental evidence to suggest that the formation of peritoneal adhesions is related to a local depression of peritoneal plasminogen activator, which is the principal peritoneal fibrin-clearing system known.[20]

Innumerable agents, including sodium citrate, heparin, olive oil, liquid paraffin, adrenocorticotropic hormone (ACTH), cortisone, pepsin, fibrinolysin, and amniotic fluid, have been used over the years to prevent adhesions, but none has accomplished this goal in an entirely successful fashion. Adhesions become collagenous and strong as the cellularity of their fibrous tissue decreases with maturation. Postoperative adhesions are the most frequent cause of intestinal obstruction today.

Extensive peritoneal fibrosis (so-called *sclerosing* or *fibrosing peritonitis*) also has been described as a reaction to asbestos, to silica in drug abusers,[22] in patients with the carcinoid syndrome, in patients with lupus,[25] in women with luteinized thecomas/thecomatosis and related proliferative stromal lesions of the ovary,[23,27] and as a complication of the administration of beta-adrenergic-blocking drugs,[21] or of compounds containing fluoropyrimidines.[24] In many instances, the etiologic agent cannot be identified; some of these 'idiopathic' cases are probably pathogenetically related to mesenteric panniculitis and – as such – are part of the spectrum of the inflammatory fibrosclerosis group of diseases (see p. 2247). A few of the cases associated with ovarian tumors have proved fatal.[27]

Reaction to foreign materials

The peritoneum reacts briskly to foreign substances. The most spectacular (and easiest to recognize) are those accompanying retained sponges and instruments after surgery, an event still haunting the laparotomy procedure and more likely to occur in emergency situations and/or in obese patients.[36] Classically, one of the better known peritoneal reactions to foreign material is *talc powder granuloma*, which is secondary to the talc (hydrated magnesium silicate) used in the past on surgical gloves. Spillage of this material into the peritoneal cavity at surgery results in nodules that can be mistaken grossly for tuberculosis or metastatic carcinoma. Microscopically, they are formed by foreign body granulomas containing birefringent crystals. The latter are made apparent with polarizing lenses or simply by lowering the condenser of the microscope.

Talc used for surgical gloves has long been recognized as a hazard and has been replaced by other substances, such as modified starch. Although these materials elicit a lesser degree of reaction, intraperitoneal granulomas may still develop,[43] on average between 10 days and 4 weeks after a laparotomy. These usually have the appearance of foreign body granulomas but sometimes exhibit tuberculoid features with caseum-like necrosis.[42] At reoperation, the findings are ascites, miliary peritoneal nodules, serosal inflammation, and adhesions. The gross appearance can closely simulate metastatic carcinoma, tuberculosis, or Crohn disease. The nature of the granulomas can be identified by the presence of granules that are periodic acid–Schiff (PAS) positive and birefringent (with a Maltese cross pattern) within the cytoplasm of histiocytes and foreign body giant cells.[33,35]

Levison et al.[40] have pointed out that the Maltese cross pattern is characteristic of corn starch, whereas other types of starch particles may have different shapes, sizes, and surface markings. The diagnosis may be suspected through the finding of starch granules in the aspirated peritoneal fluid. Fortunately, the disease is usually self-limited.

Other sources of surgical contamination are the cellulose fibers derived from disposable surgical gowns and drapes and the oxidized regenerated cellulose used as a hemostatic agent.[38,44] Sometimes the starch found in peritoneal granulomas does not originate in surgical gloves but from food starch that has gained its access to the peritoneal cavity through perforation of the bowel[34] or from the material contained in contraceptive devices.[40]

Mineral oil or paraffin placed in the peritoneal cavity in the distant past to prevent adhesions was responsible for the formation of nodules that could be grossly mistaken for metastatic carcinoma. Microscopically, these nodules exhibit foreign body giant cells, chronic inflammation, and foamy macrophages. Similar changes follow rupture of a cystic teratoma of the ovary, in which large amounts of oily material cause a profound nodular peritoneal reaction.[28] Ruptured ovarian teratomas can also be associated with peritoneal *melanosis*.[37]

Keratin from endometrioid adenocarcinomas with squamous differentiation (adenoacanthomas) of the endometrium or ovary can detach from the main tumor, reach the peritoneal cavity (through the fallopian tube in the case of uterine tumors), and elicit a brisk foreign body-type granulomatous reaction. The detection of these keratin granulomas has no prognostic significance and should not be equated with the presence of viable tumor implants.[30,39]

Peritoneal endometriosis may result in the formation of *necrotic pseudoxanthomatous nodules*. They may follow diathermy ablation of the lesion, but they may also occur spontaneously.[31,32]

Exceptionally, silicosis can involve the peritoneal serosa and simulate a tumor on gross examination.[41]

Although not a foreign body, one could mention here the curious phenomenon of implantation of normal splenic tissue in the peritoneal cavity following traumatic rupture of the spleen, a process known as *splenosis*[29] (see Chapter 22).

Cysts and loose bodies

Pseudocysts of the peritoneal cavity (lacking a mesothelial or epithelial lining) may follow inflammatory processes such as perforated colitis or perforated appendicitis.

Solitary cysts varying in size from 1 to 6 cm can be found incidentally within the peritoneal cavity, either attached to the wall or lying loose in the lower pelvis. They have a translucent wall, watery fluid in the lumen, and a lining composed of one or more layers of mesothelial cells[51] (Fig. 26.1). They probably represent acquired inclusion cysts related to chronic inflammation. A case of multilocular *melanotic* peritoneal cyst has been described.[47]

A probably related condition has been designated **cystic** or **multicystic benign mesothelioma**.[49,53,60] This process nearly always occurs in the pelvis of adult females, the average age at diagnosis being around 35 years. It has also been described involving most of the peritoneum, and a few cases have been seen in males. Often there is a history of previous pelvic surgery, endometriosis, or pelvic inflammatory disease. This entity may result in pelvic pain, present clinically as a mass, or be found incidentally at laparotomy (often at the time of a tubal ligation) or within a hernia sac. Grossly, multiple cysts are present, measuring up to 15 cm or more in diameter, attached to or engulfing pelvic organs (Fig. 26.2). Microscopically, the cysts are lined by flattened or cuboidal mesothelial cells.

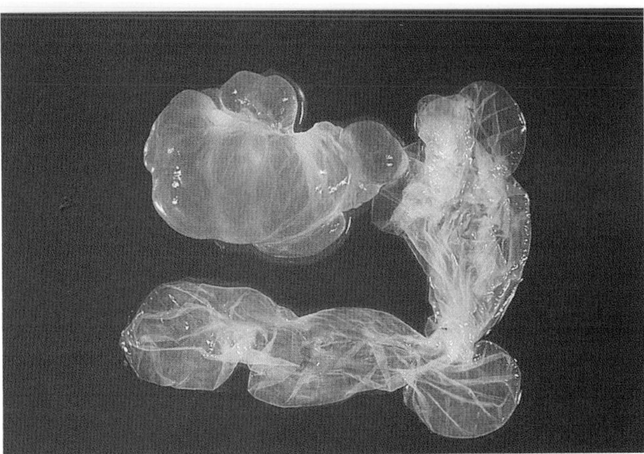

Fig. 26.1 Gross appearance of peritoneal cysts. They have a thin, translucent wall and contain a clear fluid.
(Courtesy of Dr Juan José Segura, San José, Costa Rica)

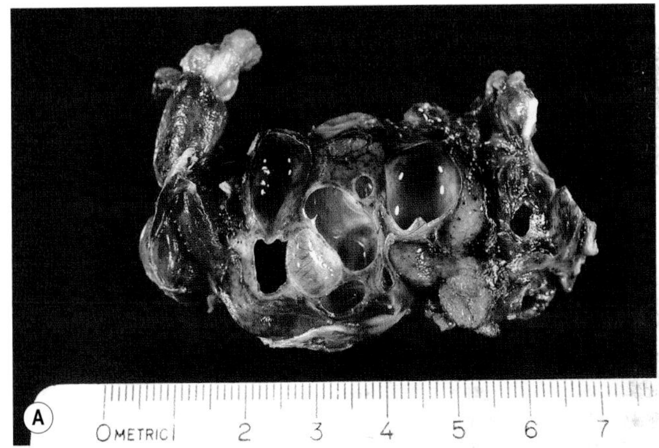

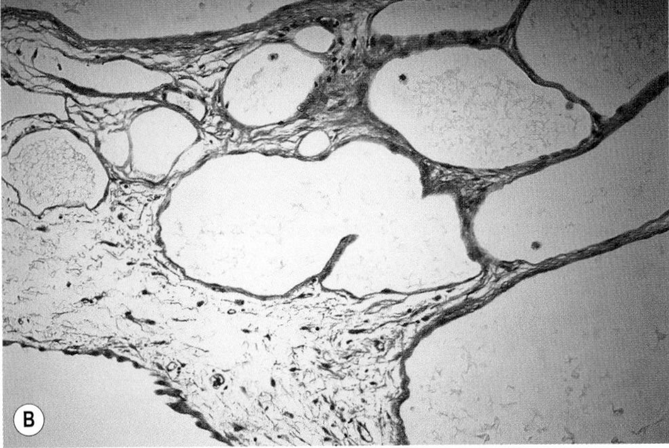

Fig. 26.2 So-called 'multicystic benign mesothelioma'. **A**, Gross appearance. **B**, Microscopic appearance. The flat shape of the mesothelium lining the cyst simulates the appearance of a lymphangioma.

When flat, the cells closely simulate the appearance of endothelial cells. Intracellular hyaline globules may be present.[50] The mesothelial cells react immunohistochemically for keratin and calretinin; are negative for factor VIII-related antigen and other endothelial markers; sometimes show focal reactivity for hormone receptors;[58] and exhibit desmosomes, tonofibrils, and slender microvilli on ultrastructural examination.[53,59] The wall, which is devoid of smooth muscle, usually shows foci of chronic inflammation, hemorrhage, and fibrin deposition. Sometimes the reactive mesothelial proliferation in the wall of these cysts is prominent enough to simulate a malignancy.[52]

The natural history of this disorder is characterized by a great tendency to local recurrence. This fact, plus the tumorlike appearance that these lesions exhibit grossly, is responsible for the assumption that they represent benign mesotheliomas. We agree with Ross et al.[56] that they probably are instead **multiple peritoneal inclusion cysts** forming as a result of peritoneal reactive proliferation. Their tendency for recurrence can be explained by persistence of the original inciting factor. Interestingly, this entity can be seen in association with adenomatoid tumor, another benign mesothelial lesion for which the neoplastic versus hyperplastic pathogenesis has been argued.[46] The main differential diagnosis is with cystic lymphangioma[45] (see pp. 2247, 2248, and 2255).

Cysts of müllerian origin can occur between the bladder and rectum in the true pelvis of males.[48] They result from persistence of müllerian duct derivatives and are usually lined by fallopian tube-type epithelium.[57] They have also been described in the mesentery and other portions of the abdominal cavity (see p. 2248). Occasionally, they may be the site of malignant transformation.[54]

Appendix epiploica may twist, undergo massive fat necrosis, and present as a sclerocalcified nodule either attached to its original site or free-floating in the abdominal cavity[61] (Fig. 26.3). Sometimes the fat necrosis has a *membranous* quality by virtue of the lining of the cysts by an eosinophilic membrane with pseudopapillary infoldings having the histochemical staining pattern of ceroid.[55]

Hyperplasia and metaplasia

The mesothelial lining surface has a great capacity to undergo florid hyperplastic changes when irritated. This hyperplasia can occur in a diffuse fashion throughout the peritoneal cavity in cases of liver cirrhosis, collagen vascular diseases (such as lupus erythematosus), and viral infections. Actually, mesothelial hyperplasia may supervene in any long-standing effusion regardless of its cause. It can also occur in a localized fashion as a response to injury. Hernia sacs can exhibit florid foci of **nodular mesothelial hyperplasia** following incarceration or some other mechanical insult; this is particularly common in children and may simulate malignancy[64,74] (Fig. 26.4). A similar change may occur in the serosa of an acutely inflamed appendix or a fallopian tube following rupture of an ectopic pregnancy, simulating implants from a serous papillary tumor of the ovary.[67] The danger of misinterpreting these reactive mesothelial changes as neoplastic is even greater when they develop in association with ovarian neoplasms, sometimes in intimate closeness to them.[65] Reactive mesothelial-lined gland-like structures also occur in association with pseudosarcomatous proliferative funiculitis (see below).[71]

Microscopically, these mesothelial hyperplastic changes may appear as papillary projections, solid nests, or tubular structures (Figs 26.5 and 26.6). They may project on the surface or interact in a complex fashion with the underlying stroma, simulating invasion.[70] Psammoma bodies may be present in the stroma of the papillary formations.[74] The cells may be vacuolated or have an entirely clear cytoplasm;[70] these vacuoles do not stain for mucin or fat. In cases of florid diffuse mesothelial hyperplasia, some of the reactive mesothelial cells can be found within the dilated ('lymphangiectatic') lumen of lymph vessels in the abdominal skin, presumably as the result of reflux.[76]

A reactive change that has acquired a notoriety out of proportion with its clinical significance is that of **nodular histiocytic/ mesothelial hyperplasia**. Among its many synonyms, the most picturesque is that of MICE (mesothelial/monocytic incidental cardiac excrescences), due to the fact that one of the sites in which it may be found is the heart[77] (see Chapter 27 for a more detailed account). Suffice it to say here that it can also present within the peritoneal cavity, nearly always as an incidental microscopic finding. It is microscopically composed of an admixture of CD68-positive histiocytes (which predominate) and keratin- and calretinin-positive mesothelial cells, the latter often appearing as clusters and micropapillae.[73] Its only importance derives from the fact that the pathologist unaware of its existence may overdiagnose it as mesothelioma, carcinoma, or worse.[63]

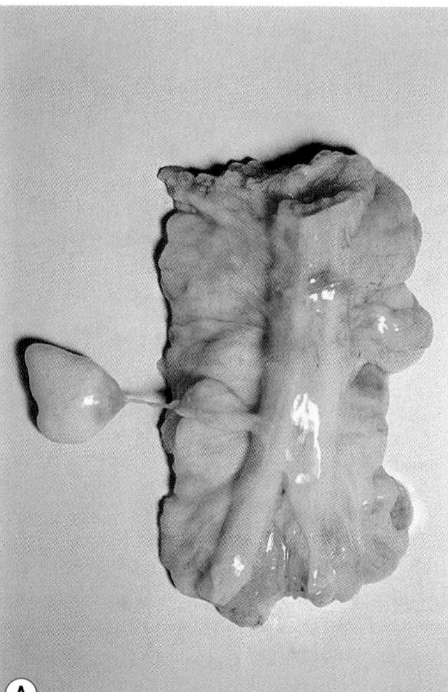

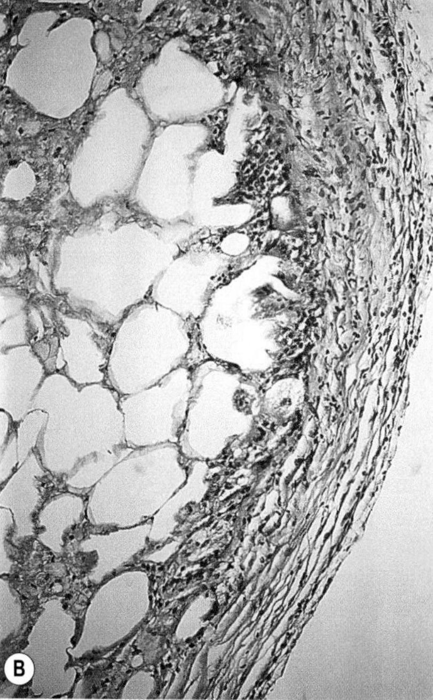

Fig. 26.3 Twisted appendix epiploica. **A**, Gross appearance. **B**, Microscopic appearance, showing inflammatory reaction to fat necrosis.

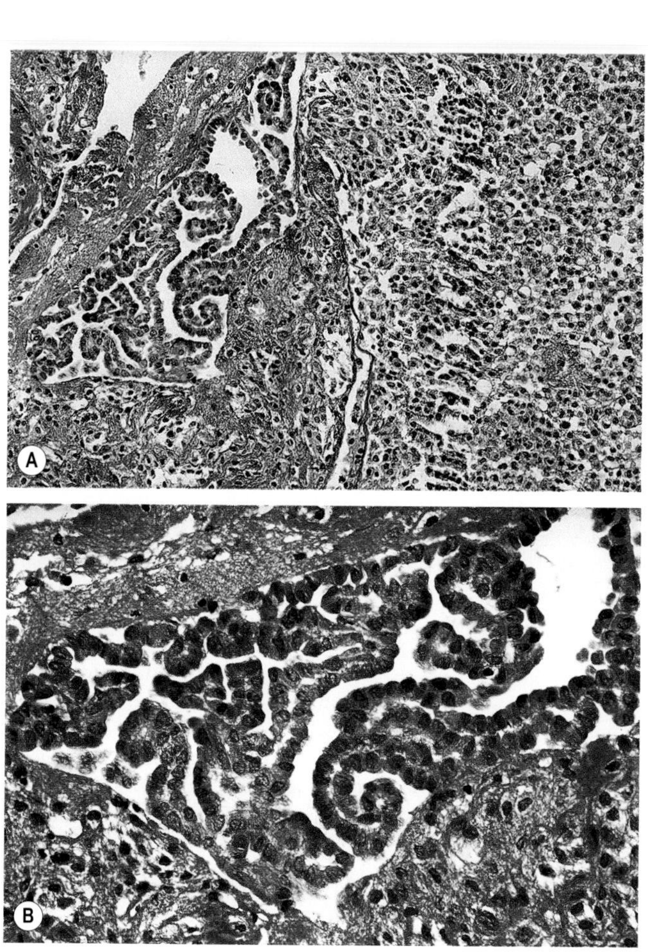

Fig. 26.4 **A** and **B**, Florid mesothelial hyperplasia in hernia sac. The complex papillary architecture may simulate a mesothelioma.

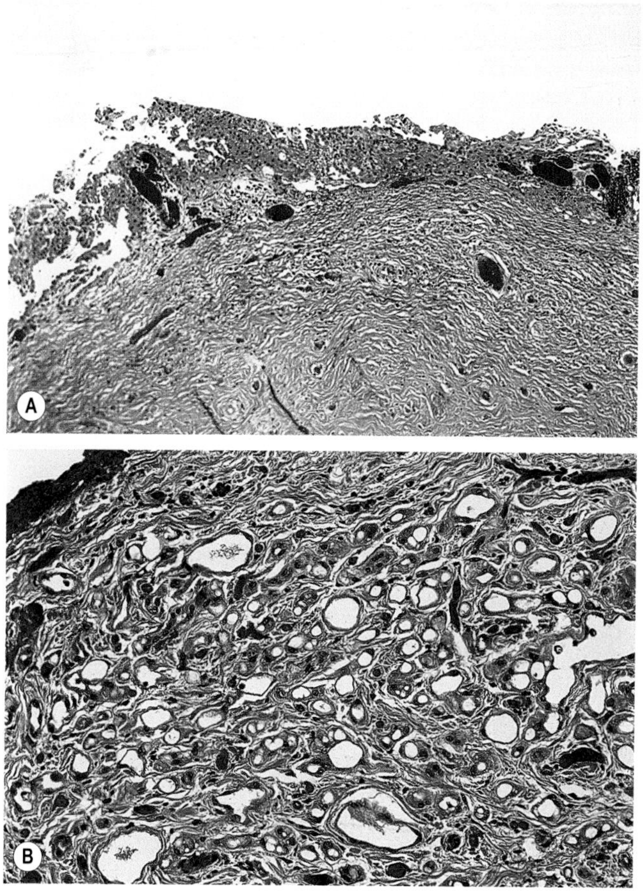

Fig. 26.6 **A** and **B**, Florid mesothelial hyperplasia with a pattern resembling adenomatoid tumor.

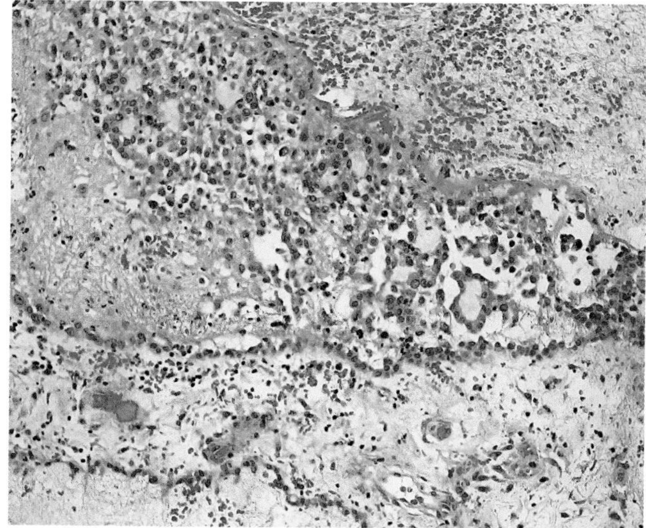

Fig. 26.5 Reactive mesothelial hyperplasia in a patient with granulosa cell tumor of the ovary. This should not be overinterpreted as a tumor implant.

The differential diagnosis between reactive mesothelial hyperplasia and mesothelioma can be very difficult. Features favoring malignancy are the presence of *grossly visible* nodular or papillary foci, marked nuclear atypia, increase in nucleocytoplasmic ratio, and presence of necrosis in the desmoplastic areas.[68,70] The latter finding is one of the most useful signs, since it is extremely unusual in reactive processes.

Immunohistochemically, reactive mesothelial cells stain strongly for keratin of various molecular weights and may regain the capacity for desmin expression normally exhibited by the developing mesothelium.[69] Reactive subserosal connective tissue cells retain their expression of vimentin but also acquire immunoreactivity for low molecular weight keratin and develop the ultrastructural features of myofibroblasts.[62] Unfortunately, these features are of little practical use in the differential diagnosis with mesothelioma.[68] Instead, immunohistochemistry can be of value in the differential diagnosis between reactive mesothelial hyperplasia and epithelial tumor implants in patients with borderline or malignant ovarian serous neoplasms, although the differences are not as sharp as those between pleural mesothelioma and lung adenocarcinoma (see under Differential diagnosis and in Chapters 7 and 19). It is important not to misinterpret as neoplastic the sometimes thick layer of keratin-positive reactive submesothelial fibroblasts that is often seen around or in between peritoneal tumor nodules of one type or another.

Mesothelial cells can also undergo metaplastic changes, the most important being *squamous metaplasia*[75] and *müllerian metaplasia*. The former is very rare and is usually seen in the context of multicystic benign mesothelioma.[72] The latter is seen almost exclusively in females, predominates in the pelvic region, and is mainly represented by endometriosis, endosalpingiosis, and ectopic decidual reaction.[78] (This is further discussed on page 2244 and in Chapter 19, Ovary.) Focal *cartilaginous metaplasia* also occurs, but this probably originates from the submesothelial mesenchymal elements rather than the mesothelium itself.[66]

Tumors

Mesothelioma

The mesotheliomas seen in the peritoneum are qualitatively similar to those occurring in the pleural cavity (see Chapter 7), but the relative proportions among the various types and the criteria used for the differential diagnosis with metastatic carcinoma (ovary and lung, respectively) are different. About 90–95% of mesotheliomas occur in the pleural cavity and only 5–10% in the peritoneal cavity.[109] Traditionally, peritoneal mesotheliomas have been divided into epithelial and fibrous, but the latter tumor is no longer considered a type of mesothelioma and is discussed separately (see p. 2243). The majority of true mesotheliomas are either solitary and benign or diffuse and malignant, but exceptions occur in both directions.

Benign mesothelioma

The benign form of mesothelioma typically presents as a solitary small papillary structure resembling grossly and microscopically the appearance of choroid plexus.[107] Most examples are incidental findings at the time of laparotomy. A few are pedunculated and may undergo torsion. We suspect that many of these lesions are reactive (i.e., examples of focal papillary mesothelial hyperplasia) rather than true neoplasms. There is no evidence that they undergo malignant transformation, and they are not related to asbestos exposure.

The above lesion is the only mesothelial proliferative process (other than the clearly reactive postinflammatory lesions) that we feel confident in regarding as benign. Solitary mesothelial proliferations having a predominantly *solid* pattern of growth and well-differentiated papillary mesothelial proliferations having a multicentric or diffuse quality are best regarded as malignant tumors[79] (see next section).

The lesion known as **multicystic benign mesothelioma** has been discussed on page 2235.

Malignant mesothelioma

General and clinical features. Most cases of peritoneal malignant mesothelioma occur in individuals past 40 years of age, but they have been described in young adults,[111] children,[82,115,132] and even neonates.[149] They occur both in males and females, with a definite predominance in the former.[87] Their frequency is on the increase.[81] About half of the cases are associated with asbestos exposure;[95,144] interestingly, peritoneal mesotheliomas are common in patients with heavy asbestos exposure, whereas pleural mesotheliomas predominate in the larger population of transiently exposed individuals. The average latency period is 15 years and over.[152] Major asbestos usage in the United States began around 1950 and continued through the 1960s, and therefore it is not unreasonable to expect a further increase in the incidence of this neoplasm. As a matter of fact, it has been estimated that the increase is likely to continue in the US and Western Europe well into the twenty-first century, at least until 2020.[92] Furthermore, the industrial expansion in Southeast Asia and China, plus the continued use of asbestos, may be harbingers of a new epidemic.[110]

The mechanism of asbestos pathogenesis seems to be related to the activation of the AP-1 pathway (which induces cell division) and to the secretion of tumor necrosis factor alpha (TNF-α) by mesothelial and other cells.[96]

Some peritoneal mesotheliomas have occurred after exposure to the contrast medium Thorotrast[130] and others following repeated mesothelial irritation.[93,143] In some instances, they have been found to coexist with pleural mesotheliomas.

The usual clinical presentation is in the form of recurrent ascites, which may be associated with abdominal cramps and increased abdominal girth.[108] Intermittent partial bowel obstruction is common. Occasionally, the disease may first manifest in a hernia sac (sometimes incarcerated), umbilicus, ovary, or large bowel wall.[90,98,101,135,145] In other instances, inguinal or cervical lymphadenopathy resulting from metastatic disease is the first sign of the tumor.[119,151] In yet other instances, the clinical presentation is in the form of a localized acute inflammatory process[116] or as a solitary distant metastasis in odd places like the palate or the lip.[89]

Gross features. Grossly, peritoneal mesothelioma usually appears as multiple plaques or nodules scattered over the visceral and parietal peritoneum.[113,156] It may be accompanied by dense intraperitoneal adhesions and shortening of the mesentery. Ascites is almost universally present. Coexisting fibrous pleural plaques are common, more so than with pleural mesotheliomas; sometimes fibrous plaques are also present within the abdominal cavity.[80] On rare occasions, the tumor presents as an isolated mass (localized mesothelioma),[79] even within the pancreas.[105] This lesion, which is much less common in the peritoneum than in the pleura, is distinguished from benign mesothelioma by virtue of its more solid appearance and the presence of atypia, which may be very subtle.[103] As already indicated, one should be very careful before making the diagnosis of benign mesothelioma in the presence of a localized mesothelial proliferation with a predominantly solid appearance. Although as a group they have a better prognosis than conventional diffuse mesotheliomas, we and others have seen several such cases in which recurrence developed in the form of disseminated peritoneal disease.[79]

Microscopic features. The microscopic pattern of malignant mesothelioma is highly variable. The most common arrangement is that of papillae or tubules lined by atypical mesothelial cells, the former having vascularized fibrous cores that may contain psammoma bodies (Figs 26.7 and 26.8).[83] In other instances, the mesothelial-like cells alternate with sarcomatoid spindle cells in a biphasic fashion. The individual cells are, in general, fairly uniform, with acidophilic or vacuolated cytoplasm and large vesicular or hyperchromatic nuclei. Mitoses may be difficult to find. Myxoid changes in the stroma may be pronounced (*myxoid mesotheliomas*).[148] Clusters of lymphoid follicles are common.[87] Exceptionally, the tumor may exhibit foci of cartilaginous or other types of stromal metaplasia.

Well-differentiated papillary mesothelioma shows a great predilection for women and is usually multifocal. Early descriptions emphasized the indolent clinical course and recommended a conservative approach,[104] but further studies have shown that it can behave in an aggressive fashion and that it should be regarded as a malignant tumor (see also under Therapy and prognosis).[94,117]

Mesothelioma with deciduoid features (*deciduoid mesothelioma*) is a morphologic variant of malignant mesothelioma in which the tumor cells resemble decidualized stroma because of their glassy acidophilic cytoplasm (Fig. 26.9). Although originally described

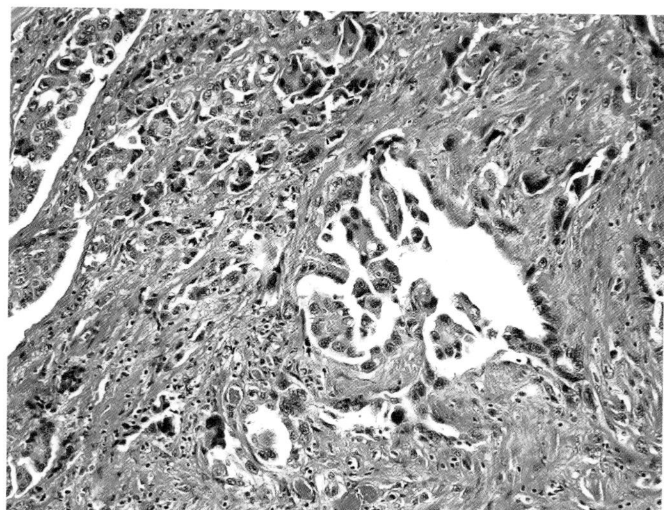

Fig. 26.7 Malignant mesothelioma with papillary formations and desmoplastic stromal reaction.

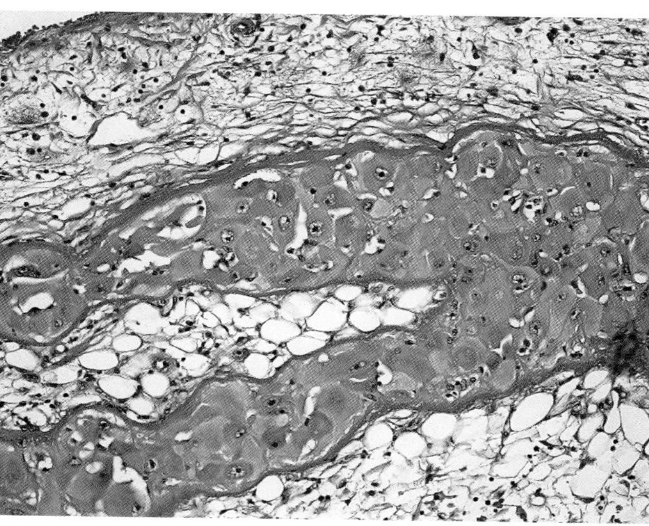

Fig. 26.9 So-called 'deciduoid mesothelioma'.

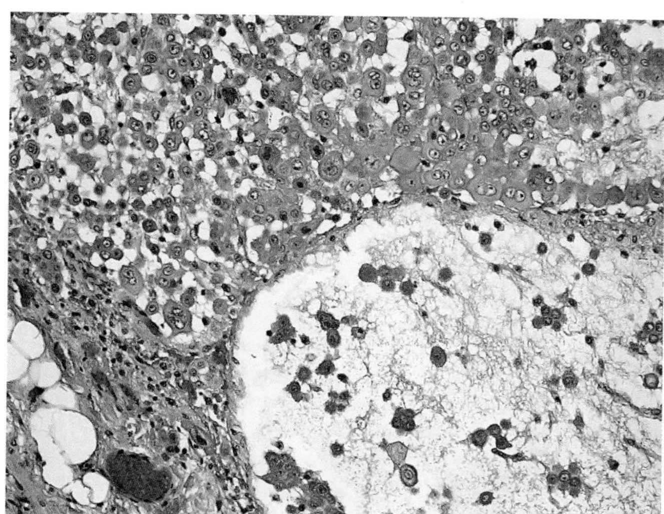

Fig. 26.8 Malignant mesothelioma with area of cystic degeneration.

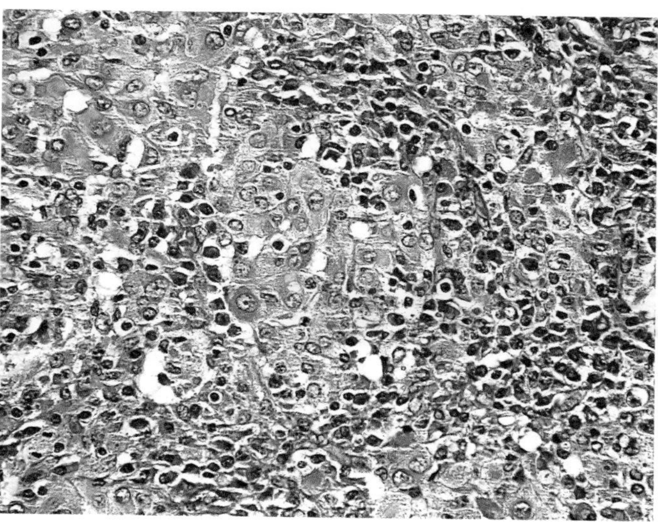

Fig. 26.10 So-called 'lymphohistiocytoid mesothelioma'. The tumor cells are admixed with numerous reactive lymphocytes and histiocytes.

in young women and unassociated with asbestos,[133] it has been shown subsequently that it can be seen in both sexes and all age groups, that it can be related to asbestos, and that it can present focally in what is otherwise a conventional tubulopapillary mesothelioma.[141,146]

Lymphohistiocytoid mesothelioma similar to its pleural counterpart has been observed in the peritoneal cavity (Fig. 26.10).

Mesothelioma with clear cell features (*clear cell mesothelioma*) is predominantly or entirely composed of tumor cells with optically clear cytoplasm.[136] This change may be due to the accumulation of glycogen, accumulation of lipids, mitochondrial swelling, presence of numerous cytoplasmic vesicles, or formation of true intracellular lumina.[135] When due to lipid surcharge, the cells may appear foamy and, if multinucleated, acquire the features of Touton giant cells.[121]

Sarcomatoid mesothelioma occurs, but not nearly as commonly as in the pleura.[122]

Mesothelioma with rhabdoid features (*rhabdoid mesothelioma*) is rare in the pleura and even more so in the peritoneum.[138] As is the case in most other sites, the rhabdoid morphology is associated with an unusually aggressive behavior.

Histochemical and immunohistochemical features. Malignant mesotheliomas usually contain extracellular mucosubstances, sometimes in large amounts. These represent acid mucopolysaccharides, since they stain with colloidal iron and Alcian blue, are removed at least partially by hyaluronidase digestion, and are PAS negative. Adenocarcinomas also may contain colloidal iron-positive material, but hyaluronidase digestion has little effect on the reaction. The detection of high levels of hyaluronic acid by histochemistry or biochemical extraction favors a diagnosis of mesothelioma, but it is not a specific finding.[99]

Immunohistochemically, the cells of malignant mesothelioma are generally positive for keratin (including keratin 5/6), EMA,

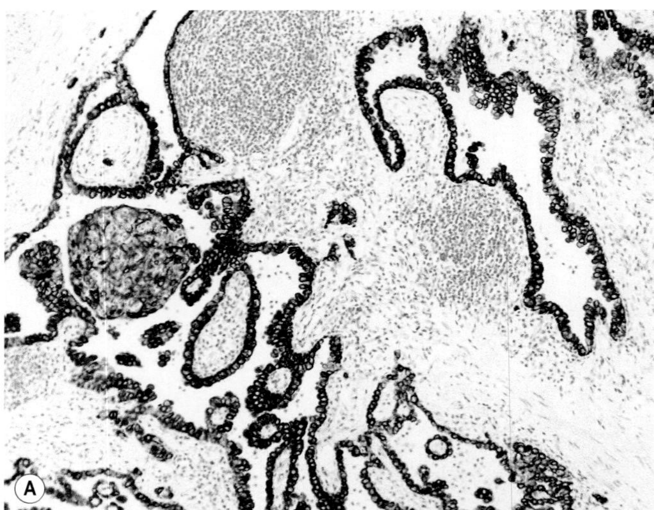

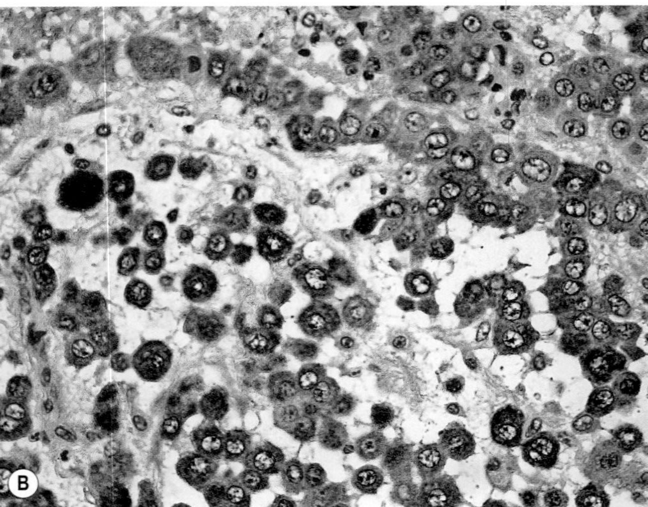

Fig. 26.11 Malignant mesothelioma cells show immunoreactivity for keratin 5/6 (**A**) and calretinin (**B**).

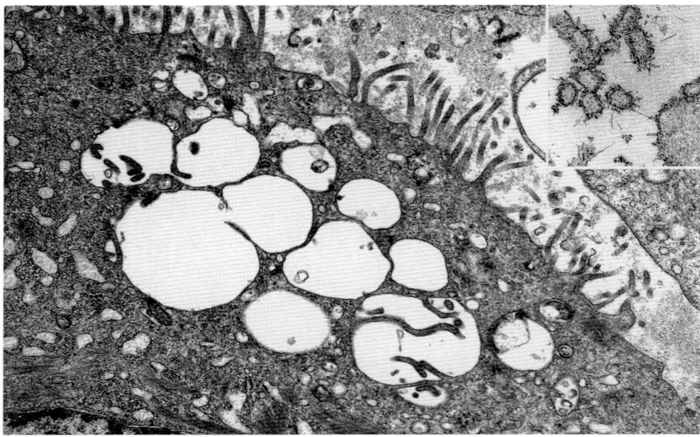

Fig. 26.12 Electron microscopic appearance of cell from malignant mesothelioma demonstrating numerous microvilli in luminal surface and intracellular vacuoles also equipped with microvilli. Inset shows microvilli coated with acid mucopolysaccharides. (×8000; inset, Hale colloidal iron, ×45 000)

(From Suzuki Y, Churg J, Kannerstein M. Ultrastructure of human malignant diffuse mesothelioma. Am J Pathol 1976, ***85:*** *241–262)*

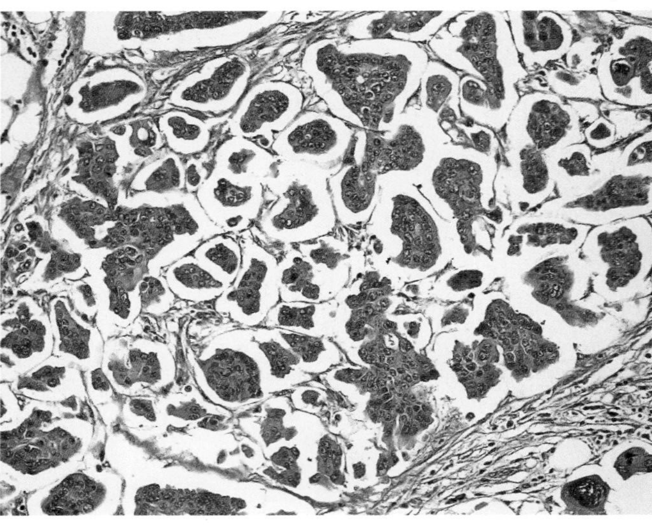

Fig. 26.13 Primary papillary serous carcinoma of peritoneum. The tumor is morphologically and immunohistochemically indistinguishable from its ovarian counterpart.

calretinin, mesothelin, the *WT1* gene product, thrombomodulin, HBME-1, podoplanin (D2-40), vimentin, neural cell adhesion molecules, and basement membrane-related proteins (type IV collagen, laminin, and laminin receptors) (Fig. 26.11). They are generally negative for CEA, B72.3, the MOC-31- and Ber-EP4-defined glycoproteins, and Leu-M1 (and related 'myelomonocytic' antigens).[112,118,124,126,137,150,155] Among the positive markers, podoplanin seems to be the best in terms of specificity, even if this specificity – like nearly all in the immunohistochemistry field – appears to be relative rather than absolute.[88,142]

Some correlation exists between the expression of these markers and the histologic appearance of the tumor.[85] In sarcomatoid mesotheliomas some or all of the markers may be lost.[84]

Some mesotheliomas have been shown to express actin and desmin;[123] when the latter is the case, the tumors have been referred to as *leiomyoid mesotheliomas*.[131]

The application of these markers to the differential diagnosis of malignant mesothelioma with metastatic carcinoma and reactive mesothelial hyperplasia is discussed below.

Electron microscopic features. By electron microscopy, the cells of a well-differentiated mesothelioma are very characteristic, to the point of them being considered at one time the diagnostic gold standard.[128] These cell exhibit polarity, abundant long and slender microvilli covered with fuzzy material, extra- and intracellular neolumina formation, glycogen granules, junctional structures, tonofilaments, and basal lamina[153] (Fig. 26.12). Transitions are found between typical mesothelial cells and cells with a mesenchymal, fibroblast-like appearance.[91] At the ultrastructural level, the cytoplasmic appearance of the mesothelioma variant known as deciduoid is seen to be due to the accumulation of cytoplasmic intermediate filaments.[147]

Molecular genetic features. Please refer to 'Malignant mesothelioma of the pleura' in Chapter 7.

Differential diagnosis. The differential diagnosis of malignant mesothelioma is mainly with reactive mesothelial hyperplasia and with primary or metastatic adenocarcinoma (Fig. 26.13). As far as the former situation is concerned, the distinction is largely based on morphologic features, since special techniques are of little use in this regard. Statistically speaking, strong immunoreactivity for EMA and overexpression of *TP53* is more common in malignant mesothelioma, but this is of no great value in the individual situation.[100] In terms of morphologic parameters, the US–Canadian Mesothelioma Reference Panel recently published a useful review article listing the most important distinguishing criteria.[100] They concluded that invasion of fat or of organ walls was the most reliable indicator of malignancy, as opposed to linear arrays of atypical mesothelial cells on the free surface, which should suggest a reactive process. They warned about the possible misinterpretation of reactive mesothelial cells in granulation tissue or between fat lobules, and emphasized the fact that cytologic atypia is not very helpful in this differential. Densely packed mesothelial cells are of no great significance if within the peritoneal space but are a feature of malignancy if present embedded within the stroma.

Regarding the differential diagnosis between mesothelioma and carcinoma, special techniques play an important role, although the differences are not as clearcut as in the pleura.[120] The reason for this is simple: whereas in the pleura the main differential diagnosis is with lung adenocarcinoma (i.e., a tumor of an endodermally derived organ with no histogenetic connection with the mesothelium), in the peritoneum the main distinction is with (papillary) serous carcinoma of müllerian type (whether metastatic from ovary/uterus or primary in the peritoneum), i.e., a neoplasm of modified mesothelial cells. Be that as it may, important clinical and therapeutic differences exist between these tumors, and a distinction among the two should always be attempted. At the morphologic level, features that favor the diagnosis of mesothelioma over serous carcinoma are a prominent tubulopapillary pattern, polygonal cells with eosinophilic cytoplasm, absence of marked nuclear pleomorphism, and absence of a high nuclear rate.[117]

Histochemically, it is generally assumed that the presence of intracytoplasmic mucin (either PAS positive after diastase digestion or Mayer mucicarmine positive) establishes the diagnosis of carcinoma. This feature is not as helpful in the peritoneum as it is in the pleura[114] and is of no absolute value, inasmuch as indubitable cases of mucin-positive mesotheliomas exist.[102]

At the immunohistochemical level, podoplanin (D2-40), calretinin and the *WT1* gene product seem to be the best mesothelioma markers, followed by thrombomodulin and keratin 5/6, whereas Ber-EP4 appears to be the best marker for carcinoma.[86,137,140] Ordóñez[140] concluded that the best evidence for mesothelioma was *negativity* for MOC-31, B72.3, Ber-EP4, CA19-9, and Leu-M1, and commented that CEA, PLAP, EMA, vimentin, HBME-1 and S-100 protein have little or no utility in this situation. As Battifora, Gown, and Ordóñez wisely stated,[88,139] the composition of any diagnostic immunohistochemical panel must be adjusted to the clinical situation to optimize its specificity. Thus, the markers chosen will be different depending on whether the differential diagnosis of a malignant mesothelioma is with müllerian-type serous carcinoma, renal cell carcinoma or squamous cell carcinoma.

As a final comment, it should be said that in cases in which the differential remains dubious, electron microscopic examination can play a decisive role.[106]

Spread and metastases. The characteristic pattern of spread of peritoneal mesothelioma is local, eventually leading to complete obliteration of the peritoneal cavity. In advanced stages, the tumor may locally invade the intestinal wall, hilum of the spleen and liver, gastric wall, pancreas, bladder, anterior abdominal wall, and retroperitoneum. Metastases to retroperitoneal or pelvic lymph nodes may develop, but metastases to lung or other distant sites are relatively rare. Peculiar instances of metastatic mesothelioma presenting as colonic polyps have been observed.[129]

Therapy and prognosis. The current therapy for malignant diffuse mesothelioma consists of debulking (cytoreductive surgery) plus adjuvant therapy (combination chemotherapy and whole-abdomen irradiation, or intraperitoneal hyperthermic perfusion).[125,134] The long-term prognosis remains extremely poor. Most patients die of the disease within 2 years of the diagnosis.[127,154] It is very difficult to predict on the basis of the histology whether the tumor will behave aggressively or not,[97,117] but nuclear grade and mitotic count, plus the extent of debulking, seem to have some prognostic significance.[117,134] In addition, there is a subset of diffuse mesotheliomas occurring in women and having well-differentiated features that behaves in an indolent fashion.[108]

Intra-abdominal desmoplastic small cell tumor

Intra-abdominal desmoplastic small cell tumor (DSCT) is a highly malignant neoplasm that characteristically presents as a single mass or multiple nodules within the abdominal cavity in adolescents and young adults, usually of the male sex.[166,174,191] However, it can also occur in the elderly.[201] One case has been reported in a patient with Peutz–Jeghers syndrome.[196] There is a definite predilection for the pelvic region, but in some instances there is extension to the entire peritoneal cavity, scrotum, and/or retroperitoneum. Sometimes the entire tumor is limited to the paratesticular region.[169,180] Accompanying ascites is the rule; malignant cells can be easily identified in the fluid.[168] Grossly, the tumor nodules are firm to hard, variously sized, and range in shape from plaque-like to spherical (Fig. 26.14). Invasion of intra-abdominal organs (such as the gastrointestinal tract) is usually restricted to the serosa. However, cases with prominent involvement of viscerae such as liver, pancreas, and ovary have been observed.[164,172,202] Lymph node metastases are rare but they have been well documented; occasionally, they represent the first manifestation of the disease.[162]

Microscopically, there are sharply outlined islands of tumor cells separated by a generally abundant stroma that tends to be very cellular ('desmoplastic') (Fig. 26.15). The tumor cells are usually small, round, and monotonous, with hyperchromatic nuclei, high mitotic activity, and very scanty cytoplasm. The abundant stroma is largely made up of fibroblasts and myofibroblasts, said to result from the secretion of various fibroblastic growth factors by the

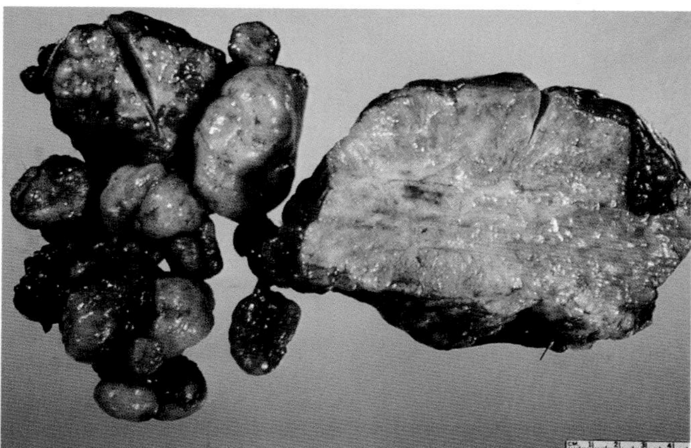

Fig. 26.14 Gross appearance of desmoplastic small cell tumor. There are multiple nodules, one of them of considerable size. Note the large areas of fibrosis.

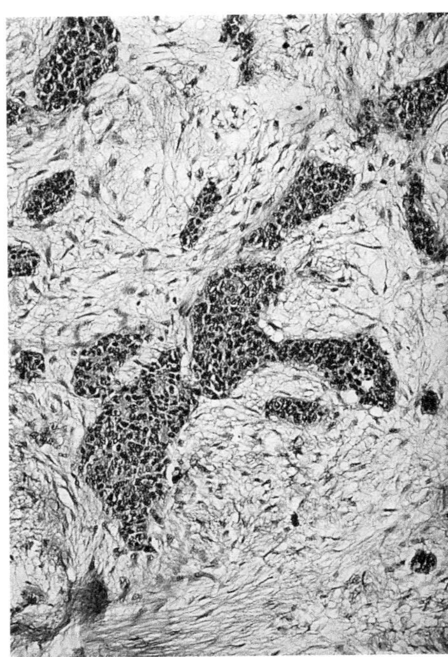

Fig. 26.15 Microscopic appearance of intra-abdominal desmoplastic small cell tumor. Low-power view showing well-defined tumor nests surrounded by cellular stroma.

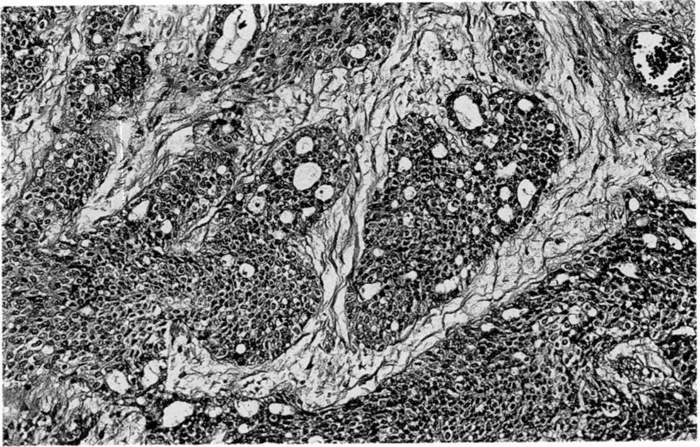

Fig. 26.16 Desmoplastic small cell tumor showing glandular formations at the periphery of the tumor nests.

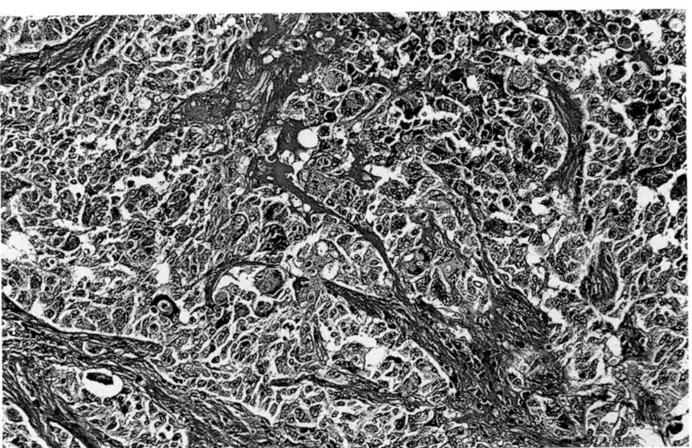

Fig. 26.17 Desmoplastic small cell tumor showing an unusual degree of pleomorphism. It was also unusual in the sense of occurring in a 76-year-old female and involving the outer uterine wall. The diagnosis was confirmed by demonstrating the *EWS–WT1* gene fusion by PCR.

tumor cells.[204] The stroma also contains proliferating vessels sometimes exhibiting a lobular configuration. These vascular structures are similar to those seen in other malignant tumors composed of primitive neuroepithelial/neuroendocrine cells and perhaps resulting from the secretion of angiogenic factor by the tumor cells.[173] Morphologic variations of DSCT include tumors with very scanty stroma, presence of tubular or glandular formations, signet ring cells, rhabdoid cells, and clusters of pleomorphic large tumor cells with bizarre nuclei[171,186,188,190] (Figs 26.16 and 26.17).

The immunohistochemical profile of this neoplasm is distinctive in the sense that it displays simultaneous expression of epithelial (keratin, EMA), muscular (desmin), and neural (neuron-specific enolase) markers (Fig. 26.18). The keratin reactivity has a diffuse cytoplasmic quality, whereas that for desmin tends to have a localized, dotlike ('globoid') quality. The tumor is also positive for *WT1*, a feature resulting from the unique gene fusion that characterizes it.[167,178] It is crucial to use the appropriate antibody for this purpose (such as WT (C-19)); i.e., that directed against the C-terminal region of the WT1 protein, since the N-terminal region of the same molecule (detected with the WT (180) antibody) is not expressed.[163,183] Vimentin is also strongly expressed, but stains for actin and myogenin are characteristically negative. CD99 (an antigen associated with Ewing sarcoma) is usually negative, although focal cytoplasmic staining may be observed. Stains for mesothelial markers such as calretinin and thrombomodulin are generally but not always negative.[189,203] Occasional reactivity for chromogranin has also been described. At the ultrastructural level, the cells have a rather primitive appearance, with a few specialized junctions, scattered membrane-bound dense-core cytoplasmic granules, and a variable amount of intermediate filaments that tend to cluster in a paranuclear location.

DSCT is associated with the unique chromosomal translocation t(11;22)(p13;q12),[194] which results in fusion of the N-terminal activation domain of *EWS* (Ewing sarcoma gene) on 22q12 with the C-terminal DNA-binding domain of *WT1* (Wilms tumor gene 1) on 11p13.[175,182,195] This finding is of practical importance in the differential diagnosis with other small round cell tumors of childhood,[161,170] particularly in the cases showing atypical morphologic or immunohistochemical features (such as negativity for keratin),[198] and also because the molecular test – such as fluorescent in situ hybridization (FISH) or reverse transcriptase polymerase chain reaction (RT-PCR) – can be carried out in the ascitic fluid.[193] Several molecular variants of the *EWS–WT1* gene fusion exist.[160,184] The involvement of these two genes may explain why the phenotypical features of this neoplasm overlap somewhat with those of Ewing sarcoma/primitive neuroectodermal tumor (PNET) and those of Wilms tumor. The peculiar topographic distribution of DSCT also suggests a relationship with the mesothelial lining and the possibility that it may represent a 'mesothelioblastoma'.[174] The transient expression of desmin by the normal developing mesothelium (see p. 2233), the selective expression of *WT1* gene products in malignant mesothelioma,[159] and the description of cases of desmoplastic small cell tumor in the pleural cavity[192] support this contention. On the other hand, the identification of typical cases of this entity in the cerebellum,[197] parotid region,[201] orbit,[165] kidney,[199] and the soft

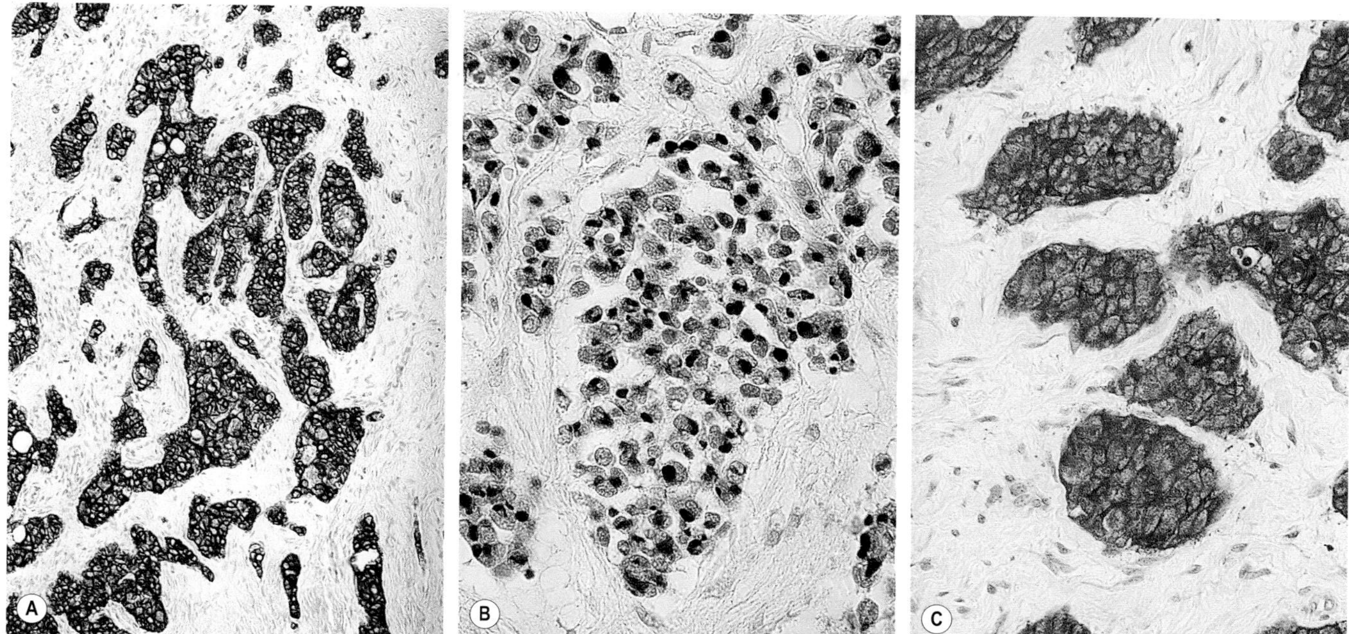

Fig. 26.18 Desmoplastic small cell tumor showing typical polyphenotypic reactivity for keratin (**A**), desmin (**B**), and neuron-specific enolase (**C**).

tissues and bone of the hand[157] casts some doubts on this hypothesis. It seems more likely that DSCT is related to the other small cell tumors of infancy, particularly Ewing sarcoma/PNET, in view of the existence of transitional or hybrid forms of these two tumors at a morphologic, immunohistochemical (DSCT with CD99 reactivity), and molecular level (DSCT with *EWS–FLI-1* or *EWS–ERG* rather than *EWS–WT1* gene fusion).[179,187]

Sometimes tumors with the *EWS-WT1* gene fusion are morphologically very different from classic DSCT, i.e., they may show a predominant component of smooth muscle-like spindle cells or produce an osteoid matrix.[158,185] It is questionable how much the morphologic spectrum of DSCT can be enlarged based on the molecular genetic findings before the entity loses its distinctiveness.

The behavior of DSCT is extremely aggressive, perhaps more so than that of any other malignant small round cell tumor of infancy.[177,191,200] The median survival is less than 3 years.[176] However, prolonged progression-free survival has been achieved in some cases with aggressive multimodality therapy.[181]

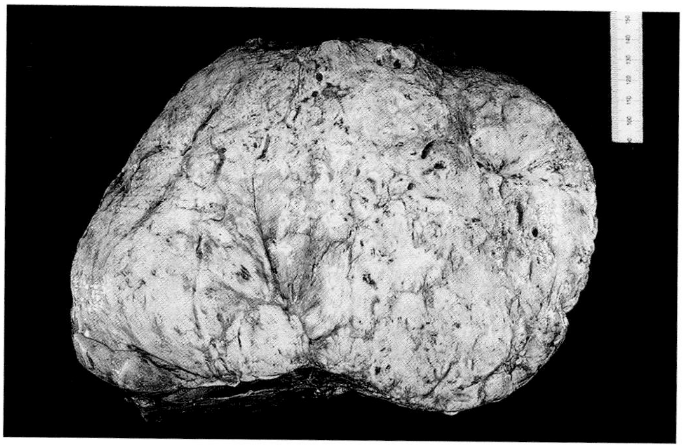

Fig. 26.19 Gross appearance of solitary fibrous tumor attached to the peritoneal side of the diaphragm.

Other primary tumors

Primary peritoneal tumors other than mesotheliomas or DSCT not connected with either the omentum or the mesentery are extremely rare.

Solitary fibrous tumor (formerly known as solitary fibrous mesothelioma) is much less common in the peritoneal than in the pleural cavity, but its morphologic features are identical (see Chapter 7) (Fig. 26.19). It presents in adulthood and – like its pleural counterpart – may be accompanied by hypoglycemia. Most cases have followed a benign clinical course,[211,222] but a malignant counterpart has been well documented.[209] The phenotype of the tumor cell is the same as that of the normal submesothelial mesenchyme.

Vascular tumors of various types occur. *Angiosarcomas* have been described, some following administration of radiation therapy[218] (Fig. 26.20). *Epithelioid hemangioendothelioma* can coat the peritoneal cavity in a diffuse fashion, simulating the pattern of growth of malignant mesothelioma, in a fashion similar to that seen in the pleural cavity[205,216,219] (Fig. 26.21). These tumors lack the herpesvirus-like DNA sequences that have been associated with Kaposi sarcoma.[215] *Cystic lymphangiomas* occur in the mesentery and retroperitoneum and simulate the appearance of so-called multicystic benign mesothelioma. They often exhibit intense superimposed reactive and inflammatory changes.[213]

Synovial sarcoma can occur within the pelvis and retroperitoneum; it needs to be distinguished mainly from biphasic mesothelioma. A molecular evaluation may be necessary for this purpose.[214] The pelvic tumors can metastasize distantly, whereas those located in the retroperitoneum tend to remain confined to the abdomen.[208]

Dendritic follicular cell tumor is being reported with an increasing frequency in the abdominal cavity; it has been claimed that it behaves more aggressively at this site than in others.[207,217,221]

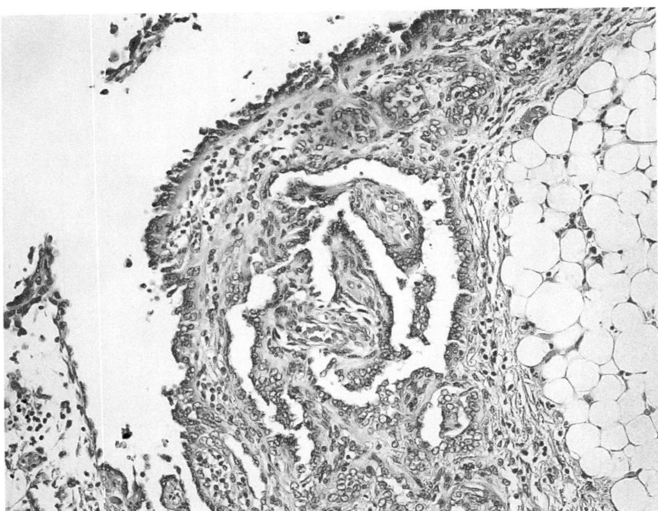

Fig. 26.20 Peritoneal angiosarcoma. The pattern of growth greatly simulates that of malignant mesothelioma.

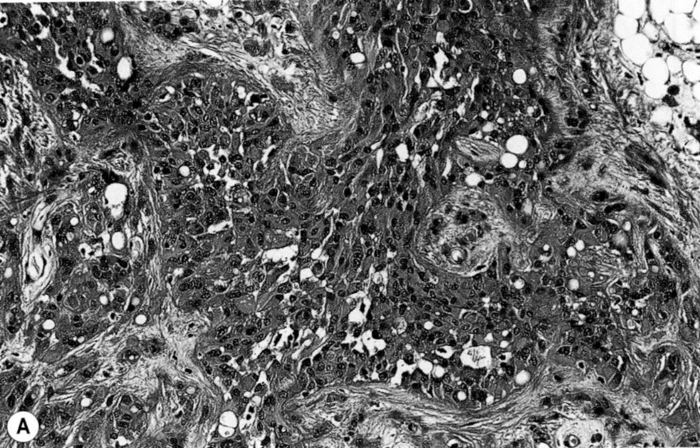

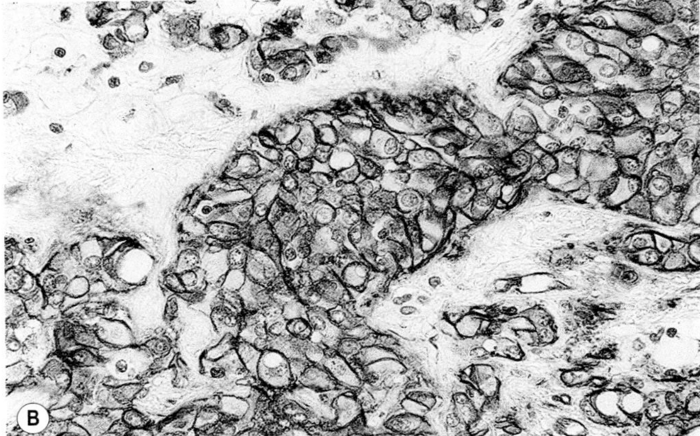

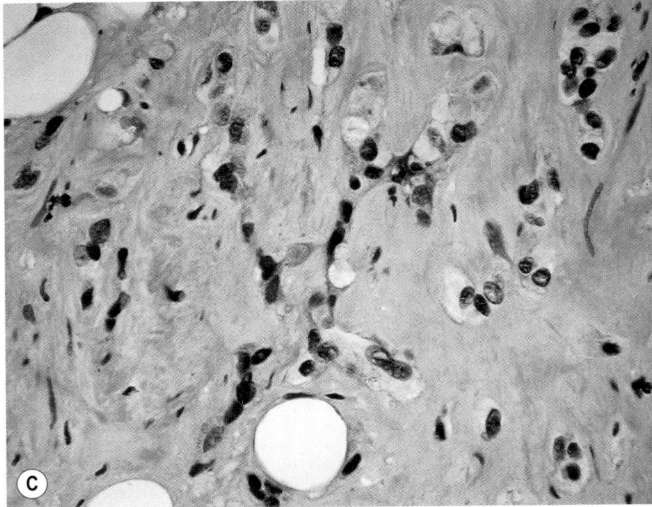

Fig. 26.21 Epithelioid hemangioendothelioma of peritoneum. **A**, Hematoxylin–eosin; **B**, CD31; **C**, FLI-1 (from another case of the same entity).

Epithelioid angiomyolipoma (PEComa) is another neoplasm that is being recognized at a heightened rate, and this includes the peritoneal cavity. Most cases have occurred in the pelvis, often with no anatomic relation with any major organ, and some have been malignant.[206] Cases described as *clear cell myomelanocytic tumor* belong to the same category.[220] PEComas can simulate microscopically renal cell carcinoma, adrenal cortical carcinoma, oncocytoma, and a variety of pleomorphic sarcomas.[212] HMB-45 positivity remains the key feature for the confirmation of the diagnosis, especially when the morphology is atypical.

Undifferentiated sarcomas of undetermined histogenesis involving the peritoneal cavity of children have been described by Gonzalez-Crussi et al.[210]

Lesions of the secondary müllerian system

The term *secondary müllerian system* has been applied to the pelvic and lower abdominal mesothelium and the subjacent mesenchyme of females, on the basis of its close embryologic relationship with the primary müllerian system (i.e., the müllerian ducts).[238] The potentiality of this tissue is manifested by the existence in the peritoneal cavity (most often in the pelvic region but also in the omentum, mesentery, and retroperitoneum) of a large variety of metaplastic and neoplastic lesions that are analogous in all regards to those more commonly found in the ovary, uterus, or other organs of the female genital tract.[243] These lesions sometimes occur in association, not surprising in view of their related histogenesis and pathogenesis.[245]

1 **Endosalpingiosis.** This is discussed in Chapter 19.
2 **Endometriosis.** This is discussed in Chapter 19 (see also p. 2250).
3 **Ectopic decidual reaction.** This is most commonly seen in the pelvis and omentum, where it appears as tiny, gray submesothelial nodules.[225,227] Microscopically, the decidual cells may exhibit bizarre hyperchromatic nuclei and be confused with metastatic squamous cell carcinoma. Vascular changes may occur as an expression of regression.[225]
4 **Leiomyomatosis peritonealis disseminata.** This is a rare benign condition in which typical uterine leiomyomas are associated with multiple small nodules of mature smooth muscle distributed throughout the omentum and both visceral and parietal layers of the peritoneum (Fig. 26.22). A mistaken diagnosis of metastatic leiomyosarcoma may result. Rarely, the disease coexists with endometriosis. Exceptionally, a sex-cord-like pattern is observed within some of the leiomyomatous nodules.[239] Its clonal pattern is similar to that

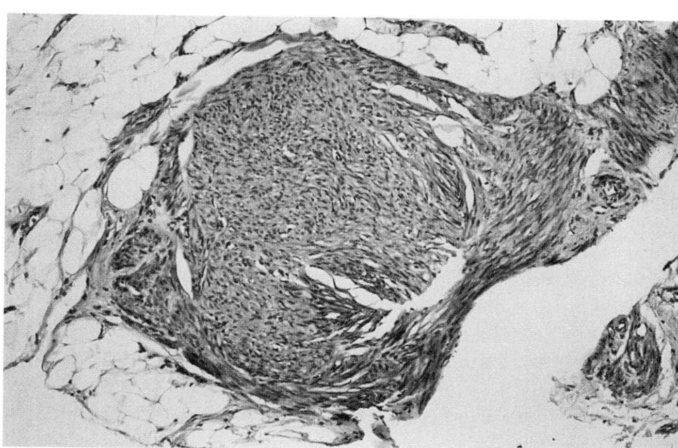

Fig. 26.22 Low-power view of leiomyomatosis peritonealis disseminata.

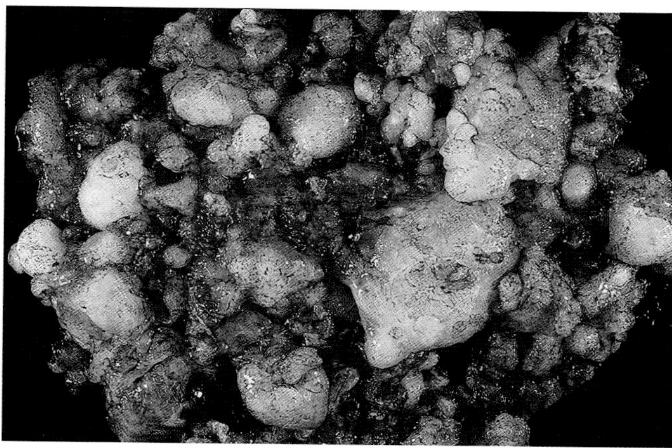

Fig. 26.23 Gross appearance of pseudomyxoma peritonei. The entire peritoneal cavity is occupied by innumerable mucinous nodules.

of uterine leiomyomas.[240] A strong association with pregnancy exists.[242] Steroid hormone receptors have been detected in the proliferating cells.[224,231] In most instances, spontaneous regression of the nodules occurs.

5 **(Papillary) serous tumors of the peritoneum.** They include morphologically conventional serous carcinomas and borderline serous tumors (including the micropapillomatosis variety) and serous psammocarcinoma[223,229,233,235–237,244] (see Fig. 26.13). They are discussed in Chapter 19.

6 **Endometrial stromal sarcoma, müllerian adenosarcoma** (with and without sarcomatous overgrowth), and **malignant mixed müllerian tumor** (with or without neuroendocrine differentiation).[226,228,230,234,241] These are discussed in Chapter 19.

Metastatic tumors

All types of metastatic tumor may involve the peritoneal cavity. The most common sites of the primary tumors are the female genital tract (particularly ovary), large bowel, and pancreas.[249,265] The ovarian and uterine tumors resulting in peritoneal carcinomatosis are usually of the serous type; the primary uterine lesion can be very superficial or even in situ.[269] The gross appearance of the peritoneal metastasis varies from single, well-defined nodules to a diffuse peritoneal thickening. Variations in consistency depend on cellularity, amount of fibrous tissue, and mucin content. Metastatic carcinoma may simulate closely the gross and microscopic appearance of malignant mesothelioma. This is particularly the case with papillary serous carcinoma of the ovary, but it can also occur with carcinoma of the lung, in conjunction with pleural spread.[266]

Pseudomyxoma peritonei is a distinctive form of tumor implant in which the peritoneal cavity contains large amounts of mucinous material[256,268] (Fig. 26.23). The viscerae are relatively spared, but polypoid mucinous masses can develop on the peritoneal surface of the small bowel.[272] Mucinous cystic lesions can also be seen in the substance of the spleen.[251] There may also be intrathoracic (pleuropulmonary) spread.[252] Traditionally, it has been stated that the primary lesion may be a borderline or malignant mucinous neoplasm of the appendix, ovary, or pancreas (see Chapters 11, 15, and 19).[258] However, several recent studies of the subject have led to the conclusion that the appendix is the primary site of origin of pseudomyxoma in the vast majority of cases in both men and women.[261,262,276,277] The further suggestion has been made that the associated mucinous ovarian tumors – when present – are most likely additional implants from the appendiceal lesions rather than independent synchronous neoplasms.[261,262,276] The subject is further discussed in Chapter 19.

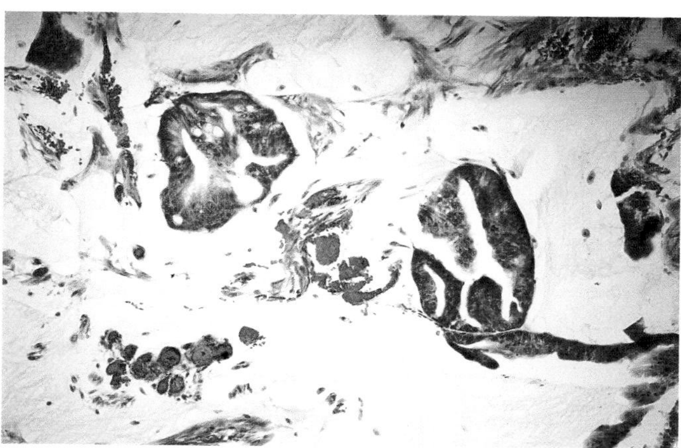

Fig. 26.24 Microscopic appearance of pseudomyxoma peritonei. Clusters of well-differentiated mucin-producing glandular cells are seen floating in a sea of mucin.

Microscopically, large pools of mucus are seen accompanied by hyperemic vessels and chronic inflammatory cells. *Viable epithelial glandular cells must be identified within the mucus to diagnose pseudomyxoma peritonei* (Fig. 26.24). These cells usually have a deceivingly bland appearance on both histologic and cytologic preparations and show no invasive properties.[255,267] Because of these features, the suggestion has been made to designate this process as *adenomucinosis,* in order to distinguish it from the *peritoneal mucinous carcinomatosis* accompanied by cytologic atypia and resulting from an invasive mucinous adenocarcinoma usually located in the gastrointestinal tract.[263] We certainly agree that these two groups are associated with a different outcome,[264,275] but we and others are afraid that the neologism *adenomucinosis* may not contribute much to the understanding of what is clearly a neoplastic condition with low-grade malignant features.[246,247]

Immunohistochemically, the cells of pseudomyxoma characteristically show expression of MUC2 (a mucin possessing the physicochemical property of being gel-forming[260]) and of CDX-2 (a marker of normal and neoplastic intestinal cells).[259]

Pseudomyxoma peritonei is characterized by a slow but relentless clinical course, with recurrent ascites that eventually reaches massive proportions ('jelly-belly syndrome'). Aggressive surgical resection is the treatment currently recommended, with most patients requiring multiple laparotomies, and in some including a total gastrectomy.[270,271]

It should be noted that mucinous cystadenomas of the ovary and appendix can rupture and pour their content into the peritoneal cavity; the resulting condition, which is self-limited and microscopically lacks tumor cells, should not be designated as pseudomyxoma peritonei.[248,254] Pseudomyxoma-like changes (pseudo-pseudomyxoma, so to speak) have also been described in the stroma of prostatic adenocarcinoma following neoadjuvant androgen ablation therapy.[274]

Another distinctive type of peritoneal tumor is *gliomatosis peritonei*. This condition has been traditionally believed to result from the selective growth of glial tissue from a ruptured ovarian teratoma,[253] but genetic studies have challenged this assumption and suggested that the glial tissue is probably derived from nonteratomatous cells, perhaps through metaplasia of submesothelial cells.[257] In exceptional circumstances gliomatosis peritonei may undergo malignant transformation;[250] this is discussed in Chapter 19 (Fig. 26.25).

Metastatic carcinoma in the peritoneal cavity (often of ovarian origin) tends to be accompanied by recurrent ascites. This is sometimes treated by peritoneovenous shunting, by which the effusion is returned to the general circulation; amazingly, this technique has not resulted in an increase in the number of extra-abdominal metastases.[273]

Cytology

The diagnosis of metastatic carcinoma in the peritoneal cavity is possible in about 75% of the cases on the basis of cytologic examination of ascitic fluid.[278] This also applies to pseudomyxoma peritonei.[283] With malignant lymphoma and leukemia, the overall yield is approximately 60%, these figures being slightly higher in the specific case of large cell lymphoma.[284]

The two most difficult problems in cytology of ascitic fluid are the distinction between reactive and neoplastic mesothelium and that between malignant mesothelioma and metastatic carcinoma (Figs 26.26–26.28). False-positive diagnoses have been caused by liver cirrhosis and other disorders associated with mesothelial hyperplasia; confusion occurs because the reactive cells may form pseudoacini closely resembling the true acini of adenocarcinoma, have multiple nuclei or a signet ring appearance, and undergo mitotic division. Evaluation of the nucleocytoplasmic ratio and of nuclear features is essential in this differential diagnosis.

Malignant mesothelioma often grows in papillary clusters.[286] It differs from metastatic adenocarcinoma by the absence of true acini, a more frequent binucleation and multinucleation, and the presence of a range of differentiation among the mesothelial cells (see Fig. 26.28). Electron microscopic and immunohistochemical techniques have been successfully applied to cytologic preparations in an effort to increase the diagnostic accuracy.[279–282,285,287]

Omentum

Hemorrhagic infarct of the omentum may result from torsion or strangulation in a hernia sac. *Primary idiopathic segmental infarction*

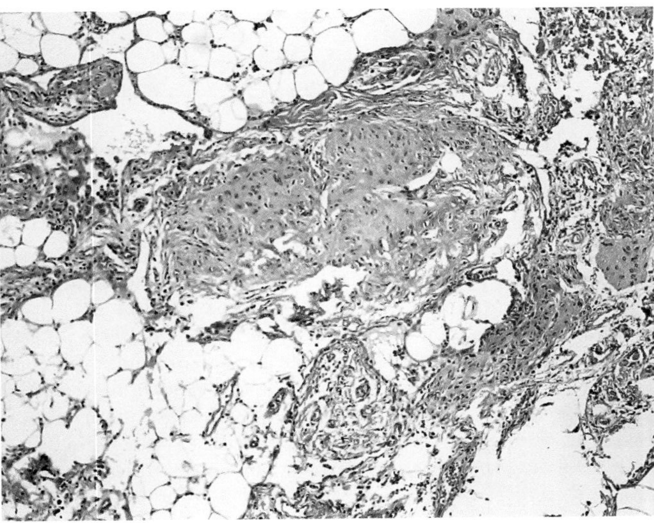

Fig. 26.25 So-called 'peritoneal gliomatosis' resulting from rupture of an ovarian teratoma.

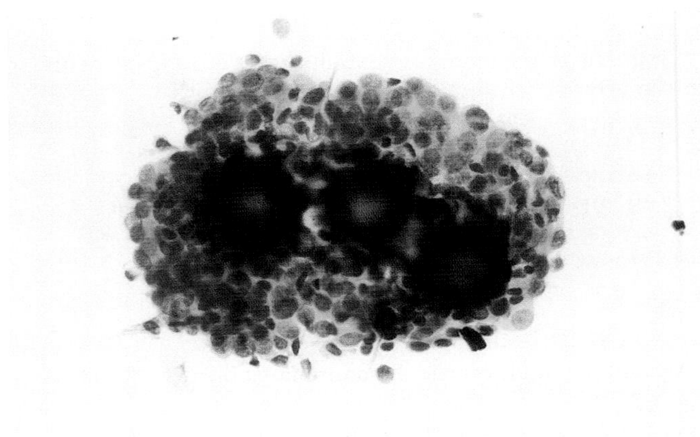

Fig. 26.26 Positive peritoneal cytology in a patient with serous carcinoma of the ovary. Note the psammomatous bodies.

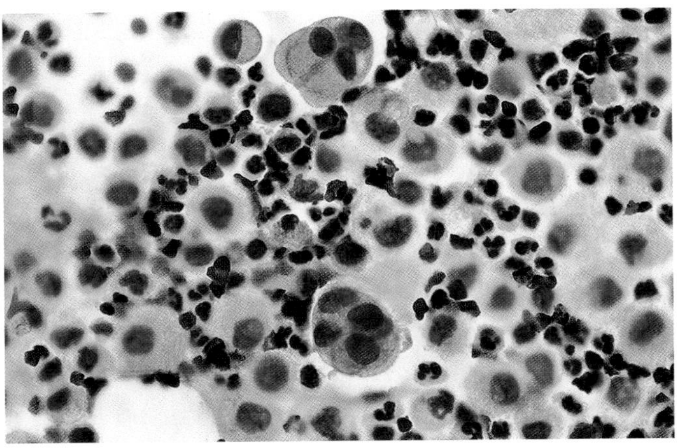

Fig. 26.27 Positive peritoneal cytology in a patient with pancreatic adenocarcinoma.

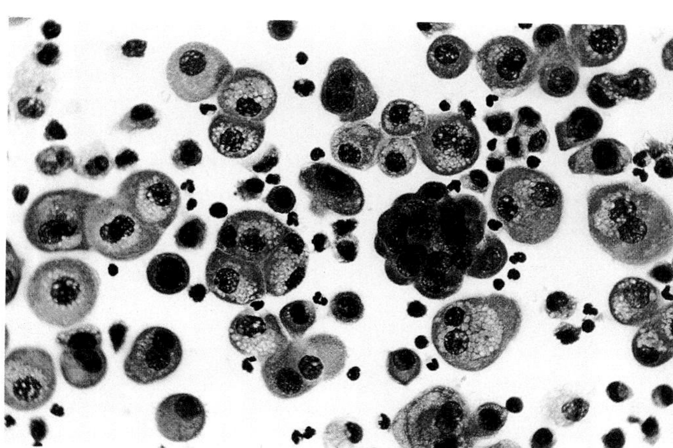

Fig. 26.28 Cytologic appearance of malignant mesothelioma. The clustering of tumor cells into morula-like structures is particularly characteristic.

of the greater omentum is an acute abdominal lesion of obscure etiology, usually mistaken clinically for acute appendicitis or cholecystitis. Characteristically, the infarcted segment of omentum is on the right side adherent to the cecum, ascending colon, and anterior parietal peritoneum.[291]

Cystic lymphangioma represents the single most frequent tumor of the omentum in children;[294] its gross and microscopic appearance recapitulates that of the more common 'cystic hygroma' of the neck.[292]

Primary solid tumors of the omentum are exceptionally rare. Smooth muscle tumors predominate among both the benign and malignant categories.[290,298] As a high percentage of these tumors are of the epithelioid (clear cell or leiomyoblastoma) type and are CD117 positive, they have therefore been incorporated into the gastrointestinal stromal tumor (GIST) category (see Chapter 11).[295,298]

Myxoid or multicentric hamartoma (omental fibromyxoid tumor) is a peculiar lesion characterized by the formation of multiple nodules in the omentum and mesentery of children;[293,294] microscopically, plump mesenchymal cells are seen in a background of prominent myxoid and inflammatory changes. The appearance is reminiscent of that of inflammatory myofibroblastic tumor.[288] Whatever the nature of this lesion may ultimately prove to be, its behavior so far has been benign.

Diffuse malignant mesothelioma of the peritoneum consistently spreads into the omentum.

Other reported primary omental lesions include *teratoma* (usually mature),[296] *elastofibroma*,[299] *follicular dendritic cell tumor*,[300] *cryptococcosis*, resulting in a tumorlike mass ('cryptococcoma'),[289] and *müllerian-type lesions* similar to those occurring in other regions of the peritoneal cavity and retroperitoneum.[297]

Metastatic carcinoma constitutes the most common malignant omental neoplasm in adults. Ovary, gastrointestinal tract, and pancreas are the most common sources of the primary tumor.

Mesentery

Mesenteric panniculitis (also called *isolated lipodystrophy of the mesentery*, *retractile mesenteritis*, and *sclerosing mesenteritis*) is a rare disorder grossly appearing as a diffuse, localized, or multinodular thickening of the mesentery of the small and/or large bowel.[313,321]

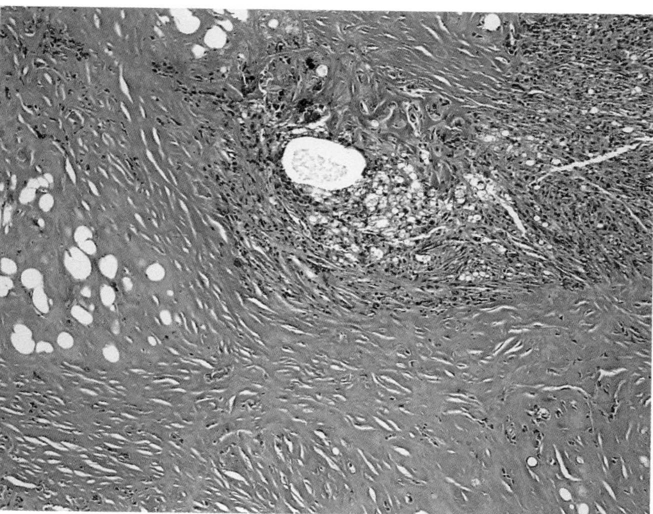

Fig. 26.29 Sclerosing mesenteritis. There is fibrosis with hyalinization, chronic inflammation, and fat necrosis surrounded by clusters of foamy macrophages.

The disease needs to be distinguished from the localized and nodular forms of panniculitis that can occur around colorectal carcinomas or diverticular disease,[302] and from the diffuse mesenteric fibrosis seen in association with chronic small bowel allograft rejection.[323] The process may lead to retraction and distortion of the intestinal loops and the formation of adhesions between them. It can also involve the pancreas and mimick pancreatic carcinoma.[344] Microscopically, there is an infiltration by inflammatory cells, myofibroblasts, and foamy macrophages, the latter probably representing a reaction to fat necrosis[337] (Fig. 26.29). The vessels traversing the lesion are often inflamed and sometimes thrombosed. The differential diagnosis includes Weber–Christian disease and Whipple disease. In eight of the 53 patients reported by Kipfer et al.,[322] a malignant lymphoma ultimately developed; other series did not show such an association. Retrospectively, some of these cases might have been malignant lymphoma with a prominent degree of sclerosis, simulating an inflammatory condition. It is likely that at least some examples of mesenteric panniculitis represent a mesenteric extension of idiopathic retroperitoneal fibrosis and, as such, members of the family of disorders collectively known as *inflammatory fibrosclerosis*, which overlaps with IgG4-related sclerosing disease.[310,313,341]

Heterotopic mesenteric ossification has a morphologic appearance similar to that of myositis ossificans of soft tissues[348] (Fig. 26.30). The condition can result in intestinal obstruction.[338] Most reported cases have occurred a short time following the performance of one or more intra-abdominal operations, such as the repair of an abdominal aortic aneurysm.[352]

Inflammatory myofibroblastic tumor presents as an intra-abdominal mass, most frequently in children and adolescents. It is often associated with fever, weight loss, and anemia, manifestations that often regress following excision of the mass.[312] Microscopically, there is a polymorphic infiltrate composed of plump oval to spindle cells arranged in a vaguely fascicular fashion, plasma cells, lymphocytes, and other inflammatory elements (Fig. 26.31). It was originally reported as a pseudoneoplastic inflammatory process and designated as *inflammatory pseudotumor* because of the rich inflammatory component and the generally favorable outcome following surgical excision. However, further experience has shown

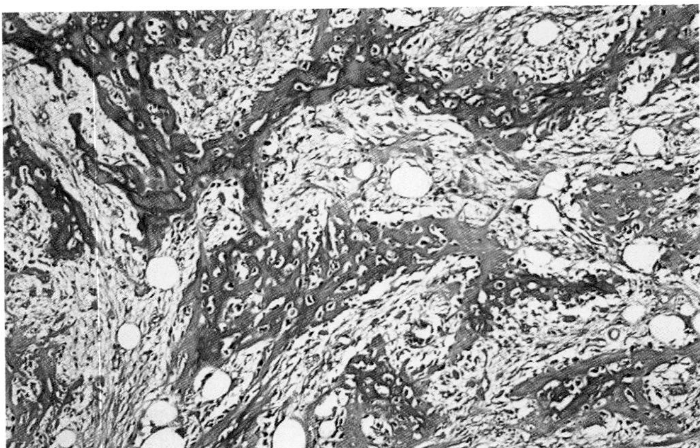

Fig. 26.30 Heterotopic mesenteric ossification. This section, which corresponds to the peripheral portion of the lesion, shows well-developed bone trabeculae.

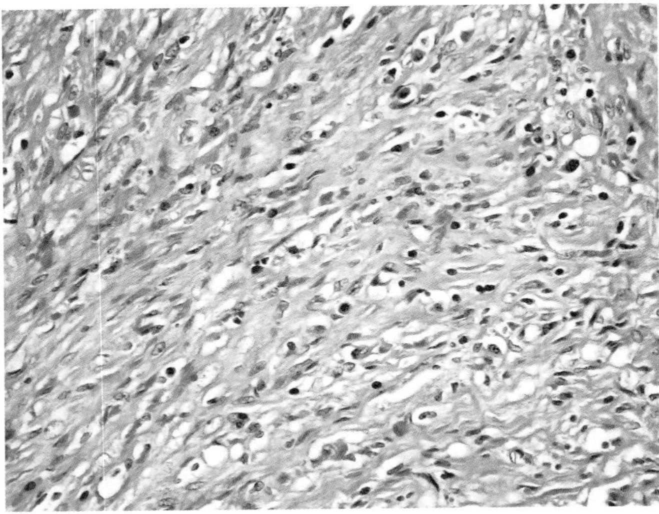

Fig. 26.31 Inflammatory pseudotumor showing an admixture of inflammatory cells in a fibrous background.

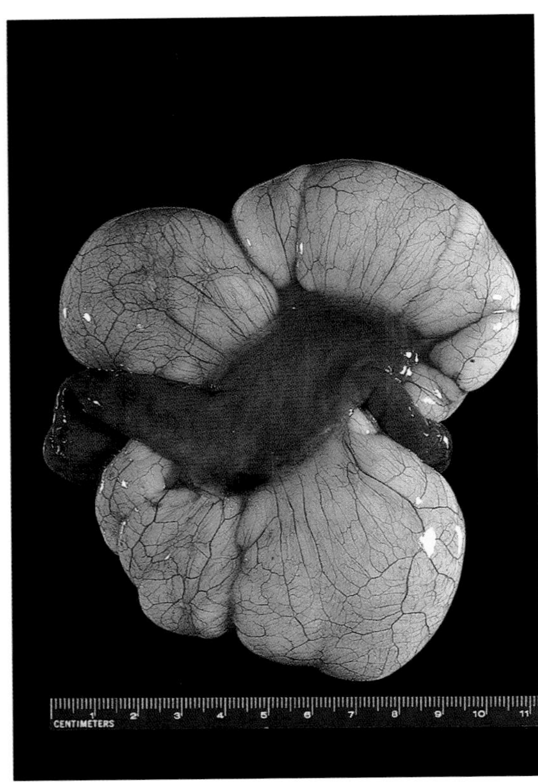

Fig. 26.32 Typical golden yellow color of chylous cyst. *(Courtesy of Dr RA Cooke, Brisbane, Australia; from Cooke RA, Stewart B. Colour atlas of anatomical pathology. Edinburgh, 2004, Churchill Livingstone)*

that these cases blend imperceptibly with others showing a more neoplastic appearance of the spindle/oval cell component and/or running an aggressive clinical course, including the development of metastases. The term *inflammatory fibrosarcoma*[330] has been proposed for the more neoplastic-appearing members of this group. There is also cytogenetic and molecular evidence that even some of the more inflammatory-appearing lesions may be neoplastic.[346] Because of these facts, the term *inflammatory myofibroblastic tumor* is currently favored for this process.[312,340] The plump oval/spindle cells of this lesion are thought to be myofibroblasts, hence the name given to this entity. However, some of the morphologic features suggest an alternative origin from so-called fibroblastic reticulum cells.[336]

It has been hypothesized that at least some of the reported cases of intra-abdominal *calcifying fibrous pseudotumor* (further discussed in Chapter 25) may represent the end stage of inflammatory myofibroblastic tumor.[311,324] However, the fact that this entity is usually immunoreactive for CD34 while negative for anaplastic lymphoma kinase (ALK) and S-100 protein, and that transitional forms are rare, is not supportive of such an association.[318] Since local recurrence can supervene in calcifying fibrous pseudotumor, it has been further suggested that it be renamed *calcifying fibrous tumor*.[334] The group of conditions recently termed reactive *nodular fibrous pseudotumor* are part of this spectrum.[350]

Mesenteric cysts are usually incidental findings, but they may be large enough to produce symptoms.[325,347] Some are seen as a component of the basal cell nevus syndrome.[314] They are round and smooth, with a thin wall and a content that may be a serous fluid resembling plasma or a white milky fluid, particularly if located near the jejunum. In the latter instance, they are referred to as *chylous cysts* (Fig. 26.32). Most of these cysts arise from lymph vessels and are lined by endothelium. When they are large and multilocular and/or have smooth muscle in their walls, we prefer to regard them as **cystic lymphangiomas**[308,329,343] and distinguish them from the HMB-45-positive **lymphangiomyomas**.[326]

Other types of mesenteric cysts occur. One is **bowel duplication**, in which the cyst is lined by intestinal mucosa, there is a layer of smooth muscle, and there is an anatomic connection with the bowel by way of an interlacing muscular wall and blood supply; over half of these are diagnosed before 6 months of age.[343] Other mesenteric cysts are lined by mesothelium and are examples of so-called **benign cystic (or multicystic) mesothelioma** (see p. 2235). Others are lined by *müllerian (fallopian tube-like) epithelium*, similar to those more commonly seen in the true pelvis[316,327] (see Chapter 19). Still others, seen in females who have had previous pelvic surgery, are lined by luteinized cells and have ovarian stroma in their wall; these are referred to as **ovarian remnant syndrome**[345] or

mesenteric cyst–ovarian implant syndrome.[339] Another peculiar abnormality of müllerian nature and disputed pathogenesis (endometriotic versus malformative) that can occur in the mesentery is the so-called *uterus-like mass.*[319]

Cystic mucinous tumors of benign and borderline type have been described in the mesentery and retroperitoneum of females.[303] They are analogous in all regards to the homonymous tumors in the ovary, of which they can be regarded as the peritoneal counterparts.[303]

Primary solid tumors of the mesentery can be of various types, most of them of mesenchymal nature.[349] *Smooth muscle tumors,* when large, usually behave in a malignant fashion even if their mitotic count is low;[317] a high proportion of the tumors reported in the past as leiomyomas or leiomyosarcomas in this location (particularly those with an epithelioid or clear cell morphology) would be reclassified as GISTs today, a statement that also applies to tumors of the omentum and retroperitoneum. If one were to split GISTs from smooth muscle tumors, as currently proposed (see Chapter 11), the large majority of the mesenteric and omental tumors would fall into the former category, in contrast to the retroperitoneal situation (see p. 2247 and Chapter 11).

Fibromatosis (*desmoid tumor*) of the mesentery should always raise the suspicion of Gardner syndrome, particularly if it develops following a surgical procedure[306,307,328] (Figs 26.33 and 26.34). During the past years we have seen several cases of fibromatosis misdiagnosed as GIST, the reasons being that they involved the bowel wall and were immunoreactive for CD34 and (questionably) for CD117 (*KIT*).[331,342,351] The reactivity for CD117 is, however, only coarse cytoplasmic and not present with some of the newer antibodies against this marker. Furthermore, it has been recently shown that mesenteric fibromatosis shows consistent nuclear immunoreactivity for β-catenin, whereas GIST does not.[332] In any event, the differential diagnosis is possible with plain hematoxylin and eosin stains in the large majority of cases.[301]

Adipose tissue tumors are usually of the atypical lipomatous tumor (well-differentiated liposarcoma) type, sometimes accompanied by secondary myxoid or inflammatory changes.

So-called malignant fibrous histiocytoma also occurs in this location, often having a polymorphous appearance and high content in foamy macrophages; it is likely that some of the cases previously reported as xanthogranulomas belong in this category.

Vascular tumors are represented by the already mentioned cystic lymphangioma, angiosarcoma, epithelioid hemangioendothelioma, and infantile hemangioendothelioma. The latter can be associated with thrombocytopenia.[315]

Peripheral nerve tumors are usually benign and represented by schwannoma, neurofibroma and perineurioma.[309,349]

Other primary mesenteric tumors of which isolated cases have been reported include an allegedly primary *carcinoid tumor,*[304] *follicular dendritic cell tumor,*[333] *paraganglioma* (Fig. 26.35), and several examples of *germ cell tumor,* including yolk sac tumor[320] and mature cystic teratoma (dermoid cyst) associated with autoimmune hemolytic anemia.[305]

Tumorlike conditions of the mesentery include, in addition to those already mentioned, *Castleman disease,* which can present as a mesenteric mass associated with hematologic disturbances,[335] and which in this location is often characterized by a rich stroma, hyalinization, and calcification (Fig. 26.36).

Metastatic carcinoma is the most common type of solid tumor of the mesentery; in most cases the primary tumor is in an intra-abdominal site.

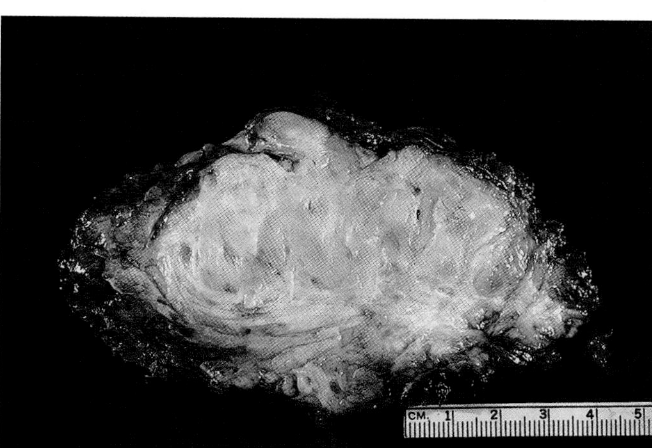

Fig. 26.33 Fibromatosis of mesentery involving the bowel wall. Cases like this are likely to be misinterpreted as GIST.

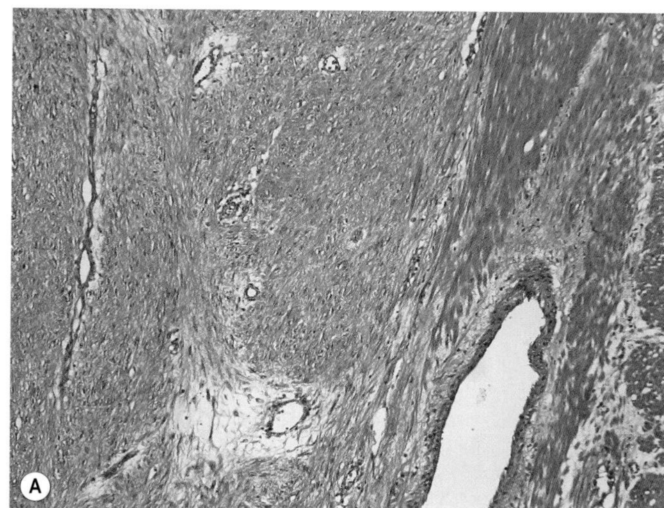

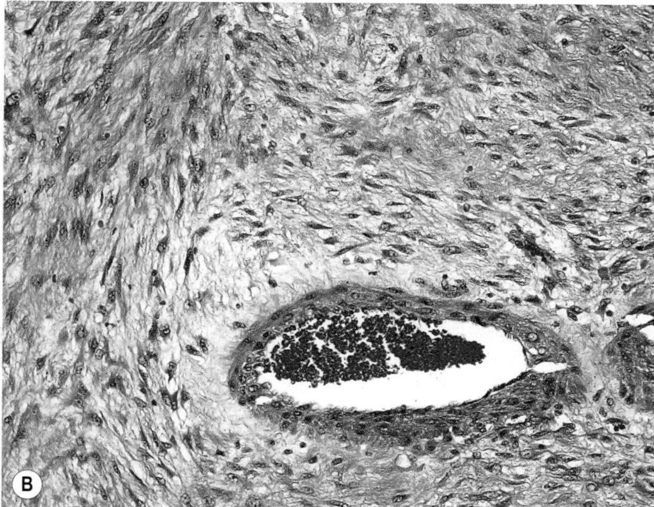

Fig. 26.34 Fibromatosis of mesentery. **A**, Entrapment of muscle fibers from bowel wall. **B**, Typical growth of myofibroblasts in a heavily collagenized background. Note the sharply etched thick-walled vessel.

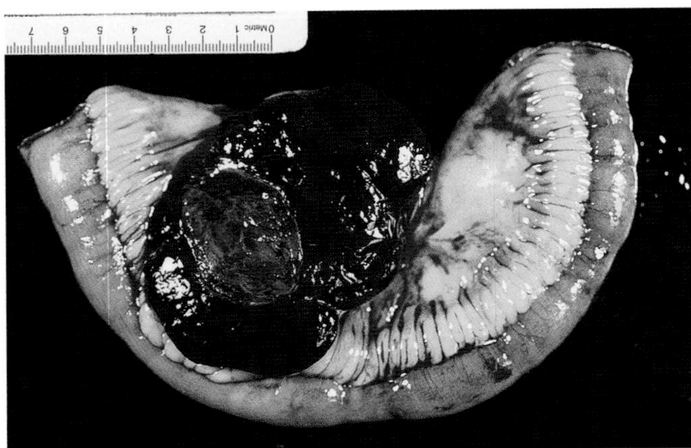

Fig. 26.35 Gross appearance of paraganglioma of the mesentery. This is a most unusual location for this tumor type. The associated hemorrhage due to the high degree of tumor vascularization is a common event.

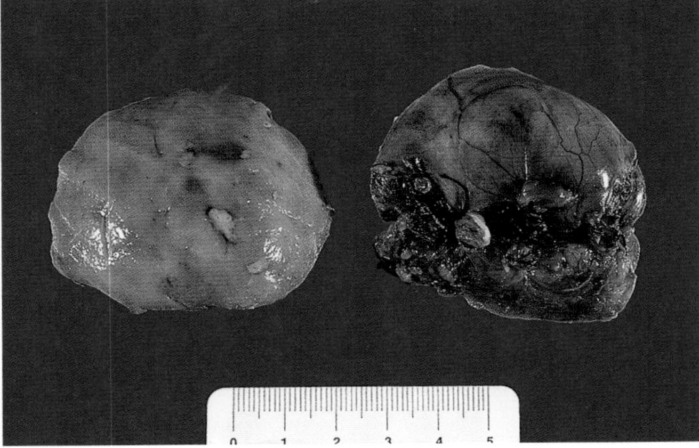

Fig. 26.36 Castleman disease in the root of the mesentery. This is a relatively common location for this entity.

Hernia sacs

This rather mundane specimen is one of the most common to be received in the surgical pathology laboratory. In most instances, there is not much of interest microscopically: an attenuated lining of mesothelial cells resting on a thin layer of connective tissue (corresponding to the processus vaginalis in indirect inguinal hernias), adipose tissue, dense fibrous tissue belonging to fascia and/or aponeurosis, and sometimes fascicles of skeletal muscle (from the transversus abdominis in the inguinal hernias). The preperitoneal fat that covers the sac may be abundant and be designated as 'lipoma' by the surgeon, but it does not represent a neoplasm. Once in a while, however, the hernial sac will show one or more startling pathologic changes. *Mesothelial hyperplasia* resulting from trauma or another injury can be so extreme as to simulate a malignancy (see p. 2236); the accompanying inflammation, hyperemia, and fibrin deposition will point toward its reactive nature (see Fig. 26.4). Sometimes a *mesothelioma* or a *metastatic carcinoma* will first become evident from the study of a herniorrhaphy specimen. The most common sources for the primary are the gastrointestinal tract, ovary, prostate, and appendix.[354,359] The pseudomyxoma peritonei that sometimes accompanies appendiceal mucinous tumors may result in filling of the hernia sac by viscid mucin (see p. 2245).[364] The finding of mucinous material within the sac at the time of the hernia repair may be the first sign of the disease.[357] A particularly exotic tumor reported within an umbilical hernia sac is an *extragonadal sex-cord tumor with annular tubules*.[353] Parenthetically, the other reported case of extragonadal tumor of this type was located in the fallopian tube and associated with endometriosis.[358]

Other changes one may encounter in a hernia sac are *endometriosis* in females and *glandular inclusions* from wolffian or müllerian remnants in prepubertal males. The latter are lined by ciliated epithelium and surrounded by a mantle of fibrous tissue; they should not be misinterpreted as portions of the vas deferens or epididymis.[360,363] Immunostaining for CD10 can provide some assistance, in the sense that the reaction is positive in the normal vas deferens and epididymis (at least focally) whereas it is always negative in the vas deferens-like inclusions and usually negative in the epididymis-like inclusions.[355] In a microscopic study of 7314 herniorrhaphies in male children, Steigman et al.[362] found these embryonal rests in 30 (0.41%), whereas they detected vas deferens in 17 (0.23%) and epididymis in 22 (0.30%). This is one of several reasons why the routine microscopic evaluation of hernia sacs remains a worthwhile procedure, as eloquently pointed out by Dehner.[356]

Crystalline foreign particulate material largely composed of talc was consistently detected in hernia sacs by polarized microscopy and X-diffraction studies by Pratt et al.[361] They suggest that the source of this talc was ingestion with food or medication, but it seems to us that they did not satisfactorily rule out the alternative possibility that the source was the surgical procedure or the processing of the specimen.

Umbilicus

The umbilicus is subject to a variety of diseases resulting from its unique anatomy and the important structures with which it is connected during development. Foraker chose this structure for some of his satirical essays on the practice of surgical pathology, by creating the mythical figure of the omphalopathologist.[367] Excluding conditions such as hernias, omphaloceles, neonatal infections, and extensive fetal malformations, the group of disorders of importance to the surgical pathologist that can affect the umbilicus are those that follow.

Urachal remnant anomalies may present as a patent sinus between the umbilicus and the bladder, as blind sinuses at any level between these two structures, and as a closed but persistently attached urachus. Steck and Helwig[373] have suggested that most cases of granulomatous omphalitis, umbilical granuloma, and pilonidal sinus of the umbilicus are related to urachal anomalies because of the fact that an attached urachus is found in nearly half of these cases (see Chapter 17, Urinary bladder).

Omphalomesenteric duct remnant anomalies include patency of the duct, 'umbilical polyp', sinus tract, attachment of Meckel diverticulum to the umbilicus by an incompletely obliterated duct, and formation of a cyst in the umbilicus or along the course of the incompletely obliterated duct[370] (see Chapter 11, Small bowel) (Fig. 26.37).

Endometriosis of the umbilicus is the most common form of cutaneous endometriosis, except for that occurring in surgical scars[371] (see Chapter 19, Uterus corpus).

Keratinous cysts of epidermal type are relatively common.[372]

Benign tumors of the umbilical region can be of various types; most of them belong to the category of benign melanocytic nevus and fibrous or fibroepithelial polyp.[372,375] The latter, which for some peculiar reason shows a marked male predominance, may be composed of dense fibrous tissue or have a nodular fasciitis-like appearance.[374]

Malignant tumors involving the umbilicus can be primary or metastatic. The most common primary malignant tumor is melanoma, followed by basal cell carcinoma and adenocarcinoma.[368,369,372] Metastatic tumors are much more common. Most of them originate in the stomach, pancreas, large bowel, or ovary.[372] The colloquial term 'Sister (Mary) Joseph's nodule' refers to umbilical metastases from malignancies of the female genital tract, usually ovarian carcinoma.[365] Several cases have been described of the peculiar phenomenon of rapid development of umbilical metastases after laparoscopic cholecystectomy for unsuspected gallbladder carcinoma.[366]

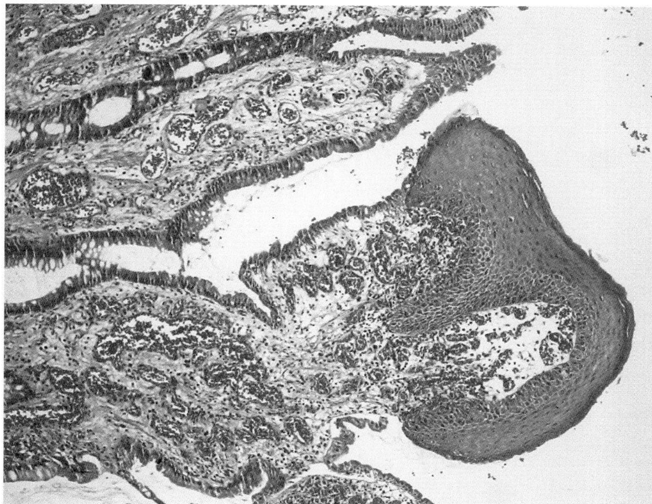

Fig. 26.37 Umbilical polyp partially lined by glandular epithelium derived from the omphalomesenteric duct.

Retroperitoneum

Normal anatomy

The retroperitoneal space is the portion of the lumboiliac region limited anteriorly by the peritoneal covering, posteriorly by the posterior abdominal wall, superiorly by the twelfth rib and vertebra, inferiorly by the base of the sacrum and iliac crest, and laterally by the side borders of the quadratus lumborum muscles. It contains, embedded in a meshwork of loose connective tissue, the adrenal glands, kidneys and ureters, aorta and its branches, inferior vena cava and its tributaries, and numerous lymph nodes.

This potentially large space allows both primary and metastatic tumors to grow silently before clinical signs and symptoms appear.

Non-neoplastic conditions

Inflammatory processes from the kidney (pyelonephritis), large bowel (diverticulitis), appendix, and pancreas may be complicated by a retroperitoneal abscess, usually resulting from coliform bacteria. In children, nontuberculous psoas abscesses are, in most cases, due to gram-positive cocci originating from a focus of tonsillitis, otitis media, or cutaneous furuncle. Perforation of the biliary system may occur within the retroperitoneum, with formation of a bile-containing cystic mass. Infection from a tuberculous vertebra may form a retroperitoneal cold abscess, which is often confined to the psoas muscle. **Malakoplakia** can involve the retroperitoneum and be confused with malignant fibrous histiocytoma[402] (Fig. 26.38). Massive retroperitoneal **hemorrhage** in the adult is most often the result of a ruptured aortic aneurysm, trauma, hemorrhagic diathesis, or anticoagulant drug therapy. Less commonly, it is of renal or

Fig. 26.38 Malakoplakia of retroperitoneum. **A**, The H&E appearance simulates malignant fibrous histiocytoma. **B**, von Kossa stain, showing numerous Michaelis–Gutmann bodies.

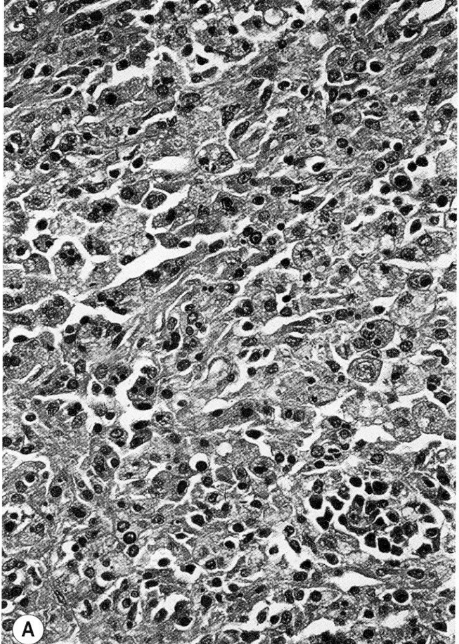

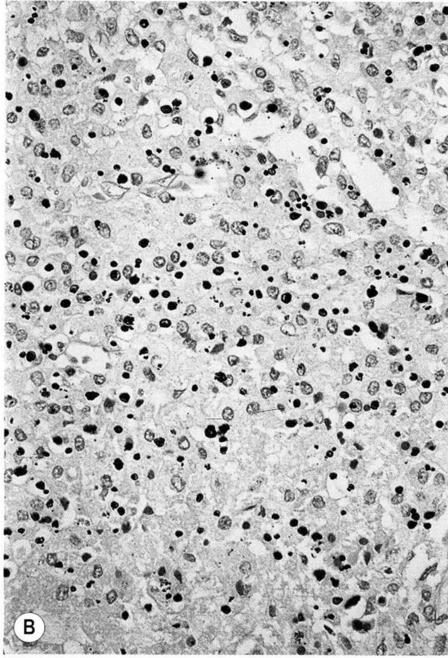

adrenal origin. In five instances reported by Lawson et al.,[392] the adrenal gland was the site of a pheochromocytoma, but in the other five there was no demonstrable abnormality. We have also seen massive retroperitoneal hemorrhage as a complication of adrenal metastases of malignant melanoma. Sometimes **perirenal hemorrhagic cysts** contain equally spaced radial striations that are probably the expression of the Liesegang phenomenon and that have been confused with parasites,[401] whereas the lesions of so-called **myospherulosis** contain clusters of darkened red blood cells within baglike formations that simulate fungal organisms (see Chapter 7).[393]

Extravasation of urine from the upper urinary tract may result in an edematous or gelatinous tumefaction in the retroperitoneum around the renal pelvis. Microscopically, the early stages are characterized by fat necrosis and inflammation and so-called 'urinary precipitates'. An important diagnostic clue is the presence of Tamm–Horsfall protein, as detected immunohistochemically.[376]

Epithelium-lined peritoneal cysts unconnected to the adrenal gland or kidney can be of various types depending on the nature of the lining: mesothelial, mesonephric,[391] müllerian (either serous or mucinous),[382,390] or bronchial. The latter, referred to as *bronchogenic cysts*, are usually found around the adrenal gland and may simulate a primary adrenal neoplasm.[383,395] They represent malformations of the embryonic foregut.

Idiopathic retroperitoneal fibrosis (Ormond disease, sclerosing fibrosis, sclerosing retroperitonitis) is a rare disease of obscure etiology that results in progressive renal failure by producing constriction and final obliteration of the ureters.[380,381,394] Grossly, an ill-defined fibrous mass occupies the retroperitoneal midline, encircles the lower abdominal aorta, and displaces the ureters medially. The latter feature is of value to the radiologist in the differential diagnosis, since most retroperitoneal neoplasms displace the ureter laterally. More localized forms exist, in which the process is sharply circumscribed in the periureteral or renal pelvic region, around one kidney, or around the bladder.[385] Microscopically, a prominent inflammatory infiltrate composed of lymphocytes, plasma cells, histiocytes, and eosinophils, often containing germinal centers, is seen accompanied by foci of fat necrosis, fibroblastic proliferation, and collagen deposition.[397] Cell marker studies have shown that a high percentage of the spindle cells present in this lesion express the immunophenotype of tissue macrophages.[386] The plasma cells, which can be very numerous, show polyclonal immunoglobulin staining,[400] with increased IgG4+ cells in more than half of the cases.[405] The fibrous tissue in the central portion tends to be more mature than that of the periphery.[377] The wall of veins is often involved by the inflammation, this *occlusive phlebitis* being another diagnostic clue to the entity.[387,396] Rarely, there is also involvement of the aorta.[397] Idiopathic retroperitoneal fibrosis may be associated with a similar process in the mediastinum, sclerosing cholangitis, Riedel thyroiditis, pseudotumor of the orbit, or generalized vasculitis. Any possible combination among these various processes has been encountered and is generically referred to as *multifocal fibrosclerosis*.[378] Several cases of retroperitoneal fibrosis were reported in the 1960s, secondary to the administration of methysergide and other drugs;[384] in many cases, cessation of therapy resulted in dramatic regression of the lesion. The available evidence strongly suggests that idiopathic retroperitoneal fibrosis represents an immunologic hypersensitivity disorder, and at least a proportion of cases represent a manifestation of IgG4-related sclerosing disease.[405] Surgical ureterolysis is the treatment of choice;[379,399] sometimes corticosteroid therapy has resulted in dramatic improvement.[398,405]

Occasionally the clinical and pathologic features of idiopathic retroperitoneal fibrosis can be simulated by malignant neoplasms accompanied by chronic inflammation and fibrosis, notably atypical lipomatous tumor, sclerosing malignant lymphoma and signet ring cell carcinoma of the stomach.[388,389,403] Immunohistochemical detection of MDM2 is useful in the differential diagnosis of atypical lipomatous tumor (positive) from idiopathic retroperitoneal fibrosis (negative).[404]

Tumors

Primary tumors of the retroperitoneal area can be of many types.[406,408] In a generic sense, neoplasms arising in the kidney, adrenal gland, and retroperitoneal lymph nodes qualify in the category and are actually the most common. However, by convention, the designation of primary retroperitoneal tumors has been reserved for tumors in this area arising outside of these structures. Most of them have been already discussed elsewhere, particularly in Chapter 25. Here, only the frequency and peculiarities of these neoplasms as they pertain to their retroperitoneal location will be considered.

Symptoms secondary to retroperitoneal neoplasms are vague and appear late in the course of the disease. They are related to displacements of organs and obstructive phenomena.[409]

The early radiologic methods for the evaluation of retroperitoneal tumors were plain roentgenograms, barium studies of the gastrointestinal tract, and intravenous/retrograde pyelograms. These were later supplemented by selective arteriography and inferior cavography, but these techniques in turn have been largely superseded by ultrasonography, CT scanning, and nuclear magnetic resonance imaging[407,410] (Fig. 26.39).

Soft tissue tumors

As a group, retroperitoneal soft tissue sarcomas are associated with a poor long-term survival rate, the main reason being the extreme difficulty encountered in performing a complete surgical removal with a rim of normal tissue around the tumor.[418,439,466] In a large series, the 5-year survival rate was 25%.[432] Complete surgical excision at the time of the initial presentation offers the best chance of long-term survival.[432,461] Local recurrence represents an ominous prognostic sign.[429]

Adipose tissue tumors are the most frequent primary retroperitoneal soft tissue neoplasms, the large majority of them being *liposarcomas*. They are particularly prone to arise and grow in the perirenal region (Figs 26.40 and 26.41). At the time of excision, they are usually extremely large. Some cases present as multiple independent tumor nodules. Retroperitoneal liposarcomas have a worse prognosis than those located in the extremities (39% versus 71% survival rate in the classic series of Enzinger and Winslow,[424] the former figure falling to 4% at 10 years). Total or near-total excision followed by radiation therapy offers the best chance of control.[441] The large majority of retroperitoneal liposarcomas are of the well-differentiated type (currently designated atypical lipomatous tumors) or of the pleomorphic type. Myxoid liposarcomas are practically nonexistent at this site; before making this diagnosis, the alternative possibility of an atypical lipomatous tumor with secondary myxoid changes should be considered.[411,433] Some atypical lipomatous tumors of the retroperitoneum (a higher number than at other sites) undergo dedifferentiation, sometimes associated with divergent differentiation in the form of rhabdomyosarcoma[416,423,430,462] (Fig. 26.42). In the presence of a pleomorphic and not easily classifiable retroperitoneal sarcoma, this possibility should be considered, and sampling of the adjacent areas looking for atypical lipomatous tumor (which may look grossly like normal fat) should be carried out. Indeed, it has been suggested that the majority

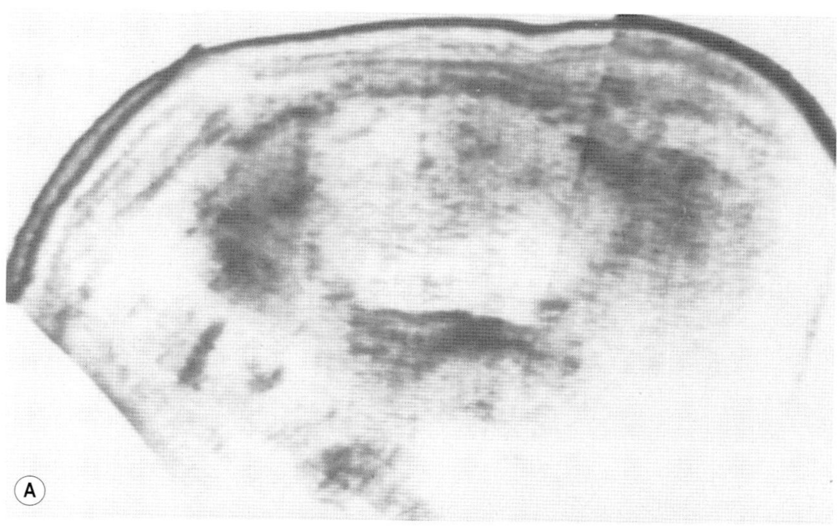

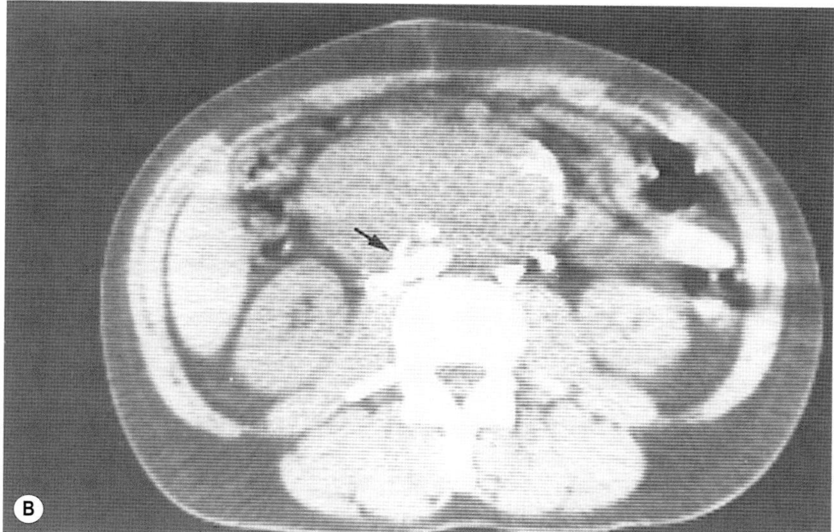

Fig. 26.39 **A**, Transverse ultrasonography in a patient with retroperitoneal metastases from testicular germ cell tumor. Echo demonstrates a massive retroperitoneal tumor lying against the spine and protruding into the abdominal cavity. Complex echo pattern within the tumor indicates areas of fibrosis, probably secondary to necrosis. **B**, Transverse computed tomography in the same patient whose sonogram is shown in **A**. The mass is again clearly shown. Its borders are better demarcated than in the sonogram, but the internal architecture is less distinct. Darker areas at the periphery of the mass (arrow) represent iodide material from previous lymphangiogram.
(Courtesy of Dr S Feinberg, Minneapolis)

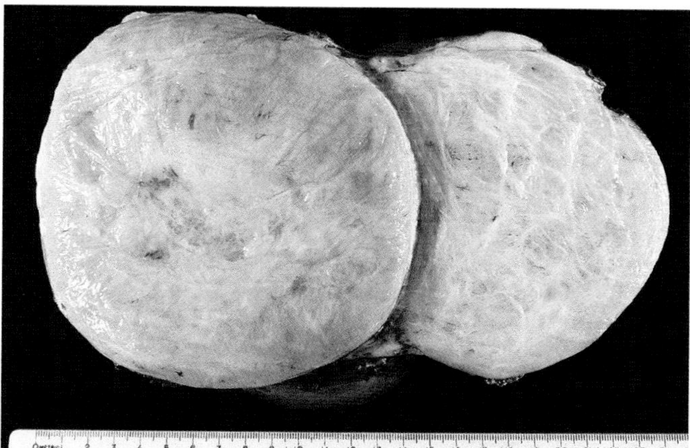

Fig. 26.40 Cut surface of atypical lipomatous tumor (well-differentiated liposarcoma) of the sclerosing subtype.

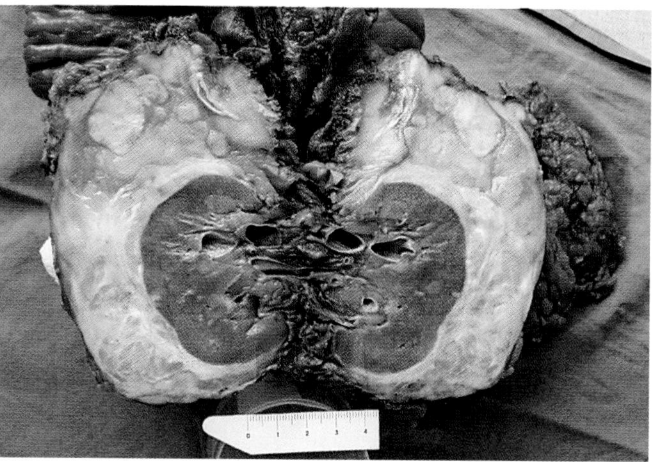

Fig. 26.41 Typical perirenal location of atypical lipomatous tumor (well-differentiated liposarcoma).

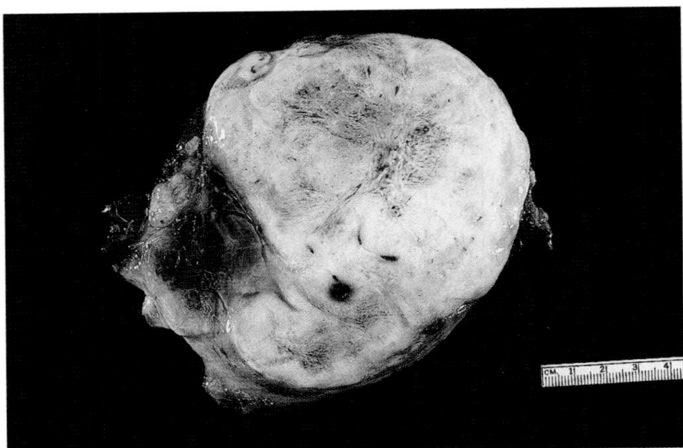

Fig. 26.42 Gross appearance of retroperitoneal atypical lipomatous tumor (well-differentiated liposarcoma) accompanied by foci of dedifferentiation, manifested by the solid whitish areas.

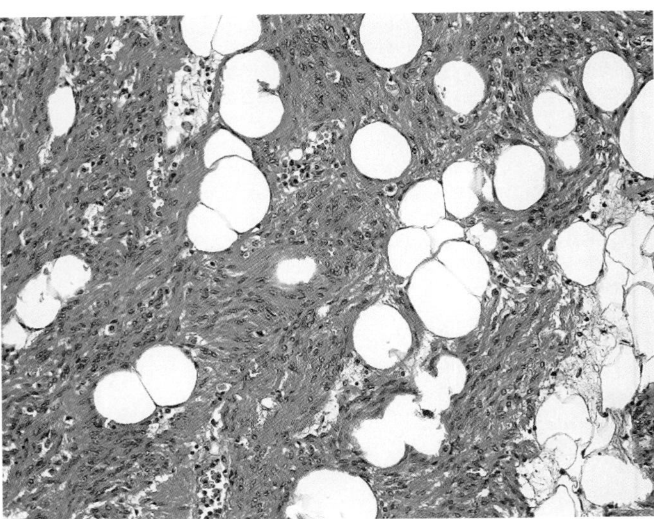

Fig. 26.43 Angiolipoma of retroperitoneum. This tumor differs from angiomyolipoma by virtue of the absence of a vascular component and its lack of reactivity to HMB-45.

of retroperitoneal tumors diagnosed in the past as malignant fibrous histiocytomas represent dedifferentiated liposarcomas (see below).[419,426] When these tumors metastasize, the clinical course is rapidly fatal.[435]

Truly benign lipomas of the retroperitoneum are extremely rare but they do exist.[438,446] Any adipose tissue tumor of the retroperitoneum with atypical nuclei and/or lipoblasts should be designated as atypical lipomatous tumor no matter how focal these features are, in view of its marked tendency for recurrence and poor long-term prognosis.[412] Many cases reported in the old literature as retroperitoneal lipomas are actually examples of atypical lipomatous tumors, particularly those in which a malignant transformation is said to have occurred. At the same time, it should be recognized that pseudoliposarcomatous changes can sometimes be seen in the perinephric adipose tissue of nephrectomy specimens.[413]

Both atypical lipomatous tumors and lipomas may contain bundles of well-differentiated smooth muscle; when benign, these tumors are referred to as *myolipomas*[447] (Fig. 26.43); angiomyolipoma is the obvious differential diagnosis (see later section).

Pleomorphic sarcoma, not otherwise specified is the second most common type of retroperitoneal sarcoma. Most of these tumors used to be diagnosed as malignant fibrous histiocytoma or one of its alleged variants, including the inflammatory type (which may be associated with marked peripheral leukocytosis[467]) but at present most of them have been reclassified as other types of soft tissue sarcoma, especially liposarcoma. It is inadvisable to classify these deep-seated lesions as benign no matter how bland their microscopic appearance may be, in view of the fact that some of them will result in repeated recurrences and even metastases. Along these lines, it should be mentioned that the majority of the cases included in the classic article by Oberling as retroperitoneal xanthogranulomas probably represent examples of soft tissue sarcomas with a prominent component of foamy macrophages.[449] This is not to say that true inflammatory processes having a prominent histiocytic component cannot occur in this region. They certainly can, specific examples being Rosai–Dorfman disease, Langerhans cell histiocytosis, the related entity known as Erdheim–Chester disease, and malakoplakia.[422] The differential diagnosis includes other types of sarcoma and sarcomatoid renal carcinoma.

Leiomyosarcoma is the third most common sarcoma in this area[431] (Fig. 26.44). This tumor has a particular tendency to undergo massive cystic degeneration when occurring in this region.

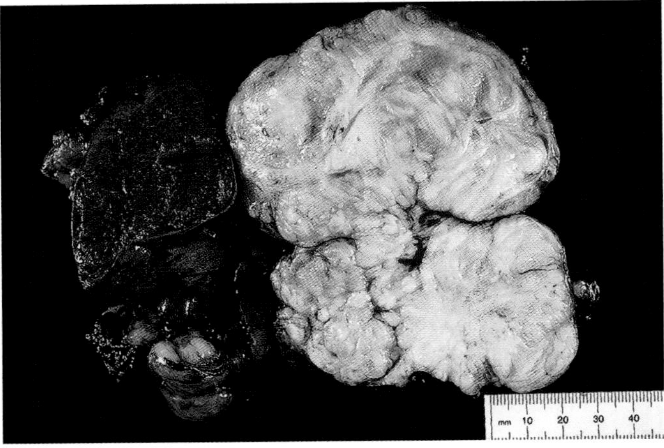

Fig. 26.44 Gross appearance of retroperitoneal leiomyosarcoma, removed in continuity with the spleen. The whorling appearance of the cut surface is characteristic.

Retroperitoneal smooth muscle tumors containing five or more mitoses per 50 high-power fields should be classified as leiomyosarcomas. Tumor cell necrosis or a tumor size greater than 10 cm is strongly suggestive of malignancy, even in the presence of a low mitotic count. When these criteria are applied to retroperitoneal tumors, it will be found that nearly all of them qualify as leiomyosarcomas (except for the tumors composed of hormonally sensitive smooth muscle, see below). The prognosis has been extremely poor in all the reported series: over 85% of the patients have died of tumor, usually within 2 years of diagnosis.[431,453,454,460]

Peculiar morphologic variations that have been reported in retroperitoneal leiomyosarcoma are granular cell changes[452] and focal skeletal muscle differentiation.[457]

A complicated issue arises from the fact that a certain proportion of retroperitoneal neoplasms traditionally regarded as leiomyosarcomas exhibit an epithelioid (clear cell) morphology, ultrastructural features suggestive of neural differentiation, CD117 (*KIT*) immunoreactivity and/or molecular evidence of *KIT* mutation, i.e., features

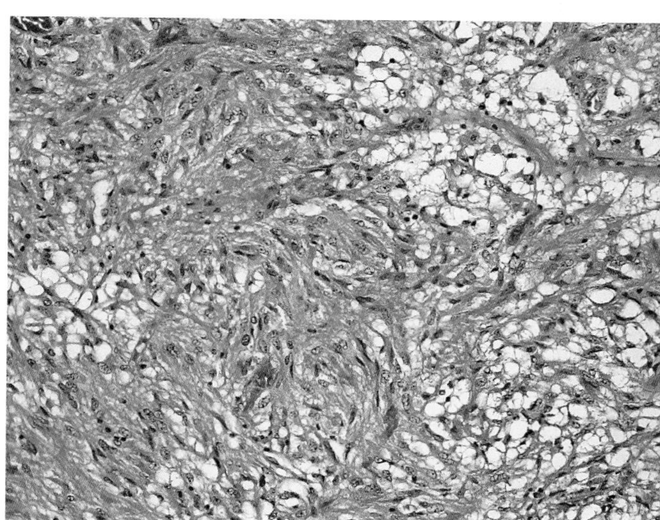

Fig. 26.45 Retroperitoneal tumor having morphologic and immunohistochemical features analogous to GIST.

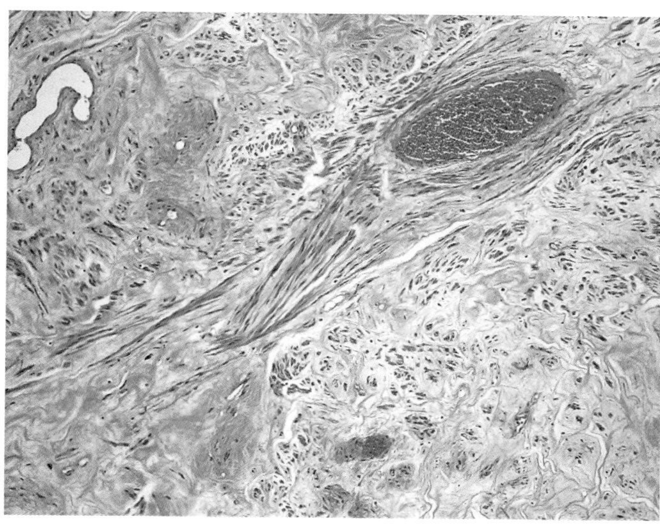

Fig. 26.46 Retroperitoneal smooth muscle tumor in pelvic region morphologically similar to uterine leiomyoma. Note the prominent hyalinization.

associated with the gastrointestinal neoplasm known as GIST[444,451,456] (Fig. 26.45). The reader is referred to Chapter 11 for a more detailed discussion of this thorny subject. Suffice it to say here that if one were to attempt to segregate these tumors sharply into leiomyosarcomas and GISTs using the proposed criteria of CD117 immunoreactivity and evidence of smooth muscle/neural differentiation, most retroperitoneal neoplasms would fall into the category of leiomyosarcomas, in sharp contrast with the situation in the gastrointestinal tract, omentum, and mesentery.

Renal angiomyolipoma is a generally benign retroperitoneal tumor that can be easily confused with liposarcoma or leiomyosarcoma in a biopsy specimen because of the atypia commonly seen in some lesional cells (see Chapter 17). The primarily intrarenal location, the admixture with mature fat and thick-walled blood vessels, and the immunoreactivity for HMB-45 should allow the recognition of this entity. It should also be noted that primary extrarenal examples of this tumor exist, some of them epithelioid and malignant.[443]

Leiomyoma is very rare as a primary retroperitoneal neoplasm. When encountering a tumor in this region with a leiomyomatous appearance, one should consider the alternative possibilities of uterine leiomyoma extending posteriorly, well-differentiated leiomyosarcoma, benign and malignant GIST, lymphangiomyoma, and the previously discussed angiomyolipoma[414] (see above). It would appear that the majority of truly benign smooth muscle tumors presenting as retroperitoneal masses are anatomically and/or functionally related to the female genital tract (such as so-called mesometrial smooth muscle, which runs parallel to the fallopian tube[469]), as suggested by the fact that there is a great predominance of females, a marked morphologic resemblance to uterine leiomyoma by virtue of hyaline change and trabecular pattern of growth, and frequent positivity for estrogen and progesterone receptors[415,440,450] (Fig. 26.46).

Rhabdomyosarcoma of retroperitoneum is usually of the embryonal type (including its botryoid variety) and rarely of the alveolar type, and is limited for all practical purposes to infants and children.[420,455] Multimodality treatment has resulted in a greater than 50% tumor response, but the long-term prognosis remains poor.[420,455] The differential diagnosis of retroperitoneal rhabdomyosarcoma in children includes malignant lymphoma, Ewing sarcoma/PNET in all its manifestations (including so-called 'paravertebral round cell tumor'),[463,471] and desmoplastic small cell tumor (i.e., the whole gamut of small cell tumors of childhood). The distinction between these various entities is often very difficult to make, to say the least, and it may be impossible in the individual case, even after performing ultrastructural and immunohistochemical studies.[421,425,464] This fact was clearly shown in a study from the Intergroup Rhabdomyosarcoma Study Committee,[420] in which almost 30% of 101 retroperitoneal soft tissue sarcomas were classified as undifferentiated or unspecified. The situation has greatly improved following the systematic evaluation of these tumors with cytogenetic and molecular genetic techniques (see Chapter 25).

Rhabdomyoma is practically nonexistent in the retroperitoneum; however, a convincing case combining features of the fetal and adult types of this tumor has been reported in a neonate.[470]

Fibromatosis may occur, sometimes in association with mediastinal involvement. In contrast to idiopathic retroperitoneal fibrosis (a disorder with which it is often confused), it lacks a prominent inflammatory component, except for perivascular lymphocytic cuffing at the growing edge.

Fibrosarcoma is one of the rarest retroperitoneal tumors in our experience. We believe that most cases so designated in the literature would today be labeled dedifferentiated liposarcomas, leiomyosarcomas, or malignant peripheral nerve sheath tumors.

Solitary fibrous tumor can present as a primary retroperitoneal mass, sometimes accompanied by hypoglycemia (Fig. 26.47). Some of the reported cases were associated with independent pleural tumors of similar appearance.[437]

Vascular tumors of several types have been described, including hemangioma, hemangiopericytoma, lymphangioma, lymphangiomyoma, and angiosarcoma.[445] Some of the angiosarcomas are of the epithelioid variety; prominent eosinophilic globules may be present in the cytoplasm of the tumor cells.[468] A peculiar variant of infantile hemangioendothelioma mimicking Kaposi sarcoma (kaposiform hemangioendothelioma) and often accompanied by thrombocytopenia and hemorrhage (Kasabach–Merritt syndrome) has a special tendency for a retroperitoneal location.[427,465]

Peripheral nerve tumors of both benign and malignant type occur; as a matter of fact, the retroperitoneum is a relatively common site for their development. Among the benign tumors, there are

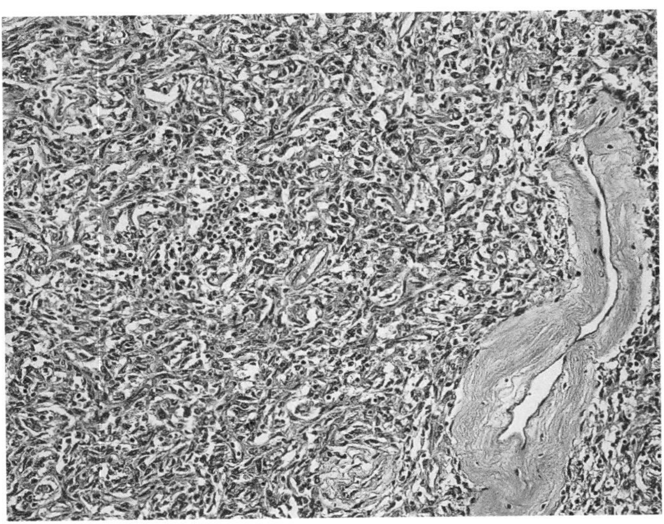

Fig. 26.47 Solitary fibrous tumor/hemangiopericytoma of the pelvic region. This is one of the most common locations for this tumor type.

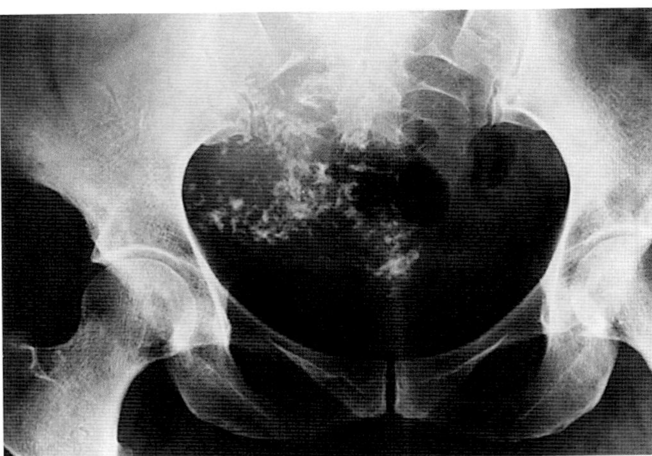

Fig. 26.49 Partially calcified retroperitoneal malignant peripheral nerve sheath tumor.

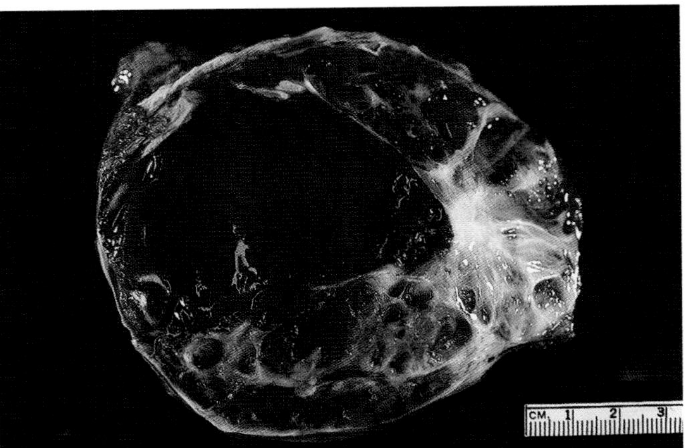

Fig. 26.48 Retroperitoneal schwannoma. The tumor is encapsulated and shows marked secondary hemorrhagic and cystic changes.

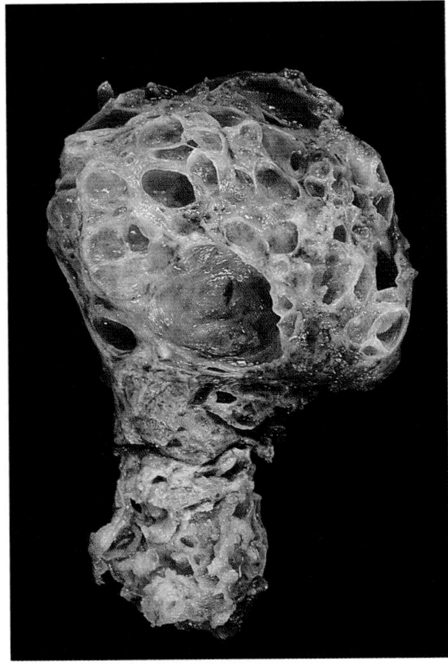

Fig. 26.50 Mature retroperitoneal teratoma. Gross appearance, showing multiple cystic spaces.

schwannomas, neurofibromas, and (rare but diagnosed with increasing frequency) *perineuriomas* (Fig. 26.48). *Malignant peripheral nerve sheath tumors* usually present as paraspinal masses and tend to behave in an aggressive fashion[442] (Fig. 26.49). They may directly invade bone and metastasize distantly. Some of these tumors have arisen from retroperitoneal ganglioneuromas,[428] and others have had the phenotypic features of a malignant perineurioma. A tumor histogenetically related to perineurioma is *meningioma*, which has been reported to present exceptionally as a primary retroperitoneal lesion.[436]

Synovial sarcoma,[459] **alveolar soft part sarcoma,**[458] **extraskeletal osteosarcoma**[417] and **endometrial stromal sarcoma**[448] can present as primary retroperitoneal neoplasms. There has also been a report of a **dendritic follicular tumor** arising extranodally from periduodenal retroperitoneal soft tissue.[434]

Germ cell tumors

Retroperitoneal germ cell tumors in children are represented by mature and immature teratoma, embryonal carcinoma, and yolk sac tumor.[473,476,478] Sometimes these occur in combination.[482] Their features merge with those of sacrococcygeal teratomas, which are discussed in more detail on page 2258.

Retroperitoneal germ cell tumors in adults can arise in this location or represent metastases from primaries in the gonads[472,474,480] (Fig. 26.50). Both types are much more common in males. The entire microscopic gamut is represented, including seminoma (germinoma), embryonal carcinoma, teratocarcinoma, mature and immature teratoma, mature teratoma with malignant transformation, yolk sac tumor, and choriocarcinoma[481] (Fig. 26.51). Their morphology mirrors that of their gonadal counterparts. OCT-4 is the most useful immunohistochemical marker for the confirmation of a diagnosis of seminoma and embryonal carcinoma, and SALL4

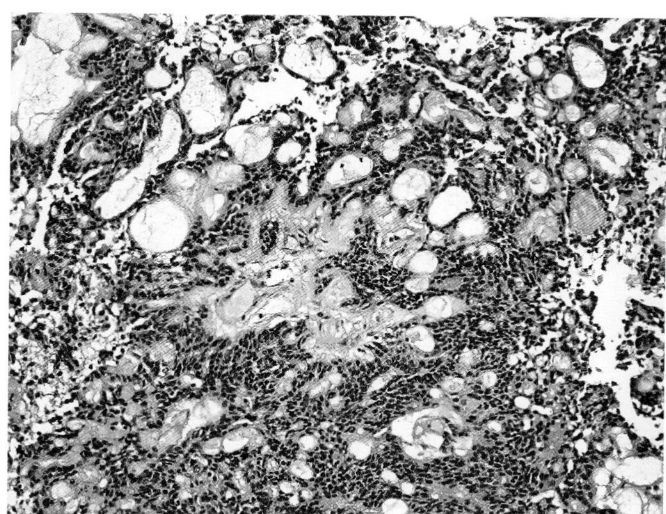

Fig. 26.51 Typical microscopic appearance of yolk sac tumor of sacrococcygeal region.

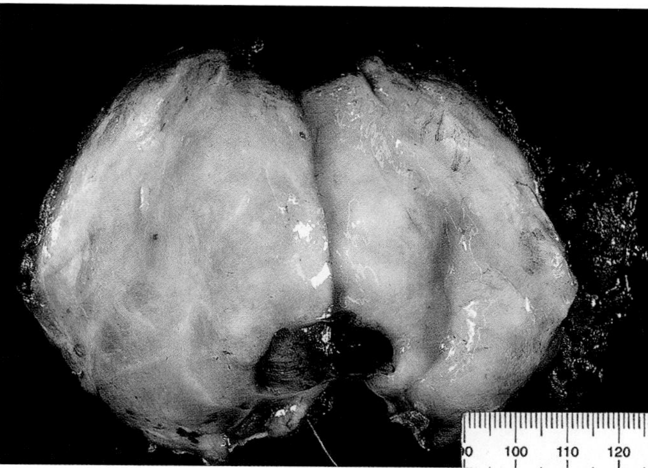

Fig. 26.52 Ganglioneuroma of retroperitoneum. The gross appearance is similar to that of neurofibroma.

is the best marker for yolk sac tumor (although seminoma and embryonal carcinoma are also positive).[483,484] Another useful procedure is the FISH technique for the detection of chromosome 12p amplification.[477]

The chances of a retroperitoneal germ cell tumor in a male being metastatic from a small testicular primary tumor are much higher than for a mediastinal tumor of the same type. The gross appearance of the tumor may give a clue in this regard: in general, primary retroperitoneal neoplasms are formed by a single mass, whereas those metastatic from the testis tend to involve several nodes, often on both sides of the peritoneum.[485] Also, seminomas are more likely to be primary than nonseminomatous germ cell tumors. The testicular primary tumor, when present, may be clinically apparent, may be occult, or may have been excised many years previously.[479] In some cases, only intratubular germ cell neoplasia is found in the testicle, suggesting the possibility of independent neoplastic events.[475] Careful palpation, roentgenograms, sonography, and scrotal thermography have been employed to detect occult testicular tumors; of these, sonography has proved to be the most useful.

Other primary tumors and tumorlike conditions

Tumors of sympathetic nervous tissue of the type more commonly seen in the adrenal gland can also be present in the retroperitoneum outside this gland, as stated in Chapter 16. This includes neuroblastoma, ganglioneuroblastoma, ganglioneuroma, and their variants (Fig. 26.52). It is important to recognize that neuroblastoma can present in adult patients and to distinguish it from Ewing sarcoma/PNET.[494]

Paragangliomas of the retroperitoneum arise outside the adrenal gland in approximately 10% of the cases. They may be located anywhere along the midline of the retroperitoneum, the best known site being the body of Zuckerkandl (situated at the origin of the inferior mesenteric artery from the aorta).[498,500] Tumors arising in **heterotopic adrenal cortex** have also been reported.

Malignant lymphomas can present initially in the retroperitoneum. The large majority are of non-Hodgkin type and B-cell nature.[491] Many of these are of follicular type and associated with extensive fibrosis that can simulate the pattern of idiopathic retroperitoneal fibrosis, as stated in the preceding section.[511] Others have a diffuse quality and run a very aggressive clinical course.[510] These tumors can be diagnosed by fine needle aspiration or core needle biopsy, supplemented by immunostains.[488]

Myelolipomas similar to those of the adrenal glands can be encountered in the presacral area. They are well circumscribed, can attain a huge size, and are composed of a mixture of fat cells and normal marrow hematopoietic elements.[486] These are usually asymptomatic, whereas mass-forming foci of extramedullary hematopoiesis (which lack fat and are ill defined) are associated with myeloproliferative diseases, hemolytic anemia, or severe skeletal diseases.[490,492]

Carcinoid tumor has been described as a retroperitoneal neoplasm; whether it represents a metastasis from an undetected primary tumor, the expression of a monodermal teratoma, or a neoplasm from endocrine cells normally present in this location remains to be determined.[512]

Tumors of müllerian type are occasionally seen as primary retroperitoneal masses in the pelvis or rectovaginal septum (see Chapter 19, Ovary). They can be of serous, mucinous, or endometrioid subtype, and can be benign, borderline, or malignant[496,499,503,506] (Fig. 26.53). They also include mixed müllerian malignant tumor (müllerian carcinosarcoma).[505] They arise either from heterotopic ovarian tissue or, more likely, from invaginations of the peritoneal mesothelial layer with concurrent or subsequent müllerian metaplasia.[489,501,502,508] Some mucinous retroperitoneal tumors have shown evidence of gastric mucosal differentiation, suggesting a totally different histogenesis.[504]

Wilms tumor has been reported in the retroperitoneum outside the kidney in the absence of teratomatous elements.[497,507,509] Some of these lesions may represent teratomas predominantly or exclusively composed of nephrogenic elements. Most of these cases have occurred in children, but they have also been recorded in adults.[493]

PEComas, i.e., tumors showing perivascular epithelioid cell features, can develop in the retroperitoneum outside the kidney. In this location they tend to be accompanied by marked sclerosis.[495]

Myoepithelioma has been described, simulating microscopically the appearance of a schwannoma.[487]

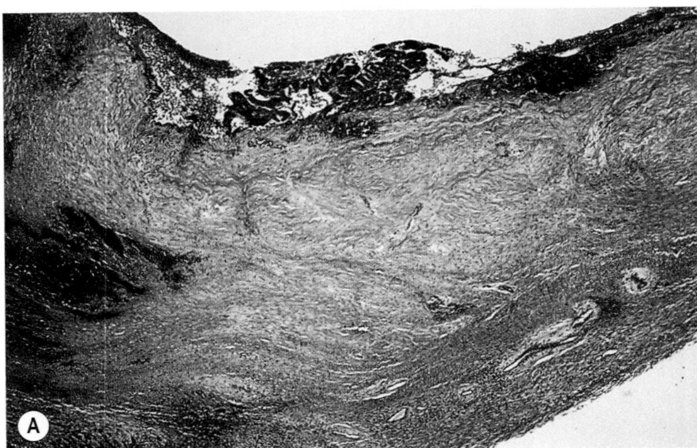

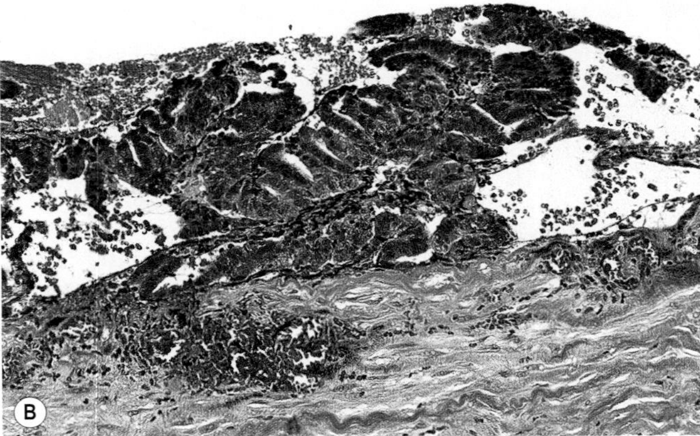

Fig. 26.53 **A** and **B**, Low-power and high-power appearance of müllerian-type cystadenocarcinoma located in the retroperitoneal region.

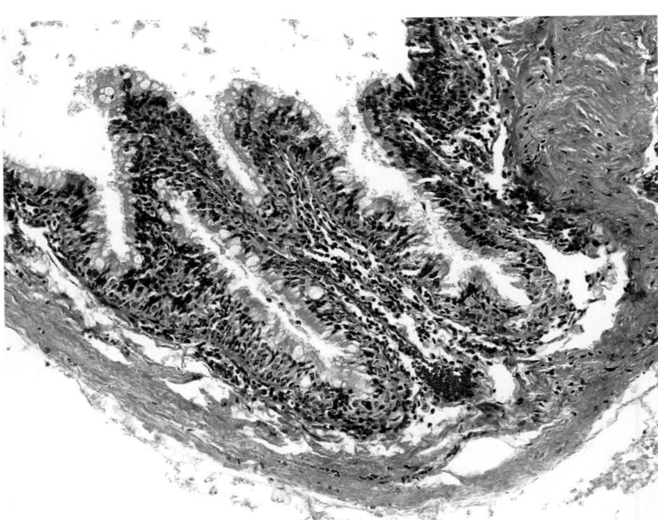

Fig. 26.54 Tailgut cyst lined by pseudostratified epithelium surrounded by a muscle wall.

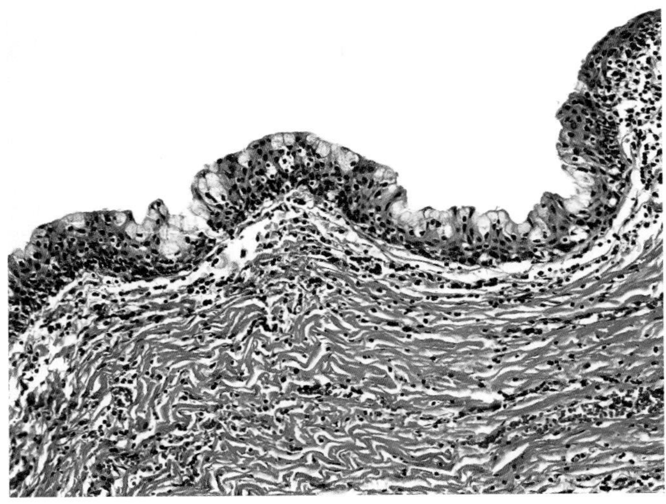

Fig. 26.55 Tailgut cyst lined by mucin-secreting well-differentiated epithelium with goblet cells.

Metastatic tumors

Secondary neoplasms may appear in the retroperitoneal space as a result of local extension or because of lymph node involvement. The former is mainly represented by pancreatic carcinoma and primary bone neoplasms, notably sacrococcygeal chordoma.

The carcinomas most commonly giving rise to retroperitoneal lymph node metastases are those originating in the testis, prostate, pancreas, uterine cervix, endometrium, and kidney.

Sacrococcygeal region

Developmental anomalies

A large and complex number of malformations can occur in the sacrococcygeal region, the most common being *meningocele* and *spina bifida*.[514,517] Some of these are discussed in Chapter 28.

Tailgut cyst (retrorectal cystic hamartoma) presents in the presacrococcygeal area, usually in adult patients but sometimes in children, as a multiloculated cyst lined by squamous, transitional, or glandular epithelium[518,519,521,523] (Figs 26.54 and 26.55). Disorganized fascicles of smooth muscle may be seen in the wall. Prominent glomus bodies, meningothelial nests and thyroid tissue may also be present.[513,522] This benign malformative lesion should be distinguished from teratoma, epidermal cyst, rectal or anal duplication, and anal gland cyst.[515,520,525] Malignant transformation can supervene in this malformation, in the form of adenocarcinoma, carcinoid tumor or Paget disease (see below).[518,524,526]

Ectopic prostatic tissue can occur in the presacral region and lead to extrinsic compression of the bowel.[516]

Germ cell tumors

Sacrococcygeal germ cell tumors in neonates and infants are nearly always primary. From 75% to 90% of the cases occur in females. They can arise in the retroperitoneum proper, be centered in the sacrococcygeal region, or involve both compartments.[532,534,543] Chromosomal analysis of these extragonadal teratomas suggests that they have arisen from postmitotic, premeiotic cells.[536] The most common type is the **mature teratoma** presenting at birth in the sacrococcygeal region or protruding through the abdominal cavity (Fig. 26.56).[529,531] It may be very large, is usually cystic and multilocular, and may appear malignant to the surgeon because of its

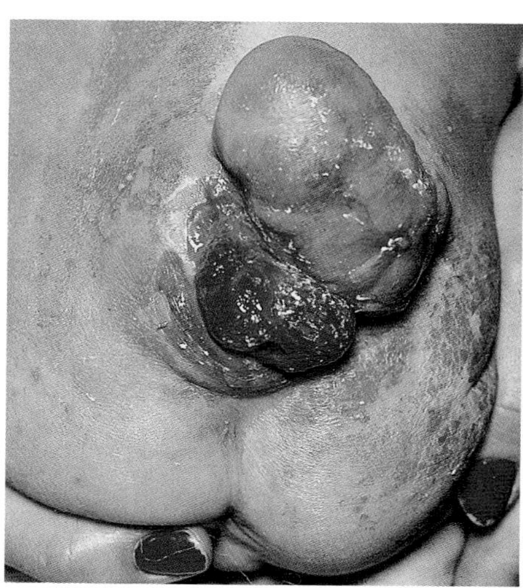

Fig. 26.56 Sacrococcygeal teratoma protruding as a polypoid, partially ulcerated mass.

stubborn adherence to neighboring structures, but this fixation is usually of an inflammatory nature, caused by reaction to extravasated material. Total excision is curative; the tip of the coccyx should be removed as part of the operation to prevent recurrence.[549] Microscopically, this tumor is composed of mature tissues throughout. Hepatic tissue is present in one-fourth of the cases.[541] The presence of immature elements in regard to amount and microscopic type should be evaluated with care.[547] If this immaturity is restricted to neuroectodermal components (which is often the case), the tendency is toward spontaneous differentiation. As a result, the behavior of this type of immature teratoma is usually benign, although occasional cases will recur or metastasize.[533,547]

Most of the clearly malignant teratomas in this age group have the appearance of **yolk sac (endodermal sinus) tumor**, either pure or associated with other germ cell components, and are accompanied by the production of oncofetal antigens[532,537,544] and expression of transcription factor GATA-4.[546] They often contain immature hepatic tissue.[541] SALL4 is a highly sensitive immunohistochemical marker that can aid in their diagnosis.[548] Yolk sac tumors run an extremely aggressive clinical course.[530,533,539] A renal component resembling Wilms tumor is sometimes found in these teratomas. It may not be easy to decide in an individual case whether the lesion represents a teratoma with predominance of nephrogenic elements or a 'teratoid' Wilms tumor.

An interesting clinical observation is that the large majority of sacrococcygeal teratomas present at birth are benign, whereas tumors in the same general location discovered after the age of 2 months are often malignant.[531,535] This has been taken by some to indicate that a malignant transformation has supervened in that short period. We doubt that this is the case. It seems to us that this clinical observation can better be explained by postulating the existence of two types of teratoma. One arises in the very distal portion of the sacrococcygeal region, is therefore clinically obvious at the time of birth, and is nearly always mature. The other arises more proximally, in the retrorectal or adjacent retroperitoneal region, is malignant from the start, and grows into the sacrococcygeal area to become clinically evident only some time after birth. It also grows within the abdominal cavity, this being responsible for the clinical observation that teratomas associated with marked bowel or bladder dysfunction are often malignant. Exceptions in both directions certainly occur, but the large majority of teratomas in this region fit into this scheme.

A sacrococcygeal presentation of teratoma in adults is exceptional.[542] Most are benign and probably have been there since birth. A few show malignant foci, either in the form of germ cell (trophoblastic, yolk sac) components or of adult-type carcinomatous tissues.[527,549] Mature teratomas excised in early life may recur in adulthood in the form of a microscopically similar neoplasm,[540] as a malignant germ cell tumor (such as yolk sac tumor),[545] or as a somatic-type malignant tumor, such as adenocarcinoma.[538]

The differential diagnosis of benign sacrococcygeal teratoma includes the already mentioned developmental abnormalities of this region, a discussion of which is beyond the scope of this book. A comprehensive review of these anomalies can be found in an article by Bale.[528]

Pilonidal disease

Pilonidal sinuses appear as small openings in the intergluteal fold about 3.5–5 cm posterior to the anal orifice. Hairs are sometimes seen protruding from them. The opening is continued by a sinus tract, which is directed upward in 93% of the cases.[554] The disease is most often seen in young white males with dark, straight hair. Although congenital anomalies related to the closure of the neural canal can certainly occur in this area, it is currently believed that the large majority of pilonidal sinuses have an acquired pathogenesis.[551] Hairs penetrate areas of inflammation from without, lodge in the dermis, and elicit a foreign body type of reaction. The sinus is lined by granulation tissue. In approximately 25% of the cases, hairs are not found within the lesion.

Pilonidal sinuses also have been described in other areas where skin folds are prominent, such as the umbilicus, clitoris, and axilla.[550] A further observation favoring the theory of the acquired origin is the fact that barbers and hairdressers occasionally develop a disease equivalent to pilonidal sinus between their fingers, the sinuses containing somebody else's hairs![556]

Cases of **squamous cell carcinoma**[552,555] and **verrucous carcinoma** (giant condyloma acuminatum)[553] developing within pilonidal sinuses have been described.

Other tumors

Neoplasms other than germ cell tumors can involve the sacrococcygeal region primarily or as an extension from adjacent sites. Many cases of **cellular blue nevus** involve this area (see Chapter 4). Cases of coccydynia have been reported secondarily to **tumors of the coccygeal glomus**, although the neoplastic nature of this process and their role in producing symptoms have been questioned[562] (see Chapter 25). Specifically, the point has been made that the normal glomus coccygeum can measure up to 4 mm in diameter and that its appearance is no different in cases of coccydynia than in those cases where it was incidentally removed in the course of operations for rectal or uterine carcinoma.[558] **Myxopapillary ependymoma** can involve the soft tissues of the buttock, unconnected with the spine[559,561] (see Chapter 28).

Carcinoid tumor can occur as a primary lesion in the presacral area. Most of these tumors probably arise from hindgut rests, as suggested by their documented association with tailgut cysts (see p. 2258).[557,560,563]

Chordoma arising in the sacrum can produce a large retrorectal or sacrococcygeal mass (see Chapter 24). Finally, **carcinomas** of the anus or rectum (particularly those of the mucinous adenocarcinoma type) can spread to this region by direct extension (see Chapter 11).

References

PERITONEUM

NORMAL ANATOMY

1 Bolen JLW, Hammar SP, McNutt MA. Reactive and neoplastic serosal tissue. A light-microscopic, ultrastructural, and immunocytochemical study. Am J Surg Pathol 1986, **10**: 34–47.

2 Carter D, True L, Otis CN. Serous membranes. In: Mills SE (ed.): Histology for pathologists, ed. 3. Philadelphia, 2007, Lippincott Williams & Wilkins, pp. 547–562.

3 Kupryjanczyk J, Karpinska G. Desmin expression in reactive mesothelium: a potential aid in evaluation of gynecologic specimens. Int J Gynecol Pathol 1998, **17**: 123–128.

4 McAuley P, Asa SL, Chiu B, Henderson J, Goltzman D, Drucker DJ. Parathyroid hormone-like peptide in normal and neoplastic mesothelial cells. Cancer 1990, **66**: 1975–1979.

INFLAMMATION

5 Bastani B, Shariatzadeh MR, Dehdashti F. Tuberculous peritonitis. Report of 30 cases and review of the literature. QJM 1985, **56**: 549–557.

6 Chen KTK. Coccidioidal peritonitis. Am J Clin Pathol 1983, **80**: 514–516.

7 Ellis H, Adair HM. Bile peritonitis. A report of fifteen patients. Postgrad Med J 1974, **50**: 713–717.

8 Forouhar F. Meconium peritonitis. Pathology, evolution, and diagnosis. Am J Clin Pathol 1982, **78**: 208–213.

9 George E, Leyser S, Zimmer HL, Simonowitz DA, Agress RL, Nordin DD. Vernix caseosa peritonitis. An infrequent complication of Cesarean section with distinctive histopathologic features. Am J Clin Pathol 1995, **103**: 681–684.

10 Gilinsky NH, Marks IN, Kottler RE, Price SK. Abdominal tuberculosis. A 10-year review. S Afr Med J 1983, **64**: 849–857.

11 Gonnella JS, Hudson EK. Clinical patterns of tuberculous peritonitis. Arch Intern Med 1966, **117**: 164–169.

12 Levine H. Needle biopsy of peritoneum in exudative ascites. Arch Intern Med 1967, **120**: 542–545.

13 Levine H. Needle biopsy diagnosis of tuberculous peritonitis. Am Rev Respir Dis 1968, **97**: 889–894.

14 Seaman WB, Wells J. Complications of the barium enema. Gastroenterology 1965, **48**: 728–737.

15 Sherman S, Rohwedder JJ, Ravikrishnan KP, Weg JLG. Tuberculous enteritis and peritonitis. Report of 36 general hospital cases. Arch Intern Med 1980, **140**: 506–507.

16 Singh MM, Bhargava AN, Jain KP. Tuberculous peritonitis. An evaluation of pathogenetic mechanisms, diagnostic procedures and therapeutic measures. N Engl J Med 1969, **281**: 1091–1094.

17 Sochocky S. Tuberculous peritonitis. A review of 100 cases. Am Rev Respir Dis 1967, **95**: 398–401.

18 Varkonyi I, Fliegel C, Rosslein R, Jenny P, Ohnacker H. Meconium periorchitis: case report and literature review. Eur J Pediatr Surg 2000, **10**: 404–407.

19 Vinuela A, Fernandez-Rojo F, Martinez-Merino A. Oxyuris granulomas of pelvic peritoneum and appendicular wall. Histopathology 1979, **3**: 69–77.

ADHESIONS

20 Bockman RF, Woods M, Sargent L, Gervin AS. A unifying pathogenetic mechanism in the etiology of intraperitoneal adhesions. J Surg Res 1976, **20**: 1–5.

21 Brown P, Baddeley H, Read AE, Davies JD, McGarry JMc. Sclerosing peritonitis. An unusual reaction to a β-adrenergic-blocking drug (Practolol). Lancet 1974, **2**: 1477–1481.

22 Castelli MJ, Armin A-R, Husain A, Orfei E. Fibrosing peritonitis in a drug abuser. Arch Pathol Lab Med 1985, **109**: 767–769.

23 Clement PB, Young RH, Hanna W, Scully RE. Sclerosing peritonitis associated with luteinized thecomas of the ovary. A clinicopathological analysis of six cases. Am J Surg Pathol 1994, **18**: 1–13.

24 Fata F, Ron IG, Maluf F, Klimstra D, Kemeny N. Intra-abdominal fibrosis after systemic and intraperitoneal therapy containing fluoropyrimidines. Cancer 2000, **88**: 2447–2451.

25 Finney AL, Spagnolo DV, Crawford GP, Shilkin KB. Pseudosarcomatous sclerosing peritonitis: A case report of an unusual form of chronic lupus peritonitis. Int J Surg Pathol 1996, **4**: 121–128.

26 Ryan GB, Grobety J, Majno G. Postoperative peritoneal adhesions. A study of the mechanisms. Am J Pathol 1971, **65**: 117–140.

27 Staats PN, McCluggage WG, Clement PB, Young RH. Luteinized thecomas (thecomatosis) of the type typically associated with sclerosing peritonitis: a clinical, histopathologic, and immunohistochemical analysis of 27 cases. Am J Surg Pathol 2008, **32**: 1273–1290.

REACTION TO FOREIGN MATERIALS

28 Auer EA, Dockerty MB, Mayo CW. Reaction to foreign material. Ruptured dermoid cyst of the ovary simulating abdominal carcinomatosis. Mayo Clin Proc 1951, **26**: 489–497.

29 Carr N, Turk E. The histological features of splenosis. Histopathology 1992, **21**: 549–554.

30 Chen KTK, Kostich ND, Rosai J. Peritoneal foreign body granulomas to keratin in uterine adenoacanthoma. Arch Pathol Lab Med 1978, **102**: 174–177.

31 Clarke TJ, Simpson RH. Necrotizing granulomas of peritoneum following diathermy ablation of endometriosis. Histopathology 1990, **16**: 400–402.

32 Clement PB, Young RH, Scully RE. Necrotic pseudoxanthomatous nodules of ovary and peritoneum in endometriosis. Am J Surg Pathol 1988, **12**: 330–397.

33 Coder DM, Olander GA. Granulomatous peritonitis caused by starch glove powder. Arch Surg 1972, **105**: 83–86.

34 Davies JD, Ansell ID. Food-starch granulomatous peritonitis. J Clin Pathol 1983, **36**: 435–438.

35 Davies JD, Neely J. The histopathology of peritoneal starch granulomas. J Pathol 1972, **107**: 265–278.

36 Gawande AA, Studdert DM, Orav EJ, Brennan TA, Zinner MJ. Risk factors for retained instruments and sponges after surgery. N Engl J Med 2003, **348**: 229–235.

37 Jaworski RC, Boable R, Greg J, Cocks P. Peritoneal 'melanosis' associated with a ruptured ovarian dermoid cyst: report of a case with electron-probe energy dispersive X-ray analysis. Int J Gynecol Pathol 2001, **20**: 386–389.

38 Kershisnik MM, Ro JY, Cannon GH, Ordóñez NG, Ayala AG, Silva EG. Histiocytic reaction in pelvic peritoneum associated with oxidized regenerated cellulose. Am J Clin Pathol 1995, **103**: 27–31.

39 Kim KR, Scully RE. Peritoneal keratin granulomas with carcinomas of endometrium and ovary and atypical polypoid adenomyoma of endometrium. A clinicopathological analysis of 22 cases. Am J Surg Pathol 1990, **14**: 925–932.

40 Levison DA, Crocker PR, Jones S, Owen RA, Barnard NJ. The varied appearances of starch particles in smears and paraffin sections. Histopathology 1988, **13**: 667–674.

41 Miranda RN, McMillan PN, Pricolo VE, Finkelstein SD. Peritoneal silicosis. Arch Pathol Lab Med 1996, **120**: 300–302.

42 Nissim F, Ashkenazy M, Borenstein R, Czernobilsky B. Tuberculoid cornstarch granulomas with caseous necrosis. A diagnostic challenge. Arch Pathol Lab Med 1981, **105**: 86–88.

43 Saxen L, Saxen E. Starch granulomas as a problem in surgical pathology. Acta Pathol Microbiol Scand 1965, **64**: 55–70.

44 Tinker MA, Burdman D, Deysine M, Teicher I, Platt N, Aufses AH Jr. Granulomatous peritonitis due to cellulose fibers from disposable surgical fabrics. Laboratory investigations and clinical implications. Ann Surg 1974, **180**: 831–835.

CYSTS AND LOOSE BODIES

45 Carpenter HA, Lancaster JR, Lee RA. Multilocular cysts of the peritoneum. Mayo Clin Proc 1982, **57**: 634–638.

46 Chan JK, Fong MH. Composite multicystic mesothelioma and adenomatoid tumour of the uterus: different morphological manifestations of the same process? Histopathology 1996, **29**: 375–377.

47 Drachenberg CB, Papadimitriou JC. Melanotic peritoneal cyst. Light-microscopic and ultrastructural studies. Arch Pathol Lab Med 1990, **114**: 463–467.

48 Eickhoff JH. Müllerian duct cyst. Report of a case and review of the literature. Scand J Urol Nephrol 1978, **12**: 89–92.

49 Katsube Y, Mukai K, Silverberg SG. Cystic mesothelioma of the peritoneum. Cancer 1982, **50**: 1615–1622.

50 Lamovec J, Sinkovec J. Multilocular peritoneal inclusion cyst (multicystic mesothelioma) with hyaline globules. Histopathology 1996, **28**: 466–469.

51 Lascano EF, Villamayor RD, Llauro JL. Loose cysts of the peritoneal cavity. Ann Surg 1960, **152**: 836–844.

52 McFadden DE, Clement PB. Peritoneal inclusion cysts with mural mesothelial proliferation. A clinicopathological analysis of six cases. Am J Surg Pathol 1986, **10**: 844–854.

53 Moore JH Jr, Crum CP, Chandler JG, Feldman PS. Benign cystic mesothelioma. Cancer 1980, **45**: 2395–2399.

54 Novak RW, Raines RB, Sollee AN. Clear cell carcinoma in a müllerian duct cyst. Am J Clin Pathol 1981, **76**: 339–341.

55 Ramdial PK, Singh B. Membranous fat necrosis in appendices epiploicae. A clinicopathological study. Virchows Arch 1998, **432**: 223–227.

56 Ross MJ, Welch WR, Scully RE. Multilocular peritoneal inclusion cysts (so-called cystic mesotheliomas). Cancer 1989, **64**: 1336–1346.

57 Sarto GE, Simpson JL. Abnormalities of the müllerian and wolffian duct systems. Birth Defects 1978, **14**: 37–55.

58 Sawh RN, Malpica A, Deavers MT, Liu J, Silva EG. Benign cystic mesothelioma of the peritoneum: a clinicopathologic study of 17 cases and immunohistochemical analysis of estrogen and progesterone receptor status. Hum Pathol 2003, **34**: 369–374.

59 Schneider V, Partridge JR, Gutierrez F, Hurt WG, Maizels MS, Demay RM. Benign cystic mesothelioma involving the female genital tract. Report of four cases. Am J Obstet Gynecol 1983, **145**: 355–359.

60 Villaschi S, Autelitano F, Santeusanio G, Balistreri P. Cystic mesothelioma of the peritoneum. A report of three cases. Am J Clin Pathol 1990, **94**: 758–761.

61 Vuong PN, Guyot H, Moulin G, Houissa-Vuong S, Berrod JL. Pseudotumoral organization of a twisted epiploic fringe or 'hard-boiled egg' in the peritoneal cavity. Arch Pathol Lab Med 1990, **114**: 531–533.

HYPERPLASIA AND METAPLASIA

62 Bolen JW, Hammar SP, McNutt MA. Reactive and neoplastic serosal tissue. A light-microscopic, ultrastructural, and immunocytochemical study. Am J Surg Pathol 1986, **10**: 34–47.

63 Chan JK, Loo KT, Yau BK, Lam SY. Nodular histiocytic/mesothelial hyperplasia: a lesion potentially mistaken for a neoplasm in transbronchial biopsy. Am J Surg Pathol 1997, **21**: 658–663.

64 Chikkamuniyappa S, Herrick J, Jagirdar JS. Nodular histiocytic/mesothelial hyperplasia: a potential pitfall. Ann Diagn Pathol 2004, **8**: 115–120.

65 Clement PB, Young RH. Florid mesothelial hyperplasia associated with ovarian tumors. A potential source of error in tumor diagnosis and staging. Int J Gynecol Pathol 1993, **12**: 51–58.

66 Fadare O, Bifulco C, Carter D, Parkash V. Cartilaginous differentiation in peritoneal tissues: a report of two cases and a review of the literature. Mod Pathol 2002, **15**: 777–780.

67 Gupta A, Bhan AK, Bell DA. Can the implants of serous borderline tumors of the ovary be distinguished from mesothelial proliferations by use of immunohistochemistry? [abstract] Mod Pathol 2003, **16**: 190A.

68 Kradin RL, Mark EJ. Distinguishing benign mesothelial hyperplasia from neoplasia: a practical approach. Semin Diagn Pathol 2006, **23**: 4–14.

69 Kupryjanczyk J, Karpinska G. Desmin expression in reactive mesothelium: a potential aid in evaluation of gynecologic specimens. Int J Gynecol Pathol 1998, **17**: 123–128.

70 McCaughey WTE, Al-Jabi M. Differentiation of serosal hyperplasia and neoplasia in biopsies. Pathol Annu 1986, **21**(Pt 1): 271–293.

71 Michal M, Hes O, Kazakov DV. Mesothelial glandular structures within pseudosarcomatous proliferative funiculitis – a diagnostic pitfall: report of 17 cases. Int J Surg Pathol 2008, **16**: 48–56.

72 Mourra N, Nion I, Parc R, Flejou JF. Squamous metaplasia of the peritoneum: a potential diagnostic pitfall. Histopathology 2004, **44**: 621–622.

73 Ordóñez NG, Ro JY, Ayala AG. Lesions described as nodular mesothelial hyperplasia are primarily composed of histiocytes. Am J Surg Pathol 1998, **22**: 285–292.

74 Rosai J, Dehner LP. Nodular mesothelial hyperplasia in hernia sacs. A benign reactive condition simulating a neoplastic process. Cancer 1975, **35**: 165–175.

75 Schatz JE, Colgan TJ. Squamous metaplasia of the peritoneum. Arch Pathol Lab Med 1991, **115**: 397–398.

76 Tomasini C, Butera AC, Pippione M. Acquired cutaneous lymphangiectasia with mesothelial cells reflux in a patient with cirrhotic ascites. Am J Dermatopathol 2008, **30**: 140–144.

77 Veinot JP, Tazelaar HD, Edwards WD, Colby TV. Mesothelial/monocytic incidental cardiac excrescences: cardiac MICE. Mod Pathol 1994, **7**: 9–16.

78 Zaytsev P, Taxy JB. Pregnancy-associated ectopic decidua. Am J Surg Pathol 1987, **11**: 526–530.

TUMORS

MESOTHELIOMA

79 Allen TC, Cagle PT, Churg AM, Colby TV, Gibbs AR, Hammar SP, Corson JM, Grimes MM, Ordóñez NG, Roggli V, Travis WD, Wick MR. Localized malignant mesothelioma. Am J Surg Pathol 2005, **29**: 866–873.

80 Andrion A, Pira E, Mollo F. Peritoneal plaques and asbestos exposure. Arch Pathol Lab Med 1983, **107**: 609–610.

81 Antman KH. Malignant mesothelioma. N Engl J Med 1980, **303**: 200–202.

82 Armstrong GR, Raafat F, Ingram L, Mann JR. Malignant peritoneal mesothelioma in childhood. Arch Pathol Lab Med 1988, **112**: 1159–1162.

83 Attanoos RL, Gibbs AR. Pathology of malignant mesothelioma. Histopathology 1997, **30**: 403–418.

84 Attanoos RL, Dojcinov SD, Webb R, Gibbs AR. Antimesothelial markers in sarcomatoid mesothelioma and other spindle cell neoplasms. Histopathology 2000, **37**: 224–231.

85 Attanoos RL, Webb R, Dojcinov SD, Gibbs AR. Malignant epithelioid mesothelioma: ant-mesothelial marker expression correlates with histological pattern. Histopathology 2001, **39**: 584–588.

86 Attanoos RL, Webb R, Dojcinov SD, Gibbs AR. Value of mesothelial and epithelial antibodies in distinguishing diffuse peritoneal mesothelioma in females from serious papillary carcinoma of the ovary and peritoneum. Histopathology 2002, **40**: 237–244.

87 Baker PM, Clement PB, Young RH. Malignant peritoneal mesothelioma in women: a study of 75 cases with emphasis on their morphologic spectrum and differential diagnosis. Am J Clin Pathol 2005, **123**: 724–737.

88 Battifora HA, Gown AM. Do we need two more mesothelial markers? Hum Pathol 2005, **36**: 451–452.

89 Beer TW, Heenan PJ. Malignant mesothelioma presenting as a lip tumor: report of two cases with one unrecognized by 166 pathologists. Am J Dermatopathol 2007, **29**: 388–391.

90 Bethwaite PB, Evans R, Naik DK, Delahunt B, Teague CA. Diffuse malignant mesothelioma arising in a paracolostomy hernial sac. Histopathology 1996, **29**: 282–284.

91 Bolen JW, Thorning D. Mesotheliomas. A light- and electron-microscopical study concerning histogenetic relationships between the epithelial and the mesenchymal variants. Am J Surg Pathol 1980, **4**: 451–464.

92 Britton M. The epidemiology of mesothelioma. Semin Oncol 2002, **29**: 18–25.

93 Brown JW, Kristensen KAB, Monroe LS. Peritoneal mesothelioma following pneumoperitoneum maintained for 12 years. Report of a case. Am J Dig Dis 1968, **13**: 830–835.

94 Butnor KJ, Sporn TA, Hammar SP, Roggli VL. Well-differentiated papillary mesothelioma. Am J Surg Pathol 2001, **25**: 1304–1309.

95 Carbone M, Kratzke RA, Testa JR. The pathogenesis of mesothelioma. Semin Oncol 2002, **29**: 2–17.

96 Carbone M, Bedrossian CW. The pathogenesis of mesothelioma. Semin Diagn Pathol 2006, **23**: 56–60.

97 Cerruto CA, Brun EA, Chang D, Sugarbaker PH. Prognostic significance of histomorphologic parameters in diffuse malignant peritoneal mesothelioma. Arch Pathol Lab Med 2006, **130**: 1654–1661.

98 Chen KT. Malignant mesothelioma presenting as Sister Joseph's nodule. Am J Dermatopathol 1991, **13**: 300–303.

99 Chiu B, Churg A, Tengblad A, Pearce R, McCaughey WTE. Analysis of hyaluronic acid in the diagnosis of malignant mesothelioma. Cancer 1984, **54**: 2195–2199.

100 Churg A, Colby TV, Cagle P, Corson J, Gibbs AR, Gilks B, Grimes M, Hammar S, Roggli V, Travis WD. The separation of benign and malignant mesothelial proliferations. Am J Surg Pathol 2000, **24**: 1183–1200.

101 Clement PB, Young RH, Scully RE. Malignant mesotheliomas presenting as ovarian masses: A report of nine cases, including two primary ovarian mesotheliomas. Am J Surg Pathol 1996, **20**: 1067–1080.

102 Cook DS, Attanoos RL, Jalloh SS, Gibbs AR. 'Mucin-positive' epithelial mesothelioma of the peritoneum: an unusual diagnostic pitfall. Histopathology 2000, **37**: 33–36.

103 Crotty TB, Myers JL, Katzenstein A-LA, Tazelaar HD, Swensen SJ, Churg A. Localized malignant mesothelioma. A clinicopathologic and flow cytometric study. Am J Surg Pathol 1994, **18**: 357–363.

104 Daya D, McCaughey WT. Well-differentiated papillary mesothelioma of the peritoneum. A clinicopathologic study of 22 cases. Cancer 1990, **65**: 292–296.

105 Espinal-Witter R, Servais EL, Klimstra DS, Lieberman MD, Yantiss RK. Localized intrapancreatic malignant mesothelioma: a rare entity that may be confused with other pancreatic neoplasms. Virchows Arch 2010, **456**: 455–461.

106 Eyden BP, Banik S, Harris M. Malignant epithelial mesothelioma of the peritoneum: observations on a problem case. Ultrastruct Pathol 1996, **20**: 337–344.

107 Goepel JR. Benign papillary mesothelioma of peritoneum. A histological, histochemical and ultrastructural study of six cases. Histopathology 1981, **5**: 21–30.

108 Goldblum J, Hart WR. Localized and diffuse mesotheliomas of the genital tract and peritoneum in women. A clinicopathologic study of nineteen true mesothelial neoplasms, other than adenomatoid tumors, multicystic mesotheliomas, and localized fibrous tumors. Am J Surg Pathol 1995, **19**: 1124–1137.

109 Hammar SP. Macroscopic, histologic, histochemical, immunohistochemical, and ultrastructural features of mesothelioma. Ultrastruct Pathol 2006, **30**: 3–17.

110 Hicks J. Biologic, cytogenetic, and molecular factors in mesothelial proliferations. Ultrastruct Pathol 2006, **30**: 19–30.

111 Kane MJ, Chahinian AP, Holland JF. Malignant mesothelioma in young adults. Cancer 1990, **65**: 1449–1455.

112 Kallianpur AR, Carstens PH, Liotta LA, Frey KP, Siegal GP. Immunoreactivity in malignant mesotheliomas with antibodies to basement membrane components and their receptors. Mod Pathol 1990, **3**: 11–18.

113 Kannerstein M, Churg J. Peritoneal mesothelioma. Hum Pathol 1977, **8**: 83–94.

114 Kannerstein M, Churg J, Magner D. Histochemistry in the diagnosis of malignant mesothelioma. Ann Clin Lab Sci 1973, **3**: 207–211.

115 Kauffman SL, Stout AP. Mesothelioma in children. Cancer 1964, **17**: 539–544.

116 Kerrigan SJA, Cagle P, Churg A. Malignant mesothelioma of the peritoneum presenting as an inflammatory lesion. Am J Surg Pathol 2003, **27**: 248–253.

117 Kerrigan SA, Turnnir RT, Clement PB, Young RH, Churg A. Diffuse malignant epithelial mesotheliomas of the peritoneum in women: a clinicopathologic study of 25 patients. Cancer 2002, **94**: 378–385.

118 Kimura N, Kimura I. Podoplanin as a marker for mesothelioma. Pathol Int 2005, **55**: 83–86.

119 King JA, Listinsky CM, Tucker JA. An intriguing case: malignant mesothelioma presenting as inguinal lymph node metastases. Ultrastruct Pathol 2004, **28**: 109–113.

120 King JE, Hasleton PS. Immunohistochemistry and the diagnosis of malignant mesothelioma [commentary]. Histopathology 2001, **38**: 471–476.

121 Kitazawa M, Kaneko H, Toshima M, Ishikawa H, Kobayashi H, Sekiya M. Malignant peritoneal mesothelioma with massive foamy cells. Codfish roe-like mesothelioma. Acta Pathol Jpn 1984, **34**: 687–692.

122 Klebe S, Brownlee NA, Mahar A, Burchette JL, Sporn TA, Vollmer RT, Roggli VL. Sarcomatoid mesothelioma: a clinical–pathologic correlation of 326 cases. Mod Pathol 2010, **23**: 470–479.

123 Kung ITM, Thallas V, Spencer EJ, Wilson SM. Expression of muscle actin in diffuse mesotheliomas. Hum Pathol 1995, **26**: 565–570.

124 Lantuejoul S, Laverriere MH, Sturm N, Moro D, Frey G, Brambilla C, Brambilla E. NCAM (neural cell adhesion molecules) expression in malignant mesothelioma. Hum Pathol 2000, **31**: 415–421.

125 Lederman GS, Recht A, Herman T, Osteen R, Corson J, Antman KH. Long-term survival in peritoneal mesothelioma. The role of radiotherapy and combined modality treatment. Cancer 1987, **59**: 1882–1886.

126 Leong A S-Y, Vernon-Roberts E. The immunohistochemistry of malignant mesothelioma. Pathol Annu 1994, **29**(Pt 2): 157–159.

127 Lerner HJ, Schoenfeld DA, Martin A, Falkson G, Borden E. Malignant mesothelioma. The Eastern Cooperative Oncology Group (ECOG) experience. Cancer 1983, **52**: 1981–1985.

128 Lloreta-Trull J. Extrathoracic mesothelial proliferations and their mimics. Ultrastruct Pathol 2006, **30**: 37–51.

129 Masangkay AV, Susin M, Baker R, Ward R, Kahn E. Metastatic malignant mesothelioma presenting as colonic polyps. Hum Pathol 1997, **28**: 993–995.

130 Maurer R, Egloff B. Malignant peritoneal mesothelioma after cholangiography with Thorotrast. Cancer 1975, **36**: 1381–1385.

131 Mayall FG, Goddard H, Gibbs AR. Intermediate filament expression in mesotheliomas. Leiomyoid mesotheliomas are not uncommon. Histopathology 1992, **21**: 453–457.

132 Moran CA, Albores-Saavedra J, Suster S. Primary peritoneal mesotheliomas in children: a clinicopathological and immunohistochemical study of eight cases. Histopathology 2008, **52**: 824–830.

133 Nascimento AG, Keeney GL, Fletcher CD. Deciduoid peritoneal mesothelioma. An unusual phenotype affecting young females. Am J Surg Pathol 1994, **18**: 439–445.

134 Nonaka D, Kusamura S, Baratti D, Casali P, Cabras AD, Younan R, Rosai J, Deraco M. Diffuse malignant mesothelioma of the peritoneum: a clinicopathological study of 35 patients treated locoregionally at a single institution. Cancer 2005, **104**: 2181–2188.

135 Ordóñez NG. Clear cell mesothelioma presenting as an incarcerated abdominal hernia. Virchows Arch 2005, **447**: 823–827.

136 Ordóñez NG. Mesothelioma with clear cell features: an ultrastructural and immunohistochemical study of 20 cases. Hum Pathol 2005, **36**: 465–473.

137 Ordóñez NG. D2-40 and podoplanin are highly specific and sensitive immunohistochemical markers of epithelioid malignant mesothelioma. Hum Pathol 2005, **36**: 372–380.

138 Ordóñez NG. Mesothelioma with rhabdoid features: an ultrastructural and immunohistochemical study of 10 cases. Mod Pathol 2006, **19**: 373–383.

139 Ordóñez NG. The diagnostic utility of immunohistochemistry in distinguishing between mesothelioma and renal cell carcinoma: a comparative study. Hum Pathol 2004, **35**: 697–710.

140 Ordóñez NG. Role of immunohistochemistry in distinguishing epithelial peritoneal mesotheliomas from peritoneal and ovarian serous carcinomas. Am J Surg Pathol 1998, **22**: 1203–1214.

141 Ordóñez NG. Epithelial mesothelioma with deciduoid features: report of four cases. Am J Surg Pathol 2000, **24**: 816–823.

142 Padgett DM, Cathro HP, Wick MR, Mills SE. Podoplanin is a better immunohistochemical marker for sarcomatoid mesothelioma than calretinin. Am J Surg Pathol 2008, **32**: 123–127.

143 Riddell RH, Goodman MJ, Moossa AR. Peritoneal malignant mesothelioma in a patient with recurrent peritonitis. Cancer 1981, **48**: 134–139.

144 Roggli VL, Sharma A, Butnor KJ, Sporn T, Vollmer RT. Malignant mesothelioma and occupational exposure to asbestos: A clinicopathological correlation of 1445 cases. Ultrastruct Pathol 2002, **26**: 55–65.

145 Shah IA, Somsin A, Wong SX, Gani OS, Chausow DD. Malignant mesothelioma presenting as colonic tumor. Hum Pathol 1998, **29**: 657.

146 Shanks JH, Harris M, Banerjee SS, Eyden BP, Joglekar VM, Nicol A, Hasleton PS, Nicholson AG. Mesotheliomas with deciduoid morphology: a morphologic spectrum and a variant not confined to young females. Am J Surg Pathol 2000, **24**: 285–294.

147 Shia J, Erlandson RA, Klimstra DS. Deciduoid mesothelioma: a report of 5 cases and literature review. Ultrastruct Pathol 2002, **26**: 355–363.

148 Shia J, Qin J, Erlandson RA, King R, Illei P, Nobrega J, Yao D, Klimstra DS. Malignant mesothelioma with a pronounced myxoid stroma: a clinical and pathological evaluation of 19 cases. Virchows Arch 2005, **447**: 828–834.

149 Silberstein MJ, Lewis JE, Blair JD, Graviss ER, Brodeur AE. Congenital peritoneal mesothelioma. J Pediatr Surg 1983, **18**: 243–246.

150 Strickler JG, Herndier BG, Rouse RV. Immunohistochemical staining in malignant mesotheliomas. Am J Clin Pathol 1987, **88**: 610–614.

151 Sussman J, Rosai J. Lymph node metastasis as the initial manifestation of malignant mesothelioma. Report of six cases. Am J Surg Pathol 1990, **14**: 819–828.

152 Suzuki Y. Diagnostic criteria for human diffuse malignant mesothelioma. Acta Pathol Jpn 1992, **42**: 767–786.

153 Suzuki Y, Churg J, Kannerstein M. Ultrastructure of human malignant diffuse mesothelioma. Am J Pathol 1976, **85**: 241–251.

154 Vogelzang NJ, Schultz SM, Iannucci AM, Kennedy BJ. Malignant mesothelioma. The University of Minnesota experience. Cancer 1984, **53**: 377–383.

155 Wick MR, Mills SE, Swanson PE. Expression of 'myelomonocytic' antigens in mesotheliomas and adenocarcinomas involving the serosal surfaces. Am J Clin Pathol 1990, **94**: 18–26.

156 Winslow DJ, Taylor HB. Malignant peritoneal mesotheliomas. Cancer 1960, **13**: 127–136.

INTRA-ABDOMINAL DESMOPLASTIC SMALL CELL TUMOR

157 Adsay V, Cheng J, Athanasian E, Gerald W, Rosai J. Primary desmoplastic small cell tumor of soft tissues and bone of the hand. Am J Surg Pathol 1999, **23**: 1408–1413.

158 Alaggio R, Rosolen A, Sartori F, Leszl A, d'Amore ES, Bisogno G, Carli M, Cecchetto G, Coffin CM, Ninfo V. Spindle cell tumor with EWS-WT1 transcript and a favorable clinical course: a variant of DSCT, a variant of leiomyosarcoma, or a new entity? Report of 2 pediatric cases. Am J Surg Pathol 2007, **31**: 454–459.

159 Amin KM, Litzky LA, Smythe WR, Mooney AM, Morris JM, Mews DJY, Pass HI, Kari C, Rodeck U, Rauscher FJ III, Kaiser LR, Albelda SM. Wilms' tumor 1 susceptibility (WT1) gene products are selectively expressed in malignant mesothelioma. Am J Pathol 1995, **146**: 344–356.

160 Antonescu CR, Gerald WL, Magid MS, Ladany M. Molecular variants of the EWS–WT1 gene fusion in desmoplastic small round cell tumor. Diagn Mol Pathol 1998, **7**: 24–28.

161 Argatoff LH, O'Connell JX, Mathers JA, Gilks CB, Sorensen PH. Detection for the EWS/WT1 gene fusion by reverse transcriptase-polymerase chain reaction in the diagnosis of intra-abdominal desmoplastic small round cell tumor. Am J Surg Pathol 1996, **20**: 406–412.

162 Backer A, Mount SL, Zarka MA, Trask CE, Allen EF, Gerald WL, Sanders DA, Weaver DL. Desmoplastic small round cell tumour of unknown primary origin with lymph node and lung metastases: histological, cytological, ultrastructural, cytogenetic and molecular findings. Virchows Arch 1998, **432**: 135–141.

163 Barnoud R, Sabourin JC, Pasquier D, Ranchere D, Bailly C, Terrier-Lacombe MJ, Pasquier B. Immunohistochemical expression of WT1 by

desmoplastic small round cell tumor: A comparative study with other small round cell tumors. Am J Surg Pathol 2000, **24**: 830–836.

164 Bismar TA, Basturk O, Gerald WL, Schwarz K, Adsay NV. Desmoplastic small cell tumor in the pancreas. Am J Surg Pathol 2004, **28**: 808–812.

165 Cao L, Ni J, Que R, Wu Z, Song Z. Desmoplastic small round cell tumor: a clinical, pathological, and immunohistochemical study of 18 Chinese cases. Int J Surg Pathol 2008, **16**: 257–262.

166 Chang F. Desmoplastic small round cell tumors: cytologic, histologic, and immunohistochemical features. Arch Pathol Lab Med 2006, **130**: 728–732.

167 Charles AK, Moore IE, Berry PJ. Immunohistochemical detection of the Wilms' tumour gene WT1 in desmoplastic small round cell tumour. Histopathology 1997, **30**: 312–314.

168 Crapanzano JP, Cardillo M, Lin O, Zakowski MF. Cytology of desmoplastic small round cell tumor. Cancer 2002, **96**: 21–32.

169 Cummings OW, Ulbright TM, Young RH, Dei Tos AP, Fletcher CDM, Hull MT. Desmoplastic small round cell tumors of the paratesticular region: a report of six cases. Am J Surg Pathol 1997, **21**: 219–225.

170 de Alava E, Ladanyi M, Rosai J, Gerald WL. Detection of chimeric transcripts in desmoplastic small round cell tumor and related developmental tumors by RT-PCR. A specific diagnostic assay. Am J Pathol 1995, **147**: 1584–1591.

171 Dorsey BV, Benjamin LE, Fauscher F, Klencke B, Venook AP, Warren RS, Weidner N. Intra-abdominal desmoplastic small round-cell tumor: expansion of the pathologic profile. Mod Pathol 1996, **9**: 703–709.

172 Fang X, Rodabaugh K, Penetrante R, Wong M, Wagner T, Sait S, Mhawech-Fauceglia P. Desmoplastic small round cell tumor (DSRCT) with ovarian involvement in 2 young women. Appl Immunohistochem Mol Morphol 2008, **16**: 94–99.

173 Gaudin PB, Rosai J. Florid vascular proliferation associated with neural and neuroendocrine neoplasms. A diagnostic clue and potential pitfall. Am J Surg Pathol 1995, **19**: 642–652.

174 Gerald WL, Miller HK, Battifora H, Miettinen M, Silva EG, Rosai J. Intra-abdominal desmoplastic small round-cell tumor. Report of 19 cases of a distinctive type of high-grade polyphenotypic malignancy affecting young individuals. Am J Surg Pathol 1991, **15**: 499–513.

175 Gerald WL, Rosai J, Ladanyi M. Characterization of the genomic breakpoint and chimeric transcripts in the EWS–WT1 gene fusion of desmoplastic small round cell tumor. Proc Natl Acad Sci USA 1995, **92**: 1028–1032.

176 Gil A, Gomez Portilla A, Brun EA, Sugarbaker PH. Clinical perspective on desmoplastic small round-cell tumor. Oncology 2004, **67**: 231–242.

177 Hassan I, Shyyan R, Donohue JH, Edmonson JH, Gunderson LL, Moir CR, Arndt CA, Nascimento AG, Que FG. Intraabdominal desmoplastic small round cell tumors: a diagnostic and therapeutic challenge. Cancer 2005, **104**: 1264–1270.

178 Hill DA, Pfeifer JD, Marley EF, Dehner LP, Humphrey PA, Zhu X, Swanson PE. WT1 staining reliably differentiates desmoplastic small round cell tumor from Ewing sarcoma/ primitive neuroectodermal tumor. An immunohistochemical and molecular diagnostic study. Am J Clin Pathol 2000, **114**: 345–353.

179 Katz RL, Quezado M, Senderowicz AM, Villalba L, Laskin WB, Tsokos M. An intra-abdominal small round cell neoplasm with features of primitive neuroectodermal and desmoplastic round cell tumor and a EWS/ FLI-1 fusion transcript. Hum Pathol 1997, **28**: 502–509.

180 Kawano N, Inayama Y, Nagashima Y, Miyagi Y, Uemura H, Saitoh K, Kubota Y, Hosaka M, Tanaka Y, Nakatani Y. Desmoplastic small round-cell tumor of the paratesticular region: Report of an adult case with demonstration of EWS and WT1 gene fusion using paraffin-embedded tissue. Mod Pathol 1999, **12**: 729–734.

181 Kushner BH, LaQuaglia MP, Wollner N, Meyers PA, Lindsley KL, Ghavimi F, Merchant TE, Boulad F, Cheung NV, Bonilla MA, Crouch G, Felleher JF Jr, Steinherz PG, Gerald WL. Desmoplastic small round-cell tumor: Prolonged progression-free survival with aggressive multimodality therapy. J Clin Oncol 1996, **14**: 1526–1531.

182 Lae ME, Roche PC, Jin L, Lloyd RV, Nascimento AG. Desmoplastic small round cell tumor: A clinicopathologic, immunohistochemical, and molecular study of 32 tumors. Am J Surg Pathol 2002, **26**: 823–835.

183 McCluggage WG. WT-1 immunohistochemical expression in small round blue cell tumours. Histopathology 2008, **52**: 631–632.

184 Murphy AJ, Bishop K, Pereira C, Chilton-MacNeill S, Ho M, Zielenska M, Thorner PS. A new molecular variant of desmoplastic small round cell tumor: significance of WT1 immunostaining in this entity. Hum Pathol 2008, **39**: 1763–1770.

185 Oshima Y, Kawaguchi S, Nagoya S, Wada T, Kokai Y, Ikeda T, Nogami S, Oya T, Hirayama Y. Abdominal small round cell tumor with osteoid and EWS/FLI1. Hum Pathol 2004, **35**: 773–775.

186 Pasquinelli G, Montanaro L, Martinelli GN. Desmoplastic small round-cell tumor: a case report on the large cell variant with immunohistochemical, ultrastructural and molecular genetic analysis. Ultrastruct Pathol 2000, **24**: 333–337.

187 Ordi J, de Alava E, Torne A, Mellado B, Pardo-Mindan J, Iglesias X, Cardesa A. Intra-abdominal desmoplastic small round cell tumor with EWS/ERG fusion transcript. Am J Surg Pathol 1998, **22**: 1026–1032.

188 Ordóñez NG. Desmoplastic small round cell tumor: I: A histopathologic study of 39 cases with emphasis on unusual histological patterns. Am J Surg Pathol 1998, **22**: 1303–1313.

189 Ordóñez NG. Desmoplastic small round cell tumor: II: An ultrastructural and immunohistochemical study with emphasis on new immunohistochemical markers. Am J Surg Pathol 1998, **22**: 1314–1327.

190 Ordóñez NG, Sahin AA. CA 125 production in desmoplastic small round cell tumor: Report of a case with elevated serum levels and prominent signet ring morphology. Hum Pathol 1998, **29**: 294–299.

191 Ordóñez NG, el-Naggar AK, Ro JY, Silva EG, Mackay B. Intra-abdominal desmoplastic small cell tumor. A light microscopic, immunocytochemical, ultrastructural, and flow cytometric study. Hum Pathol 1993, **24**: 850–865.

192 Parkash V, Gerald WL, Parma A, Miettinen M, Rosai J. Desmoplastic small round cell tumor of the pleura. Am J Surg Pathol 1995, **19**: 659–665.

193 Perez RP, Zhang PJ. Detection of EWS–WT1 fusion mRNA in ascites of a patient with desmoplastic small round cell tumor by RT-PCR. Hum Pathol 1999, **30**: 239–242.

194 Rodriguez E, Sreekantaiah C, Gerald W, Reuter VE, Motzer RJ, Chaganti RS. A recurring translocation, t(11;22)(p13;q11.2), characterizes intra-abdominal desmoplastic small round-cell tumors. Cancer Genet Cytogenet 1993, **69**: 17–21.

195 Sandberg AA, Bridge JA. Updates on the cytogenetics and molecular genetics of bone soft tissue tumors. Desmoplastic small round-cell tumors. Cancer Genet Cytogenet 2002, **138**: 1–10.

196 Shintaku M, Baba Y, Fujiwara T. Intra-abdominal desmoplastic small cell tumour in a patient with Peutz-Jeghers syndrome. Virchows Arch 1994, **425**: 211–215.

197 Tison V, Cerasoli S, Morigi F, Ladanyi M, Gerald WL, Rosai J. Intracranial desmoplastic small cell tumor. Report of a case. Am J Surg Pathol 1996, **20**: 112–117.

198 Trupiano JK, Machen SK, Barr FG, Goldblum JR. Cytokeratin-negative desmoplastic small round cell tumor: A report of two cases emphasizing the utility of reverse transcriptase-polymerase chain reaction. Mod Pathol 1999, **12**: 849–853.

199 Wang LL, Perlman EJ, Vujanic GM, Zuppan C, Brundler MA, Cheung CR, Calicchio ML, Dubois S, Cendron M, Murata-Collins JL, Wenger GD, Strzelecki D, Barr FG, Collins T, Perez-Atayde AR, Kozakewich H. Desmoplastic small round cell tumor of the kidney in childhood. Am J Surg Pathol 2007, **31**: 576–584.

200 Wills EJ. Peritoneal desmoplastic small round cell tumors with divergent differentiation. A review. Ultrastruct Pathol 1993, **17**: 295–306.

201 Wolf AN, Ladanyi M, Paull G, Blaugrund JE, Westra WH. The expanding clinical spectrum of desmoplastic small round-cell tumor: a report of two cases with molecular confirmation. Hum Pathol 1999, **30**: 430–435.

202 Young RH, Eichhorn JH, Dickersin GR, Scully RE. Ovarian involvement by the intra-abdominal desmoplastic small round cell tumor with divergent differentiation. A report of three cases. Hum Pathol 1992, **23**: 454–464.

203 Zhang PJ, Goldblum JR, Pawel BR, Fisher C, Pasha TL, Barr FG. Immunophenotype of desmoplastic small round cell tumors as detected in cases with EWS-WT1 gene fusion product. Mod Pathol 2003, **16**: 229–235.

204 Zhang PJ, Goldblum JR, Pawel BR, Pasha TL, Fisher C, Barr FG. PDGF-A, PDGF-Rbeta, TGFbeta3 and bone morphogenic protein-4 in desmoplastic small round cell tumors with EWS-WT1 gene fusion product and their role in stromal desmoplasia: an immunohistochemical study. Mod Pathol 2005, **18**: 382–387.

OTHER PRIMARY TUMORS

205 Attanoos RL, Dallimore NS, Gibbs AR. Primary epithelioid haemangioendothelioma of the peritoneum: an unusual mimic of diffuse malignant mesothelioma. Histopathology 1997, **30**: 375–377.

206 Bonetti F, Martignoni G, Manfrin E, Colato C, Gambacorta M, Faleri M, Bacchi C, Sin VC, Wong NL, Coady M, Chan JKC. Abdominopelvic sarcoma of perivascular epithelioid cells. Report of four cases in young women, one with tuberous sclerosis. Mod Pathol 2001, **14**: 563–568.

207 Cheuk W, Chan JK, Shek TW, Chang JH, Tsou MH, Yuen NW, Ng WF, Chan AC, Prat J. Inflammatory pseudotumor-like follicular dendritic cell tumor: a distinctive low-grade malignant intra-abdominal neoplasm with consistent Epstein–Barr virus association. Am J Surg Pathol 2001, **25**: 721–731.

208 Fisher C, Folpe AL, Hashimoto H, Weiss SW. Intra-abdominal synovial sarcoma: a clinicopathological study. Histopathology 2004, **45**: 245–253.

209 Fukunaga M, Naganuma H, Ushigome S, Endo Y, Ishikawa E. Malignant solitary fibrous tumour of the peritoneum. Histopathology 1996, **28**: 463–466.

210 Gonzalez-Crussi F, Sotelo-Avila C, de Mello DE. Primary peritoneal, omental, and mesenteric tumors in childhood. Semin Diagn Pathol 1986, **3**: 122–137.

211 Goodlad JR, Fletcher CD. Solitary fibrous tumour arising at unusual sites. Analysis of a series. Histopathology 1991, **19**: 515–522.

212 Gronchi A, Diment J, Colecchia M, Fiore M, Santinami M. Atypical pleomorphic epithelioid angiomyolipoma localized to the pelvis: a case report and review of the literature. Histopathology 2004, **44**: 292–295.

213 Hornick JL, Fletcher CD. Intraabdominal cystic lymphangiomas obscured by marked superimposed reactive changes: clinicopathological analysis of a series. Hum Pathol 2005, **36**: 426–432.

214 Kashima T, Matshushita H, Kuroda M, Takeuchi H, Udagawa H, Ishida T, Hara M, Machinami R. Biphasic synovial sarcoma of the peritoneal cavity with t(X:18) demonstrated by reverse transcriptase polymerase chain reaction. Pathol Int 1997, **47**: 637–641.

215 Lin BT, Chen YY, Battifora H, Weiss LM. Absence of Kaposi's sarcoma-associated herpesvirus-like DNA sequences in malignant vascular tumors of the serous membranes. Mod Pathol 1996, **9**: 1143–1146.

216 Lin BT, Colby T, Gown AM, Hammar SP, Mertens RB, Churg A, Battifora H. Malignant vascular tumors of the serous membranes mimicking mesothelioma: a report of 14 cases. Am J Surg Pathol 1996, **20**: 1431–1439.

217 Low SE, Menasce LP, Manson CM. Follicular dendritic cell sarcoma: a rare tumor presenting as an abdominal mass. Int J Surg Pathol 2007, **15**: 315–317.

218 McCaughey WTE, Dardick I, Barr JR. Angiosarcoma of serous membranes. Arch Pathol Lab Med 1983, **107**: 304–307.

219 Posligua L, Anatelli F, Dehner LP, Pfeifer JD. Primary peritoneal epithelioid hemangioendothelioma. Int J Surg Pathol 2006, **14**: 257–267.

220 Salviato T, Altavilla G, Busatto G, Pizzolitto S, Falconieri G. Diffuse intra-abdominal clear cell myomelanocytic tumor: report of an unusual presentation of 'PEComatosis' simulating peritoneal mesothelioma. Ann Diagn Pathol 2006, **10**: 352–356.

221 Shek TW, Liu CL, Peh WC, Fan ST, Ng IO. Intra-abdominal follicular dendritic cell tumour: a rare tumour in need of recognition. Histopathology 1998, **33**: 465–470.

222 Young RH, Clement PB, McCaughey WT. Solitary fibrous tumors ('fibrous mesotheliomas') of the peritoneum. A report of three cases and a review of the literature. Arch Pathol Lab Med 1990, **114**: 493–495.

LESIONS OF THE SECONDARY MÜLLERIAN SYSTEM

223 Bell DA, Scully RE. Benign and borderline serous lesions of the peritoneum in women. Pathol Annu 1989, **24**(Pt 2): 1–21.

224 Butnor KJ, Burchette JL, Robboy SJ. Progesterone receptor activity in leiomyomatosis peritonealis disseminata. Int J Gynecol Pathol 1999, **18**: 259–264.

225 Buttner A, Bassler R, Theele C. Pregnancy-associated ectopic decidua (deciduosis) of the greater omentum. An analysis of 60 biopsies with cases of fibrosing deciduosis and leiomyomatosis peritonealis disseminata. Pathol Res Pract 1993, **189**: 352–359.

226 Chang KL, Crabtree GS, Lim-Tan SK, Kempson RL, Hendrickson MR. Primary extrauterine endometrial stromal neoplasms. A clinicopathologic study of 20 cases and a review of the literature. Int J Gynecol Pathol 1993, **12**: 282–296.

227 Clement PB, Young RH, Scully RE. Nontrophoblastic pathology of the female genital tract and peritoneum associated with pregnancy. Semin Diagn Pathol 1989, **6**: 372–406.

228 Cokelaere K, Michielsen P, De Vos R, Sciot R. Primary mesenteric malignant mixed mesodermal (mullerian) tumor with neuroendocrine differentiation. Mod Pathol 2001, **14**: 515–520.

229 Dalrymple JC, Bannatyne P, Russell P, Solomon HJ, Tattersall MH, Atkinson K, Carter J, Duval P, Elliott P, Friedlander M, et al. Extraovarian peritoneal serous papillary carcinoma. A clinicopathologic study of 31 cases. Cancer 1989, **64**: 110–115.

230 Dincer AD, Timmins P, Pietrocola D, Fisher H, Ambros RA. Primary peritoneal mullerian adenosarcoma with sarcomatous overgrowth associated with endometriosis: a case report. Int J Gynecol Pathol 2002, **21**: 65–68.

231 Due W, Pickartz H. Immunohistologic detection of estrogen and progesterone receptors in disseminated peritoneal leiomyomatosis. Int J Gynecol Pathol 1989, **8**: 46–53.

232 Fox H. Primary neoplasia of the female peritoneum. Histopathology 1993, **23**: 103–110.

233 Fromm GL, Gershenson DM, Silva EG. Papillary serous carcinoma of the peritoneum. Obstet Gynecol 1990, **75**: 89–95.

234 Garamvoelgyi E, Guillou L, Gebhard S, Salmeron M, Seematter RJ, Hadji MH. Primary malignant mixed Müllerian tumor (metaplastic carcinoma) of the female peritoneum. A clinical, pathologic, and immunohistochemical study of three cases and a review of the literature. Cancer 1994, **74**: 854–863.

235 Gu J, Roth LM, Younger C, Michael H, Abdul-Karim FW, Zhang S, Ulbright TM, Eble JN, Cheng L. Molecular evidence for the independent origin of extra-ovarian papillary serious tumors of low malignant potential. J Nat Cancer Inst 2001, **93**: 1147–1152.

236 Halperin R, Zehavi S, Hadas E, Habler L, Bukovsky I, Schneider D. Immunohistochemical comparison of primary peritoneal and primary ovarian serious papillary carcinoma. Int J Gynecol Pathol 2001, **20**: 341–345.

237 Hutton RL, Dalton SR. Primary peritoneal serous borderline tumors. Arch Pathol Lab Med 2007, **131**: 138–144.

238 Lauchlan SC. The secondary müllerian system revisited. Int J Gynecol Pathol 1994, **13**: 73–79.

239 Ma KF, Chow LT. Sex cord-like pattern leiomyomatosis peritonealis disseminata. A hitherto undescribed feature. Histopathology 1992, **21**: 389–391.

240 Quade BJ, McLachlin CM, Soto-Wright V, Zuckerman J, Mutter GL, Morton CC. Disseminated peritoneal leiomyomatosis. Clonality analysis by X chromosome inactivation and cytogenetics of a clinically benign smooth muscle proliferation. Am J Pathol 1997, **150**: 2153–2166.

241 Shen D-H, Khoo US, Xue WC, Ngan HY, Wang JL, Liu VW, Chan YK, Cheung AN. Primary peritoneal malignant mixed mullerian tumors: a clinicopathologic, immunohistochemical, and genetic study. Cancer 2001, **91**: 1052–1060.

242 Tauber H-D, Wissner SE, Haskins AL. Leiomyomatosis peritonealis disseminata. An unusual complication of genital leiomyomata. Obstet Gynecol 1965, **25**: 561–574.

243 Thor AD, Young RH, Clement PB. Pathology of the fallopian tube, broad ligament, peritoneum, and pelvic soft tissues. Hum Pathol 1991, **22**: 856–867.

244 Weir MM, Bell DA, Young RH. Grade 1 peritoneal serous carcinomas: A report of 14 cases and comparison with 7 peritoneal serous psammocarcinomas and 19 peritoneal serous borderline tumors. Am J Surg Pathol 1998, **22**: 849–862.

245 Zotalis G, Nayar R, Hicks DG. Leiomyomatosis peritonealis disseminata, endometriosis, and multicystic mesothelioma: an unusual association. Int J Gynecol Pathol 1998, **17**: 178–182.

METASTATIC TUMORS

246 Bradley RF, Geisinger KR. Carcinoma by any other name: pseudomyxoma peritonei is not best viewed with an ovarian perspective. Am J Surg Pathol 2006, **30**: 1484–1485.

247 Bradley RF, Stewart JH 4th, Russell GB, Levine EA, Geisinger KR. Pseudomyxoma peritonei of appendiceal origin: a clinicopathologic analysis of 101 patients uniformly treated at a single institution, with literature review. Am J Surg Pathol 2006, **30**: 551–559.

248 Cariker M, Dockerty M. Mucinous cystadenomas and mucinous cystadenocarcinomas of the ovary. A clinical and pathological study of 355 cases. Cancer 1954, **7**: 302–310.

249 Chu DZ, Lang NP, Thompson C, Osteen PK, Westbrook KC. Peritoneal carcinomatosis in nongynecologic malignancy. A prospective study of prognostic factors. Cancer 1989, **63**: 364–367.

250 Dadmanesh F, Miller DM, Swenerton KD, Clement PB. Gliomatosis peritonei with malignant transformation. Mod Pathol 1997, **10**: 597–601.

251 Du Plessis DG, Louw JA, Wranz PA. Mucinous epithelial cysts of the spleen associated with pseudomyxoma peritonei. Histopathology 1999, **35**: 551–557.

252 Geisinger KR, Levine EA, Shen P, Bradley RF. Pleuropulmonary involvement in pseudomyxoma peritonei: morphologic assessment and literature review. Am J Clin Pathol 2007, **127**: 135–143.

253 Harms D, Janig U, Gobel U. Gliomatosis peritonei in childhood and adolescence. Pathol Res Pract 1989, **184**: 422–430.

254 Higa E, Rosai J, Pizzimbono CA, Wise L. Mucosal hyperplasia, mucinous cystadenoma and mucinous cystadenocarcinoma of appendix. A re-evaluation of appendiceal 'mucocele'. Cancer 1973, **32**: 1325–1341.

255 Jackson SL, Fleming RA, Loggie BW, Geisinger KR. Gelatinous ascites: A cytohistologic study

of pseudomyxoma peritonei in 67 patients. Mod Pathol 2001, **14**: 664–671.

256 Kahn MA, Demopoulos RI. Mucinous ovarian tumors with pseudomyxoma peritonei. A clinicopathological study. Int J Gynecol Pathol 1992, **11**: 15–23.

257 Kwan MY, Kalle W, Lau GT, Chan JK. Is gliomatosis peritonei derived from the associated ovarian teratoma? Hum Pathol 2004, **35**: 685–688.

258 Lee KR, Scully RE. Mucinous tumors of the ovary: a clinicopathologic study of 196 borderline tumors (of intestinal type) and carcinomas, including an evaluation of 11 cases with 'pseudomyxoma peritonei'. Am J Surg Pathol 2000, **24**: 1447–1464.

259 Nonaka D, Kusamura S, Baratti D, Casali P, Younan R, Deraco M. CDX-2 expression in pseudomyxoma peritonei: a clinicopathological study of 42 cases. Histopathology 2006, **49**: 381–387.

260 O'Connell JT, Hacker CM, Barsky SH. MUC2 is a molecular marker for pseudomyxoma peritonei. Mod Pathol 2002, **15**: 958–972.

261 Prayson RA, Hart WR, Petras RE. Pseudomyxoma peritonei. A clinicopathologic study of 19 cases with emphasis on site of origin and nature of associated ovarian tumors. Am J Surg Pathol 1994, **18**: 591–603.

262 Ronnett BM, Kurman RJ, Zahn CM, Schmookler BM, Jablonski KA, Kass ME, Sugarbaker PH. Pseudomyxoma peritoneum in women. A clinicopathologic analysis of 30 cases with emphasis on site of origin, prognosis, and relationship to ovarian mucinous tumors of low malignant potential. Hum Pathol 1995, **26**: 509–524.

263 Ronnett BM, Yan H, Kurman RJ, Shmookler BM, Wu L, Sugarbaker PH. Patients with pseudomyxoma peritonei associated with disseminated peritoneal adenomucinosis have a significantly more favorable prognosis than patients with peritoneal mucinous carcinomatosis. Cancer 2001, **92**: 85–91.

264 Ronnett BM. Pseudomyxoma peritonei: a rose by any other name. Am J Surg Pathol 2006, **30**: 1483–1484.

265 Sadeghi B, Arvieux C, Glehen O, Beaujard AC, Rivoire M, Baulieux J, Fontaumard E, Brachet A, Caillot JL, Faure JL, Porcheron J, Peix JL, Francois Y, Vignal J, Gilly FN. Peritoneal carcinomatosis from non-gynecologic malignancies: Results of the EVOCAPE 1 multicentric prospective study. Cancer 2000, **88**: 358–363.

266 Shah IA, Salvatore JR, Kummet T, Gani OS, Wheeler LA. Pseudomesotheliomatous carcinoma involving pleura and peritoneum: a clinicopathologic and immunohistochemical study of three cases. Ann Diagn Pathol 1999, **3**: 148–159.

267 Shin HJ, Sneige N. Epithelial cells and other cytologic features of pseudomyxoma peritonei in patients with ovarian and/or appendiceal mucinous neoplasms. A study of 12 patients including 5 men. Cancer 2000, **90**: 17–23.

268 Smith JW, Kemeny N, Caldwell C, Banner P, Sigurdson E, Huvos A. Pseudomyxoma peritonei of appendiceal origin. The Memorial Sloan-Kettering Cancer Center experience. Cancer 1992, **70**: 396–401.

269 Soslow RA, Pirog E, Isacson C. Endometrial intraepithelial carcinoma with associated peritoneal carcinomatosis. Am J Surg Pathol 2000, **24**: 726–732.

270 Sugarbaker PH. Cytoreduction including total gastrectomy for pseudomyxoma peritonei. Br J Surg 2002, **89**: 208–212.

271 Sugarbaker PH, Chang D. Results of treatment of 385 patients with peritoneal surface spread of appendiceal malignancy. Ann Surg Oncol 1999, **6**: 727–731.

272 Sugarbaker PH, Yan H, Shmookler B. Pedunculated peritoneal surface polyps in pseudomyxoma peritonei syndrome. Histopathology 2001, **39**: 525–528.

273 Tarin D, Price JE, Kettlewell MGW, Souter RG, Vass ACR, Crossley B. Mechanisms of human tumor metastasis studied in patients with peritoneovenous shunts. Cancer Res 1984, **44**: 3584–3592.

274 Tran TA, Jennings TA, Ross JS, Nazeer T. Pseudomyxoma ovariilike posttherapeutic alteration in prostatic adenocarcinoma: a distinctive pattern in patients receiving neoadjuvant androgen ablation therapy. Am J Surg Pathol 1998, **22**: 347–354.

275 Yan H, Pestieau SR, Shmookler BM, Sugarbaker PH. Histopathologic analysis in 46 patients with pseudomyxoma peritonei syndrome: failure versus success with a second-look operation. Mod Pathol 2001, **14**: 164–171.

276 Young RH, Gilks CB, Scully RE. Mucinous tumors of the appendix associated with mucinous tumors of the ovary and pseudomyxoma peritonei. A clinicopathological analysis of 22 cases supporting an origin in the appendix. Am J Surg Pathol 1991, **15**: 415–429.

277 Young RH. Pseudomyxoma peritonei and selected other aspects of the spread of appendiceal neoplasms. Semin Diagn Pathol 2004, **21**: 134–150.

CYTOLOGY

278 Cardozo PL. A critical evaluation of 3,000 cytologic analyses of pleural fluid, ascitic fluid and pericardial fluid. Acta Cytol (Baltimore) 1966, **10**: 455–460.

279 Benevolo M, Mariani L, Vocaturo G, Vasselli S, Natali PG, Mottolese M. Independent prognostic value of peritoneal immunocytodiagnosis in endometrial carcinoma. Am J Surg Pathol 2000, **24**: 241–247.

280 Chen LM, Lazcano O, Katzmann JA, Kimlinger TK, Li C-Y. The role of conventional cytology, immunocytochemistry, and flow cytometric DNA ploidy in the evaluation of body cavity fluids. A prospective study of 52 patients. Am J Clin Pathol 1998, **109**: 712–721.

281 Esteban JM, Yokota S, Husain S, Battifora H. Immunocytochemical profile of benign and carcinomatous effusions. A practical approach to difficult diagnosis. Am J Clin Pathol 1990, **94**: 698–705.

282 Hecht JL, Lee BH, Pinkus JL, Pinkus GS. The value of Wilms tumor susceptibility gene 1 in cytological preparations as a marker for malignant mesothelioma. Cancer Cytopathol 2002, **96**: 105–109.

283 Jackson SL, Fleming RA, Loggie BW, Geisinger KR. Gelatinous ascites: a cytohistologic study of pseudomyxoma peritonei in 67 patients. Mod Pathol 2001, **14**: 664–671.

284 Melamed MR. The cytological presentation of malignant lymphomas and related diseases in effusions. Cancer 1963, **16**: 413–431.

285 Nance KV, Silverman JF. Immunocytochemical panel for the identification of malignant cells in serous effusions. Am J Clin Pathol 1991, **95**: 867–874.

286 Roberts HG, Campbell GM. Exfoliative cytology of diffuse mesothelioma. J Clin Pathol 1972, **23**: 577–582.

287 Ruitenbeek T, Gouw AS, Poppema S. Immunocytology of body cavity fluids. MOC-31, a monoclonal antibody discriminating between mesothelial and epithelial cells. Arch Pathol Lab Med 1994, **118**: 265–269.

OMENTUM

288 Alaggio R, Leszl A, d'Amore ESG, Chou PM. Omental fibromyxoid tumor (OFT): a distinctive variant of inflammatory myofibroblastic tumor? A clinicopathologic and immunophenotypic variant. Lab Invest 2009, **89**(Suppl 1): 345A.

289 Chong PY, Panabokke RG, Chew KH. Omental cryptococcoma. An unusual presentation of cryptococcosis. Arch Pathol Lab Med 1986, **110**: 239–241.

290 Dixon AY, Reed JS, Dow N, Lee SH. Primary omental leiomyosarcoma masquerading as hemorrhagic ascites. Hum Pathol 1984, **15**: 233–237.

291 Epstein LI, Lempke RE. Primary idiopathic segmental infarction of the greater omentum. Case report and collective review of the literature. Ann Surg 1968, **167**: 437–443.

292 Galifer RB, Pous JG, Juskiewenski S, Pasquie M, Gaubert J. Intra-abdominal cystic lymphangiomas in childhood. Prog Pediatr Surg 1978, **11**: 173–239.

293 Gonzalez-Crussi F, de Mello DE, Sotelo-Avila C. Omental-mesenteric myxoid hamartomas. Infantile lesions simulating malignant tumors. Am J Surg Pathol 1983, **7**: 567–578.

294 Gonzalez-Crussi F, Sotelo-Avila C, de Mello DE. Primary peritoneal, omental, and mesenteric tumors in childhood. Semin Diagn Pathol 1986, **3**: 122–137.

295 Miettinen M, Sobin LH, Lasota J. Gastrointestinal stromal tumors presenting as omental masses – a clinicopathologic analysis of 95 cases. Am J Surg Pathol 2009, **33**: 1267–1275.

296 Ordóñez NG, Manning JT Jr, Ayala AG. Teratoma of the omentum. Cancer 1983, **51**: 955–958.

297 Quddus MR, Sung CJ, Lauchlan SC. Benign and malignant serous and endometrioid epithelium in the omentum. Gynecol Oncol 2000, **75**: 227–232.

298 Stout AP, Hendry J, Purdie FJ. Primary solid tumors of the great omentum. Cancer 1963, **16**: 231–243.

299 Tsutsumi A, Kawabata K, Taguchi K, Doi K. Elastofibroma of the greater omentum. Acta Pathol Jpn 1985, **35**: 233–241.

300 Yamakawa M, Andoh A, Masuda A, Miyauchi S, Kasajima T, Ohmori A, Oguma T, T'akasaki K. Follicular dendritic cell sarcoma of the omentum. Virchows Arch 2002, **440**: 660–663.

MESENTERY

301 Al-Nafussi A, Wong NACS. Intra-abdominal spindle cell lesions: a review and practical aids to diagnosis. Histopathology 2001, **38**: 387–402.

302 Bak M. Nodular intra-abdominal panniculitis: an accompaniment of colorectal carcinoma and diverticular disease. Histopathology 1996, **29**: 21–27.

303 Banerjee R, Gough J. Cystic mucinous tumours of the mesentery and retroperitoneum. Report of three cases. Histopathology 1988, **12**: 527–532.

304 Barnardo DE, Stavrou M, Bourne R, Bogomoletz W. Primary carcinoid tumor of the mesentery. Hum Pathol 1984, **15**: 796–798.

305 Buonanno G, Gonella F, Pettinato G, Castaldo C. Autoimmune hemolytic anemia and dermoid cyst of the mesentery. A case report. Cancer 1984, **54**: 2533–2536.

306 Burke AP, Sobin LH, Shekitka KM. Mesenteric fibromatosis. A follow-up study. Arch Pathol Lab Med 1990, **114**: 832–835.

307 Burke AP, Sobin LH, Shekitka KM, Federspiel BH, Helwig EB. Intra-abdominal fibromatosis. A pathologic analysis of 130 tumors with comparison of clinical subgroups. Am J Surg Pathol 1990, **14**: 335–341.

308 Carpenter HA, Lancaster JR, Lee RA. Multilocular cysts of the peritoneum. Mayo Clin Proc 1982, **57**: 634–638.

309 Castellvi J, Lloreta J, Huguet P, Plaza JA, Ramon y Cajal S. A meningiomatous perineurial tumour located in the mesentery. An ultrastructural and immunohistochemical study. Histopathology 2006, **48**: 311–312.

310 Chen TS, Montgomery EA. Are tumefactive lesions classified as sclerosing mesenteritis a subset of IgG4-related sclerosing disorders? J Clin Pathol 2008, **61**: 1093–1097.

311 Chen KTK. Intraabdominal calcifying fibrous pseudotumor. Int J Surg Pathol 1996, **4**: 9–12.

312 Coffin CM, Watterson J, Priest JR, Dehner LP. Extrapulmonary inflammatory myofibroblastic tumor (inflammatory pseudotumor). A clinicopathologic and immunohistochemical study of 84 cases. Am J Surg Pathol 1995, **19**: 859–872.

313 Emory TS, Mohihan JM, Carr NJ, Sobin LH. Sclerosing mesenteritis, mesenteric panniculitis and mesenteric lipodystrophy: a single entity? Am J Surg Pathol 1997, **21**: 392–398.

314 Gorlin RJ, Sedano HO. The multiple nevoid basal cell carcinoma syndrome revisited. Birth Defects 1971, **7**: 140–148.

315 Hansen RC, Castelino RA, Lazerson J, Probert J. Mesenteric hemangioendothelioma with thrombocytopenia. Cancer 1973, **32**: 136–141.

316 Harpaz N, Gellman E. Urogenital mesenteric cyst with fallopian tubal features. Arch Pathol Lab Med 1987, **111**: 78–80.

317 Hashimoto H, Tsuneyoshi M, Enjoji M. Malignant smooth muscle tumors of the retroperitoneum and mesentery. A clinicopathologic analysis of 44 cases. J Surg Oncol 1985, **28**: 177–186.

318 Hill KA, Gonzalez-Crussi F, Chou PM. Calcifying fibrous pseudotumor versus inflammatory myofibroblastic tumor: a histological and immunohistochemical comparison. Mod Pathol 2001, **14**: 784–790.

319 Horie Y, Kato M. Uterus-like mass of the small bowel mesentery. Pathol Int 2000, **50**: 76–80.

320 Jones MA, Clement PB, Young RH. Primary yolk sac tumors of the mesentery. A report of two cases. Am J Clin Pathol 1994, **101**: 42–47.

321 Kelly JK, Hwang WS. Idiopathic retractile (sclerosing) mesenteritis and its differential diagnosis. Am J Surg Pathol 1989, **13**: 513–521.

322 Kipfer RE, Moertel CG, Dahlin DC. Mesenteric lipodystrophy. Ann Intern Med 1974, **80**: 582–588.

323 Klaus A, Margreiter R, Pernthaler H, Klima G, Offner FA. Diffuse mesenterial sclerosis: a characteristic feature of chronic small-bowel allograft rejection. Virchows Arch 2003, **442**: 48–55.

324 Kocova L, Michal M, Sulc M, Zamecnik M. Calcifying fibrous pseudotumor of visceral peritoneum. Histopathology 1997, **31**: 182–184.

325 Kurtz RJ, Heimann TM, Holt J, Beck AR. Mesenteric and retroperitoneal cysts. Ann Surg 1986, **203**: 109–112.

326 Lamovec J, Bracko M. Infiltrating cavernous lymphangiomyoma of the mesentery: a case report. Int J Surg Pathol 1996, **3**: 275–282.

327 Lee J, Song SY, Park CS, Kim B. Mullerian cysts of the mesentery and retroperitoneum: a case report and literature review. Pathol Int 1998, **48**: 902–906.

328 Magid D, Fishman EK, Jones B, Hoover HC, Feinstein R, Siegelman SS. Desmoid tumors in Gardner syndrome. Use of computed tomography. AJR 1984, **142**: 1141–1145.

329 Mahle C, Schwartz M, Popek E, Bocklage T. Intra-abdominal lymphangiomas in children and adults: assessment of proliferative activity. Arch Pathol Lab Med 1997, **121**: 1055–1062.

330 Meis JM, Enzinger FM. Inflammatory fibrosarcoma of the mesentery and retroperitoneum. A tumor closely simulating inflammatory pseudotumor. Am J Surg Pathol 1991, **15**: 1146–1156.

331 Monihan JM, Carr NJ, Sobin LH. CD34 immunoexpression in stromal tumours of the gastrointestinal tract and in mesenteric fibromatoses. Histopathology 1994, **25**: 469–474.

332 Montgomery E, Torbenson MS, Kaushal M, Fisher C, Ahraham SC. β-Catenin immunohistochemistry separates mesenteric fibromatosis from gastrointestinal stromal tumor and sclerosing mesenteritis. Am J Surg Pathol 2002, **26**: 1296–1301.

333 Moriki T, Takahashi T, Wada M, Ueda S, Ichien M, Yamane T, Hara H. Follicular dendritic cell tumor of the mesentery. Pathol Res Pract 1997, **193**: 629–639.

334 Nascimento AF, Ruiz R, Hornick JL, Fletcher CDM. Calcifying fibrous 'pseudotumor': clinicopathologic study of 15 cases and analysis of its relationship to inflammatory myofibroblastic tumor. Int J Surg Pathol 2002, **10**: 189–196.

335 Neerhout RC, Larson W, Mansur P. Mesenteric lymphoid hamartoma associated with chronic hypoferremia, anemia, growth failure and hypoglobulinemia. N Engl J Med 1969, **280**: 922–925.

336 Nonaka D, Birbe R, Rosai J. So-called inflammatory myofibroblastic tumour: a proliferative lesion of fibroblastic reticulum cells? Histopathology 2005, **46**: 604–613.

337 Ogden WM, Bradburn DM, Rives JD. Mesenteric panniculitis. Review of 27 cases. Ann Surg 1965, **161**: 864–875.

338 Patel RM, Weiss SW, Folpe AL. Heterotopic mesenteric ossification: a distinctive pseudosarcoma commonly associated with intestinal obstruction. Am J Surg Pathol 2006, **30**: 119–122.

339 Payan HM, Gilbert EF. Mesenteric cyst–ovarian implant syndrome. Arch Pathol Lab Med 1987, **111**: 282–284.

340 Pettinato G, Manivel JC, De Rosa N, Dehner LP. Inflammatory myofibroblastic tumor (plasma cell granuloma). Am J Clin Pathol 1990, **94**: 538–546.

341 Remmele W, Muller-Lobeck H, Paulus W. Primary mesenteritis, mesenteric fibrosis and mesenteric fibromatosis. Pathol Res Pract 1988, **184**: 77–85.

342 Rodriguez JA, Guarda LA, Rosai J. Mesenteric fibromatosis with involvement of the gastrointestinal tract. A GIST simulator: a study of 25 cases. Am J Clin Pathol 2004, **121**: 93–98.

343 Ros PR, Olmstead WW, Moser RP Jr, Dachman AH, Hjermstad BH, Sobin LH. Mesenteric and omental cysts. Histologic classification with imaging correlation. Radiology 1987, **164**: 327–332.

344 Scudiere JR, Shi C, Hruban RH, Herman JM, Fishman EK, Schulick RD, Wolfgang CL, Makary MA, Thornton K, Montgomery E, Horton KM. Sclerosing mesenteritis involving the pancreas: a mimicker of pancreatic cancer. Am J Surg Pathol 2010, **34**: 447–453.

345 Shemwell RE, Weed JC. Ovarian remnant syndrome. Obstet Gynecol 1970, **36**: 299–303.

346 Treissman SP, Gillis DA, Lee CL, Giacomantonio M, Resch L. Omental-mesenteric inflammatory pseudotumor. Cytogenetic demonstration of genetic changes and monoclonality in one tumor. Cancer 1994, **73**: 1433–1437.

347 Vanek VW, Phillips AK. Retroperitoneal, mesenteric, and omental cysts. Arch Surg 1984, **119**: 838–842.

348 Wilson JD, Montague CJ, Salcuni P, Bordi C, Rosai J. Heterotopic mesenteric ossification ('intraabdominal myositis ossificans'): report of five cases. Am J Surg Pathol 1999, **23**: 1464–1470.

349 Yannopoulos K, Stout AP. Primary solid tumors of the mesentery. Cancer 1963, **16**: 914–927.

350 Yantiss RK, Nielsen GP, Lauwers GY, Rosenberg AE. Reactive nodular fibrous pseudotumor of the gastrointestinal tract and mesentery: a clinicopathologic study of five cases. Am J Surg Pathol 2003, **27**: 532–540.

351 Yantiss RK, Spiro IJ, Compton CC, Rosenberg AE. Gastrointestinal stromal tumor versus intra-abdominal fibromatosis of the bowel wall: a clinically important differential diagnosis. Am J Surg Pathol 2000, **24**: 947–957.

352 Zamolyi RQ, Souza P, Nascimento AG, Unni KK. Intraabdominal myositis ossificans: a report of 9 new cases. Int J Surg Pathol 2006, **14**: 37–41.

HERNIA SACS

353 Baron BW, Schraut WH, Azizi F, Talerman A. Extragonadal sex cord tumor with annular tubules in an umbilical hernia sac. A unique presentation with implications for histogenesis. Gynecol Oncol 1988, **30**: 71–75.

354 Bostwick D, Eble J. Prostatic adenocarcinoma metastatic to inguinal hernia sac. J Urol Pathol 1993, **1**: 193–200.

355 Cerilli LA, Sotelo-Avila C, Mills SE. Glandular inclusions in inguinal hernia sacs: morphologic and immunohistochemical distinction from epididymis and vas deferens. Am J Surg Pathol 2003, **27**: 469–476.

356 Dehner LP. Inguinal hernia in the male child: where the latest skirmish line has formed. Am J Surg Pathol 1999, **23**: 869–871.

357 Esquivel J, Sugarbaker PH. Pseudomyxoma peritonei in a hernia sac: analysis of 20 patients in whom mucoid fluid was found during a hernia repair. Eur J Surg Oncol 2001, **27**: 54–58.

358 Griffith LM, Carcangiu ML. Sex cord tumor with annular tubules associated with endometriosis of the fallopian tube. Am J Clin Pathol 1991, **96**: 259–262.

359 Nicholson CP, Donohue JH, Thompson GB, Lewis JE. A study of metastatic cancer found during inguinal hernia repair. Cancer 1992, **69**: 3008–3011.

360 Popek EJ. Embryonal remnants in inguinal hernia sacs. Hum Pathol 1990, **21**: 339–349.

361 Pratt PC, George MH, Mastin JP, Roggli VL. Crystalline foreign particulate material in hernia sacs. Hum Pathol 1985, **16**: 1141–1146.

362 Steigman CK, Sotelo-Avila C, Weber TR. The incidence of spermatic cord structures in

inguinal hernia sacs from male children. Am J Surg Pathol 1999, **23**: 880–885.

363 Walker AN, Mills SE. Glandular inclusions in inguinal hernial sacs and spermatic cords. Müllerian-like remnants confused with functional reproductive structures. Am J Clin Pathol 1984, **82**: 85–89.

364 Young RH, Rosenberg AE, Clement PB. Mucin deposits within inguinal hernia sacs: a presenting finding of low-grade mucinous cystic tumors of the appendix. A report of two cases and a review of the literature. Mod Pathol 1997, **10**: 1228–1232.

UMBILICUS

365 Brustman L, Seltzer V. Sister Joseph's nodule. Seven cases of umbilical metastases from gynecologic malignancies. Gynecol Oncol 1984, **19**: 155–162.

366 Clair DG, Lautz DB, Brooks DC. Rapid development of umbilical metastases after laparoscopic cholecystectomy for unsuspected galbladder carcinoma. Surgery 1993, **113**: 355–358.

367 Foraker AG. Job Plodd, Pathologist: his trials and tribulations. Oradell, NJ, 1975, Medical Economics Co.

368 Papalas JA, Madden JF, Selim MA. Malignant neoplasms affecting the umbilicus: clinicopathologic features of 77 tumors. Lab Invest 2009, **89**(Suppl 1): 108A.

369 Ross JE, Hill RB Jr. Primary umbilical adenocarcinoma. A case report and review of literature. Arch Pathol 1975, **99**: 327–329.

370 Steck WD, Helwig EB. Cutaneous remnants of the omphalomesenteric duct. Arch Dermatol 1964, **90**: 463–470.

371 Steck WD, Helwig EB. Cutaneous endometriosis. JAMA 1965, **191**: 101–104.

372 Steck WD, Helwig EB. Tumors of the umbilicus. Cancer 1965, **18**: 907–915.

373 Steck WD, Helwig EB. Umbilical granulomas, pilonidal disease, and the urachus. Surg Gynecol Obstet 1965, **120**: 1043–1057.

374 Vargas SO. Fibrous umbilical polyp: a distinct fasciitis-like proliferation of early childhood with a marked male predominance. Am J Surg Pathol 2001, **25**: 1438–1442.

375 Vicente J, Vazquez-Doval J, Quintanilla E. Fibroepithelial papilloma of the umbilicus. Int J Dermatol 1994, **33**: 791–792.

RETROPERITONEUM

NON-NEOPLASTIC CONDITIONS

376 Carr RA, Newman J, Antonakopulos GN, Parkinson MC. Lesions produced by the extravasation of urine from the upper urinary tract. Histopathology 1997, **30**: 335–340.

377 Catino D, Torack RM, Hagstrom JWC. Idiopathic retroperitoneal fibrosis. Histochemical evidence for lateral spread of the process from the midline. J Urol 1967, **98**: 191–194.

378 Comings DE, Skubi KB, van Eyes J, Motulsky AG. Familial multifocal fibrosclerosis. Findings suggesting that retroperitoneal fibrosis, mediastinal fibrosis, sclerosing cholangitis, Riedel's thyroiditis, and pseudo-tumor of the orbit may be different manifestations of a single disease. Ann Intern Med 1967, **66**: 884–892.

379 Cooksey G, Powell PH, Singh M, Yeates WK. Idiopathic retroperitoneal fibrosis. A long-term review after surgical treatment. Br J Urol 1982, **54**: 628–631.

380 Corradi D, Maestri R, Palmisano A, Bosio S, Greco P, Manenti L, Ferretti S, Cobelli R, Moroni G, Dei Tos AP, Buzio C, Vaglio A. Idiopathic retroperitoneal fibrosis: clinicopathologic features and differential diagnosis. Kidney Int 2007, **72**: 742–753.

381 Dehner LP, Coffin CM. Idiopathic fibrosclerotic disorders and other inflammatory pseudotumors. Semin Diagn Pathol 1998, **15**: 161–173.

382 de Peralta MN, Delahoussaye PM, Tornos CS, Silva EG. Benign retroperitoneal cysts of mullerian type. A clinicopathologic study of three cases and review of the literature. Int J Gynecol Pathol 1994, **13**: 273–278.

383 Doggett RS, Carty SE, Clarke MR. Retroperitoneal bronchogenic cyst masquerading clinically and radiologically as a phaeochromocytoma. Virchows Arch 1997, **431**: 73–76.

384 Graham JR, Suby HI, LeCompte PR, Sadowsky NL. Fibrotic disorders associated with methysergide therapy for headache. N Engl J Med 1966, **274**: 359–368.

385 Harbrecht PJ. Variants of retroperitoneal fibrosis. Ann Surg 1967, **165**: 388–401.

386 Hughes D, Buckley PJ. Idiopathic retroperitoneal fibrosis is a macrophage-rich process. Implications for its pathogenesis and treatment. Am J Surg Pathol 1993, **17**: 482–490.

387 Jones JH, Ross EJ, Matz LR, Edwards D, Davies DR. Retroperitoneal fibrosis. Am J Med 1970, **48**: 203–208.

388 Jonsson G, Lindstedt E, Rubin S-O. Two cases of metastasizing scirrhous gastric carcinoma simulating idiopathic retroperitoneal fibrosis. Scand J Urol Nephrol 1967, **1**: 299–302.

389 Kendall AR, Lakey WH. Sclerosing Hodgkin's disease vs. idiopathic retroperitoneal fibrosis. J Urol 1961, **35**: 284–291.

390 Konishi E, Nakashima Y, Iwasaki T. Immunohistochemical analysis of retroperitoneal Müllerian cyst. Hum Pathol 2003, **2**: 194–198.

391 Kurtz RJ, Heiman TM, Holt J, Beck AR. Mesenteric and retroperitoneal cysts. Arch Surg 1986, **203**: 109–112.

392 Lawson DW, Corry RJ, Patton AS, Austen WG. Massive retroperitoneal adrenal hemorrhage. Surg Gynecol Obstet 1969, **129**: 989–994.

393 Le Gall F, Huerre M, Cipolla B, Shalev M, Ramee MP. A case of myospherulosis occurring in the peritoneal adipose tissue. Pathol Res Pract 1996, **192**: 172–178.

394 Lepor H, Walsh PC. Idiopathic retroperitoneal fibrosis. J Urol 1979, **122**: 1–6.

395 Meehan SM, Scully RE. Para-adrenal bronchogenic cyst: clinical dilemma, pathologic curiosity. J Urol Pathol 1996, **4**: 51–56.

396 Meyer S, Hausman R. Occlusive phlebitis in multifocal fibrosclerosis. Am J Clin Pathol 1976, **65**: 274–283.

397 Mitchinson MJ. The pathology of idiopathic retroperitoneal fibrosis. J Clin Pathol 1970, **23**: 681–689.

398 Mitchinson MJ. Retroperitoneal fibrosis revisited. Arch Pathol Lab Med 1986, **110**: 784–786.

399 Osborn DE, Rao PN, Barnard RJ, Ackrill P, Ralston AJ, Best JJK. Surgical management of idiopathic retroperitoneal fibrosis. Br J Urol 1981, **53**: 292–296.

400 Osborne BM, Butler JJ, Bloustein P, Sumner G. Idiopathic retroperitoneal fibrosis (sclerosing retroperitonitis). Hum Pathol 1987, **18**: 735–739.

401 Sneige N, Dekmezian RH, Silva EG, Cartwright J Jr, Ayala AG. Pseudoparasitic Liesegang structures in perirenal hemorrhagic cysts. Am J Clin Pathol 1988, **89**: 148–153.

402 Terner JY, Lattes R. Malakoplakia of colon and retroperitoneum. Report of a case with a histochemical study of the Michaelis–Gutmann inclusion bodies. Am J Clin Pathol 1965, **44**: 20–31.

403 Thomas MH, Chisholm GD. Retroperitoneal fibrosis associated with malignant disease. Br J Cancer 1973, **28**: 453–458.

404 Weaver J, Goldblum JR, Turner S, Tubbs RR, Wang WL, Lazar AJ, Rubin BP. Detection of MDM2 gene amplification or protein expression distinguishes sclerosing mesenteritis and retroperitoneal fibrosis from inflammatory well-differentiated liposarcoma. Mod Pathol 2009, **22**: 66–70.

405 Zen Y, Onodera M, Inoue D, Kitao A, Matsui O, Nohara T, Namiki M, Kasashima S, Kawashima A, Matsumoto Y, Katayanagi K, Murata T, Ishizawa S, Hosaka N, Kuriki K, Nakanuma Y. Retroperitoneal fibrosis: a clinicopathologic study with respect to immunoglobulin G4. Am J Surg Pathol. 2009, **33**: 1833–1839.

TUMORS

406 Gill W, Carter DC, Durie B. Retroperitoneal tumors. A review of 134 cases. J R Coll Surg Edin 1970, **15**: 213–221.

407 Goldberg BB (ed.). Abdominal gray scale ultrasonography. New York, 1977, John Wiley & Sons.

408 Lofgren L. Primary retroperitoneal tumors. A histopathological, clinical and follow-up study supplemented by follow-up study of a series from the Finnish Cancer Register. Ann Acad Sci Fenn (Med) 1967, **129**: 5–86.

409 Parkinson MC, Chabrel CM. Clinicopathological features of retroperitoneal tumours. Br J Urol 1984, **56**: 17–23.

410 Stanley P. Computed tomographic evaluation of the retroperitoneum in infants and children. J Comput Tomogr 1983, **7**: 63–75.

SOFT TISSUE TUMORS

411 Antonescu CR, Elahi A, Humphrey M, Lui MY, Healey JH, Brennan MF, Woodruff JM, Jhanwar SC, Ladanyi M. Specificity of TLS-CHOP rearrangement for classic myxoid/round cell liposarcoma: absence in predominantly myxoid well-differentiated liposarcomas. J Mol Diagn 2000, **2**: 132–138.

412 Azumi N, Curtis J, Kempson RL, Hendrickson MR. Atypical and malignant neoplasms showing lipomatous differentiation. A study of 111 cases. Am J Surg Pathol 1987, **11**: 161–183.

413 Balzer B, Gupta R, Lazar AJ, Rao P, Amin MB. Pseudoliposarcomatous changes in the perinephric adipose tissue of nephrectomy specimens mimicking well differentiated retroperitoneal liposarcoma: evaluation in 200 nephrectomies. Lab Invest 2009, **89**(Suppl 1): 158A.

414 Bhattacharyya AK, Balogh K. Retroperitoneal lymphangioleiomyomatosis. A 36-year benign course in a postmenopausal woman. Cancer 1985, **56**: 1144–1146.

415 Billings SD, Folpe AL, Weiss SW. Do leiomyomas of deep soft tissue exist? An analysis of highly differentiated smooth muscle tumors of deep soft tissue supporting two distinct subtypes. Am J Surg Pathol 2001, **25**: 1134–1142.

416 Binh MB, Guillou L, Hostein I, Château MC, Collin F, Aurias A, Binh BN, Stoeckle E, Coindre JM. Dedifferentiated liposarcomas with divergent myosarcomatous differentiation developed in the internal trunk: a study of 27 cases and comparison to conventional dedifferentiated liposarcomas and leiomyosarcomas. Am J Surg Pathol 2007, **31**: 1557–1566.

417 Chung EB, Enzinger FM. Extraskeletal osteosarcoma. Cancer 1987, **60**: 1132–1142.

418 Cody HS III, Turnbull AD, Fortner JG, Hajdu SI. The continuing challenge of retroperitoneal sarcomas. Cancer 1981, **47**: 2147–2152.

419 Coindre J-M, Mariani O, Chibon F, Mairal A, de Saint Aubain Somerhausen N, Favre-Guillevin E, Bui NB, Stoeckle E, Hostein I, Aurias A. Most malignant fibrous histiocytomas developed in the retroperitoneum are dedifferentiated liposarcomas: a review of 25 cases initially diagnosed as malignant fibrous histiocytoma. Mod Pathol 2003, **16**: 256–262.

420 Crist WM, Raney RB, Tefft M, Heyn R, Hays DM, Newton W, Beltangady M, Maurer HM. Soft tissue sarcomas arising in the retroperitoneal space in children. A report from the Intergroup Rhabdomyosarcoma Study (IRS) Committee. Cancer 1985, **56**: 2125–2132.

421 Dickman PS, Triche TJ. Extraosseous Ewing's sarcoma versus primitive rhabdomyosarcoma. Diagnostic criteria and clinical correlation. Hum Pathol 1986, **17**: 881–893.

422 Eble JN, Rosenberg AE, Young RH. Retroperitoneal xanthogranuloma in a patient with Erdheim–Chester disease. Am J Surg Pathol 1994, **18**: 843–848.

423 Elgar F, Goldblum JR. Well-differentiated liposarcoma of the retroperitoneum: a clinicopathologic analysis of 20 cases, with particular attention to the extent of low-grade dedifferentiation. Mod Pathol 1997, **10**: 113–120.

424 Enzinger FM, Winslow DJ. Liposarcoma. A study of 103 cases. Virchows Arch Pathol Anat 1962, **335**: 367–388.

425 Erlandson RA. The ultrastructural distinction between rhabdomyosarcoma and other undifferentiated 'sarcomas'. Ultrastruct Pathol 1987, **11**: 83–101.

426 Fabre-Guillevin E, Coindre JM, Somerhausen Nde S, Bonichon F, Stoeckle E, Bui NB. Retroperitoneal liposarcomas: follow-up analysis of dedifferentiation after clinicopathologic reexamination of 86 liposarcomas and malignant fibrous histiocytomas. Cancer 2006, **106**: 2725–2733.

427 Fukunaga M, Ushigome S, Ishikawa E. Kaposiform haemangioendothelioma associated with Kasabach–Merritt syndrome. Histopathology 1996, **28**: 281–284.

428 Ghali VS, Gold JE, Vincent RA, Cosgrove JM. Malignant peripheral nerve sheath tumor arising spontaneously from retroperitoneal ganglioneuroma. A case report, review of the literature, and immunohistochemical study. Hum Pathol 1992, **23**: 72–75.

429 Gronchi A, Casali PG, Fiore M, Mariani L, Lo Vullo S, Bertulli R, Colecchia M, Lozza L, Olmi P, Santinami M, Rosai J. Retroperitoneal soft tissue sarcomas: patterns of recurrence in 167 patients treated at a single institution. Cancer 2004, **100**: 2448–2455.

430 Hasegawa T, Seki K, Hasegawa F, Matsuno Y, Shimada T, Hirose T, Sano T, Hirohashi S. Dedifferentiated liposarcoma of retroperitoneum and mesentery: varied growth patterns and histological grades – a clinicopathologic study of 32 cases. Hum Pathol 2000, **31**: 717–727.

431 Hashimoto H, Tsuneyoshi M, Enjoji M. Malignant smooth muscle tumors of the retroperitoneum and mesentery. A clinicopathologic analysis of 44 cases. J Surg Oncol 1985, **28**: 177–186.

432 Heslin MJ, Lewis JJ, Nadler E, Newman E, Woodruff JM, Casper ES, Leung D, Brennan MF. Prognostic factors associated with long-term survival for retroperitoneal sarcoma: implications for management. J Clin Oncol 1997, **15**: 2832–2839.

433 Hisaoka M, Morimitsu Y, Hashimoto H, Ishida T, Mukai H, Satoh H, Motoi T, Machinami R. Retroperitoneal liposarcoma with combined well-differentiated and myxoid malignant fibrous histiocytoma-like myxoid areas. Am J Surg Pathol 1999, **23**: 1480–1492.

434 Hollowood K, Stamp G, Zouvani J, Fletcher CDM. Extranodal follicular dendritic cell sarcoma of the gastrointestinal tract. Morphologic, immunohistochemical and ultrastructural analysis of two cases. Am J Clin Pathol 1995, **103**: 90–97.

435 Huang H-Y, Brennan MF, Antonescu CR. Distant metastasis in retroperitoneal dedifferentiated liposarcoma is rare and rapidly fatal: a clinicopathological study with emphasis on the low-grade myxofibrosarcoma-like pattern as an early sign of dedifferentiation. Mod Pathol 2005, **18**: 976–984.

436 Huszar M, Fanburg JC, Dickersin GR, Kirshner JJ, Rosenberg AE. Retroperitoneal malignant meningioma: A light microscopic, immunohistochemical, and ultrastructural study. Am J Surg Pathol 1996, **20**: 492–499.

437 Ibrahim NB, Briggs JC, Corrin B. Double primary localized fibrous tumours of the pleura and retroperitoneum. Histopathology 1993, **22**: 282–284.

438 Ida CM, Wang X, Erickson-Johnson MR, Wenger DE, Blute ML, Nascimento AG, Oliveira AM. Primary retroperitoneal lipoma: a soft tissue pathology heresy?: report of a case with classic histologic, cytogenetics, and molecular genetic features. Am J Surg Pathol 2008, **32**: 951–954.

439 Karakousis CP, Velez AF, Emrich LJ. Management of retroperitoneal sarcomas and patient survival. Am J Surg 1985, **150**: 376–380.

440 Kelley TW, Borden EC, Goldblum JR. Estrogen and progesterone receptor expression in uterine and extrauterine leiomyosarcomas: an immunohistochemical study. Appl Immunohistochem Mol Morphol 2004, **12**: 338–341.

441 Kinne DW, Chu FCH, Huvos AG, Yagoda A, Fortner JG. Treatment of primary and recurrent retroperitoneal liposarcoma. Twenty-five-year experience at Memorial Hospital. Cancer 1973, **31**: 53–64.

442 Kourea HP, Bilsky MH, Leung DHY, Lewis JJ, Woodruff JM. Subdiaphragmatic and intrathoracic paraspinal malignant peripheral nerve sheath tumors: a clinicopathologic study of 25 patients and 26 tumors. Cancer 1998, **82**: 2191–2203.

443 Lau SK, Marchevsky AM, McKenna Jr RJ, Luthringer DJ. Malignant monotypic epithelioid angiomyolipoma of the retroperitoneum. Int J Surg Pathol 2003, **11**: 223–228.

444 Lauwers GY, Erlandson RA, Casper ES, Brennan MF, Woodruff JM. Gastrointestinal autonomic nerve tumors. A clinicopathological, immunohistochemical, and ultrastructural study of 12 cases. Am J Surg Pathol 1993, **17**: 887–897.

445 Leonidas JC, Brill PW, Bhan I, Smith TH. Cystic retroperitoneal lymphangioma in infants and children. Radiology 1978, **127**: 203–208.

446 Macarenco RS, Erickson-Johnson M, Wang X, Folpe AA, Rubin BP, Nascimento AG, Oliveira AM. Retroperitoneal lipomatous tumors without cytologic atypia: are they lipomas? A clinicopathologic and molecular study of 19 cases. Am J Surg Pathol 2009, **33**: 1470–1476.

447 Michal M. Retroperitoneal myolipoma. A tumour mimicking retroperitoneal angiomyolipoma and liposarcoma with myosarcomatous differentiation. Histopathology 1994, **25**: 86–88.

448 Morrison C, Ramirez NC, Chan JKC, Wakely Jr P. Endometrial stromal sarcoma of the retroperitoneum. Ann Diagn Pathol 2002, **6**: 312–318.

449 Oberling C. Retroperitoneal xanthogranuloma. Am J Cancer 1935, **23**: 477–489.

450 Paal E, Miettinen M. Retroperitoneal leiomyomas: a clinicopathologic and immunohistochemical study of 56 cases with a comparison to retroperitoneal leiomyosarcomas. Am J Surg Pathol 2001, **25**: 1355–1363.

451 Patel R, Goldblum JR, Antonescu CR. Mutational analysis of c-kit in extragastrointestinal stromal tumors (EGIST): a molecular study of six cases [abstract]. Mod Pathol 2003, **16**: 18a–19a.

452 Piana S, Roncaroli F. Epithelioid leiomyosarcoma of retroperitoneum with granular cell change. Histopathology 1994, **25**: 90–93.

453 Rajani B, Smith TA, Reith JD, Goldblum JR. Retroperitoneal leiomyosarcomas unassociated with the gastrointestinal tract: a clinicopathologic analysis of 17 cases. Mod Pathol 1999, **12**: 21–28.

454 Ranchod M, Kempson RC. Smooth muscle tumors of the gastrointestinal tract and retroperitoneum. A pathologic analysis of 100 cases. Cancer 1977, **39**: 255–262.

455 Ransom JL, Pratt CB, Hustu O, Kumar APM, Howarth CB, Bowles D. Retroperitoneal rhabdomyosarcoma in children. Results of multimodality therapy. Cancer 1980, **45**: 845–850.

456 Reith JD, Goldblum JR, Lyles RH, Weiss SW. Extragastrointestinal (soft tissue) stromal tumors: an analysis of 48 cases with emphasis on histologic predictors of outcome. Mod Pathol 2000, **13**: 577–585.

457 Roncaroli F, Eusebi V. Rhabdomyoblastic differentiation in a leiomyosarcoma of the retroperitoneum. Hum Pathol 1996, **27**: 310–312.

458 Schmidt D, Mackay B, Sinkovics JG. Retroperitoneal tumor with vertebral metastasis in a 25-year-old female. Ultrastruct Pathol 1981, **2**: 383–388.

459 Shmookler BM. Retroperitoneal synovial sarcoma. A report of four cases. Am J Clin Pathol 1982, **77**: 686–691.

460 Shmookler BM, Lauer DH. Retroperitoneal leiomyosarcoma. A clinicopathologic analysis of 36 cases. Am J Surg Pathol 1983, **7**: 269–280.

461 Stoeckle E, Coindre JM, Bonvalot S, Kantor G, Terrier P, Bonichon F, Nguyen Bui B. Prognostic factors in retroperitoneal sarcoma: a multivariate analysis of a series of 165 patients of the French Cancer Center Federation Sarcoma Group. Cancer 2001, **92**: 359–368.

462 Tallini G, Erlandson RA, Brennan MF, Woodruff JM. Divergent myosarcomatous differentiation in retroperitoneal liposarcoma. Am J Surg Pathol 1993, **17**: 546–556.

463 Tefft M, Vawter GF, Mitus A. Paravertebral 'round cell' tumors in children. Radiology 1969, **92**: 1501–1509.

464 Triche RJ, Askin FB, Kissane JM. Neuroblastoma, Ewing's sarcoma, and the differential diagnosis of small-, round-, blue-cell tumors. In Finegold M (ed.): Pathology of neoplasia in children and adolescents, vol. 18 of Major problems in pathology. Philadelphia, 1986, W.B. Saunders.

465 Tsang WY, Chan JK. Kaposi-like infantile hemangioendothelioma. A distinctive vascular neoplasm of the retroperitoneum. Am J Surg Pathol 1991, **15**: 982–989.

466 van Doorn RC, Gallee MP, Hart AA, Gortzak E, Rutgers EJ, van Coevorden F, Keus RB, Zoetmulder FA. Resectable retroperitoneal soft tissue sarcomas. The effect of extent of resection and postoperative radiation therapy on local tumor control. Cancer 1994, **73**: 637–642.

467 Vilanova JR, Burgos-Bretones J, Simon R, Rivera-Pomar JM. Leukaemoid reaction and eosinophilia in 'inflammatory fibrous histiocytoma'. Virchows Arch [A] 1980, **388**: 237–243.

468 Vuletin JC, Wajsbort RR, Ghali V. Primary retroperitoneal angiosarcoma with eosinophilic globules. A combined light-microscopic, immunohistochemical, and ultrastructural study. Arch Pathol Lab Med 1990, **114**: 618–622.

469 Watanabe K, Tanaka M, Kusakabe T, Soeda S. Mesometrial smooth muscle as an origin of female retroperitoneal (pelvic) leiomyomas. Virchows Arch 2007, **451**: 899–904.

470 Whitten RO, Benjamin DR. Rhabdomyoma of the retroperitoneum. A report of a tumor with both adult and fetal characteristics. A study by light and electron microscopy, histochemistry, and immunochemistry. Cancer 1987, **59**: 818–824.

471 Yunis EJ. Ewing's sarcoma and related small round cell neoplasms in children. Am J Surg Pathol 1986, **10**: S54–S62.

GERM CELL TUMORS

472 Abell MR, Fayos JV, Lampe I. Retroperitoneal germinomas (seminomas) without evidence of testicular involvement. Cancer 1965, **18**: 273–290.

473 Berry CL, Keelnig J, Hilton C. Teratoma in infancy and childhood. A review of 91 cases. J Pathol 1969, **98**: 241–252.

474 Buskirk SJ, Evans RG, Farrow GM, Earle JD. Primary retroperitoneal seminoma. Cancer 1982, **49**: 1934–1936.

475 Chen KT, Cheng AC. Retroperitoneal seminoma and intratubular germ cell neoplasia. Hum Pathol 1989, **20**: 493–495.

476 Hawkins EP, Finegold MJ, Hawkins HK, Krischer JP, Starling KA, Weinberg A. Nongerminomatous malignant germ cell tumors in children. A review of 89 cases from the pediatric oncology group, 1971–1984. Cancer 1986, **58**: 2579–2584.

477 Kernek KM, Brunelli M, Ulbright TM, Eble JN, Martignoni G, Zhang S, Michael H, Cummings OW, Cheng L. Fluorescence in situ hybridization analysis of chromosome 12p in paraffin-embedded tissue is useful for establishing germ cell origin of metastatic tumors. Mod Pathol 2004, **17**: 1309–1313.

478 Lack EE, Travis WD, Welch KJ. Retroperitoneal germ cell tumors in childhood. A clinical and pathologic study of 11 cases. Cancer 1985, **56**: 602–608.

479 Maatman T, Bukowski RM, Montie JE. Retroperitoneal malignancies several years after initial treatment of germ cell cancer of the testis. Cancer 1984, **54**: 1962–1965.

480 Montague DK. Retroperitoneal germ cell tumors with no apparent testicular involvement. J Urol 1975, **113**: 505–508.

481 Moss JF, Slayton RE, Economou SG. Primary retroperitoneal pure choriocarcinoma. Two long-term complete responders from a rare fatal disease. Cancer 1988, **62**: 1053–1054.

482 Ohno Y, Kanematsu T. An endodermal sinus tumor arising from a mature cystic teratoma in the retroperitoneum in a child: is a mature teratoma a premalignant condition? Hum Pathol 1998, **29**: 1167–1169.

483 Sung MT, MacLennan GT, Cheng L. Retroperitoneal seminoma in limited biopsies: morphologic criteria and immunohistochemical findings in 30 cases. Am J Surg Pathol 2006, **30**: 766–773.

484 Wang F, Liu A, Peng Y, Rakheja D, Wei L, Xue D, Allan RW, Molberg KH, Li J, Cao D. Diagnostic utility of SALL4 in extragonadal yolk sac tumors: an immunohistochemical study of 59 cases with comparison to placental-like alkaline phosphatase, alpha-fetoprotein, and glypican-3. Am J Surg Pathol 2009, **33**: 1529–1539.

485 Weissbach L, Boedefeld EA. Localization of solitary and multiple metastases in stage II nonseminomatous testis tumor as basis for a modified staging lymph node dissection in stage I. J Urol 1987, **138**: 77–82.

OTHER PRIMARY TUMORS AND TUMORLIKE CONDITIONS

486 Brietta LK, Watkins D. Giant extra-adrenal myelolipoma. Arch Pathol Lab Med 1994, **118**: 188–190.

487 Burke T, Sahin A, Johnson DE, Ordóñez NG, Mackay B. Myoepithelioma of the retroperitoneum. Ultrastruct Pathol 1995, **19**: 269–274.

488 Cafferty LL, Katz RL, Ordóñez NG, Carrasco CH, Cabanillas FR. Fine needle aspiration diagnosis of intraabdominal and retroperitoneal lymphomas by a morphologic and immunocytochemical approach. Cancer 1990, **65**: 72–77.

489 Carabias E, Garcia Muñoz H, Dihmes FP, López Pino MA, Ballestin C. Primary mucinous cystadenocarcinoma of the retroperitoneum. Report of a case and literature review. Virchows Arch 1995, **426**: 641–645.

490 Chen KTK, Felix EL, Flam MS. Extraadrenal myelolipoma. Am J Clin Pathol 1982, **78**: 386–389.

491 Chen L, Kuriakose P, Hawley RC, Janakiraman N, Maeda K. Hematologic malignancies with primary retroperitoneal presentation: clinicopathologic study of 32 cases. Arch Pathol Lab Med 2005, **129**: 655–660.

492 Fowler MR, Williams GB, Alba JM, Byrd CR. Extra-adrenal myelolipomas compared with extra medullary hematopoietic tumors. A case of presacral myelolipoma. Am J Surg Pathol 1982, **6**: 363–374.

493 Fukutomi Y, Shibuya C, Yamamoto S, Okuno F, Nishiwaki S, Kashiki Y, Muto Y. Extrarenal Wilms' tumor in the adult patient. A case report and review of the world literature. Am J Clin Pathol 1988, **90**: 618–622.

494 Hasegawa T, Hirose T, Ayala AG, Ito S, Tomaru U, Matsuno Y, Shimoda T, Hirohashi S. Adult neuroblastoma of the retroperitoneum and abdomen: clinicopathologic distinction from primitive neuroectodermal tumor. Am J Surg Pathol 2001, **25**: 918–924.

495 Hornick JL, Fletcher CD. Sclerosing PEComa: clinicopathologic analysis of a distinctive variant with a predilection for the retroperitoneum. Am J Surg Pathol 2008, **32**: 493–501.

496 Isse K, Harada K, Suzuki Y, Ishiguro K, Sasaki M, Kajiura S, Nakanuma Y. Retroperitoneal mucinous cystadenoma: report of two cases and review of the literature. Pathol Int 2004, **54**: 132–138.

497 Koretz MJ, Wang S, Klein FA, Lawrence W Jr. Extrarenal adult Wilms' tumor. Cancer 1987, **60**: 2484–2488.

498 Kryger-Baggesen N, Kjaergaard J, Sehested M. Nonchromaffin paraganglioma of the retroperitoneum. J Urol 1985, **134**: 536–538.

499 Matsubara M, Shiozawa T, Tachibana R, Hondo T, Osasda K, Kawaguchi K, Kimura K, Konishi I. Primary retroperitoneal mucinous cystadenoma of borderline malignancy: a case report and review of the literature. Int J Gynecol Pathol 2005, **24**: 218–223.

500 Olson JR, Abell MR. Nonfunctional nonchromaffin paragangliomas of the retroperitoneum. Cancer 1969, **23**: 1358–1367.

501 Park U, Han KC, Chang HK, Huh MH. A primary mucinous cystoadenocarcinoma of the retroperitoneum. Gynecol Oncol 1991, **42**: 64–67.

502 Pennell TC, Gusdon JP. Retroperitoneal mucinous cystadenoma. Am J Obstet Gynecol 1990, **160**: 1229–1231.

503 Roma AA, Malpica A. Primary retroperitoneal mucinous tumors: a clinicopathologic study of 18 cases. Am J Surg Pathol 2009, **33**: 526–533.

504 Rothacker D, Knolle J, Stiller D, Borchard F. Primary retroperitoneal mucinous cystadenomas with gastric epithelial differentiation. Pathol Res Pract 1993, **189**: 1195–1204.

505 Shintaku M, Matsumoto T. Primary mullerian carcinosarcoma of the retroperitoneum: report of a case. J Gynecol Pathol 2001, **20**: 191–195.

506 Subramony C, Habibpour S, Hashimoto LA. Retroperitoneal mucinous cystadenoma. Arch Pathol Lab Med 2001, **125**: 691–694.

507 Tang C-K, Toker C, Wybel RE, Desai RG. An unusual pelvic tumor with benign glandular, sarcomatous, and Wilms' tumor-like components. Hum Pathol 1981, **12**: 940–944.

508 Ulbright TM, Morley DJ, Roth LM, Berkow RL. Papillary serous carcinoma of the retroperitoneum. Am J Clin Pathol 1983, **79**: 633–637.

509 Wakely PE Jr, Sprague RI, Kornstein MJ. Extrarenal Wilms' tumor. An analysis of four cases. Hum Pathol 1989, **20**: 691–695.

510 Waldron JA, Magnifico M, Duray PH, Cadman EC. Retroperitoneal mass presentations of B-immunoblastic sarcoma. Cancer 1985, **56**: 1733–1741.

511 Waldron JA, Newcomer LN, Katz ME, Cadman E. Sclerosing variants of follicular center cell lymphomas presenting in the retroperitoneum. Cancer 1983, **52**: 712–720.

512 Yajima A, Toki T, Morinaga S, Sasano H, Sasano N. A retroperitoneal endocrine carcinoma. Cancer 1984, **54**: 2040–2042.

SACROCOCCYGEAL REGION

DEVELOPMENTAL ANOMALIES

513 Andea AA, Klimstra DS. Adenocarcinoma arising in a tailgut cyst with prominent meningothelial proliferation and thyroid tissue: case report and review of the literature. Virchows Arch 2005, **446**: 316–321.

514 Bale PM. Sacrococcygeal developmental abnormalities and tumors in children. Perspect Pediatr Pathol 1984, **1**: 9–56.

515 Berry CL, Keelnig J, Hilton C. Teratoma in infancy and childhood. A review of 91 cases. J Pathol 1969, **98**: 241–252.

516 Fulton RS, Rouse RV, Ranheim EA. Ectopic prostate: case report of a presacral mass presenting with obstructive symptoms. Arch Pathol Lab Med 2001, **125**: 286–288.

517 Harrist TY, Gang DL, Kleinman GM, Mihm MC Jr, Hendren WH. Unusual sacrococcygeal embryologic malformations with cutaneous manifestations. Arch Dermatol 1982, **118**: 643–648.

518 Hjernstad BM, Helwig EB. Tailgut cysts. Report of 53 cases. Am J Clin Pathol 1988, **89**: 139–147.

519 Hood DL, Petras RE, Grundfest-Broniatowski S, Jagelman DG. Retrorectal cystic hamartoma. Report of five cases with carcinoid tumor arising in two [abstract]. Am J Clin Pathol 1988, **89**: 433.

520 MacLeod JH, Purves JKB. Duplications of the rectum. Dis Colon Rectum 1970, **13**: 133–137.

521 Marco V, Autonell J, Farre J, Fernandez-Layos M, Doncel F. Retrorectal cyst–hamartoma. Report of two cases with adenocarcinoma developing in one. Am J Surg Pathol 1982, **6**: 707–714.

522 McDermott NC, Newman J. Tailgut cyst (retrorectal cystic hamartoma) with prominent glomus bodies. Histopathology 1991, **18**: 265–266.

523 Mills SE, Walker AN, Stallings RG, Allen MS. Retrorectal cystic hamartoma. Report of three cases, including one with a perirenal component. Arch Pathol Lab Med 1984, **108**: 737–740.

524 Prasad AR, Amin MB, Randolph TL, Lee CS, Ma CK. Retrorectal cystic hamartoma: report of 5 cases with malignancy. Arch Pathol Lab Med 2000, **124**: 725–729.

525 Tagart REB. Congenital anal duplication. A cause of para-anal sinus. Br J Surg 1977, **64**: 525–528.

526 Thway K, Polson A, Pope R, Thomas JM, Fisher C. Extramammary Paget disease in a retrorectal dermoid cyst: report of a unique case. Am J Surg Pathol 2008, **32**: 635–639.

GERM CELL TUMORS

527 Ahmed HA, Pollock DJ. Malignant sacrococcygeal teratoma in the adult. Histopathology 1985, **9**: 359–363.

528 Bale PM. Sacrococcygeal developmental abnormalities and tumors in children. Perspect Pediatr Pathol 1984, **1**: 9–56.

529 Berry CL, Keelnig J, Hilton C. Teratoma in infancy and childhood. A review of 91 cases. J Pathol 1969, **98**: 241–252.

530 Chretien PB, Milam JD, Foote FW, Miller TR. Embryonal adenocarcinomas (a type of malignant teratoma) of the sacrococcygeal region. Clinical and pathologic aspects of 21 cases. Cancer 1970, **26**: 522–535.

531 Donnellan WA, Swenson O. Benign and malignant sacrococcygeal teratomas. Surgery 1968, **64**: 834–846.

532 Ein SH, Mancer K, Adeyemi SD. Malignant sacrococcygeal teratoma – endodermal sinus, yolk sac tumor – in infants and children. A 32-year review. J Pediatr Surg 1985, **20**: 473–477.

533 Gonzalez-Crussi F, Winkler RF, Mirkin DL. Sacrococcygeal teratomas in infants and children. Relationship of histology and prognosis in 40 cases. Arch Pathol Lab Med 1978, **102**: 420–425.

534 Hawkins EP, Finegold MJ, Hawkins HK, Krischer JP, Starling KA, Weinberg A. Nongerminomatous malignant germ cell tumors in children. A review of 89 cases from the pediatric oncology group, 1971–1984. Cancer 1986, **58**: 2579–2584.

535 Heerema-McKenney A, Harrison MR, Bratton B, Farrell J, Zaloudek C. Congenital teratoma: a clinicopathologic study of 22 fetal and neonatal tumors. Am J Surg Pathol 2005, **29**: 29–38.

536 Kaplan CG, Askin FB, Benirschke K. Cytogenetics of extragonadal tumors. Teratology 1979, **19**: 261–266.

537 Kuhajda FP, Taxy JB. Oncofetal antigens in sacrococcygeal teratomas. Arch Pathol Lab Med 1983, **107**: 239–242.

538 Lack EE, Glaun RS, Hefter LG, Seneca RP, Steigman C, Athari F. Late occurrence of malignancy following resection of a histologically mature sacrococcygeal teratoma. Report of a case and literature review. Arch Pathol Lab Med 1993, **117**: 724–728.

539 Lack EE, Travis WE, Welch KJ. Retroperitoneal germ cell tumors in childhood. A clinical and pathologic study of 11 cases. Cancer 1985, **56**: 602–608.

540 Lahdenne P, Heikinheimo M, Nikkanen V, Klemi P, Siimes MA, Rapola J. Neonatal benign sacrococcygeal teratoma may recur in adulthood and give rise to malignancy. Cancer 1993, **72**: 3727–3731.

541 Nakashima N, Fukatsu T, Nagasaka T, Sobue M, Takeuchi J. The frequency and histology of hepatic tissue in germ cell tumors. Am J Surg Pathol 1987, **11**: 682–692.

542 Ng EW, Porcu P, Loehrer PJ Sr. Sacrococcygeal teratoma in adults: case reports and a review of the literature. Cancer 1999, **86**: 1198–1202.

543 Noseworthy J, Lack EE, Kozakewich HPW, Vawter GF, Welch KJ. Sacrococcygeal germ cell tumors in childhood. An updated experience with 118 patients. J Pediatr Surg 1981, **16**: 358–364.

544 Olsen MM, Raffensperger JG, Gonzalez-Crussi F, Luck SR, Kaplan WE, Morgan ER. Endodermal sinus tumor. A clinical and pathological correlation. J Pediatr Surg 1982, **17**: 832–840.

545 Oosterhuis J, van Berlo R, de Jong B, Dam A, Buist J, Tamminga R, Zwierstra R. Sacral teratoma with late recurrence of yolk sac tumor. J Urol Pathol 1993, **1**: 257–268.

546 Siltanen S, Anttonen M, Heikkila P, Narita N, Laitinen M, Ritvos O, Wilson DB, Heikinheimo M. Transcription factor GATA-4 is expressed in pediatric yolk sac tumors. Am J Pathol 1999, **155**: 1823–1829.

547 Valdiserri RO, Yunis EJ. Sacrococcygeal teratomas. A review of 68 cases. Cancer 1981, **48**: 217–221.

548 Wang F, Liu A, Peng Y, Rakheja D, Wei L, Xue D, Allan RW, Molberg KH, Li J, Cao D. Diagnostic utility of SALL4 in extragonadal yolk sac tumors: an immunohistochemical study of 59 cases with comparison to placental-like alkaline phosphatase, alpha-fetoprotein, and glypican-3. Am J Surg Pathol 2009, **33**: 1529–1539.

549 Whalen TV Jr, Mahour GH, Landing BH, Woolley MM. Sacrococcygeal teratomas in infants and children. Am J Surg 1985, **150**: 373–375.

PILONIDAL DISEASE

550 Culp CE. Pilonidal disease and its treatment. Surg Clin North Am 1967, **47**: 1007–1014.

551 Davage ON. The origin of sacrococcygeal pilonidal sinuses based on an analysis of four hundred and sixty-three cases. Am J Pathol 1954, **30**: 1191–1205.

552 Lineaweaver WC, Brunson MB, Smith JF, Franzini DA, Rumley TO. Squamous carcinoma arising in a pilonidal sinus. J Surg Oncol 1984, **27**: 239–242.

553 Norris CS. Giant condyloma acuminatum (Buschke–Lowenstein tumor) involving a pilonidal sinus. A case report and review of the literature. J Surg Oncol 1983, **22**: 47–50.

554 Notaras MJ. A review of three popular methods of treatment of postanal (pilonidal) sinus disease. Br J Surg 1970, **57**: 886–890.

555 Pilipshen SJ, Gray G, Goldsmith E, Dineen P. Carcinoma arising in pilonidal sinuses. Ann Surg 1981, **193**: 506–512.

556 Schröder CM, Merk HF, Frank J. Barber's hair sinus in a female hairdresser: uncommon manifestation of an occupational dermatosis. J Eur Acad Dermatol Venereol 2006, **20**: 209–211.

OTHER TUMORS

557 Addis BJ, Rao SG, Finnis D, Carvell JE. Pre-sacral carcinoid tumour. Histopathology 1991, **18**: 563–565.

558 Gatalica Z, Wang L, Lucio ET, Miettinen M. Glomus coccygeum in surgical pathology specimens: small troublemaker. Arch Pathol Lab Med 1999, **123**: 905–908.

559 Helwig EB, Stern JB. Subcutaneous sacrococcygeal myxopapillary ependymoma. A clinicopathologic study of 32 cases. Am J Clin Pathol 1984, **81**: 156–161.

560 Horenstein MG, Erlandson RA, Gonzalez-Cueto DM, Rosai J. Presacral carcinoid tumors: report of three cases and review of the literature. Am J Surg Pathol 1998, **22**: 251–255.

561 Lemberger A, Stein M, Doron J, Fried G, Goldsher D, Feinsod M. Sacrococcygeal extradural ependymoma. Cancer 1989, **64**: 1156–1159.

562 Rahemtullah A, Szyfelbein K, Zembowicz A. Glomus coccygeum: report of a case and review of the literature. Am J Dermatopathol 2005, **27**: 497–499.

563 Song DE, Park JK, Hur B, Ro JY. Carcinoid tumor arising in a tailgut cyst of the anorectal junction with distant metastasis: a case report and review of the literature. Arch Pathol Lab Med 2004, **128**: 578–580.

Cardiovascular system

Heart, Arteries, Veins, Lymph vessels

27

Heart

CHAPTER CONTENTS

Introduction

Most operations for congenital cardiovascular malformations are directed toward improvement in the flow of oxygenated blood by such procedures as ligation or division of a patent ductus or the closure of interatrial and interventricular septal defects. Methods have been devised to relieve pulmonary, aortic, and mitral valvular stenosis. Coronary artery bypass graft surgery has become a widely used and effective procedure for the symptomatic treatment of ischemic heart disease. The reader is referred to specialized texts dealing with these various abnormalities and their methods of treatment.[1-4]

Another cardiac operation that has become almost routine in some medical centers is cardiac transplantation; here the pathologist plays a very important role in monitoring the possibility of rejection.

Normal anatomy

The major histologic components of the heart are pericardium, myocardium, endocardium, and valves.[5] The *pericardium* is divided into fibrous (parietal) and serous (visceral, also known as epicardium) portions. It is lined by a single layer of mesothelial cells resting on a basement membrane. The *myocardium* consists of bundles of cardiac muscle fibers (myocytes) separated by fibrous bands. These fibers form a syncytium with end-to-end junctions, called intercalated discs, and sometimes side-to-side junctions.[5] The nuclei of myocytes are centrally located, in contrast to those of skeletal muscle fibers. The *endocardium* consists of a single layer of endothelial cells that are continuous with those of the major blood vessels. The *semilunar (pulmonary and aortic) valves* are composed of three layers: fibrosa (made of dense collagen), spongiosa (containing large amounts of proteoglycans, loosely arranged collagen fibers, and scattered fibroblasts), and ventricularis (identified by its profusion of elastic fibers). The *atrioventricular (mitral and tricuspid) valves* are composed of the annulus (a ring of circumferentially oriented collagen and elastic fibers), leaflets, chordae tendineae, and papillary muscles. The leaflets, like those of the semilunar valves, are composed of three layers: fibrosa, ventricularis (on the ventricular side, rich in elastic fibers), and the spongiosa (on the atrial side, rich in proteoglycans).

The morphologic features of blood vessels and lymph vessels are discussed in Chapter 25.

Myocardial biopsy

The performance of myocardial or endomyocardial biopsies has become a common procedure.[7,9,14] These biopsies can be obtained through a catheter inserted in a systemic vein through a transthoracic route or at the time of surgery for congenital or acquired heart disease. Examination of multiple levels increases the sensitivity of the procedure, particularly in cases of myocarditis.[6,11] Ultrastructural examination can be of importance, especially for the evaluation of drug toxicity.[10]

The current complication rate with the intravascular procedure at specialized centers is less than 1%; the most common complication is hemopericardium (which rarely requires thoracotomy), and the most serious is cardiac perforation. The two most important indications of myocardial biopsy are monitoring of heart transplant recipients and grading of Adriamycin toxicity.[13] They can also be useful for the confirmation of the diagnosis of cardiomyopathy and myocarditis, and are essential for the diagnosis of primary and metastatic tumors.[8,9,12,15]

Cardiomyopathy and myocarditis

Idiopathic hypertrophic cardiomyopathy. This is an inherited disease of the myocardium characterized by left ventricular hypertrophy without chamber dilation in the absence of an identifiable systemic or cardiac cause.[31,43,60] It is genetically heterogeneous, with most cases caused by germline mutation in one of the many sarcomeric protein genes.[22] The main microscopic changes in this condition, as seen in whole hearts, septal myomectomy specimens, or biopsies obtained at thoracotomy, are myofiber disarray and hypertrophy and interstitial fibrosis.[39,47,48,63] Transvascular biopsy specimens are less informative, but they still show disarray of myofibrils and myofilaments within individual myocytes by ultrastructural examination. Unfortunately, these changes are not specific for this condition.[51,63] Another nonspecific change that is commonly found in idiopathic hypertrophic myocardiopathy is *basophilic degeneration* of myocardium. This appears as basophilic, finely granular material in the cytoplasm of isolated myocardial fibers and consists of polyglucosan deposits.[56,61]

Idiopathic dilated cardiomyopathy. Abnormalities in the myocardial biopsy are consistently present but, again, are of a nonspecific nature. They consist mainly of hypertrophy and degenerative changes of the myocardial fibers.[41,58,69]

A good correlation has been found between the severity of the condition clinically and the extent and degree of microscopic abnormalities, although the sometimes focal nature of the changes may be misleading. Leukocytic infiltrates are present in about one-half of the myocardial biopsies in this condition, a fact to remember in the differential diagnosis with myocarditis.[62] About 30% of cases have an inherited basis, usually autosomal dominant, due to germline mutation in a gene encoding sarcomeric protein, intermediate filament, nuclear membrane protein, cytoskeletal protein, phospholamban or ion channel protein.[36]

Restrictive (restrictive/obliterative) cardiomyopathy. In the *eosinophilic* form of this disease in its active stage, a myocarditis with a heavy component of eosinophils is present (Fig. 27.1); in the inactive stage of this form and in the *noneosinophilic* form (the most common in the United States), the biopsy findings are nonspecific.[34]

Infiltrative myocardiopathies. This is the group of cardiac diseases in which endomyocardial biopsy can be particularly rewarding. This includes amyloidosis,[53] hemosiderosis,[23] hemochromatosis, and glycogenosis. However, the diagnosis of most of these conditions can be made more readily by biopsy of another, more readily accessible organ.[40]

Other cardiomyopathies. *Ischemic cardiomyopathy* is secondary to severe coronary artery disease with myocardial infarct and is characterized by congestive heart failure and cardiac dilation. Cases with similar features occurring in the absence of a myocardial infarct have been described.[19]

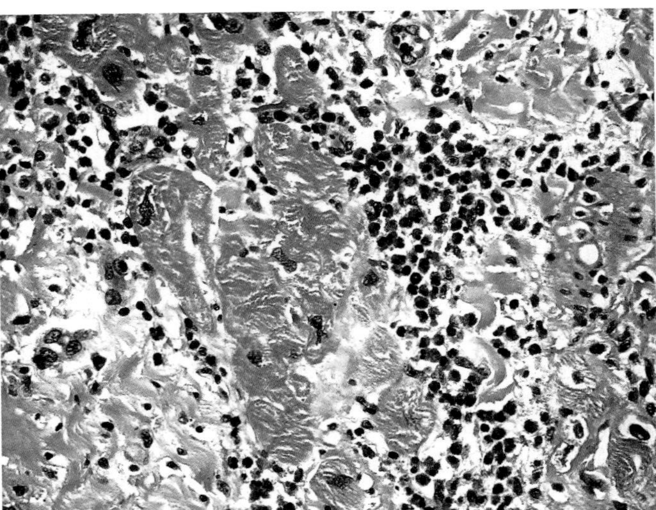

Fig. 27.1 Eosinophil-rich myocardial infiltrate in restrictive myocarditis.

Right ventricular dysplasia is a strongly familial idiopathic cardiomyopathy that mainly involves the right ventricle. The anatomic substrate is variable infiltration of the right ventricular myocardium by adipose and fibrous tissue.[46]

Myocarditis. It is agreed that the diagnosis of myocarditis requires the presence of an inflammatory infiltrate *and* myocyte necrosis or degeneration ('Dallas criteria').[17,48] The infiltrate is usually of lymphocytic nature, easily identifiable, often admixed with histiocytes, and amenable to semiquantification in routine sections.[35] The hematoxylin and eosin sections are routinely supplemented with CD3, CD4, CD20, CD45, and CD45 immunostains.[45,50,59] Most of the lymphocytes are of T-cell type.[26] In *hypersensitivity myocarditis*, the infiltrate is rich in eosinophils, is predominantly perivascular, and is accompanied by a lesser degree of necrotizing changes.[24,30,37]

The myocyte alterations can take the form of frank necrosis, vacuolization, or disruption, and are better appreciated in longitudinal sections. The presence of edema should not be used as a criterion for myocarditis. Fibrosis, if present, should be quantified (mild, moderate, or severe) and qualified (interstitial, endocardial, or replacement).

Diagnostic terms to be used in subsequent biopsies, using the first specimen as a reference point, are *ongoing* or *persistent myocarditis* when both the myocyte damage and the inflammation persist, *resolving* or *healing myocarditis* when these changes are substantially reduced, and *resolved* or *healed myocarditis* when these changes are no longer present.[17] Fenoglio et al.[38] divided their cases of myocarditis into *acute, rapidly progressive*, and *chronic*; they found a good correlation between these types and the clinical course.

The etiology of myocarditis can be viral, bacterial, fungal, parasitic (particularly Chagas disease and toxoplasmosis, the latter often seen in AIDS patients), caused by a collagen–vascular disease (especially rheumatic fever), drug-induced, radiation-induced, related to Whipple disease, or an expression of transplant rejection.[16,18,28,29,52,55,65,67,68] Rare forms of granulomatous myocarditis include tuberculosis and sarcoidosis.[54,57] In many cases of myocarditis the condition remains idiopathic, although the recently introduced molecular diagnostic approach has allowed the identification of viruses (enteroviruses and adenoviruses) in a high proportion of cases of childhood myocarditis.[25] *Giant cell myocarditis*, a different entity from sarcoidosis, is characterized by multicentric destruction

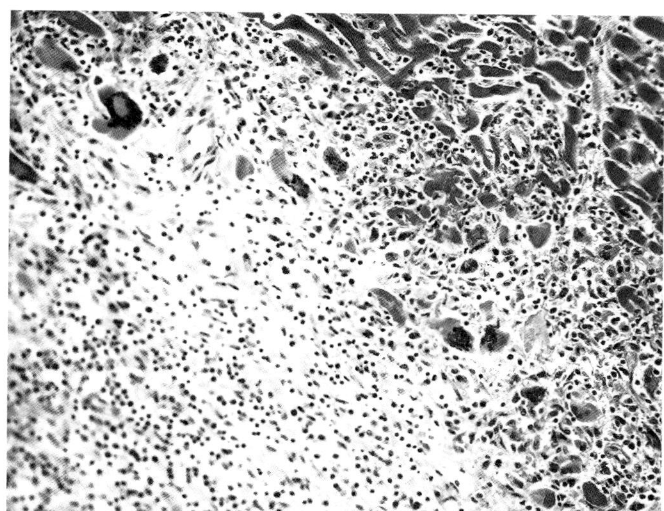

Fig. 27.2 Giant cell myocarditis. Scattered multinucleated giant cells accompanied by lymphocytes are seen in association with loss of myocardial fibers.

of the cardiac myocytes by cytotoxic T cells and the multinucleated cells that define the entity (Fig. 27.2).[27,49] The latter have the immunohistochemical profile of histiocytes.[64] Another form of myocarditis is characterized by T lymphocytes that express the gamma-delta T-cell receptor and runs a fulminant clinical course.[32]

Drug-induced and radiation-induced cardiomyopathy. The myocardial changes resulting from *Adriamycin* toxicity have been well documented.[42,44] Vacuolization of cardiac myocytes, resulting from dilation of the sarcotubular system, is the earliest change. This is followed by the appearance of the so-called 'adria cell', characterized light microscopically by loss of cross striations and myofilamentous bundles and accompanied by a homogeneous basophilic staining ('myocytolysis'). Ultrastructurally, there is dissociation of sarcomeres and fragmentation and loss of myofilaments. Immunohistochemically, cells with myocytolysis retain reactivity for myoglobin and various enzymes, suggesting that the myocyte is viable and that the change may be reversible.[33] This alteration is in no way specific for Adriamycin toxicity but can be seen in a large variety of diseases.[33] Inflammation is nil or absent, this representing an important differential feature with other myocardial lesions (Figs 27.3 and 27.4).

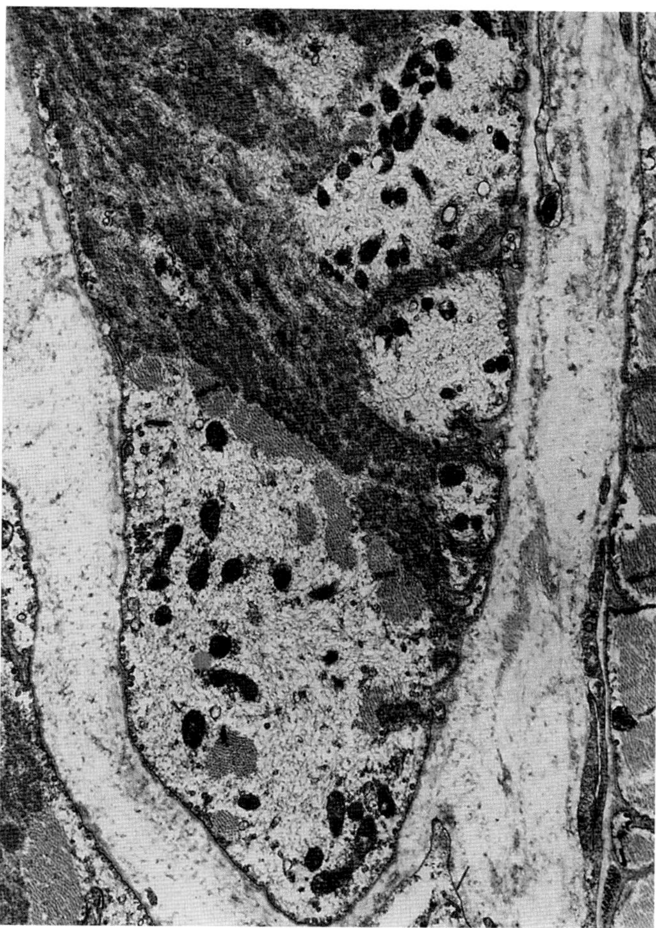

Fig. 27.3 Adriamycin cardiotoxicity. Myocyte in center ('adria cell') shows extensive pale areas of loss of myofibrils and fragmentation of myofilaments. Mitochondria (dark oval structures in same areas) are not qualitatively altered. Remnants of Z bands form a diagonal dense area in center. Note intact myocyte (right edge). (×5600)
(Courtesy of Dr LF Fajardo, Stanford, CA)

The changes are rather diffuse but seem to predominate in the subendocardial region. They are dose dependent and are enhanced if radiation therapy has also been used. In the latter instance, the changes just described are superimposed on those resulting from the radiation, which are mainly located in the capillaries.[21] It could be added here that radiation-induced heart disease also includes constrictive pericarditis, myocardial fibrosis, and appreciable valvular and coronary artery lesions.[66]

Cyclophosphamide may produce hemorrhagic necrosis, extensive capillary thrombosis, interstitial hemorrhage and fibrin deposition, and necrosis of myocardial fibers.[20]

Heart transplant

Myocardial biopsy is the most sensitive indicator of rejection.[74,77,79,84,86,90,92] The criteria used for the diagnosis depend on the immunosuppressive regimen used.[75] The main microscopic sign of rejection is a perivascular and interstitial inflammatory infiltrate, predominantly lymphocytic, accompanied by focal necrosis of myocytes and edema. Clusters of neutrophils may be present around the necrotic myocytes.[81]

One should be careful not to misinterpret a previous biopsy site as indicative of rejection; it appears as a sharply outlined area of necrotic myocytes, sometimes associated with a thrombus and granulation tissue. Rejection should also be distinguished from ischemic changes (Fig. 27.5A) and from *drug-induced hypersensitivity myocarditis*, a self-limited condition that does not cause heart failure and usually resolves without residual injury.[78]

The grading system of acute rejection episodes is a modification of the scheme originally proposed by Billingham:[72]

Early rejection (reversible) (Fig. 27.5B)
- Endocardial and interstitial edema
- Scanty perivascular and endocardial infiltrate of pyroninophilic lymphocytes with prominent nucleoli
- Pyroninophilia of endocardial and endothelial cells

Moderate rejection (reversible) (Fig. 27.5C)
- Interstitial, perivascular, and endocardial infiltrate of pyroninophilic lymphocytes with prominent nucleoli
- Early focal myocytolysis

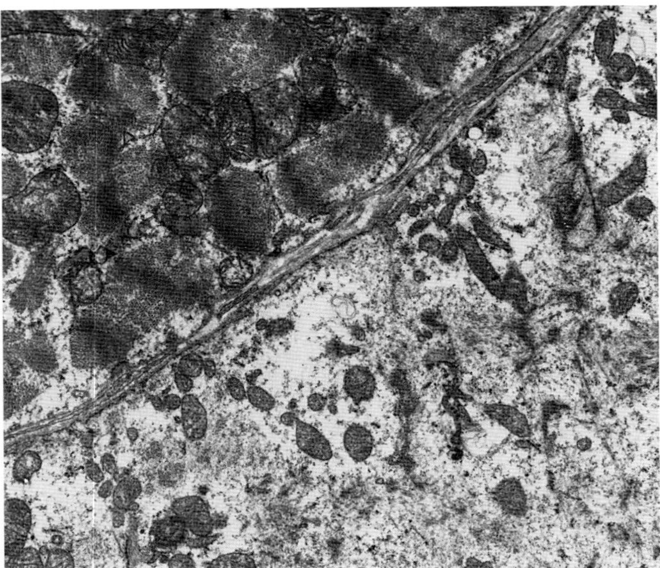

Fig. 27.4 Compare transverse section of normal cardiac myocyte (upper left) with myocyte severely affected by Adriamycin (lower right). There is complete disorganization of sarcomeres and extensive fragmentation of myofilaments. Mitochondria are small (compare with top). Remnants of Z bands are present near right edge. This complete loss of contractile elements in one myocyte, with preservation of adjacent cell, creates sharply defined amphophilic or basophilic areas that characterize 'adria cells' in paraffin sections. (×8200)
(Courtesy of Dr LF Fajardo, Stanford, CA)

Severe rejection (irreversible or very difficult to reverse)
 Interstitial hemorrhage and infiltrate of pyroninophilic lymphocytes and polymorphonuclear leukocytes, vascular and myocyte necrosis
Resolving rejection (Fig. 27.5D)
 Active fibrosis, residual small lymphocytes (nonpyroninophilic), plasma cells, and hemosiderin deposits

The system currently used is the one agreed upon by the International Society of Heart and Lung Transplantation in 1990 and revised in 2004.[88] An important addition is that of **vascular rejection**, a process that injures the endothelium in the absence of significant intramyocardial lymphocytic infiltration[83] (Fig. 27.5E).

The long-term successfully transplanted heart characteristically shows some degree of hypertrophy and fibrosis of muscle fibers.[87,89] Accelerated arteriosclerosis is now the major long-term complication of heart transplantation. Gaudin et al.[76] have shown that ischemic injury to the heart during the peritransplant period – as detected in endomyocardial biopsies – contributes to the development of this complication (Fig. 27.5F).

In about 10% of heart transplant cases, endocardial lymphoid collections develop in which the presence of the Epstein–Barr virus (EBV) genome can be demonstrated. When intense (5% of the cases), this change is referred to as *EBV-associated post-transplant lymphoproliferative disorder*.[70,80] In addition to the heart, the infiltrate may involve the lung, gastrointestinal tract, lymph nodes, and other sites.[73,82] The proliferating cells are of host origin, and the process ranges from atypical lymphoid hyperplasia to malignant lymphoma.[73,91] Some of these cases (particularly when located in the lung and gastrointestinal tract) respond to a reduction in immunosuppression.[73]

Most cases are of B-cell nature, but T-cell proliferations also occur, the latter exceptionally having the features of anaplastic large cell lymphoma.[85]

Cytomegalovirus infection can be diagnosed through the demonstration of viral inclusion bodies, with immunohistochemical or in situ hybridization techniques, or by polymerase chain reaction (PCR). The latter method is the most sensitive; however, PCR demonstration of human cytomegalovirus (HCMV) DNA in otherwise negative endomyocardial specimens is of questionable significance.[71]

Cardiac valves

Surgery to correct major defects of the valves by resection and prosthetic replacement is frequently performed (Fig. 27.6).[95,130] It should be emphasized that the most precise diagnosis will be made from the gross appearance of the valve and that usually the microscopic examination is of little value.[100,114,119,128] Photographic and radiographic examination of the specimen is also indicated. Careful examination of the gross specimen with knowledge of the clinical history often allows a distinction to be made between a rheumatic or congenital origin in a chronic valvulopathy.[115] Microscopically, both show fibrosis, calcification, occasional inflammatory cells, and sometimes foci of dystrophic amyloid deposition.[97]

The major etiologies of valvular disease, the gross morphologic assessment, and the etiologic assessment are shown in the box and Tables 27.1 and 27.2.[116]

Major etiologies of acquired mitral and aortic valve disease

Mitral valve disease

Mitral stenosis
 Postinflammatory scarring (rheumatic)
 Calcification of mitral annulus
Mitral regurgitation
 Abnormalities of leaflets and commissures
 Postinflammatory scarring (rheumatic)
 Infective endocarditis
 Floppy mitral valve
 Abnormalities of mitral apparatus
 Rupture of papillary muscle
 Papillary muscle dysfunction (fibrosis or ischemia)
 Rupture of chordae tendineae
 Left ventricular enlargement (e.g., congestive cardiomyopathy)
 Calcification of mitral annulus

Aortic valve disease

Aortic stenosis
 Calcification of congenitally deformed valve
 Senile calcific aortic stenosis
 Postinflammatory scarring (rheumatic)
Aortic regurgitation
 Abnormalities of cusps and commissures
 Postinflammatory scarring (rheumatic)
 Infective endocarditis
Aortic disease
 Syphilitic aortitis
 Ankylosing spondylitis
 Rheumatoid arthritis
 Marfan syndrome
 Aortic dissection
 Trauma

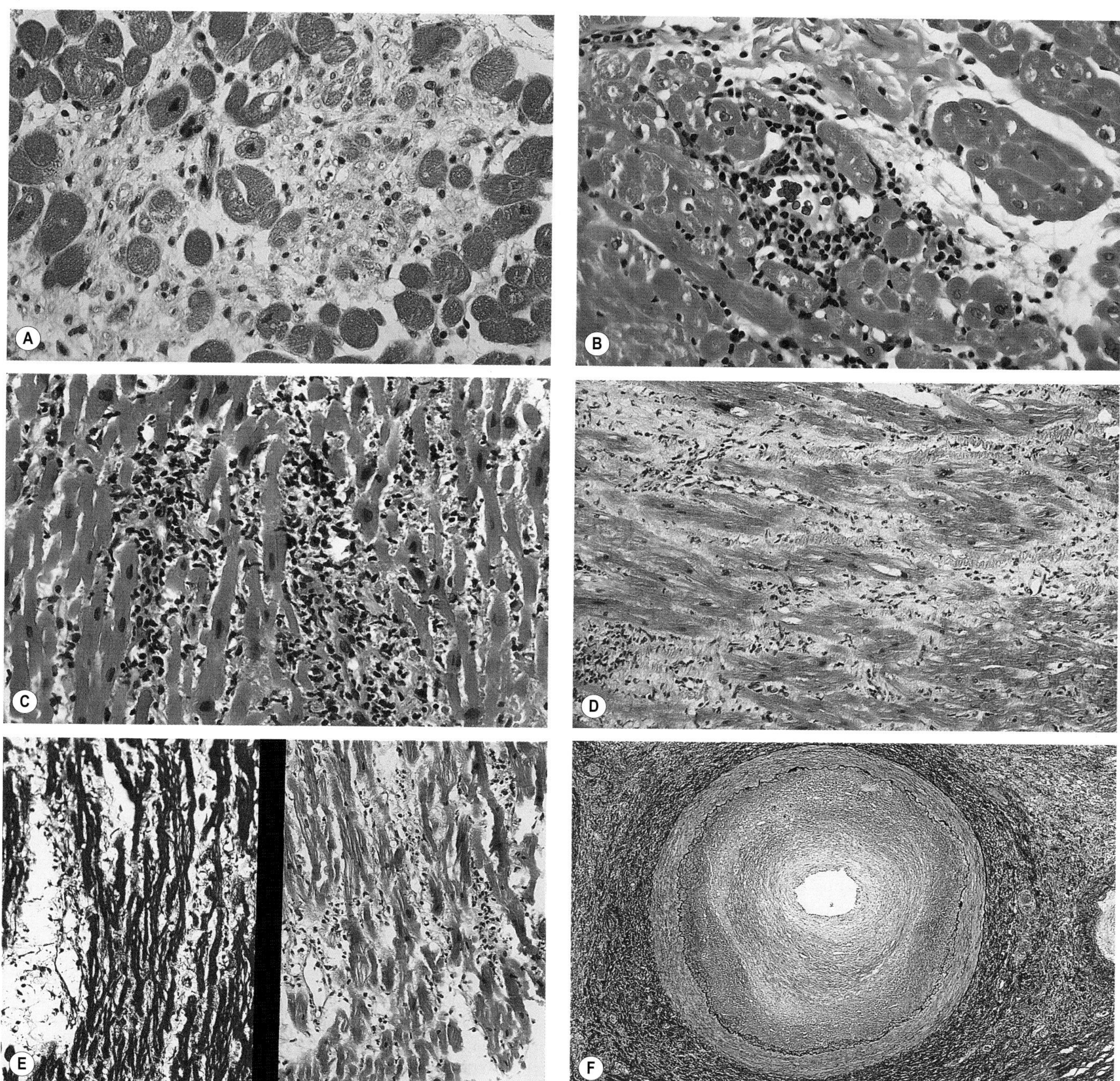

Fig. 27.5 Various microscopic appearances of heart transplant. **A**, Endomyocardial biopsy with healing ischemic changes. There is focal dropout of myofibers with sparse infiltrate of mononuclear cells, including pigment-laden histiocytes. **B**, Mild acute cellular rejection. There is patchy perivascular lymphocytic infiltrate with no myocyte injury. **C**, Moderate acute rejection showing myocyte injury or damage. **D**, Resolving rejection. There is a diminished inflammatory infiltrate with interstitial fibrosis after treatment for moderate acute rejection. **E**, Acute vascular rejection. There is a sparse inflammatory infiltrate with dilated small vessels and edema, shown with H&E (left) and trichrome (right). **F**, Chronic rejection (transplant vasculopathy). There is concentric narrowing of epicardial coronary artery by fibromuscular intimal proliferation. Note the preservation of internal elastic lamina (Elastic-van Gieson stain).
(Courtesy of Dr Richard N Eisen, Greenwich, CT)

Nearly all cases of *mitral valve* stenosis (with or without mitral insufficiency) are acquired and postinflammatory.[98] Among the cases of mitral insufficiency, Olson et al.[110] found that 38% were caused by a floppy valve (myxoid heart disease) and 31% by postinflammatory disease. They observed a floppy valve in 73% of the cases of chordal rupture and in 38% of the cases of infective endocarditis. They further noted that the relative frequency of floppy mitral valve as a cause of insufficiency had increased in recent years. Grossly, the floppy valve shows leaflet thickening and redundancy, leading to the formation of dome-like deformities reaching above the level of the annulus, which appears dilated. The chordae are often thin and attenuated, with fibrosis or fusion at the anchoring sites.[110,128,129]

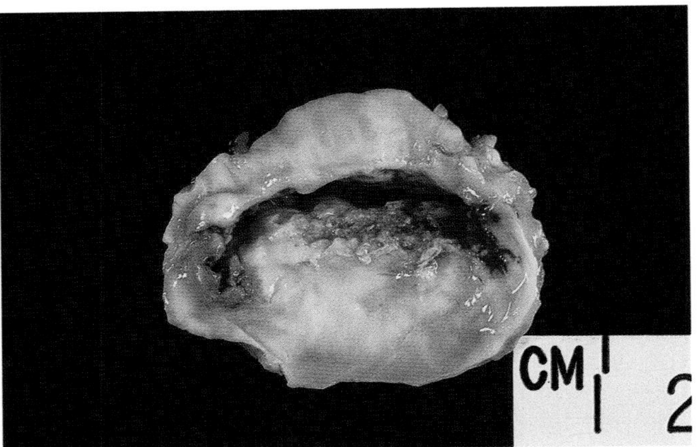

Fig. 27.6 Gross appearance of heavily fibrotic and calcified cardiac valve.

Table 27.1 Gross morphologic assessment of abnormal cardiac valvular function

PATHOLOGIC FEATURE	STENOTIC VALVE	PURELY REGURGITANT VALVE
For all valves		
Valve weight	Increased	Normal or slightly increased or decreased
Fibrous thickening	Diffuse	Diffuse, focal, or none
Calcific deposits	None to heavy	Minimal (if any)
Tissue loss (perforation, indentation)	None	May be present
Vegetations	Minimal	May be present
Commissural fusion	May be present	Minimal (if any)
Annular circumference	Normal	Normal or increased
For aortic valves		
Number of cusps	One to three	Two or three
For mitral (or tricuspid) valves		
Abnormal papillary muscles	No	May be present
Chordae tendineae		
Fusion	Usually present	Absent
Elongation	Absent	May be present
Shortening	Usually present	May be present
Rupture	Absent	May be present

Chordal rupture is seen in over one-half of the cases.[104] Microscopically, stromal accumulation of glycosaminoglycans is the distinguishing feature, leading to the appearance of 'myxoid degeneration'. A lesser degree of accumulation of this material is seen in the neural and conduction system of these patients, pointing to a more general myxoid alteration.[108] Whether this alteration is the result of a genetically determined disease or a degenerative process of nonspecific nature remains controversial. The existence of familial forms of this disorder points toward the former.[102]

Specimens of *aortic valves* removed because of stenosis may show calcification of congenitally bicuspid valves (48%), calcification of a normally tricuspid valve without commissural fusion (so-called 'senile type') (28%), calcification of an acquired bicuspid valve (13%), a fibrous (rheumatic) type valve (10%), or calcification of congenitally unicuspid valves (1%).[111,112,126] Exceptionally, osseous or cartilaginous metaplasia is encountered.[103,125] In combined aortic stenosis and insufficiency, the most common changes are those of postinflammatory disease (69%) or calcification of congenitally bicuspid (19%) and unicommissural (6%) valves.[127] Pure aortic insufficiency is not related to calcification but to causes such as aortic root dilation, bicuspid valve, and others.[99] Aortic valvulitis can be seen as a (sometimes fatal) complication of Behçet disease.[106]

Specimens of *pulmonary valve* may be received in the surgical pathology laboratory because of pure pulmonary stenosis (the majority as a component of tetralogy of Fallot), pure pulmonary insufficiency, or combined stenosis and insufficiency. Congenital heart disease accounts for 95% of the cases, and tetralogy of Fallot is the most common form. Bicuspid pulmonary valve is the most common anomaly.[93]

Specimens of *tricuspid valve* can be the result of operations for pure insufficiency (by far the most common), combined stenosis and insufficiency, and pure stenosis (very rare). The most common causes of insufficiency are postinflammatory diseases, congenital disorders, pulmonary venous hypertension, and infective endocarditis.[105]

An easy system for the identification by the pathologist of the many different types of *artificial heart valve prostheses* in existence in the mid 1970s has been developed.[124] Microscopic study of these prosthetic valves has shown that, following insertion, a neoendocardium develops at the junction with the heart wall, and from there it grows centripetally over the sewing cloth toward the valve lumen.

The pathologic changes that may be found in removed bioprosthetic heart valves include thrombosis, infection, cuspal tears and perforations, fibrous sheathing, calcification, intracuspal hematomas, and several others.[94,101,113,118,121,122] Mechanical valves may show thrombosis, infection, and various alterations associated with the valve design and the composition of the various elements.[117,123] Cuspal retraction without stenosis can also occur, leading to wide-open regurgitation.[109] Siddiqui et al.[120] listed the following complications reported post valve implantation: calcification, cusp tears, pannus growth, infectius pericarditis, valve thrombosis, and other factors specific to valve type.

At the time of the correction of a mitral stenosis, the surgeon may perform a biopsy of the *atrial appendage*. These appendages are always abnormal, showing hypertrophy of the muscle and various other alterations. About one-half of them show *Aschoff nodules*.[96] These are formed by collections of plump cells arranged in a granuloma-like fashion. The cells are positive for vimentin and negative for actin and desmin, suggesting a mesenchymal but not myocardial derivation.[107] The presence of these nodules does not correlate with the postoperative course or with clinical evidence of activity of the rheumatic process.

Table 27.2 Etiologic assessment of valvular heart disease

	SENILE DEGENERATION	MYXOMATOUS DEGENERATION	RHEUMATIC	INFECTIVE	SECONDARY
Gross features					
Leaflet/cuspal thickening	0	0/1	1	0	0
Calcification	1	0	0/1	0	0
Commissural chordal fusion	0	0	1	0	0
Leaflet cuspal redundancy	0	1	0	0	0
Leaflet cuspal defects	0	0	0	1	0
Chordal rupture	0	0/1	0	0/1	0
Histologic features					
Preservation of layered architecture	1	1	0	0/1	1
GAG accumulation in spongiosa	0	1	0	0	0/1
Thinned fibrosa	0	1	0	0	0
Neovascularization	0	0	0/1	0/1	0
Superficial fibrosis only	0/1	0/1	0	0/1	0/1

0, absent; 1, present; 0/1, present in some cases; GAG, glycosaminoglycan.
From Schoen FJ. Surgical pathology of removed natural and prosthetic heart valves. Hum Pathol 1987, **18:** 558–567.

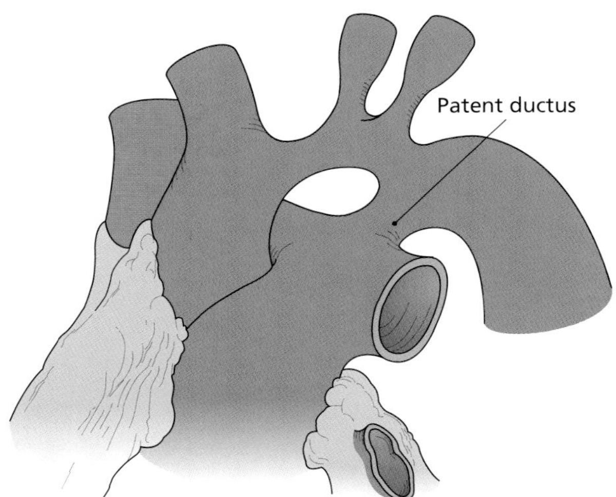

Fig. 27.7 Infantile (diffuse) type of coarctation of aorta.
(From Burford TH. Symposium on clinical surgery. Coarctation of aorta and its treatment. Surg Clin North Am 1950, ***30:*** *1249–1258)*

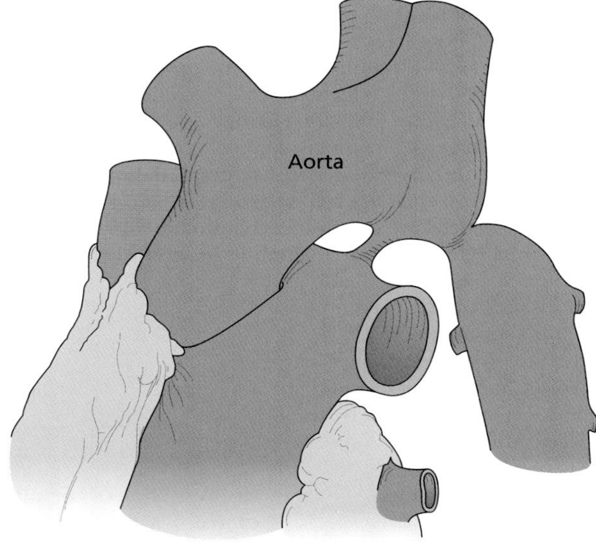

Fig. 27.8 Adult (localized) type of coarctation of aorta.
(From Burford TH. Symposium on clinical surgery. Coarctation of aorta and its treatment. Surg Clin North Am 1950, ***30:*** *1249–1258)*

Coronary artery bypass

A vast number of coronary artery bypass operations have been done during the past 50 years using a segment of saphenous vein to join the aorta to a segment of the coronary artery distal to the obstruction. The patency rate of these grafts is over 80% after 5 years. Graft failure necessitating reoperation may result from the intimal fibrous hyperplasia that develops after the first month in all grafts becoming occlusive or from atherosclerosis in older grafts.[134] This atherosclerosis is typically concentric, diffuse, without a fibrous cap, with numerous foamy and inflammatory cells (including multinucleated giant forms), and associated with erosion of the media.[132] Secondary thrombosis is common.[131,133]

Coarctation of aorta

Coarctation of aorta is divided into infantile (diffuse, preductal) and adult (localized, postductal) types (Figs 27.7 and 27.8).

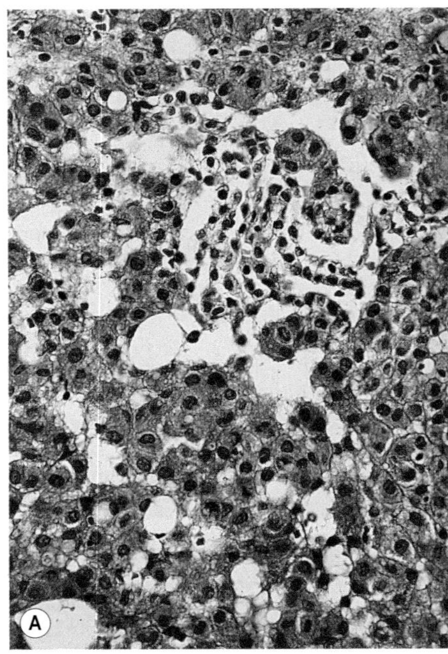

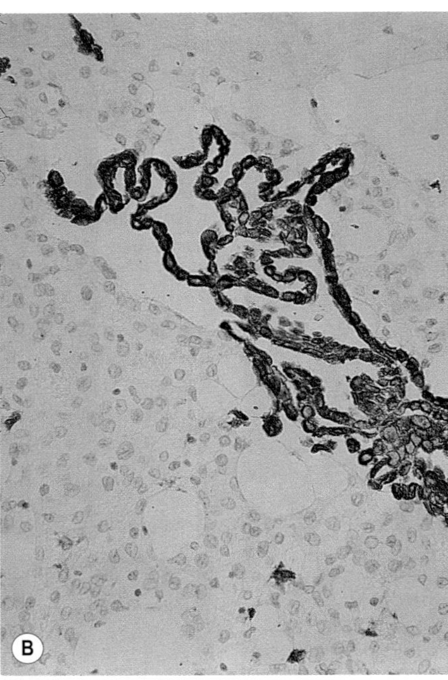

Fig. 27.13 So-called 'cardiac MICE'. **A**, This process is composed of an admixture of plump histiocytes and ribbons of small cuboidal mesothelial cells. **B**, The immunostain for keratin highlights the mesothelial cell component, which is surrounded by the negative histiocytes and other mononuclear cells.

similarities with angiomyolipoma, another HMB-45-positive lesion.[244] Rarely, cardiac rhabdomyomas in adults have a morphologic appearance similar to that of the extracardiac type of this tumor.[245]

Hamartoma of mature cardiac myocytes resembles microscopically hypertrophic cardiomyopathy but is a localized process characterized by myofiber disarray, focal scarring, and intramural coronary thickening, but no inflammation or calcification.[200,223] The usual but not exclusive location of this lesion is the left ventricle.[191,234]

Calcified amorphous tumor of the heart (cardiac CAT) is the name proposed for an endocardially based intracavitary cardiac mass characterized microscopically by nodular deposition of calcium in a background of degenerating blood cell elements and chronic inflammation.[228] The clinical course is benign. The pathogenesis is obscure, but an origin from mural thrombi has been suggested.[228]

Mesothelial/monocytic incidental cardiac excrescences ('cardiac MICE') are incidental microscopic findings at the time of cardiac surgery (usually for valvular disease) or in an endomyocardial biopsy. They may be found attached to the endocardium, free-floating in the pericardial cavity, or even inside an aortic dissecting aneurysm.[187,220,242] Ultrastructural and immunohistochemical studies have shown that the lesion is composed of an admixture of keratin-positive mesothelial cells and CD68-positive histiocytes[220] (Fig. 27.13). Microscopically, the mesothelial cells form strips, tubular and micropapillary formations surrounded by the smaller histiocytes. Huge round vacuoles are often present. Except for the latter, the appearance is very similar to that of nodular mesothelial hyperplasia as seen in hernia sacs.[230]

The process is clearly benign, non-neoplastic, and usually of no clinical significance (although a case has been reported allegedly causing severe acute cardiopulmonary failure[226]). The pathogenesis remains unclear. Ingrowth of pericardial cells along a perforation tract has been suggested.[220,242] Others have postulated an artifact produced by suctioning of the pericardial cavity during cardiac surgery,[197,243] a theory that we find difficult to accept. It has also been suggested that the process is mediated by adhesion molecules.[235] Their main practical importance resides in the fact that a pathologist unaware of their existence may mistake them for a metastatic carcinoma or some other neoplasm. We have seen a remarkable case in which a lesion of cardiac MICE contained within it a minute focus of metastatic adenocarcinoma.[186]

Cystic tumor of the atrioventricular nodal region was regarded as a mesothelioma for many years, but there is now conclusive evidence that it represents a developmental abnormality of epithelial nature and endodermal origin.[184,199,206] Specifically, it has been postulated that this condition represents a heterotopia of the ultimobranchial body analogous to solid cell rests of the thyroid gland, a very attractive hypothesis.[194] It may be associated with other congenital anomalies.[188] Because of its crucial location, it may result in complete heart block. All reported cases have been found at autopsy.

Microscopically, the lesion consists of ductular structures, cysts, and solid nests of epithelial-like cells, which on electron microscopy show desmosomes and microvilli (Fig. 27.14).[204] Immunohistochemically, the cells are reactive for keratin, CEA, and B72.3 but not for factor VIII, calretinin, WT1, or thrombomodulin.[185,188,199,219] It should be pointed out that not all nodular lesions of the atrioventricular node are examples of this entity; some are of vascular or neural nature.[210,211]

Adenomatoid tumor analogous to its more common counterpart in the male and female genital system has been reported in the heart. Here too the lesion is of mesothelial nature (as opposed to the tumor described in the preceding paragraph).[225]

Papillary fibroelastoma (fibroelastic hamartoma, fibroma, papilloma, papillary fibroblastoma) is a small papillary ('sea anemone-like') growth that usually occurs on the surface of the valves but may also be seen in other endocardial locations[183,240] (Fig. 27.15A). It is nearly always an incidental finding at surgery or autopsy[209] and is formed microscopically by a lining of hyperplastic endocardial cells covering a core of hyalinized hypocellular stroma[202,232] (Fig. 27.15B). It probably represents the end stage of the organization

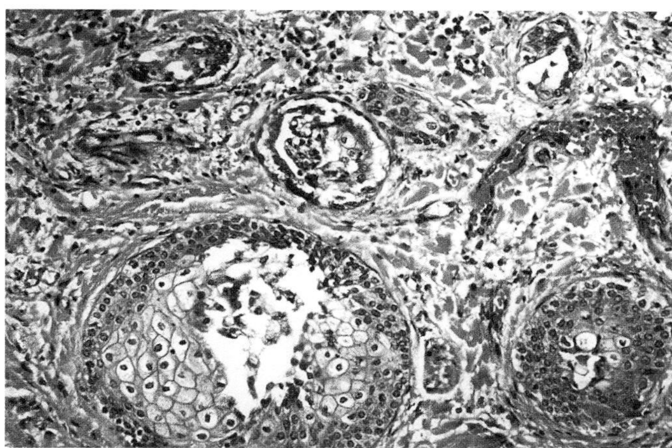

Fig. 27.14 So-called 'cystic tumor' of the atrioventricular nodal region. In this case the lining of the cysts had a definite squamoid quality.

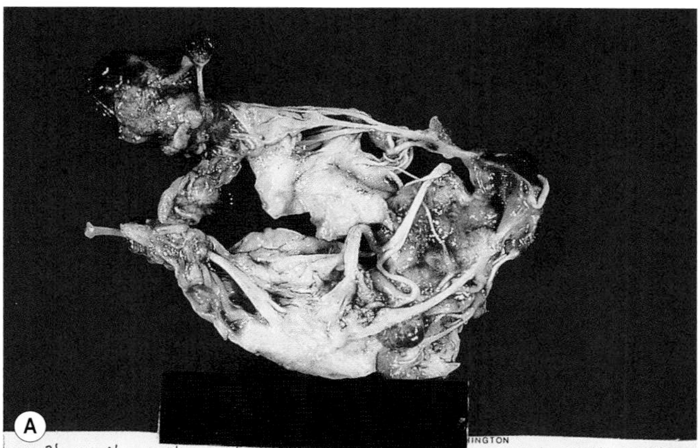

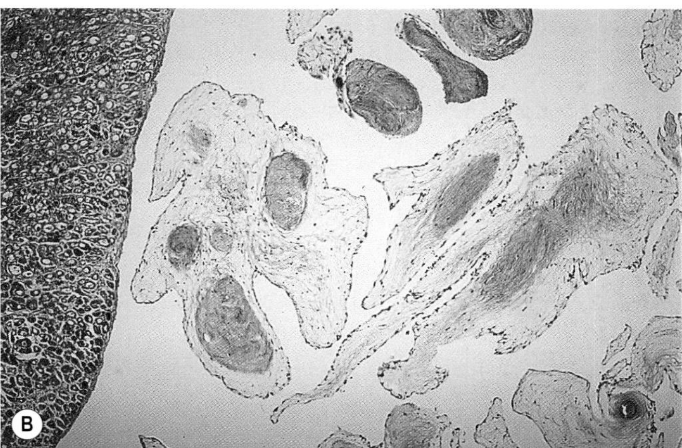

Fig. 27.15 So-called 'papillary elastofibroma'. **A**, Gross appearance. **B**, Low-power microscopic appearance. Notice the densely hyalinized central core and the flat endocardial lining.

of a mural thrombus rather than a true neoplasm, as supported by the fact that they are seen with increased frequency after cardiac surgery.[201,217]

Inflammatory myofibroblastic tumor has been reported in the heart, usually as an endocardial-based process. Its microscopic appearance is the same as that shown by this process in other

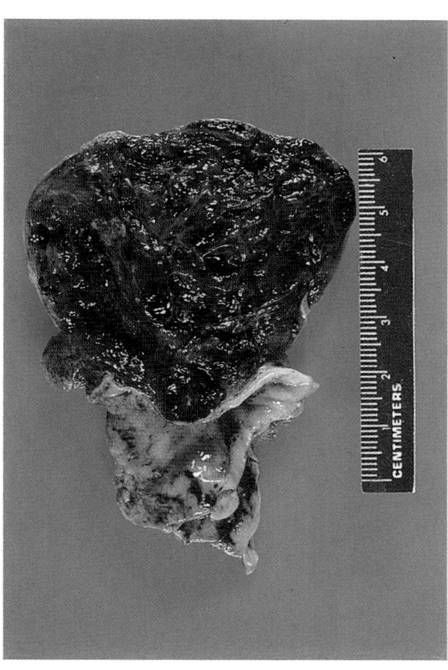

Fig. 27.16 Gross appearance of a large angiosarcoma of the heart.

locations. No metastases have been reported, but the lesion can result in myocardial infarct, syncope, and sudden death.[193,196,218,231]

Paraganglioma can present as a primary intracardiac neoplasm. The left atrium is the most common location; hypertension and elevated urine catecholamine levels are often present, in which case the term extra-adrenal pheochromocytoma has been used. The microscopic, ultrastructural, and immunohistochemical features are similar to those of paraganglioma elsewhere, including an occasional pigmented example[213,222] (see Chapter 16).

Other primary tumors of the heart include *granular cell tumor* (not to be mistaken for rhabdomyoma),[203] *hemangioma*[237] (including the epithelioid or histiocytoid variety[198,216]), *lymphangioma*,[212] *lipoma*[239,241] (to be distinguished from lipomatous hypertrophy of the atrial septum[190]), *angiolipoma*,[215] *fibroma*,[207] *schwannoma*,[224] *ganglioneuroma*,[205,227] and *benign teratoma*.[236]

Other non-neoplastic conditions reported in the heart are *ectopic thyroid*,[214] *extramedullary hematopoiesis*,[208] *inflammatory fibrosclerosis*,[238] and *Rosai–Dorfman disease*.[221,229]

Primary malignant tumors

Sarcomas of the heart are exceptionally rare.[247,249,257,269] Some of them are highly pleomorphic and unclassifiable even with the help of ultrastructural and immunohistochemical techniques. Of those that can be placed into a specific category, *angiosarcoma* is the most common.[260,263,266] It is typically located in the atrium, where it presents as a large mass (Fig. 27.16). Its microscopic appearance may be similar to that of angiosarcoma elsewhere (see Chapter 25), but the majority are poorly differentiated tumors. Ultrastructural and immunohistochemical features of endothelial differentiation can be demonstrated in some of the cases.[280] *Kaposi sarcoma* can involve the heart in its generalized form, an event that seems to be more common in the AIDS setting. The second most common category of sarcoma is that of *myosarcoma*, either *leiomyosarcoma* or

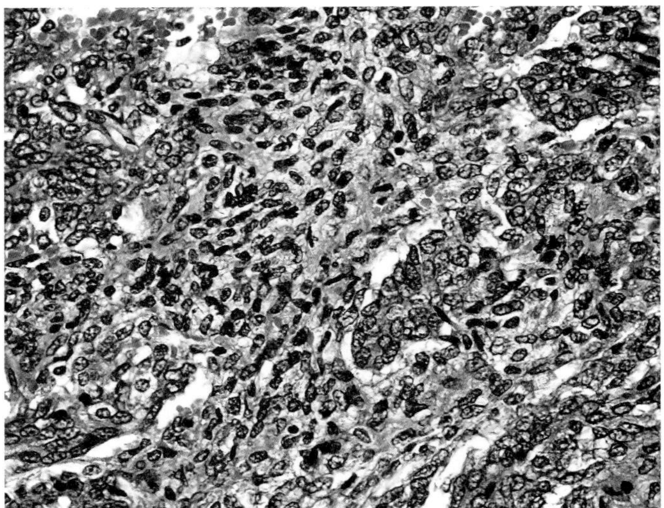

Fig. 27.17 Primary synovial sarcoma of heart showing typical biphasic appearance.

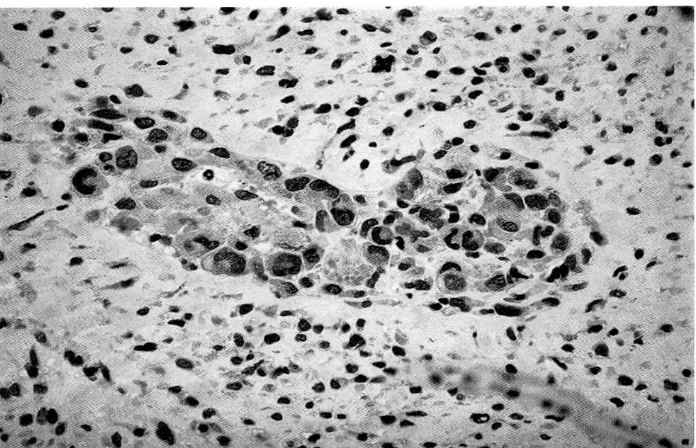

Fig. 27.18 High-grade sarcoma of heart, not further classifiable. It is not unusual for these tumors to show a ring of epithelioid large tumor cells in a perivascular location.

rhabdomyosarcoma (particularly the latter).[246] The leiomyosarcomas can have spindle cell, epithelioid, or myxoid features.[277,278] Some of them contain scattered osteoclast-like multinucleated giant cells, like those more commonly seen in leiomyosarcomas of the uterine corpus.[265] Other types described include myxofibrosarcoma,[282] so-called *malignant fibrous histiocytoma*,[270,275] *osteosarcoma*,[248,281] *fibrosarcoma, liposarcoma, synovial sarcoma*[264,274] (Fig. 27.17), *Ewing sarcoma/primitive neuroectodermal tumor* (*PNET*),[253] and *malignant peripheral nerve sheath tumor*.[276] It is possible that some of the sarcomas with prominent myxoid features represent the malignant counterpart of cardiac myxoma.[267] A feature which, although not specific, is seen often in high-grade sarcomas of the heart and large vessel, is the presence of plump epithelioid cells in a perivascular location (Fig. 27.18).

All of these tumor types occur almost always in adults, but a handful of pediatric cases are on record, including examples of *rhabdoid tumor*.[279]

Most patients with primary heart sarcomas present with intractable congestive heart failure, arrhythmias, or signs of superior vena cava obstruction. The initial diagnosis is best made with echocardiography.[251] In rare cases, a metastatic lesion is the first manifestation of the disease.[259] It has been pointed out that malignant tumors are more frequently found in the right side of the heart and that benign neoplasms are more common on the left side.[246]Surgical excision is the treatment of choice, but the prognosis remains dismal.[251,256]

Malignant lymphoma presenting as a primary heart tumor is very rare.[250,255] Most of the reported cases have been of diffuse large B-cell type.[273] AIDS and other immunocompromised patients are at an increased risk,[254,258,261] but these tumors also occur in immunocompetent individuals.[252] Some cases have been reported in association with cardiaic prostheses.[272] Secondary cardiac involvement by advanced malignant lymphoma or leukemia is a relatively common event, although it is rarely detected ante mortem; in a few instances, it constitutes the immediate cause of death.[271] The lymphoproliferative lesion associated with EBV seen in cardiac transplant recipients is discussed on page 2274. Suffice it to say here that the majority of the lymphomas developing in the transplanted heart are of B-cell type accompanied by an important reactive T-cell component.[268] It should also be mentioned that the usual type of malignant lymphoma of the heart shows no association with EBV.[262]

Metastatic tumors

Involvement of the heart by metastatic carcinoma or by generalized malignant lymphoma is a more common event than primary malignancy of this organ, by a factor of 30 to 1;[285,291] however, it is rarely seen as a biopsy or surgical specimen unless the disease affects the pericardium preferentially.[284,289] Any portion of the heart can be involved, including the conducting system, the latter exceptionally resulting in complete cardiac block.[290]

In the majority of carcinomas metastatic to the heart, the primary tumor is in the thoracic cavity or contiguous areas, and the tumor reaches the heart by metastasizing to the mediastinal lymph nodes and from there extending in a retrograde fashion to the cardiac lymph vessels.[286] Malignant tumors with a marked tendency to spread to the heart by the hematogenous route are malignant melanoma; carcinomas of kidney, lung, and breast; choriocarcinomas; and childhood rhabdomyosarcoma.[283,288] Exceptionally, the metastatic heart lesion presents as an isolated nodule, amenable to surgical therapy (Fig. 27.19).[287]

Pericardium

Pericardial (coelomic) cysts are discussed together with all other mediastinal cysts in Chapter 9.

Other congenital abnormalities are extremely rare; they include the presence of ectopic tissue such as liver.[302]

Pericarditis is of importance to the surgical pathologist for several reasons. A diagnosis of tuberculous pericarditis or sarcoidosis can be made from a pericardial open biopsy. Acute nonspecific pericarditis[306] and purulent pericarditis[303] are rarely biopsied, but the former may be troublesome because of the sometimes extreme degree of mesothelial hyperplasia that accompanies it and that can simulate malignancy. Chronic pericarditis is often accompanied by fibrosis and calcification, which may lead to constriction (so-called 'constrictive pericarditis'). This may result from tuberculosis and other infections, collagen–vascular diseases, malignant tumors, trauma, surgery, radiation therapy, or chemotherapy.[311,313] Chronic pericarditis and pericardial constriction are the most common manifestations of radiation damage to the heart.[300,313,314] The interval

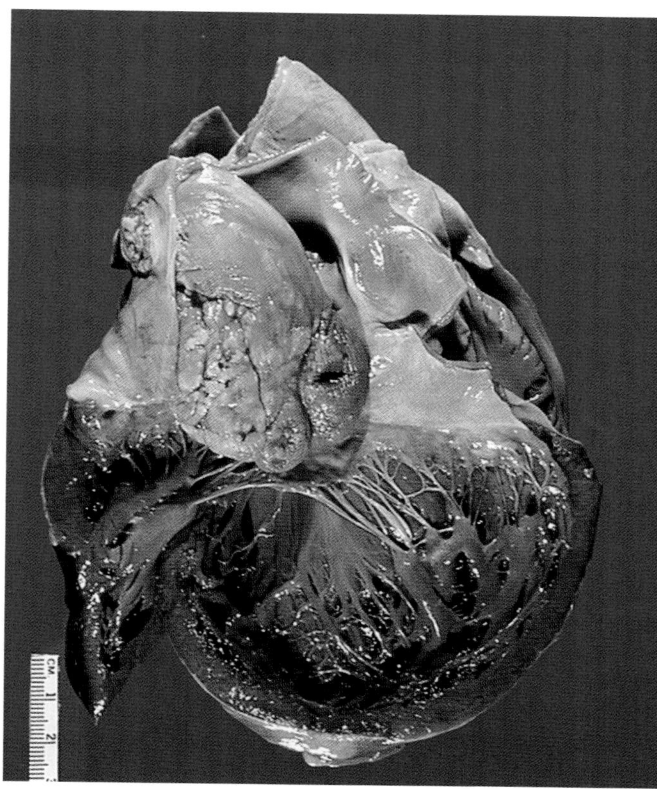

Fig. 27.19 Large metastatic carcinoma in left atrium that was continuous with tumor in left pulmonary vein. This mass simulated an atrial myxoma by echocardiography. The primary tumor was a mucoepidermoid carcinoma of left submaxillary gland.

between the radiation and the onset of the disease is usually between 50 and 125 months. Pathologic examination usually shows only dense fibrosis with deposits of calcium and a scanty inflammatory infiltrate. Residual granulomas may be found in the cases of tuberculous etiology, and atypical fibroblasts in those related to radiation.

Castleman disease located within the pericardial sac has been described.[315]

Multilocular mesothelial inclusion cyst of the pericardium is morphologically and probably pathogenetically equivalent to the condition that bears the same name in the peritoneal cavity. Although originally designated as benign multicystic mesothelioma, it probably represents a reactive change secondary to chronic irritation.[297]

Mesotheliomas of the pericardium occur, but their frequency is much less than that for similar tumors in the pleura or peritoneum. They have been reported in the setting of tuberous sclerosis[307] and may present as a single well-circumscribed mass, as multiple tumors, or as a diffuse growth encasing the heart. Sometimes, they coexist with a pleural mesothelioma. Microscopically, the appearance varies from epithelial to spindle shaped, with a frequent admixture of these elements. Pure spindle-cell (sarcomatoid) mesotheliomas are particularly unusual.[299] As in the pleura, acid mucopolysaccharides are often produced by the tumor cells. The differential diagnosis is with mesothelial hyperplasia and metastatic carcinoma. Demonstration of continuity between the tumor and the mesothelial lining cells favors a mesothelial nature for the proliferation but is not specific for it. Because of the extreme rarity of pericardial mesotheliomas and the fact that reactive mesothelial proliferation can be particularly florid in the pericardium, one should be very cautious in making a diagnosis of malignancy under these circumstances.

Most mesotheliomas of the pericardium occur in adults and are diffuse and malignant. They may locally infiltrate the superficial myocardium and even metastasize to the mediastinal lymph nodes and lungs.[298] Exceptionally, peripheral lymphadenopathy is the first manifestation of the disease.[316] Localized mesotheliomas (which are vanishingly rare) are amenable to surgical excision.[309]

Other primary tumors of the pericardium are exceptionally rare. One such group is represented by *germ cell tumors*: both mature teratoma and yolk sac tumor (endodermal sac tumor) have been reported in this location.[296,308,310] *Angiosarcoma* of pericardium may coat the pericardium in a diffuse fashion, thus simulating the pattern of growth of mesothelioma;[312] some of these have been radiation induced.[301] There have been isolated case reports of pericardial *myolipoma* (positive for estrogen receptors),[295] *ectopic thymoma* (associated with myasthenia gravis),[293]and *fibroma*.[304]

Metastatic carcinoma to the pericardium usually originates in the lung in the form of direct extension or lymphatic permeation.[304] It may result in constrictive 'pericarditis' as a result of the associated intense desmoplastic reaction (see p. 2282). Other tumors that commonly give rise to pericardial metastases are breast carcinoma, malignant melanoma, and malignant lymphoma.[292,305] Cytology is the most important technique for the evaluation of malignant pericardial effusions. Pericardial biopsy may be necessary in some cases to confirm the diagnosis. The sensitivity of DNA ploidy is too low to be of practical utility.[294]

References

INTRODUCTION

1 Cohn LH (ed.). Cardiac surgery in the adult. New York, 2008, McGraw-Hill.

2 Gardner TJ, Spray TL. Operative cardiac surgery, ed. 5. New York, 2004, Oxford University Press.

3 Kouchoukos NT, Blackstone E, Doty D, Hanley F, Karp R. Kirklin/Barratt-Boyes cardiac surgery: morphology, diagnostic criteria, natural history, techniques, results, and indications, ed. 3. Edinburgh, 2003, Churchill Livingstone.

4 Stark JF, de Leval MR, Tsang VT (eds). Surgery for congenital heart defects, ed. 3. Chichester, 2006, Wiley.

NORMAL ANATOMY

5 Berry GJ, Billingham ME. Normal heart. In: Mills SE (ed.): Histology for pathologists, ed. 3. Philadelphia, 2007, Lippincott Williams & Wilkins, pp. 527–546.

MYOCARDIAL BIOPSY

6 Burke AP, Farb A, Robinowitz M, Virmani R. Serial sectioning and multiple level examination of endomyocardial biopsies for the diagnosis of myocarditis. Mod Pathol 1991, **4**: 690–693.

7 Fenoglio JJ, Marboe CC. Endomyocardial biopsy. An overview. Hum Pathol 1987, **18**: 609–612.

8 Flipse TR, Tazelaar HD, Holmes DR Jr. Diagnosis of malignant cardiac disease by endomyocardial biopsy. Mayo Clin Proc 1990, **65**: 1415–1422.

9 Frustaci A, Pieroni M, Chimenti C. The role of endomyocardial biopsy in the diagnosis of cardiomyopathies. Ital Heart J 2002, **3**: 348–353.

10 Hammond EH. Utility of ultrastructural studies of cardiac biopsy specimens. Ultrastruct Pathol 1994, **18**: 201–202.

11 Hauck AJ, Kearney DL, Edwards WD. Evaluation of postmortem endomyocardial biopsy specimens from 38 patients with lymphocytic myocarditis. Implications for role of sampling error. Mayo Clin Proc 1989, **64**: 1235–1245.

12 Lie JT. Diagnostic histology of myocardial disease in endomyocardial biopsies and at autopsy. Pathol Annu 1989, **24**(Pt 2): 255–293.

13 Ursell PC, Fenoglio JJ. Spectrum of cardiac disease diagnosed by endomyocardial biopsy. Pathol Annu 1984, **19**(Pt 2): 197–219.

14 Veinot JP. Diagnostic endomyocardial biopsy pathology: secondary myocardial diseases and other clinical indications – review. Can J Cardiol 2002, **18**: 287–296.

15 Winters GL, Costanzo-Nordin MR. Pathological findings in 2300 consecutive endomyocardial biopsies. Mod Pathol 1991, **4**: 441–448.

CARDIOMYOPATHY AND MYOCARDITIS

16 Anderson DW, Virmani R. Emerging patterns of heart disease in human immunodeficiency virus infection. Hum Pathol 1990, **21**: 253–259.

17 Aretz HT. Myocarditis. The Dallas criteria. Hum Pathol 1987, **18**: 619–624.

18 Atkinson JB, Connor DH, Robinowitz M, McAllister HA, Virmani R. Cardiac fungal infections. Review of autopsy finding in 60 patients. Hum Pathol 1984, **15**: 935–942.

19 Atkinson JB, Virmani R. Congestive heart failure due to coronary artery disease without myocardial infarction. Clinicopathologic description of an unusual cardiomyopathy. Hum Pathol 1989, **20**: 1155–1162.

20 Billingham ME. Some recent advances in cardiac pathology. Hum Pathol 1979, **10**: 367–386.

21 Billingham ME, Bristow MR, Glatstein E, Mason JW, Masek MA, Daniels JR. Adriamycin cardiotoxicity. Endomyocardial biopsy evidence of enhancement by irradiation. Am J Surg Pathol 1977, **1**: 17–23.

22 Boss JM, Towbin JA, Ackerman MJ. Diagnostic, prognostic, and therapeutic implications of genetic testing for hypertrophic cardiomyopathy. J Am Coll Cardiol 2009, **54**: 201–211.

23 Buja LM, Roberts WC. Iron in the heart, etiology and clinical significance. Am J Med 1971, **51**: 209–221.

24 Burke AP, Saenger J, Mullick F, Virmani R. Hypersensitivity myocarditis. Arch Pathol Lab Med 1991, **115**: 764–769.

25 Calabrese F, Rigo E, Milanesi O, Boffa GM, Angelini A, Valente M, Thiene G. Molecular diagnosis of myocarditis and dilated cardiomyopathy in children: clinicopathologic features and prognostic implications. Diagn Mol Pathol 2002, **11**: 212–221.

26 Chow LH, Ye Y, Linder J, McManus BM. Phenotypic analysis of infiltrating cells in human myocarditis. An immunohistochemical study in paraffin-embedded tissue. Arch Pathol Lab Med 1989, **113**: 1357–1362.

27 Cooper LT Jr, Berry GJ, Shabetai R, for the Multicenter Giant Cell Myocarditis Study Group Investigators. Idiopathic giant-cell myocarditis – natural history and treatment. N Engl J Med 1997, **336**: 1860–1866.

28 Cooper LT Jr. Myocarditis. N Engl J Med 2009, **360**: 1526–1538.

29 d'Amati G, Di Gioia CR, Gallo P. Pathological findings of HIV-associated cardiovascular disease. Ann N Y Acad Sci 2001, **946**: 23–45.

30 Darcy T, Mullick F, Schell L, Virmani R. Distinguishing features of myocarditis. Hypersensitivity vs. idiopathic myocarditis [abstract]. Lab Invest 1988, **58**: 21A.

31 Davies MJ, McKernna WJ. Hypertrophic cardiomyopathy. Pathology and pathogenesis. Histopathology 1995, **26**: 493–500.

32 Eck M, Greiner A, Kandolf R, Schumausser B, Marx A, Müller-Hermelink HK. Active fulminant myocarditis characterized by T-lymphocytes expressing the gamma-delta T-cell receptor: a new disease entity? Am J Surg Pathol 1997, **21**: 1109–1112.

33 Edwalds GM, Said JW, Block MI, Herscher LL, Siegel RJ, Fishbein MC. Myocytolysis (vacuolar degeneration) of myocardium. Immunohistochemical evidence of viability. Hum Pathol 1984, **15**: 753–756.

34 Edwards WD. Cardiomyopathies. Hum Pathol 1987, **18**: 625–635.

35 Edwards WD, Holmes DR Jr, Reeder GS. Diagnosis of active lymphocytic myocarditis by endomyocardial biopsy. Quantitative criteria for light microscopy. Mayo Clin Proc 1982, **57**: 419–425.

36 Elliott P, Andersson B, Arbustini E, Bilinska Z, Cecchi F, Charron P, Dubourg O, Kühl U, Maisch B, McKenna WJ, Monserrat L, Pankuweit S, Rapezzi C, Seferovic P, Tavazzi L, Keren A. Classification of the cardiomyopathies: a position statement from the European Society of Cardiology Working Group on Myocardial and Pericardial Diseases. Eur Heart J 2008, **29**: 270–276.

37 Fenoglio JJ Jr, McAllister HA Jr, Mullick FG. Drug related myocarditis. I. Hypersensitivity myocarditis. Hum Pathol 1981, **12**: 900–907.

38 Fenoglio JJ Jr, Ursell PC, Kellogg CF, Drusin RE, Weiss MB. Diagnosis and classification of myocarditis by endomyocardial biopsy. N Engl J Med 1983, **308**: 12–18.

39 Ferrans VJ, Morrow AG, Roberts WC. Myocardial ultrastructure in idiopathic hypertrophic subaortic stenosis. A study of operatively excised left ventricular outflow tract muscle in 14 patients. Circulation 1972, **45**: 769–792.

40 Ferrans VJ, Roberts WC. Myocardial biopsy. A useful diagnostic procedure or only a research tool? Am J Cardiol 1978, **41**: 965–967.

41 Gravanis MB, Ansari AA. Idiopathic cardiomyopathies. A review of pathologic studies and mechanism of pathogenesis. Arch Pathol Lab Med 1987, **111**: 915–929.

42 Henderson IC, Frei E III. Adriamycin and the heart [editorial]. N Engl J Med 1979, **300**: 310–311.

43 Hughes SE. The pathology of hypertrophic cardiomyopathy. Histopathology 2004, **44**: 412–427.

44 Jaenke RS, Fajardo LF. Adriamycin-induced myocardial lesions. Report of a workshop. Am J Surg Pathol 1977, **1**: 55–60.

45 Kindermann I, Kindermann M, Kandolf R, Klingel K, Bültmann B, Müller T, Lindinger A, Böhm M. Predictors of outcome in patients with suspected myocarditis. Circulation 2008, **118**: 639–648.

46 Kollo IJ, Edwards WD, Seward JB. Right ventricular dysplasia. The Mayo Clinic experience. Mayo Clin Proc 1995, **70**: 541–548.

47 Lamke GT, Allen RD, Edwards WD, Tazelaar HD, Danielson GK. Surgical pathology of subaortic septal myectomy associated with hypertrophic cardiomyopathy. A study of 204 cases (1996–2000). Cardiovasc Pathol 2003, **12**: 149–158.

48 Lie JT. Diagnostic histology of myocardial disease in endomyocardial biopsies and at autopsy. Pathol Annu 1989, **24**(Pt 2): 255–293.

49 Litovsky SH, Burke AP, Virmani R. Giant cell myocarditis: an entity distinct from sarcoidosis characterized by multiphasic myocyte destruction by cytotoxic T cells and histiocytic giant cells. Mod Pathol 1996, **9**: 1126–1134.

50 Maisch B, Portig I, Ristic A, Hufnagel G, Pankuweit S. Definition of inflammatory cardiomyopathy (myocarditis): on the way to consensus. A status report. Herz 2000, **25**: 200–209.

51 Maron BJ, Bonow RO, Cannon RO III, Leon MB, Epstein SE. Hypertrophic cardiomyopathy. Interrelations of clinical manifestations, pathophysiology, and therapy. N Engl J Med 1987, **316**: 780–789; 844–852.

52 Mooney EE, Kenan DJ, Sweeney EC, Gaede JT. Myocarditis in Whipple's disease: an unsuspected cause of symptoms and sudden death. Mod Pathol 1997, **10**: 524–529.

53 Olson LJ, Gertz MA, Edwards WD, Li C-Y, Pellikka PA, Holmes DR Jr, Tajik AJ, Kyle RA. Senile cardiac amyloidosis with myocardial dysfunction. Diagnosis by endomyocardial biopsy and immunohistochemistry. N Engl J Med 1987, **317**: 738–742.

54 Roberts WC, McAllister HA Jr, Ferrans VJ. Sarcoidosis of the heart. A clinicopathologic study of 35 necropsy patients (group I) and review of 78 previously reported necropsy patients (group II). Am J Med 1977, **63**: 86–108.

55 Roldan EO, Moskowitz L, Hensley GT. Pathology of the heart in acquired immunodeficiency syndrome. Arch Pathol Lab Med 1987, **111**: 943–946.

56 Rosai J, Lascano EF. Basophilic (mucoid) degeneration of myocardium. A disorder of glycogen metabolism. Am J Pathol 1970, **61**: 99–116.

57 Rose AG. Cardiac tuberculosis. A study of 19 patients. Arch Pathol Lab Med 1987, **111**: 422–426.

58 Rose AG, Beck W. Dilated (congestive) cardiomyopathy. A syndrome of severe cardiac dysfunction with remarkably few morphological features of myocardial damage. Histopathology 1985, **9**: 367–379.

59 Schnitt SJ, Ciano PS, Schoen FJ. Quantitation of lymphocytes in endomyocardial biopsies. Use and limitations of antibodies to leukocyte common antigen. Hum Pathol 1987, **18**: 796–800.

60 Spirito P, Chiarella F, Carratino L, Berisso MZ, Bellotti P, Vecchio C. Clinical course and prognosis of hypertrophic cardiomyopathy in an outpatient population. N Engl J Med 1989, **320**: 749–755.

61 Tamura S, Takahashi M, Kawamura S, Ishihara T. Basophilic degeneration of the myocardium. Histological, immunohistochemical and immunoelectronmicroscopic studies. Histopathology 1995, **26**: 501–508.

62 Tazelaar HD, Billingham ME. Leukocytic infiltrates in idiopathic dilated cardiomyopathy. A source of confusion with active myocarditis. Am J Surg Pathol 1986, **10**: 405–412.

63 Tazelaar HD, Billingham ME. The surgical pathology of hypertrophic cardiomyopathy. Arch Pathol Lab Med 1987, **111**: 257–260.

64 Theaker JM, Gatter KC, Brown DC, Heryet A, Davies MJ. An investigation into the nature of giant cells in cardiac and skeletal muscle. Hum Pathol 1988, **19**: 974–979.

65 Ursell PC, Albala A, Fenoglio JJ Jr. Diagnosis of acute rheumatic carditis by endomyocardial biopsy. Hum Pathol 1982, **13**: 677–679.

66 Veinot JP, Edwards WD. Pathology of radiation-induced heart disease. A surgical and autopsy study of 27 cases. Hum Pathol 1996, **27**: 766–773.

67 Weinstein C, Fenoglio JJ. Myocarditis. Hum Pathol 1987, **18**: 613–618.

68 Wijetunga M, Rockson S. Myocarditis in systemic lupus erythematosus. Am J Med 2002, **113**: 419–423.

69 Wu LA, Lapeyre AC III, Cooper LT. Current role of endomyocardial biopsy in the management of dilated cardiomyopathy and myocarditis. Mayo Clin Proc 2001, **76**: 1030–1038.

HEART TRANSPLANT

70 Abu-Farsakh H, Cagle PT, Buffone GJ, Bruner JM, Weilbaecher D, Greenberg SD. Heart allograft involvement with Epstein–Barr virus-associated posttransplant lymphoproliferative disorder. Arch Pathol Lab Med 1992, **116**: 93–95.

71 Arbustini E, Grasso M, Diegoli M, Percivalle E, Grossi P, Bramerio M, Campana C, Goggi C, Gavazzi A, Vigano M. Histopathologic and molecular profile of human cytomegalovirus infections in patients with heart transplants. Am J Clin Pathol 1992, **98**: 205–213.

72 Billingham ME. Some recent advances in cardiac pathology. Hum Pathol 1979, **10**: 367–386.

73 Chen JM, Barr ML, Chadburn A, Frizzera G, Schenkel FA, Sciacca RR, Reison DS, Addonizio LJ, Rose EA, Knowles DM. Management of lymphoproliferative disorders after cardiac transplantation. Ann Thorac Surg 1993, **56**: 527–538.

74 Chomette G, Auriol M, Delcourt A, Karkouche B, Cabrol A, Cabrol C. Human cardiac transplants. Diagnosis of rejection by endomyocardial biopsy. Causes of death (about 30 autopsies). Virchows Arch [A] 1985, **407**: 295–307.

75 Forbes RD, Rowan RA, Billingham ME. Endocardial infiltrates in human heart transplants. A serial biopsy analysis comparing four immunosuppression protocols. Hum Pathol 1990, **21**: 850–855.

76 Gaudin PB, Rayburn BK, Hutchins GM, Kasper EK, Baughman KL, Goodman SN, Lecks LE, Baumgartner WA, Hruban RH. Peritransplant injury to the myocardium associated with the development of accelerated arteriosclerosis in heart transplant recipients. Am J Surg Pathol 1994, **18**: 338–346.

77 Hammond EH. Solid organ transplantation pathology. Major problems in pathology, **vol. 30**. Philadelphia, 1994, W.B. Saunders.

78 Hawkins ET, Levine TB, Goss SJ, Moosvi A, Levine AB. Hypersensitivity myocarditis in the explanted hearts of transplant recipients. Reappraisal of pathologic criteria and their clinical implications. Pathol Annu 1995, **30**(Pt 1): 287–304.

79 Kemnitz J, Cohnert T, Schnäfers H-J, Helmke M, Wahlers T, Herrmann G, Schmidt RM, Haverich A. A classification of cardiac allograft rejection. A modification of the classification by Billingham. Am J Surg Pathol 1987, **11**: 503–515.

80 Kottke-Marchant K, Ratliff NB. Endomyocardial lymphocytic infiltrates in cardiac transplant recipients. Incidence and characterization. Arch Pathol Lab Med 1989, **113**: 690–698.

81 Kottke-Marchant K, Ratliff NB. Endomyocardial biopsy. Pathologic findings in cardiac transplant recipients. Pathol Annu 1990, **25**(Pt 1): 211–244.

82 Morrison VA, Dunn DL, Manivel JC, Gajl-Peczalska KJ, Peterson BA. Clinical characteristics of post-transplant lymphoproliferative disorders. Am J Med 1994, **97**: 14–24.

83 Olsen SL, Wagoner LE, Hammond EH, Taylor DO, Yowell RL, Ensley RD, Bristow MR, O'Connell JB, Renlund DG. Vascular rejection in heart transplantation. Clinical correlation, treatment options, and future considerations. J Heart Lung Transplant 1993, **12**: S135–S142.

84 Pardo-Mindan FJ, Lozano MD, Contreras-Mejuto F, de Alava E. Pathology of heart transplant through endomyocardial biopsy. Semin Diagn Pathol 1992, **9**: 238–248.

85 Pitman SD, Rowsell EH, Cao JD, Huang Q, Wang J. Anaplastic large cell lymphoma associated with Epstein–Barr virus following cardiac transplant. Am J Surg Pathol 2004, **28**: 410–415.

86 Pomerance A, Stovin P. Heart transplant pathology. The British experience. J Clin Pathol 1985, **38**: 146–159.

87 Rowan RA, Billingham ME. Pathologic changes in the long-term transplanted heart. A morphometric study of myocardial hypertrophy, vascularity, and fibrosis. Hum Pathol 1990, **21**: 767–772.

88 Tan CD, Baldwin WM 3rd, Rodriguez ER. Update on cardiac transplantation pathology. Arch Pathol Lab Med 2007, **131**: 1169–1191.

89 Tazelaar HD, Gay RE, Rowan RA, Billingham ME, Gay S. Collagen profile in the transplanted heart. Hum Pathol 1990, **21**: 424–428.

90 Uys CJ, Rose AG. Cardiac transplantation. Aspects of the pathology. Pathol Annu 1982, **17**(Pt 2): 147–178.

91 Weissman DJ, Ferry JA, Harris NL, Louis DN, Delmonico F, Spiro I. Posttransplantation lymphoproliferative disorders in solid organ recipients are predominantly aggressive tumors of host origin. Am J Clin Pathol 1995, **103**: 748–755.

92 Zerbe TR, Arena V. Diagnostic reliability of endomyocardial biopsy for assessment of cardiac allograft rejection. Hum Pathol 1988, **19**: 1307–1314.

CARDIAC VALVES

93 Altrichter PM, Olson LJ, Edwards WD, Puga FJ, Danielson GK. Surgical pathology of the pulmonary valve. A study of 116 cases spanning 15 years. Mayo Clin Proc 1989, **64**: 1352–1360.

94 Billingham ME. Some recent advances in cardiac pathology. Hum Pathol 1979, **10**: 367–386.

95 Carabello BA, Crawford FA Jr. Valvular heart disease. N Engl J Med 1997, **337**: 32–41.

96 Clark RM, Anderson W. Rheumatic activity in auricular appendages removed at mitral valvoplasty. Am J Pathol 1955, **31**: 809–819.

97 Cooper JH. Localized dystrophic amyloidosis of heart valves. Hum Pathol 1983, **14**: 649–653.

98 Dare AJ, Harrity PJ, Tazelaar HD, Edwards WD, Mullany CJ. Evaluation of surgically excised mitral valves. Revised recommendations based on changing operative procedures in the 1990s. Hum Pathol 1993, **24**: 1286–1293.

99 Dare AJ, Veinot JP, Edwards WD, Tazelaar HD, Schaff HV. New observations on the etiology of aortic valve disease. A surgical pathologic study of 236 cases from 1990. Hum Pathol 1993, **24**: 1330–1338.

100 Davies MJ. Pathology of cardiac valves. London, 1980, Butterworth.

101 Ferrans VJ, Tomita Y, Hilbert SL, Jones M, Roberts WC. Pathology of bioprosthetic cardiac valves. Hum Pathol 1987, **18**: 586–595.

102 Gravanis MB, Campbell WG Jr. The syndrome of prolapse of the mitral valve. Arch Pathol Lab Med 1982, **106**: 369–374.

103 Groom DA, Starke WR. Cartilaginous metaplasia in calcific aortic valve disease. Am J Clin Pathol 1990, **93**: 809–812.

104 Hanson TP, Edwards BS, Edwards JE. Pathology of surgically excised mitral valves. One hundred consecutive cases. Arch Pathol Lab Med 1985, **109**: 823–828.

105 Hauck AJ, Freeman DP, Ackermann DM, Danielson GK, Edwards WD. Surgical pathology of the tricuspid valve. A study of 363 cases spanning 25 years. Mayo Clin Proc 1988, **63**: 851–863.

106 Lee I, Park S, Hwang I, Kim MJ, Nah SS, Yoo B, Song JK. Cardiac Behçet disease presenting as aortic valvulitis/aortitis or right heart inflammatory mass: a clinicopathologic study of 12 cases. Am J Surg Pathol 2008, **32**: 390–398.

107 Love GL, Restrepo C. Aschoff bodies of rheumatic carditis are granulomatous lesions of histiocytic origin. Mod Pathol 1988, **1**: 256–261.

108 Morales AR, Romanelli R, Boucek RJ, Tate LG, Alvarez RT, Davis JT. Myxoid heart disease. An assessment of extravalvular cardiac pathology in severe mitral valve prolapse. Hum Pathol 1992, **23**: 129–137.

109 Murphy SK, Rogler WC, Fleming WH, McManus BM. Retraction of bioprosthetic heart valve cusps. A cause of wide-open regurgitation in right-sided heart valves. Hum Pathol 1988, **19**: 140–147.

110 Olson LJ, Subramanian R, Ackermann DM, Orszulak TA, Edwards WD. Surgical pathology of the mitral valve. A study of 712 cases spanning 21 years. Mayo Clin Proc 1987, **62**: 22–34.

111 Passik CS, Ackermann DM, Pluth JR, Edwards WD. Temporal changes in the causes of aortic stenosis. A surgical pathologic study of 646 cases. Mayo Clin Proc 1987, **62**: 119–123.

112 Peterson MD, Roach RM, Edwards JE. Types of aortic stenosis in surgically removed valves. Arch Pathol Lab Med 1985, **109**: 829–832.

113 Robboy SJ, Kaiser J. Pathogenesis of fungal infection on heart valve prostheses. Hum Pathol 1975, **6**: 711–715.

114 Roberts WC, Morrow AG. Cardiac valves and the surgical pathologist. Arch Pathol 1966, **82**: 309–313.

115 Rose AG. Etiology of acquired valvular heart disease in adults. A survey of 18,132 autopsies and 100 consecutive valve-replacement operations. Arch Pathol Lab Med 1986, **110**: 385–388.

116 Schoen FJ. Surgical pathology of removed natural and prosthetic heart valves. Hum Pathol 1987, **18**: 558–567.

117 Schoen FJ, Hobson CE. Anatomic analysis of removed prosthetic heart valves. Causes of failure of 33 mechanical valves and 58 bioprostheses, 1980 to 1983. Hum Pathol 1985, **16**: 549–559.

118 Schoen FJ, Levy RJ, Piehler HR. Pathological considerations in replacement cardiac valves. Cardiovasc Pathol 1992, **1**: 29–52.

119 Schoen FJ, Sutton MSJ. Contemporary issues in the pathology of valvular heart disease. Hum Pathol 1987, **18**: 568–576.

120 Siddiqui RF, Abraham JR, Butany J. Bioprosthetic heart valves: modes of failure. Histopathology 2009, **55**: 135–144.

121 Silver MD. Cardiac pathology. A look at the last five years. II. The pathology of cardiovascular prostheses. Hum Pathol 1974, 5: 127–138.

122 Silver MD. Late complications of prosthetic heart valves. Arch Pathol Lab Med 1978, **102**: 281–284.

123 Silver MD, Butany J. Mechanical heart valves. Methods of examination, complications, and modes of failure. Hum Pathol 1987, **18**: 577–585.

124 Silver MD, Datta BN, Bowes VF. A key to identify heart valve prostheses. Arch Pathol 1975, **99**: 132–138.

125 Steiner I, Kasparová P, Kohout A, Dominik J. Bone formation in cardiac valves: a histopathological study of 128 cases. Virchows Arch 2007, **450**: 653–657.

126 Subramanian R, Olson LJ, Edwards WD. Surgical pathology of pure aortic stenosis. A study of 374 cases. Mayo Clin Proc 1984, **59**: 683–690.

127 Subramanian R, Olson LJ, Edwards WD. Surgical pathology of combined aortic stenosis and insufficiency. A study of 213 cases. Mayo Clin Proc 1985, **60**: 247–254.

128 van der Bel-Kahn J, Becker AE. The surgical pathology of rheumatic and floppy mitral valves. Distinctive morphologic features upon gross examination. Am J Surg Pathol 1986, **10**: 282–292.

129 Virmani R, Atkinson JB, Forman MB, Robinowitz M. Mitral valve prolapse. Hum Pathol 1987, **18**: 596–602.

130 Vongpatanasin W, Hillis LD, Lange RA. Prosthetic heart valves. N Engl J Med 1996, **335**: 407–416.

CORONARY ARTERY BYPASS

131 Kern WH, Wells WJ, Meyer BW. The pathology of surgically excised aortocoronary saphenous vein bypass grafts. Am J Surg Pathol 1981, **5**: 491–496.

132 Ratliff NB, Myles JL. Rapidly progressive atherosclerosis in aortocoronary saphenous vein grafts. Possible immune-mediated disease. Arch Pathol Lab Med 1989, **113**: 772–776.

133 Smith SH, Geer JC. Morphology of saphenous vein-coronary artery bypass grafts. Seven to 116 months after surgery. Arch Pathol Lab Med 1983, **107**: 13–18.

134 Yutani C, Imakita M, Ishibashi-Ueda H. Histopathological study of aorto-coronary bypass grafts with special reference to fibrin deposits on grafted saphenous veins. Acta Pathol Jpn 1989, **39**: 425–432.

COARCTATION OF AORTA

135 Bergdahl L, Bjork VO, Jonasson R. Surgical correction of coarctation of the aorta. Influence of age on late results. J Thorac Cardiovasc Surg 1983, **85**: 532–536.

136 Campbell M. Natural history of coarctation of the aorta. Br Heart J 1970, **32**: 633–640.

137 Gaynor JW. Management strategies for infants with coarctation and an associated ventricular septal defect. J Thorac Cardiovasc Surg 2001, **122**: 424–426.

138 Hornung TS, Benson LN, McLaughlin PR. Interventions for aortic coarctation. Cardiol Rev 2002, **10**: 139–148.

139 Lerberg DB, Hardesty RL, Siewers RD, Zuberbuhler JR, Bahnson HT. Coarctation of the aorta in infants and children. 25 years experience. Ann Thorac Surg 1982, **33**: 159–170.

CARDIAC TUMORS

MYXOMA

140 Acebo E, Val-Bernal JF, Gómez-Romàn JJ. Prichard's structures of the fossa ovalis are not histogenetically related to cardiac myxoma. Histopathology 2001, **39**: 529–535.

141 Berrutti L, Silverman JS. Cardiac myxoma is rich in factor XIIIa positive dendrophages: immunohistochemical study of four cases. Histopathology 1996, **28**: 529–535.

142 Bertherat J, Horvath A, Groussin L, Grabar S, Boikos S, Cazabat L, Libe R, René-Corail F, Stergiopoulos S, Bourdeau I, Bei T, Clauser E, Calender A, Kirschner LS, Bertagna X, Carney JA, Stratakis CA. Mutations in regulatory subunit type 1A of cyclic adenosine 5′-monophosphate-dependent protein kinase (PRKAR1A): phenotype analysis in 353 patients and 80 different genotypes. J Clin Endocrinol Metab 2009, **94**: 2085–2091.

143 Boxer ME. Cardiac myxoma. An immunoperoxidase study of histogenesis. Histopathology 1984, **8**: 861–872.

144 Burke AP, Virmani R. Cardiac myxoma. A clinicopathologic study. Am J Clin Pathol 1993, **100**: 671–680.

145 Carney JA. Differences between nonfamilial and familial cardiac myxoma. Am J Surg Pathol 1985, **9**: 53–55.

146 Chu PH, Jung SM, Yeh TS, Lin HC, Chu JJ. MUC1, MUC2 and MUC5AC expressions in cardiac myxoma. Virchows Arch 2005, **446**: 52–55.

147 den Bakker MA, Dinjens WNM, Bekkers JA. Cardiac myxoma with atypical glandular component: report of a case. Histopathology 2005, **48**: 206–208.

148 Deshpande A, Venugopal P, Kumar AS, Chopra P. Phenotypic characterization of cellular components of cardiac myxoma: a light microscopy and immunohistochemistry study. Hum Pathol 1996, **27**: 1056–1059.

149 Dewald GW, Dahl RJ, Spurbeck JL, Carney JA, Gordon H. Chromosomally abnormal clones and nonrandom telomeric translocations in cardiac myxomas. Mayo Clin Proc 1987, **62**: 558–567.

150 Farrell DJ, Bulmer E, Angus B, Ashcroft T. Immunohistochemical expression of endothelial markers in left atrial myxomas: a study of six cases. Histopathology 1996, **28**: 147–152.

151 Feldman PS, Horvath E, Kovacs K. An ultrastructural study of seven cardiac myxomas. Cancer 1977, **40**: 2216–2232.

152 Ferrans VJ, Roberts WC. Structural features of cardiac myxomas. Histology, histochemistry and electron microscopy. Hum Pathol 1973, 4: 111–146.

153 Fine G, Morales A, Horn RC Jr. Cardiac myxoma. A morphologic and histogenetic appraisal. Cancer 1968, **22**: 1156–1162.

154 Goldman BI, Frydman C, Harpaz N, Ryan SF, Loiterman D. Glandular cardiac myxomas. Histologic, immunohistochemical, and ultrastructural evidence of epithelial differentiation. Cancer 1987, **59**: 1767–1775.

155 Govoni E, Severi B, Cenacchi G, Laschi R, Pileri S, Rivano MT, Alampi G, Branzi A. Ultrastructural and immunohistochemical contribution to the histogenesis of human cardiac myxoma. Ultrastruct Pathol 1988, **12**: 221–233.

156 Johansson L. Histogenesis of cardiac myxomas. An immunohistochemical study of 19 cases, including one with glandular structures, and review of the literature. Arch Pathol Lab Med 1989, **113**: 735–741.

157 Kasugai T, Sakurai M, Yutani C, Hirota S, Waki N, Adachi S, Kitamura Y. Sequential malignant transformation of cardiac myxoma. Acta Pathol Jpn 1990, **40**: 687–692.

158 Kodama H, Hirotani T, Suzuki Y, Ogawa S, Yamazaki K. Cardiomyogenic differentiation in cardiac myxoma expressing lineage-specific transcription factors. Am J Pathol 2002, **161**: 381–389.

159 Landon G, Ordòñez NG, Guarda LA. Cardiac myxomas. An immunohistochemical study using endothelial, histiocytic, and smooth-muscle cell markers. Arch Pathol Lab Med 1986, **110**: 116–120.

160 Lewis CM. Clinical presentation and investigation of cardiac tumors. Semin Diagn Pathol 2008, **25**: 65–68.

161 Li Y, Pan Z, Ji Y, Sheppard M, Jeffries DJ, Archard LC, Zhang H. Herpes simplex virus type 1 infection associated with atrial myxoma. Am J Pathol 2003, **163**: 2407–2412.

162 Lie JT. Petrified cardiac myxoma masquerading as organized atrial mural thrombus. Arch Pathol Lab Med 1989, **113**: 742–745.

163 McComb RD. Heterogeneous expression of factor VIII/von Willebrand factor by cardiac myxoma cells. Am J Surg Pathol 1984, **8**: 539–544.

164 Miller DV, Tazelaar HD, Handy JR, Young DA, Hernandez JC. Thymoma arising within cardiac myxoma. Am J Surg Pathol 2005, **29**: 1208–1213.

165 Orlandi A, Ciucci A, Ferlosio A, Pellegrino A, Chiariello L, Spagnoli LG. Increased expression and activity of matrix metalloproteinases characterize embolic cardiac myxomas. Am J Pathol 2005, **166**: 1619–1628.

166 Perchinsky MJ, Lichenstein SV, Tyers GF. Primary cardiac tumors: forty years' experience with 71 patients. Cancer 1997, **79**: 1809–1815.

167 Pohost GM, Pastore JO, McKusick KA, Chiotellis PN, Kapellakis GZ, Meyers GS, Dinsmore RE, Block PC. Detection of left atrial myxoma by gated radionuclide cardiac imaging. Circulation 1977, **55**: 88–92.

168 Pucci A, Bartoloni G, Tessitore E, Carney JA, Papotti M. Cytokeratin profile and neuroendocrine cells in the glandular component of cardiac myxoma. Virchows Arch 2003, **443**: 618–624.

169 Read RC, White HJ, Murphy ML, Williams D, Sun CN, Flanagan WH. The malignant potentiality of left atrial myxoma. J Thorac Cardiovasc Surg 1974, **68**: 857–868.

170 Reed RJ, Utz MP, Terezakis N. Embolic and metastatic cardiac myxoma. Am J Dermatopathol 1989, **11**: 157–165.

171 Richardson JV, Brandt B III, Doty DB, Ehrenhaft JL. Surgical treatment of atrial myxomas. Early and late results of 111 operations and review of the literature. Ann Thorac Surg 1979, **28**: 354–358.

172 Rupp GM, Heyman RA, Martinez AJ, Sekhar LN, Jungreis CA. The pathology of metastatic cardiac myxoma. Am J Clin Pathol 1989, **91**: 221–227.

173 Salyer WR, Page DL, Hutchins GM. The development of cardiac myxomas and papillary endocardial lesions from mural thrombus. Am Heart J 1975, **89**: 14–17.

174 Samaratunga H, Searle J, Cominos D, Le Fevre I. Cerebral metastasis of an atrial myxoma mimicking an epithelioid hemangioendothelioma. Am J Surg Pathol 1994, **18**: 107–111.

175 Schmitt-Graff A, Borchard F. Cardiac myxoma with a cytokeratin-immunoreactive glandular component. Pathol Res Pract 1992, **188**: 221–225.

176 Seidman JD, Berman JJ, Hitchcock CL, Becker RL Jr, Mergner W, Moore GW, Virmani R, Yetter RA. DNA analysis of cardiac myxomas. Flow cytometry and image analysis. Hum Pathol 1991, **22**: 494–500.

177 Seo IS, Warner TFCS, Colyer RA, Winkler RF. Metastasizing atrial myxoma. Am J Surg Pathol 1980, **4**: 391–399.

178 Silverman NA. Primary cardiac tumors. Ann Surg 1980, **191**: 127–138.

179 Tanimura A, Kitazono M, Nagayama K, Tanaka S, Kosuga K. Cardiac myxoma. Morphologic, histochemical, and tissue culture studies. Hum Pathol 1988, **19**: 316–322.

180 Terracciano LM, Mhawech P, Suess K, D'Armiento M, Lehmann FS, Jundt G, Moch H, Sauter G, Mihatsch MJ. Calretinin as a marker for cardiac myxoma. Am J Clin Pathol 2000, **114**: 754–759.

181 Trotter SE, Shore DF, Olsen EG. Gamna–Gandy nodules in a cardiac myxoma. Histopathology 1990, **17**: 270–272.

182 Yin Z, Kirschner LS. The Carney complex gene PRKAR1A plays an essential role in cardiac development and myxomagenesis. Trends Cardiovasc Med 2009, **19**: 44–49.

OTHER BENIGN TUMORS AND TUMORLIKE CONDITIONS

183 Almagro UA, Perry LS, Choi H, Pintar K. Papillary fibroelastoma of the heart. Report of six cases. Arch Pathol Lab Med 1982, **206**: 318–321.

184 Aqel NM, Shousha S. Glandular inclusions in fetal myocardium. Histopathology 1994, **24**: 85–87.

185 Arai T, Kurashima C, Wada S, Chida K, Ohkawa S. Histological evidence for cell proliferation activity in cystic tumor (endodermal heterotopia) of the atrioventricular node. Pathol Int 1998, **48**: 917–923.

186 Argani P, Sternberg SS, Burt M, Adsay NV, Klimstra DS. Metastatic adenocarcinoma involving a mesothelial/monocytic incidental cardiac excrescence (cardiac MICE). Am J Surg Pathol 1997, **21**: 970–974.

187 Bando Y, Kitagawa T, Uehara H, Sano N, Satake N, Onose Y, Kitaichi T, Miki O, Katoh I, Izumi K. So-called mesothelial/ monocytic incidental cardiac excrescences obtained during valve replacement surgery: report of three cases and literature review. Virchows Arch 2000, **437**: 331–335.

188 Burke AP, Anderson PG, Virmani R, James TN, Herrera GA, Ceballos R. Tumor of the atrioventricular nodal region. A clinical and immunohistochemical study. Arch Pathol Lab Med 1990, **114**: 1057–1062.

189 Burke AP, Gatto-Weis C, Griego JE, Ellington KS, Virmani R. Adult cellular rhabdomyoma of the heart: a report of 3 cases. Hum Pathol 2002, **33**: 1092–1097.

190 Burke AP, Litovsky S, Virmani R. Lipomatous hypertrophy of the atrial septum presenting as a right atrial mass. Am J Surg Pathol 1996, **20**: 678–685.

191 Burke AP, Ribe JK, Bajaj AK, Edwards WD, Farb A, Virmani R. Hamartoma of mature cardiac myocytes. Hum Pathol 1998, **29**: 904–909.

192 Burke AP, Virmani R. Cardiac rhabdomyoma. A clinicopathologic study. Mod Pathol 1991, **4**: 70–74.

193 Burke A, Li L, Kling E, Kutys R, Virmani R, Miettinen M. Cardiac inflammatory myofibroblastic tumor: a 'benign' neoplasm that may result in syncope, myocardial infarction, and sudden death. Am J Surg Pathol 2007, **31**: 1115–1122.

194 Cameselle-Teijeiro J, Abdulkader I, Soares P, Alfonsín-Barreiro N, Moldes-Boullosa J, Sobrinho-Simões M. Cystic tumor of the atrioventricular node of the heart appears to be the heart equivalent of the solid cell nests (ultimobranchial rests) of the thyroid. Am J Clin Pathol 2005, **123**: 369–375.

195 Chan HSL, Sonley MJ, Möes CAF, Daneman A, Smith CR, Martin DJ. Primary and secondary tumors of childhood involving the heart, pericardium, and great vessels. A report of 75 cases and review of the literature. Cancer 1985, **56**: 825–836.

196 Chou P, Gonzalez-Crussi F, Cole R, Reddy VB. Plasma cell granuloma of the heart. Cancer 1988, **62**: 1409–1413.

197 Courtice RW, Stinson WA, Walley VM. Tissue fragments recovered at cardiac surgery masquerading as tumoral proliferations. Evidence suggesting iatrogenic or artefactual origin and common occurrence. Am J Surg Pathol 1994, **18**: 167–174.

198 De Nictolis M, Brancorsini D, Goteri G, Prat J. Epithelioid haemangioma of the heart. Virchows Arch 1996, **428**: 119–123.

199 Duray PH, Mark EJ, Barwick KW, Madri JA, Strom RL. Congenital polycystic tumor of the atrioventricular node. Arch Pathol Lab Med 1985, **109**: 30–34.

200 Fealey ME, Edwards WD, Miller DV, Menon SC, Dearani JA. Hamartomas of mature cardiac myocytes: report of 7 new cases and review of literature. Hum Pathol 2008, **39**: 1064–1071.

201 Fekete PS, Nassar VH, Talley JD, Boedecker EA. Cardiac papilloma. Arch Pathol Lab Med 1983, **107**: 246–248.

202 Feldman PS, Meyer MW. Fibroelastic hamartoma (fibroma) of the heart. Cancer 1976, **38**: 314–323.

203 Fenoglio JJ, McAllister HA. Granular cell tumors of the heart. Arch Pathol Lab Med 1976, **100**: 276–278.

204 Fenoglio JJ Jr, Jacobs DW, McAllister HA Jr. Ultrastructure of the mesothelioma of the atrioventricular node. Cancer 1977, **40**: 721–727.

205 Fine G. Primary tumors of the pericardium and heart. In Edwards JE, Lev M, Abell MR (eds): The heart. Baltimore, 1974, Williams & Wilkins, pp. 189–210.

206 Fine G, Raju U. Congenital polycystic tumor of the atrioventricular node (endodermal heterotopia, mesothelioma). A histogenetic appraisal with evidence for its endodermal origin. Hum Pathol 1987, **18**: 791–795.

207 Gotlieb AI. Cardiac fibromas. Semin Diagn Pathol 2008, **25**: 17–19.

208 Hill DA, Swanson PE. Myocardial extramedullary hematopoiesis: a clinicopathologic study. Mod Pathol 2000, **13**: 779–787.

209 Howard RA, Aldea GS, Shapira OM, Kasznica JM, Davidoff R. Papillary fibroelastoma: increasing recognition of a surgical disease. Ann Thorac Surg 1999, **68**: 1881–1885.

210 Hoyt JC, Hutchins GM. Angiomatous variants of so-called mesothelioma of the atrioventricular node. Arch Pathol Lab Med 1986, **110**: 851–852.

211 Jaffe R. Neuroma in the region of the atrioventricular node. Hum Pathol 1981, **12**: 375–376.

212 Jain D, Maleszewski JJ, Halushka MK. Benign cardiac tumors and tumorlike conditions. Ann Diagn Pathol 2010, **14**: 215–230.

213 Johnson TL, Shapiro B, Beierwaltes WH, Orringer MB, Lloyd RV, Sisson JC, Thompson NW. Cardiac paragangliomas. A clinicopathologic and immunohistochemical study of four cases. Am J Surg Pathol 1985, **9**: 827–834.

214 Kantelip B, Lusson JR, De Riberolles C, Lamaison D, Bailly P. Intracardiac ectopic thyroid. Hum Pathol 1986, **17**: 1293–1296.

215 Kiaer HW. Myocardial angiolipoma. Acta Pathol Microbiol Immunol Scand (A) 1984, **92**: 291–292.

216 Kuo T-T, Hsueh S, Su I-J, Gonzalez-Crussi F, Chen J-S. Histiocytoid hemangioma of the heart with peripheral eosinophilia. Cancer 1985, **55**: 2854–2861.

217 Kurup AN, Tazelaar HD, Edwards WD, Burke AP, Virmani R, Klarich KW, Orszulak TA. Iatrogenic cardiac papillary fibroelastoma: a study of 12 cases (1990 to 2000). Hum Pathol 2003, **33**: 1165–1169.

218 Li L, Cerilli LA, Wick MR. Inflammatory pseudotumor (myofibroblastic tumor) of the heart. Ann Diagn Pathol 2002, **6**: 116–121.

219 Linder J, Shelburne JD, Sorge JP, Whalen RE, Hackel DB. Congenital endodermal heterotopia of the atrioventricular node. Evidence for the endodermal origin of so-called mesotheliomas of the atrioventricular node. Hum Pathol 1984, **15**: 1093–1098.

220 Luthringer DJ, Virmani R, Weiss SW, Rosai J. A distinctive cardiovascular lesion resembling histiocytoid (epithelioid) hemangioma. Evidence suggesting mesothelial participation. Am J Surg Pathol 1990, **14**: 993–1000.

221 Maleszewski JJ, Hristov AC, Halushka MK, Miller DV. Extranodal Rosai–Dorfman disease involving the heart: report of two cases. Cardiovasc Pathol 2010, **19**: 380–384.

222 Mikolaenko I, Galliani CA, Davis GG. Pigmented cardiac paraganglioma. Arch Pathol Lab Med 2001, **125**: 680–682.

223 Miller DV, Edwards WD. Cardiovascular tumor-like conditions. Semin Diagn Pathol 2008, **25**: 54–64.

224 Monroe B, Federman M, Balogh K. Cardiac neurilemoma. Report of a case with electron microscopic examination. Arch Pathol Lab Med 1984, **108**: 300–304.

225 Natarajan S, Luthringer DJ, Fishbein MC. Adenomatoid tumor of the heart: Report of a case. Am J Surg Pathol 1997, **21**: 1378–1380.

226 Pham TT, Antons K, Shishido R, Mullvain J, Salem F, Haghighi P. A case of mesothelial/ monocytic cardiac excrescence causing severe acute cardiopulmonary failure. Am J Surg Pathol 2005, **29**: 564–567.

227 Prichard RW. Tumors of the heart. Review of the subject and report of one hundred and fifty cases. Arch Pathol 1951, **51**: 98–128.

228 Reynolds C, Tazelaar HD, Edwards WD. Calcified amorphous tumor of the heart (cardiac CAT). Hum Pathol 1997, **28**: 601–606.

229 Richter JT, Strange RG Jr, Fisher SI, Miller DV, Delvecchio DM. Extranodal Rosai–Dorfman disease presenting as a cardiac mass in an adult: report of a unique case and lack of relationship to IgG4-related sclerosing lesions. Hum Pathol 2010, **41**: 297–301.

230 Rosai J, Dehner LP. Nodular mesothelial hyperplasia in hernia sacs. A benign reactive condition simulating a neoplastic process. Cancer 1975, **35**: 165–175.

231 Rose AG, McCormick S, Cooper K, Titus JL. Inflammatory pseudotumor (plasma cell granuloma) of the heart: report of two cases and literature review. Arch Pathol Lab Med 1996, **120**: 549–554.

232 Rubin MA, Snell JA, Tazelaar HD, Lack EE, Austenfeld JL, Azumi N. Cardiac papillary fibroelastoma. An immunohistochemical investigation and unusual clinical manifestations. Mod Pathol 1995, **8**: 402–407.

233 Silverman JF, Kay S, McCue M, Lower RR, Brough AJ, Chang CH. Rhabdomyoma of the heart. Ultrastructural study of three cases. Lab Invest 1976, **35**: 596–606.

234 Sturtz CL, Abt AB, Leuenberger UA, Damiano R. Hamartoma of mature cardiac myocytes: a case report. Mod Pathol 1998, **11**: 496–499.

235 Suarez-Vilela D, Izquierdo-Garcia FM. Nodular histiocytic/mesothelial hyperplasia: a process mediated by adhesion molecules? Histopathology 2002, **40**: 299–300.

236 Swalwell CI. Benign intracardiac teratoma. A case of sudden death. Arch Pathol Lab Med 1993, **117**: 739–742.

237 Tabry IF, Nassar VH, Rizk G, Touma A, Dagher IK. Cavernous hemangioma of the heart. Case report and review of the literature. J Thorac Cardiovasc Surg 1975, **69**: 415–420.

238 Takikita-Suzuki M, Takeuchi E, Nakashima Y, Yamamoto T, Mukai K, Ogasawara K. A case of multifocal fibrosclerosis with intracardiac solid masses. Hum Pathol 2006, **37**: 493–497.

239 Tazelaar HD, Locke TJ, McGregor CG. Pathology of surgically excised primary cardiac tumors. Mayo Clin Proc 1992, **67**: 957–965.

240 Vaideeswar P, Butany JW. Benign cardiac tumors of the pluripotent mesenchyme. Semin Diagn Pathol 2008, **25**: 20–28.

241 Veinot JP. Cardiac tumors of adipocytes and cystic tumor of the atrioventricular node. Semin Diagn Pathol 2008, **25**: 29–38.

242 Veinot JP, Tazelaar HD, Edwards WD, Colby TV. Mesothelial/ monocytic incidental cardiac excrescences. Cardiac MICE. Mod Pathol 1994, **7**: 9–16.

243 Walley VM, Peters HJ, Veinot JP, Courtice RW, Venance SL. The clinical and pathological manifestations of iatrogenically produced mesothelium-rich fragments of operative debris. Eur J Cardiothorac Surg 1997, **11**: 328–332.

244 Weeks DA, Chase DR, Malott RL, Chase RL, Zuppan CW, Bekwith JB, Mierau GW. HMB-45 staining in angiomyolipoma, cardiac rhabdomyoma, other mesenchymal processes, and tuberous sclerosis-associated brain lesions. Int J Surg Pathol 1994, **1**: 191–198.

245 Yu GH, Kussmaul WG, Di Sesa VJ, Lodato RF, Brooks JS. Adult intracardiac rhabdomyoma resembling the extracardiac variant. Hum Pathol 1993, **24**: 448–451.

PRIMARY MALIGNANT TUMORS

246 Bearman RM. Primary leiomyosarcoma of the heart. Report of a case and review of the literature. Arch Pathol 1974, **98**: 62–65.

247 Burke AP, Cowan D, Virmani R. Primary sarcomas of the heart. Cancer 1992, **69**: 387–395.

248 Burke AP, Virmani R. Osteosarcomas of the heart. Am J Surg Pathol 1991, **15**: 289–295.

249 Burke A. Primary malignant cardiac tumors. Semin Diagn Pathol 2008, **25**: 39–46.

250 Cairns P, Butany J, Fulop J, Rakowski H, Hassaram S. Cardiac presentation of non-Hodgkin's lymphoma. Arch Pathol Lab Med 1987, **111**: 80–83.

251 Catton C. The management of malignant cardiac tumors: clinical considerations. Semin Diagn Pathol 2008, **25**: 69–75.

252 Chalabreysse L, Berger F, Loire R, Devouassoux G, Cordier JF, Thivolet-Bejui F. Primary cardiac lymphoma in immunocompetent patients: a report of three cases and review of the literature. Virchows Arch 2002, **441**: 456–461.

253 Charney DA, Charney JM, Ghali VS, Teplitz C. Primitive neuroectodermal tumor of the myocardium: A case report, review of the literature, immunohistochemical and ultrastructural study. Hum Pathol 1996, **27**: 1365–1369.

254 Constantino A, West TE, Gupta M, Loghmanee F. Primary cardiac lymphoma in a patient with acquired immune deficiency syndrome. Cancer 1987, **60**: 2801–2805.

255 Curtsinger CR, Wilson MJ, Yoneda K. Primary cardiac lymphoma. Cancer 1989, **64**: 521–525.

256 Cusimano RJ. Surgical management of cardiac tumors. Semin Diagn Pathol 2008, **25**: 76–81.

257 Fabian JT, Rose AG. Tumours of the heart. A study of 89 cases. S Afr Med J 1982, **61**: 71–77.

258 Guarner J, Brynes RK, Chan WC, Birdsong G, Hertzler G. Primary non-Hodgkin's lymphoma of the heart in two patients with the acquired immunodeficiency syndrome. Arch Pathol Lab Med 1987, **111**: 254–256.

259 Herhusky MJ, Gregg SB, Virmani R, Chun PKC, Bender H, Gray GF Jr. Cardiac sarcomas presenting as metastatic disease. Arch Pathol Lab Med 1985, **109**: 943–945.

260 Herrmann MA, Shankerman RA, Edwards WD, Shub C, Schaff HV. Primary cardiac angiosarcoma. A clinicopathologic study of six cases. J Thorac Cardiovasc Surg 1992, **103**: 655–664.

261 Holladay AO, Siegel RJ, Schwartz DA. Cardiac malignant lymphoma in acquired immune deficiency syndrome. Cancer 1992, **70**: 2203–2207.

262 Ito M, Nakagawa A, Tsuzuki T, Yokoi T, Yamashita Y, Asai J. Primary cardiac lymphoma: No evidence for an etiologic association with Epstein–Barr virus. Arch Pathol Lab Med 1996, **120**: 555–559.

263 Janigan DT, Husain A, Robinson NA. Cardiac angiosarcomas. A review and a case report. Cancer 1986, **57**: 852–859.

264 Karn CM, Socinski MA, Fletcher JA, Corson JM, Craighead JE. Cardiac synovial sarcoma with translocation (X; 18) associated with asbestos exposure. Cancer 1994, **73**: 74–78.

265 Katoh M, Shigematsu H. Leiomyosarcoma of the heart and its pulmonary metastasis, both with prominent osteoclast-like multinucleated giant cells expressing tartrate-resistant acid phosphatase activity. Pathol Int 1999, **49**: 74–78.

266 Kim CH, Dancer JY, Coffey D, Zhai QJ, Reardon M, Ayala AG, Ro JY. Clinicopathologic study of 24 patients with primary cardiac sarcomas: a 10-year single institution experience. Hum Pathol 2008, **39**: 933–938.

267 Klima T, Milam JD, Bossart MI, Cooley DA. Rare primary sarcomas of the heart. Arch Pathol Lab Med 1986, **110**: 1155–1159.

268 Kowal-Vern A, Swinnen L, Pyle J, Radvany R, Dizikes G, Michalov M, Molnar Z. Characterization of postcardiac transplant lymphomas: Histology, immunophenotyping, immunohistochemistry, and gene rearrangement. Arch Pathol Lab Med 1996, **120**: 41–48.

269 Lam KY, Dickens P, Chan AC. Tumors of the heart. A 20-year experience with a review of 12,485 consecutive autopsies. Arch Pathol Lab Med 1993, **117**: 1027–1031.

270 Laya MB, Mailliard JA, Bewtra C, Levin HS. Malignant fibrous histiocytoma of the heart. A case report and review of the literature. Cancer 1987, **59**: 1026–1031.

271 McDonnell PJ, Mann RB, Bulkley BH. Involvement of the heart by malignant lymphoma. A clinicopathologic study. Cancer 1982, **49**: 944–951.

272 Miller DV, Firchau DJ, McClure RF, Kurtin PJ, Feldman AL. Epstein–Barr virus-associated diffuse large B-cell lymphoma arising on cardiac prostheses. Am J Surg Pathol 2010, **34**: 377–384.

273 Nascimento AF, Winters GL, Pinkus GS. Primary cardiac lymphoma: clinical, histologic, immunophenotypic, and genotypic features of 5 cases of a rare disorder. Am J Surg Pathol 2007, **31**: 1344–1350.

274 Nicholson AG, Rigby M, Lincoln C, Meller S, Fisher C. Synovial sarcoma of the heart. Histopathology 1997, **30**: 349–352.

275 Ovcak Z, Masera A, Lamovec J. Malignant fibrous histiocytoma of the heart. Arch Pathol Lab Med 1992, **116**: 872–874.

276 Pauwels P, Dal Cin P, Sciot R, Lammens M, Penn O, Van Nes E, Kwee WS, van den Berghe H. Primary malignant peripheral nerve sheath tumor of the heart. Histopathology 1999, **34**: 56–59.

277 Pins MR, Ferrell MA, Madsen JC, Piubello Q, Dickersin R, Fletcher CDM. Epithelioid and spindle-celled leiomyosarcoma of the heart: Report of 2 cases and review of the literature. Arch Pathol Lab Med 1999, **123**: 782–788.

278 Pucci A, Gagliardotto P, Papandrea C, Di Rosa E, Morello M, di Summa M, Mollo F. An unusual myxoid leiomyosarcoma of the heart. Arch Pathol Lab Med 1996, **120**: 583–586.

279 Small EJ, Gordon GJ, Dahms BB. Malignant rhabdoid tumor of the heart in an infant. Cancer 1985, **55**: 2850–2853.

280 Yang H-Y, Wasielewski JF, Lee W, Lee E, Paik YK. Angiosarcoma of the heart. Ultrastructural study. Cancer 1981, **47**: 72–80.

281 Zanella M, Falconieri G, Bussani R, Sinagra G, Libera D. Polypoid osteosarcoma of the left atrium: report of a new case with autopsy confirmation and review of the literature. Ann Diagn Pathol 1998, **2**: 167–172.

282 Zhang PJ, Brooks JS, Goldblum JR, Yoder B, Seethala R, Pawel B, Gorman JH, Gorman RC, Huang JH, Acker M, Narula N. Primary cardiac sarcomas: a clinicopathologic analysis of a series with follow-up information in 17 patients and emphasis on long-term survival. Hum Pathol 2008, **39**: 1385–1395.

METASTATIC TUMORS

283 Gibbs P, Cebon JS, Calafiore P, Robinson WA. Cardiac metastases from malignant melanoma. Cancer 1999, **85**: 78–84.

284 Hanfling SM. Metastatic cancer to the heart. Circulation 1960, **22**: 474–483.

285 Klatt EC, Heitz DR. Cardiac metastases. Cancer 1990, **65**: 1456–1459.

286 Kline IK. Cardiac lymphatic involvement by metastatic tumor. Cancer 1972, **29**: 799–808.

287 Lagrange J-L, Despins P, Spielman M, Le Chevalier T, De Lajartre A-Y, Fontaine F, Sarrazin D, Contesso G, Génin J, Rouesse J, Grossetête R. Cardiac metastases. Case report on an isolated cardiac metastasis of a myxoid liposarcoma. Cancer 1986, **58**: 2333–2337.

288 Pratt CB, Dugger DL, Johnson WW, Ainger LE. Metastatic involvement of the heart in childhood rhabdomyosarcoma. Cancer 1973, **31**: 1492–1497.

289 Roberts WC, Glancy DL, DeVita VT Jr. Heart in malignant lymphoma (Hodgkin's disease, lymphosarcoma, reticulum cell sarcoma and mycosis fungoides). Study of 196 autopsy cases. Am J Cardiol 1968, **22**: 85–107.

290 Shehata BM, Thomas JE, Doudenko-Rufforny I. Metastatic carcinoid to the conducting system – is it a rare or merely unrecognized manifestation of carcinoid cardiopathy? Arch Pathol Lab Med 2002, **126**: 1538.

291 Smith C. Tumors of the heart. Arch Pathol Lab Med 1986, **110**: 371–374.

PERICARDIUM

292 Adenle AD, Edwards JE. Clinical and pathologic features of metastatic neoplasms of the pericardium. Chest 1982, **81**: 166–169.

293 Azoulay S, Adem C, Gatineau M, Finet JF, Bakdach H, Regnard JF, Capron F. Pericardial ectopic thymoma. Virchows Arch 2005, **446**: 185–188.

294 Bardales RH, Stanley MW, Schaefer RF, Liblit RA, Owens RB, Surhland MJ. Secondary pericardial malignancies. A critical appraisal of the role of cytology, pericardial biopsy, and DNA ploidy analysis. Am J Clin Pathol 1996, **106**: 29–34.

295 Ben-Izhak O, Elmalach I, Kerner H, Best LA. Pericardial myolipoma: a tumour presenting as a mediastinal mass and containing oestrogen receptors. Histopathology 1996, **29**: 184–185.

296 Cox JN, Friedli B, Mechmeche R, Ben Ismail M, Oberhaensli I, Faidutti B. Teratoma of the heart. A case report and review of the literature. Virchows Arch [A] 1983, **402**: 163–174.

297 Drut R, Quijano G. Multilocular mesothelial inclusion cysts (so-called benign multicystic mesothelioma) of pericardium. Histopathology 1999, **34**: 472–474.

298 Fine G. Primary tumors of the pericardium and heart. In Edwards JE, Lev M, Abell MR (eds): The heart. Baltimore, 1974, Williams & Wilkins, pp. 189–210.

299 Fukuda T, Ishikawa H, Ohnishi Y, Tachikawa S, Oguma F, Kasuya S, Sakashita I. Malignant spindle cell tumor of the pericardium. Evidence of sarcomatous mesothelioma with aberrant antigen expression. Acta Pathol Jpn 1989, **39**: 750–754.

300 Hancock EW. Heart disease after radiation [editorial]. N Engl J Med 1983, **308**: 588.

301 Killion MJ, Brodovsky HS, Schwarting R. Pericardial angiosarcoma after mediastinal irradiation for seminoma: A case report and a review of the literature. Cancer 1996, **78**: 912–917.

302 Kinnunen P, Kumala P, Kaarteenaho-Wiik R, Vuopala K. Ectopic liver in the human pericardium. Histopathology 1997, **30**: 277–279.

303 Klacsmann PG, Bulkley BH, Hutchins GM. The changed spectrum of purulent pericarditis. An 86 year autopsy experience in 200 patients. Am J Med 1977, **63**: 666–673.

304 Luk A, Ahn E, Vaideeswar P, Butany JW. Pericardial tumors. Semin Diagn Pathol 2008, **25**: 47–53.

305 Mambo NC. Diseases of the pericardium. Morphologic study of surgical specimens from 35 patients. Hum Pathol 1981, **12**: 978–987.

306 Martin A. Acute non-specific pericarditis. A description of nineteen cases. BMJ 1966, **2**: 279–281.

307 Naramoto A, Itoh N, Nakano M, Shigematsu H. An autopsy case of tuberous sclerosis associated with primary pericardial mesothelioma. Acta Pathol Jpn 1989, **39**: 400–406.

308 Nelson E, Stenzel P. Intrapericardial yolk sac tumor in an infant girl. Cancer 1987, **60**: 1567–1569.

309 Sane AC, Roggli VL. Curative resection of a well-differentiated papillary mesothelioma of the pericardium. Arch Pathol Lab Med 1995, **119**: 266–267.

310 Sicari MC, Fyfe B, Parness I, Rossi A, Unger P. Intrapericardial yolk sac tumor associated with acute myocarditis. Arch Pathol Lab Med 1999, **123**: 241–243.

311 Stewart JR, Fajardo LF. Radiation-induced heart disease. An update. Prog Cardiovasc Dis 1984, **27**: 173–194.

312 Terada T, Nakanuma Y, Matsubara T, Suematsu T. An autopsy case of primary angiosarcoma of the pericardium mimicking malignant mesothelioma. Acta Pathol Jpn 1988, **38**: 1345–1351.

313 Tötterman KJ, Pesonen E, Siltanen P. Radiation-related chronic heart disease. Chest 1983, **83**: 875–878.

314 Veinot JP, Edwards WD. Pathology of radiation-induced heart disease: A surgical and autopsy study of 27 cases. Hum Pathol 1996, **27**: 766–773.

315 Virmani R, Bewtra C, McAllister HA, Schulte RD. Intrapericardial giant lymph node hyperplasia. Am J Surg Pathol 1982, **6**: 475–481.

316 Yakirevich E, Sova Y, Drumea K, Bergman I, Quitt M, Resnick MB. Peripheral lymphadenopathy as the initial manifestation of pericardial mesothelioma: a case report. Int J Surg Pathol 2004, **12**: 403–405.

Arteries

CHAPTER CONTENTS

Normal anatomy

The reader is referred to standard textbooks and chapters on arteries, veins, capillaries, and lymph vessels for a description of the normal anatomy of these structures.[1]

Arteriosclerosis

Arteriosclerosis is a generalized progressive arterial disease associated with localized arterial occlusions and aneurysms. It is the principal cause of heart attack, stroke, and gangrene of the extremities, and is responsible for about 50% of all deaths in the United States, Europe, and Japan. The lesions result from an excessive inflammatory and proliferative response to various forms of injury to the endothelium and smooth muscle of the arterial wall.[7,9] Numerous growth factors, cytokines, and vasoregulatory molecules participate in the process.[11–13] The pathology of arteriosclerosis has gained greater surgical significance with the development of direct operative therapy for lesions of major arteries.

The pathology of arteriosclerosis primarily consists of the following:[6]

1. Formation of intimal *plaques*, composed of lipid deposits and proliferated spindle cells. The latter seem to be of heterogenous nature, fibroblasts and smooth muscle cells predominating.[10,14]
2. Reduplication and fragmentation of the internal elastic lamina.
3. Degeneration of the media indicated by fragmentation of elastic tissue network; by hyaline, mucinoid, and collagenous degeneration of the smooth muscle; and by medial calcification.
4. Adventitial fibrosis and chronic inflammatory cellular infiltration.

Arteriosclerosis may present as an occlusive process when the disease attacks the intima more rapidly than the media and adventitia, but may present as an aneurysm when the reverse is true. Occlusive disease and aneurysm may coexist in the same arterial system.[8]

The pathogenesis of arteriosclerosis is probably multifactorial, but it is currently believed that inflammation is the critical common denominator.[4,5,7,9,12] Factors thought important in its pathogenesis include changes in lipid metabolism, increased endothelial permeability to serum lipoprotein complexes, susceptibility of the intima to mechanical injury from flow turbulence at major bifurcations, and (in the presence of hypertension) elastic tissue fragmentation and thrombosis or disruption of vasa vasorum.

The areas of the arterial tree involved by arteriosclerosis that are successfully treated surgically have rapidly increased so that only occlusions of the smaller peripheral arteries of the extremities remain outside the realm of operative attack.

Surgical therapy for occlusive disease of the coronary, carotid, and mesenteric arteries is now frequently undertaken. The principal manifestations of arteriosclerosis that at present are treated surgically with some success are fusiform and saccular aneurysms of the aorta or other major arteries; dissecting aneurysm; and occlusive disease of the abdominal aorta, the iliofemoral arterial system, and, less often, the popliteal, subclavian, brachial, renal, and carotid arterial systems.[2,3,15]

Aneurysms

Aortic aneurysms

Aneurysms secondary to arteriosclerosis occur most frequently in the abdominal aorta, but the mechanism of development and the pathologic changes are similar in other portions of the aorta and in other arteries.[17]

Arterial dilation is likely initiated by a loss of elasticity or weakening of the recoil strength in the arterial wall, which results in elongation and tortuosity, as well as dilation. Initially, this dilation is most often fusiform. At the same intraluminal pressure, the larger the diameter of the artery the greater the tension in the arterial wall. The tendency for dilation thus increases rapidly after it has begun. The progressive dilation often results in a break in the arterial wall and the development of sacculation of the aneurysm.[35] The sacculations nearly always are partially filled with laminated clot, which may be the source of emboli into the arteries peripheral to the aneurysm (Fig. 27.20).

Microscopically, there are medial fibrosis and calcification, atherosclerosis, periaortic fibrosis, and thickening of the vasa vasorum. Those aneurysms located in the ascending aorta have a high incidence of fragmentation of elastic fibers and cystic medial change.[33] A mild to moderate lymphoplasmacytic infiltrate may be

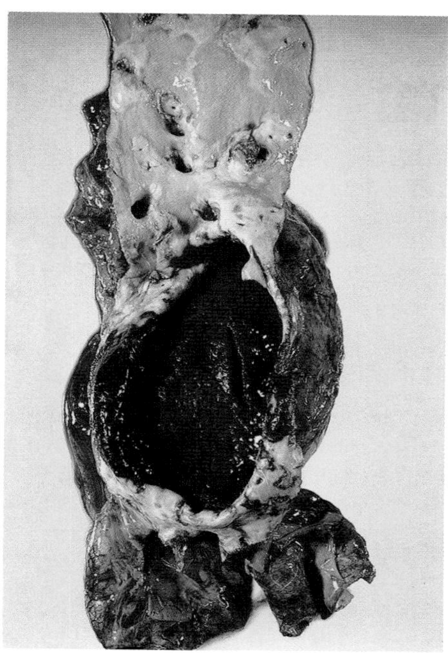

Fig. 27.20 Abdominal aortic aneurysm of arteriosclerotic origin containing a large thrombus.
(Courtesy of Dr RA Cooke, Brisbane, Australia; from Cooke RA, Stewart B. Colour atlas of anatomical pathology. Edinburgh, 2004, Churchill Livingstone)

seen in the adventitia. Although this finding is not necessarily indicative of a primary inflammatory process, aortitis is emerging as an important cause of ascending aortic aneurysms in the elderly (see p. 2296).[24,28,37,41,46] Burke et al.[22] have proposed dividing the cases of aortitis affecting the ascending aorta into necrotizing (characterized by zonal medial laminar necrosis rimmed by giant cells) and non-necrotizing (lacking necrosis and exhibiting diffuse medial inflammation). The former are usually restricted to the ascending aorta, whereas the latter are often systemic and best classified as giant cell aortitis.

Some cases of inflammatory abdominal aortic aneurysms show a mixed inflammatory infiltrate containing eosinophils, lymph follicles, perineurial inflammation, obliterative phlebitis and numerous IgG4-secreting plasma cells. These cases could represent aortic involvement by inflammatory fibrosclerosis, currently regarded as one of the IgG4-related disorders.[30,42]

Superimposed bacterial infection may complicate an aortic aneurysm of arteriosclerotic origin.[25,36] *Salmonella* is the predominant organism, followed by *Staphylococcus*.[18,19,39] Cases of aortic aneurysm have also been reported secondary to lupus erythematosus.[44]

The patient with an abdominal aneurysm may be asymptomatic and without clinical findings except for prominent abdominal aortic pulsations. The majority, however, seek treatment because of dull midabdominal or back pain associated with a pulsating, tender epigastric or retroumbilical mass that has enlarged rapidly or has been noted only recently. Painful and rapidly enlarging aneurysms will soon rupture if operative therapy is not undertaken. Retroperitoneal hemorrhages from small aneurysms may produce severe back pain with few abdominal symptoms or signs. Fistulas may develop from these aneurysms; there may be leakage into the vena cava or the duodenum or other portions of small bowel.[40] Significantly, aortoenteric fistulas also may occur as a late complication of reconstructive aortic surgery.[32] Aneurysms of the hepatic artery may rupture into the common bile duct; those of the splenic artery into the stomach, colon, or pancreatic duct; and those of the internal iliac artery into the rectosigmoid.[16,21,27]

Patients with aneurysms of the thoracic aorta survive but a short time without surgical correction.[20,35] Kampmeir[29] showed the average life expectancy after onset of symptoms to be 6–8 months. The prognosis in abdominal aneurysm appears better than that in aneurysm of the thoracic aorta.[26,31,38]

Schatz et al.[43] reviewed 141 untreated cases of abdominal aortic aneurysms at the Mayo Clinic. The prognosis was poor when the aneurysms were accompanied by symptomatic heart disease, when they were symptomatic, and when they exceeded 7.5 cm in diameter. Only 20% of the patients with aneurysm associated with symptomatic heart disease survived 5 years. Of those in whom the cause of death was known, 44% died of ruptured aneurysm.

Klippel and Butcher[34] reported 30 patients with abdominal aortic aneurysms not treated operatively: only two died of rupture. Szilagyi et al.[45] compared 223 untreated abdominal aortic aneurysms with a group of 480 treated surgically. They were able to show that modern operative mortality was significantly less than the likelihood of rupture without operation.

It may be concluded that once an aneurysm of the aortic system is of significant size, its excision and aortic reconstitution are mandatory.[23,35]

Popliteal artery aneurysms

Arteriosclerotic aneurysms of arteries in the extremities are rare except for the popliteal and femoral arteries.[48] The pathologic changes and the progressive enlargement of these aneurysms are similar to those in larger arteries, although the rate of progressive dilation usually is less. Their treatment is essential to avoid acute thrombosis, embolic phenomena, or rupture as causes of severe peripheral flow deficiency and gangrene.[49] Most patients with popliteal aneurysms are first seen because of these complications. Occasionally, such patients seek medical aid because of anterior tibial muscular necrosis. The popliteal arterial elongation associated with aneurysm formation may kink and occlude the anterior tibial artery as it passes through the interosseous membrane.[47]

Popliteal aneurysms are frequently multiple. In 69 patients having 100 popliteal aneurysms, hypertension and occlusive arterial disease were frequent.[47] Only three of these patients were women. Ninety-two of the aneurysms were considered purely arteriosclerotic; syphilis, mycotic infections, and trauma entered into the diagnosis of the remainder. In the absence of extensive gangrene, popliteal aneurysms with or without the presence of complications are best treated by excision of the aneurysm and insertion of autologous vein grafts.

Dissecting aneurysms

Dissecting aneurysms of the aorta, if untreated, are associated with a rapidly fatal course in 75–90% of the patients. Their etiology is related to an underlying degeneration of the elements of the media.[55] Factors associated with dissection are hypertension, Marfan syndrome (an autosomal dominant disorder caused by mutation in fibrillin-1 or transforming growth factor-β receptor gene),[57] Loeys–Dietz syndrome,[56] pregnancy, bicuspid aortic valve, and traumatic, atherosclerotic, or inflammatory injuries of the aortic media.[50,60] This includes procedures such as insertion of an intra-aortic balloon pump and aortic cannulation during cardiopulmonary bypass operation.

The process of dissection most commonly begins in a transverse intimal tear associated with an intimal plaque located either in the ascending aorta or in the upper descending thoracic aorta near the origin of the left subclavian artery.[53] Once this tear develops, the intramural layers of the aorta are rapidly separated by the force of the blood entering the wall. The dissection usually involves the entire circumference of the aorta as it progresses distally. Perforation often occurs through the adventitia, resulting in early death from hemorrhage into the pericardium or pleural cavity. Lower extremity symptoms and signs of acute occlusion of the abdominal aorta may be prominent because of distal aortic or iliac luminal occlusion by the leading point of the dissection. Diagnostic imaging is essential in the evaluation of suspected aortic dissection.[51]

Three major types of dissection are recognized depending on the location and extent.[53,54] Type I begins in the ascending aorta and extends beyond; type II is confined to the ascending aorta; type IIIA begins in the descending aorta and stops above the diaphragm; type IIIB also begins in the descending aorta but extends below the diaphragm. Dissecting aneurysms can also be classified according to their duration as acute, subacute, and chronic. The subacute type characteristically begins abruptly and then progresses gradually for several days before rupture and death (Fig. 27.21). The chronic form occurs in a few patients who develop a re-entry site from the dissected passage back into the lumen of the aorta. The occasional long-term survivor of dissecting aneurysm is encountered among these patients.

The objective of surgical treatment is to excise the intimal tear, obliterate entry into the false channel proximally and distally, and reconstitute the aorta, usually with the interposition of a synthetic sleeve graft; aortic valve repair or replacement may be also necessary in proximal dissections.[52,53] Medical therapy consists in lowering the arterial blood pressure and diminishing the velocity of ventricular contraction.[58,59]

There is a need for proper selection in deciding surgical versus medical therapy. There is now general agreement that acute proximal dissections should be treated surgically whenever possible, whereas the treatment of distal dissections is more controversial.

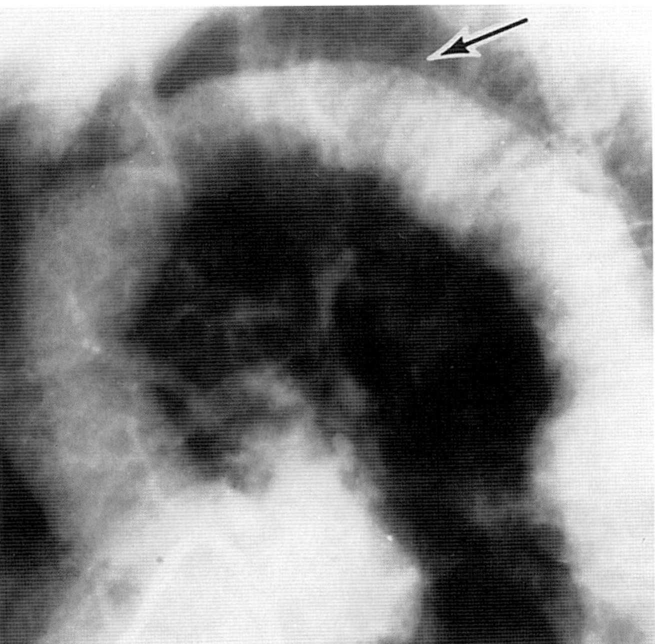

Fig. 27.21 Dissecting aneurysm in a 68-year-old man who died of rupture into pericardium on the way to the operating room. Double aortic shadow characteristic of dissecting aneurysm is indicated (arrow).

Wheat et al.[59] reported the successful treatment of patients with acute dissecting aortic aneurysm by the use of antihypertensive agents. In a series of 33 patients so treated, McFarland et al.[58] reported that the survival rate was 52%, the mean follow-up period being more than 3 years. These authors emphasized the need for proper selection in deciding a surgical versus a medical therapy.

Exceptionally, dissecting aneurysms can occur in arteries other than the aorta, such as the renal, coronary, pulmonary, and carotid vessels.[61]

Arterial substitution

Arteriosclerotic aneurysms of the abdominal aorta and the iliac arteries are best treated by excision and replacement of the involved arterial segment by synthetic prostheses.[63] Aneurysms of the popliteal arteries are probably best replaced by venous autografts. Arterial homografts are no longer used to replace diseased arterial segments because of the superiority of synthetic arterial prostheses.[62]

After implantation, homografts are partially replaced or encased by host collagenous tissue. In a few months, they lose much of their elasticity, although fragmented elastic tissue is still demonstrable histologically over a year after implantation. The evolution of the intimal surface of both homografts and synthetic cloth prostheses after implantation consists of the organization of the fibrin layer initially deposited and the development of a lining of flattened cells, which, by special staining techniques, appears nearly like normal vascular endothelium.[64] True endothelial ingrowth from the host artery occurs across the suture line for a variable distance.

Szilagyi et al.[65] reported late aneurysm formation in 2 of 55 aortic homografts and tortuous dilation in 12 of 66 femoral homografts within 3 years after insertion. Calcification may appear in the wall of homografts after long implantation. Implantation of synthetic cloth prostheses is followed by their encasement with collagen and a decline in tensile strength of some of them.

Arterial occlusive disease

Thrombotic occlusions of the major arteries are often associated with arteriosclerotic changes such as calcification, atheromatosis, and ulceration of the intima.[76] The occlusive process is often insidious, although final thrombotic obliteration of the lumen is occasionally quite rapid and may be clinically indistinguishable from embolization. Indeed, the differentiation of the two pathologically and at surgery is quite difficult in older individuals in whom arteriosclerosis of the abdominal aorta is nearly universal. The process of occlusion probably begins in the iliac arteries near the aortic bifurcation from which thrombus formation propagates cephalad in the aorta, occasionally to the level of the renal arteries. Thrombi and emboli can become secondarily infected by fungi, particularly *Aspergillus* and *Mucor*.

The syndrome of distal aortic thrombosis (Leriche syndrome) manifests itself with an insidious onset and gradual progression of symptoms of pain and easy fatigability in the legs, hips, and back; intermittent claudication; and sexual impotence.[80] In this condition, arterial insufficiency in the lower extremities usually is manifested clinically by the absence of pulses below the umbilicus. If the process is partial, weak pulsations may be felt or a characteristic systolic murmur heard over the abdominal aorta and the femoral arteries.

Despite the presence of intermittent claudication and the absence of pulses, many patients are found by arteriography to have near-normal distal arteries.[71] This patency of the peripheral arteries is probably responsible for the relative absence of muscular atrophy or of atrophy of skin appendages in the legs and feet of many of the patients despite their symptoms of peripheral blood flow insufficiency and lack of pulses.

Arteriosclerotic occlusive disease also frequently involves other major arterial bifurcations in the lower extremity such as those of the common iliac and common femoral arteries. In the latter instance, the intimal disease and thrombosis occur frequently in the external femoral artery just distal to the bifurcation. Other arterial segments in the lower extremity prone to early thrombotic occlusion are those associated with some degree of fascial fixation. Such areas exist: (1) in the external iliac artery behind the inguinal ligament; (2) in the superficial femoral artery as it passes through the fascial ring beneath the adductor longus tendon; and (3) in the anterior tibial artery where it passes through the interosseous membrane.[72]

Although arteriosclerosis is a generalized arterial disease, the tendency for occlusive complications to develop early in its evolution at the sites just noted makes possible the successful treatment of patients with marked peripheral blood flow deficiency. Surgical correction of the obstructive disease, however, often only temporarily improves the peripheral blood flow because of the progressive nature of generalized arteriosclerosis.[84] Successful operative therapy of arterial occlusive disease relieves symptoms of ischemia but actually prevents amputation of but a few extremities. However, aggressive operative therapy in properly selected patients with limited gangrene of the extremities may permit healing after amputation of only the gangrenous part.[81]

The surgical treatment of major arterial occlusive disease is performed by using two general methods: arterial substitutes and thromboendarterectomy (intimectomy).

Thromboendarterectomy is superior to arterial replacement early after treatment of arterial occlusive disease of the aorta and iliac arteries.[69] Autogenous venous bypass for femoral arterial occlusive disease appears to be associated with patency rates superior to those following endarterectomy and synthetic bypass grafts.[70,79]

Successful results in 85–95% of patients with occlusions of the aortic and iliac arteries have been reported with both methods of treatment. Postoperative aneurysm formation and vascular thrombosis have also been reported following the use of both methods. The correction of femoral occlusive disease by endarterectomy or by the bypass arterial substitution technique has proved less beneficial than for larger arteries. Approximately 70% of the patients with femoral grafts develop late thrombosis.

The incidence of late failure of both endarterectomy and arterial grafting procedures will likely always be higher in the smaller femoral artery than in the aorta and iliac arteries.

Thromboendarterectomy of major arteries is a technique in which the diseased intima and thrombotic material filling the lumen are dissected from the inner portion of the media in a smooth and uniform manner so that the remaining adventitia and media of the artery can continue to conduct blood. The remaining arterial tube is lined rapidly by a fibrinoid layer that develops a pseudoendothelial surface similar to that lining an implanted arterial substitute. Likewise, early thrombosis does not occur in these segments if the transit time of the blood through them is rapid. Endarterectomized arterial segments, examined months after the operative procedure, show a fibrous type of intima with an endothelium-like covering and preservation of the remaining media and elastic tissue.[67]

Microscopically, specimens from thromboendarterectomy may be fibrinous, mixed fibrinous and organizing, or old organized, depending on the stage of the process and reflecting various stages of remodeling of the thrombi.[68]

Arterial embolism of atheromatous origin is an important complication of arterial occlusive disease. It may occur spontaneously or following aortic surgery or angiographic procedures.[73,74,83] The complications vary according to the vessels affected and include livedo reticularis and gangrene of the lower extremities, ocular symptoms, cerebral infarct, gastrointestinal bleeding, renal hypertension, and renal failure.[66,75,77,78] The frequency of atheromatous embolism correlates with the severity of ulcerative atheromatous changes in the aorta. Simultaneous embolism to various organs may lead to a mistaken clinical diagnosis of polyarteritis nodosa.[82] Random biopsies of skeletal muscle may be diagnostic in these cases.[66]

Cystic adventitial degeneration

Cystic adventitial degeneration, a rare condition almost always affecting the popliteal artery, may cause luminal obstruction.[86,87] A collection of jelly-like material distends the wall and bulges into the lumen.[89] Most cases occur in young men without a history of trauma and without general arterial change. The microscopic appearance of the involved arterial segments is that of mucinous degeneration. The pathogenesis is probably related to that of soft tissue ganglion.[88] Other arteries may exceptionally be affected by this condition.[85]

Fibromuscular dysplasia

Fibromuscular dysplasia is a nonarteriosclerotic, noninflammatory vascular disease of unknown pathogenesis.[94] Humoral, mechanical, and genetic factors may play a role. It usually becomes manifest during the third or fourth decades of life, although it also can be seen in children.[96] It involves large and medium-sized muscular arteries, such as the renal, carotid, axillary, and mesenteric arteries, sometimes in a multicentric fashion.[92] Imaging techniques useful for the evaluation of this disease include CT scans, MRI, and angiography.[91] Morphologically, it is characterized by a disorderly arrangement and proliferation of the cellular and extracellular elements of the wall, particularly the media, with the resulting distortion of the vessel lumen. The absence of necrosis, calcification, inflammation, and fibrinoid necrosis are important negative diagnostic features. Morphologic varieties with predominant intimal or adventitial involvement have been described.[90,93] Surgical techniques for this condition include graduated or balloon intraluminal dilation (either isolated or associated with resection–anastomosis), saphenous graft, and reconstructive aneurysmorrhaphy.[95]

Mesenteric vascular occlusion

Mesenteric vascular occlusion may originate in veins or arteries. Rarely, occlusion of both occurs simultaneously. Arterial occlusion is the more frequent of the two[99] (62% of cases). After the initiation of arterial or venous thrombosis, hemorrhagic infarction of the intestine and its mesentery develops if the process is rapid in onset and extensive.

Venous mesenteric thrombosis often is associated with infection and cancer. However, infection and cancer per se are not directly related to the mesenteric venous thrombosis.

The relative reduction in the frequency of mesenteric venous occlusion is probably due to antibiotic control of many intra-abdominal infections.

Occlusion of the mesenteric arterial system may be caused by emboli from thrombi in an arteriosclerotic aorta, from a fibrillating atrium, or from a mural thrombus secondary to myocardial infarction.[104] Mesenteric arterial occlusion also may follow arteriosclerotic change in the superior mesenteric artery with local thrombosis and such rare conditions as polyarteritis, septic arteritis, and thromboangiitis obliterans.[101] Mesenteric arteries can be involved in rheumatoid disease and cause infarction.[98] Arterial and venous thrombosis, followed by ulceration and necrosis of the bowel, has been described following surgical repair of aortic coarctation.[100] The pathogenesis of this condition, which has been erroneously designated 'mesenteric arteritis', is probably related to the occurrence of hypertension during the first 2 postoperative days.

The technique of color-flow Duplex imaging can detect the presence of significant arterial stenosis in over 80% of the cases.[105]

Infarction of the small intestine or colon, perforation, and peritonitis do not always follow mesenteric vascular occlusion, either arterial or venous. As a matter of fact, many patients with significant disease of the celiac and superior mesenteric arteries as detected by Doppler sonography are asymptomatic.[103] Mesenteric infarct can be seen in the absence of arterial or venous occlusion.[102,106]

Infarction of the bowel depends on the location, extent of occlusion, rapidity of its onset, and state of the collateral circulation, as well as the general physical condition of the patient. Patients with cirrhosis of the liver and portal hypertension often have episodes of cramping abdominal pain associated with low-grade fever and moderate leukocytosis that gradually recede. Several such episodes may take place before a sufficient amount of the portal venous system is occluded to cause the clinical picture of intra-abdominal catastrophe.

The clinical diagnosis of mesenteric vascular thrombosis is difficult at times because the patient does not have the classic severe abdominal pain, distension, nausea, vomiting, leukocytosis, and shock. Such a picture depends on a massive sudden occlusion of the superior mesenteric artery or vein.

Acute occlusion of mesenteric arteries produces bowel necrosis without the early marked hypovolemic disturbances seen with extensive venous thrombosis. Bloody diarrhea is less common in arterial than in venous occlusions, but abdominal pain is generally more prominent in arterial occlusions. If the occlusion is sufficiently extensive to cause gangrene of the bowel, death from peritonitis follows if the bowel is not resected. A hypovolemic death in less than 24 hours, however, is often the outcome in the presence of massive venous occlusion.

Of the two types of occlusion, arterial embolic occlusion is more likely to be amenable to successful treatment than is venous thrombosis. The treatment of both conditions consists primarily of early abdominal exploration and resection of nonviable bowel. The determination of viability of laparotomy may be quite difficult. The extent of small bowel resection compatible with survival has been shown to be as much as three-fourths of the organ.

To date, embolectomy has but rarely remedied occlusion of the superior mesenteric artery. However, because of the serious prognosis associated with extensive small intestinal and colonic resection, this procedure should probably be attempted more often.

Chronic intestinal ischemia produces the syndrome of abdominal angina. Segmental intestinal infarction may be incident to disease of small mesenteric arteries without involvement of the proximal superior mesenteric artery. So-called 'nonocclusive intestinal infarction' is probably related to disease in these vessels in most instances.[97]

Renal artery disease and its relationship to hypertension are discussed in Chapter 17.

Traumatic and iatrogenic injuries

Rupture

Rupture of a major vessel in the absence of an aneurysm may follow open or blunt trauma; may exceptionally occur in a spontaneous fashion through an atheromatous plaque or an area destroyed by degeneration (as in Ehlers–Danlos syndrome) or inflammation;[109–111] or may be seen as a major complication of balloon dilation, surgery, or radiation therapy.[107] Fajardo and Lee[108] reviewed 11 vascular ruptures in patients who had had previous treatment for carcinoma. The vessels involved were the aorta and the carotid and femoral arteries. Most patients were men who had been subjected to surgery and radiation therapy for squamous cell carcinomas of the oropharynx, esophagus, or genitalia. In most cases, the rupture was due to surgical rather than radiotherapeutic complications, such as necrosis of skin flaps, infections, and fistulas.

Thrombosis

Nonpenetrating trauma may result in occlusive thrombosis of a major artery such as the carotid artery following blunt trauma to the paratonsillar area.[113,115] In children, trauma and arteritis constitute the two most common causes of acquired occlusions of major arteries.[112,117] Organizing and recanalizing thrombi can exhibit a papillary pattern of anastomosing channels reminiscent of angiosarcoma[114] or else acquire a myxomatous appearance with primitive mesenchymal cells, similar to that of cardiac myxoma.[116]

Pulsating hematoma

Pulsating hematoma or false aneurysm usually results from a small perforation in the artery, usually produced by a sharp instrument or a small missile.[120] Traumatic aneurysms may also follow injury to an artery by blunt trauma.[118] The defect is only a few millimeters in diameter but is sufficiently large to allow the escape of blood into the immediately surrounding tissues.

Cohen[119] emphasized the role of the adventitial layer in the development of the aneurysmal sac because of its tendency to seal off the defect in the arterial wall. Of equal importance is the nature of the surrounding tissue and the strength of its fascial structures. When strong fascial surroundings are absent, the rate of aneurysmal enlargement is quite rapid. It is slower when the area of injury is within a circumscribed fascial channel such as Hunter canal. The blood collects about the defect in the artery until the pressure within the hematoma approaches the mean blood pressure. Enlargement of the hematoma then slows because blood returns to the arterial lumen during diastole. It is this situation that produces the characteristic to-and-fro murmur heard over the pulsating hematoma. This murmur has a rather harsh systolic component and a softer diastolic component. The murmur is not constant as is the murmur of arteriovenous fistula. The walls of the pulsating hematoma contain varying amounts of laminated clot, which in turn is surrounded by a rather dense fibrous tissue reaction.

The operative treatment of pulsating hematoma is often not difficult. Usually the arterial wall defect can be closed by simple suture after evacuation of the hematoma and excision of the fibrotic aneurysmal sac. Occasionally, however, arterial substitution is required.

These lesions should be treated immediately on diagnosis to prevent continued enlargement, pain on compression of adjacent nerves and other structures, and ischemia of the tissues peripheral to them. Since ligation of the afflicted artery (if it is a major one) is no longer the treatment of choice, waiting for collateral vessels to develop is not indicated.

Acquired arteriovenous fistula

Acquired arteriovenous fistulas are seen most frequently during times of war and are produced in a manner quite similar to that of traumatic aneurysm. However, in this instance, the perforating injury involves both the artery and the adjacent vein. Such an injury usually results in a pulsating hematoma that communicates with both the arterial and venous lumina.[121]

Following trauma, the fistula may be established almost immediately. However, the communication between the arterial and venous systems is frequently delayed until the wound is partially organized and the thrombus in the hematoma surrounding the artery and vein is partially absorbed. Most patients present with a pulsating mass in the region of injury that can be differentiated from simple pulsating hematoma in several ways. The murmur over the pulsating region is usually continuous because of a continuous flow of arterial blood into the vein. In other words, during diastole the pressure in the pulsating hematoma about the arteriovenous communication is never sufficient to produce reversal of blood flow. In some slowly developing, long-standing arteriovenous communications in the absence of a pulsating hematoma, a massive sacculation of the adjacent vein may slowly develop.

Patients with an arteriovenous fistula usually show venous dilation about and peripheral to the fistula, as well as increased skin temperature in the area of the fistula. Despite increased temperature near the lesion, the extremity peripheral to it is usually cooler than normal, since the actual peripheral blood flow is less.

When arteriovenous fistulas develop between smaller arteries and veins, the sac may be excised and the vessels ligated without difficulty. Those involving the larger arteries, such as the femoral, axillary, or popliteal artery, require the maintenance of arterial continuity. Some type of arterial substitution may be necessary occasionally in larger arteriovenous aneurysms, although transvenous closure of the defect in the arterial wall usually can be accomplished satisfactorily.

The dilation of the major artery entering an arteriovenous fistula of long standing may be marked, and the degenerative changes in the arterial wall may be extensive. These changes consist of atherosclerosis, calcification, disruption of the elastic tissue network, and fibrosis. If the degeneration is sufficiently advanced, it is irreversible. In such arteries, aneurysms may develop despite the cure of the arteriovenous fistula. The dilation of the artery entering the arteriovenous fistula is thought to result from the increased flow of blood through it.

Arteriovenous fistulas are associated with increase in cardiac output, pulse rate, and blood volume, which may lead to congestive heart failure (Fig. 27.22). Such systemic results rarely, if ever, develop from a single congenital arteriovenous fistula with the exception of those that appear in the pulmonary tree. Congenital arteriovenous fistulas usually present as tumefactions containing many relatively small arteries and veins surrounded by moderately large amounts of fibrous tissue. Their treatment is primarily excisional.

Thromboangiitis obliterans

Thromboangiitis obliterans (Buerger disease) is a rare thrombotic and inflammatory disease of the arteries and veins of unknown etiology that has no single pathognomonic, clinical or pathologic sign.[122,126,131] Its inflammatory component may involve entire neurovascular bundles. Although it is a generalized vascular disease, the involvement of the arteries of the lower extremities is usually most advanced, and the resultant flow deficiency is the usual reason for the patient to seek therapy. A form preferentially involving mesenteric vessels has also been described.[132] The onset of the condition occurs most often in men between 20 and 35 years of age and may be heralded by superficial migratory acute thrombophlebitis that is precipitated by undue exertion or exposure to cold. Study of biopsies of such involved veins shows the histologic changes associated with acute intravascular thrombosis. Pathologic involvement in the arterial tree is segmental and is usually present primarily in the smaller arteries. There is a paucity of collateral flow.[123] This process has a widespread geographic distribution[128] but has been reported with increased frequency in Korea and Japan.[127]

Microscopic examination of early arterial lesions shows panarteritis often associated with thrombosis. Endothelial proliferation and periarterial fibrosis soon become prominent. The inflammatory process attacks the entire thickness of the vessel wall and perivascular tissues.[126] Where nerves are in close proximity to the vascular tree, it involves the perineurial stroma. Extension of the inflammatory process about peripheral sensory nerves may be responsible in part for the severe pain so common in afflicted extremities. Calcification in the arterial wall is absent. Arterial calcification on x-ray examination indicates arteriosclerosis rather than Buerger disease.

The arterial and venous thrombosis associated with the angiitic process becomes partially recanalized. Cellularity of the organizing fibrous tissue replacing the thrombus is often prominent. Recanalization of thrombi is incomplete and is characterized by numerous small vascular channels passing through the remaining fibrous tissue.

The pathologic process ascribed to Buerger disease may be difficult to distinguish microscopically from inflammatory and fibrotic changes that may accompany arteriosclerotic thromboses.[125]

The vascular process tends generally to be progressive, but in some instances the acute manifestation seems to subside, partially in patients who cease using tobacco.

Treatment is largely symptomatic and includes the control of pain, the avoidance of tobacco, and cleanliness of the extremity. Late in the disease, amputations may be necessary. Sympathectomy may benefit patients with cold, temperature-sensitive feet or hands and those with peripheral gangrenous ulcers.

The death of patients with Buerger disease may follow complications attending gangrene of the extremities. However, many patients with this affliction die of myocardial infarction, renal insufficiency, occlusions of mesenteric vessels, and strokes.

With the use of arteriography and careful pathologic examination, a high proportion of cases of alleged Buerger disease have actually been shown to be arteriosclerosis. This pathologic process can be mimicked with considerable exactitude by the development of embolism and thrombosis. This has led some investigators to postulate that Buerger disease is not a distinct entity but rather a peculiar manifestation of arteriosclerosis.[134] Although we agree that many cases originally diagnosed as Buerger disease are indeed examples of arteriosclerosis, there is considerable evidence that the entity thromboangiitis obliterans exists.[124,129,130,133,135]

Arteritis

Inflammatory diseases of the arteries have been classified on the basis of the etiologic agent involved, the caliber and location of the vessel affected, and the type of microscopic change observed.[136,139]

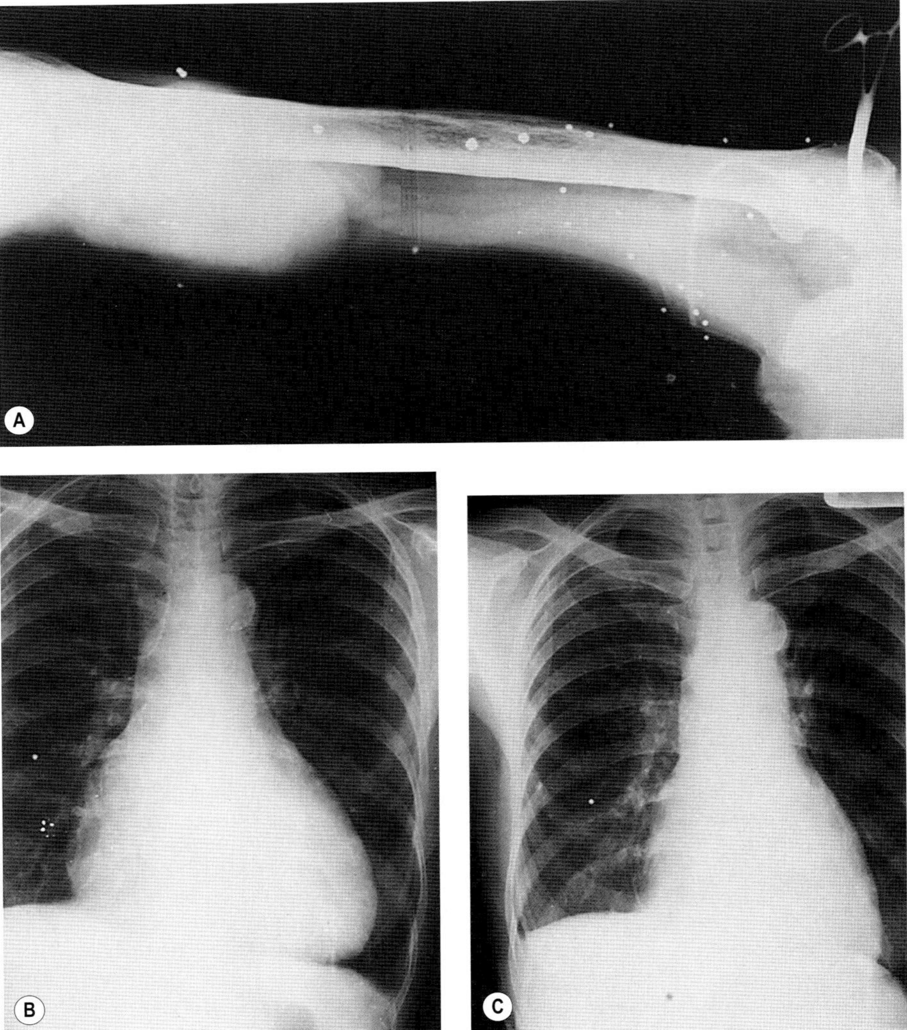

Fig. 27.22 Arteriovenous fistula in a 68-year-old woman. **A**, Arteriogram showing markedly enlarged femoral artery entering region of arteriovenous fistula. Pellets from original shotgun wound 30 years previously are visible. **B**, Radiograph before correction of arteriovenous fistula. **C**, Radiograph 5 days after operation.

The former is obviously the most desirable but, at present, impractical, since a specific etiologic agent can be detected for only a minority of the cases, such as in pneumococcal, syphilitic, mycotic, or tuberculous arteritis.[137,140] Imperfect as it is, a division based on the vessel caliber is quite useful. Within each group, the arteritides can be further subdivided into more or less specific types on the basis of the associated condition and/or pathologic appearance.[138]

Large vessel arteritis

A group of related nonsyphilitic diseases primarily affect the aorta and its main branches and are characterized by chronic inflammation and patchy destruction of the elements of the media.[144,158,162] They may result in aortic insufficiency, diffuse aortic tortuosity and elongation, the aortic arch syndrome, aneurysm formation, and dissection of the vessel (Fig. 27.23). They are more common in adults but have also been described in children.[147]

In some aortic aneurysms, there is a thick outer wall composed of fibroblasts and collagen that entrap fat, nerves, and lymph nodes, and that are accompanied by a heavy lymphoplasmacytic infiltrate.[142] These have been referred to as *inflammatory aneurysms*,[145] but it is not clear whether they represent a distinct entity or simply a variant of atherosclerotic aneurysm, perhaps induced by antigens in the atheromatous plaque, and/or mediated by adhesion molecules (see p. 2291). The latter possibility seems the most likely,[153,159] although the possibility that CMV and HIV may play a pathogenetic role in some of the cases has been suggested.[143,164]

In the variety of arteritis known as **Takayasu disease**, there is chronic inflammation and fibrosis of the arterial wall, which has a predilection for the aortic arch branches and results in the absence of pulses in the upper extremities, ocular changes, and neurologic symptoms (Figs 27.24 and 27.25).[148,155] In later stages, superimposed changes of arteriosclerosis may obscure the diagnosis.[149] In general, the possibility of an underlying arteritis should always be considered when arteriosclerotic changes in the aorta are seen in young or middle-aged individuals and when these changes are either segmental or occur at an unusual site. Most patients with Takayasu disease are young, Asian, and female. The disease is rare in the United States, but it has been well documented.[150] In a series of 16 autopsy cases reported from South

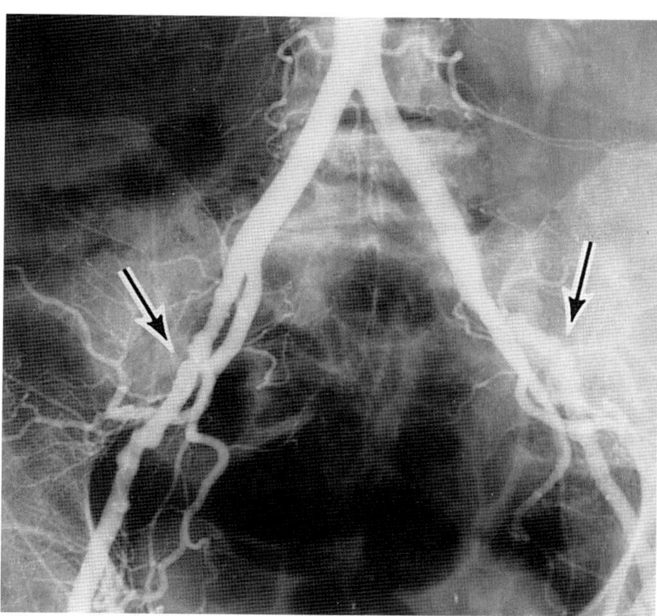

Fig. 27.23 Vasculitis in a 52-year-old woman showing scalloped irregularities limited to external iliac arteries.

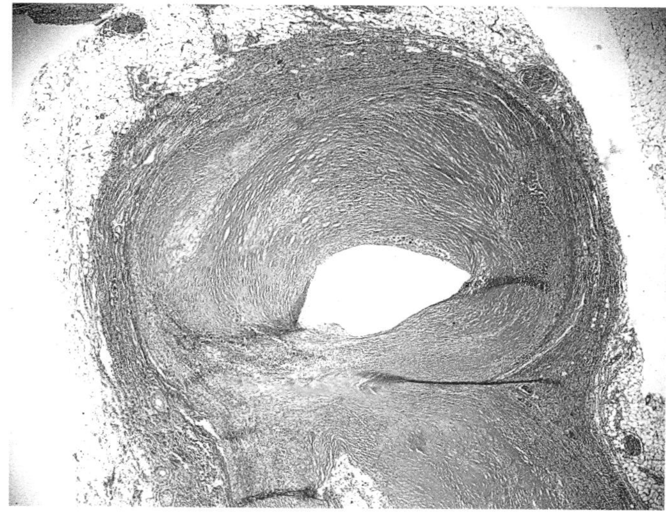

Fig. 27.24 Panoramic view of coronary artery in a case of Takayasu arteritis. The massive hyaline thickening of the wall has led to marked narrowing of the lumen.

Africa,[160] there was segmental coronary arteritis in three patients, with development of coronary aneurysms in two. There was coexistent tuberculosis in 37.5% of the patients, but this might well have been coincidental.

In **Kawasaki disease** of infants, arterial changes are prominent and may result in sudden death from acute myocardial ischemia. Microscopically, the coronary and other arteries show reactive proliferative changes in the media, panarteritis, and frequent aneurysmal dilation.[152] Marked fibrosis is present in the healed stage.[146] The etiology is unknown, but the pathologic changes are thought to be

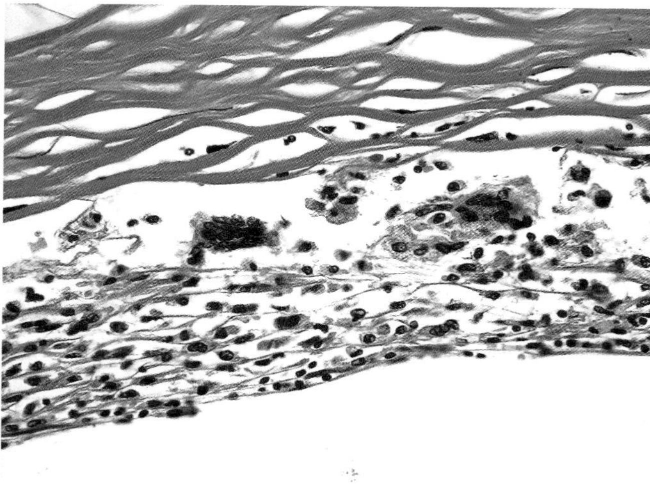

Fig. 27.25 Same case as Fig. 27.24. The high-power view shows subendothelial inflammation containing several multinucleated giant cells.

immune mediated.[141,151] Specifically, it has been suggested that the disease may be caused by a toxin that acts as a 'superantigen'.[154,157]

Aortic arteritis can be seen associated with rheumatoid arthritis, ankylosing spondylitis, and scleroderma.[161,163] There is a definite relationship between the type and location of the vessel and the frequency and etiology of the inflammatory diseases by which it may be affected. Tuberculosis characteristically involves small vessels; rarely, it may be seen in larger vessels and results in stenosis or aneurysms.[156]

Most of the reported cases of aneurysms of the superior mesenteric artery have been either syphilitic or mycotic; the majority of the latter were associated with bacterial endocarditis.

Medium-sized vessel arteritis

The classic example of medium-sized vessel arteritis is **polyarteritis nodosa**, classically described at autopsy as visible nodular lesions at the points of arterial branchings. This condition should be suspected clinically if there is a history suggesting hypersensitivity, with fever, eosinophilia, and involvement of many organ systems. Infrequently, there are skin manifestations. A muscle or peripheral nerve biopsy may be diagnostic. A biopsy is most rewarding in the presence of a nodule. Rarely, organs such as the gallbladder, appendix, or colon may show unsuspected lesions typical of polyarteritis (see respective chapters).

In **Wegener granulomatosis**, the arteritis is accompanied by necrosis and granulomatous reaction. The organs most commonly involved are the upper respiratory tract, lung, and kidney (see respective chapters).

Temporal arteritis (cranial arteritis, giant cell arteritis, Horton disease) was originally thought to be restricted to the temporal, cerebral, and retinal arteries. However, many cases with generalized arterial involvement have been described, indicating that it is a systemic disease.[175,179] This condition, which is most common in the older age group, is characterized by pain in the distribution of the temporal artery and localized tenderness. In other patients, central nervous system manifestations predominate.[173] Sometimes, nodulations can be palpated along the course of the artery.

Microscopically, partial destruction of the wall by an inflammatory infiltrate containing multinucleated giant cells is present.[174] Some of the multinucleated giant cells are of Langhans type; others are of foreign body type. Many of them are intimately associated with the internal elastic lamina, and some may even contain fragments of phagocytosed elastica in their cytoplasm. The presence of perivascular inflammation in the absence of inflammatory changes in the vessel wall is not diagnostic of temporal arteritis.[167] The pathogenesis of this disease remains unknown, but immune factors are thought to play an important role.[171]

Ultrastructurally, there is an accumulation of histiocytes, epithelioid cells, and giant cells at the intimal–medial junction, followed by fragmentation, degeneration, and dissolution of the internal elastic lamina.[178] Immunohistochemical deposition of immunoglobulins and fibrinogen occurs in the vessel wall, but this is probably the result of diffusion from the lumen rather than a primary deposit of immune complexes.[166] It is important to emphasize that the changes are often segmental and that a negative biopsy does not rule out the diagnosis. In one series, only 60% of patients with clinical evidence of temporal arteritis had positive biopsies but the other 40% (showing arteriosclerosis or atherosclerosis) also responded to steroid therapy.[165]

Serial sections should always be performed[172] and contralateral biopsies should be considered in selected cases.[169] Angiography can be useful in guiding the surgeon to biopsy the diseased area.[168]

It should also be remembered that not all cases of arteritis involving the temporal artery represent examples of the entity temporal arteritis.[176,177]

The syndrome of *polymyalgia rheumatica*, characterized by muscle pain and tenderness involving mainly the muscles of the neck, shoulder, and pelvic girdle, and accompanied by an elevated erythrocyte sedimentation rate, is often a manifestation of generalized giant cell arteritis.[170,180]

Degos disease, a progressive subendothelial fibrous thickening of the wall of medium-sized arteries and arterioles, leads to vascular occlusions in many organs, particularly the skin and the digestive system, where ischemic infarcts result.[181]

Small vessel arteritis (arteriolitis)

Small vessel arteritis is the most common variety of arterial inflammation.[182] Most examples are secondary to hypersensitivity to drugs or bacterial antigens or appear as a component of one of the collagen–vascular diseases. The two most important morphologic features to be determined are the nature of the inflammatory infiltrate (whether lymphocytic or neutrophilic) and the presence or absence of necrosis of the vessel wall. In a large majority of the cases, skin manifestations are prominent (see Chapter 4). *Sneddon syndrome* is an inflammatory syndrome of small arteries of unknown pathogenesis that is characteristically followed by smooth muscle proliferation.[183,184] The diagnosis can be suggested by skin biopsy.

Tumors

The general subject of vascular tumors is dealt with in Chapter 25. Only those neoplasms involving major vessels are discussed here.

Primary tumors of the *aorta* or *pulmonary artery* are almost invariably malignant and represent various types of sarcoma. Cases have been reported with names such as fibrosarcoma, leiomyosarcoma, rhabdomyosarcoma, fibromyxosarcoma, malignant fibrous histiocytoma, and malignant histiocytoma.[186,188,189,191,194,195,206,210] In some instances, abundant metaplastic cartilage and bone formation have been present.[185,199]

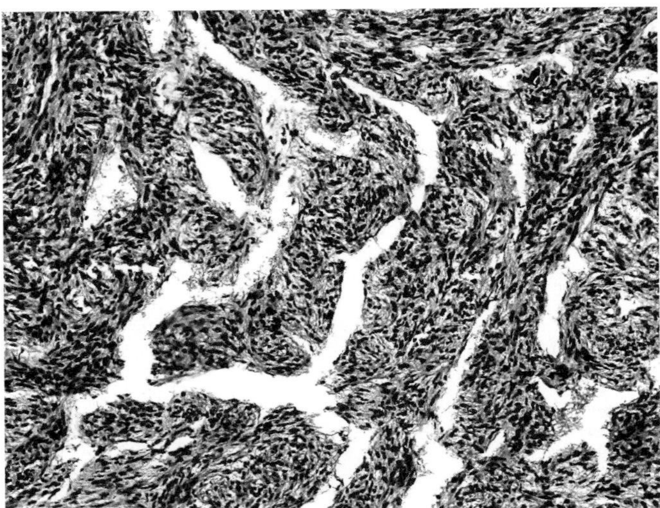

Fig. 27.26 Leiomyosarcoma of inferior vena cava. The vascular pattern of growth of the tumor is reminiscent of that seen in true hemangiopericytoma.

Some sarcomas are thought to originate from the intima and to represent a type of *angiosarcoma* (malignant hemangioendothelioma). The shape of the tumor cells ranges from spindle to epithelioid.[193] In contrast to those arising in smaller vessels, these tumors tend to have a predominantly solid pattern of growth, making the diagnosis very difficult.[207–209] Because of these interpretative problems and the fact that the clinical presentation correlates better with the location of the tumor than its microscopic type, it has been suggested that these sarcomas be simply classified as *intimal* (obstructive or nonobstructive) or *mural*.[187,198,214] Some of these tumors have arisen at the site of a vascular prosthesis,[185,190,213] and others at the site of a surgically constructed arteriovenous fistula. The latter, which represent a remarkable experiment of nature (if things done by surgeons qualify as such), have developed in the setting of chronic immunosuppression in renal transplant patients and have been of the epithelioid variety.[212]

Embolic metastases are common and the overall prognosis is dismal.[201,205] However, cases have been reported in the pulmonary artery of low-grade myxofibroblastic sarcomas (myxofibrosarcomas) with a primarily intraluminal growth and a relatively better prognosis.[211]

Most tumors arising in the inferior vena cava and other large veins are malignant and are largely represented by *leiomyosarcoma*[192,196,197,200] (see Chapter 25) (Fig. 27.26).

Additional primary tumors and tumorlike conditions that may exhibit a predominant or exclusive intravascular location are epithelioid hemangioendothelioma,[204] pyogenic granuloma, intravascular papillary endothelial hyperplasia, nodular fasciitis, so-called 'systemic or malignant angioendotheliomatosis' (which in reality is an angiotropic malignant lymphoma), and synovial sarcoma. These entities are discussed in Chapters 4 and 25. We have also seen a case of entirely intravascular Kaposi sarcoma. Arterial masses having a morphologic appearance similar to that of aneurysmal bone cyst have been recorded.[202]

Metastatic tumors can lodge in large vessels and produce occlusion. Cases of major arterial occlusion from carcinoma of lung and other sites have been well documented.[203]

References

NORMAL ANATOMY

1 Gallagher PJ, van der Wal AC. Blood vessels. In: Mills SE (ed.): Histology for pathologists, ed. 3. Philadelphia, 2007, Lippincott Williams & Wilkins, pp. 218–238.

ARTERIOSCLEROSIS

2 DeBakey ME, Crawford ES, Cooley DA, Morris GC Jr, Garrett HE, Fields WS. Cerebral arterial insufficiency. One to 11-year results following arterial reconstructive operation. Ann Surg 1965, **161**: 921–945.

3 DeBakey ME, Crawford ES, Morris GC Jr, Cooley DA. Surgical considerations of occlusive disease of the innominate, carotid, subclavian, and vertebral arteries. Ann Surg 1961, **154**: 698–725.

4 Gimbrone MA Jr. Vascular endothelium, hemodynamic forces, and atherogenesis. Am J Pathol 1999, **155**: 1–5.

5 Gimbrone MA Jr, Topper JN, Nagel T, Anderson KR, Garcia-Cardena G. Endothelial dysfunction, hemodynamic forces, and atherogenesis. Ann N Y Acad Sci 2000, **902**: 230–239.

6 Hort W. Arteriosclerosis. Its morphology in the past and today. Basic Res Cardiol 1994, **89**: 1–15.

7 Insull W Jr. The pathology of atherosclerosis: plaque development and plaque responses to medical treatment. Am J Med 2009, **122**(1 Suppl): S3–S14.

8 Kannel WB, Shurtleff D. The natural history of arteriosclerosis obliterans. Cardiovasc Clin 1971, **3**: 37–52.

9 Lamon BD, Hajjar DP. Inflammation at the molecular interface of atherogenesis: an anthropological journey. Am J Pathol 2008, **173**: 1253–1264.

10 Raines EW, Ross R. Smooth muscle cells and the pathogenesis of the lesions of atherosclerosis. Br Heart J 1993, **69**: S30–S37.

11 Ross R. Atherosclerosis. Current understanding of mechanisms and future strategies in therapy. Transplant Proc 1993, **25**: 2041–2043.

12 Ross R. The pathogenesis of atherosclerosis. A perspective for the 1990s. Nature 1993, **362**: 801–809.

13 Ross R. Rous-Whipple Award Lecture. Atherosclerosis. A defense mechanism gone awry. Am J Pathol 1993, **143**: 987–1002.

14 Stary HC, Chandler AB, Glagov S, Guyton JR, Insull W Jr, Rosenfeld ME, Schaffer SA, Schwartz CJ, Wagner WD, Wissler RW. A definition of initial, fatty streak, and intermediate lesions of atherosclerosis. A report from the Committee on Vascular Lesions of the Council on Arteriosclerosis, American Heart Association. Arterioscler Thromb 1994, **14**: 840–856.

15 Thompson JE, Kartchner MM, Austin DJ, Wheeler CG, Patman RD. Carotid endarterectomy for cerebrovascular insufficiency (stroke). Follow-up of 359 cases. Ann Surg 1966, **163**: 751–763.

ANEURYSMS

Aortic aneurysms

16 Ariyan S, Cahow CE, Greene FL, Stansel HC. Successful treatment of hepatic artery aneurysm with erosion into the common duct. Ann Surg 1975, **182**: 169–172.

17 Belkin M, Donaldson MC, Whittemore AD. Abdominal aortic aneurysms. Curr Opin Cardiol 1994, **9**: 581–590.

18 Bennett DE, Cherry JK. Bacterial infection of aortic aneurysms. A clinicopathological study. Am J Surg 1967, **113**: 321–326.

19 Bennett DE, Cherry JK. Bacterial infection of aortic aneurysms. A clinicopathological study. Am J Surg 1967, **113**: 321–326.

20 Borst HG, Laas J. Surgical treatment of thoracic aortic aneurysms. Adv Card Surg 1993, **4**: 47–87.

21 Bowers J, Koehler PR, Hammar SP, Nelson JA, Tolman KG. Rupture of a splenic artery aneurysm into the pancreatic duct. Gastroenterology 1976, **70**: 1152–1155.

22 Burke AP, Tavora F, Narula N, Tomaszewski JE, Virmani R. Aortitis and ascending aortic aneurysm: description of 52 cases and proposal of a histologic classification. Hum Pathol 2008, **39**: 514–526.

23 Darling RC, Messina CR, Brewster DC, Ottinger LW. Autopsy study of unoperated abdominal aortic aneurysms. The case for early resection. Circulation 1977, **56**(Suppl): 161–164.

24 De Vries DP, Van Schil PE, Vanmaele RG, Schoofs EL. Inflammatory aneurysms of the abdominal aorta. A five years experience. Acta Chir Belg 1994, **94**: 7–11.

25 Farkas JC, Fichelle JM, Laurian C, Jean-Baptiste A, Gigou F, Marzelle J, Goldstein FW, Cormier JM. Long-term follow-up of positive cultures in 500 abdominal aortic aneurysms. Arch Surg 1993, **128**: 284–288.

26 Hatswell EM. Abdominal aortic aneurysm surgery. I. An overview and discussion of immediate perioperative complications. Heart Lung 1994, **23**: 228–241.

27 Hirst AE Jr, Affeidt JE. Abdominal aortic aneurysm with rupture into the duodenum. A report of eight cases. Gastroenterology 1951, **17**: 504–514.

28 Imakita M, Yutani C, Ishibashi-Ueda H, Nakajima N. Atherosclerotic abdominal aneurysms. Comparative data of different types based on the degree of inflammatory reaction. Cardiovasc Pathol 1992, **1**: 65–73.

29 Kampmeir RH. Saccular aneurysm of the thoracic aorta. A clinical study of 633 cases. Ann Intern Med 1938, **12**: 624–651.

30 Kasashima S, Zen Y, Kawashima A, Konishi K, Sasaki H, Endo M, Matsumoto Y, Kawakami K, Kasashima F, Moriya M, Kimura K, Ohtake H. Inflammatory abdominal aortic aneurysm: close relationship to IgG4-related periaortitis. Am J Surg Pathol 2008, **32**: 197–204.

31 Kiell CS, Ernst CB. Advances in management of abdominal aortic aneurysm. Adv Surg 1993, **26**: 73–98.

32 Kiernan PD, Pairolero PC, Hubert JP Jr, Mucha P Jr, Wallace RB. Aortic graft-enteric fistula. Mayo Clin Proc 1980, **55**: 731–738.

33 Klima T, Spjut HJ, Coelho A, Gray AG, Wukasch DC, Reul GJ Jr, Cooley DA. The morphology of ascending aortic aneurysms. Hum Pathol 1983, **14**: 810–817.

34 Klippel AP, Butcher HR Jr. The unoperated abdominal aortic aneurysm. Am J Surg 1966, **111**: 629–631.

35 Kouchoukos NT, Dougenis D. Surgery of the thoracic aorta. N Engl J Med 1997, **336**: 1876–1888.

36 MacSweeney ST, Powell JT, Greenhalgh RM. Pathogenesis of abdominal aortic aneurysm. Br J Surg 1994, **81**: 935–941.

37 Miller DV, Oderich GS, Aubry MC, Panneton JM, Edwards WD. Surgical pathology of infected aneurysms of the descending thoracic and abdominal aorta: clinicopathologic correlations in 29 cases (1976 to 1999). Hum Pathol 2004, **35**: 1112–1120.

38 Miller DV, Isotalo PA, Weyand CM, Edwards WD, Aubry MC, Tazelaar HD. Surgical pathology of noninfectious ascending aortitis: a study of 45 cases with emphasis on an isolated variant. Am J Surg Pathol 2006, **30**: 1150–1158.

39 Oskoui R, Davis WA, Gomes MN. Salmonella aortitis. A report of a successfully treated case with a comprehensive review of the literature. Arch Intern Med 1993, **153**: 517–525.

40 Reckless JPD, McColl I, Taylor GW. Aorto-enteric fistulae. An uncommon complication of abdominal aneurysms. Br J Surg 1972, **59**: 458–460.

41 Rose AG, Dent DM. Inflammatory variant of abdominal atherosclerotic aneurysm. Arch Pathol Lab Med 1981, **105**: 409–413.

42 Sakata N, Tashiro T, Uesugi N, Kawara T, Furuya K, Hirata Y, Iwasaki H, Kojima M. IgG4-positive plasma cells in inflammatory abdominal aortic aneurysm: the possibility of an aortic manifestation of IgG4-related sclerosing disease. Am J Surg Pathol 2008, **32**: 553–559.

43 Schatz IJ, Fairbairn JF II, Juergens JL. Abdominal aortic aneurysms. A reappraisal. Circulation 1962, **26**: 200–205.

44 Stehbens WE, Delahunt B, Shirer WC, Naik DK. Aortic aneurysm in systemic lupus erythematosus. Histopathology 1993, **22**: 275–277.

45 Szilagyi DE, Smith RF, DeRusso FJ, Elliott JP, Sherrin FW. Contribution of abdominal aortic aneurysmectomy to prolongation of life. Ann Surg 1966, **164**: 678–699.

46 Yonemitsu Y, Nakagawa K, Tanaka S, Mori R, Sugimachi K, Sueishi K. In situ detection of frequent and active infection of human cytomegalovirus in inflammatory abdominal aortic aneurysms: Possible pathogenic role in sustained chronic inflammatory reaction. Lab Invest 1996, **74**: 723–736.

Popliteal artery aneurysms

47 Gifford RW Jr, Hines EA Jr, Janes JM. An analysis and follow-up study of 100 popliteal aneurysms. Surgery 1953, **33**: 284–293.

48 Huang Y, Gloviczki P. Popliteal artery aneurysms: rationale, technique, and results of endovascular treatment. Perspect Vasc Surg Endovasc Ther 2008, **20**: 201–213.

49 Roggo A, Brunner U, Ottinger LW, Largiader F. The continuing challenge of aneurysms of the popliteal artery. Surg Gynecol Obstet 1993, **177**: 565–572.

Dissecting aneurysms

50 Cavanzo FJ, Taylor HB. Effect of pregnancy on the human aorta and its relationship to dissecting aneurysms. Am J Obstet Gynecol 1969, **105**: 567–568.

51 Cigarroa JE, Isselbacher EM, De Sanctis RW, Eagle KA. Diagnostic imaging in the evaluation of suspected aortic dissection. Old standards and new directions. N Engl J Med 1993, **328**: 35–43.

52 DeBakey ME, McCollum CH, Crawford ES, Morris GC Jr, Howell J, Noon GP, Lawrie G. Dissection and dissecting aneurysms of the aorta. Twenty-year follow-up of five hundred twenty-seven patients treated surgically. Surgery 1982, **92**: 1118–1134.

53 DeSanctis RW, Doroghazi RM, Austen WG, Buckley MJ. Aortic dissection. N Engl J Med 1987, **317**: 1060–1067.

54 Guilmet D, Bachet J, Goudot B, Dreyfus G, Martinelli GL. Aortic dissection. Anatomic types and surgical approaches. J Cardiovasc Surg (Torino) 1993, **34**: 23–32.

55 Homme JL, Aubry MC, Edwards WD, Bagniewski SM, Shane Pankratz V, Kral CA, Tazelaar HD. Surgical pathology of the ascending aorta: a clinicopathologic study of 513 cases. Am J Surg Pathol 2006, **30**: 1159–1168.

56 Maleszewski JJ, Miller DV, Lu J, Dietz HC, Halushka MK. Histopathologic findings in ascending aortas from individuals with Loeys–Dietz syndrome (LDS). Am J Surg Pathol 2009, **33**: 194–201.

57 Matt P, Habashi J, Carrel T, Cameron DE, Van Eyk JE, Dietz HC. Recent advances in understanding Marfan syndrome: should we now treat surgical patients with losartan? J Thorac Cardiovasc Surg 2008, **135**: 389–394.

58 McFarland J, Willerson JT, Dinsmore RE, Austen WG, Buckley MJ, Sanders CA, DeSanctis RW. The medical treatment of dissecting aortic aneurysms. N Engl J Med 1972, **286**: 115–155.

59 Wheat MW Jr, Harris PD, Malm JR, Kaiser G, Bowman FO Jr, Palmer RF. Acute dissecting aneurysms of the aorta. Treatment and results in 64 patients. J Thorac Cardiovasc Surg 1969, **58**: 344–351.

60 Wilson SK, Hutchins GM. Aortic dissecting aneurysms. Causative factors in 204 subjects. Arch Pathol Lab Med 1982, **106**: 175–180.

61 Wychulis AR, Kincaid OW, Wallace RB. Primary dissecting aneurysms of peripheral arteries. Mayo Clin Proc 1969, **44**: 804–810.

ARTERIAL SUBSTITUTION

62 Meade JW, Linton RR, Darling RC, Menendez CV. Arterial homografts. A long-term clinical follow-up. Arch Surg 1966, **93**: 392–399.

63 Stanley JC (ed.). Biologic and synthetic vascular prostheses. New York, 1982, Grune & Stratton.

64 Stump MM, Jordan GL Jr, DeBakey ME, Halpert B. The endothelial lining of homografts and Dacron prostheses in the canine aorta. Am J Pathol 1962, **40**: 487–491.

65 Szilagyi DE, McDonald RT, Smith RF, Whitcomb JG. Biologic fate of human arterial homografts. Arch Surg 1957, **75**: 506–529.

ARTERIAL OCCLUSIVE DISEASE

66 Anderson WR, Richards AM, Weiss L. Hemorrhage and necrosis of stomach and small bowel due to atheroembolism. Am J Clin Pathol 1967, **48**: 30–38.

67 Barker WJ, Cannon JA, Zeldis LJ, Perry A. Anatomical results of endarterectomy. Surg Forum 1955, **6**: 266–269.

68 Bernard J, Yi ES. Pulmonary thromboendarterectomy: a clinicopathologic study of 200 consecutive pulmonary thromboendarterectomy cases in one institution. Hum Pathol 2007, **38**: 871–877.

69 Darling RC, Linton RR. Aortoiliofemoral endarterectomy for atherosclerotic occlusive disease. Surgery 1964, **55**: 184–194.

70 DeWeese JA, Barner HB, Mahoney EB, Rob CG. Autogenous venous by-pass grafts and thromboendarterectomies for atherosclerotic lesions of the femoropopliteal arteries. Ann Surg 1966, **163**: 205–214.

71 DeWolfe VG, Beven EG. Arteriosclerosis obliterans in the lower extremities. Correlation of clinical and angiographic findings. Cardiovasc Clin 1971, **3**: 65–92.

72 Dible JH. The pathology of limb ischaemia. St. Louis, 1966, Warren H. Green.

73 Drost H, Buis B, Haan D, Hillers JA. Cholesterol embolism as a complication of left heart catheterization. Report of seven cases. Br Heart J 1984, **52**: 339–342.

74 Harrington JT, Sommers SC, Kassirer JP. Atheromatous emboli with progressive renal failure. Renal arteriography as the probable inciting factor. Ann Intern Med 1968, **68**: 152–160.

75 Hollenhorst RW. Vascular status of patients who have cholesterol emboli in the retina. Am J Ophthalmol 1966, **61**: 1159–1165.

76 Jorgensen L. Mechanisms of thrombosis. Pathobiol Annu 1972, **2**: 139–204.

77 Kalter DC, Rudolph A, McGavran M. Livedo reticularis due to multiple cholesterol emboli. J Am Acad Dermatol 1985, **13**: 235–242.

78 Kassirer JP. Atheroembolic renal disease. N Engl J Med 1969, **280**: 812–818.

79 Kouchoukos NT, Levy JF, Balfour JF, Butcher HR Jr. Operative therapy for femoral–popliteal arterial occlusive disease. A comparison of therapeutic methods. Circulation 1967, 35(Suppl 1): 174–182.

80 Krotovsky GS, Turpitko SA, Gerasimov VB, Zabelskaya TF, Mamedov DM, Klokov KI, Uchkin IG, Papandopoulos E. Surgical treatment and prevention of vasculopathic impotence in conjunction with revascularisation of the lower extremities in Leriche's syndrome. J Cardiovasc Surg 1991, **32**: 340–343.

81 Morris GC Jr, Wheeler CG, Crawford ES, Cooley DA, DeBakey ME. Restorative vascular surgery in the presence of impending and overt gangrene of the extremities. Surgery 1962, **51**: 50–57.

82 Richards AM, Eliot RS, Kanjuh VI, Bloemendaal RD, Edwards JE. Cholesterol embolism. A multiple system disease masquerading as polyarteritis nodosa. Am J Cardiol 1965, **15**: 696–707.

83 Stout C, Hartsuck JM, Howe J, Richardson JL. Atheromatous embolism after aortofemoral bypass and aortic ligation. Arch Pathol 1972, **93**: 271–275.

84 Warren R, Gomez RL, Marston JAP, Cox JST. Femoropopliteal arteriosclerosis obliterans. Arteriographic patterns and rates of progression. Surgery 1964, **55**: 135–143.

CYSTIC ADVENTITIAL DEGENERATION

85 Blackstrom CG, Linell F, Ostberg G. Cystic myxomatous adventitial degeneration of the radial artery with development of ganglion in the connective tissue. Acta Chir Scand 1965, **129**: 447–451.

86 Flanigan DP, Burnham SJ, Goodreau JJ, Bergan JJ. Summary of cases of adventitial cystic disease of the popliteal artery. Ann Surg 1979, **189**: 165–175.

87 Haid SP, Conn I Jr, Bergan JJ. Cystic adventitial disease of the popliteal artery. Arch Surg 1970, **101**: 765–770.

88 Lewis GJT, Douglas DM, Reid W, Watt JK. Cystic adventitial disease of the popliteal artery. BMJ 1967, **3**: 411–415.

89 Terry JD, Schenken JR, Lohff MR, Neis DD. Cystic adventitial disease. Hum Pathol 1981, **23**: 639–643.

FIBROMUSCULAR DYSPLASIA

90 Crocker DW. Fibromuscular dysplasias of renal artery. Arch Pathol 1968, **85**: 602–613.

91 Furie DM, Tien RD. Fibromuscular dysplasia of arteries of the head and neck. Imaging findings. AJR Am J Roentgenol 1994, **162**: 1205–1209.

92 Harrison EG, Hung JC, Bernatz PE. Morphology of fibromuscular dysplasia of the renal artery in renovascular hypertension. Am J Med 1967, **43**: 97–112.

93 Hunt JC, Harrison EG Jr, Kincaid OW, Bernatz PE, Davis GP. Idiopathic fibrous and fibromuscular stenoses of the renal arteries associated with hypertension. Mayo Clin Proc 1962, **37**: 181–216.

94 Lüscher TF, Lie JT, Stanson AW, Houser OW, Hollier LH, Sheps SG. Arterial fibromuscular dysplasia. Mayo Clin Proc 1987, **62**: 931–952.

95 Moreau P, Albat B, Thevenet A. Fibromuscular dysplasia of the internal carotid artery. Long-term surgical results. J Cardiovasc Surg 1993, **34**: 466–472.

96 Price RA, Vawter GF. Arterial fibromuscular dysplasia in infancy and childhood. Arch Pathol 1972, **93**: 419–426.

MESENTERIC VASCULAR OCCLUSION

97 Arosemena E, Edwards JE. Lesions of the small mesenteric arteries underlying intestinal infarction. Geriatrics 1967, **22**: 122–138.

98 Bienenstock H, Minick R, Rogoff B. Mesenteric arteritis and intestinal infarction in rheumatoid disease. Arch Intern Med 1967, **119**: 359–364.

99 Flaherty MJ, Lie JT, Haggitt RC. Mesenteric inflammatory veno-occlusive disease. A seldom recognized cause of intestinal ischemia. Am J Surg Pathol 1994, **18**: 779–784.

100 Ho ECK, Moss AJ. The syndrome of 'mesenteric arteritis' following surgical repair of aortic coarctation. Report of 9 cases and review of literature. Pediatrics 1972, **49**: 40–45.

101 Kempczinski RF, Clark SM, Blebea J, Koelliker DD, Fenoglio-Preiser C. Intestinal ischemia secondary to thromboangiitis obliterans. Ann Vasc Surg 1993, **7**: 354–358.

102 Ottinger LW, Austen WG. A study of 136 patients with mesenteric infarction. Surg Gynecol Obstet 1967, **124**: 251–261.

103 Roobottom CA, Dubbins PA. Significant disease of the celiac and superior mesenteric arteries in asymptomatic patients. Predictive value of Doppler sonography. AJR Am J Roentgenol 1993, **161**: 985–988.

104 Schneider TA, Longo WE, Ure T, Vernava AM. Mesenteric ischemia. Acute arterial syndromes. Dis Colon Rectum 1994, **37**: 1163–1174.

105 Volteas N, Labropoulos N, Leon M, Kalodiki E, Chan P, Nicolaides AN. Detection of superior mesenteric and coeliac artery stenosis with colour flow Duplex imaging. Eur J Vasc Surg 1993, **7**: 616–620.

106 Williams LF, Anastasia LF, Hasiotis CA, Bosniak MA, Byrne JJ. Nonocclusive mesenteric infarction. Am J Surg 1967, **114**: 376–381.

TRAUMATIC AND IATROGENIC INJURIES

RUPTURE

107 Eeckhout E, Beuret P, Lobrinus A, Genton CY, Goy JJ. Coronary artery rupture during transluminal coronary recanalization and angioplasty in a case of acute myocardial infarction and shock. Clin Cardiol 1993, **16**: 355–356.

108 Fajardo LF, Lee A. Rupture of major vessels after radiation. Cancer 1975, **36**: 904–913.

109 Hasan RI, Krysiak P, Deiranyia AK, Hooper T. Spontaneous rupture of the internal mammary artery in Ehlers–Danlos syndrome [letter]. J Thorac Cardiovasc Surg 1993, **106**: 184–185.

110 Rodriguez HF, Rivera E. Spontaneous rupture of the thoracic aorta through an atheromatous plaque. Ann Intern Med 1961, **54**: 307–313.

111 Worrell JT, Buja LM, Reynolds RC. Pneumococcal aortitis with rupture of the aorta. Report of a case and review of the literature. Am J Clin Pathol 1988, **89**: 565–568.

THROMBOSIS

112 Bickerstaff ER. Aetiology of acute hemiplegia in childhood. J Neurosurg 1964, **2**: 82–87.

113 Houck WS, Jackson JR, Odom GL, Young WG. Occlusion of internal carotid artery in neck secondary to closed trauma to head and neck. Report of two cases. Ann Surg 1964, **159**: 219–221.

114 Kuo T, Sayers CP, Rosai J. Masson's 'vegetant intravascular hemangioendothelioma'. A lesion often mistaken for angiosarcoma. Study of seventeen cases located in the skin and soft tissues. Cancer 1976, **38**: 1227–1236.

115 Pitner SE. Carotid thrombosis due to intraoral trauma. An unusual complication of a common childhood accident. N Engl J Med 1966, **274**: 764–767.

116 Salyer WR, Salyer DC. Myxoma-like features of organizing thrombi in arteries and veins. Arch Pathol 1975, **99**: 307–311.

117 Shillito J Jr. Carotid arteritis. Cause of hemiplegia in childhood. J Neurosurg 1964, **21**: 540–551.

PULSATING HEMATOMA

118 Bennett DE, Cherry JK. The natural history of traumatic aneurysms of the aorta. Surgery 1967, **61**: 516–523.

119 Cohen SM. Peripheral aneurysm and arteriovenous fistula. Ann R Coll Surg Engl 1952, **11**: 1–30.

120 Gallen J, Wiss DA, Cantelmo N, Menzoin JO. Traumatic pseudoaneurysm of the axillary artery. Report of three cases and literature review. J Trauma 1984, **24**: 350–354.

ACQUIRED ARTERIOVENOUS FISTULA

121 Gomes MMR, Bernatz PE. Arteriovenous fistulas. A review of ten-year experience at the Mayo Clinic. Mayo Clin Proc 1970, **45**: 81–102.

THROMBOANGIITIS OBLITERANS

122 Colburn MD, Moore WS. Buerger's disease. Heart Dis Stroke 1993, **2**: 424–432.

123 Hershey FB, Pareira MD, Ahlvin RC. Quadrilateral peripheral vascular disease in the young adult. Circulation 1962, **26**: 1261–1269.

124 Ishikawa K, Kawase S, Mishima Y. Occlusive arterial disease in extremities, with special reference to Buerger's disease. Angiology 1962, **13**: 398–411.

125 Kelly PJ, Dahlin DJ, Janes JM. Clinicopathological study of ninety-four limbs amputated for occlusive vascular disease. J Bone Joint Surg 1958, **40**: 72–78.

126 Kurata A, Franke FE, Machinami R, Schulz A. Thromboangitis obliterans: classic and new morphological features. Virchows Arch 2000, **436**: 59–67.

127 McKusick VA, Harris WS. The Buerger syndrome in the Orient. Bull Johns Hopkins Hosp 1961, **109**: 241–291.

128 McKusick VA, Harris WS, Ottesen OE, Goodman RM. The Buerger syndrome in the United States. Bull Johns Hopkins Hosp 1962, **110**: 145–176.

129 McKusick VA, Harris WS, Ottesen OE, Shelley WM, Bloodwell DB. Buerger's disease. A distinct clinical and pathologic entity. JAMA 1962, **181**: 93–100.

130 Mills JL, Porter JM. Buerger's disease. A review and update. Semin Vasc Surg 1993, **6**: 14–23.

131 Olin JW. Thromboangiitis obliterans (Buerger's disease). N Engl J Med 2000, **343**: 864–869.

132 Schellong SM, Bernhards J, Ensslen F, Schafers HJ, Alexander K. Intestinal type of thromboangiitis obliterans (Buerger's disease). J Intern Med 1994, **235**: 69–73.

133 Shionoya S. Buerger's disease. Diagnosis and management. Cardiovasc Surg 1993, **1**: 207–214.

134 Wessler S, Ming S-C, Guerwich V, Greiman DG. A critical evaluation of thromboangiitis obliterans. The case against Buerger's disease. N Engl J Med 1960, **262**: 1149–1160.

135 Williams G. Recent views on Buerger's disease. J Clin Pathol 1969, **22**: 573–577.

ARTERITIS

136 Hoffman GS, Weyand CM. Inflammatory diseases of blood vessels. New York, 2002, Marcel Dekker.

137 Manion WC. Infectious angiitis. In Orbison JL, Smith DE (eds): The peripheral blood vessels. Baltimore, 1963, Williams & Wilkins, pp. 221–231.

138 Parums DV. The arteritides. Histopathology 1994, **25**: 1–20.

139 Weyand CM, Goronzy JJ. Medium- and large-vessel vasculitis. N Engl J Med 2003, **349**: 160–169.

140 Worrell JT, Buja LM, Reynolds RC. Pneumococcal aortitis with rupture of the aorta. Report of a case and review of the literature. Am J Clin Pathol 1988, **89**: 565–568.

LARGE VESSEL ARTERITIS

141 Arav-Boger R, Assia A, Jurgenson U, Spirer Z. The immunology of Kawasaki disease. Adv Pediatr 1994, **41**: 359–367.

142 Beckman EN. Plasma cell infiltrates in atherosclerotic abdominal aortic aneurysms. Am J Clin Pathol 1986, **85**: 21–24.

143 Chetty R, Batitang S, Nair R. Large artery vasculopathy in HIV-positive patients: another vasculitic enigma. Hum Pathol 2000, **31**: 374–379.

144 Domingo RT, Maramba MD, Torres LF, Wesolowski SA. Acquired aortoarteritis. A worldwide vascular entity. Arch Surg 1967, **95**: 780–790.

145 Feiner HD, Raghavendra BN, Phelps R, Rooney L. Inflammatory abdominal aortic aneurysm. Report of six cases. Hum Pathol 1984, **15**: 454–459.

146 Fujiwara H, Fujiwara T, Kao T-C, Ohshio G, Hamashima Y. Pathology of Kawasaki disease in the healed stage. Relationships between typical and atypical cases of Kawasaki disease. Acta Pathol Jpn 1986, **36**: 857–867.

147 Gonzalez-Cerna JL, Villavicencio L, Molina B, Bessudo L. Nonspecific obliterative aortitis in children. Ann Thorac Surg 1967, **4**: 193–204.

148 Hall S, Barr W, Lie JT, Stanson AW, Kazmier FJ, Hunder GG. Takayasu arteritis. A study of 32 North American patients. Medicine 1985, **64**: 89–99.

149 Ishikawa K, Maetani S. Long-term outcome for 120 Japanese patients with Takayasu's disease. Clinical and statistical analyses of related prognostic factors. Circulation 1994, **90**: 1855–1860.

150 Kerr GS, Hallahan CW, Giordano J, Leavitt RY, Fauci AS, Rottem M, Hoffman GS. Takayasu arteritis. Ann Intern Med 1994, **120**: 919–929.

151 Leung DY. Kawasaki disease. Curr Opin Rheumatol 1993, **5**: 41–50.

152 Masuda H, Shozawa T, Naoe S, Tanaka N. The intercostal artery in Kawasaki disease. A pathologic study of 17 autopsy cases. Arch Pathol Lab Med 1986, **110**: 1136–1142.

153 Mitchinson MJ. Chronic periaortitis and periarteritis. Histopathology 1984, **8**: 589–600.

154 Nadel S, Levin M. Kawasaki disease. Curr Opin Pediatr 1993, **5**: 29–34.

155 Nasu T. Pathology of pulseless disease. A systematic study and critical review of 21 autopsy cases reported in Japan. Angiology 1963, **14**: 225–242.

156 O'Leary M, Nollet DJ, Blomberg DJ. Rupture of a tuberculous pseudoaneurysm of the innominate artery into the trachea and esophagus. Report of a case and review of the literature. Hum Pathol 1977, **8**: 458–467.

157 Pariser KM. Takayasu's arteritis. Curr Opin Cardiol 1994, **9**: 575–580.

158 Restrepo C, Tejeda C, Correa P. Nonsyphilitic aortitis. Arch Pathol 1969, **87**: 1–12.

159 Rose AG, Dent DM. Inflammatory variant of abdominal atherosclerotic aneurysm. Arch Pathol Lab Med 1981, **105**: 409–413.

160 Rose AG, Sinclair-Smith CC. Takayasu's arteritis. A study of 16 autopsy cases. Arch Pathol Lab Med 1980, **104**: 231–237.

161 Roth LM, Kissane JM. Panaortitis and aortic valvulitis in progressive systemic sclerosis (scleroderma). Report of case with perforation of an aortic cusp. Am J Clin Pathol 1964, **41**: 287–296.

162 Schrire V, Asherson RA. Arteritis of the aorta and its major branches. Q J Med 1964, **33**: 439–463.

163 Valaitis J, Pilz CG, Montgomery MM. Aortitis with aortic valve insufficiency in rheumatoid arthritis. Arch Pathol 1957, **63**: 207–212.

164 Yonemitsu Y, Nakagawa K, Tanaka S, Mori R, Sugimachi K, Sueishi K. In situ detection of frequent and active infection of human cytomegalovirus in inflammatory abdominal aortic aneurysms: Possible pathogenic role in sustained chronic inflammatory reaction. Lab Invest 1996, **74**: 723–736.

MEDIUM-SIZED VESSEL ARTERITIS

165 Allsop CJ, Gallagher PJ. Temporal artery biopsy in giant-cell arteritis. A reappraisal. Am J Surg Pathol 1981, **5**: 317–323.

166 Banks PM, Cohen MD, Ginsburg WW, Hunder GG. Immunohistologic and cytochemical studies of temporal arteritis. Arthritis Rheum 1983, **26**: 1201–1207.

167 Corcoran GM, Prayson RA, Herzog KM. The significance of perivascular inflammation in the absence of arteritis in temporal artery biopsy specimens. Am J Clin Pathol 2001, **115**: 342–347.

168 Elliott PD, Baker HL Jr, Brown AL Jr. The superficial temporal artery angiogram. Radiology 1972, **102**: 635–638.

169 Goodman BW Jr. Temporal arteritis. Am J Med 1979, **67**: 839–852.

170 Hamilton CR Jr, Shelley WM, Tumulty PA. Giant cell arteritis including temporal arteritis and polymyalgia rheumatica. Medicine (Baltimore) 1971, **50**: 1–27.

171 Hunder GG, Lie JT, Goronzy JJ, Weyand CM. Pathogenesis of giant cell arteritis. Arthritis Rheum 1993, **36**: 757–761.

172 Klein RG, Campbell RJ, Hunder GG, Carney JA. Skip lesions in temporal arteritis. Mayo Clin Proc 1976, **51**: 504–510.

173 Kolodny EH, Rebeiz JJ, Caviness VS, Richardson EP. Granulomatous angiitis of the central nervous system. Arch Neurol 1968, **19**: 510–524.

174 Lie JT. Temporal artery biopsy diagnosis of giant cell arteritis: lessons from 1109 biopsies. Anat Pathol 1998, **1**: 69–97.

175 Lie JT, Failoni DD, Davis DC Jr. Temporal arteritis with giant cell aortitis, coronary arteritis, and myocardial infarction. Arch Pathol Lab Med 1986, **110**: 857–860.

176 Morgan GJ Jr, Harris ED Jr. Non-giant cell temporal arteritis. Arthritis Rheum 1978, **21**: 362–366.

177 O'Brien JP. A concept of diffuse actinic arteritis. Br J Dermatol 1978, **98**: 1–13.

178 Parker F, Healey LA, Wilske KR, Odland GF. Light and electron microscopic studies on human temporal arteries with special reference to alterations related to senescence, atherosclerosis and giant cell arteritis. Am J Pathol 1975, **79**: 57–80.

179 Parums DV. The arteritides. Histopathology 1994, **25**: 1–20.

180 Royster TS, DiRe JJ. Polymyalgia rheumatica and giant cell arteritis with bilateral axillary artery occlusion. Am Surg 1971, **37**: 421–426.

181 Strole WE Jr, Clark WH, Isselbacher KJ. Progressive arterial occlusive disease (Kohlmeier–Degos). A frequently fatal cutaneosystemic disorder. N Engl J Med 1967, **276**: 195–201.

SMALL VESSEL ARTERITIS (ARTERIOLITIS)

182 Jennette JC, Falk RJ. Small-vessel vasculitis. N Engl J Med 1997, **337**: 1512–1523.

183 Sepp N, Zelger B, Schuler G, Romani N, Fritsch P. Sneddon's syndrome. An inflammatory disorder of small arteries followed by smooth muscle proliferation. Immunohistochemical and ultrastructural evidence. Am J Surg Pathol 1995, **19**: 448–453.

184 Zelger B, Sepp N, Stockhammer G, Dosch E, Hilty E, Ofner D, Aichner F, Fritsch PO. Sneddon's syndrome. A long-term follow-up of 21 patients. Arch Dermatol 1993, **129**: 437–447.

TUMORS

185 Ben-Izhak O, Vlodavsky E, Ofer A, Engel A, Nitecky S, Hoffman A. Epithelioid angiosarcoma associated with a Dacron vascular graft. Am J Surg Pathol 1999, **23**: 1418–1422.

186 Bleisch VR, Kraus FT. Polypoid sarcoma of the pulmonary trunk. Analysis of the literature and report of a case with leptomeric organelles and ultrastructural features of rhabdomyosarcoma. Cancer 1980, **46**: 314–324.

187 Burke AP, Virmani R. Sarcomas of the great vessels. A clinicopathologic study. Cancer 1993, **71**: 1761–1773.

188 Chen KTK. Primary malignant fibrous histiocytoma of the aorta. Cancer 1981, **48**: 840–844.

189 Emmert-Buck MR, Stay EJ, Tsokos M, Travis WD. Pleomorphic rhabdomyosarcoma arising in association with the right pulmonary artery. Arch Pathol Lab Med 1994, **118**: 1220–1222.

190 Fehrenbacher JW, Bowers W, Strate R, Pittman J. Angiosarcoma of the aorta associated with a Dacron graft. Ann Thorac Surg 1981, **32**: 297–301.

191 Gaumann A, Bode-Lesniewska B, Zimmermann DR, Fanburg-Smith JC, Kirkpatrick CJ, Hofstädter F, Woenckhaus M, Stoehr R, Obermann EC, Dietmaier W, Hartmann A. Exploration of the APC/beta-catenin (WNT) pathway and a histologic classification system for pulmonary artery intimal sarcoma. A study of 18 cases. Virchows Arch 2008, **453**: 473–484.

192 Hines OJ, Nelson S, Quinones-Baldrich WJ, Eilber FR. Leiomyosarcoma of the inferior vena cava: prognosis and comparison with leiomyosarcoma of other anatomic sites. Cancer 1999, **85**: 1077–1083.

193 Hottenrott G, Mentzel T, Peters A, Schroder A, Katenkamp D. Intravascular ('intimal') epithelioid angiosarcoma: clinicopathological and immunohistochemical analysis of three cases. Virchows Arch 1999, **435**: 473–478.

194 Iwasaki I, Iwase H, Horie H, Ide G, Saito T, Furukawa Y. Leiomyosarcoma of pulmonary truncus. Acta Pathol Jpn 1984, **34**: 863–867.

195 Johansson L, Carlen B. Sarcoma of the pulmonary artery. Report of four cases with electron microscopic and immunohistochemical examinations, and review of the literature. Virchows Arch 1994, **424**: 217–224.

196 Kaiser LR, Urmacher C. Primary sarcoma of the superior pulmonary vein. Cancer 1990, **66**: 789–795.

197 Laskin WB, Fanburg-Smith JC, Burke AP, Kraszewska E, Fetsch JF, Miettinen M. Leiomyosarcoma of the inferior vena cava: clinicopathologic study of 40 cases. Am J Surg Pathol 2010, **34**: 873–881.

198 Miracco C, Laurini L, Santopietro R, De Santi MM, Sassi C, Neri E, Pepi F, Luzi P. Intimal-type primary sarcoma of the aorta. Report of a case with evidence of rhabdomyosarcomatous differentiation. Histopathology 1999, **435**: 62–66.

199 Murthy MSN, Meckstroth CV, Merkle BH, Huston JT, Cattaneo SM. Primary intimal sarcoma of pulmonary valve and trunk with osteogenic sarcomatous elements. Report of a case considered to be pulmonary embolus. Arch Pathol Lab Med 1976, **100**: 649–651.

200 Oliai BR, Tazelaar HD, Lloyd RV, Doria MI, Trastek VF. Leiomyosarcoma of the pulmonary veins. Am J Surg Pathol 1999, **23**: 1082–1088.

201 Patel KR, Niazi TBM, Griffiths AP, Hardy GJ, MacLaren CAN, Reid IN. Massive osteolytic bone metastases from a primary aortic sarcoma: a case report. Hum Pathol 1997, **28**: 1306–1310.

202 Petrik PK, Findlay JM, Sherlock RA. Aneurysmal cyst, bone type, primary in an artery. Am J Surg Pathol 1993, **17**: 1062–1066.

203 Prioleau PG, Katzenstein AA. Major peripheral arterial occlusion due to malignant tumor embolism. Cancer 1978, **42**: 2009–2014.

204 Rosai J, Gold J, Landy R. The histiocytoid hemangiomas. A unifying concept embracing several previously described entities of skin, soft tissue, large vessels, bone and heart. Hum Pathol 1979, **10**: 707–730.

205 Ruijter ET, Ten Kate FJ. Metastasising sarcoma of the aorta. Histopathology 1996, **29**: 278–281.

206 Salm R. Primary fibrosarcoma of aorta. Cancer 1972, **29**: 73–83.

207 Schmid E, Port J, Carroll RM, Freidman NB. Primary metastasizing aortic endothelioma. Cancer 1984, **54**: 1407–1411.

208 Sebenik M, Ricci A Jr, DiPasquale B, Mody K, Pytel P, Jee KJ, Knuutila S, Scholes J. Undifferentiated intimal sarcoma of large systemic blood vessels: report of 14 cases with immunohistochemical profile and review of the literature. Am J Surg Pathol 2005, **29**: 1184–1193.

209 Steffelaar JW, van der Heul RO, Blackstone E, Vos A. Primary sarcoma of the aorta. Arch Pathol 1975, **99**: 139–142.

210 Stevenson JE, Burkhead H, Trueheart RE, McLaren J. Primary malignant tumor of the aorta. Am J Med 1971, **51**: 553–559.

211 Tavora F, Miettinen M, Fanburg-Smith J, Franks TJ, Burke A. Pulmonary artery sarcoma: a histologic and follow-up study with emphasis on a subset of low-grade myofibroblastic sarcomas with a good long-term follow-up. Am J Surg Pathol 2008, **32**: 1751–1761.

212 Wehrli BM, Janzen DL, Shokeir O, Masri BA, Byrne SK, O'Connell JX. Epithelioid angiosarcoma arising in a surgically constructed arteriovenous fistula: a rare complication of chronic immunosuppression in the setting of renal transplantation. Am J Surg Pathol 1998, **22**: 1154–1159.

213 Weinberg DS, Maini BS. Primary sarcoma of the aorta associated with a vascular prosthesis. A case report. Cancer 1980, **46**: 398–402.

214 Wright EP, Virmani R, Glick AD, Page DL. Aortic intimal sarcoma with embolic metastases. Am J Surg Pathol 1985, **9**: 890–897.

Veins

CHAPTER CONTENTS

Thrombophlebitis and thromboembolism

Thrombophlebitis is a thrombotic disease of veins accompanied by varying degrees of inflammation.[3,8] Microscopically, the venous wall is edematous, the intima irregularly ulcerated, and the media infiltrated with chronic inflammatory cells. As the acute inflammatory phase of the disease subsides, varying amounts of fibrous tissue are deposited in the adventitia and in the media. During the acute phase, the thrombus becomes attached more or less firmly to the denuded intima.

The process of thrombophlebitis is associated with edema of the extremity, which may be minimal or marked. When there is but little edema and few or no clinical signs of acute inflammation in the extremity, the venous thrombosis has been termed *phlebothrombosis* or *bland noninflammatory venous thrombosis* in a classic paper coauthored by Ochsner, DeBakey and DeCamp.[9] This type of thrombophlebitis is probably more frequently associated with pulmonary emboli than is thrombophlebitis with more marked signs of inflammation. However, the rigid separation of phlebothrombosis from thrombophlebitis is neither pathologically possible nor clinically practical. In most instances, these two conditions are merely different degrees of the same process.

Thrombophlebitis may involve only the superficial veins such as the saphenous vein. Clinically, the vein is acutely inflamed and tender, and the overlying skin is red. When the thrombosis is limited to the superficial veins, there is usually little edema. However, thrombophlebitic edema may develop with marked rapidity and may be of great volume if the process extends into the deep venous system. Rapid shifts of extracellular fluid into the leg may be sufficiently massive to cause shock. In such instances, the extremity may become so swollen that cutaneous blebs develop, followed by cutaneous necrosis (*phlegmasia cerulea dolens*).[13] The usual postoperative or post-traumatic acute thrombophlebitis initially causes a painful, tender, swollen, cool, and mottled or grayish white extremity. Clinical examination is notoriously inaccurate in the diagnosis of deep vein thrombosis.

Purulent or septic thrombophlebitis is occasionally seen in association with abscess or other infection usually occurring in the peritoneal cavity or pelvis. Stein and Pruitt[14] found this complication in 4.6% of 521 burned patients who had been treated by venous catheterization. Purulent thrombophlebitis at any location is associated with marked chills and high temperature because of the bacteremia arising from the infected intravascular thrombus.

There is a statistically significant association between deep vein thrombosis and the presence of cancer in an internal organ, known as the *Trousseau syndrome.*[10] Many of the tumors are mucin-producing adenocarcinomas, and most of them have arisen from the pancreas.

Pulmonary embolism is often thought to be primarily a complication of some surgical procedure or trauma such as fracture, particularly of the lower extremity, but the incidence of this complication is as high on medical as on surgical services. Some of the factors thought to favor intravenous thrombosis and subsequent pulmonary embolism are neoplasms, cardiac disease, venous stasis from any cause, infection in the immediate area of veins, trauma, spasm of vessels, intimal injury, increased coagulability, and immobilization of the limbs.[15] The use of oral contraceptives with early regimens was found to be causally related to the presence of thromboembolic phenomena.[5,12,16] Irey et al.[6] described distinctive vascular lesions in association with thrombosis in arteries and veins of 20 young women receiving oral contraceptives. The incidence of this complication has greatly diminished with modifications in the type and dosage of contraceptive drugs.

Pulmonary embolism is seen in all forms of thrombophlebitis, but one should be aware that sudden massive pulmonary emboli frequently occur in patients without antecedent symptoms or signs of peripheral thrombophlebitis.

The greatest percentage of thrombi resulting in pulmonary embolization are thought to originate in the veins of the lower extremity. In a classic study, Rössle[11] found that 27% of patients over 20 years of age harbored thrombi in the veins of the calf at autopsy. The study of Hunter et al.[4] confirmed these observations and showed that thrombosis occurred in over 50% of middle-aged or older persons confined to bed.

McLachlin and Paterson[7] stressed the finding of intravascular thromboses arising in relationship to the valve pockets. In 100 complete dissections of the veins of the pelvis and lower extremities, they showed gross venous thrombi in 34%, and in over one-half of these there were pulmonary emboli. In their series, the thrombi found in 34 patients totaled 76: 6 in the pelvic veins, 49 in the thigh veins, and 21 in the leg veins. They found that 75% of the venous thrombi arose in the veins of the thigh and pelvis and 25% in the smaller veins of the calf and feet, with 92% arising in the lower extremities. Similar findings were reported by Beckering and Titus.[1]

Crane[2] concluded that approximately 85% of fatal pulmonary emboli arise from thrombi in the legs (90% in postsurgical patients and 80% in cardiac or medical patients).

Stasis ulcers

Whereas the chief immediate complication of thrombophlebitis is the above described pulmonary embolism, the principal long-term complication is stasis ulceration.

The treatment of acute thrombophlebitis attempts to limit the extension of the process and to prevent pulmonary embolization. Elevation, rest with the maintenance of good hydration, elastic support, and anticoagulant therapy are the initial measures. Ligation of the venous system above the area of intravascular clotting is occasionally indicated when lesser measures fail to prevent pulmonary embolus.

As the acute phase of the disease subsides, measures must be taken to avoid later stasis disease in the lower extremity. The use of elastic supports to help control any dependent edema in the extremity is imperative and may be required for many months or years. With the passage of time, collateral venous channels may develop and communicate with the superficial venous systems, resulting in secondary superficial varicosities. Recanalization of the major deep veins is usually associated with the process. Any significant varicosities in the postphlebitic extremity should be removed.

For reasons not clearly understood, the prevention and control of stasis ulceration are quite difficult in the presence of subcutaneous varicosities. The preventive measures directed toward control of dependent edema are not often carried out by patients suffering from thrombophlebitis, so after several years cutaneous pigmentation, brawny edema, dermal and subcutaneous fibrosis, extensive secondary varicosities, and ulceration of the skin in the lower one-third of the leg develop. Although stasis ulcers are seen in patients with a history of past thrombophlebitis, such a history is commonly absent. Even in patients having thrombophlebitis, the exact pathogenesis of the process leading to ulceration is unknown.

The diagnosis of stasis disease is not usually difficult. Before extensive treatment of a patient with an advanced chronic leg ulcer, careful evaluation of the arterial blood supply should be made. Any significant arterial flow deficiency will likely result in failure of surgical therapy for ulceration. Correction of major arterial occlusion should therefore be made whenever possible, before treatment of the stasis ulcer in those patients in whom both are present. Other rare causes of ulceration such as specific infections and neoplasms must be excluded. All ulcers should be cultured and any unusual-appearing ones biopsied before excisional therapy is undertaken.

If ulceration has not yet appeared, or is not extensive or chronic in nature, total removal of the varicose veins with ligation of perforating veins may control the process. If stasis ulceration is extensive, chronic, and long-standing, it is best treated by excision and stripping of all superficial varicosities of the extremity after high ligation and division of the saphena magna and its tributaries at the saphenous–femoral junction. The ulcer and its base should be excised down to normal tissue, with removal of all the inelastic thickened skin and fascia about it. The cutaneous–fascial defect should then be covered with a partial thickness cutaneous autograft.

Advanced stasis ulceration often requires extensive excision. In most instances, the depth of the excision should include the fascia overlying the muscle, as the fascial fibrosis and thickening are quite extensive in the presence of long-standing stasis ulcers. This also facilitates ligation of the perforating veins that are invariably present beneath the area of stasis fibrosis.

Varicose veins

Varicose veins occur more frequently in women than in men. They often develop in the second and third decades of life and may be present for many years without causing symptoms or complications. Their incidence is much higher in obese women, particularly those who have had several pregnancies. Varicosities developing in women after pregnancy may be secondary to deep venous thrombosis.

Larson and Smith[18] reported that 213 of 491 patients with varicose veins (43%) had a definite family history, indicating some hereditary disposition. The superficial veins of the leg become dilated and tortuous and lose valvular function. Microscopically, there is fibrosis beneath the endothelium and in the wall, with secondary elastosis and loss of muscle. Calcification may occur.

The likelihood of thrombosis with propagation into the deep venous system and the potential for the development of the post-phlebitic syndrome are sufficiently great to warrant the removal of varicose veins. The use of sclerosing agents is contraindicated because of the danger of deep venous thrombosis, as well as the temporary nature of the superficial venous occlusion obtained. The surgical removal of varicosities is best performed by venous stripping techniques and excisions.[17,19]

Tumors

Tumors of large veins are discussed together with tumors of arteries on page 2298. Tumors of smaller vessels are discussed in Chapter 25 (Soft tissues).

References

THROMBOPHLEBITIS AND THROMBOEMBOLISM

1 Beckering RE Jr, Titus JL. Femoral–popliteal venous thrombosis and pulmonary embolism. Am J Clin Pathol 1969, **52**: 530–537.

2 Crane C. Deep venous thrombosis and pulmonary embolism. N Engl J Med 1957, **257**: 147–157.

3 Gloviczki P, Yao JST. Handbook of venous disorders: guidelines of the American venous forum. London, 2001, Arnold.

4 Hunter WC, Krygier JJ, Kennedy JC, Sneedend VD. Etiology and prevention of thrombosis of the deep leg veins. Surgery 1945, **17**: 178–190.

5 Inman WHW, Vessey MP. Investigation of deaths from pulmonary coronary and cerebral thrombosis and embolism in women in childbearing age. BMJ 1968, **2**: 193–199.

6 Irey NS, Manion WC, Taylor HB. Vascular lesions in women taking oral contraceptives. Arch Pathol 1970, **89**: 1–8.

7 McLachlin J, Paterson JC. Some basic observations on venous thrombosis and pulmonary embolism. Surg Gynecol Obstet 1951, **93**: 1–8.

8 Mohr DN, Ryu JH, Litin SC, Rosenow EC III. Recent advances in the management of venous thromboembolism. Mayo Clin Proc 1988, **63**: 281–290.

9 Ochsner A, DeBakey ME, DeCamp PT. Venous thrombosis, analysis of 580 cases. Surgery 1951, **29**: 1–20.

10 Prandoni P, Lensing AW, Buller HR, Cogo A, Prins MH, Cattelan AM, Cuppini S, Noventa F, ten Cate JW. Deep-vein thrombosis and the incidence of subsequent symptomatic cancer. N Engl J Med 1992, **327**: 1128–1133.

11 Rössle R. Ueber die Bedeutung and die Entstehung der Wadenvenenthrombosen. Virchows Arch Pathol Anat 1937, **300**: 180–189.

12 Sartwell PE, Masi AT, Arthes FG, Greene GR, Smith HE. Thromboembolism and oral contraceptives. An epidemiological case-control study. Am J Epidemiol 1969, **90**: 365–380.

13 Stallworth JM, Bradham GB, Kletke RR, Price RG Jr. Phlegmasia cerulea dolens. A 10-year review. Ann Surg 1965, **161**: 802–811.

14 Stein JM, Pruitt BA Jr. Suppurative thrombophlebitis. A lethal iatrogenic disease. N Engl J Med 1970, **282**: 1452–1455.

15 Turpie AG, Chin BS, Lip GY. Venous thromboembolism: pathophysiology, clinical features, and prevention. BMJ 2002, **19**: 887–890.

16 Vessey MP, Doll R. Investigation of relation between use of oral contraceptives and thromboembolic disease. A further report. BMJ 1969, **2**: 651–657.

VARICOSE VEINS

17 Agrifoglio G, Edwards EA. Results of surgical treatment of varicose veins. JAMA 1961, **178**: 906–911.

18 Larson RA, Smith FS. Varicose veins. Evaluation of observations in 491 cases. Mayo Clin Proc 1943, **18**: 400–408.

19 Myers TT. Results of the stripping operation in the treatment of varicose veins. Mayo Clin Proc 1954, **29**: 583–590.

Lymph vessels

CHAPTER CONTENTS

With the exception of tumors of lymph vessels, such as lymphangioma and lymphangiosarcoma (see Chapter 25), the only primary lymphatic disease encountered clinically with some frequency is lymphedema. Chylothorax and chyloascites also occur, but in nearly all instances these processes are secondary to trauma, neoplastic disease, or some infectious process.

Lymphedema

All forms of lymphedema are probably associated in one way or another with inadequate lymphatic drainage Lymphedema may be classified into post-infectious, post-traumatic, obstructive, and idiopathic. In some parts of the world, lymphedema resulting from *Schistosoma* (*Filaria*) is very common.[1] Obstructive lymphedema is most often seen following obstruction of regional lymph nodes by malignant tumor or following node removal, as in radical mastectomy or in radical groin dissection. The development of lymphedema of the arm after radical mastectomy is more common in patients in whom postoperative infection has produced fibrosis in the axilla or in patients having persistent cancer in the axilla. However, lymphedema can also be seen in patients who give a history of as little trauma as a severely sprained ankle or following such infections as a furuncle.

Many patients give no history of trauma or infection associated with the onset of their lymphedema. In such instances, the lymphedema is usually termed idiopathic.[3] This type is further subdivided into *lymphedema congenita, praecox* (beginning before the age of 35 years), and *tarda*.[2,4] Congenital idiopathic lymphedema, also known as *Milroy disease*, is inherited as an autosomal dominant trait.

Postmastectomy lymphedema and, to a lesser degree, Milroy disease can be complicated by the development of lymphangiosarcoma (see Chapter 25). Curiously, this complication is extremely rare in the cases of lymphedema resulting from schistosomiasis, although several cases have been described.

Pathology

The obstructive pathogenesis of lymphedema secondary to neoplastic involvement of regional lymph nodes is self-evident. Injection techniques combined with magnification radiography have served to delineate accurately normal fine lymphatic channels, as well as those with tumor involvement[7,8,10] and have provided the scientific background for the development of the sentinel lymph node technique (Fig. 27.27).

The swelling of lymphedema is usually slowly progressive. There is dilation of the dermal lymphatics, as well as the deeper fascial lymphatics. When the degree of swelling is advanced, there is a depression of hair follicles and gross dermal edema. In such cases, the cutaneous lymphatics may be sufficiently dilated to be associated with lymphorrhea following minor cutaneous abrasions or needle punctures. Tissue sections of such skin usually show markedly dilated dermal lymph vessels.

Drinker and Yaffey[5] postulated that the increased protein content of the lymph present in chronic lymphatic stasis stimulates the deposition of fibrous tissue in the skin, subcutaneous tissue, and fascia. Such fibrosis aggravates the degree of inadequate lymphatic drainage and makes the disease slowly progressive.

Whatever the mechanism, the slowly progressive nature of lymphedema in many patients is associated with dermal thickening and collagenous deposition in the subcutaneous tissues and fascia.

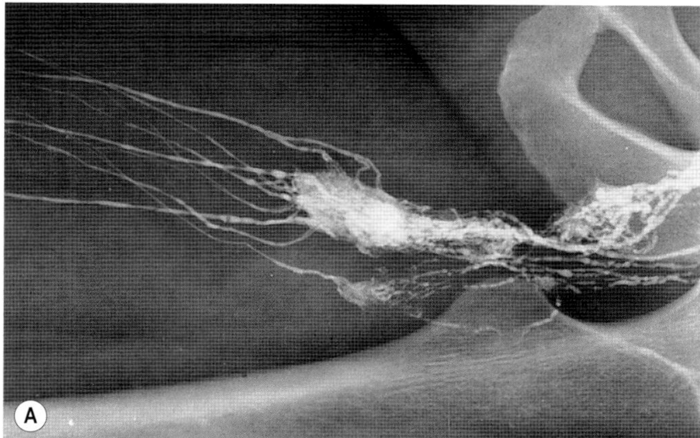

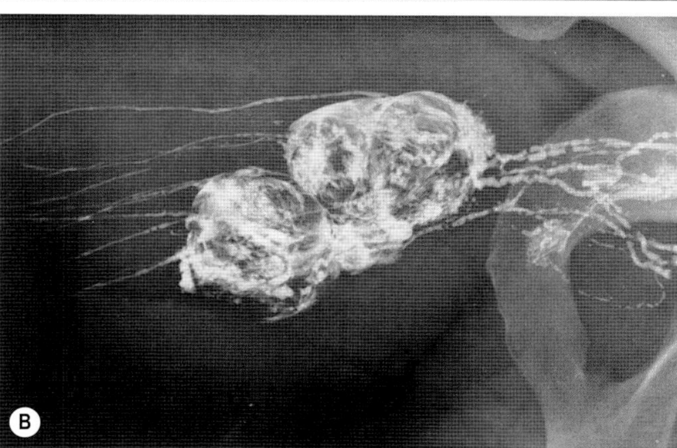

Fig. 27.27 **A**, Magnification radiograph of normal left superficial subinguinal lymph node with afferent and efferent lymphatic channels in a 40-year-old woman. **B**, Magnification radiograph of enlarged right superficial subinguinal lymph node with malignant infiltration secondary to primary melanoma of skin of heel. Same patient as shown in **A**. *(From Isard HJ, Ostrum BJ, Cullinan JE. Magnification roentgenography. A 'spot-film' technic. Med Radiogr Photogr 1962,* ***38:*** *92–109)*

Bouts of superficial cellulitis and lymphangitis often become superimposed on the lymphedema in an extremity. In some patients, recurrent bouts of such infections can become completely incapacitating. The presence of recurrent infection in such an extremity appears to hasten the deposition of collagen and may result in such a large amount of fibrotic replacement of subcutaneous fat and normal dermal structures as to make demonstration of dermal lymphatics impossible.

Kinmonth et al.[6] documented the presence of dilated, valveless, deep lymphatic channels in idiopathic lymphedema. Although many varicose-like lymphatic trunks were found in their patients, in none was a definite proximal site of lymphatic channel obstruction discovered.

In a few patients with idiopathic lymphedema having no clinical evidence or history of lymphangitis or cellulitis in the extremity, enlarged regional lymph nodes have been removed. Microscopically, these nodes exhibit a mild chronic inflammatory infiltrate, sinusoidal fibrosis, and markedly dilated lymphatic channels. Direct communication between lymph nodes and veins has been demonstrated.[9]

Treatment

Treatment of lymphedema consists primarily of elevation of the extremity, compression, and massage, which must be maintained during many years of supervision. Recurrent bouts of streptococcal lymphangitis may be prevented by daily oral administration of antibiotics. These conservative measures will control the lymphedema sufficiently to avoid operation in many patients.[11,13] Operative therapy is indicated only in about 15% of the cases when the extent of subcutaneous fibrosis, infection, and massive swelling is sufficient to markedly handicap the patient.[14,16,18]

The operation most commonly performed is the excision of the thickened fibrotic skin, the edematous subcutaneous tissue, and the thickened fascia overlying the muscles, followed by the immediate application of split-thickness cutaneous autografts.[15,17]

Gross examination of the excised portions shows dense fibrotic bands and sheets extending through the markedly swollen subcutaneous tissue. Pockets of fluid may be found in the intervening tissue spaces. The skin over the fibrotic dermis may be atrophic in some areas and hyperplastic and keratotic in others. The collagenous thickening of the dermis is often extreme. Lymphatic channels as such are not often seen histologically, especially if the process has been associated with multiple episodes of dermal infection. Dilated dermal lymphatics may instead be demonstrated histologically and by dye injection techniques in the skin of a lymphedematous extremity unassociated with long-standing episodes of infection.

Dermal and subcutaneous fibrosis similar to that seen in advanced forms of lymphedema also occurs about long-standing chronic stasis ulcers. The obliteration of dermal lymphatics, however, cannot be related primarily to the etiology of stasis ulcers since similar obliteration occurs in the fibrotic skin of long-standing lymphedema, a condition rarely associated with chronic ulceration of the lower extremity.

Perhaps the most important piece of information that the surgical pathologist must possess in this field is the fact that morbidly obese patients can develop *massive localized lymphedema* in the upper or lower limbs, and that these lesions can simulate histologically an atypical lipomatous tumor (well-differentiated liposarcoma) (see Chapter 25). Etiologically significant events include lymphadenectomy, vein stripping, and blunt trauma.[12]

Tumors

Benign and malignant tumors of lymph vessels are discussed in Chapter 25 (Soft tissues).

References

LYMPHEDEMA

1 Dandapat MC, Mohapatro SK, Mohanty SS. Filarial lymphoedema and elephantiasis of lower limb. A review of 44 cases. Br J Surg 1986, **73**: 451–453.

2 Lewis JM, Wald ER. Lymphedema praecox. J Pediatr 1984, **104**: 641–648.

3 Schirger A, Harrison EG Jr, Janes JM. Idiopathic lymphedema. JAMA 1962, **182**: 124–132.

4 Smeltzer DM, Stickler GB, Schirger A. Primary lymphedema in children and adolescents. A follow-up study and review. Pediatrics 1985, **76**: 206–218.

PATHOLOGY

5 Drinker CK, Yaffey JM. Lymphatics, lymph and lymphoid tissue. Their physiological and clinical significance. Cambridge, Mass, 1941, Harvard University Press.

6 Kinmonth JB, Taylor GW, Tracy GD, Marsh JD. Primary lymphoedema. Clinical and lymphangiographic studies of a series of 107 patients in which the lower limbs were affected. Br J Surg 1957, **95**: 1–10.

7 McPeak CJ, Constantinides SG. Lymphangiography in malignant melanoma. A comparison of clinicopathologic and lymphangiographic findings in 21 cases. Cancer 1964, **17**: 1586–1594.

8 Pomerantz M, Ketcham AS. Lymphangiography and its surgical applications. Surgery 1963, **53**: 589–597.

9 Pressman JJ, Simon MB. Experimental evidence of direct communications between lymph nodes and veins. Surgery 1961, **113**: 537–541.

10 Wallace S. Dynamics of normal and abnormal lymphatic systems as studied with contrast media. Cancer Chemother Rep 1968, **52**: 31–58.

TREATMENT

11 Browse NL. The diagnosis and management of primary lymphedema. J Vasc Surg 1986, **3**: 181–184.

12 Farshid G, Weiss SW. Massive localized lymphedema in the morbidly obese: a histologically distinct reactive lesion simulating liposarcoma. Am J Surg Pathol 1998, **22**: 1277–1283.

13 Foldi E, Foldi M, Weissleder H. Conservative treatment of lymphoedema of the limbs. Angiology 1985, **36**: 171–180.

14 Kinmonth JB. The lymphatics. Surgery, lymphography and disease of the chyle and lymph systems, ed 2. London, 1982, Edward Arnold.

15 Savage RC. The surgical management of lymphedema. Surg Gynecol Obstet 1985, **160**: 283–290.

16 Schirger A, Harrison EG Jr, Janes JM. Idiopathic lymphedema. JAMA 1962, **182**: 124–132.

17 Servelle M. Surgical treatment of lymphedema. A report of 652 cases. Surgery 1987, **101**: 485–495.

18 Thompson N. Surgical treatment of chronic lymphedema of extremities. Surg Clin North Am 1967, **47**: 445–503.

Central nervous system

28

Marc K. Rosenblum M.D.

CHAPTER CONTENTS

Normal anatomy

Dauntingly complex and characterized by extraordinary variation in regional architecture, the gross and microscopic anatomy of the human central nervous system (CNS) cannot be surveyed here in any methodic fashion. We preface this account of neurosurgical pathology with a brief review of those anatomic landmarks and topographic relationships that bear particularly on issues of differential diagnosis.[1] The cellular composition of the brain, the spinal cord, and their coverings are addressed only insofar as these topics are relevant to the current nosology of primary neoplasms arising in these locations, while considerations of traditional neurohistochemistry and immunohistology are deferred to those sections of this chapter dealing with specific tumor types and non-neoplastic conditions (e.g., demyelinating disease) that require application of such techniques for definitive classification.

Confined within the cranium and vertebral canal, the CNS is sheathed by connective tissue membranes that include a densely collagenous outer covering termed the pachymeninx or, more familiarly, dura mater and delicate inner investments known as the leptomeninges or pia-arachnoid. Under normal circumstances, these are closely apposed and loosely joined by a layer of dural border cells that are easily disrupted (artefactually or by expanding lesions such as hematomas) to yield a 'subdural space' that is, in fact, only a potential tissue compartment. A sagittal dural fold referred to as the falx cerebri lies between the cerebral hemispheres, a second such fold – the tentorium cerebelli – separating the superior cerebellar surfaces from the overlying temporal lobes of the cerebrum. Enclosed within the cranial dura, in addition to meningeal artery branches, are venous sinuses that serve both to drain the cerebral veins and to carry away cerebrospinal fluid (CSF) transported from the subarachnoid space by arachnoid villi that project into these conduits. Termed pacchionian granulations as they achieve grossly visible proportions with normal aging, these villi are draped by specialized arachnoidal cells of interest to surgical pathologists as the likely progenitors of the meningioma, a relatively common, dura-based neoplasm. Whereas the dura adheres tightly to the endosteal surfaces of the skull, at spinal levels it is attached only anteriorly to the vertebral bodies and is surrounded on its lateral and posterior aspects by a true compartment – the epidural space – which contains segments of the spinal nerve roots, blood vessels, and a very modest amount of adipose tissue.

We introduce at this juncture several localizing terms current in clinical parlance that encode information of potential utility to the pathologist and that may be encountered in neuroimaging reports and on specimen requisitions. Because the substance of the brain and spinal cord constitutes the central 'neuraxis', lesions localized to the neuroparenchyma proper are often described as intra-axial, whereas those that simply abut the CNS from a meningeal or juxtameningeal site are said to be extra-axial. The qualifiers intramedullary or extramedullary may be further invoked for masses lying within or adjacent to the spinal cord, respectively. The brain itself may be broadly but usefully parceled into supratentorial versus infratentorial components, the former situated above and the latter below the tentorium cerebelli. The cerebellum and most of the brainstem, including the pons and medulla in their entirety, are infratentorial structures that may be collectively designated the posterior fossa contents. The supratentorial CNS consists of the cerebrum (subdivided into frontal, parietal, temporal, and occipital lobes) and deep nuclei of the basal ganglia, thalamus, and hypothalamus.

Within the CNS, connective tissue is scant and essentially restricted to the adventitia of blood vessels. There are no resident lymphoid elements. The parenchyma of the brain and spinal cord is composed principally of the bodies and cytoplasmic processes of neuroepithelial cell types, including neurons and various classes of glia. Subsumed under the latter designation are supporting astrocytes, myelinating oligodendrocytes, and ependymal cells that line ventricular surfaces. These all have their neoplastic counterparts, classified generically as gliomas and subclassified as astrocytomas, oligodendrogliomas, and ependymomas, respectively. Close kin of the ependyma are the specialized epithelial elements of the choroid plexus, which are responsible for the production of CSF and are represented among brain tumors by papillomas and carcinomas. The progenitory and differentiated neurosecretory parenchymal cells of the pineal gland, situated posterior to the roof (or 'tectum') of the midbrain, may also be the targets of transformative events – thus the pineoblastoma and pineocytoma.

We close this necessarily truncated summary on a practical note. There can be no gainsaying the importance of lesion location in the formulation of differential clinical and histologic diagnoses, particularly when tumors are at issue. Meningioma, for example, should be a remote consideration for the pathologist confronted by neurosurgical material from an intra-axial mass but looms large if the lesion in question is dura-based or fills the cerebellopontine angle (where schwannoma might also be reasonably suspected). By contrast, astrocytomas of diffuse fibrillary type, oligodendrogliomas, and metastatic carcinoma account for most cerebral hemispheric tumors (particularly in adulthood). Pilocytic astrocytomas, which mainly affect young persons, exhibit a decided predilection for the cerebellum and third ventricular/hypothalamic region, whereas ependymomas frequent the fourth ventricles of children and the spinal cords of adults (where they constitute the most common intramedullary tumors). Primary CNS lymphomas are most often situated within deep, periventricular white matter structures or the basal ganglia, whereas germ cell tumors only exceptionally arise outside of a midline, pineal region–suprasellar axis, and central neurocytomas are confined within the lateral ventricles. In a similar vein, the tapering conus medullaris and filum terminale of the distal spinal cord are the nearly exclusive hosts of myxopapillary ependymomas and CNS paragangliomas. Neoplasms associated with specific locales include the papillary tumor of the pineal region, the chordoid glioma of the third ventricle and the rosette-forming glioneuronal tumor of the fourth ventricle. Many other examples of regional CNS vulnerability to particular tumor types and non-neoplastic lesions are to be found in this chapter. The foregoing should serve to underscore the potential benefits of a dialogue among pathologists, neuroradiologists, and neurosurgeons.

Congenital abnormalities

Craniospinal dysraphism

Defective midline closure of the embryonic neural tube or its mesodermally derived coverings accounts for the varied malformations collectively referred to as **dysraphic states**. Expressions of craniospinal dysraphism range from trivial skeletal abnormalities that pass undetected through life to lethal anomalies of the nervous system proper that result in intrauterine fetal demise. Considered here are those representatives of this complex group most likely to be approached by the neurosurgeon.

The large majority of dysraphic malformations occur along the spinal axis, where they are chiefly localized, although by no means restricted, to the lumbosacral region.[2,7] The minimal lesion – simple agenesis of the posterior vertebral arches – ranks among the most prevalent of congenital anomalies and is termed **spina bifida occulta**. Its presence may be suggested in otherwise asymptomatic cases by the finding of an overlying skin dimple or sinus tract, hyperpigmented patch, hairy tuft, angioma, or lipoma. **Spina bifida cystica** or **aperta** refers to the less common situation in which meningeal or neural tissues protrude through the osseous defect. The resulting lesion, generically designated a '**cystocele**', typically bulges from the posterior midline in saccular fashion and is subclassified according to the nature of its herniated elements, the major variants being **meningocele** and **myelomeningocele**. The latter, by definition, contains elements derived from the spinal cord, as well as its ensheathing meninges, and accounts for 80–90% of dysraphic cystoceles complicating spina bifida. Cystoceles may also present as ventrally positioned, pelvic, or laterally situated, paravertebral masses. The former are associated with sacral defects, the latter with hemivertebrae. It should be noted, however, that most 'lateral meningoceles' are not true dysraphic lesions; instead, they represent arachnoidal diverticula that exit the spinal canal via widened neural foramina. These are most common at thoracic levels and are often encountered in the setting of type 1 neurofibromatosis.[6] Rarely, meningomyeloceles present as finger- or tail-like appendages in the lumbosacral region.[4,13]

The resected **meningocele** is a discoid mass covered on its external aspect by skin that may be attenuated but that is not usually ulcerated or otherwise disrupted. A narrow pedicle representing the cystocele's attachment to the spinal canal may hang from its smooth, membranous inner surface. The sac proper is composed of collagenous tissue containing meningothelial cells disposed along irregular clefts, around alveolar spaces, in nests and long cords. Distinct dural and arachnoid membranes are not formed. Some examples are associated with tumorous accumulations of mature adipose tissue ('**lipomeningocele**'), and the sac wall may also exhibit a disorganized proliferation of nerve twigs, smooth muscle bundles, and blood vessels. Displaced but otherwise normal spinal nerve roots may lie within the meningocele cavity but can often be successfully repositioned and thus do not usually appear in surgical specimens. The finding of neuroglial tissue in any form mandates a diagnosis of **myelomeningocele**. This ranges in volume and organization from microscopic nests of glia embedded in the cystocele wall to recognizable, albeit deformed, spinal cord. Variants include the **lipomeningomyelocele** (which may contain, in addition to mature adipose tissue, skeletal muscle and nephrogenic tissue rests[8]) and the **syringomyelocele** (or **myelocystocele**), the latter characterized by gross distension of its included spinal cord's central canal. Rarely, meningomyeloceles are encountered in complex with intraspinal cysts lined by enteric epithelium – the so-called **split notochord syndrome**[5] – or complex teratomatous masses regarded by some as bona fide germinal neoplasms and by others as dysembryogenic growths.[9] In any of these guises, the myelomeningocele is often covered by little more than a translucent membrane that represents atretic cutis and may contain plaques of ependymoglial tissue. This is prone to ulceration and predisposes to bacterial invasion of the CSF with ascending meningoventricular infection.

The outcome for infants afflicted by spina bifida cystica depends on the size and complexity of the malformation, particularly on the extent to which spinal cord elements participate in its genesis, and is frequently influenced by the presence of associated anomalies involving the spinal cord rostral to the cystocele, the cranium, and brain. Simple meningoceles are often unassociated with neurologic debility or attended by relatively mild paraparesis, are generally closed without incident, and only exceptionally prove fatal. Unfortunately, the far more common meningomyelocele is usually complicated by significant and irreversible impairment of lower extremity and bladder function. Furthermore, nearly all affected children also suffer an associated Arnold–Chiari malformation with hydrocephalus, the main structural features of this second anomaly being caudal displacement of the medulla and cerebellar vermis, kinking of the cervicomedullary junction, widening and shallowing of the posterior fossa, and, in many instances, deformation of the midbrain with aqueductal stenosis. Untreated, few patients survive childhood, and even with aggressive surgical intervention the risk of death is considerable. The leading immediate causes of mortality are meningitis, pyelonephritis, pneumonia, and progressive hydrocephalus. Rarely, squamous carcinomas arise from the chronically irritated epidermis overlying unattended cystoceles.[3]

To the externally evident malformations just described should be added various intraspinal and juxtaspinal anomalies, often referred to as occult or 'closed' dysraphisms, that similarly occur in complex with spina bifida and its cutaneous stigmata but are imperceptible on physical examination because of their deep location. These, too, exhibit a decided predilection for the lumbosacral region, where they are typically discovered on neuroradiologic evaluation for myelopathy. It is fixation of the filum terminale or spinal roots to these abnormal structures, with resulting traction on the cord (as

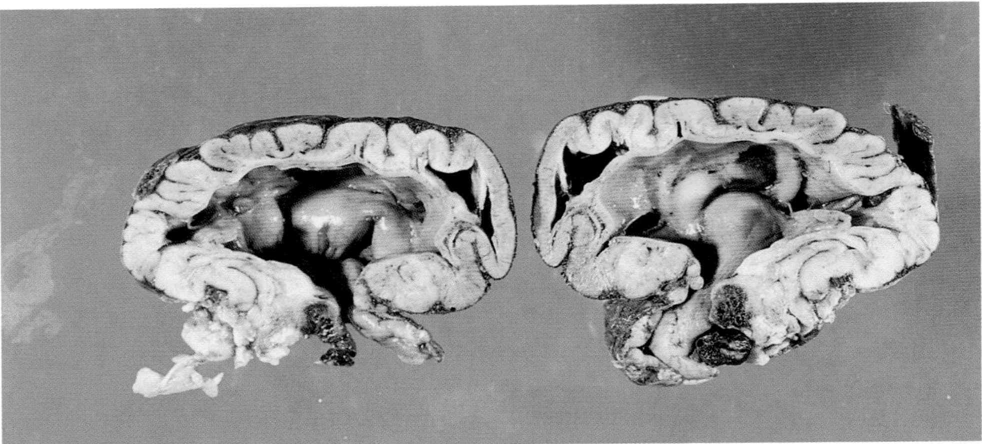

Fig. 28.1 Encephalocele. A well-developed, gyriform cortical mantle characterizes this neurosurgical specimen from the occipital region of a newborn.
(Courtesy of Dr Humberto Cravioto, New York)

evidenced by displacement of the conus medullaris below the level of the L2 vertebral body), that is often responsible for their principal neurologic manifestations – disturbed gait, bladder spasticity or hypotonia, anococcygeal and perineal pain. Maldevelopmental lesions that may present as this '**tethered cord' syndrome** include: intraspinal **lipomas**; **dermoid**, **epidermoid**, or **hindgut cysts**; **intrasacral meningeal diverticula** ('**occult meningoceles**'); and cystic intradural masses composed of neuroglial tissue ('**occult myelomeningoceles**'). The dividing collagenous or chondro-osseous septum characteristically present in cases of congenitally split spinal cord (**diastematomyelia**) is yet another potentially tethering anomaly, whereas the offending lesion in some instances is simply a short filum (typically thickened owing to fatty infiltration) or a fibrous band extending into the exposed spinal canal from the sacral subcutis. The latter is often associated with a telltale skin dimple or dermal sinus, can contain ciliated glandular elements as well as components of dermoid or epidermoid cyst, may include CNS tissue, peripheral nerve, ganglion cells, fat and muscle, and rarely exhibits a hamartomatous proliferation of included pacinian corpuscles.[2,12] Sizable **thoracolumbar hamartomas** that may contain nerves, adipose tissue, muscle, cartilage, bone, glandular structures, and primitive urinary tract-type tissues have also been described as involving the spinal canal and exerting traction on the spinal cord,[11] as have maldevelopmental lesions of müllerian derivation (further discussed as choristomas below). Fortunately, many of these associated malformations are amenable to surgical correction, division of the immobilized filum frequently resulting in substantial neurologic improvement and relief of pain.

A distant second in incidence to the dysraphic cystoceles of the lumbosacral region are those involving the cranium.[7] These, too, hug the midline and, like their spinal counterparts, may contain meningeal derivatives alone or associated neural tissues. The latter, termed **encephaloceles**, vastly predominate. Approximately 80% of encephaloceles exit the cranial cavity in the region of the occiput via defects in the posterior wall of the foramen magnum or occipital bone. These are generally covered by intact scalp, subjacent to which are recognizable dural and leptomeningeal membranes, and may contain choroid plexus, cerebellar, and brainstem elements, in addition to substantial volumes of cerebral hemispheric tissue (Fig. 28.1). The extruded brain, which encloses a central CSF-filled chamber that may communicate freely with the ventricular system, can appear remarkably well formed but commonly exhibits microscopic abnormalities of cortical architecture, if not grossly anomalous gyration, and its covering leptomeninges frequently contain islands of heterotopic neuroglial tissue. Vascular compression at the level of the encephalocele's narrow intraosseous neck may result in secondary alterations such as hemorrhage and infarction. Excision and closure can often be effected without complication, but a regrettably large percentage of occipital encephaloceles are attended by malformations of the intracranial contents, microcephaly, and mental retardation.

Extraoccipital encephaloceles may protrude through defects in other portions of the cranial vault or bulge into the anterior or posterior fontanels but are more commonly of the sincipital or basilar types. Sincipital encephaloceles present as visible facial swellings in the region of the forehead, nasal bridge, or orbit, whereas basal variants are situated in the nasal cavity, sphenoid sinus, nasopharynx, or pterygopalatine fossa and therefore are not externally evident. The latter group includes transethmoidal encephaloceles that herniate through defects in the cribriform plate and constitute the most common polypoid intranasal masses encountered in the newborn. Prior to biopsy or resection, a congenital subcutaneous or submucosal mass in any of these locations must be carefully evaluated for evidence of extension into the cranial cavity. Inasmuch as the encephalocele communicates with the subarachnoid space via its associated osseous defect, intracranial repair with dural closure is required if CSF leakage and meningitis are to be avoided. Simple neuroglial heterotopias occurring in these same regions, by contrast, are defined as maintaining no open connection to the intracranial compartment and thus may be safely approached transnasally or transorally, depending on their precise situation. These are addressed separately later in this chapter. Suffice it to say that the results of neuroimaging study are often decisive in the classification of a given lesion because both the heterotopia and true encephalocele often consist solely of aggregated astroglia embedded in fibrous tissue. Either may contain admixed neurons. Heterotopias of the nasal region rarely if ever harbor ependymal elements, a feature of some encephaloceles, but these may be encountered in examples situated in other sincipital or basilar locations. Included meninges are an inconstant feature of specimens derived from extraoccipital encephaloceles, but, when identified, exclude heterotopia from further consideration.

Although this discussion is restricted to congenital anomalies, it should be noted that meningoceles and encephaloceles may be the acquired consequences of trauma or preceding neurosurgical procedures. 'Endaural' examples may complicate chronic otitis media or mastoiditis and have been described as a late effect of cranial irradiation in childhood.[10]

Neuroglial and meningeal heterotopias

The **neuroglial heterotopia**, introduced in the preceding discussion of cranial dysraphism, is a displaced mass of mature central neuroepithelial tissue unconnected to the brain proper. Paracerebral masses of this type only rarely achieve symptomatic size.[14,24] More common are small leptomeningeal examples that constitute occasional incidental findings on post mortem examination and that are frequently noted in association with major structural anomalies of the underlying nervous system (e.g., craniospinal cystoceles).[7,20] These are of little clinical import save for their hypothesized role as progenitors of the odd primary leptomeningeal glioma. Similarly, **intrapulmonary neuroglial rests** are an autopsy curiosity virtually restricted to fetuses and neonates harboring severe neural tube defects such as anencephaly.[21] The heterotopias most likely to engage the surgical pathologist frequent the same locations favored by sincipital and basal encephaloceles – the bridge of the nose and nasal cavity, paranasal sinuses, palatal region, and nasopharynx – and are best regarded as 'sequestered' variants of their obviously dysraphic counterparts.[25,26] By far the most common of these maldevelopmental lesions, which have also been termed **glial choristomas**, is the so-called **nasal glioma**, addressed in Chapter 7. Neuroglial heterotopias may also present in the cranial bones, scalp, orbit, and submandibular region.[25,26] Their structure varies. Most consist solely of solid glial nests embedded in fibrous tissues, only about 10% containing neurons and these rarely in abundance. Astrocytes usually predominate and are often the only neuroepithelial elements present in nasal examples. Pharyngeal lesions are typically more complex, often containing ependyma-lined clefts and choroid plexus-like formations. Pigmented neuroepithelial structures suggesting retinal differentiation may also be encountered in the latter. Heterotopias composed of cerebellar tissue have been recorded to present in the anterior cranial fossa[23] and orbit,[17] among other unusual sites.[23]

The neuroglial nature of the lesions under discussion is usually obvious in routinely prepared histologic sections but may be confirmed in a questionable case by immunolabeling of matrix and included astrocytic elements with antibodies to glial fibrillary acidic protein (GFAP). The distinction of these rests from encephaloceles, a matter of considerable clinical significance, has already been addressed in the discussion of craniospinal dysraphism. It should be noted that neuroglial heterotopias occasionally exhibit worrisome cytologic abnormalities and troubling hypercellularity but are generally cured by simple excision. Even the small percentages that have reportedly recurred have been controlled with conservative local reoperation. Rare heterotopias interpreted as having undergone focal neoplastic transformation are to be found in the literature. The diminutive neoplasms purported to arise in this setting have included an oligodendroglioma,[16] a mixed glioma composed of oligodendroglial and astrocytic elements,[19] and a melanotic neuroectodermal tumor of infancy.[22] A probable instance of frontal lobe astrocytoma penetrating the cribriform plate to masquerade as a nasal glial heterotopia has also been depicted.[18]

In contrast to some sincipital and basal encephaloceles, neuroglial heterotopias do not contain elements derived from the meninges. Displaced meningothelium, however, may be encountered in curious lesions of the scalp variously interpreted as hamartomas or as meningeal dysraphias that have lost their connection to the intracranial compartment in the course of development (**'sequestered meningoceles'**).[15,27] These extracranial meningeal heterotopias are often noted at birth but may not come to surgical attention until adulthood. They are situated most often in the dermis or subcutis of the midline occipital region, at the vertex, in the posterior fontanel, or overlying the lambdoid suture. Regional alopecia is a common associated finding. The lesion consists of collagenous tissue containing irregular slit-like spaces lined by flattened meningothelial cells. These may also form solid cords or, rarely, small nests. Central neuroepithelial derivatives are not present, but islands of necrotic cellular material that could conceivably represent degenerated neuroglial components have been described in some cases. Extracranial meningeal heterotopias may be misconstrued as melanocytic lesions, lymphangiomas, or even angiosarcomas[27] but can be distinguished in problematic cases by their expression of epithelial membrane antigen (EMA) on immunohistochemical assay. These maldevelopmental lesions could theoretically serve as precursors to the rare bona fide meningiomas arising in the scalp, which are addressed along with other ectopic meningiomas in the discussion of meningothelial tumors.

The reader is referred to the section dealing with ependymal neoplasms for comment on myxopapillary ependymal rests of the sacrococcygeal region and their relationship to extramedullary ependymomas.

Choristomas and non-neuroepithelial hamartomas

Maldevelopmental rests composed of tissues foreign to the nervous system – 'choristomas' – are only rarely encountered within the confines of the dura mater (and hardly ever involve the brain proper). An exception to the last statement is the unusual lesion described as **complex choristoma of the gyrus rectus**.[29] Embedded in a gliotic matrix and containing, in addition to mature adipose tissue, benign adenosquamous epithelial components supported by myoepithelium and arranged in nests, cords or tubuloductal structures, this has been likened to the solid cell nests of the thyroid gland and cystic tumor of the atrioventricular node as sharing morphologic features and a potential derivation from neural crest progenitors. We have previously mentioned thoracolumbar hamartomas composed of various mesenchymal and epithelial components in the setting of spinal dysraphism and note that comparable lesions have rarely been identified as intramedullary growths unaccompanied by dysraphic abnormalities.[28] **Ecchordosis physaliphora** is the term used to describe an intracranial heterotopia exhibiting the histologic and ultrastructural features characteristic of the notochord and its neoplastic offspring, the chordoma.[35] Ecchordoses are typically situated just ventral to the belly of the pons, are frequently connected to notochordal remnants in the adjacent clivus via attenuated transdural stalks, and usually take the form of bosselated, gelatinous nodules loosely adherent to the basilar artery. They generally measure no more than 1–2 cm in greatest dimension and, for the most part, are autopsy curiosities. Whether some larger, symptomatic examples are best regarded as 'giant' ecchordoses or as bona fide intradural chordomas is questionable (see the section on chordoma). Neuroradiologically detected ecchordoses have been described as generally T2 hyperintense and nonenhancing on MRI, chordomas usually exhibiting contrast enhancement.[45]

Leptomeningeal rhabdomyomatosis refers to microscopic aggregates of mature striated myofibers characteristically located in the prepontine region or cerebellopontine angles.[32] These may, in addition, harbor well-differentiated adipocytes, displaced neuroglial tissue, and aberrant peripheral nerve fibers, and are usually detected in complex with major developmental anomalies of the CNS. Rarely, nodules composed of striated or smooth muscle are encountered in cranial nerve divisions.[30,37,46,47] These may contain admixed neuromatous elements and adipose tissue, can achieve considerable size and have been variously reported as **choristomas**, **neuromuscular** or **ectomesenchymal hamartomas**, **benign triton tumors**, and **rhabdomyomas**. Also on record are several **müllerian choristomas of the lumbosacral region** associated with spinal dysraphism, these potentially containing endometrium, endocervical glands, and smooth muscle bundles organized in uterus-like fashion.[42] We mention here isolated depictions of **intracerebral**[44] and **intraspinal**[38] **endometriosis**, although these are properly regarded as acquired, rather than developmental, lesions. Finally, there are the bizarre accounts of a minute adenoid cystic carcinoma arising in a cerebellopontine angle mass otherwise composed of mature salivary gland tissue[31] and a second salivary heterotopia, also in the cerebellopontine angle, associated with a solitary fibrous tumor.[41]

Meningioangiomatosis is the designation traditionally applied to what has long been regarded as an essentially hamartomatous or malformative process that usually occurs in sporadic fashion but that is clearly associated with type 2 neurofibromatosis (NF-2) as well.[40,48] Sporadic cases are nearly always solitary and found on evaluation for seizures, whereas NF-2-related examples are not infrequently multifocal and typically asymptomatic. The basic lesion (Fig. 28.2) is an en plaque proliferation of small blood vessels that dissects the cerebral cortex, halts abruptly at the gray–white junction, and is often accompanied by a spindle cell proliferation that may be tightly vasocentric or, in exuberantly cellular variants, arrayed in fascicular or storiform patterns. Loose whorling and schwannoma-like nuclear palisading may also be encountered. Extensive calcification is common, particularly conspicuous psammoma body formation, as are vascular hyalinization and regions of fibrous tissue overgrowth. A curious feature of the lesion is the tendency of entrapped neurons to develop Alzheimer-type neurofibrillary tangles.[40] Subcortical presentations have been described but are rare.[36] The term meningioangiomatosis notwithstanding, participating spindle cell populations have exhibited a meningothelial immunophenotype (specifically, labeling for EMA) or ultrastructure (e.g., interdigitating cell processes with attaching desmosomes) in only a small minority of cases, are consistently reactive for vimentin alone, and have been interpreted as being predominantly fibroblastic by some observers.[34,48]

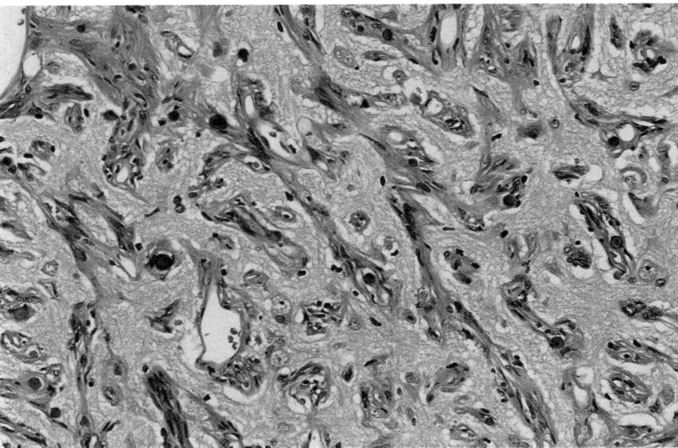

Fig. 28.2 Meningioangiomatosis. This typical example exhibits dissection of the cerebral cortex by small blood vessels with accompanying perivascular spindle cells and psammoma bodies.

Meningiomas have been described as occasionally taking root within foci of meningioangiomatosis,[33] but the interpretation of such accounts has been called into question.[40] An analysis of candidate cases for genetic abnormalities commonly associated with meningothelial tumorigenesis found that regions of apparent 'meningioangiomatosis' almost invariably shared with their neighboring meningiomas identical patterns of *NF2* and *DAL1* gene deletion,[40] such deletions (one reported example excepted[43]) being foreign to meningioangiomatosis in its uncomplicated state. This would suggest that certain meningiomas spread along the cortical microvasculature in a meningioangiomatosis-like fashion. Unusually cellular meningioangiomatoses may also be mistaken for bona fide neoplasms. The reader is referred to our discussion of meningothelial tumors for additional observations regarding this phenomenon, which must be considered in the differential diagnosis of meningeal tumors that appear to 'infiltrate' subjacent cortex. We have encountered examples of spindle cell hemangiopericytoma of the leptomeninges and high-grade cerebral fibrosarcoma in association with meningioangiomatosis, and note report of a neoplasm interpreted as an oligodendroglioma found adjacent to a focus of meningioangiomatosis as well.[39] We have also seen vascular lesions indistinguishable from meningioangiomatosis develop within irradiated cerebral cortex. Simple excision is the treatment of choice, but does not guarantee seizure control since patients with meningioangiomatosis may have complex electroencephalographic abnormalities indicative of multifocal, extralesional epileptogenic pathology.[48]

Cysts of the central neuraxis

Considered in this section are various non-neoplastic lesions, maldevelopmental or secondarily acquired, only some of which qualify as 'true' (i.e., epithelium-lined) cysts. Chief among the latter are the **colloid cysts of the anterosuperior third ventricle**.[79] These generally present in the third through fifth decades of life with manifestations of ventricular outflow obstruction, a consequence of their intimate relation to the foramen of Monro (Fig. 28.3). Thin-walled and often draped by adherent choroid plexus, colloid cysts are filled with a viscous, mucoid material that rapidly congeals on fixation. Their lining epithelium is prone to a low cuboidal attenuation resulting from pressure exerted by the cyst contents, but when well preserved is found to be of columnar type and is frequently populated by ciliated and goblet cell elements (Fig. 28.4). Only a basement membrane, inapparent at the light microscopic level, separates these from a delicate, fibrous capsule. The cyst contents are periodic acid–Schiff (PAS) positive and commonly include hyphae-like aggregates of degenerate nucleoproteins so characteristic of this entity as to be diagnostic in the absence of identifiable epithelium[89] (Fig. 28.5). An inflammatory reaction to the contents of ruptured colloid cysts is responsible for most, if not all, cases of so-called xanthogranuloma situated in the third ventricle.[81]

Ultrastructural[69] and immunocytochemical[75,101] investigations of the colloid cyst support an origin from misplaced endodermal tissues. Its constituent epithelial cell types correspond closely to those typical of respiratory mucosae, sporting an apical glycocalyx

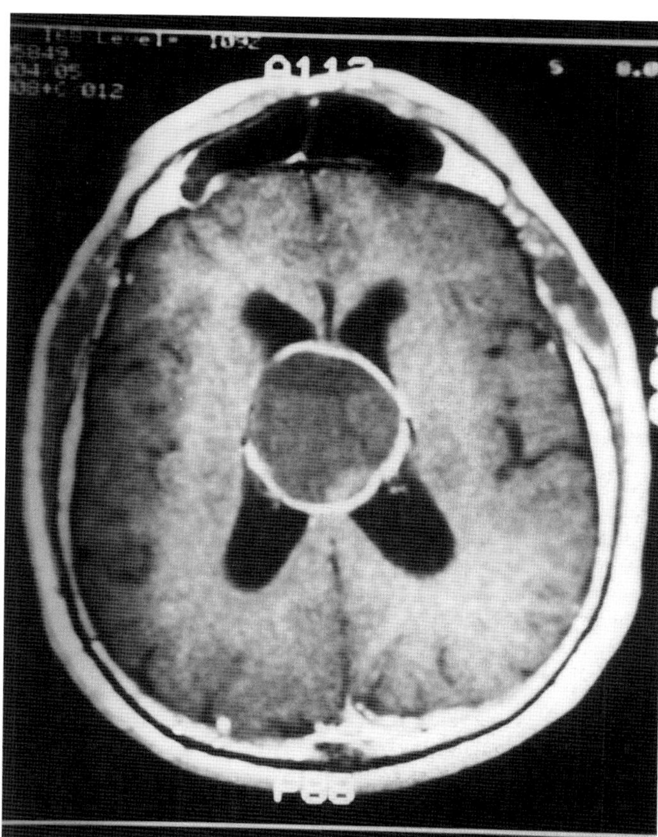

Fig. 28.3 Colloid cyst. The obstructive ventricular dilation (hydrocephalus) associated with this large example is characteristic of these lesions. Note the well-delineated cyst wall, bright in this contrast-enhanced magnetic resonance image.

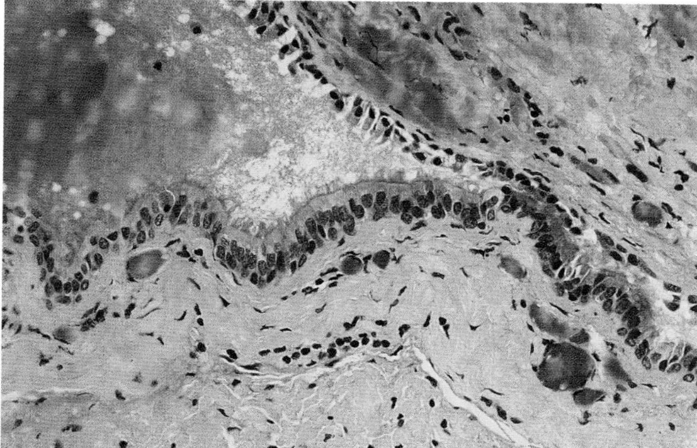

Fig. 28.4 Colloid cyst. A pseudostratified and ciliated columnar epithelium lines well-preserved colloid cysts. Note the supporting collagenous tissue of the cyst wall, yellow in this hematoxylin–phloxine–safranin preparation.

coating particularly characteristic of endodermally derived epithelia, and express cytokeratins, EMA, and carcinoembryonic antigen (CEA), but not GFAP or the choroid plexus-associated transthyretin (prealbumin). Their occasional designation as 'neuroepithelial' notwithstanding, similar histogenetic considerations apply to rare

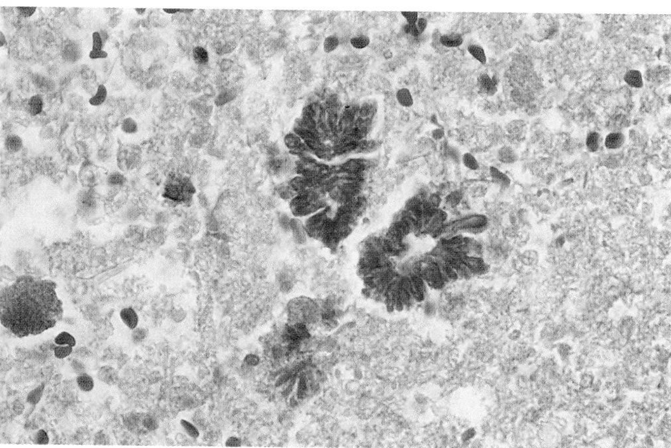

Fig. 28.5 Colloid cyst. The radiate, hyphae-like structures shown here are often found admixed with the liquid contents of colloid cysts and, for practical purposes, are diagnostic of this entity.

endodermal-type cysts[100] of comparable structure situated within the posterior fossa,[51,58] supratentorial compartment,[54] optic nerve[72] and, as discussed below, the spinal canal.[94] Adenocarcinomatous transformation of such cysts has rarely been recorded,[96] as has widespread craniospinal dissemination of histologically conventional endodermal-type cysts via the CSF.[88,100] Although properly treated in the context of pituitary disorders (see Chapter 29), the **Rathke cleft cyst**,[102] a lesion having its origin in remnants of the stomodeum, is briefly noted here for the striking resemblance of its lining epithelium to that of the colloid cyst. Curiously, however, the latter rarely contains the metaplastic squamous elements common to Rathke cleft cysts and other cystic intracranial lesions putatively of endodermal lineage.

Intraspinal cysts resulting, in all likelihood, from the incomplete separation of developing endodermal and notochordal tissues in early embryonic life have been variously designated as '**neurenteric**', '**foregut**', '**enterogenous**', and '**teratomatous**'.[100] These intradural endodermal-type cysts are typically situated anterior to the spinal cord, are often associated with local vertebral abnormalities, and may be encountered in complex with other evidences of faulty development such as intestinal malformations and dermal sinuses. An intramedullary presentation is well recognized but far less frequently encountered.[94] Most examples exhibit a simple mural structure and columnar epithelial lining similar to that of the colloid cyst, but occasional variants are endowed with a specialized respiratory or gastroenteric-type 'mucosa' and the organized supporting elements (e.g., seromucinous glands, muscularis, cartilaginous rings, ganglion cells) of the developed alimentary tract or tracheobronchial tree.[70]

Two major variants of ectodermally derived neuraxis cyst are recognized, both lined by keratinizing squamous epithelium.[61] The **epidermoid cyst**, by definition, is devoid of cutaneous-type adnexal structures and filled by friable, often lamellated keratinous debris that radiates a pearly sheen as viewed through the thin, fibrous lesional capsule. **Dermoid cysts**, by contrast, are endowed with skin appendages, including pilosebaceous units, eccrine and, occasionally, apocrine glands, as well as mural adipose tissue foreign to the epidermoid type. They may contain a greasy, yellowish-gray material admixed with hairs or just friable, keratin-rich debris similar to that of their epidermoid counterparts. Cysts of both types are, for the most part, maldevelopmental in origin, presumably arising from surface ectodermal elements trapped in association with the developing central nervous system on closure of the neural groove or formation of the secondary cerebral vesicles. The occurrence of some examples, particularly dermoids, in complex with cranio-vertebral anomalies (e.g., spina bifida), malformations of the spinal cord, and dermal sinuses attests to their dysembryogenetic basis. Well documented, however, are acquired variants, most of them epidermoid, resulting from the traumatic[99] or iatrogenic[64] implantation of cutaneous tissues in the cranial or spinal subdural space.

Epidermoid and dermoid cysts are characterized by distinctive clinical as well as histologic features.[61] The former affect subjects of all ages, most coming to attention in young adulthood or middle age, whereas the latter usually present in childhood or adolescence. Cysts of epidermoid type are widely distributed along the neuraxis, but the great majority are positioned intracranially, the cerebello-pontine angle being their single most common location. Rarely, posterior fossa examples conspicuously erode into, or lie embedded within, the cerebellum or brainstem. Supratentorial representatives exhibit a predilection for the parasellar region, but may also be situated within the ventricular system, in the cerebral hemispheres, suprasellar, or pineal regions. Intraspinal epidermoid cysts are typically intradural and extramedullary in location but may on rare occasion lie entirely within the substance of the cord.

Compared with its epidermoid counterpart, the dermoid cyst clings tightly to the midline. It, too, favors the posterior fossa but in this location characteristically occupies the cerebellar vermis or fourth ventricle. When situated above the tentorium, the dermoid cyst tends to a frontal, paramedian position on the skull base. An infantile, subgaleal variant typically resides in the anterior fontanel. Although generally outnumbered by epidermoid cysts, dermoids actually predominate at spinal levels. These exhibit a decided predilection for the lumbosacral region, where they constitute a manifestation of spinal dysraphism.

Although the clinical manifestations of dermoid and epidermoid cysts are principally referable to their local mass effects, either may present with signs and symptoms of 'chemical' or infectious meningitis. The former results from cyst rupture and the spillage of irritating keratinous and lipid-rich debris into the ventricular system and subarachnoid space.[77] Repeated episodes of bacterial meningitis are a recognized complication of cysts associated with dermal sinuses offering access to the nervous system. Patients harboring posterior fossa dermoids and occipital sinuses may also suffer cerebellar abscesses. Neoplastic transformation is a well-documented but, fortunately, rare occurrence. In most cases, the underlying lesion is a cyst of epidermoid type and the secondary cancer a squamous carcinoma.[76] The bizarre phenomenon of an osteogenic sarcoma arising in association with a cerebellar epidermoid cyst has been recorded,[52] and isolated dermoid cysts have given rise to tumors described as anaplastic sebaceous carcinoma[63] or atypical hidradenoma.[73] A temporal lobe example containing islands of keratinized, anucleate-appearing ('shadow') cells similar to those seen in pilomatricomas has been depicted.[67] Even histologically conventional cysts can recur following incomplete resection of their walls. Spontaneous seeding of the CSF by apparently benign epidermoid cysts with development of intraventricular or subarachnoid 'daughter' lesions is a recorded curiosity.[80]

Inasmuch as epidermoid cysts may arise, albeit rarely, in the suprasellar region, their differential diagnosis includes Rathke cleft cysts with extensive squamous metaplasia and craniopharyngiomas. The former will usually harbor scattered mucicarminophilic cells of cuboidal or low columnar configuration atop their squamous elements and do not evidence the advanced keratinization typical of the epidermoid cyst. The formation of cytoplasmic keratohyaline granules, typical of the epidermoid cyst's maturing squames, is generally foreign to the craniopharyngioma. Furthermore, epidermoid and Rathke cleft cysts lack the latter's islands of 'ghost cell' keratinocytes and its 'machinery oil'-like contents, and do not exhibit the basaloid elements and stellate reticulum of the adamantinomatous craniopharyngioma or the filiform architecture of its papillary variant (see Chapter 29 for details). As regards further distinction of Rathke cleft cysts from craniopharyngiomas, study of a limited number of cases found immunolabeling for cytokeratins 8 and 20 to be characteristic of the former and generally foreign to the latter.[107] Cystic craniopharyngiomas of adamantinomatous type, in addition, often manifest foci of aberrant nuclear β-catenin immunoexpression that are not encountered in metaplastic Rathke cleft cysts.[71] The exceptional dermoid cyst presenting in the pineal or suprasellar region should be separable from the mature cystic teratoma by its lack of glandular components (indicative of endodermal differentiation), muscle, or cartilage.

Glioependymal cysts are most commonly situated in the paraventricular white matter of the frontal and parietal lobes but may also lie within the cerebellum, brainstem, or spinal cord.[56,60,62] A derivation from ventricular lining elements displaced in the course of neuroembryogenesis seems most plausible for these intraparenchymal examples, rare variants positioned in the cerebellopontine angle and other extra-axial sites conceivably originating from subarachnoid neuroglial heterotopias.[68] Intramedullary lesions of this type often involve the conus medullaris, where they may actually represent cystic dilations of the ependyma-lined ventriculus terminalis.[55] As their name implies, glioependymal cysts are lined by cells resembling mature ependymocytes. Like the cells lining the more common cysts of endodermal type, these may be ciliated but differ in that they do not exhibit goblet cell differentiation, are not coated by an apical glycocalyx, and do not rest on a basal lamina, being directly apposed to fibrillary neuroglial tissue. Representatives presenting in the subarachnoid space may, however, contain 'supporting' astrocytic elements that fashion a continuous basement membrane separating them from a delicate fibrous capsule, much as the normal glia limitans are delimited from the connective tissues of the pia-arachnoid by a basal lamina.[56,68]

The limited immunocytochemical studies reported to date suggest that the cells lining glioependymal cysts can express GFAP, S-100 protein, and, possibly, cytokeratin.[56,68] Failure to elaborate CEA or transthyretin (prealbumin) may serve to distinguish these lesions from cysts of endodermal or choroid plexus type, respectively. By definition, **choroid plexus cysts** are lined by cells having the immunohistochemical and fine structural attributes of the native plexus epithelium,[83,86] considered in the discussion of this structure's epithelial neoplasms. We mention only for the sake of completeness cystic alterations that are a transient feature of some fetal choroid plexi.[53] These are of no consequence to the surgical pathologist.

Rarely, intraparenchymal brain cysts exhibit no specialized lining elements and are not associated with historical or tissue evidence of underlying trauma, hemorrhage, infarction, neoplasia, demyelinating disease, or infection that might account for their genesis. Most numerous are examples termed '**simple**' or '**gliotic**' **cysts**, presenting in the cerebellar hemispheric white matter of middle-aged or elderly adults.[98,105] That at least some of these clinically benign lesions are not congenital anomalies but represent instead 'burnt-out' pilocytic astrocytomas has been suggested in view of the latter tumor's proneness to macrocystic alterations and the presence around many simple cerebellar cysts of a dense mesh of glial processes rich in Rosenthal fibers and containing scattered atypical astrocytes.[98] Inasmuch as the neoplastic components of cerebellar cysts associated with pilocytic astrocytomas and hemangioblastomas may be confined to diminutive mural nodules, careful inspection of cystic lesions in this location following drainage at surgery is mandatory, and biopsy of various portions of their linings is prudent. Exceptional cysts arising outside the cerebellum are lined only by normal or mildly reactive neuroglial tissue, are juxtaventricular in location, and contain a fluid similar in its composition to CSF.[85,106] These likely derive from ventricular diverticula or represent collections of CSF that have dissected into the neuropil via congenital or acquired breaches in the ependyma. A congenital optic nerve cyst of simple glial type has been recorded.[74] Lesions of macrocystic neuroradiologic profile that similarly lack specialized lining elements have been reported to result from marked dilation of perivascular spaces, particularly in the cerebral hemispheric white matter.[57] It is the demonstration of traversing blood vessels that has been taken for evidence of the continuity of these pseudocysts, which are otherwise bordered by rarefied and gliotic neuroparenchyma, with the perivascular compartment.

Particularly prone to cystic change is the normal human pineal gland, but only rarely does this alteration result in a lesion of symptomatic proportions.[59] **Pineal cysts** that come to neurosurgical attention generally do so in the third through fifth decades of life, their presenting manifestations being indistinguishable from those of neoplasms in this region and including evidences of obstructive hydrocephalus, as well as disturbances of ocular motility. Like the cerebellar lesions previously described, these are lined by a dense weave of piloid astroglial processes containing Rosenthal fibers and granular bodies but do not exhibit the microcystic architecture characteristic of the pilocytic astrocytoma or approach the latter in cellularity. A second differential diagnostic consideration is the pineocytoma, as the cysts under discussion regularly contain elements of residual pineal parenchyma within their walls. These usually retain the organoid appearances typical of the normal gland, but in some cases their uniform, telltale lobularity is obscured as a result of long-standing compression. Appreciation of a given lesion's neuroradiologic features and appearance at operation is quite helpful in this regard, as pineocytomas are nearly always solid masses rather than thin-walled cysts. Simple excision is curative.

Loculated accumulations of CSF enclosed by fibroconnective tissues derived from the leptomeninges are referred to as **arachnoid cysts**.[92] Etiologically diverse, some arachnoid cysts develop as sequelae of meningitis or trauma and are circumscribed by adhesions traversing the subarachnoid space. Most, however, are considered to begin as maldevelopmental clefts in the arachnoid membrane that subsequently undergoes cystic dilation.[91] Lesions of this type are lined by an attenuated meningothelium resting on a layer of supporting fibrous tissue so thin as to be transparent at operation. These most commonly occupy the sylvian fissures, followed by the cisterna magna and cerebellopontine angles, but may occur in the suprasellar region and along the spinal neuraxis.[92] Intradiploic[104] and intramedullary[97] presentations have also been recorded. By virtue of their very gradual inflation, such lesions may produce striking deformities in neighboring neural tissues that are often unaccompanied by mass effects such as midline shifts or internal herniae and thus have a malformation-like appearance. **Dural cysts** (cystically dilated intradural clefts) are rare and described mainly as intraspinal causes of myelopathy.[65] Comparable intracranial lesions have been reported to produce sagittal sinus occlusions.[87]

Most arachnoid 'cysts' presenting at spinal levels are actually meningeal diverticula that can be shown to communicate with the subarachnoid space.[82] These may lie within or outside the dural sleeve, are potentially multifocal, and can be lined by meningothelial cells or composed solely of membranous fibrous tissue. Only a minority achieve symptomatic proportions, producing myelopathy or radicular syndromes, at times associated with erosion of adjacent vertebral bodies or the sacrum.[78] Extradural variants arising in association with the posterior spinal roots, typically at lumbosacral levels, are often eponymously designated as **Tarlov perineurial cysts**.[103] Only exceptionally do these prompt neurosurgical intervention by causing perineal pain, sciatica, or bladder or bowel dysfunction. Rarely, cystically dilated or otherwise enlarged arachnoid granulations masquerade as dermoid (or other true) cysts[50] or produce sizable lytic skull defects that arouse suspicion of neoplastic disease.[93]

Yet another cystic lesion that may impinge on the spinal neuraxis is the **juxtafacet** or **'ganglion' cyst**, a collection of acellular and often myxoid material bound within a fibrous capsule devoid of specialized lining elements.[95] The term **synovial cyst** has been employed for essentially similar lesions interpreted as containing inflamed synovium.[49] Some examples contain metaplastic chondroid elements and foci of calcification. Cysts of comparable structure may rarely arise within the ligamentum flavum.[66] A degenerative abnormality, the juxtafacet cyst typically presents at lumbar levels in association with osteoarthritic changes of the vertebral column, but may rarely occur in the cervical region.[66] Myeloradiculopathy and bony erosion are its principal complications.

Finally, we mention the intracranial extension of sinonasal mucoceles and development of intracranial mucoceles in association with frontoethmoidal osteomas,[84] as well as report of a multiloculated, cystic frontal lobe mass having the appearance of allergic nasal polyposis, the latter associated with a bony abnormality of the anterior fossa floor and complicated by CSF rhinorrhea and meningitis.[90]

Cerebrovascular disorders

Cerebral infarction

Characterized by an abrupt loss of neurologic function ('stroke') referable to a circumscribed arterial territory within the affected brain, the common variety of **cerebral infarct**[109] is an ischemic lesion of later adult life confidently diagnosed at the bedside. Occasional examples, however, are silent at onset, evolve in subacute fashion as expansile intracranial 'tumors' indistinguishable from neoplasms on conventional neuroradiologic assessment, and are consequently sampled by the neurosurgeon. Obviously, the histology of a given infarct will depend on the stage at which the dynamic cytologic and organizational alterations that follow irreversible ischemic injury are iatrogenically interrupted.[108,110] Biopsied tissues generally exhibit a spongy rarefaction reflecting the edema that is largely to blame for these lesions' associated mass effects, commonly evidence of intense vascular congestion, and may be frankly hemorrhagic. Neurons, if at all recognizable, persist only in faded, 'ghost'-like profile or appear shrunken, angulated, and abnormally eosinophilic with a loss of intranuclear detail. Neutrophilic exudates may be apparent early on, but most lesions approached surgically have evolved to the point where mononuclear phagocytes, including lipid-laden foam cells, constitute their principal reactive elements. These lend to organizing infarcts a potentially alarming hypercellularity that is all the more misleading when accompanied, as is often the case, by capillary proliferation and endothelial hypertrophy resembling glioma-associated vascular hyperplasia. Inasmuch as the cytologic features by which macrophages are recognized tend to be obscured in frozen sections but are immediately apparent in squash and smear preparations, routine use of the latter is urged for purposes of intraoperative consultation. Once a lesion has been identified as being rich in phagocytes, the major differential consideration is demyelinating disease, given detailed consideration elsewhere in this chapter. Suffice it to say that demyelinating pseudotumors only exceptionally progress to tissue necrosis, are usually characterized by perivascular lymphoid cuffing and a relative preservation of axons foreign to brain infarcts, and generally afflict patients younger than those at risk of ischemic cerebral events.

Intracranial aneurysms

The **saccular** or '**berry**' **aneurysm** ranks chief among surgically correctable cerebrovascular abnormalities and is unrivaled as a cause of massive subarachnoid hemorrhage in adults. These common lesions (their prevalence in the general population falls in the neighborhood of 2–5%) are somewhat more frequent in women and are encountered at all ages beyond puberty, although symptomatic examples cluster in the fifth through seventh decades of life.[119,122,129] Some 10–15% of cases have been estimated to occur on a familial basis.[123] The factors critical in initiating the formation of saccular intracranial aneurysms remain undefined, and the majority are unassociated with local or systemic conditions known to promote vascular injury, but hemodynamic stress probably plays the major role in their development and, on balance, the weight of evidence supports the hypothesis that these are primarily acquired, degenerative lesions rather than developmental anomalies.[109,129] Arterial hypertension is widely regarded as playing an aggravating role in their evolution and may underlie an association with the adult form of aortic coarctation, with type III polycystic kidney disease, and pheochromocytoma.[109,117,129] Connective tissue disorders that result in increased vascular fragility have mainly been associated with aneurysms of fusiform type but may also predispose to the development of saccular aneurysms, these having been described in the settings of type III collagen deficiency (Ehlers–Danlos syndrome type IV), pseudoxanthoma elasticum, and Marfan syndrome.[109,129] Aneurysms of the saccular variety occasionally occur in complex with fibromuscular dysplasia of the renal arteries, intracranial arteriovenous malformations or fistulas, and persistent primitive carotid–basilar anastomoses or other anomalies of the circle of Willis.[109,129] The latter observations notwithstanding, the localization of most saccular aneurysms (discussed below) is at odds with the theory that they commonly originate in vestigial remnants of the embryonic cerebral vasculature.

Frequently multifocal, saccular intracranial aneurysms usually lie within 3 cm of the internal carotid artery termini at the circle of Willis, and 80% involve divisions of the cerebral vasculature ventral to the posterior communicating arteries.[122] It is clear from autopsy studies that the middle cerebral arteries are most commonly affected, but most clinical series are dominated by anterior communicating and internal carotid artery examples because these are more prone to rupture.[119,120,122,129] That saccular aneurysms almost invariably bulge from points of acute angle vascular bifurcation has been interpreted by some observers as the natural consequence of increased hemodynamic impact or turbulence at these points and by others as reflecting an inherent local weakness of the vessel wall secondary to focal gaps in the arterial media known to occur near circulatory forks.[109] Although such 'defects' could theoretically influence the localization of some lesions, there actually appears to be little topographic concordance between their major distribution in the human cerebrovascular tree and that of saccular aneurysms.

On histologic examination, the walls of saccular intracranial aneurysms are composed principally of fibrous tissue, the muscular coats and elastic laminae of parent vessels typically terminating abruptly at the points of aneurysmal outpouching.[109,122] Atheromatous changes are common and may be florid but are characteristically confined to the aneurysmal sac and thus probably represent superimposed alterations of little direct etiologic significance. Much the same can be said of chronic inflammatory mural infiltration. Other secondary phenomena include partial or, in select instances, complete thrombotic occlusion, the latter presumably accounting for the occasional 'disappearance' of untreated aneurysms assessed by periodic angiographic study.

Most saccular aneurysms remain asymptomatic, and even frank rupture may be followed by spontaneous thrombotic closure of the aneurysmal sac and clinical resolution, but this is not to trivialize the associated risk of catastrophic intracranial hemorrhage. Long-term follow-up studies of patients with angiographically proven saccular aneurysms suggest a 1–2% annual incidence of rupture; approximately half of these bleeding episodes prove fatal.[120] Although subarachnoid hemorrhage alone may be lethal, it is the dissection of blood into the brain itself or ventricular system that kills in many cases. Massive intraparenchymal hematomas are most often a consequence of middle cerebral artery aneurysms, whereas anterior communicating examples are generally responsible for most episodes of fatal intraventricular hemorrhage (blood usually entering the anterior horn of the lateral ventricle after dissecting through the inferomedial frontal lobe). Another grave complication is cerebral infarction related to postrupture vasospasm, again encountered most commonly in patients harboring aneurysms of the anterior communicating arteries.

Although most observers have concluded that considerable risk of rupture is attached to saccular aneurysms exceeding 1 cm in diameter and relatively little to examples measuring 5 mm or less,[129] none of these lesions can be regarded as entirely innocent. In fact, nearly 70% of saccular aneurysms that ruptured in the course of one long-term follow-up study measured 6 mm or less in diameter on angiographic assessment.[120] Aneurysms that achieve 'giant' proportions (usually defined as having diameters of at least 3 cm) typically present with cranial neuropathies, evidence of ventricular outflow obstruction or other mass effects, rather than hemorrhage. Rarely, the surgical management of saccular aneurysms is complicated by a local granulomatous response to cotton materials employed as reinforcement following aneurysmal clipping.[113] These '**textilomas**', '**muslinomas**' or '**gauzomas**' can achieve considerable size, presenting as contrast-enhancing masses with significant accompanying edema, and may produce headache, fever, obstructive hydrocephalus, cranial nerve palsies, and endocrinopathy. In some cases a nontumorous optochiasmatic arachnoiditis provoked by these materials causes visual loss.

Although the designation of **mycotic aneurysm** would seem to specifically connote a fungal process, this term has been applied in practice to focal infectious arteritides of diverse cause having in common only an element of vascular dilation. Most mycotic intracranial aneurysms are, in fact, bacterial in nature and evolve as complications of endocarditis or, less frequently, suppurating pulmonary infection.[109,111] Streptococci and staphylococcal species are the usual offenders. The resulting lesions, often multifocal, tend to be situated on distal branches of the cerebral vasculature, are more often fusiform or irregular than berry-like in configuration, and are frequently of diminutive proportions. Fungal aneurysms are specifically addressed in the discussion of CNS mycoses. In brief, these are most often caused by *Aspergillus* and *Candida* species, generally involve the large cerebral arteries at the base of the brain, and tend to have greater diameters on presentation than their bacterial counterparts.

Atherosclerotic intracranial aneurysms generally afflict older adults, usually arise in the setting of advanced and generalized cerebrovascular atheromatosis, typically involve supraclinoid portions of the internal carotid arteries or the basilar artery, and may assume saccular, fusiform, cylindrical, or conical configurations.[109]

Fusiform lesions of the vertebrobasilar trunk are the single most common variant.[116,126] Atherosclerotic aneurysms are generally of large size and frequently achieve giant proportions. Their presenting manifestations are more often related to compression of neighboring CNS structures or ischemic complications of progressive thrombosis than to hemorrhage, although some observers assert that the associated risk of rupture is underestimated.[126] Far more common than discrete aneurysm formation is atherosclerotic '**dolichoectasia**' – diffuse dilation and tortuous elongation of the basilar or internal carotid arteries – and the two processes may coexist.

Dissecting aneurysms of the intracranial vasculature are rarities.[109] Most documented cases are without satisfactory etiologic explanation, although some have been attributed to trauma, syphilis, cystic medionecrosis, arteriosclerosis, fibromuscular dysplasia, or other local abnormalities of vascular structure. Alpha-1-antitrypsin deficiency has been linked to intracranial arteriopathy potentially complicated by dissection or aneurysm formation.[124] Luminal stenosis secondary to the intramural accumulation of blood may result in bulbar or cerebral infarction; rupture typically produces catastrophic subarachnoid hemorrhage. Symptoms referable to mass effect constitute the least frequent manifestation of intracranial arterial dissection.

Exceptionally, tumors metastatic to the CNS present as 'spontaneous' intracerebral or subarachnoid hemorrhages that ultimately prove the consequences of **neoplastic aneurysm** formation. Most neoplastic intracranial aneurysms result from the embolization of cardiac myxomas to the cerebral vasculature,[118] but examples caused by ovarian choriocarcinoma[114] and carcinomas of the lung[115] are also on record. The appearance of intracranial aneurysms years following therapeutic irradiation of the brain has also been documented.[125]

Considerable controversy surrounds the incidence of so-called **Charcot–Bouchard** (or '**miliary**') **microaneurysms** and their clinical significance.[109,121] The latter are described as saccular or fusiform lesions most commonly involving lenticulostriate, perforating pontine, and corticomedullary junction arteries measuring 25–250 microns in diameter. Said to be particularly prevalent in hypertensive subjects, their rupture is regarded by some as a major cause of basal ganglionic, bulbar, and cerebellar hemorrhage in this patient cohort. That aneurysms of Charcot–Bouchard type have received little attention in the surgical pathology literature could reflect the specialized tissue handling requisite to their identification. Studies from Japan in which surgically evacuated hematomas were subjected to meticulous examination under the dissecting microscope (and serial thin sectioning of suspect lesions) would suggest that microaneurysms are underappreciated as a factor predisposing to atraumatic lobar cerebral hemorrhage in both hypertensive and normotensive individuals.[127,128] Painstaking analysis in Caucasians, on the other hand, demonstrated most 'microaneurysms' to actually represent complex vascular tortuosities and failed to establish a link between truly aneurysmal lesions and intracerebral hemorrhage.[112] Whether these discrepancies are simply methodologic or have their basis in genetic or environmental factors is unclear. In practice, it is virtually impossible to conclusively identify microaneurysms in routinely processed paraffin sections.

Vascular malformations

Generically designated as vascular malformations are various non-neoplastic lesions resulting from focal anomalies in the development of the cerebrospinal circulation. These are usefully divided into four relatively discrete morphologic categories, namely, capillary telangiectases, angiomas of venous or cavernous type, and arteriovenous malformations.[109] Transitional or hybrid types, however, may be encountered.[135,149,158,159] Also considered in this section are arteriovenous fistulas, since these are, strictly speaking, malformations, although they are generally regarded as acquired, rather than developmental, abnormalities.

Capillary telangiectases exhibit a curious predilection for the basis pontis (particularly the region of the median raphe), but are occasionally found to involve the cerebral hemispheres and spinal cord.[109] They usually constitute incidental findings at autopsy and are only rarely complicated by symptomatic hemorrhage. On record is a massive pontomedullary case associated with a protracted history of bulbar dysfunction.[139] The lesion consists of loosely aggregated and variably ectatic capillary-type vessels (i.e., devoid of elastic or muscular mural elements) separated by normal or only mildly gliotic neuropil. A densely mineralized variant – the '**calcified telangiectatic hamartoma**' or '**hemangioma calcificans**' – is a recognized, albeit rare, cause of epilepsy, particularly of temporal lobe type.[169] Capillary telangiectases of the CNS complicate some examples of hereditary hemorrhagic telangiectasia, also known as Osler–Weber–Rendu disease.[109,162]

The **venous angioma** is a loose collection of dilated veins found typically in the digitate or deep white matter of the cerebral or cerebellar hemispheres.[109] The radial convergence of their ectatic vessels on a central draining varix lends to many of these lesions a diagnostic 'caput medusae'-like profile on angiographic study. Although venous angiomas are the most common vascular malformations of the human central nervous system, it is the exceptional example that is responsible for intracranial hemorrhage or is otherwise symptomatic.[152]

The **cavernous angioma** or '**cavernoma**' differs from all other vascular malformations in that its constituent vessels are fashioned into a compact, globose mass devoid of intervening neural elements.[109] On gross inspection, a spongy core of blood-filled channels is encircled by a thin rind of indurated (because gliotic) and rusted-appearing (because hemosiderin-laden) neural parenchyma. Histologic study will reveal closely apposed, engorged vessels composed solely of fibrous tissue (Fig. 28.6). Secondary alterations such as thrombosis and dystrophic calcification are common, some lesions undergoing extensive metaplastic ossification as well. The existence of hybrid variants exhibiting in part the structure of capillary telangiectases[158,159] has fueled speculation that cavernous angiomas may evolve from malformations of the former type,[159] but the

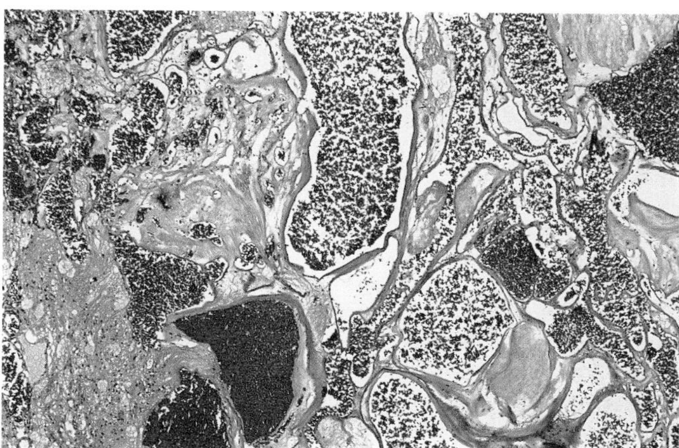

Fig. 28.6 Cavernous angioma. As illustrated, the cavernous angioma consists of ectatic and fibrous-walled vascular channels devoid of intervening neuroglial tissue. Neighboring brain parenchyma is present at lower left.

fact remains that 'mixed' lesions are exceptional. Cavernous angiomas may be situated anywhere along the neuraxis. Most examples lie above the tentorium,[166] often in cerebral white matter subjacent to the motor strip, but the posterior fossa contents and spinal cord are not immune and even the cauda equina,[156] cranial nerves,[148] and epidural compartment[171] may be involved. Multifocal cases are by no means rare. The designation of cavernous angioma has also been extended to certain extra-axial vascular malformations affecting dural venous sinuses, but these depart structurally from their counterparts positioned in the CNS proper in that they contain, in addition to compact cavernous elements, capillaries and muscular vessels of both arterial and venous type.[150] These distinctive lesions, which usually present as a consequence of cranial nerve compression and are generally mistaken for meningiomas on preoperative neuroimaging study, are not given further consideration here.

Cavernous angiomas may become manifest in childhood, but most symptomatic lesions are encountered in the third and fourth decades of life.[166] Familial cases transmitted in autosomal dominant fashion and linked to the mutation of genes involved in integrin-mediated angiogenesis and programmed cell death have been delineated,[109,144] the former including *KRIT1* abnormalities responsible for an excess of cavernous angiomas among Hispanic–American kindreds of Mexican descent. Such variants may occur in complex with cavernous angiomas of the retina,[138] hyperkeratotic venous malformations of the skin,[143] vertebral hemangiomas,[136] and café-au-lait spots.[151] That seizures are their dominant clinical manifestation reflects the proximity of most cavernous angiomas to epileptogenic cerebrocortical tissues. Less frequent complaints include focal neurologic deficits and headache. Although catastrophic hemorrhage is decidedly rare, cavernous angiomas are a recognized cause of intracranial hematomas, including both acutely symptomatic[168] and 'encapsulated' lobar types,[160] the latter resulting in all likelihood from repeated subclinical episodes of bleeding and subsequent organization. A confident preoperative diagnosis of cavernous angioma may be established by neuroradiologic means. The typical lesion, although 'angiographically occult' (i.e., not apparent on arteriographic study), appears in T2-weighted magnetic resonance images as an irregularly hyperdense nodule unassociated with significant edema or mass effect but surrounded by a hypodense penumbra resulting from the accumulation of hemosiderin in adjoining neural tissues. Focal vascular lesions having a cavernous angioma-like neuroradiologic profile may develop in the brain or spinal cord as a consequence of therapeutic CNS irradiation.[133,170] These seem more prone to hemorrhage than sporadic variants, develop most commonly in children and adolescents, and may exhibit transitional histologic features with regions of capillary and venous telangiectasis.

The most threatening of the congenital cerebrovascular anomalies under discussion is the **arteriovenous malformation** (AVM), a tangle of deformed arterial afferents and draining veins devoid of an interposed capillary bed.[109,147] AVMs may be situated in any region of the brain or spinal cord and can be restricted to the dura or choroid plexus,[134] but most lie within the distribution of the middle cerebral arteries and involve the hemispheric convexities in contiguity with their covering leptomeninges. A majority present in early and mid-adulthood as a consequence of intracranial hemorrhage, other common manifestations including seizures, focal sensorimotor deficits, and headaches not clearly referable to episodes of bleeding.[132,155] Familial cases have been described[130] and AVMs of the central neuraxis may be encountered in complex with Osler–Weber–Rendu disease (hereditary hemorrhagic telangiectasia).[162] The turbulent shunting of blood through AVMs of the brain is sometimes audible as a cranial or orbital bruit, can often be demonstrated to diagnostic advantage on angiographic study, and may

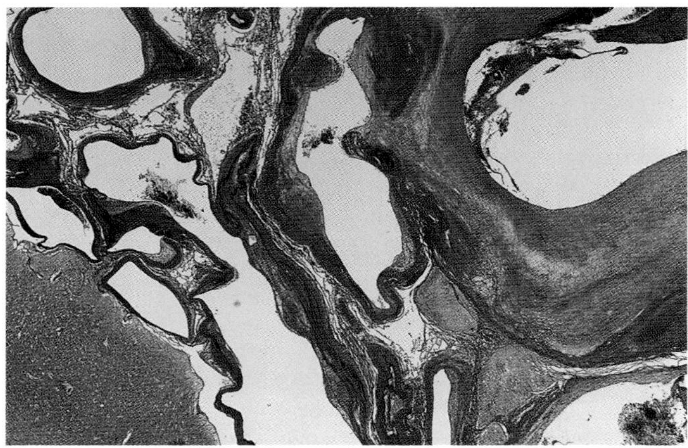

Fig. 28.7 Arteriovenous malformation. Ectatic, variably muscularized blood vessels with interrupted elastic lamina and fibrotic intimal thickening participate in this malformative lesion. (Van Gieson stain)

precipitate high output cardiac failure in afflicted infants and children, particularly those harboring extensive lesions drained by aneurysmally dilated galenic veins. Unfortunately, AVMs are complicated by fatal rupture with distressing frequency. Long-term observations suggest that symptomatic examples carry a 2–4% risk of clinically significant hemorrhage per year and, left untreated, will eventuate in the deaths of at least one-fourth of affected patients as a direct result of rupture.[132,155] Feeding arteries are prone to develop saccular aneurysms, and it is occasionally one of these, rather than the malformation itself, that is responsible for the lethal hemorrhagic ictus.

AVMs vary in size from cryptic lesions not demonstrable by angiographic means and discovered only on sampling of surgically evacuated hematomas[145] to enormous lobar examples that may focally span the full thickness of a cerebral hemisphere. As their tortuous, cirsoid vascular components form a complex network of blood-filled channels, the nature of these lesions is often apparent on casual gross inspection. Intervening neural tissues are typically attenuated, and there is evidence of rust-brown discoloration attesting to prior hemorrhage. Involved leptomeninges are thickened, opacified, and frequently siderotic as well. On histologic study (Fig. 28.7), the lesion is composed of variably ectatic and hyalinized veins, abnormally muscularized arteries, and structurally ambiguous vessels formed solely of fibrous tissue or displaying both arterial and venous characteristics.[109,147] Critical to the distinction of the true AVM from normal leptomeningeal vessels that may assume a malformative appearance in neurosurgical material as a result of artefactual compaction are the former's conspicuous mural anomalies. Chief among these are striking fluctuations in medial thickness, architectural disarray or focal disappearance of the media altogether, or its separation into inner and outer coats by a seemingly aberrant elastic lamina.[147] Cushions of fibromuscular tissue may also appear to project in polypoid fashion into the lumens of these abnormal vessels, and focal duplications and disruptions of the internal elastic lamina are common. Superimposed alterations include mural fibroplasia and atheromatosis, aneurysmal dilation, calcification, and thrombosis, which, if extensive, may preclude the visualization of even sizable malformations by angiographic methods.[145] Lesions subjected to preoperative embolization in an attempt to minimize blood loss during resection frequently exhibit an intraluminal foreign body response to the occluding material and may undergo focal necrosis,[165] radiosurgical treatment causing fibrointimal hyperplasia with progressive vaso-occlusion.[164] Entrapped neuropil usually manifests dense astrogliosis, neuronal depopulation, and ferruginous encrustation of included neuroglial elements. The reader's attention is also called to the presence, in the interstices of select AVMs, of oligodendroglioma-like regions that may be intrinsic to the underlying maldevelopmental process or the result of abnormal oligodendroglial aggregation caused by the ischemic contraction of entrapped white matter.[146,153] The association of AVMs and bona fide gliomas is discussed under the heading of 'Gliosarcoma and other gliomesenchymal tumors', as are malformation-like alterations occurring in the vascular stroma of neuroepithelial tumors.

To the sporadic and familial malformations mentioned in preceding paragraphs can be added a host of vascular anomalies constituting manifestations of so-called **neurocutaneous syndromes** (**'phakomatoses'**), some clearly heritable and others the apparent result of spontaneous mutation. The most widely recognized of these disorders is **encephalo-trigeminal angiomatosis**, known by the eponym of **Sturge–Weber syndrome** and defined as a florid venocapillary proliferation involving the leptomeninges and cortical mantle of one cerebral hemisphere in complex with a cutaneous hemangioma ('port-wine stain') lying at least in part in the ophthalmic distribution of the ipsilateral trigeminal nerve.[109,137] Progressive mineralization of the involved cortex, centered initially on its abnormal perforating vessels, results in a gyriform, 'tram-track' profile of radiologically demonstrable intracranial calcifications characteristic of the disease. Atrophy of the affected cerebral hemisphere is the rule, and patients typically suffer contralateral hemiparesis, often attended by motor seizures and mental retardation. The association of unilateral retinal angiomatosis and a cutaneous hemangioma in an ipsilateral trigeminal distribution with an AVM of the midbrain is referred to as **mesencephalo-oculo-facial angiomatosis** (also termed **neuroretinal angiomatosis**, **Bonnet–Dechaume–Blanc syndrome**, or **Wyburn–Mason syndrome**).[109] The generic designation of **cerebrofacial arteriovenous metameric syndrome** has been adopted by some observers to encompass this and other malformative vascular disorders involving the CNS, cutis, and subcutaneous tissues of the face, these including rare variants affecting the pons and cerebellum in concert with the skin of the mandibular region and upper neck.[142] Capillary telangiectases and AVMs are also recognized, albeit rare, CNS manifestations of **hereditary hemorrhagic telangiectasia (Osler–Weber–Rendu** disease).[162] **Cobb syndrome** or **cutaneomeningospinal angiomatosis** is defined by the association of a dermal angioma (often of port-wine stain type) with an intraspinal hemangioma or AVM at corresponding dermatomal levels.[141]

Arteriovenous fistulas of the craniospinal vasculature are accorded only passing consideration here because their current management – surgical clipping or selective embolic occlusion of the offending communication – does not usually yield specimens for anatomic study. It is the absence of a plexiform, angiomatous nidus interposed between its feeding arteries and venous efferents that serves to distinguish the simple fistula from the AVM on angiographic and morphologic evaluation, although the latter's participating vessels may develop fistulous connections.[167] Trauma clearly figures in the genesis of many examples (particularly carotid-cavernous sinus and vertebrovertebral types), as does neurosurgical injury, and some complicate systemic disorders such as fibromuscular dysplasia, type IV Ehlers–Danlos syndrome, and, mentioned above, Osler–Weber–Rendu disease.[109] Many arteriovenous fistulas, however, present in spontaneous fashion. Those involving the cerebral arteries proper typically come to attention in childhood or early adult life, their clinical manifestations including headache, seizures, focal sensorimotor deficits, cardiac decompensation, and intracranial hemorrhage. Catastrophic rupture, however, appears to be exceptional. Fistulas developing below the tentorium are often localized to the dural sheaths of spinal nerve roots in the low thoracic region.[131,163] Lesions of this sort afflict men far more commonly than women, usually become symptomatic in or beyond middle age, and result in progressive paraparesis, paresthesias of the lower extremities, and sphincter disturbances. Known eponymously as **Foix–Alajouanine syndrome** or as **angiodysgenetic myelomalacia** or **venous congestive myelopathy**, this disorder is typified by serpentine elongation and distension of veins coursing over the dorsal surface of the thoracic spinal cord and is likely the result of protracted local venous hypertension caused by an overlap in the vascular drainage of the adjacent dural fistula and the cord itself. Fistulas involving the perimedullary vascular plexus[167] or distantly situated in the cranial or sacral dura[157] may eventuate in a similar picture. The long-standing hemodynamic alterations[161] in such cases can produce regional expansions of the spinal cord that mimic infiltrative neoplasms and prompt biopsy. Characteristic histopathologic alterations include architectural distortion of the neuroparenchyma with gliosis, thickening and hyalinization of vascular walls, hemosiderin deposition, and varying degrees of myelin loss. Mild glial atypism can be encountered as can the formation of Rosenthal fibers (described and illustrated in our discussion of pilocytic astrocytomas), some cases also manifesting vascular thrombosis and necrosis. Dural arteriovenous fistulas drained by ectatic or aneurysmally dilated cortical veins are particularly prone to hemorrhage.[140] Dural-based arteriovenous fistulas have also been implicated in the pathogenesis of vascular malformations occupying the sigmoid and transverse sinuses.[154]

Primary angiitis

Among the less common forms of cerebrovascular disease is the idiopathic disorder variously described as **'isolated'**, **'granulomatous'**, or **'primary' angiitis of the CNS**.[173,174] Inasmuch as many histopathologically confirmed cases have not evidenced overtly granulomatous features, and as autopsy studies have disclosed exceptional instances of extraneural vascular involvement, the last of these designations would seem the most accurate and is adopted here.

Primary angiitis of the CNS can occur at any age but usually afflicts young or middle-aged adults, its principal clinical manifestations including headache, mental status changes, and focal neurologic deficits (particularly hemiparesis) that may evolve in progressive fashion or present abruptly as 'stroke'. Signs and symptoms of myelopathy occasionally dominate the clinical picture, but only rarely is morphologic evidence of vascular injury accentuated at, or confined to, spinal levels.[172,175] If not promptly diagnosed and managed, the disorder generally proves progressive and fatal.

Short of biopsy for tissue confirmation, angiography is the most useful investigative procedure and findings typical of vasculitis – particularly multifocal, segmental stenosis, dilation, or 'beading' of small- to medium-caliber leptomeningeal arteries – are considered by some to constitute sufficient grounds for the institution of corticosteroid or cytotoxic therapy in the appropriate setting (i.e., when underlying infection and other systemic processes associated with secondary CNS angiitis have been excluded from further diagnostic consideration). However, arteriograms may be unrevealing even in the face of florid vascular disease.[173] Less commonly encountered neuroradiologic abnormalities include aneurysm formation and focal 'mass' lesions secondary to infarction, often hemorrhagic.

Most observers regard biopsy as the sole means of confirming a presumptive clinical diagnosis of primary CNS angiitis, although false-negative samplings are a common consequence of the

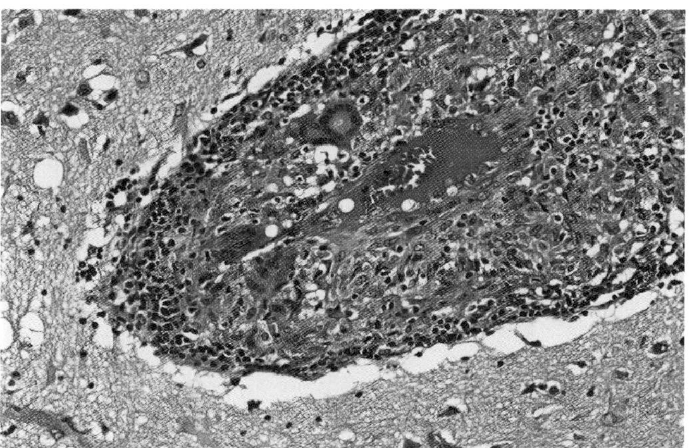

Fig. 28.8 Primary angiitis of the CNS. A frankly granulomatous inflammatory infiltrate replete with multinucleated giant cells expands the wall of this penetrating cerebrocortical blood vessel, found in biopsy material from a 34-year-old man with progressive encephalopathy.

disorder's segmental distribution. Small and midsized leptomeningeal and intracortical arteries usually bear the brunt of the injury, but neighboring veins are often involved in concert, and the process may affect the large vessels at the base of the brain as well. Rarely, however, are inflammatory alterations confined to the latter. That the histologic presentation of primary CNS angiitis is subject to considerable variation merits emphasis.[173,174] Frequently encountered are necrotizing polyarteritis-like or non-necrotizing lymphoplasmacytic variants. Mural infiltration by histiocytes, including epithelioid forms, and multinucleated giant cells of foreign body and Langhans type characterize granulomatous examples, but this is an inconstant feature (Fig. 28.8). When present, giant cells are not strictly associated with the elastic lamina and may lie in any part of the vessel wall. Secondary changes include thrombosis and, in long-standing cases, mural scarring and exuberant fibrointimal hyperplasia. The phenomenon of '**mixed' granulomatous vasculitis and amyloid deposition** is discussed below (see 'Cerebral amyloid angiopathy' below).

Notwithstanding the fact that its histologic features are shared by cerebral vasculitides complicating a variety of systemic disorders,[173,174] primary angiitis of the CNS merits distinct nosologic status on clinical grounds. This is not to deny the possibility that this curious process might be triggered by diverse offenses to the cerebrospinal circulation. Although long suspected, an infectious etiology remains unproved. Noteworthy in this regard, however, is the epidemiologic association of primary CNS angiitis with cutaneous herpes zoster infection and with underlying conditions, chiefly Hodgkin disease and other forms of hematolymphoid neoplasia, predisposing to this and other viral opportunists.[173,176] These observations are especially intriguing in view of the undisputed role of the varicella-zoster virus as agent of a large vessel cerebral arteritis, potentially indistinguishable from primary CNS angiitis, addressed in our discussion of viral disorders.

Cerebral amyloid angiopathy

The deposition of amyloid in the walls of cerebral blood vessels is a fact of aging and a conspicuous accompanying feature of varied neurologic disorders, including Alzheimer disease, Down syndrome, dementia pugilistica, and certain types of spongiform encephalopathy. It is the association of this process – **cerebral amyloid angiopathy** – with intracranial hemorrhage that compels the attention of the neurosurgeon and surgical pathologist. Cerebral amyloid angiopathy is the most common nontraumatic cause of lobar cerebral hematoma in elderly subjects (the cohort at greatest risk) and has been estimated to account for some 5–10% of all primary, atraumatic brain hemorrhages.[109,179] The disorder is not a manifestation of systemic amyloidosis and typically presents in sporadic fashion, although kindreds afflicted by heritable (autosomal dominant) syndromes of florid cerebrovascular amyloidosis and early death due to recurrent intracerebral hemorrhage have been delineated.[179] β-Amyloid peptide (Aβ), found also in the infiltrated CNS vessels and neuritic plaques of asymptomatic senescence and Alzheimer disease, constitutes the principal amyloid deposited in sporadic cases.[179] Aberrant forms of Aβ, cystatin C, transthyretin, gelsolin, and other proteins resulting from point mutations in their encoding genes are the offending amyloidogenic agents in various heredofamilial types of CNS amyloidosis with vascular involvement.[179] While a substantial proportion of sporadically affected patients evidence dementia, cerebral amyloid angiopathy, even when severe, is not necessarily associated with cognitive impairment or with Alzheimer-type cerebrocortical alterations.

The peripheral, lobar location of amyloid-associated cerebral hematomas contrasts sharply with the basal ganglionic or bulbar situation typical of hypertensive hemorrhages and reflects the particular susceptibility of superficial cortical and leptomeningeal vessels to amyloidotic infiltration. Chiefly affected are small-caliber arteries and arterioles, but veins may be involved as well. These exhibit mural expansion and, in advanced cases, effacement by acellular, eosinophilic material deposited in the adventitia and media. By definition, this possesses the histochemical properties (Fig. 28.9) and fine structural attributes common to all amyloids. Definitive identification is most readily accomplished by demonstration of a dichroic, bluish-green birefringence in Congo red-stained sections viewed under polarized light. Other defining characteristics include thioflavin S or T fluorescence under ultraviolet light. Ultrastructural study should reveal randomly arrayed, nonbranching extracellular fibrils averaging 9 nm in diameter, but is not requisite to the diagnosis if the appropriate reactions are obtained on Congo red or thioflavin assay. Amyloid-laden cerebral vessels generally maintain their patency but are subject to a variety of 'vasculopathic' alterations. These include 'double-barreling' (a targetoid, vessel-within-vessel configuration produced by what would appear to be a circumferential cleft in the media), glomeruloid arteriolar changes, obliterative fibrointimal proliferation, perivascular or intramural lymphocytic infiltration, the development of microaneurysms, and, finally, fibrinoid necrosis.[178,181] Restricted to vessels bearing a heavy amyloid burden, this last abnormality appears to play a particularly significant role in the pathogenesis of vascular rupture.[181]

As is often the case in extracranial locations, amyloid deposited in the cerebral vasculature occasionally elicits a foreign body-type response replete with multinucleated giant cells that surround affected vessels and attempt to phagocytize the offending material. Much rarer are examples of cerebral amyloid angiopathy associated with a true vasculitis of necrotizing and granulomatous type.[174,180] Such cases have been interpreted to represent, in the main, idiosyncratic host reactions to the deposited protein ('**Aβ-related angiitis**'),[180] but it is conceivable that primary cerebral vasculitides might aggravate, if not trigger, local amyloidogenic processes. Instances of cerebral amyloid angiopathy and vasculitis occurring in patients with rheumatoid arthritis are noteworthy in this regard.[177] Interestingly, most examples of angiitic cerebrovascular amyloidosis (including those reported under the rubric of combined

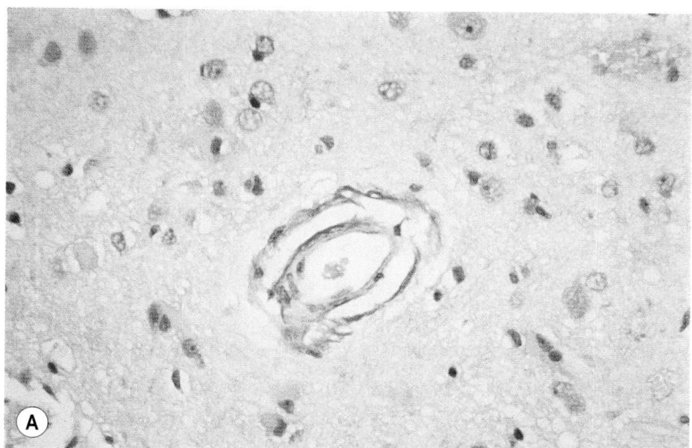

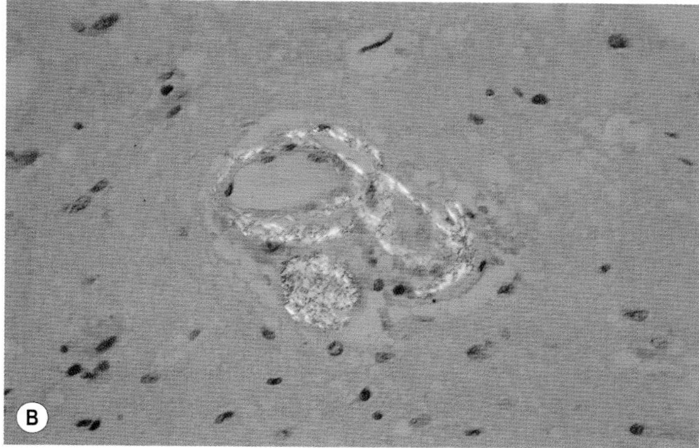

Fig. 28.9 Cerebral amyloid ('congophilic') angiopathy. As in extraneural locations, amyloid in the walls of cerebral vessels takes the Congo red stain (**A**) and exhibits an 'apple green' birefringence when sections thus prepared are viewed under polarized light (**B**). The apparent 'double-barrel' lumen evident in **A** is a common feature of amyloid-laden cerebral vessels.

granulomatous angiitis and cerebral amyloid angiopathy) have presented not with intracerebral bleeding but as nonhemorrhagic lesions, some mass-forming and radiologically taken for neoplastic, associated with alterations of mental status, headache, seizures or focal neurologic deficits of subacutely progressive nature. Sufferers are typically younger than patients with noninflammatory amyloid angiopathy.

Cerebral autosomal dominant arteriopathy with subcortical infarcts and leukoencephalopathy (CADASIL)

Cerebral autosomal dominant arteriopathy with subcortical infarcts and leukoencephalopathy (CADASIL) is, as its name implies, a heritable condition.[109,182] Hundreds of affected kindreds have been delineated worldwide. The disorder has been linked to missense mutations or, rarely, small deletions involving the *NOTCH3* gene at chromosome 19p13, the product of which is a transmembrane receptor protein and transcriptional regulator selectively expressed in vascular smooth muscle cells. Isolated nonfamilial cases seemingly due to de novo *NOTCH3* mutations have been described. Clinical manifestations of CADASIL include migraine with aura (often the earliest neurologic complaint), subcortical ischemic strokes, psychiatric symptoms, and cognitive deterioration eventuating in dementia. Most patients die within 15–25 years following their initial episodes of stroke. Nodular foci of periventricular T2 hyperintensity are characteristic and early changes seen in MR images are often apparent in presymptomatic individuals. With disease progression, lacunar white matter infarcts develop and confluent zones of increased T2-weighted MRI signal reflect a diffuse leukoencephalopathy.

CADASIL is a nonarteriosclerotic and nonamyloidotic vasculopathy that principally involves small and medium-sized arteries in the cerebral hemispheric white matter, but leptomeningeal and even systemic vessels are potentially affected by this generalized disorder.[109,182] Most recorded cases have been identified by brain biopsy, but sampling of skin, skeletal muscle, and peripheral nerve may be informative as well. The hallmark of CADASIL is accumulation of a granular, basophilic, and PAS-positive material in the tunica media of affected vessels with associated loss of medial smooth muscle cells, concentric mural sclerosis, and luminal narrowing. At the ultrastructural level, this distinctive material consists of osmiophilic, electron-dense granules 10–15 mm in size that lie free between degenerating myocytes or cluster within pericellular indentations. These deposits may be labeled by monoclonal antibodies to the NOTCH3 protein ectodomain, are specific for CADASIL, and may be identified in the presymptomatic phase of the disease. Accordingly, ultrastructural or immunohistochemical studies of small dermal or subcutaneous arteries in skin biopsy specimens have been advocated as screening procedures for family members at risk as well as diagnostic methods in suspect cases. Formal genetic assessment (e.g., single strand conformational polymorphism analysis) may also be undertaken to confirm the diagnosis.

Epidural hematoma

The great majority of **epidural hematomas** follow cranial trauma complicated by temporal bone fracture and result from laceration of middle meningeal artery branches that penetrate the skull in the region of the pterion.[183] The accumulation of blood between the calvarium and endosteal surface of the dura mater is typically rapid, associated with acute deterioration of consciousness, and soon eventuates in death as a result of transtentorial herniation with brainstem compression if not promptly evacuated. Uncommon variants become symptomatic only long after their initiating injuries. Delimited by encapsulating neomembranes formed of vascularized fibrous tissue, chronic epidural hematomas of this sort are usually of venous origin.

Subdural hematoma

Subdural hematomas result from the dissection of blood into the potential space separating the arachnoid and dura mater, closely apposed under normal circumstances.[185] Most overlie the cerebral convexities in the frontoparietal region and are thought to follow rupture of delicate bridging veins that traverse the arachnoid–dura interface en route to the superior sagittal sinus.[183] These vessels are particularly susceptible to shearing forces generated by sudden angular acceleration of the head, as commonly occurs in the setting of trauma, and many subdural hematomas are clearly associated with cranial injury. Most 'spontaneous' examples occur in the elderly, possibly because cerebral atrophy and resultant traction on these bridging vessels reduce their capacity to withstand otherwise trivial stresses. A similar phenomenon may promote the development of subdural hematomas following ventricular decompression for hydrocephalus. Patients who have received anticoagulants, who are thrombocytopenic, or who have been treated with long-term hemodialysis are also at increased risk of subdural hemorrhage.[186] A small subset of subdural hematomas result from arterial injury. These are usually associated with major craniocerebral trauma.

The pathology of the subdural hematoma is a function of its age. If evacuated within days of onset, it consists simply of clotted blood. Often, however, the original bleeding episode passes unnoticed, and the hematoma becomes symptomatic only after it has elicited an organizational response resulting in its enclosure within a discoid sac fashioned of grayish-brown, collagenous neomembranes that adhere to the dura but develop no attachments to the underlying arachnoid. The latter feature reflects the fact that the mesenchymal elements responsible for encapsulation of the hematoma derive entirely from the dura, the leptomeninges remaining curiously unmoved by the presence of blood in the subdural space and playing no part in its organization. Inasmuch as the histologic maturation of these limiting membranes proceeds in temporally predictable fashion, the chronicity of a given lesion may be estimated by thorough assessment of the membranes.[183] Suffice it to say that the outer (juxtadural) membrane, which may attain a thickness of several millimeters, consists in the early stages of proliferating spindle cells and budding capillaries that penetrate the superficial aspect of the hematoma and come to lie in a loose connective tissue matrix containing admixed siderophages, scattered lymphocytes, and, in some cases, extramedullary hematopoietic elements (normoblasts). Infiltration by eosinophils may be striking. The inner membrane, by contrast, has a simpler structure and is thinner and relatively avascular. The precise cytogenesis of the spindly, fibroblastic elements populating these neomembranes and responsible for their ensuing collagenization remains a matter of speculation, but an origin from 'dural border' cells that normally form a complex lamina apposed to the arachnoid has been suggested on the strength of fine structural observations.[184,185,187] In any event, both membranes undergo progressive hyalinization and, with complete resorption of the hematoma, fuse to form a thin fibrous rind closely resembling the adjacent dura mater on microscopic study. In exceptional instances, the hematoma sac is transformed into a calcific, even ossified, shell.

The capacity of the chronic subdural hematoma to present in clinically delayed fashion as an expanding intracranial mass would seem a paradox. Once completed, the enclosing hematoma sac could conceivably function as a semipermeable membrane and permit the ingress of fluid drawn by osmotic forces from the CSF compartment or the capillary network in its outer lamina. A prosaic (but, perhaps, more likely) explanation would incriminate these delicate vessels in episodes of rebleeding. Not infrequently, subdural hematomas that first come to attention in their chronic, encapsulated phases disclose evidence of recent, superimposed hemorrhage in the form of fresh blood layered subjacent to their vascularized outer membranes.

Inflammatory diseases

Demyelinating diseases

The idiopathic demyelinating diseases of the CNS, of which multiple sclerosis is by far the most common, are usually regarded as 'medical' disorders diagnosed on clinical grounds or at autopsy. In fact, demyelinating lesions of the cerebral hemispheric white matter and spinal cord may present as space-occupying 'tumors' associated with considerable mass effect, edema, and disruption of the blood–brain barrier evidenced, on CT or MR study, by diffuse or ring-like enhancement following administration of contrast media[191,195]

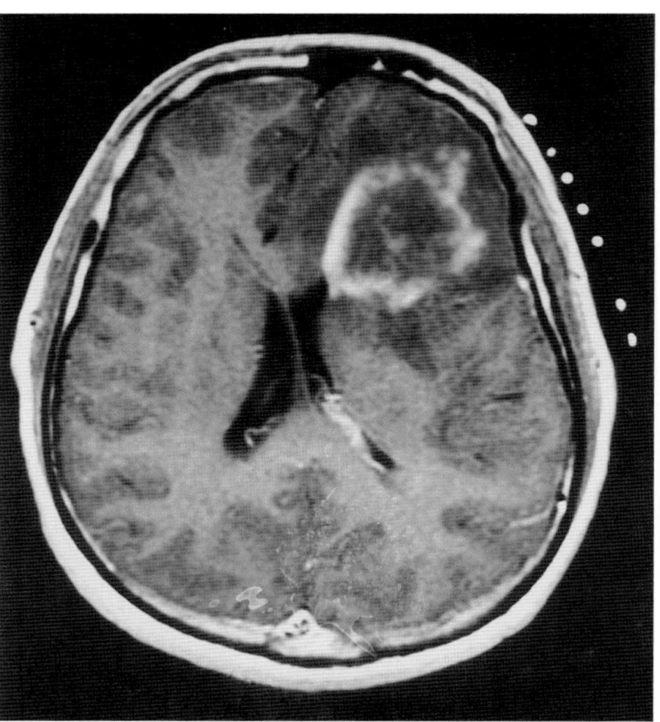

Fig. 28.10 Demyelinating pseudotumor. Taken following administration of a contrast agent that serves to delineate foci of blood–brain barrier breakdown as regions of bright signal, this magnetic resonance image demonstrates a lesion characterized by 'ring' enhancement, conspicuous hypodensity of the surrounding white matter (indicative of edema), and mass effect evidenced by obliteration of the ipsilateral ventricular angle and shift of the neighboring cingulate gyrus across the midline. The neuroradiologic diagnosis was 'probably glioblastoma, abscess also a possibility'. The patient, a 32-year-old man with subacutely progressive hemiparesis and somnolence, recovered completely following limited biopsy and a short course of corticosteroids. He remains asymptomatic 15 years after diagnosis.

(Fig. 28.10). Especially suspect on neuroradiologic grounds is the lesion that seems to fan out from a ventricular angle or that exhibits an 'open' or 'broken ring' profile characterized by the abrupt cessation of rimming contrast enhancement where it abuts a ventricular surface or overlying cortex. Few patients harboring such lesions carry a diagnosis of multiple sclerosis when they present with symptoms and signs referable to an expanding intracranial mass. Solitary examples, not surprisingly, prompt consideration of aggressive glial neoplasia or abscess formation, whereas multifocal variants suggest metastatic disease or even cerebral parasitosis when lesions exhibit cystic characteristics on scan. Such **demyelinating 'pseudotumors'** understandably occasion neurosurgical intervention for purposes of definitive diagnosis and thus enter the domain of the surgical pathologist.

The tumefactive demyelinating lesion shares with the active 'plaque' typical of subacute multiple sclerosis[193] a sharp delineation from adjacent, uninvolved white matter evident in biopsy samples that include its perimeter. Affected tissues exhibit diffuse infiltration by foamy, lipid-laden macrophages, reactive astrocytosis of variable intensity, and perivascular aggregates of small (mostly T) lymphocytes and occasional plasma cells[191,195] (Fig. 28.11). The definitive characterization of the process as a demyelinating one ultimately

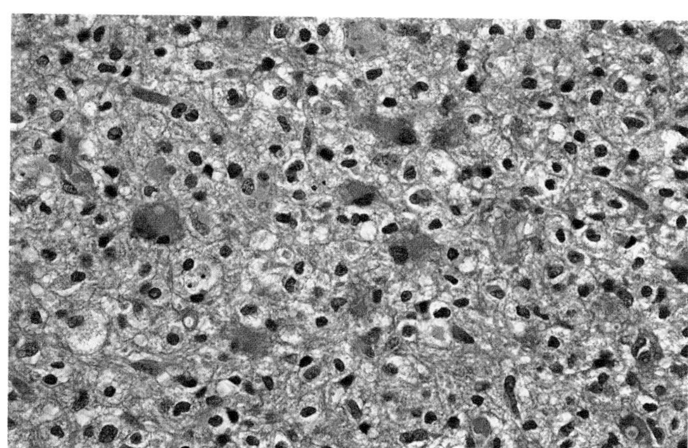

Fig. 28.11 Demyelinating pseudotumor. The hypercellularity of this lesion reflects infiltration by macrophages in large number, recognizable on careful study by their granular or foamy cytoplasm. Also apparent are several hyperplastic astrocytes.

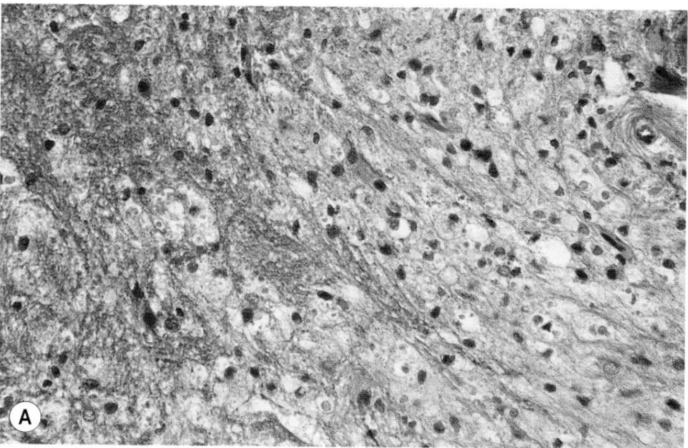

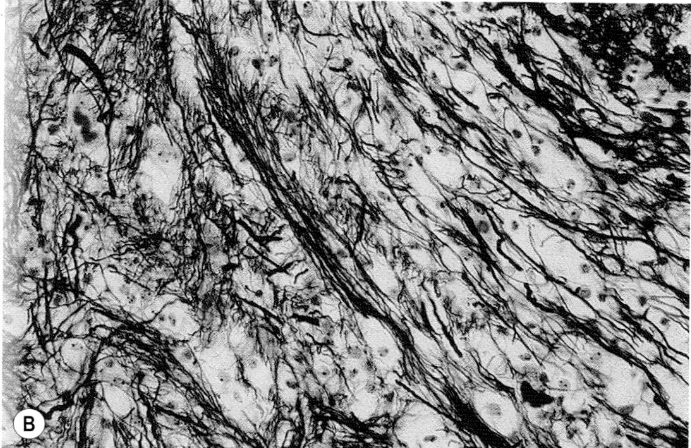

Fig. 28.12 Demyelinating pseudotumor. The interface of a demyelinated plaque (right) and normal white matter (left) is shown here in serial sections stained for myelin (**A**) and axons (**B**) by the Luxol fast blue and Bielschowsky methods, respectively. Myelin, blue in **A**, persists in the plaque only as globules present in the cytoplasm of macrophages. Axons, stained black in **B**, course uninterrupted into the region of demyelination.

requires the demonstration of relative axonal preservation in foci devoid of stainable myelin. This is readily accomplished by comparing serial sections assessed for myelin and axons by traditional neurohistochemical methods (Fig. 28.12) or assayed for components of the myelin sheath and axon using commercially available antibodies to myelin basic protein and neurofilaments, respectively. In the typical case, large numbers of axons will course uninterrupted through regions in which myelin, if at all demonstrable, persists only as phagocytized debris in the cytoplasm of macrophages. It should be pointed out, however, that a variable element of axonal depopulation is the rule, some particularly destructive examples progressing to cavitation.

In our experience, demyelinating pseudotumors are the non-neoplastic lesions most often misinterpreted on biopsy as gliomas, specifically as diffuse fibrillary astrocytomas or as oligodendrogliomas. The consequences to patients subjected to cerebral irradiation may be devastating.[194] The potential causes for error are many.[195] A diagnosis of glioma may be prompted by the florid and cytologically atypical astrogliosis that characterizes some examples – an impression likely to be reinforced by the finding of scattered mitotic figures, as well as astrocytes that appear to be in atypical mitosis by virtue of a peculiar parcellation of their nuclear material (Fig. 28.13). Perivascular lymphoid infiltrates are an inconstant feature of demyelinating lesions sampled at craniotomy and, even when conspicuous, are no guarantee that a glial proliferation is not neoplastic. Even in their absence, however, the orderly spacing of gemistocytic astrocytes typical of hyperplastic states – a 'logic' maintained in these lesions – should suggest a reactive process.

Especially confounding is failure to appreciate the high content of macrophages that lend to tissues undergoing demyelination their alarmingly hypercellular appearance. The voluminous foamy or granular cytoplasm typical of these cells when engaged in the digestion of phagocytosed myelin and useful in their distinction from glia may be obscured in suboptimally procured or processed samples. As this is particularly true of frozen sections, the use of cytologic preparations wherein these features are likely to be preserved is strongly advocated for purposes of intraoperative consultation (Fig. 28.14). Immunocytochemical assay for monocyte/macrophage markers such as HAM-56 (Fig. 28.15) and CD68 may also aid in circumventing problems of cell identification,[190]

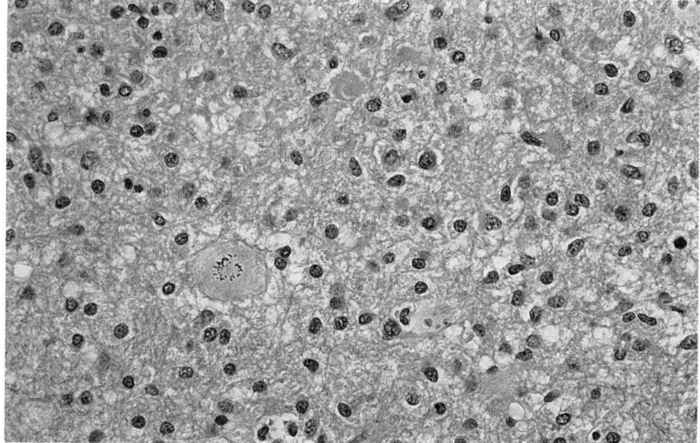

Fig. 28.13 Demyelinating pseudotumor. An apparently atypical mitotic figure and diffuse infiltrate of mononuclear cells lacking the cytoplasmic features of fully developed macrophages may lead to the incorrect diagnosis of glioma.

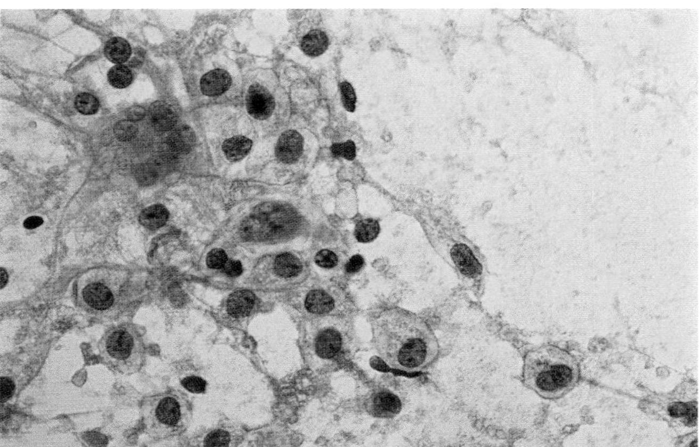

Fig. 28.14 Demyelinating pseudotumor. The presence of foamy macrophages in cytologic preparations argues strongly against a diagnosis of glioma at the time of intraoperative consultation. As shown here, somewhat atypical-appearing, multinucleate astrocytes are not uncommonly encountered in such specimens.

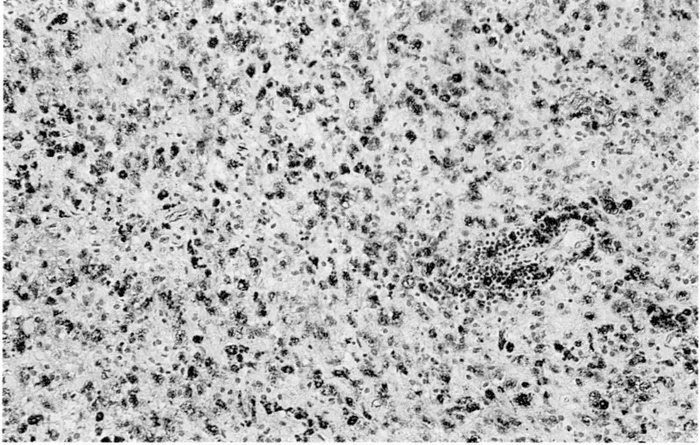

Fig. 28.15 Demyelinating pseudotumor. The density of infiltrating macrophages characteristic of demyelinating lesions is demonstrated in this immunoperoxidase assay for HAM-56.

particularly as applied to neurosurgical specimens exhibiting artefactual distortion or dominated by newly arrived mononuclear cells interrupted in their labors and thus not evidencing the cytoplasmic characteristics of fully developed, lipid-engorged phagocytes. Diffuse infiltration by macrophages in large number is so rarely a feature of the untreated glioma as to virtually exclude this diagnosis. The ready identification of such cells in smears, crush preparations, or tissue sections should instead suggest a non-neoplastic, necrotizing process (such as organizing infarction) or a selectively demyelinating disorder. Primary CNS lymphomas inadvertently treated by the preoperative administration of corticosteroids may vanish on neuroradiologic scan and can further simulate demyelinating disease by leaving behind only reactive lymphohistiocytic infiltrates but do not cause truly selective, regionally circumscribed myelin loss (see discussion of lymphoproliferative and myeloproliferative disorders for additional discussion and references). Patients suffering from multiple sclerosis on occasion do develop glial neoplasms,[192] but there is no compelling evidence that the incidence of the latter is increased in this population.

As mentioned, only exceptionally do tumefactive demyelinating lesions complicate the course of established multiple sclerosis. Interestingly, only 3 of 31 patients presenting with solitary or multifocal demyelinating pseudotumors in the series of Kepes[191] developed additional cerebral lesions during follow-up periods ranging from 9 months to 12 years. This intriguing observation has been taken as evidence that the biology of pseudotumoral demyelinating disease differs significantly from that of classic multiple sclerosis and is perhaps more akin to that of the monophasic 'allergic' encephalomyelitides triggered by viral infection or vaccination. A relapsing course, however, characterized a significant subset of cases in a smaller series.[188] Last, mention is made of a **multifocal inflammatory leukoencephalopathy** described as complicating the chemotherapy of colorectal adenocarcinoma with 5-fluorouracil and levamisole.[189] The lesions in question were demyelinative and morphologically indistinguishable from active multiple sclerosis plaques. Whether one or both of these agents was directly responsible for this condition or somehow precipitated attacks of multiple sclerosis in patients predisposed to the disorder is unclear.

Noninfectious inflammatory and reactive disorders, xanthomatous lesions, and 'histiocytoses'

The various oddities collected in this section have little in common beyond their etiologic obscurity and inflammatory or otherwise 'reactive' histologic appearances. Many are better known as systemic disorders and are given detailed consideration elsewhere in these volumes. Specific description is here accorded to only those entities unique to the nervous system.

Idiopathic hypertrophic cranial pachymeningitis is, as its name implies, an inflammatory and fibrosing disorder of unknown cause that affects the dura mater.[232,255] Clinical manifestations include headache, progressive cranial neuropathies, and cerebellar ataxia of adult onset occurring in association with radiographically demonstrable thickening and abnormal contrast enhancement of the peribulbar meninges, tentorium, and falx. The process can involve the dura over the cerebral convexities or extend into the cavernous sinus and orbit, causing painful ophthalmoplegia. **Idiopathic hypertrophic spinal pachymeningitis**, a disease of the cervicothoracic region typified by compressive myelopathy, may represent a variant of the same basic disorder.[224,245] A subset of afflicted patients evidence extradural abnormalities collected under the rubric of '**multifocal fibrosclerosis**', including inflammatory orbital pseudotumor, idiopathic mediastinal and retroperitoneal fibrosis, sclerosing cholangitis, Riedel stroma, Peyronie disease, Dupuytren contracture, fibrosing orchitis, systemic vasculitis, and fibroinflammatory lesions of the subcutaneous tissues and lungs. What may represent localized pseudotumoral variants have been recorded,[209,213] as has pachymeningitis complicating IgG4-related sclerosing disease.[207]

Dural biopsies in cases of idiopathic hypertrophic pachymeningitis disclose dispersed lymphoplasmacytic infiltrates, exuberant fibroplasia and, in some instances, necrosis and granuloma formation. Exclusion of tuberculosis, syphilis, mycotic infections, sarcoidosis, Wegener granulomatosis, rheumatoid disease, and other defined causes of chronic fibrosing meningitis is required. Secondary intracranial extension of inflammatory orbital pseudotumor may also produce a similar meningeal picture.[208] The clinical course is variable, but often inexorably progressive. Corticosteroid administration and resection of compressing fibroinflammatory meningeal masses are of benefit to some patients. The reader should note that patients undergoing craniotomy, ventricular shunting, or even lumbar puncture alone may occasionally develop neuroradiologic evidence of diffuse meningeal thickening and enhancement that is typically asymptomatic and without clinical significance. This is thought to represent a response to intracranial hypotension and may rarely occur in the absence of prior instrumentation. Biopsy material in such cases may exhibit subdural fibroplasia, neovascularization, hemosiderin deposition, and meningothelial hyperplasia.[239]

Turning from the meninges to the brain proper, we briefly mention a form of chronic encephalitis, known eponymously as **Rasmussen syndrome**, that is characterized by intractable unilateral focal seizures or epilepsia partialis continua of childhood onset, progressive cerebral hemiatrophy with hemiparesis, and cognitive decline.[200] Long suspected (but never convincingly shown) to represent a persistent viral infection, the disorder may have an autoimmune component – some afflicted patients harboring antibodies to native CNS antigens, including the glutamate GluR3 receptor. The neuropathologic substrate is nonspecific, consisting of perivascular and interstitial lymphoid infiltrates involving the cerebral cortex with microglial nodule formation, astrogliosis, and variable neuronal loss.[246] High-dose corticosteroids, intravenous gamma globulins, plasmapheresis, and surgery (including functional or actual hemispherectomy) have all been investigated in the treatment of Rasmussen syndrome and have proven beneficial to some patients. The last of these options is currently regarded as the approach of choice in typical childhood cases. More localized and clinically benign forms of idiopathic chronic encephalitis have been described, particularly in adolescents and young adults, that may mimic cerebral neoplasms.[222] Whether these represent Rasmussen variants is unclear.

Limbic encephalitis is an amnestic syndrome of adulthood typically encountered as a paraneoplastic phenomenon[220] complicating small cell carcinoma of the lung, but the disorder has also been reported in association with other tumor types (e.g., nonsmall cell lung cancers, Hodgkin disease, mammary adenocarcinomas, and testicular germ cell tumors) and, rarely, in the absence of demonstrable neoplasia.[201] Clinical manifestations progress in subacute fashion and consist principally of short-term memory loss, complex partial or generalized seizures, confusion, and disordered affect. Many examples evolve as one facet of a complex paraneoplastic disease that potentially involves the dorsal root ganglia, brainstem, cerebellum, spinal cord, autonomic ganglia, and myenteric plexi.[218] MRI studies often disclose abnormal T2 hyperintensity of the medial temporal regions (with foci of pathologic contrast enhancement in some cases) and may prompt consideration of herpes simplex encephalitis or an infiltrative process. The brunt of the injury falls on the amygdaloid nuclei, hippocampi, and entorrhinal cortices, biopsy material disclosing florid reactive astrocytosis, perivascular lymphoid cuffing, microglial or 'neuronophagic' nodule formation, and, in some cases, conspicuous neuronal depopulation. In contrast to herpes simplex encephalitis, the process is never overtly necrotizing, hemorrhagic, or attended by nuclear alterations indicative of a viral cytopathic effect.

Useful in the evaluation of suspected limbic encephalitis (the clinical manifestations of which often herald discovery of otherwise silent, low-stage tumors) is assay of serum and CSF for a specific autoantibody, designated anti-Hu, that is directed against neuronal nucleoproteins in the 35–40 kDa size range and strongly correlated with the presence of underlying small cell lung cancer.[218,220] Demonstration of this autoantibody constitutes compelling evidence for the paraneoplastic etiology of a patient's neurologic complaints and mandates a search for occult neoplastic disease that must begin with targeted investigation of the chest. Anti-Hu IgG appears to be elaborated in response to aberrant tumoral expression of this neuron-associated protein, prompting articulation of the hypothesis that an immunologic response directed initially against a triggering neoplasm comes ultimately to involve the nervous system in a cross-reaction having devastating neurologic consequences. Another neuronal autoantibody known as anti-Ta or anti-Ma2 has come to be recognized as a powerful marker of paraneoplastic limbic encephalitis in the setting of testicular germ cell neoplasia.[220] Tumor localization and treatment may effect neurologic improvement in patients with limbic encephalitis, which occasionally remits spontaneously, and is more effective than immune modulation in this regard.

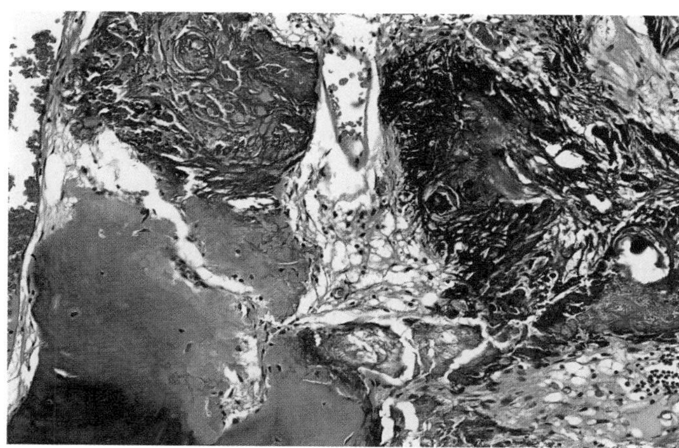

Fig. 28.16 Fibro-osseous lesion/calcifying pseudoneoplasm of the neuraxis. Fibroplasia, bone formation and the deposition of a highly characteristic basophilic matrix material in plate-like or ropey masses define this unusual process.

The histologically distinctive masses reported as '**fibro-osseous lesions**' or '**calcifying pseudoneoplasms**' **of the neural axis** (Fig. 28.16) are composed principally of nonbirefringent, basophilic matrix materials that may assume an amorphous, somewhat chondromyxoid appearance or be deposited in coarsely fibrillar, ropey or plate-like fashion.[199,250] Rimming mononuclear and foreign body-type giant cells lend a granulomatous appearance to some examples. Matrix mineralization is at least focally apparent in most cases and many exhibit mature lamellar bone formation as well. Cerebrocortical alterations of meningioangiomatosis type (discussed in the section 'Choristomas and non-neuroepithelial hamartomas') have been encountered adjacent to intracranial examples. These peculiar lesions are usually extra-axial and favor the spinal epidural compartment, but may arise from the cranial floor, within the leptomeninges or even brain. While properly regarded as non-neoplastic, they may be complicated by considerable neurologic morbidity resulting from spinal cord compression or skull base destruction with cranial nerve and cerebrovascular compromise. Ossified intracranial nodules lacking the defining matrix described above may be formed in nonspecific response to trauma, infection, or hemorrhage, and have been termed cerebral calculi or 'brain stones'. Rarely, symptomatic juxtaneural masses prove to be tophaceous lesions resulting from the crystalline deposition of sodium urate (**gout**), calcium pyrophosphate dihydrate (**pseudogout**) or calcium hydroxyapatite (**tumoral calcinosis**[217]). **Metaplastic ossification** of the leptomeninges, a common phenomenon typically unconnected to any neurologic complaints, may rarely be encountered in symptomatic forms causing progressive myelopathy associated, in some cases, with cavitation of the spinal cord.[211,236,260] While the term '**arachnoiditis ossificans**' has been used in description of such cases and many are clearly the sequelae of insults mechanical or microbial, inflammatory elements are generally not in evidence and there may be no history of a precipitating condition. Spinal cord injury can similarly be produced by ossification of the ligamentum flavum.[198]

Of those principally extraneural disorders that occasionally engage the talents of the neurosurgeon, most deserving of mention are Langerhans cell histiocytosis ('eosinophilic granuloma'), sarcoidosis, and sinus histiocytosis with massive lymphadenopathy (Rosai–Dorfman disease). CNS involvement in **Langerhans cell histiocytosis** typically follows infiltration of the calvarial floor and exhibits a striking tropism for the region of the hypothalamus and infundibulum, the eponym **Hand–Schüller–Christian disease** being applied to the classic clinical triad of diabetes insipidus, proptosis, and skull base defects on roentgenographic study. While a similar topography is characteristic of those exceptional examples restricted (on presentation, at least) to the nervous system,[219] lesions situated within the meninges, choroid plexus, and brain are on record,[256] as are instances of cerebral invasion from contiguous primary foci in the cranial vault.[252] CD1a-immunoreactive Langerhans cells may be only sparsely represented in biopsy material from affected patients. Xanthomatous masses consisting only of foamy macrophages can be encountered in this clinical setting, these possibly representing 'burned out' lesions, and a nonspecific chronic inflammatory picture with variable loss of myelin and axons may be seen (particularly in the cerebellum and brainstem).

Neurosarcoidosis most commonly assumes the form of a granulomatous basilar meningitis (Fig. 28.17) complicated by cranial neuropathies or, with extension of the process to the hypothalamic region, diabetes insipidus and other diencephalic syndromes. An accompanying granulomatous vasculitis may be apparent. While the overwhelming majority of patients have established systemic disease, primary CNS presentations have been described and can include pseudotumoral involvement of the leptomeninges,[196] dura,[225,265] cranial nerve,[251] and neuroparenchyma proper.[216] An example of necrotizing sarcoid granulomatosis presenting as a mass involving the temporal lobe and cavernous sinus has been depicted.[261] In fact, only a subset of patients evaluated for granulomatous disease of the CNS that is not demonstrably infectious will prove to have clinical manifestations (e.g., interstitial lung involvement, mediastinal lymphadenopathy) or laboratory evidence (elevated serum/CSF angiotensin converting enzyme levels) supporting a diagnosis of sarcoidosis. Unclassifiable, 'pathogen-free' granulomatous disorders were found in one study to share a tendency to diffuse neuraxial involvement, combined leptomeningeal and neuroparenchymal (particularly spinal cord) infiltration, attendant angiitis, and a poor prognosis.[264]

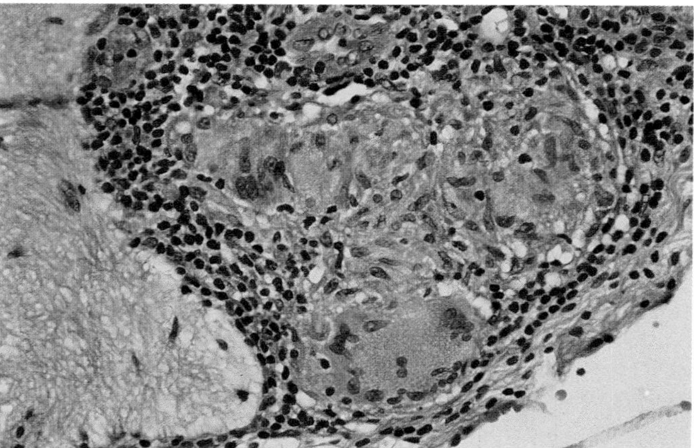

Fig. 28.17 Neurosarcoidosis. A non-necrotizing, granulomatous leptomeningitis replete with multinucleated giant cells of monocytic derivation characterizes this inflammatory disorder in its usual CNS presentation.

Dura-based masses clinically indistinguishable from meningiomas constitute the usual pattern of CNS disease in cases of **Rosai–Dorfman disease** or **extranodal sinus histiocytosis with massive lymphadenopathy (SHML)**, though lesions involving the neuroparenchyma have been communicated.[197,249] These can represent the sole manifestations of the disorder and may be multifocal. A similar predilection for the dura characterizes central neuraxial lesions that have been dubbed **inflammatory pseudotumors** or **plasma cell granulomas**,[233,234,262] though cerebral[214] and choroid plexus[204] examples have been depicted. There can be little doubt that these designations have been extended through the years to reactive lesions of disparate cause, to cases of extranodal SHML, lymphoplasmacyte-rich meningiomas, and low-grade lymphomas of mucosa-associated lymphoid tissue (MALT) type. These terms, furthermore, have been applied indiscriminately to proliferations that should be segregated as **inflammatory myofibroblastic tumors** of the nervous system.[262] The latter are given further consideration in our discussion of nonmeningothelial mesenchymal tumors. Suffice it to say that diagnoses such as inflammatory pseudotumor and plasma cell granuloma must be rendered with full acknowledgment that they do not carry specific etiologic implications and judiciously reserved for masses harboring polyclonal lymphoplasmacellular populations unaccompanied by the conspicuous spindle cell components, anaplastic lymphoma kinase (ALK) expression or *ALK* gene (2p23) rearrangements evidenced by tumors of the inflammatory myofibroblastic group. Potentially multifocal, plasma cell granulomas/inflammatory pseudotumors of the nervous system have been described in patients with systemic infections and immunologic disorders such as lupus erythematosus[262] and relapsing polychondritis.[257] IgG4-immunolabeling plasma cells may be encountered in the lesions of this group, but a link to IgG4-associated systemic autoimmune disease has not been clearly established.[234] A unique falcine mass possibly analogous to the **hyalinizing plasmacytic granuloma** of pulmonary origin contained 'raft-like' islands of acellular, hyaline connective tissue associated with a foreign body-type giant cell response.[240]

Collectively designated as 'xanthomatous' are diverse lesions sharing only a conspicuous component of foamy, lipid-laden macrophages. Mention has already been made of **xanthogranulomas** forming in relation to colloid cysts of the third ventricle. Lesions similarly composed of foamy macrophages, foreign body-type giant cells, cholesterol clefts, and reactive lymphoid infiltrates commonly occur in the glomus of the choroid plexus but only rarely attain symptomatic proportions.[205] **Cholesterol granulomas of the petrous apex** that are believed to result from chronically impaired aeration of the petrous air cells may produce headache and palsies of cranial nerves V–VIII, prompting neurosurgical intervention.[210] Dura-based masses described as **xanthomas** or **xanthogranulomas**, some of immense proportions, have been encountered in otherwise healthy subjects,[231,267] in association with abnormalities of lipid metabolism such as familial hypercholesterolemia and phytosterolemia,[202,238,242] and in the setting of systemic Weber–Christian disease (relapsing nodular nonsuppurative panniculitis[248]). Some reported examples have complicated a disorder having the clinical features of Hand–Schüller–Christian disease.[226] A remarkable case interpreted as surgical dissemination of a parasellar xanthogranuloma to the convexity dura and falx has been depicted.[215] Xanthomatous CNS infiltrates may also complicate **Erdheim–Chester disease**, an enigmatic histiocytosis, the hallmark of which is symmetric and bilateral sclerosis of the long tubular bones with colonization of the marrow spaces by lipid-laden macrophages.[244,263] On record, in addition, are xanthomas of probable traumatic etiology,[230] arguably neoplastic '**fibroxanthomas**'[227] and **juvenile xanthogranulomas**[203,247] involving the region of the Gasserian ganglion (Meckel's cave), meninges, brain, spinal cord, and ventricular system. CNS infiltration is a recognized complication of '**xanthoma disseminatum**',[221] a systemic syndrome characterized by the widespread eruption of juvenile xanthogranuloma-like lesions in normolipemic subjects, and the development of dura-based masses has been described in the setting of **necrobiotic xanthogranuloma**,[258] a similarly generalized disorder often associated with plasma cell neoplasia and other lymphoproliferative diseases. Symptomatic leptomeningeal and neuroparenchymal infiltration by foamy macrophages containing intracytoplasmic erythrocytes and lymphocytes frequently complicates the course of **hemophagocytic lymphohistiocytosis**[223] in both its primary (autosomal recessive and infantile-onset) as well as secondary (infection-triggered or paraneoplastic, particularly lymphoma-associated) forms. A possible example restricted to the CNS has been communicated.[259]

Reference has been made previously to mass-forming foreign body reactions complicating the surgical management of intracranial aneurysms. Various hemostatic substances placed within neurosurgical beds during resection of neoplasms (and other procedures) may similarly provoke a florid and potentially granulomatous inflammatory response that can mimic tumor recurrence.[243,253] The cited literature can be consulted for microscopic characteristics of the responsible agents, the reactive masses in such cases being referred to as '**gauzomas**', '**muslinomas**', '**textilomas**' or '**gossypibomas**' (from the Latin *Gossypium,* the genus of cotton plants, and the Kiswahili *boma,* meaning place of concealment).

Other odd processes that have been documented in neurosurgical material include **cerebral malakoplakia**[254,266] and the pseudoparasitic red blood cell alteration known as **myospherulosis**.[237] An isolated account depicts tumorous cerebellar infiltration by cytologically atypical histiocytes exhibiting immunoreactivity for S-100 protein and conspicuous lymphophagocytosis (emperipolesis), this possibly representing an unusual variant of extranodal SHML.[212] Lastly, we mention several described complications of systemic autoimmune (collagen vascular) disorders, including **rheumatoid meningeal nodules**,[228,229] **Wegener granulomatosis** extending to the intracranial dura from the sinonasal compartment[241] or presenting as meninges-restricted disease,[268] and a corticosteroid-responsive meningoencephalitis associated with cognitive impairment in the setting of **Sjögren syndrome**.[206,235] The term **nonvasculitic autoimmune inflammatory meningoencephalitis**[235] has been applied to this non-necrotizing process, which is characterized by perivascular lymphoid cuffing with loose aggregates of microglia in the affected cerebral cortex. This picture, also associated with corticosteroid-reversible encephalopathy, may be encountered in patients without systemic complaints, some of whom have proven to harbor circulating antibodies to Sjögren syndrome antigens, elevated rheumatoid factor or perinuclear antineutrophil cytoplasmic antibody.[235]

Infectious diseases

Bacterial infections

Bacteria are responsible for the overwhelming majority of suppurative infections involving the CNS and its coverings. Of particular concern to surgical pathologists are the common forms of localized suppuration: abscesses of the brain and spinal epidural space.

Approximately 20% of **brain abscesses** are unassociated with conditions predisposing to bacterial invasion of the nervous system, the remainder arising in patients with established pyogenic infections at extraneural sites, facilitating anatomic anomalies or histories of penetrating cranial trauma or prior neurosurgery.[273,280] Their demographic features, localization, number, and microbiologic characteristics vary with the risk factors operative in individual cases.

The extraneural bacterial infections predisposing to brain abscess are usefully divided into those involving contiguous meningeal or parameningeal sites versus those more distantly placed. Curious is the fact that cerebral abscesses rarely complicate bacterial meningitis, a notable exception to this rule being their significant association with neonatal leptomeningitides caused by *Proteus mirabilis* and *Citrobacter diversus*.[280,285] More frequently implicated among local sources of bacillary invasion are infected paranasal sinuses, middle ear cavities, and mastoids.[280] Although their pathogenesis remains imprecisely defined, abscesses associated with these various infections are commonly held to result from the retrograde thrombophlebitic carriage of organisms into the cranial cavity via emissary veins. Typically solitary, these tend to stereotyped topographic presentations. Thus, cerebral abscesses related to frontoethmoid sinusitis characteristically settle in the anterobasal frontal lobes, whereas 'otitic' examples (including those associated with chronic mastoiditis) are usually encountered in the temporal lobes or cerebellar hemispheres. Lesions complicating sphenoid sinusitis frequent both the frontal and temporal regions. The organisms most often isolated from brain abscesses in these clinical circumstances include aerobic or microaerophilic streptococci (especially members of the *Streptococcus intermedius 'milleri'* group), aerobic gram-negative bacilli (*Proteus, Escherichia coli, Klebsiella–Enterobacter,* and *Haemophilus* species), and *Bacteroides* species. Mixed infections are common. Other local suppurative processes associated with the subsequent development of brain abscess include dental sepsis and pyogenic infections of the face and scalp. Usually frontal in location, 'odontogenic' abscesses typically follow tooth extraction or other dental manipulation and harbor mixed aerobic and anaerobic populations dominated by *Fusobacterium, Bacteroides,* and *Streptococcus* species. *Staphylococcus aureus* is the main offender when facial or scalp infections are incriminated; cerebral abscesses in this setting usually occur in cases complicated by cavernous sinus thrombosis. Mandibulofacial **actinomycosis** may also eventuate in brain abscess.[287] Spinal anomalies predispose to intramedullary abscesses, as do tumors of the spinal neuraxis, but such infections are decidedly rare.[283]

Hematogenous seeding of the CNS from distant foci of infection usually results in a multiplicity of abscesses that commonly lie within the territories subtended by the middle cerebral arteries. Most germinate at the junction of the cortical mantle and underlying white matter, but the cerebellum, basal ganglia, thalami, and brainstem may also be involved. 'Metastatic' lesions of this sort most often have their origin in the thorax, chronic suppurating pulmonary disorders such as lung abscess and bronchiectasis leading the list of conditions predisposing to their development.[280] Much less common among underlying 'donors' are bacterial endocarditis (characteristically acute), empyema, osteomyelitis, and infections of deep pelvic organs or abdominal viscera. Additional risk factors of note include various conditions in which the filtering function of the lung's capillary bed is abrogated (e.g., pulmonary arteriovenous fistulas) and cyanotic congenital heart diseases when complicated by right-to-left shunts (as encountered in tetralogy of Fallot, patent foramen ovale, ventricular septal defect, and transposition of the great vessels). The secondary polycythemia that regularly attends these anomalies may further promote the genesis of abscesses from infective emboli by causing microcirculatory sludging and regional brain hypoxia. Similar mechanisms may account for the significant risk of cerebral abscess in hereditary hemorrhagic telangiectasia (Osler–Weber–Rendu disease); most patients with this complication harbor pulmonary AVMs and exhibit hypoxemia with resultant cyanosis, clubbing, and polycythemia.[278] Among iatrogenic causes of metastatic brain abscess, instrumentation of the esophagus in attempts to relieve caustic strictures or treat varices by the endoscopic injection of sclerosing agents merits citation.[286]

The microbiology of the foregoing lesions is complex, but a few generalizations are possible. *Fusobacterium*, *Bacteroides*, and streptococci are the organisms most commonly recovered from brain abscesses associated with pulmonary sepsis, actinomycotic[287] and nocardial[288] lesions (the latter often encountered in debilitated and immunosuppressed subjects) also representing secondary deposits from foci of established lung infection in a majority of cases. Streptococci and *Haemophilus* species are the typical offenders in cases related to congenital heart disease, whereas *S. aureus* dominates isolates from examples complicating acute bacterial endocarditis.

With regard to the direct inoculation of bacteria into CNS tissues, abscess formation is probably the least frequent cerebral consequence of either penetrating cranial trauma or neurosurgery.[280] *S. aureus* is the organism most often recovered from lesions arising in these circumstances, followed by *Streptococcus*, *Enterobacter*, and *Clostridium* species. *Propionibacterium acnes*, a gram-positive, anaerobic rod that causes a syndrome of shunt malfunction and immune-complex nephritis in patients with intraventricular catheters, has also emerged as an agent of traumatically and surgically acquired brain abscesses and epidural infection.[271,276] Trauma and intracranial hematoma accumulation, in addition, predispose to cerebral *Salmonella* abscess.[280]

Brain abscesses remain a diagnostic challenge to the clinician because their presenting manifestations and neuroradiologic appearances are nonspecific. Noteworthy is the fact that only 40–50% of patients are febrile on evaluation. The more common signs and symptoms are those of any expanding intracranial mass: headache, altered mental status, focal sensorimotor deficits, seizure, nausea, and vomiting.[273,280] Although central hypodensity, 'ring' enhancement, and surrounding edema are characteristic on CT or MRI studies (Fig. 28.18), these appearances may be shared by malignant neoplasms (particularly glioblastomas) and, on occasion, demyelinating disease. The enhancing pseudocapsules of abscesses tend to be thinner and of more uniform profile than the enhancing rims of glioblastomas, typically acquire a dark signal on T2-weighted MRI as they collagenize that is foreign to the perimeter of the latter, and surround contents that are bright on diffusion-weighted imaging in contrast to the centrally necrotic and dark interior of the glioblastoma in this modality. The apparent budding of smaller, 'daughter' lesions from the main mass should also suggest abscess.

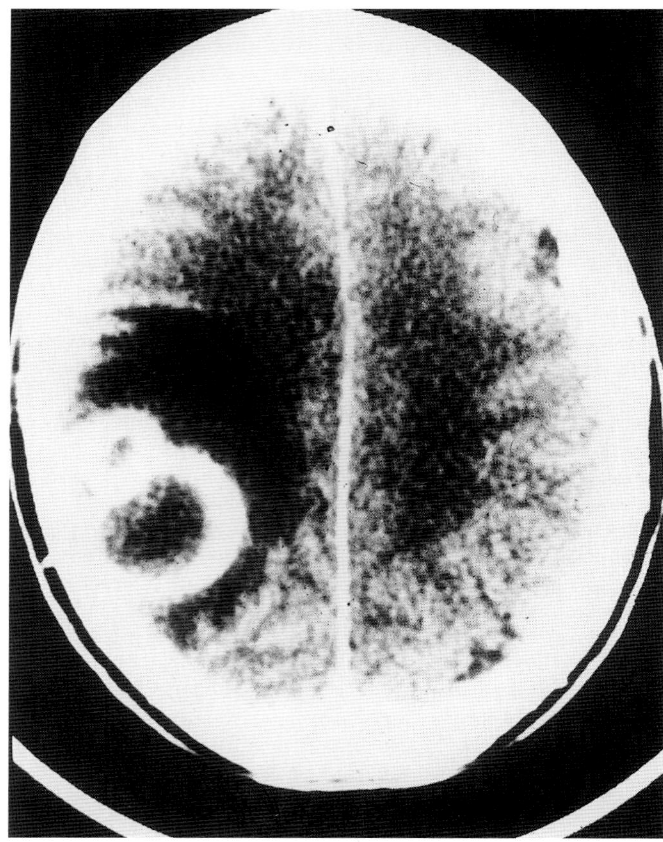

Fig. 28.18 Cerebral abscess. Ring enhancement of their developing pseudocapsules, budding of 'daughter' lesions, and marked hypodensity of adjacent white matter reflecting severe edema are all characteristic of cerebral abscesses on CT or MR study. This example complicated mandibulofacial actinomycosis.

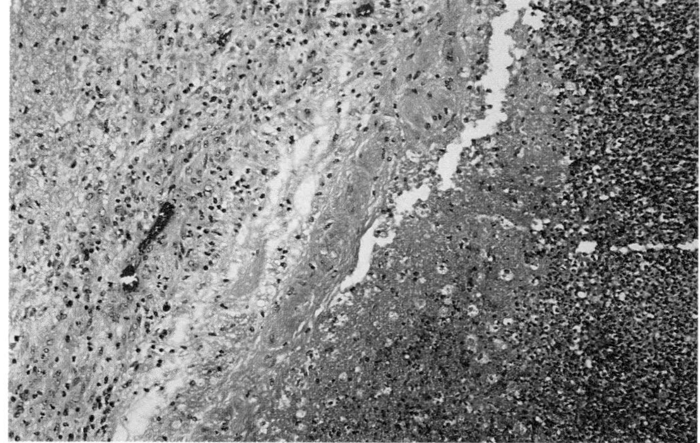

Fig. 28.19 Cerebral abscess. The lesion's purulent contents are separated from neighboring white matter by a granulation tissue-like zone of angioblastic and fibroblastic activity.

Experimental, clinical, and histopathologic observations suggest that abscesses of the human brain begin as ill-defined zones of bacterial multiplication and polymorphonuclear leukocytic infiltration (cerebritis) most commonly situated in white matter immediately subjacent to the cortical ribbon or at the gray–white junction.[280] With time, proliferating fibroblasts come to surround a central mass of fibrinopurulent debris and fashion a collagenous capsule resembling the pyogenic membranes formed in response to suppurative infections outside the nervous system (Fig. 28.19). This, in turn, is bordered by edematous, chronically inflamed, and gliotic brain tissue that may evidence foci of acute cerebritis attesting to the host's failure to entirely wall off the primary locus of infection.

The rate at which encapsulation proceeds and its completeness vary considerably. Hematogenous bacterial seeding of the brain from distant sites of suppuration generally results in abscesses with capsules less developed than those that surround examples arising secondary to contiguous pyogenic processes. Especially notorious for their poor encapsulation are nocardial lesions. That capsular organization is typically most advanced along the superficial, juxtacortical perimeter of brain abscesses is reflected in the tendency of 'daughter' lesions to bud from their deep aspects and in their tendency to rupture into the ventricular system rather than subarachnoid space. Because the mesenchymal elements responsible for capsule formation presumably derive from the adventitia of regional blood vessels and require oxygen for collagen fibrillogenesis, the relatively retarded organizational responses of paraventricular, as compared with cortical and paracortical, tissues may be a consequence of their less extensive vasculature. The intraventricular discharge of purulent material is among the most feared of all abscess-related complications, often proving fatal.

In contrast to the largely intracranial localization of bacterial abscesses involving the CNS proper, 90% of epidural examples are situated at spinal levels.[274,279] Here a 'true' (as opposed to potential) space, containing adipose tissue, nutrient arteries, and an elaborate venous plexus, expands posterior and lateral to the dura mater, whereas above the foramen magnum this fibrous sheath adheres tightly to the inner aspect of the skull. Anterior tethering of the dura to adjacent vertebral bodies presumably accounts for the fact that most **epidural abscesses** evolving along the length of the spinal cord are posteriorly or posterolaterally positioned. Approximately half of these settle in the thoracic, and one-third in the lumbar, region. Less accommodating is the epidural space at cervical levels, where the spinal canal is nearly filled by the cord itself, and sacral lesions are rare.

Roughly 30–40% of spinal epidural abscesses arise 'spontaneously', the remainder (like their neuroparenchymal counterparts) secondarily complicating infections established at contiguous or distant sites, trauma, intravenous drug abuse, spinal surgery or other invasive procedures, including epidural catheterization and lumbar puncture. Of particular importance among predisposing infections are contiguous foci of vertebral osteomyelitis, psoas and perinephric abscesses, decubitus ulcers, and other cutaneous and soft tissue suppurations. Diabetes mellitus, alcoholism, and renal failure are also recognized as significant risk factors. Presenting clinical manifestations typically include fever, malaise, and backache. If antimicrobial therapy and neurosurgical decompression are delayed, these early symptoms may progress in stepwise fashion to radiculopathy, sensorimotor and sphincter disturbances indicative of spinal cord dysfunction, and, finally, paralysis. *S. aureus* remains the most common culprit, distantly trailed by gram-negative aerobes such as *E. coli* and *Pseudomonas aeruginosa*, streptococci, and various anaerobes.

Although *Mycobacterium tuberculosis* is among the more common agents of spinal epidural abscess,[274,279,292] especially among intravenous drug abusers, the lesions it produces are typically granulomatous and caseating rather than suppurative. These usually arise in the low thoracic or lumbar region by extension from contiguous foci of tuberculous vertebral osteomyelitis or disk infection, but 'primary' examples not associated with osseous, pulmonary, or other extraskeletal disease may be encountered. Diagnosis is complicated by the fact that patients often present with back pain of insidious onset and chronic evolution unattended by fever, leukocytosis, or evidence of tuberculosis on chest film. As with nontuberculous epidural abscesses, the consequence of delayed intervention is progressive neurologic dysfunction culminating in myelopathy or 'Pott paraplegia'. Other localized forms of mycobacterial CNS infection include **tuberculoma**,[270,284,292] **focal tuberculous meningoencephalitis**,[289] and the rare **tuberculous abscess**.[291] **Subdural tuberculous empyema** has also been described.[272] Tuberculoma, defined as an encapsulated, granulomatous, and centrally caseating inflammatory mass, is by far the most common variant of neuroparenchymal tuberculosis, is usually unaccompanied by evidence of coextant meningeal infection, and may settle anywhere along the neuraxis but favors the intracranial contents. An excess of pediatric examples present in the cerebellum, constituting the posterior fossa 'tumors' encountered most frequently in some countries (e.g., India) where tuberculosis is rampant. Exceptionally, tuberculomas are dura-based,[270] rather than intra-axial, or confined to the spinal cord.[284] At substantially increased risk of developing both tuberculous meningitis and neuroparenchymal tuberculomas are human immunodeficiency virus type 1 (HIV-1)-seropositive subjects,[292] instances of CNS infection by nontuberculous mycobacteria having also been documented in this setting.[290] Mycobacteria of the avium complex characteristically evoke a nongranulomatous response that may include conspicuous spindling of infected histiocytic elements – a phenomenon that can be confused with a mesenchymal or meningothelial neoplasm.[275]

Other distinctive bacterial infections of the nervous system proper include a bulbar encephalitis ('rhombencephalitis') caused by *Listeria monocytogenes*[269] and cerebral Whipple disease, resulting from invasion of the neuropil by *Tropheryma whippelii*.[281,282] The latter process (which may rarely be confined to the CNS) is characterized in the brain, as elsewhere, by infiltrates of foamy macrophages exhibiting an intense, granular PAS positivity of their cytoplasm (which has a peculiar blue–gray tint in hematoxylin–eosin sections) and containing numerous rod-shaped bacillary forms on ultrastructural study. A florid reactive astrogliosis is the rule. *Bartonella henselae* (agent of cat-scratch disease and bacillary angiomatosis) has been described as causing space-occupying, inflammatory CNS lesions mainly in association with underlying immunodeficiency.[277]

Mycoses

The incidence of CNS mycosis has risen dramatically over the past several decades, reflecting the expanded population of immunocompromised patients susceptible to microbial opportunists. Still, neuroinvasive fungal infection only exceptionally occasions diagnostic operative intervention and thus remains a curiosity to the surgical pathologist. Most space-occupying intracranial and intraspinal lesions of mycotic etiology develop in association with diffuse meningeal or disseminated systemic infection and, consequently, are diagnosed by study of the CSF or, in the latter scenario, are treated empirically without recourse to tissue examination. Many are discovered only at autopsy. *Cryptococcus neoformans*, pathogenic molds, *Candida* species, and the dimorphic and dematiaceous fungi collectively account for the vast majority of lesions encountered in neurosurgical practice.[294]

C. neoformans, the agent of a diffuse leptomeningitis that is the single most common CNS mycosis, occasionally proliferates in localized neuroparenchymal or choroid plexus-based, intraventricular masses known as cryptococcomas.[294,303] Noteworthy is the fact that fewer than 5% of these unusual lesions arise in association with systemic disorders predisposing to opportunistic infection. Cryptococcal meningitis, by contrast, often afflicts immunosuppressed patients (e.g., HIV-1-seropositive adults, diabetics, organ transplant recipients, and patients being treated for hematologic or lymphoid neoplasia). The appearance of the cryptococcoma varies with the host's reaction, which may range from inertia to necrotizing granuloma formation and pronounced desmoplasia. When cryptococci hold the advantage, the lesion consists mainly of mucoid or gelatinous material that reflects the conspicuous elaboration of capsular mucopolysaccharides characteristic of these organisms. This is often traversed in honeycomb-like fashion by fibrous connective tissue septa. At the other extreme are sclerotic, granulomatous masses containing only rare yeast forms. Exceptional examples mimic bacterial abscesses, containing purulent debris bound by a well-developed pyogenic membrane. *Cryptococcus* is typically ovoid or spheric in profile, measures 2–15 μm in diameter, replicates by budding from a narrow base, and is reliably distinguished

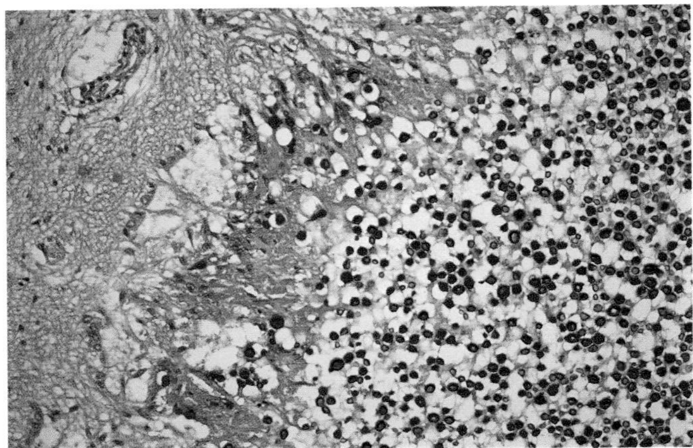

Fig. 28.20 Cryptococcoma. This neurosurgical specimen, from a previously healthy 54-year-old man with a 'tumor' primarily involving the choroid plexus and wall of the right lateral ventricle, demonstrates numerous yeast forms identifiable as *Cryptococcus neoformans* by their mucicarmine-stained capsules.

from other yeast by demonstration of its mucicarminophilic capsule (Fig. 28.20).

Fungi existing in pure hyphal form at both room temperature and 37°C are termed molds. The major CNS pathogens in this group include *Aspergillus* species, the Mucoraceae, and *Pseudallescheria boydii* (also referred to as *Scedosporium apiospermum*). *Fusarium, Paecilomyces,* and *Penicillium* species, *Streptomyces griseus,* and *Acremonium alabamensis* have also proved neuroinvasive on occasion.[294] Opportunists all, these ubiquitous organisms only rarely attack otherwise healthy individuals and share a particular predilection for patients receiving maintenance doses of broad-spectrum antibiotics through protracted periods of neutropenia, as commonly occurs in the management of leukemias and lymphomas. CNS infections that occur in such settings result from fungemia, are primarily intraparenchymal (as opposed to meningeal), are usually multifocal, and typically accompanied by evidence of systemic mycosis. The development of cerebral aspergillosis in patients treated for hematologic neoplasms, for example, is almost invariably preceded by symptomatic fungal infection of the lungs. Also at risk of blood-borne CNS seeding by pathogenic molds are patients taking corticosteroids, intravenous drug abusers, and, in the case of *P. boydii,*[299] victims of near drowning. Alcoholic liver disease and Cushing syndrome have also been associated with CNS aspergillosis.[294] A second important form of meningeal and neuroparenchymal mycosis caused by these agents follows their direct intracranial spread from foci of orbital or paranasal sinus infection. This pattern of disease is typified by rhinocerebral mucormycosis, a disorder classically associated with diabetic ketoacidosis but also complicating other acidemic states (e.g., sepsis, profound dehydration, uremia), renal transplantation, and deferoxamine therapy.[294] Prior to the application of immunosuppressive chemotherapeutic regimens to the treatment of cancer, *Aspergillus* generally invaded the CNS from primary foci of ocular, sinonasal, or middle ear infection. In addition, skull fracture, penetrating trauma, and craniotomy may set the stage for neural infection by molds.

The neurologic manifestations, distribution, and morphology of CNS lesions caused by these agents vary with the clinical circumstances surrounding infection and the immune status of the host. Particularly characteristic of cerebral disease evolving in the setting of disseminated systemic mycosis is a syndrome of multifocal stroke that reflects the shared tendency of pathogenic molds to occlude, invade, and trigger thrombosis of the leptomeningeal and perforating cerebral vasculature. The resulting lesions are basically infarcts, often hemorrhagic, that are secondarily colonized by fungi migrating through damaged blood vessel walls and that frequently exhibit little inflammatory reaction or limited superimposed suppuration. These are typically scattered in both cerebral hemispheres and often involve the deep nuclei, cerebellum, and brainstem. Contiguous fungal infiltration of the leptomeninges is common, but infection limited to these tissues is rare. Solitary lesions are exceptional, but examples produced by *Aspergillus* species,[295,309] *P. boydii,*[299] and other molds[294] are on record. These present with symptoms referable to an expanding intracranial mass, tend to occur in patients whose immune reflexes are relatively preserved, and may assume an abscess-like or even granulomatous character. Of particular note is a distinctive form of localized CNS mucormycosis characterized by a remarkably stereotypic predilection for the basal ganglia of intravenous drug abusers.[306] The more common rhinocerebral infections caused by advancing Mucoraceae are manifest as poorly delimited, necrotizing lesions again evidencing the ischemic and hemorrhagic qualities typical of these angioinvasive organisms. True mycotic aneurysm has also been described as a consequence of cerebral aspergillosis.[302]

The definitive taxonomic classification of molds requires their isolation in culture and cannot be accomplished on the basis of their morphology in tissue sections. Of the major CNS pathogens, both *Aspergillus* species and *P. boydii* appear in biopsy material as septate hyphae. *Aspergillus* species are usually somewhat stouter and branch (at acute angles) more frequently, but these are not reliably distinguishing features. By contrast, the Mucoraceae are broad, ribbon-like hyphal organisms that are nonseptate and branch at right angles.

Blastomyces dermatitidis, Histoplasma capsulatum, Coccidioides immitis, and *Paracoccidioides brasiliensis* are traditionally grouped as 'dimorphic' fungi because of their growth as filamentous mycelia at room temperature and yeast at 37°C. All are capable of infecting the CNS, usually in the form of a chronic granulomatous meningitis in patients with coextant, active systemic mycoses. Limited extension to the cerebral cortex from contiguous foci of leptomeningeal infection is common but typically of no clinical consequence. Only rarely do neuroparenchymal lesions attain symptomatic proportions.[294] Again, these unusual fungal masses are generally, although not invariably, associated with evident infection of extraneural tissues. Examples have been described both in the obviously immunodeficient and in patients with no clear risk factors for opportunistic disease.[293,301,305,307,308] Worth noting are observations that roughly half of the intracranial blastomycomas and a majority of the histoplasmomas reported to date presented as solitary lesions. Brain invasion by *C. immitis and P. brasiliensis* is, by contrast, infrequently unifocal. The interested reader is referred to the cited literature for details regarding the pathogenesis and morphology of these curious lesions and the appearances of their causative agents. Suffice it to say that these organisms as a rule evoke a necrotizing, granulomatous tissue response replete with multinucleated giant cells and, in cases of blastomycoma and histoplasmoma, foci of caseation that may prompt considerations of tuberculous infection. A suppurative infiltrate of polymorphonuclear leukocytes is also commonly observed in otherwise granulomatous masses caused by *B. dermatitidis*. Cerebral endarteritis and mycotic intracranial aneurysm caused by *C. immitis* infection have been described,[296] as has massive dural and cerebral venous thrombosis associated with coccidioidal meningitis in an AIDS patient.[300]

The dematiaceous (from the genus *Dematium*) fungi are a group of pigmented hyphal yeasts best known as the agents of chronic skin and subcutaneous infections such as Madura foot and tinea capitis. Extracutaneous disease is exceptional, but the brain is a common target in disseminated mycoses caused by these organisms. One member of the group, *Xylohypha bantiana* (*Cladosporium trichoides*), appears to be specifically neurotropic and is responsible for most CNS infections,[304] which are often classed with other deep mycoses caused by pigmented fungi under the rubric of phaeohyphomycosis. This organism is fully capable of invading the nervous systems of apparently immunocompetent hosts and, in many cases, does so in the absence of demonstrable foci of extraneural infection. Isolated patients have suffered immunosuppressive underlying conditions; exhibited preexistent phaeohyphomycotic infections of the paranasal sinuses, ear, or lungs; or have apparently acquired the infection through traumatic intracerebral implantation or intravenous drug abuse.[298] Neuroparenchymal lesions consist of necrotizing granulomas, multifocal in about 50% of cases. A similar fraction is attended by fungal meningitis. In tissue sections, the agent appears as branching, septate hyphal, and yeast-like structures with a brown or olive-green hue. Isolation in culture is required for definitive classification. Other pigmented fungi that have been reported to cause CNS disease include *Drechslera–Bipolaris–Exserohilum* and *Curvularia* species, *Fonsecaea pedrosoi*, *Wangiella dermatitidis*, *Dactylaria constricta*, *Ramichloridium obovoideum*, and *Scopulariopsis brumptii*.[294]

If *Candida* species appear to receive short shrift in these pages, it is not because the threat they pose to the nervous system is trivial in epidemiologic terms. Actually, cerebral candidiasis has emerged in recent years as one of the most common CNS mycoses encountered in immunosuppressed patients.[294] The fact remains, however, that the great majority of cerebral *Candida* infections are discovered only at autopsy, resulting from fungemia in debilitated, moribund patients. The typical lesions are diminutive foci of suppuration scattered widely in the neuropil and associated in some cases with fungal meningitis. The formation of granulomas or macroabscesses, disease limited to the meninges, and vasculitis, with resultant infarction or the development of mycotic aneurysms,[294,302] have also been described, as has the extraordinary presentation of CNS candidiasis as a localized fungal mass.[297]

Parasitoses

The CNS parasitoses include a great variety of protozoal and helminthic infections. This discussion is limited to two representatives of particular importance to the surgical pathologist – neurocysticercosis and toxoplasmosis.

Neurocysticercosis, caused by larvae of the pork tapeworm, *Taenia solium*, is the most common parasitic cerebral infection encountered in worldwide neurosurgical practice.[312] Endemic to nearly all continents, the disease is particularly prevalent in Mexico (where it is the leading cause of space-occupying intracranial lesions), Central and South America, India, Africa, and China. An increasing incidence in the United States is largely attributable to cases occurring in immigrants from these regions. Infection is acquired by ingestion of food or water contaminated by feces containing the cestode's ova. These are partially digested in the host's stomach, evolving to oncospheres and subsequently penetrating the small intestinal mucosa to disseminate throughout the body, preferentially encysting in ocular tissues, striated muscle, and brain. The ensuing clinical disorder is named for the designation given the organism at this larval stage, *Cysticercus cellulosae*.

Cysticerci actually persist in parasitized tissues for long periods without eliciting symptoms of any kind. The active clinical phase of neurocysticercosis is triggered by the host's inflammatory response to the larva's death (approximately 18 months following primary infection). The high incidence of focal or generalized seizures associated with the disorder reflects the fact that oncospheres reaching the CNS settle mainly in the epileptogenic cerebral cortex, but they may also colonize the ventricular system and basal cisterns in a distinctive pattern of infestation ('racemose' cysticercosis) resulting in obstructive hydrocephalus and consequent manifestations of elevated intracranial pressure. The presence of multifocal, rim-enhancing cerebral cysts on neuroimaging study suffices in many cases to prompt a diagnostic as well as therapeutic course of anthelmintic chemotherapy, but a substantial proportion of patients present with solitary lesions, and the host's reaction to the decaying parasite may convert the cyst to a deceptively solid inflammatory pseudotumor. Neurosurgical intervention may be obviated by CSF or serologic assay for specific anticysticercal antibodies or antigens, but false-negative results may be encountered, especially in subjects with unifocal disease.[312]

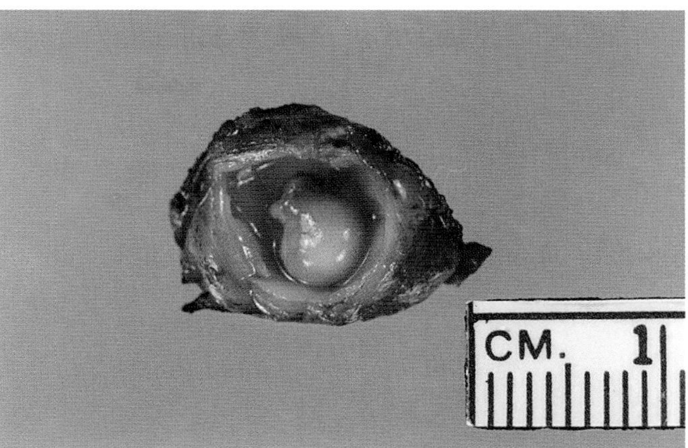

Fig. 28.21 Neurocysticercosis. Typical of cerebral *Taenia solium* infestation is the solitary, encysted scolex demonstrated in this neurosurgical specimen from the left frontal cortex of a 32-year-old Haitian man with a history of seizures.

When not completely obscured by secondary inflammatory changes, the gross appearance of cysticerci excised in toto is virtually pathognomonic (Fig. 28.21). Individual cysts are of small diameter, are circumscribed by a rubbery fibrous pseudocapsule, and contain a single larval scolex represented by a spheric or ovoid grayish-white nodule measuring no more than 3–4 mm in greatest dimension. By contrast, cestode larval cysts produced by the morphologically similar *Multiceps multiceps* contain numerous scolices and those caused by *Echinococcus granulosus* are considerably larger and endowed with a characteristically laminated wall. On histologic examination, the fibrous pseudocapsule is typically infiltrated by lymphocytes and plasma cells in large numbers, may contain eosinophils in abundance, and in some cases is the site of an active granulomatous reaction. The mummified remains of the degenerate scolex are covered by a wavy, somewhat refractile cuticle and consist largely of loose, reticular tissue containing numerous calcospherites. Relatively intact scolices possess a discernible subcuticular 'pseudoepithelial' layer, small myofiber bundles, and four suckers armed with birefringent hooklets (Fig. 28.22). Racemose cysticerci evacuated from the ventricles or subarachnoid space present as grape-like clusters of interconnected larval 'bladders' lacking organized scolices.

Toxoplasmosis is the generic designation applied to localized or systemic infections caused by the obligate intracellular protozoan *Toxoplasma gondii*. CNS involvement may assume a number of distinctive clinicomorphologic guises,[310] this discussion focusing on a 'tumefactive' variant largely confined to immunocompromised

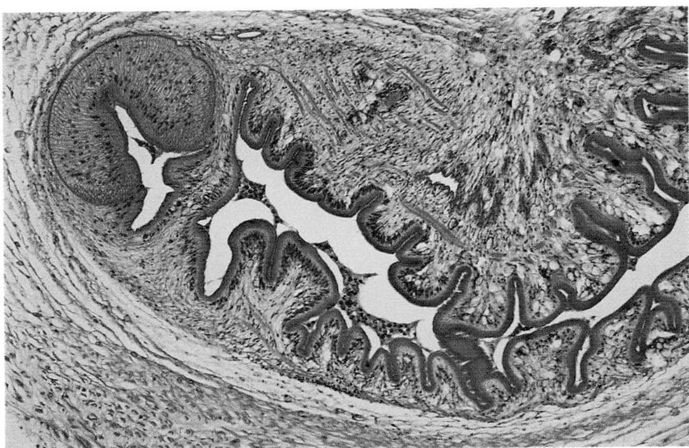

Fig. 28.22 Neurocysticercosis. The parasite's main structural features include a prominent investing tegument or 'cuticle', aggregated subcuticular cells, smooth muscle fibers, and four suckers, one of which is depicted at upper left.

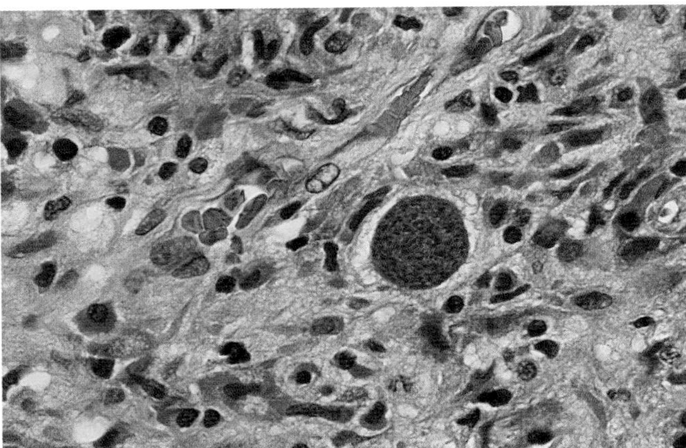

Fig. 28.23 Toxoplasmosis. Minute, basophilic structures representing bradyzoites fill a protozoal pseudocyst lying among infiltrating lymphocytes, plasma cells, and macrophages.

hosts and typically unassociated with clinical manifestations of extraneural parasitosis. Once regarded as rare and encountered principally among patients treated for hematolymphoid neoplasms (Hodgkin disease, particularly), this form of toxoplasmosis is now known to physicians the world over as a common AIDS-defining disorder and is in fact the leading cause of space-occupying intracranial lesions in the HIV-1 seropositive.[310,311] Bone marrow transplant recipients have also emerged in recent years as a population prone to CNS infections of this type. Common to the afflicted is a breakdown of cell-mediated immune surveillance thought, in most cases, to permit recrudescence of the agent in dormantly parasitized neural tissues. *T. gondii* is noted for its silent persistence in the brain following primary infection, which is usually asymptomatic and acquired by the consumption of inadequately cooked red meats containing encysted organisms or by the inadvertent ingestion of foodstuffs, soil, or other materials contaminated by protozoal oocytes shed in the feces of domestic cats.

The clinical and neuroradiologic features of CNS toxoplasmosis are quite variable, are nonspecific, and do not suffice for definitive diagnosis. Because *Toxoplasma* 'abscesses' favor neuron-rich gray matter structures such as the cerebral cortex, basal ganglia, and brainstem, it should come as no surprise that seizures, progressive hemipareses, and cranial nerve deficits figure prominently among their initial manifestations. Many patients, however, present without localizing complaints, evidencing, instead, fever, headache, lethargy, and diffuse encephalopathy, subacute in its evolution. Cranial MR imaging typically discloses multifocal, nodular lesions characterized by ring-like peripheral enhancement, surrounding edema, and mass effect, but exceptional examples are nonenhancing or diffusely so, and solitary abscesses at presentation are not rare. Isolated involvement of the spinal cord has been described.[313] Studies in the HIV-1 seropositive have demonstrated that, in this population at least, cerebral toxoplasmosis only occasionally develops in patients lacking serologic evidence of contact with the organism.[310] A negative serum anti-toxoplasma IgG titer militates against, but does not exclude, the diagnosis in this setting. It has become common practice to institute antimicrobial therapy on empiric grounds in suspect cases and to reserve neurosurgical intervention for the patient who does not respond satisfactorily to such management. Most HIV-1-seropositive individuals whose intracranial masses fail to resolve on anti-toxoplasma chemotherapy prove to harbor primary CNS lymphomas.

The *Toxoplasma* 'abscess', as it is commonly called, consists of a central mass of necrotic cellular debris surrounded by edematous and inflamed brain tissue typically exhibiting conspicuous vascular abnormalities. The latter include perivascular and intramural lymphoid infiltration, endothelial swelling, thrombosis, fibrinoid necrosis, and, in long-standing lesions, fibrous obliteration. It is within this perimeter zone that *Toxoplasma* are most numerous, the necrotic core often being devoid of identifiable organisms. Two protozoal forms are evident in active lesions. Responsible for tissue injury is the rapidly proliferating tachyzoite. This is faintly basophilic, measures approximately 4–8 µm in greatest dimension, and typically exhibits a slightly crescentic or lunate profile (the Greek *toxon* means bow or arc). Because it is often difficult to visualize tachyzoites in routine histologic preparations and to confidently distinguish them from cellular detritus, the screening of suspect biopsy material with *Toxoplasma*-specific antibodies is strongly advised. More readily apparent, although present in lesser numbers, are intracellular pseudocysts and 'true' (i.e., membrane-delimited) cysts that may attain diameters of up to 200 µm (Fig. 28.23). These are filled with minute, PAS-positive bradyzoites (named for their slow replicative cycles), are immunologically inert, and represent the form in which *Toxoplasma* chronically persist in brain and other tissues. Within the CNS, bradyzoites appear to collect preferentially within neurons and perivascular macrophages. Again, it is immune failure that is believed to somehow trigger their metamorphosis to tachyzoites and subsequent destructive invasion of neural tissues. Careful inspection of active lesions often reveals ruptured cysts that appear to be disgorging their content of protozoa into the neuropil. Like tachyzoites, bradyzoites are labeled by commercially available *Toxoplasma*-specific antibodies.

Spirochetal infections

The two major CNS spirochetoses are neurosyphilis,[315,316] caused by *Treponema pallidum*, and *neuroborreliosis* complicating infection by the agent of Lyme disease, *Borrelia burgdorferi*.[314,317] No attempt is made here to discuss the pathogenesis and varied clinical expressions of these complex syndromes, matters largely irrelevant to the surgical pathologist. Suffice it to say that intracerebral inflammatory pseudotumors (known as 'gummas' in the case of treponemal disease and accompanied by necrosis and fibroplasia in this setting) are restricted to the late stages of systemic infection by these organisms, constitute their least common manifestations, and are usually approached surgically only when the diagnosis is unsuspected on clinical grounds and so not established by the appropriate serologic methods. The reader is referred to the cited literature for further details.

Viral infections

Herpes simplex encephalitis

Herpes viruses are responsible for a wide variety of neurologic infections, our concern here being with a distinctive form of focal, necrotizing, and hemorrhagic encephalitis caused principally by *herpes simplex virus type 1* (HSV-1). **Herpes simplex encephalitis** (HSE) afflicts only 2–4 persons per 1 000 000 inhabitants a year but leads the list of potentially fatal, nonepidemic cerebral infections of viral etiology.[323] Individuals of any age may be affected. The disease is often fulminant in its evolution and is characterized by fever, disordered affect, dysphasia, seizure activity, and deterioration of consciousness. CSF pleocytosis is the rule and may be accompanied by xanthochromia, whereas abnormalities are usually localized to one or both frontotemporal regions on CT scan or MRI (Fig. 28.24). Brain biopsy is now generally obviated in the appropriate clinical circumstances by assay of CSF for HSV-specific antigens or genomic sequences. Polymerase chain reaction (PCR)-based amplification of HSV DNA has gained wide acceptance in this regard and, as the diagnostic method of choice, combines high degrees of both sensitivity and specificity.[323]

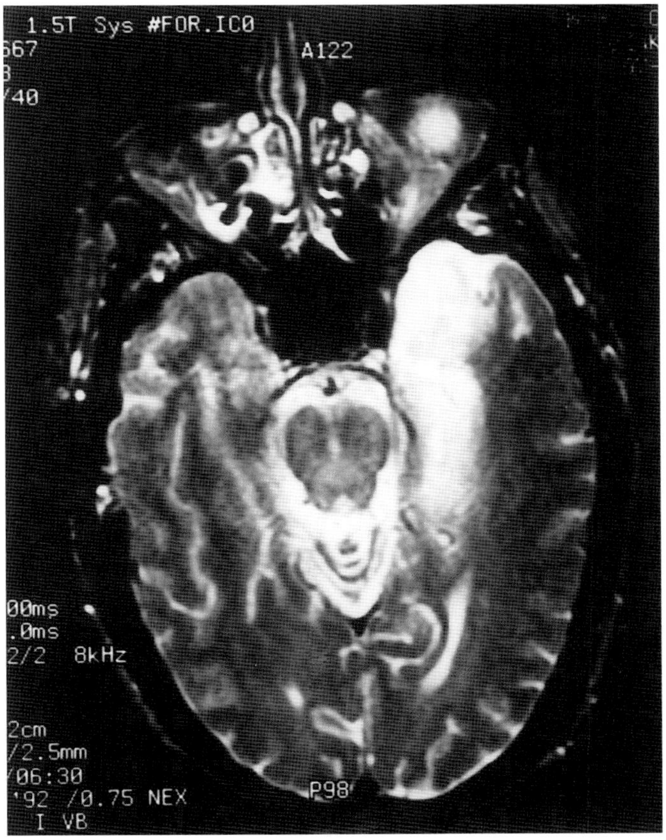

Fig. 28.24 HSE. This MRI, from a middle-aged man with headache, fever, and disordered affect, demonstrates the anteromedial temporal lobe localization of signal abnormalities ('bright' in this study) typical of HSE on neuroradiologic assessment.

A remarkably stereotypic predilection for the anteromedial temporal lobes, orbitofrontal cortex, insulae, and cingulate gyri typifies HSE.[318,319] Experimental observations support the hypothesis that this 'limbic' distribution reflects transolfactory spread of the agent to the CNS and suggest that at least some cases of HSE follow activation of virus residing latently in cerebral tissues. The histologic appearances of the disorder vary considerably with the duration of the clinical illness.[318,319] The earliest appreciable changes, evident prior to the arrival of inflammatory infiltrates, include neuronal shrinkage and eosinophilia accompanied by vascular congestion, spongy cortical rarefaction, and pallor. We have seen this picture, which closely mimics that of hypoxic–ischemic brain injury, misdiagnosed as acute cerebral infarction, although close scrutiny of these degenerating neurons often reveals a ground-glass alteration of their nucleoplasm that should suggest a viral cytopathic effect. It is during this early phase of symptomatic disease that careful search for the eosinophilic intranuclear inclusion bodies typical of herpetic infection is most likely to be rewarded (Fig. 28.25). These may be

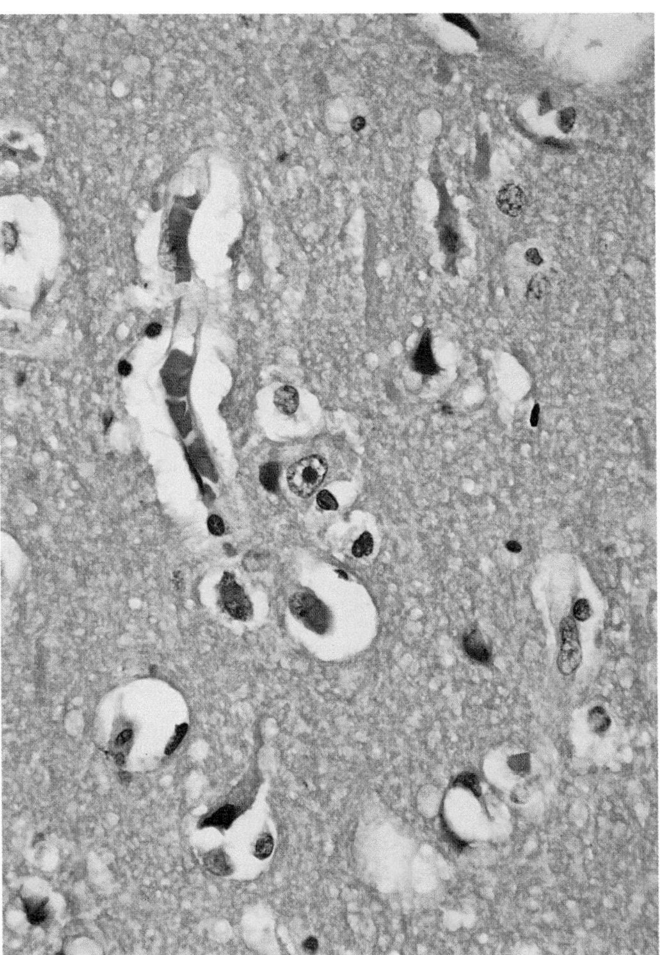

Fig. 28.25 HSE. As shown here, herpes simplex encephalitis may masquerade as a noninfectious, ischemic process (particularly if biopsied early in its clinical evolution). Note the noninflammatory appearance, neuronal shrinkage, pyknosis, and dissolution. The nucleus of an astrocyte in the center of this field contains a well-defined inclusion body.

identified in the nuclei of cortical astrocytes and satellite oligodendroglia, as well as neurons, but are an inconstant feature of the disorder.

The pronounced inflammatory reaction characteristic of fully developed HSE is usually in evidence by the second week of clinical disease. Lymphocytes and plasma cells colonize the meninges, cuff penetrating blood vessels, and migrate into the devastated cortex. Mononuclear cells may converge on infected neurons to form neuronophagic or so-called microglial nodules. These changes are often accompanied by hemorrhage and, in some cases, thrombosis and even fibrinoid necrosis of the cerebral vasculature. Foamy macrophages eventually come to dominate the invading cellular elements and ultimately clear the necrotic debris, only cavitated and gliotic remnants persisting at sites of prior infection.

Electron microscopy, immunocytochemistry and molecular genetic techniques may be profitably applied to the diagnosis of HSE and may in select cases provide evidence of HSV infection in biopsy material exhibiting little alteration at the light microscopic level. Ultrastructural study is the most laborious and least sensitive of these methods but affords direct visualization of the agent in infected cells. Assembled in the nucleus, the mature HSV particle is an icosahedral nucleocapsid averaging 100–120 nm in diameter and containing a central density representing the agent's genomic DNA (Fig. 28.26). Virions typically acquire a lipid envelope derived from the host nuclear membrane on transport into the cytoplasm. Inasmuch as similar appearances are shared by other encephalitogenic herpes viruses, electron microscopy is of limited utility in specifically identifying the offender as HSV. Commercially available antibodies to this agent are now routinely employed for this purpose, and immunohistochemical assessment is strongly recommended in all cases of clinically suspected HSE, regardless of whether inspection of biopsy material reveals evidence of an inflammatory process (Fig. 28.27). In fact, Esiri's elegant correlative studies indicate that attempts at HSV antigen detection are most likely to succeed during the first week of encephalitic symptoms.[318] Coincident with a mounting inflammatory reaction, antigen expression declines steadily through the second and third weeks of the clinical illness and is not usually demonstrable thereafter. We have noted, however, the unusual persistence of viral antigens beyond this period in cases of HSE involving immunocompromised hosts, including cancer patients and individuals with underlying infection by HIV- 1.[322] These appeared to be arrested at the noninflammatory, pseudoischemic phase characteristic of early HSE in otherwise normal individuals. HSE has also been documented in patients with primary brain tumors,[321,322] raising the question of whether a neoplasm, its surgical or adjuvant management might trigger activation of latent CNS infection by HSV.

The reader is referred elsewhere for discussion of relapsing and chronic (including granulomatous) encephalitides that have been attributed to HSV infection.[320]

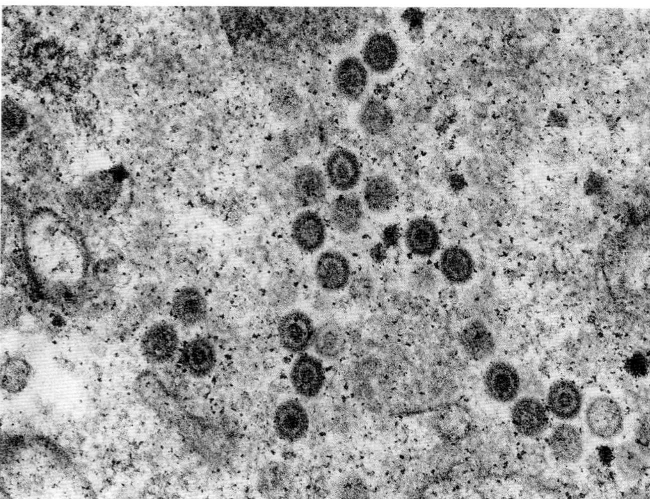

Fig. 28.26 HSE. This transmission electron photomicrograph reveals enveloped nucleocapsids with an average diameter of 100 nm in the cytoplasm of an infected cell. (×62 000)

Progressive multifocal leukoencephalopathy

Progressive multifocal leukoencephalopathy (PML) is an opportunistic demyelinating disease of the CNS caused by DNA viruses of the polyoma group. Nearly all clinical isolates responsible for the disorder have been strains of the ubiquitous *JC virus* (so designated for the initials of the first afflicted patient from whose brain the agent was recovered), with only exceptional cases linked to the related *SV-40*. Originally delineated as a paraneoplastic complication of Hodgkin disease and chronic lymphocytic leukemia,[326] PML is almost always associated with defective cell-mediated immunity, is currently encountered most frequently in the setting of underly-

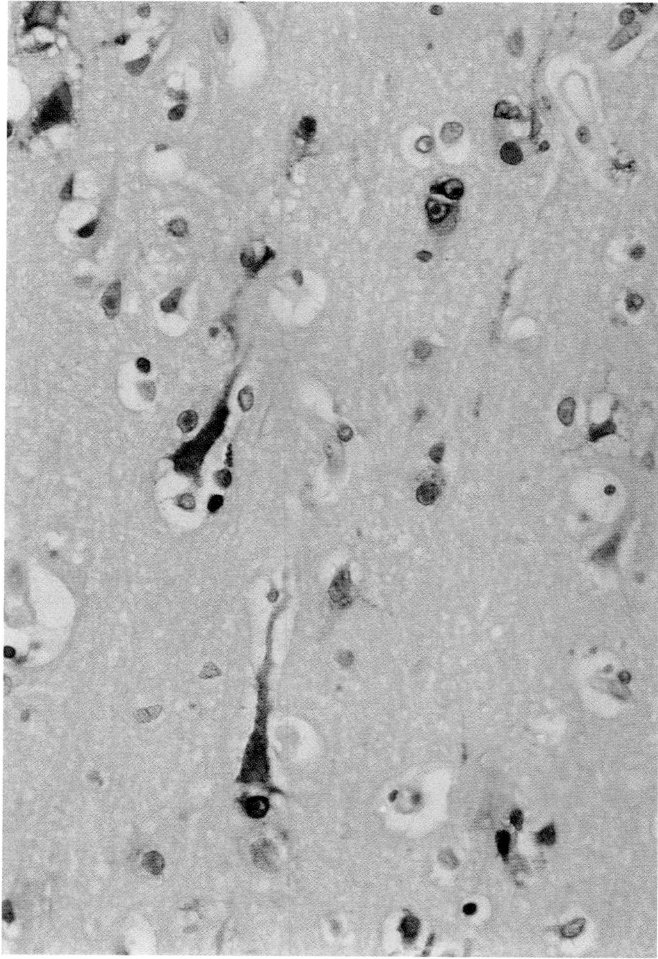

Fig. 28.27 HSE. In this immunoperoxidase preparation, the cytoplasm of neurons and inclusion bodies within the nuclei of satellite glia are labeled by antibodies to herpes simplex type 1.

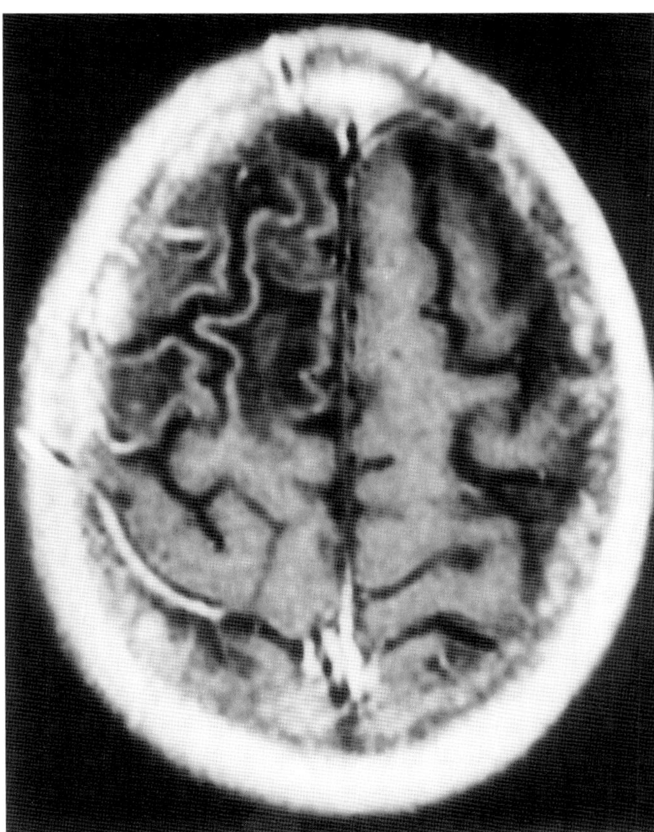

Fig. 28.28 Progressive multifocal leukoencephalopathy. A postcontrast injection MRI demonstrates the regional white matter hypodensity, absence of mass effect or abnormal enhancement, and cortical preservation that typify this demyelinating infection.

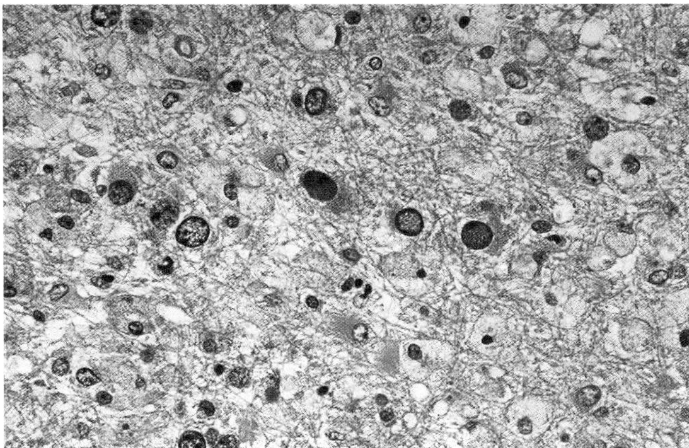

Fig. 28.29 Progressive multifocal leukoencephalopathy. JC virus-infected oligodendrocytes in the center of this field exhibit the nuclear swelling, chromatin dissolution, and replacement by amphophilic, 'ground-glass' inclusion material that are peculiar to this disorder. Note presence of scattered hyperplastic astrocytes and admixed foamy macrophages.

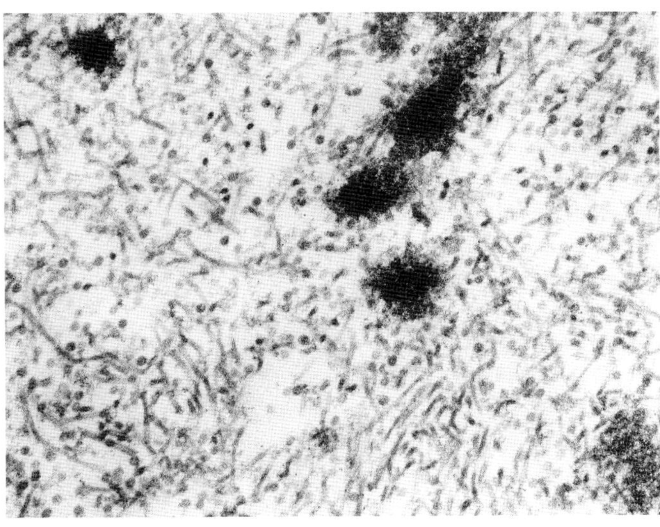

Fig. 28.30 Progressive multifocal leukoencephalopathy. This transmission electron micrograph of an oligodendrocyte's nucleus depicts nonenveloped virions of 37 nm diameter lying singly and in the filamentous arrays that are a common feature of JC infection. (×45 150)

ing HIV-1 infection, and may be the presenting manifestation of AIDS. The disease is characterized by subacutely evolving neurologic symptoms indicative of a multifocal process. Chief among these are motor deficits, cognitive decline, and visual loss. Although tumefactive variants have been described,[330,336] neuroimaging studies usually provide a clue to the nature of the process by demonstrating scattered foci of white matter hypodensity not associated with mass effect or contrast enhancement (Fig. 28.28). Amplification of JC virus-specific DNA sequences from the CSF has emerged as a useful diagnostic procedure and has lessened reliance on brain biopsy.

Any level of the central neuraxis may be affected in PML, but the cerebral hemispheric white matter generally bears the brunt of the injury. Cerebellar and bulbar localizations are less common, and the spinal cord is usually spared. It is the remarkable tropism of the JC virus for, and its replication within, oligodendroglia that are responsible for the alterations pathognomonic of PML. Productive infection of these cells results in progressive enlargement of their nuclei, dissolution of their compacted chromatin, and its replacement by homogeneously dense and basophilic or 'ground-glass', amphophilic material (Fig. 28.29). Considerably less common than this transformation of the entire nucleoplasm are demarcated eosinophilic inclusions of the sort that typify herpes virus infections. At the fine structural level, the oligodendrocytopathy characteristic of PML corresponds to a distension of the nucleus by nonenveloped, spheric or icosahedral particles measuring 33–45 nm in diameter. These are frequently aggregated in paracrystalline arrays and may be admixed with filamentous viral strands 15–25 nm in diameter (Fig. 28.30). Although immunocytochemical assay,[332] in situ hybridization,[332] and gene amplification techniques[335] may be used to confirm JC virus infection, the highly characteristic nature of the oligodendroglial karyomegaly and nucleoplasmic alterations typical of PML cannot be overemphasized.

With the ongoing infection and lysis of target cells, PML evolves as centrifugally expanding zones of oligodendroglial depletion and subsequent infiltration by foamy macrophages engaged in the scavenging and digestion of degenerating myelin sheaths. Early on, small plaques tend to a miliary clustering at the gray–white junction that probably reflects hematogenous seeding of the CNS following reactivation of the agent in sites of systemic latency. Geographic

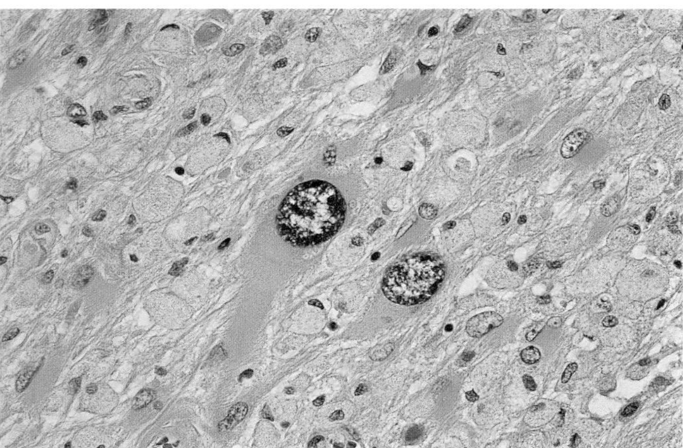

Fig. 28.31 Progressive multifocal leukoencephalopathy. Grotesque cytologic alterations may result from infection of astrocytes by the JC virus. An accompanying infiltrate of foamy macrophages should militate strongly against the diagnosis of neoplasia, despite the worrisome appearances of these bizarre cells.

zones of demyelination, resulting from the coalescence of these small lesions, become grossly evident as regions of white matter retraction, granularity, and yellowish-gray discoloration. In most cases, a relatively undisturbed cortical ribbon will span these devastated areas. This, and the characteristic persistence of axons in the face of total demyelination, reflects the resistance of neurons (cerebellar granule cells excepted) to JC virus infection. Some thinning of the axonal population, however, is the rule, and PML can progress to extensive white matter cavitation. Particularly widespread and destructive examples have been described in the setting of brain coinfection by HIV-1.[337] A most exceptional example of PML with ganglion cell-like transformation of cerebrocortical neurons possibly induced by JC virus has been communicated.[333]

A histologic feature of PML meriting further comment is atypical astrocytic hyperplasia (Fig. 28.31). In addition to florid astrogliosis – a constant finding – the demyelinating lesions of PML frequently contain greatly enlarged astrocytes exhibiting bizarre nuclear abnormalities indistinguishable from those usually associated with neoplasia. These cytologic changes (often accompanied by morphologically atypical mitotic activity, Ki-67 expression,[325] and abnormal nuclear immunoreactivity for p53[324]) are believed to reflect a form of nonpermissive infection in which the agent's genome is spliced into that of the host cell, a process integral to the recognized capacity of polyomaviruses, including JC virus isolates from patients with PML, to induce central neuroepithelial tumors in the experimental situation. The precise role, if any, of these viruses in the pathogenesis of human brain tumors remains to be clarified, but it is noteworthy that the association of PML with multifocal astrocytomas has been documented, albeit rarely.[334]

PML is usually characterized by minimal inflammatory response to the agent; however, some variants evidence intense perivascular and interstitial lymphoid infiltration. The latter often contain very few oligodendrocytes manifesting the nuclear cytopathic effects typical of JC virus infection and may prompt consideration of primary cerebral lymphoma, another recognized complication of the immunosuppressed state occurring with particular frequency in HIV-1-seropositive patients. It is this unusual form of PML that is most likely to present as a space-occupying, contrast-enhancing mass on CT or MRI study, further complicating the clinical delineation of these entities. A conspicuous inflammatory response and accompanying contrast enhancement on neuroradiologic study characterizes some examples affecting HIV-1-positive patients under highly active antiretroviral therapy (HAART)[329] and typifies biopsy material from a subset of AIDS patients surviving for considerably longer than the 3- to 6-month interval in which most cases of PML progress ineluctably to death.[328] The rare examples of spontaneously remitting PML that we have seen have been of this unusually inflammatory type and presumably reflect elimination or immunologic containment of the JC virus following a transitory abrogation of its enforced dormancy. Ironically, HAART-associated restoration of immune reflexes may precipitate exaggerated inflammatory reactions to JC virus (as well as other pathogens, including mycobacteria, cryptococci, cytomegalovirus and HIV-1) that result in paradoxic clinical deterioration while lessening systemic HIV-1 RNA levels and boosting peripheral CD4+ T-lymphocyte counts.[327] This '**immune reconstitution inflammatory syndrome (IRIS)**', which can prove fatal, is characterized by leptomeningeal and neuroparenchymal lymphoid infiltrates dominated by CD8+ T cells.[331]

Varicella-zoster virus encephalitis and cerebral vasculitis

Varicella-zoster virus (VZV), agent of chickenpox and shingles, causes a rare form of encephalitis sharing certain clinical and histologic features with PML.[341–343] The condition has to date been described exclusively in immunocompromised hosts (including patients treated for Hodgkin disease, other cancers, and AIDS) and may present months following resolution of cutaneous zoster or in the absence of a preceding exanthem. Described by some authors as a 'leukoencephalitis', this chronic infection can settle anywhere along the central neuraxis, but exhibits a striking predilection for the cerebral hemispheric white matter. It is characterized by multifocal, centrifugally expanding, and coalescent foci of demyelination and variable axonal loss with little inflammatory reaction. Many cases also evidence small infarcts resulting from VZV-mediated vascular injury as further discussed below. The nuclei of oligodendrocytes situated on the periphery of demyelinating lesions exhibit a ground-glass transformation or homogeneous filling by basophilic material superficially similar to the cytopathy induced in such cells by the JC virus but differ in not being conspicuously enlarged. Furthermore, neighboring astrocytes (and, in some cases, neurons and ependymal cells) infected by VZV contain well-demarcated Cowdry A-type intranuclear inclusions of the sort that typify herpes virus replication and are not driven to the atypical hyperplasia characteristic of PML. Fine structural study will disclose herpes-type nucleocapsids averaging approximately 100 nm in diameter within the nuclei of infected cells. These differ slightly from herpes simplex-type virions in that their core densities tend to be eccentrically positioned, but definitive identification of the agent requires immunocytochemical assay, molecular hybridization studies, or culture.

In addition to being an encephalitogen, VZV is recognized as a rare cause of cerebral vasculitis. This may involve large arteries at the base of the brain as well as smaller branches. Like the encephalitis associated with this agent, vasculitic complications of zoster typically follow resolution of the cutaneous exanthem. Two major variants have been described. One, a noninflammatory 'angiopathy' afflicting immunocompromised hosts and associated in some cases with VZV encephalitis as just described, is characterized by striking fibrointimal proliferation, thrombosis, and, in some cases, disruption of the elastica and thinning of the media without evident necrosis of mural elements.[339] The other is an overtly inflammatory and necrotizing angiitis designated by some observers as 'granulomatous' because of the presence of multinucleated histiocytes within damaged vessel walls.[338,340] This often presents as hemiplegic stroke weeks after an episode of contralateral zoster ophthalmicus in a patient with no major evidences of defective immunity.[338] In fact, we have seen several examples – all in patients seropositive for HIV-1 – displaying both angiopathic and angiitic features, depending on the portion of vessel sampled, and suspect that the former simply represent the chronic sequelae of what is primarily an inflammatory process. In addition to thrombosis with consequent cerebral infarction, VZV angiitis may result in fusiform aneurysmal dilation, mural rupture, and subarachnoid hemorrhage.[340] Definitive diagnosis requires localization of the agent by immunocytochemical assay or ultrastructural study to elements of the vessel wall, typically smooth muscle cells in the media or intimal (myo) fibroblasts. See our discussion of primary angiitis of the nervous system for further consideration of VZV as a cerebrovascular pathogen.

HIV-1 encephalomyelitis

HIV-1 encephalomyelitis is not a disorder likely to engage the surgical pathologist but demands, nevertheless, some consideration in view of the ongoing AIDS epidemic and the unique nature of the neuropathologic alterations associated with this retroviral infection.[344] HIV-1 is alone among viral encephalitogens in exhibiting no particular tropism for neuroectodermal cell types, its replication in the nervous system taking place largely within marrow-derived macrophages and microglia. CNS infection is characterized by loosely arrayed, vasocentric, or paravascular inflammatory infiltrates concentrated in the cerebral hemispheric white matter, basal ganglia, and rostral brainstem (Fig. 28.32). These are dominated by mononucleated and multinucleated macrophages, the latter reflecting a process of virally mediated cell fusion that is the characteristic cytopathic effect of this and other members of the lentivirus subfamily of retroviruses. These cells, and their mononuclear precursors, harbor and release fully formed virions, which may be found budding from their plasmalemma, aggregated in membrane-delimited intracytoplasmic vacuoles, or lying free in the cytoplasm (Fig. 28.33). The mature particle is spherical, averages 100–120 nm in diameter, and possesses a cylindrical or bar-shaped nucleoid usually positioned eccentrically and enclosed by a limiting membrane. Attendant changes include diffuse astrogliosis and microglial activation, generalized pallor of the cerebral white matter, and brain atrophy. The precise relationship of local HIV-1 replication to these indices of widespread CNS injury remains a subject of active investigation.[344]

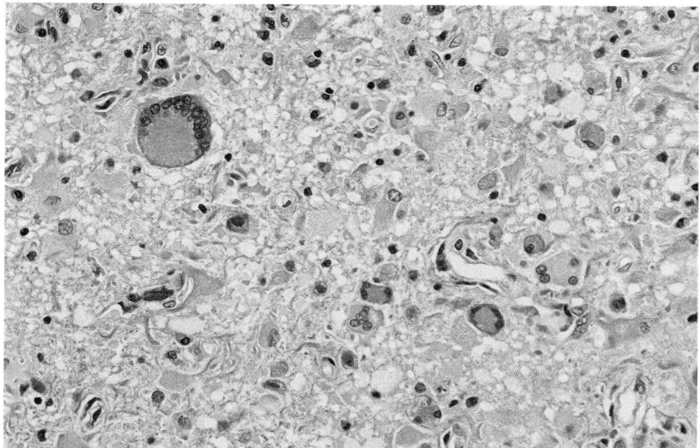

Fig. 28.32 HIV encephalitis. Nongranulomatous infiltrates centered loosely about blood vessels in the cerebral white matter (shown here) or basal ganglia and dominated by macrophages, including multinucleated forms resulting from retrovirally mediated cell fusion, characterize infection of the CNS by this agent. The associated astrogliosis and spongy rarefaction are common accompanying features.

Prion-associated diseases

Though long classed among viral disorders of the CNS, the unusual diseases collectively known as transmissible spongiform encephalopathies have resisted explication as conventional contagions and, in fact, occur in heritable and apparently sporadic, as well as clearly infectious, forms. The pathogenesis of these rare entities remains a subject of controversy and ongoing investigation, but they clearly share anomalies of a native cell membrane constituent – the prion protein (PrP) – expressed at particularly high levels by central neurons. Conformationally altered, abnormally protease-resistant and amyloidogenic PrP isoforms ('prions') characteristically accumulate in affected tissues, and there is much experimental evidence suggesting that these potentially host-derived proteins are capable of propagation and suffice for disease transmission in the absence of associated nucleic acids.[347] Prion-associated illnesses include **kuru** (linked to the practice of ritual cannibalism among the Fore tribespeople of Papua, New Guinea), **Creutzfeldt–Jakob disease (CJD)**, **'variant' CJD** (most recently described of the group and cause of great public health concern as a putative manifestation of exposure to the agent of bovine spongiform encephalopathy or 'mad cow' disease), **Gerstmann–Straussler–Scheinker disease**, and **fatal familial insomnia.**[347] The following discussion is essentially limited to practical considerations in the diagnosis of CJD, the variant most commonly encountered in clinical practice.

The iatrogenic transmission of CJD via contaminated neurosurgical instruments, human growth hormone supplements, and a variety of allografts is well documented, but the large majority of cases involve middle-aged or older adults having no evident exposure to contaminated materials or other individuals suffering the disorder. A heredofamilial variant associated with *PrP* gene

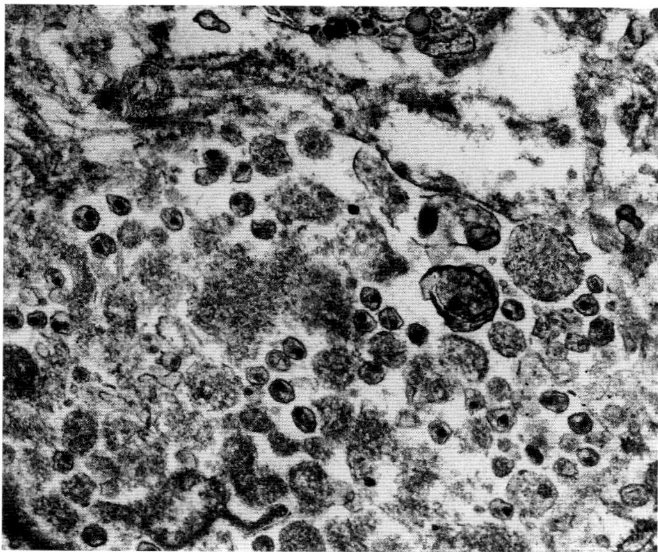

Fig. 28.33 HIV encephalitis. This transmission electron micrograph shows intracytoplasmic HIV particles measuring 110–120 nm in diameter. Note the well-defined envelopes and eccentrically positioned core densities. (×40 000)
(Courtesy of Dr Leroy Sharer, Newark, NJ)

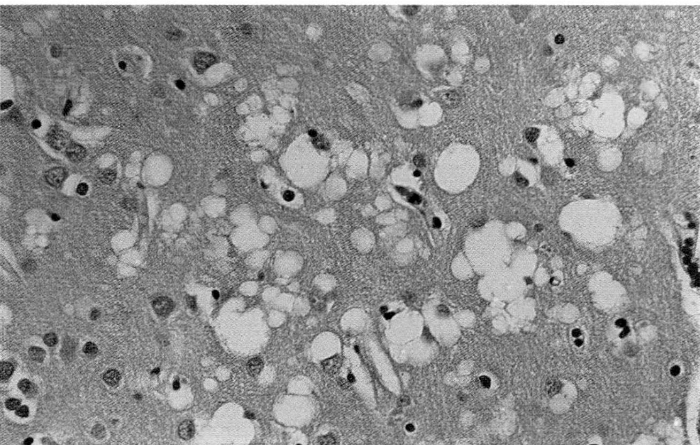

Fig. 28.34 Creutzfeldt–Jakob disease. Noninflammatory vacuolization of the cerebral cortex is the dominant alteration evident in this biopsy specimen from an elderly man with progressive dementia and myoclonus. This change typically precedes conspicuous neuronal dropout and astrogliosis, the other dominant findings in this prion-related disorder.

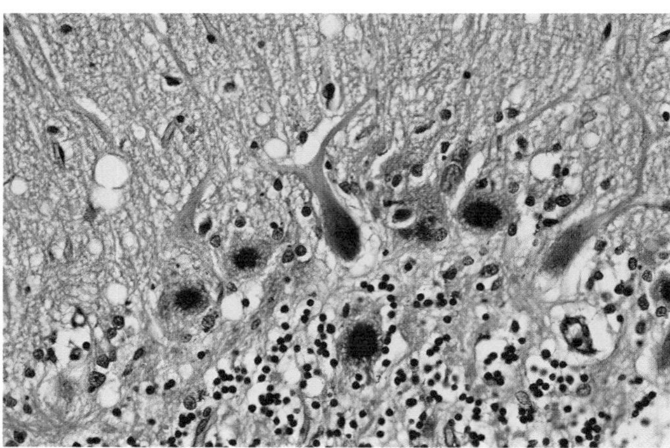

Fig. 28.35 Creutzfeldt–Jakob disease. Demonstrated in this cerebellar biopsy material are PAS-positive plaques of 'spiked ball' type ('kuru' plaques). Note the spiculate radiations at the periphery of these deposits. Mild spongiform change is present in the overlying molecular layer white matter.

mutations accounts for 10–15% of cases.[347] The course of most patients is dominated by cognitive decline that progresses relentlessly in subacute fashion to profound dementia. Particularly characteristic accompanying features are generalized myoclonus, an electroencephalographic 'burst suppression' pattern of periodic spike and wave complexes, and abnormally increased signal intensity in the basal ganglia and thalami on T2- and diffusion-weighted MRI sequences. The diagnosis is further suggested by appearance of a protein antigen (labeled 14-3-3) on CSF immunoassay. The afflicted are typically left vegetative within 6–8 months of symptom onset and rarely survive longer than a year after diagnosis.

The appearance of brain biopsy material, usually secured from the nondominant frontal lobe, depends on disease duration.[347,348] The earliest change perceptible at the light microscopic level consists of spongy vacuolization of the cortex most pronounced in deeper laminae (Fig. 28.34). Rare vacuoles may be localizable to neuronal perikarya, but most appear randomly scattered in the neuropil. The latter are situated principally within neuronal processes on fine structural study, are often traversed by membrane-derived septa, and may contain granular or curled membranous profiles. With disease progression, spongiform change becomes increasingly florid and is attended by conspicuous astrogliosis, neuronal shrinkage, and depopulation. The end-stage cortex is left virtually devoid of recognizable neurons and largely replaced by the tangled processes of hyperplastic astrocytes. At no stage of the disorder is there evidence of an inflammatory response and white matter abnormalities are limited to secondary axonal loss save for rare variants exhibiting spongy leukoencephalopathy.[346] An arresting and diagnostic feature of prion-associated diseases, but one evident in only 5% of CJD cases, is the deposition of amyloid in 'spiked ball' plaques that display radiate, spicular contours and are strongly PAS positive (Fig. 28.35). Often referred to as 'kuru' plaques, these are most often found in the cerebellar cortex (but may also be detected in cerebral gray matter) and are specifically recognized by antibodies to PrP.[347] Cerebrocortical examples may be numerous in familial CJD and have been described as a particularly conspicuous feature of 'variant' CJD cases.[347] Large, clustered deposits of PrP-immunoreactive amyloid in the cerebral and cerebellar cortices typify the dominantly inheritable Gerstmann–Straussler–Scheinker syndrome, also associated with PrP-encoding gene mutations and characterized clinically by a prominent component of progressive cerebellar ataxia.[347]

In the appropriate clinical setting (and in the absence of other potentially explanatory pathologic alterations), the presence of spongiform change alone suffices for a diagnosis of 'probable' CJD. Definitive diagnosis requires satisfaction of any one of the following criteria: (1) finding of spiked ball-type PrP amyloid plaques; (2) demonstration of protease-resistant PrP in biopsy material by specific immunohistochemical or immunoblot methods; (3) detection of a *PrP* gene mutation that is recognized as pathogenic; and (4) transmission of spongiform encephalopathy to an animal host. Readers are referred elsewhere for a fully annotated discussion of these specialized techniques.[347] A diagnosis of 'probable' CJD should not be rendered on minimal histologic criteria inasmuch as scattered intracortical vacuoles and neuronal shrinkage are common artefacts of surgical manipulation. Vacuolization that is principally pericellular may also be caused by edema, hypoxia, autolysis, poor fixation or processing, and toxic and metabolic encephalopathies. Furthermore, spongy changes that may mimic CJD (but that are often restricted to the superficial frontotemporal cortex, insula, or amygdala, and unattended by protease-resistant PrP deposition) can be encountered in otherwise typical examples of Alzheimer disease, cerebrocortical Lewy body disease, Pick disease, corticobasal degeneration, aphasic presenile dementia with lower motor neuron disease, and other dementing disorders. Conversely, an ostensibly negative biopsy should not reassure hospital staff handling tissues and fluids from suspect patients. The histopathologic alterations typical of CJD are not uniformly distributed in the involved brain and methods such as immunohistochemical assessment and Western blot analysis may reveal protease-resistant PrP in neurosurgical specimens evidencing little or no spongiform change.

Biopsy material from patients suspected to have CJD requires cautious handling, even formalinized and paraffin-embedded archival specimens retaining transmissibility. Fixation protocols have been developed that virtually eliminate infectivity while yielding histologic sections of excellent appearance and antigenic integrity (these employ formic acid immersion following initial formalinization),[345,349] but we do not recommend the processing of suspect biopsy material in general surgical pathology laboratories. Rather, these should be forwarded in formalin to facilities such as The National Prion Disease Pathology Surveillance Center of the United States (cjdsurv@po.cwru.edu) that can assess specimens for *PrP* gene mutations as well as PrP deposition.

Primary tumors

Glial tumors

Astrocytic neoplasms

Diffusely infiltrating astrocytomas

Currently classified as tumors of the astrocytic series are neoplasms varying considerably in their epidemiologic features, morphologic attributes, growth patterns, genetic profiles, and clinical behavior. **Diffusely infiltrating astrocytomas** constitute the largest group and include the astrocytic tumors most prevalent in the adult brain. These differ from other members of the astrocytoma 'family' (a fiction) not only in their insidious permeation of CNS tissues but also in an inherent tendency to biologic progression that reflects a stepwise accumulation of defined genetic abnormalities.[380] Yet to be elucidated are the events that initiate such neoplasms in their common sporadic forms. Attention has fastened recently on spontaneous mutations of the isocitrate dehydrogenase (*IDH*) gene complex, particularly *IDH1*, as lesions occurring early on and at extraordinarily high frequency in the representatives of this group (the 'primary glioblastoma' excepted, see below), in oligodendrogliomas, and in tumors of oligoastrocytic composition.[367,372,406] As detailed in the discussion to follow, the diffusely infiltrative astrocytomas have traditionally been divided on cytologic grounds into three basic variants – **fibrillary**, **gemistocytic**, and **protoplasmic**. The first of these is much the most frequently encountered species.

Named for the filamentous cytoplasmic processes that lend to their constituent cells a resemblance, however distorted, to the 'fibrous' astrocytes populating the normal brain and spinal cord, fibrillary astrocytomas collectively constitute the most common primary neoplasms of the human CNS.[380] While most are unassociated with clearly predisposing factors, radiation-related cases are clearly recognized and occasional examples complicate type 1 neurofibromatosis, or the Li–Fraumeni (germline *TP53* gene mutation) syndrome.[380] Astrocytic neoplasms of fibrillary type also occur in complex with hereditary nonpolyposis colorectal carcinoma as defining components of type 1 Turcot syndrome,[380] linked to germline DNA mismatch repair gene mutations, and have been reported in association with the multiple enchondromatosis syndromes known as Ollier or Maffucci disease.[362,380] HIV-1-infected patients may additionally be at increased risk of developing central neuroepithelial tumors, including fibrillary astrocytomas.[353]

Diffuse fibrillary astrocytomas afflict subjects of all ages and may arise at any level of the central neuraxis, but there can be no doubt of their predilection for the cerebral hemispheres of adults. Here they are characteristically centered in white matter, a minority originating in deep gray structures such as the basal ganglia and thalami. Headaches, seizures, focal sensorimotor deficits, and alterations of affect are the principal clinical manifestations of these supratentorial lesions. The common variety of brainstem glioma, encountered in childhood or adolescence as progressive cranial nerve and long tract dysfunction associated with 'pseudohypertrophic' enlargement of the pons on neuroradiologic investigation, is also an astrocytoma of diffuse fibrillary type.[361] Intraspinal examples figure prominently among primary tumors of the cervical and upper thoracic cord, but are vastly outnumbered by ependymomas at more caudal levels. Exceptional variants are situated entirely within the leptomeninges and subarachnoid space, where they may derive from heterotopic neuroglial rests.[388,396]

Neuro-oncologic practice demands that the diffuse fibrillary astrocytomas be subclassified according to their perceived biologic potential. We endorse the World Health Organization (WHO) format.[380] In this three-tiered system, fibrillary astroglial neoplasms are designated as **diffuse astrocytoma (WHO grade II)**, **anaplastic astrocytoma (WHO grade III)**, or **glioblastoma (WHO grade IV)** according to histologic indices presently outlined. The reader will note that the diagnosis of glioblastoma is generally reserved for astrocytic tumors of the highest grade and not applied to poorly differentiated gliomas that clearly exhibit oligodendroglial or ependymal features, though the revised WHO classification recognizes a 'glioblastoma with oligodendroglioma component' (see below). We would again emphasize the disheartening tendency of the diffuse fibrillary astrocytoma, however differentiated and indolent at inception, to grow increasingly alarming to the morphologist and clinically aggressive with the passage of time. A consequence of this inherent instability that bears on practical issues of diagnosis and management is the resulting regional heterogeneity for which this neoplasm is notorious, zonal variations in histologic appearance and proliferative activity potentially confounding the interpretation of observations based on limited tissue samples. The biology of astrocytoma progression is a complex topic beyond the scope of this survey, but we would be remiss to omit at this juncture mention of allelic loss and mutations involving the tumor-suppressing p53 gene (*TP53*) as early, genomically destabilizing events in the evolution of most low-grade fibrillary astrocytic neoplasms.[380]

Diffuse astrocytomas of well-differentiated (WHO grade II) fibrillary type typically present in the third or fourth decade of life and are decidedly uncommon after age 40 (beyond which the overwhelming majority of fibrillary astrocytic tumors exhibit anaplastic histologic features or are frank glioblastomas). Particularly suggestive of a slowly evolving supratentorial astrocytoma (or other low-grade neoplasm) is a protracted preoperative course characterized by intermittent seizures or headache unassociated with focal neurologic deficits. Complaints referable to such lesions may be present for years prior to their discovery, although the advent of sophisticated neuroradiologic techniques has considerably shortened the average predetection interval. As low-grade astrocytomas do not usually provoke significant neovascularization of the infiltrated neural parenchyma, they appear in CT scans and T1-weighted MR images as regions of diminished density that are not opacified ('enhanced') by contrast media employed to define foci of blood–brain barrier disruption (Fig. 28.36). The presence of such enhancement suggests that a lesion shown by biopsy to be an astrocytoma has undergone focal anaplastic progression and should prompt careful review of postoperative neuroradiologic studies to ascertain the region of tumor sampled.

At operation, WHO grade II astrocytomas of the fibrillary variety are spatially indistinct, producing a diffuse expansion and induration of permeated CNS structures along with a highly characteristic blurring or effacement of gray–white landmarks (Fig. 28.37). They may acquire a somewhat mucoid consistency as a result of myxoid change but are not prone to spontaneous hemorrhage or necrosis. Histologic study typically discloses a cellular infiltrate percolating through recognizable neuropil in a patternless array that stands in sharp contrast to the even distribution of hyperplastic astrocytes characteristic of reactive glial proliferations (Fig. 28.38). Samples of invaded cortex may disclose striking aggregation of tumor cells beneath the pia and about neurons, the latter phenomenon known as satellitosis, but it should be pointed out that these formations are shared by (and especially characteristic of) oligodendroglial tumors. A common architectural feature of immeasurable utility in

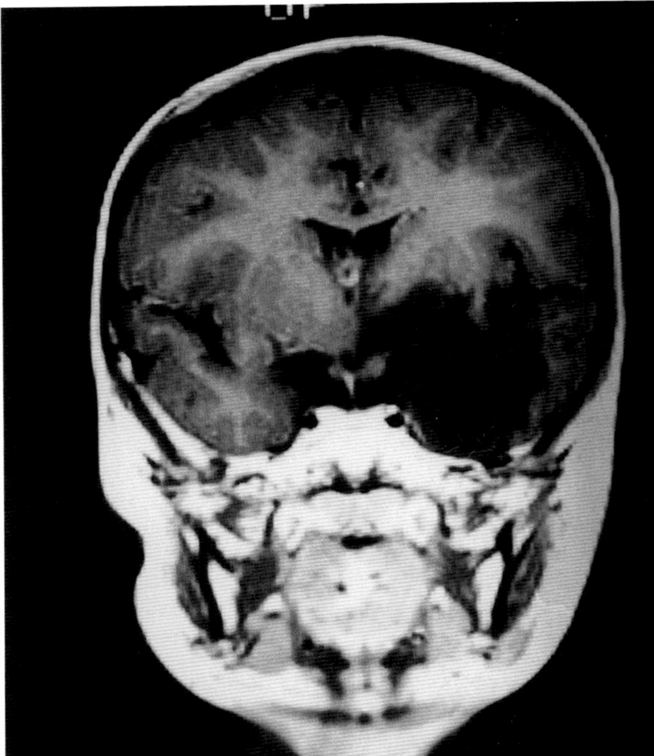

Fig. 28.36 Diffuse fibrillary astrocytoma. Neuroradiologic features common to the low-grade fibrillary astrocytoma in postcontrast MRIs, such as this temporal example, include generalized expansion and hypodensity of infiltrated regions with only modest mass effect and no foci of bright signal enhancement that would indicate blood–brain barrier disruption (see Fig. 28.43 for comparison).

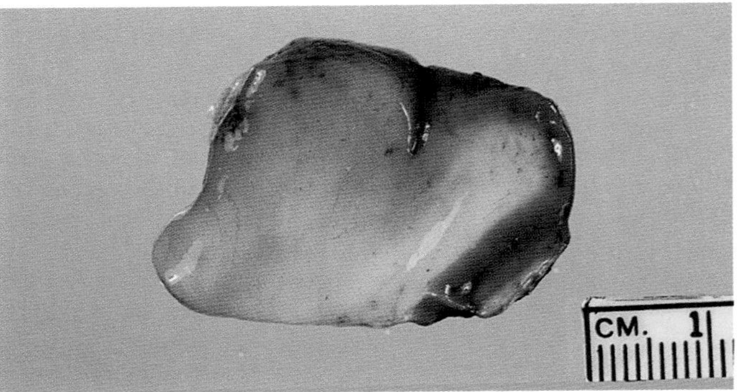

Fig. 28.37 Diffuse fibrillary astrocytoma. The insidious permeation typical of the fibrillary astrocytoma is illustrated in this anterior temporal lobectomy specimen. The gyrus at right maintains a clearly demarcated cortical ribbon over its digitate white matter. Moving to the left, there is diffuse gyral expansion and effacement of these landmarks, reflecting tumoral infiltration. No discrete mass is formed, and, as is characteristic of low-grade examples, there is no evident hemorrhage or necrosis (see Fig. 28.44 for comparison).

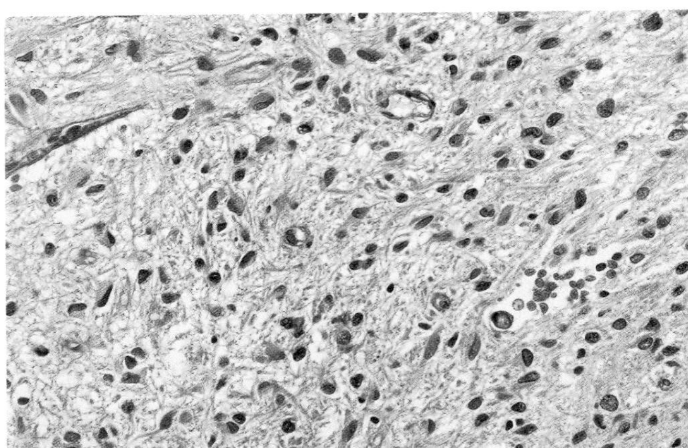

Fig. 28.38 Diffuse fibrillary astrocytoma. Conspicuous cytoplasmic processes, mild nuclear pleomorphism, and only modest hyperchromasia are evidenced by the cells of this well-differentiated astrocytoma. The absence of mitotic activity supports its classification as a low-grade lesion. Note the dyscohesive growth pattern.

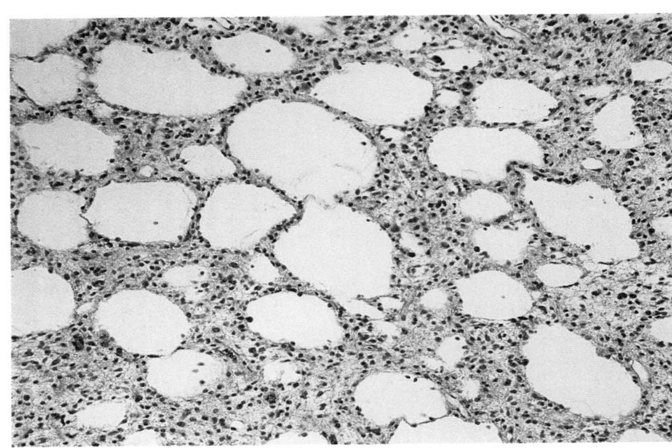

Fig. 28.39 Diffuse fibrillary astrocytoma. Foreign to reactive astroglial proliferations, microcystic change is a particularly conspicuous feature of some low-grade astrocytomas.

establishing the neoplastic nature of the process in question is microcystic change (Fig. 28.39), an alteration to which a variety of glial neoplasms (generally low grade) are prone but rarely, if ever, encountered in a reactive setting. A similar significance attaches to the finding of scattered calcospherites in biopsy material. A conspicuous admixture of foamy macrophages, on the other hand, militates strongly against the diagnosis of astrocytoma in the absence of prior therapy and should instead prompt considerations of demyelinating disease and infarction. Conspicuous lymphocytic cuffing of regional blood vessels, the hallmark of inflammatory CNS disorders, occasionally attends astrocytic neoplasms of the 'garden variety' but among neuroepithelial tumors is far more often a feature of the gemistocytic astrocytoma, pleomorphic xanthoastrocytoma, and ganglioglioma. Finally, survey of a candidate for the diagnosis of WHO grade II astrocytoma should not reveal foci of dense cellularity, proliferation of vascular elements, readily apparent mitotic activity (only rare mitoses found on patient search can be tolerated), or zones of necrosis.

At the cytologic level, astrocytomas of fibrillary type are composed, at least in part, of cells invested with delicate processes that taper from a modest perinuclear expanse of eosinophilic cytoplasm or are represented only as a background meshwork in which 'naked' nuclei appear to lie embedded (Fig. 28.38). Particularly arresting in smear or crush preparations (Fig. 28.40), which are indispens-

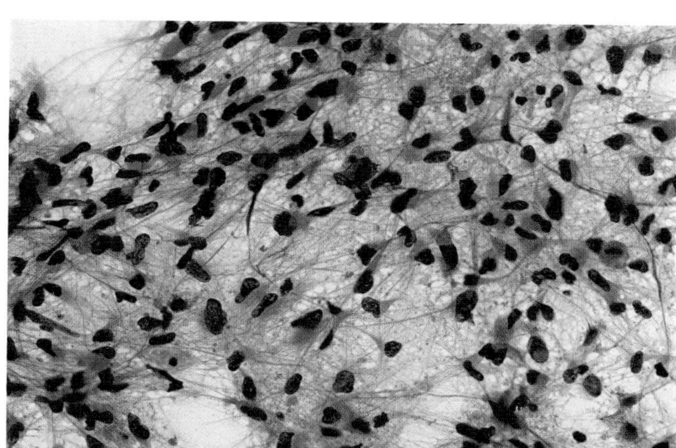

Fig. 28.40 Diffuse fibrillary astrocytoma. A lack of cellular cohesion and conspicuous cytoplasmic processes – features that serve to distinguish astrocytomas from metastatic carcinomas, lymphomas, and other neoplasms – are apparent in this intraoperative crush preparation.

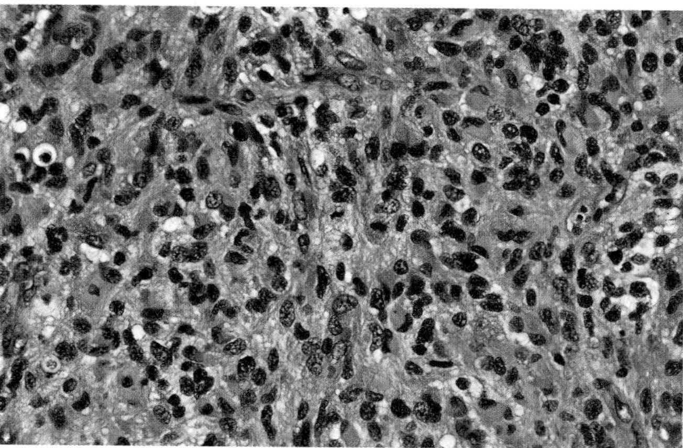

Fig. 28.42 Anaplastic astrocytoma. Compared with its low-grade counterpart (see Fig. 28.38), this lesion exhibits increased cellularity, the cytologic features of a fully malignant neoplasm, and, at center, mitotic figures.

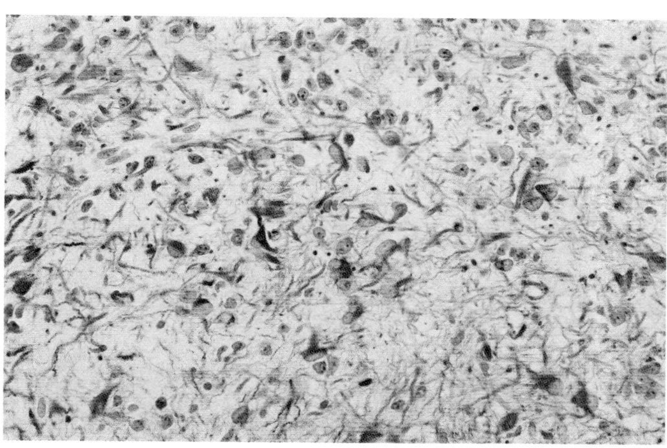

Fig. 28.41 Diffuse fibrillary astrocytoma. An immunoperoxidase preparation demonstrates labeling of tumor cell bodies and processes by a monoclonal antibody to glial fibrillary acidic protein.

able adjuncts (and expedient alternatives) to frozen section for purposes of intraoperative consultation, these may be unipolar or multipolar but, in contrast to the cytoplasmic extensions characteristic of hyperplastic astroglia, do not usually sprout from the cell body in the radial, stellate array for which the astrocyte is named. On ultrastructural study,[400] these processes contain bundles of 7–11 nm ('intermediate') filaments composed of GFAP (Fig. 28.41), the principal cytoskeletal constituent elaborated by human astrocytes, and vimentin.[359,380] Nuclei are typically oval in configuration with smooth contours, do not contain conspicuous nucleoli, often have a vesicular quality, but may be somewhat hyperchromatic. Mild variation in size and shape is to be expected, but conspicuous nuclear pleomorphism calls the diagnosis of low-grade astrocytoma into serious question.

As mentioned above, genetic events that abrogate p53 function commonly occur early in the evolution of diffuse astrocytomas.[380] Abnormal accumulation ('overexpression') of p53 in this setting is often evidenced by aberrant nuclear immunolabeling of neoplastic cells for this protein. The latter phenomenon does not necessarily reflect *TP53* mutation but, when widespread, distances infiltrating astrocytomas from the great majority of oligodendrogliomas (discussed in a later section). Diffuse and intense nuclear labeling for p53 can also be of some utility in segregating diffuse astrocytomas from the general run of reactive processes, but a variety of non-neoplastic disorders (e.g., demyelinating lesions) may evidence unanticipated reactivity on the part of astrocytes and other native cell types.[379] Aberrantly labeling cells in such conditions are usually, though not always, limited in number and manifest reactivity of modest intensity. JC virus-infected oliogdendroglia and astroctyes in progressive multifocal leukoencephalopathy commonly exhibit strong nuclear p53 expression (as well as MIB-1 reactivity). A monoclonal antibody to the dominant form of mutant IDH encountered in diffuse astrocytic (and oligodendroglial) tumors holds promise as an ideal reagent for distinguishing these neoplasms from reactive processes and other neoplastic entities.[356,357]

The **anaplastic astrocytoma (WHO grade III)** often evolves from a well-differentiated precursor lesion of the type just described, a sequence in which losses of heterozygosity involving chromosomes 10q and 19q (among others) as well as deletions affecting genes that encode p16 and other cell cycle regulators are implicated.[380] Accordingly, morphologic evidence of tumor progression may constitute a focal finding in what would otherwise qualify as a histologically favorable lesion. Microscopic examination of the prototypical case reveals an infiltrate that is at a glance more alarmingly cellular and cytologically atypical than that of the low-grade astrocytoma (Fig. 28.42), although biopsies derived from the tumor–CNS interface may contain only scattered neoplastic elements. Nuclear alterations commonly include angulation, dense hyperchromasia, and considerable variation in contour and dimension. Mitotic figures can be demonstrated and most firmly establish the diagnosis. In this regard, we would stress that the solitary mitotic figure found on close scrutiny of a generous biopsy or resection specimen does not an anaplastic astrocytoma make.[364,380] We will render this diagnosis, however, when confronted by any mitoses in a limited (e.g., stereotactic) neurosurgical sample demonstrating a fibrillary astrocytic neoplasm with pronounced nuclear abnormalities. An increase in regional blood vessels is permissible, as is hypertrophy of their lining endothelium, but complex and disorderly proliferation of vasoformative elements or zones of coagulative tumor necrosis in the setting of a cytologically malignant fibrillary astrocytic neoplasm mandate classification of the lesion as a glioblastoma. Readers should note that glioblastoma-like behavior appears to characterize certain astrocytomas that would otherwise qualify as anaplastic/WHO grade III, manifesting neither complex microvascular proliferation nor necrosis, but that are composed predominantly of poorly differentiated and mitotically hyperactive small cell elements.[391] Tumors of this profile, furthermore, often share with glioblastomas amplification of the epidermal growth factor receptor (*EGFR*) gene and expression of the strongly glioblastoma-associated mutant *EGFR-vIII* form.[380,391] We report such lesions as 'high grade astrocytomas of small cell type' and, while acknowledging that these fail to satisfy strict histologic criteria for the diagnosis of glioblastoma, comment on their grade IV biologic potential.

Although its unfortunate title would imply a neoplasm of embryonal character, the **glioblastoma (WHO grade IV)** simply represents the most aggressive of the infiltrating astrocytic tumors. 'Primary' and 'secondary' variants are recognized, the former occurring de novo (i.e., unassociated with demonstrable precursor lesions), the latter resulting from the successful expansion of particularly aggressive clones generated within preexistent, differentiated astrocytic neoplasms and often associated with chronic neurologic complaints indicative of a more protracted incubation.[380] Not surprisingly, secondary glioblastomas share with low-grade and anaplastic fibrillary astrocytomas a high incidence of *IDH1* mutation[367,372,406] and often manifest mutations or deletions affecting *TP53*.[380,401] Such abnormalities are comparatively underrepresented among primary glioblastomas (*IDH* mutations are especially unusual in this setting), these sharing a high incidence of allelic losses involving chromosome 10q but evidencing with greater frequency (among other aberrations) amplification and mutation of the *EGFR* gene on chromosome 7, mutation of the tumor suppressor *PTEN/MMAC1* gene on chromosome 10q23.3, and p16^{INK4a} deletion. *EGFR-vIII*, the major mutant form encountered in glioblastomas, seems highly associated with such tumors.[380,401] Whether predictable differences in prognosis attach to these divergent oncogenetic pathways independent of patient age at diagnosis has been controversial.[380,401] Secondary glioblastomas tend to affect a significantly younger cohort than primary variants (mean ages at presentation being approximately 40 versus 55 years, respectively) and by all accounts advancing age per se is inversely correlated with survival in the setting of fibrillary astrocytic neoplasia.[380] The presence of *IDH* mutation may emerge as a relatively favorable prognostic indicator per se in this regard.[406] Yet another member of the glioblastoma group, the **giant cell glioblastoma**, shares with the secondary glioblastoma a younger patient age at onset, frequent *TP53* mutation, and lack of *EGFR* amplification and p16^{INK4a} deletion but, like the primary variant, arises in the absence of a differentiated precursor lesion, is associated with a brief predetection clinical interval and often manifests *PTEN/MMAC1* gene mutation.[380]

That glioblastomas are biologically far more complex than their division into the foregoing types would imply has become clear through the comprehensive studies of The Cancer Genome Atlas Network,[387] as well as ongoing investigations aimed at the transcriptional and proteomic characterization of these lesions. Integrated analyses of the data generated thus far indicate that a variety of core genetic lesions and signal transduction abnormalities drive glioblastomas as biologic entities. Relatively distinct subclasses have been defined, for example, as exhibiting activation of EGFR or platelet derived growth factor (PDGF) signaling, a third subset by loss of neurofibromatosis type 1 (*NF1*) gene activity that inhibits the Ras pathway.[355,387] Profiling analyses[393] have demonstrated that glioblastomas can be segregated into a prognostically more favorable 'proneural' group that expresses genes involved in normal neurocytogenesis and differentiation versus 'proliferative' and 'mesenchymal' subtypes characterized by activation of gene programs that promote cell replication and angiogenesis, respectively. Again, these are continuing efforts that cannot be further detailed here but that promise to transform clinical approaches to these neoplasms.

Like astrocytomas of lower grade, glioblastomas may be discovered on evaluation for seizures or headache but are often attended by subacutely evolving neurologic deficits indicative of their more rapid growth and destructive invasion. A subset present in sudden, stroke-like fashion as a consequence of intratumoral hemorrhage, and occasional examples mimic metastatic disease by virtue of their multifocality.[352] Especially characteristic on CT or MR evaluation is a pattern of ring-like contrast enhancement that reflects their abnormal vascularization and tendency to spontaneous central necrosis (Fig. 28.43). On gross inspection, glioblastomas may seem relatively circumscribed and often appear to be more clearly demarcated from neighboring tissues than their better-differentiated counterparts – deceptively so, inasmuch as neoplastic cells regularly invade neuropil well beyond the apparent tumor perimeter. Hemorrhagic discoloration and foci of yellow softening indicative of coagulative necrosis impart a variegated appearance to most examples that should immediately suggest their virulent nature (Fig. 28.44).

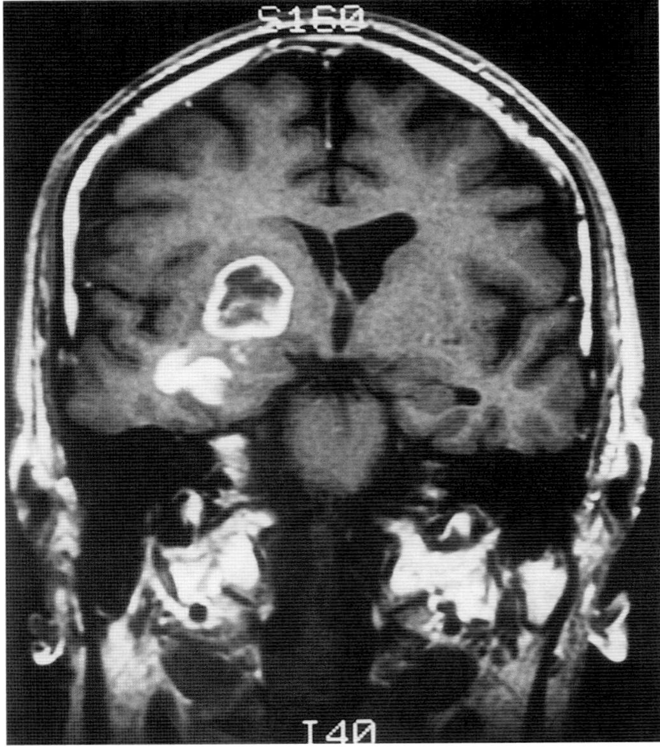

Fig. 28.43 Glioblastoma multiforme. In postcontrast injection CT or (shown here) MR studies, many glioblastomas are characterized by a bright ('enhancing') ring (representing intact, abnormally vascularized tumor tissue in which the blood–brain barrier is disrupted) that surrounds a region of hypodensity (central necrosis). The gyriform temporal lobe enhancement below this basal ganglionic example attests to neoplastic infiltration beyond the deceptively well-delimited ring margin.

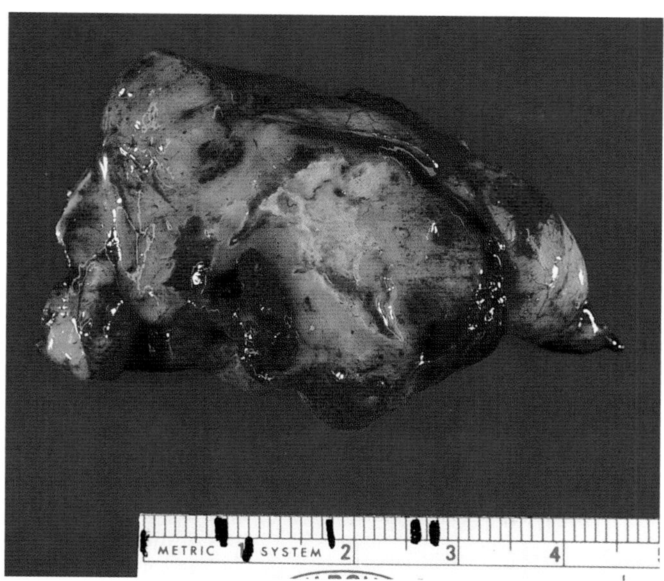

Fig. 28.44 Glioblastoma multiforme. Foci of hemorrhage and geographic yellow discoloration indicative of necrosis impart a variegated appearance to this example.

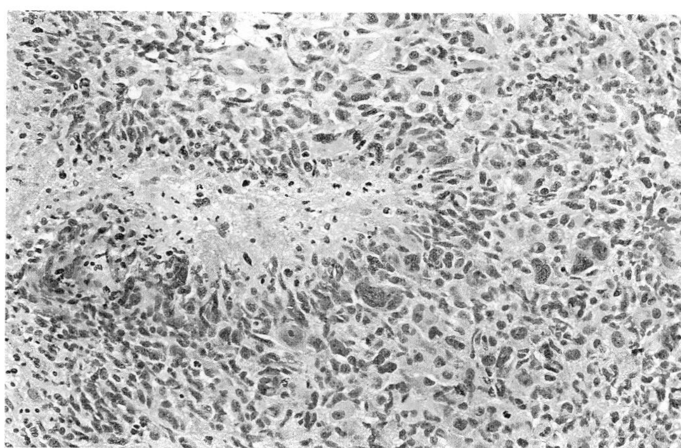

Fig. 28.45 Glioblastoma multiforme. Dense cellularity, striking pleomorphism, and zones of coagulative necrosis lined by 'palisading' tumor cells characterize the prototypical glioblastoma.

On histologic study, the glioblastoma is a highly cellular and mitotically active neoplasm. Its cytologic makeup is subject to extreme variation (thus the traditional designation of this lesion as glioblastoma 'multiforme'). Differentiated elements may be intermingled with bizarre multinucleated tumor giant cells, spindled, epithelioid,[377] rhabdoid,[363,377,405] signet ring[382] or small anaplastic forms altogether devoid of identifying astrocytic features (Fig. 28.45). The last often come to dominate the histologic picture at recurrence, selectively repopulating tumors subjected to therapy, but may also constitute the nearly exclusive elements of select **small cell glioblastomas** at presentation. EGFR amplification and mutation appear to be particularly common in the latter.[380]

A significant and controversial departure from previously endorsed practice concerns the nomenclature now recommended by the WHO for high-grade glial neoplasms having regions of both astrocytic and oligodendroglial appearance. Specifically,

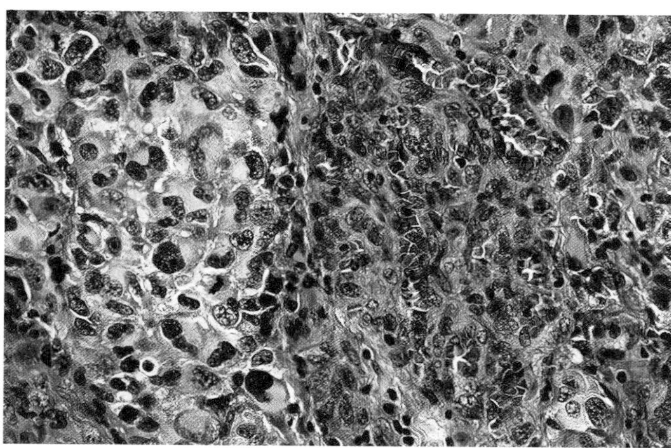

Fig. 28.46 Glioblastoma multiforme. Note the complex, 'glomeruloid' quality of the microvascular proliferation at right. Astrocytic elements are seen at left.

pathologists are advised to designate a tumor of this type as '**glioblastoma with oligodendroglioma component**' rather than anaplastic oligoastrocytoma (as formerly termed) if necrosis (with or without pseudopalisading) is identified.[380] The rationale resides in studies reporting that gliomas of this kind are associated with significantly shorter survival intervals compared to examples lacking foci of tumor necrosis (see section below on Mixed gliomas for additional citations). Affected patients, however, seem to fare somewhat better than those with glioblastomas of entirely astroctyic aspect and at least some of these tumors exhibit an oligodendroglioma-like genetic profile in their manifesting co-deletions of chromosomes 1p/19q.[370,380,401] Parenthetically, the latter alterations characterize a very small subset of histologically conventional astrocytomas, anaplastic astrocytomas, and glioblastomas that may be more responsive to treatment and associated with longer survival intervals than their genetically typical counterparts.[380]

An arresting phenomenon common to many glioblastomas is a complex form of microvascular hyperplasia, driven in paracrine fashion by tumor-derived mitogens such as vascular endothelial growth factor, in which proliferating blood vessels come to be lined by cells heaped up in disorderly fashion and are ultimately transformed into glomeruloid or solid tufts (Fig. 28.46). Although often referred to simply as 'endothelial' hyperplasia, this process involves a number of vessel-associated cell types, prominent among which are pericytic/myoid elements expressing smooth muscle-related antigens.[366,403] Its identification in neurosurgical material from patients not previously subjected to radiation therapy suffices for a diagnosis of glioblastoma by WHO criteria, as does the finding of focal coagulative tumor necrosis regardless of whether neoplastic cells align themselves about such zones in the prototypical palisades that are a 'textbook' feature of this lesion[380] (Fig. 28.45).

Irradiation induces in the glioblastoma a variety of morphologic alterations, the most predictable being widespread necrosis unrelated to regional tumor cell density (usually much reduced) and vasculopathic changes that include ectasia, fibrinoid necrosis, and obliterative mural fibroplasia (Fig. 28.47). Florid astrogliosis and infiltration by macrophages, the latter identifiable by their immunoreactivity for HAM-56, CD68, and other histiocytic 'markers', may complicate the recognition of neoplastic elements. Some re-resection specimens, in fact, consist solely of necrotic debris or contain only scattered suspect cells exhibiting cytopathic alterations, presumably treatment related, such as grotesque karyomegaly

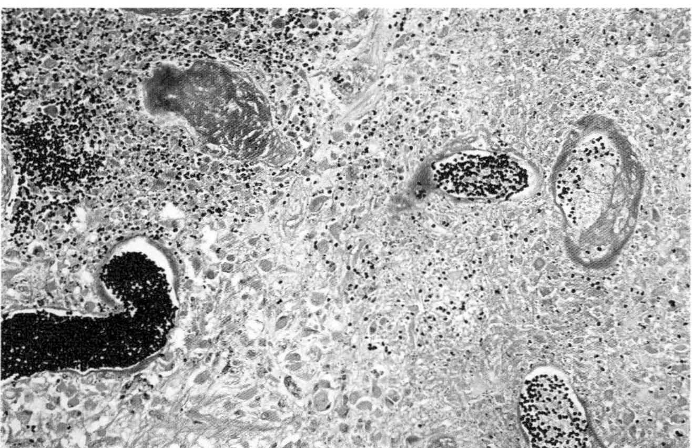

Fig. 28.47 Radiation effect. A marked reduction in cellularity, extensive necrosis, and necrotizing fibrinoid vasculopathy with vascular thrombosis and ectasia typify astrocytic neoplasms injured by irradiation.

and dense hyperchromasia with chromatin smudging and nuclear vacuolization. Although we favor the view that these cells are neoplastic, albeit damaged, it is conceivable that they represent in some cases hyperplastic astrocytes displaying radiation atypia. Whatever their origin, these elements do not imply disease progression, and we report such specimens as exhibiting treatment effect with only minimal evidence of persistent, injured tumor. The diagnosis of recurrence rests on firmest grounds when aggregates of cytologically unaltered and mitotically active tumor cells can be demonstrated, cellular palisading about foci of necrosis also constituting unimpeachable testimony to treatment failure. In some instances, the necrotizing and vasculopathic changes described here will be found to involve brain tissue (typically white matter, which is particularly susceptible to ionizing irradiation) manifesting no tumoral infiltration. This toxic process (cerebral radionecrosis) characteristically interrupts a period of apparent remission and neurologic recovery measured in months (or, in some cases, years) and may mimic post-therapy relapse to clinical and neuroradiologic perfection.

Although most of the astrocytic neoplasms under discussion are confidently distinguished from primary cerebral sarcomas and tumors metastatic to the CNS by virtue of their characteristic cytologic features and dyscohesive patterns of infiltration, select variants may occasion considerable confusion in this regard. A case in point is the **giant cell glioblastoma**, a tumor noted for its unusual circumscription, sarcomatoid cytologic features, and reticulin-rich matrix.[381,390] Once regarded as a 'monstrocellular' sarcoma, the glial nature of this neoplasm can be demonstrated by its immunohistochemical labeling for GFAP. The same can be said for spindle cell and 'xanthosarcomatous', lipid-rich variants of glioblastoma.[375] We have seen a number of high-grade astrocytic neoplasms misclassified as fibrosarcomas or malignant fibrous histiocytomas when immunohistochemical studies demonstrated cytoplasmic labeling for such nonspecific antigens as vimentin, α_1-antitrypsin, or α_1-antichymotrypsin, but failed to include examination for GFAP expression. The emergence of GFAP-negative sarcomatous components within astrocytic and other glial tumors ('gliosarcoma') is discussed below (see Gliomesenchymal tumors). Still other aggressive and poorly differentiated astrocytic tumors contain glandular or gland-like ('adenoid') formations,[374,386,398] undergo squamous metaplasia,[385] exhibit regions of adipocyte-like cellular metamorphosis[397] or assume clear cell cytologic features (owing to cytoplasmic lipidization) and a cohesive disposition in nests and sheets that bring 'balloon cell' melanoma and carcinomas of renal or adrenocortical origin to mind.[399] Immunolabeling for cytokeratin[359,360,389] and EMA[369] may further conspire to obscure the glial lineage of these and other astrocytic neoplasms. We emphasize in this regard the regular labeling of reactive and neoplastic astrocytes with the AE1/3 cytokeratin 'cocktail', these usually proving nonreactive for CAM 5.2, CK7, CK20, and the noncytokeratin epithelial marker Ber-EP4.[389] Again, assay for GFAP expression may be decisive in the unmasking of epithelioid glioblastoma variants, although the literature admittedly contains depictions of carcinomas and meningiomas that were focally decorated by antisera to this marker protein (see sections on meningothelial and secondary tumors). Glioblastomas may also harbor primitive-appearing papillary structures that invite confusion with the medulloepithelioma.[384] We further call the reader's attention to the existence of astrocytic tumors that undergo a striking granular cell metamorphosis resulting from the intracytoplasmic accumulation of engorged secondary lysosomes.[354] While these peculiar neoplasms may exhibit remarkably benign cytologic features, **granular cell astrocytomas** of this type are characterized as a group by an aggressive clinical evolution. Immunolabeling of their cytoplasm for CD68 can result in the misidentification of such tumors as reactive histiocytic infiltrates.

The astrocytic neoplasms under discussion can contain ganglion cell-like forms or small cell elements of primitive appearance that raise question of neuronal or neuroblastic differentiation. While potentially exhibiting immunoreactivity for class III β-tubulin,[373] these constituents (and their patently astroglial neighbors) generally retain at least focal GFAP expression and usually fail to label for more neuron-restricted antigens such as synaptophysin and the NeuN[404] and Hu[365] nucleoproteins. This is not to say, however, that the infiltrating astrocytomas are effectively straightjacketed in their differentiating potential. Differentiation along neuronal lines, in fact, is now recognized as an occasional attribute of neoplasms otherwise qualifying as members of the astrocytic, oligodendroglial, and ependymal series. The entity dubbed '**glioneuronal tumor with neuropil-like islands**'[351] can with much justification be viewed as a peculiar variant of infiltrating astrocytoma and is classed as such in the current WHO taxonomy.[380] Typically dominated by fibrillary and gemistocytic astroglial components, at the WHO grade II or III level, this lesion is distinguished by its content of sharply delimited micronodular collections of a delicate meshwork exhibiting intense granular immunolabeling for synaptophysin. These are rimmed in rosetted fashion or internally populated by oligodendocyte-like clear cells (neurocytes, actually) that often express NeuN and Hu. The diffuse growth pattern of this tumor, its predilection for the cerebral hemispheres of adults, the frequency with which it demonstrates aberrant p53 expression and clinical course (comparable to that of infiltrating astrocytomas matched for grade and including a capacity for biologic progression) are all consonant with the view that the glioneuronal tumor with neuropil-like islands is fundamentally of the conventional astrocytic group.

Similar considerations apply to '**glioblastomas with primitive-neuroectodermal tumor-like components**'.[392] These harbor, often disposed in relatively demarcated nodules of high density, cellular elements indistinguishable from those characterizing medulloblastomas and other embryonal neoplasms by virtue of their diminutive sizes, undifferentiated cytologic profiles, loss of GFAP expression, immunolabeling for synaptophysin (as well as other neuronal 'markers'), and alarming proliferative activity. Such components may emerge only in recurrent neurosurgical material and usually make their appearance in astrocytic tumors exhibiting the histology and genetic alterations typical of secondary glioblastomas. That this is an unusual form of biologic progression complicating glioblastomas is further suggested by the observation that widespread p53 reactivity and PTEN abnormalities (foreign to the great majority of embryonal CNS tumors) are commonly evidenced by both astroglial and primitive-looking populations, whereas the latter may selectively manifest MYC amplifications (a phenomenon unassociated with astrocytic neoplasia, but not uncommon in medulloblastomas and the like). The experience communicated to date indicates that a substantially increased risk of dissemination via the CSF attaches to glioblastomas of this kind, these generally proving refractory to regimens employed in the treatment of conventional glioblastomas and potentially showing some response to adjuvant protocols used against medulloblastomas and other neoplasms of embryonal character.

The prognosis of a given fibrillary astrocytic neoplasm is a complex function of both clinical and morphologic variables. Patient age, functional status on presentation, tumor location, and histology all affect the outcome of supratentorial examples.[380] Faring best are young subjects harboring low-grade lesions that are unassociated with focal neurologic deficits and that are situated in the cerebral hemispheres (as opposed to corpus callosum, basal ganglia, or thalami). Follow-up studies of patients identified and managed since the advent of CT and MR imaging (i.e., in the era of 'early' detection) suggest median survivals in the 6- to 10-year range under such relatively favorable circumstances, death typically following tumor progression to glioblastoma.[380] Whether attempted resection or radiotherapy prolongs the lives of patients with low-grade cerebral hemispheric astrocytomas is a contentious matter, many neuro-oncologists electing to simply follow affected individuals until there is compelling clinical or neuroradiologic evidence of tumor growth. Comparably situated anaplastic astrocytomas and glioblastomas, by contrast, are unarguably aggressive neoplasms associated with median postoperative survival periods of 24–48 and 12 months, respectively, despite irradiation and adjuvant chemotherapy.[380] Inactivation of the DNA repair enzyme O^6-methylguanine-DNA methyltransferase (MGMT), usually through promoter hypermethylation of its encoding gene, is emerging both as a predictor of enhanced tumor responsiveness to alkylating agent chemotherapy and generally favorable prognostic marker.[371] Longer post-treatment survival intervals also seem to characterize *IDH*-mutant high-grade astrocytomas compared to their *IDH*-intact counterparts.[406] Under active investigation in the treatment of glioblastomas are agents against EGFR, its major mutant form *EGFRvIII*, and downstream targets of these and other kinases. Again, young patients tend to live longer than middle-aged or elderly adults. Ultimately, however, the insidious manner in which these lesions permeate brain tissues beyond their neuroradiologically defined and grossly apparent confines frustrates operative attempts at local disease control and sets the stage for progressive infiltration of neighboring cerebral parenchyma by chemoresistant clones. This, the primary pattern of treatment failure, is occasionally complicated by the development of CSF-borne neuraxial metastases and, rarely, by spread to somatic sites, such as bone, lung, liver, or lymph node.[376,380] Most unusual, but well documented, are cases in which systemic metastases have been apparent on initial patient presentation,[376] and the bizarre phenomenon of inadvertent tumor transplantation via solid organ allografts has also been the subject of isolated reports.[350]

Similarly dismal is the prognosis attached to diffusely invasive astrocytic neoplasms of the brainstem, most of which are high grade at diagnosis.[361] It is the exceptional patient who remains alive more than 2 years from symptom onset. These lesions may mimic pilocytic astrocytomas in the generally limited biopsies secured from the bulbar region by virtue of a certain spindling imposed on their constituent cells as these infiltrate the compact fiber tracts of the pontine base. Dense hyperchromasia and conspicuous nuclear pleomorphism usually serve to distinguish these cells from well-differentiated piloid astrocytes, but in questionable cases their elongate nuclei can be shown by the appropriate histochemical methods to lie among myelinated axons rather than in a meshwork of bipolar, GFAP-immunoreactive cytoplasmic processes. It should also be pointed out that pilocytic astrocytomas (discussed later) tend at bulbar levels to a sharp circumscription and exophytic growth from the dorsal pontomedullary junction generally foreign to fibrillary astrocytic neoplasms of the brainstem. Readers are referred to our discussion of pilocytic astrocytomas below for details regarding the molecular genetic segregation of these from astrocytomas of diffuse type. Not surprisingly, patients with high-grade astrocytomas of the cerebellum and spinal cord do very poorly, whereas a subset of indolent, well-differentiated lesions occurring in the latter location appear amenable to radical resection and are compatible with long-term survival.[358]

Quantifiable methods for the determination of proliferative potential are now in wide employ as adjuncts to the conventional morphologic assessment of astrocytic and other primary CNS neoplasms. Immunohistochemical assay for the Ki-67 antigen, a non-histone nucleoprotein selectively expressed by actively cycling cells and demonstrable in paraffin-embedded material using the MIB-1 monoclonal antibody, has proven especially addicting to surgical neuropathologists in this regard (Fig. 28.48). Truth be told, the performance of this reagent is subject to all the technical vagaries that attend immunohistochemical methods, the calculation of MIB-1 labeling indices (i.e., fraction of decorated tumor cell nuclei) potentially influenced by antigen-retrieval strategies, section thickness, choice of region for quantitative analysis, number of cells assessed, use of automated versus manual counting techniques and level of nuclear staining intensity required for positive identification. Interpretation of the literature is complicated by the nonuniform manner in which studies have been conducted, but general survey[380] discloses a broad correlation of histologic grade and labeling index, and reveals (unfortunately) overlapping index ranges for low-grade astrocytomas (<5%), anaplastic astrocytomas (5–10%), and glioblastomas (>10%). Ki-67/MIB-1 labeling fractions in excess of 5–7.5% emerge from select studies[380,383] as powerful predictors of relatively shortened survival in this patient cohort, but not all

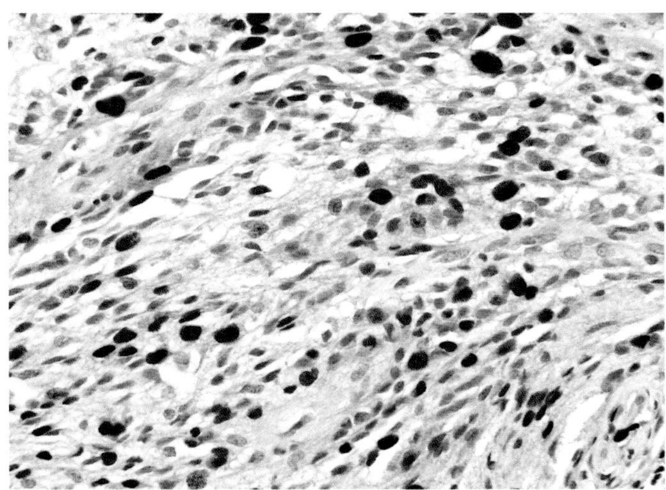

Fig. 28.48 Markers of cellular proliferation. Actively cycling tumor cells within a glioblastoma are identified in this immunoperoxidase preparation by their nuclear labeling with the MIB-1 monoclonal antibody.

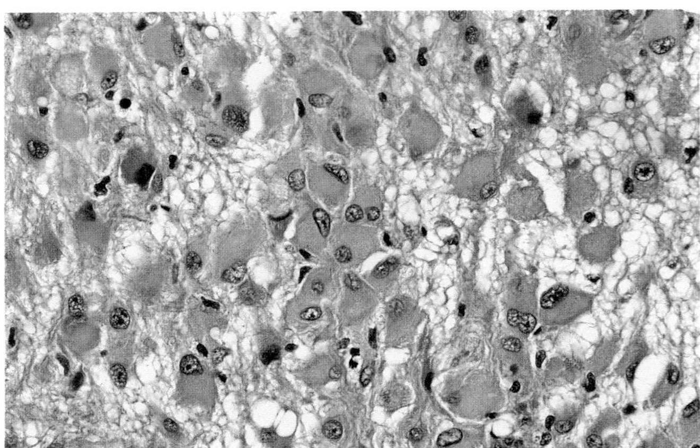

Fig. 28.49 Gemistocytic astrocytoma. Heavily dominated on initial resection by the large gemistocytes shown here, this example recurred 11 months after radiotherapy and chemotherapy. Re-resection demonstrated progression to glioblastoma. Note that these cells retain the oval and somewhat vesicular nuclei of astrocytes. For a comparison with the 'minigemistocytic' variant of oligodendroglioma, see Figure 28.63B.

investigations support their utility as independent prognostic indicators[368,380] and their significance taken on an individual case basis has been called into question. In practice, we employ MIB-1 only in the evaluation of histologically low-grade or 'borderline' fibrillary astrocytomas and simply append in our reporting of values above 5% a comment to the effect that such levels suggest a heightened proliferative potential.

Diffuse astrocytic neoplasms of fibrillary type may contain large tumor cells characterized by globose masses of glassy eosinophilic cytoplasm and peripherally displaced nuclei that seem on the verge of extrusion from their parent cell bodies (Fig. 28.49). Termed gemistocytes (from the Greek *gemistos* for laden or full), these result from an accumulation of glial-type intermediate filaments that form compacted paranuclear whorls and extend into stout cytoplasmic processes. Only exceptionally do such cells dominate the histologic picture. The designation of **gemistocytic astrocytoma** has been subjectively applied to tumors harboring these elements in varying density, current WHO guidelines[380] endorsing the suggestion[378] that gemistocytes constitute at least 20% of the neoplastic population if this diagnosis is to be entertained.

Gemistocyte-rich astrocytomas are virtually restricted to the cerebral hemispheres of adults. They often exhibit conspicuous perivascular infiltration by lymphocytes and typically contain small, poorly differentiated neoplastic cells that emerge from MIB-1 (Ki-67) immunolabeling studies as more actively proliferative than their large-bodied companions.[402] Aberrant nuclear immunolabeling for p53 is commonly seen, a phenomenon that presumably reflects the particular prevalence of *TP53* gene mutations in astrocytomas of gemistocytic type.[380] Gliovascular structuring may be apparent, radially arranged gemistocytes projecting short cytoplasmic processes towards centering blood vessels to form pseudorosettes that may bring ependymoma or astroblastoma to mind. The latter tumor types do not permeate neuroparenchyma in the diffuse fashion of the gemistocytic astrocytoma, true gemistocyte formation being foreign to the astroblastoma and only rarely encountered as a focal finding in ependymal neoplasms of otherwise conventional appearance. Care must also be taken lest the designation of gemistocytic astrocytoma be applied to oligodendroglial tumors composed of diminutive 'mini'-gemistocytes or to the exceptional oligodendroglioma undergoing macrogemistocytic change with tumor progression. These usually do not manifest perivascular lymphocytic cuffing, may exhibit a distinctively lobular or pavement-like architecture, and almost invariably harbor telltale oligodendroglial elements of classic clear cell type. Furthermore, oligodendrogliomas usually display little or no nuclear p53 immunoreactivity (*TP53* mutations are uncommon in this tumor group) and often evidence signature genetic abnormalities – specifically, combined chromosomal 1p and 19q deletions. The reader is referred to the section on oligodendrogliomas for further details and references.

Gemistocyte-rich astrocytomas that do not exhibit mitotic activity, complex microvascular proliferation or necrosis are currently accorded WHO grade II status.[380] We, however, cannot recommend the grading of these lesions without modifying comment. While acknowledging that such tumors do not necessarily behave in a highly aggressive fashion, our experience conforms to that of other observers who have found gemistocytic astrocytomas especially prone to histologic and clinical progression as compared to other ostensibly 'grade II' astrocytic neoplasms.[378,402] We append to the diagnosis a statement acknowledging this increased biologic potential. Mitotically active variants can be reported as anaplastic gemistocytic astrocytomas (WHO grade III), examples displaying microvascular hyperplasia or necrosis qualifying as gemistocytic glioblastomas (WHO grade IV).

In contrast to the fibrous astrocyte, 'protoplasmic' astrocytes principally reside in gray, rather than white, matter and fashion elongated, GFAP-rich cytoplasmic processes only in pathologic circumstances. Process-poor tumor cells resembling protoplasmic astrocytes are often apparent in foci of cortical invasion by conventional fibrillary astrocytomas and, as presently discussed, populate the microcystic regions common to astrocytomas of pilocytic type. Uncommon neoplasms that have traditionally been dubbed **protoplasmic astrocytomas** are composed exclusively of such cells.[380,395] Generally arising in the cerebral cortices of children and young adults, these present as superficially situated masses of gelatinous gray tissue. Histologic study reveals cytologically uniform cells evenly suspended in a cobweb-like matrix of short cytoplasmic fibrils and myxoid material that accumulates in microcysts of varying diameter. Nuclei, typically monomorphous, are round or slightly oval, mitotic activity is exceptional, and MIB-1 labeling indices are low (with a mean <1% in one analysis[394]). Complex microvascular hyperplasia and necrosis, furthermore, are foreign to these slow-growing, WHO grade II lesions. In practice, the diagnosis of protoplasmic astrocytoma has fallen into disuse owing to the problematic histologic distinction of this entity from diffuse astrocytomas of the usual type, from oligodendroglioma and pilocytic astrocytoma as well as the absence of any defining antigenic or genetic features.

Pilocytic astrocytomas

Pilocytic astrocytomas typically present in childhood, adolescence, or early adult life – hence their common designation by the prefacing 'juvenile' – and exhibit a decided predilection for the cerebellum, third ventricular/hypothalamic region, and anterior optic pathway.[427] They constitute the great majority of tumors collected under the traditional appellations of 'cerebellar astrocytoma' and 'optic nerve glioma', including those examples of the latter, often bilateral, complicating type 1 neurofibromatosis (NF-1 or Recklinghausen disease). NF-1 patients are also at risk of developing cerebellar, and other extraoptic, astrocytomas of pilocytic type. Pilocytic astrocytomas may arise within the cerebral hemispheres,[401,424] basal ganglia/thalami,[419] or spinal cord[420] and are overrepresented within a clinically distinctive subset of bulbar tumors that deviate

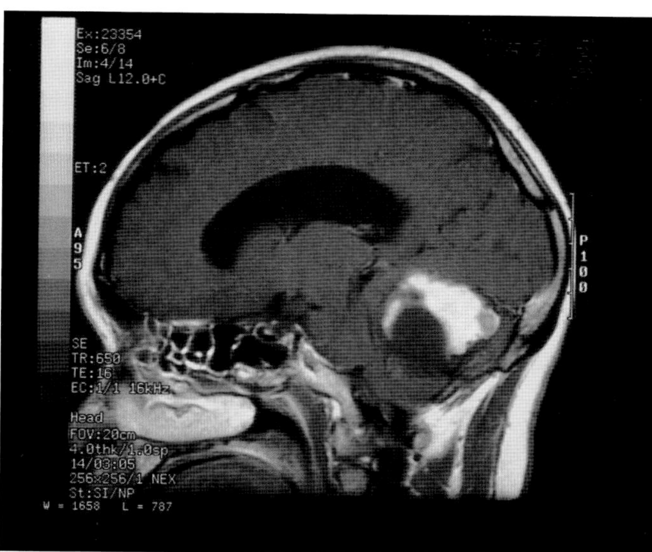

Fig. 28.50 Pilocytic astrocytoma. This typical cerebellar example is characterized by a solid, brightly contrast-enhancing mural component and associated cyst.

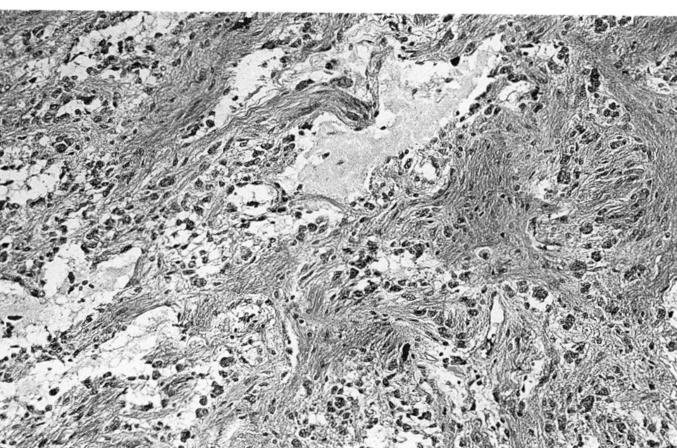

Fig. 28.51 Pilocytic astrocytoma. The biphasic cellular populations and architecture of the classic pilocytic astrocytoma are in evidence. The lesion's process-bearing spindle cell ('piloid') constituents fashion a densely fibrillar matrix, whereas its process-poor ('protoplasmic') elements aggregate in regions of myxoid change that often progress to microcyst formation.

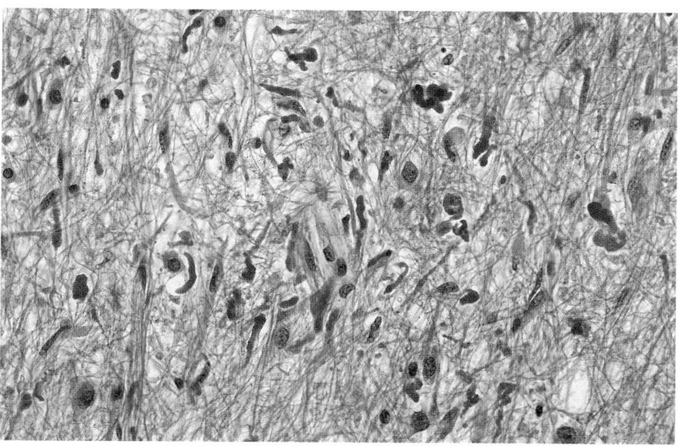

Fig. 28.52 Pilocytic astrocytoma. Varicose Rosenthal fibers lie among the otherwise delicate and hair-like cytoplasmic processes for which the pilocytic astrocytoma is named.

from the diffuse, fibrillary astrocytic neoplasms typical of the brainstem by virtue of their circumscription, by their tendency to bulge into the fourth ventricle in 'dorsally exophytic' fashion, and far more favorable prognosis.[361]

Save for those tumors positioned in the anterior visual pathway, which produce a fusiform, 'pseudohypertrophic' expansion of the optic nerve, and a subset of cerebellar examples having diffusely invasive components,[411] pilocytic astrocytomas tend to be relatively demarcated, to be nodular in contour, and frequently project into sizable cysts that may account for most of their mass effect and associated neurologic symptoms. Homogeneous contrast enhancement typifies the solid elements of the pilocytic astrocytoma, a feature serving, along with the tendency to macrocystic change and the high signal intensity often displayed on both T1- and T2-weighted MRI study, to distinguish this lesion from the diffuse fibrillary astrocytoma on neuroradiologic examination (Fig. 28.50).

The prototypical pilocytic astrocytoma is an architecturally and cytologically biphasic neoplasm composed of tumor cells in both fascicular and microcystic array (Fig. 28.51). The former component is fashioned of elements bearing the delicate, bipolar cytoplasmic processes for which the tumor is named, the adjectival pilocytic deriving from the Greek root for hair. These are typically woven in a dense fibrillar matrix in which oval or spindly tumor cell nuclei appear to lie embedded, a given cell's slender and remarkably elongated processes being optimally visualized in cytologic preparations that are useful adjuncts to the study of frozen sections during intraoperative consultation. In microcystic regions, neoplastic cells are arranged about, or float suspended in, pools of basophilic, myxoid material. Here a 'protoplasmic' cytology is assumed, tumor cells exhibiting rounded nuclear contours and manifesting little tendency to elaborate cytoplasmic extensions. It should be noted that the relative admixture of piloid and microcystic elements varies greatly from case to case. The latter are particularly likely to dominate cerebellar examples in children. Other common histologic features include oligodendroglioma-like clear cell foci and an angiomatoid vasculature characterized by complex arborization, hyaline mural fibroplasia, and ectasia. Microcalcifications may be encountered at the histologic level, though neuroradiologically evident tumoral calcification is rare. Mitotic activity is generally nil or difficult to demonstrate (some 30% of cases evidence 1–2 mitoses per 50 high-power fields[364]) and MIB-1 labeling indices usually do not exceed 1–3%.[364] A melanotic astroglial neoplasm with features of pilocytic astrocytoma has been recorded.[429]

Classically associated with the juvenile pilocytic astrocytoma are the cytoplasmic structures known as Rosenthal fibers and eosinophilic granular bodies. Vermiform acidophilic densities typically restricted to the tumor's richly fibrillated regions (Fig. 28.52), Rosenthal fibers represent masses of granular, electron-dense material surrounded by glial filaments (Fig. 28.53). They may be labeled by antisera to alpha B-crystallin and a related 27-kDa heat shock protein but are not immunoreactive in GFAP preparations.[414,418] Eosinophilic granular bodies are clustered acidophilic globules (Fig. 28.54) that probably derive from lysosomes and are immunoreactive for α_1-antitrypsin, α_1-antichymotrypsin, ubiquitin, and alpha B-crystallin.[416,421] At the ultrastructural level, granular bodies represent membrane-bound collections of amorphous

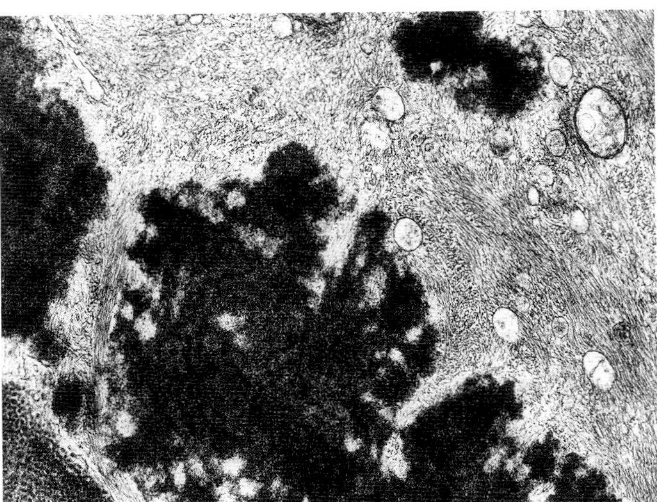

Fig. 28.53 Pilocytic astrocytoma. On transmission electron microscopic study, Rosenthal fibers are intracytoplasmic aggregates of granular, electron-dense material intimately associated with intermediate filaments, the latter composed principally of glial fibrillary acidic protein. (×25 350)

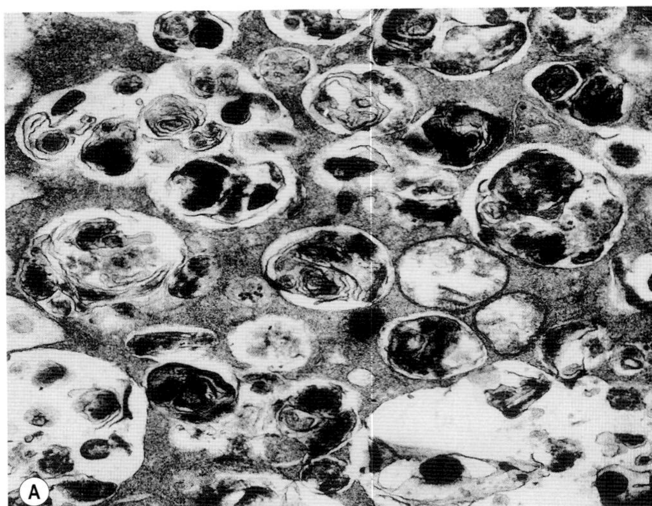

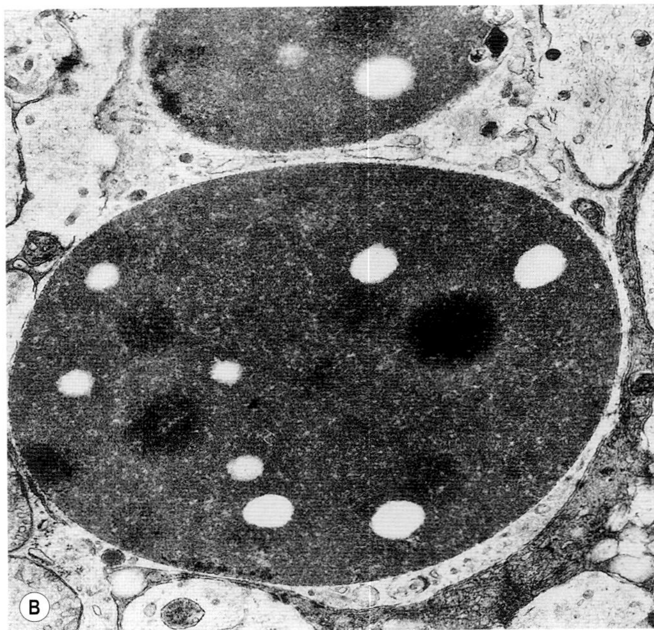

Fig. 28.55 Pilocytic astrocytoma. At the ultrastructural level, eosinophilic granular bodies appear to represent engorged lysosomes containing membranous debris ('myelin figures') (**A**) or amorphous, variably electron-dense material (**B**). (**A**, ×26 500; **B**, ×14 200)

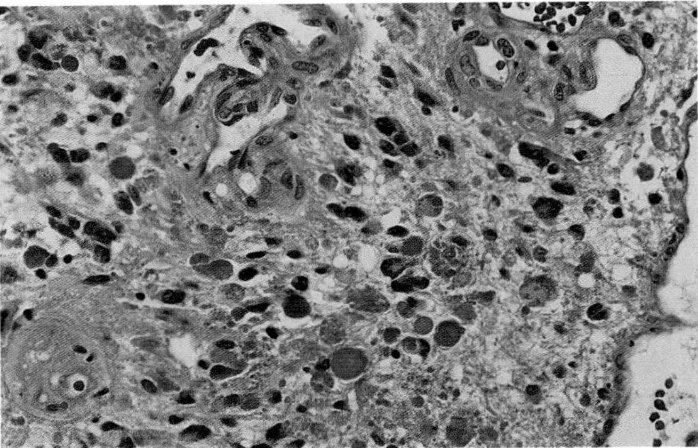

Fig. 28.54 Pilocytic astrocytoma. Eosinophilic granular bodies are typically associated with, although not restricted to, three indolent neuroepithelial tumors: the pilocytic astrocytoma, pleomorphic xanthoastrocytoma, and ganglioglioma.

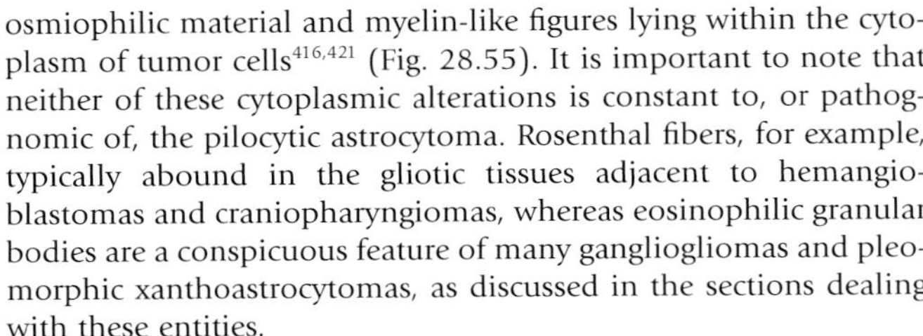

osmiophilic material and myelin-like figures lying within the cytoplasm of tumor cells[416,421] (Fig. 28.55). It is important to note that neither of these cytoplasmic alterations is constant to, or pathognomic of, the pilocytic astrocytoma. Rosenthal fibers, for example, typically abound in the gliotic tissues adjacent to hemangioblastomas and craniopharyngiomas, whereas eosinophilic granular bodies are a conspicuous feature of many gangliogliomas and pleomorphic xanthoastrocytomas, as discussed in the sections dealing with these entities.

The exacting histologic indices by which the biologic potential of the diffuse fibrillary astrocytoma is gauged simply cannot be applied to the juvenile pilocytic variant, a WHO grade I neoplasm that is among the most indolent of all central neuroepithelial tumors.[427] Isolated mitotic figures, glomeruloid vascular proliferation, multinucleated giant cell formation, and nuclear atypism (at times alarming, particularly in microcystic regions) are divorced, in this setting, from sinister prognostic import, as is the rather common finding of extension into the subarachnoid space. This is not to deny the existence of potentially aggressive lesions meriting the designation of 'anaplastic' pilocytic astrocytoma[426,428] by virtue of their conspicuous mitotic activity, dense cellularity, and foci of coagulative necrosis, but such cases are rare and actually seem somewhat more amenable to surgical control than diffuse astrocytomas exhibiting comparable features (i.e., glioblastomas).

Pilocytic astrocytomas confined to the optic nerve[407] and cerebellum[411] lend themselves to curative neurosurgical resection, as do those arising in accessible cerebral hemispheric sites,[410,424] though instances of recurrence (even decades) after radical removal are on record.[422] An increased biologic potential has been claimed for some cerebellar examples associated with NF-1.[412] A less favorable prognosis attaches, understandably, to lesions involving the optic chiasm, hypothalamus, and other regions that preclude concerted neurosurgical attack,[427] but even in these loci the clinical evolution of subtotally resected pilocytic astrocytomas is typically protracted and may extend over a decade or more. Evidence from bromodeoxyuridine studies suggests that the proliferative activity of pilocytic astrocytomas may actually diminish over time,[413] rare instances of spontaneous regression being on record.[408] Dissemination via the CSF, principally complicating opticohypothalamic lesions, is exceptional despite the fact that pilocytic astrocytomas frequently infiltrate the adjacent subarachnoid space and leptomeninges extensively.[423,425] Metastatic deposits may remain remarkably stable and are not necessarily associated with early death. 'Malignant degeneration' remains the stuff of which case reports are made.[426,428] Radiation therapy may play a role in the latter development, as many tumors evidencing such biologic progression were subjected to this treatment years prior to recurring in anaplastic and aggressive form. In fact, some may have represented independent, radiation-induced glioblastomas. Extracranial spread of opticohypothalamic pilocytic astrocytoma to the abdominal cavity via a ventriculoperitoneal shunt has been described,[425] but is a curiosity. We refer the reader to our discussion of pilomyxoid astrocytomas (see below) for further comments on a potentially aggressive glioma of childhood that has only recently been distinguished from pilocytic astrocytomas of conventional type.

We close this discussion of the clinical biology of pilocytic astrocytomas by emphasizing the importance of segregating these surgically curable neoplasms from diffuse fibrillary astrocytomas, which may arise in the cerebellum. The latter are typically resistant to all forms of therapy and, with rare exception, ultimately prove fatal. Pilocytic astrocytomas of the cerebellum occasionally consist in part of diffusely permeative elements that are indistinguishable from neoplastic cells of fibrillary astrocytic type, but these are noteworthy for their cytologic uniformity, mitotic inactivity, and lack of atypism.[411] The finding of such components, particularly in a pediatric case, should prompt a careful search for piloid or microcystic foci, but even in the absence of such tell-tale pilocytic features, the prognosis of ostensibly infiltrating astrocytomas of this kind in childhood is quite favorable.

Recent investigations of the pilocytic astrocytoma at the molecular genetic level have yielded observations that promise to revolutionize the manner in which this entity is defined and to provide novel methods for its identification.[409,415] Apparently central to the pathogenesis of pilocytic astrocytomas is upregulation of the mitogen-activated protein kinase (MAPK) pathway, which bears on cell proliferation, differentiation, and apoptosis. Whereas this is effected in the setting of NF-1 by functional loss of neurofibromin (product of the *NF1* gene and a negative regulator of MAPK pathway signaling through its inhibitory influence on Ras), it is a MAPK activator, *BRAF*, that has been implicated in the causation of most sporadically occurring astrocytomas of pilocytic type. The latter share, as their most common genetic abnormality, tandem duplications at chromosome 7q34 that result in the formation of an oncogenic *KIAA1549-BRAF* fusion gene lacking the autoinhibitory domain of wild-type *BRAF* and producing constitutive MAPK activation.[409,415] These events occur in pilocytic astrocytomas arising in varied CNS sites, but seem especially characteristic of cerebellar examples. The observation that *KIAA1549-BRAF* fusions are generally foreign to diffuse astrocytomas, coupled with the immunity of pilocytic lesions to the isocitrate dehydrogenase (*IDH1*) gene mutations common to the former, provides the rationale for a strategy of molecular diagnostic segregation in problematic cases.[417] Other MAPK activating events that have been detected in pilocytic astrocytomas include *RAF1* fusions and *KRAS* mutation.[409]

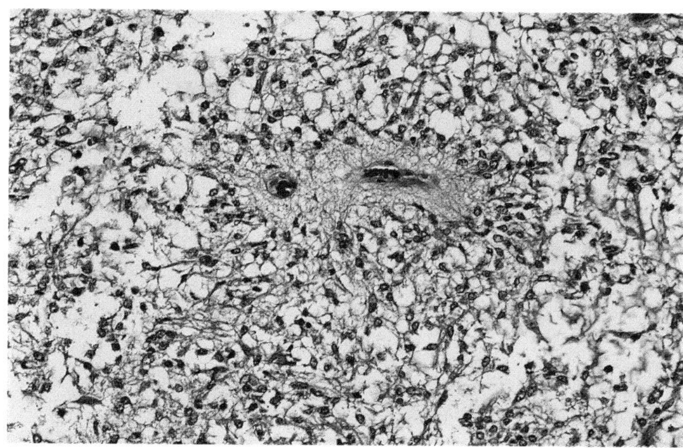

Fig. 28.56 Pilomyxoid astrocytoma. Spindled cytologic features, diffuse myxoid change, and focal perivascular pseudorosetting (center top) characterize this emerging entity.

Pilomyxoid astrocytoma

Certain tumors historically included in the pilocytic astrocytoma group have garnered attention as possibly representing a distinct biologic, as well as morphologic, entity. **Pilomyxoid astrocytoma** is the nomenclature most recently proposed for this incompletely characterized neoplasm,[427,433,434] which usually arises in the hypothalamus or optic chiasm of an infant or young child but can be encountered in other locations (including the cerebellum). The pilomyxoid lesion shares with the classic pilocytic astrocytoma a population of spindly (though less elongated), bipolar glial cells but does not evidence a biphasic alternation of solid and microcystic growth patterns, instead exhibiting diffuse and prominent myxomatous change, does not contain Rosenthal fibers, and usually lacks eosinophilic granular bodies. Many such tumors deviate further from conventional pilocytic histology in containing pseudorosette-like formations of neoplastic cells that appear to radiate from stromal blood vessels (Fig. 28.56). Mitoses are often in evidence, though not numerous, and necrosis (without pseudopalisading) may be encountered. Diffuse GFAP expression is the rule, some examples also manifesting cytoplasmic synaptophysin labeling. MIB-1 labeling indices are highly variable but often exceed the 1–3% levels encountered in pilocytic lesions of the usual type.

Precise definition of the so-called pilomyxoid astrocytoma as a biologic entity awaits additional study, as does clarification of its relationship to the classic pilocytic lesion. We have encountered tumors manifesting hybrid pilomyxoid/pilocytic features as well as neoplasms conforming in all respects to the pilomyxoid astrocytoma that evidenced more conventionally pilocytic histology on recurrence. In further attestation to a kinship, some cases placed in the pilomyxoid astrocytoma group have evidenced *BRAF* fusions of the sort just discussed as characteristic of typical pilocytic neoplasms. Readers will note that the tumors under discussion are essentially classed as pilocytic astrocytoma variants in the current WHO scheme.[427] Admittedly, a subset of pilomyxoid suprasellar neoplasms proved in one study to share certain fine structural attributes suggesting ependymal differentiation and raising question of their origin from specialized paraventricular cells known as tanycytes.[432] These included lengthy, bipolar cytoplasmic extensions with surface microvilli, rare cilia, blebs, coated vesicles and pits, 'synaptoid' complexes, intercellular junctions and foot processes terminating on delimiting, perivascular basement membranes. An origin from radial glia associated with the optic tract has also been

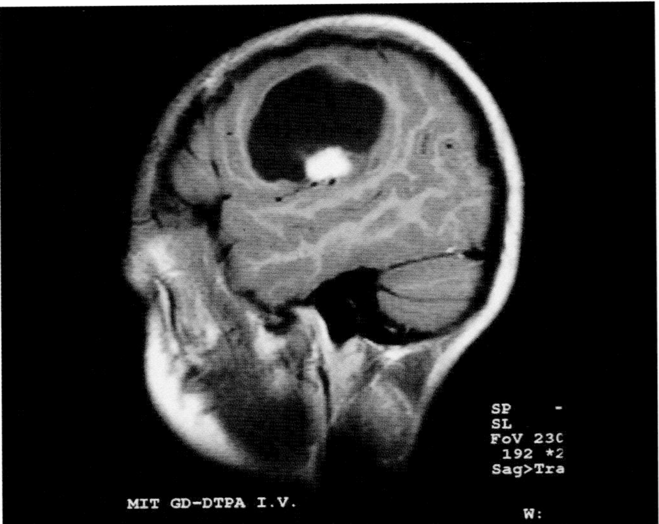

Fig. 28.57 Pleomorphic xanthoastrocytoma. This frontal lobe example is represented by a sharply delimited, intensely and homogenously contrast-enhancing nodule that projects into a large cyst. Pilocytic astrocytomas and gangliogliomas may exhibit identical neuroradiologic profiles and are the major differential diagnostic considerations in this setting.

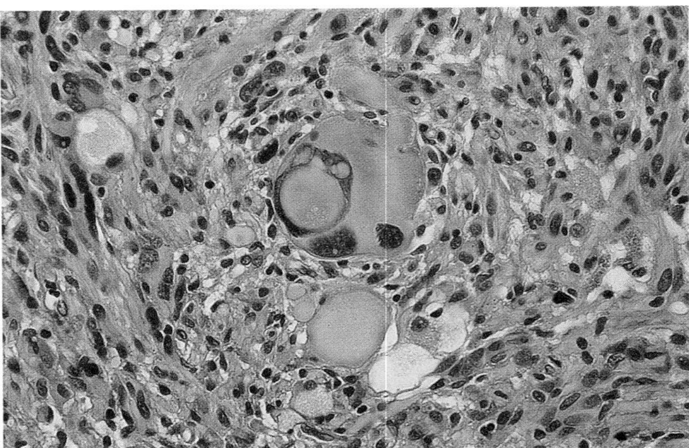

Fig. 28.58 Pleomorphic xanthoastrocytoma. Spindle and giant cells, including bizarre multinucleated forms, combine to give this relatively indolent neoplasm a most disturbing appearance. Note hyaline, granular, and vacuolar cytoplasmic alterations, the last attesting to lipid accumulation.

proposed.[430] It must be conceded that the diagnosis of pilomyxoid astrocytoma may have been extended to tumors of nonuniform cytogenesis allied by spindle cell morphology and a propensity to myxoid change. Whatever their origins, pediatric neoplasms demonstrating pure pilomyxoid astrocytoma histology carry a higher risk of local progression, symptomatic CSF seeding, and tumor-related death than pilocytic astrocytomas of the usual variety.[431,433,434] Accordingly, they have been designated as WHO grade II lesions.[427]

Pleomorphic xanthoastrocytoma

The **pleomorphic xanthoastrocytoma (WHO grade II)** is a histologically alarming, yet biologically favorable, neoplasm that typically presents in later childhood or early adult life and exhibits a predilection for the cerebral hemispheres, particularly the temporal lobes.[438,443] Cerebellar,[440] intramedullary,[447] intrasellar,[435] and retinal[455] examples have been described, as have morphologically similar tumors of the pineal region reported under the rubric of 'pleomorphic granular cell astrocytoma'.[453] Especially suggestive is neuroradiologic demonstration of a well-demarcated and partially cystic lesion containing superficially positioned, contrast-enhancing mural components of nodular or plaque-like contour (Fig. 28.57). Usually unaccompanied by significant mass effect or edema, the latter may adhere to dura and can appear at operation to lie largely above the cortical mantle.

Evaluation of surgical specimens often shows much of the pleomorphic xanthoastrocytoma to occupy the leptomeninges and subarachnoid space, but invariably discloses foci of brain parenchymal invasion in which neoplastic cells permeate Virchow–Robin spaces and the neuropil proper. The tumor is named for its potentially bizarre cytologic characteristics and the tendency of its constituent cells to intracytoplasmic lipid accumulation, although the latter is not a uniformly conspicuous feature. Most examples are composed of spindle-shaped elements in fascicular array admixed with tumor giant cells displaying worrisome, even grotesque, nuclear abnormalities (Fig. 28.58). The abundant cytoplasm of these cells may appear foamy or coarsely vacuolated – attesting to advanced lipidization – but more commonly assumes a ground-glass, finely granular or hyalin quality. Reactive lymphoid infiltrates, at times extensive, and aggregated eosinophilic granular bodies representing lysosomes distended by autophagic debris or imbibed proteinaceous material round out the histologic picture. The latter, an important clue to the diagnosis, are shared by certain other slowly growing neuroepithelial neoplasms, notably the pilocytic astrocytoma and ganglioglioma, and so likely reflect a process of cellular senescence. In fact, 'composite' tumors harboring gangliogliomatous and xanthoastrocytomatous components are on record[449] and we have rarely encountered cerebral hemispheric astrocytomas of pilocytic type with foci of leptomeningeal spread conforming to the histology of the pleomorphic xanthoastrocytoma in unalloyed form. Additional features described in select cases include a cohesive, nesting or alveolar growth pattern,[442] a hyalinizing, angiomatoid stromal vascular response,[454] and melanotic pigmentation.[452]

The sarcomatoid histologic presentation of the pleomorphic xanthoastrocytoma may be rendered all the more misleading by an intricate pericellular pattern of reticulin deposition in flagrant violation of the neurohistochemical principle that such staining in glial, as opposed to mesodermally derived, neoplasms typically remains confined to supporting vasculature. This feature actually reflects the elaboration by tumor cells of encircling basal lamina material, demonstrable at the ultrastructural level or by recourse to antibodies directed against type IV collagen or laminin,[442] and has been taken, along with the characteristically superficial location of the xanthoastrocytoma, as evidence of its derivation from a specialized class of subpial astrocytes having radially oriented cytoplasmic processes that are normally invested by basement membranes.[443] GFAP expression, mandatory for definitive diagnosis, effectively segregates this tumor from mesenchymal neoplasms,[439,443,444] though typical examples may contain relatively few immunolabeled elements. Diffuse cytoplasmic immunoreactivity for S-100 protein is the rule and tumor cells may be labeled by antisera to α_1-antitrypsin, α_1-antichymotrypsin, and other 'histiocytic' markers.[444] The latter reagents decorate a variety of neoplastic (including glial) cell types and are of notoriously little discriminatory value when applied to neurosurgical material. Noteworthy, given the association of xanthoastrocytomatous components with neuronal malformations (cortical dysplasia), hamartomas, and neoplasms,[445,449] is the observation that the tumors under discussion often harbor cells that bind antibodies to synaptophysin (among other neuronal antigens) and that can exhibit ultrastructural features of neuronal differentiation (including clear (synaptic-type) and dense core vesicles).[439] This would suggest that pleomorphic xanthoastrocytomas are capable of divergent glioneuronal differentiation and would serve, along with shared clinicobiologic features, to further ally these curious neoplasms with gangliogliomas (discussed in the section devoted to ganglion cell tumors). Noteworthy in this connection (and useful for purposes of diagnosis) is the observation that many pleomorphic xanthoastrocytomas exhibit membranous immunolabeling of tumor cells for CD34 and are further associated with cerebral cortex populated by 'dysplastic', CD34-reactive neuroepithelial cells of highly ramified appearance that cannot be appreciated in conventionally stained sections (Fig. 28.59).[451] These phenomena are common to gangliogliomas as well and, as mentioned, neoplasms having composite features of both tumor types may be encountered.[449] Tumor cell immunolabeling for neuronal antigens such as synaptophysin, NeuN, and neurofilament proteins may aid in the distinction of pleomorphic xanthoastrocytomas from giant cell glioblastomas.[446] The labeling of giant cell (and other) glioblastomas for CD34 has been reported.[437a]

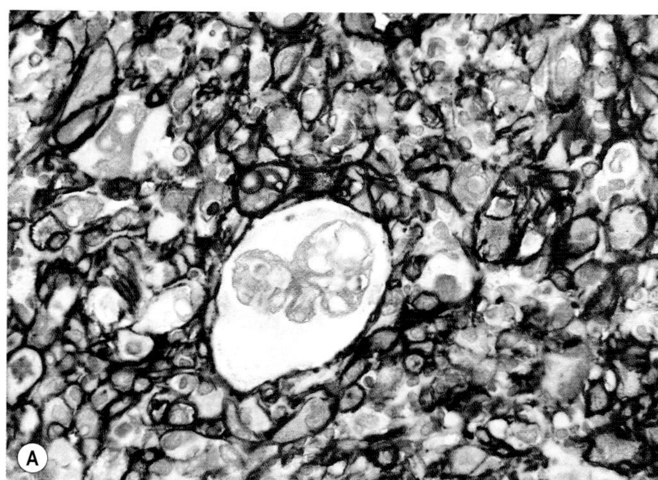

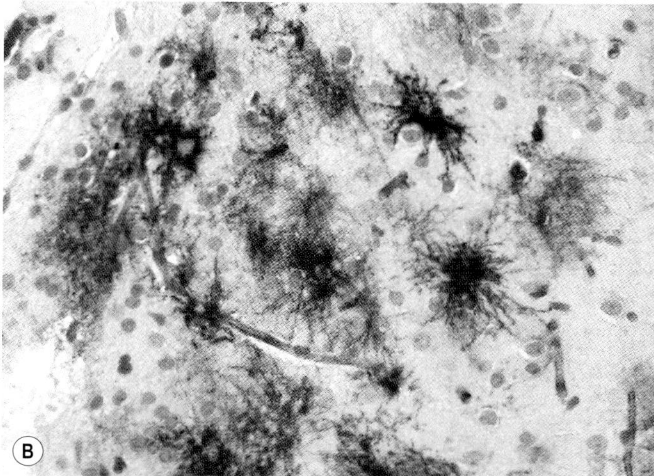

Fig. 28.59 Pleomorphic xanthoastrocytoma. Characteristic is the immunoexpression of CD34 by tumor cells (**A**) and by process-bearing neural cells in adjoining, uninvolved cerebral cortex (**B**). Note membranous quality of tumor labeling.

Despite their disturbing morphology, pleomorphic xanthoastrocytomas tend to behave in relatively benign clinical fashion, gross total resection usually sufficing to achieve long-term tumor control. A closely characterized series of 71 cases revealed recurrence-free survivals of 72% and 61% at 5 and 10 years, respectively, with overall survival figures of approximately 80% and 70% at these same postoperative intervals.[438] Extent of tumor removal bears critically on the risk of regrowth. The presence of scattered mitotic figures does not seem to constitute an ominous prognostic sign in this setting, but proliferative activity in excess of 5 mitoses per 10 high-power fields proved a predictor of shortened survival in the sizable study to which we have just referred. The emergence of poorly differentiated small cell components and the presence of necrosis have also been associated with fatal outcomes, some pleomorphic xanthoastrocytomas degenerating into glioblastoma-like histology.[438,441] Tumors exhibiting these indices of potentially aggressive evolution can be termed 'pleomorphic xanthoastrocytomas with anaplastic features'.[438,441] A recurring example with histologic evidence of anaplasia and an extensive clear cell component as well as focally papillary growth has been recorded.[450] We have encountered an example that developed sarcomatous components (pleomorphic 'xanthoastrosarcoma')[437] and a case harboring genetically confirmed elements of atypical teratoid/rhabdoid tumor has been communicated.[436] Local failure is the rule, CSF-borne spread being a rarity.[448]

Subependymal giant cell astrocytoma (tuberous sclerosis)

The **subependymal giant cell astrocytoma** typically presents in the first or second decade of life as an intraventricular mass associated with obstructive hydrocephalus, a consequence of its practically unvarying situation near the foramen of Monro (Fig. 28.60).[462,465,466] Only isolated reports describe extraventricular variants.[456,458] The lesion is virtually restricted to the setting of **tuberous sclerosis**, a

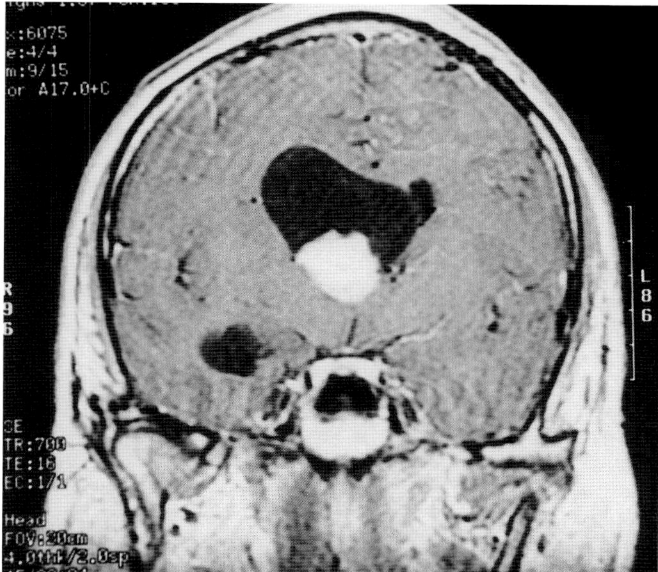

Fig. 28.60 Subependymal giant cell astrocytoma. This postcontrast injection MRI demonstrates the subependymal giant cell astrocytoma's typically intraventricular location near the foramen of Monro (with resulting obstructive hydrocephalus), as well as its characteristic circumscription. This example was not associated with other features of tuberous sclerosis.

disorder transmissible in autosomal dominant fashion via loci on chromosomes 9q34 (*TSC1*) and 16p13.3 (*TSC2*) but often encountered in a nonfamilial form resulting from spontaneous mutation.[462] Traditionally defined by the triad of mental retardation, epilepsy, and midfacial angiofibromatosis ('adenoma sebaceum'), this phakomatosis is named for distinctive foci of gyral expansion ('tubers') which are populated by dysmorphic neurons and giant astrocytes in architectural disarray and possessed of an abnormal firmness ('sclerosis') resulting from glial overgrowth. Also characteristic are periventricular 'candle gutterings', essentially miniature versions of the tumors under discussion, composed of outsized astrocytes aggregated in a fibrillary matrix prone to calcification. Dominant extracranial manifestations of the tuberous sclerosis complex include renal angiomyolipomas, cardiac rhabdomyomas, pulmonary lymphangioleiomyomatosis, fibrous dysplasia of bone, microhamartomatous rectal polyps, and various cutaneous lesions (hypopigmented macules, shagreen patches, subungual fibromas, and, as mentioned, facial angiofibromas). Some afflicted patients also harbor retinal hamartomas similar to the subependymal nodules just described or larger masses that would qualify as retinal giant cell astrocytomas. A pineal region tumor of this type in a child with tuberous sclerosis has been documented.[458]

A sharply delineated, spherical or multinodular mass of fleshy, gray–pink tissue, the subependymal giant cell astrocytoma is anchored to the ventricular wall over a broad front. Calcifications are common, some examples exhibiting foci of cystic change. Constituent cells are large, closely apposed and characterized by polygonal (ganglion cell-like), rounded (gemistocyte-like), or spindly profiles (Fig. 28.61). Their eosinophilic cytoplasm often has a glassy or hyaline appearance and their eccentrically positioned, vesicular nuclei and prominent nucleoli distinctly resemble those of large neurons or ganglion cells. An intersecting fibrovascular stroma lends a lobular architecture to many examples and tumor cell processes often condense about blood vessels in ependymomatous fashion. A curious feature of many cases is infiltration by mast cells. Immunohistochemical assessment may reveal only few GFAP-positive elements and – designation of this neoplasm as an astrocytoma notwithstanding – may show some tumor cells to colabel for (or exclusively express) such neuronal antigens as class III β-tubulin, neurofilament proteins and, rarely, synaptophysin.[460,461,465] Ultrastructural studies have demonstrated the presence of dense-core granules and synaptic formations in select cases, confirming the ability of subependymal giant cell astrocytomas to differentiate along neuronal, as well as glial, lines.[460] Accordingly, some neuropathologists prefer to designate these neoplasms simply as subependymal giant cell tumors. Ambiguous glioneuronal features also characterize the giant 'astrocytes' seen in cortical tubers, suggesting a disturbance of normal lineage commitment.[460] Subependymal giant cell astrocytomas do not exhibit immunolabeling for HMB-45 and typically evidence low MIB-1 indices.[459,464]

Subependymal giant cell astrocytomas enlarge slowly, are reluctant to invade adjacent cerebral structures and, an isolated exampled excepted,[467] have not been reported to exploit the CSF as a means of escaping their ventricular confines. Recurrence following gross total resection is rare and these indolent neoplasms are not prone to malignant transformation. Although reported examples are few, cases evidencing mitotic activity and foci of necrosis do not appear to behave in particularly sinister fashion.[457,466] Neoplasms interpreted as overtly malignant subependymal giant cell astrocytomas or glioblastomas have been described in the setting of tuberous sclerosis but are clearly exceptional.[463]

Desmoplastic infantile astrocytoma

The desmoplastic cerebral astrocytoma of infancy or desmoplastic infantile astrocytoma is a rare lesion now recognized as belonging to a tumor family capable of divergent and advanced glioneuronal differentiation. Accordingly, we address this entity along with its variant – the desmoplastic infantile ganglioglioma – in our discussion of neuronal and glioneuronal tumors.

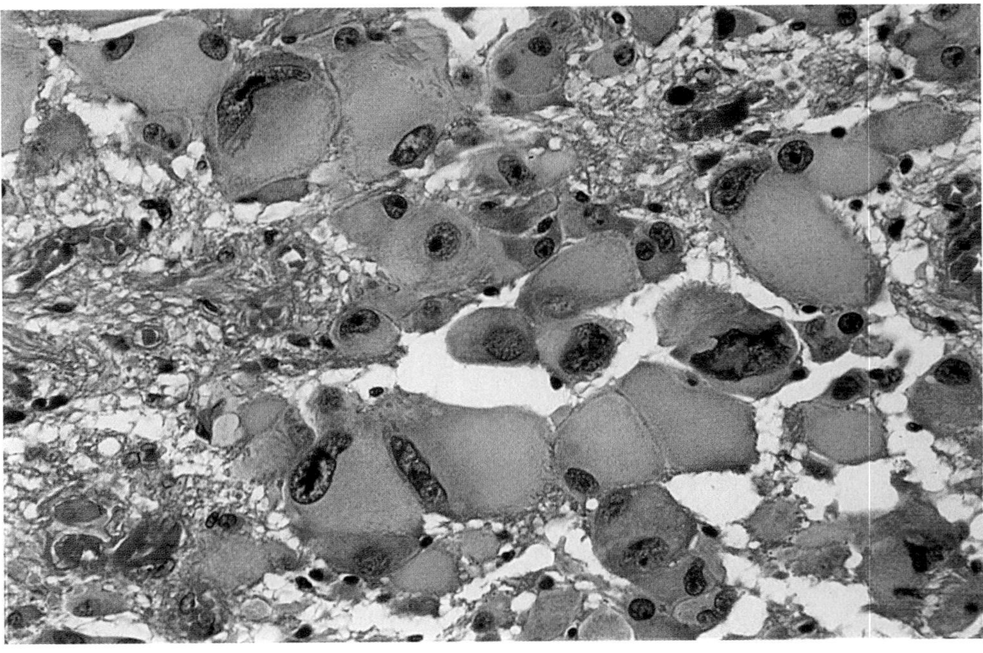

Fig. 28.61 Subependymal giant cell astrocytoma. Tumor cells that achieve truly giant proportions, often polygonal in contour and closely apposed in lobular array, are responsible for this neoplasm's name (but not evident in all cases).

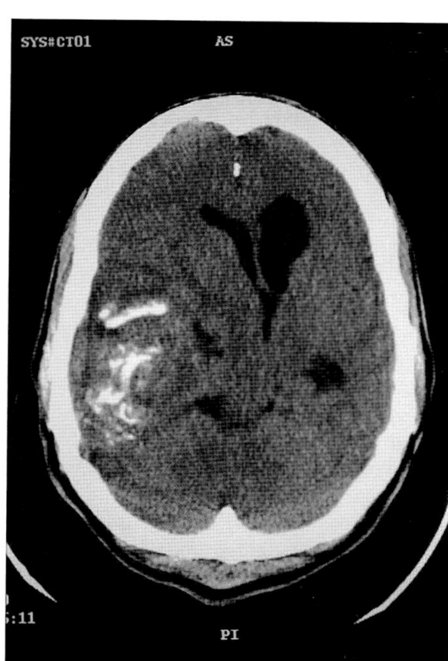

Fig. 28.62 Oligodendroglioma. The bright signal abnormalities seen in this nonenhanced CT study of a large right cerebral oligodendroglioma represent foci of intratumoral calcification. While evidenced by only a minority of oligodendroglial neoplasms, linear or plate-like calcifications of this sort are most suggestive of the diagnosis.

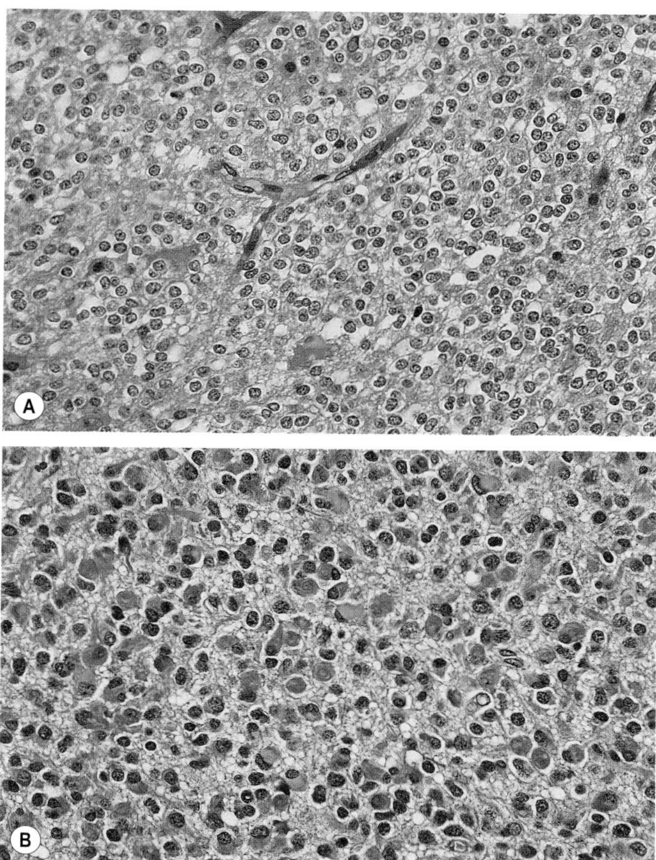

Fig. 28.63 Oligodendroglioma. Uniform, round nuclei and clear perinuclear halos (artefacts of delayed fixation) typify well-differentiated oligodendrogliomas (**A**). 'Minigemistocytic' variants (**B**) maintain oligodendroglial nuclear features while amassing globose paranuclear expanses of eosinophilic, hyaline or whorling fibrillar cytoplasm. Compare the size of these cells and their cytologic features with those of the gemistocytic astrocytoma depicted at identical magnification in Figure 28.49.

Oligodendrogliomas

The tumors of the oligodendroglioma group are named for the resemblance of their constituent cells to native oligodendrocytes, although the notion that these neoplasms derive from the latter or from progenitors committed to differentiate along oligodendroglial lines remains unsubstantiated.[490] Characteristic clinical features include a predilection for young and middle-aged adults, a cerebral hemispheric localization (the frontal and temporal lobes being principally affected), an often protracted preoperative history of intermittent seizures or headache, and partial calcification on neuroradiologic study (Fig. 28.62). As discussed under 'Gliomatosis cerebri', remarkably widespread brain infiltration is occasionally seen at diagnosis. Only exceptionally do oligodendroglial neoplasms arise below the tentorium, but no division of the CNS is immune and the literature includes accounts of tumors interpreted as oligodendrogliomas of leptomeningeal[468,492] and retinal[483] origin. To be found among the former are cases of diffuse leptomeningeal 'oligodendrogliomatosis' that seem to constitute a distinctive syndrome characterized by an onset in childhood, by remarkably widespread infiltration of the pia-arachnoid and subarachnoid space at presentation unaccompanied by involvement of the neuroparenchyma proper (or associated with only limited disease in the spinal cord), and by a surprisingly slow clinical evolution.[492] The affected leptomeninges may appear on MRI to be studded with innumerable small nodules of cystic profile. An obscuring fibroplasia that commonly attends the colonization of the pia-arachnoid by neoplastic elements in this condition can be misconstrued as evidence of a chronic sclerosing meningitis. Whether the responsible tumors are truly conventional oligodendrogliomas unconventionally situated is a matter of controversy, some observers suggesting that these are glioneuronal neoplasms of a novel variety.[473] The cited literature can be consulted for further details. We note in passing the description of oligodendroglioma-like proliferations in association with AVMs[146,153] and report of an oligodendroglioma arising adjacent to a focus of meningioangiomatosis.[39]

Oligodendrogliomas are usually found to lie mainly within white matter at operation, but extension into overlying cortex is the rule. Composed of soft, gray–pink tissue that often acquires a gelatinous consistency owing to the accumulation of myxoid matrix materials, these may evidence cystic change and can contain foci of dense calcium deposition that are palpably gritty or even rock-hard. A vulnerability to artefactual cytoplasmic dissolution accounts for the histologic presentation of classic oligodendrogliomas as permeative or, in some cases, sheet-like proliferations of uniform, small round nuclei surrounded by optically clear halos (Fig. 28.63A). A fusiform spindling of tumor cells is occasionally apparent and some high-grade, 'polymorphous' variants harbor markedly pleomorphic, giant cell subpopulations.[490] Oligodendrogliomas often contain scattered calcospherites, which may be clustered in laminar fashion within cerebral cortex along the advancing tumoral perimeter, and many are subtended by a plexiform ('chicken wire') network of thin-walled blood vessels. Of additional diagnostic utility is a tendency to perineuronal tumor cell aggregation ('satellitosis'). Perivascular and subpial growth are also commonly encountered, as are myxoid changes, microcyst formation, and nodular foci of increased cell density. In exceptional instances, tumor cells are segregated into prominent lobules by fibrovascular stromal elements or stagger across the microscopic field in rhythmic palisades.

That the 'fried egg' cellular profile of the prototypical oligodendroglioma is an artefact not seen in conventional frozen sections, intraoperative smears or crush preparations merits emphasis. The first of these techniques almost invariably produces misleading nuclear angulations, whereas the latter preserve the rounded profiles of tumor cell nuclei which appear either naked or irregularly encircled by pale eosinophilic cytoplasm in modest quantity. Distinct cytoplasmic expanses and cell membranes are also appreciable in paraffin sections prepared from very promptly fixed surgical material. Perinuclear halos, on the other hand, constitute (along with nuclear shrinkage and oligodendrocyte-like rounding) deceptive artefacts potentially imposed on astrocytomas and other non-oligodendroglial neoplasms by the common practice of ultrasonic tumor aspiration. Inspection of manually resected specimens should serve as the basis for histologic subclassification.

Oligodendrogliomas often contain intensely GFAP-positive 'minigemistocytes'[476,480] that may harbor inclusion-like, whorled intracytoplasmic bodies of filamentous substructure (Fig. 28.63B). These are of no proven prognostic significance per se but tend to be particularly numerous in high-grade oligodendroglial tumors (as defined presently) and may evidence transition to large and pleomorphic gemistocytes of astroglial type that have been associated with aggressive behavior.[480] So-called 'gliofibrillary oligodendrocytes', elements of conventional clear cell type characterized by perinuclear rims of GFAP-immunoreactive cytoplasm that may taper into short, unipolar cell processes, may also be apparent.[476] Neoplastic transformation of a glial progenitor credited with the normal spawning of oligodendroglia and a subset of astrocytes has been posited to account for these observations and could explain the frequency with which oligodendrogliomas are colonized by tumor cells evidencing transition to fibrillary astroglial morphology.[490] As discussed in the section dealing with 'mixed' gliomas, the point at which the diagnosis of oligoastrocytoma is invoked in recognition of this common phenomenon is a subjective affair. Other cytologic alterations that may be encountered in oligodendroglial neoplasms include cytoplasmic distension by a PAS-positive mucosubstance, the formation of eosinophilic granular cells stuffed with autophagic vacuoles[494] or truncated Rosenthal fibers,[477] and 'signet ring' change resulting from the intracytoplasmic accumulation of degenerating mitochondria[479] or of dilated profiles of rough endoplasmic reticulum.[485]

Unfortunately, there does not exist at present an immunocytochemical reagent that consistently and specifically identifies neoplastic cells as oligodendroglial.[490] Immunolabeling for S-100 protein, membranous Leu7 (CD57) reactivity, and cytoplasmic expression of carbonic anhydrase C and MAP-2 are characteristic but shared by other tumor types. Cytoplasmic labeling for galactocerebroside and other oligodendrocyte-associated galactolipids is inconstant and only exceptionally are tumor cells decorated by antibodies to myelin-associated glycoprotein, proteolipid protein or other differentiation antigens that mark mature oligodendroglia. While oligodendrogliomas commonly display nuclear immunoexpression of the lineage-restricted OLIG1, OLIG2, and SOX10 transcription factors,[490] this profile may be shared by other neuroepithelial neoplasms that include astrocytomas and, in the case of OLIG2, neurocytic tumors.[482] Of potentially more value as a discriminating feature (though, again, not uniformly sensitive or altogether specific) may be diffuse cytoplasmic labeling for Nogo-A,[481] a member of the reticulon family, but this requires additional investigation. In a similar vein, ultrastructural indices of oligodendroglial maturation are lacking in most cases, though careful search may rarely reveal cytoplasmic processes compacted in a concentric lamellar fashion reminiscent of myelin sheath formation.[486] Microtubules, free ribosomes, and mitochondria constitute the usual cytoplasmic contents and are unaccompanied by any unique organellar structures.

It is, in fact, what the oligodendroglioma fails to accomplish at the ultrastructural level or by way of antigen expression that often proves most useful in its distinction from certain mimickers that may assume astonishingly similar histologic guises. Specifically, it does not fashion the elaborate zonulae adherentes-type intercellular junctions, microlumens, microvillous or ciliary arrays of the clear cell ependymoma, or the clear synaptic or dense-core vesicles that betray the neuronal nature of central and extraventricular neurocytomas. The dot and ring-like immunolabeling for EMA that corresponds to ependymal microlumen formation is not displayed by oligodendroglial tumors. Neurocytic neoplasms are further (and most efficiently) distinguished by a neuronal immunophenotype that includes diffuse matrix labeling for synaptophysin and, in many instances, widespread immunoreactivity for the neuronal nuclear antigens Hu[365] and NeuN.[404] This is not to dismiss evidence that oligodendrogliomas occasionally exercise a potential for neuronal differentiation. We acknowledge the labeling of some examples (usually in focal fashion) for a variety of neuron-associated antigens,[471,495,496] including both synaptophysin and NeuN, and note particularly thought-provoking accounts of otherwise 'acceptable' oligodendrogliomas harboring unarguably neurocytic elements in rosetted array[488] and ganglion cell components.[486a] Such phenomena necessarily raise questions regarding the cytogenesis of the neoplasms currently regarded as oligodendroglial, but are exceptional and of no special clinical significance. We would emphasize that close scrutiny is required lest neoplastic infiltration of synaptophysin-rich cortex (a frequent event) be seized upon as evidence of tumoral differentiation along neuronal lines. Again, NeuN assessment is useful in this regard, as immunoreactivity for this protein is foreign to the great majority of oligodendrogliomas[472] and serves to highlight remaining native neurons in colonized gray matter. The decidedly oligodendroglioma-like dysembryoplastic neuroepithelial tumor departs from the neoplasms under discussion in its predilection for subjects younger than 20 years of age, largely cortical topography, content of intracortical nodules with a 'patterned' alveolar architecture, and intact chromosome 1p/19q status. Chromosome 1p/19q co-deletions, a common feature of histologically typical oligodendrogliomas (see below), are not harbored by central neurocytomas or clear cell ependymomas, but do characterize a subset of extraventricular neurocytic tumors.[487] Additional remarks on the latter phenomenon can be found in our discussion of neurocytomas.

Unlike clear cell meningiomas (usually extra-axial and dura-based), oligodendrogliomas are typically EMA negative, are not heavily glycogenated, and lack well-developed intercellular junctions at the electron microscopic level. Similar considerations apply to the identification of clear cell carcinomas, which may also exhibit cytokeratin reactivity. A major problem that cannot be entirely resolved by either immunohistochemical or ultrastructural assessment is appropriate subclassification of the glioma manifesting ambiguous histologic features – i.e., not falling clearly into the oligodendroglial versus diffuse astrocytic camp. Oligodendrogliomas may contain minor populations that exhibit nuclear immunoreactivity for p53, but when widespread this phenomenon is far more characteristic of the astrocytoma group and tends to an inverse correlation with the 1p/19q abnormalities to which we have just alluded.[469]

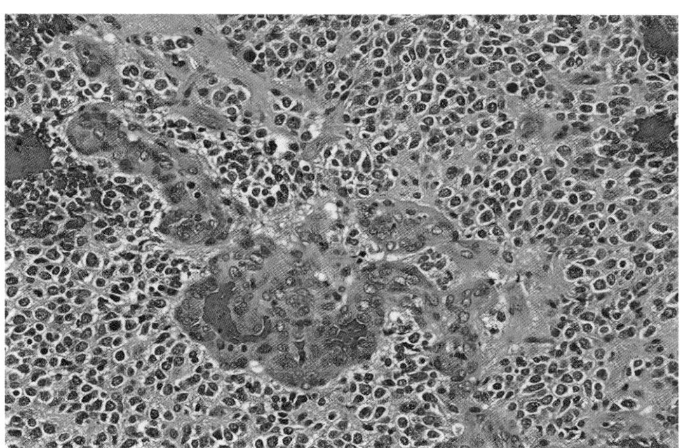

Fig. 28.64 Anaplastic oligodendroglioma. Microvascular proliferation, readily apparent mitotic activity, and cytologic atypism are features of this example.

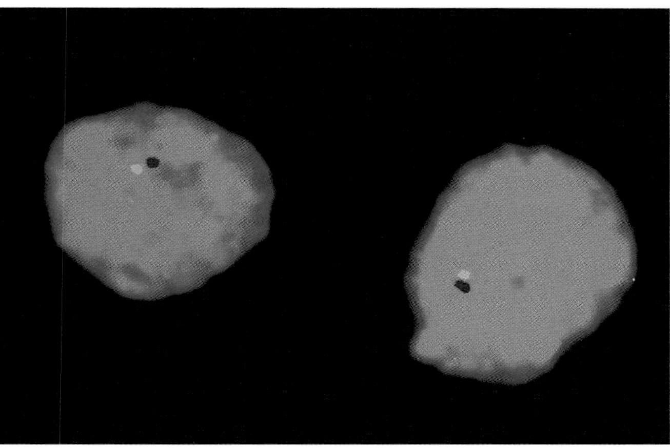

Fig. 28.65 Chromosomal deletion in oligodendrogliomas (same case as illustrated in Fig. 28.64). Fluorescence in situ hybridization utilizing centromeric (green) and telomeric (red) probes to chromosome 1p reveals only one signal pair in each of these tumor cells, indicating that both have lost the second 1p copy. This case also exhibited 19q deletion, commonly an accompanying event. The patient achieved complete remission on a regimen of procarbazine, CCNU, and vincristine.

A variety of grading strategies have emerged from correlative studies of oligodendroglioma histology and outcome,[471,475] a two-tiered segregation into low- versus high-grade variants forming the basis of the WHO classification and finding wide application among neuropathologists.[490] Reported as **'oligodendroglioma, WHO grade II'** is the well-differentiated tumor that exhibits little in the way of mitotic activity and is devoid of proliferative microvascular alterations or necrosis. Nodular foci of increased cellularity alone are compatible with this diagnosis. Endothelial hypertrophy, complex microvascular proliferation, and conspicuous mitotic activity – joined, in some cases, by necrosis and often accompanied by dense cellularity and obvious nuclear atypism – are features of the **'anaplastic oligodendroglioma, WHO grade III'** (Fig. 28.64). The latter may evolve within an underlying oligodendroglial neoplasm of low-grade character. Other variables associated with an unfavorable clinical course include advancing patient age, contrast enhancement on neuroradiologic assessment (a ring-enhancing profile seems especially ominous), and, in some studies, MIB-1 labeling indices in excess of 5%.[470,490]

Median survivals ranging from 3.5 to over 10 years for low-grade examples and from less than 1 to nearly 4 years for anaplastic lesions have emerged from retrospective surveys charting the clinical biology of oligodendroglial neoplasms.[490] A number of investigations have demonstrated that the most favorable prognosis attaches to examples harboring select molecular genetic anomalies. Specifically, combined and isolated allelic losses involving chromosomes 1p and 19q – a 'signature' strongly (though not invariably or exclusively) associated with classic oligodendrogliomatous tumor morphology[474,487,493] and usually reflecting an unbalanced translocation, i.e., t(1;19)(q10;p10)[490] – identify a subset of anaplastic oligodendroglial neoplasms that can be driven into radiation- and chemotherapy-induced remissions of gratifying durability.[474,478,490,493] Median overall survival periods exceeding 6 years have been reported following adjuvant therapy of patients with 1p/19q-deleted high-grade oligodendrogliomas, evidence also suggesting that relatively prolonged survival and treatment responsiveness characterize low-grade examples harboring such alterations.[490] A variety of methods may be applied to the demonstration of these deletions, including microsatellite analysis, comparative genomic hybridization, and fluorescence in situ hybridization (Fig. 28.65). Curiously, some workers have found chromosomal 1p/19q co-deletions to be evidenced by most oligodendrogliomas arising in the frontal, parietal, and occipital lobes, but by only a minority of histologically identical neoplasms localized to the temporal lobes, insula, or diencephalon.[490] This topographic distinction has not been observed by others, however.[474] A low incidence of 1p/19q deletion has also been described in the pediatric setting.[489] The isocitrate dehydrogenase (*IDH*) gene mutations previously mentioned in our discussion of diffuse astrocytic tumors occur at comparably high frequency in low-grade and anaplastic oligodendrogliomas, but their prognostic significance in the latter setting requires additional investigation.

Oligodendrogliomas usually kill by virtue of progressive neuroparenchymal infiltration following local recurrence. Leptomeningeal dissemination via the CSF is exceptional and distant metastasis rare.[484,490] Gliosarcomatous transformation has been recorded,[491] as further discussed under 'Gliosarcoma and other gliomesenchymal tumors'.

Ependymal tumors

Considered in this section are those neoplasms that have traditionally been classed in the ependymal series. As discussed under separate headings that follow, the astroblastoma may exhibit ependymocytic characteristics and the entities described as chordoid glioma of the third ventricle, angiocentric glioma, and papillary tumor of the pineal region unarguably manifest fine structural and immunohistochemical evidence of differentiation along this line. We follow the WHO format in segregating these distinctive lesions from the conventional ependymoma group.

Ependymomas constitute no more than 5–9% of primary CNS neoplasms, their prevalence relative to other tumor types varying considerably with patient age and presenting location.[528] A majority of intracranial examples arise in childhood, whereas intramedullary variants more commonly afflict adults. The incidence of the former peaks in the first decade of life, ependymomas comprising approximately 10% of intracranial neoplasms in the pediatric population and up to 30% of those encountered in children under 3 years of age. At least two-thirds of these childhood tumors are situated within the fourth ventricle and consequently present with evidence of increased intracranial pressure secondary to obstructive hydrocephalus. Supratentorial lesions are more evenly distributed among children and adults and are more likely to be associated with seizures and focal motor deficits.

Ependymomas of the spinal cord other than those of myxopapillary type usually arise within cervicothoracic segments and exhibit a predilection for the fourth and fifth decades of life, constituting the most common intramedullary neoplasms of adulthood.[506,528] Principal clinical manifestations include pain localized to the neck or back, numbness and paresthesias of the distal extremities, atrophy of hand musculature, and gait disturbances. An intramedullary location and multifocality characterize ependymomas complicating type 2 neurofibromatosis (NF-2), a subset of sporadic spinal cord examples sharing with these predetermined variants alterations of the *NF2* tumor suppressor gene on chromosome 22q12.[528] Ependymomas may rarely arise within cranial nerves,[523] the sella turcica,[542] and retina,[546] and have been reported to originate in the ovary and periadnexal pelvic tissues,[516] abdominal cavity,[531] liver,[552] mediastinum,[532] and lung,[505] though female genital tract and mediastinal cases may well represent 'lopsided' (i.e., monodermal) teratomas. We allude in passing to controversy over the role of simian virus 40 (SV40) in the genesis of ependymal tumors.[528] Reports that childhood ependymomas (and choroid plexus tumors) harbor SV40 or SV40-specific DNA sequences intrigue given the recognized ability of this agent to induce such neoplasms in animal hosts, but have not been replicated in all laboratories.

Wherever situated, ependymomas tend to be well circumscribed and contrast enhancing on neuroradiologic study. Supratentorial examples are often, but not invariably, found to communicate with or abut the ventricular system, lobar types frequently exhibiting cystic change and focal calcification. The latter is also a relatively common feature of posterior fossa lesions, which tend to be anchored to the floor of the fourth ventricle. Medulloblastomas, by contrast, only exceptionally undergo any appreciable mineralization and usually hang from the fourth ventricular roof when localized to the midline. Ependymomas may exploit CSF exit foramina to escape the restrictive confines of the fourth ventricle and, in so doing, can encircle the medulla and cervical spinal cord. Intramedullary variants produce a fusiform widening of involved segments and commonly precipitate syrinx formation, cystic dissection of the spinal cord usually progressing rostrally. MRI demonstration of a T2-hypointense 'hemosiderin cap' atop the rostral pole of a well-delimited and enhancing intramedullary mass is particularly suggestive.

The conventional **ependymoma (WHO grade II)** is typified by a dense meshwork of fibrillary cytoplasmic processes that condense, collar-like, about stromal blood vessels in formations known as perivascular pseudorosettes (Fig. 28.66). These are accompanied in a minority of cases by canals, tubules or actual rosettes lined by cells closely resembling normal ependymocytes (Fig. 28.67). The term '**cellular ependymoma**' may be used for densely populated examples with relatively narrow pseudorosettes but little mitotic activity, though this conveys no clinically useful information. Tumor cell nuclei are rounded or spindled, characteristically exhibit an evenly granular chromatin distribution, generally lack nucleoli, and may contain invaginated cytoplasmic pseudoinclusions or exhibit longitudinal nuclear grooving.[504] Optimally visualized in cytologic preparations, the last feature – along with the tendency of neoplastic ependymal cells to remain attached to delicate blood vessels in papillary fashion when subjected to smearing or crushing – facilitates intraoperative diagnosis. While nuclear uniformity is the rule, pleomorphic elements may be admixed and '**giant cell' ependymomas** have been described within the cranial compartment,[540] spinal cord, and filar region[555] (see discussion of myxopapillary ependymoma below). In the first of these locations, such cytologic changes are often accompanied by elevated mitotic activity and other features indicative of an aggressive biologic potential. Dystrophic calcification is a common finding in ependymomas, and some examples undergo osseous or chondroid metaplasia.[527] Melanotic ependymomas have been depicted,[501,537] as have 'xanthomatous' variants containing intracytoplasmic lipid droplets,[545] examples harboring adipocyte-like ('lipomatous') elements,[538] and 'epithelioid' subtypes characterized by the tight clustering of tumor cells in a conspicuously myxoid matrix.[519] Gemistocytic change may also be encountered in ependymomas, one report describing a case exhibiting globular, inclusion-like cytoplasmic bodies immunoreactive for GFAP.[549] Sarcomatous transformation ('ependymosarcoma') is exceptional but well documented.[535]

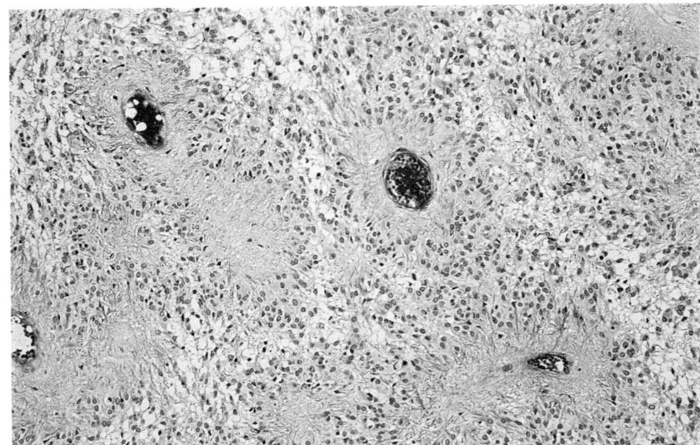

Fig. 28.66 Ependymoma. The cytoplasmic processes of ependymal tumor cells condense about blood vessels to form pseudorosettes.

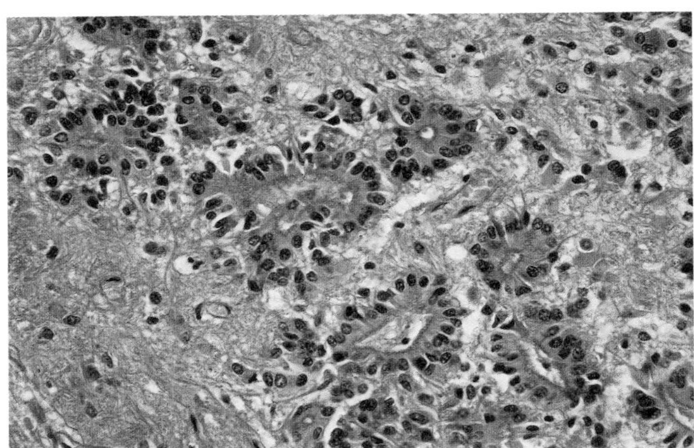

Fig. 28.67 Ependymoma. The true ependymal rosette contains a well-defined central lumen. Clustered ciliary basal bodies ('blepharoplasts') are responsible for the enhanced, granular staining of tumor cell apices.

At the ultrastructural level, ependymomas exhibit a number of specialized cytoplasmic features characteristic of non-neoplastic ependyma.[541] Elaborate, zipper-like junctional complexes (zonulae adherentes) bind their constituent cells and are likely responsible in some measure for the cohesive growth pattern and 'pushing' margins typical of such tumors. Slender microvilli and (in smaller

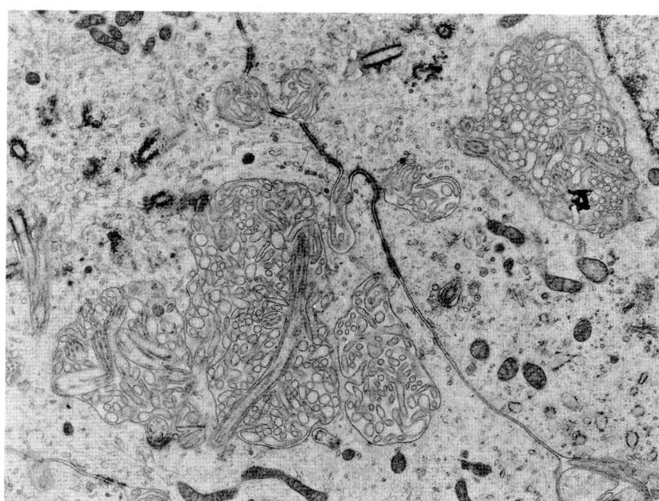

Fig. 28.68 Ependymoma. Features indicative of ependymal differentiation at the ultrastructural level include the joining of tumor cells by elongated junctional complexes and the formation of lumens filled with microvilli and, in lesser number, cilia. (×8800)

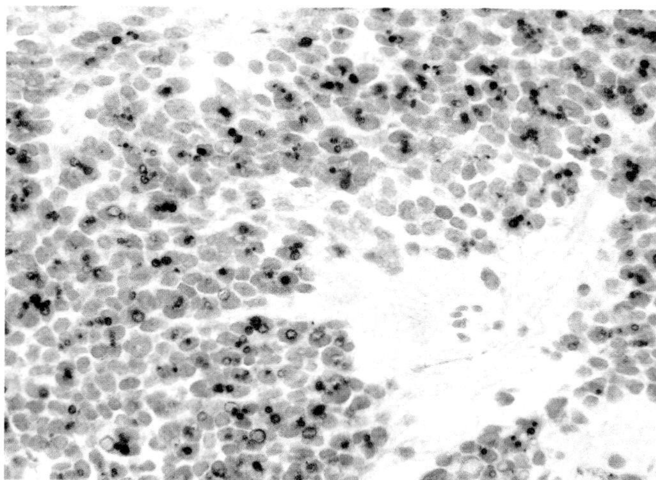

Fig. 28.69 Ependymoma. Dot- and ring-type patterns of cytoplasmic immunolabeling for EMA are diagnostically useful, though inconstant, features of this tumor group.

numbers) cilia sprout into the lumina of rosettes or intercellular clefts, again framed by membrane junctions of zonula adherens type (Fig. 28.68). Intracytoplasmic granules ('blepharoplasts') that are often apprehended by light microscopy along the apices of rosette-forming tumor cells in fact represent anchoring ciliary basal bodies. Also commonly observed on fine structural study is intracytoplasmic lumen formation, a phenomenon responsible in particularly pronounced cases for signet ring cell variants of ependymoma.[556] The phenomenon of microlumen formation by ependymocytic neoplasms has as its immunohistochemical correlate dot- and ring-type patterns of cytoplasmic EMA labeling that are of considerable diagnostic value,[512,518] though not always apparent or entirely specific if displayed by only rare tumor cells (Fig. 28.69). Intermediate filaments composed principally of (and immunoreactive for) vimentin and GFAP[528,551] are conspicuous in the cell processes of ependymal neoplasms, which, in select cases, may be coated by basal lamina material where they abut blood vessel walls.

While maintaining a diagnostic ultrastructural and immunophenotypic fidelity to the ependymal line, a subset of ependymomas exhibit distinctly confounding histologic features.[528] **Tanycytic ependymomas** (from the Greek *tanyos* – to stretch) may be confused with schwannomas, meningiomas, and fibrillary or pilocytic astrocytomas by virtue of their spindly cytologic features, fascicular growth patterns, and poorly developed, inconspicuous pseudorosettes. Such tumors are typically encountered at spinal levels.[517] Ependymomas commonly contain, in addition to admixed elements of astrocytic appearance, cells characterized by rounded nuclear profiles and perinuclear cytoplasmic clearing. Variants dominated by the latter, **clear cell ependymomas**,[509,529] are practically restricted to the supratentorial compartment and often construed as oligodendroglial, a mischance made all the more inviting by the frequent presence of intratumoral calcospherules and a plexiform vascular network. Tumors of this kind often exhibit high-grade histologic features (e.g., readily apparent mitotic activity and microvascular proliferation), are prone to recur and may do so after relatively brief postoperative intervals. Again, these retain identifying ependymal attributes at the electron microscopic level, typically manifest at least focal immunoreactivity of truncated perivascular cell processes for GFAP, and may on careful search be found to display dot-type EMA expression as described above. These attributes permit their segregation from oligodendrogliomas and other potentially clear cell neoplasms, including tumors of neurocytic type. The odd ependymoma, however, may harbor foci of neuronal differentiation.[511,536] In the latter regard, immunohistochemical labeling of some ependymomas, including clear cell forms, for synaptophysin and the NeuN neuronal nuclear protein should be noted.[472,536] Exceptional cases even exhibit overt neurocytic differentiation that can be appreciated on light microscopic assessment ('ependymoma with neuropil-like islands'),[511] but this rare phenomenon, like simple labeling for neuron-associated antigens, is typically restricted to quite minor tumoral components[511,536] and contrasts with the widespread matrix expression of synaptophysin and nuclear NeuN reactivity that characterizes many neurocytomas.

True **papillary ependymomas** – i.e., tumors in which neoplastic ependymal cells assume a columnar configuration and are supported by fibrovascular cores rather than a fibrillary glial 'stroma' – are very rare and need be distinguished from metastatic papillary carcinomas, choroid plexus papillomas, and papillary meningiomas. Immunohistochemistry may be applied to this problem and obviates more laborious electron microscopic study.[550] Like other ependymomas, papillary variants label for S-100 protein, vimentin, and GFAP. We have also seen these express CD99 in membranous fashion, as do many conventional and clear cell ependymomas.[502] Apical EMA reactivity (a feature potentially shared by ependymal rosettes) may be apparent, as may cytoplasmic decoration with the AE1/3 antikeratin 'cocktail', but ependymomas usually do not immunolabel for CAM 5.2, CK7, CK20, or CK903.[550] If present at all, tumor cells positive for such cytokeratins are typically few in number. One screening study[554] found 2 of 27 ependymomas to manifest nuclear immunoexpression of thyroid transcription factor (TTF)-1, though neither of these tumors (both localized to the third ventricle) was described as papillary. Epithelial neoplasms of the choroid plexus may harbor decidedly ependymocytic populations with elongated and tapering cytoplasmic processes that are GFAP immunoreactive, but this phenomenon (which underscores a shared neurocytogenesis) characteristically constitutes a focal finding when manifest. Choroid plexus papillomas, furthermore, generally depart from intracranial ependymomas in their reactivity for e-cadherin but not neural cell adhesion molecule (NCAM),[508] more diffuse labeling for CAM 5.2 and CK7, expression of transthyretin, Kir 7.1, and stanniocalcin-1, and elaboration of continuous basement membranes demonstrable by immunohistochemical assessment for laminin.[510] Tumors of this group are given full consideration later, as are the papillary glial neoplasm known as astroblastoma and the recently described papillary tumor of the pineal region. Select papillary meningiomas have been described as GFAP immunoreactive (see 'Meningothelial tumors'), but these are extra-axial, dural-based neoplasms and do not evidence ependymal characteristics by electron microscopy.

Location and extent of resection weigh heavily on the prognosis attaching to ependymomas. The intramedullary examples usually encountered in adults often prove amenable to control by surgical means alone in experienced hands.[506] The same cannot be said of tumors located within the cranial compartment. As posterior fossa ependymomas regularly colonize critical bulbar tissues along the floor of the fourth ventricle, few lend themselves to truly complete removal, the large majority recur despite adjuvant treatment, and approximately half kill afflicted children within 5 years of presentation (mortality rates being highest for those below 3 years of age).[528] Also prone to regrowth are supratentorial lesions, though resectable tumors may remain in remission for years after operation. Readers are referred to a recent survey[547] of published data pertaining to the question of whether histology bears independently on outcome in this setting. Unfortunately, analysis of this contradictory literature is complicated by the frequent application of nonuniform, highly subjective and consequently irreproducible grading parameters to the problem. Poorly differentiated tumors exhibiting dense cellularity and conspicuous mitotic activity (which may be accompanied by complex microvascular proliferation and necrosis with pseudopalisading) certainly merit the designation of **anaplastic ependymoma (WHO grade III)** on morphologic grounds and have proven more aggressive than their low-grade counterparts in a number of studies, but these histologic findings are not consistently predictive of an accelerated course. The prognostic implications of only regional anaplasia in the form of nodular microscopic foci of increased cellularity and mitotic activity also needs clarifying.[521,547] Interestingly, features of anaplasia are especially common in the intracranial ependymomas of young children and only rarely encountered in adult-onset ependymomas of the spinal cord. Regional necrosis without pseudopalisades is a common finding in posterior fossa ependymomas and alone does not brand a lesion as anaplastic. As regards other morphologic features of possible biologic significance, microinvasion of bordering neuroparenchyma by dyscohesive tumor cells presaged recurrence in a recent study of pediatric ependymomas.[543] Elevated MIB-1 labeling indices have been correlated with aggressive histology and poor outcome, but widely varying 'cut-off' values have been found significant (ranging from 5% to 20% or higher).[521,528,553] Molecular genetic alterations, such as chromosome 1q gains, have been identified in subsets of anaplastic ependymoma but are not currently relevant to treatment planning.[528] Despite their preferential distribution in and around the ventricular system, intracranial ependymomas only occasionally give rise to symptomatic CSF-borne metastasis; the utility of histologic assessment in predicting this complication is, again, open to question. Distant extraneural metastasis is rare, fatal ependymomas usually killing by virtue of uncontrollable progression at the primary site.

The **myxopapillary ependymoma (WHO grade I)** is a morphologically distinctive variant virtually restricted to the region of the conus medullaris and filum terminale.[544] An origin in cervicothoracic segments of the spinal cord is exceptional, an intracranial presentation exceedingly rare.[522,526] Typically of myxopapillary type are unusual extradural ependymomas that arise in the subcutaneous tissues overlying the sacrococcyx[514,520] or, less often, in the sacrum proper.[530] These curious lesions probably originate from ependymal rests representing remnants of the extradural filum terminale or coccygeal medullary vestige, a derivative of the caudal neural tube persisting beneath the skin of the postanal pit as an ependyma-lined cleft. Such rests can exhibit myxopapillary features and should not be construed as neoplastic by sole virtue of this growth pattern.[534] An ependymoma of the broad ligament having myxopapillary components has been recorded,[551] as has a retinal glioma with myxopapillary ependymal features.[513]

Myxopapillary ependymomas share with other intramedullary tumors of the ependymal series a predilection for adults in the third to fifth decades of life, though nearly one-fifth of those in a large Mayo Clinic series[544] involved patients younger than 20 years of age (some of them children). Nearly all produce low back pain, other manifestations including sciatica, sensorimotor deficits, impotence, and urinary and fecal incontinence. Neuroimaging studies usually demonstrate a sharply delimited, contrast-enhancing mass. Surgical exploration typically discloses a highly vascularized, ovoid or sausage-shaped mass that may be invested by a fibrous pseudocapsule derived from the stroma of the filum. Advanced examples can envelop the cauda equina, erode into neighboring bony structures, and infiltrate paraspinal soft tissues. A gelatinous appearance is characteristic on sectioning, many examples evidencing hemorrhagic discoloration.

The myxopapillary ependymoma is named for the manner in which cuboidal tumor cells drape themselves about a basophilic, mucinous material that in turn collars stromal blood vessels and collects in microcystic spaces (Fig. 28.70). Many examples contain, in addition, spindly elements that may engage in the formation of gliovascular pseudorosettes. Variants displaying a conspicuous complement of pleomorphic tumor giant cells may be encountered.[555] Present in select cases are eosinophilic spherules ('balloons') possibly representing amalgamated collagen fibrils, myxoid matrix components, and basal lamina materials.[544] Common degenerative alterations include vascular sclerosis, hemorrhage, and hemosiderin deposition. Long-standing cases are at times characterized by extensive fibrous tissue overgrowth and virtual obliteration of their neoplastic cellular elements.

The histologic presentation of the myxopapillary ependymoma is in most cases sufficiently distinctive as to render it instantly recognizable to the pathologist familiar with this entity. Particularly

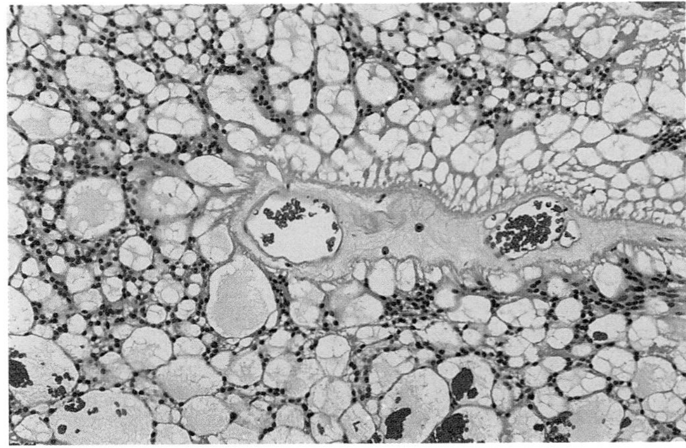

Fig. 28.70 Myxopapillary ependymoma. Note the manner in which mucinous material separates draping tumor cells from a hyalinized vascular core and accumulates in rounded microcysts.

myxomatous variants may assume a chordoma-like appearance whereas examples dominated by spindle cell elements may be mistaken for schwannomas of spinal nerve root origin. A characteristic immunophenotype, as well as a patently ependymal fine structure, distinguishes myxopapillary ependymomas from these neoplasms, from mucinous carcinomas, myxochordoid meningiomas, and paragangliomas of the cauda equina region.[503,544,550] The former share with other ependymomas the coexpression of vimentin, S-100 protein, and GFAP, but do not elaborate chromogranin or CEA, and exhibit little, if any, labeling for CAM 5.2, CK7, or CK20. Tumor labeling by the AE1/3 cytokeratin 'cocktail' may be encountered, however, while the dot and ring patterns of cytoplasmic EMA expression common to conventional ependymomas are usually not manifested by myxopapillary variants. The ultrastructural specializations previously detailed in reference to other ependymomas is faithfully evidenced by the myxopapillary type, though the latter is often less conspicuously endowed with cilia and microvilli, consistently elaborates basal lamina material that may invest cells as a continuous basement membrane, and may contain a unique and specific ultrastructural marker consisting of microtubules aggregated within cisternae of rough endoplasmic reticulum.[515]

Myxopapillary ependymomas are indolent and amenable to surgical cure, but may recur even after ostensibly complete removal. Of 77 afflicted patients described in the Mayo Clinic series,[545] five (6.5%) died of their disease but did so following repeated local recurrences over periods ranging from 12 to 15 years. The presence of cytologic atypism and modest mitotic activity did not alter the prognosis in this study, whereas lesions amenable only to subtotal resection recurred and progressed more frequently than tumors lending themselves to complete removal. Adjuvant irradiation seems to improve outcome.[497] Frankly anaplastic histology is practically never encountered and is of uncertain significance in the face of gross total excision.[499] Myxopapillary ependymomas can spread via the CSF and rarely metastasize to the lungs, liver, lymph nodes, or bone.[497,500,507] Children seem to be at particular risk for CSF-borne dissemination, which may yet be kept under control for years by surgery and irradiation.[500,507] Extraneural metastasis typically complicates stubbornly recurring tumors that have gained access to extravertebral soft tissues and is encountered at substantially increased frequency in patients with extradural variants arising in the sacrococcygeal region.[520,530] Neuroradiologic survey of the spinal axis is mandatory before a diagnosis of primary intracranial myxopapillary ependymoma can be accepted. We have seen neurosurgical intervention prompted by complaints referable to expanding cerebellopontine angle or suprasellar myxopapillary ependymomas that proved to represent secondary deposits from filar region primaries. As was the case in one reported example,[498] the patients in question only later admitted to years of lower back pain.

We defer consideration of the ependymoblastoma to our discussion of primitive neuroepithelial neoplasms and conclude this section with a brief account of the **subependymoma (WHO grade I)**, a lesion named for the resemblance of its constituent cells to, and proposed origin from, subependymal neuroglia distributed along the ventricular system. Most such tumors affect adults, are confined to the fourth ventricle and are diminutive lesions that may be discovered incidentally, but these can attain obstructing proportions.[524,539] More likely to achieve symptomatic size are those subependymomas situated in the lateral ventricles (particularly tumors originating about the foramen of Monro or from the septum pellucidum), third ventricle, cerebral aqueduct, or spinal cord.[524,533,539]

Subependymomas are usually characterized by well-delimited, lobulated contours. Small examples are typically solid and composed of rubbery or tough white tissue, whereas larger lesions often exhibit cystic change and foci of hemorrhagic discoloration.

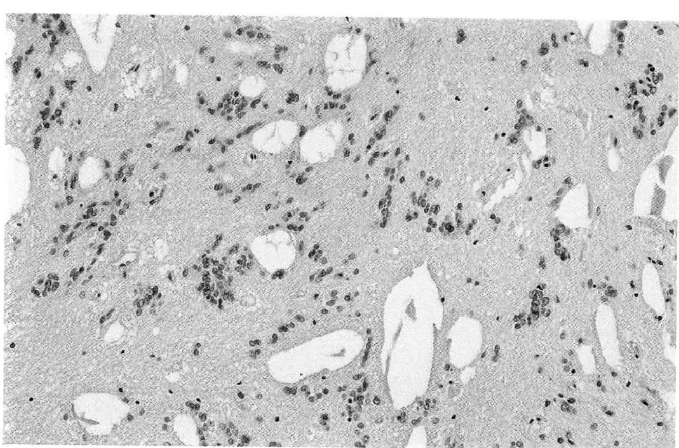

Fig. 28.71 Subependymoma. Characteristic of this entity is the huddling of small tumor cells in an expansive fibrillar meshwork. Microcystic changes commonly round out the histologic picture.

Calcification is common and may be extensive. Histologic examination discloses a multinodular growth pattern with small aggregates of tumor cells haphazardly disposed in a voluminous, hypovascular fibrillary meshwork that may be densely compacted or evidence spongy, microcystic rarefaction (Fig. 28.71). Tumor cell nuclei are generally uniform, having delicate oval contours and a punctate chromatin distribution. The occasional formation of ependymal rosettes, the occurrence of transitional or hybrid tumors containing elements of conventional ependymoma, and demonstrable ependymocytic specializations (e.g., zonulae adherentes, ciliary and microvillus arrays) on electron microscopy all serve to ally the neoplasms under discussion with other members of the ependymoma family. These evidences of ependymal differentiation notwithstanding, many subependymomas contain elements of astrocytic appearance that may assume fibrillary or gemistocytic profiles and that are devoid of prognostic import. We would emphasize that subependymomas may contain a subset of cells with conspicuously enlarged and atypical nuclei, manifest modest mitotic activity, and exhibit foci of coagulative necrosis without pseudopalisading. These findings are not predictive of an aggressive course.[524] A melanotic example has been depicted,[537] as have cases containing sarcomatous elements.[525,535,548]

Excision is the treatment of choice for subependymomas, usually sufficing for control.[524,533,539] Tumors of mixed subependymoma/ependymoma morphology are well recognized. These emerge from some studies[524] as carrying a higher risk of recurrence and are traditionally graded according to the histology of their conventionally ependymomatous components. A recent analysis[539] that included an admittedly small number of mixed lesions with available follow-up data, however, could not demonstrate significant 5-year survival differences on comparison of pure subependymomas to mixed lesions harboring elements of low-grade ependymoma with minimal mitotic activity.

Mixed gliomas

The only 'mixed' gliomas broadly recognized by both neuropathologists and the WHO[564] are those manifesting astrocytic and oligodendroglial features. These infiltrative lesions most often arise in the cerebral hemispheres of adults (the frontal and temporal lobes are favored) and are termed **oligoastrocytomas** (WHO grade II) or **anaplastic oligoastrocytomas** (WHO grade III), the latter displaying high cellularity, conspicuous nuclear atypism, readily apparent mitotic activity and, in some cases, complex microvascular hyperplasia. As noted in prior discussion of the diffusely infiltrating astrocytomas, the WHO now reserves grade IV status for the oligoastrocytic tumor evidencing necrosis and accords to this the controversial designation of glioblastoma with oligodendroglioma component. Defenders of such nomenclature point to studies[562,563] documenting the particularly ominous implications of necrosis as a histologic variable in this setting, though one widely cited investigation[562] actually found the median survival interval associated with high-grade and necrotic oligoastrocytomas to significantly exceed that characterizing glioblastomas of conventional (i.e., astrocytic) type.

Depending on the prejudices of the observer, the diagnosis of oligoastrocytoma or anaplastic oligoastrocytoma can be extended to neoplasms in which elements perceived as astrocytic or oligodendroglial in phenotype are closely and randomly intermingled as well as to those rare tumors in which these components are spatially distinct. The WHO does not endorse suggestions that either component comprises some minimum percentage of the whole.[564] Many practitioners additionally invoke these terms for diffuse gliomas populated by cells that cannot be confidently categorized as either astrocytic or oligodendroglial on morphologic grounds. We simply report the latter as infiltrating glial neoplasms with comment on their ambiguous features. Oligodendrogliomas composed in part of GFAP-positive, 'minigemistocytic' elements retaining the oligodendrocyte's rounded nuclear profile and compacted chromatin do not qualify for inclusion in the oligoastrocytoma group. In a similar vein, oligodendroglioma-like regions are not infrequently encountered in pilocytic astrocytomas and in dysembryoplastic neuroepithelial tumors (discussed in a later section) but, in these settings, are considered part of the diagnosis.

Given the subjective nature of judgments regarding just what qualifies as astrocytic versus oligodendroglial (and how much of either compels acknowledgment), it should come as no surprise that oligoastrocytoma is among the least reproducible diagnoses in surgical neuropathology even in seasoned hands[558,560] and that oligoastrocytic neoplasms as morphologically defined do not constitute a homogeneous biologic entity. Two distinct genetic variants have been delineated.[561,564] One, often composed in the main of classic oligodendrogliomatous elements, shares with the majority of pure oligodendrogliomas combined deletions of chromosomes 1p and 19q that are generally unaccompanied by *TP53* abnormalities. A second subtype, frequently astrocyte predominant or manifesting ambiguous histology, exhibits *TP53* mutations or loss of heterozygosity involving chromosome 17p with intact 1p/19q status – i.e., the genotype characterizing fibrillary and gemistocytic astrocytomas. The data collected thus far indicate that chromosome 1p/19q co-deletion, a phenomenon powerfully correlated with treatment responsiveness and extended survival in the setting of pure oligodendrogliomas, also carries relatively favorable predictive and prognostic implications when evidenced by tumors of the oligoastrocytic group.[557,558,560,562,563] Some observers have found even 1p/19q-intact oligoastrocytomas to behave less aggressively than pure astrocytomas of comparable grade, with clinical biologic profiles and survival times falling between those characterizing the latter and neoplasms of classic oligodendrogliomatous histology.[558,562]

As previously discussed, clear cell components histologically identical to oligodendroglioma may be found within otherwise conventional ependymomas, particularly supratentorial examples. The demonstration that these elements retain ependymocytic features at the ultrastructural level calls into question descriptions of mixed oligodendroglial and ependymal tumors.[559] In fact, we have not encountered a glioma that could be proved to differentiate along divergent, oligoependymal lines. The diagnosis of 'ependymoastrocytoma' should not be invoked for the common fourth ventricular ependymoma harboring minor components of astrocytic appearance or the occasional ependymoma that exhibits along its perimeter foci of astrocytoma-like neuroparenchymal permeation.

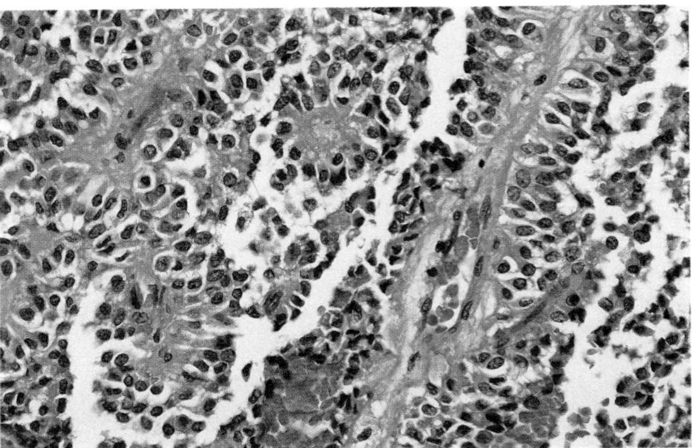

Fig. 28.72 Astroblastoma. The stout cytoplasmic processes of this papillary neoplasm's constituent cells taper rapidly toward supporting vascular cores.

Astroblastoma

The **astroblastoma** is a rare glial neoplasm that usually presents as a well-demarcated, contrast-enhancing mass in the cerebral hemisphere of a child, adolescent, or young adult.[565,566,571] The lesion is characterized by a papilliform architecture, its radially arranged cellular elements directing unipolar cytoplasmic processes toward centrally placed stromal blood vessels (Fig. 28.72). The latter are prone to progressive collagenous thickening and hyalinization, a striking feature of most cases that may advance to partial fibrous obliteration of the neoplastic tissue. Astroblastomatous cell processes are shorter, stouter, and less tapering than those forming ependymal-type pseudorosettes, differing further in their termination on target vessels as expanded footplates. Whereas ependymomatous pseudorosettes generally lie embedded in a dense fibrillar matrix, the gliovascular structures of the astroblastoma are only tenuously supported by an intervening population of astrocyte-like tumor cells or appear to float unanchored in tissue sections. Cytoplasmic immunolabeling for vimentin, S-100 protein, and GFAP are the rule, though the last may be faint or only focally demonstrable.[565–569] Reactivity for low molecular weight cytokeratins[567] and EMA[567] has also been depicted, but expression of synaptophysin has not been demonstrated.

Described ultrastructural attributes of the astroblastoma include a rich cytoplasmic complement of intermediate filaments, intercellular junctional complexes that may be well developed but that usually fall short of the elaborate zonulae adherentes characterizing ependymomas, and an investing basal lamina separating polar cell processes from adjoining stromal vessels.[565,568,570] In select cases constituent cells have been found to display certain ultrastructural features characteristic of 'tanycytes', ventricular lining elements that normally extend basal cytoplasmic processes towards regional capillaries.[570] These include 'purse string'-like constrictions of cell apices and crowning microvilli as well as lamellar cytoplasmic interdigitations ('pleats') along lateral cell borders. Evidence of neuronal differentiation has not been detected.

Inasmuch as conventional astrocytomas of diffuse type (particularly gemistocytic variants) may occasionally harbor gliovascular formations comparable to those of the astroblastoma, the latter designation is best reserved for tumors with a pure, or at least dominant, architecture of the type just described and a circumscribed, compact growth pattern. These may be divided into prognostically favorable and unfavorable types, although the correlation of histology and outcome is, admittedly, imperfect.[565,566,571] Tumors of orderly histologic aspect throughout and inconspicuous mitotic activity appear to be amenable to long-term control by surgical resection, the role of adjuvant therapy being unclear. Examples manifesting a breakdown in astroblastomatous architecture with regions of solid growth, conspicuous mitotic activity, and cellular atypia (accompanied, in some cases, by microvascular proliferation and large zones of coagulative necrosis) are overrepresented among recurring and fatal cases. These 'anaplastic astroblastomas' may develop diffusely infiltrating components, some seeding the CSF. That aggressive-looking variants may yet retain the circumscription typical of well-differentiated astroblastomas, rendering operative extirpation feasible, probably accounts for observations of unexpectedly long disease-free survival and cure in this setting, though most recorded cases have also been subjected to irradiation.

Whether astroblastomas constitute an entity sui generis is controversial, some neuropathologists viewing these as simply variants of astrocytoma or ependymoma. A recent study suggests that combined gains of chromosomes 19 and 20q, generally foreign to conventional astrocytic and ependymal neoplasms, are particularly frequent in this rare tumor group.[566] Though this does not speak to the cytogenesis of astroblastomas, it does argue for their being accorded distinct nosologic status.

Chordoid glioma of the third ventricle

The rare neoplasms reported as **chordoid gliomas of the third ventricle** have occurred almost exclusively in adults, an excess affecting women.[572–581] While tumors of comparable morphology and immunophenotype have been encountered in other locations,[576] these peculiar growths (as their name recognizes) have been nearly limited to the third ventricular/suprasellar compartment. Here they present on neuroradiologic study as large, solid, sharply circumscribed and homogeneously contrast-enhancing masses producing obstructive hydrocephalus and an array of clinical manifestations that potentially include headache, ataxia, visual and endocrine disturbances, marked fluctuations of weight, and psychotic/organic brain syndromes.

The chordoid glioma is noninfiltrative in its growth pattern and composed of epithelioid, oval to polygonal cells disposed as irregular cords or nests within a basophilic, myxoid matrix prone to coarse vacuolation (Fig. 28.73A). The latter may be PAS/DPAS positive and faintly mucicarminophilic. Tumor cells possess eosinophilic cytoplasm and round or oval nuclei with finely granular or clumped chromatin and small nucleoli. Cell cords and nests may be outlined by reticulin fibers. An additional, near constant feature of this peculiar neoplasm is interstitial and perivascular infiltration by lymphocytes and Russell body-bearing plasma cells. A unique pediatric example manifesting chondroid metaplasia has been recorded.[573] Pertinent to the differential diagnosis (which includes metastatic carcinoma, intradural chordoma, and chordoid meningioma) is the absence of true gland formation, physaliphorous cells, cellular whorls, intranuclear pseudoinclusions, and psammoma bodies. Mitoses are not found or are rare (MIB-1 labeling indices generally fall in the 0–1.5% range), conspicuous pleomorphism, microvascular proliferation, and necrosis also being foreign to these

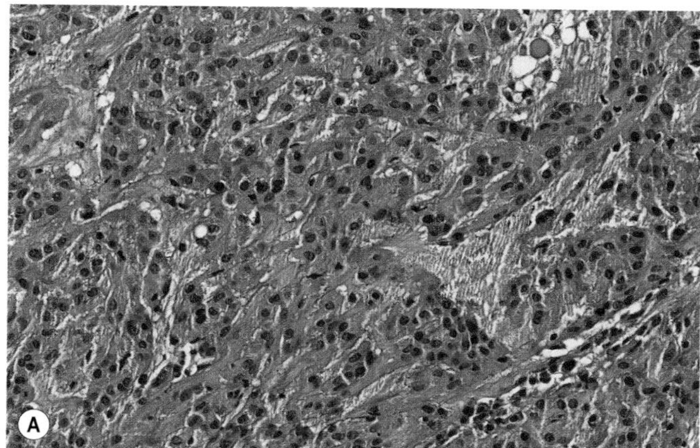

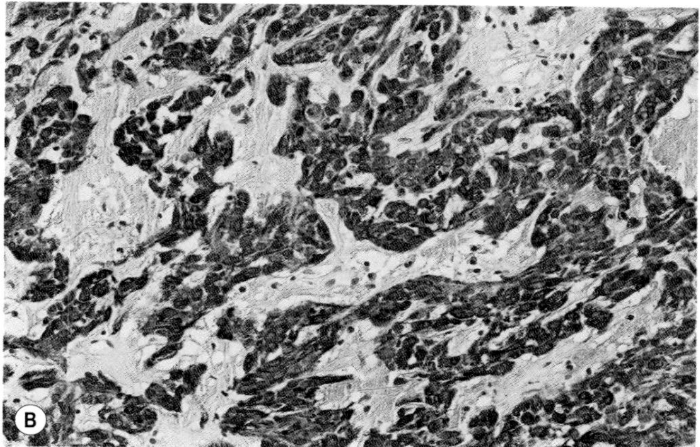

Fig. 28.73 Chordoid glioma of the third ventricle. Nests and anastomosing cords of epithelioid tumor cells arrayed against a variably myxoid stromal background typify this lesion (**A**), which is distinguished from other chordoid neoplasms by its diffuse cytoplasmic immunolabeling for GFAP (**B**). Note also in **A** the presence of plasma cells at lower right. These are often present in more conspicuous numbers.

lesions. Adjacent brain tissue typically manifests reactive gliosis with Rosenthal fiber formation.

A characteristic immunoprofile segregates chordoid gliomas from potential mimickers.[572,575,581] The former consistently evidence diffuse cytoplasmic labeling for GFAP (Fig. 28.73B) as well as vimentin, express CD34 (with cell membrane accentuation), and may be focally S-100 protein positive, but are EMA negative or only focally EMA immunoreactive. Limited labeling for a variety of cytokeratins has been reported,[572,575,581] though the AE1/3 'cocktail' may yield a pattern overlapping with that of GFAP preparations. Cytoplasmic immunolabeling for epidermal growth factor receptor and merlin/schwannomin have also been recorded,[581] as has focal synaptophysin expression in select cases,[575] but examples assessed to date have not evidenced reactivity for neurofilament proteins, estrogen or progesterone receptors, desmin, chromogranin or p53.[581] The limited ultrastructural experience communicated thus far suggests that chordoid gliomas differentiate along ependymal lines. While such pathognomonic ependymal specializations as microlumens delimited by intercellular junctional complexes of zonula adherens type have not been depicted, the formation of desmosome-like cytoplasmic attachments, microvilli, partially investing basal lamina and, in one case,[579] aberrant juxtanuclear cilia would seem to ally these unusual tumors with neoplasms of the ependymocytic series and to distance them from the astrocytic and oligodendroglial families.[572,574,576,577,580] In this connection, we would mention personal experience with an example containing papillary perivascular pseudorosettes and alveolus-like structures.[580] Chordoid gliomas have been described in one report[574] as sharing certain ultrastructural properties with specially modified ependymal cells that constitute the subcommissural organ – an ostensibly secretory body, situated in the dorsocaudal aspect of the third ventricle, that develops fully during human embryonic life and undergoes postnatal involution. Common features included zonation of cell bodies into: a perinuclear region containing prominent profiles of rough endoplasmic reticulum and Golgi apparatus; an intermediate region occupied principally by mitochondria, smooth endoplasmic reticulum, and secretory-type granules; and an apical zone displaying a rich complement of intermediate filaments and crowning microvilli. An alternative origin from specialized ependyma lining the more rostrally situated lamina terminalis has been proposed[578] and would account for the localization of relatively small tumors of this type (i.e., those not filling the entire third ventricle) to the latter region. Some workers[575] have found chordoid gliomas to consistently exhibit losses at chromosomes 9q21 and 11q13, the former alterations overlapping with those seen in select supratentorial ependymomas.

Chordoid gliomas of the third ventricle grow slowly, do not invade surrounding tissues, and have not been reported to metastasize via the CSF, but their attachment to hypothalamic/suprasellar structures complicates removal.[572,577,581] Curiously, pulmonary thromboembolism has accounted for a disproportionate share of deaths occurring in the immediate postoperative period.[572,581] Incompletely resected examples may remain relatively stable but often regrow and can eventually prove fatal.[572] The role of adjuvant therapy is undefined.

Angiocentric glioma

Angiocentric glioma is the designation adopted in the 2007 WHO formulation[582] for a distinctive entity reported as 'monomorphous angiocentric glioma'[586] and 'angiocentric neuroepithelial tumor'[584] in two defining series. Strongly associated with chronic, pharmacoresistant epilepsy having its onset in childhood or adolescence, this rare neoplasm is most often situated in the frontoparietal or temporal lobes, superficially positioned and largely cortical in topography. We have seen a possible example that arose from the tectum of the midbrain.[583] Relative circumscription, hyperintensity on T2-weighted and FLAIR sequences, and lack of contrast enhancement are regular MRI features, some examples manifesting stalk-like extensions of T2/FLAIR-hyperintense signal abnormality towards the underlying ventricular wall and rimming cortical T1 hyperintensity that may suggest the diagnosis.[584,585]

The hallmark of the angiocentric glioma is the manner in which native cerebrocortical blood vessels of all calibers are converted into a scaffolding along which bipolar spindle cells of uniform cytologic profile are disposed in multilayered sleeves and about which these neoplastic elements may also be radially arranged in pseudorosettes of decidedly ependymal aspect (Fig. 28.74). A granular, stippled chromatin distribution within slender tumor cell nuclei further suggests a lesion of ependymocytic character. Spindled cells frequently align in perpendicular palisades beneath the pia and swirl in tight ('schwannoid') micronodules, may freely diffuse into the neuroparenchyma, and can form dense and intersecting fascicles that entirely replace the affected cortex. In some cases, tumor cells of rounded and epithelioid appearance also surround vessels and lie in sheets interrupted by irregular clefts and cavities.

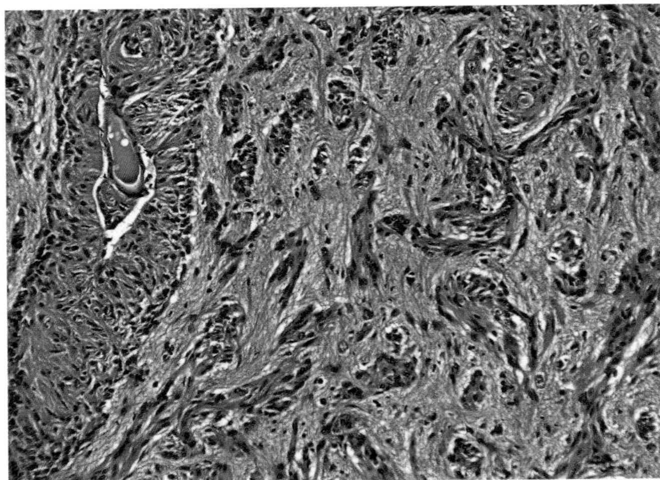

Fig. 28.74 Angiocentric glioma. Tumor cells of monomorphous, spindled profile sheath and collar cerebrocortical blood vessels in this typical example.

Immunohistochemical and ultrastructural assessments of the angiocentric glioma clearly indicate differentiation along ependymocytic lines.[584–586] Tumor cells exhibit GFAP reactivity (a finding that removes meningioangiomatosis from further diagnostic consideration) and (in contrast to the spindled, bipolar constituents of the pilocytic astrocytoma) frequently display dot-like cytoplasmic EMA labeling of the sort correlated with microlumen formation by neoplasms of the ependymal series. EMA expression along cell surfaces may also be evident. The formation of microlumens delimited by zipper-like intercellular junctions has been confirmed at the fine structural level, microvilli and cilia projecting into these structures. In explanation of a consistently extraventricular and cortex-based tumor manifesting these features, it has been proposed[584] that the angiocentric glioma derives from primitive neuroepithelial cells – the radial glia – that span the embryonic neuroepithelium and that may generate ependymocytes.

Angiocentric gliomas are mitotically inactive or display, at most, only rare mitoses. MIB-1 labeling indices are typically low, not exceeding 5% and usually falling below 1–2%. Clinical indolence is the rule, these lesions potentially remaining radiologically stable over protracted surveillance alone, and simple excision generally effecting cure.[582] Malignant progression has been described,[586] but is certainly an exception to the benign behavior that can be expected of this WHO grade I neoplasm.

Gliomatosis cerebri

Gliomatosis cerebri, as traditionally and stringently defined, is a rare condition in which large portions of the brain are permeated by neoplastic cells in such manner (i.e., without focal mass formation) as to suggest a transformative 'field effect' rather than the centrifugal spread of an initially localized glial tumor.[587,589] The WHO endorses a definition requiring that at least three cerebral lobes be involved at presentation.[589] Affected regions are typically expanded in nondestructive ('pseudohypertrophic') fashion without formation of appreciable tumor nodules. The process may be remarkably diffuse, often extending from the cerebrum into deep gray matter, as well as brainstem, and potentially involving the entire central neuraxis.[588] Formerly reserved for cases examined at autopsy, this diagnosis is now rendered on clinical grounds when biopsy material demonstrating an infiltrative glioma derives from a patient evidencing particularly widespread neuroradiologic abnormalities. Confluent multilobar and bihemispheric zones of signal hyperintensity in T2-weighted and FLAIR studies are characteristic on MRI.[590,592]

Gliomatosis cerebri is neither a uniform morphologic entity nor a condition that can be reliably identified on cytologic or histologic grounds alone. While most examples exhibit astrocytic features, oligodendrogliomatous and 'oligoastrocytic' variants are recognized.[592,593] Unusually elongated nuclear profiles in parallel array (the result of tumor cell infiltration between compacted nerve fibers) and a tendency to pronounced subpial, perivascular, and circumneuronal cellular aggregation are often emphasized as especially characteristic, but are by no means specific, or even constant, attributes.[587,591] There is, moreover, considerable variation in GFAP expression (not demonstrable in some cases), in mitotic activity and proliferative potential as assessed by MIB-1 (Ki-67) immunolabeling.[589,590] A large majority of gliomatoses qualify as WHO grade II or III lesions on histologic grounds, a small minority presenting with such grade IV features as microvascular proliferation and necrosis.[589,592]

It should come as no surprise, given the foregoing observations, that the clinical course of gliomatosis cerebri is not strictly predictable (apart from the generally poor prognosis and eventual lethality of bona fide cases).[589,590,592] A comprehensive analysis of nearly 300 reported patients found a median survival of only 14.5 months.[592] A more protracted course characterizes at least some cerebral gliomatoses of low histologic grade, the prognosis for oligodendroglial variants being better than that attaching to the more common astrocytic types.[592] Limited Ki-67 immunolabeling has also been correlated with less aggressive behavior.[590] Focal or multicentric progression may complicate otherwise well-differentiated examples and eventuate in the picture of glioblastoma. The reader interested in issues of histogenesis (unknown) and pertinent genetic data (fragmentary) is referred elsewhere.[589] Suffice it to say that the latter generally support the clonal nature of gliomatosis though signature genomic abnormalities have not been identified. Astroglial examples may evidence *TP53* mutations as well as other anomalies common to infiltrating astrocytomas of conventional type, while a subset of oligodendrogliomatoses share the chromosome 1p/19q co-deleted profile common to oligodendroglial neoplasms of the usual variety.[589,592] The presence of these deletions in the setting of oligodendroglial gliomatosis has been correlated in some analyses with treatment responsiveness and longer survival.[592] A lack of the *IDH* gene mutations common to infiltrating astrocytomas and oligodendrogliomas characterizes a subset of gliomatoses that may constitute a distinct entity.[591a]

Pituicytoma and granular cell tumor

Two unusual neoplasms, the pituicytoma and granular cell tumor of the neurohypophysis, are believed to derive from specialized glial elements ('pituicytes') native to the posterior portion of the pituitary gland and infundibulum. These entities are discussed, along with other pituitary tumors (including the spindle cell oncocytoma of the adenohypophysis, a differential diagnostic consideration), in Chapter 29 of this volume.

Gliosarcoma and other 'gliomesenchymal' tumors

CNS tumors characterized by mixed neuroepithelial and mesenchymal features are a heterogeneous lot. We have previously alluded in this connection to the emergence of sarcomatous elements from neoplasms of the astrocytic, oligodendroglial, and ependymal series. The overwhelming majority of glial tumors manifesting this phenomenon are glioblastomas and the designation of **gliosarcoma**, employed without qualification, is generally taken to connote a glioblastoma variant[380] (as opposed to 'oligosarcoma'[491] or 'ependymosarcoma'[535]). It has been suggested that approximately 2% of otherwise conventional glioblastomas spawn malignant components of mesenchymal aspect[603] and only gliosarcomatous neoplasms of this, the most common, type are accorded more extended treatment here. Passing mention is made of sarcoglioma as a term applied to tumors interpreted as primary intracranial sarcomas or meningiomas complicated by the provoked progression to neoplasia of commingled, reactive astrocytic elements.[602,604]

The clinical profile of the gliosarcoma is essentially that of the primary glioblastoma.[603,608,611] Most examples arise in the absence of recognized predisposing factors, but gliosarcomas have been associated with prior irradiation,[608] including the intracranial instillation of Thorotrast.[617] At operation, many are initially mistaken for cerebral metastases or (when attached to the dura) meningiomas, errors resulting from their characteristic circumscription and firm textures. These attributes in turn reflect the high content of connective tissue fibers typical of the gliosarcoma but foreign to most other neuroepithelial neoplasms. A marmoreal admixture of gliomatous and sarcomatous tissues lends to these tumors a strikingly biphasic architecture on histologic study (Fig. 28.75A). Mesenchymal components usually evidence appearances that would prompt the

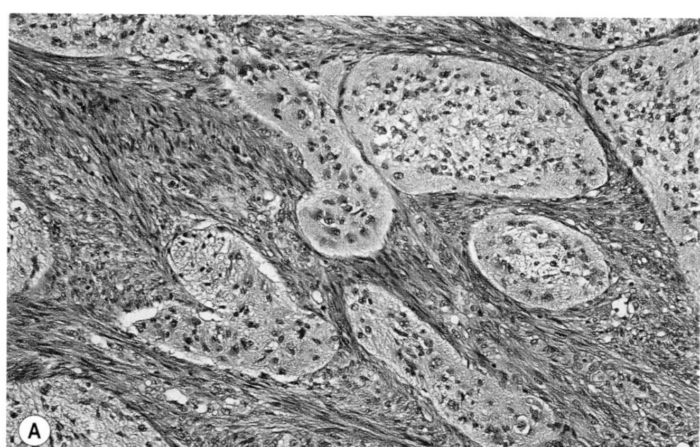

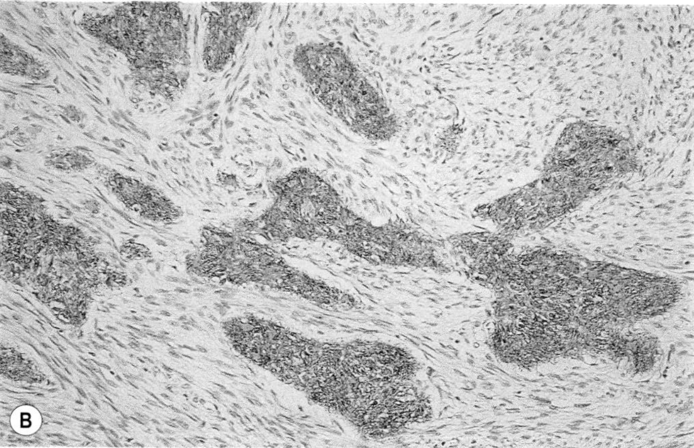

Fig. 28.75 Gliosarcoma. Islands of astrocytic tumor tissue lie embedded in what otherwise appears to be a spindle cell sarcoma (**A**). On immunoperoxidase assay (**B**), only astrocytic elements are labeled for glial fibrillary acidic protein.

diagnosis of fibrosarcoma or malignant fibrous histiocytoma in a soft tissue setting, but chondro-osteogenic and myogenic differentiation may be encountered[611] and variants harboring angiosarcomatous,[613] liposarcomatous[616] and mixed mesdodermal-type elements[607] have been reported. Squamous differentiation, 'adenoid' formations, and glandular structures may be displayed within the glial regions of select cases.[374,385,398,606]

Distinction of the gliosarcoma's dimorphic constituents can be further accomplished using a combination of traditional histochemical and immunocytochemical techniques.[598,603,608] Sarcomatous components are richly invested with connective tissue fibers demonstrable by reticulin impregnation methods and preparations for collagen, such as the Mallory trichrome stain, but do not express GFAP, the reverse being true of the glial population (Fig. 28.75B). The identification of an architecturally and cytologically distinct, GFAP-negative component is requisite to the segregation of the true gliosarcoma from collagenized, spindle cell ('desmoplastic') glioblastomas and gliomas associated with a florid fibroblastic reaction by virtue of meningeal invasion. Similarly distanced from neoplasms of gliosarcomatous character are variants of astrocytoma and ependymoma that give rise to well-differentiated, GFAP-immunoreactive cartilaginous elements,[601] as well as 'lipomatous' astroglial[596] and ependymal[538] tumors containing lipidized, adipocyte-like constituents that retain GFAP expression.

The 'malignant degeneration' of blood vessel-associated stromal elements was first held to account for the genesis of sarcomatous populations within glioblastomas.[380] The latter, as previously discussed, often manifest a florid and complex microvascular proliferation driven by the tumoral elaboration of mitogens that act on endothelium, pericytes, smooth muscle cells, and fibroblasts. Each of these cell types came to be championed as a target of transformation within evolving gliosarcomas, as did histiocytes, myofibroblasts, and uncommitted adventitial elements. That this autocrine phenomenon could eventuate in sarcomatous outgrowth – a notion originally based on perceived histologic transitions from the hyperplastic to unarguably neoplastic – was to receive only qualified support, however, from immunohistochemical and electron microscopic observations. Reports that the sarcomatous constituents of the gliosarcoma labeled for endothelial markers (factor VIII-related antigen and the UEA-1 lectin) or contained Weibel–Palade bodies on ultrastructural study[614] did not prove generally reproducible,[598] though these populations were found in many cases to exhibit focal immunoreactivity for smooth muscle actin[599,608] – a feature shared by cells of pericytic/myoid type which dominate the glioblastoma's glomeruloid microvascular formations.[366,403]

A rival histogenetic view of the gliosarcoma would have neoplastic glial cells simply undergoing phenotypic shift with tumor progression, losing GFAP expression and assuming mesenchymal attributes.[600,610] Powerful backing for this scenario derives from molecular genetic studies demonstrating that gliomatous and sarcomatous components may harbor identical *TP53* and *PTEN* mutations, p16 (*CDKN2A*) deletions and coamplifications of CDK4 and MDM2.[610] Whether a subset of tumors accorded this designation might still represent true composites, as opposed to neometaplastic lesions of clonal character, is arguable. The clonal nature of oligosarcomas and ependymosarcomas is similarly supported by shared patterns of chromosome 1p/19q deletion[491] and of NF2/protein 4.1 gene family alteration,[535] respectively.

The designation '**gliofibroma**' has been extended to a heterogeneous group of neoplasms encountered for the most part in childhood and having in common a population of astrocytes that may be invested by basal lamina material and that are embedded in a variably collagenized matrix.[595,609,612] Some appear to represent desmoplastic astrocytomas in which neoplastic glia, unaided by mesenchymal derivatives, are directly responsible for the elaboration of connective tissues,[609] whereas other examples contain a second cellular population interpreted as fibroblastic[595,605,612] or, in one study, schwannian.[615] The rarity and disparate morphologic features of the tumors reported under this rubric obviously preclude useful generalizations regarding their histogenesis and clinical biology. A number of recorded cases have evidenced conspicuous cytologic atypism and mitotic activity, pursuing an aggressive course (with CSF-borne metastasis) and ending fatally, the benign connotations of the term gliofibroma notwithstanding.[595,612] A more favorable outcome seems to be attached to those lacking features of histologic anaplasia.

This discussion of gliomesenchymal tumors is concluded with passing reference to the various uses of the term '**angioglioma**'. Originally applied to what would now be classified as the cellular variant of cerebellar hemangioblastoma, this designation has been most frequently invoked in reference to gliomas exhibiting degenerative vascular alterations resembling AVMs or cavernous angiomas.[146] Slow-growing lesions such as pilocytic astrocytomas, oligodendrogliomas, and gangliogliomas seem especially prone to such changes. These may appear hypervascular on angiographic study, exhibiting a tumoral 'blush', but as a rule do not evidence the shunting characteristic of true AVMs. Only exceptionally are the latter found in contiguity with glial neoplasms. Most such lesions are regarded as 'collision' tumors in which gliomatous and malformative tissues are fortuitously associated, but isolated reports of glial neoplasms secondarily arising at the sites of pre-existent AVMs and angiomas suggest that the gliotic reaction typical of tissues surrounding such long-standing vascular anomalies may rarely progress to neoplasia.[597] A strikingly increased concentration of oligodendrocytes in and around some AVMs appears to result from 'collapse' of chronically edematous and ischemic white matter or to represent part of the malformation process and should not necessarily prompt a diagnosis of oligodendroglioma.[146,153] Finally, we call attention to a group of exceedingly uncommon tumors interpreted as containing both gliomatous and hemangioblastomatous elements.[594] These, too, have been described as a form of 'angioglioma', a non-specific and potentially misleading term that is best abandoned.

Choroid plexus tumors

A secretory organ responsible for the production of CSF, the choroid plexus consists of a richly vascularized fibrous stroma draped by an epithelium that derives from neuroectodermal cells abutting the embryonic ventricular system. Only rarely do its specialized epithelial elements give rise to neoplasms, these generally affecting children and presenting in sporadic fashion. Carcinomas (and, rarely, papillomas) of plexus origin, however, may be encountered in the familial Li–Fraumeni (germline *TP53* mutation) syndrome, while papillomas often complicate a complex of infantile flexor spasms, agenesis of the corpus callosum, and chorioretinal anomalies known as Aicardi syndrome, and have been recorded in cases of hypomelanosis of Ito with associated X;17(q12;p13) translocation.[647] As discussed further below, reports that would link choroid plexus carcinomas to specific abnormalities of the atypical teratoid/rhabdoid tumor-associated *INI1* gene have been called into serious question.[638] That human choroid plexus tumors, like ependymomas, may harbor simian virus 40-type DNA sequences is intriguing, given the fact that expression of this agent's T antigen is specifically associated with choroid plexus neoplasia in transgenic murine models, but an etiologic link in the former scenario (as opposed to passenger effect) is yet to be established.[647]

Tumors derived from the epithelium of the choroid plexus exhibit considerable morphologic and biologic diversity. The great major-

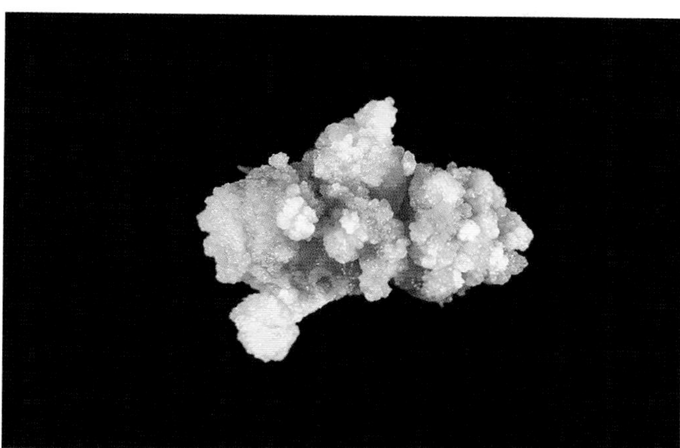

Fig. 28.76 Choroid plexus papilloma. Note the characteristically bosselated surface of this surgically resected example. Deprived of its blood supply, the tumor tissue loses its normally hyperemic appearance and may assume a tan or golden hue.

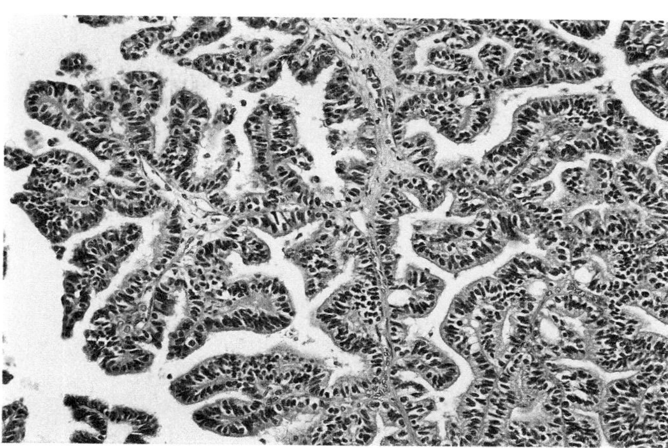

Fig. 28.77 Choroid plexus papilloma. This example's delicate fibrovascular fronds are covered by an orderly, low columnar epithelium.

ity, however, are benign neoplasms that replicate the villous architecture of the parent organ and are consequently termed **choroid plexus papillomas (WHO grade I)**.[647,648,653] Most of the latter come to attention during early childhood, displaying a predilection for the lateral ventricles. Adult cases, by contrast, are situated more often in the fourth ventricle or its lateral recesses, some presenting as tumors of the cerebellopontine angle. Multifocal presentations are on record,[629] as are ectopic neuroparenchymal,[649] suprasellar,[640] sacral nerve root-associated,[621] and sacral extradural[641] examples. Associated clinical manifestations are largely those of hydrocephalus resulting from ventricular outflow obstruction or the excessive production of CSF by these highly differentiated neoplasms. Rarely, plexus-related hydrocephalus in infancy is caused by villous hyperplasia of this organ.[651] Whether some diffuse lesions of this sort actually represent neoplasms (i.e., bilateral papillomas or papillomatosis) that can be identified by their proliferative activity as assessed in MIB-1 preparations is questionable.[625]

On gross inspection, the choroid plexus papilloma is a friable mass having a villiform or bosselated surface often likened to that of a cauliflower (Fig. 28.76). Lesions described as cystic forms of choroid plexus papilloma are most exceptional.[646] Calcification, common to these tumors, imparts to some a gritty consistency or, when extensive, stony hardness that may hinder sectioning in the undecalcified state. Histologic examination typically discloses a complex array of branching fibrovascular fronds covered by a monolayer of uniform cuboidal or columnar epithelial cells exhibiting minimal nuclear atypism and little, if any, mitotic activity (Fig. 28.77). On ultrastructural study these cells rest on an uninterrupted basement membrane, are joined at their apices by elaborate junctional complexes, are crowned by microvilli, and may be ciliated.[643] The tumoral stroma, like that of the normal choroid plexus, may be conspicuously infiltrated by foamy macrophages and is, in select cases, the site of metaplastic bone or cartilage formation.[650] The epithelial elements of some tumors undergo oncocytic change[622] (one reported example progressing to malignant 'oncocytoma'[626]) and a rare melanotic variant of the choroid plexus papilloma has also been described.[633] These neoplasms may, in addition, evidence limited ependymal differentiation, signaled by foci in which tumor cells extend tapering, GFAP-immunoreactive cytoplasmic processes toward their fibrovascular cores. This finding presumably reflects the ontogeny of the plexus epithelium as a form of specialized ependyma, but choroid plexus papillomas do not elaborate the fibrillary glial 'stroma' characteristic of ependymomas – an important differential diagnostic feature. Exceptional cases exhibit a glandular, rather than papillary, growth pattern – an arrangement for which the designations of acinar or tubular choroid plexus adenoma have been invoked.[618,628] Some of these curious variants have been mucin producing.[628] Most peculiar, but convincingly documented, is the papilloma exhibiting overt neuronal differentiation signaled by micronodular collections of synaptophysin-rich matrix ('choroid plexus papilloma with neuropil-like islands').[635]

The well-differentiated choroid plexus papilloma is usually amenable to curative resection.[647,653] Regrowth at the primary site may be encountered, particularly after subtotal removal, but progression to carcinoma is rare[637] and focally recurrent lesions often remain surgically controllable.[653] The capacity of otherwise conventional examples to seed the CSF and metastasize along the central neuraxis is a recognized but, fortunately, uncommon phenomenon.[644] More problematic is a subset of tumors, often dubbed **atypical choroid plexus papillomas**, that fall short of overt histologic malignancy while evidencing an unexpectedly complex architecture, cytologic atypism, modestly increased mitotic activity, focal necrosis or penetration of juxtatumoral brain tissue. Some have noted an increased likelihood of recurrence and progression to histologic anaplasia on the part of tumors exhibiting worrisome morphologic traits of this sort,[636,648] but this is a murky and controversial area. It has been our experience, in fact, that 'invasive' tumoral deposits are not infrequently identifiable along the perimeter of perfectly benign-appearing papillomas, where they are typically associated with a Rosenthal fiber-rich pilocytic astrogliosis attesting to a chronic and indolent process. In accord with some other observers,[642] we can attach no significance to this finding. The WHO recognizes atypical choroid plexus papillomas as grade II lesions,[647] defining these as exhibiting, at a minimum, increased mitotic activity and citing a single study[636] in which the presence of two or more mitoses per 10 high power microscopic fields emerged on multivariate analysis as independently associated with a heightened risk of recurrence.

Choroid plexus carcinoma (WHO grade III) is the appropriate designation for frankly malignant epithelial neoplasms of plexus origin.[647] The overwhelming majority of these rare tumors present in infancy or childhood and are situated in a lateral ventricle.[647,653] In contrast to their benign counterparts, choroid plexus carcinomas are highly proliferative, invasive, destructive, and typified by geographic foci of necrosis and hemorrhage. Many, while maintaining a regional fidelity to the villiform architecture of the native plexus, contain foci in which their papillary structure breaks down and is replaced by nests and patternless sheets of anaplastic cells exhibiting alarming pleomorphism and mitotic activity. Eosinophilic, PAS-positive and diastase-resistant globules are prominently displayed by some examples[645] and isolated cases have been described as containing melanotic cytoplasmic pigments.[627] These aggressive neoplasms often prove fatal, some escaping the confines of the ventricular system, seeding the subarachnoid space and even metastasizing to extraneural sites, but cure of localized examples may be effected by gross total removal and adjuvant treatment.[653]

Application of an appropriate antibody panel can be recommended for purposes of distinguishing choroid plexus tumors from potential mimickers. The former often evidence cytoplasmic colabeling for vimentin, cytokeratins (CAM 5.2 and AE1/3 reactivity are the rule, though highly variable in extent, one study[632] describing a CK7+/CK20− immunophenotype as characterizing most plexus papillomas), and S-100 protein (potentially expressed in nuclei as well).[624,648] Neoplasms of the choroid plexus may, in addition, facilitate recognition of their neuroepithelial lineage by expressing GFAP (usually in focal fashion),[624,648] and the labeling of these tumors for synaptophysin has also been depicted.[639] As previously discussed, intracranial ependymomas (including papillary variants) often exhibit widespread GFAP reactivity, contain few, if any, CAM 5.2- or CK7-positive elements, and are usually synaptophysin negative. Also noted in our prior treatment of ependymomas is the observation that the latter, unlike epithelial neoplasm of the choroid plexus, often express NCAM but not e-cadherin. As compared to primary choroid plexus tumors, metastatic carcinomas are far more likely to exhibit immunoreactivity for EMA and the surface epithelial antigens identified by monoclonal antibodies HEA125 and Ber-EP4,[631] are less often S-100 protein positive and (with rare exception) are GFAP negative. Cytoplasmic labeling for transthyretin, a 55-kDa protein involved in thyroxine and retinol transport, is a frequent feature of choroid plexus tumor immunophenotype, but is inconstant (approximately 70% of cases prove reactive) and shared by a subset of ependymomas, glioblastomas, and epithelial tumors metastatic to brain.[634]

Additional 'markers' potentially useful in the identification of choroid plexus tumors but not in general employ by neuropathologists include antibodies to the excitatory amino acid transporter-1 (EAAT-1),[620] to Kir 7.1 (an inwardly rectifying potassium channel protein),[634] and to stanniocalcin-1 (involved, among other functions, in calcium homeostasis).[634] Membraneous EAAT-1 expression characterized 66% (23/35) of choroid plexus tumors but none of 77 metastatic carcinomas (including 64 papillary adenocarcinomas of varied origin) in one study.[620] Nearly 75% (17/23) of choroid plexus neoplasms (including all 5 carcinomas) tested in a second analysis manifested membraneous cytoplasmic labeling for Kir 7.1, 100 other primary and secondary brain tumors (including 19 ependymomas, 44 metastatic carcinomas, 11 glioblastomas, and 6 atypical teratoid/rhabdoid tumors) proving nonreactive.[634] In the same study, cytoplasmic stanniocalcin-1 expression characterized 83% of choroid plexus tumors (including 3 of 5 malignant lesions) and single examples of dysembryoplastic neuroepithelial tumor (neuronal labeling) and metastatic carcinoma of thyroid origin. Kir 7.1 and stanniocalcin-1 labeling may also distinguish plexus neoplasms from papillary tumors of the pineal region, discussed later in this chapter, while EAAT-1 expression has been touted as a feature useful in distinguishing the former from native choroid plexus.[619]

Further recommended for the purpose of distinguishing anaplastic choroid plexus carcinomas from atypical teratoid/rhabdoid tumors, which share a predilection for infants and can regionally exhibit somewhat papillary or tubuloglandular growth patterns, is BAF47. This antibody recognizes the product of *INI1*, a gene situated at chromosome band 22q11.2 that encodes a ubiquitously expressed protein active in chromatin remodeling. Whereas atypical teratoid/rhabdoid tumors are left unlabeled by BAF47 in consequence of their consistent association with biallelic *INI1* inactivation (most often one copy is lost through monosomy 22 or lesser deletions, the second suffering a truncating nonsense or frameshift mutation), choroid plexus carcinomas regularly retained the expected nuclear reactivity with this reagent in a study of 20 cases classified as such by a group of experienced surgical neuropathologists.[638] Six additional neoplasms carrying referral diagnoses of choroid plexus carcinoma but reclassified as atypical teratoid/rhabdoid tumors proved BAF47 negative. While two (of four) plexus carcinomas analyzed exhibited monosomy 22, an abnormality that atypical teratoid/rhabdoid tumors have in common with varied tumor types (e.g., meningiomas), none of seven assessed manifested mutations specifically involving *INI1*. Thus, difficulties in distinguishing these entities on morphologic and other immunophenotypic grounds may account for suggestions that mutational targeting of *INI1* bears on choroid plexus carcinogenesis.[647]

We stress that the diagnosis of choroid plexus carcinoma in an adult must be regarded with considerable skepticism (regardless of tumor location, morphology, or immunohistochemical characteristics) as this entity is vanishingly rare beyond childhood and older patients presenting with intracranial carcinomas, including well-differentiated lesions of papillary configuration, almost invariably prove to harbor lung or other systemic primaries. With regard to the prognostic implications of immunophenotype in the setting of choroid plexus neoplasia, we would emphasize that the benign and malignant cannot be reliably distinguished on the basis of antigenic profile, though dampened expression of transthyretin and S-100 protein seems to be more characteristic of plexus carcinomas and of papillomas that recur following resection.[624,648] Carcinomas may also be somewhat more prone to express CEA,[624] though this is generally foreign to tumors of the choroid plexus family,[648] and are more likely to exhibit widespread nuclear p53 labeling[623] as well as MIB-1 (Ki-67) indices in excess of 5–10%.[623,652] In one recent analysis, carcinomas lacking p53 immunoexpression and *TP53* mutations were associated with far more favorable courses than their p53-labeling and *TP53*-mutant counterparts.[651a]

The reader's attention is called to a recent report describing as '**pigmented papillary epithelial neoplasm of the pituitary fossa**' a melanotic sellar tumor that underwent anaplastic spindle cell transformation following repeated resections and radiotherapy.[630] As suggested by the authors, this curiosity may represent an ectopic form of choroid plexus neoplasm.

Neuronal and glioneuronal tumors, hamartomas, and related lesions

Gangliocytoma and ganglioglioma

A biologically heterogeneous assortment of CNS tumors, including primitive neuroepithelial neoplasms of potentially aggressive character, are capable of neuronal differentiation and may spawn ganglion cell-like forms. The uncommon entities known as **gangliocytoma** and **ganglioglioma** (collectively termed 'ganglion cell tumors') share a complement of large and essentially mature neurons unassociated, by definition, with recognizably embryonal elements. Much the more prevalent species, the ganglioglioma harbors an admixed glial population of neoplastic appearance that distinguishes this lesion from the pure gangliocytoma.[658,663,669] Ganglion cell tumors usually come to neurosurgical intervention within

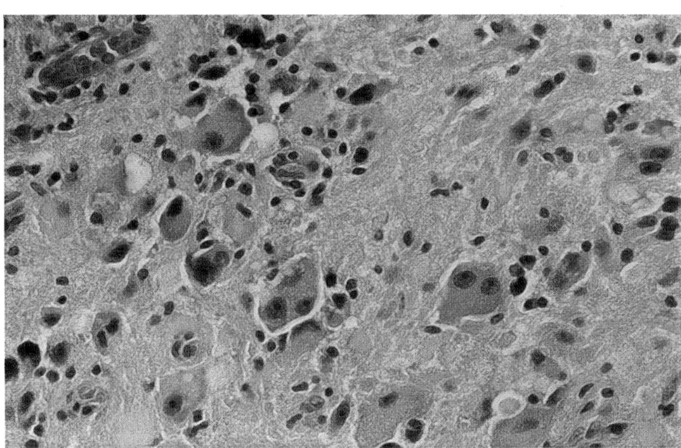

Fig. 28.78 Ganglioglioma. The neoplastic nature of the ganglion cell tumor's large neurons is readily apparent when abnormal clustering and cytologic abnormalities such as multinucleation are in evidence. Note admixed small lymphocytes, a common feature. Elsewhere this example harbored astrocytic elements.

the first three decades of life,[658,678,687,692] but may be encountered in older adults.[671] By most accounts, they favor the supratentorial compartment, but examples have been described at all levels of the central neuraxis and we concur in the observation that gangliogliomas constitute a significant percentage of pediatric tumors presenting in the brainstem and spinal cord.[358,657,676,680] Even cranial nerve cases have been depicted,[656,681] an ectopic intraorbital presentation also being on record.[672] A predilection for the temporal lobes accounts for the discovery of many ganglion cell tumors in the course of evaluation for partial complex epilepsy, often of protracted duration. Albeit nonspecific, neuroradiologic presentation as a well-demarcated, partially cystic mass evidencing contrast enhancement of its solid components and foci of calcification is especially suggestive. The cerebral hemispheric lesion presenting as a discrete mural nodule within a cyst usually proves to be a ganglion cell tumor, pilocytic astrocytoma, or pleomorphic xanthoastrocytoma (for illustration of this profile see Fig. 28.57).

Common to the gangliocytoma and ganglioglioma is the irregular distribution of variably sized neurons, some of ganglion cell-like profile, in a delicate fibrillar matrix that is prone to spongy rarefaction and that often contains scattered calcospherules (Fig. 28.78). Microcystic changes are common in regions of predominantly glial composition. Whereas native neurons trapped in an advancing glial neoplasm generally manifest little cytologic alteration and tend to an even distribution and orderly polarity, the neuronal populace of the ganglion cell tumor often displays, in addition to obvious architectural disarray and anomalous clustering, conspicuous morphologic abnormalities that can include striking pleomorphism, multinucleation, cytoplasmic vacuolization, and gigantism. Some contain Alzheimer disease-type neurofibrillary tangles and other cytoplasmic inclusions seen in neurodegenerative and neuronal storage disorders.[661] Melanotic variants have been described,[688] as have ganglion cell tumors associated with (possibly progenitory) glioneuronal hamartomas,[660] with other maldevelopmental cerebrocortical anomalies,[684] and with the curious lesions known as dysembryoplastic neuroepithelial tumors (see later discussion).

The glial component of the ganglioglioma is typically astrocytic, GFAP positive, and well differentiated, usually assuming pilocytic or fibrillary guises.[674,691] Gemistocytic elements may be encountered, but if prominent call the diagnosis into question. Gangliogliomas may contain pleomorphic xanthoastrocytomatous components, reference having previously been made in our discussion of the latter tumor type to 'composite' lesions. While gangliogliomas may harbor constituents indistinguishable from conventional oligodendroglioma, the oligodendrocyte-like clear cells present in select ganglion cell tumors actually represent 'neurocytes', i.e., diminutive neurons.[683] A remarkable example of tanycytic ependymal differentiation on the part of a ganglioglioma is also on record.[673] Only exceptionally do gangliogliomas exhibit high-grade histologic features, 'malignant degeneration' typically involving their astroglial components and potentially resulting in a glioblastoma-like picture.[664,667] **Anaplastic ganglioglioma** is the designation appropriate to the tumor densely populated by mitotically active glial cells (microvascular proliferation and necrosis may also be encountered), cytologic atypism alone, even if pronounced, not constituting grounds for this diagnosis. Elements of anaplastic oligodendrogliomatous appearance have exceptionally been observed in malignant ganglioglial tumors.[654] Some cases of this sort, however, may actually represent oligodendrogliomas with ganglion cell components.[683a] The recurrence of a ganglioglioma (3 years after subtotal resection and irradiation) as a high-grade neoplasm composed of cells exhibiting a hybrid neuronal/astrocytic phenotype on immunocytochemical and ultrastructural study has also been documented,[677] as have a neuroblastoma-like picture at relapse[665] and the emergence of sarcomatous components.[689] We have encountered a bizarre example of atypical teratoid/rhabdoid tumor that evolved within an optic pathway ganglioglioma subjected to chemotherapy and irradiation.[655]

Certain recurring histologic features merit emphasis as clues to ganglion cell tumor diagnosis. Eosinophilic granular bodies of lysosomal derivation that appear to aggregate in the matrices of many such tumors are noteworthy in this regard, only the pilocytic astrocytoma and pleomorphic xanthoastrocytoma exhibiting this presumably degenerative alteration with comparable frequency (see Fig. 28.54 for an illustration of these structures). Lymphoid infiltration can also be of some diagnostic utility to the pathologist not distracted by this common, 'pseudoencephalitic' phenomenon. In fact, a florid inflammatory reaction extending into the substance of the lesion (i.e., not simply confined to the perivascular compartment) is characteristic among central neuroepithelial tumors only of this entity and the pleomorphic xanthoastrocytoma, the more so if plasma cells are found to participate. Desmoplasia, uncommonly associated with neoplasms of neuroepithelial lineage, need be mentioned as imposing a disfiguring and deceptive spindling and fascicular or vaguely storiform architecture on the constituent cellular elements of some ganglion cell tumors. Stromal blood vessels, often prominent, frequently undergo sclerosis – ganglion cell tumors potentially masquerading as vascular malformations on angiographic and gross neurosurgical assessment.

Given their differentiated appearances, it should come as no surprise that ultrastructural studies have shown the tumoral neurons under discussion to elaborate cytoplasmic processes containing parallel microtubular arrays and clear, synaptic-type vesicles. These neurite-like extensions can terminate in well-developed synaptic complexes.[674] Neoplastic neuronal elements often harbor dense-core neurosecretory granules as well,[674] a feature generally foreign to native cortical neurons, and further depart from the latter in potentially containing spherical protein bodies characteristic of catecholaminergic neuronal populations.[675] While tumors of astrocytic lineage may assume ganglion cell-like cytologic profiles, they manifest none of these specialized neuronal features and in most instances are readily unmasked by their expression of GFAP.

The formation of aberrant axosomatic synapses is apparently responsible for the presence in many ganglion cell tumors of large neurons displaying a coarsely granular or linear deposition of

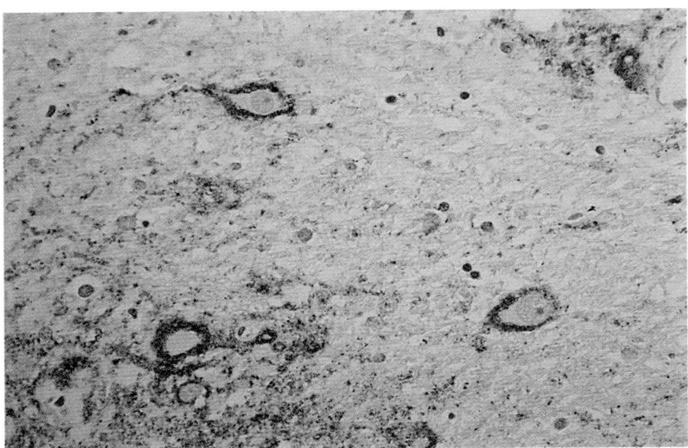

Fig. 28.79 Ganglioglioma. Surface perikaryal labeling for synaptophysin characterizes the neuronal elements of some ganglion cell tumors on immunohistochemical assay.

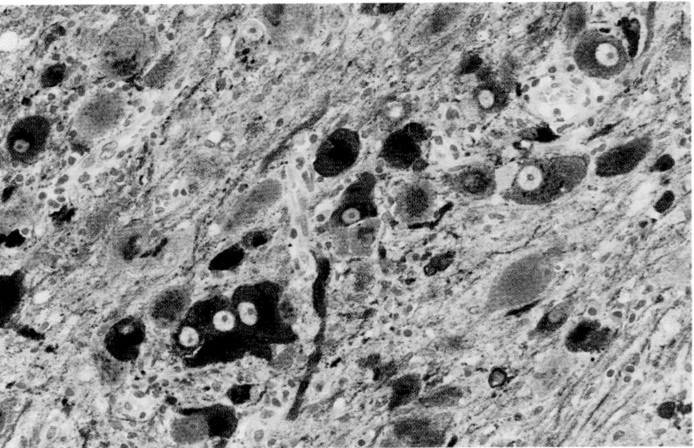

Fig. 28.80 Ganglioglioma. Diffuse and strong cytoplasmic immunoreactivity for chromogranin A, a feature foreign to native cerebrocortical neurons, characterizes the neoplastic neuronal perikarya of some ganglion cell tumors.

reaction product about their perikarya on immunocytochemical assay for synaptophysin (Fig. 28.79), a glycoprotein component of the presynaptic vesicle membrane.[674,683] This phenomenon bears significantly on the problem of distinguishing tumoral and native neurons – a comparable reaction pattern is not observed on immunoassessment of normal cerebral cortex – but must be cautiously interpreted. Circumperikaryal synaptophysin labeling is a recognized attribute of some striatal, cerebellar, bulbar, and intramedullary neurons.[686,693] Furthermore, cerebrocortical neurons entrapped within arteriovenous malformations can evidence this immunoprofile[686] and an identical labeling pattern has been depicted in a lesion of the cerebral cortex reported as postradiation neuronal gigantism,[662] suggesting that chronic, nonspecific neuronal injury may rarely provoke anomalous synaptic remodeling. Additional, and somewhat more specific (albeit inconstant), immunohistochemical evidence for the tumoral nature of a suspect neuronal population is intense and diffuse perikaryal labeling for chromogranin A (Fig. 28.80) – a reflection of the dense core granule formation noted above.[674] Native CNS neurons outside the brainstem and cerebellum, by contrast, either fail to react (as do glia) or display only punctate and relatively weak partial labeling of their perikarya for this antigen. Other aberrant immunophenotypic characteristics that can be displayed by the neurons populating ganglion cell tumors include failure to label for NeuN,[685] a nucleoprotein expressed (certain specialized neuronal subclasses, e.g., Purkinje cells, excepted) by their native counterparts throughout the CNS, and reactivity for nestin,[668] a cytoskeletal intermediate filament protein transiently elaborated by multipotent neuroepithelial stem cells but downregulated in differentiated neurons and glia. Nestin labeling may also be observed on the part of astrocytic constituents within these tumors.[668] We do not employ antibodies to nestin in clinical practice, but can attest to the paradoxically NeuN-negative immunoprofile of many gangliogliomas even when their neuronal components manifest thoroughly mature cytologic features. Some examples, however, retain entirely normal patterns of nuclear (and, at lower intensity, cytoplasmic) NeuN expression.[404] The neuronal constituents of ganglion cell tumors may also exhibit immunoreactivity for neurofilament proteins, microtubule-associated protein 2, class III β-tubulin, the neuronal nuclear protein designated as Hu,[365] α-synuclein, various neuropeptides, enzymes integral to catecholamine metabolism, and other neuron-associated antigens.[658,674,691] Restraint is advised in the interpretation of neuronal 'marker' expression limited to minor cell subsets, a phenomenon that can be encountered in otherwise astrocytic, oligodendroglial, and ependymal tumors. In these circumstances, we revert to first principles and render the diagnosis most in accord with the clinical, radiologic, and histologic features in evidence.

A final immunohistochemical feature having some utility in the identification of gangliogliomas is the fact that many exhibit regions of diffuse and intense CD34 reactivity that may include the surface labeling of neuronal perikarya as well as dense decoration of the tumoral matrix.[659,660,666] As mentioned in connection with the frequently CD34-positive pleomorphic xanthoastrocytoma, an entity exhibiting much overlap in its clinicobiologic and morphologic profiles, the expression of this antigen has been described as an attribute of neuroepithelial progenitor cells in some mammals (and is, of course, a constant property of endothelium in the CNS as elsewhere) but seems uniformly alien to differentiated neurons and glia in the human neuraxis. Gangliogliomas may further share with pleomorphic xanthoastrocytomas (and with glioneuronal hamartomas) an association with CD34-labeling cells of ramified, dendritic appearance that are only apparent in immunohistochemical preparations and that may be found to populate adjoining, ostensibly uninvolved cerebral cortex in surprising numbers.[659,660,666] These distinctive elements are illustrated in Figure 28.59B. The reader who consults the references provided on this score will find rather contradictory statements regarding CD34 expression by conventional glial neoplasms, but the demonstration of 'dysplastic' neural cells of this type in complex with intratumoral CD34 expression certainly militates against the diagnosis of an infiltrating astrocytoma or oligodendroglioma with entrapped neurons.

The WHO recognizes gangliocytomas and gangliogliomas as grade I lesions, assigning to the anaplastic ganglioglioma grade III status in what amounts to a binary formulation.[658] That there is biologic relevance to the identification of a grade II or 'atypical' ganglioglioma (i.e., one falling short of the overtly anaplastic while evidencing increased proliferative activity in complex with conspicuous microvascular hyperplasia, unexpectedly high cellularity or nuclear pleomorphism) is an assertion that awaits validating.[682] In practice, very few gangliogliomas manifest atypical characteristics of the latter sort (let alone anaplasia), the large majority are characterized by remarkable clinical indolence and their malignant transformation is a decidedly uncommon phenomenon. Supratentorial examples of the usual low-grade type, if accessible, are generally cured by resection alone.[678,680,682,687,692] Bulbar and intramedullary variants are more prone to symptomatic regrowth following operation, possibly owing to surgical limitations imposed by their physical circumstances, but run a protracted clinical course.[358,657,676] Gangliogliomas harboring atypical or patently malignant glial elements have been overrepresented among recurrent and fatal cases in some series,[682] but noteworthy are repeated observations that even frank anaplasia does not necessarily augur poorly in this setting.[679,680,683] This happy discrepancy likely reflects the tendency of gangliogliomas to expand in a compact, relatively noninvasive fashion that lends itself to the purposes of the neurosurgeon. Some observers have suggested that close neuroradiologic surveillance alone is reasonable following gross total excision of such tumors, but the optimal management of high-grade gangliogliomas remains in doubt owing to their rarity. Subtotally resected examples certainly carry a significant risk of fatal progression due to locally aggressive growth and, in some cases, leptomeningeal seeding.[687] The role of adjuvant treatment in such cases is unclear. A remarkable example of diffuse leptomeningeal gangliogliomatosis may actually have represented advanced glioneuronal maturation of a metastasizing cerebellar medulloblastoma, as noted by the authors.[690] Whether immunohistochemical assessments of proliferative activity or p53 expression bear on outcome as independent factors following gross surgical extirpation of gangliogliomas is far from clear.[674,684,691] The reader interested in these issues is encouraged to consult the cited literature. As a rule, gangliogliomas manifest low MIB-1 labeling indices, reported mean values falling in the 1–3% range.[674,684,691] Histologically anaplastic variants and recurrent lesions have been noted by some observers to evidence higher indices,[674] but, again, the independent predictive power of proliferation assays is not settled. MIB-1 reactivity is typically restricted to cells of glial appearance though, as previously mentioned, malignant elements of neuronal immunophenotype have been reported to emerge from gangliogliomas.[665,677]

Much speculation has centered on whether ganglion cell tumors represent neoplasms, hamartomatous proliferations, or combinations thereof.[658,660] A frequent association with maldevelopmental cortical abnormalities and their often remarkable clinical stability have prompted some to suggest that gangliogliomas essentially represent tumoral forms of cortical dysplasia or benign neoplasms arising in dysembryogenetic tissues.[660,684] Aberrant nestin expression by neurons in both cortical dysplasias and gangliogliomas raises further question of a link to disordered neuroembryogenetic events.[668] The shared CD34 expression alluded to previously has also been taken as evidence that gangliogliomas and glioneuronal hamartomas are linked by an origin from developmentally dysregulated neural stem cells.[659,660] One scenario would have the forces of neoplastic transformation selectively targeting glial elements residing within such hamartomas.[660] A majority of gangliogliomas assessed in one molecular genetic analysis appeared to be monoclonal,[694] supporting their neoplastic nature and the origin of their glioneuronal populations in a common, bipotential precursor. The genetic lesions responsible for transformation and malignant progression in this setting await clarification, though gains of chromosome 7, partial chromosome 9 loss, and sequence alterations in the tuberous sclerosis-associated *TSC2* gene have been identified as recurring abnormalities.[658]

We briefly call the reader's attention to the occurrence of 'intrasellar gangliocytomas' – a heterogeneous collection of benign lesions, most of which arise via neuronal transdifferentiation within growth hormone-producing (or, less commonly, other pituitary) adenomas.[670] A small minority of these curious masses may represent ganglion cell tumors ab initio or ectopic, hypothalamic-type neuronal hamartomas. Given separate consideration below are the distinctive entities known as desmoplastic infantile ganglioglioma and dysplastic gangliocytoma of the cerebellum (Lhermitte–Duclos disease).

Desmoplastic infantile ganglioglioma/desmoplastic infantile astrocytoma

Originally characterized as distinct entities,[707,708] the **desmoplastic infantile astrocytoma** and **desmoplastic infantile ganglioglioma** are allied by common (and stereotypic) clinical, neuroradiologic, morphologic, and biologic features.[696] Accordingly, they are given joint treatment in this section. Characteristic of these rare neoplasms are a presentation in the first two years of life (mean patient age at tumor discovery being 6 months, though examples in older children and teenagers have been reported), a supratentorial localization (usually frontoparietal), and associated manifestations of increased intracranial pressure that include irritability, vomiting, macrocephaly, bulging fontanels, and forced downwards deviation of the eyes (the 'sunset' sign). Virtually pathognomonic of this tumor family in the clinical setting just described is CT or MR demonstration of a superficially positioned, nodular or plaque-like mass that broadly adheres to the dura, exhibits homogeneous contrast enhancement, and is associated with a prominent subjacent cystic component of uni- or multilocular aspect (Fig. 28.81). Most examples are quite large at operation (these often measuring 10 cm or more in greatest span), are composed of tan–white tissue that is rubbery or firm to palpation owing to associated fibroplasia, and appear to lie largely outside the cerebrum proper.

Histologic study of desmoplastic infantile astrocytomas and gangliogliomas generally confirms their dural attachment and predilection for supracerebral growth, while invariably revealing tumor colonization of the adjoining cortex and frequently demonstrating spread along Virchow–Robin spaces. Common to these tumors are

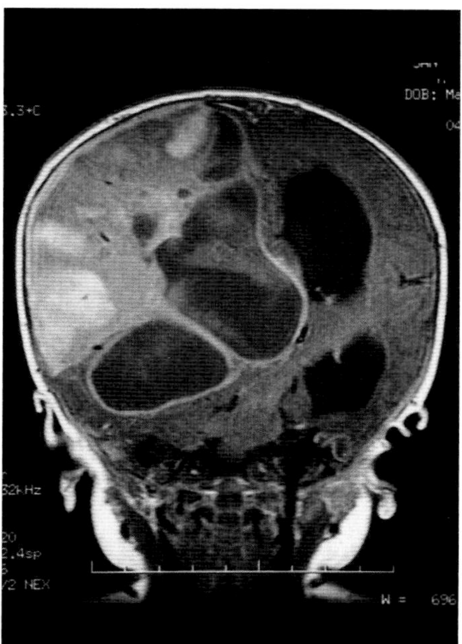

Fig. 28.81 Desmoplastic infantile ganglioglioma/astrocytoma. As demonstrated by this example in an 8-week-old boy, tumors of the desmoplastic infantile ganglioglioma/astrocytoma group are typically large cerebral growths exhibiting dural attachment of their superficially located and contrast-enhancing solid components with the formation of prominent underlying cysts.

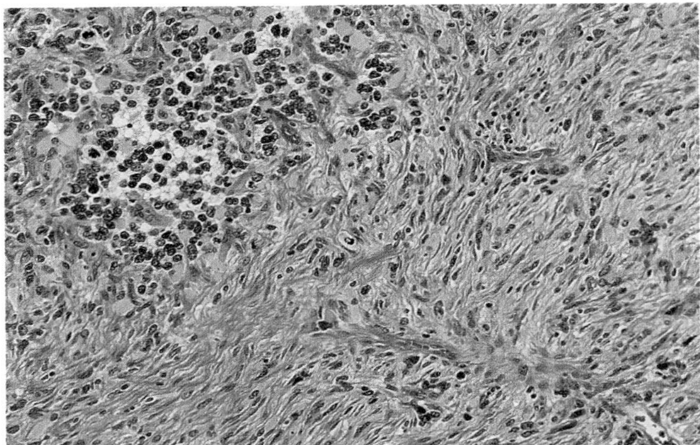

Fig. 28.82 Desmoplastic infantile ganglioglioma/astrocytoma. Distinctive features include collagenized regions dominated by spindly astrocytes in fascicular or storiform array and admixed small cells of primitive appearance in nodular aggregates.

collagenized components of pseudomesenchymal appearance as well as recognizably neuroepithelial elements (Fig. 28.82). The former, usually predominant, are populated by variably pleomorphic spindle cells in loose fascicular or storiform array, these patterns inviting confusion with bona fide fibrohistiocytic neoplasms, intracranial fibromatosis, or fibroblastic meningioma. Immunohistochemical assessment typically discloses a large complement of GFAP-positive astroglial forms within these desmoplastic regions, where they are admixed with nonlabeling elements that have proven on electron microscopic study to include fibroblasts.[695,702,707,708] Ultrastructural analyses have further shown that these neoplastic astrocytes are invested by basal lamina material, which accounts for a pericellular, reticulin-impregnable network immunoreactive for basement membrane-associated antigens such as type IV collagen.[695,702] As discussed in connection with the pleomorphic xanthoastrocytoma, this finding may signal differentiation along specialized subpial astrocytic lines.

In addition to sharing collagen-rich zones evidencing astrocytic outgrowth, the desmoplastic infantile astrocytoma and ganglioglioma are allied by the regular presence of seemingly undifferentiated small cell populations that inhabit reticulin-free islands or broader tissue expanses (Fig. 28.82). These may achieve considerable density and can exhibit mitotic activity (usually at low level), but even in areas dominated by such cells MIB-1/Ki-67 labeling indices generally remain modest. In fact, most of the tumors under discussion exhibit MIB-1 indices below 5% and the latter often fall below the 2% level.[696] High mitotic rates, microvascular proliferation and necrosis are clearly exceptional, but occasionally encountered.[698,703] Small cell components, which appear to be primitive neuroepithelial constituents capable of divergent differentiation, can exhibit cytologic transition to fibrillary astroglial, gemistocytic or neuronal morphology and may label for GFAP, various neuron-associated antigens (e.g., synaptophysin, class III β-tubulin, neurofilament proteins, MAP-2, Hu), and desmin.[696,707,708] The specific diagnosis of desmoplastic infantile ganglioglioma is reserved for tumors containing recognizable neurons, but the expression of neuron-restricted epitopes by the ostensibly uncommitted small cells populating examples devoid of patently differentiated neuronal elements exposes the artifice in so subclassifying these unusual neoplasms of early life. When present, neuronal forms include mature, atypical, and ganglion cell-sized variants. While most prevalent in noncollagenized regions, these can be detected in desmoplastic areas as well (particularly with the aid of immunoscreening for synaptophysin and neurofilament epitopes). A deep-seated example containing components of conventional ganglioglioma, gangliocytomatous foci, pilocytic astrocytoma-like regions, and elements suggesting Schwann cell differentiation has been recorded.[701]

Desmoplastic infantile gangliogliomas and astrocytomas may represent neoplasms of essentially embryonal character programmed to advanced maturation along glioneuronal lines. Their small cell components notwithstanding, a most favorable prognosis attaches to cases amenable to gross total resection and so these peculiar tumors are accorded WHO grade I status.[696] Remarkable instances of their 'spontaneous' regression following less than complete excision have been communicated.[706] Even frankly malignant histologic features (e.g., conspicuous mitotic activity and necrosis with palisading) do not necessarily augur in ominous fashion if surgical removal can be effected,[698,703] but we would caution that very few 'anaplastic' cases have been recorded to date. Recurrence following complete excision is exceptional, though subtotally removed examples may occasionally regrow over relatively brief intervals[699] and can prove fatal.[701] CSF-borne metastasis at presentation has been described,[697,704] the diagnosis in one of these reports[704] being open to question on both clinical and morphologic grounds. A second account of this phenomenon[697] detailed the virulent behavior of an example atypical by virtue of its subcortical, partly intraventricular localization and the unusually florid proliferative activity (including a MIB-1/Ki-67 labeling index of 45%) evidenced by anaplastic small cell elements that constituted one-third of the tumor bulk. Tumor recurrence and biologic progression (in the face of gross total resection) with the emergence of aggressive small cell components that manifested MIB-1/Ki-67 indices of approximately 30% and seeding of the ventricular cavities has also been depicted.[700] It would appear, however, that adjuvant therapy can be reserved for refractory lesions that cannot be extirpated by surgical means alone.[698,703,705] It has been suggested that basal lamina formation by astrocytic elements may exert a restraining influence on the proliferation of these neoplasms, basement membrane-associated proteins apparently promoting cell differentiation and growth arrest when applied to human glioma lines.[702]

Central neurocytoma and extraventricular neurocytic neoplasms

Characterized by an intraventricular location, attendant manifestations of obstructive hydrocephalus, a peak incidence in adults aged 20–40 years, and deceptively oligodendroglioma-like histology, the **central neurocytoma** is a neoplasm composed of highly differentiated, albeit diminutive, neuronal elements.[714,715] It may be situated anywhere within the ventricular confines, possibly deriving from remnants of the subependymal matrix that retain postnatal proliferative capacity, but most often inhabits anterior portions of the lateral ventricles in the foramen of Monro region and frequently involves the septum pellucidum. Common neuroradiologic features include cystic change, contrast enhancement of solid components, and conspicuous calcification (Fig. 28.83).

The central neurocytoma is remarkable for the cytologic conformity of its constituent cells (Fig. 28.84), which possess monomorphic nuclei of small diameter, rounded contour, and evenly granular chromatin content. Perinuclear clearing, a plexiform capillary microvasculature, and admixed calcospherules often conspire to render this lesion indistinguishable from the oligodendroglioma, though the central neurocytoma usually differs in its elaboration of a fine, neuropil-like fibrillar matrix that may separate streaming tumor cells, punctuate foci of sheet-like growth as

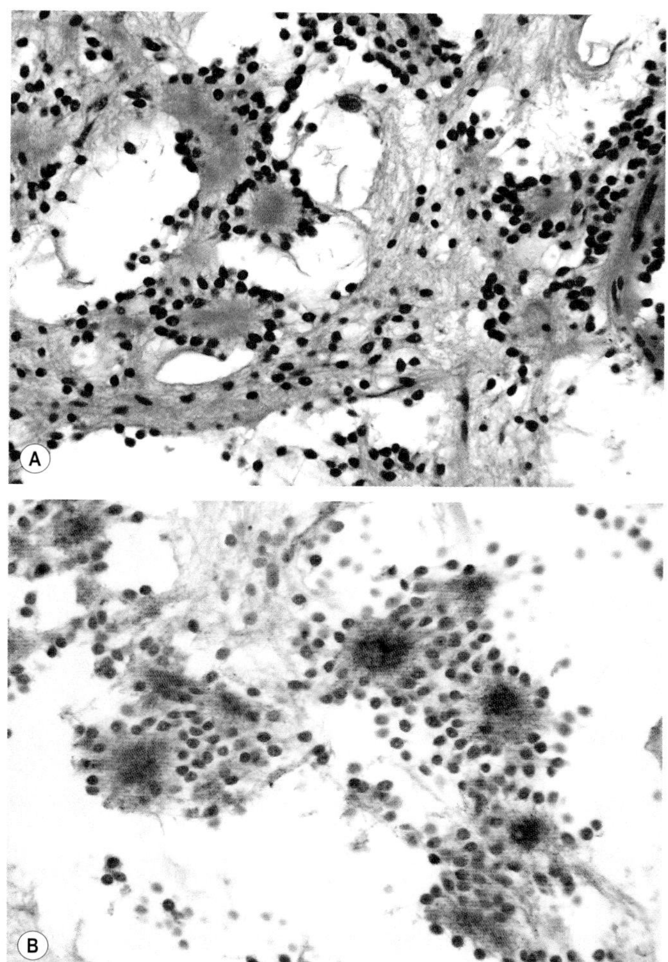

Fig. 28.90 Rosette-forming glioneuronal tumor of the fourth ventricle. Neurocytic rosettes of small diameter that often appear free-floating (**A**) and that exhibit central immunolabeling for synaptophysin (**B**) are defining components of this entity.

bromatosis. Relatively demarcated on MRI evaluation but accompanied in some cases by discrete 'satellite' lesions separate from the main mass, these neoplasms are typically T2 bright/T1 hypointense and may exhibit nodular, ring-like or linear patterns of contrast enhancement.[772,773] They are composed in biphasic fashion of glial elements resembling pilocytic astrocytoma (these often hypocellular and associated with vascular hyalinization) and neurocytic populations that engage in the formation of diminutive, synaptophysin-immunoreactive rosettes and narrow perivascular pseudorosettes that may be attended by myxoid alterations and that often seem to float within microcavities[771–773] (Fig. 28.90). Components indistinguishable from conventional oligodendroglioma and labeling for neither GFAP nor synaptophysin may be encountered. Some cases exhibit complex microvascular proliferation, but mitotic activity is inapparent, necrosis is not observed, and MIB-1 labeling indices are quite modest (not exceeding 2–3% and often no higher than 1%). Glioneuronal tumors of the fourth ventricle are indolent, WHO grade I[771] lesions that may remain stable over lengthy periods of neuroradiologic surveillance and that can be controlled by surgical means. Aggressive attempts to fully extirpate these neoplasms, however, have been complicated in a substantial number of reported cases by significant neurologic deficits. Late local recurrence following resection has been documented, as has an example evidencing intraventricular dissemination at diagnosis.[775]

Hypothalamic neuronal hamartoma

Hypothalamic neuronal hamartomas are usefully subdivided into two basic clinicoanatomic groups.[781] 'Parahypothalamic' variants – pedunculated lesions that bulge into the suprasellar cistern from attachments to the tuber cinereum or mammillary bodies – are principally associated with precocious puberty in boys. This may reflect the ectopic secretion of gonadotropic releasing factors by neurons populating hamartomas of this class.[778,780] 'Intrahypothalamic' subtypes – sessile growths broadly anchored to the tissues lining the third ventricle – characteristically produce fits of pathological laughter (known as gelastic seizures) that begin in infancy. The development of more generalized, refractory epileptic syndromes, progressive cognitive impairment, and psychiatric disturbances often complicate lesions of the latter type as well.

Most hypothalamic neuronal hamartomas measure no more than 1–2 cm in maximum dimension, though giant examples may be encountered.[781] Variably sized neurons are the dominant cellular population, these being embedded in a uniformly synaptophysin-labeling matrix that is generally indistinguishable from native neuropil and traversed in some cases by bundled axons of myelinated or nonmyelinated type. While large ganglion cell-like elements may be present, small to mid-sized neuronal forms dominate most lesions.[777,781] These are given to anomalous nodular clustering. Some cases manifest a gliotic appearance, but astrocytes and oligodendroglia are only minor cellular constituents.

Although most hypothalamic hamartomas present in isolated and sporadic fashion, the association of such lesions with a variety of malformative syndromes has been documented. Chief among the latter is the Pallister–Hall syndrome, linked in its autosomal dominant form to germline *GLI3* gene mutations[779] and characterized by a complex of anomalies that includes imperforate anus, cryptorchidism, polydactyly, pituitary aplasia, hypoplasia of the adrenal and thyroid glands, and various cardiac and renal anomalies.[776,779] In affected infants, the hypothalamic lesion may contain small, immature-appearing neuroepithelial elements and has consequentially been termed a '**hypothalamic hamartoblastoma**',[776] but the incompletely differentiated profiles of these cells (which may also populate nonsyndromic hamartomas) probably just reflect the very young age of the patients from whom they derive. Resection specimens from affected individuals surviving infancy exhibit more mature neuronal features.[782]

Glioneuronal hamartomas, cortical dysplasias, and other epileptogenic lesions

A number of published series and reviews can be recommended to readers interested in the various non-neoplastic lesions that may be associated with refractory seizure disorders compelling neurosurgical intervention.[784–787,789–791] Inasmuch as operative approaches to this problem are practiced mainly in specialized referral centers and rarely engage the general surgical pathologist, we specifically consider here only one 'tumoral' cause of pharmacoresistant epilepsy not addressed elsewhere in this text, the glioneuronal hamartoma.

Glioneuronal hamartomas figure with special prominence in surgical series addressing chronic temporal lobe epilepsy,[786,790] but occur throughout the cerebral hemispheres[789,791] and may present as intraventricular growths.[783,788] Ranging from microscopic lesions to expansile gray nodules that may be grossly evident on evaluation of lobectomy specimens and visualized by neuroradiographic means, these are sometimes found to be multifocal, are often associated with other evidences of faulty development (such as patchy cortical dysgenesis and neuronal ectopias in the temporal white matter), and may occur in complex with low-grade neuroepithelial neoplasms of varied type. Whether they serve as the progenitors of select gliomas, gangliogliomas, or dysembryoplastic neuroepithelial tumors (the more commonly associated lesions) is open to question. As noted previously, gangliogliomas do often share with these dysgenetic lesions expression of CD34, restricted in the developed human CNS to endothelial cells but displayed by neural progenitors in some species.[659,660] Populated, in most cases rather sparsely, by neurons of medium to large size and admixed astrocytes that may exhibit hyperplastic features, glioneuronal hamartomas do not evidence the cellularity, pleomorphism, or conspicuous inflammatory infiltration of the bona fide ganglioglioma, nor do they manifest alveolar patterning or the myxoid alterations characteristic of the dysembryoplastic neuroepithelial tumor. Some, like the latter, harbor oligodendrocyte-like clear cell elements (nodular aggregates of which constitute microscopic hamartomas or 'hamartias' commonly encountered in temporal lobectomies performed for epilepsy control),[786,790] but these are a minor component and further deviate in evidencing no special relationship to regional axons or the stromal vasculature. Hamartomas composed predominantly or exclusively of astrocytic forms can also be seen.[789] Spongiform change may be apparent within the lesion and can involve associated cortex in patchy fashion, this possibly representing a seizure-induced tissue disturbance. Finally, select variants contain dysmorphic cells of neuronal, astrocytic, or indeterminate lineage resembling those of the cortical tuber (the tuberous sclerosis complex is discussed in relation to subependymal giant cell astrocytomas). These include cells exhibiting a characteristically 'ballooned' appearance. Such cells are also the hallmark of a form of **focal cortical dysplasia** (known eponymously as **Taylor cortical dysplasia** or as **focal cortical dysplasia, type IIb** in the classification of Palmini et al.[785]) that is strongly associated with refractory seizures in childhood and that appears to represent a disorder of neuronal migration and differentiation.[784,787]

Dysplastic gangliocytoma of the cerebellum (Lhermitte–Duclos disease)

The **dysplastic gangliocytoma of the cerebellum**, also known by the eponymous **Lhermitte–Duclos disease**, principally affects adults in the third through fifth decades of life and usually comes to attention on evaluation for progressive ataxia or symptoms of intracranial hypertension reflecting mass effect on the fourth ventricle.[793,797] Virtually diagnostic on MRI assessment is the demonstration of regionally thickened and abnormally T2 bright cerebellar folia without associated contrast enhancement. The histologic substrate of this curious disorder is variable replacement of the internal granule cell layer by an array of large neurons with attendant expansion and aberrant myelination of the overlying molecular layer. The latter is prone to coarse spongy change and dystrophic microcalcification, often blood vessel-associated, while the subjacent folial white matter is thinned, if not cavitated. Neuronal elements are generally well differentiated in appearance, though some cases exhibit nuclear dysmorphism and hyperchromasia in scattered cellular elements.[792] Axons emanating from ganglionic constituents are oriented (relative to the pial surface) in parallel stacks within the deep molecular zone and in perpendicular array more superficially. The orientation of these axons, their appearances in Golgi preparations,[794] and observed patterns of neurofilament protein expression on immunoassay[799] indicate that the abnormal neurons in this disorder are mainly outsized caricatures of the granule cells that they would seem to replace. Immunolabeling for the NeuN neuronal nuclear protein, foreign to Purkinje cells but a consistent feature of granule cell elements, would further identify these large neurons with the latter population.[404,797] Only minor subsets have been described as manifesting Purkinje cell-like attributes that include immunoexpression of Leu4, PEP-19, L7, and calbindin as well as surface perikaryal labeling for such synaptic vesicle-associated antigens as SV2 and synaptophysin.[795,796,798]

In adult-onset form, the dysplastic gangliocytoma of the cerebellum is now recognized as a lesion virtually pathognomonic of Cowden syndrome.[793] An autosomal dominant phakomatosis linked to germline mutations of the *PTEN/MMAC1* gene on chromosome 10q23, this disease complex is chiefly characterized by multiple cutaneous tricholemmomas, oral papillomatosis, acral keratoses, macrocephaly/megalencephaly, gastrointestinal polyps of various types, thyroid abnormalities (principally goiter, but including follicular neoplasms), and a substantially increased risk of mammary adenocarcinoma (as well as benign fibroepithelial and papillomatous proliferations of the female breast). Dysplastic cerebellar gangliocytomas presenting in the adult years regularly display inactivating *PTEN* mutations, irrespective of their association with other manifestations of Cowden syndrome, and underlying germline *PTEN* mutation has been consistently demonstrated in those affected patients studied to date.[793,800] Pediatric cases, by contrast, seem divorced from these associations.[800]

The linking of dysplastic cerebellar gangliocytomas in adulthood to *PTEN* mutation has done much to clarify the pathogenesis of this entity, which has been interpreted variously as representing a compensatory hypertrophy of internal granule cells in response to faulty development of the fetal external granular layer from which they derive, as a hamartomatous growth or remarkably orchestrated neoplasm. *PTEN* acts as a regulator of cell size, survival, proliferation, and migration through its inhibitory influence on the phosphatidylinositol 3-kinase (PI3K)/AKT signaling cascade. Studies of both the human disease and murine 'knockout' models faithful to the former suggest that abrogated PTEN expression, with resulting activation of AKT and its downstream targets, suffices to produce the alterations characteristic of dysplastic cerebellar gangliocytomas in the absence of transforming events or cellular proliferation.[792,793,797,800] In fact, the enlarged internal granule cells persisting in these lesions represent in number a much reduced fraction of the normal populace, are amitotic and left unlabeled in MIB-1/Ki-67 preparations (though perivascular elements reasonably interpreted as reactive forms may exhibit immunopositivity).[792] The finding in some cases of what would appear to be granule cells aberrantly situated in the molecular layer attests to impaired migration, as well as compromised survival and dysregulated cell growth, in the evolution of this curious disorder.

Dysplastic gangliocytomas of the cerebellum behave in the manner of WHO grade I tumors, gross total excision proving curative in most instances. Late local regrowth, however, complicates the course of some patients (particularly after macroscopically incomplete resection) and has been construed as evidence for the neoplastic nature of these lesions. Such 'recurrences' may simply reflect the fact that internal granule cells in grossly normal folia remain at risk for gangliocytomatous change due to their *PTEN* mutant status. It is noteworthy in this connection that fully developed lesions are often bordered by cerebellar cortex exhibiting subtle enlargement of neurons in the superficial aspect of the internal granule cell layer,[797] a precursor abnormality not appreciable at operation. Given the germline nature of the genetic defect predisposing to dysplastic gangliocytomas, it should not surprise that patients may develop (and can present with) multifocal cerebellar involvement.

Other glioneuronal neoplasms

As we have tried to make plain in the sections devoted to these entities, the neoplasms traditionally placed in the various glioma series can exhibit neuronal 'marker' expression on immunohistochemical assessment and may on rare occasion evidence overt neuronal/neurocytic differentiation. The latter of these unanticipated phenomena merits acknowledging in surgical pathology reports, but does not alter the basic classification of such tumors as astrocytic, oligodendroglial or ependymal. In this connection, we refer readers to our discussion of the infiltrating astrocytomas for consideration of the 'glioneuronal tumor with neuropil-like islands' (essentially a diffuse, WHO grade II or III astrocytoma harboring micronodular loci of neurocytic differentiation) and 'glioblastomas with primitive neuroectodermal tumor-like components'. Oligodendrogliomas, ependymomas, and the odd choroid plexus papilloma containing neuronal populations in synaptophysin-rich, neuropil-like matrices are all cited in our foregoing treatment of these tumor groups. Described, as well, in the foregoing survey of oligodendrogliomas are diffuse subarachnoid growths of childhood that have been interpreted by some as novel glioneuronal neoplasms[473] and by others as a form of primary leptomeningeal oligodendrogliomatosis.[492]

Embryonal neuroepithelial tumors

Collectively described as 'embryonal' are neoplasms sharing, in addition to a postulated derivation from primitive neuroepithelial precursors, a peak incidence in the early years of life and an aggressive clinical biology. Most such tumors are dominated by small, anaplastic cells apparently uncommitted to any particular cytogenetic pathway on conventional histologic assessment, but the capacity of these lesions to differentiate along neuronal, glial, and, on occasion, mesenchymal lines has long been recognized and is manifest in their considerable morphologic and immunophenotypic heterogeneity.

Controversy has surrounded the nomenclature appropriate to these complex neoplasms. Their original designations were predicated on the notion that the histologic appearances of CNS tumors reflect the neoplastic transformation of specific cell types at recognizable stages of neuroembryogenesis.[804] Thus, medulloepithelioma was the name given to a tumor harboring structures resembling, and so presumed to originate from, the primitive medullary epithelium of the neural tube, whereas ependymoblastoma was used for an embryonal neoplasm seemingly committed to differentiation along ependymal lines alone, and so forth. The theoretical underpinnings of this scheme have been justly questioned and an alternative, operational approach adopted by some neuropathologists who apply the generic 'primitive neuroectodermal tumor (PNET)' to all such neoplasms with notation of the differentiating characteristics exhibited in individual cases.[803] Implied is the common origin of embryonal tumors from indifferent stem cells that either remain undifferentiated or exercise any of a number of maturational options following neoplastic transformation. Specifically, targeting of undifferentiated neuroepithelial cells known to persist in the subependymal plate and pineal anlage is hypothesized to account for the occurrence of histologically similar neoplasms of primitive character at various sites along the neuraxis.

Simply stated, the cytogenesis of these embryonal tumors remains wholly speculative, molecular genetic analyses do not support a common pathogenesis for the members of this group,[801,802] and application of the PNET brand in broad fashion fails to acknowledge significant differences in the behavior and treatment responsiveness of the lesions in question. It is our practice, in accord with WHO guidelines,[801] to employ the time-honored designations first applied to these neoplasms, flawed as they may be. The pineoblastoma is treated under pineal parenchymal neoplasms.

Medulloblastoma

The cerebellar tumors traditionally termed **medulloblastomas** are the most common of primitive neuroepithelial neoplasms arising in the CNS. These occur throughout life but are characterized by a peak incidence in children between 5 and 10 years of age.[820] Approximately 25% of afflicted patients are beyond their teenage years,[820,825] adult-onset cases clustering in the third and fourth decades, and 65% are male. At least 75% of childhood medulloblastomas arise in the cerebellar vermis, often expanding to fill the fourth ventricle and so producing manifestations of obstructive hydrocephalus (lethargy, headache, and morning emesis) in addition to truncal ataxia and disturbed gait. The relative proportion of laterally positioned, hemispheric examples increases with age. Medulloblastomas interpreted as primary leptomeningeal growths have been communicated.[836] As visualized in CT and MR images, medulloblastomas are usually solid and contrast enhancing. Unlike ependymomas, the main differential diagnostic considerations in the fourth ventricular region, they are not prone to calcification and midline examples often appear to hang from the roof of this chamber rather than bulging upwards from its floor.

While usually sporadic, medulloblastomas are known to complicate certain heritable disorders.[820] **Type 2 Turcot syndrome**, an autosomal dominant condition, is defined by the occurrence of medulloblastoma in association with adenomatous polyposis of the colon and germline mutations of the adenomatous polyposis coli (*APC*) gene (a negative regulator of the Wnt signaling pathway) on chromosome 5q21. A significantly increased risk of medulloblastoma also characterizes the **nevoid basal cell carcinoma** – or '**Gorlin**' – **syndrome**, an autosomal dominant complex caused by germline mutations of the Patched (*PTCH*) gene (chromosome 9q22.3) and including among its many manifestations odontogenic keratocysts, dyskeratotic pitting of the palms and soles, craniomegaly and other skeletal anomalies, lamellar calcium deposition in the falx cerebri and diaphragma sellae, calcifying ovarian fibromas and multifocal basal cell carcinomas notable for their early age at onset, involvement of both sun-exposed and hidden skin, melanotic pigmentation, associated calcifications, and clinical indolence. As inactivating *PTCH* mutations lead to upregulated sonic hedgehog signaling activity, it is noteworthy that medulloblastomas have also been observed in association with germline mutations of SUFU, another Hedgehog pathway inhibitor. Medulloblastomas arising in the setting of **germline *TP53* gene mutation** (including **Li–Fraumeni syndrome**), previously mentioned as predisposing to astrocytic neoplasms and other tumor types, are known to complicate subtype D1 **Fanconi anemia**, caused by *BRCA2* (13q12.3) gene mutations (these also put patients at risk for the development of mammary carcinomas, Wilms tumors, and hematologic neoplasms), and may occur at increased frequency (along with oligodendrogliomas and meningiomas) in **Rubinstein–Taybi syndrome**. The latter, due to mutations in the *CREB*-binding protein gene on chromosome 16p13.3, is typified by congenital cognitive impairment, growth retardation, and microcephaly with abnormal facies, broad thumbs and toes. Also on record is the association of medulloblastoma with **Coffin–Siris syndrome** (the complex of mental retardation, postnatal growth impairment, joint laxity, and brachydactyly of the fifth digit with absence of the nailbed) and with germline mutations of a DNA repair protein-encoding gene, designated as *NBN* or *NBS1*, that has been implicated in the cancer predisposition **Nijmegen breakage syndrome**.[809]

Given the variety of genetic aberrations associated with syndromic examples, it should come as little surprise that the sporadic neoplasms constituting the medulloblastoma group exhibit considerable genomic, as well as morphologic, diversity and do not seem to share a unifying pathogenesis. Furthermore, tumors accorded this designation may not have common cellular origins. Detailed and annotated examination of these issues can be found elsewhere.[820] Suffice it to say for purposes of the present discussion that two main variants are recognized, these being the 'classic' and 'desmoplastic/nodular' subtypes as histologically defined below. The former vastly dominate among sporadically occurring medulloblastomas and in this setting exhibit chromosome 17p losses coupled with 17q gains and isochromosome 17q formation as their most commonly associated karyotypic and molecular genetic abnormalities (30–40% of cases). Whereas a significant subset of classic medulloblastomas is characterized by mutational events that upregulate signaling in the Wnt cascade, desmoplastic/nodular variants preferentially evidence silencing mutations of *PTCH* or other lesions that activate the sonic hedgehog pathway. (As would be anticipated in view of these associations, medulloblastomas in type 2 Turcot syndrome are typically of the classic kind, while those complicating the nevoid basal cell carcinoma/Gorlin syndrome are of desmoplastic/nodular type.) Either subtype may exhibit transformation to 'large cell/anaplastic' histology, a phenomenon given full description in the paragraphs that follow and one associated with the acquisition of additional genetic anomalies that often include *MYC* amplifications. As regards histogenesis, shared patterns of gene and antigen expression have been forwarded as evidence that desmoplastic/nodular medulloblastomas derive from elements of the fetal external granular layer (these migrate to the surface of the embryonic cerebellar cortex from the roof of the fourth ventricle and are the eventual source of internal granular neurons). While at least some classic medulloblastomas exhibit activation of the granule cell differentiation program and could have similar origins, a subset manifests protein expression profiles foreign to both external granular layer cells and internal granular neurons that may link this group to pluripotent progenitors in the subependymal matrix. A class of CD133-expressing stem cells situated mainly in the postnatal cerebellar white matter are also potential candidates in the cytogenesis of medulloblastomas, which remains a speculative matter.

Classic medulloblastomas are solid masses of friable, gray–white tissue composed, at their most primitive, of small, ostensibly undifferentiated cells closely arrayed in packed sheets (Fig. 28.91). Nuclei are often densely hyperchromatic, round or angulated, invested with little or no definable cytoplasm and so prone to deformation ('molding') by their neighbors. A swirling or fascicular architecture may be encountered, as may nuclei disposed in tight perivascular pseudorosettes or regimented in compact, rhythmic palisades. Stromal elements are typically scant, consisting of small blood vessels that only exceptionally exhibit proliferative changes (and these rarely comparable to the glomeruloid alterations characteristic of high-grade gliomas). Mitotic figures may abound, MIB-1 (Ki-67) labeling indices often exceeding 50%, but most medulloblastomas exhibit surprisingly little in the way of geographic necrosis. When present, however, necrotic zones may be rimmed by pseudopalisading tumor cells in glioblastoma-like fashion. Patterns of local spread commonly evident in neurosurgical material include diffuse permeation of adjoining neuroparenchyma, arresting subpial accumulations of neoplastic cells that invite comparison to a persistent fetal external granular layer and extension into the subarachnoid compartment with reinvasion of the underlying cerebellar cortex along a broad front or via penetrating perivascular spaces. Contact with the pia-arachnoid may incite considerable fibroplasia, in florid cases forcing tumor cells into single file, trabecular or even storiform arrays.

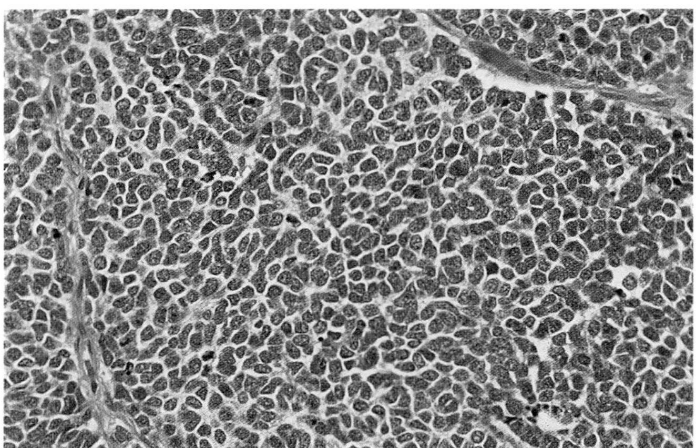

Fig. 28.91 Medulloblastoma. The classic medulloblastoma is a highly cellular neoplasm composed of diminutive, undifferentiated-looking elements possessed of little definable cytoplasm and prone to nuclear molding.

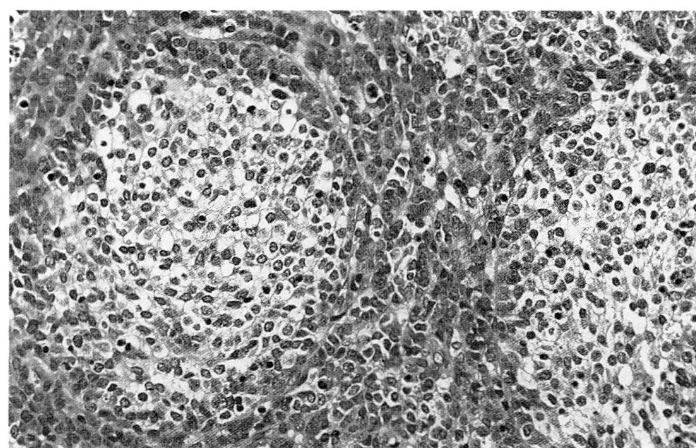

Fig. 28.92 Desmoplastic/nodular medulloblastoma. Micronodular zones of reduced cellularity ('pale islands') are a striking feature of this medulloblastoma variant.

Desmoplastic/nodular medulloblastomas may occupy the vermis and certainly afflict children, but are overrepresented among laterally situated, cerebellar hemispheric tumors occurring at all ages and particularly among those of adult onset. At operation, these neoplasms may seem leptomeninges based and are often lobulated, sharply demarcated and firm owing to the associated deposition of reticulin and collagen for which they are named. Desmoplastic/nodular medulloblastomas, however, depart from classic variants evidencing collagenization due simply to arachnoidal infiltration in their conspicuous content of 'pale islands' – micronodular, reticulin-free zones that lend to many a low magnification appearance likened to follicular lymphoid hyperplasia (Fig. 28.92). Characterized by reduced cellularity, a rarefied fibrillar matrix, the emergence of an oligodendrocyte-like (but, in fact, neurocytic) populace, and downregulated BCL2 expression with increased apoptosis and a sharp decline in mitotic activity and

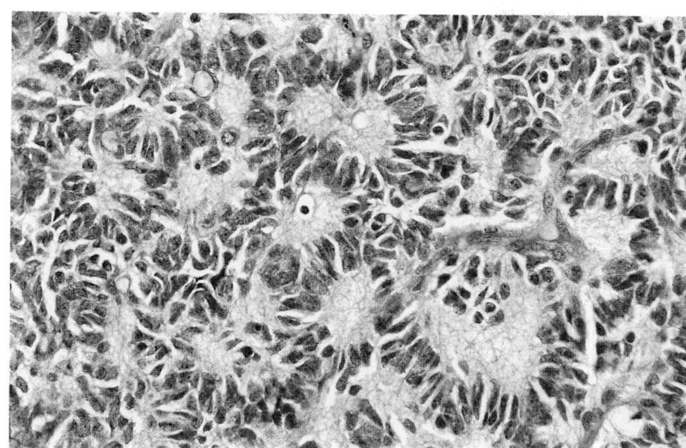

Fig. 28.93 Medulloblastoma. Homer Wright rosettes consist of tumor cell nuclei disposed in circular fashion about tangled cytoplasmic processes. These structures are indicative of differentiation along neuronal lines.

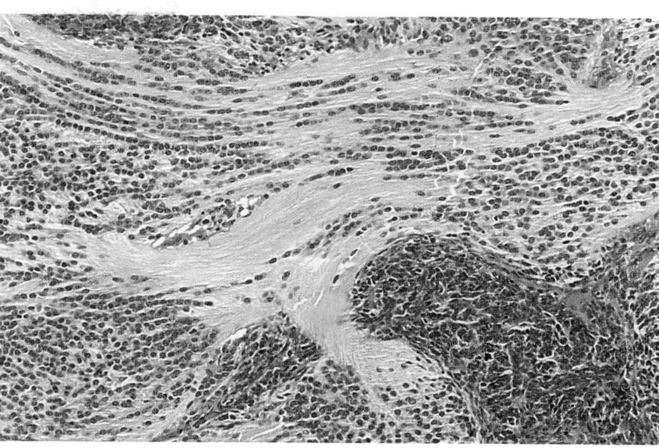

Fig. 28.94 Medulloblastoma with extensive nodularity. This variant of medulloblastoma is typified by the linear streaming of rounded, 'neurocytic' tumor cell nuclei within amassed cytoplasmic processes.

MIB-1 (Ki-67) immunolabeling,[815] the pale island is not merely free of connective tissues but represents a locus of progressive neuronal maturation and potential glial differentiation (as further addressed below). In recognition of this defining phenomenon (and to avoid confusion with collagenized medulloblastomas of otherwise classic appearance), the WHO specifically endorses the designation of these tumors as 'desmoplastic/nodular' rather than the traditional 'desmoplastic' without further qualification. Histology of this type emerges from some studies[835] as having prognostically favorable implications, but this is a debated issue.[820]

Although medulloblastomas in both classic and desmoplastic/nodular form are unarguably capable of differentiating along glial, as well as neuronal, lines, it is the latter option that is far more frequently exercised. While overt ganglion cell maturation is exceptional, the overwhelming majority of medulloblastomas (including those of thoroughly undifferentiated histologic aspect) exhibit at least focal immunolabeling for synaptophysin.[810,834] Reliable indices of neuronal differentiation that can be apprehended at the light microscopic level include, in addition to the pale islands just described, Homer Wright rosettes – radial arrangements of tumor cell nuclei about small tangles of fibrillar material devoid of a centering lumen (Fig. 28.93). Ultrastructural studies have confirmed that the cores of such structures and the neuropil-like matrix of the pale island consist of neuritic cytoplasmic processes laden with microtubules in parallel array and joined by specialized adhesion plaques, features restricted in combination to embryonal neurons.[831] Furthermore, both the Homer Wright rosette and pale island constitute loci of concentrated immunoreactivity for synaptophysin and other neuron-associated cytoplasmic antigens that include class III β-tubulin and microtubule-associated protein 2,[830] pale islands also evidencing upregulated immunoexpression of the TrkA and TrkC neurotrophin receptors.[815] Medulloblastomas may also contain populations immunoreactive for neurofilament proteins[820,828] as well as the Hu[365] and NeuN[404] neuronal nuclear antigens. Labeling for the latter reveals the oligodendrocyte-like elements of the pale island to be diminutive neuronal or 'neurocytic' forms.

Advanced neurocytic maturation characterizes the rare tumors previously referred to as **'cerebellar neuroblastomas'** or **'neuroblastic medulloblastomas'**, but now termed **'medulloblastomas with extensive nodularity'**.[820,821] These resemble desmoplastic/nodular medulloblastomas but exhibit a more strikingly lobular microarchitecture, their outsized reticulin-free zones having unusually elongated profiles, being particularly rich in synaptophysin-immunoreactive fibrillary matrix material and boasting a population of small, amitotic and uniformly rounded neurocytic cells arrayed in linear streams (Fig. 28.94). The differentiated neuronal nature of this population is apparent in that such cells elaborate cytoplasmic processes replete with clear and dense-cored secretory vesicles that may terminate in synaptic contacts. Some examples contain recognizable neurons of intermediate to large size and this embryonal neoplasm may rarely undergo sequential maturation to benign ganglioneurocytic or gangliogliomatous histology,[812,819] a phenomenon (possibly treatment-driven) recorded in isolated cases of conventional medulloblastoma as well.[808] Medulloblastomas of this sort seem to have a predilection for children younger than 3 years of age and to carry a more favorable prognosis than other subtypes (particularly in this patient cohort).[816,821] Though not all such tumors comply, neuroradiologic presentation as a cerebellar mass composed of contrast-enhancing nodules clustered in grape-like fashion is virtually diagnostic.[821]

Classic medulloblastomas are often found on immunohistochemical assessment to be colonized by GFAP-positive elements that tend to lie near stromal blood vessels and to display the stellate cytoplasmic configurations typical of reactive astroglia. These are generally taken to be entrapped, though the identification of similar cells in metastatic deposits raises the possibility that at least some represent neoplastic astrocytes of terminally differentiated nature.[820] GFAP-labeling cells of indisputably neoplastic morphology are much less frequently encountered,[820,828,834] glial differentiation sufficiently advanced as to be obvious on routine microscopic inspection being most exceptional. A conspicuous network of tumor cells having GFAP-reactive cytoplasmic rims and processes is often localized about the pale islands of desmoplastic/nodular medulloblastomas, suggesting that these micronodules are organized centers of divergent astroglial, as well as neuronal, outgrowth.[830] We mention in passing the immunolabeling of some medulloblastomas for photoreceptor-associated proteins, including rod-opsin and retinal S-antigen,[811,827,834] as well as curious variants containing neurosensory rosettes of Flexner–Wintersteiner type.[827] Shared by retinoblastomas and pineoblastomas, such evidences of photosensory differentiation have been taken to support the unified cytogenesis of these embryonal neoplasms but, as discussed previously, this is an embattled hypothesis. The immunophenotypic potential of the medulloblastoma further includes reactivity for vimentin, desmin (typically limited to minor tumor cell subsets), nestin (a class VI intermediate filament protein expressed by many embryonic cell types, including neuroepithelial progenitors in the developing CNS), neural cell adhesion molecules, nerve growth factors and their receptors.[820] Even cytoplasmic actin labeling has been described,[806] a finding that we can confirm, and exceptional cases may evidence cytokeratin (AE1/3) reactivity. The latter, when present, is usually a focal finding.

Regarding immunophenotype and its bearing on differential diagnosis, we would emphasize the labeling of nearly all medulloblastomas (including those of thoroughly undifferentiated histologic aspect) for synaptophysin as a property that may be exploited to exclude from further consideration such potentially confounding lesions as the poorly differentiated fourth ventricular ependymoma, other anaplastic gliomas, and primary cerebellar lymphoma (typified by a B-cell profile). A pertinent 'negative' is the general failure of medulloblastomas to express thyroid transcription factor-1 (TTF-1),[554] as metastatic small cell carcinoma of pulmonary origin potentially complicates the diagnostic picture when one is dealing with adult neurosurgical material (and shares synaptophysin labeling) but is usually TTF-1 reactive. We have not encountered a solitary cerebellar metastasis as the presenting manifestation of an otherwise occult small cell carcinoma. The reader must consult our section dealing with atypical teratoid/rhabdoid tumors for differential diagnostic discussion of an embryonal neoplasm that often arises in the cerebellum and frequently harbors small cell components that may mimic the medulloblastoma to histologic perfection. Bona fide medulloblastomas do not exhibit anomalies of the rhabdoid tumor-associated *INI1* gene or loss of its protein product on immunoexpression study with the BAF47 antibody.[820]

We have elected to cite here only a small sample of the many studies detailing the immunohistochemical profile of medulloblastomas and make no attempt to dissect the conflicting (and, at present, clinically immaterial) data that have emerged from efforts to correlate the expression of neuronal, glial, and photosensory antigens with tumor behavior.[811,828,834] As regards other variables that potentially bear on outcome, amplifications of the *MYCC* and *MYCN* genes are well established as auguring poorly in the setting of medulloblastoma and chromosome 17p loss, isochromosome 17q formation, and overexpression of ErbB2, PDGFR, p53 and the products of other oncogenes and cell cycle regulators have also proven adverse prognostic indicators in various studies.[820] None of these assessments, however, has found regular application to the issue of patient management. The same can be said of favorable prognostic markers that include high-level expression of the TrkC neurotrophin receptor and nuclear accumulation of β-catenin, a signal of Wnt cascade activation.[820] Medulloblastomas are classed as WHO grade IV neoplasms and are regarded collectively as potentially aggressive tumors requiring adjuvant treatment as well as surgical attack to prevent local recurrence and metastasis (particularly along CSF pathways).

At present, the therapeutic approach to medulloblastomas is predicated primarily on clinical variables.[820] The 'standard risk' patient is generally defined as a subject 3 years of age or older who has undergone complete (or near-total) resection of a tumor confined to the posterior fossa. Protocols combining chemotherapy and whole neuraxis irradiation have achieved 5-year survivals exceeding 80% in this relatively favorable clinical setting, very few such patients experiencing late relapse. Children below the age of 3 years at diagnosis and individuals of any age with evident CSF dissemination (found in approximately 30% of cases on initial evaluation), extraneural metastases or bulky (>1.5 cm^2) residual disease after surgery – 'high risk' patients – do not fare as well. Whether the excess mortality noted in the very young reflects intrinsic tumor biology or the reluctance of neuro-oncologists to expose the immature nervous system to the predictably toxic doses of radiation that have been considered requisite to achieving disease control is unclear. Certainly, the price exacted of childhood medulloblastoma survivors by conventional radiotherapy – growth failure, endocrinopathy, significant intellectual impairment, behavioral disturbances, and the induction of secondary neoplasms that include meningiomas, sarcomas, and glioblastomas – has been disheartening and continues to drive investigations aimed at reducing CNS radiation exposure in the pediatric cohort. In this connection, there is evidence to suggest that infants and young children with medulloblastomas of desmoplastic/nodular and extensively nodular type may be spared irradiation and managed with chemotherapy alone following tumor resection.[839] Whereas treatment failure in the posterior fossa or along the craniospinal axis is the rule, medulloblastomas do occasionally travel to more distant sites.[814] Skeletal deposits, often widespread, account for over 90% of systemic metastases, but the liver, lymph nodes, and lungs may be involved as may the abdominal cavity (via ventriculoperitoneal shunts placed to relieve obstructive hydrocephalus). While medulloblastomas usually conform to the principle (Collins' law) that defines the period of risk for recurrence of embryonal childhood neoplasms as equal to the patient's age at diagnosis plus 9 months, late relapse (including extraneural dissemination) may be encountered.

Particularly aggressive behavior and treatment resistance characterize '**large cell**' and '**anaplastic**' **medulloblastomas** (Fig. 28.95).[807,816,822,823,832] The former descriptor has been applied to neoplasms conspicuously or wholly populated by monomorphic cells with large, rounded and vesicular nuclei, prominent nucleoli, and variably abundant eosinophilic cytoplasm. 'Anaplastic' tumors exhibit marked variation in nuclear size and contour, multinucleated and bizarre giant cells inhabiting some examples. The cannibalistic wrapping of tumor cells about one another is a striking feature of many cases. In fact, the considerable cytologic overlap evidenced by neoplasms manifesting these alterations has prompted their consideration as a combined category (i.e., large cell/anaplastic medulloblastoma) in some studies. High mitotic rates are the rule

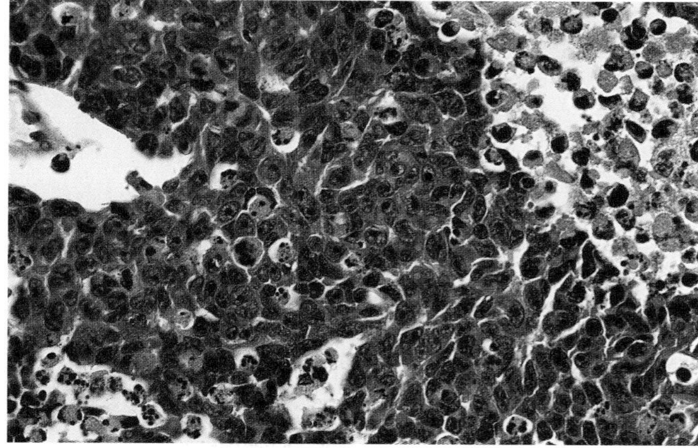

Fig. 28.95 Large cell/anaplastic medulloblastoma. Cellular enlargement, often prominent nucleoli, and pronounced mitotic and apoptotic activity are features of this virulent medulloblastoma subtype.

and apoptotic cellular remains, typically abundant, may form confluent lakes and serpiginous seams. Cytoplasmic immunolabeling for synaptophysin is generally retained (often in dot-like perinuclear form) and reactivity for neurofilament proteins and chromogranin may also be demonstrable. Focal GFAP expression has been documented, but is most uncommon. Of differential diagnostic utility are the observations that large cell/anaplastic medulloblastomas do not manifest the inclusion-like cytoplasmic bodies, EMA immunoreactivity, chromosome 22 abnormalities or loss of INI1 protein product expression characteristic of the atypical teratoid/rhabdoid tumor.[820] Large cell/anaplastic features may be apparent at presentation or appear only at relapse, are often encountered in medulloblastomas that retain classic or desmoplastic/nodular components, and can emerge within medullomyoblastomas (discussed below).[824] These observations, coupled with the demonstration that tumors characterized by large cell or anaplastic morphology may share 'background' genetic profiles (e.g., isochromosome 17q formation) with conventional medulloblastomas while harboring many additional genomic aberrations,[817,820] indicate that the representatives of this group can be regarded not as fundamentally distinct medulloblastoma subtypes but as variants exhibiting progression-associated phenomena. *MYC* oncogene amplifications, previously mentioned as an adverse prognostic indicator, are especially prevalent in this setting.[807,817,818,822]

The virulent clinical biology of large cell/anaplastic medulloblastomas has been acknowledged by some cooperative clinical trial groups in their categorizing of affected patients as 'high risk' irrespective of age at presentation, extent of disease, and completeness of resection. In this vein, we mention that the formal grading of medulloblastomas according to the extent and severity of anaplastic alterations has proven clinically relevant in some retrospective analyses and could become standard practice.[816,823,832,838] The exact criteria employed in these studies, which can be had from the cited literature, are not specifically endorsed by the WHO at the time of this writing. This is not to deny, however, that cell size, pleomorphism, mitotic and apoptotic activity constitute continuous variables when medulloblastomas are considered as a class and that reproducible morphologic criteria for identifying those tumors requiring nonstandard intervention would be most welcome.

Certain rare medulloblastoma variants merit additional comment. The **melanotic medulloblastoma** or **medulloblastoma with melanotic differentiation** (in suggested WHO parlance[820]) is defined by its content of pigmented cells disposed in tubules, papillae, or nests.[813,820,829] These are stained by conventional histochemical methods for the demonstration of melanin, can be shown to contain melanosomes in varying stages of maturation, label for HMB-45 as well as cytokeratins (AE1/3), and may reflect differentiation along the lines of the ocular pigment epithelium. Although this lesion bears some histologic resemblance to the indolent melanotic neuroectodermal tumors of infancy that arise in the maxillary and epididymal regions, it is a highly malignant neoplasm prone to early and widespread neuraxis dissemination along CSF pathways. The **medullomyoblastoma** or **medulloblastoma with myogenic differentiation** is named for its heterologous rhabdomyoblastic elements.[824,833] Medulloblastomas of classic, desmoplastic/nodular, and large cell/anaplastic types may all spawn such components.[824] This curious entity has been variously interpreted as a medulloblastoma evidencing the extreme plasticity of its multipotent neuroepithelial precursors, as a tumor derived from neural crest (ectomesenchymal) progenitors recognized for their ability to differentiate along striated muscle lines, as a composite neoplasm populated by myoblastic constituents that arise via the secondary neoplastic induction of leptomeningeal or stromal elements, and, finally, as a lopsided, bidermal teratoma. Several examples reported under this designation have harbored cystic components with the appearance of mature, tridermal teratoma.[833] Some medullomyoblastomas have been found to harbor an isochromosome 17q,[824] indicating a kinship with the conventional medulloblastoma group. Variants containing both muscular and melanotic elements have been described,[837] as has **medulloblastoma with chondroid differentiation**,[805] and a cerebellar tumor exhibiting evidence of isochromosome 17q formation and having medulloblastoma-type, ganglion cell, astrocytic, ependymal, cartilaginous, muscular, and glandular components.[826] A group of adult-onset tumors originally characterized as '**lipomatous medulloblastomas**' is now recognized to be more closely allied with neoplasms of neurocytic type. These are termed **cerebellar liponeurocytomas** in current WHO nomenclature and are discussed elsewhere under that designation (see 'Central neurocytoma and extraventricular neurocytic neoplasms'). Conventional medulloblastomas may rarely contain lipid-laden cells in conspicuous numbers, these usually proving to be foamy macrophages[721] but potentially representing lipidized tumor cells with adipocyte-like or lipoblastic profiles.[741]

Medulloepithelioma

The **medulloepithelioma** is a highly aggressive neoplasm that typically arises in the cerebrum of an infant or child younger than 5 years of age.[846] Particularly characteristic is a deep, paraventricular localization – a topography adduced in support of a postulated origin from the lining germinal matrix of the developing forebrain – but medulloepitheliomas may also originate in the third ventricular/thalamostriate regions, cerebellum, brainstem, cauda equina, optic nerves,[842] and sellar/suprasellar compartments.[849] Ocular neoplasms of comparable morphology are well recognized and rare examples presenting as sciatic nerve[847] or pelvic[844] growths are on record. These extraneural variants are not further considered here.

Often attaining massive proportions, medulloepitheliomas are usually well circumscribed and composed of friable, gray–pink tissue evidencing hemorrhage, necrosis and, in some cases, cystic change. Their defining feature is the formation of tubules, ribbons or, less frequently, papillae resembling, and believed to represent a recapitulation of, the medullary epithelial structuring of the primitive neural tube (Fig. 28.96). These are fashioned of

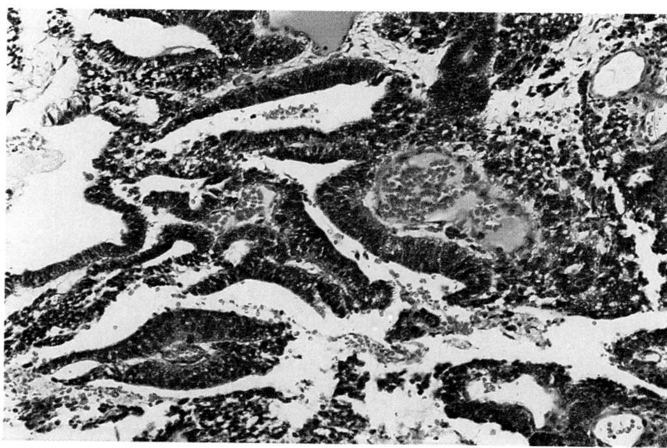

Fig. 28.96 Medulloepithelioma. A tubulopapillary disposition of its columnar elements characterizes this primitive neuroepithelial neoplasm.

pseudostratified columnar cells that rest on a continuous, PAS-positive basement membrane and are sometimes capped by apical cytoplasmic blebs. PAS-positive material may also coat luminal surfaces as an ill-defined, granular pseudomembrane. Mitotic figures are readily identifiable and generally abluminal in location, a pattern reminiscent of the juxtaventricular proliferative activity characterizing early neurocytogenesis. Selective labeling of these inner, mitotically active elements for nestin and full thickness immunoreactivity of this neoplastic neuroepithelium for vimentin and microtubule-associated protein type 5 (MAP-5) are additional antigenic features shared with the embryonic neural tube.[845] Some observers have found focal labeling for GFAP, class III β-tubulin, and neurofilament protein epitopes within these arrays, but this would appear to be exceptional.[841] Also described are instances of apical immunoreactivity for EMA and focal cytoplasmic labeling for NSE and cytokeratins.[841,845,852] It should be noted that medulloepithelial structures vary greatly in extent from case to case and may constitute only a regionally limited finding in an otherwise patternless, small cell neoplasm of thoroughly undifferentiated aspect.

In keeping with their proposed stem cell derivation, medulloepitheliomas often manifest divergent differentiation and maturation, at times advanced, along astrocytic, ependymal, neuronal and, rarely, oligodendroglial lines.[841,843,846,850] A tubulopapillary, melanotic fourth ventricular neoplasm interpreted as a pigmented medulloepithelioma is on record,[851] as is an example containing chondroid, osseous, and skeletal muscle elements.[840] The exact nosologic position of the latter in relation to the immature teratoma, which may harbor medullary-type neuroepithelial formations, is problematic. Obviously, the presence of admixed nonteratomatous germ cell components and evidence of endodermal or somatic ectodermal differentiation should be sought and excluded before a diagnosis of medulloepithelioma is rendered, particularly if neoplastic mesenchymal tissues are identified.

The differential diagnosis of the medulloepithelioma must also include the ependymoblastoma and choroid plexus carcinoma. Medulloepitheliomas may contain elements of ependymoblastoma (described below), but their neuromedullary components rest on basement membranes foreign to ependymoblastic rosettes and do not fashion at the EM level such ependymal specializations as crowning cilia, microvilli, or complex intercellular junctions of zonula adherens type.[852] Ependymoblastomas, by definition, do not manifest divergent differentiation along astrocytic or neuronal lines. The same is true of choroid plexus carcinomas which, in addition, tend to a more obviously villiform architecture than is displayed by most medulloepitheliomas and, unlike the latter, may display widespread immunoreactivity for S-100 protein and cytokeratins. We have previously cited, in our discussion of fibrillary astrocytic neoplasms, reference to glioblastomas harboring medulloepithelioma-like structures.

The medulloepithelioma is highly malignant and typically kills within 1–2 years of diagnosis, though aggressive surgical and adjuvant therapy may save some afflicted children.[848] Uncontrollable growth at the primary site is the usual cause of death, but widespread leptomeningeal metastasis is frequent as well and may occur early in the disease course.

Central neuroblastic tumors

The diagnosis of **neuroblastoma** should be reserved for extracerebellar neoplasms of embryonal appearance that can be shown to differentiate solely along neuronal lines. Neuroblastomas of the central neuraxis are typified by a presentation in the first decade of life (usually prior to age 5 years) and localization to the cerebral hemispheres,[854,857] though they may arise within the ventricular system[861] and intraspinal compartment.[858,862]

Consisting of friable gray tissue prone to necrosis, hemorrhage, and cystic change, neuroblastomas often achieve enormous proportions by the time they are discovered but tend to appear relatively circumscribed. Induction of a collagenous stroma lends to some examples a firm consistency and unusually lobulated contours. Although there is no biologic import to this division, several histologic variants are recognized. The '**classic**' **neuroblastoma** is composed of small, mitotically active cells possessed of densely hyperchromatic nuclei and disposed in highly populous sheets. Variably represented is a delicate fibrillary matrix consisting of tangled cytoplasmic processes. It is this subtype that is most likely to contain Homer Wright rosettes and large neurons of ganglion cell type. Occasional examples manifest a compact palisading of tumor cell nuclei within their neuropil-like matrices.[860] Tumor cells may also palisade about foci of necrosis, imparting a small cell glioblastoma-like histology to some examples.[859] The '**desmoplastic**' **neuroblastoma** is defined by a fibrous stroma, most developed where tumor contacts the leptomeninges, that imposes lobular, trabecular or single-file arrangements on its constituent cells. Larger than classic neuroblasts, the latter are characterized by vesicular nuclei, distinct nucleoli and, in some cases, a modest paranuclear expanse of hematoxyphilic or plum-colored cytoplasm. The '**transitional**' **neuroblastoma** combines features of both the classic and desmoplastic variants. Only exceptionally do central neuroblastic tumors evidence the graded maturational alterations so often displayed by their retroperitoneal and posterior mediastinal counterparts, meriting designation as ganglioneuroblastomas.[853,856,862–864]

In the absence of Homer Wright rosettes or an unarguably neoplastic (as opposed to entrapped) neuronal population, the diagnosis of neuroblastoma needs ultrastructural or immunocytochemical defending. Neurite-like cytoplasmic processes containing microtubules in parallel array, dense-core and clear, synaptic-type vesicles signal neuronal differentiation. Attempts at synapse formation, usually abortive, are apparent in only a small minority of cases. Immunohistochemical assessment obviates the need for electron microscopic study if cytoplasmic synaptophysin or neurofilament protein labeling can be demonstrated, nuclear NeuN expression also attesting to differentiation along neuronal lines. Synaptophysin reactivity is far the most sensitive index and typically concentrated in the fibrillar matrix. GFAP expression should be limited to cells reasonably interpreted as reactive astrocytes. These possess stellate cytoplasmic processes, are most numerous at the tumor–brain interface and, when present deeper within a lesion, usually lie near penetrating blood vessels. Some observers have credited central neuroblastic tumors with the capacity to generate GFAP-immunoreactive schwannian elements,[856] but the exact nature of the cells in question is far from clear.[863]

The interpretation of survival data reported for patients with cerebral neuroblastomas is complicated by the inclusion in some series of cases that would now be regarded as examples of central neurocytoma or desmoplastic infantile ganglioglioma, both associated with a favorable prognosis, as well as anaplastic small cell tumors not further characterized as to differentiating potential.[854,857,861] Still, neuroblastomas seem more amenable to surgical and radiotherapeutic management than other primitive extracerebellar neoplasms,[854] some observers recording a particularly gratifying outcome following resection of largely cystic examples.[855] The risks of local regrowth and CSF-borne metastasis, however, are high and spread to extraneural sites is occasionally seen.[854,857] Noteworthy are isolated instances of late local recurrence in which reoperation has demonstrated maturation of central neuroblastomas to differentiated ganglion cell tumors.[853,864]

Ependymoblastoma

A high-grade neoplasm of infancy and early childhood, the **ependymoblastoma** tends to a paraventricular localization deep within the cerebral hemispheres but may arise in the posterior fossa.[865,869] Primary leptomeningeal[871] and extradural, sacrococcygeal[870] presentations have been described, the latter associated with elevated serum alpha-fetoprotein levels. The tumor is densely populated by small, monomorphous cells disposed in sheets and broad, anastomosing cords punctuated by 'ependymoblastic' rosettes. These defining structures lack the PAS-positive basement membranes of medulloepitheliomatous arrays and are distinguished from rosettes of mature ependymal type by a multilayered stratification of their encircling nuclei and by manifest proliferative activity, mitoses often lying in a juxtaluminal position. Perivascular pseudorosettes are not in evidence or only poorly developed. Necrosis is common but not associated with cellular palisading and there is generally no microvascular proliferation – additional features separating these embryonal neoplasms from anaplastic ependymomas. Ultrastructural studies have confirmed that rosette-forming elements are ependymal in nature, sporting elaborate apical cell junctions, microvilli, and cilia.[865,868,870] These may exhibit focal GFAP immunolabeling, but this is an inconstant finding.[865,868] We have alluded to regional ependymoblastic differentiation within medulloepitheliomas. Ependymoblastomas, by definition, are devoid of medullary epithelial structures and theoretically incapable of divergent neuronal differentiation. While the latter should distinguish the ependymoblastoma from the 'embryonal tumor with abundant neuropil and true rosettes', discussed below, these may actually constitute a unified entity.[866] We would agree that the overwhelming majority of primitive neuroepithelial neoplasms harboring ependymoblastic rosettes can also be shown to contain neuroblastic elements and synaptophysin-rich matrix components when thoroughly assessed.[866] Furthermore, it would appear that a marker chromosomal anomaly consisting of amplification at 19q13.42 is shared by lesions falling into both pathologic categories.[867] Disseminated CSF-borne metastasis is common and most examples prove fatal within 1–2 years of diagnosis.

Embryonal tumor with abundant neuropil and true rosettes

The awkwardly named **embryonal tumor with abundant neuropil and true rosettes**[872] has only recently been segregated from other primitive neuroepithelial neoplasms of the CNS and is not accorded distinct status in the current WHO taxonomy, but in our practice this aggressive lesion of infancy and early childhood has proven far more prevalent than the ependymoblastoma and medulloepithelioma combined. The experience communicated to date suggests a predilection for the frontal lobes, brainstem, and cerebellum. In contrast to other CNS neoplasms of embryonal type, this primitive neuroepithelial tumor seems to afflict girls more frequently than boys and often displays little or nothing in the way of contrast enhancement on neuroradiologic study. The entity is descriptively designated for the embedding of ependymoblastic rosettes in an expansive matrix that is rich in synaptophysin and neurofilament protein on immunohistochemical assessment and that commonly exhibits broad zones of strikingly hypocellular aspect (Fig. 28.97). Also populating tumors of this group are undifferentiated and neuroblastic elements (these may fashion rosettes of Homer Wright type), some examples containing ganglion cell components or manifesting loci of neurocytic maturation in which tumor cells align in linear streams or aggregate in formations resembling the 'pale islands' of the desmoplastic/nodular medulloblastoma.

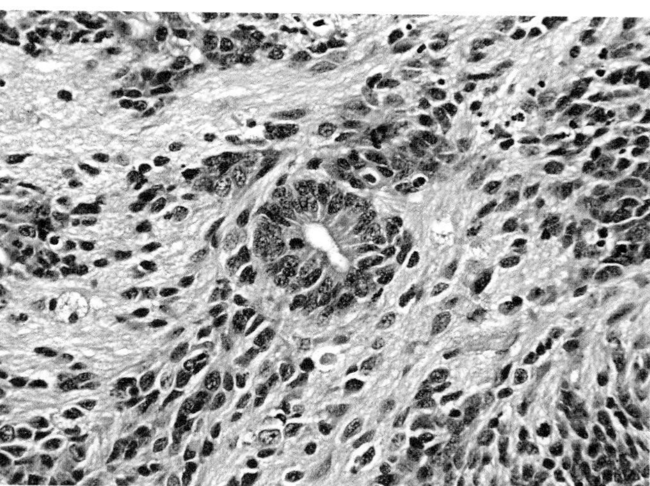

Fig. 28.97 Embryonal tumor with abundant neuropil and true rosettes. Typical is a delicate fibrillar matrix in which primitive neuroepithelial elements and ependymoblastic rosettes (center) are arrayed, the latter having well-defined (though often minute) lumens and being composed of mitotically active tumor cells with granular apical stippling.

Regions exhibiting large cell/anaplastic medulloblastoma-like histology may be encountered as well. Ependymoblastic rosettes are represented by mitotically active elements in radial, pseudostratified array about central lumens of rounded profile and often diminutive diameter. The juxtaluminal apices of participating cells typically manifest a granular stippling and are joined, at the ultrastructural level, by zonula adherens-type intercellular junctions. MIB-1 labeling activity is high in these formations and in poorly differentiated, nonrosetted components. High level genomic amplification at chromosome 19q13.42 (with upregulation of a microRNA cluster including oncomirs miRNA-372 and miRNA-373) may well constitute a 'marker' abnormality unifying this lesion with the ostensibly pure ependymoblastoma.[867,873]

The embryonal tumor with abundant neuropil and true rosettes is a virulent neoplasm that often proves resistant to surgical and adjuvant therapy. In the largest series yet published, 19 of 25 evaluable patients died of progressive disease and median survival from diagnosis was a mere 9 months.[872] Local failure is the rule, leptomeningeal dissemination further complicating some cases.

Polar spongioblastoma

It is in deference to a traditional view[876] that the so-called **polar spongioblastoma** represents a primitive neuroepithelial neoplasm of distinctive character that we briefly address it here, but there has been considerable controversy as to whether the peculiar tumors awarded this designation constitute a unified entity[877] and this diagnosis is no longer recognized in the WHO nosology. A tendency to arise in the walls of the third and fourth ventricles in childhood has been asserted,[876] but no generalizations as regards clinical course emerge from the literature. The tumor is composed of spindled cells with fusiform nuclei that appear suspended in compact palisades between delicate uni- or bipolar cytoplasmic processes in close parallel array. This arresting disposition has been likened to the radial arrangement of migrating glia ('spongioblasts') that characterizes the 16- to 18-week stage of human neuroembryogenesis.[876] Skeptics point to the fact that a comparably rhythmic architecture may be encountered in neoplasms that otherwise qualify as classic oligodendrogliomas, pilocytic astrocytomas, glioblastomas, ependymomas, neuroblastomas, and medulloblastomas.[877] To believers, however, a frequent admixture of conventional oligodendroglial and astrocytic elements has simply constituted evidence that the polar spongioblastoma derives from embryonic forbears committed to differentiate along glial lines. Uncritical acceptance of this entity is further complicated by its lack of defining immunohistochemical or ultrastructural features. The presumed spongioblastic constituents are said to be GFAP negative, consonant with their putatively primitive nature.[875,876] Whether examples reported to contain intracytoplasmic dense-core vesicles and microtubules[874] are not better regarded as neuroblastoma variants is open to question.

It is our view that the diagnosis of polar spongioblastoma, if resorted to at all, should be reserved for neoplasms that exhibit a compact, palisaded growth pattern throughout. Careful search should be made for telltale foci exhibiting the features of any of the conventional tumor types mentioned above and classification based on the histology of such areas, however limited in volume. Immunoassessment for synaptophysin expression and, if that proves negative, ultrastructural examination are required to exclude palisaded cerebral neuroblastoma.

Assorted primitive neuroectodermal tumors

The term **primitive neuroectodermal tumor (PNET)** was originally coined not as a generic appellation for embryonal neoplasms of every stripe, which it was to become, but to designate a cerebral tumor of infancy and childhood characterized by medulloblastoma-like histology and a propensity to disseminate along CSF pathways.[882] As initially defined, at least 90% of the tumor qualifying for this diagnosis had to consist of uniformly small and densely hyperchromatic cells of entirely undifferentiated appearance disposed in patternless sheets.[882] Additionally described in many cases were desmoplastic mesenchymal components, sharp tumor circumscription, high mitotic rates, necrosis, and cystic change. Often noted, as well, were limited foci of apparent glial, neuronal or bidirectional differentiation.

The problems inherent in defining a neoplasm largely on the basis of its undifferentiated appearances should be obvious. The diagnosis of PNET (more precisely designated as CNS or 'central' PNET to distinguish this from tumors of the Ewing sarcoma/'peripheral' PNET group) rests on firmest ground when applied to extracerebellar tumors of embryonal aspect exhibiting divergent neuronoglial differentiation. The demonstration of a polymorphous immunophenotype is useful in this regard, some PNETs clearly coexpressing synaptophysin and multiple intermediate filament proteins (most often the complex of vimentin–GFAP–neurofilament protein but, occasionally, cytokeratins and desmin as well[881,888,894]). Murky is the distinction of putative PNETs evidencing GFAP immunolabeling alone from highly anaplastic gliomas. In practice, we find ourselves applying the former label to largely monomorphic, small cell neoplasms of childhood containing GFAP-positive elements but manifesting neither the complex microvascular proliferation nor the perinecrotic cellular palisading that typifies high-grade glial neoplasms (particularly astrocytomas) of conventional type. Immunoreactive cells often huddle in small clusters or aggregate about stromal blood vessels, are poorly fibrillated, and may assume a microgemistocytic or miniature rhabdoid appearance. We caution the reader against the low percentage diagnosis of PNET in an adult, the neoplasm so labeled almost invariably proving to represent a glioblastoma with small cell features at reoperation or autopsy. Convincing ultrastructural or immunohistochemical evidence of divergent glioneuronal differentiation must be forwarded to support the diagnosis in this setting. Even so, the possibility must always be acknowledged that what would appear to represent a bona fide adult-onset PNET in fact represents the emergence of PNET-like elements from an underlying glioma. This phenomenon is discussed further in our consideration of glioblastomas.

Neoplasms interpreted as PNET variants have been reported to follow prophylactic cranial irradiation for childhood leukemia and lymphoma,[880] to arise in the leptomeninges,[889] spinal cord,[883] and cauda equina[858] as well as brain, to evidence choroid plexus differentiation,[884] and to contain smooth muscle,[892] rhabdomyoblastic[878] or adipocytic[887,892] elements. Central PNETs may exhibit large cell/anaplastic features (with particularly unfavorable prognostic implications) of the kind characterizing some medulloblastomas.[879] Tumors of this kind (and their conventional small cell counterparts) must be shown to retain INI1 protein expression in order to exclude atypical teratoid/rhabdoid tumor as an alternative diagnostic possibility. Use of the BAF47 antibody to this end is discussed in the section that follows.

We have encountered cerebral neoplasms similar to a unique cerebellar lesion descriptively designated as a '**desmoplastic primitive neuroectodermal tumor with divergent differentiation**'.[896] The recorded case was characterized by nests and cords of small neuroepithelial cells (some labeling for synaptophysin, neurofilament protein epitopes, GFAP, and cytokeratins) embedded in a cellular 'stroma' populated by desmin-immunoreactive elements. At recurrence, this exhibited strikingly epithelioid features and overt neuronal (ganglion cell) differentiation. Curiosities that potentially complicate the differential diagnosis of central PNETs include intracranial examples of the **melanotic neuroectodermal tumor of infancy**,[886,897] the **desmoplastic small round-cell tumor** of Gerald and Rosai,[893] and the **Ewing sarcoma/'peripheral' PNET**.[890,891,895] The last two of these entities are characterized by specific t(11;22) chromosomal translocations foreign to embryonal tumors of central neuroepithelial type[879,885] and critical to definitive tumor classification. Complete membranous immunolabeling for the *MIC2* gene product CD99, a characteristic feature of the Ewing sarcoma/'peripheral' PNET family, is only exceptionally (and focally) shared by central PNETs,[879,894] though a significant subset of these may exhibit a paranuclear dot-like pattern of reactivity.[894] Genetically confirmed intracranial examples of Ewing sarcoma/'peripheral' PNET have been described mainly as dura-based lesions.[889,890] An intramedullary case is on record.[895]

Atypical teratoid/rhabdoid tumor

The **atypical teratoid/rhabdoid tumor (AT/RT)** is a highly aggressive neoplasm encountered principally in infancy and early childhood.[900,904] Adult-onset examples are distinct rareties.[906] Over 90% of afflicted patients reported to date have been less than 5 years of age at diagnosis (mean = 20 months) and nearly 50% have harbored tumors of the cerebellum or cerebellopontine angle, often with contiguous brainstem involvement. Supratentorial (cerebral or suprasellar) examples account for at least 40% of recorded cases, trailed distantly by pineal region and intraspinal[906] variants. AT/RTs arising within cranial nerves have been depicted,[905] as have instances in which neoplasms of this kind have emerged from low-grade neuroepithelial neoplasms (pleomorphic xanthoastrocytoma[436] and ganglioglioma[655]) in what apparently represents a bizarre form of tumor progression. MRI typically discloses a bulky and contrast-enhancing mass, cystic and hemorrhagic alterations being common to this entity and its neuroradiologic profile indistinguishable from that of the medulloblastoma/PNET. Approximately 20–25% of patients have evidence of CSF dissemination at diagnosis, many succumb to disease within months of diagnosis, and survival beyond 2 years has been the exception. Intensive adjuvant protocols may ameliorate this bleak picture.[901]

AT/RTs share with rhabdoid tumors of the infantile kidney and soft tissues a linkage to biallelic inactivation of *hSNF5/INI1*, a gene mapping to chromosome 22q11.2 and encoding a ubiquitously expressed member of the SWI/SNF chromatin-remodeling complex.[898] Proteins of this family effect conformational alterations in the nucleosome that facilitate or restrict transcription factor access. Most AT/RTs demonstrate a pattern of *INI1* inactivation conforming to the 'two-hit' mechanism operative in the disabling of classic tumor-suppressing genes, loss of one copy resulting from partial deletion or monosomy 22 and the second suffering a nonsense or frameshift mutation (often in hotspot exons 5 and 9) that produces a novel stop codon. Also encountered are deletions or mutations involving both gene copies. While the majority of AT/RTs arise in sporadic fashion, germline mutations of *INI1* underlie a familial rhabdoid tumor syndrome characterized by potentially multifocal, CNS, renal, and other extraneural primaries presenting in the first year of life.[898] As presently discussed, the loss of INI1 protein product expression that is a consistent feature of AT/RTs can be exploited to facilitate the identification of these neoplasms by immunohistochemical means.

AT/RTs are so designated in acknowledgment of their potentially complex histology.[900,904] In fact, only a minority consist solely of rhabdoid cells and the latter (characterized in classic form by distinct cell borders, large and vesicular nuclei, macronucleoli, and globose, paranuclear cytoplasmic inclusions of hyalin appearance) may be only sparsely represented among tumor cells with uniformly dense and eosinophilic, finely granular, vacuolated, wispy or water-clear cytoplasm (Fig. 28.98A). These nonrhabdoid, large cell elements can include variably spindled, polygonal and bizarre, multinucleated cells disposed in nests or sheets. Bands of hyalinized collagen traverse some examples, while others exhibit pseudopapillary formations or myxoid change and a chordoid growth pattern. The adjectival 'teratoid' reflects the presence, in many tumors of this group, of varied neoplastic tissue components (Fig. 28.98B). Most prominently represented are small cell elements of embryonal appearance indistinguishable from those that typify the medulloblastoma/PNET. The latter, encountered in 60–70% of cases – and the vastly dominant component in some examples – usually assume an undifferentiated histologic profile but may fashion rosettes of Homer Wright, Flexner–Wintersteiner or ependymoblastic type, some AT/RTs containing ependymal canal- or neural tube-like structures within their primitive neuroepithelial compartment. Spindle cell mesenchymal components may be present (these often having a fetal mesenchyme-like appearance) and some examples contain epithelial elements that may be represented by cohesive cell nests, adenoid and tubuloglandular structures or keratinizing squamous islands. Differentiation along striated muscle lines has not been reported.

Immunohistochemical assessment is critical to the distinction of AT/RTs from a variety of neoplasms that may assume rhabdoid cytologic features. A complex immunophenotype is the rule.[900,904] Rhabdoid and nonrhabdoid large cell elements invariably display labeling for vimentin (with intense decoration of cytoplasmic inclusions, when present), are nearly always immunoreactive for EMA, and commonly label for GFAP and smooth muscle actin (SMA) as well. The percentage of cells reactive for each antigen is highly variable. EMA labeling may be diffuse or confined to cytoplasmic membranes, antibodies to SMA occasionally decorating a peripheral cytoplasmic ring with particular intensity (a pattern encountered in some smooth muscle tumors). In this connection, we would cite gene expression studies confirming the activation of a myogenic differentiation program in AT/RTs.[802] Also common is immunoreactivity of the large cell components for cytokeratins (AE1/3, CAM 5.2) and some may be decorated by antibodies to neurofilament protein (NFP) and synaptophysin (SYN). Desmin reactivity, present in only a minority of cases, is usually restricted to mesenchymal or PNET-like regions (which may also label for NFP, SYN, and GFAP). Epithelial elements, not surprisingly, label for cytokeratins and, less commonly, EMA. Membranous cytoplasmic immunoreactivity for claudin 6, a tight junction-associated antigen, may emerge as a phenomenon aiding in the identification of AT/RTs and their distinction from other CNS tumors.[899]

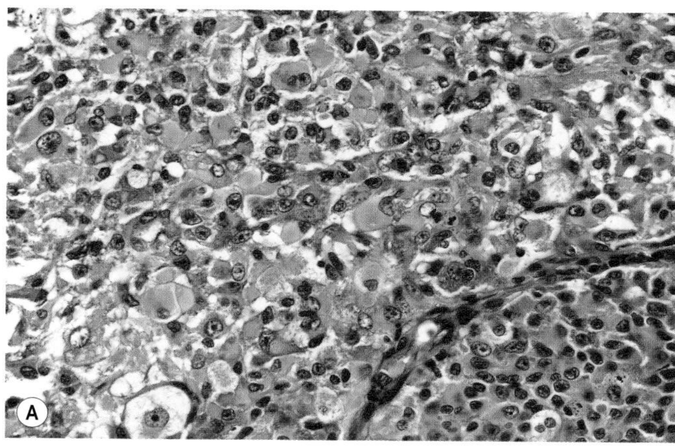

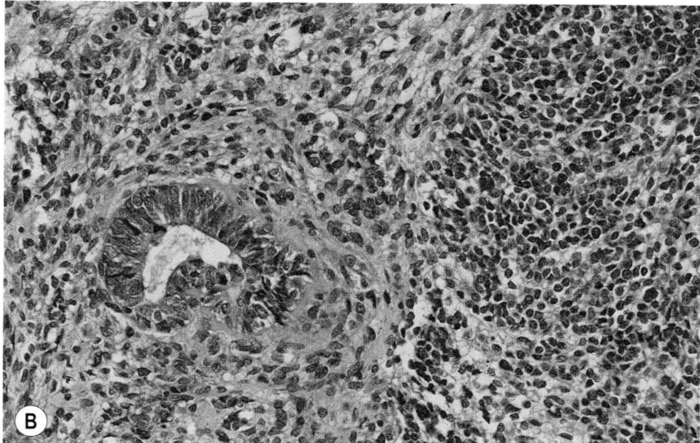

Fig. 28.98 Atypical teratoid/rhabdoid tumor. Neoplasms of this family typically contain at least some cells of large, rhabdoid phenotype (**A**). A second example (**B**) harbors, at right, small cell elements of primitive neuroepithelial appearance and a differentiated glandular structure, at left, embedded in a neoplastic component of mesenchymal aspect.

A major breakthrough in the immunohistochemical identification of AT/RTs has come with the development and marketing of a monoclonal antibody, designated as BAF47/SNF5 or BAF47 alone, that recognizes the protein product of *INI1*. The loss of gene expression at the protein level that regularly results from the *INI1*-inactivating deletions and mutations characteristic of AT/RTs is reflected in a consistent failure of tumor cells to exhibit BAF47 reactivity[902,903] (Fig. 28.99). It is a complete absence of nuclear labeling that must be demonstrated for confirmation of diagnosis (an irrelevant cytoplasmic blush may be observed), as regional loss of BAF47 immunoreactivity can be displayed by other tumor types. Results must be considered noninformative if included endothelial cells, infiltrating mononuclear elements, and native CNS

immunoreactivity for 70 and 200 kDa neurofilament proteins, or designated as grade 3 should they fail to label for the latter or manifest higher mitotic indices. Transitional (i.e., focally rosetted) tumors are placed in the grade 2 category, the mixed pineocytoma–pineoblastoma qualifying as grade 3 in this schema. Select studies have demonstrated the ability of this method to stratify affected patients in a hierarchy of increasing risk for recurrence and tumor-related death,[917] but it has not yet found wide application among neuropathologists. Some would argue that neoplasms of transitional type, to which a favorable prognosis attaches, fundamentally represent variants of pineocytoma and would be reluctant to brand the tumor evidencing more than five mitoses per 10 high-power fields as anything but a pineoblastoma. As appears to be the case for otherwise conventional pineocytomas, the presence of pleomorphic tumor giant cells does not seem to be of any prognostic import when encountered in lesions of intermediate differentiation.[912]

Papillary tumor of the pineal region

Presenting, on neuroradiologic assessment, as a circumscribed and contrast-enhancing mass producing obstructive hydrocephalus (with the expected clinical manifestations), the **papillary tumor of the pineal region** is most often encountered in young or middle-aged adults, but can afflict children and adolescents.[929–931] The entity is designated for the radial arrangement of constituent cells about supporting fibrovascular cores (Fig. 28.101A), the latter commonly exhibiting collagenous hyalinization, though regions of solid growth are frequently apparent and may vastly dominate the histologic picture. Papillary formations are composed of epithelial-looking elements, often pseudostratified, with columnar profiles, relatively well-defined cell borders, pale to slightly granular eosinophilic cytoplasm in vasocentric orientation, and peripherally displaced, rounded or oval nuclei manifesting a stippled chromatin distribution. Striking nuclear enlargement and pleomorphism may be displayed by tumor cells in areas of nested and sheet-like architecture, these solid components being punctuated in some cases by perivascular pseudorosettes, as well as true rosettes and tubules, of ependymal type. Mitotic figures are often apparent, though not in large numbers (no more than 10 per as many high-power microscopic fields is the rule), and necrosis commonly found but unattended by complex microvascular proliferation. Neurosurgical specimens that contain adjoining pineal parenchyma or other native tissues typically demonstrate a well-dermarcated, 'pushing' tumor perimeter.

Ultrastructural studies[931] have shown the papillary tumor of the pineal region to have ependymocytic characteristics. The latter include the forming of tight junctions and zonulae adherentes that bind cell apices, these crowned by microvilli and punctured by rare cilia. The presence of dense-core cytoplasmic vesicles and parallel paranuclear arrays of rough endoplasmic reticulum with cisternal dilation by granular material attest, however, to neuroendocrine and secretory functions foreign to conventional ependymal cells. These hybrid features, coupled with shared antigenic[929–931] and gene expression[910] signatures, have been taken as evidence of a tumoral origin from specially modified ependymocytes that are known to colonize the developing pineal parenchyma from the neighboring subcommissural organ.[910,931]

Morphologic evidences of ependymal differentiation notwithstanding, the neoplasms under discussion depart from the great run of ependymomas in their general failure to express GFAP (limited immunoreactivity of perivascular cell bodies has been observed in fewer than 10% of recorded cases), by the finding in only exceptional examples of dot- or ring-type EMA labeling (though diffuse and focally membranous cytoplasmic expression

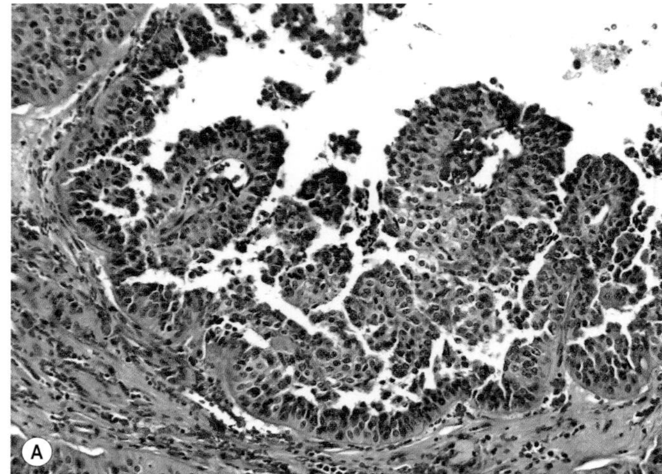

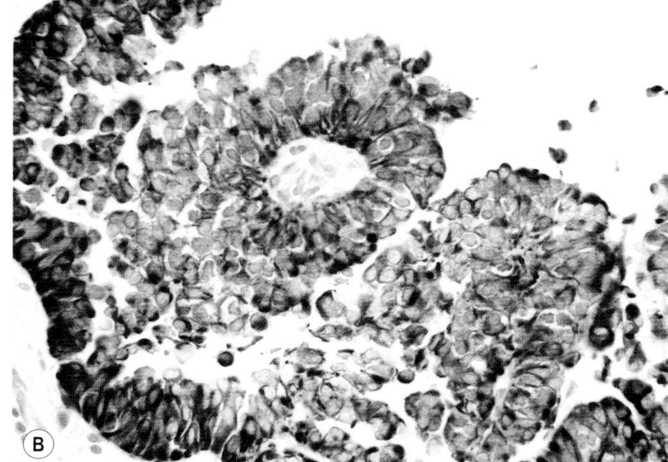

Fig. 28.101 Papillary tumor of the pineal region. Perivascular structuring (**A**) and strong immunoexpression of CK18 (**B**) typify the cellular elements of this lesion.

can be seen), and in the observation that papillary tumors of the pineal region regularly manifest reactivity for cytokeratins.[929–931] The last of these phenomena may take the form of generalized cytoplasmic immunopositivity or dot-like intracytoplasmic puncta. Most constant and often diffuse in distribution are CK18 expression (Fig. 28.101B) and labeling with the KL1 antibody (this recognizes acidic and basic keratin proteins 40–68 kDa in size), many examples exhibiting at least regional immunoreactivity with the AE1/3 and CAM 5.2 'cocktails' as well. It is the papillary component that is most likely to prove cytokeratin positive. Only a minority of communicated cases have shown focal CK5/6 or CK7 expression and CK20 negativity seems the rule. These curious neoplasms share with choroid plexus papillomas and carcinomas cytoplasmic immunolabeling, frequently widespread, for vimentin and S-100 protein (with regular nuclear expression of the latter antigen[929–931]) as well as the potential to express transthyretin,[929] but seem far more likely to exhibit MAP-2 reactivity[929,930] and far less likely to manifest Kir 7.1 or stanniocalcin-1 positivity.[930] A minority of recorded examples have evidenced synaptophysin and chromogranin A reactivity (usually focal and of weak intensity[929–931]), a small number of cases demonstrating e-cadherin and nestin expression.[929] Immunolabeling for NSE is constant, but of no discriminatory value, while all cases assessed to date have been neurofilament protein negative.[929–931]

Papillary tumors of the pineal region are prone to recurrence and can kill. A multicenter, retrospective analysis of 31 affected patients demonstrated 5-year overall and progression-free survival rates of 73% and 27%, respectively.[929] Twenty of 21 recurring tumors did so locally, one also seeding the spinal leptomeninges and a second producing such 'drop' metastases in the absence of regrowth at the primary site. Incomplete resection appears to carry a heightened risk of symptomatic relapse. The role of adjuvant therapies in the management of these lesions remains to be defined, as does a prognostically meaningful system of pathologic grading. A comparative genomic hybridization (CGH) study[930] of papillary tumors of the pineal region found a range of chromosomal imbalances comparable to those evidenced by epithelial neoplasms of the choroid plexus, including losses of 10 and 22q, as well as gains of 4, 8, 9, and 12, but their pathogenesis awaits explication.

We mention recent report of **papillary tumors of the spinal cord** that share many histologic, immunophenotypic, and ultrastructural features with the pineal region growths discussed in this section.[932] These, too, demonstrate differentiation along ependymal lines.

Meningiomas

The designation of meningioma has been extended through the years to diverse neoplasms sharing only a tendency to arise within the histogenetically complex tissues of the leptomeninges or dura mater. Thus, such dissimilar entities as the meningeal hemangiopericytoma and hemangioblastoma – currently accorded separate nosologic status among tumors of the CNS and its coverings – were once yoked under the regrettable rubric of 'angioblastic' meningioma and widely assumed to derive from a common progenitor. In a similar vein, it is recognized that most, if not all, tumors reported as melanotic or pigmented meningiomas actually represent meningeal melanocytomas. Neuropathologists now label as meningiomas only those neoplasms exhibiting morphologic or immunophenotypic evidence of an origin from meningothelial cells, specialized elements that populate the arachnoid membranes and cap the arachnoidal villi associated with intradural venous sinuses and their tributaries.

Meningiomas may make their appearance in childhood or adolescence,[981] but most are encountered in middle or later adult life.[957,966,982] Females are afflicted more commonly than males (especially at spinal levels) and some studies suggest a particularly increased prevalence in women with mammary carcinomas,[966] rare meningiomas actually harboring metastatic deposits derived from breast primaries.[1004] Coupled with their frequent expression of progesterone (and, less commonly, estrogen as well as androgen) receptors[982] and the rapid enlargement of some examples during pregnancy or the luteal phase of the menstrual cycle, these observations indicate that the growth of meningiomas is subject to hormonal influence. Noteworthy is the association of multifocal meningiomas with type 2 ('central') neurofibromatosis (NF-2),[982] the genetic locus for which resides on chromosome 22q12. Allelic loss involving this band is a frequent feature of meningiomas, including sporadic variants, as are *NF2* gene mutations (particularly common in fibroblastic and transitional variants). The presentation of a meningioma in childhood or adolescence should trigger investigation for underlying NF-2.[981] Familial examples occurring outside the setting of classic NF-2 have also been described.[982] Ionizing cranial irradiation emerges from a number of epidemiologic studies as conferring significant risk for subsequent meningioma development,[966] radiation-related lesions being more often multiple, histologically atypical, and clinically aggressive than those arising in sporadic fashion.[936,982] Less clear is the etiologic role of craniocerebral trauma,[966] but the presentation of select meningiomas in the immediate vicinity of a prior skull fracture or in close physical association with traumatically implanted foreign bodies has been convincingly documented.[938,993] Also on record are meningiomas found to lie just over glioblastomas or other gliomas.[969] Most 'collision' tumors of this sort are undoubtedly fortuitous lesions, but it is conceivable that the occasional meningioma evokes a hyperplastic glial reaction that subsequently progresses to neoplasia. As noted in our discussion of gliomesenchymal neoplasms, the term sarcoglioma has been extended to some mixed tumors postulated to have arisen in this fashion.[602] As mentioned in our prior discussion of hamartomatous lesions, tumors interpreted as meningothelial neoplasms originating in foci of meningiomatosis have been described[33] but could instead represent meningiomas with unusual patterns of perivascular growth.[40]

Most meningiomas arise within the cranial cavity, are dura-based and found in the vicinity of the superior sagittal sinus, over the cerebral convexities or in contact with the falx cerebri. Basally positioned examples favor the sphenoid ridge, olfactory grooves, tuberculum sellae, and parasellar region. Still others are anchored to the petrous ridge, presenting as cerebellopontine angle tumors when posteriorly situated. Intracranial meningiomas may also originate within the tela choroidea or stroma of the choroid plexus and rest entirely within the ventricular system. At spinal levels, meningiomas clearly favor the thoracic region, cervical examples being uncommon and lumbar lesions rare. Also recognized are epidural (intradiploic), calvarial, and intrapetrous meningiomas as well as variants located entirely outside the craniospinal confines. The latter are usually encountered in the head and neck region and include orbital (i.e., optic sheath), glabellar, sinonasal, oropharyngeal, subgaleal, juxtaparotid, and cutaneous examples.[998,999] Rarely, ectopic meningiomas are situated at even greater removes from the central neuraxis (e.g., in the mediastinum,[1002] lung,[965,992] or brachial plexus[942]). As discussed elsewhere in these volumes, the cellular aggregates originally regarded as minute pulmonary chemodectomas are actually composed of elements having the ultrastructure and immunophenotype of meningothelium.[972,973] Whether these serve as the substrate from which pulmonary meningiomas develop is unknown.

On neuroradiologic (Fig. 28.102) and gross assessment (Fig. 28.103), the typical meningioma is a solid, lobulated, or globose mass that is broadly anchored to the dura mater. Cystic variants, although uncommon, are well recognized, and the term meningioma en plaque may be invoked for the occasional lesion that presents (usually over the sphenoid ridge) as a poorly delimited, blanket-like growth. Adjoining neural tissues are generally deflected at the 'pushing' perimeters of these tumors, but grossly evident dural infiltration or invasion of nearby venous sinuses is not uncommon. Some examples insidiously permeate the neighboring skull, provoking a highly characteristic form of osteoplastic expansion and bony remodeling known as hyperostosis or, neglected, come to attention as visible masses in the scalp. None of these findings brand a meningioma as atypical or anaplastic, although involvement of the cranial floor greatly prejudices matters against the neurosurgeon and so predisposes to tumor recurrence and progression following attempted resection. Highly suspect, however, is the lesion that cannot be easily separated from the adjacent brain or spinal cord, as this implies transgression of the pia-arachnoid and invasion of the neuroparenchyma proper – traditionally regarded as prima facie evidence of aggressive biologic potential in the setting of meningothelial neoplasia. Neuroradiologic features

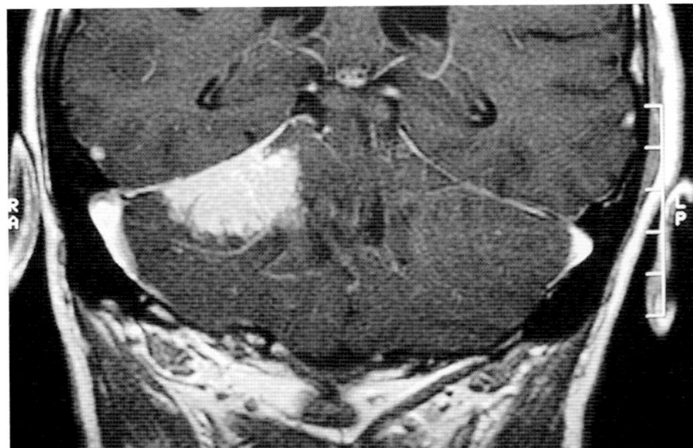

Fig. 28.102 Meningioma. Circumscription, homogeneous contrast enhancement and anchorage to the dura (in this case, the tentorium) typify the meningioma. This MRI also demonstrates thickened and abnormally enhancing dural 'tails' extending from the lesional borders – a finding suggestive, though not diagnostic, of this tumor entity.

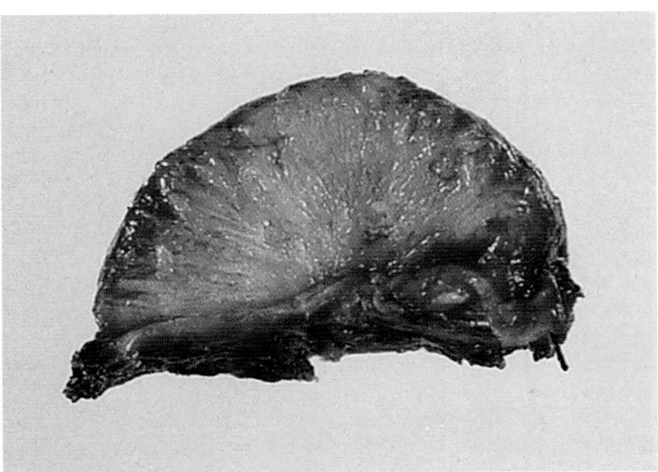

Fig. 28.103 Meningioma. The broad dural base depicted here is characteristic.

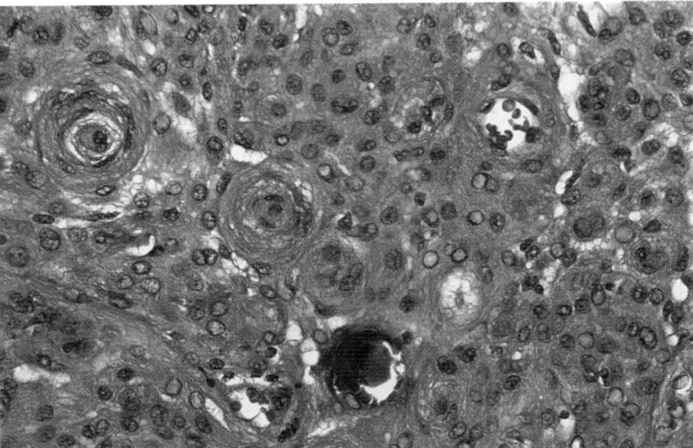

Fig. 28.104 Meningioma. Indistinct cytoplasmic boundaries, nuclear clearing ('pseudoinclusions'), cellular whorls, and a psammoma body are all apparent in this view of a meningotheliomatous (syncytial) meningioma.

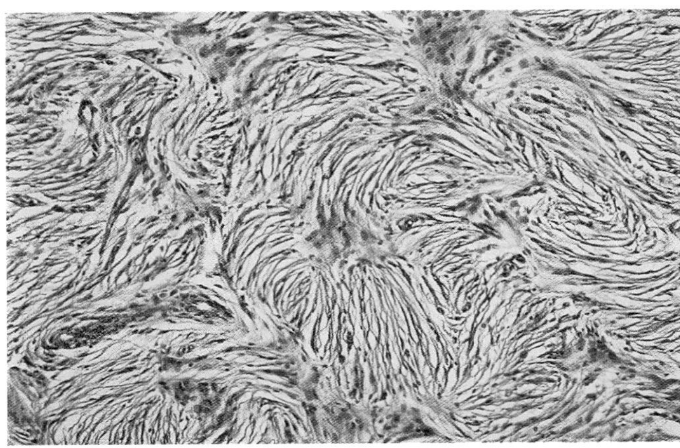

Fig. 28.105 Meningioma. Cellular spindling and a fascicular or storiform architecture are evidenced by meningiomas of 'fibroblastic' type.

that should prompt concern include indistinct tumoral margins, a 'mushrooming' growth pattern characterized by multinodular projections from the main mass, foci that fail to enhance on contrast administration (these often representing regions of necrosis), and edema of the neighboring brain on CT or MR study.[954] However, some benign meningioma subtypes (e.g., angiomatous, microcystic, and secretory variants) are recognized for their regular association with peritumoral cerebral edema.

On sectioning, most meningiomas are grayish-tan and soft, but collagenized examples have a rubbery texture and a whorled or trabeculated cut surface (resembling that of the leiomyoma), whereas variants rich in stromal mucopolysaccharides acquire a somewhat gelatinous consistency. Calcification is often readily apparent and infiltration by foamy macrophages at times results in foci of yellow discoloration, a phenomenon that may also reflect the accumulation of lipids within tumor cells. Grossly apparent regions of gray-black pigmentation characterized a unique example of meningioma colonized by hyperplastic leptomeningeal melanocytes.[975]

Meningiomas are notorious for the variety of their cytologic and histologic presentations, but most assume one of several prototypical guises.[957,982] '**Meningotheliomatous**' variants are characterized by a lobular microarchitecture and are populated by cells having delicate round or oval nuclei, inconspicuous nucleoli, lightly eosinophilic cytoplasm, and indistinct cytoplasmic borders (thus their alternative designation as syncytial meningiomas). Common to these (and other subtypes) are tumor cells concentrically wrapped in tight whorls, nuclear clearing and pale nuclear 'pseudoinclusions' consisting of invaginated cytoplasm, and the lamellated calcospherules known as psammoma bodies (Fig. 28.104). While none of these features is pathognomonic of meningioma, their demonstration in the setting of an extra-axial, dura-based mass carries considerable diagnostic weight. In contrast to the epithelioid appearances of meningotheliomatous variants, **fibrous** (or **fibroblastic**) **meningiomas** adopt a mesenchymal profile, being variably collagenized and consisting of spindly tumor cells in fascicular or storiform array (Fig. 28.105). An example containing crystalline structures rich in tyrosine has been depicted.[944] **Transitional meningiomas**, as their name implies, are hybrids, maintaining a lobular arrangement but evidencing a tendency to cellular elongation and streaming. These are often particularly rich in compact cellular whorls and endowed with psammoma bodies in conspicuous numbers. When the latter are present in profusion, the term **psammomatous meningioma** may be applied. Tumors of this type characteristically occur in middle-aged women and exhibit a particular predilection for the intraspinal compartment. It should be noted that none of the foregoing growth patterns is of any special biologic significance, most neuropathologists dispensing with these qualifying adjectives in their reporting of surgical material.

To these classic subtypes of meningioma can be added histologic variants too numerous to be accorded (and too uncommon to merit) detailed discussion or depiction here. Only the more distinctive are acknowledged. Unless otherwise stated, these depart in no way from the benign course pursued by meningiomas of more conventional appearance.

The **microcystic meningioma**[970,978] is named for its content of variably sized intercellular vacuoles, these often appearing empty but in some instances containing a lightly PAS-positive fluid derived in all likelihood via the transudation of plasma across a characteristically rich, and frequently hyalinized, stromal vasculature. Some examples actually progress to the formation of macrocysts and harbor only minor solid components. Constituent cells may exhibit cytoplasmic clearing due to glycogen or lipid accumulation and often assume spindly or stellate profiles that, along with their tendency to disaggregation, can prompt consideration of a low-grade, microcystic astrocytoma in the differential diagnosis. Nuclear pleomorphism, karyomegaly, and a smudgy hyperchromasia may be in evidence but are unattended by mitotic activity and are divorced from any sinister prognostic import, as is the common finding of severe peritumoral cerebral edema on preoperative neuroradiologic study. We mention report of a mixed testicular germ cell tumor harboring components of microcystic meningioma.[935]

The **secretory meningioma**,[987] a variant of the meningotheliomatous subtype, is distinguished by its content of 'pseudopsammoma bodies' – globular hyaline inclusions that are eosinophilic, intensely PAS positive, and diastase resistant (Fig. 28.106A). On ultrastructural study, these can be shown to lie within microvillus-lined intracellular lumina and may be immunolabeled for human secretory component, IgM, IgA, and CEA (Fig. 28.106B). Nearly always benign, the secretory meningioma may yet masquerade as a malignant neoplasm by virtue of its occasional association with elevated serum CEA levels,[967] an especially confounding phenomenon in the patient with a prior history of systemic cancer, and with subacutely progressive neurologic deficits referable to severe edema of juxtatumoral cerebral tissues.[987] The latter, generally foreign to conventional meningiomas and usually encountered as a complication of malignant meningeal neoplasms (primary or metastatic), may be associated with a curious pericytic proliferation occurring in the tumoral vascular bed.[989]

The **lymphoplasmacyte-rich meningioma** is a tumor infiltrated by chronic inflammatory elements, at times so heavily that its meningothelial (and neoplastic) nature is obscured.[939,952] There can be no doubt that at least some reported cases would be better classified as dura-based examples of inflammatory pseudotumor ('plasma cell granuloma') or sinus histiocytosis with massive lymphadenopathy (Rosai–Dorfman disease). An association with hypergammaglobulinemia has been noted.[939] Peritumoral lymphoplasmacytic infiltrates with germinal center formation are also conspicuous features of a peculiar meningeal tumor noteworthy for its **chordoid histology** and presentation in childhood or adolescence with manifestations of the **Castleman syndrome** – polyclonal dysgammaglobulinemia, iron-refractory anemia, hepatosplenomegaly, and retarded growth and sexual maturation.[958,961] Resection typically effects a remission of the systemic disorder, but this obscure

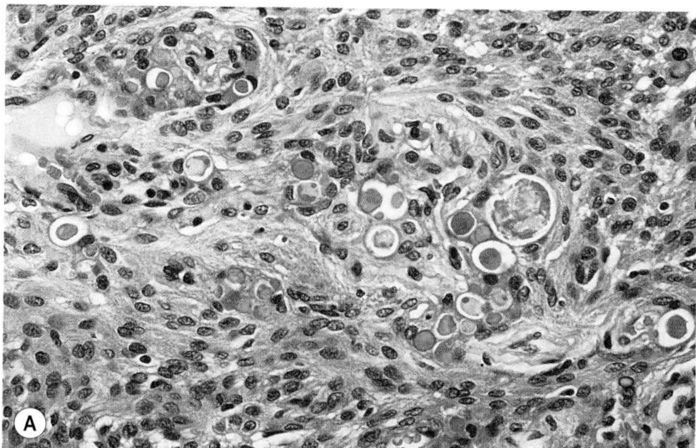

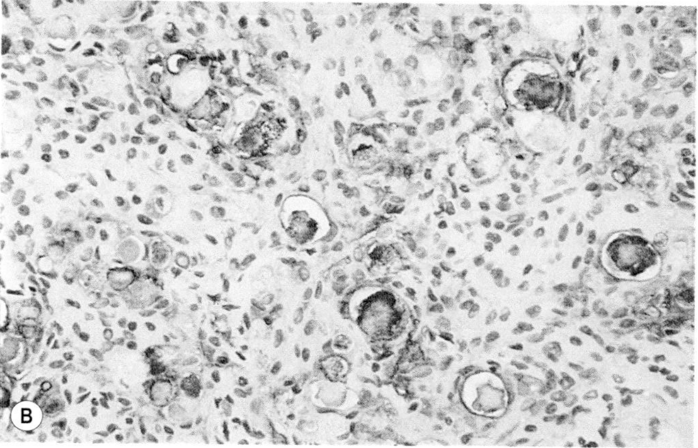

Fig. 28.106 Secretory meningioma. This variant of meningotheliomatous meningioma harbors eosinophilic globules (**A**) that label with antibodies to carcinoembryonic antigen (**B**).

neoplasm may recur and behave in locally aggressive fashion. The relationship of this lesion to adult-onset **chordoid meningiomas**,[943] which are only exceptionally accompanied by conspicuous inflammatory components or indications of Castleman syndrome,[937] and potentially masquerade as chordomas or metastatic mucinous carcinomas, is unclear. The latter, also reported as **'myxoid'** or **'mucinous' meningiomas**, proved in one analysis to be far more prone to local regrowth following subtotal resection than meningothelial tumors of conventional type.[943] We have encountered what appeared to be a primary pulmonary example.[992]

Metaplastic meningiomas can contain bone, cartilage, or adipocytic elements.[957,982] Progressive xanthomatous change, i.e., nonspecific cytoplasmic lipidization, rather than true metaplasia seems to account for so-called **lipomatous meningiomas**.[991] We would call particular attention to rare variants that may be misconstrued as sarcoma owing to potentially lipoblastic cytologic features and the occurrence in some examples of troubling nuclear abnormalities that are almost certainly degenerative in nature.[963,991] Neoplasms exhibiting meningothelial and rhabdomyosarcomatous[955] or leiomyosarcomatous[996] differentiation are also on record. Still other meningiomas evidence foci of schwannoma-like nuclear palisading; pseudoglandular structures;[959] a nesting arrangement reminiscent of paraganglioma;[957] granular cytoplasmic inclusions;[934] or a hyalinized stromal vasculature so exuberant and domineering as to suggest a malformative process or hemangioblastoma (**angiomatous meningioma**).[949] The last of these variants shares with microcystic and secretory meningiomas a generally benign clinical profile despite a tendency to cause conspicuous edema of the adjoining cerebrum. **Sclerosing meningiomas** that appear to undergo progressive fibrous obliteration are noteworthy for their frequent presentation in the pediatric group and favorable outcome despite a tendency to foci of disturbing hypercellularity, pleomorphism, and cerebrocortical infiltration.[945,953,960] Some observers have suggested that at least a subset of sclerosing childhood meningiomas are pseudoinvasive lesions arising within cortical foci of meningioangiomatoses,[33] but whether the latter entity serves as a substrate for the development of meningothelial neoplasms has been called into question.[40]

A subset of meningothelial neoplasms evidence clear cell, oncocytic or rhabdoid features. The significance of such alterations when encountered only focally is unsettled, but tumors exhibiting prominent changes of this sort merit distinct designation owing to their potential for mischief. **Clear cell meningiomas** are the most deceptive of the lot.[977,1005] These are characterized by a predilection for young subjects (including children) and are most often found in the spinal canal, cerebellopontine angle, or foramen magnum region. They are usually extra-axial and dura-based, but may be associated with cranial nerves, spinal roots, or the cauda equina. A fourth ventricular presentation has been described,[941] as has familial occurrence.[950] We have encountered a bulbar example in a 2-year-old child.[997] Composed of glycogen-rich, water-clear cells that are often disposed in patternless sheets traversed by bands of hyalinized collagen (Fig. 28.107), these unusual tumors typically manifest little or nothing in the way of classic meningothelial attributes (e.g., whorls or nuclear pseudoinclusions) and may be only focally and faintly immunoreactive for EMA, a marker of specialized arachnoidal cells expressed by most meningiomas in diffuse fashion. High recurrence rates, a potential for CSF-borne spread, and increased mortality characterize this intrinsically aggressive meningioma variant, this despite the fact that most examples do not evidence conspicuously increased mitotic activity, necrosis or other histologic features that would arouse suspicion.

That rhabdoid cytology is, in general, a marker of increased biologic potential is borne out by the discouraging behavior of most meningiomas displaying this profile, which may be evident on initial presentation or appear only in recurrent material.[983] **Rhabdoid meningiomas** in fully developed form usually retain meningotheliomatous regions but boast a prominent population of cells with vesicular nuclei, prominent nucleoli, and globose, paranuclear inclusion-like bodies representing compacted cytoplasmic vimentin filaments. These cells usually lie in lobules or sheets, but a papillary growth pattern may be encountered.[951] Conspicuously increased mitotic activity is the rule, and brain invasion common, most such tumors qualifying as atypical or frankly anaplastic by the WHO/Mayo Clinic criteria presently discussed. In one reported series, 87% of afflicted patients experienced at least one recurrence and 53% died of tumor progression.[983] The prognosis for examples evidencing rhabdoid change in the absence of elevated proliferative activity or other aggressive indicators does not appear to be as poor, but these need close watching. Similar considerations seem to apply to **oncocytic meningiomas**, i.e., meningothelial neoplasms demonstrating fine cytoplasmic granularity due to an accumulation of mitochondria.[990] High mitotic rates, necrosis, brain invasion, and recurrence have been overrepresented in the few cases recorded to date and in examples that we have encountered in consultation. A series of clinically innocent cases lacking these ominous histologic features has been communicated,[946] though the illustrated example raises questions regarding the criteria for case inclusion in the cited study.

A final variant meriting specific comment in view of its distinctive histology and clinical biology is the **papillary meningioma**, a tumor characterized by the ependymoma-like perivascular structuring of its constituent cells.[962,968] The latter can be seen to extend variably elongated cytoplasmic processes toward vessel walls, fashioning pseudorosette-like structures that disaggregate and come to float unanchored in tissue sections (Fig. 28.108). Regions exhibiting a more conventional meningothelial appearance are nearly always identifiable but usually depart from the typical in evidencing worrisome hypercellularity, mitotic activity, and, in some cases, foci of coagulative necrosis. Stubborn local recurrence, a capacity for extraneural metastasis, and often fatal outcome characterize papillary meningiomas. An excess of reported cases have presented in childhood or adolescence as compared to conventional types of meningioma.

Distinction of the meningioma from potential counterfeits occasionally requires the use of the electron microscope or immunohistochemical assay. The most constant and distinctive ultrastructural feature of meningothelial neoplasms is the complex interdigitation of tumor cell processes without intervening basal lamina material

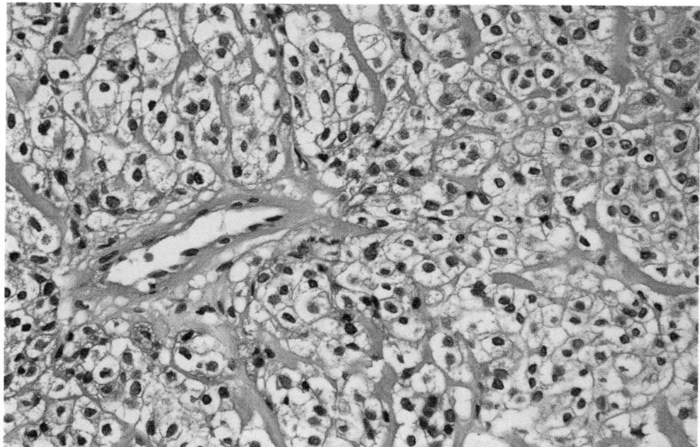

Fig. 28.107 Clear cell meningioma. The example shown here arose from the filum terminale of a 9-year-old girl. Note cytoplasmic clearing, traversing collagenous bands, and absence of meningothelial-type whorls.

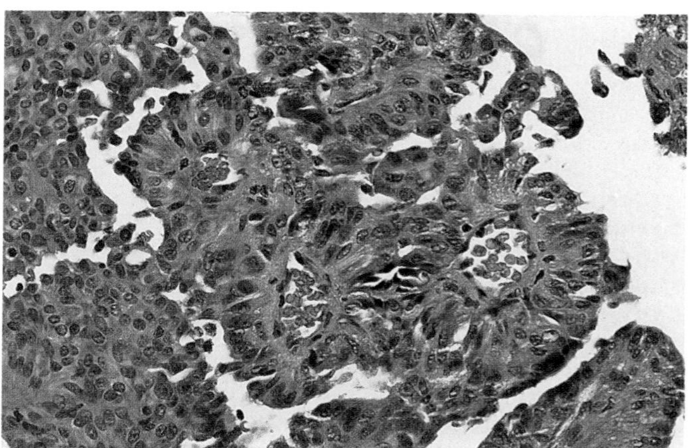

Fig. 28.108 Papillary meningioma. This intraspinal example, which elsewhere exhibited the histology of an atypical meningotheliomatous meningioma with increased mitotic activity and foci of necrosis, metastasized to lung, lymph node, and bone.

(elaborated frequently by the meningeal hemangiopericytoma and uniformly by the schwannoma), although fibroblastic variants tend to a more parallel alignment. Intercellular junctional complexes are frequent and include well-developed desmosomes, a conspicuous cytoplasmic complement of intermediate filaments rounding out the ultrastructural picture (Fig. 28.109). The latter consist of vimentin, regularly demonstrable by immunohistochemical methods regardless of tumor subtype.[982] Of particular diagnostic utility is the observation that a large majority of meningiomas exhibit (at least focally) membranous, as well as diffuse, cytoplasmic immunolabeling for EMA[982] (Fig. 28.110), a feature foreign to nerve sheath tumors other than the rare perineurioma and to most hemangiopericytomas, solitary fibrous tumors, and other fibroblastic neoplasms.[988,1003] Expression of claudin-1, though not observed as regularly as labeling for EMA, may also be of discriminatory value in distinguishing meningothelial tumors from these potential mimickers.[948,988] Unlike meningeal hemangiopericytomas, meningiomas exhibit only weak or focal labeling for CD99 and BCL2.[988] Nuclear immunoreactivity for progesterone receptors is common.[799] Reactivity for S-100 protein, if present, is usually limited to the cytoplasm of a subset of neoplastic cells but may occasionally be encountered in diffuse form (particularly in fibrous/fibroblastic meningiomas). As regards cytokeratin expression, meningiomas often share with native arachnoidal lining cells (and with epithelial cancers) immunolabeling for CK18, but are typically CK20 negative regardless of histologic pattern.[971] Focal reactivity for CK7, CK8 (CAM 5.2), CK19, and AE1/3 may be encountered (and is a consistent feature of the inclusion-bearing elements that define meningiomas of secretory type), but widespread labeling for these antigens suggests that a dura-based mass represents metastatic carcinoma.[971] One study found diffuse AE1/3 and CAM 5.2 expression by 4 of 12 high-grade/anaplastic meningiomas, but no labeling of either malignant or benign (n = 20) examples for CEA, Ber-EP4, B72.3 or CD-15 (all commonly expressed by carcinomas).[964] GFAP-labeling meningiomas of papillary,[940] rhabdoid,[951,983,995] and 'whorling–sclerosing'[947] type have been depicted but are curiosities. Whether this phenomenon actually reflects GFAP expression is open to question. In fact, one report depicting GFAP reactivity in a tumor interpreted as meningothelial[1001] seems instead to represent the first account of the neoplasm now recognized as chordoid glioma of the third ventricle. As previously noted, meningiomas rarely exercise an ability to differentiate along myogenic lines[955,996] and some otherwise conventional examples focally label for muscle-associated actins.[1000] Unlike chordomas, chordoid meningiomas do not exhibit nuclear reactivity for brachyury.[994] Rhabdoid meningioma variants do not manifest the loss of nuclear INI1 protein expression (BAF47 antibody) that is a consistent feature of atypical teratoid/rhabdoid tumors.[980]

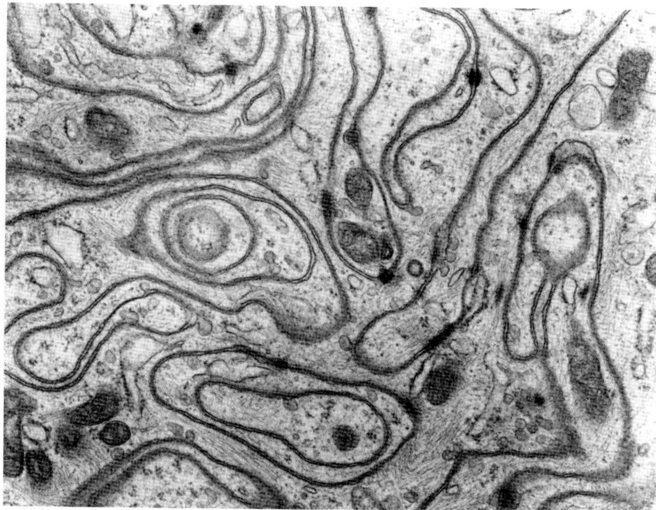

Fig. 28.109 Meningioma. Ultrastructural examination of meningiomas will often disclose complex, jigsaw puzzle-like arrays of interdigitated cytoplasmic processes laden with intermediate filaments and joined by desmosomes. As demonstrated here, neoplastic meningothelial cells are not typically coated by basement membranes (a feature of Schwann cells), nor does basal lamina material accumulate in their matrices (a characteristic of the hemangiopericytoma illustrated in Fig. 28.112). (×18 000)

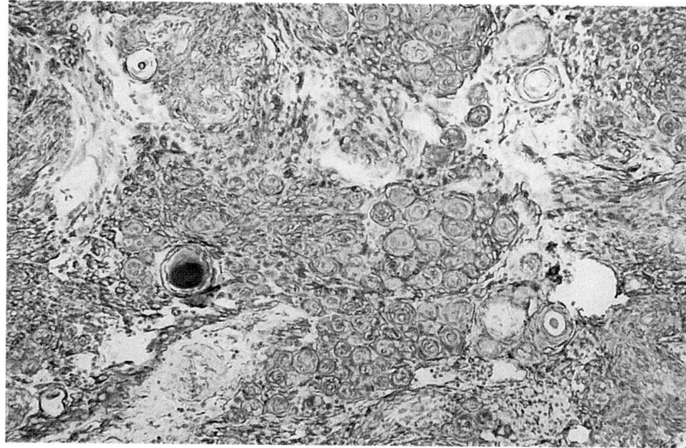

Fig. 28.110 Meningioma. Cytoplasmic labeling for epithelial membrane antigen on immunoperoxidase assay, depicted here, characterizes the overwhelming majority of meningiomas, regardless of their histologic subtype.

Meningiomas of conventional histologic type grow slowly and are amenable to surgical cure when complete excision can be effected, as is usually the case for examples arising over the cerebral convexities or along the spinal axis. Even tumors so favorably situated, however, may recur following gross total resection, the magnitude of this risk emerging only on long-term observation. In one study, for example, respective 5-, 15-, and 25-year relapse rates for histologically benign and completely excised intracranial meningiomas were 3%, 15%, and 21%.[954] By all accounts, the likelihood of regrowth is considerably higher for the less accessible olfactory groove and sphenoid wing meningiomas, en plaque examples and lesions invasive of the cranial floor proving particularly troublesome.[956] But while there can be no gainsaying the influence of tumor location on outcome in this setting, it is clear that certain morphologic features serve to independently define a subset of high-risk meningiomas to which a substantially increased likelihood of postoperative recurrence attaches. Recognizing that a number of grading strategies have proven useful in the identification of potentially aggressive meningothelial neoplasms, we can endorse with minor reservations a Mayo Clinic proposal[984,985] adopted with little modification in the 2007 WHO formulation.[982]

Application of the WHO/Mayo Clinic criteria outlined below broadly stratifies meningothelial tumors into three tiers of increasing biologic potential – **meningioma (WHO grade I)**, **atypical meningioma (WHO grade II)**, and **anaplastic meningioma (WHO grade III)**. The stated criteria are applied whether present as focal findings (often the case) or in more diffuse form. In this scheme, atypical meningiomas are defined as:

(1) containing four or more mitotic figures per 10 high-power microscopic fields (0.16 mm^2)

or

(2) exhibiting at least three of the following features:
  (a) hypercellularity
  (b) patternless, sheet-like growth
  (c) macronucleoli
  (d) small cell components with high nuclear : cytoplasmic ratio
  (e) zones of necrosis.

Anaplastic meningiomas are defined as:

(1) containing 20 or more mitoses per 10 high-power microscopic fields (0.16 mm^2)

or

(2) exhibiting a loss of differentiated features resulting in carcinoma-, melanoma-, or sarcoma-like appearances.

Readers should note that WHO grade II status is accorded clear cell and chordoid meningiomas, while papillary and rhabdoid variants are designated as WHO grade III tumors.

We would emphasize that preoperative embolization of meningiomas, undertaken to reduce their blood supplies and facilitate removal, often results in regions of necrosis with evident mitotic activity (and increased MIB-1 reactivity) in adjoining tumor tissue.[979] Potentially rendering problematic application of the foregoing criteria, this phenomenon is often, though not invariably, signaled by the presence of clearly foreign material within the tumoral vasculature. The finding of multiple zones of necrosis that appear to be at the same acute stage of development suggests such intervention but, in any case, pathologists should consult their clinical colleagues on this issue prior to releasing reports. The study cited above suggests that WHO/Mayo Clinic mitotic criteria remain valid in these circumstances, but confirmation in additional large series would be reassuring.

The reader may well wonder at our silence thus far on the issue of neuroparenchymal infiltration and tumor grading. Brain-invasive meningiomas, in fact, span the histologic spectrum, some being of otherwise typical appearance.[982,984] The demonstration of brain invasion per se adds relatively little to the predictive power of the WHO/Mayo Clinic scheme as a prognostic model once a given tumor has satisfied the listed criteria for designation as atypical or anaplastic. Meningothelial tumors of conventionally benign histologic aspect that infiltrate brain, on the other hand, appear to behave much in the manner of morphologically atypical meningiomas (see below) and so we endorse the Mayo Clinic suggestion[984] that they be so designated. This is now advocated by the WHO as well.[982]

In the experience that served as the basis for these recommendations, respective 5-year recurrence rates for conventional versus atypical meningiomas (the latter including brain-invasive but otherwise benign examples) were 12% and 41% following gross total resection.[984,985] Atypical tumors carried a 5-year mortality rate of approximately 20%. Anaplastic meningiomas, by contrast, recurred in the large majority of cases (ostensibly complete excision notwithstanding), were associated with a 68% 5-year mortality rate, and a median survival of only 18 months. Other findings that have been correlated with worrisome histology and increased biologic potential in the setting of meningothelial neoplasia include elevated MIB-1 labeling indices and, in some studies, failure to express progesterone receptors.[982] Regarding the former, meningiomas of conventional type and indolent behavior usually have MIB-1 labeling indices below 4–5% but there is overlap in the values recorded for benign, atypical, and anaplastic lesions, as well as for recurring versus nonrecurring tumors.[933,974,986] Consequently, the predictive power of this assessment in the individual case is somewhat compromised. Noteworthy is the observation that disturbing histologic features, including elevated mitotic MIB-1 indices and brain invasion, seem to be overrepresented among meningiomas occurring in the pediatric group.[981] As reviewed in the reference just cited, most studies have found these morphologic attributes to correlate with an increased risk of recurrence and fatal outcome in this patient cohort, but this has not been the experience of all. Progression-associated genetic markers, such as chromosome 1p and 14q deletions, may also be more prevalent in meningiomas of childhood and adolescence compared to adult-onset examples.[981] The reader is referred elsewhere for more comprehensive discussion of genetic alterations associated with meningioma progression.[982] At the time of this writing, these have no generally accepted role in patient management.

While application of the WHO/Mayo Clinic guidelines discussed above can be recommended as a means of stratifying affected patients into groups at increasing risk of recurrence and meningioma-related death, pathologists and attending clinicians must realize that prognostic certainty is not to be found in the proposed criteria – particularly in the mitotic thresholds that separate the typical, atypical, and anaplastic. It has long been our practice to specifically comment when confronted by any meningioma containing more than the very occasional mitosis found on careful scrutiny, close neuroradiologic surveillance being prudent in this circumstance even if a gross total excision has been effected. It also bears emphasizing that within the broad spectrum of meningiomas that qualify as merely 'atypical' by WHO/Mayo Clinic criteria are to be found examples (e.g., the tumor exhibiting 14 mitoses per 10 high-power microscopic fields, necrosis, and cerebrocortical invasion) that may not be as predictably virulent as anaplastic variants but that are capable of frankly malignant clinical behavior. The last words have not been written on these issues.

Although local regrowth is the major pattern of treatment failure, aggressive meningioma variants can spread via the CSF and, on occasion, travel to extraneural sites such as the lung, liver, bone, and lymph node.[957,982] We would point out, however, that an excess of distant metastases recorded in the literature have derived from 'angioblastic' variants that would now be classified as meningeal hemangiopericytomas. Examples of '**benign metastasizing meningioma**' have been well documented but remain curiosities.[976] As noted, venous sinus invasion is a feature of many meningiomas and is not predictive of hematogenous dissemination or germane to the designation of a given lesion as atypical or anaplastic. In a similar vein, little significance attaches to foci of pronounced nuclear pleomorphism provided that nucleolar enlargement, mitotic activity, or other atypical features are not in evidence. X-chromosome inactivation studies and *NF2* gene mutation analyses suggest that at least some sporadic cases of 'multifocal' meningioma (particularly those characterized by the presence of three or more spatially distinct tumors) actually represent clonal proliferations with dural spread.[982]

Nonmeningothelial mesenchymal tumors

Excepting the obscure process known as primary meningeal sarcomatosis and the congenital lipomatous tumors of the lumbosacral spinal canal and cranial cavity, the varied lesions surveyed in this section represent the homologs of neoplasms encountered far more frequently in the somatic soft tissues and bones than along the central neuraxis.[1006,1007] Accordingly, little attempt is made to describe or depict their histopathologic, ultrastructural, and immunophenotypic profiles, all of which are given detailed attention elsewhere in these volumes. However, we would emphasize the hazards in diagnosis occasioned by the existence of both neuroepithelial and meningothelial tumors that pretend to inclusion among the select company under discussion. Whereas CNS neoplasms exhibiting spindly or bizarre, 'monstrocellular' cytologic features were once presumed to be mesodermal in derivation if they could be shown to elaborate an intercellular reticulin network, it is now clear that candidates fulfilling this criterion must be subjected to immunohistochemical assay for evidence of cytoplasmic GFAP expression if entities such as the sarcomatoid or 'giant cell' glioblastoma, desmoplastic cerebral astrocytoma, and pleomorphic xanthoastrocytoma are to be unmasked. In addition, the possibility has always to be borne in mind, particularly in adult cases, that the biopsy ostensibly demonstrating a malignant mesenchymal tumor derives, in fact, from a gliosarcoma. Especially suspect in this regard are limited specimens evidencing the features of fibrosarcoma or malignant fibrous histiocytoma, but the gliosarcoma, as already indicated, may also contain angiosarcomatous, osteosarcomatous, chondrosarcomatous, liposarcomatous, and myosarcomatous components. Inasmuch as primitive neuroepithelial neoplasms such as the medullomyoblastoma and certain variants of pineoblastoma contain striated muscle elements, putative embryonal rhabdomyosarcomas of the CNS must be screened for telltale evidence of neural differentiation at the ultrastructural level or for the expression of synaptophysin, neurofilament proteins, GFAP, and other neuroepithelial antigens. Finally, electron microscopic study and immunocytochemical assessment for EMA and CD34 labeling may serve to distinguish the fibrosarcoma-, solitary fibrous tumor- or hemangiopericytoma-like meningioma from the genuine article. These guidelines are offered, of course, with the full realization that malignant neoplasms readily forego such luxury functions as the display of marker antigens convenient to the surgical pathologist.

Lipoma and liposarcoma

Intradural tumors composed of mature adipose tissue may be encountered anywhere along the neuraxis but are most common at spinal levels, where they can be divided into a congenital, maldevelopmental group situated principally in the lumbosacral region and a smaller, arguably neoplastic subset tending to a thoracic location. The former have already been discussed as manifestations of spinal dysraphism. Commonly occurring in complex with spina bifida and its cutaneous stigmata, **'lipomas'** of this type figure prominently among intraspinal anomalies complicated by fixation of the filum terminale, caudal displacement of the conus medullaris, and the traction-induced myelopathy known as the 'tethered cord' syndrome. These malformative lesions not infrequently contain heterotopic components such as smooth and striated muscle (**'myolipoma'**),[1012] aberrant peripheral nerve fibers, meningothelial derivatives (**'occult' lipomeningocele**), ependyma, and other neuroglial elements (**'occult' lipomeningomyelocele**).[1028] We have encountered an example that harbored mesonephroid tubules and glomeruloid structures lined by an orderly cuboidal epithelium, reference having been made to such 'nephrogenic rests' in the discussion of lipomeningomyeloceles complicating spinal dysraphism. Although entrapment of the cauda equina and permeation of the conus usually preclude thorough resection of these intraspinal masses, dramatic neurologic improvement can often be effected by debulking, division of the tethered filum, and dural reconstruction.

In contrast to the congenital lipomatous tumors of the lumbosacral canal, lipomas occurring at higher levels of the spinal axis are typically unassociated with regional anomalies of the vertebrae or intraspinal contents and usually consist of mature fat alone. Only rarely are these entirely intramedullary,[1020] one report describing a thoracic example with admixed smooth muscle (**leiomyolipoma**).[1009] Much more common are **leptomyelolipomas**,[1019] which present as subpial masses plastered over a highly variable length of the spinal cord, incorporating nerve roots and blending into the neuroparenchyma proper. These features frustrate attempts at complete excision, but, again, long-term symptomatic relief is often achieved by simple debulking. Uncommon examples contain conspicuous vascular elements and are dubbed **angiolipomas** or **angiomyolipomas**, but such lesions are more often epidural in location.[1024] An extradural location also characterized an intraspinal example of **osteolipoma** arising in the cervical region.[1021] Symptomatic accumulation of adipose tissue in this compartment is also a recognized, albeit rare, complication of natural obesity and of corticosteroid administration. Known as **spinal epidural lipomatosis**,[1018] this may consist of brown fat (**'hibernoma'**).[1022] **Intradural hibernoma** has also been described.[1014]

Intracranial lipomas are usefully segregated into a midline group and laterally situated variants, most of which involve the eighth cranial nerve. The former exhibit a decided predilection for the region of the corpus callosum but may also settle along the tuber cinereum, above the quadrigeminal plate, in the ambient cisterns, and in the third ventricle.[1013] Most are incidentally discovered at autopsy, but epileptogenic callosal examples are well recognized, tuberal variants may eventuate in hypothalamic dysfunction, and lesions impinging on the third ventricle or aqueduct of Sylvius may be complicated by progressive hydrocephalus. Sleep apnea has exceptionally been recorded in association with lipomas involving the mesencephalic tectum and rostral pons.[1025] In any of these locations, the midline lipoma is clearly maldevelopmental, being frequently associated with structural anomalies of neighboring neural tissues (e.g., agenesis of the corpus callosum) and occasionally occurring in complex with cranial defects or congenital intracranial cysts of colloid or epidermoid type. The added presence, in some instances, of cartilage, bone, smooth or striated muscle, heterotopic peripheral nerves, ganglion cells, neuroglia, and choroid plexus further attests to their malformative basis, although some observers have speculated that these more complex lesions may represent teratomas or teratoid neoplasms.[1027] As in the spinal compartment, exceptional variants merit designation as **angiolipomas**[1023] or **osteolipomas**.[1011] The latter preferentially involve the suprasellar/interpeduncular regions and tuber cinereum. A peculiar tentorial tumor having chondromatous, osseous, and lipomatous components (**'osteochondrolipoma'**) has been reported.[1008]

Intracranial lipomas situated off the midline tend to present in the cerebellopontine angle or internal auditory canal and are usually mistaken for acoustic schwannomas on clinical evaluation.[1010,1015,1029] The eighth cranial nerve is typically permeated in diffuse fashion, its fibers divided into small fascicles embedded in mature adipose tissue, and other cranial nerves may be engulfed in like manner by large lesions lying adjacent to the brainstem. These may contain dysmorphic vascular elements as well as smooth muscle bundles and striated muscle fibers, suggesting a maldevelopmental etiology (**'lipochoristoma'**). On rare occasions, intracranial lipomas settle in the region of the sylvian fissure, encasing middle cerebral artery branches and infiltrating temporal cortex.[1017] As attempts at en bloc resection may result in severe neurologic injury, it has been suggested that these and cerebellopontine angle examples be subjected to the minimum debulking required to relieve local mass effects. The intrinsically high signal characteristic of fat on T1-weighted MR study may facilitate the accurate preoperative identification of neuraxial masses as lipomas.

Liposarcomas are among the least common of all malignant mesenchymal tumors reported to involve the CNS or its coverings. Only isolated meningeal examples are on record.[1006,1016,1026] The reader is reminded that cells resembling lipoblasts or adipocytes may be encountered in hemangioblastomas as well as 'lipidized' neoplasms of meningothelial and neuroepithelial lineage.

Osseous and cartilaginous tumors

Osseous plaques adherent to the falx cerebri and undersurface of the dura in the region of the superior sagittal sinus are common incidental findings at autopsy and are generally asymptomatic. Although termed **osteomas**, these almost certainly represent reactive, metaplastic lesions and may occur with increased frequency in the setting of chronic renal failure.[1036] In a similar vein, the spinal arachnoid frequently undergoes patchy ossification but only rarely is this process so extensive as to produce myelopathy.[1037] Examples of bona fide **osteogenic sarcoma** arising from the meninges or brain have been depicted, but are most uncommon.[1033,1035,1041,1043] We have previously mentioned a case of cerebellar osteogenic sarcoma arising in association with an epidermoid cyst.

Bosselated masses of mature hyaline cartilage known as **chondromas** (or **osteochondromas** when they contain bony elements) may bulge into the cranial cavity from its floor or, much less commonly, may arise from the dura.[1034,1039] Examples complicating the generalized skeletal chondromatoses designated as **Maffucci syndrome**[1031] and **Ollier disease**[1044] have also been depicted. **Intracranial chondrosarcomas** of conventional type usually originate in the skull base, but meningeal and neuroparenchymal primaries are recognized,[1032] reports including isolated cases following cranial irradiation[1030] and evolving from chondromas.[1038] Curiously, the **mesenchymal chondrosarcoma** seems to have a special predilection for the dura among extraosseous sites.[1040] Examples arising in the leptomeninges and brain[1045] are also on record. Rarest of all cartilaginous intracranial neoplasms is the **extraskeletal myxoid chondrosarcoma**.[1042]

Fibroblastic, myofibroblastic, and 'fibrohistiocytic' tumors

Solitary fibrous tumors (SFTs) in all respects identical to those originating in the pleura and extrapleural somatic tissues constitute in our experience the most common neuraxial neoplasms composed of fibroblasts or related cell types.[1048,1068] Usually dura-based (and so taken for meningiomas on preoperative assessment), these may also arise within the lateral ventricles or the substance of the spinal cord.[1046,1068] A localization to spinal nerve root has been described,[1063] as has a postradiation example.[1067] Most such tumors are benign in appearance and clinical evolution, gross total resection usually proving curative; only exceptional cases evidencing aggressive morphologic features (e.g., conspicuous mitotic activity) or behavior (local invasion of brain or distant metastasis following repeated local recurrence) are on record.[1049,1058,1059,1068] Neuraxial SFTs share with their systemic counterparts a characteristic immunophenotype,[1048,1068] including strong and diffuse cytoplasmic labeling for CD34, frequently intense BCL2 reactivity, and failure to express S-100 protein or EMA, that facilitates their distinction from schwannomas (S-100 protein positive) and fibrous meningiomas (usually both S-100 protein and EMA reactive). More problematic in differential diagnostic terms is the meningeal hemangiopericytoma, discussed further below. CD34 expression in the latter setting is generally weaker and less widespread, but there is potential immunophenotypic overlap[1068] and these may well represent allied entities.

Benign neuraxial neoplasms of fibroblastic or myofibroblastic type reported under designations other than SFT are exceedingly rare; whether at least some such cases represent examples of the latter is arguable. The literature thus contains accounts of CNS **'fibroma'**[1062,1064] (sometimes referred to as fibromyxoma owing to mucoid stromal alterations) and **'sclerosing fibrous tumor'**[1053] as well as **angiofibroma**[1054] and **myofibroblastoma**.[1066] **Dural fibromatosis**[1057] has also been described, in some cases as a complication of neurosurgery, as has the intracranial presentation of **childhood cranial fasciitis**.[1061] Fibroblasts additionally participate in the formation of so-called intracranial **'fibroxanthomas'**, but these, often dominated by foam cells, may be reactive in nature and are considered under the rubric of xanthomatous lesions.

Fibrosarcomas of the CNS are commonly attached to the dura or leptomeninges, but some examples are situated entirely within the substance of the cerebrum or cerebellum.[1006,1051,1056] Radiation is clearly recognized as predisposing,[1051,1060] especially to sellar fibrosarcoma in patients so treated for pituitary adenomas, but spontaneous development of this tumor in the confines of the sella turcica has been described.[1055] Symptomatic local recurrence is the rule even after gross total resection of circumscribed, superficially positioned lesions, and patients with high-grade lesions usually succumb to their disease within several years of diagnosis, some developing leptomeningeal and distant, extracranial metastases. Low-grade variants seem more amenable to surgical control.[1006] Similar considerations apply to the intracranial **malignant fibrous histiocytoma** (a dubious entity from the histogenetic perspective).[1006,1052] An intracerebral **angiomatoid fibrous histiocytoma** with a t(12;22)(q13;q12) translocation resulting in a clear cell sarcoma-like type 1 *EWS/ATF-1* gene fusion has been documented.[1050] The spectrum of malignant fibroblastic tumors encountered along the neuraxis includes **low-grade fibromyxoid sarcoma** histologically similar to its soft tissue counterpart[1065] and **sclerosing epithelioid fibrosarcoma**.[1047] The latter may assume a deceptively benign, hypocellular, and amitotic appearance, but seems prone to local recurrence and distant metastasis.

As previously mentioned in our discussion of these entities, the non-neoplastic lesions that can justifiably be regarded as 'inflammatory pseudotumors' or 'plasma cell granulomas' must be distinguished from bona fide examples of **inflammatory myofibroblastic tumor** involving the CNS.[262] The last of these is a neoplasm, often meningioma-like on neuroradiologic study, that departs from the inflammatory pseudotumor group by virtue of its lack of association with underlying systemic infection or immunologic dysfunction, conspicuous content of spindle cells with cytologic atypism, frequent immunoexpression of ALK, and *ALK* gene (2p23) rearrangements. Gross total resection has been associated with a favorable course in most CNS cases communicated to date.[262]

To our opening caveats regarding neuroglial tumors that may masquerade as neoplasms of fibroblastic or fibrohistiocytic lineage, we would add the warning that astrocytic lesions routinely exhibit immunolabeling with antisera to vimentin and may also be positive on assay for α_1-antitrypsin and α_1-antichymotrypsin. No differential diagnostic significance should be attached to these findings.

Endothelial tumors

The overwhelming majority of vasoformative tumors involving the CNS are maldevelopmental anomalies (previously considered in our discussion of vascular malformations). Endothelial neoplasms of the neuraxis include **hemangiomas** (potentially multifocal and typically of capillary type with lobular growth features),[1070,1074,1077–1080] **hemangioendotheliomas** of spindled, epithelioid, and polymorphous types (the first arguably benign and the latter two best regarded as low to intermediate malignant potential lesions),[1071,1081] and aggressive **angiosarcomas** of conventional type.[1076,1084] Also on record is a unique cerebral neoplasm exhibiting hybrid components of 'angiogenic' leiomyosarcoma and epithelioid angiosarcoma,[1075] and CNS involvement by AIDS-associated **Kaposi sarcoma** has been documented.[1072] We have not encountered an example of cutaneous or visceral angiosarcoma presenting as a neuraxial mass, but metastatic atrial myxoma may masquerade as intracranial epithelioid hemangioendothelioma.[1082]

The designation of hemangioendothelioma has been extended to certain benign vasogenic meningocerebral lesions that structurally resemble the cellular ('juvenile') capillary hemangiomas encountered as cutaneous 'nevi' in infancy.[1070,1077] We have also had the opportunity to study an epileptogenic frontal lobe mass, associated with a history of antecedent cranial trauma, which exhibited the features of lobular capillary hemangioma (or so-called pyogenic granuloma) and are familiar with a case in which morphologically similar, but multifocal cerebral hemispheric lesions regressed after corticosteroid administration.[1069] Multifocal involvement of the spinal cord and cauda equina by lesions having capillary hemangiomatous features has also been described.[1073,1078] Finally, the spectrum of primary endothelial proliferations potentially involving the nervous system includes the process known as **intravascular papillary endothelial hyperplasia** or **Masson vegetant intravascular hemangioendothelioma**.[1083] Intracranial variants, which may evolve from preexisting vascular malformations or develop within dural venous sinuses, can achieve enormous proportions, may regrow if subtotally excised, and have occasionally proved fatal as a result of associated mass effects.

Meningeal hemangiopericytoma

Although their cytogenesis remains a contentious issue, select dura-based tumors long regarded as 'angioblastic' variants of meningioma are immunophenotypically, as well as morphologically, indistinguishable from hemangiopericytomas arising in the somatic soft tissues[1085–1087] (Fig. 28.111). **Meningeal hemangiopericytomas** are largely tumors of adulthood that do not exhibit the distinct predilection for women characteristic of meningiomas and that strongly favor the intracranial compartment. Their distinction from meningiomas evidencing potentially misleading pericytomatous growth patterns is usually straightforward as the latter often contain psammomatous calcospherites and tumor cells concentrically arrayed in tight whorl formations – both foreign to the hemangiopericytoma, as are the intranuclear pseudoinclusions typical of meningothelial elements and their neoplastic derivatives. Also alien to the meningioma, but a feature of many hemangiopericytomas, is a network of 'reticulin' investing individual tumor cells. This appears to represent basal lamina material at the ultrastructural level[1086,1087] (Fig. 28.112). The hemangiopericytoma further departs from the meningioma on electron microscopic study in that the cytoplasmic processes elaborated by its constituent cells, although joined by rudimentary junctions, are neither bound by well-developed desmosomes nor intertwined in complex fashion. Serving also to segregate these lesions from neoplasms of meningothelial lineage is an immunophenotype that often includes widespread and strong labeling for CD99 and BCL2 but only focal, if any, EMA or claudin-1 expression.[948,980,1003,1087,1088] Also generally foreign to hemangiopericytomas are the 1p, 14q, NF2, and 4.1B genetic deletions that may be exhibited by meningiomas.[988] Mesenchymal chondrosarcomas of dural origin routinely harbor anaplastic small cell elements in pericytomatous architectural array and thus enter the differential diagnosis, but the meningeal hemangiopericytoma lacks chondroid components. As mentioned above, meningeal hemangiopericytomas may evidence labeling for CD34 but this is usually weak and patchy as opposed to the diffuse and strong cytoplasmic reactivity typical of solitary fibrous tumors.[1068,1088] Again, these may be close kin.

Regrowth at the primary site despite seemingly complete initial resection is commonly seen in the setting of meningeal hemangiopericytoma, although this may take years to become clinically apparent. Even with the addition of postoperative radiotherapy, many afflicted patients die as a direct result of intracranial tumor progression (often after a protracted course characterized by repeated local recurrence) or extracranial metastasis (typically a late complication that develops in at least 20–25% of cases).[1085–1087] Most often seeded are the lungs, bones, and liver, but retroperitoneal organs, such as kidney and pancreas, may also be involved.[1087] While all hemangiopericytomas must be regarded as having the potential to recur locally and disseminate, histologic features may be of some efficacy in identifying the most predictably aggressive variants. Recommendations emerging from a large Armed Forces Institute of Pathology (AFIP) study[1087] are the basis for a two-tiered classification distinguishing '**anaplastic hemangiopericytomas**'

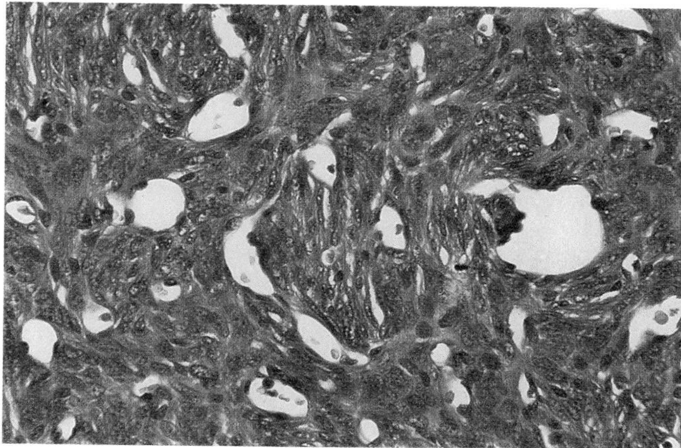

Fig. 28.111 Meningeal hemangiopericytoma. Long regarded as a form of 'angioblastic' meningioma, this lesion is now widely accepted as the homolog of its extraneural soft tissue counterpart.

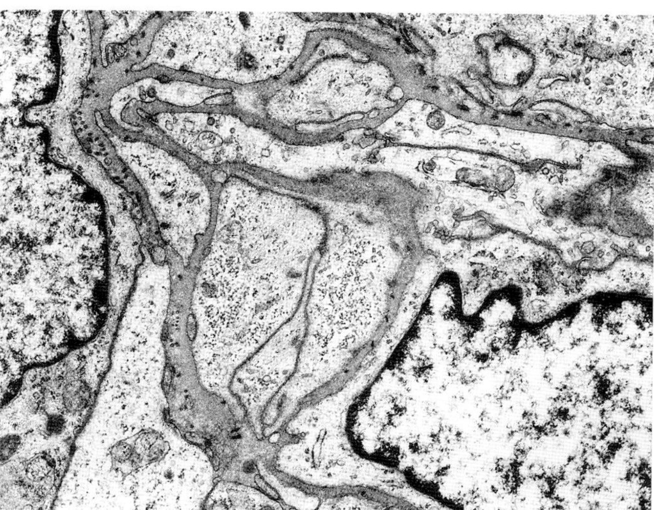

Fig. 28.112 Meningeal hemangiopericytoma. Unlike the cytoplasmic processes of meningothelial tumor cells (compare Fig. 28.109), those of the hemangiopericytoma's constituent neoplastic elements are separated by basal lamina material demonstrable on ultrastructural examination. (×11 360)

(WHO grade III) from hemangiopericytomas without other specification.[1086] The latter are accorded WHO grade II status.[1086] In this scheme, anaplastic lesions are defined as exhibiting necrosis and/or mitotic activity exceeding five per 10 high-power (400×) microscopic fields, plus at least two of the following histologic characteristics: hemorrhage, moderate to high cell density, and moderate to marked nuclear atypia. In the AFIP series, median overall survival was significantly shorter for patients with anaplastic tumors (62 months) compared to those with lower grade lesions (144 months).[1087] A more recent Mayo Clinic analysis using these criteria could not reproduce this finding but noted a significant difference in disease-free survival intervals, anaplastic hemangiopericytomas recurring on average 6.7 years earlier than their nonanaplastic counterparts.[1085] This study also suggested that the outlook for afflicted patients treated since 1990 has improved owing to reduced operative mortality and advances in the radiosurgical management of recurrent disease and the general care of those with cancer.

Myogenous tumors

Embryonal rhabdomyosarcomas account for most primary myogenous neoplasms of the CNS reported to date.[1089,1090,1093] These tend to segregate into a posterior fossa subset, characterized by a presentation in childhood and a predilection for the cerebellum, and a supratentorial group of adult onset typified by a cerebral hemispheric localization. Rare cases of **pleomorphic** and **alveolar rhabdomyosarcoma** have been documented to arise in the cerebrum as well.[1006] The midline, vermal position of many intracranial rhabdomyosarcomas arising in the pediatric population and the recognized capacity of the cerebellar medulloblastoma to differentiate along skeletal muscle lines ('medullomyoblastoma') have prompted speculation that both tumor types might originate from a common, primordial progenitor in the rhombic roof. Whatever their histogenesis, primary rhabdomyosarcomas of the CNS are high-grade neoplasms; few patients remain alive 2 years after diagnosis despite aggressive irradiation and chemotherapy. Neuraxis dissemination and extracranial metastasis may complicate local tumor progression. Mention should be made of a diffuse leptomeningeal variant unassociated with a demonstrable neuroparenchymal component,[1101] but this diagnosis requires rigorous exclusion of an occult primary focus in the orbit, paranasal sinuses, nasopharynx, or middle ear since rhabdomyosarcomas originating in these parameningeal regions frequently seed the subarachnoid space. The cited example is of note for its occurrence in a child with the neurocristopathy known as hypomelanosis of Ito. Non-neoplastic, cranial nerve-associated proliferations of skeletal and, in some instances, smooth muscle have been variously designated as **rhabdomyomas**, **neuromuscular hamartomas/choristomas**, and **benign ectomesenchymomas/Triton tumors**. These have been previously treated in our discussion of hamartomas and choristomas. **Malignant ectomesenchymoma**, a neoplasm having rhabdomyosarcomatous elements with admixed ganglion cell components, has also been described as originating in the CNS.[1007]

Sporadic instances of **leiomyoma**[1098] or **leiomyosarcoma**[1006,1091] originating from the meninges or within the neuroparenchyma have been depicted, these exceedingly rare neoplasms including such oddities as **diffuse leptomeningeal leiomyomatosis**,[1094] **angioleiomyoma**,[1092] **pleomorphic angioleiomyoma**,[1096] and the **composite leiomyosarcoma–epithelioid angiosarcoma**[1075] to which we have previously referred. Intracranial neoplasms interpreted as **myopericytomas** have also been communicated.[1097,1100] At special risk of developing neuraxial (as well as systemically situated) smooth muscle tumors are the immunocompromised, particularly patients with AIDS.[1095,1099,1102] Such tumors are usually associated with the dura or situated in juxtaneuraxial sites such as the parasellar region or cavernous sinus, but may involve the brain.[1099] They range in appearance from highly differentiated leiomyomas to frank leiomyosarcomas and, in our experience, include epithelioid variants of small, clear cell cytologic type that may be difficult to recognize as being of smooth muscle character. As is the case for their systemic counterparts arising in a background of immunosuppression, neuraxial variants consistently harbor Epstein–Barr virus (EBV) as evidenced by nuclear labeling for EBV-associated nuclear antigen 2 (EBNA-2) and EBV-encoded RNA-1 (EBER-1) on immunohistochemical and in situ hybridization assessment, respectively. EBV-associated myopericytomas have rarely been reported to complicate AIDS.[1097]

Other mesenchymal tumors

In addition to the various mesenchymal neoplasms of the CNS exhibiting specific diagnostic features, there is a disparate collection of anaplastic tumors to which only descriptive appellations such as high-grade 'spindle cell', 'pleomorphic', or 'undifferentiated' sarcoma can be given.[1006] Reported under the rubric of **primary leptomeningeal sarcomatosis** are poorly characterized variants typified by diffuse tumoral proliferation restricted to the subarachnoid space and unaccompanied by dominant foci of bulky disease.[1104] These may present with signs and symptoms of polyradiculopathy, spinal cord compression or intracranial mass effect, and are often misdiagnosed initially as chronic meningitides of infectious etiology or as manifestations of neurosarcoidosis or other inflammatory disorders. The differential diagnosis includes leptomeningeal carcinomatosis, gliomatosis, lymphomatosis, melanomatosis, and medulloblastomatosis. Neoplasms that seem to represent the intracranial equivalents of soft tissue and skeletal **myxomas** have been described,[1110] but myxoid meningioma and metastatic atrial myxoma must be excluded before this diagnosis can be accepted. Also to be found are reports of a dural **epithelioid sarcoma**,[1108] a **synovial sarcoma** originating in a spinal nerve root,[1105] a peculiar **angiomyxofibromatous tumor** of the falx[1109] and the bizarre phenomenon of **phosphaturic mesenchymal tumor** (a lesion recognized for its association with paraneoplastic osteomalacia secondary to tumor-induced renal phosphate wasting) masquerading as meningioma[1106] or spinal nerve sheath tumor.[1103] Last, we mention a primary intracranial example of **aneurysmal bone cyst** (with confirmatory 17p13 rearrangement involving the ubiquitin-specific protease 6 (USP6) locus) that presented as a cerebellopontine angle growth.[1107] The **Ewing sarcoma/peripheral primitive neuroectodermal tumor** group has been previously addressed in our discussion of embryonal neoplasms.

Nerve sheath tumors of the craniospinal axis

Inasmuch as nerve sheath tumors arising within the cranial cavity and spinal canal are the morphologic and biologic homologs of their more common, peripherally situated counterparts, the reader is referred to Chapter 25 of this text for a detailed treatment of their diagnostic, structural, and immunophenotypic features.

Schwannomas are the most frequent variant to abut the central neuraxis, usually presenting in adulthood as tumors of the cerebellopontine angle or lumbosacral spinal extramedullary space.[1145] Nearly all cerebellopontine angle tumors originate in the vestibular branch of cranial nerve VIII (acoustic schwannoma or neuroma) and produce hearing loss. Schwannomas arising at spinal levels exhibit a similar predilection for sensory divisions of the neuraxis, typically involving the posterior roots. These often assume a 'dumbbell' configuration as they squeeze through adjacent intervertebral foramina and expand into the paravertebral soft tissues. Schwannomas may involve cranial nerves other than the acoustic and lie within the central neuroparenchyma proper.[1118,1133,1137] Intraventricular[1153] and dura-based[1113] cases have been depicted as well. Bilateral eighth nerve examples are a defining feature of **neurofibromatosis type 2 (NF-2)**, an autosomal dominant disorder linked to inherited or newly acquired mutations involving a gene localized to chromosome 22q12.[1149] Affected kindreds are prone to an assortment of neoplasms, all typified in this setting by multifocality, that includes craniospinal schwannomas, meningiomas, and intramedullary ependymomas. Inactivating mutations of the *NF2* gene on chromosome 22 also characterize most acoustic schwannomas occurring in sporadic fashion.[1145] Multifocal, nonacoustic schwannomas divorced from other manifestations of NF-2 constitute a syndrome known as **schwannomatosis**.[1145]

The schwannoma's characteristic Antoni A and B structure, nuclear palisading (Verocay bodies), infiltration by foamy macrophages, and vascular hyalinization usually suffice for its recognition, NF-2-associated variants often evidencing a multilobulated growth pattern on gross and microscopic assessment.[1148] Rosenthal fibers and eosinophilic granular bodies may rarely be encountered in acoustic examples,[1115] possibly reflecting chronic stimulation of astrocytes native to the central portion of cranial nerve VIII.[1131] Meningiomas on occasion exhibit schwannoma-like features and are the most frequent counterfeit. These two tumor types may collide in patients with NF-2, 'composite' lesions of this kind only rarely occurring outside the latter clinical setting.[1138] Immunocytochemical techniques and electron microscopic study may both be usefully applied to distinguishing schwannian from meningothelial neoplasms and to the elimination of solitary fibrous tumor from the differential. Schwannomas are characterized by diffuse cytoplasmic S-100 protein expression and pericellular immunolabeling for laminin and type IV collagen,[1145] the latter (and a corresponding reticulin network) reflecting investment of their elongated cellular processes by a continuous basal lamina foreign to the typical meningioma. They may also evidence regional GFAP expression.[1139,1145] Cytoplasmic expression of EMA – a regular feature of meningothelial tumors – is usually absent from the schwannoma or restricted to normal perineurial cells incorporated into the latter's capsule and thus limited to its periphery.[1142] Admittedly, however, some observers have described EMA-reactive neoplastic elements in the substance of occasional schwannomas,[1003] these possibly manifesting differentiation along perineurial cell lines and exhibiting diffuse cytoplasmic labeling without the cell membrane accentuation characteristic of meningothelial tumors. It is worth remembering that meningiomas only rarely present in the lumbosacral regions favored by schwannomas of the spinal roots. Solitary fibrous tumors are typically nonreactive for S-100 protein, instead labeling for CD34, and their constituent fibroblastic cells do not elaborate basal lamina material.[1049] Nuclear and cytoplasmic expression of calretinin has been described as a trait segregating schwannomas from neurofibromas.[1124]

A variant of schwannoma recognized for its elaboration of melanosomal melanin exhibits a decided predilection for the spinal nerve roots.[1132,1151] An intramedullary presentation has also been recorded.[1111] Most of the **melanotic schwannomas** reported to date were stated to evolve in benign fashion, though recorded follow-up intervals for many of these cases were limited. The risk of local recurrence following incomplete resection is actually substantial,[1132] and spinal examples manifesting an aggressive course characterized by visceral and cerebral metastases have been documented.[1121,1151] A subset of melanotic schwannomas containing psammomatous concretions constitutes part of the heritable **Carney complex**,[1116] which includes cardiac, cutaneous, and mammary myxomas; spotty pigmentation; large cell calcifying Sertoli cell tumors of the testis; and evidence of endocrine hyperfunction (principally Cushing syndrome and acromegaly, the former associated with primary pigmented nodular adrenocortical disease).

A small minority of intracranial and intraspinal schwannomas are of the 'cellular' type.[1119,1122,1146] In contrast to its histologically conventional counterpart, the **cellular schwannoma** is a densely populated spindle cell tumor, typically devoid of Antoni B areas and Verocay bodies, that may contain foci of mitotic activity and is likely to be misconstrued as a sarcoma. The lesion shares with the classic schwannoma foci of vascular hyalinization, infiltration by lymphocytes and foamy macrophages, diffuse S-100 protein immunoreactivity, and highly differentiated Schwann cell features at the ultrastructural level. Such tumors may be more prone than conventional variants to recur locally following excision, but a metastasizing example has never been described. Finally, **granular cell tumors of schwannian lineage** have been noted to involve the trigeminal nerve[1117] and spinal nerve roots.[1126]

Most craniospinal **neurofibromas** represent manifestations of neurofibromatosis type 1 (NF-1; 'peripheral' or classic Recklinghausen disease), transmitted in autosomal dominant fashion by a locus on chromosome 17q11.2.[1152] This complex disorder includes, in addition to multifocal cutaneous and more deeply situated plexiform neurofibromas, dermatologic abnormalities (café-au-lait spots and axillary freckling), pigmented hamartomas of the iris (Lisch nodules), various skeletal defects, and glial neoplasms, chief among which are pilocytic astrocytomas of the anterior optic pathways. Spinal neurofibromas arising in this setting typically do so at multiple levels. Only rarely are cranial nerves involved. Curious lesions interpreted as plexiform neurofibromas of the cauda equina have been reported in patients without evidence of NF-1.[1140]

Well documented, but exceedingly uncommon, are **malignant nerve sheath tumors** originating in cranial or spinal nerve roots.[1144] These may develop de novo or from underlying schwannomas or neurofibromas, can arise spontaneously or complicate neurofibromatosis (particularly NF-1), and occasionally follow local irradiation (including radiosurgery).[1114,1120,1144] Intracerebral[1144,1147,1150] and intraventricular[1129] presentations have been described. Recorded examples include so-called **Triton tumors** (i.e., variants exhibiting rhabdomyoblastic differentiation).[1120,1127,1144] A most remarkable instance of intraspinal schwannoma spawning rhabdomyosarcomatous, primitive neuroectodermal, and epithelial elements has also been reported.[1135] Malignant paraspinal nerve sheath tumors that may invade the canal and threaten the spinal cord often originate in neurofibromas, particularly those of plexiform type, and so are strongly associated with NF-1.[1123]

Oddities that round out this brief survey include **neurothekeomas** of the craniospinal neuraxis,[1130,1141] **soft tissue-type perineuriomas** presenting as cranial nerve-associated or intraventricular growths,[1125] **intraneural perineuriomas** originating in cranial nerve divisions,[1112] and craniospinal examples of **localized hypertrophic neuropathy**.[1134,1136] Whereas the last of these entities probably represents a reactive hyperplasia characterized by the concentric wrapping of S-100 protein-expressing, EMA-negative Schwann cells about individual axons in formations known as 'onion bulbs', the intraneural perineurioma is a bona fide neoplasm in which morphologically similar structures ('pseudo-onion bulbs') reflect concentric periaxonal proliferation by EMA-labeling, S-100 nonreactive elements of perineurial cell type. Last, we mention the occurrence of **traumatic neuromas** in the CNS, most involving the spinal cord[1143] and some developing in association with tumors such as intramedullary ependymomas.[1128]

Lymphoproliferative and myeloproliferative disorders

As secondary spread of systemic lymphoproliferative and myeloproliferative disorders to the CNS does not often occasion neurosurgical intervention for diagnostic purposes, only a few general observations on this problem are offered. At greatest risk of such dissemination are patients suffering from acute leukemias,[1175] particularly of lymphoblastic type; diffuse leptomeningeal infiltration is the dominant pattern of CNS involvement encountered in this setting. In some cases, extensive permeation of cranial and spinal nerve roots accompanies the unrestrained proliferation of leukemic cells in the subarachnoid compartment. Circumscribed, dura-based, or (rarely) intracerebral masses composed of leukemic cells principally complicate the acute myelogenous leukemias but have virtually disappeared from clinical practice since the advent of modern cytoreductive therapy. Variously designated as **chloromas**, **granulocytic sarcomas**, or **myeloblastomas**, these tumors usually develop in subjects who are demonstrably leukemic[1182] but exceptionally constitute the initial manifestation of relapse following apparently successful treatment or arise in otherwise normal individuals as harbingers (with very rare exception[1222]) of subsequent bone marrow and peripheral blood involvement.[1178] Parameningeal masses of **extramedullary hematopoietic** tissue have been reported to produce neurologic dysfunction, mainly as a result of spinal cord compression, in patients with thalassemia or myelofibrosis.[1172,1209]

Involvement of the CNS in the course of node-based non-Hodgkin lymphoma is uncommon and usually limited to permeation of the leptomeninges ('lymphomatous meningitis') or, less often, infiltration of the spinal epidural space.[1191] Cerebral infiltrates are decidedly unusual in this setting and typically complicate advanced (stage IV) disease, an excess of cases occurring in patients with diffuse large cell or lymphoblastic subtypes and involvement of other extranodal sites.[1191] By contrast, patients presenting with non-Hodgkin lymphoma of the eye – an extension of the CNS – frequently develop lymphomatous lesions of the brain proper.[1211] A subset of malignant lymphomas, principally non-Hodgkin variants, are confined at diagnosis to the epidural compartment and paraspinal tissues, usually arising in the midthoracic region and prompting evaluation for compressive myelopathy.[1185,1215] Only exceptionally are the meninges colonized or the neural parenchyma penetrated in the course of systemic **Hodgkin disease**,[1216] **plasma cell myeloma**,[1180] **Waldenström macroglobulinemia**,[1205] or **mycosis fungoides**.[1163]

The designation of **primary central nervous system lymphoma (PCNSL)** is reserved for malignant lymphoid neoplasms restricted at presentation to the brain, spinal cord, or meninges.[1173] Although the association of PCNSL with states of diminished immune responsiveness has long been appreciated and its particular predilection for victims of AIDS firmly established, the majority of afflicted patients suffer no predisposing illness. Sporadic cases most often present in the sixth or seventh decades of life and manifest a 1.5 : 1 to 2 : 1 male/female ratio, whereas immunodeficiency-related examples reflect the demographics of HIV-1 infection, inherited immunologic disorders, diseases prompting organ transplantation, and other conditions necessitating iatrogenic immunosuppression. Most patients suffer the usual symptoms of an expanding intracranial mass, although PCNSLs tend to arise in the deep cerebral hemispheric white matter, corpus callosum, and basal ganglia and thus are not as prone to produce seizures as gliomas or metastatic deposits that involve epileptogenic cortical tissues. Frontocallosal and periventricular examples may prompt evaluation for personality change, depression, progressive psychomotor retardation, or frank psychosis. Rapidly progressing dementia has been associated with a distinctive subset of PCNSLs that diffusely permeate the brain rather than forming bulky masses ('**lymphomatosis cerebri**').[1213] Some tumors are discovered in the course of workup for persistent uveocyclitides unresponsive to conventional ophthalmologic treatment, a manifestation of ocular involvement that often occurs in complex with cerebral infiltration.[1211]

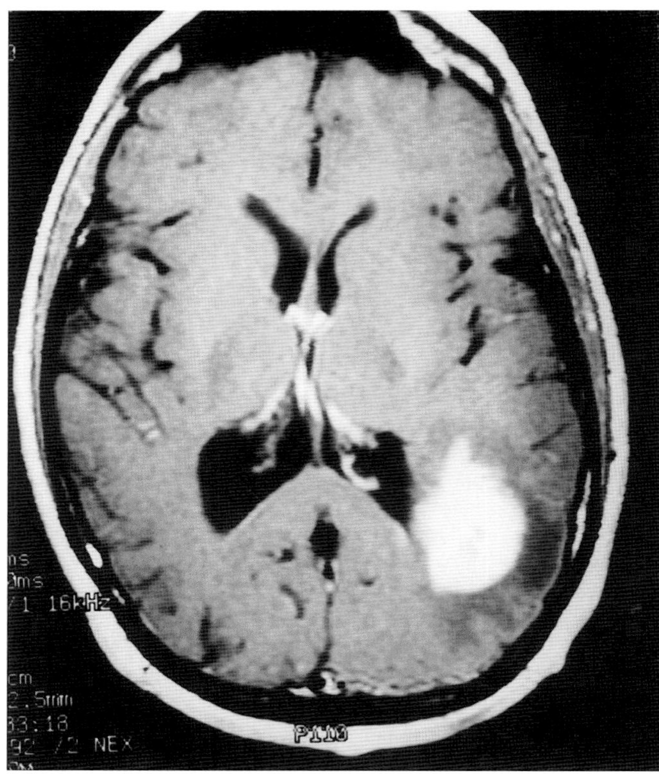

Fig. 28.113 Primary CNS lymphoma. As demonstrated in this postcontrast injection MRI, primary cerebral lymphomas exhibit a predilection for the deep, paraventricular white matter and tend to striking and fairly homogeneous enhancement in 'sporadic' (as opposed to AIDS-related) cases.

Suggestive of PCNSL on CT or MR study (Fig 28.113) are solid, nodular masses displaying hyperdensity in precontrast images, diffuse (as opposed to rim) enhancement on administration of contrast media, evidence of widespread subependymal infiltration, and multifocality. The last is apparent in some 25–40% of sporadic examples and the majority of HIV-1-associated and post-transplant cases.[1167,1173] Especially suspect in older adults are lesions that regress substantially with corticosteroid administration alone prior to biopsy, occasional lymphomas disappearing (transiently) with such treatment and masquerading as multiple sclerosis. Cases of lymphomatosis cerebri depart from the typical on MR assessment in their failure to form localized masses or enhance, characteristically demonstrating only diffuse, nonspecific white matter hyperintensity on T2-weighted and FLAIR sequences.[1213] Extensive central necrosis, a feature foreign to sporadic examples, lends to many HIV-1-associated PCNSLs a 'ring'-enhancing radiologic appearance that may be indistinguishable from *Toxoplasma* abscesses. A definitive diagnosis of PCNSL usually requires biopsy, but may be accomplished by demonstration of malignant lymphoid cells in CSF. Immunocytochemistry (for B-cell 'markers'), flow cytometry, and PCR-based molecular assessment (for immunoglobulin heavy chain (IgH) gene rearrangements) have been applied to CSF specimens as methods of facilitating nonsurgical diagnosis.[1173]

PCNSLs may arise anywhere along the neuraxis. Roughly 75% are situated in the supratentorial compartment, these favoring the deep structures enumerated above. Most of the remainder involve the cerebellum or brainstem, only rare examples being isolated to the spinal cord, cauda equina or craniospinal nerve roots.[1193,1203] The designation of '**neurolymphomatosis**' has been applied to cases of the last two types and to lymphomas of nerve more peripherally localized.[1159] A small fraction of PCNSLs present as diffuse leptomeningeal infiltrates in the absence of demonstrable intraparenchymal disease,[1201] the literature including description of **human herpesvirus 8-associated 'primary effusion lymphoma'** of the subarachnoid space as a complication of AIDS.[1179] Dura-based lymphomas are given separate consideration later in this discussion (see below). Lesions of the CNS proper are poorly defined in most instances and composed of dry, granular, tan–white or grayish-pink tissue that may evidence small foci of necrotic softening or hemorrhagic discoloration. Extensive necrosis and conspicuous hemorrhage are most commonly encountered in AIDS-related cases, which may closely mimic *Toxoplasma* abscesses on gross examination (particularly after adjuvant treatment), and in lesions complicating transplantation. Examples of lymphomatosis cerebri diffusely permeate the neuropil, particularly the cerebral hemispheric white matter, producing little architectural distortion save for a slight expansion of involved structures.[1213] A striking histologic feature of many PCNSLs is the tendency for tumor cells to aggregate in Virchow–Robin spaces and to infiltrate the walls of cerebral vessels (Fig. 28.114). This is commonly associated with reticulin deposition in concentric, ring-like patterns. Most neuroparenchymal PCNSLs are high-grade non-Hodgkin lesions of diffuse large cell type,[1165,1166,1173,1207] but all major cytologic variants have been reported in this location, including low-grade lymphomas of small lymphocytic or lymphoplasmacytic ('immunocytoma') type,[1197] anaplastic large cell lymphomas,[1184,1214] and such oddities as signet ring cell[1210] and extranodal, choroid plexus-based marginal zone lymphoma.[1199] Follicular (nodular) lymphoid neoplasms, however, are practically never encountered in this setting.[1197] Some observers have noted an overrepresentation of immunoblastic and small noncleaved Burkitt-like cell types among PCNSLs, particularly those involving AIDS patients and other immunosuppressed hosts, compared with node-based or other extranodal primary tumors.[1165] Regardless of the cytologic variety, touch preparations are useful in establishing the lymphoid nature of a given tumor at the time of intraoperative consultation (Fig. 28.115).

The overwhelming majority of PCNSLs exhibit a B-cell immunophenotype,[1165,1166,1207] including labeling for CD20 and CD79a in the absence of CD3 or CD45RO expression (Fig. 28.116). Other evidences of their B-lymphocytic lineage include clonal IgH gene rearrangements and certain characteristics shared with germinal center B cells, including recurrent translocations of the *BCL6* gene and BCL6 protein expression.[1173] PCNSLs, however, commonly evidence 'activated' (nongerminal center) B-cell features as well.[1164,1189] Thus, one sizable analysis found an activated B-cell immunophenotype in over 90% of studied examples, these labeling for CD10, BCL6, and MUM1, respectively, in 2.4%, 55.5%, and 92.6% of cases.[1164] Other characteristics shared by PCNSLs and diffuse large

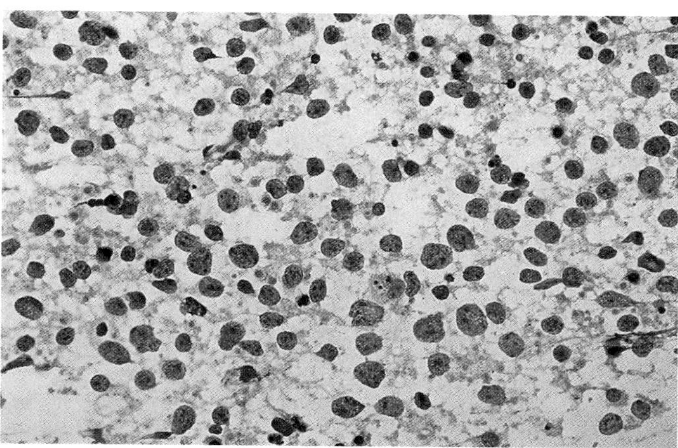

Fig. 28.115 Primary CNS lymphoma. An intraoperative smear preparation demonstrates the large cell cytology and nuclear features characteristic of CNS lymphoma. The lack of cellular cohesion or cytoplasmic processes, respectively, are useful in discriminating this tumor from metastatic carcinoma and glioblastoma multiforme, two neoplasms that commonly enter the clinical differential diagnosis.

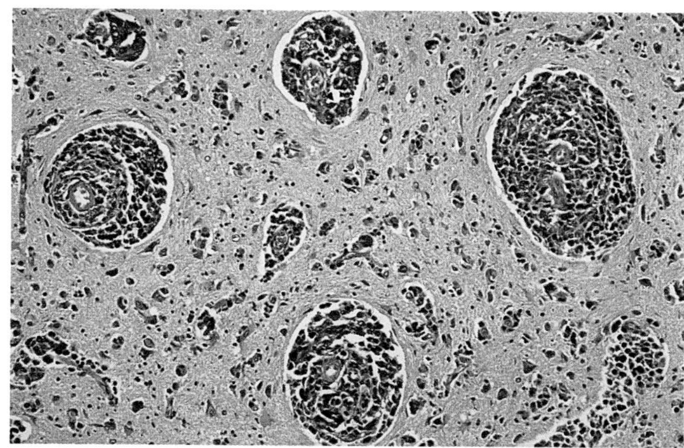

Fig. 28.114 Primary CNS lymphoma. Although not apparent in all cases, a vasocentric growth pattern with tumoral infiltration of blood vessel walls and Virchow–Robin spaces is common to primary CNS lymphomas. Systemic lymphomas secondarily involving the neuroparenchyma may also preferentially grow in this fashion.

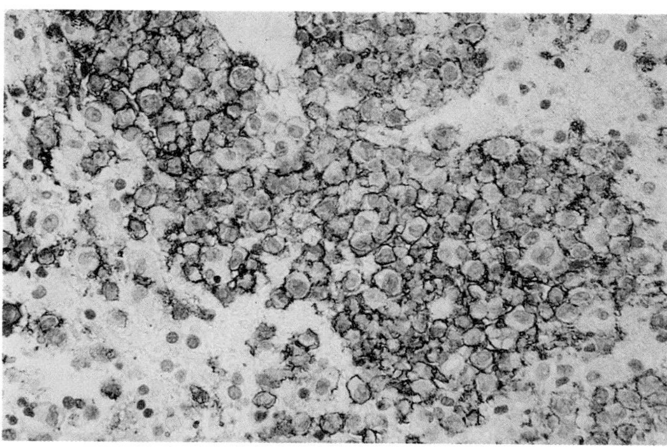

Fig. 28.116 Primary CNS lymphoma. The great majority of lymphomas arising in the CNS are of B-cell type and, as shown here, label for CD20 on immunoperoxidase (L–26) assay.

cell lymphomas of activated B-cell type arising outside the neuraxis include an IgM phenotype without evidence for immunoglobulin class switch, high-level expression of BCL2 mRNA and protein in the absence of t(14;18)(q32;q21)/*IGH–BCL2* fusion, and frequent gains of chromosome 18q21 that include the *BCL2* and *MALT1* oncogenes.[1173] The last of these phenomena constitutes the most common genetic abnormality displayed by PCNSLs and effects (with upregulated expression of other family members, upstream modulators and targets) activation of the nuclear factor kappa B (NF-κB) signaling cascade.[1171,1173] Increased NF-κB signaling could explain, at least in part, the observations that PCNSLs are highly proliferative (MIB-1/Ki-67 indices regularly exceeding 50–70% and potentially rising above 90%) while exhibiting relatively low-level apoptotic activity.[1171,1173]

It is to be emphasized that PCNSLs often harbor a conspicuous complement of admixed T cells that can confound interpretation of the histologic and immunohistochemical picture, but these reactive elements usually appear as small, well-differentiated lymphocytes that are readily distinguished from the large, atypical B cells on which the diagnosis rests. Particularly deceptive are biopsies deriving from the perimeter of PCNSLs, where reactive T lymphocytes often constitute a dominant and obscuring population, or from masses evidencing regression on preoperative corticosteroid administration. These 'sentinel lesions' may be selectively relieved of their neoplastic B-cell components, heavily infiltrated by foamy macrophages, and partially demyelinated, a phenomenon that may prompt, along with their radiologic and clinical resolution, acceptance of multiple sclerosis or demyelinating pseudotumor as the primary disease process.[1154] It is worth remembering that multiple sclerosis is, for the most part, a disorder of the young. Furthermore, it has been our experience that inadvertently 'treated' lymphomas do not leave behind the sharply demarcated zones of selective and total myelin loss with axonal preservation typical of multiple sclerosis or demyelinating pseudotumors. Clonal B-cell populations have rarely been described as participants in multiple sclerosis,[1224] but atypical B lymphocytes should not be seen in this disorder. **Primary T-cell lymphomas of the CNS** constitute no more than 2–4% of PCNSLs in series from the West, but account for a significantly higher proportion of cases afflicting Japanese and Koreans.[1170,1173,1218] These may be overrepresented among leptomeningeal and infratentorial primaries. The spectrum of variants reported to present as CNS primaries includes anaplastic large cell lymphomas[1184,1214] as well as rare examples of cytotoxic/suppressor-[1204] and natural killer (NK)-type[1198] T-cell tumors.

Neuroparenchymal PCNSLs of the usual (i.e., diffuse large B-cell) type can be driven into remission by adjuvant means but usually recur (often at CNS sites remote from the initial focus of disease) and prove fatal. High-dose, methotrexate-based chemotherapeutic regimens have achieved median survival intervals of 36–50 months and 5-year overall survival rates of approximately 30–40%.[1173] As toxic leukoencephalopathy has emerged as a frequent complication of combined radiochemotherapeutic approaches, current management strategies and ongoing clinical trials are focused on frontline chemotherapy alone (including potentially promising protocols involving autologous stem cell transplantation). The outlook for patients with intra-axial T-cell PCNSLs is similarly discouraging at present.[1218] Those exceptional examples of low-grade, small lymphocytic or lymphoplasmacytic B-cell lymphoma arising in the central neuraxis seem to be less aggressive and amenable to longer-term control.[1197] A grim prognosis attaches to AIDS-associated PCNSLs, though improvement in survival has been effected since the advent of highly active antiretroviral therapy.[1173] The usual pattern of treatment failure in the setting of PCNSL is progressive, frequently multifocal infiltration of the CNS proper, attended, in some cases, by leptomeningeal dissemination. Ocular involvement is experienced by many patients as the disease evolves,[1211] but systemic lymphomatous infiltrates develop in no more than 10% of cases.

As the central neuraxis normally lacks a resident lymphoid population, the histogenesis of PCNSLs is obscure. Specifically, whether primary neuroparenchymal and leptomeningeal lymphomas actually arise in these locales or are peripherally generated and selectively home to (or opportunistically colonize and, shielded from immune surveillance, persist within) the CNS is unclear. Infections or other inflammatory processes could summon lymphocytes to the CNS and thus set the stage for their subsequent neoplastic transformation (a particularly plausible scenario in the immunodeficient), but only exceptionally has PCNSL been described in patients with proven neurologic infections or other unarguably reactive processes characterized by lymphoid infiltration.[1158] Given the recognized ability of the Epstein–Barr virus (EBV) to immortalize B cells in vitro and to drive a polyclonal, systemic lymphoproliferation that may evolve to frank lymphoma in immunocompromised hosts, it is noteworthy that AIDS-related PCNSLs[1165] and post-transplant lymphoproliferative disease involving the CNS[1167] regularly harbor this agent whereas sporadic PCNSLs rarely do.[1166,1173] EBV has also been incriminated in a low-grade lymphoproliferative disorder resembling polymorphic B-cell hyperplasia in an HIV-1-infected child,[1200] and in a polyclonal cerebellar lymphoproliferation that progressed to lymphoma in an apparently immunocompetent adult.[1174]

Primary lymphoproliferative disorders of the CNS other than non-Hodgkin lymphoma of the neuroparenchyma and leptomeninges merit little discussion. **Primary dural lymphomas** are uncommon lesions that typically mimic meningiomas and that are usually B-cell tumors of **low-grade, marginal zone (mucosa-associated lymphoid tissue (MALT)) type**.[1220] These may evidence intratumoral amyloid deposition. Other variants have been described in this setting,[1208] including **T-cell-rich B-cell lymphoma**,[1155] small lymphocytic lymphoma, diffuse large B-cell lymphoma, anaplastic large T-cell lymphoma, and low-grade follicular lymphoma of small cleaved type.[1162,1208] Only rarely is **Hodgkin disease** confined, on presentation, to the CNS.[1166,1190,1192] PCNSLs derived from immunodeficient hosts, however, not infrequently harbor pleomorphic cellular elements that may be misconstrued as Reed–Sternberg cells. The peculiar disorder described as **neoplastic angioendotheliomatosis**, formerly regarded as an intravascular variant of angiosarcoma, is now known to be an unusual form of malignant lymphoma, typically of large B-cell type (though T-cell variants are recognized[1168]), exhibiting a remarkable tropism for blood vessels in the skin, adrenal glands, and CNS.[1161,1173] Accordingly, the disorder is now termed '**intravascular**' or '**angiotropic**' **lymphoma**. Patients often present with neurologic dysfunction – progressive encephalopathy, dementia, or stroke – that reflects multifocal cerebral infarction resulting from occlusion of vascular lumina by malignant lymphoid cells (Fig. 28.117). Cerebrovascular aneurysm formation with rupture and intracranial hemorrhage has also been reported to complicate intravascular lymphoma,[1156] as has the development of extravascular lymphomatous masses in the CNS.[1196] Rare cases have been described as limited to the brain or spinal cord,[1177] one of which occurred in a child with AIDS.[1176]

Other oddities include **Castleman disease** confined to the meninges[1186,1188] or involving spinal nerve roots,[1181] primary **plasmacytoma** of the dura,[1160] brain[1223] or spinal cord[1183] (including cases described as developing against a background of **atypical plasma cell hyperplasia**[1194]), and CNS **amyloidomas**,[1202] neither of the latter appearing to herald systemic myeloma. Amyloidomas of the gasserian ganglion are further recognized as an unusual cause

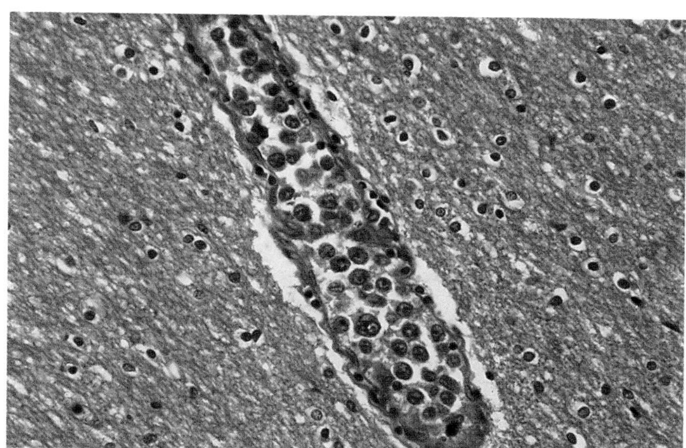

Fig. 28.117 Angiotropic lymphoma/intravascular malignant lymphomatosis. Large, highly atypical cells fill a small blood vessel in the white matter of a 63-year-old woman subjected to brain biopsy for progressive cognitive impairment. Positive immunoassays for leukocyte common antigen and CD20 confirmed their lymphoid nature and B-cell phenotype, respectively.

of trigeminal neuropathy, these also representing localized lesions and not complicating or presaging generalized plasma cell dyscrasia.[1202,1206] The vasocentric deposition in brain of type-restricted immunoglobulin light chains (amyloid forming in some cases and accompanied by modest infiltrates of small lymphocytes and mature, but monoclonal, plasma cells) has also been reported under the rubric of **CNS light chain deposition disease**[1212,1221] or as a form of **cerebral amyloid angiopathy**.[1217] The deposits in question have been almost exclusively of lambda light chain type, cerebral and gasserian amyloidomas also being composed of AL lambda light chain material and harboring clonal lambda-expressing plasma cells,[1202] but an example exhibiting kappa restriction has been communicated.[1221] Tumors interpreted as **true histiocytic neoplasms**[1169,1219] or **'microglioma'**[1195] of the brain have been depicted. Finally, there is so-called **lymphomatoid granulomatosis**, an angiocentric and necrotizing lymphoproliferative disorder historically described as a prelymphomatous condition involving the CNS in association with pulmonary disease but occasionally reported to localize in brain alone.[1157,1187] Several of these isolated cerebral variants involved patients with AIDS[1157] and a number eventuated in recognizable lymphoma. Arguably, at least some of these cases represented angiocentric forms of malignant lymphoma ab initio. The participation of EBV in this process has been documented.[1187]

Germ cell tumors

Whether **germ cell tumors** of the CNS derive, as long presumed, from primordial germ cells that aberrantly migrate to the developing central neuraxis remains a speculative matter, but the fact remains that these uncommon neoplasms are morphologically and immunophenotypically indistinguishable from germinal tumors arising in the gonads (as well as other extragonadal sites) and a subset manifests genetic abnormalities, such as X chromosome gains and isochromosome 12p formation, characteristic of testicular (and mediastinal) primaries.[1246] The latter genetic lesion, a marker alteration in the setting of testicular germ cell tumorigenesis, does not appear, however, to be as prevalent among intracranial examples.[1254] Approximately 90% of CNS germ cell tumors are discovered in the first two decades of life, case rates peaking in 10- to 12-year-olds. In Western series, these account for no more than 0.5% of all primary intracranial neoplasms and 3% of those encountered in children, but their incidence is increased some five-fold in Japan, Taiwan, and Korea.[1246] Sharing with other extragonadal germ cell tumors a predilection for the midline, at least 80% of CNS examples arise along an axis extending from the suprasellar cistern and infundibulum to the pineal gland (these constituting the most common neoplasms encountered in the latter location). A synchronous suprasellar and pineal region presentation is well recognized, though exceptional, as are cases confined to the cerebral hemispheres, basal ganglia or thalami (these may be bilateral), ventricles, spinal cord, and sella turcica. Metachronous intracranial primaries are on record, but rare.[1235] Males are afflicted more than twice as frequently as females when all sites are considered, but gender distribution varies with tumor localization: the large majority of pineal examples affect boys, suprasellar lesions occurring more often in girls.

CNS germ cell tumors generally arise in sporadic fashion, but are recognized to complicate Klinefelter syndrome[1234,1246] and their incidence may be increased in the setting of Down syndrome as well.[1228,1246] Suprasellar examples produce visual field defects, diabetes insipidus, and hypothalamopituitary failure, whereas pineal region tumors compress the tectal plate and aqueduct, presenting with symptoms and signs of obstructive hydrocephalus that are often accompanied by a vertical gaze paresis known eponymously as Parinaud syndrome. The secretion of β-human chorionic gonadotropin (β-HCG) by neoplastic syncytiotrophoblast may stimulate testosterone production in boys and result in 'precocious puberty' (isosexual pseudoprecocity), as may release of the immature testes from tonic inhibitory controls secondary to pineal and hypothalamic injury. The additional elaboration of cytochrome p450 aromatase, which catalyzes estrogen formation from C19 steroids, could explain the exceptional occurrence of precocious puberty in girls with HCG-producing intracranial germ cell tumors.[1243]

The macroscopic features, histologic and immunohistochemical criteria governing the identification and subclassification of CNS germ cell tumors differ in no way from those previously articulated in discussion of their more common gonadal counterparts and are not systematically reprised here.[1227,1246,1247] Exceeding in incidence of all other tumor types is the **germinoma**. This neoplasm is essentially identical to the seminoma in histologic appearance and antigenic profile. While the microscopic diagnosis is usually straightforward, the germinoma that has elicited a florid lymphoplasmacytic and granulomatous reaction may masquerade as tuberculosis, sarcoidosis or other inflammatory process.[1238] Immunohistochemical screening facilitates the visualization of tumor cells obscured by such an infiltrate and is mandatory when dealing with inflamed biopsy material deriving from the suprasellar–pineal axis (a unique report of apparently **idiopathic 'pinealitis'** notwithstanding[1242]). D2-40, CD117 (c-kit), and OCT4 antibodies outperform reagents against placental alkaline phosphatase (PLAP) in this regard,[1231] membranous reactivity for the first two being more germinoma specific than nuclear OCT4 expression (which is shared by embryonal carcinomas). Nuclear immunolabeling for NANOG, a homeodomain transcription factor, is a further feature of germinomas useful in their identification.[1249] We would call the reader's attention to unusual forms of 'diffuse' CNS germinoma that permeate the neuroparenchyma in glioma-like fashion rather than forming discrete tumor masses.[1248] A minority of otherwise pure germinomas harbor syncytiotrophoblastic giant cell elements that are β-HCG-immunoreactive and associated with elevated levels of this oncoprotein in serum and CSF. The prognostic implications of this phenomenon are addressed below.

Apart from germinoma, only CNS germ cell tumors of the teratoma family are likely to be encountered in pure form.[1239,1246] **Teratomas** constitute the majority of congenital CNS germ cell tumors, one account describing the remarkable discovery of a primary intracranial example in the fetus of a woman with an independent ovarian teratoma.[1244] This tumor group includes the **mature teratoma** (composed entirely of adult-type tissues), the **immature teratoma** (defined by a content of incompletely differentiated components exhibiting fetal appearances), and the **teratoma with malignant transformation** (i.e., one spawning a secondary cancer of conventional somatic type). As regards the last entity, sarcomas of undifferentiated or rhabdomyosarcomatous aspect,[1227,1239,1245] leiomyosarcoma,[1253] adenocarcinomas of enteric type,[1229] squamous carcinoma,[1239] and erythroleukemia[1230] have all been reported to arise from intracranial, teratoma-containing germ cell tumors and we have seen in consultation a mature pineal teratoma partially overgrown by malignant hemangioendothelioma. A carcinoid has been encountered within a teratomatous tumor of the spinal axis,[1233] though some argue that intraspinal 'teratomas' are complex malformations[1237] rather than true germinal neoplasms.[1225] Rarely, intracranial teratomas achieve extraordinary degrees of organization and contain fetus-like bodies.[1241] The designation of **intracranial fetus-in-fetu** has been applied to these curiosities, but is more exactingly restricted by some observers to cases of apparently abortive twinning in which one developing fetus is incorporated into the cranium of the other.[1236] While the spontaneous maturation of teratomas has been recorded,[1252] re-resection specimens composed entirely of fully differentiated somatic tissue elements usually derive from initially immature teratomatous neoplasms or mixed germ cell tumors subjected to adjuvant therapy. The apparent maturation in such circumstances may simply reflect the selective ablation of incompletely differentiated cellular components. The progressive, seemingly paradoxical enlargement of these ostensibly mature neoplasms has been referred to as the 'growing teratoma syndrome'.[1226]

Embryonal carcinoma, **yolk sac tumor**, and **choriocarcinoma** may all arise within the CNS, but only rarely are these encountered in unalloyed form. Far more frequent is their presence within mixed germ cell tumors, which often contain elements of germinoma and teratoma as well. We again emphasize the importance of immunohistochemical assessment in the evaluation of such lesions. Specifically, screening for alpha-fetoprotein is critical if minor components of yolk sac tumor are not to be overlooked (bearing in mind, however, that teratomatous glands of enteric type may also label for this antigen) and assessment for CD30 expression is of great value in distinguishing embryonal carcinomas from other germ cell tumor types. SALL4 expression is also helpful in the identification of yolk sac tumors, being a more sensitive marker than alpha-fetoprotein, but lacks comparable specificity as other germ cell tumors, including germinomas and embryonal carcinomas, also label for this stem cell transcription factor.[1240] The pathologist reporting a mixed germ cell neoplasm should specify the participating tumor types and their relative representation.

Histologic subclassification emerges from a number of multivariate analyses as bearing most heavily on CNS germ cell tumor prognosis.[1239,1250,1251] The best outcomes attach to pure germinomas in localized form (which are generally radiocurable as well as chemosensitive) and to mature teratomas that can be completely resected. The spontaneous regression of germinoma has been recorded,[1232] a phenomenon that may well be mediated by the tumor-infiltrating lymphocytes characteristic of this neoplasm. The presence of syncytiotrophoblastic giant cells within germinomas has been associated in most studies with an increased risk of local failure and decrement in survival when treated solely by irradiation.[1239,1250] Yolk sac tumors, embryonal carcinomas, choriocarcinomas, and mixtures thereof frequently resist both surgery and adjuvant treatment, carrying a high mortality, though aggressive regimens that include vigorous chemotherapy have improved matters for some patients and continue to be investigated in this setting. These virulent lesions destructively infiltrate local structures and may disseminate via the CSF, as can the germinoma. Extraneural spread is a rare complication that includes spontaneous systemic metastasis (mainly to lung and bone) as well as seeding of the peritoneal cavity via ventriculoperitoneal shunts placed for relief of obstructive hydrocephalus. Some observers have found immature teratomas and mixed tumors composed mainly of germinoma and teratomatous elements to be associated with an 'intermediate' risk of recurrence and progression.[1239] One recent analysis could not attach any prognostic significance to chromosome 12p status (either isochromosome formation or polysomy) in the setting of intracranial germ cell neoplasia.[1254]

Melanocytic tumors

We have previously mentioned melanogenesis as a function occasionally exercised by nerve sheath tumors as well as central neuroepithelial neoplasms of varying types. The CNS and its coverings also host tumors posited to derive from dendritic melanocytes of neural crest origin that normally populate the pia-arachnoid. The latter are especially numerous over the ventral medulla and high cervical spinal cord, regions that often evidence a peppery discoloration on gross inspection, but the growths for which they are held accountable are by no means restricted to these areas and, while largely leptomeninges based, may be anchored to the dura mater or situated in the substance of the brain, spinal cord, or pineal gland. Most such lesions fall into one of several fairly homogeneous diagnostic categories. As described below, these include well-differentiated and relatively indolent tumors that are termed melanocytomas as well as frankly malignant melanomas occurring in either localized or diffuse leptomeningeal form. Melanocytic neoplasms of the CNS may constitute manifestations of a generalized neurocristopathy. The syndrome of **neurocutaneous melanosis** (known also as **Touraine syndrome** in its heritable, autosomal dominant form) is defined by the association of giant or multifocal nevi of congenital type with discrete meningeal melanomas or, more commonly, an unrestrained (and ultimately fatal) proliferation of melanocytic elements, often deceptively benign in appearance, throughout the subarachnoid compartment and within Virchow–Robin spaces.[1261,1269] The spread of this process to the abdomen via ventriculoperitoneal shunts placed to relieve obstructive hydrocephalus has been described.[1258] In addition, meningeal melanocytomas[1268] and melanomas[1273] have been reported in complex with nevus of Ota, characterized by congenital cutaneous, ocular, and retrobulbar soft tissue hyperpigmentation in a maxillo-ophthalmic trigeminal nerve distribution. Intracranial melanoma has also been described in the setting of NF-1.[1263]

Melanocytomas usually present in middle age or later adult life as circumscribed, extra-axial masses attached to the leptomeninges. Most arise along the spinal neuraxis (some in association with nerve roots),[1257,1275] intracranial examples exhibiting a decided predilection for the posterior fossa and Meckel's cave.[1257] Only exceptionally do such tumors involve higher levels of the intracranial compartment,[1257,1260,1267] a remarkable case confined to the lateral ventricular system having been depicted.[1272] Characteristic MRI findings include iso/hyperintensity on T1-weighted images, a hypointense (dark) profile on T2-weighted study – these features reflecting the paramagnetic properties of melanin – and homogeneous contrast enhancement.

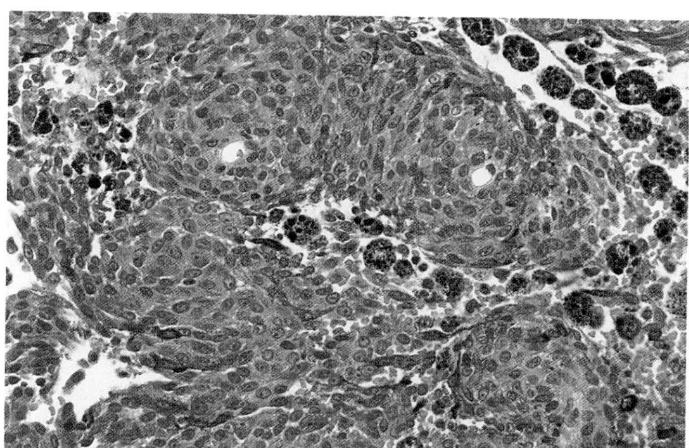

Fig. 28.118 Meningeal melanocytoma. The tendency to cellular whorling manifested by this example, resected from the cervical region of a 34-year-old man with a protracted history of neck pain and gait disturbance, accounts for the potential misclassification of melanocytomas as melanotic meningiomas. Note finely divided brown pigment in the cytoplasm of some tumor cells (as opposed to coarse pigment granules in melanophages), delicate and monomorphous nuclear features, lack of mitotic activity, and absence of necrosis.

Consisting grossly of tan–brown to coal-black tissue, melanocytomas are frequently composed of uniform spindle cells arrayed in fascicles and compactly whorled nests (the latter accounting for the once prevalent perception of these tumors as pigmented meningiomas) (Fig. 28.118). Whorling formations may be centered on delicate stromal blood vessels, cellular dehiscence often producing a pseudopapillary appearance at low magnification. Epithelioid forms may be admixed, but rarely do these dominate the histologic picture.[1257] Tumor cell nuclei may exhibit longitudinal grooving when spindled and typically contain centrally positioned eosinophilic nucleoli that are easily apprehended but of relatively small diameter. Candidates for the diagnosis of melanocytoma should not harbor macronucleoli, evidence conspicuous nuclear atypia or pleomorphism, contain more than the (very) occasional mitotic figure, or exhibit necrosis.[1257] Cytoplasmic melanization is usually advanced, particularly at the periphery of whorled nests (which are often bordered by clustered melanophages), and can obscure all cytologic detail. Virtually amelanotic examples may be encountered but are exceptional. Ultrastructural studies will confirm the presence of mature melanosomes and may show basement membrane material (also demonstrable in type IV collagen immunopreparations) to incompletely invest some cellular processes or to surround groups of neoplastic melanocytes,[1256] though the extensive basal lamina formation about individual cells and complex cytoplasmic interdigitation characteristic of the melanotic schwannoma are foreign to the melanocytoma. Immunoreactivity for vimentin, S-100 protein, and HMB-45 is regularly present, melanocytomas – in contradistinction to meningiomas – being EMA negative.[1257,1267] Tumor cells may also label for MART-1 (melan-A/A103), tyrosinase, and microphthalmia transcription factor.[1264,1272] A curious oncocytic (i.e., mitochondrion-rich) neoplasm of apparently melanocytomatous nature has been reported.[1262]

Melanocytomas are slowly expanding and generally amenable to surgical control if gross total removal can be accomplished. They have been reported to recur following resection and to invade adjoining neuroparenchyma, but the literature on this score is difficult to interpret owing to the rarity of melanocytic tumors of CNS origin and the application of nonuniform diagnostic criteria to these unusual lesions.[1257] The largest and most closely analyzed series to date included, under the rubric of melanocytoma, only well-differentiated leptomeningeal neoplasms with minimal cytologic atypism, small nucleoli, low mitotic counts (maximally one per 10 high-power fields and below this level in most cases), MIB-1 labeling indices not exceeding 2%, no necrosis or involvement of CNS proper.[1257] None regrew following gross total excision or subtotal resection, irrespective of adjuvant radiotherapy (median follow-up period of 36 months). We have encountered, however, a fatal tumor meeting all of the foregoing criteria that widely seeded the CSF. One report further describes late local recurrence and hepatic metastasis complicating the course of a foramen magnum region tumor exhibiting melanocytomatous histology.[1265] Neoplasms otherwise acceptable as melanocytomas can partially colonize the spinal cord (extending along perivascular spaces in association with florid Rosenthal fiber formation attesting to their chronicity) or may prove, in the main, to be intramedullary at operation.[1259,1264] The latter, which may cause debilitating myelopathy, are far more likely than their wholly leptomeningeal counterparts to recur after resection but nonetheless pursue a protracted course. Given the morphologic attributes and relatively favorable clinical biology of most melanocytomas, it should come as no surprise that these have been likened to ocular melanomas of spindle A and B types, as well as to cellular blue nevi. Noteworthy in this regard is the observation that primary melanocytic neoplasms of the CNS, particularly those of the melanocytoma group, may harbor activating somatic mutations of the G alpha q gene (*GNAQ*) identical to those that have been identified in uveal melanomas (as well as cellular blue nevi and nevi of Ota).[1266] Mapped to chromosome 9q21, *GNAQ* functions in melanocyte homeostasis and survival during neural crest development, encoding GTP-binding proteins that couple cell surface receptors to intracellular signaling networks that include the MAP kinase pathway.

Malignant melanomas of the CNS may present as diffuse leptomeningeal growths ('**melanomatosis**') or discrete masses. Proliferations of the former sort are particularly characteristic of childhood examples occurring as part of the **neurocutaneous melanosis** complex[1261,1269] but may be encountered at any age and in the absence of unusual dermal nevi. Clinical manifestations of intracranial hypertension, cranial nerve deficits, a meningitic or subarachnoid hemorrhage-like picture, and diffuse leptomeningeal enhancement on CT or MRI are typical of **primary leptomeningeal melanomatosis**, which can be diagnosed by demonstration in CSF samples of tumor cells that are melanin laden or immunoreactive for S-100 protein and HMB-45.[1274] Death within months of diagnosis is the rule. Solitary variants of CNS melanoma (other than those complicating neurocutaneous melanosis) mainly afflict adults and become symptomatic by virtue of their compression or invasion of neural structures. These generally share with melanocytomas an origin in the pia-arachnoid and a predilection for the posterior fossa and intraspinal compartment that stand in contrast to the intracerebral distribution characteristic of melanomas metastatic to the central neuraxis.[1257,1271] Still, meticulous search for a cutaneous, mucosal or ocular primary must prove unrevealing before a malignant melanoma can be accepted as indigenous to the CNS. Spindle cell, epithelioid, and mixed cytologic features may be encountered, evidences of malignancy including nuclear and nucleolar enlargement, coarse hyperchromatism, readily apparent mitotic activity, necrosis, and neuroparenchymal invasion.

High rates of regional recurrence, a potential for subarachnoid dissemination, and substantial mortality attach to localized CNS melanomas that cannot be surgically extirpated (unfortunately, a majority of cases). Some observers, however, have found a low incidence of CSF-borne metastasis as well as unexpectedly favorable outcomes following gross total resection in this setting, drawing parallels to the histology and behavior of spindle B, epithelioid, and mixed ocular melanomas.[1257] Again, the literature on this subject is difficult to parse owing to the almost certain inclusion in reported series of cases better classified as melanocytomas.

We close this discussion with the admission that melanocytic tumors of the central neuraxis occasionally defy ready placement in either the melanocytoma or melanoma camp, maintaining relatively reassuring cytologic profiles while exhibiting modest mitotic activity or invasive growth. These '**atypical**', '**borderline**' or '**intermediate grade' melanocytic neoplasms** are capable of recurrence, but the magnitude of this risk is unclear.[1257] In addition, cases of frankly malignant melanoma apparently evolving from lower grade tumors of melanocytomatous character have been communicated.[1270,1276] On record is an intracerebral **balloon cell melanoma** that may have arisen from a meningocortical melanocytic 'nevus'.[1255]

Paraganglioma

Primary **paragangliomas** of the craniospinal axis typically arise in the region of the cauda equina, presenting as delicately encapsulated intradural masses attached to the filum terminale or, less commonly, spinal roots.[1280,1282,1289] Afflicted patients are usually in their fifth or sixth decades and commonly complain of chronic low back pain that may be accompanied by sciatica, sensorimotor deficits, and sphincter disturbances. Functional silence is the rule, manifestations referable to the release of biogenic amines being most exceptional. Paragangliomas have also been reported to originate at cervicothoracic levels,[1282] in the pineal region,[1288] cerebellopontine angle,[1278] cerebellum,[1284] cerebrum,[1286] and sellar/suprasellar compartments.[1283] An intrasellar presentation in the setting of von Hippel–Lindau disease is on record.[1287] Simple resection usually suffices to cure these uncommon neoplasms, which are generally indolent and noninvasive, but exceptional instances of recurrence in the face of ostensibly complete removal, erosion into neighboring bone, CSF-borne spread, osseous metastasis, and tumor-related death following inadequate excision are well documented.[1282,1290] One paraganglioma of the cauda equina reported for its unusual local regrowth and metastasis to cerebellum 22 years after gross total resection was subsequently found to have occurred in a patient with germline mutation of the succinate dehydrogenase gene-subunit D (*SDHD*),[1281] an anomaly associated with heredofamilial paragangliomas of the head and neck. This example of late 'recurrence' may have represented the syndromic development of multifocal primaries.

Apart from a more frequently realized potential to express cytokeratins and to transdifferentiate along ganglion cell and, rarely, schwannian cell lines (phenomena of no clinical import but recognized in the designation of some examples as 'gangliocytic' or 'ganglioneuromatous', respectively),[1285] paragangliomas of the CNS are histologically, ultrastructurally, and immunophenotypically comparable to their systemic counterparts.[1282,1289] Accordingly, we do not describe these neoplasms here other than to emphasize that some depart from the classic arrangement of epithelioid tumor cells in cohesive nests ('Zellballen') and display, instead, spindled cytology and vaguely storiform growth or a vasocentric, pseudopapillary architecture superficially similar to that of the myxopapillary ependymoma but unaccompanied by mucoid change. Paragangliomas are readily distinguished from the latter (and from other tumors that may share a similar intraspinal topography, such as schwannomas and meningiomas) by virtue of their argyrophilia, content of dense-core granules on ultrastructural study, and immunolabeling for synaptophysin and chromogranin. A neoplasm of the cauda equina evidencing both ependymal and paraganglionic differentiation has been depicted,[1277] but is a curiosity. Paragangliomas have also been reported to variably express neurofilament proteins, GFAP, serotonin, somatostatin, and other neuropeptides.[1282,1289] Melanotic and oncocytic examples are on record,[1279,1282] one of the latter exhibiting locally aggressive growth.[1279]

Chordoma

Chordomas are familiar to all pathologists (and are given full description and differential diagnostic treatment elsewhere in these volumes) as destructive tumors of the clivus and sacrococcygeum that presumably originate from remnants of the primitive notochord persisting at these sites. Attention is called to entirely extraosseous, intradural variants that typically lie ventral to the brainstem and that present in adulthood by reason of progressive hydrocephalus, bulbar dysfunction, or intratumoral hemorrhage.[1293] Chordomas have also been described as originating in the intraspinal compartment (including a remarkable example associated with the filum terminale[1291]), as arising from the tentorium,[1294] and as occupying the anterior third ventricle[1292] (though the actual identity of the last of these reported curiosities in relation to the chordoid glioma of the third ventricle is problematic, to say the least). The relationship of the intradural chordoma to the ecchordosis physaliphora,[35] a notochordal heterotopia of comparable morphology that also favors the prepontine regions, remains a subject of debate.[1295] Although some lesions designated as intradural chordomas are clearly neoplasms and are likely derived from displaced notochordal remnants, others may simply represent outsized, symptomatic ecchordoses. Ecchordoses have been described as failing to exhibit the contrast enhancement typical of chordomas on neuroradiologic assessment,[45] but the number of studied examples has been quite limited. Gross total excision of these circumscribed masses holds the promise of cure, whatever the terminology employed in their designation. Nuclear immunolabeling for brachyury readily distinguishes chordomas from chordoid meningiomas and chordoid gliomas, as well as mucinous adenocarcinomas and chondrosarcomas (including extraskeletal myxoid types).[994] The sections dealing with these entities may be consulted for other patterns of antigen expression useful in this regard.

Hemangioblastoma (von Hippel–Lindau disease)

Hemangioblastomas are familiar to most physicians as the hallmark of **von Hippel–Lindau (VHL) disease**, variants associated with this heritable condition constituting some 20–25% of examples encountered in clinical practice.[1296,1313] An autosomal dominant disorder caused by germline mutations of a tumor suppressor gene localized to chromosome 3p25–26, the VHL complex classically includes, in addition to hemangioblastomas of the CNS and retina, visceral cysts (particularly of the kidney, liver, and pancreas), renocortical carcinomas of conventional clear cell type, adrenal pheochromocytomas, and papillary cystadenomas of the epididymis. Affected individuals may also develop endolymphatic sac tumors of the inner ear; hepatocellular adenomas and carcinomas; paragangliomas; endocrine tumors of the pancreas, thyroid gland, and gastrointestinal tract; central neuroepithelial neoplasms; visceral angiomas, and papillary cystadenomas of probable mesonephric origin involving the female genital adnexae. Sporadic hemangioblastomas may also exhibit (though less constantly than VHL-associated cases) mutations or other inactivating abnormalities of the *VHL* gene, which appears to be normally involved in aspects of angiogenesis and cell cycle regulation, and share with syndromic examples frequent losses of chromosome 6q.[1296]

The large majority of hemangioblastomas arise within the cerebellum and produce the neurologic manifestations expected of an expanding posterior fossa mass, extracerebellar examples favoring the medulla and spinal cord (including its covering leptomeninges, nerve roots, and cauda equina).[1296] No division of the central neuraxis is entirely immune and these curious neoplasms have rarely been documented to originate in the optic nerve,[1317] cerebrum,[1307] ventricular system,[1303,1310] sella turcica,[1306] spinal extradural compartment or at considerably further remove from the CNS (e.g., in association with the radial and sciatic nerves, within the pancreas, kidney, adrenal gland, bladder, retroperitoneum, soft tissues of the ankle and popliteal fossa, nasal skin, presacral region, and maxilla).[1311] Underlying VHL disease carries a special risk of multifocal (including retinal) hemangioblastomas and an increased incidence of extracerebellar primaries. The mean age at diagnosis of VHL disease-associated hemangioblastomas is approximately 30 years, sporadic examples peaking in incidence about a decade later.[1296,1313]

The hemangioblastoma often constitutes a sharply circumscribed mural nodule, at times diminutive, in what is otherwise a smooth-walled cyst or, at spinal levels, syrinx (Fig. 28.119). A clear demarcation from adjacent native tissues is typical of the hemangioblastoma, its characteristic reddish-brown and yellow coloration reflecting, respectively, a rich vasculature and high lipid content. The former component, an anastomosing network of delicate, capillary-like channels supplied by feeding vessels of larger caliber, is responsible for the naming of this entity and its traditional classification as a primary vascular neoplasm. In fact, the sole neoplastic element of the hemangioblastoma – known as the 'stromal cell' – inhabits the interstices between ramifying vascular arcades and is recognized by a pale cytoplasm often rich in neutral fats and, as a consequence, vacuolated or foamy in appearance (Fig. 28.120). Aggregation of stromal cells in cohesive nests and lobules lends to 'cellular' hemangioblastomas an epithelioid histologic presentation that invites confusion with metastatic renocortical carcinoma of clear cell type (these tumors, parenthetically, may collide in the setting of VHL disease[1314]), whereas their paucity in 'reticular' variants results in a picture that may be misconstrued as simply angiomatous. Potentially misleading as well is the tendency of stromal cells to exhibit conspicuous nuclear abnormalities, presumably degenerative, reminiscent of those encountered in neoplasms of neuroendocrine type. These changes, which may include unsettling karyomegaly, pleomorphism, and chromatin smudging, are typically unaccompanied by much, if anything, in the way of mitotic activity and are of no prognostic import. The odd hemangioblastoma will manifest mitoses in more worrisome number, but, again, this finding is not predictive of a malignant course. Regular features of additional note include infiltration by mast cells and, at the tumor–brain interface, a florid piloid astrogliosis replete with Rosenthal fibers but lacking the microcystic elements typical of the juvenile pilocytic astrocytoma. Foci of extramedullary normopoiesis may be found in hemangioblastomas, some 10% of which present with polycythemia in consequence of erythropoietin production by stromal cells.[1318] Examples of hemangioblastoma arising in association with AVM have been reported[1309] and, as mentioned in our discussion of gliomesenchymal neoplasms, the designation 'angioglioma' has been extended to rare tumors interpreted as containing a mixture of hemangioblastomatous and neoplastic glial tissues.

Investigations of stromal cell ultrastructure and immunophenotype have been the basis for widely divergent proposals regarding the cytogenesis of hemangioblastomas.[1296,1297,1299,1300,1304] Primitive 'angiomesenchymal' elements, endothelial cells, glia, arachnoidal cells, embryonic choroid plexus elements, neuroendocrine, neuroectodermal and fibrohistiocytic precursors have all been championed. Electron microscopic studies of the stromal cell have regularly disclosed only intracytoplasmic lipid droplets, microfilaments, and

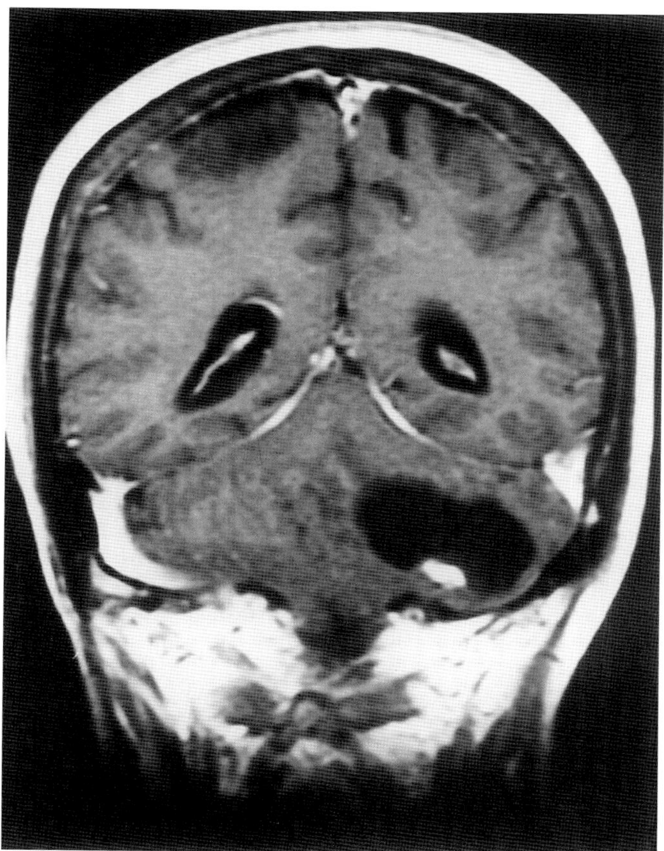

Fig. 28.119 Hemangioblastoma. Most hemangioblastomas arise in the cerebellar hemispheres, where, as emphasized in this postcontrast injection MRI, they present as diminutive, brightly enhancing, and sharply delimited mural nodules projecting into sizable cysts.

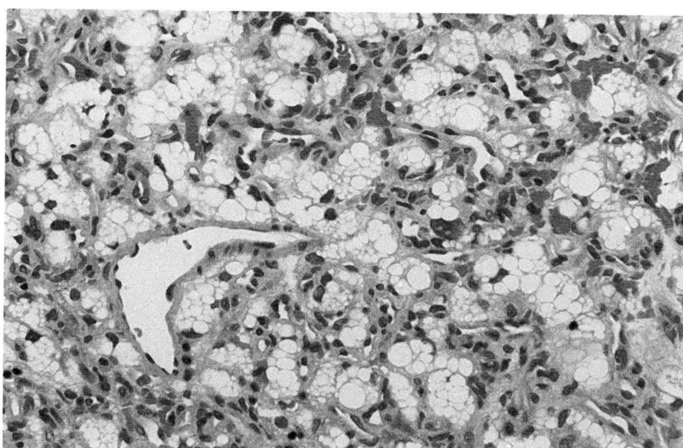

Fig. 28.120 Hemangioblastoma. The neoplasm's defining 'stromal' cells are most readily visualized when lipid accumulation imparts a foamy or vacuolated quality to their pale cytoplasm.

profiles of smooth and rough endoplasmic reticulum.[1304] Vasoformative features depicted in isolated studies[1308] have included electron-dense cytoplasmic structures resembling the Weibel–Palade bodies normally restricted to endothelial cells (some of these factor VIII-labeling by the immunogold technique), intracytoplasmic caveolae suggesting abortive capillary-type lumen formation, and such pericytic/myoid specializations as subplasmalemmal densities, pinocytotic vesicles, and cell processes partially invested by basement membrane material. Stromal cells, on the other hand, do not label for such endothelial 'markers' as CD31 and CD34 and only exceptionally have been described as expressing (and then in small numbers) factor VIII-related antigen, other endothelium-associated proteins or lectins.[1296]

A growing body of evidence would support the derivation of hemangioblastomas not from differentiated endothelium or other mature, blood vessel-associated elements but from developmentally arrested cells that normally generate in embryonic life the blood islands recognized as loci of early hematopoietic activity.[1300,1312] Stromal cells appear to share with these primitive 'hemangioblasts' and their progenitors a characteristic protein expression profile that includes the stem cell leukemia (*SCL*) gene product,[1300,1312] a specifier of hemangioblast differentiation from embryonic mesoderm that is requisite to hematopoiesis and selectively expressed in those regions of the developing CNS to which hemangioblastomas are typically localized.[1300] Under appropriate microenvironmental conditions, the cultured stromal cell similarly resembles the multipotent hemangioblast in its reported capacity to spawn erythrocytic, granulocytic, and endothelial elements.[1312] We refer the reader elsewhere for further discussion of stromal cell biology, which includes upregulated production of vascular endothelial growth factor and other promoters of angiogenesis.[1296,1313]

We emphasize certain aspects of hemangioblastoma immunophenotype that are of practical significance. GFAP reactivity (a small subset of cellular variants excepted[1301]) is typically restricted to entrapped astrocytes or to stromal cells preferentially distributed along the tumor–neuroparenchymal border, a phenomenon that could well reflect nonspecific adsorption or phagocytosis of antigen produced in adjoining gliotic tissues (the occurrence of hemangioblastomas outside the CNS (all GFAP negative) certainly militates against a glial histogenesis[1311]). That stromal cells often label for S-100 protein, NSE, and CD56/NCAM facilitates the distinction of hemangioblastomas from hemangiopericytomas and angiomas[1296,1297] (the latter phenomena, along with reported immunoreactivity for a variety of neuropeptides[1297] and sightings of dense-core intracytoplasmic granules on ultrastructural study,[1304] have been taken as evidence that stromal cells may differentiate along neuroendocrine lines). Particularly important is the observation that stromal cells can exhibit immunolabeling with some anticytokeratins but typically fail to express EMA, the latter usually distinguishing the hemangioblastoma from metastatic renocortical carcinoma and lipidized, angiomatous meningiomas.[1296,1302] Though one outlying study[1320] reported at least focal expression of EMA in 24 of 67 cases, 6 of these exhibiting labeling of 25% or more stromal cells, we have encountered this phenomenon (and then only as patchy and relatively weak reactivity) on the part of only occasional cellular hemangioblastomas. The latter further depart from clear cell carcinomas of renocortical origin in proving CD10 negative,[1305,1320] in generally remaining unlabeled by the AE1/3 anticytokeratin 'cocktail'[1320] and in being far more likely to exhibit widespread immunoexpression of inhibin-alpha[1305,1316,1320] and aquaporin 1 (a water channel protein).[1320] Nuclear expression of brachyury, another described attribute of hemangioblastomas, may also prove to be a useful 'positive' marker in suspected cases.[1300,1312] While some have found the D2-40 antibody (raised against the M2A fetal gonadal antigen) to label many hemangioblastomas but not metastatic clear cell renal carcinomas,[1316] others have found this reagent lacking in both sensitivity and specificity for purposes of this distinction.[1320]

Hemangioblastomas typically manifest only modest MIB-1/Ki-67 labeling activity, median indices in one large study being <1 (range <1–2)% for reticular and 4 (range <1–8)% for cellular subtypes.[1301] These differences achieved statistical significance, but proliferative activity as assessed by this immunohistochemical method has not been shown to bear independently on outcome.

Hemangioblastomas are benign (WHO grade I) neoplasms that usually lend themselves to curative resection. Excised examples may exceptionally recur, however, and patients afflicted with von Hippel–Lindau disease are prone to develop additional primaries.[1298,1313] Studies suggesting that cellular variants of hemangioblastoma may be somewhat more prone to recurrence than reticular forms require confirmation.[1301] CSF dissemination by histologically conventional hemangioblastomas has only rarely been recorded, this potentially occurring years after ostensibly successful resection of cerebellar examples.[1319] An example of 'multifocal' hepatic and pulmonary hemangioblastomatosis complicating VHL disease after several craniotomies for cerebellar hemangioblastoma is also on record.[1315] This could be interpreted, though, as an instance of 'benign hematogenesis metastasis' facilitated by surgery.

Other primary tumors

A unique, **tuberous sclerosis-associated papillary tumor of the hypothalamus** has been communicated.[1322] This low-grade lesion expressed cytokeratins 8/18 but not GFAP, synaptophysin, neurofilament proteins, NeuN, adenohypophyseal hormones or choroid plexus associated-antigens such as transthyretin, stanniocalcin-1 or Kir 7.1. Recently described as **cribriform neuroepithelial tumors**[1323] are intraventricular neoplasms of infancy and early childhood having ribboned, trabecular, rosetted, and variably dilated tubuloglandular formations composed of poorly differentiated cells with low columnar profiles. Apical EMA labeling as well as immunoreactivity for vimentin, MAP-2C, synaptophysin, and cytokeratins (focal) have been depicted, these cellular elements not expressing GFAP or Kir 7.1. While rhabdoid components have not been identified within these curious lesions, they fail to label for INI1 protein and can exhibit *INI/SMARCB1* gene mutation. The latter (and conspicuous proliferative activity) notwithstanding, cribriform neuroepithelial tumors seem far more amenable to control by combined surgical and adjuvant means than neoplasms of the atypical teratoid/rhabdoid tumor group. The list of neoplastic oddities that have been encountered along the central neuraxis includes a **malignant myoepithelioma** of the cranial dura,[1321] a spinal nerve root '**oncocytoma**' of indeterminate lineage,[1324] lumbar intradural masses representing misplaced **adrenocortical neoplasms**,[1327] a lesion of the sellar region described as a **heterotopic follicular carcinoma of thyroid gland type**,[1328] and a number of **ectopic, suprasellar pituitary adenomas** situated in the third ventricle/hypothalamic region.[1325,1326] A survey of intracranial sarcomas previously cited in the discussion of nonmeningothelial, mesenchymal neoplasms includes an example of cerebral **ectomesenchymoma** – a tumor composed of ganglion cell and rhabdomyosarcomatous elements.[1007]

Secondary tumors

Secondary involvement of the CNS by direct extension or hematogenous metastasis is a common complication of systemic cancer and a phenomenon that frequently prompts diagnostic, as well as palliative, neurosurgical intervention. Because we have already touched on this subject in reference to lymphoproliferative and myeloproliferative disorders, this discussion is concerned only with invasion of the central neuraxis by solid tumors.

That neoplasms arising in and around the skeletal confines of the brain and spinal cord often come to impinge on these structures should come as no surprise. Examples include the pituitary adenoma with suprasellar or retrosellar expansion, the glomus jugulare tumor (paraganglioma) that exploits neighboring foramina of the calvarial floor to present as a mass in the pontocerebellar angle, and sacrococcygeal chordomas that engulf the roots of the cauda equina. Ceruminous gland carcinomas and other neoplasms arising in the ear may occasionally billow into the middle cranial fossa to present as intracranial masses.[1333,1347] A substantial risk of local skull base destruction and invasion of contiguous meninges, potentially complicated by dissemination in the subarachnoid space, is seen in embryonal rhabdomyosarcomas originating in head and neck sites, particularly the nasopharynx, paranasal sinuses, and middle ear.[1330] Similarly situated carcinomas of mucosal or minor salivary gland derivation may behave in like fashion, but some of the latter instead track insidiously along regional nerve fiber bundles to achieve radiologically detectable proportions only within the cranial compartment.[1336,1350] Neglected, basal cell or squamous carcinomas of the face and scalp may also reach the CNS by permeating the calvarium or by propagation within perineurial spaces.[1352] The neurotropic spread of a malignant mesothelioma to the spinal cord via the brachial plexus is also on record.[1356] Cancers arising in more distant sites may secondarily infiltrate the nervous system after first metastasizing to juxtaneural structures, the vertebral column apparently serving as an especially important way station in this regard. Epidural spinal cord compression by malignant tumors, for example, is most frequently caused by carcinomas of pulmonary, prostatic, or mammary origin that have spread to the vertebrae, neoplastic cells commonly entering the spinal canal via the bony foramina traversed by vertebral veins.[1331] A similar sequence of events is postulated to account for the high incidence of vertebral and paravertebral metastases in cancer patients developing diffuse leptomeningeal carcinomatosis, principally a complication of adenocarcinomas derived from the lung and breast.[1340] This diagnosis is usually established by the demonstration of malignant cells on cytologic inspection of the CSF.

More common than instances of secondary CNS infiltration by contiguous malignant tumors are blood-borne neuraxial metastases. The principal offenders in this regard are carcinomas of the lung and breast, followed by malignant melanomas, renocortical carcinomas, and adenocarcinomas of colorectal origin.[1351] Carcinomas of the lung are the systemic cancers most likely to present initially as intracerebral tumors, accounting for roughly half of all such cases[1341] and up to 85% of lesions exhibiting adenocarcinomatous histology.[1344] Increasingly effective management of systemic disease may account for perceived rises in the incidence of intracranial deposits from ovarian carcinomas[1342] and osseous or soft tissue sarcomas,[1337,1343] but the latter remain most uncommon as neurosurgical specimens. Sarcomas typically spread to the lungs en route to the brain but may give rise to isolated cerebral or dura-based metastases that, in exceptional instances, herald discovery of the primary tumor.[1349] Noteworthy is the prominence in some series of alveolar soft part sarcoma, one of the rarest tumor types, among mesenchymal neoplasms giving rise to intracranial metastases.[1343] Mention should also be made of HIV-1-associated Kaposi sarcoma traveling to the cranial compartment,[1329] but this remains a curiosity even in the presence of widespread cutaneous and visceral involvement. Unusual, but well documented, is the transmission of maternal cancer (particularly melanoma) to the developing fetus via the placenta.[1357]

Although blood-borne tumor emboli may lodge at any level of the central neuraxis, a few useful generalizations can be made regarding the topography of metastatic lesions. Intramedullary metastases (i.e., those involving the spinal cord parenchyma) are rare,[1334,1351] the great majority of metastatic deposits coming to lie in the supratentorial or infratentorial compartments. In general, the distribution of metastases within the latter conforms to their relative volumes and blood supply.[1335,1351] Thus, most lesions settle within frontoparietal cerebral tissues subtended by the middle cerebral artery (the dominant tributary of the circle of Willis); tumor emboli often lodge within the 'watershed' zone representing the terminus of this vascular territory. For reasons that are not clear, colorectal, uterine, and renocortical carcinomas are overrepresented among cancers seeding the cerebellum.[1335] Prostatic adenocarcinomas also exhibit a curious predilection for this structure when they metastasize to the brain, but their deposits are more typically dura-based and only exceptionally involve the neural parenchyma proper.[1332,1339] Dural metastases in women most often derive from mammary carcinomas.[1339,1351,1358] As a rule, those tumors that frequently travel to the CNS (e.g., malignant melanoma and carcinomas of the lung) tend to produce multiple metastases, whereas cancers that only occasionally involve the brain (e.g., gastrointestinal adenocarcinomas) are often represented by solitary deposits. Noteworthy is a clinical study in which nearly one half of cancer patients with brain metastases were found to have unifocal lesions on neuroradiologic assessment.[1335] A particularly compelling case for neurosurgical intervention can be made in this setting because metastatic lesions are usually compact in their growth patterns and thus lend themselves to excision. Patients who undergo surgical extirpation of single metastases (usually followed by radiotherapy) may be restored to many months (or even years) of useful function, live longer, and enjoy a better quality of life than those whose tumors are simply irradiated using conventional external beam techniques.[1346,1351] Refined stereotactic and radiosurgical techniques are increasingly employed to address metastases and may improve the outlook for patients with deep-seated or multifocal lesions.

In contrast to the common glial neoplasms of adulthood, metastatic nodules tend to be sharply circumscribed and possessed of 'pushing' margins (Fig. 28.121). Much of their mass effect may be

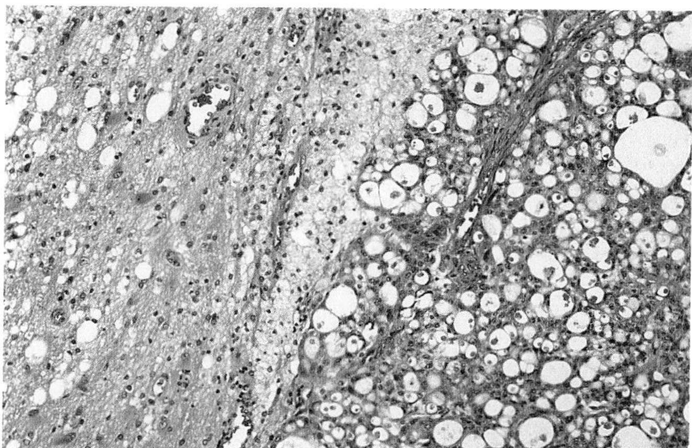

Fig. 28.121 Metastatic carcinoma. A cohesive growth pattern and clearly delimited tumor–CNS interface are hallmarks of neoplasms metastatic to the brain. The adenocarcinoma (right), derived from a primary in the left lung, 'pushes' against adjacent cerebral white matter.

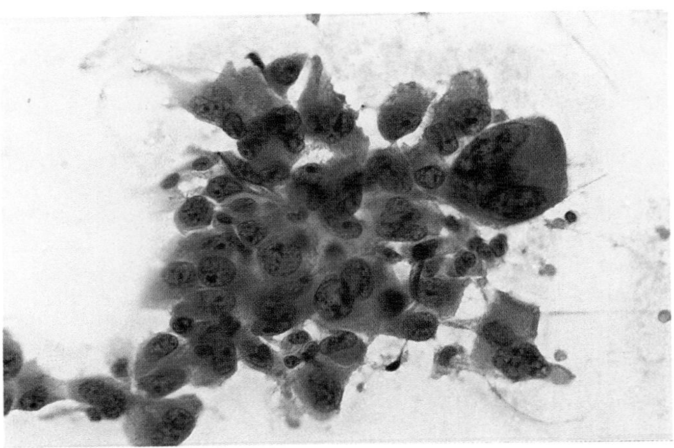

Fig. 28.122 Metastatic carcinoma. The cellular cohesion characteristic of most epithelial neoplasms and foreign to gliomas and lymphomas is generally maintained in cytology preparations, facilitating rapid intraoperative diagnosis. Note also the absence of cytoplasmic processes and presence of conspicuous nucleoli, the latter also alien to most neuroepithelial tumors, in this smear preparation of a poorly differentiated pulmonary adenocarcinoma that presented as a solitary, right frontal lobe brain mass.

derived from edematous expansion of neighboring white matter, often disproportionate to the small size of the offending deposits and usually more pronounced than the edema accompanying primary brain tumors. Most metastases are relatively superficial in location, straddling the gray–white junction to involve both cerebral cortex (thus the high incidence of associated seizures) and digitate white matter. Intralesional hemorrhage occasionally brings brain metastases to light, an especially common phenomenon in the settings of germ cell neoplasia and melanoma.[1353]

On histologic examination, most secondary cancers conform to the histology of their donor tumors and are readily distinguished from primary neoplasms of the brain or meninges on casual inspection. Features that aid in the segregation of poorly differentiated carcinomas from anaplastic gliomas include a cohesive architecture, abrupt interface with adjacent neural tissue, 'peritheliomatous' pattern of tumor cell preservation about stromal blood vessels in cases evidencing coagulative necrosis, and absence of complex microvascular hyperplasia. The last, however, is an arresting feature of some metastatic small cell carcinomas derived from the lung. A confident diagnosis of metastatic carcinoma can often be made at the time of surgery by examination of smear or crush preparations in which the cellular cohesion of most epithelial neoplasms is preserved (Fig. 28.122). The reader is reminded that glial neoplasms of varied type, including fibrillary astrocytomas, may be labeled by antibodies to cytokeratins (particularly the AE1/3 'cocktail')[359,360,389] and, on occasion, EMA.[369] It would appear that CAM 5.2, CK7, CK20, and Ber-EP4 perform in more discriminating fashion as epithelial markers in this regard.[1348] GFAP labeling of metastatic carcinomas, while documented, is an exceptional event.[389,940,1348] As metastases usually remain faithful to the donor immunophenotype, immunohistochemical assessment may focus the search for a systemic primary in the patient who does not have a history of cancer. Nuclear labeling for thyroid transcription factor-1, for example, should raise strong question of a metastatic deposit deriving from a differentiated carcinoma of the thyroid gland or nonsquamous carcinoma of the lung.[1355] Depending on the histologic findings in a given case, the differential diagnosis of a suspected metastasis may include, in addition to an epithelioid or sarcomatoid glioblastoma, the capillary hemangioblastoma, papillary ependymoma, choroid plexus tumor, and meningioma. Each of these is considered separately elsewhere in this chapter. We refer the reader to the foregoing discussion of fibrillary astrocytic neoplasms for a brief account of lipid-rich, adenoid or partially squamous glioblastomas and gliosarcomas that may masquerade as cerebral metastases.

In closing, mention is made of certain unusual forms or presentations of secondary CNS involvement by malignant neoplasms. These include diffuse seeding of the periventricular tissues by metastatic small cell carcinomas of the lung[1359] (a pattern of spread mimicking the topography of some primary CNS lymphomas), miliary or 'encephalitic' cerebral carcinomatosis or melanomatosis with widespread vascular cuffing by tumor cells on microscopic study but no conspicuous mass lesions,[1338,1354] and occlusion of major cerebral vessels by neoplastic emboli resulting in ischemic stroke.[1345] Intracardiac tumors such as myxomas are the lesions most often implicated in cerebral infarction secondary to neoplastic embolization, but this phenomenon has also been recorded in association with carcinomas arising in the head and neck, lungs, colon, and other visceral sites. As mentioned in the discussion of primary mesenchymal tumors of the CNS, deposits derived from occult atrial myxomas may be misconstrued as cerebral epithelioid hemangioendotheliomas.[1082] Atrial myxomas are also responsible for most neoplastic cerebrovascular aneurysms,[118] a metastatic complication of cancer noted in our prior treatment of vascular disorders. Yet another vascular complication of intracranial metastasis is subdural hemorrhage secondary to dura-based lesions.[1339]

Acknowledgments

Donna Bauer prepared the manuscript, hunted down references, and propped me up throughout. The photographic expertise of Allyne Manzo and Kin Kong should be plain. Dr Rosemary Purrazzella, my wife, was patience itself and will hopefully find this useful in her own practice of surgical pathology (small reward).

References

NORMAL ANATOMY

1 Fuller GN, Burger PC. Central nervous system. In Mills SE (ed.): Histology for pathologists, ed. 3. Philadelphia, 2007, Lippincott Williams & Wilkins, pp. 273–319.

CONGENITAL ABNORMALITIES

CRANIOSPINAL DYSRAPHISM

2 Bale PM. Sacrococcygeal developmental abnormalities and tumors in children. Perspect Pediatr Pathol 1984, **8**: 9–56.

3 Chadduck WM, Uthman EO. Squamous cell carcinoma and meningomyelocele. Neurosurgery 1984, **14**: 601–603.

4 Chakrabortty S, Oi S, Yoshida Y, Yamada H, Yamaguchi M, Tamaki N, Matsumoto S. Myelomeningocele and thick filum terminale with tethered cord appearing as a

human tail. Case report. J Neurosurg 1993, **78**: 966–969.

5 Ebisu T, Odake G, Fujimoto M, Ueda S, Tsujii H, Morimoto M, Sawada T. Neurenteric cysts with meningomyelocele or meningocele. Split notochord syndrome. Childs Nerv Syst 1990, **6**: 465–467.

6 Erkulvrawatr S, El Gammal T, Hawkins J, Green JB, Srinivasan G. Intrathoracic meningoceles and neurofibromatosis. Arch Neurol 1979, **36**: 557–559.

7 Harding B, Copp AJ. Malformations. In Love S, Louis DN, Ellison DW (eds): Greenfield's neuropathology, ed. 8, vol. 1. London, 2008, Arnold, pp. 335–479.

8 Ibrahim AE, Myles L, Lang DA, Ellison DW. Case of the month: June 1998 – 2 year old boy with lumbosacral mass. Brain Pathol 1998, **8**: 817–818.

9 Koen JL, McLendon RE, George TM. Intradural spinal teratoma: evidence for a dysembryogenic origin. Report of four cases. J Neurosurg 1998, **89**: 844–851.

10 Lalwani AK, Jackler RK, Harsh GR 4th, Butt FY. Bilateral temporal bone encephaloceles after cranial irradiation. Case report. J Neurosurg 1993, **79**: 596–599.

11 Morris GF, Murphy K, Rorke LB, James HE. Spinal hamartomas: a distinct clinical entity. J Neurosurg 1998, **88**: 954–957.

12 Rajpal S, Salamat MS, Tubbs RS, Kelly DR, Oakes WJ, Iskandar BJ. Tethering tracts in spina bifida occulta: revisiting an established nomenclature. J Neurosurg Spine 2007, **7**: 315–322.

13 Yamada S, Mandybur GT, Thompson JR. Dorsal midline proboscis associated with diastematomyelia and tethered cord syndrome. Case report. J Neurosurg 1996, **85**: 709–712.

NEUROGLIAL AND MENINGEAL HETEROTOPIAS

14 Abel TJ, Chowdhary A, Thapa M, Rutledge JC, Gruss J, Manning S, Avellino AM. Ectopic glioneuronal tissue in the middle cranial fossa region. Report of four cases. J Neurosurg Pediatr 2009, **3**: 188–196.

15 Bale PM, Hughes L, de Silva M. Sequestrated meningoceles of scalp: extracranial meningeal heterotopia. Hum Pathol 1990, **21**: 1156–1163.

16 Bossen EH, Hudson WR. Oligodendroglioma arising in heterotopic brain tissue of the soft palate and nasopharynx. Am J Surg Pathol 1987, **11**: 571–574.

17 Call NB, Baylis HI. Cerebellar heterotopia in the orbit. Arch Ophthalmol 1980, **98**: 717–719.

18 Chan JK, Lau WH. Nasal astrocytoma or nasal glial heterotopia? Arch Pathol Lab Med 1989, **113**: 943–945.

19 Gold AH, Sharer LR, Walden RH. Central nervous system heterotopia in association with cleft palate. Plast Reconstr Surg 1980, **66**: 434–441.

20 Hirano S, Houdou S, Hasegawa M, Kamei A, Takashima S. Clinicopathologic studies on leptomeningeal glioneuronal heterotopia in congenital anomalies. Pediatr Neurol 1992, **8**: 441–444.

21 Kershisnik MM, Kaplan C, Craven CM, Carey JC, Townsend JJ, Knisely AS. Intrapulmonary neuroglial heterotopia. Arch Pathol Lab Med 1992, **116**: 1043–1046.

22 Lee SC, Henry MM, Gonzalez-Crussi F. Simultaneous occurrence of melanotic neuroectodermal tumor and brain heterotopia in the oropharynx. Cancer 1976, **38**: 249–253.

23 Matyja E, Grajkowska W, Marchel A, Rysz A, Majkowska-Zwolinska B. Ectopic cerebellum in anterior cranial fossa: report of a unique case associated with skull congenital malformations and epilepsy. Am J Surg Pathol 2007, **31**: 322–325.

24 Oya S, Kawahara N, Aoki S, Hayashi N, Shibahara J, Izumi M, Kirino T. Intracranial extracerebral glioneuronal heterotopia. Case report and review of the literature. J Neurosurg (Pediatrics 1) 2005, **102**: 105–112.

25 Patterson K, Kapur S, Chandra RS. 'Nasal gliomas' and related brain heterotopias: a pathologist's perspective. Pediatr Pathol 1986, **5**: 353–362.

26 Sun LS, Sun ZP, Ma XC, Li TJ. Glial choristoma in the oral and maxillofacial region. A clinicopathologic study of 6 cases. Arch Pathol Lab Med 2008, **132**: 984–988.

27 Suster S, Rosai J. Hamartoma of the scalp with ectopic meningothelial elements. A distinctive benign soft tissue lesion that may simulate angiosarcoma. Am J Surg Pathol 1990, **14**: 1–11.

CHORISTOMAS AND NON-NEUROEPITHELIAL HAMARTOMAS

28 Abel TJ, Chowdhary A, Jallo G, Wang PP, Burger P, Avellino AM. Thoracic spinal cord compression by intramedullary hamartomatous tissue in a young boy: case report. Neurosurgery 2008, **62**: E1380.

29 Abel TW, Curtis M, Lin DD, Burger PC, Cummings TJ. Complex choristoma of the gyrus rectus: a distinct clinicopathologic entity? Am J Surg Pathol 2006, **30**: 625–629.

30 Apostolides PJ, Spetzler RF, Johnson PC. Ectomesenchymal hamartoma (benign 'ectomesenchymoma') of the VIIIth nerve: case report. Neurosurgery 1995, **37**: 1204–1207.

31 Curry B, Taylor CW, Fisher AW. Salivary gland heterotopia: a unique cerebellopontine angle tumor. Arch Pathol Lab Med 1982, **106**: 35–38.

32 Fix SE, Nelson J, Schochet SS Jr. Focal leptomeningeal rhabdomyomatosis of the posterior fossa. Arch Pathol Lab Med 1989, **113**: 872–873.

33 Giangaspero F, Guiducci A, Lenz FA, Mastronardi L, Burger PC. Meningioma with meningioangiomatosis: a condition mimicking invasive meningiomas in children and young adults. Report of two cases and review of the literature. Am J Surg Pathol 1999, **23**: 872–875.

34 Goates JJ, Dickson DW, Horoupian DS. Meningioangiomatosis: an immunocytochemical study. Acta Neuropathol 1991, **82**: 527–532.

35 Ho KL. Ecchordosis physaliphora and chordoma: a comparative ultrastructural study. Clin Neuropathol 1985, **4**: 77–86.

36 Kollias SS, Crone KR, Ball WS Jr, Prenger EC, Ballard ET. Meningioangiomatosis of the brain stem. Case report. J Neurosurg 1994, **80**: 732–735.

37 Lena G, Dufour T, Gambarelli D, Chabrol B, Mancini J. Choristoma of the intracranial maxillary nerve in a child. Case report. J Neurosurg 1994, **81**: 788–791.

38 Lombardo L, Mateos JH, Barroeta FF. Subarachnoid hemorrhage due to endometriosis of the spinal canal. Neurology 1968, **18**: 423–426.

39 Lopez JI, Ereno C, Oleaga L, Areitio E. Meningioangiomatosis and oligodendroglioma in a 15-year-old boy. Arch Pathol Lab Med 1996, **120**: 587–590.

40 Perry A, Kurtkaya-Yapicier O, Scheithauer BW, Robinson S, Prayson RA, Kleinschmidt-DeMasters BK, Stemmer-Rachamimov AO, Gutmann DH. Insights into meningioangiomatosis with and without meningioma: a clinicopathologic and genetic series of 24 cases with review of the literature. Brain Pathol 2005, **15**: 55–65.

41 Rodriguez F, Scheithauer BW, Ockner DM, Giannini C. Solitary fibrous tumor of the cerebellopontine angle with salivary gland heterotopia: a unique presentation. Am J Surg Pathol 2004, **28**: 139–142.

42 Sharma MC, Sarkar C, Jain D, Suri V, Garg A, Vaishya S. Uterus-like mass of mullerian origin in the lumbosacral region causing cord tethering. Report of two cases. J Neurosurg Spine 2007, **6**: 73–76.

43 Takeshima Y, Amatya VJ, Nakayori F, Nakano T, Sugiyama K, Inai K. Meningioangiomatosis occurring in a young male without neurofibromatosis: with special reference to its histogenesis and loss of heterozygosity in the NF2 gene region. Am J Surg Pathol 2002, **26**: 125–129.

44 Thibodeau LL, Prioleau GR, Manuelidis EE, Merino MJ, Heafner MD. Cerebral endometriosis. Case report. J Neurosurg 1987, **66**: 609–610.

45 Toda H, Kondo A, Iwasaki K. Neuroradiological characteristics of ecchordosis physaliphora. Case report and review of the literature. J Neurosurg 1998, **89**: 830–834.

46 Vajramani G, Devi I, Santosh V, Hegde T, Das BS, Das S, Shankar SK. Benign triton tumor of the trigeminal nerve. Childs Nerv Syst 1999, **15**: 140–144.

47 Vandewalle G, Brucher JM, Michotte A. Intracranial facial nerve rhabdomyoma. Case report. J Neurosurg 1995, **83**: 919–922.

48 Wiebe S, Munoz DG, Smith S, Lee DH. Meningioangiomatosis. A comprehensive analysis of clinical and laboratory features. Brain 1999, **122**(Pt 4): 709–726.

CYSTS OF THE CENTRAL NEURAXIS

49 Almefty R, Arnautovic KI, Webber BL. Multilevel bilateral calcified thoracic spinal synovial cysts. J Neurosurg Spine 2008, **8**: 473–477.

50 Beatty RM, Hornig GW, Hanson EJ Jr. Protruding arachnoid granulations mimicking dermoid cysts. J Pediatr Surg 1989, **24**: 411–413.

51 Bejjani GK, Wright DC, Schessel D, Sekhar LN. Endodermal cysts of the posterior fossa. Report of three cases and review of the literature. J Neurosurg 1998, **89**: 326–335.

52 Cannon TC, Bane BL, Kistler D, Schoenhals GW, Hahn M, Leech RW, Brumback RA. Primary intracerebellar osteosarcoma arising within an epidermoid cyst. Arch Pathol Lab Med 1998, **122**: 737–739.

53 Chitkara U, Cogswell C, Norton K, Wilkins IA, Mehalek K, Berkowitz RL. Choroid plexus cysts in the fetus: a benign anatomic variant or pathologic entity? Report of 41 cases and review of the literature. Obstet Gynecol 1988, **72**: 185–189.

54 Christov C, Chretien F, Brugieres P, Djindjian M. Giant supratentorial enterogenous cyst: report of a case, literature review, and discussion of pathogenesis. Neurosurgery 2004, **54**: 759–763; discussion 763.

55 Ciappetta P, D'Urso PI, Luzzi S, Ingravallo G, Cimmino A, Resta L. Cystic dilation of the ventriculus terminalis in adults. Report of 2 cases. J Neurosurg Spine 2008, **8**: 92–99.

56 Ciricillo SF, Davis RL, Wilson CB. Neuroepithelial cysts of the posterior fossa. Case report. J Neurosurg 1990, **72**: 302–305.

57 Davis G, Fitt GJ, Kalnins RM, Mitchell LA. Increased perivascular spaces mimicking frontal lobe tumor. J Neurosurg 2002, **97**: 723.

58 Del Bigio MR, Jay V, Drake JM. Prepontine cyst lined by respiratory epithelium with squamous metaplasia: immunohistochemical and ultrastructural study. Acta Neuropathol 1992, **83**: 564–568.

59 Fain JS, Tomlinson FH, Scheithauer BW, Parisi JE, Fletcher GP, Kelly PJ, Miller GM. Symptomatic glial cysts of the pineal gland. J Neurosurg 1994, **80**: 454–460.

60 Friede RL, Yasargil MG. Supratentorial intracerebral epithelial (ependymal) cysts: review, case reports, and fine structure. J Neurol Neurosurg Psychiatry 1977, **40**: 127–137.

61 Fuller G, Ribalta T. Dermoid cyst, epidermoid cyst and dermal sinus. In McLendon RE, Rosenblum MK, Bigner DD (eds): Russell and Rubinstein's pathology of tumors of the nervous system, ed. 7. London, 2006, Hodder Arnold, pp. 583–590.

62 Gherardi R, Lacombe MJ, Poirier J, Roucayrol AM, Wechsler J. Asymptomatic encephalic intraparenchymatous neuroepithelial cysts. Acta Neuropathol 1984, **63**: 264–268.

63 Gluszcz A. A cancer arising in a dermoid of the brain. A case report. J Neuropathol Exp Neurol 1962, **21**: 383–387.

64 Halcrow SJ, Crawford PJ, Craft AW. Epidermoid spinal cord tumour after lumbar puncture. Arch Dis Child 1985, **60**: 978–979.

65 Hamburger CH, Buttner A, Weis S. Dural cysts in the cervical region. Report of three cases and review of the literature. J Neurosurg 1998, **89**: 310–313.

66 Hatem O, Bedou G, Negre C, Bertrand JL, Camo J. Intraspinal cervical degenerative cyst. Report of three cases. J Neurosurg 2001, **95**: 139–142.

67 Hitchcock MG, Ellington KS, Friedman AH, Provenzaie JM, McLendon RE. Shadow cells in an intracranial dermoid cyst. Arch Pathol Lab Med 1995, **119**: 371–373.

68 Ho KL, Chason JL. A glioependymal cyst of the cerebellopontine angle. Immunohistochemical and ultrastructural studies. Acta Neuropathol 1987, **74**: 382–388.

69 Ho KL, Garcia JH. Colloid cysts of the third ventricle: ultrastructural features are compatible with endodermal derivation. Acta Neuropathol 1992, **83**: 605–612.

70 Ho KL, Tiel R. Intraspinal bronchogenic cyst: ultrastructural study of the lining epithelium. Acta Neuropathol 1989, **78**: 513–520.

71 Hofmann BM, Kreutzer J, Saeger W, Buchfelder M, Blumcke I, Fahlbusch R, Buslei R. Nuclear beta-catenin accumulation as reliable marker for the differentiation between cystic craniopharyngiomas and rathke cleft cysts: a clinico-pathologic approach. Am J Surg Pathol 2006, **30**: 1595–1603.

72 Isla A, Palacios J, Roda JM, Gutierrez M, Gonzalez C, Blazquez MG. Neuroepithelial cyst in the optic nerve. Case report. J Neurosurg 1987, **67**: 137–139.

73 Keogh AJ, Timperley WR. Atypical hidradenoma arising in a dermoid cyst of the spinal canal. J Pathol 1975, **117**: 207–209.

74 Kim KM, Kang SJ, Kim DS, Chi JG, Kim SM. Congenital intraorbital optic nerve cyst. Case report. J Neurosurg 1999, **91**: 325–327.

75 Lach B, Scheithauer BW, Gregor A, Wick MR. Colloid cyst of the third ventricle. A comparative immunohistochemical study of neuraxis cysts and choroid plexus epithelium. J Neurosurg 1993, **78**: 101–111.

76 Link MJ, Cohen PL, Breneman JC, Tew JM Jr. Malignant squamous degeneration of a cerebellopontine angle epidermoid tumor. Case report. J Neurosurg 2002, **97**: 1237–1243.

77 Lunardi P, Missori P, Rizzo A, Gagliardi FM. Chemical meningitis in ruptured intracranial dermoid. Case report and review of the literature. Surg Neurol 1989, **32**: 449–452.

78 Marbacher S, Barth A, Arnold M, Seiler RW. Multiple spinal extradural meningeal cysts presenting as acute paraplegia. Case report and review of the literature. J Neurosurg Spine 2007, **6**: 465–472.

79 Mathiesen T, Grane P, Lindgren L, Lindquist C. Third ventricle colloid cysts: a consecutive 12-year series. J Neurosurg 1997, **86**: 5–12.

80 Miyagi Y, Suzuki SO, Iwaki T, Ishido K, Araki T, Kamikaseda K. Magnetic resonance appearance of multiple intracranial epidermoid cysts: intrathecal seeding of the cysts? Case report. J Neurosurg 2000, **92**: 711–714.

81 Montaldi S, Deruaz JP, Cai ZT, de Tribolet N. Symptomatic xanthogranuloma of the third ventricle: report of two cases and review of the literature. Surg Neurol 1989, **32**: 200–205.

82 Nabors MW, Pait TG, Byrd EB, Karim NO, Davis DO, Kobrine AI, Rizzoli HV. Updated assessment and current classification of spinal meningeal cysts. J Neurosurg 1988, **68**: 366–377.

83 Nahed BV, Darbar A, Doiron R, Saad A, Robson CD, Smith ER. Acute hydrocephalus secondary to obstruction of the foramen of Monro and cerebral aqueduct caused by a choroid plexus cyst in the lateral ventricle. Case report. J Neurosurg (3 Suppl Pediatrics) 2007, **107**: 236–239.

84 Nakajima Y, Yoshimine T, Ogawa M, Takanashi M, Nakamuta K, Maruno M, Hasegawa H, Yokota J. A giant intracranial mucocele associated with an orbitoethmoidal osteoma. Case report. J Neurosurg 2000, **92**: 697–701.

85 Nakasu Y, Handa J, Watanabe K. Progressive neurological deficits with benign intracerebral cysts. Report of two cases. J Neurosurg 1986, **65**: 706–709.

86 Odake G, Tenjin H, Murakami N. Cyst of the choroid plexus in the lateral ventricle: case report and review of the literature. Neurosurgery 1990, **27**: 470–476.

87 Ojemann JG, Moran CJ, Gokden M, Dacey RG Jr. Sagittal sinus occlusion by intraluminal dural cysts. Report of two cases. J Neurosurg 1999, **91**: 867–870.

88 Perry A, Scheithauer BW, Zaias BW, Minassian HV. Aggressive enterogenous cyst with extensive craniospinal spread: case report. Neurosurgery 1999, **44**: 401–404; discussion 404–405.

89 Powers JM, Dodds HM. Primary actinomycoma of the third ventricle – the colloid cyst. A histochemical and ultrastructural study. Acta Neuropathol 1977, **37**: 21–26.

90 Reddy PK, Rao GP, Prakasham A, Purnanand A, Sulochana C, Kumar RS, Reddy YR, Chandramala MS, Indumathi D. Intracerebral polyposis. Case report. J Neurosurg 1993, **78**: 294–296.

91 Rengachary SS, Watanabe I. Ultrastructure and pathogenesis of intracranial arachnoid cysts. J Neuropathol Exp Neurol 1981, **40**: 61–83.

92 Ribalta T, Fuller GN. Arachnoid cyst. In McLendon RE, Rosenblum MK, Bigner DD (eds): Russell and Rubinstein's pathology of tumors of the nervous system, ed. 7. London, 2006, Hodder Arnold, pp. 607–609.

93 Rosenberg AE, O'Connell JX, Ojemann RG, Plata MJ, Palmer WE. Giant cystic arachnoid granulations: a rare cause of lytic skull lesions. Hum Pathol 1993, **24**: 438–441.

94 Rotondo M, D'Avanzo R, Natale M, Pasqualetto L, Bocchetti A, Agozzino L, Scuotto A. Intramedullary neurenteric cysts of the spine. Report of three cases. J Neurosurg Spine 2005, **2**: 372–376.

95 Sabo RA, Tracy PT, Weinger JM. A series of 60 juxtafacet cysts: clinical presentation, the role of spinal instability, and treatment. J Neurosurg 1996, **85**: 560–565.

96 Sahara Y, Nagasaka T, Takayasu M, Takagi T, Hata N, Yoshida J. Recurrence of a neurenteric cyst with malignant transformation in the foramen magnum after total resection. Case report. J Neurosurg 2001, **95**: 341–345.

97 Sharma A, Karande S, Sayal P, Ranadive N, Dwivedi N. Spinal intramedullary arachnoid cyst in a 4-year-old girl: a rare cause of treatable acute quadriparesis: case report. J Neurosurg 2005, **102**: 403–406.

98 Silverberg GD. Simple cysts of the cerebellum. J Neurosurg 1971, **35**: 320–327.

99 Smith CM, Timperley WR. Multiple intraspinal and intracranial epidermoids and lipomata following gunshot injury. Neuropathol Appl Neurobiol 1984, **10**: 235–239.

100 Takei H, Fuller GN, Powell SZ. Intracranial cysts of endodermal or respiratory epithelioid origin. In McLendon RE, Rosenblum MK, Bigner DD (eds): Russell and Rubinstein's pathology of tumors of the nervous system, ed. 7. London, 2006, Hodder Arnold, pp. 591–598.

101 Tsuchida T, Hruban RH, Carson BS, Phillips PC. Colloid cysts of the third ventricle: immunohistochemical evidence for nonneuroepithelial differentiation. Hum Pathol 1992, **23**: 811–816.

102 Voelker JL, Campbell RL, Muller J. Clinical, radiographic, and pathological features of symptomatic Rathke's cleft cysts. J Neurosurg 1991, **74**: 535–544.

103 Voyadzis JM, Bhargava P, Henderson FC. Tarlov cysts: a study of 10 cases with review of the literature. J Neurosurg (Spine 1) 2001, **95**: 25–32.

104 Weinand ME, Rengachary SS, McGregor DH, Watanabe I. Intradiploic arachnoid cysts. Report of two cases. J Neurosurg 1989, **70**: 954–958.

105 Weisberg LA. Non-neoplastic gliotic cerebellar cysts: clinical and computed tomographic correlations. Neuroradiology 1982, **24**: 53–57.

106 Wilkins RH, Burger PC. Benign intraparenchymal brain cysts without an epithelial lining. J Neurosurg 1988, **68**: 378–382.

107 Xin W, Rubin MA, McKeever PE. Differential expression of cytokeratins 8 and 20 distinguishes craniopharyngioma from rathke cleft cyst. Arch Pathol Lab Med 2002, **126**: 1174–1178.

CEREBROVASCULAR DISORDERS

CEREBRAL INFARCTION

108 Chuaqui R, Tapia J. Histologic assessment of the age of recent brain infarcts in man. J Neuropathol Exp Neurol 1993, **52**: 481–489.

109 Ferrer I, Kaste M, Kalimo H. Vascular diseases. In Love S, Louis DW, Ellison DW (eds): Greenfield's neuropathology, ed. 8, vol. 1. London, 2008, Arnold, pp. 121–240.

110 Mena H, Cadavid D, Rushing EJ. Human cerebral infarct: a proposed histopathologic classification based on 137 cases. Acta Neuropathol 2004, **108**: 524–530.

INTRACRANIAL ANEURYSMS

111 Bohmfalk GL, Story JL, Wissinger JP, Brown WE Jr. Bacterial intracranial aneurysm. J Neurosurg 1978, **48**: 369–382.

112 Challa VR, Moody DM, Bell MA. The Charcot–Bouchard aneurysm controversy: impact of a new histologic technique. J Neuropathol Exp Neurol 1992, **51**: 264–271.

113 Chambi I, Tasker RR, Gentili F, Lougheed WM, Smyth HS, Marshall J, Young I, Deck J, Shrubb J. Gauze-induced granuloma ('gauzoma'): an uncommon complication of gauze reinforcement of berry aneurysms. J Neurosurg 1990, **72**: 163–170.

114 Chang IB, Cho BM, Park SH, Yoon DY, Oh SM. Metastatic choriocarcinoma with multiple neoplastic intracranial microaneurysms: case report. J Neurosurg 2008, **108**: 1014–1017.

115 Cohen NR, Tan TS, Barker CS. Intracerebral haemorrhage secondary to metastasis from presumed non-small cell lung carcinoma. Neuropathol Appl Neurobiol 2004, **30**: 419–422.

116 Drake CG, Peerless SJ. Giant fusiform intracranial aneurysms. Review of 120 patients treated surgically from 1965 to 1992. J Neurosurg 1997, **87**: 141–162.

117 Erbengi A, Inci S. Pheochromocytoma and multiple intracranial aneurysms. Is it a coincidence? Case report. J Neurosurg 1997, **87**: 764–767.

118 Furuya K, Sasaki T, Yoshimoto Y, Okada Y, Fujimaki T, Kirino T. Histologically verified cerebral aneurysm formation secondary to embolism from cardiac myxoma. Case report. J Neurosurg 1995, **83**: 170–173.

119 Inagawa T, Hirano A. Ruptured intracranial aneurysms: an autopsy study of 133 patients. Surg Neurol 1990, **33**: 117–123.

120 Juvela S, Porras M, Poussa K. Natural history of unruptured intracranial aneurysms: probability of and risk factors for aneurysm rupture. J Neurosurg 2000, **93**: 379–387.

121 Lammie GA. Hypertensive cerebral small vessel disease and stroke. Brain Pathol 2002, **12**: 358–370.

122 McCormick WF, Nofzinger JD. Saccular intracranial aneurysms. An autopsy study. J Neurosurg 1965, **22**: 155–159.

123 Ronkainen A, Hernesniemi J, Tromp G. Special features of familial intracranial aneurysms: report of 215 familial aneurysms. Neurosurgery 1995, **37**: 43–46; discussion 46–47.

124 Schievink WI, Puumala MR, Meyer FB, Raffel C, Katzmann JA, Parisi JE. Giant intracranial aneurysm and fibromuscular dysplasia in an adolescent with alpha 1-antitrypsin deficiency. J Neurosurg 1996, **85**: 503–506.

125 Sciubba DM, Gallia GL, Recinos P, Garonzik IM, Clatterbuck RE. Intracranial aneurysm following radiation therapy during childhood for a brain tumor. Case report and review of the literature. J Neurosurg 2006, **105**: 134–139.

126 Shokunbi MT, Vinters HV, Kaufmann JC. Fusiform intracranial aneurysms. Clinicopathologic features. Surg Neurol 1988, **29**: 263–270.

127 Wakai S, Kumakura N, Nagai M. Lobar intracerebral hemorrhage. A clinical, radiographic, and pathological study of 29 consecutive operated cases with negative angiography. J Neurosurg 1992, **76**: 231–238.

128 Wakai S, Nagai M. Histological verification of microaneurysms as a cause of cerebral haemorrhage in surgical specimens. J Neurol Neurosurg Psychiatry 1989, **52**: 595–599.

129 Weir B. Unruptured intracranial aneurysms. A review. J Neurosurg 2002, **96**: 3–42.

VASCULAR MALFORMATIONS

130 Amin-Hanjani S, Robertson R, Arginteanu MS, Scott RM. Familial intracranial arteriovenous malformations. Case report and review of the literature. Pediatr Neurosurg 1998, **29**: 208–213.

131 Benhaiem N, Poirier J, Hurth M. Arteriovenous fistulae of the meninges draining into the spinal veins. A histological study of 28 cases. Acta Neuropathol (Berl) 1983, **62**: 103–111.

132 Brown RD Jr, Wiebers DO, Forbes G, O'Fallon WM, Piepgras DG, Marsh WR, Maciunas RJ. The natural history of unruptured intracranial arteriovenous malformations. J Neurosurg 1988, **68**: 352–357.

133 Burn S, Gunny R, Phipps K, Gaze M, Hayward R. Incidence of cavernoma development in children after radiotherapy for brain tumors. J Neurosurg (5 Suppl Pediatrics) 2007, **106**: 379–383.

134 Carleton CC, Cauthen JC. Vascular ('arteriovenous') malformations of the choroid plexus. Arch Pathol 1975, **99**: 286–288.

135 Chang SD, Steinberg GK, Rosario M, Crowley RS, Hevner RF. Mixed arteriovenous malformation and capillary telangiectasia: a rare subset of mixed vascular malformations. Case report. J Neurosurg 1997, **86**: 699–703.

136 Clatterbuck RE, Cohen B, Gailloud P, Murphy K, Rigamonti D. Vertebral hemangiomas associated with familial cerebral cavernous malformation: segmental disease expression. Case report. J Neurosurg (Spine 2) 2002, **97**: 227–230.

137 Comi AM. Pathophysiology of Sturge–Weber syndrome. J Child Neurol 2003, **18**: 509–516.

138 Dobyns WB, Michels VV, Groover RV, Mokri B, Trautmann JC, Forbes GS, Laws ER Jr. Familial cavernous malformations of the central nervous system and retina. Ann Neurol 1987, **21**: 578–583.

139 Farrell DF, Forno LS. Symptomatic capillary telangiectasis of the brainstem without hemorrhage. Report of an unusual case. Neurology 1970, **20**: 341–346.

140 Hamada J, Yano S, Kai Y, Koga K, Morioka M, Ishimaru Y, Ushio Y. Histopathological study of venous aneurysms in patients with dural arteriovenous fistulas. J Neurosurg 2000, **92**: 1023–1027.

141 Johnson WD, Petrie MM. Variety of spinal vascular pathology seen in adult Cobb syndrome. J Neurosurg Spine 2009, **10**: 430–435.

142 Kang HS, Han MH, Kwon BJ, Yoon BW, Chang KH. Cerebellopontomandibular vascular malformation: a rare type of cerebrofacial arteriovenous metameric syndrome. Case report. J Neurosurg 2005, **102**: 156–160.

143 Labauge P, Enjolras O, Bonerandi JJ, Laberge S, Dandurand M, Joujoux JM, Tournier-Lasserve E. An association between autosomal dominant cerebral cavernomas and a distinctive hyperkeratotic cutaneous vascular malformation in 4 families. Ann Neurol 1999, **45**: 250–254.

144 Laurans MS, DiLuna ML, Shin D, Niazi F, Voorhees JR, Nelson-Williams C, Johnson EW, Siegel AM, Steinberg GK, Berg MJ, Scott RM, Tedeschi G, Enevoldson TP, Anson J, Rouleau GA, Ogilvy C, Awad IA, Lifton RP, Gunel M. Mutational analysis of 206 families with cavernous malformations. J Neurosurg 2003, **99**: 38–43.

145 Lobato RD, Perez C, Rivas JJ, Cordobes F. Clinical, radiological, and pathological spectrum of angiographically occult intracranial vascular malformations. Analysis of 21 cases and review of the literature. J Neurosurg 1988, **68**: 518–531.

146 Lombardi D, Scheithauer BW, Piepgras D, Meyer FB, Forbes GS. 'Angioglioma' and the arteriovenous malformation–glioma association. J Neurosurg 1991, **75**: 589–596.

147 Mandybur TI, Nazek M. Cerebral arteriovenous malformations. A detailed morphological and immunohistochemical study using actin. Arch Pathol Lab Med 1990, **114**: 970–973.

148 Matias-Guiu X, Alejo M, Sole T, Ferrer I, Noboa R, Bartumeus F. Cavernous angiomas of the cranial nerves. Report of two cases. J Neurosurg 1990, **73**: 620–622.

149 Meyer B, Stangl AP, Schramm J. Association of venous and true arteriovenous malformation: a rare entity among mixed vascular malformations of the brain. Case report. J Neurosurg 1995, **83**: 141–144.

150 Meyer FB, Lombardi D, Scheithauer B, Nichols DA. Extra-axial cavernous hemangiomas involving the dural sinuses. J Neurosurg 1990, **73**: 187–192.

151 Musunuru K, Hillard VH, Murali R. Widespread central nervous system cavernous malformations associated with cafe-au-lait skin lesions. Case report. J Neurosurg 2003, **99**: 412–415.

152 Naff NJ, Wemmer J, Hoenig-Rigamonti K, Rigamonti DR. A longitudinal study of patients with venous malformations. Documentation of a negligible hemorrhage risk and benign natural history. Neurology 1998, **50**: 1709–1714.

153 Nazek M, Mandybur TI, Kashiwagi S. Oligodendroglial proliferative abnormality associated with arteriovenous malformation. Report of three cases with review of the literature. Neurosurgery 1988, **23**: 781–785.

154 Nishijima M, Takaku A, Endo S, Kuwayama N, Koizumi F, Sato H, Owada K. Etiological evaluation of dural arteriovenous malformations of the lateral and sigmoid sinuses based on histopathological examinations. J Neurosurg 1992, **76**: 600–606.

155 Ondra SL, Troupp H, George ED, Schwab K. The natural history of symptomatic arteriovenous malformations of the brain. A 24-year follow-up assessment. J Neurosurg 1990, **73**: 387–391.

156 Pagni CA, Canavero S, Forni M. Report of a cavernoma of the cauda equina and review of the literature. Surg Neurol 1990, **33**: 124–131.

157 Partington MD, Rufenacht DA, Marsh WR, Piepgras DG. Cranial and sacral dural arteriovenous fistulas as a cause of myelopathy. J Neurosurg 1992, **76**: 615–622.

158 Pozzati E, Marliani AF, Zucchelli M, Foschini MP, Dall'Olio M, Lanzino G. The neurovascular triad: mixed cavernous, capillary, and venous malformations of the brainstem. J Neurosurg 2007, **107**: 1113–1119.

159 Rigamonti D, Johnson PC, Spetzler RF, Hadley MN, Drayer BP. Cavernous malformations and capillary telangiectasia: a spectrum within a single pathological entity. Neurosurgery 1991, **28**: 60–64.

160 Roda JM, Carceller F, Perez-Higueras A, Morales C. Encapsulated intracerebral hematomas: a defined entity. J Neurosurg 1993, **78**: 829–833.

161 Rodriguez FJ, Crum BA, Krauss WE, Scheithauer BW, Giannini C. Venous congestive myelopathy: a mimic of neoplasia. Mod Pathol 2005, **18**: 710–718.

162 Román G, Fisher M, Perl DP, Poser CM. Neurological manifestations of hereditary hemorrhagic telangiectasia (Rendu–Osler–Weber disease). Report of 2 cases and review of the literature. Ann Neurol 1978, **4**: 130–144.

163 Rosenblum B, Oldfield EH, Doppman JL, Di Chiro G. Spinal arteriovenous malformations. A comparison of dural arteriovenous fistulas and intradural AVMs in 81 patients. J Neurosurg 1987, **67**: 795–802.

164 Schneider BF, Eberhard DA, Steiner LE. Histopathology of arteriovenous malformations after gamma knife radiosurgery. J Neurosurg 1997, **87**: 352–357.

165 Schweitzer JS, Chang BS, Madsen P, Vinuela F, Martin NA, Marroquin CE, Vinters HV. The pathology of arteriovenous malformations of the brain treated by embolotherapy. II. Results of embolization with multiple agents. Neuroradiology 1993, **35**: 468–474.

166 Simard JM, Garcia-Bengochea F, Ballinger WE Jr, Mickle JP, Quisling RG. Cavernous angioma. A review of 126 collected and 12 new clinical cases. Neurosurgery 1986, **18**: 162–172.

167 Tomlinson FH, Rufenacht DA, Sundt TM Jr, Nichols DA, Fode NC. Arteriovenous fistulas of the brain and the spinal cord. J Neurosurg 1993, **79**: 16–27.

168 Tung H, Giannotta SL, Chandrasoma PT, Zee CS. Recurrent intraparenchymal hemorrhages from angiographically occult vascular malformations. J Neurosurg 1990, **73**: 174–180.

169 Vaquero J, Manrique M, Oya S, Cabezudo JM, Bravo G. Calcified telangiectatic hamartomas of the brain. Surg Neurol 1980, **13**: 453–457.

170 Yoshino M, Morita A, Shibahara J, Kirino T. Radiation-induced spinal cord cavernous malformation. Case report. J Neurosurg (Pediatrics 1) 2005, **102**: 101–104.

171 Zevgaridis D, Buttner A, Weis S, Hamburger C, Reulen HJ. Spinal epidural cavernous hemangiomas. Report of three cases and review of the literature. J Neurosurg 1998, **88**: 903–908.

PRIMARY ANGIITIS

172 Caccamo DV, Garcia JH, Ho KL. Isolated granulomatous angiitis of the spinal cord. Ann Neurol 1992, **32**: 580–582.

173 Lie JT. Primary (granulomatous) angiitis of the central nervous system. A clinicopathologic analysis of 15 new cases and a review of the literature. Hum Pathol 1992, **23**: 164–171.

174 Miller DV, Salvarani C, Hunder GG, Brown RD, Parisi JE, Christianson TJ, Giannini C. Biopsy findings in primary angiitis of the central nervous system. Am J Surg Pathol 2009, **33**: 35–43.

175 Yoong MF, Blumbergs PC, North JB. Primary (granulomatous) angiitis of the central nervous system with multiple aneurysms of spinal arteries. Case report. J Neurosurg 1993, **79**: 603–607.

176 Yuen RW, Johnson PC. Primary angiitis of the central nervous system associated with Hodgkin's disease. Arch Pathol Lab Med 1996, **120**: 573–576.

CEREBRAL AMYLOID ANGIOPATHY

177 Mandybur TI. Cerebral amyloid angiopathy: possible relationship to rheumatoid vasculitis. Neurology 1979, **29**: 1336–1340.

178 Mandybur TI. Cerebral amyloid angiopathy: the vascular pathology and complications. J Neuropathol Exp Neurol 1986, **45**: 79–90.

179 Revesz T, Ghiso J, Lashley T, Plant G, Rostagno A, Frangione B, Holton JL. Cerebral amyloid angiopathies: a pathologic, biochemical, and genetic view. J Neuropathol Exp Neurol 2003, **62**: 885–898.

180 Scolding NJ, Joseph F, Kirby PA, Mazanti I, Gray F, Mikol J, Ellison D, Hilton DA, Williams TL, MacKenzie JM, Xuereb JH, Love S. A beta-related angiitis: primary angiitis of the central nervous system associated with cerebral amyloid angiopathy. Brain 2005, **128**: 500–515.

181 Vonsattel JP, Myers RH, Hedley-Whyte ET, Ropper AH, Bird ED, Richardson EP Jr. Cerebral amyloid angiopathy without and with cerebral hemorrhages: a comparative histological study. Ann Neurol 1991, **30**: 637–649.

CADASIL

182 Kalimo H, Ruchoux MM, Viitanen M, Kalaria RN. CADASIL. A common form of hereditary arteriopathy causing brain infarcts and dementia. Brain Pathol 2002, **12**: 371–384.

EPIDURAL AND SUBDURAL HEMATOMA

183 Blumbergs P, Reilly P, Vink R. Trauma. In Love S, Louis DW, Ellison DW (eds): Greenfield's neuropathology, ed. 8, vol. 1. London, 2008, Arnold, pp. 733–832.

184 Friede RL, Schachenmayr W. The origin of subdural neomembranes. II. Fine structure of neomembranes. Am J Pathol 1978, **92**: 69–84.

185 Schachenmayr W, Friede RL. The origin of subdural neomembranes. I. Fine structure of the dura–arachnoid interface in man. Am J Pathol 1978, **92**: 53–68.

186 Wintzen AR. The clinical course of subdural haematoma. A retrospective study of aetiological, chronological and pathological features in 212 patients and a proposed classification. Brain 1980, **103**: 855–867.

187 Yamashima T, Kida S, Kubota T, Yamamoto S. The origin of psammoma bodies in the human arachnoid villi. Acta Neuropathol (Berl) 1986, **71**: 19–25.

INFLAMMATORY DISEASES

DEMYELINATING DISEASES

188 Annesley-Williams D, Farrell A, Staunton H, Brett FM. Acute demyelination, neuropathological diagnosis, and clinical evolution. J Neuropathol Exp Neurol 2000, **59**: 477–489.

189 Hook CC, Kimmel DW, Kvols LK, Scheithauer BW, Forsyth PA, Rubin J, Moertel CG, Rodriguez M. Multifocal inflammatory leukoencephalopathy with 5-fluorouracil and levamisole. Ann Neurol 1992, **31**: 262–267.

190 Hulette CM, Downey BT, Burger PC. Macrophage markers in diagnostic neuropathology. Am J Surg Pathol 1992, **16**: 493–499.

191 Kepes JJ. Large focal tumor-like demyelinating lesions of the brain. Intermediate entity between multiple sclerosis and acute disseminated encephalomyelitis? A study of 31 patients. Ann Neurol 1993, **33**: 18–27.

192 Nahser HC, Vieregge P, Nau HE, Reinhardt V. Coincidence of multiple sclerosis and glioma. Clinical and radiological remarks on two cases. Surg Neurol 1986, **26**: 45–51.

193 Nesbit GM, Forbes GS, Scheithauer BW, Okazaki H, Rodriguez M. Multiple sclerosis: histopathologic and MR and/or CT correlation in 37 cases at biopsy and three cases at autopsy. Radiology 1991, **180**: 467–474.

194 Peterson K, Rosenblum MK, Powers JM, Alvord E, Walker RW, Posner JB. Effect of brain irradiation on demyelinating lesions. Neurology 1993, **43**: 2105–2112.

195 Zagzag D, Miller DC, Kleinman GM, Abati A, Donnenfeld H, Budzilovich GN. Demyelinating disease versus tumor in surgical neuropathology. Clues to a correct pathological diagnosis. Am J Surg Pathol 1993, **17**: 537–545.

NONINFECTIOUS INFLAMMATORY AND REACTIVE DISORDERS, XANTHOMATOUS LESIONS, AND 'HISTIOCYTOSES'

196 Abrey LE, Rosenblum MK, DeAngelis LM. Sarcoidosis of the cauda equina mimicking leptomeningeal malignancy. J Neurooncol 1998, **39**: 261–265.

197 Andriko JA, Morrison A, Colegial CH, Davis BJ, Jones RV. Rosai–Dorfman disease isolated to the central nervous system: a report of 11 cases. Mod Pathol 2001, **14**: 172–178.

198 Ben Hamouda K, Jemel H, Haouet S, Khaldi M. Thoracic myelopathy caused by ossification of the ligamentum flavum. A report of 18 cases. J Neurosurg (Spine 2) 2003, **99**: 157–161.

199 Bertoni F, Unni KK, Dahlin DC, Beabout JW, Onofrio BM. Calcifying pseudoneoplasms of the neural axis. J Neurosurg 1990, **72**: 42–48.

200 Bien CG, Granata T, Antozzi C, Cross JH, Dulac O, Kurthen M, Lassmann H, Mantegazza R, Villemure JG, Spreafico R, Elger CE. Pathogenesis, diagnosis and treatment of Rasmussen encephalitis. A European consensus statement. Brain 2005, **128**: 454–471.

201 Bien CG, Schulze-Bonhage A, Deckert M, Urbach H, Helmstaedter C, Grunwald T, Schaller C, Elger CE. Limbic encephalitis not associated with neoplasm as a cause of temporal lobe epilepsy. Neurology 2000, **55**: 1823–1828.

202 Bonhomme GR, Loevner LA, Yen DM, Deems DA, Bigelow DC, Mirza N. Extensive intracranial xanthoma associated with type II hyperlipidemia. AJNR Am J Neuroradiol 2000, **21**: 353–355.

203 Bostrom J, Janssen G, Messing-Junger M, Felsberg JU, Neuen-Jacob E, Engelbrecht V, Lenard HG, Bock WJ, Reifenberger G. Multiple intracranial juvenile xanthogranulomas. Case report. J Neurosurg 2000, **93**: 335–341.

204 Bramwit M, Kalina P, Rustia-Villa M. Inflammatory pseudotumor of the choroid plexus. AJNR Am J Neuroradiol 1997, **18**: 1307–1309.

205 Brück W, Sander U, Blanckenberg P, Friede RL. Symptomatic xanthogranuloma of

choroid plexus with unilateral hydrocephalus. Case report. J Neurosurg 1991, **75**: 324–327.

206 Caselli RJ, Scheithauer BW, Bowles CA, Trenerry MR, Meyer FB, Smigielski JS, Rodriguez M. The treatable dementia of Sjögren's syndrome. Ann Neurol 1991, **30**: 98–101.

207 Chan SK, Cheuk W, Chan KT, Chan JK. IgG4-related sclerosing pachymeningitis: a previously unrecognized form of central nervous system involvement in IgG4-related sclerosing disease. Am J Surg Pathol 2009, **33**: 1249–1252.

208 de Jesus O, Inserni JA, Gonzalez A, Colon LE. Idiopathic orbital inflammation with intracranial extension. Case report. J Neurosurg 1996, **85**: 510–513.

209 Deprez M, Born J, Hauwaert C, Otto B, Reznik M. Idiopathic hypertrophic cranial pachymeningitis mimicking multiple meningiomas. Case report and review of the literature. Acta Neuropathol (Berl) 1997, **94**: 385–389.

210 Eisenberg MB, Haddad G, Al-Mefty O. Petrous apex cholesterol granulomas. Evolution and management. J Neurosurg 1997, **86**: 822–829.

211 Faure A, Khalfallah M, Perrouin-Verbe B, Caillon F, Deschamps C, Bord E, Mathe JF, Robert R. Arachnoiditis ossificans of the cauda equina. Case report and review of the literature. J Neurosurg (Spine 2) 2002, **97**: 239–243.

212 Figarella-Branger D, Gambarelli D, Perez-Castillo M, Regis J, Peragut JC, Pellissier JF. Atypical inflammatory histiocytic tumor of the cerebellum. A histological, immunohistochemical, and ultrastructural study. Am J Surg Pathol 1990, **14**: 778–783.

213 Gilliard C, De Coene B, Lahdou JB, Boutsen Y, Noel H, Godfraind C. Cervical epidural pseudotumor and multifocal fibrosclerosis. Case report and review of the literature. J Neurosurg (Spine 1) 2000, **93**: 152–156.

214 Gochman GA, Duffy K, Crandall PH, Vinters HV. Plasma cell granuloma of the brain. Surg Neurol 1990, **33**: 347–352.

215 Goto T, Kitazawa K, Tada T, Tanaka Y, Hongo K, Kobayashi S. Surgical dissemination of intracranial xanthogranulomas. Case illustration. J Neurosurg 2001, **95**: 537.

216 Graf M, Wakhloo A, Schmidtke K, Bloss H, Volk B. Sarcoidosis of the spinal cord and medulla oblongata. A pathological and neuroradiological case report. Clin Neuropathol 1994, **13**: 19–25.

217 Grant GA, Wener MH, Yaziji H, Futran N, Bronner MP, Mandel N, Mayberg MR. Destructive tophaceous calcium hydroxyapatite tumor of the infratemporal fossa. Case report and review of the literature. J Neurosurg 1999, **90**: 148–152.

218 Graus F, Keime-Guibert F, Rene R, Benyahia B, Ribalta T, Ascaso C, Escaramis G, Delattre JY. Anti-Hu-associated paraneoplastic encephalomyelitis: analysis of 200 patients. Brain 2001, **124**: 1138–1148.

219 Grois N, Prayer D, Prosch H, Lassmann H. Neuropathology of CNS disease in Langerhans cell histiocytosis. Brain 2005, **128**: 829–838.

220 Gultekin SH, Rosenfeld MR, Voltz R, Eichen J, Posner JB, Dalmau J. Paraneoplastic limbic encephalitis. Neurological symptoms, immunological findings and tumour association in 50 patients. Brain 2000, **123**: 1481–1494.

221 Hammond RR, Mackenzie IR. Xanthoma disseminatum with massive intracranial involvement. Clin Neuropathol 1995, **14**: 314–321.

222 Hart YM, Andermann F, Fish DR, Dubeau F, Robitaille Y, Rasmussen T, Berkovic S, Marino R, Yakoubian EM, Spillane K, Scaravilli F. Chronic encephalitis and epilepsy in adults and adolescents. A variant of Rasmussen's syndrome? Neurology 1997, **48**: 418–424.

223 Henter JI, Nennesmo I. Neuropathologic findings and neurologic symptoms in twenty-three children with hemophagocytic lymphohistiocytosis. J Pediatr 1997, **130**: 358–365.

224 Ito Z, Osawa Y, Matsuyama Y, Aoki T, Harada A, Ishiguro N. Recurrence of hypertrophic spinal pachymeningitis. Report of two cases and review of the literature. J Neurosurg Spine 2006, 4: 509–513.

225 Jackson RJ, Goodman JC, Huston DP, Harper RL. Parafalcine and bilateral convexity neurosarcoidosis mimicking meningioma. Case report and review of the literature. Neurosurgery 1998, **42**: 635–638.

226 Jamjoom ZA, Raina V, al-Jamali A, Jamjoom AB, Yacub B, Sharif HS. Intracranial xanthogranuloma of the dura in Hand-Schuller–Christian disease. Case report. J Neurosurg 1993, **78**: 297–300.

227 Kamiryo T, Abiko S, Orita T, Aoki H, Watanabe Y, Hiraoka K. Bilateral intracranial fibrous xanthoma. Surg Neurol 1988, **29**: 27–31.

228 Karam NE, Roger L, Hankins LL, Reveille JD. Rheumatoid nodulosis of the meninges. J Rheumatol 1994, **21**: 1960–1963.

229 Kim RC, Collins GH. The neuropathology of rheumatoid disease. Hum Pathol 1981, **12**: 5–15.

230 Kimura H, Oka K, Nakayama Y, Tomonaga M. Xanthoma in Meckel's cave. A case report. Surg Neurol 1991, **35**: 317–320.

231 Koyama S, Tsubokawa T, Katayama Y, Hirota H. A huge intracranial xanthogranuloma in the middle cranial fossa. Case report. Neurosurgery 1991, **28**: 436–439.

232 Kupersmith MJ, Martin V, Heller G, Shah A, Mitnick HJ. Idiopathic hypertrophic pachymeningitis. Neurology 2004, **62**: 686–694.

233 Le Marc'hadour F, Fransen P, Labat-Moleur F, Passagia JG, Pasquier B. Intracranial plasma cell granuloma. A report of four cases. Surg Neurol 1994, **42**: 481–488.

234 Lui PC, Fan YS, Wong SS, Chan AN, Wong G, Chau TK, Tse GM, Cheng Y, Poon WS, Ng HK. Inflammatory pseudotumors of the central nervous system. Hum Pathol 2009, **40**: 1611–1617.

235 Lyons MK, Caselli RJ, Parisi JE. Nonvasculitic autoimmune inflammatory meningoencephalitis as a cause of potentially reversible dementia. Report of 4 cases. J Neurosurg 2008, **108**: 1024–1027.

236 Mello LR, Bernardes CI, Feltrin Y, Rodacki MA. Thoracic spine arachnoid ossification with and without cord cavitation. Report of three cases. J Neurosurg (Spine 1) 2001, **94**: 115–120.

237 Mills SE, Lininger JR. Intracranial myospherulosis. Hum Pathol 1982, **13**: 596–597.

238 Miyachi S, Kobayashi T, Takahashi T, Saito K, Hashizume Y, Sugita K. An intracranial mass lesion in systemic xanthogranulomatosis. Case report. Neurosurgery 1990, **27**: 822–826.

239 Mokri B, Parisi JE, Scheithauer BW, Piepgras DG, Miller GM. Meningeal biopsy in intracranial hypotension: meningeal enhancement on MRI. Neurology 1995, **45**: 1801–1807.

240 Nazek M, Mandybur TI, Sawaya R. Hyalinizing plasmacytic granulomatosis of the falx. Am J Surg Pathol 1988, **12**: 308–313.

241 Nishino H, Rubino FA, DeRemee RA, Swanson JW, Parisi JE. Neurological involvement in Wegener's granulomatosis: an analysis of 324 consecutive patients at the Mayo Clinic. Ann Neurol 1993, **33**: 4–9.

242 Okabe H, Ishizawa M, Matsumoto K, Ogata M, Nishioka J, Hukuda S, Hidaka H, Yasuda H, Ochi Y. Immunohistochemical analysis of spinal intradural xanthomatosis developed in a patient with phytosterolemia. Acta Neuropathol (Berl) 1992, **83**: 554–558.

243 O'Shaughnessy BA, Schafernak KT, DiPatri AJ Jr, Goldman S, Tomita T. A granulomatous reaction to Avitene mimicking recurrence of a medulloblastoma. Case report. J Neurosurg (1 Suppl Pediatrics) 2006, **104**: 33–36.

244 Oweity T, Scheithauer BW, Ching HS, Lei C, Wong KP. Multiple system Erdheim–Chester disease with massive hypothalamic–sellar involvement and hypopituitarism. J Neurosurg 2002, **96**: 344–351.

245 Pai S, Welsh CT, Patel S, Rumboldt Z. Idiopathic hypertrophic spinal pachymeningitis: report of two cases with typical MR imaging findings. AJNR Am J Neuroradiol 2007, **28**: 590–592.

246 Pardo CA, Vining EP, Guo L, Skolasky RL, Carson BS, Freeman JM. The pathology of Rasmussen syndrome: stages of cortical involvement and neuropathological studies in 45 hemispherectomies. Epilepsia 2004, **45**: 516–526.

247 Paulus W, Kirchner T, Michaela M, Kuhl J, Warmuth-Metz M, Sorensen N, Muller-Hermelink HK, Roggendorf W. Histiocytic tumor of Meckel's cave. An intracranial equivalent of juvenile xanthogranuloma of the skin. Am J Surg Pathol 1992, **16**: 76–83.

248 Pick P, Jean E, Horoupian D, Factor S. Xanthogranuloma of the dura in systemic Weber–Christian disease. Neurology 1983, **33**: 1067–1070.

249 Purav P, Ganapathy K, Mallikarjuna VS, Annapurneswari S, Kalyanaraman S, Reginald J, Natarajan P, Bapu KR, Balamurugan M. Rosai–Dorfman disease of the central nervous system. J Clin Neurosci 2005, **12**: 656–659.

250 Qian J, Rubio A, Powers JM, Rosenblum MK, Pilcher WH, Shrier DA, Stein BM, Ito M, Iannucci A. Fibro-osseous lesions of the central nervous system. Report of four cases and literature review. Am J Surg Pathol 1999, **23**: 1270–1275.

251 Quinones-Hinojosa A, Chang EF, Khan SA, McDermott MW. Isolated trigeminal nerve sarcoid granuloma mimicking trigeminal schwannoma. Case report. Neurosurgery 2003, **52**: 700–705.

252 Reznik M, Stevenaert A, Bex V, Kratzenberg E. Focal brain invasion as the first manifestation of Langerhans cell histiocytosis in an adult. Case report. Clin Neuropathol 1993, **12**: 179–183.

253 Ribalta T, McCutcheon IE, Neto AG, Gupta D, Kumar AJ, Biddle DA, Langford LA, Bruner JM, Leeds NE, Fuller GN. Textiloma (gossypiboma) mimicking recurrent intracranial tumor. Arch Pathol Lab Med 2004, **128**: 749–758.

254 Rickert CH, August C, Brandt M, Wagner V, Paulus W. Cerebral malakoplakia associated with *Escherichia coli* infection. Acta Neuropathol 2000, **99**: 595–598.

255 Riku S, Kato S. Idiopathic hypertrophic pachymeningitis. Neuropathology 2003, **23**: 335–344.

256 Rodriguez-Pereira C, Borras-Moreno JM, Pesudo-Martinez JV, Vera-Roman JM. Cerebral solitary Langerhans cell histiocytosis. Report of two cases and review of the literature. Br J Neurosurg 2005, **19**: 192–197.
257 Sato K, Kubota T, Kitai R, Miyamori I. Meningeal plasma cell granuloma with relapsing polychondritis. Case report. J Neurosurg 2006, **104**: 143–146.
258 Shah KC, Poonnoose SI, George R, Jacob M, Rajshekhar V. Necrobiotic xanthogranuloma with cutaneous and cerebral manifestations. Case report and review of the literature. J Neurosurg 2004, **100**: 1111–1114.
259 Shinoda J, Murase S, Takenaka K, Sakai N. Isolated central nervous system hemophagocytic lymphohistiocytosis. Case report. Neurosurgery 2005, **56**: E187–E190.
260 Slavin KV, Nixon RR, Nesbit GM, Burchiel KJ. Extensive arachnoid ossification with associated syringomyelia presenting as thoracic myelopathy. Case report and review of the literature. J Neurosurg (Spine 2) 1999, **91**: 223–229.
261 Strickland-Marmol LB, Fessler RG, Rojiani AM. Necrotizing sarcoid granulomatosis mimicking an intracranial neoplasm. Clinicopathologic features and review of the literature. Mod Pathol 2000, **13**: 909–913.
262 Swain RS, Tihan T, Horvai AE, Di Vizio D, Loda M, Burger PC, Scheithauer BW, Kim GE. Inflammatory myofibroblastic tumor of the central nervous system and its relationship to inflammatory pseudotumor. Hum Pathol 2008, **39**: 410–419.
263 Tashjian V, Doppenberg EM, Lyders E, Broaddus WC, Pavot P, Tye G, Liu AY, Perez J, Ghatak N. Diagnosis of Erdheim–Chester disease by using computerized tomography-guided stereotactic biopsy of a caudate lesion. Case report. J Neurosurg 2004, **101**: 521–527.
264 Thomas G, Murphy S, Staunton H, O'Neill S, Farrell MA, Brett FM. Pathogen-free granulomatous diseases of the central nervous system. Hum Pathol 1998, **29**: 110–115.
265 Tobias S, Prayson RA, Lee JH. Necrotizing neurosarcoidosis of the cranial base resembling an en plaque sphenoid wing meningioma. Case report. Neurosurgery 2002, **51**: 1290–1294.
266 Toubes-Klingler E, Prabhu VC, Bernal K, Poage D, Swindells S. Malacoplakia of the cranium and cerebrum in a human immunodeficiency virus-infected man. Case report. J Neurosurg 2006, **104**: 432–435.
267 Vaquero J, Leunda G, Cabezudo JM, De Juan M, Herrero J, Bravo G. Posterior fossa xanthogranuloma. Case report. J Neurosurg 1979, **51**: 718–722.
268 Yasuhara T, Fukuhara T, Nakagawa M, Terai Y, Yoshino K, Mizobuchi K, Fujimoto S. Wegener granulomatosis manifesting as meningitis. Case report. J Neurosurg 2002, **97**: 1229–1232.

INFECTIOUS DISEASES

BACTERIAL INFECTIONS

269 Antal EA, Loberg EM, Dietrichs E, Maehlen J. Neuropathological findings in 9 cases of *Listeria monocytogenes* brain stem encephalitis. Brain Pathol 2005, **15**: 187–191.
270 Bauer J, Johnson RF, Levy JM, Pojman DV, Ruge JR. Tuberculoma presenting as an en plaque meningioma. Case report. J Neurosurg 1996, **85**: 685–688.
271 Berenson CS, Bia FJ. *Propionibacterium acnes* causes postoperative brain abscesses unassociated with foreign bodies: case reports. Neurosurgery 1989, **25**: 130–134.
272 Cayli SR, Onal C, Kocak A, Onmus SH, Tekiner A. An unusual presentation of neurotuberculosis: subdural empyema. Case report. J Neurosurg 2001, **94**: 988–991.
273 Chun CH, Johnson JD, Hofstetter M, Raff MJ. Brain abscess. A study of 45 consecutive cases. Medicine (Baltimore) 1986, **65**: 415–431.
274 Del Curling O Jr, Gower DJ, McWhorter JM. Changing concepts in spinal epidural abscess: a report of 29 cases. Neurosurgery 1990, **27**: 185–192.
275 Di Patre PL, Radziszewski W, Martin NA, Brooks A, Vinters HV. A meningioma-mimicking tumor caused by *Mycobacterium avium* complex in an immunocompromised patient. Am J Surg Pathol 2000, **24**: 136–139.
276 Ekseth K, Broström S. Late complications of Silastic duraplasty: low-virulence infections. Case report. J Neurosurg 1999, **90**: 559–562.
277 George TI, Manley G, Koehler JE, Hung VS, McDermott M, Bollen A. Detection of *Bartonella henselae* by polymerase chain reaction in brain tissue of an immunocompromised patient with multiple enhancing lesions. Case report and review of the literature. J Neurosurg 1998, **89**: 640–644.
278 Hall WA. Hereditary hemorrhagic telangiectasia (Rendu–Osler–Weber disease) presenting with polymicrobial brain abscess. Case report. J Neurosurg 1994, **81**: 294–296.
279 Kastenbauer S, Pfister H-W, Scheld WM. Epidural abscess. In Scheld WM, Whitley RJ, Marra CM (eds): Infections of the central nervous system, ed. 3. Philadelphia, 2004, Lippincott Williams & Wilkins, pp. 509–521.
280 Kastenbauer S, Pfister H-W, Wispelwey B, Scheld WM. Brain abscess. In Scheld WM, Whitley RJ, Marra CM (eds): Infections of the central nervous system, ed. 3. Philadelphia, 2004, Lippincott Williams & Wilkins, pp. 479–507.
281 Lohr M, Stenzel W, Plum G, Gross WP, Deckert M, Klug N. Whipple disease confined to the central nervous system presenting as a solitary frontal tumor. Case report. J Neurosurg 2004, **101**: 336–339.
282 Mendel E, Khoo LT, Go JL, Hinton D, Zee CS, Apuzzo ML. Intracerebral Whipple's disease diagnosed by stereotactic biopsy: a case report and review of the literature. Neurosurgery 1999, **44**: 203–209.
283 Mohindra S, Gupta R, Mathuriya SN, Radotra BD. Intramedullary abscess in association with tumor at the conus medullaris. Report of two cases. J Neurosurg Spine 2007, **6**: 350–353.
284 Ratliff JK, Connolly ES. Intramedullary tuberculoma of the spinal cord. Case report and review of the literature. J Neurosurg (Spine 1) 1999, **90**: 125–128.
285 Renier D, Flandin C, Hirsch E, Hirsch JF. Brain abscesses in neonates. A study of 30 cases. J Neurosurg 1988, **69**: 877–882.
286 Schlitt M, Mitchem L, Zorn G, Dismukes W, Morawetz RB. Brain abscess after esophageal dilation for caustic stricture: report of three cases. Neurosurgery 1985, **17**: 947–951.
287 Smego RA Jr. Actinomycosis of the central nervous system. Rev Infect Dis 1987, **9**: 855–865.
288 Tatti KM, Shieh WJ, Phillips S, Augenbraun M, Rao C, Zaki SR. Molecular diagnosis of *Nocardia farcinica* from a cerebral abscess. Hum Pathol 2006, **37**: 1117–1121.
289 Trautmann M, Lindner O, Haase C, Bruckner O. Focal tuberculous meningoencephalitis. Eur Neurol 1983, **22**: 417–420.
290 Wallace RJ Jr. Infections due to nontuberculosis mycobacteria. In Scheld WM, Whitley RJ, Marra CM (eds): Infections of the central nervous system, ed. 3. Philadelphia, 2004, Lippincott Williams & Wilkins, pp. 461–478.
291 Whitener DR. Tuberculous brain abscess. Report of a case and review of the literature. Arch Neurol 1978, **35**: 148–155.
292 Zuger A. Tuberculosis. In Scheld WM, Whitley RJ, Marra CM (eds): Infections of the central nervous system, ed. 3. Philadelphia, 2004, Lippincott Williams & Wilkins, pp. 441–459.

MYCOSES

293 Araujo JC, Werneck L, Cravo MA. South American blastomycosis presenting as a posterior fossa tumor. Case report. J Neurosurg 1978, **49**: 425–428.
294 Cortez KJ, Walsh TJ. Space-occupying fungal lesions. In Scheld WM, Whitley RJ, Marra CM (eds): Infections of the central nervous system, ed. 3. Philadelphia, 2004, Lippincott Williams & Wilkins, pp. 713–734.
295 Goodman ML, Coffey RJ. Stereotactic drainage of Aspergillus brain abscess with long-term survival: case report and review. Neurosurgery 1989, **24**: 96–99.
296 Hadley MN, Martin NA, Spetzler RF, Johnson PC. Multiple intracranial aneurysms due to *Coccidioides immitis* infection. Case report. J Neurosurg 1987, **66**: 453–456.
297 Ilgren EB, Westmorland D, Adams CB, Mitchell RG. Cerebellar mass caused by Candida species. Case report. J Neurosurg 1984, **60**: 428–430.
298 Kasantikul V, Shuangshoti S, Sampatanukul P. Primary chromoblastomycosis of the medulla oblongata: complication of heroin addiction. Surg Neurol 1988, **29**: 319–321.
299 Kershaw P, Freeman R, Templeton D, DeGirolami PC, DeGirolami U, Tarsy D, Hoffmann S, Eliopoulos G, Karchmer AW. *Pseudallescheria boydii* infection of the central nervous system. Arch Neurol 1990, **47**: 468–472.
300 Kleinschmidt-DeMasters BK, Mazowiecki M, Bonds LA, Cohn DL, Wilson ML. Coccidioidomycosis meningitis with massive dural and cerebral venous thrombosis and tissue arthroconidia. Arch Pathol Lab Med 2000, **124**: 310–314.
301 Mendel E, Milefchik EN, Amadi J, Gruen P. Coccidioidomycosis brain abscess. Case report. J Neurosurg 1994, **81**: 614–616.
302 Mielke B, Weir B, Oldring D, von Westarp C. Fungal aneurysm: case report and review of the literature. Neurosurgery 1981, **9**: 578–582.
303 Penar PL, Kim J, Chyatte D, Sabshin JK. Intraventricular cryptococcal granuloma. Report of two cases. J Neurosurg 1988, **68**: 145–148.
304 Revankar SG, Sutton DA, Rinaldi MG. Primary central nervous system phaeohyphomycosis: a review of 101 cases. Clin Infect Dis 2004, **38**: 206–216.
305 Roos KL, Bryan JP, Maggio WW, Jane JA, Scheld WM. Intracranial blastomycoma. Medicine (Baltimore) 1987, **66**: 224–235.
306 Stave GM, Heimberger T, Kerkering TM. Zygomycosis of the basal ganglia in intravenous drug users. Am J Med 1989, **86**: 115–117.
307 Venger BH, Landon G, Rose JE. Solitary histoplasmoma of the thalamus: case report and literature review. Neurosurgery 1987, **20**: 784–787.
308 Voelker JL, Muller J, Worth RM. Intramedullary spinal Histoplasma

granuloma. Case report. J Neurosurg 1989, **70**: 959–961.

309 Yanai Y, Wakao T, Fukamachi A, Kunimine H. Intracranial granuloma caused by *Aspergillus fumigatus*. Surg Neurol 1985, **23**: 597–604.

PARASITOSES

310 Luft BJ, Sivadas R. Toxoplasmosis. In Scheld WM, Whitley RJ, Marra CM (eds): Infections of the central nervous system, ed. 3. Philadelphia, 2004, Lippincott Williams & Wilkins, pp. 755–776.

311 Navia BA, Petito CK, Gold JW, Cho ES, Jordan BD, Price RW. Cerebral toxoplasmosis complicating the acquired immune deficiency syndrome: clinical and neuropathological findings in 27 patients. Ann Neurol 1986, **19**: 224–238.

312 Pittella JE. Neurocysticercosis. Brain Pathol 1997, **7**: 681–693.

313 Resnick DK, Comey CH, Welch WC, Martinez AJ, Hoover WW, Jacobs GB. Isolated toxoplasmosis of the thoracic spinal cord in a patient with acquired immunodeficiency syndrome. Case report. J Neurosurg 1995, **82**: 493–496.

SPIROCHETAL INFECTIONS

314 Cadavid D. Lyme disease and relapsing fever. In Scheld WM, Whitley RJ, Marra CM (eds): Infections of the central nervous system, ed. 3. Philadelphia, 2004, Lippincott Williams & Wilkins, pp. 659–690.

315 Horowitz HW, Valsamis MP, Wicher V, Abbruscato F, Larsen SA, Wormser GP, Wicher K. Brief report: cerebral syphilitic gumma confirmed by the polymerase chain reaction in a man with human immunodeficiency virus infection. N Engl J Med 1994, **331**: 1488–1491.

316 Marra CM. Neurosyphilis. In Scheld WM, Whitley RJ, Marra CM (eds): Infections of the central nervous system, ed. 3. Philadelphia, 2004, Lippincott Williams & Wilkins, pp. 649–657.

317 Murray R, Morawetz R, Kepes J, el Gammal T, LeDoux M. Lyme neuroborreliosis manifesting as an intracranial mass lesion. Neurosurgery 1992, **30**: 769–773.

VIRAL INFECTIONS

Herpes simplex encephalitis

318 Esiri MM. Herpes simplex encephalitis. An immunohistological study of the distribution of viral antigen within the brain. J Neurol Sci 1982, **54**: 209–226.

319 Kennedy PG, Adams JH, Graham DI, Clements GB. A clinico-pathological study of herpes simplex encephalitis. Neuropathol Appl Neurobiol 1988, **14**: 395–415.

320 Love S, Koch P, Urbach H, Dawson TP. Chronic granulomatous herpes simplex encephalitis in children. J Neuropathol Exp Neurol 2004, **63**: 1173–1181.

321 Molloy S, Allcutt D, Brennan P, Farrell MA, Perryman R, Brett FM. Herpes simplex encephalitis occurring after chemotherapy, surgery, and stereotactic radiotherapy for medulloblastoma. Arch Pathol Lab Med 2000, **124**: 1809–1812.

322 Schiff D, Rosenblum MK. Herpes simplex encephalitis (HSE) and the immunocompromised: a clinical and autopsy study of HSE in the settings of cancer and human immunodeficiency virus-type 1 infection. Hum Pathol 1998, **29**: 215–222.

323 Whitley RJ. Herpes simplex virus. In Scheld WM, Whitley RJ, Marra CM (eds): Infections of the central nervous system, ed. 3. Philadelphia, 2004, Lippincott Williams & Wilkins, pp. 123–144.

Progressive multifocal leukoencephalopathy

324 Ariza A, Mate JL, Fernandez-Vasalo A, Gomez-Plaza C, Perez-Piteira J, Pujol M, Navas-Palacios JJ. p53 and proliferating cell nuclear antigen expression in JC virus-infected cells of progressive multifocal leukoencephalopathy. Hum Pathol 1994, **25**: 1341–1345.

325 Ariza A, Mate JL, Isamat M, Calatrava A, Fernandez-Vasalo A, Navas-Palacios JJ. Overexpression of Ki-67 and cyclins A and B1 in JC virus-infected cells of progressive multifocal leukoencephalopathy. J Neuropathol Exp Neurol 1998, **57**: 226–230.

326 Astrom KE, Mancall EL, Richardson EP Jr. Progressive multifocal leuko-encephalopathy; a hitherto unrecognized complication of chronic lymphatic leukaemia and Hodgkin's disease. Brain 1958, **81**: 93–111.

327 Di Giambenedetto S, Vago G, Pompucci A, Scoppettuolo G, Cingolani A, Marzocchetti A, Tumbarello M, Cauda R, De Luca A. Fatal inflammatory AIDS-associated PML with high CD4 counts on HAART: a new clinical entity? Neurology 2004, **63**: 2452–2453.

328 Hair LS, Nuovo G, Powers JM, Sisti MB, Britton CB, Miller JR. Progressive multifocal leukoencephalopathy in patients with human immunodeficiency virus. Hum Pathol 1992, **23**: 663–667.

329 Hoffmann C, Horst HA, Albrecht H, Schlote W. Progressive multifocal leucoencephalopathy with unusual inflammatory response during antiretroviral treatment. J Neurol Neurosurg Psychiatry 2003, **74**: 1142–1144.

330 Preskorn SH, Watanabe I. Progressive multifocal leukoencephalopathy: cerebral mass lesions. Surg Neurol 1979, **12**: 231–234.

331 Rushing EJ, Liappis A, Smirniotopoulos JD, Smith AB, Henry JM, Man YG, Nelson AM. Immune reconstitution inflammatory syndrome of the brain: case illustrations of a challenging entity. J Neuropathol Exp Neurol 2008, **67**: 819–827.

332 Schmidbauer M, Budka H, Shah KV. Progressive multifocal leukoencephalopathy (PML) in AIDS and in the pre-AIDS era. A neuropathological comparison using immunocytochemistry and in situ DNA hybridization for virus detection. Acta Neuropathol 1990, **80**: 375–380.

333 Shintaku M, Matsumoto R, Sawa H, Nagashima K. Infection with JC virus and possible dysplastic ganglion-like transformation of the cerebral cortical neurons in a case of progressive multifocal leukoencephalopathy. J Neuropathol Exp Neurol 2000, **59**: 921–929.

334 Sima AA, Finkelstein SD, McLachlan DR. Multiple malignant astrocytomas in a patient with spontaneous progressive multifocal leukoencephalopathy. Ann Neurol 1983, **14**: 183–188.

335 Ueki K, Richardson EP Jr, Henson JW, Louis DN. In situ polymerase chain reaction demonstration of JC virus in progressive multifocal leukoencephalopathy, including an index case. Ann Neurol 1994, **36**: 670–673.

336 Vanneste JA, Bellot SM, Stam FC. Progressive multifocal leukoencephalopathy presenting as a single mass lesion. Eur Neurol 1984, **23**: 113–118.

337 Vazeux R, Cumont M, Girard PM, Nassif X, Trotot P, Marche C, Matthiessen L, Vedrenne C, Mikol J, Henin D, et al. Severe encephalitis resulting from coinfections with HIV and JC virus. Neurology 1990, **40**: 944–948.

Varicella-zoster virus encephalitis and cerebral vasculitis

338 Doyle PW, Gibson G, Dolman CL. Herpes zoster ophthalmicus with contralateral hemiplegia: identification of cause. Ann Neurol 1983, **14**: 84–85.

339 Eidelberg D, Sotrel A, Horoupian DS, Neumann PE, Pumarola-Sune T, Price RW. Thrombotic cerebral vasculopathy associated with herpes zoster. Ann Neurol 1986, **19**: 7–14.

340 Fukumoto S, Kinjo M, Hokamura K, Tanaka K. Subarachnoid hemorrhage and granulomatous angiitis of the basilar artery: demonstration of the varicella-zoster-virus in the basilar artery lesions. Stroke 1986, **17**: 1024–1028.

341 Horten B, Price RW, Jimenez D. Multifocal varicella-zoster virus leukoencephalitis temporally remote from herpes zoster. Ann Neurol 1981, **9**: 251–266.

342 Kleinschmidt-DeMasters BK, Amlie-Lefond C, Gilden DH. The patterns of varicella zoster virus encephalitis. Hum Pathol 1996, **27**: 927–938.

343 Weaver S, Rosenblum MK, DeAngelis LM. Herpes varicella zoster encephalitis in immunocompromised patients. Neurology 1999, **52**: 193–195.

HIV-1 encephalomyelitis

344 Scaravilli F, Bazille C, Gray F. Neuropathologic contributions to understanding AIDS and the central nervous system. Brain Pathol 2007, **17**: 197–208.

PRION-ASSOCIATED DISEASES

345 Brumback RA. Routine use of phenolized formalin in fixation of autopsy brain tissue to reduce risk of inadvertent transmission of Creutzfeldt–Jakob disease. N Engl J Med 1988, **319**: 654.

346 Cruz-Sanchez F, Lafuente J, Gertz HJ, Stoltenburg-Didinger G. Spongiform encephalopathy with extensive involvement of white matter. J Neurol Sci 1987, **82**: 81–87.

347 Ironside JW, Ghetti B, Head MW, Piccardo P, Will RG. Prion diseases. In Love S, Louis DN, Ellison DW (eds): Greenfield's neuropathology, ed. 8. London, 2008, Hodder Arnold, pp. 1197–1273.

348 Masters CL, Richardson EP Jr. Subacute spongiform encephalopathy (Creutzfeldt–Jakob disease). The nature and progression of spongiform change. Brain 1978, **101**: 333–344.

349 Zeitner K. Safe handling of transmissible spongiform encephalopathies specimens in the histopathology laboratory. J Histotechnol 2007, **30**: 81–85.

PRIMARY TUMORS

Diffusely infiltrating astrocytomas

350 Armanios MY, Grossman SA, Yang SC, White B, Perry A, Burger PC, Orens JB. Transmission of glioblastoma multiforme following bilateral lung transplantation from an affected donor: case study and review of the literature. Neuro Oncol 2004, **6**: 259–263.

351 Barbashina V, Salazar P, Ladanyi M, Rosenblum MK, Edgar MA. Glioneuronal tumor with neuropil-like islands (GTNI): a report of 8 cases with chromosome 1p/19q deletion analysis. Am J Surg Pathol 2007, **31**: 1196–1202.

352 Barnard RO, Geddes JF. The incidence of multifocal cerebral gliomas. A histologic study of large hemisphere sections. Cancer 1987, **60**: 1519–1531.

353 Blumenthal DT, Raizer JJ, Rosenblum MK, Bilsky MH, Hariharan S, Abrey LE. Primary intracranial neoplasms in patients with HIV. Neurology 1999, **52**: 1648–1651.

354 Brat DJ, Scheithauer BW, Medina-Flores R, Rosenblum MK, Burger PC. Infiltrative astrocytomas with granular cell features (granular cell astrocytomas): a study of histopathologic features, grading, and outcome. Am J Surg Pathol 2002, **26**: 750–757.

355 Brennan C, Momota H, Hambardzumyan D, Ozawa T, Tandon A, Pedraza A, Holland E. Glioblastoma subclasses can be defined by activity among signal transduction pathways and associated genomic alterations. PLoS One 2009, **4**: e7752.

356 Capper D, Weißert S, Balss J, Habel A, Meyer J, Jäger D, Ackermann U, Tessmer C, Korshunov A, Zentgraf H, Hartmann C, von Deimling A. Characterization of R132H mutation-specific IDH1 antibody binding in brain tumors. Brain Pathol 2010, **20**: 245–254.

357 Capper D, Zentgraf H, Balss J, Hartmann C, von Deimling A. Monoclonal antibody specific for IDH1 R132H mutation. Acta Neuropathol 2009, **118**: 599–601.

358 Constantini S, Miller DC, Allen JC, Rorke LB, Freed D, Epstein FJ. Radical excision of intramedullary spinal cord tumors: surgical morbidity and long-term follow-up evaluation in 164 children and young adults. J Neurosurg 2000, **93**: 183–193.

359 Cosgrove M, Fitzgibbons PL, Sherrod A, Chandrasoma PT, Martin SE. Intermediate filament expression in astrocytic neoplasms. Am J Surg Pathol 1989, **13**: 141–145.

360 Cosgrove MM, Rich KA, Kunin SA, Sherrod AE, Martin SE. Keratin intermediate filament expression in astrocytic neoplasms: analysis by immunocytochemistry, western blot, and northern hybridization. Mod Pathol 1993, **6**: 342–347.

361 Fisher PG, Breiter SN, Carson BS, Wharam MD, Williams JA, Weingart JD, Foer DR, Goldthwaite PT, Tihan T, Burger PC. A clinicopathologic reappraisal of brain stem tumor classification. Identification of pilocystic astrocytoma and fibrillary astrocytoma as distinct entities. Cancer 2000, **89**: 1569–1576.

362 Frappaz D, Ricci AC, Kohler R, Bret P, Mottolese C. Diffuse brain stem tumor in an adolescent with multiple enchondromatosis (Ollier's disease). Childs Nerv Syst 1999, **15**: 222–225.

363 Fung KM, Perry A, Payner TD, Shan Y. Rhabdoid glioblastoma in an adult. Pathology 2004, **36**: 585–587.

364 Giannini C, Scheithauer BW, Burger PC, Christensen MR, Wollan PC, Sebo TJ, Forsyth PA, Hayostek CJ. Cellular proliferation in pilocytic and diffuse astrocytomas. J Neuropathol Exp Neurol 1999, **58**: 46–53.

365 Gultekin SH, Dalmau J, Graus Y, Posner JB, Rosenblum MK. Anti-Hu immunolabeling as an index of neuronal differentiation in human brain tumors: a study of 112 central neuroepithelial neoplasms. Am J Surg Pathol 1998, **22**: 195–200.

366 Haddad SF, Moore SA, Schelper RL, Goeken JA. Vascular smooth muscle hyperplasia underlies the formation of glomeruloid vascular structures of glioblastoma multiforme. J Neuropathol Exp Neurol 1992, **51**: 488–492.

367 Hartmann C, Meyer J, Balss J, Capper D, Mueller W, Christians A, Felsberg J, Wolter M, Mawrin C, Wick W, Weller M, Herold-Mende C, Unterberg A, Jeuken JW, Wesseling P, Reifenberger G, von Deimling A. Type and frequency of IDH1 and IDH2 mutations are related to astrocytic and oligodendroglial differentiation and age: a study of 1,010 diffuse gliomas. Acta Neuropathol 2009, **118**: 469–474.

368 Hilton DA, Love S, Barber R, Ellison D, Sandeman DR. Accumulation of p53 and Ki-67 expression do not predict survival in patients with fibrillary astrocytomas or the response of these tumors to radiotherapy. Neurosurgery 1998, **42**: 724–729.

369 Hitchcock E, Morris CS. Cross reactivity of anti-epithelial membrane antigen monoclonal for reactive and neoplastic glial cells. J Neurooncol 1987, **4**: 345–352.

370 Homma T, Fukushima T, Vaccarella S, Yonekawa Y, Di Patre PL, Franceschi S, Ohgaki H. Correlation among pathology, genotype, and patient outcomes in glioblastoma. J Neuropathol Exp Neurol 2006, **65**: 846–854.

371 Iafrate AJ, Louis DN. 'MGMT for pt mgmt': is methylguanine-DNA methyltransferase testing ready for patient management? J Mol Diagn 2008, **10**: 308–310.

372 Ichimura K, Pearson DM, Kocialkowski S, Backlund LM, Chan R, Jones DT, Collins VP. IDH1 mutations are present in the majority of common adult gliomas but rare in primary glioblastomas. Neuro Oncol 2009, **11**: 341–347.

373 Katsetos CD, Del Valle L, Geddes JF, Assimakopoulou M, Legido A, Boyd JC, Balin B, Parikh NA, Maraziotis T, de Chadarevian JP, Varakis JN, Matsas R, Spano A, Frankfurter A, Herman MM, Khalili K. Aberrant localization of the neuronal class III beta-tubulin in astrocytomas. Arch Pathol Lab Med 2001, **125**: 613–624.

374 Kepes JJ, Fulling KH, Garcia JH. The clinical significance of 'adenoid' formations of neoplastic astrocytes, imitating metastatic carcinoma, in gliosarcomas. A review of five cases. Clin Neuropathol 1982, **1**: 139–150.

375 Kepes JJ, Rubinstein LJ. Malignant gliomas with heavily lipidized (foamy) tumor cells: a report of three cases with immunoperoxidase study. Cancer 1981, **47**: 2451–2459.

376 Kleinschmidt-Demasters BK. Diffuse bone marrow metastases from glioblastoma multiforme: the role of dural invasion. Hum Pathol 1996, **27**: 197–201.

377 Kleinschmidt-DeMasters BK, Alassiri AH, Birks DK, Newell KL, Moore W, Lillehei KO. Epithelioid versus rhabdoid glioblastomas are distinguished by monosomy 22 and immunohistochemical expression of INI-1 but not claudin 6. Am J Surg Pathol 2010, **34**: 341–354.

378 Krouwer HG, Davis RL, Silver P, Prados M. Gemistocytic astrocytomas: a reappraisal. J Neurosurg 1991, **74**: 399–406.

379 Kurtkaya-Yapicier O, Scheithauer BW, Hebrink D, James CD. p53 in nonneoplastic central nervous system lesions: an immunohistochemical and genetic sequencing study. Neurosurgery 2002, **51**: 1246–1254; discussion 1254–1255.

380 Louis DN, Ohagi H, Wiestler OD, Cavenne WK (eds): WHO classification of tumours of the central nervous system. Lyon, 2007, IARC, pp. 25–49.

381 Margetts JC, Kalyan-Raman UP. Giant-celled glioblastoma of brain. A clinico-pathological and radiological study of ten cases (including immunohistochemistry and ultrastructure). Cancer 1989, **63**: 524–531.

382 Martin SE, Bonnin JM, Hall DC, Hattab EM. Glioblastoma with signet-ring morphology: a case report and review of the literature. Hum Pathol 2010, **41**: 443–446.

383 Montine TJ, Vandersteenhoven JJ, Aguzzi A, Boyko OB, Dodge RK, Kerns BJ, Burger PC. Prognostic significance of Ki-67 proliferation index in supratentorial fibrillary astrocytic neoplasms. Neurosurgery 1994, **34**: 674–679.

384 Mork SJ, Rubinstein LJ, Kepes JJ. Patterns of epithelial metaplasia in malignant gliomas. I. Papillary formations mimicking medulloepithelioma. J Neuropathol Exp Neurol 1988, **47**: 93–100.

385 Mork SJ, Rubinstein LJ, Kepes JJ, Perentes E, Uphoff DF. Patterns of epithelial metaplasia in malignant gliomas. II. Squamous differentiation of epithelial-like formations in gliosarcomas and glioblastomas. J Neuropathol Exp Neurol 1988, **47**: 101–118.

386 Mueller W, Lass U, Herms J, Kuchelmeister K, Bergmann M, von Deimling A. Clonal analysis in glioblastoma with epithelial differentiation. Brain Pathol 2001, **11**: 39–43.

387 Network CGAR. Comprehensive genomic characterization defines human glioblastoma genes and core pathways. Nature 2008, **455**: 1061–1068.

388 Ng HK, Poon WS. Primary leptomeningeal astrocytoma. Case report. J Neurosurg 1998, **88**: 586–589.

389 Oh D, Prayson RA. Evaluation of epithelial and keratin markers in glioblastoma multiforme: an immunohistochemical study. Arch Pathol Lab Med 1999, **123**: 917–920.

390 Palma L, Celli P, Maleci A, Di Lorenzo N, Cantore G. Malignant monstrocellular brain tumours. A study of 42 surgically treated cases. Acta Neurochir (Wien) 1989, **97**: 17–25.

391 Perry A, Aldape KD, George DH, Burger PC. Small cell astrocytoma: an aggressive variant that is clinicopathologically and genetically distinct from anaplastic oligodendroglioma. Cancer 2004, **101**: 2318–2326.

392 Perry A, Miller CR, Gujrati M, Scheithauer BW, Zambrano SC, Jost SC, Raghavan R, Qian J, Cochran EJ, Huse JT, Holland EC, Burger PC, Rosenblum MK. Malignant gliomas with primitive neuroectodermal tumor-like components: a clinicopathologic and genetic study of 53 cases. Brain Pathol 2009, **19**: 81–90.

393 Phillips HS, Kharbanda S, Chen R, Forrest WF, Soriano RH, Wu TD, Misra A, Nigro JM, Colman H, Soroceanu L, Williams PM, Modrusan Z, Feuerstein BG, Aldape K. Molecular subclasses of high-grade glioma predict prognosis, delineate a pattern of disease progression, and resemble stages in neurogenesis. Cancer Cell 2006, **9**: 157–173.

394 Prayson RA, Estes ML. MIB1 and p53 immunoreactivity in protoplasmic astrocytomas. Pathol Int 1996, **46**: 862–866.

395 Prayson RA, Estes ML. Protoplasmic astrocytoma. A clinicopathologic study of 16 tumors. Am J Clin Pathol 1995, **103**: 705–709.

396 Ramsay DA, Goshko V, Nag S. Primary spinal leptomeningeal astrocytoma. Acta Neuropathol 1990, **80**: 338–341.

397 Rickert CH, Riemenschneider MJ, Schachenmayr W, Richter HP, Bockhorn J,

Reifenberger G, Paulus W. Glioblastoma with adipocyte like tumor cell differentiation – histological and molecular features of a rare differentiation pattern. Brain Pathol 2009, **19**: 431–438.

398 Rodriguez FJ, Scheithauer BW, Giannini C, Bryant SC, Jenkins RB. Epithelial and pseudoepithelial differentiation in glioblastoma and gliosarcoma: a comparative morphologic and molecular genetic study. Cancer 2008, **113**: 2779–2789.

399 Rosenblum MK, Erlandson RA, Budzilovich GN. The lipid-rich epithelioid glioblastoma. Am J Surg Pathol 1991, **15**: 925–934.

400 Scheithauer BW, Bruner JM. The ultrastructural spectrum of astrocytic neoplasms. Ultrastruct Pathol 1987, **11**: 535–581.

401 Schmidt MC, Antweiler S, Urban N, Mueller W, Kuklik A, Meyer-Puttlitz B, Wiestler OD, Louis DN, Fimmers R, von Deimling A. Impact of genotype and morphology on the prognosis of glioblastoma. J Neuropathol Exp Neurol 2002, **61**: 321–328.

402 Watanabe K, Tachibana O, Yonekawa Y, Kleihues P, Ohgaki H. Role of gemistocytes in astrocytoma progression. Lab Invest 1997, **76**: 277–284.

403 Wesseling P, Schlingemann RO, Rietveld FJ, Link M, Burger PC, Ruiter DJ. Early and extensive contribution of pericytes/vascular smooth muscle cells to microvascular proliferation in glioblastoma multiforme: an immuno-light and immuno-electron microscopic study. J Neuropathol Exp Neurol 1995, **54**: 304–310.

404 Wolf HK, Buslei R, Schmidt-Kastner R, Schmidt-Kastner PK, Pietsch T, Wiestler OD, Blumcke I. NeuN: a useful neuronal marker for diagnostic histopathology. J Histochem Cytochem 1996, **44**: 1167–1171.

405 Wyatt-Ashmead J, Kleinschmidt-DeMasters BK, Hill DA, Mierau GW, McGavran L, Thompson SJ, Foreman NK. Rhabdoid glioblastoma. Clin Neuropathol 2001, **20**: 248–255.

406 Yan H, Parsons DW, Jin G, McLendon R, Rasheed BA, Yuan W, Kos I, Batinic-Haberle I, Jones S, Riggins GJ, Friedman H, Friedman A, Reardon D, Herndon J, Kinzler KW, Velculescu VE, Vogelstein B, Bigner DD. IDH1 and IDH2 mutations in gliomas. N Engl J Med 2009, **360**: 765–773.

Pilocytic astrocytomas

407 Alvord EC Jr, Lofton S. Gliomas of the optic nerve or chiasm. Outcome by patients' age, tumor site, and treatment. J Neurosurg 1988, **68**: 85–98.

408 Balkhoyor KB, Bernstein M. Involution of diencephalic pilocytic astrocytoma after partial resection. Report of two cases in adults. J Neurosurg 2000, **93**: 484–486.

409 Forshew T, Tatevossian RG, Lawson AR, Ma J, Neale G, Ogunkolade BW, Jones TA, Aarum J, Dalton J, Bailey S, Chaplin T, Carter RL, Gajjar A, Broniscer A, Young BD, Ellison DW, Sheer D. Activation of the ERK/MAPK pathway: a signature genetic defect in posterior fossa pilocytic astrocytomas. J Pathol 2009, **218**: 172–181.

410 Forsyth PA, Shaw EG, Scheithauer BW, O'Fallon JR, Layton DD Jr, Katzmann JA. Supratentorial pilocytic astrocytomas. A clinicopathologic, prognostic, and flow cytometric study of 51 patients. Cancer 1993, **72**: 1335–1342.

411 Hayostek CJ, Shaw EG, Scheithauer B, O'Fallon JR, Weiland TL, Schomberg PJ, Kelly PJ, Hu TC. Astrocytomas of the cerebellum. A comparative clinicopathologic study of pilocytic and diffuse astrocytomas. Cancer 1993, **72**: 856–869.

412 Ilgren EB, Kinnier-Wilson LM, Stiller CA. Gliomas in neurofibromatosis: a series of 89 cases with evidence for enhanced malignancy in associated cerebellar astrocytomas. Pathol Annu 1985, **20**(Pt 1): 331–358.

413 Ito S, Hoshino T, Shibuya M, Prados MD, Edwards MS, Davis RL. Proliferative characteristics of juvenile pilocytic astrocytomas determined by bromodeoxyuridine labeling. Neurosurgery 1992, **31**: 413–419.

414 Iwaki T, Iwaki A, Tateishi J, Sakaki Y, Goldman JE. Alpha B-crystallin and 27-kd heat shock protein are regulated by stress conditions in the central nervous system and accumulate in Rosenthal fibers. Am J Pathol 1993, **143**: 487–495.

415 Jones DT, Kocialkowski S, Liu L, Pearson DM, Backlund LM, Ichimura K, Collins VP. Tandem duplication producing a novel oncogenic BRAF fusion gene defines the majority of pilocytic astrocytomas. Cancer Res 2008, **68**: 8673–8677.

416 Katsetos CD, Krishna L, Friedberg E, Reidy J, Karkavelas G, Savory J. Lobar pilocytic astrocytomas of the cerebral hemispheres: II. Pathobiology – morphogenesis of the eosinophilic granular bodies. Clin Neuropathol 1994, **13**: 306–314.

417 Korshunov A, Meyer J, Capper D, Christians A, Remke M, Witt H, Pfister S, von Deimling A, Hartmann C. Combined molecular analysis of BRAF and IDH1 distinguishes pilocytic astrocytoma from diffuse astrocytoma. Acta Neuropathol 2009, **118**: 401–405.

418 Lach B, Sikorska M, Rippstein P, Gregor A, Staines W, Davie TR. Immunoelectron microscopy of Rosenthal fibers. Acta Neuropathol 1991, **81**: 503–509.

419 McGirr SJ, Kelly PJ, Scheithauer BW. Stereotactic resection of juvenile pilocytic astrocytomas of the thalamus and basal ganglia. Neurosurgery 1987, **20**: 447–452.

420 Minehan KJ, Shaw EG, Scheithauer BW, Davis DL, Onofrio BM. Spinal cord astrocytoma: pathological and treatment considerations. J Neurosurg 1995, **83**: 590–595.

421 Murayama S, Bouldin TW, Suzuki K. Immunocytochemical and ultrastructural studies of eosinophilic granular bodies in astrocytic tumors. Acta Neuropathol 1992, **83**: 408–414.

422 Pagni CA, Giordana MT, Canavero S. Benign recurrence of a pilocytic cerebellar astrocytoma 36 years after radical removal: case report. Neurosurgery 1991, **28**: 606–609.

423 Perilongo G, Carollo C, Salviati L, Murgia A, Pillon M, Basso G, Gardiman M, Laverda A. Diencephalic syndrome and disseminated juvenile pilocytic astrocytomas of the hypothalamic–optic chiasm region. Cancer 1997, **80**: 142–146.

424 Pollack IF, Claassen D, al-Shboul Q, Janosky JE, Deutsch M. Low-grade gliomas of the cerebral hemispheres in children: an analysis of 71 cases. J Neurosurg 1995, **82**: 536–547.

425 Pollack IF, Hurtt M, Pang D, Albright AL. Dissemination of low grade intracranial astrocytomas in children. Cancer 1994, **73**: 2869–2878.

426 Rodriguez FJ, Scheithauer B, Burger PC, Jenkins S, Giannini C. Anaplasia in pilocytic astrocytoma predicts aggressive behavior. Am J Surg Pathol 2010, **34**: 147–160.

427 Scheithauer B, Hawkins C, Tihan T, VandenBerg SR, Burger PC. Pilocytic astrocytoma. In Louis DN, Ohgaki H, Wiestler OD, Cavenee WK (eds): WHO classification of tumours of the central nervous system. Lyon, 2007, IARC, pp. 14–21.

428 Tomlinson FH, Scheithauer BW, Hayostek CJ, Parisi JE, Meyer FB, Shaw EG, Weiland TL, Katzmann JA, Jack CR Jr. The significance of atypia and histologic malignancy in pilocytic astrocytoma of the cerebellum: a clinicopathologic and flow cytometric study. J Child Neurol 1994, **9**: 301–310.

429 Vajtai I, Yonekawa Y, Schauble B, Paulus W. Melanotic astrocytoma. Acta Neuropathol 1996, **91**: 549–553.

Pilomyxoid astrocytoma

430 Chikai K, Ohnishi A, Kato T, Ikeda J, Sawamura Y, Iwasaki Y, Itoh T, Sawa H, Nagashima K. Clinico-pathological features of pilomyxoid astrocytoma of the optic pathway. Acta Neuropathol 2004, **108**: 109–114.

431 Fernandez C, Figarella-Branger D, Girard N, Bouvier-Labit C, Gouvernet J, Paz Paredes A, Lena G. Pilocytic astrocytomas in children: prognostic factors – a retrospective study of 80 cases. Neurosurgery 2003, **53**: 544–553.

432 Fuller CE, Frankel B, Smith M, Rodziewitz G, Landas SK, Caruso R, Schelper R. Suprasellar monomorphous pilomyxoid neoplasm: an ultastructural analysis. Clin Neuropathol 2001, **20**: 256–262.

433 Komotar RJ, Burger PC, Carson BS, Brem H, Olivi A, Goldthwaite PT, Tihan T. Pilocytic and pilomyxoid hypothalamic/chiasmatic astrocytomas. Neurosurgery 2004, **54**: 72–79.

434 Tihan T, Fisher PG, Kepner JL, Godfraind C, McComb RD, Goldthwaite PT, Burger PC. Pediatric astrocytomas with monomorphous pilomyxoid features and a less favorable outcome. J Neuropathol Exp Neurol 1999, **58**: 1061–1068.

Pleomorphic xanthoastrocytoma

435 Arita K, Kurisu K, Tominaga A, Sugiyama K, Sumida M, Hirose T. Intrasellar pleomorphic xanthoastrocytoma: case report. Neurosurgery 2002, **51**: 1079–1082.

436 Chacko G, Chacko AG, Dunham CP, Judkins AR, Biegel JA, Perry A. Atypical teratoid/rhabdoid tumor arising in the setting of a pleomorphic xanthoastrocytoma. J Neurooncol 2007, **84**: 217–222.

437 Frank S, Cordier D, Tolnay M, Rosenblum MK. A 28-year-old man with headache, visual and aphasic speech disturbances. Brain Pathol 2009, **19**: 163–166.

437a Galloway M. CD34 expression in glioblastoma and giant cell glioblastoma. Clin Neuropathol 2010, **29**: 89–93.

438 Giannini C, Scheithauer BW, Burger PC, Brat DJ, Wollan PC, Lach B, O'Neill BP. Pleomorphic xanthoastrocytoma: what do we really know about it? Cancer 1999, **85**: 2033–2045.

439 Giannini C, Scheithauer BW, Lopes MB, Hirose T, Kros JM, VandenBerg SR. Immunophenotype of pleomorphic xanthoastrocytoma. Am J Surg Pathol 2002, **26**: 479–485.

440 Gil-Gouveia R, Cristino N, Farias JP, Trindade A, Ruivo NS, Pimentel J. Pleomorphic xanthoastrocytoma of the cerebellum: illustrated review. Acta Neurochir (Wien) 2004, **146**: 1241–1244.

441 Hirose T, Ishizawa K, Sugiyama K, Kageji T, Ueki K, Kannuki S. Pleomorphic xanthoastrocytoma: a comparative pathological study between conventional and anaplastic types. Histopathology 2008, **52**: 183–193.

442 Iwaki T, Fukui M, Kondo A, Matsushima T, Takeshita I. Epithelial properties of pleomorphic xanthoastrocytomas determined in ultrastructural and immunohistochemical studies. Acta Neuropathol 1987, **74**: 142–150.

443 Kepes JJ, Rubinstein LJ, Eng LF. Pleomorphic xanthoastrocytoma: a distinctive meningocerebral glioma of young subjects with relatively favorable prognosis. A study of 12 cases. Cancer 1979, **44**: 1839–1852.

444 Kros JM, Vecht CJ, Stefanko SZ. The pleomorphic xanthoastrocytoma and its differential diagnosis: a study of five cases. Hum Pathol 1991, **22**: 1128–1135.

445 Lach B, Duggal N, DaSilva VF, Benoit BG. Association of pleomorphic xanthoastrocytoma with cortical dysplasia and neuronal tumors. A report of three cases. Cancer 1996, **78**: 2551–2563.

446 Martinez-Diaz H, Kleinschmidt-DeMasters BK, Powell SZ, Yachnis AT. Giant cell glioblastoma and pleomorphic xanthoastrocytoma show different immunohistochemical profiles for neuronal antigens and p53 but share reactivity for class III beta-tubulin. Arch Pathol Lab Med 2003, **127**: 1187–1191.

447 Nakamura M, Chiba K, Matsumoto M, Ikeda E, Toyama Y. Pleomorphic xanthoastrocytoma of the spinal cord. Case report. J Neurosurg Spine 2006, **5**: 72–75.

448 Passone E, Pizzolitto S, D'Agostini S, Skrap M, Gardiman MP, Nocerino A, Scarzello G, Perilongo G. Non-anaplastic pleomorphic xanthoastrocytoma with neuroradiological evidences of leptomeningeal dissemination. Childs Nerv Syst 2006, **22**: 614–618.

449 Perry A, Giannini C, Scheithauer BW, Rojiani AM, Yachnis AT, Seo IS, Johnson PC, Kho J, Shapiro S. Composite pleomorphic xanthoastrocytoma and ganglioglioma: report of four cases and review of the literature. Am J Surg Pathol 1997, **21**: 763–771.

450 Primavera J, Nikas DC, Zamani AA, Shafman T, Alexander E 3rd, De Girolami U, Louis DN. Clear cell pleomorphic xanthoastrocytoma: case report. Acta Neuropathol 2001, **102**: 404–408.

451 Reifenberger G, Kaulich K, Wiestler OD, Blumcke I. Expression of the CD34 antigen in pleomorphic xanthoastrocytomas. Acta Neuropathol 2003, **105**: 358–364.

452 Sharma MC, Arora R, Khanna N, Singh VP, Sarkar C. Pigmented pleomorphic xanthoastrocytoma: report of a rare case with review of the literature. Arch Pathol Lab Med 2001, **125**: 808–811.

453 Snipes GJ, Horoupian DS, Shuer LM, Silverberg GD. Pleomorphic granular cell astrocytoma of the pineal gland. Cancer 1992, **70**: 2159–2165.

454 Sugita Y, Kepes JJ, Shigemori M, Kuramoto S, Reifenberger G, Kiwit JC, Wechsler W. Pleomorphic xanthoastrocytoma with desmoplastic reaction: angiomatous variant. Report of two cases. Clin Neuropathol 1990, **9**: 271–278.

455 Zarate JO, Sampaolesi R. Pleomorphic xanthoastrocytoma of the retina. Am J Surg Pathol 1999, **23**: 79–81.

Subependymal giant cell astrocytoma (tuberous sclerosis)

456 Bollo RJ, Berliner JL, Fischer I, Miles DK, Thiele EA, Zagzag D, Weiner HL. Extraventricular subependymal giant cell tumor in a child with tuberous sclerosis complex. J Neurosurg Pediatr 2009, **4**: 85–90.

457 Chow CW, Klug GL, Lewis EA. Subependymal giant-cell astrocytoma in children. An unusual discrepancy between histological and clinical features. J Neurosurg 1988, **68**: 880–883.

458 Dashti SR, Robinson S, Rodgers M, Cohen AR. Pineal region giant cell astrocytoma associated with tuberous sclerosis: case report. J Neurosurg (Pediatrics 3) 2005, **102**: 322–325.

459 Gyure KA, Prayson RA. Subependymal giant cell astrocytoma: a clinicopathologic study with HMB45 and MIB-1 immunohistochemical analysis. Mod Pathol 1997, **10**: 313–317.

460 Hirose T, Scheithauer BW, Lopes MB, Gerber HA, Altermatt HJ, Hukee MJ, VandenBerg SR, Charlesworth JC. Tuber and subependymal giant cell astrocytoma associated with tuberous sclerosis: an immunohistochemical, ultrastructural, and immunoelectron and microscopic study. Acta Neuropathol 1995, **90**: 387–399.

461 Lopes MB, Altermatt HJ, Scheithauer BW, Shepherd CW, VandenBerg SR. Immunohistochemical characterization of subependymal giant cell astrocytomas. Acta Neuropathol 1996, **91**: 368–375.

462 Lopes MBS, Wiestler OD, Stemmer-Rachamimov AO, Sharma MC. Tuberous sclerosis complex and subependymal giant cell astrocytoma. In Louis DN, Ohgaki H, Wiestler OD, Cavenee WK (eds): WHO classification of tumours of the central nervous system. Lyon, 2007, IARC, pp. 218–221.

463 Padmalatha C, Harruff RC, Ganick D, Hafez GB. Glioblastoma multiforme with tuberous sclerosis. Report of a case. Arch Pathol Lab Med 1980, **104**: 649–650.

464 Sharma MC, Ralte AM, Arora R, Santosh V, Shankar SK, Sarkar C. Subependymal giant cell astrocytoma: a clinicopathological study of 23 cases with special emphasis on proliferative markers and expression of p53 and retinoblastoma gene proteins. Pathology 2004, **36**: 139–144.

465 Sharma MC, Ralte AM, Gaekwad S, Santosh V, Shankar SK, Sarkar C. Subependymal giant cell astrocytoma – a clinicopathological study of 23 cases with special emphasis on histogenesis. Pathol Oncol Res 2004, **10**: 219–224.

466 Shepherd CW, Scheithauer BW, Gomez MR, Altermatt HJ, Katzmann JA. Subependymal giant cell astrocytoma: a clinical, pathological, and flow cytometric study. Neurosurgery 1991, **28**: 864–868.

467 Telfeian AE, Judkins A, Younkin D, Pollock AN, Crino P. Subependymal giant cell astrocytoma with cranial and spinal metastases in a patient with tuberous sclerosis. Case report. J Neurosurg (Pediatrics 5) 2004, **100**: 498–500.

Oligodendrogliomas

468 Bourne TD, Mandell JW, Matsumoto JA, Jane JA Jr, Lopes MB. Primary disseminated leptomeningeal oligodendroglioma with 1p deletion. Case report. J Neurosurg (6 Suppl Pediatrics) 2006, **105**: 465–469.

469 Burger PC, Minn AY, Smith JS, Borell TJ, Jedlicka AE, Huntley BK, Goldthwaite PT, Jenkins RB, Feuerstein BG. Losses of chromosomal arms 1p and 19q in the diagnosis of oligodendroglioma. A study of paraffin-embedded sections. Mod Pathol 2001, **14**: 842–853.

470 Coons SW, Johnson PC, Pearl DK. The prognostic significance of Ki-67 labeling indices for oligodendrogliomas. Neurosurgery 1997, **41**: 878–884.

471 Dehghani F, Schachenmayr W, Laun A, Korf HW. Prognostic implication of histopathological, immunohistochemical and clinical features of oligodendrogliomas: a study of 89 cases. Acta Neuropathol 1998, **95**: 493–504.

472 Edgar MA, Rosenblum MK. The differential diagnosis of central nervous system tumors: a critical examination of some recent immunohistochemical applications. Arch Pathol Lab Med 2008, **132**: 500–509.

473 Gardiman MP, Fassan M, Orvieto E, D'Avella D, Denaro L, Calderone M, Severino M, Scarsello G, Viscardi E, Perilongo G. Diffuse leptomeningeal glioneuronal tumors: a new entity? Brain Pathol 2010, **20**: 361–366.

474 Giannini C, Burger PC, Berkey BA, Cairncross JG, Jenkins RB, Mehta M, Curran WJ, Aldape K. Anaplastic oligodendroglial tumors: refining the correlation among histopathology, 1p/19q deletion and clinical outcome in Intergroup Radiation Therapy Oncology Group Trial 9402. Brain Pathol 2008, **18**: 360–369.

475 Giannini C, Scheithauer BW, Weaver AL, Burger PC, Kros JM, Mork S, Graeber MB, Bauserman S, Buckner JC, Burton J, Riepe R, Tazelaar HD, Nascimento AG, Crotty T, Keeney GL, Pernicone P, Altermatt H. Oligodendrogliomas: reproducibility and prognostic value of histologic diagnosis and grading. J Neuropathol Exp Neurol 2001, **60**: 248–262.

476 Herpers MJ, Budka H. Glial fibrillary acidic protein (GFAP) in oligodendroglial tumors: gliofibrillary oligodendroglioma and transitional oligoastrocytoma as subtypes of oligodendroglioma. Acta Neuropathol 1984, **64**: 265–272.

477 Kros JM, de Jong AA, van der Kwast TH. Ultrastructural characterization of transitional cells in oligodendrogliomas. J Neuropathol Exp Neurol 1992, **51**: 186–193.

478 Kros JM, Gorlia T, Kouwenhoven MC, Zheng PP, Collins VP, Figarella-Branger D, Giangaspero F, Giannini C, Mokhtari K, Mork SJ, Paetau A, Reifenberger G, van den Bent MJ. Panel review of anaplastic oligodendroglioma from European Organization For Research and Treatment of Cancer Trial 26951: assessment of consensus in diagnosis, influence of 1p/19q loss, and correlations with outcome. J Neuropathol Exp Neurol 2007, **66**: 545–551.

479 Kros JM, van den Brink WA, van Loon-van Luyt JJ, Stefanko SZ. Signet-ring cell oligodendroglioma – report of two cases and discussion of the differential diagnosis. Acta Neuropathol 1997, **93**: 638–643.

480 Kros JM, Van Eden CG, Stefanko SZ, Waayer-Van Batenburg M, van der Kwast TH. Prognostic implications of glial fibrillary acidic protein containing cell types in oligodendrogliomas. Cancer 1990, **66**: 1204–1212.

481 Kuhlmann T, Gutenberg A, Schulten HJ, Paulus W, Rohde V, Bruck W. Nogo-A expression in glial CNS tumors: a tool to differentiate between oligodendrogliomas and other gliomas? Am J Surg Pathol 2008, **32**: 1444–1453.

482 Ligon KL, Alberta JA, Kho AT, Weiss J, Kwaan MR, Nutt CL, Louis DN, Stiles CD, Rowitch DH. The oligodendroglial lineage marker OLIG2 is universally expressed in diffuse gliomas. J Neuropathol Exp Neurol 2004, **63**: 499–509.

483 Marek J, Jakubaszko-Turkiewicz J, Oficjalska-Mlynczak J, Markowska-Woyciechowska A. Retinal oligodendroglioma. Am J Ophthalmol 1999, **128**: 389–391.

484 Merrell R, Nabors LB, Perry A, Palmer CA. 1p/19q chromosome deletions in metastatic oligodendroglioma. J Neurooncol 2006, **80**: 203–207.

485 Mikami Y, Shirabe T, Hata S, Watanabe A. Oligodendroglioma with signet-ring cell morphology: a case report with an immunohistochemical and ultrastructural study. Pathol Int 1998, **48**: 144–150.

486 Min KW, Scheithauer BW, Bauserman SC. Oligodendroglioma: the ultrastructural spectrum. Ultrastruct Pathol 1994, **18**: 47–60.

486a Perry A, Burton SS, Fuller GN, Robinson CA, Palmer CA, Resch L, Bigio EH, Gujrati M, Rosenblum MK. Oligodendroglial neoplasms with ganglioglioma-like maturation: a diagnostic pitfall. Acta Neuropathol 2010, **120**: 237–252.

487 Perry A, Fuller CE, Banerjee R, Brat DJ, Scheithauer BW. Ancillary FISH analysis for 1p and 19q status: preliminary observations in 287 gliomas and oligodendroglioma mimics. Front Biosci 2003, **8**: a1–9.

488 Perry A, Scheithauer BW, Macaulay RJ, Raffel C, Roth KA, Kros JM. Oligodendrogliomas with neurocytic differentiation. A report of 4 cases with diagnostic and histogenetic implications. J Neuropathol Exp Neurol 2002, **61**: 947–955.

489 Raghavan R, Balani J, Perry A, Margraf L, Vono MB, Cai DX, Wyatt RE, Rushing EJ, Bowers DC, Hynan LS, White CL 3rd. Pediatric oligodendrogliomas: a study of molecular alterations on 1p and 19q using fluorescence in situ hybridization. J Neuropathol Exp Neurol 2003, **62**: 530–537.

490 Reifenberger G, Kros JM, Louis DN, Collins VP. Oligodendroglial tumors. In Louis DN, Ohgaki H, Wiestler OD, Cavenee WK (eds): WHO classification of tumours of the central nervous system. Lyon, 2007, IARC, pp. 53–62.

491 Rodriguez FJ, Scheithauer BW, Jenkins R, Burger PC, Rudzinskiy P, Vlodavsky E, Schooley A, Landolfi J. Gliosarcoma arising in oligodendroglial tumors ('oligosarcoma'): a clinicopathologic study. Am J Surg Pathol 2007, **31**: 351–362.

492 Rossi S, Rodriguez FJ, Mota RA, Dei Tos AP, Di Paola F, Bendini M, Agostini S, Longatti P, Jenkins RB, Giannini C. Primary leptomeningeal oligodendroglioma with documented progression to anaplasia and t(1;19)(q10;p10) in a child. Acta Neuropathol 2009, **118**: 575–577.

493 Sasaki H, Zlatescu MC, Betensky RA, Johnk LB, Cutone AN, Cairncross JG, Louis DN. Histopathological–molecular genetic correlations in referral pathologist-diagnosed low-grade 'oligodendroglioma'. J Neuropathol Exp Neurol 2002, **61**: 58–63.

494 Takei Y, Mirra SS, Miles ML. Eosinophilic granular cells in oligodendrogliomas. An ultrastructural study. Cancer 1976, **38**: 1968–1976.

495 Wharton SB, Chan KK, Hamilton FA, Anderson JR. Expression of neuronal markers in oligodendrogliomas: an immunohistochemical study. Neuropathol Appl Neurobiol 1998, **24**: 302–308.

496 Wolf HK, Buslei R, Blumcke I, Wiestler OD, Pietsch T. Neural antigens in oligodendrogliomas and dysembryoplastic neuroepithelial tumors. Acta Neuropathol 1997, **94**: 436–443.

Ependymal tumors

497 Akyurek S, Chang EL, Yu TK, Little D, Allen PK, McCutcheon I, Mahajan A, Maor MH, Woo SY. Spinal myxopapillary ependymoma outcomes in patients treated with surgery and radiotherapy at M.D. Anderson Cancer Center. J Neurooncol 2006, **80**: 177–183.

498 al Moutaery K, Aabed MY, Ojeda VJ. Cerebral and spinal cord myxopapillary ependymomas: a case report. Pathology 1996, **28**: 373–376.

499 Awaya H, Kaneko M, Amatya VJ, Takeshima Y, Oka S, Inai K. Myxopapillary ependymoma with anaplastic features. Pathol Int 2003, **53**: 700–703.

500 Bagley CA, Kothbauer KF, Wilson S, Bookland MJ, Epstein FJ, Jallo GI. Resection of myxopapillary ependymomas in children. J Neurosurg (4 Suppl Pediatrics) 2007, **106**: 261–267.

501 Chan AC, Ho LC, Yip WW, Cheung FC. Pigmented ependymoma with lipofuscin and neuromelanin production. Arch Pathol Lab Med 2003, **127**: 872–875.

502 Choi YL, Chi JG, Suh YL. CD99 immunoreactivity in ependymoma. Appl Immunohistochem Mol Morphol 2001, **9**: 125–129.

503 Coffin CM, Swanson PE, Wick MR, Dehner LP. An immunohistochemical comparison of chordoma with renal cell carcinoma, colorectal adenocarcinoma, and myxopapillary ependymoma: a potential diagnostic dilemma in the diminutive biopsy. Mod Pathol 1993, **6**: 531–538.

504 Craver RD, McGarry P. Delicate longitudinal nuclear grooves in childhood ependymomas. Arch Pathol Lab Med 1994, **118**: 919–921.

505 Crotty TB, Hooker RP, Swensen SJ, Scheithauer BW, Myers JL. Primary malignant ependymoma of the lung. Mayo Clin Proc 1992, **67**: 373–378.

506 Epstein FJ, Farmer JP, Freed D. Adult intramedullary spinal cord ependymomas: the result of surgery in 38 patients. J Neurosurg 1993, **79**: 204–209.

507 Fassett DR, Pingree J, Kestle JR. The high incidence of tumor dissemination in myxopapillary ependymoma in pediatric patients. Report of five cases and review of the literature. J Neurosurg (Pediatrics 1) 2005, **102**: 59–64.

508 Figarella-Branger D, Lepidi H, Poncet C, Gambarelli D, Bianco N, Rougon G, Pellissier JF. Differential expression of cell adhesion molecules (CAM), neural CAM and epithelial cadherin in ependymomas and choroid plexus tumors. Acta Neuropathol 1995, **89**: 248–257.

509 Fouladi M, Helton K, Dalton J, Gilger E, Gajjar A, Merchant T, Kun L, Newsham I, Burger P, Fuller C. Clear cell ependymoma: a clinicopathologic and radiographic analysis of 10 patients. Cancer 2003, **98**: 2232–2244.

510 Furness PN, Lowe J, Tarrant GS. Subepithelial basement membrane deposition and intermediate filament expression in choroid plexus neoplasms and ependymomas. Histopathology 1990, **16**: 251–255.

511 Gessi M, Marani C, Geddes J, Arcella A, Cenacchi G, Giangaspero F. Ependymoma with neuropil-like islands: a case report with diagnostic and histogenetic implications. Acta Neuropathol 2005, **109**: 231–234.

512 Hasselblatt M, Paulus W. Sensitivity and specificity of epithelial membrane antigen staining patterns in ependymomas. Acta Neuropathol 2003, **106**: 385–388.

513 Hegyi L, Peston D, Theodorou M, Moss J, Olver J, Roncaroli F. Primary glial tumor of the retina with features of myxopapillary ependymoma. Am J Surg Pathol 2005, **29**: 1404–1409.

514 Helwig EB, Stern JB. Subcutaneous sacrococcygeal myxopapillary ependymoma. A clinicopathologic study of 32 cases. Am J Clin Pathol 1984, **81**: 156–161.

515 Ho KL. Microtubular aggregates within rough endoplasmic reticulum in myxopapillary ependymoma of the filum terminale. Arch Pathol Lab Med 1990, **114**: 956–960.

516 Idowu MO, Rosenblum MK, Wei XJ, Edgar MA, Soslow RA. Ependymomas of the central nervous system and adult extra-axial ependymomas are morphologically and immunohistochemically distinct – a comparative study with assessment of ovarian carcinomas for expression of glial fibrillary acidic protein. Am J Surg Pathol 2008, **32**: 710–718.

517 Kawano N, Yagishita S, Oka H, Utsuki S, Kobayashi I, Suzuki S, Tachibana S, Fujii K. Spinal tanycytic ependymomas. Acta Neuropathol 2001, **101**: 43–48.

518 Kawano N, Yasui Y, Utsuki S, Oka H, Fujii K, Yamashina S. Light microscopic demonstration of the microlumen of ependymoma: a study of the usefulness of antigen retrieval for epithelial membrane antigen (EMA) immunostaining. Brain Tumor Pathol 2004, **21**: 17–21.

519 Kleinman GM, Zagzag D, Miller DC. Epithelioid ependymoma: a new variant of ependymoma: report of three cases. Neurosurgery 2003, **53**: 743–747; discussion 747–748.

520 Kline MJ, Kays DW, Rojiani AM. Extradural myxopapillary ependymoma: report of two cases and review of the literature. Pediatr Pathol Lab Med 1996, **16**: 813–822.

521 Kurt E, Zheng PP, Hop WC, van der Weiden M, Bol M, van den Bent MJ, Avezaat CJ, Kros JM. Identification of relevant prognostic histopathologic features in 69 intracranial ependymomas, excluding myxopapillary ependymomas and subependymomas. Cancer 2006, **106**: 388–395.

522 Lim SC, Jang SJ. Myxopapillary ependymoma of the fourth ventricle. Clin Neurol Neurosurg 2006, **108**: 211–214.

523 Little NS, Morgan MK, Eckstein RP. Primary ependymoma of a cranial nerve. Case report. J Neurosurg 1994, **81**: 792–794.

524 Lombardi D, Scheithauer BW, Meyer FB, Forbes GS, Shaw EG, Gibney DJ, Katzmann JA. Symptomatic subependymoma: a clinicopathological and flow cytometric study. J Neurosurg 1991, **75**: 583–588.

525 Louis DN, Hedley-Whyte ET, Martuza RL. Sarcomatous proliferation of the vasculature in a subependymoma: a follow-up study of sarcomatous dedifferentiation. Acta Neuropathol 1990, **80**: 573–574.

526 Maruyama R, Koga K, Nakahara T, Kishida K, Nabeshima K. Cerebral myxopapillary ependymoma. Hum Pathol 1992, **23**: 960–962.

527 Mathews T, Moossy J. Gliomas containing bone and cartilage. J Neuropathol Exp Neurol 1974, **33**: 456–471.

528 Mclendon RE, Wiestler OD, Kros JM, Korshunov A, Ng H-K. Ependymoma and anaplastic ependymoma. In Louis DN, Ohgaki H, Wiestler OD, Cavenee WK (eds): WHO classification of tumours of the central nervous system. Lyon, 2007, IARC, pp. 74–80.

529 Min KW, Scheithauer BW. Clear cell ependymoma: a mimic of oligodendroglioma: clinicopathologic and ultrastructural considerations. Am J Surg Pathol 1997, **21**: 820–826.

530 Miralbell R, Louis DN, O'Keeffe D, Rosenberg AE, Suit HD. Metastatic ependymoma of the sacrum. Cancer 1990, **65**: 2353–2355.
531 Mogler C, Kohlhof P, Penzel R, Grenacher L, Haag GM, Schirmacher P, Mueller W. A primary malignant ependymoma of the abdominal cavity: a case report and review of the literature. Virchows Arch 2009, **454**: 475–478.
532 Nobles E, Lee R, Kircher T. Mediastinal ependymoma. Hum Pathol 1991, **22**: 94–96.
533 Orakcioglu B, Schramm P, Kohlhof P, Aschoff A, Unterberg A, Halatsch ME. Characteristics of thoracolumbar intramedullary subependymomas. J Neurosurg Spine 2009, **10**: 54–59.
534 Pulitzer DR, Martin PC, Collins PC, Ralph DR. Subcutaneous sacrococcygeal ('myxopapillary') ependymal rests. Am J Surg Pathol 1988, **12**: 672–677.
535 Rodriguez FJ, Scheithauer BW, Perry A, Oliveira AM, Jenkins RB, Oviedo A, Mork SJ, Palmer CA, Burger PC. Ependymal tumors with sarcomatous change ('ependymosarcoma'): a clinicopathologic and molecular cytogenetic study. Am J Surg Pathol 2008, **32**: 699–709.
536 Rodriguez FJ, Scheithauer BW, Robbins PD, Burger PC, Hessler RB, Perry A, Abell-Aleff PC, Mierau GW. Ependymomas with neuronal differentiation: a morphologic and immunohistochemical spectrum. Acta Neuropathol 2007, **113**: 313–324.
537 Rosenblum MK, Erlandson RA, Aleksic SN, Budzilovich GN. Melanotic ependymoma and subependymoma. Am J Surg Pathol 1990, **14**: 729–736.
538 Ruchoux MM, Kepes JJ, Dhellemmes P, Hamon M, Maurage CA, Lecomte M, Gall CM, Chilton J. Lipomatous differentiation in ependymomas: a report of three cases and comparison with similar changes reported in other central nervous system neoplasms of neuroectodermal origin. Am J Surg Pathol 1998, **22**: 338–346.
539 Rushing EJ, Cooper PB, Quezado M, Begnami M, Crespo A, Smirniotopoulos JG, Ecklund J, Olsen C, Santi M. Subependymoma revisited: clinicopathological evaluation of 83 cases. J Neurooncol 2007, **85**: 297–305.
540 Sangoi AR, Lim M, Dulai MS, Vogel H, Chang S. Suprasellar giant cell ependymoma: a rare neoplasm in a unique location. Hum Pathol 2008, **39**: 1396–1401.
541 Sara A, Bruner JM, Mackay B. Ultrastructure of ependymoma. Ultrastruct Pathol 1994, **18**: 33–42.
542 Scheithauer BW, Swearingen B, Whyte ET, Auluck PK, Stemmer-Rachamimov AO. Ependymoma of the sella turcica: a variant of pituicytoma. Hum Pathol 2009, **40**: 435–440.
543 Snuderl M, Chi SN, De Santis SM, Stemmer-Rachamimov AO, Betensky RA, De Girolami U, Kieran MW. Prognostic value of tumor microinvasion and metalloproteinases expression in intracranial pediatric ependymomas. J Neuropathol Exp Neurol 2008, **67**: 911–920.
544 Sonneland PR, Scheithauer BW, Onofrio BM. Myxopapillary ependymoma. A clinicopathologic and immunocytochemical study of 77 cases. Cancer 1985, **56**: 883–893.
545 Takahashi H, Goto J, Emura I, Honma T, Hasegawa K, Uchiyama S. Lipidized (foamy) tumor cells in a spinal cord ependymoma with collagenous metaplasia. Acta Neuropathol 1998, **95**: 421–425.
546 Tay A, Scheithauer BW, Cameron JD, Myhre MJ, Boerner MJ. Retinal ependymoma: an immunohistologic and ultrastructural study. Hum Pathol 2009, **40**: 578–583.
547 Tihan T, Zhou T, Holmes E, Burger PC, Ozuysal S, Rushing EJ. The prognostic value of histological grading of posterior fossa ependymomas in children: a Children's Oncology Group study and a review of prognostic factors. Mod Pathol 2008, **21**: 165–177.
548 Tomlinson FH, Scheithauer BW, Kelly PJ, Forbes GS. Subependymoma with rhabdomyosarcomatous differentiation: report of a case and literature review. Neurosurgery 1991, **28**: 761–768.
549 Twiss JL, Anderson LJ, Horoupian DS. Globular glial fibrillary acidic protein-reactive cytoplasmic inclusions in ependymoma: an immunoelectron-microscopic study. Acta Neuropathol 1993, **85**: 658–662.
550 Vege KD, Giannini C, Scheithauer BW. The immunophenotype of ependymomas. Appl Immunohistochem Mol Morphol 2000, **8**: 25–31.
551 Whittemore DE, Grondahl RE, Wong K. Primary extraneural myxopapillary ependymoma of the broad ligament. Arch Pathol Lab Med 2005, **129**: 1338–1342.
552 Wiendl H, Feiden W, Scherieble H, Renz T, Dichgans J, Weller M. March 2003: A 41-year-old female with a solitary lesion in the liver. Brain Pathol 2003, **13**: 421–423.
553 Wolfsberger S, Fischer I, Hoftberger R, Birner P, Slavc I, Dieckmann K, Czech T, Budka H, Hainfellner J. Ki-67 immunolabeling index is an accurate predictor of outcome in patients with intracranial ependymoma. Am J Surg Pathol 2004, **28**: 914–920.
554 Zamecnik J, Chanova M, Kodet R. Expression of thyroid transcription factor 1 in primary brain tumours. J Clin Pathol 2004, **57**: 1111–1113.
555 Zec N, De Girolami U, Schofield DE, Scott RM, Anthony DC. Giant cell ependymoma of the filum terminale. A report of two cases. Am J Surg Pathol 1996, **20**: 1091–1101.
556 Zuppan CW, Mierau GW, Weeks DA. Ependymoma with signet-ring cells. Ultrastruct Pathol 1994, **18**: 43–46.

Mixed gliomas

557 Eoli M, Bissola L, Bruzzone MG, Pollo B, Maccagnano C, De Simone T, Valletta L, Silvani A, Bianchessi D, Broggi G, Boiardi A, Finocchiaro G. Reclassification of oligoastrocytomas by loss of heterozygosity studies. Int J Cancer 2006, **119**: 84–90.
558 Fuller CE, Schmidt RE, Roth KA, Burger PC, Scheithauer BW, Banerjee R, Trinkaus K, Lytle R, Perry A. Clinical utility of fluorescence in situ hybridization (FISH) in morphologically ambiguous gliomas with hybrid oligodendroglial/astrocytic features. J Neuropathol Exp Neurol 2003, **62**: 1118–1128.
559 Hart MN, Petito CK, Earle KM. Mixed gliomas. Cancer 1974, **33**: 134–140.
560 Kros JM, Gorlia T, Kouwenhoven MC, Zheng PP, Collins VP, Figarella-Branger D, Giangaspero F, Giannini C, Mokhtari K, Mork SJ, Paetau A, Reifenberger G, van den Bent MJ. Panel review of anaplastic oligodendroglioma from European Organization For Research and Treatment of Cancer Trial 26951: assessment of consensus in diagnosis, influence of 1p/19q loss, and correlations with outcome. J Neuropathol Exp Neurol 2007, **66**: 545–551.
561 Maintz D, Fiedler K, Koopmann J, Rollbrocker B, Nechev S, Lenartz D, Stangl AP, Louis DN, Schramm J, Wiestler OD, von Deimling A. Molecular genetic evidence for subtypes of oligoastrocytomas. J Neuropathol Exp Neurol 1997, **56**: 1098–1104.
562 Miller CR, Dunham CP, Scheithauer BW, Perry A. Significance of necrosis in grading of oligodendroglial neoplasms: a clinicopathologic and genetic study of newly diagnosed high-grade gliomas. J Clin Oncol 2006, **24**: 5419–5426.
563 van den Bent MJ, Carpentier AF, Brandes AA, Sanson M, Taphoorn MJ, Bernsen HJ, Frenay M, Tijssen CC, Grisold W, Sipos L, Haaxma-Reiche H, Kros JM, van Kouwenhoven MC, Vecht CJ, Allgeier A, Lacombe D, Gorlia T. Adjuvant procarbazine, lomustine, and vincristine improves progression-free survival but not overall survival in newly diagnosed anaplastic oligodendrogliomas and oligoastrocytomas: a randomized European Organisation for Research and Treatment of Cancer phase III trial. J Clin Oncol 2006, **24**: 2715–2722.
564 von Deimling A, Reifenberger G, Kros JM, Louis DN, Collins VP. Oligoastrocytoma/anaplastic oligoastrocytoma. In Louis DN, Ohgaki HK, Wiestler OD, Cavenee WK (eds): The WHO classification of tumours of the central nervous system. Lyon, 2007, IARC, pp. 63–67.

Astroblastoma

565 Bonnin JM, Rubinstein LJ. Astroblastomas: a pathological study of 23 tumors, with a postoperative follow-up in 13 patients. Neurosurgery 1989, **25**: 6–13.
566 Brat DJ, Hirose Y, Cohen KJ, Feuerstein BG, Burger PC. Astroblastoma: clinicopathologic features and chromosomal abnormalities defined by comparative genomic hybridization. Brain Pathol 2000, **10**: 342–352.
567 Cabello A, Madero S, Castresana A, Diaz-Lobato R. Astroblastoma: electron microscopy and immunohistochemical findings: case report. Surg Neurol 1991, **35**: 116–121.
568 Jay V, Edwards V, Squire J, Rutka J. Astroblastoma: report of a case with ultrastructural, cell kinetic, and cytogenetic analysis. Pediatr Pathol 1993, **13**: 323–332.
569 Pizer BL, Moss T, Oakhill A, Webb D, Coakham HB. Congenital astroblastoma: an immunohistochemical study. Case report. J Neurosurg 1995, **83**: 550–555.
570 Rubinstein LJ, Herman MM. The astroblastoma and its possible cytogenic relationship to the tanycyte. An electron microscopic, immunohistochemical, tissue- and organ-culture study. Acta Neuropathol 1989, **78**: 472–483.
571 Thiessen B, Finlay J, Kulkarni R, Rosenblum MK. Astroblastoma: does histology predict biologic behavior? J Neurooncol 1998, **40**: 59–65.

Chordoid glioma of the third ventricle

572 Brat DJ, Scheithauer BW, Staugaitis SM, Cortez SC, Brecher K, Burger PC. Third ventricular chordoid glioma: a distinct clinicopathologic entity. J Neuropathol Exp Neurol 1998, **57**: 283–290.
573 Castellano-Sanchez AA, Schemankewitz E, Mazewski C, Brat DJ. Pediatric chordoid glioma with chondroid metaplasia. Pediatr Dev Pathol 2001, 4: 564–567.
574 Cenacchi G, Roncaroli F, Cerasoli S, Ficarra G, Merli GA, Giangaspero F. Chordoid glioma of the third ventricle: an ultrastructural study of three cases with a

histogenetic hypothesis. Am J Surg Pathol 2001, **25**: 401–405.

575 Horbinski C, Dacic S, McLendon RE, Cieply K, Datto M, Brat DJ, Chu CT. Chordoid glioma: a case report and molecular characterization of five cases. Brain Pathol 2009, **19**: 439–448.

576 Jain D, Sharma MC, Sarkar C, Suri V, Rishi A, Garg A, Vaishya S. Chordoid glioma: report of two rare examples with unusual features. Acta Neurochir (Wien) 2008, **150**: 295–300; discussion 300.

577 Kurian KM, Summers DM, Statham PF, Smith C, Bell JE, Ironside JW. Third ventricular chordoid glioma: clinicopathological study of two cases with evidence for a poor clinical outcome despite low grade histological features. Neuropathol Appl Neurobiol 2005, **31**: 354–361.

578 Leeds NE, Lang FF, Ribalta T, Sawaya R, Fuller GN. Origin of chordoid glioma of the third ventricle. Arch Pathol Lab Med 2006, **130**: 460–464.

579 Pasquier B, Peoc'h M, Morrison AL, Gay E, Pasquier D, Grand S, Sindou M, Kopp N. Chordoid glioma of the third ventricle: a report of two new cases, with further evidence supporting an ependymal differentiation, and review of the literature. Am J Surg Pathol 2002, **26**: 1330–1342.

580 Raizer JJ, Shetty T, Gutin PH, Obbens EA, Holodny AI, Antonescu CR, Rosenblum MK. Chordoid glioma: report of a case with unusual histologic features, ultrastructural study and review of the literature. J Neurooncol 2003, **63**: 39–47.

581 Reifenberger G, Weber T, Weber RG, Wolter M, Brandis A, Kuchelmeister K, Pilz P, Reusche E, Lichter P, Wiestler OD. Chordoid glioma of the third ventricle: immunohistochemical and molecular genetic characterization of a novel tumor entity. Brain Pathol 1999, **9**: 617–626.

Angiocentric glioma

582 Burger PC, Jouvet A, Preusser M, Hans VH, Rosenblum MK, Lellouch-Tubiana A. Angiocentric glioma. In Louis DN, Ohgaki H, Wiestler OD, Cavenee WK (eds): WHO classification of tumours of the central nervous system. Lyon, 2007, IARC, pp. 92–93.

583 Covington DB, Rosenblum MK, Brathwaite CD, Sandberg DI. Angiocentric glioma-like tumor of the midbrain. Pediatr Neurosurg 2009, **45**: 429–433.

584 Lellouch-Tubiana A, Boddaert N, Bourgeois M, Fohlen M, Jouvet A, Delalande O, Seidenwurm D, Brunelle F, Sainte-Rose C. Angiocentric neuroepithelial tumor (ANET): a new epilepsy-related clinicopathological entity with distinctive MRI. Brain Pathol 2005, **15**: 281–286.

585 Preusser M, Hoischen A, Novak K, Czech T, Prayer D, Hainfellner JA, Baumgartner C, Woermann FG, Tuxhorn IE, Pannek HW, Bergmann M, Radlwimmer B, Villagran R, Weber RG, Hans VH. Angiocentric glioma: report of clinico-pathologic and genetic findings in 8 cases. Am J Surg Pathol 2007, **31**: 1709–1718.

586 Wang M, Tihan T, Rojiani AM, Bodhireddy SR, Prayson RA, Iacuone JJ, Alles AJ, Donahue DJ, Hessler RB, Kim JH, Haas M, Rosenblum MK, Burger PC. Monomorphous angiocentric glioma: a distinctive epileptogenic neoplasm with features of infiltrating astrocytoma and ependymoma. J Neuropathol Exp Neurol 2005, **64**: 875–881.

Gliomatosis cerebri

587 Artigas J, Cervos-Navarro J, Iglesias JR, Ebhardt G. Gliomatosis cerebri: clinical and histological findings. Clin Neuropathol 1985, **4**: 135–148.

588 Cummings TJ, Hulette CM, Longee DC, Bottom KS, McLendon RE, Chu CT. Gliomatosis cerebri: cytologic and autopsy findings in a case involving the entire neuraxis. Clin Neuropathol 1999, **18**: 190–197.

589 Fuller GN, Kros JM. Gliomatosis cerebri. In Louis DN, Ohagaki HK, Wiestler OD, Cavenee WK (eds): WHO classification of tumours of the central nervous system. Lyon, 2007, IARC, pp. 50–52.

590 Kim DG, Yang HJ, Park IA, Chi JG, Jung HW, Han DH, Choi KS, Cho BK. Gliomatosis cerebri: clinical features, treatment, and prognosis. Acta Neurochir (Wien) 1998, **140**: 755–762.

591 Nishioka H, Ito H, Miki T. Difficulties in the antemortem diagnosis of gliomatosis cerebri: report of a case with diffuse increase of gemistocyte-like cells, mimicking reactive gliosis. Br J Neurosurg 1996, **10**: 103–107.

591a Seiz M, Tuettenberg J, Meyer J, Essig M, Schmieder K, Mawrin C, von Deimling A, Hartmann C. Detection of IDH1 mutations in gliomatosis cerebri, but only in tumors with additional solid component: evidence for molecular subtypes. Acta Neuropathol 2010, **120**: 261–267.

592 Taillibert S, Chodkiewicz C, Laigle-Donadey F, Napolitano M, Cartalat-Carel S, Sanson M. Gliomatosis cerebri: a review of 296 cases from the ANOCEF database and the literature. J Neurooncol 2006, **76**: 201–205.

593 Tancredi A, Mangiola A, Guiducci A, Peciarolo A, Ottaviano P. Oligodendrocytic gliomatosis cerebri. Acta Neurochir (Wien) 2000, **142**: 469–472.

Gliosarcoma and other 'gliomesenchymal' tumors

594 Bonnin JM, Pena CE, Rubinstein LJ. Mixed capillary hemangioblastoma and glioma. A redefinition of the 'angioglioma'. J Neuropathol Exp Neurol 1983, **42**: 504–516.

595 Cerda-Nicolas M, Kepes JJ. Gliofibromas (including malignant forms), and gliosarcomas: a comparative study and review of the literature. Acta Neuropathol 1993, **85**: 349–361.

596 Giangaspero F, Kaulich K, Cenacchi G, Cerasoli S, Lerch KD, Breu H, Reuter T, Reifenberger G. Lipoastrocytoma: a rare low-grade astrocytoma variant of pediatric age. Acta Neuropathol 2002, **103**: 152–156.

597 Goodkin R, Zaias B, Michelsen WJ. Arteriovenous malformation and glioma: coexistent or sequential? Case report. J Neurosurg 1990, **72**: 798–805.

598 Grant JW, Steart PV, Aguzzi A, Jones DB, Gallagher PJ. Gliosarcoma: an immunohistochemical study. Acta Neuropathol 1989, **79**: 305–309.

599 Haddad SF, Moore SA, Schelper RL, Goeken JA. Smooth muscle can comprise the sarcomatous component of gliosarcomas. J Neuropathol Exp Neurol 1992, **51**: 493–498.

600 Jones H, Steart PV, Weller RO. Spindle-cell glioblastoma or gliosarcoma? Neuropathol Appl Neurobiol 1991, **17**: 177–187.

601 Kepes JJ, Rubinstein LJ, Chiang H. The role of astrocytes in the formation of cartilage in gliomas. An immunohistochemical study of four cases. Am J Pathol 1984, **117**: 471–483.

602 Lalitha VS, Rubinstein LJ. Reactive glioma in intracranial sarcoma: a form of mixed sarcoma and glioma ('sarcoglioma'): report of eight cases. Cancer 1979, **43**: 246–257.

603 Meis JM, Martz KL, Nelson JS. Mixed glioblastoma multiforme and sarcoma. A clinicopathologic study of 26 radiation therapy oncology group cases. Cancer 1991, **67**: 2342–2349.

604 Montpetit VJ, Pokrupa R, Richard MT, Clapin DF. Myofibroblastic differentiation of a primary intracerebral sarcoma with gliomatous reaction. Clin Neuropathol 1988, **7**: 1–9.

605 Nomura M, Hasegawa M, Kita D, Yamashita J, Minato H, Nakazato Y. Cerebellar gliofibroma with numerous psammoma bodies. Clin Neurol Neurosurg 2006, **108**: 421–425.

606 Ozolek JA, Finkelstein SD, Couce ME. Gliosarcoma with epithelial differentiation: immunohistochemical and molecular characterization. A case report and review of the literature. Mod Pathol 2004, **17**: 739–745.

607 Paulus W, Jellinger K. Mixed glioblastoma and malignant mesenchymoma, a variety of gliosarcoma. Histopathology 1993, **22**: 277–279.

608 Perry JR, Ang LC, Bilbao JM, Muller PJ. Clinicopathologic features of primary and postirradiation cerebral gliosarcoma. Cancer 1995, **75**: 2910–2918.

609 Prayson RA. Gliofibroma: a distinct entity or a subtype of desmoplastic astrocytoma? Hum Pathol 1996, **27**: 610–613.

610 Reis RM, Konu-Lebleblicioglu D, Lopes JM, Kleihues P, Ohgaki H. Genetic profile of gliosarcomas. Am J Pathol 2000, **156**: 425–432.

611 Sarkar C, Sharma MC, Sudha K, Gaikwad S, Varma A. A clinico-pathological study of 29 cases of gliosarcoma with special reference to two unique variants. Indian J Med Res 1997, **106**: 229–235.

612 Sharma MC, Gaikwad S, Mehta VS, Dhar J, Sarkar C. Gliofibroma: mixed glial and mesenchymal tumour. Report of three cases. Clin Neurol Neurosurg 1998, **100**: 153–159.

613 Shintaku M, Miyaji K, Adachi Y. Gliosarcoma with angiosarcomatous features: a case report. Brain Tumor Pathol 1998, **15**: 101–105.

614 Slowik F, Jellinger K, Gaszo L, Fischer J. Gliosarcomas: histological, immunohistochemical, ultrastructural, and tissue culture studies. Acta Neuropathol 1985, **67**: 201–210.

615 Vazquez M, Miller DC, Epstein F, Allen JC, Budzilovich GN. Glioneurofibroma: renaming the pediatric 'gliofibroma': a neoplasm composed of Schwann cells and astrocytes. Mod Pathol 1991, **4**: 519–523.

616 Vlodavsky E, Konstantinesku M, Soustiel JF. Gliosarcoma with liposarcomatous differentiation: the new member of the lipid-containing brain tumors family. Arch Pathol Lab Med 2006, **130**: 381–384.

617 Wargotz ES, Sidawy MK, Jannotta FS. Thorotrast-associated gliosarcoma. Including comments on thorotrast use and review of sequelae with particular reference to lesions of the central nervous system. Cancer 1988, **62**: 58–66.

CHOROID PLEXUS TUMORS

618 Aquilina K, Nanra JS, Allcutt DA, Farrell M. Choroid plexus adenoma: case report and review of the literature. Childs Nerv Syst 2005, **21**: 410–415.

619 Beschorner R, Pantazis G, Jeibmann A, Boy J, Meyermann R, Mittelbronn M, Schittenhelm J. Expression of EAAT-1 distinguishes choroid plexus tumors from normal and reactive choroid plexus epithelium. Acta Neuropathol 2009, **117**: 667–675.

620 Beschorner R, Schittenhelm J, Schimmel H, Iglesias-Rozas JR, Herberts T, Schlaszus H, Meyermann R, Wehrmann M. Choroid plexus tumors differ from metastatic carcinomas by expression of the excitatory amino acid transporter-1. Hum Pathol 2006, **37**: 854–860.

621 Boldorini R, Panzarasa G, Girardi P, Monga G. Primary choroid plexus papilloma of the sacral nerve roots. J Neurosurg Spine 2009, **10**: 51–53.

622 Buccoliero AM, Bacci S, Mennonna P, Taddei GL. Pathologic quiz case: infratentorial tumor in a middle-aged woman. Oncocytic variant of choroid plexus papilloma. Arch Pathol Lab Med 2004, **128**: 1448–1450.

623 Carlotti CG Jr, Salhia B, Weitzman S, Greenberg M, Dirks PB, Mason W, Becker LE, Rutka JT. Evaluation of proliferative index and cell cycle protein expression in choroid plexus tumors in children. Acta Neuropathol 2002, **103**: 1–10.

624 Coffin CM, Wick MR, Braun JT, Dehner LP. Choroid plexus neoplasms. Clinicopathologic and immunohistochemical studies. Am J Surg Pathol 1986, **10**: 394–404.

625 D'Ambrosio AL, O'Toole JE, Connolly ES Jr, Feldstein NA. Villous hypertrophy versus choroid plexus papilloma: a case report demonstrating a diagnostic role for the proliferation index. Pediatr Neurosurg 2003, **39**: 91–96.

626 Diengdoh JV, Shaw MD. Oncocytic variant of choroid plexus papilloma. Evolution from benign to malignant 'oncocytoma'. Cancer 1993, **71**: 855–858.

627 Dobin SM, Donner LR. Pigmented choroid plexus carcinoma: a cytogenetic and ultrastructural study. Cancer Genet Cytogenet 1997, **96**: 37–41.

628 Duckett S, Osterholm J, Schaefer D, Gonzales C, Schwartzman RJ. Ossified mucin-secreting choroid plexus adenoma: case report. Neurosurgery 1991, **29**: 130–132.

629 Erman T, Gocer AI, Erdogan S, Tuna M, Ildan F, Zorludemir S. Choroid plexus papilloma of bilateral lateral ventricle. Acta Neurochir (Wien) 2003, **145**: 139–143; discussion 143.

630 Fuller CE, Smith M, Miller DC, Schelper R. Pigmented papillary epithelial neoplasm of the pituitary fossa: a distinct lesion of uncertain histogenesis. Arch Pathol Lab Med 2001, **125**: 1242–1245.

631 Gottschalk J, Jautzke G, Paulus W, Goebel S, Cervos-Navarro J. The use of immunomorphology to differentiate choroid plexus tumors from metastatic carcinomas. Cancer 1993, **72**: 1343–1349.

632 Gyure KA, Morrison AL. Cytokeratin 7 and 20 expression in choroid plexus tumors: utility in differentiating these neoplasms from metastatic carcinomas. Mod Pathol 2000, **13**: 638–643.

633 Hamilton RL. Case of the month. May 1996: Hydrocephalus in a 9 month old infant. Brain Pathol 1996, **6**: 533–534.

634 Hasselblatt M, Bohm C, Tatenhorst L, Dinh V, Newrzella D, Keyvani K, Jeibmann A, Buerger H, Rickert CH, Paulus W. Identification of novel diagnostic markers for choroid plexus tumors: a microarray-based approach. Am J Surg Pathol 2006, **30**: 66–74.

635 Hasselblatt M, Jeibmann A, Guerry M, Senner V, Paulus W, McLendon RE. Choroid plexus papilloma with neuropil-like islands. Am J Surg Pathol 2008, **32**: 162–166.

636 Jeibmann A, Hasselblatt M, Gerss J, Wrede B, Egensperger R, Beschorner R, Hans VH, Rickert CH, Wolff JE, Paulus W. Prognostic implications of atypical histologic features in choroid plexus papilloma. J Neuropathol Exp Neurol 2006, **65**: 1069–1073.

637 Jeibmann A, Wrede B, Peters O, Wolff JE, Paulus W, Hasselblatt M. Malignant progression in choroid plexus papillomas. J Neurosurg (3 Suppl Pediatrics) 2007, **107**: 199–202.

638 Judkins AR, Burger PC, Hamilton RL, Kleinschmidt-DeMasters B, Perry A, Pomeroy SL, Rosenblum MK, Yachnis AT, Zhou H, Rorke LB, Biegel JA. INI1 protein expression distinguishes atypical teratoid/rhabdoid tumor from choroid plexus carcinoma. J Neuropathol Exp Neurol 2005, **64**: 391–397.

639 Kepes JJ, Collins J. Choroid plexus epithelium (normal and neoplastic) expresses synaptophysin. A potentially useful aid in differentiating carcinoma of the choroid plexus from metastatic papillary carcinomas. J Neuropathol Exp Neurol 1999, **58**: 398–401.

640 Kimura M, Takayasu M, Suzuki Y, Negoro M, Nagasaka T, Nakashima N, Sugita K. Primary choroid plexus papilloma located in the suprasellar region: case report. Neurosurgery 1992, **31**: 563–566.

641 Kurtkaya-Yapicier O, Scheithauer BW, Van Peteghem KP, Sawicki JE. Unusual case of extradural choroid plexus papilloma of the sacral canal. Case report. J Neurosurg (Spine 1) 2002, **97**: 102–105.

642 Levy ML, Goldfarb A, Hyder DJ, Gonzales-Gomez I, Nelson M, Gilles FH, McComb JG. Choroid plexus tumors in children: significance of stromal invasion. Neurosurgery 2001, **48**: 303–309.

643 Matsushima T. Choroid plexus papillomas and human choroid plexus. A light and electron microscopic study. J Neurosurg 1983, **59**: 1054–1062.

644 McCall T, Binning M, Blumenthal DT, Jensen RL. Variations of disseminated choroid plexus papilloma: 2 case reports and a review of the literature. Surg Neurol 2006, **66**: 62–67; discussion 67–68.

645 McComb RD, Burger PC. Choroid plexus carcinoma. Report of a case with immunohistochemical and ultrastructural observations. Cancer 1983, **51**: 470–475.

646 Miyagi Y, Natori Y, Suzuki SO, Iwaki T, Morioka T, Arimura K, Maeda Y, Shono T, Matsukado K, Sasaki T. Purely cystic form of choroid plexus papilloma with acute hydrocephalus in an infant. Case report. J Neurosurg (6 Suppl Pediatrics) 2006, **105**: 480–484.

647 Paulus W, Brandner S. Choroid plexus tumours. In Louis DN, Ohgaki H, Wiestler OD, Cavenee WK (eds): WHO classification of tumours of the central nervous system. Lyon, 2007, IARC, pp. 82–85.

648 Paulus W, Janisch W. Clinicopathologic correlations in epithelial choroid plexus neoplasms: a study of 52 cases. Acta Neuropathol 1990, **80**: 635–641.

649 Pillai A, Rajeev K, Chandi S, Unnikrishnan M. Intrinsic brainstem choroid plexus papilloma. Case report. J Neurosurg 2004, **100**: 1076–1078.

650 Salazar J, Vaquero J, Aranda IF, Menendez J, Jimenez MD, Bravo G. Choroid plexus papilloma with chondroma: case report. Neurosurgery 1986, **18**: 781–783.

651 Smith ZA, Moftakhar P, Malkasian D, Xiong Z, Vinters HV, Lazareff JA. Choroid plexus hyperplasia: surgical treatment and immunohistochemical results. Case report. J Neurosurg (3 Suppl Pediatrics) 2007, **107**: 255–262.

651a Tabori U, Shlien A, Baskin B, Levitt S, Ray P, Alon N, Hawkins C, Bouffet E, Pienkowska M, Lafay-Cousin L, Gozali A, Zhukova N, Shane L, Gonzalez I, Finlay J, Malkin D. TP53 alterations determine clinical subgroups and survival of patients with choroid plexus tumors. J Clin Oncol 2010, **28**: 1995–2001.

652 Vajtai I, Varga Z, Aguzzi A. MIB-1 immunoreactivity reveals different labelling in low-grade and in malignant epithelial neoplasms of the choroid plexus. Histopathology 1996, **29**: 147–151.

653 Wolff JE, Sajedi M, Brant R, Coppes MJ, Egeler RM. Choroid plexus tumours. Br J Cancer 2002, **87**: 1086–1091.

NEURONAL AND GLIONEURONAL TUMORS, HAMARTOMAS, AND RELATED LESIONS

Gangliocytoma and ganglioglioma

654 Allegranza A, Pileri S, Frank G, Ferracini R. Cerebral ganglioglioma with anaplastic oligodendroglial component. Histopathology 1990, **17**: 439–441.

655 Allen JC, Judkins AR, Rosenblum MK, Biegel JA. Atypical teratoid/rhabdoid tumor evolving from an optic pathway ganglioglioma: case study. Neuro Oncol 2006, **8**: 79–82.

656 Athale S, Hallet KK, Jinkins JR. Ganglioglioma of the trigeminal nerve: MRI. Neuroradiology 1999, **41**: 576–578.

657 Baussard B, Di Rocco F, Garnett MR, Boddaert N, Lellouch-Tubiana A, Grill J, Puget S, Roujeau T, Zerah M, Sainte-Rose C. Pediatric infratentorial gangliogliomas: a retrospective series. J Neurosurg (4 Suppl Pediatrics) 2007, **107**: 286–291.

658 Becker AJ, Wiestler OD, Figarella-Branger D, Blümcke I. Ganglioglioma and gangliocytoma. In Louis DN, Ohgaki H, Wiestler OD, Cavenee WK (eds): WHO classification of tumours of the central nervous system. Lyon, 2007, IARC, pp. 103–105.

659 Blümcke I, Giencke K, Wardelmann E, Beyenburg S, Kral T, Sarioglu N, Pietsch T, Wolf HK, Schramm J, Elger CE, Wiestler OD. The CD34 epitope is expressed in neoplastic and malformative lesions associated with chronic, focal epilepsies. Acta Neuropathol 1999, **97**: 481–490.

660 Blümcke I, Wiestler OD. Gangliogliomas: an intriguing tumor entity associated with focal epilepsies. J Neuropathol Exp Neurol 2002, **61**: 575–584.

661 Brat DJ, Gearing M, Goldthwaite PT, Wainer BH, Burger PC. Tau-associated neuropathology in ganglion cell tumours increases with patient age but appears unrelated to ApoE genotype. Neuropathol Appl Neurobiol 2001, **27**: 197–205.

662 Caccamo D, Herman MM, Urich H, Rubinstein LJ. Focal neuronal gigantism and cerebral cortical thickening after therapeutic irradiation of the central nervous system. Arch Pathol Lab Med 1989, **113**: 880–885.

663 Choi YH, Kim IO, Cheon JE, Kim WS, Yeon KM, Wang KC, Cho BK, Chi JG. Gangliocytoma of the spinal cord: a case report. Pediatr Radiol 2001, **31**: 377–380.

664 Dash RC, Provenzale JM, McComb RD, Perry DA, Longee DC, McLendon RE. Malignant supratentorial ganglioglioma (ganglion cell-giant cell glioblastoma): a case report and review of the literature. Arch Pathol Lab Med 1999, **123**: 342–345.

665 David KM, de Sanctis S, Lewis PD, Noury AM, Edwards JM. Neuroblastomatous recurrence of ganglioglioma. Case report. J Neurosurg 2000, **93**: 698–700.

666 Deb P, Sharma MC, Tripathi M, Sarat Chandra P, Gupta A, Sarkar C. Expression of CD34 as a novel marker for glioneuronal lesions associated with chronic intractable epilepsy. Neuropathol Appl Neurobiol 2006, **32**: 461–468.

667 Di Patre PL, Payer M, Brunea M, Delavelle J, De Tribolet N, Pizzolato G. Malignant transformation of a spinal cord ganglioglioma – case report and review of the literature. Clin Neuropathol 2004, **23**: 298–303.

668 Duggal N, Hammond RR. Nestin expression in ganglioglioma. Exp Neurol 2002, **174**: 89–95.

669 Felix I, Bilbao JM, Asa SL, Tyndel F, Kovacs K, Becker LE. Cerebral and cerebellar gangliocytomas: a morphological study of nine cases. Acta Neuropathol 1994, **88**: 246–251.

670 Geddes JF, Jansen GH, Robinson SF, Gomori E, Holton JL, Monson JP, Besser GM, Revesz T. 'Gangliocytomas' of the pituitary: a heterogeneous group of lesions with differing histogenesis. Am J Surg Pathol 2000, **24**: 607–613.

671 Hakim R, Loeffler JS, Anthony DC, Black PM. Gangliogliomas in adults. Cancer 1997, **79**: 127–131.

672 Harmon HL, Gossman MD, Buchino JJ, Eberly SM, Roberts DM, Fishman PH. Orbital ganglioglioma arising from ectopic neural tissue. Am J Ophthalmol 2000, **129**: 109–111.

673 Hayashi S, Kameyama S, Fukuda M, Takahashi H. Ganglioglioma with a tanycytic ependymoma as the glial component. Acta Neuropathol 2000, **99**: 310–316.

674 Hirose T, Scheithauer BW, Lopes MB, Gerber HA, Altermatt HJ, VandenBerg SR. Ganglioglioma: an ultrastructural and immunohistochemical study. Cancer 1997, **79**: 989–1003.

675 Issidorides MR, Havaki S, Chrysanthou-Piterou M, Arvanitis DL. Ultrastructural identification of protein bodies, cellular markers of human catecholamine neurons, in a temporal lobe ganglioglioma. Ultrastruct Pathol 2000, **24**: 399–405.

676 Jallo GI, Freed D, Epstein FJ. Spinal cord gangliogliomas: a review of 56 patients. J Neurooncol 2004, **68**: 71–77.

677 Jay V, Squire J, Becker LE, Humphreys R. Malignant transformation in a ganglioglioma with anaplastic neuronal and astrocytic components. Report of a case with flow cytometric and cytogenetic analysis. Cancer 1994, **73**: 2862–2868.

678 Johnson JH Jr, Hariharan S, Berman J, Sutton LN, Rorke LB, Molloy P, Phillips PC. Clinical outcome of pediatric gangliogliomas: ninety-nine cases over 20 years. Pediatr Neurosurg 1997, **27**: 203–207.

679 Krouwer HG, Davis RL, McDermott MW, Hoshino T, Prados MD. Gangliogliomas: a clinicopathological study of 25 cases and review of the literature. J Neurooncol 1993, **17**: 139–154.

680 Lang FF, Epstein FJ, Ransohoff J, Allen JC, Wisoff J, Abbott IR, Miller DC. Central nervous system gangliogliomas. Part 2: Clinical outcome. J Neurosurg 1993, **79**: 867–873.

681 Lu WY, Goldman M, Young B, Davis DG. Optic nerve ganglioglioma. Case report. J Neurosurg 1993, **78**: 979–982.

682 Luyken C, Blümcke I, Fimmers R, Urbach H, Wiestler OD, Schramm J. Supratentorial gangliogliomas: histopathologic grading and tumor recurrence in 184 patients with a median follow-up of 8 years. Cancer 2004, **101**: 146–155.

683 Miller DC, Lang FF, Epstein FJ. Central nervous system gangliogliomas. Part 1: Pathology. J Neurosurg 1993, **79**: 859–866.

683a Perry A, Burton SS, Fuller GN, Robinson CA, Palmer CA, Resch L, Bigio EH, Gujrati M, Rosenblum MK. Oligodendroglial neoplasms with ganglioglioma-like maturation: a diagnostic pitfall. Acta Neuropathol 2010, **120**: 237–252.

684 Prayson RA, Khajavi K, Comair YG. Cortical architectural abnormalities and MIB1 immunoreactivity in gangliogliomas: a study of 60 patients with intracranial tumors. J Neuropathol Exp Neurol 1995, **54**: 513–520.

685 Preusser M, Laggner U, Haberler C, Heinzl H, Budka H, Hainfellner JA. Comparative analysis of NeuN immunoreactivity in primary brain tumours: conclusions for rational use in diagnostic histopathology. Histopathology 2006, **48**: 438–444.

686 Quinn B. Synaptophysin staining in normal brain: importance for diagnosis of ganglioglioma. Am J Surg Pathol 1998, **22**: 550–556.

687 Selch MT, Goy BW, Lee SP, El-Sadin S, Kincaid P, Park SH, Withers HR. Gangliogliomas: experience with 34 patients and review of the literature. Am J Clin Oncol 1998, **21**: 557–564.

688 Soffer D, Lach B, Constantini S. Melanotic cerebral ganglioglioma: evidence for melanogenesis in neoplastic astrocytes. Acta Neuropathol 1992, **83**: 315–323.

689 Suzuki H, Otsuki T, Iwasaki Y, Katakura R, Asano H, Tadokoro M, Suzuki Y, Tezuka F, Takei H. Anaplastic ganglioglioma with sarcomatous component: an immunohistochemical study and molecular analysis of p53 tumor suppressor gene. Neuropathology 2002, **22**: 40–47.

690 Wacker MR, Cogen PH, Etzell JE, Daneshvar L, Davis RL, Prados MD. Diffuse leptomeningeal involvement by a ganglioglioma in a child. Case report. J Neurosurg 1992, **77**: 302–306.

691 Wolf HK, Muller MB, Spanle M, Zentner J, Schramm J, Wiestler OD. Ganglioglioma: a detailed histopathological and immunohistochemical analysis of 61 cases. Acta Neuropathol 1994, **88**: 166–173.

692 Zentner J, Wolf HK, Ostertun B, Hufnagel A, Campos MG, Solymosi L, Schramm J. Gangliogliomas: clinical, radiological, and histopathological findings in 51 patients. J Neurol Neurosurg Psychiatry 1994, **57**: 1497–1502.

693 Zhang PJ, Rosenblum MK. Synaptophysin expression in the human spinal cord. Diagnostic implications of an immunohistochemical study. Am J Surg Pathol 1996, **20**: 273–276.

694 Zhu JJ, Leon SP, Folkerth RD, Guo SZ, Wu JK, Black PM. Evidence for clonal origin of neoplastic neuronal and glial cells in gangliogliomas. Am J Pathol 1997, **151**: 565–571.

Desmoplastic infantile ganglioglioma/desmoplastic infantile astrocytoma

695 Aydin F, Ghatak NR, Salvant J, Muizelaar P. Desmoplastic cerebral astrocytoma of infancy. A case report with immunohistochemical, ultrastructural and proliferation studies. Acta Neuropathol 1993, **86**: 666–670.

696 Brat DJ, VandenBerg SR, Figarella-Branger D, Taratuto AL. Desmoplastic infantile astrocytoma/ganglioglioma. In Louis DN, Ohgaki H, Wiestler OD, Cavenee WK (eds): WHO classification of tumours of the central nervous system. Lyon, 2007, IARC, pp. 96–98.

697 De Munnynck K, Van Gool S, Van Calenbergh F, Demaerel P, Uyttebroeck A, Buyse G, Sciot R. Desmoplastic infantile ganglioglioma: a potentially malignant tumor? Am J Surg Pathol 2002, **26**: 1515–1522.

698 Duffner PK, Burger PC, Cohen ME, Sanford RA, Krischer JP, Elterman R, Aronin PA, Pullen J, Horowitz ME, Parent A, et al. Desmoplastic infantile gangliogliomas: an approach to therapy. Neurosurgery 1994, **34**: 583–589; discussion 589.

699 Fan X, Larson TC, Jennings MT, Tulipan NB, Toms SA, Johnson MD. December 2000: 6 month old boy with 2 week history of progressive lethargy. Brain Pathol 2001, **11**: 265–266.

700 Hoving EW, Kros JM, Groninger E, den Dunnen WF. Desmoplastic infantile ganglioglioma with a malignant course. J Neurosurg Pediatr 2008, **1**: 95–98.

701 Komori T, Scheithauer BW, Parisi JE, Watterson J, Priest JR. Mixed conventional and desmoplastic infantile ganglioglioma: an autopsied case with 6-year follow-up. Mod Pathol 2001, **14**: 720–726.

702 Louis DN, von Deimling A, Dickersin GR, Dooling EC, Seizinger BR. Desmoplastic cerebral astrocytomas of infancy: a histopathologic, immunohistochemical, ultrastructural, and molecular genetic study. Hum Pathol 1992, **23**: 1402–1409.

703 Mallucci C, Lellouch-Tubiana A, Salazar C, Cinalli G, Renier D, Sainte-Rose C, Pierre-Kahn A, Zerah M. The management of desmoplastic neuroepithelial tumours in childhood. Childs Nerv Syst 2000, **16**: 8–14.

704 Setty SN, Miller DC, Camras L, Charbel F, Schmidt ML. Desmoplastic infantile astrocytoma with metastases at presentation. Mod Pathol 1997, **10**: 945–951.

705 Sugiyama K, Arita K, Shima T, Nakaoka M, Matsuoka T, Taniguchi E, Okamura T, Yamasaki H, Kajiwara Y, Kurisu K. Good clinical course in infants with desmoplastic cerebral neuroepithelial tumor treated by surgery alone. J Neurooncol 2002, **59**: 63–69.

706 Takeshima H, Kawahara Y, Hirano H, Obara S, Niiro M, Kuratsu J. Postoperative regression of desmoplastic infantile gangliogliomas: report of two cases. Neurosurgery 2003, **53**: 979–983; discussion 983–984.

707 Taratuto AL, Monges J, Lylyk P, Leiguarda R. Superficial cerebral astrocytoma attached to dura. Report of six cases in infants. Cancer 1984, **54**: 2505–2512.

708 VandenBerg SR, May EE, Rubinstein LJ, Herman MM, Perentes E, Vinores SA, Collins VP, Park TS. Desmoplastic supratentorial neuroepithelial tumors of infancy with divergent differentiation potential ('desmoplastic infantile gangliogliomas'). Report on 11 cases of a distinctive embryonal tumor with favorable prognosis. J Neurosurg 1987, **66**: 58–71.

Central neurocytoma and extraventricular neurocytic neoplasms

709 Aker FV, Ozkara S, Eren P, Peker O, Armagan S, Hakan T. Cerebellar liponeurocytoma/lipidized medulloblastoma. J Neurooncol 2005, **71**: 53–59.

710 Brat DJ, Scheithauer BW, Eberhart CG, Burger PC. Extraventricular neurocytomas: pathologic features and clinical outcome. Am J Surg Pathol 2001, **25**: 1252–1260.

711 Buccoliero AM, Caldarella A, Bacci S, Gallina P, Taddei A, Di Lorenzo N, Romagnoli P, Taddei GL. Cerebellar liponeurocytoma: morphological, immunohistochemical, and ultrastructural study of a relapsed case. Neuropathology 2005, **25**: 77–83.

712 Elek G, Slowik F, Eross L, Toth S, Szabo Z, Balint K. Central neurocytoma with malignant course. Neuronal and glial differentiation and craniospinal dissemination. Pathol Oncol Res 1999, **5**: 155–159.

713 Eng DY, DeMonte F, Ginsberg L, Fuller GN, Jaeckle K. Craniospinal dissemination of central neurocytoma. Report of two cases. J Neurosurg 1997, **86**: 547–552.

714 Figarella-Branger D, Pellissier JF, Daumas-Duport C, Delisle MB, Pasquier B, Parent M, Gambarelli D, Rougon G, Hassoun J. Central neurocytomas. Critical evaluation of a small-cell neuronal tumor. Am J Surg Pathol 1992, **16**: 97–109.

715 Figarella-Branger D, Soylemezoglu F, Burger PC. Central neurocytoma and extraventricular neurocytoma. In Louis DN, Ohgaki H, Wiestler OD, Cavenee WK (eds): WHO classification of tumours of the central nervous system. Lyon, 2007, IARC, pp. 106–109.

716 Friedrichs N, Vorreuther R, Fischer HP, Wiestler OD, Buettner R. Neurocytoma arising in the pelvis. Virchows Arch 2003, **443**: 217–219.

717 Fujisawa H, Marukawa K, Hasegawa M, Tohma Y, Hayashi Y, Uchiyama N, Tachibana O, Yamashita J. Genetic differences between neurocytoma and dysembryoplastic neuroepithelial tumor and oligodendroglial tumors. J Neurosurg 2002, **97**: 1350–1355.

718 George DH, Scheithauer BW. Central liponeurocytoma. Am J Surg Pathol 2001, **25**: 1551–1555.

719 Giangaspero F, Cenacchi G, Losi L, Cerasoli S, Bisceglia M, Burger PC. Extraventricular neoplasms with neurocytoma features. A clinicopathological study of 11 cases. Am J Surg Pathol 1997, **21**: 206–212.

720 Giangaspero F, Cenacchi G, Roncaroli F, Rigobello L, Manetto V, Gambacorta M, Allegranza A. Medullocytoma (lipidized medulloblastoma). A cerebellar neoplasm of adults with favorable prognosis. Am J Surg Pathol 1996, **20**: 656–664.

721 Giordana MT, Schiffer P, Boghi A, Buoncristiani P, Benech F. Medulloblastoma with lipidized cells versus lipomatous medulloblastoma. Clin Neuropathol 2000, **19**: 273–277.

722 Gonzalez-Campora R, Weller RO. Lipidized mature neuroectodermal tumour of the cerebellum with myoid differentiation. Neuropathol Appl Neurobiol 1998, **24**: 397–402.

723 Hirschowitz L, Ansari A, Cahill DJ, Bamford DS, Love S. Central neurocytoma arising within a mature cystic teratoma of the ovary. Int J Gynecol Pathol 1997, **16**: 176–179.

724 Horoupian DS, Shuster DL, Kaarsoo-Herrick M, Shuer LM. Central neurocytoma: one associated with a fourth ventricular PNET/medulloblastoma and the second mixed with adipose tissue. Hum Pathol 1997, **28**: 1111–1114.

725 Horstmann S, Perry A, Reifenberger G, Giangaspero F, Huang H, Hara A, Masuoka J, Rainov NG, Bergmann M, Heppner FL, Brandner S, Chimelli L, Montagna N, Jackson T, Davis DG, Markesbery WR, Ellison DW, Weller RO, Taddei GL, Conti R, Del Bigio MR, Gonzalez-Campora R, Radhakrishnan VV, Soylemezoglu F, Uro-Coste E, Qian J, Kleihues P, Ohgaki H. Genetic and expression profiles of cerebellar liponeurocytomas. Brain Pathol 2004, **14**: 281–289.

726 Ishiuchi S, Tamura M. Central neurocytoma: an immunohistochemical, ultrastructural and cell culture study. Acta Neuropathol 1997, **94**: 425–435.

727 Jenkinson MD, Bosma JJ, Du Plessis D, Ohgaki H, Kleihues P, Warnke P, Rainov NG. Cerebellar liponeurocytoma with an unusually aggressive clinical course: case report. Neurosurgery 2003, **53**: 1425–1427; discussion 1428.

728 Kleihues P, Chimelli L, Giangaspero F, Ohgaki H. Cerebellar liponeurocytoma. In Louis DN, Ohgaki H, Wiestler OD, Cavenee WK (eds): WHO classification of tumours of the central nervous system. Lyon, 2007, IARC, pp. 110–112.

729 Mackenzie IR. Central neurocytoma: histologic atypia, proliferation potential, and clinical outcome. Cancer 1999, **85**: 1606–1610.

730 Mierau GW, Scheithauer BW, Hukee MJ, Orsini EN. Mixed ependymoma–neuroendocrine tumor of the lateral ventricle. Ultrastruct Pathol 1996, **20**: 47–53.

731 Mrak RE. Malignant neurocytic tumor. Hum Pathol 1994, **25**: 747–752.

732 Ng TH, Wong AY, Boadle R, Compton JS. Pigmented central neurocytoma: case report and literature review. Am J Surg Pathol 1999, **23**: 1136–1140.

733 Pal L, Santosh V, Gayathri N, Das S, Das BS, Jayakumar PN, Shankar SK. Neurocytoma/rhabdomyoma (myoneurocytoma) of the cerebellum. Acta Neuropathol 1998, **95**: 318–323.

734 Park SH, Ostrzega N, Akers MA, Vinters HV. Intraventricular neurocytoma with prominent myelin figures. Ultrastruct Pathol 1999, **23**: 311–317.

735 Rades D, Fehlauer F, Lamszus K, Schild SE, Hagel C, Westphal M, Alberti W. Well-differentiated neurocytoma: what is the best available treatment? Neuro Oncol 2005, **7**: 77–83.

736 Rades D, Schild SE, Fehlauer F. Prognostic value of the MIB-1 labeling index for central neurocytomas. Neurology 2004, **62**: 987–989.

737 Robbins P, Segal A, Narula S, Stokes B, Lee M, Thomas W, Caterina P, Sinclair I, Spagnolo D. Central neurocytoma. A clinicopathological, immunohistochemical and ultrastructural study of 7 cases. Pathol Res Pract 1995, **191**: 100–111.

738 Rodriguez FJ, Mota RA, Scheithauer BW, Giannini C, Blair H, New KC, Wu KJ, Dickson DW, Jenkins RB. Interphase cytogenetics for 1p19q and t(1;19)(q10;p10) may distinguish prognostically relevant subgroups in extraventricular neurocytoma. Brain Pathol 2009, **19**: 623–629.

739 Schild SE, Scheithauer BW, Haddock MG, Schiff D, Burger PC, Wong WW, Lyons MK. Central neurocytomas. Cancer 1997, **79**: 790–795.

740 Schweitzer JB, Davies KG. Differentiating central neurocytoma. Case report. J Neurosurg 1997, **86**: 543–546.

741 Sharma MC, Agarwal M, Suri A, Gaikwad S, Mukhopadhyay P, Sarkar C. Lipomedulloblastoma in a child: a controversial entity. Hum Pathol 2002, **33**: 564–569.

742 Soylemezoglu F, Scheithauer BW, Esteve J, Kleihues P. Atypical central neurocytoma. J Neuropathol Exp Neurol 1997, **56**: 551–556.

743 Soylemezoglu F, Soffer D, Onol B, Schwechheimer K, Kleihues P. Lipomatous medulloblastoma in adults. A distinct clinicopathological entity. Am J Surg Pathol 1996, **20**: 413–418.

744 Tatter SB, Borges LF, Louis DN. Central neurocytomas of the cervical spinal cord. Report of two cases. J Neurosurg 1994, **81**: 288–293.

745 Tsuchida T, Matsumoto M, Shirayama Y, Imahori T, Kasai H, Kawamoto K. Neuronal and glial characteristics of central neurocytoma: electron microscopical analysis of two cases. Acta Neuropathol 1996, **91**: 573–577.

Dysembryoplastic neuroepithelial tumor

746 Baisden BL, Brat DJ, Melhem ER, Rosenblum MK, King AP, Burger PC. Dysembryoplastic neuroepithelial tumor-like neoplasm of the septum pellucidum: a lesion often misdiagnosed as glioma: report of 10 cases. Am J Surg Pathol 2001, **25**: 494–499.

747 Cervera-Pierot P, Varlet P, Chodkiewicz JP, Daumas-Duport C. Dysembryoplastic neuroepithelial tumors located in the caudate nucleus area: report of four cases. Neurosurgery 1997, **40**: 1065–1069; discussion 1069–1070.

748 Daumas-Duport C. Dysembryoplastic neuroepithelial tumours. Brain Pathol 1993, **3**: 283–295.

749 Daumas-Duport C, Pietsch T, Hawkins C, Shankar SK. Dysembryoplastic neuroepithelial tumour. In Louis DN, Ohgaki H, Wiestler OD, Cavenee WK (eds): WHO classification of tumours of the central nervous system. Lyon, 2007, IARC, pp. 113–114.

750 Daumas-Duport C, Scheithauer BW, Chodkiewicz JP, Laws ER Jr, Vedrenne C. Dysembryoplastic neuroepithelial tumor: a surgically curable tumor of young patients with intractable partial seizures. Report of thirty-nine cases. Neurosurgery 1988, **23**: 545–556.

751 Daumas-Duport C, Varlet P, Bacha S, Beuvon F, Cervera-Pierot P, Chodkiewicz JP. Dysembryoplastic neuroepithelial tumors: nonspecific histological forms – a study of 40 cases. J Neurooncol 1999, **41**: 267–280.

752 Elizabeth J, Bhaskara RM, Radhakrishnan VV, Radhakrishnan K, Thomas SV. Melanotic differentiation in dysembryoplastic neuroepithelial tumor. Clin Neuropathol 2000, **19**: 38–40.

753 Fernandez C, Girard N, Paz Paredes A, Bouvier-Labit C, Lena G, Figarella-Branger D. The usefulness of MR imaging in the diagnosis of dysembryoplastic neuroepithelial tumor in children: a study of 14 cases. AJNR Am J Neuroradiol 2003, **24**: 829–834.

754 Fujimoto K, Ohnishi H, Tsujimoto M, Hoshida T, Nakazato Y. Dysembryoplastic neuroepithelial tumor of the cerebellum and brainstem. Case report. J Neurosurg 2000, **93**: 487–489.

755 Gyure KA, Sandberg GD, Prayson RA, Morrison AL, Armstrong RC, Wong K. Dysembryoplastic neuroepithelial tumor: an immunohistochemical study with myelin oligodendrocyte glycoprotein. Arch Pathol Lab Med 2000, **124**: 123–126.

756 Hammond RR, Duggal N, Woulfe JM, Girvin JP. Malignant transformation of a dysembryoplastic neuroepithelial tumor. Case report. J Neurosurg 2000, **92**: 722–725.

757 Hirose T, Scheithauer BW. Mixed dysembryoplastic neuroepithelial tumor and ganglioglioma. Acta Neuropathol 1998, **95**: 649–654.

758 Hirose T, Scheithauer BW, Lopes MB, VandenBerg SR. Dysembryoplastic neuroeptihelial tumor (DNT): an immunohistochemical and ultrastructural study. J Neuropathol Exp Neurol 1994, **53**: 184–195.

759 Honavar M, Janota I, Polkey CE. Histological heterogeneity of dysembryoplastic neuroepithelial tumour: identification and differential diagnosis in a series of 74 cases. Histopathology 1999, **34**: 342–356.

760 Johnson MD, Vnencak-Jones CL, Toms SA, Moots PM, Weil R. Allelic losses in oligodendroglial and oligodendroglioma-like neoplasms: analysis using microsatellite repeats and polymerase chain reaction. Arch Pathol Lab Med 2003, **127**: 1573–1579.

761 Kurtkaya-Yapicier O, Elmaci I, Boran B, Kilic T, Sav A, Pamir MN. Dysembryoplastic neuroepithelial tumor of the midbrain tectum: a case report. Brain Tumor Pathol 2002, **19**: 97–100.

762 Prayson RA, Castilla EA, Hartke M, Pettay J, Tubbs RR, Barnett GH. Chromosome 1p allelic loss by fluorescence in situ hybridization is not observed in dysembryoplastic neuroepithelial tumors. Am J Clin Pathol 2002, **118**: 512–517.

763 Rushing EJ, Thompson LD, Mena H. Malignant transformation of a dysembryoplastic neuroepithelial tumor after radiation and chemotherapy. Ann Diagn Pathol 2003, **7**: 240–244.

764 Whittle IR, Dow GR, Lammie GA, Wardlaw J. Dysembryoplastic neuroepithelial tumour with discrete bilateral multifocality: further evidence for a germinal origin. Br J Neurosurg 1999, **13**: 508–511.

Papillary glioneuronal tumor

765 Ishizawa T, Komori T, Shibahara J, Ishizawa K, Adachi J, Nishikawa R, Matsutani M, Hirose T. Papillary glioneuronal tumor with minigemistocytic components and increased proliferative activity. Hum Pathol 2006, **37**: 627–630.

766 Javahery RJ, Davidson L, Fangusaro J, Finlay JL, Gonzalez-Gomez I, McComb JG. Aggressive variant of a papillary glioneuronal tumor. Report of 2 cases. J Neurosurg Pediatr 2009, **3**: 46–52.

767 Komori T, Scheithauer BW, Anthony DC, Rosenblum MK, McLendon RE, Scott RM, Okazaki H, Kobayashi M. Papillary glioneuronal tumor: a new variant of mixed neuronal–glial neoplasm. Am J Surg Pathol 1998, **22**: 1171–1183.

768 Nakazato Y, Figarella-Branger D, Becker AJ, Scheithauer BW, Rosenblum MK. Papillary glioneuronal tumour. In Louis DN, Ohgaki H, Wiestler OD, Cavenee WK (eds): WHO classification of tumours of the central nervous system. Lyon, 2007, IARC, pp. 113–114.

769 Tanaka Y, Yokoo H, Komori T, Makita Y, Ishizawa T, Hirose T, Ebato M, Shibahara J, Tsukayama C, Shibuya M, Nakazato Y. A distinct pattern of Olig2-positive cellular distribution in papillary glioneuronal tumors: a manifestation of the oligodendroglial phenotype? Acta Neuropathol 2005, **110**: 39–47.

Rosette-forming glioneuronal tumor of the fourth ventricle

770 Anan M, Inoue R, Ishii K, Abe T, Fujiki M, Kobayashi H, Goya T, Nakazato Y. A rosette-forming glioneuronal tumor of the spinal cord: the first case of a rosette-forming glioneuronal tumor originating from the spinal cord. Hum Pathol 2009, **40**: 898–901.

771 Hainfellner JA, Scheithauer BW, Giangaspero F, Rosenblum MK. Rosette-forming glioneuronal tumor of the fourth ventricle. In Louis DN, Ohgaki H, Wiestler OD, Cavenee WK (eds): WHO classification of tumours of the central nervous system. Lyon, 2007, IARC, pp. 115–116.

772 Komori T, Scheithauer BW, Hirose T. A rosette-forming glioneuronal tumor of the fourth ventricle: infratentorial form of dysembryoplastic neuroepithelial tumor? Am J Surg Pathol 2002, **26**: 582–591.

773 Marhold F, Preusser M, Dietrich W, Prayer D, Czech T. Clinicoradiological features of rosette-forming glioneuronal tumor (RGNT) of the fourth ventricle: report of four cases and literature review. J Neurooncol 2008, **90**: 301–308.

774 Scheithauer BW, Silva AI, Ketterling RP, Pula JH, Lininger JF, Krinock MJ. Rosette-forming glioneuronal tumor: report of a chiasmal-optic nerve example in neurofibromatosis type 1: special pathology report. Neurosurgery 2009, **64**: E771–772; discussion E772.

775 Wang Y, Xiong J, Chu SG, Liu Y, Cheng HX, Wang YF, Zhao Y, Mao Y. Rosette-forming glioneuronal tumor: report of an unusual case with intraventricular dissemination. Acta Neuropathol 2009, **118**: 813–819.

Hypothalamic neuronal hamartoma

776 Clarren SK, Alvord EC Jr, Hall JG. Congenital hypothalamic hamartoblastoma, hypopituitarism, imperforate anus, and postaxial polydactyly – a new syndrome? Part II: Neuropathological considerations. Am J Med Genet 1980, **7**: 75–83.

777 Coons SW, Rekate HL, Prenger EC, Wang N, Drees C, Ng YT, Chung SS, Kerrigan JF. The histopathology of hypothalamic hamartomas: study of 57 cases. J Neuropathol Exp Neurol 2007, **66**: 131–141.

778 Culler FL, James HE, Simon ML, Jones KL. Identification of gonadotropin-releasing hormone in neurons of a hypothalamic hamartoma in a boy with precocious puberty. Neurosurgery 1985, **17**: 408–412.

779 Johnston JJ, Olivos-Glander I, Killoran C, Elson E, Turner JT, Peters KF, Abbott MH, Aughton DJ, Aylsworth AS, Bamshad MJ, Booth C, Curry CJ, David A, Dinulos MB, Flannery DB, Fox MA, Graham JM, Grange DK, Guttmacher AE, Hannibal MC, Henn W, Hennekam RC, Holmes LB, Hoyme HE, Leppig KA, Lin AE, Macleod P, Manchester DK, Marcelis C, Mazzanti L, McCann E, McDonald MT, Mendelsohn NJ, Moeschler JB, Moghaddam B, Neri G, Newbury-Ecob R, Pagon RA, Phillips JA, Sadler LS, Stoler JM, Tilstra D, Walsh Vockley CM, Zackai EH, Zadeh TM, Brueton L, Black GC, Biesecker LG. Molecular and clinical analyses of Greig cephalopolysyndactyly and Pallister–Hall syndromes: robust phenotype prediction from the type and position of GLI3 mutations. Am J Hum Genet 2005, **76**: 609–622.

780 Price RA, Lee PA, Albright AL, Ronnekleiv OK, Gutai JP. Treatment of sexual precocity by removal of a luteinizing hormone-releasing hormone secreting hamartoma. JAMA 1984, **251**: 2247–2249.

781 Rosenblum MK. Hypothalamic neuronal hamartoma. In McLendon RE, Rosenblum MK, Bigner DD (eds): Russell and Rubinstein's tumors of the nervous system. London, 2006, Hodder Arnold, pp. 391–399.

782 Squires LA, Constantini S, Miller DC, Wisoff JH. Hypothalamic hamartoma and the Pallister–Hall syndrome. Pediatr Neurosurg 1995, **22**: 303–308.

Glioneuronal hamartomas, cortical dysplasias, and other epileptogenic lesions

783 Delalande O, Rodriguez D, Chiron C, Fohlen M. Successful surgical relief of seizures associated with hamartoma of the floor of the fourth ventricle in children: report of two cases. Neurosurgery 2001, **49**: 726–730; discussion 730–731.

784 Mischel PS, Nguyen LP, Vinters HV. Cerebral cortical dysplasia associated with pediatric epilepsy. Review of neuropathologic features and proposal for a grading system. J Neuropathol Exp Neurol 1995, **54**: 137–153.

785 Palmini A, Najm I, Avanzini G, Babb T, Guerrini R, Foldvary-Schaefer N, Jackson G, Luders HO, Prayson R, Spreafico R, Vinters HV. Terminology and classification of the cortical dysplasias. Neurology (Suppl 3) 2004, **62**: S2–8.

786 Plate KH, Wieser HG, Yasargil MG, Wiestler OD. Neuropathological findings in 224 patients with temporal lobe epilepsy. Acta Neuropathol 1993, **86**: 433–438.

787 Prayson RA, Estes ML. Cortical dysplasia: a histopathologic study of 52 cases of partial lobectomy in patients with epilepsy. Hum Pathol 1995, **26**: 493–500.

788 Sharma MS, Suri A, Shah T, Ralte A, Sarkar C, Gupta V, Mehta VS. Intraventricular glioneuronal hamartoma: histopathological correlation with magnetic resonance spectroscopy. J Neurooncol 2005, **74**: 325–328.

789 Volk EE, Prayson RA. Hamartomas in the setting of chronic epilepsy: a clinicopathologic study of 13 cases. Hum Pathol 1997, **28**: 227–232.

790 Wolf HK, Campos MG, Zentner J, Hufnagel A, Schramm J, Elger CE, Wiestler OD. Surgical pathology of temporal lobe epilepsy. Experience with 216 cases. J Neuropathol Exp Neurol 1993, **52**: 499–506.

791 Wolf HK, Zentner J, Hufnagel A, Campos MG, Schramm J, Elger CE, Wiestler OD. Surgical pathology of chronic epileptic seizure disorders: experience with 63 specimens from extratemporal corticectomies, lobectomies and functional hemispherectomies. Acta Neuropathol 1993, **86**: 466–472.

Dysplastic gangliocytoma of the cerebellum (Lhermitte–Duclos disease)

792 Abel TW, Baker SJ, Fraser MM, Tihan T, Nelson JS, Yachnis AT, Bouffard JP, Mena H, Burger PC, Eberhart CG. Lhermitte–Duclos disease: a report of 31 cases with immunohistochemical analysis of the PTEN/AKT/mTOR pathway. J Neuropathol Exp Neurol 2005, **64**: 341–349.

793 Eberhart CG, Wiestler OD, Eng C. Cowden disease and dysplastic gangliocytoma of the cerebellum/Lhermitte–Duclos disease. In Louis DN, Ohgaki H, Wiestler OD, Cavenee WK (eds): WHO classification of tumours of

the central nervous system. Lyon, 2007, IARC, pp. 113–114.
794 Ferrer I, Isamat F, Acebes J. A Golgi and electron microscopic study of a dysplastic gangliocytoma of the cerebellum. Acta Neuropathol 1979, **47**: 163–165.
795 Ferrer I, Isamat F, Lopez-Obarrio L, Conesa G, Rimbau J, Alcantara S, Espanol I, Zujar MJ. Parvalbumin and calbindin D-28K immunoreactivity in central ganglioglioma and dysplastic gangliocytoma of the cerebellum. Report of two cases. J Neurosurg 1993, **78**: 133–137.
796 Hair LS, Symmans F, Powers JM, Carmel P. Immunohistochemistry and proliferative activity in Lhermitte–Duclos disease. Acta Neuropathol 1992, **84**: 570–573.
797 Rosenblum MK, Yachnis AT. Dysplastic gangliocytoma of the cerebellum (Lhermitte–Duclos disease). In McLendon RE, Rosenblum MK, Bigner DD (eds): Russell and Rubinstein's pathology of tumors of the nervous system. London, 2006, Hodder Arnold, pp. 379–389.
798 Shiurba RA, Gessaga EC, Eng LF, Sternberger LA, Sternberger NH, Urich H. Lhermitte–Duclos disease. An immunohistochemical study of the cerebellar cortex. Acta Neuropathol 1988, **75**: 474–480.
799 Yachnis AT, Trojanowski JQ, Memmo M, Schlaepfer WW. Expression of neurofilament proteins in the hypertrophic granule cells of Lhermitte–Duclos disease: an explanation for the mass effect and the myelination of parallel fibers in the disease state. J Neuropathol Exp Neurol 1988, **47**: 206–216.
800 Zhou XP, Marsh DJ, Morrison CD, Chaudhury AR, Maxwell M, Reifenberger G, Eng C. Germline inactivation of PTEN and dysregulation of the phosphoinositol-3-kinase/Akt pathway cause human Lhermitte–Duclos disease in adults. Am J Hum Genet 2003, **73**: 1191–1198.

EMBRYONAL NEUROEPITHELIAL TUMORS

801 Louis DN, Ohgaki H, Wiestler OD, Cavenee WK (eds): The WHO classification of tumours of the central nervous system. Lyon, 2007, IARC.
802 Pomeroy SL, Tamayo P, Gaasenbeek M, Sturla LM, Angelo M, McLaughlin ME, Kim JY, Goumnerova LC, Black PM, Lau C, Allen JC, Zagzag D, Olson JM, Curran T, Wetmore C, Biegel JA, Poggio T, Mukherjee S, Rifkin R, Califano A, Stolovitzky G, Louis DN, Mesirov JP, Lander ES, Golub TR. Prediction of central nervous system embryonal tumour outcome based on gene expression. Nature 2002, **415**: 436–442.
803 Rorke LB. The cerebellar medulloblastoma and its relationship to primitive neuroectodermal tumors. J Neuropathol Exp Neurol 1983, **42**: 1–15.
804 Rubinstein LJ. Embryonal central neuroepithelial tumors and their differentiating potential. A cytogenetic view of a complex neuro-oncological problem. J Neurosurg 1985, **62**: 795–805.

Medulloblastoma

805 Anwer UE, Smith TW, DeGirolami U, Wilkinson HA. Medulloblastoma with cartilaginous differentiation. Arch Pathol Lab Med 1989, **113**: 84–88.
806 Biggs PJ, Powers JM. Neuroblastic medulloblastoma with abundant cytoplasmic actin filaments. Arch Pathol Lab Med 1984, **108**: 326–329.
807 Brown HG, Kepner JL, Perlman EJ, Friedman HS, Strother DR, Duffner PK, Kun LE, Goldthwaite PT, Burger PC. 'Large cell/anaplastic' medulloblastomas: a Pediatric Oncology Group Study. J Neuropathol Exp Neurol 2000, **59**: 857–865.
808 Cai DX, Mafra M, Schmidt RE, Scheithauer BW, Park TS, Perry A. Medulloblastomas with extensive posttherapy neuronal maturation. Report of two cases. J Neurosurg 2000, **93**: 330–334.
809 Ciara E, Piekutowska-Abramczuk D, Popowska E, Grajkowska W, Barszcz S, Perek D, Dembowska-Baginska B, Perek-Polnik M, Kowalewska E, Czajnska A, Syczewska M, Czornak K, Krajewska-Walasek M, Roszkowski M, Chrzanowska KH. Heterozygous germ-line mutations in the NBN gene predispose to medulloblastoma in pediatric patients. Acta Neuropathol 2010, **119**: 325–334.
810 Coffin CM, Braun JT, Wick MR, Dehner LP. A clinicopathologic and immunohistochemical analysis of 53 cases of medulloblastoma with emphasis on synaptophysin expression. Mod Pathol 1990, **3**: 164–170.
811 Czerwionka M, Korf HW, Hoffmann O, Busch H, Schachenmayr W. Differentiation in medulloblastomas: correlation between the immunocytochemical demonstration of photoreceptor markers (S-antigen, rod-opsin) and the survival rate in 66 patients. Acta Neuropathol 1989, **78**: 629–636.
812 de Chadarevian JP, Montes JL, O'Gorman AM, Freeman CR. Maturation of cerebellar neuroblastoma into ganglioneuroma with melanosis. A histologic, immunocytochemical, and ultrastructural study. Cancer 1987, **59**: 69–76.
813 Dolman CL. Melanotic medulloblastoma. A case report with immunohistochemical and ultrastructural examination. Acta Neuropathol 1988, **76**: 528–531.
814 Eberhart CG, Cohen KJ, Tihan T, Goldthwaite PT, Burger PC. Medulloblastomas with systemic metastases: evaluation of tumor histopathology and clinical behavior in 23 patients. J Pediatr Hematol Oncol 2003, **25**: 198–203.
815 Eberhart CG, Kaufman WE, Tihan T, Burger PC. Apoptosis, neuronal maturation, and neurotrophin expression within medulloblastoma nodules. J Neuropathol Exp Neurol 2001, **60**: 462–469.
816 Eberhart CG, Kepner JL, Goldthwaite PT, Kun LE, Duffner PK, Friedman HS, Strother DR, Burger PC. Histopathologic grading of medulloblastomas: a Pediatric Oncology Group study. Cancer 2002, **94**: 552–560.
817 Eberhart CG, Kratz J, Schuster A, Goldthwaite P, Cohen KJ, Perlman EJ, Burger PC. Comparative genomic hybridization detects an increased number of chromosomal alterations in large cell/anaplastic medulloblastomas. Brain Pathol 2002, **12**: 36–44.
818 Eberhart CG, Kratz J, Wang Y, Summers K, Stearns D, Cohen K, Dang CV, Burger PC. Histopathological and molecular prognostic markers in medulloblastoma: c-myc, N-myc, TrkC, and anaplasia. J Neuropathol Exp Neurol 2004, **63**: 441–449.
819 Geyer JR, Schofield D, Berger M, Milstein J. Differentiation of a primitive neuroectodermal tumor into a benign ganglioglioma. J Neurooncol 1992, **14**: 237–241.
820 Giangaspero F, Eberhart C, Haapasalo H, Pietsch T, Wiestler OD, Ellison DW. Medulloblastoma. In Louis DN, Ohgaki H, Wiestler OD, Cavenee WK (eds): WHO classification of tumours of the central nervous system. Lyon, 2007, IARC, pp. 132–140.
821 Giangaspero F, Perilongo G, Fondelli MP, Brisigotti M, Carollo C, Burnelli R, Burger PC, Garre ML. Medulloblastoma with extensive nodularity: a variant with favorable prognosis. J Neurosurg 1999, **91**: 971–977.
822 Giangaspero F, Rigobello L, Badiali M, Loda M, Andreini L, Basso G, Zorzi F, Montaldi A. Large-cell medulloblastomas. A distinct variant with highly aggressive behavior. Am J Surg Pathol 1992, **16**: 687–693.
823 Giangaspero F, Wellek S, Masuoka J, Gessi M, Kleihues P, Ohgaki H. Stratification of medulloblastoma on the basis of histopathological grading. Acta Neuropathol 2006, **112**: 5–12.
824 Helton KJ, Fouladi M, Boop FA, Perry A, Dalton J, Kun L, Fuller C. Medullomyoblastoma: a radiographic and clinicopathologic analysis of six cases and review of the literature. Cancer 2004, **101**: 1445–1454.
825 Hubbard JL, Scheithauer BW, Kispert DB, Carpenter SM, Wick MR, Laws ER Jr. Adult cerebellar medulloblastomas: the pathological, radiographic, and clinical disease spectrum. J Neurosurg 1989, **70**: 536–544.
826 Ismail A, Lamont JM, Tweddle AD, Pearson AD, Clifford SC, Ellison DW. A 7-year-old boy with midline cerebellar mass. Brain Pathol 2005, **15**: 261–262.
827 Jaffey PB, To GT, Xu HJ, Hu SX, Benedict WF, Donoso LA, Campbell GA. Retinoblastoma-like phenotype expressed in medulloblastomas. J Neuropathol Exp Neurol 1995, **54**: 664–672.
828 Janss AJ, Yachnis AT, Silber JH, Trojanowski JQ, Lee VM, Sutton LN, Perilongo G, Rorke LB, Phillips PC. Glial differentiation predicts poor clinical outcome in primitive neuroectodermal brain tumors. Ann Neurol 1996, **39**: 481–489.
829 Jimenez CL, Carpenter BF, Robb IA. Melanotic cerebellar tumor. Ultrastruct Pathol 1987, **11**: 751–759.
830 Katsetos CD, Herman MM, Frankfurter A, Gass P, Collins VP, Walker CC, Rosemberg S, Barnard RO, Rubinstein LJ. Cerebellar desmoplastic medulloblastomas. A further immunohistochemical characterization of the reticulin-free pale islands. Arch Pathol Lab Med 1989, **113**: 1019–1029.
831 Katsetos CD, Liu HM, Zacks SI. Immunohistochemical and ultrastructural observations on Homer Wright (neuroblastic) rosettes and the 'pale islands' of human cerebellar medulloblastomas. Hum Pathol 1988, **19**: 1219–1227.
832 Lamont JM, McManamy CS, Pearson AD, Clifford SC, Ellison DW. Combined histopathological and molecular cytogenetic stratification of medulloblastoma patients. Clin Cancer Res 2004, **10**: 5482–5493.
833 Mahapatra AK, Sinha AK, Sharma MC. Medullomyoblastoma. A rare cerebellar tumour in children. Childs Nerv Syst 1998, **14**: 312–316.
834 Maraziotis T, Perentes E, Karamitopoulou E, Nakagawa Y, Gessaga EC, Probst A, Frankfurter A. Neuron-associated class III beta-tubulin isotype, retinal S-antigen, synaptophysin, and glial fibrillary acidic protein in human medulloblastomas: a clinicopathological analysis of 36 cases. Acta Neuropathol 1992, **84**: 355–363.
835 McManamy CS, Pears J, Weston CL, Hanzely Z, Ironside JW, Taylor RE, Grundy RG, Clifford SC, Ellison DW. Nodule formation and desmoplasia in medulloblastomas

– defining the nodular/desmoplastic variant and its biological behavior. Brain Pathol 2007, **17**: 151–164.

836 Mehta RI, Cutler AR, Lasky JL 3rd, Yong WH, Lerner JT, Hirota BK, Salamon N, Mathern GW, Vinters HV. 'Primary' leptomeningeal medulloblastoma. Hum Pathol 2009, **40**: 1661–1665.

837 Polydorides AD, Perry A, Edgar MA. Large cell medulloblastoma with myogenic and melanotic differentiation: a case report with molecular analysis. J Neurooncol 2008, **88**: 193–197.

838 Rodriguez FJ, Eberhart C, O'Neill BP, Slezak J, Burger PC, Goldthwaite P, Wu W, Giannini C. Histopathologic grading of adult medulloblastomas. Cancer 2007, **109**: 2557–2565.

839 Rutkowski S, Bode U, Deinlein F, Ottensmeier H, Warmuth-Metz M, Soerensen N, Graf N, Emser A, Pietsch T, Wolff JE, Kortmann RD, Kuehl J. Treatment of early childhood medulloblastoma by postoperative chemotherapy alone. N Engl J Med 2005, **352**: 978–986.

Medulloepithelioma

840 Auer RN, Becker LE. Cerebral medulloepithelioma with bone, cartilage, and striated muscle. Light microscopic and immunohistochemical study. J Neuropathol Exp Neurol 1983, **42**: 256–267.

841 Caccamo DV, Herman MM, Rubinstein LJ. An immunohistochemical study of the primitive and maturing elements of human cerebral medulloepitheliomas. Acta Neuropathol 1989, **79**: 248–254.

842 Chavez M, Mafee MF, Castillo B, Kaufman LM, Johnstone H, Edward DP. Medulloepithelioma of the optic nerve. J Pediatr Ophthalmol Strabismus 2004, **41**: 48–52.

843 Deck JH. Cerebral medulloepithelioma with maturation into ependymal cells and ganglion cells. J Neuropathol Exp Neurol 1969, **28**: 442–454.

844 Donner LR, Teshima I. Peripheral medulloepithelioma: an immunohistochemical, ultrastructural, and cytogenetic study of a rare, chemotherapy-sensitive, pediatric tumor. Am J Surg Pathol 2003, **27**: 1008–1012.

845 Khoddami M, Becker LE. Immunohistochemistry of medulloepithelioma and neural tube. Pediatr Pathol Lab Med 1997, **17**: 913–925.

846 Molloy PT, Yachnis AT, Rorke LB, Dattilo JJ, Needle MN, Millar WS, Goldwein JW, Sutton LN, Phillips PC. Central nervous system medulloepithelioma: a series of eight cases including two arising in the pons. J Neurosurg 1996, **84**: 430–436.

847 Nakamura Y, Becker LE, Mancer K, Gillespie R. Peripheral medulloepithelioma. Acta Neuropathol 1982, **57**: 137–142.

848 Norris LS, Snodgrass S, Miller DC, Wisoff J, Garvin J, Rorke LB, Finlay JL. Recurrent central nervous system medulloepithelioma: response and outcome following marrow-ablative chemotherapy with stem cell rescue. J Pediatr Hematol Oncol 2005, **27**: 264–266.

849 Pang LM, Roebuck DJ, Ng HK, Chan YL. Sellar and suprasellar medulloepithelioma. Pediatr Radiol 2001, **31**: 594–596.

850 Scheithauer BW, Rubinstein LJ. Cerebral medulloepithelioma. Report of a case with multiple divergent neuroepithelial differentiation. Childs Brain 1979, **5**: 62–71.

851 Sharma MC, Mahapatra AK, Gaikwad S, Jain AK, Sarkar C. Pigmented medulloepithelioma: report of a case and review of the literature. Childs Nerv Syst 1998, **14**: 74–78.

852 Troost D, Jansen GH, Dingemans KP. Cerebral medulloepithelioma – electron microscopy and immunohistochemistry. Acta Neuropathol 1990, **80**: 103–107.

Central neuroblastic tumors

853 Ahdevaara P, Kalimo H, Torma T, Haltia M. Differentiating intracerebral neuroblastoma: report of a case and review of the literature. Cancer 1977, **40**: 784–788.

854 Bennett JP Jr, Rubinstein LJ. The biological behavior of primary cerebral neuroblastoma: a reappraisal of the clinical course in a series of 70 cases. Ann Neurol 1984, **16**: 21–27.

855 Berger MS, Edwards MS, Wara WM, Levin VA, Wilson CB. Primary cerebral neuroblastoma. Long-term follow-up review and therapeutic guidelines. J Neurosurg 1983, **59**: 418–423.

856 Dehner LP, Abenoza P, Sibley RK. Primary cerebral neuroectodermal tumors: neuroblastoma, differentiated neuroblastoma, and composite neuroectodermal tumor. Ultrastruct Pathol 1988, **12**: 479–494.

857 Horten BC, Rubinstein LJ. Primary cerebral neuroblastoma. A clinicopathological study of 35 cases. Brain 1976, **99**: 735–756.

858 Kepes JJ, Belton K, Roessmann U, Ketcherside WJ. Primitive neuroectodermal tumors of the cauda equina in adults with no detectable primary intracranial neoplasm – three case studies. Clin Neuropathol 1985, **4**: 1–11.

859 Ojeda VJ, Spagnolo DV, Kakulas BA. Cerebral gliomas with palisading necrosis: glioblastoma multiforme or high grade cerebral neuroblastoma? A light and electron microscopical study of three cases. Pathology 1987, **19**: 167–172.

860 Ojeda VJ, Spagnolo DV, Vaughan RJ. Palisades in primary cerebral neuroblastoma simulating so-called polar spongioblastoma. A light and electron microscopical study of an adult case. Am J Surg Pathol 1987, **11**: 316–322.

861 Rhodes RH, Cole M, Takaoka Y, Roessmann U, Cotes EE, Simon J. Intraventricular cerebral neuroblastoma. Analysis of subtypes and comparison with hemispheric neuroblastoma. Arch Pathol Lab Med 1994, **118**: 897–911.

862 Sibilla L, Martelli A, Farina L, Uggetti C, Zappoli F, Sessa F, Rodriguez y Baena R, Gaeltani P. Ganglioneuroblastoma of the spinal cord. AJNR Am J Neuroradiol 1995, **16**: 875–877.

863 Takahashi M, Ishihara T, Yokota T, Uchino F, Yokoyama T, Matsumoto N. A case of cerebral composite ganglioneuroblastoma: an immunohistochemical and ultrastructural study. Acta Neuropathol 1990, **80**: 98–102.

864 Torres LF, Grant N, Harding BN, Scaravilli F. Intracerebral neuroblastoma. Report of a case with neuronal maturation and long survival. Acta Neuropathol 1985, **68**: 110–114.

Ependymoblastoma

865 Cruz-Sanchez FF, Haustein J, Rossi ML, Cervos-Navarro J, Hughes JT. Ependymoblastoma: a histological, immunohistological and ultrastructural study of five cases. Histopathology 1988, **12**: 17–27.

866 Judkins AR, Ellison DW. Ependymoblastoma: dear, damned, distracting diagnosis, farewell! Brain Pathol 2010, **20**: 133–139.

867 Korshunov A, Remke M, Gessi M, Ryzhova M, Hielscher T, Witt H, Tobias V, Buccoliero AM, Sardi I, Gardiman MP, Bonnin J, Scheithauer B, Kulozik AE, Witt O, Mork S, von Deimling A, Wiestler OD, Giangaspero F, Rosenblum M, Pietsch T, Lichter P, Pfister SM. Focal genomic amplification at 19q13.42 comprises a powerful diagnostic marker for embryonal tumors with ependymoblastic rosettes. Acta Neuropathol 2010, **120**: 253–260.

868 Langford LA. The ultrastructure of the ependymoblastoma. Acta Neuropathol 1986, **71**: 136–141.

869 Mork SJ, Rubinstein LJ. Ependymoblastoma. A reappraisal of a rare embryonal tumor. Cancer 1985, **55**: 1536–1542.

870 Murphy MN, Dhalla SS, Diocee M, Halliday W, Wiseman NE, deSa DJ. Congenital ependymoblastoma presenting as a sacrococcygeal mass in a newborn: an immunohistochemical, light and electron microscopic study. Clin Neuropathol 1987, **6**: 169–173.

871 Wada C, Kurata A, Hirose R, Tazaki Y, Kan S, Ishihara Y, Kameya T. Primary leptomeningeal ependymoblastoma. Case report. J Neurosurg 1986, **64**: 968–973.

Embryonal tumor with abundant neuropil and true rosettes

872 Gessi M, Giangaspero F, Lauriola L, Gardiman M, Scheithauer BW, Halliday W, Hawkins C, Rosenblum MK, Burger PC, Eberhart CG. Embryonal tumors with abundant neuropil and true rosettes: a distinctive CNS primitive neuroectodermal tumor. Am J Surg Pathol 2009, **33**: 211–217.

873 Pfister S, Remke M, Castoldi M, Bai AH, Muckenthaler MU, Kulozik A, von Deimling A, Pscherer A, Lichter P, Korshunov A. Novel genomic amplification targeting the microRNA cluster at 19q13.42 in a pediatric embryonal tumor with abundant neuropil and true rosettes. Acta Neuropathol 2009, **117**: 457–464.

Polar spongioblastoma

874 de Chadarevian JP, Guyda HJ, Hollenberg RD. Hypothalamic polar spongioblastoma associated with the diencephalic syndrome. Ultrastructural demonstration of a neuroendocrine organization. Virchows Arch A Pathol Anat Histopathol 1984, **402**: 465–474.

875 Jansen GH, Troost D, Dingemans KP. Polar spongioblastoma: an immunohistochemical and electron microscopical study. Acta Neuropathol 1990, **81**: 228–232.

876 Russell DS, Rubinstein LJ. Pathology of tumours of the nervous system, ed. 5. Baltimore, 1989, Williams & Wilkins, pp. 169–172.

877 Schiffer D, Cravioto H, Giordana MT, Migheli A, Pezzulo T, Vigliani MC. Is polar spongioblastoma a tumor entity? J Neurosurg 1993, **78**: 587–591.

Assorted primitive neuroectodermal tumors

878 Abenoza P, Wick MR. Primitive cerebral neuroectodermal tumor with rhabdomyoblastic differentiation. Ultrastruct Pathol 1986, **10**: 347–354.

879 Behad A, Perry A. Central nervous system primitive neuroectodermal tumors: a clinicopathologic and genetic study of 33 cases. Brain Pathol 2010, **20**: 441–450.

880 Brustle O, Ohgaki H, Schmitt HP, Walter GF, Ostertag H, Kleihues P. Primitive neuroectodermal tumors after prophylactic central nervous system irradiation in children.

Association with an activated K-ras gene. Cancer 1992, **69**: 2385–2392.

881 Gould VE, Jansson DS, Molenaar WM, Rorke LB, Trojanowski JQ, Lee VM, Packer RJ, Franke WW. Primitive neuroectodermal tumors of the central nervous system. Patterns of expression of neuroendocrine markers, and all classes of intermediate filament proteins. Lab Invest 1990, **62**: 498–509.

882 Hart MN, Earle KM. Primitive neuroectodermal tumors of the brain in children. Cancer 1973, **32**: 890–897.

883 Jain A, Jalali R, Nadkarni TD, Sharma S. Primary intramedullary primitive neuroectodermal tumor of the cervical spinal cord. Case report. J Neurosurg Spine 2006, **4**: 497–502.

884 Janzer RC, Kleihues P. Primitive neuroectodermal tumor with choroid plexus differentiation. Clin Neuropathol 1985, **4**: 93–98.

885 Jay V, Pienkowska M, Becker L, Zielenska M. Primitive neuroectodermal tumors of the cerebrum and cerebellum: absence of t(11;22) translocation by RT-PCR analysis. Mod Pathol 1995, **8**: 488–491.

886 Kapadia SB, Frisman DM, Hitchcock CL, Ellis GL, Popek EJ. Melanotic neuroectodermal tumor of infancy. Clinicopathological, immunohistochemical, and flow cytometric study. Am J Surg Pathol 1993, **17**: 566–573.

887 Krishnamurthy S, Powers SK, Towfighi J. Primitive neuroectodermal tumor of cerebrum with adipose tissue. Arch Pathol Lab Med 2001, **125**: 264–266.

888 McLendon RE, Judkins AR, Eberhart CG, Fuller GN, Sarkar C, Ng H-K. Central nervous system primitive neuroectodermal tumours. In Louis DN, Ohgaki H, Wiestler OD, Cavenee WK (eds): WHO classification of tumours of the central nervous system. Lyon, 2007, IARC, pp. 141–146.

889 Mendal RC, Pollay M, Bobele GB, Leech RW, Brumback RA. Primary primitive neuroectodermal tumor of the leptomeninges. J Child Neurol 1996, **11**: 404–407.

890 Mobley BC, Roulston D, Shah GV, Bijwaard KE, McKeever PE. Peripheral primitive neuroectodermal tumor/Ewing's sarcoma of the craniospinal vault: case reports and review. Hum Pathol 2006, **37**: 845–853.

891 Navarro R, Laguna A, de Torres C, Cigudosa JC, Sunol M, Cruz O, Mora J. Primary Ewing sarcoma of the tentorium presenting with intracranial hemorrhage in a child. J Neurosurg (5 Suppl Pediatrics) 2007, **107**: 411–415.

892 Selassie L, Rigotti R, Kepes JJ, Towfighi J. Adipose tissue and smooth muscle in a primitive neuroectodermal tumor of cerebrum. Acta Neuropathol 1994, **87**: 217–222.

893 Tison V, Cerasoli S, Morigi F, Ladanyi M, Gerald WL, Rosai J. Intracranial desmoplastic small-cell tumor. Report of a case. Am J Surg Pathol 1996, **20**: 112–117.

894 Visee S, Soltner C, Rialland X, Machet MC, Loussouarn D, Milinkevitch S, Pasco-Papon A, Mercier P, Rousselet MC. Supratentorial primitive neuroectodermal tumours of the brain: multidirectional differentiation does not influence prognosis. A clinicopathological report of 18 patients. Histopathology 2005, **46**: 403–412.

895 Weil RJ, Zhuang Z, Pack S, Kumar S, Helman L, Fuller BG, Mackall CL, Oldfield EH. Intramedullary Ewing sarcoma of the spinal cord: consequences of molecular diagnostics. Case report. J Neurosurg 2001, **95**: 270–275.

896 Yachnis AT, Rorke LB, Biegel JA, Perilongo G, Zimmerman RA, Sutton LN. Desmoplastic primitive neuroectodermal tumor with divergent differentiation. Broadening the spectrum of desmoplastic infantile neuroepithelial tumors. Am J Surg Pathol 1992, **16**: 998–1006.

897 Yu JS, Moore MR, Kupsky WJ, Scott RM. Intracranial melanotic neuroectodermal tumor of infancy: two case reports. Surg Neurol 1992, **37**: 123–129.

Atypical teratoid/rhabdoid tumor

898 Biegel JA. Molecular genetics of atypical teratoid/rhabdoid tumor. Neurosurg Focus 2006, **20**: E11.

899 Birks DK, Kleinschmidt-DeMasters BK, Donson AM, Barton VN, McNatt SA, Foreman NK, Handler MH. Claudin 6 is a positive marker for atypical teratoid/rhabdoid tumors. Brain Pathol 2010, **20**: 140–150.

900 Burger PC, Yu IT, Tihan T, Friedman HS, Strother DR, Kepner JL, Duffner PK, Kun LE, Perlman EJ. Atypical teratoid/rhabdoid tumor of the central nervous system: a highly malignant tumor of infancy and childhood frequently mistaken for medulloblastoma: a Pediatric Oncology Group study. Am J Surg Pathol 1998, **22**: 1083–1092.

901 Chi SN, Zimmerman MA, Yao X, Cohen KJ, Burger P, Biegel JA, Rorke-Adams LB, Fisher MJ, Janss A, Mazewski C, Goldman S, Manley PE, Bowers DC, Bendel A, Rubin J, Turner CD, Marcus KJ, Goumnerova L, Ullrich NJ, Kieran MW. Intensive multimodality treatment for children with newly diagnosed CNS atypical teratoid rhabdoid tumor. J Clin Oncol 2009, **27**: 385–389.

902 Haberler C, Laggner U, Slavc I, Czech T, Ambros IM, Ambros PF, Budka H, Hainfellner JA. Immunohistochemical analysis of INI1 protein in malignant pediatric CNS tumors: lack of INI1 in atypical teratoid/rhabdoid tumors and in a fraction of primitive neuroectodermal tumors without rhabdoid phenotype. Am J Surg Pathol 2006, **30**: 1462–1468.

903 Judkins AR. Immunohistochemistry of INI1 expression: a new tool for old challenges in CNS and soft tissue pathology. Adv Anat Pathol 2007, **14**: 335–339.

904 Rorke LB, Packer RJ, Biegel JA. Central nervous system atypical teratoid/rhabdoid tumors of infancy and childhood: definition of an entity. J Neurosurg 1996, **85**: 56–65.

905 Wykoff CC, Lam BL, Brathwaite CD, Biegel JA, McKeown CA, Rosenblum MK, Allewelt HB, Sandberg DI. Atypical teratoid/rhabdoid tumor arising from the third cranial nerve. J Neuroophthalmol 2008, **28**: 207–211.

906 Zarovnaya EL, Pallatroni HF, Hug EB, Ball PA, Cromwell LD, Pipas JM, Fadul CE, Meyer LP, Park JP, Biegel JA, Perry A, Rhodes CH. Atypical teratoid/rhabdoid tumor of the spine in an adult: case report and review of the literature. J Neurooncol 2007, **84**: 49–55.

PINEAL PARENCHYMAL TUMORS

907 Amoaku WM, Willshaw HE, Parkes SE, Shah KJ, Mann JR. Trilateral retinoblastoma. A report of five patients. Cancer 1996, **78**: 858–863.

908 DeGirolami U, Zvaigzne O. Modification of the Achucarro-Hortega pineal stain for paraffin-embedded formalin-fixed tissue. Stain Technol 1973, **48**: 48–50.

909 Fauchon F, Jouvet A, Paquis P, Saint-Pierre G, Mottolese C, Ben Hassel M, Chauveinc L, Sichez JP, Philippon J, Schlienger M, Bouffet E. Parenchymal pineal tumors: a clinicopathological study of 76 cases. Int J Radiat Oncol Biol Phys 2000, **46**: 959–968.

910 Fevre-Montange M, Champier J, Szathmari A, Wierinckx A, Mottolese C, Guyotat J, Figarella-Branger D, Jouvet A, Lachuer J. Microarray analysis reveals differential gene expression patterns in tumors of the pineal region. J Neuropathol Exp Neurol 2006, **65**: 675–684.

911 Fevre-Montange M, Jouvet A, Privat K, Korf HW, Champier J, Reboul A, Aguera M, Mottolese C. Immunohistochemical, ultrastructural, biochemical and in vitro studies of a pineocytoma. Acta Neuropathol 1998, **95**: 532–539.

912 Fevre-Montange M, Szathmari A, Champier J, Mokhtari K, Chretien F, Coulon A, Figarella-Branger D, Polivka M, Varlet P, Uro-Coste E, Fauchon F, Jouvet A. Pineocytoma and pineal parenchymal tumors of intermediate differentiation presenting cytologic pleomorphism: a multicenter study. Brain Pathol 2008, **18**: 354–359.

913 Gadish T, Tulchinsky H, Deutsch AA, Rabau M. Pinealoblastoma in a patient with familial adenomatous polyposis: variant of Turcot syndrome type 2? Report of a case and review of the literature. Dis Colon Rectum 2005, **48**: 2343–2346.

914 Gudinaviciene I, Pranys D, Zheng P, Kros JM. A 10-month-old boy with a large pineal tumor. Brain Pathol 2005, **15**: 263–264, 267.

915 Illum N, Korf HW, Julian K, Rasmussen T, Herning M, Krabbe S. Concurrent uveoretinitis and pineocytoma in a child suggests a causal relationship. Br J Ophthalmol 1992, **76**: 574–576.

916 Jouvet A, Fevre-Montange M, Besancon R, Derrington E, Saint-G, Belin MF, Pialat J, Lapras C. Structural and ultrastructural characteristics of human pineal gland, and pineal parenchymal tumors. Acta Neuropathol 1994, **88**: 334–348.

917 Jouvet A, Saint-G, Fauchon F, Privat K, Bouffet E, Ruchoux MM, Chauveinc L, Fevre-Montange M. Pineal parenchymal tumors: a correlation of histological features with prognosis in 66 cases. Brain Pathol 2000, **10**: 49–60.

918 Kuchelmeister K, von Borcke IM, Klein H, Bergmann M, Gullotta F. Pleomorphic pineocytoma with extensive neuronal differentiation: report of two cases. Acta Neuropathol 1994, **88**: 448–453.

919 McGrogan G, Rivel J, Vital C, Guerin J. A pineal tumour with features of 'pineal anlage tumour'. Acta Neurochir (Wien) 1992, **117**: 73–77.

920 Mena H, Rushing EJ, Ribas JL, Delahunt B, McCarthy WF. Tumors of pineal parenchymal cells: a correlation of histological features, including nucleolar organizer regions, with survival in 35 cases. Hum Pathol 1995, **26**: 20–30.

921 Min KW, Scheithauer BW, Bauserman SC. Pineal parenchymal tumors: an ultrastructural study with prognostic implications. Ultrastruct Pathol 1994, **18**: 69–85.

922 Min KW, Seo IS, Song J. Postnatal evolution of the human pineal gland. An immunohistochemical study. Lab Invest 1987, **57**: 724–728.

923 Nakazato Y, Jouvet A, Scheithauer B. Tumours of the pineal region. In Louis DN, Ohgaki H, Wiestler OD, Cavenee WK (eds): WHO classification of tumours of the central nervous system. Lyon, 2007, IARC, pp. 121–127.

924 Plowman PN, Pizer B, Kingston JE. Pineal parenchymal tumours: II. On the aggressive behaviour of pineoblastoma in patients with

an inherited mutation of the RB1 gene. Clin Oncol (R Coll Radiol) 2004, **16**: 244–247.

925 Raisanen J, Vogel H, Horoupian DS. Primitive pineal tumor with retinoblastomatous and retinal/ciliary epithelial differentiation: an immunohistochemical study. J Neurooncol 1990, **9**: 165–170.

926 Schild SE, Scheithauer BW, Schomberg PJ, Hook CC, Kelly PJ, Frick L, Robinow JS, Buskirk SJ. Pineal parenchymal tumors. Clinical, pathologic, and therapeutic aspects. Cancer 1993, **72**: 870–880.

927 Schmidbauer M, Budka H, Pilz P. Neuroepithelial and ectomesenchymal differentiation in a primitive pineal tumor ('pineal anlage tumor'). Clin Neuropathol 1989, **8**: 7–10.

928 Sobel RA, Trice JE, Nielsen SL, Ellis WG. Pineoblastoma with ganglionic and glial differentiation: report of two cases. Acta Neuropathol 1981, **55**: 243–246.

Papillary tumor of the pineal region

929 Fevre-Montange M, Hasselblatt M, Figarella-Branger D, Chauveinc L, Champier J, Saint-G, Taillandier L, Coulon A, Paulus W, Fauchon F, Jouvet A. Prognosis and histopathologic features in papillary tumors of the pineal region: a retrospective multicenter study of 31 cases. J Neuropathol Exp Neurol 2006, **65**: 1004–1011.

930 Hasselblatt M, Blumcke I, Jeibmann A, Rickert CH, Jouvet A, van de Nes JA, Kuchelmeister K, Brunn A, Fevre-Montange M, Paulus W. Immunohistochemical profile and chromosomal imbalances in papillary tumours of the pineal region. Neuropathol Appl Neurobiol 2006, **32**: 278–283.

931 Jouvet A, Fauchon F, Liberski P, Saint-G, Didier-Bazes M, Heitzmann A, Delisle MB, Biassette HA, Vincent S, Mikol J, Streichenberger N, Ahboucha S, Brisson C, Belin MF, Fevre-Montange M. Papillary tumor of the pineal region. Am J Surg Pathol 2003, **27**: 505–512.

932 Mobley B, Kalani MY, Harsh GR IV, Edwards MS, Vogel H. Papillary tumor of the spinal cord: report of 2 cases. Am J Surg Pathol 2009, **33**: 1191–1197.

MENINGIOMAS

933 Abramovich CM, Prayson RA. Histopathologic features and MIB-1 labeling indices in recurrent and nonrecurrent meningiomas. Arch Pathol Lab Med 1999, **123**: 793–800.

934 Alexander RT, McLendon RE, Cummings TJ. Meningioma with eosinophilic granular inclusions. Clin Neuropathol 2004, **23**: 292–297.

935 Allen EA, Burger PC, Epstein JI. Microcystic meningioma arising in a mixed germ cell tumor of the testis: a case report. Am J Surg Pathol 1999, **23**: 1131–1135.

936 Al-Mefty O, Topsakal C, Pravdenkova S, Sawyer JR, Harrison MJ. Radiation-induced meningiomas: clinical, pathological, cytokinetic, and cytogenetic characteristics. J Neurosurg 2004, **100**: 1002–1013.

937 Arima T, Natsume A, Hatano H, Nakahara N, Fujita M, Ishii D, Wakabayashi T, Doyu M, Nagasaka T, Yoshida J. Intraventricular chordoid meningioma presenting with Castleman disease due to overproduction of interleukin-6. Case report. J Neurosurg 2005, **102**: 733–737.

938 Barnett GH, Chou SM, Bay JW. Posttraumatic intracranial meningioma: a case report and review of the literature. Neurosurgery 1986, **18**: 75–78.

939 Bruno MC, Ginguene C, Santangelo M, Panagiotopoulos K, Piscopo GA, Tortora F, Elefante A, De Caro ML, Cerillo A. Lymphoplasmacyte rich meningioma. A case report and review of the literature. J Neurosurg Sci 2004, **48**: 117–124; discussion 124.

940 Budka H. Non-glial specificities of immunocytochemistry for the glial fibrillary acidic protein (GFAP). Triple expression of GFAP, vimentin and cytokeratins in papillary meningioma and metastasizing renal carcinoma. Acta Neuropathol 1986, **72**: 43–54.

941 Carlotti CG Jr, Neder L, Colli BO, dos Santos MB, Garcia AS, Elias J Jr, Chimelli LC. Clear cell meningioma of the fourth ventricle. Am J Surg Pathol 2003, **27**: 131–135.

942 Coons SW, Johnson PC. Brachial plexus meningioma, report of a case with immunohistochemical and ultrastructural examination. Acta Neuropathol 1989, **77**: 445–448.

943 Couce ME, Aker FV, Scheithauer BW. Chordoid meningioma: a clinicopathologic study of 42 cases. Am J Surg Pathol 2000, **24**: 899–905.

944 Couce ME, Perry A, Webb P, Kepes JJ, Scheithauer BW. Fibrous meningioma with tyrosine-rich crystals. Ultrastruct Pathol 1999, **23**: 341–345.

945 Davidson GS, Hope JK. Meningeal tumors of childhood. Cancer 1989, **63**: 1205–1210.

946 Gallina P, Buccoliero AM, Mariotti F, Mennonna P, Di Lorenzo N. Oncocytic meningiomas: cases with benign histopathological features and a favorable clinical course. J Neurosurg 2006, **105**: 736–738.

947 Haberler C, Jarius C, Lang S, Rossler K, Gruber A, Hainfellner JA, Budka H. Fibrous meningeal tumours with extensive non-calcifying collagenous whorls and glial fibrillary acidic protein expression: the whorling-sclerosing variant of meningioma. Neuropathol Appl Neurobiol 2002, **28**: 42–47.

948 Hahn HP, Bundock EA, Hornick JL. Immunohistochemical staining for claudin-1 can help distinguish meningiomas from histologic mimics. Am J Clin Pathol 2006, **125**: 203–208.

949 Hasselblatt M, Nolte KW, Paulus W. Angiomatous meningioma: a clinicopathologic study of 38 cases. Am J Surg Pathol 2004, **28**: 390–393.

950 Heth JA, Kirby P, Menezes AH. Intraspinal familial clear cell meningioma in a mother and child. Case report. J Neurosurg 2000, **93**: 317–321.

951 Hojo H, Abe M. Rhabdoid papillary meningioma. Am J Surg Pathol 2001, **25**: 964–969.

952 Horten BC, Urich H, Stefoski D. Meningiomas with conspicuous plasma cell-lymphocytic components: a report of five cases. Cancer 1979, **43**: 258–264.

953 Im SH, Chung CK, Cho BK, Kim MK, Chi JG. Sclerosing meningioma: clinicopathological study of four cases. J Neurooncol 2004, **68**: 169–175.

954 Jaaskelainen J, Haltia M, Servo A. Atypical and anaplastic meningiomas: radiology, surgery, radiotherapy, and outcome. Surg Neurol 1986, **25**: 233–242.

955 Jacques TS, Valentine A, Bradford R, McLaughlin JE. December 2003: a 70-year-old woman with a recurrent meningeal mass. Recurrent meningioma with rhabdomyosarcomatous differentiation. Brain Pathol 2003, **13**: 229–230.

956 Kallio M, Sankila R, Hakulinen T, Jaaskelainen J. Factors affecting operative and excess long-term mortality in 935 patients with intracranial meningioma. Neurosurgery 1992, **31**: 2–12.

957 Kepes JJ. Biology, pathology and differential diagnosis. New York, 1982, Masson.

958 Kepes JJ, Chen WY, Connors MH, Vogel FS. 'Chordoid' meningeal tumors in young individuals with peritumoral lymphoplasmacellular infiltrates causing systemic manifestations of the Castleman syndrome. A report of seven cases. Cancer 1988, **62**: 391–406.

959 Kepes JJ, Goldware S, Leoni R. Meningioma with pseudoglandular pattern. A case report. J Neuropathol Exp Neurol 1983, **42**: 61–68.

960 Kim NR, Im SH, Chung CK, Suh YL, Choe G, Chi JG. Sclerosing meningioma: immunohistochemical analysis of five cases. Neuropathol Appl Neurobiol 2004, **30**: 126–135.

961 Kobata H, Kondo A, Iwasaki K, Kusaka H, Ito H, Sawada S. Chordoid meningioma in a child. Case report. J Neurosurg 1998, **88**: 319–323.

962 Kros JM, Cella F, Bakker SL, Paz YGD, Egeler RM. Papillary meningioma with pleural metastasis: case report and literature review. Acta Neurol Scand 2000, **102**: 200–202.

963 Lattes R, Bigotti G. Lipoblastic meningioma: 'vacuolated meningioma'. Hum Pathol 1991, **22**: 164–171.

964 Liu Y, Sturgis CD, Bunker M, Saad RS, Tung M, Raab SS, Silverman JF. Expression of cytokeratin by malignant meningiomas: diagnostic pitfall of cytokeratin to separate malignant meningiomas from metastatic carcinoma. Mod Pathol 2004, **17**: 1129–1133.

965 Lockett L, Chiang V, Scully N. Primary pulmonary meningioma: report of a case and review of the literature. Am J Surg Pathol 1997, **21**: 453–460.

966 Longstreth WT Jr, Dennis LK, McGuire VM, Drangsholt MT, Koepsell TD. Epidemiology of intracranial meningioma. Cancer 1993, **72**: 639–648.

967 Louis DN, Hamilton AJ, Sobel RA, Ojemann RG. Pseudopsammomatous meningioma with elevated serum carcinoembryonic antigen: a true secretory meningioma. Case report. J Neurosurg 1991, **74**: 129–132.

968 Ludwin SK, Rubinstein LJ, Russell DS. Papillary meningioma: a malignant variant of meningioma. Cancer 1975, **36**: 1363–1373.

969 Matyja E, Kuchna I, Kroh H, Mazurowski W, Zabek M. Meningiomas and gliomas in juxtaposition: casual or causal coexistence? Report of two cases. Am J Surg Pathol 1995, **19**: 37–41.

970 Michaud J, Gagne F. Microcystic meningioma. Clinicopathologic report of eight cases. Arch Pathol Lab Med 1983, **107**: 75–80.

971 Miettinen M, Paetau A. Mapping of the keratin polypeptides in meningiomas of different types: an immunohistochemical analysis of 463 cases. Hum Pathol 2002, **33**: 590–598.

972 Mizutani E, Tsuta K, Maeshima AM, Asamura H, Matsuno Y. Minute pulmonary meningothelial-like nodules: clinicopathologic analysis of 121 patients. Hum Pathol 2009, **40**: 678–682.

973 Mukhopadhyay S, El-Zammar OA, Katzenstein AL. Pulmonary meningothelial-like nodules: new insights into a common but poorly understood entity. Am J Surg Pathol 2009, **33**: 487–495.

974 Nakasu S, Li DH, Okabe H, Nakajima M, Matsuda M. Significance of MIB-1 staining indices in meningiomas: comparison of two counting methods. Am J Surg Pathol 2001, **25**: 472–478.

975 Nestor SL, Perry A, Kurtkaya O, Abell-Aleff P, Rosemblat AM, Burger PC, Scheithauer BW. Melanocytic colonization of a meningothelial meningioma: histopathological and ultrastructural findings with immunohistochemical and genetic correlation: case report. Neurosurgery 2003, **53**: 211–214; discussion 214–215.

976 Ng TH, Wong MP, Chan KW. Benign metastasizing meningioma. Clin Neurol Neurosurg 1990, **92**: 152–154.

977 Oviedo A, Pang D, Zovickian J, Smith M. Clear cell meningioma: case report and review of the literature. Pediatr Dev Pathol 2005, **8**: 386–390.

978 Paek SH, Kim SH, Chang KH, Park CK, Kim JE, Kim DG, Park SH, Jung HW. Microcystic meningiomas: radiological characteristics of 16 cases. Acta Neurochir (Wien) 2005, **147**: 965–972; discussion 972.

979 Perry A, Chicoine MR, Filiput E, Miller JP, Cross DT. Clinicopathologic assessment and grading of embolized meningiomas: a correlative study of 64 patients. Cancer 2001, **92**: 701–711.

980 Perry A, Fuller CE, Judkins AR, Dehner LP, Biegel JA. INI1 expression is retained in composite rhabdoid tumors, including rhabdoid meningiomas. Mod Pathol 2005, **18**: 951–958.

981 Perry A, Giannini C, Raghavan R, Scheithauer BW, Banerjee R, Margraf L, Bowers DC, Lytle RA, Newsham IF, Gutmann DH. Aggressive phenotypic and genotypic features in pediatric and NF2-associated meningiomas: a clinicopathologic study of 53 cases. J Neuropathol Exp Neurol 2001, **60**: 994–1003.

982 Perry A, Louis DN, Scheithauer BW, Budka H, von Deimling A. Meningiomas. In Louis DN, Ohgaki H, Wiestler OD, Cavenee WK (eds): WHO classification of tumours of the nervous system. Lyon, 2007, IARC, pp. 164–172.

983 Perry A, Scheithauer BW, Stafford SL, Abell-Aleff PC, Meyer FB. 'Rhabdoid' meningioma: an aggressive variant. Am J Surg Pathol 1998, **22**: 1482–1490.

984 Perry A, Scheithauer BW, Stafford SL, Lohse CM, Wollan PC. 'Malignancy' in meningiomas: a clinicopathologic study of 116 patients, with grading implications. Cancer 1999, **85**: 2046–2056.

985 Perry A, Stafford SL, Scheithauer BW, Suman VJ, Lohse CM. Meningioma grading: an analysis of histologic parameters. Am J Surg Pathol 1997, **21**: 1455–1465.

986 Perry A, Stafford SL, Scheithauer BW, Suman VJ, Lohse CM. The prognostic significance of MIB-1, p53, and DNA flow cytometry in completely resected primary meningiomas. Cancer 1998, **82**: 2262–2269.

987 Probst-Cousin S, Villagran-Lillo R, Lahl R, Bergmann M, Schmid KW, Gullotta F. Secretory meningioma: clinical, histologic, and immunohistochemical findings in 31 cases. Cancer 1997, **79**: 2003–2015.

988 Rajaram V, Brat DJ, Perry A. Anaplastic meningioma versus meningeal hemangiopericytoma: immunohistochemical and genetic markers. Hum Pathol 2004, **35**: 1413–1418.

989 Robinson JC, Challa VR, Jones DS, Kelly DL Jr. Pericytosis and edema generation: a unique clinicopathological variant of meningioma. Neurosurgery 1996, **39**: 700–706; discussion 706–707.

990 Roncaroli F, Riccioni L, Cerati M, Capella C, Calbucci F, Trevisan C, Eusebi V. Oncocytic meningioma. Am J Surg Pathol 1997, **21**: 375–382.

991 Roncaroli F, Scheithauer BW, Laeng RH, Cenacchi G, Abell-Aleff P, Moschopulos M. Lipomatous meningioma: a clinicopathologic study of 18 cases with special reference to the issue of metaplasia. Am J Surg Pathol 2001, **25**: 769–775.

992 Rowsell C, Sirbovan J, Rosenblum MK, Perez-Ordonez B. Primary chordoid meningioma of lung. Virchows Arch 2005, **446**: 333–337.

993 Saleh J, Silberstein HJ, Salner AL, Uphoff DF. Meningioma: the role of a foreign body and irradiation in tumor formation. Neurosurgery 1991, **29**: 113–118; discussion 118–119.

994 Sangoi AR, Dulai MS, Beck AH, Brat DJ, Vogel H. Distinguishing chordoid meningiomas from their histologic mimics: an immunohistochemical evaluation. Am J Surg Pathol 2009, **33**: 669–681.

995 Su M, Ono K, Tanaka R, Takahashi H. An unusual meningioma variant with glial fibrillary acidic protein expression. Acta Neuropathol 1997, **94**: 499–503.

996 Sugita Y, Shigemori M, Harada H, Wada Y, Hayashi I, Morimastu M, Okamoto Y, Kajiwara K. Primary meningeal sarcomas with leiomyoblastic differentiation: a proposal for a new subtype of primary meningeal sarcomas. Am J Surg Pathol 2000, **24**: 1273–1278.

997 Teo JG, Goh KY, Rosenblum MK, Muszynski CA, Epstein FJ. Intraparenchymal clear cell meningioma of the brainstem in a 2-year-old child. Case report and literature review. Pediatr Neurosurg 1998, **28**: 27–30.

998 Thompson LD, Bouffard JP, Sandberg GD, Mena H. Primary ear and temporal bone meningiomas: a clinicopathologic study of 36 cases with a review of the literature. Mod Pathol 2003, **16**: 236–245.

999 Thompson LD, Gyure KA. Extracranial sinonasal tract meningiomas: a clinicopathologic study of 30 cases with a review of the literature. Am J Surg Pathol 2000, **24**: 640–650.

1000 Tsuchida T, Matsumoto M, Shirayama Y, Kasai H, Kawamoto K. Immunohistochemical observation of foci of muscle actin-positive tumor cells in meningiomas. Arch Pathol Lab Med 1996, **120**: 267–269.

1001 Wanschitz J, Schmidbauer M, Maier H, Rossler K, Vorkapic P, Budka H. Suprasellar meningioma with expression of glial fibrillary acidic protein: a peculiar variant. Acta Neuropathol 1995, **90**: 539–544.

1002 Wilson AJ, Ratliff JL, Lagios MD, Aguilar MJ. Mediastinal meningioma. Am J Surg Pathol 1979, **3**: 557–562.

1003 Winek RR, Scheithauer BW, Wick MR. Meningioma, meningeal hemangiopericytoma (angioblastic meningioma), peripheral hemangiopericytoma, and acoustic schwannoma. A comparative immunohistochemical study. Am J Surg Pathol 1989, **13**: 251–261.

1004 Zon LI, Johns WD, Stomper PC, Kaplan WD, Connolly JL, Morris JH, Harris JR, Henderson IC, Skarin AT. Breast carcinoma metastatic to a meningioma. Case report and review of the literature. Arch Intern Med 1989, **149**: 959–962.

1005 Zorludemir S, Scheithauer BW, Hirose T, Van Houten C, Miller G, Meyer FB. Clear cell meningioma. A clinicopathologic study of a potentially aggressive variant of meningioma. Am J Surg Pathol 1995, **19**: 493–505.

NONMENINGOTHELIAL MESENCHYMAL TUMORS

1006 Oliveira AM, Scheithauer BW, Salomao DR, Parisi JE, Burger PC, Nascimento AG. Primary sarcomas of the brain and spinal cord: a study of 18 cases. Am J Surg Pathol 2002, **26**: 1056–1063.

1007 Paulus W, Slowik F, Jellinger K. Primary intracranial sarcomas: histopathological features of 19 cases. Histopathology 1991, **18**: 395–402.

Lipoma and liposarcoma

1008 Ahmadi SA, van Landeghem FK, Blechschmidt C, Lieber K, Haberl EJ, Thomale UW. Intratentorial osteochondrolipoma in a 9-year-old boy. J Neurosurg Pediatr 2009, **3**: 386–391.

1009 Arnold PM, Gust TD, Newell K. Intramedullary leiomyolipoma of the thoracic spine. Case report. J Neurosurg Spine 2007, **6**: 438–440.

1010 Bigelow DC, Eisen MD, Smith PG, Yousem DM, Levine RS, Jackler RK, Kennedy DW, Kotapka MJ. Lipomas of the internal auditory canal and cerebellopontine angle. Laryngoscope 1998, **108**: 1459–1469.

1011 Bognar L, Balint K, Bardoczy Z. Symptomatic osteolipoma of the tuber cinereum. Case report. J Neurosurg 2002, **96**: 361–363.

1012 Brown PG, Shaver EG. Myolipoma in a tethered cord. Case report and review of the literature. J Neurosurg 2000, **92**: 214–216.

1013 Budka H. Intracranial lipomatous hamartomas (intracranial 'lipomas'). A study of 13 cases including combinations with medulloblastoma, colloid and epidermoid cysts, angiomatosis and other malformations. Acta Neuropathol 1974, **28**: 205–222.

1014 Chitoku S, Kawai S, Watabe Y, Nishitani M, Fujimoto K, Otsuka H, Fushimi H, Kotoh K, Fuji T. Intradural spinal hibernoma: case report. Surg Neurol 1998, **49**: 509–512.

1015 Christensen WN, Long DM, Epstein JI. Cerebellopontine angle lipoma. Hum Pathol 1986, **17**: 739–743.

1016 Cinalli G, Zerah M, Carteret M, Doz F, Vinikoff L, Lellouch-Tubiana A, Husson B, Pierre-Kahn A. Subdural sarcoma associated with chronic subdural hematoma. Report of two cases and review of the literature. J Neurosurg 1997, **86**: 553–557.

1017 Feldman RP, Marcovici A, LaSala PA. Intracranial lipoma of the sylvian fissure. Case report and review of the literature. J Neurosurg 2001, **94**: 515–519.

1018 Haddad SF, Hitchon PW, Godersky JC. Idiopathic and glucocorticoid-induced spinal epidural lipomatosis. J Neurosurg 1991, **74**: 38–42.

1019 Harrison MJ, Mitnick RJ, Rosenblum BR, Rothman AS. Leptomyelolipoma: analysis of 20 cases. J Neurosurg 1990, **73**: 360–367.

1020 Lee M, Rezai AR, Abbott R, Coelho DH, Epstein FJ. Intramedullary spinal cord lipomas. J Neurosurg 1995, **82**: 394–400.

1021 Lin YC, Huang CC, Chen HJ. Intraspinal osteolipoma. Case report. J Neurosurg 2001, **94**: 126–128.

1022 Perling LH, Laurent JP, Cheek WR. Epidural hibernoma as a complication of corticosteroid treatment. Case report. J Neurosurg 1988, **69**: 613–616.

1023 Pirotte B, Krischek B, Levivier M, Bolyn S, Brucher JM, Brotchi J. Diagnostic and microsurgical presentation of intracranial angiolipomas. Case report and review of the literature. J Neurosurg 1998, **88**: 129–132.

1024 Preul MC, Leblanc R, Tampieri D, Robitaille Y, Pokrupa R. Spinal angiolipomas. Report of three cases. J Neurosurg 1993, **78**: 280–286.

1025 Sheridan F, Scharf D, Henderson VW, Miller CA. Lipomas of the mesencephalic tectum and rostral pons associated with sleep apnea syndrome. Clin Neuropathol 1990, **9**: 152–156.

1026 Sima A, Kindblom LG, Pellettieri L. Liposarcoma of the meninges. A case report. Acta Pathol Microbiol Scand A 1976, **84**: 306–310.

1027 Tresser N, Parveen T, Roessmann U. Intracranial lipomas with teratomatous elements. Arch Pathol Lab Med 1993, **117**: 918–920.

1028 Walsh JW, Markesbery WR. Histological features of congenital lipomas of the lower spinal canal. J Neurosurg 1980, **52**: 564–569.

1029 Wu SS, Lo WW, Tschirhart DL, Slattery WH 3rd, Carberry JN, Brackmann DE. Lipochoristomas (lipomatous tumors) of the acoustic nerve. Arch Pathol Lab Med 2003, **127**: 1475–1479.

Osseous and cartilaginous tumors

1030 Bernstein M, Perrin RG, Platts ME, Simpson WJ. Radiation-induced cerebellar chondrosarcoma. Case report. J Neurosurg 1984, **61**: 174–177.

1031 Chakrabortty S, Tamaki N, Kondoh T, Kojima N, Kamikawa H, Matsumoto S. Maffucci's syndrome associated with intracranial enchondroma and aneurysm: case report. Surg Neurol 1991, **36**: 216–220.

1032 Chandler JP, Yashar P, Laskin WB, Russell EJ. Intracranial chondrosarcoma: a case report and review of the literature. J Neurooncol 2004, **68**: 33–39.

1033 Cohen IJ, Kornreich L. Intracranial osteosarcoma: report of four cases and review of the literature. J Neurooncol 1999, **43**: 93.

1034 Cosar M, Iplikcioglu AC, Bek S, Gokduman CA. Intracranial falcine and convexity chondromas: two case reports. Br J Neurosurg 2005, **19**: 241–243.

1035 Dagcinar A, Bayrakli F, Yapicier O, Ozek M. Primary meningeal osteosarcoma of the brain during childhood. Case report. J Neurosurg Pediatr 2008, **1**: 325–329.

1036 Fallon MD, Ellerbrake D, Teitelbaum SL. Meningeal osteomas and chronic renal failure. Hum Pathol 1982, **13**: 449–453.

1037 Mello LR, Bernardes CI, Feltrin Y, Rodacki MA. Thoracic spine arachnoid ossification with and without cord cavitation. Report of three cases. J Neurosurg 2001, **94**: 115–120.

1038 Miyamori T, Mizukoshi H, Yamano K, Takayanagi N, Sugino M, Hayase H, Ito H. Intracranial chondrosarcoma – case report. Neurol Med Chir (Tokyo) 1990, **30**: 263–267.

1039 Nakayama M, Nagayama T, Hirano H, Oyoshi T, Kuratsu J. Giant chondroma arising from the dura mater of the convexity. Case report and review of the literature. J Neurosurg 2001, **94**: 331–334.

1040 Rushing EJ, Armonda RA, Ansari Q, Mena H. Mesenchymal chondrosarcoma: a clinicopathologic and flow cytometric study of 13 cases presenting in the central nervous system. Cancer 1996, **77**: 1884–1891.

1041 Saesue P, Chankaew E, Chawalparit O, Na Ayudhya NS, Muangsomboon S, Sangruchi T. Primary extraskeletal osteosarcoma in the pineal region. Case report. J Neurosurg 2004, **101**: 1061–1064.

1042 Sato K, Kubota T, Yoshida K, Murata H. Intracranial extraskeletal myxoid chondrosarcoma with special reference to lamellar inclusions in the rough endoplasmic reticulum. Acta Neuropathol 1993, **86**: 525–528.

1043 Sipos EP, Tamargo RJ, Epstein JI, North RB. Primary intracerebral small-cell osteosarcoma in an adolescent girl: report of a case. J Neurooncol 1997, **32**: 169–174.

1044 Traflet RF, Babaria AR, Barolat G, Doan HT, Gonzalez C, Mishkin MM. Intracranial chondroma in a patient with Ollier's disease. Case report. J Neurosurg 1989, **70**: 274–276.

1045 Yassa M, Bahary JP, Bourguoin P, Belair M, Berthelet F, Bouthillier A. Intra-parenchymal mesenchymal chondrosarcoma of the cerebellum: case report and review of the literature. J Neurooncol 2005, **74**: 329–331.

Fibroblastic, myofibroblastic, and 'fibrohistiocytic' tumors

1046 Alston SR, Francel PC, Jane JA Jr. Solitary fibrous tumor of the spinal cord. Am J Surg Pathol 1997, **21**: 477–483.

1047 Bilsky MH, Schefler AC, Sandberg DI, Dunkel IJ, Rosenblum MK. Sclerosing epithelioid fibrosarcomas involving the neuraxis: report of three cases. Neurosurgery 2000, **47**: 956–959.

1048 Carneiro SS, Scheithauer BW, Nascimento AG, Hirose T, Davis DH. Solitary fibrous tumor of the meninges: a lesion distinct from fibrous meningioma. A clinicopathologic and immunohistochemical study. Am J Clin Pathol 1996, **106**: 217–224.

1049 Castilla EA, Prayson RA, Stevens GH, Barnett GH. Brain-invasive solitary fibrous tumor of the meninges: report of a case. Int J Surg Pathol 2002, **10**: 217–221.

1050 Dunham C, Hussong J, Seiff M, Pfeifer J, Perry A. Primary intracerebral angiomatoid fibrous histiocytoma: report of a case with a t(12;22)(q13;q12) causing type 1 fusion of the EWS and ATF-1 genes. Am J Surg Pathol 2008, **32**: 478–484.

1051 Gaspar LE, Mackenzie IR, Gilbert JJ, Kaufmann JC, Fisher BF, Macdonald DR, Cairncross JG. Primary cerebral fibrosarcomas. Clinicopathologic study and review of the literature. Cancer 1993, **72**: 3277–3281.

1052 Hamlat A, Adn M, Caulet-Maugendre S, Guegan Y. Cerebellar malignant fibrous histiocytoma: case report and literature review. Neurosurgery 2004, **54**: 745–751; discussion 751–752.

1053 Hisaoka M, Furuta A, Rikimaru S. Sclerosing fibrous tumor of the cauda equina: a fibroblastic variant of peripheral nerve tumors? Acta Neuropathol 1993, **86**: 193–197.

1054 Iyer GV, Vaishya ND, Bhaktaviziam A, Taori GM, Abraham J. Angiofibroma of the middle cranial fossa. Case report. J Neurosurg 1971, **35**: 90–94.

1055 Lopes MB, Lanzino G, Cloft HJ, Winston DC, Vance ML, Laws ER Jr. Primary fibrosarcoma of the sella unrelated to previous radiation therapy. Mod Pathol 1998, **11**: 579–584.

1056 McDonald P, Guha A, Provias J. Primary intracranial fibrosarcoma with intratumoral hemorrhage: neuropathological diagnosis with review of the literature. J Neurooncol 1997, **35**: 133–139.

1057 Mitchell A, Scheithauer BW, Ebersold MJ, Forbes GS. Intracranial fibromatosis. Neurosurgery 1991, **29**: 123–126.

1058 Miyashita K, Hayashi Y, Fujisawa H, Hasegawa M, Yamashita J. Recurrent intracranial solitary fibrous tumor with cerebrospinal fluid dissemination. Case report. J Neurosurg 2004, **101**: 1045–1048.

1059 Ng HK, Choi PC, Wong CW, To KF, Poon WS. Metastatic solitary fibrous tumor of the meninges. Case report. J Neurosurg 2000, **93**: 490–493.

1060 Nishio S, Morioka T, Inamura T, Takeshita I, Fukui M, Sasaki M, Nakamura K, Wakisaka S. Radiation-induced brain tumours: potential late complications of radiation therapy for brain tumours. Acta Neurochir (Wien) 1998, **140**: 763–770.

1061 Pagenstecher A, Emmerich B, van Velthoven V, Korinthenberg R, Volk B. Exclusively intracranial cranial fasciitis in a child. Case report. J Neurosurg 1995, **83**: 744–747.

1062 Palma L, Spagnoli LG, Yusuf MA. Intracerebral fibroma: light and electron microscopic study. Acta Neurochir (Wien) 1985, **77**: 152–156.

1063 Piana S, Putrino I, Cavazza A, Nigrisoli E. Solitary fibrous tumor of the spinal nerve rootlet: report of a case mimicking schwannoma. Arch Pathol Lab Med 2004, **128**: 335–337.

1064 Reyes-Mugica M, Chou P, Gonzalez-Crussi F, Tomita T. Fibroma of the meninges in a child: immunohistological and ultrastructural study. Case report. J Neurosurg 1992, **76**: 143–147.

1065 Saito R, Kumabe T, Watanabe M, Jokura H, Shibuya M, Nakazato Y, Tominaga T. Low-grade fibromyxoid sarcoma of intracranial origin. Case report. J Neurosurg 2008, **108**: 798–802.

1066 Shinojima N, Ohta K, Yano S, Nakamura H, Kochi M, Ishimaru Y, Nakazato Y, Ushio Y. Myofibroblastoma in the suprasellar region. Case report. J Neurosurg 2002, **97**: 1203–1207.

1067 Slavik T, Bentley RC, Gray L, Fuchs HE, McLendon RE. Solitary fibrous tumor of the meninges occurring after irradiation of a mixed germ cell tumor of the pineal gland. Clin Neuropathol 1998, **17**: 55–60.

1068 Tihan T, Viglione M, Rosenblum MK, Olivi A, Burger PC. Solitary fibrous tumors in the central nervous system. A clinicopathologic review of 18 cases and comparison to meningeal hemangiopericytomas. Arch Pathol Lab Med 2003, **127**: 432–439.

Endothelial tumors

1069 Abe M, Tabuchi K, Takagi M, Matsumoto S, Shimokama T, Kishikawa T. Spontaneous resolution of multiple hemangiomas of the brain. Case report. J Neurosurg 1990, **73**: 448–452.

1070 Abe M, Tabuchi K, Tanaka S, Hodozuka A, Kunishio K, Kubo N, Nishimura Y. Capillary hemangioma of the central nervous system. J Neurosurg 2004, **101**: 73–81.

1071 Baehring JM, Dickey PS, Bannykh SI. Epithelioid hemangioendothelioma of the suprasellar area: a case report and review of the literature. Arch Pathol Lab Med 2004, **128**: 1289–1293.

1072 Buttner A, Marquart KH, Mehraein P, Weis S. Kaposi's sarcoma in the cerebellum of a patient with AIDS. Clin Neuropathol 1997, **16**: 185–189.

1073 Hida K, Tada M, Iwasaki Y, Abe H. Intramedullary disseminated capillary hemangioma with localized spinal cord swelling: case report. Neurosurgery 1993, **33**: 1099–1101.

1074 Karikari IO, Selznick LA, Cummings TJ, George TM. Capillary hemangioma of the fourth ventricle in an infant. Case report and review of the literature. J Neurosurg (3 Suppl Pediatrics) 2006, **104**: 188–191.

1075 Lach B, Benoit BG. Primary composite angiogenic leiomyosarcoma–epithelioid angiosarcoma of the brain. Ultrastruct Pathol 2000, **24**: 339–346.

1076 Mena H, Ribas JL, Enzinger FM, Parisi JE. Primary angiosarcoma of the central nervous system. Study of eight cases and review of the literature. J Neurosurg 1991, **75**: 73–76.

1077 Pearl GS, Takei Y, Tindall GT, O'Brien MS, Payne NS, Hoffman JC. Benign hemangioendothelioma involving the central nervous system: 'strawberry nevus' of the neuraxis. Neurosurgery 1980, **7**: 249–256.

1078 Roncaroli F, Scheithauer BW, Deen HG Jr. Multiple hemangiomas (hemangiomatosis) of the cauda equina and spinal cord. Case report. J Neurosurg 2000, **92**: 229–232.

1079 Roncaroli F, Scheithauer BW, Krauss WE. Capillary hemangioma of the spinal cord. Report of four cases. J Neurosurg (Spine 1) 2000, **93**: 148–151.

1080 Roncaroli F, Scheithauer BW, Krauss WE. Hemangioma of spinal nerve root. J Neurosurg (Spine 2) 1999, **91**: 175–180.

1081 Roncaroli F, Scheithauer BW, Papazoglou S. Primary polymorphous hemangioendothelioma of the spinal cord. Case report. J Neurosurg (Spine 1) 2001, **95**: 93–95.

1082 Samaratunga H, Searle J, Cominos D, Le Fevre I. Cerebral metastasis of an atrial myxoma mimicking an epithelioid hemangioendothelioma. Am J Surg Pathol 1994, **18**: 107–111.

1083 Stoffman MR, Kim JH. Masson's vegetant hemangioendothelioma: case report and literature review. J Neurooncol 2003, **61**: 17–22.

1084 Suzuki Y, Yoshida YK, Shirane R, Yoshimoto T, Watanabe M, Moriya T. Congenital primary cerebral angiosarcoma. Case report. J Neurosurg 2000, **92**: 466–468.

Meningeal hemangiopericytoma

1085 Ecker RD, Marsh WR, Pollock BE, Kurtkaya-Yapicier O, McClelland R, Scheithauer BW, Buckner JC. Hemangiopericytoma in the central nervous system: treatment, pathological features, and long-term follow up in 38 patients. J Neurosurg 2003, **98**: 1182–1187.

1086 Giannini C, Rushing EJ, Hainfellner JA. Haemangiopericytoma. In Louis DN, Ohgaki H, Wiestler OD, Cavanee WK (eds): WHO classification of tumours of the nervous system. Lyon, 2007, IARC, pp. 178–180.

1087 Mena H, Ribas JL, Pezeshkpour GH, Cowan DN, Parisi JE. Hemangiopericytoma of the central nervous system: a review of 94 cases. Hum Pathol 1991, **22**: 84–91.

1088 Perry A, Scheithauer BW, Nascimento AG. The immunophenotypic spectrum of meningeal hemangiopericytoma: a comparison with fibrous meningioma and solitary fibrous tumor of meninges. Am J Surg Pathol 1997, **21**: 1354–1360.

Myogenous tumors

1089 Caputo V, Repetti ML, Grimoldi N, Lazzarini G, Masini B, Radice F. Cerebral rhabdomyosarcoma with rhabdoid tumor-like features. J Neurooncol 1997, **32**: 81–86.

1090 Dropcho EJ, Allen JC. Primary intracranial rhabdomyosarcoma: case report and review of the literature. J Neurooncol 1987, **5**: 139–150.

1091 Eckhardt BP, Brandner S, Zollikofer CL, Wentz KU. Primary cerebral leiomyosarcoma in a child. Pediatr Radiol 2004, **34**: 495–498.

1092 Gasco J, Franklin B, Rangel-Castilla L, Campbell GA, Eltorky M, Salinas P. Infratentorial angioleiomyoma: a new location for a rare neoplastic entity. J Neurosurg 2009, **110**: 670–674.

1093 Herva R, Serlo W, Laitinen J, Becker LE. Intraventricular rhabdomyosarcoma after resection of hyperplastic choroid plexus. Acta Neuropathol 1996, **92**: 213–216.

1094 Janisch W, Janda J, Link I. [Primary diffuse leptomeningeal leiomyomatosis]. Zentralbl Pathol 1994, **140**: 195–200.

1095 Karpinski NC, Yaghmai R, Barba D, Hansen LA. Case of the month: March 1999 – A 26 year old HIV positive male with dura based masses. Brain Pathol 1999, **9**: 609–610.

1096 Lach B, Duncan E, Rippstein P, Benoit BG. Primary intracranial pleomorphic angioleiomyoma – a new morphologic variant. An immunohistochemical and electron microscopic study. Cancer 1994, **74**: 1915–1920.

1097 Lau PP, Wong OK, Lui PC, Cheung OY, Ho LC, Wong WC, To KF, Chan JK. Myopericytoma in patients with AIDS: a new class of Epstein–Barr virus-associated tumor. Am J Surg Pathol 2009, **33**: 1666–1672.

1098 Lin SL, Wang JS, Huang CS, Tseng HH. Primary intracerebral leiomyoma: a case with eosinophilic inclusions of actin filaments. Histopathology 1996, **28**: 365–369.

1099 Mierau GW, Greffe BS, Weeks DA. Primary leiomyosarcoma of brain in an adolescent with common variable immunodeficiency syndrome. Ultrastruct Pathol 1997, **21**: 301–305.

1100 Rousseau A, Kujas M, van Effenterre R, Boch AL, Carpentier A, Leroy JP, Poirier J. Primary intracranial myopericytoma: report of three cases and review of the literature. Neuropathol Appl Neurobiol 2005, **31**: 641–648.

1101 Xu F, De Las Casas LE, Dobbs LJ Jr. Primary meningeal rhabdomyosarcoma in a child with hypomelanosis of Ito. Arch Pathol Lab Med 2000, **124**: 762–765.

1102 Zevallos-Giampietri EA, Yanes HH, Orrego Puelles J, Barrionuevo C. Primary meningeal Epstein–Barr virus-related leiomyosarcoma in a man infected with human immunodeficiency virus: review of literature, emphasizing the differential diagnosis and pathogenesis. Appl Immunohistochem Mol Morphol 2004, **12**: 387–391.

Other mesenchymal tumors

1103 Biernat W, Kaniuka S, Stempniewicz M, Reclawowicz D, Sworczak K. Phosphaturic mesenchymal tumor of spinal nerve in a patient with osteomalacia and multiple fractures. Acta Neuropathol 2010, **119**: 379–380.

1104 Budka H, Pilz P, Guseo A. Primary leptomeningeal sarcomatosis. Clinicopathological report of six cases. J Neurol 1975, **211**: 77–93.

1105 Chu PG, Benhattar J, Weiss LM, Meagher-Villemure K. Intraneural synovial sarcoma: two cases. Mod Pathol 2004, **17**: 258–263.

1106 David K, Revesz T, Kratimenos G, Krausz T, Crockard HA. Oncogenic osteomalacia associated with a meningeal phosphaturic mesenchymal tumor. Case report. J Neurosurg 1996, **84**: 288–292.

1107 Fellig Y, Oliveira AM, Margolin E, Gomori JM, Erickson-Johnson MR, Chou MM, Umansky F, Soffer D. Extraosseous aneurysmal bone cyst of cerebello-pontine angle with USP6 rearrangement. Acta Neuropathol 2009, **118**: 579–581.

1108 Kurtkaya-Yapicier O, Scheithauer BW, Dedrick DJ, Wascher TM. Primary epithelioid sarcoma of the dura: case report. Neurosurgery 2002, **50**: 198–202; discussion 202–203.

1109 Medeiros F, Scheithauer BW, Oliveira AM, Gregory RS. Angiomyxofibromatous tumor of the falx cerebri. Am J Surg Pathol 2006, **30**: 545–547.

1110 Powers CJ, Pizzi CC, Cummings TJ, Friedman AH. Primary myxoma of the parafalcine meninges. Case report. J Neurosurg 2006, **104**: 440–443.

NERVE SHEATH TUMORS OF THE CRANIOSPINAL AXIS

1111 Acciarri N, Padovani R, Riccioni L. Intramedullary melanotic schwannoma. Report of a case and review of the literature. Br J Neurosurg 1999, **13**: 322–325.

1112 Almefty R, Webber BL, Arnautovic KI. Intraneural perineurioma of the third cranial nerve: occurrence and identification. Case report. J Neurosurg 2006, **104**: 824–827.

1113 Anton T, Guttierez J, Rock J. Tentorial schwannoma: a case report and review of the literature. J Neurooncol 2006, **76**: 307–311.

1114 Bari ME, Forster DM, Kemeny AA, Walton L, Hardy D, Anderson JR. Malignancy in a vestibular schwannoma. Report of a case with central neurofibromatosis, treated by both stereotactic radiosurgery and surgical excision, with a review of the literature. Br J Neurosurg 2002, **16**: 284–289.

1115 Brown DF, Rushing EJ. Rosenthal fibers and eosinophilic granular bodies in a classic acoustic schwannoma. Arch Pathol Lab Med 1997, **121**: 1207–1209.

1116 Carney JA. Psammomatous melanotic schwannoma. A distinctive, heritable tumor with special associations, including cardiac myxoma and the Cushing syndrome. Am J Surg Pathol 1990, **14**: 206–222.

1117 Carvalho GA, Lindeke A, Tatagiba M, Ostertag H, Samii M. Cranial granular-cell tumor of the trigeminal nerve. Case report. J Neurosurg 1994, **81**: 795–798.

1118 Casadei GP, Komori T, Scheithauer BW, Miller GM, Parisi JE, Kelly PJ. Intracranial parenchymal schwannoma. A clinicopathological and neuroimaging study of nine cases. J Neurosurg 1993, **79**: 217–222.

1119 Casadei GP, Scheithauer BW, Hirose T, Manfrini M, Van Houton C, Wood MB. Cellular schwannoma. A clinicopathologic, DNA flow cytometric, and proliferation marker study of 70 patients. Cancer 1995, **75**: 1109–1119.

1120 Comey CH, McLaughlin MR, Jho HD, Martinez AJ, Lunsford LD. Death from a malignant cerebellopontine angle triton tumor despite stereotactic radiosurgery. Case report. J Neurosurg 1998, **89**: 653–658.

1121 Cras P, Ceuterick-de Groote C, Van Vyve M, Vercruyssen A, Martin JJ. Malignant pigmented spinal nerve root schwannoma metastasizing in the brain and viscera. Clin Neuropathol 1990, **9**: 290–294.

1122 Deruaz JP, Janzer RC, Costa J. Cellular schwannomas of the intracranial and intraspinal compartment: morphological and immunological characteristics compared with classical benign schwannomas. J Neuropathol Exp Neurol 1993, **52**: 114–118.

1123 Ducatman BS, Scheithauer BW, Piepgras DG, Reiman HM, Ilstrup DM. Malignant peripheral nerve sheath tumors. A clinicopathologic study of 120 cases. Cancer 1986, **57**: 2006–2021.

Pituitary gland

29

B.K. Kleinschmidt-DeMasters M.D.

CHAPTER CONTENTS

Introduction

The pituitary gland is home to one major disease process, the pituitary adenoma, and only rarely hosts cysts, inflammatory diseases, or neoplasms of nonpituitary cell origin. However, when these do occur, they closely mimic adenoma on neuroimaging studies. Thus, correct diagnosis falls to the surgical pathologist and these exceptional entities will be referenced in some detail at the end of the chapter. This chapter will be directed towards practicing surgical pathologists, and thus figures of microscopic features of these lesions will predominate over gross images. Electron microscopy (EM) also is being required less today for classification of pituitary adenomas, and is less available in many pathology practices. Previous editions of this book,[1] as well as the World Health Organization (WHO) fascicle,[2] can be consulted for beautiful gross and EM images.

Pituitary adenomas are not homogeneous. Each subtype has its own clinical presentation, tendency for invasiveness, hormonal secretion pattern, histopathologic features, and treatment. Because adenomas are benign, generally well-differentiated tumors that closely mimic their non-neoplastic anterior pituicyte counterparts, they variably retain the ability to recapitulate normal anterior pituitary hormonal secretion. Most adenomas produce hormone products that are explainable by knowing the developmental lineage pathways taken by normal pituitary cells. A basic understanding of embryological development of pituitary gland also helps to put into perspective some of the less common entities that affect the sellar region.

Normal embryology and anatomy

The anterior lobe (pars distalis) is derived from Rathke's pouch, a tube of tissue which invaginates from the fetal oral (stomodeal) ectoderm anterior to the roof of the primitive mouth, forms by the fourth to fifth week of human gestation,[7,14] migrates dorsally towards the base of the brain, and comes in contact with the diencephalon. At the sixth fetal week, a down-pouching of the floor of the third ventricle and diencephalon forms and Rathke's pouch detaches from the oral epithelium and becomes a separate structure. Cellular proliferation begins, with the ventral part of Rathke's pouch giving rise to the pars distalis and the dorsal part to the pars intermedia[14] (Fig. 29.1, inset). The diencephalic diverticulum thereafter narrows and is obliterated. The diencephalic diverticulum is the origin of the posterior lobe of the pituitary gland (pars nervosa and infundibular stalk); these are extensions of central nervous system parenchyma. By the 14th week of human gestation, pituitary development is essentially complete.[14] After birth, the gland grows rapidly, reaching a plateau at about 3 years after birth; rapid growth again occurs between ages 10 and 13 years.[13] Modern neuroimaging allows distinction between adult anterior (adenohypophysis) and posterior (neurohypophysis) lobes (Fig. 29.2).

Remnants of the pituitary gland exist in the pharynx along the pathway of Rathke's pouch in most individuals, but the volume of tissue is approximately one-thousandth the size of the normal gland.[7] Major developmental abnormalities of the pituitary gland, such hypophyseal duplication[12] or abnormal placement in children with cleft lip and palate plus oro-ocular cleft,[10] are rare. Trisomy 21 fetuses usually have normal or only minor abnormalities in sellar bone development,[11] while fetuses with holoprosencephaly and anencephaly have more significant abnormalities in pituitary gland development.[9]

Six distinct hormone-secreting cell types appear during anterior pituitary gland development: the corticotroph (adrenocorticotrophic hormone-secreting, ACTH), somatotroph (growth hormone-secreting, GH), lactotroph (prolactin-secreting, PRL), mammosomatotroph parent cell for GH and PRL, gonadotroph (follicle stimulated hormone- and luteinizing hormone-secreting, FSH and LH, in a single cell), and thyrotroph (thyroid stimulating hormone-secreting, TSH).[5] These different cell types in the anterior gland are barely discernible on hematoxylin and eosin (H&E) in fetuses, although clear distinction from the posterior gland is seen from the earliest time points (Fig. 29.3). Cells in the anterior gland share a common Rathke pouch stem cell origin and lineage, and appear within the anterior gland in a defined order (Fig. 29.4). Pituitary-specific transcription factors, Rpx, Pitx, Lhx3, Prop-1, and

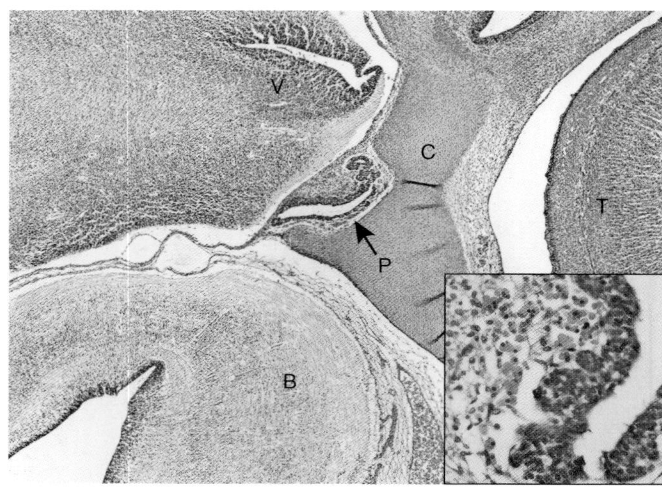

Fig. 29.1 Human fetal pituitary development, illustrated from a 20 mm crown–rump length, estimated 7 weeks' gestation; crown of head is at left of photograph. B, brain; C, cartilaginous skull base; P, pituitary gland in saddle-shaped sella; T, tongue; V, third ventricle. Inset: high magnification with early proliferation of anterior pituitary cells forming small rudimentary acini. (H&E)

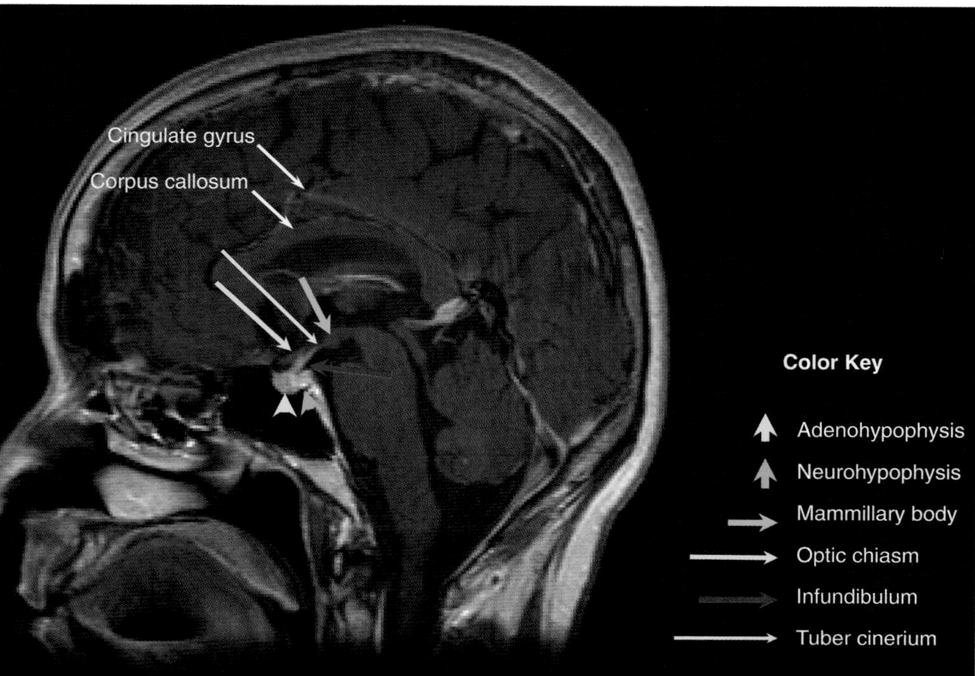

Fig. 29.2 Sagittal post-contrast, T1-weighted MRI, demonstrating normal adult anterior and posterior pituitary gland and sellar region anatomy.

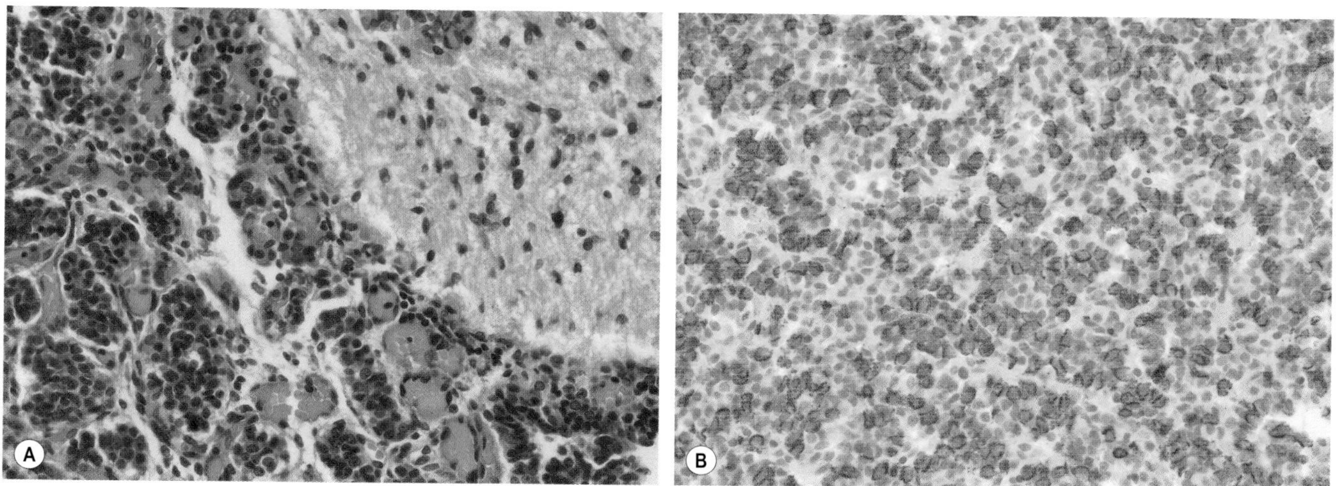

Fig. 29.3 **A,** Fetal pituitary gland at 22 weeks shows clear distinction between anterior (lower left) and posterior (upper right) gland; note rich vascularity. (H&E) **B,** Fetal pituitary gland at 22 weeks demonstrates strong diffuse immunostaining for anterior pituitary hormones at this stage of development; growth hormone immunoreactivity in the lateral wings is illustrated. (Immunoperoxidase with hematoxylin counterstain)

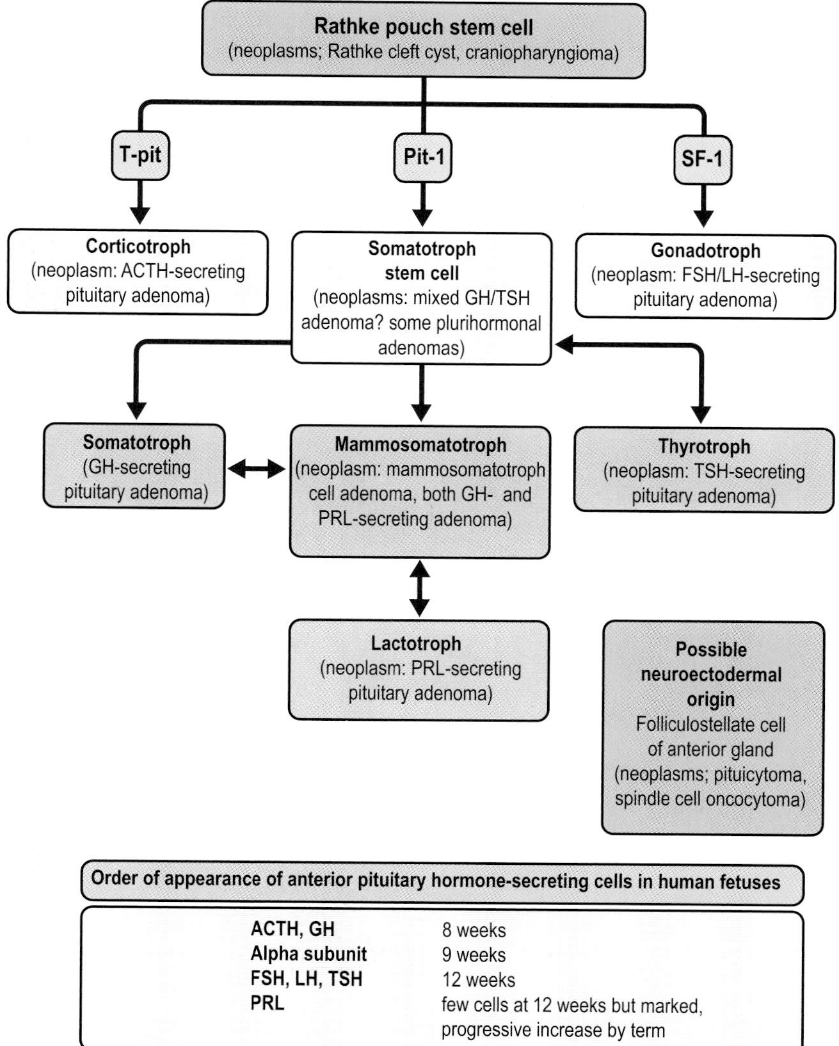

Fig. 29.4 Ontogeny and the primary transcription factors for each pituitary cell type lineage.
(Adapted from Asa SL. Practical pituitary pathology: what does the pathologist need to know? Arch Pathol Lab Med 2008, ***132:*** *1231–1240)*

Pit-1, play a role in the determination of the pituitary cell lineages.[5,6] Ontogeny and the primary transcription factors for each pituitary cell type lineage are listed in Figure 29.4, as adapted from Asa.[5] Also listed is the order of appearance of cell types during human fetal development.[3,4,8] There is fluidity between four of the cell types, GH, PRL, mammosomatotrophs, and TSH cells, which are all dependent on Pit-1 for their lineage specification; these are able to reversibly transdifferentiate under physiologic or disease conditions.[5]

An additional cell type in the anterior gland is a nonhormone-secreting folliculostellate cell thought to be of neuroectodermal origin given its immunoreactivity for glial fibrillary acidic protein (GFAP) and S-100. This cell recently has been shown to express galectin-3, as have normal prolactin and ACTH-secreting cells.[15]

Most pituitary adenomas show hormone expression profiles that recapitulate these expected developmental lineage pathways. Pituitary adenomas from those cell types that diverge early from the Rathke pouch stem cell – the corticotrophs and gonadotrophs – usually show only lineage-specific, single, more restricted hormonal expression. For example, corticotroph cell adenomas usually show immunoreactivity only for ACTH, and none of the other hormone types. Gonadotroph cell adenomas manifest immunoreactivity only for alpha subunit (αSU), FSH-β, and/or LH-β, all secreted by the same cell in the normal anterior pituitary gland, but not other hormone types. In contrast, GH and PRL immunostaining often are found together in the same adenoma due to their common precursor during fetal development – the 'parent' mammosomatotroph cell.

Normal pituitary cell types

Once the different cell types form in the anterior gland, there appears to be relatively little 'cross talk' between them in terms of physiologic function. A second curious feature is that hormone cell types are not equally distributed throughout the gland. Several cell types clustered within a single acinus, visible on H&E (Fig. 29.5A), but better appreciated with histochemical preparations such as the periodic acid–Schiff (PAS)-orange G stain, which highlights orange-staining acidophils (mostly GH-secreting cells), fuchsia-colored basophils (mostly ACTH-secreting cells), and nonstaining chromophobes (PRL, FSH/LH, and TSH-secreting cells) (Fig. 29.5B). Lateral wings are acidophil-rich with a heavy concentration of GH and PRL cells (Fig. 29.5C), while the basophil-rich 'median wedge' contains most of the ACTH and TSH immunoreactive cells. The exact role this uneven distribution has in optimal function of the gland is unclear.

The proportion of the various cell types within the lobe becomes of importance in small tissue samples, especially when the pathologist is attempting to distinguish diffuse or nodular hyperplasia, particularly in the case of ACTH hyperplasia, from normal gland. Today the outdated histochemical preparations such as PAS-orange G have been superseded by immunohistochemistry and EM, which verify the existence of multiple cell types in the anterior gland, not simply the 'three-colored' acidophil, basophil, and chromophobe cell types seen with these older histochemical preparations.

In contrast to the complex anterior pituitary gland, the posterior lobe is made up of unmyelinated axons and specialized glia. The gland has a glial, fibrillary appearance with prominent delicate blood vessels. Small fragments of normal gland are often found in surgical resection specimens of Rathke cleft cysts (Fig. 29.6A) and sometimes even adjacent to pituitary adenomas. Swellings of axons that store oxytocin or vasopressin can occasionally be discerned on H&E (Herring bodies, Fig. 29.6A, inset) and are normal findings. Antineurofilament is the single best stain for confirming the identity of the axon-rich posterior gland (Fig. 29.6B) and distinguishing it from other lesions (such as pituicytoma) that might mimic normal gland. Although alarming to the surgical pathologist when these fragments of posterior gland are found in a surgical specimen, it is important to remember that the posterior gland is a *storage* site, not *synthesis* site for these hormones. Postoperative posterior pituitary gland dysfunction after modern pituitary adenoma transsphenoidal resection is limited to transient diabetes insipidus that usually resolves after several days. Removal of these small fragments of posterior gland appears to have no long-lasting deleterious clinical effects on the patient.

The infundibular stalk is part of the posterior lobe and contains closely juxtaposed, thin-walled blood vessels that transport hypothalamic release and release-inhibiting factors to the anterior gland (Fig. 29.7). When the infundibular stalk is compressed by a mass lesion or undergoes any traumatic or circulatory disruption, the delicate, thin-walled vessels of the hypothalamic–hypophyseal portal system are pinched off (Fig. 29.7) and hypothalamic release and release-inhibiting factors do not reach the pituitary gland. Under normal physiologic conditions, the one anterior pituitary hormone which is more tonically inhibited than stimulated is PRL; the hypothalamic factor is dopamine. Interruption of the infundibular stalk by any mass lesion will abrogate passage of inhibitory dopamine to the anterior gland and result in hyperprolactinemia of a modest degree (30–200 ng/dL).[18] The histologic counterpart is

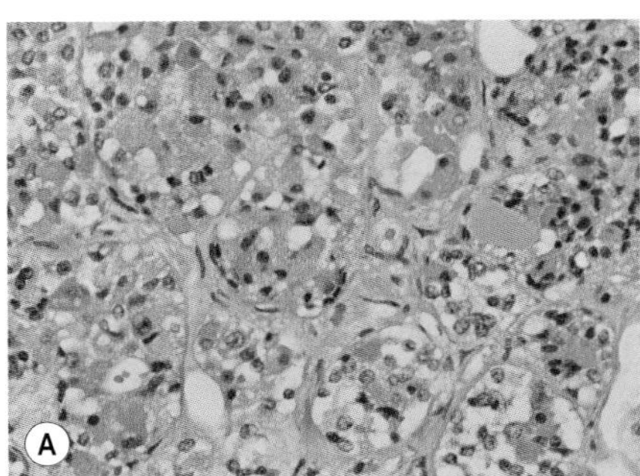

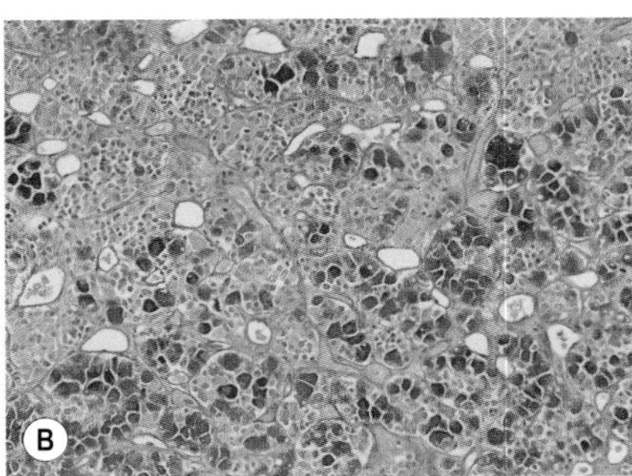

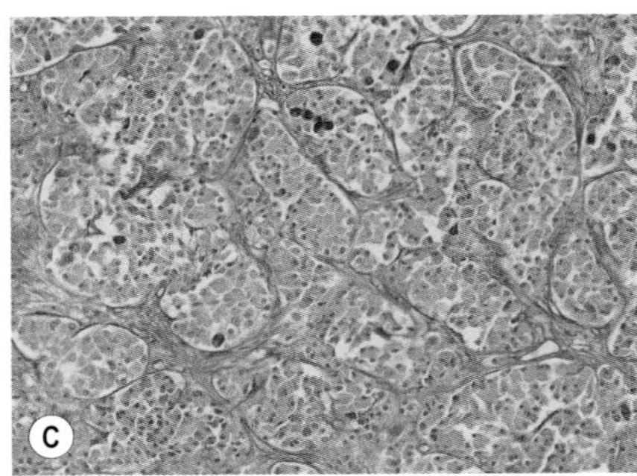

Fig. 29.5 **A,** Adult anterior pituitary gland shows different cell types on H&E. **B,** Adult anterior pituitary gland demonstrates greater distinction of cell types using histochemical preparations such as PAS-orange G; note acidophils, basophils, and chromophobes. **C,** Adult anterior pituitary gland in the lateral wings is predominantly populated by acidophilic growth hormone secreting cells; note maintenance of acinar structure. (**B** and **C,** PAS-orange G)

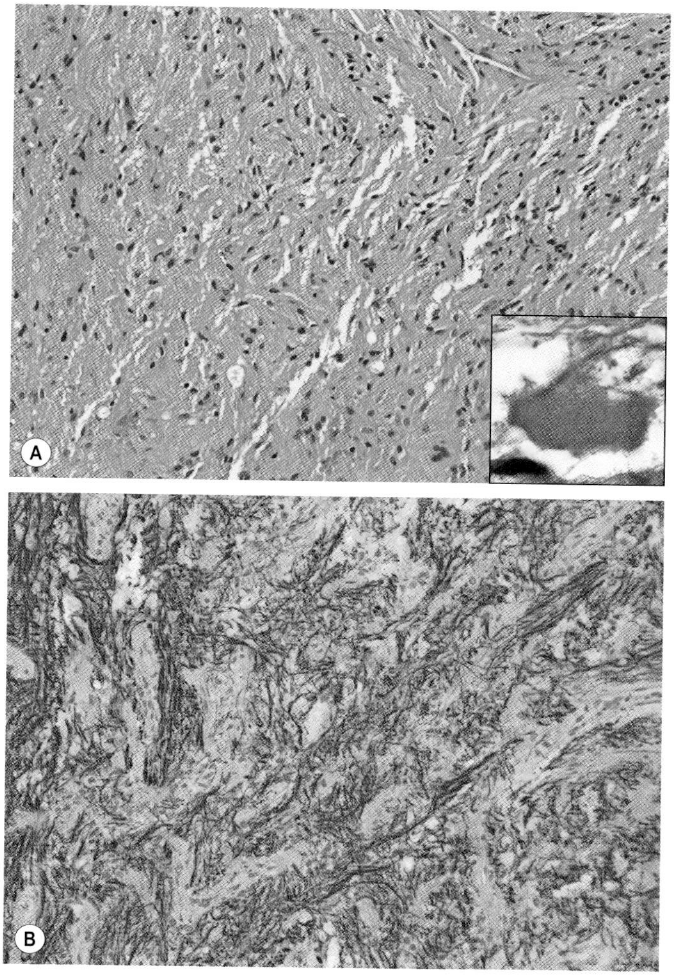

Fig. 29.6 **A,** Normal adult posterior pituitary gland manifests an eosinophilic fibrillar appearance. Inset: occasional swollen axonal processes (Herring bodies) can be found. **B,** Adult posterior pituitary gland showing abundant axons by antineurofilament staining. (Immunoperoxidase with hematoxylin counterstain)

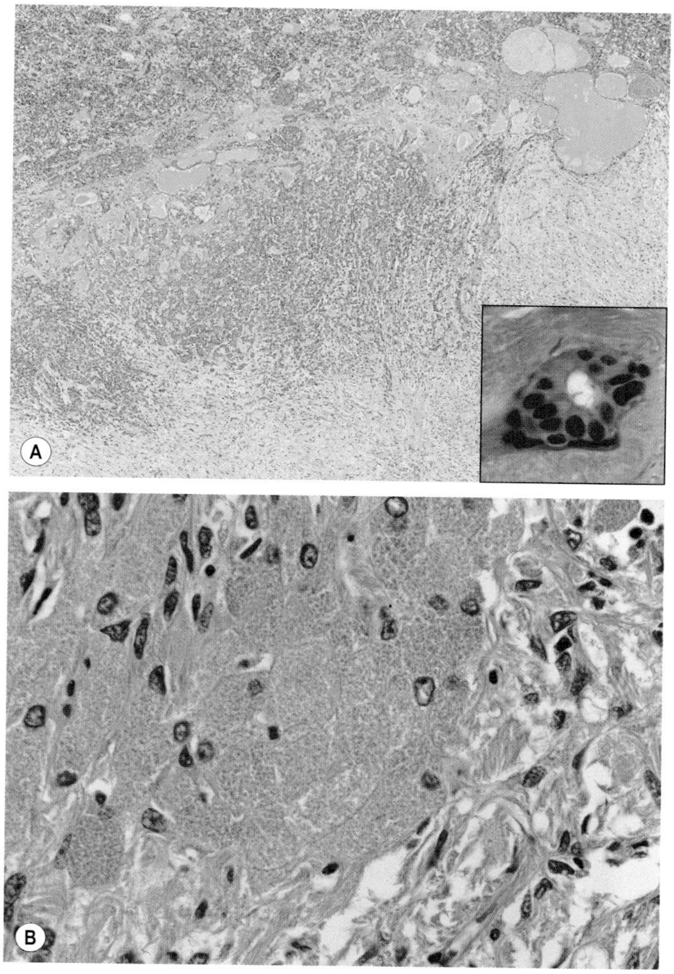

Fig. 29.8 **A,** Normal adult pituitary gland manifests a rudimentary intermediate lobe, usually containing small mucin-filled cysts (upper right) and normal physiologic 'basophil invasion' seen with aging. Inset: tubular (salivary type) glands. **B,** Incidental granular cell tumor of posterior gland.

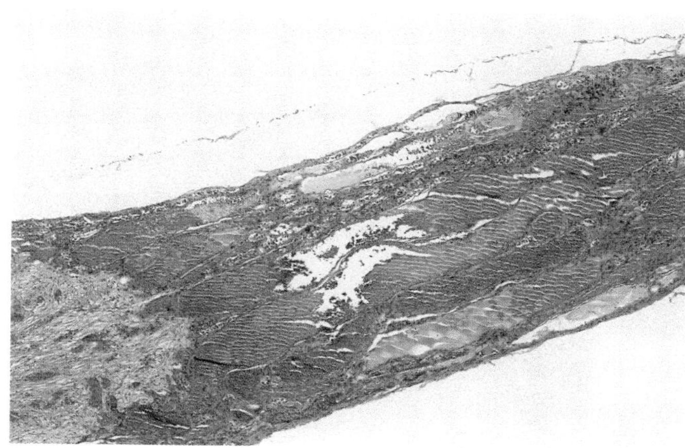

Fig. 29.7 Adult infundibular stalk showing congested, thin-walled, closely juxtaposed hypothalamic–hypophyseal portal system.

increased PRL immunostaining in the anterior gland; this physiologic response should not be misinterpreted by the surgical pathologist as a second PRL-secreting adenoma in the surgical tissue.

Normal variations in the posterior lobe include 'basophil invasion' in normal aging, represented by groups of anterior pituicytes immunoreactive for ACTH extending into the posterior gland (Fig. 29.8A) and tubular glands, known as salivary gland rests (Fig. 29.8A, inset). Salivary gland rests are incidental findings found in one study in 78 of 2300 consecutive autopsies; they occurred in all ages and closely resemble serous acinar and duct cells of the salivary gland by EM.[20] These only rarely develop cysts large enough to be symptomatic[21] or are a source for salivary gland-type neoplasms such as pleomorphic adenoma.[16] Nests of granular cells are also encountered in 6.5–17% of autopsy specimens (Fig. 29.8B), but symptomatic granular cell tumors are very uncommon.[19]

The intermediate lobe is rudimentary in humans and consists of small cyst-like structures filled with colloid. Small amounts of intermediate lobe can be found in surgical specimens (Fig. 29.8A). Larger cysts in the intermediate lobe filled with dense colloid material also occur in some surgical specimens. These intermediate lobe cysts when they occur in isolation are considered a separate entity by some workers,[17] while others lump them with Rathke cleft cysts, given their common Rathke pouch embryologic origin. Rarely, cystic hyperplasia of the intermediate pituitary lobe is associated with pituitary enlargement in patients with the *PROP1* gene-inactivating mutation.[22]

Pituitary adenomas

General features

Adenomas constitute 10–15% of all intracranial neoplasms in most neurosurgery practices. The prevalence of clinically diagnosed pituitary adenomas has recently been recognized to be 3.5–5 times more frequent than formerly thought, with a study from Belgium showing a prevalence of approximately 1 per 1000 individuals.[26]

The vast majority of adenomas are sporadic. Mutations in known oncogenes have little role in the pathogenesis of most sporadic pituitary adenomas.[31] The only somatic mutation that has been identified in a significant proportion of sporadic pituitary tumors is the *GSP* mutation which causes constitutive activation of the cAMP pathway.[31] This mutation occurs in approximately 30–40% of sporadic GH-secreting pituitary adenomas, but not other adenoma types.

Abnormalities in the signaling and feedback pathways have been demonstrated in pituitary tumors but they are unlikely to be the primary events responsible for sporadic tumors.[31] Pituitary adenomas are clonal but no specific chromosomal alterations are characteristic. Increasing chromosomal imbalances have, however, been demonstrated in recurrent tumors.[35]

Familial adenomas account for 5% or less of all adenomas,[27–29] with germline mutations in the *MEN1* gene associated with multiple endocrine neoplasia (MEN) type 1 identified in 2.7% of individuals with apparently sporadic pituitary adenomas.[36] Pituitary adenoma predisposition syndromes include MEN1 (gene *MEN1*, chromosome 11q13, results in all pituitary tumor types),[37] Carney complex (gene *PPKR1A*, chromosome 17q22–24, associated with GH- or PRL-secreting adenomas),[33] MEN4 (gene *CDKN1B*, chromosome 12p13, too few patients described to be certain of adenoma type), and familial isolated pituitary adenomas (FIPA, gene *AIP*, chromosome 11q13.32 in 15% of cases (50% of familial acromegaly), all pituitary tumor types).[25,27–29]

No strong relationship to birth control pill use has been established. Endocrine end-organ failure is not related to pituitary adenoma development except in the very rare instance of TSH hyperplasia in patients with long-standing hypothyroidism evolving into adenoma. Antecedent or concomitant hyperplasia with adenoma is exceedingly rare. Although mutations in receptors on pituitary cells is an attractive etiologic possibility for adenoma causation, at least in gonadotroph cell adenomas, no activating mutations in the gonadotropin-releasing hormone (*GNRH*) receptor gene have been identified.[24]

Pituitary adenomas usually develop in the third to sixth decades, but pediatric examples certainly occur. In a recent series of adenomas in patients less than 20 years of age, 19/20 examples were secretory and prolactinomas predominated: 9 adenomas stained solely for PRL, 5 for ACTH, 3 for GH, and 2 for both GH and PRL, and 1 did not stain with hormone antibodies.[38] Infantile pituitary adenomas are exceedingly rare; however, when they do occur, they are usually ACTH-secreting adenomas[34] (Fig. 29.9). In contrast, pituitary adenomas coming to neurosurgical resection at the other extreme of the age spectrum are not rare. In a retrospective study from 1992–2002, detailing patients aged 75 years or older who had symptomatic lesions requiring neurosurgical intervention, pituitary adenomas were the third most frequent tumor type.[32]

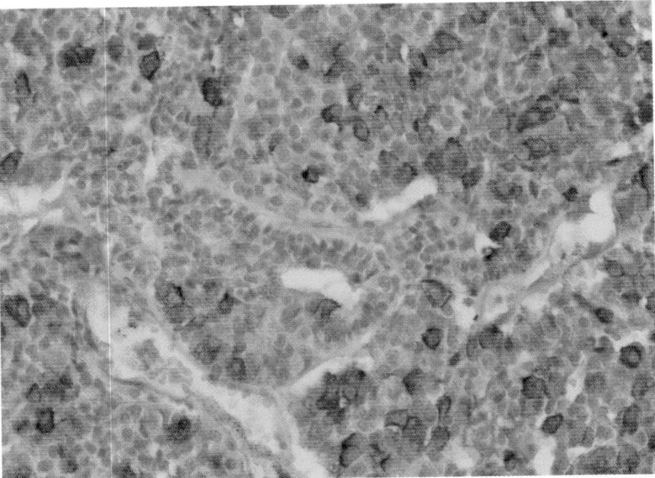

Fig. 29.9 Rare infantile pituitary adenoma with ACTH immunoreactivity.

Since pituitary adenomas are derived from endocrine-active cells, they have the potential to produce anterior pituitary hormones. Generally, only one, or rarely two, hormones are produced in sufficient quantities to result in elevated serum levels and produce clinically discernible endocrinopathies.

If the tumor is inefficient at producing hormones, the mass effects and hypopituitarism predominate because of compression of the normal gland. Clinically, loss of hormonal function in hypopituitarism occurs in an ordered fashion. GH and gonadotroph cell function is lost first, followed by TSH and ACTH. The last hormone function to be lost temporally in most people with hypopituitarism is prolactin. This ordered loss of cells due to compression of normal anterior gland can also be detected at the immunohistochemical level by the pathologist. Often a pituitary adenoma will encompass a few normal, non-neoplastic anterior pituitary cells within the adenoma as it grows. The two cell types that often survive this compression/encompassment longest before being lost are ACTH and PRL-immunoreactive cells. These cells types thus are most likely to be encountered as single or small groups of cells within an adenoma by the pathologist. If the surgical pathologist is unaware of this, these encompassed residual normal pituitary cells can serve as a considerable source of confusion when interpreting immunostaining patterns in adenoma.

The relative frequency of the various pituitary adenoma types differs depending on whether one is looking at autopsy or surgical material. The most frequently occurring adenoma found as an incidental finding at autopsy is the PRL-secreting adenoma.[30] A recent meta-analysis of the MEDLINE literature by Ezzat et al. found that 22.5% of persons harbor pituitary lesions on neuroimaging studies and 14.5% of autopsy pituitary glands contain microadenomas.[30] The WHO fascicle[2] also lists prolactinomas as being the most frequent adenoma type, based on older studies, but more recent articles[5] also note the changing demographics of adenomas coming to surgical resection.

As PRL-secreting adenomas are now routinely treated chemically with dopamine agonists such as bromocriptine, parlodel, or cabergoline, the patient no longer comes to surgery unless intolerant of the medications or there are other mitigating circumstances. In a more recent series of 3489 pituitary adenomas tumors from nine centers in Germany[39] (and in our own single-institution US experience with over 1000 cases), FSH/LH cell adenomas followed by the clinically nonsecretory adenomas clearly predominate in surgical material (Table 29.1). ACTH-producing adenomas are fourth in incidence, and TSH-secreting tumors are very rare. Most clinically nonfunctional 'null cell' adenomas show focal individual cells with immunoreactivity for gonadotrophic (FSH, LH, αSU) hormones[2] and thus occur within the same biologic spectrum and lineage pathway as gonadotroph cell adenomas. When gonadotroph adenomas are combined with nonfunctional null cell adenomas, this group constitutes 40–50% of all adenomas seen by surgical pathologists. When this same group studied a comparably large number of subclinical adenomas (3048 autopsies, 334 adenomas identified in 316 pituitary glands), the differences between cases coming to surgical excision versus autopsy material clearly became evident (Table 29.1).[23] This study also identified the incidence of double adenomas in a single autopsy gland,[23] a reported, but relatively rare, occurrence in surgically resected material.

Table 29.1 Comparison of pituitary adenoma types at surgery and postmortem exam

ADENOMA TYPE	ADENOMAS COMING TO SURGERY[a] (%) (n = 3403)	SUBCLINICAL ADENOMAS POSTMORTEM[b] (%) (n = 334)
Densely granulated GH cell adenoma	9.2	0.90
Sparsely granulated GH cell adenoma	6.3	1.20
Sparsely granulated prolactin cell adenoma	8.9	39.5
Densely granulated prolactin cell adenoma	0.3	–
Mixed bicellular GH/ prolactin cell adenoma	5.2	0.30
Mammosomatotroph adenoma	1.1	–
Acidophil stem cell adenoma	0.2	–
Densely granulated ACTH cell adenoma	7.2	8.08
Sparsely granulated ACTH cell adenoma	7.9	5.69
Crooke cell adenoma	0.03	0.30
TSH cell adenoma	1.5	0.60
FSH/LH (gonadotroph) cell adenoma	25.2	6.6
Null cell adenoma	19.8	23.1
Null cell adenoma, oncocytic variant	5.8	9.3
Plurihormonal adenoma, including 'silent adenoma, subtype 3'	1.3	2.7
Unclassified	2.1	1.8

Taken from:
[a]Saeger W, Ludecke DK, Buchfelder M, Fahlbusch R, Quabbe HJ, Petersenn S. Pathohistological classification of pituitary tumors: 10 years of experience with the German Pituitary Tumor Registry. Eur J Endocr 2007, **156:** 203–216.
[b]Buurman H, Saeger W. Subclinical adenomas in postmortem pituitaries: classification and correlations to clinical data. Eur J Endocr 2006, **154:** 753–758.

Size, spread, and grading

All pituitary adenomas, regardless of size or hormone subtype, are WHO grade I tumors. Microadenomas, defined as tumor less than or equal to 10 mm, remain confined to the sellar region (Fig. 29.10).[41]

Microadenomas may cause some degree of hypofunction of the normal anterior pituitary gland due to compression, but seldom result in compromise of posterior pituitary gland function. Indeed, diabetes insipidus is quite uncommon with pituitary adenomas of any size.

Macroadenomas, defined as greater than 1 cm in dimension, more severely distort adjacent tissues, with traction on the dura of the sellar floor or dura overlying the sella, called the diaphragma sella, causing headaches. Macroadenomas most commonly grow directly upwards (Fig. 29.11A), compressing the nearby optic chiasm in its midportion, an area containing crossing axons emanating from retinal cells within the medial retinal fields. Since these medial retinal fields are responsible for lateral visual fields, the classic symptom of optic chiasm midline compression in a pituitary adenoma is bitemporal hemianopsia. Compression of the hypothalamus directly above the gland can also occur, but hypothalamic dysfunction with pituitary adenomas is quite uncommon compared to that seen in tumors that primarily arise within suprasellar regions, such as craniopharyngiomas. Lateral growth outside the sella may compress the mesial temporal lobe, causing seizures. Adenomas may compress brain parenchyma but lack the capability of infiltrating into brain parenchyma as single cells, in contrast to gliomas, such as astrocytomas and oligodendrogliomas. Often invasive

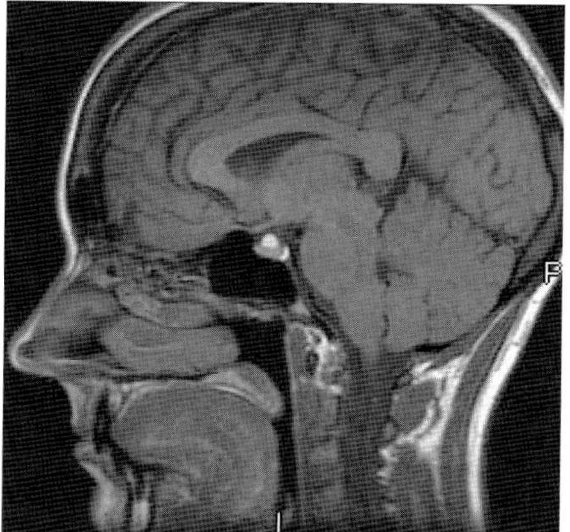

Fig. 29.10 Sagittal post-contrast, T1-weighted MRI, showing a small discrete microadenoma; this example is readily evident because of bleeding into the lesion, producing a bright signal. The more common non-hemorrhagic microadenomas are significantly more difficult to identify on neuroimaging.

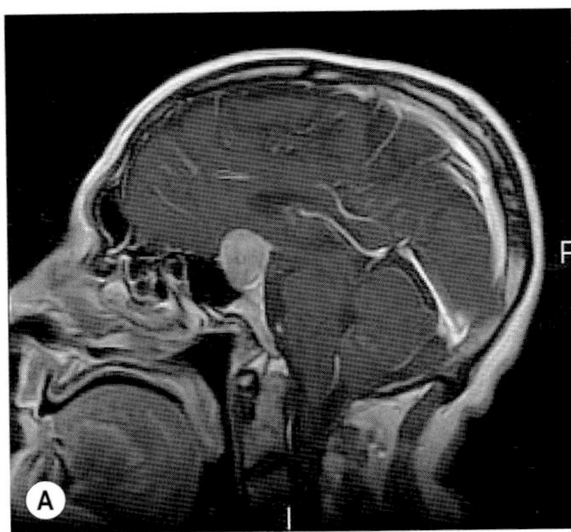

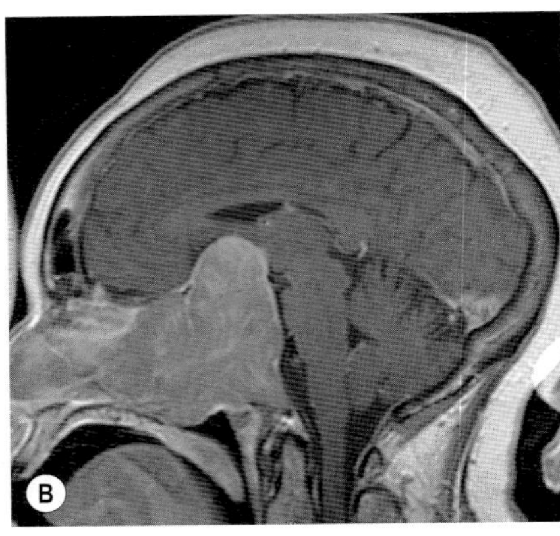

Fig. 29.11 A, Sagittal post-contrast, T1-weighted MRI, showing pituitary macroadenoma with suprasellar extension. **B,** Sagittal post-contrast, T1-weighted MRI, illustrating a giant pituitary macroadenoma with invasion of sphenoid sinus.

Table 29.2 Size of adenomas by immunophenotype

MICROADENOMAS	85% MACROADENOMAS	NEARLY 100% MACROADENOMAS
Prolactinomas in females	Densely granulated GH cell adenomas	FSH/LH adenomas
ACTH-secreting adenomas (80% microadenoma)	Sparsely granulated GH cell adenomas	TSH adenomas
	Plurihormonal adenomas	Acidophil stem cell adenomas
	Mixed GH/PRL tumors	Null cell adenomas
	Prolactinomas in males	Silent type 3 adenomas

Adapted from Saeger W, Ludecke DK, Buchfelder M, Fahlbusch R, Quabbe H-J, Petersenn S. Pathohistological classification of pituitary tumors: 10 years of experience with the German Pituitary Tumor Registry. Eur J Endocr 2007, **156:** 203–216.

adenomas extend laterally and compress the wall of the cavernous sinus. If the cavernous sinus is invaded, the macroadenoma can enwrap the carotid artery (but almost never causes vascular compromise) and distort cranial nerves III, IV, and VI, yielding cranial nerve palsies. Invasive adenomas may also extend into the sphenoid sinus and mimic primary nasopharyngeal neoplasms (Fig. 29.11B). These large invasive adenomas greater than 4 cm in diameter (Fig. 29.11B) are further designated giant adenomas.[41] Macroadenomas, and especially giant adenomas, often show cysts and hemosiderin pigment either by neuroimaging or in the tumor specimen.

Prolactinomas in premenopausal women and 80% of all ACTH-secreting adenomas are microadenomas; the remaining adenoma types are macroadenomas (Table 29.2). About 15% of GH cell adenomas, plurihormonal adenomas, and mixed GH/PRL tumors are microadenomas,[48] but virtually 100% of FSH/LH cell adenomas, TSH adenomas, null cell adenomas, and silent type 3 tumors are macroadenomas (Table 29.2). Taken together, 95–100% of hormonally inactive adenomas are macroadenomas.[48]

Grading of adenomas is performed solely on preoperative neuroimaging characteristics and not incorporated into the surgical pathologist's report. Neuroimaging grading clearly affects the neurosurgeon's ability to achieve gross surgical excision and cure. Microadenomas remain confined to the sellar space and are designated grade 0, or grade I if there is slight sellar enlargement. Macroadenomas are graded on a II–IV scale, with grade II for tumors with diffuse sellar enlargement but no bone erosion, grade III for focal bone erosion, and grade IV for extensive bone erosion including skull base and extrasellar structures.[41]

Invasiveness is defined as extension into sellar floor bone, the cavernous sinus, and/or the diaphragma sella,[48] as assessed on preoperative neuroimaging studies. The lowest rate of invasiveness is seen with ACTH adenomas (13%) due to the predominance of microadenomas.[48] Virtually 100% of acidophil stem cell, silent type 3, and TSH-cell adenomas are invasive. Thus, behavior parallels immunohistochemical subtype in adenomas and some workers feel that subtyping of pituitary adenomas by a complete immunohistochemical panel for pituitary hormones is essential in the surgical pathologist's workup.[42]

Nuclear pleomorphism is uncommon in pituitary adenomas in general and does not appear to correlate with prognosis (Fig. 29.12A). Mitoses are rare in adenomas and particularly so in microadenomas, where they were found in only 3.9% of noninvasive adenomas in one of the largest studies to date.[48] MIB-1 index in noninvasive tumors is usually <3%.[41] Mitoses can be seen in 21.4% of invasive adenomas (Fig. 29.12B) and 66.7% of carcinomas.[44] Thus, most invasive adenomas lack increased mitotic activity and carcinomas are sufficiently vanishingly rare (0.12% of all sellar masses[48]) that evaluation of mitotic index proves less helpful to the surgical pathologist than in other tumor types.

MIB-1 is generally higher in invasive adenomas[45,47–49] but does not correlate perfectly. For example, invasive adenomas were found to have a significantly higher Ki-67 index than noninvasive adenomas when those tumors with and without suprasellar extension were compared, but this difference did not hold up for tumors with cavernous sinus extension.[45] MIB-1 does correlate with hormonal subtypes of adenoma, with silent ACTH-cell and PRL-producing adenomas having the highest indices, and null cell adenomas and gonadotroph cell adenomas the lowest proliferation values, respectively.[49]

Thus, the use of MIB-1 and p53 immunohistochemistry for pituitary adenomas has been controversial. In the most recent version of the WHO fascicle on endocrine disease[41] it was mentioned that:

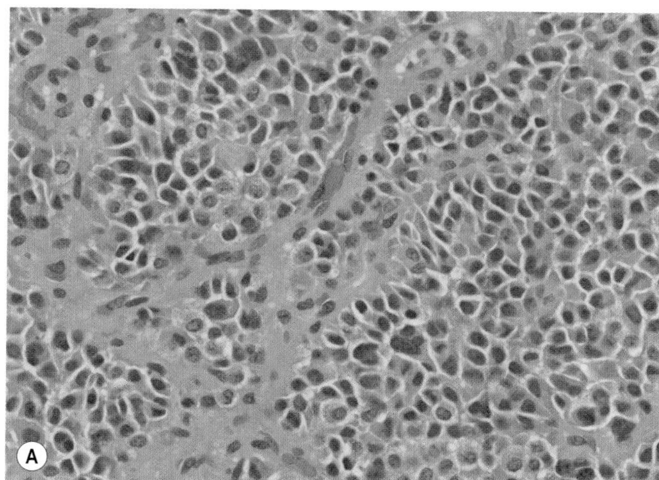

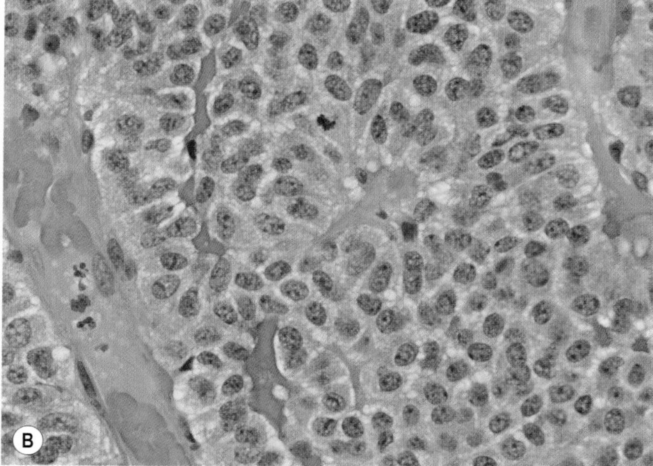

Fig. 29.12 **A,** Nuclear pleomorphism is uncommon in pituitary adenomas, but when found, has no prognostic significance. **B,** Mitoses are rare in microadenomas, but occasionally seen in macroadenomas. (H&E)

> *Some adenomas have atypical morphologic features suggestive of aggressive behavior such as invasive growth. Other features include an elevated mitotic index and a Ki-67 labeling index greater than 3%, as well as extensive nuclear staining for p53 immunoreactivity. These features are usually lacking in noninvasive adenomas and are present in nearly all pituitary carcinomas. Tumors with these features that have no documented metastases can be designated as 'atypical' adenomas.*

Despite this statement, routine use of MIB-1 and p53 immunohistochemistry is not utilized in many experienced laboratories for pituitary adenomas simply because it is unclear to the clinical team what specifically to do with the information that an adenoma is histologically 'atypical'. Specifically, few, if any, clinicians would chose to give external beam radiation therapy to a patient whose tumor was completely surgically resected, as assessed by postoperative neuroimaging, even if the MIB-1 index is elevated or p53 immunoreactivity is increased. Conversely, if the tumor is hormonally active, invasive, and not surgically curable, radiation is an option whatever the MIB-1 and p53 might show.

In a more recent 2008 publication, Asa has concurred that subtyping based on hormonal content is the most important feature for classification of pituitary adenomas.[40] She states:

> *Unfortunately, none of these [proliferation markers, antiapoptotic markers such as BCL2, DNA topoisomerase II index, galectin-3 expression] is a true marker of biologic behavior. The best predictive marker remains the tumor classification based on hormone content and cell structure. For example, among acromegalics who fail surgical resection, response to long-acting somatostatin analogues is best predicted by the subtype of somatotroph adenoma as densely or sparsely granulated. This finding renders the value of a CAM 5.2 keratin stain more important than almost any other immunostain in this setting. A silent corticotroph adenoma will recur more often and more aggressively than a silent gonadotroph adenoma. A silent subtype 3 adenoma will almost certainly behave invasively, infiltrating the base of the skull, whereas a silent adenoma of the gonadotroph lineage will usually grow by expansion upward.*

Similar to the data for invasiveness, there is a statistically significant, but numerically minimal, difference in MIB-1 labeling indices between primary (1.2%) versus recurrent adenomas (1.9%).[46] Increased chromosomal imbalances have been demonstrated in recurrent adenomas but they are not uniform; these included gains of 4q (in three of eight recurrences), 5q, and 13q (in two of eight recurrences each) as well as losses of chromosome 2 (in both primary and recurring tumors of two patients), 1p, 8q, 10, and 12q (in two of eight recurrences).[46] Recurrence in nonfunctioning adenomas has been linked to Ki-67 and TUNEL labeling indices as well as high levels of expression of phospho-Akt and phospho-p44/42MAPK.[43]

Immunohistochemical and electron microscopic features

While morphologic criteria by standard H&E usually suffice for distinguishing adenomas from other sellar region masses, such as Rathke cleft cyst, craniopharyngioma, meningioma, germinoma, metastases, and inflammatory conditions, at times the greatest challenge is distinguishing compressed and distorted normal anterior gland from adenoma. For this task, the single most informative stain is the reticulin stain, which is routinely performed on all cases. The distorted and disrupted acinar pattern of adenoma contrasts with the intact acinar pattern of the normal gland (Fig. 29.13A). Severely compressed anterior pituitary gland may form a thin rim-like crescent along the edge of some pituitary adenoma tissue fragments and the preserved acinar pattern difficult to identify for certain (Fig. 29.13B). In these instances, close attention to the immunostaining pattern will often show that the strip of compressed normal gland retains hormone staining for several different hormone types, often including prolactin (Fig. 29.13C). Another caveat for using reticulin staining to distinguish normal gland from adenoma is that some adenomas retain a large, nested pattern by reticulin and thus, while clearly abnormal, do not have a fully disintegrated reticulin framework (Fig. 29.13D).

Intraoperative touch preparations show abundant exfoliation of a monotonous population of cells and complement, or obviate the need for, actual frozen section in many cases (Fig. 29.13E).

All adenomas are immunoreactive for synaptophysin, even when they are clinically nonfunctional null cell adenomas and fail

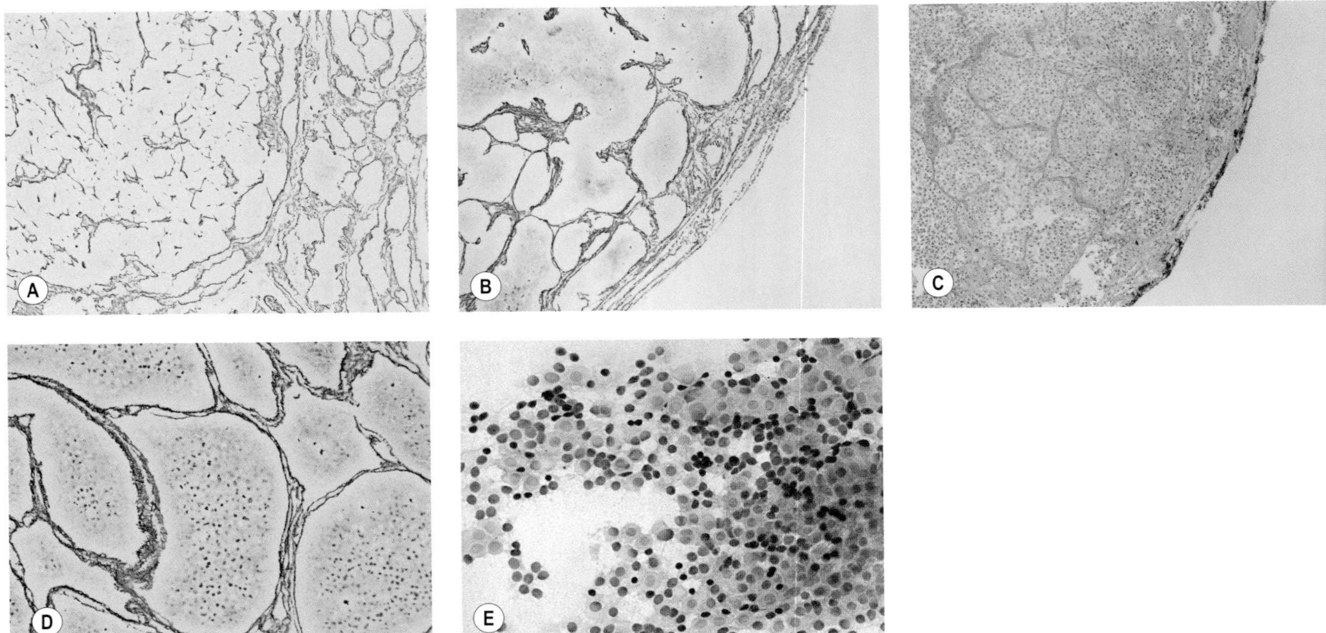

Fig. 29.13 **A,** Reticulin is the single most informative histochemical stain for adenomas and contrasts the disrupted reticulin pattern of adenoma (left), with the preserved, nested pattern in normal compressed gland (right). **B,** Severely compressed residual anterior pituitary gland at the perimeter of an adenoma is more difficult to discern by reticulin. **C,** Immunohistochemistry for prolactin from the same area of the adenoma and compressed gland as in Figure 29.13B better illustrates the residual normal anterior pituitary cells. **D,** Reticulin stain from a gonadotroph cell macroadenoma shows a nested pattern; this should not be mistaken for normal anterior gland or even hyperplasia. **E,** Intraoperative touch preparation of gonadotroph cell adenoma shows abundant exfoliation of cytologically monotonous cells. This occurs in direct parallel with acinar disruption in an adenoma, is diagnostic for pituitary adenoma and obviates the need for actual frozen section. (H&E)

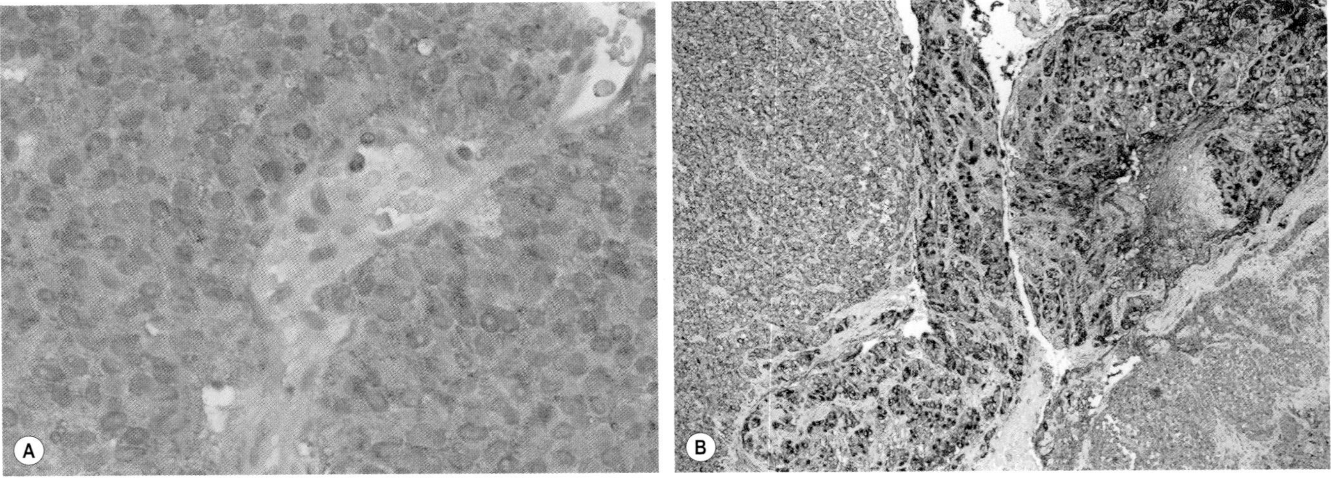

Fig. 29.14 **A,** All adenomas, including those with weak immunostaining for pituitary hormones, show synaptophysin immunoreactivity. **B,** CAM 5.2 at the edge of an adenoma shows the differential, and, in this case, stronger immunoreactivity for normal gland, compared to gonadotroph cell adenoma (left and extreme lower right) and can also aid in disclosing normal compressed gland within a specimen. (Immunoperoxidase with hematoxylin counterstain)

to show immunoreactivity for any pituitary hormone product (Fig. 29.14A). The use of synaptophysin immunohistochemistry has obviated the need for EM to document infrequent neurosecretory granules to verify adenoma diagnosis. Most adenomas will also be immunoreactive for chromogranin A and cytokeratins.[50,53] The routine use of CAM 5.2 has the added advantage that it highlights the differences between small fragments of normal compressed gland and the adenoma due to differential staining (Fig. 29.14B). Furthermore, CAM 5.2 is an essential part of the armamentarium because it identifies the signature feature of sparsely granulated growth hormone adenomas, the fibrous body (see section on sparsely granulated growth hormone adenoma), also completely replacing the need for electron microscopy[50] (see section on GH-secreting adenomas). CAM 5.2 allows separation of densely

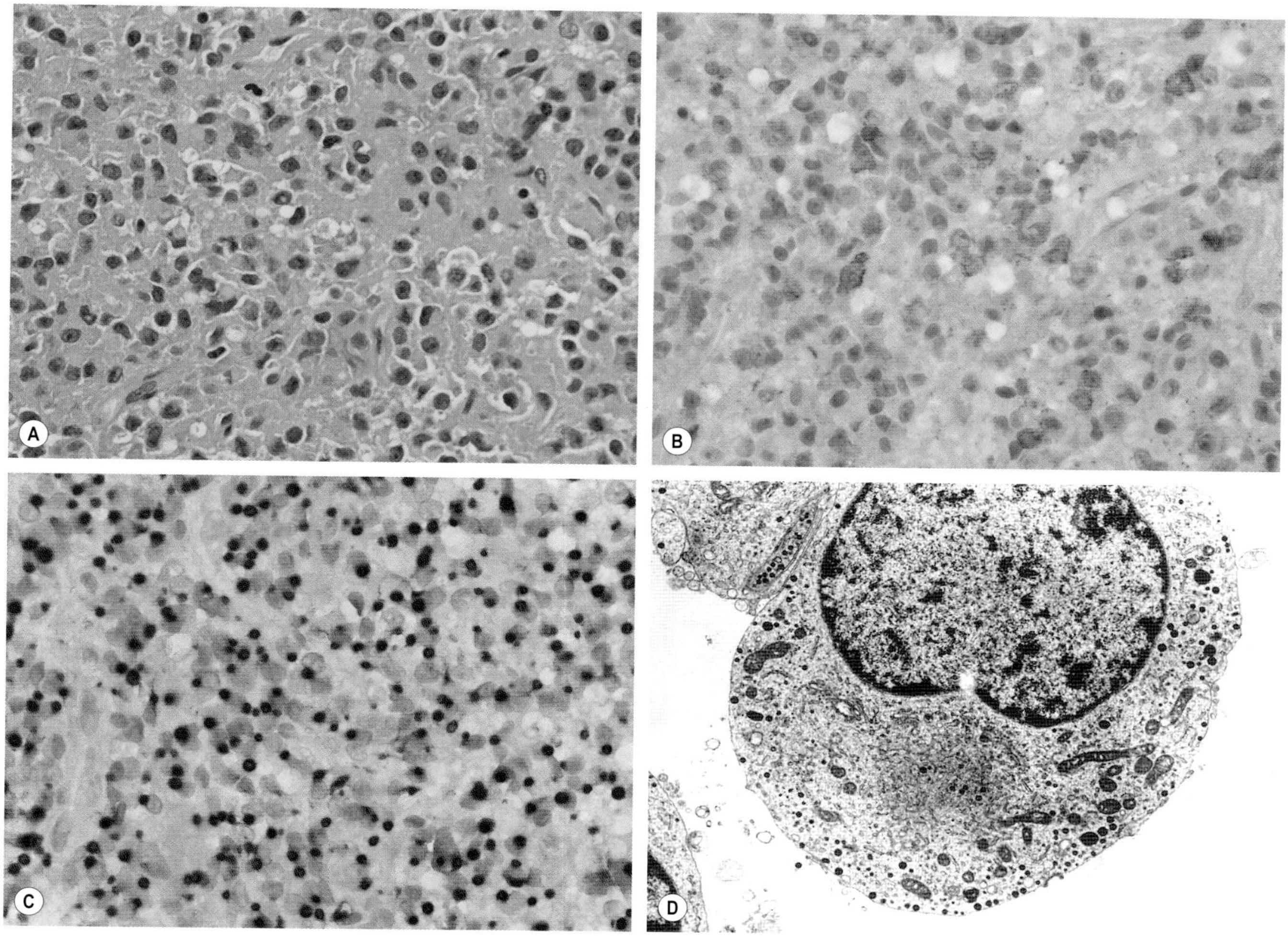

Fig. 29.22 **A,** Sparsely granulated growth hormone adenoma contains cells that lack the acidophilia of densely granulated tumors and may show more eccentrically placed nuclei and perinuclear clearing in the cytoplasm. (H&E) **B,** Sparsely granulated growth hormone adenoma manifests have weaker growth hormone immunoreactivity. (Immunoperoxidase with hematoxylin counterstain) **C,** Sparsely granulated growth hormone adenoma showing the signature feature of this adenoma type, widespread, ball-like, cytoplasmic 'fibrous bodies' on CAM 5.2. (Immunoperoxidase with hematoxylin counterstain) **D,** Sparsely granulated growth hormone adenoma on CAM 5.2 parallels the accumulation of cytoplasmic filaments seen by EM, and obviates the need for the latter in diagnosis.

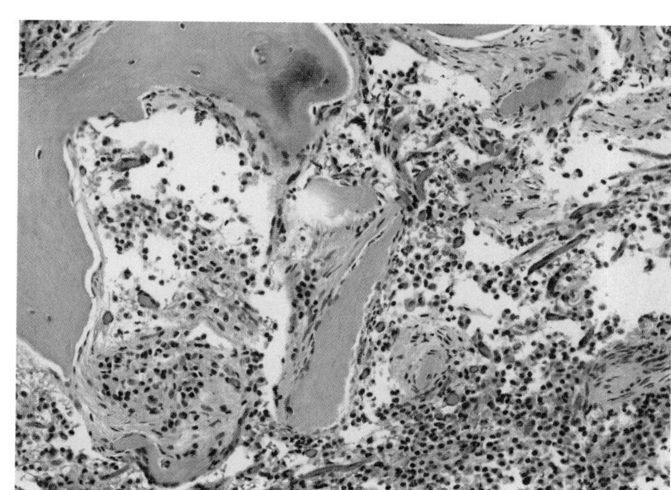

Fig. 29.23 Sparsely granulated growth hormone adenomas often invade bone, a feature easily detected by the finding of entrapped bony spicules surrounded by tumor. (H&E)

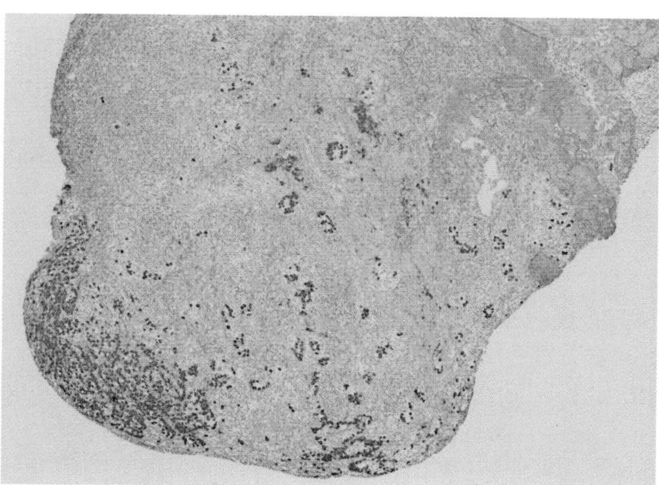

Fig. 29.24 Sparsely granulated growth hormone adenomas, as with all macroadenomas, may entrap individual anterior pituitary cells from the adjacent nonadenomatous gland; often these are PRL- or ACTH-immunoreactive cells. ACTH-immunoreactive cells are illustrated. (Immunoperoxidase for ACTH, with hematoxylin counterstain)

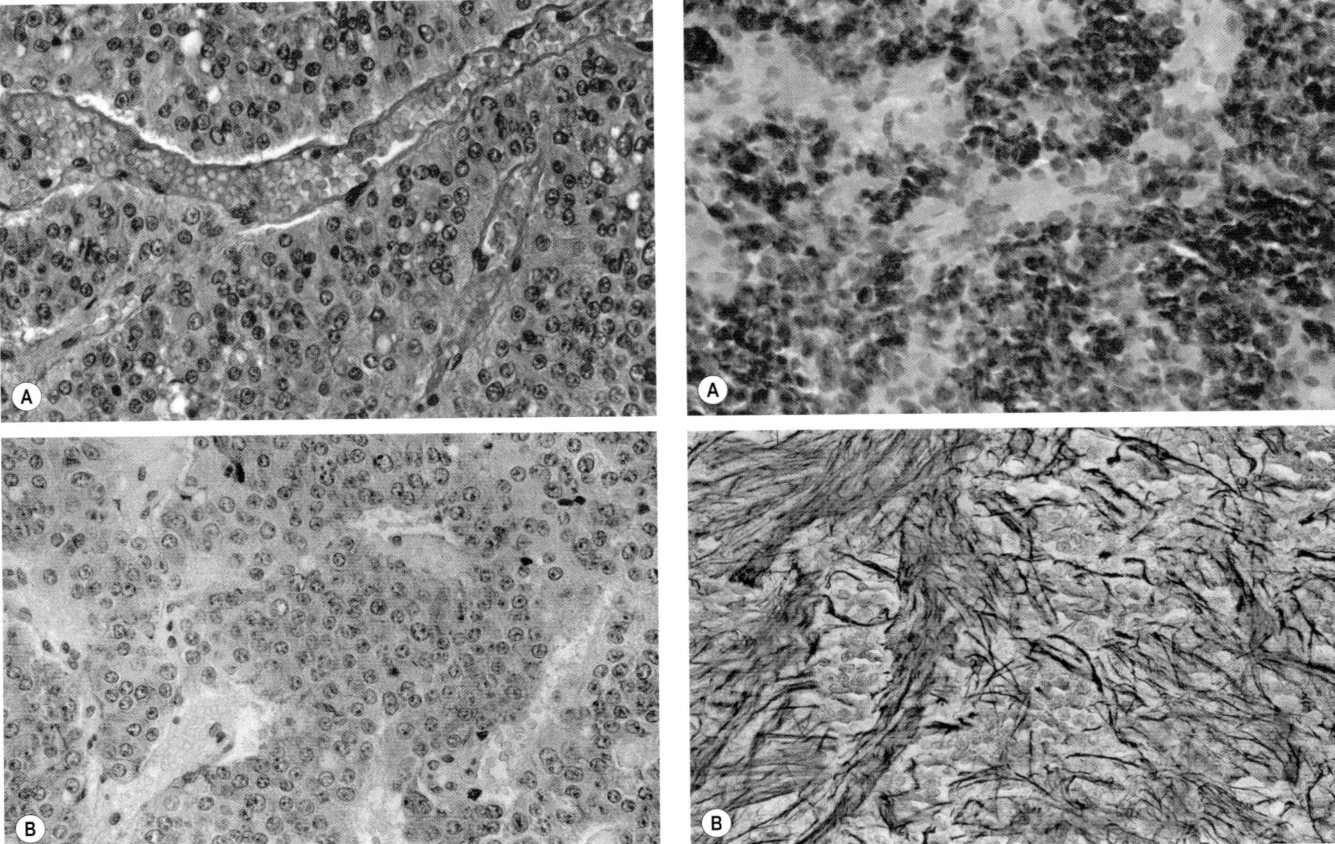

Fig. 29.25 **A,** Prolactinoma showing diffuse growth pattern, a monotonous cell population with increased nuclear chromatin content and conspicuous vasculature. (H&E) **B,** Prolactinomas usually manifest diffuse immunoreactivity for PRL only. (Immunoperoxidase for PRL, with hematoxylin counterstain)

Fig. 29.26 **A,** Prolactinoma from a patient with recent and long-term dopamine agonist treatment will demonstrate severe cytoplasmic shrinkage with near-naked nuclei that should not be mistaken for lymphocytes. (H&E) **B,** Prolactinoma from a patient with recent and long-term dopamine agonist treatment often shows fibrosis. (Reticulin)

immunostaining for PRL is demonstrable in peri-Golgi regions (Fig. 29.25B). Additional features may include psammoma body calcifications (which if they occur in adenomas are virtually confined to PRL-secreting adenomas) or amyloid derived from PRL.

Should the patient come to surgical resection proximate to taking dopamine agonists for a long time period, the peri-treatment surgical adenoma specimen will demonstrate severe cytoplasmic shrinkage with near-naked nuclei that should not be mistaken for lymphocytes (Fig. 29.26A) and a strong decrease in PRL immunoreactivity. Fibrosis will be evident in cases of long-term treatment (Fig. 29.26B). These changes may not be evident following short-term treatment.[70]

Pituitary adenomas with immunoreactivity for both GH and PRL (mixed GH and PRL immunoreactive adenoma, mammosomatotroph cell adenoma, and acidophil stem cell adenoma)

This group of mixed GH–PRL adenomas totals 6.5% of all adenomas in the German registry.[78] Mixed GH–PRL adenomas are bicellular–bihormonal adenomas that are more frequent (5.2%) than mammosomatotroph cell adenomas (1.1%).[78] The combination in bicellular adenomas is sparsely granulated PRL-secreting cells with either densely or sparsely granulated GH-secreting tumor cells. Both GH and PRL immunoreactivity is seen, and clinically both GH and PRL excess can occur.

Monocellular mammosomatotroph cell adenomas show secretion of both GH and PRL hormone products by the same cell and usually present clinically with GH excess. While confident discrimination between true bicellular mixed tumors and monocellular mammosomatotroph cell adenomas requires EM, the distinction is usually clinically unimportant.

Acidophil stem cell adenoma is rare (0.2%[78] to 4.3%[75]). The tumor is monomorphous, chromophobic, contains fibrous bodies by CAM 5.2, and may show large cytoplasmic vacuoles. This is one tumor type that does require EM for confident classification; mitochondrial accumulation with giant mitochondria is the pathognomonic feature,[77] and oncocytic change may also be seen.[75] Immunostaining shows some reactivity for PRL, with faint to absent immunoreactivity for GH. This correlates well with clinical features in that this adenoma usually is associated with hyperprolactinemia, but the blood PRL levels 'are disproportionally low for the size of the lesion'.[76] Overt acromegaly and elevated GH levels are infrequent.[75] Acidophil stem cell adenomas manifest a relatively short clinical history, are macroadenomas, and locally invasive.[75]

Eye and ocular adnexa

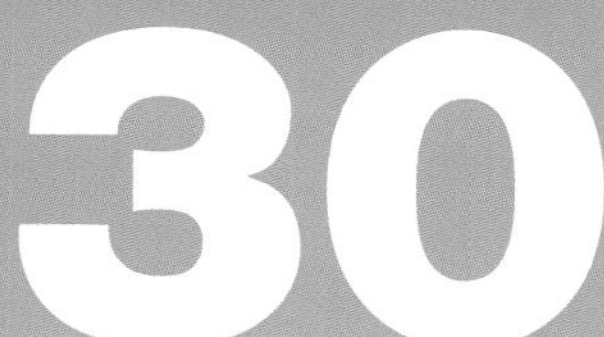

CHAPTER CONTENTS

Introduction

This chapter will cover primarily those entities that come to the attention of the surgical pathologist; therefore most non-neoplastic entities of the intraocular tissues will be excluded. For a more detailed description of these and other diseases, the reader is referred to one of the many specialized textbooks available.[1–6,8–13] As with all surgical specimens, a complete description of the lesion and a meaningful clinical history are invaluable. Clinical photographs are especially helpful in ophthalmic pathology.

Normal anatomy

The *eyelids* are divided into a cutaneous and a conjunctival portion. The former is composed of stratified squamous epithelium and the latter of a much thinner conjunctival epithelium. Skin appendages of eyelids include the sebaceous glands (glands of Zeis and meibomian glands), apocrine glands (glands of Moll), and eccrine sweat glands.[7]

The *lacrimal caruncle* is a small, reddish, fleshy protuberance that fills the triangular space between the medial margins of the upper and lower eyelids. It contains sebaceous and sweat glands.

The *lacrimal gland* is largely of serous type, with a minor mucinous component in the ductal portion and a layer of myoepithelial cells in the larger peripheral ducts.

The *lacrimal passages* allow tears produced by the lacrimal gland to be transported from the eye into the *nasal cavity*. They are represented by the *lacrimal sac* and the *nasolacrimal duct* (also known as *tear duct*), which opens in the nasal cavity. Both the lacrimal sac and the nasolacrimal duct are lined by *stratified columnar epithelium* containing mucus-secreting goblet cells. The bony passage encasing the nasolacrimal duct is called the *nasolacrimal canal*.

The *orbit* contains, in addition to the ocular globe and the lacrimal gland, the following structures: the optic nerve and its meningeal covering, Tenon's capsule, the extraocular muscles, blood vessels, and a delicate framework of fibroadipose connective tissue.

The *conjunctiva* is a thin mucous membrane that lines the inner surface of the eyelids and most of the anterior surface of the ocular globe. The conjunctival epithelium is composed of two to five layers of columnar cells that rest on a continuous basal lamina. This epithelium contains mucin-secreting goblet cells and melanocytes.

The *cornea* consists of six distinct layers: epithelium, epithelial basal lamina, Bowman's layer (an acellular structure made up of collagen fibers), stroma, Descemet membrane (a true basal lamina produced by the underlying corneal endothelial cells), and a single layer of very flat cells traditionally known as 'endothelium'.[7]

The *sclera* is mainly composed of a dense collagenous stroma admixed with occasional elastic fibers and scattered fibroblasts.

The *intraocular tissues* comprise the uveal tract (iris, ciliary body, and choroid), the retina, the crystalline lens, and the various intraocular compartments. A detailed description of these structures is beyond the scope of this book.

Eyelids

Most of the pathologic processes that involve the eyelids are those that affect the skin in general and are considered in detail in Chapter 4. Some consideration, however, is given in this chapter to those lesions that are either peculiar to the lids or present particular problems in this location.

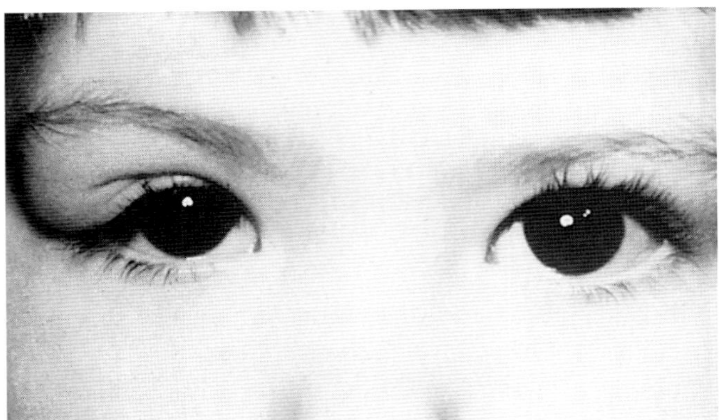

Fig. 30.1 Dermoid cyst of right upper eyelid.

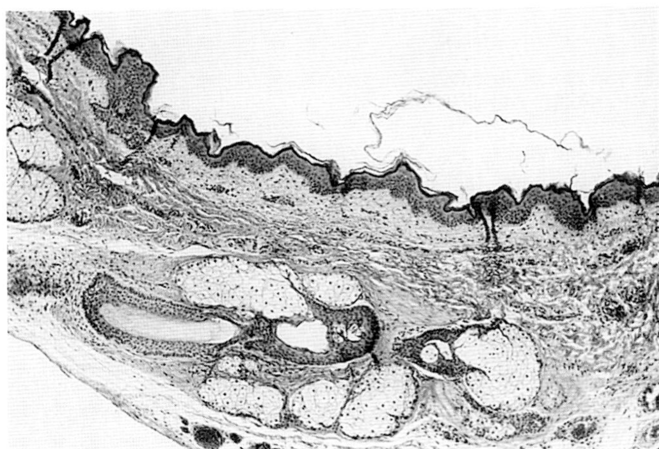

Fig. 30.2 Dermoid cyst of eyelid and brow. The cyst lumen is located in the upper right corner.

Developmental anomalies

Dermoid cysts typically involve the upper eyelid along the brow margin and may represent forward extension of a mass that is primarily intraorbital (Fig. 30.1). These lesions rest on and are often firmly attached to the periosteum of the bony orbital rim. They are soft, nontender, oval or round, and usually about 1 cm in diameter.

Microscopically, the cysts are lined by well-differentiated epidermal and dermal tissues containing all of the usual skin appendages (Fig. 30.2). The lumen is filled with keratinous debris, sebum, and hairs. In places where these contents have been extruded into the surrounding tissues, a severe foreign body inflammatory reaction may be observed.

Inflammation

Inflammation of the eyelids may be the result of viral, bacterial, rickettsial, mycotic, or parasitic infections; chemical or physical irritants; hypersensitivity states; or systemic dermatologic disorders. These inflammatory processes are rarely biopsied and are of relatively little practical significance to pathologists.

Pseudorheumatoid nodule (deep granuloma annulare) can involve the eyelid and eyebrow, and rarely the episcleral and orbital tissues.[16]

Necrobiotic xanthogranuloma with paraproteinemia is characterized by multiple nodules or plaques that involve the periorbital areas (including eyelids) along with other parts of the body. A dysproteinemia caused by an IgG paraprotein is consistently present. Microscopically, the granulomas are characterized by collagen 'necrobiosis' together with foamy macrophages and Touton giant cells.[14]

Silica granulomas are of noncaseating type and composed of epithelioid cells and multinucleated giant cells and birefringent crystals. They are surrounded by areas of fibrosis.[15]

Chalazion

Chalazion is an extremely common lesion. It represents a lipogranuloma that develops in and about a meibomian gland, presumably as a consequence of the combined effects of obstruction and nonspecific infection of the excretory passages of the gland. The sebaceous material discharged into the tarsus provokes an intense granulomatous inflammatory reaction (Fig. 30.3).

Although chalazion begins as a deep-seated process, not infrequently it erupts through the conjunctival surface of the eyelid. Ordinarily, this lesion is readily recognized and treated; however, if one or more recurrences develop after curettage, the clinician should be alerted to the possibility of a meibomian gland tumor that has escaped recognition. In such cases, excision and histopathologic study are indicated.

Microscopically, the typical chalazion reveals multiple foci of granulomatous inflammation (Fig. 30.4). In the center of many of the focal granulomas there is a small globule of fat, which in paraffin sections presents as an empty round to ovoid space (Fig. 30.5).

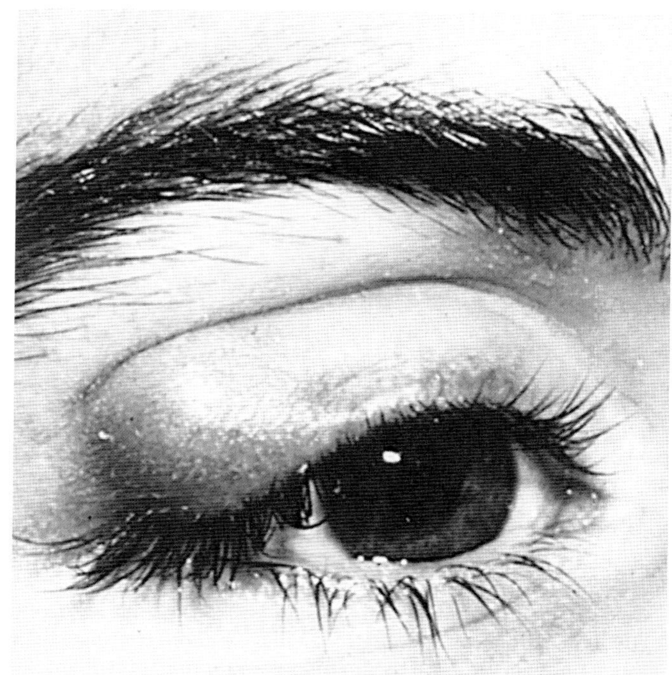

Fig. 30.3 Chalazion of right upper eyelid.

Cysts

Benign cysts of the skin of the eyelids and along the lid margins are relatively common, comprising approximately one-third of lesions removed from the lids. The most common of these are the *keratinous cysts* discussed in Chapter 4. Another relatively frequent lesion is the *cyst of Moll glands*, often referred to as sudoriferous cyst or simply ductal cyst. These present as thin-walled transparent vesicles at the lid margin. Microscopically, they are simple cysts lined by atrophic cuboidal or flattened epithelial cells with an empty lumen (Fig. 30.6). Yet another type is the *Meibomian gland cyst*, which is characteristically fixed to the tarsus (intratarsal). Microscopically, these cysts are lined by an undulating squamous epithelium possessing an inner eosinophilic cuticle that produces a peculiar refractile, strand-like intracavitary keratin. Immunohistochemically, in contrast with cutaneous keratinous cysts, there is positivity for keratin 17 and carcinoembryonic antigen (CEA).[17]

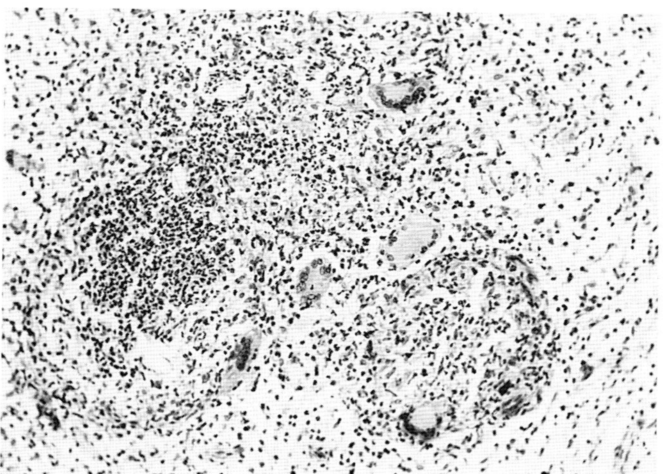

Fig. 30.4 Multiple foci of granulomatous inflammation with microabscesses and multinucleated giant cells in chalazion.

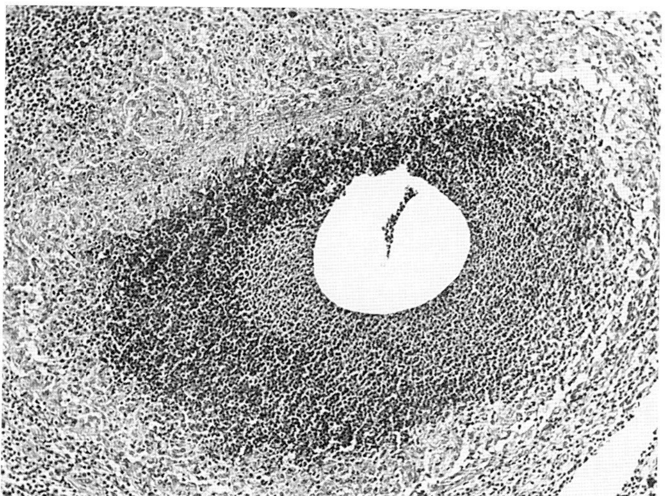

Fig. 30.5 The presence of pools of fat in the center of many of the granulomas is characteristic of chalazion.

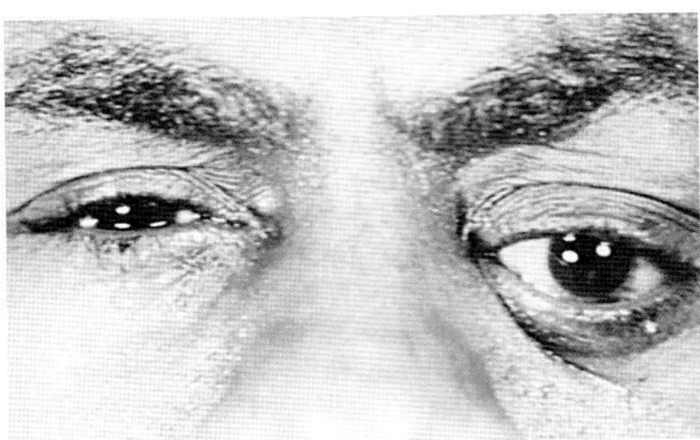

Fig. 30.16 Benign mixed tumor of left lacrimal gland in a 38-year-old man. Proptosis was accompanied by severe visual loss.

Tumors and tumorlike conditions

Most neoplasms of the lacrimal gland arise in the orbital lobe where the gland is firmly attached to the orbital rim about the lacrimal fossa. The bone tends to restrict growth in its direction. Hence the enlarging tumor characteristically displaces the eye downward and nasally (Fig. 30.16).

Epithelial tumors have, on the whole, histopathologic, ultrastructural, and immunohistochemical features very similar to those of the salivary glands[64,72,75,81] (see Chapter 12). *Benign mixed tumors* (pleomorphic adenomas) account for approximately 50–60%, *malignant mixed tumors* (carcinomas ex-pleomorphic adenomas) for 5–10%, *adenoid cystic carcinomas* for 20–30%, and *other carcinomas* for 5–10%.[67,73,77] Many of the mixed tumors have a predominant component of hyaline cells of presumed myoepithelial nature (Fig. 30.17). *Oncocytomas, epithelial–myoepithelial carcinomas,* and *myoepithelial carcinomas* (malignant myoepitheliomas) have also been reported.[71,74,76,82] Gamel and Font[70] found that adenoid cystic carcinomas with a basaloid pattern of growth had a decidedly worse prognosis than the nonbasaloid type. Because so many of these lacrimal gland tumors are not completely and adequately removed at the initial operation, there has been an excessively high recurrence rate.[79] It is even more difficult to treat the recurrences, for they are often multiple. The carcinomas have a very poor prognosis,[69,84] the outstanding exception being the carcinoma ex-pleomorphic adenoma which is noninvasive, i.e., restricted to the adenoma.[64]

The appearance of an invasive squamous cell carcinoma of the lacrimal gland can be simulated by *necrotizing sialometaplasia*, in a manner akin to that seen with greater frequency in minor (and sometimes major) salivary glands.[68]

Lymphoid tumors and tumor-like conditions (malignant lymphomas, lymphoid hyperplasias, and chronic inflammatory processes) are important causes of enlargement of the gland. In a patient who is in good general health and who presents no evidence of a systemic disease, the discovery of a lymphoid mass in the lacrimal fossa rarely heralds the development of malignant lymphoma or leukemia. In fact, in the majority of cases there is a polymorphism suggestive of a reactive inflammatory process, although in other cases the rather pure proliferation of lymphocytes makes it impossible to rule out a lymphoma or leukemia. The lacrimal glands may, of course, become involved along with other tissues in a leukemia or malignant lymphoma.

It has been recently suggested that *chronic sclerosing dacryoadenitis* may be part of the spectrum of IgG4-related sclerosing diseases.[65]

Mesenchymal tumors of the lacrimal gland are exceptional. They comprise a few case reports of solitary fibrous tumor,[66] giant cell angiofibroma (a morphologic variant of solitary fibrous tumor),[83]

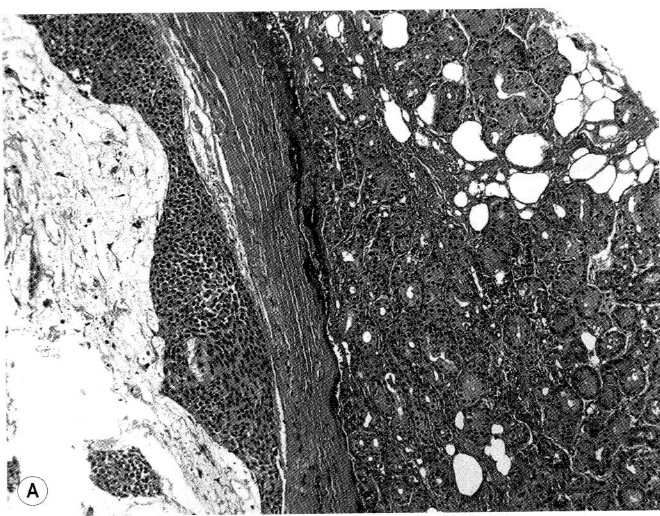

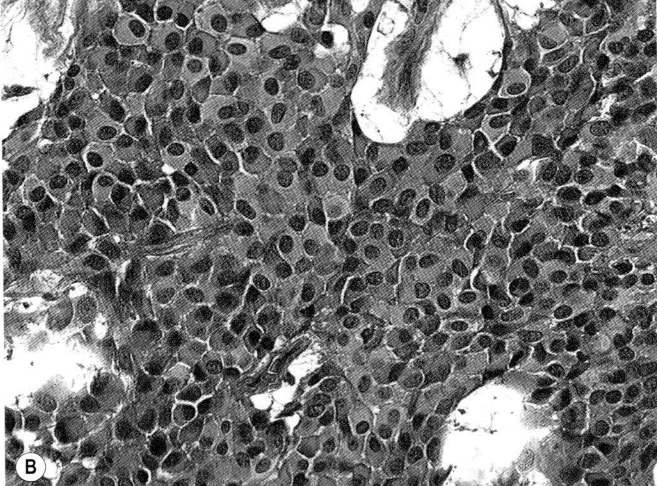

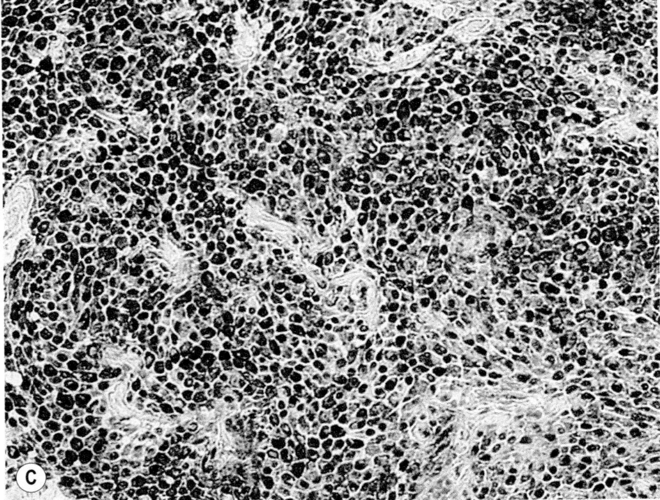

Fig. 30.17 Benign mixed tumor of lacrimal gland largely composed of so-called 'hyaline cells': **A**, low-power view showing encapsulated quality; **B**, high-power view showing a diffuse eosinophilic appearance of the cytoplasm; **C**, strong immunoreactivity for S-100 protein.

collagenous fibroma (desmoplastic fibroblastoma),[63] and granular cell tumor.[78,80]

Lacrimal passages

Diseases of the lacrimal passages that are of importance to the surgical pathologist are characterized by epiphora (the imperfect drainage of tears so that they flow over the lid margin onto the cheek) and by varying degrees of swelling, induration, and inflammation of the lower eyelid at its nasal end. Although inflammatory obstructions of these passages are common, neoplastic lesions are rare.

Canaliculitis and dacryocystitis

Canaliculitis and *dacryocystitis* may be the result of direct spread of inflammatory processes in neighboring structures such as the conjunctiva or nasal cavity, but more often their pathogenesis is obscure. Acute and chronic types are recognized, and the inflammatory reaction may be suppurative, granulomatous, or necrotizing, with the formation of fistulous tracts to the skin surface below the eyelid near the base of the nose.

The lacrimal passages become filled with purulent exudate in the acute suppurative types, whereas in the chronic forms the passages are narrowed by inflammatory thickening of the walls of the lacrimal canal or sac. Frequently there is also hyperplasia of the lining epithelium and hypersecretion of mucus. At times, the degree of papillomatous or adenomatous hyperplasia of the sac may give rise to difficulties in differential diagnosis.

Sarcoidosis may involve the lacrimal sac as an extension of upper respiratory tract disease.[85]

Mucocele

Lacrimal mucocele is another complication of chronic inflammation of the lacrimal sac. A low-grade obstructive lesion with a relatively intact and possibly hypersecreting mucosa may lead to great distention of the sac by accumulated secretions.

The contents of the cyst may be clear or milky, fluid or gelatinous, fibrinous or flocculent, sterile or infected. Microscopically, the cyst wall reveals varying degrees of atrophy, degeneration, hyperplasia, hypersecretion of the mucosa, and chronic inflammation of the subepithelial tissues.

Dacryolithiasis

Dacryolithiasis and concretions in the nasolacrimal duct ('tear stones') are of uncertain pathogenesis, but they are generally believed to be the result of low-grade inflammatory processes, including mycoses. If such concretions are crushed and examined microscopically, they will be seen to contain myriads of mycelial elements embedded in a relatively acellular matrix. Others are laminated, mineralized stones with recognizable fungal or bacterial forms.

Tumors

Neoplasms of the lacrimal passages are rare. **Papillomas** similar to those arising in the conjunctival surface of the eyelid (see p. 2469) may form in the punctum, within the nasolacrimal duct, or in the lacrimal sac. Some are of the *inverted* variety.[92] However, inflammatory hyperplasia (occasionally having pseudoepitheliomatous features) is seen more often.

On clinical grounds, it is usually not possible to distinguish malignant tumors of the lacrimal passages from benign neoplasms and pseudotumors of this structure. Dacryocystography has become an important part of the clinical evaluation of lacrimal sac tumors.

Oncocytomas (oxyphil cell adenomas) may develop in the lacrimal sac or in the caruncle. Most of the cases have been seen in elderly women, and local excision has been curative.[87]

All malignant tumors of the lacrimal passages except carcinoma are exceedingly rare, and even carcinoma is distinctly uncommon. These tumors are usually moderately well-differentiated **squamous cell carcinomas**, similar in appearance to those arising from the mucosa of the nasal cavity or in the conjunctiva. They tend to form papillary projections into the lumen and spread along natural surfaces, but they can also infiltrate directly into adjacent tissues.[93]

Other reported malignant tumors of the lacrimal sac include **mucoepidermoid carcinoma**,[91] **lymphoepithelioma-like carcinoma**,[89] **malignant melanoma**,[86,88] and **malignant lymphoma**.[90] Interestingly, and in contrast to most other ocular-related sites, the rare lymphomas of the lacrimal sac tend to be of the diffuse large B-cell type.[94]

Orbit

The clinical hallmark of disease of the orbit is *exophthalmos*. This may not necessarily be caused by a true neoplasm, and therefore the surgical pathologist may never see any specimen from the many patients who present with this finding. Thus, the most common cause of exophthalmos is *dysthyroid ophthalmopathy*, and rarely is a biopsy taken in such a circumstance.

As for the relative frequency of lesions that cause exophthalmos, many of the statistics that have been reported merely reflect the bias of the specialist involved. To the radiologist, for example, one of the most common orbital lesions producing displacement of the eye is a mucocele arising from a paranasal sinus. The ophthalmologist, however, would place mucocele far below such entities as dysthyroid ophthalmopathy, hemangioma, and inflammatory pseudotumor.[96] Procedures useful for the diagnostic evaluation of orbital masses include CT scan, MRI, and fine needle aspiration.[95,97]

Dysthyroid ophthalmopathy

The most common cause of orbital disease and of exophthalmos is dysthyroid ophthalmopathy, in which there is a dysfunction of the pituitary–thyroid axis.[98] When seen because of ocular problems, the patient may be hyperthyroid, hypothyroid, or euthyroid. There is often a history of hyperthyroidism or some form of treatment.

Unilateral orbital involvement occurs with sufficient frequency in both forms of dysthyroid ophthalmopathy to warrant this condition always being considered in the differential diagnosis of orbital tumors (Fig. 30.18).

Histopathologic changes observed in severe cases, which are most likely to come to the attention of the surgical pathologist, include widespread edema and chronic inflammation of all the orbital tissues. The most striking gross alterations are observed in the extraocular muscles, which may be massively enlarged. Muscle fibers degenerate and become hyalinized. A great increase in the interstitial connective tissue, including both cellular elements and ground substance, is observed particularly in the muscles but also in the other orbital tissues.

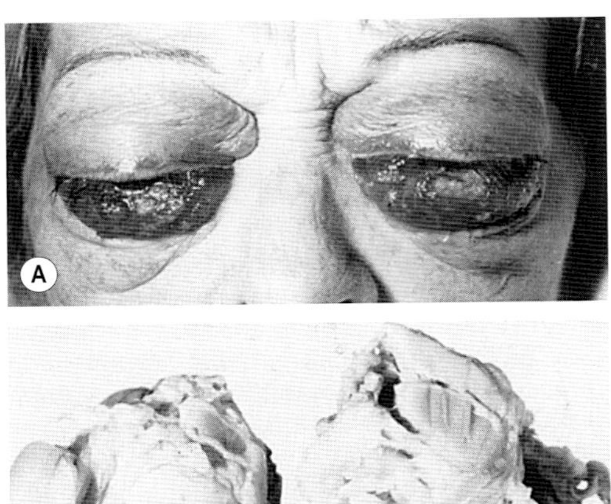

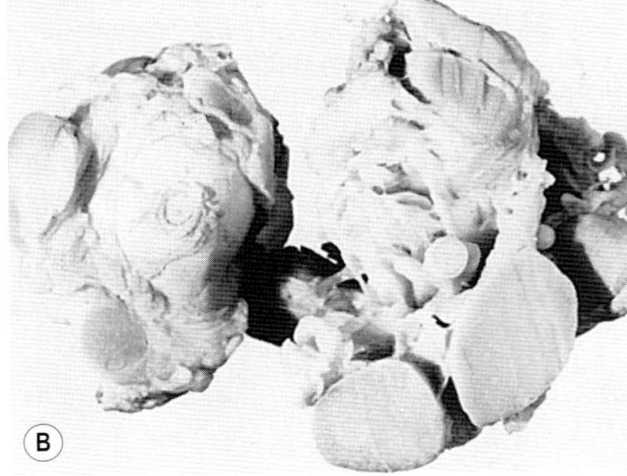

Fig. 30.18 **A**, Exophthalmos of approximately 10 months' duration in a 65-year-old woman who finally died of congestive heart failure. **B**, At autopsy, extraocular muscles were found to be massively thickened.

Inflammatory processes

Secondary inflammation of the orbit can occur from lesions arising in the face, eyes, nose, sinuses, orbital bones, blood vessels, brain, and meninges.[106] Generally, it is only when such inflammations simulate neoplasms that orbital exploration is undertaken and tissue is obtained for histopathologic diagnosis.

Specific granulomas, including those due to tuberculosis, mycosis, sarcoidosis, and Wegener granulomatosis are rare (Fig. 30.19).

Mucocele is the result of chronic inflammatory disease of the frontal and/or ethmoid sinuses. The lesion erodes through the wall of the sinus to produce an inferolateral displacement of the globe. The onset is usually insidious, and the enlargement is symptomless and slow (Fig. 30.20).

Histopathologically, this cystic mass is lined by mucus-secreting sinus mucosa with variable degrees of inflammation and scarring.

Inflammatory pseudotumors of the orbit are much more frequent than the specific infectious granulomas. These pseudotumors represent an etiologically and pathogenetically heterogeneous group.[99,107] In some instances, they have been found associated with involvement of paranasal sinuses.[101] In others, they have been the orbital manifestation of Rosai–Dorfman disease[102] (sinus histiocytosis with massive lymphadenopathy) (Fig. 30.21). Still others represent the orbital manifestation of inflammatory fibrosclerosis (idiopathic sclerosing inflammation), a process that may also involve the retroperitoneum, mediastinum, extrahepatic bile ducts, and thyroid[108] and which has recently been linked to IgG4-related sclerosing diseases.[100,109,112] The pathologic features they share include the following:

1 The formation of an indurated orbital mass often surrounding the optic nerve and incorporating one or more of the extraocular muscles.
2 A tissue reaction that includes exudation of fluid, excessive production of ground substance, mobilization of chronic inflammatory cells, vascular proliferation, and hyperplasia of connective tissue.
3 The absence of demonstrable etiologic agents or of otherwise diagnostic histopathologic alterations indicative of specific disease entities such as Hodgkin lymphoma, temporal arteritis, or lupus erythematosus.[105]

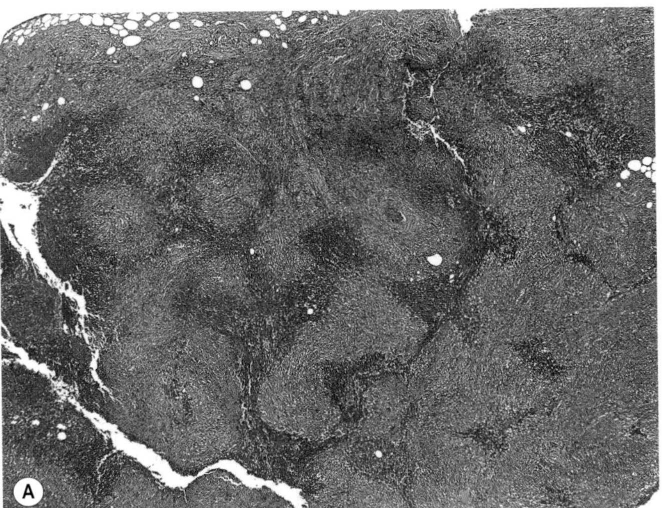

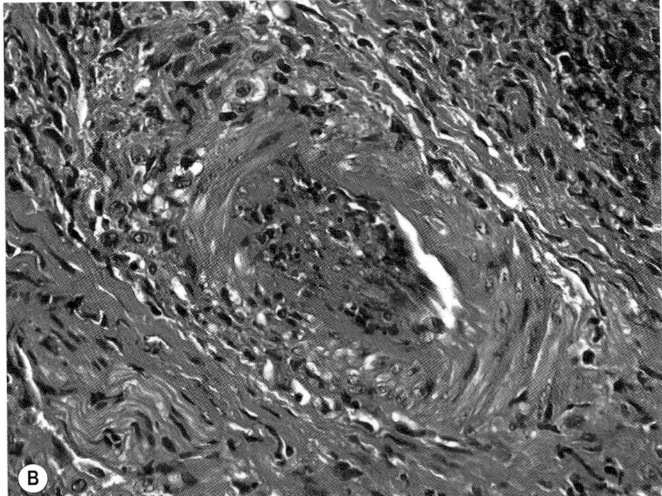

Fig. 30.19 Wegener granulomatosis involving orbit: **A**, multiple confluent granulomas; **B**, vasculitis with thrombosis.

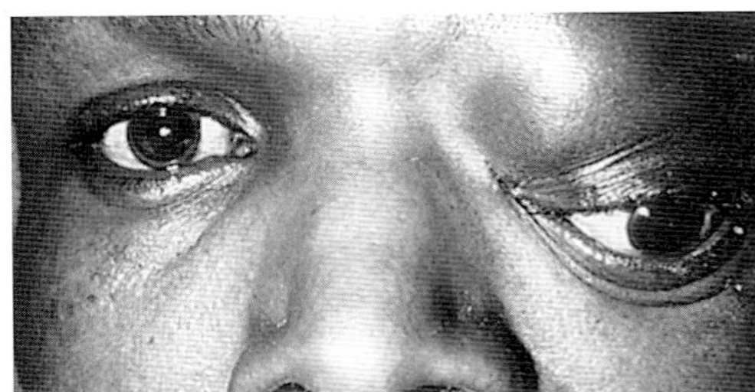

Fig. 30.20 Mucocele producing downward and lateral displacement of left eye.
(From del Regato JA, Spjut HJ. Ackerman and del Regato's cancer, ed. 6. St Louis, 1985, Mosby)

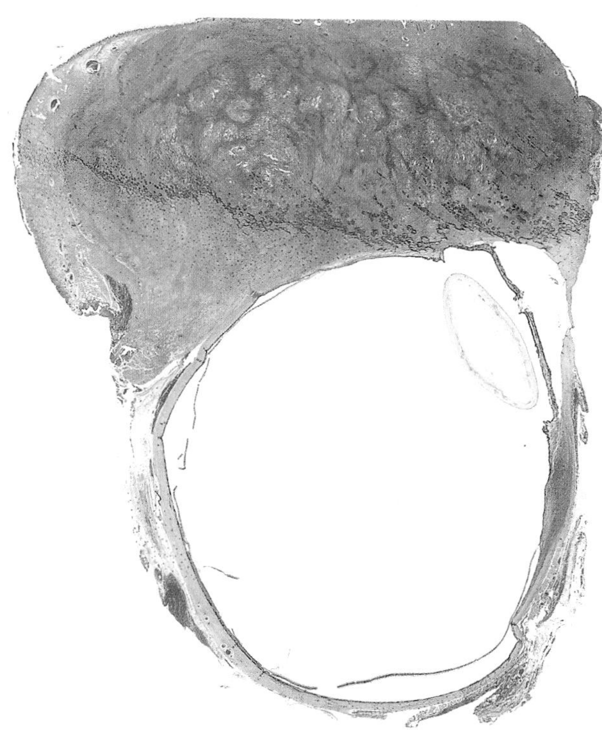

Fig. 30.21 Large intraorbital mass in a case of Rosai–Dorfman disease.

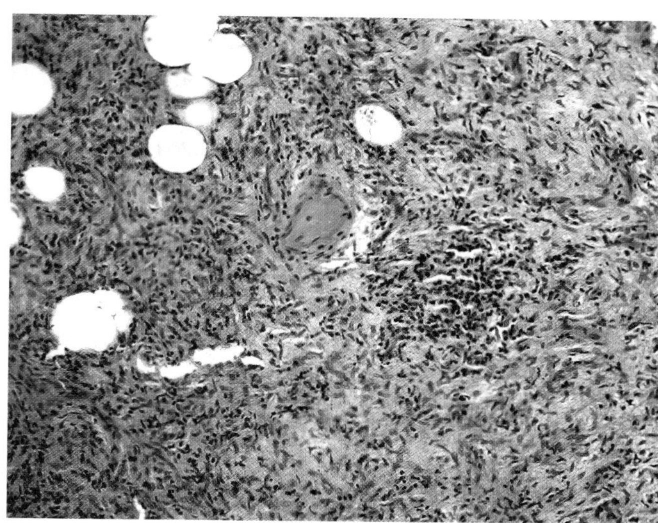

Fig 30.22 Inflammatory pseudotumor of orbit. Lymphocytes and spindle cells of fibroblastic/myofibroblastic appearance permeate the adipose tissue of the orbit.

This is not to say, however, that the microscopic features are uniform from case to case (Fig. 30.22). In some instances the proliferation of blood vessels and ground substance resembles that of exuberant granulation tissue.[104] At times, there is lymphoid hyperplasia with follicle formation (see p. 2480). Other cases with prominent involvement of extraocular muscles suggest the possibility of dysthyroid ophthalmopathy. In cases that are caused by Rosai–Dorfman disease the infiltrate is composed of large histiocytes (some exhibiting lymphocytophagocytosis), lymphocytes, and plasma cells; fibrosis can be very prominent.[102] Other types of inflammatory pseudotumors are composed of cholesterol granulomas or accumulation of keratin ('epidermoid cholesteatomas').[110,111]

A well-developed granulomatous reaction about small pools of fat is observed in certain cases. Such lesions may suggest traumatic fat necrosis. Others containing large numbers of cholesterol clefts and many foamy macrophages and giant cells suggest an area of old suppuration or hemorrhage. Periphlebitis is prominent in certain cases, and some of these may present a significant tissue eosinophilia, suggesting the possibility of a hypersensitivity angiitis, a parasitic infection, or Kimura disease.

Patients with orbital pseudotumors are usually in the third to fifth decade and in good health. The exophthalmos is of relatively sudden onset and in at least one half of the patients is associated with moderate to severe orbital pain and with lid and conjunctival edema. Diplopia is often present secondary to limitation of ocular motility in one or more fields of gaze, but visual acuity is usually unimpaired. Intracranial extension can occur.[103]

The lesion often can be palpated through the eyelids; if so, the surgeon may be able to reach it easily for a biopsy. Deeper lesions are not so readily accessible for biopsy, and if the clinical signs and symptoms are characteristic of inflammatory pseudotumor, steroids are often given without a biopsy, especially since systemic steroids often produce dramatic alleviation of signs and symptoms. The CT scan can be helpful in localizing the lesion.

Primary tumors

Mesenchymal tumors and tumorlike conditions

Rhabdomyosarcoma is the most common soft tissue sarcoma of the orbit in childhood.[130] The types seen in this age group are embryonal and alveolar, the latter being associated with a more aggressive clinical course. Some cases have occurred as a second primary tumor following irradiation for bilateral retinoblastoma.[126]

Hemangiopericytoma and **solitary fibrous tumor** are closely related and part of a morphologic continuum.[124] The former term has been used when the vascularity is prominent, while the latter has been generally employed when the tumor is solid, with keloid-like collagen and an alternation of hyper- and hypocellular areas[127,137] (Fig. 30.23). Strong immunoreactivity for CD34 and BCL2 is present, particularly in the cases with a solitary fibrous tumor pattern.[117,140] In the series reported as hemangiopericytoma by Croxatto and Font,[115] the recurrence rate was 30% and the metastatic rate was 15%, with most of the metastases developing late in the course of the disease. Some of the cases classified as solitary fibrous tumor have also followed an aggressive clinical course.[134]

Giant cell angiofibroma is characterized by a richly vascularized proliferation of spindle cells containing pseudovascular spaces and multinucleated giant cells, often of the so-called 'floret type'.[116,123] CD34 is positive. This lesion, which is not limited to the orbit,[133] may represent a variant of solitary fibrous tumor rich in giant cells.[125]

Fibrous histiocytoma used to be regarded as the most common primary mesenchymal orbital tumor in adults, the upper and nasal portions of the orbit said to be the most common sites. Font and Hidayat[118] divided their cases into benign, locally aggressive, and malignant: the 10-year survival rate was 100%, 92%, and 23%, respectively. At present, it is likely that many of these cases would be placed in another category. However, some lesions having an

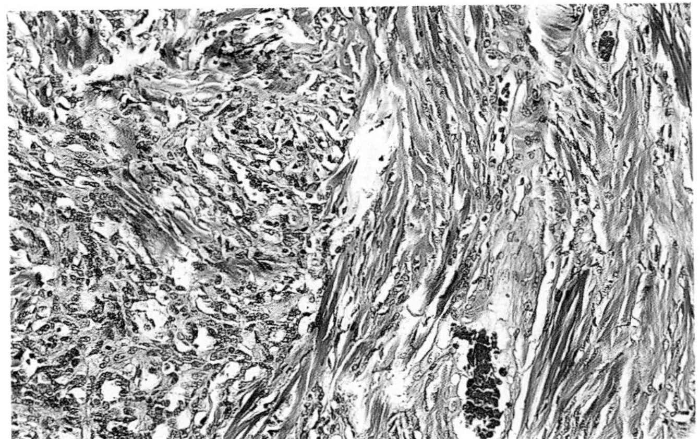

Fig. 30.23 Solitary fibrous tumor of orbit. The alternation of hypercellular and hypocellular areas is characteristic. The collagen has a keloid-type quality. This tumor was strongly immunoreactive for CD34.

admixture of fibroblast-like and histiocyte-like cells and a storiform pattern of growth remain, there being no better alternative diagnosis.

Alveolar soft-part sarcoma can present as a primary orbital tumor.[120] The age of occurrence, microscopic appearance, and evolution are similar to those seen in the other location of this tumor (see Chapter 25) (Fig. 30.24). The clinical course is indolent, distant metastases sometimes occurring 10 years or more after initial therapy.[120]

Osteosarcoma has been reported most often as a late complication of radiation therapy to the area.[122]

Other malignant mesenchymal tumors, all extremely rare, include **leiomyosarcoma**,[142,144] **liposarcoma**,[114] **fibrosarcoma**,[139] **mesenchymal chondrosarcoma**,[129] **angiosarcoma**,[128] and **Ewing sarcoma/PNET**.[141]

Angiomas are relatively common orbital tumors, with hemangiomas occurring much more commonly than lymphangiomas.[135,143]

In the infant, these soft, blue, compressible tumors are diffuse throughout the orbit and often extend forward into the eyelids (Fig. 30.25). Surgical removal is difficult; fortunately, however, most hemangiomas spontaneously regress by 4 years of age. If the tumor is so large that the visual axis of the eye is covered and the eye is at risk for the development of deprivation amblyopia, such lesions can often be reduced in size following a short course of systemic steroids or small doses of radiotherapy.

In the adult, these tumors are usually encapsulated, are situated close to the back of the eye, and can be surgically 'shelled' out. The CT scan reveals a discrete round mass that is enhanced by contrast dye (Fig. 30.26).

These tumors rarely present difficulties in histopathologic diagnosis, for they are not significantly dissimilar from angiomas elsewhere. In the infant, the lesion is usually of capillary type (the majority expressing GLUT-1, in contrast to vascular malformation) and in the adult of cavernous type.[113,132]

Schwannoma and **neurofibroma** represent a small percentage of orbital tumors. Almost all orbital schwannomas are well-encapsulated tumors that can be completely removed surgically by orbitotomy.[138] Orbital neurofibromas are usually but not always an expression of Recklinghausen disease.[131] There may be a gross deformity of the orbit and eyelid and, on palpation, the lid has been referred to as 'a bag of worms'.

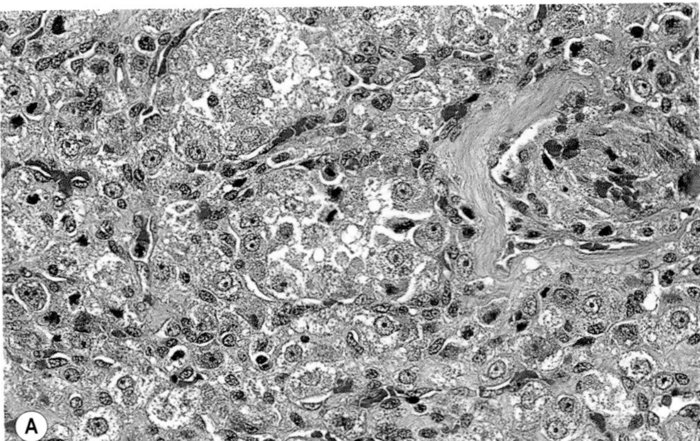

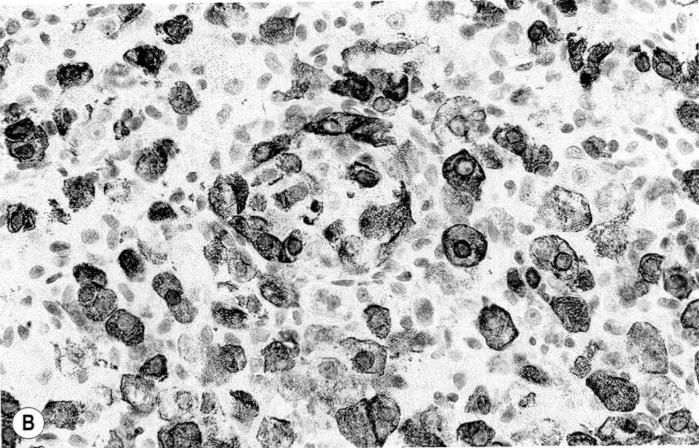

Fig. 30.24 **A** and **B**, Alveolar soft part sarcoma of orbit. **A**, Hematoxylin–eosin. **B**, Desmin immunostain. This degree of positivity for this marker is unusual but it constitutes strong evidence for muscle differentiation.

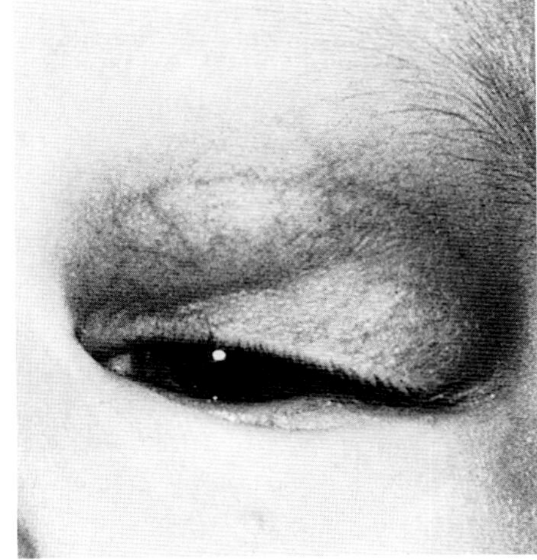

Fig. 30.25 Capillary hemangioma of left orbit and eyelid.

Other benign mesenchymal tumors that have been observed at this site are **lipoma, chondroma**, and **osteoma**.

Tumorlike proliferations also occur within the orbit, including **nodular fasciitis**[119] and **intravascular papillary endothelial hyperplasia** (Masson hemangioma).[121] A particularly interesting type of

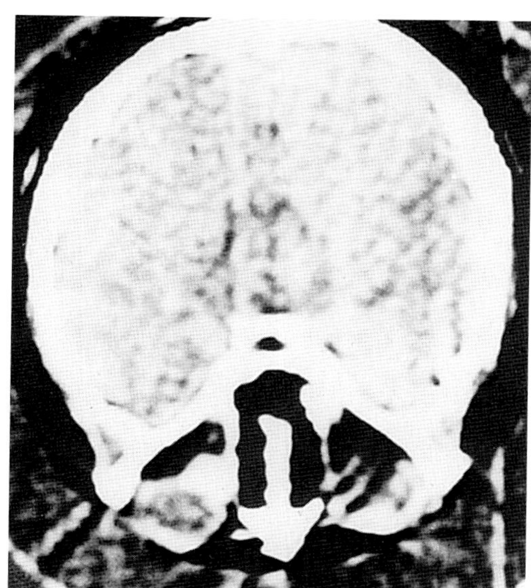

Fig. 30.26 CT scan showing hemangioma of right orbit.

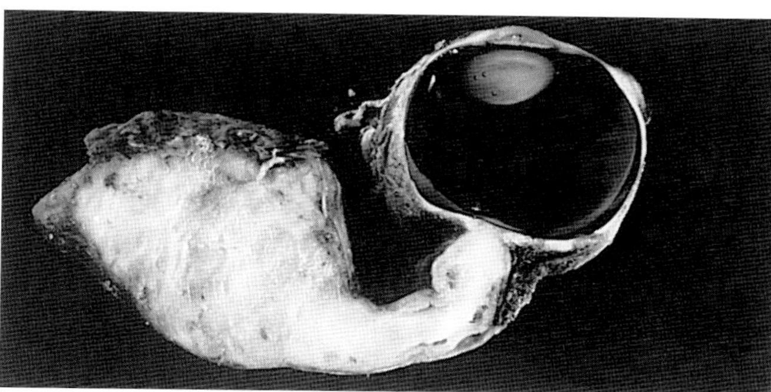

Fig. 30.27 Glioma that has produced massive enlargement of the orbital segment of the optic nerve. The tumor has completely effaced characteristic architectural features of the nerve and its meninges.

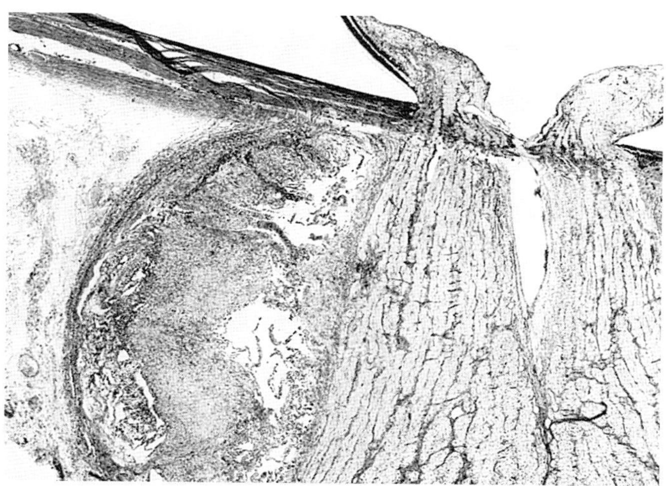

Fig. 30.28 Section through the optic nerve just anterior to the main mass of this glioma reveals minimal alteration of the parenchyma of the nerve but greatly thickened meninges. The combination of infiltrating tumor and arachnoidal proliferation is responsible for this meningeal thickening.

pseudomalignant lesion is seen as a result of prolapse of subconjunctival intraconal orbital fat, which can simulate microscopically an atypical lipomatous tumor.[136] This non-neoplastic lesion, known as **subconjunctival herniated orbital fat (SCHOF),** shows adipocytes with intranuclear vacuoles ('Lochkern'), abundant so-called floret cells (similar to those seen in pleomorphic lipoma), and inflammatory cells, but not cells with large hyperchromatic nuclei within fibrous septa, as regularly seen in true atypical lipomatous tumors.

Langerhans cell histiocytosis can involve the orbit and result in prominent exophthalmos.

Glioma of optic nerve

Gliomas of the optic nerve are relatively rare, slow-growing tumors that usually arise within the orbital segment of the nerve.

Considerable cytologic variation exists, not only from case to case but also in different portions of a given tumor. Varying degrees of cellularity are observed, but generally these neoplasms are characterized by a low degree of anaplasia. This is especially true about the margins of the tumor, where it is often impossible to be certain where reactive gliosis ends and neoplasia begins. There are typically areas of intense myxoid degeneration within the tumor. In such areas the tumor cells frequently appear to be virtually lost in the abundant hyaluronidase-sensitive mucoid accumulations.

Small tumors limited to the optic nerve can be adequately managed by resection alone; for the more extensive lesions, biopsy followed by definitive irradiation is recommended.[146,148]

As these gliomas increase in size, they tend to form a bulbous enlargement of the nerve (Fig. 30.27). They also extend along the nerve peripherally toward the eye and centrally toward the brain. In so doing, they often produce great enlargement of the optic canal, an important diagnostic sign for the radiologist. In such cases the optic nerve fibers are likely to be completely destroyed, and the optic disc typically presents the ophthalmoscopic characteristics of primary optic atrophy.

Another growth pattern exhibited by a majority of optic nerve gliomas is infiltration through the pia. This leads to great thickening of the arachnoid (Fig. 30.28). This is partly the result of more exuberant growth of the tumor cells once they have reached the arachnoid, but equally important is the reactive proliferation of arachnoidal cells. At times, this has created difficulties in differential diagnosis between glioma and meningioma.

Microscopically, almost all optic gliomas are *low-grade pilocytic astrocytomas*, similar to those occurring in the cerebellum and in the region of the third ventricle.[145,147] Rarely, malignant tumors characterized by dense cellularity, high mitotic index, marked pleomorphism, necrosis, and vascular proliferation are encountered.[147]

Gliomas of the optic nerve typically make their presence known during the first decade of life with minimal exophthalmos, optic nerve atrophy, or papilledema, and with a characteristic thickening of the nerve on CT scan. There is a distinct association of these tumors and Recklinghausen disease. The majority of optic nerve gliomas are so slow growing that surgical intervention is seldom warranted.

Meningioma

Meningiomas of the orbit arising from the meninges of the optic nerve are thought to be more aggressive tumors than the

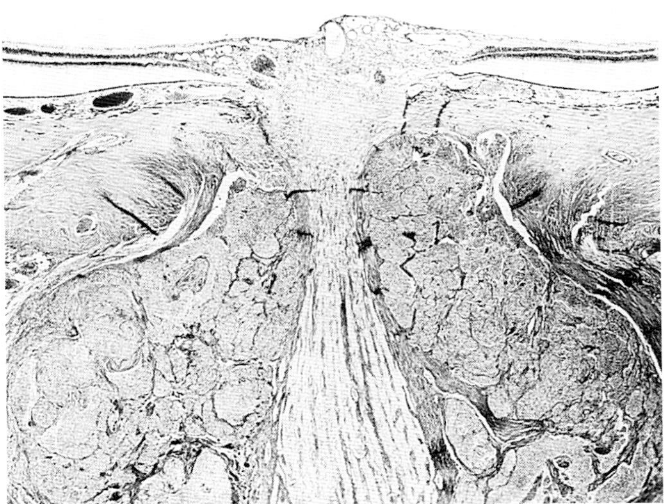

Fig. 30.29 Meningioma of optic nerve. The meninges are greatly thickened, and the optic nerve reveals severe compression atrophy.

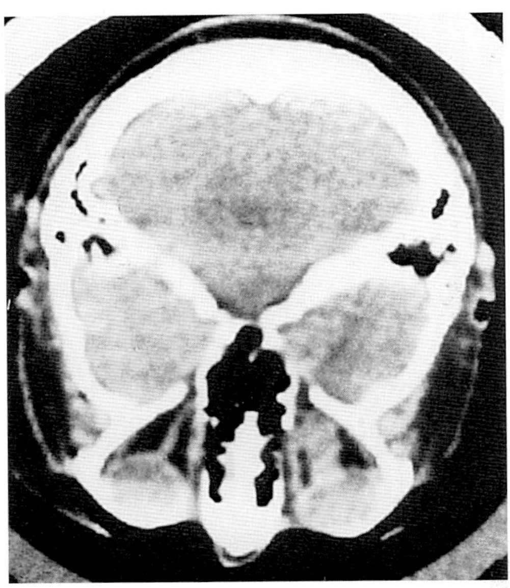

Fig. 30.30 CT scan showing perioptic meningioma of left orbit.

meningiomas of the sphenoidal ridge[150] (Fig. 30.29). However, some authors believe that they need not be operated on unless severe proptosis or proof of posterior extension occurs.

Those tumors arising from the orbital meninges generally produce some visual loss, optic atrophy, and exophthalmos. Those arising from the inner portion of the sphenoidal ridge produce more severe compression of the optic nerve within the optic canal, resulting in papilledema or optic atrophy before proptosis. The CT scan has facilitated the diagnosis and localization of these tumors (Fig. 30.30). Microscopically, most orbital meningiomas are of the meningothelial type[149] (Fig. 30.31). The differential diagnosis includes exuberant arachnoidal hyperplasia, fibrous histiocytoma, hemangiopericytoma/solitary fibrous tumor, and metastatic carcinoma.[151]

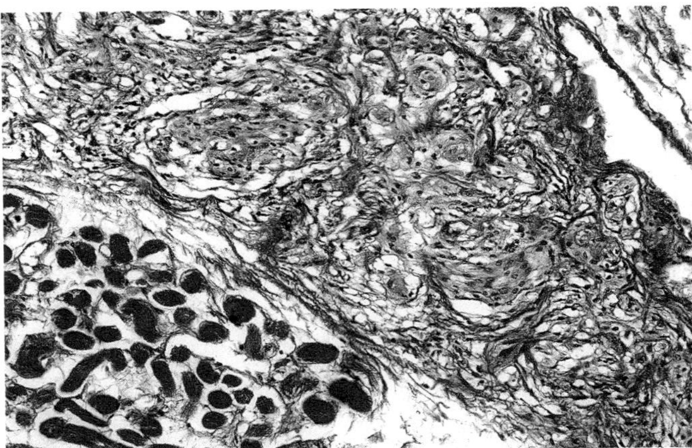

Fig. 30.31 Meningioma of orbit. The tumor has a typical meningothelial appearance.

Lymphoid tumors and tumorlike conditions

Lymphoid lesions of the orbit and other ocular sites may present great difficulties in histopathologic diagnoses. Some of these lesions develop in the course of a previously recognized malignant lymphoma or leukemia.[174] Others present initially in the orbit, but thorough clinical and laboratory examination reveals the presence of systemic involvement.[153,164] Such orbital lesions may make their appearance before peripheral blood studies are diagnostic, but bone marrow aspirates will usually furnish a conclusive answer. Still others, perhaps the majority, show disease localized to the orbit, conjunctiva, or eyelid.[171]

Microscopically, the latter lesions fall into three groups:

1 Lesions that are obviously malignant, usually non-Hodgkin lymphomas.[176] These include large B-cell lymphomas (including an Epstein–Barr virus-positive subset seen in the elderly[177]) and anaplastic large cell lymphoma (often located in the eyelid).[173]
2 Lesions that are fairly obvious examples of reactive hyperplasia with considerable polymorphism, a variety of cell types, vascular proliferation, and prominent follicles with germinal centers. IgG4-related sclerosing disease is one possible cause for the formation of such lesions.[155]
3 Lesions that are characterized by a rather uniform and monotonous but widespread proliferation of small lymphocytes, frequently associated with involvement of orbital fat, blood vessels, and nerves (Figs 30.32 and 30.33). It is this group that presents the most difficult problems in differential diagnosis.[152,160,169] Some of these lesions are accompanied by plasmacytoid differentiation, Dutcher bodies, and an associated paraproteinemia.[154] At present, most of these lesions are thought to belong to the category of extranodal marginal zone lymphoma (MALT lymphoma),[179] which thus becomes by far the most common type of lymphoma of this region, followed by follicular lymphoma[158] (except for the intraocular tissues and – curiously – the lacrimal sac, see pp. 2493 and 2474).[175] Their microscopic appearance is similar to that of MALT-type lymphomas of other sites, including the inconstant presence of plasmacytoid cells and the exceptional secondary change known as crystal-storing histiocytosis (although lymphoepithelial lesions are relatively uncommon).[163]

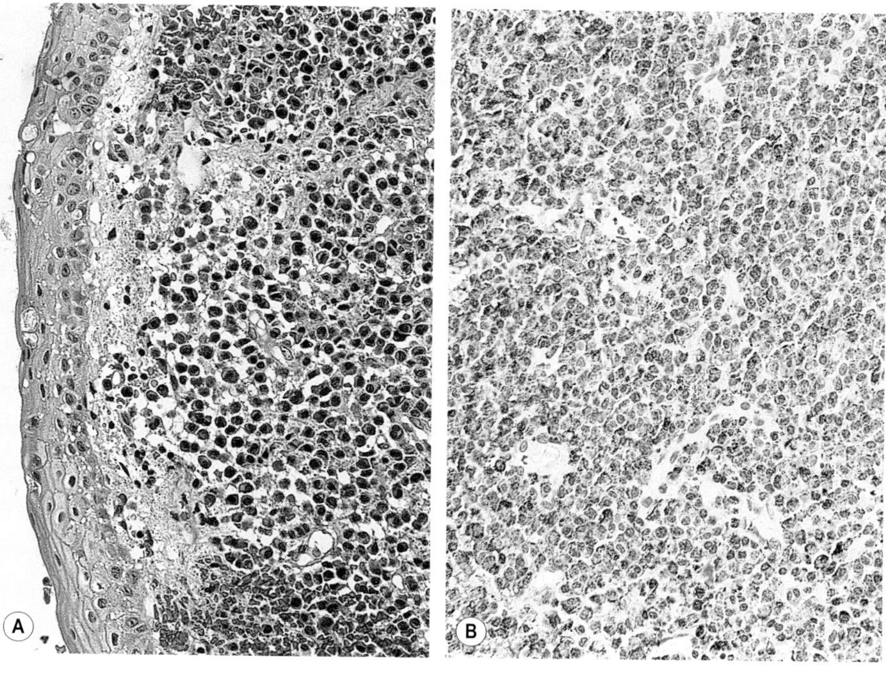

Fig. 30.32 **A** and **B**, Malignant lymphoid proliferation of conjunctiva composed of small tumor cells with prominent plasmacytoid features: **B** shows strong immunoreactivity for kappa light chain.

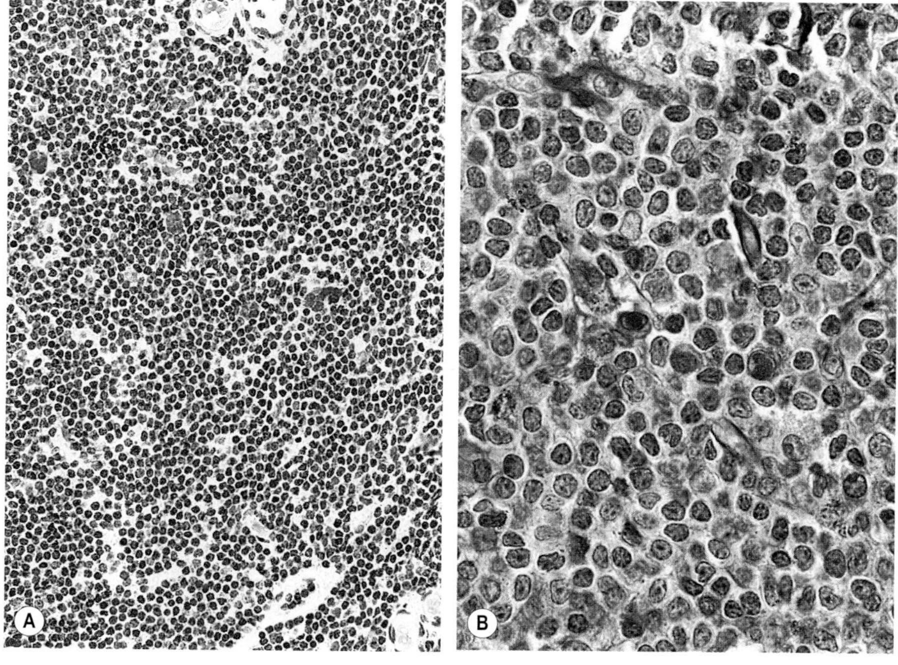

Fig. 30.33 **A** and **B**, Small lymphocytic proliferation of orbit. **A**, Low-power appearance showing a monotonous infiltrate of small lymphoid cells. **B**, PAS stain in another case, showing PAS-positive intranuclear inclusions composed of inspissated immunoglobulin (Dutcher bodies). The occurrence of these formations is strong evidence in favor of a neoplastic nature for the proliferation.

Most studies that have been carried out with the third group of lesions have shown that it is very difficult to predict which of them will develop into systemic lymphomas, whether one evaluates them by standard morphologic criteria, by cell marker analysis, or by gene rearrangement techniques.[161,166,170,178] Other studies have shown a better correlation between immunohistochemical features and outcome,[167,168] but perhaps the most important conclusion of all these studies is that the majority of patients with small lymphocytic proliferations localized to the ocular tissues enjoy an indolent clinical course and long survival with only minimal therapeutic intervention whether they are of polyclonal or monoclonal nature.[161,165] Lymphoid infiltrates of the conjunctiva are associated with a lower incidence of extraocular lymphoma (20%) than those of the orbit (35%) or eyelid (67%).[162] The most important prognostic factor is the extent of the disease at the time of presentation.[162] The claim has been made that a subset of MALT lymphomas expressing nuclear BCL10 are associated with a shorter failure-free survival.[159]

An Italian group[157] has made a provocative claim that patients with ocular adnexal lymphoma have a high prevalence of *Chlamydia*

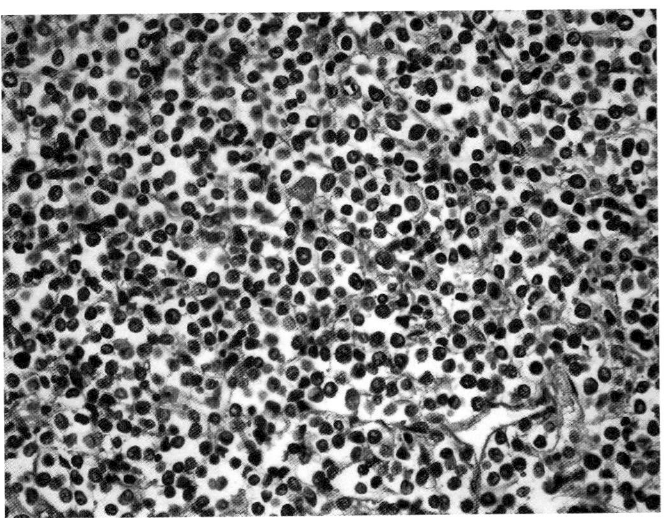

Fig. 30.34 So-called granulocytic sarcoma of orbit. This represents a localized focus of acute myelocytic leukemia.

psitacci (the etiologic agent of psittacosis) infection in both tumor tissue and peripheral blood mononuclear cells, suggesting that this organism may contribute to development of the lymphomas. However, other series from other parts of the world have given very different results.[172] Some cases of ocular lymphoma have been reported as arising against the background of IgG4-related sclerosing disease.[155,156]

Acute myeloid leukemia can involve the orbit as an initially localized lesion (granulocytic sarcoma) (Fig. 30.34).

Metastatic tumors

Direct spread to the orbit from adjacent structures can occur with primary intraocular tumors such as retinoblastoma or uveal malignant melanomas. Carcinomas of the paranasal sinuses may fail to produce diagnostic symptoms until orbital extension has occurred.

Hematogenous metastases to the orbit may be seen with many different tumors, but only rarely are these the initial manifestations of a carcinoma. Even neuroblastoma, which has a notorious reputation for metastasizing to the orbit, rarely does so before other diagnostic signs appear.

Most important in this regard is the distinct possibility that a primary embryonal rhabdomyosarcoma might be misinterpreted as a metastatic tumor. In the case of adults an orbital metastasis may, on rare occasions, be the initial manifestation of carcinoma of the breast, bronchus, kidney, or prostate.[180,181]

Carcinoid tumors of the lung or small bowel can also metastasize to the orbit or ocular globe; occasionally an orbital carcinoid tumor is found in the absence of any other disease, suggesting the possibility that it may be primary at this site.[182,183]

Conjunctiva

Specimens from the conjunctiva are thin and tend to fold into distorted patterns when placed into fixative. To prepare the tissue so that it can be oriented properly, the surgeon should spread the lesion onto a small piece of filter paper and allow it to dry for a few seconds before gently placing the filter paper with the adherent specimen into the jar with the fixative. Specimens should never be put onto sponges of any kind since these will expand when placed into the fixative, thus distorting the specimen.

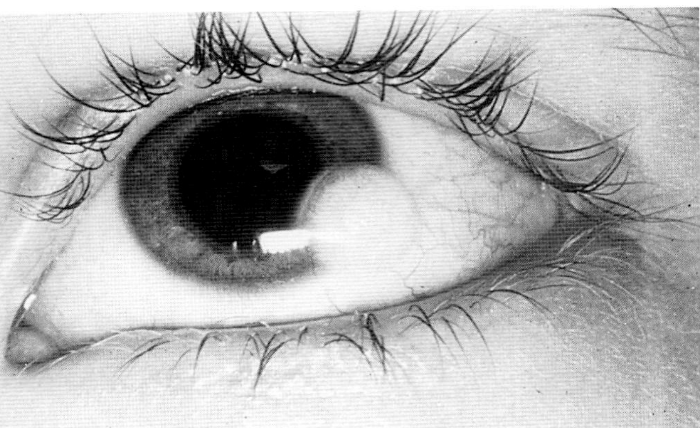

Fig. 30.35 Limbal dermoid in a child.

Developmental anomalies

Dermoid 'tumors' of the bulbar conjunctiva are firm, localized, elevated opaque masses that typically occur at the limbus, often encroaching on the cornea (Fig. 30.35). These are solid choristomatous masses, not to be confused with dermoid cysts of the orbit.

Over the lesion, the surface epithelium and the subepithelial connective tissue present the histologic features characteristic of epidermis and dermis, respectively. A few hairs typically project from the tumor. The bulk of the mass is composed of thick bundles of collagen. In some lesions, skin appendages are few, and adipose tissue is abundant. These are known as *dermolipomas*, and they are usually situated in the upper outer fornix. Ocular dermoids may be part of *Goldenhar syndrome*, in which there are extra-auricular appendages and vertebral abnormalities.

Cysts

Benign epithelium-lined inclusion cysts of the conjunctiva usually arise after accidental or surgical trauma or, rarely, de novo.

Degeneration

Pinguecula is a very common degenerative process affecting primarily the subepithelial connective tissues of the bulbar conjunctiva in the interpalpebral region. This gives rise to an elevated yellowish lesion over which the epithelium may become atrophic or thickened. Since these lesions are not progressive, they are seldom excised.

Histologically, the most characteristic feature is actinic elastosis affecting a bandlike zone beneath the epithelium. Secondary hyalinization and calcareous degeneration also may be observed. The epithelium over pingueculae typically becomes atrophic, but at times it becomes so acanthotic and dyskeratotic that the erroneous diagnosis of carcinoma may be made.

Pterygium extends into the cornea and is therefore a clinically more significant lesion than the pinguecula (Fig. 30.36). Microscopically, there is usually some actinic elastosis but also a variable amount of acute and chronic inflammation and hyperemia.

A morphologically somewhat similar lesion of the conjunctiva has been interpreted as the ocular equivalent of *elastofibroma*.[184]

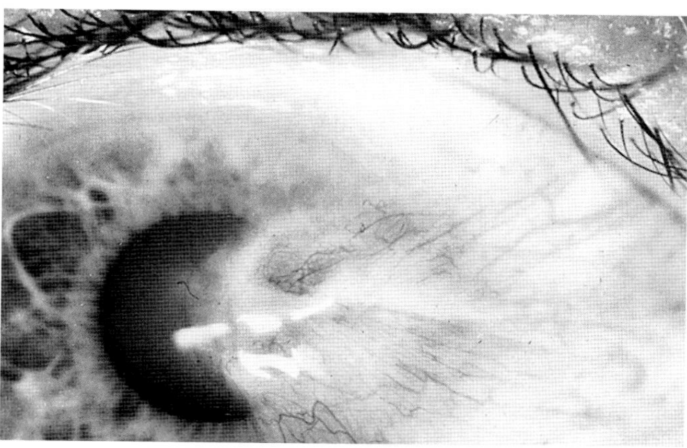

Fig. 30.36 Pterygium that has grown over the pupillary axis and has interfered with vision.

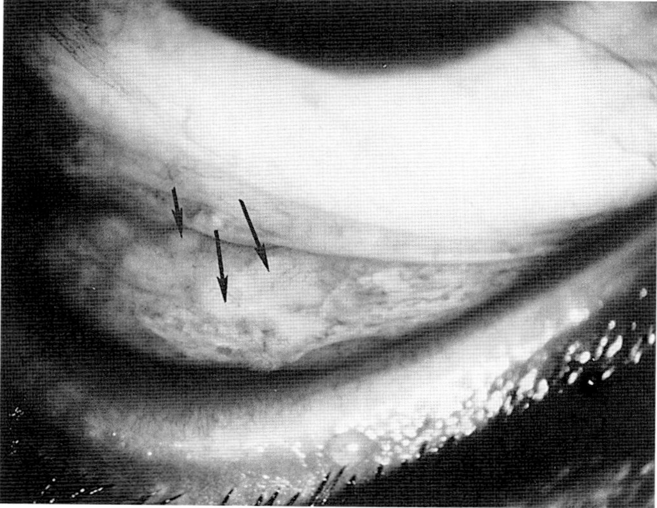

Fig. 30.37 Conjunctival granulomas in sarcoidosis (arrows).

Graft-versus-host disease

The major histopathologic changes seen in the eyes of patients undergoing bone marrow transplantation involve the conjunctiva, cornea, choroid, and lacrimal gland. The major change in the cornea is keratinization, as appreciated in biopsy specimens.[185]

Inflammation

Inflammatory lesions of the conjunctiva seldom give rise to the type of diagnostic or therapeutic problem that requires excision and histopathologic study. One lesion that deserves mention is the noncaseating granulomatous inflammation found in approximately one-fourth of patients with **sarcoidosis**[186] (Fig. 30.37). **Ligneous conjunctivitis** is a peculiar form of chronic pseudomembranous conjunctivitis that presents as a woody induration of the eyelids, together with the formation of a pseudomembrane on the tarsal conjunctiva. The cardinal feature histologically is the presence of large hyaline masses that may simulate amyloid.[187,188] The disease is thought to be due to plasminogen deficiency.[190]

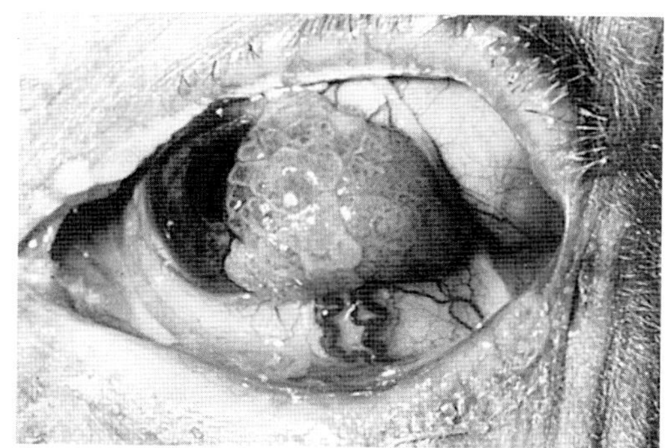

Fig. 30.38 Extensive papilloma of bulbar conjunctiva.

Inclusion (chlamydial) conjunctivitis is seen in adults as an acute or chronic infection. It is produced by *Chlamydia*, and it shows the microscopic appearance of follicular conjunctivitis indistinguishable from viral infection. The diagnosis is based on the finding of so-called 'Halberstaedter–Prowazek inclusions' on conjunctival scrapings.[192]

Actinic granuloma can develop in the conjunctiva, its microscopic appearance being equivalent to that of its more common cutaneous counterpart.[191]

Sjögren syndrome manifests itself in the conjunctiva by a polymorphic inflammatory infiltrate in the stroma, accompanied by metaplasia of the epithelium and a decreased number of goblet cells.[189]

Tumors and tumorlike conditions

Epithelial tumors

The large majority of epithelial tumors of the conjunctiva arise from the surface epithelium, but a few originate from an accessory lacrimal gland located within the conjunctiva.[194]

Papillomas are relatively common lesions of the conjunctiva with a tendency for recurrence after apparent complete excision. In children the papillomas are often multiple. The lesions have a typical papillomatous or 'mulberry' surface appearance with small vessels coming up to the surface (Fig. 30.38).

Microscopically, the typical papilloma reveals pronounced acanthosis and varying degrees of keratinization, koilocytosis, and nonspecific inflammation (see Fig. 30.7). Human papillomavirus (HPV) type 6/11 has been found in these lesions by in-situ hybridization techniques.[198]

Carcinoma in situ of the bulbar conjunctiva varies considerably in its clinical appearance. It may present as an area of leukoplakia, as a papilloma, or as a complication of pterygium or pinguecula (Fig. 30.39).

The histopathologic characteristics of carcinoma in situ of the conjunctiva and cornea are similar to those observed elsewhere in the mucous membranes, or the lesion may resemble Bowen disease or Paget disease of the skin[196] (Fig. 30.40).

There are many lesions removed from the conjunctiva that do not fall clearly into either of the categories of papilloma or carcinoma in situ. They are often not quite so benign as to be called papilloma, yet there are not enough changes to warrant a classification of carcinoma in situ. These have been traditionally referred to as *dysplasia* of the conjunctiva. Not surprisingly, the suggestion has been made that these lesions be placed within a spectrum of *conjunctival* (*or corneal*) *intraepithelial neoplasia*.[200] These lesions have been found to contain HPV type 16 in a substantial number of cases.[197]

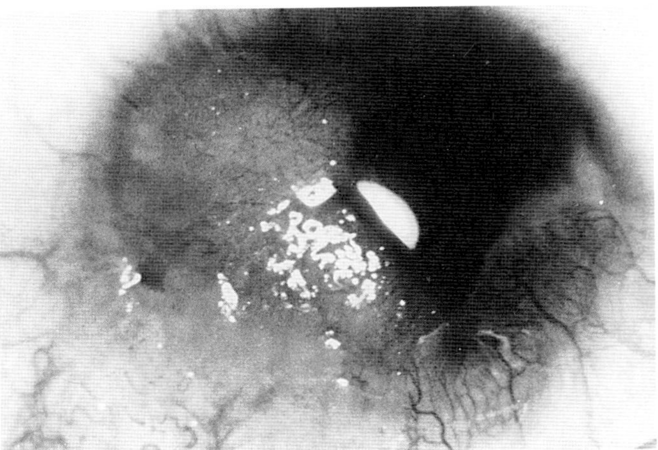

Fig. 30.39 Carcinoma in situ of conjunctiva and cornea.

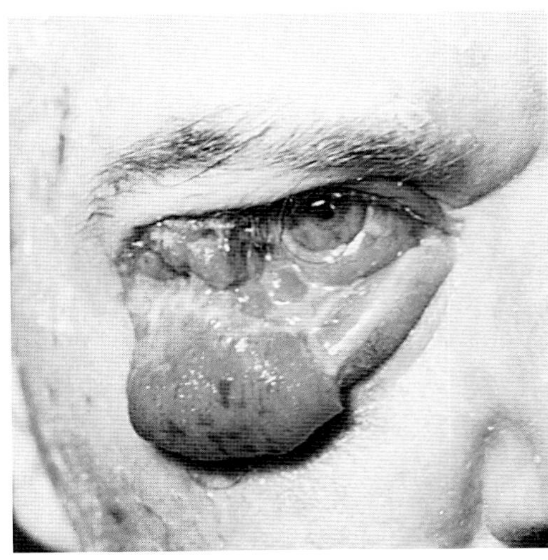

Fig. 30.41 Squamous cell carcinoma of conjunctiva. The tumor grew rapidly over a 4-month period.

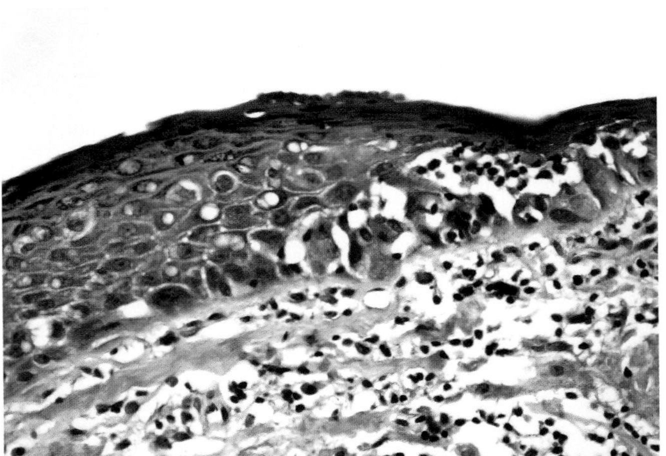

Fig. 30.40 Carcinoma of conjunctiva with pagetoid pattern of growth.

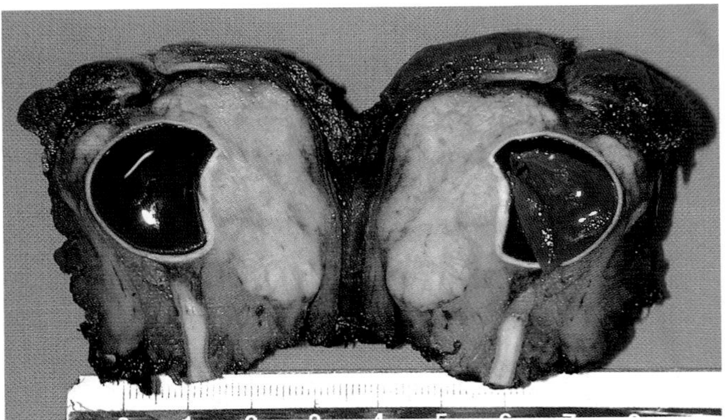

Fig. 30.42 Squamous cell carcinoma of conjunctiva growing extensively inside the orbit and compressing the ocular globe.

Invasive squamous cell carcinoma of the conjunctiva is rare but is still more common than basal cell carcinoma at this site.[193] Clinically, carcinomas of the conjunctiva with significant infiltration are seldom observed in the United States, probably because it is common practice to excise early 'precancerous' or 'in situ cancerous' lesions long before this stage occurs (Figs 30.41 and 30.42). Such lesions, as well as the majority of early invasive carcinomas of the limbal area, can be adequately controlled by excisional therapy. If untreated, these tumors will invade the anterior chamber and other portions of the ocular globe. A high proportion of the deeply invasive conjunctival carcinomas have *adenosquamous* ('mucoepidermoid') features.[195,199] Radical surgery is necessary in these cases.[196]

Melanocytic tumors and tumorlike conditions

Nevi. Nevi of the bulbar conjunctiva, like those of the skin, may be observed from birth, or they may become noticeable at any time during childhood, adolescence, or later.[210,211] At times a nevus known to have been present since infancy appears to become much larger and more pigmented at puberty (Fig. 30.43).

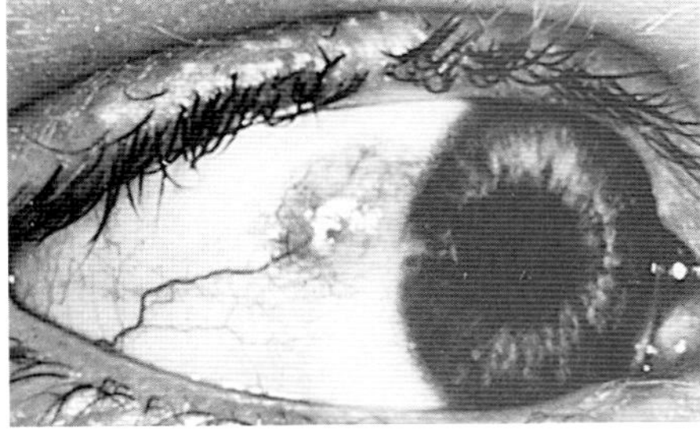

Fig. 30.43 Pigmented lesion at the limbus that proved to be a benign nevus.
(From Regato JA, Spjut HJ. Ackerman and del Regato's cancer, ed. 5. St Louis, 1977, Mosby; courtesy of the Registry of Ophthalmic Pathology, Armed Forces Institute of Pathology, Washington, DC)

Characteristically, conjunctival nevi are discrete, flat, or slightly elevated lesions located on the globe in the interpalpebral zone near the limbus, but they vary greatly in size, shape, and position. They also exhibit much variation in degree of pigmentation, approximately one-third being essentially amelanotic.

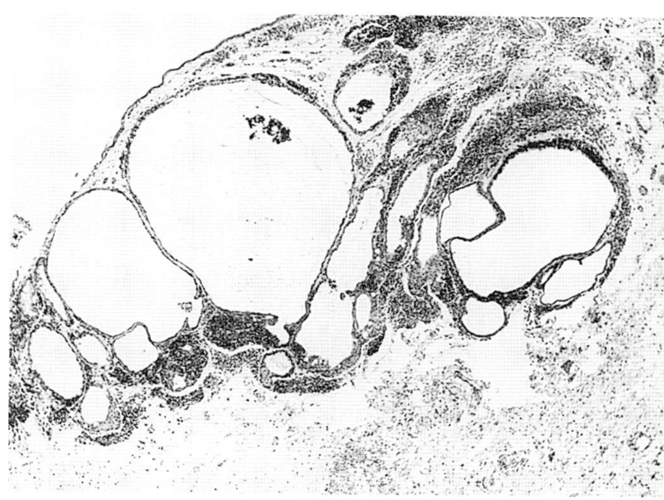

Fig. 30.44 Conjunctival nevus with many associated cystic epithelial inclusions. Small round cells about large cysts are not inflammatory cells but nevus cells. This epibulbar lesion may be analogous to hair dermal nevus of skin.

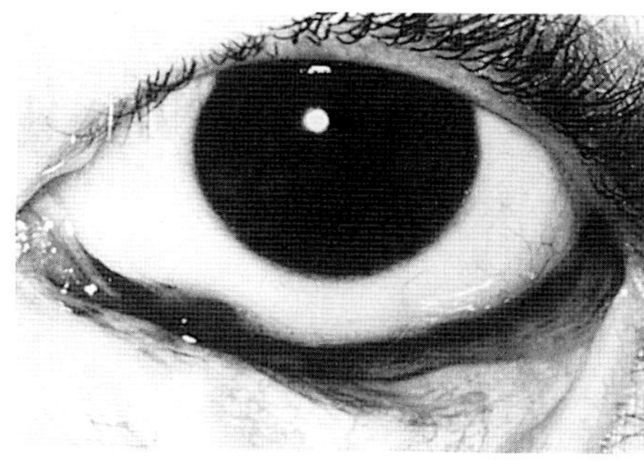

Fig. 30.45 Malignant melanoma of conjunctiva in lower cul-de-sac arising from a lesion of acquired melanosis.
(From Zimmerman LE. Discussion of pigmented tumors of the conjunctiva. In Boniuk M (ed.): Ocular and adnexal tumors. St Louis, 1964, Mosby; courtesy of the Registry of Ophthalmic Pathology, Armed Forces Institute of Pathology, Washington, DC)

Microscopically, conjunctival nevi are almost always of the junctional or compound variety. Counterparts of the common dermal nevus of the skin are rarely observed. A few of the conjunctival nevi are of Spitz type.[208] Frequently, there are numerous solid and cystic inclusions of conjunctival epithelium intimately incorporated into the subepithelial component of these nevi. At times, the epithelial inclusions may so dominate the clinical and histopathologic picture that the nevoid nature of the lesion is overlooked (Fig. 30.44). The presence of the epithelial inclusions is supportive evidence for benignity, since they are rare in melanomas. Conjunctival nevi in children, which are usually of compound type, tend to show a confluent pattern of growth and a lack maturation that may lead to overdiagnosis.[217]

Malignant melanoma. Malignant melanoma of the conjunctiva, a very rare lesion, may arise without an apparent precursor lesion, or it may be the sequela of a nevus or of so-called 'acquired melanosis' (see later discussions)[209,210,212] (Figs 30.45 and 30.46). The microscopic appearance is similar to that of its cutaneous counterpart. The prognosis is closely related to the subsite and size of the primary tumor.[218] Small localized bulbar tumors have an excellent prognosis, diffuse bulbar melanomas have an intermediate prognosis, and melanomas of the fornix and caruncle have a poor prognosis.[210] Metastatic spread is very uncommon with melanomas less than 1.5 cm in maximum thickness. In the series of 131 cases reported by Folberg et al.[206] the overall mortality was 26%; no prognostic differences were found among the melanomas arising de novo, those with an accompanying nevus, and those associated with so-called 'acquired melanosis'.

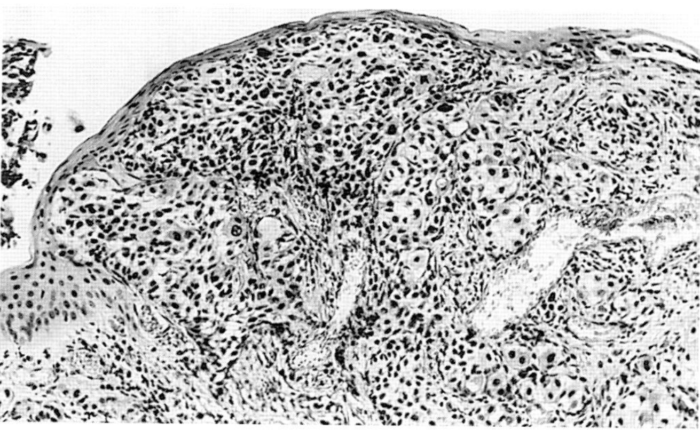

Fig. 30.46 Malignant melanoma arising in a nevus known to have been present since childhood. The patient, a 59-year-old woman, stated that the lesion suddenly became quite large several months before it was excised.

The treatment varies from local excision to exenteration of the eye, depending on the extent of the disease.

So-called 'acquired melanosis'. Acquired melanosis is a term commonly used among ophthalmologists and ophthalmic pathologists for a melanocytic proliferative lesion of the conjunctiva that has also been referred to as primary acquired melanosis, precancerous melanosis, atypical melanocytic hyperplasia, and malignant melanoma in situ.[201,204,213,215] Most cases are seen in the fifth decade of life or later, and the typical presentation is that of a diffuse nonelevated granular pigmentation of the conjunctiva. The most common site of involvement is the bulbar conjunctiva, but it can also be present in the cornea, palpebral conjunctiva, or skin of the eyelid. The extent of the lesion and the degree of pigmentation may fluctuate during the course of the years.

Microscopically, an increase in the number of melanocytes is seen along the basal layer, individually or in clusters, associated with various degrees of atypicality[205] (Fig. 30.47).

The nature and significance of this lesion have been controversial. Considerations that have been made are similar to those expressed for other acquired melanocytic proliferations of the skin, notably Hutchinson freckle. Specifically, it has been postulated that all cases of acquired melanosis (at least those exhibiting atypia) are malignant melanomas in situ.[201] Guillén and co-workers[207,214] have divided these conjunctival lesions into three groups: (1) conjunctival hypermelanosis (with or without melanocytic hyperplasia but lacking atypia); (2) atypical melanocytic hyperplasia; and (3) malignant melanoma. Sugiura et al.[216] divided their cases into a *low-risk* and a *high-risk* group, the latter showing a high association with malignant melanoma. From a practical standpoint, the important fact to remember is that the propensity for the development of invasive melanoma is directly related to the presence and degree of atypia.[203,205] In the series of Folberg et al.,[205] none of the lesions

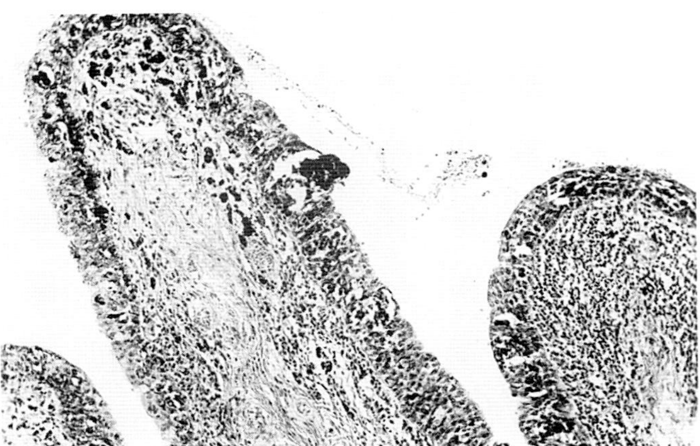

Fig. 30.47 Widespread acquired melanosis of conjunctiva.

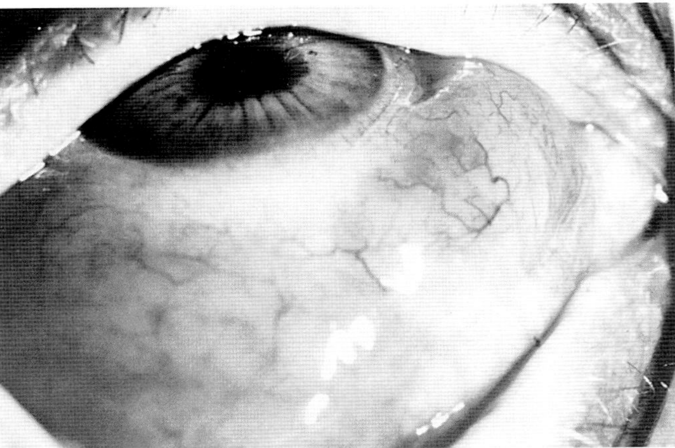

Fig. 30.48 Lymphoid infiltration of conjunctiva.

without atypia progressed to invasive melanoma, whereas 40% of those with atypia did. Accordingly, the recommendation has been made to excise all of these lesions by surgery or cryotherapy.[202,205]

Lymphoid tumors and tumorlike conditions

The morphologic appearances and diagnostic problems posed by these lesions when they present in the conjunctiva are similar to those of analogous lesions of the eyelid and orbit and are discussed on page 2480. The clinical appearance of the conjunctival lesions is that of salmon-colored, smooth masses[219] (Fig. 30.48).

Other tumors

Myxoma has been reported as a primary tumor in the conjunctiva, cornea, eyelid, and orbit. Grossly, the conjunctival lesions have a smooth, fleshy, gelatinous appearance. Local excision is curative.[223]

Intravenous pyogenic granuloma has been observed in the region of the canthus and in the lacrimal sac.[224]

Vascular tumors of various types can also involve the conjunctiva. They include hemangioma, Kaposi sarcoma,[221] and angiosarcoma.[220]

Merkel cell carcinoma has been seen as an apparently primary conjunctival tumor.[222]

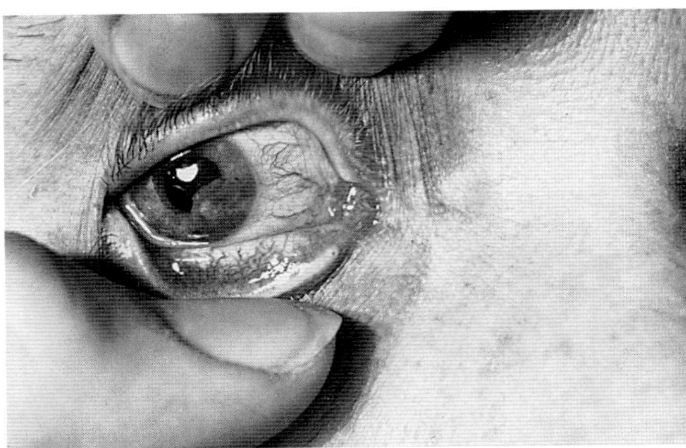

Fig. 30.49 Melanoma of iris that had been observed over a period of 10 years, during which time it became progressively larger and encroached on the pupil. Iridectomy revealed it to be of spindle A cell type. The tumor recurred and necessitated enucleation for secondary glaucoma 15 years after iridectomy.
(Courtesy of Dr ME Nugent, Bismarck, ND)

Intraocular tissues

As stated in the Introduction of this chapter, only tumors and tumor-like conditions of these structures will be discussed.

Malignant melanoma

General and clinical features

Melanomas arising from the pigmented or potentially pigment-producing cells of the uvea are the most frequent primary intraocular neoplasms in adults. They can also occur in adolescents, children, and even neonates.[225,227] It has been suggested that most of them arise on the basis of preexisting benign nevi.[235–237] A syndrome has been described in which bilateral diffuse melanocytic uveal tumors are seen in association with systemic malignant neoplasms.[226] Risk factors for uveal melanoma, in addition to uveal nevi, include a fair complexion, light irides, oculodermal and ocular melanocytosis, and Recklinghausen disease.[232]

Malignant melanoma may be located at any point in the uveal tract, with the choroid and ciliary body being more frequent locations than the iris. Melanoma of the iris presents as an elevated mass with varying degrees of pigmentation and often with distortion of the pupil and the presence of prominent vessels on the tumor (Fig. 30.49). Choroidal melanoma also may vary in pigmentation but characteristically is an irregular, slate-gray, solid, subretinal tumor producing an overlying retinal detachment and decreased vision (Figs 30.50 and 30.51). It may appear as a discoid, globular, or mushroom-shaped mass. Less commonly, it spreads diffusely and extends out along scleral canals into the orbit[231,233] (Figs 30.52–30.54).

Visual disturbance caused by retinal detachment is a much more frequent presenting complaint than the formation of an orbital tumor. Not infrequently the patient remains asymptomatic until the tumor has grown sufficiently to become necrotic and produce complications such as endophthalmitis, massive intraocular hemorrhage, and/or secondary glaucoma.

At times, malignant melanomas of the posterior uvea are not discovered until the enucleated eye is examined in the laboratory.

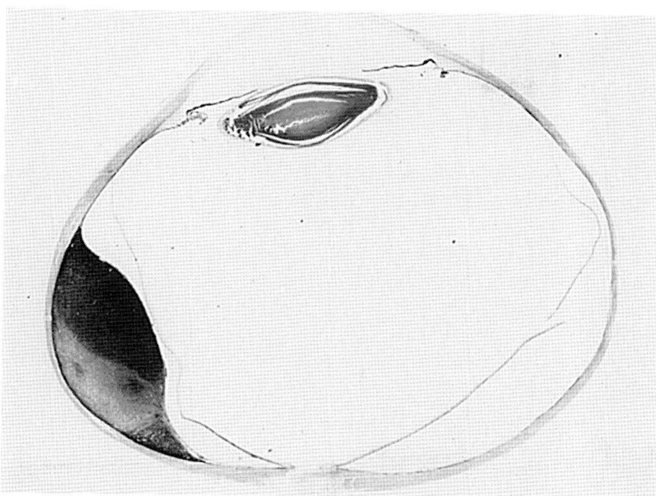

Fig. 30.50 Malignant melanoma of choroid that has not broken through Bruch's membrane but has elevated the retina. Most of the retinal separation observed in this section is artifactual.
(From Friedenwald JS, Wilder HC, Maumenee AE, Sanders TE, Keyes JEL, Hogan MJ, Owens WC, Owens EU. Ophthalmic pathology. An atlas and textbook. Philadelphia, 1952, WB Saunders)

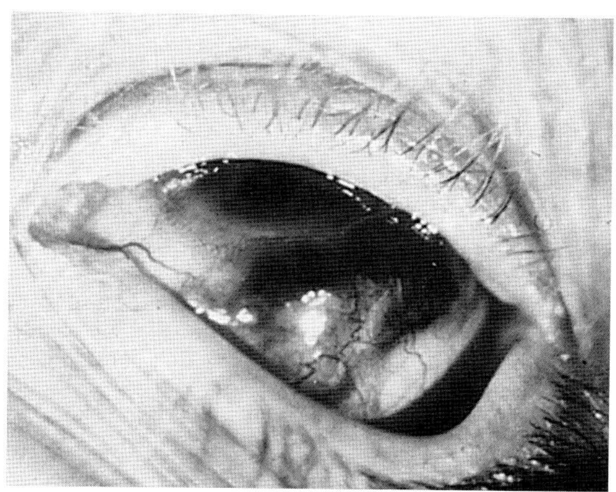

Fig. 30.52 Malignant melanoma of choroid breaking through the sclera and presenting under the conjunctiva.
(From del Regato JA, Spjut HJ. Ackerman and del Regato's cancer, ed. 5. St Louis, 1977, Mosby; courtesy of the Registry of Ophthalmic Pathology, Armed Forces Institute of Pathology, Washington, DC)

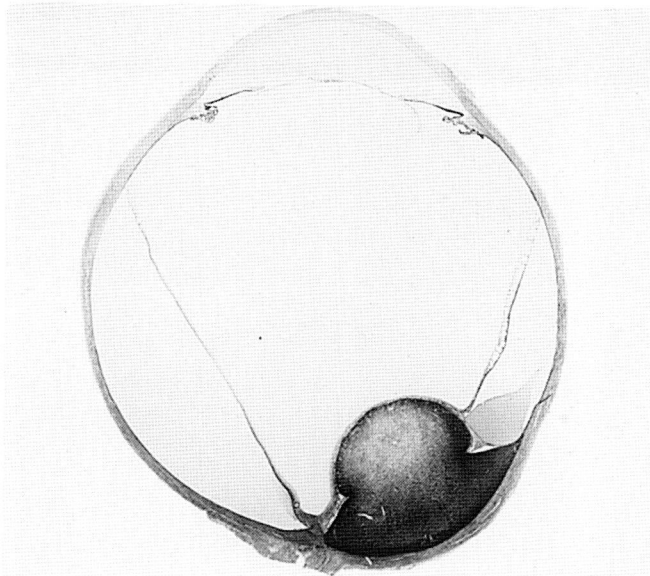

Fig. 30.51 Malignant melanoma of choroid that, by erupting through Bruch's membrane, has formed a mushroom-shaped subretinal mass.

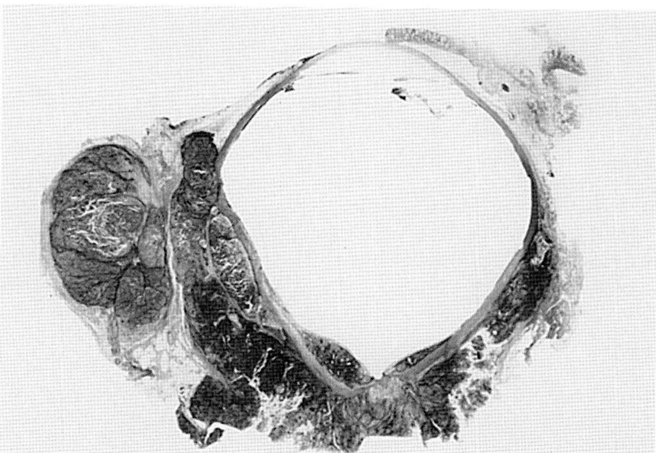

Fig. 30.53 Massive orbital extension from a small choroid melanoma that has occurred as a result of diffuse spread along natural passages through the sclera and optic nerve.
(From Friedenwald JS, Wilder HC, Maumenee AE, Sanders TE, Keyes JEL, Hogan MJ, Owens WC, Owens EU. Ophthalmic pathology. An atlas and textbook. Philadelphia, 1952, WB Saunders)

Iris tumors are more often recognized early, for they can be seen by the patient and family long before symptoms appear (Fig. 30.55).

Clinically, there are many lesions that simulate uveal malignant melanoma.[228–230,234] The most important are metastatic carcinoma, localized hemorrhage beneath the retina or between the pigment epithelium and choroid (Fig. 30.56), focal areas of proliferation of the retinal pigment epithelium (Fig. 30.57), posterior scleritis, and benign tumors such as nevi and hemangiomas.

Microscopic features

Microscopically, uveal melanomas have been traditionally divided into three types: spindle A, spindle B, and epithelioid, which may occur singly or in combination.[242] Spindle A cells are slender, benign-appearing spindle-shaped cells that have relatively small fusiform nuclei and no nucleoli. The chromatin is frequently arranged in a linear fashion along the central axis of the nucleus.

Spindle B cells are larger and more pleomorphic, merging on the one hand with spindle A cells and on the other with epithelioid cells. They typically possess large ovoid nuclei containing prominent nucleoli (Fig. 30.58). Mitotic activity may be more marked. Both spindle A and spindle B tumors tend to be quite cohesive. Some of these tumors have a distinctly fascicular pattern of growth (Fig. 30.59).

Epithelioid cells are still larger and more irregular (Fig. 30.60). They have an abundance of cytoplasm and may be truly gigantic. Multinucleated forms are not unusual. The nuclei are large, and their nucleoli are often strikingly prominent. In some tumors, many bizarre nuclei may be seen. Epithelioid cells are characteristically less cohesive than the spindle cells.

It is rather unusual for these tumors to be composed of a single cell type. Mixtures of spindle A and B cells or mixtures of spindle and epithelioid cells are common.

The microscopic differential diagnosis of primary uveal melanoma includes benign pigmented nevi.[240,243] Along these lines, it has been pointed out that the tumors traditionally designated as spindle A melanomas may actually represent spindle cell nevi (see also p. 2490). Primary uveal melanomas should also be distinguished from intraocular metastases of cutaneous malignant melanoma.[238,239,241] In addition, amelanotic melanomas raise the differential diagnosis with metastatic carcinoma, and spindle cell melanomas with a fascicular pattern of growth may resemble neurofibromas, schwannomas, or leiomyomas. The latter consideration applies particularly to tumors of the ciliary body.

Immunohistochemical and molecular genetic features

Immunohistochemically, malignant melanomas are reactive for S-100 protein, HMB-45, and Mart-1 (Melan-A). They are also positive for vimentin and sometimes for low molecular weight keratins, such as those demonstrated with CAM 5.2.[245] It has been suggested that the melanoma cells exhibiting keratin immunostaining have a greater metastatic potential.[246]

Overexpression of P53 has been observed, but this seems to represent a late event in the course of the disease.[248]

Cytogenetically, common alterations include loss of 1p, 3 (usually in the form of monosomy 3), and 6q, and gain of 6p and 8q (usually in the form of trisomy 8q).[247,249,251] Mutations in the *GNAQ* gene are found in about half of the cases, representing the most common known oncogenic mutation in this cancer, and probably an early event in oncogenesis.[250]

DNA ploidy studies have shown that all spindle A melanomas are diploid, whereas a varying number of spindle B and epithelioid melanomas are aneuploid.[244]

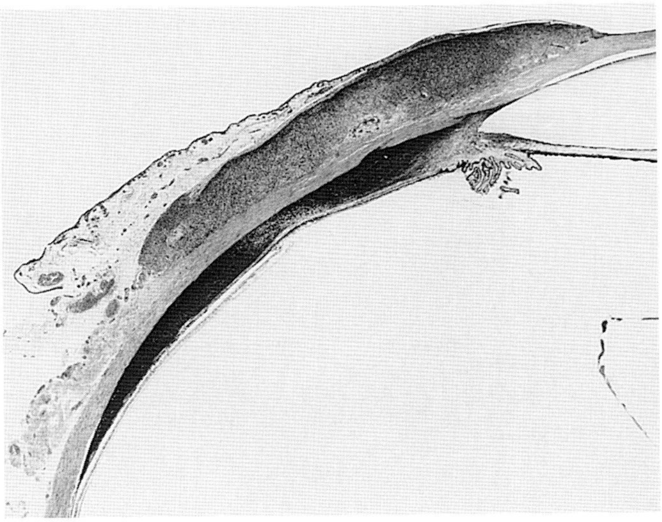

Fig. 30.54 Diffuse malignant melanoma of ciliary body and choroid that extended forward through scleral canals to form a large subconjunctival mass that encroached on the cornea.

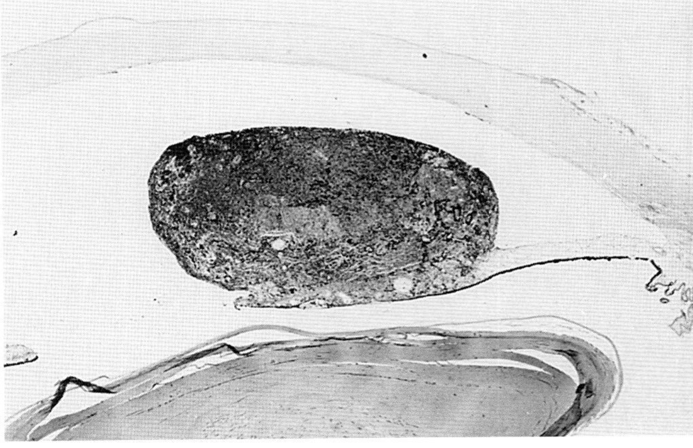

Fig. 30.55 Melanomas of iris are frequently visible through the cornea. Hence, their duration and rate of growth are often known by the patient or family long before other subjective or objective manifestations appear.

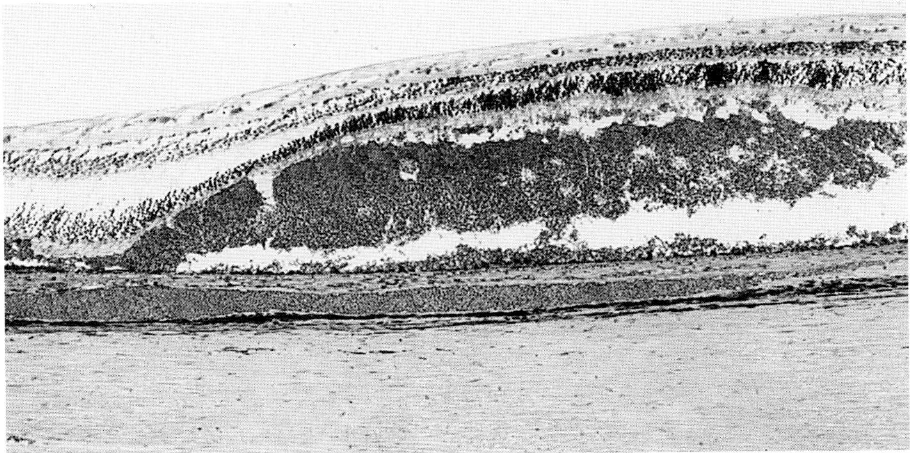

Fig. 30.56 This focal hemorrhage under the retina was clinically mistaken for melanoma.

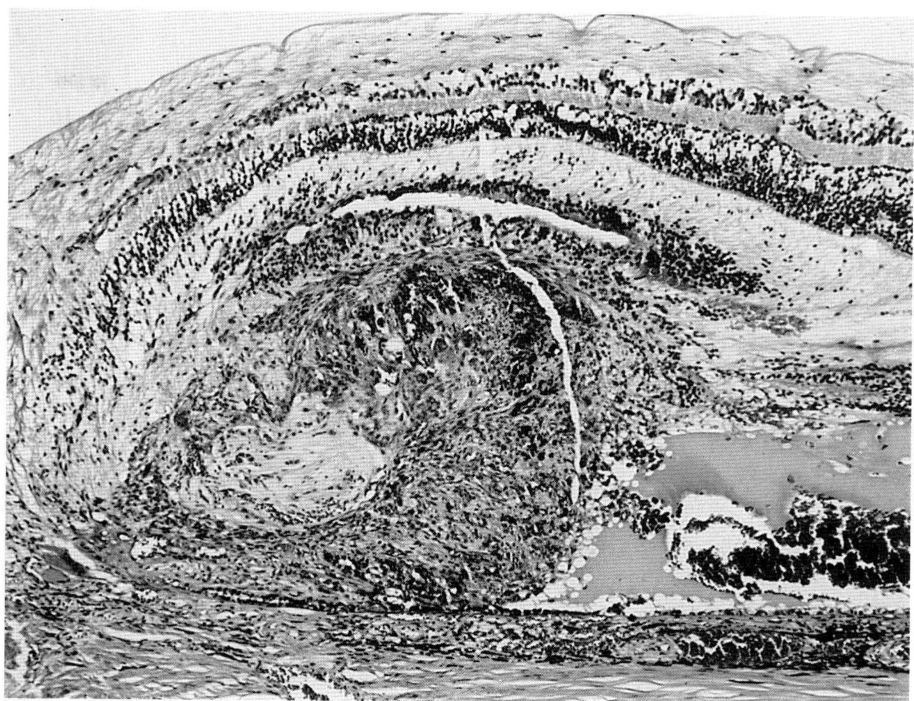

Fig. 30.57 A focal area of proliferation of retinal pigment epithelium that has elevated the retina to simulate melanoma.

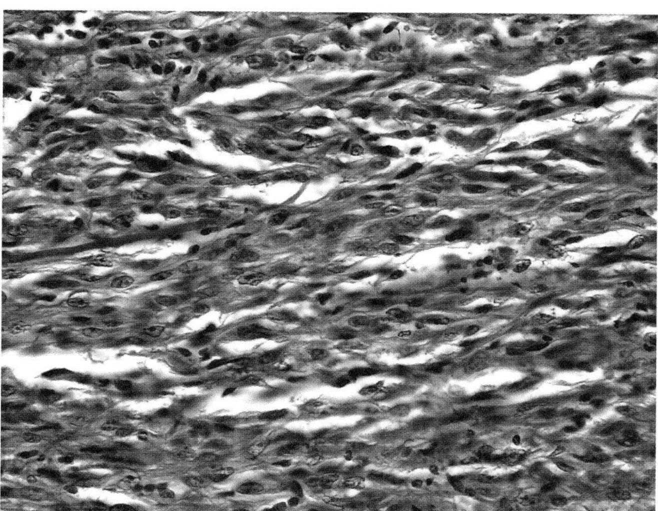

Fig. 30.58 So-called 'spindle B melanoma'. The tumor cells are spindle shaped and have conspicuous nucleoli.

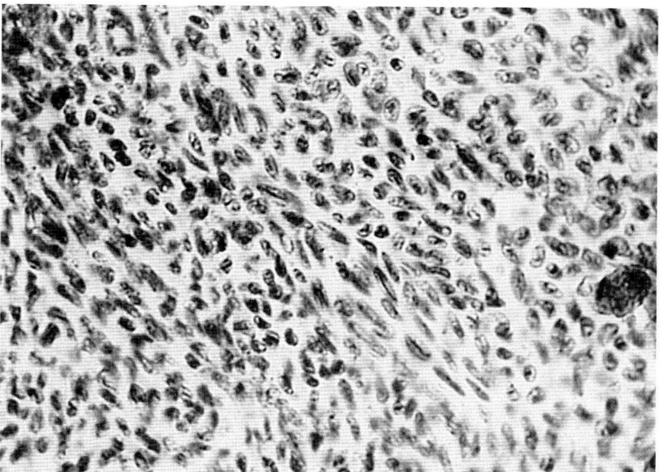

Fig. 30.59 Fascicular type of melanoma composed of spindle cells arranged about dilated capillaries.

Spread and metastases

The great tendency of uveal melanoma to spread along the course of the optic nerve has already been mentioned. The most common sites of distant metastatic involvement are liver, lung, bone, and skin.[252] The liver route is particularly common in uveal melanoma when compared to melanoma of the skin.[253] The skin metastases may simulate blue nevi clinically and pathologically.[254]

Treatment

The standard treatment of melanoma of the choroid has been enucleation of the eye, but several more conservative alternatives have gained in popularity.[258] Small melanomas of the iris can be treated by iridectomy or iridocyclectomy.[256] The suggestion has been made that enucleation may stimulate the development of metastatic disease,[259] but this has not been confirmed in other studies.[257] It is not clear whether the use of adjunctive radiation therapy improves prognosis.[255]

Prognosis

The overall mortality from metastasis of melanoma of the uveal tract 15 years after enucleation is close to 50%.[269] The prognosis of this tumor depends on several factors:

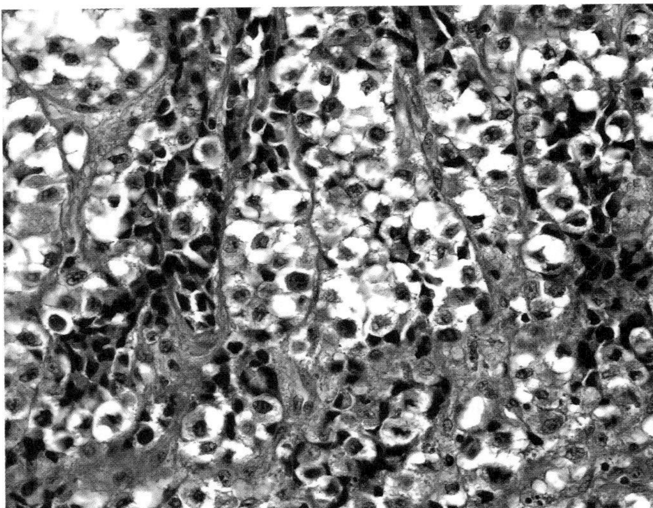

Fig. 30.60 Melanoma of epithelioid type. Some of the tumor cells have a clear cytoplasm, probably of artifactual nature.

1 *Cell type*. This is an extremely important parameter. There are no deaths with pure spindle A tumors, the proposal having therefore been made for these neoplasms to be regarded as spindle cell nevi rather than melanomas.[271] The 5-year survival rate is 66–75% for spindle B melanomas, 50% for mixed (spindle B and epithelioid) melanomas, and 25–33% for pure epithelioid melanomas.
2 *Tumor size*. Larger tumors have a worse prognosis than smaller ones.[266,269,272] It has been shown that tumor dimension is a better predictor of prognosis than height or volume.[275]
3 *Location*. Tumors located in the iris have an excellent prognosis.[276] This is in part related to their smaller size at the time of diagnosis and also to their less malignant cytologic features.[260,269] As a matter of fact, it has been suggested that most pigmented lesions of the iris traditionally designated as spindle A melanomas are benign nevi, as indicated previously.[267]
4 *Extension into the optic nerve*. This is said to be associated with a decreased survival, but there are conflicting data in this regard. A juxtapapillary location for the tumor does not result in significantly different survival rates if the optic nerve is not involved.[280]
5 *Extension into the sclera*. Extrascleral extension occurs in 10–28% of patients with choroidal melanoma.[272,274] In one series the 5-year mortality was 66% for patients with extrascleral extension and 33% for those with no extension.[278]
6 *Necrosis*. This is a sign of poor prognosis; it is usually associated with epithelioid-type tumors.
7 *Lymphocytic infiltration*. The presence of a large number of lymphocytes in the tumor stroma has been found to be significantly associated with decreased survival.[262]
8 *Neovascularization*. Melanomas with 'closed vascular loops' behave more aggressively than others, but this morphologic feature is associated with other unfavorable morphologic indicators, such as epithelioid cells.[264]
9 *Nucleolar prominence*. Nucleolar large size and pleomorphism are associated with aggressive behavior in uveal melanoma. Various methods have been devised to quantify this determination, including automated image capture and analysis of AgNOR-stained sections.[265,268,270,277]

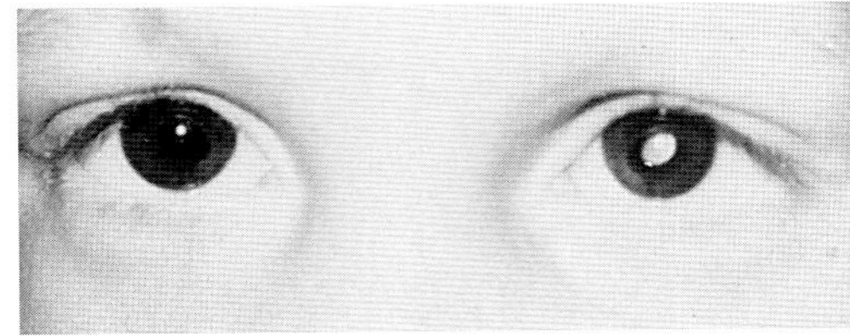

Fig. 30.61 Prominent white reflex attributed to retinoblastoma present in the dilated pupil of the left eye.

10 *Amount of pigmentation*. This feature does not have independent prognostic significance.
11 *DNA ploidy*. Most studies have found no significant correlations between DNA ploidy status and prognosis once the melanomas have been stratified into the major morphologic subtypes.[261]
12 MDR1 *expression*. Expression of the *MDR1* gene and its product P-glycoprotein seem to correlate with an adverse prognosis.[263]
13 *Gene expression profile*. Gene expression profiling studies have shown that uveal melanomas cluster into two molecular groups – tumors with the class 1 signature rarely metastasize, whereas those with the class 2 signature have a very high rate of metastasis.[273] Low expression of genes on 3p is also associated with a poor prognosis.[279]

Retinoblastoma and related lesions

General features

Retinoblastoma is the most common intraocular neoplasm of children. It is generally believed to be congenital and derived from primitive neuroectodermal cells exhibiting retinal differentiation.[284–286] However, retinoblastomas are seldom recognized until considerable growth has taken place and are usually diagnosed between the ages of 16 months and 2 years. Approximately 60% of the cases are sporadic, and the other 40% are familial, the predisposition to tumor development being transmitted in an autosomal dominant pattern. Retinoblastoma will develop in 80–90% of persons who carry any one of a variety of mutant alleles associated with a predisposition to the tumor.[288]

The responsible gene has been located in chromosome 13q14 and designated the retinoblastoma (*RB*) gene.[287] Gene mutations in both alleles are necessary to produce inactivation of the RB protein, which is a negative regulator of cell growth.[282,289,291] Patients with hereditary retinoblastoma have a germ cell mutation in one allele and develop the retinoblastoma as a result of a somatic mutation in the second allele, whereas in patients with sporadic retinoblastoma both mutations are somatic.[281,290] This model, known as Knudson's 'two-hit hypothesis', has become a paradigm of tumorigenesis.[283]

Clinical and gross features

Retinoblastomas characteristically present as a leukocoria (white pupillary reflex; Fig. 30.61) or less often as a strabismus when the tumor is in the macula. Rarely, extraocular extension with the formation of an orbital mass is the presenting manifestation.

Retinoblastomas may be flat and diffuse or elevated, and may show multicentric foci of origin, especially in the hereditary type. They may protrude into the vitreous (endophytic type; Fig. 30.62), often with vitreous seeding, or they may grow between the retina

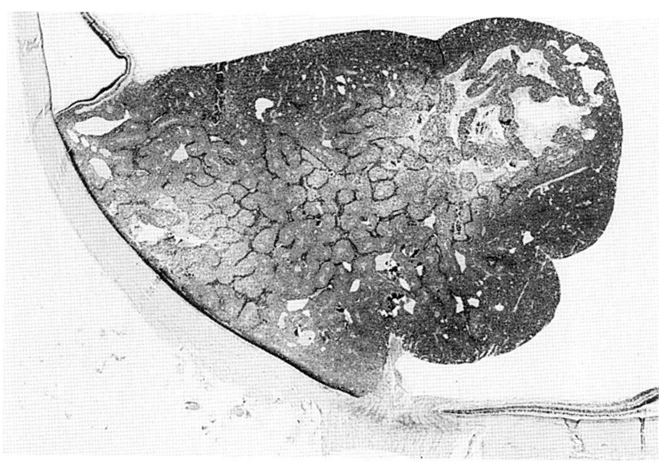

Fig. 30.62 Retinoblastoma presenting as a highly cellular neoplasm with scanty stroma. The tumor tends to outgrow its blood supply, and irregular areas of necrosis are commonly observed.

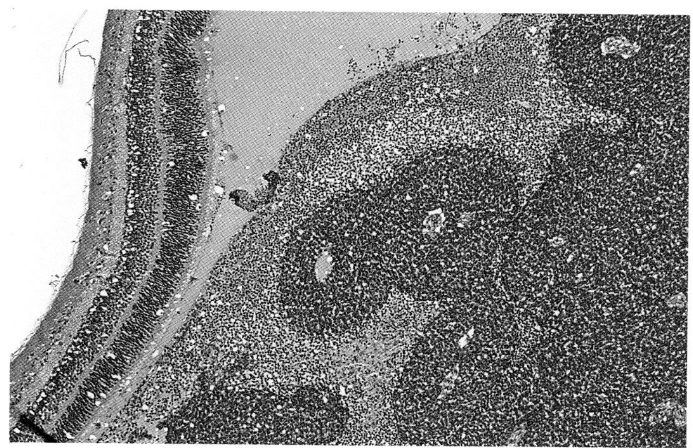

Fig. 30.63 Low-power view of retinoblastoma. There is a collar of viable cells about nutrient vessels (so-called peritheliomatous pattern). The normal retina is seen on the left.

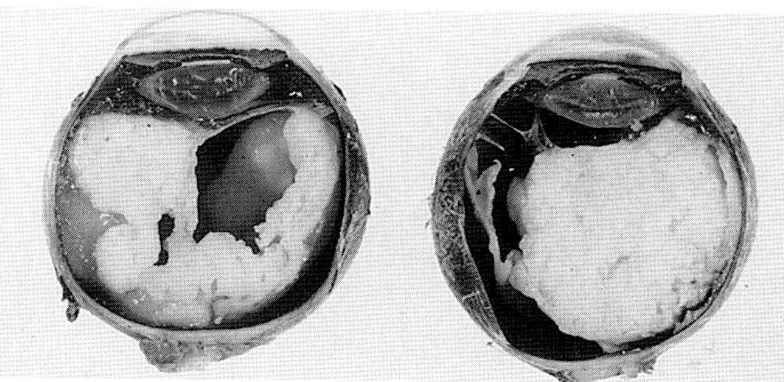

Fig. 30.64 Bilateral retinoblastoma showing a white mass consisting of detached retina and neoplastic tissue immediately behind the lens in each eye.

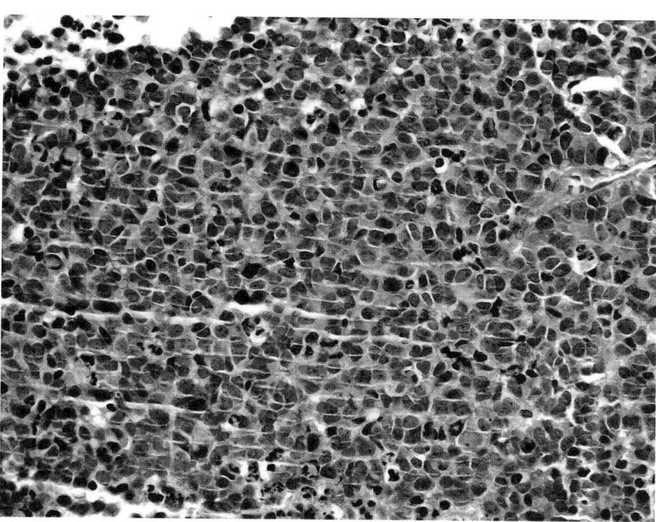

Fig. 30.65 Poorly differentiated retinoblastoma. The appearance is that of a malignant small round cell tumor.

and the pigment epithelium (exophytic type). Since the tumors tend to outgrow their blood supply, necrosis is often extensive and many minute foci of calcification are often present in these areas of necrosis (Fig. 30.63). In fact, these areas of calcification may be appreciated by x-ray examination prior to enucleation.

Bilaterality is present in 30% of all cases and in over 90% of the familial cases (Fig. 30.64). Some patients have presented with bilateral retinoblastoma and a morphologically similar intracranial neoplasm localized in the region of the pineal gland, in keeping with the 'third eye' nature of the latter structure.[295] These are referred as *trilateral retinoblastomas*[292,293] and are associated with a particularly dismal prognosis.[297]

The clinical differential diagnosis of retinoblastoma includes any disease process that leads to retinal detachment or a retrolental mass in a child under 6 years of age.[294,296] Lesions in this category include traumatic or idiopathic retinal detachments, retrolental fibroplasia, persistent hyperplastic primary vitreous, massive retinal gliosis, Coats disease, nematodiasis, astrocytomas of tuberous sclerosis, and medulloepitheliomas. Some of these disorders are discussed elsewhere in this chapter.

Microscopic features

Microscopically, retinoblastomas are composed of dense masses of small round cells with hyperchromatic nuclei and scanty cytoplasm[300] (Fig. 30.65). Trabecular and nesting formations are common.[302] Hematoxyphilic deposits in and around blood vessel walls are often seen in necrotic areas, similar to those found in pulmonary small cell carcinomas.[298] A sign of differentiation toward retinal structures is provided by the presence of so-called 'Flexner–Wintersteiner rosettes' and fleurettes (Fig. 30.66). *Differentiated retinoblastoma* is characterized by the presence of a bipolar-like cell element.[299]

Tumors showing an extreme degree of differentiation are designated as *retinocytomas* and regarded as benign.[301] These lesions carry the same genetic implications as conventional retinoblastomas; they present as small placoid, noninvasive lesions composed entirely of benign-appearing cells with numerous fleurettes, lacking necrosis or mitotic activity.[301]

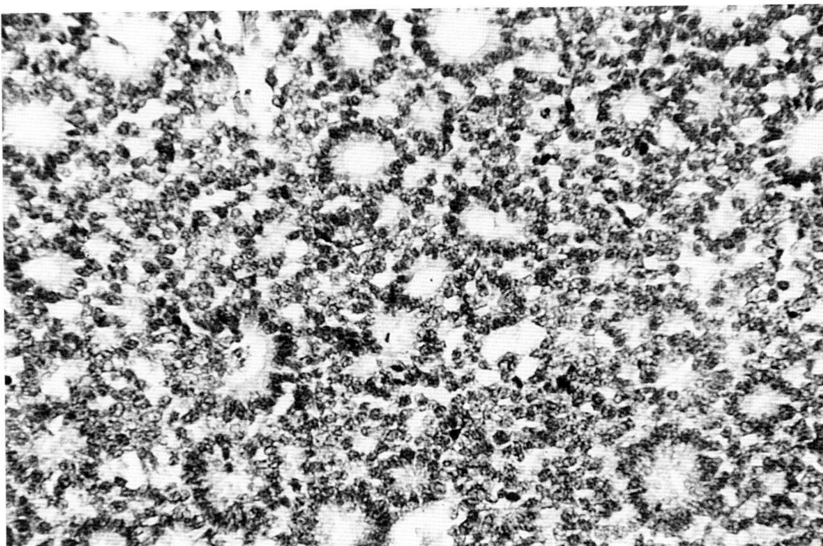

Fig. 30.66 Retinoblastoma with typical rosettes. *(From Ackerman LV, del Regato JA. Cancer, ed. 6. St Louis, 1985, Mosby)*

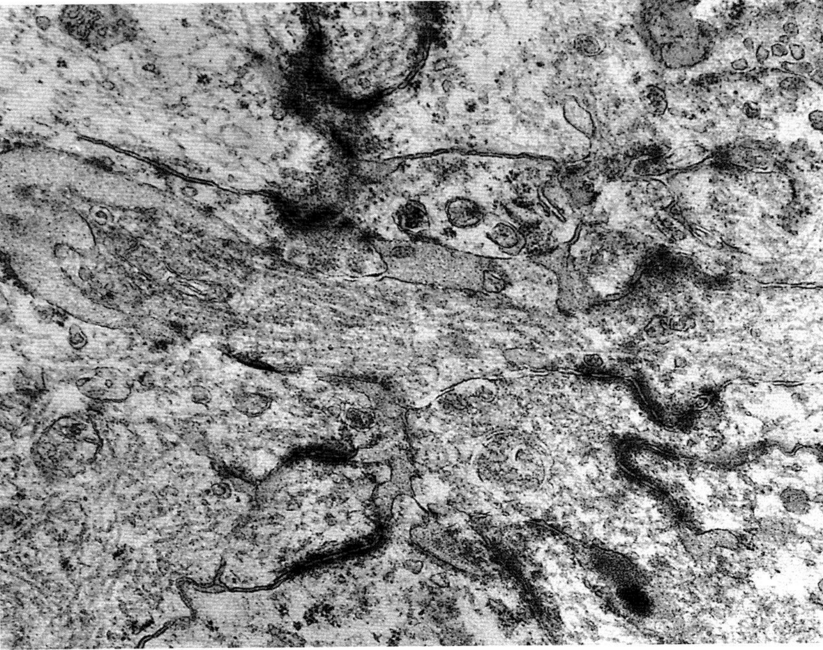

Fig. 30.67 Electron micrograph of retinoblastoma. A portion of the center of a rudimentary Flexner–Wintersteiner rosette illustrating a bulbous apical microtubule-containing cytoplasmic process and numerous cell junctions. (×20 800) *(Courtesy of Dr Robert A Erlandson, Memorial Sloan-Kettering Cancer Center)*

Electron microscopic, immunohistochemical, and molecular genetic features

Ultrastructurally, evidence of photodifferentiation has been found in the tumor cells of retinoblastoma[315,316] (Fig. 30.67). Immunohistochemically, there is reactivity for neuron-specific enolase, synaptophysin, S-100 protein, glial fibrillary acidic protein, myelin basic protein, and Leu7 (CD57), in keeping with an origin from a pluripotential neuroectodermal cell that retains neuronal and glial features.[313,314,318,319] In addition, allegedly specific markers of retinal differentiation such as retinal-binding protein, retinal S-antigen, interphotoreceptor retinal-binding protein, cone opsin, rod opsin, and MLGAPC (a mucin-like glycoprotein associated with photoreceptor cells) have been found in these tumors.[305,306,311] Interestingly, retinal S-antigen has also been detected in tumors of the pineal gland and in cerebellar medulloblastomas.[307,311] Further evidence of the retinal nature of this tumor has been obtained in vitro, where differentiation toward photoreceptors has been observed spontaneously or after the addition of differentiating agents.[317]

The MIB-1 labeling index is extremely high. Limited P53 immunostaining is present in over half of the cases. In contrast to Ewing sarcoma/PNET, most neuroblastomas are negative for CD99.[312]

Besides loss-of-function mutations in the *RB* gene, other common genetic alterations in retinoblastoma include gain of 1q, 2p, 6p, and

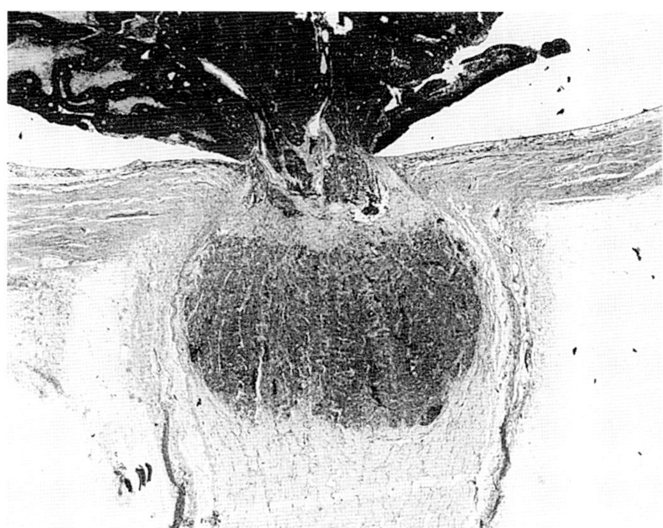

Fig. 30.68 Retinoblastomas exhibit a definite tendency to spread out of the globe by way of the optic nerve. It is therefore of utmost importance for the surgical pathologist to determine whether such optic nerve extension has occurred and, if it has, to what extent.

13q, and loss of 16q.[303,304,308,309] Some cases also show amplifications of the *NMYC*, *MDMX* or *MDM2* gene.[310]

Spread and metastases

Retinoblastoma has a tendency to invade the optic nerve, from which it can extend to the brain or be carried there by the subarachnoid fluid[321] (Fig. 30.68). Large exophytic tumors with secondary glaucoma are at highest risk for optic nerve invasion.[321] Retinoblastoma can also invade the uveal tract. Distant metastases can be limited to the cranial vault or involve distant sites, particularly the skeletal system.[320]

Treatment

The treatment of retinoblastoma depends on the extent of the disease.[327,329] Early cases can be managed with conservative measures aimed at preserving the vision, such as unilateral radiation, cryopexy, or xenon arc photocoagulation.[324] When the tumor is so large that the eye is no longer salvageable, enucleation should be performed.[330] If tumor has extended to the surgically cut end of the nerve, irradiation of the orbit and systemic chemotherapy are performed. In patients with bilateral retinoblastoma, the less affected eye is treated with radiotherapy, at times in combination with chemotherapy. Bilateral cases can also be treated with simultaneous bilateral irradiation.[322,323,325] The success rate for life of the patient and for preservation of vision is quite good. If tumor recurrences develop, they are treated with photocoagulation, cryotherapy, and cobalt discs. Chemotherapy is administered to disseminated cases, but so far with disappointing results.[326] Novel molecular targeting therapies are also being developed.[328]

Prognosis

The 5-year survival of unilateral retinoblastoma following adequate treatment is over 90% and slightly less for the bilateral cases.[339,340] Features that correlate with prognosis in retinoblastoma and which therefore need to be carefully analyzed by the pathologist[337] are as follows:

1 *Invasion of optic nerve*. In an operation for suspected neuroblastoma, the surgeon will attempt to obtain a long segment of optic nerve attached to the globe. Transverse sections of this nerve should be examined microscopically at the prelaminar and retrolaminar levels, including the surgical margin.[337] The levels of invasion of the optic nerve by retinoblastoma have been divided into prelaminar, laminar, and retrolaminar, the latter further subdivided into lesions with or without resection line involvement.[337] The prognosis decreases with each of these levels.[334–336]

2 *Invasion of meninges*. This is often associated with invasion of the optic nerve.[336]

3 *Invasion of the uveal tract*. Massive invasion of the uveal tract by retinoblastoma is an unfavorable prognostic sign.[334,335]

Long-term survivors have a greater incidence of development of malignant tumors. The incidence has ranged from 6% to 20% after 10 years, and in one series has reached 90% at 30 years. The most common types have been osteosarcoma and rhabdomyosarcoma, but several other types have been encountered, including rhabdoid tumors.[331,338] This predisposition for a second malignancy, which should be distinguished from a recurrence of the retinoblastoma,[333] is seen almost exclusively with the hereditary form of the disease.[332]

Lymphoid tumors and tumorlike conditions

Abnormalities of intraocular tissues are present in approximately 50% of patients with leukemia at autopsy.[341] These are in the form of leukemic infiltrates and hemorrhages, particularly in the choroid and retina.[341,347]

Intraocular **malignant lymphoma** is a rare disease. In contrast to other portions of the ocular apparatus, in which MALT-type lymphomas predominate, most intraocular lymphomas (also known as primary retinal lymphomas) are aggressive diffuse B-cell lymphomas.[342] In over 90% of the cases the eye lesion heralds the presence or development of extraocular lymphoma, which is located in the central nervous system in one-half or more of the cases.[344] Sometimes the lymphomatous process preferentially involves the optic nerve.[343]

Reactive lymphoid hyperplasia can also occur within the ocular globe;[345,346] the criteria for distinguishing it from lymphoma are similar to those applied elsewhere.

Other primary tumors

Fuchs adenoma (benign ciliary epithelioma, Fuchs epithelioma, coronal adenoma) is a benign tumor of the ciliary body usually found incidentally in a surgically enucleated eye or on post mortem examination. Microscopically, it is formed by interlacing trabeculae of uniform, nonpigmented ciliary epithelial cells surrounded by an amorphous, hyaline, periodic acid–Schiff (PAS)-positive material.[358]

Medulloepithelioma, also known as *diktyoma,* is a rare tumor that histologically resembles the embryonal retina; most cases arise from the ciliary epithelium, but a few have been found in the optic nerve or retina. The treatment is conservative.[351]

Leiomyomas can develop in the ciliary body or the iris. Some of these tumors are regarded as of possible neural crest origin and designated as *mesectodermal leiomyomas.*[349] Epstein–Barr virus-associated smooth muscle tumors have been reported in immunosuppressed paients.[357] **Hemangiomas, hemangioblastomas** (as a component of von Hippel–Lindau disease), **neurofibromas, astrocytomas**, and **pleomorphic xanthoastrocytomas** are sometimes found in the retina,[352,354,356,359] and a case of PEComa has been described in the ciliary body.[353]

Juvenile xanthogranuloma can occur in the iris and result in spontaneous hyphema and/or secondary glaucoma.[350] It occurs almost exclusively in young children and is associated with skin lesions of similar microscopic appearance.[360]

Glioneuroma has been described in the iris and ciliary body,[348] and **malignant mesenchymoma** (containing rhabdomyosarcomatous and liposarcomatous areas) has been reported involving the entire uveal tract.[355]

Metastatic tumors

The intraocular tissues can be involved by metastatic carcinoma and, less commonly, by metastatic cutaneous melanoma and metastatic sarcoma. In fact, if one were to do serial sections routinely on all autopsy eyes, cases of metastatic carcinoma would outnumber the primary tumors. The difference, of course, is that most of the patients were asymptomatic for ocular symptoms while alive. The most common primary lesions involved are in the breast in the female and in the lung in the male, with the gastrointestinal tract next in frequency.[361,363–366] The ocular metastasis occasionally may be the initial manifestation of the disease, and the primary lesion is discovered only after the eye has been enucleated.

The posterior choroid is the most common site for these metastases[362] (Fig. 30.69). Anterior uveal involvement is much less common, and retinal metastases are rare. Diffuse thickening of the choroid along both sides of the optic nerve is the most common presentation, but bulky tumor masses resembling malignant melanomas also may be observed.

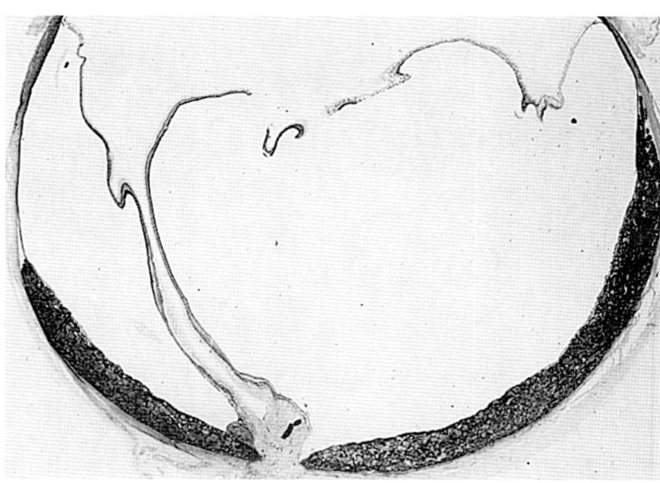

Fig. 30.69 Metastatic carcinoma from breast producing diffuse thickening of the choroid posteriorly.

Cytology

In certain cases the pathologist may be called on to examine material that has been aspirated from either the aqueous or the vitreous fluid and has been passed through a Millipore filter. Cases in which this has proved useful include large cell lymphoma,[368] retinoblastoma,[370] and phacolytic glaucoma.[369] Analysis of clonal immunoglobulin heavy chain gene rearrangements for the confirmation of a diagnosis of lymphoma can be carried out on this material.[367]

References

NORMAL ANATOMY

1 Campbell RJ. Histological typing of tumours of the eye and the adnexa. London, 1998, Springer.

2 Font RL, Croxatto JO, Rao NA. Tumors of the eye and ocular adnexa (AFIP atlas of tumor pathology). Washington, DC, 2006, American Registry of Pathology in collaboration with the Armed Forces Institute of Pathology.

3 Harry J, Misson G. Clinical ophthalmic pathology: principles of diseases of the eye and associated structures. Oxford, 2001, Butterworth Heinemann.

4 Hogan MJ, Zimmerman LE. Ophthalmic pathology. An atlas and textbook, ed. 2. Philadelphia, 1962, W.B. Saunders.

5 Hogan MJ, Alvarado JA, Weddell JE. Histology of the human eye. An atlas and textbook. Philadelphia, 1971, W.B. Saunders.

6 Jakobiec FA. Ocular and adnexal tumors. Birmingham, AL, 1978, Aesculapius.

7 Klintworth GK, Cummings TJ. Normal eye and ocular adnexia. In Mills SE (ed.): Histology for pathologists, ed. 3. Philadelphia, 2007, Lippincott Williams & Wilkins, pp. 247–270.

8 McLean IW, Burnier MN, Zimmerman LE, Jakobiec FA. Tumors of the eye and ocular adnexa. Atlas of tumor pathology, series 3, fascicle 12. Bethesda, 1994, Armed Forces Institute of Pathology.

9 Reese AB. Tumors of the eye, ed. 3. New York, 1976, Harper and Row.

10 Shields CL. Eyelid conjuctival and orbital tumors: an atlas and text, ed. 2. Philadelphia, 2007, Lippincott Williams & Wilkins.

11 Shields CL. Intraocular tumors: an atlas and text, ed. 2, Philadelphia, 2007, Lippincott Williams & Wilkins.

12 Spencer WH. Ophthalmic pathology: an atlas and textbook. Philadelphia, 1996, W.B. Saunders.

13 Yanoff M, Sassani JW. Ocular pathology, ed. 6. St Louis, 2008, Mosby.

EYELIDS

INFLAMMATION

14 Codère F, Lee RD, Anderson RL. Necrobiotic xanthogranuloma of the eyelid. Arch Ophthalmol 1983, **101**: 60–63.

15 Riddle PJ, Font RL, Johnson FB, McLean IW. Silica granuloma of eyelid and ocular adnexa. Arch Ophthalmol 1981, **99**: 683–689.

16 Ross MJ, Cohen KL, Peiffer RL Jr, Grimson BS. Episcleral and orbital pseudorheumatoid nodules. Arch Ophthalmol 1983, **101**: 418–421.

CYSTS

17 Jakobiec FA, Mehta M, Iwamoto M, Hatton MP, Thakker M, Fay A. Intratarsal keratinous cysts of the Meibomian gland: distinctive clinicopathologic and immunohistochemical features in 6 cases. Am J Ophthalmol 2010, **149**: 82–94.

TUMORS AND TUMORLIKE LESIONS

Tumors and tumorlike lesions of surface epithelium

18 Aurora AL, Blodi FC. Lesions of the eyelids. A clinicopathologic study. Surv Ophthalmol 1970, **15**: 94–104.

19 Boniuk M. Tumors of the eyelids. Int Ophthalmol Clin 1962, **2**: 239–317.

20 Boniuk M, Zimmerman LE. Eyelid tumors with reference to lesions confused with squamous cell carcinoma. II. Inverted follicular keratosis. Arch Ophthalmol 1963, **69**: 698–707.

21 Boniuk M, Zimmerman LE. Eyelid tumors with reference to lesions confused with squamous cell carcinoma. III. Keratoacanthoma. Arch Ophthalmol 1967, **77**: 29–40.

22 Caya JG, Hidayat AA, Weiner JM. A clinicopathologic study of 21 cases of adenoid squamous cell carcinoma of the eyelid and periorbital region. Am J Ophthalmol 1985, **99**: 291–297.

23 Chaflin J, Putterman AM. Frozen section control in the surgery of basal cell carcinoma of the eyelid. Am J Ophthalmol 1979, **87**: 802–809.

24 Donaldson MJ, Sullivan TJ, Whitehead KJ, Williamson RM. Squamous cell carcinoma of the eyelids. Br J Ophthalmol 2002, **86**: 1161–1165.

25 Giacomin AL, di Pietro R, Steindler P. Merkel cell carcinoma: a distinct lesion of the eyelid. Orbit 1999, **18**: 295–303.

26 Kwitko ML, Boniuk M, Zimmerman LE. Eyelid tumors with reference to lesions confused with squamous cell carcinoma. I. Incidence and errors in diagnosis. Arch Ophthalmol 1963, **69**: 693–697.

27 Searl SS, Boynton JR, Markowitch W, di Sant' Agnese PA. Malignant Merkel cell neoplasm of the eyelid. Arch Ophthalmol 1984, **102**: 907–911.

Adnexal tumors

28 Doxanas MT, Green WR. Sebaceous gland carcinoma. Review of 40 cases. Arch Ophthalmol 1984, **102**: 245–249.

29 Hassan AS, Nelson CC. Benign eyelid tumors and skin diseases. Int Ophthalmol Clin 2002, **42**: 135–149.

30 Hidayat AA, Font RL. Trichilemmoma of eyelid and eyebrow. A clinicopathologic study of 31 cases. Arch Ophthalmol 1980, **98**: 844–847.

31 Howrey RP, Lipham WJ, Schultz WH, Buckley EG, Dutton JJ, Klintworth GK, Rosoff PM. Sebaceous gland carcinoma: a subtle second malignancy following radiation therapy in patients with bilateral retinoblastoma. Cancer 1998, **83**: 767–771.

32 Izumi M, Mukai K, Nagai T, Matsubayashi J, Iwaya K, Chiu CS, Goto H. Sebaceous carcinoma of the eyelids: thirty cases from Japan. Pathol Int 2008, **58**: 483–488.

33 Langel DJ, Yeatts RP, White WL. Primary signet ring cell carcinoma of the eyelid: report of a case demonstrating further analogy to lobular carcinoma of the breast with a literature review. Am J Dermatopathol 2002, **23**: 444–449.

34 Langer K, Konrad K, Smolle J. Multiple apocrine hidrocystomas on the eyelids. Am J Dermatopathol 1989, **11**: 570–573.

35 Lee JH, Shin YW, Oh YH, Lee YJ. Trichilemmal carcinoma of the upper eyelid: a case report. Korean J Ophthalmol 2009, **23**: 301–305.

36 Pantanowitz L, Lyle S, Tahan SR. Fibroadenoma of the eyelid. Am J Dermatopathol 2002, **24**: 225–229.

37 Rao NA, Hidayat AA, McLean IW, Zimmerman LE. Sebaceous carcinomas of the ocular adnexa. A clinicopathologic study of 104 cases, with five-year follow-up data. Hum Pathol 1982, **13**: 113–122.

38 Rodgers IR, Jakobiec FA, Krebs W, Hornblass A, Gingold MP. Papillary oncocytoma of the eyelid. A previously undescribed tumor of apocrine gland origin. Ophthalmology 1988, **95**: 1071–1076.

39 Russel WG, Page DL, Hough AJ, Rogers LW. Sebaceous carcinoma of meibomian gland origin. The diagnostic importance of pagetoid spread of neoplastic cells. Am J Clin Pathol 1980, **73**: 504–511.

40 Shintaku M, Tsuta K, Yoshida H, Tsubura A, Nakashima Y, Noda K. Apocrine adenocarcinoma of the eyelid with aggressive biological behavior: report of a case. Pathol Int 2002, **52**: 169–173.

41 Snow SN, Reizner GT. Mucinous eccrine carcinoma of the eyelid. Cancer 1992, **70**: 2099–2104.

42 Tomasini C, Soro E, Pippione M. Eyelid swelling: think of metastasis of histiocytoid breast carcinoma. Dermatology 2002, **205**: 63–66.

43 Wolfe JT III, Yeatts RP, Wick MR, Campbell RJ, Waller RR. Sebaceous carcinoma of the eyelid. Errors in clinical and pathologic diagnosis. Am J Surg Pathol 1984, **8**: 597–606.

44 Wright JD, Font RL. Mucinous sweat gland adenocarcinoma of eyelid. A clinicopathologic study of 21 cases with histochemical and electron microscopic observations. Cancer 1979, **44**: 1757–1768.

Melanocytic tumors

45 Esmaeli B. Advances in the management of malignant tumors of the eyelid and conjunctiva: the role of sentinel lymph node biopsy. Int Ophthalmol Clin 2002, **42**: 151–162.

46 Henkind P, Friedman A. External ocular pigmentation. Int Ophthalmol Clin 1971, **11**: 87–111.

47 Pomeranz GA, Bunt AH, Kalina RE. Multifocal choroidal melanoma in ocular melanocytosis. Arch Ophthalmol 1981, **99**: 857–863.

48 Vaziri M, Buffam FV, Martinka M, Oryschak A, Dhaliwal H, White VA. Clinicopathologic features and behavior of cutaneous eyelid melanoma. Ophthalmology 2002, **109**: 901–908.

Lymphoid tumors and tumorlike conditions

49 Sanka RK, Eagle RC Jr, Wojno TH, Neufeld KR, Grossniklaus HE. Spectrum of CD30+ lymphoid proliferations in the eyelid lymphomatoid papulosis, cutaneous anaplastic large cell lymphoma, and anaplastic large cell lymphoma. Ophthalmology 2010, **117**: 343–351.

50 Stenson S, Ramsay DL. Ocular findings in mycosis fungoides. Arch Ophthalmol 1981, **99**: 272–277.

Mesenchymal tumors and tumorlike conditions

51 Fett DR, Putterman AM. Primary localized amyloidosis presenting as an eyelid margin tumor. Arch Ophthalmol 1986, **104**: 584–585.

52 Furusato E, Cameron JD, Newsom RW, Fujishiro T, Kojima T, Specht CS, Fetsch JF, Furusato B, Sesterhenn IA, Rushing EJ. Ocular perivascular epithelioid cell tumor: report of 2 cases with distinct clinical presentations. Hum Pathol 2010, **41**: 768–772.

53 Hassan AS, Nelson CC. Benign eyelid tumors and skin diseases. Int Ophthalmol Clin 2002, **42**: 135–149.

54 Kakizaki H, Maden A, Türe M, Yilmaz S, Chan WO. Hemangiopericytoma-solitary fibrous tumor of the eyelid. Ophthal Plast Reconstr Surg 2010, **26**: 46–48.

55 Smith ME, Zimmerman LE. Amyloidosis of the eyelid and conjunctiva. Arch Ophthalmol 1966, **75**: 42–56.

56 Sorenson RL, Spencer WH, Stewart WB, Miller WW, Kleinhenz RJ. Intravascular papillary endothelial hyperplasia of the eyelid. Arch Ophthalmol 1983, **101**: 1728–1730.

57 Tsuji H, Kanda H, Kashiwagi H, Mimura T. Primary epithelioid haemangioendothelioma of the eyelid. Br J Ophthalmol 2010, **94**: 261–262.

Metastatic tumors

58 Hood CI, Font RL, Zimmerman LE. Metastatic mammary carcinoma in the eyelid with histiocytoid appearance. Cancer 1973, **31**: 793–800.

LACRIMAL GLAND

MIKULICZ DISEASE

59 Cheuk W, Chan JK. IgG4-related sclerosing disease: a critical appraisal of an evolving clinicopathologic entity. Adv Anat Pathol 2010, **17**: 303–332.

60 Font RL, Yanoff M, Zimmerman LE. Benign lymphoepithelial lesion of the lacrimal gland and its relationship to Sjögren's syndrome. Am J Clin Pathol 1967, **48**: 365–376.

61 Godwin JT. Benign lymphoepithelial lesion of the parotid gland (adenolymphoma, chronic inflammation, lymphoepithelioma, lymphocytic tumor, Mikulicz's disease). Cancer 1952, **5**: 1089–1103.

62 Meyer D, Yanoff M, Hanno H. Differential diagnosis in Mikulicz syndrome, Mikulicz's disease, and similar disease entities. Am J Ophthalmol 1971, **70**: 516–524.

TUMORS AND TUMORLIKE CONDITIONS

63 Ahn M, Osipov V, Harris GJ. Collagenous fibroma (desmoplastic fibroblastoma) of the lacrimal gland. Ophthal Plast Reconstr Surg 2009, **25**: 250–252.

64 Bernardini FP, Devoto MH, Croxatto JO. Epithelial tumors of the lacrimal gland: an update. Curr Opin Ophthalmol 2008, **19**: 409–413.

65 Cheuk W, Yuen HK, Chan JK. Chronic sclerosing dacryoadenitis: part of the spectrum of IgG4-related sclerosing disease? Am J Surg Pathol 2007, **31**: 643–645.

66 Cho NH, Kie JH, Yang WI, Jung WH. Solitary fibrous tumour with an unusual adenofibromatous feature in the lacrimal gland. Histopathology 1998, **33**: 289–290.

67 DeRosa G, Zeppa P, Tranfa F, Bonavolontà G. Acinic cell carcinoma arising in a lacrimal gland. First case report. Cancer 1986, **57**: 1988–1991.

68 Fernando BS, Thaung C, Ataullah S, Chakravarthi R, Bonshek R, Sloan P. Necrotizing metaplasia of lacrimal gland/ necrotizing dacryometaplasia. Histopathology 2007, **51**: 578–580.

69 Forrest AW. Pathologic criteria for effective management of epithelial lacrimal gland tumors. Am J Ophthalmol 1971, **71**: 178–192.

70 Gamel JW, Font RL. Adenoid cystic carcinoma of the lacrimal gland. The clinical significance of a basaloid histologic pattern. Hum Pathol 1982, **13**: 219–225.

71 George E, Swanson PE, Newman BK, Wick MR. Oculocutaneous oncocytic tumors: clinicopathologic and immunohistochemical study of 2 cases with literature review. Am J Dermatopathol 2007, **29**: 279–285.

72 Iwamoto T, Jakobiec FA. A comparative ultrastructural study of the normal lacrimal gland and its epithelial tumors. Hum Pathol 1982, **13**: 236–262.

73 Ludwig ME, LiVolsi VA, McMahon RT. Malignant mixed tumor of the lacrimal gland. Am J Surg Pathol 1979, **3**: 457–462.

74 Morgan MB, Truitt CA, Romer C, Somach S, Pitha JV. Ocular adnexal oncocytoma: a case series and clinicopathologic review of the literature. Am J Dermatopathol 1998, **20**: 487–490.

75 Paulino AFG, Huvos AG. Epithelial tumors of the lacrimal glands: a clinicopathologic study. Ann Diagn Pathol 1999, **3**: 199–204.

76 Pecorella I, Garner A. Ostensible oncocytoma of accessory lacrimal glands. Histopathology 1997, **30**: 264–270.

77 Perzin KH, Jakobiec FA, LiVolsi VA, Desjardins L. Lacrimal gland malignant mixed tumors (carcinomas arising in benign mixed tumors). A clinico-pathologic study. Cancer 1980, **45**: 2593–2606.

78 Sabet SJ, Tarbet KJ, Lemke BN, Smith ME, Albert DM. Granular cell tumor of the lacrimal sac and nasolacrimal duct: no invasive behavior with incomplete resection. Ophthalmology 2000, **170**: 1992–1994.

79 Sanders TE, Ackerman LV, Zimmerman LE. Epithelial tumors of the lacrimal gland. A comparison of the pathologic and clinical behavior with those of the salivary glands. Am J Surg 1962, **104**: 657–665.

80 von Holstein SL, Østergaard J, Daugaard S, Toft PB, Heegaard S. Granular cell tumour of the lacrimal gland. Acta Ophthalmol 2009, **87**: 926–927.

81 Weis E, Rootman J, Joly TJ, Berean KW, Al-Katan HM, Pasternak S, Bonavolontà G, Strianese D, Saeed P, Feldman KA, Vangveeravong S, Lapointe JS, White VA. Epithelial lacrimal gland tumors: pathologic classification and current understanding. Arch Ophthalmol 2009, **127**: 1016–1028.

82 Wiwatwongwana D, Berean KW, Dolman PJ, Rootman J, White VA. Unusual carcinomas of the lacrimal gland: epithelial–myoepithelial carcinoma and myoepithelial carcinoma. Arch Ophthalmol 2009, **127**: 1054–1056.

83 Yazici B, Setzen G, Meyer DR, Williams EF, McKenna BJ. Giant cell angiofibroma of the nasolacrimal duct. Ophthal Plast Reconstr Surg 2001, **17**: 202–206.

84 Zimmerman LE, Sanders TE, Ackerman LV. Epithelial tumors of the lacrimal gland. Prognostic and therapeutic significance of histologic types. Int Ophthalmol Clin 1962, **2**: 337–367.

LACRIMAL PASSAGES

CANALICULITIS AND DACRYOCYSTITIS

85 Harris GJ, Williams GA, Clarke GP. Sarcoidosis of the lacrimal sac. Arch Ophthalmol 1981, **99**: 1198–1201.

TUMORS

86 Kuwabara H, Takeda J. Malignant melanoma of the lacrimal sac with surrounding melanosis. Arch Pathol Lab Med 1997, **121**: 517–519.

87 Lamping KA, Albert DM, Ni C, Fournier G. Oxyphil cell adenomas. Three case reports. Arch Ophthalmol 1984, **102**: 263–265.

88 Lee HM, Kang HJ, Choi G, Chae SW, Kim CH, Hwang SJ, Lee SH. Two cases of primary malignant melanoma of the lacrimal sac. Head Neck 2001, **23**: 809–813.

89 Leung SY, Chung LP, Ho CM, Yuen ST, Wong MP, Kwong WK. An Epstein–Barr virus positive undifferentiated carcinoma in the lacrimal sac. Histopathology 1996, **28**: 71–76.

90 Nakamura K, Uehara S, Omagari J, Kunitake N, Kimura M, Makino Y, Ishigami K, Masuda K. Primary non-Hodgkin's lymphoma of the lacrimal sac: a case report and a review of the literature. Cancer 1997, **80**: 2151–2155.

91 Ni C, Wagoner MD, Wang W-J, Albert DM, Fan CO, Robinson N. Mucoepidermoid carcinomas of the lacrimal sac. Arch Ophthalmol 1983, **101**: 1572–1574.

92 Raemdonck TY, Van den Broecke CM, Claerhout I, Decock CE. Inverted papilloma arising primarily from the lacrimal sac. Orbit 2009, **28**: 181–184.

93 Ryan SJ, Font RL. Primary epithelial neoplasms of the lacrimal sac. Am J Ophthalmol 1973, **76**: 73–88.

94 Sjö LD. Ophthalmic lymphoma: epidemiology and pathogenesis. Acta Ophthalmol 2009, **87**: 1–20.

ORBIT

95 Char DH. Management of orbital tumors. Mayo Clin Proc 1993, **68**: 1081–1096.

96 Shields JA, Bakewell B, Augsburger JJ, Flanagan JC. Classification and incidence of space-occupying lesions of the orbit. A survey of 645 biopsies. Arch Ophthalmol 1984, **102**: 1606–1611.

97 Zajdela A, Vielh P, Schlienger P, Haye C. Fine-needle cytology of 292 palpable orbital and eyelid tumors. Am J Clin Pathol 1990, **93**: 100–104.

DYSTHYROID OPHTHALMOPATHY

98 Bahn RS, Heufelder AE. Pathogenesis of Graves' ophthalmopathy. N Engl J Med 1993, **329**: 1468–1475.

INFLAMMATORY PROCESSES

99 Blodi F, Gass D. Inflammatory pseudotumor of the orbit. Trans Am Acad Ophthalmol Otolaryngol 1967, **71**: 303–323.

100 Cheuk W, Chan JK. IgG4-related sclerosing disease: a critical appraisal of an evolving clinicopathologic entity. Adv Anat Pathol 2010, **17**: 303–332.

101 Eshaghian J, Anderson RL. Sinus involvement in inflammatory orbital pseudotumor. Arch Ophthalmol 1981, **99**: 627–630.

102 Foucar E, Rosai J, Dorfman RF. The ophthalmologic manifestations of sinus histiocytosis with massive lymphadenopathy. Am J Ophthalmol 1979, **87**: 354–367.

103 Frohman LP, Kupersmith MJ, Lang J, Reede D, Bergeron RT, Aleksic S, Trasi S. Intracranial extension and bone destruction in orbital pseudotumor. Arch Ophthalmol 1986, **104**: 380–384.

104 Garner A. Pathology of 'pseudotumors' of the orbit. A review. J Clin Pathol 1973, **26**: 639–648.

105 Grimson BS, Simons KB. Orbital inflammation, myositis, and systemic lupus erythematosus. Arch Ophthalmol 1983, **101**: 736–738.

106 Harris GJ. Subperiosteal abscess of the orbit. Arch Ophthalmol 1983, **101**: 751–757.

107 Maalouf T, Trouchaud-Michaud C, Angioi-Duprez K, George JL. What has become of our idiopathic inflammatory pseudo-tumors of the orbit? Orbit 1999, **18**: 157–166.

108 McCarthy JM, White VA, Harris G, Simons KB, Kennerdell J, Rootman J. Idiopathic sclerosing inflammation of the orbit. Immunohistologic analysis and comparison with retroperitoneal fibrosis. Mod Pathol 1993, **6**: 581–587.

109 Mehta M, Jakobiec F, Fay A. Idiopathic fibroinflammatory disease of the face, eyelids, and periorbital membrane with immunoglobulin G4-positive plasma cells. Arch Pathol Lab Med 2009, **133**: 1251–1255.

110 Parke DW II, Font RL, Boniuk M, McCrary JA III. 'Cholesteatoma' of the orbit. Arch Ophthalmol 1982, **100**: 612–616.

111 Rosca T, Bontas E, Vladescu TG, St Tihoan C, Gherghescu G. Clinical controversy in orbitary cholesteatoma. Ann Diagn Pathol 2006, **10**: 89–94.

112 Sato Y, Ohshima K, Ichimura K, Sato M, Yamadori I, Tanaka T, Takata K, Morito T, Kondo E, Yoshino T. Ocular adnexal IgG4-related disease has uniform clinicopathology. Pathol Int 2008, **58**: 465–470.

PRIMARY TUMORS

Mesenchymal tumors and tumorlike conditions

113 Ahrens WA, Ridenour RV 3rd, Caron BL, Miller DV, Folpe AL. GLUT-1 expression in mesenchymal tumors: an immunohistochemical study of 247 soft tissue and bone neoplasms. Hum Pathol 2008, **39**: 1519–1526.

114 Cai Y-C, McMenamin ME, Rose G, Sandy CJ, Cree IA, Fletcher CD. Primary liposarcoma of the orbit: a clinicopathologic study of seven cases. Ann Diagn Pathol 2001, **5**: 255–266.

115 Croxatto JO, Font RL. Hemangiopericytoma of the orbit. A clinicopathologic study of 30 cases. Hum Pathol 1982, **13**: 210–218.

116 Dei Tos AP, Seregard S, Calonje E, Chan JK, Fletcher CD. Giant cell angiofibroma. A distinctive orbital tumor in adults. Am J Surg Pathol 1995, **19**: 1286–1293.

117 Dorfman DM, To K, Dickersin GR, Rosenberg AE, Pilch BZ. Solitary fibrous tumor of the orbit. Am J Surg Pathol 1994, **18**: 281–287.

118 Font RL, Hidayat AA. Fibrous histiocytoma of the orbit. A clinicopathologic study of 150 cases. Hum Pathol 1982, **13**: 199–209.

119 Font RL, Zimmerman LE. Nodular fasciitis of the eye and adnexa. A report of ten cases. Arch Ophthalmol 1966, **75**: 475–481.

120 Font RL, Jurco S III, Zimmerman LE. Alveolar soft-part sarcoma of the orbit. A clinicopathologic analysis of seventeen cases and a review of the literature. Hum Pathol 1982, **13**: 569–579.

121 Font RL, Wheeler TM, Boniuk M. Intravascular papillary endothelial hyperplasia of the orbit and ocular adnexa. A report of five cases. Arch Ophthalmol 1983, **101**: 1731–1736.

122 Forrest AW. Tumors following radiation about the eye. Int Ophthalmol Clin 1962, **2**: 543–553.

123 Ganesan R, Hammond CJ, Van Der Walt JD. Giant cell angiofibroma of the orbit. Histopathology 1997, **30**: 93–96.

124 Goldsmith JD, van de Rijn M, Syed N. Orbital hemangiopericytoma and solitary fibrous tumor: a morphologic continuum. Int J Surg Pathol 2003, **9**: 295–302.

125 Guillou L, Gebhard S, Coindre JM. Orbital and extraorbital giant cell angiofibroma: a giant cell-rich variant of solitary fibrous tumor? Clinicopathologic and immunohistochemical analysis of a series in favor of a unifying concept. Am J Surg Pathol 2000, **24**: 971–979.

126 Hasegawa T, Matsuno Y, Niki T, Hirohashi S, Shimoda T, Takayama J, Watanabe C, Kaneko A, Sano T, Sato M, Suzuki J. Second primary rhabdomyosarcomas in patients with bilateral retinoblastoma: a clinicopathologic and immunohistochemical study. Am J Surg Pathol 1998, **22**: 1351–1360.

127 Henderson JW, Farrow GM. Primary orbital hemangiopericytoma. An aggressive and potentially malignant neoplasm. Arch Ophthalmol 1978, **96**: 666–673.

128 Hufnagel T, Ma L, Kuo T-T. Orbital angiosarcoma with subconjunctival presentation. Report of a case and literature review. Ophthalmology 1987, **94**: 72–77.

129 Jacobs JL, Merriam JC, Chadburn A, Garvin J, Housepian E, Hilal SK. Mesenchymal chondrosarcoma of the orbit. Report of three new cases and review of the literature. Cancer 1994, **73**: 399–405.

130 Knowles D, Jakobiec F, Potter G, Jones IS. Ophthalmic striated muscle neoplasms. Surv Ophthalmol 1976, **21**: 219–261.

131 Krohel GB, Rosenberg PN, Wright JE, Smith RS. Localized orbital neurofibromas. Am J Ophthalmol 1985, **100**: 458–464.

132 Leon-Villapalos J, Wolfe K, Kangesu L. GLUT-1: an extra diagnostic tool to differentiate between haemangiomas and vascular malformations. Br J Plast Surg 2005, **58**: 348–352.

133 Mikami Y, Shimizu M, Hirokawa M, Manabe T. Extraorbital giant cell angiofibromas. Mod Pathol 1997, **10**: 1082–1087.

134 Polito E, Tosi M, Toti P, Schurfeld K, Caporossi A. Orbital solitary fibrous tumor with aggressive behavior. Three cases and review of the literature. Graefes Arch Clin Exp Ophthalmol 2002, **240**: 570–574.

135 Rosca TI, Pop MI, Curca M, Vladescu TG, Tihoan CS, Serban AT, Bontas EA, Gherghescu G. Vascular tumors in the orbit – capillary and cavernous hemangiomas. Ann Diagn Pathol 2006, **10**: 13–19.

136 Schmack I, Patel RM, Folpe AL, Wojno T, Zaldivar RA, Balzer B, Kang SJ, Weiss SW, Grossniklaus HE. Subconjunctival herniated orbital fat: a benign adipocytic lesion that may mimic pleomorphic lipoma and atypical lipomatous tumor. Am J Surg Pathol 2007, **31**: 193–198.

137 Sciot R, Goffin J, Fossion E, Wilms G, Dom R. Solitary fibrous tumour of the orbit. Histopathology 1996, **28**: 188–191.

138 Shields JA, Kapustiak J, Arbizo V, Augsburger JJ, Schnitzer RE. Orbital neurilemoma with extension through the superior orbital fissure. Arch Ophthalmol 1986, **104**: 871–873.

139 Weiner JM, Hidayat AA. Juvenile fibrosarcoma of the orbit and eyelid. A study of five cases. Arch Ophthalmol 1983, **101**: 253–259.

140 Westra WH, Gerald WL, Rosai J. Solitary fibrous tumor. Consistent CD34 immunoreactivity and occurrence in the orbit. Am J Surg Pathol 1994, **18**: 992–998.

141 Wilson WB, Roloff J, Wilson HL. Primary peripheral neuroepithelioma of the orbit with intracranial extension. Cancer 1988, **62**: 2595–2601.

142 Wojno T, Tenzel RR, Nadji M. Orbital leiomyosarcoma. Arch Ophthalmol 1983, **101**: 1566–1568.

143 Yamasaki T, Handa H, Yamashita J, Paine JT, Tashiro Y, Uno A, Ishikawa M, Asato R. Intracranial and orbital cavernous angiomas. A review of 30 cases. J Neurosurg 1986, **64**: 197–208.

144 Yeniad B, Tuncer S, Peksayar G, Mete O, Minareci O. Primary orbital leiomyosarcoma. Ophthal Plast Reconstr Surg 2009, **25**: 154–155.

Glioma of optic nerve

145 Borit A, Richardson EP Jr. The biological and clinical behaviour of pilocytic astrocytomas of the optic pathways. Brain 1982, **105**: 161–187.

146 Dosoretz DE, Blitzer PH, Wang CC, Linggood RM. Management of glioma of the optic nerve and/or chiasm. An analysis of 20 cases. Cancer 1980, **45**: 1467–1471.

147 Marquardt MD, Zimmerman LE. Histopathology of meningiomas and gliomas of the optic nerve. Hum Pathol 1982, **13**: 226–235.

148 Pierce SM, Barnes PD, Loeffler JS, McGinn C, Tarbell NJ. Definitive radiation therapy in the management of symptomatic patients with optic glioma. Survival and long-term effects. Cancer 1990, **65**: 45–52.

Meningioma

149 Jain D, Ebrahimi KB, Miller NR, Eberhart CG. Intraorbital meningiomas: a pathologic review using current World Health Organization criteria. Arch Pathol Lab Med 2010, **134**: 766–770.

150 Karp L, Zimmerman LE, Borit A, Spencer W. Primary intraorbital meningiomas. Arch Ophthalmol 1974, **91**: 24–28.

151 Marquardt MD, Zimmerman LE. Histopathology of meningiomas and gliomas of the optic nerve. Hum Pathol 1982, **13**: 226–235.

Lymphoid tumors and tumorlike conditions

152 Astarita RW, Minckler D, Taylor CR, Levine A, Lukes RJ. Orbital and adnexal lymphomas. A multiparameter approach. Am J Clin Pathol 1980, **73**: 615–621.

153 Bennett CL, Putterman A, Bitran JD, Recant W, Shapiro CM, Karesh J, Kalokhe U. Staging and therapy of orbital lymphomas. Cancer 1986, **57**: 1204–1208.

154 Brisbane JU, Lessell S, Finkel HE, Neiman RS. Malignant lymphoma presenting in the orbit. A clinicopathologic study of a rare immunoglobulin-producing variant. Cancer 1981, **47**: 548–553.

155 Cheuk W, Chan JK. IgG4-related sclerosing disease: a critical appraisal of an evolving clinicopathologic entity. Adv Anat Pathol 2010, **17**: 303–332.

156 Cheuk W, Yuen HK, Chan AC, Shih LY, Kuo TT, Ma MW, Lo YF, Chan WK, Chan JK. Ocular adnexal lymphoma associated with IgG4+ chronic sclerosing dacryoadenitis: a previously undescribed complication of IgG4-related sclerosing disease. Am J Surg Pathol 2008, **32**: 1159–1167.

157 Ferreri AJM, Guidoboni M, Ponzoni M, De Conciliis C, Dell'Oro S, Fleischhauer K, Caggiari L, Lettini AA, Dal Cin E, Ieri R, Freschi M, Villa E, Boiocchi M, Dolcetti R. Evidence for an association between *Chlamydia psittaci* and ocular adnexal lymphomas. J Natl Cancer Inst 2004, **96**: 586–594.

158 Ferry JA, Fung CY, Zukerberg L, Lucarelli MJ, Hasserjian RP, Preffer FI, Harris NL. Lymphoma of the ocular adnexa: a study of 353 cases. Am J Surg Pathol 2007, **31**: 170–184.

159 Franco R, Camacho FI, Caleo A, Staibano S, Bifano D, De Renzo A, Tranfa F, De Chiara A, Botti G, Merola R, Diez A, Bonavolontà G, De Rosa G, Piris MA. Nuclear bcl10 expression characterizes a group of ocular adnexa MALT lymphomas with shorter failure-free survival. Mod Pathol 2006, **19**: 1055–1067.

160 Knowles DM II, Jakobiec FA. Orbital lymphoid neoplasms. A clinicopathologic study of 60 patients. Cancer 1980, **46**: 576–589.

161 Knowles DM II, Jakobiec FA. Cell marker analysis of extranodal lymphoid infiltrates. To what extent does the determination of mono- or polyclonality resolve the diagnostic dilemma of malignant lymphoma *v* pseudolymphoma in an extranodal site? Semin Diagn Pathol 1985, **2**: 163–168.

162 Knowles DM, Jakobiec FA, McNally L, Burke JS. Lymphoid hyperplasia and malignant lymphoma occurring in the ocular adnexa (orbit, conjunctiva, and eyelids). A prospective multiparametric analysis of 108 cases during 1977 to 1987. Hum Pathol 1990, **21**: 959–973.

163 Kusakabe T, Watanabe K, Mori T, Iida T, Suzuki T. Crystal-storing histiocytosis associated with MALT lymphoma of the ocular adnexa: a case report with review of literature. Virchows Arch 2007, **450**: 103–108.

164 Lazzarino M, Morra E, Rosso R, Brusamolino E, Pagnucco G, Castello A, Ghisolfi A, Tafi A, Zennaro G, Bernasconi C. Clinicopathologic and immunologic characteristics of non-Hodgkin's lymphomas presenting in the orbit. A report of eight cases. Cancer 1985, **55**: 1907–1912.

165 McNally L, Jakobiec FA, Knowles DM II. Clinical, morphologic, immunophenotypic, and molecular genetic analysis of bilateral ocular adnexal lymphoid neoplasms in 17 patients. Am J Ophthalmol 1987, **103**: 555–568.

166 Mannami T, Yoshino T, Oshima K, Takase S, Kondo E, Ohara N, Nakagawa H, Ohtsuki H, Harada M, Akagi T. Clinical, histopathological and immunogenetic analysis of ocular adnexal lymphoproliferative disorders: characterization of MALT lymphoma and reactive lymphoid hyperplasia. Mod Pathol 2001, **14**: 641–649.

167 Medeiros LJ, Harris NL. Lymphoid infiltrates of the orbit and conjunctiva. A morphologic and immunophenotypic study of 99 cases. Am J Surg Pathol 1989, **13**: 459–471.

168 Medeiros LJ, Harris NL. Immunohistologic analysis of small lymphocytic infiltrates of the orbit and conjunctiva. Hum Pathol 1990, **21**: 1126–1131.

169 Morgan G, Harry J. Lymphocytic tumours of indeterminate nature. A 5-year follow-up of 98 conjunctival and orbital lesions. Br J Ophthalmol 1978, **62**: 381–383.

170 Neri A, Jakobiec FA, Pelicci P-G, Dalla-Favera R, Knowles DM II. Immunoglobulin and T cell receptor β chain gene rearrangement analysis of ocular adnexal lymphoid neoplasms. Clinical and biologic implications. Blood 1987, **70**: 1519–1529.

171 Peterson K, Gordon KB, Heinemann MH, De Angelis LM. The clinical spectrum of ocular lymphoma. Cancer 1993, **72**: 843–849.

172 Ruiz A, Reischl U, Swerdlow SH, Hartke M, Streubel B, Procop G, Tubbs RR, Cook JR. Extranodal marginal zone B-cell lymphomas of the ocular adnexa: multiparameter analysis of 34 cases including interphase molecular cytogenetics and PCR for *Chlamydia psittaci*. Am J Surg Pathol 2007, **31**: 792–802.

173 Sanka RK, Eagle RC Jr, Wojno TH, Neufeld KR, Grossniklaus HE. Spectrum of CD30+ lymphoid proliferations in the eyelid lymphomatoid papulosis, cutaneous anaplastic large cell lymphoma, and anaplastic large cell lymphoma. Ophthalmology 2010, **117**: 343–351.

174 Shome DK, Gupta NK, Prajapati NC, Raju GM, Choudhury P, Dubey AP. Orbital granulocytic sarcomas (myeloid sarcomas) in acute nonlymphocytic Leukemia. Cancer 1992, **70**: 2298–2301.

175 Sjö LD. Ophthalmic lymphoma: epidemiology and pathogenesis. Acta Ophthalmol 2009, **87**: 1–20.

176 Tewfik HH, Platz CE, Corder MP, Panther SK, Blodi FC. A clinicopathologic study of orbital and adnexal non-Hodgkin's lymphomas. Cancer 1979, **44**: 1022–1028.

177 Tsuji H, Tamura M, Yokoyama M, Takeuchi K, Mimura T. Ocular involvement by Epstein–Barr virus-positive diffuse large B-cell lymphoma of the elderly: a new disease entity in the World Health Organization classification. Arch Ophthalmol 2010, **128**: 258–259.

178 White VA, Gascoyne RD, McNeil BK, Chang WY, Brewer LV, Rootman J. Histopathologic findings and frequency of clonality detected by the polymerase chain reaction on ocular adnexal lymphoproliferative lesions. Mod Pathol 1996, **9**: 1052–1061.

179 Wotherspoon AC, Diss TC, Pan LX, Schmid C, Kerr-Muir MG, Lea SH, Isaacson PG. Primary low-grade B-cell lymphoma of the conjunctiva. A mucosa-associated lymphoid tissue type lymphoma. Histopathology 1993, **23**: 417–424.

METASTATIC TUMORS

180 Freedman MI, Folk JC. Metastatic tumors to the eye and orbit. Patient survival and clinical characteristics. Arch Ophthalmol 1987, **105**: 1215–1219.

181 Reifler DM, Kini SR, Liu D, Littleton RH. Orbital metastasis from prostatic carcinoma. Identification by immunocytology. Arch Ophthalmol 1984, **102**: 292–295.

182 Riddle PJ, Font RL, Zimmerman LE. Carcinoid tumors of the eye and orbit. A clinicopathologic study of 15 cases, with histochemical and electron microscopic observations. Hum Pathol 1982, **13**: 459–469.

183 Zimmerman LE, Stangl R, Riddle PJ. Primary carcinoid tumor of the orbit. A clinicopathologic study with histochemical and electron microscopic observations. Arch Ophthalmol 1983, **101**: 1395–1398.

CONJUNCTIVA

DEGENERATION

184 Austin P, Jakobiec FA, Iwamoto T, Hornblass A. Elastofibroma oculi. Arch Ophthalmol 1983, **101**: 1575–1579.

GRAFT-VERSUS-HOST DISEASE

185 Jabs DA, Hirst LW, Green WR, Tutschka PJ, Santos GW, Beschorner WE. The eye in bone marrow transplantation. II. Histopathology. Arch Ophthalmol 1983, **101**: 585–590.

INFLAMMATION

186 Bornstein J, Frank M, Radnec D. Conjunctival biopsy in the diagnosis of sarcoidosis. N Engl J Med 1962, **267**: 60–64.

187 Chambers J, Blodi F, Golden B, McKee A. Ligneous conjunctivitis. Trans Am Acad Ophthalmol Otolaryngol 1969, **73**: 996–1004.

188 Hidayat AA, Riddle PJ. Ligneous conjunctivitis. A clinicopathologic study of 17 cases. Ophthalmology 1987, **94**: 949–959.

189 Raphael M, Bellefqih S, Piette JC, Le Hoang P, Debre P, Chomette G. Conjunctival biopsy in Sjögren's syndrome. Correlations between histological and immunohistochemical features. Histopathology 1988, **13**: 191–202.

190 Rodríguez-Ares MT, Abdulkader I, Blanco A, Touriño-Peralba R, Ruiz-Ponte C, Vega A, Cameselle-Teijeiro J. Ligneous conjunctivitis: a clinicopathological, immunohistochemical, and genetic study including the treatment of two sisters with multiorgan involvement. Virchows Arch 2007, **451**: 815–821.

191 Steffen C. Actinic granuloma of the conjunctiva. Am J Dermatopathol 1992, **14**: 253–254.

192 Stenson S. Adult inclusion conjunctivitis. Clinical characteristics and corneal changes. Arch Ophthalmol 1981, **99**: 605–608.

TUMORS AND TUMORLIKE CONDITIONS

Epithelial tumors

193 Blodi FC. Squamous cell carcinoma of the conjunctiva. Doc Ophthalmol 1973, **34**: 93–108.

194 Font RL, Del Valle M, Avedaño J, Longo M, Boniuk M. Primary adenoid cystic carcinoma of the conjunctiva arising from the accessory lacrimal glands: a clinicopathologic study of three cases. Cornea 2008, **27**: 494–497.

195 Gamel JW, Eiferman RA, Guibor P. Mucoepidermoid carcinoma of the conjunctiva. Arch Ophthalmol 1984, **102**: 730–731.

196 Irvine AR Jr. Epibulbar squamous cell carcinoma and related lesions. Int Ophthalmol Clin 1972, **12**: 71–83.

197 McDonnell JM, Mayr AJ, Martin WJ. DNA of human papillomavirus type 16 in dysplastic and malignant lesions of the conjunctiva and cornea. N Engl J Med 1989, **320**: 1442–1446.

198 McDonnell PJ, McDonnell JM, Kessis T, Green WR, Shah KV. Detection of human papillomavirus type 6/11 DNA in conjunctival papillomas by in situ hybridization with radioactive probes. Hum Pathol 1987, **18**: 1115–1119.

199 Searl SS, Krigstein HJ, Albert DM, Grove AS Jr. Invasive squamous cell carcinoma with intraocular mucoepidermoid features. Conjunctival carcinoma with intraocular invasion and diphasic morphology. Arch Ophthalmol 1982, **100**: 109–111.

200 Waring GO III, Roth AM, Ekins MB. Clinical and pathologic description of 17 cases of corneal intraepithelial neoplasia. Am J Ophthalmol 1984, **97**: 547–559.

Melanocytic tumors and tumorlike conditions

201 Ackerman AB, Sood R, Koenig M. Primary acquired melanosis of the conjunctiva is melanoma in situ. Mod Pathol 1991, **4**: 253–263.

202 Brownstein S, Jakobiec FA, Wilkinson RD, Lombardo J, Jackson WB. Cryotherapy for precancerous melanosis (atypical melanocytic hyperplasia) of the conjunctiva. Arch Ophthalmol 1981, **99**: 1224–1231.

203 Folberg R, McLean IW. Primary acquired melanosis and melanoma of the conjunctiva. Terminology, classification, and biologic behavior. Hum Pathol 1986, **17**: 652–654.

204 Folberg R, Jakobiec FA, McLean IW, Zimmerman LE. Is primary acquired melanosis of the conjunctiva equivalent to melanoma in situ? Mod Pathol 1992, **5**: 2–8.

205 Folberg R, McLean IW, Zimmerman LE. Primary acquired melanosis of the conjunctiva. Hum Pathol 1985, **16**: 129–135.

206 Folberg R, McLean IW, Zimmerman LE. Malignant melanoma of the conjunctiva. Hum Pathol 1985, **16**: 136–143.

207 Guillén FJ, Albert DM, Mihm MC Jr. Pigmented melanocytic lesions of the conjunctiva. A new approach to their classification. Pathology 1985, **17**: 275–280.

208 Jakobiec FA, Zuckerman BD, Berlin AJ, Odell P, MacRae DW, Tuthill RJ. Unusual melanocytic nevi of the conjunctiva. Am J Ophthalmol 1985, **100**: 100–113.

209 Jay B. Naevi and melanomata of the conjunctiva. Br J Ophthalmol 1965, **49**: 169–204.

210 Jeffrey IJM, Lucas DR, McEwan C, Lee WR. Malignant melanoma of the conjunctiva. Histopathology 1986, **10**: 363–378.

211 Kabukcuoglu S, McNutt NS. Conjunctival melanocytic nevi of childhood. J Cutan Pathol 1999, **26**: 248–252.

212 Liesegang TJ. Pigmented conjunctival and scleral lesions. Mayo Clin Proc 1994, **69**: 151–161.

213 McLean IW. Differential diagnosis of the conjunctival melanoses. Ann Diagn Pathol 1998, **2**: 264–270.

214 Mihm MC Jr, Guillén FJ. Classification of non-nevoid pigmented lesions of the conjunctiva [letter to the Editor]. Hum Pathol 1985, **16**: 1078.

215 Reese AB. Precancerous and cancerous melanosis. Am J Ophthalmol 1966, **61**: 1272–1277.

216 Sugiura M, Colby KA, Mihm MC Jr, Zembowicz A. Low-risk and high-risk histologic features in conjunctival primary acquired melanosis with atypia: clinicopathologic analysis of 29 cases. Am J Surg Pathol 2007, **31**: 185–192.

217 Thiagalingam S, Johnson MM, Colby KA, Zembowicz A. Juvenile conjunctival nevus: clinicopathologic analysis of 33 cases. Am J Surg Pathol 2008, **32**: 399–406.

218 Werschnik C, Lommatzsch PK. Long-term follow-up of patients with conjunctival melanoma. Am J Clin Oncol 2002, **25**: 248–255.

Lymphoid tumors and tumorlike conditions

219 Morgan G. Lymphocytic tumours of the conjunctiva. J Clin Pathol 1971, **24**: 585–595.

Other tumors

220 Hufnagel T, Ma L, Kuo T-T. Orbital angiosarcoma with subconjunctival presentation. Report of a case and literature review. Ophthalmology 1987, **94**: 72–77.

221 Jaimovich L, Calb I, Kaminsky A. Kaposi's sarcoma of the conjunctiva. J Am Acad Dermatol 1986, **14**: 589–592.

222 Kase S, Ishijima K, Ishida S, Rao NA. Merkel cell carcinoma of the conjunctiva. Ophthalmology 2010, **117**: 637.e1–e2.

223 Patrinely JR, Green WR. Conjunctival myxoma. A clinicopathologic study of four cases and a review of the literature. Arch Ophthalmol 1983, **101**: 1416–1420.

224 Truong L, Font RL. Intravenous pyogenic granuloma of the ocular adnexa. Report of two cases and review of the literature. Arch Ophthalmol 1985, **103**: 1364–1367.

INTRAOCULAR TISSUES

MALIGNANT MELANOMA

General and clinical features

225 Barr CC, McLean IW, Zimmerman LE. Uveal melanoma in children and adolescents. Arch Ophthalmol 1981, **99**: 2133–2136.

226 Barr CC, Zimmerman LE, Curtin VT, Font RL. Bilateral diffuse melanocytic uveal tumors associated with systemic malignant neoplasms. A recently recognized syndrome. Arch Ophthalmol 1982, **100**: 249–255.

227 Broadway D, Lang S, Harper J, Madanat F, Pritchard J, Tarawneh M, Taylor D. Congenital malignant melanoma of the eye. Cancer 1991, **67**: 2642–2652.

228 Chang M, Zimmerman LE, McLean I. The persisting pseudomelanoma problem. Arch Ophthalmol 1984, **102**: 726–727.

229 Ferry AP. Lesions mistaken for malignant melanoma of posterior uvea. Arch Ophthalmol 1964, **72**: 463–469.

230 Ferry AP. Lesions mistaken for malignant melanoma of iris. Arch Ophthalmol 1965, **74**: 9–18.

231 Font RL, Spaulding A, Zimmerman LE. Diffuse malignant melanoma of the uveal tract. A clinicopathologic report of 54 cases. Trans Am Acad Ophthalmol Otolaryngol 1968, **72**: 877–895.

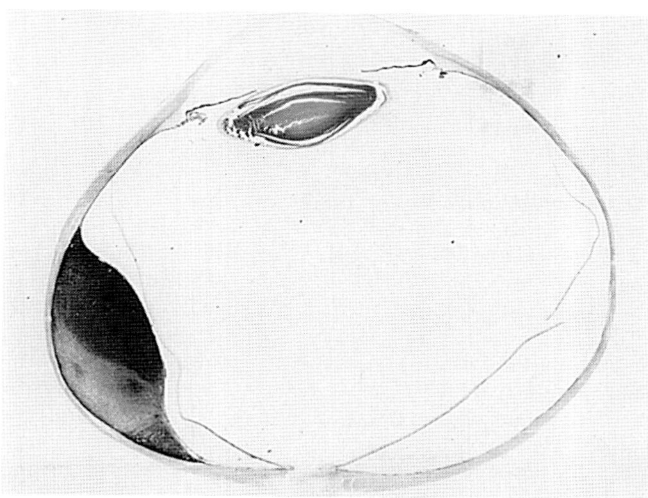

Fig. 30.50 Malignant melanoma of choroid that has not broken through Bruch's membrane but has elevated the retina. Most of the retinal separation observed in this section is artifactual.
(From Friedenwald JS, Wilder HC, Maumenee AE, Sanders TE, Keyes JEL, Hogan MJ, Owens WC, Owens EU. Ophthalmic pathology. An atlas and textbook. Philadelphia, 1952, WB Saunders)

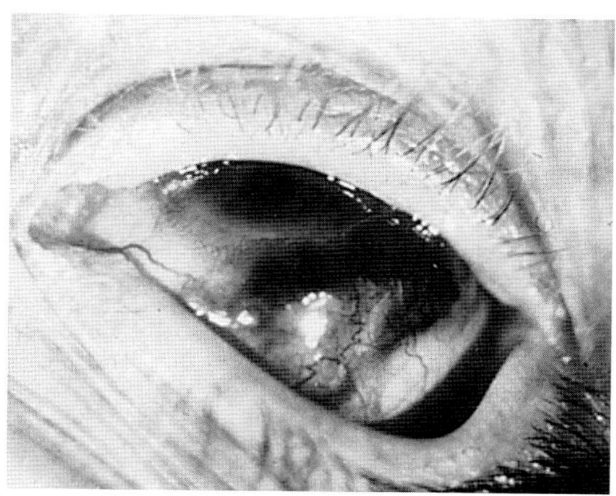

Fig. 30.52 Malignant melanoma of choroid breaking through the sclera and presenting under the conjunctiva.
(From del Regato JA, Spjut HJ. Ackerman and del Regato's cancer, ed. 5. St Louis, 1977, Mosby; courtesy of the Registry of Ophthalmic Pathology, Armed Forces Institute of Pathology, Washington, DC)

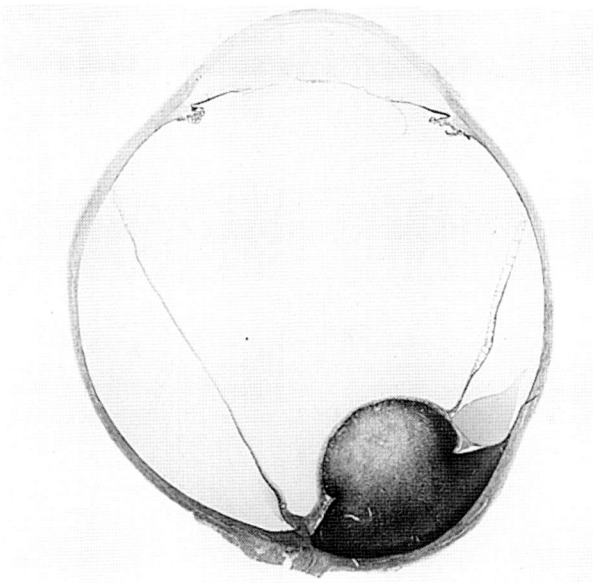

Fig. 30.51 Malignant melanoma of choroid that, by erupting through Bruch's membrane, has formed a mushroom-shaped subretinal mass.

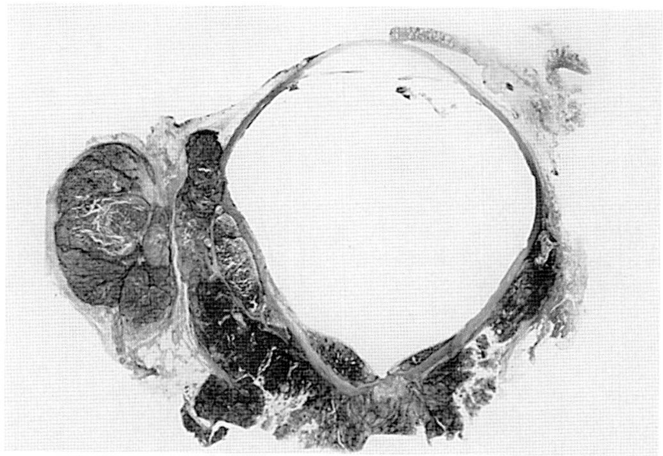

Fig. 30.53 Massive orbital extension from a small choroid melanoma that has occurred as a result of diffuse spread along natural passages through the sclera and optic nerve.
(From Friedenwald JS, Wilder HC, Maumenee AE, Sanders TE, Keyes JEL, Hogan MJ, Owens WC, Owens EU. Ophthalmic pathology. An atlas and textbook. Philadelphia, 1952, WB Saunders)

Iris tumors are more often recognized early, for they can be seen by the patient and family long before symptoms appear (Fig. 30.55).

Clinically, there are many lesions that simulate uveal malignant melanoma.[228–230,234] The most important are metastatic carcinoma, localized hemorrhage beneath the retina or between the pigment epithelium and choroid (Fig. 30.56), focal areas of proliferation of the retinal pigment epithelium (Fig. 30.57), posterior scleritis, and benign tumors such as nevi and hemangiomas.

Microscopic features

Microscopically, uveal melanomas have been traditionally divided into three types: spindle A, spindle B, and epithelioid, which may occur singly or in combination.[242] Spindle A cells are slender, benign-appearing spindle-shaped cells that have relatively small fusiform nuclei and no nucleoli. The chromatin is frequently arranged in a linear fashion along the central axis of the nucleus.

Spindle B cells are larger and more pleomorphic, merging on the one hand with spindle A cells and on the other with epithelioid cells. They typically possess large ovoid nuclei containing prominent nucleoli (Fig. 30.58). Mitotic activity may be more marked. Both spindle A and spindle B tumors tend to be quite cohesive. Some of these tumors have a distinctly fascicular pattern of growth (Fig. 30.59).

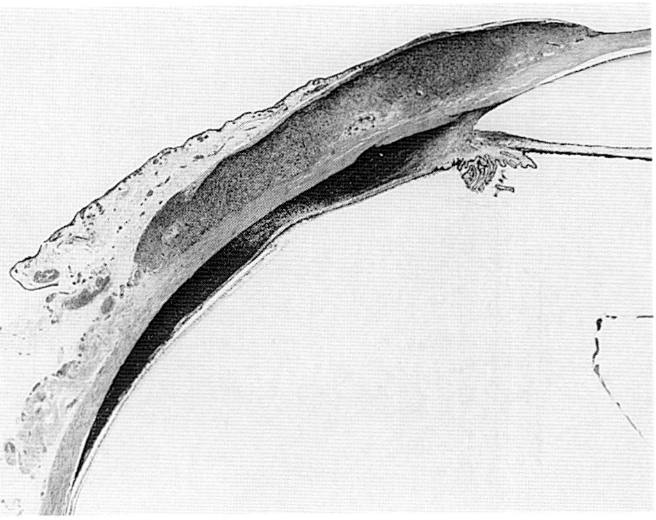

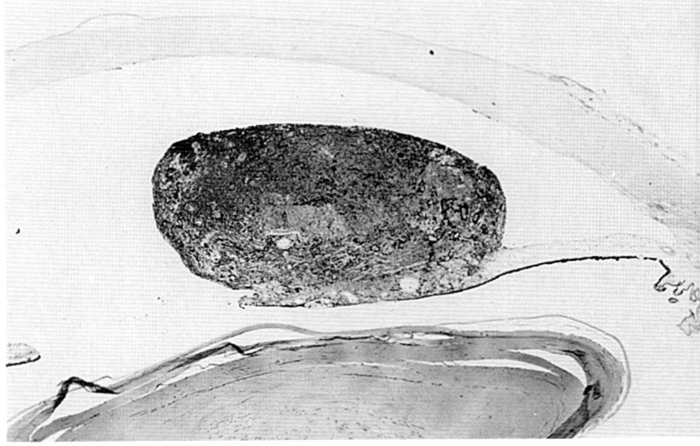

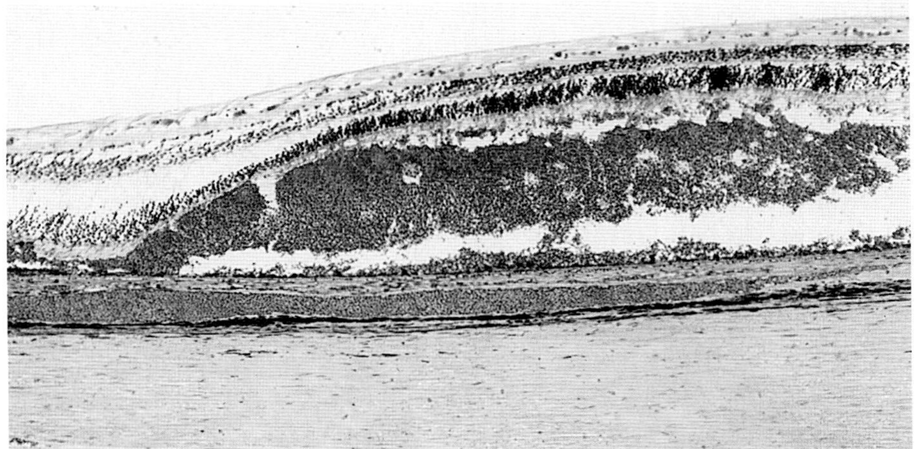

Fig. 30.62 Retinoblastoma presenting as a highly cellular neoplasm with scanty stroma. The tumor tends to outgrow its blood supply, and irregular areas of necrosis are commonly observed.

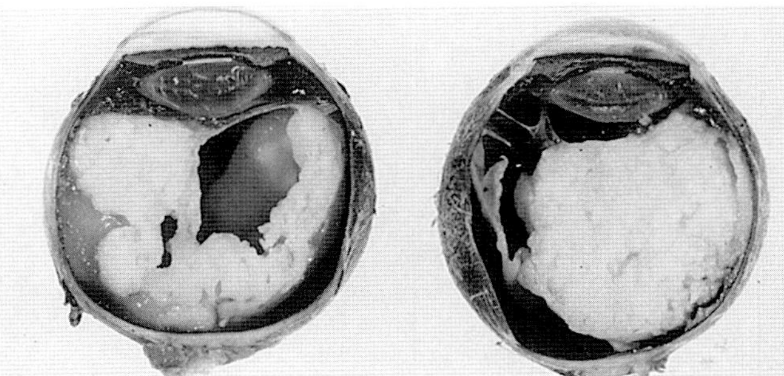

Fig. 30.64 Bilateral retinoblastoma showing a white mass consisting of detached retina and neoplastic tissue immediately behind the lens in each eye.

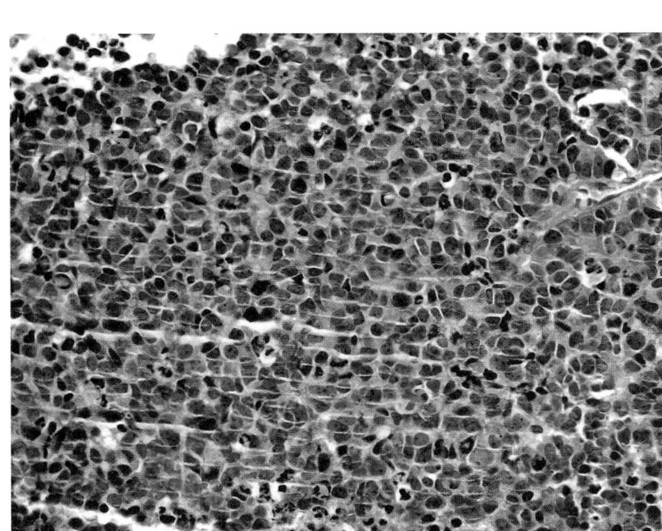

Fig. 30.65 Poorly differentiated retinoblastoma. The appearance is that of a malignant small round cell tumor.

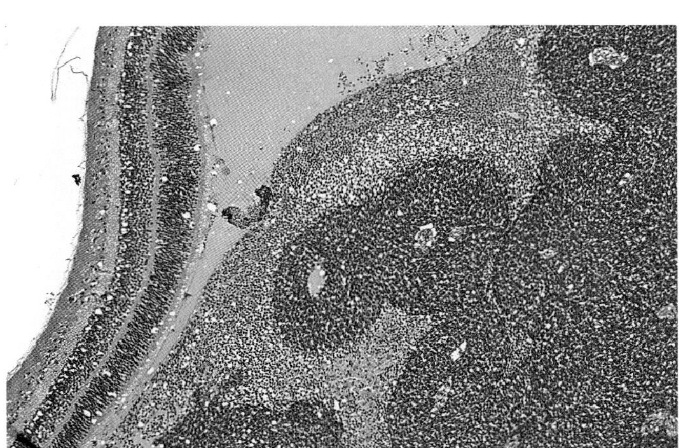

Fig. 30.63 Low-power view of retinoblastoma. There is a collar of viable cells about nutrient vessels (so-called peritheliomatous pattern). The normal retina is seen on the left.

and the pigment epithelium (exophytic type). Since the tumors tend to outgrow their blood supply, necrosis is often extensive and many minute foci of calcification are often present in these areas of necrosis (Fig. 30.63). In fact, these areas of calcification may be appreciated by x-ray examination prior to enucleation.

Bilaterality is present in 30% of all cases and in over 90% of the familial cases (Fig. 30.64). Some patients have presented with bilateral retinoblastoma and a morphologically similar intracranial neoplasm localized in the region of the pineal gland, in keeping with the 'third eye' nature of the latter structure.[295] These are referred as *trilateral retinoblastomas*[292,293] and are associated with a particularly dismal prognosis.[297]

The clinical differential diagnosis of retinoblastoma includes any disease process that leads to retinal detachment or a retrolental mass in a child under 6 years of age.[294,296] Lesions in this category include traumatic or idiopathic retinal detachments, retrolental fibroplasia, persistent hyperplastic primary vitreous, massive retinal gliosis, Coats disease, nematodiasis, astrocytomas of tuberous sclerosis, and medulloepitheliomas. Some of these disorders are discussed elsewhere in this chapter.

Microscopic features

Microscopically, retinoblastomas are composed of dense masses of small round cells with hyperchromatic nuclei and scanty cytoplasm[300] (Fig. 30.65). Trabecular and nesting formations are common.[302] Hematoxyphilic deposits in and around blood vessel walls are often seen in necrotic areas, similar to those found in pulmonary small cell carcinomas.[298] A sign of differentiation toward retinal structures is provided by the presence of so-called 'Flexner–Wintersteiner rosettes' and fleurettes (Fig. 30.66). *Differentiated retinoblastoma* is characterized by the presence of a bipolar-like cell element.[299]

Tumors showing an extreme degree of differentiation are designated as *retinocytomas* and regarded as benign.[301] These lesions carry the same genetic implications as conventional retinoblastomas; they present as small placoid, noninvasive lesions composed entirely of benign-appearing cells with numerous fleurettes, lacking necrosis or mitotic activity.[301]

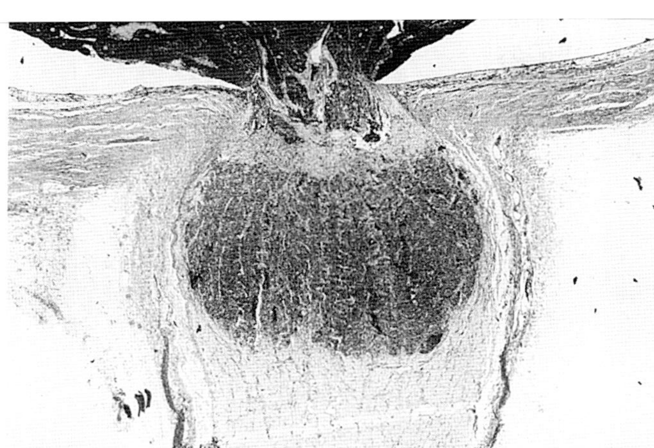

Fig. 30.68 Retinoblastomas exhibit a definite tendency to spread out of the globe by way of the optic nerve. It is therefore of utmost importance for the surgical pathologist to determine whether such optic nerve extension has occurred and, if it has, to what extent.

13q, and loss of 16q.[303,304,308,309] Some cases also show amplifications of the *NMYC*, *MDMX* or *MDM2* gene.[310]

Spread and metastases

Retinoblastoma has a tendency to invade the optic nerve, from which it can extend to the brain or be carried there by the subarachnoid fluid[321] (Fig. 30.68). Large exophytic tumors with secondary glaucoma are at highest risk for optic nerve invasion.[321] Retinoblastoma can also invade the uveal tract. Distant metastases can be limited to the cranial vault or involve distant sites, particularly the skeletal system.[320]

Treatment

The treatment of retinoblastoma depends on the extent of the disease.[327,329] Early cases can be managed with conservative measures aimed at preserving the vision, such as unilateral radiation, cryopexy, or xenon arc photocoagulation.[324] When the tumor is so large that the eye is no longer salvageable, enucleation should be performed.[330] If tumor has extended to the surgically cut end of the nerve, irradiation of the orbit and systemic chemotherapy are performed. In patients with bilateral retinoblastoma, the less affected eye is treated with radiotherapy, at times in combination with chemotherapy. Bilateral cases can also be treated with simultaneous bilateral irradiation.[322,323,325] The success rate for life of the patient and for preservation of vision is quite good. If tumor recurrences develop, they are treated with photocoagulation, cryotherapy, and

1 *Invasion of optic nerve*. In an operation for suspected neuroblastoma, the surgeon will attempt to obtain a long segment of optic nerve attached to the globe. Transverse sections of this nerve should be examined microscopically at the prelaminar and retrolaminar levels, including the surgical margin.[337] The levels of invasion of the optic nerve by retinoblastoma have been divided into prelaminar, laminar, and retrolaminar, the latter further subdivided into lesions with or without resection line involvement.[337] The prognosis decreases with each of these levels.[334–336]
2 *Invasion of meninges*. This is often associated with invasion of the optic nerve.[336]
3 *Invasion of the uveal tract*. Massive invasion of the uveal tract by retinoblastoma is an unfavorable prognostic sign.[334,335]

Long-term survivors have a greater incidence of development of malignant tumors. The incidence has ranged from 6% to 20% after 10 years, and in one series has reached 90% at 30 years. The most common types have been osteosarcoma and rhabdomyosarcoma, but several other types have been encountered, including rhabdoid tumors.[331,338] This predisposition for a second malignancy, which should be distinguished from a recurrence of the retinoblastoma,[333] is seen almost exclusively with the hereditary form of the disease.[332]

Lymphoid tumors and tumorlike conditions

Abnormalities of intraocular tissues are present in approximately 50% of patients with leukemia at autopsy.[341] These are in the form of leukemic infiltrates and hemorrhages, particularly in the choroid and retina.[341,347]

Intraocular **malignant lymphoma** is a rare disease. In contrast to other portions of the ocular apparatus, in which MALT-type lymphomas predominate, most intraocular lymphomas (also known as primary retinal lymphomas) are aggressive diffuse B-cell lymphomas.[342] In over 90% of the cases the eye lesion heralds the presence or development of extraocular lymphoma, which is located in the central nervous system in one-half or more of the cases.[344] Sometimes the lymphomatous process preferentially involves the optic nerve.[343]

Reactive lymphoid hyperplasia can also occur within the ocular globe;[345,346] the criteria for distinguishing it from lymphoma are similar to those applied elsewhere.

Other primary tumors

Fuchs adenoma (benign ciliary epithelioma, Fuchs epithelioma, coronal adenoma) is a benign tumor of the ciliary body usually found incidentally in a surgically enucleated eye or on post mortem examination. Microscopically, it is formed by interlacing trabeculae of uniform, nonpigmented ciliary epithelial cells surrounded by an amorphous, hyaline, periodic acid–Schiff (PAS)-positive material.[358]

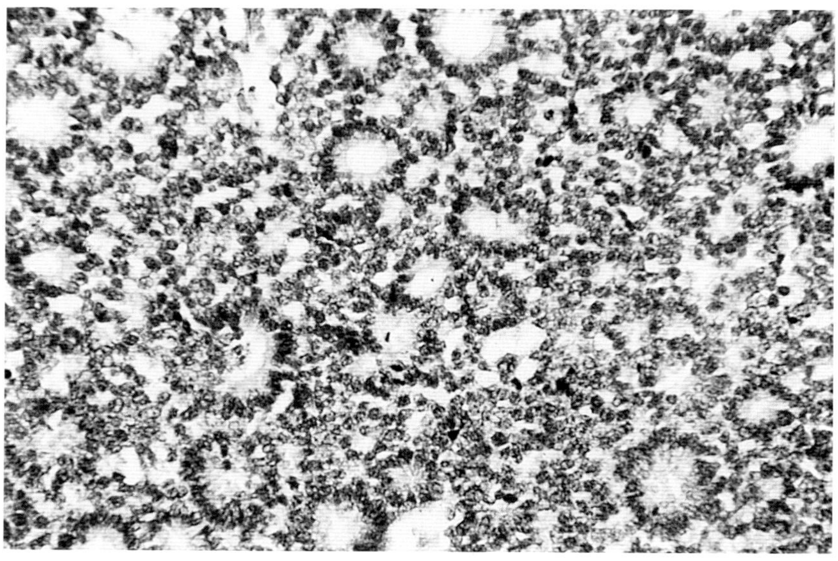

Fig. 30.66 Retinoblastoma with typical rosettes. *(From Ackerman LV, del Regato JA. Cancer, ed. 6. St Louis, 1985, Mosby)*

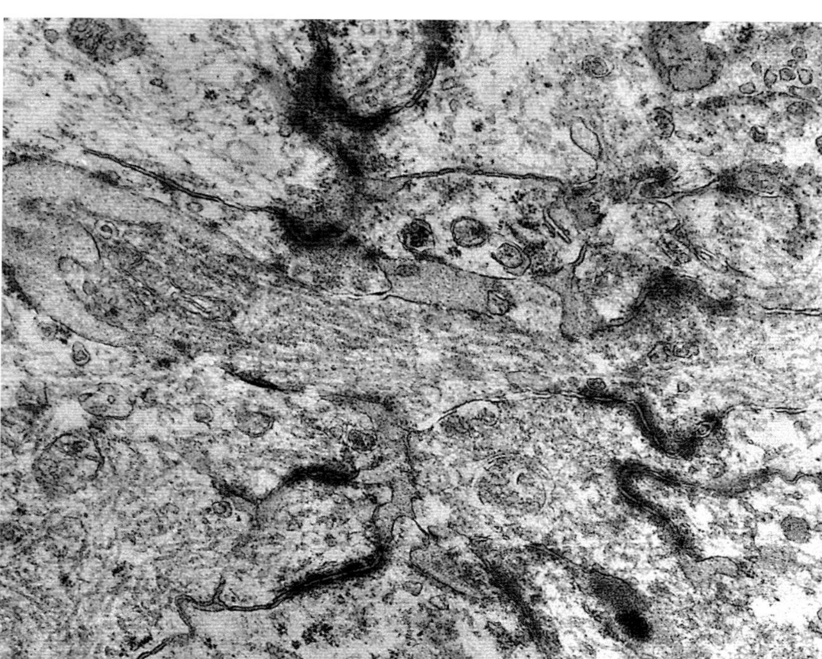

Fig. 30.67 Electron micrograph of retinoblastoma. A portion of the center of a rudimentary Flexner–Wintersteiner rosette illustrating a bulbous apical microtubule-containing cytoplasmic process and numerous cell junctions. (×20 800) *(Courtesy of Dr Robert A Erlandson, Memorial Sloan-Kettering Cancer Center)*

Electron microscopic, immunohistochemical, and molecular genetic features

Ultrastructurally, evidence of photodifferentiation has been found in the tumor cells of retinoblastoma[315,316] (Fig. 30.67).

with photoreceptor cells) have been found in these tumors.[305,306,311] Interestingly, retinal S-antigen has also been detected in tumors of the pineal gland and in cerebellar medulloblastomas.[307,311] Further evidence of the retinal nature of this tumor has been obtained in vitro, where differentiation toward photoreceptors has been

component of von Hippel–Lindau disease), **neurofibromas, astrocytomas**, and **pleomorphic xanthoastrocytomas** are sometimes found in the retina,[352,354,356,359] and a case of PEComa has been described in the ciliary body.[353]

Juvenile xanthogranuloma can occur in the iris and result in spontaneous hyphema and/or secondary glaucoma.[350] It occurs almost exclusively in young children and is associated with skin lesions of similar microscopic appearance.[360]

Glioneuroma has been described in the iris and ciliary body,[348] and **malignant mesenchymoma** (containing rhabdomyosarcomatous and liposarcomatous areas) has been reported involving the entire uveal tract.[355]

Metastatic tumors

The intraocular tissues can be involved by metastatic carcinoma and, less commonly, by metastatic cutaneous melanoma and metastatic sarcoma. In fact, if one were to do serial sections routinely on all autopsy eyes, cases of metastatic carcinoma would outnumber the primary tumors. The difference, of course, is that most of the patients were asymptomatic for ocular symptoms while alive. The most common primary lesions involved are in the breast in the female and in the lung in the male, with the gastrointestinal tract next in frequency.[361,363–366] The ocular metastasis occasionally may be the initial manifestation of the disease, and the primary lesion is discovered only after the eye has been enucleated.

The posterior choroid is the most common site for these metastases[362] (Fig. 30.69). Anterior uveal involvement is much less common, and retinal metastases are rare. Diffuse thickening of the choroid along both sides of the optic nerve is the most common presentation, but bulky tumor masses resembling malignant melanomas also may be observed.

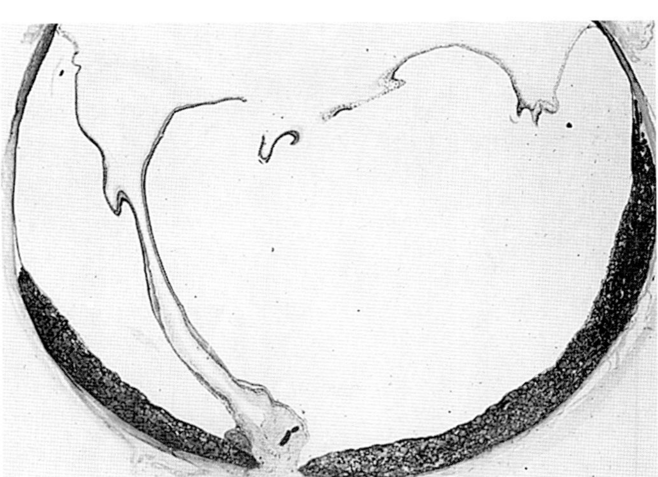

Fig. 30.69 Metastatic carcinoma from breast producing diffuse thickening of the choroid posteriorly.

Cytology

In certain cases the pathologist may be called on to examine material that has been aspirated from either the aqueous or the vitreous fluid and has been passed through a Millipore filter. Cases in which this has proved useful include large cell lymphoma,[368] retinoblastoma,[370] and phacolytic glaucoma.[369] Analysis of clonal immunoglobulin heavy chain gene rearrangements for the confirmation of a diagnosis of lymphoma can be carried out on this material.[367]

References

NORMAL ANATOMY

1 Campbell RJ. Histological typing of tumours of the eye and the adnexa. London, 1998, Springer.
2 Font RL, Croxatto JO, Rao NA. Tumors of the eye and ocular adnexa (AFIP atlas of tumor pathology). Washington, DC, 2006, American Registry of Pathology in collaboration with the Armed Forces Institute of Pathology.
3 Harry J, Misson G. Clinical ophthalmic pathology: principles of diseases of the eye and associated structures. Oxford, 2001, Butterworth Heinemann.
4 Hogan MJ, Zimmerman LE. Ophthalmic pathology. An atlas and textbook, ed. 2. Philadelphia, 1962, W.B. Saunders.
5 Hogan MJ, Alvarado JA, Weddell JE. Histology of the human eye. An atlas and textbook. Philadelphia, 1971, W.B. Saunders.
6 Jakobiec FA. Ocular and adnexal tumors. Birmingham, AL, 1978, Aesculapius.
10 Shields CL. Eyelid conjuctival and orbital tumors: an atlas and text, ed. 2. Philadelphia, 2007, Lippincott Williams & Wilkins.
11 Shields CL. Intraocular tumors: an atlas and text, ed. 2, Philadelphia, 2007, Lippincott Williams & Wilkins.
12 Spencer WH. Ophthalmic pathology: an atlas and textbook. Philadelphia, 1996, W.B. Saunders.
13 Yanoff M, Sassani JW. Ocular pathology, ed. 6. St Louis, 2008, Mosby.

EYELIDS

INFLAMMATION

14 Codère F, Lee RD, Anderson RL. Necrobiotic xanthogranuloma of the eyelid. Arch Ophthalmol 1983, **101**: 60–63.
15 Riddle PJ, Font RL, Johnson FB, McLean IW. Silica granuloma of eyelid and ocular adnexa. Arch Ophthalmol 1981, **99**: 683–689.

TUMORS AND TUMORLIKE LESIONS

Tumors and tumorlike lesions of surface epithelium

18 Aurora AL, Blodi FC. Lesions of the eyelids. A clinicopathologic study. Surv Ophthalmol 1970, **15**: 94–104.
19 Boniuk M. Tumors of the eyelids. Int Ophthalmol Clin 1962, **2**: 239–317.
20 Boniuk M, Zimmerman LE. Eyelid tumors with reference to lesions confused with squamous cell carcinoma. II. Inverted follicular keratosis. Arch Ophthalmol 1963, **69**: 698–707.
21 Boniuk M, Zimmerman LE. Eyelid tumors with reference to lesions confused with squamous cell carcinoma. III. Keratoacanthoma. Arch Ophthalmol 1967, **77**: 29–40.
22 Caya JG, Hidayat AA, Weiner JM. A

232 Mudhar HS, Parsons MA, Sisley K, Rundle P, Singh A, Rennie IG. A critical appraisal of the prognostic and predictive factors for uveal malignant melanoma. Histopathology 2004, **45**: 1–12.

233 Sassani JW, Weinstein JM, Graham WP. Massively invasive diffuse choroidal melanoma. Arch Ophthalmol 1985, **103**: 945–948.

234 Shields JA, Shields CL, De Potter P, Singh AD. Diagnosis and treatment of uveal melanoma. Semin Oncol 1996, **23**: 763–767.

235 Yanoff M, Zimmerman LE. Histogenesis of malignant melanomas of the uvea. I. Nevi of choroid and ciliary body. Arch Ophthalmol 1966, **76**: 784–796.

236 Yanoff M, Zimmerman LE. Histogenesis of malignant melanomas of the uvea. II. The relationship of uveal nevi to malignant melanomas. Cancer 1967, **20**: 493–507.

237 Yanoff M, Zimmerman LE. Histogenesis of malignant melanomas of the uvea. III. The relationship of congenital ocular melanocytosis and neurofibromatosis to uveal melanomas. Arch Ophthalmol 1967, **77**: 331–336.

Microscopic features

238 Cole EL, Zakov ZN, Meisler DM, Tuthill RJ, McMahon JT. Cutaneous malignant melanoma metastatic to the vitreous. Arch Ophthalmol 1986, **104**: 98–101.

239 de Bustros S, Augsburger JJ, Shields JA, Shakin EP, Pryor CC II. Intraocular metastases from cutaneous malignant melanoma. Arch Ophthalmol 1985, **103**: 937–940.

240 Howard GM, Forrest AW. Incidence and location of melanocytomas. Arch Ophthalmol 1967, **77**: 61–66.

241 Letson AD, Davidorf FH. Bilateral retinal metastases from cutaneous malignant melanoma. Arch Ophthalmol 1982, **100**: 605–607.

242 McLean IW, Zimmerman LE, Evans R. Reappraisal of Callender's spindle A type of malignant melanoma of choroid and ciliary body. Am J Ophthalmol 1978, **86**: 557–564.

243 Shields JA, Karan DS, Perry HD, Donoso LA. Epithelioid cell nevus of the iris. Arch Ophthalmol 1985, **103**: 235–237.

Immunohistochemical and molecular genetic features

244 Coleman K, Baak JPA, van Diest PJ, Curran B, Mullaney J, Fenton M, Leader M. DNA ploidy status in 84 ocular melanomas. A study of DNA quantitation in ocular melanomas by flow cytometry and automatic and interactive static image analysis. Hum Pathol 1995, **26**: 99–105.

245 Fuchs U, Kivela T, Summanen P, Immonen I, Tarkkanen A. An immunohistochemical and prognostic analysis of cytokeratin expression in malignant uveal melanoma. Am J Pathol 1992, **141**: 169–181.

246 Hendrix MJ, Seftor EA, Seftor RE, Gardner LM, Boldt HC, Meyer M, Pe'er J, Folberg R. Biologic determinants of uveal melanoma metastatic phenotype: role of intermediate filaments as predictive markers. Lab Invest 1998, **78**: 153–163.

247 Horsman DE, White VA. Cytogenetic analysis of uveal melanoma. Consistent occurrence of monosomy 3 and trisomy 8q. Cancer 1993, **71**: 811–819.

248 Janssen K, Kuntze J, Busse H, Schmid KW. p53 oncoprotein overexpression in choroidal melanoma. Mod Pathol 1996, **9**: 267–272.

249 Mensink HW, Kilic E, Vaarwater J, Douben H, Paridaens D, de Klein A. Molecular cytogenetic analysis of archival uveal melanoma with known clinical outcome. Cancer Genet Cytogenet 2008, **181**: 108–111.

250 Onken MD, Worley LA, Long MD, Duan S, Council ML, Bowcock AM, Harbour JW. Oncogenic mutations in GNAQ occur early in uveal melanoma. Invest Ophthalmol Vis Sci 2008, **49**: 5230–5234.

251 Singh AD, Wang MX, Donoso LA, Shields CL, De Potter P, Shields JA. Genetic aspects of uveal melanoma: a brief review. Semin Oncol 1996, **23**: 768–772.

Spread and metastases

252 Kath R, Hayungs J, Bornfeld N, Sauerwein W, Hoffken K, Seeber S. Prognosis and treatment of disseminated uveal melanoma. Cancer 1993, **72**: 2219–2223.

253 Luyten GPM, Mooy CM, Post J, Jensen OA, Luider TM, de Jong PT. Metastatic uveal melanoma: a morphologic and immunohistochemical analysis. Cancer 1996, **78**: 1967–1971.

254 Wieselthier JS, White WL. Cutaneous metastasis of ocular malignant melanoma: an unusual presentation simulating blue nevi. Am J Dermatopathol 1996, **18**: 289–295.

Treatment

255 Char DH, Phillips TL. The potential for adjuvant radiotherapy in choroidal melanoma. Arch Ophthalmol 1982, **100**: 247–248.

256 Forrest A, Keeper R, Spencer W. Iridocyclectomy for melanomas of the ciliary body. A follow-up study of pathology and surgical morbidity. Am J Ophthalmol 1978, **85**: 1237–1249.

257 Seigel D, Myers M, Ferris F III, Steinhorn SC. Survival rates after enucleation of eyes with malignant melanoma. Am J Ophthalmol 1979, **87**: 761–765.

258 Shields JA, Shields CL, De Potter P, Singh AD. Diagnosis and treatment of uveal melanoma. Semin Oncol 1996, **23**: 763–767.

259 Zimmerman LE, McLean IW, Foster W. Does enucleation of the eye containing a malignant melanoma prevent or accelerate the dissemination of tumor cells? Br J Ophthalmol 1978, **62**: 420–425.

Prognosis

260 Ashton N, Wybar K. Primary tumours of the iris. Ophthalmologica 1966, **151**: 97–113.

261 Coleman K, Baak JPA, van Diest PJ, Curran B, Mullaney J, Fenton M, Leader M. DNA ploidy status in 84 ocular melanomas. A study of DNA quantitation in ocular melanomas by flow cytometry and automatic and interactive static image analysis. Hum Pathol 1995, **26**: 99–105.

262 de la Cruz PO Jr, Specht CS, McLean IW. Lymphocytic infiltration in uveal malignant melanoma. Cancer 1990, **65**: 112–115.

263 Dunne BM, McNamara M, Clynes M, Shering SG, Larkin AM, Moran E, Barnes C, Kennedy SM. MDR1 expression is associated with adverse survival in melanoma of the uveal tract. Hum Pathol 1998, **29**: 594–598.

264 Folberg R, Pe'er J, Gruman LM, Woolson RF, Jeng G, Montague PR, Moninger TO, Yi H, Moore KC. The morphologic characteristics of tumor blood vessels as a marker of tumor progression in primary human uveal melanoma. A matched case-control study. Hum Pathol 1992, **23**: 1298–1305.

265 Gamel JW, McLean I, Greenberg RA, Naids RM, Folberg R, Donoso LA, Seddon JM, Albert DM. Objective assessment of the malignant potential of intraocular melanomas with standard microslides stained with hematoxylin-eosin. Hum Pathol 1985, **16**: 689–692.

266 Gamel JW, McLean IW, McCurdy JB. Biologic distinctions between cure and time to death in 2892 patients with intraocular melanoma. Cancer 1993, **71**: 2299–2305.

267 Jakobiec FA, Silbert G. Are most iris 'melanomas' really nevi? A clinicopathologic study of 189 lesions. Arch Ophthalmol 1981, **99**: 2117–2132.

268 McCurdy J, Gamel J, McLean I. A simple, efficient, and reproducible method for estimating the malignant potential of uveal melanoma from routine H and E slides. Pathol Res Pract 1991, **187**: 1025–1027.

269 McLean IW, Foster WD, Zimmerman LE. Uveal melanoma. Location, size, cell type, and enucleation as risk factors in metastasis. Hum Pathol 1982, **13**: 123–132.

270 McLean IW, Sibug ME, Becker RL, McCurdy JB. Uveal melanoma: the importance of large nucleoli in predicting patient outcome – an automated image analysis study. Cancer 1997, **79**: 982–988.

271 McLean IW, Zimmerman LE, Evans R. Reappraisal of Callender's spindle A type of malignant melanoma of choroid and ciliary body. Am J Ophthalmol 1978, **86**: 557–564.

272 Miller MV, Herdson PB, Hitchcock GC. Malignant melanoma of the uveal tract. A review of the Auckland experience. Pathology 1985, **17**: 281–284.

273 Onken MD, Worley LA, Harbour JW. Association between gene expression profile, proliferation and metastasis in uveal melanoma. Curr Eye Res 2010, **35**: 857–863.

274 Pach JM, Robertson DM, Taney BS, Martin JA, Campbell RJ, O'Brien PC. Prognostic factors in choroidal and ciliary body melanomas with extrascleral extension. Am J Ophthalmol 1986, **101**: 325–331.

275 Seddon JM, Albert DM, Lavin DT, Robinson N. A prognostic factor study of disease-free interval and survival following enucleation for uveal melanoma. Arch Ophthalmol 1983, **101**: 1894–1899.

276 Singh AD, Shields CL, Shields JA. Prognostic factors in uveal melanoma. Melanoma Res 2001, **11**: 255–263.

277 Sorensen FB, Gamel JW, McCurdy J. Stereologic estimation of nucleolar volume in ocular melanoma. A comparative study of size estimators with prognostic impact. Hum Pathol 1993, **24**: 513–518.

278 Starr HJ, Zimmerman LE. Extrascleral extension and orbital recurrence of malignant melanomas of the choroid and ciliary body. Int Ophthalmol Clin 1962, **2**: 369–385.

279 van Gils W, Lodder EM, Mensink HW, Kilic E, Naus NC, Bruggenwirth HT, van Ijcken W, Paridaens D, Luyten GP, de Klein A. Gene expression profiling in uveal melanoma: two regions on 3p related to prognosis. Invest Ophthalmol Vis Sci 2008, **49**: 4254–4262.

280 Weinhaus RS, Seddon JM, Albert DM, Gragoudas ES, Robinson N. Prognostic factor study of survival after enucleation for juxtapapillary melanomas. Arch Ophthalmol 1985, **103**: 1673–1677.

RETINOBLASTOMA AND RELATED LESIONS

General features

281 Gallie BL, Squire JA, Goddard A, Dunn JM, Canton M, Hinton D, Zhu XP, Phillips RA. Mechanism of oncogenesis in retinoblastoma. Lab Invest 1990, **62**: 394–408.

282 Horowitz JM, Park SH, Bogenmann E, Cheng JC, Yandell DW, Kaye FJ, Minna JD, Dryja TP, Weinberg RA. Frequent inactivation of the retinoblastoma antioncogene is restricted to a subset of human tumor cells. Proc Natl Acad Sci U S A 1990, **87**: 2775–2779.

283 Knudson A. Alfred Knudson and his two-hit hypothesis. (Interview by Ezzie Hutchinson.) Lancet Oncol 2001, **2**: 642–645.

284 Kyritsis AP, Tsokos M, Triche TJ, Chader GJ. Retinoblastoma. Origin from a primitive neuroectodermal cell? Nature 1984, **307**: 471–473.

285 Rubinstein LJ. Embryonal central neuroepithelial tumors and their differentiating potential. A cytogenetic view of a complex neuro-oncological problem. J Neurosurg 1985, **62**: 795–805.

286 Sang DN, Albert DM. Retinoblastoma. Clinical and histopathologic features. Hum Pathol 1982, **13**: 133–147.

287 Schubert EL, Hansen MF, Strong LC. The retinoblastoma gene and its significance. Ann Med 1994, **26**: 177–184.

288 Wiggs J, Nordenskjöld M, Yandell D, Rapaport J, Grondin V, Janson M, Werelius B, Petersen R, Craft A, Riedel K, Liberfarb R, Walton D, Wilson W, Dryja TP. Prediction of the risk of hereditary retinoblastoma, using DNA polymorphisms within the retinoblastoma gene. N Engl J Med 1988, **318**: 151–157.

289 Wiman KG. The retinoblastoma gene. Role in cell cycle control and cell differentiation. FASEB J 1993, **7**: 841–845.

290 Yandell DW, Campbell TA, Dayton SH, Petersen R, Walton D, Little JB, McConkie-Rosell A, Buckley EG, Dryja TP. Oncogenic point mutations in the human retinoblastoma gene. Their application to genetic counseling. N Engl J Med 1989, **321**: 1689–1695.

291 Zacksenhaus E, Bremner R, Jiang Z, Gill RM, Muncaster M, Sopta M, Philips RA, Gallie BL. Unravelling the function of the retinoblastoma gene. Adv Cancer Res 1993, **61**: 115–141.

Clinical and gross features

292 Amoaku WMK, Willshaw HE, Parkes SE, Shah KJ, Mann JR. Trilateral retinoblastoma: a report of five patients. Cancer 1996, **78**: 858–863.

293 Holladay DA, Holladay A, Montebello JF, Redmond KP. Clinical presentation, treatment, and outcome of trilateral retinoblastoma. Cancer 1991, **67**: 710–715.

294 Howard GM, Ellsworth RM. Differential diagnosis of retinoblastoma. A statistical survey of 500 children. Am J Ophthalmol 1965, **60**: 610–612.

295 Johnson DL, Chandra R, Fisher WS, Hammock MK, McKeown CA. Trilateral retinoblastoma. Ocular and pineal retinoblastomas. J Neurosurg 1985, **63**: 367–370.

296 Kogan L, Boniuk M. Causes for enucleation in childhood with special reference to pseudogliomas and retinoblastomas. Int Ophthalmol Clin 1962, **2**: 507–524.

297 Paulino AC. Trilateral retinoblastoma: is the location of the intracranial tumor important? Cancer 1999, **86**: 135–141.

Microscopic features

298 Bunt AH, Tso MOM. Feulgen-positive deposits in retinoblastoma. Incidence, composition, and ultrastructure. Arch Ophthalmol 1981, **99**: 144–150.

299 He W, Hashimoto H, Tsuneyoshi M, Enjoji M, Inomata H. A reassessment of histologic classification and an immunohistochemical study of 88 retinoblastomas. A special reference to the advent of bipolar-like cells. Cancer 1992, **70**: 2901–2908.

300 Lueder GT, Smith ME. Retinoblastoma. Semin Diagn Pathol 1994, **11**: 104–106.

301 Margo C, Hidayat A, Kopelman J, Zimmerman LE. Retinocytoma. A benign variant of retinoblastoma. Arch Ophthalmol 1983, **101**: 1519–1531.

302 Shuangshoti S, Chaiwun B, Kasantikul V. A study of 39 retinoblastomas with particular reference to morphology, cellular differentiation and tumour origin. Histopathology 1989, **15**: 113–124.

Electron microscopic, immunohistochemical, and molecular genetic features

303 Amare Kadam PS, Ghule P, Jose J, Bamne M, Kurkure P, Banavali S, Sarin R, Advani S. Constitutional genomic instability, chromosome aberrations in tumor cells and retinoblastoma. Cancer Genet Cytogenet 2004, **150**: 33–43.

304 Corson TW, Gallie BL. One hit, two hits, three hits, more? Genomic changes in the development of retinoblastoma. Genes Chromosomes Cancer 2007, **46**: 617–634.

305 Donoso LA, Hamm H, Dietzschold B, Augsburger JJ, Shields JA, Arbizo V. Rhodopsin and retinoblastoma. A monoclonal antibody histopathologic study. Arch Ophthalmol 1986, **104**: 111–113.

306 Gonzalez-Fernandez F, Lopes MB, Garcia-Fernandez JM, Foster RG, De Grip WJ, Rosemberg S, Newman SA, Vanden Berg SR. Expression of developmentally defined retinal phenotypes in the histogenesis of retinoblastoma. Am J Pathol 1992, **141**: 363–375.

307 Korf H-W, Czerwionka M, Reiner J, Schachenmayr W, Schalken JJ, de Grip W, Gery I. Immunocytochemical evidence of molecular photoreceptor markers in cerebellar medulloblastomas. Cancer 1987, **60**: 1763–1766.

308 Leiderman YI, Kiss S, Mukai S. Molecular genetics of RB1 – the retinoblastoma gene. Semin Ophthalmol 2007, **22**: 247–254.

309 Lillington DM, Kingston JE, Coen PG, Price E, Hungerford J, Domizio P, Young BD, Onadim Z. Comparative genomic hybridization of 49 primary retinoblastoma tumors identifies chromosomal regions associated with histopathology, progression, and patient outcome. Genes Chromosomes Cancer 2003, **36**: 121–128.

310 Lin P, O'Brien JM. Frontiers in the management of retinoblastoma. Am J Ophthalmol 2009, **148**: 192–198.

311 Perentes E, Rubinstein LJ. Recent applications of immunoperoxidase histochemistry in human neuro-oncology. An update. Arch Pathol Lab Med 1987, **111**: 796–812.

312 Schwimer CJ, Prayson RA. Clinicopathologic study of retinoblastoma including MIB-1, p53, and CD99 immunohistochemistry. Ann Diagn Pathol 2001, **5**: 148–154.

313 Shuangshoti S, Chaiwun B, Kasantikul V. A study of 39 retinoblastomas with particular reference to morphology, cellular differentiation and tumour origin. Histopathology 1989, **15**: 113–124.

314 Terenghi G, Polak JM, Ballesta J, Cocchia D, Michetti F, Dahl D, Marangos PJ, Garner A. Immunocytochemistry of neuronal and glial markers in retinoblastoma. Virchows Arch [A] 1984, **404**: 61–73.

315 Ts'o MO, Fine BS, Zimmerman LE. The nature of retinoblastoma. II. Photoreceptor differentiation. An electron microscopic study. Am J Ophthalmol 1970, **69**: 350–359.

316 Ts'o MO, Zimmerman LE, Fine BS. The nature of retinoblastoma. I. Photoreceptor differentiation. A clinical and histopathologic study. Am J Ophthalmol 1970, **69**: 339–349.

317 Tsokos M, Kyritsis AP, Chader GJ, Triche TJ. Differentiation of human retinoblastoma in vitro into cell types with characteristics observed in embryonal or mature retina. Am J Pathol 1986, **123**: 542–552.

318 Tsuji M, Goto M, Uehara F, Kaneko A, Sawai J, Yonezawa S, Ohba N. Photoreceptor cell differentiation in retinoblastoma demonstrated by a new immunohistochemical marker mucin-like glycoprotein associated with photoreceptor cells (MLGAPC). Histopathology 2002, **40**: 180–186.

319 Yuge K, Nakajima M, Uemura Y, Miki H, Uyama M, Tsubura A. Immunohistochemical features of the human retina and retinoblastoma. Virchows Arch 1995, **426**: 571–575.

Spread and metastases

320 MacKay CJ, Abramson DH, Ellsworth RM. Metastatic patterns of retinoblastoma. Arch Ophthalmol 1984, **102**: 391–396.

321 Shields JA, Shields CL. Current management of retinoblastoma. Mayo Clin Proc 1994, **69**: 50–56.

Treatment

322 Abramson DH, Ellsworth RM, Tretter P, Adams K, Kitchin FD. Simultaneous bilateral radiation for advanced bilateral retinoblastoma. Arch Ophthalmol 1981, **99**: 1763–1766.

323 Abramson DH, Ellsworth RM, Tretter P, Javitt J, Kitchin FD. Treatment of bilateral groups I through III retinoblastoma with bilateral radiation. Arch Ophthalmol 1981, **99**: 1761–1762.

324 Abramson DH, Marks RF, Ellsworth RM, Tretter P, Kitchin FD. The management of unilateral retinoblastoma without primary enucleation. Arch Ophthalmol 1982, **100**: 1249–1252.

325 Amendola BE, Lamm FR, Markoe AM, Karlsson UL, Shields J, Shields CL, Augsburger J, Brady LW, Woodleigh R, Miller C. Radiotherapy of retinoblastoma. A review of 63 children treated with different irradiation techniques. Cancer 1990, **66**: 21–26.

326 Antoneli CBG, Steinhorst F, Riberio K, Novaes PE, Chojniak MM, Arias V, de Camargo B. Extraocular retinoblastoma: a 13-year experience. Cancer 2003, **98**: 1292–1298.

327 Kiss S, Leiderman YI, Mukai A. Diagnosis, classification, and treatment of retinoblastoma. Int Ophthalmol Clin 2008, **48**: 135–147.

328 Lin P, O'Brien JM. Frontiers in the management of retinoblastoma. Am J Ophthalmol 2009, **148**: 192–198.

329 Shields CL, Shields JA, Baez K, Cater JR, De Potter P. Optic nerve invasion of retinoblastoma. Metastatic potential and clinical risk factors. Cancer 1994, **73**: 692–698.

330 Zelter M, Gonzalez G, Schwartz L, Gallo G, Schvartzman E, Damel A, Muriel FS. Treatment of retinoblastoma. Results obtained from a prospective study of 51 patients. Cancer 1988, **61**: 153–160.

Prognosis

331 Abramson DH, Ellsworth R, Zimmerman L. Nonocular cancer in retinoblastoma survivors. Trans Am Acad Ophthalmol Otolaryngol 1976, **81**: 454–457.

332 DerKinderen DJ, Koten JW, Nagelkerke NJD, Tan KEWP, Beemer FA, Den Otter W. Nonocular cancer in patients with hereditary

retinoblastoma and their relatives. Int J Cancer 1988, **41**: 499–504.

333 Dickman PS, Barmada M, Gollin SM, Blatt J. Malignancy after retinoblastoma: secondary cancer or recurrence? Hum Pathol 1997, **28**: 200–205.

334 Eagle RC Jr. High-risk features and tumor differentiation in retinoblastoma: a retrospective histopathologic study. Arch Pathol Lab Med 2009, **133**: 1203–1209.

335 Khelfaoui F, Validire P, Auperin A, Quintana E, Michon J, Pacquement H, Desjardins L, Asselain B, Schlienger P, Vielh P, et al. Histopathologic risk factors in retinoblastoma: a retrospective study of 172 patients treated in a single institution. Cancer 1996, **77**: 1206–1213.

336 Sang DN, Albert DM. Retinoblastoma. Clinical and histopathologic features. Hum Pathol 1982, **13**: 133–147.

337 Sastre X, Chantada GL, Doz F, Wilson MW, de Davila MT, Rodríguez-Galindo C, Chintagumpala M, Chévez-Barrios P; International Retinoblastoma Staging Working Group. Proceedings of the consensus meetings from the International Retinoblastoma Staging Working Group on the pathology guidelines for the examination of enucleated eyes and evaluation of prognostic risk factors in retinoblastoma. Arch Pathol Lab Med 2009, **133**: 1199–1202.

338 Walford N, Deferrai R, Slater RM, Delemarre JF, Dingemans KP, Van den Bergh Weerman MA, Voute PA. Intraorbital rhabdoid tumour following bilateral retinoblastoma. Histopathology 1992, **20**: 170–173.

339 Zelter M, Damel A, Gonzalez G, Schwartz L. A prospective study on the treatment of retinoblastoma in 72 patients. Cancer 1991, **68**: 1685–1690.

340 Zelter M, Gonzalez G, Schwartz L, Gallo G, Schvartzman E, Damel A, Muriel FS. Treatment of retinoblastoma. Results obtained from a prospective study of 51 patients. Cancer 1988, **61**: 153–160.

LYMPHOID TUMORS AND TUMORLIKE CONDITIONS

341 Allen R, Straatsma B. Ocular involvement in leukemia and allied disorders. Arch Ophthalmol 1961, **66**: 490–508.

342 Faia LJ, Chan CC. Primary intraocular lymphoma. Arch Pathol Lab Med 2009, **133**: 1228–1232.

343 Kline LB, Garcia JH, Harsh GR III. Lymphomatous optic neuropathy. Arch Ophthalmol 1984, **102**: 1655–1657.

344 Qualman SJ, Mendelsohn G, Mann RB, Green WR. Intraocular lymphomas. Natural history based on a clinicopathologic study of eight cases and review of the literature. Cancer 1983, **52**: 878–886.

345 Ryan S, Zimmerman LE, King FM. Reactive lymphoid hyperplasia. An unusual form of intraocular pseudotumor. Trans Am Acad Ophthalmol Otolaryngol 1972, **76**: 652–671.

346 Shields JA, Augsburger JJ, Gonder JR, MacLeod D. Localized benign lymphoid tumor of the iris. Arch Ophthalmol 1981, **99**: 2147–2148.

347 Vogel M, Font RL, Zimmerman LE, Levine R. Reticulum cell sarcoma of the retina and uvea. Am J Ophthalmol 1968, **66**: 205–215.

OTHER PRIMARY TUMORS

348 Addison DJ, Font RL. Glioneuroma of iris and ciliary body. Arch Ophthalmol 1984, **102**: 419–421.

349 Alenda C, Aranda FI, Payá A, Córdoba C. Mesectodermal leiomyoma of ciliary body. Int J Surg Pathol 2002, **10**: 309–312.

350 Bruner WE, Stark WJ, Green WR. Presumed juvenile xanthogranuloma of the iris and ciliary body in an adult. Arch Ophthalmol 1982, **100**: 457–459.

351 Cassoux N, Charlotte F, Sastre X, Orbach D, Lehoang P, Desjardins L. Conservative surgical treatment of medulloepithelioma of the ciliary body. Arch Ophthalmol 2010, **128**: 380–381.

352 Ehlers N, Jensen OA. Juxtapapillary retinal hemangioblastoma (angiomatosis retinae) in an infant. Light microscopical and ultrastructural examination. Ultrastruct Pathol 1982, **3**: 325–333.

353 Furusato E, Cameron JD, Newsom RW, Fujishiro T, Kojima T, Specht CS, Fetsch JF, Furusato B, Sesterhenn IA, Rushing EJ. Ocular perivascular epithelioid cell tumor: report of 2 cases with distinct clinical presentations. Hum Pathol 2010, **41**: 768–772.

354 Messmer E, Font RL, Laqua H, Höpping W, Naumann GOH. Cavernous hemangioma of the retina. Immunohistochemical and ultrastructural observations. Arch Ophthalmol 1984, **102**: 413–418.

355 Pe'er J, Neudorfer M, Ron N, Anteby I, Lazar M, Rosenmann E. Panuveal malignant mesenchymoma. Arch Pathol Lab Med 1995, **118**: 844–847.

356 Ulbright TM, Fulling KH, Helveston EM. Astrocytic tumors of the retina. Differentiation of sporadic tumors from phakomatosis-associated tumors. Arch Pathol Lab Med 1984, **108**: 160–163.

357 Yu L, Aldave AJ, Glasgow BJ. Epstein–Barr virus-associated smooth muscle tumor of the iris in a patient with transplant: a case report and review of the literature. Arch Pathol Lab Med 2009, **133**: 1238–1241.

358 Zaidman GW, Johnson BL, Salamon SM, Mondino BJ. Fuchs' adenoma affecting the peripheral iris. Arch Ophthalmol 1983, **101**: 771–773.

359 Zarate JO, Sampaolesi R. Pleomorphic xanthoastrocytoma of the retina. Am J Surg Pathol 1999, **23**: 79–81.

360 Zimmerman LE. Ocular lesions of juvenile xanthogranuloma. Nevoxanthoendothelioma. Trans Am Acad Ophthalmol Otolaryngol 1965, **69**: 412–442.

METASTATIC TUMORS

361 Albert DM, Rubenstein R, Scheie H. Tumor metastasis to the eye. Part I. Incidence in 213 adult patients with generalized malignancy. Am J Ophthalmol 1967, **63**(Pt 1): 724–726.

362 D'Abbadie I, Arriagada R, Spielmann M, Lê MG. Choroid metastases: clinical features and treatments in 123 patients. Cancer 2003, **98**: 1232–1238.

363 Ferry AP. Metastatic carcinoma of the eye and ocular adnexa. Int Ophthalmol Clin 1967, **7**: 615–658.

364 Ferry A, Font R. Carcinoma metastatic to the eye and orbit. Arch Ophthalmol 1974, **92**: 276–286.

365 Freedman MI, Folk JC. Metastatic tumors to the eye and orbit. Patient survival and clinical characteristics. Arch Ophthalmol 1987, **105**: 1215–1219.

366 Merrill CF, Kaufman DI, Dimitrov NV. Breast cancer metastatic to the eye is a common entity. Cancer 1991, **68**: 623–627.

CYTOLOGY

367 Baehring JM, Androudi S, Longtine JJ, Betensky RA, Sklar J, Foster CS, Hochberg FH. Analysis of clonal immunoglobulin heavy chain rearrangements in ocular lymphoma. Cancer 2005, **104**: 591–597.

368 Barr CC, Green WR, Payne JW, Knox DI, Jensen AD, Thompson RL. Intraocular reticulum-cell sarcoma. Clinicopathologic study of four cases and review of the literature. Surv Ophthalmol 1975, **19**: 224–239.

369 Goldberg MF. Cytological diagnosis of phacolytic glaucoma utilizing Millepore filtration of the aqueous. Br J Ophthalmol 1967, **51**: 847–853.

370 Wolter JR, Naylor B. A membrane filter method used to diagnose intraocular tumor. J Pediatr Ophthalmol 1968, **5**: 36–38.

Ear 31

CHAPTER CONTENTS

Introduction

Nearly all the diseases that can involve the ear also occur in other sites of the body. However, some of these diseases either have a predilection for the ear or pose special problems when occurring at this site. Only the features of these lesions as they pertain to their location in the ear will be discussed here. The general features of the various entities are dealt with in the respective chapters.

The reader is referred to the specialized books on the subject for an authoritative discussion of the specific diseases of this structure.[1–4]

Normal anatomy

The ear is divided into the external, middle, and inner segments. The external ear consists of the auricle (pinna) and the external auditory canal, which is further divided into an outer (cartilaginous) portion and an inner (osseous) portion. Microscopically, both the auricle and the canal are covered by skin that differs little from that of the skin elsewhere, except for the fact that in the inner half of the canal the epidermis is very thin and lacks rete pegs. Adnexal structures are present in both areas; they are represented by hair follicles, sebaceous glands, and eccrine sweat glands in the auricle and by hair follicles, sebaceous glands, and a special type of apocrine sweat gland (known as *ceruminous glands*) in the canal, most of which are located in the outer third of this structure.

The inner portion of the canal is separated from the middle ear by the *tympanic membrane*, a thin fibrous structure lined by an attenuated layer of keratinizing squamous epithelium on the outer surface and by a single layer of cuboidal cells on the inner surface.

The middle ear (tympanic cavity) contains the three auditory ossicles (malleus, incus, and stapes); it connects with the pharynx through the eustachian tube and with the mastoid cavity and its contiguous pneumatic spaces. The middle ear proper and the mastoid are lined by a layer of flat epithelium; the eustachian tube is covered by tall ciliated epithelium, with smooth transitions between the two types.[5,7]

The inner ear, which is located in the medial portion of the temporal bone, contains the *cochlea* and the *vestibular labyrinth*. These structures are supplied by the eighth cranial nerve, which enters the region through the internal auditory canal together with the seventh nerve. The vestibular labyrinth includes the blind *endolymphatic sac*, which is located in the middle of the posteromedial plate of the petrous bone. It has an intraosseous *rugose* portion and a *distal* portion that lies within the dura. It is lined by a flat to low columnar epithelium resting on a well-vascularized stroma.[6] The sac is connected to the *utricle* and *saccule* (the two main membranous structures of the vestibule) by the *endolymphatic duct*, which passes across the petrous bone.

Diseases of external ear

Non-neoplastic disorders

Congenital abnormalities of this region are common. *Preauricular sinuses, cysts*, and *fistulas* are derived from the first or second branchial clefts.[23,27,29] They are lined by squamous or respiratory epithelium and often contain lymphoid tissue in the wall. Cartilage and skin adnexa may also be present. Secondary inflammatory features are common.[23,29] The treatment is surgical, and recurrences are common.[11] *Accessory tragi* are unilateral or bilateral nodules present at birth, located anteriorly to the auricle in the pretragal area.[8] Like the previous lesions, they are the expression of a branchial cleft anomaly. Sometimes they are seen as a component of the oculo-auriculovertebral syndrome (Goldenhar syndrome).[15] Microscopically they are composed of a covering of skin, numerous tiny, mature hair follicles, and a core of fibrofatty tissue that may contain cartilage.[26] Depending on the relative amounts of these components, these lesions can be variously misdiagnosed as papillomas, fibromas, or soft tissue chondromas. *Ectopic salivary gland tissue* is not uncommon in the region of the middle ear; it can also be found in the external auditory canal.[21]

Keratinous cysts are common in and around the ear. Some are probably developmental anomalies related to the branchial cleft (see preceding discussion), and others are equivalent to those seen elsewhere in the skin and, as such, are either of infundibular hair follicle derivation or of epidermal inclusion type. They are all lined by keratinized squamous epithelium and filled by keratin of epidermal type. Keratinous cysts of pilar type are common in the peri-auricular area but not in the ear itself.

Cholesteatoma of the external auditory canal is composed of a cystic mass of keratinized squamous epithelium overlying an area of bone sequestration in the inner half of the canal.[24] This rare condition should not be confused with cholesteatoma of the middle ear spaces (see p. 2507) or with *keratosis obturans*, a disorder characterized by a diffuse acanthosis and hyperkeratosis of the skin of the canal associated with underlying chronic inflammation.[22,24]

Malignant external otitis, also known as necrotizing granulomatous otitis, is usually caused by *Pseudomonas aeruginosa* and affects mainly elderly patients who have diabetes. It can also be due to fungi, particularly *Aspergillus*. Microscopically, it is characterized by a necrotizing inflammatory reaction involving skin, soft tissue, cartilage, and bone, with invasion of the skull base.[31]

Chondrodermatitis nodularis chronica helicis (Winkler disease) usually involves the upper portion of the helix in older patients, but it can also occur in the antihelix and in younger individuals. Clinically, it presents as a painful, small, round nodule, often covered by a crust.[18] It is often thought clinically to be squamous cell carcinoma or actinic keratosis. Microscopically, there is marked hyperkeratosis and parakeratosis, acanthosis, and hyperplasia of the epidermis, which can reach pseudoepitheliomatous degrees (Fig. 31.1). The center is usually ulcerated and covered by granulation tissue. The underlying inflammation reaches the perichondrium and is characterized by a mononuclear infiltrate and vascular proliferation. The latter may be so pronounced as to simulate a vascular neoplasm, particularly glomus tumor.[9]

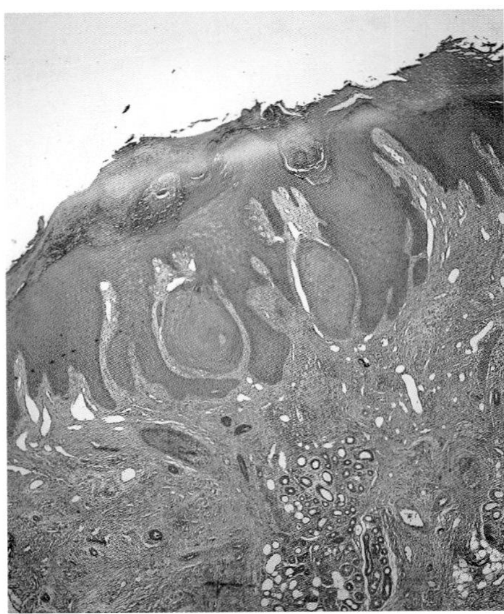

Fig. 31.1 Chondrodermatitis nodularis helicis. There is fibrosis and vascular proliferation in the dermis, accompanied by pseudoepitheliomatous hyperplasia of the overlying epithelium.

Idiopathic cystic chondromalacia (pseudocyst) results from degeneration of the auricular cartilage and is more commonly seen as a painless localized ear enlargement (sometimes bilaterally) in young males. Grossly, a cystic formation within the external auricular cartilage is filled with a watery fluid. Microscopically, the cyst has no lining, and there is no associated inflammation.[12]

Relapsing polychondritis is characterized by episodic painful inflammation of cartilage, most commonly in the outer and inner ear, nose, costochondral junctions, a variety of joints, and sometimes the cartilage of the respiratory tract.[30] Aortic insufficiency is a life-threatening complication. The external ear is affected in almost 90% of the patients, and it represents the initial site of involvement in one-third of the cases.[14,20]

Microscopically, there are degenerative changes in the cartilage (decrease in basophilic staining, loss of lacunae, and eventual replacement by collagen) and an inflammatory infiltrate that is neutrophilic initially and mononuclear in the late stages.[14] The etiology is unknown, but the detection in these patients of antibodies to type II collagen suggests an autoimmune mechanism.[13,17]

Pneumocystosis of the external ear presents as a mass microscopically composed of granulation tissue. The presence of a foamy exudate is the main diagnostic clue of this condition, usually seen in HIV-infected patients.[16]

Nodular fasciitis can involve the external ear region; its morphologic appearance is similar to that seen at other soft tissue sites (see Chapter 25).

Localized disorders of the external ear formed by the accumulation of extracellular material include *keloid* (see Chapter 4), localized *amyloidosis*, uric acid tophi of *gout*, *elastotic nodules*, and *collagenous papules*. Elastotic nodules are small papules and nodules most commonly noted on the antihelix as a result of actinic damage. Microscopically, they are composed of dermal clumps of elastic tissue.[10,28] Collagenous papules are smooth, firm, small papules, located bilaterally on the inner aspects of the aural pinnae and, in rare cases, in the external auditory canal. Microscopically, there is a dense collagenous mass in which dilated vessels and scattered fibroblasts are identified.[25] It has been suggested that auricular lesions with the microscopic features of *granuloma annulare* may be a consequence of trauma.[19]

Tumors and tumorlike conditions

Keratotic lesions

The external ear is a common site for *seborrheic keratosis* and *actinic keratosis* (see Chapter 4). Some ear lesions designated as fibroepithelial papillomas or squamous papillomas are probably variants of seborrheic keratosis. Other *squamous papillomas* present as branching complex polypoid structures in the external auditory canal. Additional types of keratotic lesion that can occur at this site are *keratoacanthoma, inverted follicular keratosis, verruca vulgaris,* and *molluscum contagiosum*. It has been estimated that 8.5% of all keratoacanthomas involve the skin of the external ear.[32] All of these entities are discussed in Chapter 4.

Basal cell carcinoma

Basal cell carcinoma is a common tumor of the auricle and external auditory canal, the ratio between the two sites being 5 : 1. In the auricle, basal cell carcinoma predominates over squamous cell carcinoma (although not as much as in the rest of the head and neck area[33]), the ratio being reversed in the external auditory canal. The microscopic features and behavior of this lesion are described in Chapter 4. If untreated, basal cell carcinomas of the canal may extend into the middle ear, mastoid, or even the cranial cavity.[35] These tumors may be treated with surgery or radiation therapy, the choice depending on the size and location.[34]

Squamous cell carcinoma

Squamous cell carcinoma of the external ear comprises one-fourth of all squamous cell cutaneous carcinomas of the head and neck region.[36] Most patients are elderly. The tumors are more common in the auricle (particularly the helix) than in the canal.[38,46,51] Many of the latter present clinically with symptoms of otitis.[48] Grossly and microscopically, they do not differ significantly from those seen elsewhere in sun-exposed skin (Fig. 31.2). Some are of the *adenoid* (*pseudoglandular*) variant, others belong to the *verrucous* type, and still others to the *spindle cell* (*sarcomatoid*) variant[43,45,50] (see Chapter 4). The pattern of local spread varies depending on the initial location of the tumor, a finding that also applies to basal cell carcinomas. Tumors of the helix spread initially along the helix and then anteriorly to the antihelix and posteriorly to the posterior surface of the ear; tumors of the antihelix spread concentrically; tumors of the posterior surface of the ear spread to the helix and along that structure.[37] Tumors at high risk for regional lymph node involvement are those with a depth of invasion >8 mm or a depth of invasion between 2 and 8 mm in conjunction with destructive cartilage invasion, lymphovascular invasion or a 'noncohesive' invasive front.[40] Tumors of the canal tend to invade bone and often destroy the tympanic membrane to penetrate into the middle ear. Like their basal cell counterparts, squamous cell carcinomas can be treated by either surgery or radiation therapy, the choice being determined by the size, location, and degree of invasiveness of the lesion.[43,44]

The prognosis is much better for tumors of the auricle than for those in the canal, a fact that is at least partially related to the earlier diagnosis of the former type of tumor.[37,42] In one series, tumor-related deaths occurred in only 1 of 17 patients with tumors of the auricle but in 11 of 21 patients with tumors of the canal.[39] Survival is directly correlated with tumor stage, the staging system generally used being that proposed by the University of Pittsburgh.[47] The prognosis is particularly ominous for tumors of the inner portion of the canal exhibiting deep involvement of the temporal bone and beyond.[41,49,52]

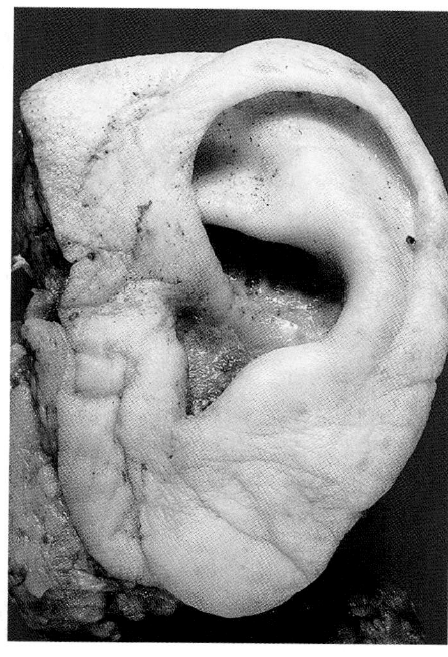

Fig. 31.2 This squamous cell carcinoma required the removal of the entire external ear.

Adnexal tumors

Almost any type of adnexal tumor can involve the skin of the external ear.[64] One of the most common is *pilomatrixoma*, often seen in children and sometimes confused microscopically with basal cell carcinoma. Reported cases of adnexal tumors of this region include other types of *hair-follicle neoplasms*[55] and *sebaceous adenoma*.[63]

Adnexal tumors of the external auditory canal are generally assumed to be of ceruminous gland origin, and the generic term *ceruminoma* has been used for them.[53] The clinical presentation is similar, although the malignant tumors are more often painful and ulcerated.[58] Four major categories are recognized.[67]

Adenoma is sharply demarcated but not encapsulated. Variously sized glandular formations lined by apocrine cells are seen microscopically (Fig. 31.3).[54] A myoepithelial layer can be discerned at the base. Mitotic figures, pleomorphism, necrosis, and invasiveness are lacking. Presence of cerumen pigment and positivity for CK7 and p63 are helpful in the differential diagnosis with other neoplasms of the region.[66]

Benign mixed tumor (pleomorphic adenoma) has an appearance similar to that of its cutaneous or salivary gland counterpart.[56] In some cases, the epithelial component exhibits apocrine features similar to those of adenoma.[65]

Syringocystadenoma papilliferum is morphologically equivalent to the tumor occurring elsewhere in the skin, particularly in the scalp (see Chapter 4). Connection with the surface of the canal is characteristic.

Adenocarcinoma may be well differentiated and therefore difficult to distinguish from adenoma. The presence of more than occasional mitotic activity, pleomorphism, the absence of a myoepithelial layer, necrosis, and invasiveness are the main identifying features.[59,60] The main problem with this tumor is local recurrence; nodal or distant metastases are exceedingly rare.[62]

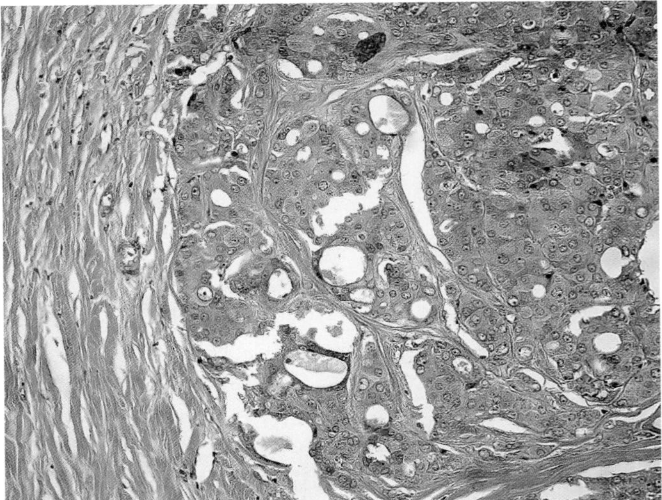

Fig. 31.3 Ceruminous adenoma. The cytoplasm of the tumor cells has an apocrine appearance.

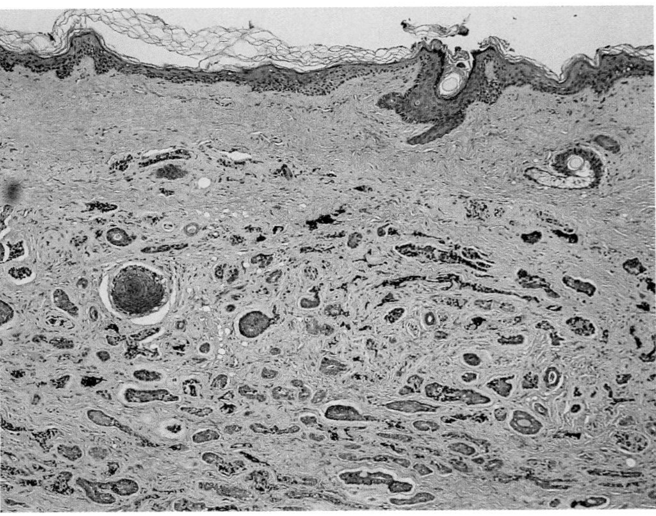

Fig. 31.4 Adenoid cystic carcinoma growing beneath the epidermis of the external ear canal.

Adenoid cystic carcinoma has an appearance similar to that of its more common equivalent in the salivary glands (see Chapter 12) (Fig. 31.4). Like the latter, it has a great tendency for local (including perineurial) invasion and distant (rather than nodal) metastases, particularly to the lungs[61] but also to brain.[57] The death rate is approximately 50%.

The differential diagnosis of these tumors includes direct invasion from so-called adenomas and paragangliomas of the middle ear and adnexal tumors of the auricle. It is particularly important to distinguish the benign eccrine dermal cylindroma arising from the conchal portion of the auricle from adenoid cystic carcinoma arising from the canal.

Melanocytic tumors

Melanocytic nevi of any of the known microscopic types can occur in the auricle or, less commonly, in the canal.[70] They may show some disturbing morphologic features, similar to those often seen in the acral, flexural, and genital areas.[70]

Malignant melanomas of the external ear comprise about 10% of all melanomas of the head and neck region.[68] Nearly all are located in the auricle rather than in the canal.[69] The most common type is superficially spreading. Nodal metastases are to the upper cervical, intraparotid, or occipital groups, depending on the exact location of the tumor in the auricle.

Other tumors

Osteoma of the external auditory canal presents as a solitary pedunculated osseous mass attached by a narrow pedicle to the tympanosquamous or tympanomastoid suture line.[73] Microscopically, it is formed by mature lamellar bone containing bone marrow and covered by keratinized squamous epithelium.[76]

Exostoses are sessile, often multiple and bilateral masses that seem to be particularly common in swimmers. Microscopically, the appearance is similar to that of osteoma except for the absence of bone marrow spaces.[76]

Myxomas of the external ear occur in patients with Carney's complex, sometimes bilaterally. Microscopically, they are nonencapsulated circumscribed nodules composed of scattered stellate and spindle cells set in a myxoid, capillary-rich matrix.[75]

Vascular tumors and tumorlike conditions include *vascular leiomyoma (angioleiomyoma)*,[71] *epithelioid (histiocytoid) hemangioma* (also known as angiolymphoid hyperplasia with eosinophilia and having a predilection for the skin of the ear, external auditory canal, and periauricular region[80]) (see Chapter 4), and the related *epithelioid angiomatous nodule*.[74] The neoplastic versus inflammatory nature of the last two entities remains debatable.

Other primary tumors of the external ear include *Merkel cell carcinoma*[78,82] and various types of soft tissue neoplasm, including *rhabdomyosarcoma* (see p. 2509), *myxoid chondrosarcoma*,[83] and *peripheral nerve sheath tumors*.[81] As already mentioned, the canal can be secondarily involved by tumors of the middle ear or salivary gland.

Exceptionally, *malignant lymphoma* presents initially as an ear lesion.[72] A peculiar lymphoid proliferation composed of CD8-positive T cells with low proliferative activity presenting as an ear nodule has been described.[77,79] Microscopically the appearance is suggestive of lymphoma, but the disease follows a very indolent clinical course. The real nature of this process remains sub judice at time of this writing.

Diseases of middle and inner ear

Non-neoplastic disorders

Developmental anomalies of the middle ear include the presence of brain tissue (as a manifestation of heterotopia or encephalocele[94,95,108] and ectopic salivary gland tissue (sometimes designated as choristoma).[103]

Inflammatory polyp ('otic polyp') arises in the middle ear on the basis of a chronic otitis media but often presents in the external auditory canal following perforation of the tympanic membrane. Microscopically, the appearance is that of chronically inflamed stroma, sometimes with the features of granulation tissue. The overlying mucosa may be of columnar ciliated type (consistent with its middle ear origin) or squamous (as a result of metaplasia). Cystically dilated glands may be present in the stroma.

Inflammations of the middle ear are usually of a nonspecific nature microscopically.[90,91,98] This structure can also be involved by specific conditions such as tuberculosis, aspergillosis, malakoplakia, and Wegener granulomatosis.[85,88,92,101,107]

Cholesteatoma usually presents during the third or fourth decade, but it may appear at any age. It is the result of chronic otitis media and may involve the middle ear, peritympanic space, mastoid cavities, and petrous portion of the temporal bone. In rare cases, it can extend into the soft tissues of the neck or the intracranial region.[84,96] Grossly, the appearance is that of a cyst filled with a granular waxy material. Microscopically, the membrane that bounds the lesion peripherally is made up of keratinizing squamous epithelium, and the content is composed of keratin squames.[99] Chronic inflammatory cells, cholesterol clefts, and foreign body-type giant cell granulomas are common. It should be noted that although *cholesterol granulomas* are often seen in the middle ear as a consequence of cholesteatoma, they may also occur independently from it as a result of hemorrhage or otitis media.

The pathogenesis of cholesteatoma is controversial; origin of the squamous epithelium from metaplasia of middle ear mucosa, migration from the external auditory canal, migration from the external surface of the tympanic membrane following a perforation, or retraction of the tympanic membrane into the middle ear have all been considered.[97,102,104,105] In the congenital form, the disease is thought to be the result of inclusions of squamous epithelium in the temporal bone. The matrix-degrading cysteine proteinase cathepsin K may be involved in the bone erosion often seen in this entity.[93]

The treatment is surgical and aimed at removal of the entire lesion, including the limiting membrane.[100]

Otosclerosis is a disorder of abnormal bone remodeling of unknown etiology. Genetic factors are clearly involved, but measles virus infection and autoimmunity may play contributory roles.[86,106] The typical and apparently unique site of involvement is the temporal bone. It is characterized by an initial bone resorption (otospongiosis) followed by bone production (otosclerosis).[99] This results in the formation of Paget disease-like woven bone with prominent cement lines.[87] The disease causes hearing loss because of fixation of the stapes footplate in the oval window. Usually, the only specimens received in the pathology laboratory are portions of the stapes head and crura, which are almost always unaffected by the disease.[87] Microscopic studies done on temporal bones at autopsy have revealed cases of 'histologic otosclerosis' that were asymptomatic, but the incidence of this finding seems much lower (about 2.5%) than previously claimed.[89]

Presbycusis (hearing loss) is a very common condition but not one likely to generate a surgical specimen. In any event, the morphologic changes described by Michaels[99] in this disorder are hair cell degeneration of the cochlea and a process that he calls *giant stereociliary degeneration*.

Tumors and tumorlike conditions

Paraganglioma

Paraganglioma of the glomus jugulare or glomus tympanicum is the most common neoplasm of the middle ear.[109] The general features of this tumor are discussed in Chapter 16. It can be found in the jugular bulb area, within the middle ear, in the external auditory canal, or around the eustachian tube.[111] In contrast to paragangliomas of other sites, those of the middle ear region have a marked predilection for females.[112] They can be familial, bilateral, or associated with paragangliomas elsewhere. Clinically, the typical presentation is that of a red mass protruding behind the tympanic membrane or extending in the canal. Profuse bleeding may be encountered at the time of biopsy. This tumor has a tendency to infiltrate adjacent bone; a few cases associated with distant metastases are on record. The initial treatment usually takes the form of local excision, but the incidence of local recurrence is over 50%.[112] Radiation therapy has also been used as an adjunct to surgery or as the primary treatment.[110]

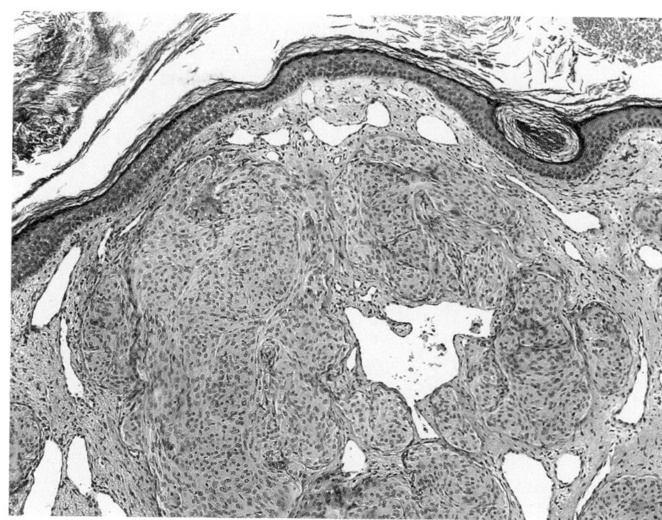

Fig. 31.5 Meningioma of ear. The appearance is identical to that of its counterpart in the central nervous system.

Meningioma

Approximately 6% of all meningiomas arise from the surface of the petrous bone, from which they may invade this structure and reach the middle ear.[113] In addition, meningiomas seemingly localized to the middle ear have been described.[114,115] The tumor may involve the external ear canal, mastoid cavity, or jugular fossa.[116] The microscopic appearance is described in Chapter 28 (Fig. 31.5). The treatment is surgical. The prognosis is substantially better for meningiomas limited to the middle ear than for those reaching this site through invasion of the petrous bone.

Schwannoma (acoustic neuroma)

The tumor traditionally known as acoustic neuroma is simply a schwannoma arising from the eighth (or sometimes the seventh) nerve, which grows within the internal auditory canal and can reach the middle ear. Its features are described in Chapters 25 and 28. These tumors are bilateral in 8% of the cases and associated with type 1 neurofibromatosis (Recklinghausen disease) in 16%.[117] The treatment is surgical.

So-called middle ear adenoma and carcinoid tumor

Middle ear adenoma is the term traditionally used for a distinctive tumor of the middle ear mostly seen in patients between 20 and 40 years of age. Grossly, the lesion is grayish white and firm, not as vascular as paraganglioma, and relatively well circumscribed. Microscopically, the pattern of growth may be solid, glandular, or trabecular (Fig. 31.6).[123,130] The tumor cells are uniform, cuboidal or cylindrical, with a moderately abundant acidophilic cytoplasm that sometimes acquires plasmacytoid features.[121,129] Mitoses are exceedingly rare, pleomorphism is minimal, and necrosis is absent.

Histochemically, there may be intraluminal positivity for mucin and intracytoplasmic argyrophilia. Ultrastructurally, the tumor cells exhibit desmosomes and microvilli; in addition, membrane-bound dense-core granules are present in many of the tumor cells.[119]

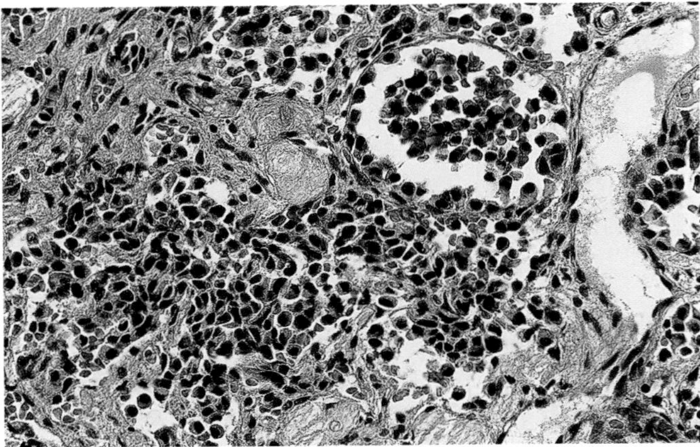

Fig. 31.6 So-called 'middle ear adenoma'. This tumor is closely related and perhaps identical to carcinoid tumor of the ear.

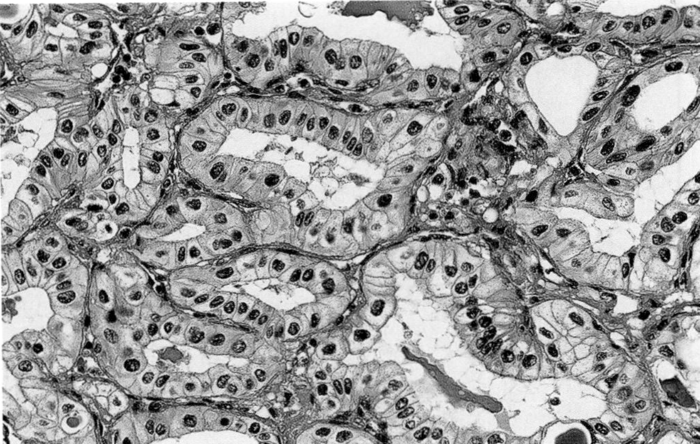

Fig. 31.7 Aggressive papillary middle ear tumor. The tumor forms glandular structures lined by clear cells. In other areas the pattern of growth was papillary.

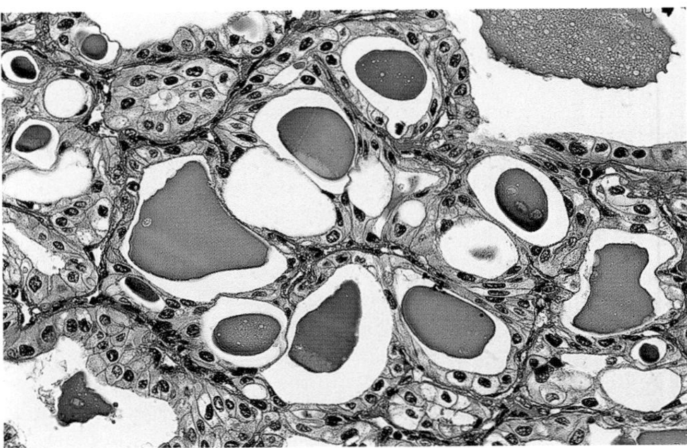

Fig. 31.8 Same case as Fig. 31.7. The cystic dilation of the glands and the presence of a colloid-like material in the lumen results in an appearance strongly reminiscent of thyroid tissue.

Immunohistochemically, positivity for keratin and lysozyme has been described.[126,127]

The histogenetic problem posed by middle ear adenoma mainly concerns its possible neuroendocrine nature and relationship with the reported cases of **carcinoid tumors** of the middle ear.[128,133] The latter tumors have many cytoarchitectural features in common with middle ear adenoma but also exhibit undeniable evidence of neuroendocrine differentiation.[125] Some authors like to view middle ear adenomas and carcinoid tumors as separate entities and regard the former as tumors of the middle ear mucosa.[127,128] However, a large number of studies performed in recent years have convincingly shown that these two tumors merge imperceptibly, in the sense of showing various degrees of combined exocrine and neuroendocrine differentiation.[118,122,131,132,134] As such, they could be regarded as analogous to adenocarcinoids or amphicrine neoplasms of other sites.[120,124] The presence of a neuroendocrine component is supported by the previously mentioned argyrophilia, demonstration of dense-core granules ultrastructurally, and reported immunoreactivity for neuron-specific enolase, chromogranin, serotonin, and numerous peptide hormones (such as pancreatic polypeptide, glucagon, cholecystokinin, and leucine-enkephalin).[122,133] Cases associated with systemic manifestations are also on record.[125]

The treatment of choice of middle ear adenoma/carcinoid tumor is surgical excision. The prognosis is excellent, with only an occasional example of local recurrence.[122,132,134]

Adenocarcinoma

Adenocarcinoma of the middle and inner ear is a somewhat confusing and controversial entity.[139,144–146] The term has sometimes been used for adenocarcinomas of the external auditory canal secondarily invading the ear and for so-called 'middle ear adenoma'.[136] However, there is a distinct form of primary adenocarcinoma of this site that is different from the entities previously mentioned. This is a *papillary adenocarcinoma* composed of uniform cuboidal cells with clear to acidophilic cytoplasm forming papillary structures that rest on a vascular stroma (Fig. 31.7). Cystic dilation of the glands often occurs, leading to a follicle-like appearance that is very reminiscent of that seen in thyroid tumors (Fig. 31.8).[135,145,147,148] Tumors with prominent cytoplasmic clearing simulate metastatic renal cell carcinoma. Gaffey et al.,[138] who refer to this neoplasm as *aggressive papillary middle-ear tumor* (APMET), favor an origin from middle ear/mastoid epithelium. In a subsequent article, they have shown that this lesion can occur in the setting of von Hippel–Lindau disease, sometimes in association with a microscopically similar tumor in the broad ligament of presumed wolffian (mesonephric) origin.[137,143] APMET is closely related if not identical to the *low-grade adenocarcinoma of probably endolymphatic sac origin* reported by Heffner[141] and referred to by some as *Heffner tumor*.[142,150] As the name indicates, the author favors an origin from endolymphatic sac epithelium. Regarding the differential diagnosis, it is well to remember that so-called 'middle ear adenoma' does not exhibit papillary formations. Cases of this tumor occurring in the setting of von Hippel–Lindau disease are associated with germline mutation of the *VHL* gene combined with loss of function of the wild-type allele through genetic deletion. Interestingly, mutations or allelic deletions of the same gene have also been found in some sporadic tumors.[140,149]

Papillary adenocarcinoma has a tendency to invade bone, from which it may spread to the cranial cavity. The treatment is surgical, but achievement of local control is difficult.[138,139]

Squamous cell carcinoma

Squamous cell carcinoma of the middle ear typically presents in older patients with a history of long-standing ear discharge, which may be hemorrhagic and is usually associated with pain and hearing

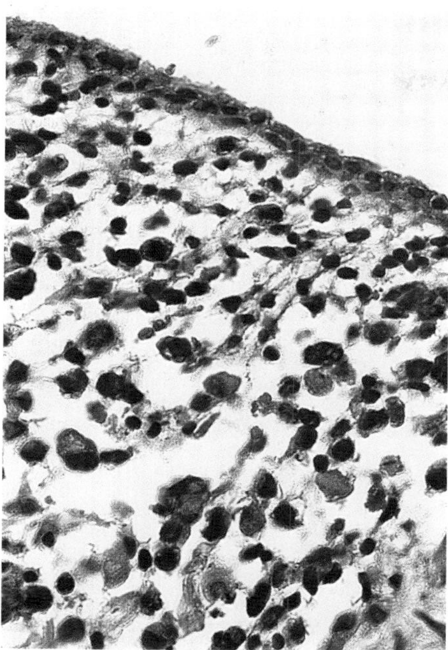

Fig. 31.9 Embryonal rhabdomyosarcoma of the middle ear. Neoplastic tumor cells are seen growing beneath a flattened epithelium. Most of the cell population is small, but there are larger elements with more abundant fibrillary acidophilic cytoplasm.

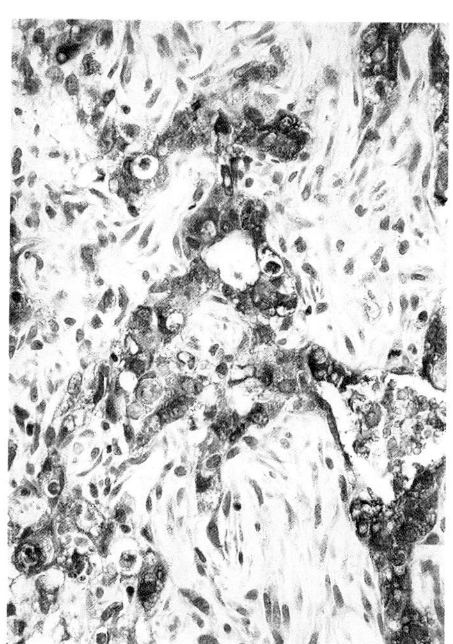

Fig. 31.10 Yolk sac tumor of the middle ear immunostained for alpha-fetoprotein.

loss.[151,154,156] Rarely, the process is bilateral.[155] An etiologic role for chronic otitis media has long been suspected.[153] Jin et al.[152] found HPV-16 genetic material in 11 of 14 cases of squamous cell carcinoma of the middle ear they studied. Grossly, the tumor fills the middle ear spaces, from where it may invade the bony walls of the mastoid ear cells, the bone septum that separates the ear from the carotid canal, the internal auditory meatus, the eustachian tube, and the external auditory canal. Eventually, it may reach the intracranial cavity and the soft tissues of the neck.[154] Microscopically, the tumor is an ordinary squamous cell carcinoma of various degrees of differentiation; in rare cases, it may be of *verrucous* type.[157] The differential diagnosis includes secondary invasion of the middle ear by squamous cell carcinomas of the external auditory canal and the eustachian tube. The preferred form of treatment is a combination of surgery and radiation therapy. In the series by Michaels and Wells,[154] the 5-year survival rate was 39%.

Rhabdomyosarcoma

Rhabdomyosarcoma of the middle ear occurs almost exclusively in children. At the time of diagnosis, the tumor has often invaded the external canal, mastoid, and meninges.[162] CT scan is the best method to delineate the tumor and to detect intracranial spread. Microscopically, the neoplasms can be of embryonal type, including the botryoid variety.[160,161] The microscopic features are described in Chapter 25 (Fig. 31.9). The treatment is a combination of surgery, radiation therapy, and multidrug chemotherapy.[159,161]

A few cases of rhabdomyosarcoma apparently localized to the external auditory canal have been reported.[158,161]

Other primary tumors

Rare benign primary tumors of the middle ear region include *lipoma, hemangioma, osteoma, ossifying fibroma, dermoid cyst* (in the eustachian tube), *teratoma*, and *'glioma'*.[163–167,169] The middle ear can also be secondarily involved in cases of *Langerhans cell histiocytosis*. A middle ear tumor with the histologic and immunohistochemical features of *yolk sac* (*endodermal sinus*) *tumor* has been reported[168] (Fig. 31.10), and another with the features of an amelanotic *malignant melanoma*.[170]

Metastatic tumors

The temporal bone can be involved by malignant tumors arising elsewhere. This involvement can be in the form of direct extension from tumors of the pharynx, salivary glands, or central nervous system, or as blood-borne distant metastases. In the latter instance, the most common sites of the primary are breast, lung, and kidney.[171,172]

References

INTRODUCTION

1 Friedmann I. Pathology of the ear. Edinburgh, 1993, Churchill Livingstone.

2 Jackler RK, Driscoll CLW (eds). Tumors of the ear and temporal bone. Philadelphia, 2000, Lippincott Williams & Wilkins.

3 Merchant SN, Nadol JB Jr. Schuknecht's pathology of the ear, ed. 3. Maidenhead, Berkshire, 2010, McGraw-Hill.

4 Nager GT. Pathology of the ear and temporal bone. Baltimore, 1993, Williams & Wilkins.

NORMAL ANATOMY

5 Lim DJ. Functional morphology of the mucosa of the middle ear and eustachian tube. Ann Otol Rhinol Laryngol 1976, **85**: 36–43.

6 Schindler RA. The ultrastructure of the endolymphatic sac in man. Laryngoscope 1980, **21**: 1–39.

7 Wenig BHM, Michaels L. The ear and temporal bone. In Mills SE (ed): Histology for pathologists, ed. 3. Baltimore, 2007, Lippincott Williams & Wilkins, pp. 371–401.

DISEASES OF THE EXTERNAL EAR

NON-NEOPLASTIC DISORDERS

8 Brownstein MH, Wanger N, Helwig EB. Accessory tragi. Arch Dermatol 1971, **104**: 625–631.
9 Calnan J, Rossatti B. On the histopathology of chondrodermatitis nodularis helicis chronica. J Clin Pathol 1959, **12**: 179–182.
10 Carter VH, Constantine VS, Poole WL. Elastotic nodules of the antihelix. Arch Dermatol 1969, **100**: 282–285.
11 Ellies M, Laskawi R, Arglebe C, Altrogge C. Clinical evaluation and surgical management of congenital preauricular fistulas. J Oral Maxillofac Surg 1998, **56**: 827–830.
12 Heffner DK, Hyams VJ. Cystic chondromalacia (endochondral pseudocyst) of the auricle. Arch Pathol Lab Med 1986, **110**: 740–743.
13 Herman JH, Dennis MV. Immunopathologic studies in relapsing polychondritis. J Clin Invest 1973, **52**: 549–558.
14 Hughes RAC, Berry CL, Siefert M, Lessof MH. Relapsing polychondritis. Three cases with a clinico-pathological study and literature review. QJM 1972, **41**: 363–380.
15 Jansen T, Romiti R, Altmeyer P. Accessory tragus: report of two cases and review of the literature. Pediatr Dermatol 2000, **17**: 391–394.
16 Mahlakwane MS, Ramdial PK, Sing Y, Calonje E, Biyana S. Otic pneumocystosis in acquired immune deficiency syndrome. Am J Surg Pathol 2008, **32**: 1038–1043.
17 McCune WJ, Schiller AL, Dynesius-Trentham RA, Trentham DE. Type II collagen-induced auricular chondritis. Arthritis Rheum 1982, **25**: 266–273.
18 Metzger SA, Goodman ML. Chondrodermatitis helicis. A clinical re-evaluation and pathological review. Laryngoscope 1976, **86**: 1402–1412.
19 Mills A, Chetty R. Auricular granuloma annulare. A consequence of trauma? Am J Dermatopathol 1992, **14**: 431–433.
20 Moloney JR. Relapsing polychondritis. Its otolaryngological manifestations. J Laryngol Otol 1978, **92**: 9–15.
21 Morimoto N, Ogawa K, Kanzaki J. Salivary gland choristoma in the middle ear: a case report. Am J Otolaryngol 1999, **20**: 232–235.
22 Naiberg J, Berger G, Hawke M. The pathologic features of keratosis obturans and cholesteatoma of the external auditory canal. Arch Otolaryngol 1984, **110**: 690–693.
23 Olsen KD, Maragos NE, Weiland LH. First branchial cleft anomalies. Laryngoscope 1980, **90**: 423–436.
24 Piepergerdes JC, Kramer BM, Behnke EE. Keratosis obturans and external auditory canal cholesteatoma. Laryngoscope 1980, **90**: 383–391.
25 Sanchez JL. Collagenous papules on the aural conchae. Am J Dermatopathol 1983, **5**: 231–233.
26 Satoh T, Tokura Y, Katsumata M, Sonoda T, Takigawa M. Histological diagnostic criteria for accessory tragi. J Cutan Pathol 1990, **17**: 206–210.
27 Skau NK, Eriksen KD. Pre-auricular fistula communicating with the external auditory meatus, combined with second branchial cleft anomalies. J Laryngol Otol 1986, **100**: 203–206.
28 Weedon D. Elastotic nodules of the ear. J Cutan Pathol 1981, **8**: 429–433.
29 Work WP. Newer concepts of first branchial cleft defects. Laryngoscope 1972, **82**: 1581–1593.
30 Yetiser S, Inal A, Taser M, Ozkaptan Y. Otolaryngological aspects of relapsing polychondritis: course and outcome. Rev Laryngol Otol Rhinol (Bord) 2001, **122**: 195–200.
31 Zaky DA, Bentley DW, Lowy K, Betts RF, Douglas RG Jr. Malignant external otitis. A severe form of otitis in diabetic patients. Am J Med 1976, **61**: 298–302.

TUMORS AND TUMORLIKE CONDITIONS

Keratotic lesions

32 Patterson HC. Facial keratoacanthoma. Otolaryngol Head Neck Surg 1983, **91**: 263–270.

Basal cell carcinoma

33 Ahmad I, Das Gupta AR. Epidemiology of basal cell carcinoma and squamous cell carcinoma of the pinna. J Laryngol Otol 2001, **115**: 85–86.
34 Avila J, Bosch A, Aristizábal S, Frias Z, Marcial V. Carcinoma of the pinna. Cancer 1977, **40**: 2891–2895.
35 Goodwin WJ, Jesse RH. Malignant neoplasms of the external auditory canal and temporal bone. Arch Otolaryngol 1980, **106**: 675–679.

Squamous cell carcinoma

36 Avila J, Bosch A, Aristizábal S, Frías Z, Marcial V. Carcinoma of the pinna. Cancer 1977, **40**: 2891–2895.
37 Bailin PL, Levine HL, Wood BG, Tucker HM. Cutaneous carcinoma of the auricular and periauricular region. Arch Otolaryngol 1980, **106**: 692–696.
38 Barnes L, Johnson JT. Clinical and pathological considerations in the evaluation of major head and neck specimens resected for cancer. Part II. Pathol Annu 1986, **21**(Pt 2): 83–110.
39 Chen KTK, Dehner LP. Primary tumors of the external and middle ear. Arch Otolaryngol 1978, **104**: 247–252.
40 Clark RR, Soutar DS, Hunter KD. A retrospective analysis of histological prognostic factors for the development of lymph node metastases from auricular squamous cell carcinoma. Histopathology 2010, **57**: 138–146.
41 Goodwin WJ, Jesse RH. Malignant neoplasms of the external auditory canal and temporal bone. Arch Otolaryngol 1980, **106**: 675–679.
42 Johns ME, Headington JT. Squamous cell carcinoma of the external auditory canal. A clinicopathologic study of 20 cases. Arch Otolaryngol 1974, **100**: 45–49.
43 Johnson WC, Helwig EB. Adenoid squamous cell carcinoma (adenoacanthoma). Cancer 1966, **19**: 1639–1650.
44 Kinney SE, Wood BG. Malignancies of the external ear canal and temporal bone. Surgical techniques and results. Laryngoscope 1987, **97**: 158–164.
45 Koso-Thomas K, Thompson LDR. Spindle cell (sarcomatoid) carcinoma of the ear: a clinicopathological study of 57 cases [abstract]. Mod Pathol 2003, **16**: 220A.
46 Lewis JS. Cancer of the ear. CA Cancer J Clin 1987, **37**: 78–87.
47 Moody SA, Hirsch BE, Myers EN. Squamous cell carcinoma of the external auditory canal: an evaluation of a staging system. Am J Otol 2000, **21**: 582–588.
48 Paaske PB, Witten J, Schwer S, Hansen HS. Results in treatment of carcinoma of the external auditory canal and middle ear. Cancer 1987, **59**: 156–160.
49 Pfreundner L, Schwager K, Willner J, Baier K, Bratengeier K, Brunner FX, Flentje M. Carcinoma of the external auditory canal and middle ear. Int J Radiat Oncol Biol Phys 1999, **44**: 777–788.
50 Proops DW, Hawke WM, van Nostrand AW, Harwood AR, Lunan M. Verrucous carcinoma of the ear. Case report. Ann Otol Rhinol Laryngol 1984, **93**: 385–388.
51 Shiffman NJ. Squamous cell carcinomas of the skin of the pinna. Can J Surg 1975, **18**: 279–283.
52 Stell PM, McCormick MS. Carcinoma of the external auditory meatus and middle ear. Prognostic factors and a suggested staging system. J Laryngol Otol 1985, **99**: 847–850.

Adnexal tumors

53 Batsakis JG, Hardy GC, Hishivama RH. Ceruminous gland tumors. Arch Otolaryngol 1967, **86**: 66–69.
54 Cankar V, Crowley H. Tumors of ceruminous glands. A clinicopathological study of 7 cases. Cancer 1964, **17**: 67–75.
55 Cohen C, Davis TS. Multiple trichogenic adnexal tumors. Am J Dermatopathol 1986, **8**: 241–246.
56 Collins RJ, Yu HC. Pleomorphic adenoma of the external auditory canal. An immunohistochemical and ultrastructural study. Cancer 1989, **64**: 870–875.
57 Conlin PA, Mira JL, Graham SC, Kaye KS, Cordero J. Ceruminous gland adenoid cystic carcinoma with contralateral metastasis to the brain. Arch Pathol Lab Med 2002, **126**: 87–89.
58 Lynde CW, McLean DI, Wood WS. Tumors of ceruminous glands. J Am Acad Dermatol 1984, **11**: 841–847.
59 Michel RG, Woodard BH, Shelburne JD, Bossen EH. Ceruminous gland adenocarcinoma. A light and electron microscopic study. Cancer 1978, **41**: 545–553.
60 Nelson BL, Thompson LDR, Barnes L. Ceruminal gland carcinomas: a clinicopathologic study of 17 cases [abstract]. Mod Pathol 2003, **16**: 221A.
61 Perzin KH, Gullane P, Conley J. Adenoid cystic carcinoma involving the external auditory canal. A clinicopathologic study of 16 cases. Cancer 1982, **50**: 2873–2883.
62 Pulec JL. Glandular tumors of the external auditory canal. Laryngoscope 1977, **87**: 1601–1612.
63 Raizada RM, Khan NU. Aural sebaceous adenomas. J Laryngol Otol 1986, **100**: 1413–1416.
64 Senturia BH, Marcus MD, Lucente SE. Disease of the external ear, ed. 2. New York, 1980, Grune & Stratton.
65 Tang X, Tamura Y, Tsutsumi Y. Mixed tumor of the external auditory canal. Pathol Int 1994, **44**: 80–83.
66 Thompson LD, Nelson BL, Barnes EL. Ceruminous adenomas: a clinicopathologic study of 41 cases with a review of the literature. Am J Surg Pathol 2004, **28**: 308–318.
67 Wetli CV, Pardo V, Millard M, Gerston K. Tumors of ceruminous glands. Cancer 1972, **29**: 1169–1178.

Melanocytic tumors

68 Byers RM, Smith JL, Russell N, Rosenberg V. Malignant melanoma of the external ear. Review of 102 cases. Am J Surg 1980, **140**: 518–521.

69 Pack GT, Conley J, Oropeza R. Melanoma of the external ear. Arch Otolaryngol 1970, **92**: 106–113.

70 Saad AG, Patel S, Mutasim DF. Melanocytic nevi of the auricular region: histologic characteristics and diagnostic difficulties. Am J Dermatopathol 2005, **27**: 111–115.

Other tumors

71 Choe KS, Sclafani AP, McCormick SA. Angioleiomyoma of the auricle: a rare tumor. Otolaryngol Head Neck Surg 2001, **125**: 109–110.

72 Darvay A, Russell-Jones R, Acland KM, Lampert I, Chu AC. Systemic B-cell lymphoma presenting as an isolated lesion on the ear. Clin Exp Dermatol 2001, **26**: 166–169.

73 Deguine C, Pulec JL. Large osteoma of the external auditory canal. Ear Nose Throat J 2001, **80**: 8.

74 Fernandez-Flores A, Montero MG, Renedo G. Cutaneous epithelioid angiomatous nodule of the external ear. Am J Dermatopathol 2005, **27**: 175–176.

75 Ferreiro JA, Carney JA. Myxomas of the external ear and their significance. Am J Surg Pathol 1994, **18**: 274–280.

76 Graham MD. Osteomas and exostoses of the external auditory canal. Ann Otol Rhinol Laryngol 1979, **88**: 566–572.

77 Li XQ, Zhou XY, Sheng WQ, Xu YX, Zhu XZ. Indolent CD8+ lymphoid proliferation of the ear: a new entity and possible occurrence of signet ring cells. Histopathology 2009, **55**: 468–470.

78 Petkovi M, Krstulja M, Radic J, Zamolo G, Muhvi D, Lovasic I, Kujundzic M, Franko A. Merkel cell carcinoma arising in the ear canal. Int J Surg Pathol 2008, **16**: 337–340.

79 Petrella T, Maubec E, Cornillet-Lefebvre P, Willemze R, Pluot M, Durlach A, Marinho E, Benhamou JL, Jansen P, Robson A, Grange F. Indolent CD8-positive lymphoid proliferation of the ear: a distinct primary cutaneous T-cell lymphoma? Am J Surg Pathol 2007, **31**: 1887–1892.

80 Thompson JW, Colman M, Williamson C, Ward PH. Angiolymphoid hyperplasia with eosinophilia of the external ear canal. Treatment with laser excision. Arch Otolaryngol 1981, **107**: 316–319.

81 Tran Ba Huy P, Hassan JM, Wassef M, Mikol J, Thurel O. Acoustic schwannoma presenting as a tumor of the external auditory canal. Case report. Ann Otol Rhinol Laryngol 1987, **96**: 415–418.

82 Virtaniemi J, Hirvikoski P, Pukkila M, Kumpulainen E, Johansson R, Kosma VM. Merkel cell carcinoma of the auricle. Eur Arch Otorhinolaryngol 2000, **257**: 558–560.

83 Worley GA, Wareing MJ, Sergeant RJ. Myxoid chondrosarcoma of the external auditory meatus. J Laryngol Otol 1999, **113**: 742–743.

DISEASES OF MIDDLE AND INNER EAR

NON-NEOPLASTIC DISORDERS

84 Arkin CF, Millard M, Medeiros LJ. Giant invasive cholesteatoma. Report of a case with cerebellar invasion. Arch Pathol Lab Med 1985, **109**: 960–961.

85 Azadeh B, Dabiri S, Moshfegh I. Malakoplakia of the middle ear. Histopathology 1991, **19**: 276–278.

86 Chole RA, McKenna M. Pathophysiology of otosclerosis. Otol Neurotol 2001, **22**: 249–257.

87 Davis GL. Pathology of otosclerosis. A review. Am J Otolaryngol 1987, **8**: 273–281.

88 Davis GL. Tumorous and inflammatory conditions of the ear. In Gnepp DR (ed.): Pathology of the head and neck, vol. 10. Contemporary issues in surgical pathology. New York, 1988, Churchill Livingstone.

89 Declau F, Van Spaendonck M, Timmermans JP, Michaels L, Liang J, Qiu JP, Van de Heyning P. Prevalence of otosclerosis in an unselected series of temporal bones. Otol Neurotol 2001, **22**: 596–602.

90 Friedmann I. Pathology of the ear. Edinburgh, 1993, Churchill Livingstone.

91 Friedmann I. Pathology of the ear. Selected topics. Pathol Annu 1978, **13**(Pt 1): 363–410.

92 Friedmann I. Nose, throat and ears. In Symmers WC St (ed.): Systemic pathology, vol. 1, ed. 3. New York, 1986, Churchill Livingstone.

93 Hansen T, Unger R, Gaumann A, Hundorf I, Maurer J, Kirkpatrick CJ, Kriegsmann J. Expression of matrix-degrading cysteine proteinase cathepsin K in cholesteatoma. Mod Pathol 2001, **14**: 1226–1231.

94 Heffner DK. Brain in the middle ear or nasal cavity: heterotopia or encephalocele? Ann Diagn Pathol 2004, **8**: 252–257.

95 Kamerer DB, Caparosa RJ. Temporal bone encephalocele. Diagnosis and treatment. Laryngoscope 1982, **92**: 878–882.

96 Kreutzer EW, DeBlanc GB. Extra aural spread of acquired cholesteatoma. Arch Otolaryngol 1982, **108**: 320–323.

97 Linde RE. Cholesterol granuloma. Ear Nose Throat J 1982, **61**: 186–189.

98 Merchant SN, Nadol JB Jr. Schuknecht's pathology of the ear, ed. 3. Maidenhead, Berkshire, 2010, McGraw-Hill.

99 Michaels L. The temporal bone. An organ in search of a histopathology. Histopathology 1991, **18**: 391–394.

100 Palva T. Surgical treatment of cholesteatomatous ear disease. J Laryngol Otol 1985, **99**: 539–544.

101 Ramages LJ, Gertler R. Aural tuberculosis. A series of 25 patients. J Laryngol Otol 1985, **99**: 1073–1080.

102 Sade J. Pathogenesis of attic cholesteatomas. J R Soc Med 1978, **71**: 716–732.

103 Saeger KL, Gruskin P, Carberry JN. Salivary gland choristoma of the middle ear. Arch Pathol Lab Med 1982, **106**: 39–40.

104 Soldati D, Mudry A. Knowledge about cholesteatoma, from the first description to the modern histopathology. Otol Neurotol 2001, **22**: 723–730.

105 Swartz JD. Cholesteatomas of the middle ear. Diagnosis, etiology, and complications. Radiol Clin North Am 1985, **22**: 15–35.

106 Van Den Bogaert K, Govaerts PJ, Schatteman I, Brown MR, Caethoven G, Offeciers FE, Somers T, Declau F, Coucke P, Van de Heyning P, Smith RJ, Van Camp G. A second gene for otosclerosis, OTSC2, maps to chromosome 7q34–36. Am J Hum Genet 2001, **68**: 495–500.

107 Wenig BHM, Michaels L. The ear and temporal bone. In Mills SE (ed): Histology for pathologists, ed. 3. Baltimore, 2007, Lippincott Williams & Wilkins, pp. 371–401.

108 Williams DC. Encephalocele of the middle ear. J Laryngol Otol 1986, **100**: 471–473.

TUMORS AND TUMORLIKE CONDITIONS

Paraganglioma

109 Alford BR, Guilford FR. A comprehensive study of tumors of the glomus jugulare. Laryngoscope 1962, **72**: 765–787.

110 Konefal JB, Pilepich MV, Spector GJ, Perez CA. Radiation therapy in the treatment of chemodectomas. Laryngoscope 1987, **97**: 1331–1335.

111 Larson TC III, Reese DF, Baker HL Jr, McDonald TJ. Glomus tympanicum chemodectomas. Radiographic and clinical characteristics. Radiology 1987, **163**: 801–806.

112 Reddy EK, Mansfield CM, Hartman GV. Chemodectoma of glomus jugulare. Cancer 1983, **52**: 337–340.

Meningioma

113 Nager GT. Meningiomas involving the temporal bone; clinical and pathological aspects. Springfield, ILL, 1964, Charles C Thomas.

114 Prayson RA. Middle ear meningiomas. Ann Diagn Pathol 2000, **4**: 149–153.

115 Salama N, Stafford N. Meningiomas presenting in the middle ear. Laryngoscope 1982, **92**: 92–97.

116 Thompson L, Bouffard JP, Sandberg G. Primary ear and temporal bone meningiomas: a clinicopathologic study of 36 cases with a review of the literature. Mod Pathol 2003, **16**: 236–245.

Schwannoma (acoustic neuroma)

117 Erickson LS, Sorenson GD, McGavran MH. A review of 140 acoustic neurinomas (neurilemmoma). Laryngoscope 1965, **75**: 601–626.

So-called middle ear adenoma and carcinoid tumor

118 Davies JE, Semeraro D, Knight LC, Griffiths GJ. Middle ear neoplasms showing adenomatous and neuroendocrine components. J Laryngol Otol 1989, **103**: 404–407.

119 El-Naggar AK, Pflatz M, Ordóñez NG, Batsakis JG. Tumors of the middle ear and endolymphatic sac. Pathol Annu 1994, **29**(Pt 2): 199–231.

120 Faverly DR, Manni JJ, Smedts F, Verhofstad AA, van Haelst UJ. Adeno-carcinoid or amphicrine tumors of the middle ear. A new entity? Pathol Res Pract 1992, **188**: 162–171.

121 Friedman I. Middle ear adenoma. Histopathology 1998, **32**: 279–280.

122 Hosoda S, Tateno H, Inoue HK, Isojima G, Kondo S, Konishi T. Carcinoid tumor of the middle ear containing serotonin and multiple peptide hormones. A case report and review of the pathology literature. Acta Pathol Jpn 1992, **42**: 614–620.

123 Hyams VJ, Michaels L. Benign adenomatous neoplasm (adenoma) of the middle ear. Clin Otolaryngol 1976, **1**: 17–26.

124 Ketabchi S, Massi D, Franchi A, Vannucchi P, Santucci M. Middle ear adenoma is an amphicrine tumor: why call it adenoma? Ultrastruct Pathol 2001, **25**: 73–78.

125 Latif MA, Madders DJ, Barton RP, Shaw PA. Carcinoid tumour of the middle ear associated with systemic symptoms. J Laryngol Otol 1987, **101**: 480–486.

126 McNutt MA, Bolen JW. Adenomatous tumor of the middle ear. An ultrastructural and immunocytochemical study. Am J Clin Pathol 1985, **84**: 541–547.

127 Mills SE, Fechner RE. Middle ear adenoma. A cytologically uniform neoplasm displaying a variety of architectural patterns. Am J Surg Pathol 1984, **8**: 677–685.

128 Murphy GF, Pilch BZ, Dickersin GR, Goodman ML, Nadol JB Jr. Carcinoid tumor of the middle ear. Am J Clin Pathol 1980, **73**: 816–823.

129 Ribe A, Fernandez PL, Ostertarg H, Claros P, Bombi JA, Palacin A, Cardesa A. Middle ear adenoma (MES): report of two cases, one with predominant 'plasmacytoid' features. Histopathology 1997, **30**: 359–364.

130 Riches WG, Johnston WH. Primary adenomatous neoplasms of the middle ear. Light and electron microscopic features of a group distinct from the ceruminomas. Am J Clin Pathol 1982, **77**: 153–161.

131 Ruck P, Pfisterer EM, Kaiserling E. Carcinoid tumour of the middle ear. A morphological and immunohistochemical study with comments on histogenesis and differential diagnosis. Pathol Res Pract 1989, **185**: 496–503.

132 Sakurai M, Mori N, Horiuchi O, Matsuura N, Kobayashi Y. Carcinoid tumor of the middle ear. An immunohistochemical and electron microscopic study. Report of a case. Acta Pathol Jpn 1988, **38**: 1453–1460.

133 Stanley MW, Horwitz CA, Levinson RM, Sibley RK. Carcinoid tumors of the middle ear. Am J Clin Pathol 1987, **87**: 592–600.

134 Wassef M, Kanavaros P, Polivka M, Nemeth J, Monteil JP, Frachet B, Tran Ba Huy P. Middle ear adenoma. A tumor displaying mucinous and neuroendocrine differentiation. Am J Surg Pathol 1989, **13**: 838–847.

Adenocarcinoma

135 Bisceglia M, D'Angelo VA, Wenig BM. Endolymphatic sac papillary tumor (Heffner tumor). Adv Anat Pathol 2006, **13**: 131–138.

136 Fayemi AO, Toker C. Primary adenocarcinoma of the middle ear. Arch Otolaryngol 1975, **101**: 449–452.

137 Gaffey MJ, Mills SE, Boyd JC. Aggressive papillary tumor of middle ear/temporal bone and adnexal papillary cystadenoma. Manifestations of von Hippel–Lindau disease. Am J Surg Pathol 1994, **18**: 1254–1260.

138 Gaffey MJ, Mills SE, Fechner RE, Intemann SR, Wick MR. Aggressive papillary middle-ear tumor. A clinicopathologic entity distinct from middle-ear adenoma. Am J Surg Pathol 1988, **12**: 790–797.

139 Glasscock ME III, McKennan KX, Levine SC, Jackson CG. Primary adenocarcinoma of the middle ear and temporal bone. Arch Otolaryngol Head Neck Surg 1987, **113**: 822–824.

140 Hamazaki S, Yoshiba M, Yao M, Nagashima Y, Taguchi K, Nakashima H, Okada S. Mutation of von Hippel–Lindau tumor suppressor gene in a sporadic endolymphatic sac tumor. Hum Pathol 2001, **32**: 1272–1276.

141 Heffner DK. Low-grade adenocarcinoma of probable endolymphatic sac origin A clinicopathologic study of 20 cases. Cancer 1989, **64**: 2292–2302.

142 Kempermann G, Neumann HP, Volk B. Endolymphatic sac tumours. Histopathology 1998, **33**: 2–10.

143 Lonser RR, Kim HJ, Butman JA, Vortmeyer AO, Choo DI, Oldfield EH. Tumors of the endolymphatic sac in von Hippel–Lindau disease. N Engl J Med 2004, **350**: 2481–2486.

144 Mills SE, Gaffey MJ, Frierson HF. Tumors of the upper aerodigestive tract and ear. Atlas of tumor pathology, series 3, fascicle 26. Washington DC, 2000, Armed Forces Institute of Pathology.

145 Pallanch JF, Weiland LH, McDonald TJ, Facer GW, Harner SG. Adenocarcinoma and adenoma of the middle ear. Laryngoscope 1982, **92**: 47–54.

146 Schuller DE, Conley JJ, Goodman JH, Clausen KP, Miller WJ. Primary adenocarcinoma of the middle ear. Otolaryngol Head Neck Surg 1983, **91**: 280–283.

147 Siedentop KH, Jeantet C. Primary adenocarcinoma of the middle ear. Report of three cases. Ann Otol Rhinol Laryngol 1961, **70**: 719–733.

148 Stone HE, Lipa M, Bell RD. Primary adenocarcinoma of the middle ear. Arch Otolaryngol 1975, **101**: 702–705.

149 Vortmeyer AO, Huang SC, Koch CA, Governale L, Dickerman RD, McKeever PE, Oldfield EH, Zhuang Z. Somatic von Hippel–Lindau gene mutations detected in sporadic endolymphatic sac tumors. Cancer Res 2000, **60**: 5963–5965.

150 Wenig BM, Heffner DK. Endolymphatic sac tumors: fact or fiction? Adv Anat Pathol 1996, **3**: 378–387.

Squamous cell carcinoma

151 Barnes L, Johnson JT. Clinical and pathological considerations in the evaluation of major head and neck specimens resected for cancer. Part II. Pathol Annu 1986, **21**(Pt 2): 83–110.

152 Jin YT, Tsai ST, Li C, Chang KC, Yan JJ, Chao WY, Eng HL, Chou TY, Wu TC, Su IJ. Prevalence of human papillomavirus in middle ear carcinoma associated with chronic otitis media. Am J Pathol 1997, **150**: 1327–1333.

153 Kenyon GS, Marks PV, Scholtz CL, Dhillon R. Squamous cell carcinoma of the middle ear. A 25-year retrospective study. Ann Otol Rhinol Laryngol 1985, **94**: 273–277.

154 Michaels L, Wells M. Squamous cell carcinoma of the middle ear. Clin Otolaryngol 1980, **5**: 235–248.

155 Milford CA, Violaris N. Bilateral carcinoma of the middle ear. J Laryngol Otol 1987, **101**: 711–713.

156 Morton RP, Stell PM, Derrick PP. Epidemiology of cancer of the middle ear cleft. Cancer 1984, **53**: 1612–1617.

157 Woodson GE, Jurco S III, Alford BR, McGavran MH. Verrucous carcinoma of the middle ear. Arch Otolaryngol 1981, **107**: 63–65.

Rhabdomyosarcoma

158 Angervall L, Dahl I, Ekedahl C. Embryonal rhabdomyosarcoma in the external ear. Acta Otolaryngol 1972, **73**: 513–520.

159 Hawkins DS, Anderson JR, Paidas CN, Wharam MD, Qualman SJ, Pappo AS, Scott Baker K, Crist WM. Improved outcome for patients with middle ear rhabdomyosarcoma: a children's oncology group study. J Clin Oncol 2001, **19**: 3073–3079.

160 Jaffe BF, Fox JE, Batsakis JG. Rhabdomyosarcoma of the middle ear and mastoid. Cancer 1971, **27**: 29–37.

161 Raney RB Jr, Lawrence W Jr, Maurer HM, Lindberg RD, Newton WA Jr, Ragab AH, Tefft M, Foulkes MA. Rhabdomyosarcoma of the ear in childhood. A report from the Intergroup Rhabdomyosarcoma Study – I. Cancer 1983, **51**: 2356–2361.

162 Tefft M, Fernandez C, Donaldson M, Newton W, Moon TE. Incidence of meningeal involvement by rhabdomyosarcoma of the head and neck in children. A report of the Intergroup Rhabdomyosarcoma Study (IRS). Cancer 1978, **42**: 253–258.

Other primary tumors

163 Cremers CW. Osteoma of the middle ear. J Laryngol Otol 1985, **99**: 383–386.

164 Gourin CG, Sofferman RA. Dermoid of the eustachian tube. Otolaryngol Head Neck Surg 1999, **120**: 772–775.

165 Roncaroli F, Scheithauer BW, Pires MM, Rodrigues AS, Pereira JR. Mature teratoma of the middle ear. Otol Neurotol 2001, **22**: 76–78.

166 Shaida AM, McFerran DJ, da Cruz M, Hardy DG, Moffat DA. Cavernous haemangioma of the internal auditory canal. J Laryngol Otol 2000, **114**: 453–455.

167 Singh SP, Cottingham SL, Slone W, Boesel CP, Welling DB, Yates AJ. Lipomas of the internal auditory canal. Arch Pathol Lab Med 1996, **120**: 681–683.

168 Stanley RJ, Scheithauer BW, Thompson EI, Kispert DB, Weiland LH, Pearson BW. Endodermal sinus tumor (yolk sac tumor) of the ear. Arch Otolaryngol Head Neck Surg 1987, **112**: 200–203.

169 Stegehuis HR, Guy AM, Anderson KR. Middle-ear lipoma presenting as airways obstruction. Case report and review of literature. J Laryngol Otol 1985, **99**: 589–591.

170 Uchida M, Matsunami T. Malignant amelanotic melanoma of the middle ear. Arch Otolaryngol Head Neck Surg 2001, **127**: 1126–1128.

Metastatic tumors

171 Hill BA, Kohut RI. Metastatic adenocarcinoma of the temporal bone. Arch Otolaryngol 1976, **102**: 568–571.

172 Schuknecht HF, Allam AF, Murakami Y. Pathology of secondary malignant tumors of the temporal bone. Ann Otol Rhinol Laryngol 1968, **77**: 5–22.

Appendix A

ADASP position papers

The Association of Directors of Anatomic and Surgical Pathology (ADASP) was founded in 1989. The membership is made up largely of directors of anatomic and/or surgical pathology from academic institutions. Originally all members were from American institutions, but subsequently the membership was enlarged to include academic centers in Canada and selected institutions from overseas.

The purposes of the Association are: (1) to promote expertise, effective administration and productive education in the practice of administering anatomic pathology laboratories; (2) to sponsor and promote the education of pathologists and others in health care related to administration of anatomic pathology and its branches; and (3) to establish and maintain appropriate relationships with other societies and groups of physicians and other scientists who share professional interests with the Association.

The main activities of the Association consist of an annual meeting held in conjunction with the annual meeting of the United States and Canadian Academy of Pathology (USCAP) and the publication of position papers, editorials, and recommendations regarding various aspects of the practice of anatomic pathology. Some of these documents are reproduced below.

Standardization of the surgical pathology report

(This document was prepared by an ad hoc committee of ADASP chaired by Richard L. Kempson, M.D. From Am J Surg Pathol 1992, **16:** 84–86.)

The Association of Directors of Anatomic and Surgical Pathology (ADASP) has concluded that a more standardized surgical pathology report may contribute positively to patient care. As the first step toward achieving this goal, ADASP has prepared the following recommendations and urges pathologists to consider adopting these for their own surgical pathology reports. The recommendations concern not only the format of the report but also provide suggestions for information to be included in the report. Widespread adoption of these recommendations should make information transfer from surgical pathology laboratories to clinicians more efficient and complete and also improve communication among surgical pathology laboratories when histologic sections are sent from one institution to another.

Demographic and specimen information

ADASP recommends the following:

1. Placing all demographic information in the top portion of the report.
2. Including in the demographic information the patient's name, location, gender, age and/or date of birth, and race, as well as the requesting physician's name, the attending physician's name (if different from the requesting physician), and the medical record or unit number.
3. Printing the name, address, telephone number, and FAX number of the laboratory at the top of the surgical pathology report.

4 Placing the surgical pathology number in the top portion of the report on every page, set off from other information so that it can be easily and quickly identified.
5 Including a summary of the pertinent clinical history as part of every surgical pathology report.
6 Including a separate 'specimens submitted' section in every report in which each separately identified tissue submitted for individual examination and diagnosis is clearly identified and listed as a separate specimen.

Gross description

ADASP recommends the following:

1 Including an adequate gross description as part of every surgical pathology report. Prerecorded gross descriptions are satisfactory, provided they include specific information about the particular specimen. Each separately identified tissue specimen submitted for individual examination and diagnosis should have its own gross description. Whether 'part' or 'all' of the specimen has been submitted for microscopic examination should always be recorded in the gross description.
2 Identifying each block with a unique number or letter. Giving multiple blocks the same identification number or letter is discouraged. A summary listing the sites from which each identified block is taken should be placed at the end of the gross description.
3 Augmenting the identification of block selections of complex specimens, when appropriate, by drawings, photographs, xerographs, etc.; but these pictorial records should *not* replace the printed block identification summary recommended in no. 2 above. Ideally, the pictorial record should accompany the chart copy, the physician copy, and the surgical pathology laboratory copy of the report.
4 Recording in the gross description the fact that margins are inked.
5 Recording the distribution of tissue for special studies in the gross description.
6 Including in the pathology report, when slides or blocks or tissues are received from another laboratory, the numbers of the slides and blocks, the referring hospital's identification numbers or letters, and the referring hospital's demographic data.

Microscopic description and comment section

For purposes of these recommendations, a microscopic description is defined as a description of the cytologic features and the architectural arrangement of the cells in a histologic section. A comment refers to all other pertinent information.

ADASP recommends the following:

1 Recording microscopic features whenever the responsible pathologist deems it appropriate, but a microscopic description need not be a part of every report.
2 Placing comments into the report whenever the responsible pathologist considers they are indicated, but a comment need not be written for every case.
3 Making it optional to place microscopic descriptions and comments in separate sections or to combine them.
4 Designating that 'special' stains have been performed, listing each stain and the results of the staining in the microscopic or comment section.
5 Listing, when immunohistochemical stains have been performed, each antibody tested and the results of the staining in the microscopic or comment section of the surgical pathology report in a separate immunohistochemical report, or both.
6 Grading all tumors for which grading has been shown to be a significant prognostic variable. When a grade is given, the grading criteria or scheme should be recorded in a comment or in the diagnosis line unless the grading scheme is standard and well understood by all clinicians.
7 Using a 'checklist' approach for recording information needed for patient treatment and prognosis. A statement relating whether each item on the checklist is positive or negative should be made. The checklist is used to ensure that all pertinent information has been included in the pathology report. Such information includes but is not limited to grade, depth of invasion, presence or absence of vascular invasion, size of the tumor, type of tumor, etc., and it is often different for different types of resection specimens. The condition of resection margins should be recorded here if clinically indicated. These checklists may be in manuals, on separate sheets, in computers, etc. It is also recommended that there be routine periodic checks of pathology reports to ensure that this information is present and summarized in an easy to find area of the comment or in the diagnosis section.
8 All information needed to formulate the pathologic state of a cancer be present in the report, but this information need not be recorded by a number or letter per se. If a stage number or letter is recorded, then the system used should be specified.

Intraoperative consultation

ADASP recommends that the intraoperative consultation report be incorporated verbatim into the final report. The persons responsible for the intraoperative report should be identified. If there is a discrepancy between the intraoperative diagnosis and the final diagnosis, this discrepancy should be recorded and discussed in a comment.

Final diagnosis

ADASP recommends the following:

1 Specifying the organ, site, and procedure as well as the diagnosis in the diagnosis section. These can be set off from the diagnosis by a dash or a colon.
2 Standardizing the format of diagnoses within each pathology department.
3 Setting off anatomic diagnoses so that they can be quickly and easily identified.
4 Listing each separately identified tissue submitted for individual examination and diagnosis in the diagnosis section along with the anatomic diagnosis for that specimen.

General considerations

ADASP recommends the following:

1 Clearly separating and identifying specimen(s) submitted, clinical information, clinical diagnosis, intraoperative diagnosis, gross description, microscopic description, comments (when they are not combined with the microscopic description), and anatomic diagnoses in such a way as to be found readily and easily in the report. Printing should be of sufficient quality to be read easily.

2 Doing a search for prior histologic and cytologic accession numbers for each case and recording pertinent prior specimen numbers in the current surgical pathology report.
3 Incorporating the results of special studies such as electron microscopy, immunohistochemistry, flow cytometry, receptor status, data, etc. into the surgical pathology report whenever possible. If this information is not a part of the surgical pathology report, the fact that tissue has been sent for the study should be recorded in the surgical pathology report.
4 Recording in the pathology report any information regarding procedures other than routine handling of tissue, such as gross photography, decalcification, specimen x-ray, freezing of samples, and placing specimens in a tissue bank.
5 Documenting intradepartmental consultations in the surgical pathology report, either by identifying the consultant in the comment section or at the end of the surgical pathology report or by having the consultant cosign the report.
6 Noting when external consultation is initiated by the pathologist in the pathology report. When the consultant's report is received, a supplemental report containing the consultant's interpretation and opinions should be issued.
7 Conveying to clinicians any clinically significant unexpected findings and documenting immediately in the surgical pathology report the fact that a call was made.
8 Citing references in the surgical pathology report when pertinent.
9 It is acceptable for the responsible pathologist to make suggestions for additional studies or procedures in the surgical pathology report if the pathologist thinks they will contribute to the case. Such information can be incorporated in the surgical pathology report as long as it is emphasized that they are only suggestions.
10 Note clearly and prominently when an amended report is issued. Changes that have been made in the report should be specified if the new report is a complete one; if only changes are recorded in the amended report, that fact should be specified.
11 Including the date the specimen was received and the date of the final report in all surgical pathology reports.

Incorporation of immunostaining data in anatomic pathology reports

(This document was prepared by an ad hoc committee of ADASP chaired by Peter M. Banks, M.D. From Am J Surg Pathol 1992, **16:** 808.)

The Council of ADASP has reviewed issues in the application of immunostains to diagnostic anatomic pathology. In selected cases this means of adding the specificity of immune mechanisms to visual microscopic appearances has become an essential adjunctive method for accurate diagnosis. It has also become evident that no immunologically defined marker is entirely specific for a disease entity. Rather, immunologically defined cellular constituents provide a dimension of resolution regarding cellular differentiation that is additive to that deriving from morphologic observations. As is the case with other ancillary methods, such as special histochemical stains or electron microscopy, immunostaining results must be integrated into a diverse mixture of data, including clinical information, gross and conventional microscopic pathologic findings and, in some cases, other types of ancillary study. It is the responsibility of the pathologist to select appropriate immunostain reagents and to render an informed interpretation of the results of these studies, based on the supplier's description of the reagents' activities, on personal experience, and on reported observations and cumulative experience in the professional literature.

For the purposes of the clarity and exchange of information among pathology laboratories and physicians, the following recommendations are offered for reporting immunostain results.

1 Immunostaining results should always be reported, regardless of perceived significance. Ideally such information should be included in the original main report (surgical, cytology, or autopsy); however, because of time constraints, it may be necessary to report immunostaining separately. When the latter method of reporting is used, it is essential that the initial report state that such studies are pending, and likewise, it is essential that the separate report refer to or even include the original report.
2 A differential diagnosis justifying immunostaining methods should be provided in the report. Reference to differential diagnosis may be very brief or general, for example, 'anaplastic large-cell neoplasm of uncertain differentiation' or 'epithelial versus lymphoid nature'.
3 In the report, or portion of the report, dealing with immunostains the following should be included:
   a The nature of the studied sample – paraffin sections, frozen sections, aspiration biopsy smears, cellular imprints, cytocentrifuge preparations, etc.
   b The immunoreagents used. These should be specifically described – 'HMB-45' rather than simply 'melanoma-related antigen'. It may be desirable with less commonly encountered reagents to provide a generic designation as well as the specific designation – muscle-specific actin ('HHF-35').
   c Results of the staining for each antibody should be reported in detail sufficient to justify the interpretation, e.g. in some cases simply *positive* or *negative*, but in others cellular patterns of staining or localization of some stain reactivity to certain cellular compartments.
4 Detailed technical information regarding the immunostaining procedures, including fixation, enhancing methods such as enzyme predigestion, and so on, need not be included in the diagnostic report but should be available in permanent laboratory records.

Consultations in surgical pathology

(This document was prepared by an ad hoc committee of ADASP chaired by Stephen G. Silverberg, M.D. From Am J Surg Pathol 1993, **17:** 743–745.)

Consultations are easier to obtain in pathology than in most other medical specialties because of the ability to cut duplicate histologic slides and forward them to any destination. Although this process has been taking place – usually with satisfactory results – for decades, there are numerous steps in the consultation process at which problems can and frequently do arise. Accordingly, ADASP has developed recommendations for consultations in anatomic pathology. Consultations may be generated for many reasons, including (but not limited to) the following:

1 Uncertainty of the referring pathologist about the diagnosis.
2 An internal disagreement between two or more pathologists in a group about the diagnosis.
3 The patient's request for a second opinion.
4 A clinician's request for a second opinion.
5 Quality assurance documentation.
6 Transfer of the patient to a different hospital or clinic, with a need for diagnosis by a pathologist at the new institution.

This section of the appendix consists of two parts: the first considers *personal consultations*, defined as consultations sent to a specific pathologist, usually for one of the first four reasons listed above; the second part deals with *institutional consultations*, in which the sixth reason is generally operative. Specifically excluded are consultations for legal purposes. ADASP recommends that the reason for the consultation be specified in the accompanying letter to the consultant.

Personal consultations

The ideal pathologic consultation proceeds from one pathologist to another; however, consultant pathologists also receive cases for consultation from clinicians, patients, patients' families, and others. ADASP makes the following recommendations:

1. The pathologist whose opinion is being solicited has the right to refuse to accept a case for consultation, if he or she believes that the interests of the patient will not be served by its acceptance.
2. The consultant who accepts a case and renders an opinion should always transmit the report to the pathologist in whose laboratory the initial diagnosis was made.

The pathologist sending a case for consultation has certain responsibilities to the consultant, and ultimately to the patient. ADASP makes the following recommendations:

1. An accompanying letter should provide the reason for the consultation, specific questions to be answered, the referring pathologist's working diagnosis or differential diagnosis, and appropriate billing information.
2. A copy of the surgical pathology report (or as much of it as has been completed) should accompany the letter and the slides; this should include pertinent demographic and clinical data and a gross description, as well as identification of the exact site of origin of each slide submitted.
3. Adequate material to solve the diagnostic problem should be submitted; in some instances, this material may consist of a single hematoxylin and eosin-stained slide, whereas in others all material available in the case – including special stains, electron micrographs, flow cytometric data, x-ray films, paraffin blocks, frozen or fixed tissue, or other special material or information – may be required. If it is anticipated that immunohistochemical stains or other additional procedures will be needed, the pertinent blocks or appropriately prepared unstained slides should be sent. Previous pathology specimens and reports from the same patient, if pertinent, should be included. If the referring pathologist has a question about a particular area on one or more slides, this question should be clearly indicated in the consultation letter and marked on the slide. The decision as to what to send should be made initially by the referring pathologist, but the consultant may request more material before making a diagnosis.

   The referring pathologist should personally assure that the material sent to the consultant is adequate to demonstrate the lesion in question and that this material is packaged to avoid breakage (Rosen PP, Am J Clin Pathol 1989, **91:** 348–354). In particular, recut slides should be inspected to ensure that they are representative. If paraffin blocks and glass slides are sent in the same container, a duplicate set of slides should be retained by the referring pathologist.
4. The referring pathologist may state the time frame in which a diagnosis is requested and in this situation attempt to determine that this schedule can be met. This may require telephoning in advance to ensure that the consultant is available, sending the consultation by an express delivery service, providing a telephone or fax number for rapid transmission of the consultant's report, and providing names and contact numbers for other physicians familiar with the case, should the referring pathologist not be available.
5. If the case is sent to more than one consultant, each should be informed of that fact, as well as of the other consultants' diagnoses.
6. If original material must be sent because no duplicates are available (for example, in the case of paraffin blocks or cytologic material), their return should be requested in the consultation letter. Whenever recut slides will suffice, they should be used and the consultant allowed to retain the slides.
7. The opinion of the consultant should be made part of the referring pathologist's report. The referring pathologist has the responsibility of making the final diagnosis and may agree or disagree with the consultant.

The consultant pathologist also has responsibilities to fulfill to optimize the consultation process. ADASP recommends the following:

1. If a case is accepted for consultation, a written report providing a diagnostic impression should be issued to identify the exact source of all material reviewed. This policy ultimately protects everyone involved in the process, including the patient.
2. Reports should be issued as expeditiously as possible. If the consultant cannot provide at least a preliminary opinion within 1 week of receipt, arrangements should be made to notify the referring pathologist.
3. When the consultant pathologist's diagnosis may alter immediate patient management, this fact should be communicated to the referring pathologist in a timely fashion.
4. If the consultant cannot make a diagnosis on the basis of the material submitted, he or she may either issue a provisional report on the basis of what is available, with suggestions for further studies to be performed by the referring pathologist, or request more or better material to perform the additional studies in the consultant's laboratory. Such a request is best made by telephone. Occasionally, the consultant may recommend a second consultant who might be more appropriate or, with permission of the referring pathologist, send the case directly to the second consultant.
5. If doing additional studies in the consultant's laboratory would generate additional charges, these charges should be authorized by the referring pathologist before the studies are undertaken.
6. Although the consultant may be asked to make recommendations for therapy and may choose to do so, it should be understood by all concerned that therapeutic recommendations made on the basis of a brief clinical summary and pathologic material alone may not always be applicable to the clinical situation.
7. The consultant should return to its source material that cannot be duplicated (e.g. paraffin blocks, cytologic slides, histologic slides showing lesions that do not persist on other cuts, original x-ray films) and otherwise should be allowed to retain and file all consultation material. The retained slides, whether placed in an institutional or a personal file, should be clearly identified and kept available for subsequent review, as should all written records related to the consultation.

8 It should be assumed that a case sent to a consultant may be published as part of a series by the consultant and that the referring pathologist can be acknowledged if permitted by the journal in which the report is published. We further recommend that publication of individual case reports by a consultant should be undertaken only with the express approval of the referring pathologist. In either of these situations, the referring pathologist may be asked by the consultant or a collaborator to contribute additional information, including follow-up, on the contributed case.

Institutional consultations

Many pathologic consultations are transmitted from one laboratory or hospital to another because the patient has been transferred to, or is seeking a second clinical opinion at, a second institution. In most such cases, the clinical consultant or the second institution (or both) will request that pertinent pathology reports and slides be reviewed by the local pathologist. Indeed, ADASP recommends that such review be standard institutional policy.

Most of the above recommendations for personal consultations also apply to institutional consultations. In the latter situation, it is even more important that the referred material be retained whenever possible in the second institution, particularly if the patient undergoes treatment there. It is also important that reports be sent directly to the patient's chart and the second institution's clinician(s) (who are more likely to be the official generators of the consultation), as well as to the referring pathologist. In the event of significant disagreement, the case should be promptly discussed with the referring pathologist. In the institutional consultation situation, institutional or departmental rules regarding turnaround time, record-keeping, quality assurance, and so on, take precedence over any mentioned above.

Immediate management of mammographically detected breast lesions

(This document was prepared by an ad hoc committee of ADASP co-chaired by Robert E. Fechner, M.D. and David L. Page, M.D. From Am J Surg Pathol 1993, **17:** 850–851.)

ADASP recommends that excisional biopsies of mammographically detected breast lesions be managed as outlined below. ADASP recognizes that special situations may lead to the management of a specimen in a manner that differs from the recommendations. Because of the special aspects of breast biopsy specimens, the recommendations for when to perform a frozen section do not necessarily apply to other types of specimens.

Until the late 1960s every breast biopsy was performed for a palpable abnormality. The biopsy specimen almost always included a lesion measuring more than 1 cm in greatest dimension. This tissue was ample for diagnosis and, with the advent of receptor studies, provided sufficient tissue when these studies were appropriate.

Presently, many biopsies are performed on women with clinically normal breasts with a mammographic abnormality. The abnormality may consist of calcifications or a density. The calcifications may or may not be associated with a grossly visible lesion in the biopsy specimen.

The purpose of a frozen section is twofold. In the case of a lesion clinically suspicious for invasive carcinoma, frozen section confirms the diagnosis and may be followed by immediate surgical therapy. In the event that no immediate surgery is planned, frozen section plays a role if a lesion is invasive carcinoma from which a fresh sample is desired for estrogen receptor (ER) and progesterone receptor (PR) assays, flow cytometry, or other studies.

The first priority in the examination of every breast biopsy specimen is to arrive at an accurate histologic diagnosis. No tissue should be used for other studies until a firm diagnosis of invasive carcinoma has been established. Depending on the reason for the biopsy and the nature of the gross specimen, different approaches are required for different breast lesions. A frozen section is not mandatory on every breast biopsy specimen and is often contraindicated. Whether to do a frozen section requires judgment. This is especially true when the gross lesion is small, i.e. less than 1 cm in greatest dimension. In this setting a frozen section may not yield a definite diagnosis. Moreover, permanent sections from the frozen block may have sufficient freezing artifact to rend the permanent sections suboptimal or even useless for diagnosis. The conservation of tissue that has never been frozen is a high priority for optimal diagnosis. Since many assays that formerly required fresh tissue can now be performed on fixed tissue, the need for frozen sections has further diminished.

Methods

The specimen should be received in the pathology laboratory uncut. This permits a specimen radiograph that retains the relationship seen on the mammogram. Ideally, the specimen margins should be inked before sectioning so that a statement can be made regarding involvement of margins if carcinoma is subsequently found. An uncut specimen also allows identification of the area in which the needle lies (if needle localization was performed).

Method for grossly visible lesions

ADASP recommends that the mammographically identified mass that is small (<1.0 cm) should not be submitted for frozen section examination. As stated previously, the first priority in any breast biopsy is to render a definitive histologic diagnosis; all other studies are secondary, e.g. tissue for ER and PR. A sample for quantitative receptors from a small mass may remove a significant portion of the lesion, which could possibly deprive the pathologist of crucial information. Incision of the mass may not only lose tissue for microscopic examination, but may distort the architecture of the surrounding tissue. This distortion could interfere with attempts to distinguish invasive cancer, radial scar, ductal adenoma, or adenosis tumor, any of which can be grossly indistinguishable from infiltrating carcinoma.

In the event that a small lesion is eventually determined to be invasive carcinoma, the lack of quantitative ER and PR information is mitigated by two factors. First, there is a close correlation between grade and receptor positivity. Second, immunohistochemical examination for receptors can be performed on the fixed tissue.

In the event that a frozen section is done and the diagnosis is suspicious for ductal carcinoma in situ, tissue should not be sent for special studies. All of the tissue should be retained for the permanent section diagnosis because detection of invasive carcinoma is the most important goal.

Methods for lesions with calcifications

Tissue removed for mammographically detected calcifications should be examined by specimen radiography to confirm that the calcified area has been excised. The biopsy specimen should remain intact to compare the specimen radiograph with the preoperative mammogram. The specimen is then sectioned as thinly as possible. If there is no grossly visible lesion suspicious of infiltrating carcinoma that measures more than 1 cm, no frozen section should be performed. The details for further sampling and processing of specimens for mammographically detected calcifications are beyond the scope of this report. The calcifications corresponding to those seen on the mammogram should be identified on slides or further steps should be taken to identify them.

In summary, the management of mammographically directed excisional biopsy specimens presents the pathologist with a number of responsibilities. The goals of immediate specimen management are:

1 To identify the area of concern on the mammogram.
2 Not to compromise the final diagnosis by freezing a small lesion or taking tissue for special studies before a definitive diagnosis has been made.

Use of human tissue blocks for research

(This document was prepared by an ad hoc committee of ADASP chaired by Virginia A. LiVolsi, M.D. From Am J Clin Pathol 1995, **105:** 260–261.)

Over the past 10–15 years, researchers working in the fields of molecular biology, genetics, and immunology have indicated that their investigations were hampered by lack of availability of human tumor tissue. In 1987, The National Cancer Institute established the Cooperative Human Tissue Network (CHTN). The tissues supplied to researchers are 'excess' (i.e. not tissue specifically removed for research or material essential for routine diagnosis and staging purposes). In addition, the research involves study of existing pathology specimens in which specific patients are not identified. These principles ('excess' tissue and not identifying the patient) form the basis of the current policy of the Department of Health and Human Services concerning exemption from informed consent. Recently, some large corporations have requested, as part of a patient acceptance into protocols, that paraffin blocks be sent to a central repository for storage. It is often a mandatory requirement that the blocks be sent for the patient to be included in the treatment protocol. However, in many cases, no specific research protocols have yet been developed for use of these blocks, and they will be placed in a repository.

For neoplastic lesions that are by nature large, such as colonic carcinomas, ovarian carcinomas, etc., this request does not seem unreasonable (i.e. that a representative block of tissue be submitted to a central repository for future studies). This can be accomplished in a prospective fashion when the specimen is processed.

This represents excess tissue, not the diagnostic material. However, for small neoplastic lesions (the area of most concern currently is breast cancer), the lesion is often so small that it is confined to only one block of tissue. Sending this block off to a repository raises several problems.

First, there are legal considerations. Various states have regulations requiring pathology departments and hospitals to maintain patient material including tissue blocks and slides for many years. The most stringent of these is New York State, which requires tissue pathology slides be kept for 20 years. Other states and the College of American Pathologists require anywhere from a 5- to 10-year period of retention of this material. Hence, it would be violating some state regulations as well as those of one major accrediting agency to send the blocks to a central repository rather than maintaining them in the hospital of origin. The legal aspects of tissue ownership, tissue block possession, and slide possession are still in flux. Some states have had cases in which regulatory decrees indicated that the information in the slides and blocks belongs to the patient, but the actual slides and blocks are the property of the original institution. Other states have indicated that everything is the property of the patient. The courts are unclear in the rulings and in some instances are frankly contradictory.

Second, there is the question of informed consent. How well are patients informed by oncologists, surgeons, or other health care providers about the nature, fragility, and irreplaceable nature of tissue blocks? It is unlikely that the 'informer' has the first-hand knowledge to explain this to the patient. In addition, the patient's privacy rights must be considered. Writing in the *Journal of NIH Research*, Charrow (Journal of NIH Research 1994, **6:** 79–81) indicated that the Institutional Review Boards (IRB) of the parent institution must approve transfer of patient material from that institution to one in which 'research' will be conducted on said material. The IRB must determine that "the research to be conducted at the transferee institution does not raise a new risk that a reasonable person would wish to know about before assenting" to send the material. If the IRB determines that the potential for "increased risk exists, the IRB should deny a request to transfer the specimen unless it first contacts the patient and obtains informed consent for the transfer". Certainly, some genetic research focusing on cancer tissue blocks in identified patients could lead to information that is potentially embarrassing, may violate privacy rights, and requires renewed specific patient consent for its use and/or transferral.

Third, who should have access to the information contained in the genetic material in these blocks? Who should have access to family data? The National Institutes of Health is currently evaluating these questions. Obviously, this situation will have to be looked at again as new legal challenges are brought and decisions rendered. Until these issues are resolved, we believe it is prudent for institutions to not release blocks for repository use.

A final issue arises: What happens when the repository is no longer funded, as funding for collaborative studies may be reduced or eliminated? Once there is no funding, how will the blocks be returned to the original institution – or will they? Will they just be lost, never to be retrieved? The legal implications of this have not been addressed. Until the many questions reviewed here are resolved, it appears inappropriate to demand that tissue blocks be stored in a repository.

Advances in computer technology will allow for an electronic repository – rather than a physical one – so that the location of specific blocks can be known. When and if specific research protocols are designed to use the tissue, unstained sections from the paraffin block for each case could be provided by the pathology department of origin (these could be provided as sections on slides or free in small tubes). The block would be maintained by the original department of pathology. With advances in polymerase chain reaction (PCR) technology, DNA and even RNA could be recovered for studies from the slides. Experienced molecular biologists have used archival material in this manner. The availability of this type of material from pathology departments should not pose a problem and certainly would conform to the legal requirements for maintaining the blocks at the institution of origin. However, the budget of the study should include funds to cover the cost of providing this material.

This position statement is not intended to oppose, and should not be interpreted as indicating that we oppose, the borrowing of blocks on a specific case as needed for an individual patient's care. An alternative of sending unstained sections is also appropriate as long as it does not completely deplete the diagnostic material. We believe that, with respect to individual patient care issues, the questions reviewed here need to be examined more fully by regulatory agencies and interested medical organizations.

Quality control and quality assurance in anatomic pathology

(This document was prepared by an ad hoc Committee of ADASP chaired by Juan Rosai, M.D. From Am J Surg Pathol 1991, **15:** 1007–1009.)

ADASP has prepared the following recommendations regarding Quality Control and Quality Assurance (QC/QA) in surgical pathology and autopsy pathology. This document does not include QC/QA issues as they apply to cytopathology and to specialized anatomic pathology laboratories such as immunohistochemistry or electron microscopy.

ADASP wishes to emphasize that the recommendations contained in this document were made taking into consideration the structure, responsibilities, and needs of academic anatomic pathology laboratories that have an active pathology residency or fellowship program. It also wishes to point out that they are to be viewed as being of a generic nature and suitable for modification depending on the specific circumstances of the individual laboratories and the respective institutions.

I It is recommended that each Department of Pathology prepare a written QC/QA plan for surgical pathology and autopsy pathology specifically devised for that Department and the respective institution. This document should be updated on a yearly basis. It should be part of the Departmental QC/QA program and, as such, should be structured along the lines of the JCAHO ten-step monitoring process as detailed in *The Accreditation Manual for Hospitals*.

II It is recommended that each Department establish a QC/QA Committee. The Committee should be appointed by the Chairman on a yearly basis. It should meet monthly, be chaired by a senior pathologist, and have as members representatives from the principal sections or divisions of the Department.

III It is recommended that the QC/QA plan for surgical pathology and autopsy pathology include the components ('indicators') listed below. The first of these indicators is of a prospective nature – i.e. to be carried out before the final report is issued. All others are of a retrospective nature – i.e. to be carried out in a regular fashion independently from the timing of the final report and usually after this has taken place.

Intradepartmental consultation

This function is to be carried out through one or both of the following mechanisms:

1 Review of selected cases by the diagnostic staff as a group, either through a periodic session ('consensus conference') or a written consultation form. The fact that this exercise has taken place should be indicated in the pathology report.

2 Review of selected cases by a second staff pathologist ('consultant'). For those cases in which the entire case is evaluated by the consultant, it is recommended that both pathologists sign the report; for cases in which only a portion of the cases has been reviewed, it is recommended that a note to that effect be added to the report.

Intraoperative consultation

It is recommended that all cases in which an intraoperative consultation has been carried out be reviewed on a regular (i.e. weekly) basis and be placed according to their final disposition in one of the following categories:

1 Agreement
2 Deferral–Appropriate
3 Deferral–Inappropriate
4 Disagreement–Minor
5 Disagreement–Major

For all cases in the 'Disagreement–Major' and 'Deferral–Inappropriate' categories, it is recommended that the reason for this occurrence be categorized as one of the following:

1 Interpretation
2 Block sampling
3 Specimen sampling
4 Technical inadequacy
5 Lack of essential clinical or pathologic data
6 Other (indicate)

It is further recommended that the medical consequences of the cases included in the 'Disagreement–Major' or 'Deferral–Inappropriate' categories be listed as one of the following:

1 None
2 Minor/questionable
3 Major

ADASP estimates that an acceptable accuracy threshold for intraoperative consultations (as measured by the number of 'Disagreement–Major' cases and determined per case) is 3%; an acceptable threshold for 'Deferred–Inappropriate' cases is 10%.

ADASP believes that it is important for each laboratory to establish its own time thresholds for intraoperative consultation, using as a standard unit the time threshold for the performance of a 'basic' frozen section, as defined by a case with a single block, with no other cases being performed by the intraoperative consultation team at the same time.

Random case review

It is recommended that the following cases be reviewed on a random basis:

1 Surgical pathology: 1% or 25/month, whichever is larger.
2 Autopsy: 10% or two/month, whichever is larger.

The review on the randomly selected cases should include all material related to them, including final report, microscopic slides, turnaround time, and special procedures, if any.

Clinical indicators

It is recommended that a Clinical Indicator be selected on a regular basis on the basis of organ/lesion (i.e. carcinoma of endometrium) or procedure (i.e. TUR), and that *all* cases belonging to that indicator in a given period be evaluated by checking them against a list of predetermined criteria. This activity should be rotated among surgical pathology and autopsy cases.

Intradepartmental and interdepartmental conferences

For all cases presented at intradepartmental and interdepartmental conferences, it is recommended that the diagnosis as listed in the final report be compared with that made by the presenter when reviewing the case for the conference.

Interinstitutional review

For cases in which an outside review has been carried out at the request of the patient, the clinician or other institution, or as part of a cooperative study, it is recommended that the diagnosis as listed in the final report be compared with that made at the outside institution. The Association estimates that an acceptable threshold for clinically significant disagreement following arbitration is 2%, as applied to those cases in which it is decided that the correct interpretation is that from the outside institution.

Surgical pathology turnaround times

ADASP believes that the following are acceptable turnaround times for surgical pathology reports, as measured in working days from the time the specimen is accessioned in the laboratory to the time the verbal report is available or the final report is signed.

TYPE OF SPECIMEN	VERBAL REPORT	WRITTEN REPORT
Rushes	1	2
Biopsies	2	3
Surgicals	2	3

Extra time should be allowed for the following procedures, to be measured in days from the time the procedure is initiated or ordered and independently from each other:

1 Overnight fixation, 1
2 Decalcification, 1
3 Resubmission, 1–2
4 Recuts, 1
5 Immunocytochemistry, 1–2
6 Electron microscopy, 2–3
7 Intradepartmental consultation, 1

ADASP estimates that an acceptable threshold for these turnaround times is 80%.

Autopsy turnaround time

ADASP believes that the following are acceptable turnaround times for autopsy reports, as measured in working days:

1 Provisional report: 1
2 Final report: 30

ADASP estimates that an acceptable threshold for the provisional report is 90%; acceptable threshold for the final report is 80%.

Specimen adequacy

It is recommended that the adequacy of submission of specimens to the laboratory be monitored in terms of fixation, safety requirements, and proper identification.

Lost specimen

This is defined as the irretrievable loss of a surgical pathology specimen that has occurred after the case has been accessioned in the laboratory and that prevents an adequate pathologic examination of that specimen. ADASP estimates that an acceptable threshold for lost specimens is one in 3000 cases.

Histology QC

It is recommended that the QC related to the histology lab include:

1 Record of time of delivery of slides.
2 Evaluation of slide quality as performed by the pathologist.
3 Evaluation of tissue adequacy as performed by the histotechnologist.

Isolated event report

It is recommended that isolated events not contemplated in any of the foregoing categories be documented through the issuing of an 'Isolated Event Report'. All such reports should be kept in a permanent log.

Quality control and quality assurance in anatomic pathology: updated recommendations

The report was prepared by an ad hoc writing committee of the Association of Directors of Anatomic and Surgical Pathology (ADASP) composed of Raouf Nakhleh, M.D., Mayo Clinic, Jacksonville, FL; Cheryl Coffin, M.D., University of Utah, Salt Lake City; and Kumarasen Cooper, MBChB, D.Phil., chair, University of Vermont, Burlington. The report was approved by the ADASP Council in February 2006.

The Association of Directors of Anatomic and Surgical Pathology (ADASP [http://www.adasp.org]), which was founded in 1989, first published recommendations for anatomic pathology quality control and quality assurance in 1991. The recommendations emphasized surgical pathology and autopsy pathology quality issues and did not address cytopathology or specialized anatomic pathology laboratories, such as those that perform immunohistochemical analysis or electron microscopy.

In the decade and a half since the original ADASP recommendations, the emphasis on quality improvement (QI) has grown tremendously, and a variety of contributions to this area of anatomic pathology have been made by ADASP, the College of American Pathologists, and single-institutional studies. The 1999 Institute of Medicine Report, *To Err Is Human: Building a Safer Health System*, further focused attention on medical errors and patient safety and also offered specific recommendations for improvement.

The present recommendations update and refine the 1991 ADASP recommendations for quality assurance (QA) and QI surgical and autopsy pathology. As in the original recommendations, these recommendations take into consideration the structure, responsibilities, and needs of academic anatomic pathology laboratories that have active residency or fellowship programs. These recommendations can be modified according to specific institutional circumstances and needs.

QA and QI plan

An annual plan should be created with the intent of monitoring quality, but also targeting specific aim(s) each year for improvement.

1 QA in surgical pathology is defined as a program for the systematic monitoring and evaluation of the various aspects of the laboratory service to ensure that standards of quality are being met.

2 QI in surgical pathology is defined as a systematic attempt to improve specific quality measures in laboratory service.

QI committee

A quality improvement committee should be formed that, depending on department size, should include most of the anatomic and surgical and autopsy pathologists, selected residents or fellows, and sufficient support staff, including key laboratory and clerical staff. In large departments (>15 faculty), the size of the committee may be limited but should include individuals from all divisions within anatomic pathology. The committee members should have clear responsibilities for specific monitors or committee assignments. Regular meetings should be held to review QI data and discuss possible changes in the QI plan or in practice.

Test cycle

Analytic diagnostic errors have been the focus of most studies; however, errors with possible patient consequences occur with equal frequency in the preanalytic and postanalytic phases of the test cycle and should be addressed with equal effort.

QA and QI monitors

A QA and QI plan should have at least one component in each of the five sections listed but could include more. Typically, more than one analytic monitor is performed annually. It is not necessary to run QA monitors all the time. If a monitor is running at a satisfactory level, it may be spot checked for a short time annually or biannually. Then resources may be directed to areas in need of improvement.

1 Preanalytic
   a Specimen fixation
   b Specimen delivery
   c Specimen and patient identification
   d Adequacy of clinical history
   e Accessioning errors
2 Analytic
   a Intraoperative: frozen section–permanent section concordance
   b Final diagnosis: peer review error rate
   c Possible histology monitors
      1 Quality of histologic sections
      2 Specimens lost in processing
      3 Turnaround time (TAT)
      4 Block labeling
      5 Slide labeling
      6 Extraneous tissue
   d Immunohistochemical analysis
      1 Frequency and causes of repeated stains
      2 TAT for immunohistochemical analysis
      3 Report audit for integration of stains with morphologic diagnosis
      4 Annual review of antibody inventory and frequency of use
      5 Enrollment in external proficiency testing should be considered, particularly for tests that directly affect patient therapy, such as HER2/neu immunostaining
   e Other ancillary study monitors may be used as needed, including monitors for fluorescence in situ hybridization, electron microscopy, and other molecular studies
3 Postanalytic
   a Transcription errors
   b Verification errors during electronic sign-out or report finalization
   c Report delivery errors
   d Incomplete reports
   e Diagnostic finding correlation with ancillary studies (immunohistochemical analysis, electron microscopy, fluorescence in situ hybridization)
4 TAT
   a Frozen section
   b Biopsy
   c Large specimen
   d Preliminary and final autopsy reports
   e Clinician satisfaction and/or complaints

Quality assurance case reviews

No single method of case reviews has been shown to be more effective in detection of errors. As a preventive measure, many departments mandate prospective review of selective cases before case verification. Depending on departmental resources, a number of methods may serve as QA case reviews including the following:

1 Review of a randomly selected percentage of cases (Past recommendations have used 1%, 2%, 5%, or 10%, depending on the size of the practice and available staff time to conduct reviews.)
2 Focused internal second review of specific organ system or malignancy type (e.g. breast cancer)
3 Interdepartmental conferences (e.g. tumor board)
4 Intradepartmental QA conference
5 Frozen section–permanent section correlation
6 Cytology–surgical pathology correlation
7 Review of previous pathology material
8 Intradepartmental review of material before release to other institutions
9 Review of outside diagnosis of in-house cases

The 'gold standard'

The only true gold standard for diagnoses is long-term follow-up and response to therapy. This, however, is impractical. Peer review has become the gold standard to judge diagnostic 'correctness' in surgical pathology. There are acceptable ways of adjudicating errors and diagnostic disagreements, e.g. external consultation.

Defining error types and quantification of effect on patient

1 Error types
   a Change in categorical interpretation (e.g. benign to malignant, malignant to benign)
      1 False-positive
      2 False-negative
   b Change within the same category of interpretation (change in type of malignancy)
   c Change in threshold (In the past, this has referred to differences of opinion such as atypical ductal hyperplasia vs ductal carcinoma in situ. This also may be used for differences in grading and staging.)

d Change in margin status
e Change in lymph node status
f Change in information unrelated to the diagnosis
g Case or patient misidentification
h Site misidentification (e.g. right vs left)

2 Effect on patient. Many institutions include some type of grading scheme to determine what harm or potential harm may result from an error.

   Consideration should be given to communicating to risk management any error that has significant harm or impact on patient care.

   a No harm or impact on patient care
   b Slight harm or impact on patient care
   c Significant harm or alteration of clinical management

Error correction

When an error is identified, this information must be communicated directly and promptly to the patient's caregiver. Because of the presence of an already erroneous report, newly distributed reports must be marked carefully with language that establishes the changes. Most changes fall into three categories.

1 Change in diagnosis. Some have used the terms amended or revised reports to indicate these changes.
2 Change of information other than the diagnosis. Some have used the term corrected report for this change.
3 Additional information, no changes to original report. Most have used the term addendum to report this change.

Acceptable error rates

Although errors causing patient harm are unfortunate, there must be acknowledgment that a certain error rate is prevalent. Error levels that may be deemed within an acceptable range should be determined based on the literature for that measure, with the goal of modification by continuous improvement.

Acceptable TAT

This should be determined based on current literature, keeping in mind that acceptable TATs also are defined by accrediting bodies. TATs are variable depending on case complexity and other factors such as the presence of a residency training program. These standards may change over time with the advent of new technologies or other factors.

Sentinel event

It is recommended that incidents in which there is significant patient harm or there is significant breach of known policies and procedures be fully investigated and reviewed and possible changes in policy or procedure be made to address the problem. A formal root cause analysis may often be helpful. These incidents and analyses also should be referred to the institutional QI committee and risk management.

Pathologist competence

The Joint Commission on Accreditation of Healthcare Organizations standards state that "at the time of renewal of privileges, the organized medical staff evaluates individuals for their continued ability to provide quality care, treatment, and services for the privileges requested as defined in the medical staff bylaws". Therefore, pathologists may be required to document evidence of acceptable performance. This may be done by collecting individual performance data on multiple parameters and always submitting these data in the context of peer group comparison. These data may include but are not limited to TAT, frozen section–permanent section concordance rates, diagnostic error rates, clinician complaints, and clinician satisfaction.

Appendix B

Quality control and quality assurance in surgical pathology

The main goals of an Anatomic Pathology Departmental Quality Control/Quality Assurance (QC/QA) program are to ensure: (1) accuracy; (2) completeness; and (3) timeliness of all the reports generated by the Division of Anatomic Pathology. These goals are achieved by the continuous monitoring of the following indicators:

Prospective:

1 Intradepartmental consultation (IDC)

Retrospective:

2 Frozen section review (FSR)
3 SP cases random review (SPRR)
4 Autopsy cases random review (ARR)
5 AP clinical indicators (CI)
6 Intradepartmental and interdepartmental conferences (CONF)
7 Interinstitutional review (IIR)
8 Specimen adequacy record (SAR)
9 Lost specimen record (LSR)
10 Single event report (SER)
11 Histology slides delivery (SD)
12 Quality control to histology (TO-H)
13 Quality control from histology (FROM-H)
14 AP turnaround times (TAT)

This activity is usually carried out by a Department Committee appointed by the Chairman, which ideally should have at least one representative from outside the Department. The Chairman of this Committee usually functions as the departmental representative to the institutional Quality Control and Quality Assurance Committee (or whatever synonym may be used for the activity at the time).

National pathology organizations such as the College of American Pathologists have published quality assurance and quality improvement manuals to assist pathologists in setting up individualized programs in their own departments.[1]

What follows is a description of the QC/QA program as it was set up in the Department of Pathology at Yale University some years ago. The elaborated printed forms that were developed on the occasion have been replaced there and elsewhere by electronic versions, but the basic procedures remain the same. This version is offered as a guideline, with the understanding that its application in other laboratories may require some modifications depending on the number of types of specimens, size of staff, and whether there is a residency and/or fellowship program or not. The program as presented here does not include cytopathology or special laboratories, such as immunohistochemistry or electron microscopy.

The meetings of the QC/QA committee are divided into two sessions: (1) one primarily concerned with QC issues, in which all committee members participate, and (2) one primarily concerned with QA issues, in which only the attendings participate.

The collection and some of the analysis of the data, organization of the monthly meetings, and all correspondence related to the QC/QA committee are carried out by a QC/QA manager working under the supervision of the Committee Chairman and having secretarial assistance.

See also section on Quality Control and Quality Assurance in Anatomic Pathology (and updated recommendations) in Appendix A, page 2520.

1 Nakhleh RE, Fitzgibbons PL. Quality improvement manual in anatomic pathology, ed. 2. Northfield, IL, 2002, College of American Pathologists.

Intradepartmental consultation (IDC)

Purpose

To provide a prospective system by which all difficult, controversial, and otherwise problematic cases can be presented by any attending for review and discussion before they are signed out.

Frequency

This collegial session is held daily using a multiheaded microscope. The collegial session is run by the director of anatomic or surgical pathology. The other participants are the anatomic pathology attendings, particularly those on service rotations. Residents, students, and visitors do not participate.

Procedure

1 The date of the conference and the names of all the attendings present should be recorded.
2 The attendings participating at the conference present for discussion cases of their choice. These cases may be selected on the basis of any of the following criteria:
   a Diagnostic difficulty
   b Controversy in interpretation among attendings and/or residents
   c Discrepancy between frozen section diagnosis and intended final diagnosis
   d Discrepancy between provisional diagnosis and intended final diagnosis
   e Management purposes, such as performance of additional biopsies, special studies, or therapeutic recommendations
   f Request on the part of the clinician or patient
   g Interesting or unusual nature of the case.
3 The material presented should include all pertinent microscopic slides, a summary of the clinical data, and, when indicated, gross specimens or gross photographs, x-rays, and electron micrographs.
4 The individual presenting the case should state their diagnostic impression and reason for presentation.
5 The case is examined simultaneously by all participants, the director of anatomic or surgical pathology leading the discussion.
6 Upon completion of the presentation and discussion of each case, the director of anatomic or surgical pathology will enter in the corresponding form the following information:
   a Pathology number
   b Name of presenter
   c Diagnostic impression of presenter and reason for presentation
   d Consensus reached.
7 If indicated, the nature of the discussion having taken place and the recommendations made.
8 All cases presented at these conferences should be so identified by entering 'Case presented at the Departmental Collegial Session of ____(date)' in the final report, immediately following the diagnosis.

Frozen section review (FSR)

Purpose

To monitor the adequacy in the performance of intraoperative consultations ('frozen sections') in surgical pathology in terms of diagnostic accuracy, timing of the procedure, and consequences of the diagnosis rendered.

Frequency

Weekly.

Procedure

1 The copy of the frozen section forms filed in surgical pathology or available through the AP information system should include the following information: time at which the specimen was received, time at which the frozen section diagnosis was given, frozen section diagnosis, and final diagnosis.
2 The QC/QA manager should collect the above information weekly and evaluate it with regard to time employed to perform the procedure and concordance between frozen section and final diagnosis. In cases in which a discordance exists (including deferred cases), the following information should be entered:
   a Pathology number
   b Frozen section diagnosis
   c Initials of resident(s) and attending(s) who performed the frozen section
   d Final diagnosis, including initials of attending
   e Final disposition, according to the following categories:
      1 Agreement
      2 Deferment – Appropriate
      3 Deferment – Inappropriate
      4 Disagreement – Minor
      5 Disagreement – Major
   f For categories 3–5, explanation for the lack of agreement according to the following categories:
      1 Interpretation
      2 Block sampling
      3 Tissue sampling
      4 Technical inadequacy
      5 Lack of important clinical or previous pathologic information
   g For categories 3–5, consequences to the patient according to the following categories:
      1 None
      2 Minor/questionable
      3 Major

h Notes, if indicated
i Action taken.

Steps **e** through **i** of this procedure should be completed by the QC/QA committee chairman. When indicated, the FS and permanent slides should be reviewed. In addition, the QC/QA manager should record the above information in a separate form, divided according to the attending who performed the procedure.

Review

1 All FS forms from the preceding month should be presented and discussed at the monthly QC/QA meeting.
2 A formal review of the FS forms should be carried out by the QC/QA committee chairman on a quarterly basis, according to the general review procedure. The results of the review are to be presented at the monthly QC/QA meeting.

SP cases random review (SPRR)

Purpose

To monitor on a random basis the adequacy of the surgical pathology report in all of its aspects.

Frequency

Weekly.

Procedure

1 The QC/QA manager should collect on a random basis one of every 50 surgical pathology cases for the purposes of this review. The material collected should consist of:
  a Copy of requisition form
  b Copy of final surgical pathology report
  c All microscopic slides
  d All material from special studies (immunohistochemistry, electron microscopy, etc.), if any
  e All gross photographs and specimen x-rays, if any
2 This material will be given to the QC/QA committee chairman, who will evaluate it for the following criteria:
  a Clinical history
  b Gross description
  c Gross photographs, if any
  d Sampling for histology
  e Quality of slides
  f Diagnosis
  g Note, if any
  h SNOMED (topography and morphology) coding
  i Special studies, if any
  j Turnaround time
  k Other.

If indicated, assistance for the evaluation should be requested from other members of the pathology department or from outside consultants. Cases in which an important deficiency is detected, especially regarding the diagnosis, should be immediately brought to the attention of the director of anatomic pathology.

Review

1 All SP forms in which deficiencies have been entered should be presented and discussed at the monthly QC/QA meeting.
2 A formal review of the SP forms should be carried out by the QC/QA committee chairman quarterly, according to the general review procedure. The results of the review are to be presented at the monthly QC/QA meeting.

Autopsy cases random review (ARR)

Purpose

To monitor on a random basis the adequacy of the autopsy report in all of its aspects.

Frequency

Monthly.

Procedure

1 The QC/QA manager should collect on a random basis one of every 10 autopsy pathology cases for the purposes of this review. The material collected should consist of:
  a Copy of autopsy requisition
  b Copy of final complete autopsy report
  c All microscopic slides
  d All material from special studies (immunohistochemistry, electron microscopy, etc.), if any
  e All gross photographs and specimen x-rays, if any
2 This material will be given to the QC/QA committee chairman, who will evaluate it for the following criteria:
  a Patient identification and history
  b Gross description
  c Gross photographs, if any
  d Sampling for histology
  e Quality of slides
  f Diagnosis
  g Clinicopathologic correlation and bibliography
  h SNOMED (topography and morphology) coding
  i Special studies, if any
  j Turnaround time
  k Other.

If indicated, assistance for the evaluation should be requested from other members of the pathology department or from outside consultants. Cases in which an important deficiency is detected, especially regarding the diagnosis, should be immediately brought to the attention of the director of anatomic pathology.

Review

1 All AUT forms in which deficiencies have been entered should be presented and discussed at the monthly QC/QA meeting.
2 A formal review of the AUT forms should be carried out by the QC/QA committee chairman on a quarterly basis, according to the general QC/QA review procedure. The results of the review are to be presented at the monthly QC/QA meeting.

AP clinical indicators (CI)

Purpose

To monitor the completeness and consistency of the information provided in the pathology report for specific specimens or diseases, and to correct any deficiencies encountered.

Frequency

Monthly.

Procedure

1 The QC/QA committee chairman should identify, on a monthly basis, a specimen or disease to be evaluated. The selection can be made on the basis of tissue received regardless of the pathology present in it (e.g., transurethral prostatectomy) or on the basis of a specific disease entity (e.g., carcinoma of large bowel). It should include, on a rotational basis, cases from surgical pathology and autopsy pathology.
2 The QC/QA manager should retrieve all consecutive reports from cases corresponding to the selected specimen/disease that had been accessioned for a predetermined period, which may vary from 2 to 12 months depending on the frequency of the selected item.
3 The reports should be given to the attending designated by the QC/QA committee chairman for this purpose, who will review them for completeness, accuracy, and consistency by cross-checking them with a predetermined list of required items. The results of the review should be tabulated, and the information obtained should be submitted to the QC/QA manager.

Review

1 The results of the review should be presented at the monthly QC/QA meeting.
2 If significant deficiencies are encountered in the review, a follow-up study should be carried out in 3–12 months depending on the nature of the material.

Intradepartmental and interdepartmental conferences (CONF)

Purpose

To monitor the degree of agreement between the final diagnosis as expressed in the pathology report (surgical, cytology, or autopsy) and the consensus reached at the intradepartmental or interdepartmental conference(s) in which the case is presented.

Frequency

Monthly.

Procedure

Attendings who present and/or discuss anatomic pathology cases at intradepartmental or interdepartmental conferences should review the diagnostic material on those cases and compare their diagnostic impressions and the consensus reached at the conference with the diagnosis as stated in the official report. This information should be entered in the CONF form. In any case in which a discrepancy exists, the nature and importance of the problem should be stated, and the case should be discussed with the attending who signed the pathology report.

Review

1 All CONF forms should be presented and reviewed at the monthly QC/QA meeting.
2 A formal review of the CONF forms should be carried out by the QC/QA committee chairman quarterly, according to the general review procedure. The results of the review are to be presented at the monthly QC/QA meeting.

Interinstitutional review (IIR)

Purpose

To monitor the degree of diagnostic agreement rate among cases that have been sent to other institutions for one of the following reasons:

1 At the clinician's or patient's request
2 At the request of another institution in which the patient is being seen
3 Because the case has been entered in a cooperative study.

If a significant discrepancy between the two diagnoses exists, the director of anatomic or surgical pathology should resolve it by subjecting the case to inside or outside arbitration and submit an addendum report with the final resolution.

Procedure

The QC/QA manager should collect and record the diagnoses made at other institutions and compare those diagnoses with those made on the same cases at our institution. All the cases in which a major discrepancy exists should be recorded, including the arbitration outcome.

Review

1 All IIR from the preceding period should be presented at the monthly QC/QA meeting.
2 A formal review of the IIR forms should be carried out by the QC/QA committee chairman biannually, according to the general review procedure. The results of the review should be presented at the monthly QC/QA meeting.

Specimen adequacy record (SAR)

Purpose

To monitor the adequacy of submission of specimens to the pathology laboratory in terms of fixation, safety requirements, and proper identification, and to correct any deficiencies encountered.

Frequency

Daily.

Procedure

1 The SP accessioner should examine all material received in the laboratory for the deficiencies listed below and record them in the SAR form if present:
   a Specimen not bagged or bagged inadequately
   b Requisition placed inside bag
   c Staples in bag

- d Lid not sealed properly and/or fluid spill contamination
- e Inadequate amount of fixative fluid
- f No clinical history
- g Requisition form missing
- h No physician name
- i No physician signature
- j No specimen
- k Discordant information between requisition form and container
- l Radioactivity detected in specimen.

If deficiencies **g** to **l** were encountered, the specimen should not be accessioned. A pathologist or pathologist assistant should be contacted to resolve the matter.

2 The QC/QA manager should review the SAR form weekly and contact the appropriate services for correction of the problem whenever indicated.

Review

1 The completed SAR forms should be filed in the SP office.
2 The QC/QA manager should review the SAR forms quarterly, tabulate the findings according to type of problem and service, and present the results at the monthly QC/QA meeting.

Lost specimen record (LSR)

Purpose

To document all incidents in which a specimen is lost, destroyed, misidentified, or otherwise mishandled so as to make impossible its pathologic interpretation, to determine their cause, and to prevent their further occurrence.

Frequency

Monthly.

Procedure

All 'lost specimen' incidents should be recorded in the LSR form, which should be sent to the QC/QA files.

Review

The review of the LSR forms should be carried out by the QC/QA committee chairman monthly, according to the general review procedure. The results of the review are to be presented at the monthly QC/QA meeting.

Single event report (SER)

Purpose

1 To document the occurrence of single events that could reflect on the delivery of care by the division of anatomic pathology and that are brought to the attention of the QC/QA committee chairman through a notification by any member of the medical or technical hospital staff, either within or outside the department.
2 To evaluate the event, and to take a corrective measure if indicated.

Frequency

Monthly.

Review

The review of the SER form should be carried out monthly, and the results of the review should be presented at the monthly QC/QA meeting.

Histology slides delivery (SD)

Purpose

To monitor the time of delivery of microscopic slides by the histology laboratory to surgical pathology, and to correct any deficiencies encountered.

Frequency

Daily.

Procedure

1 A pathology attending or resident should record the time at which the microscopic slides from biopsies and surgical cases are delivered from the histology laboratory. If there is more than one delivery of any of the categories, each should be recorded. Comments regarding any departures from the norm should be made, such as explanations for undue delays.
2 At the end of each month, the completed form should be given to the QC/QA manager, who will send copies to the director of anatomic or surgical pathology and to the histology manager. The original should be kept in the QC/QA files.

Review

1 All SD forms from the preceding month should be presented and discussed at a monthly meeting held between the supervisor of the histology laboratory and the director of anatomic or surgical pathology. Minutes from this meeting should be sent to the QC/QA manager.
2 A formal review of the SD forms should be carried out by the QC/QA committee chairman on a monthly basis, according to the general review procedure. The results of the review are to be presented at the monthly QC/QA meeting.

Quality control to histology (TO-H)

Purpose

To monitor the quality of microscopic slides produced by the histology laboratory for surgical pathology and autopsy pathology, and to correct any deficiencies encountered.

Frequency

Daily.

Procedure

1 Attendings signing out surgical and autopsy pathology material should fill out one TO-H form per diagnostic session regardless of the number of cases examined. The form should be completed even if the technical quality of all the material examined is deemed to be satisfactory. In the cases thought to be of inadequate quality, the following information should be entered: pathology number, block identification, and type of problem. An attempt should be made to be as specific as possible about the nature of technical deficiency and the time of the preliminary slide. Each attending should complete a separate form.
2 Depending on the nature of the problem, the attending may elect to submit the problem slide(s) or a photocopy of the slide(s) to the histology laboratory in conjunction with the TO-H form.
3 Once completed, the forms (and any accompanying material) should be placed by the pathologist in the histology mailbox in order for them to be hand delivered daily to the supervisor of the histology laboratory.
4 The supervisor of the histology laboratory should review the submitted forms within 48 hours of reception, evaluate independently the problem, identify the cutter if indicated, and record in the form any comments and corrective action taken. If necessary, the histology supervisor should examine personally the microscopic slides and discuss the problem with the corresponding attending. The form should be signed, dated, and filed in the histology office. A copy should be sent to the QC/QA manager.

Review

1 All TO-H forms from the preceding period should be presented and discussed at the monthly meeting held between the supervisor of the histology laboratory and the director of anatomic pathology. Minutes from this meeting should be sent to the QC/QA manager.
2 A formal review of the TO-H forms should be carried out by the QC/QA committee chairman on a monthly basis, according to the general review procedure. The results of the review should be presented at the monthly QC/QA meeting.

Quality control from histology (FROM-H)

Purpose

1 To monitor the appropriateness of the material and information supplied by the pathologists to the histology laboratory (e.g., case and block identification, size and thickness of samples, decalcification, special fixation, procedures).
2 To monitor the appropriateness of the requests made to the histology laboratory (e.g., recuts, special stains, re-embedding).
3 To correct any deficiencies encountered.

Procedure

The histology supervisor should send memos through the electronic mail system to the individuals involved. A copy should be sent to the director of anatomic or surgical pathology, and another copy should be filed in the office of the histology supervisor.

Review

1 All FROM-H forms from the preceding period should be discussed at the monthly meeting held between the supervisor of the histology laboratory and the director of anatomic or surgical pathology. Minutes from this meeting should be sent to the QC/QA manager.
2 A formal review of the FROM-H forms should be carried out by the QC/QA committee chairman monthly, according to the general review procedure. The results of this review should be presented at the monthly QC/QA meeting.

Anatomic pathology turnaround times (TAT)

Purpose

To monitor the timely reporting of surgical and autopsy pathology specimens, and to correct any deficiencies encountered.

Frequency

Daily.

Procedure

1 A computer printout should be obtained daily listing overdue cases, according to the following criteria:
   a Biopsies not finalized within 2 days of receipt
   b Surgical specimens (routines) not finalized within 3 days of receipt
   c Autopsies in which a provisional diagnosis has not been sent out in 2 days
   d Autopsies not finalized within 30 days of receipt
2 Additional time will be allowed for special procedures according to the schedule recommended by the Association of Directors of Anatomic and Surgical Pathology (see Appendix A). These extra times will be calculated by the AP information system in a noncumulative fashion and taking into account the day in which those special procedures were ordered.
3 An individual assigned to the task by the QC/QA manager should determine and record in each case the reason for the delay by checking the corresponding record as entered in the AP information system and, if necessary, by communicating with the pathologist(s) assigned to the case.
4 Once the information has been collected on all cases, the completed form should be given to the director of anatomic or surgical pathology, and a copy should be filed in the QC/QA office.
5 The director of anatomic or surgical pathology will take remedial action on the overdue cases for which no justifiable delay (i.e., waiting for a special study) has been identified.

Review

The formal review of the TAT forms should be carried out by the QC/QA committee chairman monthly, according to the general review procedure. The results of the review are to be presented at the monthly QC/QA meeting.

Appendix C

Staging of cancer

Introduction

The stage of a malignant tumor, as determined by the size of the primary tumor and the extent of local and distant spread if any, represents the single most important determinator of prognosis at most sites. The majority of the hundreds of prognostic factors that have been described in the various forms of malignancy lose most, if not all, of their significance once they are evaluated within the confines of a single stage. Because of the powerful nature of this determination, it is of the utmost importance that the criteria employed are the most pertinent and that there is uniformity throughout institutions and countries. The system now universally used, which carries the familiar TNM abbreviation (**T** for tumor, **N** for node, and **M** for metastasis), was originally developed by Pierre Denoix in France in the 1940s and adopted by the International Union Against Cancer (IUCC) in the 1950s.[2] For more than four decades the American Joint Committee on Cancer (AJCC) has played a leadership role in the USA. The joint publication of this effort (now in its seventh edition) by the IUCC and the AJCC has been a major scientific and political achievement in this regard.[1]

During the 1990s, the importance of TNM staging of cancer in the USA was heightened by the mandatory requirement that Commission on Cancer-approved hospitals use the UICC/AJCC TNM system as the major language for cancer reporting. A tribute is here due to the pathologists who have played a vital role in this effort. Among the many, a special mention should be made of W.A.D. Anderson (also the editor of a once very influential general pathology book), Leslie H. Sobin, Donald E. Henson, Carolyn C. Compton, David L. Page and most particularly Robert V.P. Hutter, to whom one of the versions of this effort was deservedly dedicated.

General rules of the TNM system

The TNM system is an expression of the anatomic extent of the disease and is based on the assessment of three components:

T The extent of the primary tumor
N The absence or presence and extent of regional lymph node metastasis
M The absence or presence of distant metastasis

Definitions of TNM

Primary tumor (T)

TX Primary tumor cannot be assessed
T0 No evidence of primary tumor
Tis Carcinoma in situ
T1, T2, T3, T4 Increasing size and/or local extent of the primary tumor

Regional lymph nodes (N)

NX Regional lymph nodes cannot be assessed
N0 No regional lymph node metastasis
N2, N2, N3 Increasing involvement of regional lymph notes

Note: Direct extension of the primary tumor into a lymph node(s) is classified as a lymph node metastasis.

Note: Metastasis in any lymph node other than regional is classified as a distant metastasis.

Distant metastasis (M)

MX Distant metastasis cannot be assessed
M0 No distant metastasis
M1 Distant metastasis

Note: For pathologic stage grouping, if sufficient tissue to evaluate the highest T and N categories has been removed for pathologic examination, M1 may be either clinical (cM1) or pathologic (pM1).

If only a metastasis has had microscopic confirmation, the classification is pathologic (pM1) and the stage is pathologic.

Histologic grade (G)

GX Grade cannot be assessed
G1 Well differentiated
G2 Moderately differentiated
G3 Poorly differentiated
G4 Undifferentiated

Staging of specific sites

The reader interested in the staging system of a particular body site should consult the latest edition (2010) of the AJCC Cancer Staging Manual, available both in a printed and an electronic format.[2]

References

1. Sobin LH. TNM: principles, history and relation to other prognostic factors. Cancer 2001, **91**(8 Suppl): 1589–1593.
2. Edge SB, Byrd DR, Compton CC, et al. (eds). AJCC cancer staging manual, ed. 7. New York, 2010, Springer.

Appendix

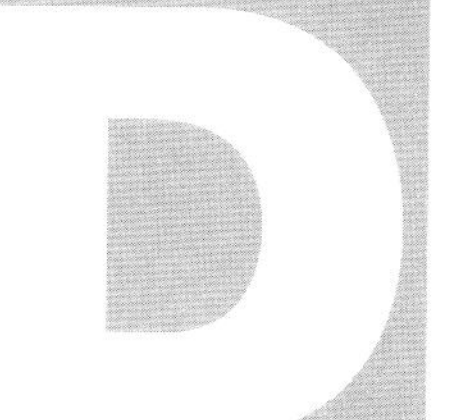

Standardized surgical pathology reporting for major tumor types

The informational content of the surgical pathology report has increased almost exponentially during the course of the last 50 years. At the time that the first edition of this book was written, a pathology report of a mastectomy specimen that read 'Invasive scirrhous carcinoma of the breast with three metastatic lymph nodes' was regarded as entirely acceptable. At present, sending out a report with only that amount of information would be almost an invitation to a malpractice suit. Many are the reasons for the need of additional pieces of information, but essentially they boil down to one fact, of which we surgical pathologists are largely responsible and should be proud: this information is clinically significant for prognostic and therapeutic reasons, which of course is the raison d'être of surgical pathology. Dr Lauren V. Ackerman would have been very happy with this development, in the sense that he thought that the most important question a pathologist had to ask himself after making a morphologic observation was: 'What does it mean for the patient?' Many of the determinations we make mean a lot to the patients and to the clinicians treating them, and therefore it is our duty to document them in a precise, clear, and consistent fashion. This becomes mandatory for patients who have been entered into protocols and for whom recording a particular piece of information becomes a requirement. Because it is virtually impossible for most individuals (except for savants of one type or another) to remember to put down all this information in the same order and with the same terminology in every instance, the use of standardized forms to be used as checklists has become an urgent necessity.[5] An objective corroboration of this was provided by a College of American Pathologists (CAP) sponsored study on the adequacy of the surgical pathology report for colorectal carcinoma among 532 pathology laboratories in the United States and Canada. Review of almost 16 000 reports showed that the single most important factor for the production of a complete report was not whether the institution in question was an academic or community type, whether it had a residency program or not, or whether its workload was light or heavy, but whether it used checklists or not.[7] Analysis of reports of other tumor types, such as lung carcinoma, has produced similar findings and led to similar conclusions.[4]

The necessity for this kind of approach has also received the strong imprimatur of the American College of Surgeons Commission on Cancer, which, beginning January 1, 2004, required that pathologists in their approved programs include *all* scientifically validated or regularly used data in their reports for each site and specimen.[2] Not everybody is happy with this trend, the point having been made that pathology reports generated with the use of these forms are impersonal and sometimes fail to transmit some unique feature of the case in the way that an old-fashioned narrative report did. Fortunately, one can have it both ways, in the sense that there is no reason why a checklist-generated report could not be followed by a 'Comment' section in which the pathologist could elaborate in his own language what it is about this case that the checklist has failed to capture or highlight. Actually, the most vitriolic criticism that has been raised against the use of these forms, written by another Dr Ackerman (A Bernard) in his inimitable style, is for the most part not a criticism of the concept itself but rather of what he views as the inclusion of erroneous categories and concepts in the form dealing with melanoma.[1] If that is the main problem, the logical solution would be to have that form corrected by the appropriate individuals rather than doing away with the whole initiative. To give every certificated pathologist "the right to issue reports of diagnoses in a manner that he or she sees fit"[1] is not an expression of academic rigor but a regressive step, an invitation to chaos, and a blow to the formidable efforts made over the years at a considerable expense by the Armed Forces Institute of Pathology, the World Health Organization and other institutions in order to promote the use of a common language in oncologic pathology, as is the norm in all other scientific disciplines.

An early attempt at report standardization was published by the members of the Pathology Department of Memorial Sloan-Kettering Cancer Center in the 1990s.[6] Currently, two major pathology organizations – the Association of Directors of Anatomic and Surgical Pathology (ADASP) and the College of American Pathologists (CAP) – are at an advanced stage of production of guidelines accompanied by checklists for the major tumor types. Those produced by ADASP are formatted according to Dr Lauren Ackerman's precept, in the sense that they are divided into two portions: one containing the information that has proved clinically useful and therefore necessary, and the other containing information that can be of interest for one reason or another but that has no proven clinical significance. The forms produced by CAP tend to be more comprehensive.[3] Those interested in going over the bibliography and background information that provides the rationale for these recommendations, as well as the names and affiliations of the various committee members, can consult the official printed versions listed below, the printed versions published in selected pathology journals (mainly the *American Journal of Surgical Pathology, American Journal of Clinical Pathology, Human Pathology,* and *Virchows Archiv*), or access them at the websites of the respective organizations:

- Association of Directors of Anatomic and Surgical Pathology (ADASP): http://www.adasp.org
- College of American Pathologists (CAP): http://www.cap.org

For practical reasons, specific recommendations from specialized societies have been inserted in the ADASP listing, while making it clear their original source.

Standards and minimum datasets for reporting common cancer have also issued by The Royal College of Pathologists and can be downloaded free of charge or ordered on line from their website, at www.rcpath.org/publications

References

1 Ackerman AB. Protocols for the reporting of cutaneous melanoma. Am J Clin Pathol 2004, **122:** 815–819. (Letter to the Editor, with reply by CN Otis and counter-reply by AB Ackerman).

2 Connolly JL, Fletcher CDM. What is needed to satisfy the American College of Surgeons Commission on Cancer requirements for the pathological reporting of cancer specimens? Hum Pathol 2003, **34:** 111.

3 Compton CC (ed.) Reporting on cancer specimens: case summaries and background documentation, 2003 edition. Northfield, IL, 2003, College of American Pathologists.

4 Gephardt GN, Baker PB. Lung carcinoma surgical pathology report adequacy: a College of American Pathologists Q-Probes study of over 8300 cases from 464 institutions. Arch Pathol Lab Med 1996, **120:** 922–927.

5 Kempson RL. The time is now. Checklists for surgical pathology reports. Arch Pathol Lab Med 1992, **116:** 1113–1119.

6 Rosai J and Members of the Department of Pathology, Memorial Sloan-Kettering Cancer Center. Standardized reporting of surgical pathology diagnoses for the major tumor types. A proposal. Am J Clin Pathol 1993, **100:** 240–255.

7 Zarbo RJ. Interinstitutional assessment of colorectal carcinoma surgical pathology report adequacy. A College of American Pathologists Q-Probes study of practice patterns from 532 laboratories and 15,940 reports. Arch Pathol Lab Med 1992, **116:** 1107–1108.

Association of Directors of Anatomic and Surgical Pathology (ADASP) recommendations for the reporting of major tumor types

In the following report, 'Recommended features' have been defined as those features that should be included in the final report because they are generally accepted as being of prognostic importance, required for staging or therapy, and/or traditionally expected. Other features are deemed 'Optional features' because they represent specific institutional preferences or are of inconclusive prognostic significance.

Bladder – carcinoma

(See also Lopez-Beltràn A, Bassi PF, Pavone-Macaluso M, Montironi R; European Society of Uropathology; Uropathology Working

Group. Handling and pathology reporting of specimens with carcinoma of the urinary bladder, ureter, and renal pelvis. A joint proposal of the European Society of Uropathology and the Uropathology Working Group. Virchows Arch 2004, **445:** 103–110.)

Final report – recommended features

Gross description

1. **Specimen identification:** labeled with name, medical record number, etc.
2. **Specimen condition:** e.g., fresh, in fixative, on ice, opened, unopened, with Foley catheter still inserted, etc.
3. **Good overall description** including nature of the specimen (chips, partial cystectomy, radical cystectomy, etc.), weight, three-dimensional measurements, etc.
4. **Describe recognizable features** if identifiable (gross evidence of carcinoma, etc.)
5. **Description of other organs:** prostate, ureters, urethra, uterus, vagina, etc.
6. **Paraffin block key** (best listed at end rather than incorporated into narrative)
7. **If ink is used,** give code

Diagnostic information

1. **Topography:** The type of specimen should be specified: bladder, bladder and prostate, bladder with vagina and uterus, etc.
2. **Type of procedure:** The type of surgical procedure should be stated: transurethral resection of bladder (TURB), partial cystectomy, total cystectomy, radical cystoprostatectomy, anterior exenteration, etc.
3. **Tumor type:** The type of carcinoma should be stated. If transitional cell carcinoma is the diagnosis, state whether it is papillary or not
4. **Tumor grade:** Use WHO or Murphy's grading system outlined in the *Third Series AFIP Fascicle* #11
5. **Tumor extent** in bladder (degree of invasion):
   - No invasion
   - Invasion of lamina propria
   - Invasion of muscularis propria
   - Invasion of paravesicular tissue
   - Presence or absence of lymphatic/vascular invasion
   - Tumor arising in diverticulum (state whether muscularis is present or not)

   Note 1: Presence of fibroadipose tissue is not an indication of paravesicular/adventitial involvement as fibroadipose tissue may be present in the lamina propria and/or between muscle bundles of the detrusor. If one is unsure whether muscle fibers associated with an invasive tumor represent invasion of the muscular wall or the muscularis mucosae of the lamina propria, then a comment explaining the problem should be included in the report
6. **Intraepithelial abnormalities**
   - Report focality or multifocality
   - If intraepithelial abnormalities are not contiguous with papillary or invasive neoplasm or are of different degrees of anaplasia, separate diagnoses are indicated
   - Report presence of pagetoid spread of carcinoma in situ (CIS) in urothelial mucosa. This is not dysplasia even though cells do not occupy the full thickness of the mucosa
7. **Tumor extent in other organs** attached to the bladder (radical cystoprostatectomies, radical cystectomies, anterior exenterations):
   - Prostate
     - Direct extension into prostate from carcinoma in bladder neck
     - Involvement of prostatic urethra
     - Involvement of prostatic ducts with or without stromal involvement
   - Ureter and urethra
     - Report any dysplastic/neoplastic change of the mucosa, including pagetoid spread of CIS
     - Report invasion into adjacent lamina propria or muscularis propria
   - Seminal vesicles
     - Report spread of carcinoma in these organs either through epithelium or by direct extension of infiltrative tumor
   - Vagina/uterus
     - Report direct extension of metastases to any of these organs
8. **Surgical margins**
   - Report status of ureteral margins, indicate which side (R or L) if one is positive
   - Report status of urethral margin
   - Report paravesicular margin involvement
9. **Report important associated conditions, e.g., adenocarcinoma of the prostate**
10. **Lymph node metastases**
    - Report presence/absence of metastases. If metastases are present, state number and size of largest one, i.e., <20 cm, 21–25 cm, or >5 cm

Final report – optional features

1. **Invasion of muscularis mucosae, if present**
2. **Genetic abnormalities**
3. **Cytometry**
4. **Morphometry**
5. **Growth factors and receptors**
6. **Stage: There are two staging systems**
   - The Marshall modification of the Jewett and Strong system (A–D)
   - The AJCC/TNM system (T1–T4, M, N)

Checklist

Specimen type
- Biopsy
- TURB
- Radical cystectomy
- Partial cystectomy
- Pelvic exenteration

Diagnosis section
Pathology report should address all applicable items
- Tumor type and grade (TCC only) (with note or comment, if necessary)
- Other mucosal abnormalities (CIS, etc.)
- Other abnormalities (e.g., changes c/w previous surgical site, cystitis glandularis et cystica)

TURB, transurethral resection of bladder; TCC, transitional cell carcinoma; CIS, carcinoma in situ; c/w, consistent with; L, left; R, right

- Pathology in other organs
  - Prostate
  - Ureters
  - Urethra
  - Seminal vesicles
  - Vasa deferentia
  - Uterus
  - Vagina
  - Rectum
  - Other
- Lymph nodes (usually submitted separately)

Muscular wall
- Present
- Not identified

Invasion
- Specimen entirely tumor
- No invasion
- Lamina propria[a]
- Muscular wall
  - Inner half
  - Outer half
- Paravesicular tissue
- Vascular
- Perineurial
- Seminal vesicles
- Prostate
  - Glands
  - Stroma

Specimen involvement
- None
- Urethra
- Ureters
  - Left
  - Right
- Paravesicular soft tissue
- Other (specify):

Lymph nodes
- No. of tumor/total nodes
- Size of largest metastasis   cm

Bone – bone tumors – resection

(From Abdul-Karim FW, Bauer TW, Kilpatrick SE, Raymond KA, Siegal GP. Recommendations for the reporting of bone tumors. Hum Pathol 2004, **35**: 1174–1177. © Elsevier Inc. All rights reserved.)

Gross description

Many of the resection specimens for skeletal neoplasms are complex, and each specimen should be thoughtfully approached and dissected with attention to providing as much information as possible concerning diagnosis, grade, and stage:

1. **State how the specimen was identified** (i.e., patient's name, medical record, surgical pathology number, etc.)
2. **Specify whether the specimen was received fresh or in fixative**
3. **Specify the type of specimen**, for example, fine or core needle biopsy, incisional biopsy, curettage, excision (segmental resection/en bloc), limb salvage, amputation, or complex resection (e.g., hemipelvectomy)
4. **Specimen description and dissection** (by specimen type)

[a]Distinguish muscularis mucosae if desired (optional)

Core needle biopsy or incisional biopsy

1. **Give a general gross description**
2. **If sufficient tissue is present**, take a sample for possible ancillary studies
3. **Submit the specimen for formalin fixation.** It requires at least 3 hours' fixation. Core needle biopsy specimens, if properly fixed, may be decalcified overnight with 5% diluted formic acid. If the core is 5 mm thick or thicker, then divide it
4. **In general, if ancillary studies are anticipated**, then a minimum of three cores may be needed. Provided that adequate material is available for morphology (touch imprint of the biopsy specimen can aid in making this determination), additional cores can be triaged for cytogenetics, molecular diagnostics, and electron microscopy in appropriate media

Curettage

1. **Give overall measurements.**
2. **Describe gross characteristics** (i.e., color, consistency, presence of bone, cartilage, fibrous tissue, necrosis, hemorrhage, myxoid change, cystic change, etc.).
3. **Attempt to separate calcified tissue** (needed for decalcification) from soft tissue fragments.
4. **If curetting was for therapeutic reasons**, then sample it extensively (i.e., about one section per centimeter).

Segmental/en bloc resection

1. **Measure the specimen.**
2. **Orient the specimen** according to radiographic/clinical information.
3. **Assess soft tissue margins**, preferably ink margins, and sample these margins using perpendicular sections from those areas where there is gross or radiographic suspicion of involvement.
4. **Examine for lymph nodes** and submit for histologic examination.
5. **Remove all soft tissues to expose tumor.**
6. **Cut bone along a plane determined by radiographs to expose most of the bone tumor.** (In general, sectioning parallel to the long axis of the bone is preferred, because it more adequately shows anatomic relationships relative to the tumor.)
7. **Alternatively, freeze the entire specimen:** cut on a bandsaw and gently remove bone dust from the cut surface with a surgical scrub brush. (Note that this may negatively impact cytomorphology.)
8. **Inspect cut surfaces,** measure the tumor, and describe its extent.
9. **Assess the distance from resection margins.**
10. **Sample the bone resection margins:** this can be done by scooping marrow from the end margin before doing any manipulation of the tumor.
11. **Describe status of the cortex** (i.e., endosteal scalloping, permeation of the cortex, penetration, breakthrough, soft tissue extension, etc.).
12. **Describe characteristics of the tumor** (i.e., color, consistency, cystic change, presence of necrosis, hemorrhage, etc.).
13. **Take a radiograph or a photograph of the cut surface** as this is often helpful for orientation and educational purposes. Cut additional 5–6 mm thick slabs parallel to the initial bisected cut.

14. **Sample an entire cut surface** of the most representative slab of tissue.
15. **Illustrate section orientation:** this is often best demonstrated by a map based on a diagram, photograph, or specimen radiograph.
16. **Cut additional random sections** from the opposite (peripheral) sides of slab, and/or cut additional sections for the remaining slabs.

Amputation or limb salvage specimens

1. **Examine the surgical margins of resection**; take sections as appropriate.
2. **Identify and dissect** major groups of lymph nodes.
3. **Inspect major vessels** (arteries and veins) and nerve trunks. Take samples if involvement by tumor is suspected.
4. **Open major joints** and describe the presence or absence of tumor involvement. Identify the location of the biopsy site.
5. **Dissect** the **specimen** and remove the soft tissues.
6. **Describe the tumor**, stating its epicenter and its relation to the cortex, periosteum, joint, and location in bone (epiphysis, metaphysis or diaphysis). Also, specify precisely whether the tumor is primarily on the surface, in the medullary cavity, or intracortical, and whether there is soft tissue extension.
7. **Examine the specimen** for coexistent and/or satellite lesions.

Examination for chemotherapeutic effect

For osteosarcomas and Ewing sarcoma, quantification of the extent of necrosis as an index of chemotherapeutic effect is indicated. This approach may also be appropriate for malignant fibrous histiocytoma of bone, because survival rates, therapy, and therapeutic response appear similar to those for osteosarcoma. Necrosis is usually expressed as a percentage of total tumor area. Prognostically significant necrosis, according to most series, appears to be roughly defined at between 90% and 97% of the microscopic tumor mass. Tumors demonstrating such massive necrosis were associated with a favorable prognosis, whereas those with less necrosis were associated with poor survival.

Defining tumor necrosis is quite difficult and can be subjective. However, specific guidelines can be applied to certain osteosarcoma subtypes. Chemotherapy tumor necrosis in osteoblastic and chondroblastic osteosarcomas is probably best defined by cell dropout (empty lacunae). Additionally, 'ghost cells', remnants of neoplastic cells appearing as minute pyknotic structures or ill-defined basophilic areas, often lie within the lacunae of postchemotherapy chondroblastic osteosarcomas. Fibroblastic and small cell osteosarcomas, as well as Ewing sarcoma, most often exhibit a tumor necrosis characterized by cellular portions of the tumor that have been largely replaced by fibrous and granulation tissue with chronic inflammatory cells. Postchemotherapy specimens of telangiectatic osteosarcoma usually reveal residual cystic spaces filled with blood and scattered hemosiderin deposition. Residual atypical cells may be evident.

In all of these specimens there may exist a population of cells that most assuredly exhibit a chemotherapy effect, although the significance of these changes is uncertain. Such cells often exhibit a marked nuclear atypia with a smudgy chromatin pattern and cytoplasmic vacuolization. In an attempt to reduce the subjectivity of determining tumor necrosis, we recommend that such cytologic changes not be considered necrosis. Taking into account all of the subtypes of osteosarcoma and Ewing sarcoma, postchemotherapy tumor necrosis is best assessed by evaluating the presence or absence of neoplastic cells.

Distinguishing spontaneous tumor necrosis from postchemotherapy tumor necrosis may not always be possible, but it is our contention that such features as absence of tumor cells accompanied by fibroblastic ingrowth and hemosiderin deposition are the result of chemotherapy and not spontaneous tumor necrosis.

We recommend the following guidelines for the evaluation of postchemotherapy osteosarcoma and Ewing sarcoma specimens:

1. An entire representative slice of the tumor should be sampled completely using a grid pattern diagram or radiograph indicating the site for each numbered block.
2. Additional blocks taken in a plane perpendicular to the previous ones are to determine the extent of the tumor in three dimensions.
3. The numbered multiple blocks systemically are obtained not only from the main tumor, but also from areas that may be 'shielded' from chemotherapy effect, such as soft tissue extension and tumor/nodal tissue interface, cortex, subcortical marrow, pericartilaginous regions, and areas surrounding hemorrhagic necrosis and ligaments.

Resection specimens from tumors other than osteosarcoma or Ewing sarcoma

Resection specimens from tumors other than osteosarcoma or Ewing sarcoma may be processed similarly, but tumor 'mapping' of an entire representative slice of tumor is probably unnecessary. Instead, we would recommend an analogous approach similar to tumors from other anatomic sites: representative sampling of the tumor (one section per cm) with meticulous attention to unusual-appearing areas, satellite lesions, anatomic relationships, and surgical margins.

Tissue for ancillary studies

Current classifications of bone tumors are based largely on light microscopy features, occasionally supported by electron microscopy and/or immunohistochemical evidence when deemed necessary. Recent advances in our understanding of the molecular biology and cytogenetics of sarcomas, especially Ewing sarcoma/peripheral neuroectodermal tumor (PNET), have already begun to impact surgical pathology reports. It is probably prudent, when possible, for the pathologist to set aside 'fresh' tissue for such studies (if available), recognizing that light microscopy must take precedence over any ancillary technique. For the present, we believe that cytogenetic studies are most appropriate for the differential diagnosis of 'small blue cell neoplasms', including Ewing sarcoma/PNET. No diagnostically specific chromosomal abnormalities have been identified in osteosarcoma.

Table App D-1 Final anatomic diagnosis checklist: Neoplastic bone

Accession No.:	Part No(s):	Date:	Patient name:
ORGAN	**SITE**	**OPERATION**	**PRIMARY TUMOR DIAGNOSIS**
Bone (Skull)	Right	Fine needle biopsy	Adamantinoma
Cranium	Left	Core needle biopsy	Conventional
Facial bones	Other_____	Incisional biopsy	Osteofibrous dysplasia-like (well-differentiated)
Jaw (gnathic bones)	Epiphyseal	Excisional biopsy	Angiosarcoma
Mandible	Metaphyseal	Curettage	Chondrosarcoma
Maxilla	Diaphyseal	Segmental resection	Conventional
Long bones (Upper limb)		En bloc resection	Clear cell
Scapula		Ray resection	Dedifferentiated
Humerus		Amputation	Mesenchymal
Radius		Complex resection	Peripheral juxtacortical (periosteal)
Ulna		Forequarter	Myxoid
Short bones (Hand)		Hindquarter	Arising in association with osteochondroma
Carpals		Hemipelvectomy	Other_____
Metacarpals		Other_____	Chordoma
Phalanges			Conventional
Long bones (Lower limb)			Chondroid
Femur			Dedifferentiated
Tibia			Ewing sarcoma/PNET
Fibula			Fibrosarcoma
Patella			Conventional
Short bones (Foot)			Periosteal
Tarsals			Giant cell tumor of bone (*specify:* conventional, malignant)
Metatarsals			Hemangioendothelioma
Phalanges			Epithelioid
Thorax			Hemangiopericytoma/solitary fibrous tumor
Clavicle			Leiomyosarcoma
Ribs			Liposarcoma
Manubrium			Malignant fibrous histiocytoma
Sternum			Malignant mesenchymoma
Spine (Vertebral column)			Malignant peripheral nerve sheath tumor
Cervical			Osteosarcoma
Thoracic			Conventional
Lumbar			Chondroblastic
Sacrum			Fibroblastic
Coccyx			Osteoblastic
Pelvis			Mixed (*specify cell types*_____)
Ilium			Low-grade central
Ischium			Intraosseous, well-differentiated
Pubis			Giant cell rich
Metastatic sites			Small cell
Lymph nodes			Telangiectatic
Regional			Epithelioid
Distant			Osteoblastoma-like
Lung			Chondroblastoma-like
Other sites__________			Associated with (*specify*: fibrous dysplasia, Paget disease of bone, __________)
			Postradiation
			Surface
			Parosteal
			Dedifferentiated parosteal
			Periosteal
			High-grade surface
			Rhabdomyosarcoma
			Other:____________________
			____________________
			____________________
			____________________

From Abdul-Karim FW, Bauer TW, Kilpatrick SE, Raymond KA, Siegal GP. Recommendations for the reporting of bone tumors. Hum Pathol 2004, **35:** 1176.

Breast – carcinoma (invasive)

Final report – recommended features

Gross description

1. **Specimen identification:** labeled with (name, number), designated as breast (right or left)
2. **Specimen condition:** fresh, in formalin, intact, cut, margins inked or not, etc.
3. **Type of procedure:** core biopsy, incisional biopsy, excisional biopsy (lumpectomy), re-excision, quadrantectomy, simple mastectomy, modified mastectomy, other
4. **Size:** the overall size of the excised specimen should be measured in three dimensions
5. **Tumor description**
   - Presence of mass(es) or absence of mass(es)
   - Margins of the mass(es) (circumscribed, infiltrative)
   - Distance of the mass(es) from nearest surgical margins (measured and recorded)
   - Location of the mass(es) (e.g., quadrant if the specimen is a mastectomy)
   - Size of the mass(es) (at least greatest diameter should be recorded, three dimensions are preferable), texture of the mass(es) (e.g., soft, fleshy, hard, gritty, etc.)
6. **Description of prior biopsy site,** if present
7. **Description of the remainder of the breast tissue,** nipple, and skin, if present
8. **Number and appearance of lymph nodes** if received
9. **Special investigations:** It is recommended that tissue submitted for special investigation (e.g., ER/PR, flow cytometry, etc.) be specified if this information is known
10. Whether a **diagnostic frozen section** was performed and the diagnosis that was made

Diagnostic information

1. **Laterality** of the breast and procedure
2. **Histologic type**
   - Ductal (usual, no special type, not otherwise specified (NOS))
   - Lobular (specify subtype)
     - Classic
     - Variant (alveolar, solid, pleomorphic, tubulolobular)
   - Tubular
   - Medullary
   - Mucinous
   - Secretory
   - Infiltrating papillary
   - Adenoid cystic
   - Metaplastic
   - Infiltrating cribriform
   - Other (specify):
3. **Histologic grade:** all ductal (NOS) carcinomas should be graded; some also advocate grading lobular carcinomas. The histologic type for the others (e.g., tubular, medullary) replaces the grade. The Scarff–Bloom–Richardson grading scheme, which evaluates the following three parameters, is recommended: degree of tubule formation, nuclear grade, and mitotic rate. Points are assigned to each parameter as follows:
   - Tubules: 75% or more of the tumor is composed of tubules = 1; 10–75% of the tumor is composed of tubules = 2; <10% of the tumor is composed of tubules = 3
   - Nuclei: small and uniform = 1; moderate variability in size and shape = 2; marked increase in size and marked irregularity = 3
   - Mitotic rate: the mitotic rate is dependent upon the area of the field selected. For a ×40 objective with a diameter of 0.33 mm (area of 0.152 mm^2), scoring of the number of mitoses per 10 fields (at the tumor edge) is as follows: 0–5 = 1; 6–10 = 2; >11 = 3. The field of the microscope used should be measured and the counts adjusted proportionately.

   The histologic grade is determined by summing the points: grade I, 3–5 points; grade II, 6–7 points; grade III, 8–9 points.
4. **Margins of resection:** the Association recognizes that, at the present time, the clinical relevance of a positive margin is not clear, and further recognizes that there is no standard definition of what constitutes a positive or negative margin. Margin involvement is, however, used by many clinicians in forming therapeutic recommendations.

   In reporting the margins of resection, state: (a) whether sections of the margins have been taken parallel (shaved) or perpendicular to the surgical margin; and (b) whether tumor is at margin (grossly or microscopically). If tumor is not present at a shaved margin or at an inked margin, the distance from the margin should be specified.
5. **Lymph node status:** given as numbers of nodes involved and the total number of nodes. If metastases are <2 mm, this fact and the size should be recorded. If any node is larger than 2 cm, it should be recorded. The presence or absence of perinodal extension of tumor into axillary fat should be recorded. If the nodes are fixed to one another or other structures, it should be recorded. The Association does not recommend immunoperoxidase techniques to detect micrometastases.
6. **Peritumoral angiolymphatic invasion:** whether tumor cells involve peritumoral vascular spaces or not should be recorded. If vascular spaces in the skin are involved, this should be recorded. Although some prefer to separate lymphatic from blood vessel invasion, it is prognostically not necessary to distinguish between lymphatic vessels and blood vessels. The Association does not recommend the routine use of immunohistochemical stains to detect intravascular invasion.
7. **Size of the carcinoma:** even though this is recorded in the gross description, the Association recommends it be reported again in the diagnosis line because of the prognostic importance of this parameter.
8. **In situ component:** the presence or absence of an in situ component should be recorded. If the in situ component is ductal and is prominent within the main tumor mass *and* is present outside the mass *or* the tumor is primarily intraductal with only focal invasion, the in situ ductal carcinoma is considered to be 'extensive' and the Association recommends recording this if the patient is to be treated by less than total mastectomy. When ductal carcinoma in situ is present, the distance of the in situ process from the nearest margin should be recorded as at the margin, or the specific distance from the margin even if the specimen also contains invasive carcinoma. Because lobular carcinoma in situ is often multifocal, the Association recommends that no specific comments on margin involvement be made.
9. **Microcalcifications:** if present on the mammogram, their presence in the sections should be sought (to be sure a

calcified lesion was not missed) and a statement made about their presence and location or their absence.

10. **Other significant disease:** atypical hyperplasias, papillomas, Paget disease of the nipple, biopsy site changes, etc.
11. **Specify** in the report if information required for prognosis or therapy is not available or cannot be adequately assessed (e.g., no nodes submitted with a mastectomy specimen, margins not assessable because specimen was cut before inking, etc.)

Final report – optional features

1. **Stage:** the data provided above should provide sufficient information for clinicians to determine stage. The Association does not consider inclusion of a specific tumor stage in the pathology report to be required.
2. **Results of ancillary investigations** (e.g., flow cytometry, ER/PR, oncogenes, p53)
3. **Specific level or location of axillary lymph nodes** unless marked and specific identification is requested by the surgeon
4. **Identification of specific margins** unless the surgeon precisely identifies them
5. **Perineurial infiltration**
6. **Microvessel quantification**

Breast – carcinoma (in situ)

Final report – recommended features

Gross description

1. **Specimen condition:** fresh, in formalin, intact, cut, margins inked or not, etc.
2. **Specimen identification:** labeled with (name, number), designated as breast (right or left)
3. **Type of procedure:** core biopsy, incisional biopsy, excisional biopsy (lumpectomy), re-excision, quadrantectomy, simple mastectomy, modified mastectomy, other
4. **Size:** the overall size of the excised specimen should be measured in three dimensions
5. **Tumor description**
   - Presence of mass(es) or absence of mass(es)
   - Margins of the mass(es) (circumscribed, infiltrative)
   - Distance of the mass(es) from nearest surgical margins (measured and recorded)
   - Location of the mass(es) (e.g., quadrant if the specimen is a mastectomy)
   - Size of the mass(es) (at least greatest diameter should be recorded, three dimensions are preferable), texture of the mass(es) (e.g., soft, fleshy, hard, gritty, etc.)
6. **Description of prior biopsy site,** if present
7. **Description of the remainder of the breast tissue,** nipple, and skin, if present
8. **Number and appearance of lymph nodes,** if received
9. **Special investigations:** it is recommended that fresh tissue should not be submitted for special investigation because the most important information is the presence or absence of invasion. Blocks may be sectioned for special investigation if that information is desirable in an individual case.
10. Whether a **diagnostic frozen section** was performed and the diagnosis that was made

Diagnostic information

1. **Laterality** of the breast and procedure
2. **Histologic type:** the Association recognizes that different terms are sometimes used for microscopically identical lesions (e.g., the term 'lobular neoplasia' includes cases of atypical lobular hyperplasia). Moreover, ADASP recognizes that although the majority of cases of in situ carcinoma are readily categorized, there are borderline lesions. The criteria for diagnosing the small borderline lesions as either lobular carcinoma in situ (LCIS) or ductal carcinoma in situ (DCIS) vary. Different authors use different qualitative and quantitative criteria in arriving at the diagnosis of LCIS or DCIS in these circumstances.

   The Association realizes that the classification system for DCIS (intraductal carcinoma) is in a state of flux; because of this, it is recommended that the lesion be graded using the traditional system based primarily upon architectural pattern, as well as assigning a specific nuclear grade.
3. **Architectural type:** ductal carcinoma in situ (intraductal carcinoma) (specify subtype):
   - Cribriform
   - Micropapillary
   - Solid (microacinar)
   - Papillary (includes most cases of intracystic)
   - Comedo (requires high-grade nuclei; necrosis usually present)
4. **Nuclear grade:** because the architectural pattern may vary from area to area in the individual case, and because nuclear grade may be important in regard to the potential for recurrence, the Association recommends that ductal carcinoma in situ be divided into high, low, or intermediate nuclear grade in addition to providing type. Lobular carcinoma in situ is not routinely graded
5. **Margins of resection:** the Association recognizes that, at the present time, the clinical relevance of a positive margin is not clear, and further recognizes that there is no standard definition of what constitutes a positive or negative margin. Margin involvement is, however, used by many clinicians in forming therapeutic recommendations

   In reporting the margins of resection, state: (a) whether sections of the margins have been taken parallel (shaved) or perpendicular to the surgical margin; and (b) whether tumor is at margin (grossly or microscopically). If tumor is not present at a shaved margin or at an inked margin, the distance from the margin should be specified. Assessment of margins for lobular carcinoma is not recommended
6. **Size:** if a mass is present, obtain this from the gross; if not, several methods can be used to measure the size of an in situ process:
   - Sectioning the biopsy from one end of the specimen to the other at 3–4 mm intervals and submitting the sections in sequence, thus allowing for an estimate of the size of the lesion based on the sections in which the lesion is present
   - In small lesions, a measurement of size of the lesion may be obtained directly from the slide
7. **Microcalcifications:** if the specimen was removed because of mammographic identification of microcalcifications, these should be identified in the tissue sections and the fact they are found should be reported. A correlation with the location of the microcalcifications in the mammogram should be reported. It should be stated in which lesion the calcifications were identified (DCIS, adenosis, etc.). If they are not found or if the microcalcifications in the sections are not in the

location indicated by the mammogram, this should be reported

8. **Other significant disease:** atypical hyperplasias, papillomas, Paget disease of the nipple, biopsy site changes, etc.
9. **Specify** in the report if information required for prognosis or therapy is not available or cannot be adequately assessed (e.g., margins not assessable because specimen was cut before inking, etc.)

Checklist

Laterality
- Breast

  —— Left —— Right

Specimen type
- Excisional (for palpable mass)
- Mammographic Loc.
- Incisional (includes core needle and FNA)
- Re-excisional
- Mastectomy
- Chest wall

Specimen size

Tumor size(s)

Tumor type
- DCIS
- Mixed NOS/ILC
- Papillary LCIS
- LCIS
- Tubular
- Cribriform
- Infiltrating ductal (NOS)
- Mucinous other (specify):
- Infiltrating lobular
- Medullary

Grade of invasion

  —— I —— II —— III

Gross margin
- Free (specify distance):
- Involved

Margins invasive (specify type of margin evaluation)
- Free (specify distance):
- Focal
- >Focal
- Nonevaluable

Margins DCIS (specify type of margin evaluation)
- Free (specify distance):
- Focal
- >Focal
- Nonevaluable

DCIS nuclear morphology
- High grade
- Intermediate grade
- Low grade

DCIS patterns (specify all that apply)
- Large areas of central necrosis (comedo)
- Small areas of central necrosis
- Cribriform
- Solid
- Micropapillary
- Papillary

Calcification in in situ
- Absent
- Prominent in DCIS
- Focal in DCIS
- In LCIS
- Prominent in benign breast tissue
- Focal in benign breast tissue

Peritumoral lymphatic invasion
- Absent
- Present
- Dermal

Peritumoral vascular invasion
- Absent
- Present

Extent DCIS within invasive tumor
- Absent
- Slight
- Moderate marked
- Tumor primarily DCIS with focal invasion

Extent DCIS adjacent to invasive tumor
- Absent
- Slight
- Moderate marked

EIC status
- Negative
- Positive
- Indeterminate

  Note 1: If a tumor is primarily DCIS with focal invasion or has a moderate or marked amount of DCIS within the infiltrating tumor and any in the adjacent tissue, it is EIC-positive

Skin
- Not sampled
- Free
- Invasive
- Dermal lymphatic

Nipple
- Not sampled
- Free
- Invasive
- Dermal lymphatic
- DCIS
- Paget

Muscle
- Not sampled
- Free
- Involved

Mastectomy tumor location
- Central
- UOQ
- UIQ
- LOQ
- LIQ

Multiple areas involved
- Central
- UOQ
- UIQ
- LOQ
- LIQ
- Only one area involved

Lymph nodes (number of involved nodes in relation to total number examined)
- Total
- Level I
- Level II
- Level III
- Other (specify):

Extranodal extension
- Absent
- Present

Metastatic cancer in
Nature of nontumorous breast tissue (describe)
Comments
Ancillary studies (results and methodology used)

Esophagus – carcinoma

Final report – recommended features

Gross description

1. **Specimen identification**: labeled with patient name, medical record number, source of specimen, etc.
2. **Specimen condition:** fresh, in fixative (specify type), unopened, opened, etc., and how designated
3. **Appropriate overall gross description,** including nature of the specimen (segmental esophagectomy, esophagogastrectomy, etc.), measurements (including overall length of specimen, length of esophagus, length of stomach), and amount and nature of periesophageal tissue included
4. **Description** of opened specimen including neoplasm (gross appearance, measurement in three dimensions, etc.), mucosal surface away from neoplasm (evidence of Barrett esophagus, other abnormalities), and distance of neoplasm from proximal and distal margins
   Note 1: If the lesion arises in the gastroesophageal junction region and involves both the esophagus and stomach, it should be classified as: (1) an esophageal carcinoma, if the epicenter of the lesion is in the esophagus; (2) a gastric carcinoma, if the epicenter is in the stomach; and (3) a gastroesophageal junction primary, if the epicenter coincides with the esophagogastric junction. For this purpose, the gastroesophageal junction is defined as the junction between the tubular esophagus and the saccular stomach
5. **Description of any additional structures included:** stomach, pericardium, etc.
6. **Paraffin block key:** ideally at end rather than incorporated into narrative
7. **If margins are inked** (proximal, distal, radial), provide code

Diagnostic information

1. **Topography:** the type of specimen should be specified (esophagus, esophagus and proximal stomach, etc.)
2. **Type of procedure**: the type of surgical procedure should be stated (total or segmental esophagectomy, esophagogastrectomy), as well as how the procedure was performed, if known (transhiatal or transthoracic)
3. **Histologic type:** use of the World Health Organization (WHO) classification is recommended:
   - Squamous cell carcinoma (including pseudosarcomatous)
   - Adenocarcinoma
   - Adenoid cystic carcinoma (basaloid squamous)
   - Mucoepidermoid carcinoma
   - Adenosquamous carcinoma
   - Undifferentiated carcinoma
   - Other
4. **Histologic grade:** use of the American Joint Committee on Cancer grading system is recommended:
   - GX: Grade cannot be assessed
   - G1 Well differentiated
   - G2 Moderately differentiated
   - G3 Poorly differentiated
   - G4 Undifferentiated
5. **Extent of invasion** of neoplasm in the esophagus, using TNM system:
   - Tis None (Tis) (see Note 2)
   - T1a Limited to lamina propria (intramucosal carcinoma)
   - T1b Into submucosa
   - T2 Into muscularis propria
   - T3 Into adventitia
   - T4 Into adjacent structures (see Note 3)

   Note 2: Although Tis refers to carcinoma in situ, the authors prefer the term high-grade dysplasia for this lesion
   Note 3: In specimens resected after radiation or chemotherapy, or both, a comment should be made regarding whether viable-appearing neoplastic tissue remains. If none is identifiable, a comment regarding the extent of the radiation/chemotherapy-induced injury should be made, i.e., its depth of extension into the esophageal wall as an indication of the probable depth of invasion of the neoplasm
6. **Mucosal abnormalities away from carcinoma**
   - Squamous epithelial dysplasia
   - Presence of Barrett metaplastic epithelium
   - Dysplasia in Barrett metaplastic epithelium
   - Other
7. **Surgical margins**
   - Status of proximal and distal surgical margins
   - Status of radial (adventitial) margin
   - If Barrett esophagus, nature of mucosa at proximal margin (squamous versus Barrett); if Barrett, comment on presence or absence of dysplasia
   - If distal mucosal margin is stomach, comment on any gastric abnormalities (*Helicobacter pylori* gastritis, etc.)
8. **Lymph nodes:** report total number of nodes/number containing metastatic carcinoma

Final report – optional features

1. **Genetic abnormalities**
2. **Flow cytometric analysis**
3. **Growth factors and receptors**
4. **Staging** using American Joint Committee on Cancer TNM system (0–IVB)

Checklist

Site of neoplasm
- Cervical esophagus (from lower border of cricoid to thoracic inlet (suprasternal notch)
- Intrathoracic esophagus (definitions given are from the AJCC manual)
- Upper portion (thoracic inlet to tracheal bifurcation)
- Mid portion (tracheal bifurcation to just above esophagogastric junction)
- Lower thoracic portion (includes intra-abdominal portion of esophagus and esophagogastric junction)
- Not specified

Type of resection
- Transthoracic
- Transhiatal
- Not specified

Resection specimen
- Esophagectomy
- Esophagogastrectomy
- Other (specify):

Dimensions of neoplasm
— cm × — cm × — cm

Distance to surgical margins
— cm to proximal margin
— cm to distal margin

Macroscopic depth of penetration of neoplasm
- Into submucosa
- Into muscularis propria
- Through esophageal wall
- Into adjacent structures (*specify*: trachea, pericardium, etc.)
- Uncertain

Barrett esophagus
- Present grossly
- Present at proximal margin grossly
- Not apparent grossly
- Uncertain

Histologic type of neoplasm
- Squamous cell carcinoma (including pseudosarcomatous)
- Adenocarcinoma
- Adenoid cystic carcinoma (basaloid squamous)
- Mucoepidermoid carcinoma
- Adenosquamous carcinoma
- Undifferentiated carcinoma

Histologic grade of carcinoma
- Grade cannot be assessed
- Well differentiated
- Moderately differentiated
- Poorly differentiated
- Undifferentiated

Depth of infiltration of neoplasm
- High-grade dysplasia only
- Limited to lamina propria
- Into submucosa
- Into muscularis propria
- Into adventitia
- Into adjacent structures (specify):

Mucosal abnormalities away from carcinoma
- Squamous epithelial dysplasia
- Barrett metaplastic epithelium
  With dysplasia
  Without dysplasia
- Other (e.g., heterotopic gastric mucosa in cervical esophagus ('inlet patch'))

Status of surgical margins
- Proximal margin free of carcinoma
  — Yes — No
- Proximal margin composed of squamous epithelium
  — Yes — No
  With dysplasia
  — Yes — No

Proximal margin composed of Barrett metaplastic epithelium
  — Yes — No
  With dysplasia
  — Yes — No

Distal margin free of carcinoma
  — Yes — No

Status of lymph nodes
- Total number of lymph nodes
- Total number involved by metastatic carcinoma

Tissue submitted for special investigative studies
- Flow cytometry
  — Yes — No
- Tissue frozen
  — Yes — No
- Other (specify):

Extra-adrenal paragangliomas

Guidelines

Extra-adrenal paragangliomas are rare neoplasms that arise in a wide variety of anatomic sites. Knowledge of the widespread anatomic distribution of the tumors and familiarity with variations in their histologic patterns will help in achieving accurate histopathologic diagnosis of these tumors. The following guidelines are offered to facilitate generation of a comprehensive surgical report, realizing of course that minor or major modifications are appropriate depending upon the features of an individual tumor. Pheochromocytomas are arbitrarily regarded as adrenal medullary paragangliomas and recommendations for reporting of adrenal tumors are covered elsewhere. Explanatory notes are appended.

Gross description

1. **Specimen identification**
   - Name, sex, age, date of birth and medical record number
   - Attending physician and/or surgeon
   - Date of surgery and date of receipt of the surgical specimen in the laboratory
   - History and/or endocrinologic data, and preoperative as well as postoperative diagnosis
2. **Specimen condition:** the date, time and state (fresh or in fixative) of specimen should be noted on receipt in the laboratory. It may be desirable to indicate in the report the approximate time elapsed between surgical removal of the specimen and receiving it for examination in the surgical pathology laboratory
3. **Tumor site:** the precise anatomic location of the tumor should be stated. Terminology of the extra-adrenal paragangliomas should be based upon anatomic site of origin (e.g., urinary bladder paraganglioma, gallbladder paraganglioma, carotid body paraganglioma). Information regarding multicentricity or bilaterality should be included (e.g., bilateral carotid body paragangliomas – familial or sporadic occurrence)
4. **Type of procedure:** the report should indicate whether the surgical specimen was a biopsy, partial excision or complete excision of the lesion or part of a more extended surgical procedure, whether a biopsy or subtotal excision was performed (or if resection was done by laparoscopy)
5. **Description of other organs:** ideally, the specimen should be given to the pathologist by the surgical team with appropriate orientation of the specimen and identification of any relevant attached tissues or organs
6. **Measure**: record tumor size (three dimensions in cm) and weight (g) following removal of extraneous tissue
7. **Specify** any other tissue or organs present
8. **Accurate and complete overall description** of the external and internal (cut) surface of the tumor, noting its color and presence of necrosis or hemorrhage
9. **Special investigations:** specimen photography, special studies and tumor dispersal (tumor bank, immunohistochemistry,

electron microscopy, DNA quantitation, cytogenetics or others) should be recorded
10. **Record** results of intraoperative consultation including frozen section and/or smear/imprint preparations

Diagnostic information

1. **Histologic type** of tumor with brief reference to clinical and/or endocrinology data if pertinent
2. **Presence and estimated extent of tumor necrosis**
3. **Presence and approximate quantitation of mitotic activity**
4. **Prognostic features** as appropriate, e.g., invasion of adjacent tissue or organs, presence of vascular/lymphatic invasion. Record status of surgical margins
5. **Status of regional lymph nodes** where pertinent, e.g., total number with metastatic tumor, if present
6. **Record** whether outside consultation is requested or desired and indicate source of consultation
7. **Record** in rare instances whether tumor has composite features with component of ganglioneuroma or malignant peripheral nerve sheath tumor. Some tumors may have areas focally resembling ganglioneuroblastoma or even neuroblastoma

Checklist

Anatomic site
- Pathologic diagnosis, with terminology based upon anatomic site of origin
- Type of resection

Tumor size (cm) and weight (g)
- Gross description, external and cut surfaces

Results of intraoperative consultation
- Microscopic examination: presence and quantitation of mitotic figures
- Presence and approximate extent of necrosis
- Invasive growth (blood vessels, adjacent tissues/organs)
- Special studies, EM, frozen tissue, immunohistochemistry
- DNA quantitation, cytogenetics, other
- Unusual pathologic features

Eye and adnexa – common malignancies

For recommendations on the reporting of tissue removed as part of the surgical treatment of common malignancies of the eye and its adnexa, see:

Folberg R, Salomao D, Grossniklaus HE, Proia AD, Rao NA, Cameron JD. Recommendations for the reporting of tissues removed as part of the surgical treatment of common malignancies of the eye and its adnexa. Am J Surg Pathol 2003, **27:** 999–1004; Mod Pathol 2003, **16:** 725–730.

Fallopian tube – resection

(From Longacre TA, Oliva E, Soslow RA. Recommendations for the reporting of fallopian tube neoplasms. Hum Pathol 2007, **38:** 1161–1163.)

Final report – recommended features

General description

1. **Specimen identification:** labeled with name, medical record, laterality
2. **Specimen condition:** intraoperative, fresh, formalin.
3. **Type of procedure:** salpingectomy, partial salpingectomy, salpingo-oophorectomy, staging procedure (specify)
4. **Relevant clinical history**

Note 1: Although these guidelines and the accompanying checklist are chiefly designed for fallopian tube malignancies, the processing of fallopian tubes from patients with known gene mutations that are associated with a predisposition to tubal carcinoma (e.g., *BRCA1*, *BRCA2*) requires special handling (see recommended sections for prophylactic salpingectomy below)

Gross description

1. **Specimen received** intact, fragmented, with (or without) attached ovary, etc.
2. **Specimen size** in three dimensions
3. **Tumor mass:** location (e.g., isthmus, ampulla, infundibulum, fimbria), size (in three dimensions), appearance, necrosis, depth of invasion (mucosal, intramural, penetrates serosal surface, etc.), relationship to contiguous structures (e.g., adhesed to ovary, pelvic peritoneum)
4. **Presence of cysts, adhesions, and nodules:** size and region of involvement (e.g., ampulla, isthmus, fimbria)
5. **Lumen:** normal, dilated, or occluded
6. **Fimbria:** normal, fused

Recommended sections

1. **Fallopian tube**
   - Fallopian tube primary tumor mass: At least three sections. Sections should be taken to demonstrate relation to uninvolved tubal mucosa, depth of invasion, and involvement of contiguous structures, if present
   - Prophylactic: Section fallopian tube(s) at 2–3 mm intervals and submit entirely for microscopic examination. Tubal fimbriae should be extensively sectioned, either by serial cross sections or preferably by serial sagittal (lengthwise) sections to maximize examination of the tubal plicae
   - Routine: Section fallopian tube(s) at 2–3 mm intervals and submit three sections to represent isthmus, ampulla, and infundibulum/fimbria (one block)
2. **Ovaries:** ovaries should be serially sectioned and carefully examined with all suspicious areas submitted to exclude stromal or surface involvement by carcinoma (possible primary site)
3. **Uterus**
   - Cervix should be serially sectioned and carefully examined with sufficient sections submitted to exclude cervical involvement by carcinoma
   - Endometrium should be serially sectioned and carefully examined with sufficient sections submitted to exclude endometrial involvement by carcinoma (possible primary site)
   - Routine sections of myometrium, serosa
4. **Omentum**
   - Sections of gross tumor, if present. Note size of largest gross tumor deposit
   - Multiple sections are optimal when no tumor is present on gross evaluation because studies in ovarian cancer have demonstrated improved tumor detection in this setting. However, there are no established guidelines regarding number of sections

5. **Lymph nodes**
   - Sample each grossly positive lymph node
   - Submit entire grossly negative lymph node(s). Bivalve through hilum if large
6. **Other staging biopsies**
   - Submit entirely, if small
   - Representative sections if grossly positive or if grossly negative and large
7. **Specify** all sections by a unique letter or number

Diagnostic information

1. **Type of procedure**
2. **Histologic type of tumor** (modified World Health Organization)
   Benign epithelial
      Papilloma
      Metaplastic papilloma (metaplastic papillary tumor)
      Cystadenoma (serous, mucinous, etc.)
   Borderline epithelial
      Serous tumor of low malignant potential
      Endometrioid tumor of low malignant potential
      Mucinous tumor of low malignant potential
   Malignant epithelial
      Carcinoma in situ
      Serous carcinoma
      Endometrioid carcinoma
      Mucinous carcinoma
      Clear cell carcinoma
      Transitional cell carcinoma
      Squamous cell carcinoma
      Mixed carcinoma
      Undifferentiated carcinoma
      Metastatic carcinoma
   Mixed epithelial–mesenchymal
      Adenofibroma
      Adenosarcoma
      Carcinosarcoma
   Germ cell tumors
      Teratoma
   Mesothelial
      Adenomatoid tumor
      Mesothelioma
   Gestational trophoblastic disease
      Hydatidiform mole
      Choriocarcinoma
      Placental site trophoblastic tumor
   Other (specify):
3. **Histologic grade of fallopian tube carcinoma:** report tumor grade and specify grading system. There is no standard grading system for tubal carcinoma. Although completely arbitrary, the Gynecologic Oncology Group (GOG) studies use a single grading system for ovary, endometrium, and fallopian tube. The chief advantage of this system is that it serves to maintain consistency in diagnosis and classification. Other grading schemes have also been proposed for gynecologic cancer, including two-tiered systems, which also have merit, particularly with respect to ovarian and extraovarian serous carcinoma. We do not recommend any one system over another; however, the ADASP does recommend use of a single grading system for all müllerian epithelial malignancies, whenever possible. The Association acknowledges that there is a need for future refinement and standardization in histologic grading of these malignancies. The ADASP Fallopian Tube Neoplasms checklist uses a modification of the GOG system
4. **Maximum dimension**
5. **Depth of invasion**
   Note 2: It is recommended that the presence of invasion into lamina propria be distinguished from invasion into muscularis mucosa, whenever possible, although current American Joint Committee on Cancer/International Federation of Gynecology and Obstetrics (AJCC/FIGO) staging systems do not distinguish between the two
6. **Presence of in situ carcinoma in adjacent uninvolved tubal mucosa**
   Note 3: The fallopian tube may exhibit a variety of epithelial proliferative changes that do not necessarily reflect a neoplastic or malignant process. Strict histologic criteria should be used before rendering a diagnosis of in situ carcinoma because this may lead to a staging procedure and prophylactic chemotherapy
7. **Involvement of ovary or endometrium:** The presence of significant ovarian parenchymal or endometrial involvement by tumor of similar histologic type excludes primary fallopian tube carcinoma. Parenchymal involvement of the ovaries, if present, should be minimal (e.g., ≤0.5 cm), predominantly confined to the surface and of significantly smaller magnitude than the tubal tumor in order for the carcinoma to be considered a primary tubal neoplasm. There are no established or recommended size criteria with respect to the presence of endometrial involvement, but myometrial invasion, cervical stromal involvement, and/or lymphovascular space invasion are more likely to be associated with a primary endometrial tumor with metastasis to the tube than a tubal primary or simultaneous tubal and endometrial primary. The above criteria are admittedly arbitrary but serve to maintain consistency in diagnosis and classification
8. **Involvement of other pelvic or intra-abdominal structures,** omentum, and lymph nodes
9. **Other findings:** salpingitis (acute/chronic/granulomatous), salpingitis isthmica nodosa, hydrosalpinx, hematosalpinx, Walthard cell rests, paratubal müllerian cysts, tubo-ovarian adhesions, endosalpingiosis, endometriosis, etc.
10. **Additional studies** (report as appropriate)
    - Cytology: Correlate with surgical findings (e.g., positive ascitic fluid or peritoneal washings should reflect the diagnosis of the primary fallopian tube tumor)
    - Immunoperoxidase studies (p53): The distinction between atypical proliferative tubal epithelial lesions and in situ carcinoma can be difficult. The presence of inflammation and admixed ciliated cells favors a benign process, but some cancers may also be associated with an inflammatory cell infiltrate. In general, carcinoma in situ is strongly immunoreactive for p53, whereas reactive processes are not
    - Receptor status (ER/PR)
    - Growth factors (HER2/neu)

Final report – optional features

In some cases, one or more of the following features may impact on the diagnosis or prognosis:

1. **Presence of endometriosis:** although not a feature of the current staging system, this may help to establish a primary site in some instances

2. **Presence of an associated mature teratoma:** this may be especially useful in establishing primary site for squamous or mucinous carcinoma
3. **Presence or absence of vascular invasion,** irrespective of vessel type

Kidney – carcinoma – resection

(From Higgins JP, McKenney JK, Brooks JD, Argani P, Epstein JI. Recommendations for the reporting of surgically resected specimens of renal cell carcinoma: The Association of Directors of Anatomic and Surgical Pathology. Hum Pathol 2009, **40:** 457–463.)

Final report – recommended features

Gross description

1. **Specimen condition:** fresh, in formalin, intact, fragmented, morcellated, etc.
2. **Specimen identification:** labeled (name, medical record number) and designated (e.g., right radical nephrectomy).
3. **Method:** If the specimen is a radical nephrectomy, inspect the external aspect of the specimen (*Gerota fascia*) for evidence of tumor. Locate the ureteral and vascular margins in the renal hilus. These may be sampled before inking the specimen when they are most easily identified. Hemostatic forceps should be placed on the ureter so that its location remains clear during and after inking. Ink the entire surface of the specimen. Cannulate the ureter using a small metal probe. Open the ureter longitudinally up to the level of the pelvis. Place the probe into a superolateral calyx and push through the renal parenchyma and perinephric soft tissue. Place a second probe in an inferolateral calyx and push through the renal parenchyma and perinephric soft tissue such that the two probes are now perpendicular to each other. Use a long, sharp knife to bivalve the kidney starting at its convex surface along the line of the metal probes. In this way, the kidney is opened along the collecting system. The renal veins should be subsequently opened in order to identify intravenous extension of tumor. Make additional cuts parallel or perpendicular to the first cut as necessary to cut the neoplasm along its greatest dimensions. In addition, cuts should be made to permit optimal viewing of the interface between the neoplasm and the perinephric fat because this is critical for assessing whether the neoplasm invades the perinephric fat and whether it approaches the margin of resection.

   A partial nephrectomy may be performed for clinical stage T1a tumors. For such specimens, ink the renal parenchymal resection margin and breadloaf the tumor perpendicular to the inked surface. Vascular and ureteral structures generally do not accompany partial nephrectomy specimens. The perinephric soft tissue will also usually not be included although sinus fat may be and must be carefully examined if it is present (see below). The important clinical information for partial nephrectomies is usually only tumor type, size, and renal parenchymal margin status, but some urologists will submit a separate specimen consisting of overlying perinephric fat for evaluation of tumor involvement
4. **Length of ureter,** other structures included (e.g., adrenal)
5. **Tumor description**
   - Site within the kidney: state whether the tumor is located at the superior or inferior pole or in the mid-portion of the kidney; if possible, determine whether the tumor is centered on the medulla or cortex. This is important for some tumor types (e.g., collecting duct carcinoma) in which the site of origin may support the diagnosis
   - Size in three dimensions
   - Gross characteristics: describe the color and consistency of the tissue and the degree of heterogeneity. State whether the tissue is friable and whether there are areas of necrosis and hemorrhage. Note and sample any areas with a homogeneous, tan bulging surface (so-called fish flesh quality), which may represent sarcomatoid dedifferentiation
   - The relationship to the perinephric soft tissue: determine whether the tumor protrudes into the perinephric soft tissue. Many renal cell carcinomas are large enough to distort the renal capsule and create a fungiform protrusion into the perinephric soft tissue. This alone is not sufficient to qualify as perinephric soft tissue invasion. Determine whether the interface between tumor and soft tissue is smooth and contoured with a pushing border (features which argue against soft tissue invasion) or irregular (a feature which suggests soft tissue invasion). The identification of separate tumor nodules in the perinephric fat by gross examination is diagnostic of pT3 disease. Under the 2002 AJCC system, extension into the renal sinus fat is also regarded as extrarenal extension (pT3a). In one study that specifically addressed extension into the sinus fat, this was a vastly more common route of perinephric soft tissue extension. In that study, no tumor penetrated the capsule that had not also invaded the sinus. In addition, the earliest evidence of macroscopic venous invasion (pT3b) is seen in the sinus fat. In fact, it has been suggested that sinus fat involvement begins as venous invasion, at least in clear cell carcinoma. In comparison to patients with only perinephric fat invasion by clear cell renal cell carcinoma, those with sinus fat invasion appear to have a worse prognosis. For these reasons, it is recommended that the sinus fat be serially sectioned at 5 mm intervals, and two sections be submitted from the interface between the tumor and the sinus tissues. It should be stated that renal oncocytomas may extend into the perinephric soft tissues, but this finding should not change the diagnosis as they still retain their excellent prognosis
   - Renal vein invasion: macroscopic invasion of veins in the renal sinus and beyond indicates a pT3b tumor. Whether the venous tumor is present only as a thrombus or invades the venous wall should also be noted, as the latter is associated with a worse prognosis. Although the only assessment required by the AJCC is whether the thrombus extends to the diaphragm, some studies have suggested that the prognosis is adversely affected by increasing distal extension of the tumor thrombus. These studies have correlated the degree of extension with the relationship to anatomic structures such as the hepatic veins. Although such correlations require clinical and/or radiologic information, it is recommended that a measurement be given from the tip of the thrombus to the renal sinus
6. **Additional pathology** (e.g., hydronephrosis, pyelonephritis, arteriolonephrosclerosis): it is recommended that an additional stain be ordered up front on the non-neoplastic renal parenchyma. This may be either a periodic acid–Schiff or a silver stain such as Jones methenamine silver. These stains enhance the review of the glomerular architecture and also serve as a prompt to address the condition of the

non-neoplastic kidney. This is important because diseases such as diabetic nephropathy and hypertensive nephrosclerosis are common in the renal cell carcinoma age group

7. **Adrenal involvement:** the adrenal can be reliably cleared of involvement by renal cell carcinoma by CT scan. As a result, adrenalectomy may not be performed as a component of a radical nephrectomy. In the current TNM classification, direct involvement of the adrenal is indicative of a pT3a tumor, whereas if the adrenal is involved by metastatic renal cell carcinoma, the finding requires a designation M1 and does not affect the pT classification. Several studies have suggested that adrenal involvement even by direct extension is an ominous finding and should warrant a designation of pT4
8. **Lymph nodes:** involvement of regional lymph nodes is an adverse prognostic indicator not otherwise specified. This appears to be true even in patients who already have distant metastases. The regional nodes may be designated renal hilar, paracaval, aortic (para-aortic, periaortic, lateral aortic), or retroperitoneal. At least 80% of the time lymph nodes are not identified in a radical nephrectomy specimen. Based on the last 1000 radical nephrectomy specimens at Stanford Hospital, renal hilar lymph nodes were identified at gross dissection in surgical pathology in only 5% of cases. Enlarged nodes from the renal hilus are often separately submitted by the urologist. According to the AJCC, if a lymph node dissection is performed, it should ordinarily include at least eight nodes
9. **Tissue submitted for special investigation:** in patients less than 20 years of age, tissue should, if possible, be submitted for cytogenetics. Although it must be acknowledged that translocation carcinomas occur across the entire age spectrum, they represent a much higher fraction of pediatric carcinomas. If a frozen section of the tumor reveals an unusual morphology in an adult patient, cytogenetics should be considered, and frozen tissue should be procured. Although karyotypic information may be helpful in the classification of common types of renal cell carcinoma, its greatest value is clearly in the diagnosis of the translocation carcinomas

Diagnostic information

1. **Laterality of tumor and type of resection.**
2. **Histologic type:** the World Health Organization 2004 classification of renal cell carcinoma is recommended:
   - Clear cell carcinoma
   - Multilocular cystic carcinoma
   - Papillary carcinoma
   - Chromophobe carcinoma
   - Mucinous tubular and spindle carcinoma
   - Collecting duct carcinoma
   - Medullary carcinoma
   - Translocation carcinomas (includes Xp11 and 6:11)
   - Tubulocystic carcinoma
   - Acquired cystic disease-associated carcinoma
   - Renal cell carcinoma, unclassified
   - Other (specify):

   Outcome for renal cell carcinoma has been strongly correlated with histologic tumor type, and accurate classification of renal cell carcinomas is essential. The different types of tumor and the features necessary for diagnosis are very well demonstrated in the 2004 World Health Organization monograph. The reader is referred to that resource for most questions of classification. Only selected topics in classification are addressed here.

   Two types of papillary renal cell carcinoma have been recognized: type 1 is composed of basophilic cells with scant cytoplasm arranged in a single layer, whereas type 2 has more abundant, often eosinophilic cytoplasm and pseudostratified nuclei. Some groups have found a better prognosis for type 1 tumors. Although the two types have been demonstrated to correlate with nuclear grade, some authors recommend that an attempt be made to separate papillary tumors into the two proposed types. A difficulty also exists with tumors that show a papillary architecture but clear cell cytology. Some such tumors have been found to have cytogenetic changes typical of clear cell carcinoma. This would support a practice of classifying these tumors as clear cell carcinoma; however, the problem is in the degree of clear cell change required in a papillary tumor for reclassification as a clear cell carcinoma. It has been suggested that 75% of the tumor cells should be clear and this appears to be a reasonable threshold. Focal or mild clear cell change may be encountered in otherwise typical papillary carcinomas. A diagnosis of papillary carcinoma remains appropriate for such tumors. Other tumors with papillary architecture and clear cells may be unclassifiable without molecular analysis; some of these will prove to be translocation carcinomas
3. **Histologic grade:** it has been acknowledged that no ideal grading scheme exists for renal cell carcinoma but that all agree that grading of renal cell carcinoma, however it is done, provides useful prognostic information and should be performed. The Fuhrman scheme is in general clinical use and has been independently validated for clear cell and papillary carcinomas. Most studies fail to show that grading of chromophobe renal cell carcinomas provides independent prediction of prognosis beyond stage. Low-stage chromophobe carcinomas, which are often Fuhrman grade 3, have an almost uniformly excellent prognosis. Until novel grading systems are developed and validated for chromophobe carcinomas, they should not be graded.

   For the remaining tumors, the overall grade should be assigned based on the highest grade that occupies at least one 400× field:
   - Small nuclei resembling those of mature lymphocytes
   - Larger nuclei with more open chromatin and small nucleoli
   - Nucleoli readily visible on examination with 10× objective
   - Marked nuclear pleomorphism, multiple macronucleoli
4. **Sarcomatoid dedifferentiation:** a malignant spindle cell pattern of growth has come to be recognized as a nonspecific pattern of dedifferentiation that may occur in any of the major types of renal cell carcinoma. The amount of sarcomatoid tissue may be of prognostic relevance and should be quantitated as a percentage. Either the underlying nonsarcomatous carcinoma component or immunohistochemical evidence of epithelial differentiation in a lesion morphologically consistent with sarcomatoid renal cell carcinoma must be identified to permit a definitive diagnosis of renal cell carcinoma. For cases with only a sarcomatoid component, consideration must also be given to the possibility of a primary or metastatic sarcoma. In patients with sarcomatoid dedifferentiation, the already poor prognosis is significantly further worsened by the presence of

necrosis. The amount of necrosis should also be estimated visually in increments of 5%

5. **Presence of necrosis:** coagulative tumor cell necrosis has been found to be of prognostic significance for both clear cell and chromophobe carcinoma and should therefore be reported
6. **Extent of local tumor spread:** this is based on the T component of the TNM classification:
   - Primary tumor cannot be assessed (TX)
   - There is no evidence of primary tumor (T0)
   - Tumor measures 7 cm or less and is confined to the kidney (T1)
   - Tumor measures less than 4 cm and is confined to the kidney (T1a)
   - Tumor measures more than 4 cm but less than 7 cm and is confined to the kidney (T1b)
   - Tumor measures more than 7 cm but is confined to the kidney (T2)
   - Tumor extends into major veins or directly invades adrenal gland or perinephric fat but not beyond Gerota fascia (T3)
   - Tumor directly invades adrenal gland or perinephric fat but not beyond Gerota fascia (T3a)
   - Tumor extends into renal vein(s) segmental (muscle-containing) branches or vena cava or its wall below the diaphragm (T3b)
   - Tumor extends into vena cava above the diaphragm or the wall of the vena cava (T3c)
   - Tumor extends beyond Gerota fascia (T4)
7. **Microscopic evidence of angiolymphatic invasion** should be assessed and documented
8. **Margins of resection**
   - No tumor identified at margins
   - Tumor is present at renal parenchymal margin of resection (partial nephrectomy)
   - Tumor present at soft tissue margin of resection
   - Intravascular tumor present at venous margin of resection
   - Tumor is present at ureter margin
   - Others: _____
9. **Lymph node metastases:** not surprisingly, the presence of lymph node metastases adversely affects the outcome of patients with renal cell carcinoma. The number of nodes sampled and the number positive should be reported. Although the prognosis may not be adversely affected by an increasing number of positive nodes (pN1 vs pN2) or the size of the largest metastatic focus, these should be reported. The prognosis appears to be significantly adversely affected by extranodal extension of the metastatic focus, and therefore it is recommended that this be assessed and reported as well

ASSOCIATION OF DIRECTORS OF ANATOMIC AND SURGICAL PATHOLOGY

Final anatomic diagnosis checklist

RENAL CELL CARCINOMA

(Excluding pediatric renal tumors and tumors of the renal pelvis)

Accession No.:	**Part No.**	**Date:**
Patient name:		
ORGAN:	**SITE:**	**OPERATION:**
Kidney	Right	Radical nephrectomy
Kidney and adrenal	Left	Radical nephrectomy and adrenalectomy
		Partial nephrectomy
Other_____	Other_____	Other_____

Specimen weight: Required_____

Tumor size: Required_____ cm × _____ cm × _____ cm

Other gross features: Required

Describe appearance of tumor, location within the renal lobe with respect to cortex versus medulla if possible, presence of necrosis, extension into the perinephric fat or the fat of the renal sinus, macroscopic invasion of veins

Tumor type (WHO 2004): Required

Clear cell carcinoma
Multilocular cystic carcinoma
Papillary carcinoma (optional: specify type 1 versus type 2)
Chromophobe cell carcinoma
Mucinous tubular and spindle carcinoma
Collecting duct carcinoma
Medullary carcinoma
Translocation carcinomas (includes Xp11 and 6;11)
Tubulocystic carcinoma
Acquired cystic disease-associated carcinoma (specify subtype)
Renal cell carcinoma, unclassified
Other: _____

Histologic grade: Required

1 Small nuclei resemble those of mature lymphocytes larger nuclei with more open chromatin and small nucleoli
2 Nucleoli readily visible on examination with 10× objective
3 Marked nuclear pleomorphism, multiple macronucleoli
4 (applies to chromophobe carcinoma)
Not applicable

Sarcomatoid dedifferentiation:

Sarcomatoid dedifferentiation is not identified
Areas of sarcomatoid dedifferentiation are identified
Specify percentage of total tumor: _____

Depth of tumor invasion: Required

Primary tumor cannot be assessed (TX)
No evidence of primary tumor (T0)
Tumor measures 7 cm or less and is confined to the kidney (T1)
Tumor measures less than 4 cm and is confined to the kidney (T1a)
Tumor measures more than 4 cm but less than 7 cm and is confined to the kidney (T1b)
Tumor measures more than 7 cm but is confined to the kidney (T2)
Tumor extends into major veins or directly invades adrenal gland or perinephric fat but not beyond Gerota fascia (T3)
Tumor directly invades adrenal gland or perinephric fat but not beyond Gerota fascia (T3a)
Tumor extends into renal vein(s) or vena cava or its segmental (muscle-containing) branches or vena cava below the diaphragm (specify presence/absence of wall invasion) (T3b)
Tumor extends into vena cava above the diaphragm or the wall of the vena cava (T3c)
Tumor extends beyond Gerota fascia (T4)

Microscopic angiolymphatic invasion: Required

Identified
Not identified

Margins of resection: Required

No tumor identified at margins
Tumor is present at renal parenchymal margin of resection (partial nephrectomy)
Tumor present at soft tissue margin of resection
Intravascular tumor present at venous margin of resection (specific presence/absence of wall invasion)
Tumor is present at ureter margin
Other: _____
Note: Retraction of vein over fully resected tumor must be excluded.

Lymph nodes (regional): Required

Number examined:_____
Number positive:_____
Comments: _____
NOTE: Regional lymph nodes include renal hilar, paracaval, para-aortic, periaortic, lateral aortic, and retroperitoneal NOS

Additional findings: Required

Acquired cystic renal disease, diabetic nephropathy, arteriolonephrosclerosis, pyelonephritis, papillary adenoma, tubulopapillary hyperplasia, cysts
Specify: _____

Adrenal gland: Optional

No histopathologic changes are present
Tumor directly invades the adrenal gland (T3a)
Adrenal involved by metastasis (M1)
Nodular/diffuse cortical hyperplasia is present
Cortical adenoma is present (specify size)
Other:_____

Ancillary studies: Optional

Slightly modified from Higgins JP, McKenney JK, Brooks JD, Argani P, Epstein JI. Recommendations for the reporting of surgically resected specimens of renal cell carcinoma: The Association of Directors of Anatomic and Surgical Pathology. Hum Pathol 2009, **40:** 461–463.

Large bowel – carcinoma

See also:

1. The updated (and very detailed) version of these recommendations (Jass JR, O'Brien MJ, Ridell RH, Snover DC, Association of Directors of Anatomic and Surgical Pathology. Recommendations for the reporting of surgically resected specimens of colorectal carcinoma. Hum Pathol 2007; **38:** 537–545)
2. An alternative set of recommendations from Leeds, UK (Quirke P, Morris E. Reporting colorectal cancer. Histopathology 2007, **50:** 103–112)

Final report – recommended features

Gross description

1. **Specimen condition:** fresh, in formalin, opened, unopened, etc.
2. **Specimen identification:** labeled with (name, number) and designated as (e.g., right colon)
3. **Part(s) of intestine included, length of each segment, other structures included** (e.g., terminal ileum, appendix, anal canal, attached/adherent organs, identified vessels)
4. **Tumor description**
   - Site within intestine
   - Proximity to nearest margin
   - Gross subtype (e.g., polypoid, annular, constricting, ulcerating, infiltrative, plaque, linitis plastica)
   - Dimensions (three if possible)
   - Macroscopic depth of penetration
   - Appearance of serosa adjacent to tumor (e.g., retracted)
5. **Presence of features of obstruction** (proximal dilation)
6. **Presence of perforation**
7. **Status of residual bowel:** polyps, inflammatory bowel disease, diverticula, ulcers, strictures
8. **Lymph nodes identified**
9. **Tissue submitted for special investigation (e.g., flow cytometry) should be specified**

Diagnostic information

1. **Site** of tumor and part of bowel resected
2. **Histologic type:** the WHO classification of invasive carcinoma is recommended:
   - Adenocarcinoma, NOS
   - Mucinous (colloid) carcinoma (>50% mucinous)
   - Signet ring cell carcinoma (>50% signet ring cells)
   - Adenosquamous carcinoma
   - Small cell undifferentiated (oat cell) carcinoma
   - Undifferentiated carcinoma
   - Other (specify):
3. **Histologic grade:** a modification of the WHO classification is recommended for adenocarcinoma NOS only:
   - Well differentiated – complex or simple tubules, easily discerned nuclear polarity, uniform sized nuclei
   - Moderately differentiated – complex, simple or slightly irregular tubules, nuclear polarity just discerned or lost
   - Poorly differentiated – highly irregular glands or an absence of glandular differentiation with loss of nuclear polarity

   Note 1: Data reported suggest strongly that the most significant prognostic information is derived from the category of poorly differentiated carcinoma versus more differentiated tumors. An alternate suggestion from the WHO is to divide adenocarcinoma into a high and low grade on this basis
4. **Depth of infiltration:** our recommendations are based on those in the TNM classification:
   - Into the submucosa but not into the muscularis propria (T1)
   - Into but not through the muscularis propria (T2)
   - Through the muscularis propria and into the subserosal fat or pericolonic or perirectal adipose tissue (T3)
   - Reaching the serosa or peritoneal surface (T4)
   - Into adjacent organs (T4)
   - With perforation if present

   Note 2: Although the TNM classification includes a level **Tis** to represent in situ carcinoma, we recommend against the use of this term for the following reasons:
   - We prefer the term *high-grade dysplasia* rather than *carcinoma in situ/severe dysplasia* (Tis in the TNM classification)
   - Intramucosal carcinoma is present when invasion of the lamina propria is present. This is also included within the category Tis. Because carcinoma of the large intestine has not been shown to have metastasizing potential until the submucosa is invaded, many individuals do not use this term in surgical pathology reports or, if they do, they state that provided the lesion has been excised completely locally no further treatment is required for that lesion
5. **Lymph node metastases:** stated as number of involved nodes and total number of nodes
6. **Presence of mesenteric deposits:** these are likely to be the equivalent of a nodal metastasis although this has not been confirmed
7. **Other sites biopsied for metastatic disease:** peritoneum, adjacent organs, liver, ovary
8. **Adequacy of local excision:** radial/proximal/distal resection margins. Assessment of proximal and distal margins is routine in the bowel as in other organs. In the rectum the deep margin (radial (lateral) margin) should be assessed. The radial margin is defined as the point at which the tumor reaches closest to a deep (lateral, circumferential) resected margin and is usually the deepest point of invasion in the rectum. Inking of the radial margin is highly recommended. For the large intestine outside of the rectum, the 'lateral' surgical resection margin is the mesenteric border of resection and is usually widely free of tumor unless dissection has deliberately been carried out close to the bowel wall. The antimesenteric serosal surface of the nonrectal large intestine is *not* a radial resection margin
9. **Other significant disease:** e.g., inflammatory bowel disease, other tumors, polyps, familial adenomatous polyposis, diverticular disease and its complications, ulcers, strictures
10. **Specify** in the report if information required for prognosis or therapy is not available or cannot be adequately assessed (e.g., no nodes found, radial margin not assessable)

Final report – optional features

1. **Stage:** the required data provided above should provide sufficient information for application of most staging systems. We in general do not recommend inclusion of a specific tumor stage in the pathology report; however, if a stage is to be included in the report the staging system used should be

specified (e.g., Astler–Collier modification of Dukes stage) rather than using the misnomer 'Dukes stage' as a generic term. We believe that the AJCC/UICC (TNM) classification is the least ambiguous and currently embodies most criteria required for prognosis and therapeutic decisions. However:
- We suggest that the stage Tis be replaced by high-grade dysplasia or intramucosal carcinoma as described above (see Depth of infiltration, above)
- We note that the derogatory effect on prognosis of perforation is not included in this system
- We are uncertain of the significance or practicality of the N3 stage (see below)

2. **Results of ancillary investigations** (e.g., flow cytometry)
3. **Specific lymph nodes**
   - Apical node if the Gabriel and Dukes modified stage or other modification requiring evaluation of this node is used
   - Nodes along a named vessel if the AJCC/UICC (TNM) classification is used and nodes along a named vessel are identified

   Based on the TNM classification:
   N0 No regional lymph node metastases
   N1 1–3 perirectal or pericolonic nodes involved
   N2 4 or more pericolic or perirectal nodes involved
   N3 Nodes specifically identified to be along the course of a named vascular trunk (e.g., ileocolic, etc.) are involved with tumor

   Note 3: While prognosis is related to the absolute number of nodes involved there is as yet little evidence that N3 has a worse prognosis than N2: some studies suggest that this division is of little prognostic value

   In most centers there is little or no attempt by the surgeon to identify these vessels and no indication that therapy is modified
4. **Nature of the advancing edge:** regular, irregular/infiltrative
5. **Inflammatory infiltrate:** e.g., Crohn-like, lymphocytic, eosinophilic
6. **Lymph vessel infiltration**
7. **Perineurial infiltration**
8. **Venous infiltration** (extramural veins only)
9. **Residual adenoma at the edge of the carcinoma**

Checklist

Tumor site
- Terminal ileum
- Transverse colon
- Descending colon
- Rectum
- Cecum
- Ascending colon
- Sigmoid colon
- Anus
- Not specified

Resection specimen
- Left hemicolectomy
- Right hemicolectomy
- Proctocolectomy
- Low anterior resection
- Not specified

Proximity to nearest margin
— cm
Dimensions — cm × — cm × — cm

Macroscopic depth of penetration of tumor
- Into submucosa
- Into muscularis propria
- Through muscularis propria
- Uncertain
- With retraction of underlying serosa

Obstruction (proximal dilation)
— Yes — No

Histologic tumor type
- Adenocarcinoma, NOS
- Signet ring cell cancer
- Small cell undifferentiated cancer
- Mucinous (colloid) cancer
- Adenosquamous cancer
- Undifferentiated cancer
- Other (specify):

Histologic grade
- Well differentiated
- Moderately differentiated
- Poorly differentiated

Depth of infiltration
- Into the submucosa but not into the muscularis propria (TI)
- Into but not through the muscularis propria (T2)
- Through the muscularis propria and into the subserosal fat or pericolonic or perirectal adipose tissue (T3)
- Reaching the serosa or peritoneal surface (T4)
- Into adjacent organs (T4)

Perforation
— Yes — No

Lymph node metastases
- Number of involved nodes
- Total number of nodes

Presence of mesenteric deposits
— Yes — No

Metastatic disease in other sites biopsied
- Yes
- No
- Specify site

Adequacy of local excision
- Proximal margin free of tumor
  — Yes — No
- Distal margin free of tumor
  — Yes — No
- One margin involved with tumor (cannot determine proximal or distal)
  — Yes — No
- Radial margin free of tumor (rectal tumors only)
  — Yes — No

Tissue submitted for special investigation
- Flow cytometry
  — Yes — No
- Other (specify):

Larynx – carcinoma

Final report – recommended features

General

1. **Topography:** type of specimen(s) received (e.g., total or partial larynx, neck contents)
2. **Type of procedure:** total or partial laryngectomy, e.g., supraglottic (horizontal) or hemilaryngectomy (vertical), radical neck dissection

3. **Exact site of tumor:** supraglottic, subglottic, glottic (see Note 1)
4. **Histologic type:** WHO classification recommended (see Note 2); comment on no tumor present post therapy
5. **Histologic grade** as appropriate: check grading systems
6. **Tumor extent:** depth of invasion with respect to landmarks. Comment on neural, vascular, cartilage, pre-epiglottic space and extralaryngeal soft tissue (muscle soft tissue, cartilage) or tracheostomy involvement as well as multifocal growth
7. **Status of surgical margins**
8. **Lymph node metastases**
   - Size of metastatic node
   - Number of involved nodes
   - Level of node involvement (diagram)
   - Comment whether or not extranodal spread of tumor is found
   - Comment on keratin debris as evidence of previous tumor
9. **Preoperative treatment effects on nodes**

Note 1: The American Joint Committee on Cancer divides the larynx into the following three regions: supraglottis, glottis, and subglottis. The supraglottis comprises the epiglottis (both its lingual and laryngeal aspects), arytenoepiglottic folds (laryngeal aspect), arytenoids, and ventricular bands (false cords). The inferior boundary of the supraglottis is a horizontal plane passing through the apex of the ventricle. The glottis comprises the true vocal cords, including the anterior and posterior commissures. The lower boundary is the horizontal plane, 1 cm below the apex of the ventricle. The subglottis is the region extending from the lower boundary of the glottis to the lower margin of the cricoid cartilage.

Note 2: Histologic type (World Health Organization classification, modified):

1. Squamous cell carcinoma, typical, keratinizing or nonkeratinizing, invasive or in situ
2. Spindle cell squamous (sarcomatoid) carcinoma
3. Verrucous carcinoma
4. Basaloid squamous carcinoma
5. Undifferentiated carcinoma (including lymphoepithelioma)
6. Salivary gland type tumors
7. Adenoid cystic carcinoma
8. Mucoepidermoid carcinoma
9. Adenosquamous carcinoma
10. Others
11. Neuroendocrine carcinoma
12. Well differentiated (carcinoid tumor)
13. Moderately differentiated (atypical carcinoma tumor)
14. Poorly differentiated (small cell carcinoma)
15. Adenocarcinoma, nonsalivary gland type
16. Other malignancies (sarcoma, melanoma, etc.)

Note 3: It is generally recognized that most masses greater than 3 cm in diameter are not single lymph nodes but represent confluent nodes or tumor in soft tissues of the neck

Gross description

1. **Specimen condition:** fresh, in formalin, opened by surgeon or pathologist, unopened, etc.
2. **Specimen identification:** labeled (with name, number) and anatomic site designation as, e.g., right partial vertical laryngectomy, modified neck dissection, etc.
3. **Describe** portions of the larynx included with specimen including other structures that may be attached: hyoid bone, adjacent pharynx, thyroid and parathyroid glands and tracheal rings
4. **Tumor description**
   - Size (give in three dimensions)
   - Shape (ulcerating, exophytic, polypoid)
   - Color
   - Necrosis
   - Multifocal growth
5. **Location of tumor:** describe all anatomic structures involved including ventricles, which cords, right and/or left, true and/or false cord (specify clearly). Distance above and/or below false and true cords respectively. Involvement of aryepiglottic folds. Does tumor cross midline or extend more than 1 cm from below true vocal cord? If tumor crosses the midline, estimate the percentage of tumor on right and left sides. Is there submucosal spread?
6. **Depth of invasion, involvement of cartilage:** note specific cartilages involved
7. **Involvement of extralaryngeal structures,** thyroid soft tissue, prelaryngeal (Delphian) lymph node, and parathyroid glands
8. **Describe tracheotomy site,** if present. Presence or absence of tumor
9. **Lymph node dissection,** if included:
   - Type: extended radical, radical, or modified radical or selective
   - Inclusion of sternomastoid muscle/submandibular and/or parotid gland/jugular vein
   - Palpable mass (solitary, matted)
   - Size and location of gross invasion of adjacent soft tissues, muscle, and jugular vein
   - Measure and describe sternomastoid muscle, major salivary glands, and internal jugular vein
   - Label lymph nodes as to levels according to anatomic location in neck dissection

Final report – optional features

1. **Interface with stroma:** infiltrating, pushing, superficial or deep invasion
2. **Extent of and location of any dysplasia:** including grade/CIS
3. **Results of ancillary investigations:** i.e., flow cytometry
4. **Type or density of inflammatory infiltrate**
5. **Distance from surgical margins**

Checklist

Topography
- Larynx
- Partial larynx
- Neck dissection

Procedure
- Total laryngectomy
- Partial laryngectomy
  - Supraglottic (horizontal)
  - Hemilaryngectomy (vertical)
- Radical neck dissection
- Partial neck dissection

Exact site of tumor
- Supraglottic
- Glottic
- Subglottic
- Transglottic

Histologic type
- CIS/severe dysplasia only
- Squamous cell carcinoma
  - Keratinizing
  - Nonkeratinizing
- Undifferentiated carcinoma
- Salivary gland carcinoma (specify):
- Neuroendocrine carcinoma
  - Well differentiated (carcinoid)
  - Moderately differentiated (atypical carcinoid)
  - Poorly differentiated (small cell carcinoma)
- Papillary (exophytic) squamous cell carcinoma
- Spindle cell carcinoma
- Verrucous carcinoma
- Basaloid squamous carcinoma
- Adenosquamous carcinoma
- Adenocarcinoma, nonsalivary type
- Other (specify):

Histologic grade
- Well differentiated
- Moderately differentiated
- Poorly differentiated
- Undifferentiated

Tumor extent
- Commissure
  — Anterior — Posterior
- Ventricle
  — Right — Left
- False cord
  — Right — Left
- True cord
  — Right — Left
- Subglottic region
  — Right — Left
- Aryepiglottic fold
  — Right — Left
- Vallecula
- Pyriform sinus
  — Right — Left
- Epiglottis
  — Right — Left

Extralaryngeal structures
- Thyroid
- Soft tissue
- Prelaryngeal (Delphian) lymph node
- Tumor invades cartilage
  — Yes — No
- Vascular invasion
  — Yes — No
- Neural invasion
  — Yes — No
- Tracheostomy invasion
  — Yes — No
- Multicentric tumor
  — Yes — No
- CIS/dysplasia present
  — Yes — No
- Verrucous hyperplasia present
  — Yes — No

Status of surgical margins (specify specimen margins or margins separately submitted)
- Free of tumor
- Involved by tumor (specify):

Lymph node metastases
- Number of nodes removed – right
- Number of nodes involved – right
- Number of nodes removed – left
- Number of nodes involved – left
- Extracapsular invasion present
- Jugular vein invasion present
- Muscle invasion present
- Keratin debris present

Preoperative treatment effects on nodes
— Yes — No

Special investigations performed
- Flow cytometry
- Electron microscopy
- Image analysis
- Molecular diagnostics
- Gross photograph

Liver – carcinoma – resection

(From Dabbs DJ, Geisinger KR, Ruggiero F, Raab SS, Nalesnik M, Silverman JF. Recommendations for the reporting of tissues removed as part of the surgical treatment of malignant liver tumors. Hum Pathol 2004, **35:** 1315–1316.)

Final report – recommended features

Gross description

1. **Specimen identification:** labeled with name, medical record number, surgical pathology number, etc.
2. **Specimen condition:** fresh or in fixative
3. **Type of procedure:** segmentectomy, trisegmentectomy, partial lobectomy, complete resection
4. **Tumor site:** exact anatomic site of the tumor in the liver
5. **Weight:** weigh the specimen and give the dimensions in length × width × thickness. Section the liver at 1.0 cm intervals
6. **Measure and describe** the lesion(s):
   - Mark the resection margin with ink
   - Describe the distribution of lesion(s):
     - Measure the lesion(s) in their greatest dimensions
     - Identify whether the lesion(s) is(are) single or multiple, superficial or deep
     - Note whether the lesion(s) involve(s) the liver capsule, hepatic vein, portal vein, or inferior vena cava
     - Note whether the biliary tract and/or the hilum is invaded
     - Identify the involved liver segment in explants
   - Measure the distance between the inked resection margin and the nearest lesion
   - Determine whether there is preexisting liver disease (e.g., cirrhosis, hepatitis, hemochromatosis, etc.)
   - Evaluate for evidence of previous chemoembolization or radiofrequency ablation
   - Investigate for evidence of locoregional lymph node metastasis
   - If the gallbladder is attached, describe it

Microscopic evaluation

1. **State whether the tumor is a primary hepatocellular or cholangiocarcinoma**, or is metastatic. Describe microscopic peritumoral satellites, if present. A satellite is defined as a tumor nodule in the same segment or less than 2 cm from a lesion and less than 50% the diameter of the larger lesion and less than 4 cm in size even if associated with a large mass. An attempt should be made to distinguish multicentric occurrence from intrahepatic metastasis when two or more nodules are present
2. **State the grade** of the hepatocellular tumor (grade I–IV)
3. **Document lymphovascular invasion**, if present
4. **Document if the resection margin is free of tumor** or not and how closely the tumor is to the inked resection margin
5. **Describe lymph node involvement or lack thereof and the site of the lymph nodes:** hilar nodes, celiac nodes, or juxtaregional (periaortic-pericaval/other intra-abdominal)
6. **Describe foci of small cell and large cell dysplasia,** if present
7. **Describe dysplastic nodules, regenerative macronodules, and their number,** if present
8. **Document underlying hepatic disease,** if present, and state the type (e.g., cirrhosis), with etiology (e.g., hepatitis B, hemosiderosis, α_1-antitrypsin)

Lung – carcinoma

Final report – recommended features

Gross description

1. **Specimen condition:** fresh, in formalin, opened, unopened etc.
2. **Specimen identification:** labeled with (name, number) and designated as (e.g., right upper lobe)
3. **Part(s) of lung included:** including measurements in three dimensions and weights, and description of other attached structures (e.g., parietal pleura, hilar lymph nodes, etc.)
4. **Tumor description**
   - Tumor location, including relationship to lobe(s), segment(s), and, if pertinent, major airway(s), and pleura. Involvement of lobar or mainstream bronchus should be specified
   - Proximity to bronchial resection margin, and to other surgical margins (i.e., chest wall soft tissue, hilar vessels) as appropriate
   - Tumor size (three dimensions if possible)
   - Presence or absence of satellite tumor nodules
5. **Description of nontumorous lung,** i.e., presence or absence of postobstructive changes or other abnormalities (e.g., bronchiectasis, mucus plugs, obstructive pneumonia, atelectasis)

Diagnostic information

1. **Tumor site:** i.e., side, lobe, specific segment if appropriate
2. **Type of procedure:** i.e., segmentectomy, lobectomy, pneumonectomy, including portion of lung resected
3. **Histologic type:** i.e., a modified World Health Organization (WHO) classification is recommended. Although the WHO classification is based on light microscopic criteria, the results of ancillary studies (i.e., histochemistry, immunohistochemistry, electron microscopy) should be reported when appropriate (e.g., large cell neuroendocrine carcinoma):
   - Squamous cell carcinoma (keratinization and/or intercellular bridges). Variant: spindle cell (squamous carcinoma)
   - Small cell carcinoma (uniform small cells, dense round or oval nuclei, diffuse chromatin, inconspicuous nucleoli, sparse cytoplasm). Variants can be mixed small cell/large cell carcinoma (spectrum of cell types ranging from typical small cells to large cells with prominent nucleoli and resembling large cell carcinoma) or combined small cell carcinoma (typical small cell carcinoma intimately admixed with areas of squamous cell carcinoma or adenocarcinoma)
   - Adenocarcinoma (tubular, acinar, or papillary growth pattern, and/or mucus production); acinar adenocarcinoma (i.e., adenocarcinoma, not otherwise specified (NOS)); papillary adenocarcinoma; solid carcinoma with mucus formation; and variants including bronchoalveolar adenocarcinoma and spindle cell (adeno)carcinoma
   - Large cell carcinoma (large nuclei, prominent nucleoli, abundant cytoplasm, without characteristic features of squamous cell, small cell, or adenocarcinoma) including variants of giant cell carcinoma and clear cell carcinoma (large cell carcinomas composed extensively (>90%) of large cells with clear or foamy cytoplasm without mucin; clear cell features also can be prominent in squamous cell carcinomas and adenocarcinomas and in metastatic renal cell carcinoma)
   - Adenosquamous carcinoma
   - Nonsmall cell neuroendocrine carcinomas, including carcinoid tumor; atypical carcinoid tumor (well-differentiated neuroendocrine carcinoma); large cell neuroendocrine carcinoma (large polygonal cells, coarse nuclear chromatin, frequent nucleoli, neuroendocrine differentiation by immunohistochemistry or electron microscopy). Classification of neuroendocrine carcinomas remains controversial, and therefore use of the category 'large cell neuroendocrine carcinoma' should be considered optional until sufficient data are available to clarify the clinical significance of this subset of large cell carcinomas
   - Bronchial gland carcinomas, adenoid cystic carcinoma, mucoepidermoid carcinoma
   - Other (specify):
4. **Histologic grade:** WHO classification (i.e., well, moderately, and poorly differentiated) recommended for squamous cell carcinoma and adenocarcinomas of acinar (i.e., adenocarcinoma, NOS) or papillary type
5. **Histologic assessment of surgical margins:** include comment regarding involvement of lobar or mainstem bronchi by invasive or in situ carcinoma, and microscopic relationship of tumor to bronchial and/or vascular margin(s)
6. **Pleural involvement:** specify whether tumor invades into but not through visceral pleura without involving parietal pleura (T2), or into parietal pleura (T3) (elastic tissue stains can be helpful in defining the limiting elastic layer of visceral pleura)
7. **Lymph node metastases:** indicate the number of involved nodes and the total number of nodes received. (Precise node counts may be difficult for fragmented specimens such as those received from mediastinoscopy.) The nodal groups (N) should be specifically identified using the American Joint Committee on Cancer intraoperative staging system for

regional lymph nodes. N2 lymph nodes (with the exception of level 11 interlobar nodes) are generally received separately and must be appropriately identified by the submitting surgeon; these are to be reported separately. Pneumonectomies are usually accompanied by attached N2 lymph nodes which should be specifically identified by location. If the nodal involvement is only by direct extension, this feature should be noted

8. **Non-neoplastic lung:** any significant abnormalities (e.g., granulomas, pneumonia, etc.) should be recorded

Final report – optional features

1. **Stage:** surgical pathology reports containing the previously listed information will contain all of the necessary data to establish the International TNM Staging System for lung carcinoma. It should be emphasized that pathologic tumor stage may be based on incomplete information and therefore may differ from clinical tumor stage
2. **Angiolymphatic invasion:** whenever possible, it should be specified whether the structures involved are blood vessels or lymphatic vessels, and whether the involved blood vessels are muscular arteries, elastic arteries, or veins
3. **Perineurial invasion**
4. **Presence or absence of perinodal (extracapsular) tumor invasion**
5. **Results of ancillary investigations:** e.g., flow cytometry

Checklist

Topography
- Right lung
  - RUL
  - RML
  - RLL
- Left lung
  - LUL
  - LLL
- Segment (specify):

Procedure
- Pneumonectomy
- Lobectomy
- Bilobectomy
- Segmentectomy
- Wedge excision
- Other (specify):

Tumor type

Tumor histologic grade
- Well differentiated
- Moderately differentiated
- Poorly differentiated/undifferentiated

Tumor location

Tumor size (greatest diameter)

Angiolymphatic invasion

Perineurial invasion

Mainstem bronchus

Bronchial margin

Visceral pleural margin

In situ carcinoma

Non-neoplastic lung
- Atelectasis
- Pneumonia
- Other (specify):

Lymph nodes with metastatic disease

This is a set of recommendations for lymph node biopsies, lymph node dissections, sentinel node biopsies, and lymph node fine needle aspiration (FNA) and core needle biopsies, intended specifically for lymph nodes being studied for metastatic neoplasms, and not to be applied to lymph nodes being evaluated for lymphoma, infections, and other disease processes. They are, however, formulated generically enough to apply regardless of whether the primary tumor is a carcinoma of the breast, carcinoma of the prostate, melanoma, or any other malignant, potentially metastasizing tumor.

Lymph node biopsies

1. In the presence of gross tumor in a biopsy of a single lymph node, one or several routine sections to demonstrate the tumor and its possible extranodal extension will suffice
2. In the absence of gross tumor, the entire node should be submitted for microscopic examination, cut into 3–4 mm slices in the longitudinal or transverse plane. If the node is so small that it cannot be sliced in this manner, it may be submitted as one piece in toto. If the node is sliced, care should be taken to process different surfaces for microscopic examination. The Association recommends the examination of several levels of each slide, stained with hematoxylin and eosin (H&E) only

Lymph node dissection

1. **Processing and staining**
   - As mentioned above, the principles presented here are generic, and may vary by site or by institution
   - Lymph node dissections are best processed fresh, although other techniques (such as fixation in Bouin solution) may be used
   - No clearing of adipose tissue is necessary, although it may represent an institutional or individual preference
   - Submit every node for microscopic examination
   - Submit the entire nodes cut as described in the preceding section unless they contain grossly visible tumor, in which case fewer slices are required, or if they are grossly largely replaced by adipose tissue, in which case processing is optional
   - Lymph node levels in a dissection specimen should be specified and submitted separately where clinically appropriate (e.g., neck dissections, colectomy specimens)
   - The summary of the sections in the surgical pathology report should include how many sections of how many nodes are submitted in each cassette. Different color inks may be used to distinguish different nodes submitted in a single cassette
   - One H&E slide per cassette is recommended
   - Immunohistochemistry and other specialized techniques may be used as part of a research study or for differential diagnosis, but are not considered mandatory at present
2. **Reporting**
   - The number of lymph nodes positive for metastatic disease and the total number of lymph nodes examined microscopically should be reported, with specific levels mentioned when appropriate

- The size of the largest metastasis (measured on the slide) should be reported if clinically indicated
- The presence of extracapsular extension may be reported, depending upon the primary site and institutional preference
- If the tumor is seen in extranodal vessels, this should be stated
- Deposits of tumor not associated with any structure recognizable as a lymph node should be separately designated
- In rare situations, the grading of nodal metastases may be important
- After preoperative chemotherapy and/or radiotherapy, the notation of necrotic versus non-necrotic tumor is recommended

Sentinel node biopsy

1. The adequacy of the sentinel node dissection depends upon the skill and experience of the surgeon. At the present time, the clinical utility of this technique is still controversial. In many institutions, this is still considered an experimental procedure
2. Where this factor has been studied, the level of radiation associated with sentinel node biopsy has not been demonstrated to pose any danger to pathologists or histotechnologists from radioactivity. However, protocols should conform to institutional and state guidelines
3. Intraoperative examination, whether by frozen section or scrape/imprint cytology, or both, is appropriate only in those clinical situations in which the results will influence immediate therapeutic management. Examination of the intraoperative specimen by other than routine (H&E) stains is experimental at the present time
4. The number of nodes received and their sizes should be noted in the gross description of the report. Each node should be processed grossly as mentioned earlier under Dissections. If any portion of the sentinel node(s) is not submitted for routine sectioning, this should be specified
5. ADASP recommends that more than one section be performed on each block in these cases, if the node or nodes are not positive grossly or at intraoperative pathologic consultation. However, it is not currently clear how many sections (and from what levels of the block) are optimal. It is also unclear whether immunostains add clinically relevant information and whether they should be substituted for additional H&E-stained sections. It should be remembered that false-positive immunostains occur, and these stains should be interpreted in the context of standard histopathology
6. If metastases are identified only by immunostains, this should be stated in the final report. Other statements on reporting provided in this document are also applicable

Fine needle aspiration and core needle biopsy

1. A negative result for tumor does not definitely exclude the presence of a metastatic tumor. Results should be correlated with the clinical situation
2. If only FNA is performed, a cell block may be useful for special studies in positive cases
3. If only a core needle biopsy is performed, all tissue should be submitted. The number of cores received should be specified in the gross description, and should be correlated with the slides received and examined
4. In many cases, it may not be possible to document on an FNA or core needle biopsy specimen that a metastatic tumor is indeed within a lymph node. In such a situation, a comment should be made to that effect

Lymphoid neoplasms

(From Jaffe ES, Banks PM, Nathwani B, Said J, Swerdlow SH. Recommendations for the reporting of lymphoid neoplasms: a report from The Association of Directors of Anatomic and Surgical Pathology. The Ad Hoc Committee on Reporting of Lymphoid Neoplams. Hum Pathol 2002, **33:** 1064–1068.)

Final report – recommended features

Background clinical information

The ADASP recommends including pertinent clinical history when this information is available. The pathologist is encouraged to obtain a clinical history, if possible. For some diseases (e.g., post-transplant-associated lymphoproliferative disease), an accurate history may be essential to diagnosis. Information should include the following:

1. Previous diagnosis of a lymphoid neoplasm, if known (with dates, site, and treatment status, if available)
2. Presence of generalized or localized lymphadenopathy
3. Evidence of organomegaly (e.g., hepatosplenomegaly)
4. Pertinent hematologic findings (e.g., lymphocytosis, pancytopenia)
5. Constitutional symptoms
6. Human immunodeficiency virus status
7. Prior immune abnormality, including congenital immune disorders
8. Autoimmune disease
9. Other pertinent serology (e.g., human T-cell lymphotropic virus-1, Epstein–Barr virus)
10. Other known cofactors (e.g., *Helicobacter pylori* infection)

Gross description

Proper handling of lymph node biopsy specimens is critical to ensure proper fixation, which is essential for the preparation of high-quality histologic sections. The Association recommends that the pathologist receive lymph node biopsies fresh and intact, and that an unsectioned lymph node biopsy never be immersed in fixative. It is recommended that each laboratory establish a protocol for handling of lymph node biopsies that ensures both optimal histologic sections and preservation of material for ancillary studies. These principles, and the procedures outlined herein, also apply to extranodal sites that may be biopsied or resected for a potential diagnosis of lymphoma. The following information should be included:

1. **Specimen identification:** labeled with patient's name, medical record number, and organ or site
2. **Specimen condition:** fresh or in fixative, intact or sectioned
3. **Type of procedure:** excisional, incisional, or core biopsy
4. **The overall dimensions of the specimen**
5. **Tumor description:** if capsule is present, whether this is intact or altered grossly. Color and consistency (firm versus fleshy); presence of nodularity, necrosis, hemorrhage

Sectioning

1. The Association recommends that lymph nodes be sectioned at 2 mm intervals, to ensure appropriate fixation
2. If the size of the lymph node permits, it is preferable to cut sections perpendicular to the long axis of the lymph node. This orientation enables best assessment of the architecture
3. If the specimen is spleen, information should include weight and description of any focal lesions (e.g., infarcts, nodules, hemorrhage) and gross abnormalities of red or white pulp
4. If the specimen is a spleen obtained for staging, the Association recommends that the spleen be sectioned at 3–5 mm intervals to look for grossly identifiable lesions. First, fixing thicker slices (1 cm) briefly in formalin may facilitate sectioning at the desired thickness. For staging laparotomy specimens for Hodgkin lymphoma, the number of grossly identifiable lesions, if less than 10, should be stated. The presence of more than four nodules has been shown to be of prognostic significance

Fixation and preservation

1. **Unique identifiers** should be used for each cassette, and the gross description should also specify the type of fixation used for each paraffin block
2. **Use more than one fixative:** It is often desirable to fix tissue in more than one fixative. Some fixatives provide excellent cytologic detail (B5, B+), but compromise the ability to extract DNA for molecular studies. Formalin is most suitable if polymerase chain reaction studies from the paraffin-embedded sections are anticipated
3. **Snap-freezing:** this is useful for preserving tissue for frozen section immunohistochemistry or future molecular studies. The following is a suitable procedure:
   - Blocks of fresh tissue approximately 1.0 × 1.0 × 0.3 cm are cut from the specimen
   - The tissue blocks are placed in a mold, cork, or other suitable form and immersed in OCT (Sakura Tissue-Tek, Torrance, CA)
   - The tissue and mold are immersed into a sludge composed of dry ice and isopentane (2-methylbutane) and snap-frozen
   - The blocks are labeled and stored at −80 °C or over liquid nitrogen
   - Blocks in OCT are suitable for frozen section immunohistochemistry and also can be used for molecular analyses. If sufficient tissue is available, blocks can be snap-frozen without OCT for molecular studies and held at −80 °C or over liquid nitrogen until needed

Diagnostic information

1. **Site of tumor:** exact anatomic site, if known, and tissue (lymph node or other)
2. **Type of procedure:** excisional, incisional, needle core
3. **Histologic tumor type:** the Association recommends using the World Health Organization (WHO) Classification of Tumors of the Hematopoietic and Lymphoid Tissues (Tables 1–4). The designation of morphologic or clinical variants is considered optional for most clinical purposes. If an alternative classification scheme is used, this should be specified in the diagnosis
4. **Tumor extent:** whether the specimen is only focally or incompletely involved
5. **Histologic type:** whether more than one histologic type is identified, such as composite lymphoma or progression to lymphoma of higher histologic grade
6. **Specimen adequacy:** a precise diagnosis may not be possible in some instances due to limitations of specimen adequacy (e.g., needle biopsy, necrotic or fibrotic specimen). If specimen adequacy is of concern, this fact should be stated explicitly
7. **Ancillary studies:** whether such studies (e.g., immunocytochemistry, molecular diagnostics) were performed, and if so, a statement regarding these studies and their diagnostic implications

Final report – optional features

Immunophenotypic information

For many subtypes of lymphoid neoplasms (e.g., peripheral T-cell lymphomas, diffuse large B-cell lymphoma, precursor B-cell lymphoblastic lymphoma/leukemia), immunophenotypic studies are essential to accurate diagnosis. In some instances (e.g., many instances of follicular lymphoma), immunophenotypic studies may not be required. If immunophenotypic studies are performed, we recommend that the results be included in an integrated single report. If ancillary studies are performed in a reference laboratory, the results should be discussed in an integrated report and the reference laboratory report appended. The report should include the following information:

1. How immunophenotypic studies were performed (flow cytometry versus immunohistochemistry)
2. Whether immunohistochemistry was performed on paraffin sections or frozen sections
3. All markers investigated, both positive and negative. Identifying antigens by the CD nomenclature is recommended. Use of the common or commercial name is optional but may be important in some cases, because different antibodies to the same CD antigen may show varying sensitivities and specificities (e.g., CD20: L26 versus Leu 16). Generic identifiers (e.g., B-cell marker, T-cell marker) should be avoided
4. The population expressing the antigen
5. Whether the antigen is only focally expressed (and, where helpful, an approximation of the percentage of positive cells)
6. Where the studies were performed, if not in the local laboratory
7. Possible significance of the immunophenotypic studies

Molecular genetic studies

Molecular genetic studies may provide useful diagnostic information about the clonality of the lymphoid infiltrate, the lineage of the lymphoid cells, or a precise molecular abnormality associated with a specific disease. As with immunophenotypic studies, if molecular analysis is performed, the Association recommends that this information be discussed in the context of the histologic findings, if possible. Important information includes:

1. Type of specimen used for the study (frozen tissue versus paraffin-embedded specimen)
2. Method used (e.g., polymerase chain reaction (PCR), Southern blot, reverse transcriptase-PCR)

3. The exact type of test performed (e.g., VJ-PCR for IgH gene rearrangement)
4. Whether the studies were done in a reference laboratory or in the local laboratory
5. Results (monoclonal, polyclonal, oligoclonal) and possible diagnostic significance

Viral studies

Viruses are important cofactors for many lymphoma types, and corroboration of a viral association may be essential for the diagnosis of some diseases (e.g., adult T-cell leukemia/lymphoma, primary effusion lymphoma). The pathologist should state the method of identification, results (positive or negative), and which cell population is affected for methods 1 and 2. Information should be included on:

1. Immunohistochemical staining
2. In situ hybridization
3. Polymerase chain reaction
4. Serology (see clinical history)

Cytogenetic studies

Cytogenetic studies may provide ancillary diagnostic information useful in the diagnosis or subclassification of lymphoma. The identification of a clonal cytogenetic abnormality supports a diagnosis of malignancy. Some cytogenetic abnormalities are highly associated with specific lymphoid malignancies (e.g., t(14;18) with follicular lymphoma). The Association recommends that the cytogenetic data be discussed in the context of the histologic findings and the complete report appended to the surgical pathology report. Information should be included on:

1. Conventional cytogenetics
2. Fluorescent in situ hybridization

Box App D-1 WHO classification of Hodgkin lymphoma (Hodgkin disease)

Nodular lymphocyte predominant Hodgkin lymphoma
Classic Hodgkin lymphoma
Nodular sclerosis Hodgkin lymphoma (Grades 1 and 2)
Lymphocyte-rich classic Hodgkin lymphoma
Mixed cellularity Hodgkin lymphoma
Lymphocyte depletion Hodgkin lymphoma

Box App D-2 Checklist for the reporting of lymphoid neoplasms

Demographics

Patient name:
Age:
Sex:
Race (optional):
Case number:

Clinical history

Prior diagnosis:
Presenting sites of disease:
Clinical symptoms:
Findings on physical examination:
Laboratory findings:

Gross assessment

Labeling of specimen:
Condition of specimen on receipt:
  Fresh
  In fixative
  Intact
  Previously sectioned
Surgical procedure:
Dimensions of the specimen:
Weight of specimen (if relevant):
Capsule:
Color and consistency:
Focal lesions:
Photography:
Allocation of tissue for special studies:
  Frozen tissue for archival storage or other studies
  Fresh tissue/cells for flow cytometry, cytogenetics
  Other tissue distribution

Diagnostic information

Anatomic site:
Tissue (lymph node or other):
Histologic tumor type:
  WHO classification:
  Other classification scheme:
Grading (if relevant, i.e., follicular lymphoma):
Adequacy:
Focal involvement:
Multiple histologic types present (composite lymphoma):
Immunophenotypic data:
Genotypic data:
Cytogenetics:
Microbiologic studies:

Special studies

Flow cytometry:
Immunohistochemistry:
  Frozen sections:
  Paraffin sections:
Molecular genetic studies:
  In situ hybridization
  Polymerase chain reaction
  Reverse transcriptase-polymerase chain reaction
  Southern blot
Cytogenetic studies:
  Conventional cytogenetics
  Fluorescent in situ hybridization

From Jaffe ES, Banks PM, Nathwani B, Said J, Swerdlow SH. Recommendations for the reporting of lymphoid neoplasms: a report from The Association of Directors of Anatomic and Surgical Pathology. The Ad Hoc Committee on Reporting of Lymphoid Neoplams. Hum Pathol 2002, **33:** 1066.

Major salivary glands

Final report – recommended features

Gross description

1. **Specimen identification:** labeled with name or medical record number
2. **Specimen condition:** fresh, in saline, or in formalin or other fixative
3. **Anatomic site and side of tumor:** parotid, submandibular or sublingual gland; left, right, or undesignated
4. **Type of procedure:** needle biopsy, open (incisional or excisional) biopsy, lobectomy, complete excision of gland, wide or radical excision
5. **Describe and measure** the entire surgical specimen (three dimensions). Identify and measure each component (i.e., total parotidectomy with attached radical neck dissection and overlying skin)
6. **Tumor characteristics:** size (three dimensions); solitary or multifocal; localized or diffusely involves the gland; confined to gland or extraglandular extension; margins (encapsulated, circumscribed, or poorly defined); color, consistency, necrosis; cyst formation; presence of apparent cartilage, calcific deposits or hyalinization
7. **Paraffin block key:** i.e., block A is from center of tumor, etc.
8. **When ink is used,** give code (i.e., black ink is inferior resection margin, blue ink is superior resection margin, etc.)

Checklist

Location
- Parotid
- Submandibular
- Sublingual

Side
- Right
- Left
- Not indicated

Procedure
- Needle
- Open biopsy (incisional or excisional)
- Lobectomy
- Complete excision of gland

Histologic type
- Benign epithelial tumors
  - Pleomorphic adenoma
  - Warthin tumor
  - Basal cell adenoma
  - Canalicular adenoma
  - Oncocytoma (oncocytic adenoma)
  - Myoepithelioma (myoepithelial adenoma)
  - Sebaceous adenoma/lymphadenoma
  - Cystadenoma
  - Intraductal papilloma
  - Sialadenoma papilliferum
  - Other
- Carcinomas
  - Acinic cell carcinoma
  - Mucoepidermoid carcinoma
  - Adenoid cystic adenoma
  - Polymorphous low-grade adenocarcinoma (terminal duct adenocarcinoma)
  - Epithelial–myoepithelial carcinoma
  - Clear cell carcinoma
  - Basal cell adenocarcinoma
  - Salivary duct carcinoma
  - Oncocytic carcinoma (malignant oncocytoma)
  - Adenocarcinoma, NOS
  - Malignant myoepithelioma (myoepithelial carcinoma)
  - Malignant mixed tumor
    - In situ/intracapsular carcinoma
    - Carcinoma ex pleomorphic adenoma
    - True malignant mixed tumor (carcinosarcoma)
    - Metastasizing pleomorphic adenoma
  - Cystadenocarcinoma
  - Mucinous adenocarcinoma
  - Squamous cell carcinoma
  - Small cell carcinoma
  - Undifferentiated carcinoma
  - Lymphoepithelial carcinoma
  - Sebaceous carcinoma/lymphadenocarcinoma
  - Sialoblastoma
  - Other
- Malignant lymphoma (specify type):
- Soft tissue neoplasms
  - Benign (specify type):
  - Malignant (specify type):
- Metastatic tumor (indicate primary if known)
- Other (specify):

Histologic grade
- Low (well differentiated)
- Intermediate (moderately differentiated)
- High (poorly differentiated)
- Undifferentiated

  Note: Grading of salivary malignancies is not standardized and may vary according to histologic type. In some instances, histologic type defines the grade; for example, epithelial–myoepithelial carcinoma and basal cell adenocarcinoma are low grade while salivary duct carcinoma is usually high grade

Tumor extent
- Confined to gland of origin
  - Intraglandular lymphatic invasion
  - Intraglandular vascular invasion
  - Intraglandular perineurial invasion
- Extraglandular extension
  - Cervical lymph nodes
  - Major nerve (facial, etc.)
  - Major blood vessel (jugular vein, etc.)
  - Bone
  - Skin
  - Other (specify):

Status of surgical margins
- Free of tumor
- Close, but technically free (specify margin and distance to margin):
- Involved by tumor (specify margin):

Lymph node metastasis
- Applies only to cervical lymph nodes. Other than for metastatic tumors, involvement of intraparotid lymph nodes by primary parotid tumors does not appear to have clinical relevance
- Cervical
  - — Right — Left
  - Number examined
  - Number positive
  - Extranodal spread
  - Size of largest positive lymph node (necessary for 'N' staging in Pathologic stage below)

- Level of lymph nodes (optional)
  - Level I (submental, submandibular)
  - Level II (upper jugular)
  - Level III (middle jugular)
  - Level IV (lower jugular)
  - Level V (posterior triangle)
  - Level VI (anterior compartment)
  - Preauricular
  - Postauricular
  - Suboccipital
  - Other

Pathologic stage

Special features
- Gross photographs
- Electron micrography
- Immunohistochemistry
- Flow cytometry
- Image analysis
- Genetic (chromosomal) analysis
- Molecular diagnostics
- Tumor tissue bank

Comments

Nasal cavity and paranasal sinuses – carcinoma

Final report – recommended features

Gross description

1. **Specimen identification:** how the specimen was labeled or identified (name, medical record number), and anatomic site designation, e.g., left maxillary sinus, left neck dissection, etc.
2. **Specimen condition:** how the specimen was received: fresh or in formalin, oriented by the surgeon, etc. Note any anatomic identifiers such as sutures or accompanying drawings
3. **Type of procedure:** maxillectomy, ethmoidectomy, etc. Describe the portions of tissue included with the specimen, including other structures that may be attached, e.g., maxillary sinus and attached tissues, such as teeth, hard palate, rim of orbit
4. **Measure** the overall dimensions of all specimens received
5. **Tumor description:** size (three dimensions), shape, color
6. **Tumor location:** anatomic site. Describe the presumed epicenter of the tumor and all the major anatomic structures involved such as sinus wall, nasal cavity, orbital rim, etc.
7. **Tumor extent:** size and depth of invasion with respect to adjacent structures, including involvement of cartilage, bone, or soft tissues
8. **Lymph node dissection,** if included: type, e.g., radical, modified, or selective; inclusion of sternocleidomastoid muscle or submandibular or parotid gland; jugular vein; measure and describe each. Describe lymph nodes – multiple solitary nodes or matted. Measure size of largest lymph node mass. Label lymph nodes as to levels according to anatomic location in the neck dissection, i.e., levels 1–5

Diagnostic information

1. **Topography:** what is included in the specimen(s) received
2. **Type of procedure:** e.g., total or partial rhinectomy, radical neck dissection
3. **Site of tumor:** e.g., lateral wall of nasal cavity, anteroinferior maxillary sinus
4. **Size**
5. **Histologic type**
6. **Histologic grade,** as appropriate
7. **Tumor extent:** size and depth of invasion with respect to adjacent structures (refer to checklist for site-specific descriptions). Note vascular, lymphatic, perineurial, bone invasion
8. **Status of surgical margins**
9. **Lymph node metastases:** nodes removed and number of nodes positive for each level examined; size of largest metastasis. Comment on whether extracapsular extension of tumor is present or absent

Final report – optional features

1. **Extent and location** of CIS or any dysplasia including grade
2. **Distance from surgical margins**
3. **Results of ancillary investigations:** immunohistochemistry, flow cytometry

Checklist

Topography
- Nose
  - Sphenoid
  - Orbital contents
- Maxillary sinus
  - Frontal
  - Soft palate
- Ethmoid sinus
  - Hard palate

Procedure
- Rhinectomy
  - — Total — Partial
- Maxillectomy
- Ethmoidectomy
- Frontal sinus excision
- Sphenoid sinus excision
- Radical neck dissection
- Partial neck dissection

Site of tumor
- Nasal cavity
  - Lateral wall
  - Floor
  - Septum
  - Roof
- Maxillary sinus
  - Anteroinferior
  - Superoposterior
  - Ethmoid
  - Sphenoid
  - Frontal

Size of tumor

— cm × — cm × — cm

Histologic type
- Carcinoma in situ only
- Squamous cell carcinoma
  - Keratinizing
  - Nonkeratinizing
- Lymphoepithelial carcinoma
- Sinonasal undifferentiated carcinoma

- Neuroendocrine carcinoma
  - Well differentiated (carcinoma)
  - Moderately differentiated (atypical carcinoid)
  - Poorly differentiated (small cell)
- Salivary gland carcinoma (specify):
- Adenocarcinoma, nonsalivary type
- Inverted (and all Schneiderian) papillomas
- Carcinoma ex Schneiderian papilloma
- Olfactory neuroblastoma
- Angiofibroma
- Chondrosarcoma
- Osteosarcoma
- Hemangiopericytoma
- Ameloblastoma
- Sarcoma
- Other malignancy

Histologic grade
- Well differentiated
- Moderately differentiated
- Poorly differentiated
- Undifferentiated

Tumor extent
- Nose/nasal cavity
- Involvement of:
  - Limited to mucosa with no destruction of bone
  - Skin
  - Columnella
  - Septum
  - Lateral wall
  - Roof (cribriform plate)
  - Ethmoid sinus involvement
  - Maxillary sinus involvement
  - Nasopharynx
  - Hard palate
  - Soft palate

Maxillary sinus
- Involvement of:
  - Limited to mucosa with no erosion or destruction of bone
  - Middle nasal meatus
  - Subcutaneous tissues or skin of cheek
  - Posterior wall of maxillary sinus
  - Orbital floor
  - Medial wall of orbit
  - Anterior ethmoid sinus
  - Orbital contents invasion
  - Cribriform plate
  - Posterior ethmoid sinus
  - Sphenoid sinus
  - Nasopharynx
  - Soft palate
  - Hard palate
  - Pterygomaxillary fossa
  - Temporal fossa
  - Base of skull

Ethmoid sinus
- Limited to sinus
- Involvement of:
  - Nasal cavity
  - Anterior orbit
  - Maxillary sinus
  - Intracranial
  - Skin of nose
  - Apex of orbit
  - Sphenoid sinus

Sphenoid
- Limited to mucosa
- Invasion beyond sinus

Other
- Vascular invasion
- Lymphatic invasion
- Perineurial invasion
- Bone invasion

Status of margins
- Margins free of tumor or estimated free margin distance from tumor
- Margins involved by tumor, list

Lymph node metastases
- Nodes removed, no. nodes positive
  - Level I
  - Level II
  - Level III
  - Level IV
  - Level V
  - Level VI
- Extracapsular extension present
- Size of largest metastasis

Special studies
- Photographs
- Electron microscopy
- Flow cytometry
- Image analysis
- Molecular studies

Neuroendocrine tumor

See Box App D-3.

Oral cavity and oropharynx – carcinoma

Final report – recommended features

Gross description

1. **Specimen identification:** labeled (with name, medical record number) and anatomic site designation, e.g., right partial glossectomy, modified neck dissection
2. **Specimen condition:** fresh, in formalin, oriented by surgeon, etc.
3. **Describe:** portions of oral cavity or oropharynx included with specimen, including other structures that may be attached, e.g., cortical bone or jaws, palate, tongue, skin of neck, maxillary sinus
4. **Measure** the overall dimensions of all specimens received
5. **Tumor description:** size (give in three dimensions), shape (ulcerating, exophytic, polypoid), color, necrosis, multifocal growth
6. **Location of the tumor:** anatomic sites and subsites
   - External upper lip (vermillion border)
   - External lower lip (vermillion border)
   - Commissures
   - Buccal mucosa
     - Mucosa of upper and lower lips
     - Cheek mucosa
     - Retromolar areas
     - Buccoalveolar sulci, upper and lower (vestibule of mouth)

Box App D-3 Minimum pathology data set: information to be included in pathology reports on neuroendocrine tumors

For resection of primary tumors

Anatomic site of tumor
Diagnosis (functional status need not be included in pathology report)
Size (three dimensions)
Presence of unusual histologic features (oncocytic, clear cell, gland-forming, etc.)
Presence of multicentric disease
(OPTIONAL: immunohistochemical staining for general neuroendocrine markers)
  Chromogranin
  Synaptophysin
  Peptide hormones, IF a specific clinical situation suggests that the correlation with a functional syndrome may be helpful
Grade (specify grading system used)
  Mitotic rate (number of mitoses per 10 high-power fields or 2 mm^2; count 50 high-power fields in the most mitotically active regions, count multiple regions)
  (OPTIONAL: Ki-67 labeling index – count multiple regions with highest labeling density, report average percentage; 'eyeballed' estimate is adequate)
Presence of nonischemic tumor necrosis
Presence of other pathologic components (e.g., non-neuroendocrine components)
Extent of invasion (use anatomic landmarks for the AJCC T-staging of analogous carcinomas of the same anatomic sites)
  Stomach: depth of invasion into/through gastric wall
  Small bowel: depth of invasion into/through bowel wall
  Large bowel: depth of invasion into/through bowel wall
  Appendix: depth of invasion into/through appendiceal wall; presence and extent of mesoappendiceal invasion
  Pancreas: the presence of extrapancreatic invasion or invasion of bile duct, duodenum, or ampulla
  All sites: involvement of serosal/peritoneal surfaces; invasion of adjacent organs or structures
Presence of vascular invasion (OPTIONAL: perform immunohistochemical stains for endothelial markers if needed)
Presence of perineurial invasion
Lymph node metastases
  Number of positive nodes
  Total number of nodes examined
TNM staging (specify staging system utilized)
Resection margins (positive/negative/close) (OPTIONAL: measure distance from margin if within 0.5 cm)
Proliferative changes or other abnormalities in non-neoplastic neuroendocrine cells

For biopsy of primary tumors

Anatomic site of tumor
Diagnosis (functional status need not be included in pathology report)
Presence of unusual histologic features (oncocytic, clear cell, gland-forming, etc.)
(OPTIONAL: immunohistochemical staining for general neuroendocrine markers)
  Chromogranin
  Synaptophysin
  Peptide hormones, IF a specific clinical situation suggests that the correlation with a functional syndrome may be helpful
Grade (specify grading system used)
  Mitotic rate (number of mitoses per 10 high-power fields or 2 mm^2; count up to 50 high-power fields)
  Ki-67 labeling index, for biopsies in which a diagnosis of high-grade neuroendocrine carcinoma cannot be excluded (count multiple regions with highest labeling density, report average percentage; 'eyeballed' estimate is adequate)
Presence of nonischemic tumor necrosis
Presence of other pathologic components (e.g., non-neuroendocrine components)

For resection of metastatic tumors

Location of metastasis(es)
Diagnosis (functional status need not be included in pathology report)
Number of metastases resected
Extent of involvement of resected tissue (percentage)
Greatest dimension of largest metastasis
Presence of unusual histologic features (oncocytic, clear cell, gland-forming, etc.)
(OPTIONAL: immunohistochemical staining for general neuroendocrine markers)
  Chromogranin
  Synaptophysin
  Peptide hormones, IF a specific clinical situation suggests the correlation with a functional syndrome may be useful
Grade (specify grading system used)
  Mitotic rate (number of mitoses per 10 high-power fields or 2 mm^2; count 50 high-power fields in the most mitotically active regions, provide separate mitotic rate for each major separate site of disease)
  (OPTIONAL: Ki-67 labeling index – count multiple regions with highest labeling density, report average percentage; 'eyeballed' estimate is adequate)
Presence of nonischemic tumor necrosis
Presence of other pathologic components
Resection margins (positive/negative/close) (OPTIONAL: measure distance from margin if within 0.5 cm)
Identification of primary site
  Immunohistochemistry for CDX2, TTF-1

For biopsy of metastatic tumors

Location of metastasis
Diagnosis (functional status need not be included in pathology report)
Presence of unusual histologic features (oncocytic, clear cell, gland-forming, etc.)
Immunohistochemical staining for general neuroendocrine markers
  Chromogranin
  Synaptophysin
  (OPTIONAL: peptide hormones, IF a specific clinical situation suggests the correlation with a functional syndrome may be useful)
Grade for adequate biopsy specimens; FNA specimens may not be adequate (specify grading system used)
  Mitotic rate (number of mitoses per 10 high-power fields or 2 mm^2; count up to 50 high-power fields)
  Ki-67 labeling index (count multiple regions with highest labeling density, report average percentage; 'eyeballed' estimate is adequate)
Presence of nonischemic tumor necrosis
Presence of other pathologic components (e.g., non-neuroendocrine components)
Identification of primary site
  Immunohistochemistry for CDX2, TTF-1

From Klimstra DS et al. Pathology reporting of neuroendocrine tumors: application of the Delphic consensus process to the development of a minimum pathology data set. Am J Surg Pathol 2010, **34:** 300–313.

- Upper alveolus and gingiva (upper gum)
- Lower alveolus and gingiva (lower gum)
- Hard palate
- Tongue
  - Dorsal surface and lateral borders anterior to vallate papillae (anterior two-thirds)
  - Inferior (ventral) surface
- Floor of mouth
- Oropharynx
  - Anterior wall (glosso-epiglottic area)
    - Base of tongue (posterior to the vallate papillae or posterior third)
    - Vallecula
  - Lateral wall
    - Tonsil
    - Tonsillar fossa and tonsillar (faucial) pillars
    - Glossotonsillar sulci (tonsillar pillars)
  - Posterior wall
  - Superior wall
    - Inferior surface of soft palate
    - Uvula

7. **Tumor extent:** based on tumor classification (AJCC, UICC) (applicable only to carcinomas of the vermillion surfaces of the lips and of the oral cavity and oropharynx, including those of minor salivary glands)
   - All sites

   Tis Carcinoma in situ
   T1 Tumor 2 cm or less in greatest dimension
   T2 Tumor more than 2 cm but not more than 4 cm in greatest dimension
   T3 Tumor more than 4 cm in greatest dimension
   T4
   Lip – tumor invades adjacent structures, e.g., through cortical bone, inferior alveolar nerve, floor of mouth, skin of face
   Oral cavity – tumor invades adjacent structures, e.g., through cortical bone, into deep (extrinsic) muscle of tongue, maxillary sinus, skin (superficial erosion alone of bone/tooth socket by gingival primary is not sufficient to classify a tumor as T4)
   Oropharynx – tumor invades adjacent structures, e.g., pterygoid muscles, mandible, hard palate, deep muscle of tongue, larynx

   Note 1: The extrinsic musculature of the tongue includes musculi hypo-, stylo-, genio-, and palatoglossus. Invasion of the intrinsic muscle alone (musculi longitudinales superior and inferior, transversus linguae and verticalis linguae) is not classified T4

   Note 2: In cases of doubt regarding the invasion through cortical bone, Paragraph 4 of the General Rules of the TNM System (TNM Booklet, p. 6) should be applied. If there is doubt concerning the correct T, N, or M category to which a particular case should be allotted, the lower (i.e., less advanced) category should be chosen. This will also be reflected in the stage grouping. If scintigraphy is feasible and the resultant finding is conclusive the tumor must be classified as T4
8. **Lymph node dissection** if included: type (extended radical, radical or modified radical or selective); inclusion of sternomastoid muscle/submandibular and/or parotid gland/jugular vein; palpable mass (solitary, matted); size and location of gross invasion of adjacent soft tissues, muscle, and jugular vein; measure and describe sternomastoid muscle, major salivary glands, and internal jugular vein; measure size of lymph nodal masses (see Notes 3a and 3b); label lymph nodes as to levels or according to anatomic location in neck dissection

   Note 3a: It is generally recognized that most masses greater than 3 cm in diameter are not single lymph nodes but represent confluent nodes or tumor in soft tissues of the neck

   Note 3b: Histologic examination of a selective neck dissection specimen will ordinarily include six or more lymph nodes. Histologic examination of a radical or modified radical neck dissection specimen will ordinarily include 10 or more lymph nodes (depending on previous RT)

Diagnostic information

1. **Topography:** type of specimen(s) received, e.g., simple excision, composite resection, neck contents
2. **Type of procedure:** e.g., total or partial glossectomy, radical neck dissection
3. **Exact site of tumor:** lip, oral cavity, oropharynx (see Checklist, Anatomic site of tumor)
4. **Histologic type:** World Health Organization (WHO) classification recommended (see Note 4) (comment on no tumor present post therapy)

   Note 4: Histologic type (WHO classification, modified) includes squamous cell carcinoma, typical, keratinizing or nonkeratinizing, invasive or in situ; spindle cell squamous (sarcomatoid) carcinoma; verrucous carcinoma; basaloid squamous cell carcinoma; papillary squamous cell carcinoma; undifferentiated carcinoma (including lymphoepithelioma); salivary gland-type tumor (adenoid cystic carcinoma, mucoepidermoid carcinoma, adenosquamous carcinoma, and others); neuroendocrine carcinoma (well-differentiated (carcinoid tumor), moderately differentiated (atypical carcinoid tumor), poorly differentiated (small cell carcinoma)); adenocarcinoma, nonsalivary gland type; other malignancies (sarcoma, melanoma, etc.)
5. **Histologic grade** as appropriate
6. **Tumor extent:** size and depth of invasion with respect to adjacent structures (e.g., tonsillar pillar, soft palate, nasal cavity, pterygoid muscles), extrinsic muscle of tongue, skin and soft tissue of neck and face. Distinguish extending to or overlying bone from gross erosion of bone and radiographic destruction of bone. Note tracheostomy involvement, as well as multifocal growth
7. **Status of surgical margins**
8. **Lymph node metastases:** size of metastatic node, number of involved nodes, level of node involvement, comment whether extranodal spread of tumor is found, comment on keratin debris and/or foreign body giant cell reaction as evidence of previous tumor
9. **Preoperative treatment:** effects on nodes

Final report – optional features

1. **Extent and location** of any dysplasia (including grade)
2. **Vascular/lymphatic invasion**
3. **Perineurial invasion**
4. **Depth of invasion**
5. **Interface with stroma:** infiltrating, pushing, **superficial or deep invasion**
6. **Inflammatory infiltrate:** type of density

7. **Results of ancillary investigations:** i.e., flow cytometry
8. **Distance** from surgical margins

Checklist

Topography
- Lip
- Oral cavity
- Oropharynx
- Neck dissection

Procedure
- Incisional biopsy
- Excisional biopsy
- Resection

Anatomic site of tumor
- External upper lip (vermillion border)
- External lower lip (vermillion border)
- Commissures
- Buccal mucosa
  - Mucosa of upper and lower lips
  - Cheek mucosa
  - Retromolar areas
  - Bucco-alveolar sulci, upper and lower (vestibule of mouth)
- Upper alveolus and gingiva (upper gum)
- Lower alveolus and gingiva (lower gum)
- Hard palate
- Tongue
  - Dorsal surface and lateral borders anterior to vallate papillae (anterior two-thirds)
  - Inferior (ventral) surface
- Floor of mouth
- Oropharynx
- Anterior wall (glosso-epiglottic area)
  - Base of tongue (posterior to the vallate papillae or posterior third)
  - Vallecula
- Lateral wall
  - Tonsil
  - Tonsillar fossa and tonsillar (faucial) pillars
  - Glossotonsillar sulci (tonsillar pillars)
- Posterior wall
- Superior wall
  - Inferior surface of soft palate
  - Uvula

Histologic type

CIS/severe dysplasia only
- Squamous cell carcinoma
  - Keratinizing
  - Nonkeratinizing
- Undifferentiated carcinoma
  - Papillary (exophytic) squamous cell carcinoma
  - Spindle cell carcinoma
  - Verrucous carcinoma
  - Basaloid carcinoma
- Neuroendocrine carcinoma
  - Well differentiated (carcinoid)
  - Moderately differentiated (atypical carcinoid)
  - Poorly differentiated (small cell carcinoma)
- Salivary gland carcinoma (specify type):
  - Adenosquamous carcinoma
  - Adenocarcinoma, nonsalivary type
  - Other malignancy (specify):

Histologic grade
- Well differentiated
- Moderately differentiated
- Poorly differentiated
- Undifferentiated

Tumor extent (see text definition)
- Tis: Carcinoma in situ
- T1: Tumor 2 cm or less in greatest dimension
- T2: Tumor more than 2 cm but not more than 4 cm in greatest dimension
- T3: Tumor more than 4 cm in greatest dimension
- T4: Tumor invades adjacent structures, e.g., through cortical bone, mandible, inferior alveolar nerve, skin or soft tissues of neck, deep (extrinsic) muscle of tongue, pterygoid muscles, maxillary sinus, hard palate, larynx
- Multicentric tumor

Status of surgical margins (specify specimen margins or margins separately submitted)
- Free of tumor
- Involved by tumor (specify):

Lymph node metastases (specify right or left)
- Number of nodes removed
- Number of nodes involved
- Size of largest involved node
- Extracapsular invasion present
- Jugular vein invasion present
- Muscle invasion present
- Keratin debris and/or foreign body giant cell reaction present

Preoperative treatment effects on nodes

— Yes — No

Special investigations performed
- Flow cytometry
- Electron micrography
- Image analysis
- Molecular diagnostics
- Gross photograph

Pancreas and periampullary region – carcinoma

Final report – recommended features

Gross description

1. **Specimen identification:** labeled with information such as name and medical record number
2. **Specimen condition:** e.g., fresh, in fixative
3. **Site:** the exact anatomic site of the tumor
4. **Type of procedure:** biopsy, local excision, standard pancreaticoduodenectomy (Whipple procedure), pylorus-preserving pancreaticoduodenectomy, total pancreatectomy, distal pancreatectomy stating specifically which organs have been removed
5. **Describe and measure** (three dimensions) the entire surgical specimen, e.g., biopsy, local excision, standard pancreaticoduodenectomy (Whipple procedure), pylorus-preserving pancreaticoduodenectomy, total pancreatectomy, distal pancreatectomy. Describe and measure each component of the specimen
6. **Describe the gross features** of the tumor: color, consistency, size, location within the pancreas (head, body, tail, or diffusely throughout the gland); encapsulated or nonencapsulated; relationship to the pancreatic and bile ducts, multicentricity; abnormalities of the pancreatic ducts

including stricture, ductal dilation; grossly visible mucin; unilocular or multilocular neoplastic cysts; cyst contents; non-neoplastic cysts in pancreatic tissue adjacent to tumor; secondary cyst formation due to tumor necrosis

7. **Describe:** for Whipple distal or total pancreatectomy specimens, describe all applicable items, e.g., status of the main pancreatic duct, accessory ducts, common bile duct, cystic duct, ampulla of Vater, duodenum, stomach, spleen, portal, superior mesenteric and splenic veins, common hepatic artery. Describe duct extension to duodenum, stomach, spleen, or colon. Report involvement of vessels, portal, superior mesenteric, and splenic veins; common hepatic artery; any other large vessels adjacent to tumor. Identify and describe surgical margins for adequacy of excision. Comment if the tumor is grossly identifiable at the margins. Describe the localization, number, and consistency of lymph nodes
8. **Paraffin block key**

Diagnostic information

1. **Type of malignancy** should be recorded. The following classification of pancreatic malignant tumors is recommended:
   - Type of neoplasm
     - Carcinoma in situ
     - Infiltrating ductal carcinoma
     - Adenosquamous carcinoma
     - Mucinous noncystic carcinoma
     - Signet ring cell carcinoma
     - Undifferentiated carcinoma
     - Spindle and giant cell type
     - With osteoclast-like giant cells
     - Small cell carcinoma
     - Mucinous cystadenocarcinoma
     - Mucinous cystic neoplasm of low malignant potential (borderline)
     - Mucinous cystic neoplasm with sarcomatous transformation of the stroma
     - Intraductal mucinous papillary carcinoma with an invasive component
     - Intraductal mucinous papillary carcinoma without an invasive component
     - Serous cystadenocarcinoma
     - Solid pseudopapillary and cystic carcinoma (malignant solid papillary and cystic tumor)
     - Acinar cell carcinoma
     - Acinar cell cystadenocarcinoma
     - Endocrine neoplasm (e.g., insulin, glucagon, somatostatin, gastrin, pancreatic polypeptide and vasoactive-intestinal peptide secreting, multihormonal)
     - Mixed acinar and endocrine carcinoma
     - Mixed ductal and endocrine carcinoma
     - Pancreatoblastoma
   - Mesenchymal tumors
     - Leiomyosarcoma
     - Osteosarcoma
   - Lymphoma
   - Others
2. **Tumor grade:** the following grading system is suggested for infiltrating ductal carcinomas:
   - Grade 1 Well differentiated, more than 95% of the tumor is composed of glands
   - Grade 2 Moderately differentiated, 50–95% of the tumor is composed of glands
   - Grade 3 Poorly differentiated, 5–49% of the tumor is composed of glands
   - Grade 4 Undifferentiated, less than 5% of the tumor is composed of glands

For papillary intraductal carcinomas, grading is optional. The grading system designed by Albores-Saavedra et al.[1] is recommended. It is based on nuclear atypia and mitotic figures. High-grade tumors are characterized by cells with vesicular or hyperchromatic nuclei and prominent nucleoli. Mitotic figures are common (>5 per 10 high-power fields). Low-grade neoplasms are composed of cuboidal or columnar pseudostratified cells with ovoid or elongated vesicular or hyperchromatic nuclei but without nucleoli and without mitotic activity. Tumors with moderate nuclear atypia and very few mitotic figures (<5 per 10 high-power fields) are included in the intermediate category. Because of the poor correlation of cytologic features, pattern of growth, and biologic behavior in most endocrine tumors, they are not graded

Checklist

Specimen type

- Biopsy
- Local excision
- Distal pancreatectomy
- Standard pancreaticoduodenectomy
- Pylorus-preserving pancreaticoduodenectomy
- Total pancreatectomy

Diagnosis section

- Pathology report should address all applicable items
- Tumor type
- Grade
- No stromal invasion
- Invasion confined to the pancreas (include size)
- Invasion of (check all applicable):
  Peripancreatic soft tissues
  Common bile duct
  Cystic duct
  Adjacent large vessels
  Portal vein
  Mesenteric
  Common hepatic artery
- Invasion of any or all of the following (check all applicable):
  Ampulla of Vater
  Duodenum
  Stomach
  Colon
  Spleen
- Invasion of:
  Small vessels
  Large vessels
  Perineurial invasion
- Other pancreatic epithelial abnormalities, such as atypical ductal hyperplasia and papillary hyperplasia, should be recorded

Pathology in other organs

- Common bile duct
- Cystic duct
- Ampulla of Vater
- Duodenum
- Stomach
- Spleen

Involvement of surgical margins
- Common bile duct
- Pancreas neck
- Pancreas uncinate
- Posterior (retroperitoneal) pancreas
- Other soft tissue margins
- Duodenum
- Stomach

Lymph nodes
- Number of lymph nodes sampled and number of lymph nodes with metastasis
- Extent of tumor
  Tumor size
  No stromal invasion present
  Invasion confined to the pancreas (include size)
  Direct extension into ampulla
  Invasion of peripancreatic soft tissues, common bile duct, cystic duct, duodenum, or invasion of adjacent large vessels (e.g., portal vein, mesenteric, or common hepatic artery)
  Invasion of spleen, colon, stomach
  Presence or absence of lymphatic or microvascular invasion
  Perineurial invasion
- Intraductal lesions: Report papillary hyperplasia, ductal hyperplasia, or carcinoma in situ adjacent to tumor. Report dysplasia or carcinoma in situ in common bile duct or ampulla of Vater
- Other lesions
  Acute or chronic pancreatitis
  Pancreatic cysts
  Calculi
  Other
- Surgical margins: Report involved or uninvolved surgical resection margins of the pancreas (e.g., neck, uncinate, posterior), bile duct, duodenum, stomach, and soft tissues, including retroperitoneal margin
- Lymph nodes: Report presence or absence of metastases in regional lymph nodes. State the number of lymph nodes sampled and the number of lymph nodes involved. Report separately submitted lymph nodes
- Report results of immunoperoxidase stains and electron microscopy in endocrine and acinal neoplasms and in combined exocrine and endocrine tumors

Optional features
- Ploidy
- Nuclear morphometry
- Genetic abnormalities
- Growth factors
- Receptors
- Stage

1 Albores-Saavedra J, Henson DE, Milchgrub S. Intraductal papillary carcinoma of the main pancreatic duct. Int J Pancreatol 1994, **16**: 223–224.

Parathyroid glands

Final report – recommended features

Primary hyperparathyroidism is a common disease, the incidence of which has increased rather dramatically over the past several decades. As a result, surgical exploration of the parathyroid has become a relatively commonplace procedure at most large institutions. Most parathyroid tumors represent either adenomas or hyperplasia. The distinction between these two entities is problematic, and usually requires pathologic examination of more than one gland as well as clinical data. This, together with the rarity of other parathyroid neoplasms, focuses this protocol on defining the information necessary to distinguish parathyroid adenoma from hyperplasia, and the features most useful in the diagnosis of parathyroid carcinoma

Gross description

1. **Specimen identification:** precisely designated site (e.g., left upper parathyroid) and whether biopsy or whole gland
2. **Specimen condition:** whether the specimen was received fresh versus in fixative (type)
3. **Describe and measure** the specimen:
   - Weight (include estimate from surgeon of percentage of gland removed, if available)
   - Size in three dimensions
   - Color and consistency
   - Presence of capsule
   - Adherence to other structures
   - Cystic elements
   - Hemorrhage
   - Necrosis
   - Nodularity
4. **Specify** when frozen section or touch imprint performed
5. **Paraffin block key**
6. **When ink is used,** so specify
7. **Special investigations:** note following if done:
   - Gross photography
   - Tissue processed for ancillary studies or stored for such potential

Diagnostic information

1. **Surgical procedure**
2. **Histologic classification**
   - Hyperplasia
   - Adenoma
   - Atypical adenoma
   - Carcinoma

   Several studies have defined histologic features important in the diagnosis of parathyroid carcinoma, including thick fibrous bands, trabecular growth pattern, and high mitotic rate. Similarly, criteria have been developed to distinguish adenoma from hyperplasia
3. **Characteristics of carcinoma**
   - Features present to make diagnosis
   - Grade (no grading currently available)
   - Extent
   - Margins
4. **Lymph nodes**

Final report – optional features

1. **Subtyping tumor:** e.g., chief cell versus clear cell
2. **Results of ancillary studies**
   - DNA ploidy
   - Proliferative activity (e.g., MIB-1, p27)
   - Nuclear morphometry
   - Genetic abnormalities
   - Growth factors and receptors
3. **Pathologic stage – proposed system** (see below)

4. **Clinical data**
   - Patient history, including family history
   - Endocrine testing results
     - Serum Ca^{2+}
     - Serum PTH
     - Other
   - Pre- and postoperative diagnoses

Proposed staging system for parathyroid carcinoma

Primary tumor (T)

T1 <3 cm
T2 >3 cm
T3 Tumor of any size with invasion of the surrounding soft tissues, such as the thyroid gland, strap muscles, etc.
T4 Massive central compartment disease invading the trachea and esophagus, or recurrent parathyroid carcinoma

Nodal involvement (N)

N0 No regional lymph node metastases
N1 Regional lymph node metastases

Metastatic involvement (M)

M0 No evidence of distant metastases
M1 Evidence of distant metastases

Checklist

Topography, procedure, and gross features

- Site
  - Left upper
  - Right upper
  - Left lower
  - Right lower
  - Other
- Procedure
  - Left upper
  - Right upper
  - Left lower
  - Right lower
  - Other
- Size
  - Left upper
  - Right upper
  - Left lower
  - Right lower
  - Other
- Weight (estimated % of entire gland)
  - Left upper
  - Right upper
  - Left lower
  - Right lower
  - Other

Histologic classification

- Hyperemia
- Adenoma
- Carcinoma
- Other

Pleural mesothelioma – resection

(From Butnor KJ, Sporn TA, Ordóñez NG, Kelly J. Recommendations for the reporting of pleural mesothelioma. Hum Pathol 2007, **38:** 1588–1589.)

Final report – recommended features

Gross description

1. **Specimen identification:** labeled with patient's name, medical record number, surgical pathology accession, number, etc. Designated as pleura (and other organs as applicable); laterality
2. **Specimen condition:** unfixed or in formalin; intact or disrupted; oriented or not
3. **Type of procedure:** core needle biopsy, thoracoscopic biopsy, thoracotomy and incisional biopsy, pleurectomy, or extrapleural pneumonectomy
4. **Measure and describe:** the overall size of the specimen should be measured in three dimensions, and the tissues included in the specimen (pleura, chest wall adipose tissue and/or skeletal muscle, ribs, diaphragm, lymph nodes, mediastinal structures, etc.) should be documented
5. **Tumor description**
   - Distribution: diffuse, nodular, localized/solitary
   - Extent of pleura involved (circumferential, subtotal) and presence or absence of involvement of fissures and interlobular septa
   - Document dominant tumor mass(es) and size
   - Appearance: color(s), texture (e.g., firm, soft, or gritty), and infiltrative capacity
   - Distance to closest resection margins: lateral soft tissue (chest wall) margin, bronchus, pulmonary vessels, mediastinal structures (if included), diaphragm
     Note 1: The closest resection margins should be inked and sampled using perpendicular sections for areas where there is gross suspicion of involvement.
   - Document appearance of excised thoracoscopic sites, if applicable (usually submitted separately)
   - Involvement of adjacent tissues (e.g., diaphragm, pericardium, lung, ribs, chest wall adipose tissue, and skeletal muscle)
   - Lymph nodes (number received (if any), site of origin, size, and description of cut surface)
   - Specific location or orientation of each tissue block taken for routine processing
   - Description of the non-neoplastic pleura, lung, and other tissues
   - Whether a diagnostic frozen section was performed and the intraoperative diagnosis

Diagnostic information

1. **Site, laterality, and procedure**
2. **Histologic type**
   - Epithelioid
   - Sarcomatoid
   - Biphasic
   - Desmoplastic
   - Other (specify):
3. **Extent of invasion:** document involvement of parietal and visceral pleura, diaphragm, lung, endothoracic fascia,

mediastinal adipose tissue and/or organs, chest wall soft tissue (solitary or diffuse involvement), and ribs

4. **Resection margin status:** positive (state which margin) or negative
5. **Lymph node status:** if present, specify the site and the number involved out of the total for each site
6. **Pathologic stage** based on pathologic features as cited

Final report – optional features

The features listed below may affect either the likelihood of recurrence or the overall prognosis. They represent specific institutional preferences or are considered to be inconclusive vis-à-vis their prognostic significance.

1. **Lymphovascular invasion**
2. **Blood vessel invasion**
3. **Findings in the non-neoplastic pleura/lung** (e.g., changes consistent with prior talc pleurodesis, plaques, fibrosis, asbestos bodies, and asbestosis)
   Note 2: Because of the etiologic association between asbestos exposure and malignant mesothelioma, quantitative fiber burden analysis may be requested in cases that include lung tissue as part of the specimen. Formalin-fixed non-neoplastic lung tissue (at least 5 g), preferably from the lower lobe, may be stored for this purpose
4. **Results of any ancillary study** (e.g., histochemical stains, immunohistochemistry, and electron microscopy)
   Note 3: Given the cytomorphologic overlap between malignant epithelioid mesothelioma and metastatic adenocarcinoma, or malignant sarcomatoid mesothelioma and primary or metastatic sarcomas, ancillary techniques (e.g., immunohistochemistry and/or electron microscopy) are routinely used to facilitate diagnosis. Because no single immunohistochemical marker is entirely sensitive or specific for malignant mesothelioma, a panel of stains should be used. The ADASP does not prescribe a particular panel of markers but recommends that at least two mesothelial-associated markers (e.g., calretinin, cytokeratins 5/6, D2-40, and WT1) be used in conjunction with two or more markers that are usually negative in malignant mesothelioma (e.g., CEA, TTF-1, Ber-EP4, and MOC-31). The results of ancillary techniques should be carefully correlated with the radiographic and gross distribution of the tumor

Prostate – carcinoma – resection

(From Epstein JI, Srigley J, Grignon D, Humphrey P. Recommendations for the reporting of prostate carcinoma. Hum Pathol 2007, **38**: 1306–1308.)

Final report – recommended features

Gross description

1. **Specimen identification:** labeled with name, medical record number, etc.
2. **Specimen condition:** fresh, in formalin, intact, cut, margins inked or not, etc.
3. **Topography:** the type of specimen should be identified, e.g., prostate
4. **Type of procedure:** core biopsy, transurethral biopsy, transurethral resection, enucleation, radical prostatectomy, radical cystoprostatectomy, other
5. **Measure the specimen:** the overall size of the excised specimen should be measured in three dimensions. TURP specimens should be weighed; needle biopsy cores should be counted and measured in length (state if multiple small fragmented cores without need for measuring)
6. **Additional organs attached:** e.g., seminal vesicles, vasa deferentia, bladder neck in radical prostatectomy specimens
7. **Tumor description**
   - Presence or absence of lesion(s)
   - Location of the lesion(s): e.g., in radical prostatectomy: posterior, posterolateral, lateral, anterior, and apex, mid, base
   - Size of the lesion(s): greatest diameter if radical prostatectomy
   - Consistency of the lesion(s): e.g., firm, fleshy
8. **Lymph nodes:** number and appearance of lymph nodes if received
9. **Frozen section:** whether a frozen section was performed and the diagnosis that was made

Diagnostic information

1. **Histologic type**
   - Adenocarcinoma (acinar, not otherwise specified)
   - Prostatic duct adenocarcinoma
   - Mucinous (colloid) adenocarcinoma
   - Signet ring cell-like carcinoma
   - Adenosquamous carcinoma
   - Small cell carcinoma
   - Sarcomatoid carcinoma
   - Undifferentiated carcinoma, not otherwise specified
   - Other (specify):
2. **Histologic grade**: all acinar adenocarcinomas should be graded using the Gleason grading system. Ductal adenocarcinomas are typically assigned a Gleason score 4 + 4 = 8, yet are diagnosed as 'ductal adenocarcinoma (Gleason score 4 + 4 = 8)' to convey the unique clinical and pathologic features of this tumor. There is no consensus as to the grading of mucinous carcinomas. Approximately one-half of urologic pathologists grade them as Gleason pattern 4 (e.g., Gleason score 4 + 4 = 8 if pure mucinous tumor). The remaining experts grade the tumor based on the underlying tumor architecture, mentally subtracting away the mucin. Regardless of the method used to grade mucinous carcinomas, most of these tumors end up being assigned a Gleason score 4 + 4 = 8. True signet ring cell carcinomas containing vacuoles of mucin that are primary in the prostate are exceedingly rare. Rather, there exist signet ring cell-like carcinomas, which contain clear vacuoles without mucin. These tumors are graded by their underlying architecture. Small cell carcinomas are not graded because they have unique clinicopathologic features and most importantly are treated differently from Gleason pattern 5 adenocarcinoma. The carcinomatous component of sarcomatoid carcinoma and adenosquamous carcinoma should be assigned a Gleason score
   For all types of specimen (needle, TURP, enucleation, radical prostatectomy), when there is a minor secondary component (<5% of tumor) and where the secondary component is of higher grade, the latter should be reported. For instance, a case showing >95% Gleason pattern 3 and <5% Gleason pattern 4 should be reported as Gleason score 3 + 4 = 7. Conversely, if a minor secondary pattern is of lower

grade, it need not be reported. For instance, where there is >95% Gleason score 4 and <5% Gleason 3, the score should be reported as Gleason score 4 + 4 = 8. These aggressive cases with only a few glands of Gleason pattern 3 should be distinguished from cases with a more prominent secondary Gleason pattern 3, which are assigned a Gleason score of 4 + 3 = 7

In needle biopsy specimens, it is recommended that separate Gleason scores be assigned for each specimen container. This is most critical for the situation where the grade for the tumor in one container is Gleason score 4 + 4 = 8 and the others are of lower grade. In these cases, the tumor behaves according to the highest grade (e.g., Gleason score 4 + 4 = 8) and not the composite (overall) score, which would be lower. Further support for assigning separate Gleason scores for different containers is that the Gleason grade factored into currently existing tables and nomograms (e.g., Partin tables, Kattan nomograms), which predict the stage and prognosis of prostate cancer, used the highest Gleason score in a case and not the composite (global) score. Providing a global or composite score reflecting the overall Gleason score in the entire specimen is optional

In needle biopsy specimens where more than two patterns are present and the worst grade is neither the predominant nor the secondary grade, the predominant and highest grade should be chosen to arrive at a score (e.g., 75% pattern 3, 20% pattern 4, and 5% pattern 5) and is assigned a Gleason score 3 + 5 = 8. It is assumed that a minor component of high-grade cancer on needle represents a sampling artifact, where it is likely that there will be a significant amount of the high-grade cancer in the prostate

In TURP or enucleation specimens, where one cannot identify separate tumor nodules, only one Gleason score is assigned. In radical prostatectomy specimens, each dominant tumor nodule is assigned a separate Gleason score. It is not necessary to assign a separate score to each small, multifocal, low-grade cancer focus in the setting of a larger higher-grade dominant nodule. In the case where there is no dominant tumor nodule, it can be stated that there are multifocal tumor nodules with a comment as to their grades. In TURP, enucleation, and radical prostatectomy specimens, the Gleason score is based on the primary (most common) and secondary (next most common) pattern. If there is a third pattern or if the second pattern occupies less than 5% of the specimen, then this pattern is reported as a tertiary pattern

3. **Tumor extent:** in core biopsies, the absolute number of involved cores should be reported out of the total number of cores received. In cases with fragmented cores where one cannot accurately derive the number of involved or total number of intact cores, one can merely state the overall percentage of the fragmented specimen involved by cancer. In addition, one should provide one other more detailed measurement of cancer, such as the linear extent of involvement in millimeters (either per core or total) or the percentage of cancer in each involved core. There is no consensus whether one should give the linear extent or percentage of involved core by either counting gaps of uninvolved tissue in the measurement or by 'collapsing' the tumor by ignoring the intervening gaps of benign tissue. As different foci of cancer along a core most likely represent the same tumor as opposed to multifocal cancer, it is preferred to record the tumor extent including the uninvolved tissue in the measurement because it more accurately represents the minimal extent of the cancer in the prostate. To distinguish small discontinuous foci from continuous cancer, one can report the following: 'Small foci of cancer discontinuously involving *X*% of the length of the core', where '*X*' is measured from one end of the cancer to the other on the core regardless of intervening benign tissue

   In TURP and enucleation specimens, the percentage of tissue involved by carcinoma is reported, with 5% the cutoff between T1a and T1b disease

   There are no uniform data that tumor volume in radical prostatectomy specimens is an independent predictive parameter of prognosis once other standard parameters are recorded. Nonetheless, it is recommended that some measurement of tumor volume be recorded even if it is a subjective quantification of 'minimal, moderate, and extensive'. If more precise measurements are required by the clinician, an 'eyeball' estimate of the percentage of the specimen involved by cancer is sufficient
4. **Margins of resection:** the entire surface of a radical prostatectomy specimen should be inked to evaluate the surgical margins. Usually, surgical margins should be designated as 'negative' if tumor is not present at the inked margin and as 'positive' if tumor cells touch the ink at the margin. When tumor is located very closely to an inked surface but is not actually in contact with the ink, it is considered negative. Positive surgical margins should not be interpreted as extraprostatic extension (EPE). Intraprostatic margins are positive in the setting of capsular incision (so-called Pt2+ or Pt2x disease). The specific locations of the positive margins are useful to report, and there should be some indication of the extent of margin positivity (e.g., unifocal versus multifocal, or focal versus extensive, or number of positive sites (blocks) or linear extent in millimeters)

   The apical and bladder neck surgical margins should be submitted entirely, preferably with a perpendicular sectioning technique. Microscopic involvement of bladder neck muscle fibers in radical prostatectomy specimens should not be equated with a Pt4 designation. The latter generally requires gross involvement of the bladder neck. A recent study has shown that patients with microscopic bladder neck involvement have recurrence rates similar to patients with seminal vesicle involvement (Pt3b)
5. **Extraprostatic extension (EPE):** this is the preferred term for the presence of tumor beyond the confines of the prostate gland. Tumor abutting on or admixed with fat constitutes EPE and in general is the only method to reliably diagnose EPE on needle biopsy. However, if one relies on the identification of tumor in fat to diagnose EPE on radical prostatectomy specimens, EPE will be underdiagnosed. One should also diagnose EPE when tumor extends beyond the condensed smooth muscle of the prostate to involve the looser connective tissue and thinner, less compact smooth muscle outside of the prostate. One can also use the overall scanning magnification to assess whether tumor has extended beyond the normal contour of the gland. Reporting EPE at the apex is controversial because the boundaries of the prostate gland in this region are vague; benign prostatic acini are seen admixed with skeletal muscle in this region. One option is merely to state whether tumor is present and whether the margins are positive or negative in the apical region while not attempting to determine if tumor is organ-confined in this area

The other option is to assume that the urologist has gone as wide as possible, and the inked margin at the apex is outside of the prostate. Tumor not extending to the ink is considered organ-confined, and tumor at the inked margin is considered as showing EPE, unless benign prostatic glands are also seen at the inked margin whereby capsular incision is diagnosed. The specific location(s) of EPE are useful to report. Descriptors of EPE (unifocal versus multifocal, or focal versus nonfocal, or focal versus extensive, or linear extent in millimeters or number of blocks) may be used

6. **Lymph node status:** indicate the number of nodes involved and the total number of nodes evaluated
7. **Angiolymphatic invasion:** this finding is independently predictive of prognosis in radical prostatectomy specimens and should be recorded. The Association does not recommend the routine use of immunohistochemical stains to detect intravascular invasion
8. **Perineurial invasion:** perineurial invasion in needle biopsy cores has been associated with EPE in most correlative radical prostatectomy studies, although its value as an independent prognostic factor has been questioned. Perineurial invasion has been found to be an independent risk factor for predicting an adverse outcome in patients treated with external beam radiation. Because it is easily measured and appears to have prognostic significance on biopsy, regardless of whether it is an independently prognostic parameter, its presence should be recorded on needle biopsy specimens. Perineurial invasion has no prognostic significance in radical prostatectomy specimens and should not be mentioned in the pathology report
9. **Prostatic intraepithelial neoplasia (PIN):** Generally, low-grade PIN is not reported. The presence of isolated high-grade PIN (HGPIN) should be reported in all biopsy specimens. The risk of cancer on repeat biopsy within 1 year of a needle biopsy diagnosis of HGPIN is not sufficiently different from the risk of cancer on repeat biopsy after a benign diagnosis on needle biopsy. Consequently, immediate repeat biopsy after a needle biopsy diagnosis of HGPIN is not necessary. Whether and when a repeat biopsy should be performed remains to be studied. The reporting of HGPIN in prostatectomy specimens is optional
10. **Staging:** It is necessary to provide the TNM staging for radical prostatectomy specimens. The subdividing of pathologically organ-confined disease whether the tumor involves less than one-half of one lobe (Pt2a), involves more than one-half of one lobe (Pt2b), or involves both lobes (Pt2c) has been criticized. This aspect of the staging system will be changed in future revisions, and many urologic pathologists do not subdivide Pt2 tumor using the current system. Adenocarcinoma of the prostate is multifocal in more than 85% of cases. In many of these cases of bilateral and/or multifocal tumor, the other tumors are small, low-grade, and clinically insignificant. Consequently, the distinction between pathologic stages T2a and T2c may reflect several very different conditions: (1) a large single tumor nodule involving both sides; (2) separate large tumor nodules on each side; (3) dominant nodule on one side with multifocal minute tumor on the other side; or (4) bilateral minute multifocal tumor. Prognostically, there are no differences between the subdivisions of Pt2. Stage Pt2b tumor almost never exists because it is almost impossible for a tumor to involve greater than one-half of the lobe without involving the other lobe. However, using the current staging system for subdividing Pt2 tumor remains an option. It is now recommended by the American College of Surgeons and will be updated in the new TNM Staging System such that pathologists do not fill in a 'Pm' (metastasis) category because that is the domain of the clinician
11. **Submission of tissue for microscopic evaluation in TURP and radical prostatectomy specimens:** TURP specimens should be sampled with 8 cassettes. In a younger man (e.g., <65 years), consideration should be given to more extensive sampling. Some experts suggest submitting additional cassettes based on the weight of the TURP. In general, random chips are submitted. If an unsuspected carcinoma is found in tissue submitted and it involves 5% or less of the tissue examined, the remaining tissue is generally submitted for microscopic examination, especially in younger patients

    Radical prostatectomy specimens may be totally submitted or partially sampled in a systematic fashion. For partial sampling in the setting of a grossly visible tumor, the sections with visible tumor along with the entire apical and bladder neck margins and samples from the base of each seminal vesicle should be submitted. If there is no grossly visible tumor, a number of systematic sampling strategies may be used. One that yields excellent prognostic information involves submitting the posterior aspect of each transverse slice along with a mid anterior block from each side. The anterior sampling detects tumors, which predominantly involve the transition zone. The entire apical and bladder neck margins and base of each seminal vesicle should also be submitted

Skin – melanoma

Final report – recommended features

Gross description

The following detailed description is most appropriate for excision biopsy specimens. Small biopsy specimens need less detail

1. **Specimen identification:** e.g., labeled with name, medical record number, etc.
2. **Specimen condition:** e.g., fresh, in fixative
3. **Site:** the exact anatomic site of the tumor
4. **Type of procedure:** excision or re-excision, incision biopsy, punch biopsy, shave biopsy, curettage, other
5. **Size:** dimensions of the specimen (length × width × thickness or, in the case of small biopsy specimens and punch biopsy specimens, maximum diameter × thickness)
6. **Measure and describe** the pigmented lesion
    - Length × width of pigmented lesion. Is the edge of the lesion regular or irregular?
    - Maximum diameter of the dominant nodule (as opposed to the diameter of dominant nodule plus the radial growth phase) (see Note 1a)
    - Ulceration or intactness of skin over the dominant nodule
    - Description of any other pigmented lesions that may be present in the specimen (diameter, elevated or flat, color(s) – uniform or variegated, ulcerated or not, regular or irregular edge)
    - Measurement of the position of additional pigmented lesion(s) relative to the dominant lesion and the nearest excision margin
    - Description of any other lesions present (e.g., scars, areas of vitiligo)

- Measurement of the minimum distance between the edge of the dominant lesion or radial growth phase (whichever is appropriate) and the nearest surgical margin (minimum clearance)

Diagnostic information

1. **Tumor type:** when possible, state whether the lesion is primary, locally recurrent, or metastatic to the site. If the lesion is not primary but lies in the dermis and/or subcutis in the area of the primary lesion it is:
   - In continuity with the primary tumor or a local scar – a persistent melanoma
   - Not in continuity with the primary tumor or a local scar – a satellite
2. **State** whether there is microscopic evidence of ulceration (see Note 3). If so, include the width of ulceration as measured with an ocular micrometer
3. **Histogenetic type:** this determination requires consideration of the gross appearance and clinical information concerning patient age, lesional site and duration, and any history of dysplastic nevi. This information is required for treatment planning and epidemiologic studies
4. **Measure** the thickness of the invasive component of the tumor in millimeters and tenths of millimeters as measured with an ocular micrometer as described by Breslow. The tumor is measured from the granular layer of the epidermis (or, when appropriate, the base of an ulcer to the deepest contiguous tumor cell, excluding tumor sheathing skin appendages) (see Note 4)
5. **Assess the depth of penetration** of the dermis relative to standard anatomic landmarks, when possible
6. **Assess the frequency of mitotic figures** per millimeter squared in the vertical growth phase (invasive nodule), if present. This is regarded as a prognostically important observation, although other authors disagree, and not all pathologists record this information
7. **Record whether there is obvious evidence of invasion** of dermal blood vessels or lymphatics. Immunohistochemical confirmation using the agglutinin of *Ulex europaeus* I or antibody to factor VIII-related antigen is optional
8. **Record desmoplasia or stromal myxoid change,** if present
9. **Report neurotropism,** if present
10. **Report whether melanoma (invasive or radial growth phase) is present** at or near the peripheral or deep 'surgical' margin and record in millimeters (using a micrometer) the minimum distance between the tumor nearest the peripheral and deep margins
11. **Record whether there is evidence of regression** subjacent to the radial growth phase or within the vertical growth phase. Regressive changes comprise foci of fibrosis that are variably cellular and variably infiltrated by lymphoid cells and macrophages and that are not due to previous surgical intervention

    Note 1a: The radial growth phase is the usually flat pigmentary abnormality that lies peripheral to the vertical growth phase (invasive component) of most primary melanomas

    Note 1b: Microscopically, a radial growth phase shows an increase in invariably atypical melanocytes, singly or in small colonies, in a basal or suprabasal position, with or without the presence of single melanoma cells in the upper papillary dermis

    Note 2: If the lesion is nonprimary, several of the items in the text are not relevant

    Note 3: It is useful to attempt to separate ulceration that is post-traumatic, i.e., secondary to a shave or punch biopsy or self-inflicted damage from ulceration that is 'nontraumatic' or 'spontaneous'. This determination requires detailed clinical information and correlation

    Note 4: It is now common to include satellites in the Breslow measurement, although some authors argue against their inclusion. If microsatellites are included in this measurement, it is important to record that the measurement has been made in this way

    Note 5: We have not included mucosal lentiginous melanoma because these recommendations refer to cutaneous melanoma

Final report – optional features

1. **Record the degree of pigmentation:** all kinds of melanoma may be amelanotic, so absence of pigment does not constitute a histogenetic subclass
2. **If a radial growth phase is present,** state whether it is pagetoid, lentiginous, or unclassifiable
3. **Record the dominant cell type:** epithelioid (round–oval) *versus* spindle (elongated) *versus* spitzoid *versus* nevocytoid *versus* balloon *versus* other. List other cell types that are present
4. **Record whether there is a nevus contiguous to the melanoma:** Is this adjacent to the melanoma? Record the type of nevus (common congenital *versus* common acquired *versus* dysplastic *versus* Spitz *versus* blue *versus* cellular blue *versus* combined nevus)
5. **Record the density and distribution** of any lymphoreticular cell infiltrate that is present:
   - Within the vertical growth phase (invasive component) and disrupting nests of melanoma cells (intratumor)
   - Peripheral to the invasive component as a band-like infiltrate
6. **Record whether necrosis is present**
   - Multicellular necrosis
7. **Record the presence of unusual features,** such as heterologous elements, e.g., bone, cartilage

Checklist

- Site
- Procedure
- Excision
- Incision biopsy (including punch)
- Shave biopsy
- Other (specify):
- Lesion is confirmed as primary
  — Yes — No
- Ulceration
- No ulceration
- Histogenetic pattern: see Note 5 above
  Malignant melanoma, no adjacent component (AC)[a] (nodular)
  With AC, superficial spreading melanoma type
  With AC, lentigo maligna type
  With AC, acral lentiginous type

[a]Adjacent component is synonymous with radial growth phase

Desmoplastic
Of the type that simulates Spitz, nevocytic nevus, other lesions
Unclassifiable

- Clark level
  — I — II — III
  — IV — V
- Breslow thickness
  — × — mm
- Mitotic rate
  — /mm^2
- Regressive fibrosis present
  — Yes — No
- Excision
  Complete
  Not complete peripherally (indicate affected margin)
  Not complete in depth
  Not complete peripherally and in depth
- Vascular invasion
  Absent
  Blood vessels
  Lymphatic vessels
  Blood and lymphatic vessels
- Microsatellites
  — Present — Absent
- Neurotropism
  — Present — Absent
- Lymph node involvement (complete as appropriate)
  Number of nodes containing tumor/total no. of nodes
  Not applicable

Skin – nonmelanocytic neoplasms

Final report – recommended features

Gross description

1. **Specimen identification:** how was specimen labeled
2. **Specimen condition:** received fresh or in fixative
3. **Specimen type:** i.e., excision, punch, shave, curetting; clinical orientation (if supplied) and measured in three dimensions
4. **Describe** the epidermis and the dermis, if present. Describe grossly identifiable lesions, their size and their extent with regards to the edges of the specimen. Note the presence or absence of subcutaneous fat and gross extent of lesion into fat
5. **If specimen is inked,** note color(s). If multiple colors are used to designate specific margins, give a key
6. **Describe** sectioning and indicate whether or not the entire specimen was submitted for histologic examination
7. **Supply paraffin block key**

Diagnostic information

1. **Tissue:** list types included in the specimen (i.e., stratum corneum only, epidermis only, skin, skin and subcutaneous tissue)
2. **Specimen type:** see Gross description
3. **Location:** as supplied by clinician
4. **Diagnosis:** there is no universally accepted classification of nonmelanocytic skin tumors. The most recent WHO classification is recommended as a general guide for the classification of epithelial and mesenchymal neoplasms which primarily arise in the skin. This can be supplemented with the more complete listing of soft tissue tumors found in the most recent WHO classification
   The classification of lymphoproliferative diseases is still evolving rapidly. In addition to the Kiel and REAL classifications, the European Organization for Research and Treatment of Cancer (EORTC) has reached consensus on a new classification for primary cutaneous lymphomas. It has the advantage of combining clinical, histologic and immunophenotypic criteria for well-defined disease entities
   The skin is frequently the site of metastasis. Whenever possible, the histology of the metastatic lesion should be compared with that of the primary (if known). In the case of an occult primary, an attempt should be made to develop a differential diagnosis and to focus it through the use of special stains, immunocytochemistry or other ancillary studies. In the case of secondary involvement of the skin by leukemic infiltrates or by extracutaneous lymphoma, the cutaneous lesion(s) should correlate with the material upon which the original diagnosis was made, and if appropriate, classified in like fashion
5. **Tumor grade:** degree of differentiation (e.g., Broder) should be indicated for invasive squamous cell carcinomas and adnexal adenocarcinomas. Basal cell carcinomas should be subtyped so as to alert the clinician to the presence of an aggressive pattern of growth. Sarcomas should be graded as low grade or high grade. Mitotic index (preferably reported as mitoses per mm^2) should be reported for tumors in which such data are useful for assessing malignant potential (e.g., smooth muscle tumors)
6. **Tumor behavior:** include the presence or absence of skin ulceration, lymphovascular involvement, perineurial invasion, involvement of skin adnexa (by squamous cell carcinoma in situ), etc. Where the clinician is unlikely to be familiar with the biologic behavior of a particular tumor, such information should be reported in a comment
7. **Tumor extent:** tumor size, extent with regards to anatomic/ histologic landmarks (e.g., extension into subcutis) should be noted
8. **Surgical margins:** these should be reported for those specimen types for which margins can be reliably assessed. Measurement by (calibrated) ocular micrometer is indicated for those instances in which the tumor approaches, but cannot be demonstrated to actually involve, a surgical margin
9. **Lymph nodes:** report the presence or absence of metastatic lesions in any lymph nodes included in the specimen. If a node dissection was performed, state the number of nodes sampled and the number of nodes involved. The presence or absence of extranodal involvement should be noted
10. **Histochemistry, immunocytochemistry, ancillary studies:** results of these studies should be included either in the 'diagnosis' section or in a separate microscopic comment
11. **Additional comments:** information relating to tumor behavior (metastatic potential), if pertinent, or association of a particular tumor with a defined clinical syndrome should be included in a comment

Stomach – carcinoma – resection

(From Robert ME, Lamps L, Lauwers GY. Recommendations for the reporting of gastric carcinoma. Hum Pathol 2008, **39:** 10–13.)

Final report – recommended features

Gross examination

Gastric biopsies

Gastric biopsies should be carefully matched with patient identification. In the case of multiple specimen containers from the same patient, great care should be taken to further identify specific sites sampled as indicated by the clinician on the specimen jar and pathology requisition form (e.g., gastric fundus, gastric antrum, gastric mass). Any discrepancy between the number of specimens, specimen labels, and the requisition sheet should be resolved immediately, before gross examination, by contacting the clinician. Documentation of specimen identification issues should be written and included with the requisition so that the pathologist is aware of the change before sign-out.

Many biopsy specimens are submitted in formalin. If tissue arrives fresh, triage of tissue for special studies, such as flow cytometry or electron microscopy, can occur as needed. Special handling is usually not needed for epithelial tumors.

The number of biopsy specimens in each container should be exactly specified in the gross dictation. This helps to properly identify each specimen when there is a question of specimen mislabeling or other issues with tissue identification. Specimens should be carefully oriented before placing in cassettes to ensure the best possible orientation on sections.

Gastric endoscopic mucosal resections

The specimen should be carefully matched with patient identification. Any concerns regarding identification or orientation should be resolved before gross dissection. The number of tissue fragments in each container should be exactly specified in the gross dictation.

If not previously done in the endoscopy suite, endoscopic mucosal resections (EMRs) should be carefully oriented (mucosa up), stretched, pinned down on a firm base, and fixed for at least 12 hours in formalin. After fixation, the surgical margins (lateral and deep) must be carefully inked. The specimen must be submitted entirely in sequential sections after ensuring the best possible orientation, routinely processed, and stained with hematoxylin and eosin. Care must be taken to orient the sections such that the circumferential (lateral) surgical margins are assessed, either 'en face' or in cross sections, depending on the size of the specimen. If provided by the clinician, further orientation as to specific margins should be documented and sections appropriately submitted.

Gastric resections for carcinoma

Gastric resections should be carefully matched with patient identification. All resections should be imaged fresh, in both the unopened and the opened state to document the most important pathologic findings. Additional images can be taken at various stages of gross examination, including after fixation and after further sectioning as needed, to document tumor location and depth. When opening the stomach, do not cut through tumor if at all possible. Cutting along the greater curvature is preferred.

When resections are sent for frozen section, it may be necessary to ink and cut certain aspects of the specimen in the fresh state. In most cases, only surgical margins need to be evaluated at the time of frozen section. The location of the tumor and distance to all surgical margins should be noted. If the tumor needs to be sampled for frozen section (a practice to be discouraged unless a true surgical decision will be made as a result), great care should be taken to cut the lesion in a manner that preserves anatomic relationships. Ink should be applied sparsely, so that it does not contaminate nonsurgical margins. After frozen sections have been completed and before fixation, tissue for special studies should be procured if needed (flow cytometry, cytogenetics, electron microscopy). Again, for gastric epithelial tumors special studies are not usually needed or can be performed on paraffin sections.

Gross examination of gastrointestinal resections takes place in two stages, before and after fixation. After the specimen has been imaged and opened, a careful gross examination and description of the mucosal and serosal surfaces should be completed. If not already accomplished, careful measurements of the tumor, its location, and the distance to all surgical margins, should be noted. The serosal surface and any surgical margins not already sampled should be inked. The specimen should then be fixed overnight (if in formalin) or for a length of time suitable to the fixative used. Before fixing, the tumor can be thinly sectioned if needed to aid fixation. This is not necessary in most cases. The tumor should not be cut completely through if this can be avoided, as retraction of the serosal margin can result in the appearance of a false-positive margin.

After fixation, the gross dissection is completed. All lesions should be serially sectioned and thoroughly examined. Additional images can be taken at this time. The depth of invasion of the tumor through the gastric wall and relationship to the serosal margin should be stated in the gross description. Any other lesions should be described. Sections should be submitted for microscopy that demonstrate the lesion, the depth of invasion, relation to adjacent benign tissue, all surgical margins, including the serosal margin, random sections of uninvolved stomach, any other lesions, and all lymph nodes. After careful gross examination for lymph nodes, a clearing solution may be used if available to ensure the retrieval of all lymph nodes present within the specimen. This practice is institution dependent and may be of questionable value in terms of identifying metastases. However, the use of clearing solutions usually increases the number of lymph nodes retrieved. At least 15 lymph nodes should be retrieved to ensure correct staging. However, the number of lymph nodes retrieved in gastrectomy specimens depends to some degree on the extent of the resection and amount of mesenteric fat included.

Summary of recommended sections

Tumor for diagnosis

- Depth of invasion
- Margins: proximal, distal, radial (see Note 1)
- Lymph nodes
- Relation of tumor to adjacent stomach

  Note 1: Radial margins in gastrectomy specimens are usually serosal-lined surfaces. Tumors that extend into the esophagus may also have a pertinent margin that is a true surgical margin transected by the surgeon. The use of the term radial margin encompasses both settings.

Sections of uninvolved stomach to assess background mucosa

- Gastritis and *Helicobacter pylori* status
- Atrophy
- Dysplasia

Other lesions (i.e., polyps)

Microscopic examination

Gastric biopsies

Gastric biopsies obtained to confirm or exclude the clinical suspicion of malignancy can be extremely challenging for the pathologist because of the usually small size of diagnostic material and the high rate of sampling error. Stated simply, biopsy results from visible gastric lesions may be: (1) positive for invasive tumor; (2) positive for in situ neoplasia (dysplasia); (3) negative for neoplasia; or (4) indeterminate for neoplasia. Each of these scenarios dictates a distinct recommendation from the pathologist. It is vital that the pathologist communicates directly with the clinician to make the correct recommendations. The following is a list of possible diagnoses on gastric biopsies from epithelial tumors and their consequences:

1. **Positive for carcinoma**
   - There should be unequivocal evidence of invasive tumor present
   - The neoplasm may be intramucosal with invasion limited to the lamina propria. The distinction from high-grade dysplasia with marked architectural changes may be challenging. Desmoplasia may be absent. This diagnosis is best made on well-oriented biopsy specimens. Alternatively, there may be evidence of submucosal invasion with well-developed desmoplasia
   - The histologic subtype should be stated if possible (e.g., intestinal type, signet ring carcinoma)
   - Implied in this diagnosis is 100% certainty. Definitive therapy will be based on the pathology report, with no need for additional biopsies to confirm the pathologic diagnosis. If there is any doubt as to the diagnosis, review by a second pathologist is encouraged. Any concerns regarding the diagnosis that preclude definitive therapy as a next step should be communicated with the clinician at least in writing and preferably verbally as well
2. **Positive for dysplasia** (intraepithelial neoplasia)
   - Dysplasia should be classified, using published criteria, as low or high grade
   - If in a visible lesion, the lesion must be completely excised to exclude an invasive component. (This must be communicated to the clinician.) Sometimes a biopsy specimen showing dysplasia is from a lesion that was obviously malignant at endoscopy, but was inadequately sampled. If the diagnosis of dysplasia is certain in this setting, there is usually no need to obtain additional biopsy specimens just to demonstrate the invasive component
   - If dysplasia is found in a random biopsy (usually in the setting of gastric atrophy), a recommendation for gastric mapping should be made. Frequent follow-up is appropriate. Gastric mapping involves extensive sampling of the body and antrum at intervals depending on the extent and severity of dysplasia discovered (low versus high grade). The decision of when to perform gastrectomy for dysplasia (low or high grade) in the setting of gastric atrophy is center dependent
3. **Negative for dysplasia or carcinoma:** in the setting of a visible lesion, a negative biopsy result raises the concern for a false negative due to sampling error. Signet ring cell carcinoma is often difficult to sample with standard biopsy forceps. Large malignant ulcers are also notoriously difficult to sample because of necrosis and inflammation. All clinically suspicious lesions must be rebiopsied, often with endoscopic ultrasound and other radiologic evaluation
4. **Indeterminate for neoplasia** (either in situ or invasive): because of ulceration and small sample size, gastric biopsies from suspicious lesions may show worrisome atypia that is insufficient for a definitive diagnosis of malignancy. In this setting, deeper sections, a second opinion, and special stains may be valuable. However, there should be no hesitation to request additional biopsies to obtain a firm diagnosis. Equivocal histology should never be 'overcalled'. A good guideline to use when deciding how to phrase the report is to ask yourself the question, 'Do I want to receive the resected stomach as a specimen?'
5. **Additional information to be included in the report:** if nonlesional gastric mucosa is present, it should be assessed for gastritis, *H. pylori*, atrophy, intestinal metaplasia, and any other changes
6. **Gastroesophageal junction (GEJ) tumors:** adenocarcinomas that straddle the GEJ can be difficult to classify as to site of origin (stomach versus esophagus). Because adenocarcinoma of the distal esophagus is treated differently from gastric cancer, it is important to clarify the site of origin if at all possible. This distinction frequently requires correlation of pathologic, endoscopic, and radiologic information. The decision cannot be made on the basis of tumor morphology at biopsy or resection alone. However, the presence of intestinal metaplasia in the esophagus adjacent to tumor (Barrett esophagus) lends support to an esophageal primary origin in ambiguous cases. Otherwise, the site of primary tumor is usually determined by location of the dominant or central portion of tumor

Gastric EMRs

Gastric EMRs are usually obtained after a diagnosis of high-grade dysplasia or malignancy has been established on biopsy. EMRs have three functions: (1) diagnostic; (2) therapeutic; and (3) guidance with regard to determination of further treatment. Because EMRs are performed with a curative intent, they should be handled and reported as surgical specimens and, therefore, the role of the surgical pathologist is crucial. Appropriate reporting is essential in guiding additional therapeutic options.

The list of possible diagnoses on gastric EMRs includes the following:

1. **Positive for carcinoma:** three features should be evaluated and reported: (1) the degree of differentiation; (2) the depth of invasion; and (3) the status of the margins (lateral and deep) and overall completeness of excision. Finally, the status of vascular invasion should also be reported, especially in cases with submucosal extension
2. **Positive for dysplasia or intraepithelial neoplasia:** dysplasia should be classified as low or high grade using published criteria. All reports should include the status of the lateral mucosal surgical margins regarding dysplasia
3. **Negative for dysplasia or intraepithelial neoplasia**

Note 2: Technical artifacts such as hemorrhage and electrodiathermic burns should be mentioned in the report if they limit the histologic interpretation.

Gastric resections

The role of the pathologist in examining gastric resections is usually not to determine the diagnosis, but to accurately stage and categorize a lesion that has been previously diagnosed by biopsy or other techniques. Nonetheless, care should be taken to ensure that tissues are adequately sampled and saved for special techniques before fixation if needed to confirm a diagnosis (e.g., flow cytometry, electron microscopy, cytogenetics). The following discussion pertains to gastric carcinoma. Refer to the AJCC staging manual and WHO classification of gastric tumors for additional detail. This guideline emphasizes the elements to be assessed and included in the pathology report for the purposes of uniformity and completeness:

1. **Tumor location**
   - Cardia, fundus, body, antrum, pylorus
   - Lesser or greater curvature, anterior wall, posterior wall

   Note 3: The distinction between gastric cardia cancer and lower esophageal adenocarcinoma arising in the setting of Barrett esophagus can be difficult. In general, if the center of the lesion is within the stomach, gastric carcinoma is favored, and vice versa. If esophageal tissue (either from previous biopsies or from the resection) reveals intestinal metaplasia, this can be used as evidence of esophageal adenocarcinoma in cases where the lesion is predominantly within the GEJ. It should be understood that there will be cases where the designation as to gastric or esophageal primary will have to be made arbitrarily, using all information available. However, a three-tiered classification scheme of GEJ tumors has been proposed. Type I tumors have an epicenter located entirely in the distal esophagus and within 1–5 cm above but not involving the GEJ. Type III cancers have epicenters entirely within the proximal stomach and 2–5 cm below the GEJ. Type II tumors have their epicenters between 1 cm above and 2 cm below the GEJ
2. **Growth pattern of advanced cancer:** this is an optional feature that may be included in pathology reports (from Bormann classification):
   - Type 1, polypoid
   - Type 2, fungating
   - Type 3, ulcerated
   - Type 4, diffusely infiltrative (linitis plastica)
3. **Tumor type** (modified from WHO classification):
   - Adenocarcinoma
     - Intestinal type
     - Diffuse type (implies a significant component of signet ring cell carcinoma; see Note 4)
   - Papillary adenocarcinoma
   - Tubular adenocarcinoma
   - Mucinous adenocarcinoma
   - Adenosquamous carcinoma
   - Squamous cell carcinoma
   - Lymphoepithelioma-like carcinoma
   - Carcinoid tumor
   - Atypical carcinoid tumor
   - Small cell carcinoma
   - Undifferentiated carcinoma
   - Other (e.g., hepatoid variant of adenocarcinoma)

   Note 4: Frequently, both intestinal and signet ring morphology are present in the same tumor
4. **Grade** (applies primarily to gland-forming variants)
   - Well differentiated – well-formed glands
   - Moderately differentiated – some gland formation and areas with single cells or islands
   - Poorly differentiated – irregular glands, single cells, nests

   Note 5: By definition, signet ring cell carcinoma is poorly differentiated
5. **TNM staging** (see ADASP checklist and AJCC staging manual)
6. **Additional studies:** certain subtypes of carcinoma may require additional studies or be associated with syndromes:
   - Epstein–Barr virus testing in lymphoepithelioma-like carcinoma
   - E-cadherin (CDH1) molecular analysis in patients with a strong family history of diffuse gastric carcinoma. This should be at the request of the clinician and with consideration for family genetic counseling
   - Microsatellite instability testing in patients with a suspicion of hereditary nonpolyposis colon cancer syndrome
   - Rarely, gastric cancer is seen in the setting of familial polyposis syndrome and Peutz–Jeghers syndrome
7. **Status of non-neoplastic stomach:** every report of gastric carcinoma should state *H. pylori* status and degree and type of gastritis (i.e., multifocal atrophic or autoimmune), if present. Specifically, the presence of intestinal metaplasia and dysplasia should be noted

Testis and adnexa

Final report – recommended features

Gross description

1. **Specimen identification:** patient's name, case number, laterality, specimen identification ('labeled as')
2. **Specimen condition:** fresh, in formalin, intact, incised by surgeon or pathologists, etc.
3. **Number of specimen containers**
4. **Structures attached to testis:** epididymis, spermatic cord, tunica vaginalis
5. **Dimensions of all the specimens**
6. **Tumor description**
   - Site in testis/paratestis: central, inferior pole, superior pole, testicular hilum, epididymis, paratesticular soft tissue, spermatic cord
   - Tumor size, shape, consistency, color, cysts, scar, necrosis, hemorrhage, calcifications
   - Relationship to tunica albuginea
   - Relationship to epididymis and spermatic cord
   - If spermatic cord involvement, distance of tumor to cord, margin. It is recommended that sections of the spermatic cord be obtained before incision of the main tumor to avoid contamination
   - Satellite tumors, if present
7. **Other lesions of the testis**
8. **Tissue submitted for special study**

Diagnostic information

1. **Topography:** left or right testis
2. **Type of procedure:** as designated by surgeon, e.g., radical or simple orchiectomy
3. **Histologic type:** a modified classification of the World Health Organization (WHO) is recommended:
   - Germ cell tumors
     - Intratubular germ cell neoplasia
       - Unclassified type (IGCNU)
       - Other forms (specify):
     - Tumors of one histologic type
       - Seminoma: variant – seminoma with syncytiotrophoblastic cells
       - Spermatocytic seminoma: variant – spermatocytic seminoma with a sarcomatous component (specify type and grade of sarcoma):
       - Embryonal carcinoma
       - Yolk sac tumor
       - Choriocarcinoma: variant – 'Monophasic' choriocarcinoma

  - Placental site trophoblastic tumor
  - Teratoma
    - Mature
    - Immature
    - With a secondary malignant component ('teratoma with malignant transformation') (specify type):
    - Monodermal variants
- Carcinoid
- Primitive neuroectodermal tumor
- Other
  - Tumors of more than one histologic type
    - Mixed germ cell tumor (specify components and provide an estimate of percentage composition):
    - Polyembryoma
    - Diffuse embryoma
  - 'Burnt-out' germ cell tumor
- Sex cord–stromal tumors
  - Leydig cell tumor
  - Sertoli cell tumor
    - Not otherwise specified type
    - Large cell calcifying type
    - Sclerosing type
  - Sertoli–Leydig cell tumor
  - Granulosa cell tumor
    - Adult type
    - Juvenile type
- Mixed sex cord–stromal tumor
- Unclassified sex cord–stromal tumor
- Mixed germ cell–sex cord–stromal tumor
  - Gonadoblastoma
  - Others
- Miscellaneous
  - Lymphoma (classify according to guidelines for nodal lymphoma)
  - Plasmacytoma and multiple myeloma
  - Granulocytic sarcoma and multiple myeloma
  - Sarcoma (specify type and grade):
  - Carcinomas and borderline tumors of ovarian type (specify type and, for carcinomas, grade):
  - Adenocarcinoma of the rete testis
  - Adenocarcinoma of the epididymis
  - Melanotic neuroectodermal tumor (retinal anlage tumor)
  - Malignant mesothelioma (specify type):
  - Desmoplastic small round cell tumor
  - Other (specify):
- Secondary tumors

4. **Other features:** for tumors in the sex cord–stromal category (with the exception of the juvenile granulosa cell tumor) specify if adverse prognostic features are present or absent. The following are included:
   - Lymphovascular space invasion
   - Coagulative tumor cell necrosis
   - Significant cytologic atypia
   - High mitotic rate (specify number of mitotic figures per 10 high-power fields, averaged from 40 high-power fields)
   - Infiltrating borders
   - Extratesticular growth (see Note 1)
   - Large tumor size

   Note 1: According to the revised TNM staging system of the American Joint Committee on Cancer, only involvement of paratesticular soft tissue, tunica vaginalis, or spermatic cord are features of extratesticular spread that merit designation as Pt2 tumors; cases with rete testis or epididymal spread or tunica albuginea invasion without penetration remain Pt1 lesions in the absence of vascular invasion
5. **Other organs:** for tumors in categories other than the sex cord–stromal group, specify if there is lymphovascular space invasion or (for testicular tumors) extratesticular extension (see above-mentioned Note)
6. **Adequacy of local excision:** assessment of resection margins
7. **Other significant testicular disease**

Final report – optional features

1. **Stage:** the data specified should facilitate application of most staging systems. In most circumstances, the pathologist will not be aware of the nodal status or other studies to permit an assignment of stage; however, accurate local staging of the testicular tumor can be accomplished, either by providing all of the requisite information (as indicated above) or by specifying a local AP stage according to the revised system of The American Joint Committee on Cancer Staging
2. **Results of ancillary studies**
3. **Association of germ cell tumors with intratubular germ cell neoplasia of the unclassified type**
4. **Presence and type of inflammatory infiltrate**
5. **Multifocal tumor**

Thymus – thymoma – resection

(From Weydert JA, De Young BR, Leslie KO. Recommendations for the reporting of surgically resected thymic epithelial tumors. Hum Pathol 2009, **40:** 919–923.)

Final report – recommended features

Clinical information

1. **Mechanism of discovery of thymic mass**
   - Incidental radiographic finding
   - Workup of thoracic problem/complaint
   - Workup of systemic disorder (see below)
2. **History of myasthenia gravis,** pure red cell aplasia, or other autoimmune/paraneoplastic process
3. **History of previous thoracic surgery** for neoplastic disease

Gross description

1. **Specimen identification:** labeled with name, medical record number, etc.
2. **Specimen condition:** fresh, fixed, etc.
3. **Specimen weight** (g) and size (centimeters) in three dimensions
4. **Anatomic orientation** (if any) as provided by surgeon; ink identifiers by pathologist (specify color and anatomic correlation)
5. **Condition of the capsule:** intact, ruptured
6. **Attached tissues** (mediastinal fat, pleura, lung, chest wall, pericardium):
   - Ink identifiers by pathologist (specify color and anatomic correlation)
   - Correlation with imaging studies
   - Correlation with intraoperative findings per surgeon
7. **Tumor size:** measure size (centimeters) in three dimensions, largest dimension listed first

Note 1: Size (greatest linear dimension) has been reported to correlate with resectability and prognosis

8. **Describe** tumor color, texture, nodularity, necrosis, fibrous bands
9. **Relationship of tumor to capsule,** attached tissues, and surgical margins

   Note 2: Consultation with the surgeon during the gross examination is optimal to determine the completeness of surgical resection. Encapsulated or minimally invasive tumors (Masaoka stage I and II, respectively) with negative surgical margins do not generally require adjuvant therapy and demonstrate very low risk of recurrence
10. **Describe** non-neoplastic thymus and/or attached tissues

    Note 3: Non-neoplastic thymus, if not involuted, will be soft, golden yellow, and lobulated. Involuted thymic tissue may be indistinguishable from adipose tissue. In cases that are involved by marked follicular thymic hyperplasia, the non-neoplastic gland may take on a gray–tan, vaguely nodular appearance similar to lymph node
11. **Sampling:** At least five sections; one section per 1 cm of greatest tumor dimension for tumors greater than 5 cm

    Note 4: Accurate histologic classification requires adequate sampling. Five sections of tumor is a reasonable starting point, and increasing the number of sections increases the likelihood of detecting microscopic transcapsular invasion. Gross extracapsular extension should be directly sampled
12. **Intraoperative consultation (frozen section):** thymoma shares the mediastinum as a primary site with other malignancies, including mediastinal Hodgkin lymphoma, non-Hodgkin lymphomas, and mediastinal germ cell tumors. If a preoperative pathologic diagnosis is not obtained, the surgeon may elect for intraoperative pathology consultation to determine the need for complete resection. Both frozen section and cytologic preparations (smear and/or touch imprint) may be useful in this setting and may assist with triage of the tissue for special studies before further handling. The most difficult issue at stake for the pathologist is distinguishing lymphoma from thymic epithelial tumors. If a definite diagnosis cannot be rendered, a portion of tissue should be saved fresh frozen and in tissue culture media in the event that molecular, flow cytometric, and/or cytogenetic studies are needed
13. **Lymph nodes**
    - Anatomic location(s) and number of pieces/nodes per location
    - Presence or absence of grossly viable tumor

    Note 5: Lymph node dissections are not performed routinely in thymectomy for thymoma. However, lymph node dissections may be performed in cases where other malignancies have not been comfortably excluded before resection of mediastinal tumor

Diagnostic information

Thymic epithelial neoplasm: thymoma

The histologic classification of thymoma is outwardly complex due to the various existing classification schemes that are in clinical use. Each classification scheme has its merits and drawbacks. For the sake of uniformity and clinical relevance, we propose that the World Health Organization (WHO) and/or the Suster–Moran systems be used in reporting of thymoma. The 2004 modification of the WHO classification was built upon the histogenetic/functional classification of Muller-Hermelink (MH). The WHO system uses letter and numerical designations (A, AB, B1, B2, B3) in an attempt to facilitate clinically relevant communication and comparison of thymoma histology across clinical studies and among pathologists. This classification scheme, like the MH scheme, is prognostically significant; however, reproducibility is an issue, particularly for those who may not encounter many thymomas in routine practice. Suster and Moran proposed a simplified schema in 1999, which essentially condensed thymic epithelial tumors into three histologic groups based on architectural morphology and epithelial cytology: thymoma, atypical thymoma, and thymic carcinoma. The Suster–Moran 'thymoma' includes WHO subtypes A, AB, B1, B2, whereas 'atypical thymoma' corresponds to WHO subtype B3. This simplified scheme has been shown to have good reproducibility and, more importantly, carries adequate prognostic power with regard to survival and recurrence. Whether one chooses to use the WHO or Suster–Moran system (or both) is a matter of local standard of practice, that is, one must pick a classification that best suits the needs of local surgeons and oncologists. Other classification systems may be used; however, we recommend that either the WHO or the Suster–Moran nomenclature (or both) be parenthetically added to the report if another classification system is being used.

Classification of thymoma (World Health Organization Classification 2004/Suster–Moran 1999)

1. **Thymoma, Type A (WHO)/Thymoma (Suster–Moran):** Type A thymoma is characterized by bland-appearing spindled-to-ovoid epithelial cells that recapitulate the appearance of involuted thymus and demonstrate few intraepithelial lymphocytes, if any. Many architectural patterns have been described, including solid sheets, rosettes, glands, and hemangiopericytoma-like patterns. This type of thymoma best corresponds to the 'medullary' thymoma of MH
2. **Thymoma, Type B1 (WHO)/Thymoma (Suster–Moran):** Type B1 thymoma is characterized by sheets and lobules of small round (cortical-like) thymic lymphocytes with single thymic epithelial cells scattered in the background; identification of these may be facilitated by cytokeratin staining. This thymoma has been referred to as 'lymphocyte-rich' thymoma and corresponds to the cortical or organoid thymoma in the MH system
3. **Thymoma, Type B2 (WHO)/Thymoma (Suster–Moran):** Type B2 thymoma is similar to B1 in that small lymphocytes dominate the histology, but in B2, the relative proportion of epithelial cells is increased, and individual cells appear more prominent, showing larger nuclei and easily discernable nucleoli compared to type B1. The epithelial cells may be found in small clusters, and perivascular palisading may be prominent. This thymoma has been referred to as 'mixed lymphoepithelial' thymoma and corresponds best to the pure cortical type thymoma of MH
4. **Thymoma, Type AB (WHO)/Thymoma (Suster–Moran):** Type AB thymoma demonstrates a mixture of type A histology and type B histology. There is usually abrupt transition from spindle cell areas (type A) to cortical-like areas (B1, B2)
5. **Thymoma, Type B3 (WHO)/Atypical thymoma (Suster–Moran):** Type B3 thymoma is characterized by increased numbers of large, round-to-polygonal epithelial cells with far fewer numbers of lymphocytes in comparison to types B1 and B2. The epithelial cells may be present in large clusters or sheets and display mild nuclear irregularities, if at all. Intraepithelial lymphocytes will be present, and this is a helpful finding in distinguishing type B3 thymoma from

thymic carcinoma. This thymoma has been referred to as 'epithelial rich' and corresponds to well-differentiated thymic carcinoma in the MH system

6. **Other (specify):**

Thymic epithelial neoplasm: thymic carcinoma

Thymic carcinoma is rare, and the reported histology of thymic carcinoma is representative of carcinomas seen outside the thymus including squamous cell carcinoma (most common), adenocarcinoma, neuroendocrine carcinoma (NEC), and special morphologic variants. Non-neuroendocrine thymic carcinoma is differentiated from type B3 thymoma (atypical thymoma) by the presence of the following: (1) overt cytologic atypia; (2) solid growth pattern; and (3) paucity or absence of intraepithelial lymphocytes. The histologic appearance of neuroendocrine thymic carcinoma generally mirrors that of pulmonary NEC: carcinoid, atypical carcinoid, small cell carcinoma, and large cell NEC. The principal difficulty with any thymic carcinoma is determining whether the carcinoma arising at the site of the thymus is primary or metastatic. This distinction may not be possible on histology alone and is best done clinically by excluding other primary cancer sites, particularly the lung. Immunohistochemistry (IHC) may be helpful in select cases. Thymic carcinoma (non-NEC types) may express CD5 and/or CD117 (c-KIT), markers that are not typically seen in carcinomas of the lung. TTF-1 may be helpful in distinguishing NEC of pulmonary origin.

- Squamous cell carcinoma
  - Keratinizing
  - Nonkeratinizing
- Adenocarcinoma
- Undifferentiated carcinoma
  - Other (specify):
- Neuroendocrine carcinoma
  - Carcinoid (well differentiated NEC)
    - Typical
    - Atypical
  - Small cell carcinoma
  - Large cell NEC
    - Angiolymphatic invasion
      - Present or absent
    - Invasion of nearby structures
      - Mediastinal fat
      - Mediastinal pleura
      - Pericardium
      - Lung
      - Chest wall
      - Other
    - Lymph nodes
      - No lymph nodes submitted
      - Lymph nodes submitted by site station
      - Number positive by site/station
    - Stage:
      - Modified Masaoka stage

  Note 6: There is no formal tumor–node–metastasis staging system for thymic epithelial neoplasms within the AJCC/UICC sixth edition. One may chose to adopt a tumor–node–metastasis style of staging based on the Masaoka staging system:

  - Stage I: Tumor completely encapsulated, grossly and microscopically; nontransmural capsular invasion is included in stage I
  - Stage II: Complete transmural (transcapsular) invasion
  - IIA Microscopic transmural (transcapsular) invasion only
  - IIB Macroscopic invasion into extracapsular soft tissue or tumor grossly adherent to mediastinal pleura or pericardium without invasion through these structures

    Note 7: The biologic and prognostic significance of distinguishing between IIA and IIB may be of little value given that most stage I and stage II tumors show excellent long-term survival. However, this distinction may be helpful for the surgeon to understand the nature of extracapsular disease that may or may not have been visually apparent at the time of surgery
  - Stage III: Macroscopic invasion into neighboring organs
  - IIIA Invasion spares the great vessels
  - IIIB Invasion includes the great vessels
  - Stage IV: Locally advanced thoracic disease or metastasis
  - IVA Pleural or pericardial dissemination
  - IVB Lymphovascular metastasis

Final report – optional features

Ancillary studies

1. **Immunohistochemistry**

   Note 8: IHC is not required routinely for the diagnosis of thymoma. IHC may be helpful in the following circumstances:
   - Confirmation of thymic epithelial cells for diagnosis and histologic subtyping
   - Excluding other potential primary sites of origin from thymic carcinoma. Although best done clinically, the exclusion of metastatic carcinoma to the mediastinum may be facilitated by the use of immunohistochemical stains for CD5 and c-KIT (CD117). These markers are expressed in a high percentage of thymic carcinomas and only rarely in the common tumors of the lungs and head and neck region

ASSOCIATION OF DIRECTORS OF ANATOMIC AND SURGICAL PATHOLOGY
Final anatomic diagnosis checklist
MEDIASTINAL THYMOMA

V1.0
Accession No.: **Part No:** **Date:**
Patient name:

ORGAN	**SITE**	**OPERATION**
Thymus	Mediastinum	Thymectomy
Other:_____		

A. Primary tumor diagnosis: Required
Thymoma
Histologic classification: World Health Organization Classification (2004)/Suster & Moran (1999):
Thymoma, type A / Thymoma
Thymoma, type AB / Thymoma
Thymoma, type B1 / Thymoma
Thymoma, type B2 / Thymoma
Thymoma, type B3 / Atypical thymoma
Other (specify)
Thymic carcinoma
Note: Primary thymic carcinoma is one of exclusion of other primary sites
Squamous cell carcinoma
Keratinizing
Nonkeratinizing
Adenocarcinoma (specify if special type)
Undifferentiated carcinoma
Other non-neuroendocrine carcinoma (specify)
Neuroendocrine carcinoma
Carcinoid (typical versus atypical)
Small cell carcinoma
Large cell neuroendocrine carcinoma
Size of tumor (three dimensions, greatest dimension listed first):
Invasion and extent of disease:
No transcapsular invasion (encapsulated thymoma)
Transcapsular invasion limited to mediastinal adipose tissue (minimally invasive)
OR
Involvement of adjacent structures (widely invasive)
Tumor invades: (circle all that apply)
Mediastinal pleura
Lung parenchyma
Pericardium
Chest wall tissue
Other (specifiy)
Completeness of resection:
Tumor is completely resected
Tumor resection is incomplete
Gross residual disease present OR
Microscopic residual disease only
Location of positive margins (specify)
Cannot assess completeness of resection (specify reason(s))

Additional tumor features
A. Angiolymphatic vessel invasion: Identified Not identified
Ancillary tumor studies: Optional Immunohistochemical studies are performed, and the immunophenotype is as follows:
A. Positive markers (tumor cells):
Negative markers (tumor cells):
Indeterminant markers:
Non-tumor associated markers:
Interpretation:
Non-neoplastic findings:
Thymic involution
Thymic follicular hyperplasia
Thymic cyst
Other (specify)
No non-neoplastic findings
B. Lymph nodes
Note: Lymph node dissections may not routinely accompany thymic resections.
Lymph nodes (anterior mediastinal, specify station(s)):
A. Positive or negative for tumor:_____
B. Comment:_____
Lymph nodes (intrathoracic, specify station(s)):
A. Positive or negative for tumor:_____
B. Comment:_____
Lymph nodes (scalene and/or supraclavicular):
A. Number examined:_____
B. Number positive:_______
C. Comment:_____
C. Stage (modified Masaoka stage): Required
Stage I:
Tumor completely encapsulated, grossly and microscopically;
non-transmural capsular invasion is included in Stage I
Stage II:
Complete transmural (transcapsular) invasion
IIA Microscopic transcapsular invasion only
IIB Macroscopic invasion into extracapsular soft tissue, or tumor grossly adherent to mediastinal pleura or pericardium without invasion through these structures
Stage III:
Macroscopic invasion into neighboring organs
IIIA Invasion spares the great vessels
IIIB Invasion includes the great vessels
Stage IV:
Locally advanced thoracic disease or metastasis
IVA Pleural or pericardial dissemination
IVB Lymphovascular metastasis

From Weydert JA, De Young BR, Leslie KO. Recommendations for the reporting of surgically resected thymic epithelial tumors. Hum Pathol 2009, **40:** 921.

Thyroid gland – carcinoma

Final report – recommended features

Gross description

1. **Specimen identification**
2. **Specimen condition:** how received (fresh or fixed, intact or previously sectioned, etc.)
3. **Type of procedure**
4. **Size:** overall dimensions and weight
5. **Outer shape, color, symmetry, and consistency** of entire specimen; presence and appearance of extrathyroid tissues
6. **Tumor description:** number, location, size, shape, consistency, color, encapsulation, secondary changes (fibrosis, calcification, cystic degeneration, hemorrhage), and distance to surgical margins
7. **Appearance of thyroid gland away from tumor;** presence of tumor multicentricity
8. **Number and appearance** of parathyroid gland(s), if any
9. **Lymph node dissection,** if included
   - Type – extended radical, radical, modified radical, selective
   - Presence of sternomastoid muscle/submandibular and/or parotid gland/jugular vein
   - Presence of a palpable mass, and whether solitary or matted
   - Size and location of gross tumor invasion of soft tissues, muscle, and jugular vein adjacent to involved lymph nodes
   - Dimensions and appearance of sternomastoid muscle, major salivary glands, and internal jugular vein
   - Size of lymph nodal masses (masses greater than 3 cm in diameter are to be regarded as confluent nodes or as extension into soft tissues)

Final report – optional features

The histologic grade can be listed as such (despite the fact that some tumor grading is implicit in the diagnosis of tumor type, i.e., poorly differentiated or undifferentiated), or the features evaluated in a grading system (such as mitotic activity or necrosis) can be listed separately. In other words, the use of 'Histologic grade' in the listing below is an alternative to using the option 'Presence and degree of mitotic activity' or 'Presence and amount of tumor necrosis'; yet another alternative is not exercising any of these options.

1. **Histologic grade**
2. **Presence and degree of mitotic activity**
3. **Presence and amount of tumor necrosis**
4. **Presence of ancillary tumor features:** such as squamous metaplasia, cytoplasmic clear cell change, mucinous features, psammoma bodies, other types of calcification, stromal (desmoplastic or 'scirrhous') reaction, and amyloid deposition

Checklist (see Note 1)

Type of specimen (see Note 2)
- Nodulectomy
- Lobectomy
- Subtotal thyroidectomy
- Total thyroidectomy
- Other

Tumor type (and subtype)
- Papillary carcinoma
  - Classic type
  - Other type
- Follicular carcinoma
  - Minimally invasive
  - Widely invasive
- Hürthle cell carcinoma
  - Minimally invasive
  - Widely invasive
- Poorly differentiated carcinoma
  - Insular type
  - Other type
- Undifferentiated (anaplastic) carcinoma
  - Without residual well-differentiated component
  - With residual well-differentiated component of type
- Medullary carcinoma
  - Classic type
  - Other type
- Mixed medullary–follicular carcinoma
- Mixed medullary–papillary carcinoma
- Other

Tumor location
- Right lobe (and isthmus)
- Left lobe (and isthmus)
- Both lobes (and isthmus)
- Isthmus

Tumor largest diameter
- — cm (see Note 3)

Encapsulation
- Absent
- Partial
- Complete

Capsular invasion
- Absent
- Present (minimal)
- Present (extensive)

Lymph vessel invasion
- Absent
- Present (minimal)
- Present (extensive)

Blood vessel invasion
- Absent
- Present (minimal)
- Present (extensive)

Extrathyroid extension
- Absent
- Present (gross)
- Present (microscopic)

Surgical margins (see Note 4)
- Negative
- Positive

Tumor multicentricity (see Note 5)
- Negative
- Positive

C cell hyperplasia (for cases of medullary carcinoma only)
- Absent
- Present

Other pathology
- None
- Adenoma(s) (specify number, location, and size)
- Nodular hyperplasia
- Lymphocytic thyroiditis
- Hashimoto thyroiditis
- Atrophy
- Fibrosis

Parathyroid gland (see Note 6)

— Yes — No

- Number
- Location
- Normal

Lymph nodes
  — Yes — No
- Number
- Location (right, left, central) and level
- Negative
- Positive

Positive (metastatic) lymph nodes
- Size of largest involved node: cm
- Perinodal (extracapsular) extension
  — Yes — No

Note 1: If the thyroid is located ectopically (mediastinal, lingual, in a thyroglossal duct cyst, or in a teratoma), this should be indicated in the report

Note 2: For nodulectomy or lobectomy specimens, the report should indicate whether the specimen is from the right or left side. (Nodulectomy is rarely, if ever, performed at present, but it is included in the checklist for the sake of completeness.) If the lobectomy specimen includes the isthmus (as is often the case), the report should make reference to this fact. For subtotal thyroidectomy specimens, the report should indicate which lobe was completely removed and which lobe was excised only partially

Note 3: Provide a size estimate for tumor bulk if the tumor is multifocal. For cases of papillary microcarcinoma (less than 1 cm in diameter), indicate in the report the exact diameter of the tumor

Note 4: If positive, specify location (capsular or isthmic), number (single or multiple), and extent (minimal/ microscopic or extensive), whenever feasible

Note 5: Specify approximate number of foci and whether these foci have the same or a different appearance. If the specimen is from a subtotal or total thyroidectomy, indicate whether the tumor foci involve one lobe or both lobes. In a case of papillary carcinoma, indicate whether psammoma bodies are present elsewhere in the gland or not, the former suggesting the presence of tumor multicentricity

Note 6: Whenever possible, the location of the gland(s) should be specified; if this gland is intrathyroidal, this fact should be noted

Uterine cervix – carcinoma

Final report – recommended features

Gross description

1. **Specimen identification:** labeled with patient name, medical record number, organ identified, etc.
2. **Specimen condition:** fresh, in fixative (formalin, Bouin, etc.), on ice, opened (by pathologist or surgeon), unopened, etc.
3. **Number of specimen containers**
4. **Type of procedure:** the type of surgical procedure should be stated (simple hysterectomy, radical hysterectomy, anterior exenteration, etc.)
5. **Topography:** the exact type of specimen should be specified (uterus, cervical cold knife core biopsy, cervical loop electrosurgical excision procedure, etc.)
6. **Brief but precise overall description:** focusing on the site and extent of the lesion and its relationship to surrounding structures:
   - Accurate overall dimensions of each specimen received
   - Exact anatomic location of cervical tumor (anterior or posterior lip, portio or endocervical canal, the 'o'clock' location, etc.)
   - Size of tumor
   - Gross estimation of depth of invasion, if any, into the cervical wall
   - Grossly apparent extension to adjacent organs and tissue, e.g., the parametrium, upper vagina, the uterine corpus, or the bladder or bowel (in exenteration specimens)
   - Comment on the proximity of the tumor to pertinent resection margins
7. **Special investigations:** flow cytometry, etc.
8. **If ink is used** for marking resection margins, provide a section code for subsequent interpretation of the microscopic findings

Diagnostic information

1. **Histologic type:** the histopathologic tumor type should be stated. The following modified terminology, as revised and adopted by the International Society of Gynecologic Pathologists (ISGP) under the auspices of the World Health Organization (WHO), is recommended
   - Squamous lesions
     - Squamous intraepithelial lesions (SIL)
       - Cervical intraepithelial neoplasia (CIN)
         - CIN 1: mild dysplasia, low-grade SIL
         - CIN 2: moderate dysplasia, high-grade SIL
         - CIN 3: severe dysplasia/carcinoma in situ, high-grade SIL

     Note 1: In the Bethesda system for cytologic classification, squamous intraepithelial lesions are divided into low grade and high grade. CIN 1 (mild dysplasia) and lesions showing clearcut evidence of papillomavirus effect are classified as low-grade lesions. CIN 2 (moderate dysplasia) and CIN 3 (severe dysplasia and carcinoma in situ) are classified as high-grade lesions
   - Squamous cell carcinoma
     - Keratinizing type
     - Nonkeratinizing type: large cell (optional); small cell (optional)
     - Verrucous carcinoma
     - Warty (condylomatous) carcinoma
     - Papillary squamous cell (transitional) carcinoma
     - Lymphoepithelioma-like carcinoma

     Note 2: Keratinizing tumors require the presence of keratin pearls. The morphologic spectrum is wide for nonkeratinizing tumors, including those having individual cell keratinization, tumor cells with clear cytoplasm, and tumor cells with eosinophilic cytoplasm and distinct cell borders. Small cell poorly differentiated carcinomas with light microscopic, immunohistochemical, and ultrastructural features of neuroendocrine differentiation are classified in the category of small cell (neuroendocrine) carcinomas
   - Glandular lesions
     - Adenocarcinoma in situ
     - Adenocarcinoma
       - Mucinous adenocarcinoma: endocervical type; intestinal type
       - Endometrioid adenocarcinoma: endometrioid adenocarcinoma with squamous metaplasia
       - Clear cell adenocarcinoma
       - Minimal deviation adenocarcinoma (adenoma malignum): endocervical type; endometrioid type

- Well-differentiated (papillary) villoglandular adenocarcinoma
- Serous carcinoma
- Mesonephric carcinoma

- Other epithelial tumors
  - Adenosquamous carcinoma
  - Glassy cell carcinoma
  - Adenoid cystic carcinoma
  - Adenoid basal carcinoma (epithelioma)

    Note 3: Some workers consider adenoid basal carcinoma to be nonmalignant and have instead proposed the term adenoid basal epithelioma
- Neuroendocrine tumors
  - Carcinoid tumor
  - Atypical carcinoid tumor
  - High-grade neuroendocrine carcinoma: small cell type; large type
- Undifferentiated carcinoma
- Mesenchymal tumors
  - Leiomyosarcoma
  - Endocervical stromal sarcoma
  - Sarcoma botryoides (embryonal rhabdomyosarcoma)
  - Alveolar soft-part sarcoma
- Mixed epithelial and mesenchymal tumors
  - Adenosarcoma
  - Malignant mixed mesodermal tumor (MMMT)
  - Wilms tumor
- Miscellaneous tumors
  - Malignant melanoma
  - Lymphoma and leukemia
  - Tumors of germ cell type
  - Yolk sac tumor

2. **Tumor grade**
   - Squamous cell carcinoma: several studies have shown that histopathologic grading systems, including the most commonly used modification of the Broder system, fail to correlate reliably with prognosis. Consequently, histopathologic grading is optional
   - Adenocarcinoma: cervical adenocarcinomas may be graded by architectural (the percentage of solid growth, excluding squamous) and cytologic (nuclear) criteria:
     - **Grade 1:** well-differentiated (10% or less solid growth). The tumor contains well-formed regular glands with papillae. The cells are elongate and columnar with uniform oval nuclei; there is minimal stratification (fewer than three cell layers in thickness). Mitotic figures are infrequent
     - **Grade 2:** moderately differentiated (11–50% solid growth). The tumor contains complex glands with frequent bridging and cribriform formation. Solid areas are more common, but these make up less than half of the tumor. The nuclei are more rounded and irregular; micronucleoli are present. Mitoses are more frequent
     - **Grade 3:** poorly differentiated (over 50% solid growth). The tumor contains sheets of malignant cells; few glands are discernible. The cells are large and irregular with pleomorphic nuclei. Occasional signet cells are present. Mitoses are abundant, with abnormal forms. Desmoplasia is pronounced, and necrosis is common
3. **Degree of invasion:** the maximum depth of invasion by tumor into the cervical stroma, in millimeters, or the proportion of the wall involved should be recorded. For purposes of staging, the International Federation of Gynecology and Obstetrics (FIGO) and the Society of Gynecologic Oncologists (SGO) subdivide squamous cell carcinomas into microinvasive and frankly invasive carcinoma:
   - An early squamous cell carcinoma with 3 mm or less of invasion from its point of origin and without angiolymphatic space invasion is classified as a microinvasive squamous cell carcinoma by SGO criteria
   - An early squamous cell carcinoma with 5 mm or less of invasion from its point of origin and no greater than 7 mm in greatest horizontal dimension is classified as a microinvasive squamous cell carcinoma by FIGO criteria. Only invasive carcinoma should be included in the measurement. Vascular space invasion is noted, if present, but does not in itself exclude a tumor from being placed in the microinvasive category
   - No consensus has been reached for the histopathologic criteria that define a 'microinvasive' cervical adenocarcinoma. The maximal deep and lateral dimensions of tumor extension, plus the presence or absence of angiolymphatic invasion, should be carefully recorded
4. **Extent of tumor:** the extent of invasion into extracervical tissues and metastases to both pelvic and extrapelvic organs should be recorded
5. **Angiolymphatic vascular space invasion:** the presence of tumor within blood vessels and/or lymphatic vessels should be noted and an attempt made to distinguish, when possible, between them
6. **Status of lymph nodes:** report the presence or absence of metastases in each submitted group of lymph nodes, recording the total number of involved lymph nodes in relation to the total number of lymph nodes identified
7. **Status of resection margins:** the adequacy of local excision should be assessed by careful examination of resection margins, the latter preferably marked by the use of ink. The distance from the deepest point of stromal invasion to the closest (inked) margin of resection may be noted in the report

Final report – optional features

1. **Stage** (see below)
2. **Glandular intraepithelial lesions:** the natural history and histopathologic criteria to define endocervical glandular lesions with atypia less than that of adenocarcinoma in situ are controversial; their reporting, therefore, is considered optional
3. **Definitions:** the following definitions are slightly modified from the *Histological Typing of Female Genital Tract Tumors*, second edition:
   - An *endocervical glandular atypia* is one that does not fulfill the criteria for glandular dysplasia–adenocarcinoma in situ, and may be associated with inflammation
   - *Glandular dysplasia* is characterized by significant nuclear abnormalities that are more striking than those encountered in glandular atypia but do not fulfill the criteria for adenocarcinoma in situ
   - In *adenocarcinoma in situ*, normally situated glands are lined by cytologically malignant glandular epithelium.

College of American Pathologists (CAP) checklists for the reporting of major tumor types

The College of American Pathologists (CAP) cancer protocols and checklists can be found on the CAP website: http://www.cap.org/cancerprotocols

Appendix E

Guidelines for handling of most common and important surgical specimens

Some general guidelines for the procedure, description, and sampling of the most common and important surgical specimens received in the laboratory are set forth in the following pages. They are mainly derived from personal experience, although the *Gross Room Manual* used for years in the Surgical Pathology Laboratory at Barnes Hospital in St Louis, and considerably expanded by the surgical pathologists at Stanford University, was freely used as a model for many of the procedures. Several other versions of these guidelines have been published over the years, either incorporated into major surgical pathology textbooks or as free-standing manuals.[1–8,10] Of them, the most detailed and up-to-date is the one published by the powerful Surgical Pathology team at Johns Hopkins, edited by William H. Westra et al, with the help of a superb medical illustrator.[10] Of course, there are also innumerable other versions which have been prepared in individual pathology laboratories for domestic use and which have never been published.

The instructions from any of these manuals can be used in a printed form, in a microfiche format or – increasingly – by incorporating them into the AP information system and making them available to the prosectors through terminals located in the dissection stations.

Naturally, not all types of specimens or eventualities can be covered. The guidelines presented herein and those from any other version will be useful only if they are taken as *general recommendations* for a typical specimen showing a typical lesion. All kinds of modifications need to be made according to the specific circumstances of the case. Each specimen is unique and thus requires variation in the dissection, description, and sampling procedures here recommended. To quote from a high source in connection with a somewhat related matter (i.e. the autopsy procedure):[9]

> *It is scarcely necessary to point out that there are many cases in which deviation from this method are not merely allowable, but also absolutely necessary. The individuality of the case must often determine the plan of the examination. But we must not begin with individualizing, nor make a rule of the exceptions. The expert may allow himself to make alterations, supposing that they are well founded, but he must be able to remember his motive for so doing, and also to state it.*

1 Fazzini EP, Waldo E, Weber DL. A manual for surgical pathologists. Springfield, IL, 1972, Thomas
2 Leong AS-Y, James CL, Thomas AC. Handbook of surgical pathology. New York, 1996, Churchill Livingstone
3 Lowe DG, Jeffrey IJM. Macro techniques in diagnostic histopathology. London, 1990, Wolfe Medical Publications
4 Nochomovitz L. Gross room and specimen handling. In Weidner N, Cote RJ, Suster S, et al (eds): Modern surgical pathology. Philadelphia, 2003, Saunders

5 Pierson KK. Principles of prosection: a guide for the anatomic pathologist. New York, 1980, Wiley
6 Rosai J. Manual of surgical pathology gross room procedures. Minneapolis, 1981, University of Minnesota Press
7 Schmidt WA. Principles and techniques of surgical pathology. Menlo Park, CA, 1983, Addison-Wesley
8 Teloh HA. Methods in surgical pathology. Springfield, IL, 1957, Thomas
9 Virchow R. Postmortem examinations and the position of pathology among biological sciences, with an introduction by Putschar WJ. The history of medicine, Series No 37. Published under the auspices of the Library of the New York Academy of Medicine, Metuchen, NJ, 1973, Scarecrow
10 Westra WH, Hruban RH, Phelps TH, Isacson C. Surgical pathology dissection. An illustrated guide, ed. 2. New York, 2003, Springer-Verlag

Adrenal gland – adrenalectomy[1]

Procedure

1. Ink the specimen
2. Measure and weigh the organ
3. Cut parallel sections at 5 mm intervals in the transverse plane
4. Look for and sample the adrenal vein

Description

1. Size and weight
2. External surface: smooth? bosselated? shape of gland preserved?
3. Cut surface: color? necrosis? hemorrhage? cystic changes? encapsulation? extension of the disease into the surrounding tissues?

Sections for histology

1. Tumor if present, trying to demonstrate relationship with normal gland, tumor capsule, and surrounding organs
2. Non-neoplastic gland, some including adrenal vein
3. Surgical margins

1 Conran RM. An approach to handling pediatric thyroid and adrenal tumors excluding neuroblastoma. Am J Clin Pathol 1998, **109**: S73–S81

Appendix – appendectomy

Appendectomy consists of the removal of the entire appendix after dividing the mesoappendix and ligating the base of the appendix that connects to the cecum.

Procedure

1. Measure organ (length and greatest diameter)
2. Divide specimen in two by cutting a cross-section 2 cm from tip
3. Cut cross-sections of proximal fragment at 5 mm intervals
4. Divide distal fragment in two by a longitudinal cut

Description

1. Length and greatest diameter
2. External surface: fibrin? pus? hemorrhage? hyperemia? perforation? condition of mesentery?
3. Wall: any localized lesions?
4. Mucosa: hyperemic? ulcerated?
5. Lumen: obliterated? dilated? Content: fecaliths? stones?

Sections for histology

1. Proximal one-third, close to surgical margin: one cross-section. If tumor is present in the specimen, paint the surgical margin with India ink and take an additional section from it
2. Mid one-third: one cross-section
3. Distal one-third: one longitudinal section

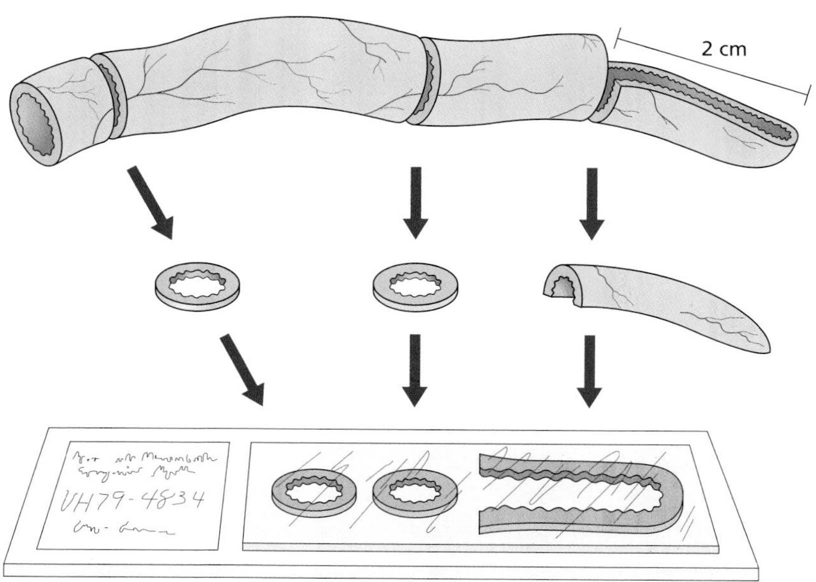

Bladder – cystectomy

Cystectomy consists in removal of the bladder. In most instances the entire organ is removed (total cystectomy). In males this may be accompanied by removal of the prostate and seminal vesicles (cystoprostatectomy). The entire length of the urethra may also be excised (cystourethrectomy). The performance of partial cystectomies for carcinoma has fallen into disfavor.

Procedure

1. Paint the entire external surface (including the prostate, if present) with India ink
2. Two options are available for the dissection depending on the type of lesion present and the status of the organ when received in the laboratory (see accompanying drawings opposite):
   a. Open with scissors in a Y shape through the anterior wall, pin on a corkboard, and fix overnight in formalin
   b. Fill with formalin, fix overnight and divide into anterior and posterior halves by first cutting the lateral bladder walls with scissors and then sectioning the prostate with a sharp knife, beginning at the bladder neck and being careful to make the cut through the urethra. See instructions for Injection of specimens – general guidelines. The injection can be performed through the urethra with a Foley catheter, with a 50 mL syringe with a large-bore needle inserted through the bladder dome after the urethra has been clamped or tied, or by filling the bladder with formalin-soaked cotton
3. Take photographs or photocopies and identify in one of them the site of the sections taken for histology

Description

1. Size of bladder; length of ureters; other organs present
2. Tumor characteristics: size (including thickness), location, extent of invasion, shape (papillary, ulcerated); multifocal lesions?
3. Appearance of non-neoplastic mucosa; thickness of bladder wall away from tumor

Sections for histology

1. Tumor: at least three sections, through bladder wall
2. Bladder neck: one section
3. Trigone: two sections
4. Anterior wall: two sections
5. Posterior wall: two sections
6. Dome: two sections
7. Any abnormal-looking area in bladder mucosa if not included in previous sections
8. Ureteral orifices, including intramural portion
9. Ureteral proximal margins
10. In males: prostate (two sections from each quadrant) and seminal vesicles (one section from each). If a prostatic carcinoma is identified, see instructions for Prostate gland – radical prostatectomy
11. Other organs present
12. Perivesical lymph nodes, if any

Bladder – stone removal

Procedure

1. Take photographs or photocopies of all stones submitted
2. Send a 1–2 g sample for crystallographic (often incorrectly referred to as chemical) analysis.[1] Specimens should be rinsed well in water and air dried. Formalin is to be avoided because uric acid is soluble therein. Heat should not be used to hasten drying because it will drive off the ammonium in magnesium ammonium phosphate, changing struvite into newberyite. Specimens should be shipped in protective containers rather than in plain envelopes. They should not be secured with a transparent tape
3. The same procedure applies to stones removed from other portions of the urinary tract, such as the renal pelvis or ureter

Description

1. Number of stones, shape, color, and consistency. *Phosphate* stones are gray or grayish white and may be hard or soft and friable. *Oxalate* stones are usually hard and smooth, rounded, or nodular (resembling mulberries) or irregularly speculated. *Urate* stones are smooth, yellow or brown, and round or oval. *Cystine* stones are hard, smooth, and yellow, with a waxy appearance. Stones associated with local bleeding may be impregnated with blood and acquire a black or dark brown color

Sections for histology

None

1 Several specialized laboratories have offered this service for many years, including the Laboratory for Stone Research, 81 Wyman Street, Newton, MA 02468, USA, and Louis C. Herring and Company, 1111 South Orange Avenue, Orlando, FL 32806–1236, USA

Bone – biopsy

Procedure

1. Trocar or needle biopsy: divide longitudinally with a fine-toothed saw if specimen is over 5 mm in diameter. Look for any soft material, dissect from rest of specimen, and process separately without decalcification
2. Open biopsy and curettage: divide calcified from noncalcified tissues and process separately

Description

1. Number and size of fragments
2. Consistency, calcification, color, cystic changes, necrosis

Sections for histology

1. Submit all material received, except for unduly large specimens. Send, separately, material to be decalcified from the rest

Bone – femoral head excision

Procedure

1. Examine articular and cut surfaces
2. Measure diameter and thickness

Breast – mammographically directed excision

(Adapted from Schnitt SJ, Connolly JL. Processing and evaluation of breast excision specimens. A clinically oriented approach. Am J Clin Pathol 1992, **98:** 125–137.)

Procedure

1 Obtain through radiograph of intact specimen
2 Measure specimen before cutting
3 Blot dry, apply India ink to surface, and blot dry again
4 Slice specimen through the equatorial plane at 1–4 mm intervals
5 Obtain radiograph of sliced specimen. Some authors have found the use of a Perspex grid useful for the subsequent localization of the lesion[1]
6 Label slices on the radiograph
7 Take a sample for hormone receptor analysis only if tumor is grossly visible and of sufficient size; do not submit tissue for this analysis if there is no grossly evident tumor

Description

1 Dimension and consistency of specimen
2 Appearance of cut sections: fibrosis, cysts (size, number, content), calcification, tumor masses (size in three dimensions, color, borders, consistency, necrosis, distance from surgical margins)

Sections for histology

Submit in its entirety. Label cassettes as in the radiograph

1 Champ CS, Mason CH, Coghill SB, Robinson M. A Perspex grid for localization of nonpalpable mammographic lesions in breast biopsies. Histopathology 1989, **124:** 311–316

Upper and middle drawings redrawn from National Cancer Institute. Standardized management of breast specimens recommended by Pathology Working Group, Breast Cancer Task Force. Am J Clin Pathol 1973, **60:** 789–798

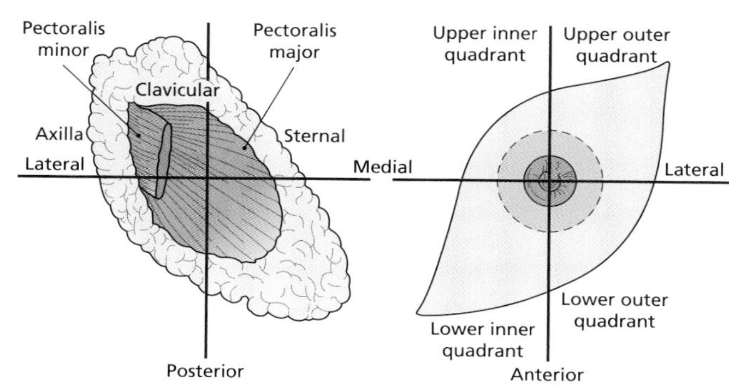

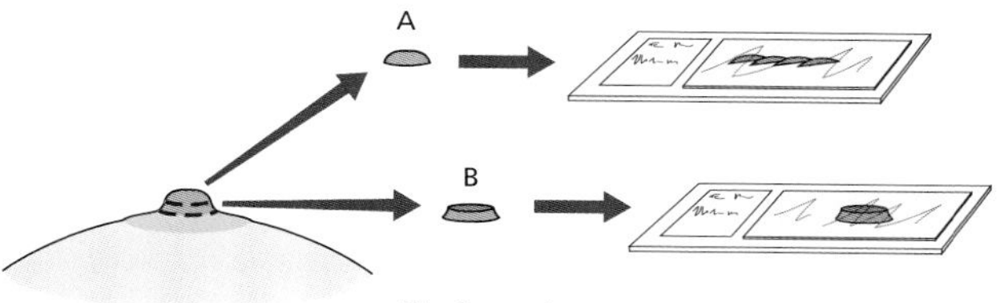

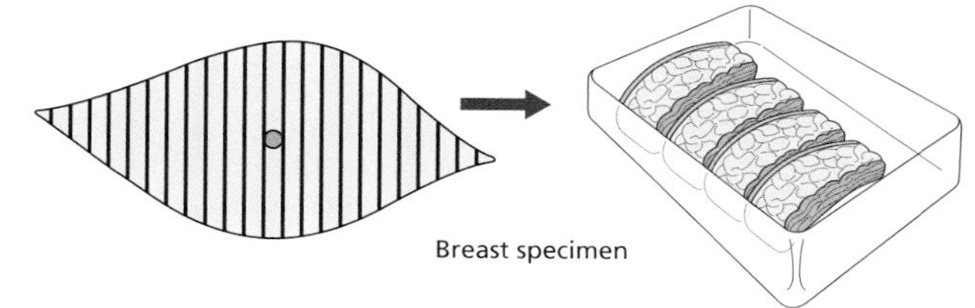

Breast – mastectomy

(Adapted from National Cancer Institute. Standardized management of breast specimens recommended by Pathology Working Group, Breast Cancer Task Force. Am J Clin Pathol 1973, **60:** 789–798.)

Several types of mastectomy procedures exist. The Halsted type *radical mastectomy*, which has been all but abandoned, consists of removal of the entire breast parenchyma, the underlying and surrounding adipose tissue, the pectoralis major and minor muscles, and the axillary contents in continuity and en bloc. A *modified radical mastectomy* (also known as extended simple mastectomy and total mastectomy) consists in removal of all the mammary tissue, including the axillary tail, together with the nipple, the surrounding skin, and a variable amount of lymph node-bearing fat from the lower axilla; the pectoralis muscles are preserved. A *simple mastectomy* consists of all or almost all of the mammary tissue, the nipple, and a variable amount of surrounding skin. A *subcutaneous mastectomy* includes most of the mammary tissue, without overlying skin or nipple and often without the axillary tail. In a quadrantectomy a portion of the breast roughly corresponding to one of the four anatomic quadrants is excised, often in combination with removal of the axillary content. A *tylectomy* (lumpectomy, excisional biopsy) consists in removal of the entire mass and a variable amount of surrounding breast tissue. A *quadrantectomy* is a form of tylectomy in which the area of excision roughly corresponds to an anatomical quadrant of the breast. Finally, there is the *supraradical mastectomy*, mentioned here only for historical reasons. It contains all the components of a radical mastectomy specimen, plus a resected segment of chest wall, usually the sternal ends of the second, third, fourth, and fifth ribs, an adjacent segment of sternum, and the subpleural connective tissue that contains the internal mammary vessels and nodes; a segment of pleura also may be present.

Procedure

First day

1 Weigh the specimen
2 Orient the specimen. In radical mastectomy cases, use the axillary fat as a marker for the lateral side and the surgical section of the muscle as a marker for the upper side. Place the specimen on the cutting board, posterior side up, with its

section from any grossly abnormal area or, if none is found, from the area closest to the tumor

laboratory is not feasible, store temporarily in the refrigerator at 4 °C.

Appendix E

Cultures – bacterial, fungal, and viral

Whenever a fresh specimen is received in the laboratory and there is some indication (clinical, gross appearance, frozen section) that it may be involved by an infectious process, cultures should be taken, unless this has already been done in the operating room.[1]

Large specimens

Several techniques can be used for large operative specimens (lung, spleen) received intact in the fresh state. In general, technique 1 (following) is recommended over technique 2

1. Technique 1
   a. Burn the surface close to the area to be cultured with a red-hot spatula
   b. Make a deep cut through this sterilized surface with a sterile blade
   c. Cut a portion of tissue from the inside using sterile forceps and scalpel or scissors. A size of 1 × 1 × 1 cm is recommended
   d. Put the specimen in a sterile container
2. Technique 2
   a. Burn the surface close to the area to be cultured with a red-hot spatula
   b. Make a deep cut through this sterilized surface with a sterile blade
   c. Introduce a sterile swab stick (such as Culturette) through the opening, push beyond the cut into the tissue, remove, and place in appropriate transport medium
3. For cystic processes that need to be cultured for anaerobic organisms: aspirate with a sterile syringe and needle (about 2–4 mL), expel air bubble from the syringe, and inject the sample into an anaerobic vial. If a vial is not available, put a rubber cork on the end of the needle

Small specimens

1. If the specimen is submitted fresh in a sterile container with the request for bacteriologic studies to be carried out:
   a. Open the container, cut a portion of tissue with sterile instruments, and transfer to a sterile container
   b. Use the rest of the specimen for histologic examination
2. If the need for culture becomes evident after the fresh specimen has been handled in a nonsterile fashion, proceed as follows:
   a. Cut a piece of the tissue (approximately 1 × 1 × 1 cm) with a sterile blade
   b. Sterilize a pair of clean forceps by dipping them in ethanol and flaming
   c. Holding the specimen with the sterilized forceps, wash thoroughly with sterile saline solution
   d. Lay specimen in a sterile container. Sterilize the forceps again and pick up the specimen in a different portion
   e. Repeat the washing with sterile solution
   f. Put the specimen in a sterile container
3. After a sample has been taken for cultures, it is advisable to make a smear from an adjacent area, fix in alcohol, and stain for the microorganisms suspected (Gram, Ziehl–Neelsen)

1 Braunstein H. The value of microbiologic culture of tissue samples in surgical pathology. Mod Pathol 1989, **2:** 217–221

DNA ploidy and cell proliferation analysis by flow cytometry – sampling

Cut viable tissue into 0.5 cm^3 cubes in the fresh state as soon as possible after excision, drop in a bottle containing culture medium (such as RPMI or DMEM), and submit to the appropriate laboratory. If immediate transportation is not feasible, store temporarily in the refrigerator at 4 °C.

Ear – temporal bone resection

Subtotal or total temporal bone resections can be carried out for carcinoma of the external auditory canal, middle ear, or mastoid.

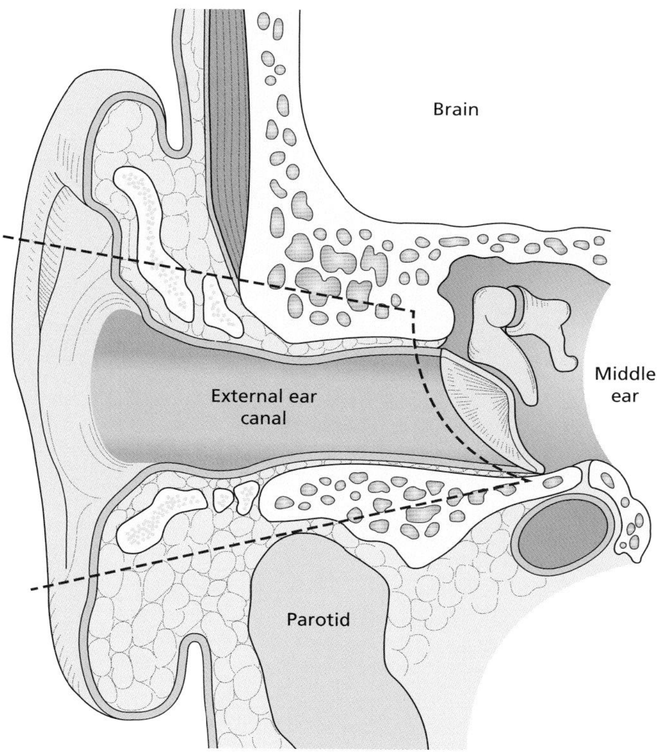

Procedure

1 Review roentgenograms if available and obtain roentgenograms of the specimen if facilities are available
2 Orient the specimen as to anteroposterior, superoinferior, and mediolateral planes
3 Mark the margins with India ink
4 Section longitudinally in two halves or in parallel cross-sections, depending on location and size of tumor

Description

1 Type of resection: subtotal or total
2 Tumor: size, gross features, and location: external ear, auditory canal, middle ear. If in the canal, does it involve the outer cartilaginous third or the inner osseous two-thirds?
3 Location within the canal: floor, walls, roof, circumferential; invasion anteriorly toward the parotid gland? superiorly toward the cranial cavity?
4 Status of tympanic membrane
5 Parotid gland, if present: invaded by tumor?

Sections for histology

1 Tumor: in its entirety
2 Surgical margins
3 Parotid gland, if present

Electron microscopy – sampling

Fixative

Several fixatives are available for electron microscopy. The most commonly used is 2.5% glutaraldehyde in Millonig phosphate buffer, in amounts of 3–4 mL per vial, which is kept refrigerated at 4 °C. The working solution can be stored for up to 1 month.

Sampling from fresh tissue

Fresh tissue is highly preferable to routinely fixed material. It is imperative for tissue to be handled *immediately* after excision.

1 Put the specimen on a clear cutting board (such as a heavy plastic card) and cut 1 mm thick slices with a sharp razor blade
2 Place several drops of electron microscopy fixative in another area of the cutting board, place the tissue slice on top, and cover with a few drops of fixative
3 Chop the slide into 1 mm cubes with a sharp razor blade, and immerse them in cold (4 °C) fixative. Five to 15 fragments of tissue are adequate. If the specimen has grossly different areas, submit for electron microscopy in separate containers
4 Submit to electron microscopy laboratory for processing; the tissue can remain in the electron microscopy fixative for several days at 4 °C

Sampling from routinely fixed tissue

In routinely fixed tissue, there is usually extensive fixation artifact, but at times recognizable diagnostic electron microscopy features are retained (such as desmosomes, neurosecretory granules, melanosomes).

1 Cut a 1 mm slice from an *edge* of the specimen that was in direct contact with the fixative
2 Proceed as for fresh tissues

Esophagus – esophagectomy

The extent of an *esophagectomy* depends on the type and location of the lesion. Most esophagectomies consist of removal of the distal portion of the organ, followed by an esophagogastric anastomosis.

For the handling of esophageal carcinomas following preoperative neoadjuvant therapy, see Chang et al.[1]

Procedure

1 Dissect the specimen in the fresh state; open longitudinally from one end to the other after marking the deep margins with India ink, trying to cut on the side opposite the tumor (see accompanying drawing **A**). If a portion of the stomach is included, open along the greater curvature in continuity with the esophageal cut (see accompanying drawing **B**)
   a Dissect the periesophageal fat and look for lymph nodes. Divide into three portions: adjacent, proximal, and distal to the tumor (the latter might include the cardioesophageal nodes)
   b Pin the specimen in a corkboard, mucosal side up, and float in a large formalin container with the specimen on the underside; fix overnight
   c Take two photographs or photocopies and identify in one of them the sites of the sections to be taken
   d Paint the surgical specimens with India ink after the specimens are fixed; this includes both mucosal ends and the soft tissue around the tumor

Description

1 Length and diameter or circumference of specimen; proximal stomach included? (if so, indicate length along lesser and greater curvature)
2 Tumor: size, appearance (fungating? rolled edges? ulcerated?); does it involve entire organ circumferentially? depth of invasion; extension into stomach and adjacent organs? distance from both lines of resection and from cardias, if present
3 Mucosa: appearance of non-neoplastic mucosa; recognizable esophageal mucosa *distal* to tumor? evidence of Barrett esophagus? (if so, length of the segment and appearance of mucosa); lumen dilated proximal to tumor?
4 Wall: thickened? varices?
5 Stomach, if present: features of cardioesophageal junction and gastric mucosa
6 Lymph nodes: number found, size of largest; do they appear grossly involved by tumor?

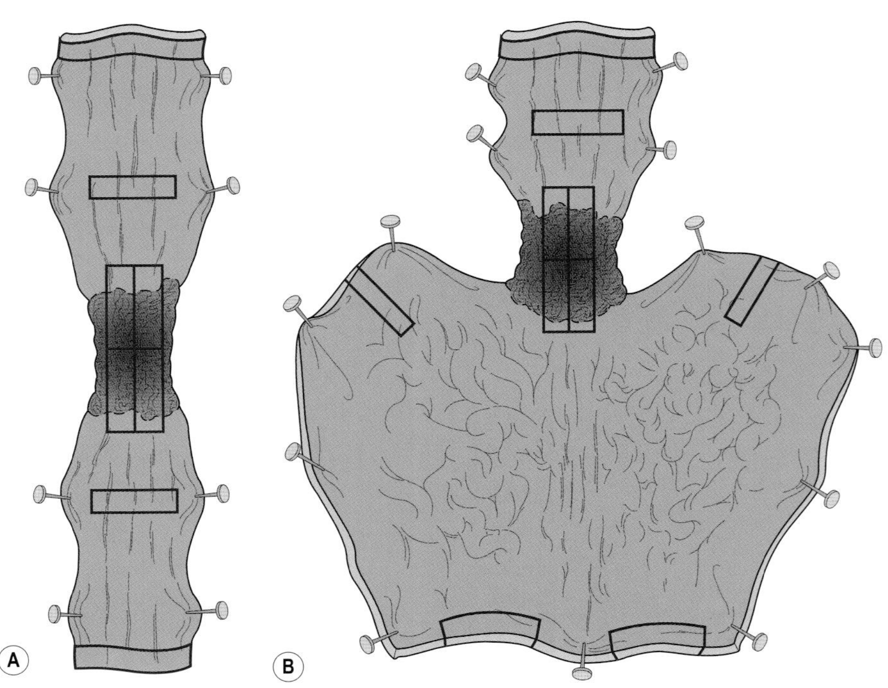

Sections for histology

1 Tumor: four longitudinal sections, one including a portion of non-neoplastic mucosa proximal to tumor and another portion distal to tumor
2 Non-neoplastic mucosa: two to three transverse sections, at different distances from tumor edge, proximally and/or distally, depending on location of tumor
3 Stomach, if present: two sections, one including gastroesophageal junction
4 Proximal line of resection
5 Distal line of resection
6 Lymph nodes:
   a Adjacent to tumor
   b Proximal to tumor
   c Distal to tumor

1 Chang F, Deere H, Mahadeva U, George S. Histopathologic examination and reporting of esophageal carcinomas following preoperative neoadjuvant therapy: practical guidelines and current issues. Am J Clin Pathol 2008, **129**: 252–262

Extremities – amputation for occlusive vascular disease

(Adapted from Rodriguez-Martinez HA, Cruz-Ortiz H, Alcantara-Vazquez A, Alcorta-Anguizola B, Burgos-Mendivil J. Dissecting technique for gangrenous lower limbs with vascular occlusions. Patologia 1972, **10**: 69–78.)

Procedure

1 Removal of femoral, popliteal, and posterior tibial neurovascular bundles and peroneal vessels:
   a Place the extremity on a dissection board with the posterior surface upward. The dissection will be completed more rapidly if an assistant holds the specimen and helps retract flaps
   b Incise longitudinally the skin over the midline of the popliteal region and the upper two-thirds of the posterior tibial region (see accompanying diagram, p. 2596)
   c Incise obliquely the skin from the lower end of the first incision to 2 cm below the posterior border of the medial malleolus (see accompanying diagram, p. 2596)
   d With a scalpel or knife, cut through the subcutaneous tissue and superficial fascia of the entire incision
   e In the posterior femoral and popliteal regions, separate, with blunt and sharp dissection, the semitendinous, semimembranous, and medial head of the gastrocnemius muscles from the biceps femoris and lateral head of the gastrocnemius. This maneuver will expose the sciatic and posterior tibial nerves and the femoral and popliteal vessels
   f Deepen the incisions made in steps **b** and **c** in the posterior tibial regions, cutting through the gastrocnemius and soleus muscles and the tendocalcaneus. This will show, underneath the intermuscular fascial septum, the posterior tibial neurovascular bundle and the peroneal vessels
   g Beginning at their upper end, dissect and excise the sciatic and posterior tibial nerves down to the place where the latter nerve joins the popliteal vessels
   h Beginning at their upper end, dissect and excise the femoral and popliteal vessels down to the place where the latter vessels join the posterior tibial nerve
   i Excise *en bloc* the popliteal vessels and the posterior tibial nerve
   j Continue with the removal of the entire posterior tibial neurovascular bundle, down to the lowest portion of the skin incision, and transect it there. The bundle should be excised together with neighboring portions of muscle fascia
   k Last, remove the peroneal vessels together with contiguous muscle fibers. These vessels are chiefly located behind the fibula and the interosseous membrane and within the muscle fibers of the flexor hallucis longus
2 Removal of the anterior tibial neurovascular bundle:
   a Place the extremity with its anterior surface upward
   b Incise longitudinally the skin from a point located between the head of the fibula and the tibial tuberosity to a joint equidistant between both malleoli (see accompanying diagram)
   c With a scalpel or knife, cut through the subcutaneous tissue and superficial fascia of the whole incision
   d In the middle portion of the incision, cut, with scissors or knife, through the fibers of the tibialis anterior muscle down to the interosseous membrane. This will uncover part of the anterior tibial neurovascular bundle
   e With sharp or blunt dissection, separate partially the regional muscular masses in the upper portion and the tendons in the lower portion, so as to expose lengthwise the anterior tibial neurovascular bundle
   f Cut across the lowest portion of the anterior tibial neurovascular bundle. Pull the bundle downward, and excise it together with portions of adjacent muscles and interosseous membrane. The upper end of the bundle becomes loose by just exerting traction downward
3 Removal of the tissue block with dorsalis pedis vessel:
   a Trace a 3–4 cm wide rectangle over the dorsum of the foot, extending from the lowest part of the anterior tibial incision to the proximal portion of the first interosseous space
   b Following the sides of the rectangle, cut through the skin, subcutaneous tissue, superficial fascia, regional muscles and tendons, and deep fascia. Actually cut down to the very dorsal surface of the regional bones
   c With a scalpel or knife, excise the whole tissue block, clearing away all the soft tissues from the underlying bones. The vessels lie very keep in this region
4 Removal of the tissue block with the medial and lateral plantar vessels:
   a Place the extremity with the posterior surface upward
   b Trace a rectangle on the sole with the following anatomic landmarks: posterior border of the medial malleolus, medial side of the foot, base of the metatarsal bones, and lateral side of the foot. The transverse limits can also be determined, approximately, dividing the sole in fifths
   c Following the sides of the rectangle, cut through the skin, subcutaneous tissue, plantar aponeurosis and fascia, and regional muscles and tendons. In fact, cut down to the very plantar surfaces of the regional bone
   d With sharp dissection, remove the entire tissue block so as to leave fully exposed the regional bones and ligaments
   e Bisect longitudinally the tissue block. The medial half represents the tissue block of the medial plantar vessels, whereas the lateral half represents the tissue block of the lateral plantar vessels

5 Take samples of skin and soft tissues from areas of ulceration, necrosis, or infection, and from bone, if indicated. Now the extremity can be disposed of
6 Fix all the excised tissues overnight in formalin. The neurovascular bundles should be pinned down on corkboard
7 Once neurovascular bundles are well fixed, cut transversely every 4–5 mm and carefully examine the wall and lumen of vessels

Description

1 Type of amputation; side of extremity
2 Length and circumference
3 Appearance of skin: ulcers (size, extent), hemorrhage, stasis dermatitis
4 Subcutaneous tissue; muscle; bone and joints
5 Appearance of major arteries and veins: atherosclerosis (degree), thrombosis

Sections for histology

1 Skin
2 Major arteries, veins, and nerves according to accompanying diagram or an abbreviated version of it
3 Skeletal muscle
4 Bone and joint (when pertinent)

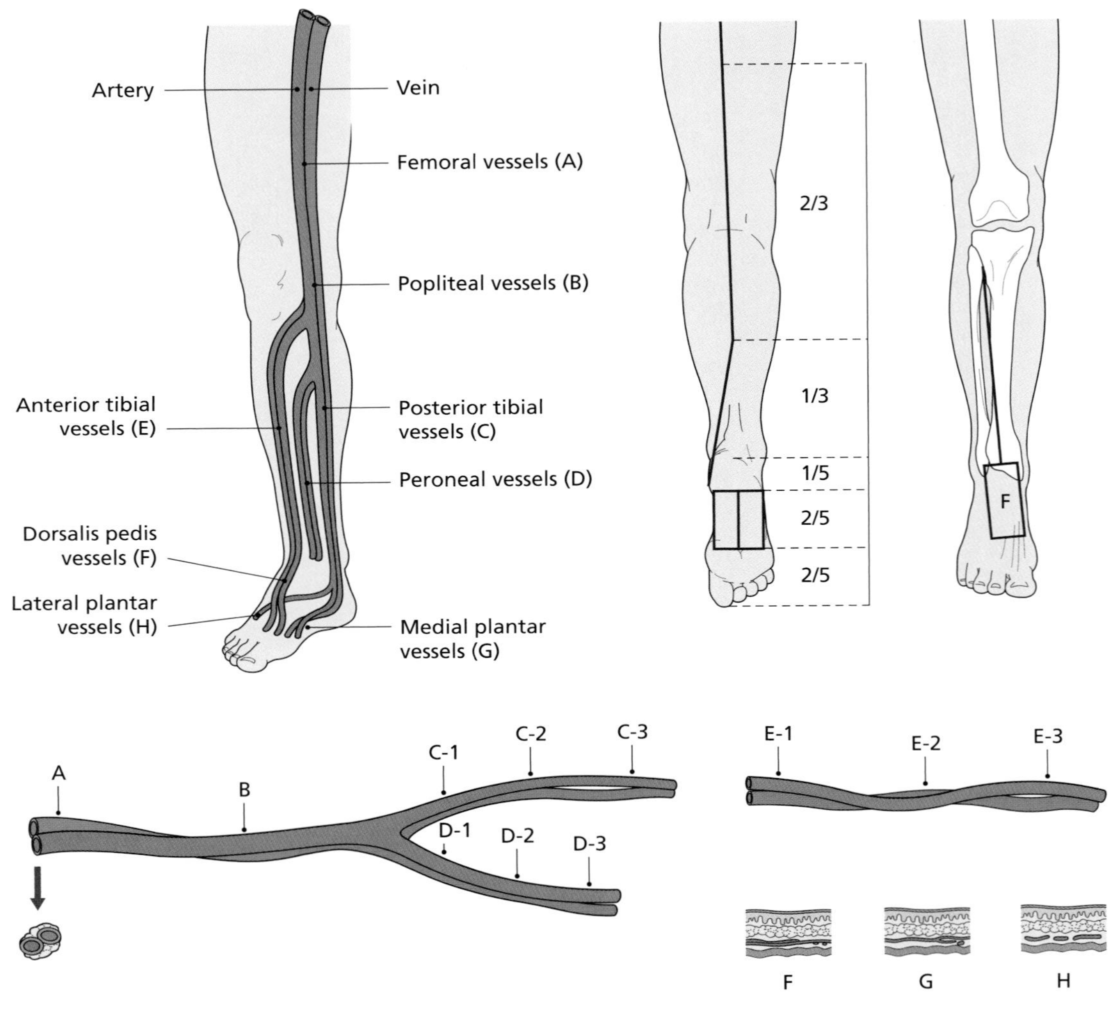

Eyes – conjunctiva

Procedure

Lesions of the conjunctiva are thin and tend to fold into distorted patterns when placed into fixative. To prepare the tissue so that the pathologist can orient it properly, the surgeon should spread the lesion onto a small piece of filter paper and allow it to dry for a few seconds before gently placing the filter paper with the adherent specimen into the jar of fixative. Specimens should never be put onto sponges of any kind since these will expand when placed into the fixative, thus distorting the specimen.

Eyes – enucleation[1–4]

Procedure

1 Fix the intact ocular globe in formalin for 24 hours before sectioning; it is not advisable to open the eye, to cut windows into the sclera, or to inject fixative into the vitreous
2 Wash in running tap water for 1 or more hours and, optionally, place in 60% ethyl alcohol for a few more hours
3 Review the summary of the clinical history and the results of the ophthalmologic examination prior to sectioning
4 Measure anteroposterior, horizontal, and vertical dimensions of the globe, length of the optic nerve, and horizontal dimensions of the cornea
5 Look for sites of accidental or surgical injuries
6 Transilluminate the globe before opening it. A substage microscope lamp in a darkened room is satisfactory. Rotate the globe over the light source; if abnormal shadows are detected, mark them on the sclera with an indelible pencil
7 Examination of the globe with a ×7 objective of a dissecting microscope can be carried out to detect minute lesions
8 If intraocular foreign bodies or retinoblastoma is suspected, take a roentgenogram of the globe before it is opened
9 If choroidal malignant melanoma is suspected, sample at least one of the vortex veins from each of the four quadrants (see accompanying drawing)
10 Open the eye with a sharp razor blade by holding the globe with the left hand, cornea down against the cutting block and the blade between the thumb and middle finger of the right hand. Open the eye with a sawing motion from back to front. The plane of section should begin adjacent to the optic nerve and end through the periphery of the cornea. The plane of section is dependent on whether a lesion has been detected in the previous steps. If it has not, cut the globe along a horizontal plane, using as surface landmarks the superior and inferior oblique insertions and the long postciliary vein (see accompanying drawing). If a lesion has been found, modify the plane of section so that the lesion will be included in the slab
11 Examine the interior of the globe

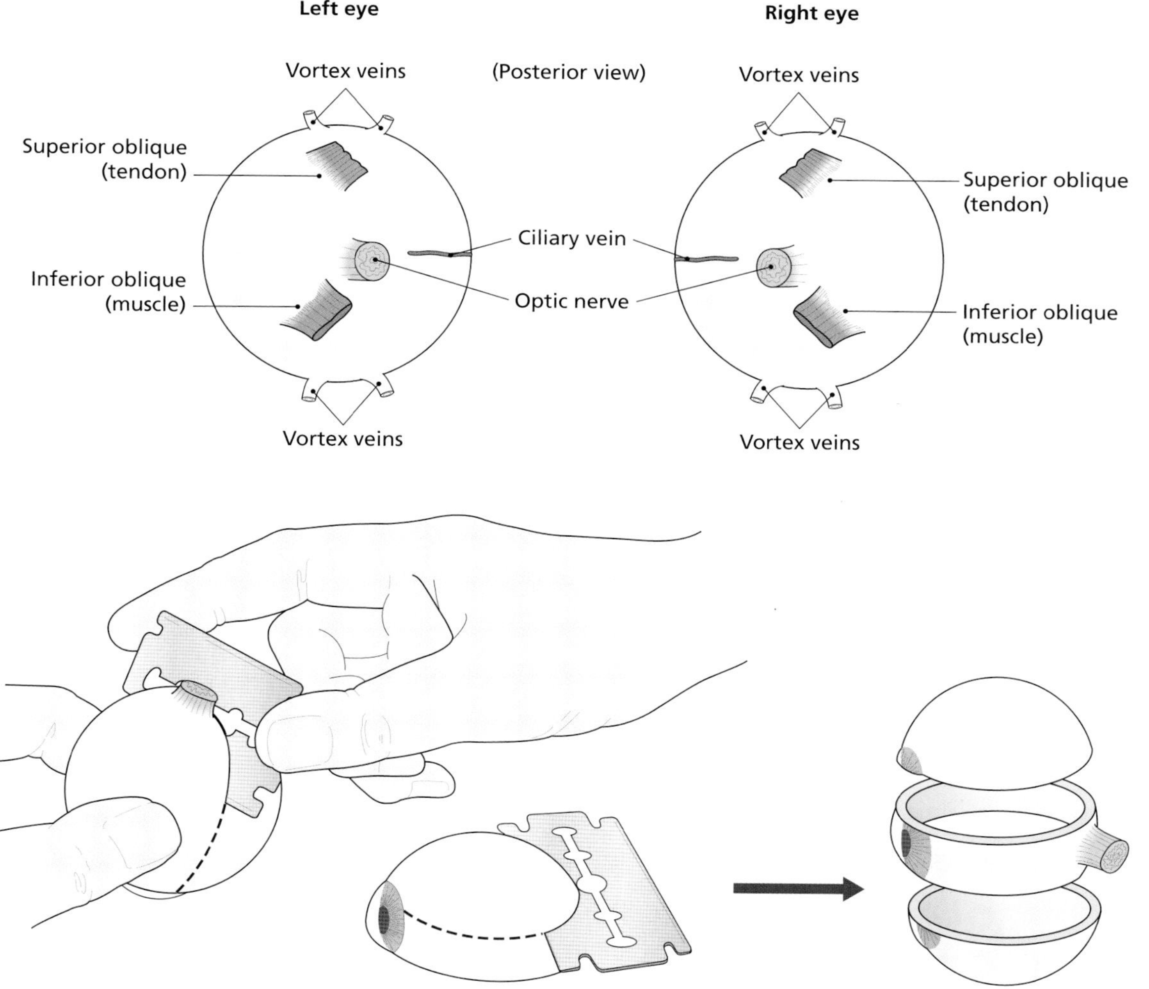

12 Place the eye flat on its cut surface, and make a second plane of section, parallel to the first, again passing from back to front
13 Examine carefully the ~8 mm disc-shaped slab thus obtained, which should contain the cornea, pupil, lens, and optic nerve. Take photographs or photocopies, if indicated

Description

Intact eye

1 Side of the globe (see accompanying drawing); anteroposterior, horizontal, and vertical dimensions
2 Length of optic nerve
3 Horizontal and vertical dimensions of cornea
4 Anterior segment: surgical incisions? corneal opacification? iris abnormalities? lens present?
5 Transillumination findings

Slab

1 Corneal thickness; anterior chamber depth; configuration of anterior chamber angle
2 Condition of iris, ciliary body, and lens
3 Condition of choroids, retina, vitreous body, and optic disc
4 If tumor present: location, size, color, edges, consistency, presence of hemorrhage or necrosis, ocular structures involved, extension into optic nerve

Sections for histology

1 Entire eye slab
2 Any (other) abnormal areas
3 In tumors, particularly retinoblastoma: cross-section of surgical margin of optic nerve
4 In suspected malignant melanoma: sample from at least one of vortex veins from each of four quadrants

1 Folberg R, Verdick R, Weingeist TA, Montague PR. The gross examination of eyes removed for choroidal and ciliary body melanomas. Ophthalmology 1986, **93:** 1643–1647
2 Herreman R, De Buen S, Cortés T. Oftalmóun Nuevo apparato para secionar los ojos en el laboratorio de anatomía patológica. Rev Fac Med (Mexico) 1965, **7:** 157–167
3 Smith ME. A method for immediate gross sectioning of enucleated globes. Am J Ophthalmol 1974, **77:** 413–414
4 Yanoff M, Fine BS. Glutaraldehyde fixation of routine surgical eye tissue. Am J Ophthalmol 1967, **63:** 137–140

Fallopian tubes – ligation[1]

In tubal ligation, an avascular segment in the midisthmic portion of the tube is made into a loop, the base is ligated, and the top of the loop is excised.

Procedure

1 Separate specimens from right and left tubes
2 Measure the length and diameter of each

Description

1 Length and diameter of each specimen
2 Do they appear to be a complete segment of each tube? lumen present?

Sections for histology

1 All tissues received, identified as to right and left tube
2 Very important that tissue be sectioned on end; instructions to histotechnician or embedding in agar may be necessary

1 Robboy SJ, Kraus FT, Kurman RJ. Gross description, processing, and reporting of gynaecologic and obstetric specimens. In Kurman RJ (ed.): Blaustein's pathology of the female genital tract, ed. 4. New York, 2002, Springer-Verlag, pp. 1319–1346

Fallopian tubes – salpingectomy[1]

Salpingectomy may be performed by itself in the case of fallopian tube pathology or – more often – as part of a total abdominal hysterectomy with unilateral or bilateral salpingo-oophorectomy.

Procedure

1. Fix the specimen before sectioning. If the tubes are attached to the uterus, they should be fixed in that position
2. Measure the length and greatest diameter
3. If the tube is relatively normal in size, serially section at 5 mm intervals and examine. Make the cuts incomplete so that the pieces remain attached by the serosa
4. If the tube is obviously enlarged, make one complete longitudinal section, followed by parallel sections, if necessary

Description

1. Length and greatest diameter
2. Serosa: fibrin? hemorrhage? fibrous adhesions to ovary or other organs?
3. Wall: abnormally thick? ruptured?
4. Mucosa: atrophic? hyperplastic? appearance of fimbriated end; inverted?
5. Lumen: patent? dilated? content; diameter, if abnormally large
6. Masses: size, appearance, invasion
7. Cysts in paraovarian region: diameter, thickness of wall, content; sessile or pedunculated?
8. In cases of suspected ectopic pregnancy: embryo or placenta identified? amount of hemorrhage; rupture?

Sections for histology

1. For incidental tubes without gross abnormalities: three cross-sections of each tube, taken from the proximal, mid, and distal portions, submitted in the same cassette (see accompanying drawing)
2. For tubes with suspected ectopic pregnancy: submit any tissue with gross appearance of products of conception. If none is grossly identified, submit any tissue with gross appearance of products of conception. If none is grossly identified, submit several sections from the wall in the area of hemorrhage as well as several from the *intraluminal clot*. If products of conception are not identified microscopically, submit additional sections
3. For tubes with other lesions: as many as needed to adequately examine any abnormal areas. If tumor is present, at least three sections must be taken to include grossly uninvolved mucosa

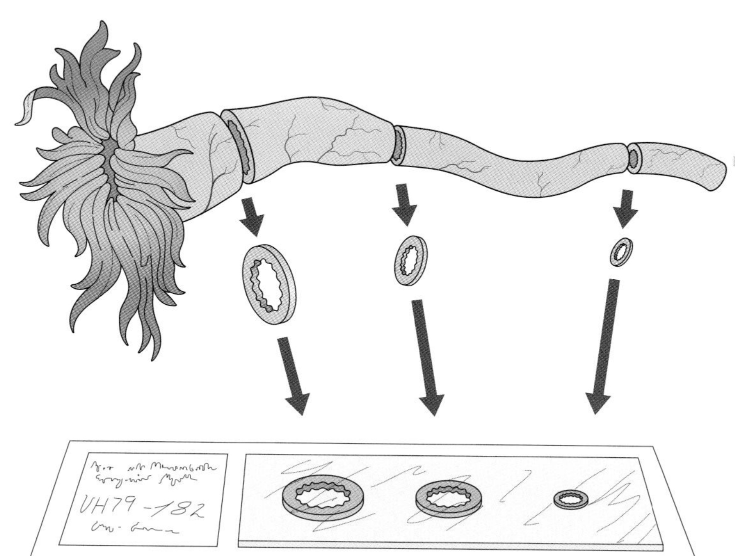

Procedure

Keep intact, cut sagittally, or dissect, depending on fetus size

1 Robboy SJ, Kraus TF, Kurman RJ. Gross description, processing, and reporting of gynaecologic and obstetric specimens. In Kurman RJ (ed.): Blaustein's pathology of the female genital tract, ed. 4. New York, 2002, Springer-Verlag, pp. 1319–1346

Fetus - abortion

Description

1 Sex; weight; crown–rump length (A), crown–heel length (B), or foot length (C) (see accompanying drawings, p. 2601)
2 Approximate length of gestation (see Table App E-1 and drawings p. 2601)
3 General condition: well preserved? macerated?
4 External and internal anomalies and other changes
5 Umbilical cord: appearance, number of vessels
6 Placental tissues accompanying fetuses:
   a Weight
   b Membranes: insertion, color, transparency, completeness; extramembranous pregnancy? marginal or membranous hemorrhage?
   c Umbilical cord: insertion, color, focal changes
   d Chorionic plate: vascular pattern, vessel caliber, color; subchorionic hemorrhage?
   e Villi: hydatidiform change? (note proportion of involved villi and size of cysts); focal lesions?

Sections for histology

1 Small embryos: submit whole embryo or one half, depending on size
2 Large fetuses: submit one section from lungs, stomach (including gastric contents), kidneys, and other organs, as indicated
3 Placental tissues:
   a Extraplacental membranes (one section)
   b Umbilical cord (one section)
   c Chorionic plate (one section)
   d Villi from chorion frondosum, including maternal surface (one section)

For a more thorough examination of specimens for fetal malformations and chromosomal abnormalities, see:

1 Klatt EC. Pathologic examination of fetal specimens from dilation and evacuation procedures. Am J Clin Pathol 1995, **103**: 415–418
2 Robboy SJ, Kraus TF, Kurman RJ. Gross description, processing, and reporting of gynaecologic and obstetric specimens. In Kurman RJ (ed.): Blaustein's pathology of the female genital tract, ed. 4. New York, 2002, Springer-Verlag, pp. 1319–1346
3 Szulman AE. Examination of the early conceptus. Arch Pathol Lab Med 1991, **115**: 696–700

Table App E-1 Relations of age, size, and weight in the human embryo

					AMOUNT OF INCREASE EACH MONTH WHEN VALUE AT START OF MONTH EQUALS UNITY	
Age of embryo	**Crown–rump (CR) length (mm)**	**Crown–heel length (mm)**	**External diameter of chorionic sac (mm)**	**Weight in grams**	**CR length**	**Weight**
One week	0.1*	–	0.2			
Two weeks	0.2*	–	3			
Three weeks	2.0	–	10			
Four weeks	5.0	–	10	0.02	49.0	40000.00
Five weeks	8.0	–	25			
Six weeks	12.0	–	30			
Seven weeks	17.0	19.0	40			
Two lunar months	25.0	30.0	50	1	3.6	49.00
Three lunar months	56.0	73.0	–	14	1.4	13.00
Four lunar months	112.0	157.0	–	105	1.0	6.50
Five lunar months	160.0	239.0	–	310	0.43	1.95
Six lunar months	203.0	296.0	–	640	0.26	1.07
Seven lunar months	242.0	355.0	–	1080	0.14	0.69
Eight lunar months	277.0	409.0	–	1670	0.14	0.55
Nine lunar months	313.0	458.0	–	2400	0.13	0.43
Full term (38 weeks)	350.0	500.0	–	3300	0.12	0.38

From Arey LB. Developmental anatomy, ed. 7, revised. Philadelphia, 1974, W.B. Saunders, p. 104.
*Total length of embryonic disc.

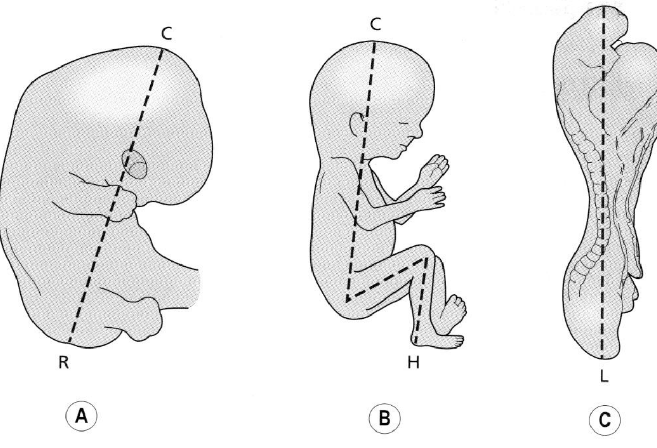

Gallbladder – cholecystectomy

Cholecystectomy consists of removal of the entire gallbladder after dissecting it from the base of the liver and suturing the cystic duct and cystic artery. At present, a high number of cholecystectomies are performed through a laparoscopic route.

Procedure

1 Open the entire organ longitudinally as soon as feasible after excision, otherwise the mucosa will quickly undergo autolytic changes
2 If stones are present, wash them, estimate the number and the size of the largest, and cut one or several of them with a scalpel
3 Search for lymph nodes along the bladder neck
4 In cases of carcinoma the organ also can be studied by extracting the bile with a syringe, filling the lumen with formalin, fixing overnight at 4 °C, and cutting the specimen with scissors and a scalpel

Description

1 Length and greatest diameter of gallbladder
2 Serosa: thickened? fibrous adhesions? fibrin?
3 Wall: thickened? (if so, focally or diffusely?) hemorrhage?
4 Mucosa: color, appearance, ulcerated? hyperplastic? cholesterosis
5 Cystic duct: dilated? impacted with stones? lymph nodes present? size and appearance
6 Approximate volume, color, and consistency of bile
7 Stones: approximate number, shape, and size range: color and appearance on cross-sections; type of stone (see accompanying table)
8 If tumor present: location, distance from fundus and neck, size; polypoid? ulcerated? infiltrative? serosal involvement?

Sections for histology

1 Three sections including entire wall: one from the fundus, one from the body, and one from the neck; additional sections from any area that appears grossly abnormal
2 In cases of suspected carcinoma in situ, the organ can be studied by embedding the entire specimen by the Swiss roll method. In addition, the bile can be decanted into a breaker or centrifuge tube and studied cytologically[1]
3 Cystic duct and lymph nodes, if they appear grossly abnormal or if the gallbladder contains a tumor

1 Albores-Saavedra J, Henson DE, Klimstra DS. Tumors of the gallbladder, extrahepatic bile ducts, and ampulla of Vater. Atlas of tumor pathology. Third series, fascicle 27. Washington DC, 2000, Armed Forces Institute of Pathology

Table App E-2 Types of gallstones

TYPE OF STONE	INCIDENCE	COMPOSITION	APPEARANCE
Pure	10%	Cholesterol Calcium bilirubinate Calcium carbonate	Solitary; crystalline surface Multiple; jet black; crystalline or amorphous Grayish white; amorphous
Mixed	80%	Cholesterol and calcium bilirubinate Cholesterol and calcium carbonate Calcium bilirubinate and calcium carbonate Cholesterol, calcium bilirubinate, and calcium carbonate	Multiple, faceted or lobulated, laminated, and crystalline on cut surfaces Hue: Yellow – cholesterol Black – calcium bilirubinate White – calcium carbonate
Combined	10%	Pure gallstone nucleus with mixed gallstone shell Mixed gallstone nucleus with pure gallstone shell	Largest of gallstones when single Hue depends on composition of shell

Slightly modified from de Schryver-Kecskemet K. Gallbladder and biliary ducts. In Kissane JM (ed.): Anderson's pathology, ed 9. St Louis, 1990, Mosby.

Procedure

1 Fix the whole specimen in formalin overnight in the refrigerator at 4 °C
2 Paint the surgical margins with India ink
3 For bone tumors: make multiple parallel sections through bone and soft tissue with a band saw, fix further in formalin, and decalcify
4 For mucosal or soft tissue tumors: separate soft tissue from the mandible with a scalpel. The direction of the dissection should be from the inferior to the superior and from the posterior to the anterior aspects
5 Take photographs or photocopies and identify in one of them the site of the sections to be taken
6 If the specimen includes a radical neck dissection, process according to instructions for Lymph node dissection – radical neck

maxillary sinus? arising from superior, medial, lateral, anterior, posterior, or inferior part of sinus? extending into intratemporal fossa, nasal cavity, ethmoid cells, or any other of aforementioned structures? presence of tumor at surgical margins?
4 Condition of ostium of maxillary sinus and any other sinuses present; fistulae present

Sections for histology

1 Tumor: as many sections as necessary, with minimum of three
2 Surgical margins

1 A very detailed set of instructions for surgical specimens from the upper aerodigestive tract is available from: Slootweg PJ, de Groot JAM. Surgical pathological anatomy of head and neck specimens: a manual for the dissection of surgical specimens from the upper aerodigestive tract. London, 1999, Springer

Heart – valve replacement

(Adapted from Roberts WC, Morrow AG. Cardiac valves and the surgical pathologist. Arch Pathol 1996, **82:** 309–313.)

Traditionally, valve replacement operations have entailed the removal of the entire diseased valve. However, in cases of mitral valve disease, there has been a tendency in recent years to remove only the anterior mitral leaflet during valve replacement and to remove only portions of the valve (usually from the posterior leaflet) during reparative procedures.

Procedure

response to chemotherapeutic agents. In some cases of metastatic cancer, it may provide some indication of the site of origin of the primary lesion. Sampling should be taken of recurrent or metastatic carcinoma, even if the original tumor had been previously assayed, to establish the continued presence or absence of the receptor.

Two methods are available for the determination of hormone receptors in tissue: biochemical and immunohistochemical. The former, based on charcoal–dextran assay, has been the standard for many years, but has been largely replaced by the immunohistochemical method. The procedure for procuring tissue for the biochemical assay if still desired is the following:

1 Examine tissue in the fresh state, immediately after excision; select a sample carefully, avoiding areas of necrosis, adipose

Appendix E

Large bowel – colectomy for tumor

The major types of large bowel resection are *total colectomy*, *right hemicolectomy* (which includes the colon up to the hepatic flexure, cecum, ileocecal valve, appendix, portion of terminal ileum, and the corresponding mesentery), *transverse colectomy* (from the hepatic to the splenic flexures), *left hemicolectomy* (from the splenic flexure to the sigmoid colon), *low anterior* (rectosigmoid) *resection*, and *abdominoperineal resection* (sigmoid colon, rectum, and anus).

Procedure

1 Dissect the lymph nodes and remove the mesentery while the specimen is fresh. (A method of injecting methylene blue into the rectal artery to improve lymph node identification in rectal carcinoma has been described[1])
2 Two options are available to study the bowel, depending on the size and location of the specimen when received in the laboratory. The first is the one usually carried out
   a Open the bowel longitudinally through its entire length, trying not to cut through the tumor. Pin the intestine on a corkboard and fix overnight in formalin
   b Inject the specimen (see Injection of specimens – general guidelines and **2b** under Procedure in the preceding section)
3 Take photographs or photocopies and identify in one of them the sites of the sections to be taken
4 In cases with deep penetration by tumor, dissect the veins carefully for possible tumor invasion
5 In general, take the sections *perpendicular* to the direction of the mucosal folds

Description

1 Part of bowel removed, length of specimen, and amount of mesentery
2 a Tumor characteristics: size (including thickness); extent around bowel; shape (fungating, flat, ulcerating); presence of necrosis or hemorrhage; extent through bowel wall; serosal involvement, satellite nodules; evidence of blood vessel invasion; invasion of adjacent organs
   b Distance of tumor to pectinate line, peritoneal reflection, each line of resection
3 Other lesions in bowel and appearance of uninvolved mucosa; if polyps absent, so state
4 Estimate of number of lymph nodes found; whether or not nodes appear involved by tumor; size of largest node

Sections for histology

1 Tumor: at least three sections (extending through the entire wall)
2 Representative section of subserosal connective tissue, fat, and blood vessel around tumor
3 Other lesions of bowel
4 Proximal line of resection
5 Distal line of resection
6 Bowel between tumor and distal line of resection (halfway or 5 cm, whichever suits the case)
7 Appendix, if included in specimen
8 Lymph nodes:
   a Around tumor
   b Distal to tumor

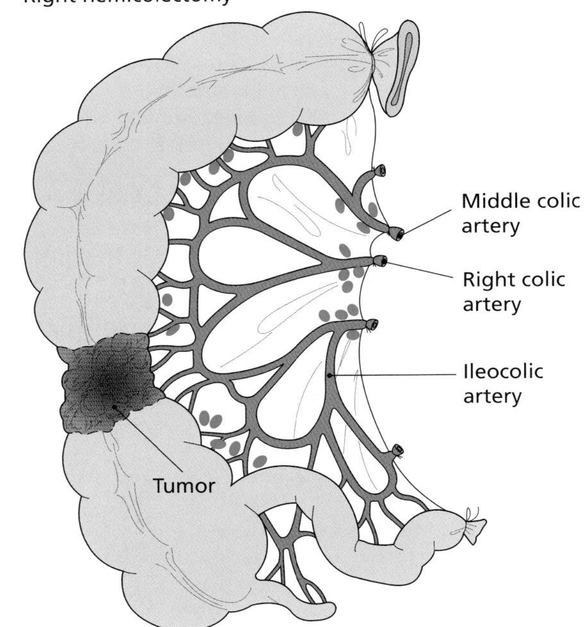

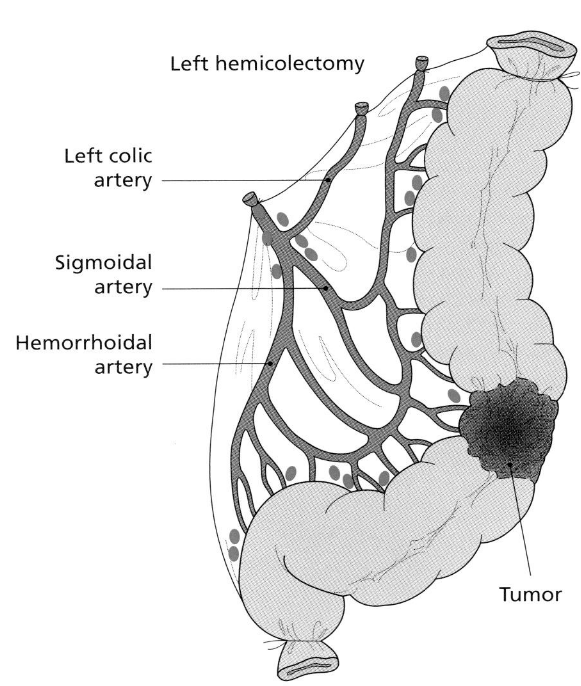

   c Proximal to tumor
   d At high point of resection (areas surrounding ligated vessels)
9 In abdominoperineal resections: anorectal junction

1 Märkl B, Kerwel TG, Wagner T, Anthuber M, Arnholdt HM. Methylene blue injection into the rectal artery as a simple method to improve lymph node harvest in rectal cancer. Mod Pathol 2007, **20:** 797–801

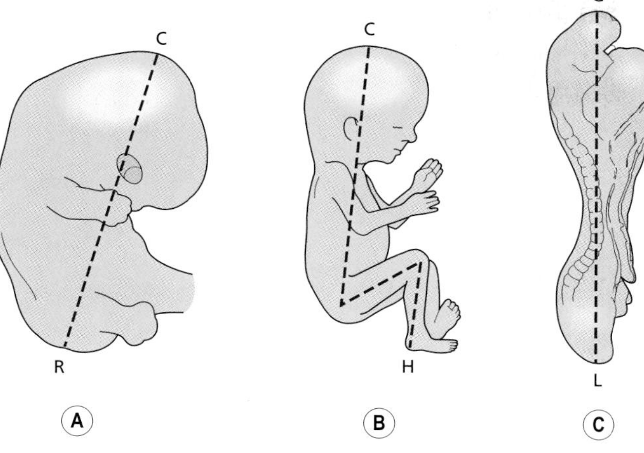

Gallbladder – cholecystectomy

Cholecystectomy consists of removal of the entire gallbladder after dissecting it from the base of the liver and suturing the cystic duct and cystic artery. At present, a high number of cholecystectomies are performed through a laparoscopic route.

Procedure

1 Open the entire organ longitudinally as soon as feasible after excision, otherwise the mucosa will quickly undergo autolytic changes
2 If stones are present, wash them, estimate the number and the size of the largest, and cut one or several of them with a scalpel
3 Search for lymph nodes along the bladder neck
4 In cases of carcinoma the organ also can be studied by extracting the bile with a syringe, filling the lumen with formalin, fixing overnight at 4 °C, and cutting the specimen with scissors and a scalpel

Description

1 Length and greatest diameter of gallbladder
2 Serosa: thickened? fibrous adhesions? fibrin?
3 Wall: thickened? (if so, focally or diffusely?) hemorrhage?
4 Mucosa: color, appearance, ulcerated? hyperplastic? cholesterosis
5 Cystic duct: dilated? impacted with stones? lymph nodes present? size and appearance
6 Approximate volume, color, and consistency of bile
7 Stones: approximate number, shape, and size range: color and appearance on cross-sections; type of stone (see accompanying table)
8 If tumor present: location, distance from fundus and neck, size; polypoid? ulcerated? infiltrative? serosal involvement?

Sections for histology

1 Three sections including entire wall: one from the fundus, one from the body, and one from the neck; additional sections from any area that appears grossly abnormal
2 In cases of suspected carcinoma in situ, the organ can be studied by embedding the entire specimen by the Swiss roll method. In addition, the bile can be decanted into a breaker or centrifuge tube and studied cytologically[1]
3 Cystic duct and lymph nodes, if they appear grossly abnormal or if the gallbladder contains a tumor

1 Albores-Saavedra J, Henson DE, Klimstra DS. Tumors of the gallbladder, extrahepatic bile ducts, and ampulla of Vater. Atlas of tumor pathology. Third series, fascicle 27. Washington DC, 2000, Armed Forces Institute of Pathology

Table App E-2 Types of gallstones

TYPE OF STONE	INCIDENCE	COMPOSITION	APPEARANCE
Pure	10%	Cholesterol Calcium bilirubinate Calcium carbonate	Solitary; crystalline surface Multiple; jet black; crystalline or amorphous Grayish white; amorphous
Mixed	80%	Cholesterol and calcium bilirubinate Cholesterol and calcium carbonate Calcium bilirubinate and calcium carbonate Cholesterol, calcium bilirubinate, and calcium carbonate	Multiple, faceted or lobulated, laminated, and crystalline on cut surfaces Hue: Yellow – cholesterol Black – calcium bilirubinate White – calcium carbonate
Combined	10%	Pure gallstone nucleus with mixed gallstone shell Mixed gallstone nucleus with pure gallstone shell	Largest of gallstones when single Hue depends on composition of shell

Slightly modified from de Schryver-Kecskemet K. Gallbladder and biliary ducts. In Kissane JM (ed.): Anderson's pathology, ed 9. St Louis, 1990, Mosby.

Heart – valve replacement

(Adapted from Roberts WC, Morrow AG. Cardiac valves and the surgical pathologist. Arch Pathol 1996, **82:** 309–313.)

Traditionally, valve replacement operations have entailed the removal of the entire diseased valve. However, in cases of mitral valve disease, there has been a tendency in recent years to remove only the anterior mitral leaflet during valve replacement and to remove only portions of the valve (usually from the posterior leaflet) during reparative procedures.

Procedure

1 Fix the specimen before sectioning
2 Take photographs or photocopies and a roentgenogram in every case. For atrioventricular valves, photograph from both atrial and ventricular aspects. For aortic valves, photograph from both aortic and ventricular aspects

Description

Atrioventricular valves

1 Leaflets fibrotic, calcified, or normal?
2 Fibrosis or calcification focal or diffuse?
3 Fibrosis or calcification distributed on leaflets? (only at margins? on one surface? on both?)
4 Leaflets immobile, shortened, stretched, or normal?
5 Commissures fused? (if so, to what extent?)
6 Chordae tendineae intact, ruptured, shortened, elongated, fused, or normal?
7 Papillary muscles normal in number, scarred, hypertrophied, or elongated?
8 Valve incompetent, stenotic, or both?
9 If incompetent: because of scanty valvular tissue, dilated annulus, or ruptured chordae or because of ruptured, scarred, or shortened papillary muscle?

Semilunar valves

Same as for atrioventricular valves in most respects plus:

1 Number of cusps present?
2 Cusps of equal or unequal size?

Sections for histology

Several sections, including free edge; decalcify, if necessary

Hormone receptor assays – sampling

(Adapted from Keffer JH. Hormone-receptor assays and cancer of the breast. The pathologist's role [editorial]. Am J Clin Pathol 1978, **70:** 719–720.)

Determination of receptors for different steroid hormones (estrogens, progesterone, androgens) has become an established technique for the evaluation of several surgically excised tissues, particularly breast carcinoma. It correlates with clinical response to hormone therapy and, according to some, also with clinical response to chemotherapeutic agents. In some cases of metastatic cancer, it may provide some indication of the site of origin of the primary lesion. Sampling should be taken of recurrent or metastatic carcinoma, even if the original tumor had been previously assayed, to establish the continued presence or absence of the receptor.

Two methods are available for the determination of hormone receptors in tissue: biochemical and immunohistochemical. The former, based on charcoal–dextran assay, has been the standard for many years, but has been largely replaced by the immunohistochemical method. The procedure for procuring tissue for the biochemical assay if still desired is the following:

1 Examine tissue in the fresh state, immediately after excision; select a sample carefully, avoiding areas of necrosis, adipose tissue, and other unsuitable areas
2 Cut a sample measuring approximately 1 cm in greatest diameter (or as large as allowable). The instruments should be clean but not necessarily sterile
3 Freeze quickly in liquid nitrogen (−70 °C) in isopentane or with freon spray
4 Store in the deep freeze until the sample is ready to be delivered (in the frozen state) to the appropriate laboratory
5 Submit for histology (for control purposes) a piece of tissue immediately adjacent to the one frozen and identify as such
6 When the lesion is so small that a 1 cm sample for biochemical assay cannot be spared, cut frozen sections and store in the freezer (−70 °C) for subsequent immunohistochemical staining for receptor

Imprints (touch preparations)

(Adapted from Berard CW, Bowling MC. Technical factors in evaluation of lymph node biopsies. Tutorial on neoplastic hematopathology, Henry Rappaport, MD, Director, Pasadena, California, Feb 5–9, 1979; presented in cooperation with The City of Hope National Medical Center and The University of Chicago Center for Continuing Education.)

1 Cut a block of tissue measuring approximately 10 × 10 × 3 mm
2 Hold the tissue gently with forceps with the freshly cut, flat surface upward (see accompanying drawing, p. 2603)
3 With the other hand, lightly touch an alcohol-clean glass slide repeatedly in serial adjacent areas with the cut surface of the tissue. Just contact – do not compress the block. If the surface touched is excessively bloody or wet, discard the slide and repeat with another slide until the touch preparations are barely opaque. Prepare an average of four slides in this fashion
4 As each slide is prepared, dry it rapidly by waving it in the air. Do not heat or blow on the slide. It should take no more than 30–60 seconds for the slide to dry; if it takes more, it means that the touches are too wet and that the resulting imprints will be unsatisfactory
5 For standard purposes, fix (after drying) in methyl alcohol, and stain two with hematoxylin–eosin and two with Wright or Giemsa stain
6 After preparation of the imprints, fix and submit for histology the block used for this purpose to correlate its appearance with that of the imprint

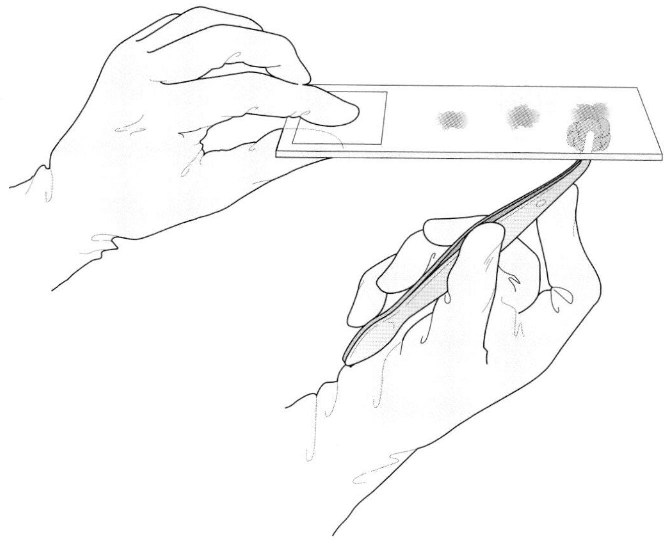

Injection of specimens – general guidelines

When feasible, the injection of surgical specimens may serve to illustrate more clearly the gross pathology present, as well as to ensure proper fixation. The procedure has been found most useful for lobectomies, pneumonectomies, cystectomies, colectomies, and pelvic exenterations.

1 Partially fill a large container with fixative
2 Prepare the specimen properly (see specific instructions for the respective organs)
3 Place in container and inject with formalin
4 Add additional fixative to the container to ensure that the entire specimen is covered by fixative
5 Place a towel or several gauze pads on the free-floating specimen to prevent the surface from drying
6 Cover the container with a lid
7 Fix for 24 hours before dissecting

Jaw resection for tumor – mandibulectomy[1]

Procedure

1 Fix the whole specimen in formalin overnight in the refrigerator at 4 °C
2 Paint the surgical margins with India ink
3 For bone tumors: make multiple parallel sections through bone and soft tissue with a band saw, fix further in formalin, and decalcify
4 For mucosal or soft tissue tumors: separate soft tissue from the mandible with a scalpel. The direction of the dissection should be from the inferior to the superior and from the posterior to the anterior aspects
5 Take photographs or photocopies and identify in one of them the site of the sections to be taken
6 If the specimen includes a radical neck dissection, process according to instructions for Lymph node dissection – radical neck

Description

1 Type of resection (partial or total) and side
2 Tumor: size, color, appearance, edges; bone invaded?
3 Non-neoplastic mucosa: leukoplakia?
4 Bone: appearance on cross-sections
5 Teeth: number and appearance

Sections for histology

1 Tumor: three sections
2 Non-neoplastic mucosa
3 Mucosal surgical margins
4 Soft tissue surgical margins
5 Bone surgical margins
6 Mandibular nerve (surgical margins)
7 Bone, if grossly involved or suspicious

1 A very detailed set of instructions for surgical specimens from the upper aerodigestive tract is available from: Slootweg PJ, de Groot JAM. Surgical pathological anatomy of head and neck specimens: a manual for the dissection of surgical specimens from the upper aerodigestive tract. London, 1999, Springer

Jaw resection for tumor – maxillectomy[1]

Procedure

1 Fix the specimen in formalin overnight in the refrigerator at 4 °C
2 Paint the surgical margins with India ink
3 Take surgical margins (anterior, posterior, external, and superior); cut the specimen with the band saw in parallel slices 0.5 cm thick. Fix them overnight. Take photographs and x-ray studies, if indicated
4 Take photographs or photocopies and identify in one of them the site of the sections to be taken

Description

1 Extent of resection
2 Presence of following structures: hard and soft palates; superior, middle, and inferior turbinates; medial and lateral pterygoid plate of sphenoid bone; air cells of ethmoid; bony floor of orbit; orbital contents; zygoma, masseter, temporalis, external and internal pterygoid muscles
3 Tumor characteristics: location, extent, size; limited to the maxillary sinus? arising from superior, medial, lateral, anterior, posterior, or inferior part of sinus? extending into intratemporal fossa, nasal cavity, ethmoid cells, or any other of aforementioned structures? presence of tumor at surgical margins?
4 Condition of ostium of maxillary sinus and any other sinuses present; fistulae present

Sections for histology

1 Tumor: as many sections as necessary, with minimum of three
2 Surgical margins

1 A very detailed set of instructions for surgical specimens from the upper aerodigestive tract is available from: Slootweg PJ, de Groot JAM. Surgical pathological anatomy of head and neck specimens: a manual for the dissection of surgical specimens from the upper aerodigestive tract. London, 1999, Springer

Kidney – needle biopsy

Procedure

The examination and sampling of this material should be carried out at the bedside or *immediately* after the specimen is received in the pathology laboratory.

1 Measure the length and diameter
2 Try to determine by gross inspection whether the cortex is present; this can be done by identifying glomeruli with a dissecting microscope or magnifying lenses. An experienced observer can do it most of the time with the naked eye on the basis of color
3 If the cortex is grossly identified:
   a Take three pieces (each 1 mm thick) from this area and fix in glutaraldehyde for electron microscopic examination
   b Take one additional piece (2 mm thick) from this area and freeze in isopentane cooled with liquid nitrogen for immunofluorescence
   c Place the remainder of the specimen in fixative for routine light microscopy
4 If the cortex cannot be identified with certainty on gross inspection, the operator may decide to perform another needle biopsy. Otherwise, the following should be done with the specimen:
   a Take two pieces (1 mm each) from *each* end and freeze for immunofluorescence
   b Take two additional pieces (2 mm) from *each* end and freeze for immunofluorescence
   c Fix the remainder for routine histology
5 If the amount of tissue is insufficient to divide for all these studies, electron microscopy and immunofluorescence have priority, one of the reasons being that a modified version of the light microscopic evaluation can be carried out on them
6 If the specimen is an open wedge biopsy, the same guidelines apply, except for the fact that the cortex is always readily identifiable and therefore double sampling is not necessary

Description

1 Number of fragments; length and diameter of each
2 Color: homogenous or not?
3 Cortex recognizable? glomeruli; size, color; prominence

Sections for histology

1 See Procedure
2 Needle renal biopsies should be routinely stained with:
   a Hematoxylin–eosin
   b Alcian blue–periodic acid–Schiff (PAS)
   c Jones silver methenamine
   d Masson trichrome

Kidney – nephrectomy for nontumoral condition

Procedure

1 Measure and weigh the organ
2 Two options are available depending on the type of abnormality present and the status of the organ when received in the laboratory:
   a Cut the kidney sagittally, strip the capsule, and carefully open the pelvis, calyces, and ureter
   b Inject with formalin through the ureter and, if possible, through the renal artery, ligate the ureter (and artery), and submerge in formalin overnight. Cut sagittally the next day, strip the capsule, and open the pelvis, calyces, and ureter. This technique is especially useful in cases of hydronephrosis
3 Take photographs or photocopies and identify in one of them the sites of the sections to be taken
4 If stones are present, submit for chemical analysis, if indicated

Description

1 Weight and size of kidney
2 Capsule: amount of pericapsular tissue, thickness of capsule, adherence to cortex
3 External surface: smooth? scars: number, size, shape (flat or V shaped?); cysts? (if so, number, size, location, content)
4 Cortex: color, width; glomeruli apparent? striations apparent and orderly?
5 Medulla: color, width; medullary rays apparent and orderly?
6 Pelvis: size; dilated? blunting of calyces? thickened? hemorrhage? crystalline deposits? stones: number, size and shape (see Bladder – stone removal); amount of peripelvic fat
7 Ureter: diameter, length, evidence of dilation or stricture
8 Renal artery and vein; appearance

Sections for histology

1 Kidney: three sections, each including cortex and medulla
2 Pelvis: two sections
3 Ureter

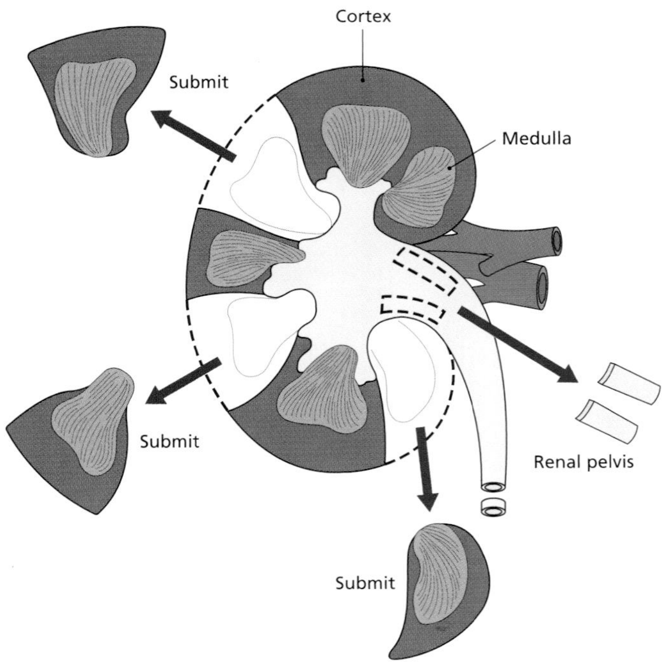

Kidney – nephrectomy for tumor[1]

Procedure

1 Look for and dissect any perirenal lymph nodes
2 Look for and open the renal vein longitudinally
3 Cut the kidney sagittally and open the pelvis, calyces, and ureter
4 Strip the capsule and look for capsular and perirenal tumor extensions
5 If stones are present, submit for chemical analysis
6 Take photographs or photocopies and identify in one of them the sites of the sections to be taken
7 Cut the kidney in thin slices, searching for additional cortical or medullary lesions

Description

1 Weight and dimensions of specimen; length and diameter of ureter
2 Tumor characteristics: size, shape, location, extent, homogenicity, necrosis, hemorrhage; invasion of capsule, perirenal tissues, calyces, pelvis, and renal vein
3 Uninvolved kidney: external surface, cortex, medulla; any additional focal lesions?
4 Pelvis: dilated? blunting of calyces? stones?
5 Presence, number, size, and appearance of perirenal lymph nodes

Sections for histology

1 Tumor: for renal cell carcinoma: minimum of three sections (including one with adjacent kidney); for pediatric tumors: minimum of one section for each centimeter of tumor diameter; for carcinoma of renal pelvis: minimum of three sections with adjacent pelvis and/or renal parenchyma
2 Kidney not involved by tumor: two sections
3 Pelvis: one section in cases of renal cell carcinoma or pediatric tumors; two sections in cases of carcinoma of renal pelvis
4 Renal artery and vein
5 Ureter: one section in cases of renal cell carcinoma or pediatric tumors; one section of every centimeter of ureter resected (and any abnormal-looking areas) in cases of carcinoma of renal pelvis
6 Lymph nodes, if present

1 Eble JN. Recommendations for examining and reporting tumor-bearing kidney specimens from adults. Semin Diagn Pathol 1998, **15**: 77–82

Large bowel – colectomy for nontumoral conditions

Procedure

1 Sample a few lymph nodes, and remove the mesentery while the specimen is fresh
2 Two options are available to study the bowel, depending on the type of abnormality present and the status of the specimen when received in the laboratory. The first is the one usually carried out
  a Open the bowel longitudinally, pin on a corkboard, and fix overnight in formalin
  b Inject the specimen (see Injection of specimens – general guidelines). Evacuate gross fecal contents by gentle external massage of the specimen. Further cleansing may be accomplished by the use of a gentle stream of formalin or saline solution (*not* water) into the bowel lumen. One end of the specimen is tied off, the specimen is injected with formalin, and the other end is tied off. If a constricting lesion is present, be sure that adequate fixative can be easily passed through the point of constriction. If this cannot be achieved, the main mass will not be properly fixed; under these circumstances, it is better to open the specimen and fix as noted in **2a** rather than to inject on both sides of the lesion. Injection is especially demonstrative in cases of diverticulosis
3 Take photographs or photocopies and identify in one of them the sites of the sections to be taken
4 In general, take the sections *perpendicular* to the direction of the mucosal folds

Description

1 Part of bowel removed, length of specimen, and amount of mesentery
2 Mucosa: type of lesions, extent, ulceration (linear or transverse), depth, pseudopolyps, hemorrhage, fissures
3 Wall: thickening (focal or diffuse), atrophy, fibrosis, necrosis
4 Serosa: fibrin, pus, fibrosis, adherence of mesentery
5 Diverticula: number, size, location in relation to teniae, content, evidence of inflammation, hemorrhage or perforation

Sections for histology

1 As many as necessary to sample abnormal areas
2 Proximal and distal lines of resection in cases of colitis
3 Appendix, if included in specimen

Large bowel – colectomy for tumor

The major types of large bowel resection are *total colectomy*, *right hemicolectomy* (which includes the colon up to the hepatic flexure, cecum, ileocecal valve, appendix, portion of terminal ileum, and the corresponding mesentery), *transverse colectomy* (from the hepatic to the splenic flexures), *left hemicolectomy* (from the splenic flexure to the sigmoid colon), *low anterior* (rectosigmoid) *resection*, and *abdominoperineal resection* (sigmoid colon, rectum, and anus).

Procedure

1 Dissect the lymph nodes and remove the mesentery while the specimen is fresh. (A method of injecting methylene blue into the rectal artery to improve lymph node identification in rectal carcinoma has been described[1])
2 Two options are available to study the bowel, depending on the size and location of the specimen when received in the laboratory. The first is the one usually carried out
   a Open the bowel longitudinally through its entire length, trying not to cut through the tumor. Pin the intestine on a corkboard and fix overnight in formalin
   b Inject the specimen (see Injection of specimens – general guidelines and **2b** under Procedure in the preceding section)
3 Take photographs or photocopies and identify in one of them the sites of the sections to be taken
4 In cases with deep penetration by tumor, dissect the veins carefully for possible tumor invasion
5 In general, take the sections *perpendicular* to the direction of the mucosal folds

Description

1 Part of bowel removed, length of specimen, and amount of mesentery
2 a Tumor characteristics: size (including thickness); extent around bowel; shape (fungating, flat, ulcerating); presence of necrosis or hemorrhage; extent through bowel wall; serosal involvement, satellite nodules; evidence of blood vessel invasion; invasion of adjacent organs
   b Distance of tumor to pectinate line, peritoneal reflection, each line of resection
3 Other lesions in bowel and appearance of uninvolved mucosa; if polyps absent, so state
4 Estimate of number of lymph nodes found; whether or not nodes appear involved by tumor; size of largest node

Sections for histology

1 Tumor: at least three sections (extending through the entire wall)
2 Representative section of subserosal connective tissue, fat, and blood vessel around tumor
3 Other lesions of bowel
4 Proximal line of resection
5 Distal line of resection
6 Bowel between tumor and distal line of resection (halfway or 5 cm, whichever suits the case)
7 Appendix, if included in specimen
8 Lymph nodes:
   a Around tumor
   b Distal to tumor
   c Proximal to tumor
   d At high point of resection (areas surrounding ligated vessels)
9 In abdominoperineal resections: anorectal junction

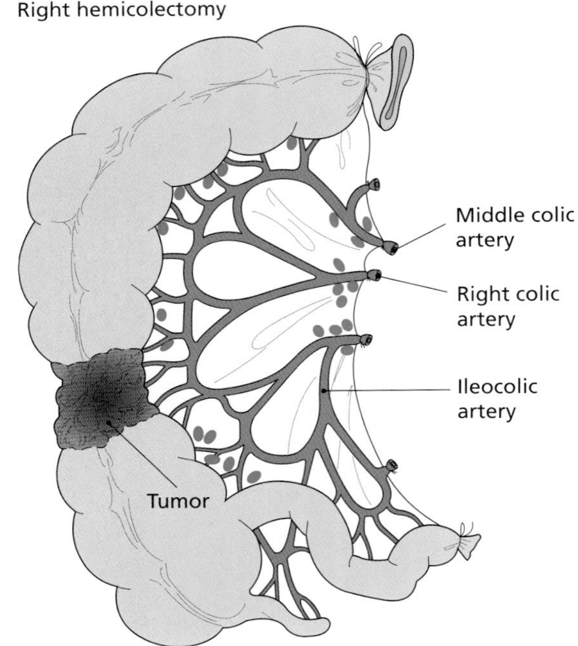

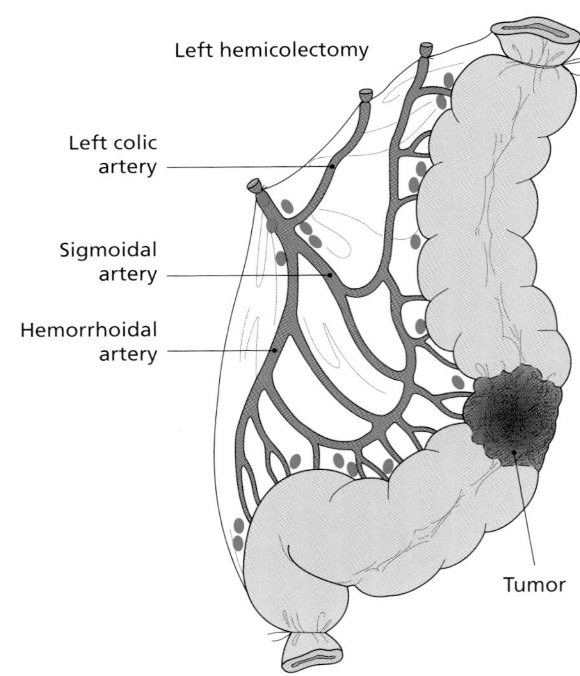

1 Märkl B, Kerwel TG, Wagner T, Anthuber M, Arnholdt HM. Methylene blue injection into the rectal artery as a simple method to improve lymph node harvest in rectal cancer. Mod Pathol 2007, **20:** 797–801

Large bowel – polypectomy

Procedure

1 Fix the specimen intact in formalin for several hours
2 Measure the diameter of the head and length of the stalk
3 For polyps with a short stalk or no stalk, identify the surgical section and cut in half longitudinally (see accompanying drawing **A**)
4 For polyps with a long stalk (1 cm or more), cut a cross-section of the stalk near the surgical margin and then cut the polyp longitudinally, leaving as long a stalk as will fit in the cassette (see accompanying drawing **B**)
5 If half the polyp head is over 3 mm, trim to this thickness on the convex side

Description

1 Dimensions of polyp; diameter of head and length of stalk
2 Polyp sessile or pedunculated? ulcerated? surface smooth or papillary? any cysts on cross-section? stalk appear normal?

Sections for histology

1 One longitudinal section (including surgical margin in polyps with short stalk or no stalk)
2 One cross-section of base of stalk (in polyps with long stalk)
3 Appendix, if included in specimen

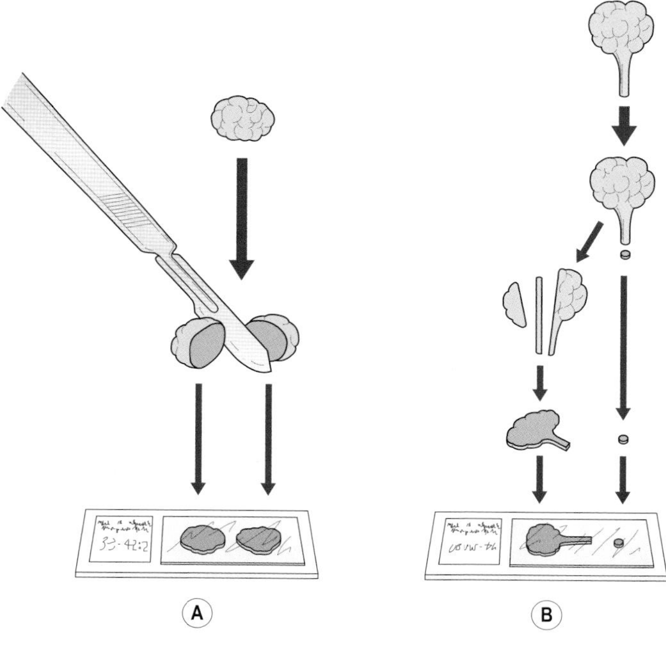

Larynx – laryngectomy[1]

(Adapted from Barnes L, Johnson JT. Pathologic and clinical consideration in the evaluation of major head and neck specimens resected for cancer. Part I. Pathol Annu 1986, **21(Pt 1)**: 173–250.)

Three types of laryngectomy are performed: hemilaryngectomy, supraglottic laryngectomy, and total. *Hemilaryngectomy* consists of dividing the thyroid cartilage in the midline and resecting in continuity the thyroid cartilage along with the corresponding true and false vocal cords and ventricle. *Supraglottic laryngectomy* consists of excising the upper half of the larynx horizontally through the ventricle. *Total laryngectomy* consists of removal of the entire larynx, including upper laryngeal rings.

Procedure

1 Separate the larynx from the radical neck dissection if accompanied by the latter
2 In total or supraglottic laryngectomy specimens, open the larynx along the posterior midline and keep it open with wires or by pinning to a corkboard
3 Photograph, if indicated
4 Fix overnight in formalin
5 Remove the hyoid bone, thyroid cartilage, and cricoid cartilage, trying to keep the soft tissue as a single piece even if the bone and cartilage need to be fragmented in the process
6 Take photographs or photocopies and identify in one of them the sites of the section to be taken
7 Paint the surgical margins (lingual, pharyngeal, and tracheal) with India ink
8 Orient as to superoinferior and anteroposterior axis
9 Handle the radical neck dissection according to instructions for Lymph node dissection – radical neck

Description

1 Type of laryngectomy: total laryngectomy, hemilaryngectomy, supraglottic laryngectomy; presence of pyriform sinus, hyoid bone, tracheal rings, thyroid and organs from neck dissection
2 Tumor characteristics: location (glottic, supraglottic, infraglottic, or transglottic?), side involved (wholly unilateral or encroaching on or crossing the midline?), size, pattern or growth (exophytic or endophytic?), ulceration, depth of invasion, presence of extralaryngeal spread, features of non-neoplastic mucosa (especially in true vocal cords)
   a For glottic tumors: length of cord involved; involvement of anterior or posterior commissures, extension to ventricle, and degree of subglottic extension as measured from the superior border of the true cord
   b For supraglottic tumors: if the hyoid bone is attached, is the tumor suprahyoid or infrahyoid? Does it involve the false cords, aryepiglottic folds, pyriform sinus (if present), or pre-epiglottic space?
   c If thyroid is included: weight, measurement, and appearance; invaded by tumor: parathyroid glands or perilaryngeal (delphian) node present? is there a tracheostomy? (if so, is there any evidence of tumor involvement?)

Sections for histology

1 Entire tumor in properly identified longitudinal strips (unless massive, in which case representative sections should be taken)
2 Representative step section of larynx, including epiglottis
3 Thyroid cartilage at the site of maximum tumor invasion, if any
4 Thyroid, parathyroid, and tracheostomy site, if present
5 Lymph nodes (see under Lymph node dissection – radical neck)

1 A very detailed set of instructions for surgical specimens from the upper aerodigestive tract is available from: Slootweg PJ, de Groot JAM. Surgical pathological anatomy of head and neck specimens: a manual for the dissection of surgical specimens from the upper aerodigestive tract. London, 1999, Springer

Lip – V excision

Procedure

1 Fix the specimen for several hours
2 Paint all surgical margins with India ink
3 Cut the specimen as shown in the accompanying drawing

Description

1 Size of specimen
2 Tumor characteristics: size, shape (ulcerated, polypoid), location (vermilion border, skin), distance to margins

Sections for histology

1 Cross-sections through center (see accompanying drawing **A**)
2 Lateral margins, without trimming (see accompanying drawing **B** and **C**)

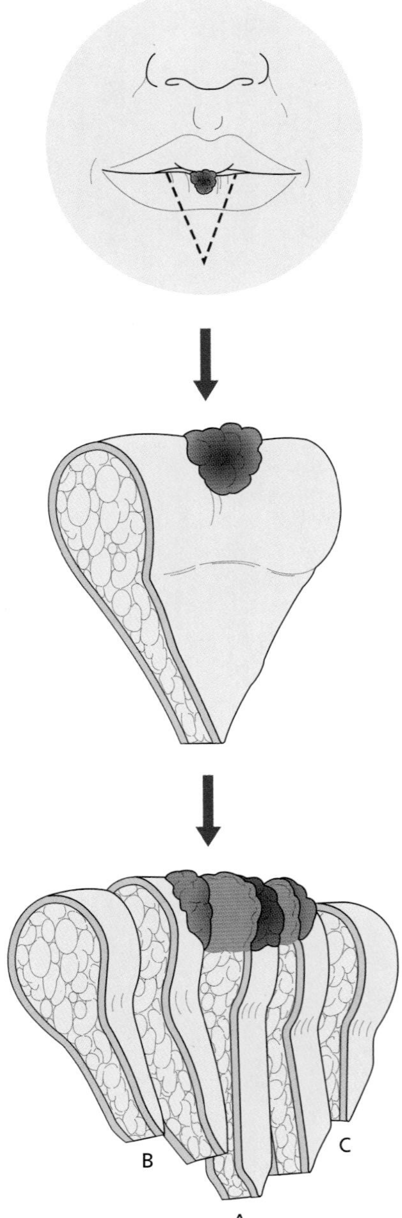

Liver – excision

Operations to remove liver masses include wedge resection, segmental resection, formal and extended right and left lobectomy, trisegmentectomy (which consists of resection of both right lobar segments and the medial segment of the left lobe), and total hepatectomy followed by liver transplant. The delineation of the various hepatic segments is difficult in the excised specimen and need not be attempted unless specifically requested by the surgeon, who may need to be consulted for assistance in the orientation of the specimen.

Procedure

1 Measure and weigh the specimen
2 *For hepatic parenchymal tumors*: paint the hepatic surgical margin and cut parallel 1 cm slices in a plane roughly corresponding to the cut of the CT scan, if one was performed and is available
3 *For tumors of major bile ducts*: identify all of the bile duct and vascular surgical margins (with the help of the surgeon, if necessary), and submit them *en face* (see later section); palpate the bile ducts for areas of induration; open the major bile ducts longitudinally with scissors; after taking photographs, serially section the bile ducts perpendicularly to their long axes; search for hilar lymph nodes

Description

1 Size and weight of specimen
2 Appearance of the capsular surface
3 *For hepatic parenchymal tumors*: size, color; consistency; margins; relationship to capsular surface, major vessels (portal and hepatic veins) and biliary tree; distance to surgical margin; multiplicity; appearance of non-neoplastic liver (congested? signs of biliary obstruction? cirrhosis?)
4 *For tumors of major bile ducts*: same as for hepatic parenchymal tumors, plus: intraductal papillary component? areas of ductal stenosis or dilation? presence of biliary stones?
5 Gallbladder: if present, describe as per instructions in Gallbladder – cholecystectomy; relationship with hepatic parenchymal or bile duct tumor
6 Hilar lymph nodes: number, size, and appearance

Sections for histology

1 Tumor: four sections or more depending on size and extent. All grossly dissimilar areas should be sampled. If several nodules are present, samples of up to five should be taken. Unless excessively large, tumors of major bile ducts should be submitted *in toto*
2 Surgical margins: these should be taken from the areas that appear grossly closer to the tumor. In the case of the tumors of major bile ducts, one of these sections should be an *en face* view of the bile duct and vascular surgical margin
3 Non-neoplastic liver: include portions distal and proximal to the tumor, if feasible
4 Gallbladder, if present; one section
5 Lymph nodes, if present: in their entirety

Lung – biopsy

(Adapted from Brody AR, Craighead JE. Preparations of human lung specimens by perfusion-fixation. Am Rev Respir Dis 1975, **112:** 645–649; Carrington CB, Gaensler EA. Clinical-pathologic approach to diffuse interstitial lung disease. In Thurlbeck WM (ed.): The lung. Baltimore, 1978, Waverley Press, pp 58–87; Churg A. An inflation procedure for open lung biopsies. Am J Surg Pathol 1983, **7:** 69–71.)

Procedure

1 Obtain cultures from lesions suspected of being infectious
2 Take samples for electron microscopy and for deep freezing, if indicated
3 Open biopsies obtained in patients with suspected interstitial lung disease are better evaluated microscopically if the specimen has been fixed in the inflated state. This can be achieved by one of three methods:
   a The surgeon should take the biopsy from a lung that is held inflated and maintain inflation by clamping the portion of the lung to be biopsied; the specimen should be placed in formalin immediately after excision
   b The small airways and/or vessels are cannulated under a dissecting microscope. This is a tedious and somewhat complicated procedure
   c The specimen is inflated slowly with formalin or other fixative (using a 25 gauge butterfly needle connected to a small syringe), sticking the needle through the pleura and gently infusing fixative until the specimen is well expanded. If the specimen is large, several punctures with the needle may be necessary. After inflation, the specimen is dropped in formalin, allowed to fix for at least 1 hour, and then cut in parallel slices

Description

1 Dimensions: weight, if specimen is large
2 Pleura: thickness; fibrosis? fibrin? other changes?
3 Lung parenchyma: consolidated? diffuse interstitial fibrosis or well-defined nodules?

Sections for histology

Submit entire biopsy

Lung – resection for nontumoral condition

Lung resections include *segmentectomy* (removal of one or more of the 18 segments in which the various pulmonary lobes are divided), *lobectomy* (removal of one or more of the five pulmonary lobes), and *pneumonectomy* (removal of one entire lung).

Procedure

1 Obtain cultures from lesions suspected of being infectious
2 Weigh the specimen
3 Two options are available depending on the type of abnormality present and the status of the organ when received in the laboratory:
   a Open the bronchi longitudinally with scissors and cut the lung parenchyma (including the lesion) in slices with a sharp knife
   b Inject with formalin through the main bronchus, tie off or clamp the bronchus, fix overnight, and section at 0.5–1 cm intervals with a sharp knife or meat cutter. The sections should be frontal, perpendicular to the hilum. The slices formed by this procedure can be kept in order by stringing them on a piece of twine
4 For lungs with tuberculosis and other contagious diseases (proven or suspected): fix in formalin for 48 hours; keep the specimen in the same container while dissecting and cutting the sections; send the contaminated instruments for sterilization; carefully wrap the contaminated material in a plastic bag and place in a scrap bucket
5 For lungs with suspected asbestosis: scrape vigorously the cut surface of the lung with a scalpel, layer 20 successive scrapings onto a glass slide, let the preparation dry, stain lightly with toluidine blue or leave unstained, apply a mounting medium and coverslip, and examine microscopically[1]
6 If a rib was submitted as part of the thoracotomy, examine according to instructions under Bone marrow – rib from thoracotomy

Description

1 Weight of specimen and type of resection (pneumonectomy, lobectomy, wedge resection)
2 Pleura: thickness; fibrosis? fibrin? other changes?
3 Bronchi: mucosa, lumen (diameter and content)
4 Parenchyma: appearance; if localized lesion is present: appearance; lobe and, if possible, bronchopulmonary segment in which located; relationships to bronchi, vessels, pleura, and lymph nodes
5 Lymph nodes: number, size, and appearance

Sections for histology

1 Main lesions: three sections
2 Uninvolved lung: one section per lobe
3 Bronchus
4 Lymph nodes, if present: at least one section

1 Mark EJ. The second diagnosis. The role of the pathologist in identifying pneumoconiosis in lungs excised for tumor. Hum Pathol 1981, **12:** 585–587

Lung – resection for tumor[1]

Procedure

1 Dissect hilar lymph nodes as a single group and take out a cross section from the bronchial line of resection while the specimen is fresh
2 Two options are available depending on the location of the tumor and the status of the organ when received in the laboratory:
   a Open all major bronchi and their branches longitudinally with scissors and follow this by cutting parallel slices of the lung, including tumor
   b Inject with formalin through the main bronchus, tie off or clamp the bronchus, fix overnight, and section at 0.5–1 cm intervals with a sharp knife or meat cutter. The sections should be frontal, perpendicular to the hilum. The slices formed by this procedure can be kept in order by stringing them on a piece of twine
3 If tuberculosis, other infections, or asbestosis is suspected in the non-neoplastic lung, proceed according to instructions listed under Lung – resection for nontumoral condition
4 If a rib was submitted as part of the thoracotomy, examine according to instructions under Bone marrow – rib from thoracotomy

Description

1 Weight of fresh specimen and type of resection (pneumonectomy, lobectomy)
2 Pleura: fibrosis, fibrin, tumor invasion; parietal pleura present (identified by presence of fat)?
3 Tumor characteristics: size, location within lobe and segment, relation with bronchi, hemorrhage, necrosis, cavitation, blood vessel invasion, extension to pleura; distance to bronchial line of resection and pleura
4 Appearance of non-neoplastic lung
5 Number and appearance of regional lymph nodes

Sections for histology

1 Tumor: three sections, including one showing relationship to bronchus, if any
2 Non-neoplastic lung, including pleura: three sections, at least one from lung distal to tumor
3 Bronchial line of resection: one cross-section comprising entire circumference
4 Lymph nodes: bronchopulmonary (hilar) and mediastinal
5 If rib submitted, process according to instructions under Bone marrow – rib from thoracotomy

1 More detailed instructions are available from: Carter D. Pathologic examination of major pulmonary specimens resected for neoplastic disease. Pathol Annu 1983, **18(Pt 2):** 315–332

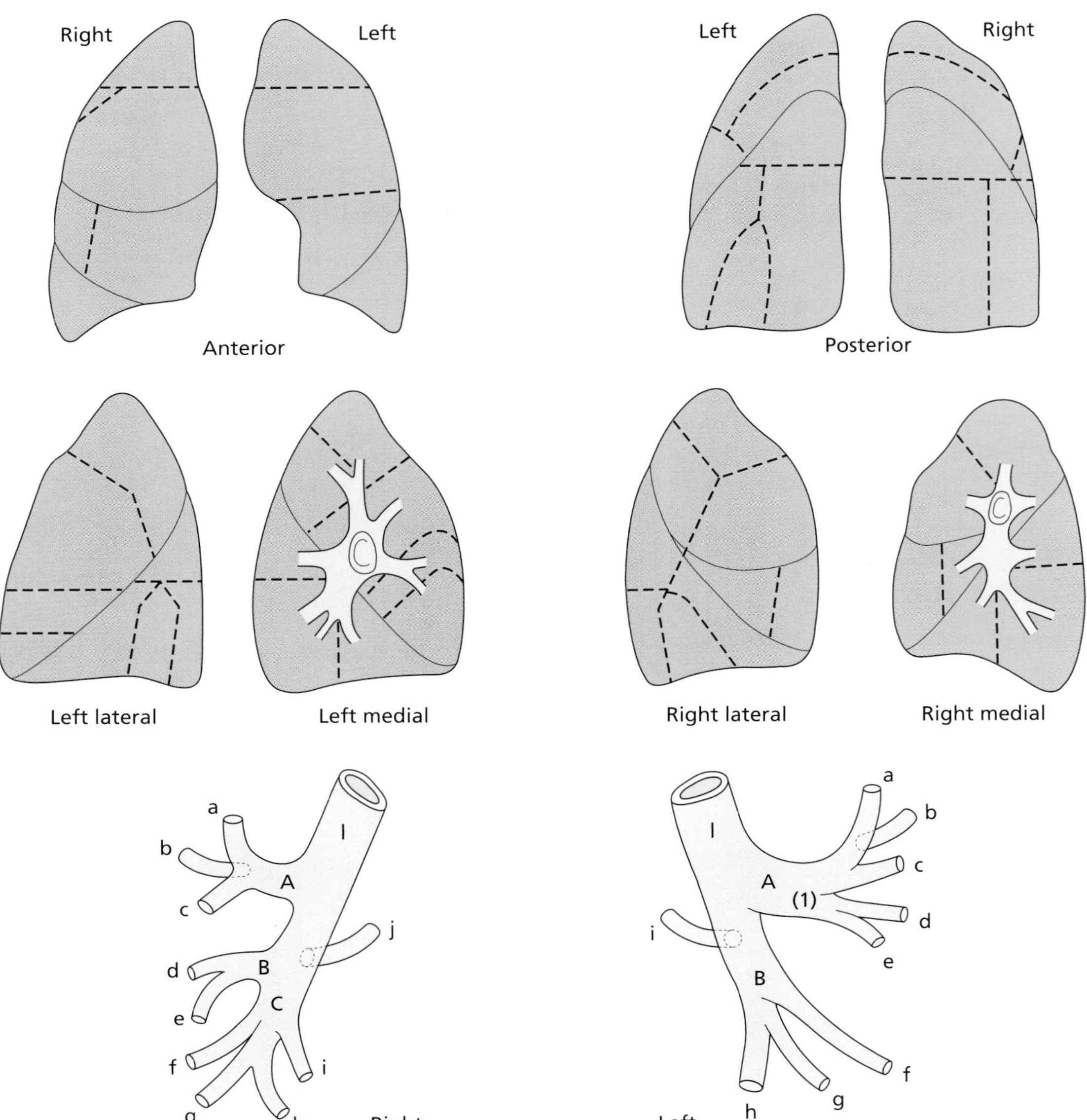

Table App E-3

BROCK'S NOMENCLATURE		JACKSON AND HUBER'S NOMENCLATURE	
Right bronchial tree (I, main bronchus; A, upper lobe bronchus; B, middle lobe bronchus; C, lower lobe bronchus)			
a	*Apical* bronchus, upper lobe	a	*Apical* bronchus, upper lobe
b	*Subapical* bronchus, upper lobe	b	*Anterior* bronchus, upper lobe
c	*Pectoral* bronchus, upper lobe	c	*Posterior* bronchus, upper lobe
d	*Medial* division, middle lobe	d	*Medial* division, middle lobe
e	*Lateral* division, middle lobe	e	*Lateral* division, middle lobe
f	*Anterior basal* bronchus, lower lobe	f	*Anterior basal* bronchus, lower lobe
g	*Middle basal* bronchus, lower lobe	g	*Lateral basal* bronchus, lower lobe
h	*Posterior* bronchus, lower lobe	h	*Posterior basal* bronchus, lower lobe
i	*Cardiac* bronchus, lower lobe	i	*Medial basal* bronchus, lower lobe
j	*Apical* bronchus, lower lobe	j	*Superior* bronchus, lower lobe
Left bronchial tree (I, main bronchus; A, upper lobe bronchus; B, lower lobe bronchus; (1), lingular bronchus)			
a	*Apical* bronchus, upper lobe	a	*Superior division*, upper lobe
b	*Subapical* bronchus, upper lobe	b	*Apical posterior*, upper lobe
c	*Pectoral* bronchus, upper lobe	c	*Anterior* bronchus, upper lobe
d	*Upper division, lingular*, upper lobe	d	*Superior lingular, inferior division*, upper lobe
e	*Lower division, lingular,* upper lobe	e	*Inferior lingular, inferior division,* upper lobe
f	*Anterior basal* bronchus, lower lobe	f	*Anterior-medial basal*, lower lobe
g	*Middle basal* bronchus, lower lobe	g	*Lateral basal*, lower lobe
h	*Posterior basal* bronchus, lower lobe	h	*Posterior basal*, lower lobe
i	*Apical* bronchus, lower lobe	i	*Superior bronchus*, lower lobe

Lymph node – biopsy

Procedure

1 If the lymph node is received in the fresh state, cut 2–3 mm slices perpendicular to the long axis and:
   a Take a small portion for culture and if an infectious disease is suspected or needs to be ruled out
   b Make four imprints of the cut surface on alcohol-cleaned slides, fix in methanol, and stain two with hematoxylin-eosin and two with Wright stain. See instructions for Imprints (touch preparations)
   c Place one of the slices in B5 fixative and submit for histology
   d In cases of suspected hematolymphoid disorders, submit tissue for cell markers (by flow cytometry), cytogenetics, and molecular genetics (see respective sections for instructions)
   e If additional tissue is available, fix in formalin, and submit for histology
2 If the specimen is received already fixed in formalin, cut in 3 mm slices and submit representative sections

Description

1 State whether node received fresh or fixed
2 Size of node and condition of capsule
3 Appearance of cut surface: color, nodularity, hemorrhage, necrosis

Sections for histology

Cross-sections of node, including at least portion of capsule: one to three sections depending on size of node

Lymph node dissection – general instructions

Procedure

1 Dissect the node-containing fat from the organ in the fresh state, using forceps and sharp scissors. Make the fat dissection as close as possible to the wall of the organ; this is where most lymph nodes are located. Divide them in groups according to specific instructions
2 Two options are available:
 a Search the fat for nodes while specimen is fresh, under a strong light and with the use of scissors, forceps, and scalpel. Avoid crushing the nodes by rough palpation. If insufficient nodes are identified, contact the senior pathologist or surgeon
 b Fix overnight in formalin or Carnoy solution, and search for nodes the next day. The latter fixative is preferred because it clears the fat somewhat

Description

1 Number of nodes in each group
2 Size of largest node in each group
3 Appearance; obvious involvement by tumor?

Sections for histology

1 *All* lymph nodes should be submitted for histology
2 Small nodes (up to 3 mm in thickness after fat is removed) are submitted as a single piece
3 Several small node groups may be submitted in the same cassette
4 Larger nodes are bisected and, if necessary, further sectioned into 2–3 mm slices. A slice as large as will fit the cassette should be submitted for each one of these larger nodes[1]
5 Store the remainder in the formalin container, properly identified as belonging to lymph node group

1 The alternative would be to submit the entirety of these large nodes, but the number of additional metastases found seems too small to justify the considerably higher cost involved (Niemann TH, Yilmaz AG, Marsh Jr WL, Lucas JG. A half node or a whole node. A comparison of methods for submitting lymph nodes. Am J Clin Pathol 1998, **109:** 571–576.)

Lymph node dissection – axillary

See under Breast – mastectomy

Lymph node dissection – inguinal

1 All lymph nodes are submitted as a single group unless the surgeon has submitted the superficial and deep groups separately. A minimum of 12 lymph nodes should be found
2 A cross-section of the internal saphenous vein also should be submitted for histology

Lymph node dissection – radical neck

The *standard* radical neck dissection includes removal of cervical lymph nodes, sternomastoid muscle, internal jugular vein, spinal accessory nerve, and submaxillary gland; the tail of the parotid is sometimes also included.

In the *modified* radical neck dissection (also known as functional or Bocca neck dissection), the sternomastoid muscle, spinal accessory nerve, and internal jugular vein are spared.

The *extended* radical neck dissection includes, in addition to the structures removed in the standard operation, the excision of retropharyngeal, paratracheal, parotid, suboccipital, and/or upper mediastinal lymph nodes.

In the *regional* (partial or selective) neck dissection, only the station of lymph nodes thought to represent the first metastatic station is removed.

The instructions following are devised for the standard radical neck dissection and need to be modified for the other three. Because of the lack of anatomic landmarks in the modified and regional procedures, the labeling of the lymph nodes according to groups needs to be done by the surgeon. The same applies to the extra lymph node groups removed in the extended operation.

Procedure

1. Orient the specimen and divide it into submaxillary gland, platysma, sternomastoid muscle, internal jugular veins, and node-containing fat
2. Divide the lymph nodes into six groups depending on whether they are on the upper or lower portion of the specimen and on their relationship with the sternomastoid muscle (see accompanying drawing). A minimum of 40 lymph nodes should be found[1]

Description

1. Site and type of primary neoplasm (see specific instructions)
2. Length of sternomastoid muscle
3. Jugular vein included? length? invaded by tumor?
4. Presence of tumor in lymph nodes, submaxillary gland, soft tissue, or muscle
5. Size of the largest node

Sections for histology

1. Superior anterior cervical lymph nodes
2. Superior jugular cervical lymph nodes
3. Superior posterior cervical lymph nodes
4. Inferior anterior cervical lymph nodes
5. Inferior jugular cervical lymph nodes
6. Inferior posterior cervical lymph nodes
7. Submaxillary gland
8. Jugular vein
9. Sternocleidomastoid muscle
10. Thyroid gland, if present

1 Other pathologists use an alternative scheme in which lymph nodes are divided into five regions: anterior (submental and submandibular), superior jugular, middle jugular, inferior jugular, and posterior (posterior triangle) (Robbins KT, Medina JE, Wolfe GT, Levine PA, Sessions RB, Pruet CW. Standardizing neck dissection terminology. Arch Otolaryngol Head Neck Surg 1991, **117:** 601–605.)

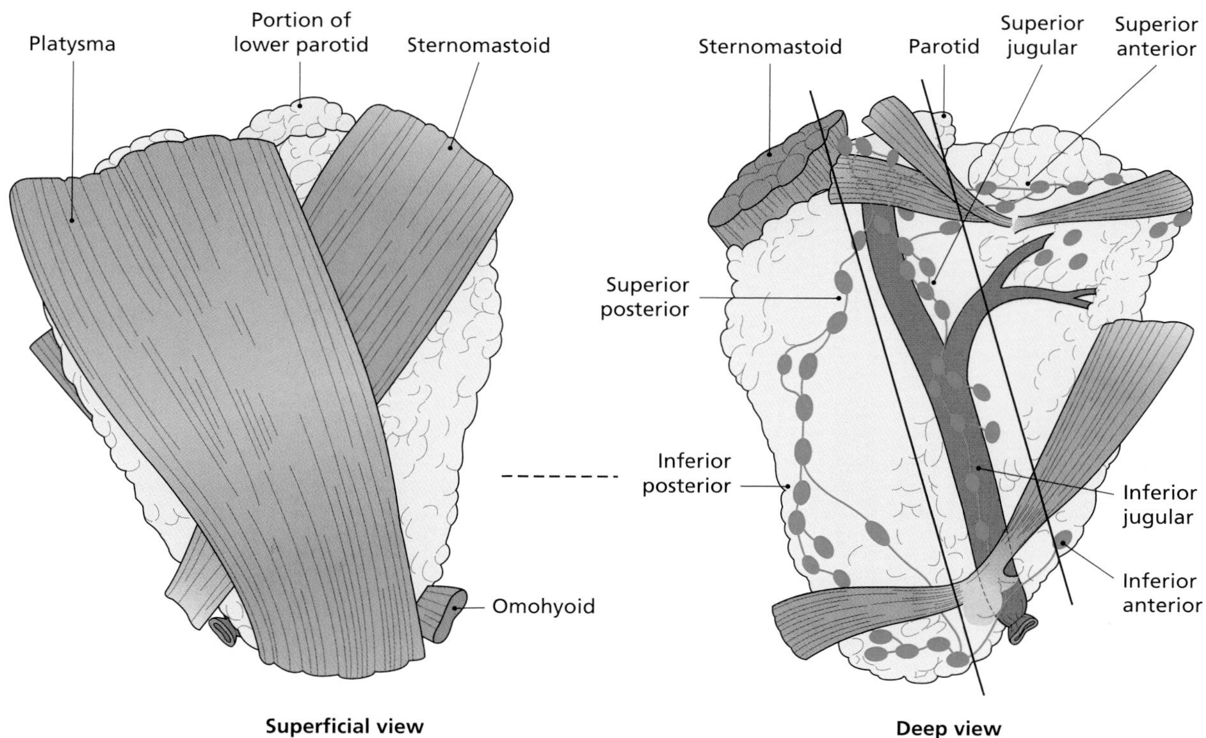

Lymph node dissection – retroperitoneal

1 For the proper evaluation of this specimen, it is essential for the surgeon to divide the lymph nodes into groups at the time the dissection is performed and submit them to the laboratory in separate containers. In most institutions, urologic surgeons divide the node groups as follows:
   - Suprahilar (above level of renal artery)
   - Superior interaortocaval
   - Pericaval
   - Periaortic
   - Common iliac (usually excised only on side of tumor)

2 If the specimen is submitted as a single piece, it is necessary to identify, with the help of the surgeon, the upper and lower borders and the periaortic and pericaval regions. When this is established, the lymph nodes can be divided in the following groups:
   - Superior periaortic
   - Middle periaortic
   - Inferior periaortic
   - Superior pericaval
   - Middle pericaval
   - Inferior pericaval
   - Common iliac (specify side)

3 If the surgeon is unavailable or unable to orient the specimen, all lymph nodes are submitted as one group. A minimum of 25 lymph nodes should be found

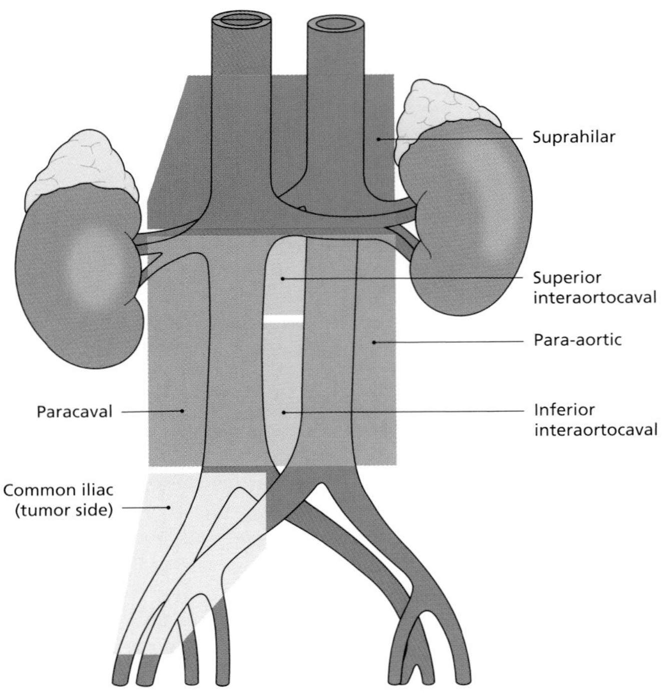

Molecular diagnosis – sampling

Evaluation of tissue using molecular techniques has become a very important diagnostic procedure, particularly for the evaluation of hematolymphoid processes and many solid tumors, particularly of soft tissue type.

Sample 1 cm^3 of fresh tumor tissue (or as much as available), drop in a Petri dish having in its bottom a layer of filter paper wet (not overly soaked) with saline solution, and submit to appropriate laboratory immediately. If prompt transportation is not feasible, freeze at −70 °C until time of use.

Needle biopsies

Procedure

1 Remove the tissue from the fixative without squeezing it with a forceps; do not use toothed forceps; handle the tissue in such a manner as to keep it intact; do not cut it transversely but rather coil it inside the cassette if overly long
2 Always search the container, including the undersurface of the lid, for tiny fragments of tissue that may be overlooked
3 Carefully wrap the tissue in a tea bag, without squeezing
4 If the amount of the tissue core permits (a core over 1 cm long or two tissue cores) and if it would be anticipated that a fat stain may be useful, save a 3–5 mm portion in formalin

Description

1 Length and diameter of core; number of fragments; color
2 Homogeneity or lack of it

Sections for histology

All material received (except if fat stains desired, see under Procedure)

Orbital exenteration

Procedure

1 Pin down the elliptic piece of orbicular skin, and fix overnight at 4 °C
2 Paint the surgical margins with India ink
3 Take surgical margins; cutaneous, soft tissue, optic nerve
4 Cut skin, soft tissue, and ocular globe

Description

1 Skin: shape and length; appearance; if lesion present: size, shape, depth of invasion, color
2 Soft tissues
3 Ocular globe: dimensions, appearance, length of optic nerve (see under Eyes – enucleation)

Sections for histology

For skin tumors

1 Tumor: three sections
2 Cutaneous surgical margins (superior, inferior, internal, and external)
3 Soft tissue surgical margins
4 Ocular globe

For ocular tumors

1 Globe with tumor
2 Orbital soft tissue adjacent to tumor
3 Surgical margin of optic nerve

Orientation of specimens with agar

1 Prepare beforehand a 3% solution of 'bacteriologic' agar, divide into 1–2 mL samples, and place in small test tubes. Keep these samples at 4 °C in the refrigerator until the time of use
2 Heat the test tube on a specially prepared hot plate until the agar acquires a semiviscid consistency. The temperature should be around 60 °C, and it is important to keep it as close as possible to this figure (otherwise, the agar will not melt or will become too fluid). The melting of the agar should take no more than 1–2 minutes. It is convenient to heat as many test tubes in the morning as will be needed during the working day. However, it is advised not to keep the agar at 60 °C longer than 24–48 hours
3 Pick up the specimen gently with a small forceps and place it in the desired position ('on edge') on top of a glass slide (see accompanying drawing)
4 While holding the specimen in this position with one hand, use the other hand to drop a small amount of melted agar on top of the specimen with a Pasteur pipette. Do not use an excessive amount. The solidifying process can be speeded up by gently blowing in the agar. When the agar has solidified just enough for the tissue to remain in the desired position without support (it should take no more than 1 minute), remove the forceps and wait an additional 1 or 2 minutes
5 Detach the tissue surrounded by the agar from the glass slide by sliding a blade beneath it (see accompanying drawing), and transfer the material to the cassette. If the size is very small, it may be necessary to wrap it in lens paper or a tea bag

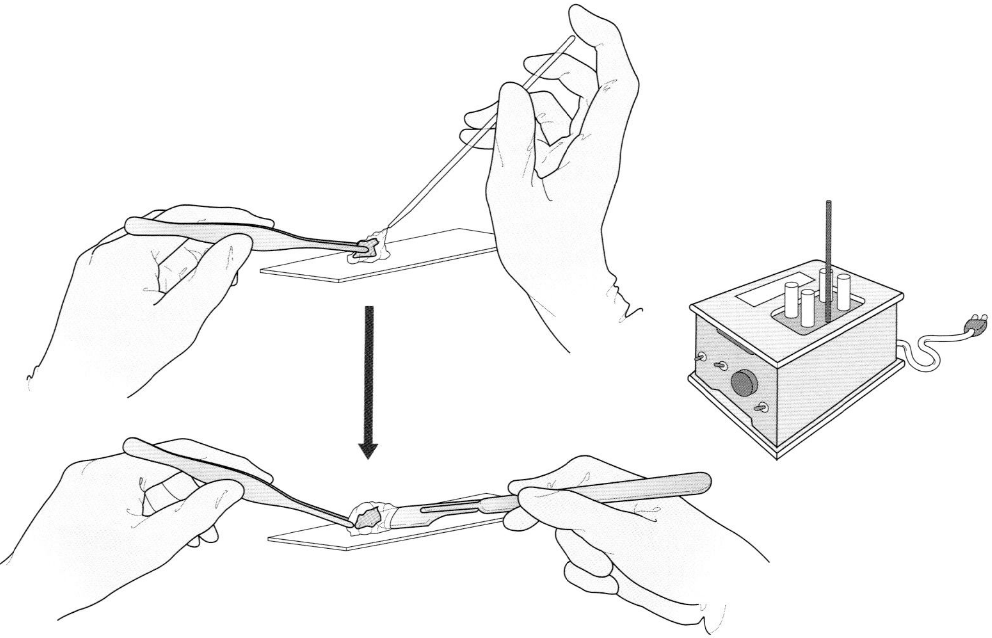

Ovary – oophorectomy[1]

Oophorectomies may be total or partial. The most common type of conservative operation is the removal of an ovarian cyst with preservation of the uninvolved parenchyma (ovarian cystectomy).

Procedure

1 Measure the organ. Weigh it if it is obviously abnormal
2 If the specimen is received fresh:
  a **Normal-sized** or nearly normal-sized organ: bivalve and fix for several hours
  b **Enlarged** organ: make several cuts and fix for several hours

Description

1 Size and shape; weight, if enlarged
2 Capsule: thickened? adhesions? hemorrhage? rupture? external surface smooth or irregular?
3 Cut section: character of cortex, medulla, and hilum; cysts (size and content); corpus luteum? calcification? hemorrhage?
4 Tumors: size; external appearance: smooth or papillary? solid or cystic? content of cystic masses; hemorrhage, necrosis, or calcification?

Sections for histology

1 For incidental oophorectomies: one sagittal section of each entire ovary, labeled as to side
2 For cysts: up to three sections of cyst wall (particularly from areas with papillary appearance)
3 For tumors: three sections or one section for each centimeter of tumor, whichever is greater; also, one section of non-neoplastic ovary, if identifiable

1 Robboy SJ, Kraus FT, Kurman RJ. Gross description, processing, and reporting of gynaecologic and obstetric specimens. In Kurman RJ (ed.): Blaustein's pathology of the female genital tract, ed. 4. New York, 2002, Springer-Verlag, pp. 1319–1346

Skin – excision for malignant tumor

Procedure

1 Paint all excision margins with India ink
2 Take photographs or photocopies in cases of large tumors and identify in one of them the site of the sections to be taken

Description

1 Shape and dimensions of specimen
2 Characteristics of lesion: size, shape, color or colors, configuration; elevated or depressed? ulceration? types of margins (sharp or ill defined? flat or elevated?); distance from margins of resection; satellite nodules?

Sections for histology

1 *Small specimens* – up to 5 cm in greatest length (see accompanying drawing **I**):

Cut parallel 3 mm slices of the entire specimen, making sure that the initial section goes from the center of the lesion to what grossly appears the narrowest surgical margin

2 *Larger specimens* (see accompanying drawing **II**):
  a Tumor: parallel 3 mm slices of the entire lesion (*T*)
  b Surgical margins: tangential sections along the entire edge (*M*)[1–5]

1 For alternative methods to evaluate surgical margins, see: Gormley DE. Evaluation of a method for controlled tissue embedding for histologic evaluation of tumor margins. Am J Dermatopathol 1987, **9:** 308–315
2 Hurt MA. The rule of halves. A method of controlling the uniform 'cutting-in' of skin biopsies. Am J Dermatopathol 1991, **13:** 7–10
3 Mondragon G, Nygaard F. Routine and special procedures for processing biopsy specimens for lesions suspected to be malignant melanomas. Am J Dermatopathol 1981, **3:** 265–272
4 Rapini RP. Comparison of methods for checking surgical margins. J Am Acad Dermatol 1990, **23:** 288–294
5 Woods JE, Farrow GM. Peripheral tissue examination for malignant lesions of the skin. Mayo Clin Proc 1991, **66:** 207–209

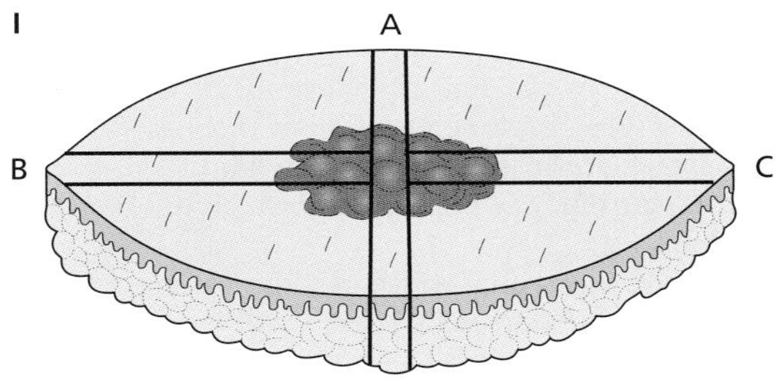

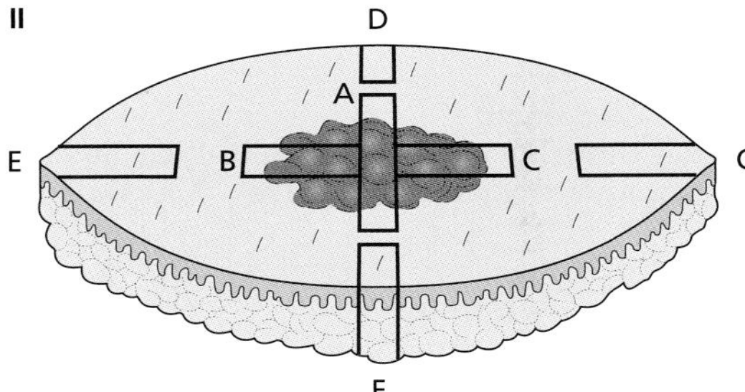

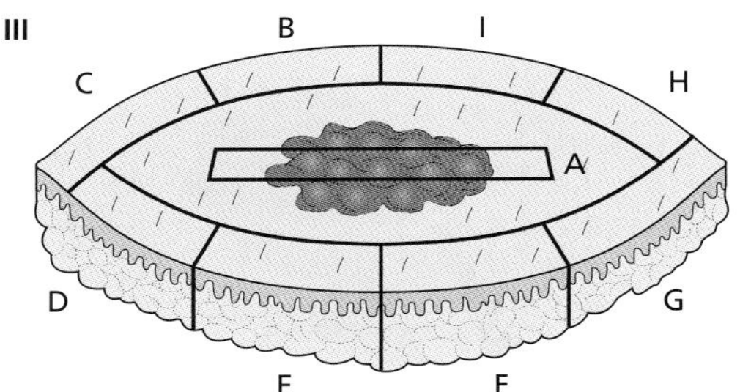

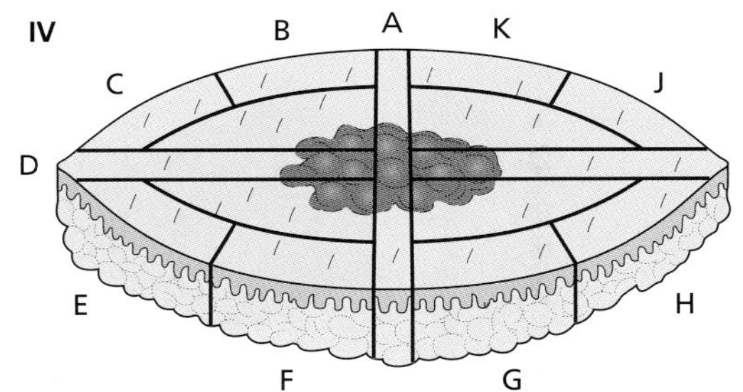

Orientation of specimens with agar

1 Prepare beforehand a 3% solution of 'bacteriologic' agar, divide into 1–2 mL samples, and place in small test tubes. Keep these samples at 4 °C in the refrigerator until the time of use
2 Heat the test tube on a specially prepared hot plate until the agar acquires a semiviscid consistency. The temperature should be around 60 °C, and it is important to keep it as close as possible to this figure (otherwise, the agar will not melt or will become too fluid). The melting of the agar should take no more than 1–2 minutes. It is convenient to heat as many test tubes in the morning as will be needed during the working day. However, it is advised not to keep the agar at 60 °C longer than 24–48 hours
3 Pick up the specimen gently with a small forceps and place it in the desired position ('on edge') on top of a glass slide (see accompanying drawing)
4 While holding the specimen in this position with one hand, use the other hand to drop a small amount of melted agar on top of the specimen with a Pasteur pipette. Do not use an excessive amount. The solidifying process can be speeded up by gently blowing in the agar. When the agar has solidified just enough for the tissue to remain in the desired position without support (it should take no more than 1 minute), remove the forceps and wait an additional 1 or 2 minutes
5 Detach the tissue surrounded by the agar from the glass slide by sliding a blade beneath it (see accompanying drawing), and transfer the material to the cassette. If the size is very small, it may be necessary to wrap it in lens paper or a tea bag

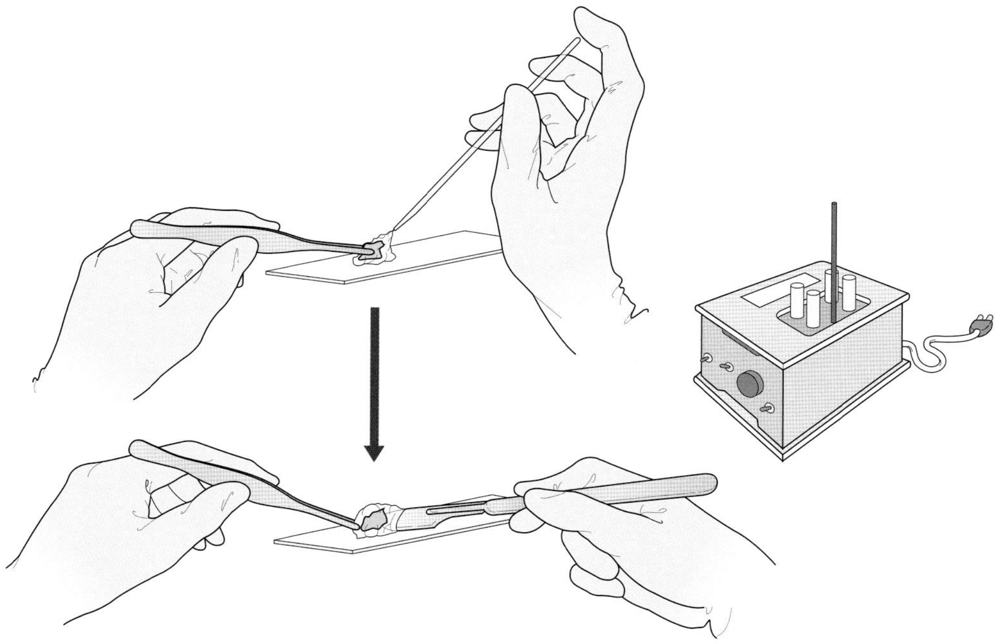

Ovary – oophorectomy[1]

Oophorectomies may be total or partial. The most common type of conservative operation is the removal of an ovarian cyst with preservation of the uninvolved parenchyma (ovarian cystectomy).

Procedure

1 Measure the organ. Weigh it if it is obviously abnormal
2 If the specimen is received fresh:
   a **Normal-sized** or nearly normal-sized organ: bivalve and fix for several hours
   b **Enlarged** organ: make several cuts and fix for several hours

Description

1 Size and shape; weight, if enlarged
2 Capsule: thickened? adhesions? hemorrhage? rupture? external surface smooth or irregular?
3 Cut section: character of cortex, medulla, and hilum; cysts (size and content); corpus luteum? calcification? hemorrhage?
4 Tumors: size; external appearance: smooth or papillary? solid or cystic? content of cystic masses; hemorrhage, necrosis, or calcification?

Sections for histology

1 For incidental oophorectomies: one sagittal section of each entire ovary, labeled as to side
2 For cysts: up to three sections of cyst wall (particularly from areas with papillary appearance)
3 For tumors: three sections or one section for each centimeter of tumor, whichever is greater; also, one section of non-neoplastic ovary, if identifiable

1 Robboy SJ, Kraus FT, Kurman RJ. Gross description, processing, and reporting of gynaecologic and obstetric specimens. In Kurman RJ (ed.): Blaustein's pathology of the female genital tract, ed. 4. New York, 2002, Springer-Verlag, pp. 1319–1346

Pancreas – pancreatectomy

The *Whipple procedure* consists of partial pancreatectomy plus partial gastrectomy and duodenectomy.[2] *Total pancreatectomy* consists of removal of the entire pancreas plus partial gastrectomy, duodenectomy, and splenectomy. *Regional pancreatectomy type I* consists of total pancreatectomy plus partial gastrectomy, cholecystectomy, duodenectomy, splenectomy, and resection of portal vein. It may also include transverse colectomy and removal of mesocolon, omentum, and regional lymph nodes. *Regional pancreatectomy type II* includes, in addition to the procedures listed under type I, the resection of mesenteric vessels, celiac axis vessels, and/or a segment of vena cava and aorta. *Distal pancreatectomy* consists in resection of the tail of the pancreas (often with a portion of the body) plus splenectomy.

Procedure

1 Dissect lymph nodes while the specimen is fresh and divide them according to groups (see accompanying drawing)
2 Fill the stomach and duodenum with gauze or cotton impregnated with formalin
3 Pin the whole specimen on a corkboard, trying to preserve the anatomic relationships
4 Place in a large container, cover with formalin, and fix overnight at 4 °C
5 Paint with India ink the common bile duct surgical margin, as well as the pancreatic surgical margin in a Whipple procedure
6 Divide the specimen into anterior and posterior halves as follows: with scissors, cut the lesser curvature of the stomach and the free border of the duodenum; with scissors, cut the gastric greater curvature up to the pancreas, as well as the fourth portion of the duodenum; with a large sharp knife, cut the peripancreatic border of the duodenum and the pancreas. The orientation of the latter cut can be better controlled by introducing a catheter through the common bile duct and by cutting in front of it. It may be necessary to postfix the two halves overnight before proceeding to further dissection, as indicated

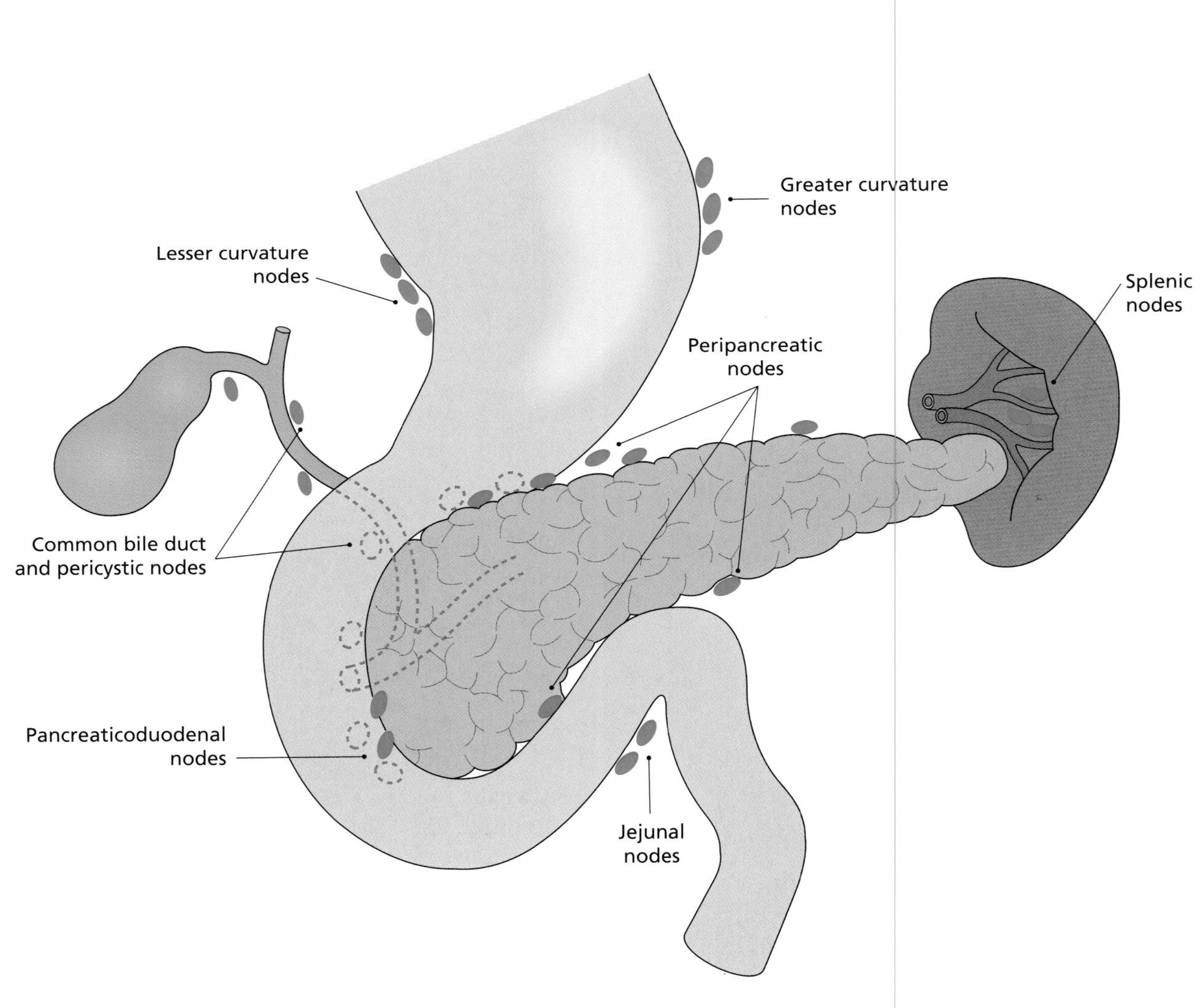

Description

1 Type of operation: Whipple procedure, total pancreatectomy, regional pancreatectomy type I or II, distal pancreatectomy
2 Organs present in specimen and their dimensions; weight of spleen
3 Tumor characteristics: involvement of ampulla, duodenal mucosa, stomach, common bile duct, pancreatic duct, and pancreas; size, shape (papillary? flat? ulcerated?), color, and consistency; if tumor is in the ampulla: intra-ampullary, periampullary, or mixed?
4 Common bile duct, main pancreatic duct, and accessory pancreatic duct: location and relationship with each other; dilated? stones? tumor?
5 Pancreas: tumor invasion? atrophy? fibrosis? ductal dilation?
6 Spleen: tumor invasion? other features
7 Location, number, and appearance of regional lymph nodes

Sections for histology

1 Tumor: up to three sections
2 Pancreas: three sections, one from distal line of resection (or proximal, depending on the type of specimen)
3 Common bile duct: two cross-sections, one from surgical margin
4 Uninvolved duodenum: two sections, one from distal line of resection
5 Stomach: two sections, including proximal line of resection
6 Lymph nodes:[1]
   - Peripancreatic (superior and inferior)
   - Pancreaticoduodenal (anterior and posterior)
   - Common bile duct and pericystic
   - Lesser curvature
   - Greater curvature
   - Splenic
   - Other groups, if present (jejunal, midcolic, omental)
7 Other organs, if present (gallbladder, spleen, portal vein, colon, omentum)

Other authors[1] divide these lymph nodes into the following five major groups:

1 Superior: superior margin of head and body of pancreas, common bile duct, and stomach (greater and lesser curvature and pylorus)
2 Inferior: inferior margin of head and body of pancreas, around mesenteric vessels, jejunal, gastrocolonic ligaments, pericolonic, and periaortic
3 Anterior (anterior pancreaticoduodenal): along the anterior surface of the head of the pancreas
4 Posterior (posterior pancreaticoduodenal): along the posterior surface of the head of the pancreas
5 Splenic: splenic hilum

1 Cubilla AL, Fitzgerald PJ. Suggested technic for examining the resected pancreas. Tumors of the exocrine pancreas, appendix A. Atlas of tumor pathology, Second series, fascicle 19. Washington DC, 1982, Armed Forces Institute of Pathology, pp 257–261
2 Young ES, Castro CY. The pancreaticoduodenectomy. Ann Diagn Pathol 2002, 6: 188–193

Parathyroid glands – parathyroidectomy

Removal of diseased parathyroid glands is usually complete, but in cases of hyperplasia a portion (approximately one half) of one gland is retained, in situ or implanted in the forearm.

Procedure

1 Accurately weigh each gland on a delicate balance after removing the surrounding fat but *before* removing any parathyroid tissue for frozen or other sections
2 Accurately label each parathyroid gland as to site

Description

Weight, color, consistency, and external appearance of *each* gland

Sections for histology

All parathyroid tissue (except for markedly enlarged gland in which minimum of three sections should be taken) accurately labeled as to site

Pelvic exenteration[1]

Most pelvic exenterations are performed on females because of postradiation persistence of carcinoma of uterine cervix. Anterior pelvic exenteration consists of removal of the vagina, uterus and adnexa, bladder, distal ureters, and urethra. Posterior pelvic exenteration consists of removal of the vagina, uterus and adnexa, and rectum. Total pelvic exenteration is a combination of the two procedures. The operation also includes removal of the pelvic lymph nodes.

Procedure

1 Gently express content from the rectosigmoid, wash with formalin or saline solution, and fill with cotton or gauze impregnated in formalin
2 Fill the vagina with the same material
3 Inject the bladder with formalin with a Foley catheter or syringe after tying the urethra
4 Suspend the specimen in anatomic position in a large container with abundant fixative
5 Inject formalin in the uterine cavity with a syringe through the fundus
6 Fix for 24 hours
7 Removal all cotton and gauze and cut sagittally in equal halves. The sections of large bowel, bladder, and vagina are made with scissors; those of the uterus are made with a knife
8 Take photographs or photocopies and identify in one of them the site of the sections to be taken
9 Remove the lymph nodes in the following groups: right parametrial, left parametrial, retrorectal, and mesosigmoid
10 Paint the surgical margins with India ink

Description

1 Type of exenteration: total, anterior, posterior; organs included; length of ureters
2 Tumor characteristics: location, invasion of other structures, size, color, consistency; fistulae: signs of radiation change?
3 Number and appearance of lymph nodes

Sections for histology

1. Tumor: three sections or one section per centimeter of tumor, whichever is greater
2. Cervix and vagina
3. Cervix and bladder
4. Cervix and rectum
5. Surgical margins (parametrial, vaginal, vesical, and rectal)
6. *In females*: vulva, vagina, cervix endometrium, tubes, ovaries (in addition to sections from tumor)
7. *In males*: prostate
8. Lymph nodes:
   - Right parametrial
   - Left parametrial
   - Retrorectal
   - Mesosigmoid

1 Robboy SJ, Kraus FT, Kurman RJ. Gross description, processing, and reporting of gynaecologic and obstetric specimens. In Kurman RJ (ed.): Blaustein's pathology of the female genital tract, ed. 4. New York, 2002, Springer-Verlag, pp. 1319–1346

Penis – penectomy

Procedure

1. If the specimen is accompanied by inguinal node dissections, separate them and handle according to specific instructions
2. Introduce a catheter through the urethra
3. Fix overnight at 4 °C
4. Paint the surgical margins (including the urethra) with India ink
5. Cut longitudinally through the center: the section should cut the urethra in two
6. Take photographs or photocopies and identify in one of them the site of the sections to be taken

Description

1. Type of operation: partial, total, with or without scrotal skin, testicles, inguinal nodes
2. Length and diameter of specimen
3. Tumor: location in relations to glans, prepuce, skin, and urethra; size, color, borders, depth of invasion
4. Glans penis: balanitis? atrophy? leukoplakia?
5. Urethra: invaded by tumor?

Sections for histology

1. Tumor: three sections
2. Glans penis and urethra
3. Surgical margin (including urethra)

1 Cubilla AL, Piris A, Pfannl R, Rodriguez I, Agüero F, Young RH. Anatomic levels: important landmarks in penectomy specimens: a detailed anatomic and histologic study based on 44 cases. Am J Surg Pathol 2001, **25**: 1091–1094

Peripheral nerve – biopsy

Procedure

1. The examination and sampling of this material should be carried out at the bedside or *immediately* after the specimen is received in the pathology laboratory. Be careful to avoid stretching or crushing
2. Measure the length and diameter (biopsies of the sural nerve usually measure between 3 and 6 cm)
3. For paraffin embedding, cut a portion 2–4 mm long from either end, fix in B5, and postfix in formalin. Divide the specimen so that a cross-section and a longitudinal section are obtained
4. For 'thick sections' and electron microscopy, fix a portion in 2.5% glutaraldehyde in 0.05 M cacodylate buffer at pH 7.4 (osmolarity ≈340). After 2 hours of fixation, the nerve is placed under a dissecting microscope and divided into 3–4 mm segments. Four to five of these pieces are submitted in large blocks, whereas the others are sectioned along a longitudinal plane. Twenty to 30 pieces are thus obtained, each having two to three fascicles. For electron microscopy, 1–2 mm^3 fragments should be submitted
5. If facilities are available for fiber teasing preparations, a 1–2 cm nerve segment should be dissected and, immediately after biopsy, fixed in formalin, postfixed in O_5O_4 in Millonig buffer at pH 7.4 for 3–5 hours at room temperature, and passed through graded glycerine, where it can be kept until time of observation
6. If indicated, a small piece of fresh nerve should be 'snap frozen' for biochemical studies, lipid staining, and immunofluorescent techniques

Description

1. Length and diameter
2. Color
3. Irregularities

Sections for histology

1. One cross-section and one longitudinal section for paraffin embedding
2. For other portions of biopsy, see under Procedure

Placenta – singleton[1,2]

Procedure and description

1. Examine as soon as possible after delivery in the fresh state; handle the specimen with great care, avoiding lacerations
2. Note the amount of blood and clots in the container and search for separate pieces of membranes, cord, or placenta
3. Examine in this order: membranes, cord, fetal surface, and maternal surface
4. Measure the distance from the placental margin to the nearest point of rupture (zero: marginal placenta previa)
5. Examine membranes for completeness (if a portion is missing, notify the obstetrician), insertion, decidual necrosis, edema, extra-amniotic pregnancy, retromembranous hemorrhage, meconium staining, color, and transparency
6. Take a long, 2–3 cm wide section of membranes beginning with the point of rupture and extending to and including a small portion of placental margin. Roll the specimen with amniotic surface inward, fix for 24 hours, take a 3 mm section from the center (taking care not to strip the amnion off), and submit for histology. Take a second section including amnion, chorion, and deciduas from the rim of the site of rupture (in vaginal deliveries)

7 Trim the remaining membranes from the placental margin
8 Measure the length of the cord and the shortest distance from the cord insertion to the placental margin
9 Examine the cord: insertion (nonmembranous or membranous; if latter, are vessels intact?), number of umbilical vessels (by sectioning the cord transversely at two or more points), color, true knots, torsion, stricture, hematoma, thrombosis
10 Remove the cord from the placenta 3 cm proximal to the insertion, and take a 2–4 cm segment from its midpoint; fix this segment for 24 hours, take a 3 mm section, and submit for histology
11 Examine the fetal surface: color, opacity, subchorionic fibrin, cysts (number and size), amnion nodosum, squamous metaplasia, thrombosis of fetal surface vessels, chorangioma
12 Examine the maternal surface: completeness, normal fissures, laceration (extent), depressed areas, retroplacental hemorrhage (size and distance from margin)
13 Measure the maximum diameter, thickness in the center, weight (after trimming cord and membranes), shape
14 Hold the placenta gently with one hand, maternal side up on a flat surface, and make parallel sections with a large sharp knife at 10 cm intervals. The fetal surface will not be cut through and will hold the specimen together
15 Remove four 2 cm pieces that include the fetal surface and intact maternal surface, selecting tissues of the placenta (within 2 cm of placental margins). Take the piece so that the fetal surface vessels are cut at right angles to their long axis; fix for 24 hours, trim a 3 mm section (through and through), and submit for histology. One section should include the chorionic plate in an area with minimal subchorionic fibrin. The other sections should include the maternal surface. Submit similar sections of lesions present
16 Examine all cross-sections for infarcts (location, size, number); intervillous thrombi (number); laminate, perivillous fibrin deposition, pallor, consistency, calcification (extent), cysts, tumors. Describe lesion location (central, lateral, or marginal), depth (parabasal, intermediate, or subchorionic), and age (recent or old)

Sections for histology

1 Placenta (as indicated previously plus abnormal areas, if present)
2 Membranes
3 Cord

1 Driscoll SG, Langston C. College of American Pathologists conference XIX on the examination of the placenta: report of the working group on methods for placental examination. Arch Pathol Lab Med 1991, **115:** 704–708

2 Robboy SJ, Kraus FT, Kurman RJ. Gross description, processing, and reporting of gynaecologic and obstetric specimens. In Kurman RJ (ed.): Blaustein's pathology of the female genital tract, ed. 4. New York, 2002, Springer-Verlag, pp. 1319–1346

Placenta – twin[1,2]

Procedure and description

1 If placentas are separate (nonfused): examine each placenta as a singleton
2 If placentas are fused:
  a Note whether the two cords are labeled twin A and twin B. If not, label them arbitrarily and make a statement to that effect
  b Determine the presence and type of dividing membranes:
    (1) If absent (monochorionic–monoamniotic), so state
    (2) If present:
      (a) Remove a square of the dividing membrane, roll it, fix it for 24 hours, take a 3 mm section, and submit for histology
      (b) Attempt to determine grossly whether the dividing membrane has chorion or not, according to the table below and on page 2620
      (c) Record the kind and number of vascular anastomoses in monochorionic–diamniotic placentas: artery-to-artery, vein-to-vein, artery-to-vein (arteriovenous shunts). The latter can be better demonstrated by injecting the artery of one twin along the plane of fusion of the placenta with 30–50 mL of saline solution containing a dye and noting whether the fluid emerges from the vein of the other twin through one or more common villous lobules. The placenta must be intact to perform this test. Arteries always run over veins
  c Divide the fused twin placenta along the 'vascular equator' (rather than through the base of the dividing membrane)
  d Examine each half as a singleton placenta

Table App E-4 Dividing membrane in twin placentas

FEATURES	DICHORIONIC–DIAMNIOTIC (FUSED)	MONOCHORIONIC–DIAMNIOTIC
Appearance	Thick and opaque	Thin and transparent
Separation of membranes by stripping	Difficult	Easy
Point of attachment to fetal surface	Ridge or tearing of chorion	Smooth and continuous, without ridge
Vascular anastomoses	Very rare	Numerous

Type	Incidence	Gross	Twin type
Dichorionic–diamniotic (separate)	35%	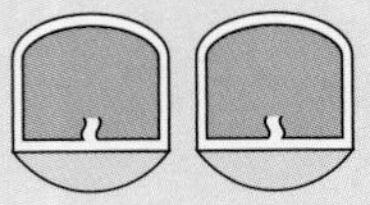	Monozygotic or dizygotic
Dichorionic–diamniotic (fused)	34%	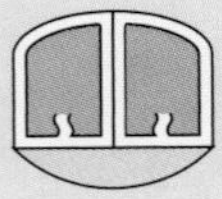	Monozygotic or dizygotic
Monochorionic–diamniotic	30%	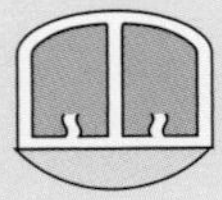	Monozygotic
Monochorionic–monoamniotic	1%	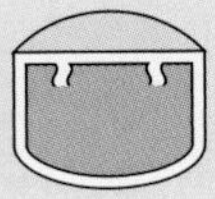	Monozygotic

Sections for histology

1 Placenta from twin A
2 Membranes from twin A
3 Cord from twin A
4 Placenta from twin B
5 Membranes from twin B
6 Cord from twin B
7 Dividing membrane, if present

1 Driscoll SG, Langston C. College of American Pathologists conference XIX on the examination of the placenta: report of the working group on methods for placental examination. Arch Pathol Lab Med 1991, **115**: 704–708

2 Robboy SJ, Kraus FT, Kurman RJ. Gross description, processing, and reporting of gynaecologic and obstetric specimens. In Kurman RJ (ed.): Blaustein's pathology of the female genital tract, ed. 4. New York, 2002, Springer-Verlag, pp. 1319–1346

Prostate gland – radical prostatectomy for tumor

This procedure can be carried out through the retropubic or the perineal route.

Procedure

1 Orient the specimen and paint the surgical margins with India ink
2 Fix the entire specimen overnight or at least for a few hours. Reduction of fixation time can be obtained by microwave treatment
3 Shave the vasa deferentia and the proximal (bladder neck) margins
4 Sample the distal (apical) margins by obtaining a thinly shaved section or amputating the distal 1 cm of the apex and sectioning the cone thus obtained perpendicularly to the cut edge
5 Serially section the prostate at 2–3 mm intervals from apex to base
6 Lay the individual slices sequentially and examine them carefully. Use the cross-section of the urethra (U-shaped, with the concavity toward the posterior lobe) as a landmark
7 Take photographs or photocopies of the slices to be submitted to histology and identify in one of them the site of the sections taken

Description

1 Weight and dimensions of specimen
2 Organs present: whole prostate? urethra (length), seminal vesicles, vas, lymph nodes
3 a Prostate: tumor (location in lobes, size, color, borders, capsular and periprostatic extension)
b Non-neoplastic prostate: nodular hyperplasia?
4 Urethra: patent? impinged by tumor?
5 Seminal vesicles: involved by tumor?

Sections for histology

1 Vasa deferentia margin
2 Proximal (bladder neck) margin
3 Distal (apical) margin, divided into right and left
4 Seminal vesicles: proximal, mid, and distal portions from each side
5 Prostate: there is no consensus on the preferred method of sampling, particularly in the absence of grossly identifiable tumor. At many institutions (particularly academic ones), the entire specimen is submitted. In others a protocol has been devised in which the specimen is partially sampled depending on the gross features of the tumor; the latter strikes the author as a more efficient alternative. The individual slices can be submitted *in toto* using extra-large cassettes (preferable if resources allow it) or by cutting the slices to fit the standard cassette (right and left halves and, if necessary, anterior and posterior quadrants)

1 Hall GS, Kramer CE, Epstein JI. Evaluation of radical prostatectomy specimens; a comparative analysis of sampling methods. Am J Surg Pathol 1992, **16**: 315–324

Prostate gland – suprapubic prostatectomy for nodular hyperplasia

Procedure

1 Step section the specimen into 3 mm slices, either in the fresh state or after formalin fixation
2 Examine *each slice* carefully for areas suspicious of carcinoma (yellow areas or foci that are harder or softer than the rest of the specimen)

Description

1 Weight of specimen
2 Shape, color, and consistency
3 Presence of hyperplastic nodules, cysts, calculi, areas suspicious of carcinoma

Sections for histology

1 Left lobe: three sections
2 Right lobe: three sections
3 Middle lobe

Prostate gland – transurethral resection (TUR)

Procedure

1 Weigh with accurate balance
2 Carefully examine all the fragments. Carcinoma of the prostate is often yellow and/or hard; submit for histology chips with these gross characteristics

Description

1 Weight of specimen
2 Size, shape, and color of chips

Sections for histology

1 *If all fragments received in a single container*
   a All of specimen until four cassettes filled
   b If an excess, one additional cassette for each additional 10 g of tissue (each cassette holds approximately 2 g)
2 *If all fragments received are identified as to lobe from which they were taken*, submit as follows for each specimen (lobe) received:
   a All of specimen until four cassettes filled
   b If an excess, one additional cassette for each additional 10 g of tissue
   c Identify in following order (not all lobes may have been biopsied in some cases):
      - Anterior lobe
      - Middle lobe
      - Posterior lobe
      - Left lateral lobe
      - Right lateral lobe
   d If carcinoma is identified microscopically in a specimen that was not entirely submitted, the remainder of the tissue should be processed in its entirety, regardless of amount

Salivary gland – resection for tumor[1]

The three most common types of operation performed because of salivary gland tumors are *superficial parotidectomy* (also known as lateral lobectomy, consisting of removal of the superficial lobe of the gland with preservation of the facial nerve), *total parotidectomy* (removal of both superficial and deep lobes, usually with sacrifice of the facial nerve), and *total submaxillectomy*.

Procedure

1. Paint surgical margins with India ink
2. Fix *in toto* or bisect in the fresh state, depending on size of specimen
3. Cut parallel sections
4. Look for intraparotid lymph nodes and for major nerves in total parotidectomy specimens
5. If the specimen includes a radical neck dissection, process according to instructions for Lymph node dissection – radical neck

Description

1. Type of specimen: parotid lobectomy, total parotidectomy without facial nerve, total parotidectomy with facial nerve, total submandibulectomy; side of operation
2. Tumor: size, location, shape, distance from closest margin; solitary or multiple? cystic or solid? encapsulated, circumscribed, or poorly defined? hemorrhage or necrosis? extraglandular extension?
3. Appearance of non-neoplastic gland
4. Appearance of intraparotid and other lymph nodes

Sections for histology

1. Tumor: four or more, depending on size; capsule or tumor margins should be included
2. Non-neoplastic gland
3. Surgical margins
4. Facial nerve margins, if included
5. Lymph nodes, if included

1 A very detailed set of instructions for surgical specimens from the upper aerodigestive tract is available from: Slootweg PJ, de Groot JAM. Surgical pathological anatomy of head and neck specimens: a manual for the dissection of surgical specimens from the upper aerodigestive tract. London, 1999, Springer

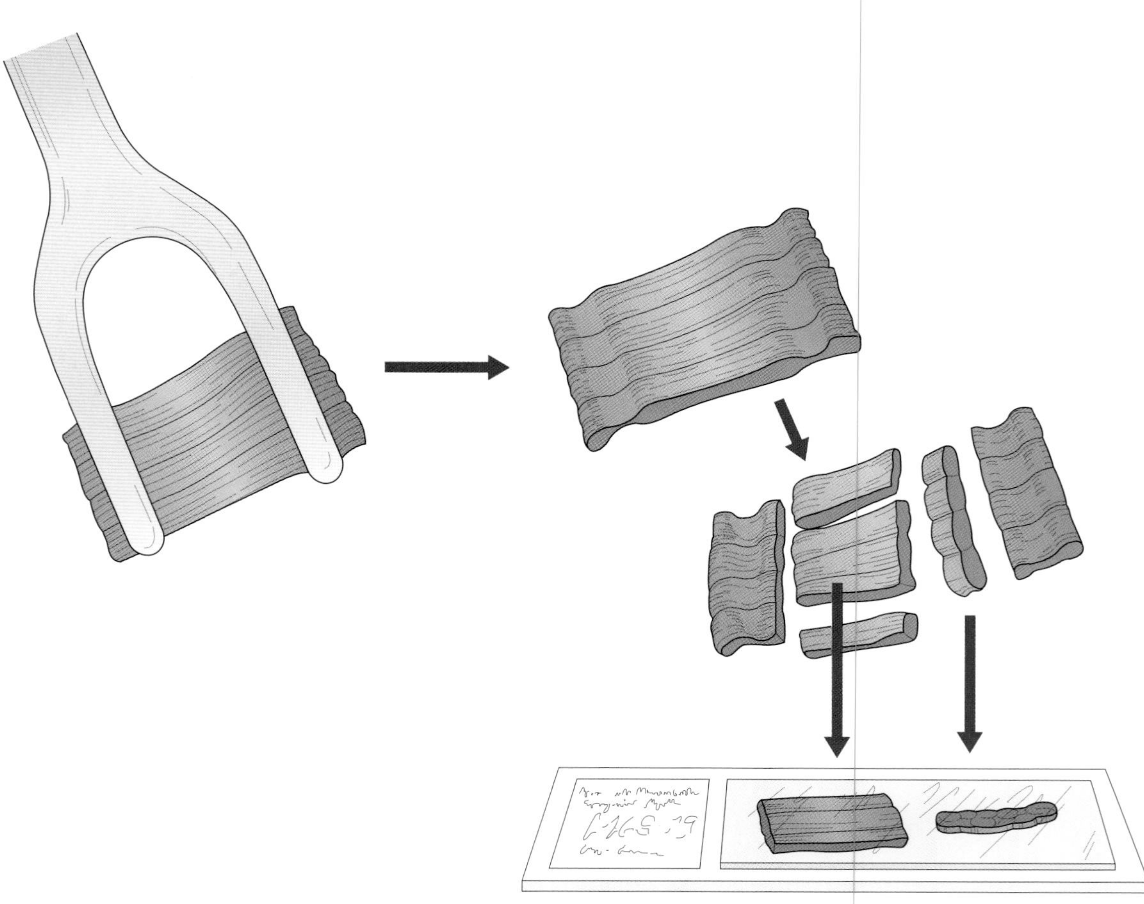

Skeletal muscle – biopsy

Procedure

The proper evaluation of a skeletal muscle biopsy includes routine processing and staining, enzyme histochemistry, and electron microscopic examination.

1 *Routine processing*: The specimen is usually received stretched on a special muscle biopsy clamp. It should remain on the clamp for overnight fixation. If the specimen is received fresh, pin it to a corkboard and fix overnight
2 *Enzyme histochemistry*: Freeze a small fragment in liquid nitrogen. It is important for this to be a cross-section. Freeze also a longitudinal section if enough tissue is available
3 *Electron microscopy*: See instructions under Electron microscopy – sampling

Description

1 Dimensions of specimen
2 Color and consistency; fibrosis? edema? necrosis?

Sections for histology

1 One longitudinal section
2 One cross-section

Skin – excision for benign lesion

Procedure

1 Pigmented nevi, seborrheic keratoses, and other benign skin conditions (as well as small basal cell carcinomas) are usually removed with narrow margins, and the size of the specimen depends mainly on the size of the lesion
2 Fix well before processing
3 If there is any clinical or gross suggestion that the tumor may be malignant, paint margins with India ink

Description

1 Size and shape of specimen; features of surface; lesion present? size, color, other features; margin grossly involved?
2 If specimen transected, description of appearance of cross-section

Sections for histology

Note: In specimens from vesicular diseases, the vesicle should be submitted intact. Do not cut through the vesicle.

1 For specimens measuring 3 mm or less (see accompanying drawing **A**): submit *in toto* without cutting
2 For specimens measuring between 4 and 6 mm in width (see accompanying drawing **B**): cut through the center and submit both halves
3 For specimens with a width of 7 mm or more (see accompanying drawing **C**): cut a 2–3 mm slice from the center for histology and save the remainder in formalin
4 Make sure that sections will be embedded on edge

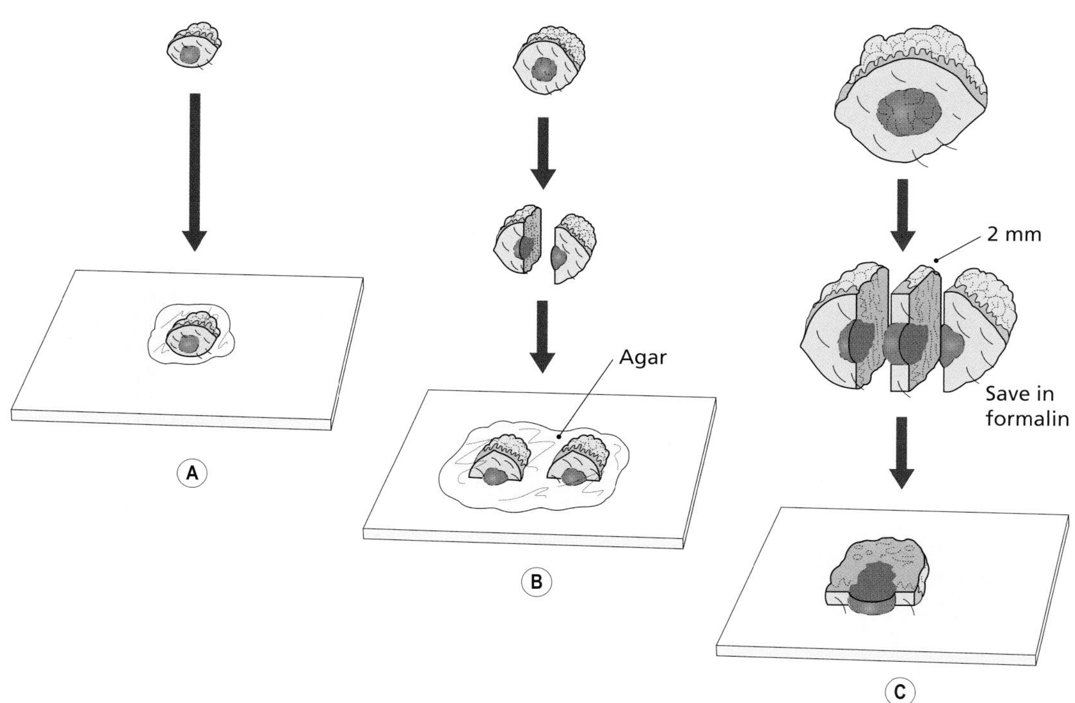

Skin – excision for malignant tumor

Procedure

1 Paint all excision margins with India ink
2 Take photographs or photocopies in cases of large tumors and identify in one of them the site of the sections to be taken

Description

1 Shape and dimensions of specimen
2 Characteristics of lesion: size, shape, color or colors, configuration; elevated or depressed? ulceration? types of margins (sharp or ill defined? flat or elevated?); distance from margins of resection; satellite nodules?

Sections for histology

1 *Small specimens* – up to 5 cm in greatest length (see accompanying drawing **I**):

Cut parallel 3 mm slices of the entire specimen, making sure that the initial section goes from the center of the lesion to what grossly appears the narrowest surgical margin

2 *Larger specimens* (see accompanying drawing **II**):
 a Tumor: parallel 3 mm slices of the entire lesion (*T*)
 b Surgical margins: tangential sections along the entire edge (*M*)[1–5]

1 For alternative methods to evaluate surgical margins, see: Gormley DE. Evaluation of a method for controlled tissue embedding for histologic evaluation of tumor margins. Am J Dermatopathol 1987, **9:** 308–315
2 Hurt MA. The rule of halves. A method of controlling the uniform 'cutting-in' of skin biopsies. Am J Dermatopathol 1991, **13:** 7–10
3 Mondragon G, Nygaard F. Routine and special procedures for processing biopsy specimens for lesions suspected to be malignant melanomas. Am J Dermatopathol 1981, **3:** 265–272
4 Rapini RP. Comparison of methods for checking surgical margins. J Am Acad Dermatol 1990, **23:** 288–294
5 Woods JE, Farrow GM. Peripheral tissue examination for malignant lesions of the skin. Mayo Clin Proc 1991, **66:** 207–209

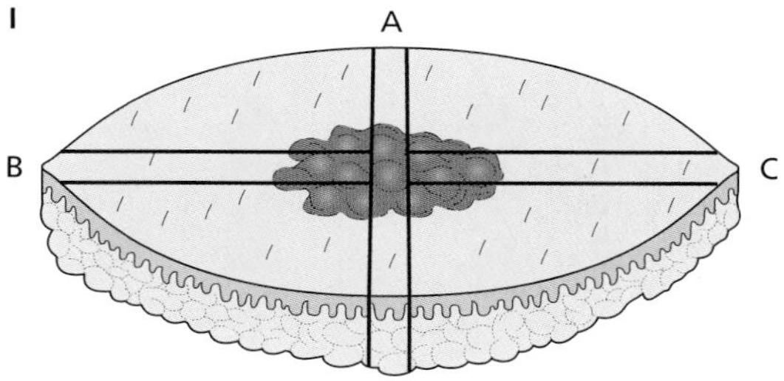

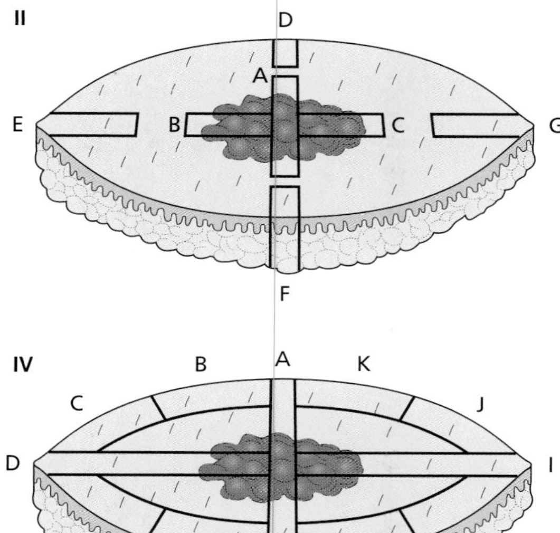

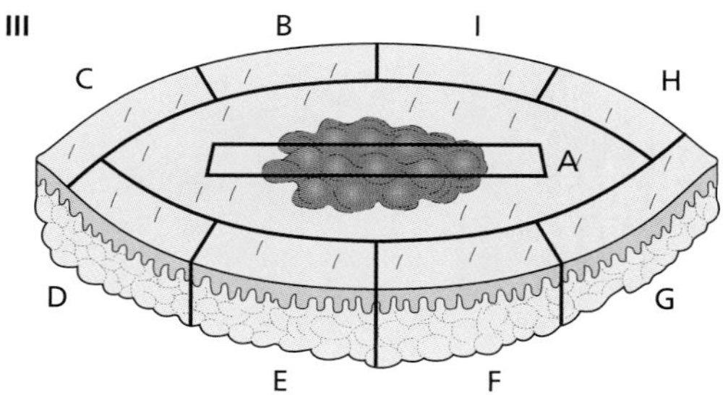

Skin – punch biopsy

Procedure

1 Submit *in toto*, if 4 mm in diameter or smaller (see accompanying drawing **A**). This prevents loss of tissue during the facing-up of the block and allows better microscopic sampling; cut in half longitudinally only if 5 mm or larger, and submit both halves for histology (see accompanying drawing **B**)
2 If the specimen is from a vesicular disease, the vesicle should be submitted *intact* for histology

Description

1 Diameter and thickness of biopsy
2 Appearance of surface; subcutis included?

Sections for histology

1 Entire biopsy (see under Procedure)
2 Make sure section oriented on edge

1 White CR Jr. Laboratory handling of skin biopsy specimens. Lab Med 1982, **13**: 211–217

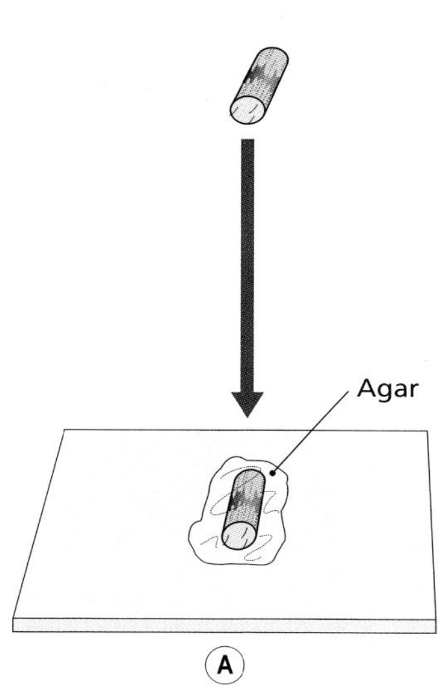

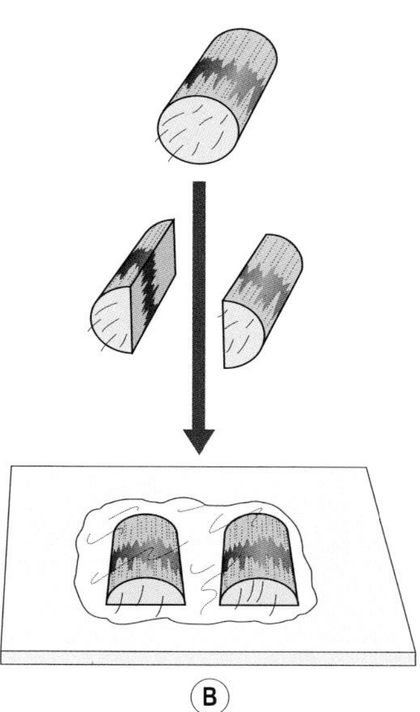

Skin – shave biopsy

Procedure

Shave biopsies of the skin, usually done for keratoses or basal cell carcinomas, can be quite thin, often of round or oval shape.

Description

1 Size of specimen
2 Number of fragments
3 Features of surface

Sections for histology

1 If width is 3 mm or less: submit *in toto* without cutting
2 If width is 4 mm or more: cut in parallel slices, about 2–3 mm thick, and submit all for histology
3 Make sure all sections are oriented on edge

1 White CR Jr. Laboratory handling of skin biopsy specimens. Lab Med 1982, **13**: 211–217

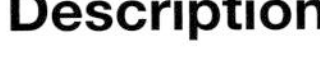

Small bowel – biopsy

Procedure

1. The specimen is usually received attached to a piece of filter paper or Gelfoam, mucosal side up; let it fix well before processing
2. Examine with dissecting microscope and determine mucosal pattern; avoid drying of the specimen and traumatizing the mucosa during this procedure. Performance of this step has lost some of the popularity it had years ago, but it still retains some usefulness as a quick predictor of the histologic appearance and as an aid for proper orientation of the specimen

Description

1. Size and color of specimen
2. Mucosal pattern with dissecting microscope (see accompanying drawings)

Sections for histology

1. The entire specimen is submitted. It is essential for it to be oriented on edge
2. If the specimen comes attached to Gelfoam, the latter can be processed together with the specimen

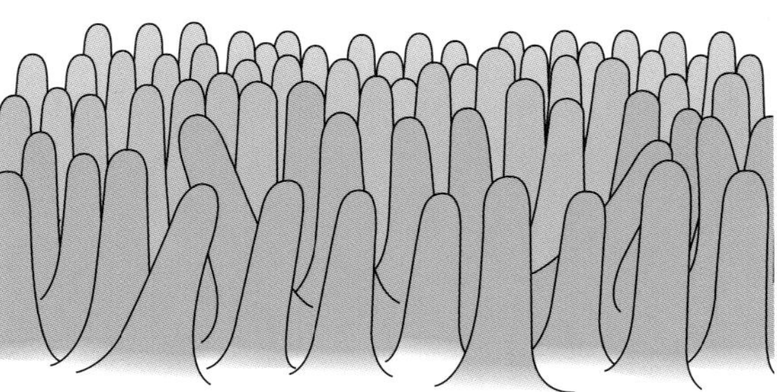

Fingerlike

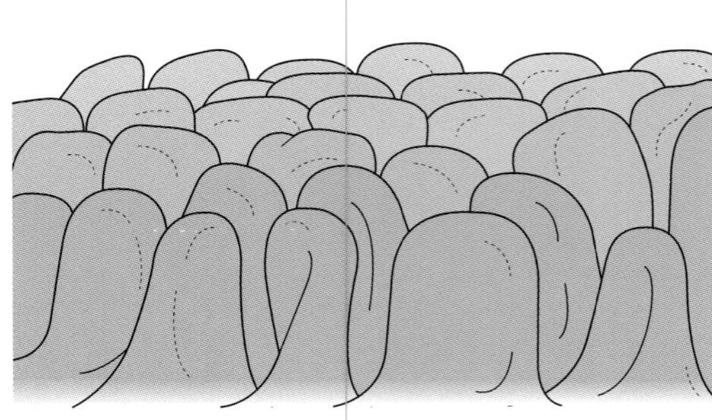

Leaflike

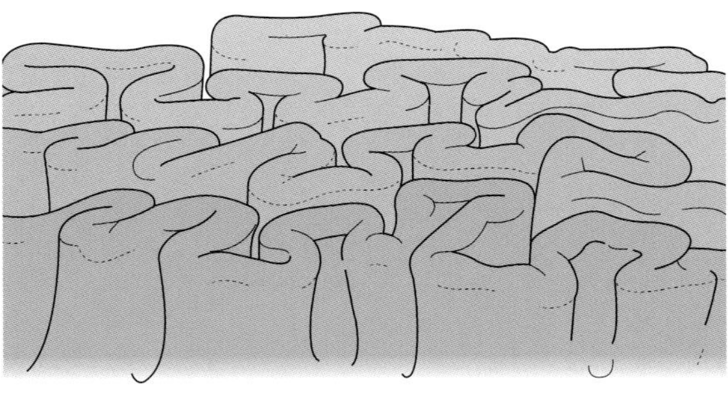

Cerebriform

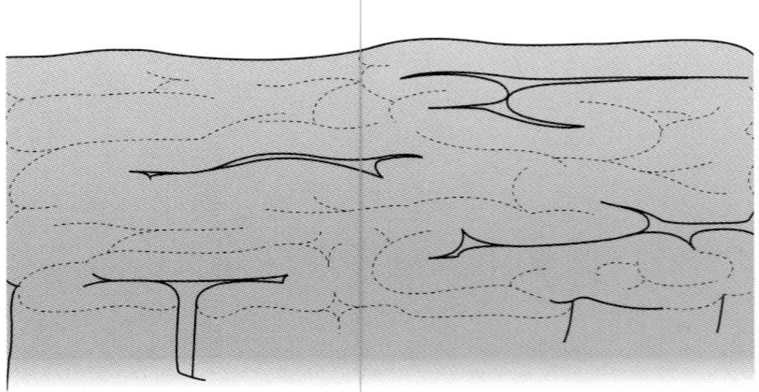

Flat

Small bowel – excision

Small bowel resections vary a great deal in length and location depending on the characteristics of the lesion. They include the regional mesentery and are usually followed by an end-to-end anastomosis.

Procedure

1. Two options are available depending on the length of the bowel and the type of pathology present:
   a. Cut longitudinally through the antimesenteric border, pin on corkboard, and fix overnight
   b. Wash out contents gently with formalin or saline solution (not with water), tie one end, fill the lumen with formalin, and tie the other end. Fix overnight and open longitudinally along the antimesenteric border

Description

1. Length and diameter of specimen
2. Mucosa: appearance; edema? hemorrhage? ulcerations? tumor? (size, location, circumferential involvement? depth of invasion)
3. Wall: thickness, abnormalities
4. Serosa: fibrosis, peritonitis, adhesions
5. Lymph nodes: size and appearance
6. Mesentery; mesenteric blood vessels

Sections for histology

1. Depends on pathology present
2. In cases of infarct: several cross-sections of mesenteric vessels

Soft tissue – resection for tumor

The procedure here described was written specifically for amputation specimens but it can be easily adapted to the lesser operations that are currently carried out for these neoplasms.

Procedure

1 Review any imaging studies (CT scans, MRIs) that may have been taken before amputation
2 Measure the length and circumference of the extremity, including a measure of the circumference at the level of the tumor
3 Determine the presence, position, and dimensions of biopsy sites
4 Search for the major lymph node groups and identify and place in separate containers
5 Cut through the skin and carefully dissect the subcutaneous fat, muscles, and major arteries, veins, and nerves *around* the tumor, avoiding cutting through the latter. Use an anatomy atlas as a guide, if necessary. Try to determine as accurately as possible the relationship of the tumor with the following structures: skin, subcutaneous fat, and specific muscles; arteries, veins, and nerves; and periosteum and bone. Mark some of the major anatomic landmarks with tags, if indicated
6 As soon as all the margins of the tumor have been determined, remove the entire area with a good margin of normal tissues using a scalpel and scissors
7 Two options, outlined later, are available for studying the specimen thus obtained. The first is used in most instances, but the second is preferable in selected cases. In either case, if a previous incision site is present, take a sample for histology at this time along the entire course of the incision
   a Divide the tumor into slices with a large, sharp knife. Continue the dissection with the forceps, scissors, and scalpel to determine the tumor relationship with the structures previously mentioned. Place several pieces from different areas in formalin, fix for several hours or overnight, and trim to place in cassettes
   b Place the entire specimen in a large pan containing formalin, cover with a towel, leave in the refrigerator at 4°C overnight, and cut parallel slices with a large sharp knife. Take x-ray studies, if pertinent. Take photographs or photocopies, and identify in one of them the site of the sections to be taken
8 Quickly dissect the soft tissues from the rest of the extremity, looking for other foci of tumor or other lesions
9 Cut the major bones of the extremities longitudinally with a band saw. Make one of the sections through the area of bone closest to the soft tissue tumor. Examine for tumor extension or other lesions
10 Open the major joints and examine them

Description

1 Type of amputation; side of extremity
2 Length and circumference of extremity, including circumference at level of tumor
3 Presence, position, and dimensions of biopsy sites
4 Tumor characteristics:
   a Primary location: subcutaneous fat; muscle compartment(s) (specify which); fascial planes
   b Tumor extension into and relation with skin, subcutaneous fat, deep fascia, muscle, periosteum, bone, joint vessels, and nerves (specify which); presence of obvious vascular or neural involvement by tumor
   c If previous incision present, is there evidence of tumor extension along it?
   d Size (three dimension), shape, color, borders (encapsulated? pushing? infiltrating?), consistency, secondary changes (cysts? necrosis? hemorrhage?)
   e Presence of myxoid changes, foci of calcification, cartilage, or bone
   f Shortest distance of tumor from margin of resection
5 Appearance of remaining extremity, if abnormal (if not, so state); skin, subcutaneous fat, muscles, major vessels and nerves, bone (tumor invasion? osteoporosis? bone marrow), joints (osteoarthritis?)
6 Appearance and approximate number of lymph nodes found

Sections for histology

1 Tumor: four sections or more, depending on size and extent. All grossly dissimilar areas should be sampled. Whenever possible, sections should be taken to include the periphery of the tumor *and* adjacent fat, muscle, skin, periosteum, vessels, and/or nerves
2 Previous incision site, if present, taken all along its course
3 Lymph nodes: if grossly normal, only representative ones; if grossly abnormal or if clinical suspicion or metastases, all of them
4 Proximal margins of resection: subcutaneous fat and muscle (plus skin and bone, if indicated)

Spleen – splenectomy

Splenectomy consists of removal of the entire spleen after ligating the splenic artery and vein.

Procedure

1 Measure and weigh the specimen
2 Cut parallel slices as thin as possible with a sharp knife or meat cutter while the specimen is fresh and examine each slice carefully for focal lesions; do not wash the cut surface in tap water. Fix each slice flat in a large container
3 Take cultures if an inflammatory condition is suspected
4 Prepare four imprints of the cut surface in all cases in which splenic pathology is suspected; stain two with hematoxylin–eosin and two with Wright stain
5 If sickle cell disease is suspected, fix a block of tissue in formalin *immediately* after it has been cut from the interior of the organ
6 Look for lymph nodes and accessory spleens in the splenic hilum
7 For the evaluation of the red pulp in diseases associated with hypersplenism, the specimen can be injected with formalin through the splenic artery. A sharp distinction between sinuses and chords will thus be obtained in the microscopic preparations
8 For the spleen removed as part of a staging procedure, see under Staging laparotomy for malignant lymphoma

Description

1 Weight and dimensions
2 Hilum: nature of vessels, presence of lymph nodes, presence of accessory spleens
3 Capsule: color, thickness, focal changes, adhesions, lacerations (location, length and depth)
4 Cut surface: color; consistency; bulging; malpighian corpuscles (size; color; conspicuous?); fibrous trabeculae; nodules or masses; diffuse infiltration?

Sections for histology

1 For incidental splenectomy: one section, including capsule
2 For traumatically ruptured spleen: one section through tear and one away from it
3 For diseased spleen: at least three sections, one to include hilum and two to include capsule

Staging laparotomy for malignant lymphoma

Procedure

1 Spleen: handle as described under Spleen – splenectomy except that *the entire spleen* should be sliced carefully, 3–4 mm apart, and each slice should be carefully examined. Any nodules, no matter how small, that differ from the adjacent normal malpighian corpuscles should be processed for histology. Square blocks containing these suspicious nodules, in addition to other obvious lesions, should be cut out and fixed separately for several hours or overnight in formalin
2 Lymph nodes: these will usually include splenic hilar, para-aortic, and possible mesenteric nodes. Dissect carefully the splenic hilum for the former
3 Liver wedge biopsy (right and left lobes): keep separate; trim into several slices, if necessary
4 Open iliac crest biopsy: fix, decalcify, and trim, if necessary

Description

1 Proceed as per instructions for the respective organs
2 Presence or absence of grossly identifiable nodes in the splenic hilum must be noted

Sections for histology

1 Spleen: all grossly abnormal or suspicious areas; if no gross abnormalities seen, four random pieces
2 Lymph nodes: all, properly identified as to site
3 Liver: all, properly identified as to lobe
4 Bone marrow: all

Stomach – gastrectomy for tumor

Gastrectomy for tumor can be *total* (including cardiac pylorus), *subtotal* (including the pylorus), and *proximal* or *inverted subtotal* (including the cardia).

Procedure

1 Open the specimen along the greater curvature (unless the lesion is in this location; if it is, open the specimen along the lesser curvature)
2 Dissect the lymph node groups according to the accompanying diagram and remove the omentum
3 If a splenectomy is included, dissect the hilar lymph nodes, measure and weigh the spleen, and cut in 1 cm longitudinal slices
4 Pin the stomach on a corkboard and fix overnight in formalin before sectioning
5 Take photographs or photocopies and identify in one of them the sites of the sections to be taken
6 Paint the surgical margins with India ink
7 In general, take the sections *perpendicular* to the directions of the mucosal folds
8 Another way to examine these specimens is as follows: inject the stomach with formalin (in cases of total gastrectomy) or fill it with gauze or cotton impregnated in formalin (in partial gastrectomies). Fix overnight. Cut the side opposite the tumor with scissors and the tumor side with a long knife
9 If a thorough mapping of the mucosal abnormalities is desired, the entire specimen can be submitted, or the Swiss roll technique can be used (see Chapter 11, Stomach)

Description

1 Type of resection (total or subtotal); length of greater curvature, lesser curvature, and duodenal cuff
2 Tumor characteristics: location, size (including thickness), shape (fungating, spreading, ulcerated); depth of invasion; presence of serosal involvement; blood vessel invasion; extension into duodenum; distance from both lines of resection
3 Appearance of non-neoplastic mucosa

Sections for histology (see accompanying drawings, p. 2629)

1 Tumor: four sections through wall and including tumor border and adjacent mucosa
2 Non-neoplastic mucosa: midstomach, two sections
3 Proximal line of resection along lesser curvature: two sections
4 Proximal line of resection along greater curvature: two sections
5 Distal line of resection (along pylorus and duodenum, if present): two sections
6 Spleen, if present
7 Pancreas, if present
8 Lymph nodes:
   a Pyloric
   b Lesser curvature
   c Greater curvature
   d Omentum
   e Perisplenic

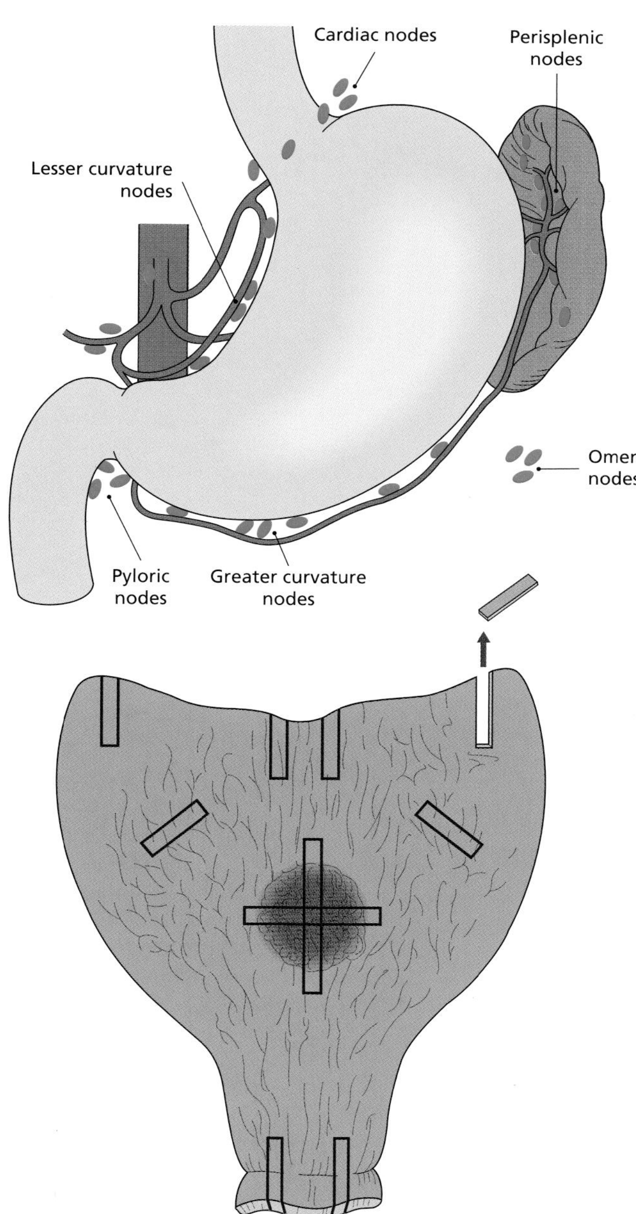

Stomach – gastrectomy for ulcer

Gastric resection for peptic ulcer, rarely done at present, includes removal of the antrum with the pylorus and a small portion of the first portion of the duodenum. For duodenal peptic ulcers, this is routinely combined with truncal vagotomy.

Procedure

1 Examine specimen in the fresh state
2 Open the specimen along the greater curvature (unless the lesion is in this location; if it is, open the specimen along the lesser curvature)
3 Dissect the lymph node groups and remove the omentum
4 Look carefully for small mucosal erosions and irregularities and for intramural or subserosal nodules
5 Pin the stomach on a corkboard and fix overnight in formalin before sectioning
6 Take photographs or photocopies and identify in one of them the sites of the sections to be taken

Description

1 Type of resection; length of greater curvature, lesser curvature, and duodenal cuff
2 Ulcer characteristics: location, size, depth of penetration, shape, and color of edges (flat or elevated? converging folds?); presence of large vessels and/or perforation at ulcer base; appearance of serosa. (If the clinicoradiographic diagnosis is peptic ulcer but no ulcer is identified in the specimen, contact the surgeon or assistant to find out whether the ulcer was not resected. Record this information as part of the gross dictation)
3 Appearance of uninvolved mucosa: atrophy, edema, hemorrhage

Sections for histology

1 Ulcer: at least four sections
2 Lesser curvature: two sections cut from proximal margin of excision (paint line of resection with India ink)
3 Greater curvature: two sections cut from proximal margin of excision (paint line of resection with India ink)
4 Pylorus and duodenum: two sections, including distal line of resection
5 Other lesions, if present
6 Lymph nodes: up to three sections

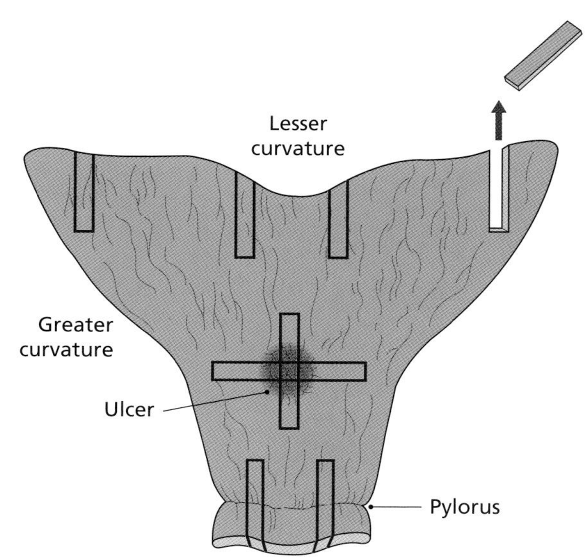

Testicle – orchidectomy

Procedure

1 Open the tunica vaginalis; weigh and measure the testicle
2 Cut the testicle sagittally while it is in the fresh state and fix in formalin
3 Take photographs or photocopies and identify in one of them the sites of the sections to be taken
4 Cut serial slices, about 3 mm thick, of each testicular half, perpendicular to the original section, stopping just at the level of the tunica albuginea (to keep them together), and examine each surface carefully
5 Cut the epididymis longitudinally throughout its entire length
6 Make several cross-sections of the spermatic cord at several levels

Description

1 Weight and dimensions of testicle
2 Length of spermatic cord
3 Features of tumor, if present: size, color; consistency; homogeneity or lack of it; presence of cysts, necrosis, hemorrhage, bone, or cartilage; tumor extension to tunica albuginea, epididymis, cord, and other structures
4 Features of non-neoplastic testicle: atrophy? fibrosis? nodules?
5 Features of rete testis and epididymis

Sections for histology

1 Tumor: at least three sections or one section for each centimeter of tumor, whichever is greater, at least one of which should include some uninvolved testicle. Most of the sections should include tunica albuginea. (Always submit sections from hemorrhagic or necrotic areas of tumor, as well as from solid or fleshy areas.)
2 Uninvolved testicle: two sections
3 Epididymis
4 Spermatic cord and surrounding soft tissue at a point about 1 cm from testicle: one cross-section
5 Spermatic cord and surrounding soft tissue at line of resection: one cross-section

Thymus gland – thymectomy

Procedure

1 Weigh the entire organ. Cut parallel slices, either in the fresh specimen or after formalin fixation
2 Look carefully for lymph nodes around the thymus

Description

1 Weight and dimensions; both lobes identifiable?
2 Relative amount of fat and thymic parenchyma
3 Tumor characteristics: size, shape, external appearance (lobulated or smooth), cut section, color, necrosis, hemorrhage, fibrous bands, calcification, cysts (size, content)
4 Attached structures (pleura, pericardium, lung, lymph nodes)

Sections for histology

1 Tumor: three or more sections, at least two of which should include capsule
2 Uninvolved thymus: two sections
3 Other organs, if present (lung, lymph nodes)

Thyroid gland – thyroidectomy

Operations on the thyroid gland include *nodulectomy* (a procedure largely abandoned that consists of enucleation of a thyroid nodule), *lobectomy* (often combined for cosmetic reasons with removal of the isthmus), *subtotal thyroidectomy* (in which the posterior capsule and a small portion of thyroid tissue – 1–2 g – are left on the side opposite to the lesion), and *total thyroidectomy* (in which the entire gland – including the posterior capsule – is removed).

Procedure

1 Weigh and measure the specimen
2 Orient the specimen and cut parallel longitudinal slices 5 mm each either in the fresh state or after formalin fixation
3 Search for parathyroid glands in the surrounding fat

Description

1 Type of specimen: lobectomy, isthmectomy, subtotal thyroidectomy, total thyroidectomy
2 Weight, shape, color, and consistency of specimen
3 Cut surface: smooth or nodular? if nodular: number, size, and appearance of nodules (cystic? calcified? hemorrhagic? necrotic?); encapsulated or invasive? distance to line of resection

Sections for histology

1 For diffuse and/or inflammatory lesions: three sections from each lobe and on from isthmus
2 For a solitary encapsulated nodule measuring up to 5 cm: entire circumference; take one additional section for each additional centimeter in diameter. Most of these sections should include the tumor capsule and adjacent thyroid tissue, if present
3 For multinodular thyroid glands: one section of each nodule (up to five nodules), including rim and adjacent normal gland; more than one section for larger nodules
4 For papillary carcinoma: block entire thyroid gland and (separately) line of resection
5 For grossly invasive carcinoma other than papillary: three sections of tumor, three of non-neoplastic gland, and one from line of resection
6 For all cases: submit parathyroid glands if found on gross inspection

Uterus – cervical biopsy[1]

Procedure

1 Do not cut the specimen unless the individual pieces are greater than 4 mm in diameter
2 It is essential that *all of the tissue* received be processed, no matter how small
3 Always carefully search the container and the underside of the lid for tiny fragments of tissue

Description

1 Number of pieces received, shape and color
2 Measurement in aggregate
3 Presence or absence of epithelium; epithelial erosions or ulcers? irregularity in epithelial thickness?
4 Any evidence of tumors or cysts?

Sections for histology

1 Submit the material in its entirety
2 If specimens are received with a specific identification (e.g. anterior lip, posterior lip), label and submit them separately
3 If a specimen from endocervical scraping is received, submit as a separate specimen in its entirety (including the endocervical mucus)

1 Robboy SJ, Kraus FT, Kurman RJ. Gross description, processing, and reporting of gynaecologic and obstetric specimens. In Kurman RJ (ed.): Blaustein's pathology of the female genital tract, ed. 4. New York, 2002, Springer-Verlag, pp. 1319–1346

Uterus – cervical conization[1]

Specimens from cervical conizations have the shape of a cone with the base toward the portio. In the *leep procedure* (loop electroexcision procedure), the cone is much smaller than that obtained with the conventional method. Orientation of the specimen is more difficult but just as important.

Procedure

1 Ideally the specimen should be received intact, in the fresh state, and with a suture or other material identifying the 12 o'clock position
2 Open the specimen by inserting a sharp pointed scissors into the cervical canal and cutting it longitudinally along the 12 o'clock position. If the specimen has not been oriented as to position, open at any site
3 Pin on a corkboard with the mucosal side up and fix in formalin for several hours
4 Paint both surgical margins with India ink, taking special care that the epithelial side of the margin is well stained along its entire length
5 Cut the entire cervix by making parallel sections, 2–3 mm apart, along the plane of the endocervical canal starting at the 12 o'clock position (or left-hand side of the specimen) and moving clockwise. Sections should be taken in such a way that the epithelium (including the squamocolumnar junction) is present in each section; some trimming of the stroma may be necessary (see accompanying drawing)

Description

1 Size (diameter and depth) and shape of cone; complete cast of cervix or fragmented?
2 Epithelium: color; presence of irregularities, erosions, healed or recent lacerations, masses (size, shape, location), cysts (size, content), previous biopsy sites

Sections for histology

1 All of the tissue must be submitted (except for trimming of the stroma)
2 If the cone has been oriented to the 12 o'clock position, identify separately:
   a Sections from 12 to 3 o'clock (**A-1** on accompanying drawings)
   b Sections from 3 to 6 o'clock (**A-2** on accompanying drawings)
   c Sections from 6 to 9 o'clock (**A-3** on accompanying drawings)
   d Sections from 9 to 12 o'clock (**A-4** on accompanying drawings)
3 If an accurate mapping of the lesions is desired, identify sequentially each section with a letter, beginning from the 12 o'clock position

1 Robboy SJ, Kraus FT, Kurman RJ. Gross description, processing, and reporting of gynaecologic and obstetric specimens. In Kurman RJ (ed.): Blaustein's pathology of the female genital tract, ed. 4. New York, 2002, Springer-Verlag, pp. 1319–1346

12 o'clock
A-4
A-1
A-3
A-2

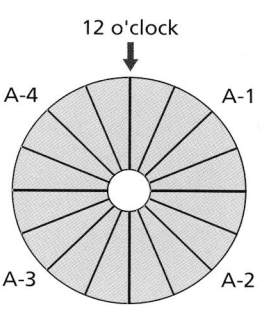

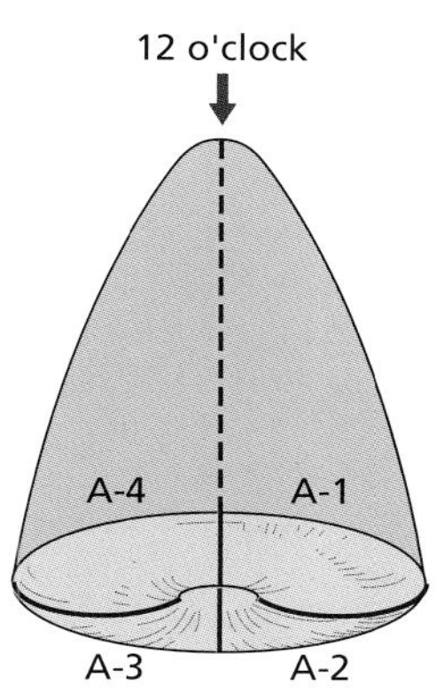

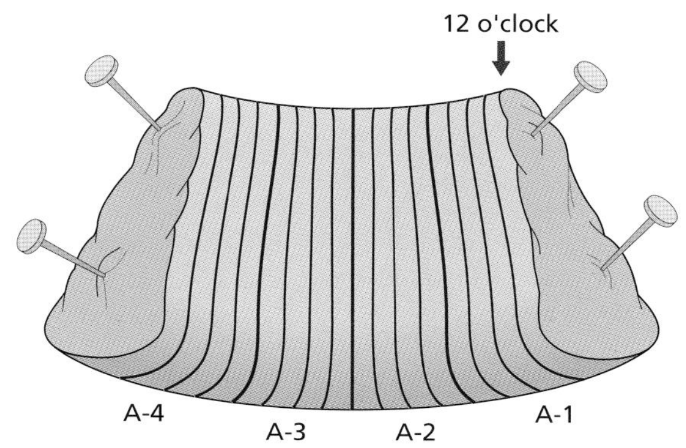

Uterus – endometrial curettings or biopsy[1]

Procedure

1 Use of metal strainer or a filter paper in a funnel to collect the specimens
2 In cases of suspected abortion, search for chorionic villi; use dissecting microscope if necessary
3 In cases of recurrent abortion, save a sample of villi for possible cytogenetic evaluation. Clean the forceps, other instruments, and the table carefully before handling the next case

Description

1 Measurement in the aggregate
2 Color and consistency; blood clots present? proportion of clots in relation to whole specimen; any unusually large or firm pieces? globular tissue? evidence of necrosis? tissue suggestive of products of conception: if so, describe the appearance of chorionic villi (a dissecting microscope may be necessary); if presence or absence of villous vessels, shape of villi (tubular, clubbed, cystic, hydatidiform); if gestational sac is present, describe as indicated under Uterus – tissue passed

Sections for histology

1 For endometrial biopsy or diagnostic curettage: submit *all* tissue. Do not fill the cassette more than half full
2 For endometrial curettage for incomplete abortion: submit representative sections of tissue with the appearance of placenta, fetal parts, and deciduas unless the entire specimen is small enough to fit into three cassettes. If the microscopic sections do not show products of conception, submit the rest of the material

1 Robboy SJ, Kraus FT, Kurman RJ. Gross description, processing, and reporting of gynaecologic and obstetric specimens. In Kurman RJ (ed.): Blaustein's pathology of the female genital tract, ed. 4. New York, 2002, Springer-Verlag, pp. 1319–1346

Uterus – hysterectomy (general instructions)[1]

Hysterectomies can be performed by either the abdominal or the vaginal route, the latter reserved for benign conditions. They consist of removal of the entire organ. Supracervical hysterectomies (in which the corpus is separated from the cervix and the latter is left in place) are no longer performed. Depending on the age of the patient and the nature of the disease, abdominal hysterectomies may be accompanied by unilateral or bilateral adnexectomy and by the removal of regional lymph nodes.

Procedure

1 If operation was done for endometrial hyperplasia, endometrial carcinoma, or cervical (in situ or invasive) carcinoma, read specific instructions before proceeding
2 Measure and weigh the specimen
3 If the uterus is received fresh and intact:
   a Open it by cutting with scissors through both lateral walls, from the cervix to the uterine cornua
   b Make a mark as to which half is anterior (e.g. by cutting a small wedge on one side) and, if the tubes are attached, by the fact that their insertion is anterior to that of the round ligament
   c Make additional cuts through any large mass in the wall
   d Fix for several hours or overnight
   e Make parallel transverse sections through each half, about 1 cm apart, beginning at the upper level of the endocervical canal and stopping short of completing them on one side to keep them together, and examine carefully each surface
   f Make several sections of the cervix along the endocervical canal
   g Make at least one cross section of every myoma present and examine carefully; larger myomas need additional cuts
   h If tubes and/or ovary accompanies the specimen, follow instructions for these organs

Description

1 Type of hysterectomy: total? radical? with salpingo-oophorectomy?
2 Shape of uterus: deformed? subserosal bulges?
3 Serosa: fibrous adhesions?
4 Wall: thickness, abnormalities
5 Endometrium: appearance; thickness; polyps? (size, shape); cysts?
6 Cervix: appearance of exocervix, squamocolumnar junction, endocervical canal; erosions? polyps? cysts?
7 Myomas: number, location (subserosal, intramural, submucosal); size; sessile or pedunculated? hemorrhage, necrosis, or calcification? ulceration of overlying endometrium?

Sections for histology

1 Cervix: one section from anterior half and one from posterior half
2 Corpus: at least two sections taken close to fundus and including endometrium, good portion of myometrium, and, if thickness permits, serosa; additional sections from any grossly abnormal areas
3 Myomas: at least one section per myoma, up to three; sections from any grossly abnormal area (e.g. soft, fleshy, necrotic, cystic)
4 Cervical or endometrial polyps: to be submitted in entirety unless extremely large

1 Robboy SJ, Kraus FT, Kurman RJ. Gross description, processing, and reporting of gynaecologic and obstetric specimens. In Kurman RJ (ed.): Blaustein's pathology of the female genital tract, ed. 4. New York, 2002, Springer-Verlag, pp. 1319–1346

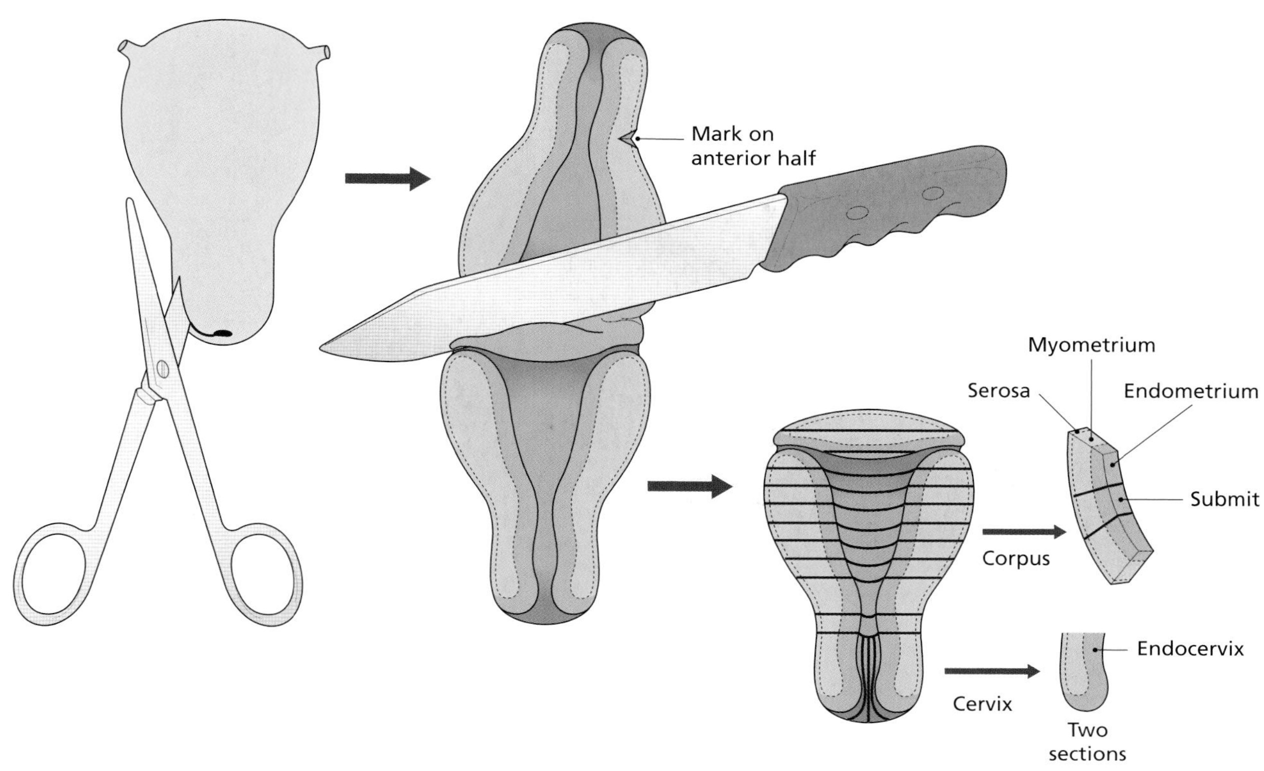

Uterus – hysterectomy for cervical carcinoma (in situ or invasive)[1]

Procedure

1 If lymph nodes are included (radical hysterectomy), dissect while fresh and separate into left and right obturator, interiliac, and left and right iliac (high nodes) groups (not all of these groups will be present in every specimen)
2 Measure and weigh the specimen; orient as to anterior and posterior sides; see under Uterus – hysterectomy (general instructions)
3 Amputate the cervix from the corpus about 2.5 cm above the external os with a sharp knife
4 Handle the uterus as described under Uterus – hysterectomy (general instructions) and the tubes and ovaries, if present, according to instructions for these organs
5 Open the cervix with scissors through the endocervical canal at the 12 o'clock position and carefully pin stretched specimen on a corkboard with the mucosal side up. Be careful to avoid tearing or rubbing the epithelial surface
6 Fix by floating for several hours or overnight with the tissue on the underside of the corkboard in a formalin container
7 Paint the vaginal surgical margin with India ink
8 Cut the entire cervix by making parallel longitudinal sections, 2–3 mm apart, along the plane of the endocervical canal starting at the 12 o'clock position and moving clockwise. Sections should be taken in such a way that the epithelium (including the squamocolumnar junction) is present in each section; some trimming of the stroma may be necessary (see accompanying drawing, p. 2634)

Description

1 Cervix: color of epithelium; presence of irregularities, erosions, healed or recent lacerations, masses (size, shape, location), cysts (size, content), previous biopsy, or conization sites
2 Rest of uterus: see under Uterus – hysterectomy (general instructions)
3 Ovaries and tubes, if present: see instructions for respective organs
4 Lymph nodes, if present: approximate number; gross appearance; seem involved by tumor?

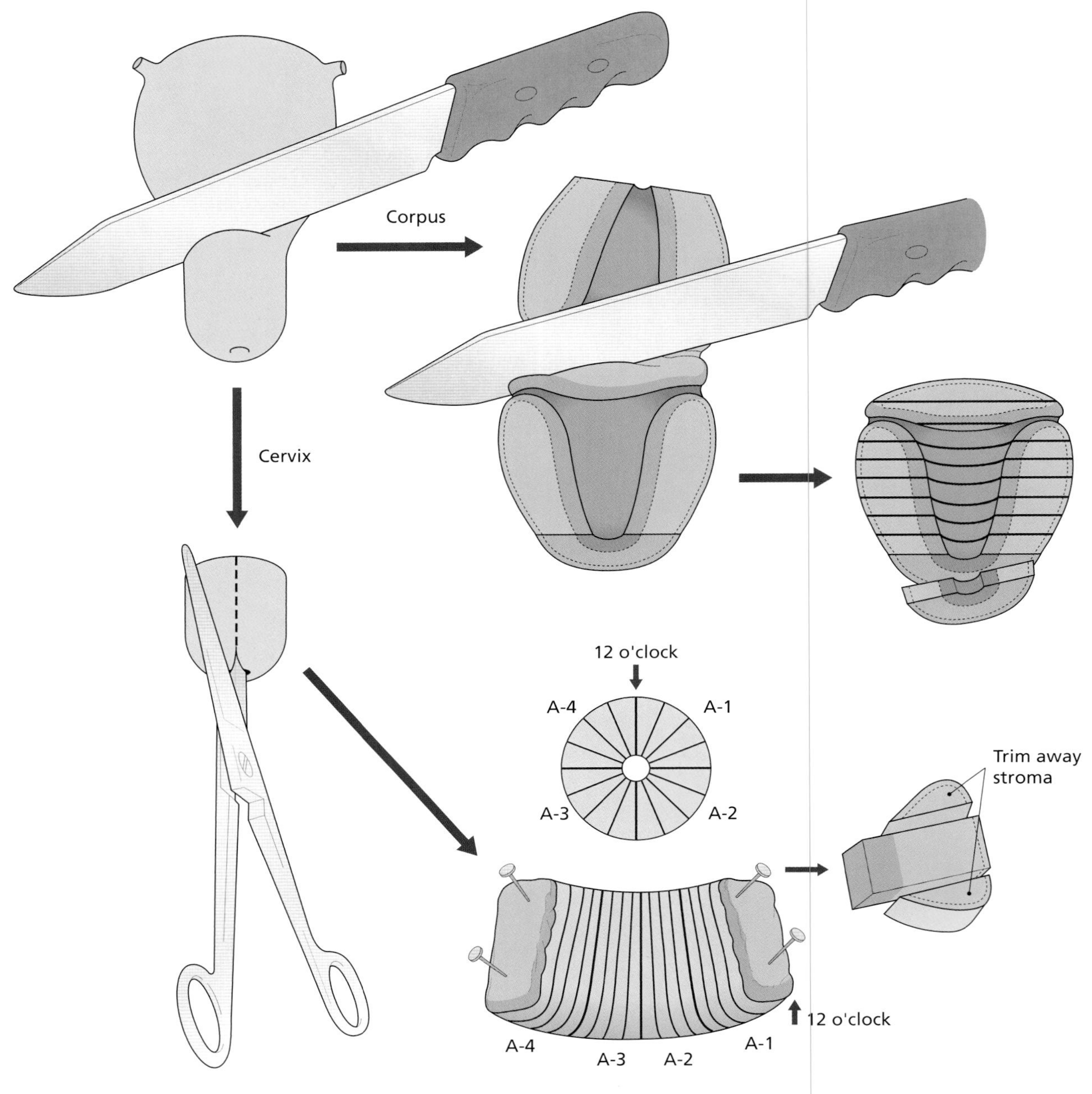

Sections for histology

1 Cervix: all tissue is submitted (except for trimming of stroma) and identified separately as follows:
   a Sections from 12 to 3 o'clock (**A-1** on accompanying drawings)
   b Sections from 3 to 6 o'clock (**A-2** on accompanying drawings)
   c Sections from 6 to 9 o'clock (**A-3** on accompanying drawings)
   d Sections from 9 to 12 o'clock (**A-4** on accompanying drawings) (If an accurate mapping of the lesions is desired, identify sequentially each section with a letter, beginning from the 12 o'clock position)
2 Vaginal cuff (entire line of resection)
3 Left soft tissue (for invasive cases only)
4 Right soft tissue (for invasive cases only)
5 Rest of uterus: see under Uterus – hysterectomy (general instructions)
6 Ovaries and tubes: see instructions for respective organs
7 Lymph nodes, if present:
   - Left obturator
   - Right obturator
   - Interiliac
   - Left iliac (high nodes)
   - Right iliac (high nodes)

1 Robboy SJ, Kraus FT, Kurman RJ. Gross description, processing, and reporting of gynaecologic and obstetric specimens. In Kurman RJ (ed.): Blaustein's pathology of the female genital tract, ed. 4. New York, 2002, Springer-Verlag, pp. 1319–1346

Uterus – hysterectomy for endometrial hyperplasia or carcinoma[1]

Procedure

1 If lymph nodes are included (radical hysterectomy), dissect while fresh and separate into left and right obturator, interiliac, and left and right iliac (high nodes) groups (not all of these groups will be present in every specimen)
2 Open and fix the uterus as indicated under Uterus – hysterectomy (general instructions)
3 If ovaries and tubes are present, handle according to respective instructions

Description

1 Type of operation: radical? total? with salpingectomy and oophorectomy?
2 Tumor: exact location; size; appearance (solid, papillary, ulcerated, necrotic, hemorrhagic); color; extent of endometrial extensions; presence of myometrial, serosal, parametrial (soft tissue), venous, cervical, or tubal extension
3 Rest of uterus: see under Uterus – hysterectomy (general instructions)
4 Ovaries and tubes: see respective instructions
5 Lymph nodes, if present: approximate number; gross appearance; seem involved by tumor?

Sections for histology

1 If obvious tumor present:
   a Three sections, one of which should be through area of deepest invasion and be complete sections from surface of endometrium through serosa (if too thick for a cassette, divide in half and identify both halves appropriately)
   b Two sections from non-neoplastic endometrium; do not need to be through entire wall
2 Soft tissue from left and eighth parametria
3 If no obvious tumor present (previous irradiation, very superficial carcinoma, endometrial hyperplasia):
   a Sample entire endometrium by making complete transverse parallel sections, 2–3 mm apart, of both uterine halves; one section should comprise entire thickness of organ, from mucosa to serosa; trim away from all others deepest two-thirds of myometrium. Label separately as anterior and posterior halves
   b Rest of uterus: see under Uterus – hysterectomy (general instructions)
   c Ovaries and tubes: see respective instructions
   d Lymph nodes, if present:
      - Left obturator
      - Right obturator
      - Interiliac
      - Left iliac (high nodes)
      - Right iliac (high nodes)

1 Robboy SJ, Kraus FT, Kurman RJ. Gross description, processing, and reporting of gynaecologic and obstetric specimens. In Kurman RJ (ed.): Blaustein's pathology of the female genital tract, ed. 4. New York, 2002, Springer-Verlag, pp. 1319–1346

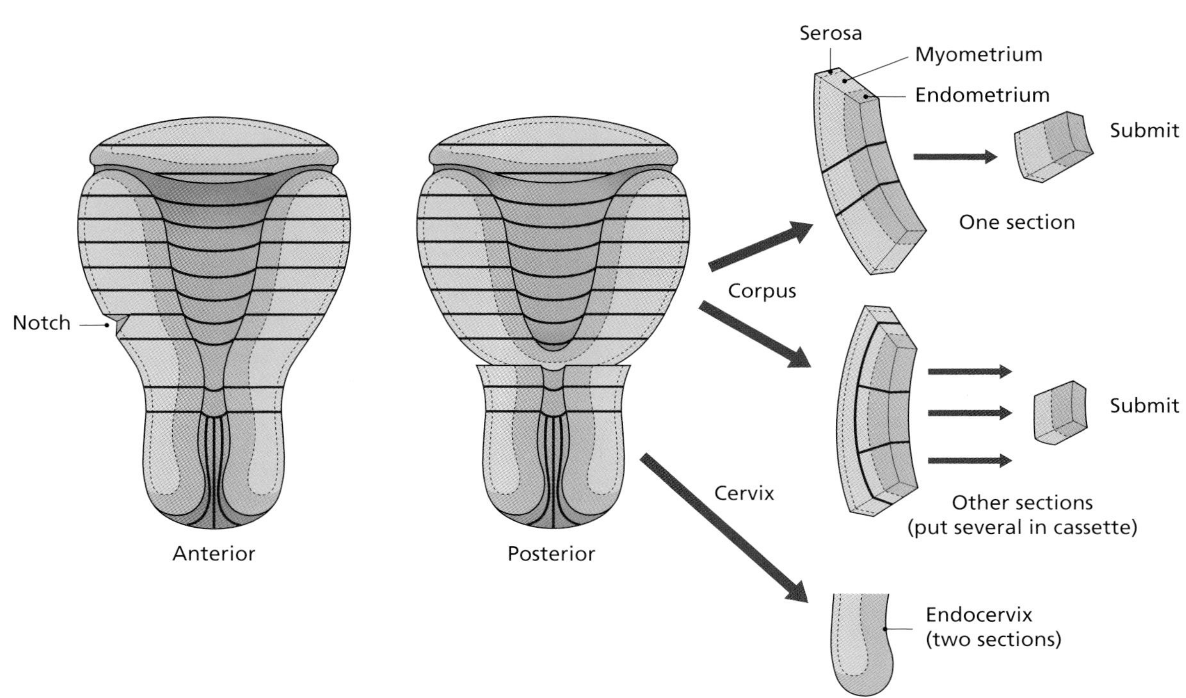

Uterus – tissue passed[1,2]

Procedure

Examine for presence of gestational sac and other evidence of conception. Use dissecting microscope, if necessary

Description

1 Measurement in the aggregate; color, consistency, appearance; decidual cast present? if so, note whether intact or ruptured, diameter, presence and size of amniotic sac, yolk sac, and embryo. If latter is present, measure and state whether it appears normal, malformed, or rudimentary, and whether there is evidence of maceration
2 If only fragments of the fetus are present, try to identify a foot and measure its length to estimate gestational age (see diagram)

Sections for histology

1 If identifiable products of conception are present: submit representative sections of the various components
2 If identifiable products of conception are absent: submit entire material

1 Berry CL (ed.) Correlation of foot length with crown–rump length of human fetuses. In: Pediatric pathology. New York, 1981, Springer-Verlag, p. 3
2 Robboy SJ, Kraus FT, Kurman RJ. Gross description, processing, and reporting of gynaecologic and obstetric specimens. In Kurman RJ (ed.): Blaustein's pathology of the female genital tract, ed. 4. New York, 2002, Springer-Verlag, pp. 1319–1346

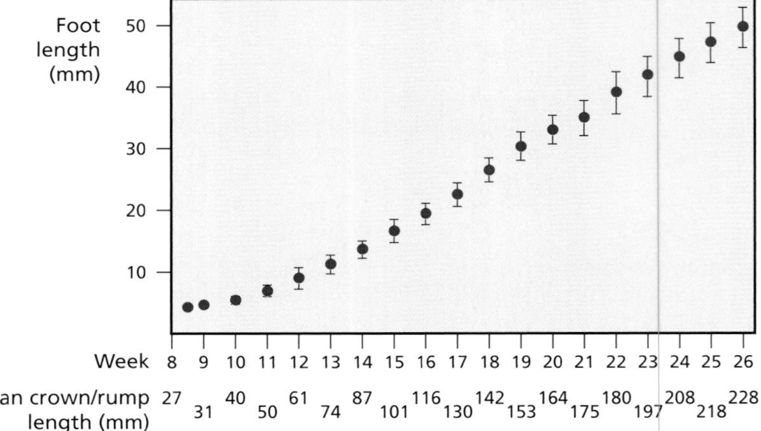

Vulva – vulvectomy[1]

Procedure

1 Measure size of the specimen, including the inguinal region, if present; also measure the size of the lesion
2 In radical vulvectomy specimens, separate lymph nodes into groups and fix overnight in separate jars; Carnoy fluid is preferable
3 Pin on a corkboard and fix overnight; be careful to pin down the entire external borders and vaginal margins. The latter are better preserved when pinned down on a cork placed in the introitus
4 Ink the circumference of the vaginal margin
5 Take photographs or photocopies and identify in one of them the sites of the sections to be taken

Description

1 Type of vulvectomy: simply, subcutaneous, radical; lymph node groups present
2 Size of specimen
3 Lesion: size, location, extent, invasion into adjacent structures or vessels, color, surface (verrucous? ulcerated?), borders (distinct? rolled?), depth of stromal invasion
4 Appearance of non-neoplastic surface: atrophy, keratosis, ulceration
5 Lymph nodes: size of largest appearing grossly involved?

Sections for histology

1 Tumor (×3)
2 Tumor and nearest deep and vaginal margins
3 Tumor and nearest cutaneous margins
4 Posterior fourchette and perineal margins
5 Section of contralateral labia majora and minora
6 Section of clitoris and anterior vaginal margin
7 Any other skin lesions, if present
8 Inguinal lymph nodes (divided into groups)

1 Robboy SJ, Kraus FT, Kurman RJ. Gross description, processing, and reporting of gynaecologic and obstetric specimens. In Kurman RJ (ed.): Blaustein's pathology of the female genital tract, ed. 4. New York, 2002, Springer-Verlag, pp. 1319– 1346

Index

The letter *t* indicates a table, *b* indicates a box, and *f* indicates a figure.

A

B

C

D

E

F

G

J

K

L

M

N

O

P

Q

R

S

T

U

V

W